THIRD EDITION
RHEUMATOLOGY
VOLUME TWO

Edited by

Marc C Hochberg, MD MPH
Professor of Medicine, Head, Division of Rheumatology
and Clinical Immunology, University of Maryland School
of Medicine, Baltimore, USA

Alan J Silman, MSc MD FRCP FMedSci
ARC Professor of Rheumatic Disease Epidemiology and
Director, Arthritis Research Campaign Epidemiology
Research Unit, University of Manchester, UK

Josef S Smolen, MD
Professor of Medicine, Chairman, Division of
Rheumatology, University of Vienna School of Medicine
and Chairman, Second Department of Medicine, Center
for the Rheumatic Diseases, Lainz Hospital, Vienna,
Austria

Michael E Weinblatt, MD
Professor of Medicine, Harvard Medical School,
Division of Rheumatology, Immunology and Allergy,
Brigham and Women's Hospital, Boston, USA

Michael H Weisman, MD
Director, Division of Rheumatology, Cedars-Sinai Medical
Center and Professor of Medicine, University College of
Los Angeles School of Medicine, Los Angeles, USA

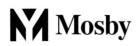 **Mosby**

Edinburgh ■ London ■ New York ■ Oxford ■ Philadelphia ■ St Louis ■ Sydney ■ Toronto 2003

MOSBY
An imprint of Elsevier Limited

First Edition published 1994
Second Edition published 1997
Third Edition published 2003
    Reprinted 2003

ISBN   0323024041

British Library Cataloguing in Publication Data
A catalogue record for this book is available from the British Library

Library of Congress Cataloging in Publication Data
A catalog record for this book is available from the Library of Congress

Notice
Medical knowledge is constantly changing. Standard safety precautions must be followed, but as new research and clinical experience broaden our knowledge, changes in treatment and drug therapy may become necessary or appropriate. Readers are advised to check the most current product information provided by the manufacturer of each drug to be administered to verify the recommended dose, the method and duration of administration, and contraindications. It is the responsibility of the practitioner, relying on experience and knowledge of the patient, to determine dosages and the best treatment for each individual patient. Neither the Publisher nor the editors nor contributors assume any liability for any injury and/or damage to persons or property arising from this publication.
The Publisher

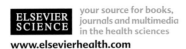
ELSEVIER SCIENCE your source for books, journals and multimedia in the health sciences
www.elsevierhealth.com

Printed in Spain

The publisher's policy is to use **paper manufactured from sustainable forests**

CONTENTS

VOLUME ONE

SECTION 1: INTRODUCTION TO THE STUDY OF RHEUMATIC DISEASES

SECTION 2: THE SCIENTIFIC BASIS OF RHEUMATIC DISEASE

SECTION 3: EVALUATION, SIGNS AND SYMPTOMS

SECTION 4: PRINCIPLES OF MANAGEMENT

SECTION 5: REGIONAL AND WIDESPREAD PAIN

SECTION 6: RHEUMATOID ARTHRITIS AND OTHER SYNOVIAL DISORDERS

SECTION 7: PEDIATRIC RHEUMATOLOGY

VOLUME TWO

SECTION 8: INFECTION-RELATED RHEUMATIC DISEASES

INFECTION

SECTION 9: SPONDYLOARTHROPATHIES

SECTION 10: CONNECTIVE TISSUE DISORDERS

SYSTEMIC LUPUS ERYTHEMATOSUS

SYSTEMIC SCLEROSIS

INFLAMMATORY MUSCLE DISEASE

SECTION 11: THE VASCULITIDES

SECTION 12: OTHER SYSTEMIC ILLNESSES

SECTION 13: OSTEOARTHRITIS AND RELATED DISORDERS

CONTRIBUTORS

David M Adlam MBBS BDS FRCS FDSRCS   CH 61
Consultant Oral and Maxillofacial Surgeon
Addenbrookes Hospital
Cambridge, UK

Kristina Åkesson MD PhD   CH 198
Associate Professor of Orthopaedics
Malmö University Hospital
Malmö, Sweden

Abdul-Wahab Al-Allaf MBChB MRCP   CH 136
(UK) MSc CCST Cert HE
Consultant Rheumatologist
Honorary Senior Lecturer
New Cross Hospital
Wolverhampton, UK

Graciela S Alarcón MD MPH   CH 47
Professor in Rheumatology
Jane Knight Lowe Chair of Medicine
University of Alabama at Birmingham
Birmingham, AL, USA

Daniel A Albert MD   CH 161
Associate Professor of Medicine and Pediatrics
University of Pennsylvania,
Philadelphia, PA, USA

Roy D Altman MD   CH 165 & 171
Professor of Medicine
Chief of Rheumatology and Immunology
University of Miami School of Medicine;
Clinical Director, Geriatric Research, Education
and Clinical Center
Miami Department of Veterans Affairs
Miami, FL, USA

Christian Antoni MD   CH 111
Rheumatologist
Department of Medicine III
University Erlangen-Nueruberg
Erlangen, Germany

Thierry Appelboom MD PhD   CH 66
Professor of Rheumatology and Physical Medicine,
University of Brussels;
Chief, Division of Rheumatology, Erasmus University of
Brussels;
Curator of the Museum of Medical History in Brussels
Erasmus Hospital
Brussels, Belgium

Cynthia Aranow MD   CH 126
Assistant Professor of Medicine
Albert Einstein College of Medicine
New York, NY, USA

Marc A Asher MD   CH 87
Professor of Orthopaedic Surgery
University of Kansas Medical Center
Kansas City, KS, USA

Lisa Badley PhD   CH 6
Director, Arthritis Community
Research and Evaluation Unit
Toronto Western Hospital Research Institute
Toronto, ON, Canada

W Timothy Ballard MD   CH 51
Director, Chattanooga Orthopaedic Group Foundation
for Research
Chattanooga, TN, USA

James E Balow MD   CH 127
Professor of Medicine
Clinical Director, NIDDK
National Institutes of Health
Bethesda, MD, USA

Gillian R Barclay DDS DrPH   CH 33
Research Fellow in Rheumatology,
Harvard Medical School;
Instructor in Health and Social Behavior,
Harvard School of Public Health
RBB Arthritis Research Center
Brigham and Women's Hospital
Boston, MA, USA

Thomas Bardin MD   CH 185, 186 & 190
Professor of Rheumatology
Hôpital Lariboisière
Paris, France

Les Barnsley BMed (Hons)   CH 53
Grad Dip Epi PhD FRACP FAFRM (RACP)
Associate Professor of Medicine
Sydney University
Head of Department of Rheumatology
Concord Hospital
Sydney, NSW, Australia

Michael J Battistone MD   CH 40
Assistant Professor of Medicine
Division of Rheumatology
University of Utah School of Medicine and Health
Sciences Center
Salt Lake City, UT, USA

Jill J F Belch MD (Hons) FRCP   CH 136
Professor of Vascular Medicine
Ninewells Hospital and Medical School
Dundee, UK

Nicholas Bellamy MD MSc MBA   CH 4   CH 170
FRCP (Glas & Edin) FRCP (C) FACP FAFRM FRACP
Professor of Rehabilitation Medicine
Director, The Centre of National Research on Disability
and Rehabilitation Medicine (CONROD)
The University of Queensland
Brisbane, Queensland, Australia

Nadia Belmatoug MD   CH 204
Senior Staff Physician and Consultant in Rheumatology
Hôpital Beaujon
Clichy, France

Basia Belza PhD RN   CH 82
Associate Professor
Department of Biobehavioral Nursing and Health
Systems
University of Washington
Seattle, WA, USA

Brian M Berman MD   CH 49
Professor of Family Medicine
Director, The Complementary Medicine Program
University of Maryland School of Medicine
Baltimore, MD, USA

Bonnie L Bermas MD   CH 48
Assistant Professor of Medicine, Harvard Medical
School;
Associate Rheumatologist, Brigham and Women's
Hospital
Boston, MA, USA

Howard A Bird MA MD FRCP   CH 37
Professor of Pharmacological Rheumatology
University of Leeds;
Clinical Pharmacology Unit
Chapel Allerton Hospital
Leeds, UK

Carol M Black CBE MD FRCP FACP F Med Sci   CH 135
Professor of Rheumatology
Royal Free and University College Medical School
London, UK

Tomás S Bocanegra MD FACP FACR   CH 95
Vice President, Development
Sankyo Pharma Inc
Edison, NJ, USA

Nikolai Bogduk MD PhD DSc Dip   CH 52
Anat Dip Pain Med FFPM (ANZCA)
Professor of Anatomy and Musculoskeletal Medicine
Newcastle Bone and Joint Institute
Royal Newcastle Hospital
Newcastle, NSW, Australia

Stefano Bombardieri MD   CH 156
Professor of Rheumatology
Instituto di Patologia Medica dell 'Universita di Pisa
Pisa, Italy

David G Borenstein MD   CH 54
Clinical Professor of Medicine
The George Washington University Medical Center
Washington, DC, USA

Dimitrios T Boumpas MD FACP   CH 127
Professor and Chairman of Medicine and
Rheumatology
University of Crete Medical School
Heraklion, Greece

F C Breedveld MD   CH 46
Professor of Rheumatology
Leiden University Medical Centre
Leiden, The Netherlands

Barry Bresnihan MD FRCP   CH 80
Professor of Rheumatology and Consultant
Rheumatologist
St Vincent's Hospital
Dublin, Ireland

Peter M Brooks MD FRACP   CH 32, 35 & 51
FAFRM FAFPHM
Executive Dean, Faculty of Health Sciences
The University of Queensland Royal Brisbane Hospital
Herston, Brisbane, Queensland, Australia

Anne C Brower MD   CH 105
Professor and Chair, Department of Radiology
Eastern Virginia Medical School
Norfolk, VA, USA

Ian N Bruce MD FRCP — CH 110
Consultant Rheumatologist and Honorary
Clinical Lecturer
Rheumatism Research Centre
Central Manchester and Manchester Children's
University Hospitals NHS Trust
Manchester, UK

W Watson Buchanan MD FRCP — CH 1
(Glasg Edin Canada) FACP FRCPI (Hon)
Emeritus Professor of Medicine
McMaster Health Sciences Centre
Hamilton, ON, Canada

Christopher Buckland-Wright BSc AKC PhD DSc — CH 168
Professor of Radiological Anatomy
Kings College
London, UK

Joseph A Buckwalter MD — CH 32 & 51
Professor and Head, Department of Orthopaedics
University of Iowa Hospitals
Iowa City, IA, USA

Peter G Bullough MB ChB — CH 169
Professor of Pathology and Laboratory Medicine
Director of Laboratory Medicine
The Hospital for Special Surgery
New York, NY, USA

Joel Buxbaum MD — CH 191
Professor, Director of Rheumatology Research
The Scripps Research Institute
La Jolla, CA, USA

Jill P Buyon MD — CH 123
Director of NIAMS Research Registry for Neonatal
Lupus
Professor of Medicine, New York University School of
Medicine
Hospital for Joint Diseases
New York, NY, USA

Eric G L Bywaters MD CBE FRCP — CH 83
Emeritus Professor of Medicine (Rheumatology)
Former Director, MRC Rheumatism Unit Taplow
Royal Postgraduate Medical School of London
London, UK

Leonard H Calabrese DO FACP — CH 98   CH 157
R. J. Fasenmyer Chair of Clinical Immunology
Vice Chairman, Department of Rheumatologic and
Immunologic Diseases
Cleveland Clinic Foundation
Cleveland, OH, USA

Jeffrey P Callen MD FACP — CH 154 & 155
Professor of Medicine (Dermatology)
Chief, Division of Dermatology
University of Louisville School of Medicine
Louisville, KY, USA

Juan J Canoso MD FACP — CH 23
Adjunct Professor of Medicine, Tufts University, Boston;
Rheumatologist, American British Cowdray Hospital
Mexico City, Mexico

Hilary Capell MB BCL BA MD FRCP — CH 39
Consultant Rheumatologist and Honorary Senior
Lecturer
Royal Infirmary
Glasgow, Scotland

Luis J Catoggio MD PhD — CH 140
Head, Rheumatology Section
Medical Services Hospital Italiano de Buenos Aires
Fundación Dr. Pedro M. Catoggio para el Progreso de la
Reumatologia
Argentina

Tim Cawston BSc PhD — CH 14
Professor of Rheumatology
The Medical School
University of Newcastle
Newcastle, UK

Michael D Chard MB BS MD FRCP — CH 56
Consultant Rheumatologist
Worthing Hospital
Worthing, West Sussex, UK

Ernest H S Choy MD MRCP — CH 43
Consultant and Senior Lecturer in Rheumathology
Academic Department of Rheumathology
Guy's and King's College Hospital (Dulwich)
London, UK

Flavia M Cicuttini MBBS FRACP PhD — CH 167
Associate Professor
Department of Epidemiology and Preventative
Medicine
Monash University
Melbourne, Australia

Philip J Clements MD MPH — CH 42
Professor of Medicine (Rheumatology)
UCLA School of Medicine
Los Angeles, CA, USA

Jonathan S Coblyn MD — CH 28
Associate Professor of Medicine, Harvard Medical
School
Director of Clinical Rheumatology
Brigham and Women's Hospital
Boston, MA, USA

Milton L Cohen MB BS MD FRACP FFPMANZCA — CH 34
Associate Professor of Medicine
Darlinghurst Arthritis and Pain Research Clinic
St Vincents Medical Centre
Sydney, NSW, Australia

Doyt L Conn MD — CH 146
Professor of Medicine
Director, Rheumatology and Immunology
Emory University School of Medicine
Atlanta, GA, USA

Cyrus Cooper MA DM FRCP FmedSci — CH 164
Professor of Rheumatology
MRC Environmental Epidemiology Unit
Southampton General Hospital
Southampton, UK

Sharon Cordner MBBS DM — CH 188
Specialist in Internal Medicine
University Hospital of The West Indies
Kingston, Jamaica

Paul Creamer — CH 173
Consultant Rheumatologist
Southmead Hospital
Bristol, UK

Mary K Crow MD — CH 121
Professor of Medicine
Hospital for Special Surgery
New York, NY, USA

Marta L Cuéllar MD — CH 112
Associate Professor
Tulane Health Sciences Center
New Orleans, LA, USA

John J Cush MD — CH 45
Chief, Rheumatology and Clinical Immunology
Presbyterian Hospital of Dallas;
Clinical Professor of Internal Medicine
The University of Texas Southwestern Medical School
Dallas, TX, USA

Vivette D'Agati MD — CH 117
Professor of Pathology
Columbia University College of Physicians and
Surgeons
New York, NY, USA

Seamus E Dalton MBBS FACRM FAFRM FACSP — CH 55
Consultant in Rehabilitation and Sports Medicine
North Sydney Orthopaedic and Sports Medicine Centre
Sydney, NSW, Australia

Lawren H Daltroy DrPH — CH 33
Associate Professor of Medicine, Harvard Medical
School;
Associate Professor of Health and Social Behaviour,
Harvard School of Public Health;
Associate Director, RBB Arthritis and Musculoskeletal
Diseases Clinical Research Center Brigham and
Women's Hospital
Boston, MA, USA

Karel De Ceulaer MD — CH 188
Consultant Rheumatologist
Daverin Medical Centre
Kingston, Jamaica

Charles Nagant de Deuxchaisnes — CH 203
Formerly Professor, The Arthritis Unit, Saint-Luc
University Hospital
Louvain University
Brussels, Belgium

Alessandra Della Rossa MD — CH 156
Rheumatologist
University of Pisa
Pisa, Italy

Pierre D Delmas MD PhD — CH 193
Professor of Medicine, Claude Bernard University
Hôpital E. Herriot
Lyon, France

Elaine Dennison MB BChir MA MRCP PhD — CH 164
Senior Research Fellow and Honorary Consultant
Rheumatologist
MRC Environmental Epidemiology Unit
Southampton General Hospital
Southampton, UK

Christopher P Denton MBBS PhD MRCP — CH 135
Senior Lecturer in Rheumatology
Centre for Rheumatology
Royal Free Hospital
London, UK

John Denton MSc   CH 22
Research Fellow in Osteoarticular Pathology
University of Manchester
Manchester, UK

Jan Dequeker MD PhD   CH 1   CH 192
Professor Emeritus of Rheumatology
University Hospitals Leuven
Leuven, Belgium

Jean-Pierre Devogelaer MD PROF   CH 203
Head, Department of Rheumatology
Director, Arthritis Unit
Saint-Luc University Hospital
Brussels, Belgium

John Dixon MA MCH (Orth) FRCS   CH 209
Consultant Orthopaedic Surgeon
Southmead Hospital
Bristol, UK

Michael Doherty MA MD FRCP ILTM   CH 179
Professor of Rheumatology
University of Nottingham
City Hospital
Nottingham, UK

Michael F Drummond PhD   CH 7
Professor of Health Economics
Centre of Health Economics
University of York
Heslington, York, UK

R M du Bois MA MD FRCP   CH 29
Professor of Respiratory Medicine
Royal Brompton Hospital
London, UK

John B Eastwood MD FRCP   CH 202
Reader in Medicine and Consultant Renal Physician
St George's Hospital Medical School
London, UK

Jonathan C W Edwards MD FRCP   CH 17
Professor of Connective Tissue Medicine
University College London
London, UK

Hani S El-Gabalawy MD   CH 108
Professor of Medicine
University of Manitoba Arthritis Centre
Winnipeg, MB, Canada

Keith B Elkon MD   CH 120
Professor of Medicine
Head, Division of Rheumatology
The University of Washington
Seattle, WA, USA

Helen Emery MD   CH 86
Professor of Pediatrics
Section Chief, Rheumatology
University of Washington Children's Hospital
Seattle, WA, USA

P Emery MA MD FRCP   CH 78
ARC Professor of Rheumatology
Leeds General Infirmary
Leeds, UK

Bryan T Emmerson MD PhD FRACP   CH 178
Emeritus Professor of Medicine
University of Queensland
Brisbane, Queensland, Australia

John M Esdaile MD CM MPH FRCP (C)   CH 70
Scientific Director, Arthritis Research Centre of Canada
Professor of Medicine, University of British Columbia
Vancouver, BC, Canada

Luis R Espinoza MD   CH 112
Professor and Chief, CSU Health Sciences Center
Louisiana State School of Medicine
New Orleans, LA, USA

John A Fairclough BM BS FRCS   CH 59
Consultant Orthopedic Surgeon
Llandough Hospital
Penarth, Vale of Glamorgan, UK

Adel G Fam MD FRCP (C) MRCP (UK) FACP   CH 57 & 60
Professor of Medicine, University of Toronto
Sunnybrook and Women's College Health Sciences
Centre
Toronto, ON, Canada

Kenneth G Faulkner PhD   CH 195
Chief Scientist, GE Medical Systems
Adjunct Associate Professor of Medicine, University of
Wisconsin
Madison, WI, USA

Gary S Firestein MD   CH 77
Professor of Medicine
Chief, Division of Rheumatology, Allergy and
Immunology
UCSD School of Medicine
La Jolla, CA, USA

Sándor S Forgács MD PhD   CH 182 & 184
Professor of Radiology
Uzsoki Hospital
Budapest, Hungary

John Forrester MB Chb FRCS (Ed and G)   CH 27
MD (Hons) FRCOphth FRCP (Ed) FAMS
Professor of Ophthalmology
University of Aberdeen School of Medicine
Aberdeen, Scotland

Victor H Frankel MD PhD   CH 10
Professor of Orthopaedic Surgery
Hospital for Joint Diseases
New York, USA

Anthony J Freemont MD FRCP FRCPath   CH 22
Professor of Osteoarticular Pathology
Head, Laboratory Medicine Academic Group
University of Manchester
Manchester, UK

Ïzzet Fresko MD   CH 151
Associate Professor of Medicine
Cerrahpasa Medical Faculty
University of Istanbul
Istanbul, Turkey

Marvin J Fritzler MD PhD   CH 120
Professor of Medicine
University of Calgary
Calgary, AB, Canada

Daniel E Furst MD   CH 42
Carl M Pearson Professor of Rheumatology
Director of Therapeutic Research
University of California in Los Angeles
Los Angeles, CA, USA

Sherine E Gabriel MD MSc   CH 2 & 7
Professor of Medicine and Epidemiology, Mayo Medical
School
Chair, Department of Health Sciences Research
Mayo Clinic
Rochester, MN, USA

Patrick Garnero PhD   CH 193
Senior Research Scientist
VP and Scientific Director, Molecular Marker, SYNARC
Lyon, France

J S Hill Gaston MA PhD FRCP   CH 75
Professor of Rheumatology
University of Cambridge Department of Medicine
Addenbrooke's Hospital
Cambridge, UK

David L George MD   CH 26
Clinical Professor of Medicine, Pennsylvania State
University
Associate Director of Medicine, Reading Hospital
Reading, PA, USA

Piet Geusens MD PhD   CH 197
Professor of Rheumatology, Linburg University Center
University Hospital, Maastricht
Maastricht, The Netherlands

Terry Gibson MD FRCP   CH 177
Consultant Physician, Guy's and St Thomas' Hospitals
Trust
Department of Rheumatology, Guy's Hospital
London, UK

Ellen M Ginzler MD MPH   CH 126
Professor of Medicine
Chief of Rheumatology, State University of New York –
Downstate Medical Center
Brooklyn, NY, USA

Dafna D Gladman MD FRCPC   CH 122
Professor of Medicine, University of Toronto;
Deputy Director, Centre for Prognosis Studies in the
Rheumatic Diseases and University of Toronto Lupus
Clinic
Toronto Western Hospital
Toronto, ON, Canada

David N Glass MD   CH 88
Professor of Pediatrics, Division of Rheumatology
Cincinnati Children's Hospital Medical Center
Cincinnati, OH, USA

Don L Goldenberg MD   CH 62
Professor of Medicine, Tufts University School of
Medicine;
Director, Arthritis – Fibromyalgia Center, Newton
Wellesley Hospital;
Chief of Rheumatology, Newton-Wellesley Hospital
Newton, MA, USA

Caroline Gordon MD FRCP   CH 125
Senior Lecturer and Consultant in Rheumatology
Division of Immunity and Infection
The University of Birmingham Medical School
Birmingham, UK

Duncan A Gordon MD FRCP MACR   CH 68
Rheumatologist
University Health Network
Toronto Western Hospital
Toronto, ON, Canada

Elena Gournelos BSc CH 49
Research Assistant
The Complementary Medicine Program
University of Maryland School of Medicine
Baltimore, MD, USA

Geoffrey P Graham MB BS FRCS CH 59
Consultant Orthopaedic Surgeon
Llandough Hospital
Penarth, Vale of Glamorgan, UK

Rodney Grahame CBE MD FRCP FACP CH 207
Emeritus Professor of Clinical Rheumatology
Hypermobility Clinic, University College London
Hospitals
London, UK

Jan T Gran MD PhD CH 102
Professor of Rheumatology
Head, Department of Rheumatology
National Hospital Rikshospitalet
Oslo, Norway

M J Green MBChB MRCP CH 78
Consultant Rheumatologist
Academic Unit of Musculoskeletal Disease
Leeds General Infirmary
Leeds, UK

Kathrin Greiner MD CH 27
Opthalmologist, Aberdeen Royal Infirmary
University of Aberdeen School of Medicine
Aberdeen, UK

Alexei A Grom MD CH 88
Assistant Professor of Pediatrics
Cincinnati Children's Hospital Medical Center
Cincinnati, OH, USA

Wolfgang L Gross MD PhD CH 145
Professor of Medicine
Poliklinik für Rheumatologie, Universitätsklinikum
Lübeck
Lübeck, Germay

Loïc Guillevin MD CH 149
Professor of Medicine
Head, Department of Internal Medicine
Hôpital Cochin
Paris, France

Poul Halberg MD PhD CH 66
Physician-in-Chief
Hvidovre Hospital
University of Copenhagen
Hvidovre, Denmark

Vedat Hamuryudan MD CH 151
Professor of Medicine
Cerrahpasa Medical Faculty
University of Istanbul
Istanbul, Turkey

Boulos Haraoui MD FRCPC CH 41
Clinical Associate Professor of Medicine, University of
Montreal
Director of Clinical Research, Rheumatic Disease Unit
CHUM, Hôpital Notre-Dame
Montreal, Quebec, Canada

John B Harley MD PhD CH 118
Professor of Medicine, University of Oklahoma
Member and Head, Arthritis and Immunology Program
University of Oklahoma Health Science Center
Oklahoma City, OK, USA

E Nigel Harris MPhil MD DM CH 131
Professor of Medicine
Dean and Senior Vice President of Academic Affairs,
Morehouse School of Medicine
Atlanta, GA, USA

Ian Haslock MD MRCP CH 107
Consultant Rheumatologist, South Tees Hospitals Trust
Visiting Professor of Clinical Bioengineering, University
of Durham
The James Cook University Hospital
Middlesborough, UK

Peter Hasselbacher MD CH 9
Professor of Medicine
University of Louisville
Louisville, KY, USA

David E Hastings MD CH 68
Professor of Surgery
University of Toronto
Toronto, ON, Canada

J Mieke Hazes MD PhD CH 81
Professor of Rheumatology
Erasmus Medical Center
Rotterdam, The Netherlands

Brian L Hazleman MA MB FRCP CH 147
Consultant Rheumatologist
Clinical Director, Rheumatology Research Unit
Addenbrooke's Hospital
Cambridge, UK

Ariane L Herrick MD FRCP CH 64
Senior Lecturer in Rheumatology, University of
Manchester
Hope Hospital
Salford, UK

Gary S Hoffman MD CH 148
Harold C Schott Chair of Rheumatologic and
Immunologic Diseases;
Director, Center for Vasculitis Care and Research
Cleveland Clinic Foundation
Cleveland, OH, USA

Tracy S Holtzman MS PT CH 91
Physical Therapist, Division of Pediatric Immunology
and Rheumatology
Washington University in St Louis
St Louis, MO, USA

Osvaldo Hübscher MD CH 19
Professor of Medicine
Section of Rheumatology and Immunology
CEMIC
Buenos Aires, Argentina

Laura K Hummers MD CH 133
Post-doctoral Fellow in Rheumatology
The Johns Hopkins University
Baltimore, Maryland
USA

Gunnar Husby MD CH 102
Professor of Medicine
Rikshospitalet University Hospital
Oslo, Norway

Robert Igwe MD CH 183 CH 201
Specialist in Endocrinology and Metabolism
William Beaumont Hospital
Berkley, MI, USA

Robert W Ike MD CH 24
Associate Professor of Internal Medicine
University of Michigan
Ann Arbor, MI, USA

Gabor G Illei MD CH 127
Senior Clinical Investigator, NIAMS
National Institutes of Health
Bethesda, MD, USA

Christopher J Jackson BAppSc MAppSc PhD CH 76
Henry Langley Research Fellow
Director, Sutton Arthritis Research Laboratories
Royal North Shore Hospital
University of Sydney
St Leonards, NSW, Australia

Dimitrios G Kassimos MD MSc CH 173
Consultant Rheumatologist
Military Hospital of Athens
Athens, Greece

Daniel Kastner MD PhD CH 11 CH 158
Chief, Genetics and Genomics Branch, NIAMS
National Institutes of Health
Bethesda, MD, USA

Tomisaku Kawasaki MD CH 152
Director, Japan Kawasaki Disease Research Center
Tokyo, Japan

Richard A Kay MB ChB PhD ILTM CH 13
Senior Research Fellow and Honorary Senior Lecturer
Department of Cell and Molecular Biology
University of Dundee Dental School
Dundee, UK

Jennifer A Kelly BS MPH CH 118
Associate Research Assistant
Oklahoma Medical Research Foundation
Oklahoma City, OK, USA

Edward Keystone MD FRCP(C) CH 41
Professor of Medicine
Director, Advanced Therapeutics
Mount Sinai Hospital
Toronto, ON, Canada

Munther A Khamashta MD FRCP PhD CH 131
Lupus Research Unit
The Rayne Institute
St Thomas' Hospital
London, UK

Muhammad Asim Khan MD FRCP MACP CH 103
Professor of Medicine, Case Western Reserve University
School of Medicine
Metro Health Medical Center
Cleveland, OH, USA

Robert P Kimberly MD CH 117
Professor of Medicine
Director, Clinical Immunology and Rheumatology
University of Alabama at Birmingham
Birmingham, AL, USA

Gabrielle H Kingsley MB FRCP CH 43
Consultant Reader in Rheumatology
GKT School of Medicine, King's College London and
University Hospital Lewisham
London, UK

John R Kirwan BSc MD FRCP   CH 36
Consultant and Reader in Rheumatology
University of Bristol Academic Rheumatology Unit
Bristol Royal Infirmary
Bristol, UK

Michael Kleerekoper MD FACP FACE   CH 183 CH 201
Professor of Medicine
Endocrine Division
Wayne State University
Detroit, MI, USA

Marisa S Klein-Gitelman MD   CH 90
Assistant Professor of Pediatrics
Feinberg School of Medicine, Northwestern University;
Interim Division Head, Pediatric Immunology and
Rheumatology
The Children's Memorial Hospital
Chicago, IL, USA

Lars Koehler MD   CH 114
Senior Lecturer and Researcher for Rheumatology
Hannover Medical School
Hannover, Germany

Brian L Kotzin MD   CH 159
Professor of Medicine and Immunology
Co-head, Division of Clinical Immunology
University of Colorado Health Sciences Center
Denver, CO, USA

Peter Kroeling MD   CH 50
Associate Professor of Physical Medicine and
Rehabilitation
Ludwig-Maximilians, University of Munich
Muenchen, Germany

Jens G Kuipers MD   CH 114
Senior Lecturer and Researcher for Rheumatology
Hannover Medical School
Hannover, Germany

Daniel Kuntz MD   CH 185, 186 & 190
Professor of Rheumatology
Hôpital Lariboisière
Paris, France

Nancy Lane MD   CH 192
Associate Professor of Medicine and Rheumatology
University of California at San Francisco
San Francisco, CA, USA

Philipp Lang MD MBA   CH 25
Associate Professor of Radiology, Harvard Medical
School;
Director, Musculoskeletal Division, Department of
Radiology
Brigham and Women's Hospital
Boston, MA, USA

Carol A Langford MD MHS   CH 150
Senior Investigator, Laboratory of Immunoregulation,
National Institute of Allergy and Infectious Diseases
National Institutes of Health
Bethesda, MD, USA

George T Lewith MA DM FRCP MRCGP   CH 49
Honorary Senior Research Fellow, University of
Southampton
Complementary Medicine Research Unit, Royal South
Hants Hospital
Southampton, UK

François Lhote MD   CH 149
Practicien Hospitalier, Service de Médecine Interne
Hôpital Delafontaine
Saint-Denis, France

Lars Lidgren MD PhD   CH 93
Professor of Orthopedics
Chairman and Professor, Department of Orthopedics
University Hospital of Lund
Lund, Sweden

Carol B Lindsley MD   CH 87
Professor and Chair, Pediatrics
Director, Pediatric Rheumatology
University of Kansas City Medical Center
Kansas City, KS, USA

Peter E Lipsky MD   CH 108
Scientific Director, National Institute of Arthritis,
Musculoskeletal and Skin Diseases
National Institutes of Health
Bethesda, MD, USA

Geoffrey Littlejohn MBBS (Hons) MD MPH   CH 172
FRACP FAFRM FRCP (Edin)
Associate Professor of Medicine, Department of
Rheumatology
Monash Medical Center
Melbourne, Victoria, Australia

Martin Lotz MD   CH 15
Professor and Head, Division of Arthritis Research
The Scripps Research Institute
La Jolla, CA, USA

James S Louie MD   CH 95
Professor Emeritus, UCLA School of Medicine
Chief of Rheumatology, Harbor-UCLA Medical Center
Torrance, CA, USA

Carlos J Lozada MD   CH 165 & 171
Associate Professor of Medicine
Director, Rheumatology Training Program, Division of
Rheumatology and Immunology
The University of Miami
Miami, FL, USA

Harvinder S Luthra MD   CH 160
John F. Finn Minnesota Arthritis Foundation
Chair, Division of Rheumatology
Mayo Clinic and Mayo Medical School
Rochester, MN, USA

Alex J MacGregor MD MA FRCP   CH 67
Consultant Rheumatologist and Honorary Senior
Lecturer
Guy's, King's and St Thomas' School of Medicine
London, UK

Rajan Madhok MBChB MD FRCP (Glasgow)   CH 39
Consultant Physician and Rheumatologist
Glasgow Royal Infirmary
Glasgow, UK

Maren Lawson Mahowald MD   CH 94
Professor of Medicine
Minneapolis Veterans Affairs Medical Center
Minneapolis, MN, USA

Walter P Maksymowych MD FRCP (C) FACP   CH 104
FRCP (UK)
Associate Professor of Medicine
University of Alberta
Edmonton, Alberta, Canada

Nisha J Manek MD   CH 167
Clinical Research Fellow
Twin Research and Genetic Epidemiology Unit
St Thomas' Hospital, London, UK

Raija Manninen MD   CH 92
Specialist in Clinical Microbiology
Satakunta Central Hospital
Pori, Finland

Susan M Manzi MD MPH   CH 116
Associate Professor of Medicine and Epidemiology
University of Pittsburgh Department of Medicine
Pittsburgh, PA, USA

Hilal Maradit Kremers MD MSc   CH 7
Assistant Professor of Epidemiology
Mayo Clinic
Rochester, MN, USA

Joan C Marini MD PhD   CH 206
Chief, Heritable Disorders Branch NICHD
National Institutes of Health
Bethesda, MD, USA

Pierre Maroteaux MD PhD   CH 205
Emeritus Director of Research CNRS
Hôpital des Enfants Malades
Paris, France

Manuel Martínez-Lavín MD   CH 162
Professor of Rheumatology, National Autonomous
University of Mexico
Chief of Rheumatology, National Institute of Cardiology
Tlalpan, Mexico

Eric L Matteson MD MPH   CH 69
Associate Professor of Medicine (Rheumatology)
Mayo Clinic and Mayo Graduate School of Medicine
Rochester, MN, USA

Bernard Mazières MD   CH 58 CH 174
Professor of Rheumatology
University Hospital of Rangueil
Toulouse, France

Rex McCallum MD   CH 163
Clinical Professor of Medicine
Duke Hospital
Durham, NC, USA

Geraldine M McCarthy MD FRCPI   CH 180
Consultant Rheumatologist, Mater Misericordiae
Hospital
Honorary Senior Lecturer, Department of Clinical
Pharmacology, Royal College of Surgeons in Ireland
Dublin, Ireland

Lachy McLean MD PhD FRACP   CH 176
Senior Lecturer in Rheumatology
University of Auckland
Auckland, New Zealand

Thomas A Medsger Jr MD   CH 139
Gerald P. Rodnan Professor of Medicine
University of Pittsburgh School of Medicine
Pittsburgh, PA, USA

L Joseph Melton, III MD   CH 194
Michael M. Eisenberg Professor
Department of Health Sciences Research
Mayo Clinic
Rochester, MN, USA

Herman Mielants MD PhD `CH 30` `CH 113`
Professor of Rheumatology
Gent University Hospital
Gent, Belgium

Frederick W Miller MD PhD `CH 138`
Chief, Environmental Autoimmunity Group
National Institute of Environmental Health Sciences
National Institutes of Health
Bethesda, MD, USA

Michael L Miller MD `CH 90`
Associate Professor
Division of Pediatric Immunology and Rheumatology
Northwestern University Medical School
Chicago, IL, USA

Marian Minor PT PhD `CH 82`
Associate Professor of Physical Therapy
University of Missouri
Columbia, MO, USA

Mila Mituszova MD `CH 175`
Consultant Rheumatologist
National Institute of Rheumatology and Physiotherapy
Budapest, Hungary

G M Mody MBChB MD FCP (SA) FRCP (London) `CH 99`
Aaron Beare Family Professor of Rheumatology
Nelson R. Mandela School of Medicine
University of Natal
Durban, South Africa

Akio Morinobu MD PhD `CH 11`
Research Fellow
National Institute of Arthritis, Musculoskeletal and Skin
Diseases
National Institutes of Health
Bethesda, MD, USA

Kathy L Moser PhD `CH 118`
Assistant Professor
University of Minnesota
Minneapolis, MN, USA

Haralampos M Moutsopoulos MD FACP `CH 130`
FRCP (Edin)
Professor and Director of Pathophysiology
University of Athens School of Medicine
Athens, Greece

Gregory R Mundy MD `CH 192`
Professor, Department of Cellular and Structural
Biology
Assistant Dean for Clinical Research
University of Texas Health Science Center at San
Antonio
San Antonio, TX, USA

Kanneboyina Nagaraju DVM PhD `CH 138`
Assistant Professor of Medicine
Johns Hopkins University School of Medicine
Baltimore, MD, USA

Stanley J Naides MD `CH 97`
Thomas B. Hallowell Professor of Medicine;
Professor of Microbiology and Immunology
Professor of Pharmacology;
Chief, Division of Rheumatology
Penn State Milton S. Hershey Medical Center
Hershey, PA, USA

David J Nashel MD FACP `CH 63`
Professor of Medicine, Georgetown and George
Washington Universities;
Chief, Medical Service, Veterans Affairs Medial Center
Washington, DC, USA

Barbara Nepom MD `CH 72`
Affiliate Research Associate Professor, Department of
Pediatrics
University of Washington School of Medicine
Seattle, WA, USA

Gerald T Nepom MD PhD `CH 72`
Director, Virginia Mason Research Center
Seattle, WA, USA

Patrick T O'Gara MD `CH 28`
Associate Professor of Medicine, Harvard Medical
School;
Director, Clinical Cardiology
Brigham and Women's Hospital
Boston, MA, USA

John J O'Shea MD `CH 11`
Chief, Molecular Immunology and Inflammation Branch
National Institute of Arthritis, Musculoskeletal and Skin
Diseases
National Institutes of Health
Bethesda, MD, USA

Chester V Oddis MD `CH 139`
Professor of Medicine
University of Pittsburgh School of Medicine
Pittsburgh, PA, USA

Bill Ollier PhD FRCPath `CH 12`
Professor of Immunogenetics
Centre for Integrated Genomic Medical Research
University of Manchester, Manchester, UK

Brad W Olney MD `CH 87`
Professor of Orthopedic Surgery, University of Kansas
School of Medicine
Wichita Clinic
Wichita, KS, USA

K Sigvard Olsson MD PhD `CH 189`
Associate Professor
Section of Hematology and Coagulation
Sahlgren's University Hospital
Göteborg, Sweden

Philippe Orcel MD PhD `CH 204`
Professor of Rheumatology
Hôpital Lariboisière
Paris, France

Lauren M Pachman MD `CH 90`
Professor of Pediatrics
Feinberg School of Medicine, Northwestern University;
Interim Director, Disease Pathogenesis Program
Children's Memorial Hospital
Chicago, IL, USA

Gabriel S Panayi ScD MD FRCP `CH 43`
ARC Professor of Rheumatology
Guy's, King's and St Thomas' School of Medicine,
King's College
London, UK

Michaelis Pazianas MD `CH 202`
Associate Professor of Medicine
University of Pennsylvania
Philadelphia, PA, USA

J David Perry MD FRCP `CH 65`
Consultant Rheumatologist
Royal London Hospital
London, UK

Michelle Petri MD MPH `CH 129`
Professor of Medicine
Johns Hopkins University School of Medicine
Baltimore, MD, USA

Ross E Petty MD PhD `CH 84`
Professor of Medicine
British Columbia Children's Hospital
Vancouver, Canada

Matthew C Pickering MBBS MRCP PhD `CH 119`
ARC Clinical Research Fellow
Imperial College School of Medicine
London, UK

Carlos Pineda MD `CH 162`
Associate Professor of Rheumatology
National Institute of Cardiology
Tlalpan, Mexico

Paul H Plotz MD `CH 138`
Chief, Arthritis and Rheumatism Branch
National Institute of Arthritis, Musculoskeletal and Skin
Diseases
National Institutes of Health
Bethesda, MD, USA

Gyula Poór MD PhD DSc `CH 175`
Professor of Rheumatology
Director General, National Institute of Rheumatology
and Physiotherapy
Budapest, Hungary

Richard Powell MBBS DM FRCP FRCPath `CH 44`
Consultant and Reader in Immunology
University Hospital
Queen's Medical Centre
Nottingham, UK

Anne-Marie F Prieur MD `CH 89`
Médecin de Hôpitaux Unité
d'Immuno-hematologie et Rhumatologie Pédiatriques
Hôpital Necker Enfantes Malades
Paris, France

M A Quinn MBChB MRCP `CH 78`
Lecturer in Rheumatology
Academic Unit of Musculoskeletal Disease
Leeds General Infirmary
Leeds, UK

Rosalind Ramsey-Goldman MD DrPH `CH 116`
Professor of Medicine
Northwestern University Medical School
Chicago, IL, USA

Elaine Remmers PhD `CH 11`
Staff Scientist
National Institute of Arthritis, Musculoskeletal and Skin
Diseases
National Institutes of Health
Bethesda, MD, USA

Donald Resnick MD `CH 71`
Professor of Radiology
Veterans Affairs Medical Center
San Diego, CA, USA

Bruce C Richardson MD PhD — CH 124
Professor of Medicine, University of Michigan
Chief, Section of Rheumatology
Ann Arbor VA Hospital
Ann Arbor, MI, USA

B Lawrence Riggs MD — CH 194
Distinguished Investigator, Mayo Foundation
Purvis and Roberta Tabor Professor of Medical
Research
Mayo Clinic and Foundation
Rochester, MN, USA

Dwight R Robinson MD — CH 16
Professor of Medicine
Massachusetts General Hospital and Harvard Medical
School
Boston, MA, USA

Drew Rowan BSc PhD — CH 14
Non-Clinical Lecturer in Molecular Rheumatology
University of Newcastle School of Medicine
Newcastle, UK

Violeta Rus MD — CH 115
Assistant Professor of Medicine
University of Maryland School of Medicine
Baltimore, MD, USA

Anthony S Russell MD FRCP(C) FRCP — CH 100
Professor of Medicine
University of Alberta
Edmonton, Alberta, Canada

Graham Russell PhD DM FRCP FRCPath FMedSci — CH 196
Norman Collisson Professor of Musculoskeletal Science
University of Oxford
Headington, Oxford, UK

Jane E Salmon MD — CH 117
Professor of Medicine
Hospital for Special Surgery
New York, NY, USA

David C Salonen BSc MD FRCP (C) — CH 105
Musculoskeletal Radiologist
University of Toronto
Toronto, ON, Canada

Philip N Sambrook MD FRACP — CH 199
Professor of Rheumatology
Royal North Shore Hospital
St Leonards, Sydney, Australia

Leslie Schrieber MBBS (Hons) MD FRACP — CH 76
Associate Professor of Medicine, University of Sydney
Royal North Shore Hospital
St Leonards, Sydney, Australia

H Ralph Schumacher Jr MD — CH 161 CH 181
Professor of Medicine, University of Pennsylvania
Director, Arthritis and Immunology Center
Veterans Affairs Medical Center
Philadelphia, PA, USA

Peter H Schur MD — CH 20
Professor of Medicine, Harvard Medical School
Director, Clinical Immunology Web
Brigham and Women's Hospital
Boston, MA, USA

David G I Scott MD FRCP — CH 143
Honorary Professor, University of East Anglia
Consultant Rheumatologist, Norfolk and Norwich
University Healthcare NHS Trust
Norfolk, UK

Peter Selby MA MD FRCP — CH 200
Honorary Senior Lecturer, University of Manchester
Consultant Physician
Manchester Royal Infirmary
Manchester, UK

Frederic Shapiro MD — CH 208
Associate Professor of Orthopedic Surgery
Harvard Medical School
Boston, MA, USA

Robert H Shmerling MD — CH 20
Associate Professor of Medicine, Harvard Medical
School
Beth Israel Deaconess Hospital
Boston, MA, USA

Alan J Silman — CH 67
ARC Professor of Rheumatic Disease Epidemiology
Director, Arthritis Research Campaign Epidemiology
Research Unit
University of Manchester, UK

Roy L Silverstein MD — CH 144
Professor of Medicine, Weill Medical College of Cornell
University
Chief, Division of Hematology and Medical Oncology
New York, NY, USA

Ronit Simantov MD — CH 144
Assistant Professor of Medicine
Weill Medical College of Cornell University
New York, NY, USA

Peter A Simkin MD — CH 8
Professor of Medicine
Adjunct Professor of Orthopaedics
University of Washington
Seattle, WA, USA

Edwin A Smith MD — CH 134
Professor of Medicine
Medical University of South Carolina
Charleston, SC, USA

Oscar Soto MD — CH 146
Assistant Professor of Medicine, Rheumatology and
Immunology
Emory University School of Medicine
Atlanta, Georgia, USA

Timothy D Spector MD MSc FRCP — CH 167
Consultant Rheumatologist
Professor of Twin Research and Genetic Epidemiology
Guys and St Thomas' Hospital
London, UK

Vida Emily Stark MS — CH 116
Research Associate
University of Pittsburgh Department of Medicine
Pittsburgh, PA, USA

E William St Clair MD — CH 163
Associate Professor of Medicine
Duke University Medical Center
Durham, NC, USA

Virginia D Steen MD — CH 132
Professor of Medicine
Georgetown University Medical Center
Washington, DC, USA

Allen C Steere MD — CH 96
Professor of Medicine, Harvard Medical School
Director, Rheumatology
Massachusetts General Hospital
Boston, MA, USA

Günter Steiner PhD — CH 74
Professor of Biochemistry, Division of Rheumatology
University Hospital of Vienna
Vienna, Austria

John H Stone MD MPH — CH 148
Associate Professor of Medicine
Director, The Johns Hopkins Vasculitis Center
Baltimore, MD, USA

Gerold Stucki MD MS — CH 50
Professor of Physical Medicine and Rehabilitation
Ludwig-Maximilians University
Muenchen, Germany

R D Sturrock MD FRCP — CH 38
McLeod ARC Professor of Rheumatology
Glasgow Royal Infirmary
Glasgow, UK

Deborah Symmons MD MFPHM FRCP — CH 3
Professor of Rheumatology and Musculoskeletal
Epidemiology
University of Manchester School of Medicine
Manchester, UK

Ilona S Szer MD — CH 153
Professor of Clinical Pediatrics
Director, Pediatric Rheumatology
Children's Hospital and Health Center
San Diego, CA, USA

Antonio Tavoni MD — CH 156
Rheumatologist
University of Pisa
Pisa, Italy

Daphne J Theodorou MD — CH 71
Musculoskeletal Radiologist
Veterans Affairs Medical Center
San Diego, CA, USA

Stavroula J Theodorou MD — CH 71
Musculoskeletal Radiologist
Veterans Affairs Medical Center
San Diego, CA, USA

Auli Toivanen MD DrMedSci — CH 109
Professor of Medicine (Emerita)
Turku University
Turku, Finland

Paavo Toivanen MD — CH 92
Professor Emeritus of Bacteriology and Serology
Turku University
Turku, Finland

Athanasios G Tzioufas MD — CH 130
Assistant Professor
University of Athens School of Medicine
Athens, Greece

Murray B Urowitz MD FRCPC   `CH 122`
Professor of Medicine, University of Toronto
Director, Centre for Prognosis Studies in The Rheumatic
Diseases and University of Toronto Lupus Clinic
Toronto Western Hospital
Toronto, ON, USA

Désirée van der Heijde MD PhD   `CH 101`
Professor of Rheumatology
University Hospital of Maastricht
Maastricht, The Netherlands

Sjef van der Linden MD PhD   `CH 101`
Professor of Rheumatology
University Hospital of Maastricht
Maastricht, The Netherlands

Anke M van Gestel MD MSc   `CH 79`
University Medical Centre, St Radboud
Nijmegen, The Netherlands

Piet L C M van Riel MD PhD   `CH 79`
Professor and Director, Clinical Research Unit
University Hospital Nijmegen
Nijmegen, The Netherlands

John Varga MD   `CH 137`
Professor of Medicine
Director, Section of Rheumatology
University of Illinois at Chicago
Chicago, IL, USA

Dimitrios Vassilopoulos MD   `CH 98`
Consultant Rheumatologist
Henry Dunant Hospital
Athens, Greece

Patrick J W Venables MD FRCP   `CH 142`
Professor of Viral Immunorheumatology
Kennedy Division, Imperial College
London, UK

Barrie Vernon-Roberts MD PhD FRCPath   `CH 106`
FRCPA FAOrth (Hons)
George Richard Marks Professor of Pathology,
University of Adelaide
Senior Visiting Pathologist, The Royal Adelaide Hospital
Director, Institute of Medical and Veterinary Science
Adelaide, Australia

Eric M Veys MD PhD   `CH 30`   `CH 113`
Professor of Rheumatology
Gent University Hospital
Gent, Belgium

Daniel J Wallace MD   `CH 128`
Clinical Professor of Medicine
UCLA School of Medicine
Los Angeles, CA, USA

Mark J Walport MA PhD FRCP FCPath FmedSci   `CH 119`
Professor of Medicine
Imperial College London
London, UK

David M Ward MBChB MRCP FRCP (G)   `CH 31`
Professor of Medicine
University of California at San Diego
San Diego, CA, USA

Richard A Watts MD FRCP   `CH 143`
Honorary Senior Lecturer, University of East Anglia;
Consultant Rheumatologist, The Ipswich Hospital NHS
Trust
Ipswich, UK

Athol U Wells MBChB MD FRACP   `CH 29`
Consultant in Respiratory Medicine
Royal Brompton Hospital
London, UK

Paco M J Welsing MD MSc   `CH 79`
Epidemiologist
University Medical Centre, St Radboud
Nijmegen, The Netherlands

Sterling G West MD   `CH 159`
Professor of Medicine
University of Colorado Health Sciences Center
Denver, CO, USA

Patience H White MD   `CH 85`
Chairman, Division of Adult and Pediatric
Rheumatology;
Professor of Medicine and Pediatrics, Children's
National Medical Center
George Washington University School of Medicine and
Health Sciences
Washington, DC, USA

Fredrick M Wigley MD   `CH 133`
Professor of Medicine
Associate Director, Division of Rheumatology
The Johns Hopkins University
Baltimore, MD, USA

Allan Wiik MD DSc (Med)   `CH 21`
Chief, Department of Autoimmunology
Statens Serum Institut
Copenhagen, Denmark

H James Williams MD   `CH 40`
Professor of Medicine
Thomas E. and Rebecca D. Jeremy Presidential
Endowed Chair for Arthritis Research
University of Utah School of Medicine
Salt Lake City, UT, USA

Frank A Wollheim MD PhD FRCP   `CH 166`
Professor of Rheumatology
Lund University Hospital
Lund, Sweden

Paul H Wooley PhD   `CH 73`
Professor of Orthopaedic Surgery, Immunology and
Biomedical Engineering
Wayne State University
Detroit, MI, USA

Anthony D Woolf BSc MBBS FRCP   `CH 18`   `CH 198`
Professor of Rheumatology, Peninsula Medical School
Consultant Rheumatologist, Royal Cornwall Hospital
Truro, Cornwall, UK

Robert L Wortmann MD   `CH 141`
Professor and Chair, Department of Internal Medicine
University of Oklahoma College of Medicine
Tulsa, OK, USA

Hasan Yazici MD   `CH 151`
Professor of Medicine
Chief, Division of Rheumatology
Cerrahpasa Medical Faculty
University of Istanbul
Istanbul, Turkey

Edward H Yelin PhD   `CH 5`
Professor of Medicine and Health Policy
University of California at San Francisco
San Francisco, CA, USA

John R York MD FRACP FRCP (Glasg)   `CH 187`
Clinical Associate Professor of Rheumatology
The Royal Prince Alfred Hospital
Camperdown, NSW, Australia

Raymond L Yung MBChB   `CH 124`
Assistant Professor of Internal Medicine
Cancer Center and Geriatrics Center
Ann Arbor, MI, USA

Sebahattin Yurdakul MD   `CH 151`
Professor of Medicine
Cerrahpasa Medical Faculty
University of Istanbul
Istanbul, Turkey

Henning K Zeidler MD   `CH 114`
Professor of Rheumatology
Hannover Medical School
Hannover, Germany

PREFACE

The third edition of *Rheumatology* is:

- The most comprehensive, authoritative rheumatology text, designed to meet the complete needs of all practicing and academic rheumatologists as well as all arthritis related health care professionals and scientists interested in disorders of the musculoskeletal system.
- Firmly grounded on modern medical science, integrating the relevant basic biology with current clinical practice.
- An easily accessible, user-friendly, beautifully illustrated colour publication.
- Consistent in style and format, each chapter is written to a strict template and rigorously edited.
- A genuinely international book, with editors, authors and material drawn from all over the world.
- Fully up-to-date, with carefully selected references to original work and key reviews up to and including 2002 publications.

THE THIRD EDITION OF *RHEUMATOLOGY* IS A TOTALLY NEW AND VERY EXCITING BOOK

A new international team of editors representing the entire spectrum of academic and clinical rheumatology and biomedical, clinical and epidemiological research, was recruited to bring you the third edition of this world famous book. The editors and publisher commissioned independent, critical reviews of the second edition from clinicians and scientists worldwide, analyzed their comments and embraced the exciting challenge of re-structuring the format and contents of the book in a way that would retain all the best features of the first and second editions of *Rheumatology*, while also striving to make a great book even better. We believe that we have succeeded and that the third edition of *Rheumatology* will become the first choice for all rheumatologists and their trainees.

As noted by prior reviewers ("*a model for other textbooks*" – NEJM; "*a departure from everything that has preceded it*" – JAMA), the success of the first and second editions owed much to the consistency of style and content, innovative use of colour illustration and user-friendly format. We have retained all of these features of the book. We have continued to use templates for each chapter, and have pursued a rigorous editorial policy in order to ensure that the content and format of the book remain both consistent and of the highest possible standard. The different sections remain colour coded (although users of the first and second editions should note that the colours have changed!).

Whilst much of what made the first and second editions so successful has therefore been retained, we have also made many major changes to the contents for this edition, the first in this new century.

The introductory section, as well as that on principles of therapy, has been extensively restructured, and many new contributors have joined the team. Every chapter has either been carefully revised (35%) or, in many cases, completely rewritten (40% of chapters). There is new information on basic biomedical science, clinical therapeutics, disease and outcome assessment, and patient management and rehabilitation. Indeed, 58 new chapters (more than one-quarter of the book) have been added to the third edition. While much new information has been added, we have also deleted some of the material found in the second edition, so that the total extent of the book is only some 146 pages longer. We have also worked hard to improve the index, in order to make it easier for the reader to find the material that he or she wants.

The new edition also includes a CDROM of the images in the book downloadable in Powerpoint ® as well as access to **www.rheumtext.com** to enable rapid electronic searches of the contents of the entire 2-volume set. You'll also find a complete library of easily downloadable electronic images, links to key society web sites, self-assessment tests, outcome measurement tools and patient information and continuous content updates.

The production of the third edition of *Rheumatology* has been a greatly enjoyable team effort. We would like to thank every one of the authors who have contributed to this or any other edition of the book, as well as the excellent team at Mosby. We look forward to bringing you a fourth edition of *Rheumatology* later this decade.

ACKNOWLEDGEMENTS

We would like to acknowledge Drs John H Klippel and Paul A Dieppe, the founding editors of *Rheumatology*, and the tremendous work of the contributors to *Rheumatology* both present and past, without whom this book would not have been possible. In addition, we would like to acknowledge our mentors: Drs. Eva Alberman, Harry Currey (deceased), Lawrence E. Shulman, Carl Steffen (deceased), Alfred D. Steinberg, Mary Betty Stevens (deceased) and Nathan Zvaifler.

We would also like to acknowledge the excellent team at Mosby led by Fiona Foley (Paul Fam, Michael Houston and Kim Murphy), and our secretaries and administrative assistants (Margarita Cook, Johanna Leibl and Robin Nichols) for all of their hard work and diligence. Last, but certainly not least, we want to acknowledge our patients.

DEDICATION

We would like to dedicate this book to our parents (living or of blessed memory), and our wives and children:

Susan Hochberg, Francine and Jennifer Hochberg

Ruth Silman, Joanna, Timothy and Daniel Silman

Alice Smolen, Eva, Nina and Daniel Smolen, and Wanda and Stefan Smolen

Barbara Weinblatt, Hillary and Courtney Weinblatt

Betsy Weisman, Greg, Nicole and Mia Colette Weisman, Lisa, Andrew and David Temple Cope, and Annie Weisman

INFECTION-RELATED RHEUMATIC DISEASES

92 Microorganisms and the locomotor system

Paavo Toivanen and Raija Manninen

Classification

- Microorganisms causing joint and bone diseases include bacteria, viruses, fungi and parasites
- Bacteria are the most important regarding diseases of the locomotor system. Bacterial diseases are septic (bacterial) arthritis, reactive arthritis, osteomyelitis and osteitis
- Viruses causing arthritis are divided into those with viral disease often accompanied by arthritis, and those only seldom associated with arthritis
- Species of fungi are recognized as human pathogens. Only a few of these are associated with joint and bone lesions
- Species of protozoa, flatworms and roundworms are associated with joint and bone lesions
- Microbial superantigens, heat shock proteins and molecular mimicry are supposed to be involved in the pathogenesis of arthritis
- Experimental microbially induced arthritides give important insights into the pathogenic mechanisms of arthritis

INTRODUCTION

Microorganisms known to cause joint and bone diseases include bacteria, viruses, fungi and parasites. They may cause diseases of the locomotor system in one of four ways:

- by being present and alive, i.e. inducing an active infection
- by being present in an inactive or degraded form
- by sending metabolites, toxins or other extracellular products from a distant focus
- via induction of immunologic mediators, which may be either cellular or humoral. Immunologic mechanisms in the pathogenesis of joint diseases potentially involve antigenic similarity or molecular mimicry between the target tissue and the inducing microorganism.

Microbially induced diseases affect either previously injured joints or primarily healthy, intact joints. The preceding injury may result from trauma, surgery, prosthesis, infection or an intra-articular injection. Reduced resistance to microbial joint and bone involvement is often associated with severe and debilitating illnesses, such as diabetes mellitus or rheumatoid arthritis (RA). Immunosuppression, induced by either disease or treatment, is also a significant cause of infectious arthritides. When a primarily healthy joint becomes infected, a predisposing factor can usually be identified.

BACTERIA

Of the four groups of microorganisms associated with diseases of the loco-motor system, bacteria are by far the most important. Bacteria of interest to rheumatologists are those which are proven causes of septic arthritis, osteomyelitis or reactive arthritis (Tables 92.1–92.3). Some of these bacteria have also been speculatively associated with the pathogenesis of RA (see Table 92.4). A rheumatologic repertoire of bacteriologic species is systematically presented here. For a more detailed bacteriologic description, several textbooks and manuals are available[1–4].

GRAM-POSITIVE COCCI

Streptococci

Streptococci are spherical or ovoid, Gram-positive cocci arranged in chains or pairs. Most streptococcal species are facultative anaerobes. The genus *Streptococcus* contains a number of species with a wide variation in pathogenicity and virulence. Regarding diseases of the locomotor system, *Streptococcus pyogenes* (β-hemolytic group A) is the most important, followed by *Streptococcus pneumoniae* and groups B and

---

TABLE 92.1 BACTERIA ASSOCIATED WITH SEPTIC ARTHRITIS

Bacteroides fragilis
Enterococcus faecium
Enterococcus faecalis
Escherichia coli
Haemophilus influenzae
Kingella kingae
Klebsiella pneumoniae
Mycobacterium tuberculosis
Neisseria gonorrhoeae
Proteus mirabilis
Pseudomonas aeruginosa
Salmonella species
Staphylococcus aureus
Staphylococcus epidermidis
Streptococcus pneumoniae
Streptococcus pyogenes

TABLE 92.2 BACTERIA ASSOCIATED WITH OSTEOMYELITIS

Bacteroides fragilis
Enterobacteriaceae species (*Escherichia coli, Salmonella, Proteus, Klebsiella*)
Mycobacterium tuberculosis
Non-group A streptococci
Peptostreptococcus anaerobius
Prevotella melaninogenica (formerly *Bacteroides melaninogenicus*)
Pseudomonas aeruginosa
Staphylococcus aureus

TABLE 92.3 BACTERIA MOST COMMONLY FOUND TRIGGERING REACTIVE ARTHRITIS

Borrelia burgdorferi
Campylobacter jejuni
Chlamydia trachomatis
Neisseria gonorrhoeae
Salmonella species
Shigella flexneri
Streptococcus pyogenes
Yersinia enterocolitica
Yersinia pseudotuberculosis

TABLE 92.4 MICROORGANISMS MOST COMMONLY IMPLICATED AS ETIOLOGIC AGENTS IN RHEUMATOID ARTHRITIS

Bacteria	Viruses
Clostridium perfringens	Adenoviruses
Enterobacteriaceae species	Cytomegalovirus
Mycobacteria	Epstein–Barr virus
Mycoplasma species	Human T cell leukemia virus type 1
Non-group A streptococci	Parvovirus B19
	Rubella virus

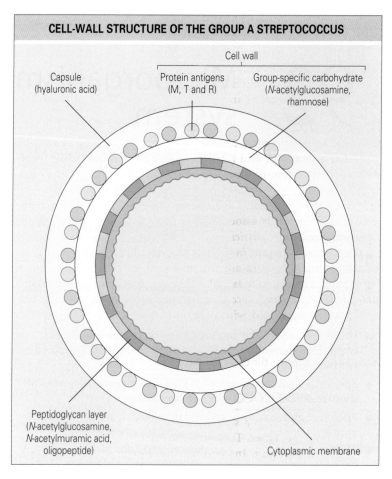

CELL-WALL STRUCTURE OF THE GROUP A STREPTOCOCCUS

Fig. 92.1 Cell wall structure of the group A streptococcus.

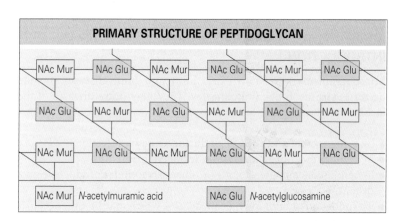

PRIMARY STRUCTURE OF PEPTIDOGLYCAN

Fig. 92.2 **Primary structure of peptidoglycan.** The peptidoglycan layer is a large bipolymer, consisting of long glycan chains with *N*-acetylmuramic acid and *N*-acetylglucosamine alternating within each chain. The muramic acid moieties are attached to a pentapeptide (vertical lines), which in turn is bound by an interpeptide bridge (diagonal lines) to a pentapeptide of another glycan chain.

G hemolytic streptococci. Streptococci of the viridans group, which is a heterogenous collection of α- and non-hemolytic streptococci, are sometimes responsible for septic arthritides.

Group A streptococci cause pyoderma, impetigo and bacterial pharyngitis. These infections, when left untreated, may lead to severe infectious complications, including mastoiditis and osteomyelitis. The most important of the streptococcal rheumatic diseases in humans is rheumatic fever, which develops as a post-infectious complication of group A streptococcal tonsillitis.

Group A streptococci are 0.5–1.0 μm in diameter and spherical in shape. They grow in chains both *in vivo* and *in vitro*. The cellular structure of group A streptococci is presented in Figure 92.1. The outermost layer, the capsule, is composed of hyaluronic acid, which is identical to the hyaluronic acid in human connective tissue. The skeleton of the streptococcal cell wall is the peptidoglycan layer, which is similar to that found in other Gram-positive bacteria.

The peptidoglycan layer is a large biopolymer, consisting of long glycan chains with *N*-acetylmuramic acid and *N*-acetylglucosamine alternating within each chain. The carboxyl groups of muramic acid moieties are substituted by penta-peptides, which in turn are bound by interpeptide bridges to penta-peptides of another glycan chain (Fig. 92.2). In streptococci and other Gram-positive bacteria a thick peptidoglycan network covers the whole bacterial cell. The network may comprise 70% of the bacterial cell wall. The glycan chain composition is almost the same in various bacteria, but the peptides vary between the species. The outer surface of the peptidoglycan layer of Gram-positive bacteria is covered by a polysaccharide layer, covalently coupled to it. This affords protection against host leukocytes.

Peptidoglycan-polysaccharide complexes from the group A streptococcal cell wall have been shown to be the crucial elements in experimentally inducing streptococcal cell-wall arthritis in the rat[5-7]. Peptidoglycan components have been demonstrated in arthritic rat joints and can be compared to the lipopolysaccharide components observed in synovial fluid cells of patients with reactive arthritis. As such, the cell-wall peptidoglycan is not a virulence factor[8], in contrast to the strepto-

coccal M protein, which is located on the bacterial fimbriae and which protects the bacteria against phagocytosis by interacting with complement[9]. Other virulence factors of streptococci include lipoteichoic acid, erythrogenic toxins, streptolysins S and O, streptokinases and DNAases.

Several examples of cross-reactions of streptococcal antigens and mammalian tissue have been demonstrated. Streptococcal cell-wall antigens, cytoplasmic membranes and M protein have been reported to cross-react with heart, glomerular basement membrane, brain, skeletal muscle, articular cartilage and synovium[9,10]. However, the exact mechanisms for induction of rheumatic fever, including synovitis, still remain unexplained (see Chapter 99). Persistence of bacterial products resistant to degradation, e.g. peptidoglycan, and capable of inducing and maintaining a local inflammatory reaction is one of the most attractive possibilities[7,11]. It is also worth noting that rheumatic fever is a late complication of only upper respiratory infections caused by group A streptococci; cutaneous infections are not followed by rheumatic fever.

Staphylococci

Staphylococci are the most common bacterial cause of septic arthritis, particularly in adults, and also hematogenous osteomyelitis[12]. They are non-motile Gram-positive cocci, 0.5–1.5μm in diameter and facultatively anaerobic. Normally, staphylococci grow on human skin and mucosal membranes. Of the 32 staphylococcal species currently recognized, commonly associated with human disease are: *S. aureus*, *S. epidermidis*, *S. saprophyticus* and *S. lugdunensis*. Of these, *S. aureus* is the usual causative agent in primary septic arthritis or septic arthritis following trauma or intra-articular injection, or as a complication of debilitating illnesses such as diabetes, RA and systemic lupus erythematosus (SLE). *Staphylococcus epidermidis* is the most common bacterial species associated with infectious complications of articular prostheses. The staphylococcal cell wall resembles that of streptococci. The complex polysaccharides bound to the peptidoglycan layer are teichoic acids specific for each staphylococcal species.

GRAM-NEGATIVE COCCI

Neisseria gonorrhoeae is a small Gram-negative diplococcus with 60 different serologic types. The surface structure of *N. gonorrhoeae* is presented in Figure 92.3. Interestingly, the cellular membrane has, in addition to peptidoglycan, a lipopolysaccharide layer. The lipopolysaccharide contains lipid A and a core polysaccharide, even though the strain-specific O side chains present in Gram-negative rods are absent. Lipopolysaccharide is responsible for tissue destruction and is a major virulence factor of *N. gonorrhoeae*.

N. gonorrhoeae may cause both septic and reactive forms of arthritis, in the same way as has been reported for *N. meningitidis*, *Haemophilus influenzae* and enterobacterial Gram-negative rods (see Chapter 94). It is quite possible that, in all cases of reactive arthritis, a shorter or longer period of septic synovitis precedes the stage when no viable bacteria are present within the synovial tissue. Likewise, a few cases of typical septic arthritis may be followed by a persistent aseptic arthritis.

N. gonorrhoeae is always pathogenic, whereas *N. meningitidis* can also be found in the upper respiratory tract without causing disease. Like gonococci, the meningococci are encapsulated Gram-negative diplococci. They cause meningitis, pneumonia or sepsis. All these can be accompanied or followed by an arthritis that may be heavily purulent or entirely reactive in nature. *N. meningitidis* is divided into 13 serogroups on the basis of the capsular polysaccharide antigens, into more than 20 serotypes on the basis of outer membrane protein antigens and into eight immunotypes on the basis of lipopolysaccharide antigens.

In addition to the *Neisseriae*, the family Neisseriaceae includes the genera *Branhamella*, *Moraxella*, *Kingella* and *Acinetobacter*. They all contain species which have rarely been associated with arthritis. Branhamellas are Gram-negative cocci, whereas moraxellas, kingellas and acinetobacters are short rods called coccobacilli. All of them – *Moraxella lacunata*, *Kingella kingae* and *Acinetobacter calcoaceticus* – are normal inhabitants of the human oral cavity. The most commonly diagnosed infections of *Kingella kingae* are endocarditis and septic arthritis.

GRAM-POSITIVE BACILLI

Anaerobes

Three bacterial genera of anaerobic Gram-positive rods are of interest to rheumatologists, *Clostridium*, *Collinsella* and *Propionibacterium*. Clostridia represent a particularly interesting chapter in the rheumatologic bacteriology: no definite proof exists that they have a role in the etiology or pathogenesis of rheumatic diseases: instead, challenging indirect evidence has been presented.

The genus *Clostridium* contains the clinically most important anaerobic, Gram-positive, spore-forming rods. They are present in soil, water, and the normal flora of the intestinal tract of animals and humans. Of the 80 species within the genus, only a few are well-recognized human pathogens, causing diseases such as tetanus, gas gangrene, botulism and other food poisonings, skin and soft tissue infections, and pseudomembranous colitis.

Two species of clostridia may have a connection with arthritis. *Clostridium difficile*, which is often a constituent of the normal gastrointestinal flora and which as a complication of antibiotic therapy may cause diarrhea and pseudomembranous colitis, has been reported to cause reactive arthritis. However, direct evidence, i.e. demonstration of bacterial antigens in the joint, is missing.

Clostridium perfringens belongs to the normal intestinal flora of animals and humans: it may cause gastroenteritis and gas gangrene. It was reported by Månsson and Olhagen in 1966[13,14] to occur in excess in the fecal flora of patients with RA. This finding has been discussed and disputed[15–17]. Månsson and co-workers also reported[18,19] an increase of bacterial counts of *C. perfringens* in feces of pigs with arthritis induced by a fish diet. It must be emphasized that even if an increased presence of *C. perfringens* can be documented in RA, it may be only secondary to or accompanying other pathogenic changes.

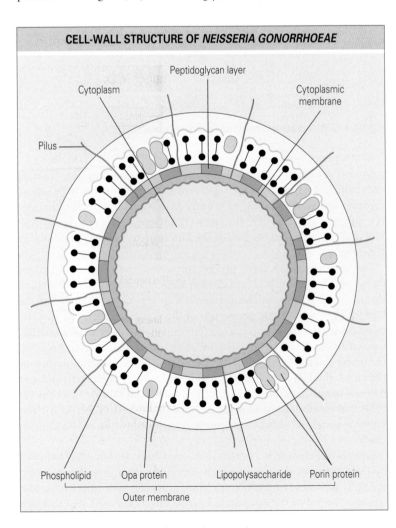

CELL-WALL STRUCTURE OF *NEISSERIA GONORRHOEAE*

Peptidoglycan layer

Cytoplasm

Cytoplasmic membrane

Pilus

Phospholipid   Opa protein   Lipopolysaccharide   Porin protein

Outer membrane

Fig. 92.3 Cell-wall structure of *Neisseria gonorrhoeae*.

Several species of genera *Eubacterium* and *Bifidobacterium* are part of the normal human intestinal flora. They are also found normally in the urogenital tract. For instance, *Collinsella aerofaciens* (formerly *Eubacterium aerofaciens*) and *Bifidobacterium adolescentis* are very low in virulence and usually do not cause disease. These two species of Gram-positive non-spore-forming anaerobic rods are of interest, however, as cell walls of both have been used to induce experimental arthritis in Lewis rats, a model very analogous to the streptococcal cell-wall arthritis in which the peptidoglycan–polysaccharide complex plays a crucial etiologic role[20–22].

Propionibacterium acnes is an anaerobic Gram-positive rod that can be isolated from the normal skin, lesions of acne vulgaris, intestinal tract, wounds, blood and abscesses. It is also a common contaminant of anaerobic cultures, causing difficulties in bacteriologic diagnosis. It is found in opportunistic infections of prosthetic devices, including articular prostheses and in synovitis associated with acne[23,24]. The infections may become chronic in nature.

Facultative anaerobes

Erysipelothrix rhusiopathiae is a Gram-positive, non-spore-forming bacillus with worldwide distribution in wild and domestic animals. The bacilli are $0.2–0.4 \times 0.5–2.5 \mu m$ in size. They are the cause of human and swine erysipelas. This skin infection sometimes becomes systemic, causing arthritis considerably more often in the pig than in humans, however. Viable *Erysipelothrix* bacteria has been isolated from synovial tissue after experimental *Erysipelothrix* arthritis in the pig[25].

Members of the genus *Actinomyces* are facultatively anaerobic Gram-positive rods that typically form delicate filaments similar to fungi. They are normal inhabitants of the respiratory, gastrointestinal and female genital tract. They cause chronic infections characterized by multiple abscesses. These are usually opportunistic infections following surgical or other procedures. Sometimes they lead to destruction of the bone, particularly after infections of the head and neck regions. Spondylitis is also a typical feature of actinomycosis.

GRAM-NEGATIVE BACILLI

Anaerobes

The family Bacteroidaceae includes 13 genera of anaerobic Gram-negative rods, of which those in the genera *Bacteroides*, *Prevotella*, *Porphyromonas* and *Fusobacterium* are most commonly associated with human disease. *Bacteroides fragilis*, *B. thetaiotaomicron*, *Prevotella melaninogenica* and *P. intermedius* are clinically the most important species[26]. They have a typical Gram-negative cell-wall structure with a surface lipopolysaccharide. The only difference is that Bacteroidaceae lipopolysaccharide has very little biological activity. Several species are natural inhabitants of the human gastrointestinal tract; fusobacteria are more commonly found in the oral cavity. Representatives of all four genera, particularly *B. fragilis*, are typical causes of endogenous infections in patients with trauma, operations, reduced host resistance, etc. Therefore they are also found in septic arthritis and hematogenous osteomyelitis.

Aerobes and facultative anaerobes

Among Gram-negative bacilli, those in the Enterobacteriaceae are the most important from the point of view of a rheumatologist. The family is divided into 14 clinically important genera (Table 92.5) and six other genera that are either clinically less important or poorly recognized. Furthermore, it includes more than 110 species that are ubiquitous worldwide in soil, water and vegetation, and are part of the normal flora of almost all animals, including humans. Some members of the family are firmly associated with septic and/or reactive arthritis, whereas others have been suspected of having a role in the etiopathogenesis of certain rheumatic diseases. Species of the family Enterobacteriaceae are closely

TABLE 92.5 CLINICALLY IMPORTANT GENERA IN THE FAMILY ENTEROBACTERIACEAE	
Citrobacter	Morganella
Edwardsiella	Proteus
Enterobacter	Providencia
Erwinia	Salmonella
Escherichia	Serratia
Hafnia	Shigella
Klebsiella	Yersinia

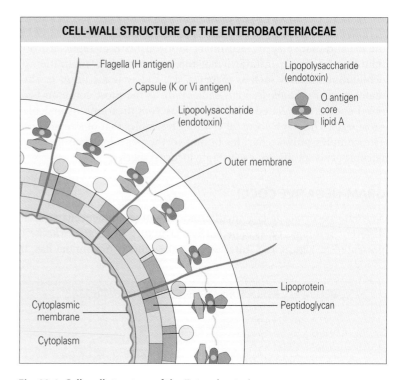

Fig. 92.4 Cell-wall structure of the Enterobacteriaceae.

related. They are $0.3–1.0 \times 1.0–6.0 \mu m$ in size, Gram-negative staining rods which do not form spores. Serologic classification is based on capsular antigens (K antigens), outer membrane lipopolysaccharides (O antigens) and flagellar structures (H antigens). The antigenic structure and cell-wall composition of the Enterobacteriaceae is presented in Figure 92.4.

The peptidoglycan layer of Enterobacteriaceae species and other Gram-negative bacteria is considerably thinner and less crosslinked than that of Gram-positive microorganisms; it comprises less than 10% of the bacterial cell wall. Toxic properties of the Gram-negative cell wall are largely due to lipopolysaccharide (endotoxin)[27]. The overall construction of lipopolysaccharides is similar in all Gram-negative bacteria, including chlamydiae (Fig. 92.5). They consist of three structural components – lipid A, core oligosaccharide and polysaccharide chain. Lipid A is the major toxic component of the lipopolysaccharide macromolecules and mostly responsible for its biological effects (Table 92.6). The serotype variation of the O antigen is determined by the polysaccharide chain.

Lipopolysaccharide is a potent inducer of fever, leukopenia (followed by leukocytosis), decreased peripheral circulation, hypotension and shock. It activates kinin and complement cascades and induces vascular leakage. Several of the lipopolysaccharide effects are mediated through macrophages and monocytes, which when stimulated by lipopolysaccharide produce interleukin-1 and tumor necrosis factor α. They are

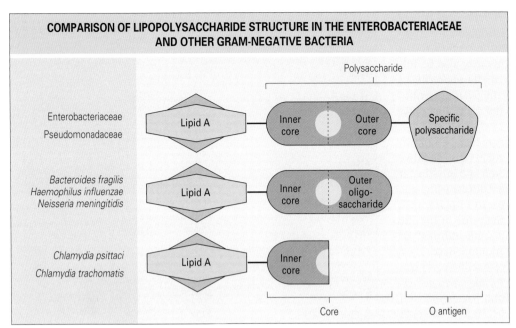

COMPARISON OF LIPOPOLYSACCHARIDE STRUCTURE IN THE ENTEROBACTERIACEAE AND OTHER GRAM-NEGATIVE BACTERIA

Fig. 92.5 Comparison of lipopolysaccharide structure in the Enterobacteriaceae and other Gram-negative bacteria. Lipopolysaccharide is anchored to the bacterial outer membrane through the lipid A component, and the polysaccharide region points to the environment.

TABLE 92.6 BIOLOGICAL EFFECTS OF LIPOPOLYSACCHARIDE (ENDOTOXIN)

- Fever
- Leukopenia, followed by leukocytosis
- Decreased peripheral circulation
- Hypotension, shock
- Activation of kinin cascade
- Activation of classic and alternative pathways of complement system
- Vascular leakage
- Activation of monocytes and macrophages
- Induction of inflammation
- Inhibition of polymorphonuclear cell functions
- Inhibition of macrophage migration

both powerful inflammatory agents, inducing local and systemic inflammation. Lipopolysaccharide is found within the synovial fluid cells in reactive arthritis triggered by enterobacteria[28–30]. Paradoxically, lipopolysaccharide may act also in an anti-inflammatory fashion. This effect works particularly after intravenous release of lipopolysaccharide, by inhibiting polymorphonuclear cell functions and macrophage migration[31].

Escherichia coli is the member of Enterobacteriaceae most frequently observed in bacterial sepsis, neonatal meningitis, urinary tract infections and travelers' diarrhea. Therefore, it is somewhat surprising that it is observed only in about 10% of cases with septic arthritis or hematogenous osteomyelitis. Reactive arthritis due to *E. coli* has been reported[32].

The genus *Shigella* includes four species: *S. dysenteriae*, *S. flexneri*, *S. boydii* and *S. sonnei*, altogether with 46 different serotypes. They all cause human shigellosis, with diarrhea, fever and bloody stools. Reactive arthritis has usually been described associated with *S. flexneri*, and only rarely with *S. sonnei*[33]. The reason for this is not known, but it is most probably due to antigenic differences between the species, Since bacteremia during the course of shigellosis is uncommon, septic arthritis due to *Shigella* species is also uncommon.

In contrast of *Shigella*, the genus *Salmonella* contains more than 2000 different serotypes. Even though most of them carry different names they can be grouped into three species (*S. typhi*, *S. enteritidis* and *S. choleraesuis*), or even into a single species (*S. enterica*) that can be divided in six subspecies. Most of the *Salmonella* serotypes are human

pathogens and therefore also an important cause of septic and reactive arthritis.

The genus *Yersinia* contains three species that are clinically important: *Y. pestis*, *Y. pseudotuberculosis* and *Y. enterocolitica*. *Y. pestis* is the cause of pneumonic and bubonic plague. *Y. pseudotuberculosis* and *Y. enterocolitica* cause gastroenteritis with fever and abdominal pains that may mimic appendicitis. The source of infection may be wild or domestic animals, contaminated food or even person-to-person contact[34]. All three *Yersinia* species can cause septic arthritis in the context of a generalized illness. In some parts of the world, *Y. pseudotuberculosis* and *Y. enterocolitica* are relatively common causes of reactive arthritis. On the basis of somatic O antigens and flagellar H antigens, 18 serogroups are known for *Y. enterocolitica* and 13 for *Y. pseudotuberculosis*[35,36]. Different serotypes are not equal in their capacity to trigger reactive arthritis. Serotypes O:3 and O:9 are common causes of reactive arthritis. For instance, serotype O:8 of *Y. enterocolitica* has very rarely been connected with human reactive arthritis. On the other hand, it is the only serotype of *Yersinia* reported to induce experimental reactive arthritis in the rat. Also, differences in the arthritogenic capacity exist even between strains of one and the same serotype[37,38].

Klebsiella pneumoniae causes lobar pneumonia, urinary tract infections and infections of wounds and soft tissue. It is sometimes found in septic arthritis, usually in patients with pre-existing urinary tract infection or other complicating disease. It does not trigger reactive arthritis, but its involvement in the pathogenesis of ankylosing spondylitis has been suggested. The suggestion is based on the reported increased occurrence of *Klebsiella*-specific serum antibodies and increased prevalence of *Klebsiella* in the fecal flora of patients with ankylosing spondylitis[39,40]. However, so far, there is no definite proof of the role of *K. pneumoniae* in the pathogenesis of rheumatic diseases[41,42].

Proteus mirabilis is a frequent cause of urinary tract infections, but has not been identified as a trigger of reactive arthritis and is only rarely implicated in septic arthritis. Patients with RA have been reported to have an increased prevalence of antibodies against *P. mirabilis*[43] and asymptomatic *P. mirabilis* bacteriuria[44]. This has led to the suggestion that *P. mirabilis* may play an etiologic role in the pathogenesis of RA based on the molecular mimicry[45–47]. So far, no further evidence for this hypothesis exists.

The family Pasteurellaceae contains three genera, *Pasteurella*, *Haemophilus*, and *Actinobacillus*. They are all Gram-negative non-spore-forming, 0.2–0.1 × 0.3–2.0μm in size, and coccoid or rods in shape. Of these *Haemophilus* species, particularly *H. influenzae* type b, was a common cause of upper respiratory tract infections and meningitis in children and also an important etiologic factor in septic arthritis before the vaccination era. *Haemophilus* meningitis may also be followed by development of reactive arthritis. *Pasteurella multocida*, a leading cause of animal bite infection, and *Actinobacillus actinomycetemcomitans*, a normal inhabitant of the oral flora, are sometimes found in septic arthritis.

Eikenella corrodens and *Streptobacillus moniliformis* are members of two clinically less important genera of facultatively anaerobic Gram-negative rods. *E. corrodens* occurs normally in the human mouth and intestine. It is probably involved in the pathogenesis of periodontal disease with bone destruction. Serious infections with abscesses may lead to peritonitis, endocarditis or septic arthritis. *S. moniliformis* is the cause of rat bite fever, complications of which may lead to persistent septic arthritis[48] or osteomyelitis. Members of the large family Pseudomonadaceae are straight or slightly curved aerobic Gram-negative bacilli ($0.5–1.0 \times 1.5–5.0\mu m$). The medically most important species *Pseudomonas aeruginosa* causes a wide variety of human infections, from bacteremia and endocarditis to chronic otitis media and musculoskeletal infections. It is a cause of septic arthritis and osteomyelitis, particularly in patients with an underlying disease. The same applies to *Pseudomonas cepacia*, which is of considerably lower virulence than *P. aeruginosa*.

Brucellas are small ($0.5–0.7 \times 0.6–1.5\mu m$) Gram-negative aerobic coccobacilli. Of the six species, four are pathogenic to man; *Brucella abortus*, *B. melitensis*, *B. suis* and *B. canis*. The clinical picture of brucellosis is characterized by localized abscesses and bacteremia, the extent of symptoms varying with the infecting species. Both *B. abortus* and *B. melitensis* are causes of septic and reactive arthritis and osteomyelitis. As far as reactive arthritis is concerned, it is of interest that *B. abortus* shows a serologic cross-reactivity with *Y. enterocolitica* and salmonellae[49,50].

The genus *Campylobacter* is completely separate and different from all the other bacterial species discussed above. *Campylobacter jejuni* occurs in the form of small tightly coiled spirals ($0.2–0.5 \times 0.5–5.0\mu m$) which grow aerobically or micro-aerophilically. Worldwide, it is a common cause of gastroenteritis. Its cell wall has the same structure as Gram-negative bacteria in general. It is a relatively frequent cause of reactive arthritis.

ACID-FAST BACILLI

Acid-fast bacilli affecting joints and bone belong to the genera *Mycobacterium* and *Nocardia*. The genus *Mycobacterium* includes 53 species of non-motile, non-spore-forming aerobic bacilli, $0.2–0.6 \times 1–10\mu m$ in size. Mycobacteria associated with human disease have been classified, on the basis of growth properties and colonial morphology, into different groups described in Table 92.7. Of human infections, 95% are due to only six species: *M. tuberculosis*, *M. leprae*, *M. kansasii*, *M. avium-intracellulare*, *M. fortuitum* and *M. chelonae*. All of these can cause joint and bone infections, which may occur in the form of spondylitis, peripheral arthritis, osteomyelitis or osteitis (see Chapter 95). The infections caused by the strictly pathogenic species, particularly by *M. tuberculosis* and *M. leprae*, are more severe and more common. Also, BCG (bacille Calmette–Guérin) vaccination may lead to osteitis[51], and BCG immunotherapy has resulted in the development of mycobacterial arthritis[52]. Among the atypical mycobacteria, *M. kansasii* and *M. marinum* are the most frequent causes of joint and bone lesions, followed by *M. avium-intracellulare*.

The mycobacterial cell wall has a peptidoglycan layer as a major component (Fig. 92.6), being one of the important factors in the pathogenesis of arthritis. In the rat (particularly in Lewis and Sprague–Dawley strains), a single intradermal injection of 0.6mg of heat-killed, dried mycobacteria leads to a generalized disease characterized by nodular

TABLE 92.7 MYCOBACTERIA ASSOCIATED WITH HUMAN DISEASE

Mycobacteria	Rate of growth*
Typical	
M. leprae	No growth *in vitro*†
M. tuberculosis	Slow
M. bovis	Slow
M. ulcerans	Slow
Atypical	
Runyon group I	
M. kansasii	Slow
M. marinum	Moderate
M. simiae	Slow
Runyon group II	
M. scrofulaceum	Slow
M. szulgai	Slow
M. xenopi	Slow
Runyon group III	Slow
M. avium-intracellulare	Slow
Runyon group IV	
M. fortuitum	Rapid
M. chelonae	Rapid

*Slow = 2–12 weeks, moderate = 8–14 days, rapid = 2–4 days. † Grown in armadillos.

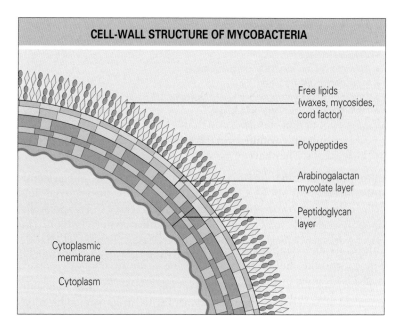

CELL-WALL STRUCTURE OF MYCOBACTERIA

Free lipids (waxes, mycosides, cord factor)

Polypeptides

Arabinogalactan mycolate layer

Peptidoglycan layer

Cytoplasmic membrane

Cytoplasm

Fig. 92.6 Cell wall structure of mycobacteria.

lesions in the skin, tendons, viscera and genitalia, as well as by arthritis and iritis. This form of adjuvant arthritis is widely used as an experimental model for RA. The disease can be induced by using protein-free wax fractions of various mycobacteria or cell-wall preparations from *Nocardia*, *Streptomyces*, *Streptococcus* and *Lactobacillus*. Also bacterial and synthetic peptidoglycans given in mineral oil induce adjuvant arthritis.

Nocardia asteroides, *N. brasiliensis* and *N. otitidis-cavarium* are the most common human pathogens within the genus *Nocardia*. They are Gram-positive although they stain quite poorly; the acid-fastness is demonstrated only when weak mineral acids are used for decolorization. Human pathogenic strains of *Nocardia* cause acute and chronic suppurative infections affecting mostly the respiratory tract and skin, but usually in immunosuppressed individuals. Joint and bone lesions as well as osteomyelitis may develop as a complication. Nocardiasis may also be complicated by mycetoma, a chronic granulomatous disease affecting connective tissues, muscle and bone, usually of the lower extremities.

Species of the genus *Rhodococcus*, taxonomically close to *Nocardia* and *Mycobacterium*, may also cause osteomyelitis. They are rare human pathogens. A distant relative of the nocardioforms is *Tropheryma whippelii*, an inculturable bacterial species associated with Whipple's disease. It is a Gram-positive actinomycete not closely related to any known genus. It can be identified only by sequencing bacterial RNA from the infected tissues[53].

SPIROCHETES

Within the family Spirochaetaceae, the genus *Borrelia* is of particular interest to rheumatologists (see Chapter 96). The genus contains 20 species; their cells are $0.2–0.5 \times 3–20\mu m$ in size and with 3–10 loose coils. They are causative agents of tick-borne and louse-borne relapsing fever in man. *Borrelia burgdorferi* is the etiologic agent of Lyme disease, characterized by erythema chronicum migrans, which is followed by a variety of chronic neurologic, cardiac and rheumatic manifestations. The bacteria stain Gram-negative, are micro-aerophilic and are difficult to culture. The development of aseptic arthritis following the initial infective erythematous skin lesion is an example of how the same disease appears as a reactive arthritis without viable microorganisms present in the synovium or as a septic arthritis.

Joint involvement is also found in congenital and acquired syphilis, due to *Treponema pallidum*. The same applies to yaws, caused by the subspecies *pertenue* of *T. pallidum*; advanced bone changes include osteoperiostitis and osteonecrosis.

CHLAMYDIAS

Chlamydia, as the only genus in the family Chlamydiaceae, contains three species of non-motile coccoid microorganisms, $0.2–1.5\mu m$ in size, which multiply only within membrane-bound vacuoles in the cytoplasm of the host cells. They have inner and outer membranes but lack a peptidoglycan layer in between. Lipopolysaccharide of the outer membrane closely resembles that of enterobacteria[54] (Fig. 92.5). Three species are known, *C. trachomatis*, *C. psittaci* and *C. pneumoniae*.

The clinical syndromes caused by *C. trachomatis* include trachoma, urinary and genital tract infections, conjunctivitis, respiratory tract infections and lymphogranuloma venereum. Several serotypes are known, and the clinical picture is dependent on the serotype. Reactive arthritis is caused by the same serotypes associated with male and female urinary and genital tract infections and respiratory tract infections. *C. pneumoniae* (known previously as *Chlamydia TWAR*) is a cause of upper respiratory tract infections. It may also cause reactive synovitis. *C. psittaci* is the cause of avian psittacosis (parrot fever); the disease can be transmitted to humans and it may be accompanied by arthralgia.

MYCOPLASMAS

The family Mycoplasmataceae has two genera, *Mycoplasma* and *Ureaplasma*. The bacteria belonging to these two genera are characterized by a complete lack of cell walls and their inability to synthesize peptidoglycan and its precursors. They are Gram-negative and usually grow facultatively anaerobically. They are pleomorphic and $0.2–0.8\mu m$ in diameter. The genus *Mycoplasma* contains 69 species and the genus *Ureaplasma* two species. *Mycoplasma pneumoniae* is a cause of respiratory tract infections: *M. hominis* and *U. urealyticum* both colonize the genital tracts of sexually active individuals and may cause genitourinary

tract infections. These three species, as well as others, have been associated with several different human diseases, but their definite etiologic contribution has remained unclear. However, their relationship with arthritis remains a worthy subject of continued research.

The interest of rheumatologists in mycoplasmas is best illustrated by the fact that 13 different species have been implicated in the etiology of arthritis in various experimental and domestic animals. Also, about 1% of patients with serologically confirmed *M. pneumoniae* infection develop mild arthritis[55].

Animal arthritides due to mycoplasmas may be spontaneous or experimental[56]. *Mycoplasma synoviae* is a common cause of joint disease in poultry, resulting in acute or chronic arthritis, tenosynovitis and lesions in periarticular tissue, mainly in the leg joints. *Mycoplasma hyorhinis* is an etiologic agent of swine arthritis, where an acute phase is followed in 6–8 months by development of chronic polyarthritis; the pathologic changes are quite similar to those in human RA. In sheep and goats, *Mycoplasma* infection may be complicated by arthritis, and the same applies to *M. bovis* and *M. alkalescens* infection in cattle. Mycoplasmal arthritis has also been reported to occur in elephants and rhesus monkeys. *Mycoplasma arthritidis* is a relatively common pathogen of laboratory and wild rats, also causing spontaneous purulent polyarthritis. Experimental *Mycoplasma*-induced arthritis has been described in chickens (*M. gallisepticum*), mice and rats (*M. pulmonis, M. arthritidis*), and rabbits (*M. arthritidis*).

The isolation of mycoplasmas and ureaplasmas from human joints has been reported. However, mycoplasmas are frequent contaminants of laboratory cultures and, in other studies, failure to isolate these organisms has also been reported[57]. *Ureaplasma urealyticum* has been described as a cause of reactive arthritis[58], and mycoplasmas and ureaplasmas have been implicated in septic arthritis, especially in immunodeficient individuals: however, their role in the pathogenesis of chronic septic arthritis remains uncertain.

OTHER MICROORGANISMS

Viruses

Viruses are replicating microorganisms with an obligate requirement for intracellular growth and dependence on host–cell interaction. Viral diseases are common human ailments, including acute respiratory and gastrointestinal infections, which quite often pass unnoticed, and chronic diseases with devastating consequences such as acquired immunodeficiency (AIDS) and poliomyelitis. Virology as a science is much younger than bacteriology, mycology and parasitology, and therefore the relationship between viruses and diseases of the locomotor system is considerably less clear[59]. It has not been possible to divide virus-induced arthritides into hematogenous and reactive arthritides as can be done for bacterially induced lesions. Likewise, pure arthritis of viral origin, without involvement of any other tissues, has not been clearly documented. For viral classification and more detailed description of viruses the reader is referred to textbooks[3,4,60].

Viral diseases that are accompanied by the development of arthritis can be divided usefully into those in which the arthritis is common and those in which the arthritis occurs only rarely (Table 92.8) (see Chapter 97). The demonstration in 1983 of parvovirus B19 as the etiologic agent of erythema infectiosum and of the accompanying joint involvement is a good example of the evolution of virologic rheumatology[61–64]. Even though parvovirus B19 is mostly a cause of acute arthritis, a putative role in the pathogenesis of RA has also been discussed; a few cases of a disease triggered by B19 and indistinguishable from RA have been described[65–67]. However, one has to conclude that so far no definite evidence for the B19 etiology of RA exists. The same can be said about some other viruses, such as herpes viruses (e.g. Epstein–Barr virus and

TABLE 92.8 VIRAL DISEASES ACCOMPANIED BY ARTHRITIS	
Virus/disease	**Virus present in joint***
Often accompanied by arthritis	
Alphaviruses	
• Chikungunya	
• Mayaro	
• O'nyong-nyong	
• Igbo-ora	
• Ross River (epidemic polyarthritis)	
• Sindbis	
– Ockelbo (Pogosta and Karelian fevers)	
– Babanki	
– Barmah Forest	
Hepatitis B virus	
Parvovirus B19	Yes
Rubella	Yes
Mumps	
Chickenpox	Yes
Seldom accompanied by arthritis	
Adenovirus	
Enteroviruses	
• Echoviruses	
• Coxsackieviruses	
Hepatitis A virus	
Hepatitis C virus	
Herpes viruses	
• Herpes simplex	Yes
• Varicella zoster	Yes
• Epstein–Barr virus	Yes
• Cytomegalovirus	Yes

*Demonstrated by culture, antigen detection or polymerase chain reaction in synovium/synovial fluid cells.

cytomegalovirus)[68,69] or adenoviruses[70], presented as possible causes of RA. On the other hand, several viral infections are known to induce autoantibodies, including rheumatoid factor.

The mechanisms by which acute viral arthritides are mediated also remains unclear, particularly as etiologic viruses cannot always be isolated from the joint tissue nor non-replicating viral particles detected. It is likely that immune complex mediated mechanisms are important; this would include the presence of viral particles within complexes in the inflamed tissue.

Alphaviruses are a remarkable group of viruses causing a variety of acute arthritides (Table 92.8). They are transmitted by different mosquito species in different parts of the world. When humans are infected, the consequences may range from subclinical or asymptomatic illness to severe disease, however, half of the patients have fibromyalgia, arthralgia or chronic arthritis as a consequence[71]. The arthritic complications due to infections with alphaviruses and other viruses are discussed in more detail in Chapter 97.

In recent years, an increasing number of patients with human immunodeficiency virus (HIV) infection and concomitant rheumatic disorders have been reported[72,73]. These range from slight arthralgias to severe diseases, including, for example psoriatic arthritis, polymyositis and HLA-B27-associated arthritides. It is unclear what role the HIV itself or the immunodeficiency state plays in the pathogenesis of arthritis. Inflammatory arthropathy has also been described in association with human T cell leukemia virus type I (HTLV-I) infections, i.e. in adult T cell leukemia and HTLV-I associated myelopathy[74,75]. Likewise, a spontaneous inflammatory synovitis occurs in mice transgenic for HTLV-I[76].

Both HIV and HTLV-I are retroviruses. The former belongs to the subfamily of lentiviruses, which in turn includes caprine arthritis–encephalitis virus and maedi-visna virus. The spontaneous caprine arthritis–encephalitis virus infection in goats represents an interesting animal model of virus-induced arthritis[77]. The arthritis is characterized by proliferative synovitis with cartilage and bone destruction closely resembling pathologic lesions in the human rheumatoid joint. The virus replicates in monocyte and/or macrophage precursors in the bone marrow. From there it seems to be transported within macrophages into the periphery, including joints. A similar type of joint involvement is also seen in the viral disease maedi-visna in sheep. The relationship between acquired immunodeficiency and rheumatic disease is discussed more fully in Chapter 98.

Fungi

Fungi include both yeasts and molds and are significantly different from bacteria[3,4]. They are eukaryotic and contain a definite nucleus with surrounding nuclear membrane. Their cell membrane is composed of chitin (glucose and mannose polymers). In clinical practice, fungi are divided in two groups based on the macroscopic appearance of the fungal colonies. Yeasts appear as creamy, moist and opaque colonies, whereas the molds or filamentous fungi produce fluffy, cotton-wool-like colonies. Historically, fungi have not been regarded as important causes of infection, and only recently has more attention been paid to them in rheumatologic microbiology. Of more than 50 000 species of fungi, only 50–75 are generally recognized as human pathogens. They live normally as saprophytes in nature and are usually not communicable by person-to-person or animal-to-person contact. A significant increase in the prevalence of mycotic infections has been introduced by the use of immunosuppressive treatment regimens and by the increasing longevity of patients with chronic debilitating illnesses. Therefore, when fungi are associated with joint and bone lesions, they are also usually found in other tissues. Fungi that have been associated with arthritis and bone lesions are listed in Table 92.9 and discussed further in Chapter 95.

Parasites

Parasites may also be involved in joint and bone lesions (Table 92.10). Human parasites are classified into five major subdivisions[3,4]. Species of three of these: the protozoa (examples are *Giardia lamblia*, *Toxoplasma gondii*, *Trypanosoma cruzi*), flatworms (*Taeniae*, *Echinococcus granulosus*, *Schistosoma mansoni*) and roundworms (*Strongyloides stercoralis*, *Trichinella spiralis*) are associated with joint and bone lesions. The fourth subdivision is arthropods, including ticks and mites known to transmit arthritis-inducing microorganisms, the best known examples

TABLE 92.9 FUNGI ASSOCIATED WITH JOINT AND BONE LESIONS
Actinomyces israelii
Actinomyces bovis
Aspergillus fumigatus
Blastomyces dermatidis
Candida albicans
Candida glabrata
Candida guilliermondi
Candida tropicalis
Cephalosporium
Coccidioides immitis
Cryptococcus neoformans
Histoplasma capsulatum
Petrilidium boydii
Sporothrix schenckii

TABLE 92.10 PARASITES ASSOCIATED WITH JOINT AND BONE LESIONS
Echinococcus granulosus
Giardia lamblia
Schistosoma mansoni
Strongyloides stercoralis
Taenia solium (larvae)
Taenia saginata (larvae)
Toxoplasma gondii
Trichinella spiralis
Trypanosoma cruzi (found in muscle)

TABLE 92.11 SUPERANTIGENS	
Exogenous	**Endogenous (mouse)**
Staphylococcal enterotoxin (for humans, mouse)	Mls antigen (minor lymphocyte stimulation)
Streptococcal M protein (humans)	Mtv (mammary tumor virus)
Mycoplasma arthritidis superantigen (mouse, rat, rabbit)	(Mls and Mtv antigens are encoded by retroviral mammary tumor virus genes)

of which are *Borrelia burgdorferi* mediated by tick *Ixodes* (several species), and alphaviruses, carried by a variety of mosquitoes and ticks.

Similar principles underlie the pathogenetic mechanisms of both parasite-induced and fungal joint and bone lesions. Joint and bone lesions associated with parasitic involvement are either manifestations of systemic disease or complications of an immunosuppressed state or another severe illness. The role of fungi and parasitic infestations in rheumatic diseases is discussed fully in Chapter 95.

MECHANISMS OF MICROBIAL-INDUCED ARTHRITIS

Superantigens

Superantigens are microbial or endogenous structures which stimulate a high proportion of T cells (5–25%) by binding in an immunologically non-specific way to the variable (V) region of certain T cell antigen receptors (Table 92.11 & Fig. 92.7). At the same time, they are also capable of binding to major histocompatibility (MHC) class II molecules; curiously, this occurs directly without antigen processing (conventional antigens undergo intracellular processing and proteolytic degradation for MHC class II binding and T cell recognition). Among the microbial superantigens, those derived from *Streptococcus pyogenes* and *Mycoplasma arthritidis*[78–80] are of rheumatologic interest, because it has been suggested that they are involved in the pathogenesis of autoimmunity. In the rheumatic diseases, experimental evidence of possible involvement of superantigens currently exists for RA[81] and psoriatic arthropathy[82]. In one study, a significant increase of T cells with a particular V type ($V_{\beta14}$) was demonstrated in synovial fluid of affected joints, these cells being virtually undetectable in the peripheral blood[83]. This could account for recruitment of T cells by a superantigen from the circulation to the site of inflammation. The nature and identity of such a potential superantigen is not known.

Heat shock proteins

Heat shock proteins (hsp or stress proteins) are molecules with a highly conserved structure and are found in all prokaryotes and eukaryotes. Their presence is ubiquitous, and they are among the most abundant

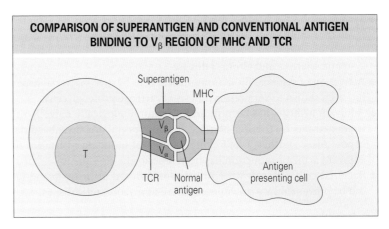

COMPARISON OF SUPERANTIGEN AND CONVENTIONAL ANTIGEN BINDING TO V_β REGION OF MHC AND TCR

Fig. 92.7 Comparison of superantigen and conventional antigen binding to V_β region of MHC and TCR. Superantigen binding to V_β region of T cell antigen receptor (TCR) and major histocompatibility (MHC) class II molecule, compared with the binding of a conventional antigen.

proteins of the biosphere. They are produced by cells in response to different physiologic and non-physiologic stimuli, and their function is to protect the cell from the deleterious effects of stress, including changes in temperature, infection and inflammation.

The hsp are divided into different classes and show a wide variety of molecular masses. Some are highly immunogenic. In rheumatology, most interest has been directed at those with a molecular weight of around 60kDa (hsp60 or 65). These function as molecular chaperones by participating in the folding, unfolding, translocation, assembly and disassembly of other proteins within the cell. hsp60 was first described in *E. coli* and has been termed GroEL. It is a common antigen in several bacterial species, including *Borrelia, Chlamydia, Mycobacterium, Pseudomonas, Salmonella, Treponema* and *Yersinia*[84]. Bacterial hsp are highly conserved, and different sequential infections lead to boosting of cellular and humoral anti-hsp responses by the host immune system. Human hsp60 shows an approximately 60% sequence homology with the mycobacterial counterpart hsp65[85]. Therefore, immune responses against the conserved sequences shared by the microbial and host hsp may potentially lead to autoimmunity[86,87].

Findings that support the possibility of hsp participating in the pathogenesis of arthritides are as follows (Table 92.12):

- Monoclonal antibodies against the mycobacterial hsp65 cross-react with human hsp60; their use has revealed increased synovial expression of hsp in adult and juvenile RA.
- T cell responses by synovial fluid T cells against the mycobacterial hsp65 are observed in adult and juvenile RA as well as in reactive arthritis.

TABLE 92.12 HEAT-SHOCK PROTEINS IN ARTHRITIS
• Increased presence of autologous hsp60 in inflamed synovium
• Response by synovial T cells against mycobacterial hsp65 in rheumatoid and reactive arthritis
• Increased level of serum antibodies specific for hsp60 in rheumatoid arthritis
• Mycobacterial hsp65 activates rheumatoid synovial mononuclear cells to suppress synthesis of cartilage proteoglycans
• Adjuvant arthritis in the rat can be included or suppressed by T cell clones specific for mycobacterial hsp65
• Several experimental models of rat arthritis can be prevented by preceding exposure to mycobacterial hsp65
Findings supporting participation of microbial heat-shock proteins (hsp60, hsp65) in the pathogenesis of arthritis.

- Serum antibodies against mycobacterial hsp65 occur at an elevated level in rheumatoid, reactive and psoriatic arthritis, ankylosing spondylitis, mixed connective tissue disease, SLE, Sjögren's syndrome, systemic sclerosis and Crohn's disease.
- Activation of synovial fluid mononuclear cells by mycobacterial hsp65 has been shown to suppress synthesis of cartilage proteoglycans.
- Adjuvant arthritis has been induced in immunologically naive X-ray irradiated rats by transfer of a T cell clone specific for mycobacterial hsp65. Also, another T cell clone capable of inducing resistance to adjuvant arthritis induction has been described.
- Bacterial cell-wall arthritis and pristane-induced arthritis in the rat can be prevented by a previous exposure to mycobacterial hsp65.

However, it has not been possible to draw definite conclusions as to which of the above findings are related to the cause and which to the consequences of the arthritic process. Participation of microbial hsp in other models of autoimmunity, including experimental and human diabetes mellitus, has also been speculated on.

Molecular mimicry

Molecular mimicry is a similarity, defined precisely at the molecular level, between a microorganism and the host. It may appear as an identity of linear or non-linear amino acid sequences, based on known DNA sequences, or as an identity of carbohydrate structures. Therefore, molecular mimicry is a better defined concept than antigenic cross-reaction, which is based on the recognition by antibodies. Antigenic cross-reactions are known to a considerably wider extent; for instance examples of those between microbes and HLA-B27 are numerous. On the other hand, molecular mimicry does not always lead to a cross-reacting immune response, because antigenicity may be dependent on the structures flanking the mimicking part of the molecule[88,89].

Several examples of microbial antigens sharing a defined similarity with molecules of human or animal origin are known[9,86,89–96]. These proteins include a minimum of four shared amino acids, and in most the similarity stretches considerably wider.

Normally, immune responses are not directed against 'self' components, due to immunologic tolerance. However, breakdown of tolerance in both B and T cell immunity may occur. It can also be seen to occur after response to microbial cross-reacting antigens. This may happen at three different levels (Fig. 92.8):

- Microbial entry leads, after or during a period of microbial proliferation, to degradation of the microbial structures. Products that are resistant to *in vivo* degradation, such as peptidoglycans and lipopolysaccharides, are retained, leading to antigen persistence within the host. Also, endogenous microorganisms, such as intestinal bacteria, may contribute to the same end result.
- Infection may be cleared but the causative microorganism remains hiding within the body, leading to microbial persistence.
- Chronic infection constitutes a persistent antigenic load.

In all of the three alternatives, continued stimulation by the cross-reacting microbial antigens provides the opportunity to break the tolerance and lead to immune response against the mimicking 'self' antigens. The final result of such reactivity against 'self' components might be an autoimmune disease.

Evidence that molecular mimicry leads to autoimmunity has been presented, for instance on the basis of studies on adjuvant arthritis (mycobacterial hsp), rheumatic fever (streptococcal M protein) and celiac disease (adenovirus). However, the evidence that this leads to autoimmune disease remains open as other explanations are possible. For example streptococcal M proteins function also as a superantigen, or in some other instances the mimicking structures are not antigenic. These suspicions do not exclude the possibility that, with increasing knowledge about the microbial and host structures involved as well as about the host immune response, a clear relationship between molecular mimicry and autoimmunity will be positively established[93–97].

Microbial transport to the joint

One of the key questions in the pathogenesis of microbe-induced arthritides is how the triggering agents are transported to the site of inflammation: via the circulation (septic infection), within immune complexes, within monocytes and/or macrophages, within polymorphonuclear cells or by entry of microbial structures alone. In septic arthritis, the route of transportation is hematogenous, with live microbes, both free and intracellularly, present in the blood. The richly vascularized subsynovium

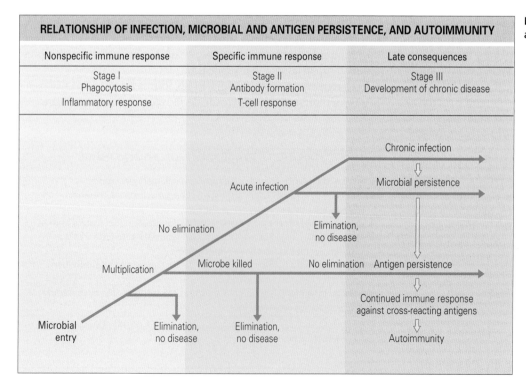

Fig. 92.8 Relationship of infection, microbial and antigen persistence, and autoimmunity.

RELATIONSHIP OF INFECTION, MICROBIAL AND ANTIGEN PERSISTENCE, AND AUTOIMMUNITY

Nonspecific immune response	Specific immune response	Late consequences
Stage I Phagocytosis Inflammatory response	Stage II Antibody formation T-cell response	Stage III Development of chronic disease

offers ample possibilities for spread of infection. The same holds true also for circulating immune complexes containing microbial antigens. In *Yersinia*-triggered reactive arthritis, these have been demonstrated both in the circulation and in the synovial fluid[98,99], and non-specific circulating immune complexes are known to correlate with severity of arthritis[100,101]. The possibility of intracellular transport applies probably to more or less degraded bacterial structures[102], and for the transport of viruses, fungi and parasites the intracellular mechanism is also the most likely.

The cells involved in the transport of microbes and microbial structures are polymorphonuclear cells, monocytes, macrophages and even lymphocytes for the transport of viruses. Polymorphonuclear cells engulf *Chlamydia* elementary bodies at the site of infection and transfer them to other tissues[103]. Mononuclear phagocytes meet the bacteria in the intestinal tract and may participate in the transport of bacterial degradation products to the synovium. In inflamed synovium, the small venules change their morphology to that of high endothelial venules (HEV). Inflammatory mediators, including lipopolysaccharide, interleukin-1 and tumor necrosis factor α, are involved in these changes, and they enhance leukocyte adhesion to the vascular endothelium. It is not known whether the appearance of HEV is a cause or a result of the increased leukocyte traffic. Of particular interest is the finding that intestinal lymphoid tissue contains immunoblasts capable of binding to HEV in inflamed synovium[104,105]. With persisting and poorly degraded antigens, such as peptidoglycans and lipopolysaccharides, some of whose antigens might mimic host tissue antigens, it is possible to envisage mechanisms which could lead to arthritis.

Entry of microbial components free in solution to the synovium is also possible. For instance, elevated levels of circulating lipopolysaccharide have been observed in patients with ankylosing spondylitis[106], and free lipopolysaccharide has been demonstrated in the synovium in RA[107].

Experimental models of microbe-induced arthritis

Spontaneous and experimentally induced animal models of arthritis have given important insights into the pathogenetic mechanisms of arthritis. They have also contributed to the development of drug research for the benefit of humans. Many of these animal disorders resemble human diseases, but none is the complete counterpart of any human disease, making conclusions sometimes extremely difficult to draw; animals do not have a spontaneous disease resembling human RA in all respects. Many of the experimental models of arthritis are based on use of microorganisms, alive, killed or fractionated (Table 92.13). Of the natural infections that are accompanied by arthritis, those caused by *Erysipelothrix rhusiopathiae*, mycoplasmas and caprine arthritis-encephalitis virus have already been discussed briefly earlier. Five experimental models of arthritis induced by microbes or microbial components are described here.

Adjuvant arthritis

Adjuvant arthritis, first described by Pearson in 1956, is the most widely used animal model of arthritis[87,108,109]. It is induced by intradermal injection of killed dried mycobacteria in mineral oil, but it can also be elicited by using a number of other bacterial extracts. After a latent period of 10–14 days, an acute inflammation appears affecting the ankles, wrists, and tarsal and interphalangeal joints. However, the disease is not limited only to the joints: the extra-articular manifestations include tendinitis, iritis, nodular lesions in the visceral organs, urethritis and diarrhea. No rheumatoid factor is produced. The symptoms reach a peak at 15–25 days after the adjuvant injection to be followed by slow resolution. The synovial lesions histologically resemble those observed in the human RA. Therefore the model has also been widely used in drug research.

The disease can be induced only in rats, Lewis and Sprague–Dawley strains being the most susceptible. Fisher rats are resistant, but if they are bred under germ-free conditions they become susceptible to arthritis

TABLE 92.13 MICROBE-INDUCED MODELS OF ARTHRITIS

Microbe/microbial component	Species
Natural infections	
Caprine arthritis–encephalitis virus	Goat
Erysipelothrix rhusiopathiae	Pig, dog, rabbit
Mycoplasma hyorhinis	Pig
Mycoplasma synoviae	Chicken
Mycoplasma arthritidis	Rat
Chlamydia psittaci	Cow, sheep
Experimental	
Bacterial DNA	Mouse
Bifidobacterium cell-wall components	Rat
Escherichia coli	Rabbit
Collinsella cell-wall components	Rat
Killed tubercle bacilli	Rat
Lactobacillus cell-wall components	Rat
Lipopolysaccharide	Rat
Mycoplasma arthritidis	Mouse, rat
Mycoplasma gallisepticum	Chicken
Mycoplasma pulmonis	Mouse, rat
Neisseria gonorrhoeae	Rabbit
Salmonella enteritidis	Rat
Staphylococcus aureus	Rabbit
Streptococcal cell-wall components	Rat
Streptococcus pyogenes	Rabbit
Yersinia enterocolitica O:8	Rat

induction. If germ-free Fisher rats are colonized with *E. coli*, they again are resistant to adjuvant arthritis. These and other similar findings indicate the importance of normal microbial flora in determining susceptibility or resistance to induction of arthritis. In similar fashion, pre-immunization of the rats with 65kDa mycobacterial hsp induces protection against adjuvant arthritis. The disease can be transferred to previously healthy naive animals by transfer of unselected T cells or T cell clones. The arthritogenic T cell clones react with a defined determinant of the 65kDa mycobacterial hsp. It is possible that molecular mimicry between the hsp and the core protein of joint cartilage is responsible for the arthritic lesions. However, mycobacterial compounds are also found in the joint tissue, and they may play a role in the pathogenesis of inflammation.

BACTERIAL CELL WALL ARTHRITIS

Cell-wall fragments from a variety of Gram-positive bacterial species are able to induce, after a single intraperitoneal injection, acute and chronic arthritis in the rat. The models studied in the most detail are those using cell walls from *Streptococcus*[5,6], *Collinsella* (formerly *Eubacterium*) *aerofaciens*[20,21,110] and *Lactobacillus*[111,112] species. Streptococcal cell walls are usually prepared from *S. pyogenes*. The other bacteria used include *Bifidobacterium* spp., *Streptococcus agalactiae*, *Enterococcus faecium*, and *Peptostreptococcus productus*[113,114]. An essential component of the cell wall preparation, particularly for induction of chronic arthritis, is intact peptidoglycan–polysaccharide complex. Evidence has been presented that the structure of peptidoglycan determines whether a bacterial cell wall is capable of inducing chronic arthritis or not[20,21]. On this basis it is understandable that closely related bacterial strains, even within a single species, have completely different arthritogenic capacity[20].

Microscopically, synovial inflammation is already present 2 days after the cell-wall injection. Acute inflammation develops in the ankles and wrists, accompanied by general illness, conjunctivitis and often diarrhea.

At this stage, up to 2 weeks after the cell-wall injection, polymorphonuclear cells are the major cell types in the synovial lesions, subsequently to be replaced by lymphocytes. Focal proliferation of the synovial lining is a consistent feature of inflamed joints. Acute symptoms are most severe at 1–3 weeks after the cell-wall injection and may wane thereafter. In most of the animals, synovitis becomes chronic and is maintained for several months, leading to joint deformation, stiffness and ankylosis. Bacterial cell-wall components can be demonstrated in the diseased joints; however, they are also demonstrable in healthy joints of arthritis-resistant rats after injection of bacterial cell walls.

In chronic bacterial cell-wall arthritis erosions are observed and spread to underlying bone tissue. Periosteal apposition of new bone and periarticular development of new bone via chondroid tissue is also observed. All these findings resemble histologic features of human RA. However, in contrast to RA, synovial plasma cells and follicle-like accumulations of lymphocytes are scarce in bacterial cell-wall arthritis, and rheumatoid factor is not produced. The disease can be transferred to naive animals by using T cell lines from arthritic animals.

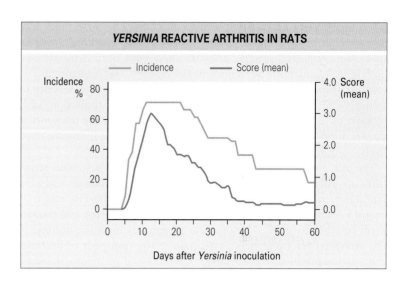

Fig. 92.9 *Yersinia* reactive arthritis in rats.

LIPOPOLYSACCHARIDE-INDUCED ARTHRITIS

Intra-articular or intravenous injection of lipopolysaccharide derived from the cell walls of Gram-negative bacteria leads to acute arthritis in the rat[114]. Bacterial species used for lipopolysaccharide preparation include *Salmonella*, *Yersinia*, *E. coli* and *N. gonorrhoeae*. The synovitis is characterized by an acute exudative reaction, with polymorphonuclear cells and fibrin in the joint space as well as by hyperplasia of the synovial lining cells. Macroscopically, the arthritis is usually found only in the ankle joints, and the symptoms are mild. If the ankles are previously injured by intra-articular injection of streptococcal cell-wall peptidoglycan–polysaccharide, intravenous injection of even minute amounts of lipopolysaccharide results in recurrence of arthritis. In this case it seems likely that the phlogistic activities of peptidoglycan and lipopolysaccharide act in synergy for the development and maintenance of synovitis.

STAPHYLOCOCCAL ARTHRITIS

Intra-articular injection of *Staphylococcus aureus* into a rabbit knee results in a progressive septic arthritis. The number of bacteria required to produce arthritis in 100% of the animals depends on the virulence of the strain used. *S. epidermidis* can also be used but considerably larger bacterial doses are needed. Thirty to sixty minutes after the inoculation, bacteria are observed in the synovial membrane adjacent to the infrapatellar and suprapatellar fat pads and elsewhere in the synovium, particularly adjacent to the articular cartilage. Usually, many of the staphylococci are intracellular. When virulent bacteria are used they induce lysis of the host cells, which may engulf them; 72 hours after the bacterial inoculation, considerable necrosis of the entire synovium may be observed[115]. Similar models have been established by using *N. gonorrhoeae*, *S. pyogenes* and *E. coli*[116]. With *S. aureus*, a hematogenously induced experimental arthritis in the mouse has also been described[117]. These and other similar models can be used to study the effect of antibiotics on septic arthritis, pathogenetic events and cellular lesions in septic arthritis, and the effect of different disease and other conditions on infectious arthritis. For the latter purposes, intra-articular injection of *S. aureus* has been used in rabbits with preceding antigen-induced arthritis[118].

YERSINIA REACTIVE ARTHRITIS

Intravenous injection of live *Y. enterocolitica* serotype O:8 leads to the development of acute arthritis at 10–20 days after the injection (Fig. 92.9) in SHR and Lewis rats[119,120]. The inflammation is characterized by diffusely distributed lymphocytes in the edematous synovia. Polymorphonuclear cells are observed only in early arthritis in low numbers. The synovial lining cell layer is slightly thickened with mild synovial ulcerations at the beginning of the disease. Erosion of the cartilaginous surface is observed also in the early stage of arthritis, but bone erosions are not found. The joint inflammation is sterile; only exceptionally can bacteria be cultured from the joint in the early phase of arthritis. The peak severity of arthritis occurs at 3–4 weeks after bacterial inoculation, followed by a decline, so that at 3 months most of the animals are symptom free. However, exacerbations may occur; these seem to depend on the persistence of live bacteria in the other organs, primarily within lymph nodes. This model of *Yersinia* reactive arthritis closely resembles human reactive arthritis and has successfully been applied to evaluate effect of antibiotics in the treatment of this disease[121,122].

Class	Infection known	Live microorganism in joint tissue	Microbial structures in joint tissue	Examples
Infective	Yes	Yes	Yes	Bacterial (septic), arthritides, infective viral arthritides
Reactive	Yes	No	Yes	Arthritides following infection with chlamydias, enterobacteria, meningococci
Inflammatory	No	No	No	Rheumatoid arthritis, ankylosing spondylitis, psoriatic arthritis

TABLE 92.14 MICROBES AND ARTHRITIS: A CLASSIFICATION

MICROBES AND ARTHRITIS: A CLASSIFICATION

On the basis of associations with microbial infection, arthritides have previously been divided into the infective, postinfective, reactive and inflammatory[123]. In this classification, postinfective arthritis was distinguished from the reactive form by the presence of microbial structures at the site of inflammation. As microbial components, e.g. *Chlamydia*, *Salmonella*, *Shigella*, *Yersinia*, are now known to be present in the inflamed synovium as well as within the synovial fluid cells in reactive arthritis[28–30,124–129], these two forms fall in the same category. On this basis, it is more accurate to classify arthritides in relation to the microbial pathogenesis as infective, reactive or inflammatory (see Fig. 92.10).

The three classes of arthritis presented in Table 92.14 are not mutually exclusive, because transient forms occur. In fact, the clinical and laboratory diagnosis between reactive and bacterial arthritis is extremely difficult or even impossible[130]. There are several examples of the same microbe causing infective and reactive arthritis; they include arthritis due to gonococci, meningococci, *Borrelia burgdorferi*, salmonellas and yersinias. In rats with experimental *Yersinia* reactive arthritis, the inflamed joints are mostly sterile and only occasionally, in the beginning of the arthritic process, are live bacteria present in the joint[119]. It is probable that many, if not all reactive arthritides, are preceded by a short phase of septic arthritis. In support of this prospect is the fact that the cellular composition of the synovial fluid is similar in septic and reactive arthritis[131]. Also, with time and increasing knowledge, one expects an increasing number of etiologic agents and of their tissue distribution to be revealed. For instance, synovitis in rheumatic fever is a typical reactive arthritis with a known etiologic agent, but the presence of microbial components within the synovium has not yet been demonstrated.

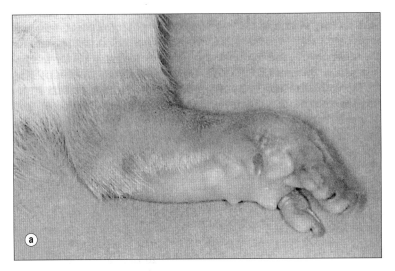
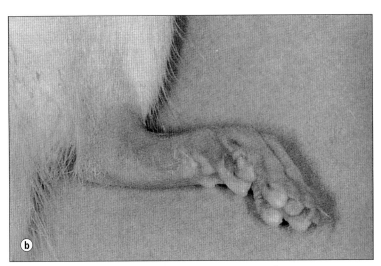

Fig. 92.10 Yersinia reactive arthritis in hindpaw of SHR rat. (a) 19 days after intravenous bacterial inoculation. (b) Control rat.

REFERENCES

1. Murray PR, Drew WL, Kobayashi GS *et al.*, eds. Medical microbiology. London: Wolfe; 1994.
2. Holt JG, Krieg NR, Sneath PHA *et al.*, eds. Bergey's manual of determinative bacteriology, 9th ed. Baltimore, MD: Williams & Wilkins; 1994.
3. Forbes BA, Sahm DM, Trevino E, eds. Bailey & Scott's diagnostic microbiology, 10th ed. St Louis, MO: Mosby; 1998.
4. Murray PR, Baron EJ, Pfaller MA *et al.*, eds. Manual of clinical microbiology, 7th ed. Washington, DC: ASM; 1999.
5. van den Broek MF. Streptococcal cell wall-induced polyarthritis in the rat. Mechanisms for chronicity and regulation of susceptibility. APMIS 1989; 97: 861–878.
6. Cromartie WJ, Craddock JG, Schwab JH *et al.* Arthritis in rats after systemic injection of streptococcal cells or cell walls. J Exp Med 1977; 146: 1585–1602.
7. Fox A. Role of bacterial debris in inflammatory diseases of the joint and eye. APMIS 1990; 98: 957–968.
8. Seidl PH, Schleifer KH, eds. Biological properties of peptidoglycan. Berlin: Walter de Gruyter; 1986.
9. Fischetti V. Streptococcal M protein; molecular design and biological behavior. Clin Microbiol Rev 1989; 2: 285–314.
10. Baird RW, Bronze MS, Kraus W *et al.* Epitopes of group A streptococcal M protein shared with antigens of articular cartilage and synovium. J Immunol 1991; 146: 3132–3137.
11. Wilder RL. Proinflammatory microbial products as etiologic agents of inflammatory arthritis. Rheum Dis Clin N Am 1987; 13: 293–306.
12. Espersen F, Frimodt-Moller N, Rosdahl VT *et al.* Changing pattern of bone and joint infections due to *Staphylococcus aureus*: study of cases of bacteremia in Denmark, 1959–1988. Rev Infect Dis 1991; 13: 347–358.
13. Månsson I, Olhagen B. Intestinal *Clostridium perfringens* in rheumatoid arthritis and other connective tissue disorders. Studies of fecal flora, serum antitoxin levels and skin hypersensitivity. Acta Rheum Scand 1966; 12: 167–174.
14. Olhagen B, Månsson I. Intestinal *Clostridium perfringens* in rheumatoid arthritis and other collagen diseases. Acta Med Scand 1968; 184: 395–402.
15. Olhagen B, Månsson I. Fecal *Clostridium perfringens* and rheumatoid arthritis. J Infect Dis 1974; 130: 444–447.
16. Sapico FL, Emori H, Smith LDS *et al.* Absence of relationship of fecal *Clostridium perfringens* to rheumatoid arthritis and rheumatoid variants. J Infect Dis 1973; 128: 559–562.
17. Shinebaum R, Neumann VC, Cooke EM *et al.* Comparison of faecal florae in patients with rheumatoid arthritis and controls. Br J Rheumatol 1987; 26: 329–333.
18. Månsson I, Norberg R, Olhagen B *et al.* Arthritis in pigs induced by dietary factors. Microbiologic, clinical and histologic studies. Clin Exp Immunol 1971; 9: 677–693.
19. Olhagen B. Arthritis in pigs induced by dietary factors. In: Mielants H, Veys EM, eds. Spondyloarthropathies: involvement of the gut. Amsterdam: Elsevier; 1987: 47–60.
20. Zhang X, Rimpiläinen M, Simelyte E *et al.* What determines arthritogenicity of bacterial cell wall? A study on *Eubacterium* cell wall-induced arthritis. Rheumatology 2000; 39: 274–282.
21. Zhang X, Rimpiläinen M, Simelyte E *et al.* Characterization of *Eubacterium* cell wall: peptidoglycan structure determines arthritogenicity. Ann Rheum Dis 2001; 60: 269–274.
22. Zhang X, Rimpiläinen M, Hoffman B *et al.* Experimental chronic arthritis and granulomatous inflammation induced by *Bifidobacterium* cell walls. Scand J Immunol 2001; 54: 171–179.
23. Schaeverbeke T, Lequen L, de Barbeyrac B *et al.* *Propionibacterium acnes* isolate from synovial tissue and fluid in a patient with oligoarthritis associated with acne and pustulosis. Arthritis Rheum 1998; 41: 1889–1893.
24. Delyle LG, Vittecoq O, Bourdel A *et al.* Chronic destructive oligoarthritis associated with *Propionibacterium acnes* in a female patient with acne vulgaris: septic-reactive arthritis? Arthritis Rheum 2000; 43: 2843–2847.
25. Franz B, Davies ME, Horner A. Localization of viable bacteria and bacterial antigens in arthritic joints of *Erysipelothrix rhusiopathiae*-infected pigs. FEMS Immunol Med Microbiol 1995; 12: 137–142.
26. Brook I, Frazier EH. Anaerobic osteomyelitis and arthritis in a military hospital: a 10-year experience. Am J Med 1993; 94: 21–28.
27. Nowotny A, Spitzer JJ, Ziegler EJ, eds. Cellular and molecular aspects of endotoxin reactions. Amsterdam: Excerpta Medica; 1990.
28. Granfors K, Jalkanen S, von Essen R *et al.* *Yersinia* antigens in synovial-fluid cells from patients with reactive arthritis. N Engl J Med 1989; 320: 216–221.

29. Granfors K, Jalkanen S, Lindberg AA et al. *Salmonella* lipopolysaccharide in synovial cells from patients with reactive arthritis. Lancet 1990; 335: 685–688.

30. Granfors K, Jalkanen S, Toivanen P et al. Bacterial lipopolysaccharide in synovial fluid cells in *Shigella* triggered reactive arthritis. J Rheumatol 1992; 19: 500.

31. Hartiala KT, Granberg I, Toivanen A et al. Inhibition of polymorphonuclear leucocyte functions in vivo by *Yersinia enterocolitica* lipopolysaccharide. Ann Rheum Dis 1989; 48: 42–47.

32. Laasila K, Leirisalo-Repo M. Recurrent reactive arthritis associated with urinary tract infection by *Escherichia coli*. J Rheumatol 1999; 26: 2277–2279.

33. Lauhio A, Lähdevirta J, Janes R et al. Reactive arthritis associated with *Shigella sonnei* infection. Arthritis Rheum 1988; 31: 1190–1193.

34. Toivanen P, Toivanen A, Olkkonen L et al. Hospital outbreak of *Yersinia enterocolitica* infection. Lancet 1973; 1: 801–803.

35. Aleksic S, Bockemühl J. Proposed revision of the Wauters et al. antigenic scheme for serotyping of *Yersinia enterocolitica*. J Clin Microbiol 1984; 20: 99–102.

36. Tsubokura M, Otsuki K, Kawaoka Y et al. Addition of new serogroups and improvement of the antigenic designs of *Yersinia pseudotuberculosis*. Curr Microbiol 1984; 11: 89–92.

37. Tertti R, Granfors K, Lehtonen O-P et al. An outbreak of *Yersinia pseudotuberculosis* infection. J Infect Dis 1984; 149: 245–250.

38. Tertti R, Vuento R, Mikkola P et al. Clinical manifestations of *Yersinia pseudotuberculosis* infection in children. Eur J Clin Microbiol Infect Dis 1989; 8: 587–591.

39. Ebringer A. Ankylosing spondylitis is caused by *Klebsiella*. Evidence from immunogenetic, microbiologic, and serologic studies. Rheum Dis Clin N Am 1992; 18: 105–121.

40. Blankenberg-Sprenkels SHD, Fielder M, Feltkamp TEW et al. Antibodies to *Klebsiella pneumoniae* in Dutch patients with ankylosing spondylitis and acute anterior uveitis and to *Proteus mirabilis* in rheumatoid arthritis. J Rheumatol 1998; 25: 743–747.

41. Russell AS, Suarez Almazor ME. Ankylosing spondylitis is not caused by *Klebsiella*. Rheum Dis Clin N Am 1992; 18: 95–104.

42. Toivanen P, Hansen DS, Mestre F et al. Somatic serogroups, capsular types, and species of fecal *Klebsiella* in patients with ankylosing spondylitis. J Clin Microbiol 1999; 37: 2808–2812.

43. Ebringer A, Cox NL, Abuljadayel I et al. *Klebsiella* antibodies in ankylosing spondylitis and *Proteus* antibodies in rheumatoid arthritis. Br J Rheumatol 1988; 27(suppl. II): 272–285.

44. Senior BW, Anderson GA, Morley KD et al. Evidence that patients with rheumatoid arthritis have asymptomatic 'non-significant' *Proteus mirabilis* bacteriuria more frequently than healthy controls. J Infection 1999; 38: 99–106.

45. Tiwana H, Wilson C, Alvarez A et al. Cross-reactivity between the rheumatoid arthritis-associated motif EQKRAA and structurally related sequences found in *Proteus mirabilis*. Infect Immun 1999; 67: 2769–2775.

46. Wilson C, Tiwana H, Ebringer A. Molecular mimicry between HLA-DR alleles associated with rheumatoid arthritis and proteus mirabilis as the aetiological basis for autoimmunity. Microbes Infect 2000; 2: 1489–1496.

47. Whiteford JR, Wilson C, Tiwana H et al. Genetic diversity in *Proteus mirabilis* isolates found in the urinary tract of rheumatoid arthritis patients. J Infection 2000; 41: 245–248.

48. Roughgarden JW. Antimicrobial therapy of rat-bite fever. Arch Intern Med 1965; 116: 39–54.

49. Granfors K, Viljanen MK, Toivanen A. Measurement of immunoglobulin M, immunoglobulin G, and immunoglobulin A antibodies against *Yersinia enterocolitica* by enzyme-linked immunosorbent assay: comparison of lipopolysaccharide and whole bacterium as antigen. J Clin Microbiol 1981; 14: 6–14.

50. Bundle DR, Gidney AJ, Perry MB et al. Serological confirmation of *Brucella abortus* and *Yersinia enterocolitica* O: 9 O-antigens by monoclonal antibodies. Infect Immun 1984; 46: 389–393.

51. Virtanen S, Lindgren I. Osteomyelitis of the femur caused by BCG. Acta Tuberc Pneum Scand 1962; 41: 260–267.

52. Ochsenkuhn T, Weber MW, Caselmann WH. Arthritis after *M. bovis* immunotherapy for bladder cancer. Ann Intern Med 1990; 112: 882.

53. Relman DA, Schmidt TM, MacDermott RP et al. Identification of the uncultured bacillus of Whipple's disease. N Engl J Med 1992; 327: 293–301.

54. Nurminen M, Leinonen M, Saikku P et al. The genus-specific antigen of *Chlamydia*: resemblance to the lipopolysaccharide of enteric bacteria. Science 1983; 220: 1279–1281.

55. Pönkä A. The occurrence and clinical picture of serologically verified *Mycoplasma pneumoniae* infections with emphasis on central nervous system, cardiac and joint manifestation. Ann Clin Res 1979; 11(suppl. 24): 1–60.

56. Jansson E, Backman A, Hakkarainen K et al. Mycoplasmas and arthritis. Z Rheumatol 1983; 42: 315–319.

57. Barile MF, Yoshida H, Roth H. Rheumatoid arthritis: new findings on the failure to isolate or detect mycoplasmas by multiple cultivation or serologic procedures and a review of the literature. Rev Infect Dis 1991; 13: 571–582.

58. Frangogiannis NG, Cate TR. Endocarditis and *Ureaplasma urealyticum* osteomyelitis in a hypogammaglobulinemic patient. A case report and review of the literature. J Infection 1998; 37: 181–184.

59. Tunn EJ, Bacon PA. Are viral arthritides reactive? In: Toivanen A, Toivanen P, eds. Reactive arthritis. Boca Raton, FL: CRC Press; 1988: 99–111.

60. Fields BN, Knipe DM, Howley PM, eds. Field's virology. New York: Lippincott-Raven; 1996.

61. Anderson MJ, Lewis E, Kidd IM et al. An outbreak of erythema infectiosum associated with human parvovirus infection. J Hyg 1984; 92: 85–93.

62. Reid DM, Reid TMS, Brown T et al. Human parvovirus-associated arthritis: a clinical and laboratory description. Lancet 1985; 1: 422–425.

63. Stierle G, Brown KA, Rainsford SG et al. Parvovirus associated antigen in the synovial membrane of patients with rheumatoid arthritis. Ann Rheum Dis 1987; 46: 219–223.

64. Scroggie DA, Carpenter MT, Cooper RI et al. Parvovirus arthropathy outbreak in southwestern United States. J Rheumatol 2000; 27: 2444–2448.

65. Nikkari S, Roivainen A, Hannonen P et al. Persistence of parvovirus B19 in synovial fluid and bone marrow. Ann Rheum Dis 1995; 54: 597–600.

66. Kerr JR, Cartron JP, Curran MD et al. A study of the role of parvovirus B19 in rheumatoid arthritis. Br J Rheumatol 1995; 34: 809–813.

67. Moore TL. Parvovirus-associated arthritis. Curr Opin Rheumatol 2000; 12: 289–294.

68. Zhang L, Nikkari S, Skurnik M et al. Detection of herpes viruses by polymerase chain reaction in lymphocytes from patients with rheumatoid arthritis. Arthritis Rheum 1993; 36: 1080–1086.

69. Tamm A, Ziegler T, Lautenschlager I et al. Detection of cytomegalovirus DNA in cells from synovial fluid and peripheral blood of patients with early rheumatoid arthritis. J Rheumatol 1993; 20: 1489–1493.

70. Nikkari S, Luukkainen R, Nikkari L et al. No evidence of adenoviral hexon regions in rheumatoid synovial cells and tissue. J Rheumatol 1994; 21: 2179–2183.

71. Laine M, Luukkainen R, Jalava J et al. Prolonged arthritis associated with sindbis-related (Pogosta) virus infection. Rheumatology 2000; 39: 1272–1274.

72. Keat A, Rowe I. Reiter's syndrome and associated arthritides. Rheum Dis Clin N Am 1991; 17: 25–42.

73. Solinger AM, Hess EV. Rheumatic diseases and AIDS – is the association real? J Rheumatol 1993; 20: 678–683.

74. Nishioka K, Maruyama J, Sato K et al. Chronic inflammatory arthropathy associated with HTLV-I (letter). Lancet 1989; 1: 441.

75. Zucker-Franklin D. Non-HIV retroviral association with rheumatic disease. Curr Rheumatol Rep 2000; 2: 156–162.

76. Iwakura Y, Tosu M, Yoshida E et al. Induction of inflammatory arthropathy resembling rheumatoid arthritis in mice transgenic for HTLV-I. Science 1991; 253: 1026–1028.

77. Peterhans E, Zanoni R, Ruff G et al. Caprine arthritis encephalitis. In: Pliska V, Stranzinger G, eds. Farm animals in biomedical research. Hamburg: Verlag Paul Parey; 1990: 147–154.

78. Tomai M, Kotb M, Majumdar G et al. Superantigenicity of streptococcal M protein. J Exp Med 1990; 172: 359–362.

79. Friedman SM, Posnett DN, Tumang JR et al. A potential role for microbial superantigens in the pathogenesis of systemic autoimmune disease. Arthritis Rheum 1991; 34: 468–480.

80. Mu HH, Sawitzke AD, Cole BC. Modulation of cytokine profiles by the *Mycoplasma* superantigen *Mycoplasma arthritidis* mitogen parallels susceptibility to arthritis induced by *M. arthritidis*. Infect Immun 2000; 68: 1142–1149.

81. Sawitzke A, Joyner D, Knudtson K et al. Anti-MAM antibodies in rheumatic disease: evidence for a MAM-like superantigen in rheumatoid arthritis? J Rheumatol 2000; 27: 358–364.

82. Yamamoto T, Katayama I, Nishioka K. Peripheral blood mononuclear cell proliferative response against staphylococcal superantigens in patients with psoriasis arthropathy. Europ J Dermatol 1999; 9: 17–21.

83. Paliard X, West SG, Lafferty JA et al. Evidence for the effects of a superantigen in rheumatoid arthritis. Science 1991; 253: 325–329.

84. Shinnick TM. Heat shock proteins as antigens of bacterial and parasitic pathogens. Curr Top Microbiol 1991; 167: 145–160.

85. Jindal S, Dudani AK, Singh B et al. Primary structure of a human mitochondrial protein homologous to the bacterial and plant chaperonins and to the 65-kiloDalton mycobacterial antigen. Mol Cell Biol 1989; 9: 2279–2283.

86. Möller G. Heat-shock proteins and the immune system. Immunol Rev 1991; 121: 1–220.

87. van Eden W, Yong DB, eds. Stress proteins in medicine. New York: Marcel Dekker; 1995.

88. Granfors K, Vuento R, Toivanen A. Host-microbe interaction in reactive arthritis. In: Toivanen A, Toivanen P, eds. Reactive arthritis. Boca Raton, FL: CRC Press; 1988: 15–49.

89. Lahesmaa R, Skurnik M, Vaara M et al. Molecular mimickry between HLA B27 and *Yersinia*, *Salmonella*, *Shigella* and *Klebsiella* within the same region of HLA α1-helix. Clin Exp Immunol 1991; 86: 399–404.

90. Toivanen P, Toivanen A. Does *Yersinia* induce autoimmunity? Int Arch Allergy Immunol 1994; 104: 107–111.

91. Mertz AKH, Daser A, Skurnik M et al. The evolutionarily conserved ribosomal protein L23 and the cationic urease α-subunit of *Yersinia enterocolitica* O:3 belong to the immunodominant antigens in *Yersinia*-triggered reactive arthritis: implications for autoimmunity. Mol Med 1994; 1: 44–55.

92. Bachmaier K, Neu N, de la Maza LM et al. *Chlamydia* infections and heart disease linked through antigenic mimicry. Science 1999; 283: 1335–1339.

93. Martin R, Gran B, Zhao Y et al. Molecular mimicry and antigen specific T cell responses in multiple sclerosis and chronic CNS Lyme disease. J Autoimmun 2001; 16: 187–192.

94. Moran AP, Prendergast MM. Molecular mimicry in *Campylobacter jejuni* and *Helicobacter pylori* lipopolysaccharides: contribution of gastrointestinal infections to autoimmunity. J Autoimmun 2001; 16: 241–256.

95. Wucherpfennig KW. Structural basis of molecular mimicry. J Autoimmun 2001; 16: 293–302.

96. Cohen I. Antigenic mimicry, clonal selection and autoimmunity. J Autoimmun 2001; 16: 337–340.

97. Lahesmaa R, Skurnik M, Toivanen P. Molecular mimicry: any role in the pathogenesis of spondyloarthropathies? Immunol Res 1993; 12: 193–208.

98. Lahesmaa-Rantala R, Granfors K, Kekomäki R et al. Circulating yersinia specific immune complexes after acute yersiniosis: a follow up study of patients with and without reactive arthritis. Ann Rheum Dis 1987; 46: 121–126.

99. Lahesmaa-Rantala R, Granfors K, Isomäki H et al. *Yersinia* specific immune complexes in the synovial fluid of patients with *Yersinia*-triggered reactive arthritis. Ann Rheum Dis 1987; 46: 510–514.

100. Manicourt DH, Orloff S. Immune complexes in polyarthritis after salmonella gastroenteritis. J Rheumatol 1981; 8: 613–620.

101. Hall RP, Gerber LH, Lawley TJ. IgA-containing immune complexes in patients with psoriatic arthritis. Clin Exp Rheumatol 1984; 2: 283–292.

102. Lehtonen L, Kortekangas P, Oksman P et al. Synovial fluid muramic acid in acute inflammatory arthritis. Br J Rheumatol 1994; 33: 1127–1130.

103. Register KB, Morgan PA. Interaction between Chlamydia spp. and human polymorphonuclear leukocytes in vitro. Infect Immun 1986; 52: 664–670.

104. Salmi M, Rajala P, Jalkanen S. Homing of mucosal leukocytes to joints. Distinct endothelial ligands in synovium mediate leukocyte-subtype specific adhesion. J Clin Invest 1997; 99: 2165–2172.

105. Salmi M, Jalkanen S. Human leukocyte subpopulations from inflamed gut bind to joint vasculature using distinct sets of adhesion molecules. J Immunol 2001; 166: 4650–4657.

106. Wagener P, Busch J, Hammer M et al. Endotoxin in the plasma of patients with inflammatory rheumatic diseases. Scand J Rheumatol 1988; 17: 301–303.

107. Wagener P, Hammer M, Schedel I. Nachweis von endotoxin im synovialgewebe von patienten mit entzündlich-rheumatischen erkrankungen. Z Rheumatol 1989; 48: 200–203.

108. Pearson CM. Development of arthritis, periarthritis and periostitis in rats given adjuvants. Proc Soc Exp Biol Med 1956; 91: 95–101.

109. Hogervorst EJM, Wagenaar JPA, Boog CJP et al. Adjuvant arthritis and immunity to the mycobacterial 65kDa heat shock protein. Int Immunol 1992; 4: 719–727.

110. Hazenberg MP, Klasen IS, Kool J et al. Are intestinal bacteria involved in the etiology of rheumatoid arthritis? APMIS 1992; 100: 1–9.

111. Simelyte E, Rimpiläinen M, Lehtonen L et al. Bacterial cell wall-induced arthritis: chemical composition and tissue distribution of four Lactobacillus strains. Infect Immun 2000; 68: 3535–3540.

112. Simelyte E, Isomäki P, Rimpiläinen M et al. Cytokine production in arthritis susceptible and resistant rats. A study with arthritogenic and non-arthritogenic Lactobacillus cell walls. Scand J Immunol 2001; 53: 132–138.

113. Stimpson SA, Esser RE, Carter PB et al. Lipopolysaccharide induces recurrence of arthritis in rat joints previously injured by peptidoglycan-polysaccharide. J Exp Med 1987; 165: 1688–1702.

114. Severijnen AJ, van Kleef R, Hazenberg MP et al. Cell wall fragments from major residents of the human intestinal flora induce chronic arthritis in rats. J Rheumatol 1989; 16: 1061–1068.

115. Johnson AH, Campbell WG, Callahan BC. Infection of rabbit knee joints after intra-articular injection of Staphylococcus aureus. Am J Pathol 1970; 60: 165–177.

116. Goldenberg DL, Chisholm PL, Rice PA. Experimental models of bacterial arthritis: a microbiologic and histopathologic characterization of the arthritis after the intraarticular injections of Neisseria gonorrhoeae, Staphylococcus aureus, group A streptococci, and Escherichia coli. J Rheumatol 1983; 10: 5–11.

117. Abdelnour A, Zhao Y-X, Holmdahl R et al. Major histocompatibility complex class II region confers susceptibility to Staphylococcus aureus arthritis. Scand J Immunol 1997; 45: 301–307.

118. Mahowald ML, Peterson L, Raskind J et al. Antigen-induced experimental septic arthritis in rabbits after intraarticular injection of Staphylococcus aureus. J Infect Dis 1986; 154: 273–282.

119. Merilahti-Palo R, Gripenberg-Lerche C, Söderström K-O et al. Long term follow up of SHR rats with experimental yersinia associated arthritis. Ann Rheum Dis 1992; 51: 91–96.

120. Gripenberg-Lerche C, Skurnik M, Toivanen P. Role of YadA-mediated collagen binding in arthritogenicity of Yersinia enterocolitica serotype O:8: experimental studies with rats. Infect Immun 1995; 63: 3222–3226.

121. Zhang Y, Gripenberg-Lerche C, Söderström K-O et al. Antibiotic prophylaxis and treatment of reactive arthritis. Lessons from an animal model. Arthritis Rheum 1996; 39: 1238–1243.

122. Zhang Y, Toivanen A, Toivanen P. Experimental Yersinia-triggered reactive arthritis; effect of a 3-week course with ciprofloxacin. Br J Rheumatol 1997; 36: 541–546.

123. Dumonde DC. Principal evidence associating rheumatic diseases with microbial infection. In: Dumonde DC, ed. Infection and immunology in the rheumatic diseases. Oxford: Blackwell Scientific; 1976: 95–96.

124. Toivanen A, Lahesmaa-Rantala R, Ståhlberg TH et al. Do bacterial antigens persist in reactive arthritis? Clin Exp Rheumatol 1987; 5(suppl. 1): 25–27.

125. Taylor-Robinson D, Thomas BJ, Dixey J et al. Evidence that Chlamydia trachomatis causes seronegative arthritis in women. Ann Rheum Dis 1988; 47: 295–299.

126. Viitanen AM, Arstila TP, Lahesmaa R et al. Application of the polymerase chain reaction and immunofluorescence techniques to the detection of bacteria in Yersinia-triggered reactive arthritis. Arthritis Rheum 1991; 34: 89–96.

127. Taylor-Robinson D, Gilroy CB, Thomas BJ et al. Detection of Chlamydia trachomatis DNA in joints of reactive arthritis patients by polymerase chain reaction. Lancet 1992; 340: 81–82.

128. Merilahti-Palo R, Pelliniemi LJ, Granfors K et al. Electron microscopy and immunolabeling of Yersinia antigens in human synovial fluid cells. Clin Exp Rheumatol 1994; 12: 255–259.

129. Nanagara R, Li F, Beutler A et al. Alteration of Chlamydia trachomatis biologic behavior in synovial membranes. Suppression of surface antigen production in reactive arthritis and Reiter's syndrome. Arthritis Rheum 1995; 38: 1410–1417.

130. Toivanen P, Toivanen A. Bacterial or reactive arthritis? Rheumatol Europe 1995; 24(suppl. 2): 253–255.

131. Kortekangas P, Aro HT, Tuominen J et al. Synovial fluid leukocytosis in bacterial arthritis vs. reactive arthritis and rheumatoid arthritis in the adult knee. Scand J Rheumatol 1992; 21: 283–288.

93 Septic arthritis and osteomyelitis

Lars Lidgren

- The skeleton is affected by a wide variety of different infections with distinct etiology, pathogenesis, clinical features and management
- Staphylococci are the most common cause of musculoskeletal sepsis
- Streptococcal and mycobacterial infections are increasing in prevalence
- Antibiotic resistance, especially in prosthetic infections of low virulence caused by coagulase-negative staphylococci, is an increasing problem
- The adherence of bacteria to biomaterials used in joint replacement remains a major unresolved problem

HISTORY

'Laudable pus' was identified by Galen as being part of the healing process in open fractures, and allowing spontaneous healing was the treatment of choice in most centers in Europe until the 19th century[1].

Hippocrates understood the importance of the reduction of fractures and the appliance of wound dressings but it was not until Lister had, as a surgeon, accepted Pasteur's findings that both antisepsis and asepsis slowly became standard practice. Bone infection in osteomyelitis is described in Greek, Roman and Arab texts from AD 500–1200, and limited sequestrectomy was an accepted treatment. Chemotherapy in osteomyelitis was first used in 1936[2] and rapidly gained popularity as penicillin was introduced.

EPIDEMIOLOGY

The annual incidence of bacterial arthritis and acute osteomyelitis in Sweden is 10/100 000[3,4]. The incidence is higher in warm and humid geographic areas and is probably also related to socioeconomic conditions. In Western Australia, among European children, there are twice as many cases of acute osteomyelitis as in, for example, Scotland or Sweden.

In New Zealand the Maori have four times, and in Australia the Aborigines 12 times, as many hospital admissions for acute osteomyelitis as Europeans in both Australia and Europe[5]. The number of acute bone infections that develop into chronic infection has been drastically reduced, by early antibiotic treatment and surgical decompression, from 10–20% to less than 2%[6].

The number of new cases of chronic osteomyelitis of post-traumatic, postoperative and hematogenous origin in various European countries during the past decade has been estimated to be 15–30/100 000 population[3,5,7]. However, the number of cases of hematogenous origin is expected to reduce substantially. In a recent study (1990–97) acute hematogenous osteomyelitis in children was found to be becoming rare, with only 2.9/100 000/year in Scotland. The annual incidence of vertebral osteomyelitis is estimated to be 0.5–1.0/100 000 population[8,9].

Postoperative diskitis occurs in about 1%[10,11] and only rarely is hematogenous diskitis seen, especially in the cervical spine in children.

Currently, at least 1.8 million joint prosthetic implants and 2 million devices for hip fractures per year are implanted all over the world. In the 1970s, before any preventive measures were taken, about 10% of all major surgical hip procedures involving an implant resulted in infection.

Improvements in surgical techniques, pre- and perioperative routines and antibiotic prophylaxis, as well as treatment against hematogenous spread from infectious foci in, for instance, the skin, have led to a reduction of the infection rate to less than 0.5% in hip surgery and 1% in knee prosthetic surgery[12].

CLINICAL FEATURES AND PATHOGENESIS

Septic arthritis

Clinical features

The presentation of septic arthritis varies with age. In infancy, the symptoms are usually systemic rather than local[13,14]. Small children develop high, septic-pattern fever (Table 93.1) and are usually ill. The clinical features are more those of sepsis than of local arthritis. Older children are also febrile and unwell but the local signs are more prominent. Distention of the joint capsule and increased intra-articular pressure contribute to pain. If the hip joint is involved it is usually held in flexion, as this position gives maximum compliance. Adults and elderly patients with osteoarthritis or rheumatoid arthritis (RA) are at greater risk of an acute septic arthritis. The lower extremities are more often

TABLE 93.1 CLINICAL FEATURES OF SEPTIC BONE AND JOINT LESIONS					
	Fever	Local pain	Inflammatory signs	Purulent drainage	Reduced function
Septic arthritis	+	+	+	− to (+)	(+) to +
Prosthetic joint infection	(+) to +	(+) to +	(−) to (+)	−	(−) to +
Septic bursitis	(+) to +	(+)	(+) to +	−	(−) to (+)
Acute osteomyelitis	+	+	(+) to +	−	− to (+)
Pelvic osteomyelitis	+	+	(−) to (+)	− to +	(+) to +
Chronic osteomyelitis	− to (+)	− to (+)	(−) to (+)	− to (+)	− to (+)
Osteitis	− to (+)	(+)	(−) to (+)	−	− to (+)
Spondylitis	(−) to +	(−) to (+)	(−)		− to +
− = avbsent (−) = low-grade (+) = moderate + = high-grade					

affected, particularly the hip and knee joints. Patients generally have severe pain and are reluctant to move and put weight on the joint[15].

The joint capsule is distended, warm and often reddened and edematous (Fig. 93.1). If the infection is detected and treated during the first 2–3 days the outcome is favorable and there is no mortality. A delay in diagnosis, particularly in septic arthritis of the hip in children, often results in joint destruction[16] (Fig. 93.2).

Pathogenesis

A prerequisite for the development of septic arthritis is that bacteria can reach the synovial membrane. This can take place in different ways (Fig. 93.3).

Firstly, bacteria may reach the joint from a remote infectious focus via the hematogenous route. Such foci are usually abscesses or infected wounds in the skin, infections in the teeth, upper or lower respiratory tract infections, urinary or intestinal tract infections or endocarditis. In some cases no obvious primary focus is noted – a common experience in septicemia. The bacteria reach the deep vascular plexus terminating in the looped capillary anastomosis (circulus articularis vasculosus)[16,17].

A second route, particularly common in small children, is a dissemination of bacteria from an acute osteomyelitic focus in the metaphysis or epiphysis. The vessels through the physis and epiphysis are not occluded as is usually the case above 1 year of age[18]. Above this age, spread of bacteria can occur from the metaphysis of the humerus and femur or in the elbow, where the joint capsule covers parts of the metaphysis, allowing bacteria to penetrate through the cortical bone and the periosteum to the joint cavity. In adults with closed growth plates there is a re-established connection between the meta-

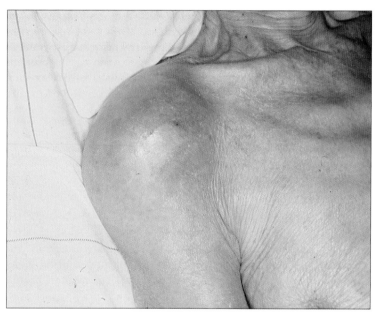

Fig. 93.1 Septic arthritis in an elderly patient, here recognized by distention, increased skin temperature and tenderness. The septic arthritis does not always differ from other kinds of arthritis.

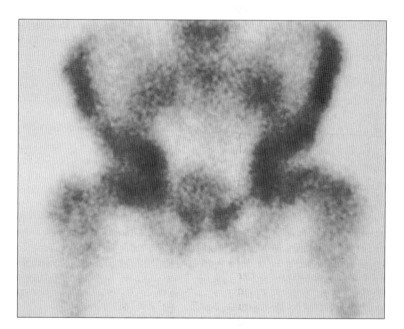

Fig. 93.2 Segmental femoral head necrosis in septic arthritis of the left hip.

Fig. 93.3 Routes by which bacteria can reach the joint.

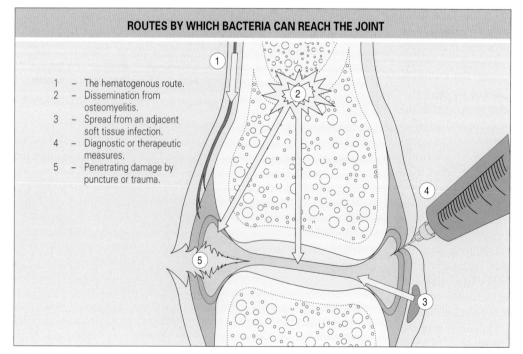

ROUTES BY WHICH BACTERIA CAN REACH THE JOINT

1 – The hematogenous route.
2 – Dissemination from osteomyelitis.
3 – Spread from an adjacent soft tissue infection.
4 – Diagnostic or therapeutic measures.
5 – Penetrating damage by puncture or trauma.

physis and the epiphysis and spread of infection to the synovial plexus is possible.

Third, an infection in the vicinity of the joint can progress to the joint or spread via the lymphogenic route. This is most often seen in non-penetrating traumatic and postoperative wound infections and in skin and soft tissue infections around the joint, particularly the knee joint.

A fourth possibility is iatrogenic infection caused by joint puncture for a diagnostic or therapeutic purpose. Although extremely rare, this has not yet been completely eradicated.

Lastly, penetrating trauma, usually caused by dirty objects or by animal or human bites, often gives rise to a severe infection because of the high inoculate of bacteria and the lacerated tissue. After joint surgery, perioperatively implanted bacteria can cause a postoperative infection.

In hematogenous infection, once the bacteria have reached the synovial membrane an inflammatory reaction starts. Leukocytes migrate to the focus and inflammatory proteins exude to the infectious focus. The synovial membrane proliferates and becomes tender, and the blood flow increases. There is exudation of bacteria, cells and proteins into the joint cavity. The bacteria in the joint fluid can be killed by phagocytes. The joint becomes swollen and the joint pressure rises and can cause cartilage damage. The enzymes elastase and collagenase are liberated from polymorphonuclear leukocytes and synovial cells degrade the cartilage. The infection and inflammation can spread in the subchondral bone[19]. Joint cartilage loses its resilience, tolerating only about a third of the normal pressure. The tissue changes become irreversible, often in a few days (Fig. 93.4)[20]. A proliferating pannus tissue will often result from persistent infection.

Prosthetic joint infection
Clinical features
The symptoms can differ in the early and late postoperative period. If an infection presents soon after surgery, staphylococci and streptococci are more common and the symptoms are more intensive, with high fever, general malaise and a wound discharging pus[21]. Later on, when the wound has healed or a sinus has developed, the patient may still have pain with soft tissue swelling (Fig. 93.5). In postoperative infections presenting late the general symptoms are usually not impressive and the local signs can be rather discrete, with slight tenderness and pain. In

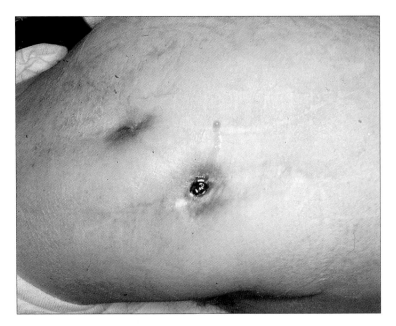

Fig. 93.5 **In spite of a severe deep infection around a prosthesis, the only external signs may be a fistula and edema.**

some cases of hip joint infection with joint effusion, the pressure can be so high that dislocation occurs[12]. In hematogenous infections the onset is usually acute, with high, septic fever and increasing pain even at rest. A hematogenous prosthetic joint infection is serious, with high morbidity and mortality, especially in fragile patients (RA) and with *Staphylococcus aureus* infection[22].

Pathogenesis
Low-virulence bacteria such as coagulase-negative staphylococci are the dominating pathogens in infections around prosthetic materials[23]. Patients with an implanted large foreign body are often elderly, which increases the risk of infection. Bacteria, particularly the staphylococci, are apt to adhere to a foreign biomaterial surface. This colonization, 'a race for the surface'[24], is the first step in a process that results in chronic infection in a prosthetic joint. Bacteria compete with host-tissue cells for the ability to produce proteins and polysaccharides and furthermore to be integrated with the surface of biomaterial. A biofilm is established. The bacteria are embedded in slime, a glycocalyx that protects them from antimicrobial agents and the cellular and humoral host defenses. Physical forces and hydrophobic interactions, non-specific chemical bindings and specific bacterial receptor–host component bindings mediated by ligands facilitate a strong attachment of bacteria to the foreign material[25,26].

Septic bursitis
The superficial subcutaneous olecranon, prepatellar and infrapatellar bursae are the most common sites affected by bacterial infections[27]. Antecedent trauma, mostly occupation-related, to the infected bursa is found in the majority of patients. Some underlying conditions, e.g. diabetes mellitus, rheumatoid arthritis, chronic alcohol abuse, may be contributing factors. Associated septicemia in cases of septic bursitis is uncommon

Acute bacterial bursitis is most common at the elbow and knee. Adults are mostly affected. The onset is rapid, often after repeated trauma. High fever, sometimes with chills, and swelling of the bursa with increased warmth, redness and pain are characteristic (Fig. 93.6). Joint function is generally not affected. In cases with olecranon bursitis without trauma, diabetes mellitus is a frequent underlying disease. The prognosis is good, with few sequelae[28].

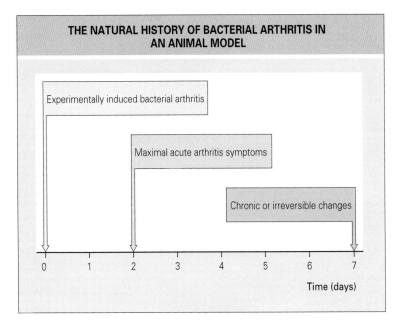

THE NATURAL HISTORY OF BACTERIAL ARTHRITIS IN AN ANIMAL MODEL

Experimentally induced bacterial arthritis

Maximal acute arthritis symptoms

Chronic or irreversible changes

0   1   2   3   4   5   6   7

Time (days)

Fig. 93.4 **The natural history of bacterial arthritis in an animal model.** This is similar to development in the clinical case. (Data from Goldenberg and Reed[20].)

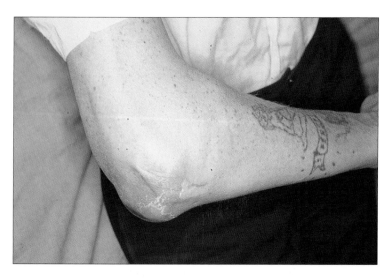

Fig. 93.6 Bursitis symptoms are similar to arthritis but a diagnostic puncture of the bursa containing purulent material in septic bursitis is easy to do.

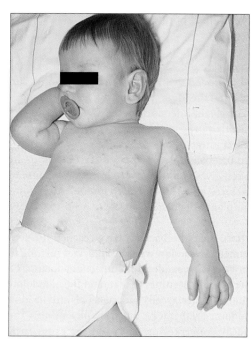

Fig. 93.7 An acute osteomyelitis in the proximal metaphysis of the left humerus. The child is not willing to move the affected limb. The roseola is consistent with a *Salmonella* infection, which was confirmed by fecal cultures.

Acute osteomyelitis

Clinical features

This type of infection principally affects children and young adults[15]. In children below 1 year of age acute osteomyelitis presents with arthritis in about 75% of cases and septicemia in almost all[14]. The epiphysis is sometimes involved[29]. Older children will not move or weight-bear on the affected limb (Fig. 93.7). The metaphysis, mostly in the lower extremities around the knee joint, in the trochanter region or in the humerus, is tender to the touch and can be swollen and warm. In the proximal humerus and femur the joint may be involved because of the insertion of the joint capsule below the metaphysis. If the infection is diagnosed and treated during the first 2–3 days after onset the prognosis is good and chronic complications are rare.

Pathogenesis

The metaphysis has a rich blood supply and a slow circulation time. By contrast, the perfusion is slow through the venous sinusoids. The endothelial cells of the sinusoids have a reduced phagocytic activity[30,31]. These factors are favorable for bacterial adherence and multiplication in the metaphysis (Fig. 93.8). The ensuing inflammatory reaction increases the intraosseous pressure, and microthrombi of the small vessels obstruct the blood flow. The result is an intraosseous inflammatory

focus with abscess formation under high pressure, and a reduced blood supply resulting in the destruction of osseous trabeculae by osteoclasts followed by osteoblastic activity forming new bone tissue[32]. In chickens it has been shown that bacteria deposit in the growth plate and bacterial proliferation occludes the blood vessels within 24 hours[33]. Abscess formation usually occurs within 2–3 days. When the purulent infection has penetrated laterally through haversian channels to the subperiosteal area and/or down to the medullary cavity, the lesion becomes chronic.

Pelvic osteomyelitis

Clinical features

In younger athletic individuals this disease presents as an acute hematogenous infection around the symphysis or the sacroiliac joints and is caused by *S. aureus*[34]. In women with obstetric or gynecologic pelvic infections a different clinical picture is seen, with subacute onset and contiguous dissemination from the pelvis.

The symptoms can be diffuse and difficult to attribute to a skeletal infection; pain and fever are the most prominent symptoms. The condition may be difficult to detect and the diagnosis is often delayed. However, the prognosis is good and sequelae are rare.

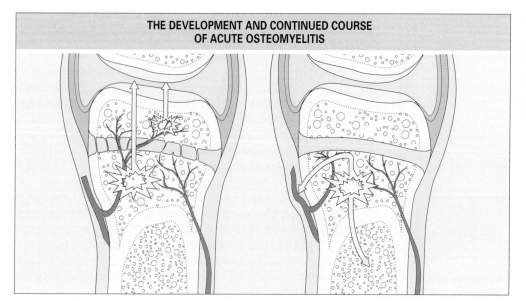

THE DEVELOPMENT AND CONTINUED COURSE OF ACUTE OSTEOMYELITIS

Fig. 93.8 The development and continued course of acute osteomyelitis. This differs with age. In infants below 1 year of age the epiphysis is nourished by penetrating arteries through the physis, allowing development of the condition within the epiphysis. In children up to 15 years of age the infection is restricted to below the epiphysis because of interruption of the vessels.

Pathogenesis

In young people, mostly men, *S. aureus* can usually reach the pelvic bones via the blood. The sacroiliac joints, the symphysis and the acetabulum are commonly affected. Osteomyelitis has been noted in athletes, and it is possible that skin lesions with colonizing *S. aureus* are the source of bacteria[34].

In women during the childbearing period, bacteria, usually Gram-negative intestinal organisms and/or anaerobes[12], may spread contiguously from an infectious focus in the pelvic region as a complication of pregnancy or gynecologic disease.

Chronic and subacute osteomyelitis
Clinical features

Chronic osteomyelitis can be intermittent or continuous. The hematogenous form caused by *S. aureus* is now mainly found in elderly people who became infected before the antibiotic era[35], and chronic osteomyelitis in adults is usually post-traumatic or postoperative. The long tubular bones in the lower extremities are most often affected in both forms. The intermittent type presents symptoms either in the form of pain, swelling and increased skin temperature around the affected area, and possibly a moderate rise in body temperature, or as a sinus continuously discharging pus without swelling and often with only slight pain. Subacute Brodie's abscess is another type of osteomyelitis that presents with pain, often without inflammatory signs (Fig. 93.9).

There is almost no mortality in chronic osteomyelitis but the relapse frequency is high (10–20%) and definitive healing is rare even after adequate treatment.

Pathogenesis

Chronic osteomyelitis can develop from an untreated acute osteomyelitis or, more commonly, as a complication of an infected fracture or postoperative infection. Often the vessels are lacerated. The massive bacterial invasion of a vast area promotes propagation of the infection, often in the whole diaphysis. Destruction of the bone tissue is prominent and sequestra and circumscribed abscesses arise. Lysis is followed by new bone deposition. This can grow centrifugally or encroach on the medullary cavity[12].

Sinus formation originating from intraosseous cavities is common, with discharge of pus, infected material and small bone pieces to the skin surface. Defective healing and skeletal malformation are common.

Osteitis
Clinical features

Infections of short and flat bones, particularly common in the feet but also occurring in the hands, and usually discrete, give rise to symptoms and are initiated by infections in the skin and/or soft tissue. The patients often have underlying diseases such as diabetes mellitus or arteriosclerosis. Because of the limited bone infection, fever is not common and pain and other symptoms commonly seen in osteomyelitis are not severe. Sometimes a thin fistula or an abrasion down to the bone surface can be the result of a penetrating infectious process. The chances of retaining the affected region intact are low as the condition usually requires varying degrees of resection or amputation[12].

Pathogenesis

If bacteria disseminate from a contiguous focus in the skin or soft tissues, the cortical bone can be affected. Most often such infections occur in the feet. The short, cancellous bones are the site of low-virulence infection. Destruction is seen but new bone formation is not as pronounced as in osteomyelitis of the long tubular bones.

Septic spondylitis
Clinical features

The symptoms of septic spondylitis are often not distinct and may be misinterpreted. However, there is often tenderness over the affected vertebrae. With the exception of postoperative diskitis[36], which rarely proceeds to spondylitis, the route of infection is hematogenous. Spondylitis is most common in the elderly (50–70 years) and located in the lumbar spine. The onset can be insidious, with increasing fever and uncharacteristic back pain or pain radiating to the thorax or abdomen. In such cases the condition is often misinterpreted as myocardial infarction, pleuropneumonia, cholecystitis or appendicitis[37]. Sometimes the onset is acute, with high body temperature, chills and severe back pain.

The process often starts at the endplate, the vertebrae often becoming affected later (Fig. 93.10) with abscess formation; the nerve roots can be involved, resulting in paresis. The purulent infection can also spread to the surrounding soft tissue, and an associated epidural abscess is also possible (Fig. 93.11). Neurologic or disabling sequelae occur in a small

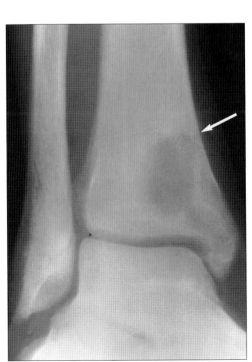

Fig. 93.9 Subacute osteomyelitis (Brodie's abscess). The well-defined oval lucency in the distal tibia shows fading sclerosis along its margins in a pattern typical of a bone abscess. Note the small projection of the upper pole of the lesion pointing to the medial metaphysis, where a subtle periosteal reaction is beginning to form (arrow). This identifies the site where this lesion may ultimately drain.

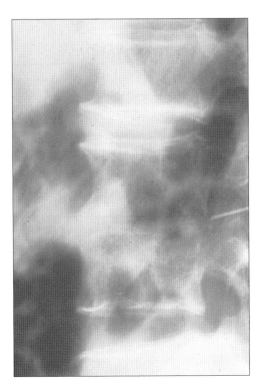

Fig. 93.10 Septic spondylitis of L3 and L4 with destruction of the disc and the adjacent end plates. The aspiration needle for culture and histology is seen. The position of the needle should always be documented with a radiograph.

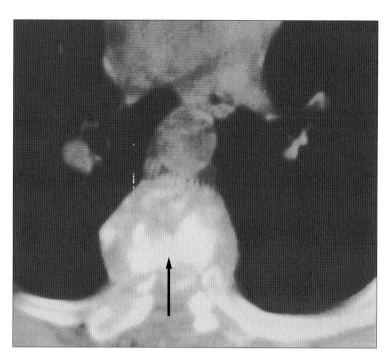

Fig. 93.11 Computed tomography scan showing osteomyelitic destruction of the fourth thoracic vertebral body with soft tissue swelling.

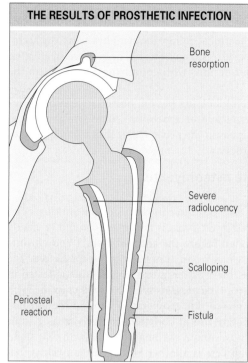

THE RESULTS OF PROSTHETIC INFECTION

Bone resorption

Severe radiolucency

Scalloping

Periosteal reaction

Fistula

Fig. 93.12 The results of prosthetic infection. Periosteal reaction, scalloping, severe radiolucency at the interface, fistula through the bone and severe bone resorption are illustrated. All these changes can also be seen in severe prosthetic mechanical loosening but do not progress as rapidly as in infection.

percentage of cases, but the prospects for complete healing of the infection are good. Serious sequelae are more likely to follow tuberculous infection.

Pathogenesis

Bacteria reach the vertebrae almost exclusively after hematogenous dissemination from a known infectious or cryptogenic focus, as in the case of acute osteomyelitis. The intervertebral space is commonly infected first, with subsequent spread to the adjacent vertebrae. Destruction of the endplate follows and the disk and the vertebrae become compressed. Later, this is often followed by spontaneous interbody vertebral fusion. Local spread of infection is common, with the formation of abscess masses localized in the epidural space or in the soft tissues.

DIAGNOSTIC PROCEDURES AND INVESTIGATIONS

The definite diagnosis of deep, late, especially hematogenous infection may sometimes be difficult. Erythrocyte sedimentation rate (ESR) together with C-reactive protein (CRP) are usually quite sensitive in non-rheumatoid patients, especially in infections associated with joint prostheses. The presence of radiographic changes indicates that an infection has been present for 2–3 weeks or more. Plain radiographs, although not specific, often show a rapidly developing irregular resorption zone around implants, sometimes with an extensive periosteal reaction (Fig. 93.12).

Scintigraphy employing sequential technetium-99m phosphate (three-phase bone scan) is diagnostic aid before radiographic changes appear. In acute hematogenous osteomyelitis with cold lesions caused by a deficient blood supply in a tubular bone, the scan can be repeated after 2–3 days. Computed tomography (CT) and magnetic resonance imaging (MRI) are helpful for the diagnosis but ideal diagnostic tests are still lacking. Indium-111-labeled leukocytes have been used in a few studies and have shown high specificity and sensitivity. In a recent study indium-111 was compared with technetium-99m nanocolloid in 35 patients with suspected infection; nanocolloid showed a sensitivity of 90% and a specificity of 80%, compared to indium[12]. In clinical prac-

tice, however, technetium-99m nanocolloid scanning has the advantage of being completed in a day, whereas indium requires the use of autologous granulocytes and a 2-day procedure (Fig. 93.13).

In acute septic arthritis the microbes are generally localized to the synovia, particularly in the initial stage. Bacteria can be killed by phagocytes and thus there is a risk of obtaining negative cultures from the aspirated joint fluid. It is advisable to dilute the aspirated material in a blood-culture bottle in a proportion of about 1:10 to inhibit the bactericidal components of the joint fluid[12]. Repeated aspiration increases both sensitivity and specificity, especially in prosthetic infection.

In addition to cultures it is advisable to make smears for direct microscopy. If it is possible to perform an arthroscopy, or when a synovectomy is indicated, tissue samples should be used for culture[38]. The same procedures are recommended in prosthetic joint infections. Quantification of cultures, with positive tissue biopsies, is important for a clinical diagnosis of infection[12].

In suspected acute osteomyelitis, pelvic osteomyelitis, sacroiliitis and spondylitis, samples for culture and direct microscopy can often be obtained by needle aspiration or open biopsy[39]. In all these acute infections cultures from blood and suspected infectious foci can facilitate the etiologic diagnosis.

In chronic osteomyelitis and osteitis with fistulae it is not adequate to take cultures from the superficial orifice. This area is usually colonized by irrelevant bacteria[12]. During the surgical exploration of the infectious focus, tissue biopsies are suitable for culture. Blood cultures and cultures from other foci in the body are not indicated, since chronic infection is restricted to the bone.

In spondylitis, puncture and aspiration of the intervertebral space (Fig. 93.10) or of a vertebra under fluoroscopy, for a smear and culture, is a rapid diagnostic method for determining the causative agent[12]. If the patient has septic fever or a focus of origin, blood cultures and a sample from the lesional area should be taken.

Recently both microscopy of frozen sections and polymerase chain reaction techniques using genetic probes for defection of infection have come into clinical use but further clinical evaluation is needed before they become general practice.

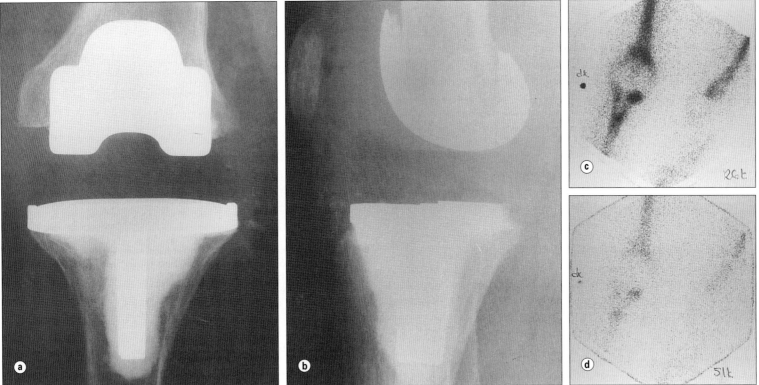
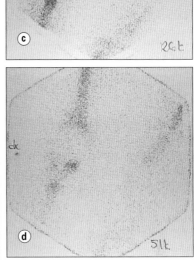

Fig. 93.13 A knee prosthesis 1 year after surgery in a patient with RA and severe pain at rest and on weight-bearing. (a, b) The radiographs show no abnormalities and no radiolucency. (c) Technetium-99m nanocolloid scintigraphy shows obviously increased uptake corresponding to the distal femur and proximal medial tibia. (d) The uptake with indium-111 leukocyte scintigraphy was increased in a similar distribution.

Recommended bacteriologic investigations for acute febrile conditions and chronic conditions are, respectively:

- blood culture, culture from primary foci, smear and culture from the local infectious focus
- representative samples from the deep infectious focus: aspirate or biopsy.

ETIOLOGY

The bacterial etiology in bone and joint infections depends on the type and route of infection. Significant factors are the course of the infection (acute or chronic), pathogenesis (hematogenous or contiguous), the localization of the infection (Table 93.2), the age of the patient and underlying disease. Of great importance also for verifying the etiology are the conditions for sampling and culturing: type and amount of material, media used, accessibility to the laboratory and the quality of the laboratory[12].

With regard to the different bacteria it is difficult to compare various patient materials and to state the relative frequency of microorganisms. *Staphylococcus aureus* is always common in all entities. It is the most common bacteria found in osteomyelitis in all ages and is almost the sole cause of chronic hematogenous osteomyelitis[35]. Coagulase-negative staphylococci and skin anaerobes are opportunistic bacteria but are common in the presence of foreign material. Beta-hemolytic Streptococcus group B is more often seen in neonatal osteomyelitis[40].

TABLE 93.2 BACTERIOLOGIC FINDINGS IN BONE AND JOINT INFECTIONS								
	Acute septic arthritis	Prosthetic joint infection	Bursitis	Acute hematogenous osteomyelitis	Chronic osteomyelitis	Pelvic osteomyelitis	Spondylitis	Diabetic osteitis
Staphylococcus aureus	+++	+++	+++	+++	+++	+++	+++	++
Coagulase-negative staphylococci		+++			+			
Hemolytic streptococcus	++	++	++	++			++	++
Other streptococci	+	+		+			+	+
Skin anaerobes	+	+++		+	+			++
Gram-negative cocci	+			+				
Haemophilus influenzae	+	+		+				
Gram-negative aerobes	+	++	+	+	+	++	++	++
Pseudomonas aeruginosa	+	+		+	+		+	
Salmonella	+	+		+	+		+	
Intestinal anaerobes		+			+	++		++
Mycobacteria	+	+			+		+	
+++ = very common (30% or more)		++ = common (5–30%)			+ = occurs in some circumstances (age, underlying disease, foreign material)			

Haemophilus influenzae is common in hematogenous arthritis in children of 1 month to 5 years of age[41]. This agent, however, is now becoming less common through vaccination of children against infections caused by capsulated *H. influenzae*. *Escherichia coli* was common some years ago in neonatal arthritis and osteomyelitis but as a result of better hygiene it is now less common and is mostly seen in neonatal arthritis[40]. Gram-negative intestinal bacteria are more frequent in the elderly in conditions such as diabetic osteitis, spondylitis and prosthetic joint infections. *Pseudomonas aeruginosa* is found in drug addicts with arthritis and spondylitis, and after trauma. In post-traumatic osteomyelitis, Gram-negative aerobes are becoming increasingly common compared to Gram-positive bacteria. *Salmonella* spp. are more common in developing countries in osteomyelitis, particularly in association with sickle cell anemia, and in arthritis in children[41]. Gonococcal arthritis is discussed separately in Chapter 94 and tuberculous arthritis is in Chapter 95. Anaerobes are found almost exclusively in diabetic osteitis and prosthetic joint infections.

Many types of microorganism are found in orthopedic infections but most of them occur only sporadically. *Mycoplasma* spp. and *Ureaplasma* spp. are rare and can cause infections in immunocompromised patients[42]. Mycobacteria, including atypical varieties, can cause arthritis, spondylitis and osteomyelitis (see Chapter 95). Overall, the global incidence of tuberculosis is rising, which will be reflected in joint and bone infections[43]. In prosthetic joint infections some unusual bacteria spread by the hematogenous route are sometimes found[44]. Moreover, in joint replacement infections, the occurrence of problematic bacteria due to high antibiotic resistance is feared. Bacteria that pose problems include methicillin-resistant *Staphylococcus aureus*, coagulase-negative staphylococci and *Enterococcus faecium*, some species of which are vancomycin-resistant.

Clavicular osteomyelitis can be caused by *S. aureus*, but *Propionibacterium acnes* is also reported as a putative agent[45].

MANAGEMENT OF BACTERIAL INFECTIONS IN BONE AND JOINTS

Prerequisites for successful antibiotic therapy in acute hematogenous osteomyelitis are susceptible causative bacteria, sufficient penetration of drugs to the bone tissue and the affected area and the availability of appropriate forms of administration, i.e. parenteral and well-absorbed oral formulations[12].

In acute hematogenous osteomyelitis, the penetration of antibiotic therapy is impaired as the intraosseous pressure rises and the blood vessels become occluded by edema and microthrombi. At the time when an abscess has developed, the access of antibiotics to the infectious focus is very limited. Therefore, the antibiotics should be instituted within 2–3 days of onset of the clinical symptoms[46].

Factors contributing to decreased efficacy of antibiotics in chronic osteomyelitis are diminished blood flow secondary to deranged bone structure, trauma and sclerosis, the presence of abscesses, sequestra and foreign material, and the development of glycocalyx[26] (Fig. 93.14). *Staphylococcus aureus* can bind to blood and tissue components such as fibrinogen, immunoglobulin G, complement, fibronectin, collagen, vitronectin, laminin and sialoprotein II[47].

Certain strains of *S. aureus*, such as phage-group I strains, are difficult to eradicate and there is an increase in penicillinase-producing or methicillin-resistant staphylococci[35]. The antimicrobial therapy recommendations made below are relevant for countries in which both the frequency of methicillin-resistant staphylococci and the bacterial resistance against antibiotics are lower than 1% (e.g. the Nordic countries). In countries where methicillin-resistance is common, drugs such as vancomycin, teicoplanin, aminoglycosides, rifampin (rifampicin), fusidic acid and

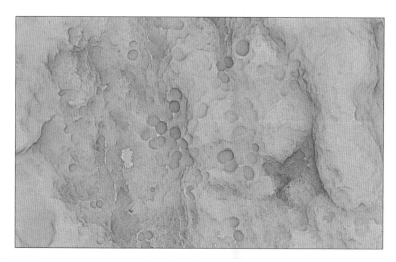

Fig. 93.14 Bone sequestra found in chronic osteomyelitis have no blood supply and function as foreign bodies with a rough, irregular surface. In this scanning electron microscopy picture adherent cocci (*S. aureus*) and a few rods (*E. coli*) are displayed.

quinolones must be used, either in single therapy or, preferably, in combination guided by susceptibility.

Septic arthritis, bursitis and prosthetic joint infections

Early and aggressive therapy is imperative to prevent destruction, especially in childhood[48], and mortality, particularly in elderly patients with RA or diabetes. The history, age and underlying diseases are valuable guides in the choice of antibiotic treatment. In all these entities *S. aureus* and other Gram-positive cocci are common and in some countries *H. influenzae* is still predominant in children under 3 years of age with acute arthritis. The occurrence of Gram-negative organisms in the elderly with predisposing diseases, as well as *S. aureus* in RA, must be taken into account[35].

Isoxazolyl penicillins in suspected Gram-positive infection and a cephalosporin in suspected Gram-negative infection are effective in the ordinary acute case. Parenteral cloxacillin 2g t.i.d. or 100mg/kg/day in Gram-positive infections, and cefuroxime 1.5g t.i.d. or 75–80mg/kg/day in Gram-negative infections is recommended. The duration of parenteral therapy should be 7–10 days and thereafter oral drugs, flucloxacillin 1.5g t.i.d. or 75–80mg/kg/day or a cephalosporin, are given for a total of up to 6 weeks[12].

In prosthetic joint infections a combination of oral clindamycin and ciprofloxacin are alternatives, depending on the bacteriologic findings. This combination may be used for the treatment of coagulase-negative staphylococci, which is the most common finding. Other useful combinations are rifampin and ciprofloxacin or rifampin and fusidic acid[49]. In such cases, which are often treated operatively, local treatment with antibiotic-containing bone cement or other vehicles could be used between the first and second operation in a two-stage procedure[12]. Because of methicillin resistance, vancomycin 1g twice daily may also be used, although its use should be restricted because of the high risk of inducing resistance among enterococci.

Bursitis can be treated with drainage and a short course of parenteral cloxacillin or benzyl penicillin, depending on the microbiological findings. In two-thirds of cases *S. aureus* or streptococci will be the dominant microorganism and subsequent oral treatment should be given for only 1–2 weeks[27].

In septic arthritis of the hip, surgical drainage of the joint is effective and necessary. In case of infection in other joints, repeated aspiration should be performed if no pus is found initially. However, if aspiration is unsuccessful or if the symptoms increase within the first 24–48 hours,

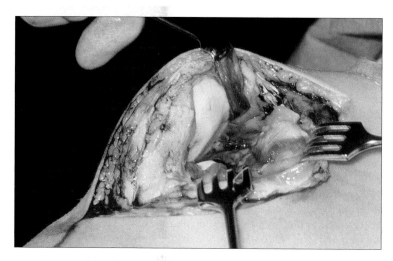

Fig. 93.15 Particularly in postoperative and post-traumatic arthritis with no response to antibiotic treatment, a pannus formation, as seen here on the femoral condyle, may develop.

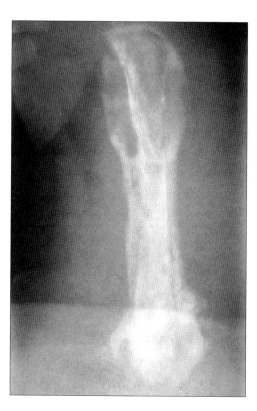

Fig. 93.16 Chronic osteomyelitis with sequestrum and involucrum in an 18-month-old boy.

an arthrotomy is necessary. Arthroscopy has been used as an alternative and is also effective for irrigation of the joint. The early use of devices for passive motion has reduced the need for surgical mobilization after bacterial arthritis. The joint is protected from weight-bearing for an average of 6 weeks. However, the patient is mobilized as soon as the pain has subsided normally within the first week. Late synovectomy has been performed in the knee joint to prevent cartilage destruction and subsequent osteoarthritis[38] (Fig. 93.15).

The treatment of infected joint implants is complicated. Factors influencing the choice of treatment include the condition of the patient and the adjacent joint soft tissue, the quality of the bone stock, the type of primary revision implants, the type and sensitivity of the infected organism, the patient's daily activity requirements and finally the rarity of the problem. The treatment of these patients should be centralized, especially decisions on definitive treatment from among long-term antibiotics, revision arthroplasty, arthrodesis and, rarely, amputation.

The surgical procedure in itself, involving meticulous removal of all foreign material in a staged procedure before the insertion of a new prosthesis, also calls for centralized treatment. The fusion rate in arthrodesis and the healing rate of an infected knee prosthesis is improved if the patient is treated at an experienced center[50]. The septic complication in a joint implant carries an overall mortality from 5% in knee prostheses up to 15% for hip prostheses[50].

Acute hematogenous osteomyelitis

Streptococci and S. aureus dominate in juveniles and adults[51]. In addition to these, H. influenzae and E. coli can also occur in neonatal osteomyelitis, and E. coli and other intestinal bacteria in the elderly.

Beta-lactam antibiotics, clindamycin, fusidic acid, certain quinolones, such as ciprofloxacin, and rifampin are known to penetrate bone tissue in sufficient amounts. Erythromycin and aminoglycosides have inadequate penetration properties[12].

Administration of parenteral antibiotics is indicated initially in acute hematogenous osteomyelitis, followed by an oral regime. Penicillins with a spectrum against Gram-positive bacteria or cephalosporins against Gram-positive and Gram-negative bacteria are the drugs of choice for acute hematogenous osteomyelitis. Clindamycin, fusidic acid and ciprofloxacin are alternatives in specified situations, based on bacteriologic findings and/or penicillin hypersensitivity. Combinations containing erythromycin, aminoglycosides and rifampin have been used but are second choices.

Staphylococcus aureus must be covered in all age groups. A combination of benzyl penicillin and isoxazolyl penicillin, or a corresponding drug, is recommended. The former is more effective against penicillin-sensitive S. aureus and streptococci and the latter against penicillinase-producing staphylococci. High doses should be used, preferably 150mg/kg/day and 100mg/kg/day respectively, in three divided doses[12].

In acute hematogenous osteomyelitis, abscesses should be drained, since decompression prevents further obstruction of blood vessels and resulting bone necrosis. Drainage also results in a dramatic improvement in the patient's general condition. If antibiotic treatment has not been started early and decompression has not been carried out, the trabecular bone may be sequestered and eventually embedded in new bone (Fig. 93.16). Weight-bearing on the extremity should be avoided until radiographic signs of bone restoration are present because there is a high risk of pathologic fracture[12].

When culture results become available, one of the two antibiotics can be withdrawn. The duration of therapy has been discussed in several articles and is proposed to be 3 weeks[33]. However, there are great difficulties involved in keeping children in hospital to receive intravenous antibiotics for such a long time. Parenteral treatment can be limited to 1 week, followed by oral treatment for up to a total of about 2 months[12].

In age groups in which H. influenzae or Gram-negative intestinal bacteria are suspected as being the cause of acute hematogenous osteomyelitis, cloxacillin should be combined with ampicillin or, preferably, a cephalosporin effective against this flora, e.g. cefuroxime, should be chosen. This drug also has sustained effect against Gram-positive bacteria. In cases of unknown etiology and in which either Gram-positive or Gram-negative bacteria are possible, cefuroxime is again the more suitable choice[12].

In elderly patients, in whom Gram-negative bacteria are common as a consequence of urinary, biliary, intestinal and lower respiratory infections or invasive diagnostic procedures at these sites, treatment with broad-spectrum antibiotics, e.g. broad-spectrum penicillins, cefuroxime, cefotaxime or trimethoprim–sulphamethoxazole, is indicated.

Parenteral treatment should be given until fever and the local signs of infection have disappeared, which usually takes 7–10 days. Laboratory variables such as ESR or CRP should be monitored, and normalization of these variables may be interpreted as evidence of the effectiveness of the antibiotic treatment. If chronic osteomyelitis with radiographic changes develops, treatment should be continued for up to 6 months, particularly in cases of staphylococcal etiology[35]. By instituting early systemic antibiotic treatment, it is possible to prevent the development of radiographic changes. The prognosis is directly related to the time at which antibiotic therapy was instituted[46]. Only when an abscess is demonstrable is operative drainage superior to antibiotic treatment[52].

Spondylitis and pelvic osteomyelitis

The evolution of spondylitis is often slow and the prognosis mostly good. There is therefore no need for haste in instituting antibiotic therapy. It is better to first attain a confirmed diagnosis and establish the etiology as far as possible. Usually, acute spondylitis with intensive symptoms such as fever, pain and disability is treated in the same way as acute hematogenous osteomyelitis, depending on disease history and bacterial findings. In the case of progressing neurology, surgical decompression is necessary. MRI is helpful in showing epidural abscess, which sometimes calls for immediate surgery. In hematogenous pelvic osteomyelitis *S. aureus* is the most common agent, particularly in patients under 50 years of age, and the onset is often more acute.

In cases of Gram-positive and *E. coli* infection, antibiotic therapy for 2–3 months is often sufficient if the radiographic findings are discrete. *Salmonella*-induced and tuberculous spondylitis are more difficult to heal, and a longer period of treatment – 6–12 months – is often needed[12].

Chronic osteomyelitis

The treatment of chronic osteomyelitis is more difficult and less well standardized than that of acute infection. Recurrences of infection are common in chronic osteomyelitis, and extensive surgery and debridement is an important part of successful therapy.

Bacteriologic and pharmacologic data make isoxazolyl penicillins the drugs of choice in chronic hematogenous osteomyelitis. They are tolerated well even in high doses, with a low rate of toxic side effects; rash and diarrhea are seen only in a few cases. There is a low risk of developing chromosomal resistance but this has not been a problem despite general long-term treatment. Generally oral drugs, such as flucloxacillin 1.5g t.i.d, could be used[12]. Probenecid, 1g b.d., enhances the serum concentration and lowers the protein binding of isoxazolyl penicillins. Clindamycin, fusidic acid and cephalosporins with effect against Gram-positive bacteria are alternatives for the treatment of patients with penicillin allergy. If the treatment fails, rifampin 0.6–0.9g daily, which penetrates into the granulocytes and kills intracellularly localized staphylococci, may be added in combination with isoxazolyl penicillin. Parenteral antibiotics should be used only for 1–2 days perioperatively in connection with the surgery, giving oral drugs for the rest of the long-term treatment period. Prolonged parenteral antibiotic therapy is not necessary but the total period of treatment should be extended. The doubling time and the metabolism of the bacteria are very slow in osteomyelitis, which necessitates prolonged treatment[53].

The long-term results are very good, and high-dose oral antibiotics for at least 6 months are tolerable and sufficient in combination with surgery. In cases where surgery is contraindicated or not accepted by the patient, antibiotics alone are usually sufficient.

Radiographic changes are already present, so careful planning is required in order to decide whether or not a sequestrum is present and whether surgical intervention is necessary. This could include procedures ranging from a simple sequestrectomy and removal of granulation tissue up to removal of an entire section of tubular bone followed by subsequent bone transplantation. Intramedullary reaming has been used for chronic hematogenous osteomyelitis with severe pain at rest, in order to re-establish a new medullary cavity and improve endosteal circulation[54].

REFERENCES

1. Bick EM. Source book of orthopedics. Hafner: New York; 1968.
2. Le Cocq JF, le Cocq E. Use of neoarsphenamine in treatment of acute *S. aureus* septicaemia and osteomyelitis. J Bone Joint Surg 1941; 23: 596–597.
3. Lidgren L, Lindberg L. Orthopedic infections during a 5-year period. Acta Orthop Scand 1972; 43: 325–334.
4. Danielsson L, Uden A. Diagnostik och behandling av akut hematogen osteit hos barn. Lakartidningen 1981; 4: 241–244.
5. Gillespie WJ, Nade S. Musculoskeletal infections. Oxford: Blackwell Scientific Publications; 1987.
6. Smith I. *Staphylococcus aureus*. In: Mandell GL, Douglas R, Bennett JE, eds. Principles and practice of infectious diseases. New York: John Wiley & Sons; 1979: 1530–1532.
7. Boda A. The problem of osteomyelitis in Hungary. In: Meeting of the European study group on bone and joint infections, Vienna, 27 August 1983.
8. Digby JM, Kersley JB. Pyogenic non-tuberculous spinal infection: an analysis of thirty cases. J Bone Joint Surg 1979; 61B: 47–55.
9. Silverthorn KM, Gillespie WJ. Pyogenic vertebrae osteomyelitis. NZ Med J 1986; 99: 62–65.
10. El-Gindi S, Aref S, Salama M, Andrew J. Infection of intervertebral discs after operation. J Bone Joint Surg 1976; 57A: 1104–1106.
11. Lindholm T S, Pylkkanen P. Discitis following removal of intervertebral disc: a report on 120 patients. Spine 1982; 7: 618–622.
12. Hedström SÅ, Lidgren L. Orthopedic infections. Lund: Studentlitteratur; 1988.
13. Fox L, Sprunt K. Neonatal osteomyelitis. Pediatrics 1978; 62: 535–542.
14. Welkon CJ, Long SS, Fischer MC, Alburger PD. Pyogenic arthritis in infants and children: a review of 95 cases. Infect Dis 1986; 5: 669–676.
15. Mitchell M, Howard B, Haller J *et al*. Septic arthritis. Radiol Clin North Am 1988; 26: 1295–1313.
16. Griffin PP. Acute septic arthritis of the hip in childhood: its pathogenesis and treatment. Hip 1979; 4: 89–104.
17. Freeland AE, Senter BS. Septic arthritis and osteomyelitis. Hand Clin 1989; 5: 533–552.
18. Alderson M, Speers D, Emslie KR, Nade S. Acute hematogenous osteomyelitis and septic arthritis – a single disease. A hypothesis based upon the presence of transphyseal blood vessels. J Bone Joint Surg 1986; 68B: 268–274.
19. Lane Smith R, Schurman DJ, Kajiyama G *et al*. The effect of antibiotics on the destruction of cartilage in experimental infectious arthritis. J Bone Joint Surg 1987; 69A: 1063–1068.
20. Goldenberg DL, Reed JI. Bacterial arthritis. N Engl J Med 1985; 312: 764–771.
21. Powers KA, Terpenning MS, Voice RA, Kauffman CA. Prosthetic joint infections in the elderly. Am J Med 1990; 88: 9N–13N.
22. Dubost JJ, Soubrier M, De Champs C *et al*. No changes in the distribution of organisms responsible for septic arthritis over a 20 year period. Ann Rheum Dis 2002; 61: 267–269.
23. Lidgren L. Join prosthetic infections: A success story. Acta Orthop Scand 2001; 72(6): 553–556.
24. Gristina AG. Biomaterial-centered infection: microbial adhesion versus tissue integration. Science 1987; 237: 1588–1595.
25. Garvin KL, Hanssen AD. Infection after total hip arthroplasty. Past, present, and future. J Bone Joint Surg 1995; 77A: 1576–1588.
26. Gristina AG, Shibata Y, Giridhar G *et al*. The glycocalyx, biofilm, microbes, and resistant infections. Semin Arthroplasty 1994; 5: 160–170.
27. Zimmerman III B, Mikolich DJ, Ho G. Septic bursitis. Semin Arthritis Rheum 1995; 24: 391–410.
28. Söderqvist B, Hedström SÅ. Predisposing factors, bacteriology and antibiotic therapy in 35 cases of septic bursitis. Scand J Infect Dis 1986; 18: 305–311.
29. Sandberg-Sørensen T, Hedeboe J, Rostgaard-Christensen E. Primary epiphyseal osteomyelitis in children. J Bone Joint Surg 1988; 70B: 818–820.
30. Fitzgerald RH. Pathogenesis of musculoskeletal sepsis. In: Hughes SPF, Fitzgerald RH, eds. Musculoskeletal infections. Chicago, IL: Year Book Medical Publishers; 1986: 14–33.
31. Wald ER. Risk factors for osteomyelitis. Am J Med 1985; 78: 206–212.
32. Peterson HA. Hematogenous osteomyelitis in children. Instr Course Lect 1983; 32: 33–37.
33. Emslie KR, Nade S. Acute hematogenous staphylococcal osteomyelitis. A description of the natural history in an avian model. Am J Pathol 1983; 110: 3333–45.
34. Hedström SÅ, Lidgren L. Acute hematogenous pelvic osteomyelitis in athletes. Am J Sports Med 1982; 1: 44–46.

35. Hedström SÅ. Staphylococcal problems in orthopedic infections. In: Hedström SÅ, ed. Advances of staphylococcal infections. Södertälje: Astra Alab AB; 1987: 87–99.

36. Dall BE, Rowe DE, Odette WG, Batts DH. Postoperative discitis. Diagnosis and management. Clin Orthop 1987; 224: 138–146.

37. Musher DM, Thorsteinsson SB, Minuth JN, Luchi RJ. Vertebral osteomyelitis: still a diagnostic pitfall. Arch Intern Med 1976; 136: 105–110.

38. Törholm C, Hedström SÅ, Sundèn G, Lidgren L. Synovectomy in bacterial arthritis. Acta Orthop Scand 1983; 54: 748–753.

39. Kasser JR. Hematogenous osteomyelitis. Untangling the diagnostic confusion. Postgrad Med 1984; 76: 79–86.

40. Jackson MA, Nelson JD. Etiology and management of acute suppurative bone and joint infections in pediatric patients. J Pediatr Orthop 1982; 2: 315–319.

41. Cavell B, Hedström SÅ. Septic *Salmonella* bone and joint infections in 2 infants. Opuscula Medica 1989; 34: 53–54.

42. Jorup-Rönström C, Ahl T, Hammarström L *et al*. Septic osteomyelitis and polyarthritis with *Ureaplasma* in hypogammaglobulinemia. Infection 1989; 17: 301–303.

43. Jellis JE. Bacterial infections: bone and joint tuberculosis. Baillière's Clin Rheumatol 1995; 9: 151–159.

44. Hedström SÅ, Lidgren L. Les infections hèmatogènes sur prothèses articulaires et leur prèvention. In: L'infection en chirurgie ortopèdique GEEIOA, ed. Expansion Scientifique Francaise (SOFCOT) no. 37: Paris; 1990: 102–105.

45. Alessi DM, Sercarz JA, Calcaterra TC. Osteomyelitis of the clavicle. Arch Otolaryngol Head Neck Surg 1988; 114: 1000–1002.

46. Vaughan PA, Newman NM, Rosman MA. Acute hematogenous osteomyelitis in children. J Pediatr Orthop 1987; 7: 652–655.

47. Rydén C. Studies on interactions between staphylococcal cells and some connective tissue components. Thesis, University of Uppsala, 1987.

48. Shaw BA, Kasser JR. Acute septic arthritis in infancy and childhood. Clin Orthop 1990; 257: 212–225.

49. Stengel D, Bauwens K, Sehouli J, Ekkernkamp A, Porzsolt F. Systematic review and meta-analysis of antibiotic therapy for bone and joint infections. Lancet Infectious Diseases 2001; 1: 175–188.

50. Knutson K, Lindstrand A, Lidgren L. Arthrodesis for failed knee arthroplasty. A report of 20 cases. J Bone Joint Surg 1985; 67B: 47–52.

51. Armstrong EP, Rush DR. Treatment of osteomyelitis. Clin Pharm, 1983; 2: 213–224.

52. LaMont RL, Anderson PA, Dajani AS, Thirumoorthi MC. Acute hematogenous osteomyelitis in children. J Pediatr Orthop 1987; 7: 579–583.

53. Zak O, Reilly TO. Animal models as predictors of the safety and efficacy of antibiotics. Eur J Clin Microbiol Inf Dis 1990; 9: 472–478.

54. Lidgren L, Törholm C. Intramedullary reaming in chronic diaphyseal osteomyelitis. Clin Orthop 1980; 151: 215–221.

94

Gonococcal arthritis

Maren Lawson Mahowald

Definition

- Syndrome of polyarthritis, tenosynovitis, dermatitis caused by the Gram-negative diplococcus, *Neisseria gonorrhoeae*

Clinical features

- Acute febrile illness with migratory or additive asymmetric polyarthralgia and tenosynovitis which may be self-limiting or evolve into purulent arthritis in one or more joints

- Diagnostic skin lesions on the trunk and distal extremities in 40–70% of patients with gonococcal bacteremia

- Patients may present with acute septic arthritis without antecedent migratory symptoms or skin lesions

- Management includes parenteral antibiotics, pain control, patient education and screening for other sexually transmitted diseases

---

HISTORY

Descriptions of gonorrhea are found in medical writings from ancient Egypt, the Old Testament (Leviticus) and the Talmud[1,2]. The term 'gonorrhea' was first used by Galen in AD 130 and comes from the Greek *gonos* (seed) and *rhoea* (flow) because urethral discharge was mistaken for semen. Houses of prostitution in Paris during the Middle Ages were called 'clapiers' (rabbit warrens), from which the word 'clap' was derived as the common name for gonorrhea[2].

In the early 18th century there was controversy as to whether gonorrhea and syphilis were the same disease. John Hunter in 1767 inoculated his urethra with pus from a patient he believed had gonorrhea. When he developed chancres, he concluded that gonorrhea and syphilis were the same. He later died from what may have been a syphilitic aortic aneurysm. In 1838 Ricord's studies established that gonorrhea and syphilis were different diseases, and Albert Neisser identified the bacterium in 1879. Lindeman recovered the gonococcal organism from a patient with septic arthritis in 1892, establishing that 'gonorrheal rheumatism' represented metastasis of infection from the genitourinary tract.

Disseminated gonococcal infection (DGI) was more common in men than in women until treatment of urethritis with sulfonamides and penicillin reduced the number of men with the condition. Women were more likely to have asymptomatic or unrecognized infections that went untreated[3–5]. During the first half of the 20th century, clinical studies failed to distinguish gonococcal urethritis from non-gonococcal urethritis and gonorrheal septic arthritis from reactive arthritis[3]. The advent of sulfonamides and penicillin, which cured gonorrhea but not non-gonococcal urethritis, established the distinction between these two.

The incidence of gonorrhea increased during and after World War II, then declined until the mid-1950s (Fig. 94.1)[6]. With the peak of the 'baby boom' in 1957, the number of individuals in the 18–24-year-old age group increased in the mid-1970s. With the 'sexual revolution' and use of non-barrier contraception in the 1960s and 1970s, the number of cases

of gonorrhea increased to more than 1 million in the USA in the early 1980s. Increased condom use, decreasing numbers of 18–24-year-olds and increased public health efforts have reduced the incidence of gonorrhea in developed countries. However, in poor urban areas and in developing countries, localized and disseminated gonococcal infections remain a serious problem.

Between 1970 and the early 1980s, isolates causing DGI had certain microbiological features: adenosine, hypoxanthine and uracil (AHU)-negative auxotype, serovar 1A, sensitivity to penicillin and resistance to normal human serum (see below: Basic Science). However, after 50 years of antibiotic therapy, *Neisseria gonorrhoeae* has adapted to evade eradication and antibiotic development is now only just ahead of the the organism's ability to develop resistance.

EPIDEMIOLOGY AND RISK FACTORS

Time trends

The epidemiology of *N. gonorrhoeae* infections has changed during the 20th century as the organism has adapted to the use of antibiotics and as the number of individuals in the high-risk 18–24-year-old age group has changed after 1945. There are 200 million cases of *N. gonorrhoeae* infections worldwide each year[7]. Substantial differences exist in regions of the world with limited public health programs and limited access to health care.

Data from the Centers for Disease Control and Prevention show that the number of reported cases of *N. gonorrhoeae* infection in the USA (half the true number) increased from approximately 250 000 per year (280 cases per 100 000) to approximately 400 000 per year between 1940 and 1947 and then decreased over the years to 1957 to prewar levels, with the availability of sulfonamides and penicillin (Fig. 94.1)[6]. In the 1960s, the incidence began increasing, to reach more than 1 million cases (468/100 000) in the late 1970s and early 1980s. During the period of increasing incidence, the male:female ratio declined from 3:1 in 1965 to 1.5:1 in 1985[2]. The dramatic increase in the incidence of gonorrhea in young white women was attributed to the sexual revolution, and the use of non-barrier contraceptives (oral contraceptives). After programs to control gonorrhea were started in the 1970s, the annual incidence declined slowly in the USA, to 123 per 100 000 in 1997 and 121/100 000 in 1998, but increased by 9.2%, to 133/100 000, in 1999 (Fig. 94.1)[6]. Possible reasons for this recent increase include expansion of screening programs, increased sensitivity of newer diagnostic tests, and a true increase in morbidity in some geographic regions and segments of the population.

Since 1985, the rate of gonococcal infections has been declining in those countries with effective control programs[5]. Intensive surveillance and treatment availability have decreased the incidence to fewer than 45/100 000 in the UK. The incidence of gonorrhea in Sweden peaked in 1970, with 487/100 000, and decreased to fewer than 5/100 000 in 1992. In Thailand, bacterial sexually transmitted diseases (STDs) decreased by

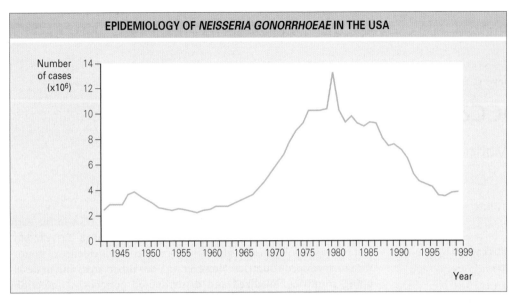

EPIDEMIOLOGY OF *NEISSERIA GONORRHOEAE* IN THE USA

Fig. 94.1 Epidemiology of *Neisseria gonorrhoeae* in the USA. Number of reported cases per year. The number of cases increased sharply in the 1970s, because of the large number of people in the 18–24 years age range (the postwar 'baby boom') and the high prevalence of unprotected sex. Increased condom use helped to reduce the incidence in the 1980s and 1990s; however, in 1999 the incidence increased 9.2% as a result of a combination of improved screening and diagnosis plus a true increase in morbidity.

79% between 1988 and 1993, against the background of an aggressive program to promote condom use. In Canada, the incidence decreased from 233/100 000 to 34/100 000 in 1992. The declining number of persons in the high-risk age group is contributing somewhat to the decreasing incidence of gonorrhea. However, gonococcal infection rates in adolescents and blacks have not declined. The greatest incidences are in developing countries, where 80% of young men have had sex with prostitutes. The prevalence of gonorrhea among gay men decreased in Seattle from 1982 to 1988, but increased again in the early 1990s, suggesting behavioral relapse.

Influences on incidence

The prevalence of gonorrhea in different regions is determined by demographic, sociologic, clinical and biological variables. Demographic risk factors (Table 94.1) associated with greater rates of *N. gonorrhoeae* infections include non-Caucasian race (black, Hispanic, Native American), lower socioeconomic status, poorer education, urban residence, prostitution, unmarried status, homosexualilty, sexual activity at a young age, and intravenous drug abuse, in both rural and urban areas[7]. Complement deficiency, especially of terminal components C5–C8, appears to be a risk factor and is found in up to 13% of persons with DGI.

Disseminated gonococcal infection

The epidemiology of DGI is dependent on the epidemiology of mucosal gonorrhea and is modified by microbiological features of the predominant infecting strains in various regions. Estimates of the proportion of gonococcal infections that disseminate are problematic, because the

actual number of asymptomatic chronic carriers is not known. Estimates of dissemination range from 0.5% to 3% of local *N. gonorrhoeae* infections. DGI is the most common form of bacterial arthritis in young adults in the USA, yet it is uncommon in Europe[8]. In the UK, DGI is rarely seen today[7], and caused fewer than 1% of all cases of septic arthritis from 1990 to 1993[8].

The majority of patients with disseminated infection are women, and the majority of these women have had no symptoms from the mucosal site of infection. There is essentially no long-lasting protective immunity to *N. gonorrhoeae*; therefore, the asymptomatic carrier population is a significant reservoir for perpetuation of infection in the community. The rate of dissemination of gonococcal infection varies; it is greatest in developing countries, where access to effective diagnosis and treatment is limited. However, recent epidemiologic studies have shown that asymptomatic chronic carriers of the gonococcus also develop DGI. In those patients with symptomatic genitourinary tract gonococcal infection, the genitourinary symptoms tend to precede arthritis onset. It has been said that symptoms of DGI typically begin 7 days after the onset of menses; however, in a series of patients studied by O'Brien *et al.*[9] (the only prospective clinical study of DGI, seven of 35 women 'were having or had just finished having menses at the time of presentation', which is approximately the proportion to be expected in any sample of young women.

The biological variables important in the epidemiology of *N. gonorrhoeae* infections are related to microbiological features of the predominant strains. The strains of *N. gonorrhoeae* typically associated with DGI have:

- AHU-negative auxotype
- serotype PorA (protein I)
- resistance to human serum
- penicillin sensitivity.

The ability of *N. gonorrhoeae* to disseminate depends on resistance to the bactericidal action of normal human sera. Gonococcal serum resistance is strongly associated with PorA and the AHU-negative auxotype. These strains are also associated with asymptomatic gonorrhea. Therefore, the incidence and prevalence of DGI have tended to parallel the prevalence of serum-resistant gonococcal strains. In the UK, where DGI is rarely seen, the prevalence of PorA, AHU-negative strains and DGI is much lower than in the USA and Scandinavia[10]. An increasing proportion of cases of DGI are associated with other auxotype or

TABLE 94.1 RISK FACTORS FOR DGI
Urban residence
Non-Caucasian
Low socioeconomic status
Low educational status
Female sex
Unmarried
Prostitution
Intravenous drug abuse
Previous gonococcal infection

serotype classes as the prevalence of serovar 1A, AHU-negative strains has declined.

The epidemiology of antimicrobial resistance in *N. gonorrhoeae* has a direct impact on the epidemiology of DGI. With increasing resistance, the number of infected individuals who do achieve prompt effective treatment responses will increase. The increasing antibiotic resistance of all gonorrhea strains has resulted in the emergence of DGI caused by antibiotic-resistant strains[11–13]. Penicillinase-producing *N. gonorrhoeae* (PPNG) strains emerged almost simultaneously in 1976 in West Africa and the Philippines. From 1976 to 1980, clusters of PPNG strains were found in Hawaii, California, Louisiana, USA, and Liverpool, UK, but now these strains are generalized throughout the world, with varying geographic prevalence. High-level chromosomal penicillin resistance emerged in North Carolina in 1983 and increased to 6% of all isolates in 1988. Similarly, 5% of isolates causing DGI were also PPNG[12]. In Durban, South Africa, PPNG prevalence had increased to 26.2% by 1994; between 1983 and 1987, 56% of isolates from gonococcal arthritis were PPNG[14]. Reduced susceptibility to fluoroquinolones has been reported in Africa, Southeast Asia, Australia and the USA. In Hong Kong, the emergence of high-level fluoroquinolone resistance has been associated with an antigenic drift from the predominant serotype PorA to PorB Bop and PorB Bpy. Fluoroquinolone resistance is chromosomally mediated and most strains are also penicillin and tetracycline resistant[15].

Two clinical series[12,13] documented that DGI can be caused by penicillin-resistant strains and, in the USA, is associated with a high rate of comorbidity factors including intravenous drug abuse, systemic lupus erythematosus (SLE), human immunodeficiency virus (HIV) infection, malignancy and diabetes. Complement deficiencies (C5–C8) also have been associated with a predisposition to gonococcal and meningococcal bacteremias. A recent review of the literature suggested that patients with SLE and low hemolytic complement activity (congenital or acquired) may have an increased incidence of neisserial infections[17] (see Chapter 119).

CLINICAL FEATURES

The time from primary gonococcal infection to initial manifestations of DGI ranges from 1 day to 3 months. Joint symptoms reach a peak within days of the onset of the first manifestation. Clinical features associated with DGI include:

- asymmetric migratory polyarthralgia
- tenosynovitis
- dermatitis
- purulent arthritis
- meningitis
- myopericarditis
- clinical sepsis.

There has been debate as to whether groupings of these features represent distinct syndromes (bacteremic form or septic arthritis form) or sequential stages of infection disseminated from a mucosal site of infection (Fig. 94.2). The most common DGI syndrome is the 'arthritis–dermatitis syndrome' (or bacteremic) form consisting of fever, asymmetric migratory or additive polyarthralgias, tenosynovitis and dermatitis lasting 3–5 days before diagnosis[13]. Tenosynovitis is most commonly seen over the dorsum of the hand (Fig. 94.3), the metacarpalphalangeal joints, wrists, ankles (Fig. 94.4) or knees. Extensor tenosynovitis often accompanies wrist involvement.

Skin lesions

The skin lesions tend to occur on the extremities in 40–70% of patients with DGI (Fig. 94.5). They are usually tiny papules, pustules or vesicles

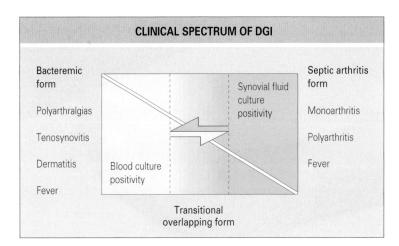

Fig. 94.2 Clinical spectrum of DGI.

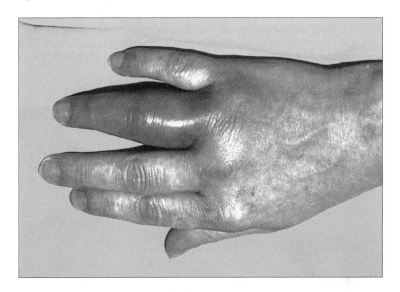

Fig. 94.3 Gonococcal arthritis. Dactylitis of the ring finger as a result of tenosynovitis in a 24-year-old woman. (Courtesy of Dr SE Thompson.)[75]

with an erythematous base; they are not painful or pruritic. The centers of the skin lesions may become necrotic or hemorrhagic and disappear within a few days after initiation of treatment. The lesions number between four and 50[9]. Erythema nodosum and erythema multiforme lesions also may be seen. Biopsy of the skin lesions shows dermal vasculitis with perivascular neutrophils, microthrombi and a neutrophilic infiltrate in the epidermis (epidermal pustules), but usually no microorganisms[16].

Joint problems

The migratory arthralgias may resolve spontaneously without treatment (possibly in 33% of patients) or evolve into a persistent septic arthritis in one or several joints. The knee, ankle, elbow or wrist are involved in 39–73% of patients with DGI. The pattern of involvement is usually asymmetric and tends to involve the upper extremity more than lower extremity joints; however, 10–15% of those affected may have symmetric polyarthritis[13]. In some patients there are no or minimal symptoms of bacteremia before the onset of acute septic arthritis in one or several joints. Purulent arthritis most commonly involves the wrists, hand joints, knees, ankles, joints of the feet, elbows, shoulders and, rarely, the hip joints.

Chronic gonococcal arthritis with joint destruction and ankylosis is rare with antibiotic therapy. With the emergence of antibiotic-resistant *N. gonorrhoeae*, infections may be more difficult to eradicate and may result in substantial joint damage or more unusual manifestations of

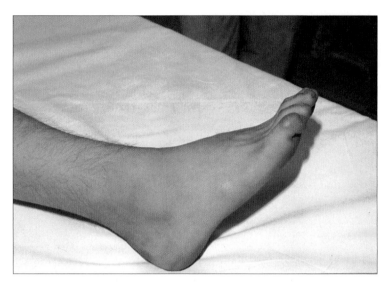

Fig. 94.4 Disseminated gonococcal infection tenosynovitis and septic arthritis. Tenosynovitis of the anterior and lateral aspect of the ankle joint. Septic arthritis in the 5th interphalangeal joint and the ankle joint. (Courtesy of Dr Peter Schlessinger.)

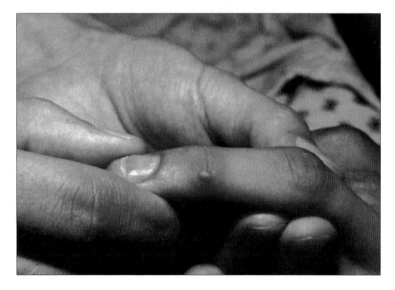

Fig. 94.5 Disseminated gonococcal infection skin lesion. Hemorrhagic vesicle over a distal interphalangeal joint. (Courtesy of Dr Peter Schlessinger.)

DGI if the initial treatment fails or the appropriate antibiotic treatment is delayed. Gonococcal osteomyelitis is extremely rare and usually occurs via direct extension from an adjacent infected joint.

Other organ involvement

In the pre-antibiotic era, gonococcal endocarditis accounted for up to 25% of bacterial endocarditis, with the aortic valve most often involved. Since 1950, there have been only infrequent reports of cases of DGI that were not recognized promptly and developed devastating complications. With gonococcal endocarditis there are abundant skin lesions and emboli to kidneys, brain and extremities, with chills; a double quotidian fever may also be seen. Other unusual manifestations of DGI that may present currently include pericarditis with electrocardiographic changes, pericardial friction rub, purulent pericardial fluid and myocarditis suggested by tachycardia and ST–T-wave changes.

Gonococcal perihepatitis, the Fitz-Hugh–Curtis syndrome, is caused by extension of infection from the Fallopian tubes via retroperitoneal lymphatic spread or via hematogenous spread (as reported in men). Acutely, the Fitz-Hugh–Curtis syndrome may mimic acute cholecystitis

with acute abdominal pain, hepatic tenderness or enlargement, and increased values in liver function tests. Reports of jaundice in patients with gonorrhea dating from before the introduction of antibiotic treatment are attributed to treatment with injections of acriflavine, an antiseptic now known to be hepatotoxic[5]. Most female patients also have evidence of salpingitis or other pelvic inflammatory disease. It is common to see transient liver function test abnormalities during the acute phases of DGI, without abdominal symptoms.

Overwhelming sepsis with Waterhouse–Friderichsen syndrome or adult respiratory distress syndrome is rare. Gonococcal meningitis is extremely rare and was reported primarily in cases seen in the preantibiotic era.

INVESTIGATIONS

Clinical suspicion for DGI should be high in any young sexually active patient who presents with acute arthritis and dermatitis. Most patients will be febrile with an increased white blood cell count (WBC), and increased erythrocyte sedimentation rate. The synovial fluid WBC count is usually greater than 30 000, but may be lower.

Bacteriological confirmation

The synovial fluid Gram stain reveals Gram-negative intracellular and extracellular cocci in fewer than 25% of purulent joint effusions[8]. All potential portals of entry such as endocervix, urethra, rectum and pharynx should be examined and cultures made (Fig. 94.6). Gonorrhea also can be detected by culturing the first 20ml of a voided urine sample. Rectal cultures should be obtained by inserting a cotton-tip swab about 2.5cm into the anal canal to sample the crypts of Morgagni, the focus of infection.

Use of the proper culture techniques is critical as the gonococcus is fragile and growth is inhibited by drying or plating on cold or dehydrated culture medium. Fluid samples should be plated immediately on fresh, prewarmed medium and incubated within 15 minutes in a moist 5% carbon dioxide atmosphere. Specimens should be inoculated at the bedside or in the clinic. Joint fluid should be plated on chocolate agar. Specimens from other mucosal surfaces with commensal organisms (pharynx, rectum, urethra and cervix) and vesicle fluid from skin lesions should be plated on selective antibiotic media such as modified Thayer–Martin medium. Synovial fluid specimens also should be plated on plain blood agar for other pathogens. Blood for culture should be inoculated into enriched broth medium. Blood culture bottle systems that contain sodium polyanetholsulfate inhibit neisserial growth.

Approximately 50% of patients with DGI will have a positive blood or synovial fluid culture, 80% will have a positive culture from a mucosal

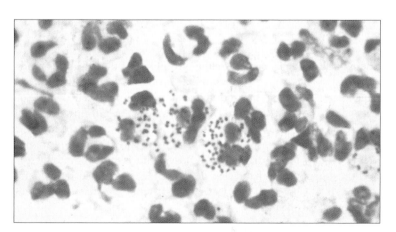

Fig. 94.6 *Neisseria gonorrhoeae:* **Gram stain of urethral exudate in gonorrhea, showing intracellular Gram-negative reniform diplococci.** (Courtesy of Dr SE Thompson.)

site, and vesicular skin lesions will uncommonly have a positive culture or Gram stain. Patients with a septic gonococcal arthritis will rarely have positive blood culture. The synovial fluid culture is usually negative if the WBC count is less than 20 000/mm³ and more often culture-positive if the WBC count is more than 40 000/mm³.

Newer molecular biology techniques are being utilized for rapid diagnosis and will undoubtedly alter current clinical teachings about active and reactive arthritis caused by fastidious organisms that are difficult to culture. Leibling et al.[18] demonstrated *N. gonorrhoeae* in synovial fluid samples using the polymerase chain reaction (PCR) technique. This technique was able to detect 10 organisms per ml of synovial fluid. In 11 of 14 cases of suspected gonococcal arthritis based on clinical presentation PCR was positive, whereas 11 cases of reactive arthritis (Reiter's syndrome) had a negative PCR[18]. Using a nested PCR technique, Muralidhar et al.[19] found PCR positivity in five of eight suspected cases of gonococcal arthritis, with 37 of 38 controls negative. All synovial fluids with positive cultures had positive PCR; two negative cultures had positive PCR. These early reports of PCR technology suggest an approximate specificity of 96%, a sensitivity of 79% and a false-positive rate of 4%. Current PCR primers do not differentiate *N. gonorrhoeae* from *N. meningitidis*, and PCR testing does not provide material for antibiotic sensitivity testing.

Radiographs

Changes on radiographs will generally include only evidence of soft tissue swelling and effusion. Cartilage destruction or evidence of osteomyelitis at the time of diagnosis suggests infection with non-gonococcal agents or prior ineffective antibiotic treatment and a resistant *N. gonorrhoeae* strain.

DIFFERENTIAL DIAGNOSIS

The differential diagnosis for a febrile illness with tenosynovitis, arthritis, arthralgias and skin lesions includes:

- reactive arthritis syndrome (arthritis, urethritis, conjunctivitis, mucosal ulcerations and dermatitis)
- non-gonococcal septic arthritis
- bacterial endocarditis
- viral hepatitis
- rheumatic fever
- meningococcemia
- Lyme disease in endemic areas
- parvovirus arthritis
- other infections.

Reactive arthritis syndrome with arthritis, urethritis, conjunctivitis, mucosal ulcerations and skin lesions is seen predominantly in men aged 20–40 years. The disease evolves over a few weeks, rather than the few days characteristic of DGI, and tends to involve joints and tendons in the lower extremities in an additive rather than a migratory manner. Conjunctivitis and painless mucosal ulcerations are prominent in reactive arthritis syndrome but rare in DGI, which has a more acute onset, usually with a greater temperature, more tenosynovitis and migratory polyarthralgias, predominantly in the upper extremities[16]. The urethritis of reactive arthritis syndrome is caused by *Ureaplasma* or *Chlamydia trachomatis* and tends to be less purulent and less painful than symptomatic gonorrhea. Patients may also have low back pain with sacroiliac involvement, typical circinate balanitis and skin lesions on the soles of the feet (keratoderma blennorrhagicum), which confirm the diagnosis (see Chapter 109).

Non-gonococcal septic arthritis must be differentiated by microbiological tests. Non-gonococcal septic arthritis is seen in men more frequently than in women, and young adults tend to be spared. Patients with non-gonococcal septic arthritis are often compromised with comorbid serious illness or have underlying chronic arthritis. Larger joints in the lower extremity are typically involved. A non-venereal infection site is usually identifiable. Tenosynovitis and rash are rare.

During the anicteric prodrome of hepatitis B infection, patients may present with urticarial skin lesions, followed by arthralgia, arthritis or tenosynovitis, which clear when the patient becomes icteric (prodrome may last up to 1 month in some cases). In those patients with less severe hepatitis B infection who do not become icteric, the polyarthritis may be migratory and tests for rheumatoid factor transiently positive. The finding of increased hepatic enzymes and a positive hepatitis B serology test are diagnostic. With hepatitis C infection, fever, arthralgias, arthritis and petechial lesions have been reported, but the distribution tends to be more symmetric and non-migratory than in DGI. These patients may have cryoglobulins and positive rheumatoid factor tests[20,21].

Acute and subacute bacterial endocarditis may be difficult to distinguish from DGI. Arthralgias, myalgias, tendonitis and back pain are common in subacute bacterial endocarditis. Skin lesions similar to those in DGI are often seen; however, splinter hemorrhages, Osler's nodes and Janeway's lesions do not occur in DGI. Rheumatoid factor is usually positive in subacute bacterial endocarditis.

Other STDs must be considered. Patients with secondary syphilis may have tenosynovitis of wrists and ankles, arthralgias and non-migratory polyarthritis, with an extensive non-pruritic papulosquamous rash, generalized lymphadenopathy, condylomata lata (perigenital mucosal plaques), oral mucosa plaques and a positive serologic test for syphilis (see Chapter 96). Symptoms resolve rapidly with penicillin treatment[22]. To date, DGI has not been a common infection in HIV-infected individuals, and only isolated case reports are available[23]. Rectal gonococcal infection in homosexual men is unlikely to be caused by the AHU-negative auxotype because it is very sensitive to fecal lipids. As the epidemiology of auxotypes changes and the population of HIV-infected individuals expands, DGI is likely to increase in this population.

Approximately 5–10% of patients with meningococcal meningitis develop an arthritis, tenosynovitis and dermatitis syndrome (synovial fluid cultures negative). In some patients a mono- or oligoarthritis may develop 5–7 days after septicemia, with sterile joint effusions and rapid resolution. With chronic meningococcemia (positive synovial fluid culture but negative blood cultures), symptoms of low-grade fever, polyarthralgias and arthritis, with a large number of skin lesions (>100) may be present for a week, but with absent meningeal signs.

In endemic areas, Lyme disease may be confused with DGI. In Lyme disease the skin lesions of erythema chronicum migrans also may develop necrotic centers, but the lesions are much larger than those seen in DGI.

The differential diagnoses for the syndrome of fever and purpuric lesions with or without arthralgias and the syndrome of tenosynovitis, arthritis and dermatitis include many other infectious and non-infectious causes. A syndrome of purpuric lesions and fever with or without arthralgias and myalgias may be caused by Gram-negative bacteremias, especially other *Neisseria* species; rickettsial infections, Rocky Mountain spotted fever and typhus fever, *Listeria monocytogenes* and staphylococcal bacteremia with endocarditis; viral infections such as enteroviruses, coxsackievirus A9 and echovirus 9, Epstein–Barr virus in children and cytomegalovirus, hepatitis B or C, and parvovirus B19 in adults; *Plasmodium falciparum*, *Vibrio vulnificus* from infected seafood and *Yersinia enterocolitica* septicemia. Non-infectious causes include polyarteritis nodosa, which also typically has abnormal urinary sediment and hypertension indicating renal involvement, SLE and rheumatoid arthritis with small vessel vasculitis, hypersensitivity vasculitis from a drug reaction, and Henoch–Schönlein purpura.

Parvovirus B19 infection in adults may present with facial flush and reticular or maculopapular rash on the trunk and extremities in association with developing joint symptoms (see Chapter 97). Polyarthralgias, joint swelling, fever, malaise and pronounced morning stiffness evolve over about 1 week, in an additive rather than a migratory pattern. Diagnosis is suggested by a history of contact with a child with fifth disease (erythema infectiosum) and confirmed by finding IgM antibody to B19[24].

BASIC SCIENCE

Structure and function

Neisseria gonorrhoeae is a Gram-negative coccus that characteristically grows in pairs. Features of clinical isolates that are associated with dissemination include the presence of pili, nutritional requirements for arginine, hypoxanthine, uracil and proline, serotype PorA, and resistance to the bactericidal activity of normal serum[25]. *N. gonorrhoeae* can produce IgA1 protease, which inactivates secretory IgA on mucosal surfaces, thus enhancing invasiveness of the gonococcus. The molecular basis for the interdependence of clinical features and microbiological features of pili and serum resistance are beginning to be understood. Cell envelope components participate in the pathogenesis of infection and host defenses. The cell envelope contains an inner cytoplasmic membrane, middle layer of peptidoglycan and an outer layer of lipo-oligosaccharide(LOS), exposed phospholipids (which accounts for permeability to hydrophobic molecules that can mutate) and outer membrane proteins (Fig. 94.7).

Cell surface proteins

Pili

Pili are cell surface proteins that are thin polymers of pilin subunits which traverse both layers of the cell envelope. Neisserial strains that contain pili are more virulent and grow as small and opaque colonies. CD46 is the pilin receptor. Pili are antigenic and enhance adhesion of the gonococcus to mucosal epithelial cells and, possibly, synovial cells. Pili interfere with phagocytosis and killing by polymorphonuclear leukocytes (PMNLs) and mononuclear cells.

Porin

Porin (Por, formerly Protein I) is the major outer membrane protein, which forms a transmembrane channel in the outer membrane. It may translocate into mucosal epithelial cells and induce endocytosis, thus triggering invasion. There are two major antigenic classes of porin: Por A and Por B. Antigenic variations in Por are the basis for serotyping. *N. gonorrhoeae* strains with Por A are resistant to the bactericidal effects of normal serum and are more prone to cause disseminated disease. Strains with Por B (high molecular weight protein 1) cause localized infections.

Opacity-associated protein

Opacity-associated protein (Opa, formerly Protein II) is exposed on the cell surface and acts as an adhesin for epithelial cell attachment, intergonococcal adhesion (producing an opaque colony) and susceptibility to bactericidal activity of normal human serum. Antibodies to Opa proteins may protect from ascending pelvic infection by preventing attachment and uptake of organisms.

Reduction-modifiable protein

Reduction-modifiable protein (Rmp, formerly Protein III) is found in all strains of gonococci and stimulates IgG-blocking antibodies, which reduce complement-mediated serum bactericidal activity in normal human serum. Rmp is closely associated with LOS and Por in the outer membrane. Resistance to the bactericidal effect of the naturally occurring IgM antibody is more common in PorA than in Por B strains, and may be mediated by an IgG-blocking antibody reacting with Rmp to interfere with the bactericidal IgM antibody activation of complement.

Lipo-oligosaccharide

Lipo-oligosaccharide is toxic to human cells and contributes to serum resistance. Serum IgM antibody directed against LOS antigens are found in normal sera and are bactericidal.

Peptidoglycan

Peptidoglycan is proinflammatory and can activate the alternative complement pathway and modulate mononuclear cell proliferation. It has direct toxicity for human Fallopian tube mucosa. Peptidoglycan fragments have been found in culture-negative synovial fluids and may play a part in inflammatory synovitis after bacteremia.

Identification of different strains

Differentiation of the various gonococcal strains for epidemiology studies is established by auxotyping, serotype identification and antibiotic sensitivities. 'Auxotyping', described in 1973, refers to the ability of different strains to grow in the absence of certain amino acids, purines, pyrimidines or other nutrients. More than 30 auxotypes have been defined. A strain unable to grow in the absence of adenosine, hypoxanthine and uracil is designated AHU-negative. Wild types with no specific nutritional requirements are referred to as prototrophic.

Earlier studies found certain auxotypes associated with different clinical features, such as asymptomatic urethritis and cervicitis or disseminated disease. In Seattle, gonococcal isolates changed from 44% AHU-negative and 54% PorA serovar in 1974–1976, to 12% AHU-negative, 24% PorA in 1981–1984. In the study by Wise *et al.*[13], penicillin-resistant organisms were identified in two of 25 isolates (8%) causing DGI at a time when the regional incidence rates in genital isolates were 6–6.5%, suggesting that penicillin-resistant strains have a similar propensity to cause DGI as penicillin-sensitive strains. In the report by Hoosen *et al.*[14] from South Africa, 56% of 34 patients with gonococcal arthritis were caused by PPNG strains and all auxotypes were prototypic, not AHU-negative.

Serovars described in 1984 refer to strain typing with monoclonal antibodies against various epitopes on the outer membrane Por (Protein I). The two serogroups, PorA and Por B, can be further classified into different serovars with monoclonal antibodies.

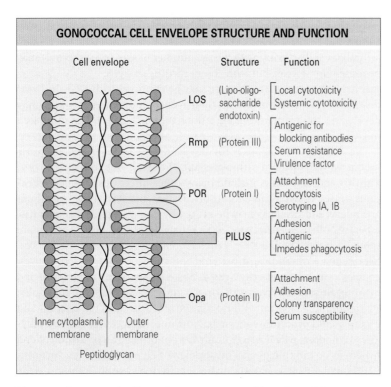

GONOCOCCAL CELL ENVELOPE STRUCTURE AND FUNCTION

Cell envelope	Structure	Function
LOS	(Lipo-oligo-saccharide endotoxin)	Local cytotoxicity / Systemic cytotoxicity
Rmp	(Protein III)	Antigenic for blocking antibodies / Serum resistance / Virulence factor
POR	(Protein I)	Attachment / Endocytosis / Serotyping IA, IB
PILUS		Adhesion / Antigenic / Impedes phagocytosis
Opa	(Protein II)	Attachment / Adhesion / Colony transparency / Serum susceptibility

Inner cytoplasmic membrane   Outer membrane

Peptidoglycan

Fig. 94.7 Gonococcal cell envelope structure and function. LOS, lipo-oligosaccharide; Rmp, reduction-modifiable protein; POR, porin; Opa, opacity-associated protein.

Epidemiology of antibiotic resistance

The epidemiology of antimicrobial susceptibility is constantly changing (Table 94.2)[25]. Gonococcal resistance to sulfonamides grew to 90% within a decade of their introduction in 1935, and clinical therapy failed. In 1944 50 000–100 000 units of penicillin cured 90% of gonococcal urethritis; however, partial penicillin resistance developed within 10 years, necessitating increased doses. Chromosomal mutations of penicillin-binding proteins and reduced membrane permeability confer resistance. Such mutations are seen in regions with high rates of antibiotic prophylaxis and use of low-dose antibiotics (Southeast Asia and Africa). It was possible to overcome the initial penicillin resistance noted between 1946 and 1976 by using higher doses. In 1976, PPNG with plasmids producing β-lactamase were found in the USA, Western Europe, the Philippines and western Africa (resistance to high-dose penicillin, cephalothin and cefazolin). By the early 1980s, 50% of isolates were PPNG strains in developing countries and in the 1990s more than 10% were PPNG in the USA[12]. High-level penicillin resistance from chromosomal mutations was reported in regional outbreaks in 1983, but is now widespread. Chromosomal resistance to β-lactam antibiotics and tetracycline alters permeability in the outer membrane, reducing the penicillin-binding affinity of Protein-II. Resistance to tetracycline is both chromosomally and plasmid mediated, and is increasing in areas in which spectinomycin has been used.

Quinolones were introduced in 1985 and resistance has emerged in Hong Kong, Japan and Rwanda[14], and in Seattle and Denver[26]. Emergence of quinolone resistance appears to be associated with antigenic drift of Por, as demonstrated by a change in serovar patterns of isolates. Most PorA serovars have been selected against, and two PorB serovars, Bo and Bpy, account for 71% and 22% of the quinolone-resistant isolates, compared with 54% and 12% of quinolone-sensitive isolates, respectively. Typically, in any geographic area only a few serovars predominate. The emerging quinolone-resistant isolates are commonly resistant to penicillin (81%), tetracycline (78%) or both (78%), but remain fully susceptible to spectinomycin, ceftriaxone and azithromycin. Multiply resistant strains have a selection advantage and may spread rapidly in the sexually active community.

The Centers for Disease Control monitors antimicrobial resistance in N. gonorrheoeae in the USA through the Gonococcal Isolate Surveillance Project. Isolates collected in 1998 were commonly resistant (29.4%) to penicillin, tetracycline or both, and 1% were resistant to ciprofloxacin. All isolates were sensitive to spectinomycin and ceftriaxone. Continuing surveillance of sentinel clinic sites can be monitored at www.cc.gov/nciod/dastlr/gcdir/Resist/gisp.html.

TABLE 94.2 *NEISSERIA GONORRHOEAE* ANTIBACTERIAL RESISTANCE

Chromosomal-mediated resistance: encoded at several loci for additive effects (requires higher doses, alters outer membrane permeability and decreases Protein II antibiotic binding)	Sulfonamides – 80% resistance within one decade Penicillin – initially noted by 1946; by 1983 MIC >8μg/ml in the USA Tetracycline – 50% resistance by 1993
Plasmid-mediated resistance	Penicillinase-producing – 1976 (β-lactamase): USA, Philippines, England, west Africa; now worldwide Tetracycline – 1985 (tet-M): MIC >10μg/ml Fluoroquinolone – 1985: Hong Kong, Japan, Rwanda; 1995, Washington, Colorado; 1999: Australia, Canada, Cleveland
MIC, minimum inhibitory concentration.	

Pathogenesis

Humans are the only natural hosts for N. gonorrhoeae infection, which requires physical contact with an infected mucosal surface. It is a highly infectious organism, with risk of infection from a single contact estimated at 60–90% for women and 20–50% for men[7]. The gonococcus attaches to mucosal epithelial cells via Opa and pili and penetrates the epithelial cells within 24–48 hours. A vigorous neutrophilic infiltration produces microabscesses, with exudation of pus in the submucosa. Neutrophils are replaced by lymphocytes and monocytes, which persist for several weeks after eradication of the organisms. Neisserial organisms can release membrane fragments into the surrounding environment, resulting in circulation of toxic or antigenic fragments that can bind to antibodies. Dissemination of gonococcal organisms is dependent on the resistance of the infecting strain to the bactericidal action of normal serum.

Gonococcal arthritis occurs secondary to bacteremic spread from a mucosal site of infection. Bacteria replicate in the synovium and provoke release of proteolytic enzymes from the synovial lining cells and PMNLs. If the infection is untreated, cartilage will be destroyed. Early in the course of infection, the synovial membrane becomes hyperplastic and the subsynovial tissue becomes infiltrated with PMNLs. After 5–7 days of antibiotic treatment, the synovial biopsy shows clearing of the acute infiltrate and, in some, a persistence of chronic inflammatory cells. The sterile chronic synovitis may persist as a 'postinfectious' arthritis. IgM-containing immune complexes are found in synovial fluid.

The pathogenesis of the 'migratory arthralgia, tenosynovitis, dermatitis' with a 'sterile' arthritis phase of DGI has been attributed to a serum sickness-like phenomenon rather than septic embolization during bacteremia. The tenosynovitis and migratory polyarthralgias are similar to immune complex-mediated serum sickness and the prodrome of hepatitis B infections. Even though 40–50% of those affected have positive blood cultures, viable organisms are rarely cultured from the skin lesions (<5%), yet immunofluorescent studies show the presence of gonococcal cell wall components or gonococcal antibody and complement in most. Circulating immune complexes have been found in serum of patients with DGI, but specific gonococcal antigens were not identified. Gonococci have been found using electron microscopic studies of synovial biopsies. The transitory nature of the arthritis dermatitis syndrome symptoms and negative cultures in some patients probably represent a combination of a successful host defense against the microorganisms and the limitations of microbiological techniques of culturing small numbers of organisms.

Activation and assembly of the terminal complement components C5–C9 are critical for Neisserial lysis. Patients with late-component complement deficiencies may not clear Gram-negative organisms readily because of an inability to kill or lyse bacteria until specific antibody develops and facilitates opsonization for phagocytosis. A small number of patients with SLE who have acquired or inherited complement deficiencies and DGI (N. meningitidis and N. gonorrhoeae) has been reported, but the pathogenic association remains to be established[17].

Natural and artifical immunity

There is little or no lasting protective immunity after N. gonorrhoeae infection, and N. gonorrhoeae are adept at evading host defenses[27]. Exogenous sialylation of gonococcal LOS glycolipid occurs on the cell surface and results in the production of a 'capsule-like' polysaccharide at sites of mucosal infection. Sialic acid confers serum resistance by inhibiting complement-mediated lysis and reduces complement-mediated opsonophagocytosis. Natural infection induces both IgG anti-LOS antibodies and anti-Rmp-blocking antibodies. IgG-blocking antibody binds to Rmp and prevents complement-mediated killing by both normal serum (IgM) and immune sera[28]. Of the N. gonorrhoeae isolates causing DGI, 50–75% are resistant to the bactericidal activity of normal human serum. Acute serum samples from patients with DGI generally lack bactericidal activity against the infecting strain, even though it may be sensitive to normal serum. Convalescent sera from DGI patients show some increased bactericidal activity. Dissemination from a local mucosal site represents a failure of the local inflammatory response to eradicate the bacteria. Gonococci also produce an IgA protease that reduces mucosal immune defenses. Antibodies to Opa proteins appear to protect against salpingitis, possibly by inhibiting attachment and uptake of gonococci at the mucosal surface.

Even though natural infection with *N. gonorrhoeae* does not confer long-lasting protective immunity, attempts to produce a vaccine to protect against gonococcal infection are under way[29]. Whole-cell vaccines with autolyzed bacteria stimulate both bactericidal and blocking antibodies, but give no protection from experimental infection. Antibodies to porin or LOS are bactericidal, and antibodies to Rmp inhibit complement-mediated lysis. Purified gonococcal components, such as porin without contaminating Rmp, are likely candidates for immune intervention. Porins also activate B cells to costimulate T cells to produce interleukin (IL)-2 and IL-4, which stimulate antibody production.

In an experimental model using rabbits, intra-articular injections of viable and non-viable *N. gonorrhoeae*, and gonococcal LOS, caused a similar early acute synovitis, with synovial cell hyperplasia and neutrophilic infiltration with persistent chronic synovitis after 5–7 days[30]. After intra-articular injection of viable *N. gonorrhoeae*, joint aspirates were sterile within a few hours, yet synovitis persisted. These studies support the concept that skin and joint manifestations of DGI are the result of dissemination of viable organisms plus an effective immune-mediated host defense.

MANAGEMENT

The management objectives in gonococcal arthritis are eradication of *N. gonorrhoeae* infection, control of pain, prevention of joint destruction and treatment of coexistent STDs. The recent increase in antibiotic-resistant strains necessitates admission to hospital for treatment so that clinical response to initial antibiotics can be monitored, joints can be drained daily and appropriate susceptibility testing carried out if the response is suboptimal. Longer courses of parenteral antibiotics may be necessary for infections caused by resistant organisms. Previous treatment recommendations for low doses of antibiotics in an outpatient setting for DGI are no longer appropriate.

Physicians treating patients with DGI and gonococcal arthritis must have a clear understanding of the changing patterns of antibiotic resistance, in addition to the co-infecting STDs (*Chlamydia*, syphilis and HIV). Some 30–50% of individuals infected with *N. gonorrhoeae* are coinfected with *Chlamydia*, which is not sensitive to ceftriaxone. Azithromycin and the quinolones ofloxacin and norfloxacin are effective against both. Determination of antibiotic sensitivity for the individual patient with DGI depends on recovery of the infecting organism.

In many patients with DGI, the diagnosis will be presumptive, and based on the clinical picture, a mucosal site of infection and prompt response to antibiotic treatment. Suboptimal response to treatment suggests incorrect diagnosis or infection with an antibiotic-resistant organism. The isolate from a mucosal site of infection often must be used for sensitivity testing. In the USA and Canada, recommended initial treatment of DGI with 1g/day parenteral ceftriaxone for 24–48 hours after clinical improvement begins (alternative treatment with cefotaxime or ceftizoxime 1g intravenously every 8 hours), followed with oral cefixime (400mg twice daily) or ciprofloxacin (500mg twice daily) to complete 7–10 days of treatment[31]. If the patient is allergic to B-lactam drugs, ciprofloxacin 500mg intravenously every 12 hours, ofloxacin 400mg intravenously every 12 hours, or spectinomycin 2g intramuscularly every 12 hours may be used. If the infecting strain proves to be penicillin sensitive, treatment can be changed to penicillin G (10^6U/day intravenously), amoxicillin (500mg four times a day) with probenecid (1g/day) or spectinomycin (1g intramuscularly twice daily).

Infected joints should be aspirated daily to remove all purulence; saline lavage may be helpful. Surgical drainage or arthroscopy are rarely needed. However, if the joint does not respond promptly or cannot be drained completely, more aggressive drainage procedures should be undertaken.

Because of the high rate of other STDs, all patients with DGI should also be treated presumptively for *Chlamydia trachomatis* with a single oral dose of 1g azithromycin (alternatives include: doxycycline 100mg twice daily by mouth for 7 days, erythromycin 500mg four times a day for 7 days, or ofloxacin 300mg twice daily by mouth for 7 days). Tetracyclines, erythromycin estolate, azithromycin, ciprofloxacin and ofloxacin should not be used during pregnancy. For pregnant women, erythromycin (500mg four times a day by mouth) or amoxicillin (500mg three times a day by mouth for 10 days) should be given instead of tetracycline to treat chlamydial infection[32]. Because gonorrheal infections are highly associated with the use of illicit drugs, patients should also be tested for syphilis and HIV. After completion of antibiotic treatment, patients should be re-evaluated within 1 week for re-culture of positive sites of infection. Repeat testing for syphilis should be performed 4–6 weeks later. The patient should be instructed to refer their sexual partner(s) of the 30 days before symptoms for treatment, to prevent reinfection and spread to other sexual partners. Education regarding sexual mode of transmission is paramount. Patient education should include advice to use condoms and a spermicide as the most effective means of preventing spread[32].

REFERENCES

1. Eisenstein BI, Masi AT. Disseminated gonococcal infection (DGI) and gonococcal arthritis (GCA): I. Bacteriology, epidemiology, host factors, pathogen factors and pathology. Semin Arthritis Rheum 1981; 10: 155–171.
2. Hook EW, Holmes KK. Gonococcal infections. Ann Int Med 1985; 102: 229–143.
3. Keefer CS, Spink WW. Gonococcic arthritis: pathogenesis, mechanism of recovery and treatment. JAMA 1937; 109: 1448–1453.
4. Wehrbein HL. Gonococcus arthritis: a study of 610 cases. Surg Gynecol Obstet 1929; 105–113.
5. Holmes KK. Human ecology and behavior in sexually transmitted bacterial infections. Proc Natl Acad Sci USA 1994; 91: 2448–2455.
6. Centers for Disease Control. Summary of notifiable diseases, United States – 1999. Morb Mort Wkly Rep 2001; 48(No. 53). <http://www2.cdc.gov/mmwr/summary.html>
7. Sherrard JS, Bingham JS. Gonorrhea now. Int J STD AIDS 1995; 6: 162–166.
8. Goldenberg DL. Septic arthritis. Lancet 1998; 351: 197–202.
9. O'Brien JP, Goldenberg DL, Rice PA. Disseminated gonococcal infection: a prospective analysis of 49 patients and review of the pathophysiology and immune mechanisms. Medicine (Baltimore) 1983; 62: 395–406.
10. Ryan MJ, Kavanagh R, Wall PG, Hazleman BL. Bacterial joint infections in England and Wales: analysis of bacterial isolates over a four year period. Br J Rheumatol 1997; 36: 370–373.
11. Easmon CSF. The changing pattern of antibiotic resistance of *N. gonorrhoeae*. Genitourin Med 1990; 66: 55–58.
12. Schwarcz SK, Zenilman JM, Achnell D *et al.* National surveillance of antimicrobial resistance in *Neisseria gonorrhoeae*. JAMA 1990; 264: 1413–1417.
13. Wise CM, Morris CR, Wasilauskas BL, Salzer WL. Gonococcal arthritis in an era of increasing penicillin resistance: presentations and outcomes in 41 recent cases (1985–1991). Arch Intern Med 1994; 154: 2690–2695.
14. Hoosen A, Mody G, Goga IE *et al.* Prominence of penicillinase-producing strains of *Neisseria gonorrhoeae* in gonococcal arthritis – experience in Durban, South Africa. Br J Rheumatol 1994; 33: 840–841.
15. Fox KK, Knapp JS, Holmes KK *et al.* Antimicrobial resistance in Neisseria gonorrhoeae in the United States, 1988–1994: the emergence of decreased susceptibility to the fluoroquinolones. J Infect Dis 1997; 175: 1396–1403.
16. Masi AT, Eisenstein BI. Disseminated gonococcal infection and gonococcal arthritis. Semin Arthritis Rheum 1981; 10: 173–198.

17. Mitchell SR, Nguyen PQ, Katz P. Increased risk of neisserial infections in systemic lupus erythematous. Semin Arthritis Rheum 1990; 20: 174–184.

18. Liebling M, Arkfeld D, Michelini G *et al*. Identification of *Neisseria gonorrhoeae* in synovial fluid using the polymerase chain reaction. Arthritis Rheum 1994; 37: 702–709.

19. Muralidhar B, Rumore P, Steinman C. Use of the polymerase chain reaction to study arthritis due to *Neisseria gonorrhoeae*. Arthritis Rheum 1994; 37: 710–717.

20. Levey JN, Bjornsson B, Banner B *et al*. Mixed cryoglobulinemia in chronic hepatitis C infection. Medicine 1994; 73: 53–67.

21. Siegel LB, Cohn L, Nashel D. Rheumatic manifestations of hepatitis C infection. Semin Arthritis Rheum 1993; 23: 149–154.

22. Reginato AJ, Schumacher HR, Jimenez S *et al*. Synovitis in secondary syphilis: clinical, light, and electronmicroscopic studies. Arthritis Rheum 1979; 22: 170–176.

23. Strongin I, Kale S, Raymond M *et al*. An unusual presentation of gonococcal arthritis in an HIV positive patient. Ann Rheum Dis 1991; 50: 572–573.

24. Naides SJ, Scharosch LL, Foto F, Howard EJ. Rheumatologic manifestations of human parvovirus B19 infection in adults: initial two years' clinical experience. Arthritis Rheum 1990; 33: 1297–1309.

25. Sparling PF, Handsfield HH. *Neisseria gonorrhoeae*. In: Principles and practice of infectious diseases. Mandell GL, Bennett JE, Dolin R, eds. Philadelphia: Churchill Livingston: 2000.

26. Meyer TF. Pathogenic Neisseria: complexity of pathogen-host cell interplay. Clin Infect Dis 1999; 28: 433–441.

27. Peeling RW. *Chlamydia trachomatis* and *Neisseria gonorrhoeae*: pathogens in retreat? Curr Opin Infect Dis 1995; 8: 26–34.

28. Rice PA, Vayo HE, Ram MR *et al*. Immunoglobulin G antibodies directed against protein III block killing of serum resistant *Neisseria gonorrhoeae* by immune serum. J Exp Med 1986; 164: 1735–1748.

29. Blake MS, Wetzler LM. Vaccines for gonorrhea: where are we on the curve? Trends Microbiol 1995; 3: 469–473.

30. Goldenberg DL, Reed JI, Rice PA. Arthritis in rabbits induced by killed *Neisseria gonorrhoeae* and gonococcal lipopolysaccharide. J Rheumatol 1984; 2: 3–8.

31. CDC 1998 guidelines for treatment of sexually transmitted diseases. Morb Mortal Wkly Rep 1997; 47(RR-1).

32. Centers for Disease Control. Treatment recommendations: disseminated gonococcal infection. Morb Mort Wkly Rep 1993; 42(RR-14): 61–62.

95 Mycobacterial, *Brucella*, fungal and parasitic arthritis

James S Louie and Tomás S Bocanegra

Definition

- Arthritis of peripheral and/or axial joints, osteomyelitis and soft tissue syndromes of muscle, bursa and tendon often result from infections with various mycobacterial, *Brucella*, fungal and parasitic organisms. Most of these musculoskeletal manifestations are due to direct infection. Other proposed consequences include reactive arthritis, immunologic injury and reactions to treatment

Clinical features

- Clinical suspicion is based on knowledge of host susceptibility factors, the organisms endemic to specific regions and the usual patterns of musculoskeletal involvement
- Diagnosis requires identification of the causative organism from infected joint, bone, muscle or other tissues by direct microscopy, culture and/or detection of pathogen specific antigens, antibodies, metabolites or nucleic acid sequences
- Successful antimicrobial and/or surgical therapy is dependent on proper identification and localization of the causative infection

TABLE 95.1 OSTEOARTICULAR TUBERCULOSIS CLINICAL SYNDROMES

- Spondylitis (Pott's disease)
- Peripheral arthritis
- Osteomyelitis and dactylitis
- Tenosynovitis and bursitis
- Poncet's disease

TABLE 95.2 CHARACTERISTICS OF OSTEOARTICULAR TUBERCULOSIS

- Slow onset chronic monoarthritis
- Weightbearing joint or thoracic spine
- Mild or no systemic symptoms
- Normal chest radiograph
- Positive purified protein derivative (PPD) skin test
- Joint space narrowing and bone erosions
- Absence of reactive bone sclerosis

OSTEOARTICULAR TUBERCULOSIS

Tuberculosis of the bone and joints due to *Mycobacterium tuberculosis* accounts for 10% of cases of extrapulmonary tuberculosis or approximately 2% of all new cases. In industrialized nations, tuberculosis is a disease of adults and the elderly, but in developing countries, it affects mostly younger individuals and children[1].

Five clinical syndromes of osteoarticular tuberculosis have been described (Table 95.1). Spondylitis, or Pott's disease, accounts for 50% of cases. Peripheral arthritis occurs in about 30% of patients, with osteomyelitis/dactylitis, tenosynovitis/bursitis and Poncet's disease accounting for the remainder.

Infection of the bone and joints follows hematogenous, lymphatic or contiguous spread of tuberculous bacilli from a primary focus of infection, most commonly located in the lungs. Yet only 30% of patients have radiographic evidence of pulmonary tuberculosis and 20% have infection in the genitourinary tract upon presentation. In the remaining 50%, a primary focus is not identified. Typically, there is a long latent period between the first episode of pulmonary infection and the development of musculoskeletal involvement. Bone seeding is the initial event in osteomyelitis, dactylitis and the intervertebral space infection in spondylitis. In peripheral arthritis, tenosynovitis and bursitis, the synovium is the primary focus of infection.

Osteoarticular tuberculosis typically develops as an insidious process affecting a single joint or bone (Table 95.2). However, in malnourished and elderly individuals, and those receiving anti-TNF monoclonal antibody or immunosuppressive therapies, the infection may be multifocal or disseminated. Considerable delay in diagnosis is the rule in tuberculosis affecting the bones and joints. In most series, the mean duration of symptoms before diagnosis is 12–18 months. Failure in the early recognition of osteoarticular tuberculosis is due to the insidious nature of the disease and the lack of clinical evidence of disease in other organs at the time of initial evaluation. With the recent increase of tuberculosis in human immunodeficiency virus (HIV) infected individuals and the ease of worldwide travel, the index of suspicion for tuberculosis has increased.

Tuberculous spondylitis

Tuberculous spondylitis, or Pott's disease, is the most common form of osteoarticular tuberculosis. Tuberculosis of the spine starts in the subchondral bone and spreads slowly to the disc space and adjoining vertebral bodies. The infection extends along the plane of the spinal longitudinal ligaments and tissues and frequently emerges as a mass or a draining sinus. The lower thoracic and the upper lumbar spine account for more than 75% of cases.

Clinical features

The first and most common symptom is spinal pain or stiffness, exacerbated by movement, which develops insidiously over months. The affected segments may be tender and demonstrate a restricted range of motion but signs of inflammation are conspicuously absent, even in advanced cases. Hence the name 'cold abscess'.

Patients with advanced disease may present with spinal deformity (gibbus) and/or neurologic deficit arising from spinal cord compression or arachnoiditis. Overall, weakness or paralysis occurs in about half of cases, particularly when the cervical spine is affected[2]. Systemic manifestations such as fever, malaise and weight loss usually indicate active tuberculosis in other organs.

Investigations

Acute phase reactants such as the erythrocyte sedimentation rate (ESR) are elevated in most cases. Radiographically, the earliest change is erosion of the anterior superior or inferior part of the vertebral body followed by erosion of the endplates and narrowing of the intervertebral disc space. As the infection spreads to the adjoining vertebrae, the collapse of the vertebral bodies results in anterior wedging and spine angulation (Fig. 95.1). Solitary lesions occur but usually more than one vertebral level is affected. A paraspinal abscess develops in up to 65% of patients, more commonly in the thoracic and cervical areas[3]. Despite extensive bone destruction, periosteal reaction, bone sclerosis or spontaneous fusion do not occur in spinal tuberculosis.

In early cases, however, plain radiographs will be normal or show equivocal changes. In such patients, computed tomography (CT) and magnetic resonance imaging (MRI) show early bone destruction, soft tissue swelling or abscesses. MRI is particularly helpful in depicting spinal cord compression. Technetium or gallium scanning and ultrasound may help localize the focus of infection or abscess but are not specific for diagnosis.

Diagnosis should be confirmed by the identification of tuberculous bacilli. From spinal lesions, cultures are positive in only 40% of paraspinal abscess fluids and 70% of caseous material from bone biopsies. Caseating granulomas in the tissue are seen in the tissue in 75%[4]. In the 50% of patients who do not demonstrate active tuberculosis at

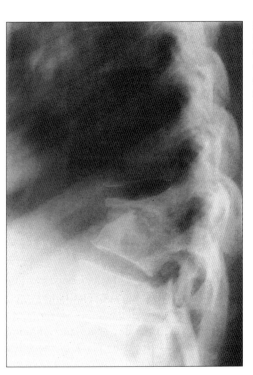

Fig. 95.1 Advanced tuberculosis of the spine. Massive collapse of T9 and T10, with absence of reactive bone sclerosis. (Courtesy of Dr A. Keat.)

another site, some clinicians would temporize for 3 months and rebiopsy. Those clinicians who choose to treat should be aware that soft tissue masses and bone destruction may persist for up to 15 months after initiation of antituberculosis therapy and should not be seen as an indication of treatment failure[3].

Differential diagnosis

Differential diagnosis includes other infections and malignancies. Unlike tuberculosis, most patients with staphylococcal and other pyogenic infections of the spine have an acute illness with prominent systemic manifestations. However, patients with *Brucella*, *Actinomyces*, *Candida*, *Aspergillus* and *Coccidioides* infections present with low-grade symptoms that simulate Pott's disease.

Several radiographic characteristics are helpful in differentiating tuberculous from non-tuberculous infections of the spine (Table 95.3). Pyogenic infections usually affect a single vertebral body, most commonly in the lumbar spine. Since the initial focus of infection is within the intervertebral disc space, the earliest radiographic change is disc space narrowing, while this is a late event in tuberculosis. In pyogenic spondylitis, collapse, spinal deformity and abscess formation are also rare, presumably because of reactive bone sclerosis. Some fungal infections such as actinomycosis, which often is accompanied by a characteristic draining sinus, may result in collapse and deformity. Calcification within or around the paraspinal abscess is pathognomonic of Pott's disease and is not seen in other types of spinal infection or malignancy.

Malignancies, including multiple myeloma, prostatic and breast carcinomas and carcinomas of the lung or gastrointestinal tract, may metastasize to the spine. In contrast to tuberculosis, the affected levels are not contiguous. In metastatic cancers, the initial lesions tend to affect the pedicles of the vertebral body. Eventually the vertebra may collapse completely but anterior wedging and deformity are uncommon. Paraspinal masses resembling a 'cold abscess' are rare.

Peripheral arthritis

Peripheral joint involvement results from hematogenous spread of the tuberculosis bacillus from the primary focus of infection. Following seeding, a low-grade granulomatous synovitis develops slowly. Trauma may play a part in some patients and explain the greater frequency of tuberculous arthritis in weight-bearing joints.

Clinical features

Tuberculous arthritis presents as an indolent process. Constitutional symptoms are usually absent unless there is active tuberculosis in other organs. The most common manifestation is monoarticular joint pain exacerbated by weight-bearing and activity. 'Soft' joint swelling is caused by marked proliferation of the synovium and joint effusion. However, other inflammatory signs are mild or absent. Range of motion is usually limited because of pain or synovial hyperplasia. Polyarticular joint involvement is seen more commonly in elderly and immunocompro-

Feature	Infectious spondylitis	Spinal tuberculosis	Malignancy
Number of vertebrae involved	One	Two or more, contiguous	One or more, non-contiguous
Segment affected	Lower lumbar	Lower thoracic, upper lumbar	Any
Location of initial lesion	Disc space	Subchondral bone	Vertebral body, pedicles
Bone destruction	Limited	Extensive, anterior, wedging	Extensive collapse
Bone sclerosis	Yes	No	Yes (with few exceptions)
Spinal deformity	No	Yes	No
Paraspinal abscess	No (with few exceptions)	Yes	No

TABLE 95.3 DIFFERENTIAL DIAGNOSIS OF SPINAL TUBERCULOSIS, INFECTIOUS SPONDYLITIS AND MALIGNANCY

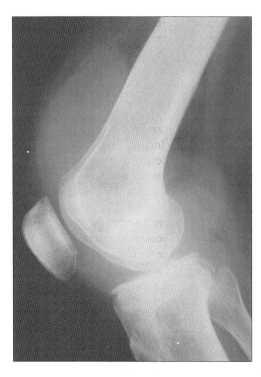

Fig. 95.2 Tuberculosis of the knee. Soft tissue swelling, blurriness of the subchondral bone and an anterior marginal erosion of the tibia. (With permission from Chapman *et al.*[5])

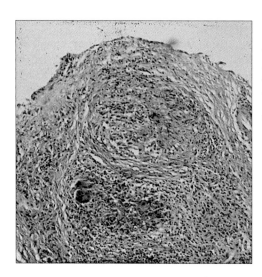

Fig. 95.3 Synovial biopsy from a patient with tuberculous arthritis, showing caseating granuloma and giant cells. (With permission from Garcia-Kutzbach[1].)

mised individuals who present with systemic symptoms and periarticular abscesses. The weight-bearing joints of the lower extremities, particularly the knee and the hip, account for 50% of peripheral tuberculous arthritis.

Investigations

Radiographic changes are mild during the early stages of the infection[4]. Soft tissue swelling and periarticular osteopenia are the initial abnormalities. Blurring of the subchondral bone surface and marginal erosions with indistinct borders develop after several weeks (Fig. 95.2). Joint space narrowing is a relatively late change. Extensive joint destruction, including joint space narrowing, occurs in patients who are not diagnosed for several months. In contrast to pyogenic arthritis, reactive bone sclerosis does not occur during the active phase of the infection but commonly develops after treatment. MRI depicts the smooth, thin borders of both the erosions and the boundaries of the abscesses, contrasting with the thick irregular rims of pyogenic abscesses[6].

Routine blood studies are not helpful for diagnosis and, although the ESR is elevated in most patients, this is non-specific.

The chest radiograph is normal or may show sequelae of prior infection without evidence of active tuberculosis. Skin testing for tuberculosis is positive in more than 90% of patients. False-negative tuberculin tests occur with general illness, protein malnutrition or corticosteroid therapy[7]. In the absence of such anergy, a persistently negative skin test makes tuberculosis unlikely.

Synovial fluid is inflammatory[8]. The synovial fluid white cell count ranges between 10 000 and 20 000 cells/mm³ with a predominance of polymorphonuclear cells. Protein levels are higher than 3.5g/dl in all fluids and the blood–synovial fluid glucose gradient is greater than 40mg/dl in most patients. Synovial biopsy shows changes consistent with tuberculosis in more than 90% of the specimens and is a quick and reliable diagnostic method[8]. Characteristically, these changes include caseating or non-caseating granulomata with multinucleated giant cells (Fig. 95.3). Arthroscopic biopsies are preferable to needle biopsies because they produce a higher yield of infected synovial tissue.

Bacteriologic confirmation of the diagnosis is of paramount importance. Ziehl–Neelsen staining of synovium and synovial fluid smear require 10 000 acid-fast bacilli per milliliter and have a low yield (10–20%). Cultures of synovial fluid are positive in about 80% of cases and cultures of synovial tissue in 94%[8]. The promise of using a mycobacterial genus-specific polymerase chain reaction (PCR) to amplify mycobacterial DNA from affected synovial fluid and tissue still requires standard primers and procedures to prove clinically useful[9].

Osteomyelitis and dactylitis

Tuberculous osteomyelitis develops following hematogenous spread from a distant focus of infection or, rarely, bacillus Calmette–Guérin (BCG) vaccination in children. It accounts for 15% of cases of chronic infectious osteomyelitis and for up to 19% of cases of osteoarticular tuberculosis[10]. A single site is usual but in 10% there may be multifocal sites. Practically any bone can be affected but tubular and flat bones are the most common sites.

Clinical features

Systemic and local clinical manifestations are modest, resulting in delayed diagnosis. In one series, the average delay in diagnosis was 28 months[10]. Swelling and tenderness are usually inconspicuous and go unattended for months. In many cases, patients present only when complications such as soft tissue abscess, extension of the infection to the neighboring joint or draining sinuses have developed. Secondary pyogenic osteomyelitis is not rare in patients with draining sinus tracts.

Investigations

Radiographs typically show lytic lesions with poorly defined margins and minimal or no reactive bone sclerosis in the epiphysis and metaphysis. Sequestrum is rare. In patients complicated with secondary pyogenic osteomyelitis, sclerosis and sequestrum formation may be prominent, masking the diagnosis of underlying tuberculosis.

Diagnosis depends on demonstration of positive cultures for tuberculosis bacilli or characteristic histologic changes on bone biopsy. Most patients have a positive purified protein derivative (PPD) skin test.

Dactylitis is a variant of tuberculous osteomyelitis affecting the long bones of the hands and feet. It occurs mainly in young children. The bones of the hands are involved more often than those in the feet and the phalanges more often than the metacarpals. The first manifestation is usually painless swelling of the diaphysis of the affected bone followed later by trophic changes in the overlying skin. The radiographic changes are known as spina ventosa, because of the ballooned-out appearance of the bone. They consist of central lytic lesions with prominent periosteal reaction and periosteal bone apposition, giving the long bone an expanded appearance[11]. Enchondroma, fibrous dysplasia, congenital syphilis, sarcoidosis and sickle cell anemia may induce similar radiographic changes in the metaphysis of long bones of hands and feet but do not cause soft tissue swelling or periosteal reaction.

Tenosynovitis and bursitis

Tenosynovitis and bursitis arising from tuberculosis are rare and are seldom discussed in clinical textbooks. They result from hematogenous spread, although direct inoculation is possible in individuals who handle infected tissues. Both are more common in adults and the elderly. Tenosynovitis is more common in the hand and wrist, especially on the dominant side[12]. Bursitis may affect any site but is more common in those bursae subjected to frequent trauma, i.e. olecranon, trochanteric, prepatellar[13].

Clinical manifestations develop insidiously and progress slowly without constitutional symptoms. The most common presenting complaint is swelling without inflammatory signs. Pain, when present, is minimal. In tenosynovitis limitation of function may be the most prominent manifestation. Radiographs are normal unless the infection has invaded the bones and joints. ESR is usually elevated and PPD is frequently positive. Diagnosis requires isolation of *Mycobacterium tuberculosis* from the tissues, or demonstration of granuloma in the synovium.

Poncet's disease

Poncet's disease is a controversial entity characterized by an aseptic polyarthritis, perhaps a reactive arthritis, developing in the presence of active tuberculosis elsewhere[14]. Any joint can be affected; however, the knees, ankles and elbows are involved more often than the small joints of the hands and feet. Cultures of synovial fluid for mycobacteria have been negative and radiographs unremarkable. In all cases, clinical manifestations resolved following eradication of the primary focus of infection with antituberculous drugs, suggesting that infective organisms and antigens were still available. The existence of Poncet's disease has been questioned because of the poor characterization of most of the patients reported. However, further support for the existence of a reactive arthritis in tuberculosis has been provided by the occurrence of a sterile polyarthritis following intravesical instillation of BCG for the treatment of bladder carcinoma[15]. PCR studies have not been reported.

Management

Chemotherapy of osteoarticular tuberculosis is highly effective using the same regimens recommended for pulmonary tuberculosis. Isoniazid, rifampin (rifampicin), ethambutol and streptomycin reach bacteriostatic concentrations in synovial tissues[16] and in 'cold abscesses', although penetration into osseous and fibrous tissue is still suspect.

Current therapeutic recommendations include three or four drug regimens (isoniazid, rifampin, pyrazinamide and ethambutol) for 12–18 months. Pyridoxine, 50mg/day, is added to regimens that include isoniazid[17].

Clinical trials with a 15-year follow-up reported that a short 6–9-month course of isoniazid and rifampin, when combined with surgical resection of the infected bone and subsequent autologous bone grafting, was as effective as an 18-month course of isoniazid with either ethambutol or para-aminosalicylic acid for the treatment of tuberculous spondylitis[18]. Recently, concerns have been raised about multi-drug-resistant tuberculosis in HIV-infected individuals and certain other groups in the population. In these cases, more than three drugs active against the resistant tuberculosis are used, including isoniazid, rifabutin or rifampin, ethambutol or streptomycin, amikacin and a quinolone such as ciprofloxacin. When resources permit, directly observed treatment is employed. In HIV-infected individuals taking protease inhibitors, a decreased dose of rifabutin is preferred over rifampin because of lower induction of the CYP 450 enzymes[17].

Immobilization, bed rest and simple debridement of the infected tissues provide no additional benefit over ambulatory chemotherapy in patients with spinal tuberculosis without neurologic deficit[19]. However, patients with tuberculosis of the spine and severe neurologic deficit or an unstable spine benefit from decompression, bone grafting and anterior fusion of the spine.

Avoidance of weight-bearing is important in tuberculosis of joints of the lower extremities but the joint should not be immobilized. A program of isometric and range of motion exercises will preserve muscle development and joint function. Surgery should be limited to patients with extensive joint destruction and functional limitation after appropriate chemotherapy. Synovectomy and debridement do not improve outcome. Arthroplasty of the hip and knee are successful in most patients, although functional outcome does not appear to be as good as for osteoarthritis. Both cemented and uncemented prostheses have been used with good results. Rates of prosthesis loosening and recurrence of tuberculosis are low, especially when the infection has been quiescent for many years. Active infection within 10 years, presence of a chronic draining sinus tract and positive culture of tissues removed during surgery are associated with a greater rate of recurrence of infection in the postoperative period. On the basis of these observations, some authors recommend prophylaxis with two or three antituberculosis drugs, starting 3 months before surgery and continuing for 6–9 months postarthroplasty[20]. Postoperative recurrence of tuberculosis is successfully treated with chemotherapy and debridement in most patients. Prosthesis removal and arthrodesis are seldom necessary except when there is a coexisting bacterial infection[21].

Chemotherapy is the treatment of choice in tuberculous osteomyelitis and dactylitis. Surgery is rarely indicated except for diagnosis and for patients who have draining sinuses or secondary pyogenic osteomyelitis. Treatment regimens similar to those for peripheral arthritis are recommended for osteomyelitis. The rate of response is high and prognosis is good. Treatment failures are rare and in most cases are due to secondary pyogenic osteomyelitis rather than to resistant organisms.

Tenosynovitis and bursitis are best treated with chemotherapy. Although synovectomy may eradicate the infection in some patients, recurrence is frequent unless followed by chemotherapy. Surgery should be limited to obtaining a tissue sample for diagnosis and for patients in whom synovial proliferation results in peripheral nerve entrapment. In Poncet's disease, treatment is aimed at eradicating the primary focus of infection.

NON-TUBERCULOUS MYCOBACTERIAL INFECTION

Non-tuberculous mycobacteria are ubiquitous organisms within the environment (for example soil, water) and in animal reservoirs. Infections of the musculoskeletal system are rare and are usually associated with predisposing factors, such as prior joint disease, trauma, use of intra-articular or oral corticosteroids, or an immunocompromised state, especially HIV infection. Most commonly, musculoskeletal infections with non-tuberculous mycobacteria result from direct inoculation, although hematogenous spread from a primary focus in the lungs may occur.

Atypical mycobacterial infection

Several species of non-tuberculous mycobacteria have been associated with musculoskeletal infections. About 70% of the cases are due to *Mycobacterium marinum*, *M. kansasii* and *M. avium–intracellulare*. However, spondylitis and peripheral arthritis due to *M. chelonei*, *M. gastri*, *M. haemophilum* and *M. terrae* have been reported[22]. The clinical manifestations, radiographic changes and histology are similar to those of tuberculosis but tenosynovitis, bursitis and polyarthritis are more common and osteomyelitis and spondylitis are less common. The most evident sites of infection are the joints and tendons of the hands and wrist, and the knees.

As in tuberculosis, diagnosis is often delayed. Chest radiograph is normal in most patients and PPD skin testing is positive in half because of cross-reaction with *M. tuberculosis*. Definite diagnosis requires isolation and characterization of the organism from drainage or biopsy material. When PCR becomes available for *M. avium–intracellulare*, time to adjunctive diagnosis and specification should be decreased compared to the current 1–3 week culture time[23].

Treatment usually requires excision of the infected tissues and chemotherapy. Clarithromycin or azithromycin added to ethambutol and rifampin or rifabutin for *M. avium*, *M. marinum* and *M. abscessus* have remarkable efficacy. Standard triple therapy is recommended for *M. kansasii* but it is important to assess drug susceptibility, since resistance and relapse is reported. Antibiotic therapy is continued for 12–18 months or until cultures are negative for 12 months.

Leprosy

Musculoskeletal manifestations develop also in leprosy, a disease caused by *Mycobacterium leprae*. The clinical manifestations of leprosy vary according to the immune status of the host. Tuberculoid leprosy develops in individuals with a high degree of cell-mediated immunity (T helper cells type 1, Th1) against the bacillus. At this pole of the leprosy spectrum, the antigen load is low, and the granuloma contain few or no bacilli. Helper T cells (CD4$^+$) predominate in the lesions. At the other end of the spectrum, lepromatous leprosy is characterized by ineffective cell-mediated immunity, a large antigen load with numerous lepra organisms in the tissues and a predominance of suppressor (CD8$^+$) T cells. Skin and peripheral nerve damage is localized in tuberculoid leprosy and widespread in the lepromatous type. Most leprosy patients have manifestations intermediate between the two polar forms (borderline leprosy) and may evolve to the tuberculoid form with treatment or to the lepromatous type if left untreated.

Acute musculoskeletal manifestations are uncommon in leprosy, with prevalence ranging from 1% to 5%. However, during the reactional states of shifting from one form to another following modifications in treatment, the prevalence may increase to 50–70%. Several musculoskeletal syndromes have been described with leprosy, including arthralgias and/or arthritis with or without erythema nodosum leprosum, the swollen hand syndrome, vasculitis and enthesitis (Table 95.4).

Erythema nodosum leprosum is a reactional state (lepra type 2 reaction) that develops in lepromatous leprosy following treatment with dapsone, clofazimine and rifampin for multibacillary leprosy. It is characterized by recurrent crops of tender subcutaneous nodules in the extremities, face and trunk, which can ulcerate, and symptoms reflective of immune complex deposition, including fever, malaise, lymphadenitis, neuritis, orchitis and glomerulonephritis. A symmetric inflammatory polyarthritis of both the upper and lower extremities develops in one-third of patients, while others develop a monoarthritis[24]. Synovial fluid is inflammatory, with a predominance of polymorphonuclear cells and an occasional foamy macrophage with intracellular lepra bacilli. The Fite stain is preferred, since the Ziehl–Neelsen stain tends to decolorize lepra bacilli.

As with the other manifestations of erythema nodosum leprosum, arthritis improves with 40–60mg/day of prednisone (prednisolone) and in severe cases with drugs that inhibit tumor necrosis factor, such as thalidomide and pentoxifylline[25,26].

TABLE 95.4 MUSCULOSKELETAL MANIFESTATIONS OF LEPROSY

- Acute polyarthritis with erythema nodosum leprosum (ENL)
- Insidious rheumatoid-like polyarthritis without ENL
- Swollen hand syndrome
- Cutaneous vasculitis with 'Lucio's phenomenon'
- Enthesitis

In contrast, arthritis not associated with erythema nodosum leprosum has an insidious onset and a persistent and progressive course, particularly in the small joints, resembling rheumatoid arthritis. Asymptomatic bilateral inflammatory sacroiliitis is frequently identified by X-rays, radionuclide imaging or CT procedures. Mononuclear cells predominate in synovial fluid. This arthritis responds variably to non-steroidal anti-inflammatory agents, chloroquine or sulfasalazine, and antimicrobials, including rifampin (600 mg) plus clofazimine (300 mg) both once monthly in conjunction with dapsone (100 mg) and clofazimine (50 mg) daily[27]. Complete resolution, however, is rare and chronic deformities (i.e. swan-neck, boutonnière) due to prior bone and nerve damage may develop over time in some patients.

Chronic deformities also result from the tropism of lepra organisms to nerve tissue, which produces the clawing of the fourth and fifth fingers related to an ulnar neuropathy, the inability to pinch related to median neuropathy, wrist drop due to radial neuropathy and foot drop related to peroneal nerve dysfunction. In addition, the loss of pain, touch, heat and cold produce an osteolysis and plantar ulceration susceptible to secondary infections and major disability.

The swollen hand syndrome is less common. It is characterized by a well-demarcated swelling of the dorsum of the hand and forearm from the metacarpophalangeal joint line to the midforearm. These changes are apparently due to granulomatous tenosynovitis and periarthritis secondary to the presence of mycobacteria in the tissues. An intermittent multiple site enthesitis may occur in some patients that is not associated with arthritis or other manifestations of a reactional state[28].

Vasculitis occurs both as part of the erythema nodosum leprosum reaction as well as of another reactional state, Lucio's phenomenon or erythema necroticans. Recurrent hemorrhagic infarcts with sharply marginated serrated margins appear on the legs. Biopsy depicts an ischemic necrosis of the epidermis, thrombosis of the larger vessels in the dermis, and numerous lepra bacilli in abnormal and normal vessels. Rheumatoid factor and antinuclear antibodies have been detected in up to 30% of patients. Occasionally patients develop a clinical syndrome similar to essential mixed cryoglobulinemia.

Diagnosis and response to therapy is supported by identification of acid-fast bacilli from skin and affected tissues, as well as by antibody to lepra-specific antigen, phonolic glycolipid (PGL)-I and specific PCR[29,30].

OSTEOARTICULAR BRUCELLOSIS

Humans acquire brucellosis mostly by ingesting contaminated milk or dairy products. Four species cause human disease, *Brucella melitensis*, *B. abortus*, *B. suis* and *B. canis*. Brucellosis typically presents as a febrile illness with hepatosplenomegaly, lymphadenopathy, and leukopenia or pancytopenia. Diagnosis is established by the clinical manifestations and recovery of *Brucella* sp. from blood or bone marrow cultures, which is the case in 15–70%. In the absence of bacteriologic confirmation, a positive serology for *Brucella* (titer >1:160), a four-fold rise in *Brucella* antibody titer by the standard tube agglutination test or a significantly increasing enzyme-linked immunosorbent assay (ELISA) level is considered definitive[31]. The 'febrile agglutinin' tests are insensitive[32].

Five musculoskeletal manifestations may occur in brucellosis: sacroiliitis, peripheral arthritis, spondylitis, osteomyelitis and bursitis (Table 95.5). Osteoarticular manifestations occur in one-third of patients, especially those infected with *B. melitensis*[33]. Children rarely develop spondylitis. Peripheral arthritis affecting the hip, knee or elbow is the most common pattern of joint involvement.

Two mechanisms of joint involvement may occur in brucellosis: a septic process, which is likely in spondylitis and leads to destructive changes, and a reactive arthritis that probably accounts for many cases

TABLE 95.5 OSTEOARTICULAR BRUCELLOSIS: CLINICAL SYNDROMES
• Sacroiliitis
• Peripheral arthritis
• Spondylitis
• Osteomyelitis
• Bursitis

of peripheral arthritis with negative synovial fluid cultures. The latter may explain the mostly benign nature of this syndrome and the spontaneous resolution of peripheral arthritis seen in some patients.

Sacroiliitis

Sacroiliitis, usually unilateral, is the most common type of articular involvement in brucellosis, occurring mainly in young adults with acute or subacute disease. Occasionally, it occurs simultaneously with peripheral arthritis.

Clinical features

Patients present with a recent-onset, poorly localized lower back pain exacerbated by weight-bearing. Standing and walking may be difficult. The sacroiliac joint is tender on palpation but there are no signs of acute inflammation.

Investigations

Erythrocyte sedimentation rate is elevated. Radiographs of the sacroiliac joints are normal during the early stages but show blurring of the joint space later. Technetium bone scan is more sensitive than conventional radiographs and allows earlier diagnosis. There are no human leukocyte antigen (HLA) associations[34].

Peripheral arthritis.

Peripheral arthritis is the second most common type of articular involvement. It occurs mainly in children and young adults with acute or subacute disease.

Clinical features

Peripheral arthritis in brucellosis is monoarticular, affecting a large, weight-bearing joint of the lower extremity such as the hip or knee; however, the shoulder and elbow joints can also be affected. Joint effusions are prominent with minimal local inflammatory signs. Some patients present with pauciarticular involvement and a few with a symmetric, 'rheumatoid-like' pattern of arthritis.

As in sacroiliitis, patients usually have acute or subacute manifestations of brucellosis, including fever, malaise, hepatosplenomegaly and lymphadenopathy.

Investigations

Erythrocyte sedimentation rate is elevated. Radiographs depict soft tissue swelling. Synovial fluid is inflammatory with protein greater than 3g/dl, white cell count is usually below 10 000 cells/ml with predominance of lymphomononuclear cells. Cultures of synovial fluid should be done in the biphasic medium of Ruiz–Castañeda. Even under these optimal conditions, only 50% of synovial fluid cultures are positive for *Brucella* spp.[33] Synovial biopsy shows non-specific chronic inflammatory changes. A specific PCR assay should be useful for identification of *Brucella* DNA from fluid or tissue.[35]

Spondylitis

Spondylitis accounts for about 10% of the cases of musculoskeletal brucellosis. It occurs mainly in the elderly and in those with chronic disease[33]. Systemic manifestations in these patients may be milder.

Clinical features

Patients present with an insidious onset of pain usually localized to the lumbar spine. There is local tenderness and limitation of mobility due to pain. Paraspinal abscesses are infrequent but neurologic compression can occur when the cervical spine is affected.

Investigations

The ESR is elevated. Radiographs usually show destructive changes at multiple levels. A characteristic finding of *Brucella* spondylitis is the Pon's sign, an erosion of the anterior and upper margin of the vertebral body with a step-like deformity or rounding-off of the corner. In contrast to tuberculous spondylitis, reactive bony sclerosis is prominent and paravertebral masses or abscesses are rare. CT may help define the anatomic changes better than plain radiographs and bone scan may show earlier changes, such as the 'Caries sign' with focal uptake at the upper and lateral margins of the vertebrae[36].

Osteomyelitis

Osteomyelitis of the ribs and long bones has been rarely reported in patients infected with *B. melitensis* and *B. suis*. Patients usually present with localized pain and tenderness. Bone scan shows increased uptake in the affected bones.

Bursitis

Bursitis is a rare manifestation of brucellosis, accounting for less than 1% of cases of osteoarticular involvement. It affects the olecranon or prepatellar bursae and resolves without sequelae following medical treatment.

Management

The prognosis of osteoarticular brucellosis is generally good. Treatment with the combination of doxycycline, 200mg/day, and rifampin, 600mg/day, for 6 weeks results in resolution of the systemic symptoms and articular manifestations in most patients and a low probability of relapse[37]. Patients with spondylitis respond better with doxycycline and streptomycin. To avoid the tooth-staining due to the tetracyclines, children are given trimethoprim–sulfamethoxazole and an aminoglycoside[38]. Abscesses may require surgical drainage, particularly when signs of neurologic compression are present. Arthrocentesis is indicated only to rule out other causes of acute peripheral arthritis but not as part of the treatment. PCR of the peripheral blood may be useful for diagnosis and in post-treatment follow-up for detection of relapse[35].

FUNGAL ARTHRITIS

Fungal infections of the bone and joints occur infrequently in those who work within endemic areas in occupations that allow increased exposure. Although primary fungal infection of the lungs or skin may be common, dissemination to other organs occurs predominantly in patients with debilitating conditions who are given corticosteroids, cytotoxics or prolonged intravenous antibiotics. Arthritis, osteomyelitis, bursitis and tenosynovitis may develop as a result of local extension of

TABLE 95.6 CHARACTERISTICS OF FUNGAL ARTHRITIS
• Treatment requires systemic antifungal plus debridement
• Geographic-distribution- or occupation-related
• Lungs and skin common port of entry
• Self-limiting polyarthritis in healthy host with primary infection
• Chronic monoarthritis and/or osteomyelitis in immunocompromised host or disseminated infection
• Diagnosis by identification of fungus in joint fluid and/or tissue

TABLE 95.7 FUNGAL ARTHRITIDES

Fungus	Underlying host status	Type of involvement	Location	Treatment
Histoplasma	Healthy	Acute polyarthritis (erythema nodosum) Osteomyelitis	Large joints Long bones, vertebrae	Self-limiting Amphotericin B
Blastomyces	Healthy	Osteomyelitis Chronic monoarthritis	Vertebrae, ribs, long bones Knee, ankle, elbow	Amphotericin B or ketoconazole plus debridement
Paracoccidioides	Malnutrition, chronic liver disease	Osteomyelitis Chronic monoarthritis	Clavicle, humerus, ribs Knee, ankle, elbow	Amphotericin B or ketoconazole plus debridement
Coccidioides	Healthy	Acute polyarthritis (erythema nodosum) Chronic monoarthritis, osteomyelitis	Large joints Knee, wrist, ankle, vertebrae, tibia, skull	Self-limiting Amphotericin B or ketoconazole plus debridement
Cryptococcus	Healthy and immunocompromised	Osteomyelitis Chronic monoarthritis	Vertebrae, pelvis, ribs Knee, ankle	Amphotericin B plus 5-fluoro-cytosine plus debridement
Aspergillus	Immunocompromised, broad-spectrum antibiotics	Osteomyelitis Chronic monoarthritis	Vertebrae, ribs Knee, wrist	Amphotericin B plus debridement
Candida	Immunocompromised, i.v. drug abusers, broad spectrum antibiotics	Osteomyelitis Chronic monoarthritis	Vertebrae Knee, hip, shoulder	Amphotericin B plus 5-fluorocytosine plus arthrocentesis
Sporothrix	Immunocompromised, alcoholism	Chronic monoarthritis Osteomyelitis Tenosynovitis/bursitis	Knee, wrist, elbow Tibia, fibula Upper extremity	Amphotericin B plus debridement

the fungal infection or by hematogenous spread from a primary focus in the lungs or soft tissues. In addition, arthralgias and arthritis may occur as a hypersensitivity reaction to a respiratory infection with certain fungi (Table 95.6).

Bone and joint infection usually present as an indolent process betrayed by a delayed diagnosis. Diagnosis requires identification of the fungus in the synovial fluid, joint or bone tissue that correlates with an appropriate clinical presentation. The latter is particularly important for fungi such as *Candida* spp. that are frequently present in the skin (Table 95.7).

Histoplasmosis

Histoplasmosis is a common infection in the Ohio and Mississippi river valleys of the USA and also in Canada and Africa. In North America it is most commonly caused by *Histoplasma capsulatum* and in Africa by *H. capsulatum* var. *duboisii*. The portal of entry is inhalation into the lung.

Clinical features

Most of the primary infections with *H. capsulatum* are asymptomatic. The symptomatic patients present with a 'flu-like' syndrome with pleuritic chest pain but not coryza or sore throat. About 10% exhibit arthralgias or arthritis of which half display erythema nodosum or erythema multiforme[39]. The joint manifestations may precede, coincide with or follow the skin lesions of erythema nodosum/multiforme. Polyarthralgias that affect large joints of the upper or lower extremities, especially the knees, ankles and wrists, are more common than actual arthritis. Some patients present with articular manifestations and hilar adenopathy resembling sarcoidosis. A few cases of carpal tunnel syndrome, flexor tenosynovitis and joint infection have been reported, especially in children and immunocompromised patients with disseminated histoplasmosis. Despite the fact that the fungus can be isolated from the bone marrow in most patients, osteomyelitis is extremely rare with *H. capsulatum*.

H. capsulatum var. *duboisii* is more prevalent in Africa. It does not produce respiratory symptoms but has a predilection for bone marrow infection. About 50% of patients develop multifocal osteomyelitis affecting mainly flat bones, but long bones and vertebrae also may be affected.

Usually the infection spreads from the bones to the soft tissues and frequently results in fistulization. When the spine is affected it may lead to spinal cord compression and paraplegia.

Identification of histoplasmosis in fluids and tissue can be achieved in 70%. Complement fixation tests support the diagnosis, particularly at titers greater than 1:32.

Management

The articular manifestations associated with primary infection with *H. capsulatum* are usually self-limited and respond well to anti-inflammatory medication. In patients with disseminated infection and those with rare 'infectious arthritis', itraconazole, 200mg/bid is given for two months or amphotericin B for three weeks followed by itraconazole. In infection with *H. capsulatum* var. *duboisii*, treatment requires amphotericin B or itraconazole 200mg three times a day for three days, then twice a day, and frequently surgical debridement[40].

Blastomycosis

Blastomycosis, caused by *Blastomyces dermatitidis*, is endemic in south-central and south-eastern USA and north-western Ontario in Canada. It is acquired by inhalation.

Clinical features

The primary lung infection is usually asymptomatic but some patients may develop non-specific influenza-like symptoms, including polyarthralgias. The blastomycosis disseminates from the lung to the skin and bones. As many as 60% of patients with disseminated disease have bone lesions[41]. Any bone can be affected but the vertebrae, ribs, long bones and skull are the most common sites. Lesions are osteolytic, with marginal sclerosis but little or no periosteal reaction and no sequestra. Vertebral lesions may invade the disc space, producing a soft tissue abscess and spinal cord compression resembling tuberculosis.

Arthritis is uncommon, occurring in 8–15% of those with disseminated disease. It is almost always a monoarthritis. The knee, ankle and elbow are the joints most commonly affected, usually as a result of direct extension from a bone lesion. However, hematogenous spread from a distant focus may occur.

Investigations

Synovial fluid is inflammatory with a predominance of polymorphonuclear cells. In over 80% of the fluids, *Blastomyces dermatitidis* is identified by direct smear or culture. The fungus can also be identified in the synovium or bone.

Management

Optimal treatment includes drainage and debridement and itraconazole 200mg b.d. for 6 months for a 95% chance of cure. In severe disease, amphotericin B 0.5mg/kg/day for a total dose of 1.5g, is the drug of choice (90% response)[42]. Fluconazole 400–800mg/day for 6 months is effective in 85% of moderate disease[43].

Paracoccidioidomycosis

Paracoccidioidomycosis, also known as South American blastomycosis, is caused by the fungus *Paracoccidioides brasiliensis*. The disease is endemic in South and Central America. Similarly to blastomycosis, the primary infection is in the lungs and may go unnoticed. Disseminated disease is uncommon and occurs mainly in patients with underlying debilitating conditions such as malnutrition or chronic liver disease. Bone involvement is uncommon, occurring in less than 10% of patients with disseminated disease. Arthritis is rare[44]. Most commonly, the disease is a result of direct extension from a contiguous bone lesion. The knee, ankle, elbow and wrist are most frequently affected.

The fungus can be identified in the synovial fluid and synovium[44]. Complement fixation and immunodiffusion testing for antibodies to the fungus are positive in sera of most of the patients. Treatment is similar to that of blastomycosis beginning with itraconazole[45].

Coccidioidomycosis

Coccidioidomycosis is prevalent in areas of the south-western USA, northern Mexico and Central America. It also occurs in a few countries of South America (Venezuela, Argentina, Paraguay). The etiologic agent, *Coccidioides immitis*, infects humans through the lungs.

Clinical features

In the great majority of the cases, the primary infection is asymptomatic. A few develop a self-limiting, influenza-like syndrome, including low-grade fevers, malaise, conjunctivitis and erythema nodosum or erythema multiforme. Disseminated infection develops in less than 1% of patients. In contrast to opportunistic fungal infections, such as aspergillosis and candidiasis, systemic coccidioidomycosis usually develops in healthy individuals. Anti-TNF monoclonal antibody therapies may be permissive.

Articular manifestations may develop in primary and disseminated disease. Mono- or polyarticular joint pain, occasionally accompanied by mild swelling, develops in 8% of patients as part of the 'hypersensitivity reaction' of primary infection. It is self-limiting and resolves leaving no sequelae[46]. A chronic granulomatous infectious arthritis occurs in about 20% of patients with disseminated disease. It usually results from local spread from a contiguous focus of osteomyelitis. This type of arthritis is monoarticular, shows modest signs of inflammation and progresses very slowly with minimal or no systemic symptoms. In many patients, arthritis is the only manifestation of systemic disease. The joints most commonly affected are the knee, wrist, ankle and elbow[47]. Joint radiographs are mostly unremarkable except for soft tissue swelling. Few patients show narrowing of the joint space but about 50% may demonstrate a para-articular focus of osteomyelitis.

Osteomyelitis is common and usually multifocal. Any bone can be affected, but most commonly the vertebrae, tibia, skull and metatarsals. Lesions are lytic surrounded by a sclerotic reaction. Bone lesions may open and drain into the surrounding tissues, resulting in a secondary bacterial arthritis or soft tissue abscess and occasionally a fistula.

Investigations

Diagnosis requires synovial biopsy for histology and tissue culture. Both allow identification of the fungus in practically all patients. Synovial fluid cultures and direct smears have a very low yield[46]. Flow cytometry assessing lymphocyte reactivity to specific antigen replaces the skin test[48]. Primers for PCR have not been validated.

Management

Treatment requires drainage, surgical debridement and an azole anti-fungal, either fluconazole, 400–800mg/day, or itraconazole, 200mg b.d., for 6 months. Because of its toxicity, amphotericin B is reserved as a second-line agent or for life-threatening disease. Intra-articular amphotericin B has been used in few patients with good results but the experience is limited. Complement fixation titers may be used to follow response to treatment. Titers lower than 1:4 are associated with a low rate of relapse after discontinuation of treatment and any rise in titer would signal a relapse[49].

Cryptococcosis

Cryptococcus neoformans infection is usually acquired by inhalation. The primary infection is pulmonary and self-limited. More than 80% of individuals with disseminated cryptococcosis have a debilitating underlying condition such as lymphoma, diabetes mellitus, sarcoidosis or acquired immunodeficiency syndrome (AIDS), or receive immunosuppressive medications. Dissemination occurs in the immunocompromised.

Clinical features

Osteomyelitis is the most common musculoskeletal manifestation, occurring in less than 10% of patients as a result of hematogenous spread. Vertebrae, pelvis, ribs and long bones are most commonly affected. Lesions may be single or, more commonly, multiple, lytic, with minimal or no bone reaction, resembling metastases[50,51].

Cryptococcal arthritis and bursitis are rare, even in patients with AIDS[52]. Most patients lack a history of prior joint disease. Monoarthritis of the knee is the most common presentation. Para-articular osteomyelitis is present in two-thirds of patients, suggesting local spread as the main mechanism of joint infection.

Investigations

Synovial fluid is inflammatory and biopsy shows acute and chronic inflammation with occasional granulomata. Diagnosis is based on isolation of the fungus from the synovial fluid or tissue. The diagnosis may also be facilitated by determining cryptococcal antigens.

Management

Treatment requires drainage, debridement and fluconazole or itraconazole for 6–12 months. Intravenous amphotericin B and 5-fluorocytosine, 25mg/kg every 6 hours for weeks, are used for meningitis and/or in AIDS. The dose and the duration for optimal results are unknown. Single-agent therapy is not recommended because of the frequency of secondary drug resistance. The total dose of amphotericin B administered to patients reported in the literature has ranged from 395mg to 4g and for 5-fluorocytosine from 2.2g to 284g[50].

Aspergillosis

Aspergillus is an opportunistic fungus that colonizes the upper respiratory tract, especially in patients with chronic obstructive pulmonary disease. In immunocompromised patients, the fungus may disseminate. The most common pathogen is *Aspergillus fumigatus*, but infections with *A. flavus*, *A. niger* and *A. terreus* may occur. Predisposing factors for disseminated disease include leukemia, leukopenia and prior treatment with broad-spectrum antibiotics, corticosteroids or cytotoxic agents.

Clinical features

Musculoskeletal involvement is rare and when it develops it is usually osteomyelitis. The most common sites are the spine and the ribs, usually resulting from contiguous spread from pulmonary infection. The symptoms are not specific: most commonly patients present with pain or tenderness and elevated ESR[53]. In the spine, the infection may extend to the intervertebral disc space, with subsequent development of a soft tissue abscess and spinal cord compression[54]. Radiographs may show narrowing of the disc space and erosion of the endplates without reactive sclerosis, similar to the findings in Pott's disease.

Arthritis and bursitis are even more infrequent and may result from extension of a contiguous bone infection or hematogenous spread. Radiographs of the affected joint usually show lytic lesions in the para-articular bone and minimal or no subperiosteal bone formation[55].

Investigations

Since *Aspergillus* is ubiquitous and frequently contaminates laboratory culture media, diagnosis of bone and joint aspergillosis must rely not only on identification of the fungus in culture but also on identification of fungal elements in the tissues and correlation with the clinical manifestations.

Management

Treatment commonly requires surgical debridement and intravenous administration of amphotericin B. Ketoconazole and itraconazole are not fungicidal for *Aspergillus* spp. at doses commonly used; therefore, they are not the treatment of choice for osteoarticular aspergillosis.

Candidiasis

Candida is another ubiquitous fungus frequently present in the mucous membranes of the gastrointestinal tract and less often in the skin. *Candida albicans* and *C. tropicalis* predominate in the former while *C. guilliermondii*, *C. parapsilosis* and other *Candida* species are more common in the skin.

Clinical features

Clinical manifestations are usually modest, consisting of pain and swelling without inflammatory signs. *Candida* species most often produce superficial infections. However, in compromised individuals, such as premature neonates, diabetics, intravenous heroin users, patients with malignancies and those receiving intravenous hyperalimentation, broad-spectrum antibiotics, chemotherapy or corticosteroids, *Candida* may disseminate to affect other organs. The kidney and the eye are the organs most commonly affected. Arthralgias and myalgias may occur occasionally during the septic phase of systemic candidiasis.

Bone and joint infection are rare, occurring in 1–2% of those who develop systemic candidiasis. *C. albicans* and *C. tropicalis* are the most common species associated with osteoarticular manifestations. However infection with other species, including *Torulopsis glabrata*, a yeast closely related to *Candida*, have been reported. Usually several weeks elapse between the diagnosis of candidemia and the development of osteomyelitis and/or arthritis. Bone and joint infection more often result from hematogenous dissemination of the fungus[56]. Extension of the infection from the bone to the adjacent joint or intervertebral space is a common mechanism of arthritis and spondylodiskitis. However, direct inoculation into the joint has been reported in a few patients[57]. Osteomyelitis is more common than arthritis. In adults, the lumbar spine is the most frequent location, while in neonates long bone involvement, usually multifocal, is more common. The knees, hips and shoulders are the joints most commonly affected in patients who develop mono- or polyarthritis. In heroin users, a syndrome of folliculitis, endophthalmitis, osteomyelitis and/or osteoarthritis develops, affecting the costochondral junctions, the spine and sacroiliac and peripheral joints. Prosthetic joints can be affected also[58].

Investigations

Synovial fluid white-cell count is variable, with polymorphonuclear leukocytes predominant. Radiographs may be normal or show changes of osteomyelitis in the adjacent bones. None of the clinical or radiographic changes are unique to candidiasis. Therefore, diagnosis must rely on the identification of the fungus in the synovial fluid or tissue biopsy. Fortunately, *Candida* grows well in regular media for bacterial cultures. For species that colonize the skin, it is necessary to confirm the diagnosis by identification of the fungus in the tissues by culture or histology.

Management

Treatment consists of the elimination of the predisposing factors and the systemic administration of amphotericin B with or without ketoconazole or fluconazole. Frequent joint aspiration is needed in peripheral arthritis. Surgical drainage and debridement are usually unnecessary. In spondylitis, surgery is indicated if there is neurologic deficit, instability of the spine or lack of response to medical treatment.

Sporotrichosis

Sporothrix schenckii is a saprophytic fungus present in decaying vegetation, timber, soil and gardening supplies. Humans become infected, most commonly, by direct inoculation through the skin.

Clinical features

Usually, sporotrichosis is an occupational disease, more frequently seen in individuals with outdoor and/or agricultural jobs. The primary lesion is a necrotic cutaneous nodule. The infection may spread along the lymphatic tracts, producing secondary lesions in the skin, regional lymphadenopathy and occasionally infection of deeper tissues. Rarely, the fungus disseminates to extracutaneous tissues. In these cases, sporotrichosis behaves like an opportunistic infection, affecting individuals with underlying diseases, such as diabetes mellitus, lympho- or myeloproliferative disorders and alcoholism, and those receiving corticosteroids or chemotherapy. Most of these cases probably result from hematogenous dissemination from a primary pulmonary infection, since about 85% of patients with disseminated sporotrichosis do not have skin lesions[59].

Disseminated disease occurs in less than 0.05% of patients. Articular and bone infections are the most common location in disseminated disease. Arthritis is monoarticular, especially when associated with neighboring cutaneous lesions. In disseminated disease, polyarticular arthritis presents as an indolent process with mild swelling and inflammatory signs[60]. Among the joints, more commonly affected are the knee, wrist, elbow and ankle. Among the bones, the tibia, fibula and the small bones of the hands and feet are the most frequent sites. Tenosynovitis has led to median and ulnar nerve entrapment[61]. Interestingly, the majority of patients with arthritis do not have cutaneous infection, but those with osteomyelitis usually have skin lesions. Synovial fluid is inflammatory.

Investigations

Diagnosis is usually delayed through lack of cutaneous lesions in most patients and the variety of joint involvement in sporotrichosis. Synovial fluid and/or synovium culture are positive in most of the patients. Synovium shows non-caseating granulomata. *Sporothrix* is rarely identified on histologic examination. Radiographs show non-specific findings such as para-articular osteopenia, narrowing of the joint space, extra-articular erosions and, occasionally, punched-out lesions. Lytic lesions with surrounding sclerosis are seen in osteomyelitis.

Management

Optimal treatment requires surgical debridement and itraconazole. Intravenous and intra-articular amphotericin are rarely required. Potassium iodide is ineffective for arthritis or osteomyelitis[62].

PARASITIC ARTHRITIS

Parasitic diseases are endemic in many developing countries and occur sporadically in industrialized nations. Once infected, the host may remain asymptomatic or develop clinical manifestations that range from minor local symptoms to multisystem and sometimes lethal disease, the latter being more common in immunocompromised and debilitated individuals.

The frequency of musculoskeletal manifestations in parasitic infections is low. Diagnosis is established by the coexistence of musculoskeletal symptoms and a parasitic infection, lack of response to conventional anti-inflammatory therapy and resolution of the symptoms upon eradication of the parasite (Table 95.8). Arthritis and bone lesions have been reported as a result of localization of the parasite in structures of the musculoskeletal system, a reaction to the presence of the parasite in neighboring tissues and secondary to an immune-mediated response to parasitic antigens and/or products released spontaneously by the parasite or following treatment (Table 95.9). Myositis and vasculitis may occur in some circumstances.

Protozoal infections

Articular manifestations have been reported rarely in protozoal infections. *Giardia lamblia*, *Cryptosporidium* sp., *Cyclospora* sp. and *Toxoplasma gondii* have been associated with arthralgias and arthritis of the knees, ankles and sacroiliac joint, even in HLA-B27-negative individuals[63–66]. Most patients have concomitant gastrointestinal manifestations and a few display hypersensitivity symptoms. Articular symptoms are characteristically refractory to anti-inflammatory agents but resolve promptly following antiparasitic treatment.

Myositis occurs with *T. gondii*, *Sarcocystis* spp., *Pleistophora* spp. and *Trachipleistophora* spp. *(Microsporida)* and infrequently in *Trypanosoma cruzi* infections[67–68]. Muscular symptoms may be focal or diffuse. In some cases, muscle wasting and contractures are prominent. Occasionally, proximal muscle weakness, elevated creatine phosphokinase and skin rash simulate polymyositis/dermatomyositis. The hypothesis that polymyositis and dermatomyositis are due to clinically unrecognized *Toxoplasma* infection is not supported (see Chapter 138). Furthermore, vasculitic reactions, which can be seen in the tissue around the invading protozoa, rarely manifest systemically[69]. As in patients with parasitic arthritis, symptoms resolve after eradication of the parasite.

Cestodes

Arthralgias and/or arthritis and bone pain seldom occur in cestode infections. Rare cases of arthritis affecting the knees or multiple joints in a rheumatoid-like pattern have been reported in patients infected with *Taenia saginata* or hydatid disease[19,70].

Muscular involvement is more frequent than arthritis. Cysticercosis, the infection with the larval stage of *T. solium*, is usually asymptomatic in muscle, although massive infections induce a diffuse, pseudohypertrophic myopathy[71]. Muscle bulk and consistency appear to be increased because of the number of cysticerci, and muscle strength is normal or decreased. Muscle enzymes are usually normal or slightly elevated. Diagnosis is confirmed by the finding of multiple cysticerci at muscle biopsy. Frequently there is evidence of cysticercosis in the brain and other organs. Treatment of patients with intramuscular cysticercosis with oral praziquantel may exacerbate fever and cause a severe myositis that requires concomitant dexamethasone administration[72].

The adult tapeworms of *Echinococcus granulosus* and *E. multilocularis* inhabit the intestine of dogs and other canids. Eggs of these worms are excreted in the feces. If humans ingest these eggs, they become accidental intermediate hosts for the larval stage, the hydatid cyst. These cysts are most commonly found in the liver and lung but may develop in other locations, including bone and muscle[73]. Surgical excision is the procedure of choice for diagnosis and treatment.

The larval tapeworm infections coenurosis and sparganosis are rare in humans. Coenurosis is caused by several species of *Taenia* (*Multiceps*). The infection is probably acquired by the ingestion of tapeworm eggs from the feces of canine definitive hosts. The subcutaneous and intramuscular forms of the infection in humans are extremely rare in North America but are seen more commonly in Africa. The larval cysts produce soft tissue masses. Surgical removal is the preferred treatment. Use of cysticidal agents such as praziquantel or albendazole may cause severe inflammatory reactions associated with the death of the parasite. A variety of carnivorous mammals, including dogs, cats and raccoons, serve as definitive hosts for tapeworms of the genus *Spirometra*. The second-stage larva, called a plerocercoid or sparganum, may infect humans, producing sparganosis. Infection is acquired by ingestion of first-stage larva in infected copepods or tissues of infected intermediate hosts such as frogs, snakes, chickens and

---

TABLE 95.8 CHARACTERISTICS OF PARASITIC ARTHRITIS

- Residence in or travel to endemic area
- Infection with intestinal or tissue-invasive parasite
- Acute or chronic mon0- or polyarthritis
- Poor response to anti-inflammatory therapy
- Resolution after eradication of parasite

TABLE 95.9 PARASITIC ARTHRITIDES

Parasite	Type of involvement	Location	Treatment
Giardia	Polyarthritis	Large joints	Tinidazole
Cryptosporidium	Polyarthritis	Large joints	Self-limiting
Toxoplasma	Polyarthritis	Large and small joints	Pyrimethamine plus sulfadiazine
Taenia	Polyarthritis	Large and small joints	Praziquantel
Echinococcus	Monoarthritis	Knee	Excision or mebendazole
	Polyarthritis	Large and small joints	
Strongyloides	Oligoarthritis	Knee, ankle	Thiabendazole
	Polyarthritis	Large and small joints	
Dracunculus	Monoarthritis	Knee, ankle	Niridazole
Filariae	Mono/oligoarthritis	Knee, ankle, hip	Diethylcarbamazine or ivermectin
Dirofilaria	Monoarthritis	Knee	Self-limiting
Schistosoma	Enthesitis	Any	Praziquantel
	Oligoarthritis	Large joints	
	Polyarthritis	Large and small joints	

pigs. The ribbon-like sparganum develops in tissues such as muscle and subcutaneous tissues. In some cases, the subcutaneous, nodular lesions are migratory. Surgical removal is the treatment of choice[74,75].

Nematodes

In *Strongyloides stercoralis* infections, a symmetric rheumatoid-like and an asymmetric oligoarthritis of the lower extremities have been described in two cases[70,76]. Larvae of *S. stercoralis* were demonstrated in the synovium of another patient[77]. The treatment of choice is oral ivermectin.

There are isolated reports of seronegative oligoarthritis of joints of the lower extremities in association with *Ankylostoma duodenale* (hookworm), *Ascaris lumbricoides* (roundworm) and *Trichuris trichiura* (whipworm) infections. These reports suggest a need for molecular and immunologic methods to describe specific DNA, RNA, antigen and/or antibodies within the articular tissues,

Dracunculus medinensis (Guinea worm) is the largest tropical nematode found in humans. It causes an infection called dracunculiasis. In the endemic regions of Africa, Asia and the Middle East, humans contract the disease by drinking water containing infected water fleas. The female parasite migrates to the subcutaneous tissues, usually in the lower extremities, and forms a bleb, which ulcerates and discharges larvae. Occasionally, the larva may invade the muscle or the joint, producing myalgias, arthralgias or monoarticular arthritis of the knee or ankle[78].

Synovial fluid is inflammatory and contains eosinophils and occasionally larvae. Radiographs may show the calcified, dead Guinea worm in deeper tissue (Fig. 95.4). In many cases, diagnosis is made by the incidental finding of Guinea worms during diagnostic arthroscopy or arthrotomy for chronic monoarthritis of unknown etiology.

Treatment consists of removal of the parasite from the joint cavity by arthroscopy or arthrotomy. Attempts to remove the worm by mechanical traction require days of continuous extraction because the length of the adult nematode can reach 80–120cm. When arthritis results from para-articular localization of the parasite, the use of anti-inflammatory agents and metronidazole may provide symptomatic relief but rarely eradicates the parasite. Mebendazole has been reported to kill the adult worm. With secondary bacterial arthritis, daily joint aspirations and appropriate intravenous antibiotics are indicated.

Joint symptoms occur in less than 10% of patients infected with *Wuchereria bancrofti*, and *Brugia malayi* (lymphatic filariasis), *Loa loa*

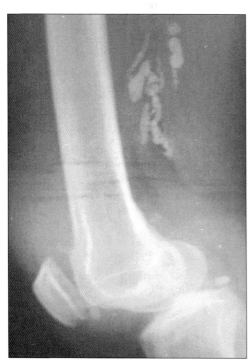

Fig. 95.4 Dracunculiasis arthritis. Calcified Guinea worms in the soft tissues of a patient with arthritis of the knee. (With permission from Garf[78].)

(Calabar swelling) and *Onchocerca volvulus*[79–81]. Arthritis may be mono- or oligoarticular, affecting mainly large joints of the lower extremities. In some patients, arthritis is the only manifestation of filariasis. Synovial fluid is inflammatory and, in many cases, contains eosinophils and microfilariae. Synovial biopsy shows mononuclear cell infiltrate and eosinophils in some patients. Diagnosis of filariasis is usually made by serology, antigen detection or identification of microfilariae in the peripheral circulation or the skin (onchocerciasis). Treatment of lymphatic filariasis consists of diethylcarbamazine, given for 2 weeks. Special care is needed in treating patients with loiasis who have high microfilaremia. Albendazole is used to lower the microfilaria count initially and diethylcarbamazine may be used subsequently. Ivermectin is considered the treatment of choice for onchocerciasis. Occasional reactions to the death of microfilaria may require administration of corticosteroids.

Dirofilariasis caused by the dog heartworm, *Dirofilaria immitis,* is a rare and self-limiting disease in humans. The clinical manifestations usually consist of lower respiratory symptoms and pulmonary nodules. Occasionally, patients may present with arthralgias or a self-limiting arthritis of the lower extremities. Treatment is not necessary.

Gnathostoma spinigerum may produce eosinophilic panniculitis and *Toxocara canis* transient myositis of the lower extremities[82]. In both cases, the clinical manifestations are due to migration of the parasite through the soft tissues.

Trematodes

Infections with *Schistosoma mansoni* and *S. haematobium* have been associated with arthritis and enthesitis[83,84]. Enthesitis commonly overlaps with arthritis and appears to be the most common musculoskeletal manifestation. Oligoarthritis of large joints of the lower extremities, unilateral sacroiliitis and polyarthritis have also been reported. Occasional patients may have rheumatoid factor at lower titers. Synovial fluid is inflammatory and synovial biopsy usually shows a mononuclear cell infiltrate. In a few patients, *Schistosoma* ova have been found (Fig. 95.5). Praziquantel will eradicate the parasites. Schistosomiasis may cause a diffuse myopathy of the shoulder and pelvic girdle muscles.

Trichinosis produces prominent myalgias and weakness of the proximal muscles of the upper and lower extremities. This infection is acquired by eating raw or undercooked meat, particularly pork, infected by the larvae of *Trichinella* spp. Horse meat has been a source of human infection in Europe. Eating the meat of scavenging carnivores such as bears may also result in infection[85]. Polymyositis is often considered initially because the creatine phosphokinase is markedly elevated without

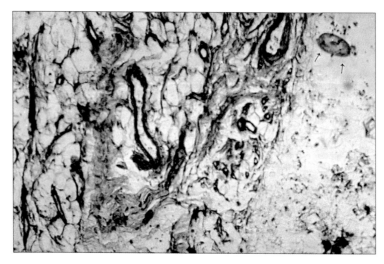

Fig. 95.5 Schistosomal arthritis. Schistosoma ovum in the synovium. (With permission from Bassiouni and Kamel[84].)

specific antibodies for more than 10 days after infection. Muscle biopsy will show eosinophilic myositis and *Trichinella* larvae[86]. Treatment consists of mebendazole 200–400mg t.i.d. for 3 days, then 400–500mg t.i.d. for 10 days, with concomitant prednisone, 40–60mg/day, or albendazole, 400mg b.d., for 14 days.

Few cases of vasculitis associated with nematode infections have been reported. Leukocytoclastic vasculitis has been described during strongyloidiasis and loiasis. Systemic necrotizing vasculitis mimicking polyarteritis nodosa and Churg–Strauss angiitis has occurred in patients with trichinosis and ascariasis[87,88].

REFERENCES

1. Garcia-Kutzbach A. Tuberculosis arthritis. In: Espinoza LR, Goldenberg DL, Arnett F, Alarcón GS, eds. Infections in the rheumatic diseases. A comprehensive review of microbial relations to rheumatic disorders. New York: Grune & Stratton; 1988: 131–138.
2. Janssens JP, de Haller R. Spinal tuberculosis in a developed country. A review of 26 cases with special emphasis on abscesses and neurologic complications. Clin Orthop 1990; 257: 67–75.
3. Sharif HS, Morgan JL, Al Shahed MS, Al Thagafi MYA. Role of CT and MR imaging in the management of tuberculous spondylitis. Radiogr Clin North Am 1995; 33: 787–804.
4. Medical Research Council Working Party on Tuberculosis of the Spine. A controlled trial of anterior fusion and debridement in the surgical management of tuberculosis of the spine in patients on standard chemotherapy. Tubercle 1978; 58: 79–105.
5. Chapman M, Murray RO, Stoker DJ. Tuberculosis of the bones and joints. Semin Roentgenol 1979; 14: 266–282.
6. Hong SH, Kim SM, Ahn JM et al. Tuberculous versus pyogenic arthritis: MR imaging evaluation. Radiology 2001; 218: 848–853.
7. Haas DW. Mycobacterium tuberculosis. In: Mandell GL, Bennett J, Dolin R, eds. Principles and practice of infectious disease, 5th ed. Edinburgh: Churchill Livingstone; 2000: 2576–2607.
8. Wallace R, Cohen AS. Tuberculous arthritis. A report of two cases with review of biopsy and synovial fluid findings. Am J Med 1976; 61: 277–282.
9. Van der Heijden IM, Wilbrink B, Schouls LM et al. Detection of mycobacteria in joint samples from patients with arthritis using genus specific polymerase chain reaction and sequence analysis. Rheumatology 1999; 38: 547–553.
10. Martini M, Adjrad A, Boudjemaa A. Tuberculous osteomyelitis. A review of 125 cases. Int Orthop 1986; 10: 201–207.
11. Wessels G, Hesseling PB, Beyers N. Skeletal tuberculosis: dactilitis and involvement of the skull. Pediatr Radiol 1998; 28: 234–236.
12. Jackson RH, King JW. Tenosynovitis of the hand: a forgotten manifestation of tuberculosis. Rev Infect Dis 1989; 11: 616–618.
13. Schickendantz MS, Watson JT. Mycobacterial prepatellar bursitis. Clin Orthop 1990; 258: 209–212.
14. Pugh MT, Southwood TR. Tuberculous rheumatism. Poncet's disease – a sterile controversy? (Editorial) Rev Rheum 1993; 60: 735–740.
15. Keat A. TB or not TB? That is the question. Br J Rheumatol 1993; 32: 769–773.
16. Wu QQ, Na XC, Tian WC. The concentration of four antituberculous drugs in cold abscesses of patients with bone and joint tuberculosis. Chin Med J 1987; 100: 819–822.
17. Small PM, Fujiwara PI. Medical progress: management of tuberculosis in the United States. N Engl J Med 2002; 345: 189–200.
18. Medical Research Council working party on tuberculosis of the spine. A 15 year assessment of controlled trials of the management of tuberculosis of the spine in Kora and Hong Kong. Thirteenth report. J Bone Joint Surg 1998; 80B: 456–462.
19. Buskila D, Sikenik S, Klein M, Horowitz J. Polyarthritis associated with hydatid cyst (Echinococcosis) of the liver. Clin Rheumatol 1992; 11: 286–287.
20. Berbari EF, HanssenAD, Duffy MC et al. Prosthetic joint infection due to Mycobacterium tuberculosis: a case series and review of the literature. Am J Orthop 1998; 27: 219–227.
21. Spinner RJ, Sexton DJ, Goldner RG, Levin LS. Periprosthetic infections due to Mycobacterium tuberculosis in patients with no prior history of tuberculosis. J Arthroplasty 1996; 11: 217.
22. Hirsch R, Miller SM, Kazi S et al. Human immunodeficiency virus-associated atypical mycobacterial skeletal infections. Semin Arthritis Rheum 1996; 25: 347–356.
23. Kulski JK, Khinsoe C, Pryce T, Christianssen K. Use of a multiplex PCR to detect and identify Mycobacterium avium and M. intracellulare in blood culture fluids of AIDS patients. J Clin Microbiol 1995; 33: 668–674.
24. Cossermelli-Messina W, Net CF, Cossermelli W. Articular inflammatory manifestations in patients with different forms of leprosy. J Rheumatol 1998; 25: 111–119.
25. Iyer CGS, Languillon J, Ramanujam K et al. WHO co-ordinated short term double blind trial with thalidomide in the treatment of acute lepra reaction in male lepromatous patients. Bull WHO 1971; 45: 719–732.
26. Sampio EP, Moraes MO, Nery JAC et al. Pentoxifylline decreases in vivo and in vitro tumor necrosis factor-alpha (TNF-α) production in lepromatous leprosy patients with erythema nodosum leprosum (ENL). Clin Exp Immunol 1998; 111: 300–308.
27. WHO Expert Committee on Leprosy. Seventh Report. WHO Tech Rep Ser No 874. Geneva: WHO; 1998
28. Atkin SL, El-Ghobary A, Kamel M et al. Clinical and laboratory studies in patients with leprosy and enthesitis. Ann Rheum Dis 1990; 49: 715–717.
29. Cho SN, Cellona RV, Villahermosa LG et al. Detection of phenolic glycolipid I of Mycobacterium leprae in sera from leprosy patients before and after start of multidrug therapy. Clin Diagn Lab Immunol 2001; 8: 138–142.
30. Williams DL, Pittman TL, Gillis TP et al. Simultaneous detection of Mycobacterium leprae and its susceptibility to dapsone using DNA heteroduplex analysis. J Clin Microbiol 2001; 39: 2083–2088.
31. Ariza J. Brucellosis. Curr Opin Infect Dis 1996; 9: 126–131.
32. Young EJ. Brucella species. In: Mandell GL, Bennett J, Dolin R, eds. Principles and practice of infectious disease, 5th ed. Edinburgh: Churchill Livingstone; 2000: 2386–2393.
33. Gotuzzo E, Alarcón GS, Bocanegra TS et al. Articular involvement in human brucellosis: a retrospective analysis of 304 cases. Semin Arthritis Rheum 1982; 12: 245–255.
34. Alarcon GS, Gotuzza E, Hinostroza SA et al. HLA studies in brucellar spondylitis. Clin Rheum 1985; 4: 312–314.
35. Morata P, Queipo-Ortuno MI, Reguera JM et al. Post treatment follow-up of Brucellosis by PCR assay. J Clin Microbiol 1999; 37: 4163–4166.
36. Bahar RH, Al-Suhaila AR, Mousa AM et al. Brucellosis: appearance on skeletal imaging. Clin Nucl Med 1987: 13: 102–104.
37. Ariza J, Gudiol F, Pallares R et al. Treatment of human brucellosis with doxycycline plus rifampin or doxycycline plus streptomycin. Ann Intern Med 1992; 117: 25–30.
38. Lubani MM, Dudin KI, Sharda DC et al. A multicenter therapeutic study of 1100 children with brucellosis. Pediatr Infect Dis J 1989; 8: 75–78.
39. Rosenthal J, Brandt KD, Wheat LJ, Salama TG. Rheumatologic manifestations of histoplasmosis in the recent Indianapolis epidemic. Arthritis Rheum 1983; 26: 1065–1070.
40. Cockshot WP, Lucas AO. Histoplasmosis duboisii. Q J Med 1964; 33: 223–328.
41. MacDonald PB, Black GB, MacKenzie R. Orthopaedic manifestations of blastomycosis. J Bone J Surg 1990; 72A: 860–864.
42. Bradsher RW Histoplasmosis and blastomycosis. Clin Infect Dis 1996; 22: S102–S111.
43. Pappas PG, Bradsher RW, Kauffman CA. Treatment of blastomycosis with higher doses of fluconazole. Clin Infect Dis 1997; 25: 200–205.
44. Castañeda OJ, Alarcón GS, Garcia MT, Lumbreras H. Paracoccidioides brasiliensis arthritis. Report of a case and review of the literature. J Rheum 1985; 12: 356–358.
45. Borgia G, Reynaud L, Ceerini R et al. A case of paracoccidioidomycosis: experience with long term therapy. Infection 2000; 28: 119–120.
46. Koster FT, Galgiani JN. Coccidioidal arthritis. In: Espinoza LR, Goldenberg DL, Arnett F, Alarcón GS, eds. Infections in the rheumatic diseases. A comprehensive review of microbial relations to rheumatic disorders. New York: Grune & Stratton; 1988: 165–171.
47. Bayer AS, Guze LB. Fungal arthritis II. Coccidioidal synovitis: clinical, diagnostic, therapeutic and prognostic considerations. Semin Arthritis Rheum 1979; 8: 200–211.
48. Ampel N, Kramer LA, Li L et al. In vitro whole-blood analysis of cellular immunity in patients with active coccidioidomycosis by using the antigen preparation T27K. Clin Diagn Lab Immunol 2002; 9: 1039–1043.
49. Stevens DA. Coccidioidomycosis N Engl J Med 1995; 332: 1077–1082.
50. Behrman RE, Masci JR, Nicholas P. Cryptococcal skeletal infections: case report and review. Rev Infect Dis 1990; 12: 181–190.
51. Liu PY. Cryptococcal osteomyelitis: case report and review. Diagn Microbiol Infect Dis 1998: 30: 33–35.
52. Farr RW, Wright RA. Cryptococcal olecranon bursitis in cirrhosis. J Rheumatol 1992; 19: 172–173.
53. Barnwell PA, Jelsma LF, Raff MJ. Aspergillus osteomyelitis. Report of a case and review of the literature. Diagn Microbiol Infect Dis 1985; 3: 515–519.
54. Rahman NU, Jamjoon ZA, Jamjoon A. Spinal aspergillosis in a nonimmunocompromised host mimicking Pott's paraplegia. Neurosurg Rev 2000; 23: 107–111.
55. Steinfeld S, Durez P, Hauzeur JP et al. Articular aspergillosis: two case reports and review of the literature. Br J Rheumat 1997; 36: 1331–1334.
56. Edwards JE. Candida species. In: Mandell GL, Bennett J, Dolin R, eds. Principles and practice of infectious disease, 5th ed. Edinburgh: Churchill Livingstone; 2000: 2656–2672.
57. Silveira LH, Cuellar ML, Citera G et al. Candida arthritis. Rheum Dis Clin N Am 1993; 19: 427–437.
58. Hansen BL, Andersen K. Fungal arthritis. Scand J Rheumatol 1995; 24: 248–250.
59. Kwon-Chung KJ, Bennett JE. Sporotrichosis. In: Medical mycology. Philadelphia, PA: Lea & Febiger; 1992: 707.
60. Chang AC, Destouet JM, Murphy WA. Musculoskeletal sporotrichosis. Skeletal Radiol 1984; 12: 23–238.
61. Atdjian M, Granda JL, Ingberg HO, Kaplan BL. Systemic sporotrichosis polytenosynovitis with median and ulnar nerve entrapment. JAMA 1980; 243: 1841.
62. Sharkey-Mathis PK, Kauffman CA, Graybill JR et al. Treatment of sporotrichosis with itraconazole. Am J Med 1993; 95: 279.
63. Shaw RA, Stevens MB. The reactive arthritis of giardiasis. A case report. JAMA 1987; 258: 2734–2735.
64. Cron RQ, Sherry DD. Reiter's syndrome associated with cryptosporidial gastroenteritis. J Rheumatol 1995; 22: 1962–1963.
65. Connor BA, Johnson E, Soave R. Reiter syndrome following protracted symptoms of Cyclospora infection. Emerg Infect Dis 2001; 7: 453–454.
66. Gemou V, Messaritakis J, Karpathios T, Kingo A. Chronic polyarthritis of toxoplasmic etiology. Helv Paediatr Acta 1983; 38: 295–296.

67. Field AS, Marriott DJ, Milliken ST *et al*. Myositis associated with a new described microsporidian, *Trachipleistophora hominis*, in a patient with AIDS. J Clin Microbiol 1996; 34: 2803–2811.

68. Cossermelli W, Friedman H, Pastor EH *et al*. Polymyositis in Chagas' disease. Ann Rheum Dis 1978; 37: 277–280.

69. Carmenini G, Toto A, Martusciello S *et al*. Vascular involvement and toxoplasma infection. Br J Dermatol 1991; 124: 114.

70. Bocanegra TS, Espinoza LR, Bridgeford PH *et al*. Reactive arthritis induced by parasitic infection. Ann Intern Med 1981; 94: 207–209.

71. Sawhney BB, Chopra JS, Banerji AK, Wahi PL. Pseudohypertrophic myopathy in cysticercosis. Neurology 1976; 26: 270–272.

72. Takayanagui OM, Chimelli L. Disseminated muscular cysticercosis with myositis induced by praziquantel therapy. Am J Trop Med Hyg 1998; 59: 1002–1003.

73. García Picazo D, Vasquez Aragón P, Palomares Ortiz G *et al*. Multiple hydatidosis of the liver, bones and muscles. Rev Esp Enferm Dig 1995; 87: 267–268.

74. Templeton AC. Human coenurosis. A report of 14 cases from Uganda. Trans R Soc Trop Med Hyg 1968; 62: 251–255.

75. Nakamura T, Hara M, Matsuoka M *et al*. Human proliferative sparganosis. A new Japanese case. Am J Clin Pathol 1990; 94: 224–228.

76. Doury P. Parasitic arthritis and parasitic rheumatism. Sem Hop Paris 1994; 7: 522–528.

77. Akôglu T, Tuncer I, Erken E *et al*. Parasitic arthritis induced by *Strongyloides stercoralis*. Ann Rheum Dis 1984; 43: 523–525.

78. Garf AE. Parasitic rheumatism: rheumatic manifestations associated with calcified guinea worm. J Rheumatol 1985; 12: 976–979.

79. Salfield S. Filarial arthritis in the Sepik district of Papua New Guinea. Med J Aust 1975; 1: 264–267.

80. Carme B, Mamboueni JP, Copin N, Noireau F. Clinical and biological study of Loa-Loa filariases in Congolese. Am J Trop Med Hyg 1989; 41: 331–337.

81. Commandre F, Lapeyre L, Viani JL *et al*. Arthritis associated with filarioses. Rheumatologie 1976; 18: 27–33.

82. Ruiz-Maldonaldo R, Mosqueda-Cabrera M. Human gnathostomiasis (nodular migratory eosinophilic panniculitis). Int J Dermatol 1999; 38: 56–57.

83. Atkin SL, Kamel M, El-Hady AM *et al*. Schistosomiasis and inflammatory polyarthritis: a clinical, radiological and laboratory study of 96 patients infected by *S. mansoni* with particular reference to the diarthrodial joint. Q J Med 1986; 59: 479–487.

84. Bassiouni M, Kamel M. Bilharzial arthropathy. Ann Rheum Dis 1984; 43: 806–809.

85. Dworkin MS, Gamble HR, Zarlenga DS, Tennican PO. Outbreak of trichinellosis associated with eating cougar jerky. J Infect Dis 1996; 174: 663–666.

86. Ferraccioli GF, Mercadanti M, Salaffi F *et al*. Prospective rheumatological study of muscle and joint symptoms during *Trichinella nelsoni* infection. Q J Med 1988; 69: 973–984.

87. Frayha RA. Trichinosis-related polyarteritis nodosa. Am J Med 1981; 71: 307–312.

88. Chanhan A, Scott DGI, Neuberger J *et al*. Churg–Strauss vasculitis and *Ascaris* infection. Ann Rheum Dis 1990; 49: 320–322.

96 Lyme disease and syphilitic arthritis

Allen C Steere

LYME DISEASE

Definition

- A tick-borne infection caused by the spirochete *Borrelia burgdorferi*, *B. afzelii* or *B. garinii* leading to multisystem illness primarily in the skin, joints, nervous system and/or heart

Clinical features

- Peak onset in the summer months in endemic areas in North America, Europe or Asia

- First clinical sign usually a slowly expanding skin lesion, erythema migrans, which occurs at the site of the tick bite

- Disseminated infection often associated with characteristic manifestations in the skin, joints, nervous system and/or heart

- Diagnosis usually based on characteristic clinical findings and a positive IgG serologic test for *B. burgdorferi*

- Treatment with oral antibiotics except for objective neurologic abnormalities, which seem to require intravenous antibiotic therapy

SYPHILITIC ARTHRITIS

Definition

- Osteoarticular lesions occurring in congenital, secondary and tertiary syphilis caused by infection with *Treponema pallidum*

Clinical features

- Diagnosis based on typical clinical patterns of joint involvement, rash and lymphadenopathy, in addition to serologic testing

LYME DISEASE

History

Lyme disease was described as a separate entity in 1976 because of geographic clustering of children in Lyme, Connecticut who were believed to have juvenile rheumatoid arthritis[1]. The rural setting of the case clusters and the identification of erythema migrans as a feature of the illness suggested that the disorder was transmitted by an arthropod. It soon became apparent that Lyme disease was a multisystem illness that affected primarily the skin, nervous system, heart or joints[2]. Epidemiologic studies of patients with erythema migrans implicated certain *Ixodes* ticks as vectors of the disease[3].

In addition to providing clues about the cause of the illness, erythema migrans linked Lyme disease with certain syndromes in Europe. Early in this century, Afzelius in Sweden and Lipschutz in Austria[4] described a characteristic expanding skin lesion, called erythema migrans or erythema chronicum migrans, which they attributed to *Ixodes ricinus* tick bites. Many years later, it was recognized that erythema migrans could be followed by a chronic skin disease, acrodermatitis chronica atrophicans, which had already been described as a separate entity[5]. In the 1940s, Bannwarth in Germany defined a syndrome, also called tick-borne meningo-polyneuritis, that consisted of radicular pain followed by chronic lymphocytic meningitis and sometimes cranial or peripheral neuritis[6]. These various syndromes were brought together conclusively in 1982 and 1983 with the recovery of a previously unrecognized spirochete from the tick vector[7] and from infected patients[8].

Lyme disease or Lyme borreliosis is now recognized as an important infectious disease in North America, Europe and Asia[9]. In the USA, the infection is caused by *Borrelia burgdorferi*, whereas in Europe it is caused primarily by *Borrelia afzelii* and *Borrelia garinii*, and only these two species are responsible for the illness in Asia[10].

Epidemiology

Since surveillance for Lyme disease was begun by the Centers for Disease Control and Prevention in 1982, the number of reported cases has increased dramatically. Currently, about 15 000 cases are reported each year, making Lyme disease the most common vector-borne disease in the USA[11]. The disorder occurs primarily in three distinct foci: in the northeast from Maine to Maryland, in the midwest in Wisconsin and Minnesota, and in the west in northern California and Oregon (Fig. 96. 1). In Europe, Lyme borreliosis is widely established in forested areas[12]. The highest reported frequencies of the disease are in middle Europe and Scandinavia, particularly in Germany, Austria, Slovenia and Sweden. The infection also occurs in Russia, China and Japan.

Lyme borreliosis is transmitted by ticks of the *Ixodes ricinus* complex, including *I. scapularis* in the northeastern and north central USA, *I. pacificus* in the western states, *I. ricinus* in Europe and *I. persulcatus* in Asia[13]. These ticks, which are nearly identical in appearance, have larval, nymphal and adult stages; they require a blood meal at each stage (Fig. 96.2). The risk of infection in a given area depends largely on the density of these ticks, and on their feeding habits and animal hosts, which have evolved differently in different geographic locations.

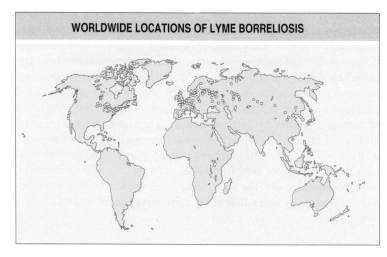

WORLDWIDE LOCATIONS OF LYME BORRELIOSIS

Fig. 96.1 Worldwide locations of Lyme borreliosis. The yellow dots show affected locations in North America, Europe and Asia.

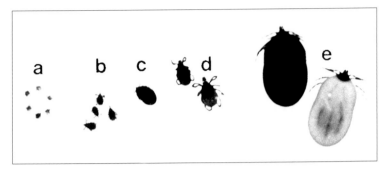

Fig. 96.2 The life-cycle stages of *Ixodes scapularis*, the tick that transmits Lyme disease in the northeastern and north central USA. (a) Tiny larval ticks, which are <1mm in diameter. (b) Unengorged nymphal ticks, which are only 1–2mm in diameter. This stage of the tick is primarily responsible for transmission of the spirochete to humans during the late spring and early summer. (c) An engorged nymphal tick. (d) Unengorged adult male (black) and female (orange) ticks. (e) Engorged adult male and female ticks.

In the north eastern and north central USA, *I. scapularis* (also called *I. dammini*) ticks are abundant, and a highly efficient cycle of *B. burgdorferi* transmission occurs between immature larval and nymphal *I. scapularis* and white-footed mice[14], resulting in high infection rates in nymphal ticks and a high frequency of human Lyme disease during the late spring and summer months[11]. The vector ecology of *B. burgdorferi* is quite different on the West coast in northern California and Oregon[15]. There, the frequency of Lyme disease is low because nymphal *I. pacifius* ticks often feed on lizards rather than rodents, and lizards are not susceptible to *B. burgdorferi* infection. Similarly, in the southeastern USA, nymphal *I. scapularis* feed primarily on lizards, and *B. burgdorferi* infection occurs rarely, if at all, in that part of the country. There, a skin rash resembling erythema migrans, which is not caused by *B. burgdorferi*, has been associated with the bite of the Lone-Star tick[16].

Etiologic agent

As with all spirochetes, the *Borrelia* species have a protoplasmic cylinder surrounded by periplasm containing the flagella, which is surrounded, in turn, by an outer membrane (Fig. 96.3).[17] The unique feature of *Borrelia* species is that a number of their outer membrane proteins are encoded by plasmid genes. Recently, the complete genome of *B. burgdorferi* sensu stricto (strain B31) was sequenced[18]. The genome is quite small (approximately 1.5 megabases) and consists of a highly unusual linear chromosome of 950kb, in addition to nine linear and 12 circular plasmids.

The remarkable aspect of the *B. burgdorferi* genome is the large number of sequences for predicted or known lipoproteins[18], including the plasmid-encoded outer-surface proteins (Osp) A–F. These and other differentially expressed outer-surface proteins presumably help the spirochete to adapt to and survive in markedly different arthropod and mammalian environments[19]. In addition, during early, disseminated infection, a surface-exposed lipoprotein, called VlsE, has been reported to undergo extensive antigenic variation[20]. The organism has a minimal number of proteins with biosynthetic activity and apparently depends on the host for much of its nutritional requirements[18]. The genome contains no homologs for systems specialized in the secretion of toxins or other virulence factors. The only known virulence factors of *B. burgdorferi* are surface proteins that allow spirochetal attachment to mammalian cells.

Pathogenesis

To maintain its complex life enzootic cycle, *B. burgdorferi* must adapt to two markedly different environments, the tick and the mammalian

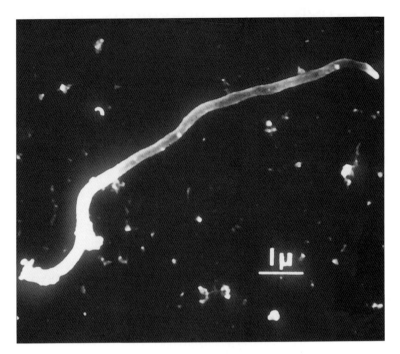

Fig. 96.3 Scanning electron micrograph of *Borrelia burgdorferi*. The *Borrelia* spp. are longer and more loosely coiled than the other spirochetes. Of the *Borrelia* spp., *B. burgdorferi* is the longest (20–30μm) and narrowest (0.2–0.3μm).

host[21]. In the midgut of the tick, the spirochete expresses OspA and OspB, two closely related proteins[22]. When the blood meal is taken, OspC is upregulated as the organism traverses to the tick salivary gland and to the mammalian host[23]. After injection by the tick, the spirochete usually spreads locally in the skin, and within days to weeks it may disseminate. *B. burgdorferi* has a number of mechanisms that may aid dissemination. For example, OspC sequences vary considerably among strains, and only a few of the OspC sequence groups are associated with disseminated disease[24]. Spread through skin and other tissue matrices may be facilitated by the spirochete's binding of human plasminogen and its activators to its surface[25]. The organism migrates through the endothelium primarily at intracellular junctions, but may also penetrate through the cytoplasm of the cell[26]. During dissemination and homing to specific sites, the organism attaches to certain host integrins[27], matrix glycosaminoglycans[28] and extracellular matrix proteins[29]. For example, *Borrelia* decorin binding proteins A and B bind decorin, a glycosaminoglycan on collagen fibrils, which may explain why the organism is commonly aligned with collagen fibrils in the extracellular matrix in the heart, nervous system or joints[30]. Decorin-deficient mice have lesser bacterial colonization of joints and milder arthritis than normal mice of the same strain that express decorin[31].

As shown definitively in murine models, proinflammatory innate immune responses are critical in the control of early, disseminated infection[32,33]. Spirochetal lipoproteins, which bind the CD14 molecule and Toll-like receptor-2 on macrophages, are potent activators of the innate immune response, leading to the production of macrophage-derived proinflammatory cytokines[34]. In addition, T helper 1 cells (Th1), which are a part of the adaptive immune response, are prominent early in the murine infection[35]. In humans, infiltrates of macrophages and T cells in erythema migrans lesions express mRNA for both proinflammatory (Th1) and anti-inflammatory (Th2) cytokines[36]. Particularly in disseminated infection, adaptive T and B cell responses in lymph nodes lead to antibody production to many components of the organism[37,38].

Spread of *B. burgdorferi* within the nervous system has been demonstrated in non-human primates[39], which are the only known animal model of neuroborreliosis. In immunosuppressed monkeys, which had a larger spirochetal burden than immunocompetent animals, *B. burgdorferi* localized to the leptomeninges, motor and sensory nerve roots and dorsal root ganglia, but not to the brain parenchyma[40]. In the peripheral nervous system, spirochetes were seen in the perineurium, the connective tissue sheath surrounding each bundle of peripheral nerve fibers.

During attacks of arthritis in human patients, innate immune responses are found to *B. burgdorferi* lipoproteins, and $\gamma\delta$ T cells in joint fluid may aid in this response[41]. In addition, marked adaptive immune responses are seen to many spirochetal proteins[38,42]. A borrelia-specific, proinflammatory Th1 response is concentrated in joint fluid[43,44], but anti-inflammatory (Th2) cytokines are also present[44]. Furthermore, patients with Lyme arthritis usually have higher borrelia-specific antibody titers than patients with any other manifestation of the illness, including late neuroborreliosis[38,45]. In the murine infection, antibody responses are critical in the resolution of arthritis[46,47], whereas cellular responses are the dominant factor in resolution of the cardiac lesion[48,49].

Compared with patients with treatment responsive arthritis, those with a treatment-resistant course have an increased frequency of HLA-DRBI*0401 or related alleles, and they more often have cellular and humoral immune responses to OspA[42,50]. It has been proposed that autoimmunity may develop within the proinflammatory milieu of affected joints in patients with treatment-resistant arthritis because of molecular mimicry between an immunodominant T cell epitope of OspA (OspA$_{165-173}$) of *B. burgdorferi* and a similar sequence in a human protein, perhaps human lymphocyte function associated antigen-1 (hLFA-1$\alpha_{332-340}$)[51], an adhesion molecule that is highly expressed on T cells in synovium[52]. OspA$_{165-173}$-reactive T cells are concentrated in the joints of these patients[53]. When hLFA-1$\alpha_{332-340}$ is processed and presented by the DRB1*0401 molecule, this self peptide may behave as a partial agonist for such cells[54]. However, hLFA-1 may not be the only, or even the most important, autoantigen in treatment-resistant Lyme arthritis.

Clinical features

As with syphilis, Lyme disease generally occurs in stages, with different clinical manifestations at each stage. Early infection consists of stage 1 (localized erythema migrans), followed within days to weeks by stage 2 (disseminated infection particularly affecting the nervous system, heart or joints), followed within weeks to months by late infection (stage 3, persistent infection)[55]. The basic outlines of the disease are similar worldwide, but there are regional variations, primarily between America and Eurasia (Table 96.1).

Skin manifestations

Erythema migrans and early disseminated infection, and acrodermatitis

In 80% or more of American patients, Lyme disease begins with a slowly expanding skin lesion, erythema migrans, which occurs at the site of the tick bite (Fig. 96.4)[56]. As the area around the center expands, most lesions develop bright red outer borders with partial central clearing. The centers of early lesions sometimes become intensely erythematous and indurated, vesicular or necrotic. In Europe, erythema migrans is often an indolent, localized infection, whereas this lesion in the USA is associated with more intense inflammation and signs that often

---

TABLE 96.1 COMPARISON OF LYME DISEASE IN NORTH AMERICA AND EURASIA

Systems affected	North America (*B. burgdorferi*)	Europe and Asia (*B. afzelii* or *B. garinii*)
Skin		
Acute phase	Erythema migrans faster spreading, more intensely inflamed, and of briefer duration; frequent, possibly widespread hematogenous dissemination	Erythema migrans slower spreading, less intensely inflamed and of longer duration; less frequent hematogeneous dissemination, but possible regional or contiguous spread to other sites
Chronic phase	Acrodermatitis rarely reported	Acrodermatitis chronica atrophicans, caused primarily by *B. afzelii*
Nervous system		
Acute phase	Meningitis, severe headache, mild neck stiffness, less prominent radiculoneuritis	Severe radicular pain and pleocytosis, less prominent headache and neck stiffness, caused particularly by *B. garinii*
Chronic phase	Subtle sensory polyneuropathy without acrodermatitis Subtle encephalopathy, cognitive disturbance, slight intrathecal antibody production	Subtle sensory polyneuropathy within areas affected by acrodermatitis Severe sensory polyneuropathy within areas affected by acrodermatitis Severe encephalomyelitis, spasticity, cognitive abnormalities, and marked intrathecal antibody production, caused primarily by *B. garinii*
Cardiac		
Acute phase	Atrioventricular block and subtle myocarditis	Atrioventricular block and subtle myocarditis
Chronic phase	None reported	Dilated cardiomyopathy
Arthritis		
Acute phase	More frequent oligoarticular arthritis, more intense joint inflammation	Less frequent oligoarticular arthritis, less intense joint inflammation
Chronic phase	Treatment-resistant arthritis in about 10 percent of patients, probably due to autoimmune mechanism	Persistent arthritis rare, probably not due to an autoimmune mechanism
Asymptomatic infection		
	In about 10 percent of patients	In more than 10 percent of patients
Antibody response		
	Expansion of response to many spirochetal proteins	Expansion of response to fewer spirochetal proteins

(With permission from Steere[9].)

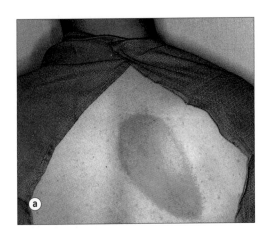

Fig. 96.4 Erythema migrans of Lyme disease. Lyme disease usually begins with a slowly expanding skin lesion, erythema migrans, that occurs at the site of a tick bite. (a) Classic erythema migrans skin lesion (10cm in diameter) on the back. The lesion has a redder outer border, with slight central clearing. (b) Pale lesion (7cm in diameter) with several vesicles in the center, near the groin. (c) Pale lesion (5cm in diameter) with a target center over the iliac crest. In each instance, *B. burgdorferi* was isolated from a skin biopsy sample of the lesion. (Courtesy of Dr Vijay Sikand, East Lyme, CT, USA.)

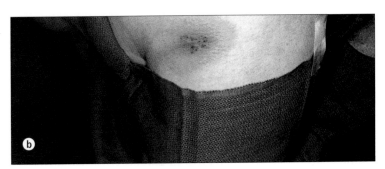

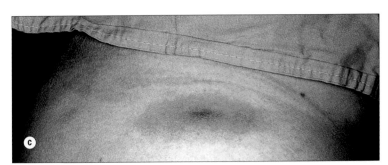

suggest dissemination of the spirochete[57]. In one study, spirochetes were cultured from plasma samples in 50% of American patients with erythema migrans[58].

Although the list of the possible manifestations of the disease is long (Table 96.2), disseminated infection is often associated with characteristic symptoms in the skin, nervous system or musculoskeletal sites[55,56]. Excruciating headache, particularly in the back of the head, and mild neck stiffness are common – a picture that raises the possibility of meningitis. Among 12 patients who had such symptoms associated with erythema migrans, eight had a positive test for *B. burgdorferi* DNA in cerebrospinal fluid, but none had a spinal fluid pleocytosis at that time[59]. The musculoskeletal pain is often migratory in joints, bursae, tendons, muscle or bone, lasting only hours in a given location. Fever, if present, is typically low grade, except in young children. At this stage, patients often have debilitating malaise and fatigue.

In European patients, especially elderly women with *B. afzelii* infection, a chronic, slowly progressive skin condition called acrodermatitis chronica atrophicans may develop on sun-exposed acral surfaces[60]. These lesions, which may be the presenting manifestation of the disease, may last for many years, and *B. burgdorferi* has been cultured from such lesions as late as 10 years after disease onset[61].

Neurologic manifestations

Within weeks, during or shortly after the period of early disseminated infection, about 15% of untreated patients in the USA develop objective signs and symptoms of acute neuroborreliosis[55,62]. Possible manifestations include lymphocytic meningitis with episodic headache and mild neck stiffness, subtle encephalitis with difficulty with mental functioning, cranial neuropathy (particularly unilateral or bilateral facial palsy), motor or sensory radiculoneuritis, mononeuritis multiplex, cerebellar ataxia or myelitis[62–64]. In Europe, the first neurologic sign is often radicular pain, which is followed by the development of a pleocytosis in cerebrospinal fluid, but meningeal or encephalitic signs are more often absent[65]. In children, the optic nerve may also be affected because of inflammation or increased intracranial pressure, which may lead to blindness[66]. However, even in untreated patients, acute neurologic involvement typically improves or resolves within weeks to months.

In 5% or fewer of untreated patients, *B. burgdorferi* may cause chronic neuroborreliosis, sometimes after long periods of latent infection[67]. In both America and Europe, a chronic axonal polyneuropathy may develop, manifested primarily as spinal radicular pain or distal paresthesias[65,67,68]. Electromyograms typically show diffuse involvement of both proximal and distal nerve segments. In Europe, *B. garinii* may cause chronic encephalomyelitis, characterized by spastic paraparesis, cranial neuropathy, or cognitive impairment with marked intrathecal antibody production to the spirochete[65]. In the USA, a mild, late neurologic syndrome has been reported, called Lyme encephalopathy, manifested primarily by subtle cognitive disturbances[67,69,70]. Although inflammatory changes are lacking in cerebrospinal fluid, intrathecal production of antibodies to the spirochete can often be demonstrated. One unusual case of *B. burgdorferi*-induced meningoencephalitis and cerebral vasculitis has been reported that was unresponsive to antibiotics[71]. In this case, a T cell clone recovered from cerebrospinal fluid responded both to spirochetal epitopes and autoantigens.

Carditis

Within several weeks after disease onset, about 5% of untreated patients have acute cardiac involvement, most commonly fluctuating degrees of atrioventricular block, or occasionally acute myopericarditis, mild left ventricular dysfunction or, rarely, cardiomegaly or fatal pancarditis[55,72]. The duration of cardiac abnormalities is usually brief (between 3 days and 6 weeks); complete heart block usually does not persist for longer than 1 week, and insertion of a permanent pacemaker is not necessary[73]. One elderly patient, who was co-infected with *B. burgdorferi* and *Babesia microtii*, died from cardiac involvement of the infection[74]. In Europe, *B. burgdorferi* has been isolated from endomyocardial biopsies of several patients with chronic dilated cardiomyopathy[75,76]. However, this complication has not been observed in the USA[77].

Joint involvement

Months after the onset of illness, about 60% of untreated patients in the USA have intermittent attacks of joint swelling and pain, primarily in large joints, especially the knee, over a period of several years (Fig. 96.5)[55,78]. However, other large and small joints, the temporomandibular joint or

TABLE 96.2 MANIFESTATIONS OF LYME DISEASE BY STAGE

System	Early infection Localized Stage 1	Early infection Disseminated Stage 2	Late infection Persistent Stage 3
Skin	Erythema migrans	Secondary annular lesions Malar rash Diffuse erythema or urticaria Evanescent lesions Lymphocytoma	Acrodermatitis chronica atrophicans Localized scleroderma-like lesions
Musculoskeletal		Migratory pain in joints, tendons bursae, muscle, bone Brief arthritis attacks Myositis Osteomyelitis Panniculitis	Prolonged arthritis attacks Chronic arthritis Peripheral enthesopathy Periostitis or joint subluxations below lesions of acrodermatitis
Neurologic		Meningitis Cranial neuritis, Bell's palsy Motor or sensory radiculoneuritis Subtle encephalitis Mononeuritis multiplex Myelitis Chorea Cerebellar ataxia	Chronic encephalomyelitis Subtle encephalopathy Chronic axonal polyradiculopathy
Lymphatic	Regional lympadenopathy	Regional or generalized Lymphadenopathy Splenomegaly	
Heart		Atrioventricular nodal block Myopericarditis Pancarditis	
Eyes		Conjunctivitis Iritis Choroiditis Retinal hemorrhage or detachment Panophthalmitis	Keratitis
Liver		Mild hepatitis	
Respiratory		Non-exudative sore throat	
Kidney		Microscopic hematuria or proteinuria	
Genitourinary		Orchitis	
Constitutional symptoms	Minor	Severe malaise and fatigue	Fatigue

The systems are listed from the most to the least commonly affected. The staging system provides a guideline for the expected timing of the different manifestations of the illness, but this may vary in an individual case. (With permission from Steere[55].)

periarticular sites are sometimes affected (Table 96.3). Affected knees may be very swollen and warm, but not particularly painful. Baker's cysts may form and rupture early. Attacks of arthritis, which usually affect only one or a few joints at a time, last from a few weeks to months, separated by longer periods of complete remission. The total number of patients who continue to have recurrent attacks of arthritis decreases by about 10–20% each year. A clinical course with arthritis as the only feature of the illness may be more common in children than in adults, and joint involvement may be milder in young children than in older children[79–81].

Usually, after several brief attacks of arthritis, about 10% of untreated patients develop chronic Lyme arthritis, defined as 1 year or more of continuous joint inflammation[78]. Similarly, in about 10% of patients, particularly those with human leukocyte antigen-DRB1*0401 or related alleles[82,83], the arthritis persists in knees for months or even several years after intravenous or oral antibiotic treatment for 30 or 60 days, respectively[84]. Polymerase chain reaction (PCR) tests for *B. burgdorferi* DNA in synovium or joint fluid are usually negative after this treat-

ment[85,86], suggesting that live spirochetes have been eradicated by it. An autoimmune pathogenesis has been proposed to explain this treatment-resistant course[42,51]. However, even chronic Lyme arthritis eventually remits spontaneously[78].

In Europe, the pattern of arthritis is similar with that in the USA, but the frequency of arthritis and the intensity of joint inflammation are less, and chronic arthritis is rare[87,88].

Investigations

B. burgdorferi can be cultured in a complex liquid medium called Barbour–Stoenner–Kelly medium[8], which permits definitive diagnosis. However, except in a few cases, positive cultures have been obtained only early in the illness, primarily from biopsies of erythema migrans lesions[89], less often from plasma samples[58] and only occasionally from cerebrospinal fluid samples in patients with meningitis[64]. The principal role for PCR testing in Lyme disease is in the detection of *B. burgdorferi* DNA from joint fluid[85], which is greatly superior to culture for this purpose. Although *B. burgdorferi* DNA has been detected in cere-

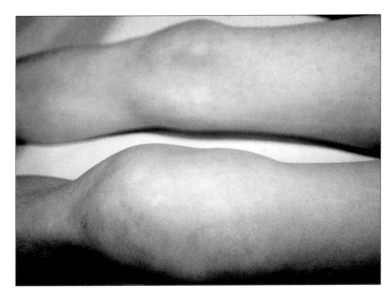

Fig. 96.5 The swollen knee of a 9-year-old child with Lyme arthritis. In the USA, affected knees may be very swollen and warm, but not particularly painful. In Europe and Asia, the amount of joint swelling is often less.

TABLE 96.3 JOINT AND PERIARTICULAR INVOLVEMENT IN LYME DISEASE. JOINTS AND PERIARTICULAR SITES AFFECTED IN 28 UNTREATED PATIENTS WITH LYME DISEASE

Joint	No. of patients (*n*=28)	Periarticular site	No. of patients (*n*=28)
Knee	27	Tendons	
Shoulder	14	Back	9
Ankle	12	Neck	6
Elbow	11	Bicipital	4
Temporomandibular	11	Lateral epicondyle	2
Wrist	10	Lateral collateral	1
Hip	9	De Quervain's	1
Metacarpophalangeal	4	Bursae	
Proximal interphalangeal	4	Prepatellar	4
Distal interphalangeal	4	Subacromial	2
Metatarsophalangeal	4	Infraspinatus	2
Sternoclavicular	1	Olecranon	2
		Sausage digits	2
		Heel pain	2

(With permission from Steere[78].)

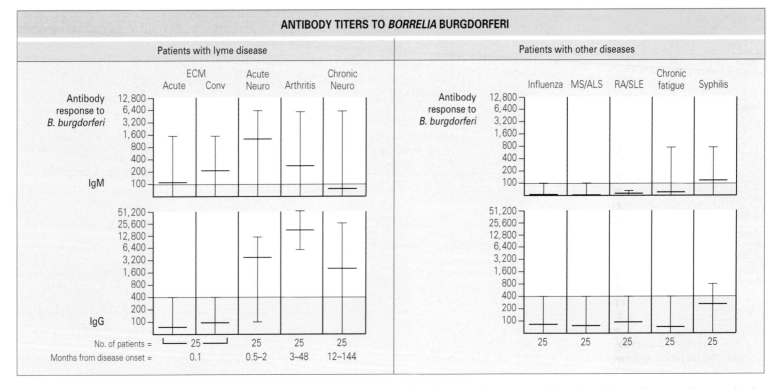

Fig. 96.6 Antibody titers to *Borrelia burgdorferi*. Titers acquired by ELISA in patients from the USA with various manifestations of Lyme disease and in control individuals. Horizontal bars, mean; vertical bars, range; hatched bars, normal range derived from sera from 50 normal control individuals. Acute neuro, meningitis; ALS, amyotrophic lateral sclerosis; Chronic neuro, encephalopathy or polyneuropathy; Conv, convalescent phase; EM, erythema migrans; MS, multiple sclerosis; RA, rheumatoid arthritis; SLE, systemic lupus erythematosus. (With permission from Dressler *et al.*[45])

brospinal fluid by PCR among patients with acute or chronic neuroborreliosis[90,91], it is a low-yield procedure. The Lyme urine antigen test, which has given grossly unreliable results[92], should not be used to support the diagnosis of Lyme disease.

In patients in the USA, the diagnosis is usually based on the recognition of a characteristic clinical picture, together with exposure in an endemic area and, except in those with erythema migrans, a positive antibody response to *B. burgdorferi* by enzyme-linked immunosorbent assay (ELISA) and western blot, interpreted according to the Centers for Disease Control/Association of State and Territorial Public Health

Laboratory Directors' criteria (Figs 96.6 & 96.7, Table 96.4)[45,93,94]. In Europe, where there is less expansion of the antibody response, no single set of criteria for immunoblot interpretation give high levels of sensitivity and specificity in all countries[95].

Serodiagnosis is insensitive during the first several weeks of infection. In the USA, approximately 20–30% of patients have positive responses, usually of the IgM isotype, during this period[45,96], but by convalescence 2–4 weeks later, about 70–80% have seroreactivity, even after antibiotic treatment. After 1 month, the great majority of patients with active infection have positive IgG antibody responses[45]. In persons with illness

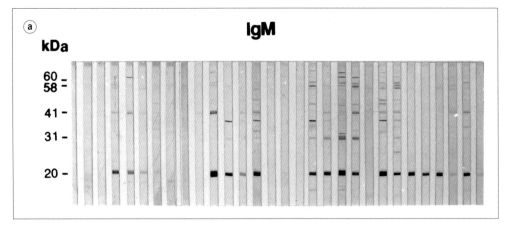

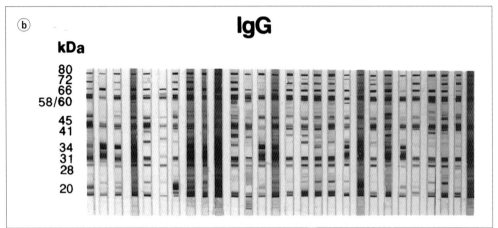

Fig. 96.7 Western blots showing positive responses for antibody to *B. burgdorferi*. (a) IgM western blot in 25 patients with erythema migrans. (b) IgG western blot in 25 patients with Lyme arthritis. In patients with erythema migrans, the IgM response is directed particularly against the 23kDa OspC protein and the 41kDa flagellar protein of the spirochete. Months to years after disease onset, in patients with Lyme arthritis, the IgG response is directed against many spirochetal proteins. Molecular mass markers (kDa) are shown at the left. (With permission from Dressler *et al.*[45])

TABLE 96.4 LYME DISEASE NATIONAL SURVEILLANCE CASE DEFINITION*

A case of Lyme disease is defined as follows:
1. A person with erythema migrans, observed by a physician.
   This skin lesion expands slowly over days to weeks to form a large round lesion, often with central clearing. To be counted for surveillance purposes, a solitary lesion must reach a size of at least 5cm
2. A person with at least one later manifestation and laboratory evidence of infection.
   Nervous system: Lymphocytic meningitis, cranial neuritis, radiculoneuropathy or, rarely, encephalomyelitis, alone or in combination. For encephalomyelitis to be counted for surveillance purposes, there must be evidence of intrathecal antibody production against *B. burgdorferi* in cerebrospinal fluid
   Cardiovascular system: Acute-onset, high-grade (2nd or 3rd degree) atrioventricular conduction defects that resolve in days to weeks and are sometimes associated with myocarditis
   Musculoskeletal system: Recurrent, brief attacks (weeks to months) of objective joint swelling in one or a few joints, sometimes followed by chronic arthritis in one or a few joints
3. Laboratory evidence.
   Isolation of *B. burgdorferi* from tissue or body fluid or detection of diagnostic levels of antibody to the spirochete by the two-test approach of ELISA and western blot, interpreted according to the Centers for Disease Control/Association of State and Territorial Public Health Laboratory Directors' criteria.*

* In a person with acute disease of less than 1 month duration, IgM and IgG antibody responses should be measured in acute and convalescent serum samples. An IgM western blot is considered positive if at least two of the following three bands are present: 23, 39 or 41kDa. An IgG blot is considered positive if at least five of the following 10 bands are present: 18, 23, 28, 30, 39, 41, 45, 58, 66 or 93kDa. Only the IgG response should be used to support the diagnosis after the first 1 month of infection. After that time, an IgM response alone is likely to be a false-positive result

(Adapted from recommendations made by the Centers for Disease Control and Prevention[92,93]; with permission from Steere[9].)

---

for longer than 1 month, a positive IgM test alone is likely to be a false-positive result, and therefore this response should not be used to support the diagnosis of Lyme disease after the first 1 month of infection. Several second-generation tests that use recombinant spirochetal proteins or synthetic peptides have shown promising results[97,98].

In patients with neuroborreliosis, especially in those with meningitis, intrathecal production of IgM, IgG or IgA antibody to *B. burgdorferi* may often be demonstrated by antibody capture enzyme immunoassay[99]. In patients with peripheral nervous system involvement, electromyograms typically show an axonal polyneuropathy or radiculoneuropathy, with diffuse involvement of both proximal and distal nerve segments[68]. Neither single photon emission computed tomography scanning of the brain[100] nor neuropsychological tests of memory[101] have sufficient specificity to be helpful in diagnosis.

Patients with Lyme carditis usually have fluctuating degrees of atrioventricular nodal block or, sometimes, more generalized repolarization abnormalities, including ST segment or T-wave changes[72,73]. Occasionally, they may have radionuclide evidence of mild left ventricular dysfunction and, rarely, chest radiographs may reveal cardiomegaly.

Among patients with Lyme arthritis, joint fluid white cells counts range from 500 to 110 000 cells/mm³, most of which, in patients with high white cell counts, are polymorphonuclear leukocytes[78]. Although tests for rheumatoid factor and antinuclear antibodies are usually negative, small amounts of rheumatoid factor[102] or antinuclear antibodies in low titer[81] may be detected. The most common radiographic finding is knee joint effusion[103]. Later in the illness, the joints of some patients with chronic arthritis show the typical changes of an inflammatory arthritis, including juxta-articular osteoporosis, cartilage loss and cortical or marginal bone erosions. Before antibiotic treatment, PCR tests for *B. burgdorferi* DNA in joint fluid are usually positive[85]. *B. burgdorferi* DNA may be detected more readily in synovial tissue than in synovial fluid[104,105]. The spirochete has been cultured only rarely from affected joints[106].

After antibiotic treatment, antibody titers decrease slowly, but IgG and even IgM responses may persist for many years after treatment[107]. Thus even a positive IgM response cannot by interpreted as showing recent infection or reinfection unless the appropriate clinical picture is present. *B. burgdorferi* may also cause asymptomatic infection in approximately 10% of patients in the USA[108], and in a greater percentage in Europe[109]. In tests that use whole sonicated spirochetes as the antigen preparation, vaccination for Lyme disease may cause positive IgG results by ELISA, but vaccine-induced or infection-induced antibody responses may usually be differentiated by western blotting[108]. If patients with past or asymptomatic infection or vaccine-induced immunity have symptoms caused by another illness, the danger is that they may be attributed incorrectly to Lyme disease.

Differential diagnosis
Coinfection

I. scapularis ticks transmit not only *B. burgdorferi*, but also other infectious agents, including a red blood cell parasite, *Babesia microtii*, and the agent of human granulocytic ehrlichiosis, *Anaplasma phagocytophila* Ehrlichiosis may cause a flu-like illness associated with high fever, particularly in elderly individuals[110]. *Babesia microti* usually causes only mild or asymptomatic infection, but in elderly or asplenic individuals, it may result in a severe, malaria-like illness[111]. Of 240 patients diagnosed with Lyme disease in Connecticut, 26 (11%) were coinfected with *Babesia*[112]. Of 52 persons with IgG titers positive for *B. burgdorferi*, two (4%) had IgG antibodies to the human granulocytic ehrlichia agent[113]. When patients are coinfected with *B. burgdorferi* and one or both of these other tick-borne pathogens, they may have more severe illness[112].

Evidence for these infections includes the identification of ehrlichia or babesia DNA by PCR in blood tests or IgG seroconversion between acute and convalescent serum samples, determined by indirect immunofluorescence. Serologic diagnosis is confounded by the fact that ehrlichia infection may produce a false-positive IgM western blot for Lyme disease[114]. Neither *Babesia* nor *Ehrlichia* is known to cause chronic disease such as occurs with untreated *B. burgdorferi* infection.

Positive Lyme serology and non-specific symptoms

Patients may develop pain, fatigue or neurocognitive syndromes soon after contracting Lyme disease, and in some cases these symptoms may persist for years[115,116]. These patients have an array of subjective symptoms, including debilitating fatigue, diffuse musculoskeletal pain, cognitive difficulty and sleep disturbance, usually accompanied by normal neurologic and neurocognitive test results. This clinical picture, which is sometimes called post-Lyme disease or chronic Lyme disease syndrome, is similar to chronic fatigue syndrome or fibromyalgia. This postinfectious syndrome occurs more frequently in patients whose symptoms are suggestive of early dissemination of the spirochete to the nervous system, particularly if treatment is delayed[117,118]. However, in one large study, the frequency of symptoms of pain and fatigue was no greater in patients who had had Lyme disease than in age-matched individuals who had not had this infection[119]. In contrast with the experience with chronic neuroborreliosis, these syndromes are not cured by further antibiotic treatment[120].

Lyme arthritis or other rheumatic disease?

Lyme arthritis typically causes marked joint swelling and pain in one or a few joints at a time, with minimal systemic symptoms[78]. This clinical picture is most like reactive arthritis (Reiter's syndrome) in adults, or pauciarticular juvenile rheumatoid arthritis in children. Lyme arthritis does not cause chronic, symmetrical polyarthritis and therefore distinguishing Lyme arthritis from rheumatoid arthritis is not difficult. Fibromyalgia and chronic fatigue syndrome are commonly

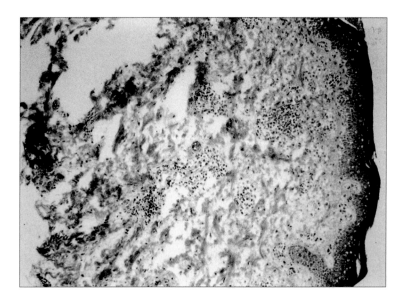

Fig. 96.8 Histopathology of lesional skin in patient with erythema migrans. The lesion shows a moderate infiltration of mononuclear cells, primarily lymphocytes, macrophages and, sometimes, a few plasma cells in the papillary rather than the reticular dermis. Section stained with hematoxylin and eosin. Original magnification ×100.

misdiagnosed as Lyme disease[115,121,122]. In contrast with Lyme arthritis, patients with fibromyalgia often have marked fatigue, severe headache, diffuse musculoskeletal pain, stiffness and pain in many joints, diffuse dysesthesias, difficulty with concentration and sleep disturbance. On physical examination, such patients have several symmetric tender points in characteristic locations, but they lack evidence of joint inflammation.

Histology

B. burgdorferi has been seen in small numbers in most affected tissues. Histologically, these tissues usually show an infiltration of lymphocytes and macrophages with some plasma cells (Fig. 96.8)[36,123,124]. Synovial tissue from patients with chronic Lyme arthritis shows synovial hypertrophy, vascular proliferation, stromal deposition of fibrin and infiltration of mononuclear cells, sometimes with pseudolymphoid follicles (Fig. 96.9)[125,126]. This picture is similar to that found in the various forms of chronic inflammatory arthritis, including rheumatoid arthritis. However, compared with other synovial diseases, some degree of vascular damage, including obliterative microvascular lesions, seem to be found only in Lyme synovia.

Management

Evidence-based treatment recommendations for Lyme disease were recently presented by the Infectious Diseases Society of America[127] (Table 96.5). In general, Lyme disease can be treated effectively with appropriate oral antibiotic agents, except for neurologic abnormalities, which seem to require treatment with intravenous antibiotics. The American College of Physicians has also developed an algorithm to guide testing and treatment, depending on the pretest probability of Lyme disease[128]. According to this algorithm, empirical antibiotic therapy without serologic testing is recommended for patients with a high pre-test probability of Lyme disease (such as those with erythema migrans), two-step testing (by ELISA and, if positive, by western blot) is recommended for patients with an intermediate pre-test probability (such as those with recurrent oligoarticular arthritis), and neither testing nor treatment is recommended for those with a low pre-test probability (such as those with non-specific symptoms of myalgia, arthralgias and fatigue).

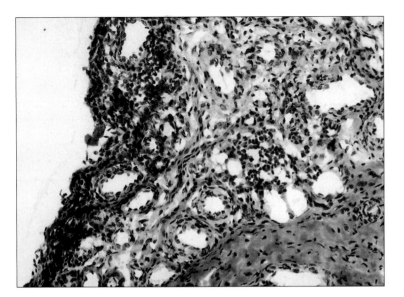

Fig. 96.9 Cellular architecture and infiltrating cells in synovial tissue from a patient with treatment-resistant Lyme arthritis. The tissue shows villous hypertrophy, synovial cell hyperplasia, vascular proliferation and an infiltration of mononuclear cells. Section stained with hematoxylin and eosin. Original magnification ×200.

Early localized or disseminated infection

For early localized or disseminated infection, doxycycline for 14 to 21 days is recommended in persons older than 8 years of age, except for pregnant women (Table 96.5). An advantage of doxycycline is its efficacy against the agent of human granulocytic ehrlichiosis, a possible coinfecting agent. Amoxicillin, the second-choice alternative, should be used in children or pregnant women. In case of allergy, cefuroxime axetil is a third-choice alternative. Erythromycin or its cogeners, which are fourth-choice alternatives, are recommended only for patients who are unable to take doxycycline, amoxicillin or cefuroxime axetil. Because maternal–fetal transmission of *B. burgdorferi* seems to occur rarely, if at all[129], standard treatment for the manifestation of the illness is recommended.

In multicenter studies of patients with erythema migrans, similar results were obtained with doxycycline, amoxicillin and cefuroxime axetil, and more than 90% of patients had satisfactory outcomes[130,131]. Although some patients had subjective symptoms after treatment, objective evidence of persistent infection or relapse was rare, and retreatment was usually not needed. Intravenous ceftriaxone, although effective, was not superior to oral agents as long as the patient did not have objective neurological involvement[132]. In contrast with second- and third-generation cephalosporin antibiotics, first-generation cephalosporins, such as cephalexin, were ineffective[133].

Neurologic abnormalities

For patients with objective neurologic abnormalities, 2- to 4-week courses of intravenous ceftriaxone are most commonly given[67,70,134] Parenteral treatment with cefotaxime or penicillin G may be a satisfactory alternative[135]. The signs and symptoms of acute neuroborreliosis usually resolve within weeks, but those of chronic neuroborreliosis improve slowly over a period of months. Objective evidence of relapse is rare after a 4-week course of treatment. In Europe, oral doxycycline may be adequate treatment for acute neuroborreliosis[136]. Although this medication may be used successfully in patients with facial palsy alone in the USA, it is important to assess whether such patients have more diffuse involvement of the nervous system, which is best treated with intravenous therapy. Lyme encephalopathy may be treated successfully with a 1-month course of intravenous ceftriaxone[70], but immune-mediated or postinfectious phenomena may also play a part in the pathogenesis of these syndromes.

TABLE 96.5 TREATMENT REGIMENS FOR LYME DISEASE

Early infection (local or disseminated)

Adults
    Doxycycline, 100mg orally twice daily for 14–21 days
    Amoxicillin, 500mg orally three times daily for 14–21 days
or (alternatives in case of doxycycline or amoxicillin allergy):
    Cefuroxime axetil, 500 mg orally twice daily for 14–21 days
    Erythromycin, 250 mg orally 4 times a day for 14–21 days

Children (age 8 years or less)
    Amoxicillin, 250mg orally three times a day or 50mg/kg per day in three divided doses for 14–21 days
or (alternatives in case of penicillin allergy):
    Cefuroxime axetil, 125mg orally twice daily or 30mg/kg per day in two divided doses for 14–21 days
    Erythromycin, 250mg orally three times a day or 30mg/kg per day in three divided doses for 14–21 days

Neurologic abnormalities (early or late)

Adults
    Ceftriaxone 2g i.v. once a day for 14–28 days
    Cefotaxime, 2g i.v. every eight hours for 14–28 days
    Na penicillin G, 3.3×10^6U i.v. every 4h for 14–28 days
or (alternative in case of ceftriaxone or penicillin allergy):
    Doxycycline, 100mg orally three times a day for 30 days, but this regimen may be ineffective for late neuroborreliosis
    Facial palsy alone: oral regimens may be adequate

Children (age 8 years or less)
    Ceftriaxone, 75–100mg/kg per day (maximum 2g) i.v. once a day for 14–28 days
    Cefotaxime, 150mg/kg per day in three or four divided doses (maximum 6g) for 14–28 days
    Na penicillin G, 200 000–400 000U/kg per day in six divided doses for 14–28 days

Arthritis (intermittent or chronic)

    Oral regimens listed above for 30–60 days
or
    i.v. regimens listed above for 14–28 days

Cardiac abnormalities

    First-degree atrioventricular block: oral regimens, as for early infection
    High-degree atrioventricular block (P–R interval >0.3s): i.v. regimens and cardiac monitoring
    Once the patient has stabilized, the course may be completed with oral therapy

Pregnant women

    Standard treatment for manifestation of the illness. Avoid doxycycline

i.v., intravenous

Antibiotic recommendations are based on the guidelines from the Infectious Diseases Society of America[127]. (With permission from Steere[9]) .

Carditis

In patients with high-degree atrioventricular nodal block (P–R interval >0.3s), intravenous treatment for at least part of the course and cardiac monitoring are recommended, but insertion of a permanent pacemaker is not necessary. Once the patient's condition has stabilized, the course may be completed with oral treatment.

Arthritis

Either oral or intravenous regimens are usually effective for the treatment of Lyme arthritis[84,134]. Oral treatment is easier to administer, it is associated with fewer side effects and it is considerably less expensive[137]. Its disadvantage is that some patients treated with oral agents have subsequently manifested overt neuroborreliosis, which may require intravenous therapy for successful treatment[84]. Despite treatment with either oral or intravenous antibiotics, about 10% of patients in the USA have persistent joint inflammation for months or even several years after at least 2 months of oral antibiotics or at least 1 month of intravenous antibiotics[84]. If patients have persistent arthritis despite this treatment, and if the results of PCR testing of joint fluid are negative, such patients may be treated with anti-inflammatory agents or arthroscopic synovectomy.

Post-Lyme disease syndrome

Patients with post-Lyme disease syndrome are best treated symptomatically, rather than with prolonged courses of antibiotics. In a study of patients with this syndrome who received either intravenous ceftriaxone for 30 days followed by oral doxycycline for 60 days or intravenous and oral placebo preparations for the same duration, there were no significant differences between the groups in the percentage of patients who felt that their symptoms had improved, worsened or stayed the same[119]. Prolonged ceftriaxone therapy for unsubstantiated Lyme disease has resulted in biliary complications[138] and, in one reported case, prolonged cefotaxime administration resulted in death[139].

Prevention

Protection against tick bites

The risk of tick bites in high-risk areas may be reduced by simple measures. These include avoidance of tick infested areas, protective clothing, use of repellants and acaracides, tick checks and landscape modifications of periresidential environments[140].

Studies have shown the frequency of Lyme disease after a recognized tick bite to be only about 1%[141], perhaps because at least 24 hours of tick attachment seems to be necessary for transmission to occur[142]. Thus, if an attached tick is removed quickly, no other treatment is usually necessary. However, a single 200mg dose of doxycycline effectively prevents Lyme disease when given within 72 hours after the tick bite occurs[143].

Vaccination

A vaccine for Lyme disease, consisting of recombinant OspA in adjuvant, was commercially available in the USA, but it was recently withdrawn by the manufacturer. In a phase III efficacy and safety trial, vaccine efficacy in the prevention of definite Lyme disease was 49% after two injections, and 76% after three injections[108]. The most important factor in protection was the strength of the antibody response to the protective antibody epitope of OspA. Injection of the vaccine was associated with mild-to-moderate local or systemic reactions lasting a median duration of 3 days. Although T cell responses to OspA have been associated with treatment-resistant Lyme arthritis[42,51], vaccine or placebo recipients did not differ significantly in the development of arthritis or any other late syndrome after vaccination. Thus, the conditions necessary for the induction of autoimmunity in joints in the natural infection seemed not to be duplicated with vaccination. Although the vaccine is no longer available, the experience gained with it has proven the feasibility of vaccination for the prevention of this complex, tick-borne infection.

SYPHILITIC ARTHRITIS

Clinical manifestations

Osteoarticular manifestations may accompany congenital, secondary or tertiary syphilis (Table 96.6), but such manifestations are now seen most commonly in association with secondary syphilis[144]. During this phase of the infection, approximately 4–8% of patients have subacute or chronic arthritis. Knees or other large joints may show mild-to-moderate inflammation, but small joints and tendons may also be involved.

TABLE 96.6 OSTEOARTICULAR MANIFESTATIONS OF *T. PALLIDUM* INFECTION	

Congenital syphilis
  Osteitis
  Periostitis
  Gummata of bone
	Osteochondritis

Secondary syphilis
  Polyarthritis and tenosynovitis
  Osteitis
  Periostitis
	Polyarthralgias

Tertiary syphilis Gumma of bone and joints	Charcot arthropathy

Arthralgias are common. Joint fluid white blood cell counts range from 4000 to 13 000cells/mm^3. In addition, these patients may have several osteolytic lesions, with or without periostitis, most commonly in the skull, but also in the spine. Such lesions may be associated with headache or back pain. Important clues to diagnosis are that patients with secondary syphilis commonly have maculopapular rashes, particularly in the upper extremities, including on the palms and soles, mucous patches in the mouth and non-painful generalized lymphadenopathy[144]. Affected women may have condyloma lata in the genital area.

Although rare today, Charcot joints, which occur in 5–10% of patients with tabes dorsalis, are the most common joint manifestation of tertiary syphilis[144]. The destruction of joints results from loss of sensation and trauma, rather than spirochetal infection. During this stage, rare patients may have gummatous synovitis, affecting primarily large joints. When surrounding bones are affected, radiographs show erosion of subchondral bone, areas of bone reabsorption and reactive changes like those observed in other chronic infections.

The most common osteoarticular manifestation of early congenital syphilis is osteochondritis, which affects areas of enchondral ossification symmetrically[144]. Bone involvement occurs during the first 3–6 weeks of life, and is rarely seen after 3 months of age. Years later, patients may develop chronic symmetric synovitis of larger joints, usually knees or elbows – so-called Clutton's joints.

Syphilis and human immunodeficiency virus infection

Syphilis has again become a significant clinical problem because of co-infection with *T. pallidum* and human immunodeficiency virus (HIV). In such patients, syphilis may have an atypical presentation, blunted serologic response, an aggressive course and incomplete response to standard antibiotic regimens[144]. One patient was reported who presented with symmetric polyarthritis, positive tests for rheumatoid factor, antinuclear antibodies, antibodies to double-stranded DNA and initially negative syphilis serologies[145]. When skin lesions developed that were suggestive of HIV, he was found to be HIV-positive and, by that time, his syphilis serologies were strongly positive. More commonly, syphilitic arthritis in patients with HIV needs to be differentiated from that caused by HIV itself, in addition to reactive arthritis or psoriatic arthritis, which may have a more severe course in patients with HIV.

Serodiagnosis

As in Lyme disease, the diagnosis of syphilis usually depends on recognition of a characteristic clinical picture, with serologic confirmation. The standard non-treponemal screening test is the Venereal Disease Research Laboratory (VDRL) slide test. If this test is positive, the principal specific anti-treponemal test is the fluorescent treponemal antibody-absorbed (FTA-absorbed) test. Even after treatment, this test usually remains positive for life. Although syphilis and systemic lupus erythematosus are associated with antibodies against phospholipid, the epitope is different, and anti-phospholipid antibodies in syphilis are not associated with thrombosis[146]. Infection with the Lyme disease agent, *B. burgdorferi*, may result in a positive FTA-absorbed test, but it does not cause a positive VDRL test[147].

Treatment

The standard treatment for secondary syphilis is benzathine penicillin G, 2.4×10^6U intramuscularly weekly for two or three doses; for tertiary

syphilis it is intravenous pencillin G, $2-4 \times 10^6$U every 4 hours for 10 days[148]. Alternate regimens include treatment with doxycycline, amoxicillin or ceftriaxone. Some physicians prefer to use intravenous regimens for the treatment of secondary syphilis in patients who are coinfected with HIV.

REFERENCES

1. Steere AC, Malawista SE, Snydman DR et al. Lyme arthritis: an epidemic of oligoarticular arthritis in children and adults in three Connecticut communities. Arthritis Rheum 1977; 20: 7–17.
2. Steere AC, Malawista SE, Hardin JA et al. Erythema chronicum migrans and Lyme arthritis: the enlarging clinical spectrum. Ann Intern Med 1977; 86: 685–698.
3. Steere AC, Broderick TF, Malawista SE. Erythema chronicum migrans and Lyme arthritis: epidemiologic evidence for a tick vector. Am J Epidemiol 1978; 108: 312–321.
4. Lipschutz B. Uber eine seltene Erythemform (Erythema chronicum migrans). Arch Dermatol Syph 1913; 118: 349–356.
5. Buchwald A. Ein fall von diffuser idiopathischer Hautatrophie. Arch Dermatol Syph 1883; 10: 553.
6. Bannwarth A. Zur Klinik und Pathogenese der 'chronischen lymphocytaren Meningitis'. Arch Psychiatr Nervenkrankh 1944; 117: 161–185.
7. Burgdorfer W, Barbour AG, Hayes SF et al. Lyme disease – a tick-borne spirochetosis? Science 1982; 216: 1317–1319.
8. Steere AC, Grodzicki RL, Kornblatt AN et al. The spirochetal etiology of Lyme disease. N Engl J Med 1983; 308: 733–740.
9. Steere AC. Lyme disease. N Engl J Med 2001; 345: 115–125.
10. Baranton G, Postic D, Saint Girons I et al. Delineation of *Borrelia burgdorferi* sensu stricto, *Borrelia garinii* sp. nov., and group VS461 asssociated with Lyme borreliosis. Int J Syst Bacteriol 1992; 42: 378–383.
11. Orloski KA, Hayes EB, Campbell GL, Dennis DT. Surveillance for Lyme disease – United States, 1992–1998. MMWR Morb Mortal Wkly Rep 2000; 49: 1–11.
12. Stanek G, Satz N, Strle F, Wilske B. Epidemiology of Lyme borreliosis. In: Weber K, Burgdorfer W, eds. Aspects of Lyme borreliosis. Berlin, Heidelberg: Springer-Verlag; 1993: 358–370.
13. Lane RS, Piesman J, Burgdorfer W. Lyme borreliosis: relation of its causative agent to its vectors and hosts in North America and Europe. Annu Rev Entomol 1991; 36: 587–609.
14. Spielman A. The emergence of Lyme disease and human babesiosis in a changing environment. Ann NY Acad Sci 1994; 740: 146–156.
15. Brown RN, Lane RS. Lyme disease in California: a novel enzootic transmission cycle of *Borrelia burgdorferi*. Science 1992; 256: 1439–1442.
16. Campbell GL, Paul WS, Schriefer ME et al. Epidemiologic and diagnostic studies of patients with suspected early Lyme disease, Missouri, 1990–1993. J Infect Dis 1995; 172: 470–480.
17. Barbour AG, Hayes SF. Biology of Borrelia species. Microbiol Rev 1986; 50: 381–400.
18. Fraser CM, Casjens S, Huang WM et al. Genomic sequence of a Lyme disease spirochete, *Borrelia burgdorferi*. Nature 1997; 390: 580–586.
19. de Silva AM, Fikrig E. Arthropod- and host-specific gene expression by *Borrelia burgdorferi*. J Clin Invest 1997; 100: S3–S5.
20. Zhang J-R, Norris SJ. Genetic variation of the *Borrelia burgdorferi* gene VlsE involves cassettes-specific, segmental gene conversation. Infect Immun 1998; 66: 3698–3704.
21. Akins DR, Bourell KW, Caimaro MJ et al. A new animal model for studying Lyme disease spirochetes in a mammalian host-adapted state. J Clin Invest 1998; 101: 2240–2250.
22. Montgomery RR, Malawista SE, Feen KJM, Bockenstedt LK. Direct demonstration of antigenic substitution of *Borrelia burgdorferi* ex vivo: exploration of the paradox of the early immune response to outer surface proteins A and C in Lyme disease. J Exp Med 1996; 183: 261–269.
23. Schwan TG, Piesman J, Golde WT et al. Induction of an outer surface protein on *Borrelia burgdorferi* during tick feeding. Proc Natl Acad Sci USA 1995; 92: 2909–2913.
24. Seinost G, Dykhuizen DE, Dattwyler RJ et al. Four clones of *Borrelia burgdorferi* sensu stricto cause invasive infection in humans. Infect Immun 1999; 67: 3518–3524.
25. Coleman JL, Gebbia JA, Pieman J et al. Plasminogen is required for efficient dissemination of *B. burgdorferi* in ticks and for enhancement of spirochetemia in mice. Cell 1997; 89: 1111–1119.
26. Thomas DD, Comstock LE. Interaction of Lyme disease spirochetes with cultured eucaryotic cells. Infect Immun 1989; 57: 1324–1326.
27. Coburn J, Chege W, Magoun L et al. Characterization of a candidate *Borrelia burgdorferi* β3-chain integrin ligand identified using a phage display library. Mol Microbiol 1999; 34: 926–940.
28. Parveen N, Leong JM. Identification of a candidate glycosaminoglycan-binding adhesin of the Lyme disease spirochete *Borrelia burgdorferi*. Mol Microbiol 2000; 35: 1220–1234.
29. Probert WS, Johnson BJB. Identification of a 47 kDa fibronectin-binding protein expressed by *Borrelia burgdorferi* isolate B31. Mol Microbiol 1998; 30: 1003–1015.
30. Guo BP, Brown EL, Dorward DW et al. Decorin-binding adhesins from *Borrelia burgdorferi*. Mol Microbiol 1998; 30: 711–723.
31. Brown EL, Wooten M, Johnson BJB et al. Resistance to Lyme disease in decorin-deficit mice. J Clin Invest 2001; 107: 845–852.
32. Weis JJ, McCracken BA, Ma Y et al. Identification of quantitative trait loci governing arthritis severity and humoral responses in the murine model of Lyme disease. J Immun 1999; 162: 948–956.
33. Barthold SW, de Souza M. Exacerbation of Lyme arthritis in beige mice. J Infect Dis 1995; 172: 178–184.
34. Hirschfeld M, Kirschning CJ, Schwandner R et al. Cutting edge: inflammatory signaling by *Borrelia burgdorferi* lipoproteins is mediated by Toll-like receptor 2. J Immunol 1999; 163: 2382–2386.
35. Kang I, Barthold SW, Persing DH, Bockenstedt LK. T-helper-cell cytokines in the early evolution of murine Lyme arthritis. Infect Immun 1997; 65: 3107–3111.
36. Muellegger RR, McHugh G, Ruthazer R et al. Differential expression of cytokine mRNA in skin specimens from patients with erythema migrans or acrodermatitis chronica atrophicans. J Invest Derm 2000; 115: 1115–1123.
37. Krause A, Brade V, Schoerner C et al. T cell proliferation induced by *Borrelia burgdorferi* in patients with Lyme borreliosis. Arthritis Rheum 1991; 34: 393–402.
38. Akin E, McHugh GL, Flavell RA et al. The immunoglobin (IgG) antibody response to OspA and OspB correlates with severe and prolonged Lyme arthritis and the IgG response to P35 correlates with mild and brief arthritis. Infect Immun 1999; 67: 173–181.
39. Roberts ED, Bohm RPJ, Lowrie RCJ et al. Pathogenesis of Lyme neuroborreliosis in the rhesus monkey: the early disseminated and chronic phases of disease in the peripheral nervous system. J Infect Dis 1998; 178: 722–732.
40. Cadavid D, O'Neill T, Schaefer H, Pachner AR. Localization of *Borrelia burgdorferi* in the nervous system and other organs in a nonhuman primate model of Lyme disease. Lab Invest 2000; 80: 1043–1054.
41. Vincent MS, Roessner K, Sellati T et al. Lyme arthritis synovial $\gamma\delta$ T cells respond to *Borrelia burgdorferi* lipoproteins and lipidated hexapeptides. J Immun 1998; 161: 5762–5771.
42. Chen J, Field JA, Glickstein L et al. Association of antibiotic treatment-resistant Lyme arthritis with T cell responses to dominant epitopes of outer-surface protein A (OspA) of *Borrelia burgdorferi*. Arthritis Rheum 1999; 42: 1813–1822.
43. Gross DM, Steere AC, Huber BT. Dominent T helper 1 response is antigen specific and localized to synovial fluid in patients with Lyme arthritis. J Immun 1998; 160: 1022–1028.
44. Yin Z, Braun J, Neure L et al. T cell cytokine pattern in the joints of patients with Lyme arthritis and its regulation by cytokines and anticytokines. Arthritis Rheum 1997; 40: 69–79.
45. Dressler F, Whalen JA, Reinhardt BN, Steere AC. Western blotting in the serodiagnosis of Lyme disease. J Infect Dis 1993; 167: 392–400.
46. Barthold SW, Feng S, Bockenstedt LK et al. Protective and arthritis-resolving activity in sera of mice infected with *Borrelia burgdorferi*. Clin Infect Dis 1997; 25: S9–S17.
47. Feng S, Hodzic E, Barthold SW. Lyme arthritis resolution with antiserum to a 37-kilodalton *Borrelia burgdorferi* protein. Infect Immun 2000; 68: 4169–4173.
48. Kelleher Doyle M, Telford SR, Criscione L et al. Cytokines in murine Lyme carditis: Th 1 cytokine expression follows expression of proinflammatory cytokines in susceptible mouse strain. J Infect Dis 1998; 177: 242–246.
49. Barthold SW, Beck DS, Hansen GM et al. Lyme borreliosis in selected strains and ages of laboratory mice. J Infect Dis 1990; 162: 133–138.
50. Kalish RA, Leong JM, Steere AC. Association of treatment resistant chronic Lyme arthritis with HLA-DR4 and antibody reactivity to OspA and OspB of *Borrelia burgdorferi*. Infect Immun 1993; 61: 2774–2779.
51. Gross DM, Forsthuber T, Tary-Lehman M et al. Identification of LFA-1 as a candidate autoantigen in treatment-resistant Lyme arthritis. Science 1998; 281: 703–706.
52. Akin E, Aversa J, Steere AC. Expression of adhesion molecules in synovia of patients with treatment- resistant Lyme arthritis. Infect Immun 2001; 69: 1774–1780.
53. Meyer AL, Trollmo C, Crawford F et al. Direct enumeration of *Borrelia*-reactive CD4[+] T cells ex vivo by using MHC class II tetramers. Proc Natl Acad Sci USA 2000; 97: 11433–11438.
54. Trollmo C, Meyer AI, Steere AC et al. Molecular mimicry in Lyme arthritis demonstrated at the single cell level: LFA-1α L is a partial agonist for OspA-reactive T cells. J Immunol 2001; 166: 5286–5291.
55. Steere AC. Lyme disease. N Engl J Med 1989; 321: 586–596.
56. Steere AC, Bartenhagen NH, Craft JE et al. The early clinical manifestations of Lyme disease. Ann Intern Med 1983; 99: 76–82.

57. Strle F, Nadelman RB, Cimperman J et al. Comparison of culture-confirmed erythema migrans caused by Borrelia burgdorferi sensu stricto in New York state and by Borrelia afzelii in Slovenia. Ann Intern Med 1999; 130: 32–36.

58. Wormser GP, Bittker S, Cooper D et al. Comparison of the yields of blood cultures using serum or plasma from patients with early Lyme disease. J Clin Microbiol 2000; 38: 1648–1650.

59. Luft BJ, Steinman CR, Neimark HC et al. Invasion of the central nervous system by Borrelia burgdorferi in acute disseminated infection. JAMA 1992; 267: 1364–1367.

60. Asbrink E, Hovmark A. Early and late cutaneous manifestations of Ixodes-borne borreliosis (erythema migrans borreliosis, Lyme borreliosis). Ann NY Acad Sci 1988; 539: 4–15.

61. Asbrink E, Hovmark A. Successful cultivation of spirochetes from skin lesions of patients with erythema chronica migrans afzelius and acrodermatitis chronica atrophicans. Acta Pathol Microbiol Immunol Scand 1985; 93: 161–163.

62. Pachner AR, Steere AC. The triad of neurologic manifestations of Lyme disease: meningitis, cranial neuritis, and radiculoneuritis. Neurology 1985; 35: 47–53.

63. Reik L, Steere AC, Bartenhagen NH et al. Neurologic abnormalities of Lyme disease. Medicine (Baltimore) 1979; 58: 281–294.

64. Coyle PK, Goodman JL, Krupp LB et al. Lyme disease: continuum: lifelong learning in neurology, vo. 5, No.4, part A. Philadelphia: Lippincott Williams & Wilkins; 1999.

65. Oschmann P, Dorndorf W, Hornig C et al. Stages and syndromes of neuroborreliosis. J Neurology 1998; 245: 262–272.

66. Rothermel H, Hedges TR III, Steere AC. Optic neuropathy in children with Lyme disease. Pediatrics 2001; 108: 477–481.

67. Logigian EL, Kaplan RF, Steere AC. Chronic neurologic manifestations of Lyme disease. N Engl J Med 1990; 323: 1438–1444.

68. Logigian EL, Steere AC. Clinical and electrophysiologic findings in chronic neuropathy of Lyme disease. Neurology 1992; 42: 303–311.

69. Halperin JJ, Luft BJ, Anand AK et al. Lyme neuroborreliosis: central nervous system manifestations. Neurology 1989; 39: 753–759.

70. Logigian EL, Kaplan RF, Steere AC. Successful treatment of Lyme encephalopathy with intravenous ceftriaxone. J Infect Dis 1999; 180: 377–383.

71. Hemmer B, Gran B, Zhao Y et al. Identification of candidate T-cell epitopes and molecular mimics in chronic Lyme disease. Nat Med 1999; 5: 1375–1382.

72. Steere AC, Batsford WP, Weinberg M et al. Lyme carditis: cardiac abnormalities of Lyme disease. Ann Intern Med 1980; 93: 8–16.

73. McAlister HF, Klementowicz PT, Andrews C et al. Lyme carditis: an important cause of reversible heart block. Ann Intern Med 1989; 110: 339–345.

74. Marcus LC, Steere AC, Duray PH et al. Fatal pancarditis in a patient with coexistent Lyme disease and babesiosis: demonstration of spirochetes in the myocardium. Ann Intern Med 1985; 103: 374–36.

75. Stanek G, Klein J, Bittner R, Glogar D. Isolation of Borrelia burgdorferi from the myocardium of a patient with longstanding cardiomyopathy. N Engl J Med 1990; 322: 249–252.

76. Lardieri G, Salvi A, Camerini F et al. Isolation of Borrelia burgdorferi from myocardium [letter]. Lancet 1993; 342: 8869.

77. Sonnesyn SW, Diehl SC, Johnson RC et al. A prospective study of the seroprevalance of Borrelia burgdorferi infection in patients with severe heart failure. Am J Cardiol 1995; 76: 97–100.

78. Steere AC, Schoen RT, Taylor E. The clinical evolution of Lyme arthritis. Ann Intern Med 1987; 107: 725–731.

79. Szer IS, Taylor E, Steere AC. The long-term course of children with Lyme arthritis. N Engl J Med 1991; 325: 159–163.

80. Huppertz H-I, Karch H, Suschke H-J et al. Lyme arthritis in European children and adolescents. Arthritis Rheum 1995; 38: 361–368.

81. Eichenfield AH, Goldsmith DP, Benach JL et al. Childhood Lyme arthritis: experience in an endemic area. J Pediatr 1986; 109: 753–758.

82. Steere AC, Dwyer E, Winchester R. Association of chronic Lyme arthritis with HLA-DR4 and HLA-DR2 alleles. N Engl J Med 1990; 323: 219–223.

83. Steere AC, Baxter-Lowe LA. Association of chronic, treatment-resistant Lyme arthritis with rheumatoid arthritis (RA) alleles [abstract]. Arthritis Rheum 1998; 41: S81.

84. Steere AC, Levin RE, Molloy PJ et al. Treatment of Lyme arthritis. Arthritis Rheum 1994; 37: 878–888.

85. Nocton JJ, Dressler F, Rutledge BJ et al. Detection of Borrelia burgdorferi DNA by polymerase chain reaction in synovial fluid in Lyme arthritis. N Engl J Med 1994; 330: 229–234.

86. Carlson D, Hernandez J, Bloom BJ et al. Lack of Borrelia burgdorferi DNA in synovial samples in patients with antibiotic treatment-resistant Lyme arthritis. Arthritis Rheum 1999; 42: 2705–2709.

87. Herzer P, Wilske B, Preac-Mursic V et al. Lyme arthritis: clinical features, serological, and radiographic findings of cases in Germany. Klin Wochenschr 1986; 64: 206–215.

88. Hovmark A, Asbrink E, Olsson I. Joint and bone involvement in Swedish patients with Ixodes ricinus-borne Borrelia infection. Zentralbl Bakt Hyg 1986; A263: 275–284.

89. Berger BW, Johnson RC, Kodner C, Coleman L. Cultivation of Borrelia burgdorferi from erythema migrans lesions and perilesional skin. J Clin Microbiol 1992; 30: 359–361.

90. Nocton JJ, Bloom BJ, Rutledge BJ et al. Detection of Borrelia burgdorferi DNA by polymerase chain reaction in cerebrospinal fluid in patients with Lyme neuroborreliosis. J Infect Dis 1996; 174: 623–627.

91. Lebech AM, Hansen K, Rutledge BJ et al. Diagnostic detection and direct genotyping of Borrelia burgdorferi by polymerase chain reaction in cerebrospinal fluid in Lyme neuroborreliosis. Mol Diagn 1998; 3: 131–141.

92. Klempner MS, Schmid C, Hu L et al. Intralaboratory reliability of serologic and urine testing in Lyme disease. Am J Med 2001; 110: 217–219.

93. Case definitions for public health surveillance. MMWR Morb Mortal Wkly Rep 1990; 39: 19–21.

94. Second International Conference on serologic diagnosis of Lyme disease. Recommendations for test performance and interpretation. MMWR Morb Mortal Wkly Rep 1995; 44: 590–591.

95. Robertson J, Guy E, Andrews N et al. A European multicenter study of immunoblotting in serodiagnosis of Lyme borreliosis. J Clin Microbiol 2000; 38: 2097–2102.

96. Engstrom SM, Shoop E, Johnson RC. Immunoblot interpretation criteria for serodiagnosis of early Lyme disease. J Clin Microbiol 1995; 33: 419–427.

97. Gomes-Solecki MJ, Dunn JJ, Luft BJ et al. Recombinant chimeric Borrelia proteins for diagnosis of Lyme disease. J Clin Microbiol 2000; 38: 2530–2535.

98. Liang FT, Steere AC, Marques AR et al. Sensitive and specific serodiagnosis of Lyme disease by enzyme-linked immunosorbent assay with a peptide based on an immunodominant conserved region of Borrelia burgdorferi VlsE. J Clin Microbiol 1999; 37: 3990–3996.

99. Steere AC, Berardi VP, Weeks KE et al. Evaluation of the intrathecal antibody response to Borrelia burgdorferi as a diagnostic test for Lyme neuroborreliosis. J Infect Dis1990; 161: 1203–1209.

100. Logigian EL, Johnson KA, Kijewski MF et al. Reversible cerebral hypoperfusion in Lyme encephalopathy. Neurology 1997; 49: 1661–1670.

101. Kaplan RF, Jones-Woodward L. Lyme encephalopathy: a neuropsychological perspective. Semin Neurol 1997; 17: 31–37.

102. Axford JS, Rees DH, Mageed RA et al. Increased IgA rheumatoid factor and V(H)1 associated cross reactive idiotype expression in patients with Lyme arthritis and neuroborreliosis. Ann Rheum Dis 1999; 58: 757–761.

103. Lawson JP, Steere AC. Lyme arthritis: radiologic findings. Radiology 1985; 154: 37–43.

104. Jaulhac B, Chary-Valckenaere I et al. Detection of Borrelia burgdorferi by DNA amplification in synovial tissue samples from patients with Lyme arthritis. Arthritis Rheum 1996; 39: 736–745.

105. Priem S, Burmester GR, Kamradt T et al. Detection of Borrelia burgdoferi by polymerase chain reaction in synovial membrane, but not in synovial fluid from patients with persisting Lyme arthritis after antibiotic therapy. Ann Rheum Dis 1998; 57: 118–121.

106. Snydman DR, Schenkein DP, Berardi VP et al. Borrelia burgdorferi in joint fluid in chronic Lyme arthritis. Ann Intern Med 1986; 104: 798–800.

107. Kalish RA, McHugh G, Granquist J et al. Persistence of IgM or IgG antibody responses to Borrelia burgdorferi 10 to 20 years after active Lyme disease. Clin Infect Dis 2001; 33: 780–785.

108. Steere AC, Sikand VK, Meurice F et al. Vaccination against Lyme disease with recombinant Borrelia burgdorferi outer-surface lipoprotein a with adjuvant. N Engl J Med 1998; 339: 209–215.

109. Gustafson R, Svenungsson B, Gardulf A et al. Prevalence of tick-borne encephalitis and Lyme borreliosis in a defined Swedish population. Scand J Infect Dis 1990; 22: 297–306.

110. Goodman JL, Nelson C, Vitale B et al. Direct cultivation of the causative agent of human granulocytic ehrlichiosis. N Engl J Med 1996; 334: 209–215.

111. Ruebush TK 2nd, Juranek DD, Chisholm ES et al. Human babesiosis on Nantucket Island. Evidence for self-limited and subclinical infections. N Engl J Med 1977; 297: 825–827.

112. Krause PJ, Telford SR, Spielman A et al. Concurrent Lyme disease and babesiosis: evidence for increased severity and duration of illness. JAMA 1996; 275: 1657–1660.

113. DeMartino SJ, Carlyon JA, Fikrig E. Coinfection with Borrelia burgdorferi and the agent of human granulocytic ehrlichiosis. N Engl J Med 2001; 345: 150–151.

114. Wormser GP, Horowitz HW, Nowakowski J et al. Positive Lyme disease serology in patients with clinical and laboratory evidence of human granulocytic ehrlichiosis. Am J Clin Pathol 1997; 107: 142–147.

115. Sigal LH. Summary of the first 100 patients seen at a Lyme disease referral center. Am J Med 1990; 88: 577–581.

116. Dinerman H, Steere AC. Lyme disease associated with fibromyalgia. Ann Intern Med 1992; 117: 281–285.

117. Shadick NA, Phillips CB, Sangha O et al. Musculoskeletal and neurologic outcomes in patients with previously treated Lyme disease. Ann Intern Med 1999; 131: 919–926.

118. Kalish RA, Kaplan RF, Taylor E et al. Evaluation of study patients with Lyme disease, 10–20 year follow-up. J Infect Dis 2001; 183: 453–460.

119. Seltzer EG, Gerber MA, Cartter ML et al. Long-term outcomes of persons with Lyme disease. JAMA 2000; 283: 609–616.

120. Klempner MS, Hu LT, Evans J et al. Two controlled trials of antibiotic treatments in patients with persistent symptoms and a history of Lyme disease. N Engl J Med 2001; 345: 85–92.

121. Steere AC, Taylor E, McHugh GL, Logigian EL. The overdiagnosis of Lyme disease. JAMA 1993; 269: 1812–1816.

122. Burdge DR, O'Hanlon DP. Experience at a referral center for patients with suspected Lyme disease in an area of nonendemicity: first 65 patients. Clin Infect Dis 1993; 16: 558–560.

123. Duray PH. The surgical pathology of human Lyme disease: an enlarging picture. Am J Surg Path 1987; 11: 47–60.

124. Vallat JM, Hugon J, Lubeau M et al. Tick-bite meningoradiculoneuritis: clinical, electrophysiologic, and histologic findings in 10 cases. Neurology 1987; 37: 749–753.

125. Johnston YE, Duray PH, Steere AC et al. Lyme arthritis: spirochetes found in synovial microangiopathic lesions. Am J Path 1985; 118: 26–34.

126. Steere AC, Duray PH, Butcher EC. Spirochetal antigens and lymphoid cell surface markers in Lyme synovitis: comparison with rheumatoid synovium and tonsillar lymphoid tissue. Arthritis Rheum 1988; 31: 487–495.

127. Wormser GP, Nadelman RB, Dattwyler RJ et al. Practice guidelines for the treatment of Lyme disease. Clin Infect Dis 2000; 31: S1–S14.

128. Nichol G, Dennis DT, Steere AC et al. Test-treatment strategies for patients suspected of having Lyme disease: a cost-effectiveness analysis. Ann Intern Med 1998; 128: 37–48.

129. Williams CL, Stobino B, Weinstein A et al. Maternal Lyme disease and congenital malformations: a cord blood serosurvey in endemic and control areas. Paediatr Perinat Epidemiol 1995; 9: 320–330.

130. Dattwyler RJ, Volkman DJ, Conaty SM *et al*. Amoxycillin plus probenecid versus doxycycline for treatment of erythema migrans borreliosis. Lancet 1990; 336: 1404–1406.

131. Nadelman RB, Luger SW, Frank E *et al*. Comparison of cefuroxime axetil and doxycycline in the treatment of early Lyme disease. Ann Intern Med 1992; 117: 273–280.

132. Dattwyler RJ, Luft BJ, Kunkel MJ *et al*. Ceftriaxone compared with doxycycline for the treatment of acute disseminated Lyme disease. N Engl J Med 1997; 337: 289–294.

133. Nowakowski J, McKenna D, Nadelman RB *et al*. Failure of treatment with cephalexin for Lyme disease. Arch Fam Med 2000; 9: 563–567.

134. Dattwyler RJ, Halperin JJ, Volkman DJ, Luft BJ. Treatment of late Lyme borreliosis – randomized comparison of ceftriaxone and penicillin. Lancet 1988; 1: 1191–1194.

135. Pfister HW, Preac-Mursic V, Wilske B, Einhaupl KM. Cefotaxime vs penicillin G for acute neurologic manifestations of Lyme borreliosis: a prospective randomized study. Arch Neurol 1989; 46: 1190–1194.

136. Karlsson M, Hammers-Berggren S, Lindquist L *et al*. Comparison of intravenous penicillin G and oral doxycycline for treatment of Lyme neuroborreliosis. Neurology 1994; 44: 1203–1207.

137. Eckman MH, Steere AC, Kalish RA, Pauker SG. Cost effectiveness of oral as compared with intravenous antibiotic therapy for patients with early Lyme disease or Lyme arthritis. N Engl J Med 1997; 337: 357–363.

138. Ettestad PJ, Campbell GL, Weibel SF *et al*. Biliary complications in the treatment of unsubstantiated Lyme disease. J Infect Dis 1995; 171: 356–361.

139. Patel R, Grogg KL, Edwards WD *et al*. Death from inappropriate therapy for Lyme disease. Clin Infect Dis 2000; 31: 1107–1109.

140. Centers for Disease Control and Prevention. Recommendations for the use of Lyme disease vaccine. MMWR Morb Mortal Wkly Rep 1999; 48: 1–21.

141. Shapiro ED, Gerber MA, Holabird NB *et al*. A controlled trial of antimicrobial prophylaxis for Lyme disease after deer-tick bites. N Engl J Med 1992; 327: 1769–1773.

142. Piesman J. Dynamics of *Borrelia burgdorferi* transmission by nymphal *Ixodes dammini* ticks. J Infect Dis 1993; 167: 1082–1085.

143. Nadelman RB, Nowakowski J, Fish D *et al*. Single dose doxycycline prophylaxis for prevention of Lyme disease after an *Ixodes scapularis* tick bite. N Engl J Med 2001; 345: 79–84.

144. Reginato AJ. Syphilitic arthritis and osteitis. Rheum Dis Clin N Am 1993; 19: 379–398.

145. Burgoyne M, Agudelo C, Pisko E. Chronic syphilitic polyarthritis mimicking systemic lupus erythematosus/rheumatoid arthritis as the initial presentation of human immundeficiency virus infection. J Rheum 1992; 19: 313–315.

146. Colaco CB, Male DK. Anti-phospholipid antibodies in syphilis and a thrombotic subset of SLE: distinct profiles of epitope specificity. Clin Exp Immunol 1985; 59: 449–456.

147. Craft JE, Grodzicki RL, Steere AC. The antibody response in Lyme disease: evaluation of diagnostic tests. J Infect Dis 1984; 149: 789–795.

148. Tramont EC. Treponema pallidum (syphilis). In: Mandell GL, Bennett JE, Dolin R, eds. Principles and practice of infectious diseases, 5E. Philadelphia: Churchill Livingstone; 2000: 2474–2490.

97 Viral arthritis

Stanley J Naides

Definition

- A host of different viruses may cause arthritis through various pathogenetic mechanisms, including direct infection of synovial cells, immune complex formation and others
- The most common arthritogenic viruses in N. America and Western Europe include parvovirus B19, rubella and hepatitis B, while a variety of mosquito-borne viruses cause epidemics of polyarthritis in Africa, the western Pacific and South America

Clinical features

- The majority of virally caused arthritides are acute and self-limiting illnesses, usually accompanied by fever, distinctive cutaneous manifestations, hematologic abnormalities (especially B19 infection) and other clinical features
- Chronic polyarthritis mimicking rheumatoid arthritis may occur, especially in adults with parvovirus B19 or rubella infections but also in several other infections
- Diagnosis requires knowledge of the epidemiology of these viral infections and laboratory investigations of the disease process

INTRODUCTION

Viruses are attractive candidates for etiologic agents of various idiopathic rheumatic diseases. Although data to support a direct role for viruses in diseases such as classical seropositive erosive rheumatoid arthritis are tenuous, arthralgia and frank arthritis are often prominent features of acute viral infection (Table 97.1). Several viruses have been shown to be the etiologic agents of epidemics of febrile arthritis affecting thousands of individuals. Describing the mechanisms by which specific viruses cause acute and chronic rheumatic symptoms may offer insights into pathogenesis and identify specific etiological agents for subsets of idiopathic disease.

Host factors including age, genetic background and immune response are important determinants of clinical expression of viral infection. Viral factors include mode of viral entry, tissue tropism, replication strategies, cytopathological effects, ability to establish persistent infection, viral expression of host-like antigens and ability to alter host antigens. Several viruses directly infect the cells of the synovium. Target cells may die by classic cell necrosis (karyorrhexis), the virus may initiate programmed cell death (apoptosis) or the virus may express virally encoded antigens on the cell surface that target the cell for immune-mediated attack.

Viral infection also may result in non-lytic mechanisms of arthritis pathogenesis. Transactivation of host genes by viral gene products may activate the infected cell or induce cytokines that elicit an immune response. Viral antigens expressed on the cell surface may be seen as foreign and elicit an immune response. Alternatively, molecular mimicry of host autoantigens may break immune tolerance, resulting in autoimmunity, or infection may elicit 'danger signals' that induce an immune response. The humoral immune response may generate antibody that deposits in immune complexes, either locally at the site of viral infection or systemically with deposition of circulating immune complex in the synovium.

PARVOVIRUS B19

History

'Parvo-' derives from the Greek, meaning 'small'. B19 is a member of the family Parvoviridae, subfamily Parvovirinae, genus *Erythrovirus*,

TABLE 97.1 VIRUS INFECTIONS WITH PROMINENT JOINT INVOLVEMENT	
Erythrovirus	
Parvovirus B19	Symmetric polyarthralgia/polyarthritis lasting days to weeks Prolonged, about 12% lasting months to years
Togaviruses	
Rubella virus	Morbilliform rash and symmetric polyarthritis in women and children following natural infection or immunization
Chikungunya virus	Explosive onset fever, polyarthralgia/polyarthritis and rash in epidemics in Africa and Asia
O'nyong-nyong virus	Epidemic fever, polyarthralgia/polyarthritis and rash in Africa
Igbo-ora virus	An epidemic of fever, myalgia, arthralgia and rash in the Ivory Coast
Ross River virus (epidemic polyarthritis)	Fever, rash and polyarthritis in Australia, New Zealand, New Guinea and the Pacific islands, in sporadic and epidemic occurrence
Sindbis virus	Epidemic rash and arthritis in Sweden, Finland and the Karelian isthmus
Mayaro virus	Epidemic febrile polyarthritis in South American rain forest
Hepadnavirus	
Hepatitis B virus	Urticarial rash and small and large joint arthritis preceding icterus
Flavivirus	
Hepatitis C virus	Acute polyarthritis in acute infection; cryoglobulinemia in chronic infection, including essential mixed cryoglobulinemia
Retroviruses	
Human T-lymphocyte leukemia virus (HTLV)-1	Nodular rash and oligoarthritis associated with abnormal cellular infiltrates
Human immunodeficiency virus (HIV)	See Chapter 98

consisting of the small, non-enveloped, single-stranded DNA viruses, autonomously replicating in erythroid precursors. B19 measures approximately 23nm in diameter. Although infection occurs in a variety of tissue types, reproduction is most efficient in erythroid progenitors. Numerous autonomous mammalian parvoviruses are known, but parvoviruses are extremely species-specific and are not known to readily cross species. While many of the clinical syndromes associated with B19 infection have been well known for many years and may mimic known animal diseases caused by their species-specific parvoviruses, B19 was first associated with disease only in 1981.

Epidemiology

Parvovirus B19 infection is common and widespread. Transmission is via nasopharyngeal secretions. A large proportion of B19 infections in community outbreaks remains asymptomatic or presents as undiagnosed non-specific viral illnesses. Up to 60% of adults show serologic evidence of past B19 infection. Outbreaks occur in late winter and spring, although epidemics also have been reported in summer and fall. Within a community, outbreaks tend to occur every 3–5 years, representing the period of time for a fresh cohort of susceptible children to enter the school system. With multiple exposures, the risk of infection in susceptible adults may be as high as 50%. Workers in occupations with increased exposure to children, such as schoolteachers, day-care workers and hospital personnel, have an increased risk of infection[1]. Sporadic cases occur between outbreaks.

The incubation period following natural infection is 7–18 days. In human volunteers, introduction of B19 nasally was followed in 7 days by a flu-like illness associated with viremia, viral shedding in nasal secretions and a reticulocytosis. Onset of the IgM antibody response 4–6 days later was associated with clearing of viremia, cessation of nasal shedding of virus and a second phase of clinical illness characterized by rash, arthralgia and arthritis. Onset of the anti-B19 IgG antibody response occurred almost concurrently with the IgM response[2]. In natural infections, the two phases of clinical illness often overlap.

Clinical features

The most common manifestation is erythema infectiosum, or 'fifth disease', a common rash illness in children characterized by bright red 'slapped cheeks' and a macular, maculopapular and occasionally vesicular or hemorrhagic eruption on the torso or extremities[3] (Fig. 97.1). While infection in children may be asymptomatic, mild flu-like symptoms may occur, including sore throat, headache, fever, cough, anorexia, vomiting, diarrhea and arthralgia. In adults, the rash tends to be subtler and the bright red 'slapped cheeks' are often absent. Uncommon dermatologic manifestations include vesiculopustular eruption, purpura with or without thrombocytopenia, Henoch–Schönlein purpura and a 'socks and gloves' erythema.

Parvovirus B19 infection may be associated with paresthesia in the fingers. Rarely, progressive arm weakness may occur, as may numbness of the toes. In such instances, nerve conduction studies may show mild slowing of nerve conduction velocities and decreased amplitudes of motor and sensory potentials.

Parvovirus B19 causes transient aplastic crisis in the setting of chronic hemolytic anemia. It may also cross the placenta to infect the fetus. Affected fetuses develop hydrops fetalis due to B19-induced aplastic crisis resulting in a high-output cardiac failure, or to viral cardiomyopathy. In children and adults, B19 has been reported to less commonly cause pancytopenia, isolated anemia, thrombocytopenia, leukopenia, myocarditis, neuropathy and hepatitis. Patients with congenital or acquired immune deficiencies, including prior chemotherapy for lymphoproliferative disorders, immunosuppressive therapy for transplantation or human acquired immune deficiency syndrome (AIDS) may fail to clear B19 infection. Such individuals may have chronic or recurrent

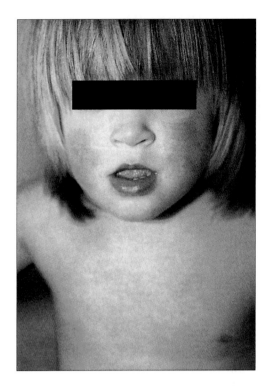

Fig. 97.1 Classic 'slapped cheeks' of a child with erythema infectiosum, or fifth disease, caused by parvovirus B19. A lacy macular erythematous eruption is also present on the trunk but is not in focus. (With permission from Feder[4]; copyright © Massachusetts Medical Society, 1994.)

anemia, thrombocytopenia or leukopenia. B19 infection is the leading cause of pure red cell aplasia in patients with AIDS. It has been reported in association with vasculitis in some cases.

In outbreaks of 'slapped cheek' rash, arthralgia occurs in about 5% and joint swelling in 3% of children under 10 years of age. In adolescents, joint pain and swelling occurs in 12% and 5% respectively. However, in adults 20 years of age or older, joint pain and swelling occurs in 77% and 60% respectively. B19 infection in adults may be associated with a severe flu-like illness in which polyarthralgia and joint swelling are prominent. The distribution of involved joints is rheumatoid-like, with prominent symmetric involvement of the metacarpophalangeal, finger proximal interphalangeal, wrist, knee and ankle joints. Onset of joint symptoms may or may not be preceded by a viral prodrome consisting of fever, malaise, chills and myalgias. Most patients present with acute, moderately to markedly severe, symmetric polyarthritis that usually starts in the hands or knees and within 24–48 hours spreads to include the wrists, ankles, feet, elbows and shoulders. Spinal involvement is uncommon.

Joint symptoms in adults are usually self limiting but a minority of adults may have symptoms for prolonged periods of time, falling into one of two patterns. Approximately two-thirds of patients have continuous symptoms of morning stiffness and arthralgias with intermittent flares. The other third are symptom-free between flares. Morning stiffness is prominent.

Rheumatoid factor may be present in low to moderate titer during the acute phase of infection but usually resolves. Low to moderate titer anti-DNA, antilymphocyte, antinuclear and antiphospholipid antibodies may be present acutely.

Chronic B19 arthropathy may last for up to 9 years, the longest follow-up to date; however, signs of acute synovitis tend to resolve several weeks after the initial infection. Pain remains a prominent feature in patients who continue to report morning stiffness. Approximately 12% of patients presenting with 'early synovitis' had B19-induced rheumatoid-like arthropathy; the majority are women[5].

The distribution and symmetry of B19 arthropathy may suggest a diagnosis of rheumatoid arthritis[5]. About half of all patients with chronic B19 arthropathy meet American College of Rheumatology criteria for a diagnosis of rheumatoid arthritis – morning stiffness that may last for more than an hour, symmetric involvement, involvement of at least three joints and involvement of the hand joints. Joint erosions and rheumatoid nodules are absent. While an initial report suggested that chronic B19 arthropathy may be associated with HLA-DR4, as is seen in classic erosive rheumatoid arthritis, subsequent studies by the same group have demonstrated no increased association with HLA-DR4[3]. The absence of rheumatoid nodules or joint destruction aids in the differential diagnosis of B19 arthropathy from classical, erosive rheumatoid arthritis.

Investigations

A number of approaches and methodologies have been used in the laboratory to confirm B19 infection. Immune electron microscopy, detection of B19 DNA during viremia, and detection of anti-B19 immunoglobulin (IgM antibody) may be used. However, the most useful modality in the rheumatology clinic is the IgM serology because patients usually have anti-B19 IgM antibodies at the time of presentation with polyarthralgia and/or polyarthritis.

Both radioimmunoassays (RIA) and enzyme-linked immunoabsorbent assays (ELISA) have been used to detect B19 antigen and specific antibody to B19 capsid[3,5]. The anti-B19 IgM antibody response is usually positive for at least 2 months following onset of joint symptoms but may wane shortly thereafter. However, the IgM antibody may be detectable in occasional patients for 6 months or longer. Because of the high seroprevalence of anti-B19 IgG in the adult population, detection of anti-B19 IgG antibody in the absence of anti-B19 IgM shortly after presentation of acute onset joint symptoms suggests past B19 infection and other diagnoses should be entertained.

Since there is a brief window of diagnostic opportunity, B19 infection should be considered in all patients presenting with sudden onset symmetric polyarthralgia and/or polyarthritis, because failure to obtain B19 serologic testing at presentation may result in failure to detect diagnostic anti-B19 IgM in those patients in whom joint symptoms persist.

Pathogenesis

Anti-B19 IgM antibody and acute phase IgG antibody (less than 1 week postresponse) recognize the major capsid protein, VP2. After about 1 week, anti-B19 IgG antibody also recognizes determinants unique to the minor capsid protein VP1. VP1 and VP2 are encoded in the same open reading frame but VP2 uses a downstream transcription start site. Thus VP1 contains a unique N-terminal 227 amino acid sequence not present in VP2. VP1 therefore contains unique determinants either in the unique non-overlapping N-terminal region or resulting from conformational differences in the sequences shared between the two proteins. Patients with B19-associated bone marrow suppression in the setting of congenital immune deficiency, prior chemotherapy or AIDS often lack convalescent anti-VP1 IgG antibodies and are unable to neutralize B19 virus in experimental bone marrow culture systems. While this work suggests that neutralizing determinants are unique to VP1 (since antibodies from immune-deficient patients recognized VP2), recent work with synthetic peptides suggests that neutralizing determinants may be found on VP2 as well[3]. In the absence of neutralizing antibodies to B19, B19 persists in the bone marrow and may cause chronic or intermittent suppression of one or more hematopoietic lineages.

Management

There is no specific treatment or vaccine for B19 infection currently available. Treatment remains symptomatic with non-steroidal anti-inflammatory drugs (NSAIDs). Neutralizing antibody to B19 is contained in commercial pooled immunoglobulin since seroprevalence of anti-B19 IgG antibody in the adult population is approximately 50%. Intravenous immunoglobulin has been successful in the treatment of bone marrow suppression and of B19 persistence in immunocompro-

mised patients but initial studies suggest that this is not applicable to chronic arthropathy patients.

TOGAVIRUSES

Rubella virus

Rubella is the 'third disease' of childhood described by German physicians in the late 19th century. Rubella virus is the sole member of the genus *Rubivirus* in the Togaviridae family of enveloped single-stranded RNA viruses. The spherical rubella virion measures 50–70nm in diameter with a 30nm dense core. Envelope glycoproteins form spike-like projections measuring 5–6nm and contain the hemagglutination activity[6].

Epidemiology

Rubella is transmitted by nasopharyngeal secretions. Peak incidence occurs in late winter and spring, although vaccination has reduced the incidence of rubella outbreaks that previously occurred in 6–9-year cycles, mostly in children. Recent rubella outbreaks have occurred in college students and in adults, suggesting that, with widespread vaccination, the age profile has shifted towards young adults, whose risk of infection is 10–20%, comparable to the prevaccine era.

Rash occurs 14–21 days after infection (Fig. 97.2). Viremia precedes rash by 6–7 days, peaks immediately prior to onset of rash and clears within 48 hours of the appearance of rash. Viral shedding in nasopharyngeal secretions may be detected from 7 days before until 14 days after onset of rash, but is maximal from just before eruption until 5–6 days posteruption[6].

Clinical features

Infection in children and adults may be asymptomatic. A classic syndrome consists of rash, low-grade fever, malaise, coryza and prominent posterior cervical, postauricular and occipital lymphadenopathy. Constitutional symptoms may precede onset of rash by 5 days. The rash may vary during a brief 2–3 day period, presenting as a morbilliform facial eruption before spreading to the torso, upper and then lower extremities. The facial rash may coalesce and clear as the extremities become involved. In some cases, the rash is only a transient blush.

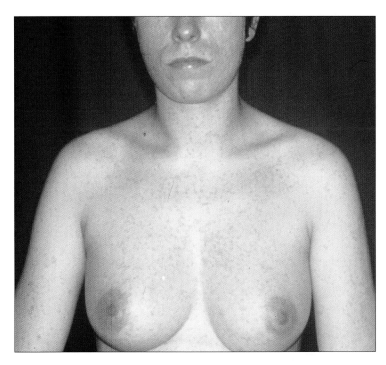

Fig. 97.2 The morbilliform rash of rubella infection.

Joint symptoms are common in women, occurring 1 week before or after onset of the rash. Like B19 arthropathy, arthralgias are more common than frank arthritis, and stiffness is prominent. Joint involvement, which is symmetric or migratory, usually resolves over a few days to 2 weeks. The metacarpophalangeal and finger proximal interphalangeal, wrist, elbow, ankle and knee joints are most frequently affected. Periarthritis, tenosynovitis and carpal tunnel syndrome may be seen. In some patients, symptoms may persist for several months or years.

Live attenuated rubella vaccines have a high frequency of postvaccination arthralgia, myalgia, arthritis and paraesthesias. The HPV77/DK12 strain is the most arthritogenic of the vaccine strains, causing joint involvement similar to natural infection, usually 2 weeks postinoculation and lasting less than a week. However, in some patients symptoms may persist for more than a year. The currently used vaccine, RA27/3, may cause postvaccination joint symptoms in as many as 15% or more of recipients.

In children, two rheumatologic syndromes may occur following natural infection or vaccination. In the 'arm syndrome', brachial radiculoneuropathy causes arm and hand pain and dysesthesias that are worse at night. The 'catcher's crouch' syndrome is a lumbar radiculoneuropathy characterized by popliteal fossa pain on arising in the morning that is exacerbated by knee extension and minimized in a 'catcher's crouch' position (Fig. 97.3). The pain gradually subsides through the day. Both syndromes occur 1–2 months postvaccination. The initial episode may last up to 2 months but recurrences are usually shorter in duration. Episodes may recur for up to 1 year, eventually resolving without permanent sequelae[7].

Investigations

Rubella is readily cultured from tissues and body fluids, including throat swabs. Virus is detected in tissue culture by cytopathic effects or by interference of enterovirus growth in primary African green monkey kidney cell cultures. Antirubella IgM antibody positivity or anti-IgG antibody seroconversion is diagnostic of rubella infection. Antirubella IgM and IgG are usually present at onset of joint symptoms. IgM antibody peaks

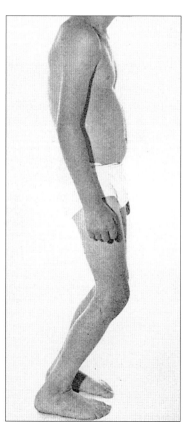

Fig. 97.3 Catcher's crouch syndrome in a child following rubella immunization. (With permission from Kilroy et al.[7])

8–21 days after symptom onset and is undetectable in most patients after about 5 weeks. Therefore, antirubella IgM positivity indicates recent infection, usually in the previous 1–2 months. A diagnosis of rubella infection based on IgG serology can only be made with paired acute and convalescent sera. Antirubella IgG rises rapidly over a period of 7–21 days after symptom onset and is long-lived. A positive IgG screen without titer or an isolated single serum sample only documents immunity[6].

Pathogenesis

An inadequate humoral immune response to specific epitopes may allow rubella virus to persist in patients with rubella arthritis[8]. Rubella may be detected in synovial fluid during arthritis flares and in lymphocytes years after symptoms resolve. Onset of rash and arthritis is coincident with antibody production, including neutralizing antibodies to whole virus, which suggests a role for either antibody or immune complexes in the synovitis[6].

Management

Non-steroidal anti-inflammatory drugs may be used for symptom control. Some investigators have suggested that low to moderate doses of corticosteroids may be needed to control symptoms and viremia[9].

Alphaviruses

Chikungunya virus

History

Chikungunya virus was isolated during an epidemic of febrile arthritis in Tanzania in 1952–53. Chikungunya, in local dialect meaning 'that which twists or bends up', was applied to the virus and the disease. Similar epidemics probably occurred in Africa, Asia, India, Indonesia and possibly the southern USA from 1779 to 1828[10].

Epidemiology

Chikungunya virus is transmitted from its reservoir in baboons, monkeys and, in Senegal, *Scotophilus* bat species to man by *Aedes* mosquitoes. *Mansonia africana* and mosquitoes from other genera also may act as vectors. In a 1964 epidemic in Bangkok, Thailand, an estimated 40 000 patients out of an urban area of 2 million were infected. The seroconversion rate was 31%. Urban centers that have not encountered Chikungunya fever either endemically or epidemically for a prolonged period and that have large susceptible school age populations are at risk of significant outbreaks. Recently, increased travel associated with globalization may have led to reintroduction of the virus into new human populations[11]. The reinfestation of *Aedes aegypti* and the introduction of *Aedes albopictus* into the western hemisphere raise the specter of an expanded geographic distribution.

Clinical features

The incubation period is usually 2–3 days but ranges over 1–12 days. Typically, intense viremia occurs within 48 hours following a mosquito bite. Chikungunya fever has an explosive onset characterized by fever and severe arthralgia[12]. Fever quickly reaches 39–40°C with rigors and may last 2–3 days with a range of 1–7 days. Viremia begins to wane around day 3. Facial and neck flushing followed by macular or maculopapular rash begins 1–10 days after fever onset. Typically, the rash begins on days 2–5 of the illness and is associated with defervescence. The rash may last 1–5 days and may recur with fever. It is located on the torso, extremities and occasionally the face, palms and soles. It may be pruritic. Suffusion of the conjunctiva is prominent. Isolated petechiae and mucosal bleeding may occur. In some patients, involved skin desquamates. Sore throat, pharyngitis, headache, photophobia, retroorbital pain, anorexia, nausea, vomiting and abdominal pain may accompany the acute illness. Lymphadenopathy may be tender but is usually not massive. Following the acute illness, the patient may remain afebrile for 1–2 days before fever recurs.

Diffuse myalgia and back and shoulder pain are common. Migratory polyarthralgia, stiffness and swelling predominantly affect the small joints of the hands, wrists, feet and ankles. Large joints are less severely affected. Previously injured joints may be disproportionately affected. Large effusions are uncommon. In some cases, symptoms may persist for months before resolution. Approximately 10% of patients have joint symptoms at 1 year postinfection[13]. A destructive arthropathy may occur in a few adult patients with chronic symptoms[14]. Low titer rheumatoid factor may be found in those with long-standing symptoms. Symptoms in children tend to be milder. In symptomatic children nausea and vomiting, pharyngitis and facial flushing are prominent features but arthralgia, arthritis and rash are uncommon and when present are milder and briefer in duration than in adults. Children may present with a mild dengue-like hemorrhagic fever, headache, pharyngeal injection, vomiting, abdominal pain, constipation, diarrhea, cough or lymphadenopathy.

Investigation

A diagnosis of Chikungunya fever should be entertained in any febrile patient resident in or returning from an endemic area. A history of epidemic in the locale of exposure is helpful. Synovial fluid shows decreased viscosity, poor mucin clot and 2000–5000 white cells/mm^3.

The diagnosis requires laboratory confirmation. Virus may be isolated from serum during days 2–4 of illness. In some patients the viremia is sufficiently intense as to allow detection of Chikungunya viral antigen by hemagglutination. As viremia is cleared, hemagglutination inhibition antibody develops. Neutralizing antibody production parallels hemagglutination inhibition activity. Antibodies capable of fixing complement develop by the third week and slowly decrease over the subsequent year. Chikungunya-virus-specific IgM antibodies may be found for 6 months or longer, which is helpful in establishing the diagnosis in patients dwelling in endemic areas[10].

Pathogenesis

Little is known regarding the pathogenesis of Chikungunya fever or arthritis. Involved skin shows erythrocyte extravasation from superficial capillaries and perivascular cuffing. In one patient with chronic arthropathy, the synovium appeared to be atrophic on arthroscopy and was histologically normal[13]. A few patients may have chronic arthralgia. Case reports suggest that a few patients with chronic arthropathy develop destructive joint lesions. Synovitis in Chikungunya fever probably results from direct viral infection of synovium.

Management

Management is supportive. During the acute attack, range of motion exercises decrease stiffness. NSAIDs are useful. Chloroquine phosphate (250mg/day) has been used when NSAIDs failed.

O'nyong-nyong virus

History

O'nyong-nyong virus was first described in an outbreak in the Acholi province of northwestern Uganda in February 1959. The name derives from the Acholi word meaning 'joint breaker'. Within 2 years the virus had spread through Uganda and the surrounding region, affecting 2 million people. Serologically determined attack rates ranged from 50% to 60% with 9–78% of infected individuals becoming symptomatic[15]. Disease spread at a rate of 2–3km daily. After the epidemic, the virus was not detected again until it was isolated from *Anopheles funestus* mosquitoes in Kenya in 1978. *Anopheles gambiae* also serves as a vector. In 1996, O'nyong-nyong virus infection recurred in northwestern Uganda in a large outbreak[16]. Serologic surveys indicate that O'nyong-nyong virus is endogenous. The non-human vertebrate reservoir for O'nyong-nyong virus is not known.

Clinical features

O'nyong-nyong fever is clinically similar to Chikungunya fever[10,16,17]. The incubation period lasts at least 8 days and is followed by sudden-onset polyarthralgia and/or polyarthritis. Rash typically begins 4 days later as the joints improve. The rash, which tends to be uniform, lasts 4–7 days before fading. The fever is less prominent than that in Chikungunya fever but posterior cervical lymphadenopathy may be marked. While residual joint pain may persist, there appears to be no long-term sequelae.

Diagnosis

Viral isolation by intracerebral injection into suckling mice produces runting, rash and alopecia. Hemagglutination inhibition or complement fixation tests identify O'nyong-nyong virus[10], which is closely related to Chikungunya virus. Mouse antisera raised against Chikungunya virus or O'nyong-nyong virus react equally well with O'nyong-nyong virus, but O'nyong-nyong antisera do not react well with Chikungunya virus. The pathogenetic mechanism of O'nyong-nyong virus is unknown.

Management

Management during the acute attack is symptomatic and includes the use of NSAIDs and range-of-motion exercises. Patients recover without sequelae.

Igbo-ora virus

Igbo-ora is 'the disease that breaks your wings'. Igbo-ora virus is serologically similar to Chikungunya and O'nyong-nyong viruses[18]. A single patient with fever, sore throat and arthritis was initially identified. In 1984, an epidemic of fever, myalgias, arthralgias and rash occurred in four villages in the Ivory Coast. The virus can be isolated from *Anopheles funestus* mosquitoes, *Anopheles gambiae* mosquitoes and ill patients.

Ross River virus (epidemic polyarthritis)

History

Epidemics of fever and rash have occurred in Australia since 1928[10]. Allied soldiers stationed in Australia during World War II were affected. Ross River virus was isolated from mosquitoes and serologically associated with epidemic polyarthritis; finally the virus was isolated from epidemic polyarthritis patients in Australia, confirming Ross River virus as the etiologic agent of epidemic polyarthritis.

Epidemiology

Weber's line is a hypothetical demarcation separating the Australian geographic zone from the Asiatic zone. West of Weber's line, antibodies to Ross River virus are not found. Antibodies to Ross River virus have been observed in endogenous populations in Papua New Guinea, West New Guinea, the Bismarck Archipelago, Rossel Island and the Solomon Islands. A major epidemic of febrile polyarthritis occurred in the Fiji Islands from 1979–80, affecting over 40 000. Judging from serologic surveys, a low level of Ross River virus infection was endogenous in the Fiji Islands before 1979 but, following the 1979–80 epidemic, up to 90% of the residents of some communities developed antibody. Another epidemic occurred in the Cook Islands in 1980.

In Australia, both endemic cases and epidemics occur in tropical and temperate regions. Queensland and New South Wales are the territories with the greatest incidence but outbreaks and sporadic cases also occur in other regions. Seroprevalence is 6–15% in temperate coastal zones but 27–39% in the plains of the Murray Valley river system. High rainfall with increased mosquito populations usually precedes epidemic periods. Cases occur from spring through fall.

Aedes vigilax, which breeds in salt marshes, is the major vector on the east Australian coast (Table 97.2)[10]. *Aedes camptorhynchus* breeds in salt marshes of southern Australia. *Culex annulirostris* breeds in fresh water. Other Australian *Aedes* species and *Mansonia uniformus* may also serve as vectors. Several mammalian species may serve as intermediate hosts,

TABLE 97.2 MOSQUITO VECTORS OF ALPHAVIRUSES		
Virus	**Mosquito**	**Disease occurrence**
Chikungunya virus	*Aedes* species	Africa, Asia
	Mansonia africana	Africa, Asia
O'nyong-nyong virus	*Anopheles funestus*	Africa
	Anopheles gambiae	
Igbo-ora virus	*Anopheles funestus*	Ivory Coast (west Africa)
	Anopheles gambiae	
Ross River virus	*Aedes vigilax*	Australia, New Zealand, New Guinea, Pacific islands
	Aedes camptorhynchus	
	Culex annulirostris	
	Mansonia uniformus	
	Aedes polynesiensis	
	Aedes aegypti	
Barmah Forest virus	*Aedes* species	Australia
	Anopheles species	
	Culex species	
Sindbis virus	*Aedes* species	Sweden, Finland, Karelian isthmus of Russia
	Culex species	
	Culiseta species	
Mayaro virus	*Haemagogus* species	Bolivia, Brazil

A list of the mosquitoes serving as vectors for alphavirus transmission and location of disease occurrence.

including domestic animals, rodents and marsupials. In the Pacific islands outbreaks, *Aedes polynesiensis*, *Aedes aegypti*, *Aedes vigilax* and *Culex annulirostris* have served as vectors.

Infection rates in Australia range from 0.2% to 3.5% per year. While male and female infection rates are similar, there is a predominance of women in presenting cases. During epidemics in Fiji and New South Wales, the majority of those infected were symptomatic. Children have a lower proportion of infections that are symptomatic compared to adults.

Clinical features

Polyarthralgia occurs abruptly after a 7–11-day incubation period. A macular, papular or maculopapular rash, which may be pruritic, usually follows onset of arthralgia by 1–2 days but may precede joint symptoms by 11 days or follow joint symptoms by 15 days. Vesicles, papules or petechiae are typically seen on the trunk and extremities, although involvement of the palms, soles and face may occur. The rash resolves by fading to a brownish discoloration or by desquamation. Despite its name, half the patients have no fever, and those who do may have only modest fevers lasting 1–3 days. Nausea, headache and myalgia are common. Respiratory symptoms, mild photophobia and lymphadenopathy may occur.

Arthralgia is severe and incapacitating in a majority of patients. Joint distribution is often migratory and asymmetric, with metacarpophalangeal and finger interphalangeal joint, wrist, knee and ankle involvement. Shoulders, elbows, and toes also may be involved. Axial, hip and temporomandibular involvement occasionally occurs. Arthralgias are worse in the morning and after periods of inactivity. Mild exercise tends to improve joint symptoms. One-third of patients have frank synovitis. Polyarticular swelling and tenosynovitis are common. Up to a third have paresthesias and palm or sole pain. Classic carpal tunnel syndrome may be seen. Half of all patients are able to resume their daily activities within 4 weeks, although residual polyarthralgia may be present. Joint symptoms may recur but episodes of relapse gradually resolve. A few patients will continue to have joint symptoms for up to 3 years[19].

Diagnosis

The diagnosis of Ross River virus infection should be considered in anyone with a febrile arthritis in the appropriate geographic setting.

Patients may present without a rash, which may confound the differential diagnosis. Synovial fluid white blood cell counts range from 1500 to 13 800 cells/mm³, predominately monocytes and vacuolated macrophages. The virus has been isolated only from antibody-negative sera. In the Australian epidemics prior to 1979, patients were antibody-positive at the time of presentation. In contrast, patients in the Pacific Islands epidemics of 1979–80 remained viremic and seronegative for up to 1 week following onset of the symptoms[20].

Pathogenesis

Ross River virus antigen may be detected early in monocytes and macrophages by immunofluorescence, but intact virus is not identifiable by electron microscopy or cell culture. Both erythematous and purpuric rashes show mild dermal perivascular mononuclear cell infiltrates, mostly T-lymphocytes. Purpuric areas also show erythrocyte extra-vasation. Viral antigen may be detected in epithelial cells in both erythematous and purpuric skin lesions, and in perivascular zones in erythematous lesions[21].

Management

Management of the acute infection is symptomatic. NSAIDs provide relief for joint pain. Occasional patients develop more prolonged joint symptoms but usually recover fully.

Barmah Forest virus

Barmah Forest virus, an alphavirus newly described in Australia, may present in a fashion similar to epidemic febrile polyarthritis[22].

Sindbis virus

Sindbis virus was named after the Egyptian village where it was first isolated from local mosquitoes in 1952. Sindbis virus is now the prototype alphavirus studied in the laboratory.

Epidemiology

Sindbis virus infection presents as Okelbo disease, Pogosta disease or Karelian fever in Sweden, Finland and the neighboring Karelian isthmus of Russia, respectively[12]. *Aedes*, *Culex* and *Culiseta* mosquito species transmit the virus to humans from birds. Cases are confined to predominately forested areas, where individuals involved in outdoor activities or occupations are at risk. Sindbis virus infection also has been reported from Uganda, South Africa, Zimbabwe, central Africa and Australia, as sporadic cases or small outbreaks[10].

Clinical features

Rash and arthralgia are the presenting symptoms although one may precede the other by a few days. A low-grade fever may be present. Constitutional symptoms are usually mild and include headache, fatigue, malaise, nausea, vomiting, pharyngitis and paresthesias. A macular rash typically begins on the torso then spreads to the arms and legs, palms, soles and occasionally the head. Macules evolve to form papules, which tend to vesiculate. Vesiculation is prominent on pressure points, including the palms and soles. As the rash fades, a brownish discoloration is left. Vesicles on the palms and soles may become hemorrhagic. The rash may recur during convalescence[23].

Arthralgia and arthritis involve the small joints of the hands and feet, wrists, elbows, ankles and knees. Occasionally, the axial skeleton becomes involved. Tendinitis is common, often involving the extensor tendons of the hand and the Achilles tendon. Non-erosive chronic arthropathy is common, with up to one third of patients having arthropathy 2 or more years after onset. A smaller number have symptoms for as long as 5–6 years[24].

Diagnosis

Hemagglutination inhibition and complement fixation tests for Sindbis virus antibodies confirm the diagnosis. Antibodies appear during the first week of illness.

Pathogenesis

Sindbis virus has been isolated from a skin vesicle in the absence of viremia. Skin lesions show perivascular edema, hemorrhage, lymphocytic infiltrates and areas of necrosis. Anti-Sindbis-virus IgM may persist for years, raising the possibility that Sindbis virus arthritis is associated with viral persistence[24].

Mayaro virus

Mayaro virus was first recognized in Trinidad in 1954 and has caused epidemics in Bolivia and Brazil. Mayaro virus is transmitted from monkeys to man by *Haemagogus* mosquitoes. Mayaro virus was responsible for an outbreak in Belterra, Brazil in 1988 characterized by sudden onset of fever, headache, dizziness, chills and arthralgias in the wrists, fingers, ankles and toes. Of 4000 exposed latex gatherers, 800 were infected, with a clinical attack rate of 80%. One fifth had joint swelling. Unilateral inguinal lymphadenopathy was seen in some patients. Leukopenia was common. Viremia was present during the first 1–2 days of illness. After 2–5 days, fever resolved but a maculopapular rash on the trunk and extremities appeared, lasting about 3 days. Recovery was complete, although some patients had persistent arthralgias at 2-month follow-up[25].

Several cases of imported Mayaro virus infection have presented in the USA after travel from an area of endemicity in the Brazil–Bolivia–Peru border region[26]. Interestingly, Mayaro virus has been isolated from a bird in Louisiana[27]. Introduction of togaviruses into the USA has recently been demonstrated by the West Nile virus outbreak in New York and Connecticut, and its spread to other states.

HEPATITIS B VIRUS

History

Hepatitis B virus (HBV), a member of the family Hepadnaviridae, genus *Orthohepadnavirus*, is an enveloped double-stranded DNA icosahedral virus measuring 42nm in diameter[28,29].

Epidemiology

Transmitted by parenteral and sexual routes, HBV infection occurs worldwide, but prevalence is higher in Asia, the Middle East and sub-Saharan Africa. The prevalence in China may be as high as 10%, compared to 0.01% in the USA. Most acute infections in endemic regions occur at an early age with many acquired perinatally. Early HBV infection is usually asymptomatic. The annual incidence of infection in children may be as high as 5%. The rate of HBV carriage and specific antibody declines with age. In the West, most infections are acquired during adulthood through sexual or needle exposures, and are more often associated with acute hepatitis. Of those with hepatitis, 5–10% develop persistent infection. In endemic regions, HBV is a common cause of chronic liver disease and a leading cause of hepatocellular carcinoma[30].

Clinical features

The incubation period from infection to hepatitis is usually 45–120 days. A preicteric prodromal period lasts several days to a month and may be associated with fever, myalgia, malaise, anorexia, nausea and vomiting. Significant viremia occurs early in infection. Soluble immune complexes with circulating hepatitis B surface antigen (HB_sAg) form as antihepatitis-B-surface-antigen antibodies (HB_sAb) are produced. An immune-complex-mediated arthritis is usually sudden in onset and often severe. Joint involvement is typically symmetric with simultaneous involvement of several joints at onset but arthritis may be migratory or additive[31]. The joints of the hands and knees are most often affected but wrists, ankles, elbows, shoulders and other large joints may be involved as well. Fusiform swelling may be seen in the small joints of the hands. Morning stiffness is common. Arthritis and urticaria may precede jaundice by days to weeks and may persist several weeks after jaundice. However, arthritis and rash usually subside soon after onset of clinical jaundice. While arthritis is usually limited to the preicteric prodrome, those who develop chronic active hepatitis or chronic HBV viremia may have recurrent polyarthralgia or polyarthritis. Polyarteritis nodosa may be associated with chronic hepatitis B viremia.

Diagnosis

Urticaria in the presence of polyarthritis should raise the possibility of HBV infection. Acute hepatitis may be asymptomatic but elevated bilirubin and transaminases are usually present when the arthritis appears. At the time of arthritis onset, peak levels of serum HB_sAg are detectable. Virions, viral DNA, polymerase and hepatitis B e antigen may be detectable in serum. Antihepatitis-B core antigen IgM antibodies are present and indicate acute HBV infection as opposed to past or chronic infection.

Pathogenesis

It is thought that HBV arthritis is mediated by immune complex deposition in synovium. Immune complexes containing HB_sAg, antibody and complement components may be detected.

HEPATITIS C VIRUS

History

Hepatitis C virus (HCV), a member of the family Flaviviridae, is an enveloped, single-stranded RNA spherical virus measuring 38–50nm in diameter[32].

Epidemiology

Infection with HCV occurs worldwide. Seroprevalence is less than 1% in developed Western countries but is higher in Africa and Asia, where it may cause a quarter of the acute and chronic hepatitides. In Japan, this figure may reach 50%.

Hepatitis C virus is transmitted by the parenteral route. Sexual transmission appears to be rare. HCV is responsible for 95% of post-transfusion hepatitis in countries routinely screening donated blood for HBV. More than half of all cases of non-A, non-B hepatitis are attributable to HCV infection[33]. Genotypic variants of HCV have been described and these differ in their pathogenicity, including severity of disease and response to an interferon. HCV is currently grouped into six major genotypes or clades, with over 50 genotypic subtypes[34].

Clinical features

Acute HCV infection is usually benign. Up to 80% of post-transfusion infections are anicteric and asymptomatic. Prior to cirrhosis, liver enzyme elevations are usually minimal when present. Community-acquired cases present as a more symptomatic illness in which significant enzyme elevations occur. However, fulminant HCV hepatitis is rare. HCV is strongly associated with HBV-negative hepatocellular carcinoma, especially in Africa and Japan.

Acute onset polyarthritis in a rheumatoid distribution, including the small joints of the hands, wrists, shoulders, knees and hips, may occur in acute HCV infection[35]. In established disease, HCV is often associated with type II cryoglobulinemia. It may present as essential mixed cryoglobulinemia, a triad of arthritis, palpable purpura and cryoglobulinemia. Indeed, a majority of patients with essential mixed cryoglobulinemia have HCV infection. Less commonly, HCV infection may be seen in secondary cryoglobulinemia. The presence of anti-HCV antibodies in essential mixed cryoglobulinemia is associated with more severe cutaneous involvement, e.g. Raynaud's phenomenon, purpura, livedo reticularis, distal ulcers and gangrene. HCV RNA may be found in 75% of cryoprecipitates from patients with essential mixed cryoglobulinemia and anti-HCV antibodies[36].

Diagnosis

Serologic tests use an array of antigens in an enzyme immunoassay. A recombinant strip immunoblot assay (RIBA) is confirmatory. Second generation RIBA-2 tests for reactivity to four viral antigens: c33c, c22-3, c100-3 and 5-1-1. A positive RIBA-2, especially to c33c and c22-3, is a sensitive test for HCV infection[37]. C33c positivity is associated with viremia. Patients may have HCV RNA detectable by reverse transcription polymerase chain reaction (RT-PCR) amplification methods in the absence of a positive serology.

Pathogenesis

Chronic HCV infection leads to cirrhosis, end-stage liver failure and hepatocellular carcinoma but the frequency of these sequelae and the mechanisms by which they occur are not known. Infection with HCV persists despite vigorous antibody response to an array of viral epitopes. A high rate of mutation in the envelope protein is responsible for the emergence of neutralization escape mutants and development of quasispecies[38]. Why HCV elicits cryoglobulins remains to be fully delineated. However, it has been proposed that HCV envelope glycoproteins are capable of binding IgG Fc. Antibodies to IgG Fc develop though epitope spreading from initial response directed to virus[39].

Management

Interferon α has been shown to be efficacious in the treatment of chronic HCV hepatitis and HCV-associated cryoglobulinemia. Interferon-α2b at a dose of 3 million units thrice weekly for 6 months suppresses viral titers and ameliorates clinical disease in about half of patients[40]. Some protocols call for slightly higher doses. Those with symptomatic cryoglobulinemia failing interferon therapy require immunosuppressive therapy. Relapse after completion of the initial course of interferon therapy is common. Addition of ribavirin to therapeutic regimens has improved the rate of viral clearing. There is controversy whether interferon therapy precipitates autoimmune disease such as autoimmune thyroiditis.

RETROVIRUSES

Human T-lymphocyte leukemia virus-1

Endemic in Japan, HTLV-1 has been observed to be associated with oligoarthritis and a nodular rash. The patients have positive serology for anti-HTLV antibodies. Type C viral particles are seen in skin lesions. Atypical synovial cells with lobulated nuclei and T-cell synovial infiltrates suggest direct involvement of the synovial tissue by the leukemic process[41].

OTHER VIRUSES

Apart from specific viral infections described above in which arthralgia and/or arthritis are typically prominent manifestations, there are a host of commonly encountered viral syndromes in which joint involvement occasionally occurs. Children with varicella rarely develop brief monoarticular or pauciarticular arthritis that is thought to be viral in origin. Adults with mumps occasionally develop small or large joint synovitis lasting up to several weeks. Arthritis may precede or follow parotitis by up to 4 weeks.

Infection with adenovirus and Coxsackieviruses A9, B2, B3, B4 and B6 have been associated with recurrent episodes of polyarthritis, pleuritis, myalgia, rash, pharyngitis, myocarditis and leukocytosis. Epstein–Barr-virus-induced mononucleosis is frequently accompanied by polyarthralgia, but occasional monoarticular knee arthritis occurs. A few cases of polyarthritis, fever and myalgias due to echovirus 9 infection have been reported. Arthritis associated with herpes simplex virus or cytomegalovirus infections is also rare, although severe cytomegalovirus polyarthritis may occur following bone marrow transplantation[42]. Herpes simplex virus occasionally causes arthritis of the knee, known as 'herpes gladiatorum' because it is seen in wrestlers. Vaccinia virus has been associated with postvaccination knee arthritis in only two reported cases.

REFERENCES

1. Bell LM, Naides SJ, Stoffman P et al. Human parvovirus B19 infection among hospital staff members after contact with infected patients. N Engl J Med 1989; 321: 485–491.
2. Anderson MJ, Higgins PG, Davis LR et al. Experimental parvoviral infection in humans. J Infect Dis 1985; 152: 257–265.
3. Naides SJ. Parvoviruses. In: Specter S, Hodinka R L, Young SA, eds. Clinical virology manual, 3rd ed. New York: Elsevier Science 2000: 487–500.
4. Feder HM Jr. Fifth disease. N Engl J Med 1994; 331: 1062.
5. Naides SJ, Scharosch LL, Foto F, Howard EJ. Rheumatologic manifestations of human parvovirus B19 infection in adults. Initial two-year clinical experience. Arthritis Rheum 1990; 33: 1297–1309.
6. Chantler J, Wolinsky JS, Tingle A. Rubella virus. In: Knipe DM, Howley PM, Griffin DE et al. Fields virology, 4th ed. Philadelphia, PA: Lippincott Williams & Wilkins 2001: 963–990.
7. Kilroy AW, Schaffner W, Fleet WF Jr et al. Two syndromes following rubella immunization. Clinical observations and epidemiological studies. JAMA 1970; 214: 2287–2292.
8. Williams LL, Wolinsky JS, Cao S-N et al. Antibody response to rubella virus antigen and structural proteins in retinitis pigmentosa. J Infect Dis 1992; 166: 525–530.
9. Mitchell LA, Tingle AJ, Shukin R et al. Chronic rubella vaccine-associated arthropathy. Arch Intern Med 1993; 153: 2268–2274.
10. Griffin DE. Alphaviruses. In: Knipe DM, Howley PM, Griffin DE et al. Fields virology, 4th ed. Philadelphia, PA: Lippincott Williams & Wilkins 2001: 917–962.
11. Lam SK, Chua KB, Hooi PS et al. Chikungunya infection – an emerging disease in Malaysia. Southeast Asian J Trop Med Public Health 2001; 32: 447–451.
12. Tesh RB. Arthritides caused by mosquito-borne viruses. Ann Rev Med 1982; 33: 31–40.
13. Brighton SW, Prozesky OW, De la Harpe AL. Chikungunya virus infection. A retrospective study of 107 cases. S Afr Med J 1983; 63: 313–315.
14. Brighton SW, Simson IW. A destructive arthropathy following Chikungunya virus arthritis – a possible association. Clin Rheumatol 1984; 3: 253–258.
15. Williams MC, Woodall JP, Gillett JD. O'nyong-nyong fever: an epidemic in East Africa. VII. Virus isolations from man and serological studies up to July 1961. Trans R Soc Trop Med Hyg 1965; 59: 186–197.

16. Kiwanuka N, Sanders EJ, Rwaguma EB *et al*. O'nyong-nyong fever in south-central Uganda, 1996–1997: clinical features and validation of a clinical case definition for surveillance purposes. Clin Infect Dis 1999; 29: 1243–1250.

17. Shore H. O'nyong-nyong fever: an epidemic virus disease in East Africa. III. Some clinical and epidemiological observations in the northern province. Trans R Soc Trop Med Hyg 1961; 55: 361–373.

18. Moore DL, Causey OR, Carey DE *et al*. Arthropod-borne viral infections of man in Nigeria, 1964–1970. Ann Trop Med Parasitol 1975; 69: 49–64.

19. Fraser JRE. Epidemic polyarthritis and Ross River virus disease. Clin Rheum Dis 1986; 12: 369–388.

20. Aaskov JG, Mataika JU, Lawrence GW *et al*. An epidemic of Ross River virus infection in Fiji, 1979. Am J Trop Med Hyg 1981; 30: 1053–1059.

21. Fraser JR, Ratnamohan VM, Dowling JP *et al*. The exanthem of Ross River virus infection: histology, location of virus antigen and nature of inflammatory infiltrate. J Clin Pathol 1983; 36: 1256–1263.

22. Lindsay MDA, Johansen CA, Broom AK *et al*. Emergence of Barmah Forest virus in western Australia. Emerging Infect Dis (online) 1995; 1: 1–6.

23. Tesh RB. Arthritides caused by mosquito-borne viruses. Annu Rev Med 1982; 33: 31–40.

24. Niklasson B, Espmark A, Lundstrom J. Occurrence of arthralgia and specific IgM antibodies three to four years after Ockelbo disease. J Infect Dis 1988; 157: 832–835.

25. Hoch AL, Peterson NE, LeDuc JW, Pinheiro FP. An outbreak of Mayaro virus disease in Belterra, Brazil. III. Entomological and ecological studies. Am J Trop Med Hyg 1981; 30: 689–698.

26. Tesh RB, Watts DM, Russell KL *et al*. Mayaro virus disease: an emerging mosquito-borne zoonosis in tropical South America. Clin Infect Dis 1999; 28: 67–73.

27. Calisher CH, Gutierrez E, Maness KS, Lord RD. Isolation of Mayaro virus from a migrating bird captured in Louisiana in 1967. Bull Pan Am Health Organ 1974; 8: 243–248.

28. Hollinger FB, Liang, TJ. Hepatitis B virus. In: Knipe DM, Howley PM, Griffin DE *et al*. Fields virology, 4th ed. Philadelphia, PA: Lippincott Williams & Wilkins 2001: 2971–3036.

29. Seeger C. Hepatitis B viruses: molecular biology (human). In: Webster RG, Granoff A, eds. Encyclopedia of virology. San Diego, CA: Academic Press; 1994: 560–544.

30. Robinson WS. Hepatitis B viruses: General features (human). In: Webster RG, Granoff A, eds. Encyclopedia of virology. San Diego, CA: Academic Press; 1994: 554–9.

31. Alarcon GS, Townes AS. Arthritis in viral hepatitis. Report of two cases and review of the literature. Johns Hopkins Med J 1973; 132: 1–15.

32. Purcell RH. Hepatitis C virus. In: In: Webster RG, Granoff A, eds. Encyclopedia of virology. San Diego, CA: Academic Press; 1994: 569–74.

33. Bhandari BN, Wright TL. Hepatitis C: an overview. Annu Rev Med 1995; 46: 309–317.

34. Major ME, Rehermann B, Feinstone SM. Hepatitis C virus. In: Knipe DM, Howley PM, Griffin DE *et al*. Fields virology, 4th ed. Philadelphia, PA: Lippincott Williams & Wilkins 2001: 1127–1161.

35. Siegel LB, Cohn L, Nashel D. Rheumatic manifestations of hepatitis C infection. Semin Arthritis Rheum 1993; 23: 149–154.

36. Munoz-Fernandez S, Barbado FJ, Martin Mola E *et al*. Evidence of hepatitis C virus antibodies in the cryoprecipitate of patients with mixed cryoglobulinemia. J Rheumatol 1994; 21: 229–233.

37. Van der Poel CL. Hepatitis C virus: into the fourth generation. Vox Sang 1994; 67(suppl 3): 95–98.

38. Shimizu YK, Hijikata M, Iwamoto A *et al*. Neutralizing antibodies against hepatitis C virus and the emergence of neutralization escape mutant viruses. J Virol 1994; 68: 1494–1500.

39. Wunschmann S, Medh JD, Klinzmann D *et al*. Characterization of hepatitis C virus (HCV) and HCV E2 interactions with CD81 and the low-density lipoprotein receptor. J Virol 2000; 74: 10055–10062.

40. Jenkins PJ, Cromie SL, Bowden DS *et al*. Chronic hepatitis C and interferon alfa therapy: predictors of long term response. Med J Aust 1996; 164: 150–152.

41. Nishioka K, Nakajima T, Hasunuma T, Sato K. Rheumatic manifestation of human leukemia virus infection. Rheum Dis Clin North Am 1993; 19: 489–503.

42. Burns LJ, Gingrich RD. Cytomegalovirus infection presenting as polyarticular arthritis following autologous BMT. Bone Marrow Transplant 1993; 11: 77–79.

98

Rheumatic aspects of human immunodeficiency virus infection and other immunodeficient states

Dimitrios Vassilopoulos and Leonard H Calabrese

HUMAN IMMUNODEFICIENCY VIRUS INFECTION

Definition

- Human retroviral infection with the human immunodeficiency virus (HIV)
- Infectious state characterized by progressive immunodeficiency and immunodysregulation
- Frequently associated with a wide range of clinical findings, including opportunistic infections and malignancies
- Occasionally associated with a variety of autoimmune-like and rheumatic manifestations including arthritis, myositis, Sjögren's-like syndrome and vasculitis

Clinical features

- Arthritis including reactive arthritis (Reiter's syndrome), psoriatic arthritis and idiopathic articular disease
- Myositis including polymyositis, non-inflammatory myopathies and drug-induced disease
- Vasculitic disease representing the spectrum of vascular inflammation
- Sjögren's-like disease characterized by diffuse lymphocytic infiltration

HYPOGAMMAGLOBULINEMIA

Definition

- Can be congenital or acquired
- Associated with arthritis, often infectious, and several autoimmune syndromes

Clinical features

- Hypogammaglobulinemia is often complicated by recurrent pyogenic infections
- Occasionally, hypogammaglobulinemia is complicated by infective or non-infective arthritis, echovirus and a polymyositis-like illness, and autoimmune disorders

HISTORY

The first cases of acquired immunodeficiency syndrome (AIDS) were identified in 1981, when previously healthy individuals were observed to develop a variety of unusual and dramatic opportunistic infections and cancers known to thrive in an immunosuppressive milieu. Throughout the early 1980s, the absence of an identifiable etiology for the syndrome necessitated recognition primarily on clinical grounds. Although the spectrum of reported opportunistic infections continued to enlarge, there were no substantive reports of significant rheumatic disease. In 1984, the etiology of AIDS was discovered in the form of the human lentivirus named human immunodeficiency virus, or HIV. Following this discovery came the development of a powerful system of serologic detection that quickly led to two clinical revelations. First, the study of

the asymptomatic carrier state revealed that HIV induced far more than a state of immunologic unresponsiveness or deficiency but, more importantly, a state of profound immunodysregulation. Secondly, a series of clinical observations and disease associations quickly followed, greatly enlarging the spectrum of HIV-induced illness. Among these clinical observations were a variety of autoimmune-like and rheumatic diseases. In 1987, Winchester and colleagues[1] described a series of 13 patients from New York City with HIV infection and reactive arthritis (Reiter's syndrome), stimulating further systematic investigations of rheumatic disease in HIV infection. Beginning in late 1995, a dramatic change occurred in the management of HIV disease, with the advent and widespread use of combination antiretroviral therapy now commonly referred to as 'highly active anti-retroviral therapy' (HAART). This regimen, using a minimum of three drugs, from the current and growing armamentarium of 16 widely approved and available agents in the industrialized world, has resulted in dramatic reductions in mortality and a changing pattern of morbidity[2]. To date, although many questions regarding epidemiology, pathogenesis and treatment remain unanswered, the coexistence of a distinct spectrum of rheumatic disease and HIV has become of great practical importance to both the clinical and research rheumatologist.

EPIDEMIOLOGY

Human immunodeficiency virus infection is a worldwide epidemic that grew from an estimated 100 000 infections in 1980 to an estimated 35 million by December of 2000[3,4]. The epidemic is far more extensive than predicted by the World Health Organization a decade ago, exceeding these estimates by 50%. Africa continues to lead the world in bearing the burden of HIV disease, with 70% of the world's infected adults and 80% of the children living there. Furthermore, Africa has been the source of 75% of all HIV-related deaths since the beginning of the epidemic. Table 98.1 provides regional statistics demonstrating the global nature of the epidemic and its predominant mode of regional transmission. For the first time, small examples of aggressive prevention programs appear to be paying off noticeably in countries such as Uganda and Thailand, but these pockets of good news are offset by dramatic increases in new infections in regions of Eastern Europe and Asia.

The transmission of HIV is accomplished through three routes. First, it is a sexually transmitted disease that is bidirectionally transmitted from men to men, men to women, women to men and, rarely, even women to women. Secondly, it is a blood-borne pathogen that can be transmitted through the sharing of intravenous (i.v.) needles and syringes among drug users, or through contaminated blood or blood products. Thirdly, it can be transmitted perinatally from an infected mother to her unborn child. Several patterns of transmission have been noted on a worldwide basis, with Pattern I being predominantly among homosexual or bisexual men and i.v. drug users in Western Europe, North America, some areas of South America, Australia and New Zealand. Pattern II is predominantly heterosexual transmission in

TABLE 98.1 WORLDWIDE DISTRIBUTION OF HIV INFECTION					
Region	Epidemic started	Adults and children living with HIV/AIDS	Adult prevalence rate (%)	HIV-positive adults who are women (%)	Main mode(s) of transmission for adults living with HIV/AIDS
Sub-Saharan Africa	late '70s–early '80s	25.3 million	8.8	55	Hetero
North Africa and Middle East	late '80s	400 000	0.2	40	Hetero, IDU
South and South-East Asia	late '80s	5.8 million	0.56	35	Hetero, IDU
East Asia and Pacific	late '80s	640 000	0.07	13	IDU, hetero, MSM
Latin America	late '70s–early '80s	1.4 million	0.5	25	MSM, IDU, hetero
Caribbean	late '70s–early '80s	390 000	2.3	35	Hetero, MSM
Eastern Europe and Central Asia	early '90s	700 000	0.35	25	IDU
Western Europe	late '70s–early '80s	540 000	0.24	25	MSM, IDU
North America	late '70s–early '80s	920 000	0.6	20	MSM, IDU, hetero
Australia and New Zealand	late '70s–early '80s	15 000	0.13	10	MSM
TOTAL		36.1 million	1.1	47	

Hetero, heterosexual transmission; IDU, transmission through injecting drug use; MSM, sexual transmission among men who have sex with men
Regional HIV/AIDS statistics and features – December 2000. (Data from UNAIDS/WHO[3].)

Africa, the Caribbean and some areas of South America. Pattern III is the most recently detected and describes transmission among persons with several sex partners. This is being observed in Asia, the Pacific region, the Middle East, Eastern Europe and some rural areas of South America.

The epidemiology of rheumatic disease and HIV infection is an area of significant controversy. It is undeniable that patients with HIV infection often develop a variety of rheumatic syndromes; however, many of these reports have been anecdotal. Series of prospective epidemiologic investigations, primarily studying articular disease, have reported highly disparate results[5]. From the extremes of these observations, it would appear that HIV may either confer a dramatic risk for the development of certain rheumatic syndromes or alternatively be protective. The differences between these epidemiologic studies may be explained by several observations including:

- the radically different types of research design (point prevalence estimates by examination, questionnaires, prospective longitudinal cohort design, study endpoints)
- varying case mix (homosexuals or i.v. drug users, etc.)
- differing stages of HIV infection among individuals
- possible regional differences in the virus.

Table 98.2 presents the frequency of various rheumatic manifestations in a large number of HIV-positive patients (458) seen in an outpatient rheumatology clinic[6].

CLINICAL FEATURES

Articular disease

Arthralgia

A wide variety of articular clinical syndromes have been identified in HIV-infected individuals (Table 98.3), but the most commonly observed symptoms are simple arthralgias. These are generally intermittent, mild and polyarticular. In our experience, they occur most frequently in the later stages of HIV infection. The significance of their presence is hard to ascertain, as most of these individuals are infected with several opportunistic agents and have profound constitutional symptoms at the time.

TABLE 98.2 FREQUENCY OF RHEUMATIC DISEASE MANIFESTATIONS IN HIV-POSITIVE PATIENTS	
Diagnosis	No. of patients (%)
Diffuse Infiltrative lymphocytosis syndrome (DILS)	94 (21)
Bursitis/tenosynovitis	86 (19)
Low back pain	34 (7)
Osteoarthritis	31 (7)
HIV-associated arthralgia	28 (6)
Increased creatine kinase	26 (6)
Parotid enlargement	21 (6)
Reactive arthritis/psoriatic arthritis	19 (4)
HIV-associated arthritis	17 (4)
Fibromyalgia	17 (4)
Hepatitis B/C syndromes	15 (3)
HIV-associated polymyositis	10 (2)
Gout	8 (2)
Infectious arthritis	6 (1)
Systemic lupus erythematosus	5 (1)
Sicca symptoms	4 (1)
Vasculitis	4 (1)
Ankylosing spondylitis	2 (0.5)

An assessment of the distribution of rheumatic diagnoses in 458 HIV-positive patients seen at an outpatient clinic betwee 1994 and 2000 (Adapted with permission from Reveille[6].)

TABLE 98.3 RHEUMATIC SYNDROMES FREQUENTLY OBSERVED WITH HIV INFECTION	
Articular syndromes	Arthralgia
	Reactive arthritis (Reiter's syndrome)
	Psoriatic arthritis
	Undifferentiated spondyloarthropathy
	Idiopathic or HIV-associated arthritis
	Septic arthritis
	Osteonecrosis
Connective tissue diseases	Sjögren's-like syndrome
	Inflammatory and non-inflammatory myopathy
	Systemic vasculitis
	Lupus-like syndrome

Reactive arthritis (Reiter's syndrome)

An aseptic peripheral arthritis occurs in HIV-infected individuals and has been reported predominantly among homosexual men. In many of these patients there are accompanying extra-articular features suggestive of reactive arthritis, including urethritis, ocular inflammation and skin lesions[7]. The skin disease reported in such individuals ranges from seborrhea to frank keratoderma blennorrhagica. The propensity of HIV-infected individuals to have several different skin lesions simultaneously, and for patients with clear-cut reactive arthritis to have frank psoriasis, illustrates the continuing difficulty with nosology of articular disease in HIV infection. Solomon et al.[7] have stressed that HIV-infected patients are frequently best classified as suffering from undifferentiated spondyloarthropathy[7].

Many HIV patients with reactive arthritis and undifferentiated spondyloarthropathy developed their disease in the wake of identifiable infection such as *Shigella flexneri* or *Campylobacter jejuni* and, rarely, *Yersinia pseudotuberculosis* or *Y. enterocolitica*. Surprisingly, despite a high frequency of history of urethritis, there are no reported cases of infection with *Chlamydia trachomatis*[8]. The articular disease in these patients primarily involves knees, ankles and feet, although a small minority may also have involvement of the hands, wrists and upper extremities. Solomon et al.[7] have stressed the frequent presence of multi-digit dactylitis, which at times can be relatively painless and may give the appearance of edema of the foot. Axial disease is unusual, and radiographic sacroiliitis is extremely rare. Enthesopathy in the distribution of the Achillis tendon, plantar fascia, anterior and posterior tibial tendons and extensor tendons are also seen. These lesions collectively may cause patients to walk on the outside margins of the feet in a broad-based manner, giving a characteristic gait and stance referred to as 'AIDS foot', which may simulate peripheral neuropathy[7].

The clinical course in such patients is highly variable and probably reflects the underlying clinical heterogeneity. The disease may be relatively mild, not associated with radiographic changes, and easily controlled by non-steroidal anti-inflammatory drugs (NSAIDs). At times, however, it may be unusually severe, associated with radiographic periostitis and erosions[9,10], and highly refractory to anti-inflammatory medications. A more severe course of reactive arthritis with persistent polyarticular involvement accompanied by erosive changes and progression to joint fusion has been reported recently in African blacks[10].

The risk of reactive arthritis may have, at least in part, an immunogenetic basis. Thus, in white HIV-infected patients with reactive arthritis, there is a strong association with human leukocyte antigen (HLA)-B27[6]. The same is true for patients with peripheral psoriatic arthritis. However, in several studies in African blacks no association with HLA-B27 has been detected[11].

Treatment with NSAIDs will usually suffice for the majority of patients, whereas for refractory cases sulfasalazine, etretinate, hydroxychloroquine and even methotrexate have been administered[6].

Psoriatic arthritis

There is a spectrum of papulosquamous dermopathy associated with HIV infection. These changes range from seborrheic dermatitis at the mild end, through frank psoriasis vulgaris (Fig. 98.1) to pustular psoriasis at the severe end. The latter is indistinguishable from keratoderma blennorrhagica. The exact prevalence of psoriasis in HIV-infected patients is difficult to ascertain, given the overlap of skin diseases in the continuous spectrum of involvement mentioned above. Overall, although its prevalence is not different than that of the general population, its severity is increased[8,12]. Regardless of prevalence, the acute onset of papulosquamous dermopathy in an adult with or without arthritis should warrant consideration of possible HIV infection, especially in individuals at high risk.

Arthritis and enthesopathy similar to that described in patients with reactive arthritis is also seen concomitantly with psoriasis. The relative frequency of psoriatic arthritis in patients with HIV infection varies in different populations. Although earlier studies did not show a significantly greater prevalence in white HIV-infected patients[8,11], recent studies in black Africans have demonstrated an increase[13]. Psoriatic arthritis in the presence of HIV appears to follow a more severe course, as with psoriasis infection *per se*. In a recent study of 27 HIV-infected patients with psoriatic arthritis from Zambia, Njobvu and McGill[13] reported an asymmetric polyarticular pattern of involvement in the majority of patients (~80%). Joints of the lower extremities were more frequently involved, and enthesitis was present in 50% of cases[13]. Skin and joint disease appeared simultaneously in most patients (65%) – an unusual pattern of presentation, at least for white patients[13]. Sacroiliitis was suspected clinically in 20% of patients but that was not confirmed radiologically[13].

Immunogenetic studies in small number of psoriatic HIV-positive patients have found that HLA-B27 is significantly associated with peripheral arthritis. Indeed, compared with HIV-unrelated psoriasis, HLA-B27 is encountered in increased frequency in HIV-infected individuals with skin disease (23% in HIV infection compared with 8% in controls), giving further support to the notion of a disease continuum[14]. Although these data have not been reproduced in larger number of patients, other HLA alleles associated with psoriasis *per se*, particularly Cw*0602, are associated with the development of psoriatic skin lesions in HIV-infected patients[15].

The clinical course of psoriatic arthritis is heterogeneous, with variable progression of both the skin and joint disease. Data regarding the efficacy of various therapeutic interventions are limited. Antiretroviral treatment appears to have a beneficial effect on skin disease[16–18], but its effect on joint manifestations is unclear. Oral gold[19], cyclosporine[20] and methotrexate (7.5–15mg/week)[21,22] have been tried successfully in small number of HIV-infected patients with psoriatic arthritis. Recently, case reports of psoriatic arthritis treated with biologic agents that target the action of specific cytokines such as tumor necrosis factor (TNF)-α[23] and interleukin (IL)-1[24] have been published. Despite clinical improvement of joint and skin disease with anti-TNF-α treatment, infectious complications were noted[23]. Carefully performed studies involving larger number of patients are needed in order to evaluate the efficacy and safety of such promising agents in the treatment of psoriasis and psoriatic arthritis in HIV-infected individuals.

Other forms of HIV-associated arthritis

In most prospective series investigating the presence of articular disease in HIV infection, the most frequently encountered condition, aside from

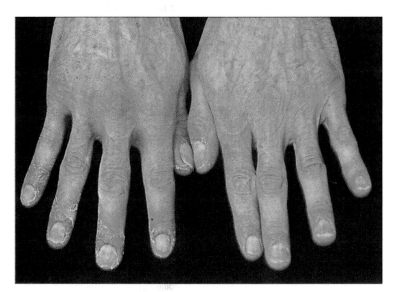

Fig. 98.1 The hands of a patient with psoriatic arthritis and HIV infection.

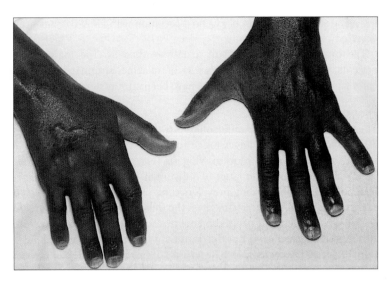

Fig. 98.2 The hands of a 35-year-old man with advanced HIV infection fulfilling the American College of Rheumatology criteria for rheumatoid arthritis.

arthralgias, is idiopathic seronegative arthritis. Within this group, Rynes[25] has described a subgroup of patients presenting with exquisite pain in the knees or ankles lasting from hours to a few days. The syndrome has been labeled the 'painful articular syndrome'[26]. The synovial fluid white blood cell count often reveals a minimally inflammatory state, with counts in the range of 50–2600 cells/mm³. Narcotics are often required for relief of symptomatic pain.

More frequently, though, an inflammatory asymmetric oligoarthritis involving the large joints of the lower extremities has been reported[27,28]. Radiologically there is absence of erosive bone changes and clinically the arthritis follows a self-limiting course, with the majority of symptoms resolving in 2–6 weeks[6,27,28]. In few cases, a symmetric polyarthritis resembling rheumatoid arthritis (RA) has been reported[9,28]. Given the self-limited course of this condition, most patients do not require long-term anti-inflammatory treatment. It has been reported anecdotally that hydroxychloroquine, oral gold and sulfasalazine have been tried with success[6].

The relationship between HIV infection and RA has been the subject of considerable debate. The observation of clinical remission occurring in several patients with RA who subsequently became infected with HIV prompted some observers to suggest that RA and HIV cannot coexist. Ornstein et al.[29] have reported a patient with coexisting RA and HIV infection and identified four additional cases associated with destructive radiographic manifestations, all occurring with a CD4 cell count of fewer than 20 cells/mm³ (Fig. 98.2). Other reports have also documented progressive joint destruction despite depletion of CD4 cells[30].

Musculoskeletal infections

Considering the remarkable array of opportunistic infections and increased incidence of pyogenic infections in HIV-infected individuals, it is surprising that there are so few cases of musculoskeletal infectious complications[31]. In large series of HIV-infected patients, the incidence of musculoskeletal infections has been less than 1%[6,31–34]. These infectious complications include septic arthritis, osteomyelitis, pyomyositis (see below) and, rarely, septic bursitis[31].

Most cases of septic arthritis that have been reported in the literature were caused by *Staphylococcus aureus*[31]. Other frequently encountered agents include *Streptococcus* and *Salmonella* species, and atypical *Mycobacteria*[31]. Opportunistic joint infections caused by various microorganisms have sporadically been reported[31]. Despite the rarity of these reports, their existence emphasizes the importance of approaching all new articular disease, especially that which is acute and monoarticular,

as potentially infectious with both routine and opportunistic pathogens. In general, the clinical presentation, course and prognosis of septic arthritis in HIV-positive individuals does not differ from that of septic arthritis in HIV-negative individuals[31].

Osteomyelitis usually develops at advanced stages of HIV infection and is most commonly due to *Mycobacteria* (atypical species and *M. tuberculosis*) and *Staphylococcus aureus*[31]. Its prognosis, despite appropriate antimicrobial treatment, appears to be worse than that of septic arthritis.

Connective tissue disease
Sjögren's-like syndrome

Sjögren's syndrome is characterized by multiple exocrine gland dysfunction, leading principally to keratoconjunctivitis sicca and xerostomia (see Chapter 130). The clinical situations in which the diagnosis is made range from primary Sjögren's syndrome, an autoimmune disease in itself with or without an associated connective tissue disease, to isolated sicca complaints not associated with other autoimmune phenomena and frequently detected in elderly women. Histopathologically, the architecture of minor salivary glands is not specific in Sjögren's syndrome. Pathologically, several conditions, including graft-versus-host disease, lymphoma, hepatitis C virus and HIV infection, must be excluded for the pathologic diagnosis of primary Sjögren's syndrome. In patients with known HIV infection who are receiving treatment with protease inhibitors, the possibility of parotid lipomatosis must also be excluded[35].

The presence of sicca symptoms and parotid gland enlargement, and a light microscopic picture compatible with Sjögren's syndrome, have been noted in HIV-infected individuals. The distinct nature of this condition, from both the immunopathologic and genetic perspectives, was elucidated recently[36] and clearly demonstrated that the sicca complex occurring in HIV-infected individuals is a distinct entity, despite its superficial similarity to primary Sjögren's syndrome. The name 'diffuse infiltrative lymphocytosis syndrome' (DILS) has been proposed, because of the diffuse lymphocytic visceral infiltration demonstrated in these patients.

It has now become clear that DILS represents a syndrome characterized by salivary gland enlargement (often massive) with associated sicca symptoms (more than 60% of the cases), CD8 lymphocytosis and a number of extraglandular complications as a result of lymphocytic infiltration of various organs[6]. Involved organs include the lungs (lymphocytic interstitial pneumonitis), nerves (peripheral neuropathy, aseptic meningitis, VIIth nerve palsy), kidneys (interstitial nephritis, renal tubular acidosis), liver (hepatitis), muscles (polymyositis) and hematopoietic system (lymphoma). The prevalence of DILS in large series of HIV-infected patients has ranged between 3% and 8%[37,38].

The light microscopic picture is often indistinguishable from primary Sjögren's syndrome, with intense lymphocytic infiltrations, but examination by immunohistochemistry reveals that, in contrast to the CD4 predominance of Sjögren's syndrome, the infiltrates in patients with DILS are predominantly CD8 (Fig. 98.3). Recently, histological analysis of salivary glands revealed the frequent presence of cystic duct dilatation with associated CD8⁺ cell infiltration (lymphoepithelial cysts)[6]. CD8⁺ cells are occasionally found diffusely throughout the viscera and display an array of post-thymic maturation markers, including major histocompatibility complex (MHC) class II, CD29 and leukocyte function antigen-l[39]. Biopsies from involved nerves in patients with DILS-associated peripheral neuropathy revealed marked CD8 angiocentric infiltration of vessel walls in epi- and endo-neurium, in addition to muscles, without fibrinoid necrosis[40]. Clonal analysis of the infiltrating cells revealed a polyclonal T cell population, excluding the possibility of a T cell lymphoma[41].

Immunogenetically, these patients are distinctive, with an increased frequency of HLA-DR5 in black patients (86% compared with 7% in

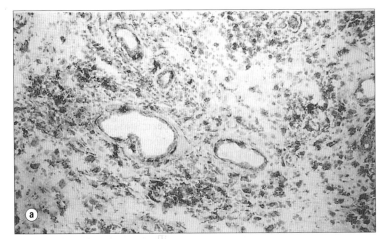

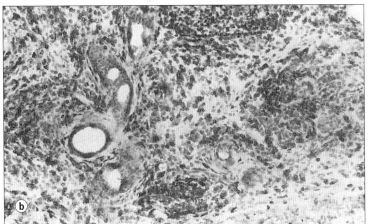

Fig. 98.3 Biopsy samples of the salivary glands of a patient with HIV.
(a) A heavy infiltrate of CD8+ cells and atrophy of the gland are seen.
(b) Scattered CD4+ cells are evident. (Original magnification × 3100). (With permission from Calabrese LH, Wilke WS, Perkins AD, *et al*. Rheumatoid arthritis complicated by infection with the human immunodeficiency virus and the development of Sjögren's syndrome. Arthritis Rheum 1989; 32: 1453–1457.)

controls) and an increase in HLA-DR6 and -DR7 in whites. This is in contrast to the HLA-DR2 and HLA-DR3 predominance in primary Sjögren's syndrome. Molecular genetic analysis of these HLA-DR alleles in patients with DILS has revealed that the associated DR5 sub-type in Africans is DR5 JVM (DRB1*1102). Further, this subtype, together with the other reported associated DRB1 alleles: DR6 (DRB1*1102), DR6 (DRB1*1301) and DR7 (DRB1*0701), all share a common amino acid sequence in the third hypervariable region of the DR molecule.

These data suggest that the predisposition to DILS in both blacks and whites is associated with specific polymorphic residues in the α-helical third diversity region of the MHC class II molecule. Serologically, in contrast to patients with primary Sjögren's syndrome, these patients are routinely negative by immunodiffusion techniques for antinuclear antibodies including anti-Ro and anti-La, although an older study had suggested that low levels of these antibodies may be detected by more sensitive techniques[39]. Earlier studies have also suggested that patients with DILS have a slower progression of their HIV disease, with reduced overall mortality. Further studies are needed in order to confirm these early observations and the effect of the newer antiviral agents.

In patients with DILS, salivary gland enlargement and sicca symptoms are the most commonly encountered problems. Zidovudine and, more recently, moderate doses of corticosteroids (prednisone 30–40mg/day), have been reported to be successful in ameliorating these signs and symptoms[6]. More ominously in patients with DILS, extraglandular complications, including progressive lymphocytic interstitial pneumonitis, interstitial nephritis, cranial neuropathies and aseptic meningitis, are occasionally encountered. In patients with progressive disease, Itescu[39]

has reported that high-dose corticosteroid treatment (40–60mg prednisone daily for 8–12 weeks) is effective in controlling disease. These investigators administered zidovudine (AZT) also, with the theoretic goal of inhibiting HIV replication in CD4 cells while nonselectively inducing lympholysis with high-dose prednisone. Similar encouraging results with corticosteroids in patients with DILS-associated peripheral polyneuropathy have been recently reported by Moulignier *et al*.[40]. The toxicity observed in this group of patients has been acceptable, considering the high degree of morbidity of extraglandular disease. It is possible that patients with DILS may represent a more benign subset of HIV infection and thus may tolerate higher doses of immunosuppressive treatment. In patients with lymphoepithelial parotid cysts, a favorable response to combination antiretroviral and prednisone treatment has been reported[42].

Myopathy

Muscle disease was one of the first rheumatic complications to be noted in HIV-infected individuals, and there now is a recognized spectrum of muscle disease associated with the infection (Table 98.4).

Numerous cases of myopathies that are clinically and histologically indistinguishable from polymyositis and dermatomyositis have also been reported[43]. At times, the muscle disease is both the presenting problem (as opposed to HIV) and the dominant source of morbidity. Clinically, as in idiopathic polymyositis, the presenting symptoms are generally proximal muscle weakness involving both upper and lower extremities but predominating in the lower. In several patients, the classic rash of facial heliotrope and Gottron's papules on the knuckles have been noted[43]. Pathologically, there is generally an interstitial inflammatory infiltrate with CD8+ lymphocytes, with varying degrees of individual cell degeneration and regeneration (Fig. 98.4). The infiltrating

---

TABLE 98.4 SPECTRUM OF MUSCLE DISEASE IN HIV INFECTION

- Polymyositis/dermatomyositis
- Nemaline rod disease
- Wasting myopathy
- Pyomyositis
- HIV/HTLV-I myositis
- Fibromyalgia
- AZT myopathy

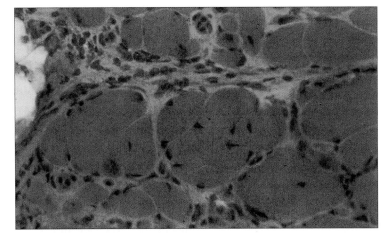

Fig. 98.4 A section of muscle demonstrating prominent lymphocytic interstitial infiltrate in an HIV-infected patient. (Hematoxylin and eosin; original magnification × 3400.)

CD8[+] T cells display a memory phenotype, whereas muscle fibers express MHC-I and the costimulatory molecule BB-1, indicating that they may act, not only as target cells, but also as antigen-presenting cells[44]. Increased muscle enzyme concentrations are frequent and at times extremely high, whereas the electromyogram is reflective of an active necrotizing myopathy. In addition, abnormalities of nerve conduction are often noted. An active inflammatory myopathy associated with prominent peripheral neuropathy should make the clinician suspicious of several diseases, including systemic necrotizing vasculitis, inclusion body myositis and HIV infection.

Another myopathic syndrome reported in HIV-infected patients includes the presence of nemaline rods without significant inflammation (nemaline rod myopathy)[43]. These ultrastructural findings may be observed in both congenital and acquired myopathy, but their presence should raise the possibility of an underlying HIV infection.

The 'wasting' syndrome, a condition characterized by progressive weight loss in HIV infection, has been associated with an active non-inflammatory myopathy[45]. Biopsies from patients with HIV-associated wasting syndrome have revealed heterogeneous findings and the frequent coexistence of malnutrition[46]. In a series of five patients with this condition, most were noted to have increased muscle enzyme concentrations and biopsy pictures showing individual cell degeneration and regeneration without significant inflammation. Several of these individuals appeared to respond to corticosteroid treatment. Other forms of treatment, including anabolic steroids, human growth hormone, nutritional supplements and cytokine antagonists, have been tried in patients with HIV-associated wasting syndrome, with variable success[47].

Pyomyositis is a rare condition characterized by single or multiple muscle abscesses not formed by contiguous spread from outside muscle tissues. Numerous cases of pyomyositis have been reported in HIV-infected patients[31]. The infection is seen almost exclusively in men at advanced stages of the disease. The majority of reported cases were caused by *Staphylococcus aureus*, although occasionally opportunistic pathogens such as *Citrobacter freudii* and *Microsporidia* have been identified[31]. Most patients present with localized tender swelling of muscles, usually in the thighs, with or without fever and constitutional symptoms[31]. Diagnosis usually requires computed tomographic or magnetic resonance imaging of the affected muscles and drainage, for identification of the responsible organism. The majority of patients improve with appropriate antimicrobial therapy, but recurrences are not uncommon.

Treatment-related muscle diseases

The use of nucleoside analogs for the treatment of HIV infection has been occasionally associated with myopathy. Most cases have been reported in patients receiving AZT, but recently a few cases were identified in patients taking stavudine[48]. Between 15% and 40% of patients receiving AZT develop increased serum concentrations of creatine kinase, whereas a much smaller percentage develop clinical myositis with myalgias or weakness, or both. The duration of AZT treatment has ranged from a few months to several years, and it is often difficult to differentiate this syndrome from HIV-associated polymyositis. Dalakas et al.[43] have demonstrated that AZT-associated myopathy is pathologically distinct. They showed, in a comparison of muscle pathology in HIV-infected patients with inflammatory myopathy, that numerous ragged-red fibers indicative of abnormal mitochondria with paracrystalline inclusions were found only in AZT-treated patients. Other investigators have reported direct AZT-incuced mitochondrial damage, with cytochrome c oxidase deficiency[49]. The disease may or may not respond to dose reduction, but frequently improves if the drug can be discontinued.

Recently, a syndrome of hepatic steatosis, lactic acidosis and myopathy with increased concentrations of creatine kinase was reported in four patients receiving stavudine[48]. Similarly to AZT-induced myopathy, muscle damage was attributed to direct mitochondrial injury. Biopsies of affected muscles revealed abundance of lipid droplets without associated muscle inflammation.

Investigation and treatment of muscle diseases

Patients with HIV-associated myopathy do not have the characteristic autoantibodies seen in idiopathic inflammatory myopathies (see Chapter 138??). Extensive studies of biopsied muscles have revealed only occasional evidence of HIV in degenerating myocytes but, more frequently, infiltrating macrophages and lymphocytes are noted. A single case report of polymyositis associated with a dual infection of both HIV and human T cell leukemia/lymphoma virus (HTLV-I) revealed diffuse infection of myocytes with HTLV-I but not HIV. Subsequent studies of dual-infected cases have failed to reproduce this finding.

Collectively, the extremely broad nature of muscle disease associated with HIV infection suggests that HIV infection should be considered in patients with possible muscle disease, particularly for those patients at high risk. Treatment of myopathy in the setting of HIV infection must be directed at the specific cause of the disorder.

If the patient is receiving treatment with nucleoside analogs (AZT or stavudine), the drug(s) should be stopped, because the condition may be difficult to distinguish from drug-induced disease. If the patient does not improve or is not receiving nucleoside analogs, the cautious use of immunosuppressive agents should be attempted. Patients with HIV infection and inflammatory myopathy tend to respond to much lower doses of corticosteroids than do patients with idiopathic polymyositis. For patients with clinically significant weakness that is compromising quality of life, initial treatment should be prednisone in a dose of about 0.5mg/kg/day and maintained until muscle enzymes and strength are normalized, generally for about 4–8 weeks. After this initial treatment, the prednisone can be tapered to the lowest possible dose to control symptoms.

For patients with non-inflammatory myopathy complicated by wasting, there is no satisfactory treatment. Aggressive nutritional support is essential. The use of immunosuppressive drugs should be avoided, given the advanced stage of immunodeficiency and disability in such patients. The role of other more specific treatments (human growth hormone, anti-TNF-based treatments, anabolic steroids, etc.) has yet to be defined.

Vasculitis

Although some of the rheumatic syndromes described in HIV-infected patients are clinically distinctive, the vasculitic conditions reported in this setting in general appear to represent a microcosm of the entire spectrum of systemic vasculitis occurring sporadically (Table 98.5). With the exception of the recently reported large-vessel aneurysmal vasculitis, seen nearly exclusively in Africa[50,51], it is impossible to ascertain whether any or most of these are causally associated or merely represent a chance occurrence between a common condition (HIV) and a rare condition (vasculitis). Alternatively, their co-occurrence may be due to associated factors such as coinfections (hepatitis C virus, cytomegalovirus, etc.) or treatment.

Within the spectrum of reported cases, several groups stand out. The angiocentric immunoproliferative lesions encompass a group of disorders including benign lymphocytic angiitis, lymphomatoid granulomatosis and angiocentric lymphoma. These diseases are all characterized by angiocentric and angiodestructive lymphocytic inflammation, primarily from T lymphocytes (Fig. 98.5). Numerous cases of angiocentric immunoproliferative lesions have been reported in the setting of HIV infection, and appear to be largely CD8[+] T cell in nature. This contrasts with the vast majority of lymphoproliferative diseases associated with HIV infection, which are B cell in origin. HIV infection should be

TABLE 98.5 CLASSIFICATION OF SYSTEMIC VASCULITIS AND RELATIONSHIP TO HIV INFECTION

Vasculitis		Reported in association with HIV infection
Systemic necrotizing vasculitis	Polyarteritis	Yes
	Churg–Strauss	Yes
	Polyangiitis or overlap	Yes
Hypersensitivity vasculitis group	Hypersensitivity vasculitis	Yes
	Henoch–Schönlein purpura	Yes
	Essential cryoglobulinemia	No
	Urticarial vasculitis	No
Granulomatous angiitis	Wegener's granulomatosis	No
	Lymphomatoid granulomatosis	Yes
Giant cell arteritis	Temporal arteritis	No
	Takayasu's arteritis	No
Primary angiitis of the nervous system		Yes

strongly considered in all cases of lymphocytic angiitis, particularly in those individuals at high risk.

A polyarteritis nodosa-like condition has also been reported in the setting of HIV infection. Muscle and nerve involvement are quite common, in addition to digital ischemia leading to gangrene. Leucocytoclastic vasculitis involving the small vessels of the skin has also been reported, including cases of Henoch–Schönlein purpura[6].

Primary angiitis of the central nervous system is a rare disorder characterized by angiitis confined to the tissues of the central nervous system. Considering the rarity of this disorder, it is noteworthy that there are numerous cases reported in association with HIV infection[52]. These cases have been both granulomatous and non-granulomatous in their pathology. It has been postulated that the etiology of the condition may be the reactivation of a latent herpes virus such as varicella zoster, although this is unproven.

More recently, a series of interesting case reports, coming largely from South Africa, have described a unique vasculitic complication that is best described as large vessel in distribution, and frequently demonstrating aneurysm formation leading to vascular occlusion[50,51]. In the largest cohort of patients described to date, 20 patients of median age 37 years and predominantly men were described. All patients had critical ischemia involving the upper and lower limbs. Large aneurysms involving primary branches of the aorta such as carotid, femoral and superior mesenteric arteries, in addition to the aorta itself, were described. Pathologically, acute and chronic inflammatory changes were found

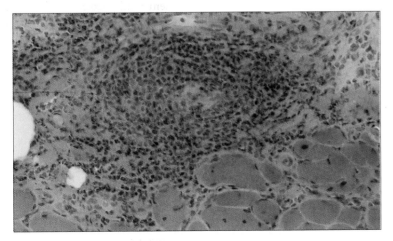

Fig. 98.5 A section of skeletal muscle from an HIV-infected patient, demonstrating severe vasculitis with infiltration of the vascular wall and obliteration of the vascular lumen by lymphoplasmacytic infiltrate. (Hematoxylin and eosin, original magnification × 3200.)

within the aneurysm walls, with a unique inflammatory infiltrate often demonstrating leucocytoclastic features within the vasa vasorum. Furthermore, a unique proliferation of slit-like vascular channels was noted in the adventitial layer[50]. The nature of this aneurysmal vasculitic condition is unclear at the present time, because the necessary technically demanding studies to search for microbial pathogens have not been performed. It is curious that all cases have been reported in patients with advanced disease who are largely untreated, which may account for the fact that this syndrome has rarely been described in Western countries. In contrast, aneurysmal disease primarily involving cerebral vessels, but occasionally involving other vessels such as the coronaries, has been described in pediatric HIV disease[53,54]. In some of these cases, opportunistic pathogens have been identified, such as varicella zoster virus or fungal pathogens, but in others no microbial agent has been detected. Aneurysmal vasculitic disease in the setting of HIV infection clearly warrants further investigation.

The issue of whether HIV itself is culpable in the pathogenesis of systemic vasculitis is still unsettled. Gherardi et al.[55] have reported a large clinicopathological series of 34 cases in which they demonstrated HIV antigen and genome within the vascular inflammatory infiltrate in two patients. In some of their patients, evidence for opportunistic pathogens such as cytomegalovirus was found. The authors concluded that inflammatory vascular disease in the setting of HIV infection was heterogeneous and results from multifactorial pathogenic mechanisms.

From a practical perspective, considering the importance of underlying HIV infection when therapeutic strategies are being planned for patients with systemic vasculitis, serologic testing should routinely be performed. In addition, given the strong association of small and large vessel vasculitis with other blood-borne pathogens, a complete battery of serologic testing for HIV, hepatitis C virus and hepatitis B virus should be included in the initial evaluation of such vasculitic syndromes.

The complexities of treating systemic necrotizing vasculitis in HIV infection are similar to those of treating other connective tissue diseases in this context. These conditions frequently require high-dose immunosuppressive treatment and, unfortunately, appear to occur in patients with advanced HIV infection. No prospective trials of any therapeutic agents in any of the vasculitic syndromes have been reported to date. HIV-associated vasculitis appears to respond to traditional measures but, unfortunately, most patients have been highly immunocompromised at the outset. Non-immunosuppressive modalities, although unproven, should be seriously considered (e.g. apheresis, i.v. gammaglobulin) in the setting of advanced immunosuppression and progressive arteritis[56]. As always, aggressive antiretroviral and antimicrobial

TABLE 98.6 CLINICAL AND LABORATORY FEATURES OF HIV INFECTION THAT MAY MIMIC SLE	
Constitutional	Fever, malaise, weight loss
Dermatologic	Butterfly rash due to seborrhea Alopecia Cutaneous vasculitis Oral aphthosis
Musculoskeletal	Arthralgia/arthritis Myalgia/myositis
Neurologic	Psychosis Seizures Peripheral neuropathy
Renal	Azotemia Proteinuria/hematuria
Lymphadenopathy	
Hematologic	Immune thrombocytopenia Leukopenia/lymphopenia Coombs-positive hemolytic anemia
Immunologic	Antinuclear antibodies Hypergammaglobulinemia Circulating immune complexes

prophylaxis should be coadministered with any immunosuppressive regimen. There are no reports on the efficacy of antiviral therapy in treating any of the vasculitic syndromes.

Lupus-like syndrome

Human immunodeficiency virus infection and systemic lupus erythematosus (SLE) are both multisystem diseases with many similar clinical and laboratory phenomena, and at times they are difficult to differentiate (Table 98.6). Clinically, patients with both conditions may have constitutional symptoms, including fever, malaise and weight loss, and have a wide variety of cutaneous diseases with similar appearances. The seborrheic rash of HIV may appear in a butterfly distribution, and alopecia has been reported in the context of HIV. The musculoskeletal manifestations with arthralgia and myalgia are similar, and both groups of patients have similar neurologic findings. HIV may at times be accompanied by a nephropathy causing hematuria and proteinuria, and lymphadenopathy is seen in both diseases. In addition, these conditions share many serological findings, including antinuclear antibodies. Awareness of these facts is important to the practicing rheumatologist, particularly when confronted with a patient at high risk for HIV infection with symptoms and signs of SLE. Rarely, cases of concomitant SLE and HIV disease have been reported[57]. As will subsequently be discussed, differentiating these from the laboratory point of view may at times be difficult: for example, there will be a high number of false-positive HIV tests in patients with *bona fide* connective tissue disease.

METABOLIC COMPLICATIONS OF HIV INFECTION

Aggressive treatment with HAART has extended life expectancy of HIV-infected individuals by decades, but also has created a series of new clinical challenges in dealing with HIV infection. Presumably as a consequence of the HAART regimen or the new longevity, HIV-infected patients are experiencing profound metabolic complications, including insulin resistance, hyperlipidemia, body fat redistribution, lactic acidosis and other problems[58]. In addition, certain newly recognized rheumatic disorders would appear to fall within this metabolic spectrum of complications: namely, osteonecrosis of bone and osteoporosis.

Osteonecrosis in HIV infection

Osteonecrosis or avascular necrosis of bone is a final common pathway of a number of conditions, most of which lead to impairment of the blood supply to bone. Tissue necrosis takes place in the subchondral bone, which may ultimately lead to compression fractures and deformity of the articular surface. Numerous risk factors have been associated with avascular necrosis of bone, including glucocorticoid use, hemoglobinopathies, metabolic conditions such as Gaucher disease, and heavy use of alcohol and tobacco.

Isolated reports of avascular necrosis of bone in the setting of HIV infection have long been noted, but have generally involved small numbers of cases and conclusions regarding an etiologic link have been difficult to establish. More recently, several larger series including a case–control study[59] have been published that have demonstrated a dramatically increased incidence of avascular necrosis of bone. These studies have estimated that the relative risk of avascular necrosis of bone may be 50 times greater than that of the non-infected population. Not surprisingly, it has been difficult to identify precisely the key epidemiological risks in this setting, given the numerous potential confounders found in the HIV-infected population. Varying studies have demonstrated significant associations with the use of glucocorticoids, lipid-decreasing agents, anabolic steroid use, protease-based HAART treatment, alcohol abuse and hypercoagulability. In summary, HIV infection may represent an additional predisposing factor to traditional risks for the development of avascular necrosis of bone.

From the practical perspective, these data suggest that physicians who treat HIV-infected patients must be aware of the symptoms and maintain a high index of suspicion for avascular necrosis of bone. As with non-HIV-infected patients, early detection remains the best prognostic factor in the successful treatment of avascular necrosis of bonei regardless of its cause.

Osteoporosis in HIV Infection

It is perhaps not surprising, given the wide range of metabolic complications now being observed in the HIV-infected population, that osteopenia and osteoporosis have been reported by numerous investigators[60]. In a cross-sectional study of 112 men with HIV infection, a high incidence of osteopenia and osteoporosis with a relative risk of 2.2 has been demonstrated. Individuals receiving protease inhibitor-based HAART had greater bone loss than those not receiving such therapy. Several other reports, most in abstract form, confirm this finding, but have not conclusively demonstrated a relationship to HAART treatment. They have, however, raised other possible etiologic issues, such as duration of HIV infection, age, the presence of mild degrees of lactic acidosis, and other factors.

The observation that 20% of male patients, aged about 40 years, have a bone mineral density T-score of less than −2, is not in itself particularly alarming. The concern is that, as this is potentially a progressive disease over many decades, bone loss may represent a growing and important clinical complication in this population. At the present time, firm recommendations regarding screening and treatment cannot be made.

INVESTIGATIONS AND DIFFERENTIAL DIAGNOSIS

The laboratory profiles of HIV-infected patients bear many similarities to those of patients with idiopathic autoimmune disease and connective tissue disease syndromes (Table 98.7). This is important to rheumatologists for two reasons. First, the recognition that such laboratory phenomena occur in the setting of other common conditions is important, because it alters the specificity of diagnostic tests for rheumatic disease. Secondly and similarly, the fact that a human retrovirus infection can result in such a broad array of laboratory phenomena has important theoretic implications regarding the part these viruses play in the pathogenesis of connective tissue disease.

TABLE 98.7 AUTOIMMUNE LABORATORY PHENOMENA ASSOCIATED WITH HIV INFECTION	
Polyclonal hypergammaglobulinemia	
Circulating immune complexes	
Autoantibodies	Antinuclear
	Rheumatoid factor
	Anticardiolipin
	Cryoglobulins
Anticellular antibodies	Antiplatelet
	Anti-red-blood-cell
	Antilymphocyte
	Antibrain
	Anti-parietal-cell
Miscellaneous	β_2-microglobulin
	Acid-labile interferon-α
	Serum lysozyme
	Urinary neopterin
	IL-2 receptors (serum)

For the clinician, several points regarding these laboratory observations must be emphasized. First, the majority of these laboratory abnormalities tend to increase in prevalence and magnitude over time and in parallel with the severity of the underlying HIV infection. Secondly, although the majority of HIV-infected individuals, at the endstages of their HIV infection, will display some of these laboratory abnormalities – for example, polyclonal hypergammaglobulinemia (nearly 100%), circulating immune complexes (approximately 60–80%) and anticardiolipin antibodies (approximately 50–80%) – other findings, such as antinuclear antibodies and rheumatoid factor, are detected far less often.

In recent years there has been disagreement in the literature regarding the frequency with which autoantibodies occur in the setting of HIV infection. High-titer autoantibodies characteristic of connective tissue disease are relatively infrequent when detected by clinical assays, but a large spectrum of autoantibodies can be detected by alternative techniques. Utilizing an enzyme-linked immunosorbent assay (ELISA) against a series of synthetic antigens (double-stranded DNA, Sm, U1 RNP and 60kDa Ro or SSA) known to be recognized in a variety of disorders such as SLE, mixed connective tissue disease and Sjögren's syndrome, Muller et al.[61] found reactivity in 44–95% of HIV-infected patients. There was no evidence of such reactivity in the sera of high-risk HIV-uninfected homosexual men. Most intriguingly, the presence in HIV infection of sustained concentrations of serum interferon (IFN)-α of the acid-labile subtype is similar in magnitude and duration to that detected in certain connective tissue diseases such as SLE, Sjögren's syndrome and systemic necrotizing vasculitis. This shared feature between connective tissue disease and HIV infection provides one of the strongest inferential supports for a viral etiology of traditional autoimmune diseases.

It should be recognized that any of these rheumatic syndromes may be the presenting manifestation and occur in advance of recognized HIV infection. Accordingly, it is exceedingly important to take candid and non-judgmental sexual histories on all patients, to determine who is at the greatest risk and in need of HIV testing. In addition, the subtle physical clues of underlying HIV infection must be recognized. These include oral thrush, hairy leukoplakia, recurrent dermatomal zoster, molluscum contagiosum and seborrheic dermatitis. A second issue worthy of emphasis is that patients with idiopathic connective tissue disease undergoing HIV testing are prone to develop false-positive HIV serologies, particularly with the ELISA. Thus, as in all HIV testing situations, no results should be considered final or discussed with patients, until a confirmatory test is performed and is positive. These confirmatory assays are most widely done at present by the western blot technique, but other reliable techniques are now becoming available.

THE HIV VIRION

Structure

Human immunodeficiency virus is a human retrovirus and a member of the lentivirus family. Lentiviruses characteristically cause indolent infections, and are notable for involvement of the nervous system, long periods of clinical latency and persistent viremia. All retroviruses are RNA viruses, which by definition replicate through a DNA intermediate. Retroviruses all share common sets of protein that are physically contained within the virion (Fig. 98.6). High-resolution electron microscopy has revealed the HIV-1 virion to be icosahedral in structure, containing 72 external spikes. The spikes are formed by two major viral envelope proteins, gp120 and gp41. Within the lipid bilayer there are a number of host-associated proteins, including MHC antigens acquired during viral budding. The core of the virus contains a variety of structural proteins, which probably stabilize the exterior and interior integrity of the virion. Most importantly, the core also contains two copies of single-stranded RNA associated with various preformed viral enzymes, including reverse transcriptase, integrase and protease.

The genomic structure of all retroviruses contains three protypic genes: *gag* (nuclear core proteins), *pol* (virally associated enzymes including reverse transcriptase and protease), and *env* (envelope glycoproteins). These genomic regions are flanked by two long terminal repeat regions, one at each end, containing promoter and enhancer regions. HIV-1 contains no less than six open reading frames in addition to the protypic *gag-*, *pol-* and *env*-coding sequences (Fig. 98.7). Two of these accessory genes, *tat* and *rev*, are essential for viral growth. *Tat* is a major transactivator that interacts with the proviral long terminal repeat, and *rev* acts post-transcriptionally, assisting in the shift from early- to late-phase viral expression. In contrast, the other accessory genes, such as *nef*, *vpu*, *vif*, *vpr* and *vpx*, encode factors that are not essential for viral production in certain *in vitro* systems, and thus are commonly referred to as 'accessory proteins'. The biological significance of these accessory proteins is only now becoming more clearly understood.

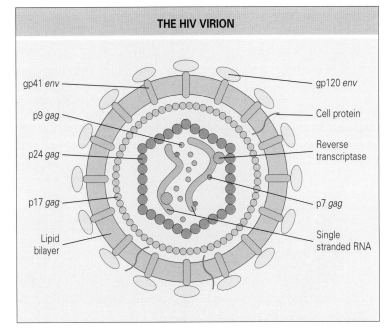

THE HIV VIRION

gp41 *env* — gp120 *env* — Cell protein — Reverse transcriptase — p9 *gag* — p24 *gag* — p17 *gag* — p7 *gag* — Lipid bilayer — Single stranded RNA

Fig. 98.6 The HIV virion. The *env* (envelope) (gp120, gp41), *gag* (nucleocapsid) (p24, p17) and *pol* (reverse transcriptase) structures are shown. The gp120 surface glycoprotein serves as the recognition unit for the CD4 epitope on mononuclear cells.

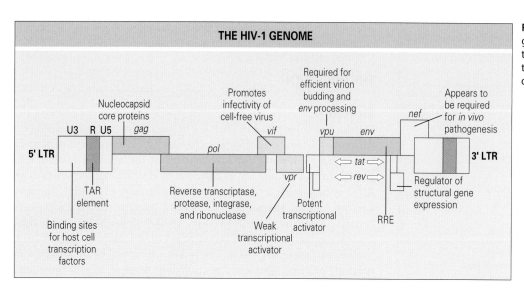

Fig. 98.7 The HIV-1 genome. The nine known genes and their recognized functions. LTR, long terminal repeat; RRE, *rev* response element; TAR, transactivation response element; R, U3, U5, domains in the retroviral 5′ LTR.

Viral life cycle

The human CD4-bearing T cell and monocyte are the major cellular targets of HIV-1 infection in humans. HIV-1 preferentially infects cells via a binding of envelope glycoprotein to the CD4 receptor. To enter the cell, HIV utilizes a coreceptor in addition to the CD4 receptor: namely, CCR4 on T cells and CCR5 on macrophages, monocytes and some T cells; these are both members of the chemokine family of receptors[62,63]. After internalization, the virion is partially uncoded in preparation for replication (Fig. 98.8). Each single strand of viral RNA is transcribed into a double-stranded DNA replica of the original RNA genome, flanked by long terminal repeat regions. This is accomplished primarily through the virally encoded enzyme, reverse transcriptase, working in concert with other virally encoded enzymes. The viral DNA copy or provirus is then inserted into the host genome by viral integrase, another enzyme encoded by the *pol* gene. Varying quantities of unintegrated viral DNA may persist in cells that may represent replication defective mutants. Full integration of the proviral genome into the host's DNA may require a variety of cofactors, in particular cellular activation. After viral integration, the virus may remain in a clinically quiescent or latent form or, after appropriate signaling, may actively transcribe itself into new viral progeny.

IMMUNOLOGICAL ASPECTS OF HIV INFECTION

HIV pathogenesis and the role of immune activation

After the primary infection with HIV, a burst of viral proliferation can be detected by high levels of HIV RNA in blood and in peripheral lymphoid organs. In the first few weeks (Fig. 98.9), this is accompanied by a robust and integrated immune response, including both humoral and cell-mediated elements[62,63]. The viremia reaches a peak and within weeks to months progressively recedes, presumably as a result of the vigorous immune response, until a hypothesized viral set-point is reached that reflects a balance between viral production and destruction. Both humoral and cellular elements contribute to the overall control of viral infection, but it is believed that HIV-specific cytotoxic T cells are the most important, and temporally correlate with the control of viremia[63]. After this phase, the host enters a largely asymptomatic phase during which viremia persists and CD4 cells are destroyed at a slow, steady

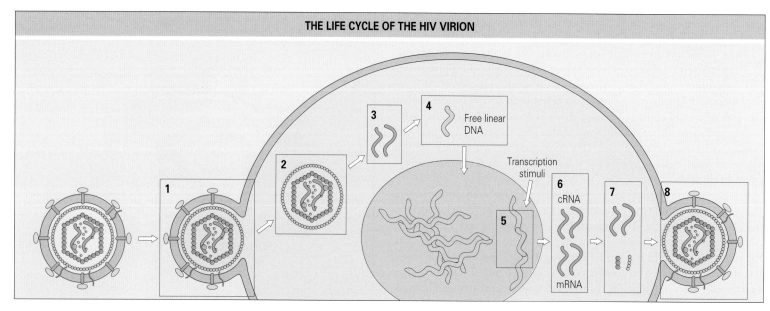

Fig. 98.8 The life cycle of the HIV virion. (1) First, the virus binds and penetrates the cell, followed (2) by uncoating and (3) synthesis of cDNA within the cytoplasm. (4) The viral DNA duplex is transported to the nucleus and inserted into the host genome or (5) translocated to the nucleus to be integrated into the genomic DNA of the host. The infection can remain latent (non-expressing) or, after appropriate stimuli (cellular activation signals, other host transcription factors), convert to a productive infection. (6) The transcribed viral RNA then reassembles in the cytoplasm and (7) combines with translated viral structural glycoproteins at the inner cell membrane. (8) Finally, the newly formed virion buds off, potentially to infect another cell.

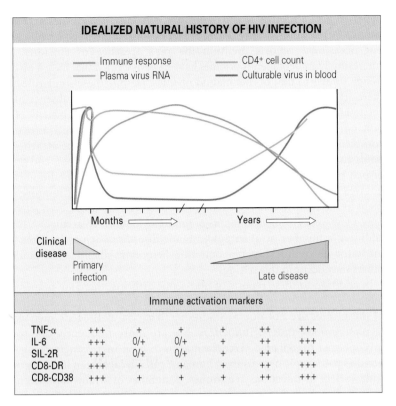

IDEALIZED NATURAL HISTORY OF HIV INFECTION

— Immune response — CD4+ cell count
— Plasma virus RNA — Culturable virus in blood

Months ⇒   Years ⇒

Clinical disease

Primary infection   Late disease

Immune activation markers

TNF-α	+++	+	+	+	++	+++
IL-6	+++	0/+	0/+	+	++	+++
SIL-2R	+++	0/+	0/+	+	++	+++
CD8-DR	+++	+	+	+	++	+++
CD8-CD38	+++	+	+	+	++	+++

Fig. 98.9 Idealized natural history of HIV infection: viral, immune activation and clinical features. (Adapted with permission from Calabrese and Galperin[62].)

pace. Eventually, progression to disease occurs, characterized by decreasing CD4 cell counts, increasing levels of viremia and, ultimately, profound immunosuppression.

A feature of HIV infection shared by only a small number of other chronic viral infections (such as hepatitis C, hepatitis B and HTLV-I) is a state of persistent and prolonged viral replication. It was previously believed that the prolonged period of clinical latency referred to above reflected underlying viral latency. More recently, progressive HIV replication both in blood and lymphoid tissues has been described, with estimates that at least 10^{10} virions are produced and cleared each day throughout the life of an infected person. The half-life of virions in the circulation is less than 6 hours, and that of actively infected CD4+ T cells is approximately 1.5 days. In addition to the active and rapid replication of the virus, its primary replicative enzyme, reverse transcriptase, is highly error-prone and produces new mutations each day. The diversity within the viral genome increases throughout the life of the host, leading to escape from the host's integrated immune response, in addition to resistance to antiviral agents.

A sentinel feature of HIV infection, and one which may explain the array of autoimmune laboratory and clinical phenomena, is a state of persistent and prolonged immune activation. This activation is manifest by a variety of indicators including: increased T cell activation, particularly among CD8 and CD4 cells (HLA-DR, CD38); a number of soluble markers of immune activation, including increased plasma concentrations of β_2-microglobulin, IL-2 receptors and serum and urinary neopterin; increased concentrations of numerous inflammatory cytokines, including TNF-α, IL-6, IFN-γ and IL-12[62].

Cytokine production is believed to be important in HIV pathogenesis, and possibly a contributor to the development of autoimmune complications. During the primary phase of the infection, numerous inflammatory cytokines such as TNF, IL-6, IL-12 and IFN-γ can be detected in either serum or lymphoid tissue, or both. In later stages of the disease, increased concentrations of TNF have correlated with increasing amounts of viral replication. This state of persistent immune activation

may have numerous deleterious effects on the host, including its general enhancing effects on viral proliferation. Inflammatory cytokines such as TNF and IL-1 are both capable of releasing the intracellular messenger, nuclear factor (NF) κB. NFκB is also an activator of HIV transcription, by binding to the long terminal repeat region of the viral RNA. Clinical correlates of the link between immune activation and viral production can be seen after vaccinations or in association with opportunistic infections such as mycobacteria, which are both capable of increasing viral loads. This state of immune activation may also compromise the host immune response, by rendering the immune system less capable of responding to new antigenic challenge, thus enhancing the immunosuppressive state. Persistent immune activation has been also linked to progressive depletion of CD4+ T cells[64]. Finally, it may be hypothesized that persistent immune activation may favor the development of a multitude of clinical and laboratory phenomena with autoimmune features.

Mechanisms of autoimmunity in HIV infection

The mechanisms whereby human retrovirus may induce autoimmune laboratory or clinical phenomena are beyond the scope of this Chapter, but have been reviewed elsewhere[62]. Potential mechanisms that may be involved in this process include:

1. Molecular mimicry, in which there is some evidence of homology between viral and host species leading to a breakdown of immunologic tolerance.

2. Augmentation of cryptic self-referring to cryptic epitopes, which are antigens for which self-reactive lymphocytes exist, but for varied reasons do not undergo immune activation. In the setting of a chronic retroviral infection with persistent immune activation, this could lead to an upregulation of enhanced antigen processing by upregulation of costimulatory molecules on antigen-presenting cells, leading to an aberrant immune response.

3. 'Retrovirus-induced hypersensitivity' refers to a phenomenon whereby the immune system makes a response to an appropriate antigen but, in so doing, damages normal bystander tissues. Again, the chronic state of immune activation associated with chronic viral replication could lead to innocent bystander immune damage at anatomic sites of HIV infection. Similar mechanisms have been postulated for chronic infection such as hepatitis C and hepatitis B.

4. Immune regulatory genes or autogenes have been postulated as a mechanism whereby retroviruses, either exogenous or endogenous, may alter the expression of genes that have a critical role in immune regulation and, thus, have been dubbed 'autogenes'. In HTLV-I infections, a related human retrovirus, an accessory gene known as *tax*, has been demonstrated to upregulate the expression of several oncogenes contributing to synovial proliferation in an arthritis with unique features that has been described in that setting. In addition, HTLV-I *tax*-transfected synoviocytes display upregulation of numerous inflammatory cytokines, including TNF-α, IL-1β and IL-6. The homologue of *tax* in HIV is *tat* and, although there are no examples of *tat*-transgenic autoimmune diseases in animals, *tat* has been demonstrated to be capable of transforming human keratinocytes and upregulating the expression of IL-6, in addition to modulating apoptosis. These data suggest that *tat* could play a part in such diseases as psoriasis in addition to other inflammatory diseases, via altering the expression of host cellular genes controlling inflammation or immunoproliferation.

The effects of HAART on the immune response

The introduction of HAART therapy in the past 6 years has resulted in dramatic declines in mortality from HIV disease. This has been attributed to immune restoration as a result of suppression of HIV replication. Although immune restoration is rarely complete after HAART therapy, it can be dramatic, with tangible reductions in opportunistic infections and malignancies. Furthermore, along with increasing CD4 cell counts, HAART therapy does reduce concentrations of inflammatory cytokines such as TNF-α in serum[65] and other inflammatory cytokines in lymphoid tissues[66]. This reduction of immune activation may explain the clinical observation that non-infectious rheumatic complications have also declined in the period after treatment with HAART. Careful epidemiologic studies are needed to support this conclusion. In the longitudinal experience at the Cleveland Clinic, where HIV-infected patients are routinely examined for rheumatic manifestations, among 53 cases of non-infectious rheumatic complications (reactive arthritis, psoriatic arthritis, vasculitis, Sjögren's-like syndrome), 50 were noted to occur in the pre-HAART period and only three in patients receiving HAART treatment.

HYPOGAMMAGLOBULINEMIA AND ARTHRITIS

Clinical features

The congenital form of hypogammaglobulinemia or agammaglobulinemia is genetically transmitted in an X-linked fashion, presenting after several months of life, when maternal antibody has dissipated[67,68]. Patients generally begin to develop frequent sinus and pulmonary infections with bacterial organisms including *S. pneumoniae* and *Haemophilus influenzae*, although other pathogens, including non-bacterial and opportunistic agents, may be seen. The acquired form of hypogammaglobulinemia, referred to as common variable immunodeficiency (CVID), can present at any age and is characterized by recurrent bacterial infections, autoimmune manifestations and granulomatous disease affecting different organs[67-69]. Almost 25% of patients with CVID develop autoimmune diseases – mainly autoimmune cytopenias (thrombocytopenia, hemolytic anemia, neutropenia) and autoimmune thyroid disease[69]. Granulomatous disease in different organs, including lymphoid tissues, skin and solid organs (lungs, kidneys, liver), has been described in 5–10% of patients with CVID[70]. Furthermore, a greater incidence of non-Hodgkin lymphomas (mainly B cell) has also been noted, and represented the most common cause of death in a large cohort of patients with CVID[69].

Arthritis

There is a high prevalence of arthritis with hypogammaglobulinemia. In a series of 281 patients with the disease from the UK, 22% of boys with the X-linked variety and 7% of those with CVID presented with arthritis that was described as 'non-septic'. The patients were nearly equally divided between groups with monoarticular, oligoarticular and polyarticular disease[71]. In the most recent series of 248 patients with CVID from the USA, 3.6% of patients developed an 'RA-like' picture[69]. The medical literature describing arthritis and antibody-deficiency states is complex, because most authors attempt to separate articular disease into 'septic' and 'non-septic' varieties. The difficulty in this type of analysis emanates from the fact that many joint infections observed in this population are caused by highly fastidious organisms such as *Mycoplasma* or *Ureaplasma*, or even viral agents. Older case reports using less sophisticated microbiological techniques [not based on polymerase chain reaction (PCR)], and investigations not carefully searching for such organisms, may inadvertently misclassify their patients. In addition, there appears to be a significant degree of clinical overlap between these varieties of arthritis.

A polyarthritic, non-septic arthritis of obscure etiology has been repeatedly described in hypogammaglobulinemia in both the X-linked and CVID varieties[69,71]. Some investigators have claimed the disease is identical to RA, although rheumatoid factor is universally absent. Synovial histology has occasionally demonstrated marked lymphocytic hypertrophy, although plasma cells are generally absent and frank pannus formation is lacking. There are no detailed radiographic studies, but occasional reports mention the rare presence of erosions[72]. Interestingly, subcutaneous nodules have been described that have a histology similar to that of rheumatoid nodules. Despite these similarities, there are differentiating features in most cases, including the absence of rheumatoid factor, the low prevalence of bony erosions, the paucity of polymorphonuclear leukocytes in synovial fluid and tissues, and normal complement concentrations in synovial fluid. Clinically, the arthritis tends to affect the large joints and spare the fingers and toes, and to display prominent tenosynovitis. The natural history of this condition is not well described, but there are numerous reports of dramatic improvement in the arthritis and regression of subcutaneous nodules, even after only a few weeks of small amounts of immunoglobulin replacement[73]. In addition, a number of other autoimmune disorders such as immune-mediated thrombocytopenia, immune hemolytic anemia, SLE and others may occur in this setting.

In addition to these reports of non-septic arthritis, there are numerous cases of arthritis of infectious origin. Interestingly, the vast majority of these cases are not due to traditional bacterial pathogens such as *S. pneumoniae* and *H. influenzae*, but are more frequently due to mycoplasma organisms. Mycoplasmas have been increasingly recognized as pathogenic organisms in humans, and are capable of inducing a wide variety of infectious syndromes. A number of strains have been identified in the joint tissues of patients with hypogammaglobulinemia, including *Mp. pneumoniae*, *Mp. hominis*, *Mp. salivarium* and *Ureaplasma urealyticum*[74,75]. These septic syndromes have been, at times, highly destructive monoarticular, oligoarticular or polyarticular arthropathies, and usually occur in patients undergoing gamma globulin replacement therapy. The formation of subcutaneous nodules is not uncommon. Other features associated with mycoplasmal septic arthritis include low-grade fever, urethritis, conjunctivitis and low synovial fluid glucose, making this syndrome suggest the differential diagnosis of reactive arthritis. A few patients have been reported to have osteomyelitis in addition to arthritis. Although appropriate culture techniques can allow the identification of these organisms in affected joints and soft tissues, more recently, PCR testing has allowed identification of such infections in the face of negative cultures[75]. At present, every effort must be made to document the presence of an infecting pathogen in such settings, including the use of PCR. In the absence of such investigations, empiric treatment is clearly warranted.

Polymyositis and dermatomyositis

In patients with hypogammaglobulinemia of the X-linked variety, a cutaneous muscular syndrome has been described that closely resembles polymyositis and dermatomyositis[76,77]. The syndrome is nearly always accompanied by an echovirus infection of the central nervous system that ranges from being asymptomatic to being clinically devastating. The muscle disease may be easily overlooked because of its insidious nature. Occasionally a non-pitting edema of the lower legs is the first sign of the condition, and a transient erythematous rash, at times with a violaceous hue, may be reminiscent of classic dermatomyositis. The degree of muscle disease varies greatly, and for prolonged periods of time patients may often complain only of stiffness, rather than weakness. Over time there can be severe wasting of the muscles, with flexion contractures of the knees, elbows and hips. Histologically, within the muscle there is a lymphocytic infiltration that is predominantly CD8[+]. Serum muscle enzymes are frequently normal in the chronic cases, increasing only during acute exacerbation. Electromyography may reveal a patchy myopathic process.

Nearly all patients with the muscular syndrome eventually develop central nervous system disease, but occasional patients have been noted to have positive viral cultures in the cerebrospinal fluid for up to 10 years before neurologic symptoms or signs. Headache, hearing impairment and convulsions are all common features of the syndrome.

The diagnosis is best made by culturing echovirus from the cerebrospinal fluid. Virus may occasionally be retrieved from muscle tissues, but this appears to be less reliable. The pathogenesis of the muscle disease remains obscure. Even though virus may occasionally be retrieved from muscle biopsies, there are no studies using *in situ* hybridization or immunohistochemical techniques that demonstrate the infection to be primarily myopathic.

Management

The overall management of patients with hypogammaglobulinemia is based on prevention and prompt treatment of accompanying infections. Patients with either the X-linked or CVID varieties of disease are prone to frequent upper and lower respiratory tract infections, which frequently lead to severe pulmonary disease and cor pulmonale in later life. Awareness of an increased incidence of autoimmune disease in CVID is also important for long-term management. The use of immunoglobulin replacement therapy, particularly with i.v. preparations, has revolutionized the care of these patients.

Arthritis

The patient with hypogammaglobulinemia and arthritis must be carefully assessed to determine whether infection is present within the joints. Virtually all patients with hypogammaglobulinemia and arthritis are candidates for i.v. immunoglobulin replacement therapy. Clinical reports of dramatic improvement of arthritis, including resolution of subcutaneous nodules, with minimal immunoglobulin replacement have suggested that this may be a highly treatable form of polyarthritis. Although the pathogenesis of the arthritis is unclear, one theory is that it may be due to antigenic overload similar to the arthritis seen in patients after intestinal bypass surgery. Standard treatment is 200mg/kg immunoglobulin given i.v. once per month. For patients with severe disease, higher doses may be indicated, in the range of 400–600mg/kg per month. I.v. immunoglobulin treatment can generally be given quite safely in an outpatient setting, although both infusion-rate-dependent and hypersensitivity reactions may occur.

Patients with infectious arthritis and hypogammaglobulinemia not only require i.v. immunoglobulin therapy, but should probably be treated with the higher-dose regimens. Not all batches of i.v. immunoglobulin have high titers of specific antibodies for mycoplasmal organisms, and doses in excess of 600mg/kg per month may be needed.

Antimicrobial treatment for mycoplasmal infections is of paramount importance. I.v. or oral tetracycline for a minimum of 10 weeks in combination with i.v. immunoglobulin has been reported to be successful in a number of patients. Others have been successfully treated with only a few weeks of treatment. As with all cases of infectious arthritis, careful clinical monitoring is necessary.

Polymyositis and dermatomyositis

The treatment of the polymyositis or dermatomyositis-like syndrome in patients with hypogammaglobulinemia is problematic. As virtually all these cases are believed to be due to chronic echovirus infection, treatment has been primarily directed at this pathogen, as opposed to the host response to it. There have been reports of both success and lack of success for high-dose i.v. immunoglobulin treatment in this syndrome[76]. The use of intrathecal immunoglobulin for central nervous system involvement has also been reported to be successful on occasion. Efforts to use immunoglobulin preparations that are enriched for anti-echovirus activity have been advocated. The outcome for the syndrome is poor, particularly when complicated by meningoencephalitis, but factors contributing to favorable clinical outcome in a few patients include a short duration of symptoms before initiation of treatment, the use of extremely high doses of gammaglobulin, and the administration

of intrathecal treatment in addition to i.v. treatment. The lymphocytic infiltrates in muscular tissues suggest the role of host immune factors may be important, but attempts to treat this disease with immunosuppressive drugs have generally been unrewarding[76].

Autoimmune diseases

Most patients with CVID and autoimmune cytopenias are treated with a combination of i.v. immunoglobulin and short courses of corticosteroids[69]. In refractory cases, splenectomy was associated with a good outcome in a recent retrospective study[69].

OTHER IMMUNE DEFICIENCY STATES

The application of modern molecular and biological techniques has resulted in the discovery and earlier diagnosis of various genetic defects leading to the development of immune deficiency states (primary immunodeficiencies). These genetically determined defects can affect different elements of the normal immune system, including T or B lymphocytes[67], phagocytes[78] and complement components[79,80], causing a number of distinct immunodeficiency syndromes. The majority of clinical manifestations of primary immunodeficiencies appear early in life, but certain immunodeficiencies, including CVID, IgG subclass deficiencies, IgA deficiency and deficiencies of the late components of complement, can present during adulthood.

Most patients with primary immunodeficiencies present with recurrent infections in different sites and from various microorganisms, depending on the specific arm of the immune system that is not functioning correctly. Furthermore, certain immune deficiencies are associated with autoimmune manifestations as a result of dysregulation of the physiologic homeostatic mechanisms of the immune system. Although a complete description of the various autoimmune syndromes developing in the setting of primary immunodeficiencies is beyond the scope of this chapter, some of these associations that can present in adulthood will be presented.

There appears to be an increased incidence of a wide variety of autoimmune disorders, such as SLE, juvenile chronic arthritis and others, in the setting of selective IgA deficiency[81,82]. This is the most common primary immunodeficiency disorder, occurring with a reported prevalence of from 1 in 330 to 1 in 2200. Parenteral immunoglobulin replacement therapy is not indicated unless there is concomitant IgG subclass deficiency. Even in this setting, such patients may be at risk for anaphylactic reactions by virtue of a high frequency of anti-IgA antibodies, particularly of the IgE type.

Patients with Wiskott–Aldrich syndrome (thrombocytopenic purpura with small platelets, eczema and susceptibility to infection) who survive the first years of life can develop a number of autoimmune manifestations, including autoimmune cytopenias and vasculitis[83]. Recently, cases of vasculitis with aneurysm formation involving branches of the aorta or mesenteric arteries have been reported in adult patients with this syndrome[84,85].

Hyper-IgM syndrome is an X-linked disorder characterized by molecular defects in the CD154 (or CD40 ligand) molecule, which is present on the surface of activated CD4⁺ T cells and plays a crucial role in T cell–B cell interactions[86]. Mutations in the CD154 gene lead to limited production of IgG, IgA and IgE immunoglobulins; at the same time, serum concentrations of IgM are increased. This molecular defect causes a clinical syndrome characterized by recurrent infections (including *Pneumocystis carinii* pneumonia), diarrhea, chronic neutropenia and, in approximately 10% of the cases, arthritis[87]. Webster *et al.*[88] reported an aggressive polyarthritis with a distribution similar to RA, accompanied by erosions and subcutaneous nodules in an adult patient with hyper-IgM syndrome. Rheumatoid factor was absent, and there was characteristic development of large periarticular cysts. The arthritis followed an unremitting course despite therapy and, later in life, aneurysmal arterial disease ensued.

Mutations in the genes that regulate apoptosis, including Fas (CD 95) and Fas-ligand, lead to the development of an autoimmune syndrome characterized by non-malignant lymphoproliferation (lymphadenopathy, hepatosplenomegaly), increased numbers of CD3[+] double-negative (CD4[−]CD8[−]) T cells and a number of autoimmune manifestations (mainly autoimmune cytopenias) [89]. The syndrome has been termed 'autoimmune lymphoproliferative syndrome' and its molecular and immunologic characteristics have been thoroughly investigated. An accumulation of autoreactive T cells that do not undergo physiologic programmed cell death or apoptosis in lymphoid tissues is the central pathophysiologic event that is responsible for the development of autoimmunity. These expanded populations of T cells display a predominant T helper 2 phenotype characterized by increased concentrations of IL-10 that may contribute to the autoimmune characteristics of these patients[89]. Patients with autoimmune lymphoproliferative syndrome

and autoimmune cytopenias have been treated successfully with immunosuppressive drugs (corticosteroids) and i.v. immunoglobulin.

Recently, a syndrome resembling Wegener's granulomatosis with necrotizing granulomatous lesions of the upper respiratory tract and skin has been reported[90]. These patients had also history of recurrent bacterial infections, bronchiectases and small-vessel vasculitis involving the skin. Molecular and immunological studies revealed decreased expression of MHC-I molecules as a result of mutations in genes encoding proteins that transport peptide antigens from the cytoplasm to the cell surface ('transporters associated with antigen processing')[90]. Increased numbers of autoreactive natural killer and γδ T cells have been detected in the peripheral blood and granulomatous lesions of these patients, implying a direct pathogenetic role[90]. Immunosuppressive therapy did not lead to clinical improvement when it was instituted in these patients[90].

REFERENCES

1. Winchester R, Bernstein DH, Fischer HD et al. The co-occurence of Reiter's syndrome and aquired immunodeficiency. Ann Intern Med 1987; 106: 19–26.
2. Hogg RS, O'Shaughnessy MV, Gataric N et al. Decline in deaths from AIDS due to new antiretrovirals. Lancet 1997; 349: 1294.
3. UNAIDS/WHO. AIDS epidemic update. December 2000; 1–28.
4. Piot P, Bartos M, Ghys PD et al. The global impact of HIV/AIDS. Nature 2001; 410: 968–973.
5. Calabrese LH. Human immunodeficiency virus (HIV) infection and arthritis [published erratum appears in Rheum Dis Clin North Am 1993; 19: ix]. Rheum Dis Clin North Am 1993; 19: 477–488.
6. Reveille JD. The changing spectrum of rheumatic disease in human immunodeficiency virus infection. Semin Arthritis Rheum 2000; 30: 147–166.
7. Solomon G, Brancato L, Winchester R. An approach to the human immunodeficiency virus-positive patient with a spondyloarthropathic disease. Rheum Dis Clin North Am 1991; 17: 43–58.
8. Keat A. HIV and overlap with Reiter's syndrome. Baillières Clin Rheumatol 1994; 8: 363–377.
9. Rosenberg ZS, Norman A, Solomon G. Arthritis associated with HIV infection: radiographic manifestations. Radiology 1989; 173: 171–176.
10. Njobvu P, McGill P, Kerr H et al. Spondyloarthropathy and human immunodeficiency virus infection in Zambia. J Rheumatol 1998; 25: 1553–1559.
11. Cuellar ML, Espinoza LR. Human immunodeficiency virus associated spondyloarthropathy: lessons from the Third World. J Rheumatol 1999; 26: 2071–2073.
12. Samet JH, Muz P, Cabral P et al. Dermatologic manifestations in HIV-infected patients: a primary care perspective. Mayo Clin Proc 1999; 74: 658–660.
13. Njobvu P, McGill P. Psoriatic arthritis and human immunodeficiency virus infection in Zambia. J Rheumatol 2000; 27: 1699–1702.
14. Reveille JD, Conant MA, Duvic M. Human immunodeficiency virus-associated psoriasis, psoriatic arthritis, and Reiter's syndrome: a disease continuum? Arthritis Rheum 1990; 33: 1574–1578.
15. Mallon E, Young D, Bunce M et al. HLA-Cw*0602 and HIV-associated psoriasis. Br J Dermatol 1998; 139: 527–533.
16. Berthelot P, Guglielminotti C, Fresard A et al. Dramatic cutaneous psoriasis improvement in a patient with the human immunodeficiency virus treated with 2′,3′-dideoxy,3′-thyacytidine [correction of 2′,3′-dideoxycytidine] and ritonavir. Arch Dermatol 1997; 133: 531.
17. Duvic M, Crane MM, Conant M et al. Zidovudine improves psoriasis in human immunodeficiency virus-positive males. Arch Dermatol 1994; 130: 447–451.
18. Fischer T, Schworer H, Vente C et al. Clinical improvement of HIV-associated psoriasis parallels a reduction of HIV viral load induced by effective antiretroviral therapy. AIDS 1999; 13: 628–629.
19. Shapiro DL, Masci JR. Treatment of HIV associated psoriatic arthritis with oral gold. J Rheumatol 1996; 23: 1818–1820.
20. Tourne L, Durez P, Van Vooren JP et al. Alleviation of HIV-associated psoriasis and psoriatic arthritis with cyclosporine. J Am Acad Dermatol 1997; 37: 501–502.
21. Masson C, Chennebault JM, Leclech C. Is HIV infection contraindication to the use of methotrexate in psoriatic arthritis? J Rheumatol 1995; 22: 2191.
22. Maurer TA, Zackheim HS, Tuffanelli L, Berger TG. The use of methotrexate for treatment of psoriasis in patients with HIV infection. J Am Acad Dermatol 1994; 31: 372–375.
23. Aboulafia DM, Bundow D, Wilske K, Ochs UI. Etanercept for the treatment of human immunodeficiency virus-associated psoriatic arthritis. Mayo Clin Proc 2000; 75: 1093–1098.
24. Takebe N, Paredes J, Pino MC et al. Phase I/II trial of the type I soluble recombinant human interleukin-1 receptor in HIV-1-infected patients. J Interferon Cytokine Res 1998; 18: 321–326.
25. Rynes RI. Painful rheumatic syndromes associated with human immunodeficiency virus infection. Rheum Dis Clin North Am 1991; 17: 79–87.
26. Berman A, Espinoza LR, Diaz JD et al. Rheumatic manifestations of human immunodeficiency virus infection. Am J Med 1988; 85: 59–64.

27. Berman A, Cahn P, Perez H et al. Human immunodeficiency virus infection associated arthritis: clinical characteristics. J Rheumatol 1999; 26: 1158–1162.
28. Stein CM, Davis P. Arthritis associated with HIV infection in Zimbabwe. J Rheumatol 1996; 23: 506–511.
29. Ornstein MH, Kerr LD, Spiera H. A reexamination of the relationship between active rheumatoid arthritis and the acquired immunodeficiency syndrome. Arthritis Rheum 1995; 38: 1701–1706.
30. Muller-Ladner U, Kriegsmann J, Gay RE et al. Progressive joint destruction in a human immunodeficiency virus-infected patient with rheumatoid arthritis. Arthritis Rheum 1995; 38: 1328–1332.
31. Vassilopoulos D, Chalasani P, Jurado RL et al. Musculoskeletal infections in patients with human immunodeficiency virus infection. Medicine 1997; 76: 284–294.
32. Belzunegui J, Gonzalez C, Lopez L et al. Osteoarticular and muscle infectious lesions in patients with the human immunodeficiency virus. Clin Rheumatol 1997; 16: 450–453.
33. Ventura G, Gasparini G, Lucia MB et al. Osteoarticular bacterial infections are rare in HIV-infected patients: 14 cases found among 4,023 HIV-infected patients. Acta Orthop Scand 1997; 68: 554–558.
34. Hughes RA, Rowe IF, Shanson D, Keat AC. Septic bone, joint and muscle lesions associated with human immunodeficiency virus infection. Br J Rheumatol 1992; 31: 381–388.
35. Olive A, Salavert A, Manriquez M et al. Parotid lipomatosis in HIV positive patients: a new clinical disorder associated with protease inhibitors. Ann Rheum Dis 1998; 57: 749.
36. Itescu S, Brancato LJ, Buxbaum J et al. A diffuse infiltrative CD8 lymphocytosis syndrome in human immunodeficiency virus (HIV) infection: a host immune response associated with HLA-DR5. Ann Intern Med 1990; 112: 3–10.
37. Kordossis T, Paikos S, Aroni K et al. Prevalence of Sjögren's-like syndrome in a cohort of HIV-1-positive patients: descriptive pathology and immunopathology. Br J Rheumatol 1998; 37: 691–695.
38. Williams FM, Cohen PR, Jumshyd J, Reveille JD. Prevalence of the diffuse infiltrative lymphocytosis syndrome among human immunodeficiency virus type 1-positive outpatients. Arthritis Rheum 1998; 41: 863–868.
39. Itescu S. Diffuse infiltrative lymphocytosis syndrome in human immunodeficiency virus infection – a Sjögren's-like disease. Rheum Dis Clin North Am 1991; 17: 99–115.
40. Moulignier A, Authier FJ, Baudrimont M et al. Peripheral neuropathy in human immunodeficiency virus-infected patients with the diffuse infiltrative lymphocytosis syndrome. Ann Neurol 1997; 41: 438–445.
41. Gherardi RK, Chretien F, Delfau-Larue MH et al. Neuropathy in diffuse infiltrative lymphocytosis syndrome: an HIV neuropathy, not a lymphoma. Neurology 1998; 50: 1041–1044.
42. Craven DE, Duncan RA, Stram JR et al. Response of lymphoepithelial parotid cysts to antiretroviral treatment in HIV-infected adults. Ann Intern Med 1998; 128: 455–459.
43. Dalakas MC. Retroviruses and inflammatory myopathies in humans and primates. Baillières Clin Neurol 1993; 2: 659–691.
44. Murata K, Dalakas MC. Expression of the costimulatory molecule BB-1, the ligands CTLA-4 and CD28, and their mRNA in inflammatory myopathies. Am J Pathol 1999; 155: 453–460.
45. Simpson DM, Bender AN, Farraye J et al. Human immunodeficiency virus wasting syndrome may represent a treatable myopathy. Neurology 1990; 40: 535–538.
46. Miro O, Pedrol E, Cebrian M et al. Skeletal muscle studies in patients with HIV-related wasting syndrome. J Neurol Sci 1997; 150: 153–159.
47. Moldawer LL, Sattler FR. Human immunodeficiency virus-associated wasting and mechanisms of cachexia associated with inflammation. Semin Oncol 1998; 25: 73–81.
48. Miller KD, Cameron M, Wood LV et al. Lactic acidosis and hepatic steatosis associated with use of stavudine: report of four cases. Ann Intern Med 2000; 133: 192–196.
49. Yerroum M, Pham-Dang C, Authier FJ et al. Cytochrome c oxidase deficiency in the muscle of patients with zidovudine myopathy is segmental and affects both mitochondrial DNA- and nuclear DNA-encoded subunits. Acta Neuropathol (Berl) 2000; 100: 82–86.

50. Chetty R, Batitang S, Nair R. Large artery vasculopathy in HIV-positive patients: another vasculitic enigma. Hum Pathol 2000; 31: 374–379.

51. Nair R, Robbs JV, Chetty R *et al*. Occlusive arterial disease in HIV-infected patients: a preliminary report. Eur J Vasc Endovasc Surg 2000; 20: 353–357.

52. Calabrese LH. Vasculitis and infection with the human immunodeficiency virus. Rheum Dis Clin North Am 1991; 17: 131–147.

53. Dubrovsky T, Curless R, Scott G *et al*. Cerebral aneurysmal arteriopathy in childhood AIDS. Neurology 1998; 51: 560–565.

54. Fulmer BB, Dillard SC, Musulman EM *et al*. Two cases of cerebral aneurysms in HIV+ children. Pediatr Neurosurg 1998; 28: 31–34.

55. Gherardi R, Belec L, Mhiri C *et al*. The spectrum of vasculitis in human immunodeficiency virus-infected patients. A clinicopathologic evaluation. Arthritis Rheum 1993; 36: 1164–1174.

56. Gisselbrecht M, Cohen P, Lortholary O *et al*. Human immunodeficiency virus-related vasculitis. Ann Med Interne 1998; 149: 398–405.

57. Daikh BE, Holyst MM. Lupus-specific autoantibodies in concomitant human immunodeficiency virus and systemic lupus erythematosus: case report and literature review. Semin Arthritis Rheum 2001; 30: 418–425.

58. Wanke CA. Epidemiological and clinical aspects of the metabolic complications of HIV infection the fat redistribution syndrome. AIDS 1999; 13: 1287–1293.

59. Scribner AN, Troia-Cancio PV, Cox BA *et al*. Osteonecrosis in HIV: a case–control study. J Acquir Immune Defic Syndr 2000; 25: 19–25.

60. Tebas P, Powderly WG, Claxton S *et al*. Accelerated bone mineral loss in HIV-infected patients receiving potent antiretroviral therapy. AIDS 2000; 14: F63–F67.

61. Muller S, Richalet P, Laurent-Crawford A *et al*. Autoantibodies typical of non-organ-specific autoimmune diseases in HIV-seropositive patients. AIDS 1992; 6: 933–942.

62. Calabrese LH, Galperin C. Autoimmune and rheumatic aspects of infection with human immunodeficiency virus. Semin Clin Immunol 1997; 2: 5–16.

63. Hogan CM, Hammer SM. Host determinants in HIV infection and disease. Part 1: cellular and humoral immune responses. Ann Intern Med 2001; 134: 761–776.

64. Hazenberg MD, Hamann D, Schuitemaker H, Miedema F. T cell depletion in HIV-1 infection: how CD4+ T cells go out of stock. Nat Immunol 2000; 1: 285–289.

65. Aukrust P, Muller F, Lien E *et al*. Tumor necrosis factor (TNF) system levels in human immunodeficiency virus-infected patients during highly active antiretroviral therapy: persistent TNF activation is associated with virologic and immunologic treatment failure. J Infect Dis 1999; 179: 74–82.

66. Andersson J, Fehniger TE, Patterson BK *et al*. Early reduction of immune activation in lymphoid tissue following highly active HIV therapy. AIDS 1998; 12: F123–F129.

67. Buckley RH. Primary immunodeficiency diseases due to defects in lymphocytes. N Engl J Med 2000; 343: 1313–1324.

68. Ten RM. Primary immunodeficiencies. Mayo Clin Proc 1998; 73: 865–872.

69. Cunningham-Rundles C, Bodian C. Common variable immunodeficiency: clinical and immunological features of 248 patients. Clin Immunol 1999; 92: 34–48.

70. Mechanic LJ, Dikman S, Cunningham-Rundles C. Granulomatous disease in common variable immunodeficiency. Ann Intern Med 1997; 127: 613–617.

71. Hansel TT, Haeney MR, Thompson RA. Primary hypogammaglobulinaemia and arthritis. BMJ 1987; 295: 174–175.

72. Pipitone N, Jolliffe VA, Cauli A *et al*. Do B cells influence disease progression in chronic synovitis? Lessons from primary hypogammaglobulinaemia. Rheumatology (Oxford) 2000; 39: 1280–1285.

73. Lee AH, Levinson AI, Schumacher HRJ. Hypogammaglobulinemia and rheumatic disease. Semin Arthritis Rheum 1993; 22: 252–264.

74. Schaeverbeke T, Vernhes JP, Lequen L *et al*. Mycoplasmas and arthritides. Rev Rhum (Engl Ed) 1997; 64: 120–128.

75. Puechal X, Hilliquin P, Renoux M, Menkes CJ. Ureaplasma urealyticum destructive septic polyarthritis revealing a common variable immunodeficiency. Arthritis Rheum 1995; 38: 1524–1526.

76. Crennan JM, Van Scoy RE, McKenna CH, Smith TF. Echovirus polymyositis in patients with hypogammaglobulinemia. Failure of high-dose intravenous gammaglobulin therapy and review of the literature. Am J Med 1986; 81: 35–42.

77. Webster AD. Inflammatory disorders of muscle. Echovirus disease in hypogammaglobulinaemic patients. Clin Rheum Dis 1984; 10: 189–203.

78. Lekstrom-Himes JA, Gallin JI. Immunodeficiency diseases caused by defects in phagocytes. N Engl J Med 2000; 343: 1703–1714.

79. Walport MJ. Complement. First of two parts. N Engl J Med 2001; 344: 1058–1066.

80. Walport MJ. Complement. Second of two parts. N Engl J Med 2001; 344: 1140–1144.

81. Hammarstrom L, Vorechovsky I, Webster D. Selective IgA deficiency (SIgAD) and common variable immunodeficiency (CVID). Clin Exp Immunol 2000; 120: 225–231.

82. Itescu S. Adult immunodeficiency and rheumatic disease. Rheum Dis Clin North Am 1996; 22: 53–73.

83. Akman IO, Ostrov BE, Neudorf S. Autoimmune manifestations of the Wiskott–Aldrich syndrome. Semin Arthritis Rheum 1998; 27: 218–225.

84. McCluggage WG, Armstrong DJ, Maxwell RJ *et al*. Systemic vasculitis and aneurysm formation in the Wiskott–Aldrich syndrome. J Clin Pathol 1999; 52: 390–392.

85. van Son JA, O'Marcaigh AS, Edwards WD *et al*. Successful resection of thoracic aortic aneurysms in Wiskott–Aldrich syndrome. Ann Thorac Surg 1995; 60: 685–687.

86. Ramesh N, Seki M, Notarangelo LD, Geha RS. The hyper-IgM (HIM) syndrome. Springer Semin Immunopathol 1998; 19: 383–399.

87. Notarangelo LD, Duse M, Ugazio AG. Immunodeficiency with hyper-IgM (HIM). Immunodefic Rev 1992; 3: 101–121.

88. Webster EA, Khakoo AY, Mackus WJ *et al*. An aggressive form of polyarticular arthritis in a man with CD154 mutation (X-linked hyper-IgM syndrome). Arthritis Rheum 1999; 42: 1291–1296.

89. Straus SE, Sneller M, Lenardo MJ *et al*. An inherited disorder of lymphocyte apoptosis: the autoimmune lymphoproliferative syndrome. Ann Intern Med 1999; 130: 591–601.

90. Moins-Teisserenc HT, Gadola SD, Cella M *et al*. Association of a syndrome resembling Wegener's granulomatosis with low surface expression of HLA class-I molecules. Lancet 1999; 354: 1598–1603.

99 Acute rheumatic fever

G M Mody

Definition

- Acute rheumatic fever is a systemic inflammatory disease that occurs 2–3 weeks after a pharyngeal infection with group A β-hemolytic streptococci
- The disease is mediated by an autoimmune response to antigenic components of the organism that cross-react with similar epitopes in human tissues such as the heart, joints, brain and skin

Clinical features

The acute form of the illness is characterized by:

- Fever
- Arthritis, which is usually migratory and affects predominantly the large joints
- Cardiac manifestations due to involvement of the pericardium, myocardium, endocardium and heart valves
- Neurological involvement, which manifests as Sydenham's chorea
- Cutaneous involvement consisting of erythema marginatum and subcutaneous nodules, which are less common

INTRODUCTION

The term acute rheumatic fever describes the usual presentation of the disease; it may not be acute, rheumatic or febrile. Arthritis is common in acute rheumatic fever but the morbidity and mortality of the disease is usually related to involvement of the heart. These observations were made as early as 1884 by Lasegue, who noted that 'Rheumatic fever is a disease that licks the joints but bites the heart'.

EPIDEMIOLOGY

Acute rheumatic fever was common in Europe and North America at the beginning of the 20th century. Since then there has been a rapid decline in the incidence of the disease and this was further accelerated by the introduction of antibiotics in 1950. These observations are best illustrated from Denmark where the annual incidence was over 200/100 000 population between 1862 and 1900 but by 1948 it had fallen to approximately 55/100 000 population. The decline continued, and by 1962 the incidence was just over 10/100 000 population (Fig. 99.1). At present the average incidence recorded in most affluent or developed communities is less than 5/100 000 population[1,2].

A reduction in the incidence of acute rheumatic fever in industrialized countries in Europe, North America and also in Japan suggested that improvement in living conditions with less overcrowding and better hygiene as well as the widespread availability and use of antibiotics were responsible. In the USA the incidence of rheumatic fever was as low as 0.23–1.88/100 000/year among children and adolescents in the early 1980s[3], although it had risen nearly tenfold in some areas by the mid-

1980s. A large outbreak in Utah, USA[4] was followed by smaller outbreaks in Pennsylvania[5] and Ohio[6] and in military bases in San Diego and Missouri[7,8]. During the Utah outbreak most of the affected children were from upper middle class homes with access to medical care, emphasizing the importance of factors other than poverty and overcrowding in its pathogenesis[4].

The prevalence rate of rheumatic heart disease in developed countries is approximately 0.2–0.5/100 000[9]. By contrast, there is still an unacceptably high prevalence of rheumatic fever and rheumatic heart diseases in developing countries[9,10]. A survey of schoolchildren in South Africa in 1996 reported a prevalence of 6.9/1000 children, rising to 20/1000 children in the 12–14 age group[11]. A prevalence of 9.6/1000 was also reported among Aborigines in Northern Australia, with a rate of 24/1000 in a large rural community. The prevalence rate per 1000 in other developing countries is 2.06 in Samoan children, 1.42 in Sri Lankans aged 5–14 years and 1.25 in Maori children in New Zealand[9]. In India, the prevalence of rheumatic heart disease is between 1.5 and 5.6 cases per 1000[12].

At the time of the resurgence of acute rheumatic fever in the USA, cases of invasive, life threatening streptococcal infection were reported in the USA[13–15], UK[16], Scandinavia[17] and other parts of Europe. This toxic streptococcal syndrome was characterized by localized or generalized rash, hypotension and multiorgan failure. It occurred mainly in adults and resulted from cutaneous or soft tissue infections with streptococci of M type I and strains producing pyrogenic toxin A. It has been proposed that changes in streptococcal epidemiology are related to changes in the virulence of the streptococcus strains.

PATHOLOGY

Rheumatic fever can cause pathological changes throughout the body, especially in the connective tissue and around blood vessels.

Cardiac involvement

In the heart, the pericardium, myocardium and endocardium can be affected, resulting in a pancarditis.

In the acute phase, there may be diffuse myocardial involvement leading to conduction disturbances and heart failure. Death may result in a small proportion of patients and, at post mortem, there is dilatation of the chambers and the myocardium is pale, flabby and edematous.

The histological changes in the myocardium may consist of a nonspecific myocarditis with edema of the muscle fibers and focal collections of inflammatory cells in the interstitial connective tissue, or a specific granulomatous myocarditis with the presence of the characteristic Aschoff nodules[18]. The typical acute and subacute inflammatory foci seen in heart muscle are shown in Figure 99.2. The Aschoff nodules are composed of a central area of fibrinoid necrosis surrounded by specialized histiocytes called Aschoff giant cells and Anitschkow cells (caterpillar cells), which in turn are mixed with lymphocytes. Silver[19] and Stollerman[20] defined three phases in the progression of Aschoff nodules:

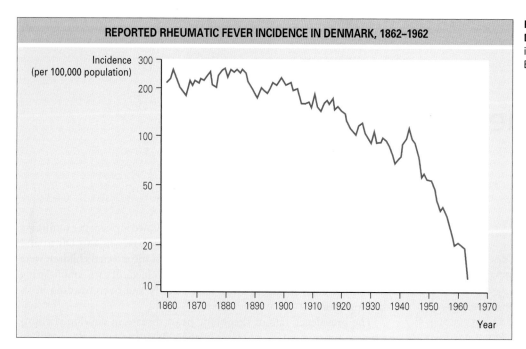

REPORTED RHEUMATIC FEVER INCIDENCE IN DENMARK, 1862–1962

Incidence (per 100,000 population)

Fig. 99.1 Reported incidence of rheumatic fever in Denmark 1862–1962. Serial changes in reported incidence over a century. (Data from Public Health Board of Denmark.)

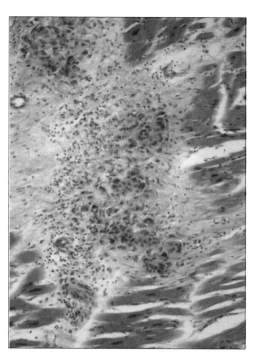

Fig. 99.2 Photomicrograph showing extensive mononuclear cell infiltration and adjacent cardiac muscle fiber destruction and dissolution in a region of active rheumatic carditis. Many activated monocytoid cells with large asymmetric nuclei and abundant cytoplasm are seen. (Hematoxylin and eosin stain, original magnification ×350.)

- the early stage with central fibrinoid necrosis, edema and an infiltrate of lymphocytes and plasma cells (non-specific or exudative–degenerative phase)
- the specific granulomatous stage with accumulation of characteristic Aschoff giant cells and Anitschkow cells
- the late stage with diminution of the cellular infiltrate and replacement by scar tissue.

The presence of Aschoff nodules indicates that there has been an episode of acute rheumatic fever. They can persist for many years and may be identified at the time of valve replacement surgery even in patients who do not have any clinical or laboratory evidence of rheumatic activity[21]. The persistence of the Aschoff nodules seems to correlate with the tendency of the host to develop progressive stenosis and fibrosis of the mitral value[22].

In the early stages, endocarditis is associated with thickening of the valves as a result of edema, and a row of vegetations or verrucous lesions are present along the free borders of the cusps. These tiny vegetations are platelet-rich microthrombi, which do not become dislodged and therefore do not produce the embolic phenomena seen with the larger vegetations of infective endocarditis[18]. The mitral valve is most commonly affected, followed by the aortic valve, either alone or with the mitral valve. During healing, vascularization takes place, with an increase in fibroblastic activity resulting in fibrosis. The degree of fibrosis is variable and in most cases it does not affect the function of the valve. In other patients the scarring is progressive over years and may affect the subendocardial tissue, as well as the annulus, cusp and chordae tendineae. These changes can lead to contraction of the cusp or thickening and stiffening of the cusp leading to valvular incompetence or fusion of commissures resulting in stenosis.

The reason why some patients have progressive scarring while others do not is not known. Some patients have recurrent episodes of streptococcal infection resulting in further immunological injury while others may develop small mural thrombi on the damaged valves and the release of growth factors from the platelets and other components of the thrombi may lead to further fibrosis[18].

Pathological analysis of heart valves obtained at the time of valve replacement show foci of abundant mononuclear or lymphocytic infiltrates within tissues (Fig. 99.3). Immunological study of the inflammatory cell types has shown a predominance of T cells of the OKT4 (CD4) or T-helper lineage[23,24]. The prominence of T-helper cells suggests that local production of potent lymphokines, such as interleukin (IL)-2, tumor necrosis factor (TNF) or even IL-6, contributes to the chronic pathological changes.

Pericarditis affects both layers of the pericardium, which may be thickened and covered by a fibrin-rich exudates. There may also be serosanguineous fluid in the pericardial cavity. The pericarditis resolves completely with fibrosis and adhesions but constriction does not occur.

Articular involvement

Pathological changes in the joints consist of exudative changes with edema of the synovial membrane, focal necrosis in the joint capsule, edema and inflammation in the periarticular tissues and joint effusion. These changes are completely reversible.

Other changes

The subcutaneous nodules (Fig. 99.4) that are seen in the acute phase resemble Aschoff nodules. The pathological changes in the brain in

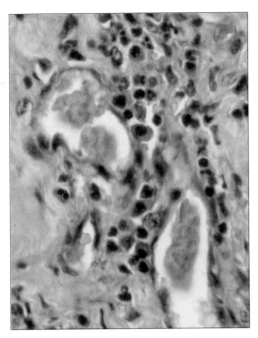

Fig. 99.3 Typical interstitial perivascular lymphocytic infiltrates noted in a rheumatic mitral valve removed during mitral valve replacement 12 years following the initial attack of acute rheumatic fever. Such areas of chronic low-grade inflammation are frequently present in rheumatic heart valvular tissues 10–20 years after the last clinically detectable episode of rheumatic activity. (Hematoxylin and eosin stain , original magnification ×350.)

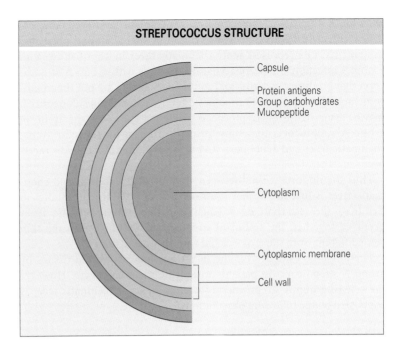

Fig. 99.5 Streptococcus structure. A schematic representation of the streptococcus organism shows the cytoplasm in the center surrounded by the cytoplasmic membrane, the three layers of the cell wall (protein, carbohydrate and mucopeptide) and the outer capsule.

A cross-section of the streptococcus is shown schematically in Figure 99.5. It has a core of cytoplasm surrounded by a cytoplasmic membrane, a cell wall and a capsule on the external surface[25].

The capsule is composed of *N*-acetylglucosamine and glucuronic acid, and is structurally identical to the hyaluronic acid of mammalian tissues. The presence of a large mucoid capsule is one of the important characteristics of certain 'rheumatogenic' strains of streptococcus[26].

The cell wall is made up of three layers, the outermost protein layer, the middle carbohydrate layer and the innermost mucopeptide protoplast. The outer protein layer contains proteins that are designated M, R and T. The most important is the M protein, which determines the virulence of the organism. It stimulates the formation of opsonizing and precipitating antibodies and may impede phagocytosis. The group A streptococci are classified into serologic types on the basis of their M protein. The carbohydrate layer consists of a polysaccharide chain, components of which may cross-react with the glycosides of the heart valves[27]. The role of the mucopeptide portion of the cell wall in the pathogenesis of rheumatic fever is not known.

The cytoplasmic membrane is made up of antigenic lipoprotein that cross-reacts with the glomerular basement membrane and sarcolemmal antigen.

Streptococcal toxins

The streptococcus produces many extracellular products, which include the erythrogenic toxin, streptolysin O, streptolysin S, streptokinase, diphosphopyridine nucleotidase and deoxyribonucleases. Streptolysin O elicits an antibody response, antistreptolysin (ASO) which is the basis of the antibody assay. The antigenicity of streptolysin O is inhibited by lipid in the skin and this may account for the lack of association between streptococcal skin infections and rheumatic fever.

The streptococcus has many antigens that are similar to mammalian tissue and may cross-react with the joint, heart (myocardium, valvular tissue), skin, kidney and brain[28].

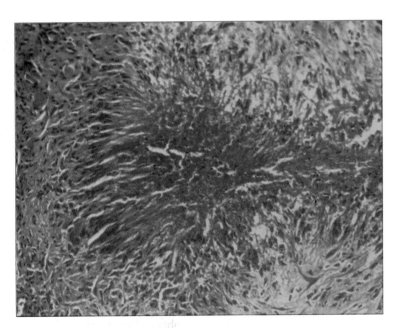

Fig. 99.4 Typical histologic picture of a rheumatic fever nodule. Evidence of fibrous tissue, a number of fibroblasts and a few interstitial lymphocytes are noted. A similar histologic appearance might also be seen in subcutaneous nodules associated with rheumatoid arthritis. (Hematoxylin and eosin stain, original magnification ×350.)

patients with chorea are not well defined, as patients with active chorea rarely die from this complication and brain tissue is rarely available for post-mortem examination.

GROUP A STREPTOCOCCUS

Structure

Streptococci are a group of Gram-positive microorganisms that are arranged in chains on culture. They are able to hemolyze erythrocytes and this property forms the basis for their classification. The α-hemolytic streptococci do not produce complete hemolysis and form colonies surrounded by a greenish halo, while the β-hemolytic streptococci produce a clear zone of hemolysis. The γ-streptococci do not have any effect on blood-containing media.

Rheumatic fever and the streptococcus

Epidemiological studies have shown a causal relationship between group A streptococcal pharyngitis and acute rheumatic fever[29,30]. However not all group A streptococcal infections cause rheumatic fever even if the site of the antecedent infection is pharyngeal. A survey among untreated military recruits reported acute rheumatic fever in 3% of those with group A infection[26]. Extrapharyngeal infections with group A streptococci that produce pyoderma and soft tissue infection are not rheumatogenic and do not produce rheumatic fever. Acute glomerulonephritis may be associated with streptococcal pyoderma due to certain strains of group A streptococci that show primary tropism for the skin. Acute rheumatic fever and acute post-streptococcal glomerulonephritis rarely occur together.

Thus the important link between streptococcal infection and rheumatic fever is that the former must occur within the throat. Studies in Trinidad showed that, even when impetigo and rheumatic fever occurred together, the strains of streptococci identified from the skin were different from those associated with rheumatic fever[31].

There is little evidence for the direct invasion of affected tissues by group A streptococci in patients with acute rheumatic fever. However the role of group A streptococcal infection in acute rheumatic fever is supported by the following observations[27].

- Outbreaks of rheumatic fever follow epidemics of either streptococcal sore throats or scarlet fever[26].
- Treatment of documented streptococcal pharyngitis markedly reduces the incidence of subsequent rheumatic fever[32].
- Antimicrobial prophylaxis prevents recurrence in known patients with acute rheumatic fever[33].
- Most patients have elevated titers of antistreptococcal antibodies (streptolysin O, hyaluronidase and streptokinase) regardless of whether or not they recall an antecedent streptococcal sore throat[34].

PATHOGENESIS

The pathogenesis of acute rheumatic fever has been reviewed in detail[1,27,35,36]. Carapetis suggested in 1996 that the pathogenesis could be considered on the basis of factors related to the host (genetic susceptibility), the organism (rheumatogenicity) and the immune response[35].

The current concept of the pathogenesis of acute rheumatic fever is that it is due to group A streptococcal pharyngitis occurring in a susceptible host, which leads to an autoimmune response to epitopes in the organism that cross-react with similar epitopes in human tissues (e.g. in the joints, heart, brain and skin)[27,35,37].

Organism factors

The observation that only infection with some strains of group A streptococcus leads to the development of acute rheumatic fever has led to the recognition of the concept of 'rheumatogenicity'[35]. Rheumatogenic strains are primarily tropic for the throat and not the skin[9].

A large amount of M protein can be extracted from the rheumatogenic strains, which helps in their identification. The role of the surface M protein in the pathogenesis of acute rheumatic fever is supported by the observation that rheumatogenic strains tend to be rich in M protein, express certain epitopes associated with acute rheumatic fever, induce an intense M-type-specific immune response and also share M epitopes with human tissue. They cannot produce lipoprotein lipase, the opacity factor, the latter being characteristic of strains associated with skin infection[35]. Rheumatogenic strains are also highly contagious and are rapidly transmitted by close person-to-person contact[9]. Many authors have reported associations of rheumatic fever with certain M types of group A streptococcus, including types 1, 3, 5, 6, 14, 18, 19, 24, 27 and 29[38]. Bessen et al. reported that there were two classes of M protein[39]. The rheumatogenic strains have M protein with distinct epitopes, which they called Class I M protein, and the M protein of non-rheumatogenic strains is called Class II M protein[39].

The emphasis on the M protein in the pathogenesis of acute rheumatic fever has recently been questioned. Some strains of group A streptococcus associated with acute rheumatic fever in an endemic area were not M-typeable or were from M types that are usually associated with skin disease[40]. The rheumatogenicity of group A streptococci is now considered to be associated with the strain per se rather than the M type and it is thought that any group A streptococcus can acquire the ability to cause disease. Group A streptococci have the ability to horizontally transfer genetic material so that the epitopes that cross-react with human tissue may be transferred between strains[35,41]. These observation may explain why, in endemic areas, rheumatic-fever-associated strains come from M types that are not usually associated with rheumatic fever or are not M-typeable[42].

Other potential mechanisms that have been implicated in the pathogenesis of acute rheumatic fever are the properties of components and products of group A streptococci to act as superantigens and can stimulate the T cells without requiring antigen presentation[35]. However, this view has been questioned recently, as these properties may be due to contamination[35,43]. The role of co-pathogens has also been suggested and Coxsackie virus has been suggested as a possible co-pathogen[35,44].

Host factors

There is a high prevalence of streptococcal pharyngitis in many populations but only a small percentage develop acute rheumatic fever. Acute rheumatic fever occurs in 2–3% of people during outbreaks of pharyngitis and the incidence is lower with sporadic pharyngitis[45,46]. The disease is familial but the transmission of the disease has been variously suggested as being autosomal recessive[47] or autosomal dominant with limited penetrance[48]. Studies of monozygotic and dizygotic twins have failed to show strong concordance for expression of the disease[48].

Since autoimmune responses have been postulated in the pathogenesis of acute rheumatic fever, an immunogenetic predisposition has been sought. An earlier study using serological methods showed an association with human leukocyte antigen (HLA) DR4 in Caucasians and DR2 in African-Americans[49]. Subsequent associations with HLA DR4 have been reported in Caucasians[50–52], with DR2 in African-Americans[50], with DR3 in Indians[53] and with DR1 and DRw6 in South African Blacks[54]. Studies using molecular HLA typing techniques[55,56] have led to a re-evaluation of the MHC class II associations with rheumatic fever and rheumatic heart disease. It is now suggested that DRB1*0701, DR6 and DQB1*0201 confer susceptibility to rheumatic fever; such observations are in agreement with those reported in Turkey[57], Mexico[58], South Africa[54] and Japan[59]. An association of rheumatic fever with HLA DR7 was recently reported in a Brazilian study[60].

Recent studies have identified a non-HLA B-cell marker that is present in patients with acute rheumatic fever. A monoclonal antibody (D8/17) was prepared by immunizing mice with B cells from a patient with rheumatic fever[61]. The B-cell antigen was expressed on an increased number of B cells in 100% of patients from different ethnic groups and in only 10% of normals[27,61]. This marker was, however, absent in one third of north Indian patients[62]. A new monoclonal antibody developed against the B cells of north Indians patients with rheumatic fever, PGI/MNII, was positive in 86% and 94% of patients with rheumatic fever and rheumatic heart disease respectively[62].

Family studies have shown marked elevations of the B-cell antigens defined by the D8/17 monoclonal antibody in unaffected family members (Fig. 99.6)[1,61]. The B-cell alloantigen D8/17 has been shown to be of value in differentiating Sydenham's chorea from lupus chorea.

In summary, it is likely that the susceptibility to acute rheumatic fever is polygenic, with the reported HLA class antigens being close to or in linkage with the rheumatic fever susceptibility gene; the D8/17 antigen may be associated with one of the genes[27].

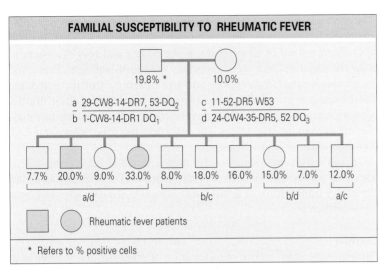

FAMILIAL SUSCEPTIBILITY TO RHEUMATIC FEVER

a 29-CW8-14-DR7, 53-DQ$_2$
b 1-CW8-14-DR1 DQ$_1$

c 11-52-DR5 W53
d 24-CW4-35-DR5, 52 DQ$_3$

Rheumatic fever patients

* Refers to % positive cells

Fig. 99.6 Familial susceptibility to rheumatic fever. Representative distribution of percentages of B cells bearing the D8/17 marker in kindred of a patient with previous acute rheumatic fever. Many as yet unaffected members of the family show marked elevations in numbers of B cells staining with monoclonal antibody D8/17. (Adapted with permission from Khanna et al.[61])

Immune response

Rheumatic fever is recognized as one of the diseases where there is molecular mimicry between a foreign agent (group A streptococci) and host tissue (e.g. heart, brain). Many antigens or components of group A streptococci have been shown to cross-react directly with various human tissues, as shown in Table 99.1. It was postulated that components of streptococci, such as streptococcal membrane, group-specific glycoprotein or carbohydrate components, induce both a humoral and cell-mediated immune response that cross-reacts with the host tissues. The detection of antibodies to streptococcal antigens that are similar to human tissues suggested that humoral immunity played a major role in the pathogenesis of acute rheumatic fever[63,64]. Recent evidence, however, suggests that the primary damage may be mediated by cellular immunity and that the antibodies are produced in response to antigens released from damaged tissues[35].

Immunopathological studies of heart tissue showed that infiltrates of the heart valve consisted mainly of T lymphocytes and the Aschoff body, which is the characteristic cardiac lesion of rheumatic fever and is derived from macrophage lineage[23,65,66]. The T cells and macrophages are present in cell-mediated immune responses. B cells, which are associated with humoral immunity, are uncommonly found.

The role of cellular immunity is also supported by the detection of increased levels of several markers of cellular immune activation such

TABLE 99.1 CROSS-REACTIONS BETWEEN STREPTOCOCCAL COMPONENTS AND HUMAN TISSUE

Streptococcal antigenic component	Cross-reactive human tissue
Cell walls and membranes	Myocardium
Plasma membranes	Myocardial cell membranes
Polysaccharide and glycoproteins	Heart valves
Cell membranes	Cytoplasmic components of caudate and subthalamic neurons
Membranes	Cardiac myosin
M protein	Cardiac myosin; heart sarcolemmal membrane

Documented antigenic cross-reactions between various group A streptococcal components and autologous human host tissue.

as circulating CD4$^+$ lymphocytes, IL-1 and IL-2, IL-2-receptor-positive T cell, TNF-α receptors, leukocyte migration inhibition, natural killer (NK) cell cytotoxicity, mononuclear cell cytotoxicity, T-cell responsiveness to streptococcal antigens, neopterin and oxygen free-radical production by phagocytes[35]. The response by T cells to an epitope on the M protein of group A streptococci and cardiac myosin epitopes was reported by Prukasakom et al.[67]

A hypothesis of the pathogenesis of rheumatic fever that includes some of the above observations has been proposed by Carapetis et al.[35] The cross-reactive antigens of streptococci are presented to helper T-cells (Th) by antigen presenting cells in conjunction with MHC II antigens. Abnormal presentation or recognition of these antigens leads to uncontrolled Th activation and proliferation, possibly mediated by IL-2. This leads to the release of lymphokines, activation of NK cells and cytoxic T cells, and secondary activation of macrophages and neutrophils. As a result there is eradication of the streptococci and damage to the host tissue due to cross-reactivity. Antigens released from the host tissue induce an antibody response, which may further damage the tissue or serve as a marker of damaged tissue.

Measurements of T-cell responsiveness in rheumatic fever have shown increased reactivity during acute episodes[63,68,69]. The ability of T cells to amplify and perpetuate the chronic rheumatic process is unknown[70].

CLINICAL MANIFESTATIONS

The clinical manifestations of acute rheumatic fever are variable and there is no single clinical feature or laboratory test that is diagnostic. The Jones criteria, originally proposed in 1944 and revised in 1992[71] (Table 99.2) are used to establish a diagnosis.

TABLE 99.2 GUIDELINES FOR THE DIAGNOSIS OF INITIAL ATTACK OF RHEUMATIC FEVER

Major manifestations	Minor manifestations	Supporting evidence of antecedent group A streptococcal infection
Carditis	Clinical findings	Positive throat culture or rapid streptococcal infection test
Polyarthritis	Arthralgia	
Chorea	Fever	Elevated or rising streptococcal antibody titer
Erythema marginatum	Laboratory findings:	
Subcutaneous nodules	Elevated acute-phase reactants	
	Erythrocyte sedimentation rate	
	C-reactive protein	
	Prolonged P–R interval	

If supported by evidence of preceding group A streptococcal infection, the presence of two major manifestations or of one major and two minor manifestations indicates a high probability of acute rheumatic fever.

(Jones criteria, updated 1992).

The typical attack of acute rheumatic fever follows an episode of streptococcal pharyngitis after a latent period of 2–3 weeks (average of 18.6 days)[72]. During the latent period there is no clinical or laboratory evidence of active inflammation. About one-third of patients cannot remember having an upper respiratory tract infection preceding the onset of the first attack of acute rheumatic fever.

Acute rheumatic fever occurs most commonly in children between the ages of 4 and 9 years. In developing countries such as India, juvenile mitral stenosis may occur at the age of 3–4 years[73].

The prevalence of the various major criteria varies in different studies depending on whether the patients are studied prospectively or in retrospective studies. The illness usually begins with a high fever but in some patients the fever may be low-grade[74] or absent. The commonest of the major criteria is polyarthritis, which occurs between two-thirds and three-quarters of patients, followed by carditis and chorea.

Major criteria

Arthritis

Arthritis is the most common presenting symptom of acute rheumatic fever. Joint involvement is usually more common (nearly 100%)[75], and more severe, in young adults than in teenagers (82%) and children (66%)[76]. The joint pain is typically described as migratory, which implies that the pain may spread to involve other joints in quick succession without having completely resolved in the preceding joints. Thus the arthritis of rheumatic fever has also been called additive. In untreated patients the number of joints involved may vary from six to 16[77].

The affected joints may be painful and swollen, although many patients have joint pain and tenderness with little objective evidence of inflammation. The affected joint may be inflamed for only a few days to a week before it begins to subside. In about two-thirds of patients the polyarthritis is severe for about a week and may last another 1–2 weeks in the remainder before it resolves completely. If there is persistent swelling of the joints after 4 weeks, it is then necessary to consider other conditions such as juvenile idiopathic arthritis or systemic lupus erythematosus.

At the onset of the illness the joint involvement is asymmetrical and usually affects the lower limbs initially before spreading to the upper limbs. Monoarthritis has been reported in 17–25% of patients[74,76]. The large joints such as the knees, ankles, elbows and wrists are most frequently involved. The hip, shoulder and the small joints of the hands and feet are less frequently involved.

The clinical pattern of joint involvement in a large series of patients was as follows:

- one or both knees in 76%
- one or both ankles in 50%
- elbows, wrists, hips or small joints of the feet in 12–15%
- shoulder or small joints of the hand in 7–8%
- lumbo-sacral in 2%
- cervical in 1%
- sternoclavicular in 0.5%
- temporomandibular in 0.5%[27,76].

In clinical practice most patients who develop joint pain will be treated empirically with aspirin or non-steroidal anti-inflammatory drugs (NSAIDs). The progression of the arthralgia or arthritis may thus be prevented and the typical migratory pattern of acute rheumatic fever may not be seen.

Analysis of the synovial fluid has shown the presence of sterile inflammatory fluid. There may be a reduction in complement components C1q, C3 and C4, suggesting their consumption by immune complexes[78].

Radiographs may show the presence of effusion but no other abnormalities are noted.

Jaccoud's arthritis or Jaccoud's arthropathy (also called chronic post-rheumatic fever arthropathy) is a rare manifestation of acute rheumatic fever characterized by deformities of the fingers and toes[79,80]. There is ulnar deviation of the fingers, especially the fourth and fifth, flexion of the metacarpophalangeal joints and hyperextension of the proximal interphalangeal joints. The hand is usually painless and there are no signs of inflammation. The deformities are usually correctible but may become fixed in the later stages. There are no true erosions on X-ray and rheumatoid factor is usually negative.

Jaccoud's arthropathy may occur after repeated attacks of rheumatic fever and results from recurrent inflammation of the fibrous articular capsule. A similar form of arthropathy is seen in patients with systemic lupus erythematosus[81].

Carditis

Carditis is the most serious manifestation of acute rheumatic fever as it may lead to chronic rheumatic heart disease and sometimes severe heart failure. However, it is usually less severe, although it may produce scarring of the heart valve. In some patients the carditis is asymptomatic and is only detected during clinical examination of a patient with arthritis or chorea. The incidence of carditis during the initial attack of acute rheumatic fever varies from 40–91% depending on the selection of patients and whether the diagnosis is made on clinical assessment alone or combined with echocardiography.

The incidence of carditis in rheumatic fever varies with the age of the patient. It is reported in 90–92% of children under the age of 3 years[82], in 50% of children aged 3–6 years, in 32% of teenagers aged 14–17 years[76], and only in 15% of adults with a first attack of rheumatic fever[75]. In Bland and Jones's[83] review of 1000 patients in 1951, 65% of patients were diagnosed as having carditis. In the recent Utah outbreak in the USA[4], 91% had carditis when clinical examination was combined with echocardiography.

The symptoms and signs of carditis depend on whether there is involvement of the pericardium, myocardium or a heart valve. The clinical diagnosis of carditis is based on the detection of an organic murmur that was not previously present, presence of a pericardial friction rub or signs of pericardial effusion, cardiomegaly or congestive heart failure.

Patients with myocarditis may develop cardiomegaly and congestive heart failure, which may be severe and life-threatening. They require aggressive treatment with diuretics and anti-inflammatory drugs, which may include corticosteroids. Myocardial damage may manifest with electrocardiographic changes, which include varying degrees of heart block. Patients with first-degree heart block are usually asymptomatic. Patients with second-degree and third-degree heart block may be symptomatic and require a pacemaker if they develop congestive heart failure.

Pericarditis is associated with anterior chest pain and a pericardial friction rub may be detected on clinical examination. Pericarditis can be detected clinically in about 10% of patients. The pericardial effusion may sometimes be large but cardiac tamponade is rare. Constrictive pericarditis does not occur.

The mitral valve is involved most often, followed by the aortic valve. Mitral stenosis is a classical finding in acute rheumatic fever. Mitral incompetence is also common and may occur alone or with mitral stenosis or other valvular lesions. When the aortic valve is involved, aortic incompetence is commoner than aortic stenosis.

Echocardiography is more sensitive than clinical examination alone for the detection of valvular abnormalities[84]. The significance of the milder lesions detected in echocardiography is uncertain but it is possible that some of them may heal without any sequence[84]. In 1992 when the Jones criteria for the diagnosis of acute rheumatic fever were revised, the American Heart Association recommendation stated that 'at present there is insufficient information to allow the use of echocardiography, including Doppler, to document valvular regurgitation without accompanying auscultatory findings as the sole criteria for valvulitis in acute rheumatic fever'.

Echocardiography is widely available in most developed countries and is likely to be used for detection of valvular involvement or the assessment of severity.

Congestive heart failure may be due to myocarditis or severe involvement of one or more heart valves. It occurs in 5–10% of the initial episodes and is more frequent during recurrences of rheumatic fever.

If patients do not have a high fever, arthritis, chest pain due to pericarditis, or chorea, they may not seek medical attention and may later present with rheumatic heart disease without an antecedent history of rheumatic fever. A survey of 12 000 Black schoolchildren in South Africa reported a prevalence of rheumatic heart disease in 6.9/1000 and 82.5% of the affected children were previously undiagnosed[11].

Sydenham's chorea
Chorea may be the only presenting manifestation of acute rheumatic fever. It is commoner in females and after puberty there is an even greater female predominance. The latent period between the episode of streptococcal pharyngitis and the development of chorea is considerably longer (6–8 weeks) than for arthritis and carditis. Chorea is characterized by the presence of involuntary, purposeless and jerky movements of the hands, arms, shoulders, feet, legs, face and trunk. The purposeless movements interfere with voluntary activity and disappear during sleep. Initially chorea may be confined to the face or one arm and sometimes it may be completely unilateral (hemichorea).

Chorea may last for a week to 2 years but usually lasts 8–15 weeks. When chorea occurs alone, the erythrocyte sedimentation rate (ESR), C-reactive protein and streptococcal antibody titers may be normal, because of the long latent period and resolution of the original infection. Chorea does not occur simultaneously with arthritis but may coexist with carditis. Some of the patients with chorea may have a cardiac murmur while others may only later manifest involvement of the mitral valve.

Subcutaneous nodules
The subcutaneous nodules of acute rheumatic fever resemble the nodules of rheumatoid arthritis and may be detected over the occiput, elbows, knees, ankles and Achilles tendons. In rheumatic fever, the nodules around the elbow tend to occur over the olecranon while rheumatoid nodules tend to occur more distally along the extensor aspect of the upper forearm. They are usually firm, painless and freely movable over the subcutaneous tissue. They vary in size from 0.5–2cm and tend to occur in crops. They are usually smaller, more discrete and less persistent than rheumatoid nodules.

They were detected in only 1.5% of patients in a recent series of 786 patients[85], but a higher prevalence was reported in earlier studies. Nodules are usually seen in children with prolonged active carditis rather than in the early stages of acute rheumatic fever. They may persist for a few weeks but seldom for more than a month. Multiple crops of nodules may be related to the severity of the rheumatic carditis.

Erythema marginatum
Erythema marginatum is a less common manifestation of acute rheumatic fever and occurs on the upper arms or trunk but not the face. It has a characteristic appearance and is therefore helpful in the diagnosis of acute rheumatic fever but is not pathognomonic. The rash is evanescent, pink in color and non-pruritic. It extends centrifugally while the skin at the center returns to normal – hence the name 'erythema marginatum'. It has an irregular serpiginous border. The rash may also become more prominent after a hot shower. Erythema marginatum usually occurs only in patients with carditis and may occur early or later in the course of the disease.

Other manifestations
The temperature is usually raised during attacks of acute rheumatic fever and ranges from 38.4–40°C[27]. A recent survey of patients with acute rheumatic fever noted a low-grade fever of 38°C or less in 29%[35]. The temperature usually decreases in a week and rarely lasts more than 4 weeks.

Abdominal pain may be severe and may mimic acute appendicitis. Epistaxis was reported as a common manifestation in the past but is now uncommon. Rheumatic pneumonia is uncommon and is difficult to distinguish from pulmonary edema and other causes of alveolitis.

A recent survey has shown that patients with Sydenham's chorea and rheumatic fever have a high risk of developing neuropsychiatric symptoms. Obsessive compulsive disorder is more common and attention deficit hyperactivity disorder is a risk factor for Sydenham's chorea in children with rheumatic fever[86]. The association with obsessive compulsive disorder is interesting in view of the finding of increased D8/17 B-cell positivity in these patients.

INVESTIGATIONS

The investigation of a patient with suspected acute rheumatic fever includes seeking evidence of streptococcal infection, acute phase reactants such as ESR and C-reactive protein, electrocardiography, chest X-ray and other supporting tests.

Throat cultures
Throat cultures should be taken at presentation to isolate the organism. They are usually negative by the time patients present with arthritis or carditis. A positive throat culture may be due to convalescent carriage of the original rheumatogenic strain or a new infection with a different strain.

Streptococcal antibody tests
The antibody tests are directed against the extracellular products of streptococci and include antistreptolysin O, anti-DNAse B, anti-hyaluronidase, anti-NADase (anti-DPNase) and antistreptokinase. Antistreptolysin O is the most widely used test. Streptococcal antibody tests are useful because they usually reach a peak at the time of clinical presentation of acute rheumatic fever; the presence of a high titer indicates a true infection and a significant rise in the titer on repeat testing supports the diagnosis of a recent infection[27].

The antibody levels usually reach a peak at about 4–5 weeks after the pharyngeal infection. They decrease rapidly over the next few months and then more slowly after 6 months[27]. As only about 80% of the patients have a rise in the titer of antistreptolysin O, it may be necessary to perform other antibody tests such as anti-DNAse B and antihyaluronidase.

Acute phase reactants
The ESR and C-reactive protein are usually elevated during the acute illness with arthritis or carditis. They may, however, be normal when chorea is the only clinical manifestation. They usually respond to salicylates or NSAIDs. They may also be useful in monitoring recurrences of acute rheumatic fever.

Chest X-ray
Moderate or massive cardiomegaly may be present, depending on the severity of the carditis. Heart failure may occur with severe myocarditis or valvular involvement. Pericarditis with an effusion may produce a globular heart.

Electrocardiography
There may be features of pericarditis with diffuse elevation of the ST segments. Myocarditis may be associated with tachycardia and

prolongation of the P–R interval. Some patients may have second-degree heart block and, rarely, complete heart block. An earlier series of 700 patients reported electrocardiographic abnormalities in 21% with 60% of them having varying degrees of heart block[87].

Echocardiography

The role of echocardiography in acute rheumatic fever has not been clearly defined and was not included in the 1992 revised Jones criteria[71]. However it is likely to be used widely in clinical practice. The long-term significance of subclinical abnormalities that are detected on echocardiography is unknown. In the Utah epidemic, carditis was detected on auscultation in 68% of patients[88]. Doppler ultrasound examination detected inaudible valvular incompetence in 47% of patients with only polyarthritis at onset and in 57% of patients with chorea alone[88].

Other tests

A mild normocytic normochromic anemia may be present. Antibodies to cardiac tropomyosin are elevated in most patients with acute rheumatic fever and can be detected by ELISA assays. Using a monoclonal antibody (D8/17), patients with acute rheumatic fever show increased levels of D8/17-positive cells. They have been detected in 100% of patients of diverse ethnic origins and only in 10% of normals[61]. The latter tests are not widely available at present.

DIAGNOSIS

The original Jones criteria for rheumatic fever were proposed in 1944 and have been modified in 1992 (Table 99.2)[71]. They serve as a guideline for the diagnosis of the initial attack of rheumatic fever and include a combination of clinical and laboratory features. It is important to try and establish a diagnosis so that the patient can be treated with antibiotics and a decision can be made on the need for long-term prophylaxis. By contrast, overdiagnosis can lead to unnecessary anxiety for patients and their families and subject patients to long-term therapy.

The basic requirement is documented evidence of a preceding streptococcal infection such as a positive throat culture, rapid streptococcal antigen test or elevated or rising streptococcal antibody titer. There is then high probability of the diagnosis of acute rheumatic fever if there are two major or one major and two minor criteria in association with evidence of a streptococcal infection.

In certain circumstances, a diagnosis of rheumatic fever is likely even in the absence of evidence of a preceding streptococcal infection. Lone chorea occurs after a long latent period when there is no evidence of a streptococcal infection. Some patients with indolent carditis may manifest late in the course of the illness and carditis may be the only manifestation.

The polyarthritis of rheumatic fever can also present diagnostic difficulty when it is the only major manifestation. When fever is also present, it is necessary to consider other diagnoses such as gonococcal arthritis, Lyme disease or a connective tissue disease.

A comparison of the prevalence of the various major criteria in different series is shown in Table 99.3.

TREATMENT

The treatment of acute rheumatic fever will depend on the spectrum of clinical manifestations present and their severity, as well as the stage of the illness at the time of presentation. One of the major determinants of the nature and duration of therapy is the presence and severity of carditis. The treatment of rheumatic fever has been reviewed recently[90].

Bed rest

All patients should have a period of bed rest during an attack of acute rheumatic fever. They will require monitoring for the presence or progression of carditis. Once the symptoms and signs of acute inflammation have resolved, patients are allowed to be ambulatory. A 4-week period of bed rest is recommended for patients with carditis[91].

Antimicrobial therapy

Adequate treatment of the streptococcal pharyngeal infection is essential to avoid prolonged and repetitive exposure to streptococcal antigen. The treatment of choice is penicillin, which is best given as a single intramuscular dose of benzathine penicillin. If penicillin is given orally, a 10-day course is necessary (see also Primary prevention, below).

Analgesics and non-steroidal anti-inflammatory drugs

Patients with mild symptoms of fever and joints without carditis may respond to analgesics alone. Patients with moderate or severe arthritis should be treated with salicylates in a dose of 80–100mg/kg/day to maintain a blood level of 20–30mg/dl. Salicylate doses of 4g or more may be required in adults. Patients on high-dose salicylates will require monitoring for adverse effects, including nausea, vomiting, abdominal pain and gastrointestinal bleeding. Treatment should be continued until the symptoms and signs of inflammation have resolved. The higher dose of salicylates should be continued for 2 weeks and then reduced. Use of other NSAIDs is also likely to be of value and naproxen has been reported to be effective and well tolerated[92].

Steroid therapy

Steroids have a potent anti-inflammatory effect but are not superior to salicylates in altering the course of the illness and preventing the development of heart disease. They should not be used routinely but have been used in the presence of severe carditis and heart failure. If the heart failure is due to active carditis, then steroids may be of value. They are not helpful if the heart failure is due to severe valvular damage.

Treatment of heart failure

Heart failure is treated with bed rest and steroids are used if there is active carditis. Conventional management may also include the use of

TABLE 99.3 PREVALENCE OF THE MAJOR MANIFESTATIONS OF ACUTE RHEUMATIC FEVER[83,85,88,89]				
	São Paulo, Brazil $n = 786$	Utah, USA $n = 274$	Boston, USA $n = 1000$	Konya, Turkey $n = 274$
Carditis	50.4	68.2	65.3	60.9
Polyarthritis	57.6	36.1	41.0	81.4
Chorea	34.8	36.4	51.8	17.9
Erythema marginatum	1.6	4.0	7.1	0.4
Subcutaneous nodules	1.5	2.6	8.8	0.7

A comparison of the prevalence of the major criteria for acute rheumatic fever in different populations (figures are percentages).

diuretics, digoxin or vasodilators, depending on the nature of the underlying abnormalities.

Sydenham's chorea

Chorea is usually a self-limiting and benign manifestation that does not require specific therapy. It may be protracted and disabling in some patients and responds to haloperidol.

PREVENTION

Primary prevention

Primary prevention refers to the prevention of the first attack of rheumatic fever by early treatment of the streptococcal pharyngeal infection. In 1950, Denny and colleagues showed that rheumatic fever can be prevented if the preceding pharyngeal infection due to group A streptococci is adequately treated with penicillin[93]. Penicillin is the treatment of choice, as it is bactericidal. Ideally, the streptococcal infection should be confirmed by throat culture, which requires overnight incubation, or by using a rapid diagnostic antigen detection kit. A positive throat culture does not differentiate between active streptococcal pharyngeal infection and an asymptomatic carrier with viral pharyngitis. Many of the kit tests are specific and, if the test is positive, the patient should be treated. The kit tests are also less sensitive than culture and the American Heart Association has recommended that a negative antigen test is confirmed with a throat culture[93]. In developing countries the above guidelines are not always practical and patients often receive empirical penicillin therapy during episodes of pharyngitis.

The most effective treatment is a single injection of benzathine penicillin G intramuscularly. The recommended dose is 600 000 units in children less than 27kg (60lb) and 1.2 million units in those who are more than 27kg (60lb)[93]. The alternative is to use oral penicillin V (phenoxymethyl penicillin) for 10 days (250mg in children and 500mg in adolescent and adults, two to three times daily)[93]. The use of intramuscular penicillin obviates the need for oral medication to be taken for 10 days and overcomes the problem of compliance, as patients may stop treatment when they feel better after a few days. Patients who are allergic to penicillin should be treated with oral erythromycin for 10 days with a maximum dose of 1g/day (erythromycin estolate 20–40mg/kg/day in two to four divided doses or erythromycin ethylsuccinate 40mg/kg/day in two to four divided doses)[93].

During an epidemic, mass penicillin prophylaxis is of value and intramuscular penicillin has been effective in military camps[94].

Secondary prevention

Secondary prevention refers to the prevention of recurrences of rheumatic fever by the use of continuous prophylaxis against streptococcal infection. The most effective regimen is the use of benzathine penicillin G 1.2 million units by intramuscular injection once every 4 weeks. In developing countries, where there is a high incidence of acute rheumatic fever and an increased risk of recurrence, intramuscular penicillin G should be given once every 3 weeks, as the levels of penicillin are low in the fourth week. The alternative treatment is penicillin V 250mg twice daily orally or sulfadiazine 0.5g once a day if less than 27kg (60lb) or 1g/day if more than 27kg (60lb)[93]. Patients who are allergic to penicillin and sulfadiazine should be treated with erythromycin 250mg twice a day.

A large survey of 1790 patients who received 32 000 injections of benzathine penicillin G showed a recurrence rate of rheumatic fever of 0.45% in patients on intramuscular penicillin G compared to 11.5% in patients who were not compliant[95].

There are no clear guidelines for the duration of the treatment that would apply to children as well as to young adults. Patients who have significant rheumatic heart disease, history of a recent attack or a history of recurrence should receive prophylactic treatment. The risk of an attack of acute rheumatic fever following a group A streptococcal infection increases from 1–3% during the first attack of streptococcal pharyngitis to 25–75% in subsequent attacks[96]. The risk of recurrence depends on many factors, such as the presence of carditis, the severity of cardiac involvement, the time interval since the most recent attack and the risk of streptococcal throat infections, depending on living conditions and occupation. Patients with previous carditis have an increased risk of carditis during recurrence of rheumatic fever. It is necessary for the treatment to be individualized and it can vary from 5 years' to lifelong prophylaxis.

Patients with rheumatic heart disease should receive prophylactic antibiotics to prevent infective endocarditis when they undergo surgical procedures on the mouth (dental extractions), eyes, ears, nose, throat and the gastrointestinal and genitourinary tracts.

Vaccines

Rheumatic fever and rheumatic heart disease are the commonest cause of cardiac-associated deaths in young adults in developing countries. The high prevalence of rheumatic fever in developing countries, the resurgence of rheumatic fever in the USA and the occurrence of a severe illness such as the toxic streptococcal syndrome have further emphasized the need to develop an effective vaccine.

Strategies for the development of vaccines have been reviewed[9,35,97]. Most of them have focussed on either the N-terminal region or the carboxy-terminal region of the M protein. The characterization of the M protein molecule has already been completed[9].

Some of the important considerations in the development of the vaccine are as follows.

- The vaccine should not exacerbate the rheumatic disease it is designed to prevent. M protein sites that are associated with tissue cross-reactivity or infiltrates should be avoided and therefore thorough testing in animals is necessary.
- There are more than 80 different M protein serotypes that cause infection and only a few of the serotypes can be used for a type-specific vaccine. M protein serotypes are also cyclic and different serotypes produce rheumatic fever in different parts of the world.
- The immune response should produce lasting protection.

Efforts to produce the ideal vaccine have been going on for over three decades since the development of a partially purified M3 vaccine[98]. Research on M protein vaccines has taken place since the 1970s and, although there has been considerable experience and improvement in our knowledge of vaccines, there has been little success. Other potential targets for vaccines are $C5\alpha$ peptidase, streptococcal proteinase (pyrogenic exotoxin B) and carbohydrate–protein conjugates. Current research is promising and hopefully vaccines will be available for clinical trials in the future.

REFERENCES

1. Williams RC Jr. Acute rheumatic fever. In: Klippel JH, Dieppe PA eds. Rheumatology, 2nd ed. London: Mosby 1997; 6.8.1–6.8.10.
2. Gordis L. The virtual disappearance of rheumatic fever in the United States: lessons in the rise and fall of disease. T. Duckett Jones memorial lecture 1985; 72: 1155–1162.
3. Bisno AL. The resurgence of acute rheumatic fever in the United States. Annu Rev Med 1990; 41: 319–329.
4. Veasy LG, Wiedmeier SE, Orsmond GS et al. Resurgence of acute rheumatic fever in the intermountain area of the United States. N Engl J Med 1987; 316: 421–427.
5. Hosier D, Craenen JM, Teske DW, Wheller JJ. Resurgence of acute rheumatic fever. Am J Dis Child 1987: 141: 730–733.
6. Wald ER, Dashefsky B, Feidt C et al. Acute rheumatic fever in western Pennsylvania and tristate area. Pediatrics 1987; 80: 371–4.

7. Centers for Disease Control. Acute rheumatic fever at a navy training center – San Diego, California. Morbid Mortal Wkly Rep 1988; 37: 101–104.

8. Centers for Disease Control. Acute rheumatic fever among army trainees – Fort Leonardwood, Missouri 1987–1988. Morbid Mortal Wkly Rep 1988; 37: 519–526.

9. Stollerman GH. Rheumatic fever. Lancet 1997; 349: 935–942.

10. McLaren MJ, Marcowitz M. Rheumatic heart disease in developing countries : the consequence of inadequate prevention. Ann Intern Med 1994; 120: 243–245.

11. McLaren MJ, Hawkins DM, Koornhof HJ et al. Epidemiology of rheumatic heart disease in black school children of Soweto, Johannesburg. Br Med J 1975; 3: 474–478.

12. Agarwall BL. Rheumatic fever and rheumatic heart disease in developing countries. New Delhi: Arnold Publishers; 1988: 24–75.

13. Bartter T, Dascal A, Carroll K, Curley FJ. 'Toxic strep syndrome.' A manifestation of group A streptococcal infection. Arch Intern Med 1988; 148: 1421–1424.

14. Stollerman GH. Changing group A streptococci. The reappearance of streptococcal 'toxic shock'. Arch Intern Med 1988; 148: 1268–1270.

15. Stevens DL, Tanner MH, Winship J et al. Severe group A streptococcal infections associated with a toxic shock-like syndrome and scarlet fever toxin A. N Engl J Med 1989; 321: 1–7.

16. Francis J, Warren RE. Streptococcus pyogenes bacteraemia in Cambridge – a review of 67 episodes. Q J Med 1988; 68: 603–613.

17. Martin PR, Holby EA. Streptococcal serogroup A epidemic in Norway 1987–1988. Scand J Infect Dis 1990; 22: 421–429.

18. Woolf N. Acute rheumatic fever. In: Woolf N, ed. Pathology. Basic and systems. London: WB Saunders; 1998: 355–358.

19. Silver MD. Blood flow obstruction related to tricuspid, pulmonary and mitral valves. In: Silver MD, ed. Cardiovascular pathology. New York: Churchill Livingstone; 1991: 933–984.

20. Stollerman GH. Pathology of rheumatic fever. In: Stollerman GH, ed. Rheumatic fever and streptococcal infection. New York: Grune & Stratton; 1975: 123–145.

21. Stollerman GH. Rheumatic fever. In: Kelley WN, Harris EJ, Ruddy S, Sledge CB, eds. Textbook of rheumatology. Philadelphia, PA: WB Saunders; 1989: 1312–1324.

22. Virmani R, Roberts WC. Aschoff bodies in operatively excised atrial appendages and in papillary muscles. Frequency and clinical significance. Circulation 1977; 55: 559–563.

23. Husby G, Arora R, Williams RC Jr et al. Immunofluorescence studies of florid rheumatic Aschoff lesions. Arthritis Rheum 1986; 29: 207–211.

24. Chopra P, Tandon HD, Raizada V et al. Comparative studies of mitral valves in rheumatic heart disease. Arch Intern Med 1983; 143: 661–666.

25. El-Said GM. Rheumatic fever. In: Oski FA, eds. Principles and practice of pediatrics. Philadelphia, PA: JB Lippincott; 1994: 1626–1631.

26. Stollerman GH. Rheumatic fever and streptococcal infection. Philadelphia, PA: Grune & Stratton; 1975: 70.

27. Gibofsky A, Kerwar S, Zabriskie JB. Rheumatic fever. The relationships between host, microbe and genetics. Rheum Dis Clin North Am 1998; 24: 237–259.

28. Fraude J, Gibofsky A, Buskisk DR et al. Cross reactivity between streptococcus and human tissue: a model of molecular mimicry and autoimmunity. Curr Top Microbiol Immunol 1989; 145: 5–26.

29. Coburn AF, Young D. The epidemiology of hemolytic streptococcus during World War II in the United States Navy. Baltimore, MD: Williams & Wilkins; 1949.

30. Rammelkamp CH, Denny FW, Wannamaker LW. Studies on the epidemiology of rheumatic fever in the armed services. In: Thomas L, ed. Rheumatic fever. A symposium. Minneapolis, MN: University of Minnesota Press; 1952: 72–89.

31. Potter EV, Swartman M, Mohammed I et al. Tropical acute rheumatic fever and associated streptococcal infections compared with concurrent acute glomerulonephritis. J Pediatr 1978; 92: 325–333.

32. McCarty M. The role of immunological mechanisms in the pathogenesis of rheumatic fever. In: Read SE, Zabriskie JB, eds. Streptococcal disease and the immune response. New York: Academic Press; 1980: 13–21.

32. Denny FW Jr, Wannamaker LW, Brink WR et al. Prevention of rheumatic fever: treatment of the preceding streptococcal infection. JAMA 1950; 143: 151–153.

33. Markowitz M, Gordis L. Rheumatic fever, 2nd ed. Philadelphia, PA: WB Saunders; 1972.

34. Stollerman GH, Lewis AJ, Schultz I et al. Relationship of the immune response to group-A streptococci to the causes of acute, chronic and recurrent rheumatic fever. Am J Med 1956; 20: 163–169.

35. Carapetis JR, Currie BJ, Good MF. Towards understanding the pathogenesis of rheumatic fever. Scand J Rheumatol 1996; 25: 127–131.

36. Cunningham MW. Pathogenesis of Group A streptococcal infections. Clin Microbiol Rev 2000; 13: 470–511.

37. Zabriskie JB, Kerwar S, Gibofsky A. The arthritogenic properties of microbial antigens. Their implications in disease states. Rheum Dis Clin North Am 1998; 24: 211–226.

38. Stollerman GH. Rheumatogenic streptococci and autoimmunity. Clin Immunopathol 1991; 61: 131–142.

39. Bessen D, Jones KF, Fischetti VA. Evidence for two distinct classes of streptococcal M-protein and their relationship to rheumatic fever. J Exp Med 1989; 169: 269–283.

40. Martin DR, Single LA. Molecular epidemiology of group A streptococcus M type 1 infections. J Infect Dis 1993; 167: 112–117.

41. Bessen DE, Hollingshead SK. Allelic polymorphism of emm loci provides evidence for horizontal gene spread in group A streptococci. Proc Natl Acad Sci USA 1994; 91: 3280–3284.

42. Tran PO, Johnson DR, Kaplan EL. The presence of M protein in the nontypeable group A streptococcal upper respiratory tract isolates from South East Asia. J Infect Dis 1994; 169: 658–661.

43. Schmidt KH, Gerlach D, Wollweber L et al. Mitogenicity of M5 protein extracted from Streptococcus pyogenes cells is due to streptococcal pyrogenic exotoxin C and mitogenic factor MF. Infect Immun 1995; 63: 4569–4575.

44. Kotb M. Infection and autoimmunity: a story of the host, the pathogen, and the copathogen. Clin Immunol Immunopathol 1995; 74: 10–22.

45. Rammelkamp CH, Wannamaker LW, Denny FW. The epidemiology and prevention of rheumatic fever. Bull NY Acad Med 1952; 28: 321–334.

46. Siegel AC, Johnson EE, Stollerman GH. Controlled studies of streptococcal pharyngitis in a pediatric population 1: factors related to the attack rate of rheumatic fever. N Engl J Med 1961; 265: 559–566.

47. Wilson M, Schweitzer MD, Lubschez R. The familial epidemiology of rheumatic fever. J Pediatr 1943; 22: 468–492.

48. Taranta A, Torosdag S, Metrakos JD et al. Rheumatic fever in monozygotic and dizygotic twins. Circulation 1959; 20: 778–792.

49. Ayoub EM, Barrett DJ, Maclaren NK, Krischer JP. Association of class II human histocompatibility leukocyte antigens with rheumatic fever. J Clin Invest 1986; 77: 2019–2026.

50. Anastasiou-Nana MI, Anderson JL, Carlquist JF, Nanas JN. HLA-DR typing and lymphocyte subset evaluation in rheumatic heart disease: a search for immune response factors. Am Heart J 1986; 112: 992–997.

51. Rajapakse CN, Halim K, Al-Orainey I et al. A genetic marker for rheumatic heart disease. Br Heart J 1987; 58: 659–662.

52. Carlquist JF, Ward RH, Meyer KJ et al. Immune response factors in rheumatic heart disease: meta-analysis of HLA-DR associations and evaluation of additional class II alleles. J Am Coll Cardiol 1995; 26: 452–457.

53. Jhinghan B, Mehra NK, Reddy KS et al. HLA blood groups and secretor status in patients with established rheumatic fever and rheumatic heart disease. Tissue Antigens 1986; 27: 172–178.

54. Maharaj B, Hammond MG, Appadoo B et al. HLA-A, B, DR, and DQ antigens in black patients with severe chronic rheumatic heart disease. Circulation 1987; 76: 259–261.

55. Ahmed S, Ayoub EM, Scornik JC et al. Post-streptococcal reactive arthritis: clinical characteristics and association with HLA DR alleles. Arthritis Rheum 1998; 41: 1096–1102.

56. Guedez Y, Kotby A, El-Demellawy M et al. HLA class II associations with rheumatic heart disease are more evident and consistent among clinically homogenous patients. Circulation 1999; 99: 2784–2790.

57. Ozkan M, Carin M, Sonnez G et al. HLA antigens in Turkish race with rheumatic heart disease. Circulation 1993; 87: 1974–1978.

58. Debaz H, Olivio A, Perez-Luque E et al. DNA analysis of HLA class II alleles in rheumatic heart disease in Mexicans. Hum Immunol 1996; 53: 206–215.

59. Koyanagi T, Koga Y, Nishi H et al. DNA typing of HLA class II genes in Japanese patients with rheumatic heart disease. J Mol Cell Cardiol 1996; 28: 1349–1353.

60. Jeane EL, Visentainer, Fatima C et al. Association of HLA-DR7 with rheumatic fever in the Brazilian population. J Rheumatol 2000; 27: 1518–1519.

61. Khanna AK, Buskirk DR, Williams RC Jr et al. Presence of a non-HLA B cell antigen I rheumatic fever patients and their families as defined by a monoclonal antibody. J Clin Invest 1989; 83: 1710–1716.

62. Kaur SD, Kumar A, Grover KL et al. Ethnic differences in expression of susceptibility marker(s) in rheumatic fever/rheumatic heart disease patients. Int J Cardiol 1998; 64: 9–14.

63. Stollerman GH. Rheumatogenic streptococcus and autoimmunity. Clin Immunol Immunopathol 1991; 61: 131–142.

64. Kaplan MH. Immunologic relation of streptococcal and tissue antigens. I. Properties of an antigen in certain strains of group A streptococci exhibiting an immunologic crossreaction with human heart tissue. J Immunol 1963; 90: 595–606.

65. Raizada V, Williams RC Jr, Chopra P et al. Tissue distribution of lymphocytes in rheumatic heart valves as defined by monoclonal anti-T cell antibodies. Am J Med 1983; 74: 90–96.

66. Kemeny E, Grieve T, Marcus R et al. Identification of mononuclear cells and T cell subsets in rheumatic valvulitis. Clin Immunol Immunopathol 1989; 52: 225–237.

67. Pruksakorn S, Currie B, Brandt E et al. Identification of T cell autoepitopes that cross-react with the C-terminal segment of the M protein of group-A streptococci. Int Immunol 1994; 6: 1235–1244.

68. Read SE, Fischetti VA, Utermohlen V et al. Cellular reactivity studies to streptococcal antigens. Migration inhibition studies in patients with streptococcal infections and rheumatic fever. J Clin Invest 1974; 54: 439–450.

69. Sapry RP, Ganguly NK, Sharma S et al. Cellular reaction to group A beta-hemolytic streptococcal membrane antigen and its relation to complement levels in patients with rheumatic heart disease. Br Med J 1977; 1: 422–422.

70. Williams RC. Understanding rheumatic fever. Scand J Rheumatol 199; 25: 132–133.

71. Special Writing Group of the Committee on Rheumatic Fever, Endocarditis and Kawasaki Disease of the Council on Cardiovascular Disease in the young. Guidelines for the diagnosis of rheumatic fever: Jones Criteria, updated 1992. American Heart Association. Circulation: 1993; 87: 302–307.

72. Rammelkamp CH Jr, Stolzer B. The latent period before the onset of acute rheumatic fever. Yale J Biol Med 1961/62; 34: 386–398.

73. Roy SB, Bhatia ML, Lazaro J, Ramalingawami V. Juvenile mitral stenosis in India. Lancet 1963; 2: 1193–1196.

74. Carapetis JR, Currie BJ. Rheumatic fever in a high incidence population: the importance of monoarthritis and low grade fever. Arch Dis Childhood 2001; 85: 223–227.

75. Barnett AL, Jerry EE, Persellin RH. Acute rheumatic fever in adults. JAMA 1975; 232: 925–928.

76. Feinstein AR, Spagnulo M. The clinical patterns of rheumatic fever : a reappraisal. Medicine 1986; 164: 762–776.

77. Graef B, Parent S, Zitron W, Wyckoff J. Studies in rheumatic fever: the natural course of acute manifestations of rheumatic fever uninfluenced by 'specific' therapy. Am J Med Sci 1933; 185: 197–210.

78. Swartman M, Potter EV, Poon-King T. Immunoglobulin components in synovial fluids of patients with acute rheumatic fever. J Clin Invest 1975; 56: 111–117.

79. Bird JA, Perloff JK. Chronic post rheumatic fever arthropathy of Jaccoud. Am Heart J 1983; 105: 515–517.

80. Girigis FL, Popple AW, Bruckner FE. Jaccoud's arthropathy: a case report and necropsy study. Ann Rheum Dis 1978; 37: 561–565.

81. Esdaile JM, Danoff D, Rosenthall L, Gutkowski A. Deforming arthritis in systemic lupus erythematosus. Ann Rheum Dis 1981; 40: 124–126.

82. Rosenthal A, Czoniczer G, Messel BF. Rheumatic fever under three years of age. A report of 10 cases. Pediatrics 1968; 41: 612–619.

83. Bland EF, Jones TD. Rheumatic fever and rheumatic heart disease: a twenty year report on 1,000 patients followed since childhood. Circulation 1951; 4: 836–843.

84. Vasan RS, Shrivastava S, Vijayakumar MD et al. Echocardiographic evaluation of patients with acute rheumatic fever and rheumatic carditis. Circulation 1996; 94: 73–82.

85. Da Silva CH. Rheumatic fever: a multicenter study in the state of Sao Paulo. Pediatric Committee – Sao Paulo Pediatric Rheumatology Society. Rev Hosp Clin Fac Med Univ Sao Paulo 1999; 54: 85–90.

86. Mercadante MT, Busatto GF, Lombroso PJ et al. The psychiatric symptoms of rheumatic fever. Am J Psychiatry 2000; 157: 2036–2038.

87. Sokolow M. Significance of electrocardiographic changes in rheumatic fever. Am J Med 1948; 5: 365–378.

88. Veasy LG, Tani LY, Hill HR. Persistence of acute rheumatic fever in the intermountain area of the United States. J Pediatr 1994; 124: 9–16.

89. Karaaslan S, Oran B, Reis I, Erkul I. Acute rheumatic fever in Konya, Turkey. Pediatr Int 2000; 42: 71–75.

90. Thatai D, Turi ZG. Current guidelines for the treatment of patients with rheumatic fever. Drugs 1999; 57: 545–555.

91. Da Silva NA, Pereira BA. Acute rheumatic fever; still a challenge. Rheum Dis Clin North Am 1997; 23: 545–568.

92. Uziel Y, Hashkes PJ, Kassem E et al. The use of naproxen in the treatment of children with rheumatic fever. J Pediatrics 2000; 137: 269–271.

93. Dajani A, Taubert K, Ferrieri P et al. Treatment of acute streptococcal pharyngitis and prevention of rheumatic fever. A statement for health professionals. Pediatrics 1995; 96: 758–764.

94. Frank PF, Stollerman GH, Miller LF. Protection of a military population from rheumatic fever. JAMA 1965; 193: 755.

95. Markowitz M, Kaplan E, Cuttica R et al. Allergic reactions to long-term benzathine penicillin prophylaxis for rheumatic fever. Lancet 1991; 337: 1308–1310.

96. Denny FW. T Duckett Jones and rheumatic fever in 1986. Circulation 1987; 76: 963–970.

97. Fischetti VA. Streptococcal M protein: molecular design and biological behaviour. Clin Microbiol Rev 1989; 2: 285–314.

98. Massel BF, Michael JG, Amezcua J, Siner M. Secondary and apparent primary antibody responses after group A streptococcal vaccination of 21 children. Appl Microbiol 1968; 16: 509–518.

SPONDYLOARTHROPATHIES

SPONDYLOARTHROPATHIES

100 History

Anthony S Russell

Definition

- A chronic systemic inflammatory disorder that mainly affects the axial skeleton
- Two forms of the disease are recognized – primary (idiopathic) and secondary, associated with reactive arthritis, psoriasis or inflammatory bowel diseases

Clinical features

- Typical presentation is with low back pain of insidious onset
- Arthritis of hips and enthesopathies are common
- Extraskeletal complications include acute anterior uveitis, aortic valvular disease and the cauda equina syndrome

INTRODUCTION

In developed Western societies, ankylosing spondylitis (AS) typically presents during the third decade of life, whereas in developing countries it presents much earlier, in late childhood, and is often a much more disabling disease. Moreover, AS is a disease in which genetic factors (e.g. human leukocyte antigen (HLA)-B27) play a part. It is surprising, therefore, that such genes should have persisted through millenia, unless, like genes for sickle cell disease, they also have some positive survival value. No such effect has yet been shown, and therefore the antiquity of AS is of some interest.

EARLIEST CASES

The very first clinical description of AS is generally agreed to be that by Connor in 1691 but whether or not the disease was present earlier

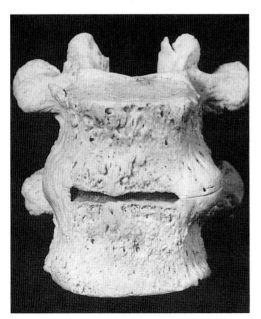

Fig. 100.1 A lumbar spine, dating from around the 15th century, apparently showing a unilateral syndesmophyte.

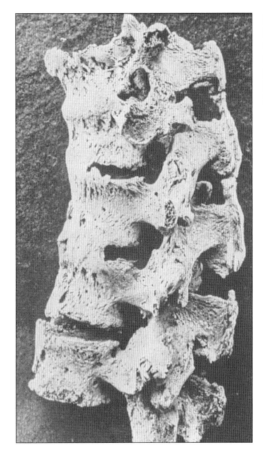

Fig. 100.2 Anterior interosseous fusion in an early Nubian skeleton. (With permission of the British Library from Wood-Jones[3].)

remains controversial. The difficulty is in the distinction between AS and Forestier's disease (diffuse idiopathic skeletal hyperostosis, DISH)[1] and other causes of intervertebral fusion[2]. Radiographically, the appearances can at times be remarkably similar, as has been recognized[1], although generally the two disorders are easily distinguishable. Unfortunately, extrapolation from the skeletal remains with which the paleopathologists are faced to the presumptive radiographic appearances is difficult, and this makes interpretation even more complex and uncertain.

The difficulty of clearly recognizing AS in such specimens is illustrated in Figure 100.1, which shows part of a lumbar spine dating approximately from the 15th century, and Figure 100.2, which shows anterior interosseous fusion of L1–L4, with good disc space preservation, in an early Nubian skeleton[3]. The description in the pathologic report of this study indicated that the most frequent disease seen is

> rheumatoid arthritis, and the most common manifestation is spondylitis deformans … may be present as mere lipping of the adjacent edges of individual vertebrae or may involve many vertebrae and even ankylose whole series together. It is very common to find in the prehistoric bodies two or more lumbar vertebrae fused by irregular osseous bridges connecting their bodies and frequently these

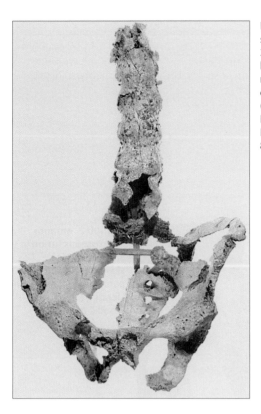

Fig. 100.3 Part of a skeleton dating from 3500 BC, clearly showing bony bridging, but with minimal preservation of the sacroiliac joints. (With permission from Dastugue J. L'Anthropologie 1976; 80: 625–653.)

osseous bridges are limited to one side of the anterior surface. Its site of election is in the lower lumbar region: so very common is this disease that in a prehistoric cemetary in the main street of Shellal no adult body failed to show some traces of its presence ….

Although the features seen in Figure 100.2 are certainly compatible with AS, the prevalence of the associated apophyseal involvement would seem extremely high for this disease; despite the unusual lumbar predominance, I would interpret it as DISH. The same conclusion was reached by Rogers et al.[4] in 13 of 15 examples of spinal fusion they found. In the two others, an asymmetric sacroiliitis was associated.

Dastugue[5] described an even older skeleton (3500 BC) (Fig. 100.3), found in a neolithic grave in Calvados. Again, bony bridging is clearly present, but the sacroiliac joints are minimally preserved, and whether the degree of fusion still observable is abnormal is difficult to judge.

Although the appearances shown in Figure 100.4 look very much like those that would be expected in a patient with AS, both Fauré and I share reservations regarding this diagnosis. However, if it is indeed AS,

then Rameses II is certainly the first specific individual known to have had this disease.

The skeleton from medieval Geneva described by Kramar[6] does have radiographs, but the sacroiliac abnormalities described are not convincing. Nevertheless, in 1691 Connor presented a diagram of a relatively contemporary skeleton that is very likely to be from a patient with AS. He even guessed at some of the clinical features that this patient may have had. Other descriptions and collections of affected skeletal remains followed. As described by O'Connell[7], Lyon's clinical description in 1831 was followed by an autopsy, obtained with difficulty, that substantiated the retrospective diagnosis, and by 1850 Rokitansky was clearly aware of the difference between AS and DISH. He described DISH, 'as if a quantity of bony matter had been poured over a bone and coagulated as it flowed …'.

Many isolated, but in retrospect clear-cut, descriptions of patients with AS were made before the 'discoveries' by Strumpell (1897 in Berlin), Marie (1898 in Paris) and von Bechterew (1893 in St Petersburg). Brodie's patient (1841) had concomitant iritis and Fagge's (1877) had apophyseal fusion rather than anterior syndesmophytes. Fagge also described that the lungs showed bronchiectasis of both upper lobes. Pierre Marie provided the most detailed of the major reports and was followed by Leri, his trainee, who provided autopsy material to illustrate the pathologic features[7,8].

THE CONTRIBUTION OF RADIOGRAPHY

Involvement of the sacroiliac joints was soon noted, but its critical importance was appreciated only after the radiographic studies had become more standardized. In 1931, Buckley described 60 patients with AS and reviewed the topic well[9], pointing out that the categorization into Bechterew and Marie–Strumpell types appeared invalid. He also described seven among 60 patients whose symptoms clearly began after an accident – an association that is often discussed in this age of litigation, but which remains unsettled. The work by Romanus and Yden[10] produced new descriptions, including 'shining corners'.

MORE RECENT INSIGHTS

In the USA, AS was often thought of as rheumatoid arthritis affecting the spine that is, rheumatoid spondylitis; this term was never prevalent in the UK, Canada or Europe. A number of factors led to its final abandonment: for example, the widespread acceptance of the clinical relevance of the rheumatoid factor test for rheumatoid arthritis and the persistent seronegativity of patients with AS. Even as late as 1960, however, Graham from Canada argued that the term 'rheumatoid spondylitis' was unhelpful[11]. The development of the Rome criteria perhaps ended the use of rheumatoid spondylitis as a descriptive term, even by its most diehard supporters.

In 1974 Moll et al.[12] introduced the concept of 'seronegative spondylarthropathy' on the basis of overlapping clinical and radiologic features within a number of different diseases. Although this concept has been modified, and for example Behçet's and Whipple's disease have been excluded, overall the concept has been progressively accepted and, indeed, there are now classification criteria by Amor et al.[13] and by the European Spondylarthropathy Study Group[14]. There are some significant differences between these classifications, but the overall principles have been well accepted. The term 'spondylarthropathy' evolved, via an error in spelling, to 'spondyloarthropathy' which, primarily because of its more agreeable sound, has become the accepted term in this field.

It was during the period leading to the publication by Moll et al. (1971–1974) that the associations were noted between HLA-B27 and, firstly, AS and, subsequently, reactive arthritis, acute anterior uveitis and psoriatic arthritis. These associations were clearly in accord with the

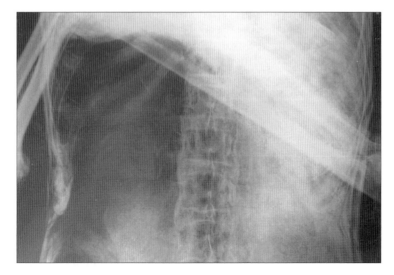

Fig. 100.4 Radiograph of the dorsolumbar spine from the mummy of Rameses II. (Courtesy of Professor C. Fauré.)

clinical description of the spondyloarthropathies and, indeed, have been included in Amor's classification system, but we still need an understanding of how HLA-B27 predisposes to disease susceptibility. Perhaps the most dramatic experimental studies in this area involve the development of HLA-B27 transgenic rats which, in the presence of normal bowel flora, develop an analogous spondyloarthropathy. This resolved any doubts that the critical gene was B27, and not a gene at some closely linked locus. It is possible that modern techniques of DNA amplification may allow a re-examination of some early skeletal remains, to determine the HLA type of those early putative spondylitic skeletons.

REFERENCES

1. Yagan R, Khan MA. Confusion of roentgenographic differential diagnosis of ankylosing hyperostosis (Forestier's disease) and ankylosing spondylitis. Spine 1990; 4: 561–575.
2. Russell AS, Percy JS, Lentle BC. Vertebral sclerosis in adults. Ann Rheum Dis 1978; 37: 18–22.
3. Wood-Jones F. Archaeological survey of Nubia. Bulletin 2. 1907–1908: 55–69.
4. Rogers J, Watt I, Dieppe P. Paleopathology of spinal osteophytosis, vertebral ankylosis, ankylosing spondylitis and vertebral hyperostosis. Ann Rheum Dis 1985; 44: 113–120.
5. Dastugue J. Les maladies de nos ancêtres. La Recherche 1982; 13: 980–988.
6. Kramar C. A case of ankylosing spondylitis in medieval Geneva. Ossa 1981; 8: 115–129.
7. O'Connell D. Ankylosing spondylitis. The literature up to the close of the nineteenth century. Ann Rheum Dis 1956; 15: 119–123.
8. Bywaters EGL. Historical introduction. In: Moll JMH, ed. Ankylosing spondylitis. Edinburgh: Churchill Livingstone; 1980: 1–15.
9. Buckley CW. Spondylitis deformans. BMJ 1931; i: 1108–1112.
10. Romanus R, Yden S. Pelvo-spondylitis ossificans. Copenhagen: Munksgaard; 1955.
11. Graham W. Is rheumatoid arthritis a separate entity? Arthritis Rheum 1960; 3: 88–90.
12. Moll J, Haslock I, MacRae IF, Wright V. Association between ankylosing spondylitis, psoriatic arthritis, Reiter's disease, the intestinal arthropathies, and Behçet's syndrome. Medicine 1974; 53: 343–364.
13. Amor B, Dougados M, Mijijawa M. Critères de classification des spondylarthropathies. Rev Rhum 1990; 57: 85–89.
14. Dougados M, van der Linden S, Juhlin R et al. The European spondylarthropathy study group. Preliminary criteria for the classification of spondylarthropathies. Arthritis Rheum 1991; 1218–1226.

101 Classification of spondyloarthropathies

Sjef van der Linden and Désirée van der Heijde

- Spondyloarthropathies are a family of related diseases
- Diagnostic and classification criteria serve different purposes: diagnostic criteria apply to individual patients, classification criteria apply to groups of patients. They should not be used interchangeably
- For any given disease and a given diagnostic test, sensitivity and specificity show an inverse relationship: an increase in one is associated with a decrease in the other

HISTORY

About 50 years ago it was still common practice to consider rheumatic diseases as idiopathic non-specific syndromes that could be triggered by many different etiologic factors, for example psoriasis or urethritis. This reasoning was analogous to the triggering of rheumatic fever by streptococci. The nosological approach at that time is reflected by the classification of rheumatic diseases proposed by the International League Against Rheumatism in 1957 (Table 101.1)[1]. Diseases now considered as spondyloarthropathies – such as ankylosing spondylitis, reactive arthritis and psoriatic arthritis – were then classified as 'atypical' or 'special forms of rheumatoid arthritis'. 'Lumpers' preferred to group these so-called 'variants of rheumatoid arthritis' with rheumatoid arthritis, whereas 'splitters' favored the idea that all so-called 'variants of rheumatoid arthritis' are in fact entirely separate entities.

In the 1960s, Wright and colleagues drew attention to possible interrelationships among certain rheumatoid factor negative ('seronegative') variants of rheumatoid arthritis. They then formulated the concept of 'seronegative spondarthritides' as a group of rheumatic disorders sharing in common many clinical, radiologic and serologic features, in addition to familial and genetic relationships. This concept had been formulated before the association of human leukocyte antigen (HLA)-alleles with certain rheumatic diseases had been described; indeed, the striking association between HLA-B27 and ankylosing spondylitis was not reported until 1973. The nosological implication of the plural form of the term 'spondarthritides' (as opposed to 'spondarthritis') was intended to emphasize the idea of a group of similar and strongly interrelated conditions, rather than a single disease entity with different clinical manifestations[2].

Initially, it was felt that the principal diseases qualifying for inclusion in the seronegative spondarthritides (nowadays referred to by a variety of other terms, including: spondylarthritides, spondylarthropathies or spondyloarthropathies) should be idiopathic ankylosing spondylitis, psoriatic arthritis, Reiter's disease, ulcerative colitis, Crohn's disease, Whipple's disease and Behçet's syndrome[2]. On the basis of additional findings, including the lack of association with HLA-B27, Whipple's disease and Behçet's syndrome are now not considered to belong to this group. However, juvenile-onset ankylosing spondylitis and unspecified spondyloarthropathies are now incorporated (Table 101. 2).

Inclusion of diseases among the spondyloarthropathies is based on their many and often striking points of similarity, the most important of which include: negative tests for rheumatoid factor, absence of subcutaneous rheumatoid nodules, peripheral inflammatory arthritis, radiological sacroiliitis with or without clinical ankylosing spondylitis, tendency to familial aggregation, and a tendency to exhibit clinical inter-relationships between individual members of the group[2]. Such inter-relationships are considered to be present when two or more of the following clinical features coexist: (1) psoriatic skin or nail lesions; (2) other lesions such as ocular or genitourinary inflammation; (3) buccal, genital or bowel ulceration. Clearly, this group of disorders constitute a *family* of interrelated, but heterogeneous conditions, rather than a single disease with different clinical manifestations (Table 101.3).

TABLE 101.1 PROPOSED CLASSIFICATION OF RHEUMATIC DISEASES BY THE INTERNATIONAL LEAGUE AGAINST RHEUMATISM (ABBREVIATED) (ADAPTED FROM COPEMAN[1].)

Articular

Inflammatory
  Idiopathic
    Rheumatic fever
    Rheumatoid arthritis
    Atypical forms of rheumatoid arthritis
    – Arthritis with psoriasis
    – Juvenile rheumatoid arthritis
    – Felty's syndrome
    – Reiter's syndrome
    Specific forms of rheumatoid arthritis
    – Ankylosing spondylitis
    – Intermittent hydrarthrosis
    – Palindromic rheumatism
  Infectious
    Arthritis due to specific infection
Degenerative
  Osteoarthritis
  Intervertebral disc disease
  Osteochondrosis

Note that arthritis with psoriasis, Reiter's syndrome and ankylosing spondylitis were classified as atypical or special forms of rheumatoid arthritis

---

TABLE 101.2 DISEASES BELONGING TO THE SPONDYLOARTHROPATHIES

- Ankylosing spondylitis
- Reactive arthritis
- Arthropathy of inflammatory bowel disease (Crohn's disease, ulcerative colitis)
- Psoriatic arthritis
- Undifferentiated spondyloarthropathies
- Juvenile chronic arthritis: juvenile-onset ankylosing spondylitis

TABLE 101.3 CLINICAL CHARACTERISTICS OF SPONDYLOARTHROPATHIES
• Pattern of peripheral arthritis: predominantly of lower limb, asymmetric • Tendency to radiographic sacroiliitis • Absence of rheumatoid factor • Absence of subcutaneous nodules and other extra-articular features of rheumatoid arthritis • Overlapping extra-articular features characteristic of the group (such as anterior uveitis) • Significant familial aggregation • Association with HLA-B27

CLASSIFICATION

Criteria

Classification as a general term means separating certain issues into classes. Criteria are used to define those issues that belong to a specific class or category and those that do not belong to it. Indeed, different types of criteria are needed for different functions[3]. Classification, therefore, makes use of criteria and may address a whole spectrum of specific purposes.

One function of classification is to provide a *taxonomy* for disorders, whereby signs and symptoms can be attributed to separate diseases or related groups of diseases. It is in this field that one encounters the terms *diagnostic* and *classification* criteria. Although the main purpose of both sets of criteria is to ensure comparability across patients or studies, it is important to keep in mind that diagnostic and classification criteria have quite distinct features.

Diagnostic and classification criteria are examples of *discriminative* instruments. Both diagnostic and classification criteria must be insensitive to changes in disease activity. Apart from this, test characteristics such as sensitivity and specificity of both types of criteria might differ considerably[4].

Classification criteria apply to *groups* of patients. These groups should be homogeneous and not include many false positives – that is, they should have *high specificity* (although usually at some loss of sensitivity, because, for a given diagnostic test, specificity and sensitivity show an inverse relationship). Such criteria enable comparisons and are mainly applied in clinical studies. Patients who do not fulfil a certain set of classification criteria will usually not be included in clinical trials assessing the efficacy or safety of a particular intervention. Of course, the generalizability of study results to all patients in clinical practice with that particular disease might be limited if one applies strictly classification criteria.

Diagnostic criteria primarily apply not to groups, but to individual persons. In order to establish a correct diagnosis and ensure that cases are not missed, such criteria should have *high sensitivity* (especially for *early* cases of a particular disease; e.g. early ankylosing spondylitis). This will result in lower specificity – that is, more false-positives might be expected than with classification criteria. Therefore, in clinical practice diagnostic criteria are mainly applied to individual patients. Clearly, patients who do not (yet) fulfil a certain set of diagnostic criteria should not be withheld appropriate treatment.

Classification criteria, although clearly not intended for diagnostic purposes, are frequently used in clinical practice as an aid to identify somewhat atypical or undifferentiated cases.

Classification criteria for spondyloarthropathies

The spectrum of spondyloarthropathies is wider than the sum of the disorders mentioned in Table 101.2. Seronegative oligoarthritis, dactylitis, or polyarthritis of the lower extremities, heel pain due to enthesitis,

TABLE 101.4 EUROPEAN SPONDYLOARTHROPATHY STUDY GROUP CLASSIFICATION CRITERIA
Inflammatory spinal pain *or* Synovitis (asymmetric, predominantly in lower limbs) *and any one of the following:* • Positive family history • Psoriasis • Inflammatory bowel disease • Alternate buttock pain • Enthesopathy Sensitivity, 77%; specificity, 89% *Adding:* • Sacroiliitis Sensitivity, 87%; specificity, 87%
(From Dougados *et al.*[5])

TABLE 101.5 CRITERIA FOR ANKYLOSING SPONDYLITIS
Rome, 1961 *Clinical criteria* 1. Low back pain and stiffness for more than 3 months, not relieved by rest 2. Pain and stiffness in the thoracic region 3. Limited motion in the lumbar spine 4. Limited chest expansion 5. History or evidence of iritis or its sequelae *Radiological criterion* 6. Roentgenogram showing bilateral sacroiliac changes characteristic of ankylosing spondylitis (this would exclude bilateral osteoarthritis of the sacroiliac joints) *Definite ankylosing spondylitis if:* 1. Grade 3–4 bilateral sacroiliitis with at least one clinical criterion 2. At least 4 clinical criteria **New York, 1966** *Clinical criteria* 1. Limitation of motion of the lumbar spine in all 3 planes: anterior flexion, lateral flexion, and extension 2. Pain at the dorsolumbar junction or in the lumbar spine 3. Limitation of chest expansion to 2.5cm or less measured at the level of the 4th intercostal space *Grading of radiographs* Normal, 0; suspicious, 1; minimal sacroiliitis, 2; moderate sacroiliitis, 3; ankylosis, 4 *Definite ankylosing spondylitis if:* 1. Grade 3–4 bilateral sacroiliitis with at least 1 clinical criterion 2. Grade 3–4 unilateral or grade 2 bilateral sacroiliitis with clinical criterion 1 or with both clinical criteria 2 and 3 *Probable ankylosing spondylitis* Grade 3–4 bilateral sacroiliitis with no clinical criteria **Modified New York, 1984** *Criteria* 1. Low back pain for at least 3 months' duration improved by exercise and not relieved by rest 2. Limitation of lumbar spine motion in sagittal and frontal planes 3. Chest expansion decreased relative to normal values for age and sex 4a. Unilateral sacroiliitis grade 3–4 4b. Bilateral sacroiliitis grade 2–4 *Definite ankylosing spondylitis if* (4a OR 4b) AND any clinical criterion (1–3)
(Data from van der Linden *et al.*[8])

and other undifferentiated cases of spondyloarthropathies have been ignored in epidemiologic studies because of the inadequacy of existing criteria. To encompass patients with undifferentiated spondyloarthropathies, classification criteria for the entire group of spondyloarthropathies have been developed (Table 101.4)[5]. These European Spondyloarthropathy Study Group (ESSG) criteria for spondyloarthropathy resulted in a sensitivity of 87% and a specificity of 87%. In the subgroup of early cases (those in whom signs and symptoms had developed within the previous year), the sensitivity declined to 68%, although the specificity increased to 93% These criteria, although clearly not intended for diagnostic purposes, might be useful for the identification of atypical and undifferentiated forms of spondyloarthropathies before additional studies, such as radiography of sacroiliac joints or – on rare occasions – an HLA-B27 test, are requested. Despite differences in the sociocultural and geographic characteristics, this set of criteria performed quite well in other populations, with a sensitivity of 99% and a specificity of 89%[6].

Classification criteria for ankylosing spondylitis

As in many other diseases in which the etiology is not clearly defined (for example by the isolation of a specific causative pathogen), the diagnosis of ankylosing spondylitis must rest on clinical features alone. The disease is 'primary' or 'idiopathic' if no associated disorder is present and 'secondary' if the disease is associated with psoriasis or chronic inflammatory bowel disease.

In daily practice, a presumptive clinical diagnosis of ankylosing spondylitis is usually supported by radiologic evidence of sacroiliitis. Indeed, many think of ankylosing spondylitis as 'symptomatic sacroiliitis.' However, the presence of sacroiliitis *per se* does not necessarily mean the presence of ankylosing spondylitis. Moreover, although radiographic sacroiliitis is very frequent in ankylosing spondylitis, it is by no means an early or obligate manifestation of the disease[7].

Lack of both sensitivity and specificity in the original New York criteria led to a *modification* of these criteria for ankylosing spondylitis (Table 101.5)[8]. With this adaptation, the sensitivity increased from 76% to 83%, whereas the specificity decreased only from 99% to 98%. The New York criteria of 'limitation of the lumbar spine' and of 'limitation of chest expansion' appear to reflect disease duration; they are usually not present in early disease[9]. Indeed, it should be stressed that, contrary to what the title of this paper suggests these criteria are in fact *classification* criteria and not well suited for *early* diagnosis[8].

Classification criteria for other spondyloarthropathies

For other forms of spondyloarthropathies such as psoriatic arthritis or inflammatory bowel disease-associated spondyloarthropathy, no specific widely accepted classification criteria exist yet. Difficulties in establishing consensus on the definition of reactive arthritis have been reviewed recently elsewhere[10]. Therefore, in that instance one could apply the ESSG classification criteria. However, conversely, it is not satisfactory to apply these criteria, for example, to all subgroups of patients with psoriasis who also have articular manifestations.

REFERENCES

1. Copeman WSC. Introductory note on the nomenclature and classification of the rheumatic diseases. In: Copeman WSC, ed. Textbook of the rheumatic diseases, 4E. Edinburgh and London: Livingstone; 1969: 12–18.
2. Wright V, Moll JMH. Seronegative polyarthritis. Amsterdam, New York, Oxford: North Holland Publishing Company; 1976.
3. Fries JF, Hochberg MC, Medsger TA *et al*. Criteria for rheumatic disease. Different types and different functions. Arthritis Rheum 1994; 37: 454–462.
4. Hunder GG. The use and misuse of classification and diagnostic criteria for complex diseases. Ann Rheum Dis 1998; 129: 417–418.
5. Dougados M, van der Linden S, Juhlin R *et al*. The European Spondylarthropathy Study Group: preliminary criteria for the classification of spondylarthropathy. Arthritis Rheum 1991; 34: 1218–1227.
6. Cury SE, Vilar MJP, Ciconelli RM *et al*. Evaluation of the European Spondylarthropathy Study Group (ESSG) preliminary classification criteria in Brazilian patients. Clin Exp Rheumatol 1997; 15: 79–82.
7. Khan MA, van der Linden SM, Kuhner I *et al*. Spondylitis disease without radiologic evidence of sacroiliitis in relatives of HLA-B27 positive ankylosing spondylitis patients. Arthritis Rheum 1985; 28: 40–43.
8. Van der Linden SM, Valkenburg HA, Cats A: Evaluation of diagnostic criteria for ankylosing spondylitis: a proposal for modification of the New York criteria. Arthritis Rheum 1984; 27: 361–368.
9. Goei Thé HS, Steven MM, van der Linden S *et al*. Evaluation of diagnostic criteria for ankylosing spondylitis: a comparison of the Rome, New York and modified New York criteria in patients with a positive clinical history screening test for ankylosing spondylitis. Br J Rheumatol 1985; 24: 242–249.
10. Sieper J, Braun J, Kingsley G. Report on the Fourth International Workshop on Reactive Arthritis. Arthritis Rheum 2000: 43: 720–734.

102 Epidemiology of ankylosing spondylitis

Jan T Gran and Gunnar Husby

- The link between ankylosing spondylitis (AS) and human leukocyte antigen (HLA)-B27 holds in all populations: those with a low frequency of HLA-B27 have a low frequency of AS
- Both HLA-B27 and AS are rare in black populations
- In whites, AS occurs with a prevalence of 0.5–1.0%
- The male to female ratio is 5:1
- The annual incidence of AS in white Americans is approximately 6.6/100 000
- Variants of AS, lacking classic features, are not uncommon

INTRODUCTION

Ankylosing spondylitis (AS) was, for many years, regarded as a severe, crippling rheumatic disease, affecting males only and occurring in perhaps fewer than 0.10% of the general white population[1]. Recent studies, however, have clearly shown that the demographic and clinical spectrum of AS is much wider. The disease affects women not infrequently and is of greater prevalence than previously appreciated.

DIAGNOSTIC CRITERIA

Basic to all epidemiologic research is the concept of disease definition, and the use of appropriate diagnostic criteria. The development of classification criteria for AS is discussed in detail in Chapter 101, although the key principles are worth emphasizing here, as they influence the interpretation of the published data. Such diagnostic criteria for AS were first introduced in 1961 (Rome criteria; Table 102.1)[2] and revised in 1966 (New York criteria; Table 102.2)[3]. Both sets of criteria were based on the concomitant occurrence of one or more clinical features and sacroiliitis. However, the Rome criteria permitted a diagnosis of AS to be made in the absence of definite arthritic changes of the sacroiliac joints.

According to Calin *et al.*[4], the consideration of five disease history variables may prove useful: age at onset less than 40 years; insidious onset of disease; morning stiffness of the back; back pain improving with exercise;

and, finally, back pain lasting for at least 3 months. Unfortunately, these criteria have been found to be insufficiently discriminatory by recent population surveys of AS[5,6], and hence cannot be recommended for use in research. The criteria have also been tested in primary care[7]. In one study of 313 patients with back pain, 46 (15%) of 313 patients had four or more positive replies to the screening questionnaire[7]. Of these, only two suffered from definite AS, but 18 (39%) exhibited clinical features often associated with spondyloarthropathy. The study again emphasizes the limited use of these criteria for diagnostic purposes, but their use for 'inflammatory back pain' in clinical practice may, however, be supported provided other criteria are used for a final diagnosis.

In the early phase of AS, that is the time from onset of symptoms before development of changes typical of the disease, the criteria may be used to select those cases that may be classified as AS on follow-up. Some of the patients giving at least two affirmative responses to the five clinical criteria and exhibiting human leukocyte antigen (HLA)-B27 positivity

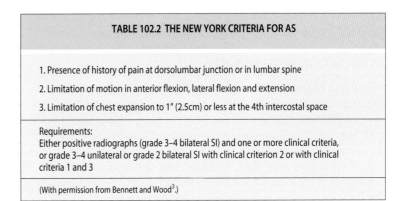

TABLE 102.2 THE NEW YORK CRITERIA FOR AS
1. Presence of history of pain at dorsolumbar junction or in lumbar spine
2. Limitation of motion in anterior flexion, lateral flexion and extension
3. Limitation of chest expansion to 1" (2.5cm) or less at the 4th intercostal space
Requirements: Either positive radiographs (grade 3–4 bilateral SI) and one or more clinical criteria, or grade 3–4 unilateral or grade 2 bilateral SI with clinical criterion 2 or with clinical criteria 1 and 3
(With permission from Bennett and Wood[3].)

TABLE 102.1 THE ROME CRITERIA FOR AS
Low back pain and stiffness for more than 3 months not relieved by rest
Pain and stiffness of the thoracic region
Limited motion in lumbar spine
Limited chest expansion
Evidence or history of iritis or its sequelae
Requirements: Either positive radiographs (bilateral SI) and one or more clinical criteria, or four out of five clinical criteria
SI, sacroiliitis. (With permission from Kellgren et al.[2])

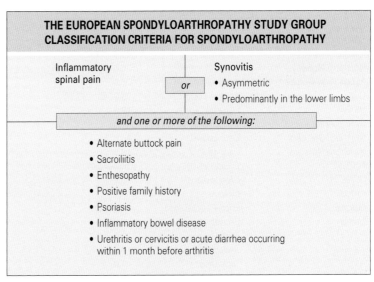

Fig. 102.1 The European Spondyloarthropathy Study Group classification criteria for spondyloarthropathy.

may, in due time, develop definite AS. However, definite arthritic changes in the sacroiliac joints remain an essential finding for the diagnosis of this disorder, and only patients exhibiting such features should be regarded as having AS, in the context of epidemiologic surveys.

In Europe, classification criteria for spondyloarthropathy have been developed[8] and successfully evaluated in population surveys[9]. The European Spondyloarthropathy Study Group (ESSG) criteria[8] (Fig. 101.1) provide an opportunity to classify patients as suffering from spondyloarthropathy in the absence of a specific diagnosis. Consequently, the use of such criteria offers advantages to epidemiologists involved in the study of spondyloarthropathies by allowing analyses of rather large groups of diseased persons. However, the ESSG criteria should not be used as diagnostic criteria. Clearly, a patient with synovitis and psoriasis (Fig. 102.1) is classified as a seronegative spondyloarthropathy, although the specific diagnosis of the patient would still be psoriatic arthritis.

ASSOCIATION WITH HLA-B27

A well-established feature of AS is the association with the histocompatibility antigen HLA-B27[10,11], which is demonstrated in about 90–95% of cases. The prevalence of HLA-B27 in the general population does, however, show considerable geographic variation (Table 102.3), occurring in 50% of Haida Indians of northern Canada[25] but being virtually absent among black Africans[25] and Guatemalan Indians[26]. At present, there exists no satisfactory explanation of the great variation in the frequency of this genetic marker among such groups. It has been hypothesized, however, that the presence of HLA-B27 might have conferred some advantages to the host, in particular regarding resistance to specific infections[27]; after an outbreak of epidemic infections, the survivors will consequently exhibit an increased frequency of HLA-B27. However, this does not explain the outstanding rarity of this histocompatibility antigen among inhabitants of the African continent, the populations of which have been repeatedly attacked by various epidemic infections. Other possible explanations may be the effects of genetic drift and the coincidental founder effect.

The prevalence of HLA-B27 in the population has a significant impact on the occurrence of B27-related disorders. If the prevalence of HLA-B27 in the population is low, the overall prevalence rate of AS will be significantly decreased, with a decreased proportion of cases that are B27-positive. A high prevalence of HLA-B27 in a population will have the opposite effects: B27-related diseases will be seen rather frequently and their association with HLA-B27 will be very strong.

During the past few years it has become evident that HLA-B27 can be divided into at least 20 different subtypes. These are designated HLA B*2701 to HLA B*2720[28], with only small variations in amino acid sequences distinguishing the various subtypes. HLA B*2705 is the most frequently occurring subtype among most non-black populations studied. No particular allele appears to confer susceptibility to AS, and the occurrence of AS or related spondyloarthropathy has been documented in individuals possessing any of the first 10 alleles[28]. It has been suggested that the occurrence of spondyloarthropathy in multiple HLA B27 subtypes supports the involvement of the HLA B27 antigen itself directly in the disease process[29].

In the Fula ethnic group in Gambia, West Africa, HLA B*2703 is also of significant prevalence and the overall prevalence of HLA-B27 is 6%[30]. In one study of 900 Fula men, however, none suffered from AS[30]. Moreover, in a study of 82 persons in Mali, a West African country with North Arab genetic admixture, a 9.7% prevalence of HLA-B27 was reported[31]. Similar to the findings in Gambia[30], AS appears to be extremely rare in Mali.

These findings show that the correlation between population frequency of HLA-B27 and occurrence of AS is not always present, and may also suggest the presence of some non-B27 protective factors. Further epidemiologic and immunogenetic studies of HLA B27 subtypes may shed new light on the pathogenesis of spondyloarthropathy.

PREVALENCE

There have been three methods of ascertaining cases to determine the prevalence of AS. The first is to study the medical records of patients admitted to the hospital of the region being investigated. The second is to examine clinically a random sample of B27-positive persons, most often blood donors, and then extrapolate the results to the general population. Thirdly, prevalence can be determined by performing population surveys involving a large number of unselected persons.

Hospital-based studies

There are some evident advantages of using hospital records to study the prevalence of AS. Large numbers of cases are usually available to provide robust estimates of the distribution by age and sex, in addition to the frequency of disease complications. Furthermore, the patients being diagnosed by specialists in the field may have a greater chance of conforming to established diagnostic criteria. Having been admitted to hospital, the patients often undergo full examinations, which may create greater chances for detecting new disease associations. However, recruitment based on patients attending hospital may reveal only the more severe and typical cases, giving a rather false impression of both disease manifestations and severity of the disorder studied. A greater chance of suffering from coexistent diseases is observed in patients who have been admitted to hospital, thereby possibly introducing a bias when estimating the mortality of actual cases. Furthermore, such an approach will fail to capture the patients with less severe disease who do not attend hospital, resulting in an underestimation of the prevalence of AS.

Studies based on hospital records in Western countries (Table 102.4) have concluded that the prevalence of AS is about 0.10%, with, surprisingly, remarkably little variation between the different studies. It seems as if the prevalence of HLA-B27 in the population only slightly influences the rate of admission to hospital because of AS, although this was not observed in a comparison of black and white inhabitants of the USA[36]. Furthermore, it is somewhat surprising that the prevalence rates of AS, obtained by studying hospital records, appear to have remained stationary at 0.10–0.20% throughout the past five decades; no significant decrease or increase in the frequency of AS seems to have occurred. Indeed, an increase in the rate of AS diagnosed would have been expected, but did not happen.

TABLE 102.3 HLA-B27 PREVALENCE IN VARIOUS POPULATIONS

Region	Ethnicity	Prevalence of HLA B27 (%)
Papua New Guinea	Pawaian[12]	52.9
Canada	Haida Indians[13]	50.0
USA	Yupic Eskimos[14]	40.0
USA	Navajo Indians[15]	36.0
Russia	Chukhsas[16]	33.9
Northern Norway	Lapps (Samis)[17]	26.0
Papua New Guinea	Karimui[18]	25.9
USA	Inupiat Eskimos[14]	25.0
USA	Pima Indians[13]	18.0
United Arabian Emirates	Yemini Arabs[19]	17.0
Northern Sweden	Caucasians[20]	16.6
Northern Norway	Caucasians[21]	15.9
Finland	Caucasians[22]	14.0–16.0
USA	Cree Indians[23]	13.9
Africa	Malians[24]	9.7
Europe	Euro-Caucasians[25]	4.0–13.0
China	Chinese[25]	2.0–9.0
–	Arabs[25]	3.0
–	Jews[25]	3.0
–	Japanese[25]	<1.0
Guatemala[26]	–	0.0
Africa	Blacks[25]	0.0

TABLE 102.4 THE PREVALENCE OF ANKYLOSING SPONDYLITIS IN HOSPITALIZED PATIENTS

Region	Prevalence of AS (%)			Prevalence of B27 in the population (%)	Diagnostic criteria
	Males	Females	Total		
England[1]	–	–	0.05–0.10	–	–
Norway[32]	0.31	0.60	–	10.00	–
USA[33]	0.40	0.05	0.23	8.00	–
Bulgaria[34]	0.30	0.07	–	–	–
Romania[35]	–	–	0.11	–	–
USA[36]	0.03	–	–	8.00	–
USA[36]	0.01	–	–	0–2.00	–
Holland[37]	–	–	0.08	7.80	–
Iraq[38]	–	–	0.07	2.10	NY
USA[39]	0.20	0.07	0.13	8.00	NY
Norway[40]	–	–	0.08	15.90	NY
Alaska (Inuit)[41]	0.20	0	0.10	25.00	–
Alaska (Yupik)[42]	0.30	0.10	0.20	40.00	Rome

During this period, the availability of radiography in the diagnosis of AS has improved and the use of computed tomography and magnetic resonance imaging has been introduced to detect AS at an earlier stage. One explanation could be that only those with more classic and advanced cases of AS attend hospital clinics, and that these cases of AS have rarely represented any diagnostic problem. In addition, the earlier reports of greater prevalence rates of AS may be explained by changes in approach to disease classification. Thus the more recent patient populations reported are restricted to a greater degree, to primary or idiopathic AS. Since the introduction of the term 'spondyloarthropathy complex'[43], patients with other B27-related disorders, such as reactive arthritis and psoriatic spondylitis, have been excluded from groups considered to have AS.

Studies of hospital patients have further documented a clear male predominance in AS. However, earlier reports on a male to female ratio of 10–20:1 should be interpreted with caution. Many of these reports were based on records from military or veteran administration hospitals, in which the overwhelming majority of patients were male. In addition, there may have been a negative bias towards females, who have a lesser chance of being referred to hospital because of back complaints.

Blood donor studies

Blood donors have been used as a sample of the general popualation in which an initial screen for HLA B27 was followed by further examination of both B27-positive and -negative individuals. However, such studies (Table 102.5) have revealed conflicting results regarding the occurrence of AS. The prevalence of AS among B27-positive donors has varied from 0% to 25.00%, and among B27-negative individuals between 0% and 5.60%. The reasons for the apparent discrepancies include observer variation in the interpretation of sacroiliac joint radiographs and the selection issues involved in the use of blood donors. It can be argued that blood donors are not likely to be representative of the general population. They are often selected because of absence of known disease, and classic cases of AS may be unlikely to volunteer for such medical services. Thus some of the groups studied may have revealed prevalence rates lower than those being found in the general population. This renders even more surprising the original results of Calin and Fries[44] and Cohen et al.[46,] who found extremely high prevalence rates of AS among such cases (Table 102.5). Even more remarkable was the reported increased frequency of AS among cases not possessing HLA-B27[44] – results that have not been supported by population surveys. The prevalence of AS in the general population as based on studies of blood donors will consequently vary from 0.10% to 2.00%. A recent study from Berlin, Germany, revealed a frequency of spondyloarthropathy among blood donors of

TABLE 102.5 OCCURRENCE OF ANKYLOSING SPONDYLITIS AMONG INDIVIDUALS WITH HLA-B27

Author	Number of subjects studied		Prevalence of AS (%)	
	B27-positive	B27-negative	B27-positive	B27-negative
Blood donor studies				
Calin and Fries[44]	78	126	20.00	5.60
Truog et al.[45]	41	147	19.50	0.70
Cohen et al.[46] (a)	24	31	25.00	0
Thorel et al.[47]	39	40	12.80	2.50
Chappel et al.[48]	32	22	3.10	0
Christiansen et al.[49]	61	35	0	0
Population studies				
Gofton[13] (b)	104	–	8.20	–
Gömör et al.[50]	–	–	1.80	0.02
Contu et al.[51]	26	50	15.40	0
Alcalay et al.[52]	40	40	7.50	0
Dawkins et al.[53]	168	–	1.60	–
Hollingsworth et al.[54]	125	–	6.00–21.00	–
LeClerq and Russell[55]	84	–	1.20	–
Van der Linden[56] (c)	230	2727	1.30	0.15
Gran et al.[40] (d)	–	–	6.70	0.20
Johnsen et al.[17] (e)	–	–	5.20	0

(a) Males only.
(b) Based on population frequency of AS of about 4.00%.
(c) Figures based on a population frequency of AS of 7.80% and the findings of three B27-positive and four B27-negative cases of AS.
(d) Based on a prevalence of AS and B27 in the general population of 1.10% and 15.90%, respectively.
(e) Based on a prevalence of AS and B27 in the general population of 1.30% and 26.00%, respectively.

TABLE 102.6 PREVALENCE OF ANKYLOSING SPONDYLITIS BASED ON POPULATION SURVEYS

Region	Prevalence of AS (%)			Number of AS found			Number of persons studied			HLA-B27 in the population (%)
	Males	Females	Total	Males	Females	Total	Males	Females	Total	
Canada [58]	6.20	–	–	13	–	–	209	–	–	50.00
Hungary [50]	0.40	0.08	0.23	12	3	15	–	–	6469	12.90
Turkey [59]	0.14	–	–	2	–	–	1436	–	–	–
USA (Cree Indian) [23]	–	0	0	0	0	0	–	–	103	13.60
Finland [60]	–	–	0.40–1.60	–	–	–	–	–	–	14.00–16.00
Holland [56]	–	–	0.1	–	–	3	–	–	2947	7.80
Finland [61]	–	–	1.03	2	4	6	76	120	196	14.00
North Norway [40]	2.20	0.60	1.10–1.40	22	5	27	216	159	375	15.90
Papua New Guinea [18]	–	–	0.90	0	1	1	–	–	109	25.90
Norway (Lapps) [17]	–	–	1.32	6	4	10	–	–	207	26.00

13.6%, yielding a prevalence of AS of 0.86% in the general population[57]. To date, most studies on blood donors have, however, not contributed significantly to the estimation of the true prevalence of AS. Moreover, some blood donor studies[44] have indicated an almost equal sex distribution in AS, whereas others have found a significant excess of males.

Population surveys

Population surveys involve unselected groups of individuals, thereby estimating the true prevalence of the disorder in addition to yielding a greater chance of studying the natural disease course. Furthermore, such studies may offer a greater insight into the full disease spectrum and allow a more accurate calculation of the incidence of disease complications and associations. However, most, if not all, population surveys are hampered by high non-response – a number of individuals not volunteering to participate in the survey, particularly if X-rays are required. Thus the studied sample may not be representative of the general population. Another limiting factor is the relatively high financial cost of such investigations, which may explain the relatively small number of population surveys performed in AS (Table 102.6).

In general, epidemiologic surveys on AS in North America, North Scandinavia, Siberia and Asia indicate that 4–7% of the HLA-B27-positive population will have the disease, and that the prevalence of AS will roughly correlate with the population frequency of the antigen.

North American populations

The greatest prevalence of AS has been found among male Haidas[58], native inhabitants of northern Canada, of whom 4–6% have AS. Given a population frequency for HLA-B27 of 50% in this community, approximately 8.00% of these individuals have developed AS. Unfortunately, the occurrence of AS among female Haidas remains unknown.

Epidemiologic studies of circumpolar populations in Alaska have been performed by Boyer et al.[62]. They studied the occurrence of spondyloarthropathy among two Eskimo populations, the Inupiat and the Yupik, by means of available medical registers followed by clinical examinations. Radiographs were obtained when clinically indicated. Most patients with spondyloarthropathy were classified as having undifferentiated spondyloarthropathy, whereas the prevalence of AS among adults aged 20 years and older was 0.1–0.4%. If all those with possible spondyloarthropathy and radiologic sacroiliitis were regarded as having AS, the prevalence of AS would amount to 1.2%. HLA-B27 is found in 25% and 40% of the

Inupiat and Yupik Eskimo populations, respectively[28]. Thus fewer than 5% of B27-positive Alaskan Eskimos contract AS, which is strikingly less than the anticipated 10% risk among Haida Indians[13].

European populations

A population survey of AS among whites in Tromsø, North Norway, revealed a prevalence of this disorder of 1.1–1.4%, with a sex ratio of 5:1 in favor of males[40]. Of the 27 persons diagnosed as having AS, 95% possessed HLA-B27, compared with just under 16.0% in the general population. Thus 6.7% of all B27-positive individuals appeared to have contracted AS, whereas the corresponding figure for B27-negative individuals was 0.2%. Thus the calculated risks of having AS, for both groups and based on previous studies of blood donors[44,46], were not supported by this population survey. Conversely prevalence rates estimated in this population study were much greater than those obtained by reviewing hospital records. Furthermore, the overwhelming majority of those with AS found in the population survey could not be traced in the medical records of the corresponding local hospitals. In fact, almost 80% of the individuals with AS were unaware of the diagnosis, although almost all of them had visited a physician because of back problems. A study of the hospital records of this population would have revealed a falsely low prevalence rate of AS.

A population study of Norwegian Lapps (Samis) has confirmed the impression of a high prevalence of AS in populations with a high frequency of HLA-B27[17]. The prevalence of HLA-B27 among Norwegian Lapps is about 25%[63], whereas that of AS is 1.8%, all sufferers possessing HLA-B27[17]. Consequently, approximately 5% of the B27-positive individuals were afflicted by AS.

The circumpolar population of Chukotka, Russia, has also been subjected to epidemiologic investigation[16]. The prevalence of HLA-B27 among Chukhsas is 34%, and it was estimated that 1.3% suffered from AS[16]. Although the number of cases found with AS was small, the risk of having AS in B27-positive Chukhsas appears to be less than 5%.

The results of population surveys in the northern-most parts of the world[17,40,63] contrast sharply with the conclusions reached by population surveys in other parts of Europe, including Holland[56], Hungary[50] and Turkey[59], in which the prevalences determined were in the range 0.10–0.23%. As 7.80–12.90% of these ethnic groups[44,46,58] possess HLA-B27, a frequency of AS among B27-positive individuals of about

1.50% should be expected. The Dutch study[56] was based on examination of an older population (44 years and older) previously subjected to radiographic examination. The Hungarian workers[50] examined only clinically suspected cases and may have missed a significant number of AS cases because of the absence of reliable clinical criteria for AS[64]. In the Turkish study[59], classic cases of AS had been excluded before the survey, which included only male soldiers considerably younger than the average age at onset of AS.

Asian populations

Unfortunately, too few studies on the occurrence of AS in Asia have been performed to date. However, two epidemiologic surveys, in China[65] and Taiwan[66], have estimated prevalence rates of AS to be between 0.2% and 0.5%. On the basis of a prevalence of HLA-B27 of approximately 6% in the general population, about 6% of B27-positive Chinese have contracted AS.

Summary of population surveys

Although the study designs of these surveys vary considerably, making valid comparisons rather difficult, there seems to exist regions with high population frequencies of both AS and HLA-B27, in contrast to areas of moderate to low population prevalences of both AS and HLA-B27. However, the estimates of the prevalence of AS of 0.10%[56] are about the same as those obtained by studies based on hospital inpatients. Indeed, such a finding indicates that a population prevalence of AS of 0.10% is much too low, as it is rather unlikely that all cases with AS present in a population would be found in the medical records under a diagnosis of AS. Consequently, among white populations, a prevalence of AS of 0.50–1.00% should be expected, whereas some particular populations may exhibit prevalence rates of 1.00–2.00%. Among black populations, both AS and HLA-B27 are very infrequently encountered. Population studies of AS have yet to be performed in developing countries. Reports from African hospitals[67–69] indicate, however, that AS is a rare but severe disease, presenting rather late and infrequently associated with extra-articular involvement and HLA-B27.

The population surveys have also shown that AS should not be regarded as a rare disease among women. Perhaps a sex ratio of 5:1 in favor of males is a more likely figure than the earlier estimated ratio of males to females of 10–20:1. The population surveys have, however, failed to support the proposals arising from blood donor studies[44] of an almost equal sex distribution of this rheumatic disorder.

Unfortunately, no population survey has yet been performed that includes a sufficient number of cases of AS to allow the distribution of AS among different age groups to be estimated. So far, both population surveys[17,40] and studies of hospital inpatients[8] indicate that the greatest prevalence of AS may be found in the age group of 40–45 years. Moreover, the prevalence rate of AS after age 60 years may show a significant decrease[8].

INCIDENCE OF ANKYLOSING SPONDYLITIS

The incidence rate of AS is most easily ascertained from hospital-based studies and, according to Carter et al.[39], the overall annual incidence rate of AS among American whites is 6.6 cases per 100 000 inhabitants. The age- and sex-adjusted incidence for primary AS for the years 1935–1989 in the same area was 6.3/100 000 population, indicating no substantial increase or decrease in occurrence of the disease[70]. In a recent study from Finland using the nationwide sickness insurance

TABLE 102.7 PROPOSED CLINICAL EXPRESSIONS OF ANKYLOSING SPONDYLITIS

Classic AS
  Inflammatory back symptoms and SI
  IBD, SI and spinal changes

Spinal AS

Clinical AS

Asymptomatic AS

AS associated with:
  Psoriasis
  Ulcerative colitis
  Crohn's disease
  Whipple's disease

scheme, an annual incidence of AS among adults aged 16 years and older was 6.9 per 100 000 for the years 1980, 1985 and 1990[71]. Although the rates calculated were strikingly similar to those reported by Carter et al.[39], the authors emphasized that the figures represented minimum calculations.

CLINICAL VARIANTS OF ANKYLOSING SPONDYLITIS

In the Tromsø study[40], it was shown that cases with AS selected from the general population may exhibit clinical and radiographic features different from those of hospital inpatients. Less restriction of spinal mobility, a lower incidence of peripheral arthritis and less pronounced manifestations were noted among patients selected through the population survey, compared with hospital inpatients with AS[43,44]. The clinical and radiographic picture of AS may therefore reflect only the most severe and typical cases of this disease.

Another interesting finding, observed in both population surveys[45] and studies of hospital inpatients[75,76] is the existence of variants of AS (Table 102.7). Thus a few patients with AS may develop radiographic features of AS entirely restricted to the spine and sparing the sacroiliac joints. Additional prospective studies are evidently needed to further understanding of such cases of spinal AS. It has also been suggested that AS may exist without any radiographic abnormalities at all[77], but at present little evidence has accumulated to support this notion. Such a widening of the diagnostic spectrum may produce more confusion rather than providing new insight into the pathogenesis of true AS. Moreover, population studies have produced little evidence to support the inclusion of asymptomatic sacroiliitis as part of the disease spectrum of AS. Studies of patients with inflammatory bowel disease[78] have shown that radiographic sacroiliitis is not uncommon in this population and, moreover, is not associated with the disease susceptibility antigen HLA-B27.

SUMMARY

Clearly, there is a need for further epidemiologic studies of AS. The development of clinical criteria, precluding the need for sacroiliac X-ray is highly desirable, to make such studies more feasible. Many aspects of the epidemiology of AS such as the influence of social classes and occupation have scarcely been investigated. Of particular interest is the suggestion that AS may develop at an earlier age among those in countries with poor living conditions and that, as these improve, the age at onset of AS increases[76].

REFERENCES

1. West HF. The aetiology of ankylosing spondylitis. Ann Rheum Dis 1949; 8: 143–148.
2. Kellgren JH, Jeffrey MR, Ball J, eds. The epidemiology of chronic rheumatism, vol 1. Oxford: Blackwell; 1963: 326.
3. Bennett PM, Wood PHN. In: Bennet PM, Wood PHN, eds. Population studies of the rheumatic diseases. Amsterdam International Congress Series No. 148. Amsterdam: Excerpta Medica Foundation; 1966: 456.
4. Calin A, Kaye B, Sternberg M et al. The prevalence and nature of back pain in an industrial complex. A questionnaire and radiographic and HLA analysis. Spine 1980; 5: 201–205.
5. van der Linden S, Valkenburg HA, Cats A. Evaluation of diagnostic criteria for ankylosing spondylitis. Arthritis Rheum 1984; 27: 361–368.
6. Gran JT. An epidemiological survey of the signs and symptoms of ankylosing spondylitis. Clin Rheumatol 1985; 4: 161–169.
7. Underwood MR, Dawes P. Inflammatory back pain in primary care. Br J Rheumatol 1995; 34: 1074–1077.
8. Dougados M, van der Linden S, Juhlin R et al. The European Spondyloarthropathy Study Group preliminary criteria for the classification of spondyloarthropathy. Arthritis Rheum 1991; 34: 1218–1227.
9. Boyer GS, Templin DW, Goring WP. Evaluation of the ESSG preliminary classification criteria in Alaskan Eskimos. Arthritis Rheum 1993; 36: 534–538.
10. Brewerton DA, Hart FD, Nicholls A et al. Ankylosing spondylitis and HLA-A27. Lancet 1973; i: 904–907.
11. Schlosstein T, Terasaki PI, Bluestone R, Pearson CM. High association of an HLA antigen, w27, with ankylosing spondylitis. N Engl J Med 1973; 288: 704–706.
12. Bhatia K, Prasad ML, Barnish G, Koki G. Antigen and haplotype frequencies at three human leucocyte antigen loci (HLA-A, -B, -C) in the Pawaia of Papua New Guinea. Am J Phys Anthropol 1988; 75: 329–340.
13. Gofton JP. Epidemiology, tissue type antigens and Bechterew's syndrome (ankylosing spondylitis) in various ethnical populations. Scand J Rheumatol 1980; 9(suppl 32): 166–168.
14. Hansen JA, Lauier AP, Nisperos B et al. The HLA system in Inupiat and Central Yupik Alaskan Eskimos. Hum Immunol 1986; 16: 315–328.
15. Rate RG, Morse HG, Bonnell MD, Kuberski TT. 'Navajo arthritis' reconsidered. Arthritis Rheum 1980; 23: 1299–1302.
16. Alexeeva L, Krylov M, Vturin V et al. Prevalence of spondyloarthropathies and HLA B27 in the native population of Chukotka, Russia. J Rheumatol 1994; 21: 2298–2300.
17. Johnsen K, Gran JT, Dale K, Husby G. The prevalence of ankylosing spondylitis in a Norwegian Sami population. J Rheumatol 1992; 19: 1591–1594.
18. Clunie GPR, Koki G, Prasad ML et al. HLA-B27, arthritis and spondylitis in an isolated community in Papua New Guinea. Br J Rheumatol 1990; 29: 97–100.
19. Al-Attia HM, Al-Amiri N. HLA B27 in healthy adults in UAE. Scand J Rheumatol 1995; 24: 225–227.
20. Bjelle A, Cedergren B, Dahlquist SR. HLA-B27 in the population of northern Sweden. Scand J Rheumatol 1982; 11: 23–26.
21. Gran JT, Mellby AS, Husby G. The prevalence of HLA-B27 in northern Norway. Scand J Rheumatol 1984; 13: 173–176.
22. Nissilä M, Isomäki H, Koota K et al. HLA-B27 and rheumatoid arthritis. Scand J Rheumatol 1975; 4(suppl 8): 30.
23. Russell AS, Davis P, Schlaut J. Prevalence of ankylosing spondylitis and HLA-B27 in a North American Indian population: a pilot study. Can Med Assoc J 1977; 116: 148–149.
24. Kalidi I, Fofana Y, Rahly A. Study of HLA antigens in a population of Mali (West Africa). Tissue Antigens 1988; 31: 98–102.
25. Khan MA. HLA and ankylosing spondylitis. In: Calabro JJ, Carson Dick W, eds. Ankylosing spondylitis. New clinical applications. Rheumatology, vol 1. Lancaster: MTP; 1987: 23–44.
26. Masi AT, Medsger TA. A new look at the epidemiology of ankylosing spondylitis and related syndromes. Clin Orthoped Rel Res 1979; 143: 15–29.
27. Gofton JP. HLA-B27 and ankylosing spondylitis in BC Indians. J Rheumatol 1984; 11: 572–573.
28. Khan MA. Update: the twenty subtypes of HLA-B27. Curr Opin Rheum 2000; 12: 235–238.
29. Maclean L. HLA-B27 subtypes: implications for the spondyloarthropathies. Ann Rheum Dis 1992; 51: 929–931.
30. Brown MA, Jepson A, Young A et al. Ankylosing spondylitis in West Africa – evidence for a non-HLA-B27 protective effect. Ann Rheum Dis 1997; 56: 68–70.
31. Kalidi I, Fofana Y, Rahly AA et al. Study of HLA antigens in a population of Mali (West Africa). Tissue Antigens 1988; 31: 98–102.
32. Holst H, Iversen PF. On the incidence of spondylarthritis ankylopoetica in a Norwegian county. Acta Med Scand 1952; 142: 333–338.
33. Mikkelsen WM, Dodge H, Duff IF. Estimates of the prevalence of rheumatic diseases in the population of Tecumseh, Michigan, 1959–1960. J Chron Dis 1967; 20: 351–359.
34. Tzonchev VT, Pilosoff T, Kanev K. Prevalence of inflammatory arthritis in Bulgaria. In: Bennett PM, Wood PMN, eds. Population studies of the rheumatic disease. Amsterdam International Congress Series No. 148. Amsterdam: Excerpta Medica Foundation; 1968: 60–63.
35. Stoia I, Ramnaeantu P, Stocescu M, Dragomir M. Epidemiologische und Familienuntersuchungen bei drei chronischen Reumatischen Erkrankungen. Zeitschr Rheumaforsch 1969; 28: 201–207.
36. Baum J, Ziff M. The rarity of ankylosing spondylitis in the black race. Arthritis Rheum 1971; 14: 12–18.
37. De Blecourt JJ. 533 patients with ankylosing spondylitis seen and followed in the period 1948–1971. Ann Rheum Dis 1973; 32: 383–385.
38. Al-Rawi ZS, Il-Shakarchi HA, Hasan F, Thewaini AJ. Ankylosing spondylitis and its association with the histocompatibility antigen HLA-B27: an epidemiological and clinical study. Rheumatol Rehabil 1978; 17: 72–75.
39. Carter ET, McKenna CH, Brian DD, Kurland LT. Epidemiology of ankylosing spondylitis in Rochester, Minnesota 1935–1973. Arthritis Rheum 1979; 22: 365–370.
40. Gran JT, Husby G, Hordvik M. Prevalence of ankylosing spondylitis in males and females in a young middle-aged population in Tromsø, Northern Norway. Ann Rheum Dis 1985; 44: 359–367.
41. Boyer GS, Lanier AP, Templin DT. Prevalence rates of spondyloarthropathies, rheumatoid arthritis and other rheumatic diseases in an Alaskan Inupiat Eskimo population. J Rheumatol 1988; 15: 678–683.
42. Boyer GS, Lanier AP, Templin DW, Bulkow L. Spondylarthropathy and rheumatoid arthritis in Alaskan, Yupik Eskimos. J Rheumatol 1990; 17: 489–496.
43. Wright V. Relationship between ankylosing spondylitis and other spondarthritides. In: Moll JMH, ed. Ankylosing spondylitis. London: Churchill Livingston; 1980: 42–51.
44. Calin A, Fries JF. Striking prevalence of ankylosing spondylitis in 'healthy' w27 positive males and females. A controlled study. N Engl J Med 1975; 293: 835–839.
45. Truog P, Dolivo P, Steiger U. Etude de l'incidence des sacroiliitis chez les porteurs de l'antigène HLA-B27 (rapport préliminaire). Med Hyg 1975; 33: 1889–1891.
46. Cohen LM, Mittal KK, Schmid FR et al. Increased risk for spondylitis stigmata in apparently healthy HLA-Aw27 men. Ann Int Med 1976; 84: 1–7.
47. Thorel JB, Cavelier B, Bonneau JC et al. Etude d'une population porteuse de l'antigène HLA-B27 comparée à celle d'une population témoin non-B27 à la recherche de la spondylarthrite ankylosante. Rev Rheumatol 1978; 45: 275–282.
48. Chappel R, Muylle L, Mortier G et al. Risque de développer une spondylarthrite ankylosante chez des personnes «en bonne santé» porteuses de l'antigène HLA-B27. Acta Rhumatol 1979; 3: 319–328.
49. Christiansen FT, Hawkins BR, Dawkins RL et al. The prevalence of ankylosing spondylitis among B27 positive normal individuals – a reassessment. J Rheumatol 1979; 6: 713–718.
50. Gömör B, Gyodi E, Bakos L. Distribution of HLA-B27 and ankylosing spondylitis in the Hungarian population. J Rheumatol 1977; 4(suppl 3): 33–35.
51. Contu L, Capelli P, Sale S. HLA-B27 and ankylosing spondylitis: a population and family study in Sardinia. J Rheumatol 1977; 4(suppl 3): 18–23.
52. Alcalay M, Amor B, Haider F et al. Ankylosing spondylitis and chlamydial infection in apparently healthy B27 blood donors. J Rheumatol 1979; 6: 439–446.
53. Dawkins RL, Owen ET, Cheah DS. Prevalence of ankylosing spondylitis and abnormalities of the sacroiliac joints in HLA-B27-positive individuals. J Rheumatol 1981; 8: 1025–1026.
54. Hollingsworth PN, Cheah PS, Dawkins RL et al. Observer variation in grading sacroiliac radiographs in HLA-B27-positive individuals. J Rheumatol 1983; 10: 247–254.
55. LeClercq SA, Russell AS. The risk of sacroiliitis in B27-positive persons: a reappraisal. J Rheumatol 1984; 11: 327–329.
56. van der Linden SM, Valkenburg HA, de Jongh BM, Cats A. The risk of developing ankylosing spondylitis in HLA-B27 positive individuals. Arthritis Rheum 1984; 27: 241–249.
57. Braun J, Bollow M, Remlinger G et al. Prevalence of spondyloarthropathies in HLA-B27 positive and negative blood donors. Arthritis Rheum 1998; 41: 58–67.
58. Gofton JP, Robinson HS, Trueman GE. Ankylosing spondylitis in a Canadian Indian population. Ann Rheum Dis 1966; 25: 525–527.
59. Yenal O, Usman ON, Yassa K et al. Zur epidemiologische rheumatischer Syndrome in der Türkei. Z Rheumatol 1977; 36: 294–298.
60. Julkunen H. Rheumatoid spondylitis. Thesis. Acta Rheumatol Scand 1962; (suppl 4).
61. Julkunen H, Korpi J. Ankylosing spondylitis in three Finnish population samples. Prostatovesiculitis and salpingoopheritis as aetiological factors. Scand J Rheumatol 1984; 13(suppl 52): 16–18.
62. Boyer GS, Templin DW, Cornoni-Huntley JC et al. Prevalence of spondyloarthropathies in Alaskan Eskimos. J Rheumatol 1994; 21: 2292–2297.
63. Thorsby E, Bratlie A, Teisberg P. HLA polymorphism of Norwegian Lapps. Tissue Antigens 1971; 1: 137–146.
64. Gran JT, Husby G. Clinical aspects, comparisons, men versus women, hospitalized versus epidemiological patients. In: Calabro JJ, Carson Dick W, eds. Ankylosing spondylitis, new clinical applications, rheumatology. Lancaster: MTP; 1987: 79–108.
65. Wigley RD, Zhang N, Zeng Q et al. Rheumatic diseases in China: ILAR-China study comparing the prevalence of rheumatic symptoms in Northern and Southern rural populations. J Rheumatol 1994; 21: 1484–1490.
66. Chou C, Pei L, Chang D et al. Prevalence of rheumatic diseases in Taiwan: a population study of urban, suburban, rural differences. J Rheumatol 1994; 21: 302–306.
67. Adebajo A, Davis P. Rheumatic diseases in African blacks. Semin Arthritis Rheum 1994; 24: 139–153.
68. Mijiyawa M. Spondyloarthropathies in patients attending the rheumatology unit of Lome Hospital. J Rheumatol 1993; 20: 1167–1169.
69. Muamba JM, Molanda N, Yuma O. Ankylosing spondylitis in two Zairian brothers. Clin Rheumatol 1993; 12: 268–270.
70. Carbone LD, Cooper C, Michet LJ et al. Ankylosing spondylitis in Rochester, Minnesota, 1935–1989. Arthritis Rheum 1992; 35: 1476–1482.
71. Kaiplainen-Seppanen O, Aho K, Heliovaara M. Incidence and prevalence of ankylosing spondylitis in Finland. J Rheumatol 1997; 24: 496–499.

72. Gran JT, Husby G. Ankylosing spondylitis: a comparative study of patients in an epidemiological survey, and those admitted to a department of rheumatology. J Rheumatol 1984; 11: 788–793.

73. Gran JT, Hordvik M, Husby G. Roentgenological features of ankylosing spondylitis. A comparison between patients attending hospital and cases selected through an epidemiological survey. Clin Rheumatol 1984; 3: 467–472.

74. Gran JT, Husby G, Hordvik M. Spinal ankylosing spondylitis: a variant form of ankylosing spondylitis or a distinct disease entity? Ann Rheum Dis 1985; 44: 368–371.

75. The HSG, Cats A. Follow-up findings in three patients with spinal ankylosing spondylitis. Scand J Rheumatol 1988; 15: 221–223.

76. Calin A. Ankylosing spondylitis *sine* sacroiliitis. Arthritis Rheum 1979; 22: 303–304.

77. Khan MA, van der Linden SJ, Valkenburg HA *et al.* Symptomatic ankylosing spondylitis without radiographic sacroiliitis in HLA-B27-positive relatives. Arthritis Rheum 1985; 28: 40–43.

78. Dekker-Sayes BJ, Meuwissen SGM, van den Bergloonen EM *et al.* Prevalence of peripheral arthritis, sacroiliitis and ankylosing spondylitis in patients suffering from inflammatory bowel disease. Ann Rheum Dis 1978; 37: 33–35.

103 Clinical features of ankylosing spondylitis

Muhammad Asim Khan

Definition

- A chronic systemic inflammatory rheumatic disorder with predilection for axial skeletal involvement, and inflammation at sites of bony insertions for tendons and ligaments (enthesitis)
- Sacroiliitis is its hallmark
- Strong genetic predisposition associated with HLA-B27

Clincal features

- Chronic inflammatory low back pain and stiffness
- Limitation of spinal mobility and chest expansion
- Acute anterior uveitis or other less common extra-articular manifestations in some patients
- Association with psoriasis, chronic inflammatory bowel disease and reactive arthritis in some patients
- Characteristic radiographic findings
- Generally good symptomatic response to anti-inflammatory doses of non-steroidal anti-inflammatory drugs

INTRODUCTION

Ankylosing spondylitis (AS) is a chronic systemic inflammatory rheumatic disorder of uncertain etiology that primarily affects the axial skeleton (sacroiliac joints and spine); sacroiliac joint involvement (sacroiliitis) is its hallmark[1-3] (Fig. 103.1). The name is derived from the Greek roots *angkylos* = 'bent' (although the word ankylosis now means joint stiffening or fusion) and *spondylos* = spinal vertebra. However, spinal ankylosis appears only in late stages of the disease and may not occur at all in some patients with mild disease.[1-12] Hip and shoulder joints and less commonly the peripheral (limb) joints may also be involved. There can also be involvement of some extra-articular structures. The disease is approximately two to three times more common in males than females in developed countries[2,12].

Historical aspects

This disease has affected mankind since antiquity,[4] but the earliest anatomical descriptions of skeletons with abnormalities typical of AS are attributed to Realdo Colombo in 1559, and Bernard Connor in 1693[6]. Bernard Connor described an ankylosed skeleton consisting of fused pelvis, spine and ribs that was unearthed by French farmers in a cemetery. He wrote that the bones were 'so straitly and intimately joined, their ligaments perfectly bony, and their articulations so effaced, that they really made but one uniform continuous bone'.

The first clinical descriptions of the disease were reported in the mid to late 19th century and medical interest in AS was stimulated by a series of publications between the years 1893 and 1899 by Vladimir von Bechterew (1857–1927) in St Petersburg, Russia[6]. Other clinical reports on AS were published by Adolf Strümpell (1853–1926) and Pierre Marie

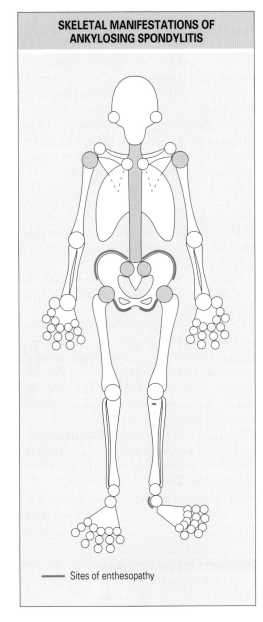

SKELETAL MANIFESTATIONS OF ANKYLOSING SPONDYLITIS

— Sites of enthesopathy

Fig. 103.1 Skeletal manifestations of ankylosing spondylitis. The axial skeletal sites frequently involved in AS are colored pink, while the blue coloration marks some of the sites of enthesopathy, such as the heels, iliac crest and gluteal and tibial tuberosities.

(1853–1940). Therefore, AS has been known by many different names, including 'morbus Bechterew' (Bechterew's disease), 'Marie–Strümpell disease' and 'morbus Strümpell–Marie–Bechterew'. The earliest X-ray examination of a patient with AS was described in 1899, and Walter Geilinger[7] in 1917 provided one of the first clear radiographic descriptions of the typical syndesmophytes that lead to spinal fusion in AS. Krebs, Scott, Forestier and others, many years later in the 1930s, clearly delineated other radiographic manifestations of AS, including sacroiliitis[6].

During the first half of the 20th century the disease was inappropriately also known as 'rheumatoid spondylitis', particularly in the USA, because of the false belief that it was a variant of rheumatoid arthritis (RA). It was only in 1963 that the American Rheumatism Association officially adopted the term ankylosing spondylitis in preference to rheumatoid spondylitis. In Europe, on the other hand, the term ankylosing spondylitis, or its variants 'spondylitis ankylosans' and 'spondylarthritis ankylopoietica', have been in wide use for more than 100 years[6–9].

Spondyloarthropathies

Ankylosing spondylitis mostly occurs alone without any associated disease but it may sometimes be associated with inflammatory bowel disease (IBD; ulcerative colitis and Crohn's disease), psoriasis or reactive arthritis – so-called 'secondary' AS. The arthritis observed in AS or in association with these related diseases is frequently referred to collectively as 'spondyloarthropathy' because sacroiliitis, spondylitis and inflammatory peripheral arthritis are their frequent manifestations[5,10–15]. By definition, the term 'primary', 'uncomplicated' or 'pure' AS implies exclusion of the other spondyloarthropathies; it is typically a disease predominantly involving the axial skeleton and is generally considered to be the commonest and most typical form of spondyloarthropathy in developed countries[10–12]. Some authors add a prefix 'seronegative' to the term 'spondyloarthropathy' to denote the lack of association of this group of diseases with IgM rheumatoid factor in the serum of patients.

CLINICAL FEATURES

Ankylosing spondylitis usually begins with back pain and stiffness in late adolescence and early adulthood. The average age of onset in developed countries varies between 24 and 26 years, and disease onset after age 45 is very rare[1,2,5,6,9,13]. A variety of clinical presentations due to enthesitis, peripheral arthritis or acute anterior uveitis may antedate back symptoms in some patients[11–26] (Table 103.1).

About 15% of patients have onset of their disease in childhood (before age 16) but this percentage may be as high as 40% in some developing countries[14,15,23–26]. Many of these children, often boys, have 5–10 years of persistent or recurrent bouts of enthesitis and/or lower extremity oligoarthritis (seronegative enthesopathy and arthritis, SEA syndrome) before definite symptoms and signs of axial disease develop. The SEA syndrome and juvenile-onset forms of AS and related spondyloarthropathies account for about 20% of all cases of juvenile arthritis seen by pediatric rheumatologists[24,25]. They are relatively more commonly observed among North American native populations and Mexican mestizos, and in many developing countries[14,15,23,26].

The clinical features of AS can be divided into musculoskeletal and extraskeletal manifestations (Table 103.1). The earliest, most typical

TABLE 103.1 CLINICAL FEATURES OF AS	
Skeletal	Axial arthritis, e.g. sacroiliitis and spondylitis
	Arthritis of 'girdle joints' (hips and shoulders)
	Peripheral arthritis uncommon
	Others: enthesitis, osteoporosis, vertebral fractures, spondylodiscitis, pseudoarthrosis
Extraskeletal	Acute anterior uveitis
	Cardiovascular involvement
	Pulmonary involvement
	Cauda equina syndrome
	Enteric mucosal lesions
	Amyloidosis, miscellaneous

and consistent findings of AS result from sacroiliitis and enthesitis (Fig. 103.2)[27–32]. There is often associated inflammation of discovertebral, apophyseal, costovertebral and costotransverse joints of the spine, and of the paravertebral ligamentous structures. This can result in fibrous and bony ankylosis after many years, perhaps as a secondary consequence of the primary inflammatory process[29,30,32] (Fig. 103.3).

Musculoskeletal manifestations
Chronic low back pain and stiffness

The most common and characteristic initial symptoms are chronic low back pain and stiffness, usually of insidious onset and dull in character. Many patients complain of pain in the buttock region as their earliest symptom but are unable to localize it precisely[5,6,12,16]. The pain probably represents sacroiliac joint involvement and is felt deep in the gluteal region, but some patients may note radiation of pain down the upper part of posterior thigh region, which can be misdiagnosed as 'lumbago' or 'sciatica', although neurologic examination is within normal limits. The pain may be unilateral or intermittent at first, or may alternate, first in one buttock and then the other, but it generally becomes persistent and bilateral within a few months, and the lower lumbar area becomes stiff and painful. This may be accompanied by sacroiliac and/or spinal tenderness.

The back pain and stiffness can be quite severe at this early stage and the pain tends to be accentuated on coughing, sneezing or maneuvers that cause a sudden twist of the back. Sometimes, pain and stiffness in the midthoracic or cervical region, or chest pain, may be the initial symptom, rather than the more typical low backache[10–12,17]. Back symptoms tend to worsen after prolonged periods of inactivity ('gel phenomenon'), and are therefore worse in the morning. The pain and stiffness tend to be eased by moving about ('limbering up') and with mild physical activity or exercise, and a hot shower. Some patients may wake-up at night to exercise or move about for a few minutes before returning to bed. The patient often experiences difficulty in getting out of bed because of pain and stiffness and may roll sideways off the bed, trying not to flex or rotate the spine.

Because of the high prevalence of back pain in the population at large, it is helpful to elicit from the patient's clinical history certain features that help in differentiating the non-inflammatory causes from the inflammatory back pain of AS and related spondyloarthropathies[6,16]. Characteristically, the onset of inflammatory back symptoms is insidious rather than abrupt, and the patient often cannot precisely date the onset of symptoms because they may be trivial or fleeting aches and pains in the beginning. The onset is usually in young individuals in their late teens and early twenties. It is very uncommon for the disease to begin after 45 years of age[6,13]. As the symptoms become chronic (defined as persistence for at least 3 months), the patient notices prominent back pain and stiffness in the morning that usually lasts for half an hour or more. The symptoms improve with physical activity or exercise but not with rest, and they get worse on prolonged rest.

Occasionally, back pain may be absent or too mild to impel the patient to seek medical care. Some may complain only of back stiffness, fleeting muscle aches or musculotendinous tender spots. These symptoms may become worse on exposure to cold or dampness[2,16,33], and some of these patients may be misdiagnosed as having fibromyalgia. Mild constitutional symptoms, such as anorexia, malaise, weight loss and low-grade fever, may occur in some patients in the early stages of their disease, and are relatively more common among patients with juvenile-onset AS, especially in developing countries[2,16,23,25,26].

Sleep disturbance and daytime fatigue

In many patients the back pain and stiffness may interrupt sleep, especially in the early morning hours, rather than at earlier times in the

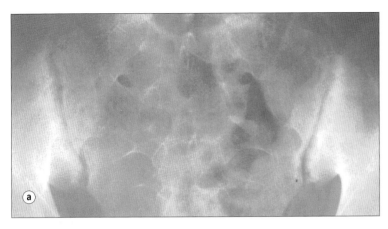

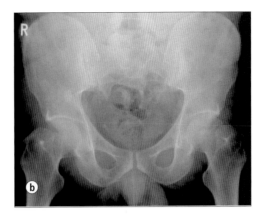

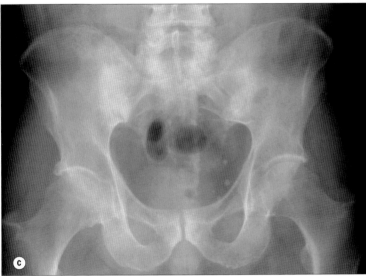

Fig. 103.2 Radiographic changes of sacroiliitis. (a) Early radiographic changes of sacroiliitis in AS consist of bony erosions ('postage stamp serrations') and adjacent bony sclerosis. These changes are typically seen first, and tend to be more prominent, on the iliac side of the sacroiliac joints. (b) Pelvic radiograph showing bilateral sacroiliitis (grade 2–3), with erosions, bony sclerosis and joint width irregularities. (c) Pelvic radiograph showing bilateral sacroiliitis (grade 3), with definite erosions, severe juxta-articular bony sclerosis and blurring of the joint. Radiographic changes of osteitis pubis are also present. (b & c Courtesy of M Rudwaleit and J Sieper.)

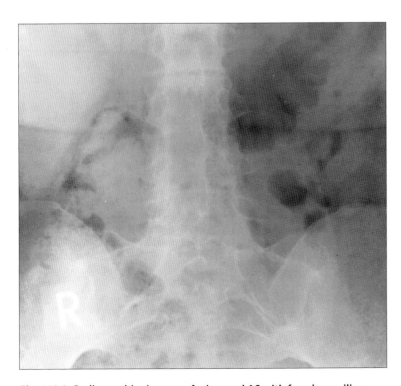

Fig. 103.3 Radiographic changes of advanced AS with fused sacroiliac joints. The ankylosis has also involved the lower lumbar spine ('bamboo spine'). Discogenic disease with end-plate bone changes is present at the L2, L3 level.

night. Therefore inadequate sleep and daytime somnolence and fatigue can be major complaints, and they are closely related to pain and stiffness at bedtime and during the night. A recent study found that 80% of the female and 50% of the male AS patients complained of too little sleep, primarily because of pain, compared to less than 30% of the general population[34].

Enthesitis

Enthesitis can result in extra-articular or juxta-articular bony tenderness, a major or presenting complaint in some patients, especially among those with juvenile-onset AS[20–30]. Enthesitis may appear alone or with arthritis, and can cause tenderness of costosternal junctions, spinous processes, iliac crests, greater trochanters, ischial tuberosities, tibial tubercles or sites of attachments of ligaments and tendons to calcaneus and tarsal bones of the feet. Plantar fasciitis or less often Achilles tendinitis can result in heel pain and tenderness over the inferior and posterior surfaces of the calcaneus respectively[20–24].

Hip and shoulder involvement

Sometimes the first symptoms may result from involvement of 'root' or 'girdle' joints (the hips and the shoulders). An accurate assessment of the range of motion of these joints should be recorded, because their involvement can result in severe functional limitation and disability. These joints may be involved at some stage of disease in one-third of the patients but this is relatively more common among those with juvenile-onset of AS[24–26,29]. If hip involvement has not occurred in the first 10 years of disease, it is very unlikely to occur later. However, some degree of fixed flexion contracture may be noted at later stages of the disease, and that can give rise to a characteristic rigid gait with some flexion at the knees to maintain an erect posture.

Hip joint involvement is usually bilateral, insidious in onset and potentially more crippling than involvement of any other joint of the extremities. It typically results in symmetric concentric joint space narrowing[29] (Fig. 103.4). The pain is typically felt in the groin but in some it may be felt in the ipsilateral knee or the thigh. Some patients with juvenile onset of AS may present with recurrent episodes of unilateral or bilateral painful but reversible contractures of their hip flexor muscles.

Involvement of the shoulder girdle (glenohumeral, acromioclavicular or sternoclavicular joints) may only lead to relatively minor limitations, mostly resulting from some loss of shoulder joint and thoracoscapular movement[35]. Erosive enthesitis of the supraspinatus tendon insertion is the characteristic shoulder lesion in AS patients[29] (Fig. 103.5). Primary involvement of the glenohumeral joint is rare but it can result in complete ankylosis of the joint[29].

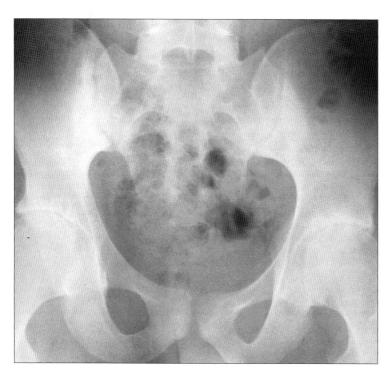

Fig. 103.4 Radiographic changes resulting from bilateral hip joint involvement in moderately advanced stages of AS.

Peripheral joint involvement

Involvement of peripheral joints other than hips and shoulders is infrequent in primary AS in developed countries, although sites affected may include the knees, wrists, elbows and feet. When present, involvement is usually asymmetric, monoarticular or oligoarticular; it is normally mild, rarely persistent or erosive and tends to resolve without any residual joint deformity in most patients[1,2,6,11,12]. However, peripheral joint involvement is relatively more frequent in developing countries, and also among patients who have associated psoriasis or inflammatory bowel disease, or those with juvenile onset of AS[13–15, 21–26]. Peripheral joint involvement can occasionally occur after the axial disease has become inactive. Rare occurrence of inflammatory edema of distal extremities together with peripheral arthritis and enthesitis has been reported[13].

Intermittent knee hydroarthrosis is occasionally the presenting manifestation of juvenile-onset AS[23,25]. Tarsal joint involvement in the feet, primarily reported in Mexican mestizo children, can be an unusual presenting manifestation of juvenile AS. It can ultimately lead to bony ankylosis of joints of the feet and is therefore called 'tarsal ankylosing enthesitis' or 'ankylosing tarsitis'[23].

Chest and spinal involvement

Involvement of the thoracic spine (including the costovertebral and costotransverse joints), enthesitis at costosternal areas and inflammation of manubriosternal junction or sternoclavicular joints may cause chest pain[17,21,29]. The pain may be accentuated on coughing or sneezing and at times may even mimic symptoms of atypical angina or pericarditis. Many patients give a history of having complained of chest pain to a physician before AS has been diagnosed. Some patients notice an inability to expand the chest fully on inspiration. Stiffness and pain in the cervical spine generally tend to develop after some years but occasionally occur in the early stages of the disease. Some patients may get recurrent episodes of stiff neck (torticollis).

Physical examination

As in other diseases where the etiology is not clearly defined, the diagnosis of AS is based on clinical and radiographic features[16,29–31,36–39]. A thorough physical examination, particularly of the musculoskeletal system, is needed. Clinical signs are sometimes minimal in the early stages of the disease. Examination of the sacroiliac joints and the spine (including the neck), measurement of chest expansion and range of motion of the hip and shoulder joints, and a search for signs of enthesitis are critical in making an early diagnosis of AS[16,31,39]. Important physical findings due to enthesitis that can be present in many patients but are often overlooked include tenderness over vertebral spinal processes, iliac crest, anterior

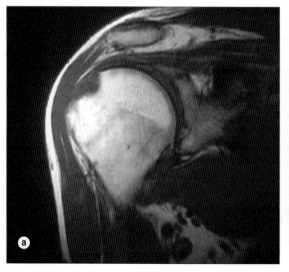

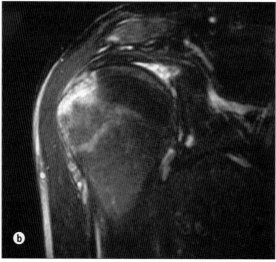

Fig. 103.5 Magnetic resonance images showing enthesitis at the rotator cuff insertion into the superolateral aspect of the humeral head. (a) T1-weighted image, coronal section, demonstrating loss of the marrow fat signal in the greater tuberosity of the humeral head. (b) T2-weighted image, coronal section, demonstrating diffuse edema in the greater tuberosity of the humerus adjacent to the supraspinatus enthesis. (Courtesy of W Maksymowych.)

chest wall, calcaneus (plantar fasciitis and/or Achilles tendinitis), ischial tuberosities, greater trochanters and sometimes tibial tubercles[5,22–25].

Direct pressure over the sacroiliac joint frequently, but not always, elicits pain if there is active sacroiliitis (Fig. 103.6). Sometimes sacroiliac pain may be elicited by pressure over the anterior superior iliac spines and on compressing the two iliac bones towards each other or forcing them away from each other. The pain can also be elicited by pressure over the lower half of the sacrum, with the patient lying prone, or by compressing the pelvis with the patient lying on one side. Hyperextension of the lumbar spine or hyperextension of one hip joint while applying counterpressure on the iliac crest by the other hand, with the patient lying supine, can also be painful. Other maneuvers include maximal flexion of one hip joint and hyperextension of the other, or maximal flexion, abduction and external rotation of the hip joints (Figs 103.7 & 103.8). All these maneuvers are then repeated on the opposite side. However, these tests will also elicit pain in the presence of hip joint involvement by itself.

If two or more of these maneuvers elicit pain in the region of the sacroiliac joints, the likelihood of the presence of active sacroiliitis (in the presence of appropriate clinical symptoms) is quite strong, and this must be confirmed by radiographic imaging[29–31] (Fig. 103.2). These clinical signs, however, may be absent in some patients despite sacroiliitis because the sacroiliac joints have strong ligaments that limit their

motion, and also these tests are not specific for sacroiliitis. In addition, these physical signs become negative in late stages of the disease, as fibrosis and bony ankylosis replace inflammation. Clinical detection of flexion contracture of the hip joint is illustrated in Figure 103.9 and limitation of shoulder range of motion in Figure 103.10.

Tenderness and stiffness of the paraspinal muscles often accompany the inflammation of the axial skeleton, and the initial loss of spinal mobility is usually due to pain and muscle spasm rather than bony ankylosis. Therefore, marked improvement in spinal mobility can occur

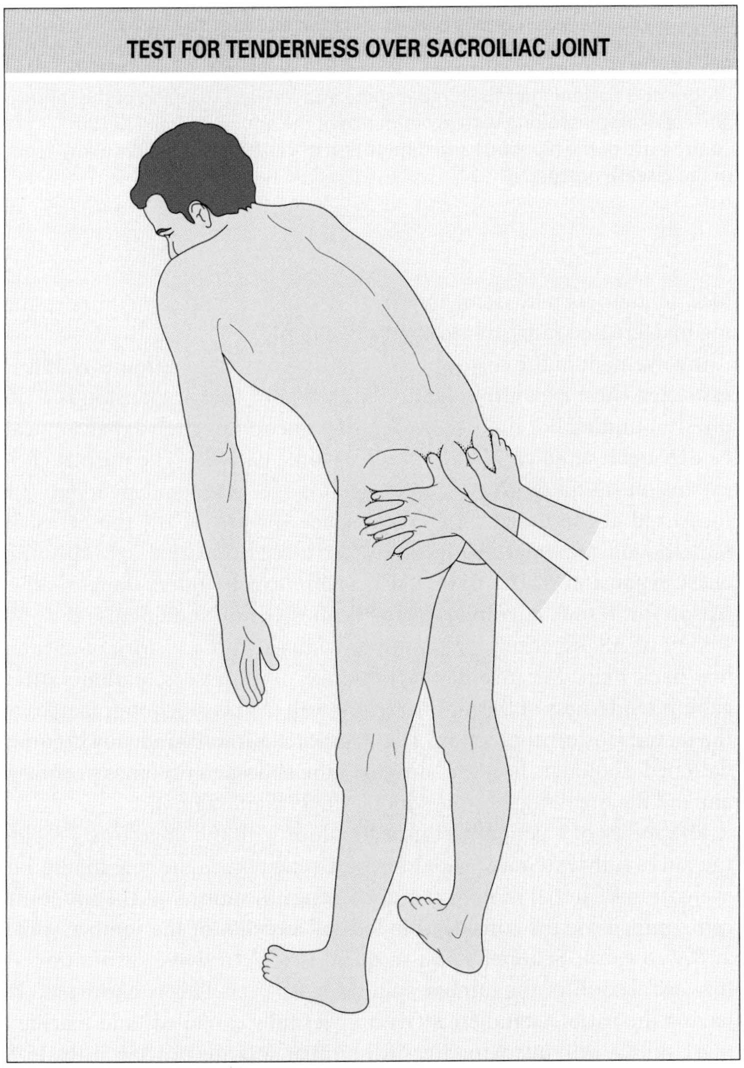

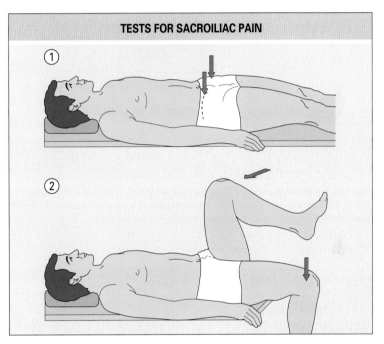

Fig. 103.7 Tests for sacroiliac pain. Two procedures that may cause pain in the sacroiliac area in patients with sacroiliitis. Application of direct pressure on the anterior superior iliac spines, along with attempts to force the iliac spines laterally apart (1); and forced flexion of one hip maximally towards the opposite shoulder, with hyperextension of the contralateral hip joint (2).

TEST FOR TENDERNESS OVER SACROILIAC JOINT

Fig. 103.6 Test for tenderness over sacroiliac joint. Application of firm pressure by thumb (or fist) directly over the sacroiliac joints can elicit tenderness in many patients. The figure also illustrates the patient's inability to touch the floor. The decrease in spinal mobility is often more readily recognized on hyperextension (dorsiflexion) or lateral flexion of the spine.

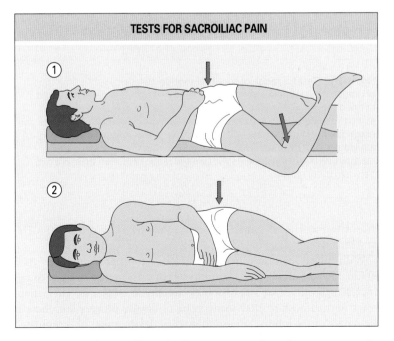

Fig. 103.8 Tests for sacroiliac pain. Two more procedures that may cause pain in the sacroiliac area in patients with sacroiliitis. Application of downward pressure on the flexed knee, with hip flexed, abducted and externally rotated (1); and compression of the pelvis with the patient lying on one side (2).

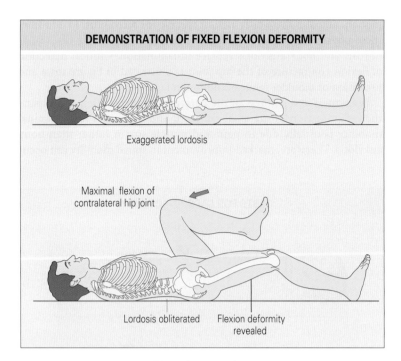

DEMONSTRATION OF FIXED FLEXION DEFORMITY

Exaggerated lordosis

Maximal flexion of contralateral hip joint

Lordosis obliterated   Flexion deformity revealed

Fig. 103.9 Demonstration of fixed flexion deformity. Fixed flexion deformity of the hip joint can be revealed as the contralateral hip joint is maximally flexed to obliterate the exaggerated compensatory lumbar lordosis.

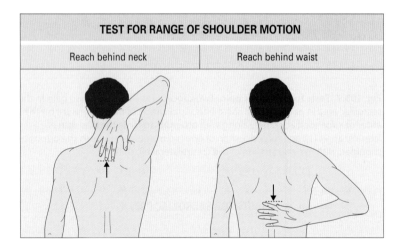

TEST FOR RANGE OF SHOULDER MOTION

Reach behind neck	Reach behind waist

Fig. 103.10 Test for range of shoulder motion. Relatively subtle limitation of motion of the shoulder joint can easily be detected. The patient is asked to bring the arm behind the waist (to test internal rotation) and reach up along the spine as high as possible, then to bring the arm behind the neck and reach down along the spine as far as possible (to test external rotation). In individuals with the normal range of motion of the shoulder joints, these reaches overlap, but in patients with limited range of motion there is a gap between these reaches.

after treatment with non-steroidal anti-inflammatory drugs (NSAIDs) and intensive physical therapy at an early stage of the disease.

With longer disease duration and disease progression, there is a gradual loss of mobility of the lumbar spine. The entire spine becomes increasingly stiff, with loss of spinal mobility in all planes. The patient loses normal posture after many years of disease progression; there is flattening of the lumbar spine and gradual development of accentuated dorsal (thoracic) spinal kyphosis (Fig. 103.11). The inflammatory process can extend to involve the cervical spine, and assessment of its range of motion, particularly the lateral flexion, axial rotation and hyperextension, should not be neglected[39]. Temporomandibular joint pain and

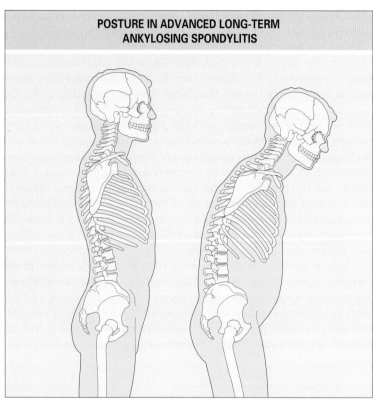

POSTURE IN ADVANCED LONG-TERM ANKYLOSING SPONDYLITIS

Fig. 103.11 Posture in advanced long-term ankylosing spondylitis. Progressive flattening of the lumbar spine and forward stooping of the thoracic and cervical spine, along with prominence of the abdomen, mild flexion contracture of the hip joints and diminution of vertical height after many years of the disease process.

local tenderness may occur in about 10% of patients, sometimes resulting in decreased range of motion of this joint.

Involvement of the costovertebral and costotransverse joints results in restricted chest expansion. Severe limitation of chest expansion is a late physical finding but mild to moderate reduction of chest expansion can be detectable at an early stage of AS in some patients. The normal chest expansion is 5cm or greater, although it is age- and sex-dependent. It is measured at the fourth intercostal space (or just below the breast in females) on maximal inspiration after forced maximal expiration. A chest expansion of less than 2.5cm is abnormal (unless there is other reason for it, such as emphysema or scoliosis), and should raise the possibility of AS, especially in young individuals with a history of chronic low back pain. Because of the presence of enthesitis, patients often exhibit tenderness of the anterior chest wall over costochondral areas or the manubriosternal junction. The anterior chest wall gradually becomes flattened, shoulders become 'stooped', the abdomen becomes protuberant and the breathing becomes increasingly diaphragmatic.

The ability of a patient to touch the floor with the fingertips, keeping the knees fully extended, should not be relied on as the sole method of evaluation of spinal mobility. A good range of motion of the hip joints can compensate for considerable loss of mobility of the lumbar spine, and *vice versa*. Schober's test is quite useful to detect limitation of forward flexion of the lumbar spine (Fig. 103.12). This is performed by having the patient stand erect (with knees fully extended) and placing a mark on the skin overlying the fifth lumbar spinous process at the level of the posterior superior iliac spines (the 'dimples of Venus'). A second mark is placed 10cm above in the midline. The patient is then asked to maximally bend the spine forward without bending the knees. The 10cm distance between the two marks on the skin expands by 5cm or more in normal healthy individuals through stretching of the skin overlying the

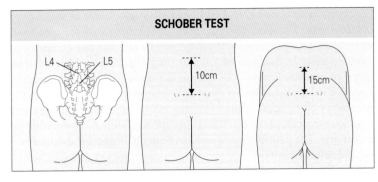

SCHOBER TEST

L4   L5

10cm

15cm

Fig. 103.12 Schober test. This measures the ability to flex the lumbar spine (see text).

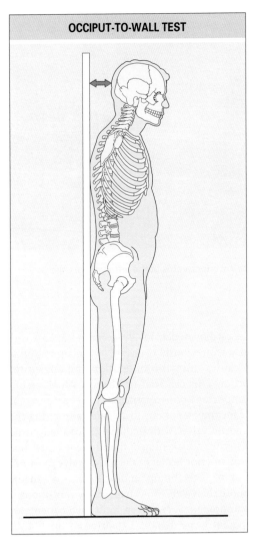

OCCIPUT-TO-WALL TEST

Fig. 103.13 Occiput-to-wall test.

mobile lumbar spine. An increase of less than 3cm indicates diminished lumbar spinal mobility. Limitations of lateral flexion as well as hyper-extension of the spine also accompany and often precede this diminished spinal mobility on forward flexion.

Although spinal ankylosis develops at a variable rate and pattern, the typical spinal deformities of AS usually evolve after 10 or more years. However, the disease may occasionally remain confined to one part of the spine. Involvement of the cervical spine, usually one of the last musculoskeletal manifestations, results in progressive limitation of neck motion with a decreased ability to turn or extend the neck fully and a gradual development of forward stooping of the neck after many years (Fig. 103.11). The stooping of the neck can be measured by the occiput-to-wall test (Fig. 103.13). The patient, while standing erect with the buttocks against a wall and the back of the heels touching the wall, attempts to touch the wall with the back of the head while keeping a horizontal gaze. Any gap between the occiput and the wall is measured.

At this advanced stage the presence of disease is readily apparent because of the characteristic gait and posture and the way the patient sits or rises from the examining table. At this stage the pain from spinal involvement diminishes and there is less morning stiffness, but some degree of inflammatory pain is usually present. In extreme cases, the entire spine may be fused in a flexed position and the field of vision becomes limited, making it difficult for some patients to look ahead as they walk. Similarly, the hip joints may become ankylosed and the patient may need to stand with knees flexed to maintain posture. Such patients may injure themselves more readily because the rigid spine impairs their ability to balance themselves after sudden changes of position.

The deep tendon reflexes in the lower extremities are normal and the straight-leg-raising test is negative. Convincing evidence for involvement of skeletal muscles in AS is lacking. The muscle weakness and sometimes marked muscle wasting seen in some patients with advanced disease probably results from disuse, although some ultrastructural changes in muscle and a persistent modestly raised level of serum creatine kinase have occasionally been observed[2,16]. However, in addition to any myopathy, one should not overlook the presence of any myelopathy in such patients.

Extraskeletal manifestations

Ocular manifestations

Acute anterior uveitis is the most common extra-articular feature of AS, occurring in 25–40% of patients at some time in the course of their disease[40–45]. It is an acute inflammation of the iris and ciliary body and is therefore also called 'acute iritis' or 'iridocyclitis'. It is relatively more common in those AS patients who possess HLA-B27, or have peripheral joint involvement[41,45]. In North America and western Europe, close to 95% of patients with AS and acute anterior uveitis possess HLA-B27,

and approximately 50% of all patients with isolated acute anterior uveitis are HLA-B27-positive. It is the most common definable type, representing about 15% of all kinds of uveitis. Occasionally, the uveitis may be the presenting symptom that draws attention to the diagnosis of AS or related spondyloarthropathy[40,42].

It is typically unilateral, but has a tendency to recur, not infrequently in the contralateral eye. The symptoms usually begin acutely with eye pain, increased lacrimation, photophobia and some blurring of vision. The eye is inflamed, there is circumcorneal congestion (Fig. 103.14), the pupil is small, the iris is edematous and it may appear slightly discolored compared to the contralateral side. There is copious exudate in the anterior chamber of the eye, which can be seen on slit-lamp examination. The inflammatory cells adhere to the endothelial lining cells of the cornea, forming small aggregates called keratitic precipitates. Ophthalmologists characterize these findings as 'non-granulomatous' to distinguish them from what is usually seen in uveitis of sarcoidosis and some of the other granulomatous diseases.

The individual attack of acute uveitis usually subsides within a few weeks without any sequelae, but residual visual impairment may occur if treatment is inadequate or delayed. The pupil may become irregular if the inflamed iris gets stuck to the cornea (anterior synechiae) or to the lens (posterior synechiae). This can result in secondary glaucoma and cataract in the long run. In rare cases, the posterior chamber may also be involved, resulting in cystoid macular edema; and one should look for the presence of associated IBD or psoriais if the uveitis begins insidiously, lasts longer than 6 months, is bilateral or involves the posterior uveal tract[43,44].

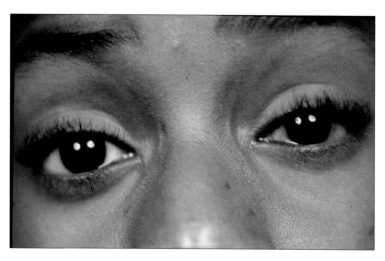

Fig. 103.14 Untreated acute anterior uveitis of the left eye. Note the circumcorneal congestion.

Cardiac manifestations

Recent studies suggest that cardiovascular involvement in patients with AS is more common than was previously realized[46–48]. Inflammation at the aortic root (aortitis) causes intimal proliferation and adventitial scarring of the vasa vasorum. This can lead to fibrosis, which results in hemodynamically unimportant consequences. However, in some patients, it results in aortic incompetence due to a dilated aortic ring and thickened and shortened aortic valves with nodularities of their cusps. The fibrotic process can also cause thickening of the adjacent ventricular septum and the basal part of anterior leaflet of the mitral valve to form a characteristic 'subaortic bump'. This 'bump' and/or thickened valvular cusps can be detected in more than 30% of AS patients by transthoracic and transesophageal echocardiography. However, most such patients are without any clinically apparent heart disease. Extension of the fibrotic process into the atrioventricular conduction bundle can, however, cause partial or complete heart block[47].

The risk of occurrence of aortic insufficiency and cardiac conduction disturbances increases with the age of the patient, the duration of AS, the presence of HLA-B27 and peripheral joint involvement[47]. For example, cardiac conduction disturbances occur in up to 3% of those with disease of 15 years' duration but up to 9% after 30 years. Complete heart block causing Stokes–Adam's attacks may supervene in some patients, necessitating implantation of cardiac pacemakers. The aortic regurgitation follows a chronic but relentless course to heart failure, usually over several years, necessitating valvular replacement. Sometimes acute aortic (and rarely even mitral) insufficiency with rapid deterioration of cardiac function can occur in relatively young patients with minimal spondylitis[46].

Studies in Sweden have described the occurrence of the cardiac syndrome of 'lone aortic incompetence plus pacemaker-requiring bradycardia' in men without spondyloarthropathy as an HLA-B27-associated inflammatory condition[47]. Among 91 patients with the combination of heart block and aortic insufficiency, 88% had HLA-B27 but only about 20% of them had AS or related spondyloarthropathy. There is no association between HLA-B27 and lone aortic incompetence in the absence of complete heart block or spondyloarthropathy. However, HLA-B27 was found to be more prevalent (17%) among 83 patients with isolated complete heart block (without any clinical or radiographic evidence of associated spondyloarthropathy) than the 6% prevalence in normal controls.

Pulmonary manifestations

Rigidity of the chest wall in patients with AS results in inability to expand the chest fully on inspiration and can result in mild restrictive lung func-

tion impairment. However, this does not usually result in ventilatory insufficiency because of increased diaphragmatic contribution. Pleuropulmonary involvement can occur as a rare and late extraskeletal manifestation, in the form of a slowly progressive and usually bilateral apical pulmonary fibrobullous disease in 1–2% of patients. It appears as linear or patchy opacities on chest radiographs and they can eventually become cystic[49]. These cavitations may mimic tuberculosis lesions and may become colonized by *Aspergillus* species, with the formation of mycetoma. The patient may complain of cough, increasing dyspnea and occasionally hemoptysis.

Newer imaging modalities, such as thin-section high-resolution computed tomography (CT), indicate that there is general under-recognition of the pulmonary parenchymal involvement in AS[50,51]. An uncontrolled study of 26 AS patients revealed a high incidence of lung abnormalities on high-resolution CT of the lungs, including four patients with interstitial lung disease that has hitherto not been associated with AS[51]. The abnormalities observed are usually subtle and subclinical, mostly comprising thickening of the interlobular septa, mild bronchial wall or pleural thickening, pleuropulmonary irregularities and linear septal thickening. Moreover, they do not correlate with functional and clinical impairment.

Gastrointestinal manifestations

Apart from the well known association of chronic IBD with AS, there is also a high prevalence of other forms of spondyloarthropathies, unrelated to the extent of the bowel disease[52–55]. However, sacroiliitis, both symptomatic and asymptomatic, is related to the disease duration. In a recent study of a population-based cohort of 521 patients with IBD seen 6 years after diagnosis, 6% of patients with Crohn's disease and 2.6% of those with ulcerative colitis were found to have AS[54]. The overall prevalence of spondyloarthropathy was 22%, and 2% had radiological sacroiliitis without clinical features of spondyloarthropathy.

Clinically 'silent' (asymptomatic) enteric mucosal inflammatory lesions, both macroscopic and microscopic, have been detected in the terminal ileum and proximal colon on ileocolonoscopic studies in more than 50% of AS patients with no gastrointestinal symptoms[52]. Follow-up studies of such patients indicate that 6% of them will develop IBD and, among those with histologically 'chronic' inflammatory gut lesions, between 15% and 25% will develop clinically obvious Crohn's disease[52]. This suggests that the latter group of patients initially had a subclinical form of Crohn's disease when they presented with arthritis, and supports the existence of a pathogenic link between gut inflammation and AS that is independent of HLA-B27.

Osteoporosis

Spinal osteoporosis is frequently observed, especially in patients with severe AS of long duration, partly as a result of lack of spinal mobility due to ankylosis, but it may also be related to mineralization defect[56,57] (Fig. 103.15). A marked reduction in bone mineral density of the lumbar spine and femoral neck has been reported by dual energy X-ray absorptiometry (DEXA) measurement in a group of young patients with early AS. It may result from proinflammatory cytokines and contributes to spinal fractures and progressive spinal deformity in some patients. Bone biopsies and assessment of biochemical markers of bone metabolism have shown that both diminished bone formation and enhanced bone resorption are involved[56,57].

Spondylodiscitis and spinal fractures

An aseptic spondylodiscitis, mostly in the midthoracic spine and usually asymptomatic, can occur without any physical trauma and is relatively more common in the patients whose spondylitis also involves the cervical spine[58]. There is also an increased prevalence of anterior compression of the vertebral body, discovertebral destructive lesions (so-called Andersson lesions) and spinal fractures[59–65].

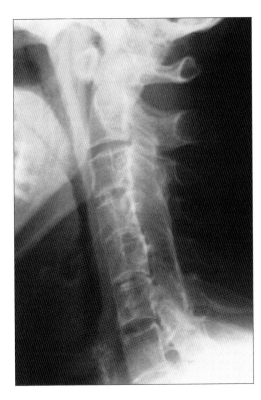

Fig. 103.15 Radiograph of cervical spine, lateral view, showing marked osteopenia and bony fusions at multiple levels. Osteitis of the corners of the vertebral bodies is best demonstrated at C6–C7 level anteriorly, causing 'shiny corners' (Romanus lesions) due to reactive bone sclerosis. There is associated bony resorption that results in 'squared' vertebral bodies and formation of a vertical bony 'bridging' (syndesmophyte formation) between the two vertebral bodies. There is extensive fusion of the apophyseal joints posteriorly from C3 to C7 level. There is no subluxation at the atlantoaxial junction.

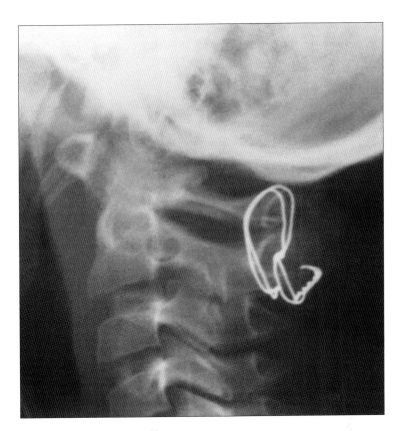

Fig. 103.16 Radiograph of the cervical spine, lateral view, of a young boy with juvenile ankylosing spondylitis. He had undergone surgery for spontaneous severe atlantoaxial subluxation, and the radiograph shows incomplete reduction of the subluxation following surgery.

The ankylosed spine breaks like a long bone and the fracture line is usually transverse; it is more often transdiscal (i.e. across syndysmophytes) than transvertebral. The rigid osteoporotic spine is unduly susceptible to fracture even after a relatively minor trauma, including events that may not be remembered or recalled by the patient[59,60]. One should exclude the possibility of spinal fracture in any patient with advanced AS who complains of new onset of neck or back pain, even in the absence of a definite trauma.

The fracture of cervical spine, usually at the C5–6 or C6–7 level, can result in quadriplegia, especially if associated with dislocation, and is a very serious complication with a high morbidity and mortality[59,65]. Sometimes the undiagnosed or improperly treated fracture results in spondylodiscitis and pseudoarthrosis, and can lead to severe kyphotic deformities[59–64]. The diagnosis of these fractures may be difficult in a 'bamboo spine', and focal spinal abnormalities on bone scans can be a clue to the presence of fracture or pseudarthrosis[60,63]. Magnetic resonance imaging (MRI) is important in detecting and evaluating complications of fractures or pseudoarthrosis, as well as changes in the dura mater, soft tissue and longitudinal ligaments[64].

Atlantoaxial subluxation

Erosions of the odontoid process and the transverse ligament can result in spontaneous atlantoaxial subluxation, usually anteriorly (Fig. 103.16). It can present as occipital pain, with or without signs of spinal cord compression, and is relatively more commonly observed in those with peripheral joint involvement, and also possibly among Mexican patients[66]. It generally occurs in the later stages of the disease, although it can be an early manifestation[67]. Rarely vertical (upward migration of the odontoid process into the brainstem (platybasia)), rotatory, posterior atlantoaxial, or subaxial subluxations, and fracture of the odontoid process have been reported[29,68].

Neurological manifestations

Neurological involvement may occur in patients with AS and is related most often to fracture dislocation of the spine, cauda equina syndrome or atlantoaxial subluxation. A slowly progressive cauda equina syndrome is a rare but significant complication of long-standing AS and results from fibrous entrapment and scarring of the sacral and lower lumbar nerve roots resulting from chronic adhesive arachnoiditis[69,70]. It is associated with dural calcification, erosions of the spinal canal associated with enlarged dural sacs (dural ectasia), and dorsal dural diverticula, which are characteristic of this condition and can be demonstrated by CT and MRI. It can result in sensory loss in the sacral and lower lumbar dermatomes ('saddle anesthesia') and decreased rectal and/or urinary sphincter tone, and may also cause some pain and weakness in the legs. Occurrence of a multiple-sclerosis-like syndrome has also been reported in AS patients but proper epidemiological studies are needed to verify if there is any association[71–73].

Renal manifestations

Renal disease, with or without any impairment of renal function, can occur in patients with AS for various reasons and usually presents with proteinuria and microscopic hematuria, sometimes detected on routine urinalysis[74–79]. Secondary amyloidosis (AA type) is now rarely observed among patients with AS or related spondyloarthropathies in the USA and is also decreasing in some other countries. This is possibly because of more widespread use of NSAIDs and other drugs now available to better control chronic inflammation[78,79]. However, amyloidosis often remains undiagnosed until late in its course because of its slow evolution and relative rarity. This complication should, however, be considered in the differential diagnosis of proteinuria with or without progressive azotemia. Biopsies of abdominal fat pad or rectal mucosa in one European study detected presence of amyloidosis in 10 of 137 unselected patients with AS (approximately 7%), but only two had clinical amyloidosis with proteinuria[77]. However, three more patients developed clinical amyloidosis after a mean of 5.4 years of follow-up.

An increased incidence of IgA nephropathy has also been reported in patients with AS and related spondyloarthropathies[76,80]. Interestingly, an elevated level of serum IgA is frequently observed in patients with AS[81].

Renal disease can also result from chronic NSAID use, and there are a few old reports of a somewhat higher incidence of chronic non-specific prostatitis among patients with AS.

Other clinical manifestations

Preliminary reports indicate that patients with AS and related spondyloarthropathies have an increased incidence of Sjögren's syndrome[82,83]. A possible association with vitiligo has also been suggested[84]. There are a few case reports of co-occurrence of relapsing polychondritis, sarcoidosis, familial Mediterranean fever, Behçet's disease, or retroperitoneal fibrosis in patients with AS and related spondyloarthropathies[85-88], and there is one study suggesting a higher incidence of varicoceles in AS patients[89]. Some spondylitis patients with associated IBD may get pyoderma gangrenosum, erythema nodosum, or sclerosing cholangitis, which are well-recognized extraintestinal manifestations of IBD[90].

INVESTIGATIONS

The most useful investigations are from musculoskeletal imaging (see below), although a number of other laboratory tests are informative. An elevated erythrocyte sedimentation rate (ESR) or serum C-reactive protein (CRP) is present in up to 70% of patients with active AS[6]. However, there is a lack of clear correlation with clinical disease activity, and levels of these acute phase reactants seem to have only limited clinical usefulness[6,91]. A normal ESR and/or CRP does not exclude the presence of clinically active AS. Both may relate more to peripheral arthropathy than the axial disease in AS. Generally speaking, the finding of an elevated ESR or serum CRP in a person with inflammatory back pain increases the likelihood of AS.

A mild normocytic normochromic anemia is present in 15% of patients, depending on the severity of the inflammatory process. Mild to moderate elevations of serum concentration of IgA are observed in 50–60% of patients with AS, and the serum IgA level correlates with acute phase reactants, disease activity and the presence of peripheral arthritis in particular[2,16,81]. Serum complement levels are normal or elevated. Some investigators have detected circulating immune complexes in the serum of patients with AS, while others have not confirmed these findings.

Positive tests for rheumatoid factor and antinuclear antibodies do not occur more frequently in patients with AS than in healthy controls[2,8]. Modest elevations of serum alkaline phosphatase (primarily derived from bone) are seen in some patients but are unrelated to the activity or the duration of the disease and their clinical significance is unclear[16]. The synovial fluid in AS patients does not show markedly distinctive features compared to other inflammatory arthropathies. Mild elevation of cerebrospinal fluid protein has been noted in some patients, perhaps as a result of mild arachnoiditis.

Pulmonary function tests show no ventilatory insufficiency even in advanced cases of AS; an increased diaphragmatic contribution helps to compensate for the rigidity of the chest wall. Vital capacity and total lung capacity are moderately reduced, reflecting the restricted chest wall movement; residual lung volume and functional residual capacity are usually, but not always, increased; and airflow measurements are normal.

Musculoskeletal imaging

Characteristically, the radiographic changes of AS are seen in the axial skeleton, especially in the sacroiliac, discovertebral, apophyseal, costovertebral and costotransverse joints, and they evolve slowly over many years[21,29,30]. The earliest, most consistent and most characteristic radiographic findings are seen in the sacroiliac joints. Various methods have been used to examine the sacroiliac joints radiographically; none is ideal because of the complex configuration and individual variations of these joints. The radiographic interpretation of early sacroiliitis can be difficult, party due to the presence of degenerative changes. A plain anteroposterior radiograph of the pelvis or one aimed 30° cephalad (Ferguson's view) is usually adequate to visualize these joints, and an oblique view is not recommended.[92]

The radiographic findings of sacroiliitis are usually bilateral and symmetric. They are first seen in the lower third (synovial part) of the joint, mostly on the iliac side and consist of blurring of the subchondral bone plate[29]. In more advanced disease, erosions ('postage stamp serrations') and sclerosis of the adjacent bones are seen at both joint margins (Fig. 103.2). Progressive subchondral bone erosions at both joint margins can result in 'pseudo-widening' of the sacroiliac joint space. Later erosions become less obvious but the subchondral sclerosis persists and may become more prominent.

There is gradual fibrosis, calcification, interosseous bridging and ossification of the sacroiliac joints. Ultimately (usually after several years) there may be complete bony fusion across the joint and resolution of the adjacent bony sclerosis (Fig. 103.3). Other pelvic abnormalities that may occur include sclerosis and bony erosions at the pubic symphysis (osteitis pubis), and cortical irregularities and osteitis ('whiskering') at sites of osseous attachment of tendons and ligaments (enthesitis), particularly at the ischial tuberosities, iliac crest and femoral trochanters[29].

The evaluation of the sacroiliac joints has been studied by infrared thermography, radionuclide scintigraphy (bone scan), conventional tomography and single photon emission CT (SPECT) in patients with early disease in whom standard radiography of the sacroiliac joints may show normal or equivocal changes. CT of the sacroiliac joint is a more sensitive technique than conventional radiography but both only detect chronic changes (Fig. 103.17). Infrared thermography is not useful and conventional tomography and scintigraphy also need not be performed for diagnosis in such patients because conventional tomography is inferior to CT, and scintigraphy is too non-specific to be of much clinical value in this situation[29,30,93].

Sacroiliac plane radiographs are less reliable in detecting sacroiliitis in children and adolescents, and these patients may require dynamic (gadolinium-enhanced) MRI, which produces, without any ionizing radiation, excellent but more costly computer-generated imaging[6,9,30,94-96]. Dynamic MRI and the use of 'STIR' and other fat suppression techniques can demonstrate the inflammatory response associated with enthesitis[9,20,30,96] (Figs 103.18–103.20). The inflammatory reaction involves not only the adjacent soft tissues but also the under-

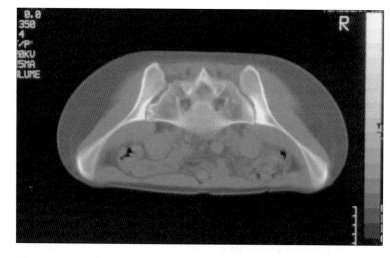

Fig. 103.17 CT of the sacroiliac joints demonstrating definite bilateral sacroiliitis (erosions and sclerosis). (Courtesy of M Rudwaleit and J Sieper.)

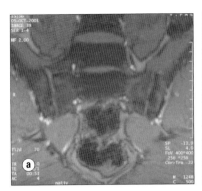
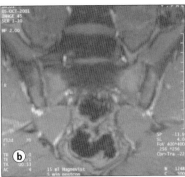
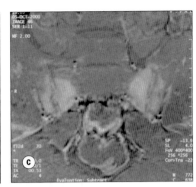

Fig. 103.18 Imaging of inflammatory changes. (a) MRI of the sacroiliac joints. (b) Bilateral inflammatory changes visualized by gadolinium enhancement (5 minutes after gadolinium injection). (c) MRI subtraction evaluation; enhancement of synovial part of sacroiliac joints and juxta-articular bone (reflecting inflammatory changes in the bone, the so called 'bone edema') are clearly visible. (Courtesy of M Rudwaleit and J Sieper.)

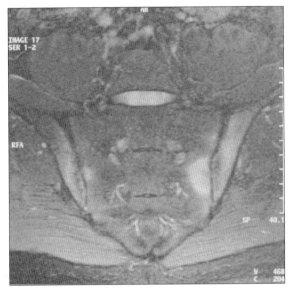

Fig. 103.19 MRI of the sacroiliac joints. This image uses a fat suppression technique (STIR) to visualize inflammatory changes in the bone ('bone edema'), which are more marked on one side. (Courtesy of M Rudwaleit and J Sieper.)

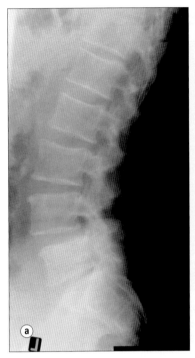
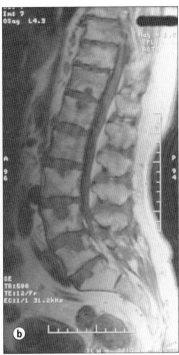

Fig. 103.20 Imaging of AS. (a) Radiograph (lateral view) of the lumbar spine showing a typical Andersson lesion (spondylodiscitis) of the 4th lumbar vertebra. (b) Sagittal T1-weighted MRI of the same patient reveals multisegmental involvement that was not visible on plain radiographs. Moreover, it also shows fat deposition in several vertebral bodies, reflecting degenerative or postinflammatory changes. (Courtesy of M Rudwaleit and J Sieper.)

lying bone marrow, and it can sometimes extend to a considerable distance away from the involved enthesis insertion. This utilisation of MRI in detecting the inflammatory response at an early stage is not sufficiently well characterised to recommend its widespread use at present[36].

Studies of families with AS have demonstrated that HLA-B27-positive individuals who have typical inflammatory back symptoms or chest pain can lack any radiographic evidence of sacroiliitis or spondylitis[97]. It may take an average of 9 years before sacroiliitis can be detected by plain radiography in such patients, according to one study[98]. In a study of long-term follow-up of undifferentiated spondyloarthropathy, a majority (68%) of such patients developed AS[99]. Dynamic MRI is more sensitive than CT in detecting early sacroiliitis in such patients[9,30,96], and it is also very helpful in detecting spinal fractures and dural diverticuli associated with cauda equina syndrome in AS[63,70].

A study compared CT and MRI in 24 patients with clinical evidence of AS but uncertain radiologic findings, and 12 controls[100]. CT was found to be more specific but less sensitive than MRI; contrast-enhanced MRI especially is more likely to detect early lesions. CT detected sacroiliitis in 38% of the 24 patients and none of the controls. MRI detected sacroiliitis in 54% of the patients, but 17% of controls. Additional studies are required before dynamic MRI can be accepted as a substitute for conventional radiography for detecting sacroiliitis or for monitoring disease activity or progression[95,101]. Ultrasonography is useful in detecting enthesitis and associated bursitis, tendinitis and tenosynovitis (Fig. 103.21), but its accuracy varies, depending on the operator's experience[13,102].

The inflammatory lesions in the vertebral column affect the apophyseal (posterior intervertebral) joints, the superficial layers of the annulus fibrosus at their attachment to the corners of vertebral bodies, and the intervertebral ligaments. Marginal erosive lesions of the corner of the vertebral body with adjacent reactive bone sclerosis can be seen radiographically as 'highlighted corners' (Romanus lesion) (Figs 103.15 & 103.22), but they are better demonstrated by contrast-enhanced (dynamic) MRI[9,20,29,30,94]. Subsequent bone resorption (erosions) can result in 'squaring' of the vertebral body, and this can be followed by a gradual ossification of the superficial layers of the annulus fibrosus and eventually 'bony bridging' between the adjacent vertebrae[29,32]. These vertical bony bridges are called syndesmophytes (Figs 103.23 & 103.24). They begin at the angles of the involved vertebral bodies and are called 'marginal' syndesmophytes. They usually start forming initially in the lower thoracic and the adjacent lumbar spine and then start appearing in the upper thoracic and ultimately the cervical spine.

Radiographic changes identical to those seen in 'primary' AS are generally also seen in those with 'secondary' AS in association with

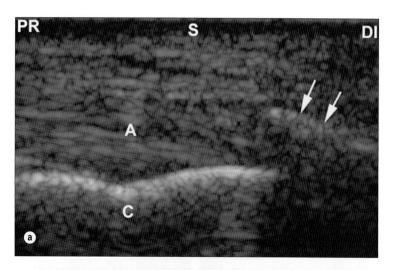

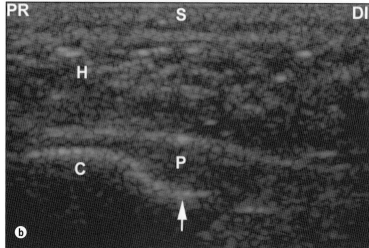

Fig. 103.21 Imaging of the foot. (a). Longitudinal ultrasound scan showing Achilles tendinitis (enthesitis); the tendon is marked as A, and the arrows indicate the presence of an enthesophyte. PR, proximal part of the tendon; DI, distal part; C, calcaneus; S, skin. (b). Longitudinal ultrasound scan showing plantar fasciitis; the enthesophyte is marked by an arrow. C, calcaneus; H, heel fat pad; S, skin. (Courtesy of P Balint and D Kane.)

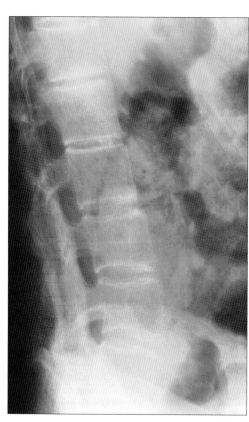

Fig. 103.22 Radiograph of lumbar spine. Lateral view, showing 'shiny corners' (Romanus lesions) and 'squared' vertebral bodies. Mild discogenic disease (discitis) is present between the T12 and L1 vertebrae.

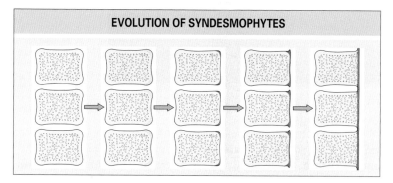

EVOLUTION OF SYNDESMOPHYTES

Fig. 103.23 Evolution of syndesmophytes. Lateral view of lumbar spinal vertebral bodies. Osteitis of the corners of the vertebral bodies anteriorly, causing reactive sclerosis ('shiny corners'), shown in red, leads to local bone resorption and resultant 'squared' vertebral bodies. This is followed by vertical bony 'bridging' (syndesmophyte formation), resulting from ossification of the superficial layers of the annulus fibrosus. (Modified from Khan[102].)

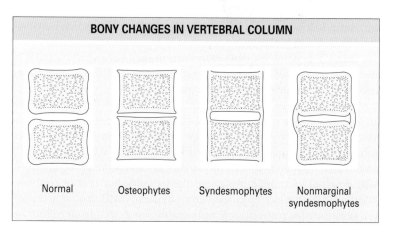

BONY CHANGES IN VERTEBRAL COLUMN

Normal | Osteophytes | Syndesmophytes | Nonmarginal syndesmophytes

Fig. 103.24 Bony changes in vertebral column. Evolution of bony changes observed in degenerative disc disease (osteophytes), ankylosing spondylitis (syndesmophytes) and psoriatic spondylitis (non-marginal syndesmophytes), affecting the lumbar spine (anteroposterior view).

ulcerative colitis and Crohn's disease[1,2,29]. In contrast, patients with spondylitis in association with reactive arthritis and psoriasis tend to develop random, asymmetric and bulky syndesmophytes (Figs 103.24 & 103.25). These are often called 'non-marginal' syndesmophytes because they do not just extend from one vertebral angle to the other but may start from the middle of one vertebral body and extend to the same area of the adjacent vertebral body. Differentiation of the various forms of spondyloarthropathy in the end, of course, is based on accompanying clinical features rather than any radiographic differences[5,16,31,103,104] (Table 103.2).

There are often concomitant inflammatory changes and resultant ankylosis in the apophyseal joints, and ossification of some of the spinal ligaments. There is involvement of the costovertebral and costotransverse joints, which can gradually result in limitation of chest expansion. Patients with long-standing severe AS ultimately develop a virtually complete fusion of the vertebral column ('bamboo spine'), which often includes the cervical spine (Fig. 103.26). Some patients may develop spondylodiscitis at one or multiple levels in the spine; it causes discovertebral destructive changes (Andersson lesion), a circumscribed aseptic destructive process and sclerosis affecting intervertebral discs and the adjacent bone plates of the vertebral bodies[29,58,105] (Fig. 103.3).

Spinal osteopenia is frequently observed, which increases the risk of vertebral compression and/or transverse spinal fracture and pseudo-

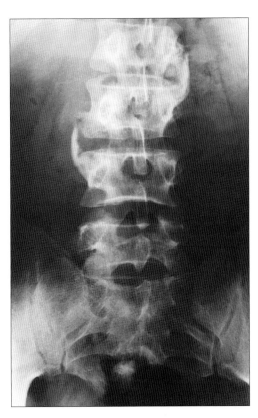

Fig. 103.25 Radiograph of lumbar spine, antero-posterior view, showing bulky, asymmetric non-marginal syndesmophytes in a patient with reactive arthritis. These non-marginal syndesmophytes are identical to those seen in some patients with psoriatic spondylitis, and they can occur in the absence of radiologically ascertainable sacroiliitis. The sacroiliac joints do not show any erosive disease in this patient.

Hip joint involvement has been correlated with early age at onset for AS and is a bad prognostic sign[106] (Fig. 103.4). It leads to symmetric concentric joint space narrowing, irregularity of the subchondral bone plate with subchondral sclerosis, osteophyte formation at the outer margins of the articular surfaces (both the acetabulum and the femoral head) and ultimately bony ankylosis[29]. Shoulder girdle involvement can result in erosions on the superolateral aspect of the humeral head due to erosive enthesitis of the supraspinatus tendon (Fig. 103.5). Involvement of the glenohumeral joint is less common, and it causes concentric joint space narrowing and can lead to bony fusion. There is a relative absence of periarticular osteopenia in the involved hip or shoulder girdles in early stages, as compared to RA. There can be erosive abnormalities or osseous ankylosis of the acromioclavicular joint. Periosteal osseous proliferation leads to a shaggy contour of the marginal bone, and also at sites of bony attachment of ligaments and tendons ('enthesophytes'), such as at the acromial attachment of the acromioclavicular ligament ('bearded acromion')[29].

DIAGNOSIS

The clinical diagnosis of AS depends primarily on the history and physical examination and is confirmed by radiographic examination[5,16,30]. The patient's symptoms, the family history and the articular and extra-articular physical findings offer the best clues to diagnosis. On initial evaluation of a patient, certain features of the patient's history and physical examination raise the index of suspicion, and finding radiographic evidence of bilateral sacroiliitis markedly heightens the probability of AS[16].

It needs to be emphasized, however, that sacroiliitis is not unique to AS and does occur in other spondyloarthropathies. Therefore, although radiography of the pelvis is a useful test for differentiating AS from other causes of back pain, the occurrence of sacroiliitis alone does not necessarily represent definite AS, which requires the added presence of one or more clinical feature(s).

The first internationally accepted classification criteria for AS were proposed in Rome in 1961 and were revised 5 years later in New York, when the presence of radiographic evidence of sacroiliitis was proposed to be necessary for the diagnosis[12,36,107]. These criteria have subsequently been modified[108] (Table 103.3) but there may be a need to further revise them in light of recent progress in our understanding of the broader spectrum of disease. All these criteria greatly depend on the radiographic evidence of sacroiliitis, which is the best non-clinical indicator of the presence of AS. A patient can be classified as having AS if sacroiliitis is associated with at least one clinical criterion, other causes of sacroiliitis having been excluded. These criteria are designed to be highly specific and they may therefore lack sensitivity if used for clinical diagnosis because not all patients with mild or early disease may meet the criteria[9–12,109–113].

The diagnosis of AS is unfortunately often delayed, usually by 5 or more years[109–113]. Some patients may not have any chronic inflammatory low back pain or sacroiliitis at an early stage, when they may present with symptoms resulting from enthesitis or acute iritis[5,24,42]. Others may get intermittent episodes of stiff neck, shoulder pain or chest tenderness[5,16,17]. This is more likely to occur in children/adolescents and women because of an atypical or incomplete clinical picture due to arthritis and/or enthesitis[5,12,25,110–113]. For example, the presenting symptom in some children may be intermittent knee effusions, pain in the groin (hip joint), or painful ankle or foot and resultant limp[23–25]. Some patients may suffer from psoriasis or IBD, or have a family history of these diseases, or of AS and related diseases, including acute iritis. Multiple referrals of such patients for the same complaint often do not result in a correct diagnosis, and during this prolonged diagnostic delay many unnecessary and invasive investigations are performed[5].

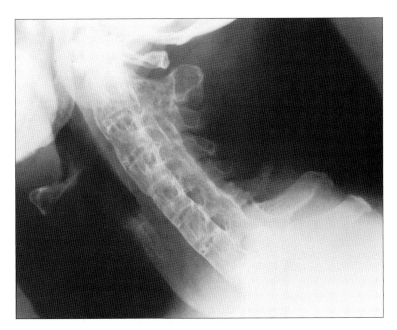

Fig. 103.26 Spinal fusion. Radiograph (lateral view) of the cervical spine showing complete fusion in a patient who had suffered from ankylosing spondylitis for more than 40 years. He later sustained a neck fracture (C6–7 level) after a relatively trivial fall.

arthrosis[56–65]. DXA, quantitative CT and quantitative ultrasound measurements can detect the presence of decreased bone mineral density of the lumbar spine and the femoral neck[57]. However, the presence of marked syndesmophytes in advanced disease may yield normal or increased value for the bone mineral density of the lumbar spine.

Magnetic resonance imaging is important in detecting and evaluating complications of fractures or pseudoarthrosis, as well as changes in the duramater, soft tissue and spinal ligaments[64]. The fractures or pseudoarthrosis give a pattern of either low signal on T1-weighted and high signal on T2-weighted images, or low signal on both T1- and T2-weighted images.

TABLE 103.2 COMPARISON OF ANKYLOSING SPONDYLITIS AND RELATED DISORDERS

Characteristic	Disorder				
	Ankylosing spondylitis	Reactive arthritis	Juvenile spondyloarthropathy	Psoriatic arthropathy*	Enteropathic arthropathy†
Usual age at onset	Young adult age <40	Young to middle-aged adult	Childhood onset, ages 8–16 years	Young to middle-aged adult	Young to middle-aged adult
Sex ratio	Three times more common in males	Predominantly males	Predominantly males	Equally distributed	Equally distributed
Usual type of onset	Gradual	Acute	Variable	Variable	Gradual
Sacroiliitis or spondylitis	Virtually 100%	<50%	<50%	~20%	<20%
Symmetry of sacroiliitis	Symmetric	Asymmetric	Variable	Asymmetric	Symmetric
Peripheral joint involvement	~25%	~90%	~90%	~95%	15–20%
HLA-B27 (in Whites)	~90%	~75%	~85%	<50%‡	~50%‡
Eye involvement§	25–30%	~50%	~20%	~20%	≤15%
Cardiac involvement	1–4%	5–10%	Rare	Rare	Rare
Skin or nail involvement	None	<40%	Uncommon	Virtually 100%	Uncommon
Role of infectious agents as triggers	Unknown	Yes	Unknown	Unknown	Unknown

* About 5–7% of patients with psoriasis deveop arthritis, and psoriatic spondylitis accounts for about 10% of all patients with psoriatic arthritis. † Associated with chronic inflammatory bowel disease. ‡ B27 prevalence is higher in those with spondylitis or sacroiliitis. § Predominantly conjunctivitis in reactive and psoriatic arthritis, and acute anterior uveitis in the other three disorders listed. (Adapted from Arnett et al.[104])

TABLE 103.3 THE MODIFIED NEW YORK CRITERIA FOR AS
1. Low back pain of at least 3 months duration improved by exercise and not relieved by rest
2. Limitation of lumbar spinal motion in sagittal (sideways) and frontal (forward and backward) planes
3. Chest expansion decreased relative to normal values for the same sex and age
4. Bilateral sacroiliitis grade 2–4 *or* unilateral sacroiliitis grade 3 or 4
Definite ankylosing spondylitis is present if criterion 4 *and* any one of the other criteria is fulfilled.

Use of HLA-B27 typing as an aid to diagnosis

The radiographic evidence of sacroiliitis is the best non-clinical indicator of the disease presence. However, the status of the sacroiliac joints on routine pelvic radiographs may not always be easy to interpret in the early phase of the disease, especially in adolescents. There is a place for a less expensive and non-invasive laboratory test in such clinical situations to help minimize the degree of uncertainty of the diagnosis. HLA-B27 typing can be of value in such a situation, or where an unusual or atypical clinical presentation of AS is suspected, or in the diagnosis of early undifferentiated spondyloarthropathy[112,113] (Fig. 103.27).

However, the clinical usefulness of this test may differ appreciably among ethnic and racial groups[2,16,112]. HLA-B27 is present in approximately 8% of the normal white population (of western European extraction) and in more than 90% of patients with 'primary' AS, indicating that HLA-B27 typing as a test for AS is highly specific (100 − 8 = 92%) and also highly sensitive (more than 90%)[5,45,112]. In other words, the test is 8% 'false-positive' (i.e. presence of HLA-B27 is unrelated to the clinical problem) and less than 10% 'false-negative' (i.e. fewer than 10% of patients with 'primary' AS lack HLA-B27). Therefore, as with other clinical tests that are neither 100% sensitive nor 100% specific, the clinical usefulness (predictive value) of HLA-B27 test depends on the clinical situation in which it is ordered[112]. The test is most useful when the physician faces a clinical 'toss-up' situation, i.e. the pretest probability of AS is approximately 0.5, in the presence of equivocal findings on sacroiliac radiography[16,112,113] (Table 103.4).

The clinical usefulness (predictive value) of a positive test result will be highest in those population groups that have a low general prevalence of HLA-B27, and yet HLA-B27 has a strong association with AS in such a population. This is the case among the Japanese; they show a strong association (>85%) of HLA-B27 with AS but this gene is present in less than 1% of the population[112–114]. On the other hand, a positive test result will be relatively less useful among Inuits – in spite of a strong association of HLA-B27 (>90%) with AS – because there is a high prevalence of HLA-B27 (25–40%) in the Inuit population[112–114]. If the HLA-B27 test is ordered in an Inuit patient in whom the pretest probability of AS or a related spondyloarthropathy is very low, and the test result is positive, the probability that the patient has the disease still remains relatively low.

Among African-Americans, on the other hand, HLA-B27 is present in 2–4% of the general population but in only about 50% of AS patients[16,112–114]. Therefore, if the HLA-B27 test were ordered because of a reasonable suspicion of AS ('toss-up' situation), the likelihood of the disease being present would be markedly strengthened by a positive test result. However, a negative test result would not be of value in excluding the disease because 50% of African-American patients with AS lack this gene.

The HLA-B27 test cannot be thought of as a 'routine', 'diagnostic', 'confirmatory' or 'screening' test for AS in patients presenting with back pain or arthritis. As a rule, in those patients in whom history and physical examination suggest AS but whose radiographic findings do not

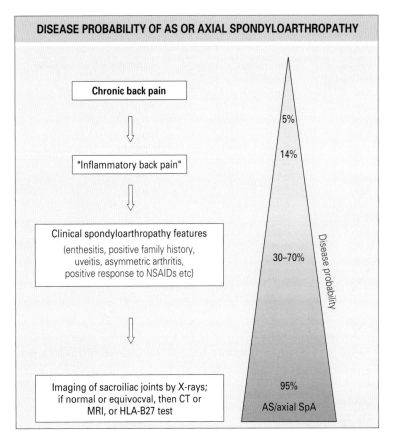

DISEASE PROBABILITY OF AS OR AXIAL SPONDYLOARTHROPATHY

Fig. 103.27 Disease probability of AS or axial spondyloarthropathy. A single clinical feature is not sufficient to make the diagnosis: the more features typical of the disease are present the higher the diagnostic probability. In the typical chronic low back pain population presenting to their primary care physician, presence of at least two of the following four features increases the probability of AS or axial spondyloarthropathy by a factor of three, rising from less than 5% at baseline to more than 14%. These clinical features are: (a) back pain and stiffness every morning that lasts at least 30 minute; (b) symptoms improve with exercise but not with rest; (c) presence of alternating or bilateral buttock pain; and (d) the symptoms interrupt sleep in the early morning hours more so than at other times in the night. Then on top of that, if the patient manifests additional clinical feature(s) (some of them are listed in this figure), the probability of disease presence easily reaches or can even exceed a 'toss-up' clinical situation, i.e. 30–70% range. The diagnosis can be established when radiographic evidence of sacroiliitis is present. However, back pain due to AS often precedes unequivocal radiographic signs of sacroiliitis by several years. Therefore, the status of the sacroiliac joints on a pelvic radiograph may not always be easy to interpret in the early phase of the disease, particularly in adolescent patients. Newer imaging modalities (see text) can help to detect early sacroiliitis in this clinical situation. Alternatively, an early diagnosis of AS or axial spondyloarthropathy can be made with much less uncertainty when test for HLA-B27 is positive in this 'toss-up' situation (Table 103.4), although the diagnosis will be a little presumptive because the criteria for AS (Table 103.3) greatly depend on the radiographic evidence of sacroiliitis, which is the best non-clinical indicator of the disease presence[112,113]. (Courtesy of M Rudwaleit and J Sieper [Adapted with permission]).

permit this diagnosis to be made, the HLA-B27 test may allow the presumptive diagnosis of AS to be accepted or rejected with less uncertainty[112–114]. In patients with back pain or arthritis in whom AS is suggested neither by the history nor by physical examination, HLA-B27 testing is inappropriate because a positive result would still not permit the diagnosis of AS to be made.

An overwhelming majority of patients with AS can be readily diagnosed clinically on the basis of the history, physical examination and radiographic findings, and they do not need to be tested for HLA-B27. Moreover, it does not help to distinguish between AS, reactive arthritis and other spondyloarthropathies, because all these diseases are associated with HLA-B27, although the strength of the association varies

TABLE 103.4 POST-TEST PROBABILITIES OF ANKYLOSING SPONDYLITIS IN WHITES

Pre-test probability	Probability given positive test result	Probability given negative test result
0.01	0.100	0.001
0.05	0.380	0.005
0.10	0.560	0.010
0.20	0.740	0.020
0.30	0.830	0.030
0.40	0.880	0.050
0.50	0.920	0.080
0.60	0.950	0.120
0.70	0.960	0.170
0.80	0.980	0.260
0.90	0.990	0.440
0.95	0.995	0.620
0.99	0.999	0.900

(Adapted from Khan and Khan[112].)

TABLE 103.5 ASSOCIATION OF HLA-B27 AND SPONDYLOARTHROPATHIES (IN WHITES)

Disease	Approximate HLA-B27 prevalence (%)
Ankylosing spondylitis	~90
Reactive arthritis	40–80
Juvenile spondyloarthropathy	~70
Enteropathic spondyloarthritis	35–75
Psoriatic spondyloarthritis	40–50
Undifferentiated spondyloarthropathy	~70
Acute anterior uveitis (acute iritis)	~50
Aortic incompetence with heart block	~80
General healthy population	~8

among them (Table 103.5). Differentiation between these diseases is based primarily on clinical features (Table 103.2).

Although HLA-B27 typing can define the population at higher risk of AS and related spondyloarthropathies, it is of very limited practical value for that purpose because no effective means of prevention are currently available. Moreover, most HLA-B27-positive people in the general population never develop AS or a related disease. HLA-B27 typing may help ophthalmologists to better define a patient presenting with acute uveitis and refer HLA-B27-positive patients for rheumatology consultation, especially those with associated musculoskeletal symptoms, because up to 75% of them have or will develop AS or a related spondyloarthropathy[40,42,43,113].

Familial aggregation of AS and related spondyloarthropathies, acute anterior uveitis, aortic incompetence plus heart block, and hip joint involvement are more common in patients with HLA-B27 and they tend to have a younger age of onset[2,41]. Moreover, the presence of HLA-B27 is associated with the development of more severe and prolonged joint symptoms in reactive arthritis and an increased risk of sacroiliitis and spondylitis. However, knowledge of HLA-B27 status at disease onset is of uncertain value in predicting the patient's long-term prognosis.

HLA-B27 itself is not an allele but a family of at least 26 different alleles – HLA-B*2701 to HLA-B*2725 (there is no B*2722 allele, and B*2705 itself comprises three variants: B*27052, B*27053, B*27054), based on sequence-based typing methods[31,114,115]. These alleles, also called subtypes, differ from each other by one or more amino-acid substitutions, mostly resulting from changes in exons 2 and 3, which encode the α1

and α2 domains, respectively, that from the peptide-binding cleft. Their assignment to the HLA-B27 family is based on nucleotide sequence homology, and nearly all members of the family can by typed by the traditional serologic methods. However, certain subtypes, such as B*2712, B*2715 and B*2723 may show no serological reactions with B27-specific antisera; but they can be detected by polymerase chain reaction sequence-specific primer (PCR-SSP) method updated to enable the detection of all the subtypes, or by sequence-based typing.

The most widely distributed subtype around the world is HLA-B*2705, and it is clearly associated with AS and related spondyloarthropathies except in the west African population of Senegal and Gambia. HLA-B*2704, another strongly disease-associated subtype, is predominant among the Chinese and Japanese[114,115]. Occurrence of AS has been observed in individuals possessing any one of the first 10 relatively more common HLA-B27 subtypes except HLA-B*2706 and HLA-B*2709[116,117]. Disease occurrence has not been studied in most of the remaining subtypes that are all quite rare, but occurrence of AS has been documented in individuals possessing B*2713, B*2714, B*2715 or B*2719. Data from south-east Asia indicate that HLA-B*2706 may not be associated with AS and related spondyloarthropathies, but occurrence of AS has been documented in HLA-B*2706 individuals who also have one of the disease associated subtypes, B*2705 or B*2704[117]. HLA-B*2709, a subtype primarily observed among residents of the island of Sardinia, seems to lack any association with AS among Sardinians, although a few patients with undifferentiated spondyloarthropathy have been reported from the Italian mainland[118,119].

Differential diagnosis

Low back pain with stiffness is the most common presenting symptom in patients with AS, although a variety of other presentations may antedate back symptoms in many patients. However, backache is one of the most common health problems and results from multiple causes, and AS is not its most common cause in the general population[18,19,120]. These various causes may be divided into two main subtypes:

- spondylogenic: traumatic, structural (degenerative and discogenic), inflammatory, metabolic, infective and neoplastic or other bone lesions
- non-spondylogenic: neurologic, vascular, viscerogenic, psychogenic.

Fibromyalgia, which affects 2–4% of women between 20 and 60 years of age, can also cause diagnostic confusion because the primary complaint in some AS patients, especially women, may be fleeting muscle aches and pains or musculotendinous tender areas in the back, fatigue and disturbed sleep. Moreover, just as in many patients with fibromyalgia, these symptoms may become worse on exposure to cold or dampness[33].

The back pain from many of the non-inflammatory spondylogenic causes that can be confused radiologically with AS, particularly in patients with widespread degenerative disc disease (at multiple discovertebral junctions and apophyseal joints) and ankylosing hyperostosis. However, the non-inflammatory type of back pain is generally aggravated by physical activity and relieved by rest. Moreover, there is generally no limitation of chest expansion (corrected for age), the lateral spinal flexion is usually within normal limits and the ESR is frequently normal. The sacroiliac joint radiographs are usually normal or show only mild degenerative changes; the typical bony erosions and marked subchondral sclerosis of sacroiliitis are absent.

The typical osteophytes of severe degenerative disc disease are easily distinguishable from syndesmophytes[21,29] (Fig. 103.24). However, diagnostic confusion can occur in some AS patients who have concomitant degenerative disc disease at the time the syndesmophytes are forming. In some elderly patients with severe degenerative changes of the sacroiliac joint, such as joint space narrowing, subchondral bone sclerosis and

TABLE 103.6 FEATURES DIFFERENTIATING BETWEEN ANKYLOSING HYPEROSTOSIS AND AS

Feature	Ankylosing hyperostosis	Ankylosing spondylitis
Usual age of onset (years)	>50	<40
Thoracolumbar kyphosis	±	++
Limitation of spinal mobility	±	++
Pain	±	++
Limitation of chest expansion	±	++
Radiographic features:		
Hyperostosis	++	+
Sacroiliac joint erosion	– –	++
Sacroiliac joint (synovial) obliteration	±	++
Sacroiliac joint (ligamentous) obliteration	±	++
Apophyseal joint obliteration	– –	++
Anterior longitudinal ligament ossification	++	±
Posterior longitudinal ligament ossification	+	?
Syndesmophytes	– –	++
Enthesopathies (whiskerings) with erosions	– –	++
Enthesopathies (whiskerings) without erosions	++	+

(Adapted from Yagan and Khan[121].)

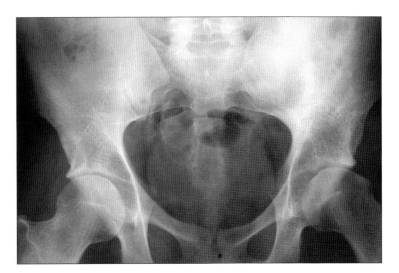

Fig. 103.28 Radiograph of the pelvis (anteroposterior view) of a patient with SAPHO syndrome. Osteitis involving the left sacroiliac joint.

bridging osteophytes in the lower part of the joints may erroneously suggest sacroiliitis on pelvic radiography, but not on CT.

The posture of patients with spinal stenosis may be confused with AS; this condition is usually seen in elderly patients with degenerative disc disease[120]. These patients have varying degrees of pain, worsened by standing erect, walking downhill or lying on the back, and eased by forward stooping or lying on the side with the hip flexed. There is pseudoclaudication, often involving the L4 nerve root, and neurologic findings are variable.

Ankylosing hyperostosis, also called Forestier's disease or diffuse idiopathic skeletal hyperostosis (DISH), usually occurs in elderly individuals and is characterized by hyperostosis affecting the anterior longitudinal ligament and bony attachments of tendons and ligaments; there is no association with HLA-B27[121]. The differentiating features between AS and DISH are listed in Table 103.6. Ossification of the posterior longitudinal ligament has on rare occasion been observed in DISH as well as in AS[122]. Occasionally, severe hyperostotic and degenerative changes of the sacroiliac joints can occur, such as capsular ossifications, joint space narrowing and subchondral bone sclerosis. These changes can give an appearance superficially resembling sacroiliitis or fused sacroiliac joints on the anteroposterior pelvic radiogram. Chronic treatment with retinoids (synthetic derivatives of vitamin A) for skin diseases such as acne and psoriasis can sometimes cause bone abnormalities mimicking spondyloarthropathies or DISH[123]. The sacroiliac joints, however, are typically unaffected.

Osteitis condensans ilii, a self-limiting and often asymptomatic condition that is seen primarily in young multiparous women and shows no association with HLA-B27, should not be confused with sacroiliitis[19,29]. It is characterized by radiographic evidence of a triangular area of dense sclerotic bone adjacent to the lower half of the sacroiliac joints, primarily on the iliac side. The sacroiliac joint itself, however, is normal.

Infections of the spine such as septic (pyogenic) sacroiliitis or disc space infection, tuberculous spondylitis and spondylitis due to brucellosis should not be confused with AS[120,124,125]. Sacroiliac joint changes suggesting sacroiliitis, and even complete fusion of these joints, can sometimes be observed in paraplegics and quadriplegics[126]. The osteoarticular manifestations of sternocostoclavicular hyperostosis and chronic aseptic osteomyelitis, often multifocal and recurrent, sometimes in association with acne conglobata, acne fulminans, hidradenitis suppurativa or palmoplantar pustulosis, can involve several spondyloarthropathic features, especially on long-term follow-up[127,128]. These include anterior chest wall involvement, seronegative asymmetric oligoarthritis and enthesopathies, but sacroiliac joint involvement is primarily unilateral and there is no association with HLA-B27 and no familial aggregation (Fig. 103.28). An eponym, SAPHO syndrome (synovitis–acne–pustulosis–hyperostosis–osteitis), is now being widely used for this clinical condition[127].

Miscellaneous other conditions that might be confused radiographically with AS because of sacroiliac joint abnormalities or syndesmophyte-like appearance of the spine include primary and secondary hyperparathyroidism, dialysis-associated spondyloarthropathy, Scheuermann's disease, congenital kyphoscoliosis, fluorosis, chondrocalcinosis, ochronosis and Paget's disease affecting pelvis or spine[29,120,129,130]. Other causes of back pain include spinal osteoporosis with or without compression fractures and sacral insufficiency fractures, axial osteomalacia, multiple myeloma, metastatic prostate cancer and other malignancies, chronic pelvic inflammatory disease, referred pain from abdominal viscera and retroperitoneal fibrosis[29,120,131,132].

A late-onset undifferentiated spondyloarthropathy syndrome that occurs in men that are over 50 years of age has recently been described[13]. This arthropathy may sometimes resemble the syndrome of remitting seronegative symmetric synovitis with pitting edema (RS3PE). At onset, the patients may show little or no clinical involvement of the axial skeleton, but many of them later develop bilateral sacroiliitis or even go on to develop AS.

The distinction of AS from RA is usually not difficult. Patients with RA usually have polyarthritis that is symmetric in distribution and affects small and large joints of the extremities; involvement of the sacroiliac, apophyseal and costovertebral joints is very rare. In AS, on the other hand, any involvement of peripheral joints (other than hip and shoulder joints) is usually oligoarticular and asymmetric, affecting more often the larger joints of lower extremities; serologic tests for rheumatoid factor are negative; and subcutaneous nodules are absent. There are rare instances of concurrent AS and RA, primarily seen in individuals who have co-inherited the genetic predisposing factors for both diseases, i.e. HLA-B27 for AS and HLA-DR4 for RA.

NATURAL HISTORY

The course of AS is highly variable, with no predictable pattern of progression[6,12,134,135]. It can be characterized by spontaneous remissions and exacerbation, particularly in early disease[2,134]. Daily pain and stiffness generally persist for many decades for most patients, rarely going into long-term remission. However, the outcome can be generally favorable in many patients because the disease may remain relatively mild or limited to the sacroiliac joints and the lumbar spine. Those who have mild disease with only limited spinal involvement maintain good functional ability. Patients with persistent severe disease can get progressive functional impairment associated with spinal fusion, including the cervical spine, and associated kyphosis.

Although the axial disease is more severe in males, the overall pattern seems to be similar in both sexes[6,12,135]. Pregnancy does not improve the symptoms of AS; either no change or only temporary aggravation of activity is observed during pregnancy[135]. Hormonal status, fertility and course of pregnancy and childbirth have been reported to be normal in women with AS.

The clinical assessment of disease activity in patients with AS is difficult, especially in uncomplicated disease confined to the sacroiliac joints and spine. However, the newly developed composite assessment criteria, now known as the WHO/ILAR/OMERACT core set for clinical and functional assessment of AS, have been found to be very useful[36,133] (Table 103.7). They can be used for evaluating therapy with symptom-modifying and disease-controlling antirheumatic drugs and physical therapy, and for clinical record keeping in daily practice. A preliminary definition of short-term improvement in AS has also been published[36]. Moreover, a recently proposed instrument (18 item questionnaire that takes about 4 minutes to complete) for assessing quality of life (ASQoL) provides a valuable tool for assessing the impact of therapeutic interventions for AS.

Disability

Most with AS patients remain gainfully employed, despite having severely restricted spinal mobility[6,137–142]. A recent large study of age- and sex-matched German patients with AS and RA seen at tertiary rheumatological centers shows that they have similar levels of pain and impaired wellbeing, but AS less often leads to early termination of gainful employment[137]. Only 3% of AS patients in one European study were unable to work after 2 decades of disease[138]. The disease in women was somewhat milder, but the patients' self-ratings did not show a more favorable overall outcome because their self-ratings of pain and impaired activities of daily living were worse than those in men[137].

Although it is difficult to predict the ultimate outcome for an individual patient, some factors, particularly occurring during the first 10 years of the disease, are particularly important with respect to subsequent outcome[6,106,135]. Patients with hip joint involvement, who more often have a younger age of onset, or those with a completely ankylosed cervical spine with kyphosis, are more likely to become disabled. The results of total hip arthroplasty in recent years have been very gratifying in preventing partial or total disability in many such patients. Poor response or intolerance to NSAIDs, and the presence of severe extra-articular complications worsen the prognosis. The stage of AS at the time of its diagnosis and initiation of the appropriate therapy, severity of early stages of the disease, the quality of medical management, and the degree of patient compliance with the suggested treatment, also influence the overall prognosis.

A recent American study indicates that functional disability in AS progresses more rapidly in older patients and smokers, and less rapidly in those who have better social support and are able to perform back exercises regularly[141]. In a Norwegian study, cessation of work was associated with low level of education, complete ossification of the spine, acute anterior uveitis, female sex and the co-existence of non-rheumatic diseases[134]. Patients with physically demanding jobs are more likely to change their type of work, decrease their work hours or experience temporary or permanent work disability than those with jobs that are physically less demanding[139]. Functional disability is the most important predictor of total healthcare (direct and indirect).

Disease heterogeneity

There is ample evidence to suggest disease heterogeneity of AS, best exemplified by the difference between the HLA-B27-positive and HLA-B27-negative patients[41,45,114,143]. Even although there are many similarities, generally speaking, HLA-B27-negative AS is somewhat later in its onset, significantly less often complicated by acute anterior uveitis and more frequently accompanied by psoriasis, ulcerative colitis and Crohn's disease, and less often shows familial aggregation[41,45,114,144]. In fact, it is unusual among people of northern European extraction to observe families with two or more first-degree relatives affected with HLA-B27-negative AS in the absence of psoriasis or chronic IBD in the family.

Detailed studies are under way to understand the genetic aspects of susceptibility, severity, and clinical expression in ankylosing spondylitis[114,144]. HLA-B27-positive twins show more than 50% pairwise concordance rate for AS if they are monozygotic versus only 20% if they are dizygotic[2,144]. The ongoing genome-wide studies indicate that, besides HLA-B27 and some additional genes in the MHC region on the short arm of chromosome 6, a few more genes on other chromosomes seem to be involved as well[114,143–146]. Thus it is very likely that several genes may influence susceptibility to AS, and others may influence disease severity and phenotypic expression[144].

Life span

An excess mortality was observed in the past, primarily ascribed to amyloidosis and complications of spinal irradiation (excess malignancies, especially a fivefold increase in leukemias)[147,148]. In subsequent studies an excess mortality was observed among non-irradiated patients seen at tertiary care centers, primarily due to cardiopulmonary causes, but only

TABLE 103.7 ASSESSMENT OF DISEASE ACTIVITY IN PATIENTS WITH AS	
Domain	**Instrument**
Physical function	BASFI *or* Dougados Functional Index
Pain	Visual analog scale (VAS) – last week/spine/ at night/due to AS *and* VAS – last week/spine/ due to AS
Spinal mobility	Chest expansion test *and* modified Schober's test *and* occiput to wall distance test
Patient global	VAS – last week
Stiffness	Duration of morning stiffness – spine/last week
Peripheral joints	Number of swollen joints (44 joint count)
Entheses	No preferred instrument is yet available
Acute phase reactants	ESR
X-ray spine	Anteroposterior + lateral lumbar spine *and* Lateral cervical spine *and* X-ray pelvis (sacroiliac and hip joints)
X-ray pelvis	(see under X-ray spine above)
Fatigue	No preferred instrument is yet available

The SM-ARD/PT core set comprises the following five components: Physical function, Pain, Spinal mobility, Patient global, Stiffness. These components are also included in the other two core sets, i.e. for DC-ART and clinical record keeping. The additional components for clinical record keeping are: Peripheral joints, Entheses, Acute phase reactants. The core set for DC-ART, in addition to the above mentioned eight components, requires: X-ray spine, X-ray pelvis and Fatigue.
Specific instruments for each domain in core sets for symptom-modifying (SM-ARD) and disease controlling antirheumatic drugs (DC-ART), and for physical therapy (PT) and clinical record-keeping.

more than 20 years after their disease diagnosis[149–151]. These studies consisted of patients with disease severe enough to both impel the patients to seek specialized care and to be correctly diagnosed at a time when AS was felt to be a rare disease[150]. It is quite likely that the survival of those patients with mild disease, who form the majority of patients with AS, is comparable to that of the general population. However, spinal fracture, cardiopulmonary involvement, associated medical conditions, including ulcerative colitis and Crohn's disease, as well as complications of medical and surgical treatment, may contribute to premature mortality in some patients.

REFERENCES

1. Moll JMH, ed, Ankylosing spondylitis. Edinburgh: Churchill Livingstone; 1980.
2. Calin A, Taurog J, eds. The spondylarthritides. Oxford: Oxford University Press; 1998.
3. Braun J, Khan MA, Sieper J. Entheses and enthesopathy: what is the target of the immune response. Ann Rheum Dis 2000; 59: 985–994.
4. Feldtkeller E, Lemmel E-M, Russell AS. Ankylosing spondylitis in the pharaohs of ancient Egypt. Rheumatol Int 2003; 23: 1–5.
5. Khan MA. Update on spondyloarthropathies. Ann Intern Med 2002; 135: 896–907.
6. Sieper J, Braun J, Rudwaleit M, Boonen A, Zink A. Ankylosing spondylitis: an overview. Ann Rheum Dis 2002; 61 (Suppl 3): iii 8–iii 18.
7. Geilinger W. Ankylosierenden Spondylitis. Druck Der Union Deutsche Verlagsgesellschaft, Stuttgart, [German Edition] 1917.
8. Khan MA. Five classical clinical papers on ankylosing spondylitis. In Dieppe P, Wollheim FA, Schumacher HR (Eds.). Classical Papers in Rheumatology. Martin Dunitz Ltd., London, 2002, pp. 118–133.7.
9. Braun J, Sieper J (Eds). Spondylitis ankylosans. Unimed Verlag AG, Bremen [German Edition] 2002.
10. Khan MA, van der Linden SM. A wider spectrum of spondyloarthropathies. Semin Arthritis Rheum 1990; 20: 107–113.
11. Khan MA (Ed.): Spondyloarthropathies. Rheum Dis Clin North Am. 1992; 18: 1–276.
12. van der Linden SJ, van der Heijde D. Spondylarthopathies. Ankylosing spondylitis. In: Ruddy S, Harris ED, Sledge CB, (Eds). Kelly's textbook of rheumatology, 6th ed. Philadelphia, PA: WB Saunders; 2000: 1039–1053.
13. Olivieri I, Ciancio G, Pedula A et al. Ankylosing spondylitis and undifferentiated spondyloarthropathies: a clinical review and description of a disease subset with older age at onset. Curr Opin Rheumatol 2001; 13: 280–284.
14. Boyer GS, Templin DW, Bowler A et al. Spondyloarthropathy in the community: clinical syndromes and disease manifestations in Alaskan Eskimo populations. J Rheumatol 1999, 26: 1537–1544.
15. Boyer GS, Templin DW, Bowler A et al. A comparison of patients with spondyloarthropathy seen in specialty clinics with those identified in a community wide epidemiologic study: has the classic case misled us? Arch Intern Med 1997; 157: 2111–2117.
16. Khan MA, Kushner I. Diagnosis of ankylosing spondylitis. In: Cohen AS, ed. Progress in clinical rheumatology 1. Orlando, FL: Grune & Stratton; 1984: 145–178.
17. Van der Linden SM, Khan MA, Rentsch HU et al. Chest pain without radiographic sacroiliitis in relatives of patients with ankylosing spondylitis. J Rheumatol 1988; 15: 836–839.
18. Blackburn WD Jr, Alarcón GS, Ball GV. Evaluation of patients with back pain of suspected inflammatory nature. Am J Med 1988; 85: 766–770.
19. Khan MA. Back and neck pain. In: Fitzgerald F, ed. Current practice of medicine, 2nd ed. Philadelphia, PA: Current Medicine; 1999: 187–203.
20. McGonagle D, Khan MA, Marzo-Ortega H et al. Entheitis in ankylosing spondylitis and related spondyloarthropathies. Curr Opin Rheumatol 1999; 11: 244–250.
21. Khan MA, ed. Ankylosing spondylitis and related spondyloarthropathies. Spine: state of the art reviews. Philadelphia, PA: Hanley & Belfus; 1990.
22. Yu D, ed. Spondyloarthropathies. Rheum Dis Clin North Am 1998; 24: 663–915.
23. Burgos-Vargos R, Vasquez-Mellado J. The early clinical recognition of juvenile-onset ankylosing spondylitis and its differentiation from juvenile rheumatoid arthritis. Arthritis Rheum 1995; 38: 835–844.
24. Rosenberg AM, Petty RE. A syndrome of seronegative enthesopathy and arthropathy in children. Arthritis Rheum 1982; 25: 1041–1047.
25. Cassidy JT, Petty RE, eds. Textbook of pediatric rheumatology, 4th ed, Philadelphia, PA: WB Saunders; 2001.
26. Baek HJ, Shin KC, Lee YJ et al. Juvenile onset ankylosing spondylitis (JAS) has less severe spinal disease course than adult onset ankylosing spondylitis (AAS): clinical comparison between JAS and AAS in Korea. J Rheumatol 2002; 29: 1780–5.
27. Maksymowych W. Ankylosing spondylitis: at the interface of bone and cartilage. J Rheumatol 1999; 27: 2295–2301.
28. François RJ, Braun J, Khan MA. Entheses and enthesitis: a histopathological review and relevance to spondyloarthropathies. Curr Opin Rheumatol 2001; 13: 255–264.
29. Resnick D, Niwayama G. Ankylosing spondylitis. In: Resnick D, ed. Diagnosis of bone and joint disorders. 3rd Edition. Philadelphia: WB Saunders; 1995:1008–74.
30. Braun J, Bollow M, Sieper J. Radiologic diagnosis and pathology of the spondyloarthropathies. Rheum Dis Clin North Am 1998; 24: 697–735.
31. Khan MA: Spondyloarthropathies. In: Hunder G, ed. Atlas of Rheumatology. 3rd Edition. Philadelphia, PA: Current Medicine 2002, pp. 141–167.
32. Aufdermaur M. The morbid anatomy of ankylosing spondylitis. Doc Rheumatol Geigy 1957: 1–70.
33. Challier B, Urlacher F, Vancon G et al. Is quality of life affected by season and weather conditions in ankylosing spondylitis? Clin Exp Rheumatol 2001; 19: 277–281.
34. Hultgren S, Broman JE, Gudbjornsson B et al. Sleep disturbances in outpatients with ankylosing spondylitis: a questionnaire study with gender implications. Scand J Rheumatol 2000; 29: 365–369.
35. Will R, Kennedy G, Elswood J et al. Ankylosing spondylitis and the shoulder: commonly involved but infrequently disabling. J Rheumatol 2000; 27: 177–182.
36. Braun J, van der Heijde D, Dougados M et al. Staging of patients with ankylosing spondylitis: a preliminary proposal. Ann Rheum Dis 2002; 61 (Suppl 3): iii19–iii23.
37. Deyo RA, Jarvik JG. Diagnostic evaluation of low back pain with emphasis on imaging. Ann Intern Med. 2002; 137: 586–597.
38. Blower PW, Griffin AJ. Clinical sacroiliac tests in ankylosing spondylitis and other causes of back pain – 2 studies. Ann Rheum Dis 1984; 43: 192–195.
39. Viitanen JV, Kokko ML, Heikkila S, Kautiainen H. Neck mobility assessment in ankylosing spondylitis: a clinical study of nine measurements including new type methods for cervical rotation and lateral flexion. Br J Rheumatol 1998; 37: 377–381.
40. Banares A. Hernandez-Garcia C, Fernandez-Gutierrez B, Jover JA. Eye involvement in the spondyloarthropathies. Rheum Dis Clin North Am 1998; 24: 771–784.
41. Khan MA, Braun WE, Kushner I. Comparison of clinical features of HLA-B27 positive and negative patients with ankylosing spondylitis. Arthritis Rheum 1977; 20: 909–912.
42. Pato E, Banares A, Jover JA et al. Undiagnosed spondyloarthropathy in patients presenting with anterior uveitis. J Rheumatol 2000; 27: 2198–2202.
43. Smith JR. HLA-B27–associated uveitis. Ophthalmol Clin North Am 2002; 15: 297–307.
44. Uy HS, Christen WG, Foster CS. HLA-B27 associated uveitis and cystoid macular edema. Ocul Immunol Inflamm 2001; 9: 177–183.
45. Feldtkeller E, Khan MA, van der Heijde D, van der Linden S, Braun J. Age at disease onset and diagnosis delay in HLA-B27 negative vs. positive patients with ankylosing spondylitis. Rheumatol Int 2003 in press.
46. Lautermann D, Braun J. Ankylosing spondylitis – cardiac manifestations. Clin Exp Rheumatol 2002; 20 (Suppl. 28) S11–S15.
47. Bergfeldt L. HLA-B27 associated cardiac disease. Ann Intern Med 1997; 127: 621–629.
48. Sun JP, Khan MA, Farhat AZ, Bahler RC: Alterations in cardiac diastolic function in patients with ankylosing spondylitis. Intl J Cardiol 37; 65–72, 1992.
49. Boushea DK, Sundstrom WR. The pleuropulmonary manifestations of ankylosing spondylitis. Semin Arthritis Rheum 1989; 18: 277–281.
50. Turetschek K, Ebner W, Fleischmann D et al. Early pulmonary involvement in ankylosing spondylitis: assessment with thin-section CT. Clin Radiol 2000; 55: 632–636.
51. Casserly IP, Fenlon HM, Breatnac HE, Sant SM. Lung findings on high-resolution computed tomography in idiopathic ankylosing spondylitis. Correlation with clinical findings, pulmonary function testing and plain radiography. Br J Rheumatol 1997; 36: 677–682.
52. De Keyser F, Baeten D, Van Den Bosch F et al. Gut inflammation and spondyloarthropathies. Curr Rheumatol Rep. 2002; 4: 525–532.
53. Baeten D, De Keyser F, Mielants H, Veys EM. Immune linkage between inflammatory bowel and spondyloarthropathies. Curr Opin Rheumatol 2002; 14: 342–347.
54. Palm Oyvind, Moum B, Ongre A, Gran JT. Prevalence of ankylosing spondylitis and other spondyloarthropathies among patients with inflammatory bowel disease: a population study (The IBSEN Study). J Rheumatol 2002; 29: 511–515.
55. Salvarani C, Vlachonikolis IG, van der Heijde DM et al. Musculoskeletal manifestations in a population based cohort of inflammatory bowel disease patients. Scand J Gastroenterol 2001; 36: 1307–1313.
56. Gratacos J, Collado A, Pons F et al. Significant loss of bone mass in patients with early, active ankylosing spondylitis: a followup study. Arthritis Rheum 1999; 42: 2319–2324.
57. Toussirot E, Michel F, Wendling D. Bone density, ultrasound measurement and body composition in early ankylosing spondylitis. Rheumatol 2001; 40: 882–888.
58. Kabaskal Y, Garrett SL, Calin A. The epidemiology of spondylodiscitis in ankylosing spondylitis, a controlled study. Br J Rheumatol 1996; 35: 660–663.
59. Hitchon PW, From AM, Brenton MD, Glaser JA, Torner JC. Fractures of the thoracolumbar spine complicating ankylosing spondylitis. J Neurosurg 2002; 97(2 Suppl): 218–222.
60. Finkelstein JA, Chapman JR, Mirza S. Occult vertebral fractures in ankylosing spondylitis. Spinal Cord 1999; 37: 444–447.
61. Mitra D, Elvins DM, Speden DJ, Collins AJ. The prevalence of vertebral fractures in mild ankylosing spondylitis and their relationship to bone mineral density. Rheumatology (Oxford) 2000; 39: 85–89.
62. Cooper C, Carbone L, Michet CJ et al. Fracture risk in patients with ankylosing spondylitis: a population based study. J Rheumatol 1994; 21: 1877–1882.
63. Resnick D, Williamson S, Alazraki N. Focal spinal abnormalities on bone scans in ankylosing spondylitis: a clue to the presence of fracture or pseudarthrosis. Clin Nucl Med 1995; 6: 213–217.
64. Shih TT, Chen PQ, Li YW, Hsu CY. Spinal fractures and pseudoarthrosis complicating ankylosing spondylitis: MRI manifestation and clinical significance. J Comput Assist Tomogr 2001; 25: 164–170.

65. Tico N, Ramon S, Garcia-Ortun F *et al*. Traumatic spinal cord injury complicating ankylosing spondylitis. Spinal Cord 1998; 36: 349–352.
66. Ramos-Remus C, Gomez-Vargas A, Guzman-Guzman JL *et al*. Frequency of atlantoaxial subluxation and neurologic involvement in patients with ankylosing spondylitis. J Rheumatol 1995; 22: 2120.
67. Thompson GH, Khan MA, Bilenker RM. Spontaneous atlantoaxial subluxation as a presenting manifestation of juvenile ankylosing spondylitis. Spine 1982; 7: 78–79.
68. Little H, Swinson DR, Cruickshank B. Upward subluxation of the axis in ankylosing spondylitis. Am J Med 1976; 60: 279–285.
69. Tullous MW, Skerhut HEI, Story JL *et al*. Cauda equina syndrome of long-standing ankylosing spondylitis. Case report and review of the literature. J Neurosurg 1990; 73: 441–447.
70. Bilgen IG, Yunten N, Ustun EE *et al*. Adhesive arachnoiditis causing cauda equina syndrome in ankylosing spondylitis: CT and MRI demonstration of dural calcification and a dorsal dural diverticulum. Neuroradiology 1999; 41: 508–511.
71. Khan MA, Kushner I. Ankylosing spondylitis and multiple sclerosis: a possible association. Arthritis Rheum 1979; 22: 784–786.
72. Hanrahan PS, Russell AS, McLean DR. Ankylosing spondylitis and multiple sclerosis: an apparent association. J Rheumatol 1988; 15: 1512–1514.
73. Cellerini M, Gabbrielli S, Bongi SM. Cerebral magnetic resonance imaging in a patient with ankylosing spondylitis and multiple sclerosis-like syndrome. Neuroradiology 2001; 43: 1067–1069.
74. Strobel ES. Fritschka E. Renal diseases in ankylosing spondylitis: review of the literature illustrated by case reports. Clin Rheumatol 1998; 17: 524–530.
75. Vilar MJP, Cury SE, Ferraz MB *et al*. Renal abnormalities in ankylosing spondylitis. Scand J Rheumatol 1997; 26: 19–23.
76. Lai KN, Li PKT, Hawkins B, Lai FM-M. IgA nephropathy associated with ankylosing spondylitis: occurrence in women as well as in men. Ann Rheum Dis 1989; 48: 435–437.
77. Gratacos J, Orellana C, Sanmarti R *et al*. Secondary amyloidosis in ankylosing spondylitis: a systematic survey of 137 patients using abdominal fat aspiration. J Rheumatol 1997; 24: 912–925.
78. Ahmed Q, Chung-Park M, Mustafa K, Khan MA. Psoriatic spondyloarthropathy with secondary amyloidosis. J Rheumatol 1996; 23: 1107–1110.
79. Laiho K, Tiitinen S, Kaarela K *et al*. Secondary amyloidosis has decreased in patients with inflammatory joint disease in Finland. Clin Rheumatol 1999; 18: 122–123.
80. Satko SG, Iskandar SS, Appel RG. IgA nephropathy and Reiter's syndrome. Report of two cases and review of the literature. Nephron 2000; 84: 177–182.
81. Mackiewicz A, Khan MA, Reynolds TL *et al*. Serum IgA and acute phase proteins in ankylosing spondylitis. Ann Rheum Dis 1989; 48: 99–103.
82. Scotto di Fazano C, Grilo RM, Vergne P, *et al*. Is the relationship between spondyloarthropathy and Sjogren's syndrome in women coincidental? A study of 13 cases. Joint Bone Spine 2002; 69: 383–387.
83. Brandt J, Rudwaleit M, Eggens U *et al*. Increased frequency of Sjogren's syndrome in patients with spondyloarthropathy. J Rheumatol 1998; 25: 718–724.
84. Padula A, Ciancio G, La Civita L *et al*. Association between vitiligo and spondyloarthritis. J Rheumatol 2001; 28: 313–314.
85. Pazirandeh M, Ziran BH, Khandelwal BK *et al*. Relapsing polychondritis and spondyloarthropathies. J Rheumatol 1988; 15: 630–632.
86. Abouzahir A, El Maghraoui A, Tabache F *et al*. Sarcoidosis and ankylosing spondylitis. A case report and review of the literature. Ann Med Interne (Paris) 2002; 153: 407–10. [Article in French]
87. LeBlanc CM, Inman RD, Dent P *et al*. Retroperitoneal fibrosis: An extra-articular manifestation of ankylosing spondylitis. Arthritis Rheum 2002; 47: 210–214.
88. Bezza A, Maghraoui AE, Ghadouane M *et al*. Idiopathic retroperitoneal fibrosis and ankylosing spondylitis. A new case report. Joint Bone Spine. 2002; 69: 502–505.
89. Ozgocmen S, Kocakoc E, Kiris A, Ardicoglu A, Ardicoglu O. Incidence of varicoceles in patients with ankylosing spondylitis evaluated by physical examination and color duplex sonography. Urology. 2002; 59: 919–922.
90. Bernstein CN, Blanchard JF, Rawsthorne P, Yu N The prevalence of extraintestinal diseases in inflammatory bowel disease: a population based study. Am J Gastroenterol 2001; 96: 1116–1122.
91. Spoorenberg A, van der Heijde D, de Klerk E *et al*. Relative value of erythrocyte sedimentation rate and C-reactive protein in assessment of disease activity in ankylosing spondylitis. J Rheumatol 1999; 26: 980–984.
92. Battistone MJ, Manaster BJ, Reda DJ, Clegg DO. Radiographic diagnosis of sacroiliitis – Are sacroiliac views really better? J Rheumatol 1998; 25: 2395–401.
93. Miron SD, Khan MA, Wiesen E *et al*. The value of quantitative sacroiliac scintigraphy in detection of sacroiliitis. Clin Rheumatol 1983; 2: 407–414.
94. Jevtic V, Kos-Golja M, Rozman B, McCall I. Marginal erosive discovertebral 'Romanus' lesions in ankylosing spondylitis demonstrated by contrast enhanced Gd-DTPA magnetic resonance imaging. Skeletal Radiol 2000; 29: 27–33.
95. Yu W, Feng F, Dion E *et al*. Comparison of radiography, computed tomography and magnetic resonance imaging in the detection of sacroiliitis accompanying ankylosing spondylitis. Skeletal Radiol 1998; 27: 311–320.
96. Bollow M, Braun J, Biedermann T *et al*. Use of contrast-enhanced MR imaging to detect sacroiliitis in children. Skeletal Radiol 1998; 27: 606–616.
97. Khan MA, van der Linden S, Kushner I *et al*. Spondylitic disease without radiographic evidence of sacroiliitis in relatives of HLA-B27 positive ankylosing spondylitis patients. Arthritis Rheum 1985; 28: 40–43.
98. Mau W, Zeidler H, Mau R *et al*. Clinical features and prognosis of patients with possible ankylosing spondylitis: results of a 10 year follow-up. J Rheumatol 1988; 15: 1109–1114.
99. Kumar A, Bansal M, Srivastva DN *et al*. Long-term outcome of undifferentiated spondyloarthropathy. Rheumatol Int 2001; 20: 221–224.
100. Hanly, JG, Mitchell, MJ, Barnes DC *et al*. Early recognition of sacroiliitis by magnetic resonance imaging and computed tomography. J Rheumatol 1994; 21: 2088.
101. Oostveen J, Prevo R, den Boer J, van de Laar M. Early detection of sacroiliitis on magnetic resonance imaging and subsequent development of sacroiliitis on plain radiography. A prospective, longitudinal study. J Rheumatol 1999; 26: 1953–1958.
102. Balint PV, Kane D, Wilson H, McInnes IB, Sturrock RD. Ultrasonography of entheseal insertions in the lower limb in spondyloarthropathy. Ann Rheum Dis. 2002; 61: 905–910.
103. Khan MA. Ankylosing spondylitis: the facts. Oxford University Press, Oxford, UK, 2002; pp. 1–193.
104. Arnett FC, Khan MA, Wilkens RF. Are you missing ankylosing spondylitis? Patient Care 1986; 20: 51–78.
105. Dihlmann W, Delling G. Disco-vertebral destructive lesions (so-called Andersson lesions) associated with ankylosing spondylitis. Skeletal Radiol 1983; 3: 10–16.
106. Amor B, Santos RS, Nahal R *et al*. Predictive factors for the longterm outcome of spondyloarthropathies. J Rheumatol 1994; 21: 1883–1887.
107. Kellgren JH, ed. The epidemiology of chronic rheumatism, vol. II. Oxford: Blackwell Scientific; 1963.
108. van der Linden S, Valkenburg HA, Cats A. Evaluation of diagnostic criteria for ankylosing spondylitis. A proposal for modification of the New York criteria. Arthritis Rheum 1984; 27: 361–367.
109. Kidd BL, Cawley MI. Delay in diagnosis of spondarthritis. Br J Rheumatol 1988; 27: 230–232.
110. Mader R. Atypical clinical presentation of ankylosing spondylitis. Semin Arthritis Rheum 1999; 29: 191–196.
111. Gran JT, Ostensen M. Spondyloarthritides in females. Baillière's Clin Rheumatol 1998; 12: 695–715.
112. Khan MA, Khan MK. Diagnostic value of HLA-B27 testing in ankylosing spondylitis and Reiter's syndrome. Ann Intern Med 1982; 96: 70–76.
113. Khan MA. Thoughts concerning the early diagnosis of ankylosing spondylitis and related diseases. Clin Exp Rheumatol 2002; 20 (Suppl. 28): S6–S10.
114. Khan MA, Ball EJ. Ankylosing spondylitis and genetic aspects. Baillière's Best Pract Res Clin Rheumatol 2002 (in press).
115. Ball E, Khan MA. HLA-B27 polymorphism. Joint Bone Spine 20001; 68: 378–382.
116. Ramos M, De Castro JA. HLA-B27 and the pathogenesis of spondyloarthritis. Tissue Antigens 2002; 60: 191–205.
117. Feltkamp TEW, Mardjuadi A, Huang F, Chou C-T. Spondyloarthropathies in eastern Asia. Curr Opin Rheumatol 2001; 13: 285–290.
118. D'Amato M, Fiorillo MT, Galeazzi M *et al*. Frequency of the new HLA-B*2709 allele in ankylosing spondylitis patients and healthy individuals. Dis Markers 1995; 12: 215–217.
119. Olivieri I, Ciancio G, Padula A *et al*. The HLA-B*2709 subtype confers susceptibility to spondylarthropathy. Arthritis Rheum 2002; 46: 553–554.
120. Deyo RA, Weinstein JN. Low back pain. N Engl J Med 2001; 344: 363–370.
121. Yagan R, Khan MA. Confusion of roentgenographic differential diagnosis of ankylosing hyperostosis (Forestier's disease) and ankylosing spondylitis. Spine: State of the Art Reviews 1990; 4: 561–575.
122. Yagan R, Khan MA, Bellon EM. Spondylitis and posterior longitudinal ligament ossification in the cervical spine. Arthritis Rheum 1983; 26: 226–230.
123. Kaplan G, Haettich B. Rheumatological symptoms due to retinoids. Baillière's Clin Rheumatol 1991; 5: 77–97.
124. Hetem SF, Schils JP. Imaging of infections and inflammatory conditions of the spine. Semin Musculoskeletal Radiol 2000; 4: 329–347.
125. Stabler A, Reiser MF. Imaging of spinal infection. Radiol Clin North Am 2001; 39: 115–135.
126. Khan MA, Kushner I, Freehafer AA. Sacroiliac joint abnormalities in paraplegics. Ann Rheum Dis 1979; 38: 317–319.
127. Kahn M-F, Khan MA. SAPHO syndrome. Baillière's Clin Rheumatol 1994; 8: 333–326.
128. Hayem G, Bouchaud-Chabot A, Benali K *et al*. SAPHO syndrome: a long-term follow-up study of 120 cases. Semin Arthritis Rheum 1999; 29: 159–171.
129. Theodorou DJ, Theodorou SJ, Resnick D. Imaging in dialysis spondyloarthropathy. Semin Dial 2002; 15: 290–6.
130. Wenger DR, Frick SL. Scheuermann kyphosis. Spine 1999; 24: 2630–2639.
131. Nelson AM, Riggs BL, Jowsey JO. Atypical axial osteomalcia: report of four cases with two having features of ankylosing spondylitis. Arthritis Rheum 1978; 21: 715–722.
132. Akkus S, Tamer MN, Yorgancigil H. A case of osteomalacia mimicking ankylosing spondylitis. Rheumatol Int 2001; 20: 239–242.
133. Dougados M, van der Heijde D. Ankylosing spondylitis: how should the disease be assessed? Best Pract Res Clin Rheumatol. 2002; 16: 605–18.
134. Gran JT, Skomsvoll JF. The outcome of ankylosing spondylitis: a study of 100 patients. Br J Rheumatol 1997; 36: 766–771.
135. Ostensen M, Ostensen H. Ankylosing spondylitis – the female aspect. J Rheumatol 1998; 25: 120–124.
136. Doward LC, Spoorenberg A, Cook SA *et al*. Development of the ASQoL: a quality of life instrument specific to ankylosing spondylitis. Ann Rheum Dis 2003; 62: 20–26.
137. Zink A, Braun J, Listing J, Wollenhaupt J. Disability and handicap in rheumatoid arthritis and ankylosing spondylitis–results from the German Rheumatological database. J Rheumatol 2000; 27: 613–622.
138. Boonen A, de Vet H, van der Heijde D, van der Linden S. Work status and its determinants among patients with ankylosing spondylitis. A systematic literature review. J Rheumatol 2001; 28: 1056–1062.
139. Ward MM, Kuzis S. Risk factors for work disability in patients with ankylosing spondylitis. J Rheumatol 2001; 28: 315–321.
140. Chorus AM, Boonen A, Miedema H, van der Linden S. Employment perspective in patients with ankylosing spondylitis. Ann Rheum Dis 2002; 61: 693–699.
141. Ward MM. Predictors of the progression of functional disability in patients with ankylosing spondylitis. J Rheumatol 2002; 29: 1420–1425.

142. Boonen A, Severens JL. Ankylosing spondylitis: what is the cost to society, and can it be reduced? Best Pract Res Clin Rheumatol 2002; 16: 691–705.

143. Lopez-Larrea C, Mijiyawa M, Gonzalez S *et al.* Association of ankylosing spondylitis with HLA-B*3403 in a West African population. Arthritis Rheum 2002; 46: 2968–2971.

144. Brown MA, Crane AM, Wordsworth BP. Genetic aspects of susceptibility, severity, and clinical expression in ankylosing spondylitis. Curr Opin Rheumatol 2002; 14: 355–360.

145. Brown MA, Wordsworth BP, Reveille JD. Genetics of ankylosing spondylitis. Clin Exp Rheumatol 2002; 20(Suppl. 28): S43–S49.

146. Laval SH, Timms A, Edwards S *et al.* Whole-genome screening in ankylosing spondylitis: evidence of non-MHC genetic-susceptibility loci. Am J Hum Genet 2001; 68: 916–926.

147. Kaprove RE, Little AH, Graham DC, Rosen PS. Ankylosing spondylitis. Survival in men with and without radiotherapy. Arthritis Rheum 1980; 23: 57–61.

148. Smith PG, Doll R. Mortality among patients with ankylosing spondylitis after a single treatment course with x-rays. Br Med J 1982; 284: 449–460.

149. Lehtinen K. Cause of death in 79 patients with ankylosing spondylitis. J Rheumatol 1980; 9: 145–147.

150. Khan MA, Khan MK, Kushner I. Survival among patients with ankylosing spondylitis: a life-table analysis. J Rheumatol 1981; 8: 86–90.

151. Braun J, Pincus T. Mortality, course of disease and prognosis of patients with ankylosing spondylitis. Clin Exp Rheumatol 2002; 20(Suppl. 28): S16–S22.

104 Etiology and pathogenesis of ankylosing spondylitis

Walter P Maksymowych

- Subchondral bone marrow inflammation in the sacroiliac joints and at peripheral sites adjacent to certain entheses is a characteristic histopathologic feature

- Inflammation has a predilection for fibrocartilaginous sites rich in aggrecans and type II collagen

- Population variance is largely explained by genetic factors, most likely oligogenic, which may also influence disease severity and phenotype

- Human leukocyte antigen (HLA)-B27 is directly involved in the pathogenesis of disease and acts in a permissive manner, although it contributes only 20–30% of the entire genetic risk

- Certain B27 subtypes, B2706 and B2709, may be only weakly disease-associated and differ from disease-associated subtypes, B2705 and B2704, in their ability to bind peptides with different C-terminal amino acid residues, favoring the arthritogenic peptide hypothesis of disease

- Additional HLA loci, B60 and DRB1 0101 in whites and B39 in Japanese, and non-HLA loci on chromosome 22, specifically the cytochrome P450 *CYP2D6* gene, and on chromosome 2, have been associated with disease, although contributions of individual non-HLA loci are weak

- A high level of B27 expression on bone marrow derived cells, CD4+ and CD8+ T cells, specific non-MHC genes, certain B27-bound peptides and intestinal bacteria are required for development of disease in B27-transgenic rats

- A propensity for B27 to misfold, to form homodimers through pairing of cysteine residues at position 67 and to participate in signal transduction events are additional specific aspects of B27 biology that may be related to disease

- The association with intestinal inflammation reinforces the importance of exposure to intestinal bacteria, which may lead to altered processing of the B27 molecule and alterations in the B27-bound peptide repertoire

- Impaired Th1 cytokine expression is typical in ankylosing spondylitis (AS), in both peripheral blood and colonic lamina propria, whereas expression of tumor necrosis factor (TNF)-α in sacroiliac joints and the description of a TNF-α-overexpressing mouse transgenic model of spondylitis highlight the pathophysiologic role of this cytokine in causing inflammation.

INTRODUCTION

Ankylosing spondylitis (AS) and other human leukocyte antigen (HLA)-B27 associated forms of arthritis (e.g. reactive arthritis) constitute a relatively common group of arthritides (spondyloarthropathies) that affect up to 2% of white individuals. There is marked geographic variation in both the prevalence and the phenotypic manifestations. Pathologic hallmarks include sacroiliitis, enthesopathic lesions and specific extra-articular lesions such as acute anterior uveitis. Concomitant lesions that

may precede the development of AS include inflammatory bowel disease and psoriasis. There is a predilection for males, and disease onset is typically in the third and fourth decades of life, although it may present in juveniles, either with asymmetric involvement of large joints in the lower limbs or a syndrome of enthesopathy and involvement of the tarsal joints. Epidemiologic and familial data have established a strong disease association with the HLA class I antigen, B27, but also suggest that additional genes modify both susceptibility to AS and the phenotypic expression of disease. Other studies have highlighted the important role of intestinal bacteria, both invasive and commensal, and of mucosal inflammation in the pathogenesis of disease. Considerable progress has also been made in our understanding of immunologic effector mechanisms perpetuating chronic inflammation, which has led to major advances in treatment. This chapter will discuss the current state of knowledge regarding the pathogenesis of AS in the context of several broad themes that address the nature and evolution of the target lesion, the association with B27 and other genetic factors, the pathophysiologic role of B27, the consequences of host encounter with bacteria and the nature of immunologic effector mechanisms that drive chronic inflammation.

EVOLUTION OF THE PRIMARY LESION

Histopathologic studies

Detailed histopathologic studies of articular lesions in early disease are limited and primarily describe the findings in the sacroiliac and hip joints. Early case reports described central erosion of the femoral head,

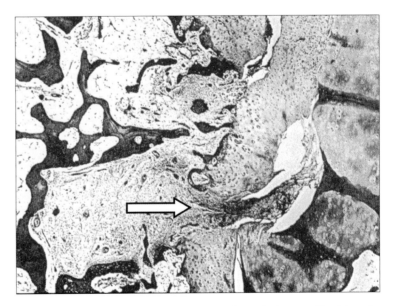

Fig. 104.1 Coronal histopathological section through the sacroiliac joint of a patient with ankylosing spondylitis, demonstrating subchondral granulation tissue (arrow) eroding through the iliac cartilage into the joint cavity. (With permission from Schichikawa *et al.*[1])

acetabular erosion, denuded articular cartilage and penetration of the calcified zone of cartilage by vascular fibrous tissue originating from subchondral bone marrow. Examination of the sacroiliac joints has also revealed subchondral granulation tissue eroding through the joint cartilage into the joint cavity (Fig. 104.1). Schichikawa et al.[1] described five patients with disease duration varying from 10 to 32 months who underwent open biopsy of the sacroiliac joints. Granulation tissue in subchondral bone marrow was noted in all the patients, with iliac cartilage being replaced by fibrous tissue. A more recent study compared sacroiliac joint biopsies from 12 cases of AS with those from 22 autopsy specimens studied as controls[2]. Prominent and early features included synovitis and subchondral bone marrow inflammation; later features included widespread destruction of cartilage and subchondral bone. Enthesitis did not appear to be prominent at any stage of disease. Histopathologic evidence for marrow inflammation has also been found in the os ischium and vertebral body.

Similar observations have now been recorded at peripheral sites of involvement in AS. Examination of biopsy specimens of the cruciate ligament enthesis in the knee and the vastus lateralis attachment to the femur obtained at arthroplasty from patients with spondyloarthropathies, rheumatoid arthritis (RA) and osteoarthritis controls has revealed that the presence of subchondral bone marrow inflammation and infiltration with CD8+ T cells and macrophages was confined to patients with spondyloarthropathy[3].

Imaging studies

Novel techniques in magnetic resonance imaging (MRI) have demonstrated that subchondral edema is an early pathologic finding in sacroiliitis, consistent with histopathologic reports. In particular, the introduction of fat-suppressed MRI sequences allows the detection of bone marrow edema that is usually obscured by marrow fat in conventional MRI (Fig. 104.2). Several reports have now described subchon-

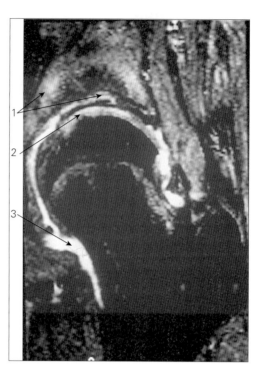

Fig. 104.3 Coronal T1-weighted gradient echo magnetic resonance image with gadolinium augmentation of the left hip of a 19-year-old man with sacroiliitis and a 3-year history of left groin pain. Gadolinium uptake is seen in: the acetabulum (1), the subchondral region of the femoral head (2) and the synovium (3).

dral edema on MRI of sacroiliac joints in patients with inflammatory low back pain, but normal or only suspicious changes of sacroiliitis on plain radiography[4]. Furthermore, MRI of juveniles with arthritis has shown sacroiliitis, primarily consisting of capsulitis and subchondral bone marrow edema, in 10% of those who were HLA-B27-positive and had synovitis of the hips, knees, or both, despite the absence of back symptoms. These observations have been verified using an additional refinement of MRI, namely dynamic imaging with gadolinium augmentation[5]. Gadolinium accumulates at sites of increased vascular permeability and the rate and degree of augmentation can be quantified, thereby providing several measures of the severity of inflammation (Fig. 104.3). Correlation has been documented between clinical variables of disease activity, histopathologic severity of inflammation and degree of gadolinium augmentation noted on MRI.

As for peripheral sites, fat suppression MRI of knee joints from individuals attending a clinic for patients with early arthritis has shown enthesitis with adjacent bone marrow edema in those patients who ultimately developed spondyloarthropathy rather than RA[6].

Candidate target lesion(s)

These observations raise the question as to why the characteristic propensity is for inflammatory lesions in axial joints and certain entheses (e.g. tendo Achillis). Furthermore, what might constitute the primary target antigen(s), for the development of extra-articular manifestations (e.g. acute anterior uveitis, aortitis) and the extensive osteitis and adjacent enthesopathy?

Anatomical predilection

The peculiar predilection for disease in fibrocartilaginous sites such as the symphysis pubis, the manubriosternal junction and the intervertebral discs, is widely accepted and led several investigators to conclude, several decades ago, that the primary pathologic site affected in AS is, in fact, cartilage. Fibrocartilage is also found in the root and wall of the aorta, in addition to the central fibrous body of the heart. Furthermore, immunologic cross-reactivity has been demonstrated between molecules within cartilage and those in both the anterior uvea and the media of arterial vessels. Detailed anatomic evaluation of entheses has revealed two anatomical categories:

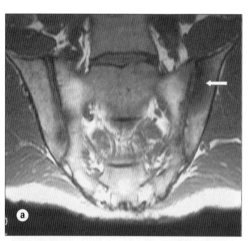

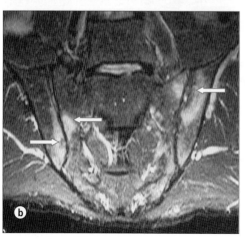

Fig. 104.2 MRI of sacroiliac joints of 31-year-old patient with ankylosing spondylitis. (a) Coronal T1-weighted MRI section demonstrates diffuse erosion of the upper half of the iliac side of the left sacroiliac joint (arrow). Bilaterally, subtle erosion is present inferiorly. Intense inflammation is associated with loss of marrow fat signal around the erosions. (b) Coronal T2 STIR MRI of same patient as in 1a. Fat signal from bone marrow is suppressed with this MRI technique allowing water associated with marrow inflammation to be detected as a white signal on a dark background. The STIR sequence demonstrates high intensity signal typical of bone marrow edema/inflammation which is more extensive in distribution but otherwise corresponds to the findings on T1 images (arrows).

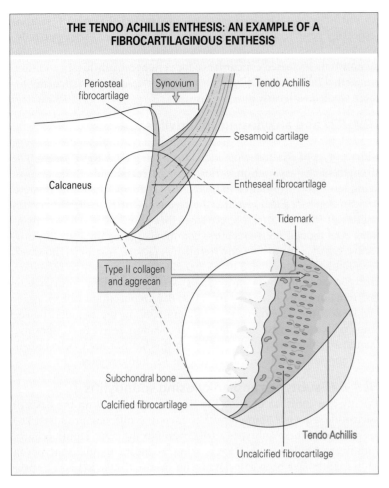

THE TENDO ACHILLIS ENTHESIS: AN EXAMPLE OF A FIBROCARTILAGINOUS ENTHESIS

Fig. 104.4 **The tendo Achillis enthesis: an example of a fibrocartilaginous enthesis.**

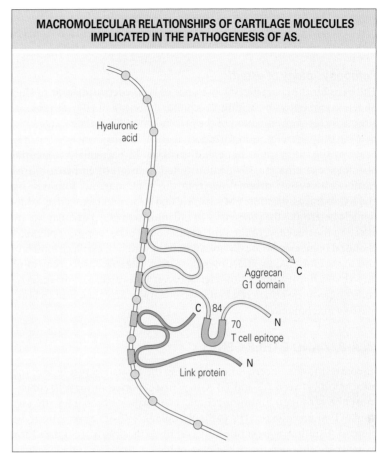

MACROMOLECULAR RELATIONSHIPS OF CARTILAGE MOLECULES IMPLICATED IN THE PATHOGENESIS OF AS.

Fig. 104.5 **Macromolecular relationships of cartilage molecules implicated in the pathogenesis of AS.** Development of T cell immunity to a certain epitope of aggrecan (residues 70–84) is associated with joint inflammation in Balb/c mice[8].

1. Fibrous entheses, which attach to metaphyses or diaphyses, do not contain fibrocartilage, and do not appear to be inflamed in AS (e.g. deltoid attachment to the humerus)
2. Fibrocartilaginous entheses attach to the epiphyses of long or short bones (e.g. tendo Achillis enthesis) and fibrocartilage is found at several sites within this complex structure (Fig. 104.4). In addition, fibrocartilage may be found where tendons wrap around bony or fibrous pulleys and are subject to compression (e.g. peroneus longus tendon within the cuboid groove). At these sites, the adjacent bone will also contain a layer of fibrocartilage – the periosteal fibrocartilage (e.g. the plantar aspect of the cuboid). Sesamoid fibrocartilage is found on the deep surface of tendons and protects tendons from compressive forces on adjacent bone. The transitional zone at the site of attachment of enthesis to bone includes fibrous connective tissue continuous with the tendon and a layer of uncalcified fibrocartilage separated by the tidemark from calcified fibrocartilage that sits on top of subchondral bone (Fig. 104.4). Immunohistochemical and biochemical examination of human tendo Achillis has shown that aggrecan, the major proteoglycan found in cartilage, and type II collagen are almost exclusively confined to the fibrocartilaginous portion of the enthesis.

Target antigen(s): animal models

Several animal models of spondyloarthropathies have been developed on the basis of the induction of autoimmunity to antigens present in cartilage and fibrous tissue. These include a murine model of polyarthritis and spondylitis that resembles human AS. In this model, humoral and cellular immunity to aggrecan is induced in Balb/c mice after immunization with fetal human cartilage proteoglycan[7]. Adult or bovine cartilage proteoglycans can also be used, provided the keratan sulfate side chains have been removed (the side chains may impair T cell responses by decreasing antigen uptake or antigenic processing in antigen-presenting cells). Passive transfer from arthritic to naïve mice requires both CD4+ T and B cells[8]. Immunization with either the isolated G1 globular domain of aggrecan or the link protein that interacts with aggrecan and hyaluronic acid (Fig. 104.5) can also induce polyarthritis and spondylitis. Immunization with versicans, a proteoglycan containing a G1 domain found in the intervertebral disc and produced by smooth muscle cells in arterial vessel walls and by osteoblasts, induces sacroiliitis and spondylitis without peripheral arthritis.

An ossifying enthesopathy, particularly involving the tendo Achillis and the patellar tendon, can be induced in Wistar Furth rats after immunization with native human fetal type II collagen and muramyl dipeptide[9]. These animals also develop spondylodiscitis, with early lesions involving the angles of the vertebral plates, reminiscent of the Romanus lesion of AS, ultimately leading to syndesmophytes. However, there are no inflammatory lesions in the sacroiliac joints, anterior chamber of the eye or the heart, and immunity to collagen has been described in RA in addition to AS.

Target antigen(s): human studies

Cellular immunity to both proteoglycan and link protein has been reported in patients with AS and, to a lesser extent, in those with RA[10]. Conversely, cellular and humoral immunity to type II collagen have been observed more commonly in RA and much less so in AS. A specific CD4+ T cell response to the G1 domain of aggrecan has also been demonstrated in AS, in both peripheral blood and synovial fluid, by enumerating activated T cells with intracellular staining for gamma interferon (IFNγ) and tumor necrosis factor (TNF-α) after exposure to antigen. The demonstration of similar T cell responses in RA suggests that cellular immunity to these antigens may reflect cartilage damage, with exposure of neoantigens.

Pathophysiology of osteitis

The basis for the characteristic presence of bone edema adjacent to sites of active enthesitis and within subchondral bone is unclear at present, although recent examination of the rat tendo Achillis enthesis suggests a mechanism whereby immunization against cartilage antigen(s) may occur at the interface of bone and cartilage. In particular, sequential histologic examination has demonstrated invasion of entheseal fibrocartilage by vessels originating from the bone marrow, followed by endochondral ossification[11]. Mechanical and structural factors may additionally determine the propensity to inflammation at a particular site by affecting the thickness of the subchondral bony plate. For example, subchondral bone may be locally absent both in vertebral cartilage endplate and at certain tendon attachments, so that marrow spaces may abut directly on fibrocartilage. Contact between fibrocartilaginous antigens and antigen-presenting cells in the bone marrow may then lead to bone marrow inflammation.

HLA-B27 AND OTHER GENES

In contrast to the uncertainties regarding the primary target lesion, the association between AS and HLA-B27, first reported in 1973[12,13], constitutes the strongest immunogenetic association observed with any human immune disease. The pathophysiologic role of B27 remains to be defined. Familial aggregation of cases of AS has been recognized for many years, although the risk of developing AS decreases dramatically in increasingly distantly related individuals. Recurrence–risk modeling in relatives of patients with AS suggests an oligogenic model, with three to nine genes operating in addition to B27[14]. The degree of clustering can be estimated by the risk ratio, λ (frequency of disease in relatives divided by the disease frequency in the general population). In AS, the sibling recurrence risk (λ_S) is greater than 50 in AS. A large study of twins in the UK has described disease concordance of 75% in identical twins, compared with 13% in non-identical twins[15]. This study also suggests that 97% of the population variance can be explained by additive genetic effects. Furthermore, this work suggests that any environmental influences are likely to be ubiquitous, in that most of the population is exposed to the environmental trigger(s) and, hence, is non-contributory to population variance. In contrast, there appears to be a high degree of concordance for calendar year of disease onset, but discordance for age at onset, suggesting that environmental factors have a greater role in the timing of disease onset than do genetic factors. Genetic factors may play a more important part in influencing disease severity, affected sibling pairs having closer scores for disability, pain and radiological damage than expected. There is also increasing evidence for at least two distinct AS phenotypes, so that patients with extra-articular manifestations (especially peripheral arthritis, enthesitis and psoriasis) segregate independently from those without these manifestations. Twin studies also demonstrate increased concordance for peripheral arthritis. In addition, a maternal influence on disease risk has been described, particularly for those women with early onset of disease.

HLA-B27 and ankylosing spondylitis

The risk for AS in HLA-B27-positive individuals is of the order of 2–5%, with 90–95% of affected white individuals being HLA-B27-positive. The strength of the association varies amongst racial and ethnic groups, being less evident in native Indonesians, Lebanese, Thais and Western African Blacks[16]. Furthermore, the frequency of HLA-B27 in certain regions of Western Africa approaches that observed in white populations even though AS is much less common, arguing for a role for protective genetic, or possibly environmental, factors. In general, however, the population prevalence of AS parallels the frequency of HLA-B27. Only 60–80% of those individuals with concomitant psoriasis or inflammatory bowel disease carry HLA-B27, implicating a role for genes involved in the development of inflammation in the skin and bowel. Some evidence suggests that disease may be more severe in B27-positive than in B27-negative patients, although this has not been well studied. There appears to be no increased risk for B27 homozygotes.

HLA-B27 subtypes and ankylosing spondylitis

Twenty-five subtypes of HLA-B27 have been assigned on the basis of nucleotide sequence homology; they encode 23 different products. The prevalence of these subtypes varies amongst different ethnic groups, with B*2705, followed by B*2702, being the most common subtypes in whites. Both have been associated with disease (Table 104.1). The predominant subtype in Asia among the Chinese and Japanese is B*2704, whereas B*2706 is generally the most common subtype in other Asians. B*2704 is clearly associated with disease, and B*2706 may be neutral or weakly associated[17]. B*2703 occurs in Western Africa, and although it does not appear to be associated with disease, there appears to be no increased risk for B*2705 individuals, either. B*2709 has been primarily observed among Sardinians and does not seem to be associated with AS[18]. Because of the rarity of the remaining subtypes, there are insufficient epidemiological data to address potential disease associations.

Determination of the crystal structure of HLA B*2705 and characterization of the peptide binding properties of B*2705 and other subtypes suggest a mechanism for the B27 disease association (Fig. 104.6). Analysis of the B27 antigen binding groove has focused on the associated pockets (A to F), which accommodate the side chains and amino and carboxyl terminals of the bound peptide. This has shown that the B pocket (or '45' pocket), highlighted by the position 45 glutamine residue at the apex of the pocket, is conserved between the various B27 subtypes

TABLE 104.1 GEOGRAPHIC/ETHNIC DISTRIBUTION OF HLA-B27 SUBTYPES THAT HAVE BEEN EXAMINED FOR THEIR ASSOCIATION WITH ANKYLOSING SPONDYLITIS		
HLA-B27 subtype	**Ethnic/geographic distribution**	**Disease association**
B*2702	Semitic, Iberian, Northern European	Yes
B*2703	Western Africa	? Non-associated*
B*2704	Chinese, Japanese	Yes
B*2705	Worldwide (especially circumpolar regions)	Yes
B*2706	Asia	Non-associated
B*2707	India, Europe	Yes
B*2709	Sardinia	Non-associated
* Detailed epidemiological data are lacking.		

TABLE 104.2 *HLA-B27* SUBTYPE AMINO ACID SEQUENCE VARIATIONS

	HLA-B27 alpha 1 domain amino acid variations							*HLA-B27* alpha 2 domain amino acid variations														
	59	63	67	69	70	71	74	77	80	81	82	83	94	95	97	103	113	114	116	131	152	163
B*2705	Tyr	Glu	Cys	Ala	Lys	Ala	Asp	Asp	Thr	Leu	Leu	Arg	Thr	Leu	Asn	Val	Tyr	His	Asp	Ser	Val	Glu
B*2701	–	–	–	–	–	–	Tyr	Asn	–	Ala	–	–	–	–	–	–	–	–	–	–	–	–
B*2702	–	–	–	–	–	–	–	Asn	Ile	Ala	–	–	–	–	–	–	–	–	–	–	–	–
B*2703	His	–	–	–	–	–	–	–	–	–	–	–	–	–	–	–	–	–	–	–	–	–
B*2704	–	–	–	–	–	–	–	Ser	–	–	–	–	–	–	–	–	–	–	–	–	Glu	–
B*2706	–	–	–	–	–	–	–	Ser	–	–	–	–	–	–	–	–	Asp	Tyr	–	–	Glu	–
B*2707	–	–	–	–	–	–	–	–	–	–	–	–	–	–	Ser	–	His	Asp	Tyr	Arg	–	–
B*2708	–	–	–	–	–	–	–	Ser	Asn	–	Arg	Gly	–	–	–	–	–	–	–	–	–	–
B*2709	–	–	–	–	–	–	–	–	–	–	–	–	–	–	–	–	–	–	His	–	–	–

and yet differs from most other HLA B molecules[20]. Most naturally bound peptides eluted from *B27* share an arginine at position 2 that interacts with the position 45 glutamine in the B pocket[21]. These observations suggest that the B pocket may convey specificity for the binding of a putative arthritogenic peptide(s). In addition, both non-disease-associated subtypes, B*2709 and B*2706, differ from the disease-associated B*2705 subtype at position 116, located in the F pocket, which binds the peptide C-terminal amino acid (Table 104.2 & Fig. 104.6). This alters the binding specificity of *B27*, in addition to cytotoxic T cell recognition. B*2709 does not bind peptides with C-terminal arginine or tyrosine, indicating that sites other than the B pocket may also influence the binding of an arthritogenic peptide(s). One study has shown that differential peptide binding affinity for a self epitope, vasoactive intestinal peptide receptor 1, between B*2705 and B*2709 was associated with CD8+ T cell autoreactivity for that epitope that correlated with disease[22]. Although the role of this particular self epitope in disease remains speculative, this observation reinforces the paradigm favoring the involvement of an arthritogenic peptide(s) in disease pathogenesis.

Non-B27 *HLA* genes and ankylosing spondylitis

Population studies and examination of families with several affected members have implicated *HLA-B60* in risk for disease in *B27*-positive individuals[23], although this is not evident in non-white individuals. An increased risk associated with *B39* has been observed in the Japanese, in whom the prevalence of *B27* is low. This has not been demonstrated in white patients. Interestingly, *HLA-B39* shares the same amino acid residues that make up the B pocket in *B27*, and is capable of binding the same peptides.

Genome-wide screening has demonstrated an extensive region of linkage with disease within the *HLA* region, suggesting that this may reflect the presence of extended *HLA* haplotypes containing two or more genes relevant to disease susceptibility. Several groups have examined polymorphisms in the *TNFα* gene located within the *HLA* class III region, 250kb centromeric to the *HLA* class I region (Fig. 104.7). The *TNFα* locus polymorphisms investigated include several promoter polymorphisms and five microsatellite genetic markers. The most frequently studied have been the two G/A nucleotide substitutions at positions −308 and −238 relative to the transcriptional start site. A significant decrease in the rare A allele at position −308 has been found in patients with AS from Germany and Scotland, but not in three other populations[24]. Differences in ancestral *HLA* haplotypes could account for the population differences observed with these polymorphisms, reflecting linkage disequilibrium with another disease-associated *HLA* allele.

Several reports have examined the major histocompatibility complex (MHC) class I chain related genes A and B (*MICA* and *MICB*), which are located centromeric to HLA-B and telomeric to the *TNFα* locus

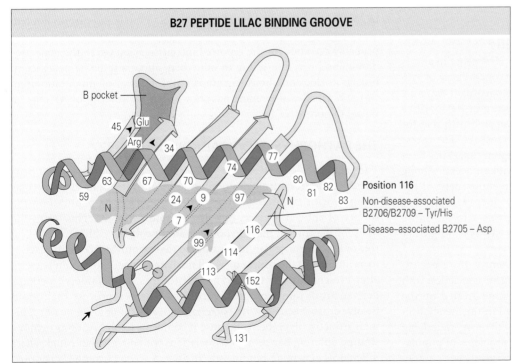

B27 PEPTIDE LILAC BINDING GROOVE

Fig. 104.6 The HLA B27 peptide-binding groove, with peptide. The amino acid residue at position 116 distinguishes disease-associated (B*2705) from non-associated (B*2706/B*2709) *B27* subtypes. (Modified with permission from Maksymowych[19].)

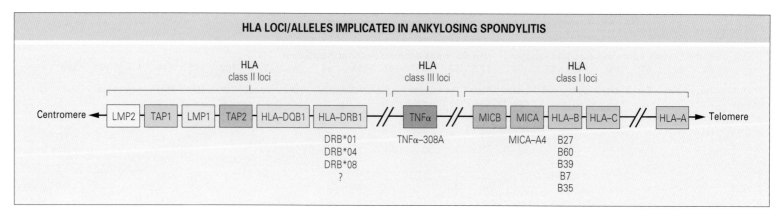

Fig. 104.7 HLA loci/alleles implicated in ankylosing spondylitis.

(Fig. 104.7). *MICA* resembles other HLA class I molecules with respect to overall structure and is highly polymorphic, being expressed primarily on fibroblasts and epithelial cells. In general, no *B27*-independent associations have been described. However, one *MICA* allele (*MICA* 008), which is in linkage disequilibrium with B*2706, carries a frameshift mutation in the transmembrane segment that could cause the production of a truncated secreted product. In addition, an increased frequency of the *MICA-A4* allele has been noted in *B27*-negative patients from Sardinia.

A large case–control study of HLA class II associations in white patients in the UK has demonstrated a weak but significantly increased risk associated with *HLA DRB1*01* and *HLA DRB1*08* alleles, independent of *B27*[25]. An additional locus at or near *DRB1* has also been implicated using linkage analysis and genome-wide screening by the North American AS gene consortium. Other work has examined the potential contribution of *HLA* class II genes involved in antigen processing and transport. These are located centromeric to *HLA DQ* and include two genes (*LMP2* and *LMP7*) that encode IFNγ-inducible subunits of the proteasome (a multicatalytic proteinase that degrades cytoplasmic proteins into peptides) and two genes (*TAP1* and *TAP2*) that encode peptide transporters (which transfer peptides from the cytoplasm into the endoplasmic reticulum for binding to *HLA* class I molecules). Associations between polymorphisms in these genes and disease have not been consistently reported.

Non-HLA genes and ankylosing spondylitis

There is strong evidence to support the role of non-*HLA* genes in ankylosing spondylitis. First, there is an increased disease concordance of 75% in identical twins, compared with 27% in *HLA-B27*-concordant dizygotic twins. Secondly, there is an increased risk for disease in *B27*-positive first-degree relatives of AS probands (10–20%) compared with that for *B27*-positive individuals in the general population (2–5%)[26]. The excess recurrence in sibs that is attributable to the *HLA* region (λ_{HLA}) has been estimated at 5.2 by linkage analysis, as compared with an overall sibling recurrence:risk ratio (λ_S) of 82[27]. In contrast, the component of the increased risk in siblings attributable to non-*HLA* loci ($\lambda_{non-HLA}$) has been estimated at 14, which is approximately equivalent to the entire genetic component of insulin-dependent diabetes (λ_S=15) and greater than that for RA (λ_S=6) (Table 104.3).

Case–control studies have been largely inconsistent with respect to non-*HLA* markers aside from two reports describing an association with polymorphism in the cytochrome P450 *CYP2D6* gene located on the long arm of chromosome 22[28]. This gene is involved in the metabolism of a variety of drugs and chemicals, although the mechanism underlying this association is not understood. To address the problems of population stratification inherent to case–control studies, several gene consortia have undertaken whole-genome screens on multicase families, using microsatellite markers to identify potential regions linked to AS. Non-*HLA* regions showing 'suggestive' or stronger linkage with disease have been reported on chromosomes 1p, 2q, 9q, 10q, 16q and 19q, although contributions of individual loci are weak ($\lambda<1.9$)[27]. The most consistent linkage has been noted with markers on chromosome 2q. Loci on chromosome 16q have also demonstrated linkage with inflammatory bowel disease, although these loci are in a region distinct from that implicated in AS. The power to detect linkage to genes of moderate effect is limited, requiring large numbers of families and affected sib-pairs, and this most probably accounts for the reported inconsistencies. Given the male predominance, it is interesting to note there appears to be no evidence of linkage to loci on the X chromosome for genes of moderate effect (≥ 1.5)[29]. Finally, one report has shown that the severity of AS may be linked to non-*MHC* loci[30].

THE PATHOPHYSIOLOGICAL ROLE OF HLA-B27

The primary role of HLA class I molecules, such as B27, is to bind peptides, derived from proteolysis of intracellular proteins, in a trimolecular complex with β_2-microglobulin and to present these peptides on the surface of antigen-presenting cells to cytotoxic T cells. This forms the basis for the current main hypothesis addressing the pathophysiological role of B27. In particular, it is proposed that cytotoxic T cell autoreactivity is induced in the course of T cell mediated defence to certain bacteria after presentation by B27 of an arthritogenic self peptide(s), perhaps derived from joint/entheseal cartilage. This is a process that could involve cross-reactivity with bacterial-derived peptides (Fig. 104.8). This is an attractive hypothesis, because it conforms to observations demonstrating differing B27 subtype associations with disease that could reflect differences in peptide-binding specificities. A second hypothesis has pro-

TABLE 104.3 CONTRIBUTION OF GENETIC RISK FACTORS TO PREDISPOSITION FOR AS IN COMPARISON WITH OTHER GENETIC DISEASES

Risk factor	Risk ratio (λ)*
AS in sibling	82
Total HLA contribution	5.2
Total non-HLA contribution	14
Individual non-HLA loci	<1.9
RA in sibling	6
Diabetes in sibling	15

*Frequency of disease in siblings divided by disease frequency in the general population

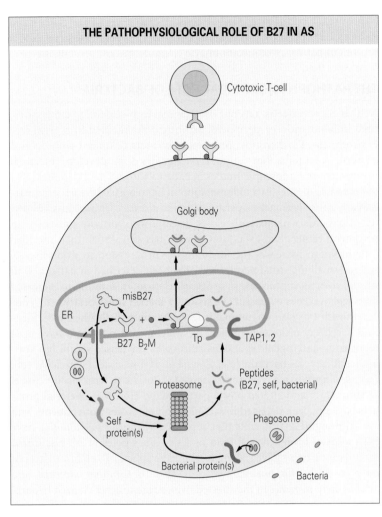

THE PATHOPHYSIOLOGICAL ROLE OF B27 IN AS

Fig. 104.8 The pathophysiological role of B27 in AS. An altered host–pathogen interaction is associated with aberrant antigenic processing of self protein(s), which could include B27 itself after misfolding of the heavy chain (misB27) and retrograde transport from the endoplasmic reticulum (ER). B27-restricted presentation of an arthritogenic self peptide(s) may trigger activation of cytotoxic T cells through cross-reactivity with a bacterial peptide(s). β_2m, β_2-microglobulin; TAP1,2, transporters associated with peptide transport; Tp, tapaisin.

posed that peptides derived from B27 itself may be 'arthritogenic' when presented by B27 to cytotoxic T cells or on class II molecules to CD4$^+$ T cells[31]. A third hypothesis proposes that the B27 molecule has additional specific biologic properties, unrelated to antigen presentation, that promote inflammation on exposure to pathophysiologic stimuli. Several animal models have explored these hypotheses.

B27-transgenic animal models

The development of the human *HLA-B27*-transgenic rat model has increased our understanding of the direct role of *B27* in disease pathogenesis. These animals develop chronic intestinal inflammation similar to Crohn's disease at 16 weeks of age, followed by axial and peripheral arthritis in 70% of animals by 20 weeks[32]. As in humans, disease is more commonly observed, and is particularly severe, in males. Disease expression is related to high *B27* copy number, does not require a thymus, but does require T cells and *B27* expression on a bone marrow derived cell (Fig. 104.9). Adoptive transfer experiments in nude mice indicate that disease can be transferred with CD4$^+$ T cells, but not thymus-derived CD8$^+$ T cells. However, depletion of extrathymically derived CD8$^+$ T cells by administration of an anti-CD8α monoclonal antibody does ameliorate disease. Impaired antigen-presenting function of dendritic cells in disease-prone animals has also been described, despite normal cell surface expression of molecules important for T cell activation. The importance of multiple non-*B27* genes is highlighted by the abrogation of disease when animals are back-crossed onto a DA strain genetic background. Animals maintained in a germ-free environment do not develop either colitis or arthritis until introduced into the normal laboratory environment[33].

Mutation of the cysteine residue with serine at position 67, which constitutes part of the B pocket, and subsequent transgene expression of the mutant B27 molecule in rats leads to a substantially decreased incidence of arthritis. In addition, breeding of *B27*-transgenic rats with rats transgenic for a B27-binding influenza nucleoprotein-derived peptide results in alteration of the B27-bound peptide repertoire, with displacement of 90% of endogenous B27-bound peptides by the influenza peptide and a marked decrease in the incidence of arthritis[33]. These data are consistent with the notion that the unique structural characteristics of the B pocket convey specificity for the binding of a putative arthritogenic peptide.

The introduction of the human *B27* transgene with or without the human β_2-microglobulin gene into a β_2-microglobulin-knockout mouse also results in the development of peripheral arthritis, primarily in

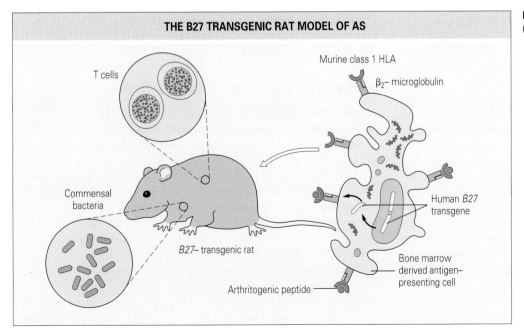

THE B27 TRANSGENIC RAT MODEL OF AS

Fig. 104.9 The B27 transgenic rat model of AS.
(Modified with permission from Maksymowych[19].)

males[34]. This can occur in the absence of class II molecules, requires the class I heavy-chain $\alpha 1$ and $\alpha 2$ antigen-binding domains, and can be ameliorated by a monoclonal antibody to the class I heavy chain. Animals maintained in a barrier facility do not develop disease until transferred to conventional housing. The apparent absence of surface B27 expression casts doubt on the role of cytotoxic T cells in disease pathogenesis. However, the B27 heavy chain alone can be efficiently recognized by B27-allospecific cytotoxic T cells, suggesting that the class I restricted antigen presentation capability of B27 is not severely compromised without β_2-microglobulin. When these mice are exposed to a synthetic B27-binding peptide there is a decreased incidence of disease, consistent with a role for a B27-bound arthritogenic peptide. B27 heavy chains can form a disulfide-bonded homodimer, requiring the cysteine residue at position 67, that can bind peptide[35]. This may allow antigen presentation in the absence of β_2-microglobulin. The precise role of B27 in disease pathogenesis in this particular experimental model is uncertain, however, in view of the fact that other class I molecules expressed as transgenes in the β_2-microglobulin-knockout mouse may also precipitate peripheral arthritis with a frequency similar to that of B27.

HLA-B27: an autoantigen

The polymorphic region of B27 spanning residues 169–179 demonstrates homology with bacterial proteins and is one of the endogenous peptides presented *in vivo* by B27 in B27-transfected lymphoblastoid cell lines[36,37]. However, this epitope is equally bound by disease-associated (B2705, B2704) and non-associated (B2706) B27 subtypes, raising doubts as to its relevance to disease. Peripheral blood T cell reactivity to B27-derived synthetic peptides has been preferentially observed in B27-positive patients with AS as compared with controls, but this is associated with the expansion of γ/δ T cells. These cells may have a regulatory rather than a primary pathogenic role in disease.

HLA-B27 biology unrelated to antigen presentation

Normal folding of the B27 molecule is dependent on its association with β_2-microglobulin and peptide. Tapaisin is an endoplasmic reticulum resident protein that facilitates peptide loading of class I molecules after transport of peptides (mediated by the transporter of antigenic peptides, TAP) from the cytoplasm (Fig. 104.8). B27 may differ from other class I molecules in being less dependent on tapaisin for peptide loading and may then bind certain peptides rather weakly through a tapaisin-independent pathway, rendering these B27 molecules unstable and, therefore, liable to misfold. Mutational and peptide binding analyses of the B27 antigen-binding pocket suggest that the propensity of B27 to misfold as compared with other class I molecules is dependent on its unique structural properties[38]. Misfolding of B27 may in turn lead to accumulation of B27 heavy chains in the endoplasmic reticulum, triggering a stress response and activation of a variety of genes, including those for transcriptional factors (e.g. nuclear factor κB) that activate various proinflammatory cytokines (e.g. interleukin (IL)-1 and TNF-α). Alternatively, misfolded B27 molecules may be transported in a retrograde fashion out of the endoplasmic reticulum to the cytoplasm, where they are degraded by cytoplasmic proteasomes (Fig. 104.8). This represents the most likely mechanism whereby peptides derived from B27 are generated *in vivo*, as noted in B27-transfected lymphoblastoid cell lines. Misfolded B27 heavy chains may also form homodimers by pairing of cysteine residues at position 67, which may then present neoantigens. Although these properties are likely to be relevant in animals expressing high copy numbers of *B27* or deficient in β_2-microglobulin, these phenomena have yet to be demonstrated in human disease.

Finally, there is evidence that B27 can participate in signal transduction events involving a serine residue in the cytoplasmic domain.

Exposure of cultured epithelial cells (HeLa) to invasive *Salmonella* induces B27-specific expression of *c-fos*, a rapid response gene, and a proinflammatory cytokine, monocyte chemoattractant protein-1[39].

THE PATHOPHYSIOLOGICAL ROLE OF BACTERIA

Neither B27-transgenic rats nor B27-transgenic mice develop either intestinal inflammation or peripheral arthritis if maintained in a germ-free environment. Furthermore, only transgenic rats colonized with defined bacterial cocktails that contain *Bacteroides* spp. develop intestinal inflammation. Endoscopic studies in patients with AS have demonstrated the presence of intestinal inflammation in up to 60% of the patients, particularly those with active peripheral joint disease[40]. Prospective follow-up of patients with juvenile onset disease, who initially present with peripheral rather than axial joint disease, has also shown that intestinal inflammation increases the likelihood of progression to axial disease. Altered small intestinal permeability has been described in patients with AS and their asymptomatic first-degree relatives, in addition to increased numbers of B cells expressing CD45Ro+, a marker for memory cells, consistent with exposure to luminally derived antigens[41]. Furthermore, identical T cell expansions in the colonic mucosa and synovium have been reported in enterogenic spondyloarthropathy. Increased serum IgA antibodies to several bacteria (e.g. *Klebsiella pneumoniae*, *Escherichia coli*, *Proteus mirabilis*) have been observed, consistent with occult bowel inflammation and altered bowel permeability. However, bacterial products have not been detected in sacroiliac joint biopsies from patients with AS. Although CD4+ T cells that recognize *Klebsiella pneumoniae* have been derived from synovial fluid in active AS, studies in AS-discordant monozygotic twins have shown decreased peripheral T cell reactivity, not only to *Klebsiella pneumoniae*, but also to *Candida albicans* and *Streptococcus pyogenes* in the affected twin, suggesting generalized hyporesponsiveness to common bacterial antigens[42]. Furthermore, HLA-B27-restricted CD8+ T cells with specificity for bacterial antigen have not yet been observed in AS, in contrast to reactive arthritis. The precise role of bacteria, therefore, remains to be determined.

Several consequences of bacterial invasion of cultured cell lines have been described, including alternative processing of B27 associated with removal of the transmembrane segment and secretion of soluble B27, decreased expression of serological B27 epitopes on the cell surface as detected by peptide-dependent monoclonal antibodies, upregulation of the IFNγ-inducible proteasome subunits, LMP2, LMP7 and PA28, and alterations in the B27-bound peptide repertoire[43]. These observations provide circumstantial evidence for an effect of bacteria on modulation of B27-restricted antigen presentation, particularly self antigen(s), in keeping with the finding of autoreactive B27-restricted CD8+ T cell clones in AS synovial fluid.

IMMUNOLOGICAL EFFECTOR MECHANISMS

Immunohistological analyses of computed tomography-guided synovial biopsies from sacroiliac joints of patients with AS with relatively short disease duration (mean 4.6 years) have revealed the presence of macrophages, CD4+ and CD8+ T cells, and mRNA for TNF-α but not for IL-1β[44]. Similar results for cellular infiltrates have been reported in immunohistologic analyses of peripheral joint synovium, with the addition of large numbers of plasma cells. Data analyzing cytokine expression in peripheral synovium of patients with AS are lacking, however, and reports describing a Th2 cytokine profile primarily include patients with reactive arthritis. The pathophysiologic significance of excess TNF-α is highlighted in the phenotype of a transgenic mouse model in which overexpression of TNF-α occurs as a consequence of a deletion in the 3′ regulatory region of a murine TNF-α transgene that controls translation of TNF protein. This results in a form of spondylitis resembling human disease. In addition, several uncontrolled and controlled studies have now reported significant efficacy of anti-TNF-α treatments in patients with AS.

Examination of peripheral blood T cells has shown decreased numbers of T cells staining for the Th1 cytokines, IL-2 and IFNγ, in addition to decreased TNF-α^+ T cells in both patients with AS and B27-positive healthy controls, as compared with B27-negative controls[45]. Conversely, the percentage of IL-10$^+$/CD8$^+$ T cells is greater in patients with AS than in B27-positive or -negative controls, whereas there are no differences for the Th2 cytokine, IL-4. Similar findings are evident in colonic lamina propria lymphocytes from patients with AS compared with controls, indicating that AS is characterized by impaired Th1 cytokine responses. Treatments directed against TNF-α restore normal Th1 responses, commensurate with clinical improvement and consistent with prior observations that persistently high concentrations of TNF-α impair T cell production of IL-2 and IFNγ. The impaired Th1 cytokine response is also likely to be of pathophysiologic significance, because this may be associated with impaired T cell defence against bacteria, particularly in the gut, leading to chronic inflammation, autoimmunity, or both.

FUTURE PERSPECTIVES

International collaborations are needed to facilitate the large-scale collection of family data required for the discovery of additional regions in the human genome harboring disease-associated genes. In addition, further mapping of the human genome with single nucleotide polymorphisms spaced once per 1000 nucleotides, together with high-throughput DNA genotyping methodologies, will allow further refinement of regions of interest, with fewer families and by analyses of unrelated populations. Increasing characterization of gene-coding regions with the availability of expressed sequence tag databases and the sequence of the human genome will ultimately lead to a more realistic approach to candidate gene analysis. The availability of the increasingly sophisticated imaging technologies that are required for early diagnosis, together with the availability of microchip gene expression technologies and tools for proteomic analysis, will allow more detailed dissection of pathophysiologic pathways relevant to disease. Finally, greater understanding of the rules determining antigenic processing *in vivo*, the availability of sensitive ELISPOT and B27 tetramer technology and the information obtained from candidate gene studies will lead to a more realistic examination of candidate disease antigens and CTL reactivity in vivo.

REFERENCES

1. Schichikawa K, Tsyimoto M, Nishioka J et al. Histopathology of early sacroiliitis and enthesitis in ankylosing spondylitis. In: Ziff M, Cohen SB, eds. Advances in inflammation research, vol 9: the spondyloarthropathies. New York: Raven Press; 1985: 15–24.
2. Francois RJ, Gardner DL, Degrave EJ, Bywaters EGL. Histopathologic evidence that sacroiliitis in ankylosing sondylitis is not merely enthesitis. Arthritis Rheum 2000; 43: 2011–1124.
3. Laloux L, Voisin M-C, Allain J et al. Immunohistological study of entheses in spondyloathropathies: comparison in rheumatoid arthritis and osteoarthritis. Ann Rheum Dis 2001; 60: 316–321.
4. Oostveen J, Prevo R, den Boer J, van de Laar M. Early detection of sacroiliitis on magnetic resonance imaging and subsequent development of sacroiliitis on plain radiography. A prospective, longitudinal study. J Rheumatol 1999; 26: 1953–1958.
5. Braun J, Bollow M, Eggens U et al. Use of dynamic magnetic resonance imaging with fast imaging in the detection of early and advanced sacroiliitis in spondyloarthropathy patients. Arthritis Rheum 1994; 37: 1039–1045.
6. McGonagle D, Gibbon W, O'Connor P et al. Characteristic magnetic resonance imaging entheseal changes of knee synovitis in spondyloarthropathy. Arthritis Rheum 1998; 41: 694–700.
7. Glant T, Mikecz K, Arzoumanian A, Poole AR. Proteoglycan-induced arthritis in Balb/c mice. Arthritis Rheum 1987; 30: 201–212.
8. Zhang Y, Guerassimov A, Leroux JY et al. Arthritis induced by proteoglycan aggrecan G1 domain in BALB/c mice. Evidence for T cell involvement and the immunosuppressive influence of keratan sulfate on recognition of T and B cell epitopes. J Clin Invest 1998; 101: 1678–1686.
9. Gillet P, Bannwarth B, Charriere G et al. Studies on Type II collagen induced arthritis in rats: an experimental model of peripheral and axial ossifying enthesopathy. J Rheumatol 1989; 16: 721–728.
10. Mikecz K, Arzoumanian A, Poole AR. Isolation of proteoglycan-specific T lymphocytes from patients with ankylosing spondylitis. Cell Immunol 1988; 112: 55–63.
11. Benjamin M, Rufai A, Ralphs JR. The mechanism of formation of bony spurs (enthesophytes) in the achilles tendon. Arthritis Rheum 2000; 43: 576–583.
12. Brewerton DA, Hart FD, Nicholls A et al. Ankylosing spondylitis and HL-A 27. Lancet 1973; 1: 904–907.
13. Schlosstein L, Terasaki PI, Bluestone R, Pearson CM. High association of an HL-A antigen, W27, with ankylosing spondylitis. N Engl J Med 1973; 288: 704–706.
14. Brown MA, Laval SH, Brophy S, Calin A. Recurrence risk modeling of the genetic susceptibility to ankylosing spondylitis. Ann Rheum Dis 2000; 59: 268–270.
15. Brown MA, Kennedy LG, MacGregor AJ et al. Susceptibility to ankylosing spondylitis in twins: the role of genes, HLA, and the environment. Arthritis Rheum 1997; 40: 1823–1828.
16. Lau CS, Burgos-Vargas R, Louthrenoo W et al. Features of spondyloarthritis worldwide. Rheum Dis Clin North Am 1998; 24: 753–770.
17. Gonzalez-Roces S, Alvarez MV, Gonzalez S et al. HLA-B27 and worldwide susceptibility to ankylosing spondylitis. Tissue Antigens 1997; 49: 116–123.
18. D'Amato M, Fiorillo MT, Carcassi C et al. Relevance of residue 116 of HLA-B27 in determining susceptibility to ankylosing spondylitis. Eur J Immunol 1995; 25: 3199–3201.
19. Maksymowych WP. Ankylosing spondylitis. In: Tannenbaum H, Russell AS, eds. Mechanisms in rheumatology. Concord, Ontario: Core Health Services; 2001: 87–92.
20. Bjorkman PJ, Parham P. Structure, function, and diversity of class I major histocompatibility complex molecules. Ann Rev Biochem 1990; 59: 253–288.
21. Jardetzky TS, Lane WS, Robinson RA et al. Identification of self peptides bound to purified HLA-B27. Nature 1991; 353: 326–329.
22. Fiorillo MT, Maragno M, Butler R et al. CD8$^+$ T cell autoreactivity to an HLA B27-restricted self-epitope correlates with ankylosing spondylitis. J Clin Invest 2000; 106: 47–53.
23. Robinson WP, van der Linden SM, Khan MA et al. HLA-Bw60 increases susceptibility to ankylosing spondylitis in HLA-B27+ patients. Arthritis Rheum 1989; 32: 1135–1141.
24. Rudwaleit M, Hohler T. Cytokine gene polymorphisms relevant for the spondyloarthropathies. Curr Opin Rheumatol 2001; 13: 250–254.
25. Brown MA, Kennedy LG, Darke C et al. The effect of HLA-DR genes on susceptibility to and severity of ankylosing spondylitis. Arthritis Rheum 1998; 41: 460–465.
26. Calin A, Marder A, Becks E, Burns T. Genetic differences between B27 positive patients with ankylosing spondylitis and B27 positive healthy controls. Arthritis Rheum 1983; 26: 1460–1464.
27. Laval SH, Timms A, Edwards S et al. Whole-genome screening in ankylosing spondylitis: evidence of non-MHC genetic-susceptibility loci. Am J Hum Genet 2001; 68: 918–926.
28. Brown MA, Edwards S, Hoyle E et al. Polymorphisms of the CYP2D6 gene increase susceptibility to ankylosing spondylitis. Hum Mol Genet 2000; 9: 1563–1566.
29. Hoyle E, Laval SH, Calin A et al. The X-chromosome and susceptibility to ankylosing spondylitis. Arthritis Rheum 2000; 43: 1353–1355.
30. Hamersma J, Cardon LR, Bradbury L et al. Is disease severity in ankylosing spondylitis genetically determined? Arthritis Rheum 2001; 44: 1396–1400.
31. Sieper J, Braun J. Pathogenesis of spondyloarthropathies. Persistent bacterial antigen, autoimmunity, or both? Arthritis Rheum 1995; 38: 1547–1554.
32. Hammer RE, Maika SD, Richardson JA et al. Spontaneous inflammatory disease in transgenic rats expressing HLA-B27 and human beta 2m: an animal model of HLA-B27-associated human disorders. Cell 1990; 63: 1099–1112.
33. Taurog JD, Richardson JA, Croft JT et al. The germfree state prevents development of gut and joint inflammatory disease in HLA-B27 transgenic rats. J Exp Med 1994; 180: 2359–2364.
34. Zhou M, Sayad A, Simmons WA et al.The specificity of peptides bound to human histocompatibility leukocyte antigen HLA-B27 influences the prevalence of arthritis in HLA-B27 transgenic rats. J Exp Med 1998; 188: 877–886.
35. Khare SD, Luthra HS, David CS. Spontaneous inflammatory arthritis in HLA-B27 transgenic mice lacking beta 2-microglobulin: a model of human spondyloarthropathies. J Exp Med 1995; 182: 1153–1158.
36. Allen R, O'Callaghan CA, McMichael AJ, Bowness P. HLA-B27 can form a novel β_2-microglobulin-free heavy chain homodimer structure. J Immunol 1999; 162: 5045–5048.
37. Schofield H, Kurien B, Gross T et al. HLA-B27 binding of peptide from its own sequence and similar peptides from bacteria: implications for spondyloarthropathies. Lancet 1995; 345: 1542–1544.
38. Boisgerault F, Tieng V, Stolzenberg MC et al. Differences in endogenous peptides presented by HLA-B*2705 and B*2703 allelic variants. Implications for susceptibility to spondyloarthropathies. J Clin Invest 1998; 98: 2764–2770.
39. Mear JP, Schreiber KL, Munz C et al. Misfolding of HLA-B27 as a result of its B pocket suggests a novel mechanism for its role in susceptibility to spondyloarthropathies. J Immunol 1999; 163: 6665–6670.

40. Ikawa T, Ikeda M, Yamaguchi A *et al*. Expression of arthritis-causing HLA-B27 on HeLa cells promotes induction of *c-fos* in response to *in vitro* invasion by *Salmonella typhimurium*. J Clin Invest 1998; 101: 263–272.

41. Mielants H, Veys EM, Goemaere S *et al*. Gut inflammation in the spondyloarthropathies: clinical, radiologic, biologic and genetic features in relation to the type of histology. A prospective study. J Rheumatol 1991; 18: 1542–1551.

42. Vaile JH, Meddings JB, Yacyshyn BR *et al*. Bowel permeability and CD45Ro expression on circulating CD20+ B cells in patients with ankylosing spondylitis and their relatives. J Rheumatol 1999; 26: 128–135.

43. Hohler T, Hug R, Schneider PM *et al*. Ankylosing spondylitis in monozygotic twins: studies on immunological parameters. Ann Rheum Dis 1999; 58: 435–440.

44. Maksymowych WP, Kane K. Bacterial modulation of antigen processing and presentation. Microbes Infect 2000; 2: 199–211.

45. Braun J, Bollow M, Neure L *et al*. Use of immunohistologic and in situ hybridization techniques in the examination of sacroiliac joint biopsy specimens from patients with ankylosing spondylitis. Arthritis Rheum 1995; 38: 499–505.

46. Rudwaleit M, Siegert S, Yin Z *et al*. Low T cell production of TNFα and IFNγ in ankylosing spondylitis: its relation to HLA-B27 and influence of the TNF–308 gene polymorphism. Ann Rheum Dis 2000; 60: 36–42.

105 Seronegative spondyloarthropathies: imaging

David C Salonen and Anne C Brower

- The radiographic hallmarks of the spondyloarthropathies include normal bone mineralization, erosion, periostitis and bone proliferation at entheses
- The spondyloarthropathies may be separated from each other by the extent of erosions and bone proliferation, together with their distribution and symmetry of involvement
- Ankylosing spondylitis – bilateral symmetrical involvement of sacroiliac joints with early ankylosis, squaring of vertebral bodies, symmetric syndesmophytes and peripheral involvement of shoulders and hips
- Reactive arthritis – bilateral asymmetrical sacroiliac involvement, bulky asymmetrical paravertebral ossification and typical involvement of lower extremity joints
- Psoriatic arthritis – spinal and sacroiliac changes similar to reactive arthritis and common involvement of wrists, hands, feet and shoulders

INTRODUCTION

The seronegative spondyloarthropathies are a group of inflammatory arthritides that include ankylosing spondylitis, psoriatic arthritis, reactive arthritis and the enteropathic arthropathies. They share common clinical, laboratory and radiographic features. The radiographic hallmarks common to all spondyloarthropathies are normal mineralization, erosion, bone proliferation and spinal and sacroiliac involvement.

While they share radiographic features with rheumatoid arthritis (RA), the radiographic differences are sufficient to separate them into a distinct category of arthritis[1-4]. The fundamental differences between RA and the seronegative spondyloarthropathies lie in the distribution of the disease and the morphologic changes observed around a specific joint. While RA affects primarily synovial joints, the seronegative spondyloarthropathies affect not just the synovial joints but also the fibrocartilaginous joints and the entheses, or sites of attachment of tendons, ligaments and capsules (see Chapter 106). Further, the seronegative spondyloarthropathies commonly involve the axial system which, except for the cervical spine is rarely involved in RA. The single most important radiographic change that distinguishes seronegative spondyloarthropathies from RA, however, is the presence of bone proliferation. The latter is manifested as bone excrescences adjacent to erosions, bone proliferation at entheses, periostitis and bone ankylosis[5].

Multiple imaging modalities are available to evaluate the spondyloarthropathies. These include conventional radiography, conventional tomography, bone scintigraphy, computed tomography (CT), ultrasound and magnetic resonance imaging (MRI). The appropriate imaging modality must be chosen for accurate evaluation of the joint involved.

IMAGING THE SACROILIAC JOINT

The sacroiliac joint is perhaps the most difficult joint in the body to image. This is because of its complex anatomy and undulating articular surfaces. Conventional radiographs are the first-line imaging approach to the diagnosis and progression of disease. Accurate interpretation requires the expertise of interested radiologists. CT has become more frequently used, as the presence of erosions may be more easily detected in routine clinical practice. Conventional tomography and bone scintigraphy are useful adjuncts. The role of MRI of the sacroiliac joint has increased over the last decade.

Conventional radiography
Technique
The true synovial component of the sacroiliac joint is the anterior inferior one-half to two-thirds. This area is best imaged on a modified Ferguson view[6] (Fig. 105.1). The patient is placed in a supine position and, when possible, the knees and hips are flexed. The X-ray tube is centered at L5/S1 and then angled 25–30° towards the head. If the tube is angled too steeply, the pubic symphysis will overlie the anterior inferior aspect of the sacroiliac joints and obscure them from accurate evaluation. If the patient is placed in a prone position, the X-ray tube is angled 15° towards the feet.

Radiographic changes
The earliest radiographic change, visualized in all spondyloarthropathies, is erosion of the iliac side of the sacroiliac joint, where the

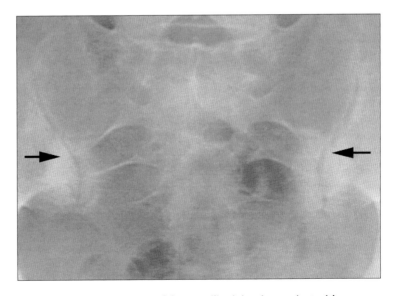

Fig. 105.1 AP Ferguson view of the sacroiliac joints in a patient with ankylosing spondylitis. The area of the sacroiliac joint inferior to the arrows is imaged by the Ferguson view and not by an AP view. Note the bilateral, symmetric involvement with erosions and eburnation.

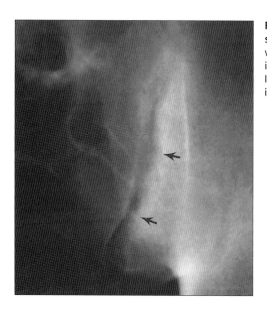

Fig. 105.2 AP view of sacroiliac joint. The white cortical line is intact on the sacral side. It is ill-defined on the iliac side (arrows).

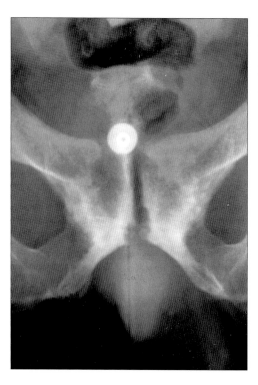

Fig. 105.3 AP view of the pubic symphysis in a patient with ankylosing spondylitis. There is extensive erosive change surrounded by reparative change.

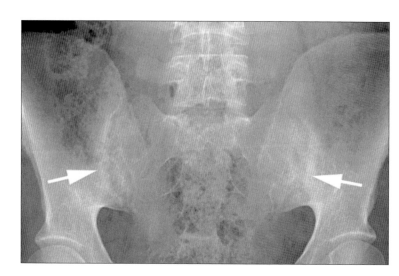

Fig. 105.4 AP Ferguson view of the sacroiliac joints in a patient with ankylosing spondylitis. There is bilateral, symmetric involvement with succinct erosions (arrows).

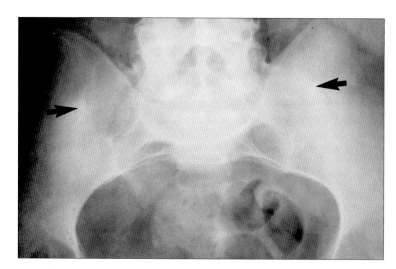

Fig. 105.5 AP view of the sacroiliac joints in long-standing ankylosing spondylitis shows total ankylosis. Ossification of the ligaments connecting the posterior superior aspect of the sacroiliac joints is evident (arrows).

cartilage is thinner (Fig. 105.2). The edge of the joint looks poorly defined and somewhat frayed, with loss of the white cortical line. As erosive disease progresses, there is apparent ('pseudo') widening of the joint. Reparative bone is laid down behind the erosive change and eventually dominates the radiographic picture. Finally, bone ankylosis may occur across the sacroiliac joint. Once the sacroiliac joint is ankylosed, the surrounding bone becomes osteoporotic secondary to loss of normal mechanical stress across the joint.

When imaging the sacroiliac joints, it is generally beneficial to obtain an anteroposterior (AP) view of the pelvis, for often other areas of the pelvis are involved[1,3,4]. The pubic symphysis, being a cartilaginous joint, is uniquely involved in all spondyloarthropathies. Erosive change is followed by reparative change and sometimes ankylosis (Fig. 105.3). In addition, all the spondyloarthropathies involve the entheses; ossification of ligamentous attachments to the ischial tuberosities, the iliac crest and the femoral trochanters gives the pelvis a whiskered appearance.

The task of the conventional radiographic diagnosis is further complicated by significant inter- and intraobserver variation, both in recogniz-

ing and in grading sacroiliitis in cases in which the diagnosis was clinically suspected[7].

Ankylosing spondylitis

In ankylosing spondylitis[8–9], the sacroiliac joints are frequently the first joints to show radiographic abnormality. Erosive and reparative changes occur in a bilateral and symmetric fashion (Fig. 105.4); bone ankylosis occurs early in the disease (Fig. 105.5). By contrast, the posterior superior aspect of the sacroiliac joint comprises the apposition of two bones joined together by ligaments. There is no cartilage, capsule or synovium present. In ankylosing spondylitis, these ligaments ossify, first causing poor definition of this area before becoming totally ankylosed.

Other spondyloarthropathies

Involvement of the sacroiliac joints in the enteropathic arthropathies is radiographically indistinguishable from that of ankylosing spondylitis. Again there is bilateral symmetric involvement with early progression to bone ankylosis.

Sacroiliitis occurs in at least 60% of patients with reactive arthritis and in 10–25% of patients with psoriatic arthritis[10–12]. The radiographic changes differ from those of ankylosing spondylitis, both in extent and distribution (Fig. 105.6). Both the erosions and reparative bone response

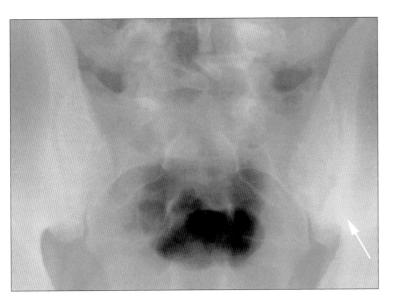

Fig. 105.6 AP Ferguson view of the sacroiliac joints in a patient with psoriatic arthritis. There is bilateral, asymmetric involvement. There is blurring and eburnation of the sacroiliac joints. This is most evident on the left side (arrow).

are more extensive. Ankylosis of the joint is not as common. There may be blurring and eburnation of the posterior aspect of the joint due to ligamentous involvement. The changes occur most commonly bilaterally and asymmetrically. Therefore, early in the disease, changes may appear to be unilateral. However, as changes become obvious in one sacroiliac joint, there should be subtle changes involving the opposite sacroiliac joint (Fig. 105.7).

Conventional tomography

The size, orientation and obscuration of the sacroiliac joint by overlying structures may cause occasional imaging problems on the conventional radiograph. In the past, conventional tomography was a useful adjunct although this has been increasingly replaced by CT, although the former modality still provides accurate assessment. A 'zonographic' technique, which produces sections of increased thickness, is preferred, as it gives more contrast to the image[2].

Bone scintigraphy

Bone scintigraphy[2] is a useful adjunct to the evaluation of sacroiliac disease. It confirms the presence of hyperemia and inflammation that

may not be apparent radiographically. For example, if a patient demonstrates unilateral sacroiliac disease on the conventional radiograph (Fig. 105.7a), this might suggest possible infection. However, the subsequent detection of bilateral disease on bone scintigraphy confirms the correct diagnosis of a seronegative spondyloarthropathy. Serial scintigraphy may also help to define the activity of the disease.

The relative benefits of qualitative analysis versus quantitative analysis of the scintigraphic image have been widely discussed[13,14]. Quantitative analysis is based on comparing sacroiliac joint to sacral activity. A sacroiliac joint:sacral activity ratio greater than 1.32–1.45 is generally considered to be abnormal. Some have questioned using sacral activity as a normal reference point, given that the sacrum is too close to the inflammatory process. Most radiologists feel that qualitative analysis is easier and just as accurate as quantitative analysis.

Many studies have demonstrated that, although quantitative bone scintigraphy is very sensitive to abnormalities in the sacroiliac joints, the findings are too non-specific to consistently diagnose inflammatory sacroiliitis[15–17]. Specifically, one comparison study has shown that sacroiliitis may be diagnosed too frequently in patients who lack clinical and laboratory findings suggestive of an inflammatory condition and who turn out to have mechanical causes of lower back pain[18].

Computed tomography

Many clinicians advocate the use of CT for evaluation of sacroiliac disease[19,20]. The patient is easily positioned and any abnormality is relatively easily seen (Fig. 105.8). With the advent of the new scanners, CT is superior to both conventional radiography and bone scintigraphy in the assessment of sacroiliac joint pathology. CT allows multiple continuous or overlapped, thin (2.5–5mm), well collimated slices through the sacroiliac joints. This affords early detection of sacroiliitis, including cortical erosions and subchondral sclerosis. CT should not, however, be the initial imaging approach for evaluation of sacroiliac disease. It should be used only as an adjunct to conventional radiography where the diagnosis and/or grade of disease involvement remains in question.

Magnetic resonance imaging

Since the early 1990s the utility of MRI in the assessment of sacroiliitis has been widely investigated. Its capabilities for direct multiplanar imaging and soft tissue resolution make it an excellent choice for evaluating the sacroiliac joints. Perhaps the most valuable quality of MRI is the flexibility it offers for manipulating imaging pulse sequences to optimize visualization of specific tissue characteristics. Users vary in the imaging sequences employed in the assessment of the sacroiliac joints

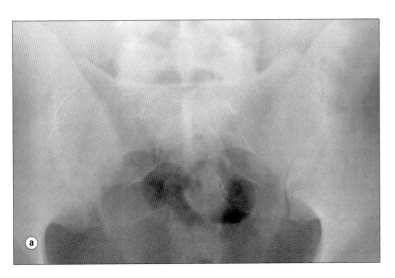

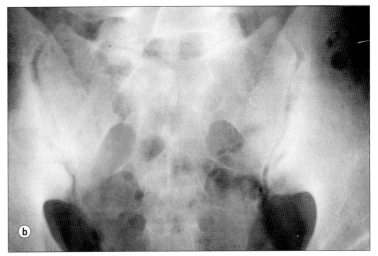

Fig 105.7 Sacroiliac disease. (a) Routine anteroposterior view shows equivocal changes in left sacroiliac joint. (b) Ferguson view demonstrates clearcut bilateral sacroiliitis.

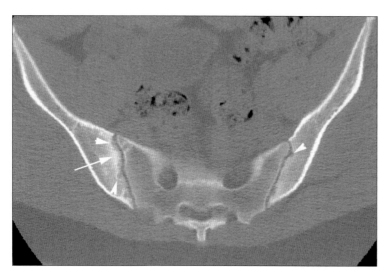

Fig. 105.8 Axial CT image of the sacroiliac joints in a patient with psoriatic arthritis. There is bilateral, asymmetric joint involvement. Erosions are noted bilaterally (arrow-heads) and there is eburnation (arrow).

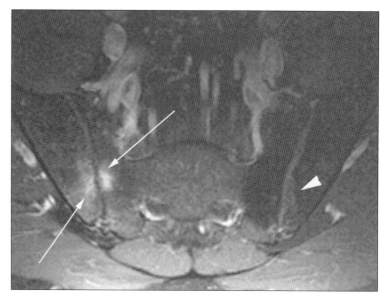

Fig. 105.9 MR image of the sacroiliac joints in a patient with undifferentiated spondyloarthropathy. Axial T1-weighted image with fat suppression following intravenous administration of Gd-DTPA demonstrates increased signal intensity in the subchondral bone marrow within the iliac and sacral sides of the right joint (arrows) and early erosions of the left joint (arrowhead).

but all usually include parameters for the detection of anatomic (short TE), and water-sensitive (T2 with fat saturation or short tau inversion recovery, STIR) imaging.

Magnetic resonance imaging is excellent at depicting the normal sacroiliac joint and clearly distinguishes the synovial and ligamentous compartments. In normal subjects, direct visualization of cartilage on both sides of the synovial compartment of the joint is possible; this appears as a thin line of intermediate signal on T1-weighted images. A thin, linear band of low signal intensity is present on both sacral and iliac sides of the joint, corresponding to normal subchondral bone. The bone marrow is composed of fat and parallels the signal of fat elsewhere in the imaging field.

Early studies showed that MRI was able to demonstrate abnormalities in the subchondral bone and periarticular bone marrow[21]. Two types of lesion were identified. Type I lesions were characterized by low signal intensity in T1-weighted images and high signal intensity in STIR and T2-weighted images. These lesions were located close to the joint space and were diffusely distributed in the bone marrow. They probably represent subchondral edema and indicate the acute, or active, phase of inflammation and were associated with erosions on CT. Type II lesions were characterized by high signal on T1-weighted images in the periarticular marrow, reflecting fatty replacement and an absence of marrow edema. Areas of low signal intensity on all pulse sequences were also noted, which were associated with erosions and subchondral sclerosis on CT. Such changes were felt to represent the later changes of fibrosis and bony sclerosis. On the basis of these findings, MRI can potentially differentiate between acute and chronic changes. Interpretation of these findings was supported by published data from an open biopsy study of patients with early sacroiliitis, which indicated that early histopathologic changes occurred in the subchondral bone[22]. Thus subchondral bone marrow edema would be the earliest non-contrast MRI finding.

In more recent studies, MRI has been shown to be more sensitive and specific than conventional radiography, bone scintigraphy and CT in diagnosing sacroiliitis[23–25]. MRI specificity has been reported to be between 90% and 100% with the development and implementation of newer sequences. Sensitivity has also been improved with the use of contrast-enhanced MRI employing gadolinium-diethylenetriaminepentaacetic acid (Gd-DTPA), which is administered intravenously as a bolus prior to image acquisition[26–29]. Contrast-enhanced MRI studies demonstrated abnormalities in those patients clinically suspected to have sacroiliitis in whom imaging studies, even including unenhanced MRI, were normal or equivocal (Fig. 105.9).

Recently, MRI has also been shown to be an excellent imaging technique for monitoring inflammatory changes in patients with seronegative spondyloarthropathy receiving powerful disease-modifying therapies such as anti-tumour-necrosis-factor (TNF) therapy[30].

Another recent advance is the assessment of sacroiliitis with a perfusion MRI. This involves a rapid injection of Gd-DTPA intravenously followed by fast imaging of the area of interest. This technique can produce not only qualitative but quantitative assessment of the sacroiliac joints, which may be the future method of choice for diagnosing seronegative spondyloarthropathy and evaluation of therapeutic efficacy.

IMAGING THE SPINE

The seronegative spondyloarthropathies involve the spine at the diskovertebral, apophyseal, costovertebral and atlantoaxial joints, as well as the posterior ligamentous attachments. Initial imaging should be performed with conventional radiography, although CT and MRI play significant roles in imaging various parts of the spine. All other modalities play a lesser role.

Conventional radiography

Technique

Anteroposterior and lateral views of the spine are adequate for imaging diskovertebral joints and all ligamentous problems. Oblique views may be needed for the apophyseal joints. Flexed lateral and odontoid views of the cervical spine are important in evaluating atlantoaxial joints.

Diskovertebral joint

Ankylosing spondylitis

In ankylosing spondylitis[1–4,31–33], the first changes observed in the spine are small erosions with adjacent repair at the corners of the vertebral bodies, resulting in loss of the normal concave contour of the anterior border of the vertebral bodies. The vertebral bodies appear square, with shiny corners (Fig. 105.10). In general, changes start in the lower lumbar spine and ascend the spine, eventually including the cervical spine. The shiny corner is called a Romanus lesion. This is accompanied or followed by ossification of the outer layer of the annulus fibrosus of the

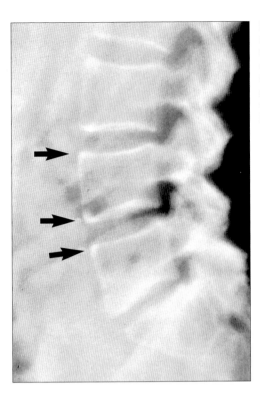

Fig. 105.10 Lateral view of the lumbosacral spine showing shiny corners in a patient with ankylosing spondylitis (arrows). (With permission from Brower and Colon[3].)

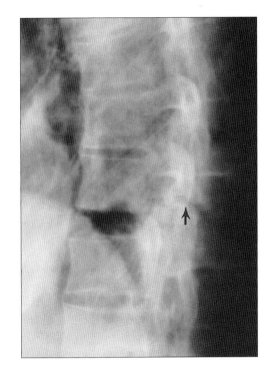

Fig. 105.12 Lateral view of the lower thoracic and upper lumbar area. There is ankylosis of the entire spine except at T12–L1. Here there is distraction of the disc space and fracture (arrow) through the posterior elements. (Courtesy of Dr C S Resnick.)

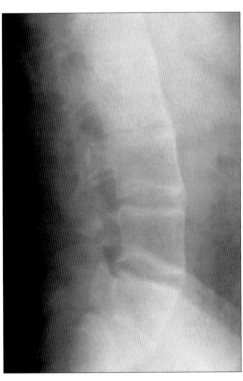

Fig. 105.11 Lateral view of the lumbosacral spine showing syndesmophytes of ankylosing spondylitis, giving it a bamboo appearance.

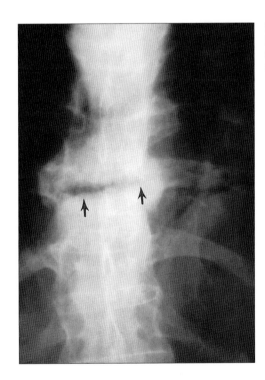

Fig. 105.13 Pseudoarthrosis in ankylosing spondylitis (arrow).

disc (Sharpey's fibers) and the deep layers of the longitudinal ligaments. This ossification, called a syndesmophyte, is thin and succinct, and syndesmophytes ascend the spine in a symmetric fashion to produce a bamboo appearance (Fig. 105.11). Although the cervical spine is usually last to be involved, females occasionally demonstrate disease first in the cervical spine. Once the spine is ankylosed and immobile, the discs may calcify, especially if there is apophyseal ankylosis as well.

In the ankylosed spine, erosive changes at the diskovertebral junction (Andersson lesions) may develop. These changes may be secondary to inflammation or infection but are most commonly secondary to fracture (Fig. 105.12). A fracture through the ankylosed spine becomes the single point of motion in the entire spine, resulting in a pseudoarthrosis (Fig. 105.13). The disc degenerates and disintegrates; the adjacent bone erodes and repairs. The radiographic changes may resemble severe degenerative disc disease, septic discitis and osteomyelitis, or neuropathic osteoarthropathy.

Other spondyloarthropathies

The changes around the discovertebral joints in reactive arthritis and psoriasis[11,12,34–36] differ from those of ankylosing spondylitis. The Romanus lesion and squaring of the vertebral bodies are not present. Instead of succinct, symmetric syndesmophytes that ascend the spine, there is thick paravertebral ossification. Large bulky bone outgrowths, located further away from the vertebral column, occur with no predictable pattern (Fig. 105.14). Calcification of discs is much rarer. Spine involvement is more common in psoriatic arthritis than in reactive arthritis; however, it is still less common than in ankylosing spondylitis.

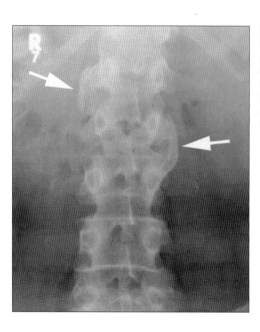

Fig. 105.14 AP view of the lumbar spine in a patient with psoriatic arthritis. There is bulky, asymmetric paravertebral ossification at multiple levels (arrows).

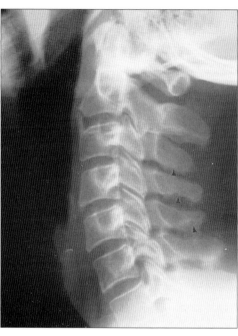

Fig. 105.15 Lateral view of the cervical spine in a patient with psoriatic arthritis. The posterior spinous processes show erosive changes at ligamentous attachments (arrowheads). (With permission from Brower and Colon[3].)

Only rarely does an Andersson lesion or pseudoarthrosis occur in psoriatic arthritis.

Other spine changes

Erosive changes and ankylosis of the apophyseal joints may occur in any of the spondyloarthropathies. The apophyseal joints are commonly involved in ankylosing spondylitis, although rarely in psoriatic arthritis except in the cervical spine.

The posterior ligamentous attachments may ossify in ankylosing spondylitis, causing ankylosis of one spinous process to another. In psoriatic arthritis, especially in the cervical spine, erosive and bone proliferative changes at these ligamentous attachments are more common than ankylosis[37] (Fig. 105.15). The atlantoaxial joints may be involved in any of the spondyloarthropathies. The changes are indistinguishable from those of RA. This means that there may be subluxation of the atlantoaxial joint in any direction, as well as erosive changes of the odontoid peg.

Computed tomography

Most of the radiographic changes previously described can be imaged by conventional radiography, so CT should be reserved for cases with equivocal changes. It is excellent for detecting spinal fractures, spinal stenosis, thecal diverticula and atlantoaxial instability. One complication of ankylosing spondylitis best diagnosed with CT is involvement of the cauda equina. Also, CT with contrast demonstrates widening of the neural canal, dilatation of the dural sac and thecal diverticula[1].

Magnetic resonance imaging

In the spine, MRI is the modality of choice to image any soft tissue structures. It ascertains intrusion of the neural canal by disc, ligament, synovium and inflammatory processes. As in RA, it is the modality of choice in a patient with neurologic symptoms[1–2]. MRI is highly sensitive for marrow abnormalities, such as metastatic disease, infection and fracture.

Recently, Gd-DTPA-enhanced MRI of the spine has been shown to successfully demonstrate the Romanus lesion as low signal intensity areas on T1-weighted images and as high signal on T2-weighted images and postcontrast T1-weighted images. These findings represent edema and hyperemia of inflammatory tissue. Contrast enhancement was absent in cases in which there was radiographic evidence of syndesmophyte formation. As in sacroiliitis, the presence of contrast enhancement may reflect the more active and early phase of inflammation. Contrast-enhanced MRI can not only facilitate early diagnosis, it also may play a role in documenting the stage of disease[38].

IMAGING THE APPENDICULAR SYSTEM

There is wide variation in the degree of appendicular involvement between the spondyloarthropathies[3,4,39,40]. Ankylosing spondylitis rarely involves joints other than the shoulders and hips. By contrast, the other spondyloarthropathies rarely involve the hips, and only psoriasis occasionally involves the shoulder. Reactive arthritis preferentially affects the lower extremities, primarily the feet, ankles and knees, while psoriatic arthritis involves the hands, then the feet and finally the ankles, knees and shoulders. The enteropathic arthropathies may cause inflammation of one or a few joints, which is self-limiting. There is usually soft tissue swelling and juxta-articular osteoporosis but rarely permanent damage.

Conventional radiography

In the appendicular system, conventional radiography remains the imaging modality of choice at the present time. Other modalities are primarily used as an adjunct. The positioning and techniques used for conventional radiography are the same as those discussed in Chapter 25.

The hand and wrist

Of patients with psoriatic arthritis, 75% will have involvement of the hand and wrist[41–43]. There are several patterns of distribution within this area:

- involvement of distal interphalangeal (DIP) and proximal interphalangeal (PIP) joints;
- involvement of wrist and isolated rays;
- involvement of multiple joints similar to RA.

Disease in the wrist is not as frequent as disease in the DIP and PIP joints. When a single ray is involved, the entire digit may be swollen and resemble a cocktail sausage or 'hot-dog' (Fig. 105.16). Mineralization of affected digits remains normal. Erosions occur first at the margins of the joint and then progress towards the center. Accompanying erosion is bone production, giving the eroded edge a spiculated, frayed or paint-brush appearance (Fig. 105.17). Erosion may become so extensive as to give an appearance of a widened rather than a narrowed joint space. A widened joint space helps to distinguish confusing changes from osteoarthritis. Erosion may produce a blunt, tapered, osseous surface on the proximal bone of a joint, which may protrude into an expanded base of the distal bone of the joint. This appearance is likened to 'a pencil in a

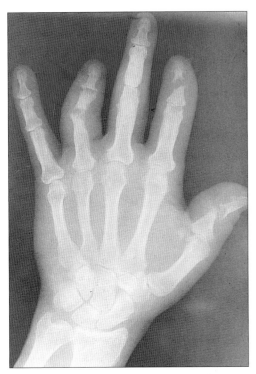

Fig. 105.16 **Posteroanterior view of the hand in a patient with psoriatic arthritis.** There is sausage-like swelling of the first, second and fourth digits. Normal mineralization is present. Severe erosive changes create apparent widened joint spaces of the thumb interphalangeal, the index DIP and the ring finger PIP joints. Periosteal new bone has been incorporated into the cortex of the proximal phalanx of the index digit, and the middle and proximal phalanges of the middle digit, thus widening the shaft. (With permission from Brower[44].)

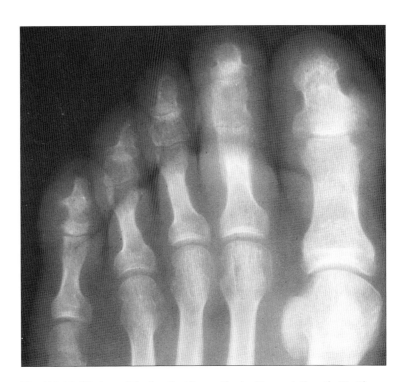

Fig. 105.18 **AP view of the forefoot in a patient with psoriatic arthritis.** There is juxta-articular osteoporosis. There are erosive changes with accompanying bone productive changes at the IP joint of the big toe. There is soft tissue swelling and periostitis along the proximal phalanx of the second digit. (With permission from Brower and Colon[3].)

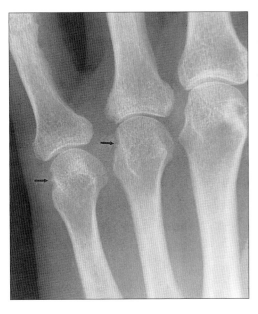

Fig. 105.17 **Posteroanterior view of the metacarpophalangeal joint showing erosive changes accompanied by bone production giving the erosion a spiculated or frayed appearance (arrows).**

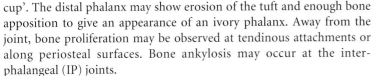

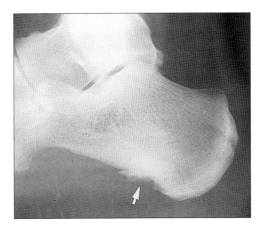

Fig. 105.19 **Lateral view of the heel in a patient with psoriatic arthritis.** Erosion and bone proliferation at the attachment of the plantar aponeurosis (arrow) is seen. (With permission from Brower[44].)

The foot

In psoriatic arthritis[34,46], the feet are involved almost as commonly as the hands, with similar radiographic changes (Fig. 105.18). An entire toe may be swollen. Mineralization is maintained, despite severe erosive changes. Bone proliferation is similar to that seen in the hands. The IP joints are the most frequently involved joints, with the IP joint of the great toe being affected more frequently than in any other arthropathy. Bone ankylosis may be seen in the IP joints. Other changes observed are at the attachments of the plantar aponeurosis or the Achilles tendon to the calcaneus. At these sites, erosive and bone productive changes occur, producing irregular, ill-defined spurs (Fig. 105.19). These changes should not be confused with the well defined, well corticated, traumatic ossification often occurring at these sites.

In reactive arthritis[34,46,47] the foot is the most commonly affected site. The radiographic changes are quite similar to those of psoriatic arthritis. Slight differences may be:

- persistence of juxta-articular osteoporosis
- presence of a periostitis without articular abnormality

cup'. The distal phalanx may show erosion of the tuft and enough bone apposition to give an appearance of an ivory phalanx. Away from the joint, bone proliferation may be observed at tendinous attachments or along periosteal surfaces. Bone ankylosis may occur at the interphalangeal (IP) joints.

Reactive arthritis[34,45] rarely affects the hand but when it does the radiographic changes are indistinguishable from psoriatic arthritis. However, unlike psoriatic arthritis, involvement of the hand tends to be monoarticular and to involve a PIP joint more frequently than a metacarpophalangeal or DIP joint. The thumb, including the sesamoids of the thumb, is a frequent site of the monoarticular arthropathy. Carpal involvement is rare. Radiographic changes in the hand in ankylosing spondylitis[40] are extremely rare. When present, small erosions with minimal bone repair soon give way to bone ankylosis. The enteropathic arthropathies do not tend to produce permanent damage of the joints.

- decreased occurrence of ankylosis of the IP joints
- preference for involvement of the metatarsophalangeal over the IP joints.

Calcaneal involvement occurs in more than 50% of patients with reactive arthritis; often this may be the only bone involved. Changes at the Achilles tendon attachment are less frequent than in psoriatic arthritis. The entire inferior aspect of the calcaneus may demonstrate erosion and hyperostosis. This is a manifestation of the waxing and waning course of the disease.

Ankylosing spondylitis and the enteropathic arthropathies[39,40] rarely affect the feet. Ankylosing spondylitis tends to ankylose and the enteropathic arthropathies tend to have soft tissue swelling and juxta-articular osteoporosis without permanent damage.

The hips

After the sacroiliac joints and spine, the hip is the joint most commonly affected by ankylosing spondylitis[47]. The hips are involved bilaterally and symmetrically with uniform loss of joint space, which may progress to acetabular protrusion. Erosive disease is not, however, a prominent feature. A cuff of osteophytes forms at the junction of the head and neck of the femur and at the superior and inferior margin of the acetabulum (Fig. 105.20). Usually, bone ankylosis occurs at the peripheral portion of the joint. Radiographically, a normal femoral head and joint space may be observed through the bone ankylosis (Fig. 105.21). Once the hips are ankylosed, the bone structures become osteoporotic. In reactive arthritis and psoriasis[34] the hips are rarely involved. However, when they are involved, there is uniform joint space narrowing, erosion and bone production, but seldom ankylosis.

The shoulder

Shoulder involvement may be seen in ankylosing spondylitis and psoriatic arthritis. Of patients with long-standing ankylosing spondylitis[40], 30% will have shoulder involvement. The involvement is bilateral and symmetric with joint space narrowing and small erosive changes on the superior lateral aspect of the humeral head. Some patients will have a deep erosion called the 'hatchet sign'. Bone proliferation may be seen in ligamentous attachments. However, these changes are transient and bone ankylosis of the joint will take over. In patients with psoriatic arthritis, shoulder involvement tends to be more erosive and bone production is less than in ankylosing spondylitis[34] (Fig. 105.22).

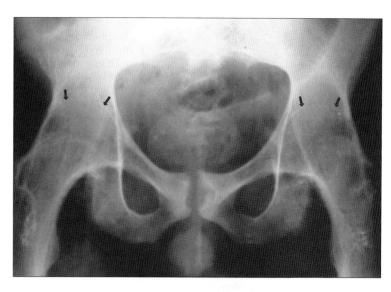

Fig. 105.21 AP view of the pelvis in a patient with long-standing ankylosing spondylitis. There is generalized osteoporosis. There is ankylosis of the sacroiliac joints, pubic symphysis and both hips. A normal rounded contour of the femoral head is seen through the bone ankylosis (arrows).

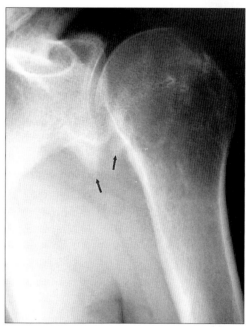

Fig. 105.22 AP view of the shoulder shows loss of the joint space with ossification of various ligamentous attachments around the shoulder joint (arrows). (With permission from Brower and Colon[3].)

Other appendicular sites

The knees and ankles are frequently affected in patients with reactive arthritis, less frequently in patients with psoriatic arthritis and rarely in patients with ankylosing spondylitis. Reactive arthritis and psoriasis tend to present with asymmetric disease, while ankylosing spondylitis presents with symmetric disease. Joint effusion, bone erosion and bone proliferation are the classic findings. Since all the spondyloarthropathies may involve the cartilaginous joints, the sternomanubrial joint should be observed in addition to the pubic symphysis and the discovertebral joint. All of the spondyloarthropathies affect the entheses; ossifications occur at the medial and lateral malleoli, the ulnar olecranon, the anterior surface of the patella, the inferior clavicular margin and the humeral tuberosities.

Bone scintigraphy

Bone scintigraphy is an extremely useful additional approach to conventional radiography[2]. It will confirm the presence of disease, illustrate its distribution and determine its activity. For example, in the patient who

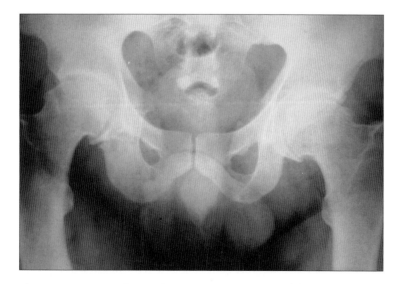

Fig. 105.20 AP view of the pelvis of a patient with ankylosing spondylitis. Normal mineralization is present. There is uniform loss of both hip joints with axial migration. A cuff of osteophytes is present at the junction of the head and neck as well as at the inferior and superior aspects of the acetabulum.

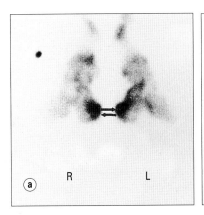
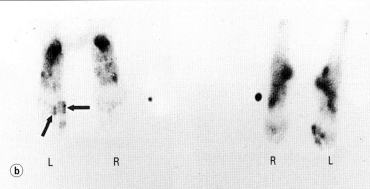

Fig. 105.23 Technetium-99m scan of the feet of a patient with reactive arthritis. Although conventional radiographs were normal, this scan demonstrates the distribution of uptake in a patient with reactive arthritis. (a) There is uptake at the inferior aspect of the calcanei, at the attachment of the plantar aponeuroses (arrows). (b) There is also uptake along the outside of the proximal phalanges in the periosteal area of the first and second digit of the left foot (arrows).

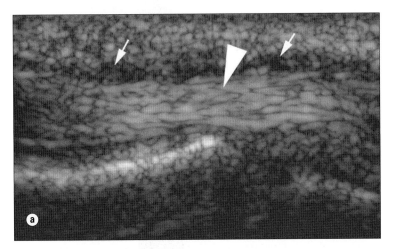

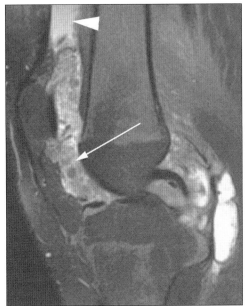

Fig. 105.25 MRI of the knee in a patient with psoriatic arthritis. Sagittal T2-weighted image with fat suppression demonstrates marked synovitis (arrow) and a joint effusion (arrowhead).

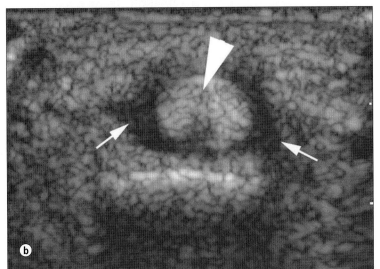

Fig. 105.24 Ultrasound images: tenosynovitis of the finger. (a) Longitudinal and (b) axial images demonstrate fluid in the tendon sheaths (arrows) of the flexor tendons (arrowheads).

presents with foot pain and normal conventional radiographs, the bone scan may demonstrate increased activity in a distribution typical of reactive arthritis (Fig. 105.23). It is possible to make such a diagnosis from the bone scan alone.

Other imaging modalities

Ultrasonography, CT and MRI are being used more frequently for diagnosis as well as evaluation of therapy in seronegative spondyloarthropathies.

The small size of the peripheral joints and their superficial location (as opposed to the difficult-to-access sacroiliac joints in the pelvis) allows

for easy ultrasonographic examination. Ultrasound and power Doppler ultrasound are excellent at depicting early inflammatory soft tissue changes in the joint such as fluid collections, synovitis and tenosynovitis[48,49] (Fig. 105.24). Furthermore, ultrasound is relatively inexpensive and does not convey radiation exposure that is inherent in conventional radiography or CT.

Magnetic resonance imaging may be employed for the evaluation of peripheral joints and soft tissues (Fig. 105.25), including the assessment of dactylitis, synovitis and tenosynovitis. In cases of dactylitis, MRI can detect not only erosions in the characteristic locations but other evidence of fluid collections in the flexor and extensor tendon sheaths that indicate tenosynovitis not apparent on conventional radiographs[50] (Fig. 105.26). MRI may be used to assess active enthesitis. Marrow edema can be detected adjacent to ligamentous and tendinous attachments[51,52].

Comparison of ultrasound versus MRI found that both modalities were sensitive to the presence of effusion around small joints but that MRI was more sensitive and specific for the detection of pathology in tendon sheaths[53] and superior in the detection of calcaneal bursitis[54].

SUMMARY

The seronegative spondyloarthropathies can be separated radiographically from RA by the presence of bone proliferation and involvement of the sacroiliac joints and spine. In turn, they can be separated from each other by observing the extent of erosion and/or bone proliferation within the joint involved, the symmetry or asymmetry of disease and the

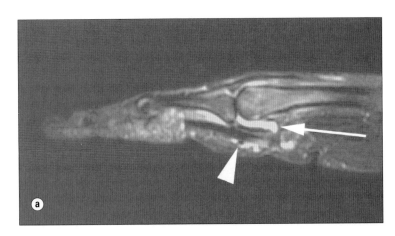
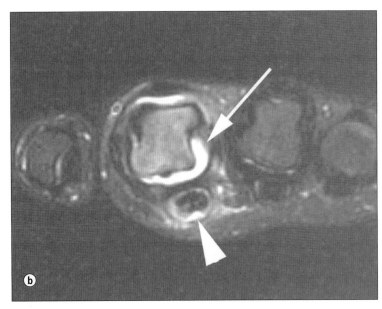

Fig. 105.26 MRI of a finger in a patient with psoriatic arthritis. (a) Sagittal and (b) axial T2-weighted image with fat suppression of the index finger demonstrate an effusion in the metacarpophalangeal joint (arrow) and tenosynovitis of the flexor tendons (arrowhead).

distribution of disease within the individual. All imaging should begin with conventional radiography. Additional information may often be obtained through bone scintigraphy. CT effectively displays cortical erosions and subchondral sclerosis as well as the late findings of joint space narrowing and bony ankylosis. MRI has emerged as a valuable modality in the diagnosis of sacroiliitis. It is both sensitive and highly specific, and demonstrates abnormalities in articular cartilage, synovium and subchondral bone marrow. Its ability to demonstrate these changes is highly advantageous to the diagnosis with early disease, when findings on other modalities are normal to equivocal, and in monitoring therapy.

REFERENCES

1. Resnick D. Section IV: Rheumatoid arthritis and related diseases. In: Resnick D, ed. Bone and joint imaging. Philadelphia, PA: WB Saunders; 1989: 244–258, 299–343.
2. Brower AC. Arthritis in black and white. Philadelphia, PA: WB Saunders; 1988.
3. Brower AC, Colon E. Spondyloarthropathies. Postgrad Radiol 1989; 9: 203–220.
4. McEwen C, Ditata D, Lingg C et al. Ankylosing spondylitis and the spondylitis accompanying ulcerative colitis, regional enteritis, psoriasis, and Reiter's disease. A comparative study. Arthritis Rheum 1971; 14: 291–318.
5. Resnick D, Niwayama G. On the nature and significance of bony proliferation in rheumatoid variant disorders. AJR 1977; 129: 275–278.
6. Brower A. Disorders of the sacroiliac joint. Radiology 1978; 1: 3–26.
7. Luong AA, Salonen DC. Imaging of the seronegative spondyloarthropathies. Current Rheumatology Reports 2000, 2: 288–296.
8. Berens DL. Roentgen features of ankylosing spondylitis. Clin Orthop 1971; 74: 20–33.
9. Resnick D, Niwayama G, Goergen TG. Comparison of radiographic abnormalities of the sacro-iliac joint in degenerative disease and ankylosing spondylitis. AJR 1977; 128: 189–196.
10. Russell AS, Davis P, Percy JS, Lentle BC. The sacroiliitis of acute Reiter's syndrome. J Rheumatol 1977; 4: 293–296.
11. Jajic I. Radiological changes in the sacroiliac joints and spines of patients with psoriatic arthritis and psoriasis. Ann Rheum Dis 1968; 27: 1–6.
12. Killebrew K, Gold RH, Sholkoff SD. Psoriatic spondylitis. Radiology 1973; 108: 9–16.
13. Goldberg RP, Genant HK, Shimshak R, Shames D. Applications and limitations of quantitative sacroiliac joint scintigraphy. Radiology 1978; 128: 683–689.
14. Vyas K, Eklem M, Seto H et al. Quantitative scintigraphy of sacroiliac joints: effect of age, gender, and laterality. AJR 1981; 136: 589–592.
15. Ho G Jr, Sadovnikoff N, Malhotra CM et al. Quantitative sacroiliac joint scintigraphy: a critical assessment. Arthritis Rheum 1979, 22: 837–844.
16. Chase WF, Houk RW, Winn RE et al. The clinical usefulness of radionuclide scintigraphy in suspected sacro-iliitis: a prospective study. Br J Rheumatol 1983; 22: 67–72.
17. Miron SD, Wiesen EJ, Kushner I et al. The value of quantitative sacroiliac scintigraphy in detection of sacroiliitis. Clin Rheumatol 1983, 2: 407–414.
18. Fam AG, Rubenstein JD, Ching-Sang H et al. Computed tomography in the diagnosis of early ankylosing spondylitis. Arthritis Rheum 1985, 28: 930–937.
19. Kozin F, Carrera GF, Ryan LM et al. Computed tomography in the diagnosis of sacroiliitis. Arthritis Rheum 1981; 24: 1479–1485.
20. Volger JB III, Brown WH, Helms CA, Genant HK. The normal sacroiliac joint: a CT study of asymptomatic patients. Radiology 1984; 151: 433–437.
21. Ahlstrom H, Feltelius N, Nyman R et al. Magnetic resonance imaging of sacroiliac joint inflammation. Arthritis Rheum 1990; 33: 1763–1769.
22. Shichikawa K, Tsujimoto M, Nishioka J et al. Histopathology of early sacroiliitis and enthesitis in ankylosing spondylitis. In: Ziff M, Cohen SB, eds. Advances in inflammation research. New York: Raven Press; 1985: 15–24.
23. Murphey MD, Wetzel LH, Bramble JM et al. Sacroiliitis: MR imaging findings. Radiology 1991, 180: 239–244.
24. Docherty P, Mitchell MJ, MacMillan L et al. Magnetic resonance imaging in the detection of sacroiliitis. J Rheumatol 1992, 19: 393–401.
25. Battafarano DF, Sterling GW, Rak KM et al. Magnetic resonance imaging in the diagnosis of active sacroiliitis. Semin Arthritis Rheum 1993, 23: 161–176.
26. Braun J, Bollow M, Eggens U et al. Use of dynamic magnetic resonance imaging with fast imaging in the detection of early and advanced sacroiliitis in spondyloarthropathy patients. Arthritis Rheum 1994, 37: 1039–1045.
27. Bollow M, Braun J, Hamm B et al. Early sacroiliitis in patients with spondyloarthropathy: evaluation with dynamic gadolinium-enhanced MRI. J Rheumatol 1996, 23: 2107–2115.
28. Blum U, Buitrago-Tellez C, Mundinger A et al. Magnetic resonance imaging (MRI) for detection of active sacroiliitis: a prospective study comparing conventional radiography, scintigraphy, and contrast enhanced MRI. J Rheumatol 1996, 23: 2107–2115.
29. Yu W, Feng F, Dion E et al. Comparison of radiography, computed tomography and magnetic resonance imaging in detection of sacroiliitis accompanying ankylosing spondylitis. Skeletal Radiol 1998, 27: 311–320.
30. Stone M, Salonen D, Lax M et al. Clinical and imaging correlates of response to treatment with infliximab in patients with ankylosing spondylitis. J Rheumatol 2001, 28: 1605–1614.
31. Cawley MID, Chalmers TM, Kellgren JH, Ball J. Destructive lesions of vertebral bodies in ankylosing spondylitis. Ann Rheum Dis 1972; 31: 345–358.
32. Gelman MI, Umber JS. Fractures of the thoracolumbar spine in ankylosing spondylitis. AJR 1978; 130: 485–491.
33. Rivelis M, Freiberger RH. Vertebral destruction at unfused segments in late ankylosing spondylitis. Radiology 1969; 93: 251–256.
34. Peterson CC Jr, Silbiger ML. Reiter's syndrome and psoriatic arthritis. Their roentgen spectra and some interesting similarities. AJR 1967; 101: 860–871.
35. Cliff JM. Spinal bony bridging and carditis in Reiter's disease. Ann Rheum Dis 1971; 30: 171–179.
36. Sundaram M, Patton JT. Paravertebral ossification in psoriasis and Reiter's disease. Br J Radiol 1975; 48: 628–633.
37. Kaplan D, Plotz CM, Nathanson L, Frank L. Cervical spine in psoriasis and in psoriatic arthritis. Ann Rheum Dis 1964; 23: 50–56.
38. Jevtic V, Kos-Golja M, Rozman B et al. Marginal erosive discovertebral 'Romanus' lesions in ankylosing spondylitis demonstrated by contrast enhanced Gd-DTPA magnetic resonance imaging. Skeletal Radiol 2000; 29: 27–33.
39. Dekker-Sacys BJ, Meuwissen SGM, Van Den BergLoonen EM et al. Ankylosing spondylitis and inflammatory bowel disease. II. Prevalence of peripheral arthritis, sacroiliitis and ankylosing spondylitis in patients suffering from inflammatory bowel disease. Ann Rheum Dis 1978; 37: 36–41.

40. Resnick D. Patterns of peripheral joint disease in ankylosing spondylitis. Radiology 1974; 110: 523–532.
41. Forrester DM. The 'cocktail sausage' digit. Arthritis Rheum 1983; 26; 664–667.
42. Martel W, Stuck KJ, Dworin AM, Hylland RG. Erosive osteoarthritis and psoriatic arthritis: a radiologic comparison in the hand, wrist, and foot. Am J Rheumatol 1980; 134: 125–135.
43. Resnick D, Broderick RW. Bony proliferation of terminal phalanges in psoriasis. The 'ivory' phalanx. J Can Assoc Radiol 1977; 28: 664–667.
44. Brower AC. The radiographic features of psoriatic arthritis. In: Gerber L, Espinoza L, eds. Psoriatic arthritis. Orlando, FL: Grune & Stratton; 1985: 125–127.
45. Martel W, Braunstein EM, Borlaza G et al. Radiologic features of Reiter's disease. Radiology 1979; 132: 1–10.
46. Resnick D, Feingold ML, Curd J et al. Calcaneal abnormalities in articular disorders. Rheumatoid arthritis, ankylosing spondylitis, psoriatic arthritis and Reiter's syndrome. Radiology 1977; 125: 355–366.
47. Dwosh IL, Resnick D, Becker MA. Hip involvement in ankylosing spondylitis. Arthritis Rheum 1976; 19; 683–692.
48. Stone M, Bergin D, Whelan B, et. al. Power doppler ultrasound assessment of rheumatoid hand synovitis. J Rheumatol 2001, 28: 1979–1982.
49. Backhaus M, Kamradt T, Sandrock D et al. Arthritis of finger joints: a comprehensive approach comparing conventional radiography, scintigraphy, ultrasound, and contrast enhanced magnetic resonance imaging. Arthritis Rheum 1999, 42: 1232–1245.
50. Olivieri I, Barozzi L, Pierro A et al. Toe dactylitis in patients with spondyloarthropathy: assessment by magnetic resonance imaging. J Rheumatol 1997, 24: 926–930.
51. McGonagle D, Kahn MA, Marzo-Ortega H et al. Enthesitis in spondyloarthropathy. Curr Opin Rheumatol 1999, 11: 244–250.
52. Olivieri I, Barozzi L, Padula A. Enthesopathy: clinical manifestations, imaging and treatment. Baillière's Clin Rheumatol 1998, 12: 665–681.
53. Coari G, Iagnocco A, Mastrantuono M et al. Sonographic and NMR imaging study of sausage digit. Acta Derm Venereol (Stockh) 1994; 186(S): 33–34.
54. Olivieri I, Barozzi L, Padula A et al. Retrocalcaneal bursitis in spondyloarthropathy: assessment by ultrasound and magnetic resonance imaging. J Rheumatol 1998; 25: 1352–1357.

SPONDYLOARTHROPATHIES

106 Ankylosing spondylitis: pathology

Barrie Vernon-Roberts

- Key initial chronic inflammatory lesions occur at ligamentous attachments to bone (entheses)
- Ankylosis of synovial and spinal joints results from healing of enthesis lesions with capsular ossification and bony bridging
- Bony ankylosis of the synovial (inferior) portion of the sacroiliac joint in ankylosing spondylitis (AS) results from capsular and non-inflammatory endochondral ossification
- Synovial membrane histology is similar to that in rheumatoid arthritis
- Aortic regurgitation is associated with characteristic fibrous scarring affecting the aortic root
- Lung and kidney pathology is not specific to AS, but amyloidosis may lead to renal failure

INTRODUCTION

Ankylosing spondylitis (AS) is rarely a fatal disease, and patients infrequently undergo autopsy because the great majority die from diseases not causally related to AS. Therefore, tissue for pathologic examination seldom becomes available. However, pathologic findings in sufficient numbers of cases of unequivocal AS have been published such that the articular and extra-articular pathology of the condition can now be reviewed with a significant degree of confidence.

LIGAMENTOUS ATTACHMENTS

Much, but not all, of the skeletal pathology of AS is explained by the changes that take place at entheses (see Chapter 114). Therefore, AS may affect: the capsules and intracapsular ligaments of large synovial (diarthrodial) joints and the apophyseal joints; the ligamentous structures of cartilaginous joints, commonly including the intervertebral discs, manubriosternal joints and the symphysis pubis; and the ligamentous attachments in sites as diverse as the spinous processes of the vertebrae, the iliac crests, trochanters, patellae, calcanei and the clavicle.

Convincing histopathologic evidence has shown that there is an initial inflammatory erosive process involving the enthesis, followed by healing during which new bone is formed[1] (Figs 106.1 & 106.2). The findings indicate that the inflammatory phase may be patchy and brief, and that the bone forms in fibrous tissue without preceding cartilage formation. The new bone tends to fill the defect in the eroded bone, joining the deeper bone to the eroded end of the ligament (Fig. 106.2), thus forming a new enthesis above the original level of the cortical surface. Therefore, the final outcome of healing is an irregular bony prominence, with sclerosis of the adjacent cancellous bone[1] (Fig. 106.3).

There is some evidence that ligamentous lesions are not confined to the enthesis zone, and that focal inflammation and edema may adjoin small blood vessels elsewhere within the ligaments. In some instances, this leads to the development of fibrosis and new bone formation[1] at some distance from the ligamentous attachment to the bone.

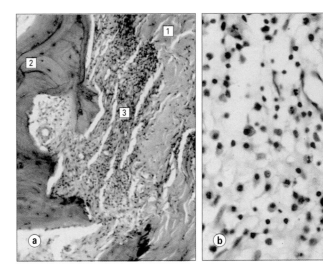

Fig. 106.1 Active inflammatory erosive enthesopathy of a ligamentous attachment to the iliac crest. (a) Low-power microscopy shows that the attachment between the ligament (1) and the bone (2) has been destroyed by an inflammatory focus (3). (b) High-power microscopy shows that the inflammatory infiltrate consists mainly of chronic inflammatory cells, with occasional neutrophils, in an edematous matrix containing new blood vessels. (Hematoxylin and eosin). (Courtesy of Professor J Ball.)

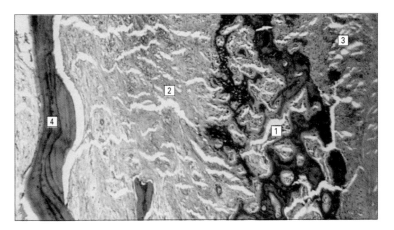

Fig. 106.2 Low-power microscopy of a healing erosive enthesopathy involving the ligamentous attachment to the greater trochanter. This shows newly woven repair bone (1) and fibrous scar tissue (2) occupying the zone between the ligament (3) and the original bone of the trochanter (4). (Hematoxylin and eosin). (Courtesy of Professor J Ball.)

CARTILAGINOUS JOINTS

The pathology of AS differs from that of rheumatoid disease in having a much greater tendency for the involvement of cartilaginous joints, including the intervertebral discs, the manubriosternal joints and the symphysis pubis.

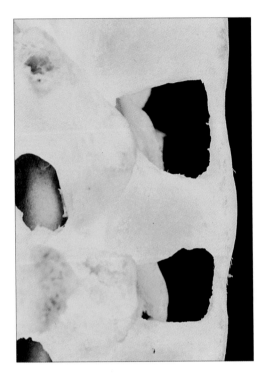

Fig. 106.3 Ossification of the supraspinous ligament resulting from healing of zones involved by earlier inflammation.

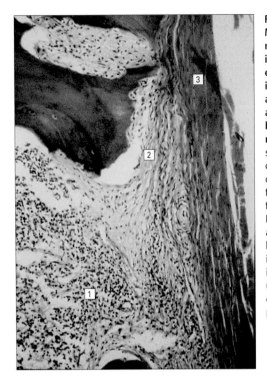

Fig. 106.5 Medium-power microscopy of an active inflammatory erosive enthesopathy involving the attachment of the anterior annulus to the bone of the vertebral rim. Although there are substantial numbers of chronic inflammatory cells (1) present, early fibrous repair tissue (2) formation has occurred. Note that, typically, the anterior longitudinal ligament (3) is not involved in the inflammatory process. (Hematoxylin and eosin). (With permission from Ball[1].)

Intervertebral discs

Early reports on the pathology of AS were dominated by descriptions of the characteristic macroscopic changes in the spine in the advanced stages of the disease. The rare early histologic accounts of spinal pathology, involving predominantly tissues from the region of the disc obtained from a single or a few cases in each report, described the presence of chronic inflammation and granulation tissue[2–8], fibrosis[2,3,7], chondroid metaplasia and calcification[9], and new bone formation[2,3,5,7,9–11]. However, Ball[1] should be accorded the credit for emphasizing that the spinal manifestations of the disease are explicable on the basis of a sequence (Fig. 106.4) involving an initial inflammatory and destructive enthesopathy, followed by a healing process during which new bone formation may result in ankylosis between adjoining vertebrae.

The most common initial feature is the appearance of erosive lesions involving the ligamentous insertion into the bone at the anterior or anterolateral attachment of the outer annulus at or just below the junction of the annular flange and the corner of the vertebral body, and sometimes at both sites[1]. Occasionally, lesions of a similar kind are seen in the posterior attachments of the outer annulus[1]. Microscopically, the erosive lesions demonstrate infiltration by lymphocytes and plasma cells, and these inflammatory cells tend to spread in a narrow band between the fibers of the outer annulus[1] (Fig. 106.5).

The erosive lesions at the attachment of the annulus heal by the initial formation of woven repair bone which, in due course, is remodeled to form mature lamellar bone. The extension of this new bone across, and for the most part firmly attached to, the outer layers of the annulus pro-

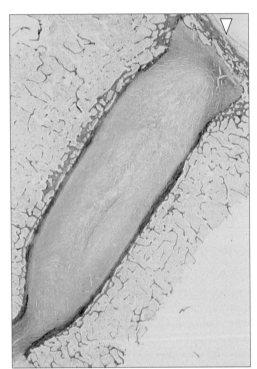

Fig. 106.6 Low-power microscopy of a syndesmophyte (arrow) replacing the outer layers of the anterior annulus and uniting the vertebral bodies. Note that the disc is otherwise normal in appearance. (Hematoxylin & eosin). (Courtesy of Professor J Ball.)

vides the basis for the appearance of the familiar syndesmophytes (Fig. 106.6). The stimulus to the progressive growth of syndesmophytes

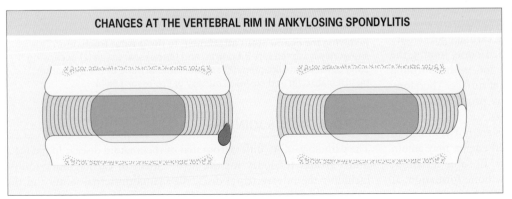

CHANGES AT THE VERTEBRAL RIM IN ANKYLOSING SPONDYLITIS

Fig. 106.4 Changes at the vertebral rim in ankylosing spondylitis. An inflammatory enthesopathy destroys the attachment region of the outer annulus and a syndesmophyte results from healing by ossification.

ally enclose an otherwise normal joint, and this suggests that these capsular changes are the apophyseal equivalent of syndesmophytes[1].

SACROILIAC JOINTS

It is important to note, in considering the pathology of AS, that the sacroiliac joints of normal individuals differ from other synovial joints. Thus there are clear differences between the structure of the articular cartilage of the opposing surfaces, and the joints commonly exhibit synostosis in late adult life, even in the absence of AS. Specifically, the iliac cartilage normally is much thinner than that of the sacral surface. The chondrocytes of the iliac cartilage are clumped in the deeper layers and run in column formations at right angles to the surface, whereas the chondrocytes of the sacral cartilage are spindle- or oval-shaped, with their long axes arranged parallel to the surface. In addition, the collagen fibers of the iliac cartilage are arranged in arcades, as in the hyaline cartilage of other synovial joints, whereas those of the sacral cartilage run parallel to the surface. From the age of 40 years onwards, bony ankylosis occurs with increasing frequency[26–28], with up to 80% of men and 30% of women showing partial or complete ankylosis by the age of 60 years. Age-related bony ankylosis always involves the ligamentous (superior) portion of the sacroiliac space, but intra-articular ankylosis of the synovial (inferior) portion has been claimed to occur only in AS[28].

There have been few opportunities to study the pathology of the sacroiliac joints early in the course of the disease. The initial radiologic features of patchy periarticular osteoporosis, widening of the interosseus space, superficial erosions and focal sclerosis of the subchondral bone can be accounted for by irregular endochondral ossification. This results in the replacement of the dense subchondral bone plate and densely calcified cartilage by more porous cancellous bone, with no evidence of inflammatory osteitis in recent-onset or long-standing disease[1]. Thus there is no pathologic confirmation that the radiologic erosions are inflammatory in nature, but they can be explained by the finding of focal areas of bone porosity (Figs 106.13 & 106.14). The bone sclerosis on the iliac side is the result of appositional lamellar bone formation[1]. Although there are no reports of inflammatory capsular attachment lesions or synovitis[1], these may occur only in the early stages of the disease, long before the joints become available for pathologic study.

In long-standing AS, there is general agreement that capsular ossification commonly produces an outer shell of bone similar to that seen in the apophyseal joints. This shell may enclose normal articular cartilage, cartilage showing endochondral ossification (especially on the iliac side) or a joint ankylosed by fibrous and bony bridges spanning the

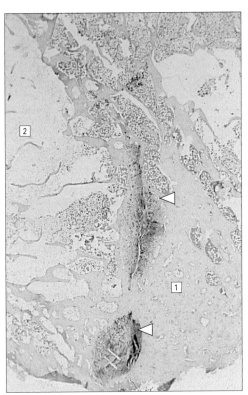

Fig. 106.14 Low-power microscopic view of the sacroiliac joint shown in Fig. 106.13. It shows islands of residual articular cartilage (arrows) separated by bony bridges, and zones of osteosclerosis (1) and osteoporosis (2). (Hematoxylin and eosin.)

joint. In advanced cases, the joint may sometimes be totally obliterated by bone[29], but it is often the case that scattered islands[1,9,29,30] (Figs 106.13 & 106.14) or more extensive areas of intact articular cartilage may remain. As the ligamentous (superior) portion also commonly undergoes ossification, bony fusion of the entire (synovial and ligamentous) sacroiliac space may result[29].

EXTRASKELETAL LESIONS

The occurrence in AS of lesions, possibly specific to the disease, of the heart and aorta and of the lungs is well established. Pathologic changes in other tissues, most frequently the kidney, appear not to be specific to AS.

Heart and aorta

Autopsy studies of patients with AS who have had symptoms resulting from aortic regurgitation[4,31–33] have shown that characteristic cardiovascular pathology exists in such cases.

Frequently, the heart is enlarged as a result of hypertrophy of the left ventricle, and the ascending aorta may show a wrinkled appearance to its lining, similar to that of the 'tree bark' changes seen in syphilis. Typically, there is a distinctive fibrous scarring, limited to the aortic wall behind and immediately above the sinuses of Valsalva, particularly behind and adjacent to the commissures of the aortic valve. A dense adventitial scar extends below the base of the aortic valve to form a characteristic subvalvular ridge. The fibrous tissue extends into the base of the anterior mitral leaflet to form an elevation that may be associated with mitral regurgitation, usually of a mild degree. Further extension of this fibrous tissue may also involve the interventricular septum, and this explains the associated conduction disturbances that are encountered. The aortic valve cusps are shortened, and are usually diffusely thickened.

The microscopic evidence suggests that the sequence of pathologic changes involves areas of patchy destruction of aortic tissue being replaced by granulation tissue and fibrous tissue formation. Fibrous scarring is associated with the accumulation of lymphocytes and plasma cells around small blood vessels, which may show marked thickening of their walls.

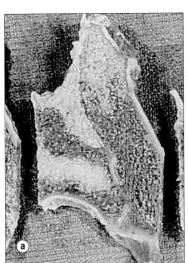 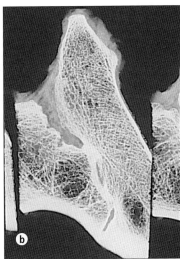

Fig. 106.13 (a) Macroscopic and (b) radiographic views of a slab from the center of a sacroiliac joint in long-standing AS. They show dense capsular ossification, residual articular cartilage and focal osteoporosis.

Aortic regurgitation appears to result from a combination of thickening of the valve cusps, caudal displacement of the cusps by fibrous tissue located behind the commissures, and dilatation of the aortic root[32]. Mitral regurgitation, although rare, appears to result from dilatation of the left ventricle and fibrous thickening at the basal portion of the anterior mitral leaflet. Bundle branch block and complete heart block appear to result from fibrous tissue extensions into the conducting system[32].

Lungs

There have been relatively few pathologic studies of pulmonary involvement in AS[34], and there is insufficient evidence as to whether the disease begins in or around the bronchi, or in alveolar tissue. From the evidence of biopsy and material obtained at autopsy, the early changes consist of patchy pneumonic changes, with chronic inflammatory cell and fibroblast infiltration, progressing to extensive interalveolar fibrosis with areas of hyalinization. Later, dense pleural and pulmonary fibrosis cause distortion of the lung parenchyma, with development of many cysts, some of which may be large. Usually, the end result is dense fibrosis, bronchiectasis and cavity formation. The pulmonary pathology is not restricted to AS, and may be seen in a variety of diseases.

Kidneys

Arteritis occurring in AS is rare, and appears to be restricted to single case descriptions of Wegener-type changes or widespread inflammatory arteritis; however, non-hypertensive renal vascular disease is common[35]

and occurs as either amyloidosis or fibrinoid-type arteriolar hyalinosis. Renal arteriolar hyalinosis is accompanied by the deposition of immunoglobulin, fibrinogen and complement in the walls of arterioles, and in the basement membrane regions of glomeruli and tubules, with ultrastructural deposits of electron-dense material in these locations[36].

CAUSE OF DEATH

Ankylosing spondylitis is usually compatible with long survival despite disability, and few patients are entirely immobilized. Clearly, the rigidity of a completely ankylosed cervical spine carries a substantial risk of fracture-dislocation as a result of minor trauma, and there is an immediate mortality in about 50% of such cases. Patients may also sustain spinal cord damage after spontaneous atlantoaxial subluxation or dislocation.

The occurrence of leukemia or aplastic anemia in patients heavily irradiated for treatment of AS, when that form of therapy was fashionable, has been well documented. In these patients the incidence of leukemia is 10 times, and that of aplastic anemia 40 times, that expected in an unselected population. However, the incidence of cancer and leukemia in patients not treated by irradiation does not differ from that in the remainder of the population[37]. As treatment by irradiation is no longer favored, amyloidosis leading to renal failure has become the most important cause of death directly attributable to AS. In fact, renal failure in AS should be suspected as being caused by amyloidosis until proved otherwise[4].

REFERENCES

1. Ball J. Enthesopathy of rheumatoid and ankylosing spondylitis. Ann Rheum Dis 1971; 30: 213–223.
2. Cruickshank B. Lesions of cartilaginous joints in ankylosing spondylitis. J Pathol Bact 1956; 71: 73–84.
3. Cruickshank B. Pathology of ankylosing spondylitis. Bull Rheum Dis 1960; 10: 211–214.
4. Cruickshank B. Pathology of ankylosing spondylitis. Clin Orthop Rel Res 1971; 74: 43–58.
5. Engfeldt B, Romanus R, Ydén S. Histological studies of pelvo-spondylitis (ankylosing spondylitis) correlated with clinical and radiological findings. Ann Rheum Dis 1954; 13: 219–228.
6. Kanefield DG, Mullins BP, Freehafer AA et al. Destructive lesions of the spine in ankylosing spondylitis. J Bone Joint Surg Am 1969; 51: 1369–1375.
7. Rivelis M, Freiberger RH. Vertebral destruction at unfused segments in late ankylosing spondylitis. Radiology 1969; 93: 251–256.
8. Wholey MH, Pugh DG, Bickel WH. Localized destructive lesions in rheumatoid spondylitis. Radiology 1960; 74: 54–56.
9. Collins DH. The pathology of articular and spinal diseases. London: Edward Arnold; 1949.
10. Aufdermauer M. The morbid anatomy of ankylosing spondylitis. Documenta Rheumatologica. Basle: Geigy: 1957; No 2.
11. Schmorl G, Junghanns H. The human spine in health and disease. New York: Grune & Stratton; 1971.
12. Vernon-Roberts B. Disc pathology and disease states. In: Ghosh P, ed. The biology of the intervertebral disc, vol 2. Boca Raton: CRC Press; 1988: 73–120.
13. Cawley MID, Chalmers TM, Kellgren JH, Ball J. Destructive lesions of vertebral bodies in ankylosing spondylitis. Ann Rheum Dis 1972; 31: 345–358.
14. Vernon-Roberts B. Pathology of intervertebral discs and apophyseal joints. In: Jayson MIV, ed. The lumbar spine and back pain, 3E. London: Churchill Livingstone; 1987: 37–55.
15. Cooper NS, Soren A, McEwen C, Rosenberger JL. Diagnostic specificity of synovial lesions. Hum Pathol 1981; 12: 314–328.
16. Cruickshank B. Histopathology of diarthrodial joints in ankylosing spondylitis. Ann Rheum Dis 1951; 10: 393–404.
17. Revell PA, Mayston V. Histopathology of the synovial membrane of peripheral joints in ankylosing spondylitis. Ann Rheum Dis 1982; 41: 579–586.
18. Soren A. Histodiagnosis and clinical correlation of rheumatoid and other synovitis. Philadelphia: JB Lippincott; 1978.
19. Baeten D, Demetter P, Cuvelier C et al. Comparative study of the synovial histology in rheumatoid arthritis, spondyloarthropathy, and osteoarthritis: influence of disease duration and activity. Ann Rheum Dis 2000; 59: 945–953.

20. Cunnane G, Bresnihan B, FitzGerald O. Immunohistologic analysis of peripheral joint disease in ankylosing spondylitis. Arthritis Rheum 1998; 41: 180–182.
21. Smith MD, O'Donnell J, Highton J et al. Immunohistochemical analysis of synovial membranes from inflammatory and non-inflammatory arthritides: scarcity of CD5 positive B cells and IL2 receptor bearing T cells. Pathology 1992; 24: 19–26.
22. Kidd BL, Moore K, Walters MT et al. Immunohistological features of synovitis in ankylosing spondylitis: a comparison with rheumatoid arthritis. Ann Rheum Dis 1989; 48: 92–98.
23. Laloux L, Voisin MC, Allain J et al. Comparative histological study of enthesitis in spondyloarthropathies [abstract]. Arthritis Rheum 1999; 42: S402.
24. Julkunen H. Rheumatoid spondylitis – clinical and laboratory study of 149 cases compared with 182 cases of rheumatoid arthritis. Acta Rheum Scand 1962; (suppl 4): 1–110.
25. Kendall MJ, Farr M, Meynell MJ, Hawkins CF. Synovial fluid in ankylosing spondylitis. Ann Rheum Dis 1973; 32: 487–492.
26. Sashin D. A critical analysis of the anatomy and the pathological changes of the sacroiliac joints. J Bone Joint Surg 1930; 12: 891–910.
27. Horwitz T, Manges Smith R. An anatomical, pathological and roentgenological study of the intervertebral joints of the lumbar spine and of the sacroiliac joints. Am J Roentgenol 1940; 43: 173–186.
28. Resnick D, Niwayama G, Goergen TG. Degenerative disease of the sacroiliac joint. Invest Radiol 1975; 10: 608–621.
29. Resnick D, Niwayama G, eds. Ankylosing spondylitis. In: Diagnosis of bone and joint disorders, 2E. Philadelphia: WB Saunders; 1988: 1103–1170.
30. François RF, Gardner D, Degrave E, Bywaters E. Sacroiliitis in ankylosing spondylitis is not merely enthesitis. Arthritis Rheum 2000; 43: 2011–2024.
31. Ansell BM, Bywaters EGL, Doniach I. The aortic lesion of ankylosing spondylitis. Br Heart J 1958; 20: 507–515.
32. Bulkley BH, Roberts WC. Ankylosing spondylitis and aortic regurgitation. Circulation 1973; 18: 1014–1027.
33. Schilder DP, Proctor Harvey W, Hufnagel CA. Rheumatoid spondylitis and aortic insufficiency. N Engl J Med 1956; 255: 11–17.
34. Davies D. Ankylosing spondylitis and lung fibrosis. Q J Med 1972; 164: 395–410.
35. Pasternack A, Tallqvist G, Martio J. Renal vascular changes in ankylosing spondylitis. Acta Med Scand 1970; 187: 519–523.
36. Pasternack A, Törnroth T, Martio J. Ultrastructural studies of renal arteriolar changes in ankylosing spondylitis. Acta Pathol Microbiol Scand 1971; 79: 591–603.
37. Smith PG, Doll R, Radford EP. Cancer mortality among patients with ankylosing spondylitis not given X-ray therapy. Br J Radiol 1977; 50: 728–734.

107 Ankylosing spondylitis: management

Ian Haslock

- Early diagnosis, patient education and physical therapy are essential for the successful management of ankylosing spondylitis
- The goals of physical therapy are to restore and maintain posture and movement to as near normal as possible
- Self-management with exercises must be continued on a lifelong basis
- Non-steroidal anti-inflammatory drugs relieve pain and stiffness and facilitate physical therapy
- Sulfasalazine and methotrexate have some effect, particularly in peripheral joint disease
- Anti-tumor necrosis factor-α therapy appears to offer both symptom relief and the possibility of true disease modification

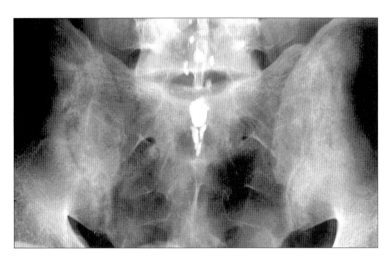

Fig. 107.1 Sacroiliac joint radiograph of a man with AS. Sacroiliitis is shown, along with residual contrast material from a previous myelogram.

INTRODUCTION

The cornerstones of treatment of all rheumatic diseases are early, accurate diagnosis and effective patient education. These are probably more important in ankylosing spondylitis (AS) than in any other condition. Early diagnosis enables treatment before permanent rigidity and deformity have taken place. It also enables patients to develop an appropriate lifestyle as early as possible. The patient's long-term cooperation is the single most crucial factor leading to successful management of AS. It is unlikely that the degree of long-term cooperation and commitment needed to develop a therapeutic lifestyle will be achieved unless the patient has a thorough understanding of the disease and the rationale behind its management.

As soon as the diagnosis of AS is made, the patient must be given a clear description of the nature of spondylitis. In particular, AS must be differentiated from mechanical back pain, and the differences in therapeutic approach to these conditions must be clearly stated. The advice can be reinforced with written material, such as that produced by the Arthritis Research Campaign (ARC) and National Ankylosing Spondylitis Society (NASS) in the UK and the Arthritis Foundation and the Spondylitis Society of America in the USA. Evaluation of the ARC leaflets confirmed their effectiveness in conveying information[1], but it is also important that this is reinforced by other members of the multidisciplinary team, especially the clinic nurses and physical therapists. Many patients now look for information on the internet. All the organisations mentioned above have informative, accurate web sites, but not all information given on the web is unbiased and accurate[2] and healthcare professionals managing patients with spondylitis must be prepared both to give advice regarding appropriate web sites and to refute misinformation given by others.

Unfortunately, many patients suffer from delay in diagnosis[3] and may have been given alternative diagnoses before the accurate one is made. The patient whose radiograph is shown in Figure 107.1 is typical of many patients with AS. His sacroiliac pain had been diagnosed as 'sciatica' and he had investigations including myelography and exploratory surgery in

order to find the cause of his symptoms. His sacroiliitis was clearly visible, but unreported, on many previous films. Such patients are justifiably suspicious of a totally new diagnosis, especially one which requires a radically different approach to treatment compared with previous advice. There is evidence that delays in diagnosis are decreasing. A survey of the 14 000 members of the German ankylosing spondylitis society, the Deutsche Vereinigung Morbus Bechterew (DVMB), showed that the average time to diagnosis had decreased from 15 years in those with a disease onset in the 1950s to 7.5 years for those with disease onset in 1975–79. It did not appear that further improvements were occurring at later dates[4].

OBJECTIVES OF TREATMENT

Initially, the objective is to reduce the patients' pain and stiffness, if possible by self-management. Where movement has been lost, there is an urgent need to restore as much as possible. The long-term objectives are to maintain symptom relief, maintain posture and movement, including chest wall and peripheral joint movement, and enable a full work capacity unimpeded by sickness absenteeism. In enabling these objectives, medication should be minimal and self-care maximal.

MANAGEMENT TECHNIQUES

Physical therapy

Physiotherapy is widely recognized as the single most important aspect of management of AS. There is some evidence that exercise alone can produce adequate symptom relief in many patients with AS; 178 of 236 patients from the armed forces followed long-term achieved symptom control by this means alone[5]. Controlled studies of physical therapy are

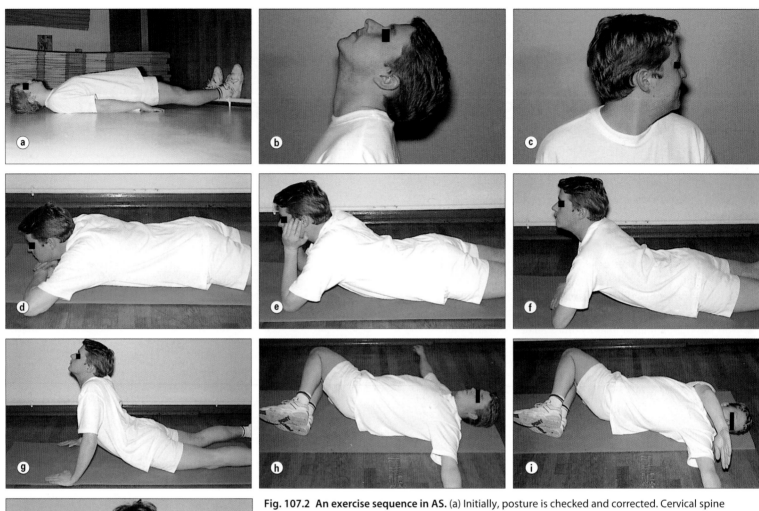

Fig. 107.2 An exercise sequence in AS. (a) Initially, posture is checked and corrected. Cervical spine exercises include full flexion (b), extension (c) and rotation (d–g). A full sequence of back extension is followed by rotation in (h, i) lying and (j) upright kneeling positions. Finally, breathing using thoracic muscles is checked and practiced.

has also been shown to increase range of movement in the short term[7]. Physical therapy takes two forms; that provided within the physical therapy department, and the patients' own home exercise regimes.

At the time of diagnosis of AS, the patient should have an immediate referral to a physical therapist, whose aims will be to restore posture and movement to as near normal as possible. Hydrotherapy is particularly valuable in producing the appropriate environment in which movement can be maximized[8]. A variety of pain relief methods such as pulsed short-wave therapy, local heat or cold, interferential therapy, local ultrasound or transcutaneous nerve stimulation[9] may be useful in facilitating movement. Non-steroidal anti-inflammatory drugs (NSAIDs) in high doses also may be needed during this phase of treatment, again with the objective of diminishing pain to a degree sufficient to allow full mobilization. Regaining lost movement at this time may cause discomfort, which results in apprehension in many patients, especially those who have been previously misdiagnosed and instructed to rest if pain increases. The attending physician must be sensitive to the patient's anxieties and willing to produce the greatest possible degree of analgesia to facilitate increased range of movement. Chest expansion and breathing exercises are also important. Local enthesopathy may need systemic drug treatment, local corticosteroid injection or local treatment by the physical therapist, using modalities such as ultrasound.

The initial period of treatment must be combined with an intensive education program. The patient must be told repeatedly that long-term success in disease management is dependent on the regularity of their

rare, although significant benefit from exercise and education can be demonstrated over relatively short periods[6] and manipulative therapy

home exercise regime; extra discomfort must be seen as a need for extra exercise, not extra rest. In teaching patients their home exercise regime, it is essential that therapists recognize that doing regular exercises is time-consuming and boring. It is therefore essential to try to incorporate as much appropriate exercise as possible into the patient's lifestyle by encouraging recreational exercises such as swimming and lighter sports such as badminton. Postural correction often involves undoing ingrained habits, particularly sitting in slouched positions. Good chest movement and breathing technique have to be taught, not assumed, and all these patients should be strongly advised not to smoke.

The initial period of physical therapy is a time of intense activity for the therapist and the patient. If treatment has been started before a significant amount of fixed deformity has occurred, and if the patient has proved cooperative with the treatment program, both therapist and patient will be rewarded by improved movement and decreased symptoms. The fact that this period of disease management is short and that the gains made are often quite dramatic, makes it a popular time for all concerned. However, unless the instant gratification of this exciting period can be translated into commitment to a long-term management program, the progess made is likely to be transient.

The patient's own efforts are the key to long-term success. Persuading all patients with AS that a daily exercise program must become as automatic a part of their day as cleaning their teeth or combing their hair calls for a major educational effort and constant reinforcement. The program the therapist teaches must be realistic physically, taking into account the degree of deformity that has already become fixed, and must have a time commitment that can be accommodated within the patient's everyday life (Fig. 107.2). Unrealistic expectations produce negative reactions that sabotage the entire program. The exercise and lifestyle program should also aim at cardiovascular fitness, as this has been shown to be important in maintaining work capacity, even if chest wall rigidity has occurred[10].

Lifelong regular exercise

Supervision of exercise regimes long-term by physical therapists has been shown to improve persistence with exercises and result in better outcomes than simple encouragement to persist with a home exercise regime[11]. Internal self-motivation involves frequent reinforcement of the need to exercise, coupled with clear explanation of its value in disease management. External motivation from spouses and family members is important. Joining a self-help group such as NASS often provides the spur needed to undertake regular exercise, although objective evidence of benefit from membership in a self-help group is lacking[12]. The provision of devices giving feedback regarding the effectiveness of home exercises can also be helpful in maintaining the impetus to continue them effectively[13].

Reinforcement of the exercise program is the responsibility of all health professionals coming into contact with the patient. The understanding, help and support of family members is also important, and securing their cooperation is a vital part of the educational process. Every consultation, for whatever purpose, should include the questions, 'Are you still doing all the exercises the physical therapist showed you?' and 'How often are you doing them?'. Any deterioration in posture should also be noted and commented on, with an attempt made to find the cause and remedy the problem.

Many patients with AS do not require regular prescriptions, and some mechanism must exist to ensure that they are seen and assessed regularly by their physical therapist, or family or hospital doctor. A chart showing progressive change in objective measurements, which the patient keeps, is a good method of documenting progression for both the patient and the clinical team. Even patients with late disease benefit from techniques such as appropriately applied passive stretching[14], and once demonstrated to be effective, techniques such as this can be taught to the

patient for use with the assistance of a helper. Supervised training periods, including sessions in a hydrotherapy pool undertaken at weekly intervals, have also been shown to maintain mobility and function over prolonged periods, although no untreated control group was available for comparison[15]. However, the measured retention of movement and posture over a 5-year period using this regime provides a useful benchmark for alternative strategies.

A particularly intensive approach to physical treatment has been used in the AS unit at Bath, England[16]. Patients there were admitted to hospital each year for an intensive 3-week period of physiotherapy and hydrotherapy, accompanied by an educational program and reinforcement of their home exercise regime. Short-term benefit was found by comparing measurements made at the beginning with those at the end of each in-patient period. It was concluded that, even in advanced disease, small but worthwhile benefits could be achieved. A similar regime provided similar results over a slightly longer follow-up period[17], but whether such a highly expensive use of resources is justified, especially in comparison with intensive outpatient regimes, remains open to question.

For more everyday practice, one reliable way of reinforcing exercises and lifestyle is through a patient-run group. Most branches have arrangements for regular assessment and exercise sessions, usually staffed by volunteer physical therapists. Each session incorporates a warm-up and stretching period followed by exercise sessions, including hydrotherapy where available, and often culminating in light-heartedly competitive games. The meetings give the opportunity for discussion of problems with the therapist, and more formal educational sessions to improve the patient's knowledge of their disease and its management. Also, patient groups such as NASS provide a rich source of knowledge[4] and opinion, in addition to a focus of pressure for better diagnostic and treatment facilities.

The end-product of these efforts should be knowledgeable, active patients with a postural and exercise program built in to their daily lives, enabling them to be fit and active with minimal symptoms.

OCCUPATIONAL THERAPY

In the case of patients with early disease, occupational therapists will probably limit their interventions to the educational part of patient management. This will particularly involve advice about posture, especially appropriate seating, and recreation. The psychologic training of occupational therapists often makes them the most appropriate team member to lead the development of pain control strategies with patients[18].

For those in whom disease is more advanced, assessment of activities of daily living and ergonomic assessment of the home and the work place become more important, and may lead to the provision of aids if deformity produces significant practical problems. Patients with spondylitis often find that their decreased bending ability causes problems with dressing, and items such as elastic laces and stocking aids become essential for independence. Raised chair seats and toilet seats, showers in place of baths and other more complex home modifications may be needed as disease advances. Mobility is vital to all patients with arthritis; and car adaptations including wide-view mirrors, and modified controls may be required by those with more advanced spondylitis. For patients with very severe fixed spinal deformity, prismatic spectacles may be the only method of achieving an adequate amount of forward vision.

Other members of the multidisciplinary team, such as podiatrists and social workers, will also become involved with any patient whose disease progresses. Work is an area of particular importance to patients with AS, as many are on the thresholds of their careers when the diagnosis is made, and a realistic discussion about the possibility of disease progression may be an important part of their career choice. Those in employment may need skilled career advice to facilitate changing to more suitable occupations, but for most this can be achieved without a significant diminution in their job satisfaction or income[19]. Studies undertaken in the armed forces demonstrate the ability of fit, active, well-motivated people to follow a physically demanding career despite AS. Unfortunately, the persuasive talents of the Marine drill sergeant regarding regular exercise have no equal in civilian life. In general, the greatest problems for AS patients lie in jobs involving prolonged work in a single position, especially desk or computer work. Work posture is vital, as is the need to change position regularly and, preferably, to undertake some form of exercise such as a brisk walk, during the lunchbreak.

DRUG TREATMENT

Simple analgesics are usually considered to have a limited role in treating inflammatory rheumatic diseases. They are, however, quite widely used, about 33% of patients taking them, often as over-the-counter rather than prescribed medication. This reflects patients' desire for pain relief as their most important objective of drug treatment[20]. Health professionals are not good at appreciating the severity of patients' pain. Aggregated data from clinical trials suggested that both doctors and nurses assessed the patients pain as about 20% less than the patients did. This is probably because of a combination of the poverty of the tools used to assess pain routinely, coupled with a societal prejudice to applaud stoicism, and difficulty by the professional in accepting the inadequacies of their prescribed treatments. Patients also desire their medication to be as risk-free as possible[21], and the extensive publicity regarding NSAID-induced gastrointestinal bleeding seems to have had a considerable effect on patients' perceptions of these drugs, which enhances the desire to stick with simple analgesics, or no drugs at all, whenever possible. It also contributes to the popularity of 'alternative' therapy, which promises safety in addition to a degree of efficacy unobtainable by allopathic means.

Non-steroidal anti-inflammatory drugs

The NSAIDs are used extensively to provide symptom relief to patients with AS. Overall, the objective of NSAIDs is to relieve pain sufficiently to allow free movement, especially for the exercise program essential to the spondylitic patient. During early stages of the disease they are often used in full dosage to cover the entire day. This schedule is particularly important when initial physical therapy is being used to maximize movement. Subsequently, morning stiffness is often the only symptom, or the predominant one, and a single sustained-release or long-acting night-time dose such as modified-release indomethacin 75mg, modified-release diclofenac 100mg or naproxen 500mg is often the preparation of choice, allowing freedom of movement in the morning. Many patients find that even this level of medication is needed only on an occasional basis, provided they maintain their regular exercises. Others will require either prolonged night-time medication or the continued use of divided doses to give more sustained symptom relief.

Choice of NSAID

The traditional 'best' NSAID is phenylbutazone, which has been claimed for many years to have particular benefit in patients with AS. For this reason, although phenylbutazone has been banned for general use in many countries, some may still permit its prescription by hospital consultants only, specifically in the treatment of AS. Despite the continuing availability of this medication for AS, it is now little used in the UK and USA and there is no convincing evidence that its 'special' efficacy has been missed. This view is not shared in much of continental Europe, where it remains the treatment of choice in AS for many physicians.

Indomethacin is probably the most widely used NSAID in AS, and has adopted the role of phenylbutazone as being especially valuable for patients with seronegative spondyloarthritis. A large study of more than 1300 British patients with AS showed that indomethacin was both the NSAID most commonly and continuously used, and the one that was most likely to be taken over a prolonged period[22]. It has the advantage of several dosage forms and sizes, making it flexible in use. Single modified-release 75mg doses at night are an effective way of diminishing morning stiffness. Suppositories have been used for this purpose in the mistaken belief that they deliver a sustained action by virtue of slower absorption; this is untrue, the morning activity being related to the greater dose in the suppositories (100mg) rather than to differences in absorption rate. Indomethacin has a reputation as a drug with a high incidence of side effects. Central nervous system toxicities, especially headache, do limit its use. These appear to be associated with peak plasma concentrations, and are reduced by modified-release preparations. The belief that indomethacin is particularly toxic as far as the upper gastrointestinal tract is concerned is not borne out by endoscopic studies[23] and, in any case, spondylitic patients are usually in a younger age group, with less risk of serious side effects in the gut, at their time of maximal NSAID need.

Naproxen is the second most popular NSAID[22]. It has a long half-life, giving relief of morning stiffness from a 500mg night-time dose, or whole-day symptom relief from a twice-daily dosage. The dose may be increased to 1.5g daily to relieve symptoms from acute exacerbations.

Almost all other NSAIDs are also used in treating AS. Selection is always a balance of effectiveness and tolerance. Patients' responses, both positive and adverse, are highly individual and far exceed the overall statistical differences between drugs. It has been suggested that summation of these apparently idiosyncratic differences can result in an overall 'pecking order' of NSAIDs being constructed that might give guidance for selection, taking into account factors such as age and sex in addition to individual diagnoses[24].

The effects of NSAIDs have been attributed to their ability to inhibit prostaglandins involved in the inflammatory process, with the side effects relating to the simultaneous inhibition of protective prostaglandins. It has been demonstrated that the target enzyme cyclo-oxygenase (COX) exists in two isoforms: a constitutive form, COX1, being responsible for the protective action in areas such as maintenance of gastric defences, and an inducible form, COX2, involved in the inflammatory process. This observation has enabled an understanding of differences in toxicity in the conventional NSAIDs, with higher ratios of COX1:COX2 inhibition being associated with greater toxicity. It has also led to the development of so-called 'specific' COX2 inhibitors or 'coxibs', which, in normal therapeutic doses, have little or no COX1-inhibiting activity. Two such compounds are now available – rofecoxib and celecoxib – and they appear to have borne out the theoretical prediction that their efficacy would be similar to that of conventional NSAIDs while the amount of serious upper gastrointestinal toxicity would be diminished. Experience of their use in AS is limited, but there is evidence of short-term efficacy in this disease[25]. Long-term studies in AS and comparisons with a range of NSAIDs, including newer ones with higher COX2:COX1 ratios than current drugs, and comparisons between individual coxibs, are still required before their definitive role can be assessed.

Two aspects of NSAID use in AS deserve particular attention. First, their proven action is restricted to relief of symptoms such as pain and stiffness. Any increase in spinal movement is related to an increased ability to exercise because of this symptom relief, rather than to any intrinsic action of the drug. Secondly, clinical trials of NSAIDs in AS must be studied with considerable attention to the details of the trial procedures. Many trials allow physical therapy to continue during drug treatment if the patient was being treated with it on entry to the study. Physical therapy is such an important part of AS management that the results of any study that allows inconsistent physical therapeutic input should be rejected. Many trial procedures are also of insufficient duration to give optimal information regarding efficacy and tolerability[26].

There are also two ways in which NSAIDs might have a more specific role in AS. A retrospective analysis of a small number of patients taking phenylbutazone suggested that this drug inhibited the calcification of syndesmophytes[27]. Similar suggestions have been made regarding indomethacin[28]. These observations have not been explored using prospective placebo-controlled studies, but it has been suggested that AS has become less severe since the introduction of NSAIDs[29]. It is thus unknown whether NSAIDs should be used in the symptomatic fashion outlined above, or whether they should be taken on a long-term basis irrespective of symptoms The effects of NSAIDs on the upper gastrointestinal tract are well recognized, but more recently their effects in the small bowel have been recognized as being both common and important. When these observations are coupled with the observation of silent lesions in the same area observed by ileocolonoscopy and scintigraphy[30] in patients with seronegative spondyloarthropathies, the potential for NSAIDs to have an adverse effect on the disease must be considered.

Disease-modifying treatment

In contrast to the claims made in rheumatoid arthritis (RA), no claim has yet been made that any drug has a true disease-modifying effect on AS. Almost all the second line drugs used in the management of RA have been tried at some time in AS. The majority have been disappointing, with gold, penicillamine and antimalarials proving ineffective.

Sulfasalazine

Sulfasalazine has particular properties that command attention, with interest based on its widespread use in the treatment of inflammatory bowel disease. Although it was generally accepted that AS is an hereditary accompaniment to inflammatory bowel disease[31], rather than being caused by it, as is the case with enteropathic arthritis, this view received challenge from the work of Mielants and colleagues (see Chapter 113). They undertook colonoscopy and visual examination of the terminal ileum, initially in patients with reactive arthritis after enteric infection. They observed inflammatory lesions in the small bowel, and later extended their observations to idiopathic AS, in which similar lesions were again demonstrated[32]. Although clinically silent, these lesions bear a striking histologic similarity to Crohn's disease, and some of the patients who have them go on to develop florid clinical Crohn's disease. Their relationship to etiology is thus a continuing source of speculation. Under these circumstances, use of sulfasalazine combines the serendipitous logic of extrapolation from RA to AS with a scientific logic suggested by these observations.

Several studies of sulfasalazine have now been undertaken both in patients with peripheral joint synovitis and in those with spinal disease alone. An initial meta-analysis confirmed both the efficacy and safety of sulfasalazine in AS in the short term[33]. A more recent re-evaluation of published trials suggested that the spinal and peripheral joints are affected differently, and that sulfasalazine should be considered as a safe and well-tolerated therapy for persistent, active peripheral synovitis[34]. There is some evidence that the effect is greater in those with early disease than those in whom disease is more advanced, this being defined by the presence of fixed or bony deformity[35]. There is also some evidence that clinical improvement is accompanied by decreases in C-reactive protein (CRP) concentration and erythrocyte sedimentation rate (ESR), a combination of events that in RA is considered indicative of disease-modifying action. As sulfasalazine is a drug with which there is considerable clinical experience, including its safe use over many years, it would seem reasonable to introduce it early in the treatment of patients whose disease shows signs of poor control by physical treatment coupled with NSAIDs. Incremental doses starting at 0.5g twice daily and increasing to 1.5g twice daily have been used, although slightly higher doses are sometimes used to treat inflammatory bowel disease and are logical if partial response occurs.

Sulfasalazine may reduce the sperm count, and a warning about this is part of the information given to all men taking it. In practice,there seems to be little effect except in those in whom infertility is proving a problem. In contrast, sulfasalazine is probably the safest drug treatment for a woman contemplating pregnancy.

Methotrexate

Methotrexate has been given to patients with AS in low dosages (7.5–25mg oral or intramuscular weekly pulsed doses) similar to those used in RA, and appears to have a beneficial effect on both peripheral joints and spinal disease[36], although few placebo-controlled studies have yet been published. Many of the patients to whom methotrexate might be of particular value are young people with severe, active disease that is unremittingly progressive despite cooperation with an exercise regime. Some of these patients wish to start a family, and the potentially teratogenic effect in both men and women taking this drug has proved a significant practical problem.

All patients taking methotrexate must be warned explicitly about its teratogenic risks. Men must be reminded of the need to ensure adequare contraceptive precautions during intercourse while they are taking methotrexate and for 3 months thereafter. Women taking methotrexate must ensure they take reliable contraceptive precautions during treatment and for 3 months after stopping treatment, and must also be warned that termination of pregnancy may be needed should they accidentally conceive. In practice, these constraints have proved an inhibition to many patients contemplating the use of methotrexate.

Other immunosuppressive agents

Cyclophosphamide, given intravenously in 200mg doses on alternate days for 3 weeks, followed by a 100mg oral dose weekly for 3 months, has been used successfully on an open basis, producing a reduction in peripheral joint synovitis and spinal pain, although no improvement in spinal movement[37]. This was accompanied by a significant decrease in ESR, but no controlled studies have been undertaken. There is also anecdotal evidence that azathioprine is helpful in intractable enthesopathy, but again controlled observations do not exist.

Pamidronate

The major use of bisphosphonates has been in the treatment of osteoporosis and other bone disorders such as Paget's disease. Recent work suggests that they may suppress the formation of proinflammatory cytokines such as interleukin (IL)-1, IL-6 and tumor necrosis factor (TNF)-α. An open study in patients with AS used two regimes of intravenous pamidronate, 30mg monthly for 3 months then 60mg monthly for a further 3 months, compared with 60mg monthly for 3 months. Both groups showed clinical improvement and the 6-month regime also produced a reduction in ESR[38]. The only significant side effect of treatment was a post-injection flare, especially after the first infusion. This occurred in 50% of patients, which will produce difficulty with double-blind evaluation against placebo. This form of treatment could also have an effect on the osteoporosis found in AS, mediated both by its antiinflammatory and antiresorptive actions.

Thalidomide

Thalidomide also affects proinflammatory cytokines, particularly IL-12 and TNF-α. Open studies in AS at doses of up to 300mg daily produced both significant clinical improvement and a decrease in CRP[39].

Tumor necrosis factor-α blockade

The TNF-α blocking drugs, infliximab and etanercept, have proved dramaticaly effective in the treatment of rheumatoid arthritis and also Crohn's disease. There is less experience in AS, but the findings of a number of studies are now available[40,41] that suggest a high level of effectiveness in AS. The short-term efficacy demonstrated in early studies[42] appears to be maintained after follow-up for 1 year[43]. These drugs appear to act on both spinal and peripheral joints, and offer hope of genuine disease retardation, with prevention or delay of spinal ankylosis. This possibility is supported by the improvement in magnetic resonance imaging (MRI) appearances of both sacroiliitis and enthesitis during etanercept treatment[44]. A clinical and MRI study using infliximab also showed improvement in MRI appearance in both early and advanced disease[45]. Experience of early treatment, which would be predicted to be of maximum benefit, is small at present, but the 11 patients in one study[46] had a mean disease duration of 5 years (range 0.5–13 years), and showed very considerable improvement. Of the 10 patients who completed the regimen of three infliximab infusions, nine showed improvement of 50% or more in activity, function and pain scores. There were significant decreases in both CRP and IL-6. SF36 scores showed improvement, and two of three patients with MRI evidence of inflammation showed improvement.

The potential for effective, truly disease-modifying, but expensive and potentially toxic, therapy in AS produces some important questions[47]. Who should be treated? The majority of patients with AS do well with regular exercises and non-steroidal drugs. It would seem inappropriate to introduce anti-TNF treatment at an early stage in these patients. However, prognostic factors in early AS are not well defined, so picking an appropriate cohort for early aggressive treatment rationally is at present difficult. A 10-year longitudinal study of 151 patients with AS was carried out in an attempt to determine poor prognostic factors[48]. It found that hip arthritis, increased ESR (more than 30mm in the first 1 hour), poor response to NSAIDs, limitation of spinal movement and oligoarthritis, occurring in the first 2 years of disease, plus onset at age 16 years or less, were poor prognostic factors. At present, the criterion used for any extension of therapy is the failure of simple treatment, which might be inappropriately vague if optimal gain is to be achieved from these drugs. How early is early? Delays in diagnosis of AS are still measured in years, with little sign of recent improvement. If timely early treatment is the most effective, there will be difficulty recruiting patients for convincing clinical trials and, if successful, difficulty improving early diagnosis at primary care level. In summary, the exact place of this treatment remains to be defined, but this definition is needed urgently, as it offers what is, at present, the best potential treatment for a disease that can have catastrophic long-term consequences.

Corticosteroids

Long-term treatment with systemic corticosteroids has little part to play in the management of AS, although rare patients exist in whom no other form of treatment proves effective. Despite its appearance of overossification, the spine in AS contains vertebrae that are significantly osteoporotic, possibly as a result of diversion of mechanical stress from the vertebral bodies to the surrounding syndesmophyte bridges, in addition to the effect of proinflammatory cytokines. The effect of long-term corticosteroids on this osteoporosis is unproved, but on theoretic grounds might be expected to increase it. Figure 107.3 shows the bone mineral density (BMD) of an active man with AS who had a good exercise record and had been treated with low-dose corticosteroids for 21 years. The osteoporosis seen puts him at significant risk of spinal fracture.

Parenteral low-dose corticotropin proved ineffective when added to an inpatient rehabilitation regime[49]. Intravenous pulsed methylprednisolone is undoubtedly effective in reducing severe symptoms[50]. The indications for its use are poorly defined, but experience suggests it is an extremely effective way of controlling symptoms on a short-term basis. The period of reduced symptoms produced by this treatment should always be utilized for intensive physical therapy, in order to maximize movement and correct posture as much as possible. Local corticosteroid injections are useful both for peripheral joint disease and for local treatment of enthesopathy.

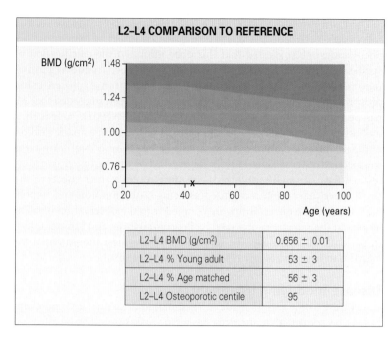

L2–L4 BMD (g/cm²)	0.656 ± 0.01
L2–L4 % Young adult	53 ± 3
L2–L4 % Age matched	56 ± 3
L2–L4 Osteoporotic centile	95

Fig. 107.3 Bone mineral density with corticosteroid treatment. Result from dual-energy X-ray absorptiometer scan of a 42-year-old man with AS. He had been treated with prednisolone for 21 years. His Z score for vertebral height was −2.44.

Radiation therapy

Radioactive synovectomy, using yttrium-90 especially, is a useful treatment for chronic synovitis, particularly in the knee. This treatment should be reserved for those who have completed their family, because of the small risk of chromosome change through irradiation of the groin lymphatics.

External radiotherapy aimed at the spine and sacroiliac joints was widely used until the publication of work by Court-Brown and Doll[51], which demonstrated an increased incidence of leukemia in patients treated in this way. Since then, radiotherapy has been largely discarded, although it is possible that carefully targeted treatment using modern equipment would give benefit with a degree of safety comparable to that of some disease-modifying antirheumatic drugs – certainly the doses and frequency of treatment used in the 1940s were well in excess of those that would be used now. Patients who had been treated with radiotherapy also illustrate the need for persisting with exercises, irrespective of the quality of symptom control. Many of these patients were told they had been cured, and hence their regular exercise regimes were no longer needed. Although many remained pain-free, the progression of spinal fusion and the disability caused by it continued unabated.

Local radiotherapy is still accepted as having a small place in the management of AS. Any isolated joints or entheses unresponsive to systemic and local treatment might be considered for this form of treatment, but in practice it is almost exclusively reserved for the treatment of painful heels. Although an apparently 'minor' problem, painful heels can be the source of considerable disability. Enthesitis at the insertion of the tendo Achillis or the plantar fascia into the calcaneum may also be accompanied by calcaneal periostitis (Fig. 107.4). Although this usually occurs in established AS, it may be either the presenting symptom or, rarely, the sole manifestation of the disease. Treatment with sorbo insoles and local physiotherapy may be effective. Local steroid injections can be dramatically effective, although injection of Achilles tendinitis and paratendinitis may lead to tendon rupture[52]. Resistant cases usually respond rapidly to local radiotherapy[53], preferably with superficial orthovoltage radiation or, if this is unavailable, electrons of appropriate energy (6–9McV) from a suitable linear accelerator. The localized area treated and the relatively

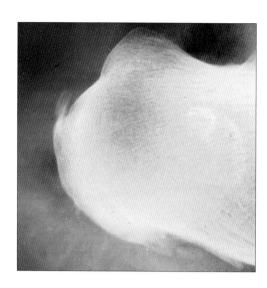

Fig. 107.4 Radiographic features in the heel of a patient with spondyloarthropathy. 'Whiskering' is present at the insertion of the tendo achillis, and plantar aponeurosis periostitis can be seen along the inferior and posterior aspects of the calcaneus.

small dose needed (6–12Gy) mean that complications are extremely unlikely, and this form of treatment can, therefore, be recommended under these circumstances.

OSTEOPOROSIS IN ANKYLOSING SPONDYLITIS

The development of thick bony bridges between vertebrae and the apparent tendency of patients with AS to be prone to heterotopic new bone formation after surgery have given the impression that AS is a disease characterized by thick and excessive bone. In addition, treatment with prolonged weight-bearing exercise should provide the stimulus for maximal bone formation. Despite this, many patients with AS show evidence of significant spinal osteoporosis[54]. This is presumably related to deviation of mechanical stresses away from the vertebral bodies by the syndesmophytic bridges, although the local relationship between bridging and porosis has not yet been ascertained. Local inflammatory disease may also contribute to local bone loss from a mechanism similar to the juxta-articular bone loss in RA[55]. There is certainly an association with active inflammation[56], but there is still some doubt as to the exact mechanisms involved, as most patients show normal markers of bone formation and resorption[57]. Osteoporosis may contribute to the vulnerability of the AS spine when subjected to trauma.

It would seem reasonable for all patients with AS to undergo bone densitometry, usually by dual-energy X-ray absorptiometry scanning, to ascertain their degree of osteoporosis, with follow-up scans at regular intervals of not less than 2 years. Hip measurement is especially important in those in whom the presence of syndesmophytes artificially increases the spinal density. Where significant osteoporosis is found, the usual investigations of this condition, remembering that many of the patients are male, should be undertaken. Treatment recommendations are at present speculative, but if a patient has osteoporosis, and no non-spondylitic cause for this has been found, the treatment of choice is probably a bisphosphonate such as alendronate or risedronate in postmenopausal women and in men. There is at present no information on the effect that inflammatory lesions in the gut of the spondylitic patient have on either calcium absorption or the development of osteoporosis, although idiopathic inflammatory bowel disease is associated with excess bone loss[58].

NON-LOCOMOTOR DISEASE

Eye disease is the most common extralocomotor complication of AS with at least 20% of patients suffering isolated or repeated attacks of iritis (anterior uveitis). As there is no close temporal relationship between the severity of iritis and spondylitis, the eye disease is usually treated as a separate entity, although there is some evidence that sulphasalazine may produce a reduction in both the severity and frequency of anterior uveitis[59]. The most important aspect of treatment is to ensure that the patients seek immediate medical advice on developing a painful red eye. The consequences of delayed or inadequate treatment are the formation of synechiae, which are adhesions from the back of the iris. Secondary glaucoma may then supervene.

Anterior uveitis associated with AS is usually unilateral. In most cases, topical treatment with corticosteroid eye drops and mydriatics is all that is required. The eye may need to be protected from the light to ensure comfort during the period of pupillary dilatation. Administration of corticosteroids orally or by intraocular injection is required when local treatment fails to relieve the inflammation. In children with treatment-resistant uveitis, etanercept has been shown to be beneficial[60], but a retrospective study in adults with a variety of rheumatic diseases, including AS and psoriatic spondylitis, showed that, in contrast to 100% showing a decrease in articular inflammation, only 38% showed improvement of their uveitis. Neither of the patients with spondylitis showed improvement in their eyes, the patient with psoriatic spondylitis actually developing eye disease during etanercept treatment[61]. Three patients with chronic unilateral anterior uveitis were included in one study of infliximab[45]. Two were described as showing 'noticeable improvement', whereas the third suffered a flare after initial improvement. More work is obviously needed to define the role of anti-TNF drugs in the management of this potentially serious condition.

Iritis is, on occasions, the presenting symptom of AS, especially in those in whom back pain is mild or stiffness has occurred insidiously. Those treating apparently idiopathic anterior uveitis, especially when unilateral, should always consider the possibility of this diagnosis. One study of 514 consecutive patients with anterior uveitis attending a specialist uveitis clinic[62] showed that 117 (22.7%) had a seronegative spondyloarthritis, with ankylosing spondylitis being the most common (75 patients). In 62 of the spondylarthritis patients, including 35 with AS, uveitis was the presenting symptom.

The two major internal organs involved in AS are the heart and the lungs. Diseases such as aortic valve disease are treated identically to similar diseases in non-spondylitic patients. Extra precautions may be needed at the time of any surgery, as neck rigidity can produce difficulties for anesthesia. Long-term anticoagulation after valve surgery complicates the treatment of the joint disease because of interactions with NSAIDs, which displace warfarin from protein binding and thus alter anticoagulant need. Also, patients who are in need of cardiac surgery, and hence anticoagulation, are usually older, and so come into the age group in which the risk of major bleeding produced by NSAIDs is increased. It is prudent in these patients to avoid non-selective NSAIDs if at all possible, and if symptom relief cannot be obtained in any other way, to use COX2-selective inhibitors. These may be useful in this situation, as they do not inhibit platelet function and have been shown to be associated with a lower risk of gastrointestinal bleeding. An alternative approach is cotherapy with proton-pump inhibitors.

Upper zone lung fibrosis is, at least in part, caused by inadequate aeration of this area, especially in those with rigid chest walls who rely on diaphragmatic breathing. Inclusion of breathing exercises in the routine for patients with AS is an important part of prevention of this complication. When it occurs, diagnostic confusion with tuberculosis may occur, especially where cavitation occurs (Fig. 107.5). Such cavities may become colonized with *Aspergilla*.

No specific treatment is available for the lung disease of AS. Stopping smoking and regular breathing exercises are obviously essential. Incidental infections and fungal colonization require appropriate specific treatment, which should be given promptly in order to minimize further lung damage.

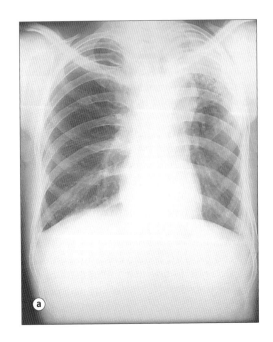
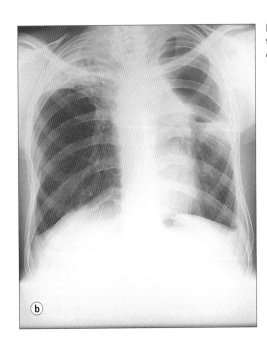

Fig. 107.5 (a) Upper lobe lung fibrosis leading to (b) cavitation in AS. This cavity became colonized with *Aspergilla*.

MANAGEMENT OF WOMEN WITH ANKYLOSING SPONDYLITIS

Until relatively recently, conventional teaching was that ankylosing spondylitis is rare in women. This led to situations typified by the patient shown in Figure 107.6. When she presented with symptoms typical of AS, that diagnosis was not considered as it was 'well known' that this disease did not occur in women. As a result, she was treated with a corset, which certainly made her spinal rigidity worse. Despite her clinically obvious AS, this diagnosis had still not been considered because she was able to touch her toes – as she illustrates, this is easily

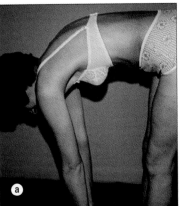

Fig. 107.6 AS in women.
(a) This woman with AS was misdiagnosed because of her ability to touch her toes. Thorough examination revealed (b) her full range of extension (c) and her side flexion to be virtually nil. More accurate observation and the performance of a Schober test (Fig. 107.12) revealed that her forward flexion took place almost entirely from her hips.

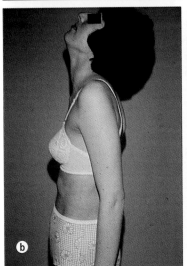
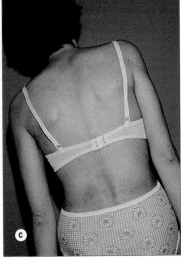

possible for someone with a rigid back who has mobile hips and well-stretched hamstrings, and is a perfect example of the reason why finger–floor distance is an inappropriate measure.

Pregnancy in women with AS requires particular consideration for five reasons:

● Genetic counselling. AS is known to be a disease with a strong genetic component. Many patients require discussion of the implications of this before embarking on pregnancy
● Effects of treatment on conception. AS itself does not appear to affect fertility adversely, but some drugs used to treat AS, such as methotrexate, are potentially teratogenic, and appropriate advice about this must be given to all women of childbearing age
● Effects of pregnancy on disease activity. About 75% of women with RA have amelioration of their disease during pregnancy. This is not the case in AS, when at most 25% improve during pregnancy, the majority being the same or worse at this time[63]. Carefully planned physical therapy based on that used for all AS patients is important for these patients, in addition to the usual regime of antenatal exercises. All medication should be kept to a minimum, but many will need at least intermittent NSAIDs in order to maintain function
● Delivery. Given that the sacroiliac joints, and sometimes the hips, are targets for inflammation in AS, some problems with delivery might be anticipated. Although the majority of women with AS are able to have normal vaginal deliveries, the cesarean section rate does appear to be greater than in women who do not have AS, with the AS cited as the reason for section in more than 50%[64].
● Postpartum disease flares. Over 50% of the patients surveyed by Ostensen and Ostensen[64] reported a flare of their disease during the 6 months postpartum. This was sufficient to interfere with baby care in many of them. There was a strong correlation between flares of disease postpartum and active disease at the time of conception. This raises the question as to whether women with AS should be advised not to become pregnant during periods of disease activity.

The underlying principles of management of men and women with AS are identical although, compared with men, women report more pain and more need for medication, especially sulphasalazine and corticosteroids, despite having less severe spinal X-ray changes overall and a lesser incidence of iritis[4]. It is apparent, however, that women with AS require more awareness amongst heathcare professionals that they do suffer from AS, and that their disease presents some specific problems in management that require specific interventions over and above those of their male counterparts.

ANKYLOSING SPONDYLITIS ASSOCIATED WITH OTHER DISEASES

As the central member of the seronegative spondyloarthropathies, AS may be associated with other diseases in the group, particularly psoriasis and inflammatory bowel disease. The treatment of the skin and joint components of AS associated with psoriasis are separate, except that methotrexate might have a beneficial effect on both aspects of the disease (see Chapter 112). When AS is associated with inflammatory bowel disease, it must be remembered that NSAIDs may cause exacerbation of the bowel disease[65] and must be used with care. The propensity for fenamates to cause diarrhea makes them particularly unsuitable. There is speculation that modified-release formulations, which are designed to release small quantities of drug throughout the length of the gut, might be particularly problematic, although at present this is unproved. The effect of sulfasalazine on both gut and joints makes it a particularly good choice under these circumstances, although the salicylate-only medications such as mesalamine (mesalazine) that are now being used to treat inflammatory bowel disease have no direct effect on joint disease.

SURGERY

The rigid, flexed cervical spine and immobile chest wall of the patient with AS may produce significant technical difficulties for the anesthesiologist and a need for immaculate perioperative management by the physical therapist. Prolonged recumbancy is a time of great danger to the AS patient. Despite this, surgery can be an extremely valuable part of their management. Spinal surgery involves two areas particularly: the cervical spine, where atlantoaxial subluxation may require attention or where osteotomy can improve posture and forwards vision; and the dorsolumbar spine, where the paradoxical operation of spinal fusion may be needed for a 'last joint' problem, or where osteotomy may be used to improve spinal posture.

Atlantoaxial subluxation is less common in AS than in RA. Patients with RA can have significant degrees of atlantoaxial slip with no symptoms, because of the general ligamentous laxity and erosion of bones

that accompany this pathology. In contrast, the bone and ligaments in AS are rigid and unyielding, with neurologic sequelae being consequently more common. In such patients, cervical fusion may be necessary in order to retain neurologic integrity and control symptoms such as referred occipital pain (Fig. 107.7).

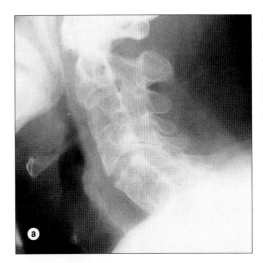

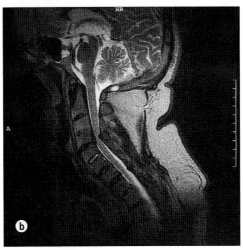

Fig. 107.8 Last-joint syndrome in AS. Although this usually occurs in the dorsolumbar spine, the example shown here is in the cervical spine. (a) On X-ray. (b) On MRI.

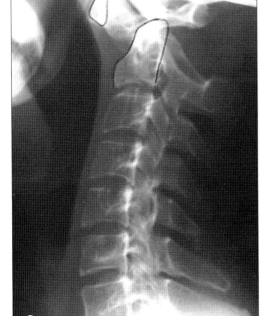

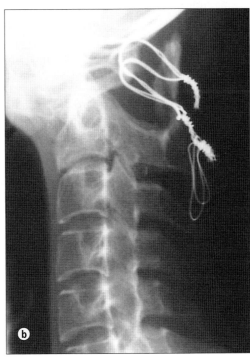

Fig. 107.7 Before and after cervical fusion. (a) The atlantoaxial subluxation seen preoperatively was accompanied by severe pain and numbness over the occiput. (b) The symptoms were completely relieved by cervical fusion.

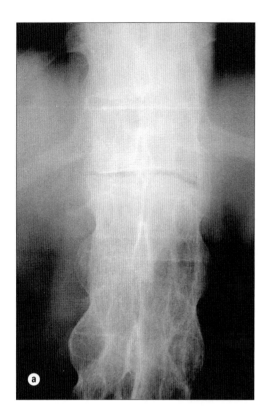
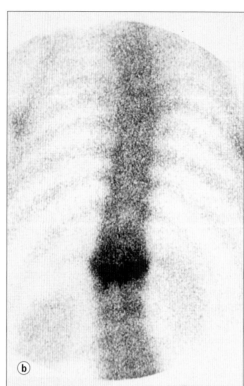

Fig. 107.9 Last-joint syndrome in AS.
(a) X-ray appearance showing the 'last joint' with discitis. (b) Discitis demonstrated by isotope scanning.

The 'last-joint' syndrome, in which bridging ossification of syndesmophytes has taken place at every level except one (Fig. 107.8), presents a cruel dilemma: on the one hand, exercise continues to be important in maintaining posture, even when extensive fusion has taken place; on the other, the sole mobile segment is exposed to considerable stresses during activity, with pain, which may be severe, and sometimes the development of discitis (Fig. 107.9). Treatment is initially by rest, sometimes by the use of a corset or brace[66]. Surgical fusion is required where the pain is unrelieved by conservative means, or where diskitis is so severe that healing under external immobilization fails to occur.

Spinal surgery may also be indicated when the posture of a fixed spondylitic spine is so extreme that forward vision can only be achieved with prismatic spectacles. A wedge osteotomy produces a less stooped posture, with a consequent ability to see ahead. This surgery may be sited at the cervical or dorsolumbar area, and is accompanied by a risk of neurologic damage, which must be balanced against the potential improvement in lifestyle produced by postural correction and enhanced forward vision. This type of surgery should only be undertaken by a skilled spinal surgeon, anesthesiologist, nursing and physical therapy team in theatres equipped for intraoperative spinal monitoring. In this and all surgery on AS patients, the period of postoperative immobilization should be kept to a minimum and the physical therapist should ensure that the patient maintains the fullest possible range of movements compatible with any necessary postoperative fixation. Attention to breathing is particularly important if postoperative chest infection is to be avoided. New techniques for the insertion of cement into osteoporotic wedged vertebrae to restore their anatomy are now available, but there is as yet insufficient experience with them to know if they have any place in spondylitis.

The root joints (those at the 'roots' of the limbs – i.e. the shoulders and hips), particularly the hips, are frequently involved in AS, and total hip replacement is indicated in those in whom severe pain or severe limitation of movement occurs. Loss of range at the hips may reveal a greater than expected degree of disability caused by spinal fusion, forward flexion, in particular, being entirely dependent on hip movement in some patients.

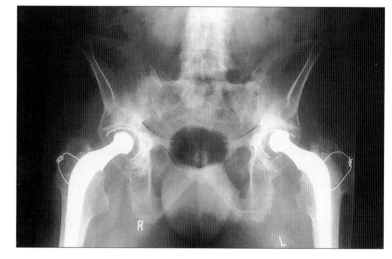

Fig. 107.10 Total hip replacement in AS. These prostheses had been inserted 13 years before this X-ray was taken.

Two anxieties have been expressed regarding hip replacement in patients with AS. As many are young and active, it has been suggested that mechanical failure produced by high use might be a major problem. There is also anxiety that patients with AS may be particularly prone to extra-articular ossification, causing loss of movement in the replaced joint. Long-term follow-up suggests that these are not common problems, with a high degree of short-term and long-term value accruing from the operation[67]. It should be noted, too, that patients followed long-term in these studies had replacement with conventional cemented hips (Fig. 107.10), rather than the cementless ones that are now sometimes selected for younger, more active patients, or the more limited resurfacing prostheses such as the McMinn.

DETERMINATION OF IMPROVEMENT OR DETERIORATION

There are many approaches to assessing treatment response in AS. As with many inflammatory diseases, determination of ESR, plasma

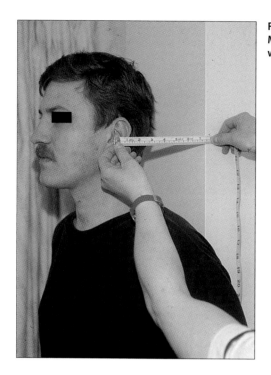

Fig. 107.11
Measurement of
wall–tragus distance.

viscosity or CRP may be valuable in the initial diagnosis and in following subsequent progress. However, the relationships between these measurements and disease progression are imprecise and insufficient to produce an adequate description of disease state[68]. Symptoms are mainly pain and stiffness, which can be measured by a variety of techniques such as visual analog scales. No technique exists for measuring spinal stiffness objectively.

Clinical measures

Posture is easier to visualize than to quantify. Serial photographs may produce a telling record of disease progression. Simpler methods include wall–occiput or wall–tragus measurements (Fig. 107.11), which are easy to undertake with a tape measure and have a reasonable level of intra- and interpersonal reliability. Interobserver error is particularly impor-

tant in AS, as measurements will be needed over long periods of time and are unlikely to be undertaken by the same observer throughout.

Measurement of movement should ideally cover all areas of the spine, in addition to peripheral joints, and incorporate all planes of movement. Because the different planes are affected to the same extent, measurement of one usually suffices as a surrogate for the others in everyday practice. The simplest technique is Macrae's modification of Schober's technique[69], which measures forward flexion of the lumbar spine. The lumbosacral junction is identified between the dimples of Venus, and marks are made 5cm below it and 10cm above. Because the lower point is adjacent to the tethered skin over the coccyx and the upper point is free to move, flexion causes distraction of the two marks (Fig. 107.12). The result is usually expressed as the amount of skin distraction, this in turn being related to true spinal motion in a linear fashion. Methods of measuring side flexion and rotation have been devised but are rarely used, most assessments being by eye or by simple clinical means such as the distance reached by the fingertips down the lateral thigh. Provided precautions are taken to ensure that no flexion takes place simultaneously, measurement of this distance using a tape measure is reliable and correlates well with instrumental measurement using an inclinometer. One frequently used measure that deserves unequivocal condemnation is measuring the fingertip–floor distance on forward flexion. This measures an inconsistent combination of spinal and hip movement, although it is frequently suggested as being a useful measure of spinal flexion. In some patients, the fingertips or even the full palm can be placed on the floor in the absence of any true spinal flexion, and this measurement should be discarded because of its practical imprecision and the imprecision in thought that often accompanies its use.

Chest expansion is reduced when the costovertebral joints are involved in the inflammatory process. Simple measurement with a tape measure at the level of the 4th rib anteriorly provides useful and simple quantification. Although an arbitrary 2.5cm expansion is used in some epidemiologic definitions of AS, there is considerable overlap between AS patients and controls (Fig. 107.13), and a significant decrease in

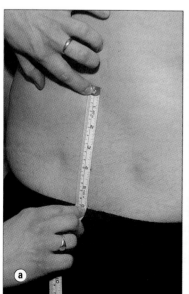
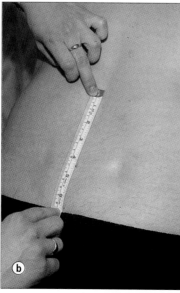

Fig. 107.12 Macrae's modification of Schober's test. (a) The lumbosacral junction is identified between the dimples of Venus, and measurement made 5cm below and 10cm above. (b) The distraction of these marks is proportional to true lumbar flexion. In the example shown, the patient has AS and skin distraction is limited.

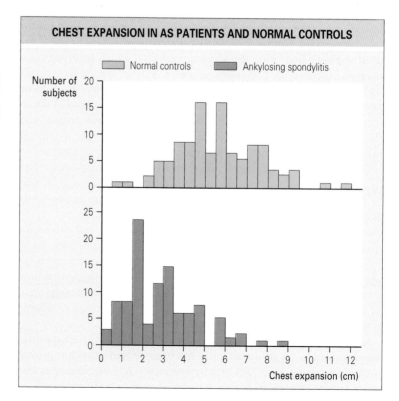

Fig. 107.13 Chest expansion in AS patients and normal controls. Although patients with AS have significantly less chest expansion than normal controls, the overlap is considerable. (Data from Moll and Wright[70].)

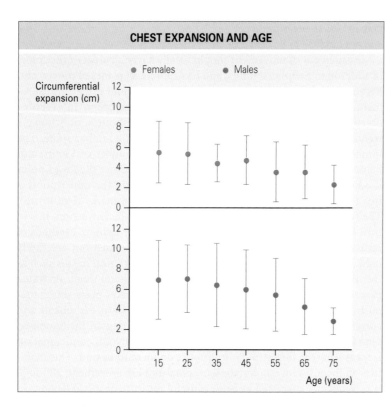

Fig. 107.14 Chest expansion and age. Chest expansion decreases with age, and this must be taken into account when considering the normality of an individual clinical measurement. (Data from Moll and Wright[71].)

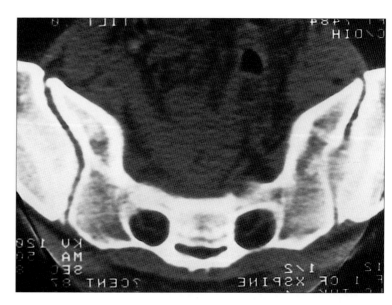

Fig. 107.15 Sacroiliac MRI. Sacroiliitis in a woman with a normal X-ray. This shows both small erosions and early fusion.

normal chest expansion with age (Fig. 107.14). These factors make chest expansion a more useful measure of progression than an absolute point measurement.

Some relatively simple instruments have been designed that facilitate measurement of spinal movement. The spondylometer, introduced in 1949[72], is a protractor with a long articulated arm. Flexion produces a composite measure of lumbar and dorsal movement, the design of the instrument automatically giving more weight to flexion in the clinically more important lumbar area. Inclinometers have also been used, the most sophisticated being the arthrospinometer, which incorporates a magnetic compass as a standard reference, thus increasing its versatility[73]. Although used episodically in drug trials, none of these has become part of routine use. However, there is now an increasing need to document the long-term results of the treatment of rheumatic disease, and the low intraobserver errors of instruments such as the spondylometer may produce a resurgence of interest in them as everyday clinical tools.

Flexion of the dorsal spine is incorporated into spondylometer and inclinometer measurements, and the arthrospinometer may also be used to measure dorsal rotation, although the technique is too cumbersome and time consuming to be used other than for research. Cervical spine movement has proved difficult to measure except by eye, and although a number of gadgets to enhance measurement have been devised, none has yet found a place in routine clinical practice. As neck rotation appears to be an important parameter contributing to overall disability, a simple measure of it may be an important facet of overall assessment of the patient with AS. Use of a protractor has proved a reliable method[74], and should probably be more widely used.

Enthesopathy is a characteristic of all the seronegative spondyloarthropathies. An enthesitis index has been devised[75] that has proved useful in assessing the results of drug treatments. It is suggested that this index reflects changes in disease activity better than traditional anthropometric measures, although the Assessment of Ankylosing Spondylitis working group were unable to recommend any currently available instrument for measuring enthesitis[76].

Imaging

Sacroiliac inflammation is an important feature of AS, but its measurement has proved difficult. There are many clinical tests for the presence of sacroiliitis, but these prove unreliable in practice[77] and at best facilitate only a 'present or absent' judgment, rather than allowing gradation of response. Scintigraphy has advocates as a diagnostic method, although it has not achieved universal acceptance. Personal experience suggests that it is a useful aid to diagnosis in carefully selected patients, but there is no evidence of its utility in measuring progression. Thermography has been shown to be capable of detecting sacroiliac inflammation and of detecting change in response to drugs. It is, however, an expensive, cumbersome and time-consuming technique, and is unsuited to routine practice. MRI is a sensitive way of detecting sacroiliitis before radiological change is apparent (Fig. 107.15)[78]. Its cost has hitherto made it more useful for early diagnosis rather than evaluation of disease progression, but the need for rigorous evaluation of expensive treatments such as anti-TNF-α has changed this balance, and it has been used successfully to demonstrate improvement using such treatment[44,45].

Radiological changes are characteristic features of AS. A number of radiological assessment instruments have been developed, including the Stoke Ankylosing Spondylitis Spine Score (SASSS)[79] and the Bath Ankylosing Spondylitis Radiology Index (BASRI)[80]. Overall radiological assessments are of more value over long rather than short time periods[81] and it is probably now inappropriate to rely on measures involving repeated exposure to ionizing radiation, despite their convenience and relatively low cost, when alternatives exist.

Patient-centered outcomes

A number of newer indices have patient questionnaires at their heart. This approach combines economy, as an external metrologist is not required, with an increasing appreciation of the importance of the patient's perception of their own disease. The Health Assessment Questionaire, which is widely used in evaluating RA, has been modified (HAQ-S) with the aim of extending its role into the management of patients with spondyloarthritis[82]. The Dougados Functional Index (DFI) combines both a questionnaire and an articular index specifically designed for spondyloarthritis. This provides an evaluation of both the disease and its response to treatment[83].

The Bath group have developed an extensive repertoire of indices that explore different aspects of the patient's disease[84]. Three self-administered questionnaires evaluate disease status (Bath Ankylosing

Spondylitis Disease Activity Index, BASDAI), disability (Bath Ankylosing Spondylitis Functional Index, BASFI) and the patient's perception of the effects of disease on their well-being (Bath Ankylosis Spondylitis Patient Global Score, BAS-G). A set of physical measures are added (Bath Ankylosis Spondylitis Metrology Index, BASMI), and the package gives a broad view of the patient's disease, and also gives insight into the complexity of comprehensiveness in assessment. The full set of Bath indices seems likely to have more of a place in research than in routine practice.

The BASFI has been compared with the DFI and the HAQ-S, and was shown to be more responsive than the other two indices in situations both of improvement and of deterioration in functional performance[85]. This must be interpreted with some caution, as all three indices showed means towards the lower end of the scale. A comparison of the DFI and the HAQ-S suggested that the HAQ-S showed greater construct validity and sensitivity to change than the DFI, although it showed little advantage over the unmodified HAQ[86]. One important finding of this study was that the six measures of physical function (cervical rotation, occiput to wall distance, chest expansion, Schober test, Smythe's test and intermalleolar straddle) that were used to assess construct validity explained a maximum of 24% (HAQ-S) of the instruments they were evaluating. This illustrates well the importance of looking beyond pure physical measurements in evaluating AS. The literature regarding the DFI and the BASFI was reviewed on behalf of the Assessments in Ankylosing Spondylitis working group[87]. The conclusion was that each had value, but that there were insufficient head-to-head comparisons under different circumstances to choose an overall 'best' instrument. A modification of the DFI, replacing its 3-point Likert scale with a 5-point one, was evaluated for the same working party, and no significant differences were found between it and the BASFI[88]. Both are, therefore, included as recommended tools by the Assessments in Ankylosing Spondylitis working group[76].

QUALITY OF LIFE

Despite its reputation as a mild disease, AS can have considerable effects on the quality of life of those who have it. Even in those with mild disease, the intrusive effects of regular exercises, however 'good for you' they may be, coupled with the need to take medication with its consequent side effects, and the knowledge that there is a strong genetic component to the disease, all take their toll. Severe disease with constant pain, restriction of movement, social dysfunction, work loss, deformity and fatigue has an all too obvious effect. There have been few attempts to measure this aspect of AS, although a review for the Outcome Measures in Rheumatology group (OMERACT) showed that they have been used more frequently recently[89] and the need to justify the increased cost of expensive new therapies has meant that evaluations such as the SF36 before and after treatment are now being used increasingly[46]. Despite this, the totality of the disease burden to the individual, their family and society is still relatively unexplored.

CONCLUSION

Epidemiologic studies of AS have suggested that the disease is becoming milder and its age of onset later. This conflicts with anecdotal experience by the author from a general rheumatology department, which suggests that an increasing number of people have severe, aggressive disease that is failing to respond to the simple NSAID plus exercise programs that have appeared to be so successful in the past. The team approach to treatment, often utilizing the physical therapist as the focal point for the patient, remains a valid way of delivering care. However, there is a need to develop better prognostic markers early in the course of the disease, so that intensive drug treatment can be started early in those patients for whom it is appropriate. Development of strategies based on this need, while maintaining the primacy of physical treatment and patient education, remains a priority for the development of AS therapy. Research is still needed regarding all aspects of treatment, from the optimum use of NSAIDs and the most effective physical therapy and exercise regimes to the place of modern, expensive treatments in this disease. The burden of disease needs more formal evaluation, and, above all, professional education must be a priority if genuine early diagnosis of AS is to become a reality.

REFERENCES

1. Lubrano E, Helliwell P, Moreno P et al. The assessment of knowledge in AS patients by a self-administered questionnaire. Br J Rheumatol 1998; 37: 437–41.
2. Suarez-Almazor M, Kendall CJ, Dorgan M. Surfing the net – information on the world wide web for persons with arthritis: patient empowerment or patient deceit? J Rheumatol 2001; 28: 185–191.
3. Kidd BL, Cawley MID. Delay in diagnosis of spondarthritis, Br J Rheumatol 1988; 27: 230–232.
4. Feldtkeller E, Bruckel J, Khan MA. Scientific contributions of ankylosing spondylitis patient advocacy groups. Curr Opin Rheumatol 2000; 12: 239–247.
5. Wynn Parry CB. Physical measures of rehabilitation. In: Moll JMH, ed. Ankylosing spondylitis. Edinburgh: Churchill Livingstone; 1980: 214–226.
6. Kraag G, Stokes B, Groh J et al. The effects of comprehensive home physiotherapy and supervision on patients with ankylosing spondylitis – a randomised controlled trial. J Rheumatol 1990; 17: 228–233.
7. Ormos G, Domjan L, Balint G. A controlled trial for assessing the effect of manual therapy on cervical spine mobility. Hung Rheumatol 1987; (suppl): 177–180.
8. Tishier M, Brotovski Y, Yaron M. Effect of spa therapy on patients with ankylosing spondylitis. Clin Rheumatol 1995; 14: 21–25.
9. Gemignani G, Olivieri I, Rujo G, Pasero G. Transcutaneous elecrical nerve stimulation in ankylosing spondylitis: a double-blind study. Arthritis Rheum 1991; 34: 788–789.
10. Fisher LR, Cawley MID, Holgate ST. Relation between chest expansion, pulmonary function, and exercise tolerance in patients with ankylosing spondylitis. Ann Rheum Dis 1990; 49: 921–925.
11. Hidding A, van der Linden S, Gielen X et al. Continuation of group physical therapy is necessary in ankylosing spondylitis. Arthritis Care Res 1994; 7: 90–96.
12. Russell P, Unsworth A, Haslock I. The effect of exercise on ankylosing spondylitis: a preliminary study. Br J Rheumatol 1993; 32: 498–506.
13. Kraag G, Stokes B, Groh J et al. The effects of comprehensive home physiotherapy and supervision on patients with ankylosing spondylitis – an 8-month follow up. J Rheumatol 1994; 21: 261–263.
14. Bulstrode SJ, Barefoot J, Harrison RA, Clarke AK. The role of passive stretching in the treatment of ankylosing spondylitis. Br J Rheumatol 1987; 26: 40–42.
15. Rassmussen JO, Hansen TM. Physical training for patients with ankylosing spondylitis. Arthritis Care Res 1989; 2: 25–27.
16. Roberts WN, Larson MG, Liang MH et al. Sensitivity of anthropometric techniques for clinical trials in ankylosing spondylitis. Br J Rheumatol 1989; 28: 40–45.
17. Vitanen JV, Lehtinen K, Suni J, Kantiainen H. Fifteen months follow-up of intensive in-patient physiotherapy and exercise in ankylosing spondylitis. Clin Rheumatol 1995; 14: 413–419.
18. Buckelew SP, Parker JC. Coping with arthritis pain. Arthritis Care Res 1989; 2: 136–145.
19. Wordsworth BP, Mowat AG. A review of 100 patients with ankylosing spondylitis with particular reference to socio-economic effects. Br J Rheumatol 1986; 25: 175–180.
20. Pal B. Use of simple analgesics in the treatment of ankylosing spondylitis. Br J Rheumatol 1987; 26: 207–209.
21. O'Brien BJ, Elswood J, Calin A. Perception of prescription drug risks: a survey of patients with ankylosing spondylitis. J Rheumatol 1990; 17: 503–507.
22. Calin A, Elswood J. A prospective nationwide cross-sectional study of NSAID usage in 1331 patients with ankylosing spondylitis. J Rheumatol 1990; 17: 801–803.
23. Henry D, Lim LL-Y, Rodriguez LAG et al. Variability in risk of gastrointestinal complications with individual non-steroidal anti-inflammatory drugs: results of a collaborative meta-analysis. BMJ 1996; 312: 1563–1566.
24. Cox NL, Doherty SM. Non-steroidal anti-inflammatories: out-patient audit of patient preferences and side-effects in different diseases. In: Rainsford KD, Velo GP, eds. Side effects of anti-inflammatory drugs. Part 1: Clinical and epidemiological aspects. Lancaster: MTP Press; 1987: 137–150.
25. Dougados M, Behier JM, Jolchine et al. Efficacy of Celecoxib, a COX-2 specific inhibitor, in ankylosing spondylitis: a placebo and conventional NSAID controlled study. Arthritis Rheum 2001; 44: 180–185.
26. Dougados M, Gueguen A, Nakache J-P et al. Ankylosing spondylitis: what is the optimum duration of a clinical study? A one year versus a 6 weeks non-steroidal anti-inflammatory drug trial. Rheumatology 1999; 38: 235–244.

27. Boersma JW. Retardation of ossification of the lumbar vertebral column in ankylosing spondylitis by means of phenylbutazone. Scand J Rheumatol 1976; 5: 60–64.

28. Lehtinen R. Clinical and radiological features of ankylosing spondylitis in the 1950s and 1976 in the same hospital. Scand J Rheumatol 1979; 8: 57–61.

29. Saraux A, Guedes C, Allain J et al. Prevalence of rheumatoid arthritis and spondyloarthropathy in Brittany, France. J Rheumatol 1999; 26: 22–27.

30. Alonso J C, Soriano A, Rubio C et al. Technetium-99m-HMPAO-labeled leukocyte imaging in patients with seronegative spondylarthropathies. J Nucl Med Technol 1999; 27: 204–206.

31. Moll JMH, Haslock I, Macrae IF, Wright V. Associations between ankylosing spondylitis, psoriatic arthritis, Reiter's disease, the intestinal arthropathies and Behçet's syndrome. Medicine (Baltimore) 1974; 53: 343–364.

32. Mielants H, Veys EM, de Vos M, Cuvelier C. Gut inflammation in the pathogenesis of idiopathic forms of reactive arthritis and in the peripheral joint involvement of ankylosing spondylitis. In: Spondyloarthropathies: involvement of the gut. Mielants H, Veys EM, eds Amsterdam: Excerpta Medica; 1989: 11–12.

33. Ferraz MB, Tugwell P, Goldsmith CH, Atra E. Meta-analysis of sulfasalazine and ankylosing spondylitis. J Rheumatol 1990; 17: 1482–1486.

34. Clegg DO, Reda D J, Abdellatif M. Comparison of sulfasalazine and placebo for the treatment of axial and peripheral articular manifestations of the seronegative spondylarthropathies: a Department of Veterans Affairs cooperative study. Arthritis Rheum 1999; 42: 2325–2329.

35. McConkey B. Sulphasalazine and ankylosing spondylitis. Br J Rheumatol 1990; 29: 2–5.

36. Creemers MCW, Franssen MJAM, van der Putte LBA et al. Methotrexate in severe ankylosing spondylitis: an open study. J Rheumatol 1995; 22: 1104–1107.

37. Sadowska-Wroblewska M, Garwolinska H, Maczynska-Rusiniak B. A trial of cyclophosphamide in ankylosing spondylitis with involvement of peripheral joints and high disease activity. Scand J Rheumatol 1986; 15: 259–264.

38. Maksymowych WP, Jhangri GS, Leclercq S et al. An open study of pamidronate in the treatment of refractory ankylosing spondylitis. J Rheumatol 1998; 25: 714–717.

39. Breban M, Gombert B, Amor B, Dougados M. Efficacy of thalidomide in the treatment of refractory ankylosing spondylitis. Arthritis Rheum 1999; 42: 580–581.

40. Gorman J D, Sack K E, Davis J C. Etanercept in the treatment of ankylosing spondylitis: a randomised double-blind placebo-controlled study. Arthritis Rheum 2000; 43(suppl): Abstract 2020.

41. Brandt J, Haibel H, Thriene W et al. Quality of life improvement in patients with severe ankylosing spondylitis upon treatment with anti-TNF-α. Arthritis Rheum 2000; 43(suppl): Abstract 2001.

42. Van den Bosch P, Kruithof E, Baeten D et al. Effects of a loading dose regimen of three infusions of chimeric monoclonal antibody to tumour necrosis factor α (infliximab) in spondyloarthropathy: an open pilot study. Ann Rheum Dis 2000; 59: 428–433.

43. Kruithof E, Van den Bosch F, Baeten D et al. TNF-α blockade with infliximab in patients with active spondyloarthropathy: follow up of one year maintenance regimen. J Rheumatol 2001; 28(suppl 63): Abstract T88.

44. Marzo-Ortega H, McGonagle D, O'Connor P et al. A clinical and MRI assessment of the efficacy of the recombinant TNF alpha receptions: Fc fusion protein etancercept in the treatment of resistant spondyloarthropathy. Arthritis Rheum 2000; 43(suppl): Abstract 209.

45. Stone M, Salonen D, Lax M et al. Clinical and imaging correlates of response to treatment with infliximab in patients with ankylosing spondylitis. J Rheumatol 2001; 28: 1605–1614.

46. Brandt J, Haibel H, Cornely D et al. Successful treatment of active ankylosing spondylitis with the anti-tumour necrosis factor α monoclonal antibody infliximab. Arthritis Rheum 2000; 43: 1346–1352.

47. Braun J, Sieper J. Anti-TNF-α: a new dimension in the pharmacotherapy of the spondyloarthropathies? Ann Rheum Dis 2000; 59: 404–406.

48. Amor B, Silva-Santos R, Nahal R et al. Predictive factors of the long term outcome of spondylarthopathies. J Rheumatol 1994; 21: 1883–1887.

49. Wordsworth BP, Pearcy MJ, Mowat AG. In-patient regime for the treatment of ankylosing spondylitis: an appraisal of improvement in spinal mobility and the effects of corticotrophin. Br J Rheumatol 1984; 23: 39–43.

50. Peters N D, Ejstrup L. Intravenous methylprednisolone pulse therapy in ankylosing spondylitis. Scand J Rheumatol 1992; 21: 134–138.

51. Court-Brown WM, Doll R. Mortality from cancer and other causes after radiotherapy for ankylosing spondylitis. BMJ 1965; ii: 1327–1332.

52. Gibson T. Is there a place for corticosteroid injection in the management of Achilles tendon lesions? Br J Rheumatol 1991; 30: 436.

53. Grill V, Smith M, Ahern M, Littlejohn G. Local radiotherapy for pedal manifestations of 2 HLA B27 related arthopathies. Br J Rheumatol 1988; 27: 390–392.

54. Will R, Palmer R, Bhalla A et al.et al. Osteoporosis in early ankylosing spondylitis: a primary pathological event? Lancet 1989; ii: 1483–1485.

55. Marhoffer W, Stracke H, Masoud I et al. Evidence of impaired cartilage/bone turnover in patients with active ankylosing spondylitis. Ann Rheum Dis 1995; 54: 556–559.

56. Gratacos J, Collado A, Pons F et al. Significant loss of bone mass in patients with early, active ankylosing spondylitis. Arthritis Rheum 1999; 42: 2319–2324.

57. Bronson WD, Walker SD, Hillman LS et al. Bone mineral density and biochemical markers of bone metabolism in ankylosing spondylitis. J Rheumatol 1998; 25: 929–935.

58. Roux C, Abitbol V, Chaussade S et al. Bone loss in patients with inflammatory bowel disease: a prospective study. Osteoporos Int 1995; 5: 156–160.

59. Dougados M, Berenbaum F, Maetzel A, Amor B. The use of sulfasalazine for the prevention of attacks of acute anterior uveitis associated with spondylarthropathy. Rev Rheum (Engl Ed) 1993; 60: 80–82.

60. Reiff A, Takei S, Sadeglic S et al. Etanercept therapy in children with treatment-resistant uveitis. Arthritis Rheum 2001; 44: 1411–1415.

61. Smith JR, Levinson RD, Holland GN et al. Differential efficacy of tumor necrosis factor inhibition in the management of inflammatory eye disease and associated rheumatic disease. Arthritis Care Res 2001; 45: 252–257.

62. Pato E, Banares A, Jover JA et al. Underdiagnosis of spondyloarthropathy in patients presenting with anterior uveitis. J Rheumatol 2000; 27: 2198–2202.

63. Ostensen M, Husby G. Ankylosing spondylitis and pregnancy. Rheum Dis Clin N Am 1989; 15: 241–254.

64. Ostensen M, Ostensen H. Ankylosing spondylitis; the female aspect. J Rheumatol 1998; 25: 120–124.

65. Somerville RW, Hawkey CJ. Non-steroidal anti-inflammatory drugs and the gastrointestinal tract. Postgrad Med J 1986; 62: 23–28.

66. Dunn N, Preston B, Lloyd Jones K. Unexplained acute backache in longstanding ankylosing spondylitis. BMJ 1985; 291: 1632–1634.

67. Calin A, Elswood J. The outcome of 138 total hip replacements and 12 revisions in ankylosing spondylitis: high success rate after a mean follow-up of 7.5 years. J Rheumatol 1989; 16: 955–958.

68. Ruof J, Stucki G. Validity aspects of erythrocyte sedimentation rate and C-reactive protein in ankylosing spondylitis: a literature review. J Rheumatol 1999; 26: 966–970.

69. Macrea IF, Wright V. Measurement of back movement. Ann Rheum Dis 1969; 28: 584–593.

70. Moll JMH, Wright V. The pattern of chest and spinal mobility in ankylosing spondylitis. Rheumatol Rehab 1973; 12: 115–134.

71. Moll JMH, Wright V. An objective study of chest expansion. Ann Rheum Dis 1972; 31: 1–8.

72. Dunham WF. Ankylosing spondylitis: measurement of hip and spinal movements. Br J Phys Med 1949; 12: 126–129.

73. Domjan L, Balint G. A new goniometer for measuring spinal and peripheral joint mobility. Hung Rheumatol 1987; 71–76.

74. Pile RD, Laurent MR, Salmond CE et al. Clinical assessment of ankylosing spondylitis: a study of observer variation in spinal measurements. Br J Rheumatol 1991; 17: 29–34.

75. Mander N, Simpson JN, McLellan A et al. Studies with an enthesis index as a method of clinical assessment in ankylosing spondylitis. Ann Rheum Dis 1987; 46: 197–202.

76. van der Heijde D, van der Linden S, Dougados M, Bellamy N, Russel AS, Edmonds J. Ankylosing spondylitis: plenary discussion and results of voting on selection of domains and some specific instruments. J Rheumatol 1999; 26: 997–1002.

77. Rudge SR, Swannel AJ, Rose DH, Todd JH. The clinical assessment of sacro-iliac joint involvement in ankylosing spondylitis. Rheumatol Rehab 1982; 21: 15–20.

78. Oostveen J, Prevo R, den Boer J, van de Laar M. Early detection of sacroiliitis on magnetic resonance imaging and subsequent development of sacroiliitis on plain radiography. A prospective, longitudinal study. J Rheumatol 1999; 26: 1953–1958.

79. Dawes P. Stoke Ankylosing Spondylitis Spine Score. J Rheumatol 1999; 26: 993–996.

80. Calin A, Mackay K, Santos H, Brophy S. A new dimension to outcome: application of the Bath Ankylosing Spondylitis Radiology Index. J Rheumatol 1999; 26: 988–992.

81. Spoorenberg A, de Vlam K, van der Heijde D et al. Radiological scoring methods in ankylosing spondylitis: reliability and sensitivity to change over one year. J Rheumatol 1999; 26: 997–1002.

82. Daltroy LH, Larson MG, Roberts WN, Liang MH. A modification of the Health Assessment Questionnaire for the spondyloarthropathies. J Rheumatol 1990; 17: 946–950.

83. Dougados M, Gueguen A, Nakache J-P et al. Evaluation of a functional index and an articular index in ankylosing spondylitis. J Rheumatol 1988; 15: 302–307.

84. Calin A. The individual with ankylosing spondylitis: defining disease status and the impact of the illness. Br J Rheumatol 1995; 34: 663–672.

85. Ruof J, Sangha O, Stucki G. Comparative responsiveness of 3 functional indices in ankylosing spondylitis. J Rheumatol 1999; 26: 1959–1633.

86. Ward MM, Kuzis S. Validity and sensitivity to change of spondylitis-specific measures of functional disability. J Rheumatol 1999; 26: 121–127.

87. Ruof J, Stucki G. Comparision of the Dougados Functional Index and the Bath Ankylosing Spondylitis Functional Index. A literature review. J Rheumatol 1999; 26: 955–960.

88. Spoorenberg A, van der Heijde D, de Klerk E et al. A comparative study of the usefulness of the Bath Ankylosing Spondylitis Functional Index and the Dougados Functional Index in the assessment of ankylosing sponylitis. J Rheumatol 1999; 26: 961–965.

89. Ortiz Z, Shea B, Dieguez M G et al. The responsiveness of generic quality of life instruments in rheumatic diseases. A systematic review of randomized controlled trials. J Rheumatol 1999; 26: 210–216.

108 Reactive arthritis: etiology and pathogenesis

Hani S El-Gabalawy and Peter E Lipsky

- The pathogenesis of spondyloarthropathies is unclear; however, an interaction of host HLA-B27 and certain bacteria plays a central role
- The potential roles of HLA-B27 structure, function, molecular mimicry and/or other effects in relation to these bacteria are discussed
- It is hypothesized that an interaction of host HLA-B27 and certain bacteria play a central role in the spondyloarthropathies
- Current evidence points to an amino acid cluster associated with the B pocket of HLA-B27 as critical in pathogenesis
- The spondyloarthropathies appear to be triggered by CD8+ T cells responding to peptides derived from bacteria which are bound to HLA-B27

INTRODUCTION

Reactive arthritis is one of the spondyloarthropathic disorders which share a number of common features, of which the most salient is an association with the Class I histocompatibility antigen, HLA-B27[1,2]. Understanding the etiopathogenesis of reactive arthritis is dependent on a detailed understanding therefore of the nature of the association with HLA B27 and its interaction with infection. These components are considered in turn.

ASSOCIATION WITH HLA-B27

Class I antigens of the major histocompatibility complex (MHC) are 44kDa polymorphic molecules that are noncovalently associated with a monomorphic 12kDa protein, β_2-microglobulin, and expressed as a heterodimer on the surface of many cell-types[3,4]. The function of these molecules is to bind specific peptides generated from cytoplasmic proteins by proteolysis, and present the peptides to CD8+ T cells expressing appropriate T cell receptors. Allelic variations in the amino acids of class I MHC molecules have traditionally been identified by antisera. HLA-B27 is a serologically defined allele of the HLA-B locus, one of the three classic loci encoding class I MHC molecules. Examination of HLA-B gene products that react with HLA-B27 typing allo-antisera has revealed a family of allelic subtypes[5]. These have been designated by the World Health Organization HLA Nomenclature Committee as *HLA-B*2701* through *HLA-B*2712* with the ordering based on charge determined by isoelectric focusing and not their frequency in the population. More recently, additional subtypes have been described on the basis of detailed nucleotide sequencing, but the biological and clinical significance of these minor variations remains uncertain[5]. One HLA-B27 subtype (B*2708) has been identified that originally was thought to be an HLA-B7 subtype because of its reactivity with B7-specific antisera[6]. HLA-B*2705 is the predominant subtype in all populations except certain Asian populations in which B*2704 or B*2706 may be more common. HLA-B*2701, B*2707, B*2708, B*2709, B*2710, B*2711, and B*2712 are rarely encountered, whereas HLA-B*2703 is found relatively commonly in West Africa, but is infrequent elsewhere[5]. The amino acids that vary among the different HLA-B27 subtypes are shown in Table 108.1.

An association between many, but not all, of the HLA-B27 subtypes and the spondyloarthropathies has been demonstrated. This has been most comprehensively analyzed for ankylosing spondylitis[5]. Several of the HLA-B27 subtypes, including HLA-B*2701 and HLA-B*2707 are rare,

TABLE 108.1 NOMENCLATURE AND AMINO ACID DIFFERENCES OF THE HLA-B27 SUBTYPES

Domain					α_1						α_2		
Amino acid	59	74	77	80	81	82	83	97	113	114	116	131	152
POCKET	A	C/F	C/F	C/F	C/F	E,C/F	D	D,E	C/F	E			
Subtype													
B*2705	Tyr	Asp	Asp	Thr	Leu	Leu	Arg	Asn	Tyr	His	Asp	Ser	Val
B*2701	—	Tyr	Asn	—	Ala	—	—	—	—	—	—	—	—
B*2702	—	—	Asn	Ile	Ala	—	—	—	—	—	—	—	—
B*2703	His	—	—	—	—	—	—	—	—	—	—	—	—
B*2704	—	—	Ser	—	—	—	—	—	—	—	—	—	Glu
B*2706	—	—	Ser	—	—	—	—	—	—	Asp	Tyr	—	Glu
B*2707	—	—	—	—	—	—	—	Ser	His	Asn	Tyr	Arg	—
B*2708	—	—	Ser	Asn	—	Arg	Gly	—	—	Asn	—	—	—
B*2709	—	—	—	—	—	—	—	—	—	—	His	—	—
B*2710	—	—	—	—	—	—	—	—	—	—	—	—	Glu
B*2711	—	—	Ser	—	—	—	—	Ser	His	Asn	Tyr	Arg	—
B*2712	—	—	Ser	Asn	—	Arg	Gly	—	—	—	—	—	—

The extracellular domain of HLA-B27 consists of receptor-like polymorphic α_1 and α_2 domains that bind peptides. Six pockets (A–F) project from the cleft under the alpha–helices and serve to accommodate side chains of individual amino acids of the bound peptides.

and thus have not been amenable to population studies. However, patients with these HLA-B27 subtypes and ankylosing spondylitis have been described. Association of ankylosing spondylitis with three of the other subtypes, HLA-B*2705, B*2702 and B*2704 has been observed in many populations[5]. It remains uncertain, however, whether HLA-B*2706 is associated. Although individual cases with HLA B*2706 in Thailand or Indonesia have been reported[7], a clear association has not been found in these populations where this subtype is common[8]. It also is uncertain whether there is an association between HLA-B*2703 and ankylosing spondylitis. In West Africa, HLA-B*2703 is relatively common, but ankylosing spondylitis is extremely rare[8,9]. Other factors may play a role in this apparent lack of association, however, as ankylosing spondylitis is not associated with either HLA-B*2703 or the more common HLA-B*2705 in West African populations. Finally, HLA-B*2708, a rare subtype, and HLA-B*2709 found in Italians on the island of Sardinia do not appear to be associated with ankylosing spondylitis[5,8].

There is an association of HLA-B27 with the other spondyloarthropathies, but the association does not appear to be as strong. In reactive arthritis, for example, the frequency of HLA-B27 ranges between 60% and 90%[2,10–13]. In reactive arthritis initiated by certain microorganisms, such as *Salmonella*, however, it is much lower, with the frequency of HLA-B27 positive affected persons ranging between 20% and 33%[11,12]. In *Chlamydia*-associated arthritis, the frequency of HLA-B27 positivity ranges between 40% and 50%[13,14], whereas 70–80% of *Yersinia*-induced[15] and 80–90% of *Shigella*-induced[16,17] reactive arthritis patients are HLA-B27 positive. Of note, however, and of potential importance when considering pathogenesis, the frequency of HLA-B27 positivity in all chronic forms of reactive arthritis is much higher (>90%) than in those with short-lived disease, regardless of the initiating microorganism. Indeed, it has been suggested that reactive arthritis syndromes could be classified on the basis of the triggering organism and the presence of HLA-B27[10]. The non-HLA-B27 related syndromes would simply be classified as 'post-infectious'. The inability to identify a specific triggering organism in a substantial proportion of patients with otherwise typical reactive arthritis clinical features continues to be highly problematic in any attempt to classify this syndrome more completely[18].

An important question is whether HLA-B27 itself is a direct disease susceptibility factor or, alternatively, merely a marker for a disease susceptibility gene in close linkage disequilibrium with HLA-B27. Indirect evidence from clinical epidemiology strongly suggests that HLA-B27 itself is the disease susceptibility gene[1]. Moreover, analyses of families with multiple cases has clearly shown significant genetic linkage of HLA-B27 and ankylosing spondylitis[19,20]. Finally, direct evidence that the HLA-B27 molecule itself can predispose to the spondyloarthropathies has come from studies of transgenic rats expressing HLA-B*2705[21]. These animals spontaneously develop a broad spectrum of disease manifestations closely resembling human HLA-B27-associated disease[21,22]. Clinical features include peripheral arthropathy, gastrointestinal, genitourinary tract and cutaneous inflammation, as well as sacroiliitis (Fig. 108.1). Furthermore, an HLA-B27 transgenic mouse bred into a strain lacking MHC class II molecules developed spontaneous inflammatory disease, arguing against a role for MHC class II molecules in these diseases and specifically for a role of presentation of HLA-B27 derived peptides by MHC class II molecules[23]. The association of the HLA-B27 molecule and susceptibility to the development of spondyloarthropathy, therefore is likely to relate to one or more unique features of its structure or function.

STRUCTURE OF HLA-B27

The three-dimensional structure of HLA class I molecules, including HLA-B*2705, has been determined[24,25]. The extracellular domains of these molecules consist of a membrane proximal immunoglobulin-like structure encoded by the α_3 domain of the molecule and a receptor-like peptide binding domain encoded by the polymorphic α_1 and α_2 domains. The α_3 domain is similar in each class I MHC molecule and is involved in the noncovalent association with β_2 microglobulin. The unique features of each HLA-A, -B and -C allele are, in general, determined by the amino acids of the α_1 and α_2 domains of the molecule. These appear to alter the peptide binding capacity of the molecule.

The α_1 and α_2 domains are folded into a peptide-binding cleft, with antiparallel α-helical regions from each domain creating the two walls that are 10–18Å apart and eight antiparallel β-pleated sheets forming the floor (Fig. 108.2). Most of the polymorphic amino acid residues in class I MHC molecules are clustered along this cleft, projecting into it either from the two α-helices or from the floor of the β-pleated sheet.

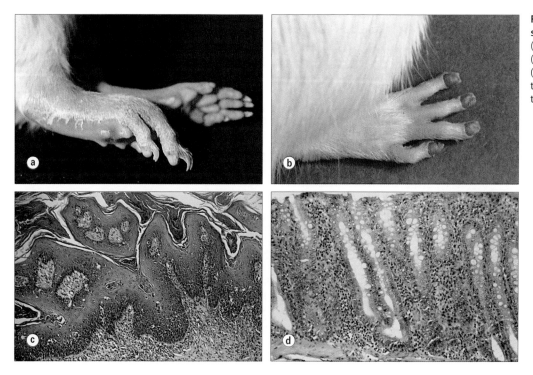

Fig. 108.1 Clinical manifestations of spondyloarthropathy in HLA-B27 transgenic rats.
(a) Peripheral arthritis, (b) nail changes,
(c) psoriasiform skin lesions and
(d) gastrointestinal inflammation characteristic of the spondyloarthropathies are found in HLA-B27 transgenic rats.

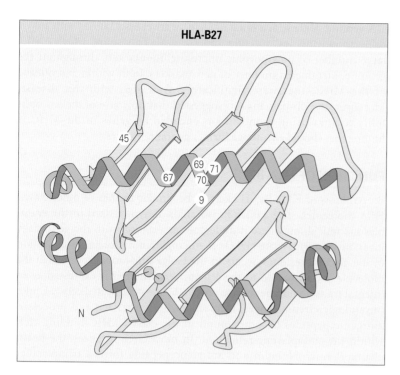

HLA-B27

Fig. 108.2 HLA-B27 – presumed structure. Highlighted are the amino acids that are thought to be involved in binding of specific antigenic peptides by HLA-B27 (N: amino terminal).

Six pockets (A–F) project from the cleft under the α-helices and serve to accommodate side chains of individual amino acids of bound peptides[26,27]. The A and F pockets bind the amino and carboxy termini of the antigenic peptide, respectively, and are highly conserved in HLA-class I molecules[27,28]. HLA-B*2703 is unique in that the tyrosine that is found in all other HLA class I molecules at position 59 in the A pocket is exchanged for a histidine[27]. This change might play a role in the possibly altered susceptibility of HLA-B*2703 positive persons to ankylosing spondylitis[9]. It was initially suggested that peptides binding HLA-B*2703 are only modestly different from those binding HLA-B*2705[29]. A more recent study showed that an endogenous peptide with sequence homology to proteins from enteric bacteria is presented by the spondylitis associated HLA-B*2705 (and HLA-B27*2702), but not by HLA-B*2703[30]. Other pockets contain additional polymorphic amino acids and contribute to binding of specific peptides. For HLA-B27, the pocket projecting under the superior α-helix to residue 45, the B pocket, is thought to play a critical role in the binding of peptide[25,26].

Class I MHC molecules function to bind antigenic peptides, largely derived from intracellular protein synthesis[31]. Such peptides are generated from partial proteolytic cleavage of endogenously synthesized proteins by a multicatalytic protease complex in the cytosol, termed the proteosome[32]. The peptides generated from proteosome-mediated proteolysis are transported from the cytoplasm into the endoplasmic reticulum where they bind to newly synthesized HLA-class I heavy chains. Transport of peptides into the endoplasmic reticulum is accomplished by components of a peptide pump known as transporters associated with antigen processing (TAP1 and TAP2)[33]. In man, there is minimal polymorphism of these peptide transporters and they, therefore, do not appear to limit the availability of peptides for binding to class I MHC molecules[34]. The binding of peptide by the newly synthesized HLA class I heavy chain and its association with β2 microglobulin stabilizes the complex permitting it to appear on the cell surface.

The amino acids of the pockets of class I MHC molecules are primarily responsible for the capacity of different class I MHC molecules to bind specific peptides[25,26]. In the case of HLA-B27, the B pocket is largely responsible for specificity, with the A and F pockets contributing stability[35]. Because of the amino acids of the B pocket, HLA-B27 molecules usually bind peptides with a positively charged amino acid, most often arginine, in the dominant anchor positions which is the second amino acid (P2) of the antigenic peptide. Typically, peptides consisting of nine amino acids are bound by class I MHC molecules[36], usually in an extended conformation[25], although larger or smaller peptides also may bind[27]. After reaching the cell surface, endogenously synthesized peptide, bound in the peptide-binding cleft of class I MHC molecules, is presented to CD8+ T-lymphocytes expressing specific clonally distributed antigen receptors capable of recognizing the combination of polymorphic class I MHC molecule plus antigenic peptide[37].

Each of the known HLA-B27 subtypes differ at specific amino acids. These amino acids are likely to be involved in the binding of specific antigenic peptides (see Fig. 108.2). Peptide binding capability may explain some of the association of specific HLA-B27 subtypes with ankylosing spondylitis. Thus, HLA-B*2706 and HLA-B*2709, which may not be associated with ankylosing spondylitis, have amino acid substitutions that are likely to alter the nature of the peptides they can bind compared to those which bind HLA-B*2705[29,38,39]. If peptide binding is important, it is likely that susceptibility to ankylosing spondylitis is unrelated to the portions of the molecules that differ among the associated subtypes.

Comparison of the HLA-B27 subtypes with other HLA class I sequences indicates that one amino acid residue is unique to all of the B27 subtypes[40] (Fig. 108.2). The lysine at position 70 is at the mouth of the B pocket pointing inward towards the peptide binding cleft and, therefore, is a candidate to be involved in peptide binding. The consensus HLA-B27 sequence shares a cluster of six amino acids within the peptide-binding cleft, including the HLA-B27-unique residue, Lys70, as well as His9, Glu45, Cys67, Ala69 and Ala71[41]. Besides HLA-B27, no other known class I HLA sequence possesses more than two of these residues. It is likely, therefore, that this portion of the HLA-B27 molecule is the disease susceptibility element. Since these amino acids are arrayed in the antigen binding cleft and the B pocket of the molecule, it is reasonable to conclude that disease susceptibility relates to the unique capacity of these amino acids to permit HLA-B27 to bind a specific peptide or set of peptides capable of triggering or propagating the disease. Of considerable interest is the recent demonstration that gorillas exhibiting features indistinguishable from those of human spondyloarthropathies had MHC class I molecules that bound peptides similar to those bound by HLA-B27[42]. Notably, despite major differences in the amino acid sequence of human HLA-B27 and the MHC class I molecule of the affected gorillas, including differences in the amino acids in the respective B pockets of these molecules, both these molecules demonstrated a requirement for the presence of a positively charged amino acid, particularly arginine, in the P2 position of the bound peptides. Indeed, the gorilla MHC class I molecule, Gogo-B*0101, effectively bound HLA-B27 associated peptides. Thus, although the identity of arthritogenic peptides in HLA-B27 associated human spondyloarthropathies remains to be delineated, evidence is mounting that such peptides feature a positively charged amino acid such as arginine or glutamine at the P2 position[43-45].

The cysteine residue at position 67 of HLA-B27 may be of particular importance because it is unpaired and oriented opposite lysine at position 70 that is at the mouth of the B pocket. Biochemical evidence indicates that the Cys67 of HLA-B27 contains a reactive sulfhydryl group[40]. This indicates that HLA-B27 is unique in having a reactive sulfhydryl group oriented into the peptide-binding cleft. Although HLA-B14 and HLA-B65 also contain a Cys at 67[40], the surrounding environment in these molecules differs from HLA-B27, thereby making the Cys67 in these molecules less available for disulfide formation. The presence of this reactive thiol in the binding cleft may alter peptide binding or the recognition of HLA-B27 itself. It has been suggested that homocysteine produced by arthritigenic bacteria may selectively modify the cysteine at position 67, and thereby alter its immunogenicity making it a target of cytotoxic T cells in patients[46]. It remains uncertain whether oxidation of the cysteine at position 67 alters its recognition by antibodies[47]. Position 67 of HLA-B27 is not only important because of its potential to bind peptides covalently, but also because it influences the conformation of the molecule so that it can be recognized, for example, by specific monoclonal antibodies[48].

In summary, current information supports the conclusion that the amino acid cluster associated with the portion of the B pocket of HLA-B27, shown in Figure 108.2, forms a critical part of the structure of the molecule that is likely to be involved in the pathogenesis of the spondyloarthropathies.

INVOLVEMENT OF OTHER GENES

The frequency of ankylosing spondylitis in unselected HLA-B27+ individuals is less than 2%, whereas that in HLA-B27+ family members of an HLA-B27+ patient with ankylosing spondylitis approaches 20%[49]. Although this might be explained by shared environmental factors, an alternative explanation for these results is that another gene or genes may play a role in determining disease susceptibility. One set of genes potentially contributing to susceptibility to ankylosing spondylitis are other genes in the MHC region. Other HLA-B alleles may contribute to disease susceptibility. Thus, the presence of HLA-B60 increases the risk of ankylosing spondylitis threefold in both HLA-B27 positive[19,50] and HLA-B27 negative individuals. Similarly, HLA-B39 may be associated with HLA-B27 negative ankylosing spondylitis[51]. It is interesting to note that HLA-B39 may bind some peptides in common with HLA-B27, but HLA-B60 appears to bind a separate set of peptides[51,52]. Thus, HLA-B60 may be an independent susceptibility gene for ankylosing spondylitis. The HLA-B7 cross-reacting group of HLA antigens also may be associated with HLA-B27 negative ankylosing spondylitis and undifferentiated spondyloarthropathy[53]. Because of the close proximity of the TNF locus to the HLA-B locus in the MHC complex and the pivotal role that TNF plays in inflammation, a number of studies have attempted to associate spondyloarthropathies with polymorphisms in the TNF genes or their promotors[54–57]. Although these studies have yielded conflicting results, in general, the associations that have been identified likely result from linkage disequilibrium with HLA-B27 rather than an independent effect on disease susceptibility.

Only weak associations between class II MHC molecules, and especially HLA-DR1, and ankylosing spondylitis have been reported[58]. Polymorphisms at the TAP genes do not appear to play a role in ankylosing spondylitis[59,60], but peripheral arthritis and iritis may be associated with a particular TAP1 polymorphism[61]. An association with polymorphism of both TAP1 and TAP2 alleles, independent of HLA-B27, has been reported in reactive arthritis[62]. As with TAP genes, polymorphisms of the proteosome components do not appear to be associated with ankylosing spondylitis, but may influence the presence of extraspinal disease[59,63,64]. Another candidate gene product that could be involved in susceptibility to ankylosing spondylitis is the T cell receptor (TCR) for antigen, since the specificity of the TCR involved in recognition of HLA-B27 and HLA-B27-bound peptides is likely to be an important determinant in the pathogenesis of the spondyloarthropathies. It is probable that specific residues of the HLA-B27 molecule recognized by T cells or binding peptides that are recognized by specific T cells play an essential role in determining the specific TCR involved. Nonrandom usage of the various segments of the β chain of the TCR has been found in human T cell clones recognizing HLA-B27[65,66], supporting the conclusion that limited numbers of TCR gene products may be involved in recognizing HLA-B27 and, perhaps, HLA-B27-bound peptides.

A genome-wide scan aiming to identify novel associations with ankylosing spondylitis was recently undertaken[67]. This study, which used a large number of polymorphic microsatellite markers throughout the genome, identified a number of new markers, both within and outside of the MHC, that were significantly associated with this disease. Moreover, the sib-pair analysis suggested that only 31% of the susceptibility to ankylosing spondylitis is encoded by genes in the MHC, a finding that should encourage further genomic studies.

FUNCTION OF HLA-B27

Biosynthesis of HLA-B27 is likely to be similar to that of other class I HLA molecules. The 44kDa heavy chain is synthesized in the endoplasmic reticulum, where it undergoes association with the genetically invariant nonglycosylated 12kDa β_2 microglobulin protein. Modification of the glycosyl residues occurs in the Golgi apparatus, from which the molecule is transported to the cell surface, where it is expressed as an integral transmembrane surface protein by most nucleated cells[31]. Under physiologic circumstances, intracellularly synthesized and processed antigenic peptides become bound in the class I MHC binding cleft within the endoplasmic reticulum. In most circumstances, the heavy chain, β_2 microglobulin and antigenic peptide form a trimolecular complex within the endoplasmic reticulum that permits stable association on the cell surface[31]. Most peptides that are presented by class I MHC molecules are synthesized within the antigen presenting cell, and encoded either by endogenous genes or by intracellular viruses or bacteria[31,68]. It is the peptide–MHC molecular complex expressed on the cell surface that is recognized by CD8+ T-lymphocytes[37]. Class I MHC molecules expressed within the thymic cortex also have been shown to influence the T cell repertoire by exerting both positive and negative selective influences on the CD4+CD8+ thymocyte precursors of mature T cells[69]. Thus, class I MHC molecules play a dual role with regard to antigen recognition by T cells. On the one hand, class I MHC molecules serve to select the TCR repertoire of CD8+ T cells in the thymus and, on the other, they function to bind and present antigen to CD8+ T cells in peripheral tissues.

THE BACTERIAL TRIGGER

There is considerable evidence that an antecedent bacterial infection is involved in the initiation of reactive arthritis as well as other spondyloarthropathies[1–3]. Reactive arthritis is frequently initiated by urogenital or enteric infection with one of a number of obligate or facultative intracellular bacteria, including *Chlamydia trachomatis*, *Yersinia enterocolitica*, *Shigella flexneri*, *Campylobacter jejuni* or *Salmonella typhimurium*. After a mucosal infection with one of these organisms there is dissemination of bacterial material[70,71] and, in the case of *Chlamydia*, living microorganisms[72,73] to synovial tissues. *C. trachomatis* nucleic acid has been detected not only in the synovial fluid and tissue of patients with reactive arthritis and undifferentiated oligoarthritis[74], but also in the synovium of some asymptomatic individuals[75]. Perhaps surprisingly, there was not a good correlation between the detection of synovial *Chlamydia*, and the presence of an anti-chlamydial immune response[74]. Moreover, there has been a suggestion that the gene expression profile of *C. trachomatis* in the synovium of patients with reactive arthritis may be aberrant[76]. These data raise the possibility that cells in the synovium may serve as reservoirs for *Chlamydia*, while the behavior of this microorganism under these circumstance may alter the host's immune response to allow an ongoing synovitis without effective clearance. In support of this, a rat model of *C. trachomatis* synovitis demonstrated that synoviocytes served as reservoirs for chlamydial antigens sustaining an intense chronic synovitis[77].

Within the synovial membrane and synovial fluid, T cells reactive to bacterial antigens can be detected at increased frequency compared to autologous blood or within synovial tissues or fluid of patients with other forms of arthritis[78]. This appears to result from local expansion of T cells in response to bacterial antigens residing with synovial tissues. An analysis of the TCR beta chain repertoire in synovial fluid compared to peripheral blood in individuals with reactive arthritis demonstrated frequent oligoclonality and shared sequences in the CDR3 region between the T cells of different patients[79]. Most of these responding T cells are CD4+ T cells that are responsive to bacterial antigenic peptides presented by MHC class II molecules. A number of specific proteins appear to trigger responsive CD4+ T cells, including the ribosomal proteins, L2 and L23 of Yersinia and Chlamydia, a subunit of Yersinia urease and the conserved 18kDa histone-like protein and 60kDa heat shock protein of Chlamydia[78]. A 12 amino acid sequence derived from Yersinia hsp60 was shown to be a dominant antigen for both CD4 and CD8 responses in patients with Yersinia-triggered reactive arthritis[80]. Although less frequent, HLA-B27 restricted CD8+ T cell responses to bacterial antigens can also be found in synovial fluid of some patients with reactive arthritis[81].

A critical role for normal enteric bacterial flora has been shown in the HLA-B27 transgenic rat[82,83]. When these rats were re-derived in a germ-free environment, no evidence of enteric or articular inflammation was observed, although typical psoriasiform skin lesions developed. When germ-free rats were reconstituted with enteric flora from specific pathogen free rats, gastrointestinal inflammation and arthritis rapidly developed. Anaerobic organisms appeared to be especially important in the development of arthritis.

The role of a specific bacterial trigger in ankylosing spondylitis is less certain. A possible role of Klebsiella has been suggested, especially in those patients with enteric lesions that are common in ankylosing spondylitis. A correlation between elevated titers of anti-Klebsiella antibodies and the presence of enteric lesions in ankylosing spondylitis has been noted[84]. However, T cell responses have been difficult to detect[85], even though increased numbers of CD4+ T cells have been noted in the synovial membrane of the sacroiliac joints of patients with ankylosing spondylitis[86].

It has been suggested that the expression of HLA-B27 plays a role in altering bacterial elimination[87]. HLA-B27 transgenic mice given Yersinia intragastrically retained the organisms in the gastrointestinal tract and the spleen for a persistent period of time compared to control mice[88]. Persistence was mediated by a Yersinia-specific protein, Yad-A. Similar results have been shown with Salmonella on human monocytic cell lines[89]. Whether bacterial persistence might enhance the likelihood of a pathogenic immune response remains unclear. Of relevance, it was recently demonstrated that HLA-B27 plays an important role in modulating immune recognition and CTL responses against Chlamydia in a transgenic rat model of infection[90].

Most organisms that trigger reactive arthritis are cleared relatively quickly[73,88]. Therefore, persistence of bacterial products is unlikely to explain the ongoing inflammatory response in the majority of patients with a persistent arthropathy. Interestingly, a detailed study of one patient demonstrated what appeared to be an articular reactivation of a persistent Yersinia infection months after the initial episode of reactive arthritis[91]. A number of studies have demonstrated bacterial antigens derived from the triggering organisms in the synovial fluid and tissues of some reactive arthritis patients, but these are typically detected early in the course of the arthropathy and only in a minority of affected individuals[91–93]. Of note, chronic reactive arthritis is much more highly associated with HLA-B27 than acute disease[22], suggesting that ongoing inflammation may depend on persistent T cell stimulation by either persistent bacterial antigens, or cross-reactive autoantigens, or perhaps both.

MOLECULAR MIMICRY

Several hypotheses can be constructed to account for the observation that infectious agents can trigger chronic reactive arthritis in HLA-B27 positive individuals. One hypothesis is that a small region of a human antigen is identical to amino acid sequences of proteins encoded by the triggering microorganism. This hypothesis has been termed molecular mimicry[94]. The mimicry may be of a structural gene product or the HLA-B27 molecule itself. Although it is not clear how mimicry of a class I MHC molecule would lead to an anatomically localized disease with characteristics of the spondyloarthropathies, there is considerable evidence for the sharing of antigenic determinants between HLA-B27 and different bacterial products. Most of this evidence depends upon cross-reactivities of various antibodies. Evidence of T cell cross-reactivity to epitopes shared between initiating microorganisms and self-proteins has been more difficult to document. A recent study documented cross reactivity between mouse hsp60 and an antigen derived from the Salmonella GroEL molecule presented in the context of an MHC class 1b molecule and recognized by CD8 T cells[95].

A computer search for bacterial proteins with amino acid sequence homology to HLA-B27 has yielded positive results[96,97]. Thus, the nitrogenase enzyme in Klebsiella pneumoniae contains a six amino acid region that is homologous with HLA-B*2705 residues[72–77]. Similarly, a 2mDa plasmid, termed pHS-2, was identified in several arthritogenic S. flexneri isolates but was absent from nonarthritogenic Shigella[17,98]. The nucleotide sequence of this plasmid revealed a predicted open reading frame encoding a 22 amino acid peptide potentially encoding an eight-amino-acid stretch (Ala-Gln-Thr-Asp-Arg-His-Ser-Leu), seven residues of which are identical to residues 71–78 of the HLA-B*2704 and HLA-B*2706 sequences (Ala-Gln-Thr-Asp-Arg-Glu-Ser-Leu). Residues 1–5 and 8 of this sequence are shared by all HLA-B27 subtypes known to be associated with the spondyloarthropathies. T cell reactivity to these peptides has not been examined and, therefore, their role in the pathogenesis of the spondyloarthropathies, including reactive arthritis remains unknown.

THE ROLE OF T CELLS

The association of HLA-B27 implies a role for CD8+ T cells in the pathogenesis of these conditions, since the only known functions of the polymorphic portions of class I MHC molecules are selection of the TCR repertoire of CD8+ T cells in the thymus and presentation of antigen to CD8+ T cells in the periphery[31,41,69]. Direct evidence that CD8+ T cells are likely to be involved in the pathogenesis has come from observations made in individuals with acquired immune deficiency syndrome (AIDS). Despite suppression of the function of CD4+ T cells, these individuals are capable of developing reactive arthritis[99]. Of note, ankylosing spondylitis has not been reported in AIDS patients, although this may relate to the extended length of time required to develop symptomatic spondylitis. Reactive arthritis developing in patients with AIDS frequently follows a gastrointestinal or genitourinary infection, is usually associated with HLA-B27 and can be extremely aggressive. CD8+ T cell function is usually normal, although the number and function of CD4+ T cells can be severely depleted. Moreover, the finding that reactive arthritis is extremely aggressive in AIDS patients, although not occurring at increased frequency, suggests that CD4+ T cells may function to suppress the development of reactive arthritis.

As shown in Figure 108.3, reactive arthritis appears to be triggered by CD8+ T cells responding to a bacterially derived antigenic peptide bound to HLA-B27. In this model, CD4+ T cells function to regulate this response by recognizing other bacterially encoded antigenic peptides presented in the context of class II MHC molecules. As a result of

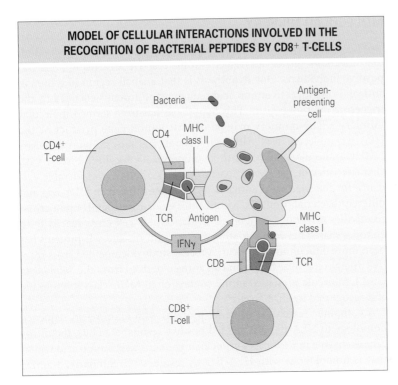

Fig. 108.3 Model of cellular interactions involved in the recognition of bacterial peptides by CD8⁺ T cells.

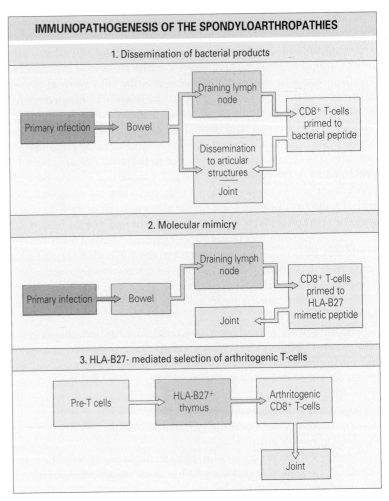

Fig. 108.4 Immunopathogenesis of the spondyloarthropathies. Potential immunopathogenic mechanisms. The primary infectious process is shown in the bowel, although it could involve the genitourinary tract as well.

this response, CD4⁺ T cells may produce high levels of interferon-γ and other cytokines which activate the macrophages[100–102], and thereby limit intracellular growth of the triggering microorganisms and the production of peptides that can associate with HLA-B27 and initiate arthritogenic responses of CD8⁺ T cells. Interestingly interleukin-4 (IL-4) mRNA and interferon-γ (IFN-γ) mRNA have been found to be produced by the synovial membrane of patients with reactive arthritis[103], suggesting the possibility that IL-4 might limit the action of interferon-γ, thereby facilitate the persistence of initiating bacteria and perhaps increase the likelihood of inducing an ongoing immune response mediated by CD8⁺ T cells.

T cells clearly play a role in the inflammatory disease manifested by HLA-B27 transgenic rats. Thus, T cell deficient nude rats expressing HLA-*B*2705 do not develop disease unless reconstituted with T cells[104]. Disease develops most reproducibly upon transfer of CD4⁺ T cells to T cell deficient rats, although CD8⁺ T cells also can transfer disease. On the basis of data from the HLA-B27 transgenic rat model, it appears that a critical cell in the induction of the disease is an antigen-presenting cell expressing abundant HLA-B27[105].

POTENTIAL IMMUNOPATHOGENIC MECHANISMS

Although the role of the HLA-B27 molecule in the pathogenesis of reactive arthritis is not completely known, an understanding of its function suggests ways in which it may be involved in these conditions (Fig. 108.4). One hypothesis is that infection with particular gastrointestinal or genitourinary microorganisms triggers an immune response by CD8⁺ T cells. These organisms are intracellular pathogens and would, therefore, generate peptides within infected host antigen presenting cells. The arthritogenic response would involve those bacterial peptides that bind to HLA-B27 and are presented to CD8⁺ T cells. In addition to triggering immune responses, there is dissemination of microbial antigens, including the ones restricted by HLA-B27 to distant tissue, including the synovium, which is richly endowed with phagocytic cells. In this model, joint inflammation would result from persistent

reactivity to those slowly cleared microbial products located within synovial tissue.

An alternative hypothesis is that the pathogenesis of the disease involves the induction of autoreactivity to autoantigens because of molecular mimicry between epitopes on the infecting microorganism and host tissues. In this model, infection with a bacterium expressing an HLA-B27 mimetic peptide might result in priming of CD8⁺ T cells to the endogenous HLA-B27 derived amino acid sequences. During the infection with the microorganism, an immune response to a variety of other bacterial antigens or perhaps the adjuvant effect of the microorganism might provide sufficient help to overcome normal tolerance to self-peptides. Subsequently, endogenous HLA-B27 itself could be the source of the antigenic peptide. This could be produced within the synovium in increased amounts after a variety of traumatic or stressful insults that result in the local production of cytokines and might account for the tendency of the disease to exacerbate and remit. In this model, HLA-B27 or another class I MHC molecule could serve as the presenting element. The critical role of HLA-B27 would therefore be to provide the endogenously derived peptide that is the target of persistent stimulation of autoreactive CD8⁺ T cells.

Finally, it is possible that the role of HLA-B27 in the development of the spondyloarthropathies is less direct. HLA-B27 may function at the level of the thymus to select a repertoire of TCR expressed by CD8⁺ T cells that includes receptors uniquely capable of responding to microbial antigens in a pathogenic manner.

The involvement of CD4⁺ T cells suggested by the presence of CD4⁺ T cells in the synovium reactive to bacterial antigens, the accentuation of disease by human immunodeficiency virus (HIV) infection and the ability of CD4$^+$ T cells to transfer disease to T cell depleted HLA-B27 transgenic rats remains unexplained. It is possible that the CD4$^+$ T cell response is a first line, largely protective, response in acute disease. Only when this fails to eliminate bacterial antigens by the production of cytokines, such as interferon-γ, can priming of CD8$^+$ cells occur effectively with the subsequent development of chronic, highly HLA-B27 associated inflammatory arthritis. Consistent with this is the exuberant disease noted in CD4$^+$ T cell immunodeficient AIDS patients and the capacity of CD4$^+$ T cells to transfer colonic inflammation but rarely arthritis to T cell depleted HLA-B27 transgenic rats.

It is important to recognize that each of these hypotheses is tenable. Moreover, none is mutually exclusive of the others. A combination of the above events may be involved in the development of the spondyloarthropathies. Finally, the hypotheses do not address a number of issues, including the unique tissue distribution of the disease, its immunopathogenesis in HLA-B27 negative individuals, and the immunopathologic relationship between reactive arthritis on the one hand and ankylosing spondylitis on the other.

REFERENCES

1. Calin A, Taurog JD. The spondyloarthropathies. Oxford: Oxford University Press, 1998.
2. Hughes R, Keat A. Reactive arthritis. Semin Arthritis Rheum 1994; 24: 190–210.
3. Spencer Wells R, Parham P. HLA class I genes: structure and diversity. In: Browning M, McMichael A, eds. HLA and MHC: genes, molecules and function. Oxford: BIOS Scientific Publishers; 1996: 77–96.
4. Cerundolo V, Braud V. Cell biology of MHC class I molecules. In: Browning M, McMichael A, eds. HLA and MHC: genes, molecules and function. Oxford: BIOS Scientific Publishers; 1996: 193–223.
5. Reveille JD, Ball EJ, Khan MA. HLA-B27 and genetic predisposing factor in spondylathropathies. Curr Opin Rheumatol 2001; 13: 265–272.
6. Hildebrand W, Domena J, Shen S et al. The HLA-B7 Qui antigen is encoded by a new subtype of HLA-B27 (B*2708). Tissue Antigens 1994; 44: 47–51.
7. Lopez-Larrea C, Sujirachato K, Mehra NK et al. HLA-B27 subtypes in Asian patients with ankylosing spondylitis. Evidence for new associations. Tissue Antigens 1995; 45: 169–176.
8. Gonzalez-Roces S, Alvarez MV, Gonzalez S et al. HLA-B27 polymorphism and worldwide susceptibility to ankylosing spondylitis. Tissue Antigens 1997; 49: 116–123.
9. Hill AVS, Allsopp CEM, Kwaitkowski D et al. HLA-class I typing PCR: HLA-B27 and an African B27 subtype. Lancet 1991; 337: 640–642.
10. Toivanen P, Toivanen A. Two forms of reactive arthritis? Ann Rheum Dis 1999; 58: 737–741.
11. Thomson GTD, DeRubeis DA, Hodge MA et al. Post-Salmonella reactive arthritis: late clinical sequelae in a point source cohort. Am J Med 1995; 98: 13–21.
12. Mattila L, Leirisalo-Repo M, Koskimies S et al. Reactive arthritis following an outbreak of Salmonella infection in Finland. Br J Rheumatol 1994; 33: 1136–1141.
13. Kvien TK, Glennas A, Melby K et al. Reactive arthritis: incidence, triggering agents and clinical presentation. J Rheumatol 1994; 21: 115–122.
14. Zeidler H, Wollenhaupt J. Chlamydia-induced arthritis: the clinical spectrum, serology and prognosis. In: Lipsky PE, Taurog JD, eds. HLA-B27$^+$ spondyloarthropathies. New York: Elsevier; 1991: 175–187.
15. Herrlinger JD, Asmussen JU. Long-term prognosis in Yersinia arthritis: Clinical and serological findings. Ann Rheum Dis 1992; 51: 1332–1334.
16. van Bohemen CG, Lionarons RJ, vanBodegom P et al. Susceptibility and HLA-B27 in post-dysenteric arthropathies. Immunology 1985; 56: 377–379.
17. Stieglitz H, Fosmire S, Lipsky P. Identification of a 2Mda plasmid from Shigella flexneri associated with reactive arthritis. Arthritis Rheum 1989; 32: 937–948.
18. Inman RD. Classification criteria for reactive arthritis. J Rheumatol 1999; 26: 1219–1221.
19. Rubin LA, Amos CI, Wade JA et al. Investigating the genetic basis for ankylosing spondylitis. Linkage studies with the major histocompatibility complex region. Arthritis Rheum 1994; 37: 1212–1220.
20. Martinez-Borra J, Gonzalez S, Lopez-Larrea C. Genetic factors predisposing to spondylarthropathies. Arthritis Rheum. 2000; 43: 485–492.
21. Hammer RE, Maika SD, Richardson JA et al. Spontaneous inflammatory disease in transgenic rats expressing HLA-B27 and human a$_2$m: an animal model of HLA-B27-associated human disorders. Cell 1990; 63: 1099–1112.
22. Taurog JD, Maika SD, Simmons WA et al. Susceptibility to inflammatory disease in HLA-B27 transgenic rat lines correlates with the level of B27 expression. J Immunol 1993; 150: 4168–4178.
23. Khare SD, Bull MJ, Hanson J et al. Spontaneous inflammatory disease in HLA-B27 transgenic mice is independent of MHC class II molecules: a direct role for B27 heavy chains and not B27-derived peptides. J Immunol 1998; 160: 101–106.
24. Bjorkman PJ, Saper MA, Samraoui B et al. The foreign antigen binding site and T cell recognition regions of class I histocompatibility antigens. Nature 1987; 329: 512–518.
25. Madden DR, Gorga JC, Strominger JL, Wiley DC. The structure of HLA-B27 reveals nonamer self-peptides bound in an extended conformation. Nature 1991; 353: 321–325.
26. Madden DR, Gorga JC, Strominger JL, Wiley DC. The three-dimensional structure of HLA-B27 at 2.1 A resolution suggests a general mechanism for tight peptide binding to MHC. Cell 1992; 70: 1035–1048.
27. Urban RG, Chicz RM, Lane WS et al. A subset of HLA-B27 molecules contains peptides much longer than nonamers. Proc Natl Acad Sci USA 1994; 91: 1534–1538.
28. Rotzschke O, Falk K, Stevanovic S et al. Dominant aromatic/aliphatic C-terminal anchor in HLA-B*2702 and B*2705 peptide motifs. Immunogenetics 1994; 39: 74–77.
29. Colbert RA, Rowland-Jones SL, McMichael AJ, Frelinger JA. Differences in peptide presentation between B27 subtypes: the importance of the P1 side chain in maintaining high affinity peptide binding to B*2703. Immunity 1994; 1: 121–130.
30. Boisgerault F, Tieng V, Stolzenberg MC et al. Differences in endogenous peptides presented by HLA-B*2705 and B*2703 allelic variants. Implications for susceptibility to spondyloarthropathies. J Clin Invest 1996; 98: 2764–2770.
31. Germain RN. MHC-dependent antigen processing and peptide presentation: providing ligands for T lymphocyte activation. Cell 1994; 76: 287–299.
32. Hilt W, Wolf D. Proteasomes: destruction as a programme. Trends Biochem Sci 1996; 21: 96–102.
33. Powis SJ, Tonkss, Mockridge I et al. Alleles and haplotypes of the MHC-encoded ABC transporters TAP1 and TAP2. Immunogenetics 1993; 37: 373–380.
34. Obst R, Armandola E, Nijenhuis M et al. TAP polymorphism does not influence transport of peptide variants in mice and humans. Eur J Immunol 1995; 25: 2170–2176.
35. Colbert RA, Rowland-Jones SL, McMichael AJ, Frelinger JA. Allele-specific B pocket transplant in class I major histocompatibility complex protein changes: requirement for anchor residue at P2 of peptide. Proc Natl Acad Sci USA 1993; 90: 6879–6883.
36. Jardetsky TS, Lune WS, Robinson RA et al. Identification of self peptides bound to purified HLA-B27. Nature 1991; 353: 326–329.
37. Townsend A, Bodmer H. Antigen recognition by class I-restricted T lymphocytes. Ann Rev Immunol 1989; 7: 601–624.
38. Rudwaleit M, Bowness P, Wordsworth P. The nucleotide sequence of HLA-B*2704 reveals a new amino acid substitution in exon 4 which is also present in HLA-B*2706. Immunogenetics 1996; 43: 160–162.
39. Fiorillo MT, Greco G, Maragno M et al. The naturally occurring polymorphism Asp116→His116, differentiating the ankylosing spondylitis-associated HLA-B*2705 from the non-associated HLA-B*2709 subtype, influences peptide-specific CD8 T cell recognition. Eur J Immunol 1998; 28: 2508–2516.
40. Parham P, Lomen CE, Lawlor DA et al. Nature of polymorphism in HLA, -B, and -C molecules. Proc Natl Acad Sci USA 1988; 85: 4005–4009.
41. Benjamin R, Parham P. Guilt by association: HLA-B27 and ankylosing spondylitis. Immunol Today 1990; 11: 137–142.
42. Urvater JA, Hickman H, Dzuris JL et al. Gorillas with spondyloarthropathies express an MHC class I molecule with only limited sequence similarity to HLA-B27 that binds peptides with arginine at P2. J Immunol 2001; 166: 3334–3344.
43. Simmons WA, Summerfield SG, Roopenian DC et al. Novel HY peptide antigens presented by HLA-B27. J Immunol 1997; 159: 2750–2759.
44. Raghavan M, Lebron JA, Johnson JL, Bjorkman PJ. Extended repertoire of permissible peptide ligands for HLA-B*2702. Protein Sci 1996; 5: 2080–2088.
45. Zhou M, Sayad A, Simmons WA et al. The specificity of peptides bound to human histocompatibility leukocyte antigen (HLA)-B27 influences the prevalence of arthritis in HLA-B27 transgenic rats. J Exp Med 1998; 188: 877–886.
46. Gao X-M, Wordsworth P, McMichael AJ et al. Homocysteine modification of HLA antigens and its immunological consequences. Eur J Immunol 1996; 26: 1443–1450.
47. MacLean IL, Lowdell MW, Blake DR et al. Absence of a specific effect of free radicals on HLA-B27. Ann Rheum Dis 1990; 51: 963–964.
48. Taurog JD, El-Zaatari FAK. In vitro mutagenesis of HLA-B27. Substitution of an unpaired cysteine residue in the alpha 1 domain causes loss of antibody-defined epitopes. J Clin Invest 1988; 82: 987–992.
49. van der Linden SM, Valkenburg HA, de Jongh BM, Cats A. The risk of developing ankylosing spondylitis in HLA-B27 positive individuals. A comparison of relatives of spondylitis patients with the general population. Arthritis Rheum 1984; 27: 241–249.
50. Robinson WP, van der Linden S, Khan MA et al. HLA-Bw60 increases susceptibility to ankylosing spondylitis in HLA-B27(+) patients. Arthritis Rheum 1989; 32: 1135–1141.
51. Yagamuchi A, Tsuchiya N, Mitsui H et al. Association of HLA-B39 with HLA-B27-negative ankylosing spondylitis and pauciarticular juvenile rheumatoid arthritis in Japanese patients. Evidence for a role of the peptide anchoring pocket. Arthritis Rheum 1995; 38: 1672–1677.

52. Rammensee H, Friede T, Stevanovic S. MHC ligands and peptide motifs: first listing. Immunogenetics 1995; 41: 178–228.
53. Cedoz, JP, Wendlin, D, Viel, JF. The B-7 cross-reactive group and spondyloarthropathies: an epidemiological approach. J Rheumatol 1995; 22: 1184–1190.
54. Verjans GM, Brinkman BM, Van Doornik CE et al. Polymorphism of tumour necrosis factor-alpha (TNF-alpha) at position -308 in relation to ankylosing spondylitis. Clin Exp Immunol 1994; 97: 45–47.
55. Kaijzel EL, Brinkman BM, van Krugten MV et al. Polymorphism within the tumor necrosis factor alpha (TNF) promoter region in patients with ankylosing spondylitis. Hum Immunol 1999; 60: 140–144.
56. Fraile A, Nieto A, Beraun Y et al. Tumor necrosis factor gene polymorphisms in ankylosing spondylitis. Tissue Antigens 1998; 51: 386–390.
57. Hohler T, Schaper T, Schneider PM et al. Association of different tumor necrosis factor alpha promoter allele frequencies with ankylosing spondylitis in HLA-B27 positive individuals. Arthritis Rheum 1998; 41: 1489–1492.
58. Brown MA, Kennedy LG, Darke C et al. The effect of HLA-DR genes on susceptibility to and severity of ankylosing spondylitis. Arthritis Rheum 1998; 41: 460–465.
59. Burney RO, Pile KD, Gibons K et al. Analysis of the MHC class II encoded components of the HLA class I antigen processing pathway in ankylosing spondylitis. Ann Rheum Dis 1994; 53: 58–60.
60. Westmann P, Partanen J, Leirisalo-Repo M, Koskimies S. TAP1 and TAP2 polymorphism in HLA-B27-positive subpopulations – no allelic differences in ankylosing spondylitis and reactive arthritis. Hum Immunol 1995; 44: 236–242.
61. Maksymowych WP, Tao S, Li Y et al. Allelic variation at the TAP1 locus influences disease phenotype in HLA-B27 positive individuals with ankylosing spondylitis. Tissue Antigens 1995; 45: 328–332.
62. Barron KS, Reveille JD, Carrington M et al. Susceptibility to Reiter's syndrome is associated with alleles of TAP genes. Arthritis Rheum 1995; 38: 684–689.
63. Maksymowych WP, Suarez-Almazor M, Chou C-T, Russell A. Polymorphism in the LMP2 gene influences susceptibility to extraspinal disease in HLA-B27 positive individuals with ankylosing spondylitis. Ann Rheum Dis 1995; 54: 321–324.
64. Hohler T, Schaper T, Schneider PM et al. No primary association between LMP2 polymorphisms and extraspinal manifestations in spondyloarthropathies. Ann Rheum Dis 1997; 56: 741–743.
65. Bragado R, Lauzurica P, Lopez D, Lopez de Castro JA. T cell receptor Vβ– gene usage in a human alloreactive response. Shared structural features among HLA-B27 specific T cell clones. J Exp Med 1990; 171: 1189–1204.
66. Duchmann R, May E, Ackermann B et al. HLA-B27-restricted cytotoxic T lymphocyte responses to arthritogenic enterobacteria or self-antigens are dominated by closely related TCRBV gene segments. A study in patients with reactive arthritis. Scand J Immunol 1996; 43: 101–108.
67. Brown MA, Pile KD, Kennedy LG et al. A genome-wide screen for susceptibility loci in ankylosing spondylitis. Arthritis Rheum 1998; 41: 588–595.
68. Yewdell JW, Bennink JR. The binary logic of antigen processing and presentation of T cells. Cell 1990; 62: 203–206.
69. von Boehmer H, Kisielow P. Self–nonself discrimination by T cells. Science 1990; 248: 1369–1372.
70. Gransfors K, Jalkanen S, Lindberg AA et al. Salmonella lipopolysaccharide in synovial cells from patients with reactive arthritis. Lancet 1990; 33: 685–686.
71. Nikkari S, Merilahti-Palo R, Saario R et al. Yersinia-triggered reactive arthritis. Use of polymerase chain reaction and immunocytochemical staining in the detection of bacterial components from synovial specimens. Arthritis Rheum 1992; 35: 682–687.
72. Bas S, Griffais R, Kvien TK et al. Amplification of plasmid and chromosome chlamydia DNA in synovial fluid of patients with reactive arthritis and undifferentiated seronegative oligoarthropathies. Arthritis Rheum 1995; 38: 1005–1013.
73. Nanagara R, Li F, Beutler A et al. Alteration of Chlamydia trachomatis biologic behavior in synovial membranes. Arthritis Rheum 1995; 38: 1410–1417.
74. Wilkinson NZ, Kingsley GH, Sieper J et al. Lack of correlation between the detection of Chlamydia trachomatis DNA in synovial fluid from patients with a range of rheumatic diseases and the presence of an antichlamydial immune response. Arthritis Rheum 1998; 41: 845–854.
75. Schumacher HRJ, Arayssi T, Crane M et al. Chlamydia trachomatis nucleic acids can be found in the synovium of some asymptomatic subjects. Arthritis Rheum 1999; 42: 1281–1284.
76. Gerard HC, Branigan PJ, Schumacher HRJ, Hudson AP. Synovial chlamydia trachomatis in patients with reactive arthritis/Reiter's syndrome are viable but show aberrant gene expression. J Rheumatol 1998; 25: 734–742.
77. Inman RD, Chiu B. Synoviocyte-packaged chlamydia trachomatis induces a chronic aseptic arthritis. J Clin Invest 1998; 102: 1776–1782.
78. Burmester GR, Daser A, Kamradt T et al. Immunology of reactive arthritis. Ann Rev Immun 1995; 13: 229–250.
79. Dulphy N, Peyrat MA, Tieng V et al. Common intra-articular T cell expansions in patients with reactive arthritis: identical beta-chain junctional sequences and cytotoxicity toward HLA-B27. J Immunol 1999; 162: 3830–3839.
80. Mertz AK, Wu P, Sturniolo T et al. Multispecific CD4+ T cell response to a single 12-mer epitope of the immunodominant heat-shock protein 60 of Yersinia enterocolitica in Yersinia-triggered reactive arthritis: overlap with the B27-restricted CD8 epitope, functional properties, and epitope presentation by multiple DR alleles. J Immunol 2000; 164: 1529–1537.
81. Hermann E, Yu DTY, Meyer zum Büschenfelde K-H, Fleischer B. HLA-B27-restricted CD8 T cells derived from synovial fluids of patients with reactive arthritis and ankylosing spondylitis. Lancet 1993; 342: 646–650.
82. Taurog JD, Richardson JA, Croft JT et al. The germfree state prevents development of gut and joint inflammatory disease in HLA-B27 transgenic rats. J Exp Med 1994; 180: 2359–2364.
83. Rath HC, Herfarth, HH, Ikeda JS et al. Normal luminal bacteria, especially Bacteroides, mediate chronic colitis, gastritis and arthritis in HLA-B27/human b₂ microglobulin transgenic rats. J Clin Invest 1966; 98: 945–953.
84. Granfors K, Mäki-Ikola O, Leirisala-Repo M. Association of gut inflammation with the increased serum Klebsiella pneumoniae-specific antibody levels in patients with axial type of ankylosing spondylitis. Arthritis Rheum 1995; 38: S348.
85. Hermann E, Sucke B, Droste U et al. Klebsiella pneumoniae-reactive T cells in blood and synovial fluid of patients with ankylosing spondylitis. Arthritis Rheum 1995; 38: 1277–1282.
86. Braun J, Bollow M, Neure L et al. Use of immunohistologic and in situ hybridization techniques in the examination of sacroiliac joint biopsy specimens from patients with ankylosing spondylitis. Arthritis Rheum 1995; 38: 499–505.
87. Kapasi K, Inman RD. HLA-B27 expression modulates gram-negative bacterial invasion into transfected L cells. J Immunol 1992; 148: 3554–3559.
88. Heesemann J, Gaede K, Autenrieth IB. Experimental Yersinia enterocolitica infection in rodents: A model for human yersiniosis. APMIS 1993; 1: 417–429.
89. Laitio P, Virtala M, Salmi M et al. HLA-B27 modulates intracellular survival of Salmonella enteritidis in human monocytic cells. Eur J Immunol 1997; 27: 1331–1338.
90. Popov I, Dela Cruz CS, Barber BH et al. The effect of an anti-HLA-B27 immune response on CTL recognition of Chlamydia. J Immunol 2001; 167: 3375–3382.
91. Gaston JS, Cox C, Granfors K. Clinical and experimental evidence for persistent Yersinia infection in reactive arthritis. Arthritis Rheum 1999; 42: 2239–2242.
92. Nikkari S, Rantakokko K, Ekman P et al. Salmonella-triggered reactive arthritis: use of polymerase chain reaction, immunocytochemical staining, and gas chromatography-mass spectrometry in the detection of bacterial components from synovial fluid. Arthritis Rheum 1999; 42: 84–89.
93. Granfors K, Merilahti-Palo R, Luukkainen R et al. Persistence of Yersinia antigens in peripheral blood cells from patients with Yersinia enterocolitica O:3 infection with or without reactive arthritis. Arthritis Rheum 1998; 41: 855–862.
94. Albert LJ, Inman RD. Molecular mimicry and autoimmunity. N Engl J Med 1999; 341: 2068–2074.
95. Lo WF, Woods AS, DeCloux A et al. Molecular mimicry mediated by MHC class Ib molecules after infection with gram-negative pathogens. Nat Med 2000; 6: 215–218.
96. Schwimmbeck PL, Yu DT, Oldstone MB. Autoantibodies to HLA-B27 in the sera of HLA-B27 patients with ankylosing spondylitis and Reiter's syndrome. Molecular mimicry with Klebsiella pneumoniae as potential mechanism of autoimmune disease. J Exp Med 1987; 166: 173–181.
97. Tsuchiya N, Husby G, Williams RCJ. Studies of humoral and cell-mediated immunity to peptides shared by HLA-27.1 and Klebsiella pneumoniae nitrogenase in ankylosing spondylitis. Clin Exp Immunol 1989; 76: 354–360.
98. Tsuchiya N, Husby G, Williams RC et al. Autoantibodies to HLA-B27 sequence cross-react with the hypothetical peptide from the arthritis-associated Shigella plasmid. J Clin Invest 1990; 85: 1193–1203.
99. Winchester R, Bernstein DH, Fischer HD et al. The co-occurrence of Reiter's syndrome and acquired immunodeficiency. Ann Intern Med 1987; 106: 19–26.
100. Beatty WL, Byrne GI, Morrison RP. Morphological and antigenic characterization of interferon-γ medicated persistent Chlamydia trachomatis infection in vitro. Proc Natl Acad Sci USA 1993; 85: 4000–4004.
101. Autenrieth IB, Beer M, Bohn E et al. Immune responses to Yersinia enterocolitica insusceptible BALB/c and resistant C57BL/6 mice: an essential role for gamma interferon. Infect Immun 1994; 62: 2590–2599.
102. Bohn E, Heesemann J, Ehlers S, Autenrieth IB. Early gamma interferon mRNA expression is associated with resistance of mice against Yersinia enterocolitica. Infect Immun 1994; 62: 3027–3032.
103. Simon AK, Seipelt E, Sieper J. Divergent T cell cytokine patterns in inflammatory arthritis. Proc Natl Acad Sci USA 1994; 91: 8562–8566.
104. Breban M, Fernandez-Sueiro JL, Simmons WA et al. T cells but not thymic exposure to HLA-B27 are required for the inflammatory disease of HLA-B27 transgenic rats. Immunology 1996; 256: 794–803.
105. Breban J, Hammer RE, Richardson JA, Taurog JD. Transfer of the inflammatory disease of HLA-B27 transgenic rats by bone marrow engraftment. J Exp Med 1993; 178: 1606–1616.

109 Reactive arthritis: clinical features and treatment

Auli Toivanen

Definition

- A sterile joint inflammation that develops after a distant infection
- The disease is systemic and not limited to the joints
- Triggering infections most commonly originate in the throat, urogenital organs or gastrointestinal tract
- The disease also occurs without obvious preceding infection, e.g. in association with inflammatory bowel disease

Clinical features

- Arthritis, enthesopathy, tendinitis, tenosynovitis, osteitis and muscle pains
- Skin and mucous membrane lesions are frequent
- Eye inflammations, e.g. uveitis and conjunctivitis
- Visceral involvement, such as nephritis or carditis, is relatively rare
- Severity ranges from mild arthralgia to disabling disease
- Spontaneous recovery is common and the prognosis is, in general, good
- Later, many patients suffer arthralgias and recurrences, and some develop ankylosing spondylitis
- Susceptibility to the disease is strongly linked to possession of the HLA-B27 antigen

HISTORICAL BACKGROUND

Reiter's syndrome, frequently considered as the most typical example of reactive arthritis was named after Hans Reiter (1881–1969) who, in 1916, described an officer suffering from a dysenteric illness with arthritis, urethritis and conjunctivitis[1]. Reiter did not actually recognize that the arthritis and conjunctivitis were related to the dysentery, but called the disease 'spirochaetosis arthritica'. However, as early as the 16th century, Pierre van Forest, and in the 17th century, Martinière, had recognized arthritis as a complication of urethritis. The first description of 'reactive arthritis' is attributed to Sir Benjamin Brodie (1783–1862)[2].

At the end of the Second World War, in Finland, Ilmari Paronen observed 344 cases of arthritis in connection with an outbreak of *Shigella* that occurred on the Karelian isthmus[3]. In 1969, Sairanen and coworkers published a follow-up study of 100 of these patients, detailing the prognosis of the disorder[4]. The term 'reactive arthritis' was introduced in 1976 by Aho *et al.*[5], and has gained wide use, even though it does not indicate the systemic character of the disease. The term 'Reiter's syndrome' is still in general use and refers to the triad of arthritis, urethritis and conjunctivitis, with 'incomplete Reiter's syndrome' used to describe conditions in which only two of these features are present. Both complete and incomplete Reiter's syndrome should be considered to be identical with reactive arthritis.

Observations of family clustering were soon confirmed by the finding that reactive arthritis is strongly associated with human leukocyte antigen (HLA)-B27. Great research interest has been focused on reactive arthritis, partly because the information gained may elucidate pathogenetic processes involved in the development of other rheumatic diseases, such as rheumatoid arthritis and ankylosing spondylitis.

EPIDEMIOLOGY

Because the clinical severity of reactive arthritis varies greatly and milder cases apparently go unnoticed, the true incidence of reactive arthritis is hard to assess. Certainly, growing awareness of reactive arthritis as a diagnostic possibility has increased the number of cases recognized. According to a Finnish estimation[6,7], the annual incidence of arthritis after bowel or urogenital infection is 30 per 100000 adults, to which must be added a proportion of cases of seronegative oligoarthritis, some of which are probably reactive arthritis, the incidence of which is 40/100 000 (Table 109.1). Reactive arthritis apparently affects all populations. Typically, it is a disorder of young adults, rare in small children and in older people; most patients are aged between 20 and 40 years[2,8]. Rheumatic fever, which also can be considered a type of reactive arthritis, occurs often in developing countries, but has practically disappeared elsewhere.

Reactive arthritis affects males and females with the same frequency. Genetic factors play a part in susceptibility to the disease, most patients reporting a family history of a similar disease. Between 65% and 96% of those affected are positive for HLA-B27. Indeed, HLA-B27 is a strong risk factor for developing reactive arthritis[9–12], with the increase in risk as high as 50-fold[5]. However, the association is not absolute: HLA-B27-positive individuals do not always develop reactive arthritis, even after a suitable infection, and the arthritis can occur also in HLA-B27-negative individuals. This is illustrated by observations by van Bohemen *et al.*[13] in connection with an outbreak of bacillary dysentery in The Netherlands: in three families, some but not all HLA-B27-positive members developed reactive arthritis after verified infection. The disease is more severe and the tendency to chronic development is greater in HLA-B27-positive individuals (see Chapter 108)[12,14,15], although HLA-B27-negative individuals can have a chronic or

---

TABLE 109.1
EPIDEMIOLOGY OF REACTIVE ARTHRITIS

- Most commonly affects young adults
- Equally frequent in males and females
- Annual incidence 30–40/100 000
- Probably worldwide
- Genetic associations
  Family clustering
  Strongly associated with HLA-B27
- Frequency in connection with infection,
  (e.g. enteric) varies

prolonged course of the disease[16]. Recently, it has been suggested that two forms of the disease – HLA-B27 associated and non-associated – should be distinguished[17]. These two forms also are triggered by different infectious agents, as discussed below.

The frequency of reactive arthritis after enteric infections caused by *Salmonella, Shigella* and *Campylobacter* has been reported to be 1–4% in unselected populations[18–20]. In some *Yersinia* outbreaks, the frequency of this complication has been quite high and in others negligible[21,22]. The fact that bacteria of the same genus, or species even, vary in their capacity to trigger reactive arthritis is of considerable interest.

CLINICAL FEATURES

Reactive arthritis has generally been defined as sterile synovitis developing after a distant infection. The detection of microbial components, including microbial DNA and RNA in the joints of patients with this disease has led to worldwide reconsideration of the definition. However, at present there are no generally accepted diagnostic criteria available for use by clinicians[23,24].

History

Typically, the first symptoms are of joint discomfort. A careful history may indicate symptoms of enteric or urogenital infection a few days to a couple of weeks previously, and often the patient reports such symptoms in other family members. Sometimes, abdominal pains in the few days before the appearance of joint symptoms may be suspected to be due to acute appendicitis or salpingo-oophoritis; this is especially the case in young adults. They may even have undergone laparotomy, in which case usually only mesenteric lymphadenitis has been found. Yet it is remarkable that patients requiring hospital care for severe enteritis caused by, for example, *Yersinia*, have rarely developed reactive arthritis. A common clinical experience is that the symptoms of the triggering infection have often been mild and, in about 10% of cases, the infection has passed unnoticed[25,26].

Infections most commonly preceding reactive arthritis are those caused by *Salmonella, Shigella, Yersinia, Campylobacter, Chlamydia trachomatis* or *C. pneumoniae, Borreliae, Neisseria* and streptococci. Several viruses have been implicated; those most often mentioned in connection with joint inflammation are rubella, hepatitis and parvovirus. It is apparent that the disease triggered by enteric or urogenital infection is usually HLA-B27-associated, but this is not the case for reactive arthritis caused by several other infectious agents such as *Borrelia*, meningococci, streptococci or viruses[17,27,28]. It is important to note that *Salmonella, Borrelia* and *Neisseria* can cause true septic arthritis in addition to reactive arthritis. It is not unusual, however, that a triggering infection cannot be identified, and in these cases the diagnosis remains uncertain. Non-infectious inflammatory bowel diseases may be associated with reactive arthritis[29,30] – for example, after intestinal bypass operation for morbid obesity. It is obvious, however, that in these conditions the intestinal microbial flora or the mucosal defense mechanisms are altered[26]. The same may apply to reactive arthritis occurring after a pseudomembranous colitis associated with overgrowth of *Clostridium difficile*[31].

General symptoms

Reactive arthritis is a systemic disease (Fig. 109.1), although the severity varies greatly. Frequently, general symptoms such as malaise, fatigue and fever are seen.

Joint and musculoskeletal symptoms

The most prominent symptoms are usually those in the joints. They vary from mild arthralgias to severely disabling polyarthritis[2,12,15,25]. Typically, there is asymmetric monoarthritis or oligoarthritis. The weight-bearing joints are most often affected: knees (Fig. 109.2), ankles

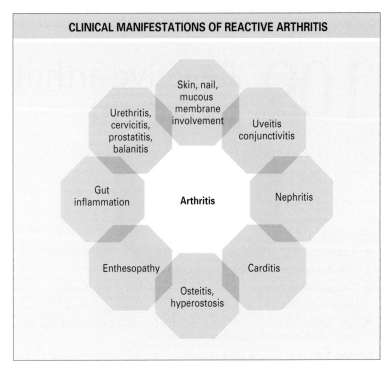

CLINICAL MANIFESTATIONS OF REACTIVE ARTHRITIS

Fig. 109.1 Clinical manifestations of reactive arthritis.

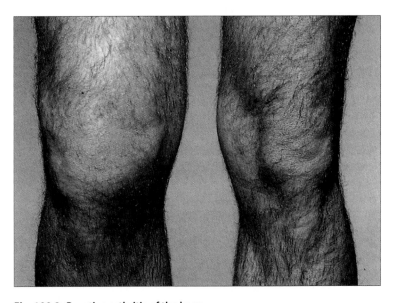

Fig. 109.2 Reactive arthritis of the knee.

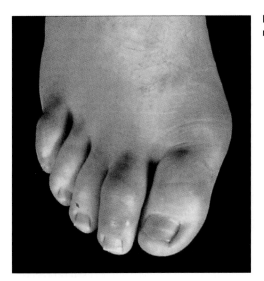

Fig. 109.3 Dactylitis in reactive arthritis.

and hips – but quite commonly other large joints, such as the shoulders, elbows and wrists, and small joints of the hands and feet may also be involved. The inflammation may vary from day to day and shift from one joint to another. The joints involved may be red and warm, and occasionally there is also *erythema nodosum*. Dactylitis is not uncommon (Fig. 109.3), and sometimes the condition may mimic rheumatoid arthritis, with stiffness on inactivity. Especially in the later stages, patients often complain of pains in the sacroiliac region.

A diagnosis cannot be made on the basis of physical examination alone, because the findings vary greatly and may mimic any other disease involving joint inflammation, including gout, rheumatoid arthritis or true purulent arthritis[32].

Reactive arthritis is not limited to the joints: enthesopathies, tenosynovitis, or both, are present in a high proportion of cases. Thus plantar fasciitis, Achilles tendinitis or bursitis of the ankle region often results in difficulties in walking. Pain on palpation is frequent at the sites where tendons attach to bones, and this enthesopathy may also limit movement. In severe cases, muscle wasting may be quite prominent. Unusually severe cases may become bedridden. Rarely, the disease renders the patient quite helpless and disabled. The outcome, however, is not related to the initial severity of the disease.

Skin and mucous membrane symptoms

The skin lesion most commonly attributed to reactive arthritis is *keratoderma blenorrhagicum* (Fig. 109.4), often referred to as '*pustulosis palmoplantaris*'. The lesions are indistinguishable from psoriasis, both clinically and histologically. The same holds for the nail lesions seen in both reactive arthritis and psoriasis. This similarity has not gained wide attention, but may be of interest when the pathogenesis of reactive arthritis and psoriatic arthropathy are considered. *Erythema nodosum*, often seen after *Yersinia* infection, is not common in the course of reactive arthritis and is not associated with HLA-B27.

When reactive arthritis is triggered by urogenital infection such as gonorrhea or chlamydial urethritis, it is called uroarthritis. Sterile urogenital inflammation can also be part of the reactive disease. Thus 'sterile urethritis' has been tacitly included in the triad classically recognized as Reiter's syndrome. Circinate balanitis (Fig. 109.5), which is also psoriatic in nature, and cystitis and prostatitis may be present, and can sometimes lead to complications such as shrinking of the bladder. Further, it seems that pelvic inflammatory disease, including salpingitis, may arise in women with reactive arthritis[33]. Inflammation of the urogenital tract has a tendency to relapse.

Various lesions are seen in the mouth. Wright and Moll[2] describe these as painless shiny patches, occurring on the palate, tongue and

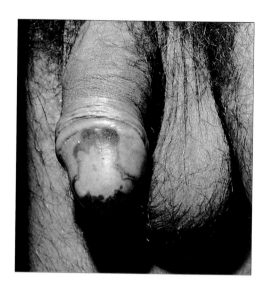

Fig. 109.5 Circinate balanitis in a man with reactive arthritis. (Courtesy of Professor VK Havu, Department of Dermatology, University of Turku.)

mucosa of the cheeks and lips. Erythema of the soft palate, uvula and tonsillar region has been described occasionally.

Gastrointestinal symptoms

Enteric infections or inflammatory diseases can, like urogenital infections, be the etiologic triggering event. It has become apparent that, as in the urogenital system, the epithelium of the intestine may form part of the reactive disease itself. Patients may complain of occasional abdominal pains and diarrhea, but at this stage no pathogens can be isolated from stool cultures. When ileocolonoscopy has been carried out in patients with established reactive arthritis, either macroscopically or microscopically detectable lesions resembling ulcerative colitis or Crohn's disease have been seen[29,30].

Ocular lesions

Inflammatory eye lesions form a classic part of the clinical picture. They may be either unilateral or bilateral. Conjunctivitis with sterile discharge is frequently seen. It usually subsides, but may progress to produce episcleritis, keratitis or even corneal ulcerations[2]. Acute uveitis, especially anterior uveitis (iritis), is also common. The ocular lesions may be the only or the first manifestation of reactive arthritis. They have a strong tendency to recur. Patients with reactive iritis most commonly complain of redness, photophobia and pain, and some have diminution of vision and increased lacrimation[34]. In patients with ocular complaints, it is advisable to undertake careful ophthalmologic examination, because if ocular lesions are left undiagnosed and untreated, permanent damage to the vision may follow.

Other systemic manifestations

Carditis is classically associated with rheumatic fever, and in developing countries valvular disease as a late sequel is a major problem. In reactive arthritides seen after enteric or urogenital infections, cardiac involvement is not as prominent. With increasing awareness it has become apparent, however, that conduction disturbances, even requiring pacemaker treatment, may occur[2,12].

Mild renal and urinary pathology, such as proteinuria, microhematuria and aseptic pyuria, are seen in about 50% of patients with reactive arthritis. Severe glomerulonephritis and IgA nephropathy are rare and hardly ever lead to permanently impaired renal function.

INVESTIGATIONS

In most cases of reactive arthritis, the patient seeks medical help for joint symptoms or for eye inflammation. The history and findings at the physical examination may immediately suggest the diagnosis, but confirmation requires laboratory and radiologic investigations (Table 109.2).

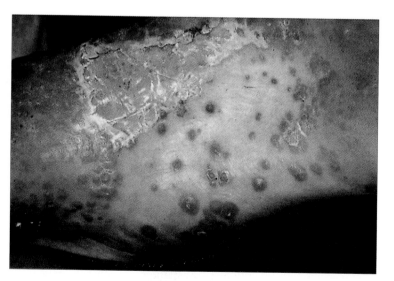

Fig. 109.4 Skin lesions (keratoderma blenorrhagicum) in reactive arthritis.

TABLE 109.2 INVESTIGATION OF REACTIVE ARTHRITIS

- ESR
- C-Reactive protein
- Blood cell count
- Liver function tests, e.g. ALT, AST, GGT
- Kidney function tests, e.g. serum creatinine or blood urea nitrogen
- Rheumatoid factor tests
- Urine analysis
- Electrocardiogram
- Joint fluid sample with analysis of:
  Cell count
  Exclusion of crystals
  Gram stain
  Bacterial culture
- Bacterial culture of:
  Feces
  Urine or urethral swab
  Cervical sample
  Throat
- Blood culture (not always necessary)
- Antibody determination at admission
- HLA-B27 antigen (or HLA typing) after 2–4 weeks
- Radiograph of affected joints
- Ophthalmologic examination if eye symptoms present

ALT, serum alanine-aminotransferase; ESR, erythrocyte sedimentation rate; GGT, serum gamma glutamyltransferase.

Laboratory investigations

The erythrocyte sedimentation rate is markedly increased in most cases of acute reactive arthritis, and values exceeding 60mm/h are commonly seen. The C-reactive protein is similarly increased at the onset of the disease. At a later stage, patients with chronic symptoms nevertheless have normal erythrocyte sedimentation rate and C-reactive protein values. The blood cell count may reveal moderate leukocytosis and mild anemia.

Urine analysis should be carried out at diagnosis and should be repeated during the follow-up, in order to detect possible aseptic pyuria resulting from urethritis. It is advisable to check renal function, for example by serum creatinine or blood urea nitrogen tests, and liver function by serum alanine aminotransferase or serum gamma glutamyltransferase. Tests for rheumatoid factor are usually negative.

Electrocardiography should be performed and repeated in patients who have a prolonged disease course, to exclude possible conduction disturbances. When endocarditis is suspected, especially in cases of rheumatic fever, it is essential also to assess cardiac function by echocardiography.

Joint fluid should always be aspirated when possible. Gram stain and bacterial culture should be performed to exclude septic arthritis[32]. In reactive arthritis, bacteria are not demonstrable either by staining or even extensive culturing. Microbial components have been detected, however, in the synovial membrane or in synovial fluid, by the use of special techniques not suitable for routine clinical work; these include immunofluorescence, immunoelectronmicroscopy, immunoblotting and polymerase chain reaction (PCR) techniques. In the early stages of reactive arthritis, the cell count in the synovial fluid can be quite high, and polymorphonuclear leukocytes can dominate the picture[32,35]. Later, lymphocytosis can develop. Demonstrations of specific antibodies in the synovial fluid, and of synovial mononuclear cells specifically responding to an infectious agent may be of diagnostic significance. However, these methods require elaborate techniques not available in most hospitals. Microscopy under polarized light should be performed, to exclude gout or pseudogout. Blood culture is not routinely necessary, but should be undertaken if joint infection is suspected.

Microbiologic and serologic studies form a cornerstone of diagnosis. Every effort should be made to isolate the causative microorganism from the throat, feces or urogenital tract. For detection of *Chlamydia*, application of PCR to first voided urine samples is a practical method. Isolation of *Yersinia* requires special methods, and it is easily missed in routine fecal culture. In most cases, however, results are negative, which emphasizes the role of serology. The serologic tests to be considered include antibody assays against *Salmonella*, *Yersinia*, *Campylobacter*, *Chlamydia*, *Neisseria gonorrhoeae*, *Borrelia burgdorferi* and β-hemolytic streptococci. Increase in and persistence of IgA class antibodies are especially characteristic, and these antibodies are not reliably detected by bacterial agglutination[36].

Depending on the infection history of the patient, antibodies against various viruses may yield a specific diagnosis.

It should be stressed that the list of microorganisms triggering reactive arthritis is steadily growing, and it is assumed that more remain to be identified. Thus negative serology does not rule out a diagnosis of reactive arthritis; furthermore, in some patients the antibodies increase slowly and yield a positive result only a few weeks after the onset of disease.

Detection of the HLA-B27 antigen is helpful in the diagnosis and in considering the treatment and follow-up of the patient. As noted before, however, the disease may also occur, and even have a chronic course, in HLA-B27-negative individuals.

Radiography and other imaging

Radiographic studies of symptomatic joints should be undertaken not so much to confirm the diagnosis of reactive arthritis as to rule out erosive disease, for example rheumatoid arthritis. The findings in reactive arthritis are usually rather scant, such as juxta-articular osteoporosis and soft tissue swelling. In patients with recurrent and chronic disease, erosions may be observed. More often, periosteal reaction and proliferation, especially at the insertion sites of tendons, are seen. Thus plantar spurs are a common sign in chronic cases. Magnetic resonance imaging has proved useful for the detection of joint effusion, enthesitis and tendinitis, but the benefit for routine clinical practice is small.

Chronic or recurring reactive arthritis also often leads to sacroiliitis and spondylitis that may be radiographically indistinguishable from ankylosing spondylitis, which is more easily detected by magnetic resonance imaging.

Radionuclide scintigraphy is a sensitive technique for demonstrating inflammation and is superior to radiography, especially in cases of enthesopathy, periostitis or early sacroiliitis[2,37].

Other investigations

Synovial biopsy is not of diagnostic value, as the inflammation is nonspecific. On occasion, exclusion of alternative diagnoses such as pigmented villonodular synovitis or tuberculous arthritis may be valuable.

In patients with reactive arthritis, inflammatory bowel disease (ulcerative colitis or Crohn's disease) may be a background factor. Ileocolonoscopy has revealed that, in many patients, either macroscopic or microscopic lesions of these conditions are present, in the absence of subjective symptoms[29,30]. Scintigraphy using radiolabeled leukocytes is used to search for inflammatory sites in the bowel area, especially in the terminal ileum. Neither this procedure nor endoscopy or radiographic investigation of the colon are routinely recommended.

In those with eye symptoms, it is advisable to refer the patient to an ophthalmologist, because uveitis requires rapid diagnosis for prompt and correct treatment. Without a slit-lamp examination, the uveitis may remain undiagnosed and result in permanent damage to the vision.

DIFFERENTIAL DIAGNOSIS

The most important question at presentation is whether the patient has reactive arthritis or true septic infection of the joint[32]. This may be extremely difficult to resolve, but it is especially crucial to do so in children, in whom a purulent arthritis may rapidly lead to destruction of the joint. Therefore it is advisable to proceed with blind antimicrobial treatment on the basis of a presumptive diagnosis of septic arthritis in uncertain cases. Joint inflammation may be sufficiently intense to produce redness reminiscent of erysipelas.

Gout or pseudogout may present with symptoms and findings similar to those of reactive arthritis, but careful history taking, analysis of crystals in the joint fluid and serum urate determination clarify the situation in most instances.

Rheumatoid arthritis, psoraitic arthritis and ankylosing spondylitis can often only be differentiated from reactive arthritis on prolonged follow-up.

ETIOLOGY

There is no disagreement that infection is central to the etiology of reactive arthritis. A previously healthy but genetically predisposed individual contracts a suitable triggering infection and, after some time, reactive arthritis develops. This pathogenetic process spans the incubation time of the triggering infection and its clinically overt phase, and thereafter a few days to a couple of weeks until the full-blown reactive arthritis[17]. With increasing awareness of this condition, the list of the causative agents is still growing. Although efforts have been made to characterize the microorganisms linked to reactive arthritis, no common or definite feature has so far emerged. Many of the bacteria implicated are Gram-negative, have cell membranes that contain lipopolysaccharide and peptidoglycan, and are intracellularly invasive – that is, able to enter cells and to survive (and even multiply) intracellularly[38]. Many are quite common in the environment, and infection does not necessarily lead to reactive arthritis. In most instances, the triggering infection affects the throat, the intestine or the urogenital tract. Therefore it appears that mucosal immune defense mechanisms must be of importance – but how and why are not known[39]. The frequency of reactive arthritis with outbreaks of Yersinia, Salmonella and Shigella varies quite considerably. The fact that several different microbes lead to a similar clinical entity demonstrates that the classical Koch postulates do not apply in this instance.

The available evidence implies that some features of a microbe are important for its arthritogenicity[13,38,39]. Such features are discussed in more detail in Chapter 108.

PATHOGENESIS

The pathogenesis of reactive arthritis is interesting not only in itself but also, given the time course, as a putative model of other inflammatory diseases of the joints and connective tissue. By contrast, rheumatoid arthritis and ankylosing spondylitis develop slowly, and when the diagnosis can be established with the accuracy necessary for research work, several months and even years have lapsed. At such a late stage, it is difficult to gain information on the early triggering or pathogenetic events. Reactive arthritis has a sudden onset, within days or a few weeks of the triggering infection, which often can be identified, and thus studies on its pathogenesis are possible. The joint inflammation develops some time after the actual triggering infection and it is apparent that immunologic defense mechanisms have a central role. Much new information has been gained, and several groups are working on the pathogenesis.

Role of HLA-B27

An important factor associated with the susceptibility to reactive arthritis is the HLA-B27 antigen. Although not all HLA-B27-positive individuals develop reactive arthritis after a suitable triggering infection, and some B27-negative individuals may do so, this tissue antigen indisputably has an important role. For more than two decades, extensive efforts have been devoted by several groups to clarify the mechanisms

behind this association. The different HLA-B27 loci have been characterized in minute detail and the peptides bound by this structure have been analysed. Yet it remains unknown how HLA-B27 works in the pathogenetic process.

A theory that has gained wide attention is that of molecular mimicry – that is, 'trigger' microorganisms share a structure with the HLA-B27 molecule[40]. Sequencing of genes for HLA-B27 and microbial antigens has further made it possible to carry out comparisons at the nucleotide and amino acid levels. Indeed, molecular mimicry in the form of amino acid homology has been observed between HLA-B27 and microbial antigens[41]; however, this apparently is not restricted to disease-associated microorganisms. Work using synthetic peptides and their capacity to generate a response by either B or T cells has raised suspicions about the biological importance of this homology. Therefore the role of molecular mimicry in the pathogenesis of reactive arthritis or ankylosing spondylitis needs critical re-evaluation[38,42].

Recently, mouse and rat strains carrying a transgene for HLA-B27 have been developed. These may help to elucidate the role of HLA-B27 in the pathogenesis of reactive arthritis and ankylosing spondylitis. The role of HLA-B27 is also discussed in Chapter 108.

Immune response

In studies of the immune reaction against the triggering microorganisms, several interesting findings have been obtained. As an example, the results for Yersinia-triggered reactive arthritis are presented in Table 109.3.

In follow-up studies, the immune responses of patients developing reactive arthritis have been compared with those recovering without postinfectious complications[12,36]. The most characteristic feature of patients with reactive arthritis is a strong and persisting IgA antibody response. With time, the antibodies increase in avidity, indicating a maturation of the response. Considering the short half-life of IgA, this indicates prolonged antigenic stimulation. The observation that the antibodies recognize a multitude of antigenic epitopes of Yersinia suggests that the driving force might be either whole microbes or large components of them.

The T cell responses against Yersinia antigens are weak in peripheral blood samples of patients with reactive arthritis, compared with those of persons who do not develop postinfectious complications[36]. However, at the synovial level, a strong but relatively non-specific response of T cells is seen[43]. It seems that T cells with slightly different specificities can be cloned from the synovial fluid, indicating that local stimulation may play a part[44-46].

Yersinia infection always causes formation of immune complexes. Such complexes composed of Yersinia antigen and specific antibody have been demonstrated in the blood and synovial fluid of patients with reactive arthritis[47].

All these observations suggest that, in patients with reactive arthritis, the microorganism may persist somewhere in the body, for example in

---

TABLE 109.3

IMMUNE RESPONSE IN YERSINIA-TRIGGERED REACTIVE ARTHRITIS

- Initially, weak IgM-class antibody production
- Later, strong and persisting IgG and especially IgA antibody production
- IgA antibodies increase in avidity with time
- Antibodies are directed against several antigenic epitopes of Yersinia
- Non-specific immune complexes are always found in serum
- Specific immune complexes containing Yersinia and anti-Yersinia antibody may be found in serum and in synovial fluid
- Peripheral blood T cells show weak response to Yersinia
- T cells in the synovial fluid show vigorous but somewhat non-specific response to Yersinia (or other arthritis-triggering microorganism)

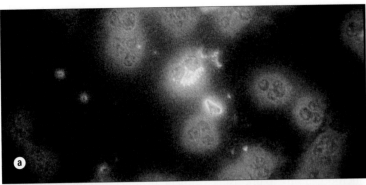
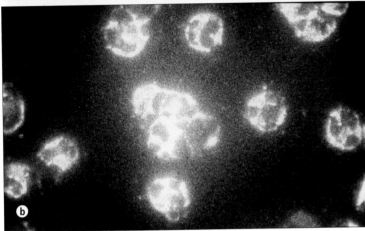

Fig. 109.6 Microbial material in synovial fluid cells. (a) In a patient with *Yersinia*-triggered reactive arthritis. (b) In a patient with chronic *Yersinia*-triggered reactive arthritis. There is positive immunofluorescence staining by an antiserum obtained by immunizing a rabbit with live *Yersinia*. Most of the cells are polymorphonuclear granulocytes and, in the chronic case, nearly all are strongly positive. (With permission from Granfors *et al.*[46])

TABLE 109.4
TREATMENT OF ACUTE REACTIVE ARTHRITIS

- Antibiotics if infection is still present
- Rest
- Non-steroidal anti-inflammatory drugs
- Intra-articular corticosteroids
- Systemic corticosteroids
- Rarely, disease modifying antirheumatic drugs

the intestinal mucosa or in the mesenteric lymph nodes. Furthermore, microbial components might actually enter the site of inflammation itself – that is, the synovium or the synovial fluid. Using immunofluorescence (Fig. 109.6) and immunoblotting techniques, in addition to immunoelectronmicroscopy, positive reactions have been obtained in reactive arthritis triggered by *Chlamydia*, *Salmonella*, *Yersinia* and *Shigella*[48–54]. Moreover, PCR methodology has resulted in positive demonstration of chlamydia DNA and RNA in the synovial fluid of patients with reactive arthritis[55–57]. It must be stressed, however, that viable organisms have not been isolated, in spite of extensive efforts.

Currently it seems, therefore, that reactive arthritis involves persistence of the triggering microorganism in the host, and the spread of its components either as parts of immune complexes or within phagocytosing cells into the joints, where they activate the inflammatory cascade[58–61].

MANAGEMENT

Acute reactive arthritis

There are some general considerations in the management of reactive arthritis. First, the disease most commonly affects previously healthy, young adults. Secondly, the severity of the disease varies from mild arthralgias to a severe arthritis, and hence treatment has to be adjusted accordingly[62,63]. The patient may be afraid of having a chronic, progressively destructive disease. Correct information is the cornerstone of the treatment, to relieve unnecessary anxiety and to achieve the patient's compliance with suggested treatments.

Obviously, suitable rest is advisable. Even within a few weeks after recovery, the patient should not use the joints too vigorously, as non-specific factors and minor traumas may lead to recurrences. When several joints are affected, muscle wasting may occur unless physiotherapy is given.

Non-steroidal anti-inflammatory drugs (NSAIDs) form the basis of treatment (Table 109.4). They should be used regularly over some time in order to achieve maximum anti-inflammatory effect, and patients should be informed of this, otherwise they consider the drug as an analgesic. During recovery, insufficient analgesia may lead to limited use of the joints and actually prolong the rehabilitation. There is no definite drug of choice, because patients' responses differ (see Chapter 35). In the case of enthesopathies, locally applied NSAID ointments may be useful.

Corticosteroids are a valuable asset in the treatment of reactive arthritis. In many cases, intra-articular administration gives prompt relief. However, septic arthritis must be excluded before the injection. Systemic treatment with corticosteroids has also proved effective. They should be used in patients in whom NSAIDs have not had a sufficient effect and in whom many joints are affected. The treatment can be started with a relatively high dose, 30–50mg daily of prednisolone or its equivalent, tapering down according to the improvement. Oral corticosteroids should be withdrawn slowly, but with NSAIDs continuing. Corticosteroids should not be used for more than 2–4 months (see Chapter 36).

Antibiotic treatment

As persistence of the triggering microbe and presence of microbial components at the sites of inflammation have been demonstrated, the role of antibiotic treatment has become a central question. Many physicians do indeed give the patients with reactive arthritis at least a short course of antibiotics. However, there is no clinical evidence supporting this practice.

Antibiotic treatment should be given if a microbe is isolated. This is more to diminish spread of the infection than to influence the continuing course of the disease. In two instances antibiotics have been proven to be useful. In rheumatic fever they are used for primary or secondary prevention. However, they do not have a role in the treatment of the rheumatic fever itself. The treatment of borreliosis to minimize the impact of Lyme disease is discussed in Chapter 96. Clinical and experimental data exist to indicate that, if antibacterial treatment of reactive arthritis can be started very early during the pathogenetic process, the disease can be prevented or the prognosis improved. However, it is obvious that, at the time of the first joint symptoms – which is when the patient usually comes to the physician – the pathogenic process is probably not reversible. All available clinical evidence indicates that, in fully developed reactive arthritis, short term antibacterial treatment has no beneficial effect, and overall the results with long-term administration of antibacterial agents are also poor[63–66]. Studies using an experimental model of reactive arthritis in rats have yielded similar results[66,67]. In some instances, sulphasalazine has proven beneficial, probably because of its antirheumatic effect rather than its antibacterial effect. In addition, tetracyclines have sometimes been found to have an effect on reactive arthritis, but, again, this is probably due to their anti-inflammatory action rather than any antibacterial effect[63,66,68].

Cases with chronic symptoms

Recurrences of reactive arthritis are treated in the same way as the acute disease. Chronic arthralgias are a difficult therapeutic problem. With time, the patients often derive less and less benefit from the various NSAIDs, and side effects become more common with prolonged use. Nevertheless, these drugs are the best of the alternatives. Physical therapy may give some patients relief, but does not have a long-term effect. In chronic cases, corticosteroids are not advisable, because their therapeutic effect in this situation is not very good, and the prognosis is in any case good in almost all patients.

As in acute reactive arthritis, in chronic reactive arthritis antibiotics have also not proven useful, even when administered for a 3-month period[66,69]. Sulfasalazine is of interest because of the observation that patients with reactive arthritis often have more or less asymptomatic inflammation of the bowel. However, results regarding the effect of sulphasalazine are somewhat contradictory[70–73]. In some instances, it may give good results. The drug should be started at low dose, increasing to 2g/day, or even 3g/day if tolerated by the patient. Unfortunately, some patients cannot continue with the drug because of gastrointestinal intolerance.

When the symptoms of chronic reactive arthritis resemble rheumatoid arthritis, classic antirheumatic treatment, for example gold salts (injected or by mouth), may prove quite useful and lead to rapid improvement. In these patients the treatment can be stopped after some months without the disease relapsing. There have been some reports regarding the use of methotrexate or azathioprine, but the results of controlled trials with a large number of patients are not yet available[63].

Extra-articular disease

Ocular inflammation must be diagnosed and treated promptly, otherwise irreversible damage to eyesight may occur. If possible, the patient should be referred to an ophthalmologist, because the diagnosis of uveitis requires the use of a slit-lamp. Treatment consists of corticosteroids in the form of eye drops or even systemically, and of mydriatics. The patient should be informed about the strong possibility of recurrence.

Excluding the endocarditis of rheumatic fever, discussed in Chapter 99, the most common cardiac complications are conduction disturbances. In these instances, a cardiac pacemaker may be indicated.

The nephritis that can be associated with reactive arthritis is usually mild, subsides spontaneously and does not require any treatment. Skin lesions, which are considered identical to psoriasis by many dermatologists, are treated accordingly. In mild cases, keratinolytic agents such as salicylic acid ointment or topical corticosteroid may be used. In more severe cases, methotrexate or retinoids are often beneficial.

PROGNOSIS

The prognosis of reactive arthritis is generally good. The duration of the of an episode varies from a few days to several weeks. Even patients who are severely incapacitated and bedridden can look forwards to full recovery. However, recurrences are frequent, and they can be triggered not only by new infections but also by non-specific stress factors. Urogenital and eye inflammations, particularly, have a tendency to recur. Many patients complain of abdominal discomfort and occasional diarrhea for months and even years after the initial attack of the disease. Back pain and arthralgia are common, and also frank synovitis may be seen. Tendinitis and enthesopathy may lead to erosion or proliferation of bone at the tendon insertions. These joint symptoms may be precipitated by rather non-specific factors, such as changes in the weather, and many patients report discomfort during the fall and winter seasons. Conversely, a new infection by bacteria known to trigger the disease may pass without any sequelae. The non-symptomatic period between recurrences may last for several years. It remains an open question whether degenerative changes, such as osteoarthritis, develop more readily in a joint that has been affected by reactive arthritis.

Follow-up studies of reactive arthritis suggest that 20–70% of patients later suffer some joint discomfort or other symptoms[74,75]. For the individual patient, it is important to know that, in spite of unpleasant symptoms, severe destructive disease as a sequel of reactive arthritis is extremely rare. Similarly, follow-up has not revealed reactive arthritis to be a precurser of rheumatoid arthritis. Thus, of 100 patients who were studied 20 years after a *Shigella*-triggered reactive arthritis, none had rheumatoid arthritis[4], and in another follow-up study of 60 patients, only one definite case of rheumatoid arthritis was found[74]. Although both clinical and radiographic sacroiliitis typical of ankylosing spondylitis can occur on follow-up, even in these cases the disease usually remains mild. With this knowledge, the patient may tolerate the discomfort and learn to live with the disease rather well.

REFERENCES

1. Reiter H. Uber eine bisher unerkannte Spirochäteninfektion (*Spirochaetosis arthritica*). Dtsch Med Wochenschr 1916; 42: 1535–1536.
2. Wright V, Moll JMH, eds. Seronegative polyarthritis. Amsterdam: North Holland Publishing Company; 1976.
3. Paronen I. Reiter's disease. A study of 344 cases observed in Finland. Acta Med Scand 1948; (suppl 212): 1–112.
4. Sairanen E, Paronen I, Mähönen H. Reiter's syndrome: a follow-up study. Acta Med Scand 1969; 185: 57–63.
5. Aho K, Ahvonen P, Lassus A et al. *Yersinia* arthritis and related diseases: clinical and immunogenetic implications. In: Dumonde DC, ed. Infection and immunology in the rheumatic diseases. Oxford: Blackwell Scientific Publications; 1976: 341–344.
6. Isomäki H, Raunio J, von Essen R et al. Incidence of inflammatory rheumatic diseases in Finland. Scand J Rheumatol 1978; 7: 188–192.
7. Aho K. Bowel infection predisposing to reactive arthritis. In: Rooney PJ, ed. Baillière's clinical rheumatology, vol 3. London: Baillière Tindall; 1989: 303–319.
8. Leino R, Kalliomäki JL. Yersiniosis as an internal disease. Ann Intern Med 1974; 81: 458–461.
9. Aho K, Ahvonen P, Lassus A et al. HLA-B27 in reactive arthritis: a study of *Yersinia* arthritis and Reiter's disease. Arthritis Rheum 1974; 17: 521–526.
10. Laitinen O, Leirisalo M, Skylv G. Relation between HLA-B27 and clinical features with *Yersinia* arthritis. Arthritis Rheum 1977; 20: 1121–1124.
11. Keat A. HLA-linked disease susceptibility and reactive arthritis. J Infect 1982; 5: 227–239.
12. Lahesmaa-Rantala R, Toivanen A. Clinical spectrum of reactive arthritis. In: Toivanen A, Toivanen P, eds. Reactive arthritis. Boca Raton: CRC Press; 1988: 1–13.
13. van Bohemen CG, Lionarons RJ, van Bodegom P et al. Susceptibility and HLA-B27 in post-dysenteric arthropathies. Immunology 1985; 56: 377–379.
14. Calin A, Fries JF. An 'experimental' epidemic of Reiter's syndrome revisited. Follow-up evidence on genetic and environmental factors. Ann Intern Med 1976; 84: 564–566.
15. Leirisalo M, Skylv G, Kousa M et al. Follow-up study on patients with Reiter's disease and reactive arthritis with special reference to HLA-B27. Arthritis Rheum 1982; 25: 249–259.
16. Laivoranta S, Ilonen J, Tuokko J et al. HLA frequencies in HLA-B27 negative patients with reactive arthritis. Clin Exp Rheumatol 1995; 13: 637–640.
17. Toivanen P, Toivanen A. Two forms of reactive arthritis? Ann Rheum Dis 1999; 58: 737–741.
18. Håkansson U, Löw B, Eitrem R et al. HLA-B27 and reactive arthritis in an outbreak of salmonellosis. Tissue Antigens 1975; 6: 366–367.
19. Simon DG, Kaslow RA, Rosenbaum J et al. Reiter's syndrome following epidemic shigellosis. J Rheumatol 1981; 8: 969–973.
20. Eastmond CJ, Rennie JAN, Reid TMS. An outbreak of *Campylobacter* enteritis – a rheumatological follow-up survey. J Rheumatol 1983; 10: 107–108.
21. Tertti R, Granfors K, Lehtonen O-P et al. An outbreak of *Yersinia pseudotuberculosis* infection. J Infect Dis 1984; 149: 245–250.
22. Tertti R, Vuento R, Mikkola PGK et al. Clinical manifestations of *Yersinia pseudotuberculosis* infection in children. Eur J Clin Microbiol Infect Dis 1989; 8: 587–591.
23. Gran JT. Classification and diagnosis of seronegative spondylarthropathies. Scand J Rheumatol 1999; 28: 332–335.
24. Toivanen A, Toivanen P. Reactive arthritis. Curr Opin Rheumatol 2000; 12: 300–305.
25. Ahvonen P. Human yersiniosis in Finland. II. Clinical features. Ann Clin Res 1972; 4: 39–48.

26. Leino R, Toivanen A. Arthritis associated with gastrointestinal disorders. In: Toivanen A, Toivanen P, eds. Reactive arthritis. Boca Raton: CRC Press; 1988: 77–86.
27. Toivanen P, Toivanen A. Role of micro-organisms in the pathogenesis of arthritis: lessons from reactive and Lyme arthritis. Scand J Rheumatol 1995; 24(suppl 101): 191–197.
28. Toivanen A, Toivanen P. Aetiopathogenesis of reactive arthritis. Rheumatol Eur 1995; 24: 5–8.
29. De Vos M, Cuvelier C, Mielants H et al. Ileocolonoscopy in seronegative spondylarthropathy. Gastroenterology 1989; 96: 339–344.
30. Mielants H, Veys EM. The gut and reactive arthritis. Rheumatol Eur 1995; 24: 9–11.
31. Nikkari S, Yli-Kerttula U, Toivanen P. Reactive arthritis in a patient with simultaneous parvovirus B19 infection and Clostridium difficile diarrhoea. Br J Rheumatol 1997; 36: 143–144.
32. Toivanen P, Toivanen A. Bacterial or reactive arthritis? Rheumatol Eur 1995; 24(suppl 2): 253–255.
33. Yli-Kerttula UI, Vilppula AH. Reactive salpingitis. In: Toivanen A, Toivanen P, eds. Reactive arthritis. Boca Raton: CRC Press; 1988: 125–131.
34. Saari KM. The eye and reactive arthritis. In: Toivanen A, Toivanen P, eds. Reactive arthritis. Boca Raton: CRC Press; 1988: 113–124.
35. Shmerling RH, Delbanco TL, Tosteson ANA et al. Synovial fluid tests. What should be ordered? JAMA 1990; 264: 1009–1014.
36. Toivanen A, Granfors K, Lahesmaa-Rantala R et al. Pathogenesis of Yersinia-triggered reactive arthritis: immunological, microbiological and clinical aspects. Immunol Rev 1985; 86: 47–70.
37. Isomäki H, Anttila P. Radiology of reactive arthritis. In: Toivanen A, Toivanen P, eds. Reactive arthritis. Boca Raton: CRC Press; 1988: 133–138.
38. Sieper J, Braun J. Pathogenesis of spondylarthropathies. Persistent bacterial antigen, autoimmunity, or both? Arthritis Rheum 1995; 38: 1547–1554.
39. Toivanen A, Toivanen P. Epidemiologic aspects, clinical features, and management of ankylosing spondylitis and reactive arthritis. Curr Opin Rheumatol 1994; 6: 354–359.
40. Oldstone MBA. Molecular mimicry and autoimmune disease. Cell 1987; 50: 819–820.
41. Schwimmbeck PL, Oldstone MBA. Klebsiella pneumoniae and HLA B27-associated diseases of Reiter's syndrome and ankylosing spondylitis. Curr Topics Microbiol Immunol 1989; 145: 45–56.
42. Lahesmaa R, Skurnik M, Toivanen P. Molecular mimicry: any role in the pathogenesis of spondyloarthropathies? Immunol Res 1993; 12: 193–208.
43. Gaston JSH, Life PF, Granfors K et al. Synovial T lymphocyte recognition of organisms that trigger reactive arthritis. Clin Exp Immunol 1989; 76: 348–353.
44. Hermann E, Mayet W-J, Poralla T et al. Salmonella-reactive synovial fluid T-cell clones in a patient with post-infectious salmonella arthritis. Scand J Rheum 1990; 19: 350–355.
45. Hermann E, Yu DT, Meyer zum Büschenfelde K-H et al. HLA-B27-restricted CD8 T cells derived from synovial fluids of patients with reactive arthritis and ankylosing spondylitis. Lancet 1993; 342: 646–650.
46. Herrmann E. T cells in reactive arthritis. APMIS 1993; 101: 177–186.
47. Lahesmaa-Rantala R, Granfors K, Isomäki H et al. Yersinia specific immune complexes in the synovial fluid of patients with Yersinia-triggered reactive arthritis. Ann Rheum Dis 1987; 46: 10–14.
48. Granfors K, Jalkanen S, von Essen R et al. Yersinia antigens in synovial-fluid cells from patients with reactive arthritis. N Engl J Med 1989; 320: 216–221.
49. Toivanen A, Lahesmaa-Rantala R, Ståhlberg T et al. Do bacterial antigens persist in reactive arthritis? Clin Exp Rheum 1987; 5(suppl 1): 25–27.
50. Keat A, Thomas B, Dixey J et al. Chlamydia trachomatis and reactive arthritis – the missing link. Lancet 1987; i: 72–74.
51. Schumacher HR Jr, Magge S, Cherian PV et al. Light and electron microscopic studies on the synovial membrane in Reiter's syndrome. Immunocytochemical identification of chlamydial antigen in patients with early disease. Arthritis Rheum 1988; 31: 937–946.
52. Granfors K, Jalkanen S, Lindberg AA et al. Salmonella lipopolysaccharide in synovial cells from patients with reactive arthritis. Lancet 1990; 335: 685–688.
53. Hammer M, Zeidler H, Klimsa S et al. Yersinia enterocolitica in the synovial membrane of patients with Yersinia-induced arthritis. Arthritis Rheum 1990; 33: 1795–1800.
54. Merilahti-Palo R, Söderström K-O, Lahesmaa-Rantala R et al. Bacterial antigens in synovial biopsy specimens in Yersinia-triggered reactive arthritis. Ann Rheum Dis 1991; 50: 87–90.
55. Taylor-Robinson D, Gilroy CB, Thomas BJ et al. Detection of Chlamydia trachomatis DNA in joints of reactive arthritis patients by polymerase chain reaction. Lancet 1992; 340: 81–82.
56. Gérard HC, Branigan PJ, Schumacher HR Jr et al. Synovial Chlamydia trachomatis in patients with reactive arthritis/Reiter's syndrome are viable but show aberrant gene expression. J Rheumatol 1998; 25: 734–742.
57. Hughes RA, Keat AC. Reiter's syndrome and reactive arthritis: a current view. Semin Arthritis Rheum 1994; 24: 190–210.
58. Lipsky PE, Davis LS, Cush JJ et al. The role of cytokines in the pathogenesis of rheumatoid arthritis. Springer Semin Immunopathol 1989; 11: 123–162.
59. Ziff M. Role of endothelium in chronic inflammation. Springer Semin Immunopathol 1989; 11: 199–214.
60. Toivanen A, Toivanen P. Pathogenesis of reactive arthritis. In: Toivanen A, Toivanen P, eds. Reactive arthritis. Boca Raton: CRC Press; 1988: 167–178.
61. Simon AK, Seipelt E, Sieper J. Divergent T-cell cytokine patterns in inflammatory arthritis. Proc Natl Acad Sci USA 1994; 91: 8562–8566.
62. Toivanen A, Toivanen P. Epidemiologic, clinical, and therapeutic aspects of reactive arthritis and ankylosing spondylitis. Curr Opin Rheumatol 1995; 7: 279–283.
63. Toivanen A. Managing reactive arthritis. Rheumatology 2000; 39: 117–121.
64. Sieper J, Fendler C, Laitko S et al. No benefit of long-term ciprofloxacin treatment in patients with reactive arthritis and undifferentiated oligoarthritis. Arthritis Rheum 1999; 42: 1386–1396.
65. Yli-Kerttula T, Luukkainen R, Yli-Kerttula U et al. Effect of a three-month course of ciprofloxacin on the outcome of reactive arthritis. Ann Rheum Dis 2000; 59: 565–570.
66. Toivanen A. Bacteria-triggered reactive arthritis. Implications for antibacterial treatment. Drugs 2001; 61: 343–351.
67. Zhang Y, Toivanen A, Toivanen P. Experimental Yersinia-triggered reactive arthritis; effect of a 3-week course with ciprofloxacin. Br J Rheumatol 1997; 36: 541–546.
68. Lauhio A, Leirisalo-Repo M, Lähdevirta J et al. Double-blind, placebo controlled study of three-month treatment with lymecycline in reactive arthritis, with special reference to Chlamydia arthritis. Arthritis Rheum 1991; 34: 6–14.
69. Toivanen A, Yli-Kerttula T, Luukkainen R et al. Effect of antimicrobial treatment on chronic reactive arthritis. Clin Exp Rheumatol 1993; 11: 301–307.
70. Mielants H, Veys EM. HLA-B27 related arthritis and bowel inflammation. Part 1. Sulphasalazine (Salazopyrin) in HLA-B27 related reactive arthritis. J Rheumatol 1985; 12: 287–293.
71. Trnavský K, Pelisková Z, Vácha J. Sulphasalazine in the treatment of reactive arthritis. Scand J Rheumatol 1988; (Suppl 67): 76–79.
72. Egsmose C, Hansen TM, Andersen LS et al. Limited effect of sulphasalazine treatment in reactive arthritis. A randomised double blind placebo controlled trial. Ann Rheum Dis 1997; 56: 32–36.
73. Clegg DO, Reda DJ, Abdellatif M. Comparison of sulphasalazine and placebo for the treatment of axial and peripheral articular manifestations of the seronegative spondylarthropathies. Arthritis Rheum 1999; 42: 2325–2329.
74. Kalliomäki JL, Leino R. Follow-up studies of joint complications in yersiniosis. Acta Med Scand 1979; 205: 521–525.
75. Yli-Kerttula T, Tertti R, Toivanen A. Ten-year follow up study of patients from a Yersinia pseudotuberculosis III outbreak. Clin Exp Rheumatol 1995; 13: 333–337.

110 Psoriatic arthritis: clinical features

Ian N Bruce

- Definition: An inflammatory arthritis associated with psoriasis, which is usually negative for rheumatoid factor
- Prevalence: 0.04–0.1%
- Sex distribution: equal
- 15% develop psoriasis AFTER onset of arthritis
- Nail changes have the strongest association with arthropathy, particularly affecting the distal interphalangeal joints
- Typical clinical features:
  — Distal interphalangeal joint involvement
  — Asymmetric sacroiliitis/spondylitis
  — Dactylitis
  — Enthesitis
- Number of joints involved can increase with disease duration
- Polyarticular involvement tends to have poorer long-term outcomes

HISTORY

Psoriatic arthritis can be defined as 'an inflammatory arthritis associated with psoriasis, which is usually negative for rheumatoid factor' (RF)[1]. Alibert first described the association between psoriasis and arthritis in 1818, although the term 'psoriasis arthritique' was first used by Bazin in 1860. Bourdillon developed a more detailed description of the condition in 1888[1]. It has only been since the 1950s that psoriatic arthritis has been systematically studied. Wright[2] noted that patients with psoriasis and erosive arthritis had a low frequency of RF positivity. In addition, he also pointed out the predilection for involvement of the distal interphalangeal (DIP) and sacroiliac joints, the frequent asymmetric nature of the arthritis and the tendency to severe joint destruction – 'arthritis mutilans'.

In 1964, the American Rheumatism Association recognized psoriatic arthritis as a distinct entity[3]. In the past 40 years, our understanding of the clinical spectrum of psoriatic arthritis has expanded as a result of detailed analysis of large clinic series and improvements in imaging techniques. Considerable controversy continues, however, as to the distinctiveness of psoriatic arthritis as a discrete entity.

EPIDEMIOLOGY

The association of psoriasis and arthritis (Tables 110.1 and 110.2) Several studies have demonstrated that psoriasis is more common in patients with inflammatory arthritis and also that inflammatory arthritis occurs more commonly in cases with psoriasis than in the background population. In a retrospective clinic series, Dawson and Tyson[4] noted psoriasis in 2.6% of patients with inflammatory polyarthritis, compared with 0.3% of those with osteoarthritis. In a population study, Hellgren[5] found psoriasis in 4.5% of patients with 'rheumatoid arthritis (RA)', compared with 2.7% of controls. When RF status is taken into account, the association between psoriasis and inflammatory arthritis is greatest

TABLE 110.1 INCREASED PREVALENCE OF INFLAMMATORY POLYARTHRITIS IN PSORIASIS

Author	Year	IPA in psoriasis (%)	IPA in controls (%)	Comments
Leczinsky[8]	1948	6.8	0.7	Controls had other skin conditions
Hellgren[5]	1969	9	2.3	IPA defined as possible – classic RA
Van Romunde et al.[9]	1984	5	2.2	Only 41 psoriasis patients studied

IPA, inflammatory polyarthritis.

TABLE 110.2 INCREASED PREVALENCE OF PSORIASIS IN INFLAMMATORY POLYARTHRITIS, ESPECIALLY SERONEGATIVE ARTHROPATHIES

Author	Year	Controls (%)	All IPA (%)	Seropositive IPA (%)	Seronegative IPA (%)
Dawson and Tyson[4]	1938	0.3	2.6		
Baker[6]	1966	1.5		1.2	20.2
Mongan and Atwater[7]	1968			2.8	12.5
Hellgren[5]	1969	2.7	4.5		
Harrison et al.[10]	1997		5	1.7	5.6

IPA, inflammatory polyarthritis.

TABLE 110.3 PREVALENCE AND INCIDENCE OF PSORIATIC ARTHRITIS				
Author	Year	Country	Prevalence (%)	Incidence/year
Lomholt[13]	1963	Faroe Islands	0.04	
Van Romunde[9]	1984	Netherlands	0.05	
Shbeeb et al.[14]	2000	USA	0.1	
Kaipiainen-Seppanen[15]	1996	Finland		6/100 000
Harrison et al.[10]	1997	UK		3.6/100 000 (males)
				3.4/100 000 (females)
Shbeeb et al.[14]	2000	USA		6/100 000

amongst seronegative patients[6,7]. In one study psoriasis occurred in 1.3% of controls and 1.2% of those with seropositive arthritis, whereas 20.2% of patients with seronegative inflammatory arthritis had psoriasis[6] (Table 110.2). With regard to the presence of inflammatory arthritis in patients with psoriasis, a similar association has been noted. In Hellgren's study[5], 9% of patients with psoriasis had 'RA', compared with 2.3% of controls. Similarly, Leczinsky[8] found that 6.8% of patients with psoriasis had inflammatory arthritis, compared with 0.7% of controls with other skin complaints (Table 110.1). Other uncontrolled clinic surveys of patients with psoriasis have suggested a 30–35% prevalence of inflammatory arthritis[11,12]. These higher estimates may reflect the more detailed evaluation of axial and peripheral joints undertaken, although awareness and selection biases cannot be excluded. Overall, there is an increased association between inflammatory arthritis and psoriasis. Several explanations for this association can be suggested. First, psoriasis may be a risk factor for inflammatory arthritis. Secondly, psoriasis and inflammatory arthritis may share a common etiologic trigger. Finally, a distinct entity of psoriatic arthritis may exist. The last of these is generally accepted to be true, but until more is known about psoriatic arthritis, the first two explanations cannot be completely discounted.

Incidence and prevalence of psoriatic arthritis

There have only been a few studies estimating the prevalence of psoriatic arthritis in the general population, giving rates of between 0.04 and 0.1%[9,13,14] (Table 110.3). These likely underestimate the true prevalence of psoriatic arthritis, because the dermatological or rheumatological criteria applied will often lead to exclusion of some cases. In addition, it is difficult to account for patients who have minimal or no psoriasis at the time of study. The incidence of psoriatic arthritis has recently been estimated in Europe and the USA[10,14,15]. In the Norfolk Arthritis Registry of recent onset inflammatory arthritis (a community-based cohort), the incidence of psoriatic arthritis was estimated to be 3.6 per 100 000 per annum in men and 3.4 per 100 000 per annum in women. This study did not include patients presenting with monoarthritis or spondyloarthropathy only. The incidence in Olmsted County, Minnesota, USA was reported as 6.6 per 100 000 per annum, for both sexes combined[14]. Again, only patients with a dermatologist-confirmed diagnosis of psoriasis were included.

Additional observations

In contrast to RA, which has a female preponderance, the overall sex distribution of psoriatic arthritis is 1:1[10,14,16]. The mean age at onset of psoriatic arthritis is in the range of 30–55 years[10,16,17]. With regard to the timing of skin and joint disease, approximately 67% of patients develop psoriasis before the onset of arthritis[11,16,17]. In about 16%, the two conditions occur within 12 months of each other[11,16], and in the remainder, arthritis precedes the onset of psoriasis by more than 1 year[11,16]. The timing of onset may not be randomly distributed across all patients with psoriasis. Rahman et al.[18] found that, in patients with type 1 psoriasis (age of onset <40 years old), the skin disorder preceded the onset of arthritis by a

mean of 9 years. In contrast, in older patients with type 2 psoriasis (age of onset >40 years old), arthropathy developed at a mean period of 1 year after the onset of skin disease, suggesting that a greater proportion of older patients have a near synchronous onset of the two conditions.

Relationship to HIV infection

An association of HIV infection with susceptibility to psoriatic arthritis has long been suggested. Indeed, the prevalence of psoriatic arthritis in HIV infection is greater than expected in the general population[19]. This has particular implications for the incidence and prevalence of psoriatic arthritis in Africa. Historically, seronegative arthropathies are uncommon in sub-Saharan Africa because of the low prevalence of human leukocyte antigen (HLA)-B27[20]. A recent study from Zambia found that spondyloarthropathies are now the most common group of inflammatory arthritis observed in this population[21]. The prevalence of spondyloarthropathies was 180/100 000 among HIV-positive populations, compared with 15/100 000 in HIV-negative populations[21]. A subsequent study from the same region found that 27 of 28 patients (96%) with psoriatic arthritis were HIV-positive, compared with 30% of the background population[22]. Several studies in North American HIV cohorts have found a prevalence of psoriatic arthritis of 0.4–2%[19,23,24]. In the context of HIV infection, severe skin and polyarticular joint disease, which often occur simultaneously, have been reported[22,25,26]. The spectrum of severity is wide, and in some cases improvement of arthritis with the onset of AIDS has been observed[22].

CLINICAL FEATURES

Psoriatic arthropathy is classified within the group of seronegative spondyloarthropathies (see Chapter 101), on the basis of work by Moll and Wright[1] and others that has demonstrated many clinical and familial associations between psoriatic arthritis and other conditions in this group, such as reactive arthritis and ankylosing spondylitis. The inclusion of psoriatic arthritis within the spondyloarthropathies is also reflected in the European Spondylarthropathies Study Group (ESSG) criteria[27].

Articular involvement

Joint involvement in psoriatic arthritis can vary considerably, from an isolated monoarthritis to extensive destructive arthritis. It can involve peripheral joints and the axial spine with varying frequencies. The most

TABLE 110.4 THE MOLL AND WRIGHT CLASSIFICATION OF PSORIATIC ARTHRITIS[1]
• Arthritis with distal interphalangeal joint involvement predominant
• Arthritis mutilans
• Symmetric polyarthritis – indistinguishable from RA
• Asymmetric oligoarticular arthritis
• Predominant spondylitis

Author	Disease duration (years)	Frequency (%)				
		DIP predominant	Oligoarticular	Polyarticular	Spondyloarthropathy	Arthritis mutilans
Jones et al.[17]	Onset	2*	63†	25	10	0
Veale et al.[28]	4 (median)	16	43	33	4	2
Gladman et al.[16‡]	9 (mean)	12	14	40	2	16
Jones et al.[17]	12 (mean)	1*	26	63	6	4

TABLE 110.5 RELATIVE FREQUENCY OF VARIOUS SUBTYPES OF PSORIATIC ARTHRITIS

* Defined as DIP only, in this series. † Includes mono- and oligoarticular onset. ‡ The balance in this series had overlapping patterns.

Findings of selected clinic series are displayed according to disease duration of the cohort studied. (Note: Jones et al.[17] described patterns at onset and follow-up.)

widely used classification is that proposed by Moll and Wright[1], which identifies five major subtypes of psoriatic arthritis (Table 110.4). There have been many further attempts to revise and modify this system, but these have not been widely adopted. Applying this system has, however, provided some valuable insights into the nature of psoriatic arthritis and provides a framework in which to consider many of the key features of psoriatic arthritis. There is a high degree of overlap between categories within this classification, and hence it has limitations in practice. For example, spondyloarthropathy may be the dominant feature in only a minority of patients, whereas clinical and radiological involvement of the spine can be detected in approximately one-third of cases[16]. Similarly, exclusive involvement of the DIP joint is less common than involvement of this joint as part of a general peripheral arthritis[17,28]. It is thus not surprising that series have shown quite marked differences in their relative proportions of these subtypes. This is partly related to the entry criteria to these cohorts, as well as to some differences in the definitions for each subgroup used. In addition, the disease duration at the time of study has a significant influence (Table 110.5, Fig. 110.1). Thus Jones et al.[17] found that, whereas the majority of patients described mono- or oligoarticular disease at onset, after a mean follow-up of 12.1 years, 63% of patients had polyarthritis. Marsal et al.[29] also found that the median number of joints affected at onset of disease was 2 (range 0–8), compared with a median of 10 (range 2–19) after a follow-up period of 8 years. Arthritis mutilans is also a feature of prolonged disease[17]. In addition, there is a tendency for the frequency of spinal involvement to increase with time[30]. A more pragmatic classification based simply on peripheral or axial involvement has therefore been suggested, and may be justified[29].

Symmetry of involvement in psoriatic arthritis

Wright[2] identified asymmetry as a common feature of psoriatic arthritis. In particular, asymmetric involvement was typical of the oligoarticular pattern[1]. Other investigators have also found that the majority of patients with oligoarticular arthritis have an asymmetric pattern[16,17]. In contrast, the majority of patients with polyarticular disease have symmetric involvement[17,31]. Symmetry may, however, be largely a function of the total number of joints involved in the inflammatory process. In a comparison of patients with early and late RA and psoriatic arthritis, after correction for the total number of involved joints there was no difference in the degree of joint symmetry observed between these conditions[32].

Distal interphalangeal joint involvement

Involvement of the DIP joints in psoriatic arthritis is considered a distinctive feature of this condition (Fig. 110.2). These joints are thus involved more frequently in those with psoriatic arthritis than in patients with inflammatory arthritis without psoriasis[33]. In a community-based survey of early inflammatory arthritis, a DIP-predominant pattern at onset was found in 3.9% of patients with psoriasis, compared with 0.3% of patients without psoriasis[10]. Several large hospital series have noted *involvement* of the DIP joints, as part of a polyarthritis, in up to 54% of patients with psoriatic arthritis[16,17,28]. In contrast, the 'DIP-predominant' subgroup of those with psoriatic arthritis represents a much smaller proportion of cases (1–16%). As the DIP joints may be the first to be involved, the DIP predominant pattern can occur early in the disease course[1,28]. DIP joint involvement is also commonly associated with two other significant features of psoriatic arthritis, namely dactylitis[16,28] and nail dystrophy[2].

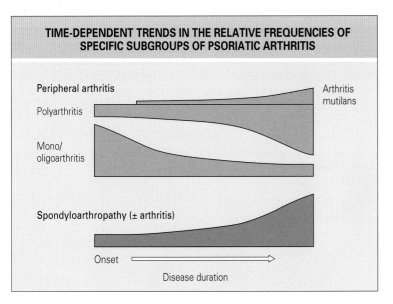

TIME-DEPENDENT TRENDS IN THE RELATIVE FREQUENCIES OF SPECIFIC SUBGROUPS OF PSORIATIC ARTHRITIS

Peripheral arthritis

Polyarthritis

Arthritis mutilans

Mono/ oligoarthritis

Spondyloarthropathy (± arthritis)

Onset

Disease duration

Fig 110.1 Time-dependent trends in the relative frequencies of specific subgroups of psoriatic arthritis. ±, with or without.

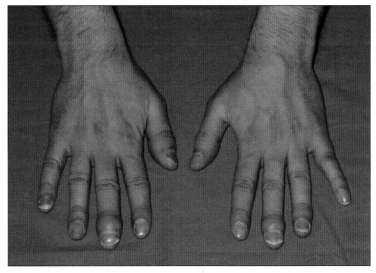

Fig. 110.2 Psoriatic arthritis with predominant involvement of the DIP joints. (Copyright University of Manchester.)

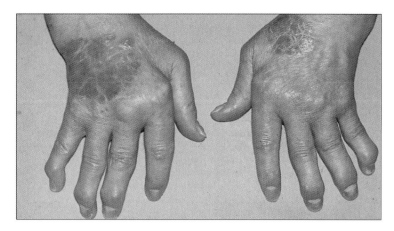

Fig. 110.3 Symmetric polyarthritis resembling RA.

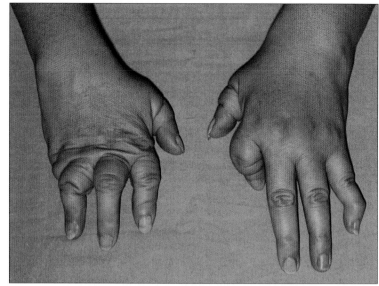

Fig. 110.4 Arthritis mutilans. Note shortening of the thumbs and left index finger (the right 5th finger has been amputated). (Copyright University of Manchester.)

Mono- and oligoarticular arthritis

The frequency of these forms of psoriatic arthritis is highly variable across different series, ranging in prevalence from 11% to 70%[1,16]. Indeed, in a community-based study of psoriatic arthritis in Olmsted County, Minnesota USA, 90% of patients with psoriatic arthritis had an oligoarticular pattern at onset[14]. As pointed out earlier, mono- and oligoarthritis are the most common presenting patterns[14,17,29]. A high proportion will, however, progress towards additional joint involvement[17]. In addition to involvement of the lower limb joints, this pattern of arthritis can frequently affect the small joints of the hands, including the proximal interphalangeal and DIP joints. This pattern also has a male predominance[28].

Symmetric polyarthritis

Symmetric polyarthritis involves the small joints of the hands and feet, in addition to larger joints (Fig. 110.3). It has a female preponderance[16,28,34] and can be clinically indistinguishable from RA[2,31]. The exact frequency of this pattern is again controversial. Shbeeb *et al.*[14] described a 3% prevalence of polyarthritis at onset. The frequency in hospital clinics can range from 15% to 61%, and may in part reflect the referral base that these clinics serve[1,16,34]. Polyarthritis also tends to develop over time, and patients with polyarticular disease have a longer disease duration than the other more discrete patterns[17,28]. Regardless of the precise frequency of the polyarthritis, it is patients with this condition who have more evidence of erosive joint damage[28,29].

Arthritis mutilans

There is no clear definition of this commonly used term. In general, it describes the end stage of a destructive erosive arthritis, with disorganization of joints leading to subluxation, 'flail' joints and digital telescoping – the so-called 'doigt en lorgnette' (opera glass finger)[2] (Figs 110.4 & 110.5). In most series, the prevalence is less than 5%[1,17,28]. Arthritis mutilans is associated with long-standing disease and a female preponderance[17,29]. An association with sacroiliac joint involvement has also been described[1,29].

Spondyloarthropathy

The spondyloarthropathy of psoriatic arthritis is uncommon as a predominant feature, and only accounts for approximately 5% of cases[1,16]. Careful clinical and radiological assessment, however, reveals involvement of the axial spine in 20–40% of cases[16,28,34], increasing to as many as 51% at long-term follow-up[30]. Involvement of the sacroiliac joints can be symmetric or asymmetric. In patients with bilateral sacroiliitis, there is a stronger association with HLA B27[34]. During follow-up, although the radiographic changes in the spine tend to progress, spinal mobility is preserved or improves, and this form of spinal disease carries a better prognosis than pure ankylosing spondylitis[35]. This may partly reflect the

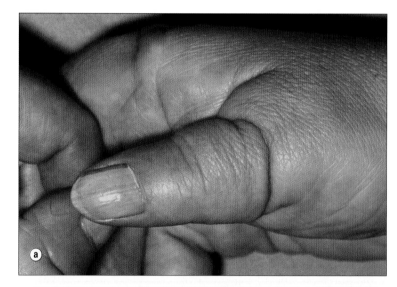

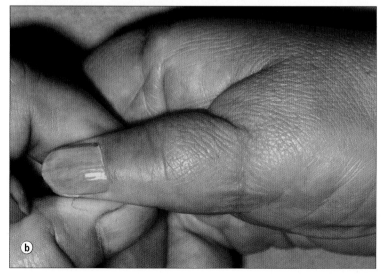

Fig. 110.5 Digital telescoping in arthritis mutilans. (Copyright University of Manchester.)

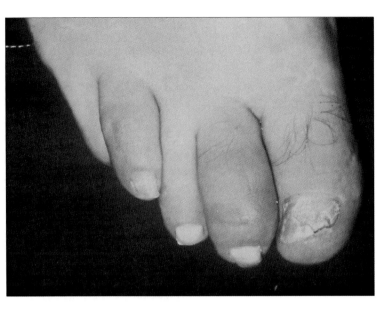

Fig. 110.6 Dactylitis of the second toe.

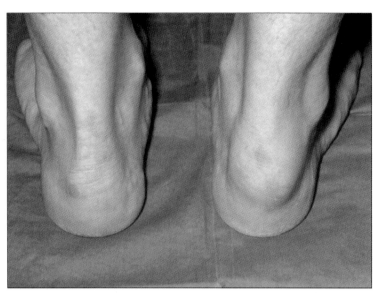

Fig. 110.7 Enthesitis involving the insertion of the right tendo Achilles.

random nature of spinal involvement that is observed, in addition to a lower frequency of zygoapophyseal joint fusion seen in psoriatic arthritis[36,37]. The cervical spine is also a common site of involvement in psoriatic arthritis. This can occur as part of a more widespread axial disease or as the sole site of axial involvement. Cervical spine disease becomes more frequent with time[38]. Two main types of cervical spine changes are described[38,39]: an ankylosing type, similar to that seen in ankylosing spondylitis, and an erosive/inflammatory type that can result in atlantoaxial or subaxial instability. Since cervical spine involvement can be clinically silent, patients with psoriatic arthritis, particularly those with long-standing disease, should have cervical spine radiographs before a general anesthetic[38].

Other musculoskeletal features
Dactylitis
Dactylitis or 'sausage digit' is a feature of the seronegative spondyloarthropathies in general. It represents a complete swelling of a single digit in the hand or foot. Dactylitis is a common feature of psoriatic arthritis, occurring in 30–40% of patients during the course of their disease[16,28]. It most commonly involves one or two digits at a time, and the feet are affected more commonly than the hands[40] (Fig. 110.6). There is an association with DIP joint involvement[16,28]. Radiologically, patients with a history of dactylitis more frequently develop erosive damage[29,40]. Magnetic resonance imaging (MRI) has revealed dactylitis to be strongly associated with flexor tenosynovitis, whereas active synovitis during an episode is not a universal finding[41,42].

Enthesitis
Inflammatory lesions at the insertion of tendon into bone are a hallmark clinical feature of spondyloarthropathies and, indeed, it has been postulated that it is this inflammatory lesion that is the key central pathogenic process in all seronegative spondyloarthropathies[43] (see Chapter 114). Symptomatic enthesitis occurs in 20–40% of patients with psoriatic arthritis[44,45]. It has been reported to be a presenting feature in 4%[44]. Common sites of enthesitis include the tendo Achilles (Fig. 110.7), the plantar fascia insertion into the calcaneum, and ligamentous insertions into pelvic bones.

Peripheral edema
Peripheral edema of one or more distal extremities is an increasingly recognized feature of several inflammatory conditions, including psoriatic arthritis. In contrast to the remitting seronegative symmetric synovitis with peripheral edema syndrome, distal extremity swelling in psoriatic arthritis is frequently asymmetric and preferentially affects the lower limbs. It can occur at any time and may be a presenting feature of the disease[45]. Clinically and radiologically, it is associated with extensor tenosynovitis and local enthesitis, and the edema is often along the course of the involved tendon[45]. Peripheral edema is usually responsive to oral steroids. Several cases of lymphedema associated with psoriatic arthritis have also been reported[46,47]. Although generally less painful, lymphedema can become more extensive, and has been associated with progression of erosive damage[46]. The response to steroids and disease-modifying antirheumatic drugs is varied, and it can be an additional source of disability in these patients[46,47].

Synovitis, acne, pustulosis, hyperostosis and osteitis syndrome
The syndrome of synovitis, acne, pustulosis, hyperostosis and osteitis (SAPHO; see Chapter 161) is an uncommon but recognized subgroup of psoriatic arthritis. Clinically, fewer than 3% of patients with psoriatic arthritis present in this fashion. Nevertheless, at least 67% of all patients with SAPHO have psoriasis vulgaris or palmoplantar pustulosis[48]. Scintigraphy suggests that involvement of the anterior chest wall may occur with a much greater frequency in patients with psoriatic arthritis than is clinically recognized[31].

Psoriatic onycho-pachydermo-periostitis
Several case reports of the rare manifestation of psoriatic arthritis known as psoriatic onycho-pachydermo-periostitis have been described. The key features include severe involvement of one or more terminal phalanges, with associated severe nail dystrophy, soft tissue swelling and marked periosteal reaction of the distal phalanx radiologically. The involvement of the DIP joint appears variable, but is difficult to assess because of the marked local inflammation[49,50]. Involvement of the great toe had been particularly described in this condition, and marked periostitis may eventually result in the radiological phenomenon of the 'ivory phalanx'[51].

Associated nail and skin changes
Skin changes
There is a suggestion that patients with psoriatic arthritis may have more extensive psoriasis than patients with uncomplicated psoriasis only[52], but, in general, most patients with psoriatic arthritis have only mild to moderate skin disease[53]. There is also no correlation between the extent of skin disease and total joint scores in patients with psoriatic arthritis[17,53]. Nevertheless, 30–40% of patients with psoriatic arthritis report

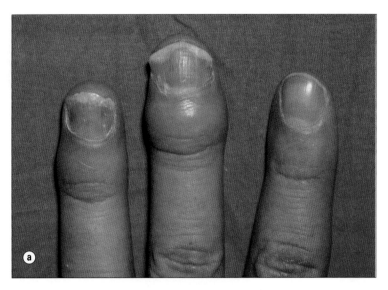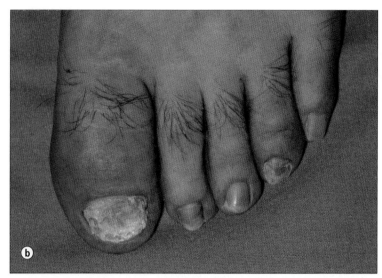

Fig.110.8 Involvement of the joint and adjacent nail. (a) In the right hand. (b) In the foot. Note the lack of involvement of the right 4th finger and nail. (Copyright University of Manchester.)

synchronicity of flares of their joint and skin disease, although the validity of this observation has not been formally tested[2,16,52]. No subtype of psoriasis is over-represented in patients with psoriatic arthritis, although an association between palmoplantar pustulosis and the SAPHO syndrome is described.

Nail involvement

In contrast to skin disease, there is a close association between nail and joint involvement in psoriatic arthritis. Anatomically, the nail is closely related to the distal phalanx by Sharpey's fibers that insert into bone in a manner similar to an enthesis. This close association may help explain the clinical observations. Nail involvement is seen in 20–40% of patients with uncomplicated psoriasis, whereas 60–80% of patients with psoriatic arthritis have nail involvement[16,17,28]. All the typical nail changes of psoriasis can be observed in psoriatic arthritis, including pitting, ridging, hyperkeratosis and onycholysis[1]. A closer temporal association between the onset of nail and joint disease has been described compared with the onset of skin and joint disease. Although skin disease may precede arthropathy by an average of 7–10 years, the onset of nail changes often occurs only 1–2 years before the onset of arthropathy[2]. The association between nails and joints is particularly marked in the presence of DIP joint arthritis, and 80–100% of such patients have nail involvement that frequently occurs at the adjacent nail[2,17,28] (Fig. 110.8). Patients with DIP joint involvement also have more severe nail changes[17,33], and patients with nail disease have more DIP joint involvement[53]. There is also a closer synchronicity between flares of DIP joint disease and worsening of nail involvement than is reported for flares of skin and joint disease[2].

Other extra-articular features

There is an overlap between the extra-articular features observed in psoriatic arthritis and those of the other seronegative spondyloarthropathies. Ocular inflammation can occur, most frequently presenting as conjunctivitis. However, iritis has also been described in 7% of those affected by psoriatic arthritis[16]. Additional uncommon complications such as oral ulceration, urethritis and aortic valve disease have also been reported[54].

JUVENILE PSORIATIC ARTHRITIS

Psoriatic arthritis developing in those younger than 16 years is relatively uncommon, and appears to account for less than 10% of chronic arthritis in childhood[55,56]. In contrast to adult-onset psoriatic arthritis, in juvenile-onset psoriatic arthritis the arthropathy precedes psoriasis in up to

TABLE 110.6 PROPOSED CRITERIA FOR THE DIAGNOSIS OF JUVENILE PSORIATIC ARTHRITIS	
Diagnosis	**Criteria**
Definite psoriatic arthritis	Arthritis onset before age 16 years *and either* Typical psoriasis *or* three minor criteria from: Dactylitis Nail pitting Psoriasis-like rash Family history of psoriasis (first- or second-degree relative)
Probable psoriatic arthritis	Arthritis onset before age 16 years *and* two minor criteria
(After Southwood *et al.*[57])	

50% of cases[55,57]. In view of this, careful attention needs to be paid to examination of the nails and taking an accurate family history in children with arthritis, as reflected in the criteria proposed by Southwood *et al.*[57] (Table 110.6). Juvenile psoriatic arthritis has a female preponderance of 2–3:1[55,57]. It frequently presents as a mono- or oligoarthritis, and the knee is often the first joint affected. As with the adult form, progression toward polyarthritis occurs in a significant proportion of those affected, and involvement of the small joints of the hands and feet occurs commonly during the disease course[55,57,58]. The other typical musculoskeletal features of adult psoriatic arthritis, such as dactylitis, enthesitis and DIP joint involvement, are all recognized. In addition, chronic uveitis is reported in 10–15% of patients, and may be associated with antinuclear antibodies[55,57]. The prognosis of juvenile psoriatic arthritis is good. It can, however, persist into adulthood, and 10–15% of those affected have significant residual disabilities[55,59].

INVESTIGATIONS

Laboratory investigation

There are no diagnostic laboratory tests for psoriatic arthritis. Several studies have shown that the acute-phase reactants display typical inflammatory changes when the disease is active. In particular, anemia of chronic disease, hypoalbuminemia, and increased erythrocyte sedimentation rate (ESR), C-reactive protein and fibrinogen are described[60]. Hypergammaglobulinemia with increased IgG and IgA is observed[16,61]. Increased IgA is especially associated with spondyloarthropathy[34]. Overall, the ESR and C-reactive protein show a good correlation with inflammatory disease activity, particularly in polyarticular disease[31,34,61]. Because, in most series of patients, a positive RF is not taken as an absolute exclusion criteria for the case definition of psoriatic arthritis, an RF-positive status has been reported in 5–10% of patients[16,34]. In a community cohort of patients with recent-onset inflammatory polyarthritis, patients with psoriasis were significantly less likely to be RF-positive compared with those without psoriasis (13% compared with 31%)[10]. Positivity for antinuclear antibody is also found in 10–14% of patients with psoriatic arthritis[16,34]. Hyperuricemia is present in up to 20% of patients with psoriatic arthritis[62]. A prospective study of patients with psoriatic arthritis found that the best predictors of hyperuricemia were renal impairment and increased total cholesterol. There was no correlation with the extent or severity of skin involvement. This suggests that hyperuricemia in the context of psoriatic arthritis is not the result of increased epidermal cell turnover, but rather reflects other relevant metabolic changes[62].

Radiographic changes
Peripheral joint features

Many radiological features reflect the clinical distribution of psoriatic arthritis described above. Therefore, involvement of the DIP joints (Fig. 110.9) and an asymmetric distribution when few joints are affected are well described. In addition, the involvement of entheseal sites can

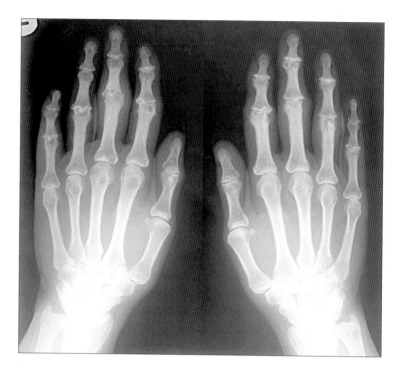

Fig. 110.9 Radiograph of the hands, showing erosive changes at the DIP and PIP joints, with sparing of the MCP joints and wrists. (Copyright Dr R Whitehouse.)

result in proliferative new bone formation in sites of predilection – for example, the plantar fascia and tendo Achillis insertions. With regard to the onset of erosive change in peripheral joints, in a community survey

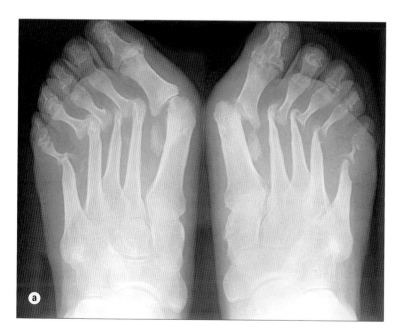

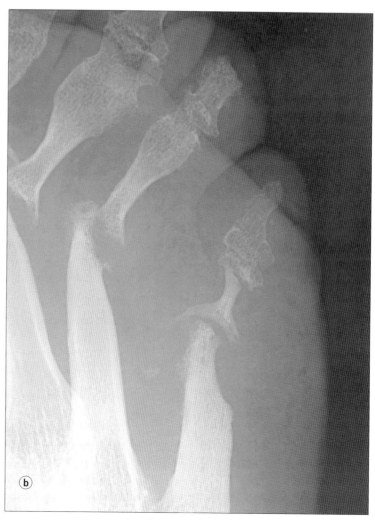

Fig. 110.10 Arthritis mutilans. Marked osteolysis and 'pencilling', resulting in complete disorganization of the metatarsophalangeal (MTP) joints. There is also a 'pencil-in-cup' deformity of the right 5th MTP joint (b). (Copyright Dr R Whitehouse.)

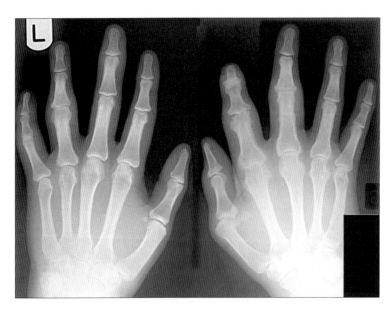

Fig. 110.11 Asymmetric involvement of the hands. Soft tissue swelling and periosteal reaction in the right 2nd and 3rd fingers in the typical 'ray' distribution. (Copyright Dr R Whitehouse.)

of early inflammatory arthritis, patients with psoriasis had a reduced risk of erosions developing at 1 year, compared with patients without psoriasis[10]. This reduced risk was explained by the lower incidence of RF positivity in the psoriasis group. Nevertheless, 22% of patients with psoriasis

and early arthritis had evidence of erosions at 1 year[10]. In more established hospital cohorts, the prevalence of erosions can range from 35% to 70%[16,28,29]. Erosions are most frequent in patients with polyarthritis and in those with longer disease duration[28,29]. As mentioned earlier, there is an association between dactylitis and erosions. With regard to the distribution of erosions, in a case–control study comparing patients with psoriatic arthropathy and patients with seropositive arthritis without psoriasis, erosions were less frequent at the wrist and more common in the DIP joints of those with psoriatic arthritis[63]. In addition to erosions, soft tissue swelling can be seen around sites of active inflammation, although periarticular osteopenia is not a feature in psoriatic arthritis[64]. The other radiographic features of psoriatic arthritis in peripheral joints can be broadly grouped into destructive and proliferative changes.

Destructive changes

● Osteolysis may result in whittling or 'pencilling' of a phalanx. This can occur alone or in association with an erosion at the base of the adjacent phalanx, which causes the classic 'pencil in cup' deformity[65]. Such destruction is typical of the arthritis mutilans pattern of disease (Fig. 110.10).

Proliferative changes[65]

● Periostitis. Proliferative new bone formation can occur along the shaft of the metacarpal and metatarsal bones (Figs 110.11 & 110.12a). When this change occurs adjacent to an erosion, the term 'whiskering' is often used (Fig. 110.12b)

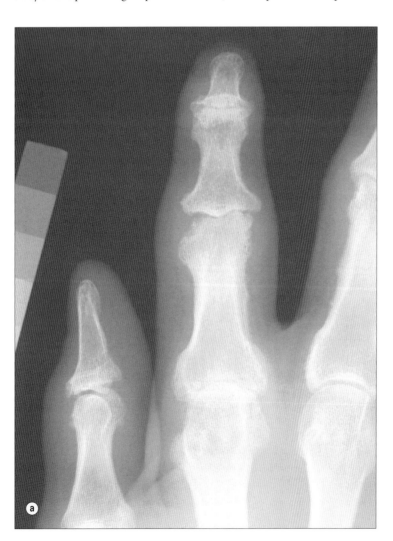

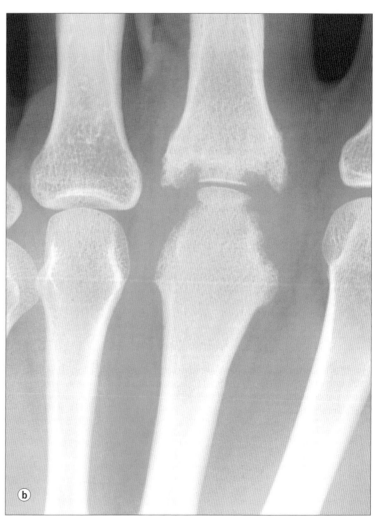

Fig. 110.12 Examples of periosteal reactions. (a) Along the shaft of the proximal phalanx. (b) Adjacent to a large erosion, producing 'whiskering'. (Copyright Dr R Whitehouse.)

- Ivory phalanx (see Psoriatic onycho-pachydermo-periostitis, above)
- Bony ankylosis and joint fusion (Fig. 110.13).

Spinal changes

Radiographic evidence of sacroiliitis in psoriatic arthritis can be symmetric or asymmetric. Asymmetric sacroiliitis is more common in psoriatic arthritis than in ankylosing spondylitis[37] (Fig. 110.14). Many of the classic features of ankylosing spondylitis can be observed in psoriatic arthritis, but patients with psoriatic arthritis tend to have less frequent involvement of the zygapophyseal joint and less severe and extensive involvement of the lumbar spine[37,66]. Overall, the spinal involvement in psoriatic arthritis tends to be more 'spotty' and asymmetric in nature, with frequent involvement of the cervical spine[37,66]. An additional feature in the spine is paravertebral ossification or 'chunky' syndesmophytes[67]. These appear distinct from the classic 'marginal' syndesmophytes observed in ankylosing spondylitis. The chunky syndesmophytes again occur in a patchy and asymmetric fashion throughout the axial spine (Fig. 110.15).

Other imaging modalities

There is increasing interest in the use of MRI and ultrasonography to delineate the clinical manifestation of diseases such as psoriatic arthritis. MRI studies have demonstrated that, in psoriatic arthritis, there is frequent involvement of extra-articular tissue such as ligaments, periarticular soft tissue and tendon sheaths, and bone (Fig. 110.16)[41,68]. In addition to delineating clinical joint involvement, MRI has also demonstrated evidence of 'subclinical' musculoskeletal changes in a significant proportion of patients with apparently uncomplicated psoriasis[69]. Scintigraphy in patients with psoriatic arthritis has also demonstrated more extensive involvement than is appreciated clinically, particularly

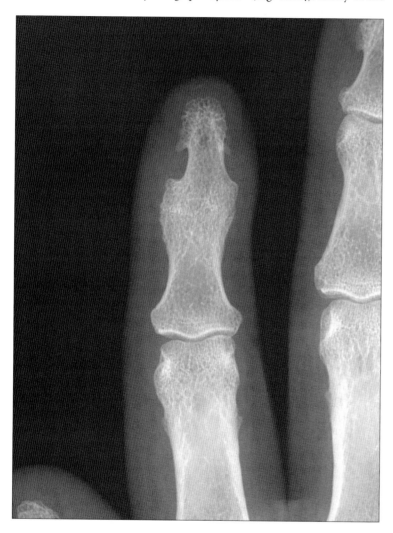

Fig. 110.13 Bony ankylosis of the DIP joint. (Copyright Dr R Whitehouse.)

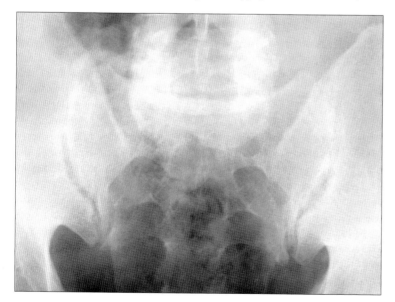

Fig. 110.14 Early asymmetric sacroiliitis, with erosion and sclerosis of the left sacroiliac joint. (Copyright Dr R Whitehouse.)

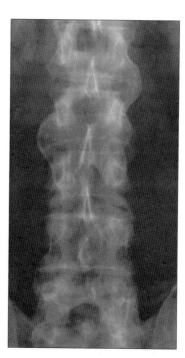

Fig. 110.15 Non-marginal 'chunky' syndesmophytes.

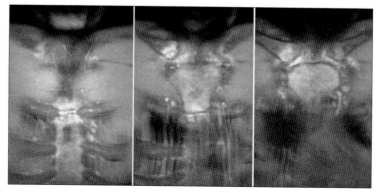

Fig. 110.16 Involvement of extra-articular tissues in psoriatic arthritis. Magnetic resonance images (coronal fat-suppressed proton-density-weighted) showing osteitis and bone edema as high signal in the clavicles, manubrium and upper sternum of a patient with SAPHO. (Copyright Dr R Whitehouse.)

in the anterior chest wall and large peripheral joints[31]. Such techniques can therefore facilitate the clinical evaluation of patients with psoriasis and articular complaints.

DIFFERENTIAL DIAGNOSIS AND CLINICAL EVALUATION

Differential diagnosis

Psoriatic arthritis poses an important diagnostic challenge to the physician. There are no clear diagnostic criteria, and the wide range of clinical presentations from isolated enthesitis or monoarthritis through polyarthritis and spondylitis means that the differential diagnosis is quite extensive. Given the frequency of hyperuricemia, crystal arthropathies also need to be excluded. In this instance, joint fluid analysis may be the only reliable way to exclude this possibility. The distinctions between psoriatic arthritis and RA or psoriatic arthritis and ankylosing spondylitis have been discussed and are summarized in Tables 110.7 and 110.8. In patients in

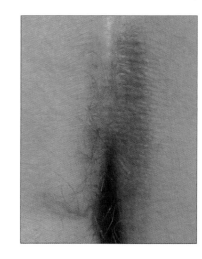

Fig. 110.17 Flexural psoriasis in the natal cleft, a typical 'hidden' site for psoriasis.

whom there is no clinical evidence of skin or nail disease, distinguishing psoriatic arthritis from other arthropathies is particularly difficult.

Clinical evaluation

When assessing joint involvement in psoriatic arthritis, it is important to bear in mind that patients with this condition can be less tender over affected joints than are patients with RA[70]. In addition, effusions can be more difficult to detect in patients with psoriatic arthritis[71]. For these reasons, it is easy to underestimate the extent of joint involvement in psoriatic arthritis. Examination for other musculoskeletal features such as enthesitis, tenosynovitis and axial spine involvement is also necessary. Limitations in spinal movement may not follow the classic pattern observed in ankylosing spondylitis, and may be confined to the neck or thoracic spine in the absence of lumbar spine or sacroiliac joint involvement. Radiological evaluation complements the clinical examination, particularly when there has been a history of previous joint symptoms, as residual joint damage may be detectable radiologically in the absence of current symptoms. Similarly, previous or current inflammatory back symptoms suggest spondylitis and require radiological examination. Finally, a detailed examination of the skin and nails to include 'hidden areas' such as the scalp, perineum and periumbilical area is important (Fig. 110.17). The choice of therapeutic agent(s) is determined by the extent and severity of the skin *and* joint disease, and by an estimation of the risk of disease progression.

PROGNOSIS

Functional impairment

There have been only a few prospective studies of prognosis in psoriatic arthritis. The general impression is that the condition is associated with less long-term disability than is observed in RA[1]. Several hospital clinic series have, however, shown that between 11% and 42% of patients with psoriatic arthritis have American College of Rheumatology grade III or IV functional impairment at time of study[16,28,29,34]. All studies are agreed that there is an association between polyarthritis and functional disability. With regard to disease progression, studies from the University of Toronto Psoriatic Arthritis Clinic have shown that patients with at least five joint effusions at the time of presentation to the clinic are significantly more likely to develop progressive joint deformity at follow-up. Additional predictive factors include the presence of HLA-B27, -B39 or -DQw3[72,73].

Mortality

With regard to mortality, a community-based study in Olmsted County, Minnesota, USA showed no difference in survival for patients with psoriatic arthritis compared with members of the general popula-

TABLE 110.7 KEY FEATURES THAT HELP DISTINGUISH BETWEEN PSORIATIC ARTHRITIS AND RHEUMATOID ARTHRITIS

Feature	Psoriatic arthritis	Rheumatoid arthritis
Sex M:F	1.1	2:1
RF	<10%	80%
DIP joints	30–50%	Uncommon
Pattern of joint involvement	Asymmetric 'Ray' pattern	Symmetric 'Row' pattern
Sacroiliac joints/axial spine	35% – any level	Cervical spine in late disease
Other musculoskeletal	Enthesitis Dactylitis Periarticular erythema	
Extra-articular	Skin Nail dystrophy	Nodules Sicca Vasculitis
Radiology	Erosion (DIP joints) Periostitis/bony proliferation	Periarticular osteopenia Erosion (wrists)

TABLE 110.8 KEY FEATURES THAT HELP DISTINGUISH BETWEEN PSORIATIC ARTHRITIS AND ANKYLOSING SPONDYLITIS

Feature	Psoriatic arthritis	Ankylosing spondylitis
Sex M:F	1:1	9:1
Sacroiliac joints/ axial spine	35%	100%
Spinal movements	↓	↓↓
Peripheral joint involvement	90–95%	40%
Peripheral joint pattern	Upper and lower limbs Large and small joints	Lower limbs Large joints
Dactylitis	Common	Uncommon
HLA-B27	10–25%	90%
Spinal radiology	Random distribution Asymmetric 'Chunky' syndesmophytes	Contiguous involvement Symmetric Classic syndesmophytes

tion[14]. In contrast, in a hospital cohort an increased mortality rate compared with that in the general population was observed, with standardized mortality ratio values of 1.65 and 1.59 for males and females, respectively[74]; this likely reflects the spectrum of disease under long-term follow-up in hospital clinics. In this series, there was a particular excess of deaths as a result of diseases of the respiratory system such as pneumonia and obstructive airways disease[74]. The most significant predictive factors for mortality in this study were radiological damage, increased ESR and prior use of disease-modifying drugs, with nail lesions being identified as a 'protective factor'[75]. From these studies, one can conclude that patients with polyarthritis are most likely to have functional impairment and progression of disease. In addition, extensive and progressive disease may also be associated with an excess mortality.

REFERENCES

1. Moll JMH, Wright V. Psoriatic arthritis. Semin Arthritis Rheum 1973; 3: 55–78.
2. Wright V. Rheumatism and psoriasis. A re-evaluation. Am J Med 1959; 27: 454–462.
3. Blumberg BS, Bunim JJ, Calkins E et al. ARA nomenclature and classification of arthritis and rheumatism (tentative). Arthritis Rheum 1964; 7: 93–97.
4. Dawson MH, Tyson TL. Psoriasis arthropathica. With observations on certain features common to psoriasis and rheumatoid arthritis. Trans Assoc Am Physicians 1938; 53: 303–309.
5. Hellgren L. Association between rheumatoid arthritis and psoriasis in total populations. Acta Rheumatol Scand 1969; 15: 316–326.
6. Baker H. Epidemiological aspects of psoriasis and arthritis. Br J Dermatol 1966; 78: 249–261.
7. Mongan ES, Atwater EC. A comparison of patients with seropositive and seronegative rheumatoid arthritis. Med Clin North Am 1968; 52: 533–538.
8. Leczinsky CG. The incidence of arthropathy in a ten-year series of psoriasis cases. Acta Dermatoken 1948; 28: 483–487.
9. van Romunde LKJ, Valkenburg HA, Swart-Bruinsma W et al. Psoriasis and arthritis. I: A population study. Rheumatol Int 1984; 4: 55–60.
10. Harrison BJ, Silman AJ, Barrett EM et al. Presence of psoriasis does not influence the presentation or short term outcome of patients with early inflammatory polyarthritis. J Rheumatol 1997; 24: 1744–1749.
11. Scarpa R, Oriente P, Pucino A et al. Psoriatic arthritis in psoriatic patients. Br J Rheumatol 1984; 23: 246–250.
12. Little H, Harvie JN, Lester RS. Psoriatic arthritis in severe psoriasis. Can Med Assoc J 1975; 112: 317–319.
13. Lomholt G. Psoriasis. Prevalence, spontaneous course and genetics. A census study of the prevalence of skin diseases on the Faroe Islands. GEC GAD; Copenhagen: 1963.
14. Shbeeb M, Uramoto KM, Gibson LE et al. The epidemiology of psoriatic arthritis in Olmsted County, Minnesota, USA, 1982–1991. J Rheumatol 2000; 27: 1247–1250.
15. Kaipiainen-Seppanen O. Incidence of psoriatic arthritis in Finland. Br J Rheumatol 1996; 35: 1289–1291.
16. Gladman DD, Shuckett R, Russell ML et al. Psoriatic arthritis (PSA) – an Analysis of 220 patients. Q J Med 1987; 238: 127–141.
17. Jones SM, Armas J, Cohen M et al. Psoriatic arthritis: outcome of disease subsets and relationship of joint disease to nail and skin disease. Br J Rheumatol 1994; 33: 834–839.
18. Rahman P, Schentag CT, Gladman DD. Immunogenetic profile of patients with psoriatic arthritis varies according to the age at onset of psoriasis. Arthritis Rheum 1999; 42: 822–823.
19. Solinger AM, Hess EV. Rheumatic diseases and AIDS – is the association real? J Rheumatol 1994; 20: 678–683.
20. Mijiyawa M, Oniankitan O, Khan MA. Spondyloarthropathies in sub-Saharan Africa. Curr Opin Rheumatol 2000; 12: 281–286.
21. Njobvu P, McGill P, Kerr H et al. Spondyloarthropathy and human immunodeficiency virus infection in Zambia. J Rheumatol 1998; 25: 1553–1559.
22. Njobvu P, McGill P. Psoriatic arthritis and human immunodeficiency virus infection in Zambia. J Rheumatol 2000; 27: 1699–1702.
23. Calabrese LH, Kelley DM, Myers A et al. Rheumatic symptoms and human immunodeficiency virus infection. The influence of clinical and laboratory variables in a longitudinal cohort study. Arthritis Rheum 1991; 34: 257–263.
24. Berman A, Espinoza LR, Diaz JD et al. Rheumatic manifestations of human immunodeficiency virus infection. Am J Med 1988; 85: 59–64.
25. Espinoza LR, Berman A, Vasey FB et al. Posriatic arthritis and acquired immunodeficiency syndrome. Arthritis Rheum 1988; 31: 1034–1040.
26. Duvic M, Johnson TM, Rapini RP et al. Acquired immunodeficiency syndrome-associated psoriasis and Reiter's syndrome. Arch Dermatol 1987; 123: 1622–1632.
27. Dougados M, Van der Linden S, Juhlin R et al. The European Spondylarthropathy Study Group preliminary criteria for the classification of spondylarthropathy. Arthritis Rheum 1991; 34: 1218–1227.
28. Veale D, Rodgers S, Fitzgerald O. Classification of clinical subsets in psoriatic arthritis. Br J Rheumatol 1994; 33: 133–138.
29. Marsal S, Armadans-Gil L, Martinez M et al. Clinical, radiographic and HLA associations as markers for different patterns of psoriatic arthritis. Br J Rheumatol 1999; 38: 332–337.
30. Gladman DD, Brubacher B, Buskila D et al. Psoriatic spondyloarthropathy in men and women: a clinical, radiographic and HLA study. Clin Invest Med 1992; 15: 371–375.
31. Helliwell P, Marchesoni A, Peters M et al. A re-evaluation of the osteoarticular manifestations of psoriasis. Br J Rheumatol 1991; 30: 339–345.
32. Helliwell P, Hetthen J, Sokoll K et al. Joint symmetry in early and late rheumatoid and psoriatic arthritis. Arthritis Rheum 2000; 43: 865–871.
33. Van Romunde LKJ, Cats A, Hermans J, Valkenburg HA. Psoriasis and arthritis. II. A cross-sectional comparative study of patients with psoriatic arthritis and seronegative and seropositive polyarthritis: clinical aspects. Rheumatol Int 1984; 4: 61–65.
34. Torre Alonso JC, Rodriguez Perez A, Arribas Castrillo JM et al. Psoriatic arthritis (PA): a clinical, immunological and radiological study of 180 patients. Br J Rheumatol 1991; 30: 245–250.
35. Gladman DD, Brubacher B, Buskila D et al. Differences in the expression of spondyloarthropathy: a comparison between ankylosing spondylitis and psoriatic arthritis. Clin Invest Med 1992; 16: 1–7.
36. Hanly JG, Russell ML, Gladman DD. Psoriatic spondyloarthropathy: a long term prospective study. Ann Rheum Dis 1988; 47: 386–393.
37. Helliwell P, Hickling P, Wright V. Do the radiological changes of classic ankylosing spondylitis differ from the changes found in the spondylitis associated with inflammatory bowel disease, psoriasis, and reactive arthritis? Ann Rheum Dis 1998; 57: 135–140.
38. Jenkinson T, Armas J, Evison G et al. The cervical spine in psoriatic arthritis: a clinical and radiological study. Br J Rheumatol 1994; 33: 255–259.
39. Salvarani C, Macchioni P, Cremonesi T et al. The cervical spine in patients with psoriatic arthritis: a clinical, radiological and immunogenetic study. Ann Rheum Dis 1992; 51: 73–77.
40. Brockbank J, Stein M, Schentag CT et al. Characteristics of dactylitis in psoriatic arthritis (PsA). Arthritis Rheum 2000; 43(suppl): S105.
41. Olivieri I, Barozzi L, Favaro L et al. Dactylitis in patients with seronegative spondylarthropathy. Assessment by ultrasonography and magnetic resonance imaging. Arthritis Rheum 1996; 39: 1524–1529.
42. Olivieri I, Barozzi L, Pierro A et al. Toe dactylitis in patients with spondyloarthropathy: assessment by magnetic resonance imaging. J Rheumatol 1997; 24: 926–930.
43. McGonagle D, Gibbon W, Emery P. Classification of inflammatory arthritis by enthesitis. Lancet 1998; 352: 1137–1140.
44. Scarpa R. Peripheral enthesopathies in psoriatic arthritis. J Rheumatol 1998; 25: 2259–2290.
45. Cantini F, Salvarani C, Olivieri I et al. Distal extremity swelling with pitting edema in psoriatic arthritis: a case–control study. Clin Exp Rheumatol 2001; 19: 291–296.
46. Mulherin DM, FitzGerald O, Bresnihan B. Lymphedema of the upper limb in patients with psoriatic arthritis. Semin Arthritis Rheum 1993; 22: 350–356.
47. Salvarani C, Cantini F, Olivieri I et al. Distal extremity swelling with pitting edema in psoriatic arthritis: evidence of 2 pathological mechanisms. J Rheumatol 1999; 26: 1831–1834.
48. Hayem G, Bouchaud-Chabot A, Benali K et al. SAPHO syndrome: a long-term follow-up study of 120 cases. Semin Arthritis Rheum 1999; 29: 159–171.
49. Goupille P, Laulan J, Vedere V et al. Psoriatic onycho-periostitis. Scand J Rheumatol 1995; 24: 53–54.
50. Boisseau-Garsaud A-M, Beylot-Barry MD, Doutre M-S et al. Psoriatic onycho-pachydermo-periostitis. Arch Dermatol 1996; 132: 176–180.
51. Resnick D, Broderick TW. Bony proliferation of terminal toe phalanges in psoriasis: the 'ivory' phalanx. J Can Assoc Radiol 1977; 28: 187–189.
52. Stern RS. The epidemiology of joint complaints in patients with psoriasis. J Rheumatol 1985; 12: 315–320.
53. Cohen MR, Reda JD, Clegg DO. Baseline relationship between psoriasis and psoriatic arthritis: analysis of 221 patients with active psoriatic arthritis. J Rheumatol 1999; 28: 1752–1756.
54. Gladman DD. Psoriatic arthritis. Spine 1990; 4: 637–656.
55. Lambert JR, Ansell BM, Stephenson E, Wright V. Psoriatic arthritis in childhood. Clin Rheum Dis 1976; 2: 339–352.
56. Ansell BM. Juvenile psoriatic arthritis. Baillière's Clin Rheumatol 1994; 8: 317–332.
57. Southwood TR, Petty RE, Malleson PN et al. Psoriatic arthritis in children. Arthritis Rheum 1989; 32: 1007–1013.
58. Hamilton ML, Gladman DD, Shore A et al. Juvenile psoriatic arthritis and HLA antigens. Ann Rheum Dis 1990; 49: 694–697.
59. Shore A, Ansell BM. Juvenile psoriatic arthritis: an analysis of 60 cases. J Pediatr 1982; 100: 529–535.
60. Troughton PR, Morgan AW. Laboratory findings and pathology of psoriatic arthritis. Ballière's Clin Rheumatol 1994; 8: 439–463.
61. Laurent MR, Panayi GS, Shepherd P. Circulating immune complexes, serum immunoglobulins and acute phase protein in psoriasis and arthritis. Ann Rheum Dis 1981; 40: 66–69.
62. Bruce IN, Schentag CT, Gladman DD. Hyperuricemia in psoriatic arthritis prevalence and associated features. J Clin Rheumatol 2000; 6: 6–9.
63. Van Romunde LKJ, Cats A, Hermans J et al. Psoriasis and arthrisis. III: A cross-sectional comparative study of patients with psoriatic arthritis and seronegative and seropositive polyarthritis: radiological and HLA aspects. Rheumatol Int 1984; 4: 67–73.
64. Resnick D, Niwayama J. Psoriatic arthritis. In: Diagnosis of bone and joint disorders, 2nd edn. Philadelphia: WB Saunders 1988: 1171–1198.
65. Wright V. Psoriasis and arthritis. A study of the radiographic appearances. Br JRadiol 1957; 30: 113–119.

66. McEwen C, DiTata D, Lingg C *et al*. Ankylosing spondylitis and spondylitis accompanying ulcerative colitis, regional enteritis, psoriasis and Reiter's disease. A comparative study. Arthritis Rheum 1971; 14: 291–318.

67. Bywaters EGL, Dixon AStJ. Paravertebral ossification in psoriatic arthritis. Ann Rheum Dis 1965; 24: 313–331.

68. Jevtic V, Watt I, Rozman B *et al*. Distinctive radiological features of small hand joints in rheumatoid arthritis and seronegative spondyloarthritis demonstrated by contrast-enhanced (Gd-DTPA) magnetic resonance imaging. Skeletal Radiol 1995; 24: 351–355.

69. Offidani A, Cellini A, Valeri G, Giovagnoni A. Subclinical joint involvement in psoriasis: magnetic resonance imaging and X-ray findings. Acta Derm Venereol (Stockh) 1998; 78: 463–465.

70. Buskila D, Langevitz P, Gladman DD *et al*. Patients with rheumatoid arthritis are more tender than those with psoriatic arthritis. J Rheumatol 1992; 19: 1115–1119.

71. Bruce IN, Gladman DD. Psoriatic arthritis. Recognition and management. BioDrugs 1998; 9: 271–278.

72. Gladman DD, Farewell VT, Nadeau C. Clinical indicators of progression in psoriatic arthritis: multivariate relative risk model. J Rheumatol 1995; 22: 675–679.

73. Gladman DD, Farewell VT. The role of HLA antigens as indicators of disease progression in psoriatic arthritis. Arthritis Rheum 1995; 38: 845–850.

74. Wong K, Gladman DD, Husted J *et al*. Mortality studies in psoriatic arthritis. Arthritis Rheum 1997; 40: 1868–1872.

75. Gladman DD, Farewell VT, Wong K, Husted J. Mortality studies in psoriatic arthritis. results from a single outpatient center. II. Prognostic indicators for death. Arthritis Rheum 1998; 41: 1103–1110.

111 Psoriatic arthritis: etiology and pathogenesis

Christian Antoni

- The genetic diversity in psoriatic arthritis (PsA) suggests a polygenic influence. PsA is associated with genes that are also associated with psoriasis (e.g. *HLA-Cw6*) and with arthritis (e.g. *HLA B27*). A newly recognized class I related gene A (*MICA*) is more strongly associated with PsA itself and correlates with the susceptibility for developing PsA

- The role of environmental factors such as infection, trauma and stress is still unclear

- The importance of the T cell in the pathogenesis of PsA is demonstrated by the association of PsA with human immunodeficiency virus infection, the expansion of T cell clones from synovial membrane, which expand in an autoantigen-driven manner, and the efficacy of anti-T cell treatment on the skin lesion and the synovitis

- In addition to the role of the T cells, the histopathology of PsA, with its distinct vascular pattern and thickening of the vessel walls, differentiates it from rheumatoid arthritis

- In PsA, monocyte derived cytokines such as tumor necrosis factor (TNF)-α are expressed both in the synovial membrane and in the psoriatic lesions. They differ in the level of expression, but the pattern is similar

- Anti-TNF-α treatment is effective in PsA and leads to a reduction in synovitis and psoriatic lesions. The magnitude and the time course of the effect on both symptoms demonstrate the pathogenic role of this cytokine in PsA.

ETIOLOGY OF PSORIATIC ARTHRITIS

Psoriatic arthritis (PsA) is part of the heterogeneous group of diseases, unified in the concept of spondyloarthropathies (see Chapter 101). The common etiology of ankylosing spondylitis, reactive arthritis, enteropathic arthritis, undifferentiated arthritis and PsA is poorly understood. Recently, an enthesitis-based model for the pathogenesis of spondyloarthropathy as pathogenic link between these diseases and their differentiation from rheumatoid arthritis (RA) has been proposed[1]. Nevertheless, the concept of PsA is not universally accepted. It is clear that PsA is more common than the random co-occurrence of psoriasis and inflammatory arthritis, supporting the existence of PsA as a disease entity[2]. The diagnostic criteria are still debated. For example: do patients with psoriasis, rheumatoid factor and polyarthritis have PsA, or RA with psoriasis? Because the understanding of the clinical nature and the pathology of the disease is not precise, and because PsA is not clearly distinguished from other entities, defining its etiology is difficult[2].

Genetics

In a primary care setting, the prevalences of psoriasis and PsA are 1.7% and 0.3%, respectively[3]. Familial aggregation of PsA suggests a genetic contribution to the etiology[4], and recently a strong paternal transmission in PsA was described[5]. In psoriasis, monozygotic twins showed a concordance of 65–72%, compared with 15–30% in dizygotic twins[6]. Whether the same findings are observed in twins with PsA has yet to be determined. Many studies have investigated human leukocyte antigen (*HLA*) class I alleles in PsA and showed an association of *HLA-B13, -B17* and *-Cw6* in comparison with the normal population[7]. Detailed molecular typing showed that the *Cw6* association is with the *Cw*0602* allele, which is also found in psoriasis alone[8]. Studies have been undertaken that contrasted the association of *HLA* class I in psoriasis alone with PsA and with the general population. The results have been inconsistent. Some studies suggest that the effects are weaker with PsA[9,10]; in contrast, however, *HLA-B27* and *-B7* have been associated with PsA independently of psoriasis[9]. The former antigen was more strongly associated with the presence of sacroiliitis, whereas other HLA antigens showed no correlation with the clinical or radiologic picture of the patients[10]. A newer study investigated the class I major histocompatibility complex (MHC) chain related gene A (*MICA*) comparing both psoriasis and PsA patients with healthy controls[11]. This showed that *MICA-A9* polymorphism, corresponding to the allele *MICA-002*, was only increased in PsA, whereas the *Cw*0602* allele was significantly increased in both psoriasis and PsA. Thus *MICA-002* may be a possible candidate gene for the development of PsA. The same authors have since obtained further evidence in favor of this hypothesis[12]. In conclusion, although PsA has been associated with genes known to be associated with psoriasis (e.g. *HLA-Cw6*) and with arthritis (e.g. *HLA-B27*), apart from *MICA* there is little evidence of a separate genetic influence on PsA itself.

Environmental factors

Infection

The suggestion that infection has a possible role in the pathogenesis of PsA is suggested by the facts, firstly, that other forms of seronegative arthropathy are often associated with infections and, secondly, that guttate psoriasis is linked to streptococcal upper respiratory tract infection. In the peripheral blood from seven of 19 patients with PsA, 16S rRNA from group A streptococci could be detected. Two of these patients were also positive for 26S rRNA from group B streptococci[13]. In one patient, the synovial fluid was also positive. In contrast, in all 17 patients with RA, blood samples were negative ($p=0.006$)[13]. This study supports the hypothesis that infection has a role in the etiology of PsA, although proof is difficult. The presence of bacteria or related antigens was not demonstrated in a large number of joints examined from patients with PsA. A recent study showed no disease-specific role of the synovial T lymphocytes when PsA, RA and osteoarthritis were compared[14]: T cell clones proliferated in response to group A streptococci in a similar pattern in all three diseases. Although the immunoreactivity to streptococcal antigens is accepted, it remains unclear if the infection triggers PsA, or if the breakage of the skin barrier because of the psoriasis leads to streptococcal exposure and finally to a form of reactive arthritis.

Acquired immunodeficiency syndrome

Infection with human immunodeficiency virus (HIV) is associated with the development of psoriasis and PsA. In Zambia, 94% of the population of patients with PsA were HIV-positive, compared with 30% of the background population[15]. The association of the HIV infection and PsA may hint at a viral trigger of PsA, but it is also possible that infection with HIV increases the risk for other infections that may trigger PsA. It is also possible that the reduction in the number of CD4 cells changes the balance of the T cells. CD8$^+$ T cells may play an important part in the pathogenesis of PsA.

Trauma

The mechanism of the Köebner phenomenon, the appearance of psoriatic lesions after skin injury, is well known. In case–control studies, the possibility of a 'deep Köebner phenomenon' has been investigated[16]. In one study, 9% of patients with PsA had an acute injury before the onset of the disease, compared with only 1% of the patients with RA. In a second study, 8% of the patients with PsA experienced some kind of trauma within 3 months before the onset of the disease, compared with only 2% of those with RA[17]. In general, however, a history of trauma has been described in only a minority of patients with PsA. It is possible that recurrent minor trauma, which might be difficult to ascertain, causes inflammation in the involved joints such as the distal interphalangeal joints. It has recently been proposed by McGonagle et al.[1] that biomechanical stresses lead to tissue microtrauma, with the consequent activation of stress genes and upregulation of adhesion molecules. The healing and inflammatory responses are closely linked, and mediated by the same inflammatory cells and cytokines, particularly interleukin (IL)-1 and tumor necrosis factor (TNF). McGonagle et al.[1] postulated that, in susceptible patients, for example those with HLA-B27 antigen, the microtrauma and the microbial factor at the diseased site upregulate the proinflammatory cytokines until the homeostasis has shifted from repair to inflammation. In support of this, the neuropeptide, substance P, and vasoactive intestinal peptide are both overexpressed in skin lesions and in the synovium of patients with PsA[18]. In a patient with hemiplegia, substance P was prevented from release in the paretic extremities and the motor nerve damage resulted in sparing of developing psoriasis and PsA in those paralysed extremities[19].

Stress

The greater frequency of PsA in patients with severe psoriasis has been used as an argument that psychological stress can cause skin and joint involvement[2]. The role of psychological stress is well described, but the pathogenesis remains unclear[20]; Fearon and Veale[21] recently stated that it may be linked to neuropeptide release by the nervous system.

PATHOGENESIS OF PSORIATIC ARTHRITIS

The predominant role of the T cells

Recent studies have shown that T cells and the proinflammatory cytokines have important roles in the pathogenesis of both psoriasis and PsA. Such evidence came from examination of T cells both from active skin lesions and the joints, and from results of T cell targeting or cytokine modulating treatments, which are efficacious in PsA in skin and joint lesions. Costello and colleagues[22] were able to show that CD8$^+$ T cell clones (predominantly, but also some CD4$^+$ T cell clones) from the synovial fluid expanded in a selective, although not identified, autoantigen-driven manner. They also described a predominance of CD8$^+$ T cells in synovial fluid from patients with PsA compared with that from patients with RA[23]. The majority of these cells are activated memory T cells expressing CD45RO and HLA-DR antigens. In addition, Tassiulas and colleagues[24] showed similarities of expanding T cell clones from skin and synovial fluid.

A more specific approach was recently described using two T cell directed biological agents. The humanized monoclonal IgG$_1$ antibody, efaluzimab, directed against the α subunit of the lymphocyte function-associated antigen (LFA)-1 CD11a showed efficacy in two double-blind trials in psoriasis. The binding blocks interaction of LFA-1 with its ligands, the intercellular adhesion molecules 1, 2 and 3. The beneficial effect on psoriasis is most probably attributable to inhibition of (a) the binding of T cells to endothelial cells, (b) the trafficking of T cells from the circulation into the dermis and (c) the activation of the T cells[25].

A third approach has been to use a human fusion protein, alefacept, consisting of the first extracellular domain of LFA-3 fused with the hinge and second and third constant domain (C$_H$2 and C$_H$3) sequences of the heavy chain of IgG$_1$. The LFA-3 domain of alefacept binds to CD2 on T cells. CD2 is upregulated on memory T cells (CD45Ro$^+$). The IgG$_1$ domain interacts with FcγRIII receptors and leads to selective T cell apoptosis. Alefacept has shown to produce a reduction in psoriasis lesions and synovitis in patients with PsA[26].

The effect of both the above drugs, which selectively target T cells, on psoriasis, and of alefacept on PsA have showed that the T cell, most probably the memory-effector T cell, has an important role in the pathogenesis of the disease. Another clinical observation that supports the importance of T cells in PsA is that patients with PsA went into remission after allogeneic bone marrow transplantation, whereas another patient developed new PsA after receiving a bone marrow transplant from a donor who suffered from PsA[27].

Vascular patterns in the skin and synovium of patients with PsA

The morphological vascular changes in the synovial membrane and skin lesions in patients with PsA are different from the changes in RA. Thus, in contrast to RA, in PsA, hyperplasia and hypertrophy of synoviocytes are minimal and the walls of capillaries and small arteries show marked thickening and inflammatory perivascular infiltrates[28]. In a recent arthroscopy study, 73% of patients with PsA and with reactive arthritis had predominantly tortuous, bushy vessels, whereas 89% of the patients with RA had mainly straight, branching vessels. The distinct vascular patterns in PsA and reactive arthritis compared with those in RA may reflect different specific vascular factors in the pathogenesis of these arthritides[29]. In psoriatic lesions, molecules such as TNF-α, transforming growth factor-β, vascular endothelial growth factor and platelet-derived growth factor have been isolated and are perhaps responsible for the changes in endothelial function[30]. The clonal expansion of the T cells occurs after the migration through the endothelium. The specific vascular pattern in PsA and the high concentrations of specific growth factors may suggest that the angiogenesis and the altered vascular function have important roles in the initiation of inflammation in the skin and the joints[21]. In contrast, investigation of in situ apoptosis in PsA, reactive arthritis and RA showed no differences between the diseases[31].

Proinflammatory cytokines

In psoriatic skin and in synovial membrane of patients with PsA, the concentrations of proinflammatory cytokines such as TNF-α or IL-1 are increased[32,33]. Danning and colleagues[34] investigated biopsies from synovial membrane from patients with PsA, RA and osteoarthritis, and skin biopsies from lesional and perilesional areas from patients with PsA. They showed that TNF-α, IL-1, IL-15 and IL-10 are expressed both in skin and in synovial membrane of patients with PsA in greater concentrations than in patients with osteoarthritis. The pattern of expression of monokines is similar in PsA and RA, although quantitative differences have been observed[34]. The expression of TNF-α, IL-1 and IL-15 is lower in the synovial membrane of PsA than in RA. The same was true for nuclear factor κB (NFκB), which is regulated by proinflammatory cytokines such as TNF-α. The reduced expression of TNF-α and NFκB may be due to the reduced number of macrophages in the synovial membrane of patients with PsA. These data suggest that the same cytokines trigger the inflammation in the skin and in the synovial mem-

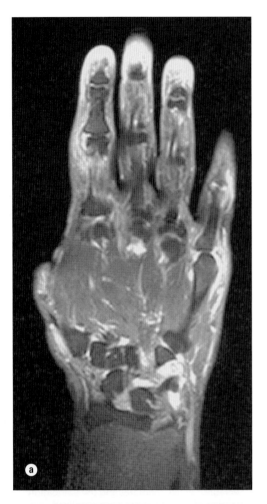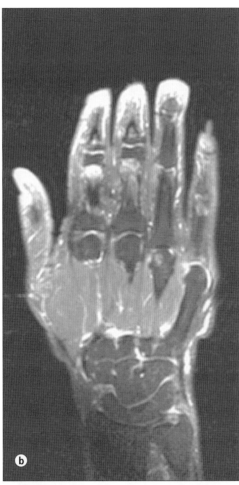

Fig. 111.1 Magnetic resonance images (with gadolinium uptake) showing the effect of infliximab treatment in the right hand of a patient with PsA. (a) The hand before treatment. (b) The hand after 10 weeks of anti-TNF-α treatment with infliximab. Synovitis of the fifth metacarpophalangeal and second proximal interphalangeal joints cleared during treatment.

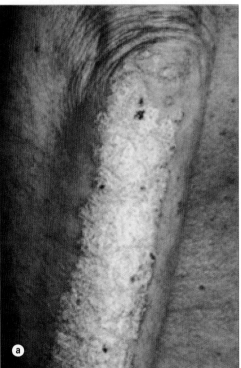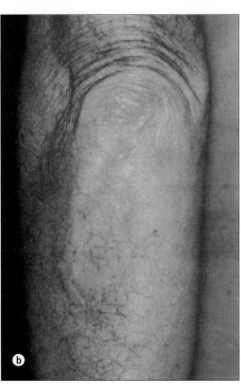

Fig. 111.2 Psoriatic lesion of the left elbow. (a) Before treatment. (b) After 10 weeks of anti-TNF-α treatment with infliximab.

brane in PsA. Despite the important role of T cells in the pathogenesis of PsA, cytokines are important in perpetuating the effector phase in the synovial membrane and the skin, and it was postulated that anti-TNF-α treatment would show efficacy in PsA, as it does in RA[34].

The occurrence of the skin lesion and the synovitis does not correlate in all patients. Anti-T cell treatment with cyclosporin A showed efficacy on both, but the skin and synovitis do not necessarily respond in the same manner. The success of anti-TNF treatment in RA and the scientific rationale of the role of proinflammatory cytokines in PsA led to open and double-blind trials investigating the efficacy of anti-TNF-α treatment in PsA. Mease and colleagues[35] showed, in a double-blind trial, that blockade of TNF with etanercept led not only to an impressive reduction in synovitis, but also to an improvement in skin lesions. In a small magnetic resonance imaging study, the efficacy of infliximab was

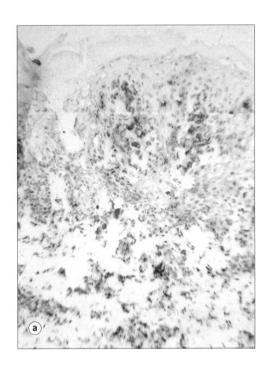
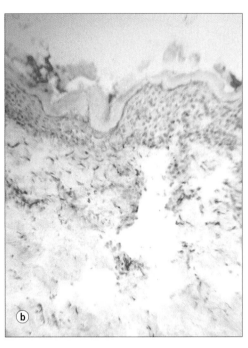

Fig. 111.3 Expression of HLA-DR. (a) Before anti-TNF-α treatment, expression is upregulated. (b) At week 10, expression is normalized.

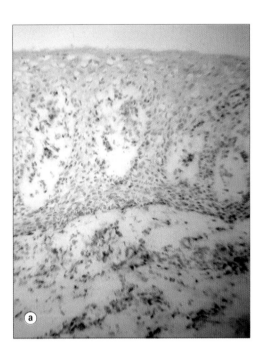
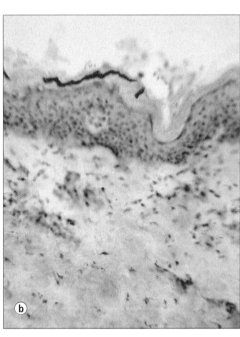

Fig. 111.4 Histology showing the effect of infliximab treatment in PsA. (a) Before initiation of anti-TNF-α treatment there is marked expression of TNF-α and inflammatory infiltrates. (b) At week 10 of treatment, TNF-α expression is no longer detectable. Cellular infiltrates and the elongation and fusion of the rete ridges are normalized.

demonstrated[36]. A reduction in synovitis during treatment was demonstrated using magnetic resonance imaging with gadolinium uptake (Fig. 111.1), and there was an improvement in skin lesions (Fig. 111.2). Skin biopsies taken at the same time points as the magnetic resonance images, before and 10 weeks after start of the infliximab treatment, also demonstrated a reduction of inflammation and cellular infiltrates and normalization of the skin. Histology also revealed marked reductions in the expression of HLA-DR (Fig. 111.3) and TNF-α (Fig. 111.4).

SUMMARY

The pathogenesis of PsA is complex. Because the manifestations of the skin and the joint can occur independently, different factors must be involved. Beside clinical similarities, the immunological features are comparable at both sites of the disease. The immunogenetics, histopathology and the role of the T cells, which may respond to a yet unidentified autoantigen, are disease specific. The cytokine expression is similar to that in RA, and anti-TNF-α treatment is efficacious. Whether the lower expression of proinflammatory cytokines in the synovial membrane has a pathogenic role has yet to be proven.

REFERENCES

1. McGonagle D, Stockwin L, Isaacs J et al. An enthesitis based model for the pathogenesis of spondyloarthropathy. Additive effects of microbial adjuvant and biomechanical factors at disease sites. J Rheumatol 2001; 28: 2155–2159.

2. Bruce IN, Silman AJ. The aetiology of psoriatic arthritis. Rheumatology (Oxf) 2001; 40: 363–366.

3. Kay LJ, Parry-James JE, Walker DJ. The prevalence and impact of psoriasis and psoriatic arthritis in the primary care population in North East England. Arthritis Rheum 1999; 42(suppl): S299.

4. Moll JM, Wright V. Familial occurrence of psoriatic arthritis. Ann Rheum Dis 1973; 32: 181–201.

5. Rahman P, Gladman DD, Schentag CT et al. Excessive paternal transmission in psoriatic arthritis. Arthritis Rheum 1999; 42: 1228–1231.

6. van Steensel MA, Steijlen PM. Genetics of psoriasis. Clin Dermatol 1997; 15: 669–675.

7. Eastmond CJ. Psoriatic arthritis. Genetics and HLA antigens. Baillières Clin Rheumatol 1994; 8: 263–276.

8. Gladman DD, Cheung C, Ng CM et al. HLA-C locus alleles in patients with psoriatic arthritis (PsA). Hum Immunol 1999; 60: 259–261.

9. Gladman DD, Anhorn KA, Schachter RK et al. HLA antigens in psoriatic arthritis. J Rheumatol 1986; 13: 586–592.

10. Marsal S, Armadans-Gil L, Martinez M et al. Clinical, radiographic and HLA associations as markers for different patterns of psoriatic arthritis. Rheumatology (Oxf) 1999; 38: 332–337.

11. Gonzalez S, Martinez-Borra J, Torre-Alonso JC et al. The MICA-A9 triplet repeat polymorphism in the transmembrane region confers additional susceptibility to the development of psoriatic arthritis and is independent of the association of Cw*0602 in psoriasis. Arthritis Rheum 1999; 42: 1010–1016.

12. Gonzalez S, Martinez-Borra J, Lopez-Vazquez A et al. MICA rather than MICB, TNFA, or HLA-DRB1 is associated with susceptibility to psoriatic arthritis. J Rheumatol 2002; 29: 973–978.

13. Wang Q, Vasey FB, Mahfood JP et al. V2 regions of 16S ribosomal RNA used as a molecular marker for the species identification of streptococci in peripheral blood and synovial fluid from patients with psoriatic arthritis. Arthritis Rheum 1999; 42: 2055–2059.

14. Thomssen H, Hoffmann B, Schank M et al. There is no disease-specific role for streptococci-responsive synovial T lymphocytes in the pathogenesis of psoriatic arthritis. Med Microbiol Immunol (Berl) 2000; 188: 203–207.

15. Njobvu P, McGill P. Psoriatic arthritis and human immunodeficiency virus infection in Zambia. J Rheumatol 2000; 27: 1699–702.

16. Scarpa R, Del Puente A, di Girolamo C et al. Interplay between environmental factors, articular involvement, and HLA-B27 in patients with psoriatic arthritis. Ann Rheum Dis 1992; 51: 78–79.

17. Punzi L, Pianon M, Bertazzolo N et al. Clinical, laboratory and immunogenetic aspects of post-traumatic psoriatic arthritis: a study of 25 patients. Clin Exp Rheumatol 1998; 16: 277–281.

18. Eedy DJ, Johnston CF, Shaw C et al. Neuropeptides in psoriasis: an immunocytochemical and radioimmunoassay study. J Invest Dermatol 1991; 96: 434–438.

19. Veale D, Farrell M, Fitzgerald O. Mechanism of joint sparing in a patient with unilateral psoriatic arthritis and a longstanding hemiplegia. Br J Rheumatol 1993; 32: 413–416.

20. Fortune DG, Main CJ, O'Sullivan TM et al. Quality of life in patients with psoriasis: the contribution of clinical variables and psoriasis-specific stress. Br J Dermatol 1997; 137: 755–760.

21. Fearon U, Veale DJ. Pathogenesis of psoriatic arthritis. Clin Exp Dermatol 2001; 26: 333–337.

22. Costello PJ, Winchester RJ, Curran SA et al. Psoriatic arthritis joint fluids are characterized by CD8 and CD4 T cell clonal expansions appear antigen driven. J Immunol 2001; 166: 2878–2886.

23. Costello P, Bresnihan B, O'Farrelly C et al. Predominance of CD8+ T lymphocytes in psoriatic arthritis. J Rheumatol 1999; 26: 1117–1124.

24. Tassiulas I, Duncan SR, Centola M et al. Clonal characteristics of T cell infiltrates in skin and synovium of patients with psoriatic arthritis. Hum Immunol 1999; 60: 479–491.

25. Papp K, Bissonnette R, Krueger JG et al. The treatment of moderate to severe psoriasis with a new anti-CD11a monoclonal antibody. J Am Acad Dermatol 2001; 45: 665–674.

26. Ellis CN, Krueger GG. Treatment of chronic plaque psoriasis by selective targeting of memory effector T lymphocytes. N Engl J Med 2001; 345: 248–255.

27. Daikeler T, Gunaydin I, Einsele H et al. Transmission of psoriatic arthritis by allogeneic bone marrow transplantation for chronic myelogenous leukaemia from an HLA-identical donor. Rheumatology (Oxf) 1999; 38: 89–90.

28. Espinoza LR, Vasey FB, Espinoza CG et al. Vascular changes in psoriatic synovium. A light and electron microscopic study. Arthritis Rheum 1982; 25: 677–684.

29. Reece RJ, Canete JD, Parsons WJ et al. Distinct vascular patterns of early synovitis in psoriatic, reactive, and rheumatoid arthritis. Arthritis Rheum 1999; 42: 1481–1484.

30. Creamer D, Jaggar R, Allen M et al. Overexpression of the angiogenic factor platelet-derived endothelial cell growth factor/thymidine phosphorylase in psoriatic epidermis. Br J Dermatol 1997; 137: 851–855.

31. Ceponis A, Hietanen J, Tamulaitiene M et al. A comparative quantitative morphometric study of cell apoptosis in synovial membranes in psoriatic, reactive and rheumatoid arthritis. Rheumatology (Oxf) 1999; 38: 431–440.

32. Olaniran AK, Baker BS, Paige DG et al. Cytokine expression in psoriatic skin lesions during PUVA therapy. Arch Dermatol Res 1996; 288: 421–425.

33. Partsch G, Steiner G, Leeb BF et al. Highly increased levels of tumor necrosis factor-alpha and other proinflammatory cytokines in psoriatic arthritis synovial fluid. J Rheumatol 1997; 24: 518–523.

34. Danning CL, Illei GG, Hitchon C et al. Macrophage-derived cytokine and nuclear factor kappaB p65 expression in synovial membrane and skin of patients with psoriatic arthritis. Arthritis Rheum 2000; 43: 1244–1256.

35. Mease PJ, Goffe BS, Metz J et al. Etanercept in the treatment of psoriatic arthritis and psoriasis: a randomised trial. Lancet 2000; 356: 385–390.

36. Antoni C, Dechant C, Lorenz HM et al. Open-label study of infliximab treatment for psoriatic arthritis: clinical and magnetic resonance imaging measurements of reduction of inflammation. Arthritis Rheum 2002; 47: 506–512.

112 Psoriatic arthritis: management

Marta L Cuéllar and Luis R Espinoza

- Management of psoriatic arthritis should be comprehensive and includes non-pharmacological, pharmacological, rehabilitative and surgical reconstructive therapies with concomitant skin management

- Most patients with psoriatic arthritis – particularly those with peripheral joint involvement – exhibit excellent clinical response to traditional or non-selective non-steroidal anti-inflammatory drugs (NSAIDs). Selective cyclo-oxygenase-2 inhibitors also appear to be effective, but prospective controlled studies regarding their efficacy are not yet available

- Disease-modifying agents, including methotrexate and leflunomide alone or in combination, are effective in the management of psoriatic arthritis refractory to NSAIDs

- The use of biological agents (infliximab, etanercept) is being shown to be highly efficacious and their use accompanied by a high remission rate and decreased progression of radiographic damage

TABLE 112.1 THERAPEUTIC MANAGEMENT OF PSORIATIC ARTHRITIS

Patient education	Assistive devices and educational material
Rehabilitation and physical therapy	Early and aggressive active and passive physical therapy Dynamic strengthening exercises Preservation of a normal upright posture Avoidance of contact sports and heavy physical activity
Pharmacologic measures	Non-steroidal anti-inflammatory drugs Selective COX-2 inhibitors Disease-modifying drugs
Dermatologic measures	Photochemotherapy with psoralen Steroids
Surgical measures	Synovectomy Joint arthroplasty

Early institution of an aggressive comprehensive medical management program may prevent the development of serious joint deformity and disability

INTRODUCTION

The introduction, in recent years, of more powerful and specific anti-inflammatory agents with improved efficacy or decreased toxicity, or both, is having a major impact in the way rheumatologists manage patients with chronic arthritis, including rheumatoid arthritis (RA) and psoriatic arthritis. The use of cyclo-oxygenase (COX)-2-selective non-steroidal anti-inflammatory drugs (NSAIDs), leflunomide, and specific tumor necrosis factor (TNF)-α inhibitors has expanded the therapeutic armamentarium for the management of these chronic rheumatic disorders[1–3]. Although it has become quite clear that treatment with methotrexate, sulfasalazine and cyclosporin is efficacious and associated with a fairly acceptable safety profile in patients with psoriatic arthritis[4,5], it is increasingly being demonstrated, particularly in RA, that the use of the newer compounds, especially the biologic agents etanercept and infliximab, is accompanied by a high rate of remission and decreased progression of radiographic damage[6,7].

These major advances in drug development are ameliorating the care provided to patients with psoriatic arthritis. More importantly, the early use of these agents allows better suppression of skin and joint inflammation, maintenance and improvement of musculoskeletal function, prevention of joint deformity and disability, and emotional adjustment to the presence of skin rash and arthritis[8,9]. A multidisciplinary approach involving the close collaboration of rheumatologists, dermatologists, primary care physicians, orthopedists and rehabilitation specialists is needed in order to accomplish these objectives.

The management of psoriatic arthritis should be a comprehensive one, and includes pharmacological, rehabilitative and surgical reconstructive treatments, with concomitant management of skin involvement[10] (Tables 112.1–112.3).

PHARMACOLOGIC MANAGEMENT

Non-steroidal anti-inflammatory treatment

Most patients with psoriatic arthritis exhibit excellent clinical response of their peripheral joint involvement while receiving NSAIDs. With the exception of aspirin, the great majority of traditional or non-selective NSAIDs, given at full doses, have been shown to be beneficial for patients with psoriatic arthritis presenting with the oligoarticular or monoarticular pattern of joint involvement[11]. In contrast, patients with psoriatic

TABLE 112.2 DISEASE-MODIFYING DRUGS IN PSORIATIC ARTHRITIS

- Methotrexate
- Sulfasalazine
- Cyclosporin A
- Azathioprine
- Leflunomide
- Biological agents
  - Etanercept (Enbrel)
  - Infliximab (Remicade)
  - Alefacept
- Gold compounds
- Retinoid treatment
- Corticosteroids
- Colchicine

The most common agents used in treatment of psoriatic arthritis – alone or in combination

TABLE 112.3 MISCELLANEOUS AGENTS USED IN THE TREATMENT OF PSORIATIC ARTHRITIS

- Antimalarials
- Vitamin D derivatives
- D-penicillamine
- Apheresis
- Antibiotics
- Non-selective inhibitors of TNF-α
  - Pamidronate?
  - Thalidomide?
- Alternative treatment?
- Autologous stem cell transplantation

The use of some of these agents and treatment modalities, such as alternative therapy, autologous stem cell transplantation and non-selective inhibitors of TNF-α, requires further investigation

arthritis exhibiting polyarticular, spondylitic or more severe forms of joint involvement usually require a more aggressive form of treatment, including the use of second-line agents alone or in combination.

There is still no great body of evidence regarding the use of celecoxib and rofecoxib, both COX-2-selective inhibitors, in patient with psoriatic arthritis. COX-2-selective inhibitors are replacing non-selective NSAIDs because of their better gastrointestinal safety[12], but their role in the management of psoriatic arthritis is not yet established. There is a need for prospective and controlled studies with selective COX-2 inhibitors in psoriatic arthritis, in order to define their precise role.

Disease-modifying agents

It is well established that psoriatic arthritis may not be benign, but can lead to significant functional limitation and deforming destructive arthropathy in up to 20–30% of patients[13]. Risk factors associated with poor prognosis have been identified (Table 112.4), and early use of more aggressive treatment, including disease-modifying agents, is widespread, with the added advantage that most of these agents also have a beneficial effect on psoriasis. A variety of disease-modifying agents have been used, including sulfasalazine, methotrexate, antimalarials, gold compounds, azathioprine, retinoids and cyclosporin A. More recently, the use of biologic agents such as etanercept and infliximab, and other agents such as leflunomide, has been shown to have an excellent beneficial effect for both skin and joint involvement, accompanied by a good safety profile.

Methotrexate

Methotrexate is the agent of choice for a large proportion of patients with psoriatic arthritis unresponsive to NSAIDs[14]. Its use in early psori-

TABLE 112.4 PSORIATIC ARTHRITIS: RISK FACTORS FOR A POOR PROGNOSIS

- Juvenile onset
- Young adult onset
- Extensive skin involvement
- Polyarticular involvement
- Failed response to non-steroidal anti-inflammatory drugs
- Association with HIV infection
- Association with certain HLA antigens
  - HLA-B27, correlates with spondylitic involvement
  - HLA-B27, -B39 and -DQw3 correlate with progressive disease
  - HLA-DR3, -DR4 correlate with erosive disease.

Recognition of these risk factors associated with disease severity allows better and prompt planning of an early and aggressive therapeutic program

atic arthritis with or without NSAIDs or in combination with other disease-modifying agents, particularly sulfasalazine or cyclosporin A, has been recommended. The average dose is between 7.5 and 15mg per week, given as a single dose or divided into two doses taken 12h apart on the same day; we prefer the former. The dosage can be increased to 25–30mg per week until improvement occurs, and then it should be tapered down to a maintenance dose, which varies from patient to patient. Methotrexate given at these dosages has been shown to be effective for both skin and joint inflammatory involvement in most studies, both control and uncontrolled. Some studies, however, have failed to demonstrate its efficacy in the treatment of psoriatic arthritis.

Lacaille et al.[15] recently reported on their experience with long-term treatment with intramuscular gold and methotrexate. They reviewed medical records from all patients with psoriatic arthritis attending the gold and methotrexate clinics at the Vancouver Mary Pack Arthritis Centre between 1971 and 1995. The odds of a clinical response (defined as at least 50% reduction in active joint count from initial to last visit or for at least 6 months) and the relative risk of discontinuing treatment (methotrexate or intramuscular gold) were estimated after controlling for significant baseline covariates, using logistic regression and Cox regression analyses, respectively. The frequency of side effects and the reasons for treatment cessation were also compared. Eighty-seven patients received 111 treatment courses, 43 of methotrexate and 68 of intramuscular gold. The likelihood of a clinical response was 8.9 times greater [95% confidence interval (CI) 1.8 to 44.0] with methotrexate than with intramuscular gold. The frequency of side effects was similar for both treatments, but patients were 5 times more likely (95% CI 2.4 to 10.4) to discontinue treatment with intramuscular gold than with methotrexate. No major or severe toxicity occurred. Of interest, patients with psoriatic arthritis with a longer duration of disease before initiation of study treatment were less likely to achieve a clinical response. The authors concluded that methotrexate was well tolerated and superior to intramuscular gold, and that their data supported the notion that earlier treatment may be associated with a better clinical response.

In general, methotrexate is well tolerated and has a very good safety profile. It is necessary, however, to monitor carefully liver and renal function, hematological indexes and other predisposing risk factors, such as low serum albumin, concomitant use of antibiotics, in order to prevent serious toxicity[16]. Serious side effects may occur, but appear to be relatively infrequent, particularly if monitoring is performed every 6–8 weeks (Table 112.5). At present, there are no adequate evidence-based guidelines for monitoring liver toxicity in patients with psoriatic arthritis who are receiving methotrexate treatment. Therefore, it is recommended that each patient's need for liver biopsy should be evaluated individually and that patients should undergo biopsy only if a specific cumulative dose of methotrexate has been reached (>3g) or a persistent significant increase in liver enzymes is present (more than three times the upper limit of normal). The American College of Rheumatology guidelines for monitoring liver toxicity in methotrexate-treated patients with RA recommend that liver biopsies need not be

TABLE 112.5 RISK FACTORS ASSOCIATED WITH METHOTREXATE TOXICITY

- Renal insufficiency
- Low serum albumin
- Concomitant use of antibiotics
- Folate deficiency
- Older age
- Cumulative dose

Predisposing factors most commonly associated with methotrexate toxicity

performed before methotrexate administration or routinely thereafter. These suggestions were based on the incidence of clinically significant liver disease, the factors predictive of its occurrence, the cost of the procedure and the complications arising from it[17].

Sulfasalazine

Evidence accumulated over the past several years has provided support for a beneficial effect of sulfasalazine in patients with psoriatic arthritis. Both controlled and uncontrolled studies have demonstrated a good clinical response of the peripheral arthritis in patients with psoriatic arthritis. Its main limiting factor is its well-recognized gastrointestinal intolerance, with up to 40% of patients unable to tolerate full doses because of severe gastrointestinal distress.

Clegg et al.[18] have published their experience with sulfasalazine in the treatment of psoriatic arthritis. Their objective was to determine whether sulfasalazine at a dosage of 2g/day was effective for the treatment of active psoriatic arthritis unresponsive to NSAIDs. They recruited 221 patients with psoriatic arthritis from 15 clinics, allocated them randomly to groups to receive sulfasalazine or placebo, and followed them for 36 weeks. Treatment response was based on joint pain/tenderness and swelling scores, and physician and patient global assessment. Longitudinal analysis revealed a trend favoring sulfasalazine treatment, although this did not reach statistical significance. At the end of treatment, response rates were 58% for sulfasalazine, compared with 45% for placebo ($p = 0.05$). In addition, the Westergren erythrocyte sedimentation rate declined more in the group taking sulfasalazine than in those taking placebo ($p < 0.0001$). Adverse reactions were few and were mainly non-specific gastrointestinal complaints such as dyspepsia, nausea, vomiting and diarrhea.

In a subsequent analysis, Clegg et al.[19] examined the data comparing the effects of sulfasalazine 2g/day and placebo on the axial and peripheral articular manifestations of psoriatic arthritis. Patients were classified as treatment responders on the basis of meeting predefined improvement criteria in four outcome measures: both patient and physician global assessments in all patients, morning stiffness and back pain in patients with axial manifestations, and joint pain/tenderness scores and joint swelling scores in patients with peripheral articular manifestations. Of the patients with axial disease, 40% of the sulfasalazine group and 43% of the placebo group met the predefined response criteria ($p = 0.67$). Of the patients with peripheral arthritis, 59% of the sulfasalazine-treated patients and 43% of the placebo-treated patients showed a response ($p = 0.0007$). Therefore, it appears that the response to sulfasalazine of patients with seronegative spondyloarthropathy including psoriatic arthritis is related to the peripheral articular manifestations of their disease. Axial and peripheral articular manifestations of seronegative spondyloarthropathy appear to respond differently to sulfasalazine. In patients with persistently active peripheral arthritis, sulfasalazine is safe, well tolerated, and effective.

Rahman et al.[20] also published their experience of the use of sulfasalazine in patients with psoriatic arthritis attending their psoriatic arthritis clinic at the University of Toronto. For patients who were able to tolerate sulfasalazine for at least 3 months, a matched control was identified who did not receive sulfasalazine. The primary outcome measures were the tolerability of sulfasalazine, clinical response of the actively inflamed joints at 6 and 12 months, and the change in radiograph score at 24 months. Thirty-six patients received sulfasalazine. Fourteen patients discontinued sulfasalazine because of one or more side effects occurring within 3 months of initiation of treatment. For the remaining 20 patients, a 50% reduction in actively inflamed joint count was seen in seven of 20 patients at 6 months and 11 of 15 patients at 12 months, compared with seven of 19 patients in the control group at 6 months and 10 of 20 at 12 months. No change in radiographic score at 24 months was observed in either group. In this study, sulfasalazine treatment was accompanied by a high frequency of side effects, did not show beneficial effect over the control group, and did not halt radiographic progress in psoriatic arthritis.

There is a high rate of discontinuation of sulfasalazine secondary to gastrointestinal intolerance. In order to minimize this, a 'start low, go slow' approach is recommended. In addition, the use of enteric-coated formulations of sulfasalazine should improve gastrointestinal tolerability and thus patient acceptance. It is recommended to start with 500mg of sulfasalazine twice daily for the first 10–14 days, and then to increase it gradually over, the next 2–3 weeks, to 2g daily. Some patients may require doses up to 3g daily.

Cyclosporin A

The use of cyclosporin A alone or in combination with other disease-modifying antirheumatic drugs (DMARDs), most commonly methotrexate, sulfasalazine, or both, has been shown to be an effective therapeutic agent for the treatment of severe, recalcitrant psoriasis and its related arthritis. Cyclosporin A has also been shown to be effective in patients with palmoplantar pustulosis, and in the presence of certain extra-articular and dermatological complications, including lymphedema[21].

The efficacy of cyclosporin A in the treatment of these disorders has been demonstrated in several placebo-controlled studies[22]. Most recently, Raffayova et al.[23] conducted an open 18-week study with cyclosporin A administered to patients with psoriatic arthritis and confirmed its therapeutic efficacy. A significant improvement in psoriatic symptoms was observed during the study. As early as 2 weeks after administration of an average daily dose of cyclosporin A 4.8mg/kg, skin symptoms improved by 66%. Arthritis also improved after 18 weeks. In this study, the lowest optimal effective maintenance dose was 3.3mg/kg. Improvement was achieved after an average of 10 weeks of administration of cyclosporin A.

In general, the clinical response of both skin and joint involvement is dose related, and may occur with doses of cyclosporin A appreciably lower than those used in transplantation – for example, 2.5–5mg/kg per day – and improvement is seen at 3–4 weeks in most patients. Some concern, however, remains about serious side effects, particularly renal, even with low doses. The exact rate of relapse upon discontinuation of the drug, its long-term side effects, and its high costs are issues that remain unsolved.

Leflunomide

Leflunomide is a relatively new agent in the antirheumatic treatment of RA[24]. The active metabolite, A-77-1726, inhibits the enzyme dihydro-orotate dehydrogenase, which has a critical role in de novo production of pyrimidine. It controls mitogen-induced T cell proliferation, as the presence of pyrimidine is needed for this process to proceed. Psoriasis and its related arthritis are believed to be mediated by T cell dependent mechanisms[25,26].

Liang and Barr[27] recently evaluated the efficacy and toxicity of this compound in the treatment of both psoriasis and psoriatic arthritis. Twelve consecutive patients with psoriatic arthritis who had failed to respond to at least one DMARD were started on a regimen of leflunomide alone or in addition to their previous disease-modifying medication. Global assessment of improvement in psoriasis and psoriatic arthritis was scored on a 0–3 scale after 2–3 months of treatment. Modified tender and swollen joint counts, patients' and physicians' global assessments and grip strength before and after treatment were available for analysis in 50% of these patients. Eight patients had combined moderate-to-marked improvement in both psoriasis and psoriatic arthritis. Three patients in whom toxicity necessitated the temporary discontinuation of the drug were able to resume the drug at lower dosage with a good clinical benefit. Three patients discontinued the treatment, but in none of them was this because of toxicity. Effect on radiological progression of the disease was not evaluated. These data suggest that leflunomide alone or in combination with another DMARD may be effective in controlling both skin and joint disease in patients with psoriasis and psoriatic arthritis. Improvement was seen within 4–8 weeks, and arthritis appeared to have a better and more rapid response than skin involvement. There is a need, however, for placebo-controlled trials of leflunomide in psoriatic arthritis.

The correct place of leflunomide in the management of psoriatic arthritis remains to be determined. Extrapolating from the experience seen in RA, it appears that leflunomide may be indicated initially in those patients with psoriatic arthritis who have suboptimal responses to methotrexate, or in combination with methotrexate. This combination – leflunomide and methotrexate – is well tolerated by RA patients and there are no significant pharmacokinetic interactions between the drugs[28]. The potential risk of serious liver damage should be kept in mind, however, when combination treatment with leflunomide and methotrexate is used[29].

Leflunomide is contraindicated during pregnancy and lactation. Contraception is mandatory for women of childbearing age who are receiving this drug. Women receiving leflunomide who are suspected to be pregnant should stop it immediately and be carefully monitored by their physician. A negative pregnancy test before initiation of treatment is recommended. Men receiving leflunomide should also use adequate contraception.

Gold therapy

Chrysotherapy is beneficial in a subset of patients with psoriatic arthritis[30]. Patients with psoriatic arthritis exhibiting polyarticular involvement present a better clinical response to gold compounds than do patients with psoriatic arthritis presenting with the oligoarticular and spondylitic types. It has been shown, however, to be much less effective than methotrexate treatment[15].

Azathioprine

Azathioprine has been shown to be effective in psoriasis for both skin and joint involvement[31]. Doses ranging from 2 to 3mg/kg per day are recommended, with close monitoring of bone marrow function, because of the potential of the drug for serious marrow toxicity. Patients receiving long-term azathioprine treatment should also be screened for underlying malignancy. Azathioprine hypersensitivity reactions may also occur[32].

Retinoid treatment

Retinoid compounds, particularly etritinate, have been shown to be highly effective in the management of psoriasis and psoriatic arthritis[33]. A main limitation in the use of these compounds, however, is the high incidence of side effects. In addition, the teratogenic potential of these compounds remains a serious limitation for their use in women of childbearing age.

Mycophenolate mofetil

Mycophenolate mofetil is widely used as an immunosuppressant in organ transplantation, and also in some autoimmune disorders such as pyroderma gangrenosum, systemic lupus erythematosus and dermatomyositis[34]. It has recently been used with great effectiveness in psoriasis and psoriatic arthritis. Grundman-Kollman et al.[35] reported their experience in five patients with moderate to severe chronic plaque psoriasis and six patients with psoriatic arthritis refractory to conventional systemic or topical antipsoriatic treatment and who were treated with mycophenolate mofetil monotherapy (2g/day) in a 10-week study. Patients with moderate psoriasis and psoriatic arthritis responded well to treatment, whereas those with severe psoriasis did not respond to this

drug. It was well tolerated, and this compound may develop into a therapeutic alternative in patients with psoriatic arthritis.

Meta-analysis of DMARDs

Jones et al.[36] performed a meta-analysis in psoriatic arthritis, with the objective of determining the relative efficacy and toxicity of pharmacological agents in the treatment of the condition. The main outcome measures included individual component variables derived from the Outcome Measures in Rheumatology Clinical Trials Core Set for RA. These include acute-phase reactants, disability, pain, patient global assessment, swollen joint count, tender joint count and radiographic changes of joints in any trial of 1 year or longer, and the change in pooled disease index. Nineteen randomized trials were identified, of which 11 were included in the quantitative analysis with data from 777 individuals. All agents were better than placebo, but only parenteral high-dose methotrexate, salazopyrin, azathioprine and etretinate achieved statistical significance for the global index of disease activity. Analysis of response in individual disease activity markers was more variable, with considerable differences between different medications and responses. In all trials, the placebo group improved over baseline. There were insufficient data to allow examination of toxicity. It was concluded that parenteral high-dose methotrexate and salazopyrin are the only two agents with well-demonstrated published efficacy in psoriatic arthritis. The magnitude of the effect with etretinate, oral low-dose methotrexate and azathioprine suggests that they may be effective, but that further multicenter clinical trials are needed to establish their efficacy.

Biologic agents

Two biologic agents, etanercept and infliximab – both TNF-α inhibitors – have been approved for their use in the treatment of RA[37,38]. Inhibition of the proinflammatory cytokine, TNF, is associated with a marked decrease in the signs and symptoms of RA in the majority of patients.

Both psoriasis and its related arthritis are pathological processes mainly mediated by activated T cells, which appear to be responsible for the epidermal and synovial hyperproliferation seen, and also inflammatory infiltration in the epidermis, dermis and subsynovial space[25,26]. These activated T cells release a variety of cytokines, including TNF-α, interleukin (IL)-6, IL-8, granulocyte-macrophage colony-stimulating factor (GM-CSF), and interferon gamma. The proinflammatory cytokine TNF-α has a major role in this process, and has been detected in increased concentrations in both psoriatic skin and synovial lesions. TNF-α, through activation of nuclear factor (NF) κB, induces synthesis of several cytokines, particularly IL-6, IL-8 and GM-CSF. In addition, TNF-α favors the accumulation of inflammatory cells in both skin and synovium, by upregulating the expression of intracellular adhesion molecule-I on endothelial cells and keratinocytes[39]. Therefore, it is quite logical to assume a potential role for TNF-α in both psoriasis and psoriatic arthritis, and also infer that use of inhibitors of TNF-α may result in amelioration of disease activity in these disorders.

Evidence is rapidly accumulating, from both controlled and uncontrolled trials, that inhibition of TNF-α results in significant clinical response of both psoriasis and psoriatic arthritis.

The first randomized, double-blind, placebo-controlled trial of etanercept, a TNF-α inhibitor, in patients with psoriatic arthritis was a 12-week study undertaken to assess the efficacy and safety of etanercept 25 mg twice weekly by subcutaneous injection or placebo, in 60 patients with psoriasis and psoriatic arthritis[40]. Psoriatic arthritis endpoints included the proportion of patients who met the Psoriatic Arthritis Response Criteria and who met the American College of Rheumatology preliminary criteria for improvement (ACR20). Psoriasis endpoints included improvement in the psoriasis area and severity index (PASI), and improvement in prospectively identified individual target lesions. Most psoriatic arthritis patients (87%) fulfilled the Psoriatic Arthritis Response Criteria, compared with seven (23%) of patients in the placebo-controlled group. The ACR20 was achieved by 22 (73%) of etanercept-treated patients, compared with four (13%) of placebo-treated patients. Of the 19 patients in each treatment group assessed for psoriasis, five (26%) of the etanercept-treated patients achieved a 75% improvement in the PASI, compared with none of the placebo-treated patients ($p = 0.015$). The median improvement in PASI was 46%, compared with 9% in etanercept-treated and placebo-treated patients, respectively; similarly, median target lesion improvements were 50% and 0, respectively. Etanercept was well tolerated.

Several pilot studies have shown similar result[41–43]. In our experience with more than 20 patients with psoriatic arthritis treated in this manner, etanercept has been shown to be highly effective for both skin and nails, and also joint involvement – both peripheral and spinal. Some of our patients with psoriatic arthritis have also experienced a significant radiologic improvement in their erosive involvement, in a manner similar to that described for RA patients. Etanercept has also been shown to be effective in human immunodeficiency virus-associated psoriatic arthritis refractory to DMARDs[44]. Its use in this situation, however, should be carefully monitored, in view of the fatal sepsis that occurred in that particular patient[44].

An open trial of infliximab, the second inhibitor of TNF-α approved for the treatment of RA, has shown this agent to be highly effective in the treatment of severe psoriatic arthritis, and well tolerated over 1 year of use. As already shown with etanercept, skin involvement also responds well[45].

Data on the use of these agents in psoriasis are also relevant for consideration. Chaudhari et al.[46] recently published their experience with infliximab in a group of patients with psoriasis who had moderate to severe plaque psoriasis involving at least 5% of the body surface area. Their objective was to assess the clinical benefit and safety of infliximab monotherapy and to determine the role of TNF-α in the pathogenesis of psoriasis. Thirty-three patients were randomly assigned to receive intravenous placebo ($n = 11$) or infliximab 5mg/kg ($n = 11$) or infliximab 10mg/kg ($n = 11$) at weeks 0, 2 and 6. Patients were assessed at week 10 for the primary endpoint (score on the physician's global assessment). Three patients withdrew from the study. Both groups of infliximab-treated patients experienced significant and similar clinical improvement when compared with those receiving placebo. The median time to response was 4 weeks for patients in both infliximab groups. Infliximab was well tolerated and no serious side effects were noted. These findings confirm the efficacy of inhibition of TNF-α in the treatment of psoriasis, and also provide support for an important role of TNF-α in the pathogenesis of these disorders.

Accumulated evidence strongly suggests that both available inhibitors of TNF-α are powerful anti-inflammatory agents and extremely effective for both psoriasis and psoriatic arthritis. Issues that remain to be defined include whether or not they should be used in patients refractory to other DMARDs, whether they should be used alone or in combination with other DMARDS, and for how long they should be used. Their place in the management of these disorders, however, remains to be defined. There is a need for long-term studies to determine their safety profile, especially given the recent reports of rare but serious infectious complications in patients with RA[47].

A highly promising disease-remitting agent, alefacept, has recently been shown to be effective in the treatment of chronic plaque psoriasis. Alefacept exerts a pronounced inhibitory effect on CD45RO$^+$ T lymphocytes and was shown in a multicenter, randomized, placebo-controlled, double-blind study to be associated with significant and, in some patients, sustained clinical response after the cessation of treatment.

Patients with psoriatic arthritis were not included in the study, however[48].

Other drugs

Corticosteroid treatment

Systemic corticosteroids should be used only in extreme situations such as in patients with severe exacerbation of both skin and joint disease refractory to conventional treatment. Their topical use, however, is recommended for control of skin disease. Their use in children should be avoided because of the high relapse rate, and toxicity upon reduction or discontinuation of their use. Intra-articular corticosteroid use may be of great benefit in patients with mono- or oligoarticular psoriatic arthritis. The use of high-frequency ultrasonography may provide great guidance when approaching small joints[49].

Colchichine treatment

Colchicine at a dose of 1.5 mg/day in divided doses may be of benefit to a subset of patients with psoriatic arthritis, such as those presenting with arthro-osteitis and SAPHO syndrome[50]. It has been reported that colchicine may be beneficial for renal amyloidosis associated with psoriatic arthritis[51].

Miscellaneous agents

A variety of agents, including antimalarials, apheresis, vitamin D derivatives, D-penicillamine and photochemotherapy with methoxypsoralen, have been used to treat patients with psoriatic arthritis[52,53]. The use of these agents, however, has almost been abandoned in favor of methotrexate or newer DMARDs or biologic agents, because of their limited clinical response, or their high frequency of side effects.

It would be of great interest to assess the clinical response of patients with psoriatic arthritis to less selective inhibitors of TNF-α. Both pamidronate – a bisphosphonate synthetic analog of pyrophosphate – and thalidomide have been shown to inhibit the action of TNF-α. To date, clinical experience with these compounds has shown promising clinical responses in patients with ankylosing spondylitis[54,55]. Autologous stem cell transplantation is a promising therapeutic option in some refractory autoimmune disorders. To date, however, there is only limited experience in psoriatic arthritis, and further studies are needed to define its indications and effectiveness in the management of psoriatic arthritis[56].

NON-DRUG TREATMENTS

Balneotherapy

Balneotherapy (mud packs and sulfur baths) at the Dead Sea has been shown to benefit patients with psoriatic arthritis[57]. More recently, Elkayan et al.[58] reported on their experience in a total of 42 patients with psoriatic arthritis treated for 4 weeks. Patients were randomly allocated to two groups. Both groups received daily sun exposure and regular bathing at the Dead Sea; one group was also treated with mud packs and sulfur baths. Patients were assessed 3 days before arrival, at the end of 4 weeks, and at weeks 8, 16 and 28 from the start of treatment. Comparison between groups revealed a similar statistically significant improvement for variables such as PASI, morning stiffness, patient self-assessment, right and left grip, Schober test and distance from finger to floor when bending forward. Improvement in other variables such as number of tender and swollen joints, and inflammatory neck and back pain, was statistically significant only in the group receiving balneotherapy. Thus the addition of balneotherapy to sun exposure and Dead Sea baths appears to prolong beneficial effects and improves inflammatory neck and back pain. Sukenik et al.[59] obtained similar results in patients with psoriatic arthritis and concomitant fibromyalgia.

REHABILITATION

The indications for rehabilitation management follow the same guidelines as those for any other chronic inflammatory articular disorder. Rehabilitation therapy should be considered in every patient with psoriatic arthritis, and should be aimed at maximizing the potential for normal physical and emotional activities.

Most patients with psoriatic arthritis will benefit from a combination of rest, exercise and, when appropriate, selective joint immobilization. The implementation of any of these measures alone or in combination will depend on the degree of active synovitis and the type and size of joint involvement. Early joint mobilization after surgery, particularly of small joints of the hands, is necessary because rapid development of joint/bone fusion is characteristically seen in psoriatic arthritis. Local heat facilitates implementation of exercise therapy in the postoperative phase.

Cryotherapy in the form of ice packs, ethyl chloride or fluromethane sprays, or ice massage is more beneficial and physiologic in the presence of enthesitis and joint inflammation.

In patients with spondylitis, implementation of exercise designed to preserve a normal upright posture is recommended. Treatment to prevent or to treat osteoporosis should be instituted as early as possible and prolonged use of corsets or bed rest should also be avoided. Patients with psoriatic arthritis should be counseled and advised to avoid heavy physical activity and contact sports, but swimming should be encouraged.

The use of orthotic devices including crutches, walkers, canes and splints should be advised in order to improve both ambulation and the functional capacity of a given joint.

SURGICAL MANAGEMENT

Considerable progress in the medical management of psoriasis and psoriatic arthritis has occurred. This is expected to translate into an improved morbidity and other related complications in these disorders. With the advent of newer therapeutic modalities, particularly the use of biologic agents, it is anticipated that there will be a greater rate of remission and, more importantly, preservation of joint function and prevention of joint destruction and deformity, in patients with psoriatic arthritis. Synovectomy may still be used in highly selected cases, and major reconstructive surgery, including joint replacement, is to be performed when necessary.

REFERENCES

1. Dougados M, Behier JM, Jolchine I et al. Efficacy of celecoxib, a COX-2 specific inhibitor in ankylosing spondylitis: a placebo and conventional NSAID controlled study. Arthritis Rheum 2001; 44: 180–185.
2. Weinblatt ME, Kremer JM, Coblyn JS et al. Pharmacokinetics, safety, and efficacy of combination treatment with MTX and leflunomide in patients with active rheumatoid arthritis. Arthritis Rheum 1999; 42: 1322–1328.
3. Jones RE, Moreland LW.Tumor necrosis factor inhibitors for rheumatoid arthritis. Bull Rheum Dis 1999; 48: 1–4.
4. Cuellar ML, Espinoza LR. Management of the spondyloarthropathies. Curr Opinion Rheumatol 1996; 8: 288–295.
5. Salvarani C, Olivieri I, Cantini F et al. Psoriatic arthritis. Curr Opinion Rheumatol 1999; 11: 251–256.
6. Moreland LW, Schiff MH, Baumgartner SW et al. Etanercept therapy in rheumatoid arthritis. A randomized, controlled trial. Ann Intern Med 1999; 130: 478–486.
7. Antoni C, Kalden JR. Combination therapy of the chimeric monoclonal anti-tumor necrosis factor alpha antibody (infliximab) with methotrexate in patients with rheumatoid arthritis. Clin Exp Rheumatol 1999; 17(suppl 18): S73–S77.
8. Cuellar ML, Citera G, Espinoza LR. Treatment of psoriatic arthritis. Baillières Clin Rheumatol 1994; 8: 483–498.
9. Gladman DD. Natural history of psoriatic arthritis. Baillières Clin Rheumatol 1994; 8: 379–394.
10. Cuellar ML, Espinoza LR. Psoriatic arthritis: current development. J Fla Med Assoc 1995; 82: 338–342.
11. Gladman DD, Brockbank J. Psoriatic arthritis. Exp Opinion Invest Drugs 2000; 9: 1511–1522.
12. Lipsky PE, Abramson SB, Breedveld FC et al. Analysis of the effect of COX-2 specific inhibitors and recommendations for their use in clinical practice. J Rheumatol 2000; 27: 1338–1340.
13. Gladman DD, Schuckett R, Russell ML et al. Psoriatic arthritis (PSA) – an analysis of 220 patients. Q J Med 1987; 238: 127–141.
14. Espinoza LR, Zakraoui L, Espinoza CG et al. Psoriatic arthritis: clinical responses and side effects to methotrexate therapy. J Rheumatol 1992; 12: 872–877.
15. Lacaille D, Stein HB, Raboud J, Klinkhoff AV. Longterm therapy of psoriatic arthritis: intramuscular gold or methotrexate? J Rheumatol 2000; 27: 1922–1927.
16. Gutierrez-Urena S, Molina JF, Garcia C et al. Pancytopenia secondary to methotrexate therapy in rheumatoid arthritis. Arthritis Rheum 1996; 39: 272–276.
17. Kremer JM, Alarcon GS, Lightfoot RW Jr et al. Methotrexate for rheumatoid arthritis: suggested guidelines for monitoring liver toxicity. Arthritis Rheum 1994; 37: 316–328.
18. Clegg DO, Reda DJ, Mejias E et al. Comparison of sulfasalazine and placebo in the treatment of psoriatic arthritis. A Department of Veterans Affairs Study. Arthritis Rheum 1996; 39: 2013–2020.
19. Clegg DO, Reda DJ, Abdellatif M. Comparison of sulfasalazine and placebo for the treatment of axial and peripheral articular manifestations of the seronegative spondyloarthropathies: a Department of Veterans Affairs cooperative study. Arthritis Rheum 1999; 42: 2325–2329.
20. Rahman P, Gladman DD, Cook RJ et al. The use of sulfasalazine in psoriatic arthritis: a clinic experience. J Rheumatol 1998; 25: 1957–1961.
21. Vaccaro M, Borgia F, Guarneri F et al. Successful treatment of pustulotic arthro-osteitis (Sonozaki syndrome) with systemic cyclosporin. Clin Exp Dermatol 2001; 26: 45–47.
22. Mahrle G, Schulze HJ, Farber L et al. Low-dose short-term cyclosporine versus etretinate in psoriasis: improvement of skin, nail, and joint involvement. J Am Acad Dermatol 1995; 32: 78–88.
23. Raffayova H, Rovensky J, Malis F. Treatment with cyclosporin in patients with psoriatic arthritis: results of clinical assessment. Int J Clin Pharmacol Res 2000; 20: 1–11.
24. Kremer JM. Methotrexate and leflunomide: biochemical basis for combination therapy in the treatment of rheumatoid arthritis. Semin Arthritis Rheum 1999; 29: 14–26.
25. Gottlieb AB. Immunopathogenesis of psoriasis. Arch Dermatol 1997; 133: 781–782.
26. Espinoza LR, van Solingen R, Cuellar ML, Angulo J. Insights into the pathogenesis of psoriasis and psoriatic arthritis. Am J Med Sci 1998; 316: 271–276.
27. Liang GC, Barr WG. Leflunomide for psoriasis and psoriatic arthritis. J Clin Rheumatol 2001; 7: 366–370.
28. Fox RI. Mechanism of action of leflunomide in rheumatoid arthritis. J Rheumatol 1998; 25: 5306–5326.
29. Mroczkowski PJ, Weinblatt ME, Kremer JM. MTX and leflunomide combination therapy for patients with active rheumatoid arthritis. Clin Exp Rheumatol 1999; 17: S66–S68.
30. Bruckle W, Dexel T, Grasedyck K, Schatten Kirchner M. Treatment of psoriatic arthritis. Clin Rheumatol 1994; 13: 209–216.
31. Levy J, Paulus H, Eugene V et al. A double-blind controlled evaluation of azathioprine treatment in rheumatoid arthritis and psoriatic arthritis. Arthritis Rheum 1992; 15: 116–117.
32. Fields CL, Robinson JW, Roy JM et al. Hypersensitivity reaction to azathioprine. South Med J 1998; 91: 471–474.
33. Klinkhoff AV, Gertner E, Chalmers A et al. Pilot study of etretinate in psoriatic arthritis. J Rheumatol 1989; 16: 789–791.
34. Gelber AC, Nousari HC, Wigley FM. Mycophenolate mofetil in the treatment of severe skin manifestations of DM: a series of 4 cases. J Rheumatol 2000; 27: 1542–1545.
35. Grundman-Kollman M, Mooser G, Schraeder P et al. Treatment of chronic plaque-stage psoriasis and psoriatic arthritis with mycophenolate mofetil. J Am Acad Dermatol 2000; 42: 835–837.
36. Jones G, Crotty M, Brooks P. Psoriatic arthritis: a quantitative overview of therapeutic options. The psoriatic arthritis meta-analysis study group. Br J Rheumatol 1997; 36: 95–99.
37. Moreland LW, Baumgartner SW, Schiff MH et al. Treatment of rheumatoid arthritis with a recombinant human tumor necrosis factor receptor (p75)–Fc fusion protein. N Engl J Med 1997; 337: 141–147.
38. Maini RN, Breedveld FC, Kalden JR et al. Therapeutic efficacy of multiple i.v. infusions of anti-tumor necrosis factor alpha monoclonal antibody combined with low-dose weekly methotrexate in rheumatoid arthritis. Arthritis Rheum 1998; 41: 1552–1563.
39. Ettehadi P, Greaves MW, Wallach D et al. Elevated tumor necrosis-alpha biological activity in psoriatic skin lesions. Clin Exp Immunol 1994; 96: 146–151.
40. Mease PJ, Goffe BS, Metz J et al. Etanercept in the treatment of psoriatic arthritis and psoriasis: a randomized trial. Lancet 2000; 356: 385–390.
41. Elkayam O, Yaron M, Caspi D. From wheels to feet: a dramatic response of severe chronic psoriatic arthritis to etanercept. Ann Rheum Dis 2000; 59: 839.
42. Yazici Y, Erkan D, Lockshin MD. A preliminary study of etanercept in the treatment of severe, resistant psoriatic arthritis. Clin Exp Rheumatol 2000; 18: 732–734.
43. Cuellar ML, Mendez EA, Collins RD et al. Efficacy of etanercept in refractory psoriatic arthritis. Arthritis Rheum 2000; 43:(suppl): S106.
44. Aboulafia DM, Bundow D, Wilkse K, Ochs UI. Etanercept for the treatment of human immunodeficiency virus-associated psoriatic arthritis. Mayo Clin Proc 2000; 75: 1093–1098.

45. Dechant C, Antoni C, Wendler J *et al*. One year outcome of patients with severe psoriatic arthritis treated with infliximab. Arthritis Rheum 2000; 43 (suppl): S102.

46. Chaudhari U, Romano P, Mulcahy LD *et al*. Efficacy and safety of infliximab monotherapy for plaque-type psoriasis: a randomized trial. Lancet 2001; 357: 1842–1847.

47. Keane J, Gershon S, Wise RP *et al*. Tuberculosis associated with infliximab, a tumor necrosis factor α-neutralizing agent. N Engl J Med 2001; 345: 1098–1104.

48. Ellis CN, Krugeger GG. Treatment of chronic plaque psoriasis by selective targeting of memory effector T lymphocytes. N Engl J Med 2001; 345: 248–255.

49. Grassi W, Lamanna G, Farina A, Cervini C. Synovitis of small joints: sonographic guided diagnostic and therapeutic approach. Ann Rheum Dis 1999; 58: 595–597.

50. McKendry RJ, Kraag G, Seigel S, al-Awadhi A. Therapeutic value of colchicines in the treatment of patients with psoriatic arthritis. Ann Rheum Dis 1993; 12: 826–828.

51. Kagan A, Husza'r M, Frunkin A, Rapoport J. Reversal of nephrotic syndrome due to AA amyloidosis in psoriatic patients on longterm colchicine treatment. Case report and review of the literature. Nephron 1999; 82: 348–353.

52. Huckins D, Felson DT, Holick M. Treatment of psoriatic arthritis with oral 1,25-dihydroxyvitamin D_3: a pilot study. Arthritis Rheum 1990; 33: 1723–1727.

53. Jorstad S, Bergh K, Iversen OJ *et al*. Effects of cascade apheresis in patients with psoriasis and psoriatic arthropathy. Blood Purif 1998; 16: 37–42.

54. Maksymowych WP, Jhangri GS, Leclercq S *et al*. An open study of pamidronate in the treatment of refractory ankylosing spondylitis. J Rheumatol 1998; 25: 714–717.

55. Moreira AL, Sampaio EP, Zmudzinas A *et al*. Thalidomide exerts its inhibitory action on tumor necrosis factor alpha by enhancing mRNA degradation. J Exp Med 1993; 177: 1675–1680.

56. Burt RK, Traynor AE, Pope R *et al*. Treatment of autoimmune disease by intense immunosuppressive conditioning and autologous hematopoietic stem cell transplantation. Blood 1998; 92: 3505–3514.

57. Sukenik S, Giryes H, Halevy S *et al*. Treatment of psoriatic arthritis at the Dead Sea. J Rheumatol 1994; 21: 1305–1309.

58. Elkayam O, Ophir J, Brener S *et al*. Immediate and delayed effects of treatment at the Dead Sea in patients with psoriatic arthritis. Rheumatol Int 2000; 19: 77–82.

59. Sukenik S, Baradin R, Codish S *et al*. Balneotherapy at the Dead Sea area for patients with psoriatic arthritis and concomitant fibromyalgia. Israel Med Assoc J 2001; 3: 147–150.

113 Enteropathic arthropathies: diagnosis, pathophysiology and treatment

Eric M Veys and Herman Mielants

Definition

- Arthropathies associated with diseases of the large and small intestines: inflammatory bowel disease (Crohn's disease, ulcerative colitis), infectious enteritis, Whipple's disease, intestinal bypass surgery and celiac disease

Clinical features

- Inflammatory bowel disease, infectious enteritis: axial involvement, peripheral enthesitis, association with human leukocyte antigen (HLA)-B27

- Intestinal bypass surgery, celiac disease, Whipple's disease: polyarticular symmetric peripheral joint involvement, no axial involvement, no association with HLA-B27

- The enteropathic arthropathies are not restricted to adults.

HISTORY

A relationship between the gut and arthritis was postulated by Smith[1], who performed segmental bowel surgery to treat patients with rheumatoid arthritis. Bargen[2] recognized arthritis as a complication of ulcerative colitis. Hench[3] described a peripheral arthritis in patients with inflammatory bowel disease (IBD) and observed a tendency of the arthritis to flare with exacerbations of the colitis and to subside with remission of the gut symptoms. The introduction of the concept of spondyloarthropathies by Wright and Moll[4] generated further study of the relationship between arthritis and bowel inflammation.

ENTEROPATHIC ARTHROPATHIES IN INFLAMMATORY BOWEL DISEASES

From the early description of the association of peripheral arthritis and sacroiliitis with ulcerative colitis and Crohn's disease, the idea emerged that IBD might belong to the spondyloarthropathy group of disorders[5]. The distinction between rheumatoid arthritis and the arthropathies related to IBD was highlighted by clinical surveys showing that patients with IBD-related arthropathies had a pauciarticular, asymmetric pattern of peripheral joint involvement, the occurrence of sacroiliitis and spondylitis (Fig. 113.1) and peripheral enthesopathy, and the absence of rheumatoid factor and subcutaneous nodules.

Epidemiology

The prevalence of ulcerative colitis ranges between 50 and 100 per 100 000 population. The disease seems to be more frequent in whites than in non-whites, and more frequent in persons of Ashkenazic Jewish background. The prevalence of Crohn's disease has increased during the past few decades, to about 75 per 100 000 population. Arthritis is the most common extra-intestinal manifestation of either type of IBD and appears in 2–20% of the patients with either ulcerative colitis or Crohn's disease[6]. Moreover, the occurrence of peripheral arthritis is increased both in patients with colonic involvement and in those with more extensive bowel disease.

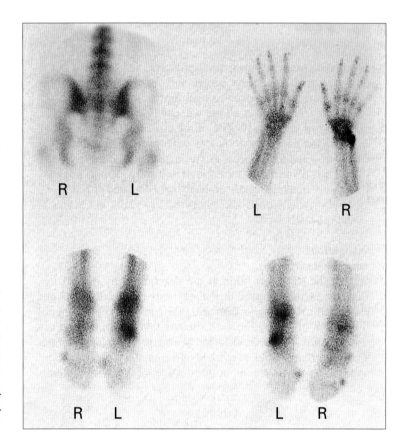

Fig. 113.1 Technitium scan showing pauciarticular asymmetric joint involvement in a patient with spondyloarthritis associated with inflammatory bowel disease. There is increased uptake at the left wrist, right Fascia Plantaris, first metatarsophalangeal right and third and fourth metatarsophalangeal left.

Sacroiliitis and ankylosing spondylitis (AS) are also related to IBD. The reported frequency of AS varies between studies, from 1 to 25% in ulcerative colitis and from 2 to 7% in Crohn's disease[6]. If radiographic sacroiliitis is considered as the sole criterion, the prevalence in Crohn's disease increases to 30%, suggesting that subclinical axial involvement in patients with IBD is more common than reported in many studies[7]. Conversely, the frequency of true IBD (ulcerative colitis or Crohn's disease) in AS is less than 4%; but if the occurrence of subclinical bowel inflammation is considered, the prevalence of gut involvement in a group of patients with spondyloarthropathy increases to 60%[8].

Genetic markers

Familial aggregation of both Crohn's disease and ulcerative colitis has been documented, as has the occurrence of both diseases within the same family[9,10]. There is a genetic predisposition to both diseases. An association with human leukocyte antigen (HLA) antigens is not obvious, but in some studies increased frequencies of HLA-B16, -B18 and -B62 have been reported in patients with Crohn's disease. More recently, two independent groups described disease-predisposing variants (alleles) of the *NOD2* gene in the region of chromosome 16, which shows strong linkage to Crohn's disease[11,12]. NOD 2 is a cytosolic protein the expression of which is restricted to monocytes/macrophages, with no expression detected in lymphocytes; it detects bacteria in the gut and helps to control the inflammatory response they induce[13].

Genetic studies in patients with IBD-associated arthropathy showed that peripheral arthritis occurring in IBD is not associated with HLA-B27. Sacroiliitis and especially spondylitis, however, are associated with HLA-B27 (respectively 40% and 60%), but to a lesser degree than in uncomplicated AS (90%).

Family studies in patients with IBD have revealed that HLA-B27 is rarely responsible for axial involvement in relatives; another gene, HLA-linked or not, seems likely. HLA-B62 was reported in a high proportion of patients with Crohn's disease and spondyloarthropathy in one study[8].

Clinical features
Peripheral arthritis and tendinitis
Clinically, the arthritis that is associated with IBD is characterized by its pauciarticular and asymmetric pattern; indeed, a monoarthritis is not uncommon. Men and women are equally represented. Large and small joints are involved, predominantly those of the lower limbs (knees, ankles and metatarsophalangeal joints). Arthritis of the hips and shoulders is less frequent and tends to be associated with sacroiliitis and spondylitis. The arthritis is generally migratory and transient, but recurrent. Evolution to chronicity may occur, together with radiographically demonstrable erosive lesions. A flare of the gut symptomatology, especially in ulcerative colitis, is frequently accompanied by recurrence of peripheral arthritis. Indeed, surgical removal of the colon in ulcerative colitis has been reported to have a curative effect on the peripheral joint symptoms[14]. Enthesopathies can occur at the heel (insertion of the tendo Achillis or the plantar fascia) or at the knee (insertion of the patellar tendon).

The timing of the first attack of arthritis seems to be independent of the duration of colitis in ulcerative colitis. In Crohn's disease, the joints can be affected before the onset of the intestinal symptoms[14]. Intestinal symptoms can also remain absent, although ileocolonoscopic biopsy specimens taken from the terminal ileum reveal mild to severe inflammatory lesions, indicating the presence of subclinical Crohn's disease in these patients[15].

Sacroiliitis and spondylitis
The prevalence of axial involvement in patients with IBD is estimated to be between 5 and 12%[16], but these percentages could be greater, because of the existence of silent axial involvement[7]. This particularly applies to sacroiliitis. The male:female ratio is 3:1, which is comparable to that for uncomplicated AS. The clinical features and the radiographic signs of spinal disease cannot be distinguished from those of idiopathic AS. Axial involvement can precede the bowel disease by many years.

Inflammatory low back pain, buttock pain and chest pain are the most common subjective complaints; they are frequently accompanied by limitation of lumbar spine mobility and chest expansion. As in uncomplicated AS, the limitation of cervical spine mobility is a hallmark of progression of the disease to generalized ankylosis. The axial symptoms are independent of exacerbations of the gut inflammation, and surgical treatment of the gut is not followed by improvement of the spinal symptoms. Consequently, it has been suggested that peripheral arthritis is a manifestation of IBD *per se*, whereas the spondylitis is an associated disease.

Other extraintestinal manifestations of IBD
Acute anterior uveitis is the most common ocular manifestation in IBD, occurring in 3–11% of patients. It is associated with HLA-B27 and with axial joint involvement. Acute at onset, it is unilateral and transient, but frequently recurrent and spares the cornea and retina. Conjunctivitis and episcleritis are other rare ocular manifestations occurring in IBD and are characterized by a red eye without pain and photophobia.

Skin lesions occur in 10–25% of the patients. Erythema nodosum is most common and coincides with exacerbations of the gut inflammation and thus tends to occur in patients with active peripheral synovitis. Pyoderma gangrenosum is less frequent, is not related to the gut inflammation and is probably an associated disorder.

Secondary amyloidosis is encountered occasionally, especially in Crohn's disease, and is usually fatal.

Investigations
Laboratory tests
The laboratory findings are determined by the activity of the bowel disorder. Iron deficiency anemia, leukocytosis and a marked thrombocytosis with platelet counts greater than 700 000/mm³ are not uncommon. The erythrocyte sedimentation rate and other acute-phase reactants are increased. Rheumatoid factor is absent. The synovial fluid is not characteristic: mild to marked inflammatory changes can be found, with a white blood cell count ranging from 1500 to 50 000/mm³, and glucose concentrations are not reduced. Microbiologic cultures are negative.

Radiographic findings
The sacroiliac and axial involvement in IBD cannot be distinguished from those seen in uncomplicated AS (Fig. 113.2). Sacroiliitis is typically bilateral, as are syndesmophytes, which usually show marginal insertions on vertebral bodies. Peripheral joint involvement is generally not accompanied by radiographic changes, but erosive lesions, mainly of the metatarsal joints, have been described. These lesions show some differences from those in rheumatoid arthritis; for example, an absence of osteoporosis and the presence of adjacent bone proliferation. Rarely, a destructive granulomatous synovitis may be seen in Crohn's disease. Enthesopathies do not differ radiographically from those seen in other spondyloarthropathies (Fig. 113.3).

Differential diagnosis
Initially, the clinical signs of spondyloarthropathy must be recognized and differentiated from those of rheumatoid arthritis and other connec-

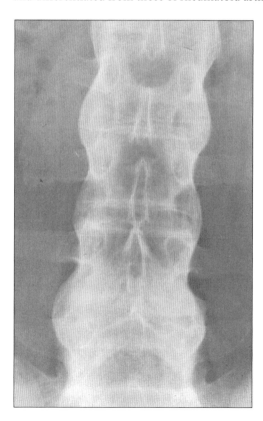

Fig. 113.2 Bamboo spine in a woman with severe Crohn's disease.

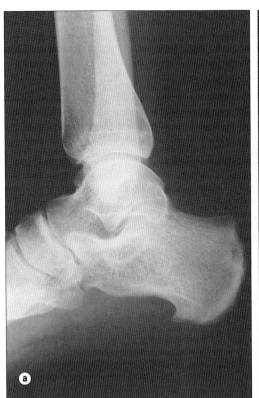
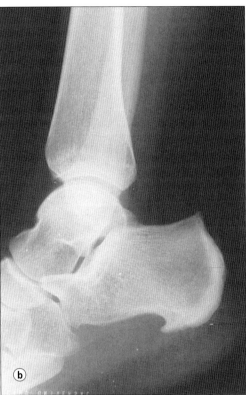

Fig. 113.3 Enthesopathy at the heel. (a) Erosive lesion at the insertion of the tendo Achillis and the beginning of bone apposition at the insertion of the plantar fascia. (b) The same foot 2 years later, with spur formation at the insertions of the Achilles tendon and the plantar fascia.

TABLE 113.1 DIFFERENCES BETWEEN RHEUMATOID ARTHRITIS AND SPONDYLOARTHROPATHY

	Rheumatoid arthritis	Spondyloarthropathy
Peripheral arthritis	Polyarticular	Pauciarticular
Sacroiliitis		●
Spondylitis		●
Enthesitis		●
Subcutaneous nodules	●	
Rheumatoid factor	●	
Symmetry	●	

TABLE 113.2 THE SPECTRUM OF SPONDYLOARTHROPATHY

Ankylosing spondylitis

Reactive arthritis
 Urogenital
 Enterogenic

Psoriatic arthritis

Inflammatory bowel diseases
 Crohn's disease
 Ulcerative colitis

Juvenile chronic arthritis

Uveitis

SAPHO* syndrome

Undifferentiated spondyloarthropathies

*Synovitis, acne, pustulosis, hyperostosis, osteitis.

tive tissue diseases (Table 113.1). When a patient presents with the clinical signs of spondyloarthropathy, IBD should be considered (Table 113.2) as the gut symptoms may be very mild. The presence of spondylitis in an HLA-B27-negative patient increases the risk of IBD.

The clinical and subjective intestinal signs of both IBD and infectious enterocolitis are not always clear-cut, and may even remain absent. Furthermore, many patients in whom the clinicoradiographic features conform very well to the major criteria of spondyloarthropathies cannot be classified under one of the specific entities belonging to this concept. These patients are mainly classified as having undifferentiated spondyloarthropathies. Ileocolonoscopic studies have revealed the presence of gut

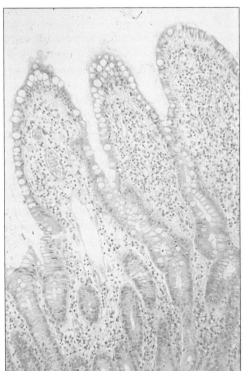

Fig. 113.4 Histologic appearance of acute inflammatory lesions in the terminal ileum. The architecture of the villi and the crypts is preserved, the epithelial layer is infiltrated by mononuclear cells, and the lamina propria is enlarged and infiltrated by polymorphonuclear and mononuclear cells.

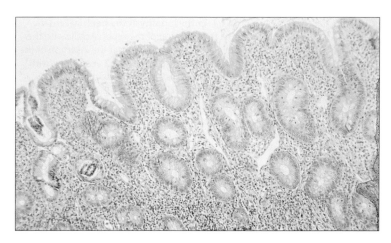

Fig. 113.5 Histology of chronic lesions in the terminal ileum. There is flattening and fusion of the villi, branching of the crypts and enlargement of the lamina propria, which is infiltrated by a large number of mononuclear cells.

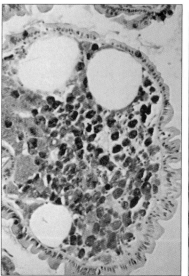
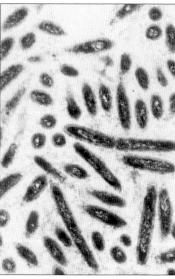

Fig. 113.6 The typical histologic features of Whipple's disease. (a) Small intestinal mucosal appearance, with large vacuoles and macrophages filled with periodic acid-Schiff reagent (×180). (b) Electron micrograph showing the rod-shaped organisms that lie free in the lamina propria (×17 000). (With permission from Dieppe PA *et al., Atlas of Clinical Rheumatology,* London: Gower Medical Publishing;1986. Courtesy of Dr AB Price.)

inflammation in about 67% of these patients, even in the absence of clinical intestinal symptoms[15,17,18].

The histologic lesions can be subdivided into acute inflammatory lesions similar to those encountered in acute infectious enterocolitis (Fig. 113.4), and chronic lesions similar to those found in the terminal ileal loop in patients with early IBD[17] (Fig. 113.5). Consequently, spondyloarthritic joint symptoms may be the only manifestations of subclinical Crohn's disease or of an unrecognized infectious enterocolitis.

Treatment

Treatment of the IBD should be the prime consideration, as this will quiet the peripheral arthritis. As in the other spondyloarthropathies, non-steroidal anti-inflammatory drugs (NSAIDs) may be effective in the treatment of the peripheral arthritis and the spondylitis associated with IBD. However, these drugs may cause an exacerbation of the gut symptoms of ulcerative colitis.

It is generally accepted that NSAIDs, even if they improve the inflammation in peripheral joints and in tendons, rarely induce a total remission at these locations. Sulfasalazine, which appears to be an effective treatment for the colonic involvement in ulcerative colitis and Crohn's disease, has been used with some success in the spondyloarthropathies[19,20].

Corticosteroids should only be used systemically if they are indicated to control the bowel disease; they have no effect on axial involvement. Intra-articular injections can be useful, especially if only a small number of joints is involved.

Methotrexate has been reported recently to be effective in treating Crohn's disease, but its efficacy in the associated arthritis remains unknown[21].

Recently, the use of biological treatments that block tumor necrosis factor (TNF)-α has opened new perspectives for the treatment of patients with inflammatory bowel disease. Infliximab is a chimeric anti-TNF-α monoclonal antibody that neutralizes the soluble cytokine in addition to blocking the membrane-bound cytokine[22]. It has been approved by the health authorities in the USA (FDA) and Europe (EMEA) for use as a treatment for therapy-resistant moderate to severe Crohn's disease and fistules[23,24]. More recently a significant improvement of articular as well as axial inflammation was described in patients with spondyloarthropathy associated with Crohn's disease with infliximab[25]. Observation of these patients suggested that refractory joint manifestation in Crohn's disease might be a potential indication for infliximab treatment, and warranted further investigation of the therapeutic potential of TNF-α blockade in patients with other subtypes of spondyloarthropathy (see further).

ARTHROPATHIES ASSOCIATED WITH WHIPPLE'S DISEASE

Whipple's disease is a rare chronic systemic disease that is difficult to diagnose. It potentially involves any organ system, but the small intestine is affected in the majority of patients. Confirmation of the diagnosis is obtained on biopsy of the small intestine or involved lymph node. The presence of macrophages containing glycoprotein granules staining with periodic acid-Schiff in the lamina propria of the small intestine and mesenteric nodes, and of rod-shaped free bacilli in the lamina propria, are the most typical findings (Fig. 113.6)[26]. Relman *et al.*[27] used the polymerase chain reaction to amplify the sequences of bacterial 16S rRNA from tissues of five patients with Whipple's disease, and detected a unique 1321 base sequence from these tissues, but in none of those from 10 controls. This sequence indicated the presence of a previously uncharacterized bacillus, called *Tropheryma Whippelii.* A test based on the polymerase chain reaction can now be used in diagnosing the disease, using affected tissues or even peripheral blood[28].

The relationship between Whipple's disease and HLA-B27 is not clear, and the findings of recent studies do not support the inclusion of Whipple's disease in the spondyloarthropathy concept[29].

Clinical features

Whipple's disease is much more frequent in men than in women (ratio 9:1). The most common complaints are diarrhea, severe weight loss, fever and arthritis[26]. Axillary and cervical lymphadenopathy, generalized hyperpigmentation and serositis are also common features. Rarely, the nervous system may be involved.

Peripheral arthritis is observed in 80% of cases, and may antedate the intestinal complaints by up to 5 years. Flares of the articular signs are not related to the intestinal symptoms. The pattern of joint involvement is mainly polyarticular and symmetric.

Investigations

Low serum carotene concentrations and anemia, hypoalbuminemia and low serum iron concentrations are the most frequent laboratory abnormalities, together with an increase of fat in stool samples[26].

Synovial fluid contains variable numbers of cells (4000–100 000 cells/mm³), which are predominantly polymorphonuclear cells (up to

100%). Erosive lesions on radiographs are generally absent, although destructive arthritis has been reported. The incidence of axial involvement is controversial, varying from 8 to 20%.

Treatment
The administration of appropriate antibiotics, usually tetracyclines, for at least 1 year generally is curative, but the disease may relapse.

ARTHROPATHIES ASSOCIATED WITH CELIAC DISEASE

Celiac disease, or gluten-sensitive enteropathy, is known to be associated with abnormal intestinal permeability. Many disorders, such as dermatitis herpetiformis, hyposplenism and autoimmune disorders have been associated with the disease. More recently, several reports have focused on the occurrence of arthritis related to celiac disease in a limited number of cases[30,31]. Several patients in whom pathology of the gut has been diagnosed also present a prominent arthritis that resolves on a gluten-free diet.

The absence of any other disease and the striking response of the joint manifestations to a gluten-free diet support the causal relationship between celiac disease and arthritis. The absence of bowel symptoms in 50% of the patients with arthritis and the variable pattern of arthritis in these patients render the identification of celiac disease difficult. Malaise, weight loss and low serum folate concentrations are the most common features.

Clinical features
The distribution of arthritis varies. The lumbar spine, hips, knees and shoulders are most commonly affected[30], followed by the elbow, wrist and ankle in fewer than 50% of the patients. Peripheral joint involvement is relatively symmetric and is accompanied by morning stiffness and joint swelling. Radiographic changes are rare.

Pathogenesis
The pathogenesis of the arthritis is unclear. The high frequency of HLA-B8, DR3 in patients with celiac disease has been repeatedly reported. Results of HLA typing, however, are only available in a small number of patients with arthritis. Bourne et al.[30] found HLA-A1, B8, DR3 in five of their six patients, whereas HLA-B27 was found in two.

The pathogenesis of celiac disease, although not completely clarified, thus seems to indicate marked genetic susceptibility, with an immunologically mediated mucosal injury and the presence of antibodies to gliadin[32].

Treatment
Institution of a gluten-free diet resolves both the articular problems and the alterations in intestinal permeability. The fact that patients do not have a relapse of their arthritis after rechallenge with gluten is difficult to explain, but suggests that gluten may not be directly involved in the pathogenesis of arthritis in these patients[31].

ARTHROPATHIES ASSOCIATED WITH INTESTINAL BYPASS SURGERY

Between 1954 and 1983, more than 100 000 individuals underwent jejunoileal bypass surgery as a treatment for morbid obesity. Initially, jejunocolic bypass procedures were performed, but because of severe metabolic complications, they were abandoned and replaced by jejunoileal bypass surgery. However, these techniques also led to postoperative complications in more than 25% of the patients, so they are no longer performed. This iatrogenic arthritis associated with jejunoileal bypass surgery, recognized as the 'arthritis–dermatitis' syndrome, led to important advances in the understanding of inflammatory joint disease[33,34]. A bypass-like arthritis also can occur in patients who have not undergone intestinal bypass surgery but instead have intestinal derangements causing bacterial overgrowth from postoperative, inflammatory or diverticular conditions.

RELATION BETWEEN GUT PATHOLOGY AND ARTICULAR INFLAMMATION

Clinical evidence
Many clinical observations indicate that the gut has an important role in the pathogenesis of several disorders classified as spondyloarthropathies (Table 113.3). The mechanisms by which gut pathology can lead to articular inflammation is the subject of intense research. In AS, a higher fecal carriage of *Klebsiella pneumoniae* has been related to active manifestations of the disease[35]. It has been postulated that Gram-negative enteric bacteria crossing the gut wall stimulate antigen–antibody reactions with the HLA-B27 structure[9] or with HLA-B27-associated structures on cells of the target organs[10], by molecular mimicry. An increase of IgG-containing cells in the lamina propria of the rectal mucosa in patients with AS has been demonstrated[36], suggesting an immune response to a local antigen in the bowel.

Ileocolonoscopic studies have suggested that subclinical IBD might exist in some cases of AS[17,18,37]. Evidence of gut inflammation, mainly unrelated to clinical intestinal symptoms, was found in nearly 65% of a large cohort of patients whose symptoms corresponded to the classification criteria for spondyloarthropathy as proposed by the European Spondyloarthropathy Study Group[38], and in only 5% of the control groups. The incidence of gut inflammation was 80% in patients with enterogenic reactive arthritis, 70% in those with undifferentiated spondyloarthropathy and in patients with AS with combined peripheral joint involvement, and 34% in patients with AS with axial involvement alone.

Follow-up studies of these patients have demonstrated that most patients with normal gut histology or acute inflammatory lesions exhibited transient arthritis, whereas the majority of those with chronic lesions had persistent inflammatory joint symptoms; 6% of these patients developed Crohn's disease[39]. Repeat ileocolonoscopy demonstrated that the remission of the rheumatic disease was always associated with the disappearance of the gut inflammation, 50% of the patients with chronic joint disease presented persistent gut inflammation, and 40% of those patients developed IBD[40,41].

These studies underline the close relationship between gut and joint inflammation in spondyloarthropathies, and indicate that some patients with spondyloarthropathy may have a form of subclinical Crohn's disease in which the joint symptoms are the only clinical expression[42].

TABLE 113.3 CLINICAL EVIDENCE AND ANIMAL MODELS SUPPORTING THE ROLE OF THE GUT IN THE PATHOGENESIS OF DISORDERS CLASSIFIED WITHIN THE SPONDYLOARTHROPATHIES
Clinical evidence
Ankylosing spondylitis: Klebsiella infection?
Enterogenic reactive arthritis
Inflammatory bowel diseases
Subclinical gut inflammation in spondyloarthropathies
Whipple's disease
Celiac disease
Intestinal bypass surgery
Animal models
Protein-rich diet in pigs
Oral challenge with bovine serum albumin in mice
HLA-B27 and b$_2$-microglobulin transgenic rats

Enterogenic reactive arthritis is included in the spondyloarthropathies because of the pattern of peripheral joint involvement, the occurrence of enthesopathies and sacroiliitis, and the increased prevalence of HLA-B27. The peripheral synovitis and the tendinitis in reactive arthritis may be initiated by an infectious enteritis, triggered by *Salmonella*, *Shigella*, *Yersinia* or *Campylobacter* spp., although in many cases the intestinal manifestations are minimal or even absent. In *Yersinia*, *Salmonella* and *Shigella* reactive arthritis, antigenic material has been shown in synovial fluid and in the synovial membrane[43,44]. The persistence of secretory immunoglobulin A class serum antibodies and the demonstration of *Yersinia* antigen in the gut tissue suggest an impaired elimination of these bacteria from the gut wall[45-47]. The subject of enteropathic reactive arthritis is dealt with in more detail in Chapters 108 and 109.

Animal models

Oral challenge of laboratory animals can induce peripheral arthritis in different models. Pigs fed a protein-rich diet develop an abnormal intestinal microbial flora, with an increase of *Clostridium perfringens* and increased titers of antibody to this microorganism, along with an asymmetric peripheral arthritis[48]. In mice with unilateral chronic bovine serum albumin-related arthritis, a flare-up of the arthritis may be induced with an oral challenge with the mouse bovine serum albumin antigen[49]. By local or systemic injection of primary structural components of bacterial cell membranes[50-53], some authors were able to induce acute and chronic arthritis in rats.

Investigators also have introduced the human *HLA-B27* and human β_2-microglobulin genes into rats of different lines[54] to investigate the role of the HLA-B27 molecule in the pathogenesis of the spondyloarthropathies. Rats from two transgenic lines (LEW 21-4H and 33-3) spontaneously developed a multiorgan inflammatory disease, involving the gastrointestinal tract, the peripheral and axial joints, male genital tract, skin, nails and heart, comparable to the HLA-B27-associated human diseases. The most prevalent site of involvement appeared to be the gastrointestinal tract. The histologic appearance described in the model is similar to that found on ileocolonoscopy in human spondyloarthropathies and IBD[15].

The role of bacteria in triggering the disease in B27-transgenic rats has been addressed by maintaining the animals in a germ-free environment. Under these conditions, the B27 lines remain free from joint and gut disease, but may have skin and genital lesions. As gut and joint disease were suppressed in germ-free conditions, it cannot be concluded whether joint disease arises as a consequence of an intestinal process, or whether both are parallel consequences of one or more processes related to gut bacteria. Nevertheless, direct evidence is provided that commensal enteric bacteria have a primary role in the pathogenesis of HLA-B27-related diseases and of IBD also[55].

PATHOGENIC MECHANISMS OF ENTEROGENIC ARTHROPATHIES

In humans, there is compelling evidence that gut inflammation and increased gut permeability have roles not only in reactive arthritis, but also in other types of spondyloarthropathies[39,41,42,56], whereas both bacterial antigens and T cells reactive with those antigens have been demonstrated in the joint[43,44,57,58]. Correlating the bacterial hypothesis with the major histocompatibility complex class I linkage, it has been proposed that HLA-B27 is involved in the activation of cytotoxic T lymphocytes by presenting either specific bacterial peptides or arthritogenic self peptides cross-reacting with bacterial antigens. Alternatively, HLA-B27 itself could share peptide sequence homologies with bacterial antigens that could trigger cytotoxic T lymphocytes (molecular mimicry)[59]. However, HLA-B27 also has effects that are independent of its antigen-presenting function: it impairs bacterial elimination, leading to defective host defense, with persistence of bacterial antigens[60], and it alters intracellular signaling and the secretion of proinflammatory cytokines[61]. Finally, HLA-B27 appears to be particularly sensitive to misfolding during the intracellular assembly process[62,63], thereby triggering inflammation through two different pathways. First, misfolding can induce the activation of nuclear factor (NF)-κB and the secretion of proinflammatory cytokines[64], or lower the threshold of NF-κB activation by other stimuli such as lipopolysaccharides[65]. Secondly, misfolding can lead to the formation of HLA-B27 heavy-chain homodimers and, consequently, potentially immunogenic structures that could be recognized by T helper cells[66,67].

In summary, interactions at several levels between bacterial infections and genetic factors appear to activate both the innate and the acquired immunity in spondyloarthropathy. Emerging insights into these interactions, the role of defective host defense and the etiopathogenic relationship between joint and gut will allow better understanding of the disease and provide new opportunities for experimental therapeutic intervention in spondyloarthropathy[68].

REFERENCES

1. Smith R. Treatment of rheumatoid arthritis by colectomy. Ann Surg 1922; 76: 515–578.
2. Bargen JA. Complications and sequelae of chronic ulcerative colitis. Ann Intern Med 1929; 3: 335.
3. Hench PS. Acute and chronic arthritis. In: Whipple GH, ed. Nelson's looseleaf of surgery. New York: Thomas Nelson Sons; 1935: 104.
4. Wright V, Moll JMH. Seronegative polyarthritis. Amsterdam: North Holland Publishing Company; 1976.
5. Wright V. Seronegative polyarthritis. A unified concept. Arthritis Rheum 1978; 21: 618–633.
6. Gravallese EM, Kantrowitz FG. Arthritic manifestations of inflammatory bowel disease. Am J Gastroenterol 1988; 83: 703–709.
7. de Vlam K, Mielants H, Cuvelier C et al. Spondyloarthropathy is underestimated in inflammatory bowel disease: prevalence and HLA association. J Rheumatol 2000; 27: 1860–1865.
8. Mielants H, Veys EM. The gut in the spondyloarthropathies. J Rheumatol 1990; 17: 7–10.
9. Ebringer A. Ankylosing spondylitis, immune response genes and molecular mimicry. Lancet 1979; 1: 1186.
10. Seager K, Bashri HV, Geczy AF. Evidence for a specific B27-associated cell surface marker in lymphocytes of patients with ankylosing spondylitis. Nature 1979; 277: 68–70.
11. Hugot JF, Chamaillard M, Zouali H et al. Association of NOD-2 leucine-rich repeat variants with susceptibility to Crohn's disease. Nature 2001; 411: 599–603.
12. Ogura Y, Bonen DK, Inohara N et al. A frameshift mutation in NOD2 associated with susceptibility to Crohn's disease. Nature 2001; 411: 603–606.
13. Ogura Y, Inohara N, Benito A et al. NOD2, a Nod1/Apaf-1 family member that is restricted to monocytes and activates NF-κB. J Biol Chem 2001; 276: 4812–4818.
14. Wright V, Watkinson G. The arthritis of ulcerative colitis. BMJ 1965; 2: 670–675.
15. Mielants H, Veys EM, Cuvelier C, De Vos M. Subclinical involvement of the gut in undifferentiated spondyloarthropathies. Clin Exp Rheumatol 1989; 7: 499–504.
16. Moll JMH. Inflammatory bowel disease. Clin Rheum Dis 1985; 11: 87–111.
17. Mielants H, Veys EM, Goemaere S et al. Gut inflammation in the spondyloarthropathies: clinical, radiological, biological and genetic features in relation to the type of histology. A prospective study. J Rheumatol 1991; 18: 1542–1551.
18. Simenon G, Van Gossum A, Adler M et al. Macroscopic and microscopic gut lesions in seronegative spondyloarthropathies. J Rheumatol 1990; 17: 1491–1494.
19. Dougados M, Van Der Linden S, Leirisalo-Repo M et al. Sulfasalazine in the treatment of spondylarthropathies. A randomized, multicenter, double-blind, placebo-controlled study. Arthritis Rheum 1995; 38: 618–627.
20. Clegg DO, Reda DJ, Abdellatif M. Comparison of sulfasalazine and placebo for the treatment of axial and peripheral articular manifestations of the seronegative spondyloarthropathies. Arthritis Rheum 1999; 42: 2325–2329.
21. Kozarek RA. Methotrexate for refractory Crohn's disease: preliminary answers to definitive questions. Mayo Clin Proc 1996; 71: 104–105.
22. Knight DM, Trinh H, Le T et al. Construction and initial characterization of a mouse–human chimeric anti-TNF antibody. Mol Immunol 1993; 30: 1443–1453.
23. Targan SR, Hanauer SB, Van Deventer SJ et al. A short-term study of chimeric monoclonal antibocy CA2 to tumor necrosis factor alpha for Crohn's disease. Crohn's Disease CA2 Study Group. N Engl J Med 1997; 337: 1029–1035.

24. Present DH, Rutgeerts P, Targan S et al. Infliximab for the treatment of fistulas in patients with Crohn's disease. N Engl J Med 1999; 340: 1398–1405.

25. Van den Bosch F, Kruithof E, De Vos M et al. Crohn's disease associated with spondyloarthropathy: effect of TNF-α blockade with infliximab on the articular symptoms. Lancet 2000; 356: 1821–1882.

26. Fleming JL, Wiesner RH, Shorter RG. Whipple's disease: clinical, biochemical and histopathologic features and assessment of treatment in 29 patients. Mayo Clin Proc 1988; 63: 539–551.

27. Relman DA, Schmidt TM, MacDermott RP et al. Identification of the uncultured bacillus of Whipple's disease. N Engl J Med 1992; 327: 293–301.

28. Lowsky R, Archer GL, Fyles G et al. Brief report: diagnosis of Whipple's disease by molecular analysis of peripheral blood. N Engl J Med 1994; 331: 1343–1346.

29. Olivieri I, Brandi G, Padula A et al. Lack of association with spondyloarthritis and HLA-B27 in Italian patients with Whipple's disease. J Rheumatol 2001; 28: 1294–1297.

30. Bourne JT, Kumar P, Huskisson EC et al. Arthritis and celiac disease. Ann Rheum Dis 1985; 44: 592–598.

31. Pinals RS. Arthritis associated with gluten-sensitive enteropathy. J Rheumatol 1986; 13: 201–204.

32. McPherson RA. Commentary: advances in the laboratory diagnosis of celiac disease. J Clin Lab Anal 2001; 15: 105–107.

33. Stein HE, Schlapper OLA, Boyko W et al. The intestinal bypass arthritis–dermatitis syndrome. Arthritis Rheum 1981; 24: 684–690.

34. Clegg DO, Zone JJ, Samuelson CO Jr et al. Circulating immune complexes containing secretory IgA in jejunoileal bypass disease. Ann Rheum Dis 1985; 44: 239–244.

35. Ebringer RW, Caudell DR, Cowling P et al. Sequential studies in ankylosing spondylitis. Association of Klebsiella pneumoniae with active disease. Ann Rheum Dis 1978; 37: 146–151.

36. Stodell MA, Butler RS, Zemelman VA et al. Increased numbers of IgG-containing cells in rectal lamina propria of patients with ankylosing spondylitis. Ann Rheum Dis 1985; 43: 172–176.

37. Leirisalo-Repo M, Turunen V, Stenman S et al. High frequency of silent inflammatory bowel disease in spondyloarthropathy. Arthritis Rheum 1994; 37: 23–35.

38. Dougados M, Van der Linden S, Juhlin R et al. The European Spondylarthropathy Study Group preliminary criteria for the classification of spondylarthropathy. Arthritis Rheum 1991; 34: 1218–1227.

39. Mielants H, Veys EM, De Vos M et al. The evolution of spondylarthropathies in relation to gut histology. I. Clinical aspects. J Rheumatol 1995; 22: 2266–2272.

40. Mielants H, Veys EM, Cuvelier C et al. The evolution of spondylarthropathies in relation to gut histology. II. Histological aspects. J Rheumatol 1995; 22: 2273–2278.

41. Mielants H, Veys EM, Cuvelier C et al. The evolution of spondylarthropathies in relation to gut histology. III. Relation between gut and joint. J Rheumatol 1995; 22: 2279–2284.

42. De Vos M, Mielants H, Cuvelier C et al. Long-term evolution of gut inflammation in patients with spondylarthropathy. Gastroenterology 1996; 110: 1696–1703.

43. Granfors K, Jalkanen S, Von Essen R et al. Yersinia antigens in synovial fluid cells from patients with reactive arthritis. N Engl J Med 1989; 320: 216–221.

44. Granfors K, Jalkanen S, Lindberg A et al. Salmonella lipopolysaccharides in synovial cells from patients with reactive arthritis. Lancet 1990; 335: 6985–6988.

45. De Koning J, Heeseman J, Hoogkamp-Korstanje JAA et al. Yersinia in intestinal biopsy specimens from patients with seronegative spondyloarthropathy: correlation with specific serum IgA antibodies. J Infect Dis 1989; 159: 109–112.

46. Granfors K, Toivanen A. IgA anti Yersinia antibodies in Yersinia triggered reactive arthritis. Ann Rheum Dis 1986; 45: 561–565.

47. Mäko-Ikola O, Hill JL, Lahesmaa R et al. IgG and IgA antibody responses in Yersinia-triggered reactive arthritis. Br J Rheumatol 1992; 31: 315–318.

48. Mansson I, Norberg R, Olhagen B et al. Arthritis in pigs induced by dietary factors. Microbiologic, clinical and histologic studies. Clin Exp Immunol 1971; 9: 677–683.

49. Lens JW, Van den Berg WB, Van de Putte LA. Flare-up of antigen-induced arthritis after challenge with oral antigen. Clin Exp Immunol 1984; 58: 364–371.

50. Lehman TA, Allen JB, Plotz PH et al. Polyarthritis in rats following the systemic injection of Lactobacillus casei cell walls in aqueous suspension. Arthritis Rheum 1983; 26: 1259–1265.

51. Stimpson SA, Brown RR, Anderig K. Arthropathic properties of cell wall polymers from normal flora bacteria. Infect Immun 1986; 51: 240–249.

52. Severijnen AJ, Hazenberg MP, Van De Merwe JP. Induction of chronic arthritis in rats by cell wall fragments of anaerobic coccoid rods isolated from the faecal flora of patients with Crohn's disease. Digestion 1988; 39: 118–125.

53. Severijnen AJ, Van Kleef R, Hazenberg MP et al. Cell wall fragments from major residents of the human intestinal flora induce chronic arthritis in rats. J Rheumatol 1989; 16: 1061–1068.

54. Hammar RE, Maika SD, Richardson JA et al. Spontaneous inflammatory disease in transgenic rats expressing HLA-B27 and human β_2-microglobulins: an animal model of HLA-B27-associated human disorders. Cell 1990; 63: 1099–1112.

55. Taurog J, Richardson JA, Croft JAT et al. The germfree state prevents development of gut and joint inflammatory disease in HLA-B27 transgenic rats. J Exp Med 1994; 180: 2359–2364.

56. Mielants H, Veys EM, Cuvelier C et al. Ileocolonoscopic findings in seronegative spondylarthropathies. Br J Rheumatol 1988; 27: S95–S105.

57. Hermann E, Fleischer B, Mayet WJ et al. Response of synovial fluid T cell clones to Yersinia enterocolitica antigens in patients with reactive arthritis. Clin Exp Immunol 1989; 75: 365–370.

58. Hermann E, Yu D, Meyer zum Buschenfelde KH et al. HLA-B27 restricted CD8 T cells derived from synovial fluids of patients with reactive arthritis and ankylosing spondylitis. Lancet 1993; 342: 645–650.

59. Lopez-Larrea C, Gonzalez S, Martinez-Borra J. The role of HLA-B27 polymorphism and molecular mimicry in spondyloarthropathy. Mol Med Today 1998; 4: 540–549.

60. Laitio P, Virtala M, Salmi M et al. HLA-B27 modulates intracellular survival of Salmonella enterides in human monocytic cells. Eur J Immunol 1997; 27: 1331–1338.

61. Ikawa T, Ikeda M, Yamaguchi A et al. Expression of arthritis-causing HLA-B27 on HeLa cells promotes induction of c-fos in response to in vitro invasion by Salmonella typhimurium. J Clin Invest 1998; 101: 263–272.

62. Colbert RA. HLA-B27 misfolding: a solution to spondyloarthropathy conundrum? Mol Med Today 2000; 6: 224–230.

63. Mear JP, Schreiber KL, Munz C et al. Misfolding of HLA-B27 as a result of its B pocket suggests a novel mechanism for its role in susceptibility to spondyloarthropathies. J Immunol 1999; 163: 6655–6670.

64. Baeuerle PA, Henkel T. Function and activation of NF-kappa B in the immune system. Annu Rev Immunol 1994; 12: 141–149.

65. Pentinen MA, Holmberg CI, Sistonen L et al. MHC class I molecules modulate LPS-induced NF-κB activation in U937 human monocytic cells. Arthritis Rheum 1999; 42: S385.

66. Allen RL, O'Callaghan CA, McMichael AJ et al. Cutting edge: HLA-B27 can form a novel beta2-microglobulin-free heavy chain homodimer structure. J Immunol 1999; 162: 5045–5048.

67. Khare SD, Hansen J, Luthra HS et al. HLA-B27 heavy chains contribute to spontaneous inflammatory disease in B27/human beta2-microglobulin (beta2m) double transgenic mice with disrupted mouse beta2m. J Clin Invest 1996; 98: 2746–2755.

68. De Keyser F, Van Damme N, De Vos M et al. Opportunities for immune modulation in the spondyloarthropathies with special reference to gut inflammation. Inflamm Res 2000; 49: 47–54.

114 Enthesopathy

Lars Koehler, Jens G Kuipers and Henning K Zeidler

- Anatomically, two different types of enthesis should be discriminated. The *fibrous entheses* are characterized by pure dense fibrous connective tissue that links the tendon or ligament to the bone, whereas *fibrocartilaginous entheses* have a transitional zone of fibrocartilage at the bony interface

- The term 'enthesopathy' comprises all pathological alterations at an enthesis of whatever origin: degenerative, metabolic, traumatic, infective, inflammatory; the term 'enthesitis' is more restricted to inflammatory conditions

- Enthesitis is a hallmark of the spondyloarthropathies, although numerous other conditions and diseases have to be distinguished in given enthesopathic symptoms

- The clinical features are variable depending on the location, severity and underlying disease, although pain, loss of function and disability are common signs and symptoms

- Clinical examination and imaging techniques are the key procedures for diagnosis and follow-up

- The therapeutic spectrum includes physical modalities, analgesics, non-steroidal anti-inflammatory drugs, local injections (e.g. corticosteroids) and radiation

INTRODUCTION

The enthesis is a site of insertion of a tendon, ligament or articular capsule into bone. Thus a great variety of anatomical sites can be affected in pathological disorders (Fig. 114.1). However, some entheseal structures are more often affected in rheumatic diseases, such as the tendo Achillis, fascia plantaris, pes anserinus, greater trochanter of the hip, ischial tuberosities, iliac crest and medial epicondyle of the elbow.

Any pathologic alteration of the enthesis, whether traumatic or degenerative or caused by inflammatory and metabolic diseases, is termed 'enthesopathy'; ossification at this site is termed an 'enthesophyte'. By contrast, the term 'enthesitis' is restricted to inflammatory disease.

HISTORY

The term enthesopathy was first used by Niepel[1]. Ball, in his 1971 Heberden Oration lecture discussing enthesopathy of rheumatoid and ankylosing spondylitis, initiated the important view that the enthesis is centrally affected in ankylosing spondylitis, in contrast to rheumatoid arthritis, in which predominantly synovial structures are inflamed[2]. In the following years, the primarily pathoanatomical concept of enthesitis was introduced into the clinical terminology of undefined conditions such as the syndrome of seronegative enthesopathy and arthropathy in children, in addition to a constitutive feature of spondyloarthropathy as defined by the preliminary European Spondylarthropathy Study Group classification criteria[3,4].

More recently, the hypothesis was put forward that the synovitis in psoriatic arthritis, and perhaps spondyloarthropathy in general, is secondary to entheseal inflammation, in contrast to the primary synovitis of rheumatoid arthritis[5]. Thus enthesitis is now a generally accepted major manifestation and pathology of ankylosing spondylitis and the other spondyloarthropathies.

EPIDEMIOLOGY

With advancing age, enthesopathies are commonly observed at tendon or ligament attachment sites. These bony outgrowths presumably relate to a degenerative enthesopathy, but most occur in healthy individuals. Enthesophytes were noted as a skeletal phenomenon in up to 18% of iliac crests and 25% of patellae examined[6]. In addition to age-related degeneration, other factors such as mechanical overuse, traumatic effects, local ischemia and metabolic changes may also have a causative role, but the inflammatory etiology of the spondyloarthropathies has generated most interest recently.

Between 10% and 60% of patients with spondyloarthropathies have clinically overt enthesitis, usually in combination with peripheral arthritis[7]. In a study describing the disease manifestation of spondyloarthropathy in an Alaskan Eskimo population, the medical records revealed an even greater frequency (94%) of symptoms consistent with tendinitis or enthesopathy at some time in the patient's history, compared with 63% in the controls[8]. In *juvenile spondyloarthropathy*, enthesitis is very common and a more obvious initial feature than sacroiliitis[9]. The reported incidence of enthesitis in acute *reactive arthritis* varies between 10% and 30%, usually in association with arthritis[10]. Moreover, enthesitis can be the only musculoskeletal symptom, in about 5–10% of patients with reactive musculoskeletal complications. Most recently, a Spanish study noted talalgia (pain in the heel or ankle) in 38% as the key enthesopathic manifestation in a group of patients with possible spondyloarthropathy. Those patients who also fulfilled the Amor or European Spondylarthropathy Study Group criteria had a frequency of talalgia of 65% and 54%, respectively, whereas the patients who failed to fulfil criteria had frequencies of talalgia of only 13% and 3%, respectively[11].

Although the genetics of such isolated reactive enthesitis has not been studied in detail, a number of studies suggest a weaker association between human leukocyte antigen (HLA)-B27 and reactive arthritis than in the classical spondyloarthropathy.

ANATOMY AND PATHOLOGY

Anatomy

The enthesis is defined as the site of insertion of a tendon, ligament, joint capsule or fascia to bone. Two major types of entheses are known: the fibrocartilaginous and the fibrous type (Table 114.1). The latter is characterized by dense fibrous connective tissue that attaches the tendon or ligament directly to the bone, whereas the fibrocartilaginous type is characterized by a transitional zone of fibrocartilage at the bony interface and is mostly involved in the spondyloarthropathies.

COMMON ENTHESOPATHIES

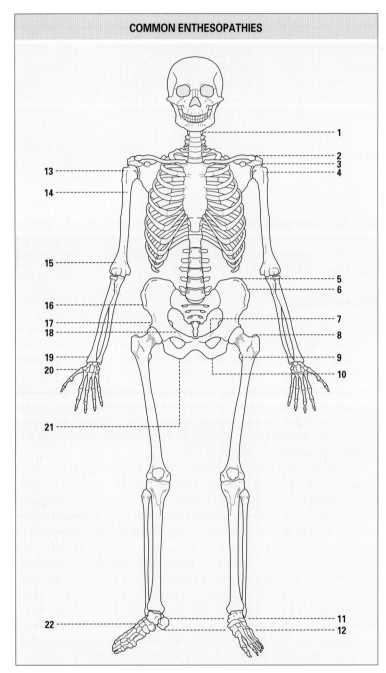

Fig. 114.1 Common enthesopathies. Associated muscles (M.) and ligaments (Lig.) are given in parentheses. **(1)** Enthesiopathia processorum spinosorum; **(2)** Enthesiopathia acromii (Mm. trapezius, deltoideus; Lig. Acromio-claviculare); **(3)** Enthesiopathia proc. coracoideii (Mm. biceps, coracobrachialis, pectoralis minor; Lig. coracoacromiale); **(4)** Enthesiopathia tuberculi maioris humeri (Mm. supraspinatus, infraspinatus, teres minor, rotator-cuff); **(5)** Enthesiopathia ligamenti iliolumbalis; **(6)** Enthesiopathia cristae ilicae (Mm. obliqui abdominis); **(7)** Enthesiopathia spinae ischii (Mm. gemellus spinalis; Lig sacrospinalis); **(8)** Enthesiopathia trochanteris maioris (Mm. gluteus medius, obturatores, piriformis, vastus lateralis); **(9)** Enthesiopathia trochanteris minoris (M. iliopsoas); **(10)** Enthesiopathia tuberis ischii (Mm. semimembranaceus, caput longum bicipitis femoris, quadratus femoris, adductor magnus); **(11)** Enthesiopathia retrocalanea (Mm. triceps surae; tendo achillis); **(12)** Enthesiopathia subcalcanea (Mm. abductor gigiti quinti, flexor digiti quanti brevis, quadratus plantae, adductor hallucis; aponeurosis plantae); **(13)** Enthesiopathia tuberculi minoris humeri (Mm. subscapularis); **(14)** Enthesiopathia m. deltoidea; **(15)** Enthesiopathia m. triceps brachii, calcar olecrani, patella cubiti; **(16)** Enthesiopathia spinae iliacae anterioris (Mm. sartorius, tensor fasciae latae); **(17)** Enthesiopathia tuberculi ilii (M. rectus femoris; ligamenta); **(18)** Enthesiopathia pectinei; **(19)** Enthesiopathia epiphyseos distalis radii (Mm. brachioradialis, flexor carpi radialis, abductor pollicis brevis, opponens policis, adductor digiti minimi); **(20)** Enthesiopathia abductoris pollicis longi; **(21)** Enthesiopathia m. gracilis, calcar m. gracilis; **(22)** Enthesiopathia tuberositatis metatarsi quinti (M. abductor digiti V).

TABLE 114.1 THE TWO TYPES OF ENTHESIS		
	Fibrocartilaginous enthesis	**Fibrous enthesis**
Origin	Cartilage	Tendon, ligament, periosteal
Attachment site	Epiphyses, apophyses	Metaphyses, diaphyses
Glycosaminoglycans	Present	Absent
Locations	Achilles tendon, anulus fibrosus, sacroiliac joint ligament, joint capsule insertions	Perivertebral ligaments, sacroiliac joint ligament

The fibrocartilaginous entheses are composed of:

- the tendon with dense fibrous connective tissue and some longitudinally orientated fibroblasts
- a zone of uncalcified fibrocartilage
- an abrupt transition to calcified fibrocartilage
- bone.

Uncalcified and calcified fibrocartilage are separated by a sharp borderline called the 'tidemark', whereas the junction between calcified fibrocartilage and bone is highly irregular, with interdigitations and some collagen fibers (Sharpey fibers), which penetrate directly into the bone trabeculae, holding together bone and fibrocartilage.

Fibrocartilage is a dynamic tissue with the ability to promote bone formation, as shown in histological analyses during postnatal growth[13]. This is of relevance, given the characteristic occurrence of ankylosis in the spondyloarthropathies.

Fibrous entheses are typical of the metaphyses and diaphyses of long bone, whereas fibrocartilaginous entheses are characteristic of the tendon insertions into the epiphyses, where the direction of force transmitted by the tendon is changing throughout the range of joint movement.

Entheses are well innervated with both pain and proprioceptive receptors. Numerous blood vessels are present in entheses and are derived from the peritenon, perichondrium, periostium and the adjacent bone marrow.

Histopathology

Enthesitis is histopathologically characterized by bony erosions and destruction, with inflammatory fibroblastoid cell infiltrates invading the bone that is adjacent to the entheseal site[14] and the subchondral bone[12] (Fig. 114.2). Inflammatory cells, predominantly T lymphocytes, and edema in the bone marrow close to the enthesis have been observed[15]. This is followed by capsular ossification, myxoid bone marrow changes, chondroid metaplasia, synchondrosis and ossification (Fig. 114.3). The new bone formation takes the form of desmal ossification at the enthesis junction with bone, and also by enchondral ossification at sites where cartilage is present[16,17]. Transforming growth factor β, bone morphogenic proteins and tumor necrosis factor (TNF)-α are probably involved in bone destruction and ossification of entheses[12].

ETIOLOGY AND PATHOGENESIS

The concept that enthesitis is the hallmark in the spondyloarthropathies has recently been supported by fat-suppressed magnetic resonance imaging (MRI) analysis in patients with spondyloarthropathies of recent onset. Knee effusions in these patients exhibited enthesitis, with a preponderance of focal peri-entheseal high signal compatible with fluid or

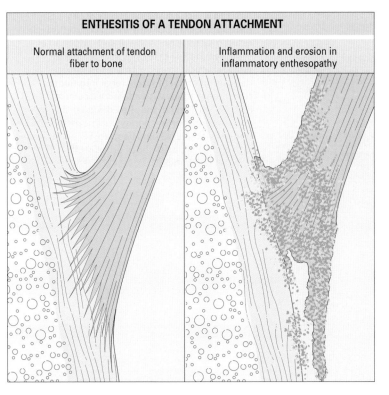

ENTHESITIS OF A TENDON ATTACHMENT

Normal attachment of tendon fiber to bone	Inflammation and erosion in inflammatory enthesopathy

Fig. 114.2 Enthesitis of a tendon attachment. The invagination of the tendon fiber into bone in a normal patient contrasts with the inflammation and erosion noted in enthesitis.

edema, and bone marrow edema maximal at entheseal insertions, in contrast to findings in rheumatoid arthritis[18]. In comprehensive histopathological studies of sacroiliitis in ankylosing spondylitis, mild but destructive synovitis and myxoid subchondral bone marrow were the earliest changes identified. These lesions destroyed the adjacent articular tissues, a loss that was followed by fibrous scaring, woven bone formation and new cartilage, with fusion of cartilage leading to ankylosis. Active enthesitis occurred in the advanced and late cases, but was not observed in the earliest cases of sacroiliitis[19].

Fibrocartilage has been found at major sites of spondyloarthropathy pathology such as the iliac part of the sacroiliac joint, entheses and both the aortic root and wall. It is thus of interest that murine models with

humoral and cellular immunity to the major cartilage proteoglycan, aggrecan, resemble human ankylosing spondylitis. Furthermore, in such models, destruction of the hip and sacroiliac joints is very often characterized by subchondral granulation tissue. Thus the hypothesis was brought forward that subchondral osteiitis and autoimmunitiy to fibrocartilage-derived autoantigens constitute the basis for bone and joint erosions and destruction in the spondyloarthropathies[20].

Different mechanisms, depending on the location affected by spondyloarthropathy and the time, early or late, in the disease process, may explain these different phenomena, although the latter are not mutually exclusive. Currently therefore, enthesitis, although common and characteristic for spondyloarthropathies, has not been accepted in general as the unifying concept, but could be viewed rather as part of the pathophysiology of the spondyloarthropathies.

The precise etiology and pathophysiology of enthesitis is not understood. A potential explanation for the entheseal tropism of inflammation is that small particles (0.02–1.1μm in diameter) such as bacteria localize to certain transitional zones, including entheses, where highly and scarcely vascularized areas come close[21]. Bacteria may then induce fibrocartilage degeneration by activating chondrocytes, resulting in the development of autoimmunity to previously unexposed antigens[20]. Persisting bacterial infection, well documented in patients with reactive arthritis, may also occur at enthesal insertion; however, until now there are no data supporting this hypothesis.

As biomechanical stress occurs at entheses in addition to other locations involved in spondyloarthropathy (aorta, lung apex, uvea), it has been suggested that such stress with microtrauma and subsequent healing, together with the deposition of bacterial products, may be important. Relevant features include the special vascularity of entheses, with subsequent activation of Toll-like receptors by CpG motifs, lipopolysaccharide or bacterial heat-shock protein. These may, either directly or indirectly, induce nuclear factor (NF)-κB activation, which may serve as a costimulatory signal in major histocompatibility complex class I antigen/arthritogenic peptide presentation to T cells, leading to inflammation[22]. The recently demonstrated misfolding and accumulation of HLA-B27 in the endoplasmic reticulum may additionally activate NF-κB, inducing production of proinflammatory cytokines[23]. This therefore exceeds the threshold at which subclinical inflammation resulting from microtrauma after biomechanical stress will lead to clinically overt enthesitis.

These hypotheses are presented schematically in Figure 114.4.

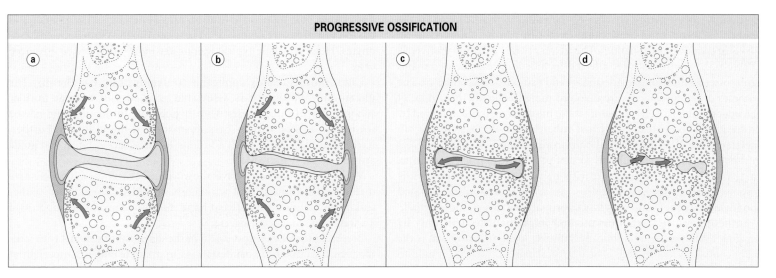

PROGRESSIVE OSSIFICATION

Fig. 114.3 Progressive ossification. (a) Initially, inflammmatory changes are noted at attachments to bone. (b) This progresses to bone erosions. (c) Capsular ossification leads to peripheral bone ankylosis. (d) The central articular cartilage is then replaced by enchondral ossification, leading to intra-articular ankylosis of bone.

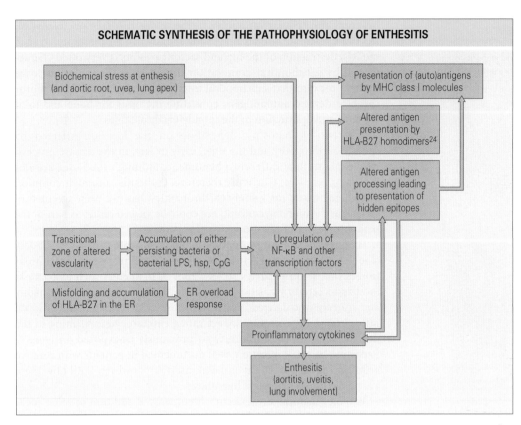

SCHEMATIC SYNTHESIS OF THE PATHOPHYSIOLOGY OF ENTHESITIS

Fig. 114.4 Schematic synthesis of the pathophysiology of enthesitis. Enthesitis is the result of activation of NF-κB and induction of proinflammatory cytokines in response to biomechanical stress, with microtrauma, deposition of bacteria/bacterial fragments at transitional zones with altered vascularity, HLA-B27 misfolding, and altered antigen processing and presentation in spondyloarthropathy. CpG, unmethylated CpG dinucleotide; ER, endoplasmic reticulum; hsp, heat-shock protein; LPS, lipopolysaccharide.

TABLE 114.2 FREQUENCY OF ENTHESITIS IN THE DIFFERENT SPONDYLOARTHROPATHIES	
Spondyloarthropathy	Frequency of enthesitis (%)
Ankylosing spondylitis	25–28
Reactive arthritis	13–58
Psoriatic arthritis	20
Spondarthritis associated with IBD	7–33
Undifferentiated spondarthritis	27
IBD, irritable bowel disease	

CLINICAL FEATURES

Enthesitis, inflammatory changes of the enthesis, is a hallmark of the spondyloarthropathies. Peripheral enthesitis can be observed in all forms of spondyloarthropathies. The frequency ranges from 13% to 60% (Table 114.2). Entheseal sites affected include joint capsules, cartilaginous–osseous junctions, syndesmoses and extra-articular entheses. The entheses of the lower limb are involved more frequently than those of the upper limb[24–27]. Heel enthesis is the most frequent site, followed by enthesitis of the patella, the tibial tubercle and the base of the 5th metatarsal bone[25,26]. Severe heel pain from plantar fasciitis or Achilles enthesitis, or both, was found in 39% of patients with reactive arthritis, in 33% with either psoriatic arthritis or with ankylosing spondylitis associated with ulcerative colitis, in 27% with undifferentiated spondyloarthropathy and in 15% with primary ankylosing spondylitis[28].

Enthesitis can be asymptomatic and might be detectable only by imaging techniques[27,29,30]. Clinically, however, pain on movement is the main complaint in enthesitis. The degree of pain can vary from mild to disabling. The pain is often pronounced after a period of rest, especially in the morning, and improves gradually with movement. Soft tissue swelling may be visible at superficial sites such as the tendo Achillis.

Physical examination of deep-seated entheses such as those on the greater trochanter may reveal tenderness and palpable swelling.

Enthesitis can antedate the occurrence of other spondyloarthropathy-related symptoms such as inflammatory back pain or peripheral arthritis. This constellation occurs especially in juvenile-onset forms of spondyloarthropathy[31]. Like other manifestations of spondyloarthropathy, enthesitis may sometimes occur as the only long-standing clinically apparent symptom of the HLA-B27-asociated disease process.

DIAGNOSTIC INVESTIGATIONS

The imaging methods used for diagnosing peripheral enthesitis include conventional radiography, bone scintigraphy, ultrasound and MRI.

The combination of erosion and bone proliferation are the radiographic hallmarks of enthesitis (Fig. 114.5). In the acute inflammatory phase, osteopenia at the site of entheseal insertion into bone is common, and erosions may develop. Subsequently, when the repair process predominates, soft tissue calcification and bone cortex irregularities at tendon insertions are observed[32]. These can progress into bony enthesophytes. However, these typical lesions are mostly detected in advanced cases.

Ultrasound is readily applicable to demonstrating enthesitis. The ultrasound appearance is associated with loss of normal fibrillar echogenicity of the entheses, with hypoechoic thickening, and edema with bone erosion or new bone formation at the insertion. Further, ultrasound may reveal small effusions in the adjacent bursa and guide arthrocentesis (Fig. 114.6).

Various recent studies have shown that MRI is the most sensitive method for identification of active enthesitis. MRI can show peri-entheseal inflammation with adjacent bone marrow edema in fat-suppressed T2-weighted sequences (Fig. 114.7).

Bone scintigraphy is most useful in the diagnosis of patients with multilocular inflammatory manifestations in multiple enthesis, especially at locations difficult to investigate by clinical examination (Fig. 114.8).

No systematic study has compared the different imaging techniques for diagnosis of enthesitis, either individually or in combination. We

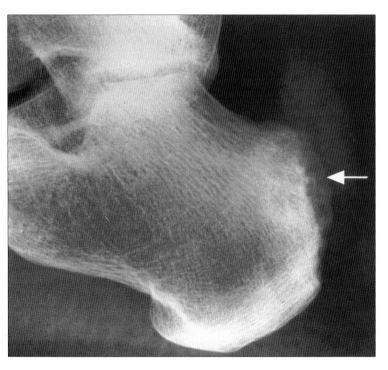

Fig. 114.5 Radiograph of enthesitis at the attachment of the plantar aponeurosis (arrow). (Courtesy of Dr Freyschmidt, Bremen, Germany).

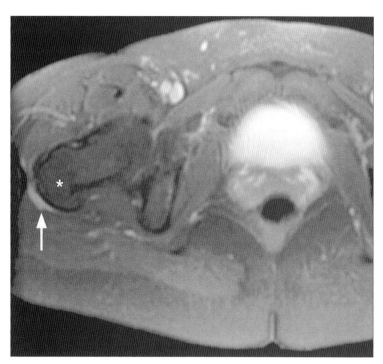

Fig. 114.7 MRI of an enthesitis. Coronal T2-weighted fat-suppressed MRI of the right hip. An enthesitis of the iliopsoas tendon (arrow) at its attachment to the greater trochanter (*) can be seen. (Courtesy of Drs Kirchhoff and Galanski, Department of Radiology, Medical School, Hannover, Germany.)

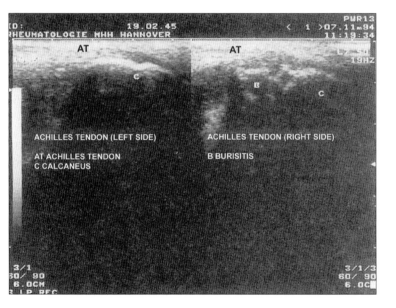

Fig. 114.6 Ultrasound image of an erosive enthesitis at the site of insertion of the right tendo Achillis. When compared with the healthy site, erosions (note the irregularity of the corticalis) and a bursitis subachilleae are visible. (Courtesy of Dr Huelsemann, Department of Rheumatology, Medical School, Hannover, Germany.)

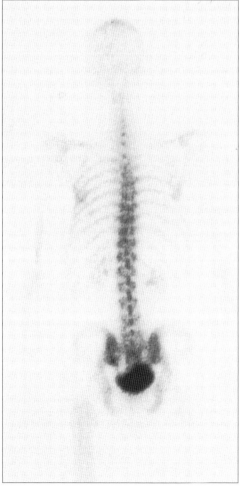

Fig. 114.8 Scintigraphy of enthesitis of the processi spinosorum. An increased enhancement at the attachment of the processi spinosorum and of the iliac joint was detected by scintigraphy. (Courtesy of Drs Boerner and Gratz, Department of Nuclear Medicine, Medical School, Hannover, Germany.)

therefore present our own strategy. In any patient with suspected enthesitis, plain radiographs of the affected site should be performed. In the case of typical radiographic changes, no further imaging is required. However, in cases without typical changes, further imaging should be undertaken. Thus both ultrasound and MRI have improved early diagnosis and also enabled more accurate detection of pathology at various anatomic sites of the musculoskeletal system predominantly involved in spondyloarthropathy. If this imaging technique fails to yield a definite and unequivocal result, scintigraphy is the next choices for imaging. This provides the advantage of imaging other manifestions of spondyloarthropathies, such as arthritis or spinal involvement.

TABLE 114.3 DIFFERENTIAL DIAGNOSIS OF ENTHESOPATHY
Traumatic or degenerative
Diffuse idiopathic skeletal hyperostosis
Calcium pyrophosphate dihydrate or hydroxyapatite deposition disease
Chronic fluoride intoxication
Chronic retinoid toxicity
Endocrine disorders (acromegaly)

DIFFERENTIAL DIAGNOSIS

Numerous diseases can lead to the clinical presentation of entheseopathy and have to be considered as potential differential diagnosis of enthesitis related to the spondyloarthropathies (Table 114.3).

MANAGEMENT

A stepwise approach to treatment of enthesitis usually results in remission of this important manifestation of spondyloarthropathies (Fig. 114.9). Refractory enthesitis, defined by persistence of symptoms after a period of 2 years despite adequate treatment, occurs only in a minority of cases (6%)[33].

The first-line treatment of enthesitis consists of non-steroidal anti-inflammatory drugs (NSAIDs), physical therapy and orthoses[34,35]. Various NSAIDs have been shown to be effective in the treatment of spondarthritides, including indomethacin, diclofenac, naproxen, piroxicam and, most recently, meloxicam[36,37]. However, NSAIDs can cause clinically important side effects, especially in the gastrointestinal tract. Increasing evidence suggests that a selective new class of NSAIDs, the cyclo-oxygenase (COX)-2 inhibitors, have no deleterious effect on the gastrointestinal tract. The value of celecoxib, a COX-2 inhibitor, in the anti-inflammatory treatment of ankylosing spondylitis, and its potency to relieve spinal pain in comparison with diclofenac have been demonstrated recently[38]. At present, no data are available concerning the efficacy of COX-2 selective inhibitors for the treatment of enthesitis.

If disease is refractory to this treatment, the number of entheses involved is important with regard to further treatment (stage 2 in Figure 114.9). Local injections of steroid should be tried for patients with enthesitis at one or a limited number of sites. Conflicting data exist with respect to the use of sulphasalazine as a second-line drug[39,40]. Therefore, treatment with sulphasalazine is recommended for patients

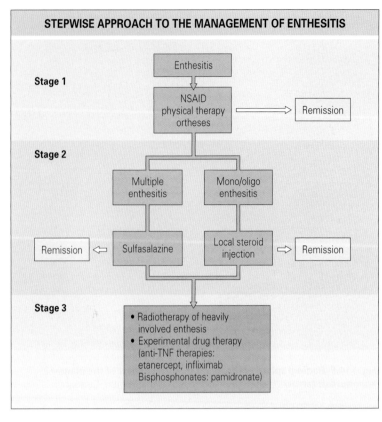

Fig. 114.9 Stepwise approach to the management of enthesitis.

with multiple enthesitis and increased acute-phase reactants. The efficacy of this treatment should be evaluated after 3–4 months.

Low-dose anti-inflammatory radiotherapy and experimental drug treatment are reserved for those patients with persistent enthesitis despite physiotherapy and appropriate drug treatment (stage 3). Because of the superficial location of most entheses, orthovoltage beams are the appropriate choice. The recommended dose consists of 6–12Gy given in two to six fractions. Possible long-term hazards such as leukemia, or local side effects such as bone sarcoma or osteonecrosis, have not been reported to date. Anti-TNF-α treatment, for example with etanercept or infliximab, in addition to the bisphosphonate, pamidronate, have been used with success in open trails in ankylosing spondylitis and the other spondyloarthropathies. The effect of these drugs on this specific manifestation has not yet been investigated in controlled trials.

Surgery does not provide any benefical effect in enthesitis[40,41].

REFERENCES

1. Niepel G, Kostka D, Kopecky S, Manca S. Enthesopathy. Acta Rheum Balneolog Pistiniana 1966; 1: 1–64.
2. Ball J. Enthesopathy of rheumatoid and ankylosing spondylitis. Ann Rheum Dis 1970; 30: 213–223.
3. Rosenberg AM, Petty RE. A syndrome of seronegative enthesopathy and arthropathy in children. Arthritis Rheum 1982; 25: 1041–1047.
4. Dougados M, van der Linde S, Juhlin R et al. The European Spondylarthropathy Study Group preliminary criteria for the classification of spondylarthropathy. Arthritis Rheum 1991; 34: 218–227.
5. McGonagle D, Gibbon W, Emery P. Classification of inflammatory arthritis by enthesitis. Lancet 1998; 352: 1137–1140.
6. Shaibani A, Workman R, Rothschild BM. The significance of enthesopathy as a skeletal phenomenon. Clin Exp Rheum 1993; 5: 428–435.
7. Braun J, Sieper J. The sacroiliac joint in the spondylarthropathies. Curr Opin Rheumatol 1996; 7: 275–283.
8. Boyer G, Templin DW, Bowler A et al. Spondylarthropathy in the community: clinical syndromes and disease manifestations in Alaskan Eskimo populations. J Rheumatol 1999; 26: 1537–1544.
9. Burgos-Vargas R, Vazquez-Mellado J. The early clinical recognition of juvenile-onset ankylosing spondylitis and its differentiation from juvenile rheumatoid arthritis. Arthritis Rheum 1995; 38: 835–844.
10. Leirisalo-Repo M. Enthesitis and reactive arthritis. Ann Rheum Dis 2000; 59: 998.
11. Collantes E, Veroz R, Escudero A, et al. Can some cases of 'possible' spondyloarthropathy be classified as 'definite' or 'undifferentiated' spondyloarthropathy? Value of criteria for spondyloarthropathies. Joint Bone Spine 2000; 67: 516–520.
12. Braun J, Khan MA, Sieper J. Enthesitis and ankylosis in spondyloarthropathy: what is the target of the immune response? Ann Rheum Dis 2000; 59: 985–994.
13. Gao J, Messner K, Ralphs JR, Benjamin M. An immunohistochemical study of enthesis development in the medial collateral ligament of the rat knee joint. Anat Embryol (Berlin) 1996; 194: 399–406.
14. Braun J, Bollow M, Eggens U et al. Use of dynamic magnetic resonance imaging with fast imaging in the detection of early and advanced sacroiliitis in spondylarthropathy patients. Arthritis Rheum 1994; 37: 1039–1045.
15. Laloux L, Voisin MC, Allain J et al. Comparative histological study of enthesitis in spondylarthropathies [abstract]. Arthritis Rheum 1999; 42: S402.
16. Fassbender HG, Fassbender R. Synovial characteristics of seronegative spondarthritides. Clin Investig 1992; 70: 706.
17. Ceponis A, Konttinen YT, Imai S et al. Synovial lining, endothelial and inflammatory mononuclear cell proliferation in synovial membrane in psoriatic and reactive arthritis: a comparative quantitative morphometric study. Br J Rheumatol 1998; 37: 170–178.

18. McGonagle D, Gibbon W, O'Connor P *et al.* Characteristic magnetic resonance imaging entheseal changes of knee synovitis in spondylarthropathy. Arthritis Rheum 1998; 41: 694–700.

19. Francois RJ, Gardner DL, Degrave EJ, Bywaters EGL. Histopathologic evidence that sacroiliitis in ankylosing spondylitis is not merely enthesitis. Systematic study of specimens from patients and control subjects. Arthritis Rheum 2000; 43: 2011–2024.

20. Maksymowych WP. Ankylosing spondylitis – at the interface of bone and cartilage [editorial]. J Rheumatol 2000; 27: 2295–2301.

21. Schulz LC, Schaening U, Pena M, Hermanns W. Borderline-tissues as sites of antigen deposition and persistence – a unifying concept of rheumatoid inflammation. Rheumatol Int 1985; 5: 221–227.

22. McGonagle D, Emery P. Enthesitis, osteitis, microbes, biomechanics, and immune reactivity in ankylosing spondylitis [editorial]. J Rheumatol 2000; 27: 2302–2304.

23. Colbert RA. HLA-B27 misfolding: a solution to the spondyloarthropathy conundrum? Molec Med Today 2000; 6: 224–230.

24. Paolaggi JB, Goutet MC, Strutz PH *et al.* Les enthésopathies des spondyloarthropathies inflammatoires: fréquence, description clinique, radiologique et anatomique. Etat actuel de la question. Rev Rhum Mal Ostéoartic 1984; 51: 457–462.

25. Olivieri I, Foto M, Ruju GP *et al.* Low frequency of axial involvement in Caucasian pediatric patients with seronegative enthesiopathy and arthropathy syndrome after 5 years of disease. J Rheumatol 1992; 19: 469–475.

26. Olivieri I, Padula A, Pierro A. Late onset undifferentiated seronegative spondyloarthropathy. J Rheumatol 1995; 22: 899–903.

27. Lethinen A, Taavitsainen M, Leirisalo-Repo M. Sonographic analysis of enthesopathy in the lower extremities of patients with spondyloarthropathy. Clin Exp Rheumatol 1994; 12: 143–148.

28. Gerster JC. Plantar fasciitis and Achilles tendinitis among 150 cases of seronegative spondarthritis. Rheumatol Rehab 1980; 18: 218–222.

29. Lopez-Bote LP, Humbria-Mendiola A, Ossorio-Castellanos C *et al.* The calcaneus in ankylosing spondylitis: a randomized study of 43 patients. Scand J Rheumatol 1989; 18: 143–148.

30. Secundini R, Scheines EJ, Gusis SE *et al.* Clinico-radiological correlation of enthesitis in seronegative spondyloarthropathies (SNSA). Clin Rheumatol 1997; 16: 129–132.

31. Burgos-Vargas R, Pacheo-Tena C, Vázques-Mellado J. Juvenile onset spondyloarthropathies. Rheum Dis Clin North Am 1997; 23: 569–598.

32. Watt I. Basic differential diagnosis of arthritis. Eur Radiol 1997; 7: 344–351.

33. Dougados M, Contreras L, Maetzel A, Amor, B. Les tarsalgies des spondylarthropathies: présentation clinique et traitement. Rev Rheum Mal Osteoartic 1992; 59: 611 (abstract A1112).

34. Olivieri I, Barozzi L, Padula A. Enthesiopathy: clinical manifestations, imaging and treatment. Baillières Clin Rheumatol 1998; 12: 665–681.

35. Koehler L, Kuipers JG, Zeidler H. Managing seronegative spondarthritides. Rheumatology 2000; 39: 360–368.

36. Toussirot E, Wendling D. Current guildlines for drug treatment of ankylosing spondylitis. Drugs 1998; 56: 225–240.

37. Dougados M, Gueguen A, Nakache JP *et al.* Ankylosing spondylitis: what is the optimum duration of a clinical study? A one year versus a 6 weeks non-steroidal anti-inflammatory drug trial. Rheumatology 1999; 38: 235–244.

38. Dougados M, Béhier J-M, Jolchine I *et al.* Efficacy of celecoxib, a cyclooxygenase 2-specific inhibitor in the treatment of ankylosing spondylitis. Arthritis Rheum 2001; 44: 180–185.

39. Lethinen A, Leirosalo-Repo M, Taavitsainen M. Persistence of enthesopathic changes in patients with spondylarthropathy during a 6-month follow-up. Clin Exp Rheumatol 1995; 13: 733–736.

40. Amor B, Dougados M, Khan MA. Management of refractory ankylosing spondylitis and related spondylarthropathies. Rheum Dis Clin North Am 1995; 21: 117–128.

41. Gerster JC, Saudan Y, Fallet GH. Talalgia. A review of 30 severe cases. J Rheumatol 1978; 5: 210–216.

CONNECTIVE TISSUE DISORDERS

115 History

Violeta Rus

- The term 'lupus' means 'wolf' in Latin and originally denoted wolf-bite-like facial lesions
- Cazenave in France coined the term 'lupus erythematosus' (1833)
- Von Hebra in Vienna published the first illustration of the facial skin changes (1856) and pointed to the 'butterfly'-like appearance (1846)
- Kaposi in Vienna recognized the systemic nature of the disease (1872) which was later described in detail by Jadassohn (1904)
- Libman and Sacks in New York described the typical endocarditis (1923), Baehr the typical glomerular changes (1935), and Klemperer, Pollack and Baehr coined the terms 'diffuse collagen disease' (1941) and 'diffuse connective tissue disease'
- Reinhart and Hauck from Germany demonstrated the first false-positive test for syphilis in SLE (1909) and Hargraves detected the LE cell phenomenon (1948) as the first anti-nuclear antibody reactivity, to be followed by respective research until today
- The LE anticoagulant was described in 1952 and the antiphospholipid syndrome recognized by Hughes *et al.* in 1986
- Experimental models have allowed more pathogenetic insights
- First successful therapies consisted of quinine (1894, Payne) and salicilin and the use of glucocorticoids (Hench, 1952) led to a significant change of prognosis

HISTORY

Early descriptions

The history of systemic lupus erythematosus (SLE) dates back at least to the Middle Ages. Until the beginning of the 19th century, the term 'lupus' had been used for various types of lesions or conditions, but none of its descriptions included sufficient detail to suggest a modern diagnosis of lupus. After standardization of the dermatologic terminology at the turn of the 19th century, major landmarks divided the history of lupus into three periods. The classical period saw the description of the cutaneous features of the disease, at that time the most obvious clinical manifestation. The neoclassical period saw the recognition of lupus as a distinct disease with systemic and visceral manifestations. The modern period, which was initiated by the discovery of the 'LE' cell in 1948, is characterized by developments that have exponentially expanded our knowledge about the pathophysiology, clinical and laboratory features, and treatment of this disorder.

The history of lupus has been the subject of a number of excellent reviews[1-5]. The term 'lupus' (Latin for 'wolf') was first used to designate cutaneous diseases during the Middle Ages. It was used generically to describe erosive skin lesions that ate away the flesh and were evocative of a wolf's bite. The first known medical use of the term lupus appeared in the description of the healing of Eraclius, Bishop of Liège, at the shrine of St Martin in Tours, c. 916 AD, by Herbernus of Tours[1]:

He (Eraclius) was seriously affected and almost brought to the point of death by the disease called lupus … . The location of the disease … was not to be seen, nonetheless, a sort of red line remained as a mark of the scar.[1]

In the 13th century, a physician from the school of Salerno, Rogerius Frugardi, mentioned that 'Sometimes lupus arises in the thighs and the lower legs [and is] distinguished from cancer …'[6]. He introduced the term *noli me tangere* ('touch me not') to describe facial ulcers. The association of 'lupus' with ulcerated lesions of the legs persisted until the 16th century, when physicians started to use the term primarily for facial lesions. However, a great deal of confusion still persisted until Robert Willan (1757–1812), a physician working in London, proposed a classification of skin disorders based entirely on clinical observation, and standardized the dermatologic terminology. Willan clearly differentiated *noli me tangere*, lupus and herpes. Under the heading of lupus were described destructive or ulcerative skin diseases of the face and nose, whereas vesicular diseases were classified under the heading of herpes. Because of his premature death, Willan's work was finished and published by his student Thomas Bateman (1757–1812) who wrote in 1810[7]:

Of this disease (lupus) I shall not treat at any length; for I can mention no medicine, which has been of any essential service in the cure of it, and it requires the constant assistance of the surgeon, in consequence of the spreading ulcerations, in which the original tubercles terminate. The term was intended by Dr. Wilan to comprise together with the *noli me tangere* (do not touch me) affecting the nose and lips, other slow tubercular affections, especially about the face, commonly ending in ragged ulcerations of the cheeks, forehead, eyelids, and lips, and sometimes occurring in other parts of the body where they gradually destroy the skin and muscular parts to considerable depth. Sometimes the disease appears in the cheek circularly, or in the form of a sort of ringworm, destroying the substance, and leaving a deep and deformed cicatrix.

In Willan's classification, lupus vulgaris and other cutaneous disorders were also classified under the heading lupus. Later authors separated lupus into lupus vulgaris and lupus erythematosus.

'Lupus erythematosus'

Although Willan and Bateman described cases of what appear to be cutaneous lupus, it was the French physician, Pierre L Cazenave (1802–1877), who reported the observations of his mentor, Laurent Theodore Biett (1781–1840), and published in 1833 the first description of lupus erythematosus under the name of 'erythema centrifugum'[8]:

It is often of very rare occurrence, and appears more frequently in young people, especially in females, whose health is otherwise excellent. It attacks the face chiefly. It generally appears in the form of round red patches, slightly elevated, and about the size of a shilling: these patches generally begin by a small red spot, slightly papular, which gradually increases in circumference, and sometimes spreads over the greater part of her face. The edges of the patches are prominent, and the center, which retains its natural colour, is depressed. There is considerable degree of heat and redness, but no pain or itching, and each patch leaves a slight depression on the skin. The causes of this variety are unknown. It sometime coexists with dysmenorrhea; it is essentially a chronic affection, although its appearance would indicate the reverse.

Later on, he described skin lesions such as atrophy, telangectasia, fixed erythema, adherent scaling and follicular plugging[9]. After observing more advanced cases, Cazenave renamed 'erythema centrifugum' as 'lupus erythemateux', terminology that was accepted by his colleagues. Although Cazenave and his successors clearly differentiated lupus erythematosus from lupus vulgaris (i.e. acute cutaneous tuberculosis), the term lupus used without any other descriptor continued to refer to lupus vulgaris, which was much more prevalent than lupus erythematosus.

In 1846, Ferdinand von Hebra (1816–1880), a Viennese physician, described lupus under the heading of 'seborrhea congestiva' and first introduced the butterfly metaphor to describe the malar rash[10]:

> One sees at the beginning of this illness – mainly on the face, on the cheeks and the nose in a distribution not dissimilar to a butterfly … and finally presents with sharply demarcated, vividly red and scaling lesions non-itching, non-oozing, and non-eroded.

Hebra also published the first illustrations of lupus erythematosus in 1856 in his *Atlas of Skin Diseases*, and changed the term lupus erythemateux into the Latin 'lupus erythematosus'. Although reports by Cazenave and others indicated that this chronic disease may become severe, it seemed established that it remained localized to the skin.

Moriz Kaposi (born Kohn) (1837–1902) is credited with recognizing, in 1872, the systemic nature of the disease: 'lupus erythematosus may also appear as a disseminated or generalized acute or subacute febrile eruption and in such circumstances intense local and constitutional symptoms may affect the organism and may even endanger or destroy the life of the patient.' A student and also the son-in-law of Hebra, Kaposi wrote in his textbook published in 1875[11]:

> experience has shown that lupus erythematosus … may not only extend more deeply locally, and may be attended by altogether more severe pathological changes … but that also various grave and even dangerous constitutional symptoms may be intimately associated with the process in question, and the death may result from conditions which must be considered to arise from local malady. Of late, therefore, Lupus erythematosus has become more important affection, and it has become necessary to modify, in some measure, the description usually given of the clinical character of the disease.

Kaposi noted two types of lupus erythematosus: the first one appeared as 'characteristic large discs' which he called the discoid form, and the second one as 'disseminated and aggregated small spots' which he called the disseminated form[11]. Furthermore, he described various 'concomitant symptoms' that characterized the disseminated form, including subcutaneous nodules, arthritis with synovial hypertrophy of both small and large joints, lymphadenopathy, fever, weight loss, anemia and central nervous system involvement[11]. He noted also the possibility of a fatal outcome: 'In the course of 2–3 weeks death ensues being preceded by increased mental disturbance, sopor or by pleuropneumonia'[11].

Kaposi emphasized the distinction between lupus vulgaris and lupus: 'the disease called lupus erythematosus does not have the least in common with lupus vulgaris', and criticized those who confused them: 'No confusion in our ideas regarding lupus need be caused by the circumstance that, since 1851, a cutaneous affection, thoroughly distinct from Lupus vulgaris, has been included under the designation of Lupus, after the example of Cazenave, with the title of Lupus Erythematosus'[12].

Kaposi firmly believed that lupus is not a manifestation of tuberculosis, and shared Hebra's opinion that lupus is the result of changes in the sebaceous gland[11]:

we are unable to adduce any very satisfactory data bearing on the cause of Lupus Erythematosus … . In some cases, we recognize a distinctively local cause for lupus erythematosus i.e. severe local seborrhoea … . The condition, therefore represents a 'Seborrhoea Congestiva' (Hebra) as evinced by the chronic congestion around the orifices of the follicles, the dilation of the latter, and the hypersecretion from the glands.

After Kaposi's description of SLE in 1872, a number of reports illustrated other features of lupus. Jonathan Hutchinson published the description of lupus marginatum, which resembles the subset of lupus now called subacute cutaneous lupus. Fox, in 1890, described the involvement of the mucous membranes and Sequira and Balean, in 1902, described acroasphyxia (Raynaud's phenomenon).

The existence of a disseminated or systemic form was firmly established by the work of Osler in Baltimore[13] and Jadassohn in Vienna[14]. In a series of publications, Osler described, under the term 'erythema exudativum multiforme', systemic manifestations of a variety of diseases involving the skin. From 29 cases summarized by Osler, it can be surmized that a large number had Henoch–Schönlein purpura, a few probably had erythema multiforme, angioedema and gonococcal septicemia, and only two patients clearly had lupus. Certainly, Osler realized he had 'jumbled together a motley group of cases'. To this criticism, he replied: 'I did so on purpose for I was seeking similarities, not diversities'[13]. Osler recognized that lupus can occur without cutaneous findings: 'The attacks may not be characterized by skin manifestations; the visceral symptoms alone may be present, and to the outward view the patient may have no indication whatever of erythema exudativum'[15]. However, this concept was accepted only three decades later, when a postmortem diagnosis of SLE was established in a patient who had no cutaneous manifestations. Although Osler's contribution to the description of systemic lupus erythematosus has been the subject of controversy, his carefully described cases emphasized the concept of multisystem involvement.

In 1904, Jadassohn, in Vienna, summarized the contemporary dermatologic experience in the recognition of clinical features of lupus erythematosus and called attention to certain organ manifestations. In his comprehensive review, he referred to joint symptoms, ulcerations of the mucous membranes, glandular swelling and, particularly, renal involvement. He also emphasized the etiology, pathogenesis, pathology, diagnosis, prognosis and treatment of lupus[14]. He believed the disease could be a result of 'flooding of the organism with infectious and toxic material'. Although the reports of Osler and Jadassohn established lupus as a separate disease entity, considerable confusion still persisted, and many thought SLE was a variant of tuberculosis.

The 20th century: clinicopathologic advances

Autopsy reports on lupus were first presented by Kaposi in 1872[16]. Death was attributed to intercurrent pneumonia in some of the cases and to tuberculosis in others. In the following decades, a considerable number of autopsy studies were performed on patients who had died of lupus, but apparently no unique pathologic abnormalities were noted. This lack of progress was largely due to the excessive preoccupation of the anatomic investigations with proving or disproving the presence of tuberculous foci.

In contrast, the first half of the 20th century marked a prolific phase in the history of lupus, characterized by important pathologic observations and clinicopathologic correlations. New advances in our understanding of SLE were made at Mount Sinai hospital in New York City by Libman and Sacks, who described an 'endocarditis of a peculiar type, particularly because of the unusual manner of spread of the endocardial lesions along the posterior wall of the left ventricle'[17]. Furthermore, they made the important contribution of distinguishing the associated clinical syndrome from rheumatic fever on one hand, and from subacute bacterial endocarditis on the other. The authors noted the similarity of their cases to lupus erythematosus, but did not establish a definitive diagnosis. Only in 1940 was the non-bacterial valvular and mural endocarditis unequivocally attributed to lupus. The same authors also noted the characteristic 'onion skin' changes of periarterial splenic fibrosis, described as 'a broad zone of hyaline-like connective tissue' and with 'the arteriolar lumen in each instance … diminished in caliber'. The findings of Libman and Sachs were extended in a series of articles by Gross[18], who described the hematoxylin stained bodies of SLE. In 1935, in a pathological study of 23 cases of SLE, Baehr described the wire-loop glomerular capillary lesions in patients with glomerulonephritis[19]. In 1936, Friedberg, Gross and Wallach made a postmortem diagnosis of SLE in four cases in which cutaneous lesions were not present, confirming Osler's clinical observation that SLE can occur without cutaneous features[20].

Despite the absence of tuberculous foci in most autopsy examinations, it was still speculated by some that lupus was induced by 'toxic substances of tuberculous origin'. Observations at the autopsy table by Keil in 1933 finally rejected the idea that tuberculosis was a major factor in the pathogenesis of the disease. Keil reviewed autopsy cases of systemic lupus and reported that only 20% showed evidence of active or remote tuberculosis[21]. Two other main observations contributed to the modern pathogenetic concept of SLE. The first was the demonstration by the German pathologist, Fritz Linge (1892–1974), that rheumatic fever involves diffusely the connective tissue, and not only the synovium and the heart[22]. The second was the description of ubiquitous fibrinoid degeneration and staining alterations in the ground substance and connective tissue, made by Klemperer and colleagues in 1941[23]:

> The apparent heterogeneous involvement of various organs in this disease had no logic until it became apparent that the widespread lesions were identical in that they were mere local expression of a morbid process affecting the entire collagenous tissue system. The most prominent of these alterations is fibrinoid degeneration – a descriptive morphologic term indicating well defined optical and tinctorial alterations in the collagen fibers and ground substance.

This observation led Klemperer, Pollack and Baehr to the theory of collagen disease as the pathologic basis of SLE, and the concept of 'diffuse collagen disease'. Initially limited to SLE and scleroderma, this label has been rapidly accepted and, according to Klemperer and colleagues, misused: 'There is a danger that it may become a catch-all term for maladies with puzzling clinical and anatomic features. It is not a term applicable to diagnosis and certainly does not define the morbid process of the diseases grouped together'. The more preferred term, 'diffuse connective tissue disease', persists in use to this day[24].

Autoantibodies

Although the hematoxylin bodies have proved to be virtually specific for SLE, they were of little benefit for the antemortem diagnosis of SLE. Therefore, the next major breakthrough in the understanding of SLE was the discovery of autoantibodies and their value in the diagnosis of SLE.

Historically, the oldest immunologic finding in SLE was the biologic false-positive (BFP) serological test for syphilis. In 1906, Wasserman described a serologic test for syphilis and, 1 year later, Landsteiner devised the non-treponemal test that rapidly gained widespread use. In 1909 and 1910, the German physicians Reinhart and Hauck separately reported the first cases of false-positive tests for syphilis in patients with disseminated lupus erythematosus who did not have syphilis. In 1941, Pangborn made the observation that the agent in the beef-heart extract that was used in the complement fixation test for syphilis was a phospholipid, and Coburn and Moore related BFP to hypergamma-globulinemia. Haserick and Long were first to report that BFP tests for syphilis preceded the diagnosis of SLE. Dr Moore at Johns Hopkins Hospital reported his long-term follow-up of 148 individuals with

chronic false-positive test for syphilis. Systemic lupus developed in 7% of them, and a further 30% had symptoms consistent with collagen diseases[25]. A chronic BFP reaction continues to be recognized as a serologic feature of SLE, and has been included among the diagnostic criteria for the condition.

The major serologic breakthrough in the diagnosis of SLE was the discovery of the 'LE' cell by Hargraves, Richmond and Morton at the Mayo Clinic in 1948[26]. Hargraves and colleagues were intrigued by the discovery of 'peculiar, rather stuctureless globular bodies taking purple stain' both intracellularly and extracellularly in the bone marrow of patients with acute disseminated lupus erythematosus, and postulated that the phenomenon '… is the end result of … phagocytosis of free nuclear material with a resulting round vacuole containing this partially digested and lysed nuclear material… .' Pursuing the observation that LE cells were present only in specimens that were not immediately fixed, Hargraves realized that LE cells represented an *in vitro* phenomenon. Shortly thereafter, Hargraves and Haserick had independently adapted the test to peripheral blood.

The discovery of the LE phenomenon, considered by Hargraves an 'unexpected bonus to immunopathology from morphologic hematology'[27], marks the foundation of a new discipline that has greatly contributed to the study of lupus erythematosus. More than any other discovery in the 20th century, the LE test has changed our concept of SLE. By identifying occult, mild cases, it transformed SLE from a rare, fulminant disease to a chronic pleomorphic condition with a wide spectrum of forms and outcomes.

Although initially believed to be pathognomonic for SLE, after a few years LE cells were demonstrated in 16% of patients with rheumatoid arthritis. The sensitivity of the test was also diminished by the observation that only 50–70% of patients with SLE have detectable LE cells. However, LE positivity has been widely used for the diagnosis of lupus, and later on was included among the classification criteria for SLE.

The discovery of the LE phenomenon has stimulated an intense search for other serological abnormalities, and ultimately led to the detection of autoantibodies. John Haserick showed that the factor that induces the formation of LE cells is a gamma globulin present in the blood of patients with SLE[28]. In 1954, Miescher and Fauconnet[29] reported that isolated cell nuclei could absorb the serum factor that induces LE phenomena and postulated that the LE factor is an antibody against a nuclear component. In 1957, the American physician, George Friou, developed the technique of antibody detection by indirect immunofluorescence[30]. Thus was born the fluorescent antinuclear antibody test, which is positive in 95–98% of the SLE cases. Subsequently, the recognition of antibodies to DNA[31] and the description of antibodies to extractable nuclear antigens[32] expanded the range of immunodiagnostic laboratory tests in lupus. Some of these antibodies could be correlated with newly recognized subsets of lupus. Neonatal lupus, produced by the transplacental transfer of anti-Ro antibodies and manifested by skin lesions and potentially fatal heart block, was first described in 1954. Subacute cutaneous lupus erythematosus, a distinct form of annular, photosensitive skin lesions seemingly produced by anti-Ro antibodies, was described by Sontheimer *et al.* in 1979[33].

The more recent discovery of a set of antibodies that are identified functionally by prolongation of *in vitro* coagulation tests has helped identify a new subgroup of patients with SLE with a distinct phenotype. In 1952, Conley and Hartmann noticed that some patients with SLE had an uncommon coagulation abnormality called 'lupus anticoagulant'[34]. In 1957, Laurel and Nilsson found that the lupus inhibitor was frequently associated with BFP and that the factor responsible for its activity was an immunoglobulin that could be absorbed by cardiolipin[35]. In 1963, Bowie made the observation that the anticoagulant was not associated with bleeding as initially believed, but with thrombosis[36]. Beaumont, and later on Nilsson, noted the association of lupus anticoagulant with spontaneous abortion. The association of these clinical features with anticardiolipin antibodies could be confirmed only when, in 1983, Harris and colleagues at Hammersmith Hospital in London, UK, designed a sensitive assay for the detection of antiphospholipid antibodies using cardiolipin as antigen[37]. This led to the recognition in 1986 of the antiphospholipid syndrome[38].

Recent advances

Two major advances that mark the modern era made a significant contribution to the understanding of SLE pathogenesis: the development of animal models of lupus and the recognition of the role of genetic predisposition to the development of lupus. The first animal model of systemic lupus was the hybrid New Zealand Black/New Zealand white mouse[39]. This murine model has provided many insights into the pathogenesis of autoantibody formation, mechanisms of immunologic tolerance, the development of glomerulonephritis, the role of sex hormones in modulating the course of the disease, and evaluation of treatments.

The familial occurrence of systemic lupus was first noted by Leonhardt in 1954 and later studied by Arnett and Shulman at Johns Hopkins Hospital[40]. Subsequently, familial aggregation of lupus, the concordance of lupus in monozygotic twin pairs, and the association of genetic markers with lupus have been described over the past 30 years[41]. In association studies of human lupus, the contributions of the major histocompatibility complex loci, Fcγ receptors, various cytokines, components of the complement cascade, and proteins involved in apoptosis have been explored. Most recently, genome screens by linkage analysis have indicated candidate susceptibility genes on chromosome 1 and several other chromosomal regions[42-44].

TREATMENT

No discussion of lupus is complete without a review of the development of treatment. Payne, in 1894, first reported the usefulness of quinine in the treatment of lupus[45]. Four years later, Radcliffe-Crocker noted the beneficial effect of the use of salicylates in conjunction with quinine: 'In violent inflammatory cases he has observed good results from salicilin,

as well as from quinine'[46]. It was not until the middle of this century that the treatment of systemic lupus was revolutionized by the discovery of the efficacy of adrenocorticotrophic hormone and cortisone by Hench[47]. Currently, corticosteroids are the primary treatment for many patients with lupus. Chloroquine was first used for discoid SLE in 1954[48] and antimalarial drugs have become the main treatment for patients with skin and joint involvement.

CLASSIFICATION

Systemic lupus erythematosus has been increasingly recognized as a disorder characterized by heterogenous clinical and laboratory features. Therefore, comparison between studies of patients with lupus required a standardized definition of disease to assure homogeneity of the case population. Influenced by the Jones criteria for acute rheumatic fever established in 1944[49], the American Rheumatism Association (later the American College of Rheumatology) published the preliminary criteria for the classification of SLE in 1971[50]. Fourteen criteria were selected on the basis of evaluation of 74 manifestations of SLE in a group of 245 patients with unequivocal SLE in comparison with 234 patients with rheumatoid arthritis and 217 patients with other diseases. The criteria were revised in 1982 and 11 criteria were chosen. The presence of at least four criteria was required in both sets. Although classification criteria were intended to be used mainly for the purpose of classifying patients in clinical, epidemiologic, therapeutic and pathogenetic studies of SLE, they also served to facilitate education and to guide clinical practice.

CONCLUSION

The history of lupus evolved from the clinical description of a distinct cutaneous disease to that of a multisystem disease associated with pathologic lesions of the blood vessels and connective tissue and characteristic immunologic markers. The explosion of the immunologic and molecular genetic research during the modern era has tremendously advanced our knowledge and understanding of the disease. It is hoped that this exponential growth of knowledge will reveal the still elusive etiology, and will allow the development of more effective treatments.

REFERENCES

1. Smith CD, Cyr M. The history of lupus erythematosus from Hippocrates to Osler. Rheum Dis Clin North Am 1988; 14: 1–14.
2. Benedek TG. Historical background of discoid and systemic lupus erythematosus. In: Wallace DJ, Hahn BH, eds. Dubois' lupus erythematosus, 5E. Baltimore: Williams & Wilkins; 1997: 3–16.
3. Blotzer JW. Systemic lupus erythematosus 1. Historical aspects. Md Med J 1983; 32: 439–441.
4. Skinner A. The origin of medical terms. Baltimore: Williams and Wilkins Co.; 1949: 219.
5. Hochberg MC. The history of lupus erythematosus. Md Med J 1991; 40: 871–873.
6. Neuburger M. Geschichte der Medizin, vol II. Enke F, ed. Stuttgart: 1911: 307.
7. Bateman T. A practical synopsis of cutaneous diseases. Philadelphia: Collins & Croft; 1818: 305.
8. Cazenave A, Schedel HE. Manual of the diseases of the skin, 2E (American). New York: S&S Wood; 1852: 35–36.
9. Cazenave A, Chausit M. Annales des maladies de la peau et de la syphilis. 1851: 297–299.
10. von Hebra F. Jahresbericht uber die Forschritte der gesammten Medicin in allen Landern im Jahre 1845. Canstatt BF, Eisenmann G, eds. Erlangen: F Enke; 1846: 226–227.
11. Kaposi M. Lupus erythematosus. In: Hebra F, Kaposi M, eds. On diseases of the skin including the exanthemata, vol IV. London: The New Sydenham Society; 1880: 14–37.
12. Kaposi M. Lupus vulgaris. In: Hebra F, Kaposi M, eds. On diseases of the skin including the exanthemata, vol IV (1875). London: The New Sydenham Society; 1880: 49–63.
13. Osler W. On the visceral manifestations of the erythema group of skin diseases (third paper). Am J Med Sci 1904; 127: 1–23.
14. Jadassohn J. Lupus erythematodes. In: Mracek F, ed. Handbuch der Hautkrankheiten. Wien: Alfred Holder; 1904: 298–404.
15. Osler W. The visceral lesions of the erythema group. Br J Dermatol 1900; 12: 227–245.
16. Kaposi M. Neue Beitrage zur Kenntnis des Lupus Erythematosus. Arch Derm Syph 1872; 4: 36–78.
17. Libman E, Sacks B. A hitherto underdescribed form of valvular and mural endocarditis. Trans Assoc Am Physicians 1923; 38: 46–61.
18. Gross L. The heart in atypical verucous endocarditis (Libman-Sacks). Contributions to the medical sciences in honor of Dr Emanuel Libman by his pupils, friends, and colleagues, vol 2. New York: The International Press; 1932: 527–550.
19. Baehr G. A diffuse disease of the peripheral circulation usually associated with lupus erythematosus and endocarditis. Trans Assoc Am Physicians 1935; 50: 139–155.
20. Friedberg CK, Gross L, Wallach K. Nonbacterial thrombotic endocarditis associated with prolonged fever, arthritis, inflammation of serous membranes and wide-spread vascular lesions. Arch Intern Med 1936; 58: 662–684.
21. Keil H. Relationship between lupus erythematosus and tuberculosis. Arch Derm Syph 1933; 28: 765–779.
22. Klinge F. Der Rheumatismus; pathologische-anatomische und experimentell-pathologische Tatsachen. Ergeb Path Path Anat 1933; 27: 1–355.
23. Klemperer P, Gueft B, Lee SL et al. Cytochemical changes of acute lupus erythematosus. Arch Pathol 1950; 49: 503–516.
24. Klemperer P, Pollack AD, Baehr G. Diffuse collagen disease. Acute disseminated lupus erythematosus and diffuse scleroderma. JAMA 1942; 119: 331–332.
25. Moore JE. The natural history of systemic lupus erythematosus: an approach to its study through chronic biologic false positive reactors. J Chron Dis 1955; 2: 297–316.
26. Hargraves MM, Richmond H, Morton R. Presentation of two bone marrow elements: the tart cell and the 'L.E.' Cell. Mayo Clin Proc 1948; 23: 25–28.
27. Hargraves MM. Discovery of the LE cell and its morphology. Mayo Clin Proc 1969; 44: 579–599.
28. Haserick JR. Blood factor in acute disseminated lupus erythematosus. II. Induction of specific antibodies against LE factor. Blood 1950; 5: 718–722.

29. Miescher P, Fauconnet M. L'absorption du facteur 'LE' par des noyaux cellulaire isoles. Experientia 1954; 10: 252–254.

30. Friou GJ. Clinical application of lupus serum nucleoprotein reaction using fluorescent antibody technique. J Clin Invest 1957; 109: 890A.

31. Deicher HR, Holman HR, Kunkel JB. The precipitin reaction between DNA and a serum factor in SLE. J Exp Med 1959; 109: 97–114.

32. Tan EM, Kunkel HG. Characteristics of a soluble nuclear antigen precipitating with sera of patients with systemic lupus erythematosus. J Immunol 1966; 96: 464–471.

33. Sontheimer RD, Thomas JR, Gilliam JN. Subacute cutaneous lupus erythematosus. A cutaneous marker for a distinct lupus erythematosus subset. Arch Dermatol 1979; 115: 1409–1415.

34. Conley CL, Hartmann RC. A hemorrhagic disorder caused by circulating anticoagulant in patients with disseminated lupus erythematosus. J Clin Invest 1952; 31: 621–622.

35. Laurel AB, Nilsson IM. Hypergammaglobulinemia, circulating anticoagulant and biologic false positive Wasserman reaction: a study of 2 cases. J Lab Clin Med 1957; 49: 416–430.

36. Bowie EJ, Thompson JH, Pacussi CA, Owen CA. Thrombosis in systemic lupus erythematosus despite circulating anticoagulants. J Lab Clin Med 1963; 62: 153–159.

37. Harris EN, Gharavi AE, Boey ML et al. Anticardiolipin antibodies: detection by radioimmunoassay and association with thrombosis in systemic lupus erythematosus. Lancet 1983; 2: 1211–1214.

38. Hughes GRV, Harris EN, Gharavi AE. The antiphospholipid syndrome. J Rheumatol 1986; 13: 486–489.

39. Bielschowsky M, Helyer BJ, Howie JB. Spontaneous hemolytic anemia in mice of NZB/BL strain. Proc Univ Otago Med School 1959; 37: 9–11.

40. Arnett FC, Shulman LE. Studies in familial systemic lupus erythematosus. Medicine (Baltimore) 1976; 55: 313–322.

41. Hochberg MC. The application of genetic epidemiology to systemic lupus erythematosus. J Rheumatol 1987; 14: 867–869.

42. Gaffney PM, Ortmann WA, Selby SA et al. Genome screening in human systemic lupus erythematosus: results from a second Minnesota cohort and combined analyses of 187 sib-pair families. Am J Hum Genet 2000; 66: 547–556.

43. Moser KL, Neas BR, Salmon JE et al. Genome scan of human systemic lupus erythematosus: evidence for linkage on chromosome 1q in African-American pedigrees. Proc Natl Acad Sci USA 1998; 95: 14869–14874.

44. Tsao BP, Cantor RM, Kalunian KC et al. Evidence for linkage of a candidate chromosome 1 region to human systemic lupus erythematosus. J Clin Invest 1997; 99: 725–731.

45. Payne JF. A post-graduate lecture on lupus erythematosus. Clin J 1894; 4: 223–230.

46. Radcliffe-Crocker. Discussion on lupus erythematosus. Br J Dermatol 1898; 10: 375.

47. Hench PS. The reversibility of certain rheumatic conditions by the use of cortisone or of the pituitary adrenocorticotrophic hormone. Ann Intern Med 1952; 36: 1–38.

48. Pillsbury DM, Jacobson C. Treatment of chronic discoid lupus erythematosus with chloroquine (Aralen). JAMA 1954; 154: 1330–1333.

49. Jones TD. The diagnosis of rheumatic fever. JAMA 1944; 126: 481–484.

50. Cohen AS, Reynolds WE, Franklin EC et al. Preliminary criteria for the classification of systemic lupus erythematosus. Bull Rheum Dis 1971; 21: 643–648.

116 Epidemiology and classification of systemic lupus erythematosus

Susan M Manzi, Vida Emily Stark and Rosalind Ramsey-Goldman

- The incidence and prevalence of systemic lupus erythematosus (SLE) vary among different racial/ethnic groups

- Survival in patients with SLE has improved significantly over the past five decades, but patients still have a three to five times increased mortality compared with the general population

- Early deaths are due to severe disease manifestations (renal, central nervous system, vasculitis) or infections, whereas late deaths (myocardial infarction, cerebrovascular event) are due to complications from disease damage or treatment toxicity

- African-American patients with SLE appear to have poorer survival than do white patients, but this observation may be confounded by socioeconomic factors or disease severity at presentation

- The American College of Rheumatology criteria for the classification of SLE serve as helpful reminders of those features that distinguish SLE from other connective tissue diseases

- The spectrum of clinical manifestations in SLE is much greater than described by these criteria, and disease severity may vary widely among patients with SLE.

EPIDEMIOLOGY

Incidence and prevalence

Systemic lupus erythematosus (SLE) is one of the most common autoimmune disorders in women during their childbearing years, and it is being recognized increasingly throughout the world's population. Because SLE is a debilitating disease that affects young people in the prime of life, refining the estimates of who is affected and predicting their outcomes are essential in decreasing the mortality and morbidity associated with this disease.

Rigorous interpretation of the differences in previously reported incidence and prevalence rates of SLE is hampered by limitations in study methodology. These limitations include the lack of standardized criteria for case detection and the absence of any formal estimate of the proportion of all cases in the population that are actually detected. In addition, passive methods of case ascertainment, such as medical records review, may not be ideal for smaller populations. For example, many studies that have used a review of inpatient medical records for case ascertainment may be overlooking patients with SLE who may not have been hospitalized early in the disease course; they may also be excluding patients with less severe disease. Multiple sources of ascertainment should be used for maximum accuracy. Moreover, capture–recapture methods may improve the accuracy of reported incidence rates for SLE and allow meaningful comparisons between studies.

In the USA (1950–1990), the overall average incidence of SLE has been estimated to range between 1.8 and 7.6 cases per 100 000 person-years (Table 116.1)[1-6]. Similar incidence rates, ranging from 3.3 to 4.8 per 100 000 person-years, were observed in four European cohorts from Iceland, England, and Sweden[7-10]. In a study examining the average annual incidence of SLE from 1985 to 1990, capture–recapture methodology was used to provide a more accurate estimate of the total number of cases in the population[5]. Using this technique, the estimated ascertainment was 85% (95% confidence interval (CI) 78 to 92), which resulted in an adjusted incidence rate of 2.4 per 100 000 person-years (95% CI 2.6 to 3.2 per 100 000 person-years). In total, 269 incident cases of SLE (191 definite and 78 probable by 1982 American College of Rheumatology criteria) were identified. The race- and sex-specific incidence rates of definite SLE per 100 000 persons were 0.4 (95% CI 0.2 to 0.7) for white males, 3.5 (95% CI 2.9 to 4.2) for white females, 0.7 (95% CI 0.0 to 2.0) for African-American males, and 9.2 (95% CI 6.8 to 12.5) for African-American females. These rates were in accordance with previous reports of a greater incidence of SLE among females compared with males and among African-Americans compared with whites.

The prevalence of SLE in the USA ranges from 14.6 to 50.8 per 100 000 persons (Table 116.2)[1-3]. Recent data suggest an increased prevalence in North American Indians compared with whites[11-13]; however, results are inconclusive when Asians and whites are compared[9,14]. There are no studies of prevalence among US Hispanic populations.

Study	Date	Location	Incidence rates per 100 000 person-years				
			WM	WF	AAM	AAF	Total
Siegel[1]	1956–65	New York, NY Jefferson County, AL	0.3	2.5	1.1	8.1	2.0
Fessel[2]	1965–73	San Francisco, CA	ND	ND	ND	ND	7.6
Michet[3]	1950–79	Rochester, MN	0.9	2.5	ND	ND	1.8
Michet[3]	1970–79	Rochester, MN	0.8	3.4	ND	ND	2.2
Hochberg[4]	1970–77	Baltimore, MD	0.4	3.9	2.5	11.4	4.6
McCarty[5]	1985–90	Pittsburgh, PA	0.4	3.5	0.7	9.2	2.4

TABLE 116.1 INCIDENCE OF SLE IN SEX AND RACE SUBSETS IN THE USA

WM, white male; WF, white female; AAM, African-American male; AAF, African-American female.

TABLE 116.2 PREVALENCE OF SLE IN SEX AND RACE SUBSETS THE USA

Study	Date	Location	Incidence rates per 100 000 person-years				
			WM	WF	AAM	AAF	Total
Siegel[1]	1965	New York, NY					
		Jefferson County, AL	3	17	3	56	14.6
Fessel[2]	1973	San Francisco, CA	7	71	53	283	50.8
Michet[3]	1980	Rochester, MN	19	54	ND	ND	40.0

WM, white male; WF, white female; AAM, African-American male; AAF, African-American female.

Overall statistics for the incidence and prevalence of SLE can be misleading. More information may be gleaned from a breakdown of a study population into subsets such as those based on sex and race/ethnicity. For example, the incidence of lupus is dramatically higher in women than in men. The peak incidence occurs between the ages of 15 and 45 years, the childbearing years, when the female-to-male ratio is about 12:1. In pediatric and older-onset patients the female-to-male ratio is closer to 2:1. Also, the contribution of race/ethnicity to the incidence and prevalence of SLE is increasingly apparent. Evidence suggests that SLE is more common in African-American than in white populations. Results from studies of two urban cohorts using capture–recapture methodology revealed that African-American and Afro-Caribbean women had a three- to fivefold greater incidence of disease when compared with whites[5,9]. In addition, Afro-Caribbean women were significantly younger at disease onset compared with white women: median ages 26 and 33 years, respectively. When the prevalence of SLE was stratified by race, the Afro-Caribbean prevalence rate was approximately five times that for whites[9]. In the USA, prevalence rates of SLE in female African-Americans range from 17.9 to 283 per 100 000[1,2]. In a West Indian study of female patients with SLE, a prevalence rate of 83.8 per 100 000 was reported[15].

Although SLE is more common in African-American than white populations in the USA, there are no population-based studies of the prevalence of SLE in Africa. The available data, consisting primarily of case reports and reports of series of hospital inpatients, imply that this disease is rare[16]. The prevalence of SLE increases from Africa to Europe, a phenomenon termed the 'prevalence gradient hypothesis'[16,17]. Potential initiators of a prevalence gradient include genetic factors and environmental triggers such as nutritional differences or exposures to pathogens. There is also a suggestion of an increased prevalence of SLE from Africa to North America, but the data are limited and not directly comparable because of different study criteria such as those for diagnosis and disease severity. Interestingly, the rate in African-Europeans (197–207 per 100 000) exceeds that of African-Americans[8,9].

Information regarding the incidence and prevalence of SLE in other non-white populations is scant. Few studies of SLE in Native Americans have been performed, even though there appears to be an increased risk of SLE in this population. A study using the Indian Health Services Database reported an overall annual incidence of SLE, ranging from 1 to 4 per 100 000 person-years in different tribes of American Indians[11]. The prevalence of SLE among Eskimos was reported to be 11 per 100 000 persons[13]. The incidence of SLE in Hawaii is 41.8 per 100 000 person-years, although a lower incidence was found in native Hawaiians (0.8-fold that of whites); comparison of Asian subgroups with whites revealed that the incidence rate of SLE was 1.3-fold greater in Japanese, 1.5-fold greater in Filipinos, and 2.5-fold greater in Chinese[18]. In England, increased incidence (fivefold greater) and prevalence (twofold greater) of SLE were noted in Asians compared with those in whites[9], although no increased prevalence was noted among Asians (predominantly Chinese) residing in the San Francisco area[2].

The prevalence of SLE was found to be 40–70 per 100 000 persons in Mainland China and 54 per 100 000 persons in Taiwan[19]. The apparent variability in epidemiological data describing SLE in Asians may be due to genetic heterogeneity, environment or study methodology. The Lupus in Minority Populations Nature versus Nurture (LUMINA) study reported initial data describing the characteristics and severity of SLE within the US Hispanic population[20], but there have been no rigorous studies of the incidence or prevalence of SLE in this group, despite a suggestion of increased morbidity and mortality. The major difficulty lies in the heterogeneity of the term 'Hispanic'. In the USA, Hispanics comprise 11.7% of the total population, but consist of several distinct groups, with 65% Mexican-Americans, 4.3% Cuban-Americans, 9.6% Puerto-Rican Americans, 14.3% Central- and South- Americans, and 7.3% listed as 'other'[21].

In summary, although most studies of the incidence and prevalence of SLE have been performed using white population cohorts, it appears that individual races/ethnicities may exhibit differences in disease susceptibility. Further studies are needed to clarify potential reasons, such as genetic factors with regional variation in gene pools caused by selection or admixture, and environmental factors including toxins, infections and diet. In the future, a multicenter international study using rigorous methods for case ascertainment and refined definitions of race will be essential for examining sex- and race-specific prevalence and incidence rates[22,23]. The results obtained may guide research efforts towards an understanding of the modifiable risk factors, which may also differ among racial/ethnic groups.

Mortality

Over the past 50 years, the survival of patients with SLE has improved dramatically (Table 116.3). In 1955, the 5-year survival rate was only 50%[24], whereas in the 1990s, the 10-year survival rate approached or exceeded 90%, and the 20-year survival rate approached 70%[36,37,43]. Factors contributing to this improvement include earlier diagnosis, more potent pharmaceutical agents, and improved treatments such as dialysis and kidney transplantation. Nonetheless, despite better survival, mortality rates for patients with SLE remain three to five times greater than those in the general population[40,44]. As with studies of incidence and prevalence, research investigating factors that may be predictive of mortality in patients with SLE focuses on age at disease onset, sex, race/ethnicity, and socioeconomic status.

Host factors

The association of age at disease onset with increased mortality appears to be significant. In two recent studies in urban populations, older age at diagnosis of SLE correlated with decreased survival[39,40]. Patients with SLE who were older than 50 years at diagnosis displayed significantly decreased survival rates[40], and the risk of SLE-related mortality was estimated to increase by 28% with each 10-year increase in age[39]. Using Cox proportional hazards modeling, the adjusted 5-, 10- and 15-year survival estimates were 83%, 79% and 79% for the age group 2–13 years; 84%,

TABLE 116.3 SLE SURVIVAL RATES (PUBLISHED STUDIES FROM 1955 TO 1995)

Study	Year	Center	Survival rate (%) 5 years	10 years	15 years	20 years
Merrell and Shulman[24]	1955	Baltimore	50	–	–	–
Kellum and Hasericke[25]	1964	Cleveland	69	54	–	–
Urman and Rothfield[26]	1968	New York	70	63	–	–
Estes and Christian[27]	1971	New York	77	60	50	–
Urowitz et al.[28]	1974	Toronto	75	63	53	–
Urman and Rothfield[26]	1976	Farmington	93	84	–	–
Wallace et al.[29]	1981	Los Angeles	88	79	74	–
Ginzler et al.[30]	1982	Multicenter	86	76	–	–
Jonsson et al.[31]	1985	Sweden	97	–	–	–
Malaviya et al.[32]	1986	India	68	50	–	–
Stafford-Brady et al.[33]	1988	Toronto	84	75	64	–
Swaak et al.[34]	1989	Holland	92	87	–	–
Reveille et al.[35]	1990	Alabama	89	83	79	–
Gripenberg and Helve[36]	1991	Finland	–	91	81	–
Pistiner et al.[37]	1991	Los Angeles	97	93	83	–
Seleznick and Fries[38]	1991	Stanford	88	64	–	–
Ward et al.[39]	1993	Durham	82	71	63	–
Abu-Shakra et al.[40]	1993	Toronto	93	85	79	68
Nossent[41]	1993	Curacao	56	–	–	–
Massardo et al.[42]	1994	Chile	92	77	66	–
Tucker et al.[43]	1995	London	93	85	79	–

(Adapted with permission from Gladman[50].)

75%, and 67% for the age group 14–54 years and 69%, 47%, and 36% for the age group 55–80 years. In contrast, another study found no differences in mortality rates between childhood-onset and adult-onset SLE[43].

The sex of patients with SLE has also been implicated as a factor affecting mortality. In most studies, decreased survival is associated with male sex[39,40,45–48]. Compared with female SLE patients, SLE males had greater all-cause mortality rates (hazard ratio 1.55; 95% CI 1.02 to 2.35), but not SLE-related mortality (hazard ratio 1.37; 95% CI 0.76 to 2.48)[39]. A significantly increased 1-year crude mortality rate was seen in male patients with SLE (8.23%) compared with that in SLE females (4.6%)[49]. In general, however, when differences in age distribution between male and female patients with SLE are considered, sex does not emerge as a significant predictor of survival.

Race/ethnicity appear to be associated with mortality rates in SLE, although it has been difficult to separate race itself from socioeconomic status, particularly among African-Americans and whites in the USA[50]. Generally, African-American and Hispanic patients with SLE in the USA have a worse prognosis than white patients[20,30,35,51]. Similarly, patients with SLE who are of Asian, Indian, Afro-Caribbean, and Hispanic race have a worse prognosis than either North American or European whites[32,42,52,53]. In the Multicenter Lupus Survival study, calculation of survival rates based on race subsets revealed that the most important predictors of mortality were disease severity at study entry and insurance status, not African-American race[30]. In this study, the distribution of race differed significantly between the center with the highest survival (85% whites and 7.3% African-Americans) and the center with the lowest survival rate (22.3% whites and 61.1% African-Americans); this finding was consistent across centers, with greater survival in white patients. Nonetheless, at study entry, African-American patients with SLE had more severe disease (as measured by increased serum creatinine, hematocrit less than 30%, proteinuria greater than 1+, and greater frequency of neuropsychiatric involvement) and were more likely to carry public rather than private medical insurance; these factors dictated the survival outcome. In contrast to these findings, African-American

patients with SLE seen at the University of Alabama between 1975 and 1985 fared worse than white patients, with 26% and 20% mortality, respectively (p=0.002), medical insurance status notwithstanding[35]. In a recent study of patients with SLE at Duke University, African-American patients had poorer survival than whites at 5, 10 and 15 years (76%, 65% and 55% compared with 87%, 76% and 70%, respectively; p=0.005). However, after determining the interrelationships among age, sex, race, and socioeconomic status (insurance and median household income), the association of race with mortality was no longer significant, whereas the other variables remained significant[39]. Similar observations were noted in two other studies. In a recent multicenter analysis of Hispanic, African-American, and white SLE patients with 5 or fewer years of disease at study entry, survival rates were associated with disease severity at study entry, socioeconomic status, and Systemic Lupus International Cooperating Clinics score, whereas race was not a significant factor[20]. In a study using nationwide cause-of-death data collected by the National Center for Health Statistics from 1968 to 1991, African-American and white SLE women who were younger than 45 years had different survival rates, which continued to widen during the study period[54]. Among white women, overall SLE mortality was constant at 4.6 deaths per million, with a decline in younger women and an increase in older women, whereas among African-American women, overall SLE mortality rose 30% to a mean annual rate of 18.7 per million, with a constant rate in younger women and an increasing rate in older women. Proposed reasons for these discrepancies included an increased predisposition for SLE and more severe, treatment-resistant disease in young African-American women. Asian women in the USA and China exhibit similar mortality rates for SLE[2,55], although Asians in England have a worse prognosis[52,56].

Causes of death

Early mortality usually occurs because of active disease, especially in the renal and central nervous systems. Later deaths are frequently the result of complications of SLE or its treatment. This bimodal pattern of mortality suggests that improved treatment does not cure lupus, but postpones death from a related or other cause at an older age[28]. The most critical predictor of mortality in SLE is renal disease, measured by either serum creatinine or qualitative urine protein excretion[30,40,41,43,57,58]. In one study of patients with lupus nephritis, survival at 5, 10, and 20 years was 80%, 69%, and 53%, respectively[59]. In a study of patients with lupus nephritis after kidney transplantation, the 5-year survival was reported to be 85.9%[60]. The contribution of race to the occurrence and severity of renal disease has also been assessed; in a recent study, African-American women had the greatest rates of lupus renal disease and worse renal survival compared with white women[61].

Another critical parameter for predicting mortality from SLE is believed to be the degree of disease in the central nervous system. Overall, patients with neuropsychiatric symptoms exhibit decreased survival[35]. It has been suggested that central nervous system involvement predicts mortality only in patients with active disease in other organs[62], although it is not clear if this represents an independent predictor, because severe multisystem disease itself (as measured by SLE Disease Activity Index scores >20) can predict mortality[40].

A leading cause of death in patients with SLE is infection. In a recent European study, 28.9% of patients with SLE died from infection, primarily bacterial sepsis[63]. As reported in several East Indian studies, infection represented 20% of the overall mortality, after irreversible renal damage (44%) and uncontrolled disease activity (35%)[53,64,65]. In a Brazilian study, a mortality of 58% resulted from infection[66].

The contribution of race to mortality is under investigation. The results of the LUMINA study indicate differences in causes of death among ethnic groups[20]: in Hispanic patients, active disease secondary to SLE was the cause of death in 80%; in the African-American patients, infections caused death in 50%; in white patients, death was attributed to other causes in 50%.

The distinction between race and ethnicity was recently described[23,24]. The challenge for investigators is to appreciate that observations related only to race may not apply to an entire ethnic group. Future studies must incorporate emerging information about race and ethnicity in order to identify those at risk for more severe disease and death, and to understand the spectrum of disease phenotypes across race and ethnic groups.

In summary, patients with SLE of African or Hispanic descent appear to have greater mortality rates, but there are conflicting data on survival rates among other non-white groups such as Asians and American-Indians. The precise contributions of race/ethnicity, socioeconomic status, or disease severity warrant further intensive investigation.

DEFINITION AND CLASSIFICATION

Systemic lupus erythematosus is the prototypic inflammatory auto-immune disease, with multiorgan involvement, a wide variety of manifestations, and an unpredictable course. The dynamic nature of the disease, with changeable and intermittent signs and symptoms, makes the diagnosis particularly challenging. Often, unequivocal diagnosis is not made initially, requiring prolonged observation. In addition, there are other diseases with multisystem involvement that may mimic SLE. Both clinical presentation and laboratory testing must be combined in diagnosing SLE, with special attention paid to family history of autoimmune disease, in addition to the patient's drug history.

Criteria for disease classification, intended to ensure comparability of patients from different geographical locations, were developed in 1971, revised in 1982, and revised again in 1997 (Table 116.4)[67]. They include malar rash (non-scarring rash across the bridge of the nose and cheeks), discoid rash (scarring rash), photosensitivity, oral ulcers, arthritis, serositis (pleuritis or pericarditis), renal involvement, central nervous system involvement (seizures or psychosis), hematologic abnormalities

---

TABLE 116.4 CLASSIFICATION OF SLE – 1997 REVISED CRITERIA

1. Malar rash
   Fixed erythema, flat or raised, over the malar eminences, tending to spare the nasolabial folds
2. Discoid rash
   Erythematosus raised patches with adherent keratotic scaling and follicular plugging; atrophic scarring occur in older lesions
3. Photosensitivity
   Skin rash as a result of unusual reaction to sunlight, by patient history or physician observation
4. Oral ulcers
   Oral or nasopharyngeal ulceration, usually painless, observed by a physician
5. Arthritis
   Non-erosive arthritis involving 2 or more peripheral joints, characterized by tenderness, swelling or effusion
6. Serositis
   (a) Pleuritis – convincing history of pleuritic pain or rub heard by a physician or evidence of pleural effusion
       or
   (b) Pericarditis – documented by ECG or rub or evidence of pericardial effusion
7. Renal disorder
   (a) Persistent proteinuria greater than 0.5g per day or greater than 3+ if quantitation not performed
       or
   (b) Cellular casts – may be red cell, hemoglobin, granular, tubular or mixed
8. Neurological disorder
   (a) Seizures – in the absence of offending drugs or known metabolic derangements (e.g. uremia, ketoacidosis, or electrolyte imbalance)
       or
   (b) Psychosis – in the absence of offending drugs or known metabolic derangements (e.g. uremia, ketoacidosis or electrolyte imbalance)
9. Hematologic disorder
   (a) Hemolytic anemia – with reticulocytosis
       or
   (b) Leukopenia – less than 4000/mm³ total on 2 or more occasions
       or
   (c) Lymphopenia – less than 1500/mm³ on 2 or more occasions
       or
   (d) Thrombocytopenia – less than 100 000/mm³ in the absence of offending drugs
10. Immunologic disorder
    (a) Anti-DNA – antibody to native DNA in abnormal titer
        or
    (b) Anti-Sm – presence of antibody to Sm nuclear antigen
        or
    (b) Positive finding of antiphospholipid antibodies based on (1) an abnormal serum concentrationof IgG or IgM anticardiolipin antibodies, (2) a positive test result for lupus anticoagulant using a standard method or (3) a false-positive serologic test for syphilis known to be positive for at least 6 months and confirmed by *Treponema pallidum* immobilization or fluorescent treponemal antibody absorption test
11. Antinuclear antibody
    An abnormal titer of antinuclear antibody by immunofluorescence or an equivalent assay at any point in time and in the absence of drugs known to be associated with 'drug-induced lupus' syndrome

These criteria have been revised on the basis of recommendations made by the Diagnostic and Therapeutic Criteria Committee of the American College of Rheumatology[67].

(hemolytic anemia, leukopenia, thrombocytopenia), immunologic markers (antibodies to native DNA, Smith antigen, anticardiolipin IgG, IgM, lupus anticoagulant or a false-positive serologic test for syphilis), and antinuclear antibody. Positivity for at least four of the 11 criteria allows classification of a patient as having SLE. Although these criteria were established primarily for research purposes, they serve as helpful reminders of those features that distinguish SLE from other connective tissue diseases. However, the clinical manifestations in SLE are much greater than described by these criteria, and disease severity may vary widely, even in patients with the same clinical criteria.

Some of the most common symptoms of SLE are not specific for the disease. Constitutional symptoms such as fatigue, malaise, fever in the absence of infection, and weight loss may be seen in many chronic illnesses. Other disease manifestations not included in the criteria are lymphadenopathy, myositis, ocular inflammation, cutaneous and mesenteric vasculitis, and pneumonitis. Central nervous system dysfunction and renal disease are two of the most critical manifestations. Various central nervous system abnormalities include cognitive impairment, mood disorders, strokes, movement disorders, headache, and aseptic meningitis. There is great variability in the expression, course, and histopathology of renal disease, with virtually all patients with SLE displaying some degree of glomerular abnormality by renal biopsy, but only 40–70% with clinically apparent disease. Early detection of renal involvement is essential, because early intervention may prevent or delay end-stage renal disease.

SUMMARY

SLE is a chronic disease that affects young people in the prime of life. Refining the estimates of who is affected and predicting their outcomes are essential in decreasing mortality and morbidity. Interpretation of the differences between previously reported rates of incidence and prevalence of SLE is hampered by limitations in study methodology and case definition. Although most studies of the incidence and prevalence of SLE have been performed using white population cohorts, it appears that individual races/ethnicities may possess differences in disease susceptibility. Further studies are needed to clarify potential reasons for this, such as genetic factors with regional variation in gene pools caused by selection or admixture, and environmental factors.

Survival in SLE has improved significantly over the past five decades, but patients still have a three- to fivefold increased mortality compared with the general population. African-American patients with SLE appear to have poorer survival than white patients, but this finding may be confounded by socioeconomic factors or disease severity at presentation. Early deaths are generally caused by severe disease manifestations (renal, central nervous system, vasculitis) or infections, whereas late deaths (myocardial infarction, cerebrovascular event) are the result of complications from disease damage or treatment toxicity.

Diagnosis of SLE is generally not problematic when many typical symptoms and signs are present, but may be more troublesome when the disease manifests with only a few complaints or when problems evolve over time. The American College of Rheumatology criteria for the classification of SLE serve as helpful reminders of those features that distinguish SLE from other connective tissue diseases, but the spectrum of clinical manifestations in SLE is much greater than they describe, and disease severity may vary widely among patients with SLE.

REFERENCES

1. Siegel M, Holley HL, Lee SL. Epidemiologic studies on systemic lupus erythematosus. Comparative data for New York City and Jefferson County, Alabama, 1956–1965. Arthritis Rheum 1970; 13: 802–811.
2. Fessel WJ. Systemic lupus erythematosus in the community. Incidence, prevalence, outcome, and first symptoms; the high prevalence in black women. Arch Int Med 1974; 134: 1027–1035.
3. Michet CJ, McKenna CH, Elveback LR et al. Epidemiology of systemic lupus erythematosus and other connective tissue diseases in Rochester, Minnesota, 1950 through 1979. Mayo Clin Proc 1985; 60: 105–113.
4. Hochberg MC. The incidence of systemic lupus erythematosus in Baltimore, Maryland, 1970–1977. Arthritis Rheum 1985; 28: 80–86.
5. McCarty DJ, Manzi S, Medsger TA et al. Incidence of systemic lupus erythematosus. Race and gender differences. Arthritis Rheum 1995; 38: 1260–1270.
6. Siegel M, Lee SL. The epidemiology of systemic lupus erythematosus. Semin Arthritis Rheum 1973; 3: 1–54.
7. Gudmundsson S, Steinsson K. Systemic lupus erythematosus in Iceland 1975 through 1984. A nationwide epidemiological study in an unselected population. J Rheumatol 1990; 17: 1162–1167.
8. Hopkinson ND, Doherty M, Powell RJ. Clinical features and race-specific incidence/prevalence rates of systemic lupus erythematosus in a geographically complete cohort of patients. Ann Rheum Dis 1994; 53: 675–680.
9. Johnson AE, Gordon C, Palmer RG, Bacon PA. The prevalence and incidence of systemic lupus erythematosus in Birmingham, England. Relationship to ethnicity and country of birth. Arthritis Rheum 1995; 38: 551–558.
10. Stahl-Hallengren C, Jonsen A, Nived O, Sturfelt G. Incidence studies of systemic lupus erythematosus in Southern Sweden: increasing age, decreasing frequency of renal manifestations and good prognosis. J Rheumatol 2000; 27: 685–691.
11. Acers TE, Acers-Warn A. Incidence patterns of immunogenetic diseases in the North American Indians. J Okla State Med Assoc 1994; 87: 309–314.
12. Atkins C, Reuffel L, Roddy J et al. Rheumatic disease in the Nuu-Chah-Nulth native Indians of the Pacific Northwest. J Rheumatol 1988; 15: 684–690.
13. Boyer GS, Templin DW, Lanier AP. Rheumatic diseases in Alaskan Indians of the southeast coast: high prevalence of rheumatoid arthritis and systemic lupus erythematosus. J Rheumatol 1991; 18: 1477–1484.
14. Serdula MK, Rhoads GG. Frequency of systemic lupus erythematosus in different ethnic groups in Hawaii. Arthritis Rheum 1979; 22: 328–333.
15. Nossent JC. Systemic lupus erythematosus on the Caribbean island of Curacao: an epidemiological investigation. Ann Rheum Dis 1992; 51: 1197–1201.
16. Bae SC, Fraser P, Liang MH. The epidemiology of systemic lupus erythematosus in populations of African ancestry: a critical review of the 'prevalence gradient hypothesis'. Arthritis Rheum 1998; 41: 2091–2099.
17. Symmons DP. Frequency of lupus in people of African origin. Lupus 1995; 4: 176–178.
18. Maskarinec G, Katz AR. Prevalence of systemic lupus erythematosus in Hawaii: is there a difference between ethnic groups? Hawaii Med J 1995; 54: 406–409.
19. Nai-Cheng C. Rheumatic diseases in China. J Rheumatol 1976; 3: 186–190.
20. Alarcon GS, McGwin G Jr, Bastian HM et al. Systemic lupus erythematosus in three ethnic groups. VII [correction of VIII]. Predictors of early mortality in the LUMINA cohort. LUMINA Study Group [erratum appears in Arthritis Rheum 2001; 45: 306]. Arthritis Rheum 2001; 45: 191–202.
21. Escalante A, del Rincon I. Epidemiology and impact of rheumatic disorders in the United States Hispanic population. Curr Opin Rheumatol 2001; 13: 104–110.
22. Lin SS, Kelsey JL. Use of race and ethnicity in epidemiologic research: concepts, methodological issues, and suggestions for research. Epidemiol Rev 2000; 22: 187–202.
23. Brooks K, Fessler BJ, Bastian H, Alarcon GS. Sociocultural issues in clinical research. Arthritis Rheum 2001; 45: 203–207.
24. Merrell M, Shulman LE. Determination of prognosis in chronic disease, illustrated by systemic lupus erythematosus. J Chron Dis 1955; 1: 12–32.
25. Kellum RE, Hasericke JR. Systemic lupus erythematosus, a statistical evaluation of mortality based on a consecutive series of 299 patients. Arch Int Med 1964; 113: 200–207.
26. Urman JD, Rothfield NF. Corticosteroid treatment in systemic lupus erythematosus. Survival studies. JAMA 1977; 238: 2272–2276.
27. Estes D, Christian CL. The natural history of systemic lupus erythematosus by prospective analysis. Medicine (Baltimore) 1971; 50: 85–95.
28. Urowitz MB, Bookman AA, Koehler BE et al. The bimodal mortality pattern of systemic lupus erythematosus. Am J Med 1976; 60: 221–225.
29. Wallace DJ, Podell T, Weiner J et al. Systemic lupus erythematosus – survival patterns. Experience with 609 patients. JAMA 1981; 245: 934–938.
30. Ginzler EM, Diamond HS, Weiner M et al. A multicenter study of outcome in systemic lupus erythematosus. I. Entry variables as predictors of prognosis. Arthritis Rheum 1982; 25: 601–611.
31. Jonsson H, Nived O, Sturfelt G. Outcome in systemic lupus erythematosus: a prospective study of patients from a defined population. Medicine 1989; 68: 141–150.
32. Malaviya AN, Misra R, Banerjee S et al. Systemic lupus erythematosus in North Indian Asians. A prospective analysis of clinical and immunological features. Rheumatol Int 1986; 6: 97–101.
33. Stafford-Brady FJ, Urowitz MB, Gladman DD, Easterbrook M. Lupus retinopathy. Patterns, associations, and prognosis. Arthritis Rheum 1988; 31: 1105–1110.
34. Swaak AJ, Nossent JC, Bronsveld W et al. Systemic lupus erythematosus. I. Outcome and survival: Dutch experience with 110 patients studied prospectively. Ann Rheum Dis 1989; 48: 447–454.
35. Reveille JD, Bartolucci A, Alarcon GS. Prognosis in systemic lupus erythematosus. Negative impact of increasing age at onset, black race, and thrombocytopenia, as well as causes of death. Arthritis Rheum 1990; 33: 37–48.
36. Gripenberg M, Helve T. Outcome of systemic lupus erythematosus. A study of 66 patients over 7 years with special reference to the predictive value of anti-DNA antibody determinations. Scand J Rheumatol 1991; 20: 104–109.
37. Pistiner M, Wallace DJ, Nessim S et al. Lupus erythematosus in the 1980s: a survey of 570 patients. Semin Arthritis Rheum 1991; 21: 55–64.

38. Seleznick MJ, Fries JF. Variables associated with decreased survival in systemic lupus erythematosus. Semin Arthritis Rheum 1991; 21: 73–80.

39. Ward MM, Pyun E, Studenski S. Long-term survival in systemic lupus erythematosus. Patient characteristics associated with poorer outcomes. Arthritis Rheum 1995; 38: 274–283.

40. Abu-Shakra M, Urowitz MB, Gladman DD, Gough J. Mortality studies in systemic lupus erythematosus. Results from a single center. II. Predictor variables for mortality. J Rheumatol 1995; 22: 1265–1270.

41. Nossent JC. Course and prognostic value of Systemic Lupus Erythematosus Disease Activity Index in black Caribbean patients. Semin Arthritis Rheum 1993; 23: 16–21.

42. Massardo L, Martinez ME, Jacobelli S et al. Survival of Chilean patients with systemic lupus erythematosus. Semin Arthritis Rheum 1994; 24: 1–11.

43. Tucker LB, Menon S, Schaller JG, Isenberg DA. Adult- and childhood-onset systemic lupus erythematosus: a comparison of onset, clinical features, serology, and outcome. Br J Rheumatol 1995; 34: 866–872.

44. Uramoto KM, Michet CJ Jr, Thumboo J et al. Trends in the incidence and mortality of systemic lupus erythematosus, 1950–1992. Arthritis Rheum 1999; 42: 46–50.

45. Iseki K, Miyasato F, Oura T et al. An epidemiologic analysis of end-stage lupus nephritis. Am J Kidney Dis 1994; 23: 547–554.

46. Miller MH, Urowitz MB, Gladman DD, Killinger DW. Systemic lupus erythematosus in males. Medicine 1983; 62: 327–334.

47. Kaufman LD, Gomez-Reino JJ, Heinicke MH, Gorevic PD. Male lupus: retrospective analysis of the clinical and laboratory features of 52 patients, with a review of the literature. Semin Arthritis Rheum 1989; 18: 189–197.

48. Inman RD, Jovanovic L, Markenson JA et al. Systemic lupus erythematosus in men. Genetic and endocrine features. Arch Int Med 1982; 142: 1813–1815.

49. Prete P, Majlessi A, Gilman S, Hamideh F. Systemic lupus erythematosus in men: a retrospective analysis in a Veterans Administration healthcare system population. J Clin Rheumatol 2001; 7: 142–150.

50. Gladman DD. Prognosis and treatment of systemic lupus erythematosus. Curr Opin Rheumatol 1996; 8: 430–437.

51. Studenski S, Allen NB, Caldwell DS et al. Survival in systemic lupus erythematosus. A multivariate analysis of demographic factors. Arthritis Rheum 1987; 30: 1326–1332.

52. Samanta A, Feehally J, Roy S et al. High prevalence of systemic disease and mortality in Asian subjects with systemic lupus erythematosus. Ann Rheum Dis 1991; 50: 490–492.

53. Kumar A, Malaviya AN, Singh RR et al. Survival in patients with systemic lupus erythematosus in India. Rheumatol Int 1992; 12: 107–109.

54. Walsh SJ, Algert C, Gregorio DI et al. Divergent racial trends in mortality from systemic lupus erythematosus. J Rheumatol 1995; 22: 1663–1668.

55. Mok CC, Lee KW, Ho CT et al. A prospective study of survival and prognostic indicators of systemic lupus erythematosus in a southern Chinese population. Rheumatology 2000; 39: 399–406.

56. Feehally J, Burden AC, Mayberry JF et al. Disease variations in Asians in Leicester. Q J Med 1993; 86: 263–269.

57. Esdaile JM, Abrahamowicz M, MacKenzie T et al. The time-dependence of long-term prediction in lupus nephritis. Arthritis Rheum 1994; 37: 359–368.

58. McLaughlin JR, Bombardier C, Farewell VT et al. Kidney biopsy in systemic lupus erythematosus. III. Survival analysis controlling for clinical and laboratory variables. Arthritis Rheum 1994; 37: 559–567.

59. Donadio JV, Hart GM, Bergstralh EJ, Holley KE. Prognostic determinants in lupus nephritis: a long-term clinicopathologic study. Lupus 1995; 4: 109–115.

60. el-Shahawy MA, Aswad S, Mendez RG et al. Renal transplantation in systemic lupus erythematosus: a single-center experience with sixty-four cases. Am J Nephrol 1995; 15: 123–128.

61. Dooley MA, Hogan S, Jennette C, Falk R. Cyclophosphamide therapy for lupus nephritis: poor renal survival in black Americans. Glomerular Disease Collaborative Network. Kidney Int 1997; 51: 1188–1195.

62. Sibley JT, Olszynski WP, Decoteau WE, Sundaram MB. The incidence and prognosis of central nervous system disease in systemic lupus erythematosus. J Rheumatol 1992; 19: 47–52.

63. Cervera R, Khamashta MA, Font J et al. Morbidity and mortality in systemic lupus erythematosus during a 5-year period. A multicenter prospective study of 1,000 patients. European Working Party on Systemic Lupus Erythematosus. Medicine 1999; 78: 167–175.

64. Malaviya AN, Khan KM, Tiwari SC, Bhuyan UN. Systemic connective tissue disease in India. VII. Deaths in systemic lupus erythematosus. J Assoc Physicians India 1984; 32: 313–316.

65. Malaviya AN, Chandrasekaran AN, Kumar A, Shamar PN. Systemic lupus erythematosus in India [erratum appears in Lupus 1998; 7: 370]. Lupus 1997; 6: 690–700.

66. Iriya SM, Capelozzi VL, Calich I et al. Causes of death in patients with systemic lupus erythematosus in Sao Paulo, Brazil: a study of 113 autopsies. Arch Int Med 2001; 161: 1557.

67. Hochberg MC. Updating the American College of Rheumatology revised criteria for the classification of systemic lupus erythematosus. Arthritis Rheum 1997; 40: 1725.

117 Immunopathology

Jane E Salmon, Robert P Kimberly and Vivette D'Agati

- A prototypic immune complex disease involving excess antibody formation and immune complex deposits in tissue

- Characteristic lesions include hematoxylin bodies, Libman–Sacks endocarditis, vasculitis, thrombotic microangiopathy and glomerulonephritis

- Antibody properties are important in determining the pathogenic potential of immune complexes

- Complement deficiencies may alter immune complex handling

- Genetic variations in receptors for immunoglobulin (Fcγ receptors) influence antibody binding and pathologic effects of immune complexes

INTRODUCTION

Systemic lupus erythematosus (SLE) is the prototypic immune complex disease, characterized by excessive autoantibody production, immune complex formation and immunologically mediated tissue injury. Tissue pathology in all organs reflects a variety of aberrant immunologic mechanisms, but tissue damage in patients with lupus may also reflect non-immunologic processes. Some of these, such as early atherosclerosis, may, however, be initiated and accelerated through immunologic effector mechanisms.

The complexity of abnormal immunoregulation observed in patients with SLE has made it difficult for the clinical investigator to identify clearly the critical elements underlying the immunopathogenesis of SLE. However, several inter-related immunologic elements may be central. B cell and T cell abnormalities, including defects in B cell tolerance, autoantigen specific T helper cells and intrinsic T cell functional and biochemical irregularities[1,2], result in the production of autoantibodies. Production of at least some of these autoantibodies is driven by increased levels of nucleosomes, perhaps reflecting accelerated apoptosis of lymphocytes[3,4], and by abnormal cytokine concentrations. The sum of these abnormalities is an array of autoantibodies and circulating immune complexes. Taken together with deficiencies in mononuclear phagocyte function and immune complex clearance, SLE is a critical model for our understanding of immune complex mediated immunopathogenesis.

Unlike some autoimmune diseases, such as Hashimoto's thyroiditis and myasthenia gravis, which are highly organ-specific, SLE affects many different organs in a systemic fashion and is not organ-specific (Fig. 117.1). In this regard, the autoimmune mechanisms in SLE may be more similar to those found in diseases such as Sjögren's syndrome, rheumatoid arthritis (RA), dermatomyositis and scleroderma, as suggested by Klemperer *et al.* in their studies of the 'connective tissue' diseases[5]. Certainly, autoantibody formation, immunoglobulin deposition and primary or secondary infiltration of tissues with mononuclear cells are cardinal features of the disease. Both antigen-specific and antigen-non-specific immunologic targeting may be important. These processes

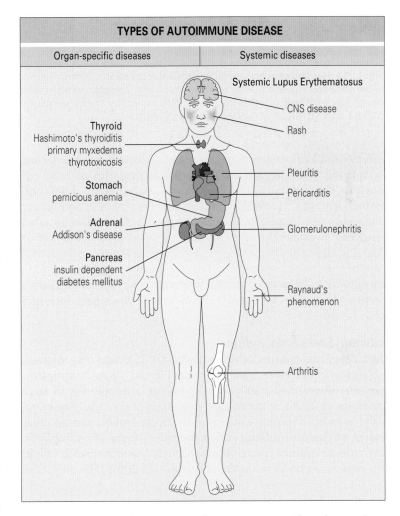

TYPES OF AUTOIMMUNE DISEASE

Organ-specific diseases	Systemic diseases

Systemic Lupus Erythematosus

CNS disease

Rash

Thyroid
Hashimoto's thyroiditis
primary myxedema
thyrotoxicosis

Pleuritis

Stomach
pernicious anemia

Pericarditis

Adrenal
Addison's disease

Glomerulonephritis

Pancreas
insulin dependent
diabetes mellitus

Raynaud's phenomenon

Arthritis

Fig. 117.1 Two types of autoimmune disease: organ-specific and systemic. Although the systemic autoimmune diseases produce symptoms in several organs, each disease may be marked by characteristic patterns of organ involvement. CNS, central nervous system.

eventually become apparent through a broad range of pathologic manifestations, including fibrinoid necrosis, hematoxylin bodies, vascular injury, disruption of the dermal–epidermal junction of skin, and glomerulonephritis.

PATHOLOGY

Characteristic lesions
Hematoxylin bodies
Several pathologic findings are characteristic of SLE. Hematoxylin bodies are usually oval or spindle-shaped basophilic structures that may approach the size of an intact cell. Also known as 'LE bodies',

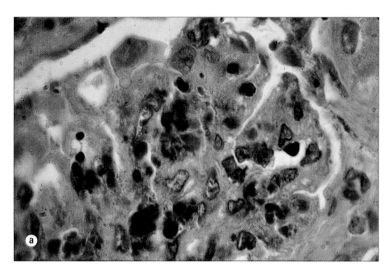
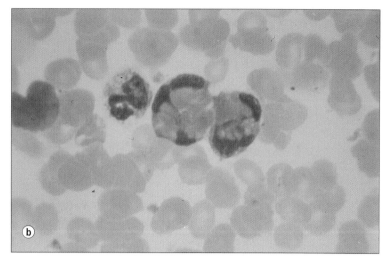

Fig. 117.2 Hematoxylin bodies. (a) A glomerulus containing several lilac hematoxylin bodies, corresponding to exposed nuclei in which the chromatin has undergone swelling and clumpy transformation after complexing with ambient antinuclear antibody. (Hematoxylin and eosin stain.) (b) LE cells. Two phagocytic cells have ingested large basophilic inclusions. The inclusions, termed hematoxylin bodies when seen before ingestion, contain DNA and IgG. (Wright stain.) (With permission of Professor IM Roitt.)

hematoxylin bodies resemble aggregates of chromatin and degenerated cytoplasmic organelles and can be formed *in vitro* with epithelial cell nuclei[6]. Biochemically, they appear to contain both DNA and immunoglobulin[7], probably reflecting the interaction of antinuclear antibodies with degenerating nuclear material. Although most often described in glomeruli and endocardium, hematoxylin bodies can be found in almost any organ (Fig. 117.2a). They are found in only a small number of biopsy specimens, but are highly suggestive of SLE. Engulfment of hematoxylin bodies by phagocytes produces the characteristic 'LE cell' – a phagocyte with a large basophilic inclusion (Fig. 117.2b).

Libman–Sacks endocarditis

At autopsy, the majority of patients who had SLE have non-bacterial, verrucous endocarditis, also known as Libman–Sacks endocarditis. Grossly, these small friable vegetations are often present in large numbers, especially at the forward-flow edges of the valve. The mitral valve is most commonly affected, but verrucae may be seen on other valves, on chordae tendineae and on the endocardium. Microscopically, the verrucae consist of proteinaceous deposits and mononuclear cells in the context of platelet thrombi and necrotic cell debris (Fig. 117. 3). The

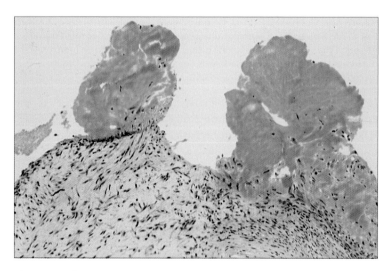

Fig. 117.3 Libman–Sacks endocarditis. Two verrucae on the surface of this valve contain fibrin and necrotic cell debris. Inflammatory cells are localized primarily at the endocardial surface. (Hematoxylin and eosin stain.)

occurrence of valvular lesions in association with antiphospholipid antibodies raises interesting speculations about pathogenesis of verrucous endocarditis, but the valvular abnormalities in primary antiphospholipid syndrome appear to be distinct, with valvular thickening but no vegetations[8,9]. For verrucous endocarditis, it is possible that circulating immune complexes may adhere to the valvular surface, contribute to initial endocardial damage and serve as a nidus for the deposition of fibrin and platelets.

Cutaneous immunopathology

The pathology of skin lesions illustrates the basic pathophysiologic mechanisms in SLE: immune complex formation with consequent tissue damage, acute vascular and perivascular inflammation, and more chronic mononuclear cell infiltration. Each of these features can be found in the histopathology of cutaneous lupus, although immunoglobulin deposition at the dermal–epidermal junction is the most consistent.

Analysis of lesional skin in SLE may demonstrate liquefactive degeneration of the basal cell layer of the epidermis, fibrinoid necrosis of the dermis, and perivascular and perifollicular infiltrates of inflammatory cells. In chronic lesions, there is prominent hyperkeratosis and follicular plugging, although these features are less evident in subacute cutaneous lupus, and usually absent in acute cutaneous lesions. Disorganization of the basal cell layer of the epidermis is found in chronic cutaneous and subacute cutaneous lesions; it may also be found in acute cutaneous lesions, although it may be more subtle. The mononuclear cell infiltrate, typically with T cell predominance, in the upper regions of the dermis may disrupt the dermal–epidermal junction in chronic lesions, but tends to be more localized to perivascular and periappendageal areas in other lesions[10]. Edema of the upper dermis with extravasation of erythrocytes can be found in all SLE skin lesions.

In less common forms of lupus skin lesions, the histologic picture is somewhat different. In bullous SLE, there are subepidermal bullae without vacuolar degeneration, but with an inflammatory infiltrate (mostly neutrophils) in the dermal papillae[11]. In lupus profundus, or lupus erythematosus panniculitis, there is deep dermal and subcutaneous involvement with nodules. Lesions in the epidermis may or may not accompany nodule formation[12].

In almost all cases, deposits of immunoglobulin (IgG, IgA and IgM) and complement components from the classic and alternative pathways are observed along the dermal–epidermal junction at the site of cutaneous lesions. In a majority of patients with systemic disease,

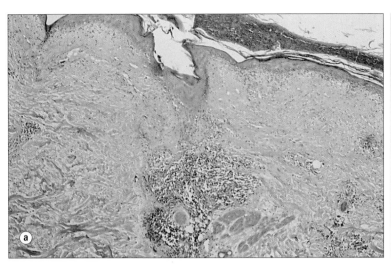
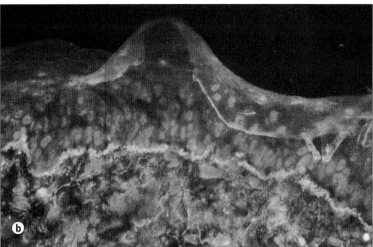

Fig. 117.4 Cutaneous immunopathology and the lupus band test, demonstrating immunoglobulin and complement deposition in non-sun-exposed skin. (a) Light microscopy reveals thickening of the dermal–epidermal junction, and inflammatory cells associated with a dermal appendage. (Hematoxylin and eosin stain.) (b) At a higher power, immunofluorescence demonstrates IgM and C3b at the dermal–epidermal junction (bright green horizontal band, seen midway through this section). (With permission from Brostoff J *et al.* Clinical Immunology. London: Gower; 1991.)

immunofluorescence reveals similar deposits at the dermal–epidermal junction in normal non-sun-exposed skin and at sites of cutaneous lesions. This characteristic immunofluorescence, the lupus band test (Fig. 117.4), may be helpful in diagnosis, although it can also be positive in RA, Sjögren's syndrome, dermatomyositis, progressive systemic sclerosis and other clinical conditions[13].

The dermal–epidermal localization of immunoglobulin and complement may result from nuclear material in the subepidermal space derived from apoptotic keratinocytes[14]. At the highly vascular dermal–epidermal junction, these nuclear antigens may have the opportunity to react with circulating autoantibodies, to form antigen–antibody complexes and precipitate as immune aggregates and to initiate tissue injury. This model suggests a basis for photosensitivity in SLE in which ultraviolet irradiation leads to increased apoptosis of keratinocytes, increased nuclear debris, and subsequent immune complex

material precipitating at the dermal–epidermal junction. Although attractive, this model does not fully reconcile the presence of immunoglobulin at the dermal–epidermal junction with the absence of accompanying tissue damage and the presence of a lymphocytic infiltrate suggestive of cell-mediated immunity.

Vascular immunopathology

Several types of vascular lesions may occur in SLE. The most common lesion is immune complex deposition in the walls of small arteries and arterioles[15] (Fig. 117.5). In some instances, the vascular immune deposits occur without associated inflammatory response and can only be demonstrated by immunofluorescence and electron microscopy. In others, the vascular immune deposits are accompanied by perivascular infiltrates of mononuclear leukocytes. Necrotizing large or small vessel vasculitis with fibrinoid necrosis and neutrophil infiltration resembling that seen in polyarteritis nodosa or Wegener's granulomatosis are relatively uncommon (Fig. 117.6). Necrotizing vasculitis occurring in SLE can be distinguished from that of polyarteritis nodosa and Wegener's granulomatosis by the presence of vascular wall immune deposits and the absence of antineutrophil cytoplasmic antibodies. Presumably, these

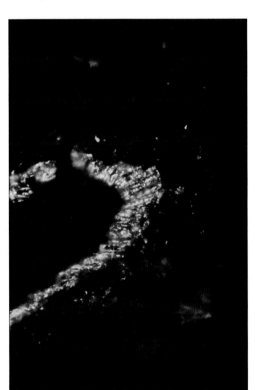

Fig. 117.5 Vascular immune deposits in SLE. Immune complex deposition is demonstrated in the wall of a small intrarenal artery, using antibody to human IgG. (Immunofluorescence, anti-IgG.)

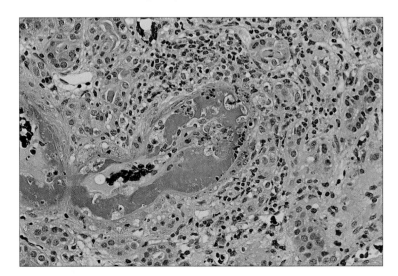

Fig. 117.6 Necrotizing small vessel vasculitis in SLE. The vasculitis resembles the lesions seen in polyarteritis nodosa/microscopic polyangiitis. There is transmural infiltration by lymphocytes and neutrophils, with endothelial degeneration and intimal fibrinoid necrosis. (Hematoxylin and eosin stain.)

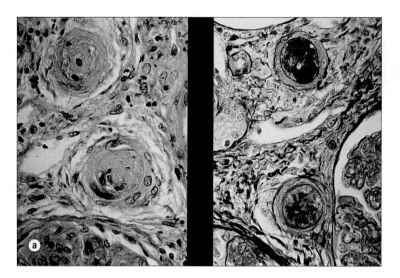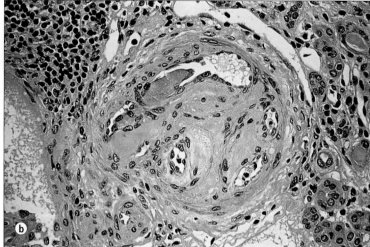

Fig. 117.7 Vascular lesions of thrombotic microangiopathy associated with lupus anticoagulant in SLE. (a) Acute thrombotic lesions with occlusion of the arteriolar lumen by fibrin thrombus that stains eosinophilic (left panel). This intraluminal fibrin gives an orange staining reaction with the Lendrum stain for fibrin (right panel). The endothelium appears necrotic and desquamated; however, there is no leukocyte infiltration of the vessel wall. (b) An organized thrombus with recanalization severely narrows a small artery of the kidney. (Hematoxylin and eosin stain.)

pathologic and serologic distinctions reflect different pathophysiologic mechanisms.

Vascular lesions of thrombotic microangiopathy may occur in patients with lupus who have circulating anticardiolipin antibodies, lupus anticoagulant, or both, and less commonly in those who develop a syndrome of hemolytic uremic syndrome in association with autoantibody to the von Willebrand factor cleaving protease[16]. Lesions of thrombotic microangiopathy in SLE are morphologically indistinguishable from those occurring in hemolytic uremic syndrome or thrombotic thrombocytopenic purpura. They are characterized by intraluminal fibrin thrombi that may be acute or organizing, without accompanying vascular immune deposits (Fig. 117.7).

Renal immunopathology

The renal manifestations of SLE, collectively termed 'lupus nephritis', are extremely heterogeneous[17]. All four renal compartments – the glomeruli, tubules, interstitium and blood vessels – may be affected. The incidence of clinical renal disease underestimates the prevalence of pathologic renal involvement, especially if routine light microscopy is supplemented by the more sensitive techniques of immunofluorescence and electron microscopy. The morphologic features of lupus nephritis are also extremely protean, with the capacity to transform over time, either spontaneously or in response to treatment.

Lupus nephritis is one of the few renal diseases in which immune deposits can be detected in any or all renal compartments, including glomeruli, tubules, interstitium and blood vessels. IgG is found almost universally (>98%) and is usually dominant in intensity. Co-deposits of IgM and IgA are common. When all three immunoglobulin classes are found, the designation 'full house' staining is often applied. Deposits of complements C1 and C3 and properdin can be demonstrated in the majority of cases, consistent with activation of both the classic and alternative complement pathways.

Investigators have attempted to define and quantify the many morphologic lesions of lupus nephritis in a comprehensive, systematic fashion[18]. Widespread use of the World Health Organization (WHO) classification has improved the uniformity and reproducibility of biopsy interpretation and provided the standardized nomenclature essential for clinicopathologic studies addressing outcome and prognosis[19] (Table 117.1).

Although tubular, interstitial and vascular lesions are common in lupus nephritis and may contribute significantly to overall disease sever-

ity, activity and chronicity, the WHO classification is based entirely on evaluation of the glomerular alterations. Accurate classification requires careful assessment of the glomerular alterations by light microscopy, followed by integration of the immunofluorescence and electron microscopic findings. The first step is to determine whether there is glomerular hypercellularity in the mesangial, endocapillary or extracapillary zones. The distribution of the endocapillary hypercellularity is assessed (focal: <50%; diffuse: >50% of glomeruli affected). Attention is given to the presence of infiltrating leukocytes, necrotizing lesions and glomerular basement membrane thickening. These light microscopic findings are then interpreted in the context of the distribution of the glomerular immune deposits in mesangial, subendothelial and subepithelial locations as detected by light microscopy, immunofluorescence and electron microscopy.

The overall distribution of immune deposits detected by immunofluorescence can be refined further at the ultrastructural level. Mesangial electron-dense deposits are typically observed in all classes of lupus nephritis with the exception of class I. They are the defining feature of class II and can be considered the common substratum upon which the higher classes are built. Class III and class IV lupus nephritis display subendothelial and mesangial deposits. The distribution of the subendothelial deposits is more focal and segmental in class III and more diffuse and global in class IV, corresponding to the general distribution of the endocapillary proliferative lesions. Although scattered subepithelial deposits may also be detected in class III and class IV, regular subepithelial deposits are a distinguishing feature of class V.

TABLE 117.1 WHO CLASSIFICATION OF LUPUS NEPHRITIS	
Class I	Normal glomeruli (by LM, IF, EM)
Class II	Purely mesangial disease
	a. Normocellular mesangium by LM but mesangial deposits by IF and/or EM
	b. Mesangial hypercellularity with mesangial deposits by IF and/or EM
Class III	Focal proliferative glomerulonephritis
Class IV	Diffuse proliferative glomerulonephritis
Class V	Membranous glomerulonephritis
Class VI	Chronic sclerosing glomerulonephritis

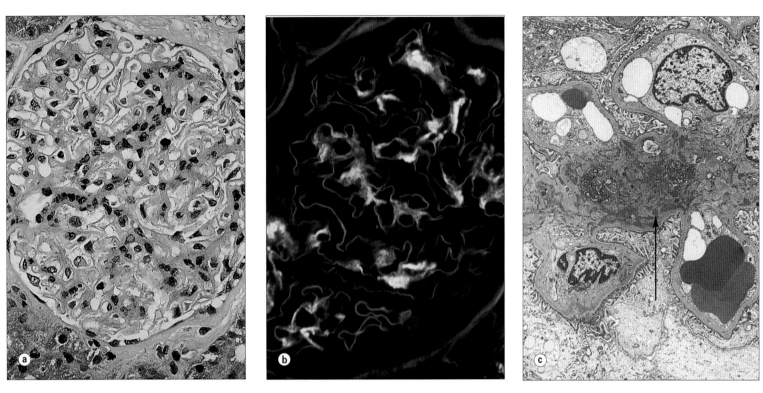

Fig. 117.8 Lupus nephritis class IIb (mesangial proliferative lupus nephritis). (a) Mild mesangial hypercellularity without compromise of the glomerular capillary lumina. (Hematoxylin and eosin stain.) (b) Granular deposits of IgG are confined to the mesangial stalk, with sparing of the peripheral glomerular capillary walls (Immunofluorescence, anti-IgG.) (c) Electron micrograph showing four individual glomerular capillaries oriented around a central mesangial stalk. Electron dense deposits are present within the central mesangial region (arrow), but do not extend into the peripheral glomerular basement membranes.

Class II designates glomerular disease limited to the mesangium (Fig. 117.8). In class IIa, the glomerular mesangium is normocellular; however, immune deposits confined to the mesangium can be detected by fluorescence microscopy and electron microscopy. In class IIb, these purely mesangial immune deposits are accompanied by mesangial proliferation (defined as more than three mesangial cells in mesangial areas away from the vascular pole, assessed in histologic sections 3μm thick).

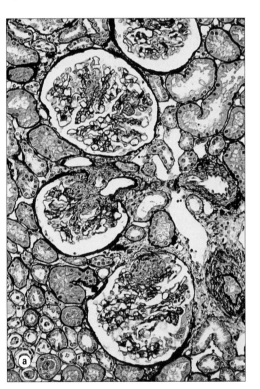
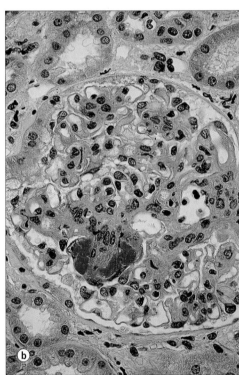
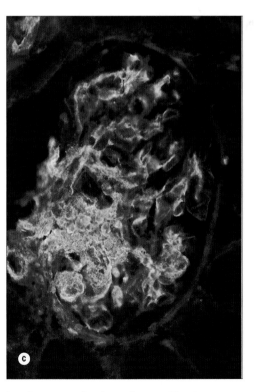

Fig. 117.9 Lupus nephritis class III (focal proliferative lupus nephritis). (a) Low power view shows three glomeruli with segmental endocapillary proliferation causing obliteration of the glomerular capillary lumina in a portion of the glomerular tuft. Adjacent glomerular capillaries are patent. (Jones methenamine silver.) (b) Individual glomerulus with segmental occlusion of the glomerular capillaries by endocapillary proliferation with infiltrating leukocytes and fibrinoid necrosis. The remainder of the glomerular tuft displays mesangial hypercellularity. (Hematoxylin and eosin stain.) (c) Deposits of IgG are identified in the peripheral glomerular capillaries of a segment of the tuft (corresponding to an area of endocapillary proliferation). Mesangial deposits are present in the adjacent glomerular lobules. (Immunofluorescence, anti-IgG.)

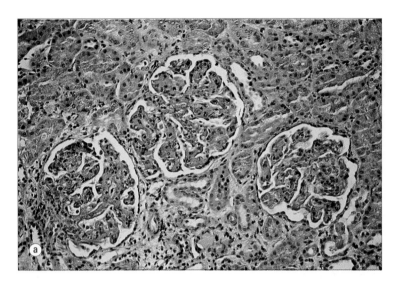
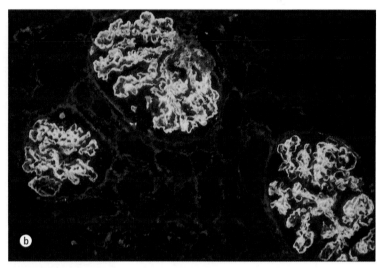

Fig. 117.10 Lupus nephritis class IV (diffuse proliferative lupus nephritis). (a) Low power view shows the diffuse and global distribution of the endocapillary proliferation. (Hematoxylin and eosin stain.) (b) Diffuse and global deposition of IgG throughout the glomerular mesangium and outlining the peripheral capillary walls. (Immunofluorescence, anti-IgG.)

Most investigators consider class III and class IV lupus nephritis to be qualitatively similar glomerular lesions that differ only in severity and distribution. Class III lupus nephritis consists of a focal and segmental endocapillary proliferative glomerulonephritis that affects fewer than 50% of glomeruli (Fig. 117.9). Class IV lupus nephritis is distinguished from class III arbitrarily, on the basis of involvement of more than 50% of glomeruli by endocapillary proliferation. Typically, the endocapillary proliferation in class IV is relatively diffuse and global (Fig. 117.10). Glomerular endothelial cells, monocytes, lymphocytes and neutrophils may contribute to the endocapillary hypercellularity (Fig. 117.11a). As in class III, lobules without endocapillary proliferation usually manifest varying degrees of mesangial proliferation (Fig. 117.9b).

Common light microscopic features of active class III and class IV lupus nephritis include wire loop (subendothelial) deposits, hyaline thrombi, necroses, hematoxylin bodies, and cellular crescents. *Subendothelial immune deposits* are the *sine qua non* of active class III and IV lupus nephritis and are typically detectable by immunofluorescence and electron microscopy in the distribution of the endocapillary proliferation. When large enough to be detected by light microscopy, subendothelial deposits may form 'wire loop' thickenings of the glomerular capillary walls (Fig. 117.11b–d). Some cases of class III or class IV lupus nephritis manifest large intracapillary deposits forming '*hyaline thrombi*' (Fig. 117.11b). This term is a misnomer, inasmuch as these do not represent true fibrin thrombi, but massive intracapillary immune deposits. Glomerular *necrosis* consists of a focus of smudgy fibrinoid degeneration of the glomerular tuft (Fig. 117.9b). Necrosis may be accompanied by any or all of the following: deposition of intracapillary fibrin, glomerular basement membrane rupture, and apoptosis of infiltrating neutrophils producing pyknotic or karyorrhectic nuclear debris ('nuclear dust'). Although they are the only truly pathognomonic lesions of lupus nephritis, *hematoxylin bodies* are extremely uncommon, affecting fewer than 2% of biopsy specimens of lupus nephritis. These smudgy, lilac-staining structures are the tissue equivalent of the LE body and consist of naked nuclei in which the chromatin has been altered by binding to ambient antinuclear antibodies (Fig. 117.2a). *Cellular crescents* are a feature of active lupus nephritis that may be encountered frequently in both class III and class IV disease. They are common overlying necrotizing lesions, but also may occur in glomeruli with non-necrotizing endocapillary proliferative lesions.

Active glomerular lesions that persist over time or do not respond to treatment may lead to *glomerular scarring* (or *sclerosis*), a feature of chronic and irreversible glomerular injury. In class III, the glomerular scarring is often initially focal and segmental, mirroring the distribution of the proliferative and necrotizing lesions. Associated fibrous crescents may form synechiae to the sclerotic segments. Similarly, in chronic class IV lupus nephritis, the glomerular sclerosis is typically more global and diffuse. Of course, glomerular obsolescence is not restricted to class III and class IV, but also can supervene on class V. Glomerular sclerosis in lupus nephritis may also occur in the course of aging or as a complication of hypertensive arterionephrosclerosis, and does not necessarily imply scarring in the course of immunologically mediated injury.

Membranous lupus nephritis (class V) is characterized by diffuse thickening of the glomerular capillary walls as a result of numerous subepithelial electron-dense deposits separated by basement membrane spikes (Fig. 117.12). This lesion usually occurs on a background of mesangial hypercellularity and mesangial immune deposits. Because scattered subepithelial deposits may also be encountered in class III and class IV lupus nephritis, the designation membranous lupus nephritis should be reserved for those cases in which the subepithelial deposits predominate.

The modified WHO classification recognizes a sixth class, in which the findings are those of extremely chronic advanced glomerulonephritis with widespread glomerular scarring affecting most glomeruli[19]. Most of these examples of class VI lupus nephritis undoubtedly represent advanced class IV disease. In some cases, the process is so 'endstage' that a diagnosis of chronic lupus nephritis is difficult on morphologic grounds. Immunofluorescence and electron microscopy may reveal residual small granular electron-dense deposits in the thickened glomerular capillary walls, tubulointerstitial compartment or vessel walls.

Tubulointerstitial lesions can be encountered in all classes of lupus nephritis, particularly class IV, and correlate closely with the degree of renal functional impairment. Active lesions include interstitial inflammation by lymphocytes, monocytes and plasma cells, in addition to immune deposits in tubular basement membranes, interstitial collagen and the walls of interstitial capillaries (Fig. 117.13). There is a poor correlation between the severity of interstitial inflammation and the presence or amount of tubulointerstitial immune deposits, implicating a more complex role for cell mediated immunity[20].

Prognosis correlates with the class of lupus nephritis, and with measures of activity and chronicity. Prognosis is excellent in class II, more guarded in class III and V, and poorest in class IV (particularly in patients in whom there is high chronicity and persistent activity that is resistant to treatment). Attempts to quantify the degree of activity and chronicity in lupus nephritis are predicated on the intuitive assumption that active lesions are more amenable to treatment and chronic lesions

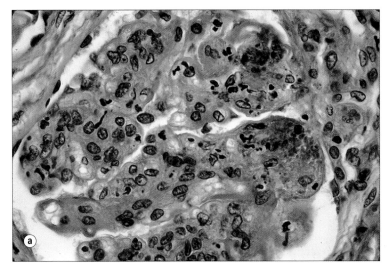

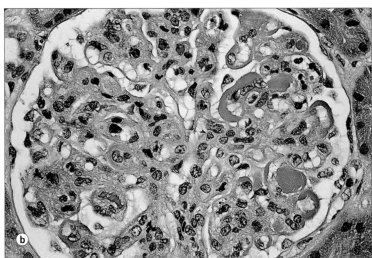

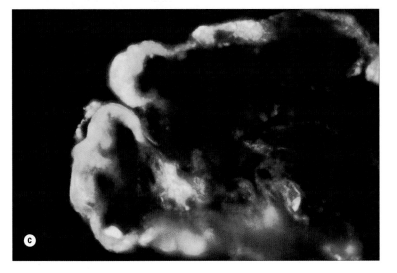

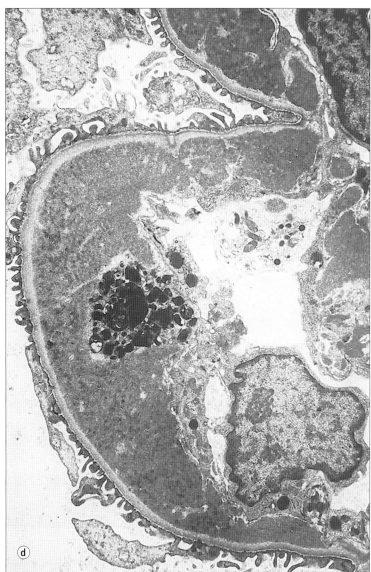

Fig. 117.11 Lupus nephritis class IV (diffuse proliferative lupus nephritis). (a) The glomerular capillary lumina contain many infiltrating leukocytes, including neutrophils. Some of these neutrophils are undergoing apoptosis, forming pyknotic or karyorrhectic nuclear debris. (Hematoxylin and eosin stain.) (b) Several glomerular capillary walls are thickened by eosinophilic deposits that form thick 'wire loops'. Some of the immune deposits are so large that they obliterate the glomerular capillary lumina, forming 'hyaline thrombi'. (Hematoxylin and eosin stain.) (c) By immunofluorescence, the wire loop deposits correspond to large peripheral capillary wall immune deposits that are located in the subendothelial region. These deposits are comma-shaped because they conform to the smooth outer glomerular basement contour. (Immunofluorescence, anti-IgG.) (d) Seen on electron microscopy, the wire loop consists of a large circumferential subendothelial electron-dense deposit that forms along the inner aspect of the glomerular capillary wall, between the glomerular endothelium and the glomerular basement membrane.

represent largely irreversible damage. Assessment of disease activity and chronicity provides a helpful, albeit inexact, guide to prognosis and treatment. Activity indices, first formulated in the 1960s, have been recently refined and popularized by Austin's group as the National Institutes of Health (NIH) activity and chronicity index[21,22]. According to the NIH schema, activity index is calculated by summing the score for each of six histologic features (glomerular endocapillary proliferation, glomerular leukocyte infiltration, glomerular subendothelial hyaline deposits, glomerular fibrinoid necrosis or karyorrhexis, cellular crescents and interstitial inflammation), which are graded individually on a scale of 0–3+: 0 = absent, 1+ = less than 25% of glomeruli affected, 2+ =25–50% of glomeruli affected, 3+ = more than 50% of glomeruli affected. The scores for glomerular necrosis and cellular crescents are accorded double weight because of their more ominous importance. Interstitial inflammation is graded as 1+ = mild, 2+ = moderate, 3+ = severe. The sum of these values gives a total possible activity score of 0–24. Similarly, chronicity is graded on a scale of 0–12 by summing each of four features of chronicity (each scored as 0–3+): glomerular sclerosis, fibrous crescents, tubular atrophy and interstitial fibrosis.

The NIH group initially found an activity index greater than 12 and a chronicity greater than 4 to be predictors of poor outcome[22]. In subsequent analyses, the combination of cellular crescents and moderate to

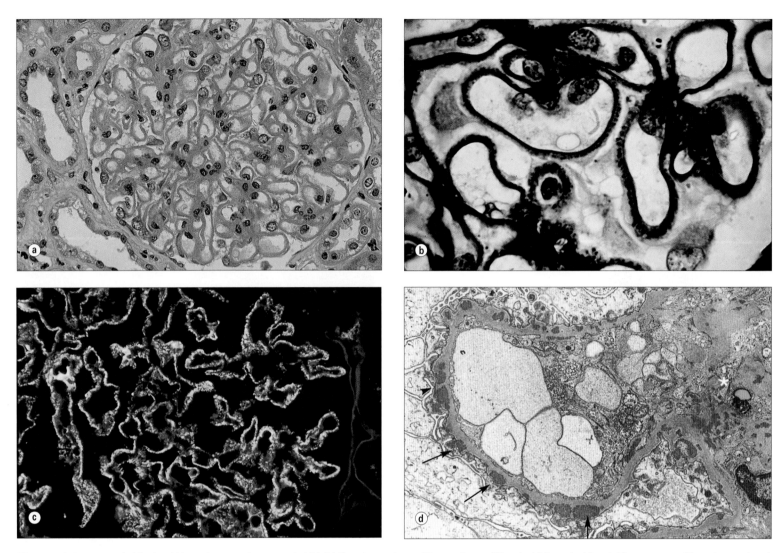

Fig. 117.12 Lupus nephritis class V (membranous lupus nephritis). (a) The glomerular capillary walls are diffusely thickened with a rigid appearance. There is associated mild mesangial hypercellularity, but without evidence of endocapillary proliferation. (Hematoxylin and eosin stain.) (b) Silver stain delineates the characteristic 'spikes' that project at right angles from the glomerular basement membranes, like bristles on a comb. (Jones methenamine silver.) (c) The immunofluorescence pattern is finely granular, corresponding to deposits along the outer aspect of the glomerular capillary walls. (Immunofluorescence, anti-IgG.) (d) Electron micrograph showing subepithelial electron-dense deposits (arrows) located on the outer aspect of the glomerular capillary wall, between the visceral epithelial cells (podocytes) and the glomerular basement membrane. Some of these deposits are separated by intervening projections of glomerular basement membrane material, forming 'spikes' (arrowhead). Deposits are also seen in the adjacent mesangial matrix (*), deep to the glomerular capillary lumen.

severe interstitial fibrosis was a sensitive predictor of doubling of serum creatinine[23]. The value and reproducibility of these indices has been debated. Schwartz and coworkers have noted problems in intra- and interobserver reproducibility[24]. Although there does not appear to be a precise cut-off for activity and chronicity that predicts outcome, there is general agreement that greater chronicity portends a worse prognosis. Despite their limitations, activity and chronicity indices are of particular value when repeat biopsies are performed in individual patients to monitor disease evolution and response to treatment.

The morphologic subtypes of lupus nephritis are defined according to the distribution of immune deposits within the glomerular tuft. However, we know surprisingly little about the factors that govern the localization of immune deposits within the glomerular filter. It is likely that the diverse morphologic expressions of lupus nephritis reflect differences in the composition and properties of immune complexes, including immune complex load, specificity, size, avidity, affinity, charge and immunoglobulin isotype (see below). It has been proposed that a mesangial pattern of immune deposition is favored by relatively small immune complex load of intermediate-sized, high-avidity complexes that resist elimination by mesangial clearing mechanisms. Larger quantities of intermediate-sized or large immune complexes could overwhelm the mesangium and spill out into the subendothelial zones. There is experimental evidence to support the formation of subepithelial deposits from smaller, low-avidity, cationic immune complexes in relative antigen excess, which may dissociate and reform *in situ*, perhaps favored by electrostatic interactions with the polyanionic constituents of the glomerular capillary wall.

In the past, the paradigm for lupus nephritis has been a classic type III hypersensitivity reaction mechanism of glomerular deposition of circulating autoantibody-containing immune complexes, followed by complement activation and subsequent neutrophil-mediated tissue injury. In recent years, emphasis has shifted away from the exclusive role of renal deposition of preformed circulating immune complexes to recognize the importance of local formation of immune deposits[17,25,26]. Charge interactions favor the local binding of positively charged nucleosomes to fixed anionic sites in the glomerular capillary wall. Once planted in the glomerular filter, these autoantigens may interact with circulating autoantibody, leading to *in situ* formation of immune complexes. Some anti-DNA antibodies exhibit a range of cross-reactivities to normal glomerular constituents, such as heparan sulfate proteoglycans, laminin and type IV collagen, suggesting another potential mechanism of *in situ* immune complex formation. Finally, the poor correlation between the

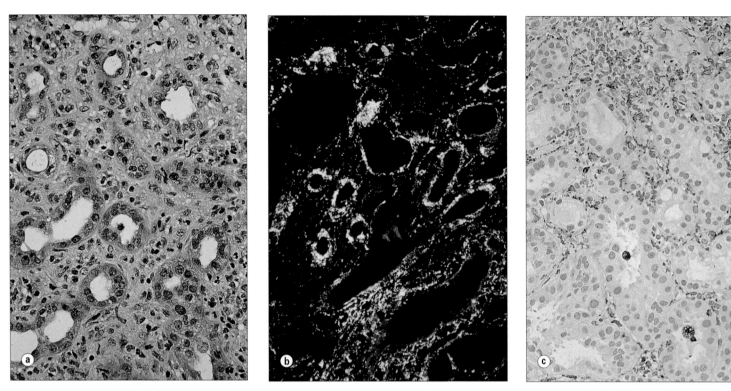

Fig. 117.13 Tubulointerstitial lesions in active lupus nephritis. (a) The renal interstitium is expanded by edema and dense inflammatory infiltrates (Hematoxylin and eosin stain). (b) An example with extensive immune deposits within the interstitial connective tissue and outlining the tubular basement membranes. (Immunofluorescence, anti-IgG.) (c) Immunostaining for CD68 shows many monocytes within the renal interstitium between tubules. (Immunocytochemistry, anti-CD68.)

quantity of circulating immune complexes and the activity of the glomerulonephritis implies a potential role for local antigen presentation at the level of the glomerulus by activated macrophages or T cells. Fcγ receptor (FcγR)-bearing monocytes appear to be essential effector cells in glomerulonephritis, as demonstrated by the protection of Fcγ-deficient mice from the development of nephritis, but not from the glomerular deposition of immune complexes or complement[27].

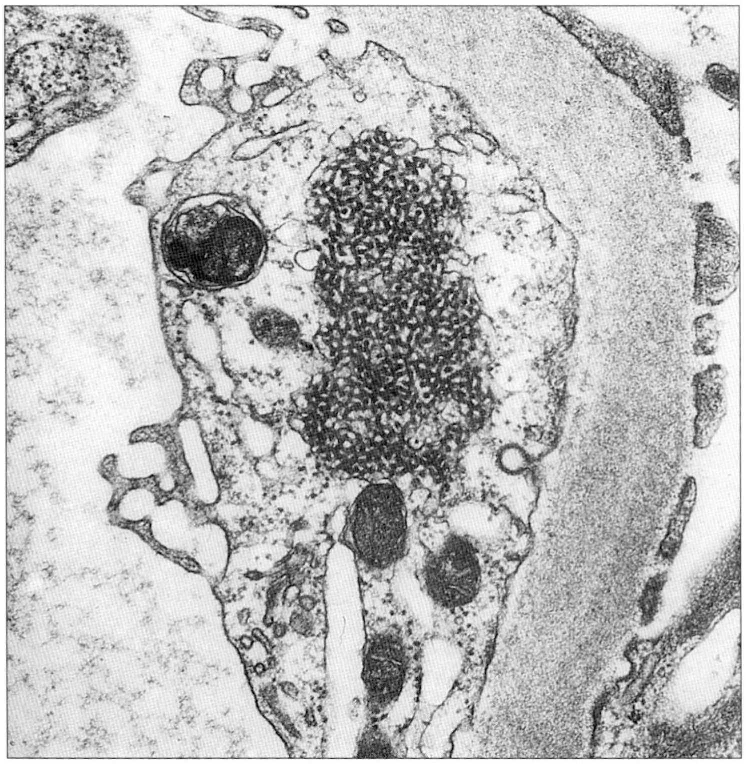

Neutrophil and monocyte recruitment is particularly marked in active lupus nephritis. A complex network of cytokine activation appears to mediate their influx and to promote downstream effects on mesangial proliferation, matrix production and crescent formation[17]. Inflammatory and fibrogenic cytokines that have been demonstrated to be upregulated in lupus nephritis include monocyte chemoattractant protein type 1 (MCP-1), interleukin (IL)-1, IL-2 receptor, IL-6, interferon (IFN)-γ, IFN-α, tumor necrosis factor (TNF)-α, and transforming growth factor (TGF)-β. The morphologic correlate of increased interferon concentrations is the presence of tubuloreticular inclusions ('interferon footprints') in the endothelial cell cytoplasm of all classes of lupus nephritis (Fig. 117.14). Renal tubular expression of intercellular adhesion molecule-1, class II molecules (DR and DQ) and costimulatory molecule CD40 has correlated with disease activity. A number of procoagulant factors such as increased prothrombin, reduced plaminogen activator and increased local formation of thromboxane A$_2$ and platelet-derived growth factor are important mediators of endothelial injury and crescent formation.

Central nervous system immunopathology

Involvement of the central nervous system in SLE is common and can assume diverse clinical and morphologic manifestations. Neurologic involvement directly attributable to the immunopathologic derangements of SLE must be distinguished from the effects of drugs (such as steroids), hypertension and infections that complicate immunosuppressive therapy. Although the term 'lupus cerebritis' is used in common medical parlance to describe the pathologic manifestations of SLE in the brain, most cerebral involvement is actually attributable to vascular lesions[28]. In the past, the majority of vascular pathology in the central nervous system was believed to represent lupus vasculitis, a vascular inflammation caused by deposition of immunoglobulin and complement in vessel walls, as may occur in other organs. It is now recognized that, although such necrotizing or inflammatory vasculitis does account

Fig. 117.14 Endothelial tubulo-reticular inclusion. Electron micrograph of a large endothelial tubuloreticular inclusion is identified within a glomerular endothelial cell. This intracytoplasmic inclusion consists of interanastomosing tubular structures located within the dilated endoplasmic reticulum of the endothelial cell cytoplasm.

for less than 15% of the vascular lesions of central nervous system lupus, more than 70% of vascular pathology is attributable to thrombotic lesions of small intracranial vessels, with or without associated endothelial proliferation and perivascular inflammation[29]. Most patients with thrombotic vasculopathy have associated anticardiolipin or antiphospholipid antibodies and lack immune complex deposition in the vessel walls. There are also rare reports of arterial thromboemboli that have been linked to Libman–Sacks endocarditis.

The parenchymal injury that occurs secondary to lupus vascular lesions (whether of inflammatory, thrombotic, or thromboembolic nature) usually takes the form of micro- or macroinfarcts, sometimes complicated by hemorrhage in subarachnoid, subdural or intracerebral locations[30]. Hemorrhage may also result from bleeding tendencies caused by thrombocytopenia or hypoprothrombinemia in the context of anticardiolipin/antiphospholipid antibody syndrome, immune thrombocytopenic purpura, or thrombotic thrombocytopenic purpura. Depending on the location of the vascular lesions and the distribution and extent of the parenchymal injury, clinical presentations vary widely from localized neurologic deficits (such as paresis, cranial nerve palsy, movement disorder and seizure) to more generalized manifestations (such as headache, altered consciousness, psychosis and impaired cognition). Interestingly, deposition of immune complexes may occur in the choroid plexus, a specialized vascular structure with filtration functions that bears some similarities to the renal glomerulus.

Central nervous system disease of non-vascular origin appears to be less common and less well understood. In most cases there are no identifiable pathological lesions. A potential role for antineuronal and antiglial antibodies has been proposed. Some of these antibodies have specificity for neurofilaments or brain synaptic plasma membrane antigen and can be demonstrated using complement-dependent cytotoxicity assays on cultured human neuronal cell lines. A subset of anti-lymphocyte antibodies also has been shown to cross-react with neurons. Recent evidence suggests that antibodies to the glutamate receptor may contribute to neurocognitive dysfunction. There is also an association between anti-ribosomal P protein and the development of lupus psychosis, although the underlying pathophysiology and anatomic correlates remain to be defined.

Cardiopulmonary immunopathology

Pathologic changes can occur in the lung parenchyma, endocardium, myocardium and pleuropericardial membranes[31–34]. In lupus lung, with intra-alveolar hemorrhage, typical deposits of immunoglobulin and complement support immune-mediated injury mechanisms consonant with those in the kidney and other organs. The occurrence of non-bacterial verrucous endocarditis, characteristic of SLE, also suggests a role for autoantibodies, and perhaps immune complexes. Pericarditis is commonly seen in postmortem series, whether or not patients had symptomatic evidence of pericarditis. Gross morphology reveals a fibrinous exudate, whereas microscopic examination shows a perivascular mononuclear cell infiltration with edema and fibrinoid necrosis. A granular pattern of immunofluorescence for IgG is consistent with immune complex deposition.

Clinically significant inflammatory myocardial disease is uncommon, but increasingly early atherosclerotic coronary artery disease is being recognized. The role of vasculitis as an initiating event, and the roles of continuing vasculitis, corticosteroids and hypertension as accelerating factors, are unclear[33,34].

PROPERTIES OF IMMUNE COMPLEXES

Although not all manifestations of SLE can be attributed to immune complexes, these complexes do appear to have a central role in the pathology and immunopathology of SLE. Thus critical questions in pathogenesis focus on the nature of immune complexes and their handling, the nature of the autoantibodies that make up the complexes and the basis for the increased production of these autoantibodies. Complement and complement receptors are discussed in Chapter 119, autoantibodies in Chapter 120 and cellular immunity in Chapter 121.

Antibodies and antigens

Of the five classes of human immunoglobulins (IgG, IgM, IgA, IgE and IgD), IgG is the most common constituent of immune complexes found in SLE. IgM is more typically associated with lower-affinity antibodies, and IgA often reflects stimulation of mucosal immunity. IgG has four subclasses, each of which have distinct physicochemical and immunologic properties (Table 117.2), reflecting differences both in primary amino acid sequence and in glycosylation of the subclass-specific heavy chains Fig. 117.15)[35]. The genes encoding immunoglobulin heavy chains are located on the long arm of human chromosome 14. Allelic polymorphisms in heavy-chain genes (recognized as Gm allotypes) lead to variation in the primary amino acid sequence of the heavy chain, but the role of these variants in SLE is currently unknown.

IgG1 is the most common immunoglobulin in serum, and both IgG1 and IgG3 are produced primarily against protein antigens. IgG2, the second most common immunoglobulin, is typically produced in response to polysaccharide antigens. IgG4 production is associated with prolonged antigenic stimulation. In addition to the nature of the antigen, regulation of IgG subclass production is influenced by the antigen-presenting cell and the cytokines released at the time of antigen presentation. The significance of the relationship between the biochemical nature of the antigen, the IgG subclass produced and the biological properties of these

TABLE 117.2 PROPERTIES OF HUMAN IgG SUBCLASSES				
	IgG1	IgG2	IgG3	IgG4
Serum levels (% of total)	60–65	20–25	5–10	3–6
Complement fixation	+++	+	++++	±
Cryoprecipitation	++	+	+++	+
Rheumatoid factor binding	+++	+++	±	+++
Placental transfer	++	±	++	++
Fractional catabolic rate (%)	7–9	7–9	17	7–9
Staph. protein A binding	+	+	−	+
Strep. protein G binding	+	+	+	+
Allotypic variants 'Gm markers'	some	few	many	none

TABLE 117.3 IMPORTANT PROPERTIES OF IMMUNE COMPLEXES

Property	Influenced by
Lattice size	Valence of antibody and antigen Molar ratio of antibody and antigen Absolute concentration of antibody and antigen Association constant of antibody for antigen
Net charge	Charge of antibody and antigen
Complement fixation	Class and subclass of antibody Lattice size Availability of complement components
Complement receptor binding	Quantitative complement fixation Processing of C3b to iC3b and C3d,g Availability of complement receptors
Fcg receptor binding	Lattice size Antibody class and subclass Phenotype of host Fcg receptors
Glomerular deposition	Lattice size (large.small) Net cationic (positive) charge

TABLE 117.4 MEASUREMENT OF IMMUNE COMPLEXES

Detection strategy	Assay used	Limitations
Cryoprecipitability	Cryoglobulins	Insensitive, semiquantitative Includes non-specific proteins
Solubility	Polyethylene glycol	Insensitive, semiquantitative Includes non-specific proteins
Complement fixation binding of C1q	Fluid-phase C1q binding assay Solid-phase C1q binding assay	IC must actively bind C1q
Complement components bound to IC	Raji cell assay	IC must contain C3d False-positive with lymphocytotoxic antibodies to B cells
	Conglutinin assay	IC must contain iC3b
	Erythrocyte binding	IC must contain C3b
Immunoglobulin aggregates: multivalent binding	Rheumatoid factor assay	IgM, not IgG, detected Hypergammaglobulinemia may interfere
	Staph protein A binding assay	IgG, not IgM, detected Hypergammaglobulinemia may interfere

IC, immune complex
Note that several of these properties will vary with the subclass of immunoglobulin involved.
Circulating immune complexes may also be bound to erythrocytes via CR1 (see text) and be unavailable for measurement in the serum.

subclasses remains incompletely understood. There is no doubt, however, that the nature of the IgG subclass in an immune complex influences both the biological properties of the immune complex *in vivo* (Table 117.3) and the ability to detect the immune complex *in vitro* (Table 117.4).

One of the most striking differences among the IgG subclasses is found in the structure of the hinge region (Fig. 117.15). The lower hinge region participates in the binding of the early complement component C1q to IgG and in the binding of IgG to its corresponding cell receptors (FcγRs)[36,37]. The binding of IgG to different FcγRs is sensitive to specific residues within this region in the second constant domain of the heavy chain (C$_H$2). It is likely that C1q and FcγRs interact with composite sites on IgG – that is, a tertiary structure comprised of several different linear regions, conformational determinants, or both.

The antigens are also critical constituents of immune complexes, not only because they influence the nature of the humoral immune response, but also because their own physicochemical properties strongly influence the nature of the complex (Table 117.3). In addition to size and valence, discussed in the next section, the antigen may also have unique properties that influence its handling. For example, complexes containing an antigen asialo-orosomucoid with available galactose may bind to galactose receptors on hepatocytes. Nucleosomes, which may bind both C reactive protein and specific antibody as opsonins, may also bind directly to the negatively charged basement membrane of the glomerulus. In most instances, our knowledge of the antigen component of an immune complex is limited.

Critical properties of immune complexes

The formation and the fate of soluble immune complexes depend on the biophysical and immunologic properties of the antigen and the antibody (Table 117.3). These properties include the size, net charge and valence of the antigen, the class and the subclass of the antibody, the affinity of the antibody–antigen interaction, net charge and concentration of antibody, the molar ratio of available antigen and antibody, and the ability of the immune complex to interact with the proteins of the complement system[38]. The lattice size of the immune complex is strongly influenced by the physical size and valence of the antigen, by the association constant of antibody for that antigen, by the molar ratio of antigen and antibody and by the absolute concentration of the reactants. Complement fixation is more efficient with larger complexes. Larger complexes also present a broader multivalent array of ligands for complement and FcγRs to bind. Finally, of course, the class and subclass of antibody are important in complement activation and determining which FcγRs can be engaged.

In the clinical setting, it is difficult to evaluate all these variables, but in experimental models there is ample evidence that they are very important. Many examples are available. Large complexes are cleared more rapidly

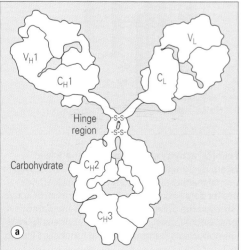
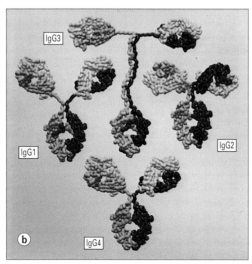

Fig. 117.15 Human IgG immunoglobulin molecules.
(a) Domains, hinge region and the carbohydrate moiety are shown in diagram form. (b) Computer-generated space-filling models of the four IgG subclasses. (Reprinted from Shakib F. The human IgG subclasses, 1990, with permission from Elsevier Science Ltd.)

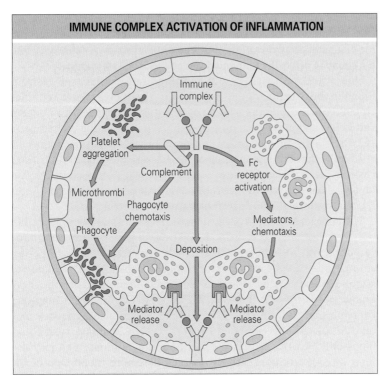

Fig. 117.16 Immune complex activation of inflammation. Immune complexes activate complement, releasing C3a and C5a. In turn, C3a and C5a stimulate neutrophils, mononuclear phagocytes, basophils and mast cells and cause release of inflammatory mediators. Immune complexes deposited on the vessel wall cause further deposition of complement and lead to both Fcγ receptor-mediated and complement-mediated stimulation of phagocytic cells.

than small ones, complexes between antibody and double-stranded DNA bind to a receptor for a complement fragment (C3b) on erythrocytes (complement receptor type 1, or CR1) differently than do certain antibody–protein complexes, and complexes with net positive charge localize to the glomerulus more efficiently than those with neutral charge. Most immedi-

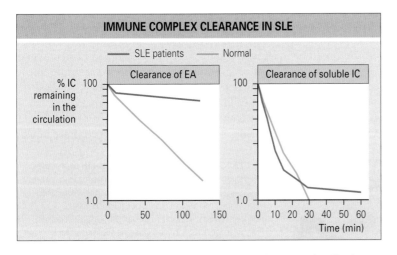

Fig. 117.17 Immune complex clearance in SLE. The clearance of antibody opsonized erythrocytes (EA) is dramatically decreased in patients with active SLE. The EA probe is a sensitive measure of mononuclear phagocyte system FcγR function. In contrast to the initial clearance of EA, the clearance of soluble immune complexes (IC) is more rapid in patients with SLE. Some data indicate that this more rapid disappearance from the circulation does not correspond to an increase in uptake of immune complexes by the mononuclear phagocyte system, but rather reflects greater deposition of immune complexes in the capillary beds as a result of deficiencies in the complement system (see text). However, at later times (15min), there is delayed clearance of soluble immune complexes, which may reflect the same FcγR dysfunction observed with the EA probe.

ately, it is important to be aware of the properties of immune complexes that can influence their measurement *in vitro* (Table 117.4).

Pathogenetic mechanisms

Once deposition of an immune complex in tissue has occurred, either through *in situ* formation or by direct immune complex deposition, FcγR-mediated uptake by antigen-presenting cells can lead to amplification of the humoral immune response, and FcγR-mediated activation of mast cells and phagocytes, in addition to complement activation, leads to an inflammatory response through the generation of soluble mediators, including complement fragments C3a and C5a. These mediators attract and activate polymorphonuclear leukocytes and mononuclear phagocytes, cause release of additional inflammatory mediators from these cells, mast cells and basophils, and activate large granular lymphocytes (Fig. 117.16). Activation of platelets may cause platelet aggregation and microthrombi, in addition to release of vasoactive compounds increasing vascular permeability. The production of reactive oxygen metabolites, release of hydrolytic enzymes and secretion of cytokines can cause direct destruction of local tissue and further stimulation of leukocytes. Thus the continued presence of immune complexes in chronic immune-complex-mediated diseases can lead to prolonged tissue damage, which may result in clinically evident vasculitis, pleuropericarditis, cutaneous lesions and glomerulonephritis.

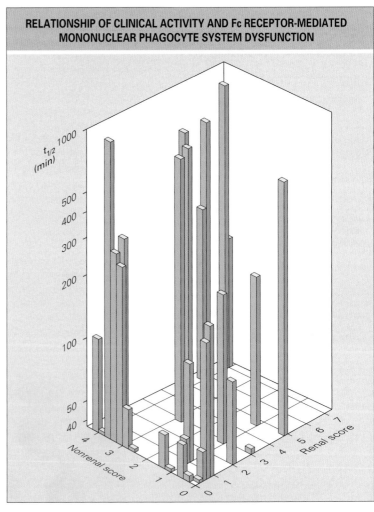

Fig. 117.18 Relationship of clinical activity and Fc receptor-mediated mononuclear phagocyte system dysfunction. Clinical activity was assessed in terms of both renal and non-renal manifestations. Longer (taller) clearance half-time values represent greater degrees of dysfunction. Patients with active renal and non-renal disease showed the greatest degree of FcR-mediated clearance impairment. (Adapted from Kimberly RP, Salmon JE, Edberg JC *et al*. The role of Fcγ receptors in mononuclear phagocyte system function. Clin Exp Rheumatol 1989; 75: 103–108.)

BIOLOGY OF IMMUNE COMPLEX HANDLING

Normally, antigen–antibody immune complexes are quickly and safely removed by the mononuclear phagocyte system, a collective term for fixed tissue phagocytes found primarily in liver and spleen. However, when both the antigen and antibody are present for prolonged periods of time and when defects in the immune complex clearance mechanisms are present, immune complexes may deposit in host tissues, with subsequent tissue damage. *In vivo* and *in vitro* abnormalities in both FcγR- and complement-mediated clearance of immune complexes have been described in SLE[39–42]. For example, patients with SLE display delayed clearance kinetics of certain IgG-coated erythrocytes, a model immune complex that is used to assess FcγR-mediated clearance (Fig. 117.17). Interestingly, some soluble immune complexes disappear from the circulation of patients with SLE more rapidly than from that of normal individuals, but this difference may reflect rapid deposition in peripheral tissues as a result of inefficient complement-mediated immune complex solubilization, rather than enhanced complement-mediated removal by the mononuclear phagocyte system. Abnormal receptor-mediated clearance contributes to immune complex deposition and is correlated with disease activity (Fig. 117.18), but many other factors also influence immune complex handling. These factors include the size and composition of the complex, pre-existing tissue inflammation and the opportunity for charge–charge interactions. The vascular endothelium and the glomerular basement membrane are highly susceptible tissue targets for immune complex damage.

Role of complement in immune complex handling

In order to prevent disease mediated by immune complex deposition, a number of protective mechanisms have evolved that effectively eliminate immune complexes both from the circulation and from tissues. Central to these protective mechanisms is the complement system, the same system implicated in the pathogenic destruction of tissue[43]. In addition, C reactive protein, which can mediate complement fixation, also has an important role, especially in the handling of nuclear debris. The complement system is discussed in detail in Chapter 119, but several fundamental points deserve emphasis here. Immune complex handling (and clearance) is influenced strongly by three roles of the complement system:

● Complement C1q binds to immune complex, and receptors for C1q are important in the uptake of these complexes
● Complement activation maintains immune complex solubility by preventing the formation of large insoluble immune aggregates, and by transforming insoluble complexes into smaller soluble ones
● Complement activation leads to the opsonization of complexes with complement components or fragments for recognition by complement receptors on phagocytes.

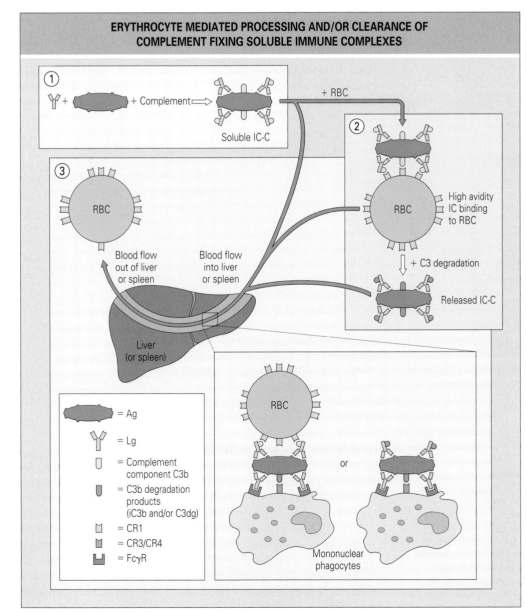

ERYTHROCYTE MEDIATED PROCESSING AND/OR CLEARANCE OF COMPLEMENT FIXING SOLUBLE IMMUNE COMPLEXES

Soluble IC-C

+ RBC

High avidity IC binding to RBC

+ C3 degradation

Released IC-C

Blood flow out of liver or spleen

Blood flow into liver or spleen

Liver (or spleen)

Mononuclear phagocytes

or

= Ag
= Lg
= Complement component C3b
= C3b degradation products (iC3b and/or C3dg)
= CR1
= CR3/CR4
= FcγR

Fig. 117.19 Erythrocyte-mediated processing and clearance of complement-fixing soluble immune complexes. The clearance of complement-fixing soluble immune complexes can be divided into three distinct phases. (1) In the first phase, immune complex formation, complement activation and opsonization occur. (2) In the second phase, after the soluble immune complexes have fixed complement and have bound C3b fragments, the complement-opsonized immune complex (IC-C) can bind to erythrocytes (the immune adherence reaction). Once the immune complex is bound to the erythrocyte, complement-mediated processing of the complex can occur. In this series of events, the erythrocyte complement receptor for C3b (CR1) facilitates the proteolytic degradation of C3b to iC3b and C3dg, which leads to release of the immune complex from the erythrocyte. Immune complex at each of these stages in the immune complex processing cascade may be recognized and cleared by the macrophages of the mononuclear phagocyte system. (3) In the final phase, complexes from either phase 1 or phase 2 enter the mononuclear phagocyte system and are recognized by macrophages via Fc receptors for IgG (FcγRI, FcγRII and FcγRIII) and complement receptors for the degradation products of C3b (CR3 and CR4), and are removed from the circulation. Some data suggest that removal (stripping) of erythrocyte-bound immune complexes by macrophages of the mononuclear phagocyte system results in a decrease in the level of CR1 on the erythrocyte. In this model, the erythrocyte would then acquire reduced CR1 levels after transit through the mononuclear phagocyte system. Ag, antigen; RBC, red blood cell.

Receptors for both C1q and C3 degradation products (C3b, iC3b and C3dg) are important in immune complex binding, internalization and subsequent release of inflammatory mediators.

The opsonization of complexes with C3b can also lead to immune adherence – the binding of C3b to a specific receptor for C3b (CR1) on erythrocytes – as originally observed in 1953 by Nelson[44]. Later, Cornacoff and colleagues showed that a significant fraction of immune complexes formed *ex vivo* and injected into the circulation of primates became bound to erythrocytes via CR1[45]. Similarly, nascent immune complexes, formed *in vivo* in the circulation from free antibody and free antigen, fix complement and bind to erythrocytes. On the basis of these experimental models and more recent observations in humans[41,46,47], the role of the erythrocyte in immune complex handling has become more clearly understood. Circulating complement-fixing immune complexes interact with erythrocytes, which express the bulk of the available complement receptors in the circulation.

The potential biological roles for immune adherence in complex handling are several (Fig. 117.19). One role includes the erythrocytes serving as a 'buffering' system, which can bind complement-opsonized immune complexes and decrease the probability of their deposition[47,48]. This role would probably be most important in chronic immune complex conditions, in which small differences in this buffering capacity could be multiplied over time. Another role may be to act as an immune complex 'shuttle', which can facilitate immune complex presentation to the mononuclear phagocyte system. Although this is an attractive idea, available data cannot distinguish between the influence of the intrinsic properties of the immune complex and the role of immune adherence *per se* on clearance kinetics. Finally, the immune adherence reaction may accelerate complement-mediated immune complex processing. CR1 on erythrocytes serves as a cofactor for factor I, which facilitates the degradation of immune-complex-bound C3b to iC3b and C3dg. Degradation of C3b decreases binding affinity between the immune complex and the erythrocyte CR1, with release of the immune complex from the erythrocyte. Other complement receptors on the macrophages of the mononuclear phagocyte system bind to these C3 degradation products. Thus immune adherence via the erythrocyte CR1 may lead to more efficient complement-mediated recognition of the immune complex by phagocytes, and to more efficient complement-mediated solubilization.

Complement deficiencies in SLE

One might anticipate that a complement deficiency with decreased generation of proinflammatory fragments might be beneficial in SLE, but both inherited and acquired deficiencies in complement and complement receptors have been described in patients with SLE[49,50]. These are discussed in detail in Chapter 119. Several different mechanisms can lead to homozygous complement component deficiency, and homozygous deficiencies in the early components of the complement cascade (C1q, C4, C2 and C3) are often associated with SLE. The association of C4 deficiency with SLE is particularly interesting, because the genes that encode C4A and C4B are located within the major histocompatibility complex on human chromosome 6. Historically, the significance of the increased prevalence of C4A null allele, especially in white patients, has been confounded by strong linkage disequilibrium between C4A null alleles and human leukocyte antigen (HLA)-DR3. However, the association of the C4A null allele with SLE has been found in other ethnic populations in the absence of an HLA-DR3 association. The physiologic basis for an association between SLE and the C4A null genotype, but not the C4B null genotype, is uncertain, but it is notable that the C4A gene product is more efficient at forming amide links with amino groups. Some data suggest that the C4A gene product is especially important in immune complex processing (solubilization and opsonization). Early complement component deficiencies may lead to a marked decrease in the ability to opsonize or solubilize immune complexes (Fig. 117.20) and a persistence of autoantigens, and thus may predispose to the development of SLE by promoting cycles of tissue deposition, inflammation and, over long periods of time, tissue destruction.

Complement receptors in SLE

Four distinct complement receptors, each with preferential binding for different fragments of C3, have been identified (see Chapter 119)[49]. Complement receptors types 1 and 2 (CR1 and CR2) are members of a family of molecules termed the regulators of complement activation (RCA)[51]. Sequence analysis of the RCA family has shown that all these proteins share certain structural features, suggesting that they probably originated from a single ancestral gene through gene duplication. CR1 is widely distributed (erythrocytes, polymorphonuclear leukocytes, mononuclear phagocytes, B cells, some T cells and mesangial phagocytes) and binds C3b, the initial degradation product of C3, C4b, and to

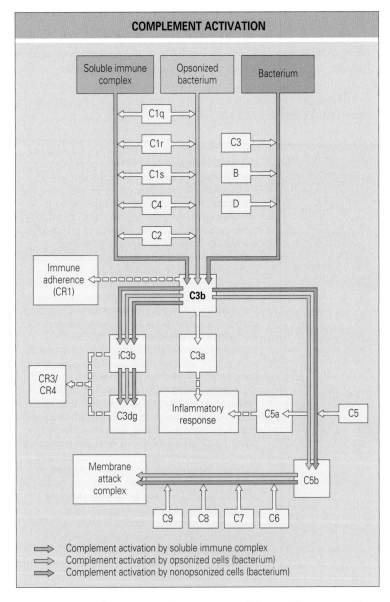

Fig. 117.20 Complement activation. Activation of the complement cascade by soluble immune complexes and antibody-opsonized bacterium (the classic pathway) and by non-opsonized bacterium (the alternative pathway) are shown. The common component, C3b, mediates the immune adherence reaction with the receptor for C3b (called complement receptor type 1 or CR1), whereas the C3b degradation products, iC3b and C3dg, bind to complement receptors 3 and 4 (CR3 and CR4). The bacterium can activate further components of the complement cascade to result in formation of the membrane attack complex. All three activation pathways can result in C3a generation, and the bacterium can also result in C5a production. These components are vasodilators and potent chemotactic peptides, which can initiate an inflammatory response.

a lesser degree iC3b, the further degradation product of C3b. CR1 on erythrocytes is clearly important in binding and processing immune complexes, but its expression on and role in fixed tissue macrophages is less certain. CR2 is expressed on B cells, follicular dendritic cells and some cells of the T cell lineage. It binds iC3b and C3dg, a degradation product of iC3b. Although CR2 is important in antibody production by B cells, it is not involved in immune complex processing[52]. CR2 also acts as a receptor for the Epstein–Barr virus. CR3 and CR4 are structurally distinct from CR1 and CR2. They are members of a group of adhesion receptors known as β_2 integrins, and are composed of two chains: an α chain of variable size and a common β chain[49]. Both CR3 and CR4, which bind the C3 degradation product iC3b, are found on fixed tissue macrophages, mononuclear phagocytes, polymorphonuclear leukocytes and follicular dendritic cells. CR3 and CR4 are probably important in immune complex uptake after erythrocyte CR1-mediated processing of the immune-complex-bound C3. Deficiency of the family of β_2 integrins is associated with loss of adhesive and phagocytic capacity, with severe impairment of host defenses, but not with SLE.

In SLE, there may be reduced amounts of CR1 on erythrocytes. This reduction is acquired, although an inherited polymorphism of CR1 expression on erythrocytes may contribute in some patients. The acquired reduction in CR1 number has been demonstrated by transfusion of normal erythrocytes into patients with SLE; normal erythrocytes with high levels of CR1 'acquire' lower levels of CR1 expression with time after transfusion[53]. This phenomenon also occurs in non-human primates after infusion of a bolus of immune complexes. The CR1 are most probably stripped from erythrocytes, as the immune complexes are taken up by phagocytes in the liver in a process facilitated by FcγRs[54] (Fig. 117.19). Therefore, the combined presence of genetically determined deficiencies in the complement system, amplified by further acquired deficiencies, leads to a condition of continued complex formation and deposition.

Receptors for the Fc region of IgG

Structure

Immune complexes containing IgG antibodies engage receptors for the Fc region of IgG (FcγRs). In contrast to the complement receptors, which bind fragments of complement components, FcγRs bind IgG ligand in its native form. FcγRI and FcγRIIa also bind C reactive protein and serve as its receptors in humans. Cross-linking of FcγR triggers internalization by FcγR-expressing cells and leads to degranulation by phagocytes and mast cells, immediate release of inflammatory mediators, and synthesis and release of cytokines[52]. The three families of Fcγ receptors – FcγRI, FcγRII, FcγRIII (Table 117.5, Fig. 117.21) – are encoded by distinct genes on human chromosome 1. Each family member has distinct ligand-binding properties and is differentially expressed on various cell types (Tables 117.6 & 117.7)[54,55]. As members of the immunoglobulin supergene family, all share the common structural motif of two or three immunoglobulin-like disulfide-linked domains in the extracellular portion of the receptor (Fig. 117.21). Although these receptors share similar but not identical extracellular domains, the transmembrane and cytoplasmic tails are highly divergent. This diversity is responsible for the variety of functions that these receptors can elicit

TABLE 117.5 HUMAN Fcγ RECEPTOR FAMILIES

Structural Isoforms	FcγRI			FcγRII			FcγRIII	
Distinct genes	A	B	C	A	B	C	A	B
Splice variants	?	?	?	a1, a2	b1, b2, b3			
Allelic variants	+			H131/R131	(+)	(+)	V176/F176	NA1/NA2
Membrane anchor	TM γ-chain	TM	TM	a1: TM a2: secreted	TM	TM	γ/ζ complex	GPI

TM: conventional transmembrane protein
γ/ζ complex: although FcgRIIIA is a transmembrane protein, a member of this family of signal transducing molecules is required for cell surface expression of FcγRIIIA
GPI: glycosylphosphatidylinositol membrane anchor
By convention, distinct genes within an FcγR family are designated with an uppercase letter, whereas the protein products from these genes are designated with the corresponding lowercase letter.

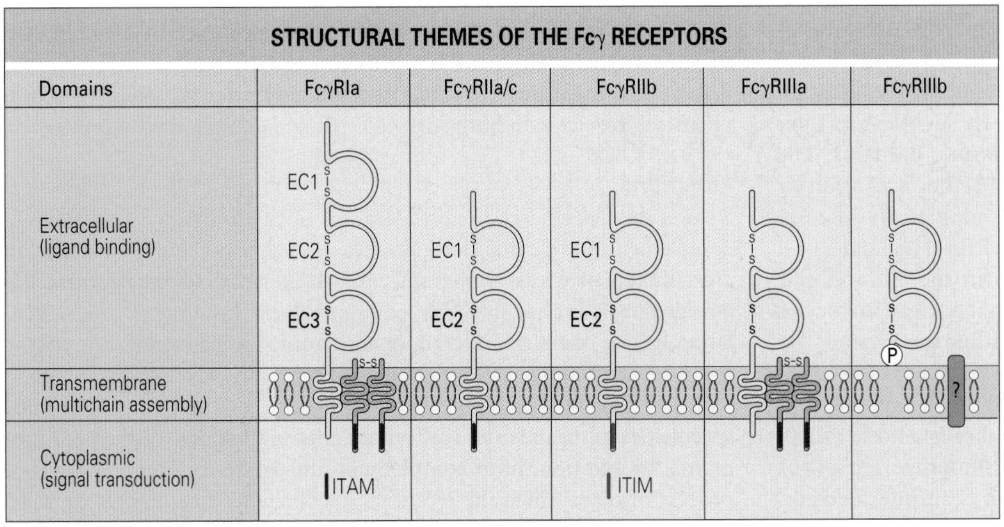

STRUCTURAL THEMES OF THE Fcγ RECEPTORS

Domains	FcγRIa	FcγRIIa/c	FcγRIIb	FcγRIIIa	FcγRIIIb
Extracellular (ligand binding)	EC1 EC2 EC3	EC1 EC2	EC1 EC2		
Transmembrane (multichain assembly)					
Cytoplasmic (signal transduction)	ITAM		ITIM		

Fig. 117.21 Structural themes of the Fcγ receptors. All FcγRs have extracellular domains composed of two (or three for FcγRIA) disulfide-bonded immunoglobulin superfamily motifs. FcγRIa and FcγRIIIa share the same γ-chain. The signaling motif used by FcγRIIb is an immunoreceptor tyrosine inhibitory motif that is similar to the immunoreceptor tyrosine activation motif (ITAM) but has only one tyrosine, which forms a docking site for molecules including an src-homology domain type 2-containing tyrosine phosphatase. The signaling motifs engaged by FcγRIIIb are not completely understood.

TABLE 117.6 Fcγ RECEPTOR CELLULAR DISTRIBUTION

Gene family	Isoform	Cell types
FcγRI	a	Monocytes, Mφ, IFN-γ- or G-CSF-stimulated PMN, IFN-γ-stimulated eosinophils
	b/c	(mRNA encoding FcγRIb is present in monocytes, Mφ, IFN-γ-stimulated PMN)
FcγRII	a	Platelets, PMN, monocytes, Mφ, Langerhans cells, mast cells (?B cells, NK cells)
	b	B cells, monocytes, Mφ, and PMN
	c	(mRNA present in monocytes, Mφ, PMN, platelets, NK cells and B cells)
FcγRIII	a	NK cells, Mφ (including mesangial cells), subpopulation of monocytes, mast cells, (subset of T cells)
	b	PMN, IFN-γ-stimulated eosinophils

G-CSF, granulocyte-colony-stimulating factor; Mφ, macrophage; NK, natural killer; PMN, polymorphonuclear leukocytes
FcγRs are expressed in myeloid and lymphoid lineages. Data on protein expression are not complete.

TABLE 117.7 HUMAN Fcg RECEPTORS AND IgG SUBCLASS SPECIFITY

FcgR family	FcgR gene	Glycoprotein (kDa)	Affinity for IgG (K_a)	IgG subclass specificity
FcgRI	FcgRIA	72	10^8–10^9 M[21]	1,3.4..2
	FcgRIB	??	??	unknown
FcgRII	FcgRIIA-R131	40–50	,10^7 M[21]	1,3..4,2
	FcgRIIA-H131	40–50	,10^7 M[21]	1,2,3..4
	FcgRIIB,C	40–50	,10^7 M[21]	1,3..4,2
FcgRIII	FcgRIIIA-V176	60–70	;7×10^6 M[21]	1,3..4,2
	FcgRIIIA-F176	60–70	;3×10^6 M[21]	1,3..4,2
	FcgRIIIB	50–80	,10^7 M[21]	1,3..4,2

(Fig. 117.21, Table 117.6)[55]. Interestingly, through the use of data generated through the Human Genome Project, additional homologues have been identified and their unique expression on B cells raises a possible role in autoantibody production.

FcγRI, expressed on monocytes, macrophages and IFN-γ-stimulated polymorphonuclear leukocytes, is distinguished by its three extracellular immunoglobulin-like domains and its high affinity for IgG (Table 117.7). It associates non-covalently in the membrane with a homodimer of the γ-accessory chain, a member of the γ/ζ family of signal transducing molecules. The γ-chain is also found in association with the high-affinity receptor for IgE (FcεRI), the high-affinity receptor for IgA (FcαR), FcγRIIIa (see below), and the T cell receptor–CD3 complex (although it is distinct from CD3γ). ζ-Chain is found in association with the CD3 complex and FcγRIIIa on natural killer (NK) cells (see below). Data suggest that two or three highly homologous genes may encode for distinct isoforms of FcγRI, but the biological significance of these genes is uncertain. FcγRI, the high-affinity receptor for IgG, is the only FcγR that binds monomeric IgG. It is also a receptor for C reactive protein. FcγRI may play a part in antigen processing on monocytes and/or macrophages.

FcγRII is a low-affinity receptor with two immunoglobulin-like extracellular domains. It is widely distributed and is found on most leukocytes and platelets. It interacts most effectively with multivalent IgG immune complexes and IgG-opsonized particles. The FcγRII family has three distinct yet highly homologous genes (FcγRIIA, FcγRIIB and FcγRIIC) and several alternative splice products, resulting in expression of six protein isoforms. The three genes are nearly identical in their extracellular domains, but differ in their cytoplasmic domains. The divergence in cytoplasmic domains determines whether activation or inhibition results from engagement by ligand. In addition to different isoforms, there are at least two allelic forms of FcγRIIa (H131 and R131). These alleles, which differ in two amino acids in the extracellular domain, are expressed codominantly on polymorphonuclear leukocytes and monocytes and have differing IgG subclass binding specificities.

FcγRIII is encoded for by two distinct genes. These genes are selectively expressed in specific cell types, with FcγRIIIa found on NK cells and mononuclear phagocytes (including mesangial cells) and FcγRIIIb found on polymorphonuclear leukocytes and eosinophils. These isoforms bind IgG with different affinities: FcγRIIIa is an intermediate-

affinity receptor that can bind monomeric IgG at physiologic concentrations, whereas FcγRIIIb is a low-affinity receptor that binds immune complexes (like FcγRII). FcγRIIIa is a transmembrane glycoprotein that associates in the membrane with a dimer composed of members of the γ/ζ family of signal transduction molecules. On NK cells, both γ- and ζ-chains have been found to associate with FcγRIIIa, but on macrophages only γ-chain is found. FcγRIIIb provides a dramatic example of structural divergence. It lacks both the transmembrane and cytoplasmic domains and is anchored to the membrane through a glycosyl-phosphatidylinositol moiety. Both FcγRIIIa and FcγRIIIb have allelic forms that are biologically important. Alleles differ in their capacity to bind ligand, and the alleles of FcγRIIIb (called NA1 and NA2, reflecting their initial description as neutrophil-associated antigens) have quantitatively different capacities for neutrophil priming, despite comparable expression and equivalent ligand binding[56]. Like the H131 and R131 polymorphic alleles of FcγRIIA, the FcγRIII alleles differ by only a few amino acids and are expressed in a codominant fashion (Fig. 117.22).

Normal sera contain soluble FcγRII and FcγRIII, which are derived either from alternative splicing of mRNA (FcγRIIa) or from proteolytic release from circulating cells (FcγRIII)[57]. One proposed biological function of plasma FcγR is to suppress IgG production by B cells[58]. A striking property of soluble FcγRII is the ability to suppress completely the inflammation induced by immune complex, in the reverse passive Arthus reaction[59]. Soluble FcγRIIIb may also modulate neutrophils through interactions between carbohydrates on the soluble receptor and the lectin-like domain of CR3. However, the physiologic significance of these circulating IgG binding proteins for IgG production, immune complex handling or other functions is not yet clear. Soluble FcγR binding to immune complexes might affect clearance by changing the size of complexes, altering their solubility, modifying their ability to activate complement and capture C3b, and thus alter the ability of complexes to interact with both surface FcγR and complement receptors.

Function

Several themes emerge in consideration of the functional properties of complement and FcγRs. Both families of receptors require clustering or cross-linking of at least two receptors on the same cell to initiate intracellular signaling[60]. Presumably, this requirement for clustering prevents circulating IgG or complement components from stimulating effector cells in the absence of antigen. Both families of receptors have several members with cell-type specific expression, with some distinct yet overlapping specificities for ligands and with some capacity to initiate distinct cell programs. In addition, both complement and FcγRs can be activated – a process through which the receptors may enhance quantitative capacity,

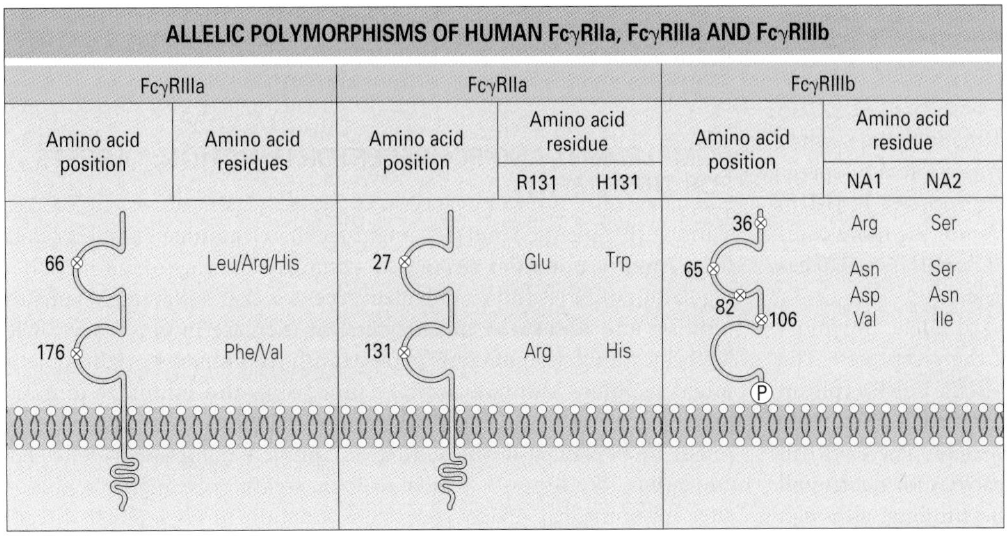

Fig. 117.22 Allelic polymorphisms of human FcγRIIa, FcγRIIIa and FcγRIIIb. The R131 and H131 alleles of FcγRIIa have markedly different binding capacities for human IgG2 and murine IgG1 as a consequence of an amino acid substitution in position 131 in the second extracellular domain. Polymorphic forms of FcγRIIIa have been described, but the total number of alleles is not known. Changes in the sequence at amino acid positions 66 and 176 have been reported to result in different binding capacities for all IgG subclasses. The NA1 and NA2 polymorphism of FcγRIIIb, the glycosyl-phosphatidylinositol linked protein expressed exclusively in neutrophils, reflects four amino acid substitutions resulting in a different number of potential N-linked glycosylation sites (NA1 = 4, NA2 = 6). In contrast to the FcγRIIa and FcγRIIIa polymorphisms, the difference in phagocytic function of the NA1 compared with NA2 alleles does not reflect differences in ligand binding.

ALLELIC POLYMORPHISMS OF HUMAN FcγRIIa, FcγRIIIa AND FcγRIIIb

FcγRIIIa		FcγRIIa			FcγRIIIb		
Amino acid position	Amino acid residues	Amino acid position	Amino acid residue		Amino acid position	Amino acid residue	
			R131	H131		NA1	NA2
66	Leu/Arg/His	27	Glu	Trp	36	Arg	Ser
					65	Asn	Ser
					82	Asp	Asn
176	Phe/Val	131	Arg	His	106	Val	Ile

acquire new functional capabilities, or both. Unlike CR3 and CR4, however, FcγRs are able to internalize ligand without prior cell priming or activation through other pathways. Both families have the potential to modify immune complex properties – CR1 through its cofactor activity and immune complex solubilization and FcγR, perhaps, through soluble forms binding to immune complex. Taken together, these themes outline an intricate network of mechanisms for immune complex handling.

Three strategies for signal transduction and the initiation of effector functions by phagocyte FcγRs are now apparent. FcγRIa and FcγRIIIa associate in the membrane with the γ/ζ family molecules, which express a tyrosine-based activation motif in their cytoplasmic domains (the immunoreceptor tyrosine activation motif, ITAM) (Fig. 117.21). This motif, which is utilized by numerous immunologically important receptors, including the T cell receptor and B cell receptor for antigen, is characterized by a tyrosine–X–X–leucine repeat (X is any amino acid) that is separated by seven to nine amino acids[61]. Within the motif, the tyrosines can become phosphorylated by a member of the *src* family of tyrosine kinases. Activation is initiated when FcγR are clustered at the cell surface by multivalent immune complexes. The phosphorylated tyrosine–X–X– leucine forms a docking site for other signaling intermediates that contain an srchomology domain type 2. Each ITAM-containing molecule differs in the flanking amino acids, which provides specificity in the recruitment of additional signaling intermediates and in subsequent downstream signaling events.

In contrast to the γ/ζ-associated FcγR, FcγRIIa incorporates an ITAM in its cytoplasmic domain. This ITAM has an additional five amino acids separating the tyrosine repeat. The insertion of these additional amino acids alters the functional properties of the ITAM[62]. The mechanism by which the glycosyl-phosphatidylinositol-linked FcγRIIIb engages intracellular signaling molecules remains unknown. Among the possibilities are an interaction with another transmembrane protein, direct association with an *src* family kinase residing in lipid domains within the membrane, or an extracellular carbohydrate–lectin interaction with CR3. There is evidence for each of these possibilities.

In addition to these activating FcγRs, there are inhibitory FcγRs, FcγRIIb, which modulate the thresholds for activation of cells and terminate stimulating signals. FcγRIIb is a single-chain, low-affinity receptor with an extracellular domain highly homologous to its activating counterparts and a cytoplasmic domain containing an immunoreceptor tyrosine inhibitory motif (ITIM) (Fig. 117.21). Inert when self-aggregated, inhibitory FcγRs abolish cellular signals when coligated with stimulatory receptors, such as ITAM-bearing FcγRs. The ITIM (valine/isoleucine–X–tyrosine–X–X–leucine) is phosphorylated by protein tyrosine kinases and then recruits phosphatases, which are involved in transducing the inhibitory signals. In cells that express both stimulatory and inhibitory FcγRs, such as human phagocytes, the relative amounts of these two types of receptors determine the state of cell activation after interaction with immune complexes[55,60,63].

Although FcγRs on lymphoid cells (NK cells, B cells and T cells) may not be directly involved in immune complex handling, they are important modulators of the immune response. NK cell FcγRIIIa mediates antibody-dependent cellular cytotoxicity; B cell FcγRIIb downmodulates B cell function when co-cross-linked with the B cell receptor for antigen (surface immunoglobulin, sIg) (e.g. by an immune complex that has antigen also bound to sIg). This function is initiated by an ITIM in the cytoplasmic domain of FcγRIIb. Recruitment of phosphatases and other molecules to the ITIM decreases the intensity of signal generated by sIg. Reduced expression of FcγRIIb is associated with increased susceptibility to the development of autoimmunity and autoimmune disease, suggesting that FcγRIIb functions *in vivo* to maintain peripheral tolerance[64]. A role for FcγR in T cell maturation has been suggested in the mouse, but no comparable function in humans has been found.

Fcγ receptors and SLE

The importance of FcγRs in immune complex clearance has been shown in a number of different *in vivo* models (Fig. 117.17); it is likely that both intrinsic (genetic) differences and acquired differences for all three families of FcγR contribute to net function. For example, experimental blockade of FcγRIIIa by infusion of an anti-FcγRIII monoclonal antibody in both human and non-human primates (chimpanzee) inhibits the clearance of IgG anti-D-sensitized erythrocytes, of soluble DNA–anti-DNA immune complexes and, to a lesser degree, of erythrocyte-bound DNA–anti-DNA immune complexes[65]. The prolongation of FcγR-mediated mononuclear phagocyte system clearance of IgG-opsonized erythrocytes in normal disease-free donors with HLA-DR2 and DR3 (the same DR alleles associated with SLE) relative to other normal disease-free donors[38] is associated with a decreased FcγRI-specific phagocytosis.

Acquired differences in receptor expression and function contribute to disease-associated differences in immune complex clearance (Fig. 117.18). Various cytokines, including TGF-β, IL-10 and IFN-γ, can alter FcγR expression and function: IFN-γ and IL-10 upregulate FcγRI expression, TGF-β upregulates macrophage FcγRIIIa, and IL-4 decreases FcγR expression. Anti-FcγR autoantibodies (especially anti-FcγRIII) in patients with SLE, scleroderma and other autoimmune diseases may also be important; high titers of these autoantibodies appear to correlate with immune complex levels.

Review of FcγR deficiencies[66–68] reveals an initial report of complete FcγRIIIb deficiency on neutrophils in a patient with SLE. FcγRIIIb deficiency has been associated with neonatal neutropenia when FcγRIIIb-deficient mothers, alloimmunized during a previous pregnancy, have given birth to an infant with the appropriate FcγRIIIb epitopes. Neither the very rare deficiency of FcγRIa nor the more commonly evident variations in the quantitative level of FcγRIIa1 in platelets has yet been associated with clinically evident sequelae.

Currently, three different FcγRs have recognized allelic polymorphisms that influence the functional capacity of the receptors[55]. The FcγRIIa polymorphism (H131, R131) and the FcγRIIIa polymorphism (F176, V176) affect ligand binding – the FcγRIIa H131 allele is the only FcγR that binds human IgG2 to any appreciable extent. The FcγRIIIb alleles (NA1, NA2) have different quantitative capacities for neutrophil priming. This difference is independent of ligand binding, although some evidence suggests a difference in the binding of IgG3 (NA1>NA2). Each of these polymorphisms establishes the precedent for genetically determined, functionally important alleles of FcγRs, each of which influences cell triggering and may provide important models for risk factors in disease pathogenesis.

Genetic linkage studies in families in which several members have SLE indicate linkage of the SLE phenotype with a region of human chromosome 1 (1q20–23), the same region that contains the genes that encode all of the FcγRs and the associated γ-chain (see Chapter 118). Indeed, the alleles of FcγRIIa and FcγRIIIa represent risk factors for the SLE diathesis. A multicenter study of African-American patients with SLE has shown a significantly reduced distribution of H131 homozygosity for FcγRIIa compared with controls without SLE[69]. This difference was particularly pronounced in patients with lupus nephritis. As the H131 allele is the predominant FcγR binding IgG2, it may be especially important in handling immune complexes that contain IgG2 autoantibodies. FcγRIIa alleles may not be a risk factor for all patients with SLE, as demonstrated by differing results in white patients from The Netherlands, USA and UK[70]. FcγRIIa alleles appear to be disease modifiers in patients with pathogenic IgG2 autoantibodies, conferring inherited risk for disease severity or phenotypes. For example, in patients with anti-C1q autoantibodies, FcγRIIa-R131 genes are associated with renal disease[71]. Most autoantibodies are not of the IgG2 isotype, but rather of the IgG1 and IgG3 isotypes. Recent studies of ethnically diverse patients with SLE have shown a significant skewing in the FcγRIIIa-158F/V alleles[72,73]. In patients with SLE and nephritis, the homozygous 158V (high-affinity allele) is under-represented compared with those without nephritis. Continuing studies have demonstrated model-dependent linkage, significant transmission disequilibrium and

confirmed case–control associations of FcγRIIIa alleles and SLE. Nonetheless, it is highly likely that there are additional polymorphic candidate genes within this region of chromosome 1.

COMPLEMENT AND FCγ RECEPTOR FUNCTION: TARGETS FOR TREATMENT

Various therapeutic strategies might facilitate immune complex handling. Among potential strategies, tissue-specific, cytokine-mediated regulation of FcγR and complement receptor expression might enhance binding and uptake by phagocytes. An increase in erythrocyte CR1 levels by stimulation of erythropoiesis with recombinant erythropoietin might facilitate immune complex processing and minimize immune complex deposition[74]. Administration of complement components might be beneficial in the setting of complete component-deficiency and lupus-like illness[75]. Pharmacologic treatments might be able to alter mononuclear phagocyte system function *in vivo*, either directly or in concert with certain cytokines. Open studies of intravenous infusion of gamma globulin have been reported for SLE and other rheumatic diseases, but the mechanisms (e.g. blockade of FcγRs, induction of inhibitory FcγRs, or idiotypic interactions with autoantibodies), the indications and the efficacy of this approach require further study[76,77].

The striking observations that soluble FcγRs[59] and CR1[78] block active inflammatory reactions indicate the potential for these soluble receptors as therapeutic agents. Interventions in the effector stage of immune complex diseases could be accomplished by blocking FcγR. Early components of complement do not seem to be *required* for the initiation of inflammatory responses, whereas later components amplify injury and may act downstream of FcγR activation. By exploiting the intrinsic properties of different FcγRs (e.g. the H131 allele of FcγRIIa, which binds IgG2, or the V158 allele of FcγRIIIa, which binds IgG with a greater affinity), one could develop a panel of soluble FcγRs with differing affinities and subclass preferences that would allow more specific targeting of disease-associated autoantibodies.

Alternatively, by changing the balance of stimulatory and inhibitory FcγRs expressed on phagocytes with cyokines or pharmacologic agents, one could modulate immune complex-triggered inflammation[27,55,63]. Because immune complexes can either enhance or suppress the humoral immune response, depending upon the type of Fcγ receptor engaged (stimulatory or inhibitory) and the cell type involved (B cells or antigen-presenting cells), alterations in balance of FcγR expression can also influence afferent responses. The opportunities for therapeutic intervention are indeed many.

REFERENCES

1. Hohan C, Datta SK. Lupus. Key pathogenic mechanisms and contributing factors. Clin Immunol Immunopath 1996; 77: 209–220.
2. Dayal AK, Kammer GM. The T cell enigma in lupus. Arthritis Rheum 1995; 39: 23–33.
3. Emlen W, Niebur J, Kadera R. Accelerated *in vitro* apoptosis of lymphocytes from patients with systemic lupus erythematosus. J Immunol 1994; 152: 3685–3692.
4. Mountz JD, Wu J, Cheng J, Zhou T. Autoimmune disease: a problem of defective apoptosis. Arthitis Rheum 1994; 37: 1415–1420.
5. Klemperer P, Pollack AD, Baehr G. Diffuse collagen disease. Acute disseminated lupus erythematosus and diffuse scleroderma. JAMA 1942; 119: 331–332.
6. Cruickshank, B. The basic pattern of tissue damage and pathology of systemic lupus erythematosus. In: Wallace DJ, Dubois EL, eds. Dubois' lupus erythematosus. Philadephia: Lea and Febiger; 1987: 53–104.
7. Godman GC, Deitch AD, Klemperer P. The composition of the LE and hematoxylin bodies of systemic lupus erythematosus. Am J Pathol 1957; 34: 1–17.
8. Ford PM, Ford SE, Lillicarp DP. Association of lupus anticoagulant with severe valvular heart disease in systemic lupus erythematosus. J Rheumatol 1988; 15: 597–600.
9. Galve E, Ordi J, Barquinero J *et al.* Valvular heart disease in the primary antiphospholipid syndrome. Ann Intern Med 1992; 116: 293–298.
10. Clark WH Jr, Reed RJ, Mimm MC. Lupus erythematosus. Histopathology of cutaneous lesions. Human Pathol 1973; 4: 157–163.
11. Tani M, Shimizu R, Ban M *et al.* Systemic lupus erythematosus with vesiculobullous lesions. Arch Dermatol 1984; 120: 1497–14501.
12. Winkelmann RK. Panniculitis and SLE. JAMA 1970; 22: 472–475.
13. Douglas Smith C, Marino C, Rothfield N. Clinical utility of the lupus band test. Arthritis Rheum 1984; 27: 382–387.
14. Gilliam JN. The significance of cutaneous immunoglobulin deposits in lupus erythematosus and NZB/NZW hybrid mice. J Invest Dermatol 1975; 65: 154–161.
15. Appel GB, Pirani CL, D'Agati VD. Renal vascular involvement in systemic lupus. J Am Soc Nephrol 1994; 4: 1499–1515.
16. D'Agati V, Kunis C, Williams G, Appel GB. Anticardiolipin antibody and renal disease. J Am Soc Nephrol 1990; 1: 777–784.
17. D'Agati V. Renal disease in systemic lupus erythematosus, mixed connective tissue disease, Sjogren's syndrome, and rheumatoid arthritis. In: Jennette JC, Olson JL, Schwartz MM, Silva FG, eds. Heptinstall's Pathology of the Kidney, 5E, ch 13. Philadelphia: Lippincott Raven Publishers; 1998: 514–624.

18. Appel GB, Silva FG, Pirani CL *et al*. Renal involvement in systemic lupus erythematosus (SLE): a study of 56 patients emphasizing histologic classification. Medicine (Baltimore) 1978; 57: 371–410.

19. Churg J, Bernstein J, Glassock R. Renal disease: classification and atlas of glomerular diseases, 2E. New York: Igaku-Shoin, 1995; 152.

20. Park MH, D'Agati VD, Appel GB, Pirani CL. Tubulointerstitial disease in lupus nephritis: relationship to immune deposits, interstitial inflammation, glomerular changes, renal function and prognosis. Nephron 1986; 44: 309–319.

21. Austin HA, Muenz LR, Joyce KM *et al*. Prognostic factors in lupus nephritis: contribution of renal histological data. Am J Med 1983; 75: 382–391.

22. Austin HA, Muenz LR, Joyce KM *et al*. Diffuse proliferative lupus nephritis: identification of specific pathologic features affecting renal outcome. Kidney Int 1984; 25: 689–695.

23. Austin HA, Boumpas DT, Vaughan EM, Balow JE. Predicting renal outcomes in severe lupus nephritis: contributions of clinical and histologic data. Kidney Int 1994; 45: 544–550.

24. Schwartz MM, Lan SP, Bernstein J *et al*. Irreproducibility of the activity and chronicity indices limits their utility in the management of lupus nephritis. Lupus Nephritis Collaborative Study Group. Am J Kidney Dis 1993; 21: 374–377.

25. Foster MH, Cinzman B, Madaio MP. Nephritiogenic autoantibodies in systemic lupus erythematosus: immunochemical properties, mechanisms of immune deposition and genetic origins. Lab Invest 1993; 69: 494–507.

26. Berden JH, Licht R, van Bruggen MC, Tax WJ. Role of nucleosomes for induction and glomerular binding of autoantibodies in lupus nephritis. Curr Opin Nephrol Hypertens 1999; 8: 299–306.

27. Clynes R, Dumitru C, Ravetch JV. Uncoupling of immune complex formation and kidney damage in autoimmune glomerulonephritis. Science 1998; 279: 1052–1054.

28. Johnson RT, Richardson EP. The neurological manifestations of systemic lupus erythematosus. A clinical-pathological study of 24 cases and review of the literature. Medicine (Baltimore) 1968; 47: 337–369.

29. Ellis SG, Verity MA. Central nervous system involvement in systemic lupus erythematosus: a review of neuropathologic findings in 57 cases 1955–1977. Semin Arthritis Rheum 1979; 8: 212–221.

30. Harris EN, Gharavi AE, Asherson RA *et al*. Cerebral infarction in systemic lupus: association with anticardiolipin antibodies. Clin Exp Rheumatol 1984; 2: 47–51.

31. Purnell DC, Baggenstoss AH, Olsen AM. Pulmonary lesions in disseminated lupus erythematosus. Ann Intern Med 1955; 42: 619–628.

32. Bidani AK, Roberts JL, Schwartz JL, Lewis EJ. Immunopathology of cardiac lesions in fatal SLE. Am J Med 1980; 69: 849–850.

33. Doherty NE, Siegel RJ. Cardiovascular manifestations of systemic lupus erythematosus. Am Heart J 1985; 110: 1257–1265.

34. Bulkley BH, Roberts WC. The heart in systemic lupus erythematosus and the changes induced in it by corticosteroid therapy. Am J Med 1975; 58: 243–264.

35. Jefferis R. Molecular structure of human IgG subclasses. In: Shakib F, ed. The human IgG subclasses. Oxford: Pergamon Press; 1990: 15–30.

36. Duncan AR, Winter G. The binding site for Clq on IgG. Nature 1988,332: 738–40.

37. Duncan AR, Woof JM, Partridge LJ, Burton DR, Winter G. Localization of the binding site for the human high-affinity Fc receptor for IgG. Nature 1988; 332: 563–4.

38. Mannik M. Immune complexes. In: Lahita, RG, ed. Systemic lupus erythematosus, 2E. Churchill Livingstone: New York; 1992: 327–341.

39. Kimberly RP, Gibofsky A, Salmon JE, Fotino M. Impaired Fc-mediated mononuclear phagocyte system clearance in HLA-DR2 and MTl-positive healthy young adults. J Exp Med 1983; 157: 1698–1703.

40. Salmon JE, Kimberly RP, Gibofsky A, Fotino M. Defective mononuclear phagocyte function in systemic lupus erythematosus: dissociation of Fc receptor–ligand binding and internalization. J Immunol 1984; 133: 2525–2531.

41. Madi N, Steiger G, Estreicher J, Schifferli JA. Immune adherence and clearance of hepatitis B surface Ag/Ab complexes is abnormal in patients with system lupus erythematosus. Clin Exp Immunol 1991; 85: 373–378.

42. Lobatto S, Daha MR, Breedveld FC *et al*. Abnormal clearance of soluble aggregates of human immunoglobulin G in patients with systemic lupus erythematosus. Clin Exp Immunol 1988; 72: 55–59.

43. Walport MJ. Complement. New Engl J Med 2002; 344: 1058–1065, 1140–1144.

44. Nelson RA. The immune adherence phenomenon: an immunologically specific reaction between micro-organisms and erythrocytes leading to enhanced phagocytosis. Science 1953; 118: 733–737.

45. Cornacoff JB, Hebert LA, Smead WL. Primate erythrocyte-immune complex-clearing mechanism. J Clin Invest 1983; 71: 236–247.

46. Schifferli JA, Ng YC, Estreicher J, Walport MJ. The clearance of tetanus/anti-tetanus toxoid immune complexes from the circulation of humans. Complement- and erythrocyte complement receptor I-dependent mechanisms. J Immunol 1988; 140: 899–904.

47. Hebert L. The clearance of immune complexes from the circulation of man and other primates. Am J Kidney Dis 1991; 17: 352–361.

48. Schifferli JA, Taylor RP. Physiological and pathological aspects of circulating immune complexes. Kidney Int 1989; 35: 993–1003.

49. Holers VM. Complement. In: Rich R, ed. Complement deficiencies on clinical immunology. London: Harcourt Health Sciences Inc; 2001: 21.1–21.18.

50. Pickering MC, Botto M, Taylor PR *et al*. Systemic lupus erythematosus, complement deficiency and apoptosis. Adv Immunol 2000; 76: 227–324.

51. Ahearn JM, Fearon DT. Structure and function of the complement receptors, CRI (CD35) and CR2 (CD21). Adv Immunol 1989; 46: 183–219.

52. Carroll MC. The role of complement in B cell activation and tolerance. Adv Immunol 2000; 74: 61–88.

53. Walport M, Ng YC, Lachmann PJ. Erythrocytes transfused into patients with SLE and haemolytic anaemia lose complement receptor type I from their cell surface. Clin Exp Immunol 1987; 69: 501–507.

54. Salmon JE, Pricop L. Human receptors for immunoglobulin. Key elements in the pathogenesis of rheumatic disease. Arthritis Rheum 2001; 44: 739–750.

55. Bolland S, Ravetch JV. Inhibitory pathways triggered by ITIM-containing receptors. Adv Immunol 1999; 72: 149–177.

56. Salmon JE, Edberg JC, Kimberly RP. Fcgamma receptor III on human neutrophils: allelic variants have functionally distinct capacities. J Clin Invest 1990; 85: 1287–1295.

57. Huizinga TWJ, De Haas M, Kleijer M *et al*. Soluble Fcgamma receptor III in human plasma originates from release by neutrophils. J Clin Invest 1990; 86: 416–423.

58. Sautes C, Varin N, Hogarth PM *et al*. Molecular and functional studies of recombinant soluble Fc gamma receptors. Mol Immunol 1990; 27: 1201–1207.

59. Ierino FL, Powell MS, McKenzie IF *et al*. Recombinant soluble human Fc gamma RII: production, characterization, and inhibition of the Arthus reaction. J Exp Med 1993; 178: 1617–1628.

60. Daeron M. Fc receptor biology. Annu Rev Immunol 1997; 15: 203–234.

61. Cambier J. Antigen and Fc receptor signaling. The awesome power of the immunoreceptor tyrosine-based activation motif (ITAM). J Immunol 1995; 155: 3281–3285.

62. Edberg JC, Lin CT, Lau D *et al*. The Ca²⁺ dependence of human Fcgamma receptor-initiated phagocytosis. J Biol Chem 1995; 270: 22301–22307.

63. Pricop L, Redecha P, Teillard J-L *et al*. Differential modulation of stimulatory and inhibitory Fcgamma receptos on human moncytes by TH1 and TH2 cytokines. J Immunol 2001; 166: 531–537.

64. Bolland S, Ravtech JV. Spontaneous autoimmune disease in FcgammaRII deficient mice results from strain-specific epistasis. Immmunity 2001; 13: 277–285.

65. Kimberly RP, Edberg JC, Merriam LT *et al*. *In vivo* handling of soluble complement fixing Ab/dsDNA immune complexes in chimpanzees. J Clin Invest 1989; 84: 962–970.

66. Ceuppens JL, Baroja ML, Van Vaeck F, Anderson CL. A defect in the membrane expression of high affinity 72 kD Fc receptors on phagocytic cells in four healthy subjects. J Clin Invest 1988; 82: 571–578.

67. Huizinga TWJ, Kuijpers RWAM, Kleijer M *et al*. Maternal genomic neutrophil FcRIII deficiency leading to neonatal isoimmune neutropenia. Blood 1990; 76: 1927–1932.

68. Clark MR, Lui L, Clarkson SB *et al*. An abnormality of the gene that encodes neutrophil Fc receptor III in a patient with systemic lupus erythematosus. J Clin Invest 1990; 86: 341–346.

69. Salmon JE, Milard S, Schacter LA *et al*. Fcγ RIIA alleles are heritable risk factors for lupus nephritis in African-Americans. J Clin Invest 1996; 97: 1348–1354.

70. Lehrnbecher T, Foster CB, Zhu S *et al*. Variant genotypes of the low-affinity Fcgamma receptors in two control populations and a review of low-affinity Fcgamma receptor polymorphisms in control and disease populations. Blood 1999; 94: 4220–4232.

71. Haseley LA, Wisnieski JJ, Denburg MR *et al*. Antibodies to C1q in systemic lupus erythematosus: characteristics and relation to Fc gamma RIIA alleles. Kidney Int 1997; 52: 1375–1380.

72. Wu J, Edberg JC, Redecha PB *et al*. A novel polymorphism of FcgammaRIIIa (CD16) alters receptor function and predisposes to autoimmune disease. J Clin Invest 1997; 100: 1059–1070.

73. Koene HR, Kleijer M, Swaak AJ *et al*. The Fc gammaRIIIA-158F allele is a risk factor for systemic lupus erythematosus. Arthritis Rheum 1998; 41: 1813–1818.

74. Hebert LA, Birmingham DJ, Shen X-P, Cosio FG. Stimulating erythropoiesis increases complement receptor expression on primate erythrocytes. Clin Exp Immunol 1992,62: 301–306.

75. Steinsson K, Erlendsson K, Valdimarsson H. Successful plasma infusion treatment of a patient with C2 deficiency and system lupus erythematosus. Clinical experience over forty-five months. Arthritis Rheum 1989; 32: 906–913.

76. Salmon JE, Kapur S, Meryhew NL *et al*. High-dose, pulse intravenous methylprednisolone enhances Fcgamma receptor-mediated mononuclear phagocyte function in systemic lupus erythematosus. Arthritis Rheum 1989; 32: 717–725.

77. Samuelsson A, Towers TL, Ravtech JV. Anti-inflammatory activity of IVIG mediated through the inhibitory Fc receptor. Science 2001; 291: 445–446.

78. Weisman HF, Bartow MK, Leppo MP *et al*. Recombinant soluble CR1 suppressed complement activation, inflammation and necrosis associated with reperfusion of ischemic myocardium. Trans Assoc Am Physicians 1990; 103: 60–72.

118 Genetics of lupus

John B Harley, Jennifer A Kelly and Kathy L Moser

- Genetic susceptibility to lupus is strongly supported by linkage and association studies, in addition to familial aggregation and twin concordance studies
- Several genes are involved
- Known genetic associations implicate HLA genes, including complement components and Fc receptor genes
- Murine models of lupus provide clues to the genetic basis of human lupus
- Human genome studies have revealed many linkages and promise to change our understanding of lupus dramatically.

INTRODUCTION

In complicated biological situations, use of a genetic approach to identify the components that are important in pathogenesis has proved to be a powerful tool. The means now available with which to tackle the genetics of common diseases have led to important progress in complex genetic conditions such as breast cancer and juvenile-onset diabetes. The promise of the genetic approach is to transform our understanding of disease fundamentally. Upon this premise, a major effort is under way to find and explain the susceptibility genes in lupus.

The more traditional genetic approaches using families of lupus patients and cohort comparisons have yielded some provocative findings. Familial aggregation has been well recognized in systemic lupus erythematosus, and efforts to understand the mode of inheritance have suggested that the segregation of autoimmunity in pedigrees containing a lupus proband follows an autosomal-dominant mode of inheritance, with 92% penetrance in women and 49% penetrance in men[1]. The cohort comparison approach, focusing on a gene (or biological process) and its association with disease in a cross-sectional sample of patients, has been most extensively used in studying human leukocyte antigen (HLA) class II polymorphisms. There are clearly other important genes, including those for complement, complement receptors, immunoglobulins, immunoglobulin receptors, T cell receptors (TCRs) and the apoptosis (programmed cell death)-related genes such as the resistance gene, bcl-2.

The new tools of human genetics used to screen the genome for disease-associated regions include microsatellite polymorphisms detected by polymerase chain reaction expansion of DNA, more powerful computer software and analytic tools, and informatic systems capable of managing large data collections. Studies in lupus have only recently begun to use these tools, with several studies indicating genetic linkages in chromosomes 1, 2, 4, 6, and 16[2–7].

A few principles appear to be emerging for the genes identified with lupus. On the basis of the perspective that lupus is a disease generated by humoral autoimmunity, most investigators anticipate genetic contributions on several levels (Table 118.1). The genes that influence the interaction with the environmental factor(s) leading to the development of

TABLE 118.1 CLASSES OF GENES POTENTIALLY IMPORTANT IN SYSTEMIC ERYTHEMATOSUS (SLE)

Gene function	Some candidate examples
Susceptibility (induction of autoimmunity)	Acute-phase reactants
	C-reactive protein
	Mannose-binding protein
	Complement components
	Cytokine genes
	IL-1α
	TNF-α
Specificity of the immune response	MHC Class II
	T cell receptor genes
	B cell receptor genes
Host response	Complement components
	Complement receptors
	Receptors for immunoglobulin (Fc receptors)

humoral autoimmunity are likely to be important. Genes that have a role in the immune regulation and in shaping the characteristic specificity of the autoantibody repertoire (such as *HLA* class II genes) are clearly important. Finally, the genes that influence the host response to humoral autoimmunity, including complement and Fc receptor genes responsible for immune complex processing, probably mediate much of the tissue injury and influence specific disease expression.

Most likely, some of the genes that contribute to murine lupus will also be important in human lupus and will provide a useful framework within which to guide investigations in man. The individual inbred experimental models in mice are expected to be simpler to explore than the complex outbred genetic events leading to lupus in man.

POTENTIAL FOR GENES IN LUPUS

Familial aggregation of disease raises the suspicion that a particular disease has a genetic basis. When inheritance follows predictable patterns, the mode of inheritance and the relationship between the genetic polymorphisms conferring risk and the disease phenotype can be established. In lupus, the pattern of inheritance does not follow a simple pattern such as autosomal recessive, autosomal dominant or sex-linked recessive. Nonetheless, there is about a 10% chance that any given patient with lupus will have another family member who also has lupus. This represents a more than 100-fold greater risk for lupus than is found in the general population[8].

The incidence and prevalence of lupus vary by sex and race[8]. African-American women have a 2.5- to sixfold increase in risk relative to white women. With estimates of prevalence as high as 1:250 for African-American women[8], lupus is a relatively common disease in this subpopulation in North America. In contrast, lupus is believed to be almost non-existent in West and Central Africa[8–10]. This result suggests two possibilities. The combination of African with European or Native

American genes may generate risk for lupus not found in an African genetic background when not admixed. Alternatively, the environmental exposure between North America and Central Africa is different in a way that is important for the envriomental risk factor(s) that generate lupus. Other examples of the incidence of lupus changing with geography are known[8,10].

Women have a 2.5- to 12-fold increase in incidence of disease over men[8]. The female preponderance for lupus extends across all populations studied. Indeed, the risk of lupus in patients with Klinefelter's syndrome, who usually have XXY sex chromosomes, seems to be greater than in normal XY men and, perhaps, similar to that of normal XX women[11].

The risk to an identical twin of a patient with lupus has been variously estimated. The largest study shows a concordance rate of about 24%[12], whereas the concordant occurrence of lupus in fraternal (non-identical) twins is much lower, about 2% or 3%. In lupus, the sibling recurrence rate (λ_s) is approximately 20, indicating that the disease is likely to have complex genetics[13]. The inability to define a simple mode of genetic segregation in multiplex pedigrees also argues that multiple genetic effects are required for expression of the lupus phenotype. Thus the genetics of lupus are most likely to be complex, analogous to juvenile diabetes mellitus and breast cancer, rather than simple Mendelian inheritance, as in Huntington's disease or cystic fibrosis.

LUPUS-RELATED LOCI AND ALLELES

Association studies comparing groups of patients and controls are susceptible to experimental artifact, perhaps because of variation between populations compounded by the complexity of the genetic contributions to lupus. Much of the literature concerning the genetics of lupus is based on such studies, and is therefore somewhat confusing. Nonetheless, some associations have been confirmed, at least in part (Table 118.2).

HLA genes

The histocompatibility region on the short arm of human chromosome 6 is arguably the most intensively studied collection of genes in the mammalian genome (see Chapter 12). Spanning approximately 3 500 000 bases (3.5 megabases) of DNA, this region contains some 120 identified human genes. The HLA gene products from this region provide the interface between the efferent and afferent immune responses by specifically interacting with antigen and presenting processed antigen to the TCRs. This presentation, in turn, can generate a spectrum of cellular responses ranging from death of the responding cell to inactivation (anergy) to extraordinary proliferation and maturation of the lymphocytes producing the specific immunoglobulin or TCR. Costimulatory signals, concentration of the antigen and density of

the derivative surface peptides all appear to determine what the response of the immune system will be, perhaps also influencing the autoimmune responses found in lupus.

The specificity of immune responses, however, seems to be mainly determined by the particular HLA molecules that present peptides to TCRs. The HLA genes are divided into three classes: I, II and III. The HLA class I gene products, known as A, B and C, usually present peptides from the cytoplasm to CD8+ cytotoxic T cells. The HLA class II gene products, known as DR, DQ and DP, present peptides from the extracellular milieu to CD4+ helper T cells. Class III genes include the complement component genes C2 and C4 and TNF. As the HLA genes have an important role in the immune response and are among the most highly variable genes known in the human genome, it is not surprising that their alleles are related to the risk of developing disorders of the immune response[14].

An example is the relationship between HLA-B27 and the risk of developing ankylosing spondylitis. In North America, among people of European descent, the odds ratio for the relationship between B27 and ankylosing spondylitis is more than 40[14], and animals transgenic for human B27 develop a similar disease[15,16], implying that B27 itself is responsible for the observed relationship.

In contrast, the associations of HLA antigens with lupus are less powerful and more confusing. The variable relationships and occasional multiple associations may reflect differing population ethnicities, different patient characteristics (clinical phenotype), changing technologies and some methodologic issues[17]. For example, the HLA class II nomenclature and methodology have evolved with time and, although the serologically determined DR3 and DR2 correspond to the DNA sequence-defined DRB1*0301 and DRB1*0201, earlier studies cannot always be directly translated into current nomenclature. Despite these problems, the HLA class II allele DR3 is associated with lupus in patients of European descent. The allele DR2 is also associated with lupus in many studies, although this association appears to have a more global distribution. The associations of DR2 and DR3 have odds ratios of 1.5–4, when considered individually[14].

A true association does not establish the direct participation of the gene product in pathogenesis and may reflect linkage disequilibrium between the marker and another unidentified gene. The 3.5 megabase HLA region, although large, comprises only about 0.1% of the human genome. In outbred human populations, the alleles at most neighboring genes have been shuffled so much that they are random in most situations. Recent data suggest that an average of 60 000 bases (or ~0.002% of the human genome) is sufficient largely to extinguish the linkage disequilibrium effect in European-derived populations. An even smaller piece of the genome is needed to find the average linkage disequilibrium effect in Africans[18].

The most extreme example of linkage disequilibrium within the HLA region is the linkage of the DR3 allele among individuals of Northern European descent who tend to have paticular alleles at neighboring loci over a few centiMorgans of the genome, including A1-Cw7-B8-TNFB*1-C2C-Bfs-C4AQ0-C4B1-DRB1*0301-DQA1*0501-DQB1*0201. (TAP2 and DP genes are towards the centromere and make much less consistent contributions to the haplotype.) The occurrence of linkage disequilibrium among individual alleles at neighboring loci is sometimes referred to as a 'persistent haplotype'. Linkage disequilibrium extending across such a great distance is very unusual in an outbred population. Even though only B8 and DR3 are measured in most studies, this haplotype is associated with an increased risk of lupus. It is important to note, however, that in some studies individual alleles at particular loci, such as DR3, DQ2 or C4A0, are more closely associated than is the haplotype. DQA1*0501 is on the B8-DR3 haplotype and may be more closely related to lupus than is DR3 or C4AQ0. Other alleles at DQA1 and DQB1 appear to be related to the risk of lupus with similar or greater effects than alleles at DR genes.

TABLE 118.2 GENETIC FACTORS IN LUPUS

Risk factor	Odds ratio	Population
Female risk	3–10	Global
Race	~4	African-American over European
C4AQ0-DR3-DQ2	~3	European
DR3	~3	European
DR2	1.5–4	European, Asian, African-American
DQA1*0501	3–6	European
C4AQ0/C4AQ0[†]	1.5–5	European, Asian, African-American
C2Q0/C2Q0[†]	~4.5	European
FcγRIIA, R131/R131[†]	≤4	African-American, European (?)
FcγRIIIA, F176/F176[†]	2–2.5	European, Korean

[†] Homozygous state.

'European' in this context means people of European extraction, wherever they now live. 'African-Americans' are people of African ancestry who are now in North America.

The alleles and loci responsible for the associations observed between lupus and the *HLA* region have yet to be established. Perhaps, this is a reflection of the relatively weak effect at *HLA*, where even *DR3* usually has an odds ratio for association with lupus of less than 3. Given the complexity of the observed phenomena and the high frequency of the disease-associated alleles in the normal population, the difficulty establishing linkage at this locus is not surprising. As the association of lupus with *DR3* is consistently found, however, this association almost certainly reflects an important genetic effect somewhere in the *HLA* region.

Complement components and TNF

The presence of linkage disequilibrium in *HLA* means that it is not possible to be confident that the *HLA-DR* locus *per se* is responsible for the increased risk of lupus. Other candidate genes, such as tumor necrosis factor (TNF), are in the *HLA* region. The allele *TNFB*1* is increased in patients with lupus, but it is in disequilibrium with alleles at *DR* and *DQ* and with the *B3-DR3* haplotype. *TNFB*1* may make an independent contribution towards the risk of lupus[19]. In African-Americans, several genes have been associated with lupus. These genes include not only the genetic associations reported with *HLA-DR2*[20], *DR3*[21] and *DR4*[22], but also other genes in the *HLA* region, including the *C4A* null allele[23], *TNF-α* promoter[24] and the heat-shock protein 70-2 (*Hsp70-2*) polymorphism detected with the *PstI* restriction enzyme[25]. None of these associations has been convincingly confirmed, which leaves substantial doubt that they are truly increased in the population of patients with lupus when compared to normal controls.

There is strong evidence that null alleles of the early components of the classical complement pathway, alleles at the genes for *C1*, *C4* or *C2*, increase the risk of lupus[17]. *TNF*, *C2* and *C4* are all part of the *HLA* class III region on human chromosome 6 at p21. Other alleles, such as *A1*, *A3*, *B7*, *B8*, *B18*, *B35*, *B39*, *DRw52*, *DR4*, *DR4–DR2* heterozygotes, *DR7*, *SC01*, *GLO2*, *DQ6*, *DPB1*0301* and *DPB1*1401* have also been associated with lupus in some studies[17].

Clearly, the risk of lupus is increased among patients who are deficient for any of the components of the early part of the classical pathway, *C1*, *C2* or *C4*[26,27] (see Chapter 119). Complete complement deficiencies are rare. The most common is homozygous C2 deficiency, which is present in about one in 10 000 individuals of European ancestry. The relative risk for homozygous C2 deficiency in lupus appears to be greater than 3.5[28,29]. Complete C4 deficiency requires the absence of a functional gene product from both of the *C4* genes, *C4A* and *C4B*, which is very rare. Conversely, most of the known C4-deficient individuals have developed lupus[26]. In patients with lupus who are of Northern European origin, the null allele *C4AQo* is as common as it is on the *B8-DR3* haplotype[26]. More than 25 studies have found an association between lupus and *C4AQo* or *C4BQo*. Attempts to differentiate the effects between *C4A*, *DR* and *DQ* appear to be underpowered and by themselves are inconclusive. Considered in aggregate, however, the data appear to support the existence of independent genetic risk factors for lupus in the *HLA* region, one or more among the complement genes and others at either *DR* or *DQ*, or at both.

Immunoglobulin receptors

There is evidence relating decreased function of the Fc receptors to increased risk of lupus. Not only do tissue expression and affinity for various forms of immunoglobulin vary among the Fc receptors; in addition, the form of the Fc receptor determines whether binding to the receptor serves to enhance or suppress antigen-specific responses. Rare null defects in the FcγRIIIB gene, which is expressed on neutrophils, have been found in individuals taken from populations of patients with lupus[30,31]. As null alleles at this locus are quite unusual in the general population, it is possible that they have increased the risk of developing lupus in the few patients in whom these genetic abnormalities have been observed.

Recent work has shown a convincing and reproducible association of an allele of *FcγRIIIA* with lupus[32,33]. There are two common alleles in the population that vary between phenylalanine and valine at amino acid position 176 in this Fc receptor; the allele with phenylalanine at this position is associated with lupus[32,33]. This change reduces the affinity of the receptor FcγRIIIA for immune complexes containing IgG isotypes 1 and 3. Their disposal or processing must, therefore, proceed by an alternate mechanism, one that increases the risk of lupus. However, at present, the nature of the relevant biological activity of FcγRIIIA that generates risk for lupus, or even whether *FcγRIIIA* is the responsible gene, instead of a locus in linkage disequilibrium, remains unproven.

The findings of a well-performed multicenter cohort study strongly suggested that *FcγRIIA* is important in African-American patients with lupus nephritis[34]. The odds ratio of greater than 4 for an association between lupus nephritis and the homozygous presence or absence of particular alleles of this receptor suggest an important contribution to the genetic risk of either developing lupus or having lupus nephritis. Although these investigators found no relationship between this allele and lupus or lupus nephritis in white patients, another study of this polymorphism in a Dutch cohort found an increased risk for lupus nephritis among whites[34]. Therefore, the observation that the *FcγRIIA* alleles (or alleles at a locus in disequilibrium with *FcγRIIA*) are related to lupus nephritis can be considered to be confirmed. The populations in which this effect operates remain to be clearly resolved.

FcγRIIA alleles differ at a single nucleotide in the coding region for the extracellular domain, which changes a histidine (H) at amino acid position 131 to an arginine (R). This change reduces the affinity of this Fc receptor for immune complexes containing IgG2. In both studies[34,35], the homozygotes for the low-affinity form (R[131]) were enriched in the patients with lupus nephritis. Immune complexes containing IgG2 may not be processed by the cells of individuals with these receptors, thereby allowing the immune complexes to remain available to cause lupus nephritis.

Other genes

Any gene that influences the immune system is a potential contributor to the genetic risk of lupus, and many different genes have been explored. Acetylator phenotypes, immunoglobulin allotypes, TCRs, complement receptors, complement-binding proteins and a number of cytokines have been evaluated in association studies that usually did not have the statistical power to find a reliable difference, had one truly been present.

The available experimental tools and resources are not yet adequate to examine each of the possible genes one at a time. It is believed that such genetic association studies would be more sensitive and powerful for the discovery of genetic effects[36]. Accordingly, the strategy of 'scanning' the genome for linkage between microsatellite markers and the disease phenotype is being pursued. After regions containing genetic effects are identified, then further analysis with additional pedigrees and more closely spaced markers can be used to narrow the region responsible for the observed genetic effect. Ultimately, alleles of particular candidate genes are identified and evaluated for being the genetic differences that create the genetic risk for lupus. This paradigm is being applied to most disorders in which a genetic effect is known, and lupus is no exception.

GENETIC LINKAGE IN LUPUS

A substantial advantage for genetic linkage or association studies is that prior knowledge of a specific gene is not required, because the disease gene is isolated on the basis of its location in the genome, rather than its specific function. Systematic searches throughout the human genome for genetic components related to lupus have been completed.

A variety of factors make it more difficult to elucidate the genetic factors in complex polygenic diseases, such as lupus. Classification of affected individuals in the pedigree can be problematic and lead to errors in the detection of linkage. Limitations intrinsic to the classification criteria (established in 1982) used to identify lupus as consistently as possible, in addition to failure of investigators to apply these criteria uniformly can contribute to misspecifications of the phenotype and reduce the power to discover genetic effects.

The preponderance of available evidence suggests that several genes are likely to be important. The entire repertoire of susceptibility genes is not likely to be uniform across all families and, especially, across those in different racial groups. Genetic heterogeneity may even operate within families, where the precise combination of genetic factors varies from one affected individual to another. Incomplete penetrance is also almost certain to be present, some individuals carrying the correct milieu of susceptibility genes, but not necessarily expressing disease. We already know from twin studies that incomplete penetrance occurs. Environmental influences and epistatic influences from other loci may also cloud the ability to detect genetic effects.

The analytical methods available to detect linkage also have limitations. Traditional maximum-likelihood model-based (logarithm of the odds score) methods are sensitive to specification of an inheritance model, which has been particularly difficult to determine for lupus. Allele-sharing methods (usually of affected siblings or other relatives) are less powerful and generally require hundreds of affected sib-pairs in order to detect linkage. Transmission disequilibrium tests are being used increasingly often for establishing genetic association in complex disease studies, but require allelic association (i.e. genetic disequilibrium) to be present. Further development of genetic analysis methods are likely to play an important part in studies of linkage in lupus and many other complex diseases.

Despite these obstacles, linkage studies in human lupus are currently in progress and their initial results have been reported. The most convincing linkages (Table 118.3) provide an early glimpse of the genetic complexity of this disorder[3-7,37,38].

FcγRIIA is in a linked region, although linkage at this locus has been detected in only one study. The effect at FcγRIIA appears to be of greater magnitude in African-American pedigrees multiplex for lupus – a result that is consistent with the previous demonstration of genetic association at this locus[34,35].

A linkage at 1q41 has also been identified and has subsequently been supported by several studies[2,4–6]. This type of consistency with mutually reinforcing results is unusual for complex genetic disorders. A candidate gene to explain this effect was initially shown to have close genetic association[39], but efforts to confirm the association have failed[40,41], and the role of this candidate is controversial.

A linkage toward the bottom of chromosome 2, at 2q37, has been detected in Icelandic and Swedish pedigrees[37]. The presence of this linkage effect has been confirmed by the same study in an extended set of Nordic pedigrees[38].

Chromosome 4 contains a lupus susceptibility gene near the telomere of its short arm, at 4p15, that operates in European-Americans. This effect has been detected in two independent collections of pedigrees multiplex for lupus[7].

With so many studies demonstrating genetic associations at HLA, the absence of a linkage in this region would be worrisome. The collection of pedigrees multiplex for lupus collected in Minnesota shows a strong linkage effect here[4,5], one that is confirmed by the Oklahoma pedigrees (unpublished observations). Perhaps, the linkage approach and the large collections now available will provide the power to sort through the genetic disequilibrium effects and identify the responsible genes with confidence.

Finally, a linkage has been established on chromosome 16. As for the linkages on chromosome 2 and 4, the responsible gene may be any one of literally hundreds of genes in the linked region and identifying it will be the lucky result of many more years work.

Perhaps, before leaving genetic linkage of lupus, the reader should be reminded that this effort is in its infancy. Not only are there many linkages with lupus still to discover, but in addition each one will require a serious effort to find the responsible susceptibility gene(s). Morever, only the results of genome scan linkage obtained using lupus as the phenotype have been published. Linkage with subgroups using clinical and laboratory findings will each hold the possibility of genetic discovery. Finally, newer tools such as DNA chip technologies and high-throughput single polymorphism genotyping may make genome scanning for genetic association practical. The theoretically improved power of genetic association compared with genetic linkage[36] suggests that another set of genetic effects will be found using this approach.

LESSONS FROM THE MOUSE

Lupus-like disease can arise spontaneously in outbred murine populations. Certain manipulations, such as graft-versus-host disease, l-canavanine ingestion and peptide immunization, may also generate disease[42–44]. In addition, many genetically manipulated mouse strains develop a lupus-like phenotype[45]. The frequency with which such animals have been found suggests that lupus-like systemic autoimmunity is a common phenotype for immune dysregulation and abnormalities of apoptosis. The most intensively studied models of lupus, however, are murine strains that have a genetic predisposition for humoral autoimmunity and lupus nephritis.

The MRL lpr/lpr mouse develops lymphadenopathy, antinuclear antibodies, anti-double stranded DNA (anti-dsDNA), nephritis and other clinical features of lupus. The lpr defect markedly affects expression of the fas gene, a critical element in the regulation of apoptosis. In the context of the MRL genetic background, a defective fas gene accelerates expression of disease characteristic of human lupus. A few individuals are heterozygous for defects in the fas gene. These individuals have anemia, thrombocytopenia, intermittent lymphadenopathy and a predilection for neoplasms in midlife[46]. However, defects in fas are only rarely associated with lupus in man[47]. Other genes affecting apoptosis continue to attract interest. For example, the gene product of bcl-2 prevents apoptosis, and mice with the bcl-2 gene eliminated from their genome are predisposed to lupus-like disease[48]. Many of the mechanisms at work to produce this model of lupus are not known.

The BXSB mouse has a gene on the Y chromosome, called Yaa for 'Y chromosome autoimmunity accelerating factor', which confers the risk for lupus in males. These mice develop anti-dsDNA, other autoantibodies, glomerulonephritis, lymphadenopathy, myocardial infarcts and thymic abnormalities.

The most intensively studied mouse model of lupus is the F1 cross of NZB × NZW. This mouse develops positive antinuclear antibodies, anti-dsDNA antibodies and nephritis. Female mice are more severely affected

TABLE 118.3 CONVINCING LINKAGES IN LUPUS

Location	Marker	LOD score*
1q21.3	FcγRIIA	3.37[3]
1q41	D1s2860-D1s213	3.30[39]
2q37	D2s125	4.51[38]
4p16-15	D4s2366	3.84[7]
6p21-11	D6s426	4.19[5]
16q13	D16s415	3.85[5]

* Maximum published LOD score, and source reference. (LOD score ≥3.3).

than are males. This model may be the murine model most similar to human lupus. Like human lupus, the NZB × NZW F1 mouse is also genetically complex. A number of ongoing studies are attempting to define the genes that mediate lupus nephritis, anti-dsDNA, IgM hyper-gammaglobulinemia, splenomegaly and other features in this model[49–54]. The initial work has established the presence of multiple genetic effects, which best fit an additive model for lupus nephritis[49,52,54]. An additive model suggests that alleles at different genetic loci make independent, but cumulative, contributions towards expression of the phenotype.

The genetic complexity already known in murine lupus does not auger well for there being simple genetics for lupus in man. For example, *sle1* on mouse chromosome 4 is a subject of recent intense scrutiny. Upon careful genetic dissection, this effect was further divided into four separable genetic effects, found very close to one another in a region syntenic to human chromosome 1q21-44[45]. The many genetic effects now known to originate with the NZB × NZW F1 model of lupus alone show the extraordinary complexity that lupus presents[55,56].

The genetics of mouse lupus may be extremely important to the understanding of human lupus. Indeed, some of the same genes may be conferring risk both in the mouse and in man. For example, histocompatibility genes are important risk factors both in human (*HLA* genes) and in mouse, in which histocompatibility genes (*H-2* genes) influence the expression of the lupus phenotype in the NZB × NZW F1[53], BSXB[57] and MRL *lpr/lpr*[58] murine models of lupus. This consistency suggests that mouse genetics will provide other important insights for those studying lupus in man. Furthermore, identifying the particular gene is much more practical in the mouse, in which breeding is controlled and generation times are much shorter. Because the organization of genes is nearly identical for large regions of the human and murine genomes, an effect localized to a particular region of the mouse genome can be explored in the analogous region of the human genome (the syntenic region). Once this is accomplished, the particular gene can then be evaluated for a role in man. This strategy promises to accelerate the location of linkages and the identification of many of the genes that cause human lupus.

GENETIC EFFECTS IN OTHER ASPECTS OF LUPUS

Genetic risk factors may be associated with the diagnosis of lupus, with individual clinical manifestations or with particular immune abnormalities such as specific autoantibodies. Indeed, the common precipitins are associated with particular *HLA* alleles (Table 118.4). Perhaps, the strongest of these is the association of *HLA* class II genes with anti-Ro(SS-A) autoantibodies. Associations include *DR3, DR2, DQ1* and *DQ2* heterozygotes, and heterozygotes of *HLA-DQA1*0101, -0102* or *-0103* and *DQB1*0201*, among others[59]. Complement component C2 deficiency and a TCR β-chain polymorphism have been associated with anti-Ro[59,60].

TABLE 118.4 *HLA* ASSOCIATIONS WITH LUPUS AUTOANTIBODIES

Precipitating antibody	*HLA* allele
Anti-Ro(SS-A)	DR3, DR2, DQ1–DQ2 heterozygotes
Anti-nRNP	DR4, DQw8
Anti-DNA	DR2
Anticardiolipin	DR4, DQw7
Antiphospholipid	DR4, DQw7

Indeed, the TCR β-chain polymorphism has been shown to be synergistic with the heterozygous *DQ1–DQ2* state[59].

Other autoantibody specificities may also have relationships with specific *HLA* alleles. The relationship of these autoantibodies to *HLA* class II alleles provides an important insight into the determinants of autoantibody specificity. Anti-Sm and anti-nRNP autoantibodies are directed against the spliceosome (see Chapter 120). These antibodies have been most frequently associated with DR4 in peoples of European descent[17]. The *HLA* associations with anti-dsDNA are weak and often not present although, when found, have been associated most frequently with *DR2*[17]. The lupus anticoagulant, anticardiolipin and antiphospholipid antibodies have been most frequently associated with *DR4* or *DQw7*[17] (see Chapter 131).

Simultaneous consideration of the relationships between the *HLA* alleles, autoantibodies and clinical expression of disease has led to a model of disease expression in lupus. In these experiments, the autoantibodies were more closely related to clinical manifestations than were the *HLA* class II alleles[61], which suggests that the genetics of lupus probably operate at several levels. Several genes that appear to increase the risk of disease are in the *HLA* region. There are also genes that appear to be related to the particular autoantibody specificities. Although these appear to be different genes, some are also in the *HLA* region. The greater concordance between identical twins for autoantibodies than for the diagnosis of lupus[62] supports this formulation.

CONCLUSIONS

Lupus is the most studied prototype for systemic autoimmunity. Clearly, a large number of genes are important and have the potential to define clinically important variation in the human population and to identify disease risk. These genes include those in the histocompatibility region, especially the class II *HLA* genes, complement component genes and immunoglobulin receptor genes. Genetic linkage and genetic association studies in man, in addition to work with murine models of lupus, promise to provide important new insight that will fundamentally change our understanding of this disorder.

REFERENCES

1. Bias WB, Reveille JD, Beaty TH *et al.* Evidence that autoimmunity in man is a Mendelian dominant trait. Am J Hum Genet 1986; 39: 584–602.
2. Tsao BP, Cantor RM, Kalunian KC *et al.* Evidence for linkage of a candidate chromosome 1 region to human systemic lupus erythematosus. J Clin Invest 1997; 99: 725–731.
3. Moser KL, Neas BR, Salmon JE *et al.* Genome scan of human systemic lupus erythematosus: evidence for linkage on chromosome 1q in African-American pedigrees. Proc Natl Acad Sci USA 1998; 95: 14869–14874.
4. Gaffney PM, Kearns GM, Shark KB *et al.* A genome-wide search for susceptibility genes in human systemic lupus erythematosus sib-pair families. Proc Natl Acad Sci USA 1998; 95: 14875–14879.
5. Gaffney PM, Ortmann WA, Selby SA *et al.* Genome screening in human systemic lupus erythematosus: results from a second Minnesota cohort and combined analyses of 187 sib-pair families. Am J Hum Genet 2000; 66: 547–556.
6. Moser KL, Gray-McGuire C, Kelly J *et al.* Confirmation of genetic linkage between human systemic lupus erythematosus and chromosome 1q41. Arthritis Rheum 1999; 42: 1902–1907.
7. Gray-McGuire C, Moser KL, Gaffney P *et al.* Genome scan of human systemic lupus erythematosus by regression modeling: evidence of linkage and epistasis at 4p16–15.2. Am J Hum Genet 2000; 67: 1460–1469.
8. McCarty DJ, Manzi S, Medsger TA *et al.* Incidence of systemic lupus erythematosus. Race and gender differences. Arthritis Rheum 1995; 38: 1260–1270.
9. Fessel W. Systemic lupus erythematosus in the community: incidence, prevalence, outcome, and first symptoms. Arch Int Med 1974; 134: 1027–1035.
10. Citera G, Wilson WA. Ethnic and geographic perspectives in SLE. Lupus 1993; 2: 351–353.
11. Ortiz-Neu C, Leroy EC. The incidence of Klinefelter's syndrome and systemic lupus erythematosus. Arthritis Rheum 1969; 12: 241–246.
12. Deapen D, Escalante A, Weinrib L *et al.* A revised estimate of twin concordance in systemic lupus erythematosus. Arthritis Rheum 1992; 35: 311–318.
13. Risch N. Linkage strategies for genetically complex traits. I. Multilocus models. Am J Hum Genet 1990; 46: 222–228.
14. Tiwari JH, Terasaki PI. Connective tissue diseases. In: HLA and disease associations. New York: Springer-Verlag; 1985: 363–369.

15. Khare SD, Luthra HS, David CS. Spontaneous inflammatory arthritis in HLA-B27 transgenic mice lacking beta 2-microglobulin: a model of human spondyloarthropathies. J Exp Med 1995; 182: 1153–1158.

16. Breban M, Hammer RE, Richardson JA et al. Transfer of the inflammatory disease of HLA-B27 transgenic rats by bone marrow engraftment. J Exp Med 1993; 178: 1607–1616.

17. Schur P. Genetics of systemic lupus erythematosus. Lupus 1995; 4: 425–437.

18. Reich DE, Cargill M, Bolk S et al. Linkage disequilibrium in the human genome. Nature 2001; 411: 199–204.

19. Bettinotti MP, Hartung K, Deicher H et al. Polymorphism of the tumor necrosis factor beta gene in systemic lupus erythematosus: TNFB–MHC haplotypes. Immunogenetics 1993; 37: 449–454.

20. Kachru RB, Sequeira W, Mittal KK et al. A significant increase of HLA-DR3 and DR2 in systemic lupus erythematosus among blacks. J Rheumatol 1984; 11: 471–474.

21. Alarif LI, Ruppert GB, Wilson R et al. HLA-DR antigens in blacks with rheumatoid arthritis and systemic lupus erythematosus. J Rheumatol 1983; 10: 297–300.

22. Wilson WA, Scopelitis E, Michalski JP. Association of HLA-DR7 with both antibody to SSA(Ro) and disease susceptibility in blacks with systemic lupus erythematosus. J Rheumatol 1984; 11: 653–657.

23. Petri M, Watson R, Winkelstein JA et al. Clinical expression of systemic lupus erythematosus in patients with C4A deficiency. Medicine 1993; 72: 236–244.

24. Sullivan KE, Wooten C, Schmeckpeper BJ et al. A promoter polymorphism of tumor necrosis factor alpha associated with systemic lupus erythematosus in African-Americans. Arthritis Rheum 1997; 40: 2207–2211.

25. Jarjour W, Reed AM, Gauthier J et al. The 8.5-kb PstI allele of stress protein gene, Hsp70-2. Human Immunol 1996; 45: 59–63.

26. Agnello V. Complement deficiency and systemic lupus erythematosus. In: Lahita RG, ed. Systemic lupus erythematosus. New York: Wiley; 1987: 565–589.

27. Walport MJ. Complement. Second of two parts. N Engl J Med 2001; 344: 1140–1144.

28. Truedson L, Sturfelt G, Nived O. Prevalence of the type I complement C2 deficiency gene in Swedish systemic lupus erythematosus patients. Lupus 1993; 2: 325–327.

29. Sullivan KE, Petri MA, Schmeckpeper BJ et al. Prevalence of a mutation causing C2 deficiency in systemic lupus erythematosus. J Rheumatol 1994; 21: 1128–1133.

30. Clark MR, Liu L, Clarkson SB et al. An abnormality of the gene that encodes neutrophil Fc receptor III in a patient with systemic lupus erythematosus. J Clin Invest 1990; 86: 341–346.

31. Enenkel B, Jung D, Frey J. Molecular basis of IgG Fc receptor III defect in a patient with systemic lupus erythematosus. Eur J Immunol 1991; 21: 659–663.

32. Wu J, Edberg JC, Redecha PB et al. A novel polymorphism of Fcgamma RIIIa (CD16) alters receptor function and predisposes to autoimmune disease. J Clin Invest 1997; 100: 1059–1070.

33. Edberg JC, Langefeld C, Moser KL et al. Linkage and association of a functional SNP in the FcγRIIIA gene with SLE. Abstracts of the 65th Annual Scientific Meeting of the American College of Rheumatology, San Francisco, CA, 11–15 November, 2001.

34. Salmon JE, Millard S, Schacter LA et al. FcγRIIA alleles are heritable risk factors for lupus nephritis in African-Americans. J Clin Invest 1996; 97: 1348–1354.

35. Duits AJ, Bootsma H, Derksen RHWM et al. Skewed distribution of IgG Fc receptor IIa (CD32) polymorphism is associated with renal disease in systemic lupus erythematosus patients. Arthritis Rheum 1995; 39: 1832–1836.

36. Risch NJ. Searching for genetic determinants in the new millennium. Nature 2000; 405: 847–856.

37. Lindqvist AKB, Steinsson K, Johanneson B et al. A susceptibility locus for human systemic lupus erythematosus (hSLE1) on chromosome 2q. J Autoimmun 2000; 14: 169–178.

38. Magnusson V, Lindqvist AKB, Castillejo-Lopez C et al. Fine mapping of the SLEB2 locus involved in susceptibility to systemic lupus erythematosus. Genomics 2000; 70: 307–314.

39. Tsao BP, Cantor RM, Grossman JM et al. PARP alleles within the linked chromosomal region are associated with systemic lupus erythematosus. J Clin Invest 1999; 103: 1135–1140.

40. Criswell LA, Moser KL, Gaffney PM et al. PARP alleles and SLE: failure to confirm association with disease susceptibility. J Clin Invest 2000; 105: 1501–1502.

41. Delrieu O, Michel M, Frances C et al. Poly(ADP-ribose) polymerase alleles in French Caucasians are associated neither with lupus nor with primary antiphospholipid syndrome. GRAID Research Group. Group for Research on Auto-Immune Disorders. Arthritis Rheum 1999; 42: 2194–2197.

42. van Rappard-van der Veen FM, Kiesel U, Poels L et al. Further evidence against random polyclonal antibody formation in mice with lupus-like graft-vs host disease. J Immunol 1984; 132: 1814–1820.

43. Malinow MR, Bardana EJ, Pirofsky B et al. Systemic lupus erythematosus-like syndrome in monkeys fed alfalfa sprouts: role of a nonprotein amino acid. Science 1982; 216: 415–417.

44. James JA, Gross T, Scofield RH et al. PPPGMRPP immunization generates anti-Sm humoral autoimmunity and induces systemic lupus erythematosus. J Exp Med 1995; 181: 453–462.

45. Morel L, Blenman KR, Croker BP et al. The major murine systemic lupus erythematosus susceptibility locus, Sle1, is a cluster of functionally related genes. Proc Natl Acad Sci USA 2001; 98: 1787–1792.

46. Drappa J, Vaishnaw AK, Sullivan KE et al. Fas gene mutations in the Canale–Smith syndrome, an inherited lymphoproliferative disorder associated with autoimmunity. N Engl J Med 1996; 335: 1643–1649.

47. Wu J, Wilson J, He J et al. Fas ligand mutation in a patient with systemic lupus erythematosus and lymphoproliferative disease. J Clin Invest 1996; 98: 1107–1113.

48. Strasser A, Whittingham S, Vaux DL et al. Enforced BCL2 expression in B-lymphoid cells prolongs antibody responses and elicits autoimmune disease. Proc Natl Acad Sci USA 1991; 88: 8661–8665.

49. Hirose S, Tsurui H, Nishimura H et al. Mapping of a gene for hypergamma-globulinemia to the distal region on chromosome 4 in NZB mice and its contribution to systemic lupus erythematosus in (NZB×NZW)F1 mice. Int Immunol 1994; 6: 1857–1864.

50. Kono DH, Burlingame RW, Owens DG et al. Lupus susceptibility loci in New Zealand mice. Proc Natl Acad Sci USA 1994; 91: 10168–10172.

51. Drake CG, Babcock SK, Palmer E et al. Genetic analysis of the NZB contribution to lupus-like autoimmune disease in (NZB×NZW)F1 mice. Proc Natl Acad Sci USA 1994; 91: 4062–4066.

52. Morel L, Rudofsky UH, Longmate JA et al. Polygenic control of susceptibility to murine systemic lupus erythematosus. Immunity 1994; 1: 219–229.

53. Drake CG, Rozzo SJ, Vyse TJ et al. Genetic contributions to lupus-like disease in (NZB×NZW)F$_1$ mice. Immunol Rev 1995; 144: 51–74.

54. Drake CG, Rozzo SJ, Hirschfeld HF et al. Analysis of the New Zealand Black contribution to lupus-like renal disease. Multiple genes that operate in a threshold manner. J Immunol 1995; 154: 2441–2447.

55. Kono DH, Theofilopoulos AN. Genetics of systemic autoimmunity in mouse models of lupus. Int Rev Immunol 2000; 19: 367–387.

56. Vyse TJ, Kotzin BL. Genetic susceptibility to systemic lupus erythematosus. Annu Rev Immunol 1998; 16: 261–292.

57. Merino R, Iwamoto M, Fossanti L et al. Prevention of systemic lupus erythematosus in autoimmune BXSB mice by a transgene encoding I-E alpha chain. J Exp Med 1993; 178: 1189–1197.

58. Jevnikar AM, Grusby MJ, Glimcher LH. Prevention of nephritis in major histocompatibility complex class II-deficient MRL-lpr mice. J Exp Med 1994; 179: 1137–1143.

59. Scofield RH, Frank MB, Neas BR et al. Cooperative association of T cell β receptor and HLA-DQ alleles in the production of anti-Ro in systemic lupus erythematosus. Clin Immunol Immunopathol 1994; 72: 335–341.

60. Provost TT, Arnett FC, Reichlin M. Homozygous C2 deficiency, lupus erythematosus and anti-Ro(SS-A) antibodies. Arthritis Rheum 1983; 26: 1279–1282.

61. Harley JB, Sestak AS, Willis LG et al. A model for disease heterogeneity in systemic lupus erythematosus. Relationships between histocompatibility antigens, autoantibodies and lymphopenia or renal disease. Arthritis Rheum 1989; 32: 826–836.

62. Reichlin M, Harley JB, Lockshin M. Serologic studies on monozygotic twins with systemic lupus erythematosus. Arthritis Rheum 1993; 35: 457–464.

119

The complement system

Matthew C Pickering and Mark J Walport

- The biological functions of complement proteins include (1) killing of microbes mediated by leukocyte activation, opsonization and target cell lysis, (2) augmentation of antibody responses and (3) resolution of inflammatory responses through the clearance of immune complexes and apoptotic cells

- Complement can be activated through three distinct pathways: the classical pathway, the lectin pathway and the alternative pathway

- The classical pathway is activated by IgG or IgM bound to antigens and directly by certain microorganisms

- The lectin pathway is triggered by the binding of the serum protein, mannose-binding lectin, to arrays of terminal mannose groups on the surface of certain bacteria

- The alternative pathway is in a continuous state of 'tick-over' activation as a result of the constant activation of complement C3 in plasma by hydrolysis

- The complement system is tightly regulated in the fluid-phase and on host cell surfaces by a series of proteins that serve to limit damage to host tissues during complement activation

- Inherited and acquired deficiencies of complement proteins and regulators in humans may be associated with disease

- Examples of inherited complement deficiency and disease include the association between classical pathway component deficiency and systemic lupus erythematosus (SLE) and the association between C1 inhibitor deficiency and hereditary angioedema

- Acquired complement deficiency may occur in rheumatological conditions such as SLE and rheumatoid vasculitis as a result of either high levels of complement activation or the presence of autoantibodies to complement proteins: for example, anti-C1q antibodies found in approximately 33% of patients with SLE

- Serial measurements of complement proteins, commonly C3 and C4, may serve as useful indicators of disease activity in patients with SLE, whereas functional assays such as total hemolytic activity (CH50) are a useful screening investigation for inherited complement deficiency.

INTRODUCTION

The complement system is part of the innate immune system and consists of more than 20 different proteins (Fig. 119.1). Complement is a major effector mechanism of inflammatory responses, has an important role in the physiological removal of immune complexes and has an accessory role in the induction of antibody responses. It can be activated through three distinct pathways: the classical, alternative and lectin pathways. The classical pathway is a predominantly antibody-dependent pathway, activated principally by aggregated IgG or IgM in immune complexes. The lectin pathway is antibody-independent and is principally activated by the binding of mannose-binding lectin (MBL) to terminal mannose groups on the surface of bacteria. The alternative

pathway is in a constant steady state of low-level activation, continuously generating fluid-phase complement C3b through a pathway termed the C3 'tick-over' pathway. Each of these three pathways generates C3b convertases, which cleave native C3 to form the active product C3b. C3 deposited on foreign surfaces is rapidly amplified through a pathway termed the alternative pathway amplification loop. Binding of C3b to C3 convertases generates a trimolecular complex capable of binding and cleaving C5. This complex is called a C5 convertase enzyme and initiates the terminal complement pathway. This culminates in the formation of the membrane attack complex (MAC), which disrupts target cell membrane integrity and can result in cell lysis.

Complement regulatory proteins tightly regulate complement activation, preventing both depletion of complement proteins and limiting complement-mediated host-cell damage. Protein deficiency affecting either the complement activation pathways or the complement regulatory proteins, can cause disease in humans. In the following sections, we will describe the pathways of complement activation and outline the role of the complement system in rheumatologic diseases.

COMPLEMENT ACTIVATION

The classical pathway

Activation: predominantly by antibody-mediated mechanisms

The initial step in classical pathway activation is the binding of two or more of the six globular domains of C1q to the Fc portions of antibody bound to antigen. C1q is comprised of six subunits, each of which consists of a carboxyl terminal globular head attached to a collagenous tail[1]. Each subunit is formed by three polypeptide chains (A, B and C chains), which are encoded by separate genes. C1q binds to the second constant domains of the heavy chain (C_H2) of the Fc region of IgG that is aggregated, for example in an immune complex[2]. In contrast, the interaction between C1q and non-aggregated IgG is very weak. The various IgG isotypes have different capacities to bind to and activate C1q. In humans, IgG3 is the most potent activator, followed by IgG1 and then IgG2. IgG4 does not bind C1q and thus cannot activate the classical pathway. C1q also binds to the C_H3 domain of IgM that has adopted a stable configuration after binding of antigen. The classical pathway may also be activated in an antibody-independent manner by the direct binding of C1q to certain other host or pathogen ligands, for example C-reactive protein (CRP) complexed to its phospholipid ligands and pathogens including retroviruses and *Mycoplasma pneumoniae*.

Sequence of events during classical pathway activation

The classical pathway activation cascade is illustrated in Figure 119.2. Two molecules of C1r and two molecules of C1s interact to form a calcium dependent tetramer ($C1r_2$–$C1s_2$) complexed with C1q. Binding of C1q to complexed IgG or IgM results in a conformational change in the C1 complex. This causes one of the C1r molecules to activate first itself (autocatalysis), and then the other, to generate two active C1r

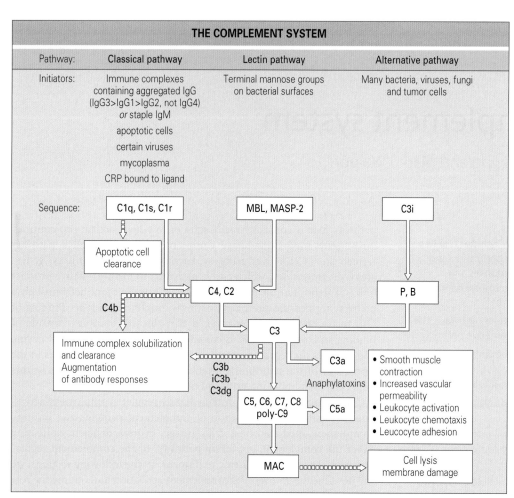

Fig. 119.1 The complement system. Complement can be activated by three pathways: the classical, lectin and alternative pathways. The principal functions of complement are: (1) host defense against infection (opsonization, chemotaxis and activation of leukocytes, cell lysis), (2) disposal of waste (immune complex and apoptotic cell clearance) and (3) augmentation of antibody responses. CRP, C-reactive protein; MAC, membrane attack complex, MBL, mannose-binding lectin; MASP, MBL-associated serine protease.

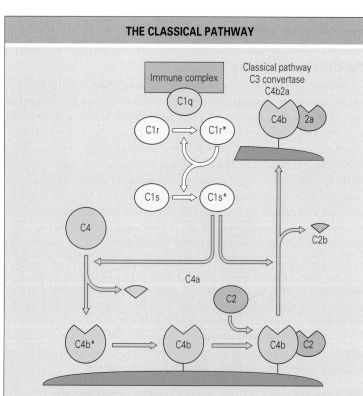

Fig. 119.2 The classical pathway. After the binding of C1q to immune complexes, C1r catalyzes its own activation (autocatalysis) and then the activation of C1s. Activated C1s (C1s*) cleaves C4a from native C4 to form activated C4 (C4b*). Surface-bound C4b then binds C2. C1s* cleaves the C2 molecule attached to C4b to release C2b, leaving the larger product (C2a) attached to C4b. This remaining complex, C4b2a, represents the classical pathway C3 convertase.

enzymes. These then cleave the C1s molecules to generate active C1s serine esterases[3]. The next step in the activation sequence is the cleavage of C4 by the activated C1s enzymes contained within the C1 complex. C4 is cleaved to release two products: C4b and C4a. C4a has weak anaphylatoxic activity (see below), but it is the C4b fragment that is critical in the generation of the classical pathway C3 convertase. C4 contains an internal thioester bond ($-[C=O]-S-$) that becomes highly unstable during the generation of C4b[4]. (C3 is homologous to C4 and also contains an internal thioester bond.) Activation of the internal thioester bond allows the covalent binding of a small proportion of C4b to proteins and carbohydrates at sites of complement activation. This bound C4b may now act as an acceptor site for fluid phase C2. C2 bound to C4b (the C4bC2 complex) becomes susceptible to cleavage by activated C1s. This releases C2b, leaving the larger C2a fragment bound to C4b. This complex, C4b2a, is an enzyme named the classical pathway C3 convertase. This surface-bound classical pathway C3 convertase enzyme cleaves C3, causing the generation of large amounts of C3b, which coats the activating surface, a phenomenon termed opsonization. C4b2a is also able to bind C3b, forming the classical pathway C5 convertase, C4b2aC3b[5].

The alternative pathway

The alternative pathway comprises six plasma proteins: C3, factor B, factor D, factor H, factor I and properdin. The fundamental feature of the alternative pathway is that it can be activated by means of antibody-independent pathways by potential pathogens such as bacteria, fungi, viruses and parasites, and by abnormal host tissues, including virus-infected cells and tumor cells.

Activation: the C3 'tick-over' pathway

The alternative pathway is in a constant state of activation or 'tick-over' that results in the generation of low levels of activated C3 (C3b*) in the fluid-phase.

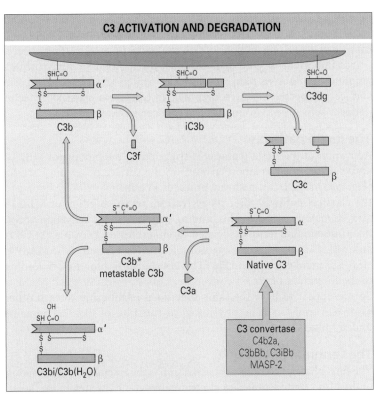

Fig. 119.3 C3 activation and degradation. C3 convertases cleave the α-chain of C3, releasing the anaphylatoxin C3a, and generating C3b*. The majority of the fluid-phase C3b* is inactivated through hydrolysis by water to generate C3bi or C3b(H₂O). However, some of the C3b* will bind to host cells, where it becomes inactivated by factor I. This inactivation takes place in two steps. The first involves two cleavage sites within the α-chain, which releases a small peptide (termed C3f) and generates iC3b. The second inactivation step involves a further cleavage of the α-chain, releasing C3c and leaving C3dg bound to the cell surface. The first inactivation step utilizes factor H in the fluid phase and membrane cofactor protein (MCP) and complement receptor 1 (CR1) on cell surfaces. CR1 is the sole cofactor for the second inactivation step.

After the first isolation of C3, it was observed that its hemolytic activity decayed spontaneously in aqueous solution[6]. The explanation for this decay came with the discovery that native C3 contains an unstable internal thioester bond (–[C=O]-S-) (Fig. 119.3)[7,8]. Spontaneous hydrolysis of the thioester bond of native C3 *in vivo* provides a steady source of 'C3b-like' C3 (referred to as C3(H₂O) or C3i) that can form an efficient C3 convertase (C3iBb) in the presence of factors B and D and magnesium. The formation of this convertase enzyme is described in more detail in the next section of this chapter. This fluid-phase C3 convertase enzyme cleaves C3 into two fragments, C3a and C3b. The internal thioester bond in C3b is highly unstable, and causes the covalent binding of a small amount C3b to hydroxyl groups on carbohydrates and some amino acids (Fig. 119.3). This pathway for the generation of small amounts of surface-bound C3b is known as the C3 'tick-over' pathway (Fig. 119.4).

The alternative pathway of complement activation is regulated by two plasma proteins named factor H and factor I. Factor H inactivates the C3 convertase enzyme by promoting the dissociation of C3i and Bb. It also acts as a cofactor to the serine esterase enzyme factor I, which cleaves C3i to products that can no longer participate in the formation of C3 convertase enzymes.

Sequence of events during alternative pathway activation

The sequence of events after activation of the alternative pathway is shown in Figure 119.5. The first step in the alternative pathway activation sequence is the non-covalent interaction of factor B with C3i in the fluid-phase or with C3b on target surfaces (Fig. 119.4). Factor B is a pro-

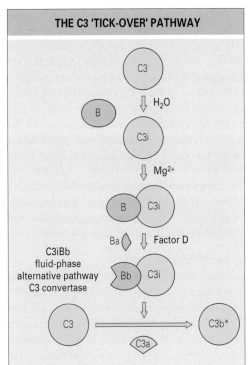

Fig. 119.4 The C3 'tick-over' pathway. The thioester bond of native C3 becomes hydrolyzed by water, forming C3i, which binds factor B in the presence of magnesium. This complex is then cleaved by factor D to generate the fluid-phase alternative pathway C3 convertase: C3iBb. This C3 convertase can directly cleave native C3 in the fluid-phase, producing C3b* and releasing the anaphylatoxin, C3a. C3b* denotes metastable C3b – that is, C3b in which the internal thioester bond is exposed.

enzyme (zymogen), containing serine esterase activity that is only expressed when factor B is activated by proteolytic cleavage. Factor B is only a substrate for such proteolytic cleavage when it is bound to C3b or C3i. When bound in this way, factor B can be cleaved by the serine protease, factor D, releasing a small inactive fragment, Ba, whereas the larger fragment with serine esterase activity, known as Bb, remains bound to C3b. The C3bBb complex has C3 cleaving activity and is known as the alternative pathway C3 convertase[9]. It spontaneously decays unless stabilized by the addition of a serum protein named properdin. However, even the properdin-stabilized C3 convertase decays spontaneously, and this decay is accelerated by the action of the complement regulatory protein, factor H[10]. After the release of Bb, C3b is inactivated by cleavage by the enzyme, factor I, in conjunction with its cofactor, factor H[11].

Importance of the reactive surface

The fate of surface-bound C3b is critically dependent on the nature of the reactive surface.

The capacity of C3b* to bind covalently to proteins and carbohydrates is very transient – estimated to be 60μs[12] – because of the rapid hydrolysis of the exposed thioester bond by water (Fig. 119.3). Although the majority of C3b* generated is inactivated by hydrolysis, a small amount binds covalently to proteins and carbohydrates in the immediate vicinity of the site of C3 activation. The fate of this covalently bound C3 is determined by the nature of the surface to which it binds. C3b bound to foreign (i.e. non-self) surfaces can act as an acceptor site for factor B and initiate the amplification loop of the alternative pathway (Fig. 119.5). Such surfaces are commonly referred to as 'protected surfaces' because the bound C3b is protected from proteolytic inactivation by factor I and factor H, and hence able to interact with factor B to generate the surface-bound alternative pathway C3 convertase, C3bBb. In contrast, C3b bound to the host's own cells does not bind factor B but, instead, preferentially binds to factor H or to one of a family of intrinsic cell membrane proteins (such as complement receptor 1 (CR1; CD35) and membrane cofactor protein (MCP; CD46)), which act as cofactors to enzyme factor I that cleaves C3b to inactive products (iC3b and C3dg). These inactive C3 products cannot bind factor B and are therefore incapable of participating in further complement activation.

To recapitulate, the fate of surface-bound C3b is controlled by two factors. The first of these is the affinity of surface-bound C3b for factor H. On activating surfaces (e.g. many bacteria) the affinity of factor H for surface C3b is low, rendering the bound C3b resistant to inactivation by factors H and I and allowing amplification to proceed. In contrast, the affinity of factor H for C3b bound to the body's own cells and tissues is high, causing rapid inactivation of C3b by factor I[13]. The high affinity of factor H for C3b on host cells and tissues is partially explained by the presence of surface sialic acid and other polyanions that promote factor H binding. For example, removal of cell surface sialic acid from sheep erythrocytes converts them from a non-activating to an activating surface[14]. Secondly, there are membrane-bound complement regulatory molecules, including CD35 and CD46, which serve to protect host cells by inhibiting the formation of C3 convertases, promoting both their dissociation and the subsequent proteolytic inactivation of C3b by factor I.

The alternative pathway amplification loop

In vivo evidence for the existence of a C3b amplification loop was provided by studies of the first human identified with complete factor I deficiency[15–17]. This individual was demonstrated to have chronically low concentrations of both C3 and factor B, an observation consistent with chronic alternative pathway activation. Furthermore, immunochemical depletion of factor I *in vitro* resulted in rapid conversion of both C3 (to C3b) and factor B (to Bb)[18]. Thus, *in vitro* factor I depletion mimicked the *in vivo* complement profile described in the factor I-deficient patient. These findings were consistent with the hypothesis that lack of inactivation of C3b by factor I resulted in uncontrolled generation of C3b

because of the existence of a positive feed-back loop – that is, a C3b amplification pathway[19]. It is now known that amplification is rapid, and capable of depositing millions of C3b molecules on an activating surface.

It is important to note that, although the term 'alternative pathway amplification loop' is used, amplification will proceed on a permissive surface irrespective of the source of C3b (e.g. from classical or lectin pathway activation). C3 amplification is depicted in Figure 119.5.

The lectin pathway

Activation of the lectin pathway is triggered by the binding of MBL to arrays of terminal mannose groups on the surface of certain bacteria (Fig. 119.1). The lectin pathway proceeds in a manner closely similar to the classical pathway after its activation, by the binding of MBL to arrayed mannose groups. This binding step leads to the activation of two mannose-binding lectin-associated serine proteases, known as MASP-1 and MASP-2, that are closely homologous to C1r and C1s. MASP-2 cleaves C4 and C2 sequentially in a very similar fashion to C1s, leading to the formation of the C3 convertase, C4b2a[20,21]. MASP-1 and MASP-2 do not appear to have the same functional relationship to each other as do C1r and C1s. The physiological function of MASP-1 remains undetermined.

The terminal pathway

The final phase of complement activation is the assembly and formation of the MAC, first identified in electron micrographs as membrane 'holes' and 'hollow cylinders' (Fig. 119.6)[22]. The first stage is the enzymatic cleavage of C5 to release C5a, whilst the larger fragment, C5b, binds sequentially and non-enzymatically to the plasma proteins, C6, C7, C8 and C9. As a result of the polymerization of C9, the final MAC takes the form $C5bC6C7C8(C9_n)$, commonly denoted as $C5b-9_n$, where n represents the number of polymerized C9 molecules. The polymerization of

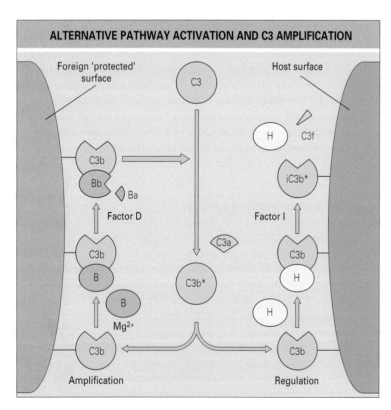

Fig. 119.5 Alternative pathway activation and C3 amplification. The fate of C3b deposited on a surface is dependent on its affinity for factor B or factor H. On foreign surfaces (known as 'protected', because they are permissive for the activation of complement), deposited C3b binds factor B, which is then cleaved by factor D, to generate the surface-bound alternative pathway C3 convertase: C3bBb. This C3 convertase then converts further C3 in the vicinity of the activating surface and, through this positive feedback, amplification of C3 deposition occurs. In contrast, on non-activating surfaces, for example host cells, deposited C3b binds to factor H and is inactivated by the action of factor I. C3b* denotes metastable C3b – that is, C3b in which the internal thioester bond is exposed.

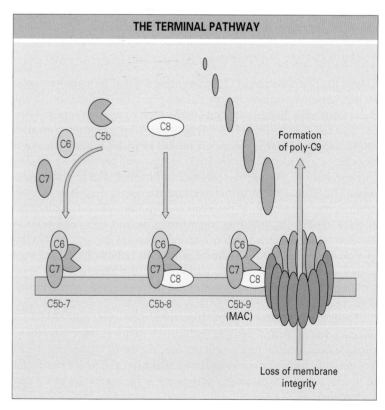

Fig. 119.6 The terminal pathway. After the generation of C5b by the C5 convertases, the assembly of the MAC proceeds non-enzymatically. C5b binds first C6 then C7, to form a hydrophobic complex that can insert into bilayers. C8 then binds, followed by the stepwise addition of up to 19 C9 monomers. This results in the formation of the lytic plug, which compromises membrane integrity.

C9 produces a hydrophobic complex that forms 'holes' in lipid bilayers, resulting in target lysis.

Sequence of events during terminal pathway activation

The C3 convertases of both the classical pathway (C4b2a) and the alternative pathway (C3bBb), on binding a further C3b molecule, generate the C5 convertases: C4b2aC3b and C3bBbC3b, respectively. The classical pathway C5 convertase is formed after the covalent binding of one C3b molecule to C4b within the C4b2a convertase, forming the complex: C4b2aC3b. The C4b–C3b dimer within this complex serves as a high-affinity receptor for fluid-phase C5[23]. An analogous situation occurs for the alternative pathway C5 convertase, in which a C3b–C3b dimer is generated[24].

The cleavage of C5 by a C5 convertase enzyme generates two fragments, C5a and C5b. C5a is a 74 amino acid peptide known as an anaphylatoxin, because it causes a reaction similar to anaphylaxis after injection into experimental animals. C5b possesses a metastable binding site for C6 which is believed to be the result of transient exposure of hydrophobic sites[25]. The C5b–C6 interaction forms a stable, hydrophilic bimolecular complex that remains bound to C3b within the C5 convertase until it interacts with C7. The interaction of native C7 with the C5b-6 complex results in the transient exposure of phospholipid binding sites on C7, so that the C5b-7 trimolecular complex is able to insert into lipid bilayers by hydrophobic interactions. The membrane-bound C5b-7 complex then interacts with fluid-phase C8. C8 consists of three polypeptide chains (α, β and γ) and binds to C5b-7 via its β-chain. After this binding has occurred, the α-chain of C8 inserts into the lipid membrane. The final stage in the formation of the MAC is the interaction between C5b-8 and C9. C9 is a single-chain serum protein that interacts with C8 in the membrane-bound C5b-8 complex, which, in turn, initiates polymerization of C9 so that one C5b-8 complex binds up to 12–15 C9 molecules[26].

Regulation of complement activation

The activation of complement is tightly regulated in both the fluid-phase and on cell surfaces; this prevents complement activation by autologous host tissues and protects the host from the bystander effects of complement activation as part of host defense responses against pathogenic microorganisms. The evolution of the complement system has been accompanied by the development of a sophisticated regulatory system consisting of fluid-phase and membrane-bound regulatory proteins (Table 119.1). We will discuss these regulatory proteins under two headings: those that act principally in the fluid-phase (C1 inhibitor, C4b-binding protein, factor I, factor H, vitronectin, clusterin) and those that are membrane-bound (MCP; CD46), decay-accelerating factor (DAF, CD55), CR1 (CD35), CD59 (sometimes known as homologous restriction factor).

Fluid-phase complement regulatory proteins

C1 inhibitor and C4b-binding protein inhibit classical pathway activation, whereas factor H downregulates alternative pathway activation. Factor I is responsible for the proteolytic inactivation of C4b and C3b which, in the fluid-phase, requires the plasma cofactors C4b-binding protein and factor H, respectively.

C1 inhibitor is a member of the family of serine proteinase inhibitors (serpins) that inactivates C1 by binding to and inactivating the catalytic sites of enzymatically active C1r and C1s. C1 inhibitor prevents uncontrolled fluid-phase C1 activation. It is also a physiological inhibitor of other important serine proteinases, including kallikrein, factor XIIa and plasmin. Inherited heterozygous deficiency of C1 inhibitor is associated with the disease hereditary angioedema (discussed later in this chapter). **C4b-binding protein** has decay-accelerating activity against the classical pathway C3 convertase, C4b2a[27] and is able to bind to C4b, preventing the binding of C2. It is an essential fluid-phase cofactor for factor I-mediated proteolytic inactivation of C4b[28].

Factor H inhibits alternative pathway activation by binding to C3b (thus preventing binding of factor B). It also has decay-accelerating activity for both C3bBb and C3iBb, and is an essential fluid-phase cofactor for the factor I-mediated proteolytic inactivation of C3b to iC3b[29]. Its importance in vivo is illustrated by the complement profile of individuals genetically deficient in factor H. In such cases, the fluid-phase generation of C3b by the tick-over pathway proceeds unhindered, resulting in complete fluid-phase consumption of C3.

TABLE 119.1 COMPLEMENT REGULATORY MOLECULES

	M_r (kDa)	Serum concentration (µg/ml)	Chromosomal location	Function
Fluid-phase				
C1 inhibitor	105	120–200	11	Inhibits enzymatically active C1r and C1s
C4-binding protein	560	200	RCA – 1q32	Binds to C4b, preventing binding of C2 Dissociates classical pathway C3 convertase: C4b2a Cofactor for factor I-mediated inactivation of C4b
Factor I	88	40	4	Proteolytic inactivation of C3b and C4b; requires cofactor
Factor H	150	500	RCA – 1q32	Binds to C3b, preventing binding of factor B Dissociates alternative pathway C3 convertase: C3bBb Cofactor for the factor I-mediated inactivation of C3b
Vitronectin (S-protein)	80	250–450	17q	Binds fluid-phase C5b-7, preventing insertion into lipid membranes
Clusterin	80	35–105	8	Binds fluid-phase C5b-7, preventing insertion into lipid membranes
Membrane-bound				
DAF (CD55)	70	–	RCA – 1q32	Accelerates the decay of the C3 and C5 convertases
MCP (CD46)	45–70	–	RCA – 1q32	Cofactor for the factor I-mediated cleavage of C3b and C4b in C3 and C5 convertases
CR1 (CD35)	190–280	–	RCA – 1q32	Cofactor for factor I-mediated inactivation of C4b, C3b and iC3b Accelerates the decay of the C3 and C5 convertases
CD59	18–25	–	11p13	Binds to C5b-8, preventing binding of C9 Binds to C5b-9, preventing polymerization of C9

Factor I is a serine protease that is responsible for the inactivation of C3b and C4b. The factor I-mediated proteolytic inactivation of C3b occurs in two steps. Initially, factor I cleaves the α-chain of C3b, forming iC3b[30]. Essential cofactors for this reaction include factor H in the fluid-phase[29] and MCP and CR1 on cell surfaces. Factor I degrades iC3b further, with the aid of CR1 as cofactor, to produce C3dg and C3c.

Vitronectin (previously known as S-protein) is a single-chain glycoprotein that is able to bind to the metastable reactive site within the C5b-7 complex, preventing its insertion into lipid bilayers from the fluid-phase[31]. Fluid-phase C5b-7 also binds strongly to serum lipoproteins, which again prevents insertion of the complex into cell membranes. The importance of vitronectin and serum lipoproteins is that they prevent the diffusion of active C5b-7 complexes to sites distant from the immediate vicinity of complement activation. This restricts MAC insertion to membranes at the site of complement activation, and prevents bystander lysis of normal host cells.

Membrane-bound complement regulatory proteins
Membrane-bound complement regulatory proteins fall into two functional categories. The first is proteins that prevent the assembly and promote the destruction of cell-bound C3 and C5 convertases, including MCP, DAF and CR1. The second category is a protein that prevents the assembly of the MAC in cell membranes, known as CD59.

MCP (CD46) is a widely expressed cell-surface protein that expresses cofactor activity for the proteolytic degradation of C3b and C4b to iC3b and iC4b, respectively, by factor I[32]. **DAF** (CD55) accelerates the dissociation of the classical pathway C3 convertase, C4b2a, and also promotes the dissociation of Bb from the alternative pathway C3 convertase and the C5 convertases. The molecule does not prevent formation of the C3 or C5 convertases, nor does it possess factor I cofactor activity for the inactivation of C3b and C4b.

CR1 differs from MCP and DAF in having important receptor activities for the large fragments of C3 and C4, in addition to its cofactor activities for the cleavage of these proteins by factor I. It is present on erythrocytes, neutrophils, eosinophils, monocytes, B lymphocytes, follicular dendritic cells and glomerular epithelial cells (podocytes). CR1 has a major role in the transport of opsonized immune complexes to the fixed cells of the mononuclear phagocytic system and functions as an opsonic receptor on neutrophils, monocytes and macrophages for C3b and C4b. CR1 also has complement-regulatory activities. It acts as a cofactor for the factor I-mediated inactivation of C4b and for both inactivation steps of C3b: C3b to iC3b, releasing C3f, and iC3b to C3dg, releasing C3c. In addition, CR1 possesses decay-accelerating activity for the classical and alternative pathway C3 convertases.

CD59 is a membrane-bound inhibitor of the MAC[33]. It is a single-chain glycoprotein that, like DAF, is anchored to plasma membranes by a particular anchoring moiety, known as a glycosylphosphatidylinositol anchor. It is widely expressed in human tissues and cells. CD59 inhibits the MAC by binding to C8 in the C5b-8 complex, and prevents the binding of C9 and subsequent C9 polymerization.

BIOLOGICAL FUNCTIONS OF COMPLEMENT

The biological functions of complement can be divided into three categories. First, complement has a role in the killing of microorganisms through opsonization, activation of leukocytes and target-cell lysis. The second activity of complement is as a bridge between the humoral adaptive immune system (antibody) and innate immunity. Many of the effector activities of antibody are mediated by the activation of complement by antibodies bound to antigens (immune complexes). Activation of complement also augments antibody responses and thereby enhances host defense against pathogens. The third activity of complement is in the resolution of inflammatory responses. It is in this role that comple-

ment may prevent the development of systemic lupus erythematosus (SLE) by promoting the clearance of tissue debris.

Opsonization, leukocyte activation and target-cell lysis
Complement activation promotes the killing of pathogens through opsonization, leukocyte activation and target-cell lysis. Fixed C4b, C3b and iC3b on bacterial surfaces or immune complexes are ligands for complement receptors present on phagocytic cells and promote the uptake of pathogens for killing by phagocytes. Coating of a target with these fragments is referred to as opsonization.

Complement activation also results in the production of the anaphylatoxins, C3a and C5a, which are potent inducers of inflammation. These are small peptides that are released after cleavage of the α-chain of their respective parent proteins (C3 and C5). This occurs predominantly during complement activation, but can also occur by the direct action of some host enzymes that are expressed as part of inflammatory responses – for example, neutrophil elastase, plasmin and kallikrein. The anaphylatoxins produce degranulation of mast cells, basophils, eosinophils and phagocytic cells, and cause smooth muscle contraction and increased vascular permeability. C5a is a more potent anaphylatoxin than C3a. C4a, which is cleaved from C4b by the action of C1s, has very weak anaphylatoxic activity.

The anaphylatoxins mediate their actions by ligation of specific G-protein-coupled receptors. The C5a receptor belongs to the rhodopsin superfamily of G-protein-coupled receptors and is expressed on cells derived from the myeloid lineage (neutrophils, eosinophils, basophils, mast cells, monocytes and macrophages). Rapid internalization of C5a occurs after ligation to its receptor, followed by intracellular degradation. Furthermore, the circulating enzyme, carboxypeptidase N, cleaves the C-terminal arginine from C5a to form the less potent C5a-des-Arg molecule. These mechanisms regulate C5a activity and account for its very short biological half-life. Deletion of these receptors in mice has aided the understanding of the roles of C5a and C3a in inflammatory responses in vivo. For example, mice with targeted deletion of the C5a receptor showed impaired mucosal lung defence and were completely protected from injury using an experimental model for the study of inflammation mediated by immune complexes, known as the pulmonary reverse passive Arthus model[34,35], whereas C3a-receptor-deficient mice were protected against pulmonary injury in a murine model of allergic airways disease[36]. In contrast, only partial protection was seen in the C5a-receptor-deficient mice using models of immune complex formation in the peritoneal cavity and skin, suggesting that other mechanisms contribute to the inflammatory response to immune complexes formed at these sites[37].

Immune complex processing and clearance of apoptotic cells
Fcγ receptors and complement mediate the normal processing of immune complexes. One important role of complement is to maintain immune complexes in solution. Deposition of C3b on antigen precipitated by antibody-mediated classical pathway activation within the immune complex (i.e. opsonization) modifies the lattice structure of the complex, maintaining solubility[38]. Complement is also important in enabling the recognition and capture of immune complexes by complement receptors on cells of the mononuclear phagocytic system (Table 119.2). In primates, CR1 on erythrocytes is predominantly responsible for binding to C3b-bearing immune complexes in the circulation. CR1 and other complement receptors also serve to promote immune responses by binding antigens in the form of immune complexes to B-lymphocytes and follicular dendritic cells. In the absence of complement, the clearance of immune complexes is abnormal, a phenomenon that has been demonstrated in many studies of patients with SLE (reviewed by Walport et al.[39]). Thus complement deficiency states may

TABLE 119.2 COMPLEMENT RECEPTORS

Receptor	Ligands	Cellular distribution	Function
CR1 (CD35)	C3b>iC3b C4b	Erythrocytes Neutrophils B cells Monocytes/macrophages Follicular dendritic cells Glomerular epithelial cells	*Opsonic* receptor (i.e. mediates phagocytosis of particles opsonized with C4b, C3b and iC3b) Mediator of *immune adherence* – phenomenon in which organisms opsonized with antibody and complement (C4b, C3b, iC3b) adhere to erythrocytes (via surface CR1) Cofactor for factor I-mediated inactivation of C3b (see also Table 119.1) Mediates binding of opsonized immune complexes to erythrocytes, allowing transportation to fixed cells of mononuclear phagocytic system
CR2 (CD21)	iC3b C3dg Epstein–Barr virus (EBV)	B cells Follicular dendritic cells Epithelial cells of nasopharynx and cervix	Lowers threshold for B ell activation after ligation of antigen-specific B cell receptor Mediates EBV entry to cells
CR3 (CD18/CD11b)	iC3b Zymosan Fibrinogen Factor X ICAM-1	Monocytes/macrophages Neutrophils Natural killer cells Follicular dendritic cells	Member of the β_2-integrin family Leukocyte adhesion Mediates phagocytosis of particles opsonized with iC3b

ICAM-1, intercellular cell adhesion molecule 1.

result in impaired clearance of immune complexes, allowing subsequent deposition in tissues, with injury via ligation of Fcγ receptors on neutrophils and other leukocytes.

There is a mounting body of evidence that suggests that the complement system, particularly C1q, is important in the physiological clearance of apoptotic cells (reviewed by Pickering *et al.*[40]). This first followed the observation that apoptotic, but not viable, human keratinocytes bind C1q directly *in vitro*[41]. An *in vivo* defect in clearance of apoptotic cells has been demonstrated in C1q-deficient mice, generated by gene-targeting[42]. These mice spontaneously developed antinuclear antibodies and a proliferative glomerulonephritis, characterized by increased numbers of glomerular apoptotic bodies. Moreover, C1q-deficient mice were shown to have impaired clearance of apoptotic cells in a model of sterile peritonitis[43].

Complement and the immune response

Complement was first shown to play a part in the generation of an antibody response by the demonstration that transient depletion of C3 using cobra venom factor resulted in an impaired antibody response to T cell dependent antigens[44]. It was then shown that mice treated with cobra venom factor were also unable to localize antigen to the germinal centers of the spleen or lymph nodes[45]. However, later studies of guinea-pigs with genetic deficiency of either C2, C4 or C3 showed that the impaired antibody response to antigen (in these studies, bacteriophage φx174) was strictly dependent on the dose of antigen[46]. More recently, studies in C3-deficient, C4-deficient and C1q-deficient mice, immunized with T cell dependent antigens, have shown impaired germinal center formation, impaired B cell response and failure to class-switch[47,48]. In addition, mice deficient in the complement receptors, CR1 (CD35) and CR2 (CD21), also demonstrated a reduction in antibody response to T cell dependent antigens and in germinal center formation[49,50].

The role of complement in the generation of antibody responses has been dramatically illustrated by the demonstration that C3d coupled to antigen enhanced the immune response, behaving as a natural adjuvant[51]. The fusion of either two or three molecules of murine C3d to recombinant hen egg lysozyme, was respectively, 1000 and 10 000 times more immunogenic than antigen alone. The mechanism by which the complement system plays a critical part in the generation of humoral responses to low-dose antigen has been explained in two different ways. First, opsonization of the antigen by complement enhances the targeting of antigen to follicular dendritic cells, which express CD35 (CR1) and CD21 (CR2), leading to more efficient antigen presentation to B cells. Secondly, the threshold for B cell activation is lowered if the cognate antigen is opsonized with complement. The mechanism by which this occurs is believed to be mediated by the binding of C3d on antigen to CD21 of the CD19/CD21 membrane protein complex on B cells[52].

COMPLEMENT AND DISEASE

Both inherited and acquired complement deficiency are associated with disease. Studies of individuals with inherited complement deficiency are particularly important to the rheumatologist, because of the strong association between classical pathway deficiency and SLE. Furthermore, acquired complement deficiency is commonly seen in SLE, rheumatoid vasculitis and mixed essential cryoglobulinemia and serial measurement of complement provides a useful index of disease activity in SLE. In the following sections, we will discuss inherited complement deficiency, acquired complement deficiency and measurement of complement in disorders relevant to rheumatology.

Inherited complement deficiency and disease

Inherited complement deficiency although rare can be efficiently screened for during the diagnostic work-up, by performing functional complement assays such as total hemolytic activity or 'CH50' assay. Absent or unmeasurable CH50, particularly in the presence of normal or high concentrations of C3 and C4 (unless it is either of these proteins that is deficient), suggests hereditary complement deficiency. The finding of absent or unmeasurable CH50 should be confirmed by repeating the assay on freshly collected serum. Complement components are not stable at room temperature for long periods, and functional assays, such as the CH50, are particularly sensitive in this regard. A normal CH50 requires an intact classical pathway, the presence of C3 and an intact terminal pathway. Individuals with SLE and absent CH50 with normal or increased C3 and C4 concentrations should be screened for classical pathway component (C1q, C1r, C1s, C4 and C2) deficiency. The presence or absence of individual components can be tested using widely available antigenic assays. It is notable that, even in very active lupus, in which diminished C4 and C3 are commonly seen, complete absence of these proteins is rare and, if present, suggests hereditary deficiency. Table 119.3 summarizes the relationships between various forms of

TABLE 119.3 HEREDITARY COMPLEMENT DEFICIENCY AND DISEASE

Component	Functional defect or consequence	Disease association
Classical pathway components		
C1q, C1r, C1s, C4 and C2	Inability to activate the classical pathway	SLE
Alternative pathway components		
Factor B* and Factor D	Alternative pathway activation blocked	Neisserial infection
Properdin (X-linked)	Failure to stabilize alternative pathway C3 convertase	Recurrent pyogenic infections, particularly Neisserial infections
C3	Inability to produce opsonic fragments (C3b, iC3b, C3dg)	Recurrent pyogenic infections, MPGN
	Alternative pathway activation blocked	
	Inability to form the MAC	
Lectin pathway components		
MBL	Inability to activate the lectin pathway (opsonic defect)	Recurrent pyogenic infections, particularly in childhood
Terminal pathway components		
C5, C6, C7, C8 and C9	Inability to form the MAC	Neisserial infection
		Many C9-deficient cases healthy
Deficiency of complement regulators		
Fluid-phase		
C1 inhibitor	Uncontrolled fluid-phase C1 activation	Angioedema
Factor H	Uncontrolled fluid-phase C3 activation	MPGN
	Secondary C3 depletion	HUS
		Recurrent pyogenic infection
Factor I	Uncontrolled fluid-phase C3 activation	Recurrent pyogenic infection
	Secondary C3 depletion	Nephritis rare
		(HUS not reported)
Membrane-bound		
CD59*	Inability to regulate MAC assembly on host cells	Anemia
DAF	Loss of decay-accelerating activity on host cell membranes	Healthy
DAF and CD59 on erythrocytes	As for CD59 and DAF	PNH – an acquired disorder

* Single case reported.

HUS, hemolytic uremic syndrome; PNH, paroxsymal nocturnal hemoglobinuria; MPGN, membranoproliferative glomerulonephritis.

TABLE 119.4 COMPLEMENT PROFILES AND INHERITED COMPLEMENT DEFICIENCY

C3	C4	CH50	AP50	Possible deficiency
Normal or increased	Normal or increased	0	Normal	Classical pathway (C1q, C1r, C1s, C2)
Normal or increased	0	0	Normal	C4
0	Normal	0	0	C3
Very low	Normal	0	0	Factor H or I deficiency*
Normal	Normal	0	0	Terminal pathway C5, C6, C7, C8, C9
Normal	Normal	Normal	0	Factor B or D deficiency
Normal	Low	Low or normal	Normal	C1 inhibitor deficiency

* C3 nephritic factor can cause complement activation, giving a pattern of results very similar to those of factor H or I deficiency.

hereditary complement deficiency and disease, and complement profiles suggestive of inherited deficiency are illustrated in Table 119.4, using the most commonly performed complement assays: C3, C4, CH50 and the alternative pathway hemolytic activity assay (AP50).

Deficiency of classical pathway components: C1q, C1s, C1r, C2 and C4

Homozygous hereditary deficiency of each of the classical pathway components (C1q, C1r, C1s, C4 and C2) is associated with an increased sus-

ceptibility to SLE[40]. Both the severity of disease and strength of this association are greatest for homozygous C1q deficiency, followed in turn by homozygous C4 and C2 deficiency. Homozygous C1q deficiency is the strongest genetic susceptibility factor for SLE that has been identified in humans. Thirty-nine of the 42 recorded patients with homozygous C1q deficiency have developed a clinical syndrome closely similar to SLE. In the affected patients, rash occurred in 37, glomerulonephritis in 16 and cerebral disease in eight. Antinuclear antibodies were reported in 24 of the 35 patients tested. Notably, the incidence of anti-double stranded

DNA antibodies was low: only five of the 25 patients tested were positive. No clinical phenotype has been observed amongst any of the heterozygous C1q-deficient relatives of the homozygous cases.

Hereditary deficiency of C1s and C1r is more rare than that of C1q deficiency and, in the majority of cases, deficiencies of both components coincide. In such individuals, C1r concentrations are usually absent, with those of C1s less than 50% of normal. As in homozygous C1q deficiency, SLE occurs in the majority of these individuals (eight of the 14 reported cases). The finding of normal C3 and C4 concentrations in a young woman with severe lupus and absent CH50 raises the suspicion of classical pathway component deficiency. Antigenic assays may confirm the presence of C2 and C4, but show complete absence of, for example, C1q. In homozygous C4 deficiency, the prevalence of SLE is approximately 75% (18 of 24 cases) and the lupus illness is of moderate severity, often developing at an early age and associated with increased frequency of pyogenic infections.

Homozygous C2 deficiency is the most common inherited classical pathway complement deficiency, with an approximate prevalence in the Western European white populations of 1:20 000. In contrast to homozygous C1q deficiency, the majority of affected individuals are probably healthy. SLE has been reported in up to 33% of C2-deficient individuals, although this figure is likely to be an overestimate as a result of ascertainment artifact, with a more realistic incidence approaching 10%.

In addition to standard treatment regimens for SLE, definitive treatment strategies in patients with SLE caused by classical pathway component deficiency include measures to replace the 'missing' component. Fresh frozen plasma can be used as a source of components such as C1q and C2, but only anecdotal evidence of this is available[53–55] and this approach should only be considered in a specialist unit. There is a theoretical danger that complement repletion could cause disease exacerbation, because of the potential for large-scale complement activation caused by immune complexes previously deposited and ineffectively cleared from tissues. Concentrates of specific complement components are not available, with the sole exception of C1 inhibitor concentrates used for the treatment of angioedema.

There is a strong association between the presence of C4A null alleles and SLE among Western European white individuals (reviewed by Pickering et al.[40]). C4 is encoded by duplicated genes termed C4A and C4B, located within the major histocompatibility complex class III region. These genes are highly polymorphic and variants include null alleles termed *C4AQ*o* or *C4BQ*o*. A single C4 null allele may be seen in up to 30% of healthy white individuals, with approximately 4% having homozygous C4A deficiency and 1%, homozygous C4B deficiency. The association between *C4AQ*o* alleles and SLE is complicated by the observation that, in white patients with lupus, such alleles are in strong linkage dysequilibrium with *HLA-DR3* on the extended haplotype: *HLA-A1, B8, DR3, C4AQ*o*. This creates a fundamental difficulty in determining whether the presence of *C4AQ*o* alleles directly represents disease susceptibility alleles or is associated with lupus by virtue of linkage dysequilibrium with a susceptibility gene(s) on the extended haplotype. Evidence that the presence of *C4AQ*o* alleles predisposes to SLE independently of *HLA-DR3* comes from the finding that *C4AQ*o* alleles are associated with SLE among populations in which the incidence of *HLA-DR3* is low – for example among Japanese patients with lupus. In contrast to *C4AQ*o*, *C4BQ*o* alleles have a very weak association with lupus.

Alternative pathway components: C3, factor B, factor D and properdin

Homozygous C3 deficiency is strongly associated with recurrent and severe bacterial infections, particularly those caused by encapsulated organisms such as *Neisseria meningitidis*, *Streptococcus pneumoniae* and *Haemophilus influenzae* (reviewed by Botto and Walport[56]). This serves to illustrate the major importance *in vivo* of C3 as an opsonin. Major infections in patients with C3 deficiency are most prominent in childhood, and are less of a clinical problem in adults. This presumably reflects the lesser importance of complement in host defense against pyogenic bacteria, as antibody responses mature in response to repeated infectious challenges. Homozygous C3 deficiency has been reported in 23 individuals from 16 families (reviewed by Pickering et al.[40]). Unlike inherited deficiency of the classical pathway components, the incidence of SLE is low. Membranoproliferative glomerulonephritis has been described in one homozygous and one heterozygous C3-deficient individual.

Factor B deficiency has been reported in only one individual, who presented with meningococcal septicemia[57]. Factor D deficiency has been reported in two families, and is associated with absent alternative pathway hemolytic activity. The index case in one family presented with recurrent infections caused by *Neisseria gonorrhoea*[58]. The index case in the second family was a patient with a history of serious *Neisseria meningitidis*, but three other factor D-deficient individuals in the family were healthy[59]. Properdin deficiency is also associated with recurrent and severe childhood pyogenic infections (particularly neisserial infection) and is inherited as an X-linked trait[60].

Terminal pathway components

Deficiency of any of the terminal pathway components (C5, C6, C7, C8 and C9) results in a particular increased susceptibility to Neisserial infections. This provides evidence that extracellular lysis by the MAC is critical in host defense against these organisms. C9 deficiency is rare in white individuals, but surprisingly frequent in Japanese, with an incidence of approximately 1/1000[61]. These individuals are at an increased risk of Neisserial infection, but otherwise have normal health.

Lectin pathway components

The physiological importance of the lectin pathway in humans can be appreciated from the phenotype described in individuals with MBL deficiency. MBL deficiency is associated with an opsonic defect and recurrent infections, particularly in childhood. Several polymorphisms that result in reduced serum concentrations of MBL have been identified. These include three point mutations in exon 1 and two linked promoter polymorphisms[62,63]. One of the point mutations (resulting in the substitution of aspartic acid for glycine in codon 54: Asp[54] mutation), is associated with severe, recurrent infections in children and adults[64] and the mutant MBL protein is unable to activate complement[65]. It should be noted that certain ethnic groups have a high incidence of dominant alleles that result in low serum concentrations of MBL. This may be partially explained by the observation that low concentrations of MBL afford protection, although incomplete and weak, against mycobacterial infection[66].

Deficiency of fluid-phase complement regulators: C1 inhibitor, factor I and factor H

Hereditary C1 inhibitor deficiency is transmitted as an autosomal dominant trait and heterozygous individuals experience episodic recurrent subcutaneous and submucosal swelling (hereditary angioedema)[67]. Involvement of the upper airways may result in life-threatening airway obstruction. Involvement of the bowel mucosa may produce severe abdominal pain mimicking common surgical emergencies. In normal circumstances, C1 inhibitor binds to and inactivates enzymatically active C1r and C1s. It also inhibits plasmin, kallikrein and activated coagulation factors XIIa and XIa. Deficiency results in uncontrolled fluid-phase classical pathway activation and consequently reduced concentrations of both C4 and C2. Acute angioedema attacks are caused by increased vascular permeability at the affected sites. This is believed to relate to increased bradykinin concentrations as a consequence of uncontrolled cleavage of kininogen by kallikrein[68]. Plasmin activation may be important in the precipitation of attacks, by consuming the reduced amounts of available C1 inhibitor in individuals with only half normal functional expression of the protein, caused by the presence of one defective allele. Hereditary deficiency may be due to absence of the protein (type I deficiency, 85%) or due to a dysfunctional circulating protein (type II, 15%). It is important to note that the latter subtype may be missed if antigenic detection assays alone are used in screening; functional C1 inhibitor assays are necessary to detect this particular deficiency, as the abnormal protein may be present in normal serum concentrations. Treatment of acute angioedema relies on replacing the C1 inhibitor, traditionally using fresh frozen plasma, but more recently using C1 inhibitor concentrates[69].

Hereditary deficiency of factor I, has been reported in 27 individuals from 26 families[70–74]. Factor I deficiency is associated with recurrent pyogenic infections, most likely a consequence of secondary C3 deficiency. In contrast to the phenotype associated with factor H deficiency, only one factor I-deficient individual has developed glomerulonephritis, which histologically was focal segmental glomerulonephritis[71]. Deficiency of factor H is also very rare, with only 29 cases from 12 families reported. Only three of these individuals were healthy at the time of reporting[75–77]. Two major phenotypic manifestations have been described in factor H-deficient humans: hemolytic uremic syndrome[75,77–79] and membranoproliferative glomerulonephritis (MPGN)[78,80,81]. Hemolytic uremic syndrome has also been reported in individuals with heterozygous factor H deficiency. The mechanism by which factor H deficiency results in these phenotypes is not understood. Deficiency of either factor H or I is associated with uncontrolled fluid-phase, alternative pathway complement activation. This results in secondary and severe C3 deficiency, together with depletion of the alternative pathway components (properdin and factor B). The typical associated complement profile is that of absent alternative pathway hemolytic activity, in addition to absent total hemolytic activity (CH50), the latter a consequence of secondary C3 depletion.

Deficiency of membrane-bound complement regulators: DAF and CD59

Lack of regulation of MAC assembly on host cells would be predicted to predispose to cell injury through lysis. In paroxysmal nocturnal hemoglobinuria, an acquired condition, a clone of erythrocytes that lack both CD59 and DAF develops. This defect is due to a somatic mutation in a clone of erythrocyte precursors, which results in deficiency of phosphatidylinositol phospholipid glycan class A[82]. This protein is required for synthesis of glycosylphosphatidylinositol phospholipid, which provides a 'lipid membrane anchor' for many proteins, including both DAF and CD59. As one might expect, the abnormal red cells in this condition are susceptible to lysis by autologous complement activation. It is notable that the few genetically DAF-deficient individuals described appear healthy, with no evidence of significant red cell hemolysis *in vivo*. In contrast, the single reported case of CD59 deficiency was associated with a paroxysmal nocturnal hemoglobinuria-like phenotype[83]. Thus, in paroxysmal nocturnal hemoglobinuria, lack of CD59 is likely to be the major contributor to the excessive susceptibility to lysis of red cells by autologous complement.

Acquired complement deficiency

Examples of acquired complement deficiency and disease are summarized in Table 119.5. In some conditions (e.g. SLE and rheumatoid vasculitis), there is excessive classical pathway activation, whereas in others (e.g. partial lipodystrophy and MPGN type II), there is excessive alternative pathway activation. Acquired abnormalities of complement have been described in association with a series of autoantibodies to complement proteins, which are discussed first.

Acquired hypocomplementemia caused by autoantibodies to complement proteins

The most important of the autoantibodies causing acquired hypocomplementemia include C3 nephritic factor[84] and anti-C1q antibodies[85].

C3 nephritic factor is an IgG autoantibody directed against a neoepitope on the fluid-phase and cell-bound alternative pathway C3 convertase (C3iBb and C3bBb respectively)[86]. The binding of C3 nephritic factor to the C3 convertase renders it resistant to inactivation by factor H. The consequent uncontrolled alternative pathway activation results in secondary C3 deficiency. C3 nephritic factor is most commonly associated with partial lipodystrophy and MPGN type II[87].

Anti-C1q antibodies are IgG autoantibodies that are directed against neoepitopes on the collagen-like region of the C1q molecule[85]. These antibodies, found in approximately 33% of patients with lupus, show a significant inverse correlation with concentrations of C1q, C3 and C4[88]. The mechanism of the hypocomplementemia associated with the presence of anti-C1q antibodies is not certain. Anti-C1q antibodies do not cause complement activation in the fluid-phase when added to fresh serum samples. The most likely mechanism is that they amplify complement activation by immune complexes in tissues, by binding to C1q fixed to immune complexes, thereby enlarging the complexes and promoting further complement activation. The presence of anti-C1q antibodies in SLE has been found to correlate strongly with the presence of proliferative nephritis[89,90]. Increases in anti-C1q antibody titers have been shown to precede renal involvement in SLE[90] and, in contrast to increases in anti-DNA antibody titers, appear to increase specifically before renal relapse[91]. These antibodies have been recovered from renal biopsies of patients with lupus with proliferative nephritis in greater concentrations than that of serum, supporting the hypothesis that they have a direct role in the pathogenesis of the nephritis[92].

Antibodies to C1 inhibitor (associated with acquired angioedema)[93] and a classical pathway nephritic factor (an autoantibody to the classical pathway C3 convertase: C4b2a) have also been reported[94]. Acquired angioedema has an important association with lymphoproliferative

---

TABLE 119.5 EXAMPLES OF ACQUIRED COMPLEMENT DEFICIENCY AND DISEASE

C3 low, C4 normal *Predominantly alternative pathway activation*	C4 low, C3 normal or low *Predominantly classical pathway activation*
MPGN type II with C3 nephritic factor	Active SLE
Partial lipodystrophy with C3 nephritic factor	Mixed essential cryoglobulinemia
Post-streptococcal glomerulonephritis	Acquired C1 inhibitor deficiency
	Rheumatoid vasculitis
	Felty's syndrome
	Chronic infection, e.g.
	• Subacute bacterial endocarditis
	• Infected ventriculoatrial shunts
	Hypocomplementemic urticarial vasculitis syndrome (HUVS)

disorders, particularly B cell lymphoma, and typically presents late in life compared with inherited C1 inhibitor deficiency.

Rheumatologic disorders characterized by hypocomplementemia

Systemic lupus erythematosus, rheumatoid vasculitis and Felty's syndrome, hypocomplementemic urticarial vasculitis (HUVS) and mixed essential cryoglobulinemia are among the rheumatologic disorders characterized by hypocomplementemia.

Hypocomplementemia is frequently seen in patients with SLE who have active disease. Concentrations of classical pathway proteins are low (e.g. C4) and in severe disease, particularly renal involvement, reduction in serum C3 may also occur. Furthermore, a normal C3 concentration is unusual in lupus nephritis (reviewed by Lloyd and Schur[95]). It should be noted that, in patients with lupus who are homozygous for C4A deficiency, C4 concentrations may remain low even during disease remission. However, despite these observations, serial complement measurements only approximately correlate with disease activity. One reason for this is that the concentrations of complement proteins are influenced by both synthetic and catabolic rates, and both may be abnormal in disease. Activation products of complement components such as the C3 degradation products (e.g. C3a, iC3b and C3d) have been measured in an attempt to predict and counteract this difficulty[96–98]. Although there is some evidence that measurement of these products correlate more strongly with disease activity, such assays are not routinely available and still provide only a crude marker of disease activity. The presence of antibodies to complement proteins further complicates the measurement of complement activity in patients with SLE; these include anti-C1q antibodies, which have been discussed above. Anti-C1q antibodies are correlated with hypocomplementemia independently of disease activity and, in such cases, fluctuation of complement concentrations over time are likely to reflect changes in the autoantibody concentration. However, as mentioned earlier, there is some evidence that the presence of these antibodies is associated with the development of lupus nephritis. Patients with SLE should have functional complement assays performed (e.g. total hemolytic activity) to screen for inherited complement deficiency.

Although serum complement concentrations are typically normal in patients with rheumatoid arthritis, uncontrolled complement activation within inflamed joints is likely to contribute significantly to joint damage. Evidence for this includes the demonstration of increased complement degradation products in synovial fuid from affected joints, including C3 and C4 fragments[99]. Furthermore, complement inhibition has been partially successful in ameliorating experimental arthritis in animal models (reviewed by Linton and Morgan[100]). One important instance in rheumatoid disease in which abnormal serum complement concentrations may be found is in individuals with rheumatoid vasculitis. In this condition, depression of serum C4 concentrations is fre-quently seen and may correlate with disease activity[101]. Rheumatoid vasculitis predominantly occurs in individuals with long-standing rheumatoid arthritis, nodules, severe erosive disease and high titers of circulating rheumatoid factor, and in those individuals with Felty's syndrome.

Hypocomplementemic urticarial vasculitis syndrome (HUVS) is a rare condition characterized clinically by urticarial vasculitis (which, histologically, is usually a leukocytoclastic vasculitis) and polyarthritis or polyarthralgia together with hypocomplementemia, with reduction in both C4 and C3 concentrations, together with marked depression in C1q concentrations[102]. Rarely, C3 concentrations may be normal, but a low C4 is invariably found. This condition is characterized by the presence of C1q precipitins, which form in agarose gels containing HUVS sera and C1q. These are now known to be caused by the presence of IgG autoantibodies to C1q[103]. The concentration of these anti-C1q antibodies correlates inversely with those of C3, C4 and C1q. Other important clinical features associated with HUVS include angioedema, obstructive pulmonary disease and renal disease (typically, MPGN type I)[104].

Cryoglobulins are immunoglobulins that reversibly precipitate in the cold and have been classified into three groups[105]. Type I cryoglobulins are homogenous, being composed of monoclonal immunoglobulin (e.g. IgM or IgG paraproteins seen in lymphoproliferative and myeloproliferative disorders). Type II cryoglobulins are comprised of monoclonal immunoglobulin and polyclonal immunoglobulin, typically monoclonal IgM rheumatoid factor with polyclonal IgG, whereas in type III cryoglobulins, both components are polyclonal immunoglobulins. Patients with type II cryoglobulins or mixed essential cryoglobulinemia typically have evidence of classical pathway activation with reduction in serum C4 concentrations, whereas C3 concentrations remain normal[106]. Characteristic clinical features include dependent palpable purpuric lesions, renal disease (frequently MPGN), arthralgia and sensorimotor peripheral neuropathy. Cryoglobulins should be tested in patients presenting with unexplained renal disease or peripheral neuropathy and low C4. Type II cryoglobulinemia is known to be strongly associated with chronic infections, particularly chronic hepatitis C virus infection, which should be tested for in such patients[107].

There is one extremely important clinical association of both hereditary and acquired hypocomplementemia from any cause in patients with SLE. Patients with chronic hypocomplementemia are at particular risk of developing serious infection with encapsulated organisms such as *Streptococcus pneumoniae* and *Neisseria meningitidis*. These patients can be considered to be 'functionally asplenic', because the hypocomplementemia, in addition to causing defective opsonization and local phagocytosis, also results in reduced splenic clearance of these organisms[108]. There is a strong case that, analogous to patients receiving standard post-splenectomy prophylaxis, such patients should receive prophylactic penicillin treatment and be considered for both pneumococcal and meningococcal vaccination[109].

REFERENCES

1. Sim RB, Reid KB. C1: molecular interactions with activating systems. Immunol Today 1991; 12: 307–311.
2. Cooper NR. The classical complement pathway: activation and regulation of the first complement component. Adv Immunol 1985; 37: 151–216.
3. Dodds AW, Sim RB, Porter RR et al. Activation of the first component of human complement (C1) by antibody-antigen aggregates. Biochem J 1978; 175: 383–390.
4. Law SK, Lichtenberg NA, Holcombe FH et al. Interaction between the labile binding sites of the fourth (C4) and fifth (C5) human complement proteins and erythrocyte cell membranes. J Immunol 1980; 125: 634–639.
5. Vogt W, Schmidt G, Von Buttlar B et al. A new function of the activated third component of complement: binding to C5, an essential step for C5 activation. Immunology 1978; 34: 29–40.
6. Muller-Eberhard HJ, Nilsson U, Aronsson T. Isolation and characterisation of two β1-glycoproteins of human serum. J Exp Med 1960; 111: 201–215.
7. Pangburn MK, Muller-Eberhard HJ. Relation of putative thioester bond in C3 to activation of the alternative pathway and the binding of C3b to biological targets of complement. J Exp Med 1980; 152: 1102–1114.
8. Tack BF, Harrison RA, Janatova J et al. Evidence for presence of an internal thiolester bond in third component of human complement. Proc Natl Acad Sci USA 1980; 77: 5764–5768.
9. Vogt W, Dames W, Schmidt G et al. Complement activation by the properdin system: formation of a stoichiometric C3 cleaving complex of properdin factor B with C36. Immunochemistry 1977; 14: 201–205.
10. Weiler JM, Daha MR, Austen KF et al. Control of the amplification convertase of complement by the plasma protein beta1H. Proc Natl Acad Sci USA 1976; 73: 3268–3272.
11. Lachmann PJ, Muller-Eberhard HJ. The demonstration in human serum of conglutinogen-activating factor and its effect on the third component of complement. J Immunol 1968; 100: 691–698.

12. Sim RB, Twose TM, Paterson DS et al. The covalent-binding reaction of complement component C3. Biochem J 1981; 193: 115–127.
13. Fearon DT, Austen KF. Activation of the alternative complement pathway with rabbit erythrocytes by circumvention of the regulatory action of endogenous control proteins. J Exp Med 1977; 146: 22–33.
14. Pangburn MK, Muller-Eberhard HJ. Complement C3 convertase: cell surface restriction of beta1H control and generation of restriction on neuraminidase-treated cells. Proc Natl Acad Sci USA 1978; 75: 2416–2420.
15. Alper CA, Abramson N, Johnston RB et al. Studies in vivo and in vitro on an abnormality in the metabolism of C3 in a patient with increased susceptibility to infection. J Clin Invest 1970; 49: 1975–1985.
16. Abramson N, Alper CA, Lachmann PJ et al. Deficiency of C3 inactivator in man. J Immunol 1971; 107: 19–27.
17. Alper CA, Rosen FS, Lachmann PJ. Inactivator of the third component of complement as an inhibitor in the properdin pathway. Proc Natl Acad Sci USA 1972; 69: 2910–2913.
18. Nicol PA, Lachmann PJ. The alternate pathway of complement activation. The role of C3 and its inactivator (KAF). Immunology 1973; 24: 259–275.
19. Lachmann PJ, Nicol P. Reaction mechanism of the alternative pathway of complement fixation. Lancet 1973; 1: 465–467.
20. Thiel S, Vorup-Jensen T, Stover CM et al. A second serine protease associated with mannan-binding lectin that activates complement. Nature 1997; 386: 506–510.
21. Matsushita M, Fujita T. Activation of the classical complement pathway by mannose-binding protein in association with a novel C1s-like serine protease. J Exp Med 1992; 176: 1497–1502.
22. Humphrey JH, Dourmashkin RR. The lesions in cell membranes caused by complement. Adv Immunol 1969; 11: 75–115.
23. Takata Y, Kinoshita T, Kozono H et al. Covalent association of C3b with C4b within C5 convertase of the classical complement pathway. J Exp Med 1987; 165: 1494–1507.
24. Kinoshita T, Takata Y, Kozono H et al. C5 convertase of the alternative complement pathway: covalent linkage between two C3b molecules within the trimolecular complex enzyme. J Immunol 1988; 141: 3895–3901.
25. Muller-Eberhard HJ. The membrane attack complex of complement. Annu Rev Immunol 1986; 4: 503–528.
26. Podack ER, Tschoop J, Muller-Eberhard HJ. Molecular organization of C9 within the membrane attack complex of complement. Induction of circular C9 polymerization by the C5b-8 assembly. J Exp Med 1982; 156: 268–282.
27. Gigli I, Fujita T, Nussenzweig V. Modulation of the classical pathway C3 convertase by plasma proteins C4 binding protein and C3b inactivator. Proc Natl Acad Sci USA 1979; 76: 6596–6600.
28. Fujita T, Gigli I, Nussenzweig V. Human C4-binding protein. II. Role in proteolysis of C4b by C3b-inactivator. J Exp Med 1978; 148: 1044–1051.
29. Pangburn MK, Schreiber RD, Muller-Eberhard HJ. Human complement C3b inactivator: isolation, characterization, and demonstration of an absolute requirement for the serum protein beta1H for cleavage of C3b and C4b in solution. J Exp Med 1977; 146: 257–270.
30. Harrison RA, Lachmann PJ. The physiological breakdown of the third component of human complement. Mol Immunol 1980; 17: 9–20.
31. Podack ER, Kolb WP, Muller-Eberhard HJ. The SC5b-7 complex: formation, isolation, properties, and subunit composition. J Immunol 1977; 119: 2024–2029.
32. Seya T, Turner JR, Atkinson JP. Purification and characterization of a membrane protein (gp45-70) that is a cofactor for cleavage of C3b and C4b. J Exp Med 1986; 163: 837–855.
33. Sugita Y, Nakano Y, Tomita M. Isolation from human erythrocytes of a new membrane protein which inhibits the formation of complement transmembrane channels. J Biochem 1988; 104: 633–637.
34. Bozic CR, Lu B, Hopken UE et al. Neurogenic amplification of immune complex inflammation. Science 1996; 273: 1722–1725.
35. Hopken UE, Lu B, Gerard NP et al. The C5a chemoattractant receptor mediates mucosal defence to infection. Nature 1996; 383: 86–89.
36. Humbles AA, Lu B, Nilsson CA et al. A role for the C3a anaphylatoxin receptor in the effector phase of asthma. Nature 2000; 406: 998–1001.
37. Hopken UE, Lu B, Gerard NP et al. Impaired inflammatory responses in the reverse arthus reaction through genetic deletion of the C5a receptor. J Exp Med 1997; 186: 749–756.
38. Lachmann PJ, Walport MJ. Deficiency of the effector mechanisms of the immune response and autoimmunity. Ciba Found Symp 1987; 129: 149–171.
39. Walport MJ, Davies KA, Botto M. C1q and systemic lupus erythematosus. Immunobiology 1998; 199: 265–285.
40. Pickering MC, Botto M, Taylor PR et al. Systemic lupus erythematosus, complement deficiency, and apoptosis. Adv Immunol 2000; 76: 227–324.
41. Korb LC, Ahearn JM. C1q binds directly and specifically to surface blebs of apoptotic human keratinocytes: complement deficiency and systemic lupus erythematosus revisited. J Immunol 1997; 158: 4525–4528.
42. Botto M, Dell'Agnola C, Bygrave AE et al. Homozygous C1q deficiency causes glomerulonephritis associated with multiple apoptotic bodies. Nat Genet 1998; 19: 56–59.
43. Taylor PR, Carugati A, Fadok VA et al. A hierarchical role for classical pathway complement proteins in the clearance of apoptotic cells in vivo. J Exp Med 2000; 192: 359–366.
44. Pepys MB. Role of complement in induction of antibody production in vivo. Effect of cobra factor and other C3-reactive agents on thymus-dependent and thymus-independent antibody responses. J Exp Med 1974; 140: 126–145.
45. Papamichail M, Gutierrez C, Embling P et al. Complement dependence of localisation of aggregated IgG in germinal centres. Scand J Immunol 1975; 4: 343–347.
46. Bottger EC, Metzger S, Bitter-Suermann D et al. Impaired humoral immune response in complement C3-deficient guinea pigs: absence of secondary antibody response. Eur J Immunol 1986; 16: 1231–1235.
47. Fischer MB, Ma M, Goerg S et al. Regulation of the B cell response to T-dependent antigens by classical pathway complement. J Immunol 1996; 157: 549–556.
48. Cutler AJ, Botto M, van Essen D et al. T cell-dependent immune response in C1q-deficient mice: defective interferon gamma production by antigen-specific T cells. J Exp Med 1998; 187: 1789–1797.
49. Ahearn JM, Fischer MB, Croix D et al. Disruption of the Cr2 locus results in a reduction in B-1a cells and in an impaired B cell response to T-dependent antigen. Immunity 1996; 4: 251–262.
50. Molina H, Holers VM, Li B et al. Markedly impaired humoral immune response in mice deficient in complement receptors 1 and 2. Proc Natl Acad Sci USA 1996; 93: 3357–3361.
51. Dempsey PW, Allison ME, Akkaraju S et al. C3d of complement as a molecular adjuvant: bridging innate and acquired immunity. Science 1996; 271: 348–350.
52. Fearon DT, Carter RH. The CD19/CR2/TAPA-1 complex of B lymphocytes: linking natural to acquired immunity. Annu Rev Immunol 1995; 13: 127–149.
53. Erlendsson K, Traustadottir K, Freysdottir J et al. Reciprocal changes in complement activity and immune-complex levels during plasma infusion in a C2-deficient SLE patient. Lupus 1993; 2: 161–165.
54. Steinsson K, Erlendsson K, Valdimarsson H. Successful plasma infusion treatment of a patient with C2 deficiency and systemic lupus erythematosus: clinical experience over forty-five months. Arthritis Rheum 1989; 32: 906–913.
55. Hudson-Peacock MJ, Joseph SA, Cox J et al. Systemic lupus erythematosus complicating complement type 2 deficiency: successful treatment with fresh frozen plasma. Br J Dermatol 1997; 136: 388–392.
56. Botto M, Walport MJ. Hereditary deficiency of C3 in animals and humans. Int Rev Immunol 1993; 10: 37–50.
57. Densen P, Weiler J, Ackerman L et al. Functional and antigenic analysis of human factor B deficiency [abstract]. Mol Immunol 1996; 33(suppl 1): 68.
58. Hiemstra PS, Langeler E, Compier B et al. Complete and partial deficiencies of complement factor D in a Dutch family. J Clin Invest 1989; 84: 1957–1961.
59. Biesma DH, Hannema AJ, van Velzen-Blad H et al. A family with complement factor D deficiency. J Clin Invest 2001; 108: 233–240.
60. Sjoholm AG, Braconier JH, Soderstrom C. Properdin deficiency in a family with fulminant meningococcal infections. Clin Exp Immunol 1982; 50: 291–297.
61. Fukumori Y, Yoshimura K, Ohnoki S et al. A high incidence of C9 deficiency among healthy blood donors in Osaka, Japan. Int Immunol 1989; 1: 85–89.
62. Madsen HO, Garred P, Thiel S et al. Interplay between promoter and structural gene variants control basal serum level of mannan-binding protein. J Immunol 1995; 155: 3013–3020.
63. Lipscombe RJ, Sumiya M, Summerfield JA et al. Distinct physicochemical characteristics of human mannose binding protein expressed by individuals of differing genotype. Immunology 1995; 85: 660–667.
64. Summerfield JA, Ryder S, Sumiya M et al. Mannose binding protein gene mutations associated with unusual and severe infections in adults. Lancet 1995; 345: 886–889.
65. Super M, Gillies SD, Foley S et al. Distinct and overlapping functions of allelic forms of human mannose binding protein. Nat Genet 1992; 2: 50–55.
66. Bellamy R, Ruwende C, McAdam KP et al. Mannose binding protein deficiency is not associated with malaria, hepatitis B carriage nor tuberculosis in Africans. Q J Med 1998; 91: 13–18.
67. Cicardi M, Bergamaschini L, Cugno M et al. Pathogenetic and clinical aspects of C1 inhibitor deficiency. Immunobiology 1998; 199: 366–376.
68. Nussberger J, Cugno M, Amstutz C et al. Plasma bradykinin in angio-oedema. Lancet 1998; 351: 1693–1697.
69. Waytes AT, Rosen FS, Frank MM. Treatment of hereditary angioedema with a vapor-heated C1 inhibitor concentrate. N Engl J Med 1996; 334: 1630–1634.
70. Naked GM, Florido MP, Ferreira de Paula P et al. Deficiency of human complement factor I associated with lowered factor H. Clin Immunol 2000; 96: 162–167.
71. Sadallah S, Gudat F, Laissue JA et al. Glomerulonephritis in a patient with complement factor I deficiency. Am J Kidney Dis 1999; 33: 1153–1157.
72. Amadei N, Baracho GV, Nudelman V et al. Inherited complete factor I deficiency associated with systemic lupus erythematosus, higher susceptibility to infection and low levels of factor H. Scand J Immunol 2001; 53: 615–621.
73. Vyse TJ, Spath PJ, Davies KA et al. Hereditary complement factor I deficiency. Q J Med 1994; 87: 385–401.
74. Leitao MF, Vilela MM, Rutz R et al. Complement factor I deficiency in a family with recurrent infections. Immunopharmacology 1997; 38: 207–113.
75. Thompson RA, Winterborn MH. Hypocomplementaemia due to a genetic deficiency of beta 1H globulin. Clin Exp Immunol 1981; 46: 110–119.
76. Brai M, Misiano G, Maringhini S et al. Combined homozygous factor H and heterozygous C2 deficiency in an Italian family. J Clin Immunol 1988; 8: 50–56.
77. Pichette V, Querin S, Schurch W et al. Familial hemolytic-uremic syndrome and homozygous factor H deficiency. Am J Kidney Dis 1994; 24: 936–941.
78. Rougier N, Kazatchkine MD, Rougier JP et al. Human complement factor H deficiency associated with hemolytic uremic syndrome. J Am Soc Nephrol 1998; 9: 2318–2326.
79. Ohali M, Shalev H, Schlesinger M et al. Hypocomplementemic autosomal recessive hemolytic uremic syndrome with decreased factor H. Pediatr Nephrol 1998; 12: 619–624.
80. Lopez-Larrea C, Dieguez MA, Enguix A et al. A familial deficiency of complement factor H. Biochem Soc Trans 1987; 15: 648–649.
81. Levy M, Halbwachs-Mecarelli L, Gubler MC et al. H deficiency in two brothers with atypical dense intramembranous deposit disease. Kidney Int 1986; 30: 949–956.
82. Bessler M, Mason PJ, Hillmen P et al. Paroxysmal nocturnal haemoglobinuria (PNH) is caused by somatic mutations in the PIG-A gene. EMBO J 1994; 13: 110–117.

83. Yamashina M, Ueda E, Kinoshita T *et al*. Inherited complete deficiency of 20-kilodalton homologous restriction factor (CD59) as a cause of paroxysmal nocturnal hemoglobinuria. N Engl J Med 1990; 323: 1184–1189.

84. Spitzer RE, Vallota EH, Forristal J *et al*. Serum C´3 lytic system in patients with glomerulonephritis. Science 1969; 164: 436–437.

85. Antes U, Heinz HP, Loos M. Evidence for the presence of autoantibodies to the collagen-like portion of C1q in systemic lupus erythematosus. Arthritis Rheum 1988; 31: 457–464.

86. Daha MR, Fearon DT, Austen KF. C3 nephritic factor (C3NeF): stabilization of fluid phase and cell-bound alternative pathway convertase. J Immunol 1976; 116: 1–7.

87. Sissons JG, West RJ, Fallows J *et al*. The complement abnormalities of lipodystrophy. N Engl J Med 1976; 294: 461–465.

88. Siegert C, Daha M, Westedt ML *et al*. IgG autoantibodies against C1q are correlated with nephritis, hypocomplementemia, and dsDNA antibodies in systemic lupus erythematosus. J Rheumatol 1991; 18: 230–234.

89. Trendelenburg M, Marfurt J, Gerber I *et al*. Lack of occurrence of severe lupus nephritis among anti-C1q autoantibody-negative patients. Arthritis Rheum 1999; 42: 187–188.

90. Siegert CE, Daha MR, Tseng CM *et al*. Predictive value of IgG autoantibodies against C1q for nephritis in systemic lupus erythematosus. Ann Rheum Dis 1993; 52: 851–856.

91. Coremans IE, Spronk PE, Bootsma H *et al*. Changes in antibodies to C1q predict renal relapses in systemic lupus erythematosus. Am J Kidney Dis 1995; 26: 595–601.

92. Mannik M, Wener MH. Deposition of antibodies to the collagen-like region of C1q in renal glomeruli of patients with proliferative lupus glomerulonephritis. Arthritis Rheum 1997; 40: 1504–1511.

93. Jackson J, Sim RB, Whelan A *et al*. An IgG autoantibody which inactivates C1-inhibitor. Nature 1986; 323: 722–724.

94. Daha MR, Hazevoet HM, Vanes LA. Regulation of immune complex-mediated complement activation by autoantibodies (F-42) isolated from sera of patients with systemic lupus erythematosus. Clin Exp Immunol 1983; 53: 541–546.

95. Lloyd W, Schur PH. Immune complexes, complement, and anti-DNA in exacerbations of systemic lupus erythematosus (SLE). Medicine (Baltimore) 1981; 60: 208–217.

96. Hopkins P, Belmont HM, Buyon J *et al*. Increased levels of plasma anaphylatoxins in systemic lupus erythematosus predict flares of the disease and may elicit vascular injury in lupus cerebritis. Arthritis Rheum 1988; 31: 632–6341.

97. Negoro N, Okamura M, Takeda T *et al*. The clinical significance of iC3b neoantigen expression in plasma from patients with systemic lupus erythematosus. Arthritis Rheum 1989; 32: 1233–1242.

98. Perrin LH, Lambert PH, Miescher PA. Complement breakdown products in plasma from patients with systemic lupus erythematosus and patients with membranoproliferative or other glomerulonephritis. J Clin Invest 1975; 56: 165–176.

99. Perrin LH, Nydegger UE, Zubler RH *et al*. Correlation between levels of breakdown products of C3, C4, and properdin factor B in synovial fluids from patients with rheumatoid arthritis. Arthritis Rheum 1977; 20: 647–652.

100. Linton SM, Morgan BP. Complement activation and inhibition in experimental models of arthritis. Mol Immunol 1999; 36: 905–914.

101. Scott DG, Bacon PA, Allen C *et al*. IgG rheumatoid factor, complement and immune complexes in rheumatoid synovitis and vasculitis: comparative and serial studies during cytotoxic therapy. Clin Exp Immunol 1981; 43: 54–63.

102. Zeiss CR, Burch FX, Marder RJ *et al*. A hypocomplementemic vasculitic urticarial syndrome. Report of four new cases and definition of the disease. Am J Med 1980; 68: 867–875.

103. Wisnieski JJ, Naff GB. Serum IgG antibodies to C1q in hypocomplementemic urticarial vasculitis syndrome. Arthritis Rheum 1989; 32: 1119–1127.

104. Wisnieski JJ, Baer AN, Christensen J *et al*. Hypocomplementemic urticarial vasculitis syndrome. Clinical and serologic findings in 18 patients. Medicine (Baltimore) 1995; 74: 24–41.

105. Brouet JC, Clauvel JP, Danon F *et al*. Biologic and clinical significance of cryoglobulins. A report of 86 cases. Am J Med 1974; 57: 775–788.

106. Tarantino A, Anelli A, Costantino A *et al*. Serum complement pattern in essential mixed cryoglobulinaemia. Clin Exp Immunol 1978; 32: 77–85.

107. Agnello V, Chung RT, Kaplan LM. A role for hepatitis C virus infection in type II cryoglobulinemia. N Engl J Med 1992; 327: 1490–1495.

108. Davies KA. Complement, immune complexes and systemic lupus erythematosus: Michael Mason Prize Essay 1995. Br J Rheumatol 1996; 35: 5–23.

109. Davies KA, Beynon HL, Walport MJ. Long-term management after splenectomy. Consider prophylaxis in systematic lupus erythematosus. BMJ 1994; 308: 133.

120 Autoantibodies in SLE

Marvin J Fritzler and Keith B Elkon

- Some autoantibodies have a high diagnostic specificity for systemic lupus erythematosus (SLE), particularly anti-Sm, anti-dsDNA and anti-ribosome P
- The levels of some autoantibodies parallel disease activity
- Certain autoantibodies are associated with clinical subsets of disease
- Some autoantibodies may directly or indirectly cause cell or tissue injury
- Autoantibodies provide important clues to the etiology of SLE
- Autoantibodies are useful tools for cell biologists to use in exploring the function of the cellular antigens

HISTORICAL PERSPECTIVE

Discovery of the 'LE cell' in 1948 and the subsequent identification of the plasma requirement for the LE cell phenomenon in the following year, the detection of antiphospholipid antibodies in 1952 and the recognition of antiDNA antibodies and the 'antinuclear factor' in 1957 provided the first clues to the striking serologic abnormalities present in the blood of patients with systemic lupus erythematosus (SLE) and led to the concept of SLE as an autoimmune disease (reviewed by Christian and Elkon[1]). Identification of other autoantibodies with different specificities distinguished on the basis of 'lines of identity' by immunodiffusion soon followed. By the early 1970s, autoantibodies to histones, Sm, ribonucleoprotein (RNP), Ro(SS-A), La(SS-B) antigens and ribosomes had also been described. When the nature of the antigen was unknown (Sm, Ro and La), the autoantibodies were named after the patients in whom they were first described.

In the 1980s, technological advances in immunoprecipitation of radiolabeled cell extracts and Western blotting provided the tools to elucidate the molecular nature of the nucleic acid and protein antigens in SLE and other diseases. The Sm, Ro and La antigens were found to be RNP complexes, each comprising one or more proteins and several small RNAs. In the 1990s, advances in recombinant DNA technology enabled most of the protein autoantigens to be molecularly cloned and to be synthesized in large quantities. In several instances, identification of the antigenic sites or epitopes on the protein has enabled relevant parts of the antigen to be chemically synthesized. Immunoassays utilizing recombinant or synthetic antigens are replacing conventional tests for the detection of autoantibodies.

ANTIBODIES, ANTIGENS AND THE NORMAL IMMUNE RESPONSE

At present, it is uncertain whether the autoantibodies produced in SLE result from an immune response that is appropriate to an initial immunizing antigen, or whether the antibodies are produced because of a defect in immune regulation (see Mechanisms of autoantibody production, below). Regardless of the mechanisms involved, many attributes of autoantibodies can best be understood in the context of an immune response.

Autoantibodies are immunoglobulins that bind via their combining sites to antigens originating in the same individual or species (autoantigen). The specificity of the antibody is conveyed by the variable regions of the heavy (V_H) and light (V_L) chains, whereas the biological properties (e.g. complement fixation, binding to Fc receptors) are dictated by the constant region of the heavy chains (C_H). These biological effects depend on the immunoglobulin isotype (IgM, IgG, IgA, IgD, IgE) and subclass/isotype (IgG1–4, IgA1–2). Although any antibody binding to a 'self' antigen becomes by definition an autoantibody, the binding may or may not be relevant to autoimmune diseases. Natural antibodies are immunoglobulins, predominantly of the IgM isotype, that occur in normal individuals and bind to a variety of self proteins[2]. The function of these autoantibodies is uncertain, but they may serve a beneficial role in helping to clear self molecules from the circulation.

An idiotype is an antigenic determinant present on the variable region of an antibody molecule. As such, it is made up of a region of V_H, V_L or the V_H–V_L structure (Fig. 120.1). Jerne has proposed that anti-idiotype antibodies regulate the production of the immunoglobulin bearing the idiotype[3]. Idiotypes may be private (present in a single individual) or public and cross-reactive (present in many individuals, usually of the same strain or species).

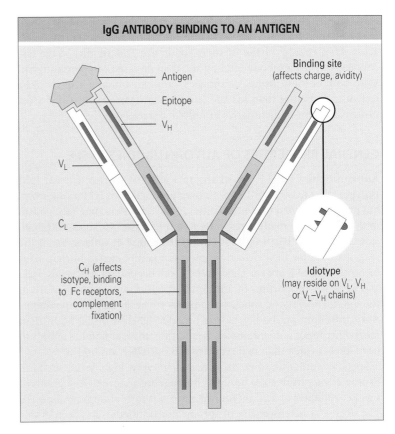

IgG ANTIBODY BINDING TO AN ANTIGEN

Antigen
Epitope
V_H
V_L
C_L
Binding site (affects charge, avidity)
C_H (affects isotype, binding to Fc receptors, complement fixation)
Idiotype (may reside on V_L, V_H or V_L–V_H chains)

Fig. 120.1 Schematic diagram of an IgG antibody binding to an antigen. C, constant region; H, heavy chain; L, light chain; V, variable region.

The significance of an autoantibody should be evaluated by considering the antibody, the antigen and the assay used for detection. Important features of the antibody are its class, valence, titer, clonality and affinity. IgM antibodies reflect a primary immune response, are pentavalent (hence, much more efficient in hemagglutination assays) and are usually of low affinity (therefore much more likely to bind non-specifically). In contrast, bivalent IgG antibodies indicate persistent antigen stimulation analogous to secondary immunization. These antibodies are usually of high affinity and, after binding to their cognate antigen, produce precipitin lines in agarose gels (immunodiffusion and counter-immunoelectrophoresis assays). This type of autoantibody is prominent both in multisystem and in most organ-specific autoimmune diseases.

The autoantigen may be a protein, nucleic acid, carbohydrate, lipid or a multimolecular complex. Although any self molecule that is bound by an antibody is an antigen, this does not necessarily imply that the antigen is the immunogen (the molecule that induced the production of the antibody). The relationship between the antigen and the immunogen is one of the central questions in autoimmunity.

The immune response to foreign protein antigens is polyclonal (derived from many B cell clones). Monoclonal antibodies arise from neoplastic proliferation of a single B cell clone, or are produced by *in vitro* fusions of individual B cells in the laboratory. The failure of monoclonal antibodies to form precipitin lines in agarose gels, and their frequent cross-reactivity or 'polyspecificity'[4], may make the specificity of monoclonal autoantibodies difficult to establish. A large proportion of monoclonal autoantibodies, especially those obtained from humans, have the properties of natural autoantibodies, namely IgM class, low affinity and polyspecificity.

Solid phase immunoassays, such as hemagglutination, enzyme-linked immunosorbent assays (ELISA) and radioimmunoassays, are influenced by total immunoglobulin concentrations, and readily detect low-affinity antibodies. Consequently, these assays are more likely to give false positive tests for autoantibodies than are agarose gels, immunoprecipitation or western blots. Finally, the nature of the antigen should be considered. Highly charged molecules such as DNA, histones and IgG itself may be bound by antibodies with oppositely charged clusters of amino acids. Haptens, by virtue of their small size and rigidity, have less contact with the antibody binding site than do large complex antigens. With both of these groups of antigens, antibody binding is likely to be less discriminating than for the complex tertiary structures of most protein antigens in their native or unfolded state.

GENERAL PROPERTIES OF AUTOANTIBODIES IN SLE

Autoantibodies in SLE are of the IgG and, to a lesser extent, IgM isotypes[5]. The reason for the continuing production of IgM is unknown, but it may be related to abnormalities in the class-switching mechanism in the B cell or, perhaps, a response to mitogens or cytokines. Although subclass analysis has been more difficult because of differences in the reagents used for their detection, most autoantibodies to nucleic acids or proteins in SLE are enriched in the T cell dependent subclasses, IgG1 and IgG3[6]. A proportion of anti-Sm and anti-P autoantibodies are of the IgG2 subclass, a subclass believed to be T cell independent[7]. Anticardiolipin antibodies have a broader subclass distribution than most other lupus autoantibodies. In addition, these antibodies appear to be of lower avidity than that reported for anti-DNA antibodies[8].

Specific autoantibodies are present at very high levels in SLE. Estimates vary from a few hundred micrograms to several milligrams of IgG per milliliter of serum (equivalent to 0.1–20% of total serum IgG). The degree of heterogeneity of specific autoantibodies has been evaluated by isoelectric focusing (separation of proteins according to their charge) and by determining the light-chain distribution of the antibody.

These studies indicate that there is a polyclonal immune response to each autoantigen. In general, therefore, the properties of autoantibodies in SLE resemble the properties of antibodies to foreign protein antigens. The relevance of these findings in relation to the etiology of the disease is discussed in the section on Mechanisms of Autoantibody Production.

Several public idiotypes on anti-DNA antibodies have been described in both human and murine SLE. In some cases, the titers of the idiotype and anti-idiotype[9] suggest a regulatory role for the anti-idiotype. Some idiotypes appear to be strongly associated with tissue injury and therefore may serve as additional serologic markers of disease activity.

In most autoimmune diseases, autoantibodies are polyclonal. This is more obvious in multisystem autoimmune diseases in which individual patient sera react with several nucleic acid and protein antigens and therefore must be derived from different clonal precursors. Moreover, when the humoral immune response to individual protein antigens has been analyzed in detail, most sera have been found to contain antibodies to several epitopes (antigenic sites) on each protein. Most evidence suggests that autoantibodies are produced as a focused immune response to a relatively select group of structurally or functionally related nucleoprotein antigens. The autoantibodies themselves have the characteristics of a secondary immune response – high-titer antibodies of the IgG isotype, evidence of extensive somatic mutation typical of an antigen-driven immune response and restriction in the idiotypes, particularly anti-DNA antibodies.

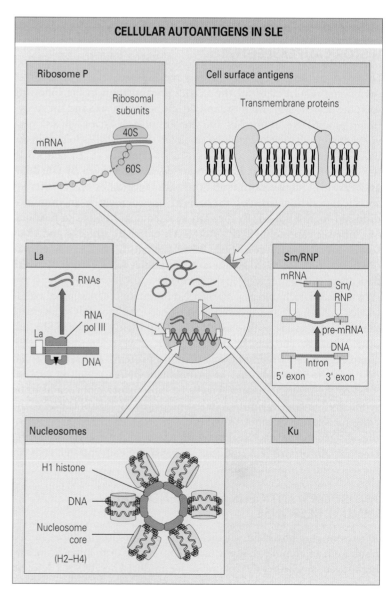

Fig. 120.2 Cellular autoantigens in SLE.

The reasons why the patient should mount an immune response to acetylcholine receptors in myasthenia gravis, to nucleosomes and RNP complexes in SLE and to nucleolar components in scleroderma remain unknown. This may in part reflect the major histocompatibility complex (MHC) type of the patient group, but this is not the entire explanation.

SPECIFIC AUTOANTIBODIES

Autoantibodies in SLE primarily target intranuclear nucleic acids, proteins and nucleoprotein complexes and are often referred to as antinuclear antibodies (ANA). SLE autoantibodies also bind to cell surface antigens that are expressed on certain cell types, including lymphocytes, and neuroblastoma cell lines, in addition to various plasma and extracellular components. In some cases, the antigen may be located at several sites; for example, negatively charged phospholipids are normally located on the inner surface of cell membranes and in the mitochondria. The locations of these antigens are shown in Figure 120.2, and their structure and function (where known) are summarized in Table 120.1.

Antibodies to DNA and DNA-binding proteins

Anti-DNA

The genetic information of all living organisms is contained in DNA. When intact, DNA forms a double-stranded helix as a result of pairing between complementary bases on each strand. DNA in higher animals is carried on chromosomes. Within the nucleus, DNA is compacted and surrounded by proteins. Some of these proteins, such as histones, are predominantly structural, whereas other proteins regulate transcription (synthesis of RNA) or DNA replication. DNA–histone complexes are called chromatin, and chromatin is packed in repeating structures called nucleosomes. Each nucleosome comprises 200 base pairs of DNA twisted around an octamer of histones (two molecules each of H2A, H2B, H3 and H4) (Fig. 120.2). The histone H1 is believed to bind on the surface and stabilize the nucleosome by linking adjacent nucleosomes.

As anti-DNA antibodies were discovered about 40 years ago, a voluminous literature describing their properties and associations now exists[10,11]. At least three forms of DNA are antigenic in SLE: single-stranded (ss)DNA, double-stranded (ds)DNA and left-handed (Z)DNA. Many lupus sera contain antibodies that bind to more than one form of DNA. However, anti-dsDNA antibodies are rarely found in diseases other than SLE. Anti-DNA antibodies bind predominantly to the sugar phosphate backbone of DNA and therefore bind to DNA obtained from any species.

Anti-dsDNA antibodies are detected in approximately 60% of patients with SLE (Table 120.2), although the exact frequency depends on the test used for detection. In general, anti-dsDNA levels reflect disease activity, but sufficient exceptions occur to make antibody levels of limited value in many patients. The strongest clinical association of anti-DNA has been with nephritis. Once again, however, anti-DNA antibodies are not a *sine qua non* for the development of nephritis, and patients may have high levels of anti-DNA antibodies without overt renal disease. There are many possible explanations for these discrepancies that may be related to the antibody (affinity, fine specificity, subclass), the antigen (size, conformation, accessory proteins) or the test used to detect anti-DNA. Tests that utilize solution-phase binding to radiolabeled DNA, such as the Farr assay, detect relatively high-affinity antibodies, whereas solid phase immunoassays, such as ELISA and the Crithidia lucilliae immunofluoresence assays, also detect low-affinity interactions.

TABLE 120.1 THE STRUCTURE AND FUNCTION OF SLE AUTOANTIGENS

Antigen	Structure	Function
Intracellular		
DNA	Double helix	Template for transcription and replication
Histones	H1, H2A, H2B, H3, H4	Components of chromatin
Ro (SS-A)	52, 60kDa proteins	Unknown
	? Calreticulin	Calcium binding protein
La (SS-B)	48kDa phosphoprotein	Transcription termination factor
Sm	B, B', D and E proteins	Spliceosome components
RNP	68kDa, A and C proteins	Spliceosome components
U1 RNA	Small nuclear RNA	Spliceosome component
P	P0, P1, P2 ribosomal proteins	Factor binding for protein synthesis
28S RNA	Ribosomal RNA	GTPase domain
Ku/Ki	70 and 80kDa proteins	Repair DNA breaks
Cell membrane		
Lymphocyte	CD45 (and others)	Phosphotyrosine phosphatase
Red cell	?	
Platelet	?	
Neuroblastoma	? 97kDa protein	Unknown
Stress proteins	hsp 73, 90	Protein transport/folding
Serum		
Phospholipid	Acidic phospholipids	Coagulation
		Cell membrane component
IgG*	see Fig. 120.1	Antibody

* IgG aggregates or immune complexes are the antigens recognized by rheumatoid factor

TABLE 120.2 CLINICAL ASSOCIATIONS OF AUTOANTIBODIES IN SLE

Antibody	Frequency (%)*	Specificity† for SLE	Clinical subset
dsDNA	60–90	++	Nephritis
ssDNA	90	–	
Histones	50–70	+	
H2A, H2B		+	Drug-induced lupus
Ro(SS-A)	20–60	+	Subacute cutaneous lupus,
La(SS-B)	15–40	+	congenital heart block
Sm	10–30	++	? Nephritis, ? CNS
RNP	10–30	+	Mixed connective tissue disease§
U1 RNP	10	+	
P	10–15	++	Lupus psychosis
28S RNA	8–12	++	
Ku/Ki	10	+	
Cardiolipin	10–30	–	Thrombosis, fetal loss, thrombocytopenia

* The frequency depends upon the sensitivity of the test used to detect the antibodies. The higher frequencies are usually observed in ELISAs or radioimmunoassays. In the case of anti-Sm antibodies, higher frequencies are observed in blacks

† ++ = highly specific; + = antibody present in other autoimmune disorders; – = antibody present in other inflammatory diseases

§ An overlap syndrome of SLE, polymyositis and scleroderma occurring in higher frequency in patients with anti-RNP and anti-Sm antibodies: (see Chapter 142)

Systemic lupus erythematosus has been considered to be the human equivalent of experimental serum sickness, and DNA–anti-DNA immune complexes are believed to be responsible for glomerulonephritis. Considerable evidence supports this model, including detection of free DNA in the plasma, changes in serum anti-DNA and complement concentrations consistent with the formation of immune complexes, and detection of anti-DNA antibodies in the kidneys[12]. As described later, more recent studies have challenged the traditional explanation for glomerulonephritis in SLE. Although it seems likely that DNA–anti-DNA immune complexes are, in part, responsible for glomerulonephritis in many patients with lupus, in situ formation of immune reactants and other mechanisms of tissue injury are also likely to be involved[13].

Increasing evidence suggests that anti-DNA and antihistone autoantibodies (see below) reflect a dominant immune response to nucleosomes. This is important in relation to evolving concepts of apoptosis in SLE (see Mechanisms of Autoantibody Production).

Antihistone

Autoantibodies to histones have been detected in up to 90% of patients with idiopathic and drug-induced lupus. The correlation of clinical features and disease activity with histone antibody titers or classes is not clearly established. Depending on the antigen used (intact nucleosomes, purified histones, synthetic peptides) and the method used for detection of antibodies, binding to all histone components, particularly H1 and H2B, and the higher-order structures of chromatin has been reported in SLE. It has been shown that the LE cell formed in vivo, and the LE cell phenomenon demonstrated in vitro, were dependent on the histone H1 and mediated by histone antibodies[14].

The specificities of antihistone autoantibodies differ in lupus induced by different drugs. Procainamide and quinidine induce IgG antibodies reactive with an (H2A–H2B)DNA complex, although these antibodies do not bind to dsDNA. In contrast, hydralazine and chlorpromazine induce IgM antibodies that bind to H1, H3–H4, H2A–H2B and ssDNA[15]. Antihistone antibodies have also been detected in other diseases such as adult and juvenile rheumatoid arthritis and systemic sclerosis.

As discussed above, a pathogenic role for anti-dsDNA and anti-dsDNA-DNA complexes in the development of lupus nephritis has been considered. More recent evidence has suggested a key role for histone-DNA-anti-DNA complexes also. This is supported by studies showing that the binding of anti-DNA antibodies to glomerular basement membranes is enhanced by the sequential perfusion of purified histones and then DNA[16].

Anti-Ku (Ki/nuclear factor IV)

Ku is a heterodimer comprising two proteins of 70kDa and 86kDa. It preferentially binds to the termini of dsDNA and has a role in DNA repair, although it may also function in DNA replication and recombination[17]. Anti-Ku antibodies produce both diffuse nuclear and nucleolar immunofluorescence staining. Evidence for enhanced binding to human rather than mouse antigen has been reported. Anti-Ku antibodies have been detected in scleroderma–myositis overlap, scleroderma and SLE.

Anti-PCNA (cyclin)

Proliferating cell nuclear antigen (PCNA) is a 36kDa protein known to be an auxiliary protein of DNA polymerase δ. Although the antibody is observed in fewer than 5% of SLE patients, the antigenic specificity of the antibody is of interest, because it produces positive nuclear immunofluorescence only in dividing cells. This observation is due to the fact that there is enhanced expression of the protein in the late G and early S phases of the cell cycle.

Antibodies to RNA and to ribonucleoproteins

Anti-RNA

Within the cell nucleus, DNA is transcribed into RNA by enzymes called RNA polymerases (pols). There are three different pols: pol I synthesizes ribosomal (r)RNA, pol II synthesizes messenger (m)RNA, and pol III synthesizes most small nuclear and cytoplasmic RNAs. In some cases, especially with small RNAs, the structure is characterized by intramolecular base pairing, whereas the structure of larger RNAs is also influenced by binding of RNA to proteins.

Autoantibodies reactive against single- and double-stranded RNA have been reported in up to 60% of patients with SLE[18]. No unique clinical associations with these antibodies have been observed. Anti-RNA antibodies are also found in lower frequency in patients with other autoimmune disorders.

Anti-Sm, anti-RNP and anti-U1 RNA

The Sm (B, B′, D and E) and RNP (A, C and 68kDa) proteins are complexed with uridine-rich (U) small nuclear RNAs1–3, 5 and 6 to form small nuclear (sn)RNPs (Fig. 120.2). Each snRNP particle consists of one (or two, U2/U4) U RNAs bound to Sm proteins. The Sm proteins are present on all the snRNPs, whereas the RNP proteins are present only on the U1 snRNP. The U2 snRNP contains the Sm proteins in addition to the unique proteins designated A′ and B″. snRNPs form part of the spliceosome, a much larger RNP that splices the introns out of pre-messenger RNA (Fig. 120.2)[19]. Anti-Sm antibodies bind preferentially to the B, B′ and D proteins.

Anti-Sm is detected in 3–10% of white and up to 30% of black and Chinese patients with SLE. The antibody is highly specific for SLE. Apart from its diagnostic utility, the clinical relevance of this autoantibody is controversial. Associations with renal and nervous system involvement have been reported and it has been suggested that levels of anti-Sm are useful indicators of disease activity.

Almost all sera containing anti-Sm also contain anti-RNP[20]; the converse, however, is not true. Patients with high titers of anti-RNP without anti-Sm frequently have an overlap syndrome (mixed connective tissue disease) characterized by clinical features of lupus, polymyositis and scleroderma (see Chapter 142). Most anti-Sm/RNP sera target several components of the snRNP. On immunoblots, SmB and B′ (two proteins that are identical except for the addition of 10 amino acids at the carboxyl terminus of SmB′, resulting from alternative splicing of a single RNA transcript) are immunodominant. In addition, approximately 40% of anti-RNP sera bind to U1 RNA. These sera appear to be remarkably specific, as they do not bind to the other U RNAs, despite the high degree of sequence homology. Immunoassays utilizing recombinant SmB and a carboxyl-terminal synthetic peptide that bears a dominant epitope appear to be sensitive alternatives for detection of anti-Sm antibodies.

Anti-Ro(SS-A) and anti-La(SS-B)

La is a nuclear phosphoprotein that binds to precursor transfer (t)RNAs and 5S rRNA (but not the mature RNA products), and to certain small RNAs encoded by viruses[21]. Recent studies suggest that La is a transcription termination factor. The most thoroughly characterized Ro proteins are Ro 60 and Ro 52 (the numbers are based on their molecular weights). These proteins do not have any sequence homology and are encoded by separate genes. Different isoforms of Ro 52 have been reported in different cell types. Both Ro 60 and Ro 52 are known to be present in both cytoplasmic and nuclear compartments. Ro 60 is complexed to small RNAs, Y1–5, that reside in the cytoplasm, although their presence in the nucleus has been described. Human cells contain four Ro RNAs: hY1, and hY3–5. Calreticulin, a protein involved in calcium binding in the endoplasmic reticulum, has been reported to be a Ro antigen. At present, anti-calreticulin antibodies are considered a separate population of antibodies that are sometimes detected in autoimmune diseases The structural or functional relationships between Ro and La remain uncertain.

The frequency of anti-Ro and anti-La in SLE depends upon the test used for detection. Anti-Ro is present in approximately 60% of SLE sera by immunodiffusion techniques but less than 20% by Western blots. These results are most likely explained by reactivity of anti-Ro sera to conformational epitopes, protein–RNA complexes, or both, which are dissociated on immunoblots. Conversely, anti-La is detected in approximately 20% of sera by immunodiffusion and 50–60% of sera by Western blots. When both tests are used, anti-Ro and anti-La are almost always both present in the same sera. Although most anti-Ro/La-positive patients with either SLE or Sjögren's syndrome have antibodies that bind to both Ro 60 and Ro 52, approximately 40% of Sjögren's anti-Ro sera recognize only Ro 52, and 20% of SLE sera bind to Ro 60, but not to Ro 52 in an immunoblot assay[22].

Anti-Ro/La antibodies are important clinically because they are associated with subacute cutaneous lupus erythematosus and with the neonatal lupus erythematosus syndrome. Subacute cutaneous lupus erythematosus is an annular form of cutaneous lupus that is exacerbated by exposure of the skin to sunlight[23]. Anti-Ro antibodies are present in approximately 70% of such patients. Anti-Ro antibodies are also detected more frequently in mothers of infants with the transient skin rash of neonatal lupus erythematosus. More importantly, anti-Ro/La antibodies are present in more than 80% of mothers of infants with congenital heart block (see Chapter 123) when sensitive tests such as ELISA or immunoblotting are used. The potential mechanisms of such associations are discussed below.

Antiribosomal antibodies

Soon after the discovery of antinuclear antibodies, it became evident that some autoantibodies in SLE and related diseases were directed against cytoplasmic constituents. One of the best defined anticytoplasmic antibodies are antiribosomal antibodies, which occur in approximately 10% of randomly selected SLE patients, but in up to 40% of patients with active disease. Antiribosomal antibodies are most frequently directed against three phosphoproteins (P proteins) – P0, P1 and P2 – located on the large ribosomal subunit (see Fig. 120.2). The shared, conserved carboxyl terminus of the P proteins contains the dominant antibody epitope in almost all sera tested[24]. Anti-P antibodies appear to be a highly specific diagnostic marker for SLE, as they are rarely detected in other multisystem autoimmune disorders. They increase in titer in patients with active disease and have been reported to be detected more frequently in patients with severe behavioral disturbances. This may be particularly true of patients with affective disorders. Other antiribosomal antibodies have been detected in patients with SLE. These antibodies include anti-28S rRNA, anti-S10 and anti-L12. In all cases, the frequencies with which these antibodies are detected are increased in sera containing anti-P. Despite the very large size of 28S rRNA (approximately 4 kilobases), the epitope recognized by anti-28S sera has been mapped to a 59 nucleotide fragment between nucleotide 1943 and 2002. This region of 28S rRNA is also highly conserved, and is believed to represent the guanine triphosphatase (GTPase) center of the ribosome. Guanosine triphosphate cleavage is an essential step for the activities of initiation, elongation and termination on the ribosome. The P proteins are also known to play essential, but as yet undefined, roles in GTPase activity on the ribosome. These findings indicate that some SLE patients produce autoantibodies directed against multiple components of a functionally related GTPase domain on the ribosome.

Antibodies to other intracellular antigens

Antibodies to a variety of other intracellular antigens have been described[25]. These include antibodies that react with components of the Golgi complex, endosomes, the mitotic spindle apparatus, onco-fetal antigens, RNA helicase and the proteasome α-type subunit. The frequency of each of these antibodies in SLE is very low, and large clinical cohorts of patients will need to be studied before clear-cut clinical correlations can be established.

Antibodies to cell membrane components
Antibodies to blood cells

Cold reactive lymphocytotoxic antibodies, predominantly of the IgM class, occur in up to 80% of patients with SLE. IgG and warm reactive antibodies have also been described. Antilymphocyte antibodies are produced in other autoimmune diseases as well as in virus infections. The specificities of antilymphocyte antibodies have been difficult to establish, because SLE sera frequently contain alloreactive antibodies induced by pregnancy or blood transfusions. In addition, many 'antilymphocyte' antibodies also bind to other cell types (e.g. neurons, erythrocytes). However, some antigens that are predominantly or exclusively located on lymphocytes, namely CD45 (a protein tyrosine phosphatase), and a glycoprotein of 46kDa, have been identified[26]. Antilymphocyte antibodies are potentially of pathogenetic significance, because they may be responsible for the lymphopenia characteristic of active SLE and, if targeted to certain receptors, could modulate lymphocyte function.

Approximately 10% of patients with SLE have a positive IgG Coomb's test. Although a positive test is generally interpreted to reflect the presence of anti-red cell antibodies, the demonstration that immune complexes bind to CR1 receptors on red cells (see Chapter 117) has made evaluation of the Coomb's test difficult. Erythrocyte-bound IgG is, in some cases, responsible for hemolytic anemia in patients with SLE.

Immune complexes also bind to platelets by the Fc receptor present on the platelet membrane. The presence and specificities of antiplatelet antibodies on SLE have therefore also been difficult to establish. Antiplatelet antibodies may contribute to thrombocytopenia.

Antineuronal antibodies

IgG and IgM antibodies that bind to the surface of neuroblastoma cells *in vitro* have been detected in the serum of patients with SLE. It has been suggested that the presence of IgG antineuronal antibodies in the cerebrospinal fluid correlate best with central nervous system involvement in SLE[27]. The association is strongest in patients with generalized central nervous system disease (psychosis, generalized seizures and 'organic brain syndrome'). It remains to be determined whether antineuroblastoma antibodies bind to neurons in the adult human brain. As in the case of antilymphocyte antibodies, the significance of autoantibodies binding to specific receptors on the cell surface is, potentially, considerable.

Antibodies to stress proteins

Stress or heat-shock proteins (hsp) are a family of highly conserved proteins that are induced by thermal and other noxious stimuli. Although these proteins are predominantly located within mitochondria and the endoplasmic reticulum, the proteins or their peptide fragments may be present on cell surfaces under certain circumstances. IgM antibodies to the 73kDa member of the hsp70 family and IgG antibodies to hsp90 have been identified in a small proportion of patients with SLE[28]. These proteins were localized to the lymphocyte plasma membrane. There is considerable interest in the immune response to stress proteins, in view of the strong proliferative response to hsp65 of T cells derived from several autoimmune diseases. Antibodies to calreticulin may also represent a response to stressed or dying cells.

Antiphospholipid antibodies

A false-positive test for syphilis and the lupus anticoagulant were among the first serologic abnormalities identified in patients with SLE. These antibodies bind to the acidic phospholipids cardiolipin, phosphatidylserine, phosphatidylinositol and phosphatidic acid. Because cardiolipin, and phosphatidylserine, are located within the cell (Fig. 120.2), these antigens are inaccessible on normal intact cells. Phospholipids are also present in serum bound to proteins (lipoproteins) and have important roles in the coagulation, and possibly other, cascades. Two important points relevant to antigenic specificity are noteworthy: first, most SLE antibodies that bind to cardiolipin recognize the complex of cardiolipin with β_2-glycoprotein I, a plasma protein; secondly, anti-cardiolipin antibodies bind more avidly to the oxidized than to the non-oxidized form of cardiolipin. Further details of the antigenic specificity and the association of anti-cardiolipin antibodies with thrombosis, fetal loss and thrombocytopenia are discussed in Chapter 131.

DETECTION OF AUTOANTIBODIES

Autoimmune diseases are frequently considered in the differential diagnosis of skin, kidney, joint, lung, hematologic, nervous system and other disorders. The most economical screening test and practical starting point is the ANA test. This test detects many autoantibodies that bind to non-tissue-specific intracellular antigens. The methods for detecting autoantibodies are illustrated in Figure 120.3 and their sensitivities and specificities compared in Table 120.3. Most commonly, the ANA test is performed by indirect immunofluorescence using an epithelial cell line, HEp-2, as a substrate. This substrate is far better than mouse kidney or liver in terms of sensitivity and ability to distinguish staining patterns produced by different autoantibodies seen in SLE. The patterns obtained by immunofluorescence provide a clue to the autoantibody specificity. For example, anti-DNA and antihistone give relatively homogeneous nuclear fluorescence; anti-Sm/RNP antibodies produce a coarse speckled nuclear staining, with sparing of the nucleoli (see also Chapter 21). However, autoantibody specificities cannot be diagnosed with certainty by the immunofluorescence pattern. Gel precipitation or other immunoassays using purified antigens are used for a more precise determination of autoantibody specificity. Immunoprecipitation of radiolabeled cell extracts and Western blots remain predominantly research applications but are both highly specific and sensitive tests.

There is growing use of commercially available ELISA kits that provide economical and rapid detection of ANA and related specific autoantibodies such as Sm, U1-RNP, Ro, La and ribosomal P proteins, but there are significant differences between the performance of kits provided by various manufacturers[29]. This is compounded further by interlaboratory variation of results, even when the same sera are tested with the same commercial kit. As an approach to increasing the accuracy and reliability of autoantibody testing, highly characterized consensus prototype sera have been made available through the Center for Disease Control in Atlanta, and standardization is being attempted by a number of organizations. Clinicians are encouraged to be familiar with the advantages and limitations of the various diagnostic tests being used in their setting . Newer technology based on advanced solid-phase systems (i.e. antigen arrays) and microfluidics hold promise for increased specificity and decreased intermanufacturer and interlaboratory variation of test results.

DIAGNOSTIC VALUE AND CLINICAL UTILITY

Some autoantibodies, such as rheumatoid factors and anti-ssDNA, are produced in infections and in a variety of autoimmune disorders and

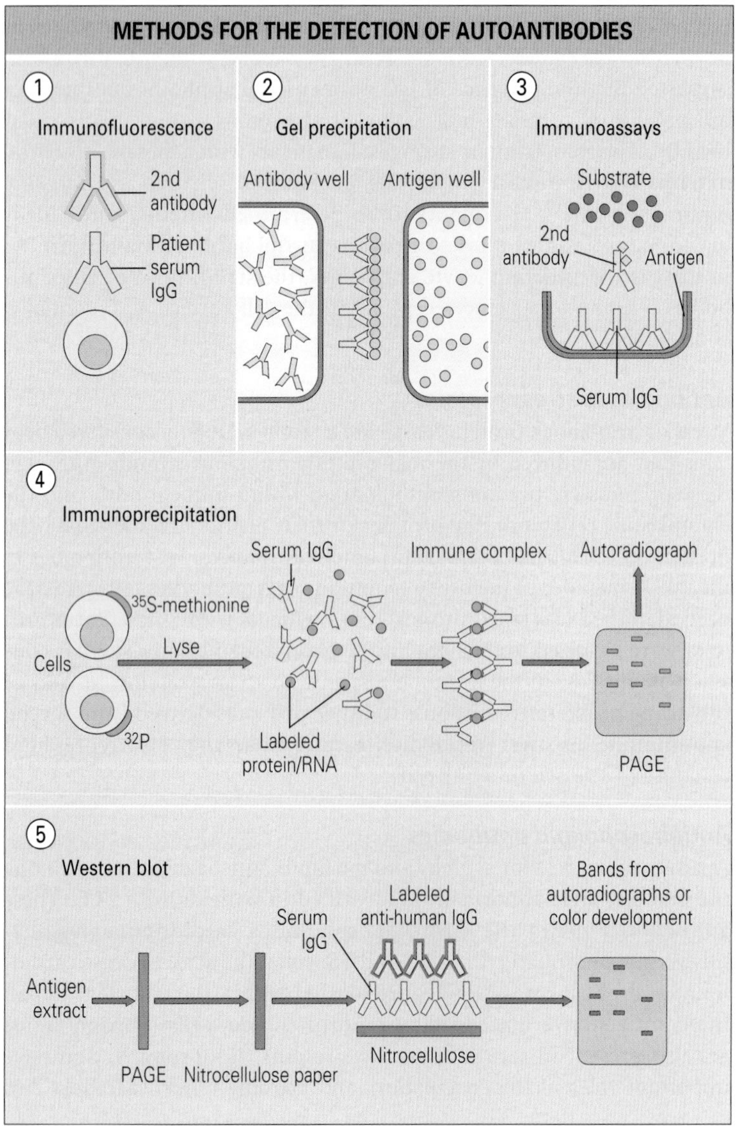

Fig. 120.3 Methods for the detection of autoantibodies.
(1) *Immunofluorescence*. The standard ANA test is performed by incubating fixed, permeabilized cells (usually HEp-2) on a glass slide with a dilution of the patient's serum, followed by conjugated anti-human IgG (or IgM). The slide is then viewed by microscopy and the intensity and pattern of fluorescence evaluated.
(2) *Gel precipitation*. Patient serum is placed in one (antibody) well and a saline-soluble extract (usually from rabbit thymus) in the other (antigen) well of an agarose gel on a glass slide. Either the antigen and antibody are allowed to diffuse (Ouchterlony immunodiffusion) or they are driven together by electrophoresis (counter-immunoelectrophoresis). If antibodies bind to an antigen in the extract, a line of precipitation forms. This precipitin line can be identified by applying known reference sera on either side of the patient serum.
(3) *Immunoassays*. ELISA: a purified antigen is coated onto the wells of a polystyrene microtiter plate. The plate is blocked with albumin and incubated with the patient's diluted serum, followed by anti-human IgG to which an enzyme such as alkaline phosphatase or horseradish peroxidase has been conjugated. A substrate for the enzyme is then added to each well and, depending on the amount of second antibody remaining on the plate, a color reaction develops. The color reaction is quantified spectrophotometrically. Solid-phase radioimmunoassays work on similar principles, except that the second antibody is radiolabeled and the bound antibody is quantified in a gamma counter.
(4) *Immunoprecipitation*. Cells in culture are incubated with ^{35}S-methionine (to radiolabel proteins) or ^{32}P (to label nucleic acids). The cells are lysed and incubated with patient IgG adsorbed to protein-A beads. The antibodies bind to the labeled antigens and these antigens are eluted from the beads and applied to polyacrylamide gels to separate the components by size (polyacrylamide gel electrophoresis; PAGE). The gels are exposed to radiographic film (autoradiography) and bands corresponding to the labeled antigens are seen on the autoradiograph. (5) *Western blot*. An antigen extract is applied to a polyacrylamide gel and the components separated by PAGE. After electrophoresis, the proteins are electrophoretically blotted to nitrocellulose paper. Strips of nitrocellulose paper are then sequentially probed with a dilution of patient serum followed by an enzyme-labeled or radiolabeled second antibody. The molecular weight of the protein is then determined by comparison with molecular weight standards.

TABLE 120.3 SENSITIVITY AND SPECIFICITIES OF TESTS USED TO DETECT SLE AUTOANTIBODIES

Method	Test Antigen	Sensitivity	Specificity	Application
Immunofluorescence	Whole cells Kinetoplast (Crithidia) Specific cell lines	+++ +++ +++	+ ++++ +	Screening for ANA Detect anti-DNA Detect antimembrane antibodies
Gel precipitation	Soluble cell extract	+	+++	Screening specific antibodies
ELISA	Recombinant proteins* Synthetic peptides† DNA Cardiolipin	++++ ++++ +++ +++	+++ +++ +++ ++++	Specific detection and quantitation
RIA	DNA (Farr)	++++	+++	Specific detection and quantitation

* The following protein antigens have been cloned and used for detection of antibodies: Ro, La, SmB, RNP (68, A, C), ribosomal P proteins, Ku

† The following synthetic peptide antigens have been used successfully for detection of antibodies: ribosomal P proteins, calreticulin, SmB

RIA, radiommunoassay

are therefore of little help in the differential diagnosis of disease. In contrast, most of the autoantibodies found in SLE are not detected in chronic infections. A negative ANA test result makes the diagnosis of SLE or any other systemic autoimmune disease highly unlikely, whereas a positive test (especially a titer greater than 1/160) strongly supports the diagnosis. Exceptions to this rule are the vasculitides, in which the ANA is positive in only about 33% of cases. Antineutrophil cytoplasmic autoantibodies are, however, more frequently detected in these diseases when neutrophils are used as a cell substrate (see Chapters 143 & 145). Although the exclusive presence of anti-Ro antibodies was, at one time, believed o be associated with ANA-negative lupus, most patients with anti-Ro have positive ANAs on HEp-2 or other tissue culture cells. Some SLE sera with exclusive antiribosomal activity are ANA-negative in a strict sense, but show strong cytoplasmic staining on HEp-2 cells.

Few, if any, autoantibodies can be used alone to diagnose an autoimmune disease, because autoantibodies may be detected in individuals without overt clinical disease (particularly relatives of patients with autoimmune diseases[5]. Furthermore, some autoantibodies, although highly specific, are present in a minority of patients (e.g. anti-Sm occurs in only 5–30% of patients with SLE). For these reasons, detection of autoantibodies is usually used to confirm a clinical diagnosis or to help to define a subset of patients within the diagnostic category of SLE (Table 120.2). Detection of anti-dsDNA, Sm or ribosomal P protein strongly supports a clinical diagnosis of SLE.

For the majority of autoantibodies, it is uncertain whether variations in circulating antibody concentrations have any prognostic significance. This has, in part, been due to the absence of sensitive and quantitative immunoassays with which to measure antibody concentrations. However, even when these requirements have been met (e.g. for anti-DNA in SLE or antiacetylcholine receptor antibodies in myasthenia gravis), it has become apparent that antibody levels rarely show a simple correlation with disease activity. This is likely due to the fact that many biological variables, such as class and subclass of the antibody, the purity and homogeneity of the test autoantigen, epitope specificity of the antibody and variation between individuals in the effector phase of the inflammatory response, influence pathogenicity. Despite current limitations, some autoantibodies clearly have important implications, as discussed above and shown in Table 120.2. The presence of anti-Ro (SS-A), and anti-La(SS-B) antibodies in pregnant women with or without a full-blown autoimmune disease conveys a significantly increased risk of the neonatal lupus syndrome[30]. Similarly, prospective studies of anticardiolipin antibodies in pregnant women have shown a significantly increased frequency of midtrimester fetal loss in women with high levels of anticardiolipin antibodies[31]. Certain autoantibodies are also helpful in defining subsets of patients within a disease category. Patients with SLE and anti-La antibodies are reported to have a lower incidence of renal disease[32]. Quantitative immunoassays utilizing the newer synthetic and recombinant antigens[33] may allow the predictive value of changes in antibody levels to be established; for example, studies of antiribosomal P protein antibodies against a synthetic peptide antigen suggested that antibody levels parallel the clinical activity of certain neuropsychiatric manifestations in SLE[34,35].

AUTOANTIBODIES AS A CAUSE OF TISSUE INJURY

It is well known that autoantibodies can be produced in response to tissue breakdown induced by trauma or infection, but these antibodies are usually short lived. It is possible that autoantibodies in autoimmune diseases are also initiated by a response to dying cells, but that the immune response is not regulated appropriately (see below). Whereas most autoantibodies in autoimmune diseases do not directly cause tissue injury, there are many clear-cut examples of autoantibodies causing disease. The different mechanisms (established and proposed) for autoantibody-mediated disease are discussed in this section and illustrated in Figure 120.4.

A direct role for autoantibody-mediated injury is particularly obvious for antibodies directed against cell surface membranes, e.g. anti-erythrocyte, antiplatelet or antilymphocytotoxic antibodies in SLE. Autoantibodies that bind to surface membranes eliminate the cells either by complement-mediated lysis or by enhancing phagocytosis by the mononuclear phagocyte system. Several studies have suggested that some autoantibodies to intracellular proteins bind to cell surface membranes. This may be due to cross-reactivity or may be explained by translocation of intracellular antigens after injury to the cell[36]. It is possible that the association between anti-Ro/La antibodies and photosensitive skin rashes may be explained by this mechanism.

Another well-described mechanism of tissue injury in autoimmune diseases is deposition of antigen–antibody complexes. Autoantibodies directed against intracellular proteins and nucleic acids bind to antigens released from dead cells within the circulation and deposit in vessels (causing vasculitis) or the kidneys (causing glomerulonephritis). This model has been very well studied in experimental animals and is, at least in part, responsible for nephritis in SLE[12]. Other possible mechanisms include binding of cationic autoantibodies to antigens such as nucleosomes *in situ*, deposition of virus–antivirus immune complexes and cell-mediated immunity.

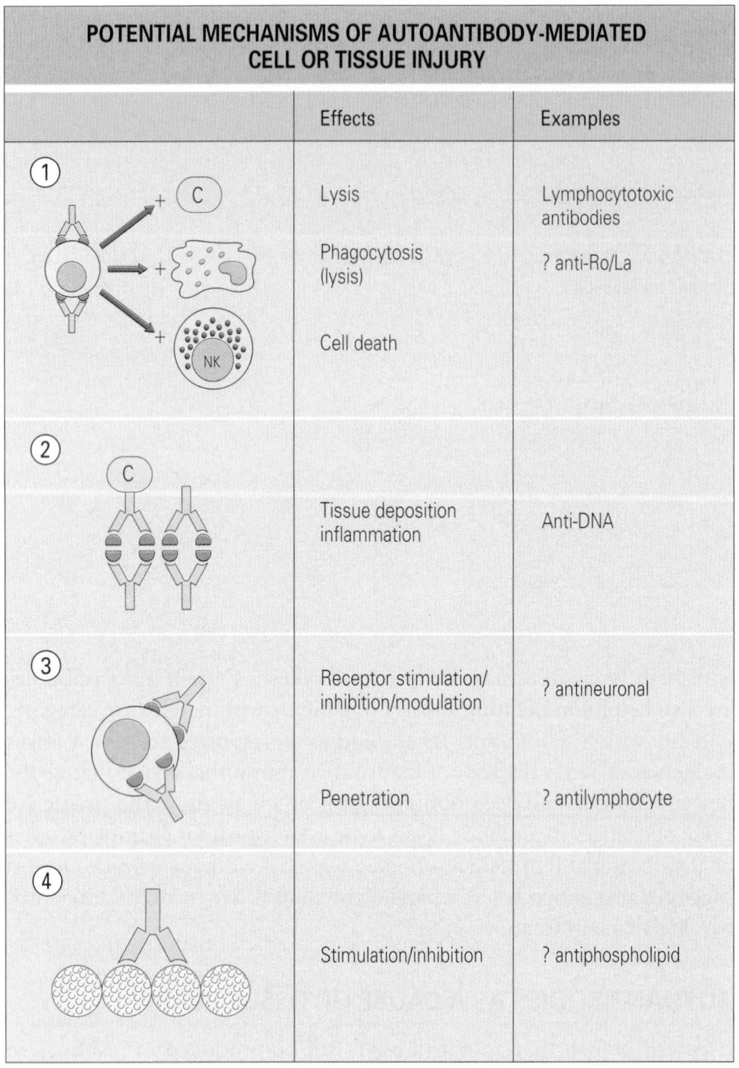

POTENTIAL MECHANISMS OF AUTOANTIBODY-MEDIATED CELL OR TISSUE INJURY		
	Effects	Examples
(1)	Lysis	Lymphocytotoxic antibodies
	Phagocytosis (lysis)	? anti-Ro/La
	Cell death	
(2)	Tissue deposition inflammation	Anti-DNA
(3)	Receptor stimulation/ inhibition/modulation	? antineuronal
	Penetration	? antilymphocyte
(4)	Stimulation/inhibition	? antiphospholipid

Fig. 120.4 Potential mechanisms of autoantibody-mediated cell or tissue injury. (1) Antibody targets may be normal cell surface antigens, altered antigens or intracellular antigens transported to the cell surface (e.g. by ultraviolet light or infection). Antibody may initiate complement (C)-mediated lysis, Fcγ receptor-mediated phagocytosis by mononuclear phagocytes (Mφ) or neutrophils leading to inflammation, or receptor-mediated cell death by natural killer (NK) cells. (2) *Immune complex deposition.* Inflammation is caused by complement split products and by recruitment of phagocytes. (3) Autoantibodies may bind to cell surface receptors and may be internalized. (4) Antibodies may inhibit or facilitate the coagulation cascade by binding directly to phospholipids or, indirectly, by modulating expression of procoagulant factors.

More controversial mechanisms of autoantibody-mediated injury are penetration into living cells, interference with complex extracellular cascades and antibody-dependent cellular cytotoxicity. The evidence for antibody penetration into living cells consists of detection of IgG within epidermal cells on skin biopsies of some patients with SLE[37] and IgG within a subpopulation of T lymphocytes in patients with high-titer anti-RNP antibodies[38]. Many other examples of antibody penetration[39] have been discussed. Antibodies directed against cell surface receptors could also potentially stimulate, inhibit or modulate the receptor from the cell surface. The ultimate fate of autoantibodies within the cell remains uncertain. It is clear from *in vitro* studies with monoclonal antiphospholipid antibodies[4] and the association between prolonged clotting times and antiphospholipid antibodies that autoantibodies can interfere with the coagulation cascade, but the explanation for increased thrombosis *in vivo* remains a major challenge. Immunoconglutinins (antibodies to complement components) are another example of autoantibodies to components of an intravascular cascade. The patho-genic effects of these autoantibodies are uncertain. The final mechanism, antibody-dependent cellular cytotoxicity, could potentially cause cell injury *in vivo*. Whether natural killer cells amplify the cytotoxic potential of autoantibodies directed against cell surface antigens is not known.

For most autoantibodies in SLE, a direct pathogenic effect and the mechanism whereby they cause disease remain to be proven. The most clear-cut way to establish a cause–effect relationship is to administer the antibody in question passively to an experimental animal and test for the effect. Such an approach has shown that antiacetylcholine receptor antibodies are sufficient to induce myasthenia gravis[40] and that IgG fractions from patients with pemphigus and pemphigoid induce damage to keratinocytes *in vitro* and *in vivo*[41,42]. This mode of experimental verification is more difficult in multisystem autoimmune diseases, because each patient's serum usually contains several autoantibodies. In addition, the possibility that human antibodies will have different phlogistic properties in an experimental animal, and difficulties in maintaining high levels of antibody (and possibly antigen) in the animal, are further experimental problems.

MECHANISMS OF AUTOANTIBODY PRODUCTION

Tolerance, autoimmunity and anti-DNA antibodies

Tolerance is discussed elsewhere in this volume, and detailed reviews of this topic in relation to autoimmunity have been addressed previously[43,44]. In brief, *central tolerance* refers to the deletion of high-affinity self-reactive lymphocytes in the thymus (T cells) or bone marrow (B cells) in the process of negative selection; *peripheral tolerance* refers to the further inactivation of self-reactive lymphocytes in the periphery through the induction of anergy, active inhibition or apoptosis[43]. Furthermore, negative regulatory circuits are operational in cells of the innate immune system such as macrophages and natural killer cells. Despite the elimination or functional inactivation (anergy) of self-reactive cells, there is compelling evidence that low-affinity potentially autoreactive cells persist in the peripheral immune system, and that very low affinity reactivity to self antigens is required for survival of lymphocytes in the peripheral immune system. It is therefore not surprising that neoplastic proliferation of B cell clones (in some cases of myeloma or Waldenström's macroglobulinemia) results in the production of monoclonal autoantibodies (e.g. rheumatoid factors, the red blood cell antigen, I, and anti-myelin-associated glycoprotein) or that autoimmune diseases are relatively common in the population.

Immunization of mice, even those predisposed to lupus, with autoantigens such as DNA, fails to induce an immune response. This indicates that autoimmunity does not simply result from exposure to high quantities of self antigen. Recent studies suggest provocative ideas about mechanisms whereby immunity to highly conserved antigens such as DNA could arise:

- Bacterial DNA is immunogenic[11]
- Bacterial DNA contains unmethylated DNA and the CpG motif has been shown to exert a powerful proinflammatory effect on B cells and macrophages[45]
- Anti-DNA antibodies can be induced in mice by immunization with a specific peptide in a polylysine-containing conjugate[46].
- Mammalian DNA-anti-DNA complexes can activate rheumatoid factor producing B cells through Toll Like Receptors (TLR)[47].

Do autoantibodies result from an inappropriate immune response to dying cells?

One phenomenon that has attracted considerable interest in SLE is apoptosis – the appearance of cells undergoing programmed cell death (Figure 120.5). A characteristic feature of apoptosis is the release of nucleosomes (comprising DNA and histones) from the nucleus into the

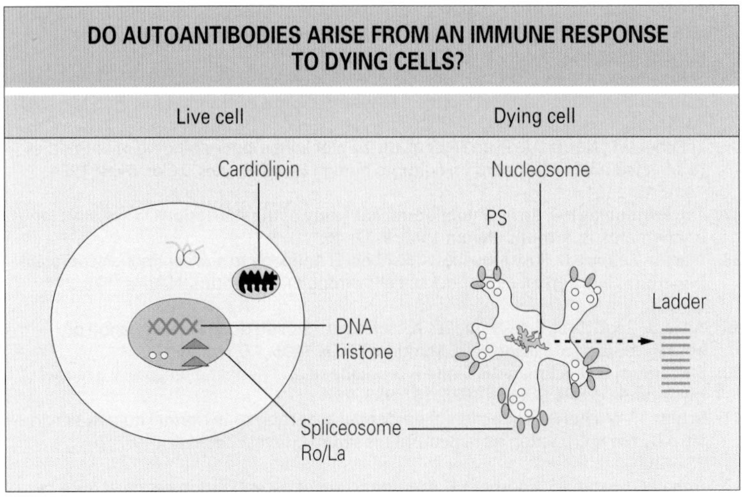

DO AUTOANTIBODIES ARISE FROM AN IMMUNE RESPONSE TO DYING CELLS?

Fig. 120.5 Do autoantibodies arise from an immune response to dying cells? As discussed in the text, one possible explanation for autoantigen selection in SLE is an immune response to dying cells. In this model, the generation of specific autoantibodies (which are detected on extracts derived from living cells) may be explained by immunization with dying cells as follows: anticardiolipin antibodies (cardiolipin is a normal component of mitochondrial membranes) cross-react with negatively charged phospolipids such as phosphatidylserine (PS) that are exposed on the outside of the cell membrane on dying cells; anti-DNA and anti-histone antibodies are targeted to nucleosomes that are released from the nucleus of apoptotic cells (can be detected as a 'ladder' when analyzed by gel electrophoresis); anti-Sm/RNP and anti-Ro/La autoantibodies translocate from the nucleus into apoptotic blebs.

cytoplasm of a dying cell. As the serologic hallmark of SLE is the presence of autoantibodies against nucleosomes, and nucleosomes have been detected in the circulation of patients with clinically active SLE, the hypothesis that patients are immunized by apoptotic cell fragments is attractive. It was reported some time ago that ultraviolet irradiation of keratinocytes induces the cell surface expression of certain lupus autoantigens[36]. This phenomenon is now believed to be explained by translocation of proteins and nucleoprotein complexes to 'apoptotic blebs' on the periphery of dying keratinocytes[48]. Enhanced susceptibility of SLE cells to ultraviolet (and perhaps other forms of injury) could, therefore, explain increased immunization, not only by nucleosomes, but also by antigens such as Ro, U1 RNP and ribosomes. However, apoptosis is a normal physiologic event in the thymus and bone marrow and the products of apoptotic cells would be predicted to tolerize lymphocytes, therefore apoptosis *per se* is not sufficient to explain autoantibody production in SLE. It is possible that impaired removal of the dying cells or an abnormal form of cell death caused by cytotoxic T cells breaks tolerance. There is evidence in support of both of these concepts. For example, autoantibodies may be relatively selective for proteins that are cleaved by granzyme B[49], a serine protease released by cytotoxic T cells. A number of studies suggest that failure to remove dying cells rapidly, for example as a result of lack of opsonins or defects in

macrophage function, may promote an inflammatory response to self antigens (discussed by Gershov et al.[50]).

The role of environmental factors and molecular mimicry

It is clear from drug-induced lupus syndromes that environmental factors can induce autoantibodies and autoimmune diseases, although these syndromes are reversible upon withdrawal of the drugs. As susceptibility to both drug-induced and idiopathic autoimmune diseases are influenced by age, sex, race and MHC type, it has frequently been proposed that idiopathic autoimmune diseases arise from an environmental agent (such as a virus) in genetically predisposed hosts. Such an agent could induce autoantibodies either because it induces antibodies that cross-react with self proteins (molecular mimicry) or because the agent could directly modify host (self) antigens. Recent experimental models suggest that foreign antigens break B and T cell tolerance after immunization by generating cross-reactive lymphocytes or altered antigen processing, or both, in the context of costimulatory molecule upregulation[51-53].

Alternatively, an environmental agent could induce autoantibodies by modifying self MHC determinants, by inducing aberrant MHC class II expression and presentation of self antigens[54], or by interfering with more complex mechanisms of lymphocyte function. In such cases, autoantibody specificity may be influenced by host MHC, the physiochemical nature of self antigens and the T and B cell repertoire. For example, in one model of autoimmunity, graft-versus-host disease (caused by donor T helper cells stimulating host B cells), autoantibodies with specificities similar to those of SLE are observed (reviewed by Shustov et al.[55]). It has been suggested that, in graft-versus-host disease, multivalency of antigens (e.g. DNA and cardiolipin) provides the necessary second signal to activate B cells to produce autoantibodies. As different mouse strains produce different autoantibodies, other host factors must influence autoantibody specificity.

Whether autoantibodies and autoimmune disease are generated by the idiotype–anti-idiotype network in response to a foreign antigen remains to be determined.

Antigen and epitope spreading

How do antibodies become polyclonal, and why do autoantibodies in SLE target different proteins and RNA in the same particle? Studies in experimental animals demonstrate how an initial highly restricted immune response can develop a pattern of diversity. Immunization of animals with a peptide antigen leads initially to a humoral immune response targeted towards a single epitope, followed by spreading to involve several epitopes on the same protein – 'epitope spreading'[56] – and even different non-cross-reacting proteins in the same particle – 'antigen spreading'. Spreading results from uptake of immune complexes, processing and presentation of peptides derived from the particle. Presentation of peptides to T cells results in the expansion of autoreactive T cell populations which, in turn, activate B cells through expression of CD40 ligand and cytokines to generate high-affinity autoantibodies.

REFERENCES

1. Christian CL, Elkon KB. Autoantibodies to intracellular proteins: clinical and biological implications. Am J Med 1986; 80: 53–61.
2. Boes M. Role of natural and immune IgM antibodies in immune responses. Mol Immunol 2000; 37: 1141–1149.
3. Jerne NK. Towards a network theory of the immune system. Ann Immunol (Paris) 1974; 125C: 373–389.
4. Lafer E, Rauch J, Andrzejewski C et al. Polyspecific monoclonal lupus autoantibodies reactive with both polynucleotides and phospholipids. J Exp Med 1981; 153: 897–904.
5. Talal N, Pillarisetty RJ, DeHoratius RJ et al. Immunologic regulation of spontaneous antibodies to DNA and RNA I. Significance of IgM and IgG antibodies in SLE patients and asymptomatic relatives. Clin Exp Immunol 1976; 25: 377–382.
6. Rubin RL, Tang FL, Chan EK et al. IgG subclasses of autoantibodies in systemic lupus erythematosus, Sjögren's syndrome, and drug-induced autoimmunity. J Immunol 1986; 137: 2528–2534.
7. Bonfa E, Chu JL, Brot N et al. Lupus anti-ribosomal antibodies show limited heterogeneity and are predominantly of the IgG1 and IgG2 subclasses. Clin Immunol Immunopathol 1987; 45: 129–138.

8. Gharavi AE, Harris EN, Lockshin MD et al. IgG subclass and light chain distribution of anticardiolipin and anti-DNA antibodies in SLE. Ann Rheum Dis 1988; 47: 286–290.
9. Isenberg DA, Shoenfeld Y, Madaio MP et al. Anti-DNA antibody idiotypes in systemic lupus erythematosus. Lancet 1984; 2: 417–422.
10. Schwartz RS, Stollar BD. Origins of anti-DNA autoantibodies. J Clin Invest 1985; 75: 321–327.
11. Pisetsky DS. Anti-DNA and autoantibodies. Curr Opin Rheumatol 2000; 12: 364–368.
12. Cochrane CG, Koffler D. Immune complex disease in experimental animals and man. Adv Immunol 1973; 16: 185–264.
13. Kramers C, Hylkema MN, van Bruggen MCJ et al. Anti-nucleosome antibodies complexed to nucleosomal antigens show anti-DNA reactivity and bind to rat glomerular basement membrane in vivo. J Clin Invest 1994; 94: 568–577.
14. Schett G, Steiner G, Smolen JS. Nuclear antigen histone H1 is primarily involved in lupus erythematosus cell formation. Arthritis Rheum 1998; 41: 1446–1455.
15. Burlingame RW, Rubin RL. Drug-induced anti-histone autoantibodies display two patterns of reactivity with substructures of chromatin. J Clin Invest 1991; 88: 680–690.
16. Kramers K, Hylkema M, Termaat RM et al. Histones in lupus nephritis. Exp Nephrol 1993; 1: 224–228.
17. Tuteja R, Tuteja N. Ku autoantigen: a multifunctional DNA-binding protein. Crit Rev Biochem Mol Biol 2000; 35: 1–33.
18. Schur PH, Monroe M. Antibodies to ribonucleic acid in systemic lupus erythematosus. Proc Natl Acad Sci USA 1969; 63: 1108–1112.
19. Guthrie C. The spliceosome is a dynamic ribonucleoprotein machine. Harvey Lect 1994; 90: 59–80.
20. Van Venrooij WJ, Sillekens PT. Small nuclear RNA associated proteins: autoantigens in connective tissue diseases. Clin Exp Rheumatol 1989; 7: 635–645.
21. Maraia RJ, Intine RV. Recognition of nascent RNA by the human La antigen: conserved and divergent features of structure and function. Mol Cell Biol 2001; 21: 367–379.
22. Ben-Chetrit E, Fox RI, Tan EM. Dissociation of immune responses to the SS-A (Ro) 52-kd and 60-kd polypeptides in systemic lupus erythematosus and Sjögren's syndrome. Arthritis Rheum 1990; 33: 349–355.
23. Sontheimer RD, Maddison PJ, Reichlin M et al. Serologic and HLA associations in subacute cutaneous lupus erythematosus, a clinical subset of lupus erythematosus. Ann Intern Med 1982; 97: 664–671.
24. Elkon KB, Skelly S, Parnassa AP et al. The identification and synthesis of a ribosomal protein antigenic determinant in systemic lupus erythematosus. Proc Natl Acad Sci USA 1986; 83: 7419–7423.
25. von Muhlen CA, Chan EK, Angles-Cano E et al. Advances in autoantibodies in SLE. Lupus 1998; 7: 507–514.
26. Mimura T, Fernsten P, Jarjour W et al. Autoantibodies specific for different isoforms of CD45 in systemic lupus erythematosus. J Exp Med 1990; 172: 653–656.
27. Bluestein HG, Williams GW, Steinberg AD. Cerebrospinal fluid antibodies to neuronal cells: association with neuropsychiatric manifestations of systemic lupus erythematosus. Am J Med 1981; 70: 240–246.
28. Minota S, Koyasu S, Yahara I et al. Autoantibodies to the heat-shock protein hsp90 in systemic lupus erythematosus. J Clin Invest 1988; 81: 106–109.
29. Tan EM, Smolen JS, McDougal JS et al. A critical evaluation of enzyme immunoassays for detection of antinuclear autoantibodies of defined specificities. I. Precision, sensitivity, and specificity. Arthritis Rheum 1999; 42: 455–464.
30. Buyon JP, Winchester R. Congenital complete heart block. A human model of passively acquired autoimmune injury. Arthritis Rheum 1990; 33: 609–614.
31. Lockshin MD, Druzin ML, Goei S et al. Antibody to cardiolipin as a predictor of fetal distress or death in pregnant patients with systemic lupus erythematosus. N Engl J Med 1985; 313: 152–156.
32. Wasicek CA, Reichlin M. Clinical and serological differences between systemic lupus erythematosus patients with antibodies to Ro versus patients with antibodies to Ro and La. J Clin Invest 1982; 69: 835–843.
33. Meheus L, van Venrooij WJ, Wiik A et al. Multicenter validation of recombinant, natural and synthetic antigens used in a single multiparameter assay for the detection of specific anti-nuclear autoantibodies in connective tissue disorders. Clin Exp Rheumatol 1999; 17: 205–214.
34. Bonfa E, Golombek SJ, Kaufman LD et al. Association between lupus psychosis and anti-ribosomal P protein antibodies: measurement of antibody using a synthetic peptide antigen. N Engl J Med 1987; 317: 265–271.
35. Schneebaum AB, Singleton JD, West SG et al. Association of psychiatric manifestations with antibodies to ribosomal P protein in systemic lupus erythematosus. Am J Med 1991; 90: 54–62.
36. LeFeber WP, Norris DA, Ryan SR et al. Ultraviolet light induces binding of antibodies to selected nuclear antigens on cultured human keratinocytes. J Clin Invest 1984; 74: 1545–1551.
37. Tan EM, Kunkel HG. An immunofluorescent study of the skin lesions in systemic lupus erythematosus. Arthritis Rheum 1966; 9: 37–46.
38. Alarcon-Segovia D, Ruiz-Arguelles A, Fishbein E. Antibody to nuclear ribonucleoprotein penetrates live human mononuclear cells through Fc receptors. Nature 1978; 271: 67–69.
39. Alarcon-Segovia D, Ruiz-Arguelles A, Llorente L. Broken dogma: penetration of autoantibodies into living cells. Immunol Today 1996; 17: 163–164.
40. Satyamurti S, Drachman DB, Slone F. Blockade of acetylcholine receptors: a model of myasthenia gravis. Science 1975; 187: 955–957.
41. Schiltz JR, Michel B. Production of epidermal acantholysis in normal human skin in vitro by the IgG fraction from pemphigus serum. J Invest Dermatol 1976; 67: 254–260.
42. Anhalt GJ, Labib RS, Voorhees JJ et al. Induction of pemphigus in neonatal mice by passive transfer of IgG from patients with the disease. N Engl J Med 1982; 306: 1189–1196.
43. Elkon K. Immunologic tolerance and apoptosis. In: Rich RR, Kotzin B, Shearer W, Schroeder HW, eds. Clinical immunology, 2E. London: Harcourt International; 2001: 11.11–11.18.
44. Elkon KB. Apoptosis. In: Ruddy S, Sledge CB, eds. Kelley's textbook of rheumatology, 6E. Philadelphia: WB Saunders Company; 1999: 1–8.
45. Krieg AM. The role of CpG motifs in innate immunity. Curr Opin Immunol 2000; 12: 35–43.
46. Putterman C, Diamond B. Immunization with a peptide surrogate for double-stranded DNA (dsDNA) induces autoantibody production and renal immunoglobulin deposition. J Exp Med 1998; 188: 29–38.
47. Leadbetter EA, Rifkin IR, Hohlbaum BC et al. Chromatin-IgG complexes activate B cells by dual engagement of IgM and toll-like receptors. Nature 2002; 416: 603–607.
48. Casciola-Rosen LA, Anhalt G, Rosen A. Autoantigens targeted in systemic lupus erythematosus are clustered in two populations of surface structures on apoptotic keratinocytes. J Exp Med 1994; 179: 1317–1330.
49. Casciola-Rosen L, Andrade F, Ulanet D et al. Cleavage by granzyme B is strongly predictive of autoantigen status: implications for initiation of autoimmunity. J Exp Med 1999; 190: 815–826.
50. Gershov D, Kim S, Brot N et al. C-reactive protein binds to apoptotic cells, protects the cells from assembly of the terminal complement components, and sustains an antiinflammatory innate immune response. Implications for systemic autoimmunity. J Exp Med 2000; 192: 1353–1364.
51. Mamula MJ, Fatenejad S, Craft J. B cells process and present lupus autoantigens that initiate autoimmune T cell responses. J Immunol 1994; 152: 1453–1461.
52. Dong X, Hamilton KJ, Satoh M et al. Initiation of autoimmunity to the p53 tumor suppressor protein by complexes of p53 and SV40 large T antigen. J Exp Med 1994; 179: 1243–1252.
53. Matzinger P. Tolerance, danger, and the extended family. Annu Rev Immunol 1994; 12: 991–1045.
54. Londei M, Lamb JR, Bottazzo GF et al. Epithelial cells expressing aberrant MHC class II determinants can present antigen to cloned human T cells. Nature 1984; 312: 639–641.
55. Shustov A, Luzina I, Nguyen P et al. Role of perforin in controlling B-cell hyperactivity and humoral autoimmunity. J Clin Invest 2000; 106: R39–R47.
56. James JA, Gross T, Scofield RH et al. Immunoglobulin epitope spreading and autoimmune disease after peptide immunization: Sm B/B´-derived PPPGMRPP and PPPGIRGP induce spliceosome autoimmunity. J Exp Med 1995; 181: 453–462.

121 Cellular immunology

Mary K Crow

- Systemic lupus erythematosus is associated with a myriad of cellular immune system abnormalities that directly contribute to autoantibody secretion, immune complex formation, tissue damage and disease

- An essential role for excessive or poorly controlled activity of T helper cells in the activation and differentiation of autoantibody-forming B cells is likely to be a final common pathway

- Viruses, particularly infectious or endogenous retroviral products, are likely candidates as triggers that initiate the cellular immune dysfunction

- Alternatively, ultraviolet radiation and certain drugs can trigger SLE, indicating that cell damage may provoke a sufficient immunologic challenge to induce autoimmunity in the genetically susceptible host

- Individual variability in genomic sequence may prove to be the most important factor that underlies the immune defects of lupus

---

TABLE 121.1 PROPOSED BENEFICIAL ROLES FOR AUTOREACTIVE LYMPHOCYTES

T Lymphocytes
Autoreactive T cells may inhibit excessive activity by autologous B or T cells
Autoreactive T cells may contribute to immune surveillance of emerging malignant autologous cells
T cells reactive with TCR determinants on autologous T cells may downregulate excessive T cell activity

B Lymphocytes
B cells specific for autoantigens may bind and present those antigens, in the context of self MHC molecules, to self-reactive T cells in the thymus. This process might result in deletion of those T cells with high affinity for the autoantigen/self-MHC complex
B cells reactive with IgG (i.e. those with rheumatoid factor specificity) may bind and process antigen-bearing immune complexes and present antigenic peptides to antigen-specific T cells
B cells specific for the antigen binding region on autologous antibodies may differentiate and secrete 'anti-idiotype' antibodies, thus contributing to an internally regulated antibody network

INTRODUCTION

The clinical manifestations of systemic lupus erythematosus (SLE) are readily attributable to the activity of antibodies reactive with human antigens or the deposition of immune complexes, resulting in complement activation, inflammation and tissue damage. Cell-mediated processes may also directly contribute to tissue pathology. The autoantibody specificities involved in this process (reviewed in Chapter 120) characteristically have reactivity with DNA, RNA or phospholipids, or with proteins that bind to these molecules, whereas T lymphocyte specificities are most likely restricted to protein antigens.

Hypergammaglobulinemia, autoantibody production and immune complex deposition suggest excess, abnormal or poorly regulated B cell function in SLE, but the important and challenging question remains: what drives this B cell activity? The answer must lie in the complex interactions among T lymphocytes, B lymphocytes and antigen-presenting cells, the host (genetic and hormonal) factors affecting these interactions and environmental triggers that perturb the balance in this system.

AUTOREACTIVE CELLS IN THE NORMAL IMMUNE SYSTEM

'Horror autotoxicus', an expression originally coined by Paul Ehrlich, reflects the horror of an organism that is damaging to itself, as occurs in autoimmune disease. However, it is now known that B lymphocytes with specificity for autoantigens are not only present in healthy individuals, but may have a beneficial role early in life (Table 121.1). Autoreactive B cells may help to expand the numbers of memory T cells specific for a wide range of foreign antigens, and may also act in an immunoregulatory capacity[1]. B cells with the potential to secrete immunoglobulin specific for DNA have been documented among the B cell repertoire of normal individuals, and sequence analysis of immunoglobulin genes encoding anti-DNA antibodies indicates that these specificities can be encoded in the germline. There is no convincing evidence to support an inherited

difference between the specificities of B cells from normal individuals and those from patients with SLE.

Similarly, some autoreactivity normally occurs within the T cell compartment of the immune system. T cells will proliferate *in vitro* in response to determinants on autologous non-T cells. This response may reflect the recognition of self peptides in association with major histocompatibility complex (MHC) class II antigens. The generation of suppressor cells, now most often referred to as regulatory cells, in that system has been proposed to contribute to immune surveillance of abnormal cells or control of excess T or B cell activity[2]. T cells specific for defined autoantigens are far less common, although such cells have occasionally been described, as in the case of rare myelin basic protein reactive T cells in normal individuals. Many potentially autoreactive T cells, however, are carefully eliminated early in development, whereas T cells with low affinity for autoantigens may become part of the peripheral T cell repertoire. Autoreactive cells are, then, a part of the normal immune system, although more common in the B cell compartment than in the T cell compartment. These cells may even play an active part in controlling the immune system, and must themselves be tightly regulated. The secretion of autoantibodies in SLE is increasingly seen as the result of abnormal regulation by T lymphocytes, resulting in an impairment of the carefully monitored response to autoantigens.

NORMAL TOLERANCE TO AUTOANTIGENS

In order to avoid excessive or destructive reactivity with autoantigens, the immune system must tailor its repertoire of specificities to react primarily with foreign antigens. This process is termed the generation of immunologic tolerance. Although highly effective in the T cell compart-

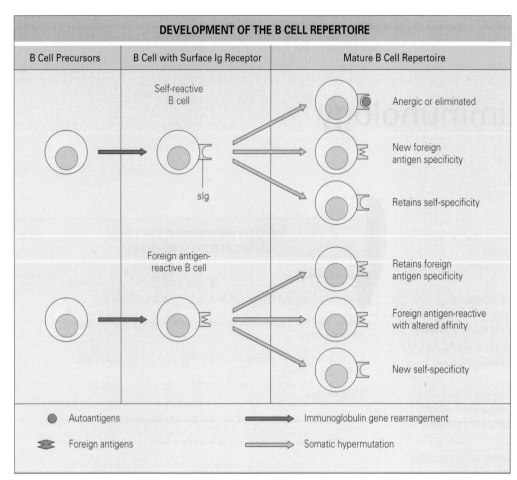

DEVELOPMENT OF THE B CELL REPERTOIRE

B Cell Precursors	B Cell with Surface Ig Receptor	Mature B Cell Repertoire

Self-reactive B cell

sIg

Anergic or eliminated

New foreign antigen specificity

Retains self-specificity

Foreign antigen-reactive B cell

Retains foreign antigen specificity

Foreign antigen-reactive with altered affinity

New self-specificity

● Autoantigens

✹ Foreign antigens

➜ Immunoglobulin gene rearrangement

⇨ Somatic hypermutation

Fig. 121.1 Development of the B cell repertoire. B cell precursors undergo immunoglobulin gene rearrangement to generate a population of mature B cells bearing surface immunoglobulin (sIg) with a range of specificities, including some reactive with autoantigens. Under the influence of T helper cells, the immunoglobulin genes of B cells that have interacted with their specific antigen undergo mutation, resulting in alterations of affinity and, in some cases, specificity of their protein products. Self-reactive specificities may be lost, or new self-reactivities may be gained by the B cell repertoire.

ment, the induction of B cell tolerance to autoantigens is not complete (Fig. 121.1). In addition to the autoantibody specificities encoded in the germline, the normal process of B cell ontogeny can result in self-reactive B cells. Bone marrow-derived precursors differentiate by the productive rearrangement of heavy- and light-chain gene segments, yielding an immunoglobulin (Ig) molecule. The random rearrangement of these gene segments results in a population of B cells bearing surface immunoglobulin with a wide spectrum of antigen specificities, including some reactive with autoantigens. Although there is evidence to support the clonal elimination or induction of anergy in some self-reactive B cells, other self-specific B cells persist and remain potentially active. In addition, B cells undergo somatic hypermutation of the hypervariable regions of immunoglobulin genes, resulting in alterations in the structure of the antigen-binding region of antibody and the generation of new antibody reactivities. This phenomenon allows the evolution of higher-affinity antibodies over the course of an immune response, but may also lead to the development of self-reactive B cells. For example, a single point mutation leading to an amino acid substitution in the antigen-binding domain has been shown to transform a phosphocholine-specific antibody into an anti-DNA antibody[3].

Tolerance in the B cell pool is maintained by the stringent requirement of those cells for several signals before achieving the capacity to differentiate to antibody-forming cells (Fig. 121.2). Those signals include, first, the binding of specific antigen to B cell surface Ig receptors and, second, T cell help. The strength of the surface Ig-mediated B cell signal is determined by many factors, including the valency of the antigen, the affinity of the antigen for the surface Ig receptor, and both positive and negative supplementary signals, delivered through transmembrane molecules such as CD19, CD22 and FcγRIIb. The coordinated function of intracellular kinases and phosphatases, activated after ligation of these transmembrane molecules, determines the 'threshold' for B cell activation through surface Ig[4]. Antigen-non-specific T cell help is

provided by T cell derived growth and differentiation factors (lymphokines), and survival signals delivered by soluble and cell surface molecules produced by macrophages also contribute to B cell differentiation. It is the requirement of the B cell for direct cell–cell interaction with antigen-specific T helper (Th) cells that permits tight regulation of the antibody specificities secreted during the course of an immune response. The T cell surface molecules that mediate this direct T cell help include the T cell receptor (TCR), which binds to antigenic peptides associated with MHC molecules on the B cell surface, and cell surface adhesion and costimulatory molecules, which tighten the physical interaction between T and B cells (Table 121.2).

The binding together of T and B cell surface molecules not only permits the delivery of T cell derived lymphokines directly to the B cell, but also facilitates the generation of membrane-mediated activation signals in the B cell. Members of the tumor necrosis factor (TNF) and TNF receptor molecular families have emerged as essential mediators of cell–cell interactions. Binding of T cell CD40 ligand to B cell CD40 is required for Th cell mediated B cell activation and differentiation, whereas binding of T cell Fas ligand to B cell Fas receptor can result in pruning of the B cell repertoire and downregulation of B cell function through induction of programmed cell death – apoptosis[5]. Another member of the TNF superfamily, BLyS (also called BAFF or TALL1), is produced by macrophages and provides positive signals to the B cell, supporting B cell maturation and survival[6]. Even when autoantigen-specific B cells persist, these demanding requirements for coordinated signals from both antigen and antigen-activated T cells make their differentiation into autoantibody-secreting plasma cells unlikely.

The primary responsibility for regulating self-reactivity in the immune system, then, falls to the T lymphocyte. Several mechanisms operate to refine the T cell repertoire and assure that autoreactive T cells are eliminated or tightly controlled. T cells are rendered tolerant to self in any of three ways (Fig. 121.3): first, self-reactive T lymphocytes may be elimi-

GROWTH AND DIFFERENTIATION OF B CELLS REQUIRES SEVERAL SIGNALS

Anergy

sIg binds antigen in the absence of T cell help resulting in anergy or elimination of B cell

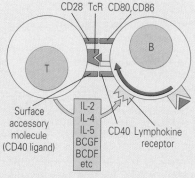

B Cell Growth and Differentiation

sIg binds antigen; TcR binds antigenic peptide/MHC complex; T and B cell surface accessory molecules interact; T cell secretes lymphokines, lymphokines bind to B cell receptors resulting in proliferation and differentiation of B cell

B Cell Apoptosis

Antigen-specific T cell binds to B cell bearing antigenic peptide in the absence of sIg signal. CD40 ligation results in Fas expression. Ligation of Fas may result in apoptosis

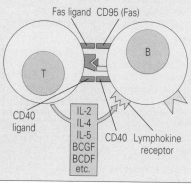

Fig. 121.2 Growth and differentiation of B cells requires several signals. Full activation of a B cell, resulting in proliferation and differentiation to antibody-forming cells, requires both an sIg-mediated signal, usually delivered by the binding of antigen to its specific cell surface receptor, and T cell help, mediated by the binding of TCR to antigenic peptide on B cell surface MHC molecules, the interaction of T and B cell surface accessory molecules (CD28 with CD80 or CD86; CD40 ligand with CD40), and the delivery of T cell derived lymphokines, including interleukins (IL) and B cell growth and differentiation factors (BCGF, BCDF), to the B cell. Survival factors from macrophages, such as BLyS, are also important. When a B cell receives these signals in coordinated and timely fashion, growth and maturation occur (middle panel). An sIg-mediated signal, in the absence of T cell help, results in B cell anergy or death (top), whereas specific T cell help, in the absence of a recent sIg-mediated signal, is inadequate for induction of B cell proliferation and differentiation, but may prepare the B cell for death by inducing CD95 (Fas receptor) (bottom).

TABLE 121.2
CELL SURFACE MOLECULES IMPORTANT IN IMMUNE RESPONSES

Molecule	Proposed Function
T cells	
T cell receptor for antigen – α chain and β chain	Binds antigenic peptide in association with MHC molecules
CD3	Transduces activation signal to T cell after TCR binds antigen
CD4	Identifies many Th cells; binds to MHC class II molecules
CD8	Identifies many T suppressor and T cytotoxic cells; binds to MHC class I molecules
CD2	Binds to LFA-3; sheep red blood cell receptor
LFA-1 (CD11a)	Binds to ICAM-1
CD45 RA	Regulates T cell activation by its tyrosine protein phosphatase activity
CD28	Binds to CD80 and CD86 molecules on B cells; delivers accessory activation signal to T cells
CD40 ligand	Delivers activation signal through CD40 on B cells, macrophages, dendritic cells and endothelial cells
Fas ligand	Initiates cell death program after binding CD95 (Fas) on activated lymphocytes
CD95 (Fas)	Signals cell death program
IL-2 receptor (α chain is CD25)	On activated T cells and T regulatory cells; binds IL-2
IL-1 receptor	On some Th cells; binds IL-1
B cells	
sIg	Specific receptor for antigen
MHC class I	Associates with antigenic peptides; binds to CD8
MHC class II	Associates with antigenic peptides; binds to CD4
CD5	On subset of B cells associated with secretion of IgM autoantibodies
CD40	Binds CD40 ligand on Th cells; delivers secondary activation signal to B cells
TACI, BCMA, BR3	Receptors for BLyS
CD21 (CR2)	B cell receptor for C3d and EBV
CD19, CD22	Modulate sIg signals
CD45	Provides phosphatase activity needed for B cell activation
CD95 (Fas)	Signals cell death program
CD32 (FcγRII)	Fc receptor for IgG; ligation inhibits sIg signals
CD54 (ICAM-1)	Binds to LFA-1
CD80, CD86	Binds to CD28
LFA-1 (CD11a)	Binds to ICAM-1
Macrophages	
MHC class I	Associates with antigenic peptides; binds to CD8
MHC class II	Associates with antigenic peptides; binds to CD4
CD54 (ICAM-1)	Binds to LFA-1
LFA-3	Binds to CD2
BLyS	Provides maturation and survival signals to B cells
CD11b (CR3)	iC3b receptor
CD16 (FcγRIII)	Fc receptor for IgG; ligation activates cells
CD32 (FcγRII)	Fc receptor for IgG; FcγRIIa activates and FcγRIIb inhibits cells
CD64 (FcγRI)	Fc receptor for IgG; recognizes monomeric IgG

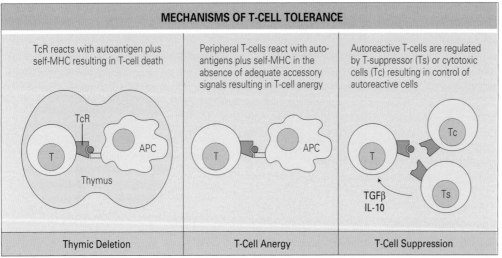

MECHANISMS OF T-CELL TOLERANCE

Thymic Deletion	T-Cell Anergy	T-Cell Suppression
TcR reacts with autoantigen plus self-MHC resulting in T-cell death	Peripheral T-cells react with auto-antigens plus self-MHC in the absence of adequate accessory signals resulting in T-cell anergy	Autoreactive T-cells are regulated by T-suppressor (Ts) or cytotoxic cells (Tc) resulting in control of autoreactive cells

Fig. 121.3 Mechanisms of T cell tolerance. The elimination or inactivation of potentially self-reactive T cells is assured by any of three mechanisms: first, the interaction of T cell TCR with autoantigens bound to self MHC molecules in the thymus early in the development of the immune system, resulting in death of those T cells ('negative selection') (left panel); second, partial activation of peripheral T cells by interaction of TCR with autoantigens bound to self-MHC molecules, but in the absence of certain accessory cell-mediated secondary activation signals, resulting in T cell anergy (middle panel); third, the control or elimination of self-reactive T cells by regulatory T cells, suppressor or cytotoxic, that recognize TCR on the autoreactive T cells (right panel).

nated in the thymus early in ontogeny, resulting in clonal deletion[7]. Second, self-reactive T cells that escape from the thymus may remain ignorant of antigen or be rendered anergic after interaction of the TCR with low-affinity antigen or in the absence of adequate secondary accessory signals[2,8]. Finally, autoreactive cells in the peripheral pool may remain potentially active, but are controlled by other components of the immune system, such as cytotoxic or regulatory T cells[9]. Impairment in any of these mechanisms might allow self-reactive T cells to expand within the peripheral immune system. In addition, excess availability of self-antigen, self-antigen presented in association with foreign antigen or in an altered form, or a generally immunostimulatory adjuvant-like microenvironment, might trigger activation of those low-affinity self-reactive T cells in the mature immune repertoire.

Although the cellular immune mechanisms that account for the initiation of SLE are not understood, the T lymphocyte is likely to be in good part responsible for driving the B cell hyperactivity that is observed. As the B cell repertoire, even in the normal individual, includes cells with the potential for the secretion of autoantibody, those cells may be vulnerable to induction of differentiation should appropriate T cell help become available. At the level of the B cell, an altered threshold for activation through surface Ig receptors could also contribute to autoantibody production.

ANIMAL MODELS OF SLE

Spontaneous lupus-like disease models

Spontaneous and experimental animal models of SLE have been used to elucidate the relative roles of the cellular components of the immune system in the pathogenesis of SLE. Studies of spontaneous murine SLE-like disease have focused on two strains: New Zealand Black (NZB) and the F1 hybrids (B/W F1) that result from mating NZB mice with New Zealand White (NZW) mice, and the MRL lpr/lpr strain (Table 121.3).

New Zealand Black and F1 hybrids

The predominant clinical manifestation observed in NZB mice is hemolytic anemia, with chronic glomerulonephritis occurring in most older mice. These mice produce IgM antinuclear antibodies, but do not secrete IgG antibodies reactive with double-stranded DNA (dsDNA), those autoantibodies which are most damaging to glomeruli. However, after NZB mice are mated with phenotypically normal NZW mice, an F1 is generated that develops early renal disease characterized clinically by proteinuria and pathologically by chronic obliterative glomerulonephritis. High levels of antibodies to nuclear antigens and cationic IgG anti-dsDNA antibodies are detected in the serum, granular deposits of IgG and C3 are observed in the renal mesangium, and antibodies reactive with dsDNA have been eluted from these kidneys. The cellular defects

TABLE 121.3 SPONTANEOUS MODELS OF MURINE LUPUS	
NZB x NZW F1	
Clinical	
NZB	Hemolytic anemia Late-onset glomerulonephritis IgM anti-DNA antibody
NZW	Phenotypically normal
B/W F1	Early proteinuria and chronic obliterative glomerulonephritis High levels of cationic IgG anti-dsDNA antibodies Mesangial deposits of IgG and C3
Immunologic	
NZB	Spontaneous B cell hyperactivity Increased B cell response to T cell-derived growth factors Accelerated thymic atrophy
NZW	Deletion of a segment of TCR b chain gene Different pattern on restriction fragment length polymorphism analysis of TCR a chain gene when compared with other strains Bears unusual H-2^Z haplotype Macrophages secrete low levels of TNFa activity (TNFa gene is encoded in MHC)
B/W F1	Spontaneous B cell hyperactivity Increased B cell response to T cell-derived growth factors Accelerated thymic atrophy Th cells from older mice induce IgG anti-dsDNA antibody in vitro May be decreased T suppressor mechanisms Disease ameliorated by anti-CD4 antibody Administration of TNFa may delay onset of disease
MRL lpr/lpr	
Clinical	
MRL 1/1	Anti-DNA antibodies Late-onset renal disease
lpr gene	Mutation in CD95, Fas receptor Associated with massive lymphadenopathy and impaired apoptosis
MRL lpr/lpr	Early-onset immune complex-mediated glomerulonephritis High levels of IgG anti-dsDNA antibody Massive lymphadenopathy
Immunologic	
MRL 1/1	Th cells can induce production of cationic IgG anti-dsDNA antibodies
lpr gene	Contributes to capacity of B cells to secrete antichromatin antibody Results in abundant T cells with unusual phenotype in peripheral lymphoid organs
MRL lpr/lpr	Th cells induce production of cationic IgG anti-dsDNA antibodies Age-dependent loss of certain CD4[1] T cell responses Poor IL-2 production by Th cells Disease ameliorated by anti-CD4 antibody

that account for this clinical picture have been studied in detail[10]. B cells from both NZB and B/W F1 mice spontaneously proliferate and secrete immunoglobulin *in vitro*, and show increased numbers of B cell colony-forming units. When compared with B cells from normal mice, these B cells have increased responses to T cell derived B cell growth factors, including interleukin(IL)-5, and have increased mRNA for *c-myc*, an oncogene expressed in activated and proliferating cells. In addition, NZB B cells have enhanced capacity to stimulate the proliferation of syngeneic T cell populations, a property that does not appear to be accounted for by increased expression of MHC class II molecules. This evidence for B cell hyperactivity in NZB and B/W F1 mice was initially interpreted to support a maturation defect that accelerates B cell activity. Endogenous B stem cell hyperactivity may be one component of the predisposition to autoimmune disease in these mice, but the additional abnormalities that are characteristic of the B/W F1, but not of the NZB parent – high levels of cationic IgG autoantibodies reactive with dsDNA – suggest that the genetic contribution of NZW mice is reflected in altered T cell function[11].

Excessive T cell help, impaired T cell mediated suppression, or both, may contribute to B cell hyperactivity in B/W F1 mice. The IgG isotype of the pathogenic antinuclear antibodies suggests that T cell help has been necessary for the production of these autoantibodies. Experimental evidence for a role for excessive T cell help includes the amelioration of disease severity in B/W F1 mice by treatment with anti-CD4 monoclonal antibodies reactive with Th cells[12], and the capacity of T cells from 7-month-old, but not 2-month-old, B/W F1 mice to induce IgG anti-dsDNA autoantibody production by B/W F1 B cells *in vitro*[13]. A recent study of a related murine lupus strain has characterized Th cells that drive anti-DNA autoantibody secretion[14]. The long-lasting ameliorization of disease in these animals, after therapeutic interruption of Th cell interaction with anti-CD40 ligand antibody, supports the important role of T cell help in this model, and suggests a potential therapeutic target in human disease. Evidence for impaired T regulatory mechanisms after the onset of autoimmunity includes decreased IgG anti-DNA antibody secretion by B/W F1 splenocytes cultured with young, but not old, B/W F1 T cells with suppressor phenotype[13]. In addition, abnormalities of the thymus, the lymphoid organ responsible for the fine-tuning of the composition of the T cell repertoire, have been described in NZB and B/W F1 mice. Thymic epithelial cells are abnormal and accelerated thymic atrophy is observed. Although subtle impairments in thymic 'education' may account for the excessive T cell help and impaired T suppression that have been described, no global abnormalities in the generation of self-tolerance by the B/W F1 thymus have been detected, at least as assessed by the analysis of TCR variable region gene products reactive to autoantigens. Data demonstrating that B/W F1 athymic mice do not develop kidney disease, whereas those mice engrafted with a thymus do develop autoimmune disease, support the requirement for T cells in the development of the full-blown lupus-like disease[15]. Whether the thymus bears intrinsic abnormalities or whether thymic atrophy and other defects are secondary to stem cell abnormalities that are manifest after maturation of those cells in the thymus is not clear. However, data demonstrating the transfer of lupus-like disease by the donation of T-cell-depleted bone marrow or fetal-liver-derived stem cells to normal recipients support the concept of the thymus being one of the sites in which autoimmunity develops, rather than primarily responsible for abnormal immune function[16].

Recent studies using microsatellite analysis have assigned loci on at least five chromosomes that are associated with immunologic and clinical manifestations of murine lupus, and support a multigenic etiology for human lupus[17–19]. Loci on the long arm of chromosome 1 have generated particular interest, and members of the CD2 immunoglobulin superfamily, complement receptors and an interferon-inducible gene are targets of recent study in lupus-susceptible mice[20–22].

MRL lpr/lpr

Lupus-like disease in MRL lpr/lpr mice is also characterized by high levels of anti-dsDNA autoantibodies and early onset of immune complex-mediated glomerulonephritis. The congenic MRL +/+ strain does produce anti-DNA antibodies and can develop late-onset renal disease, but the breeding of the recessive lpr gene, associated with massive lymphadenopathy, into the MRL genome provides an accelerating effect on the autoimmune disease. The contribution of the background MRL strain to lupus-like disease appears to depend on the capacity of Th cells to induce the production of highly cationic antibodies reactive with dsDNA[11]. Only Th cells from older mice (at least 5 months of age) permit secretion of these pathogenic antibodies.

The accelerating effects associated with the lpr gene have been definitively attributed to the insertion of a retrotransposon within the gene encoding the Fas receptor, CD95, a member of the TNF receptor molecular family[23]. Fas is expressed on activated T and B cells, and ligation of this receptor can initiate a cell death program, resulting in apoptosis. Normally, interaction between T cell Fas ligand and Fas receptor on activated lymphocytes mediates activation-induced cell death of T cells and contributes to elimination of B cells activated by Th cells in the absence of recent antigen-induced surface Ig signals. In lpr mice, the structural abnormality in Fas results in impaired peripheral immune tolerance and in uncontrolled lymphoproliferation[24].

Although altered Th activity may drive the production of the pathogenic autoantibodies in these mice, this T cell help does not go unchecked. An age-dependent loss of certain CD4+ T cell responses specific for hapten-altered self and for allogeneic determinants presented in association with self-MHC class II molecules has been described in MRL lpr/lpr, but not the congenic MRL +/+, mice[25]. This loss of self-restricted Th cell function has been attributed to CD4+ T suppressor cells that can inhibit IL-2 production by the Th cells. This suppression may represent an attempt of the immune system to downregulate excessive T cell help. In the MRL lpr/lpr mouse, this effort at suppression is evidently only partially effective, serving to impair IL-2 production, but failing to inhibit B cell activation.

Experimental lupus-like disease

The autoimmune manifestations of chronic graft-versus-host disease (GVHD), which may emerge following the adoptive transfer of parental T cells into F1 recipient mice, have been particularly useful in understanding the cellular interactions which may result in SLE (Fig. 121.4)[26]. In that model, as in human SLE, a role for genetic predisposition is clear, as only selected inbred strains of non-autoimmune mice develop an SLE-like illness. The autoantibody responses generated are very analogous to those observed in human SLE, and include anti-dsDNA, antiphospholipid and anti-red blood cell specificities. The high proportion of autoantibodies generated in these mice suggests an antigen-driven response, not merely polyclonal B cell activation. Experiments in which isolated parental T cell subsets, either helper or suppressor/cytotoxic, are transferred into the F1 recipients have demonstrated that it is the Th cell that drives autoantibody production. Specifically, parental Th cells, recognizing MHC class II antigens contributed by the other parent and expressed on the F1 recipient's B cells, interact with and activate those B cells. As all recipient B cells, regardless of their specificity for antigen, express the MHC class II alloantigen recognized by the donor Th cells, every B cell is a potential target of direct, cognate T cell help. Presumably, the continuous presence of certain multivalent autoantigens selectively drives autoantibody production. In the early stage of GVHD, donor Th cells are highly activated, and secrete abundant lymphokines, including IL-2. This phase of Th cell activity is followed, as in the MRL lpr/lpr model, by selective suppression of certain Th cell functions[27]. This occurs after the onset of autoimmunity and probably accounts for the impaired secretion of IL-2 by the Th cell that is observed in these animals.

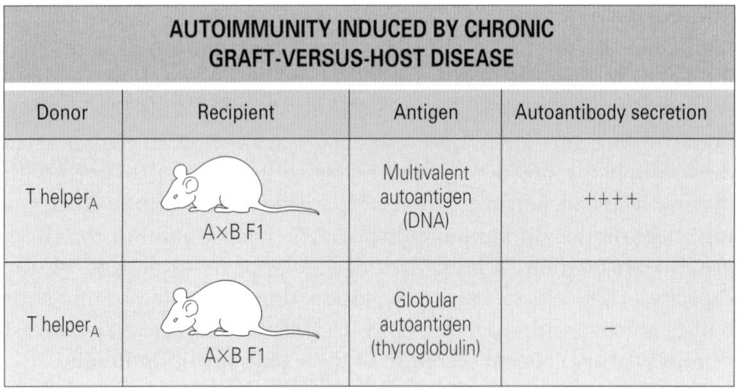

AUTOIMMUNITY INDUCED BY CHRONIC GRAFT-VERSUS-HOST DISEASE			
Donor	Recipient	Antigen	Autoantibody secretion
T helper$_A$	A×B F1	Multivalent autoantigen (DNA)	++++
T helper$_A$	A×B F1	Globular autoantigen (thyroglobulin)	–

Fig. 121.4 Autoimmunity induced by chronic graft-versus-host disease. The transfer of parental Th cells ('A') into F1 recipients ('A × B F1') bearing cells expressing cell surface histocompatibility antigens ('B') foreign to 'A', results in secretion of autoantibodies and a clinical syndrome similar to SLE. The interaction of 'A' T cell TCR with 'B' determinants on 'A × B F1' B cells, regardless of the antigen specificity of those B cells, mediates the disease. As B cells require both sIg-mediated and T-cell-mediated help in order to undergo growth and differentiation (Fig. 121.2), only those B cells which have received a recent sIg signal will be induced to secrete antibodies. Multivalent autoantigens, such as DNA, are more effective than globular autoantigens, such as thyroglobulin, at inducing autoantibody secretion in this model, perhaps reflecting a capacity of multivalent antigens to mediate an sIg signal that is 'stronger' or of greater duration.

The role of IL-2 in lupus-like disease has also been studied in an experimental model that utilizes the MRL lpr/lpr mouse. These mice were vaccinated with live recombinant vaccinia virus expressing the human IL-2 gene[28]. Decreased production of autoantibodies, attenuation of renal pathology and prolonged survival were observed in the inoculated mice, but not in those that had received wild-type vaccinia virus lacking the IL-2 gene. Although the mechanisms of these salutory effects were not elucidated, the results suggest that restoration of adequate concentrations of IL-2 may permit improved regulation of the autoimmune process.

With the advent of technology to generate 'knockout' and transgenic mice, either deficient or overexpressing a particular gene, it has become clear that lupus-like disease, or at least production of anti-DNA antibodies and renal deposition of immune complexes, can readily occur when the threshold for activation of the immune system is lowered. Alteration of cell surface accessory proteins such as CD19, CD21, CD45, PD-1, or BLyS, or intracellular signaling molecules such as PTEN or SHP-1, modifies immune system activity such that self-antigens are more immunogenic. Additionally, overexpression of proteins that inhibit apoptosis, as in bcl-2 transgenic mice, has been demonstrated to promote SLE-like disease. Unfortunately, the experimental results from these murine models have not been readily transferred to human lupus, as genetic defects in these threshold-setting molecules have only very rarely been detected in patients.

Taken together, the pieces of information gleaned from both spontaneous and experimentally induced models of murine lupus strongly support an essential, although not exclusive, role for Th cells in the induction of pathogenic autoantibody secretion by B cells, in addition to a failure of secondary immunoregulatory mechanisms. Moreover, the various knockout models clearly demonstrate that animals of diverse genetic backgrounds can develop at least some manifestations of lupus when lymphocyte activation is perturbed. These *in vivo* models may be giving us the message that a clue to the etiology of lupus lies in the factors that mediate generalized immune system activation, rather than in the presence of a unique self-antigen or antigen-specific lymphocyte receptor. These animal systems have the significant advantage of allowing analysis of the cellular mechanisms that are active early in the

disease, in addition to the later efforts of the immune system to control the emerging autoimmunity.

CELLULAR IMMUNE FUNCTION IN SLE

A host of immunologic abnormalities, encompassing all components of the immune system, have been thoroughly described in patients with SLE (Table 121.4)[29–31]. Many of these cellular immune abnormalities are likely to be secondary to the autoimmune process, rather than intrinsic defects, as they are more pronounced during flares of the disease and may be improved or undetectable when the disease is in remission. The characterization of these functional impairments has contributed to our understanding of the susceptibility of these patients to infection, but has not provided the answer to the essential issue of the etiologic trigger for SLE. In general, the immunologic abnormalities in patients with SLE are analogous to those of lupus-prone mice after the onset of autoimmune disease. That is, we are seeing the alterations of immune function that are the sum of the organism's attempt, or failed attempt, to regulate current autoimmunity. We rarely have the opportunity to study cellular immune function at the preclinical stage of SLE, but the similarities between the lymphocyte abnormalities observed in the murine systems after the onset of autoimmunity and those abnormalities observed in patients with active SLE suggest that the very early events in the murine and human systems may also be comparable. As in the spontaneous murine models and in chronic GVHD, impaired regulation of Th cell activity is likely to be an important factor in human SLE.

T cell function

The lymphocyte count in general, and T cell number particularly, may be decreased in patients with SLE. This lymphopenia has traditionally been attributed to the effects of T cell reactive autoantibodies, although recent data support a contribution of activation-induced cell death. Studies of CD4:CD8 (helper:suppressor) ratios among patients have yielded variable results. More dramatic than alterations in numbers

TABLE 121.4 ABNORMALITIES IN CELLULAR IMMUNE FUNCTION IN SLE
T cell functions
Decreased T cell number
Alterations in T cell subset ratios
Cutaneous anergy
Impaired T cell proliferation in response to mitogens, antigens and in autologous and allogeneic mixed lymphocyte reactions
Impaired secretion of IL-2
Impaired expression of IL-2 receptors
Reduced natural killer cell activity
Reduced antibody-dependent cellular cytotoxicity
Enhanced interferon and IL-10 production
Impaired T cell capping
Variable T suppressor cell function
Increased CD40 ligand expression
Spontaneous apoptosis in vitro
B cell functions
Activated cell morphology
Spontaneous proliferation and antibody secretion
Secretion of polyclonal immunoglobulins and high levels of antibodies specific for a restricted group of defined intracellular autoantigens
Increased responses to T-cell-derived growth and differentiation factors
Accessory cell functions
Defective Fcγ receptor function
Impaired secretion of IL-1
Impaired delivery of accessory signals to T cells; may be partially overcome by addition of protein kinase C activators to cell cultures.
Increased production of BLyS

of T cells or T cell subsets are deficits in their function, particularly those that depend on the secretion of IL-2. T cell proliferative responses to mitogens, soluble recall antigens such as tetanus toxoid, and autologous non-T-cells in the autologous mixed lymphocyte reaction are all severely impaired. These deficits are most marked in patients with active disease, but are also noted in most patients with inactive disease. In contrast, the T cell proliferative responses induced by monoclonal antibodies reactive with the CD3 molecular complex, comprising the chains of the TCR that transduce activation signals to the T cell, are of similar magnitude in patients with SLE and normal individuals. The responses that are impaired in patients with SLE are known to be highly dependent on the secretion of IL-2, whereas anti-CD3-induced T cell proliferation is less IL-2 dependent and is a property mainly of helper inducer T cells – those which secrete IL-4 and deliver help to B cells. The T cell proliferative defects in SLE are, then, consistent with those seen in the murine models, in which IL-2 secretion is selectively impaired after the onset of autoimmunity. In fact, deficient IL-2 production has been documented in in vitro studies of SLE T cell function. Some investigators have found that supplementing in vitro cultures with IL-2 will increase the responses of SLE T cells to mitogens or antigens, but the addition of IL-1 or phorbol myristate acetate, often used to substitute for macrophage-derived accessory signals in T cell responses, will also partially correct the defective responses of SLE T cells. These results suggest a possible role for impaired accessory cell function in the poor T cell responses seen in SLE.

Regulatory T cell function, now felt to reside in the CD4$^+$CD25$^+$ T cell population and associated with production of transforming growth factor β and IL-10, has not been carefully studied in SLE patients. However, some data support a role for suppressor cells in the impaired IL-2 production of SLE T cells. In contrast, T cell mediated inhibition of B cell differentiation is decreased in SLE patients compared with normal individuals. These results may again be similar to those observed in the murine models, in which T suppressor cells may inhibit the function of those T cells that secrete IL-2, but not those that provide help for B cell differentiation.

These numerous abnormalities in SLE T cell function in such predominantly in vitro assays may not be directly linked to the primary disease process, whereas several observations of augmented function may more closely reflect the underlying mechanisms of autoimmunity in SLE. Th cells that specifically respond to lupus autoantigens have been documented, and Th cell lines and clones, which deliver help for anti-dsDNA autoantibody in vitro, have been characterized[32,33]. In addition to this antigen-specific T cell help, non-specific mechanisms of Th cell function are augmented, particularly in active SLE. CD40 ligand, an essential mediator of direct T cell help to B cells, macrophages and other cell types, such as endothelial cells, is normally tightly regulated and is expressed briefly following TCR-mediated T cell activation. In contrast to T cells from healthy individuals, T cells from patients with SLE with active disease have detectable T cell surface CD40 ligand and most lupus T cells show prolonged CD40 ligand expression after in vitro activation[34,35]. Augmented expression of CD40 ligand may contribute to increased T cell help for B cell activation, in addition to the activation of endothelial cells, with subsequent vascular damage. Another indication of current T cell autoreactivity in SLE may be the observation of increased spontaneous lymphocyte apoptosis in patients with active disease[36,37]. Reversal of the spontaneous in vitro apoptosis of SLE T cells by neutralizing antibody to Fas ligand suggests that this process may be a function of activation-induced cell death, and that underlying the many observed abnormalities in SLE T cell function is a more primary process of both antigen-specific and generalized T cell activation. In contrast to the MRL lpr/lpr murine lupus model, no significant deficit in the function of the Fas–Fas ligand system has been documented in patients with SLE. On the contrary, Fas receptor expression is increased on SLE lymphocytes, reflecting activation, and Fas ligand-mediated apoptosis is intact, if not increased, on the basis of its role in the spontaneous apoptosis observed in vitro[37,38].

B cell function

B lymphocyte function in SLE is most simply characterized as hyperactive. A high proportion of peripheral blood B cells are activated by morphologic criteria. SLE B cells in vitro proliferate and differentiate to antibody-secreting cells spontaneously, without the addition of traditional mitogens. The spectrum of B cells that secrete antibody in patients with SLE represents a polyclonal assortment, but characteristic of SLE is the selective and high-level secretion of a restricted population of autoantibody specificities (described in Chapter 120).

As in the case of SLE T cells, an important issue is whether the B cell abnormalities observed represent primary, intrinsic B lineage defects or, alternatively, are secondary to excessive T cell help or impaired immunoregulation mediated by T cells or macrophages. The spontaneous models of murine lupus described above would suggest that intrinsic B cell defects play a permissive role in the pathogenesis of SLE, but that the full-blown clinical syndrome, with the secretion of high-affinity IgG anti-dsDNA autoantibodies and immune complex-mediated glomerulonephritis, requires Th cells. In the human system, this question is more difficult to study. Increased responsiveness of SLE B cells to T cell derived growth and differentiation factors has been documented[39] and may result from intrinsic B cell activity or, more likely, be attributable to previous in vivo activation by interaction of sIg with antigen or by cognate interaction with Th cells. An altered 'set point' or threshold for activation of SLE B cells through sIg could contribute to B cell activity. The functions of B cell protein kinases, phosphatases and the cell surface receptors that trigger activity of these second messenger molecules are being actively investigated in SLE B cells.

Accessory cell function

The mononuclear phagocyte system is essential for the inactivation of pathogenic infectious organisms and for the clearance of potentially pathogenic immune complexes and senescent or apoptotic cells (described in Chapter 117). In terms of cellular immune function, macrophages bind, process and present antigenic peptides to T cells; they physically interact with T cells, delivering secondary activation signals to those cells through cell surface adhesion and costimulatory molecules; and macrophages secrete a panoply of soluble products, including IL-1, IL-10, IL-12, TNFα, IL-6, and BLyS, that provide important accessory and regulatory signals to both T and B cells.

Although T and B cells appear to be the major cellular immune players generating pathogenic autoantibodies, impairments in the capacity of macrophages to activate T cells and abnormal secretion of monokines have been documented, and may contribute to the characteristic poor T cell proliferative function in SLE. In this regard, IL-10, a monocyte-derived product that is increased in patients with active SLE and has T cell inhibitory and B cell differentiative properties, is of particular interest.

POTENTIAL ETIOLOGIES FOR CELLULAR IMMUNE DYSFUNCTION IN SLE

Genetic and hormonal influences clearly predispose to and accelerate the autoimmune diathesis, but an environmental factor appears necessary to trigger the process. The often abrupt, febrile onset, constitutional features and waxing and waning course of many autoimmune diseases suggest that infection represents the relevant environmental trigger, yet there is little evidence of current infection in patients with SLE. A mechanism of current popular appeal is an augmentation or impaired clearance of apoptotic cells, resulting in increased availability of self antigens that trigger immune system activation. Exposure to ultraviolet light is one possible stimulus for apoptosis and exposure of self antigens. Other environmental factors, such as drugs that demethylate DNA, may modify the structure or function of the genome of the lupus-susceptible individual to permit transcription of immunostimulatory genomic products, including endogenous virus-like sequences. Microbial products could play a part in exacerbating immune system activity through their production of superantigens that non-specifically trigger T and B cell activation.

Role of cell damage and apoptotic cells

The documented capacity of ultraviolet radiation and certain drugs to initiate or exacerbate autoimmunity, or at least autoantibody production, suggests mechanisms through which autoantigen-specific Th cells can be activated. These and other stimuli can mediate cellular damage and apoptosis, potentially resulting in the augmented expression of costimulatory molecules, exposure of previously cryptic autoantigenic determinants or generation of cellular debris enriched in potential autoantigens. Of particular interest is the demonstration that initiation of the apoptotic process in epidermal keratinocytes by ultraviolet radiation is followed by concentration of fragments of small nuclear ribonucleoproteins and other classic lupus autoantigens in apoptotic 'blebs' on the cell surface[40]. These self proteins and phospholipids may be cleaved to generate previously unexposed epitopes. These observations have led to suggestions from several investigators that apoptotic cells might themselves represent a trigger for induction of autoimmunity. Typically, apoptotic cells are immediately coated with complement products and cleared by cells of the reticuloendothelial cell system. Should this clearance pathway be impaired, because of either deficiencies of complement components or phagocytic cells, the load of apoptotic debris and associated cleaved products might be sufficient to trigger immune system activation. Under these circumstances, autoreactive T cells present in low frequency or expressing TCR with low avidity for autoantigen might become activated. If followed by efficient delivery of T cell help to B cells, these events would lead to spreading of the autoreactive T cell response to additional determinants of the immunizing cell-derived particles, resulting in secretion of the classic spectrum of lupus autoantibody specificities. This scenario is attractive, and has garnered some support in studies in which administration of apoptotic cells to healthy mice generated autoantibodies. However, a full-blown lupus syndrome has not developed in those experiments. Moreover, it has been proposed that the uptake and presentation of self antigens derived from apoptotic cells may be a normal occurrence and even contribute to maintenance of immune homeostasis. Support for a triggering role for apoptotic cells in lupus will await direct demonstration of pathogenic T cell activation by products of apoptotic cells.

A role for apoptotic cells or debris in the induction of SLE remains speculative. However, the importance of adequate regulation of immune system homeostasis through apoptosis of activated lymphocytes is clear. The defective expression of Fas in MRL/lpr lupus mice accounts for the accelerated emergence of lupus in those autoimmune-prone mice.

Autoimmunity is also seen in some patients with autoimmune lymphoproliferative syndrome who have mutations in Fas. Inadequate removal of self-reactive lymphocytes through apoptosis permits induction of autoantibodies, a defect that may also have a pathogenic role in some cases of human lupus.

Microbial superantigens

Microbial superantigens identified to date include several staphylococcal enterotoxins, the pyrogenic enterotoxin of group A streptococcus and a soluble product of *Mycoplasma arthritidis*[41]. Certain endogenous murine retroviral-encoded gene products [e.g. minor lymphocyte stimulating (mls) antigens] are also categorized as superantigens[42]. As a group, superantigens share several remarkable characteristics that distinguish them from conventional antigens (Fig. 121.5). First, superantigen recognition is a function of TCRβ chain variable (Vβ) gene usage, with little influence from other TCR gene elements, or cell surface expression of the CD4 or CD8 antigens. Thus a particular superantigen is recognized by virtually all T cells that utilize a single or small group of TCR V gene families. Also, superantigens bind selectively and with high affinity to MHC class II molecules. In the absence of antigen processing and in an MHC non-restricted manner, superantigen–MHC class II antigen complexes on the antigen-presenting cell surface trigger the proliferation of T cells expressing the relevant TCR V gene products. Finally, the microbial superantigens are among the most potent T cell mitogens known, functioning at concentrations of less than 10^{-11}M.

The unique properties of microbial superantigens suggest at least three mechanisms by which these substances could activate the immune system, contributing to autoimmunity (Fig. 121.6)[43]. First, the dual affinity of superantigens for MHC class II molecules and selected TCR Vβ gene products could allow these microbial toxins to perturb the immune system in a manner analogous to that seen in GVHD. A microbial superantigen may bind to MHC class II antigens on the surface of any B cell, regardless of its specificity for antigens, and render that B cell a target of cognate T cell help by superantigen-specific Th cells. This model predicts that, *in vivo*, given the requirement for several signals in order to induce B cell differentiation (Fig. 121.2), the presence of multivalent autoantigens and a superantigen 'bridge' mediating abnormal Th–B cell interaction could result in the spectrum of autoantibodies that characterize GVH-mediated and, by extension, spontaneously arising autoimmunity.

Second, the binding of microbial superantigen to MHC class II molecules may in itself deliver activation signals to the B cell that mimic those induced by Th cell TCR–MHC class II antigen interaction, preparing the B cells that have interacted with antigen to respond more efficiently to lymphokines. Evidence of monocyte and B cell activation induced by superantigen binding has been documented.

Third, microbial superantigen may activate quiescent T cells that recognize autoantigens. The spectrum of superantigen-activated autoreactive T cells may include those recognizing autoantigens selectively expressed in particular anatomic sites, resulting in organ-specific

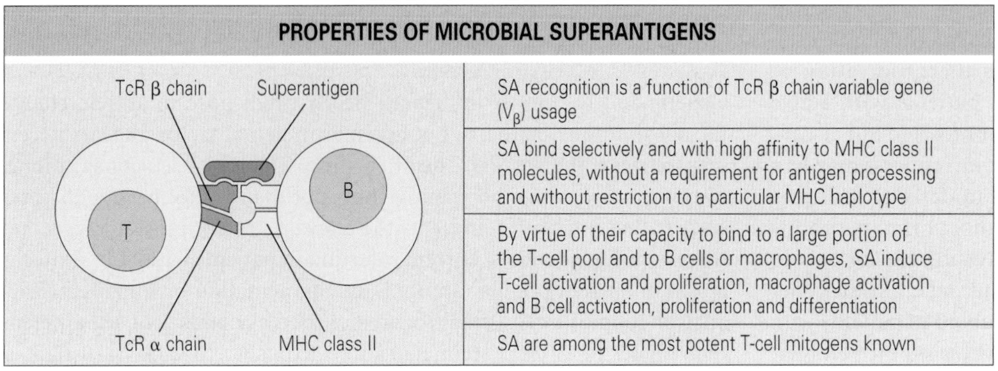

PROPERTIES OF MICROBIAL SUPERANTIGENS

	SA recognition is a function of TcR β chain variable gene (V$_\beta$) usage
	SA bind selectively and with high affinity to MHC class II molecules, without a requirement for antigen processing and without restriction to a particular MHC haplotype
	By virtue of their capacity to bind to a large portion of the T-cell pool and to B cells or macrophages, SA induce T-cell activation and proliferation, macrophage activation and B cell activation, proliferation and differentiation
	SA are among the most potent T-cell mitogens known

Fig. 121.5 Microbial superantigens. Superantigens (SA) are the soluble products of bacteria or mycoplasma species with the unique capacity to bind to the β chain of the TCR and to non-polymorphic determinants on MHC class II antigens, at sites distinct from those bound by antigenic peptides. Each superantigen binds to certain common amino acid sequences expressed by the protein products (TCR β chain) of one or several TCR β chain variable gene families. Thus a superantigen will bind to a set of T cells bearing TCR with a spectrum of antigen specificities, yet having a high degree of amino acid sequence homology.

MECHANISMS BY WHICH MICROBIAL SUPERANTIGENS MIGHT RESULT IN AUTOIMMUNITY

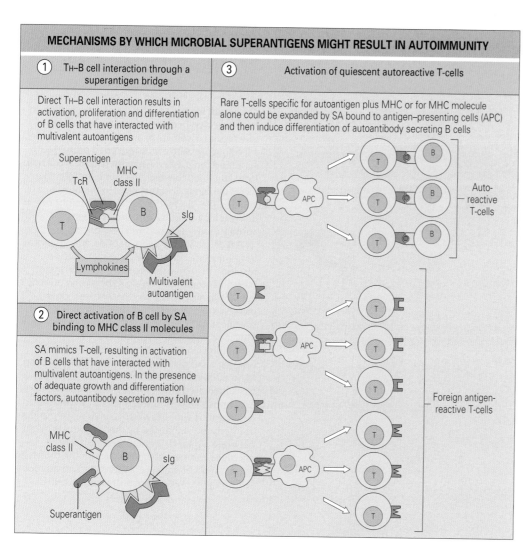

① TH–B cell interaction through a superantigen bridge

Direct TH–B cell interaction results in activation, proliferation and differentiation of B cells that have interacted with multivalent autoantigens

② Direct activation of B cell by SA binding to MHC class II molecules

SA mimics T-cell, resulting in activation of B cells that have interacted with multivalent autoantigens. In the presence of adequate growth and differentiation factors, autoantibody secretion may follow

③ Activation of quiescent autoreactive T-cells

Rare T-cells specific for autoantigen plus MHC or for MHC molecule alone could be expanded by SA bound to antigen–presenting cells (APC) and then induce differentiation of autoantibody secreting B cells

Fig. 121.6 Mechanisms by which microbial superantigens might result in autoimmunity. Superantigens (SA) could mediate the activation of autoreactive T or B cells in three ways. First, by facilitating Th–B cell interaction through a superantigen bridge. Second, by direct activation of autoreactive B cells after binding of superantigens to B cell surface MHC class II antigens. Finally, by the activation and expansion of rare quiescent autoreactive T cells present among the population of superantigen-reactive T cells. sIg, surface immunoglobulin.

disease, or T cells reactive to self-MHC class II antigens, triggering an autologous GVH-like reaction and systemic autoimmunity. Although most superantigen-reactive cells would revert to resting after clearance of the superantigen-producing microbe, the superantigen-activated autoreactive T cells may be sustained in the active state by the presence of the relevant autoantigen.

The superantigen model could be compatible with the episodic course that characterizes human SLE. After a virus or microbial infection initiates the immune system activation in SLE, the inciting microbial agent and its superantigen may be cleared. At this point, the GVH-like stimulus to the B cell pool is eliminated, autoantibody production ceases and a period of clinical remission ensues. The immune system of the patient with SLE would, however, not be normal. As a consequence of the initial episode, autoantibody-forming B cells are now represented in the memory B cell pool, which is more easily triggered by antigen and non-specific lymphokines, without a requirement for direct Th–B cell interaction. The accumulation of easily activated autoreactive B cells in the memory population could account for 'flares' of SLE during intercurrent infections or physical or physiologic stress (e.g. pregnancy). Although support for a role for superantigens in exacerbating inflammatory arthritis has been demonstrated in animal models, experimental documentation of a pathogenic role for superantigen in human or murine lupus has not yet been provided.

Viruses

A role for viruses in the pathogenesis of SLE has long been postulated. Direct evidence for the involvement of specific viruses is lacking, but striking similarities in the clinical picture and immunologic abnormalities common to patients with SLE and to a subset of those infected by ubi-

quitous agents, such as cytomegalovirus and Epstein–Barr virus (EBV), suggest that these or other viruses may trigger SLE. The mechanisms by which viruses might induce the cellular immune system to generate autoantibody secretion are not known, but a recent study in the murine system provided clues[44]. Mice that express a protein encoded by the vesicular stomatitis virus on the surface of their B cells, in association with MHC class II molecules, are induced to secrete autoantibody in the presence of cognate T cell help. Thus the alteration of class II proteins by viral antigens may result in the preferential activation by altered self MHC class II-reactive T cells or B cells that have recently bound autoantigen via their surface immunoglobulin receptors. In vitro evidence of the potential for altered self-reactive Th cells to activate autologous B cells has been presented[45]. Alternatively, the virus-altered MHC class II molecules may present autoantigenic peptides to autoantigen-specific T cells that were not deleted from the T cell repertoire in the thymus, because they recognize antigen bound to non-self MHC determinants, not to self MHC determinants (Fig. 121.7). These proposed mechanisms that might account for T cell dependent induction of autoantibody production in SLE have been previously discussed by Eisenberg and Cohen[46]. Viruses can also promote an immunostimulatory microenvironment that can contribute to generalized immune system activation, with an antigenic preference for proteins and nucleic acids associated with the virus. This adjuvant-like milieu could be generated by CpG-rich viral sequences that promote maturation of antigen presenting cells, by interferon-α, a cytokine induced by viral RNA, or by virus-stimulated augmentation of MHC class II molecule expression on accessory cells, resulting in the potential for augmented T cell activation, including excessive helper activity[47,48]. Another mechanism supported by experimental data is 'molecular mimicry', in which peptide sequences

1355

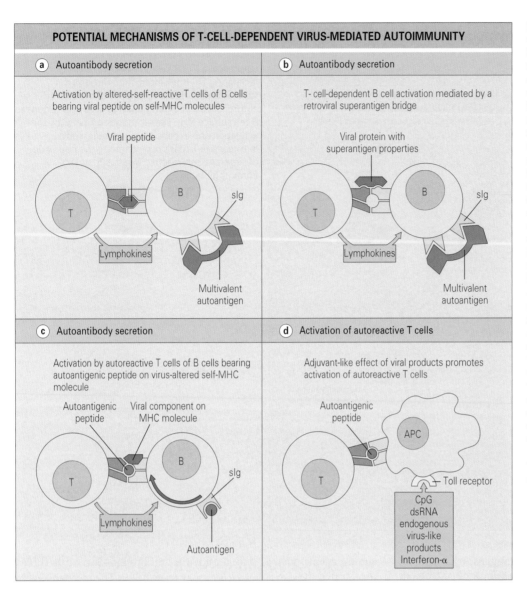

Fig. 121.7 Potential mechanisms of T cell dependent virus-mediated autoimmunity. The interaction or infection of B cells with a virus could result in T cell mediated induction of autoantibody secretion by at least three potential mechanisms. (a) A B cell to which a viral peptide or fragment has bound via surface MHC class II molecules might receive T cell help from a virus-altered self-specific T cell. (b) In a variation of this model, a B cell expressing a virus-encoded protein with superantigen properties might receive T cell help from any T cell to which that superantigen-like molecule binds. In either case, in the presence of an adequate sIg-mediated signal, as might be delivered by a multivalent autoantigen, autoantibody secretion will be induced. (c) A B cell to which a viral peptide or fragment has bound via surface MHC class II molecules, resulting in a 'non-self' class II molecule, might bind an autoantigen via sIg, process and present autoantigenic peptides on the 'non-self' class II molecule and receive T cell signals from T cells specific for autoantigen in the context of 'non-self' MHC. Such T cells, unlike those reactive with autoantigen in the context of 'self'-MHC, would have escaped deletion during thymic maturation. (d) In addition to these antigen-specific modes of virus-mediated autoimmunity, endogenous or exogenous viral products, such as CpG motifs, endogenous viral-like mRNAs or viral-like proteins, or interferon-α induced by those products might generate a generally immunostimulatory microenvironment that would lower the threshold for initiation of immune responses to ubiquitous self-antigens. APC, antigen-presenting cell.

common to a virus (an EBV protein, for example) and a target lupus autoantigen (Sm, for example) can induce autoantibodies specific for that autoantigen and, in some cases, glomerulonephritis. Many mechanisms by which viruses might induce lupus can thus be proposed and are reasonable, but it remains difficult to document definitively an etiologic role for any particular virus. A recent intriguing report provides epidemiologic evidence for increased exposure to EBV among patients with SLE compared with carefully matched controls[49]. These data keep alive the hope that specific etiologic triggers will eventually be defined.

Retroviruses

In many vertebrate species, endogenous type-C retroviruses (via transcription of viral RNA into DNA) are transmitted vertically. In humans, mRNA transcripts related to full-length endogenous retroviral DNA are expressed in cell lines and placenta. The potential for those transcripts to encode functional proteins is suggested by detection of type-C retrovirus-related p30 and p75 proteins in human placenta. Moreover, electron microscopy and measurements of reverse transcriptase activity have revealed human placentas to contain type-C virus-like particles. Infectious human retroviruses are now well described, including human T lymphotrophic virus-1, which induces adult T cell leukemia, and human immunodeficiency virus (HIV)-1, causing acquired immune deficiency syndrome, a disease often accompanied by clinical features characteristic of autoimmunity.

In addition to endogenous retroviral sequences with the capacity to encode virus-like particles, another class of genomic elements with virus-like DNA sequence, the long interspersed nuclear elements (LINEs), are occasionally present in full-length form that can be transcribed into mRNA that encodes an RNA-binding protein and a reverse transcriptase[50]. These LINE RNA and protein products are enriched in ribonucleoprotein particles and could promote immune responses to associated proteins.

A potential role for endogenous retroviral sequences, virus-like LINE elements, or infectious retroviruses in the pathogenesis of SLE is supported by studies in both murine and human systems[51]. Evidence for enhanced expression of endogenous type-C retroviruses is seen in murine lupus strains, and recent data demonstrate that these full-length polytropic endogenous retroviral sequences are preferentially expressed in bone marrow cells of lupus-prone, but not control[52], murine strains. In human studies, 30% of SLE sera, but not normal sera, were found to react with the p24 gag protein of HIV-1[53]. These SLE patients were not infected with HIV-1, and the p24 antibody activity was associated with anti-Sm autoantibody activity. A potential role for 'molecular mimicry' in the induction of autoantibodies is suggested by amino acid homology and antibody cross-reactivity between the p30 gag sequence of type-C retroviruses and the 69kDa protein of U1 small nuclear ribonuclear proteins[54].

In common with bacterial superantigen, mls determinants that are expressed on murine B cells have the capacity to delete interacting T cells during thymic development or, alternatively, to stimulate the proliferation of certain populations of mature T cells. The mls determinants, protein products of vertically transmitted retroviruses, selectively activate and expand populations of T cells bearing the products of selected TCR variable gene families. If comparable retroviral proteins are expressed on human cells, most likely in association with MHC class II molecules, those products could trigger the expansion of rare auto-reactive T cells among those T cells bearing the reactive TCR V gene product, or they might mediate T–B cell interaction, resulting in preferential autoantibody formation similar to that observed in experimental GVHD (Fig. 121.4)[43]. Recent data documenting selective TCR Vβ gene family usage by pathogenic T cells in murine autoimmune diseases (experimental autoimmune encephalomyelitis, type II collagen arthritis and in the induction of autoantibody production in MRL lpr/lpr mice) are consistent with a potential role for microbial products with super-antigen properties in the induction of the cellular immune dysfunction that initiates and mediates murine lupus. However, confirmation of an etiologic role for superantigens in human systemic autoimmune disease is currently lacking.

CONCLUSION

Clearly, SLE is associated with a myriad of cellular immune system abnormalities. Some of the impaired immune functions directly contribute to the secretion of the autoantibodies that form immune complexes, mediate tissue damage and lead to disease. Many of the observed abnormalities, however, are secondary effects and are unlikely to be essential for the disease process. The investigation of spontaneous and experimental models of murine lupus-like disease has been invaluable in developing our current understanding of the immune events that mediate SLE. Taking all of the available data together, an essential role for excessive or poorly controlled activity of T helper cells in the activation and differentiation of autoantibody-forming B cells is likely to be a final common pathway. The characterization of those T helper cells that mediate this process, and the mechanisms by which tolerance of SLE T cells is 'broken', are active and important areas for current and future investigation.

Finally, the environmental triggers that initiate the cellular immune dysfunction must be identified. Environmental factors, whether they be viruses, hormones, demethylating drugs or ultraviolet light, may act on the genome to induce an immunostiumatory milieu that mimics the effect of adjuvants on immune system activation. The common outcome is the generation of both generalized immune system activity and a specific focus on antigenic targets that are involved in genome-related functions. It will be important to characterize the mechanisms used by each of these potential triggers to provoke a sufficient immunologic stimulus to surpass the threshold for induction of autoimmunity in the genetically susceptible host.

REFERENCES

1. Carson DA, Chen PP, Kipps JP. New roles for rheumatoid factor. J Clin Invest 1991; 87: 379–383.
2. Shevach EM. Regulatory T cells in autoimmunity. Annu Rev Immunol 2000; 18: 423–449.
3. Giusti AM, Chien NC, Zack DJ et al. Somatic diversification of S107 from an antiphosphocholine to an anti-DNA antibody is due to a single base change in its heavy chain variable region. Proc Natl Acad Sci USA 1987; 84: 2926–2930.
4. Justement LB, Campbell KS, Chien NC, Cambier JC. Regulation of B cell antigen receptor signal transduction and phosphorylation by CD45. Science 1991; 252: 1839–1842.
5. Schattner E, Elkon KB, Tumang JR et al. CD40 ligation induces Apo-1/Fas expression on human B lymphocytes and facilitates apoptosis through the Apo-1/Fas pathway. J Exp Med 1995; 182: 1557–1565.
6. Gross JA, Dillon SR, Mudri S et al. TACI-Ig neutralizes molecules critical for B cell development and autoimmune disease. Impaired B cell maturation in mice lacking BlyS. Immunity 2001; 15: 289–302.
7. Kappler JW, Roehm N, Marrack P. T-cell tolerance by clonal elimination in the thymus. Cell 1987; 49: 273–280.
8. Jenkins MK, Schwartz RH. Antigen presentation by chemically-modified splenocytes induces antigen-specific T-cell unresponsiveness in vitro and in vivo. J Exp Med 1987; 165: 302–319.
9. Miller RD, Calkins CE. Suppressor T-cells and self tolerance: active suppression required for normal regulation of anti-erythrocyte autoantibody response in spleen cells from non-autoimmune mice. J Immunol 1988; 140: 3779–3785.
10. Yoshida S, Castles JJ, Gershwin ME. The pathogenesis of autoimmunity in New Zealand mice. Semin Arthritis Rheum 1990; 19: 224–242.
11. Datta SK, Patel H, Berry D. Induction of a cationic shift in IgG anti-DNA autoantibodies: role of T helper cells with classical and novel phenotypes in three murine models of lupus nephritis. J Exp Med 1987; 165: 1252–1268.
12. Wofsy D, Seaman WE. Successful treatment of autoimmunity in NZB/NZW F1 mice with monoclonal antibody to L3T4. J Exp Med 1985; 161: 378–391.
13. Sekigawa I, Okada T, Noguchi K et al. Class-specific regulation of anti-DNA antibody synthesis and the age-associated changes in (NZB × NZW) F1 hybrid mice. J Immunol 1987; 138: 2890–2895.
14. Mohan C, Shi Y, Laman JD, Datta SK. Interaction between CD40 and its ligand gp39 in the development of murine lupus nephritis. J Immunol 1995; 154: 1470–1480.
15. Mihara M, Ohsugi Y, Saito K et al. Immunologic abnormality in NZB/NZW F1 mice: thymic independent occurrence of B cell abnormality and requirement for T-cells in the development of autoimmune disease, as evidenced by an analysis of the athymic nude individuals. J Immunol 1988; 141: 85–90.
16. Sardina EE, Sagiura K, Ikehara S, Good RA. Transplantation of wheat germ agglutinin-positive hematopoietic cells to prevent or induce systemic autoimmune disease. Proc Natl Acad Sci USA 1991; 88: 3218–3222.
17. Drake CG, Kotzin BL. Genetic and immunologic mechanisms in the pathogenesis of systemic lupus erythematosus. Curr Opin Immunol 1992; 4: 733–740.
18. Morel L, Rudofsky UH, Longmate JA et al. Polygenic control of susceptibility to murine systemic lupus erythematosus. Immunity 1994; 1: 219–229.
19. Kono DH, Burlingame RW, Owens DG et al. Lupus susceptibility loci in New Zealand mice. Proc Natl Acad Sci USA 1994; 91: 10168–10172.
20. Morel L, Blenman KR, Croker BP, Wakeland EK. The major murine systemic lupus erythematosus susceptibility locus, Sle1, is a cluster of functionally related genes. Proc Natl Acad Sci USA 2001; 98: 1787–1792.
21. Boackle SA, Holers VM, Chen X et al. Cr2, a candidate in the murine SLE 1c lupus susceptibility locus, encodes a dysfunctional protein. Immunity 2001; 15: 775–785.
22. Rozzo SJ, Allard JD, Choubey D et al. Evidence for an interferon-inducible gene, Ifi202, in the susceptibility to systemic lupus. Immunity 2001; 15: 435–443.
23. Chu JL, Drappa J, Parnassa A, Elkon KB. The defect in Fas mRNA expression in MRL/lpr mice is associated with insertion of the retrotransposon, Etn. J Exp Med 1993; 178: 723–730.
24. Watanabe-Fukunaga R, Brannan CI, Copeland NG et al. Lymphoproliferation disorder in mice explained by defects in Fas antigen that mediates apoptosis. Nature 1992; 356: 314–317.
25. Via CS, Shearer GM. Functional heterogeneity of L3T4+ T-cells suppress major histocompatibility complex-self-restricted L3T4+ T helper cell function in association with autoimmunity. J Exp Med 1988; 168: 2165–2181.
26. Gleichmann E, Pals ST, Rolink AG et al. Graft-versus-host reactions: clues to the etiopathology of a spectrum of immunological diseases. Immunol Today 1984; 5: 324–332.
27. Moser M, Mizuochi T, Sharrow SO et al. Graft-versus-host reaction limited to a class II MHC difference results in a selective deficiency in L3T4+ but not in Lyt-2 T cell function. J Immunol 1987; 138: 1355–1362.
28. Gutierrez-Ramos JC, Andreu JL, Revilla Y et al. Recovery from autoimmunity of MRL/lpr mice after infection with an interleukin 2 vaccinia recombinant virus. Nature 1990; 346: 271–274.
29. Kammer GM, Stein RL. T-lymphocyte immune dysfunctions in systemic lupus erythematosus. J Lab Clin Med 1990; 115: 273–282.
30. Alpert SD, Koide J, Takada S, Engleman EG. T-cell regulatory disturbances in the rheumatic diseases. Rheum Dis Clin North Am 1987; 13: 431–445.
31. Tsokos GC. An overview of cellular immune function in systemic lupus erythematosus. In: Lahita RG, ed. Systemic lupus erythematosus, 2E. New York: Churchill Livingstone; 1992: 15–50.
32. Crow MK, DelGiudice-Asch G, Zehetbauer JB et al. Autoantigen-specific T-cell proliferation induced by the ribosomal P2 protein in patients with systemic lupus erythematosus. J Clin Invest 1994; 94: 345–352.
33. Desai A, Mao C, Rajagopalan S et al. Structure and specificity of T-cell receptors expressed by potentially pathogenic anti-DNA autoantibody-inducing T-cells in human lupus. J Clin Invest 1995; 95: 531–541.
34. Desai-Mehta A, Lu L, Ramsey-Goldman R, Datta SK. Hyperexpression of CD40 ligand by B and T-cells in human lupus and its role in pathogenic autoantibody production. J Clin Invest 1996; 97: 2063–2073.
35. Koshy M, Berger D, Crow MK. Increased expression of CD40 ligand on systemic lupus erythematosus lymphocytes. J Clin Invest 1996; 98: 826–837.
36. Emlen W, Niebur J, Kadera R. Accelerated in vitro apoptosis of lymphocytes from patients with systemic lupus erythematosus. J Immunol 1994; 152: 3685–3692.
37. Georgescu L, Vakkalanka RK, Nagata S et al. Interleukin-10 promotes activation-induced cell death of SLE lymphocytes mediated by Fas ligand. J Clin Invest 1997; 100: 2622–2633..
38. Mysler E, Bini P, Drappa J et al. The apoptosis-1/Fas protein in human systemic lupus erythematosus. J Clin Invest 1994; 93: 1029–1034.
39. Veda Y, Sakane T, Tsunematsu T. Hyperreactivity of activated B cells to B cell growth factor in patients with systemic lupus erythematosus. J Immunol 1989; 143: 3988–3993.

40. Casciola-Rosen LA, Anhalt G, Rosen A. Autoantigens targeted in systemic lupus erythematosus are clustered in two populations of surface structures on apoptotic keratinocytes. J Exp Med 1994; 179: 1317–1330.

41. Marrack P, Kappler JW. The staphylococcal enterotoxins and their relatives. Science 1990; 248: 705–711.

42. Choi Y, Kappler JW, Marrack P. A superantigen encoded in the open reading frame of the 3′ long terminal repeat of mouse mammary tumor virus. Nature 1991; 350: 203–207.

43. Friedman SM, Posnett DN, Tumang JR et al. A potential role for microbial superantigens in the pathogenesis of systemic autoimmune disease. Arthritis Rheum 1991; 34: 468–480.

44. Zinkernagal RM, Cooper S, Chambers J et al. Virus-induced autoantibody response to a transgenic viral antigen. Nature 1990; 345: 68–71.

45. Principato MA, Thompson GS, Friedman SM. A cloned major histocompatibility complex restricted trinitrophenyl reactive human helper T-cell line which activates B cell subsets via two distinct pathways. J Exp Med 1983; 158: 1444–1458.

46. Eisenberg RA, Cohen PL. Class II major histocompatibility antigens and the etiology of systemic lupus erythematosus. Clin Immunol Immunopathol 1983; 29: 1–6.

47. Krug A, Rothenfusser S, Homung V et al. Identification of CpG oligonucleotide sequences with high induction of IFN-alpha-beta in plasmacytoid dendritic cells. Eur J Immunol 2001; 31: 2154–2163.

48. Van Uden JH, Tran CH, Carson DA, Raz E. Type I interferon is required to mount an adaptive response to immunostimulatory DNA. Eur J Immunol 2001; 3281–3290.

49. James JA, Neas BR, Moser KL et al. Systemic lupus erythematosus in adults is associated with previous Epstein–Barr virus exposure. Arthritis Rheum 2001; 44: 1122–1126.

50. Kimberland ML, Divorky V, Prchal J et al. Full-length human L1 insertions retain the capacity for high frequency retrotransposition in cultured cells. Hum Mol Genet 1999; 8: 1557–1560.

51. Krieg AM, Steinberg AD. Retroviruses and autoimmunity. J Autoimmun 1990; 3: 137–166.

52. Krieg AM, Gourley MF, Steinberg AD. Association of murine lupus and thymic full-length endogenous retroviral expression maps to a bone marrow stem cell. J Immunol 1991; 146: 3002–3005.

53. Talal N, Garry RF, Schur PH et al. A conserved idiotype and antibodies to retroviral proteins in systemic lupus erythematosus. J Clin Invest 1990; 85: 1866–1871.

54. Query CC, Keene JD. A human autoimmune protein associated with UI RNA contains a region of homology that is cross-reactive with retroviral p30 gag antigen. Cell 1987; 51: 211–220.

122 Clinical features

Dafna D Gladman and Murray B Urowitz

Definition

- An inflammatory multisystem disease of unknown etiology with protean clinical and laboratory manifestations and a variable course and prognosis
- Immunologic aberrations give rise to production of excessive amounts of autoantibodies, some of which cause cytotoxic damage, whereas others participate in immune complex formation resulting in immune inflammation

Clinical features

- Clinical manifestations may be constitutional or result from inflammation in various organ systems, including skin and mucous membranes, joints, kidney, brain, serous membranes, lung, heart and, occasionally, the gastrointestinal tract
- Organ systems may be involved singly or in any combination
- Involvement of vital organs, particularly the kidneys and central nervous system, accounts for significant morbidity and mortality
- Morbidity and mortality result from tissue damage due to the disease process or its treatment

HISTORY

The term 'lupus', Latin for wolf, was used in the 18th century to describe a variety of skin conditions. However, the first historical account of lupus erythematosus was by Biett, in 1833[1]. For a number of decades the disease was considered a chronic dermatologic disorder, but in 1872 Kaposi described the systemic nature of lupus erythematosus. Indeed, many of the manifestations of systemic lupus erythematosus (SLE) were recognized by Kaposi.

Current understanding of SLE has evolved from the clinical descriptions that followed, and was enhanced by the discovery of the LE cell phenomenon by Hargraves et al. in 1948[2]. The subsequent recognition of the antinuclear factor by Friou[3] provided some insight into the pathogenesis of the disease, whereas recognition of the inflammatory and immunologic features of the disease provided insight into therapeutic modalities.

Subsequently, late causes of mortality and morbidity not immediately related to immunologic abnormalities of SLE have been described, such as premature atheroscelrosis[4], neurocognitive dysfunction and avascular necrosis[5].

EPIDEMIOLOGY

Systemic lupus erythematosus is recognized worldwide. Estimates of its prevalence vary widely and range from 15–124/100 000 population in the USA[6,7], 12–24.7/100 000 in Britain[8], and 22.1/100 000[9] in the province of Manitoba, Canada, to 39/100 000 in Sweden[10] (Fig. 122.1). This variation may reflect true differences in the prevalence of the disease in different geographic areas, or differences in case selection in various studies. On the basis of the most recent studies in the USA, it is likely that the true prevalence is close to the often quoted prevalence rate of 1:1000. Incidence rates have also varied, from 1.8/100 000 per year in Rochester to 7.6/100 000 per year in San Francisco[7,10]. In Scandinavia, the incidence rates lie between these extremes at 4.5/100 000 per year[11], whereas the incidence rate in the Nottingham study was 4.0/100 000[8].

Systemic lupus erythematosus is clearly more prevalent in women, particularly in their reproductive years. In most studies of SLE, 90% of patients are women. For the 14–64 years age group, the ratios of age-specific and sex-specific incidence rates show a 6- to 10-fold female excess, which is not noted in patients younger than 14 years, or older than 65 years of age. This effect of age and sex on the incidence and prevalence rates of SLE suggests a role for hormonal factors in its pathogenesis.

In the USA, SLE is three times more common among blacks than whites. A study in Hawaii demonstrated a greater frequency of SLE among Orientals than among whites. Nonetheless, a high frequency of SLE was noted in Sweden in a population that is strictly white. The highest prevalence rates for SLE in Nottingham, England, were noted for Afro-Caribbeans (207/100 000) followed by Asians (48.8/100 000), and whites (20.3/100 000)[8]. The study from Manitoba, Canada, demonstrated a greater frequency of SLE among North American Indians (42.3/100 000) than in the remainder of the population (20.6/100 000)[9].

In addition to their effect on prevalence and incidence, age, sex, race and socioeconomic status have been suggested to have an influence on disease expression. Black patients with SLE have been shown more commonly to have Sm and RNP antibodies, discoid skin lesions, cellular casts and serositis[12]. These were not related to age, sex or socioeconomic status. Conversely, socioeconomic factors have been identified as important prognostic indicators.

Genetic epidemiology

Genetic factors have long been considered to have a role in the etiopathogenesis of SLE. Support for this concept has come from the observation that there is a high prevalence of SLE among monozygotic twins[13]. Further evidence for a hereditary predisposition to SLE comes from family studies. It is estimated that 5–12% of relatives of patients with SLE develop the condition[14,15].

Human leukocyte antigen (HLA) studies have allowed a more detailed analysis of genetic epidemiology in SLE, and the further determination of the mode of inheritance and the number of genes that might contribute to disease susceptibility. In population studies, class II antigens, particularly HLA-DR2 and -DR3, were found to occur more frequently among patients with SLE[16]. Several investigators have identified an association between SLE and the C4A null allele. Although Schur et al.[17] found a significantly increased frequency of the alleles C4AQ0 and DR3 and the complotype SC01 only in patients of English/Irish descent, others have shown an association between C4A null alleles in white and black populations in the USA, and in Chinese and Japanese patients[18–21].

Population studies have demonstrated associations between several HLA genes and SLE, but the associations have not been uniform, suggesting that, in this complex condition, different genes are responsible

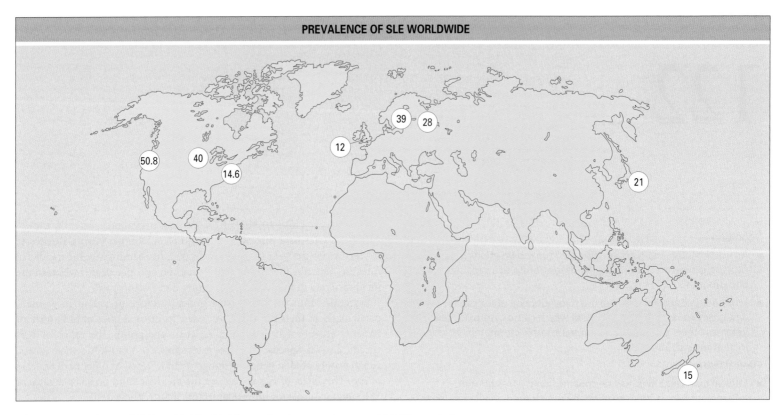

Fig. 122.1 Prevalence of SLE worldwide. World map showing prevalence per 100 000 population.

for the development of a variable disease pattern. For example a study of patients with clinical evidence of lupus nephritis identified an increased frequency of DR2, DQw1, and especially DQb1.AZH, and a decreased frequency of HLA-DR4 in these patients[22]. Another study suggested an interaction between C4A*Q0 and DQA*0501[23]. Associations with other polymorphic genes, including immunoglobulin and T cell receptor genes, have also been reported[24]. Indeed, data from genome scans in families with several members affected with SLE identified a number of genetic loci to be associated with SLE and suggest a multigene theory as an explanation for the inheritance of lupus[25,26].

CLINICAL FEATURES

Clinical manifestations at onset and at any time in the course of the disease in three of the largest reported SLE series in the English literature, the University of Toronto Clinic, the University of Southern

TABLE 122.1 FREQUENCY OF LUPUS MANIFESTATIONS (%)					
Manifestation	Toronto (*n* = 994)		Europe (*n* = 1000)		USC (*n* = 464)
	Onset	Ever	Onset	Ever	Ever
Constitutional	53	80	36	52	41
Arthritis	42	64	69	84	91
Skin	66	86	40	58	55
Mucous membranes	21	50	11	24	19
Pleurisy	14	27	17	36	31
Lung	6	14	3	7	7
Pericarditis	11	20	?	?	12
Myocarditis	1	3	?	?	2
Raynaud's	32	61	18	34	24
Thrombophlebitis	1	5	4	14	11
Vasculitis	12	32	?	?	?
Renal	42	73	16	39	28
Nephrotic syndrome	6	13	?	?	14
Azotemia	7	17	?	?	?
CNS	20	49	12	27	11
Cytoid bodies	2	2	?	?	2
Gastrointestinal	15	39	?	?	?
Pancreatitis	1	2	?	?	2
Lymphadenopathy	15	30	7	12	10
Myositis	3	4	4	9	5

CNS, central nervous system; USC, University of Southern California; ?, information not available

Frequencies at onset, and at any time, in three large series of lupus patients.

California at Los Angeles Clinic and the 'Euro-Lupus' project are displayed in Table 122.1[27].

General

Constitutional complaints such as malaise, overwhelming fatigue, fever and weight loss are common presenting features of SLE. The presence of these features does not help the physician in the diagnosis of the disease, or in the identification of a flare, because they are just as likely to represent the development of infection or of fibromyalgia.

Fever in SLE is a challenging clinical problem. Many patients develop fever during the course of their disease as a manifestation of active lupus. However, patients with lupus are highly prone to developing infections, which account for a large proportion of the deaths from the disease. In addition, other causes of fever should be considered, including drug-related or malignancy. A diligent history and physical examination, with particular attention to specific features of SLE or to a source of infection, will help guide the physician, and appropriate laboratory tests and radiographs should be ordered. At times it may be necessary to treat for an infection empirically until results of laboratory cultures have been received.

Although some organ system involvements such as skin disease or arthritis are common in SLE, any system may be involved and present in variable combinations with other organ systems. Thus SLE may have such diverse clinical presentations as rash and arthritis, or pleurisy and proteinuria, or Raynaud's phenomenon and seizures or pyrexia of unknown origin. It is only with a high index of suspicion, a careful history and physical examination, and by obtaining appropriate laboratory confirmation, that the diagnosis will become obvious.

Skin manifestations

The skin lesions seen in patients with lupus can be classified into those that are lupus-specific histologically, and those that are lupus-non-specific[28] (Table 122.2). The lupus-specific lesions may be further divided into those that are acute, subacute and chronic.

Lupus-specific lesions

Acute lesions

The most recognized skin manifestation of SLE is the 'butterfly' rash (Fig. 122.2), which usually presents acutely as an erythematous, elevated

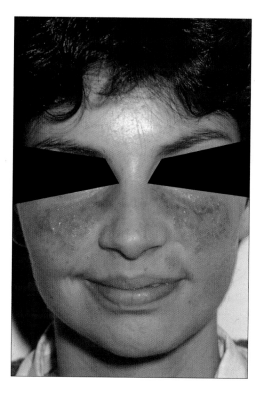

Fig. 122.2 Erythematous malar rash of SLE. Note that the rash does not cross the nasolabial fold.

lesion, pruritic or painful, in a malar distribution, commonly precipitated by exposure to sunlight. The rash may last from days to weeks. Its presence facilitates the diagnosis of SLE and is commonly accompanied by other inflammatory manifestations of the disease. Pathologically, the lesions may show only non-specific inflammation, although by immunofluorescence the classic immune deposits at the dermal–epidermal junction may be seen. The presence of immune deposits in uninvolved skin in patients with SLE has been believed to be helpful in diagnosis[29]. Other acute cutaneous lesions include generalized erythema and bullous lesions. The latter lesions are uncommon cutaneous manifestations of SLE; their histology is characterized by acute inflammation, which may be immune-complex mediated, and which differentiates them from primary vesiculobullous disease[30].

More than 50% of patients with SLE demonstrate photosensitivity. In addition to the skin reaction, patients may develop exacerbations of their systemic disease. The mechanism for the photosensitivity is unknown, but it has been suggested that lymphocytes from patients with SLE are sensitive to 360–400nm light, related to a clastogenic factor in these cells[31]. The damaged chromatin may then provide a substrate for autoantibody production, with the development of a local, or systemic, inflammatory response. Indeed, a recent study showed that ultraviolet B light increased the binding of antibody probes for Ro(SS-A) and La(SS-B) on keratinocytes in a dose-dependent manner[32,33].

Subacute cutaneous lupus erythematosus

Subacute cutaneous lupus erythematosus (SCLE) refers to a distinct cutaneous lesion that is non-fixed, non-scarring, exacerbating and remitting. This lesion is thus intermediate between the evanescent malar rash of active lupus, and the chronic lesions of the disease, which usually cause scarring. These lesions commonly occur in sun-exposed areas and may be generalized. The lesions originate as erythematous papules or small plaques with a slight scale, and may evolve further into a plaque and scale, the papulosquamous variant, which mimics psoriasis or lichen planus, or merge and form polycyclic or annular lesions, which may mimic erythema annulare centrifugum (Fig. 122.3). SCLE may be accompanied by musculoskeletal complaints and serologic abnormalities, the most common of which is the antibody to Ro(SS-A), which has been demonstrated in the lesion. Many patients with antinuclear antibody (ANA)-negative lupus have demonstrated the annular lesions of

TABLE 122.2
CLASSIFICATION OF CUTANEOUS LESIONS
Lupus-specific lesions
Acute
Malar 'butterfly' rash
Generalized erythema
Bullous lupus erythematosus
Subacute cutaneous lupus
Annular – polycyclic
Papulosquamous (psoriasiform)
Chronic lupus
Localized discoid
Generalized discoid
Lupus profundus
Lupus-non-specific lesions
Panniculitis
Urticarial lesions
Vasculitis
Livedo reticularis
Oral lesions
Non-scarring alopecia
Associated skin conditions (psoriasis, lichen planus, porphyria)

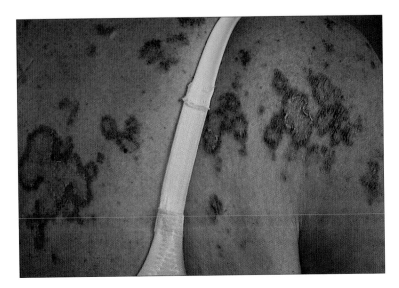

Fig. 122.3 Subacute cutaneous lupus lesions.

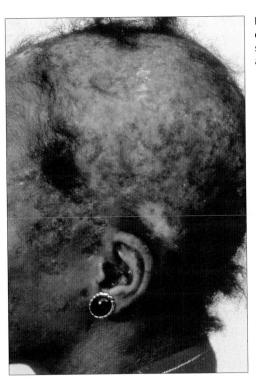

SCLE. The overall prognosis for patients with SCLE is generally better than that for patients with acute cutaneous lesions, although the skin lesions may be more refractory.

Chronic lupus

Discoid lesions are chronic cutaneous lesions that may occur in the absence of any systemic manifestations, as discoid lupus, or may be a manifestation of SLE. These lesions often begin as erythematous papules or plaques, with scaling that may become thick and adherent, with a hypopigmented central area. As the lesion progresses, follicular plugging occurs, with the development of scarring with central atrophy (Fig. 122.4). Discoid lesions may occur in the malar region, or in other sun-exposed areas. Lesions in the scalp lead to extensive, and often permanent, alopecia. Discoid lupus may be localized or generalized, the latter being more likely to be associated with systemic features and serologic abnormalities. Pathologically, the discoid lesion typically demonstrates hyperkeratosis, follicular plugging, edema and mononuclear cell infiltration at the dermal–epidermal junction. On the basis of the pathologic differences between SCLE and discoid skin lesions, different pathogenetic mechanisms contribute to the development of these lesions, such that antibody-mediated cytotoxicity leads to SCLE lesions, whereas chronic cutaneous lesions result from T cell mediated cytotoxicity[28].

Lupus-non-specific lesions

Panniculitis is a rare cutaneous manifestation of SLE. The lesion presents as a deep, firm nodule, with or without a surface change. A biopsy may

show perivascular infiltration of mononuclear cells and fat necrosis. There may be a skin lesion over the nodule, which may demonstrate the perivascular infiltrate without fat necrosis that is known as lupus profundus.

Alopecia is a common feature of SLE. Hair loss may be diffuse or patchy. It may be associated with exacerbations of the disease, in which case it tends to regrow when the disease is under control. Alternatively, it may result from the extensive scarring of discoid lesions, in which case it may be permanent (Fig. 122.5). Alopecia may also be drug-induced, for example by corticosteroids or cytotoxic drugs.

Mucous membrane lesions may result in ulcers of the mouth (Fig. 122.6) or vagina, or produce nasal septal erosions. The latter occasionally lead to nasal septal perforation (Fig. 122.7). Such lesions have been reported to result from vasculitis.

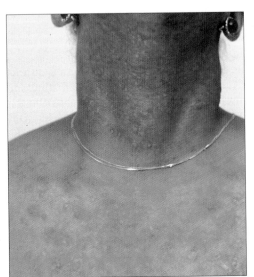

Fig. 122.4 Discoid lupus involving neck and upper chest. The lesions have characteristic central scarring.

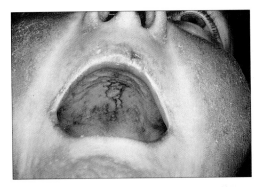

Fig. 122.6 Mouth ulcers in a patient with SLE.

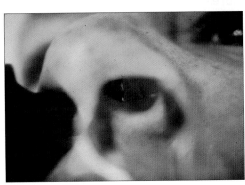

Fig. 122.7 Nasal septal perforation in a patient with SLE.

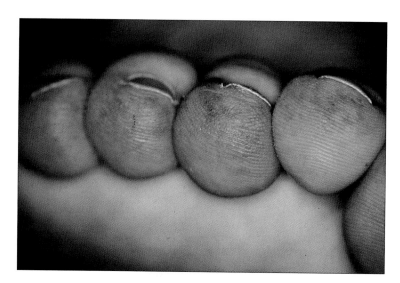

Fig. 122.8 Early vasculitic lesions over the tips of the toes in a patient with active SLE.

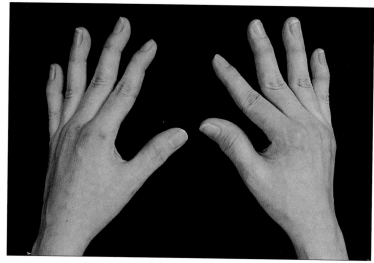

Fig. 122.10 Swan-neck deformities in a patient with SLE.

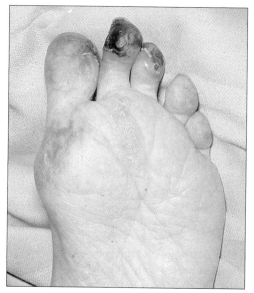

Fig. 122.9 Gangrene of the toe in a patient with SLE and vasculitis.

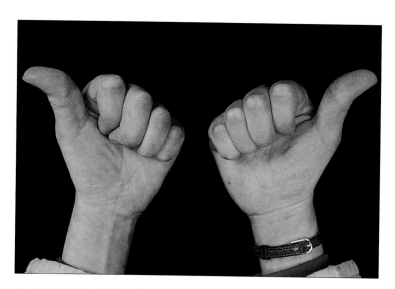

Fig. 122.11 Fists of the patient in Figure 122.10, showing the deformities reduced.

Urticarial lesions occur in 5–10% of patients, are often chronic and typically represent cutaneous vasculitis. Vasculitic lesions may also manifest as palpable purpura, nailfold or digital ulcerations, subcutaneous nodules, livedo reticularis, splinter hemorrhages, pulp space and palmar or plantar lesions (Fig 122.8), simulating Osler's nodes and Janeway's lesions. Vasculitic lesions at the tip of a digit may result in gangrene (Fig. 122.9). Raynaud's phenomenon occurs in more than 50% of patients. Unlike scleroderma, the Raynaud's phenomenon of lupus is not commonly associated with pulp-space pits or ulcerations.

Musculoskeletal features

Arthritis

Arthralgias or arthritis, or both constitute the most common presenting manifestation of SLE[34]. The acute arthritis may affect any joint but, typically, the small joints of the hands, wrists and knees are involved. Most cases are symmetric, but a significant percentage may have an asymmetric polyarthritis. Swelling is usually soft tissue, with effusions tending to be minimal. The acute inflammation may be migratory in nature or persistent and become chronic. Nodules similar to those found in rheumatoid arthritis (RA) are found in approximately 10% of patients with lupus. Synovial fluid analysis reveals mild inflammatory changes and may reveal LE cells, ANA positivity and diminished complement concentrations.

Unlike RA, the arthritis of systemic lupus is typically not erosive or destructive of bone. However, clinically deforming arthritis does occur, and may take a number of different forms[35]. There may be mild synovial thickening about proximal interphalangeal joints or over tendon sheaths, ulnar deviation of the fingers, and subluxations and contractures. When subluxations occur in the small joints of the hands, they are initially reversible (Figs 122.10 & 122.11), but can become fixed. This pattern of non-erosive but deforming disease has been called Jaccoud's arthritis[34]. Other authors have noted flexion contractures of the elbows[36], and deforming arthropathy of the feet[37]. Often, patients who go on to develop deforming arthropathy have had continuous low-grade active arthritis, sometimes in the absence of other signs of SLE. Histologic examination of synovium in the acute stage reveals mild, usually perivascular inflammatory cell infiltrate, mild synovial cell proliferation and mild fibrinous deposition in synovial lining cells. In the more chronic stage, more synovial cell proliferation may be seen, but not approaching the intensity seen in RA. Radiographic findings in SLE arthritis are usually minimal, but may be found in up to 50% of patients[34,35]. There may be periarticular or diffuse osteoporosis and soft tissue swelling, but, unlike RA, there are no erosions even when severe deformities from subluxations are present. Occasionally, one may see hook-like erosions of the metacarpal heads late in the disease, similar to the erosions described in post-rheumatic fever Jaccoud's syndrome.

These changes are more likely a result of bone trauma, due to misplaced tendon sheaths, rather than to erosions from a proliferative synovitis.

As tenosynovitis is an early manifestation of the synovitis of SLE, it is not surprising that tendon rupture syndromes have been reported in a number of different sites in the body, including the patellar tendons, the long head of the biceps, the triceps and the extensor tendons of the hands. Patients who present with tendon ruptures may give a history of the sudden onset of pain or inability to move a joint. Dramatic traumas are not often a part of the history and most patients have a history of long-standing use of corticosteroids. Histologic examination of the ruptured tendons has revealed inflammation in some instances, but not invariably. Thus one may incriminate either inflammation or corticosteroid-induced tendon degeneration as the mechanism for tendon damage.

Two complications of SLE or its treatment, septic arthritis and osteonecrosis, may confuse the diagnosis of acute synovitis in SLE. Although septic arthritis is not common in SLE, despite the immuno-suppressed state, it should be suspected when one joint is inflamed out of proportion to all others. This state necessitates aspiration and culture of the synovial fluid to rule out infection.

Osteonecrosis

Acute joint pain presenting in the later stages of SLE, especially localized to a very few areas, most commonly the hips, may indicate the development of osteonecrosis. In most large series now, osteonecrosis is recognized as an important cause of disability in late lupus, occurring in about 10% of patients followed over a long period of time[38]. Patients with osteonecrosis are generally in the younger age group and have an interval between diagnosis of lupus and osteonecrosis of about 4 years. The hip is the joint most commonly involved, although most joints in the body have been reported to have been affected. From 50% to 67% of patients with osteonecrosis will have several affected sites and, typically, will have been taking high-dose corticosteroids at some time during the course of their illness.

There is no general agreement as to the predictive role of any specific manifestation of SLE, such as Raynaud's phenomenon or vasculitis, in the subsequent development of osteonecrosis, and there is currently no general consensus on pathogenesis. Findings of a recent nested

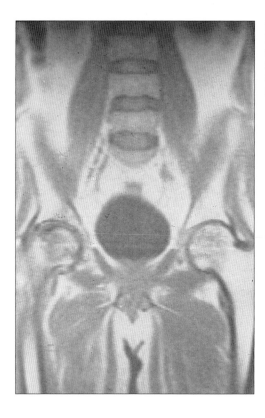

Fig. 122.13
MRI showing advanced changes of osteonecrosis of the right hip and early changes on the left.

case–control study suggests that osteonecrosis is related to previous arthritis, steroid use and treatment with cytotoxic drugs[38].

Diagnosis of osteonecrosis in patients presenting with focal pain can be difficult. Changes in the routine radiographs (Fig. 122.12) are late findings. Earlier diagnosis can be made using radionuclide bone scans or magnetic resonance imaging (MRI) to demonstrate bone abnormality (Fig. 122.13). Although many patients with osteonecrosis have a poor outcome with respect to pain and disability, leading to joint replacement, some patients do respond to decreased weight bearing and the passage of time. These patients may be left with some joint irregularity, but with joint space adequate to avoid surgery. The size and exact location of the avascular area may determine the future necessity for joint replacement. Core decompression with or without bone grafting has not yet been demonstrated to be a useful treatment. Osteonecrosis is not associated with decreased survival, but is associated with physical disability[39].

Myositis

Patients with SLE may complain of muscle pain and weakness. The nature of the myalgia is not always clear. It may be secondary to joint inflammation, in which case the arthritis will be easily demonstrable on physical examination. Patients with SLE may develop a drug-related myopathy, secondary to corticosteroid use or as a complication of anti-malarials. In addition, true muscle inflammation may be seen in patients with SLE. However, the histologic features of myositis in SLE may not be as striking as in idiopathic polymyositis[34]. Finol et al.[40] described the ultrastructural pathology in patients with SLE. Findings included myositis, with muscle atrophy, microtubular inclusions and a mononuclear cell infiltrate and, in one patient with an increased creatine phosphokinase concentration, fiber necrosis. Vacuolar myopathy was found in one patient not treated with antimalarials.

Fibromyalgia

In the differential diagnosis of musculoskeletal complaints in patients with SLE one must consider the possibility of fibromyalgia, which is common in this patient population[41]. Fibromyalgia may be distinguished from true arthritis or myositis by the presence of tender points, and the absence of true inflammatory arthritis or evidence of muscle weakness.

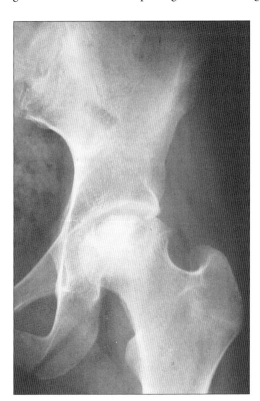

Fig. 122.12
Radiograph demonstrating advanced osteonecrosis of the hip.

On the other hand, fibromyalgia may accompany true arthritis, and its presence needs to be taken into consideration when planning a treatment program for the patient. Fibromyalgia has been shown to contribute to reduced quality of life in patients with SLE[42].

Renal disease

Specific symptoms referable to the kidney are not volunteered by the patient until there is advanced nephrotic syndrome or renal failure. The revised criteria for the classification of SLE recognizes proteinuria of more than 0.5g per 24 hours (or a qualitative dipstick score of >3+ if a quantitative evaluation is not done) or the presence of casts (including red blood cells, heme, granular, tubular or mixed) as evidence of renal disease. In addition, the presence of hematuria (>5 red blood cells/high power field) or pyuria (>5 white blood cells/high power field), or both, in the absence of infection, and the detection of an increased serum creatinine concentration, have been recognized as evidence for clinical renal disease[43]. It is important to appreciate that, in order to identify the presence of renal disease, urine analysis, in addition to a serum creatinine test, must be performed regularly. A renal biopsy may provide a more accurate documentation of renal disease. Most patients with lupus manifest some abnormality on renal biopsy, although in some cases it is possible to document this only with special techniques, such as immunofluorescence or electron microscopy.

The World Health Organization (WHO) has classified lupus nephritis according to the presence of changes on light, immunofluorescence and electron microscopy (Table 122.3) [44]. Mesangial alterations (WHO class II, Fig. 122.14) including mesangial widening or hypercellularity are most common. Proliferative changes may be either focal (WHO class II, Fig. 122.15) or diffuse glomerulonephritis (WHO class IV, Fig. 122.16). Membranous lesions (WHO class V, Fig. 122.17), and glomerulosclerosis (WHO class VI, Fig. 122.18) may also be seen. Renal biopsies may demonstrate hematoxylin bodies, which are the tissue equivalent of the LE cell phenomenon (Fig. 122.19). Most patients with mesangial lesions do not demonstrate clinical renal disease, as might be demonstrated by the presence of an active sediment or increased serum creatinine. However, patients with mesangial lesions may, on occasion, have promi-

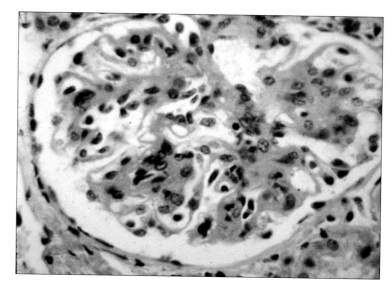

Fig. 122.14 Kidney biopsy specimen showing mesangial lesions (WHO class II).

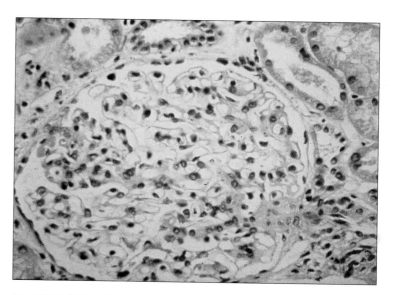

Fig. 122.15 Kidney biopsy showing focal proliferative glomerulonephritis (WHO class III).

nent clinical evidence of renal involvement, and without a biopsy may be treated more aggressively than is perhaps indicated by the lesion itself[45]. Patients with class III and class IV disease tend to have evidence of clinical renal disease and impaired renal function; however, this is not universal. Knowledge of the various morphologic patterns contributes to decisions regarding treatment[44]. Further information may be derived from the renal biopsy with regards to the site of immune deposits, seen by either immunofluorescence (Fig. 122.20) or electron microscopy (Figs 122.21 & 122.22).

The role of kidney biopsy in the assessment of lupus nephritis has been controversial. Several studies have supported the concept that diffuse proliferative lupus nephritis is associated with poor prognosis, both in terms of renal function and in terms of patient survival. Other reports, however, have repudiated the usefulness of renal biopsy in predicting outcome, and claimed that the renal morphology does not add to the clinical information obtained before biopsy[44]. Using a quantitative classification system (Table 122.4), it is clear that these morphologic features seen on kidney biopsies have both prognostic and therapeutic implications[44]. The presence of chronic lesions is clearly associated with lower survival, both for the patient and for the kidney. Moreover, the presence of active lesions would suggest that aggressive anti-inflammatory immunosuppressive treatment, or both, should be considered.

TABLE 122.3 WHO CLASSIFICATION OF LUPUS NEPHRITIS IN 148 BIOPSIES	
I Normal glomeruli	12
a) Nil (by all techniques)	3
b) Normal by light but deposits on electron microscopy or immunofluorescence	9
II Pure mesangial alterations (mesangiopathy)	62
a) Mesangial widening and/or mild hypercellularity	51
b) Moderate hypercellularity	11
IIIA Focal segmental glomerulonephritis	19
a) 'Active' necrotizing lesions	14
b) 'Active' and sclerosing lesions	5
IIIB Focal proliferative glomerulonephritis	3
a) 'Active' necrotizing lesions	1
b) 'Active' and sclerosing lesions	2
IV Diffuse glomerulonephritis	37
a) Without segmental lesions	9
b) With 'active'necrotizing lesions	13
c) With 'active' and sclerosing lesions	14
d) With sclerosing lesions	1
V Diffuse membranous glomerulonephritis	11
a) Pure membranous glomerulonephritis	2
b) Associated with lesions of category II	7
c) Associated with lesions of category III	0
d) Associated with lesions of category IV	2
VI Advanced sclerosing glomerulonephritis	4

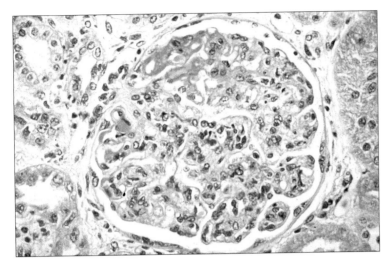

Fig. 122.16 Kidney biopsy showing diffuse proliferative glomerulonephritis (WHO class IV).

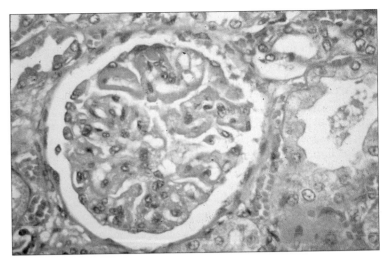

Fig. 122.17 Kidney biopsy showing membranous glomerulonephritis (WHO class V).

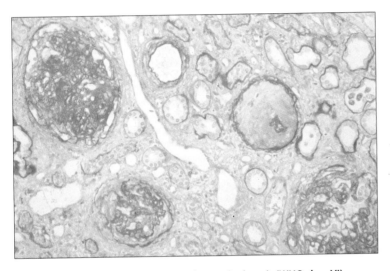

Fig. 122.18 Kidney biopsy showing advanced sclerosis (WHO class VI).

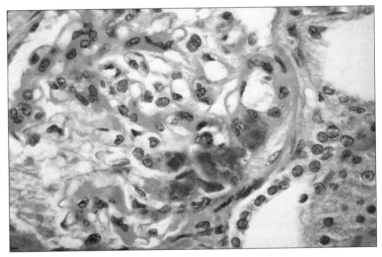

Fig. 122.19 Hematoxylin bodies in a glomerulus of a patient with lupus nephritis.

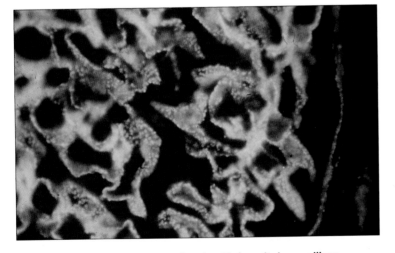

Fig. 122.20 Immunofluorescence showing C3 deposits in a capillary distribution.

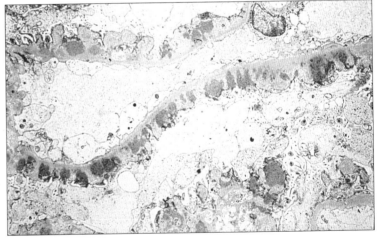

Fig. 122.21 Electron micrograph of a glomerulus showing intramembranous immune deposits.

Several studies have looked at the predictive value of clinical manifestations of renal disease using renal insufficiency as the outcome measure. Austin et al.[46] found increased risk of renal failure to be associated with younger age, male sex and an increased serum creatinine concentration. This model was enhanced by including the renal chronicity index. Nossent et al.[47] concluded that a chronicity index greater than 3

(Table 122.4), especially in young patients, is the most important factor associated with decreased renal survival. Indeed, their findings suggest that, unlike a histologic evaluation, renal function tests alone cannot distinguish between reversible and irreversible renal disease. McLaughlin et al.[48] demonstrated the prognostic value of renal biopsy in patients with normal serum creatinine at the time of the biopsy. In patients with

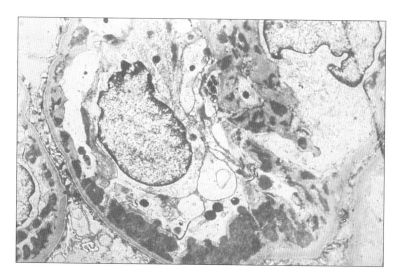

Fig. 122.22 Electron micrograph of a glomerulus showing subendothelial immune deposits.

TABLE 122.4 ACTIVITY AND CHRONICITY INDICES FOR LUPUS NEPHRITIS

	Activity	Chronicity
Glomerular lesions	1. Proliferation	1. Sclerotic glomeruli
	2. Necrosis/karyorrhexis	2. Fibrous crescents
	3. Hyaline thrombi	
	4. Cellular crescents	
	5. Leukocytic exudation	
Tubulointerstitial lesions	1. Mononuclear cell infiltration	1. Tubular atrophy
		2. Interstitial fibrosis

evidence of diffuse proliferative glomerulonephritis with glomerular thrombosis, there may be improved prognosis through the use of ancrod[49]. Jacobson *et al.*[50] retrospecively studied 94 patients with normal serum creatinine at the time of biopsy and analyzed the prognostic value of renal biopsy and clincial variables for the development of end-stage renal disease. They found that duration of renal disease of more than 1 year at the time of biopsy, and the presence of WHO class IV glomerulonephritis, hyaline thrombi, leukocyte infiltration and an active urinary sediment were associated with the development of end-stage renal disease.

Repeat renal biopsies also have a role in the management of patients with SLE. Morphological changes have been observed, and the majority of patients have had changes in treatment based on the biopsy results[51].

Several investigators had suggested that patients with lupus nephritis who develop renal insufficiency have decreased lupus disease activity. However, more recent studies refute this notion. Patients with renal insufficiency, whether undergoing dialysis or transplantation, continue to demonstrate current disease activity measured by the SLE disease activity index (SLEDAI)[52,53].

Neuropsychiatric manifestations

The diagnosis of neuropsychiatric involvement in SLE has been difficult. The American College of Rheumatology (ACR) Ad Hoc Committee on Neuropsychiatric Lupus Nomenclature has proposed a standardized nomenclature for the neuropsychiatric syndromes of SLE[54]. The relationship of neuropsychiatric features to the lupus disease process is not always clear[55]. There is a wide spectrum of clinical manifestations (Table 122.5), which may be grouped into neurologic, including the central nervous system (CNS), cranial and peripheral nerves, and

TABLE 122.5 NEUROPSYCHIATRIC MANIFESTATIONS OF SLE

Neurologic
Seizures – grand mal, petit mal, focal, temporal lobe
Stroke syndrome
Movement disorder
Headache
Transverse myelitis
Cranial neuropathy
Peripheral neuropathy

Psychiatric
Organic brain syndrome
Psychosis
Psychoneurosis
Neurocognitive dysfunction

psychiatric, including psychosis and severe depression[56]. Many patients present with mixed neurologic and psychiatric manifestations[55,56]. Furthermore, patients may have more than one manifestation at a time, a fact that makes their classification more difficult.

Neurologic features

Intractable headaches, unresponsive to narcotic analgesics, are the most common feature of neurologic disease in patients with lupus[57]. The headaches may be migrainous in type[58], and may accompany other neuropsychiatric features. Seizure may be either focal or generalized. The occurrence of chorea in SLE has also been recognized. Chorea occurs early in the course of the disease and resembles Sydenham's chorea. Its association with the anticardiolipin antibody has been suggested[55]. Cerebrovascular accidents, including paresis or subarachnoid hemorrhage, may be associated with vasculitis or, like chorea, related to the anticardiolipin syndrome, resulting in vessel occlusion. Cranial neuropathies may present with visual defects, blindness, papilledema, nystagmus or ptosis, tinnitus and vertigo, or facial palsy. By far the most common are those related to the function of the eye. The retinopathy seen in patients with SLE is likely to be secondary to vasculitis[59]. The majority of these patients have cotton-wool spots (cytoid bodies) (Fig. 122.23), hemorrhages or areas of vasculitis (Fig. 122.24). Abnormalities of the optic nerve head manifested by papilledema or optic atrophy may also be seen.

Peripheral neuropathy is uncommon, and may include motor, sensory (stocking glove distribution) or mixed motor and sensory polyneuropathy or mononeuritis multiplex. An acute ascending motor paralysis indistinguishable from Guillain–Barré syndrome has been reported.

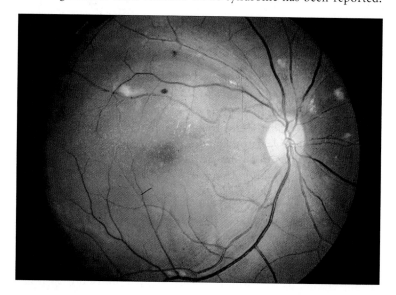

Fig. 122.23 Funduscopic examination in a patient with SLE demonstrating cytoid bodies.

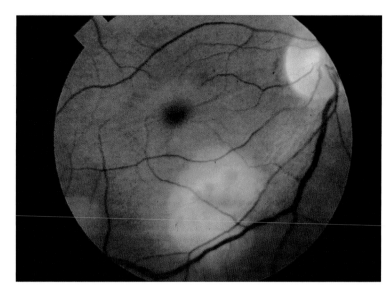

Fig. 122.24 Funduscopic examination in a patient with SLE demonstrating choroidal vasculitis.

Transverse myelitis, presenting with lower extremity paralysis, sensory deficits and loss of sphincter control, has rarely been reported in patients with SLE[55].

Psychiatric features

Frank psychosis has long been recognized as a manifestation of SLE[55,56]. The use of corticosteroids has been implicated in causing psychosis in some patients; however, stopping the drug in these patients and demonstrating that the psychosis gets worse confirms its relationship to the lupus process. The reported association between antiribosomal P protein antibodies and lupus psychosis in some studies, and severe depression in others, suggests a pathogenic relationship, but these findings are not consistent. Therefore the use of antiribosomal P antibody in diagnosis or monitoring patients is not useful, and the exact role of this antibody in SLE remains to be determined[60].

Organic brain syndrome in SLE is defined as a state of disturbed mental function with delirium, emotional inadequacy, and impaired memory or concentration, in the absence of drugs, infection or a metabolic cause. The prevalence of cognitive impairment in SLE is likely to be underestimated. Kremer et al.[61] attempted a systematic definition of the broader range of psychiatric symptoms in patients with lupus, using a combination of a standard psychiatric interview and several well-validated measures, and reported a high prevalence of psychopathology. There was a lack of correlation between the presence of non-organic non-psychotic psychopathology and underlying organic CNS disease or SLE disease activity. No correlation was found with non-organic non-psychotic psychopathology and use of corticosteroids.

In a similar study of neurocognitive function in SLE, it has been found that more than 80% of patients with SLE who had either active or inactive neuropsychiatric involvement, and 42% of patients who had never had neuropsychiatric manifestations, demonstrated significant cognitive impairment, as compared with 17% of patients with RA and 14% of the normal controls. However, a variety of cognitive deficits were present in patients with SLE, without a significant association with emotional disturbances[62].

In a study from São Paulo, Brazil[63], 63% of patients with active SLE were diagnosed with a psychiatric disorder. Patients with a psychiatric disorder were more likely to have neurologic abnormalities and subjective cognitive impairment than patients who did not have psychiatric manifestations. Patients with major psychiatric features (e.g. delirium, dementia, organic hallucinations, delusional syndromes, major depressive episodes) had more severe neurocognitive abnormalities, more ophthalmologic abnormalities and calcifications on computed tomography (CT) scanning than did patients with mild depressive symptoms or patients without psychiatric manifestations.

Pathogenesis

The pathogenesis of CNS lupus is not well understood, but it is generally believed that more than one mechanism must be postulated, to encompass the wide spectrum of clinical findings. The most common finding in postmortem series is the presence of several microinfarcts[55,56]. Non-inflammatory thickening of small vessels by intimal proliferation is also seen, which may result from the reaction of antibodies with the phospholipids in the vascular endothelial cell membranes. Other pathologic findings include thrombotic occlusion of major vessels, which are the likely cause of some cerebrovascular accidents, whereas others may be related to the anticardiolipin antibody, intracerebral hemorrhage or embolism from mitral valve endocarditis. The pathologic findings do not always correlate with the clinical picture. A true vasculitis with inflammatory cell infiltrate and fibrinoid necrosis has rarely been demonstrated in brain pathology. However, it should be remembered that, unlike skin and renal disease, in which biopsies are readily available, most of the available pathology in the CNS comes from postmortem studies, and therefore vasculitis would be difficult to demonstrate, even if it existed.

Support for vascular inflammation comes from studies showing enhanced cerebral blood flow during episodes of CNS activity[55,59]. Autoantibodies that cross-react with neuronal membrane antigens, and lymphocytotoxic antibodies, have been found in both the serum and cerebrospinal fluid of patients with SLE. These antibodies may be produced locally or pass through an immunologically damaged cerebral circulation or choroid plexus. Changes in antineuronal antibodies frequently parallel concurrent changes in anti-DNA antibodies and overall disease activity, in addition to cognitive dysfunction[56]. These antibodies may exert their effects by binding to molecules on neuronal membranes, preventing signal responses or propagation. Potentially important target molecules on the cell surface include the very late antigens family of integrins and heat shock proteins[64].

An increased incidence of antineurofilament antibody has been found in patients with SLE who have 'diffuse' neuropsychiatric manifestations, and was frequently negative in 'focal' neuropsychiatric disease[65]. Patients with SLE and diffuse neuropsychiatric disease were more likely to have an increased IgG index, oligoclonal bands and antineuronal antibodies in the cerebrospinal fluid than were patients with focal lesions[63]. The association between antiribosomal P protein and psychiatric manifestations of SLE may have a similar mechanism[62,66]. Patients with focal lesions had evidence of peripheral vasculitis, lupus anticoagulant or anticardiolipin antibody, or both, and lesions on cranial MRI, perhaps suggesting immune complex vasculitis with resultant vascular occlusion as the mechanism for these manifestations[66].

Diagnosis

The diagnosis of neuropsychiatric lupus is primarily clinical. Exclusion of possible etiologies such as sepsis, uremia and severe hypertension is mandatory. Evidence of disease activity in other organs is helpful, but not always present. Non-specific cerebrospinal fluid abnormalities such as increased cell count, increased protein or reduced glucose may be present in 33% of the patients. Increases in IgG, IgA or IgM indices have been described in patients with CNS lupus, and proposed as evidence of CNS disease activity[55,65,66]. Electroencephalogram abnormalities are common in patients with neuropsychiatric lupus, but are non-specific[67]. The development of computerized quantitative electroencephalography may be more sensitive in detecting subtle electrophysiologic changes associated with lupus, and requires evaluation. Evoked potentials have been proposed as a sensitive measure of CNS involvement in SLE.

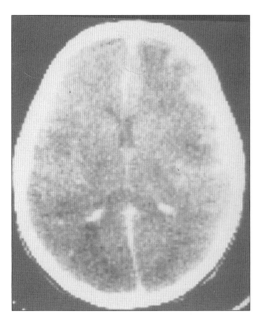

Fig. 122.25
CT scan of the brain, demonstrating microinfarcts.

Radionuclide scans have not uniformly been helpful. However, positron emission tomography, showing areas of low attenuation that may represent areas of disturbed cerebral circulation and metabolism, appears promising[67]. CT findings such as evidence of cerebral infarction (Fig. 122.25) and hemorrhage may reflect specific pathologic processes. Cortical atrophy may be found in SLE, but does not necessarily reflect CNS disease[55,65,66]. Single photon emission computed tomography has been increasingly used to identify abnormalities in patients with neuropsychiatric lupus[68,69]. This technique still requires further study into its sensitivity and specificity in patients whose symptoms are not easily discernible clinically.

Magnetic resonance imaging appears to be superior to conventional CT, and particularly useful in the evaluation of patients with diffuse presentations[67]. Some of the lesions seen on MRI, particularly the small focal areas of increased signal intensity in both the cerebral white matter and the cortical gray matter, tend to disappear after treatment with corticosteroids. These lesions may therefore represent either areas of local edema or inflammatory infiltrates that resolve with treatment. A more advanced technique, magnetic resonance spectroscopy, using either phosphorus-31 or hydrogen-1, may provide better demonstration of brain lesions in neuropsychiatric lupus[67,70] . Further research is clearly indicated before any of these techniques becomes the 'gold standard' for the diagnosis of neuropsychiatric lupus.

Serositis

Serositis in SLE is common and may present as pleurisy, pericarditis or peritonitis. Pleural manifestations have been variously reported in 30–60% of patients with SLE[71,72]. A clinical history of pleuritic pain is more common than radiographic change. Pleural rubs are found less frequently than either clinical pleurisy or radiographic abnormalities. However, autopsy findings of pleural involvement are more common than in clinical diagnoses.

Pleural effusions may occur and are usually small, but can occasionally be massive. They are also frequently bilateral. Pleural effusions are seen more frequently in the aged and in drug-induced lupus. When pleural effusions are significant, other causes of effusion such as infection must be ruled out by thoracocentesis before treatment is initiated. The fluid is usually an exudate and the glucose concentration is usually normal, in contrast to RA in which it is low. The white blood cell count is moderately increased and the differential count commonly reveals neutrophils in the acute stage and lymphocytes in the later stages of the illness. LE cells have been described in the pleural fluid. Some investigators have suggested that ANA positivity in the pleural fluid is the most sensitive test for lupus pleuritis[73], although others have not found this test helpful[74].

Pericarditis is the most common presentation of heart involvement in SLE, but is less frequent than pleurisy as a feature of serositis. Clinical pericarditis has an incidence of 20–30% in most large series, but may be found in more than 60% of patients with lupus, at autopsy[75–77]. The clinical diagnosis is frequently difficult and depends on a constellation of clinical findings, including typical precordial chest pain and a pericardial rub. However, pericarditis may also be painless and clinically silent[76]. Conversely, posterior pericardial effusions may be found on echocardiography in patients who have no suspected history of pericarditis. Pericardial effusions (Fig. 122.26) are seen frequently as a feature of pericarditis in lupus, but cardiac tamponade is rare. However, this complication does occur, and on rare occasions may be the presenting manifestation of SLE[78]. Pericardial fluid has been examined in only a small number of cases. Most samples demonstrated a leukocytosis, with a high percentage of neutrophils. Glucose concentrations are significantly lower than in the serum samples, and several reports have documented reduced complement activity in addition to increased ANA concentrations and positive LE cells, and the presence of immune complexes in the pericardial effusions.

Certain patients may be more predisposed to large pericardial effusions because of concomitant diseases such as uremia. In addition, infectious pericarditis in SLE has been reported both with bacteria and with fungi[79,80] Pericardiocentesis should be performed in patients with cardiac tamponade or in patients in whom infection is suspected. Constrictive pericarditis can occasionally develop in patients with pericardial involvement, although this is very uncommon.

The gastrointestinal syndrome of acute SLE usually manifested by diffuse abdominal pain, anorexia, nausea and occasionally vomiting, and a pseudo-obstruction presentation has a number of possible etiologies,

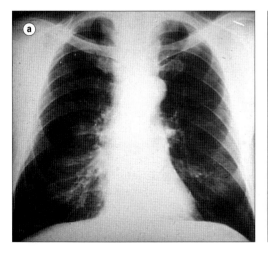
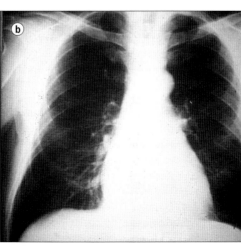

Fig. 122.26 Pericardial effusion. Change in cardiac silhouette from (a) normal baseline in (b) a patient with SLE and acute pericarditis.

including diffuse peritonitis, bowel vasculitis, pancreatitis or inflammatory bowel disease[81]. It is likely that, in the majority of such cases, peritoneal inflammation is the cause of the symptoms. Ascites may be associated with peritonitis in about 11% of cases. However, at autopsy, evidence of peritoneal inflammation may be found in up to 60% of cases[82]. When ascites is present in conjunction with abdominal pain and active lupus elsewhere, it generally follows the course and response to treatment of the other features of lupus. However, in a small number of patients, ascites may become chronic. In those circumstances it may be painless and associated with only minimal or no other manifestations of active lupus. The peritoneum may also be thickened with adhesions.

Acute lupus peritonitis must be differentiated from bowel infarction with perforation, acute pancreatitis or bacterial peritonitis. Chronic lupus peritonitis must be differentiated from congestive heart failure, constrictive pericarditis, nephrotic syndrome, Budd–Chiari syndrome, intra-abdominal malignancy and intra-abdominal sepsis with a chronic infectious agent such as tuberculosis. When infection or malignancy is suspected, aspiration of ascitic fluid is required.

Pulmonary involvement

Pulmonary involvement in SLE may consist of lupus pleuritis, lupus pneumonitis, pulmonary hemorrhage, pulmonary embolism or pulmonary hypertension[56,83].

Pneumonitis

Lupus pneumonitis may present either as an acute or as a chronic illness. The acute illness simulates pneumonia and may present with classic symptoms of fever, dyspnea, cough and occasionally hemoptysis. The pulmonary infiltrates are usually associated with other signs of active SLE. The chronic form of lupus pneumonitis presents as a diffuse interstitial lung disease and is characterized by dyspnea on exertion, non-productive cough and basilar rales. The acute pneumonitis syndrome must be differentiated from infection and, when doubt persists, invasive investigation is indicated, including bronchoalveolar lavage. In chronic lupus pneumonitis, the major clinical question revolves around whether the pulmonary fibrosis has an active component. Gallium scanning of the lung may help differentiate active from inactive disease.

On occasions, lupus pneumonitis may present as a lymphocytic interstitial pneumonia simulating a lymphangitic pulmonary malignancy. Usually, this lesion is associated with active disease and will respond to the treatment of active lupus. Lung involvement in SLE may be more common than may be appreciated by plain radiography. A recent prospective CT study of 48 patients with SLE without previously known lung involvement identified 38% of patients with normal plain radiographs to have abnormal CT findings. These correlated with disease duration and decreased single-breath diffusing capacity for carbon monoxide[84].

Pulmonary hemorrhage

Pulmonary hemorrhage presenting with cough and hemoptysis or as a pulmonary infiltrate is an uncommon but very serious feature of SLE[85]. It is presumed to be due to pulmonary vasculitis. Other causes of hemorrhagic pneumonia, such as some forms of viral pneumonia, must be considered in differential diagnoses.

Pulmonary hypertension

Lupus pulmonary involvement may also give rise to a syndrome of pulmonary hypertension that is similar to idiopathic pulmonary hypertension[86]. In this syndrome, patients present with dyspnea and a normal chest radiograph. They are mildly hypoxic and have a restrictive pattern on pulmonary function testing. Carbon dioxide diffusion capacity is reduced and Raynaud's phenomenon is frequently present. Doppler studies and cardiac catheterization confirm pulmonary hypertension. Pulmonary hypertension was found in 14% of 28 patients enrolled in an

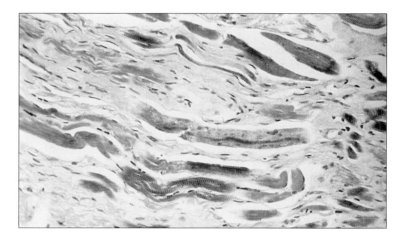

Fig. 122.27 Micrograph of the diaphragm in a patient with a shrinking lung syndrome demonstrating fibrosis.

echocardiographic study in patients with SLE[87]; over a period of 5 years, the prevalence of pulmonary hypertension increased to 43%. An increase in pulmonary artery resistance was documented in patients with SLE compared with controls[87]. Patients are frequently treated with systemic vasodilators, and more recently with epoprostenol[88]; however, the prognosis is generally grave. One must always exclude secondary pulmonary hypertension by searching for sites of deep venous thrombosis and for multiple pulmonary emboli. When there is any doubt, pulmonary angiography should be performed, as a diagnosis of multiple pulmonary emboli might lead to potential life-saving treatment. One must also exclude the antiphospholipid antibody syndrome with intrapulmonary clotting (see Chapter 131).

Shrinking lung syndrome

Unexplained dyspnea, small lung volumes with restrictive pulmonary function studies and an elevated diaphragm can signal an acute shrinking lung syndrome[89]. The syndrome responds to acute treatment of SLE with corticosteroids.

Patients may present in the late stages of lupus with the symptom of increasing dyspnea in the face of a normal chest examination. Chest radiographs may reveal increased diaphragms, but normal lung fields. Pulmonary function tests will usually reveal small lung volumes and a restrictive pattern. This chronic form of the shrinking lung syndrome is a result of altered respiratory mechanics, on the basis of either impaired respiratory muscle or diaphragmatic function, or problems in the respiratory skeletal apparatus. Some studies have demonstrated specific intercostal muscle weakness or diaphragmatic weakness[90]. One postmortem study revealed the diaphragm in a patient with shrinking lung syndrome in late lupus to be fibrotic and thinned[91] (Fig. 122.27). When shrinking lung syndrome occurs in the face of late stage lupus without other signs of active disease, the prognosis is grave.

Cardiac involvement

Cardiac involvement in SLE may consist of pericarditis, myocarditis, endocarditis and coronary artery disease.

Myocarditis

Myocarditis should be suspected in patients who present with arrhythmias or conduction defects, unexplained cardiomegaly with or without congestive heart failure or an unexplained tachycardia. Such patients usually have associated pericarditis and other features of active SLE. Peripheral myositis may be an associated feature. Congestive heart failure is a less common feature of SLE and is usually secondary to a combination of factors, which may include myocarditis. However, associated hypertension and the use of corticosteroids are usually more important contributing factors.

The myocardial involvement may be subtle in systemic lupus, with abnormalities only being detected with non-invasive testing. Sasson et al.[92], using pulsed Doppler echocardiography, demonstrated impaired left ventricular diastolic dysfunction in 64% of patients with active SLE and 14% of patients with inactive SLE, all of whom did not have any clinical evidence of cardiac disease, had normal electrocardiograms and no evidence for pericardial or valvular disease. Repeat Doppler echocardiographic studies at 7 months showed a trend towards improvement in left ventricular function in patients whose SLE became inactive. Badui et al.[93] found 16 of 100 consecutive patients with SLE to have evidence of ischemic heart disease as judged by electrocardiography, echocardiography, or both. Hosenpud et al.[94] described abnormal thallium scans in 10 of 26 patients with SLE selected randomly. These abnormalities included reversible defects suggesting ischemia, in addition to persistent defects suggesting scarring. These findings may suggest either previous myocarditis or coronary artery disease. In patients with suspected myocarditis, endomyocardial biopsy may help confirm the diagnosis[95].

Endocarditis

The true incidence of endocarditis is very difficult to discern in lupus, because the majority of murmurs heard clinically are not associated with any organic valvular disease on investigation or at autopsy. Non-bacterial verrucous vegetations described by Libman and Sacks[75] are found in 15–60% of patients at autopsy. Vegetations may vary from mere valvular thickening detected by two-dimensional echocardiography, to very large lesions causing significant valvular dysfunction[75,96]. Valvular replacement has been required on occasion, with significant mortality. Acute and subacute bacterial endocarditis may occur on previously involved valves. For this reason, prophylactic antibiotics for certain surgical procedures are advisable in patients with lupus endocarditis.

Coronary heart disease

Coronary artery disease in lupus is primarily a manifestation of generalized atherosclerosis, which is discussed in greater detail in the section on late-stage lupus. Coronary vasculitis, in contrast, is much less common in SLE[97], and when it occurs is usually associated with other features of active disease, in contradistinction to atherosclerotic coronary artery disease, which is usually associated with inactive lupus. Coronary artery occlusion may also occur in association with a circulating anticoagulant (see Chapter 131).

Gastrointestinal involvement

The gastrointestinal tract may be involved in many different ways in systemic lupus[98]. Many patients complain of a nondescript dyspepsia and nausea associated with active disease, without clear evidence of involvement of the gastrointestinal tract. However, this may represent low-grade peritoneal inflammation or vascular disease of the bowel, or be related to medication. Gastrointestinal involvement may, in addition, present as esophageal disease, mesenteric vasculitis, inflammatory bowel disease, pancreatitis and liver disease. Esophageal complaints, especially dysphagia, are uncommon in systemic lupus, but may be associated with esophageal dysrhythmias seen in those patients who frequently also manifest Raynaud's phenomenon.

Mesenteric vasculitis

The gastrointestinal presentation of greatest significance is that associated with mesenteric vasculitis[99]. Patients generally present with lower abdominal pain, which may be insidious and may be intermittent over a period of weeks or months. Arteriography may reveal the presence of vasculitis. Bleeding per rectum may occur and both small bowel and colonic ulcerations may be seen on colonoscopy. Intestinal perforations from mesenteric vasculitis have been described. Although patients with mesenteric vasculitis often have evidence of vasculitis elsewhere, this is not always the case[100]. Thus, if mesenteric vasculitis is suspected, intensive investigation should be undertaken and treatment instituted to abort perforation. However, if perforation is suspected or does occur, surgical intervention is necessary.

Inflammatory bowel disease

Inflammatory bowel disease has been rarely reported in SLE[101]. Clinically, it may be difficult to distinguish between idiopathic inflammatory bowel disease and lupus enteritis. If it is caused by SLE, other features of that illness are usually present.

Pancreatitis

Acute pancreatitis occurs in about 8% of patients with lupus. Presentation includes the typical symptoms of abdominal pain, nausea and vomiting and an increased serum amylase. Although one may question whether the pancreatitis is due to lupus or corticosteroids, pancreatitis has been described in some patients not receiving corticosteroids[102,103].

Liver involvement

Although hepatomegaly occurs commonly in SLE, overt clinical liver disease is uncommon. The most common abnormality is increased liver enzymes, including aspartate aminotransferase, alanine aminotransferase, lactate dehydrogenase and alkaline phosphatase. These abnormalities have been associated with active SLE and the administration of non-steroidal anti-inflammatory medications, especially salicylates. So striking is this coincidence that, if a young woman presents with a polyarthritis, is treated with aspirin and develops increased liver enzyme, one should suspect SLE. Liver enzyme abnormalities return to normal when the lupus is under control and the anti-inflammatory medications are stopped.

Lupoid hepatitis is a subset of chronic active hepatitis, with an array of immunologic phenomena, both serologically and clinically. However, in that condition the liver is the primary organ of involvement, and this may result in liver damage and its consequences. An association between primary biliary cirrhosis and autoimmune disease has been suggested, and several patients with primary biliary cirrhosis who present with a multisystem disease consistent with SLE have been reported. Whether this is a chance coexistence of the two diseases or a direct relationship is not clear.

Reticuloendothelial system involvement

Periarterial fibrosis, or 'onion-skin lesions' in the spleen, has been considered pathognomonic of SLE. It has been suggested that saturation of the reticuloendothelial system contributes to the prolonged circulation of immune complexes and their subsequent tissue deposition[104]. Indeed, defective Fc receptor function in patients with SLE has been demonstrated and varies with disease activity. Splenic atrophy has been reported in patients with SLE[105] and the occurrence of splenic lymphoma has also been recognized[106].

Lymphadenopathy is a common non-specific feature of SLE. The nodes are usually soft, non-tender and vary in size. In some patients there may be fluctuation of the lymphadenopathy with disease exacerbations. Pathologically, the lymph nodes demonstrate reactive hyperplasia[107].

LABORATORY FEATURES

Hematologic abnormalities

Cytopenias, including anemia, leukopenia or lymphopenia, and thrombocytopenia, are frequent manifestations of SLE, and are included in the revised criteria for classification.

Anemia

Although anemia in SLE may have many different etiologies, including those secondary to chronic inflammatory disease, renal insufficiency, blood loss or drugs, the most significant in acute SLE is the autoimmune hemolytic anemia caused by autoantibodies directed against RBC antigens[108], detected by Coombs' test. Occasionally, the hemolytic anemia in lupus is Coombs' negative. Similarly, one may find a positive Coombs' test in the absence of any evidence of hemolysis.

Leukopenia/lymphopenia

Leukopenia generally ranges between 2500 and 4000/mm³ and is often associated with active disease. One must always consider other causes for leukopenia, such as drugs and infection. When the leukopenia is secondary to active lupus, the bone marrow is usually normal. The white blood count rarely decreases to less than 1500/mm³ in active SLE, unless there is an additional cause. In some instances, when the total white count does reach these values, patients have been noted to have high spiking fevers requiring significant doses of corticosteroids to suppress the active disease. Lymphocytopenia is usually associated with antibodies to lymphocytes and is associated with active SLE.

Thrombocytopenia

As with anemia, other etiologies such as infection or drugs must be ruled out as a cause of thrombocytopenia in patients with lupus. Although antiplatelet antibodies are a frequent finding in SLE, they are not always associated with thrombocytopenia.

Two distinct subsets of patients with thrombocytopenia have been identified in SLE: a subset in whom the thrombocytopenia is one feature of a severely active patient with SLE, and a second subset in whom the thrombocytopenia is an isolated finding. In the former, the thrombocytopenia tends to be refractory and follows the course of the acute lupus and its response to treatment. In the latter subset, patients usually present with a platelet count of less than 50 000/mm³, without serious bleeding. In both groups, patients may present with mild petechiae or purpura[109].

In some instances of refractory thrombocytopenia with SLE, often without platelet antibodies, the antiphospholipid syndrome should be suspected (see Chapter 131). In addition, thrombocytopenia may be a feature of thrombotic thrombocytopenic purpura (TTP) syndrome, which may complicate SLE[110]. TTP is characterized by thrombocytopenia, microangiopathic hemolytic anemia, CNS deficits, renal dysfunction and fevers. Recognition of this form of microangiopathy in patients with SLE has increased over the past two decades. TTP may occur in either quiescent or active lupus disease states. A high level of suspicion for TTP is appropriate when a patient with SLE presents with multiorgan system deterioration and microangiopathy. Because of similarities in presentation, it is often difficult to distinguish between active SLE and TTP on clinical grounds. As treatment of TTP differs from that of SLE, prompt diagnosis is crucial.

Pancytopenia

Pancytopenia in SLE may result from the effects of drugs, particularly immunosuppressive drugs. It may also complicate infections in patients with SLE. In addition, patients with SLE may develop pancytopenia as a result of the hemophagocytic syndrome[111].

Other findings

A variety of hemostatic abnormalities have been reported in lupus, the most common being the lupus anticoagulant. This phenomenon is dealt with in detail in Chapter 131 on the antiphospholipid antibody syndrome. The most frequent laboratory accompaniments of this syndrome include a prolonged partial prothrombin time, the presence of anticardiolipin antibody, thrombocytopenia, a positive Coombs' test and a false-positive Venereal Disease Research Laboratories (VDRL) test for syphilis. The false-positive VDRL test may precede the onset of the other symptoms of SLE by many years.

The erythrocyte sedimentation rate is frequently increased during the course of active SLE, but it does not mirror the activity of the disease, and in lupus in remission may remain increased for long periods of time. A positive C reactive protein test, at one time purported to measure infection in lupus, has not been proven to be a constant indicator of a superimposed infection. However, C reactive protein has now been associated with a predisposition to coronary artery disease in otherwise healthy individuals, and with a poor prognosis in patients with myocardial infarction[112]. Its role in predicting coronary artery disease in SLE is currently under intensive study.

Serologic abnormalities

Complement concentrations, measured as either total hemolytic complement or complement components C3 and C4, have been shown to be depressed in active SLE, most commonly from consumption by immune complexes. Alternatively, depressed concentrations of serum complement may reflect inherited deficiencies of complement components, decreased production by as yet unidentified mechanisms or protein loss in the urine when there is nephrotic syndrome.

Some of the antibodies seen in SLE (see Chapter 120) are more specific for certain disease states and may therefore be useful in diagnosis. These include anti-Sm, which is seen primarily in systemic lupus, antihistone antibody, which is seen primarily in drug-induced lupus, and anti-Ro and anti-La antibodies, which are seen in Sjögren's syndrome and in systemic lupus. Antibodies to double-stranded (ds)DNA are seen primarily in lupus.

Antibodies such as anti-DNA antibodies were initially believed to reflect disease activity in SLE and therefore to be monitors of treatment in this disease[113]. However, clinical experience indicates that DNA antibodies and depressed concentrations of serum complement are an imperfect predictor of clinical disease activity. Increased concentrations do not appear to correlate consistently with any clinical feature except renal disease. In some patients, these abnormalities may persist for many years, and on occasion return to normal without any intervening flare of disease[114].

Approximately 5% of patients with SLE do not demonstrate the classic antibody systems for SLE, namely ANA and LE cells, and have been referred to as having 'ANA-negative lupus'. These patients have clinical evidence of SLE and tend to have more skin rash, photosensitivity, Raynaud's phenomenon and serositis. Some of these patients have subsequently been shown to have the anti-Ro(SS-A) antibody[115].

Complement deficiency and SLE

In a patient with SLE and possible complement deficiency, such as one in whom the C3 and C4 concentrations are normal but the CH50 is low (or C3 or C4 concentrations are low even in the absence of active disease or high autoantibody levels), results first need to be confirmed with a correctly collected sample before evaluation for a possible complement deficiency is begun. Because complement components are not stable at room temperature for more than a few hours, one cause of spurious low CH50 concentrations in the face of normal C3 and C4 concentrations is improper sample handling.

Complete complement deficiency from a congenital cause is very unusual in patients with SLE – it usually accounts for fewer than 2% of patients in large series. Therefore, the great majority of low complement values that are measured in patients are acquired as part of the disease process. A common genetic deficiency affects the C2 gene. About 1 in 3 C2-deficient individuals have an autoimmune disease, most commonly SLE.

In complete deficiencies of the early classic pathway components (C1, C4 and C2) or C3, the risk of SLE or autoimmune disease is very high (from around 33% for C2 to >90% for C1). In contrast, individuals with deficiencies of later components (C5–C9) generally have far fewer autoimmune manifestations, but a much greater risk of recurrent infection, particularly with *Neisseria* species. Patients with complete complement deficiencies are believed, in general, to have a more benign SLE disease course that is characterized by an earlier age at disease onset, decreased incidence of renal and CNS disease, lower-titer or negative ANA and, usually, no anti-dsDNA antibodies. For example, patients with C2 deficiency typically have prominent cutaneous disease and high-titer SS-A/Ro antibodies, whereas patients with C1q deficiency frequently have severe nephritis with or without CNS disease, even in the face of low-titer ANAs and negative dsDNA antibodies. (See also Chapter 119.)

THE EVOLVING SPECTRUM OF SLE

Disease patterns

The many different combinations of organ system involvement in SLE have long been known in medicine. Current concepts of pathogenesis implicate an immune complex inflammation in a variety of tissues, giving rise to clinical symptoms. However, patients may present with signs and symptoms loosely tied to SLE, but with a different underlying pathogenesis and natural history, thus requiring different therapeutic approaches. One must be aware of these presentations so that not all patients are painted with the same therapeutic brush. Some of these altered patterns include latent lupus, drug-induced lupus, antiphospholipid antibody syndrome and late-stage lupus (Fig. 122.28).

Latent lupus

The term 'latent lupus' is used to describe a group of patients who present with a constellation of features suggestive of SLE, but who do not qualify by 'criteria' or by a rheumatologist's intuition as having classic SLE[116,117]. These patients usually present with either one or two of the ACR classification criteria for SLE, plus a number of additional and much less specific features suggestive of lupus. These features may include lymphadenopathy, fever, headache, nodules, Sjögren's syndrome, fatigue, neuropathy, few active joints, an increase in partial prothrombin time, hypergammaglobulinemia and an increased erythrocyte sedimentation rate, depressed complement, positive rheumatoid factor or aspirin-induced hepatotoxicity.

Many of these patients will persist with their constellation of signs and symptoms over many years, without ever developing classic lupus. They generally do not respond well to treatment for lupus and are best followed with symptomatic treatment. Although a small number do eventually develop classic lupus, none of the presenting clinical or laboratory features are sufficiently predictive to identify such patients in advance. Patients with latent lupus tend to have a milder form of disease, not presenting with CNS involvement or renal disease.

Drug-induced lupus

Drug-induced lupus (see also Chapter 124) may be diagnosed in a patient in whom there is no prior history suggestive of SLE, in whom the clinical and serologic manifestations of lupus appear while they are receiving the drug concerned, and in whom improvement in clinical symptoms occurs quickly on stopping the drug, with a more gradual resolution of the serologic abnormalities[118,119].

The drugs associated with drug-induced lupus can be classified into three categories: those for which proof of the association is definite and for which appropriate, controlled, prospective studies have been performed, those drugs that are only possibly associated and, finally, drugs for which the association is still questionable. Examples of drugs in the first category include chlorpromazine, methyldopa, hydralazine, procainamide and isoniazid. Examples of drugs in the second category include dilantin, penicillamine, minocycline and quinidine; the third category is represented by a wide variety of drugs, including gold salts, a number of antibiotics, and griseofulvin and infliximab[120].

The clinical features of drug-related lupus are usually less severe than those of idiopathic SLE. The most commonly reported clinical features are constitutional symptoms, fever, arthritis and serositis. Central nervous system and renal involvement are distinctly uncommon. Laboratory tests reveal the presence of cytopenias, and positive LE cell preparation, ANA and rheumatoid factor tests. Antibodies to single-stranded DNA are commonly found, but antibodies to dsDNA are not. Complement concentrations are generally not depressed. Antihistone antibodies occur in more than 90% of cases. However, antihistone antibodies are not specific, as they are also found in 20–30% of patients with idiopathic SLE.

An interesting clinical question arises when patients with idiopathic SLE require drugs known to induce drug-induced lupus in other instances. The general practice is to use these drugs in such patients when they are necessary, because, generally, they pose no increased problems in patients with idiopathic lupus.

Late-stage lupus

Although short-term prognosis in lupus has improved dramatically over the past three decades, the mortality rates in patients surviving more than 5 years, and especially more than 10 years, have not shown a similar dramatic improvement. Patients with disease duration of more than 5 years tend to die of causes other than active SLE[121]. In such patients, mortality and morbidity are affected by long-term complications in SLE that are either the result of the previous SLE itself or a consequence of its treatment (Table 122.6).

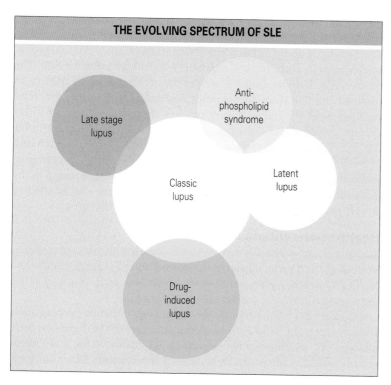

THE EVOLVING SPECTRUM OF SLE

Late stage lupus — Anti-phospholipid syndrome — Classic lupus — Latent lupus — Drug-induced lupus

Fig. 122.28 The evolving spectrum of SLE.

TABLE 122.6 LATE COMPLICATIONS OF SLE	
Acute episodes	**Chronic morbidity**
Glomerulonephritis	End-stage renal disease, dialysis, transplantation
Vasculitis	Atherosclerosis, venous syndromes, pulmonary emboli
Arthritis	Osteonecrosis
Cerebritis	Neuropsychiatric dysfunction
Pneumonitis	Shrinking lung syndrome

Atherosclerosis

Atherosclerosis manifests in patients with SLE as coronary artery disease, cerebral vascular disease and peripheral vascular disease. Patients best studied to date have been those who presented with atherosclerotic heart disease. These patients have usually demonstrated a significantly increased frequency of pericarditis, myocarditis, congestive heart failure and hypertension in their earlier active phase of systemic lupus[122]. Furthermore, metabolic risk factors such as hyperlipidemia, hyperglycemia and frank diabetes are more common among patients who develop atherosclerosis than in lupus patients in general[122]. There has been no reported difference in the use of corticosteroids in patients with or without atherosclerosis, although the average corticosteroid dose and the duration of use have generally been found to be greater. Vasculitis has not been shown to be increased in patients who later present with atherosclerosis, and cigarette smoking has also not been shown to be a clear predisposing factor.

Population and cohort studies have indicated that the prevalence of coronary artery disease and the incidence of myocardial infarction are significantly greater in patients with SLE, even in the face of a lesser number of traditional risk factors, compared with the general population. This suggests that SLE itself is a risk factor for accelerated atherosclerosis[122].

Thrombophlebitis/pulmonary emboli

Approximately 10% of patients with systemic lupus may demonstrate acute thrombophlebitis as a feature of their illness, either as a manifestation of lupus vasculitis or associated with a circulating anticoagulant[123]. In the former instance, there will usually be other signs of active systemic lupus. However, either early or late in the course of the lupus, patients may present with a bland phlebothrombosis (Fig. 122.29), with or without pulmonary emboli. In some patients, multiple pulmonary emboli may be the first indication that there is a venous problem. In such instances, one may presume that previous venous inflammation gave rise to secondary thrombosis, followed by multiple pulmonary emboli. The relationship between clotting and the antiphospholipid syndrome is discussed elsewhere.

Neurologic disorders

Assessments of cognitive function changes in SLE patients have demonstrated unequivocal deterioration in mental function. In the acute illness, both active systemic lupus and corticosteroids have been implicated as causative factors in organic brain dysfunction, as discussed previously. However, in late-stage lupus, when there is no longer any evidence of active disease and the patient is taking little or no corticosteroid, neurocognitive disabilities remain a frequent complaint. Patients often complain of decreased memory, decreased ability to do mathematical chores and increased speech disabilities. When such patients are submitted to a battery of neurocognitive tests, they are indeed shown to have significant impairment.

In addition, patients with systemic lupus undergoing neurologic investigation have been shown to demonstrate significant cortical atrophy on CT scanning. This has been shown both in patients who have had previous CNS disease caused by lupus and in those who have not, in addition to those who have current neurocognitive symptoms and in those who do not. Thus the exact pathogenesis of the neurocognitive disabilities that occur in latent lupus are not clear at present. They may be a feature of SLE in general, CNS disease of SLE in particular, related to the corticosteroids used to treat SLE or a combination of these factors.

CRITERIA FOR THE CLASSIFICATION OF SLE

For a disease with such protean manifestations and variable course as SLE, the need for classification criteria that would allow comparison of patients from different centers is quite clear[124]. The 1997 modification[125] of the 1982 revised ACR criteria for SLE are listed in Table 122.7. The ACR criteria for the classification of SLE help distinguish patients with SLE from patients with other connective tissue diseases, and thus enable this comparison.

Criteria for disease activity in SLE

More than 60 systems to assess clinical disease activity in SLE have been devised, but there have only been a handful of instruments that have been validated[126]. Three of these, the SLE Disease Activity Index, the British Isles Lupus Assessment Group and the SLE Activity Measure all distinguished among patients, and correlate highly with each other[126]. The SLE Disease Activity Index was recently modified and used to define flare[127]. Regardless of the instrument used to score the disease activity, a full history, physical examination and laboratory tests including serologic markers for SLE are required[128].

Criteria for damage in SLE

As patients with SLE live longer, they accumulate organ damage both as a result of previous inflammation and from complications of treatment. The Systemic Lupus International Collaborating Clinics (SLICC) group, in conjunction with the ACR, developed a damage index for SLE. The SLICC/ACR Damage Index describes the accumulation of damage in patients with SLE since disease onset, and includes items that may have resulted from the inflammatory process, disease treatment or intercurrent events without attribution[129]. The SLICC/ACR Damage Index has been validated and used in a number of studies[126]. It has been found to predict mortality[130]. The Damage Index may thus provide an important outcome measure in SLE, both for studies of prognosis, and in the assessment of long-term effects of treatment. It may also be used to stratify patients for therapeutic trials.

Health status criteria in SLE

Measurements of health status include quality-of-life assessments, psychologic and social impact of the disease, and physical disability. The Medical Outcome Survey Short-Form-36 has been recommended as the instrument of choice to assess quality of life in SLE[131,132].

It is clear that some patients with lupus have difficulty keeping a job and are depressed. Most patients note some effect of the disease on their lifestyle. The relationship between impaired quality of life and disease activity and damage is not clear. Several investigators have found no correlation between health status and disease activity or damage, and consider these to be independent domains in the assessment of patients

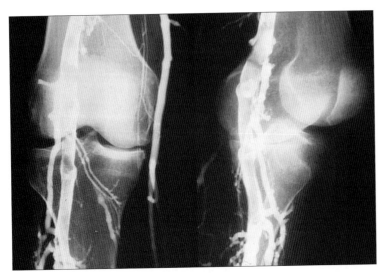

Fig. 122.29 A venogram showing venous thrombosis in a patient with SLE of the right leg and early changes on the left.

TABLE 122.7 THE 1997 REVISED ACR CRITERIA FOR THE CLASSIFICATION OF SLE

Item	Definition
Malar rash	Fixed erythema, flat or raised, over the malar eminences, sparing the nasolabial folds
Discoid rash	Erythematous raised patches with adherent keratotic scaling and follicular plugging: atrophic scarring may occur in older lesions
Photosensitivity	Skin rash as a results of unusual reaction to sunlight, by patient history or physician observation
Oral ulcers	Oral or nasopharyngeal ulceration, usually painless, observed by a physician
Non-erosive arthritis	Involving two or more peripheral joints, characterized by tenderness, swelling, or effusion
Pleuritis or pericarditis	(a) Pleuritis – convincing history of pleuritic pain or rub heard by a physician or evidence of pleural effusion or (b) Pericarditis – documented by electrocardiogram or rub or evidence of pericardial effusion
Renal disorder	(a) Persistent proteinuria >0.5g/day or >3+ if quantitative not performed or (b) Cellular casts – may be red cell, hemoglobin, granular, tubular or mixed
Seizures or psychosis	(a) Seizures – in the absence of offending drugs or known metabolic derangement: e.g. uremia, ketoacidosis or electrolyte imbalance or (b) Psychosis – in the absence of offending drugs or known metabolic derangement: e.g. uremia, ketoacidosis or electrolyte imbalance
Hematologic disorder	(a) Hemolytic anemia with reticulocytosis or (b) Leukopenia – less than 4000/mm³ on two occasions or (c) Lymphopenia – less than 1500/mm³ on two occasions or (d) Thrombocytopenia – less than 100 000/mm³ in the absence of offending drugs
Immunologic disorder	(a) Anti-DNA: antibody to native DNA in abnormal titer or (b) Anti-Sm: presence of antibody to Sm nuclear antigen or (c) Positive finding of antiphospholipid antibodies based on: (1) an abnormal serum concentration of IgG or IgM anticardiolipin antibodies (2) a positive test for lupus anticoagulant using a standard method or (3) a false-positive test for at least 6 months and confirmed by *Treponema pallidum* immobilization or fluorescent treponomal antibody absorption test
Positive ANA	An abnormal titer of ANA by immunofluorescence or an equivalent assay at any point in time in the absence of drug

with SLE, whereas others found that it is related to disease activity and damage[132–134]. The role of formal education in the assessment of health status in patients with SLE was studied by Callahan and Pincus[135]. They administered a clinical status questionnaire to 124 patients with SLE, and found that those with more than 12 years of formal education were more likely to be working full-time than those with 11 years or less of formal education. Moreover, patients with a lower level of education had poorer clinical status on all five self-report scales than did patients with 12 or more years of formal education.

PROGNOSIS

Our understanding of the prospects of recovery from SLE has evolved in the past four decades, both because of better comprehension of the disease process itself, and through the development of methods with which to assess outcome. Survival rates have increased over the past four decades, from less than 50% in 5 years in 1955, to more than 90% survival at 5 years in the 1990s (Table 122.8[136–144]). Recent studies provide survival rates of close to 70% at 20 years[145]. Several reasons have been cited for this improved survival. These include earlier diagnosis, which allows inclusion of milder cases, better therapeutic modalities for lupus, including better use of corticosteroids and immunosuppressive agents,

and advances in medical treatment in general, such as improved antibiotics, antihypertensive agents, availability of renal dialysis and transplantation. However, the pattern of disease in SLE has not changed significantly over the past two decades[146]. A specific study of the reasons for improved survival in SLE also showed that, over a 24-year period, the disease expression did not change, nor did the medications, and yet improved survival in patients with SLE was noticeable above that of the general population. This was believed to reflect more judicious use of currently available medications and better management of the complications of SLE[147].

Despite the improved survival, patients with SLE still die at a rate three times that of the general population[138,147]. The causes of death may be divided into those related to the SLE disease process itself, those related to treatment, and deaths from unrelated causes. The causes related to the SLE include active disease, vasculitis leading to CNS disease or intestinal perforation, intractable bleeding and end-organ failure, such as renal, cardiac or pulmonary. Treatment for SLE may in itself result in fatal complications such as fulminant infection (which may just as likely be associated with active disease), perforation or peptic ulcer disease and, possibly, vascular disease.

In addition to the general principles for improved survival in SLE, there may be specific factors that affect mortality (Table 122.9). These

TABLE 122.8 SURVIVAL RATES IN SLE

Study	No. of patients	Outcome year	Center	Survival (%)			
				5	10	15	20
Estes and Christian[136]	150	1971	New York	77	60	50	–
Wallace et al.[137]	609	1979	Los Angeles	88	79	74	–
Reveille et al.[138]	389	1990	Alabama	89	83	79	–
Pistiner et al.[139]	570	1990	Los Angeles	97	93	83	–
Ward et al.[140]	408	1991	Durham	82	71	63	–
Massardo et al.[141]	218	1993	Chile	92	77	66	–
Abu-Shakra et al.[121]	665	1993	Toronto	93	85	79	68
Tucker et al.[142]	165	1993	London	93	86	78	–
Blanco et al.[143]	306	1993	Spain	90	85	80	–
Jacobsen et al.[144]	513	1999	Denmark	91	76	64	53

Findings in large series (>100 patients) with data for at least 15 years.

TABLE 122.9 FACTORS THAT AFFECT MORTALITY IN SLE

Study	Year	Time	Age	Race	Sex	SES	Renal	CNS	BP	Plat	DA
Estes and Christian[136]	1955	A	–	–	–	?	+	+	?	?	?
Wallace et al.[137]	1981	D	+	–	–	?	+	–	–	–	?
Reveille et al.[138]	1990	D	+	+	–	–	+	?	+	+	?
Pistiner et al.[139]	1991	D	–	–	+	–	+	?	?	+	?
Ward et al.[140]	1993	A	+	–	–	+	?	?	?	?	?
Massardo et al.[141]	1993	A	–	–	–	–	+	–	–	+	+*
Abu-Shakra et al.[148]	1993	A	+	–	–	–	+	–	–	+	+*
Blanco et al.[143]	1993	A	–	–	+	?	+	+	?	?	?
Jacobsen et al.[144]	1999	A	+	NA	+	?	–	+	?	?	?

A, any time before death; BP, blood pressure; D, at diagnosis; DA, disease activity; NA, not applicable; Plat, platelets; SES, socioeconomic status; –, negative association; +, positive association; ?, not studied; *at study entry

include general features that are unrelated to the disease process itself, such as race, sex, age at onset and socioeconomic status.

Racial differences

Black patients with SLE have been considered to have a poorer prognosis than white patients. Although race did not appear as an important prognostic factor in a logistic regression analysis in the multicenter study published by Ginzler et al.[149], it was found to be a factor adversely affecting survival in SLE when a Cox multivariate analysis was applied to a group of 389 patients studied by Reveille et al.[138]. It has been difficult to separate out the effects of race and socioeconomic status, particularly with reference to differences between white and black patients in the USA. In Reveille's study, white patients with private insurance fared better than black patients with private insurance[138]. However, there was no difference in outcome when black patients with and without private insurance were compared. This supports the notion that there may be racial differences in the expression of this disease and its outcome. However, Ward et al.[140] demonstrated that, although survival was better for whites than for blacks, it was related to socioeconomic status, which was poorer among blacks. In Malaysia, Indian patients were found to fare worse than Chinese[150].

Sex

The relationship between sex and prognosis has been controversial. A higher mortality in females than males with SLE has been suggested by some, whereas others demonstrated a better prognosis for women than for men. Sex did not appear as a significant predictor in the statistical analysis performed by Ginzler et al.[149], or in the University of Toronto cohort[148] Thus the issue of the effect of sex on prognosis in SLE remains unanswered.

Age at onset

Age at onset of SLE was found to be a significant predictor of survival at both 1 and 5 years in the multicenter study, with better survival in the older patients[149]. In contrast, Reveille et al.[138] found that increasing age of onset adversely affected survival, and Abu-Shakra et al.[148] found age older than 50 years at diagnosis to be a risk for death. Onset of SLE in the pediatric age group has been associated with worse prognosis, but a study of childhood SLE found the 5-year survival to be the same as for the adult populations, at 85.3%[151]. Indeed, a comparison with the estimated survival of the age-matched segment of the US population showed that SLE patients fared worse in all age groups[140].

Socioeconomic status

Patients with better education and higher socioeconomic status seem to fare better than the poorer population. Patients of a lower education level, which may reflect lower socioeconomic status, do less well than those of a higher education level.

Disease factors

The association between specific disease manifestations and outcome in SLE has been well recognized. The presence of CNS disease has been found commonly in patients who die with active lupus[121], and has been found to be associated with decreased survival. Similarly, the presence of nephritis carries a poor prognosis for patients with lupus. The predictive value of serum creatinine concentration for overall mortality in SLE has been recognized for some time. A recent 10-year case–control study demonstrated that, compared with patients with SLE but no nephritis matched for age and sex, patients with lupus nephritis had a greater prevalence of hyperlipidemia (44% compared with 2%, $P<0.001$), hypertension (44% compared with 9%, $P<0.001$) and antiphospholipid antibodies (45% compared with 22%, $P=0.01$) at study onset. More patients with lupus nephritis patients died (16% compared with 2% $P=0.02$), the majority from cardiovascular complications[152].

Early studies of the relationship of renal morphology based on light microscopy suggested that advanced lesions, such as diffuse proliferative glomerulonephritis, were associated with greater mortality than was seen with the milder lesions, such as mesangial or minimal lesion. Conversely, several investigators have suggested that, as new predictive information, renal biopsy adds only a limited value to already available clinical variables. McLaughlin et al.[48], using univariate analysis, found a trend for the association of WHO classes with mortality. However, it was the presence of proliferative lesions that was associated with a significantly greater risk of dying. The presence of chronic lesions, such as glomerular sclerosis and interstitial fibrosis, was also significantly associated with reduced survival rates. Moreover, the predictive value of proliferative and chronic

lesions was particularly useful in patients with normal serum creatinine concentrations. Nossent et al.[47] also demonstrated that a high chronicity index was associated with patient mortality in both univariate and multivariate analyses. Thus, although renal biopsy may not be of additional help in patients who already demonstrate clinical evidence of renal damage (increased creatinine), it provides useful information in patients who are studied before damage occurs[153]. Moreover, the presence of proliferative lesions on the biopsy is prognostically significant. Renal damage (increased serum creatinine, dialysis or transplantation) has been found to be a risk factor for mortality[150].

Aside from the association of neuropsychiatric manifestations and renal disease with increased mortality, other disease manifestations have been found to affect prognosis. In the multicenter study[149], anemia from any cause was found to be a predictor for mortality. In the University of Alabama study[138], and in the Toronto cohort[150], thrombocytopenia emerged as an important predictor of mortality. Lung involvement was also found to be a risk factor for mortality. Overall disease activity at presentation measured by the SLEDAI has also been identified as a risk factor for poor outcome[150]. Moreover, a high SLEDAI over follow-up is also associated with death within 6 months[154]. Early damage, within the first year of diagnosis of SLE, is also associated with mortality[130].

REFERENCES

1. Smith CD, Cyr M. The history of lupus erythematosus. From Hippocrates to Osler. Rheum Dis Clin North Am 1988; 14: 1–14.
2. Hargraves MM, Richmond H, Morton R. Presentation of two bone marrow elements. The 'tart' cell and the 'L.E.' cell. Proc Mayo Clin 1948; 23: 25–28.
3. Friou GJ. Identification of the nuclear component of the interaction of lupus erythematosus globulin and nuclei. J Immunol 1958; 80: 476–481.
4. Urowitz MB, Bookman AAM, Koehler BE et al. The bimodal mortality in systemic lupus erythematosus. Am J Med 1976; 60: 221-225.
5. Gladman DD, Urowitz MB. Morbidity in systemic lupus erythematosus. J Rheum 1986; 14(suppl 13): 223–226.
6. Hochberg MC, Perlmutter SL, Medsger TA et al. Prevalence of self-reported physician-diagnosed systemic lupus erythematosus in the USA. Lupus 1995; 4: 454–456.
7. Uramoto KM, Michet CJ, Thumboo J et al. Trends in the incidence and mortality of systemic lupus erythematosus (SLE) 1950–1992. Arthritis Rheum 1999; 42: 46–50.
8. Hopkinson ND, Doherty M, Powell RJ. Clinical features and race-specific incidence/prevalence rates of systemic lupus erythematosus in a geographically complete cohort of patients. Ann Rheum Dis 1994; l53: 675–680.
9. Peschken CA, Esdaile JM. Systemic lupus erythematosus in North American Indians: a population based study. J Rheumatol 2000; 27: 1884–1891.
10. Hochberg MC. Systemic lupus erythematosus. Rheum Dis Clin North Am 1990; 16: 617–639.
11. Stahl-Hallengren C, Jonsen A, Nived O, Sturfelt G. Incidence studies of systemic lupus erythematosus in Southern Sweden: increasing age, decreasing frequency of renal manifestations and good prognosis. J Rheumatol 2000; 27: 685–691.
12. Ward MM, Studenski S. Clinical manifestations of systemic lupus erythematosus. Identification of racial and socioeconomic influence. Arch Intern Med 1990; 150: 849–953.
13. Block SK, Winfield JB, Lockshin MC et al. Studies of twins with systemic lupus erythematosus. A review of the literature and presentation of 12 additional sets. Am J Med 1975; 59: 533–552.
14. Lawrence JS, Martins L, Drake G. A family survey of lupus erythematosus. J Rheumatol 1987; 14: 913–921.
15. Hochberg MC. The application of genetic epidemiology to systemic lupus erythematosus. J Rheumatol 1987; 14: 867–869.
16. Reinersten JL, Klippel JH, Johnson AH et al. B-lymphocyte alloantigens associated with systemic lupus erythematosus. N Engl J Med 1978; 299: 515–518.
17. Schur PH, Marcus-Bagley D, Awdeh Z et al. The effect of ethnicity on major histocompatibility complex complement allotypes and extended haplotypes in patients with systemic lupus erythematosus. Arthritis Rheum 1990; 33: 985–992.
18. Olsen ML, Goldstein R, Arnett FC et al. C4A gene deletion and HLA associations in black Americans with systemic lupus erythematosus. Immunogenetics 1989; 30: 27–33.
19. Petri M, Watson R, Winkelstein HA, McLean RH. Clinical expression of systemic lupus erythematosus in patients with C4A deficiency. Medicine 1993; 72: 236–244.
20. Hartung K, Fontana A, Klar M et al. Association of class I, II, and III MHC gene products with systemic lupus erythematosus. Results of a central European multicenter study. Rheumatol Int 1989; 9: 13–18.
21. Dunckley J, Gatenby PA, Hawkins B et al. Deficiency of C4A is a genetic determinant of systemic lupus erythematosus in three ethnic groups. J Immunogenet 1987; 14: 209–218.
22. Fronek A, Timmerman LA, Alper CA et al. Major histocompatibility complex genes and susceptibility to systemic lupus erythematosus. Arthritis Rheum 1990; 33: 1542–1553.
23. Davies EJ, Steers G, Ollier WER et al. Relative contributions of HLA-SQA and complement C4A loci in determining susceptibility to systemic lupus erythematosus. Br J Rheumatol 1995; 34: 221–225.
24. Huang DF, Siminovitch KA, Liu XY et al. Population and family studies of three disease-related polymorphic genes in systemic lupus erythematosus. J Clin Invest 1995; 95: 1766–1772.
25. Gaffney PM, Kearns GM, Shark KB et al. A genome-wide search for susceptibility genes in human systemic lupus erythematosus sib-pair families. Proc Natl Acad Sci USA 1998; 95: 14875–14879.
26. Moser KL, Neas BR, Salmon JE et al. Genome scan of human systemic lupus erythematosus: evidence for linkage on chromosome 1q in African-American pedigrees. Proc Natl Acad Sci USA 1998; 95: 14869–14874.
27. Cervera R, Khamashta M, Font J et al. Systemic lupus erythematosus: clinical and immunologic patterns of disease expression in a cohort of 1000 patients. Medicine 1993; 72: 113–124.
28. Boumpas DR, Fessler BJ, Austin HA et al. Systemic lupus erythematosus: emerging concepts. Part 2: Dermatologic and joint disease, the antiphospholipid antibody syndrome, pregnancy and hormonal therapy, morbidity and mortality, and pathogenesis. Ann Int Med 1995; 123: 42–53.
29. Cardinali C, Caproni M, Fabbri P. The utility of the lupus band test on sun-protected non-lesional skin for the diagnosis of systemic lupus erythematosus. Clin Exp Rheumatol 1999; 17: 427–432.
30. Gammon RW, Briggaman RA, Inman AO et al. Evidence supporting a role for immune complex-mediated inflammation in the pathogenesis of bullous lesions of systemic lupus erythematosus. J Invest Dermatol 1983; 81: 320–325.
31. Emerit I, Michelson AM. Mechanism of photosensitivity in systemic lupus erythematosus patients. Proc Natl Acad Sci USA 1984; 78: 2537–2540.
32. Furukawa P, Kshihara-Sawami M, Lyons MB, Norris DA. Binding of antibodies to the extractable nuclear antigens SS-A/Ro and SS-B/La is induced on the surface of human keratinocytes by ultraviolet light (UVL): implications for the pathogenesis of photosensitive cutaneous lupus. J Invest Dermatol 1990; 94: 77–85.
33. Nyberg F, Hasan T, Skoglund C, Stephansson E. Early events in ultraviolet light-induced skin lesions in lupus erythematosus: expression patterns of adhesion molecules ICAM-1, VCAM-1 and E-selectin. Acta Dermato-Vener 1999; 79: 431–436.
34. Cronin ME. Musculoskeletal manifestations of systemic lupus erythematosus. Rheum Dis Clin North Am 1988; 14: 99–116.
35. Reilly PA, Evison G, McHugh NJ, Maddison PJ. Arthropathy of hands and feet in systemic lupus erythematosus. J Rheumatol 1990; 17: 777–784.
36. Esdaile JM, Danoff D, Rosenthal L, Gutowsko A. Deforming arthritis in systemic lupus erythematosus. Ann Rheum Dis 1981; 40: 124–126.
37. Morley KD, Leung A, Rynes RI. Lupus foot. BMJ 1982; 284: 557–558.
38. Gladman DD, Urowitz MB, Chaudhry-Ahluwalia V et al. Predictive factors for symptomatic osteonecrosis in systemic lupus erythematosus. J Rheumatol 2001; 28: 761–765.
39. Gladman DD, Urowitz MB, Chaudhry-Ahluwalia V et al. Outcome of symptomatic osteonecrosis in 95 patients with systemic lupus erythematosus. J Rheum 2001; 28: 2226–2269.
40. Finol HR, Montagnani S, Marquez A et al. Ultrastructural pathology of skeletal muscle in systemic lupus erythematosus. J Rheumatol 1990; 17: 210–219.
41. Smythe H, Lee D, Rush P, Buskila D. Tender shins and steroid therapy. J Rheumatol 1991; 18: 1568–1572.
42. Gladman D, Urowitz M, Gough J, MacKinnon A: Fibromyalgia is a major contributor to quality of life in lupus. J Rheumatol 1997; 24: 2145–2149.

43. Rahman P, Gladman DD, Dominique Ibanez, Urowitz MB. Significance of isolated hematuria and isolated pyuria in systemic lupus erythematosus. Lupus 2001; 10: 418–423.

44. Golbus J, McCune WJ. Lupus nephritis. Classification, prognosis, immunopathogenesis and treatment. Rheum Dis Clin North Am 1994; 20: 213–242.

45. Gladman DD, Urowitz MB, Cole E et al. Kidney biopsy in SLE. I. A clinical–morphologic evaluation. Q J Med 1989; 73: 1125–1153.

46. Austin HA, Muenz LR, Joyce KM et al. Prognostic factors in lupus nephritis. Contribution of renal histologic data. Am J Med 1983; 75: 382–3891.

47. Nossent HC, Nenzen-Logmans SC, Vroom TM et al. Contribution of renal biopsy data in predicting outcome in lupus nephritis. Arthritis Rheum 1990; 33: 970–977.

48. McLaughlin J, Gladman DD, Urowitz MB et al. Renal biopsy in SLE. II: Survival analyses according to biopsy results. Arthritis Rheum 1991; 34: 1268–1273.

49. Hariharan S, Pollak VE, Kant KS et al. Diffuse proliferative lupus nephritis: long-term observations in patients treated with ancrod. Clin Nephrol 1990; 34: 61–69.

50. Jacobsen S, Starklint H, Petersen J et al. Prognostic value of renal biopsy and clinical variables in patients with lupus nephritis and normal serum creatinine. Scand J Rheumatol 1999; 28: 288–299.

51. Bajaj S, Albert L, Gladman DD et al. Serial renal biopsy in systemic lupus erythematosus. J Rheumatol 2000; 27: 2822–2826.

52. Bruce IN, Gladman DD, Urowitz MB. Extra-renal disease activity in SLE is not suppressed by chronic renal insufficiency or renal replacement therapy. J Rheumatol 1999; 26: 1490–1494.

53. Krane NK, Burjak K, Archie M, O'Donovan R. Persistent lupus activity in end-stage renal disease. Am J Kid Dis 1999; 33: 872–879.

54. ACR Ad Hoc Committee on Neuropsychiatric Lupus Nomenclature. The American College of Rheumatology nomenclature and case definitions for neuropsychiatric lupus syndromes. Arthritis Rheum 1999; 42: 599–608.

55. Kovacs JAJ, Urowitz MB, Gladman DD. Dilemmas in neuropsychiatric lupus. Rheum Dis Clin North Am 1993; 19: 795–814.

56. Boumpas DT, Austin HA, Fessler BJ et al. Systemic lupus erythematosus: emerging concepts. Part 1: Renal, neuropsychiatric, cardiovascular, pulmonary and hematologic disease. Ann Int Med 1995; 122: 940–950.

57. Amit M, Molad Y, Levy O, Wisenbeek AJ. Headache in systemic lupus erythematosus and its relation to other disease manifestations. Clin Exp Rheumatol 1999; 17: 467–470.

58. Glanz BI, Venkatezan A, Schur PH, Lew RA et al. Prevalence of migraine in patients with systemic lupus erythematosus. Headache 2001; 41: 285–289.

59. Stafford-Brady FJ, Urowitz MB, Gladman DD, Easterbrook M. Lupus retinopathy. Patterns, associations and prognosis. Arthritis Rheum 1988; 31: 1105–1110.

60. Teh L, Isenberg DA. Antiribosomal P protein antibodies in systemic lupus erythematosus. A reappraisal. Arthritis Rheum 1994; 37: 307–315.

61. Kremer JM, Rynes RI, Bartholomew LE et al. Non-organic non-psychotic psychopathology (NONPP) in patients with systemic lupus erythematosus. Semin Arthritis Rheum 1981; 11: 182–189.

62. Denburg SD, Denburg JA, Carbotte RM, Fisk JD et al. Cognitive deficits in systemic lupus erythematosus. Rheum Dis Clin North Am 1993; 19: 815–831.

63. Miguel EC, Rodriques Pereira RM, de Bragança Pereira CA et al. Psychiatric manifestations of systemic lupus erythematosus: clinical features, symptoms, and signs of central nervous system activity in 43 patients. Medicine 1994; 73: 224–232.

64. Minota S, Koyasu S, Yahara I, Winfield J. Autoantibodies to the heat shock protein hsp90 in systemic lupus erythematosus. J Clin Invest 1988; 81: 106–109.

65. Robbins ML, Kornguth SE, Bell CL et al. Antineurofilament antibody evaluation in neuropsychiatric systemic lupus erythematosus. Combination with anticardiolipin antibody assay and magnetic resonance imaging. Arthritis Rheum 1988; 31: 623–631.

66. West SG, Emlen W, Wener MH, Kotzin BL. Neuropsychiatric lupus erythematosus: a 10-year prospective study on the value of diagnostic tests. Am J Med 1995; 99: 153–163.

67. Sibbitt WL Jr, Sibbitt RR, Brooks WM. Neuroimaging in neuropsychiatric systemic lupus erythematosus. Arthritis Rheum 1999; 42: 2026–2038.

68. Kovacs JAJ, Urowitz MB, Gladman DD, Zeman R. The use of SPECT in neuropsychiatric SLE: a pilot study. J Rheumatol 1995; 22: 1247–1253.

69. Kodama K, Okada S, Hino T et al. Single photon emission computed tomography in systemic lupus erythematosus with psychiatric symptoms. J Neurol Neurosurg Psychiatry 1995; 58: 307–311.

70. Griffey RH, Brown MS, Bankhurst AD et al. Depletion of high-energy phosphates in the central nervous system of patients with systemic lupus erythematosus, as determined by phosphorus-31 nuclear magnetic resonance spectroscopy. Arthritis Rheum 1990; 33: 827–833.

71. Segal AM, Calabrese LH, Ahmad M et al. The pulmonary manifestations of systemic lupus erythematosus. Semin Arthritis Rheum 1985; 14: 202–224.

72. Orens JB, Martinez FJ, Lynch III JP. Pleuropulmonary manifestations of systemic lupus erythematosus. Rheum Dis Clin North Am 1994; 20: 159–193.

73. Good Jr JT, King TE, Antony VB, Sahn SA. Lupus pleuritis: clinical features and pleural fluid characteristics with special reference to pleural fluid antinuclear antibodies. Chest 1983; 84: 714–718.

74. Wang DY, Yang PC, Yu WL et al. Serial antinuclear antibodies titre in pleural and pericardial fluid. Eur Resp J 2000; 15: 1106–1110.

75. Leung WH, Wong KL, Lau CP et al. Cardiac abnormalities in systemic lupus erythematosus: a prospective M-mode, cross-sectional and Doppler echocardiographic study. Int J Cardiol 1990; 27: 367–375.

76. Sturfelt G, Eskilsson J, Nived O, Truedsson L et al. Cardiovascular disease in systemic lupus erythematosus. A study of 75 patients from a defined population. Medicine 1992; 71: 216–223.

77. Bulkley BH, Roberts WC. The heart in systemic lupus erythematosus and the changes induced in it by corticosteroid therapy. Am J Med 1975; 58: 243–264.

78. Zashin SJ, Lipsky PE. Pericardial tamponade complicating systemic lupus erythematosus. J Rheumatol 1989; 16: 374–377.

79. Kaufman LD, Seifert FC, Eilbott DJ et al. Candida pericarditis and tamponade in a patient with systemic lupus erythematosus. Arch Intern Med 1988; 148: 715–717.

80. Coe MD, Hamer DH, Levy CS et al. Gonococcal pericarditis with tamponade in a patient with systemic lupus erythematosus. Arthritis Rheum 1990; 33: 1438–1441.

81. Mok MY, Wong RW, Lau CS. Intestinal pseudo-obstruction in systemic lupus erythematosus: an uncommon but important clinical manifestation. Lupus 2000; 9: 11–18.

82. Schoshoe JT, Koch AE, Chang RW. Chronic lupus peritonitis with ascites: review of the literature with a case report. Semin Arthritis Rheum 1988; 18: 121–126.

83. Carette S. Cardiopulmonary manifestations of systemic lupus erythematosus. Rheum Dis Clin North Am 1988; 14: 135–147.

84. Bankier AA, Kiener HP, Wiesmayr MN et al. Discrete lung involvement in systemic lupus erythematosus: CT assessment. Radiology 1995; 196: 835–840.

85. Zamora MR, Warner ML, Tuder R, Schwarz MI. Diffuse alveolar hemorrhage and systemic lupus erythematosus. Clinical presentation, histology, survival, and outcome. Medicine 1997; 76: 192–202.

86. Asherson RA, Oakley CM. Pulmonary hypertension in a lupus clinic: experience with twenty-four patients. J Rheumatol 1990; 17: 1292–1298.

87. Winslow TM, Ossipov MO, Fazio GP et al. Five-year follow-up study of the prevalence and progression of pulmonary hypertension in systemic lupus erythematosus. Am Heart J 1995; 129: 510–515.

88. Robbins IM, Gaine SP, Schilz R et al. Epoprostenol for treatment of pulmonary hypertension in patients with systemic lupus erythematosus. Chest 2000; 117: 14–18.

89. Walz-Leblanc BA, Urowitz MB, Gladman DD, Hanly PJ. The 'shrinking lungs syndrome' in systemic lupus erythematosus – improvement with corticosteroid therapy. J Rheumatol 1992; 19: 1970–1972.

90. Warrington KJ, Moder KG, Brutinel WM. The shrinking lung syndrome in systemic lupus erythematosus. Mayo Clin Proc 2000; 75: 467–472.

91. Rubin LA, Urowitz MB. Shrinking lung syndrome in SLE – a clinical pathologic study. J Rheumatol 1983; 10: 973–976.

92. Sasson Z, Rasooly Y, Chow CW et al. Impairment of left ventricular diastolic function in systemic lupus erythematosus. Am J Cardiol 1992; 69: 1629–1634.

93. Badui E, Garcia-Rubi D, Robles E et al.. Cardiovascular manifestations in systemic lupus erythematosus. Angiology 1985; 36: 431–441.

94. Hosenpud JD, Montanaro A, Hart MV et al. Myocardial perfusion abnormalities in asymptomatic patients with systemic lupus erythematosus. Am J Med 1984; 77: 286–292.

95. Tamburino C, Fiore C, Foti R et al. Endomyocardial biopsy in diagnosis and management of cardiovascular manifestations of systemic lupus erythematosus. Clin Rheumatol 1989; 8: 108–112.

96. Straaton KV, Chatham WW, Reveille JD et al. Clinically significant valvular heart disease in systemic lupus erythematosus. Am J Med 1988; 85: 645–650.

97. Korbet SM, Schwartz MM, Lewis EJ. Immune complex deposition and coronary vasculitis in systemic lupus erythematosus. Am J Med 1984; 77: 141–145.

98. Hallegua DS, Wallace DJ. Gastrointestinal manifestations of systemic lupus erythematosus. Curr Opin Rheumatol 2000; 12: 379–385.

99. Zizic TM, Classen JN, Stevens MB. Acute abdominal complications of systemic lupus erythematosus and polyarteritis nodosa. Am J Med 1982; 73: 525–531.

100. Gladman DD, Ross T, Richardson B, Kulkarni S. Bowel involvement in systemic lupus erythematosus: Crohn's disease or lupus vasculitis. Arthritis Rheum 1985; 28: 466–470.

101. Nagata M, Ogawa Y, Hisano S, Ueda K. Crohn's disease in systemic lupus erythematosus: a case report. Eur J Pediatr 1989; 148: 525–526.

102. Reynolds JC, Inman RD, Kimberly RP et al. Acute pancreatitis in systemic lupus erythematosus: report of twenty cases and a review of the literature. Medicine 1982; 61: 25–32.

103. Saab S, Corr MP, Weisman MH. Corticosteroids and systemic lupus erythematosus pancreatitis: a case series. J Rheumatol 1998; 25: 801–806.

104. Haakenstad AO, Mannik M. Saturation of the reticuloendothelial system with soluble immune complexes. J Immunol 1974; 112: 1939–1948.

105. Dillon AM, Stein HB, English RA. Splenic atrophy in SLE. Ann Intern Med 1982; 96: 40–43.

106. Buskila D, Gladman DD, Hanna W, Kahn HJ. Primary malignant lymphoma of the spleen in systemic lupus erythematosus. J Rheumatol 1989; 16: 993–996.

107. Kojima M, Nakamura S, Morishita Y et al. Reactive follicular hyperplasia in the lymph node lesions from systemic lupus erythematosus patients: a clinicopathological and immunohistological study of 21 cases. Pathol Int 2000; 50: 304–312.

108. Voulgarelis M, Kokori SI, Ioannidis JP et al. Anaemia in systemic lupus erythematosus: aetiological profile and the role of erythropoietin. Ann Rheum Dis 2000; 59: 217–222.

109. Miller MH, Urowitz MB, Gladman DD: The significance of thrombocytopenia in systemic lupus erythematosus. Arthritis Rheum 1983; 26: 1181–1186.

110. Musio F, Bohen EM, Yuan CM, Welch PG. Review of thrombotic thrombocytopenic purpura in the setting of systemic lupus erythematosus. Semin Arthritis Rheum 1998; 28: 1–19.

111. Papo T, Andre MH, Amoura Z et al. The spectrum of reactive hemophagocytic syndrome in systemic lupus erythematosus. J Rheumatol 1999; 26: 927–930.

112. Ridker PM, Hennekens CH, Buring JE, Rifai NC. C-Reactive protein and other markers of inflammation in the prediction of cardiovascular disease in women. N Engl J Med 2000; 342: 836–843.

113. Lloyd W, Schur PH. Immune complexes, complement, and anti-DNA in exacerbations of systemic lupus erythematosus (SLE). Medicine 1981; 60: 208–207.

114. Walz-Leblanc B, Gladman DD, Urowitz MB, Goodman PJ. Serologically active clinically quiescent SLE. J Rheumatol 1994; 21: 2239–2241.

115. Reichlin M. ANA negative systemic lupus erythematosus sera revisited serologically. Lupus 2000; 9: 116–119.

116. Ganczarczyk L, Urowitz MB, Gladman DD. Latent lupus. J Rheumatol 1989; 16: 475–478.
117. Swaak AHG, van de Bring H, Smeenk RJT et al. Incomplete lupus erythematosus: results of a multicentre study under the supervision of EULAR Standing Committee on International Clinical Studies Including Therapeutic Trials (ESCISIT). Rheumatology 2001: 40: 89–94.
118. Hess EV. Drug-related lupus. N Engl J Med 1988; 318: 1460–`1462.
119. Rubin RL. Etiology and mechanisms of drug-induced lupus. Curr Opin Rheumatol 1999; 11: 357–363.
120. Schaible TF. Long term safety of infliximab. Can J Gastroenterol 2000; 14(suppl C): 29–32.
121. Abu-Shakra M, Urowitz MB, Gladman DD, Gough J. Mortality studies in systemic lupus erythematosus. Results from a single centre. I. Causes of death. J Rheumatol 1995; 22: 1259–1264.
122. Bruce IN, Gladman DD, Urowitz MB. Premature atherosclerosis in SLE. Rheum Dis Clin North Am 2000; 26: 257–278.
123. Gladman DD, Urowitz MB. Venous syndromes and pulmonary embolism in systemic lupus erythematosus. Ann Rheum Dis 1980; 39: 340–343.
124. Tan EM, Cohen AS, Fries JF et al. The 1982 revised criteria for the classification of systemic lupus erythematosus. Arthritis Rheum 1982; 25: 1271–1277.
125. Hochberg MC. Updating the American College of Rheumatology revised criteria for the classification of systemic lupus erythematosus [letter]. Arthritis Rheum 1997; 40: 1725.
126. Urowitz MB, Gladman DD. Assessment of disease activity and damage in SLE. Baillière's Clinical Rheumatology 1998; 12: 405–413.
127. Gladman DD, Ibañez D, Urowitz MB. Systemic lupus erythematosus disease activity index 2000. J Rheumatol 2002; 29: 288–291.
128. Gladman DD, Urowitz MB, Esdaile JM et al. American College of Rheumatology Ad Hoc Committee on SLE Guidelines. Guidelines for referral and management of systemic lupus erythematosus in adults. Arthritis Rheum 1999; 42: 1785–1796.
129. Gladman D, Ginzler E, Goldsmith CH et al. The development and initial validation of the SLICC/ACR damage index for SLE. Arthritis Rheum 1996; 39: 363–369.
130. Rahman P, Gladman DD, Urowitz MB et al. Early damage as measured by the SLICC/ACR Damage Index is a predictor of mortality in SLE. Lupus 2001; 10: 93–96.
131. Gladman DD, Urowitz M, Fortin P et al. Workshop Report: Systemic Lupus Erythematosus International Collaborating Clinics (SLICC) Conference on Assessment of Lupus Flare and Quality of Life Measures in SLE. J Rheumatol 1996; 23: 1953–1535.
132. Gordon C, Clarke AE. Quality of life and economic evaluation in SLE clinical trials. Lupus 1999; 8: 645–654.
133. Hanly JG. Disease activity, cumulative damage and quality of life in systematic lupus erythematosus: results of a cross-sectional study. Lupus 1997; 6: 243–247.
134. Wang C, Mayo NE, Fortin PR. The relationship between health related quality of life and disease activity and damage in systemic lupus erythematosus. J Rheumatol 2001; 28: 525–532.
135. Callahan LF, Pincus T. Associations between clinical status questionnaire scores and formal education level in persons with systemic lupus erythematosus. Arthritis Rheum 1990; 33: 407–411.
136. Estes D, Christian CL. The natural history of systemic lupus erythematosus by prospective analysis. Medicine 1971; 50: 85–95.
137. Wallace DJ, Podell T, Weiner J et al. Systemic lupus erythematosus survival patterns. Experience with 609 patients. JAMA 1981; 245: 934–938.
138. Reveille JD, Bartolucci A, Alarcón-Segovia D. Prognosis in systemic lupus erythematosus. Negative impact of increasing age at onset, black race, and thrombocytopenia, as well as causes of death. Arthritis Rheum 1990; 33: 37–48.
139. Pistiner M, Wallace DJ, Nessim S et al. Lupus erythematosus in the 1980s: a survey of 570 patients. Semin Arthritis Rheum 1991; 21: 55–64.
140. Ward MM, Pyun E, Studenski S. Long-term survival in systemic lupus erythematosus. Patient characteristics associated with poorer outcomes. Arthritis Rheum 1995; 38: 274–283.
141. Massardo L, Martinez ME, Jacobelli S et al. Survival of Chilean patients with systemic lupus erythematosus. Semin Arthritis Rheum 1994; 24: 1–11.
142. Tucker LB, Menon S, Schaller JG, Isenberg DA. Adult and childhood onset systemic lupus erythematosus: a comparison of onset, clinical features, serology and outcome. Br J Rheumatol 1995; 34: 866–872.
143. Blanco FJ, Gomez-Reino JJ, de la Mata J et al. Survival analysis of 306 European Spanish patients with systemic lupus erythematosus. Lupus 1998; 7: 159–163.
144. Jacobsen s, Petersen J, Ulman S et al. Mortality and causes of death of 513 Danish patients with systemic lupus erythematosus. Scand J Rheumatol 1999; 28: 75–80.
145. Urowitz MB, Gladman DD. How to improve morbidity and mortality in systemic lupus erythematosus. Rheumatology 2000; 39: 237–243.
146. Swaak AJG, Nieuwenhuis EJ, Smeenk RJT. Changes in clinical features of patients with systemic lupus erythematosus followed prospectively over 2 decades. Rheumatol Int 1992; 12: 71–75.
147. Urowitz MB, Gladman DD, Abu-Shakra M, Farewell VT. Mortality studies in systemic lupus erythematosus. Results from a single centre. III. Improved survival over 24 years. J Rheumatol 1997; 24: 1061–1065.
148. Abu-Shakra M, Urowitz MB, Gladman DD, Gough J. Mortality studies in systemic lupus erythematosus. Results from a single centre. II. Predictor variables for mortality. J Rheumatol 1995; 22: 1265–1270.
149. Ginzler EM, Diamond H, Weiner M et al. A multicenter study of outcome in systemic lupus erythematosus. I. Entry variables as predictors of prognosis. Arthritis Rheum 1982; 25: 601–611.
150. Wang F, Wang CL, Tan CT, Manivasagar M. Systemic lupus erythematosus in Malaysia: a study of 539 patients and comparison of prevalence and disease expression in different racial and gender groups. Lupus 1997; 6: 248–253.
151. Lacks S, White P. Morbidity associated with childhood systemic lupus erythematosus. J Rheumatol 1990; 17: 941–945.
152. Font J, Ramos-Casals M, Cervera R et al. Cardiovascular risk factors and the long-term outcome of lupus nephritis. Q J Med 2001; 94: 19–26.
153. McLaughlin JR, Bombardier CB, Farewell VT et al. Kidney biopsy in systemic lupus erythematosus. III. Survival analysis controlling for clinical and laboratory variables. Arthritis Rheum 1994; 37: 559–567.
154. Cook RJ, Gladman DD, Pericak D, Urowitz MB. Prediction of short-term mortality in SLE with time-dependent measures of disease activity. J Rheumatol 2000; 27: 1892–1895.

123 Neonatal lupus

Jill P Buyon

Definition of the problem

- Congenital heart block detected before or at birth, in the absence of structural abnormalities, is strongly associated with maternal autoantibodies to Ro(SS-A) and La(SS-B) ribonucleoproteins, independent of whether the mother has systemic lupus erythematosus, Sjögren's syndrome or is totally asymptomatic

- Autoimmune-associated congenital heart block is considered to result from the transplacental passage of autoantibodies into the fetal circulation resulting in tissue injury, most often clinically detected between 18 and 24 weeks of gestation

- Congenital heart block carries a substantial morbidity and mortality: 60% of affected children require pacemakers and nearly a third die

- Other neonatal abnormalities, including cutaneous manifestations, cholestasis and cytopenias, are also associated with anti-Ro(SS-A) and La(SS-B) antibodies in the maternal and fetal circulation and are now grouped under the heading of neonatal lupus syndromes (NLS)

- The non-cardiac manifestations of NLS are transient, resolving at about 6 months of life, coincident with the disappearance of maternal autoantibodies from the neonatal circulation.

THE TYPICAL CASE

A 32-year-old white woman was 21 weeks pregnant when her fetus was noted to have a heart rate of 60 beats/min during a routine obstetric evaluation. A sonogram done at 16 weeks (at the time of amniocentesis) had revealed a normal fetal heart rate of 140 beats/min. The patient's past medical history was significant only for rare arthralgias of her hands, which she attributed to extensive typing, and an occasional sensation of grittiness of her eyes making the use of contact lenses difficult.

Her family history was notable for two male first cousins with systemic lupus erythematosus (SLE). The fetus was evaluated by echocardiography and the presumptive diagnosis of congenital heart block (CHB) was confirmed (Fig. 123.1a). There were no apparent structural abnormalities. A moderate pericardial effusion was noted. The mother's serum was found (by commercial enzyme-linked immunosorbent assay, ELISA) to contain high titers of antibodies to both Ro(SS-A) and La(SS-B). On immunoblot, reactivities to 48kDa La(SS-B) and 52kDa Ro(SS-A) were detected. Dexamethasone was prescribed at 4mg/day. Weekly echocardiograms revealed a gradual disappearance of the pericardial effusion and no signs of left ventricular failure; heart block persisted. At 34 weeks there was a marked decrease of amniotic fluid, and an elective cesarean section was done at 35 weeks gestation. At 15 months of age a pacemaker was implanted because of decreasing heart rate and signs of mild left ventricular dysfunction.

The mother remained healthy and became pregnant again. No prophylactic prednisone was advised; however, weekly fetal echocardiograms were performed from weeks 18 to 26, and thereafter every 2–3 weeks. Auscultation was done weekly. A healthy girl was delivered vaginally at 38 weeks. One month later the mother noted an erythematous rash around the infant's eyes and annular lesions in the scalp after taking the child out to the park on a sunny spring day. The diagnosis of neonatal lupus was made. A mild topical corticosteroid cream was prescribed and avoidance of sunlight recommended; no systemic therapy was prescribed. The rash disappeared at 6 months of age. The mother has remained healthy at 13 years of follow-up.

DIAGNOSTIC PROBLEMS

The identification of fetal bradycardia by either auscultation or routine obstetric ultrasound should prompt two immediate responses. The first

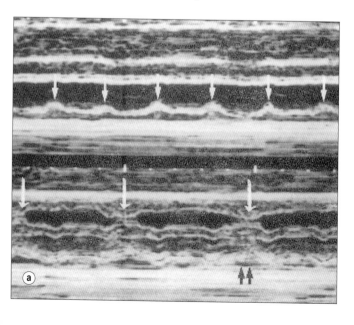

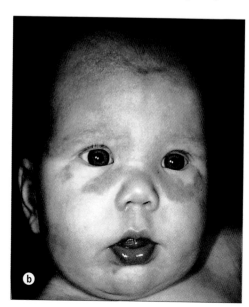

Figure 123.1 Congenital heart block. (a) Dual M-mode echocardiograph, simultaneously displaying discordant atrial (A) and ventricular (V) systolic excursion (single white arrows). A pericardial effusion (double black arrows) is seen. (b) Typical skin rash with predilection for the periorbital area. This rash resolved completely, without scarring. (Photograph courtesy of Dr Susan Manzi.)

is to obtain a two-dimensional and M-mode fetal echocardiographic and Doppler ultrasound to document whether there is an atrial arrhythmia or atrioventricular block (and to what degree; note that only second or third degree block will be clinically manifest as bradycardia). These studies will also ascertain whether there are any structural abnormalities of the heart such as atrioventricular septal defects, left atrial isomerism or abnormalities of the great arteries. An associated myocarditis is supported by the finding of decreased contractility in addition to secondary changes such as an increase of cardiac size, pericardial effusions and tricuspid regurgitation. The second response is an evaluation of the mother's serum for the presence of anti-Ro(SS-A) with or without La(SS-B) antibodies. Most commercial testing is by ELISA, which is a sensitive method for detection of these antibodies (see also Chapters 20 & 21). An immunoblot may be performed for evaluation of the fine specificity of the anti-Ro(SSA) response; this does not alter the management of an identified case of CHB, but it may be useful for deciding on the management of a pregnant woman in whom there is concern regarding the possibility of having an infant with CHB. In most women with affected children the anti-Ro(SSA) titers are quite high; immunoblot reveals reactivity to either the 52kDa or 60kDa Ro antigen (although the former is more common), and anti-La(SSB) antibodies are also present. Stated another way, low titer anti-Ro(SSA) antibodies that do not blot any component (presumably because they react only with native 60kDa Ro) are only rarely encountered in mothers whose children have CHB. The mother's serum should be similarly evaluated if her offspring develops a characteristic rash, i.e. involvement of the face, particularly around the eyes, and scalp (Fig. 123.1b). In some instances the rash is present in other locations and can cover virtually the entire body. The lesions are superficial inflammatory plaques resembling subacute cutaneous lupus erythematosus of the adult and are typically annular or elliptic with erythema and scaling. Hypopigmentation is frequent and may be a prominent feature.

THERAPEUTIC OPTIONS

Since CHB is most often identified between 18 and 24 weeks of gestation, intrauterine therapy is possible. The clinical approach to cardiac manifestations of neonatal lupus includes obstetric and rheumatologic management of both the fetus identified with CHB and the fetus with a normal heart beat but at high risk of developing CHB. In either situation, the critical decision is whether any treatment is necessary.

Guidelines are not well established and are based empirically on anecdotal evidence. For the former situation (as in the case above) the clinician needs to know if the presence of bradycardia represents an irreversible fibrotic process and if continued autoimmune tissue injury will cause progressive damage. The rationale for treatment of identified heart block and prevention of potential heart block is to diminish a generalized inflammatory insult and lower the titer of maternal autoantibodies. Several intrauterine therapeutic regimens have been tried, including dexamethasone, which is not metabolized by the placenta and is available to the fetus in an active form, and plasmapheresis. A proposed therapeutic approach is outlined in Table 123.1. Maternal risks of dexamethasone are similar to those of any glucocorticoid and include infection, osteoporosis, osteonecrosis, diabetes, hypertension and preeclampsia. Fetal risks include oligohydramnios, intrauterine growth retardation and adrenal suppression. Recently in the United States, an NIH-funded multicenter double-blind placebo-controlled prospective trial has been initiated to evaluate the efficacy of 4 mg of dexamethasone in the treatment of newly identified second or third degree block (PRIDE, or PR interval and dexamethasone evaluation, in CHB).

With regard to prophylactic therapy of the high-risk mother (documentation of high titer anti-Ro(SS-A) and La(SS-B) antibodies, anti-48kDa La(SS-B) and 52kDa Ro(SS-A) on immunoblot, and a previous child with NLS), there is no role for initiation of either prednisone or dexamethasone. Maternal prednisone (at least in low and moderate doses) early in pregnancy does not prevent the development of CHB. This might be anticipated since prednisone given to the mother is not active in the fetus and levels of anti-Ro(SS-A) and anti-La(SS-B) antibodies remain relatively constant during corticosteroid therapy. In our experience, mothers who do not have anti-La(SS-B) antibodies, and only have anti-Ro(SS-A) antibodies of low titer that do not recognize either the 60kDa or 52kDa component on sodium dodecyl sulfate (SDS)-immunoblot, appear to be at lower risk (see above). We recommend that the fetuses of all women with anti-Ro(SS-A) antibodies be evaluated by serial echocardiography, but especially for women with high titer antibodies that recognize the 52kDa component on SDS-immunoblot and have associated anti-La antibodies. A recent major advance in echocardiography has now made possible the detection of first degree block. This is done by measurement of the mechanical PR interval. Normative data have already been published. A second USA-based multicenter NIH-funded trial is currently under way to address the frequency of first degree block in mothers with anti-Ro(SS-A) and

---

TABLE 123.1 THERAPEUTIC APPROACH TO CHB DIAGNOSED *IN UTERO*

Situation	Treatment
1. Degree of block at presentation	
• 3rd degree (>3 weeks from detection)	• Evaluate by serial echocardiography and obstetrical sonography; no therapy is initiated.
• 3rd degree (<3 weeks from detection)	• 4mg p.o. dexamethasone daily for 6 weeks. If no change, taper dose to discontinue. If reversal to 2nd degree or better, continue until delivery, then taper.
• Alternating 2nd/3rd degree	• 4mg p.o dexamethasone for 6 weeks. If progression to 3rd degree, taper. If reversal to 2nd degree or better, continue until delivery, taper.
• 2nd degree • Prolonged mechanical PR interval (1st degree)	• 4mg p.o. dexamethasone daily until delivery, then taper. If progresion to 3rd degree, taper after 3rd degree persists for 6 weeks.
2. Block associated with signs of myocarditis, CHF and/or hydropic changes	• 4mg p.o. dexamethasone daily until improvement, then taper.
3. Severely hydropic fetus	• 4mg p.o. dexamethasone daily apheresis as a last resort rapidly to remove maternal antibodies, or deliver if lungs are mature.

CHF, congestive heart failure.

whether it is a marker for more advanced block (component of the PRIDE in CHB Trial, discussed above). Echocardiograms are done weekly from 16 to 26 weeks and every other week until 32 weeks. The rationale is to evaluate during the period of presumed vulnerability.

All neonates (both healthy infants and those with CHB) whose mothers have anti-Ro(SS-A) or La(SS-B) antibodies should be protected from excessive exposure to the sun, since they may develop skin lesions up to 6 months of age. Treatment is generally conservative, and in many cases no intervention is required. Topical corticosteroids, preferably those that are not fluorinated, may be used. High-potency topical corticosteroids can produce systemic effects. Since the lesions are transient and generally benign, systemic therapies such as antimalarials are not recommended in young children, in whom the therapeutic dose approaches the toxic dose.

Mothers who have had children with NLS (cardiac and/or cutaneous manifestations) need to be aware of several important points to guide future management. If the mother has no signs or symptoms of a rheumatic disease, she should be reassured that she does not have SLE. Her prognosis is likely to be excellent and, even if she does develop symptoms, severe life-threatening SLE is rare. Of 157 women we evaluated, 52 (33%) were asymptomatic, 28 (18%) had an undifferentiated autoimmune syndrome, 29 (18%) had SLE, 31 (20%) had Sjögren's syndrome, 11 (7%) had SLE/Sjögren's syndrome, and one (<1%) had rheumatoid arthritis/Sjögren's syndrome at the time NLS was identified (prior to or at birth). Mean follow up was 7.5 years. Of the 52 initially asymptomatic mothers, 21 (40%) developed symptoms of a rheumatic disease: three (6%) developed undifferentiated autoimmune syndrome, nine (18%) Sjögren's syndrome and nine (18%) SLE. Of the 28 mothers initially categorized as having undifferentiated autoimmune syndrome, three (11%) developed SLE and four (14%) Sjögren's syndrome. Four (13%) of 31 mothers with Sjögren's syndrome progressed to SLE. Notably, the majority of patients with SLE at the time of the affected pregnancy have not experienced disease progression. Only one patient has developed central nervous system involvement and none has developed end-stage renal disease. The one maternal death was due to a myocardial infarction. There was no significant association between the presence of antibodies to the 48kDa La(SS-B), 52kDa Ro(SS-A) or 60kDa Ro(SS-A) antigens, as measured by immunoblot, and the final maternal clinical status.

The recurrence rate of CHB is low – 15% – but does exceed the rate of 1% for primigravidas with anti-Ro(SS-A). In our series, of 79 subsequent pregnancies after having a child with CHB, 12 (15%) resulted in CHB. One of these mothers gave birth to another child with CHB despite taking 30mg of prednisone daily from 9 weeks of gestation to delivery. Seven (9%) subsequent children without CHB had rashes consistent with NLS. Importantly, mothers who have given birth to a child with cutaneous manifestations can subsequently give birth to a child with CHB. In our series, of 30 pregnancies subsequent to the birth of a child with NLS rash, seven (23%) resulted in CHB and 11 (37%) in a second child with rash. To date, there is no gender-based difference in the frequency of either CHB or NLS rash.

CONCLUSIONS

Approximately 1% of mothers with anti-Ro(SS-A) antibodies have a baby with NLS independent of whether the mother has a rheumatic disease or is totally asymptomatic. All women with SLE, Sjögren's syndrome, rheumatoid arthritis or only the history of a positive antinuclear antibody test who are planning a pregnancy should be screened for anti-Ro(SS-A) and La(SS-B) antibodies by ELISA. If these antibodies are present, prophylactic therapy is not indicated but serial echocardiographic analysis (preferably with inclusion of the mechanical PR interval) is suggested. Treatment of CHB identified *in utero* is not established but guidelines are provided. With the establishment of an NIH-supported National Research Registry for Neonatal Lupus, we have been able to report morbidity, mortality, recurrence rates and maternal progression of disease more accurately.

REFERENCES

Buyon JP. The heart and skin of neonatal lupus: does maternal health matter? Am J Med 2000; 108: 741–743.

Buyon JP. Neonatal lupus syndromes. In: Lahita R, ed. Systemic lupus erythematosus, 3rd ed. New York: Academic Press; 1998: 337–359.

Buyon JP, Hiebert R, Copel J et al. Autoimmune-associated congenital heart block: mortality, morbidity, and recurrence rates obtained from a national neonatal lupus registry. J Am Coll Cardiol 1998; 31: 1658–1666.

Buyon JP, Waltuck J, Kleinman C, Copel J. In utero identification and therapy of congenital heart block (CHB). Lupus 1995; 4: 116–121.

Buyon JP, Winchester RJ, Slade SG et al. Identification of mothers at risk for congenital heart block and other neonatal lupus syndromes in their children. Arthritis Rheum 1993; 36: 1263–1273.

Eronen M, Siren MK, Ekblad H et al. Short- and long-term outcome of children with congenital complete heart block diagnosed in utero or as a newborn. Pediatrics 2000; 106: 86–91.

Glickstein JS, Buyon JP, Friedman D. Pulsed Doppler echocardiographic assessment of the fetal PR interval. Am J Cardiol 2000; 86: 236–239.

Julkunen H, Eronen M. Long-term outcome of mothers of children with isolated heart block in Finland. Arthritis Rheum 2001; 44: 647–652.

Julkunen H, Eronen M. The rate of recurrence of isolated congenital heart block: a population-based study. Arthritis Rheum 2001; 44: 487–488.

Lawrence S, Luy L, Laxer R et al. The health of mothers of children with cutaneous neonatal lupus erythematosus differs from that of mothers of children with congenital heart block. Am J Med 2000; 108: 705–709.

Lee LA. Neonatal lupus erythematosus. J Invest Dermatol 1993; 100: 9–13.

Neiman AR, Lee LA, Weston WL, Buyon JP. Cutaneous manifestations of neonatal lupus without heart block: characteristics of mothers and children enrolled in a national registry. J Pediatr 2000; 37: 674–680.

Saleeb S, Copel J, Friedman D, Buyon JP. Comparison of treatment with fluorinated glucocorticoids to the natural history of autoantibody-associated congenital heart block: retrospective review of the Research Registry for Neonatal Lupus. Arthritis Rheum 1999; 42: 2335–2345.

Silverman ED. Congenital heart block and neonatal lupus erythematosus: prevention is the goal. J Rheumatol 1993; 20: 1101–1104.

Waltuck J, Buyon JP. Autoantibody-associated congenital heart block: outcome in mothers and children. Ann Intern Med 1994; 120: 544–551.

124 Drug-induced lupus

Raymond L Yung and Bruce C Richardson

- Drug-induced lupus (DIL) remains an underrecognized clinical entity
- Most of the reported associations are case reports or case series and have not been examined carefully in epidemiological studies
- Some of the newer biologic and anticytokine therapies appear to be associated with an increased incidence of DIL
- Drugs more recently associated with DIL have clinical pictures that are quite different from 'classic' DIL, including autoantibody profiles that more resemble idiopathic lupus
- Understanding the mechanisms behind DIL will probably provide important insights into the pathogenesis of autoimmunity

INTRODUCTION – HISTORICAL ASPECTS

Lupus develops when people with the appropriate predisposing genes are exposed to certain environmental factors, and drug-induced lupus (DIL) represents the clearest example of a defined environmental agent triggering lupus in genetically susceptible individuals. The first definite association between ingestion of a drug and the onset of lupus was reported in 1953, when it was noted that approximately 7% of hydralazine-treated patients developed a lupus-like illness. In the decade that followed, procainamide and anticonvulsants were added to the list of lupus-inducing drugs. With the advent of modern autoantibody testing it has become clear that diverse therapeutic agents are capable of inducing ANAs in patients. Depending on the agent, a proportion of these patients will also develop clinical features resembling idiopathic lupus. Over 100 drugs have now been reported to cause DIL (Table 124.1), including a number of newer biologics and antiviral therapeutics.

EPIDEMIOLOGY

Despite the common association, DIL remains an underappreciated and understudied problem. The annual incidence of DIL in the United States has been estimated to be 15 000–20 000 new cases per year. Approximately 30 000–50 000 patients are affected at any given time, representing 6–12% of all lupus cases. The frequency of DIL is probably underreported, as many cases are mild and self-limiting once the offending drug is removed. The epidemiology of DIL reflects the population taking the particular lupus-inducing drug. For example, because older males are more likely to require procainamide and hydralazine for cardiovascular disease, there are more cases of procainamide- and hydralazine-induced lupus in men. Nevertheless, women receiving these agents are two to four times more likely to develop DIL than their male counterparts. The reason for this is unclear, but may involve both hormonal and non-hormonal gender-associated factors. Little is known about racial susceptibility to DIL. Whites have been reported to be affected up to six times more frequently than blacks and to have a more severe disease. However, this may simply represent demographic bias in the populations studied.

TABLE 124.1 DRUGS IMPLICATED IN DRUG-INDUCED LUPUS

Drugs with good evidence of association

Carbamazepine	Isoniazid	Phenytoin
Chlorpromazine	Methyldopa	Procainamide
Ethosuximide	Minocycline	Quinidine
Hydralazine	Penicillamine	Sulfasalazine

Case reports

Acebutolol	Ibuprofen	Phenylbutazone
Aminoglutethimide	Infliximab	Phenylethylacetylurea
Amiodarone	Interferon (α,γ)	Practolol
Amoproxan	Interleukin 2	Prazosin
Anthiomaline	Labetalol	Primidone
Atenolol	Lamotrigine	Prinolol
Benoxaprofen	Leuprolide acetate	Promethazine
Canavanine (L-)	Levo-Dopa	Propylthiouracil
Captopril	Levomepromazine	Psoralen
Chlorprothixene	Lithium carbonate	Pyrathiazine
Cimetidine	Lovastatin	Pyrithoxine
Cinnarizine	Mephenytoin	Quinine
Clonidine	Mesalazine	Rifamycin
Clozapine	Methimazole	(5-amino)salicylic acid
COL-3	Methysergide	Simvastatin
Danazol	Methylthiouracil	Spironolactone
Dapsone	Metrizamide	Streptomycin
Debrisoquin	Minoxidil	Sulindac
Diclofenac	Nalidixic acid	Sulfadimethoxine
1,2-dimethyl-3-hydroxypyride-4-1 (L1)	Nitrofurantoin	Sulfamethoxypyridazine
	Nomifensine	Terbinafine
Disopyramide	Oral contraceptives	Tetracycline
Estrogens	Olsalazine	Tetrazine
Etanercept	Oxyphenisatin	Thionamide
Flutamide	Para-aminosalicylic acid	Thloridazine
Fluvastatin	Penicillin	Timolol eye drops
Gold salts	Perazine	Tolazamide
Griseofulvin	Perphenazine	Tolmetin
Guanoxan	Phenelzine	Trimethadione
Hydrazine	Phenopyrazone	Zafirlukast

GUIDELINES FOR DEFINING DRUG-INDUCED LUPUS

There is no consensus on the diagnostic criteria for DIL and many cases of DIL do not fulfill the current American College of Rheumatology criteria for idiopathic lupus. In addition, most reported associations are either case reports or case series with no epidemiologic or long-term clinical/laboratory studies to confirm a causal effect. DIL should be suspected in patients who do not have a history of idiopathic lupus, who develop a positive ANA and at least one clinical feature of lupus after an appropriate duration of drug exposure, and whose symptoms resolve after discontinuation of the drug. Thus, the clinician should determine whether there is a temporal relationship between the onset of the drug therapy and the development of the clinical and serological signs of lupus. Although rarely done, reintroduction of the drug should result in the reappearance of the disease.

The diagnosis of DIL can be particularly difficult in patients with underlying systemic rheumatic diseases. Unless the managing physician has a high index of suspicion, the patient's complaints could either be dismissed or an unnecessarily expensive workup may be initiated. Drug-induced rheumatic complaints may also be misinterpreted as an exacerbation of the underlying illness. The physician may then intensify the treatment regimen, perpetuating the real problem. Examples include the use of minocycline, sulfasalazine or anti-TNF therapy in rheumatoid arthritis patients (see below).

CLINICAL FEATURES

It is not possible to distinguish DIL from idiopathic lupus by clinical features, although patients with DIL generally have a milder illness. The clinical features of procainamide and hydralazine-induced lupus are presented in Table 124.2. More than 80% of patients with DIL have musculoskeletal complaints, including arthralgias and myalgias. However, frank arthritis is less common and a significant joint effusion is rare. Although less common than in idiopathic lupus, discoid and malar rash can occur in DIL, particularly in hydralazine-induced lupus. A positive 'lupus band' test and Sweet's syndrome have also been described in DIL. Pleuropulmonary involvement is particularly common in procainamide-induced lupus. Pericarditis and, rarely, significant pericardial effusion or tamponade have been reported in DIL associated with procainamide, hydralazine, isoniazid and sulfasalazine. Central nervous system and significant renal involvement is considered unusual in DIL. However, more severe cases with immune complex glomerulonephritis have been reported with hydralazine, procainamide, quinidine, penicillamine, sulfasalazine and interferon treatment. It is important to remember that deteriorating renal function in these patients may also be due to other underlying medical conditions (e.g. hypertension, diabetes) or drugs (e.g. non-steroidal anti-inflammatories).

A number of new clinical associations have been described in recent years with features that are distinct from the 'classic' DIL involving procainamide and hydralazine. Although it will be impossible to consider every drug, a few will be discussed in this chapter.

Treatment with a number of the newer biologic agents has been associated with the development of autoimmunity, including DIL. Interferons (IFN) have antitumor, antiviral and immunomodulating properties, and both α- and γ-IFN have been linked to the development of a positive ANA and clinical lupus. In one study of 135 patients receiving IFN treatment for carcinoid tumors, 14% developed a newly positive ANA and 19% developed an autoimmune disorder, including one patient with arthritis, leukopenia, and antinuclear and anti-dsDNA antibodies. Other studies showed the frequency of IFN-induced lupus to be between 0.15 and 0.7%, and up to 8% of patients receiving long-term IFN therapy will develop anti-dsDNA antibodies. Treatment of lupus-prone mice with IFN worsens the disease. In addition, lupus patients have elevated IFN levels that correlate with their ANA and anti-DNA antibody titers and disease activity.

Anti-TNF agents are now standard treatment for both early and established rheumatoid arthritis. In a large clinical trial 23% of rheumatoid arthritis patients treated with infliximab, a chimeric IgG1κ anti-TNF monoclonal antibody, developed a positive ANA between screening and last evaluation, compared to 6% of placebo-treated patients. Depending on the assay used, up to 7% of the infliximab-treated patients also developed anti-dsDNA antibodies, which were mostly IgM. The experience in Crohn's disease is similar. Approximately one-third of infliximab-treated Crohn's disease patients develop a positive ANA, and anti-dsDNA antibodies are found in approximately 9% of treated patients. Crohn's disease patients taking baseline immunosuppressants have a reduced incidence of anti-DNA antibodies (3%) compared to those who do not (21%). In addition, patients are twice as likely to develop anti-dsDNA antibodies if they were ANA-positive at study entry. At least three patients (two with rheumatoid arthritis and one with Crohn's disease) have developed clinical DIL. The experience with etanercept, a recombinant TNF receptor:Fc fusion protein, is similar to that of infliximab in rheumatoid arthritis. An increased incidence of ANA and anti-dsDNA antibodies has been described. Interestingly, some patients have developed anti-dsDNA antibodies with a negative ANA. There have been occasional reports of seropositive rheumatoid arthritis patients who developed additional autoantibodies and subacute cutaneous lupus or discoid lupus. It is unclear how anti-TNF therapies induce lupus in susceptible individuals, but studies in lupus-prone mice suggest that suppression of TNF levels may contribute to disease progression. This may also happen in people with an underlying autoimmune disease such as rheumatoid arthritis.

Minocycline, a synthetic tetracycline, is a popular treatment for acne vulgaris in some countries, including the United Kingdom. This drug is also a useful treatment for rheumatoid arthritis and other autoimmune diseases. Minocycline has increasingly been associated with a number of immune and autoimmune phenomena, including serum sickness, autoimmune hepatitis, vasculitis and lupus. Not surprisingly, the average age of patients with minocycline-induced lupus (22 years) is younger than those with procainamide- or hydralazine-induced lupus. The majority of patients received the drug for over a year prior to the onset of their lupus symptoms. Small joint polyarthralgia and arthritis are the most common complaints, often associated with diffuse myalgia. About half the affected patients have laboratory evidence of liver involvement and 20% have skin rashes. Pleuropulmonary and hematological involvements are uncommon, and the nervous system and kidneys are usually spared.

LABORATORY FEATURES

Cytopenias are less common in DIL than in idiopathic lupus, and severe hematological abnormalities are unusual. A positive Coombs' test has been reported in association with procainamide, methyldopa and chlorpromazine. Rarely, methyldopa may induce hemolytic anemia as well.

By definition, DIL patients are ANA positive. However, most patients who develop a positive ANA while receiving a known lupus-inducing drug do not develop clinical disease. The specificity of the ANA is more restrictive in DIL than in idiopathic lupus. Most of the antibodies react

TABLE 124.2 CLINICAL FEATURES OF PROCAINAMIDE AND HYDRALAZINE-INDUCED LUPUS		
Clinical features	Procainamide-induced lupus (%)	Hydralazine-induced lupus (%)
Arthralgia	77	85
Myalgia	44	57
Fever	41	38
Skin rash	9	27
Adenopathy	8	14
Hepatomegaly	25	24
Splenomegaly	12	14
Pleuropulmonary	75	30
Pericarditis	16	5
Neuropsychiatric	1	4
Renal	<1	13

with histone or histone–DNA complexes. However, antihistone antibodies lack specificity and are also found in many other autoimmune disorders, including idiopathic lupus, adult and juvenile rheumatoid arthritis, Felty's syndrome, and undifferentiated connective tissue disease. There has been considerable interest in defining the fine specificity of antihistone antibodies in DIL. For example, patients with procainamide-induced lupus tend to produce IgG antibodies with specificity against an (H2A-H2B)–DNA complex, whereas asymptomatic patients receiving procainamide are more likely to have IgM antibodies to H2A-H2B dimers lacking DNA. However, this restricted activity is not specific for DIL: IgG antibodies against the H2A-H2B dimer have been found in the sera of 15–20% of antihistone-positive idiopathic lupus patients. Although studies of antihistone antibodies may provide important insights into the mechanisms behind DIL, their diagnostic value is limited.

Antiphospholipid antibodies, including the lupus anticoagulant and anticardiolipin antibodies, have been reported in association with a number of drugs, including chlorpromazine, procainamide, hydralazine, perphenazine, quinidine, quinine and sulfasalazine. The antibodies are mostly of the IgM subclass, and are generally not associated with thrombotic events.

THERAPEUTIC OPTIONS

The most important aspect of DIL management involves recognizing that a drug is responsible for the illness. As a rule, symptoms of DIL are self-limiting once the offending drug is stopped. The development of a positive ANA while receiving a drug is not sufficient reason to discontinue the drug, although careful monitoring for subsequent clinical illness is important. Constitutional and musculoskeletal symptoms are usually adequately controlled with aspirin or other NSAIDs. Low-dose prednisone is occasionally necessary, and higher doses may be used for resistant or symptomatic pericardial effusion. The rare case of biopsy-proven renal disease or vasculitis should be treated as for idiopathic lupus. Although most symptoms of DIL resolve within weeks of discontinuing the offending drug, occasional patients may take up to 1 year to recover completely.

PATHOGENESIS

The mechanisms causing DIL are not well understood. Drugs most commonly implicated contain aromatic amines, hydrazines, sulfhydryl groups or a phenol ring. The diversity of these chemical structures suggests that no single configuration is responsible. Recent data suggest that some drugs implicated in DIL, including procainamide and hydralazine, may alter gene expression by inhibiting T-cell DNA methylation. Pharmacological levels of these drugs induce overexpression of lymphocyte function-associated antigen (LFA)-1 by this mechanism, causing autoreactivity in CD4$^+$ T cells. The drug-treated T cells will then proliferate in response to autologous antigen-presenting cells, inducing macrophage apoptosis. Adoptive transfer of the drug-treated cells (or T cells made autoreactive by LFA-1 transfection) into mice causes a lupus-like disease with anti-DNA antibodies, immune complex glomerulonephritis, interstitial pneumonitis and a liver disease resembling primary biliary cirrhosis, confirming the importance of these effects. More recent work suggests that some drugs implicated in DIL may induce T-cell DNA hypomethylation via inhibition of the ERK signaling pathway, leading to altered expression of enzymes regulating T-cell DNA methylation. Interestingly, similar T-cell changes, including LFA-1 overexpression, autoreactivity, DNA hypomethylation and ERK signaling pathway abnormalities, have all been described in T cells from patients with idiopathic lupus.

CONCLUSIONS

The practicing physician needs to be aware of the potential problem of DIL. Prompt recognition and effective countermeasures are associated with an excellent outcome in most cases. The number of reported associations is expected to increase as new drugs are developed. Because some of these case reports may represent idiosyncratic reactions or the coincidental development of idiopathic lupus, rigorous epidemiologic, clinical and laboratory testing should be done to confirm the association. Finally, physicians need to be aware that many patients with chronic diseases ingest over-the-counter alternative medicines that could potentially induce the development of autoimmune diseases, including lupus.

FURTHER READING

Miller FW, Hess EV, Clauw DJ et al. Approaches for the identification and defining environmentally associated rheumatic disorders. Arthritis Rheum 2000; 43: 243–249.

Schlienger RG, Bircher AJ, Meier CR. Minocycline-induced lupus. A systemic review. Dermatol 2000; 200: 223–231.

Ioannou Y, Isenberg DA. Current evidence for the induction of autoimmune rheumatic manifestations by cytokine therapy. Arthritis Rheum 2000; 43: 1431–1442.

Charles PJ, Smeenk RJT, De Jong J, Feldmann M, Maini RN. Assessment of antibodies to double-stranded DNA induced in rheumatoid arthritis patients following treatment with infliximab, a monoclonal antibody to tumor necrosis factor α: findings in open-label and randomized placebo-controlled trials. Arthritis Rheum 2000; 43: 2383–2390.

Ronnblom LE. Alm GV. Oberg KE. Autoimmunity after alpha-interferon therapy for malignant carcinoid tumors. Ann Intern Med 1991; 115: 178–183.

Quddus J, Johnson KJ, Gavalchin J et al. Treating activated CD4$^+$ T cells with either of two distinct DNA methyltransferase inhibitors, 5-azacytidine or procainamide, is sufficient to cause a lupus-like disease in syngeneic mice. J Clin Invest. 1993; 92: 38–53.

Yung RL, Richardson BC. Drug-induced lupus. Rheum Dis Clin North Am 1994; 20: 61–86.

125 Assessing disease activity and outcome in systemic lupus erythematosus

Caroline Gordon

- Disease activity needs to be distinguished from chronic damage
- The patient's perception of their disease does not depend on disease activity alone
- Fatigue is common and may be due to lupus, comorbid disease such as fibromyalgia, or psychosocial factors
- It is important to screen for infection, especially if the CRP is raised

INTRODUCTION

Systemic lupus erythematosus (SLE) is a condition with very heterogeneous manifestations that requires careful assessment. It does not matter whether the patient is being assessed (1) as part of routine care to plan the future therapeutic strategy, (2) to decide if they are fit enough to consider pregnancy, (3) to determine whether they are eligible for a clinical trial, or (4) to assess their response to therapy within the context of a clinical trial. Understanding the factors that can determine the symptoms reported by the patient and the signs observed by the physician is essential. Blood tests are helpful but need to be interpreted in the light of clinical features and past history. Only after careful assessment can the physician discuss with the patient what options are available for the management of their disease.

Outcome used to be measured in terms of survival but this is no longer sufficient, as over 90% of patients survive for at least 5 years after diagnosis, and over 80% survive at least 10 years[1]. Morbidity in these survivors may still be considerable, however, and all the factors influencing the patients' sense of wellbeing need to be assessed and discussed, whether or not the patient is being followed up as part of an outcome observational study or a clinical trial. Assessment of the effects of lupus disease on a patient can be divided into three components: disease activity, chronic damage and health status[2]. The assessment of potentially reversible disease activity is what most people will think of when 'assessment of lupus' is mentioned. However, it is most important to distinguish chronic damage from active disease, or else the patient may be overtreated for a clinical feature that is no longer reversible[2]. Finally, the effects of the disease on the patient should be assessed in some objective way. This involves the determination of the patient's health status or quality of life and functional ability[3]. This is not necessarily related to disease activity and will not respond to simple therapeutic strategies such as a change in steroid dose. In fact, studies have shown that what is measured by quality of life or health status surveys and standardized indices for disease activity and damage are all different from each other and reflect distinct outcomes of the disease. It was recently agreed that the core outcome domains for randomized clinical trials and longitudinal observational studies should be disease activity, damage, health-related quality of life and an assessment of toxicity/adverse events[4]. Assessment of the economic costs involved in caring for lupus patients is likely to become increasingly important. Methodology has been developed to assess this, but this will not be discussed further here[3].

ASSESSMENT OF DISEASE ACTIVITY

Systematic approach to assessment

Active SLE can present in diverse ways. In order to assess a patient fully it is essential to recognize that there is more to lupus than the American College of Rheumatology (ACR) criteria. All the systems of the body need to be screened, so patients should be assessed literally from head to foot, with both direct questioning and full physical examination, as patients may not report all relevant features. Details of the clinical features that may be found in each system are discussed in Chapter 122. Appropriate investigations such as ECG, echocardiography, lung function tests and imaging with X-rays, CT scans, MRI and other modalities may be required to help establish the nature of abnormalities detected on clinical assessment, and for monitoring for improvement and deterioration.

Whatever feature is being considered it is important to determine how long it has been present, whether it has occurred before, and if so, whether it resolved spontaneously or as the result of a particular intervention. Is it currently getting worse, better, or is it stable? It is essential to decide whether or not the feature is likely to be due to active lupus, a complication of lupus (such as chronic lung fibrosis or infection), or other comorbid disease, whether autoimmune or not. For example, a patient may complain of increasingly severe fatigue, diffuse hair loss and myalgia. Do they have a flare of active lupus and/or fibromyalgia and/or autoimmune hypothyroidism? Evidence for each condition must be sought by careful questioning, clinical examination and laboratory testing, as any of these may be present alone or in combination in a patient with lupus. Features of active lupus may be additive or migratory, with different parts of the body being affected on different days (for example a malar rash followed by arthritis in a wrist lasting 2 days, then arthritis in an ankle and multiple mouth ulcers).

It is necessary to determine the circumstances around and prior to the onset of the lupus flare. Was the patient exposed to sunlight; did they suffer an infection; had they reduced therapy and, if so, from what dose and over what timespan? Symptoms, particularly rashes, triggered by sunlight may resolve spontaneously with assiduous avoidance of further UV exposure, increased use of sunblock to protect against unavoidable sun exposure, and/or local steroid therapy. In other cases increased systemic therapy may be required, particularly if this was the patient's previous experience. If an infection triggered the flare of disease activity it is most unlikely that the symptoms will settle without adequate treatment of the infection as well as immunosuppression appropriate to the lupus feature(s). Sometimes, if a disease flare will not settle it is important to look for a persistent, subclinical infectious trigger. Occasionally the patient may have drug-induced features as well as idiopathic lupus which improves with a change in drug therapy, such as a change in anticonvulsant. If the flare is limited to one or two systems and came on soon after a particular reduction in steroids, it may be possible to regain control with a modest increase in steroid dose and restoration of the dose that was previously adequate. But the number of systems involved, the extent and severity of each feature and the rate of deterioration in symptoms is also important in the assessment, in order to guide the physician in deciding what type of therapy is likely to control the disease from now onwards. It may also be important to consider psychosocial issues that need addressing, for reasons that will become clearer.

Neuropsychiatric manifestations of lupus can be difficult to categorize and to distinguish from non-SLE neurological disease. The American College of Rheumatology has produced specific guidelines for diagnosing and reporting neuropsychiatric manifestations that are helpful when assessing patients with such problems: http://www.rheumatology.org/ar/1999/aprilappendix.html[5].

Use of laboratory tests in the assessment of disease activity

When assessing disease activity in lupus it is essential to consider the results of hematologic and biochemical tests. These are often more important than the immunologic tests, although serological tests are useful not only for diagnosis but also for following disease activity. The results of the basic full blood count with white count differential is fundamental in the assessment of a lupus patient. Lymphopenia is the commonest manifestation of lupus. Some patients have leukopenia and neutropenia regularly with active disease. This needs to be borne in mind when following patients on cytotoxic therapy, as a reduced count may mean the need for more therapy not less. Testing the response to increased steroids can be helpful in demonstrating that there is a functional reserve in the bone marrow. Thrombocytopenia may be low grade and chronic as part of the antiphospholipid syndrome, or sudden and serious with an acute lupus flare. Erythrocyte sedimentation rate (ESR) is often raised in SLE but is not very helpful for monitoring disease activity. C-reactive protein (CRP) is usually normal or only slightly raised, for example in serositis or arthritis. The discrepancy between ESR and CRP in SLE can be useful in screening patients in whom a diagnosis has not been made. When the CRP is raised, particularly above 50g/l, infection is usually present and the patient with SLE should be screened carefully for this.

Renal assessment at the very least requires a urine dipstick to screen for proteinuria, hematuria, leukocyturia, and nitrates to screen for infection. When assessing hematuria it is important to exclude infection, stones and menstrual blood loss. Microscopic examination of the urine to look for casts is still the best way of identifying active renal disease. Proteinuria and renal function can be assessed more reliably on a 24 hour urine specimen with well motivated patients than by urine dipstick and serum creatinine. However, urine protein/creatinine ratios and measurement of serum cystatin C are gaining favor, particularly for clinical trials in lupus nephritis, as they are more robust tests and less dependent on patient cooperation. The best way of distinguishing renal activity from damage and establishing the type of renal involvement is by a renal biopsy (see Chapters 117 and 127).

The value of serological tests in lupus disease activity assessment has been much debated[6]. About 60% of lupus patients have antidouble-stranded (ds) DNA antibodies. This test can only therefore be used in those known to manifest these antibodies. It is rare for levels to rise steadily without a disease flare eventually developing. The problem is that at the peak of clinical disease activity the level may fall rather than continuing to rise, probably owing to deposition of antibodies in the tissues[7]. When the flare will occur and whether a fall in the level of anti-dsDNA antibodies is seen with the clinical flare probably depends on how often the test is performed in the individual patient. Patients with changing anti-dsDNA antibody levels should be reviewed more frequently and caution should be exercised over reducing therapy. A disease flare, often involving the kidneys, hematology or vasculitis, is most likely if the C3 and C4 levels are falling steadily or a complement degradation product (for example C3d or C4d) is rising steadily, especially if the levels are well outside the normal range[8]. However, isolated mucocutaneous disease flares are rarely associated with any serological change and persistently slightly abnormal serological tests do not usually predict a disease flare. In an individual patient it often becomes clear what serological changes precede a flare, and such observations can be used to guide therapeutic decisions in that patient in the future. Studies have not consistently shown benefit from serological testing in lupus because which tests change, how quickly and by how much, varies between patients and depends on which systems are involved.

With CNS disease a lumbar puncture is often necessary to exclude infection. It is important to screen for atypical infections, including TB and fungi, in immunosuppressed patients. Lymphocytes and raised CSF protein may be observed, making it difficult to distinguish aseptic meningitis due to lupus from viral meningitis. Other evidence of active lupus will help to support the diagnosis of active SLE, especially in the presence of oligoclonal bands, with IgG specific to the CSF indicating intrathecal antibody formation. This test is not specific for multiple sclerosis and is useful in SLE.

Recording of disease activity

Because lupus can vary so much, standardized methods of recording disease activity have been devised. The best known of these are the Systemic Lupus Erythematosus Disease Activity Index (SLEDAI), the British Isles Lupus Assessment Group (BILAG) index, and the Systemic Lupus Activity Measure (SLAM)[6]. These indices are valid, reliable, and show sensitivity to change in disease activity. They correlate well with each other and they can be used in children[9]. It is fundamental to all of these indices that the features which are recorded are attributed to lupus. Thus fatigue and myalgia associated with fibromyalgia should not be recorded as lupus activity in the BILAG and SLAM indices. Details about the clinical features to be recorded in each index are defined in a glossary. The definitions are not necessarily the same in each index, therefore the appropriate glossary must be used when using the indices. For example, BILAG distinguishes arthralgia without signs of synovitis, from arthritis in one or more joints with normal function, and severe polyarthritis with loss of function in two or more joints. In the SLEDAI, arthritis with joint tenderness and swelling or effusion must be present in more than two joints to score. It is essential when undertaking outcome studies or clinical trials that one of these validated indices is used, rather than just describing certain clinical features without reference to a defined index of disease activity. The indices are also very useful for following disease activity and response to therapy in the routine management of lupus patients. Summary tables can be generated, especially by specifically designed computer programs such as the British Lupus Integrated Prospective System (BLIPS)[10].

The choice of index to use for a clinical study depends on the aims of the study. Many people find SLEDAI the easiest to use[2,9,11]. There are only 24 features to record, covering the most common and most serious manifestations of lupus (Table 125.1). A weighted score is given so that the more serious manifestations, such as vasculitis, renal manifestations and neurological features, score more highly than others such as skin rashes and abnormal serological tests. However, some relatively mild vasculitic features score the same as more extensive disease (for example splinter hemorrhages, and gangrene of several digits). The maximum potential score is 105, but in practice scores are rarely above 40. The original SLEDAI predominantly records features which are new or deteriorating, but records any abnormal anti-dsDNA antibody level and abnormal C3 or C4 level. This caused some concern as there was no way of recording ongoing disease activity in certain systems or changes in serological tests. In the last few years modifications have been proposed (SELENA-SLEDAI and SLEDAI 2001) which do record ongoing disease activity[6]. These changes are likely to make SLEDAI more useful for clinical trials when the assessment of any disease activity needs to be

TABLE 125.1 SYSTEMIC LUPUS ERYTHEMATOSUS DISEASE ACTIVITY INDEX (SLEDAI)

Weighted score	*SLEDAI score	Descriptor	Definition
8		Seizure	Recent onset. Exclude metabolic, infectious or drug-related causes.
8		Psychosis	Altered ability to function in normal activity due to severe disturbance in the perception of reality. Includes hallucinations; incoherence; marked loose associations; impoverished thought content; marked illogical thinking; bizarre, disorganized or catatonic behavior. Exclude the presence of uremia and offending drugs
8		Organic brain syndrome	Altered mental function with impaired orientation or impaired memory or other intellectual function, with rapid onset and fluctuating clinical features. Includes a clouding of consciousness with a reduced capacity to focus and an inability to sustain attention on environment, and at least two of the following: perceptual disturbance, incoherent speech, insomnia or daytime drowsiness, increased or decreased psychomotor activity. Exclude metabolic, infectious and drug-related causes
8		Visual	Retinal changes from systemic lupus erythematosus: cytoid bodies, retinal hemorrhages, serous exudate or hemorrhages in the choroid, optic neuritis (not due to hypertension, drugs or infection)
8		Cranial nerve	New onset of a sensory or motor neuropathy involving a cranial nerve.
8		Lupus headache	Severe, persistent headache; may be migrainous; unresponsive to narcotic analgesia
8		Cerebrovascular accident	New syndrome. Exclude arteriosclerosis
8		Vasculitis	Ulceration, gangrene, tender finger nodules, periungual infarction, splinter hemorrhages. Vasculitis confirmed by biopsy or angiogram
4		Arthritis	More than two joints with pain and signs of inflammation (such as tenderness, swelling or effusion)
4		Myositis	Proximal muscle aching or weakness associated with elevated creatine phosphokinase/aldolase levels, electromyographic changes, or a biopsy showing myositis
4		Casts	Heme, granular or erythrocyte
4		Hematuria	More than 5 erythrocytes per high-power field. Exclude other causes (stone, infection)
4		Proteinuria	More than 0.5g of urinary protein excreted per 24h. New onset or recent increase of more than 0.5g per 24h
4		Pyuria	More than 5 leukocytes per high-power field. Exclude infection
2		New malar rash	New onset or recurrence of an inflammatory type of rash
2		Alopecia	New or recurrent. A patch of abnormal, diffuse hair loss
2		Mucous membrane	New onset or recurrence of oral or nasal ulcerations
2		Pleurisy	Pleuritic chest pain with pleural rub or effusion, or pleural thickening
2		Pericarditis	Pericardial pain with at least one of rub or effusion. Confirmation by electrocardiography or echocardiography
2		Low complement	A decrease in CH_{50}, C3 or C4 level (to less than the lower limit of the laboratory-determined normal range)
2		Increased DNA binding	More than 25% binding by Farr assay (to more than the upper limit of the laboratory-determined normal range, e.g. 25%)
1		Fever	More than 38°C after the exclusion of infection
1		Thrombocytopenia	Fewer than 100 000 platelets
1		Leukopenia	Leukocyte count of < 3000/mm³ (not due to drugs)

Total SLEDAI score * Enter the weighted score for each descriptor in the SLE-DAI score column if the descriptor was present at the time of the visit or in the preceding 10 days.

recorded, but studies showing that these modifications are valid and reliable have yet to be published.

The BILAG index is more comprehensive and records clinical disease activity in each of eight systems separately[6]. It includes renal and hematological manifestations of lupus but no immunological tests. Although a graded score for each system can be calculated manually, from A for the most severe disease to E for a system that has never been involved, it is more reliable to use a computerized database devised for the purpose[10]. It is considered by many too long to be practical, because there are 86 features to record and the score for each system is less obvious than with other indices. However, it is the most comprehensive index and the features to be recorded should be part of the routine assessment of any lupus patient. It is most suited to use in clinical trials, where the effects of an intervention on each system need to be identified. It is also the only index that considers whether features are new, worse, the same or improving. Thus features which are improving before a treatment starts cannot appear to improve as much with a new therapy as those features which were initially new or deteriorating. Despite the extensive number of features covered by the BILAG there are some omissions. It does not cover retinal or eye manifestations that are covered by SLEDAI and SLAM, nor abdominal pain due to serositis, unlike SLAM. In many respects SLAM and BILAG are similar, in that both have some degree of inbuilt assessment of disease severity and exclude immunology. The most frequently used modification of SLAM, SLAM-R, only covers 30 defined items, with the option to add one additional feature[6]. SLAM and SLAM-R are felt by some to put too much weight on subjective features reported by the patient, rather than simply recording objective signs observed by the physician (as in SLEDAI), and they cover renal disease less well than SLEDAI and BILAG.

ASSESSMENT OF DAMAGE AND OTHER COMPLICATIONS OF LUPUS

The SLICC/ACR damage index

As survival and disease control have improved in lupus patients there has been an increasing awareness that patients are succumbing to complications of the disease and/or its therapy. Urowitz was the first to report the bimodal pattern of deaths in lupus, with early deaths being predominantly due to disease activity and late deaths to cardiovascular disease. Over the last 15 years there has been increasing recognition of premature vascular disease affecting the coronary, cerebrovascular and peripheral circulations of lupus patients[1]. Consequently, when a group of investigators, the Systemic Lupus International Collaborating Clinics (SLICC) group, interested in outcome measures in lupus produced a clinical index of chronic damage, these features were included[2]. In addition, the damage index includes features that can be related more closely to the after-effects of disease activity, such as pulmonary fibrosis and scarring of the skin, and features probably more related to therapy than disease, such as osteoporotic fractures and diabetes mellitus. Some features defy accurate attribution to disease, therapy or comorbid disease, but this does not matter. Features should be recorded if they develop after the onset of lupus and fulfill the criteria stated in the glossary, irrespective of attribution. In general, damage features should persist continuously for at least 6 months to score, or should be associated with an immediate pathological scar such as myocardial infarction or stroke.

The derivation of a single index for recording chronic damage in lupus for use in outcome studies and clinical trials was a major achievement. It was endorsed by the American College of Rheumatology, such that the full title of the index is the SLICC/ACR damage index[2]. There are 41 items covering 12 systems (Table 125.2). Some features may score 2 points if they occur more than once, so the maximum score is theoretically 47, but scores above 12 are rare. In most cohorts about half the patients have at least one item of damage. The score can only increase with time. Once damage has occurred it cannot subsequently be discounted, as there will always be an associated pathological scar even if function belatedly improves. The SLICC/ACR damage index has been shown to be valid and reliable. It is distinct from disease activity, and early accumulation of damage is associated with a poor prognosis and increased mortality[6]. Thus it is an important outcome measure in lupus studies to complement the assessment of current disease activity. All physicians managing patients with lupus should be aware of the risk of the complications covered by the SLICC/ACR damage index (DI). They should try to prevent their development, or should treat them promptly if they occur. As features have to be present for 6 months to be recorded, and because risk factors for some items of damage may accumulate over several years (for example myocardial infarction), the SLICC/ACR damage index can only be used reliably in clinical trials where therapy will be continued for more than 1 year and patients have short disease duration at entry. However, the DI score at trial entry is likely to be important in stratifying patients.

Other complications of lupus

There are some outcomes of interest that are not covered by the damage index. Infection requiring hospital admission is a potentially reversible complication but causes a significant number of deaths in lupus patients. It could be covered by drug toxicity/adverse events monitoring, but there are no specific recommendations for lupus beyond the current advice for drugs used to treat SLE patients. Similarly, gastrointestinal bleeding is only recorded if surgical resection results. Sicca symptoms

TABLE 125.2 SLICC/ACR DAMAGE INDEX FOR SLE

Damage (non-reversible change, not related to active inflammation) occurring since onset of lupus, ascertained by clinical assessment and present for at least 6 months unless otherwise stated. Repeat episodes must occur at least 6 months apart to score 2; the same lesion cannot be scored twice.

Item	Score
Ocular (either eye, by clinical assessment)	
Any cataract ever	0, 1
Retinal change or optic atrophy	0, 1
Neuropsychiatric	
Cognitive impairment (e.g. memory deficit, difficulty with calculation, poor concentration, difficulty in spoken or written language, impaired performance level) or major psychosis	0, 1
Seizures requiring therapy for 6 months	0, 1
Cerebravascular accident ever (score 2 if >1)	0, 1, 2
Cranial or peripheral neuropathy (excluding optic)	0, 1
Transverse myelitis	0, 1
Renal	
Estimated or measured glomerular filtration rate <50%	0,1
Proteinuria >3.5g/24h	0,1
or End-stage renal disease (regardless of dialysis or transplantation)	or 3
Pulmonary	
Pulmonary hypertension (right ventricular prominence, or loud P2)	0, 1
Pulmonary fibrosis (physical and radiograph)	0, 1
Shrinking lung (radiograph)	0, 1
Pleural fibrosis (radiograph)	0, 1
Pulmonary infarction (radiograph)	0, 1
Cardiovascular	
Angina or coronary artery bypass	0, 1
Myocardial infarction ever (score 2 if >1)	0, 1, 2
Cardiomyopathy (ventricular dysfunction)	0, 1
Valvular disease (diastolic murmur, or systolic murmur >3/6)	0, 1
Pericarditis for 6 months, or pericardiectomy	0, 1
Peripheral vascular	
Claudication for 6 months	0, 1
Minor tissue loss (pulp space)	0, 1
Significant tissue loss ever (e.g. loss of digit or limb) (score 2 if > 1 site)	0, 1, 2
Venous thrombosis with swelling, ulceration or venous stasis	0, 1
Gastrointestinal	
Infarction or resection of bowel below duodenum, spleen, liver or gallbladder ever, for cause any (score 2 if > 1 site)	0, 1 ,2
Mesenteric insufficiency	0, 1
Chronic peritonitis	0, 1
Stricture or upper gastrointestinal tract surgery ever	0, 1
Chronic pancreatitis	0, 1
Musculoskeletal	
Muscle atrophy or weakness	0, 1
Deforming or erosive arthritis (including reducible deformities, excluding avascular necrosis)	0, 1
Osteoporosis with fracture or vertebral collapse (excluding avascular necrosis)	0, 1
Avascular necrosis (score 2 if > 1)	0, 1, 2
Osteomyelitis	0, 1
Tendon rupture	0, 1
Skin	
Scarring chronic alopecia	0, 1
Extensive scarring of panniculum other than scalp and pulp space	0, 1
Skin ulceration (excluding thrombosis for > 6 months)	0, 1
Premature gonadal failure	0, 1
Diabetes (regardless of treatment)	0, 1
Malignancy (exclude dysplasia) (score 2 if > 1 site)	0, 1, 2

due to secondary Sjögren's syndrome and chronic hypertension in the absence of active renal disease are not recorded unless ventricular dysfunction is caused.

ASSESSMENT OF HEALTH STATUS, QUALITY OF LIFE AND FUNCTIONAL ABILITY

It is important to assess the patient's perception of their own health and to be aware of the factors that may influence this. There is no specific lupus measure of health status and a number of generic health surveys are available. One of the most comprehensive and best validated for use in lupus is the Short-Form-36 (SF36). This covers eight domains, namely physical function, social function, role limitations due to physical or emotional factors, mental health, vitality, pain, and general health perception[6,11]. More detailed questionnaires for assessing quality of life, physical disability, depression, psychological distress, stress and fatigue are available and have been used in lupus[3]. Many studies have shown that health status measures are significantly impaired in lupus patients. Health status (especially fatigue) is most strongly correlated with psychosocial factors and less consistently with disease activity and chronic damage[3,12,13]. This suggests that physicians need to consider non-drug modalities of therapy if their patients are to feel well and be more active. It may be hard to change some social predictors of poor health status, such as educational level, socioeconomic group, and access to health insurance. However, it may be possible to find ways of helping patients to have better social support, to be more satisfied with their medical care and to cope better with their disease. Methodology is available for measuring such outcomes and there is some evidence that such measures might help to reduce disease activity and the accumulation of damage. Future studies will assess whether such interventions are helpful in practice.

CONCLUSION

The assessment of lupus patients requires three components of disease to be considered: activity, damage and health status. Based on this assessment, the physician can plan appropriate therapy to control active disease, limit the accumulation of damage and other complications of lupus and its therapy, and improve the patient's perception of their disease. This approach should improve the outcome of the disease in terms of morbidity, mortality and patient satisfaction with medical care.

REFERENCES

1. Trager J, Ward MM. Mortality and causes of death in systemic lupus erythematosus. Curr Opin Rheumatol 2001; 13: 345–351.
2. Urowitz MB, Gladman DD. Measures of disease activity and damage in SLE. Baillières Clin Rheumatol 1998; 12: 405–413.
3. Gordon C, Clarke AE. Quality of life and economic evaluation in SLE clinical trials. Lupus 1999; 8: 645–654.
4. Smolen JS, Strand V, Cardiel M et al. Randomized clinical trials and longitudinal observational studies in systemic lupus erythematosus: consensus on a preliminary core set of outcome domains. J Rheumatol 1999; 26: 504–507.
5. The American College of Rheumatology nomenclature and case definitions for neuropsychiatric lupus syndromes. Arthritis Rheum 1999; 42: 599–608.
6. Isenberg D, Ramsey-Goldman R. Assessing patients with lupus: towards a drug responder index. Rheumatology (Oxford) 1999; 38: 1045–1049.
7. Ho A, Magder LS, Barr SG, Petri M. Decreases in anti-double-stranded DNA levels are associated with concurrent flares in patients with systemic lupus erythematosus. Arthritis Rheum 2001; 44: 2342–2349.
8. Ho A, Barr SG, Magder LS, Petri M. A decrease in complement is associated with increased renal and hematologic activity in patients with systemic lupus erythematosus. Arthritis Rheum 2001; 44: 2350–2357.
9. Brunner HI, Feldman BM, Bombardier C, Silverman ED. Sensitivity of the Systemic Lupus Erythematosus Disease Activity Index, British Isles Lupus Assessment Group Index, and Systemic Lupus Activity Measure in the evaluation of clinical change in childhood-onset systemic lupus erythematosus. Arthritis Rheum 1999; 42: 1354–1360.
10. Isenberg DA, Gordon C. From BILAG to BLIPS – disease activity assessment in lupus past, present and future. Lupus 2000; 9: 651–654.
11. Strand V, Gladman D, Isenberg D, Petri M, Smolen J, Tugwell P. Outcome measures to be used in clinical trials in systemic lupus erythematosus. J Rheumatol 1999; 26: 490–497.
12. Sutcliffe N, Clarke AE, Levinton C, Frost C, Gordon C, Isenberg DA. Associates of health status in patients with systemic lupus erythematosus. J Rheumatol 1999; 26: 2352–2356.
13. Wang C, Mayo NE, Fortin PR. The relationship between health related quality of life and disease activity and damage in systemic lupus erythematosus. J Rheumatol 2001; 28: 525–532.

126 Treatment of constitutional symptoms, skin, joint, serositis, cardiopulmonary, hematologic and central nervous system manifestations

Cynthia Aranow and Ellen M Ginzler

- The management of patients with systemic lupus erythematosus (SLE) is decided on an individual basis, guided by the degree and severity of specific symptoms and organ system involvement
- Non-steroidal anti-inflammatory drugs are an important first-line therapy for the treatment of constitutional signs, musculoskeletal symptoms and mild serositis
- Antimalarials are frequently effective for chronic constitutional signs and cutaneous and musculoskeletal manifestations, with an excellent therapeutic benefit to toxicity profile
- Most clinical manifestations of SLE respond well to corticosteroids, with a wide dose range depending upon the organ systems involved and the degree of severity. However, short- and long-term corticosteroid toxicities account for substantial morbidity
- Immunosuppressive agents are useful in patients with life- or organ-threatening manifestations, as well as for steroid sparing in patients who are either steroid dependent or refractory

INTRODUCTION

Systemic lupus erythematosus (SLE) is an autoimmune inflammatory multisystem disease with diverse manifestations and a course characterized by flares (increases in disease activity) and remissions. Treatment will vary between patients and from flare to flare even within the same patient, depending upon the severity and the particular manifestation(s)

of the increased disease activity (Table 126.1). Although useful for epidemiologic studies of lupus cohorts, disease activity indices such as SLEDAI, SLAM and BILAG may not be useful guides upon which to base therapeutic interventions. Some clinical flares may be life threatening, whereas others consist predominantly of constitutional symptoms. Activity scores may not accurately capture the severity of the flares. For example, using the SLEDAI alopecia and a malar rash will score equivalently to an increase in proteinuria. Disease management after achieving control of the inflammatory features typically includes tapering of the immunosuppression required to suppress disease activity while closely monitoring for evidence of a potential relapse. In many instances long-term maintenance therapy may be required. This chapter reviews the management of the heterogenous (non-renal) features of SLE. Although new interventions have recently become available, the approach to many of these manifestations has changed little. This chapter will not discuss the management of the potential adverse effects associated with corticosteroid treatment or with the use of other anti-inflammatory and immunosuppressive medications. Similarly, treatment of associated medical conditions (i.e. hypertension in lupus nephritis, dialysis, infections) seen by rheumatologists caring for lupus patients will not be covered.

PATIENT EDUCATION

A knowledgeable patient who understands the disease is more likely to be compliant with appointments and medications. There is abundant

	Manifestations of SLE				
Agents	**Constitutional**	**Musculoskeletal**	**Serositis**	**Cutaneous**	**Major organ**
NSAIDs	✓	✓	✓		
Corticosteroids					
Topical				✓	
Low dose (i.e. prednisone <0.5mg/kg/day)	✓	✓	✓	✓	
High dose (i.e. prednisone 1.0mg/kg/day or 1g IV methylprednisolone)					✓ ✓
Antimalarials	✓	✓	✓	✓	✓
Dapsone				✓	
Thalidomide				✓	
Immunosuppressives					
Azathioprine	✓	✓	✓	✓	✓
Cyclophosphamide					✓
Chlorambucil					✓
Cyclosporin					✓
Methotrexate		✓	✓		
Immunoglobulins					✓
Danazol					✓

TABLE 126.1 DRUGS USED IN THE MANAGEMENT OF SYSTEMIC LUPUS ERYTHEMATOSUS

literature available from sources such as the Lupus Foundation of America and the Arthritis Foundation. Patient support groups are another valuable source of information and are also a forum through which patients may share the skills they have acquired for coping with this chronic disease. Establishing a good doctor–patient relationship is fundamental to the management of any chronic disease.

THERAPEUTIC INTERVENTION: NON-STEROIDAL ANTI-INFLAMMATORY DRUGS (NSAIDs)

Although NSAIDs are not specifically approved by the Food and Drug Administration for use in SLE they are approved for arthritis and soft tissue complaints and are ubiquitously used in lupus. NSAIDs are usually used for mild lupus activity before low-dose corticosteroids are initiated, or with antimalarials. NSAIDs are additionally combined with corticosteroids in an effort to minimize the corticosteroid dose, or to suppress lupus activity when alternate-day corticosteroids are used. They are commonly administered for the symptomatic treatment of musculoskeletal manifestations, mild serositis and systemic features such as fever. NSAIDs prevent the formation of prostaglandins by inhibiting the cyclo-oxgenases COX-1 and COX-2. As with other rheumatic diseases, there seem to be differences in patient responsiveness to individual NSAIDs, and drugs from different chemical classes may need to be tried before settling on the single best drug for a particular patient.

Adverse effects from NSAIDs may occur in lupus patients. Deleterious effects on the kidneys, liver and CNS may pose diagnostic dilemmas, as they may mimic features of active lupus. Renal dysfunction may result from impairment of glomerular filtration, tubular function or renal blood flow. Nephrotic syndrome, interstitial nephritis, acute tubular necrosis and minimal change disease are also reported to occur rarely with NSAID administration[1]. Lupus patients taking NSAIDs who present with renal abnormalities should be taken off the NSAID and monitored before assuming the presence of lupus nephritis. Similarly, NSAID-induced hepatitis must be considered in a patient taking NSAIDs who develops liver enzyme abnormalities before concluding the presence of autoimmune hepatitis. Lupus patients taking NSAIDs, particularly ibuprofen, have an increased susceptibility to developing aseptic meningitis, characterized by headache, meningismus, fever with a lymphocytosis and elevated protein in cerebrospinal fluid[2]. This syndrome may be confused with features of CNS lupus. Rechallenging with ibuprofen may result in a recurrence within 24 hours. Headaches, dizziness, confusion or depression are other neuropsychiatric symptoms that may result from NSAID administration.

Although treatment with the newer COX-2 specific inhibitors has the advantage of less gastrointestinal toxicity, other potential adverse effects of NSAIDs are not limited. Additionally, as the COX-2 specific inhibitors do not affect platelet function, certain subsets of lupus patients, such as those with antiphospholipid antibodies, may be prone to developing thrombosis after exposure to COX-2 inhibition. There is a report of four patients with high-titer anticardiolipin antibodies who experienced thrombotic events after treatment with a COX-2 specific inhibitor[3].

CORTICOSTEROIDS

Corticosteroids are clearly the cornerstone of SLE treatment. Their rapid onset of action reduces inflammation and results in resolution of the inflammatory manifestations of lupus activity. They are typically prescribed orally in low, medium (0.5mg/kg) or high doses (1mg/kg), depending upon the targeted manifestation(s) (Table 126.2). Although usually given as a single morning dose, corticosteroids may be given in split doses (2–4 times a day) for enhanced effectiveness. Pulse steroids (intravenous methylprednisonone 1g, usually given for 3 consecutive days) may be useful for treatment of severe or life- or organ-threatening features of disease. After control of disease activity is achieved, tapering of the prednisone dose is initiated. The rapidity of the dose reduction varies significantly and is dependent upon the initial disease manifestations, the duration of corticosteroid treatment, the responsiveness of the patient's disease (does the disease remain under control, or do new or recurrent symptoms re-emerge as the dose is lowered?) and the patient's tolerance of steroids (do steroid toxicities develop?), as well as the experience and practice patterns of the individual rheumatologist. Typically, the dose is not lowered by more than 25% decrements. Although total discontinuation of corticosteroids is a goal desired by both patients and physicians, many patients require maintenance with low-dose corticosteroids (5–10mg/day) to prevent recurrence. One small retrospective study suggests that continuation of low-dose prednisone may be protective for patients initially treated for major disease activity[4].

As corticosteroids are associated with multiple toxicities, monitoring of blood pressure, cholesterol, glucose, bone density and ocular pressure is an important adjunctive measure taken by most rheumatologists. Maintaining a high index of suspicion for the development of other toxicities, including gastrointestinal ulceration, avascular necrosis, atherosclerosis and steroid myopathy, is also important in the management of patients on corticosteroids.

ANTIMALARIALS

Antimalarial agents are commonly used to treat non-life threatening manifestations of SLE which either do not respond to non-steroidal anti-inflammatory drugs and/or low-dose corticosteroids, or which recur when these agents are tapered or discontinued. Typically these features include constitutional symptoms such as fatigue, musculoskeletal symptoms, skin rashes and pleuritic chest pain (Table 126.3). Hydroxychloroquine, a 4-aminoquinolone derivative, is the most commonly used antimalarial, generally begun at a dose of 400mg daily. Clinical response may be expected within 4–6 weeks, and in some patients this is sustained even with a dose reduction to 200mg daily.

TABLE 126.2 CORTICOSTEROIDS IN SLE

Indication	Corticosteroid regimen	
Rashes	Topical	Short-acting: hydrocortisone (0.125–1.0%) Intermediate-acting: triamcinolone (0.025–0.5%) Long-acting: betamethasone (0.01–0.1%)
	Intralesional (discoid lupus)	Triamcinolone acetonide
Minor disease activity	Oral prednisone (or equivalent) <0.5mg/kg/day in single or divided daily dose	
Major disease activity	Oral prednisone (or equivalent) 1.0mg/kg/day in single or divided daily dose or Intravenous methylprednisolone (1g or 15mg/kg), usually repeated for 3 consecutive days	

TABLE 126.3 ANTIMALARIALS USED IN LUPUS

Drug		Daily dose
4-Aminoquinolone derivatives	Hydroxychloroquine	200–400mg*
	Chloroquine	250mg*
9-Aminoacridine derivatives	Quinacrine (mepacrine)	100mg*

* In patients weighing less than 45kg, dose reductions are necessary: 5–7mg/kg for hydroxy-chloroquine, 4mg/kg for chloroquine, 1–2mg/kg for quinacrine.

Chloroquine, also an aminoquinolone derivative, is less commonly used than hydroxychloroquine. Patients who do not demonstrate a benefit from an aminoquinolone may respond to the 9-aminoacridine compound quinacrine in a dose of 100mg/day. In some cases in which only a partial response to a single antimalarial agent has been achieved, the combination of two or more of these agents may prove to be synergistic[5,6]. A recent uncontrolled report on six SLE patients suggests that the combination of hydroxycloroquine and quinacrine may be beneficial not only for chronic cutaneous lupus manifestations, but also for maintenance of remission of major organ involvement[7]. It should be noted that the production of Atabrine® was discontinued in the United States in 1992, but quinacrine hydrochloride is available from compounding pharmacies.

Antimalarials were used in the treatment of rheumatic diseases many years before any knowledge of their mechanism of action was available. It is now generally accepted that they have important immunomodulatory effects (Table 126.4), decreasing antigen processing and presentation by both macrophages and lymphoid dendritic cells. This appears to result from an increase in intracytoplasmic pH, which in turn alters the molecular assembly of α-ϵ-peptide complexes of class II MHC molecules. Subsequent decreased stimulation of CD4 T cells ultimately leads to a downregulation of responses, including decreased production of cytokines such as IL-1, IL-2, IL-4, IL-5, IL-6 and tumor necrosis factor[8]. Although a number of potential side effects of antimalarials are well described, in practice toxicity does not significantly limit their usefulness. Antimalarials may induce a hemolytic anemia in individuals (most often those of black race) with glucose-6 phosphate dehydrogenase

TABLE 126.4 IMMUNOMODULATORY EFFECTS OF ANTIMALARIALS

Mechanism	Effect
Accumulation in lysosomes, resulting in increase in intracellular pH	Delays recycling of proteins such as enzymes and surface receptors from lysosomes to the cell surface Disrupts normal assimilation of peptides with class II MHC molecules, resulting in decreased interaction between antigen presenting cells and T cells Decreases cytokine production (eg. IL-1, IL-6, TNF-α)
Inhibits activity of phospholipases A_2 and C	Decreases production of leukotrienes and prostaglandins, resulting in decreased phagocytosis and chemotaxis
Bind to DNA by intercalation between adjacent base pairs	Stabilizes DNA, inhibiting its denaturation Blocks the LE cell phenomenon

deficiency; therefore, it is advisable to screen for the presence of this enzyme prior to instituting therapy. Decreased levels in patients with a heterozygous trait do not appear to trigger hemolysis.

Ocular toxicity is responsible for the most significant concern with regard to antimalarial therapy. Deposition of these agents in the melanin of the pigmented epithelial layer of the retina may damage rods and cones. Early damage is usually reversible but is most often asymptomatic, necessitating regular ophthalmologic examination, including visual acuity, slit-lamp, fundoscopic and visual field testing, usually every 6–12 months. The initial retinal changes are noted in the macula, with edema, increased stippling pigmentation, and loss of the foveal reflex to bright light. Visual field defects are generally associated with more severe retinal changes, including optic disc pallor and atrophy, attenuation of retinal arterioles, fine granular pigmentary changes in the peripheral retina, and prominent choroidal patterns in the advanced stages. The development of retinopathy is generally dose and duration dependent. Chloroquine has been clearly shown to have an increased risk of ocular toxicity compared to hydroxychloroquine; 95% of long-term chloroquine users will develop corneal deposits, compared to less than 10% of hydroxychoroquine users[9]. In a Canadian study of 156 SLE patients receiving antimalarials, one developed retinopathy after 6 years at a dose of 6.5mg/kg/day (0.95 cases/1000 patient years of hydroxychloroquine)[10]. Nevertheless, reports of hydroxychloroquine macular toxicity continue to appear, underscoring the need for careful follow-up and detection of early lesions[11,12].

The toxicity associated with chronic antimalarial therapy should not be confused with early side effects related to deposition of drug in the cornea, occasionally resulting in blurred vision, photophobia or visual halos. These visual problems generally resolve within several weeks.

Other manifestations of antimalarial toxicity are uncommon. Gastrointestinal distress often resolves with continued administration. Other early side effects include headache, malaise, and rarely erythematous pruritic rashes. Long-term antimalarial therapy may be associated with a reversible neuromyopathy which may be confused with symptoms of active lupus; muscle biopsy may be necessary to confirm the diagnosis[13]. A single case report of the institution of hydroxychloroquine in a young SLE patient with a history of complex partial seizure suggests that this agent may have precipitated a tonic–clonic seizure[14]. Case reports of the development of cardiac conduction disorders, including complete heart block, in one instance associated with a hypertrophic cardiomyopathy, have been described in patients receiving both short- and long-term treatment with antimalarials for SLE. Both patients improved with discontinuation of antimalarial therapy[15,16]. Ototoxicity secondary to antimalarials remains a controversial issue, and is generally attributed to chloroquine. Two patients receiving several years of hydroxychloroquine therapy are reported to have suffered irreversible sensorineural hearing loss; however, this is also a well-recognized manifestation of autoimmune disease itself[17].

Antimalarials are generally considered to be contraindicated in pregnancy, and conventional wisdom holds that it is not advisable to institute antimalarial therapy in a woman who intends to become pregnant. Rare cases of congenital defects such as cleft palate, sensorineural hearing loss and posterior column defects have been reported, generally associated with chloroquine or quinacrine. The decision regarding discontinuation of antimalarials in a patient who has had a therapeutic benefit and who is now contemplating pregnancy, is more difficult. The half-life of hydroxcholorquine is about 8 weeks, and it may remain detectable in urine for up to 6 months after discontinuation, so that fetal exposure to the agent is not avoided by discontinuation at the time when pregnancy is confirmed. Many rheumatologists opt to continue antimalarials during pregnancy, considering the danger to the fetus of an exacerbation of disease activity in the mother to be greater than the risk of fetal abnormalities[18]. Several reports have documented series of

16–36 SLE pregnancies in patients receiving 4-aminoquinolones; none were associated with congenital abnormalities[19–21].

In addition to the therapeutic effects of antimalarials on SLE disease manifestations, beneficial effects have been reported with regard to improvement in lipoprotein profiles. This is particularly important in patients treated with corticosteroids or those with nephrotic syndrome and secondary hypercholesterolemia. Chloroquine is known to inhibit cholesterol synthesis through its effect on 2,3-oxidosqualene-lanesterol cyclase[22]. It also stimulates LDL receptor activity in cultured fibroblasts[23] and increases the activity of HMG-CoA reductase[22]. Although a recent study of 44 Chinese patients with mild or inactive disease receiving hydroxychloroquine showed no significant effect of the antimalarial therapy on serum lipid profiles[24], many other investigators have demonstrated significant reductions in total cholesterol, triglycerides and LDL cholesterol in association with antimalarial therapy, whether the patient was receiving concomitant steroid therapy or not[25–28]. In her cohort of 264 lupus patients with repeated measures of serum cholesterol during 3027 visits, Petri[29] demonstrated that hydroxychloroquine was able to counteract the adverse effect of 10mg of prednisone on cholesterol level.

Another potential benefit of antimalarials is in prophylaxis against thromboembolic events. Since the 1970s some British orthopedic surgeons have used hydroxychloroquine immediately prior to and after surgery to prevent deep venous thrombosis and pulmonary emboli, with generally beneficial results reported in both uncontrolled and randomized series. Petri reported in her SLE cohort that hydroxychloroquine was protective against future thrombosis in prospectively ascertained venous and arterial thrombotic events[29]. She suggested that this phenomenon might be due to an inhibitory effect on platelet aggregation, an immunosuppressive effect resulting in the lowering of procoagulant antiphospholipid antibody levels, or secondary to either reduction of SLE activity in general or a decrease in atherosclerotic risk factors such as hypercholesterolemia.

Despite the widespread use of antimalarials in SLE, no randomized controlled studies of their efficacy exist. Similarly, information regarding the appropriate duration of therapy after therapeutic success or even disease remission was lacking, until a 1991 study of the effect of discontinuing hydroxychloroquine therapy was carried out by the Canadian Hydroxychloroquine Study Group[30]. In a 24-week randomized double-blind placebo-controlled study in 47 patients with clinically stable SLE, 25 were assigned to continue their same dose of hydroxychloroquine and 22 were assigned to the placebo group. The relative risk of a disease exacerbation was 2.5 times higher (16 of 22 vs. 9 of 25) in the patients taking placebo than in those continuing to take hydroxychloroquine, and 6.1 times greater for severe exacerbations (5 of 22 vs. 1 of 25); the time to flare was also shorter in the placebo group ($p=0.02$)[30]. In an additional 3-year follow-up period of the same patients, the primary outcome measure was the time to a major flare, defined as the institution or increase in dose of prednisone of 10mg/day or the institution of an immunosuppressive agent. Overall, hydroxychloroquine discontinuation reduced major disease flares by 57%, suggesting that this antimalarial agent has a long-term protective effect[31].

IMMUNOSUPPRESSIVE DRUGS

Immunosuppressive drugs have been used to treat SLE for at least three decades, often borrowed from the oncology and transplantation experience, and became part of the therapeutic regimen for lupus manifestations long before much was known about their mechanism of action in suppressing autoimmunity. Most of these agents are used acutely primarily for life-threatening lupus manifestations, and will be discussed in more detail in relation to specific organ system involvement. In exchange for their immunosuppressive potency they have many and varied toxicities, but virtually all cause a high frequency of gastro-intestinal complaints. The potential for suppression of both erythroid and myeloid elements of the bone marrow and an increased risk of infection require vigilance when monitoring patients receiving these agents.

Azathioprine

Azathioprine is probably the most common immunosuppressive drug used not specifically for acute treatment of active disease manifestations but as a steroid-sparing agent in SLE patients who are steroid dependent or who have repeated disease exacerbations necessitating reinstitution of steroids[32]. Maintenance treatment with azathioprine in doses of 1.5–2.5mg/kg/day has been shown to be associated with a lower rate of development of severe forms of SLE, such as nephritis, or central nervous system involvement[33]. Azathioprine is a purine analog generated by the attachment of an imidazole group to 6-mercaptopurine. Its immunosuppressive action appears to be derived from a suppression of DNA synthesis by the nucleoprotein metabolites of 6-mercaptopurine which inhibit the enzymatic conversion of inosinic acid to xanthylic acid and of adenylsuccinic acid to adenylic acid.

In addition to its effects on the bone marrow, azathioprine can cause hepatotoxicity, usually when given in doses higher than 2.5g/kg/day. Drug hypersensitivity may also result in an acute hepatitis, with elevated transaminases and hepatocellular necrosis and mild biliary stasis on liver biopsy. This syndrome may be accompanied by fever, abdominal pain and a maculopapular rash. The findings are generally reversible upon discontinuation of the drug[34]. Pancreatitis has also been reported to occur in SLE patients receiving azathioprine, but its occurrence may have been associated with other features of disease activity.

Individual case reports have suggested an association of azathioprine with an increased risk of malignancy. An increase in the development of cervical atypia has been documented in women receiving azathioprine[35], thereby indicating the need for regular follow-up with PAP smears. Although it has been suggested that prolonged treatment with azathioprine results in an increase in hematologic and lymphoproliferative malignancies, a large study documenting a higher than expected rate of such malignancies in SLE patients concluded that none of the affected patients had received azathioprine or other immunosuppressive agents[36].

Potential teratogenic effects on the fetus have limited the use of most immunosuppressive agents in pregnant lupus patients. For many years this prohibition included azathioprine. Nevertheless, uncomplicated pregnancies resulting in normal infants have been reported since the 1970s, and only a single case report of an infant born with preaxial polydactyly to a mother taking azathioprine implicates the drug as teratogenic[37]. It is now widely accepted among rheumatologists and obstetricians that azathioprine can be safely continued during pregnancy in women with lupus[38], and may in fact help to preserve the pregnancy by preventing a disease exacerbation.

TREATMENT OF SPECIFIC DISEASE OR ORGAN SYSTEM MANIFESTATIONS: CONSTITUTIONAL SYMPTOMS

Constitutional symptoms such as fatigue, arthralgia, myalgia, weight loss and low-grade fevers are frequent in patients with SLE and can occur alone or may accompany or herald the onset of a more severe organ flare. As fever, arthralgias and myalgias are also symptoms of infections, the appearance of constitutional symptoms should prompt an investigation for an infectious etiology as well as for features of an active lupus flare. NSAIDs are often effective treatment for constitutional symptoms, particularly arthralgias, myalgias and low-grade fevers. Low-dose steroids may be useful if intervention with NSAIDs is unsuccessful or if their use is contraindicated (e.g. in a patient with renal insufficiency). It is worth noting that secondary fibromyalgia has been reported to occur in up to one-third of lupus patients[39]. Fatigue with aches and pains may be difficult to treat in this subset of non-inflammatory patients, but may respond to low-dose tricyclic antidepressants, muscle relaxants and increased aerobic conditioning.

SKIN RASH

Malar rashes and other mild photosensitive rashes associated with mild to moderate exacerbations of SLE activity usually respond to the avoidance of ultraviolet light, coupled with the use of sunscreens and topical or low-dose oral corticosteroids (doses up to 20mg/day), commonly resolving with no sequelae. Intralesional steroids may be appropriate for isolated lesions, especially in the absence of other systemic manifestations of active disease. More persistent rashes requiring higher doses of steroids, or those that recur when steroids are tapered, including both erythematous inflammatory lesions and discoid lupus lesions, are most often treated with antimalarial agents.

Before a patient is considered to be resistant to antimalarial therapy several other possibilities should be considered, including failure to avoid excessive ultraviolet light exposure, or that the continuing or worsening rash is actually the result of a lichenoid drug reaction secondary to the antimalarial itself[40]. It has also been suggested that smoking decreases the efficacy of antimalarial therapy in cutaneous lupus through the induction of hepatic cytochrome P450, thus altering the metabolism of antimalarials[41]. In a study of 61 patients with discoid lupus or subacute cutaneous lupus rashes, 90% of the non-smokers and only 40% of the smokers ($p<0.0002$) responded to antimalarial therapy[42].

In patients who fail to respond to low- to moderate-dose steroids and antimalarials despite attention to the above caveats, the antilepromatous agent dapsone in oral doses of 25–100mg/day has been beneficial, especially for cutaneous manifestations such as bullous lupus, lupus panniculitis ('lupus profundus'), vasculitic lesions and oral ulcers[43–45]. A positive response is often observed within 1–4 weeks. Some patients with antimalarial-refractory discoid lupus and subacute cutaneous lupus rashes may also respond to dapsone. The most common side effect is hemolytic anemia; however, many other rare toxic manifestations have been described, most notably agranulocytosis and toxic epidermal necrolysis.

For patients with refractory skin manifestations of systemic and isolated discoid lupus there has been a renewed interest in the use of thalidomide, a drug developed as a sedative in the 1950s and subsequently withdrawn from the market in 1961 because of its severe teratogenic effects. Thalidomide has known immunologic effects, which provide the rationale for its use in treating autoimmune disease (Table 126.5).

TABLE 126.5 IMMUNOMODULATORY EFFECTS OF THALIDOMIDE

Mechanism	Action
Suppresses neutrophil function *in vitro*	Decreases chemotaxis and phagocytosis
Suppresses production of Th1-dependent cytokines	Decreases monocyte TNF-α production Inhibits interferon-γ production by cultured peripheral blood mononuclear cells
Enhances production of Th2-dependent cytokines	Enhances production of IL-4 and IL-5
Co-stimulates human T cells *in vitro*	Increases IL-2-mediated T-cell proliferation Greater effect on CD8+ cells results in decreased CD4:CD8 ratio
Inhibits basic fibroblast growth factor	Suppresses angiogenesis

It reduces TNF-α production by human monocytes, decreases peripheral CD4:CD8 lymphocyte ratios, enhances the production of TH2-dependent cytokines, suppresses in vitro neutrophil function, inhibits angiogenesis (probably the effect responsible for its teratogenicity), and modulates lipopolysaccharide induction of adhesiveness in postcapillary venules[46].

In 1983, a series of 60 patients with refractory discoid lupus treated with high starting doses of thalidomide (400mg/day) was reported[47]. The response rate was 90%, but the development of peripheral neuropathy was common and limited its continued use. Although it has been difficult to obtain in the United States, thalidomide is now being produced in Germany. No controlled studies of thalidomide in lupus skin disease have been reported, but a number of recent uncontrolled low-dose open-label series of 10–22 patients have been described[48–52]. The starting dose is usually 100mg/day, tapering to 25–50mg/day after a clinical response is achieved. A complete response was observed in 44–72% of patients in these series, and a partial response in 18–37%. Discontinuation of thalidomide was reported in 0–14% of patients, predominantly for severe drowsiness or paresthesias and documented peripheral neuropathy. Relapses of skin disease were common (65–75%) upon discontinuation, but reinstitution of therapy generally resulted in a return of benefit. Because of the severe potential for birth defects, women of childbearing age must be carefully counseled before therapy is instituted, and effective contraception must be ensured. In order to prescribe thalidomide, both patient and physician must comply with a program guaranteeing safety, the System for Thalidomide Education and Prescribing Safety (STEPS).

Beneficial effects of other agents have been reported in small series of steroid and antimalarial-resistant cutaneous lupus. These include high-dose intravenous immunoglobulin, immunosuppressive agents (azathioprine, methotrexate, cyclophosphamide, cyclosporine, cytarabine, mycophenolate mofetil), the oral gold agent auranofin, and both topical and oral retinoids[53,54]. Severe disfiguring skin lesions which appear to be irreversible may in fact respond to aggressive immunosuppressive therapy, sometimes initiated for more life-threatening manifestations of lupus activity such as nephritis or cerebritis (Fig. 126.1).

ARTHRITIS

The classic description of the musculoskeletal involvement in SLE is non-erosive, non-deforming arthralgias and/or arthritis in a distribution similar to that of rheumatoid arthritis, primarily affecting the small joints of the hands and the wrists. It may be the presenting symptom of SLE or accompany other manifestations of an active disease exacerbation. Acutely, a response to NSAIDs or low-dose steroids is not uncommon. Antimalarials are frequently the drug of choice for SLE patients whose musculoskeletal symptoms are chronic, particularly if they are associated with palpable synovitis.

In SLE patients whose arthritis is chronic and antimalarial resistant or who develop radiologic evidence of erosive disease, treatment with agents more frequently used in rheumatoid arthritis has become well accepted. Despite its potential for renal toxicity, especially proteinuria, which might be confused with active lupus nephritis, in our own experience parenteral gold injections have been used with beneficial results and an acceptable safety profile. In recent years, as weekly oral methotrexate has become the first-line disease-modifying antirheumatic drug for rheumatoid arthritis, it has been shown to be efficacious for antimalarial resistant lupus arthritis as well. Wilke *et al.*[55] described methotrexate's steroid-sparing ability as well as its usefulness for lupus arthritis in 17 patients studied retrospectively, but concluded that side effects were more common in SLE than among 87 similarly dosed rheumatoid arthritis patients. Leukopenia, oral ulcers and parenchymal hepatotoxicity were the most common side effects. Rahman *et al.*

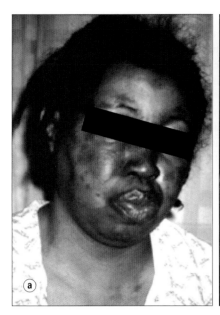 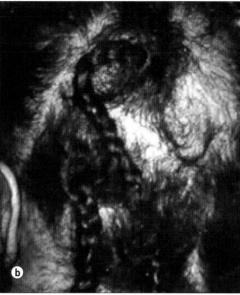 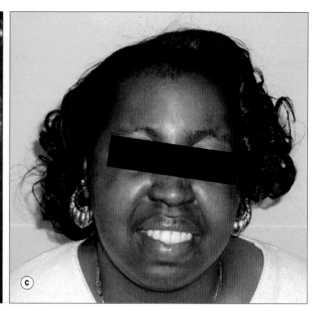

Fig. 126.1 Severe discoid lupus. This patient with severe discoid lupus lesions and cutaneous vasculitis involving her face, trunk and extremities (a) and generalized alopecia (b) failed to respond to moderate doses of corticosteroids (up to 40mg prednisone/day, hydroxychloroquine 400mg/day, and dapsone 100mg/day) over a period of at least 6 months. She subsequently developed central nervous system involvement and nephritis with the nephrotic syndrome and azotemia. Aggressive therapy with pulse methylprednisolone followed by oral steroids in doses up to 120mg prednisone/day and monthly doses of intravenous cyclophosphamide resulted not only in a dramatic improvement in her CNS and renal manifestations but also in complete resolution of her cutaneous manifestations, with no scarring sequelae (c).

subsequently described a series of 17 antimalarial-resistant SLE patients who received methotrexate for persistently active arthritis; during a mean 3.5-year follow-up period, toxicity leading to termination of therapy was infrequent, occurring in only two patients[56]. Compared to a control group, the methotrexate-treated patients had a higher mean joint count at baseline $(p = 0.003)$. After 6 months the 15 of 17 patients in the methotrexate group showed at least a 60% improvement in joint count compared to only 2 of 17 in the control group $(p < 0.001)$. A greater decrease in steroid dose and SLEDAI score were also observed in the methotrexate group. Similarly, in a series of 24 SLE Australian patients treated with 25 courses of methotrexate principally for arthritis over a mean period of 14.4 months, only two terminated therapy because of toxicity[57]. The median initial and peak methotrexate doses were 7.5 and 10mg/week, respectively. A reduction in steroid dose was successful in 36% of patients, but the change was not statistically significant. In the only prospective controlled study reported to date, Sato[58] found a significant improvement in SLEDAI score, steroid requirement and frequency of articular involvement after 6 months of methotrexate therapy. None of these studies have commented on the incidence or progression of radiographic erosions in methotrexate-treated SLE patients with chronic arthritis.

CARDIOPULMONARY

There has been little change in the treatment of serositis over the years in patients with SLE. Many episodes of pleuritis or pericarditis respond to NSAIDs; corticosteroids in moderate doses are useful in refractory cases. Hydroxychloroquine may be added as adjunctive therapy in patients with recurring episodes of serositis. Intravenous immunoglobulin has also been used anecdotally for life-threatening pericarditis[59,60].

Pulmonary hemorrhage requires treatment with high-dose corticosteroids in combination with a cytotoxic agent, typically cyclophosphamide. Plasmapheresis[61] may offer additional benefit in these patients with severe life-threatening disease.

Lupus pneumonitis is an additional manifestation of severe life-threatening disease requiring aggressive therapeutic intervention.

Although controlled trials are not available for this clinical feature, high-dose corticosteroid therapy with the addition of azathioprine, cyclophosphamide or intravenous immunoglobulin (IVIG) is warranted and may improve morbidity and mortality[32,61,62].

Pulmonary hypertension is usually treated with a variety of vasodilatory agents and anticoagulants, in addition to immunosuppression with corticosteroids and cytotoxics, in an effort to alleviate clinical symptoms and improve hemodynamic abnormalities. Vasodilatory agents have included calcium channel blockers and prostaglandin analogs, such as intravenous epoprostenol (prostaglandin I_2)[63] and monthly low-dose infusion of iloprost, a prostaglandin I_2 analog[64]. There has been a preliminary report of the effectiveness of continuous infusion of treprostinil, another prostaglandin I_2 analog, in patients with connective tissue disease, including SLE, which demonstrated improved symptoms and hemodynamics in these patients[65]. Bosentan, an oral endothelin-receptor antagonist, has recently become available for the treatment of pulmonary hypertension. It increases exercise capacity and improves hemodynamics in patients with pulmonary hypertension[66]. Its role in SLE remains to be determined. Pulmonary thromboendarterectomy has been reported to be successful in three patients with pulmonary hypertension in association with the antiphospholiplid syndrome[67].

Myocarditis is an uncommon cardiac manifestation of SLE which usually requires high-dose prednisone (1mg/kg/day) for treatment. Cytotoxic intervention with azathioprine or cyclophospamide has been useful in some patients; intravenous immunoglobulin has also been used successfully for this feature[68–70].

HEMATOLOGIC

Immune-mediated cytopenias occur commonly in SLE and when mild require no treatment. When low counts become clinically significant, corticosteroids in moderate or high doses usually result in a beneficial response. However, there are patients who are either unresponsive to high-dose corticosteroids or in whom high-dose steroids are unable to be tapered; in these circumstances other interventions are necessary.

Other measures used for patients with hemolytic anemia include azathioprine[32,71], danazol[72,73], IVIG[74] and plasmapheresis.[75,76] Splenectomy may be beneficial but its efficacy may not be sustained. Severe neutropenia in the febrile patient is usually responsive to treatment with granulocyte-stimulating factor[77,78]. Lymphopenia per se does not require treatment. Lymphocyte counts usually rise as the patient's overall activity is treated. However, patients with CD4 counts below 200 may be prone to opportunistic infections such as *Pneumocystis carinii*[79] and may require prophylaxis while they are at risk. Adjunctive measures in corticosteroid-resistant or -dependent patients with thrombocytopenia have included IVIG. The effect although prompt, is often only temporary, requiring the administration of other agents. Cyclosporin, danazol, dapsone and cyclophosphamide have been used successfully in anecdotal and case series[80–84]. Newer biologic agents may eventually play a role in this arena; there is a report of refractory thrombocytopenia in a lupus patient responding to interleukin-11[85]. The role of splenectomy in refractory thrombocytopenia in lupus remains unclear, with some series demonstrating long-term effectiveness whereas others show the necessity for continued immunosuppression despite surgical removal of the spleen.

Thrombotic thrombocytopenic purpura (TTP) is a rare feature that may occur with lupus. Treatment of TTP in lupus has been similar to that for primary TTP, i.e. steroids with plasma exchange. There are reports of improved survival in lupus when cyclophosphamide is added to the treatment regimen[86,87].

NEUROPSYCHIATRIC

There are numerous neuropsychiatric symptoms that occur in patients with lupus resulting from a multitude of etiologies. These include adverse events due to medications (e.g. NSAID-induced aseptic meningitis, corticosteroid psychosis or mood swings), infections, and features of the antiphospholipid antibody syndrome, i.e. strokes, seizures and chorea. Management of these symptoms requires the ability to identify the causative factor, followed by appropriate interventions directed at the specific etiology (removal of the offending medication, administration of antibiotics, anticoagulation etc.). Neuropsychiatric symptoms that are believed to respond to anti-inflammatory and immunosuppressive agents include organic brain syndromes, pyschoses, some seizures, some headaches, peripheral neuropathies and myelopathy. These features almost always require high-dose corticosteroids, and often pulse methylprednisolone. Pulse cyclophosphamide administered every 3–6 weeks may be efficacious in steroid-resistant cases[88–90]; intravenous immunoglobulin[91,92] and intrathecal methotrexate[93] are other therapies that have been reported to be of benefit. The outcomes of some neuropsychiatric manifestations such as transverse myelitis have been shown to be favorably affected by the prompt initiation of cyclophosphamide[94].

Despite the lack of a 'gold standard' for diagnosing central nervous system manifestations of SLE, cognitive deficit is easier to identify than to treat. Some patients will demonstrate reversible manifestations of cognitive dysfunction which appear to be associated with other manifestations of disease activity, especially organic brain syndrome, but also in the presence of electrolyte disturbances or azotemia and during episodes of infection. Treatment of the underlying SLE activity or infection should result in improvement of cognitive impairment. Medications such as anticonvulsants may also have side effects that appear as cognitive impairments.

In other lupus patients cognitive impairment appears to be slowly progressive and irreversible, even in the absence of other manifestations of disease activity. This is frequently associated with the presence of antiphospholipid antibodies, even in the absence of other evidence of thromboembolic disease. Long-term anticoagulation may halt the progression of cognitive deficit in such patients. When no inciting factor can be found, therapeutic intervention may be directed at lifestyle changes, including occupational therapy and the involvement of family members in enhancing the patient's daily environment.

HORMONE THERAPY

The safety of hormone (estrogen) therapy in SLE remains an area of controversy. Premenopausal patients could benefit from the positive effects of hormones given as oral contraceptive agents or as estrogen replacement therapy in the perimenopausal and menopausal years. However, there are theoretical concerns that estrogen administration to lupus patients may trigger an increase in disease activity, including the exacerbation of lupus-like disease in animal models and epidemiologic data in humans. Epidemiologic data include the strong female predominance observed in lupus, onset occurring primarily in the childbearing years, and the association between postmenopausal hormone therapy and an increased risk for subsequent development of SLE[95]. There are clearly lupus patients in whom estrogens are contraindicated, i.e. those with antiphospholipid antibodies. However, it is uncertain whether a majority of lupus patients might receive estrogen without potential harm. A case–control study comparing 16 postmenopausal patients on hormone replacement therapy (HRT) with 32 controls not receiving HRT showed no difference in the rate of flares over a follow-up period of 1 year[96]. In another small study of 34 patients, the rate of flare was equivalent in a group of patients given hormonal replacement therapy ($n = 11$) to that in patients ($n = 23$) not receiving replacement; the magnitude of the observed flares was also not significantly different between the two groups[97]. A preliminary report of hormone replacement given to a larger group of postmenopausal lupus patients ($n = 106$) also showed no exacerbation of disease activity in the 52 patients randomized to receive therapy compared to patients receiving placebo[98]. There are no reports of the safety of hormone therapy as oral contraception in premenopausal lupus patients. The results of an ongoing trial assessing the safety of hormone contraception as well as hormone replacement therapy are eagerly anticipated.

INNOVATIVE THERAPIES: AVAILABLE DRUGS NOT APPROVED FOR SLE INDICATIONS

Many of the immunosuppressive agents used to treat SLE in general or specific organ system manifestations have been 'borrowed' from the oncology or transplant experience. In fact, the only class of drugs specifically approved by the Food and Drug Administration (FDA) for the treatment of lupus is the 4-aminoquinolone antimalarials, despite the absence of controlled randomized clinical trials. Given the knowledge that SLE is predominantly a disease of women of childbearing age, it has become clear that a number of hormonal mechanisms may be important in its pathogenesis and hence a potential target for new therapies. Drugs approved and marketed for other indications are being used in uncontrolled series and controlled clinical trials.

Bromocriptine

Prolactin, a peptide hormone synthesized by the pituitary gland, as well as at multiple other sites including lymphocytes, has been found to be elevated in the serum of some women with SLE[99]. As a cytokine, prolactin has many immunologic effects on T cells, B cells, macrophages and natural killer cells, including induction of interleukin (IL)-2 receptors on lymphocytes[99]. Circulating prolactin binds to prolactin receptors distributed throughout the immune system.

Bromocriptine is a dopamine agonist that selectively inhibits secretion of prolactin by the pituitary gland. Bromocriptine therefore has the capacity to inhibit the immune functions stimulated by prolactin, resulting in decreased antibody formation and cell-mediated immune

TABLE 126.6 IMMUNOMODULATORY EFFECTS OF BROMOCRIPTINE

Mechanism	Action
Suppresses prolactin secretion by the pituitary receptors on lymphocytes	Decreases prolactin induction of IL-2 Decreases circulating autoantibody levels (e.g. antipituitary antibodies, anti-dsDNA) in hyperprolactinemic individuals
Direct suppressive effects on T and B cells	Decreases early stages of T-cell activation Inhibits proliferation and immunoglobulin production of mitogen-stimulated human B cells *in vitro*

TABLE 126.7 IMMUNOMODULATORY EFFECTS OF DEHYDROEPIANDROSTERONE

- Enhances IL-2 production by T lymphocytes *in vitro*
- Partially reverses the decreased IL-2 production by SLE T lymphocytes *in vitro*

responses (Table 126.6). It has also been suggested that bromocriptine may act directly to suppress the early phases of human T-cell activation and the proliferation and immunoglobulin production in mitogen-stimulated B lymphocytes[100].

Initial observations suggesting the possible benefit of bromocriptine in SLE occurred during its use in patients with SLE and concomitant prolactinomas, in which the lupus symptoms resolved[101] and subsequently recurred with discontinuation of the drug[102]. Despite the fact that some investigators have failed to show a correlation between prolactin levels and SLE disease activity[103,104], uncontrolled series in patients with both normal and elevated prolactin levels[105], and later randomized controlled double-blind studies, have shown improvement in SLE symptoms and serologic measures of disease activity in prolactin-treated patients[99,105]. Therapeutic benefit was noted for fatigue, headache, arthralgias, skin rash, and anti-dsDNA titers. Steroid-sparing effects, a decreased number of flares and an increased time to flare similar to that achieved with hydroxychloroquine were observed[99]. The dose of bromocriptine in most reported studies was 2.5–3.75mg/day, but doses up to 30mg/day have been used to normalize prolactin levels. Bromocriptine is not teratogenic, has no significant drug interactions, and has been used safely in combination with steroids, antimalarials and other immunosuppressive agents[106].

Dehydroepiandrosterone

Dehydroepiandrosterone (DHEA, prasterone), a naturally occurring weak male androgen, has also shown promise in ameliorating symptoms and serologic abnormalities in SLE. The rationale for its use is based on the known hormonal influence of estrogens and androgens on SLE activity. Decreased serum levels of DHEA have been demonstrated in some SLE patients, unrelated to levels of disease activity[107]. DHEA has also been shown to have immunomodulatory effects on T lymphocytes (Table 126.7)[108]. An uncontrolled trial of DHEA in 50 lupus patients in doses ranging from 50 to 200mg/day demonstrated improvement in SLEDAI scores and decreased steroid requirement among the 21 patients who completed 12 months of treatment[109]. In a subsequent double-blind, randomized placebo-controlled trial in 191 female patients receiving 10–30mg prednisone/day at onset, treatment with 200mg/day of DHEA was significantly associated with a sustained reduction in prednisone dose <7.5mg/day while maintaining stabilization or improvement in disease activity[110].

In a subset of 37 patients treated in the above controlled study, the effect of DHEA on bone density was examined[111]. Bone mineral density was significantly improved in patients receiving DHEA compared to those on placebo, particularly in the postmenopausal group. As an anabolic steroid, DHEA has also been shown to ameliorate the deleterious effects of glucocorticoids, such as diabetes, amino acid deamination and hypertension[112]. It may have a benefit in diminishing the severity of steroid-induced myopathy and avascular necrosis as well. In fact, Robinzon and Cutolo suggest that as SLE patients with chronic glucocorticoid administration have suppression of ACTH secretion resulting in a further decrease in DHEA levels, DHEA replacement therapy should be considered in order to prevent glucocorticoid side effects. Side effects of DHEA are minimal, most commonly the development or worsening of acne.

Lipid-lowering statins

Premature atherosclerosis is now a well recognized complication of SLE, and recommendations for reducing known risk factors for atherogenesis should be part of the therapeutic regimen for all lupus patients. This includes measures to minimize glucose intolerance, hypertension and hyperlipidemia. Recently, the properties of statins have been shown to extend beyond their lipid-lowering ability to include immunomodulatory activity, probably related to effects on endothelial cell function, which may be beneficial even in lupus patients with normal lipid levels[113]. Controlled trials of statins aimed at assessing their ability to decrease disease activity in lupus are currently in the design phase.

REFERENCES

1. Clive DM, Stoff JS. Renal syndromes associated with nonsteroidal antiinflammatory drugs. N Engl J Med 1984; 310: 563–572.
2. Bouland DL, Specht NL, Hegstad DR. Ibuprofen and aseptic meningitis. Ann Intern Med 1986; 104: 731 [letter].
3. Crofford LJ, Oates JC, McCune WJ et al. Thrombosis in patients with systemic lupus erythematosus treated with specific cyclooxygenase 2 inhibitors. A report of four cases. Arthritis Rheum 2001; 43: 1891–1896.
4. Aranow C, Emy J, Barland P. Reactivation of inactive systemic lupus erythematosus. Scand J Rheumatol 1996; 25: 282–286.
5. Tye MJ, White H, Appel B. Lupus erythematosus treated with a combination of quinacrine, hydroxychoroquine and chloroquine. N Engl J Med 1959; 260: 63–66.
6. Feldmann R, Salomon D, Saurat JH. The association of the two antimalarials chloroquine and quinacrine for treatment-resistant chronic and subacute cutaneous lupus erythematosus. Dermatology 1994; 189: 425–427.
7. Toubi E, Rosner I, Rozenbaum M et al. The benefit of combining hyroxycholoroquine with quinacrine in the treatment of SLE patients. Lupus 2000; 9: 92–95.
8. Fox RI, Kang H-I. Mechanism of action of antimalarial drugs: Inhibition of antigen processing and presentation. Lupus 1993; 2 (Suppl 1): S9–S12.
9. Easterbrook M. Is corneal deposition of antimalarial any indication of retinal toxicity? Can J Ophthalmol 1990; 25: 249–225.
10. Wang C, Fortin PR, Li Y et al. Discontinuation of antimalarial drugs in systemic lupus erythematosus. J Rheumatol 199; 26: 808–815.
11. Bienfang D, Coblyn JS, Liang MH. Corzillius M. Hydroxychloroquine retinopathy despite regular ophthalmologic evaluation: a consecutive series. J Rheumatol 2000; 27: 2703–2706.
12. Warner AE. Early hydroxychloroquine macular toxicity. Arthritis Rheum 2001; 44: 1959–1961.
13. Avina-Zubeta JA, Johnson ES, Suarez-Almozar ME, Russell AS. Incidence of myopathy in patients treated with antimalarials. A report of three cases and a review of the literature. Br J Rheumatol 1995; 34: 166–170.
14. Malcangi G, Fraticelli P, Palmieri C et al. Hydroxychloroquine-induced seizure in a patient with systemic lupus erythematosus. Rheumatol Int 2000; 20: 31–33.
15. Baguet JP. Tremel F, Fabre M. Chloroquine cardiomyopathy with conduction disorders. Heart 1999; 81: 221–223.
16. Comin-Colet J, Sanchez-Corral MA, Alegre-Sancho JJ et al. Complete heart block in an adult with systemic lupus erythematosus and recent onset of hydroxychloroquine therapy. Lupus 2001; 10: 59–62.

17. Johansen PB, Grant JT. Ototoxicity due to hydroxychloroquine: report of two cases. Clin Exp Rheumatol 1998; 16: 472–474.
18. Schulzer M, Esdaile JM. The use of antimalarial treatment in lupus pregnancy and lactation. Arthritis Rheum 2000; 43 (Suppl): S272.
19. Parke A, West B. Hydroxychloroquine in pregnant patients with systemic lupus erythematosus. J Rheumatol 1996; 23: 1715–1718.
20. Buchanan NM, Toubi E, Khamashta MA et al. Hydroxychloroquine and lupus pregnancy. Ann Rheum Dis 1996; 55: 486–488.
21. Tincani A, Faden D, Lojacono A et al. Hydroxychloroquine in pregnant patients with rheumatic disease. Gestational and neonatal outcome. Arthritis Rheum 2001; 44 (Suppl): S397.
22. Chen HW, Leonard DA. Chloroquine inhibits cyclization of squalene oxide to lanosterol in mammalian cells. J Biol Chem 1984; 259: 8156–8162.
23. Oram JF, Albers JJ, Cheung MC, Bierman EL. The effects of subfractions of high density lipoprotein on cholesterol efflux from cultured fibroblasts. Regulation of low density lipoprotein receptor activity. J Biol Chem 1981; 256: 8348–8356.
24. Tam LS, Li EK, Lam CW, Tomlinson B. Hydroxychloroquine has no significant effect on lipids and apolipoproteins in Chinese systemic lupus erythematosus patients with mild or inactive disease. Lupus 2000; 9: 413–416.
25. Wallace DJ, Metzger AL, Stecher VJ et al. Cholesterol-lowering effect of hydroxychloroquine in patients with rheumatic disease: reversal of deleterious effects of steroids on lipids. Am J Med 1990; 89: 322–326.
26. Hodis HN, Quismorio FP Jr, Wickham E, Blankenhorn DH. The lipid, lipoprotein and apolipoprotein effects of hydroxychloroquine in patients with systemic lupus erythematosus. J Rheumatol 1993; 20: 661–665.
27. Tam LS, Gladman DD, Hallett DC et al. Effect of antimalarial agents on the fasting lipid profile in systemic lupus erythematosus. J Rheumatol 2000; 27: 2142–2145.
28. Borba EF, Bonfa E. Longterm beneficial effect of chloroquine diphosphate on lipoprotein profile in lupus patients with and without steroid therapy. J Rheumatol 2001; 28: 780–785.
29. Petri M. Hydroxychloroquine use in the Baltimore Lupus Cohort: effects on lipids, glucose and thrombosis. Lupus 1996; 5 (Suppl 1): S16–S22.
30. The Canadian Hydroxychloroquine Study Group. A randomized study of the effect of withdrawing hydroxychloroquine sulfate in systemic lupus erythematosus. N Engl J Med 1991; 324: 150–154.
31. The Canadian Hydroxychloroquine Study Group. A long-term study of hydroxy-chloroquine withdrawal on exacerbations in systemic lupus erythematosus. Lupus 1998; 7: 80–85.
32. Abu-Shakra M, Shoenfeld Y. Azathioprine therapy for patients with systemic lupus erythematosus. Arthritis Rheum 2001; 10: 152–153.
33. Ginzler E, Sharon E, Diamond H, Kaplan D. Long-term maintenance therapy with azathioprine in systemic lupus erythematosus. Arthritis Rheum 1975; 18: 27–34.
34. Jeurissen MEC, Boerbooms AM Th, van de Putte LBA, Kruijsen MWM. Azathioprine induced fever, chills, rash, and hepatotoxicity in rheuamtoid arthritis. Ann Rheum Dis 1990; 49: 25–27.
35. Nyberg G, Eriksson O, Westberg NG. Increased incidence of cervical atypia in women with systemic lupus erythematosus treated with chemotherapy. Arthritis Rheum 1981; 24: 649–650.
36. Abu-Shakra M, Gladman DD, Urowitz MB. Malignancy in SLE. Arthritis Rheum 1996; 39: 1050–1054.
37. Williamson RA, Karp LE. Azathioprine teratogenicity: review of the literature and case report. Obstet Gynecol 1981; 58: 247–250.
38. Ramsey-Goldman R, Schilling E. Immunosuppressive drug use during pregnancy. Rheum Dis Clin North Am 1997; 23: 149–167.
39. Akkasilpa S, Minor M, Goldman D et al. Association of coping responses with fibromyalgia tender points in patients with systemic lupus erythematosus. J Rheumatol 2000; 27: 671–674.
40. Callen JP. Management of antimalarial-refractory cutaneous lupus erythematosus. Lupus 1997; 6: 203–208.
41. Rahman P, Gladman DD, Urowitz MB. Smoking interferes with efficacy of antimalarial therapy in cutaneous lupus. J Rheumatol 1998; 25: 1716–1719.
42. Jewell ML, McCauliffe DP. Patients with cutaneous lupus erythematosus who smoke are less responsive to antimalarial treatment. J Am Acad Dermatol 2000; 42: 983–987.
43. Neri R, Mosca M, Bernacchi E, Bombardieri S. A case of SLE with acute, subacute and chronic cutaneous lesions successfully treated with Dapsone. Lupus 1999; 8: 240–243.
44. Nishijima C, Hatta N, Inaoki M et al. Urticarial vasculitis in systemic lupus erythematosus: fair response to prednisolone/dapsone and persistent hypocomplementemia. Eur J Dermatol 1999; 9: 54–56.
45. Cotell S, Robinson ND, Chan LS. Autoimmune blistering skin diseases. Am J Emerg Med 2000; 18: 288–299.
46. Karim MY, Ruiz-Irastorza G, Khamashta MA, Hughes GRV. Update on therapy – thalidomide in the treatment of lupus. Lupus 2001; 10: 188–192.
47. Knop J, Bonsmann G, Happle R et al. Thalidomide in the treatment of sixty cases of chronic discoid lupus erythematosus. Br J Dermatol 1983; 108: 461–466.
48. Walchner M, Meurer M, Plewig G, Messer G. Clinical and immunologic parameters during thalidomide treatment of lupus erythematosus. Int J Dermatol 2000; 39: 383–388.
49. Ordi-Ros J, Cortes F, Cucurull E et al. Thalidomide in the treatment of cutaneous lupus refractory to conventional therapy. J Rheumatol 2000; 27: 1429–1433.
50. Kyriakos PK, Kontochristopoulos GJ, Panteleos DN. Experience with low-dose thalidomide therapy in chronic discoid lupus erythematosus. Int J Dermatol 2000; 39: 218–222.
51. Duong DJ, Spigel GT, Moxley RT, Gaspari AA. American experience with low-dose thalidomide for severe cutaneous lupus erythematosus. Arch Dermatol 1999; 135: 1079–1087.
52. Stevens RJ, Andujar C, Edwards CJ et al. Thalidomide in the treatment of the cutaneous manifestations of lupus erythematosus: experience in sixteen consecutive patients. Br J Rheumatol 1997; 36: 353–359.
53. Callen JP. New and emerging therapies for collagen-vascular diseases. Dermatol Clin 2000; 18: 139–146.
54. Goyal S, Nousari HC. Treatment of resistant discoid lupus erythematosus of the palms and soles with myophenolate mofetil. J Am Acad Dermatol 2001; 45: 142–144.
55. Wilke WS, Krall PL, Scheetz RJ et al. Methotrexate for systemic lupus erythematosus: a retrospective analysis or 17 unselected cases. Clin Exp Rheumatol 1991; 9: 581–587.
56. Rahman P, Humphrey-Murto S, Gladman DD, Urowitz MB. Efficacy and tolerability of methotrexate in antimalarial resistant lupus arthritis. J Rheumatol 1998; 25: 243–246.
57. Kipen Y, Littlejohn GO, Morand EF. Methotrexate use in systemic lupus erythematosus. Lupus 1997; 6: 385–389.
58. Sato EI. Methotrexate therapy in systemic lupus erythematosus. Lupus 2001; 10: 162–164.
59. Hjortkjoer Petersen H, Nielsen H, Hansen M, Stensgaard-Hansen F, Helin P. High-dose immunoglobulin therapy in pericarditis caused by SLE. Scand J Rheumatol 1990; 19: 91–93.
60. Meissner M, Sherer Y, Levy Y, Chwalinska-Sadowska H, Langevitz P, Shoenfeld Y. Intravenous immunoglobulin therapy in a patient with lupus serositis and nephritis. Rheumatol Int 2000; 19: 199–201.
61. Erickson RW, Franklin WA, Emlen W. Treatment of hemorrhagic lupus pneumonitis with plasmapheresis. Semin Arthritis Rheum 1994; 24: 114–123.
62. Eiser AR, Shanies HM. Treatment of lupus interstitial lung disease with intravenous cyclophosphamide. Arthritis Rheum. 1994; 37: 428–431.
63. Robbins IM, Gaine SP, Schilz R, Tapson VF, Rubin LJ, Loyd JE. Epoprostenol for treatment of pulmonary hypertension in patients with systemic lupus erythematosus. Chest. 2000 ; 117: 14–18.
64. Mok MY, Tse HF, Lau CS. Pulmonary hypertension secondary to systemic lupus erythematosus: prolonged survival following treatment with intermittent low dose iloprost. Lupus. 1999; 8: 328–331.
65. Oudiz RJ, Schilz RJ, Arneson C, Jeffs RA. Treprostinil (Remodulin) in connective tissue disease associated pulmonary hypertension. Presented at the American College of Rheumatology Annual Meeting, "Late Breaking Abstract #4," San Francisco, November, 2001.
66. Channick RN, Simonneau G, Sitbon O et al. Effects of the dual endothelin-receptor antagonist bosentan in patients with pulmonary hypertension: a randomised placebo-controlled study. Lancet. 2001; 358: 1113–1114.
67. Sato N, Kyotani S, Sakamaki F, Nagaya N, Oya H, Nakanishi N. Pulmonary thrombo-endarterectomy for chronic pulmonary thromboembolism in three patients with systemic lupus erythematosus and antiphospholipid syndrome. Nihon Kokyuki Gakkai Zasshi 2000; 38: 958–964.
68. Naarendorp M, Kerr LD, Khan AS, Ornstein MH Dramatic improvement of left ventricular function after cytotoxic therapy in lupus patients with acute cardio-myopathy: report of 6 cases. J Rheumatol 1999; 26: 2257–2260.
69. Fairfax MJ, Osborn TG, Williams GA, Tsai CC, Moore TL Endomyocardial biopsy in patients with systemic lupus erythematosus. J Rheumatol 1988; 15: 593–596.
70. Sherer Y, Levy Y, Shoenfeld Y. Marked improvement of severe cardiac dysfunction after one course of intravenous immunoglobulin in a patient with systemic lupus erythematosus. Clin Rheumatol 1999; 18: 238–240.
71. Pirofsky B. Immune haemolytic disease: the autoimmune haemolytic anaemias. Clin Haematol. 1975; 4: 167–80.
72. Ahn YS, Harrington WJ, Mylvaganam R, Ayub J, Pall LM. Danazol therapy for auto-immune hemolytic anemia. Ann Intern Med. 1985; 102: 298–301.
73. Cervera H, Jara LJ, Pizarro S et al. Danazol for systemic lupus erythematosus with refractory autoimmune thrombocytopenia or Evans' syndrome. J Rheumatol 1995; 22: 1867–1871.
74. Majer RV, Hyde RD. High-dose intravenous immunoglobulin in the treatment of autoimmune haemolytic anaemia. Clin Lab Haematol 1988; 10: 391–395.
75. von Keyserlingk H, Meyer-Sabellek W, Arntz R, Haller H. Plasma exchange treatment in autoimmune hemolytic anemia of the warm antibody type with renal failure. Vox Sang. 1987; 52: 298–300.
76. al-Shahi R, Mason JC, Rao R, Hurd C, Thompson EM, Haskard DO, Davies KA. Systemic lupus erythematosus, thrombocytopenia, microangiopathic haemolytic anaemia and anti-CD36 antibodies. Br J Rheumatol 1997; 36: 794–798.
77. Euler HH, Harten P, Zeuner RA, Schwab UM.Recombinant human granulocyte colony stimulating factor in patients with systemic lupus erythematosus associated neutropenia and refractory infections. J Rheumatol 1997; 24: 2153–2157.
78. Hellmich B, Schnabel A, Gross WL. Treatment of severe neutropenia due to Felty's syndrome or systemic lupus erythematosus with granulocyte colony-stimulating factor. Semin Arthritis Rheum 1999; 29: 82–99.
79. Godeau B, Coutant-Perronne V, Le Thi Huong D et al. Pneumocystis carinii pneumonia in the course of connective tissue disease: report of 34 cases. J Rheumatol. 1994; 21: 246–251.
80. Morton SJ, Powell RJ. An audit of cyclosporin for systemic lupus erythematosus and related overlap syndromes: limitations of its use. Ann Rheum Dis 2000; 59: 487–489.
81. Sugiyama M Ogasawara H, Kaneko H et al. Effect of extremely low dose cyclosporin on the thrombocytopenia in systemic lupus erythematosus. Lupus 1998; 7: 53–56.
82. Blanco R, Martinez-Taboada VM, Rodriguez-Valverde V, Sanchez-Andrade A, Gonzalez-Gay MA. Successful therapy with danazol in refractory autoimmune thrombocytopenia associated with rheumatic diseases. Br J Rheumatol 1997; 36: 1095–1099.
83. Nishina M, Saito E, Kinoshita M. Correction of severe leukocytopenia and thrombocy-topenia in systemic lupus erythematosus by treatment with dapsone. J Rheumatol 1997; 24: 811–812.

84. Boumpas DT, Barez S, Klippel JH, Balow JE. Intermittent cyclophosphamide for the treatment of autoimmune thrombocytopenia in systemic lupus erythematosus. Ann Intern Med 1990; 112: 674–677.

85. Feinglass S, Deodar A. Treatment of lupus-induced thrombocytopenia with recombinant human interleukin-11. Arthritis Rheum 2001; 44: 170–175.

86. Vaidya S, Abul-ezz S, Lipsmeyer E. Thrombotic thrombocytopenic purpura and systemic lupus erythematosus. Scand J Rheumatol 2001; 30: 308–310.

87. Perez-Sanchez I, Anguita J, Pintado T. Use of cyclophosphamide in the treatment of thrombotic thrombocytopenic purpura complicating systemic lupus erythematosus: report of two cases. Ann Hematol 1999; 78: 285-287.

88. Boumpas DT, Yamada H, Patronas NJ, Scott D, Klippel JH, Balow JE. Pulse cyclophosphamide for severe neuropsychiatric lupus. QJ Med 1991; 81: 975–984.

89. Neuwelt CM, Lacks S, Kaye BR, Ellman JB, Borenstein DG. Role of intravenous cyclophosphamide in the treatment of severe neuropsychiatric systemic lupus erythematosus. Am J Med 1995; 98: 32–41.

90. Ramos PC, Mendez MJ, Ames PR, Khamashta MA, Hughes GR. Pulse cyclophosphamide in the treatment of neuropsychiatric systemic lupus erythematosus. Clin Exp Rheumatol 1996; 14: 295–299.

91. Viertel A, Weidmann E, Wigand R, Geiger H, Mondorf UF. Treatment of severe systemic lupus erythematosus with immunoadsorption and intravenous immunoglobulins. Intensive Care Med 2000; 26: 823–824.

92. Levy Y, Sherer Y, Ahmed A et al. A study of 20 SLE patients with intravenous immunoglobulin – clinical and serologic response. Lupus 1999; 8: 705–712.

93. Valesini G, Priori R, Francia A et al. Central nervous system involvement in systemic lupus erythematosus: a new therapeutic approach with intrathecal dexamethasone and methotrexate. Springer Semin Immunopathol 1994; 16: 313–321.

94. Harisdangkul V, Doorenbos D, Subramony SH. Lupus transverse myelopathy: better outcome with early recognition and aggressive high-dose intravenous corticosteroid pulse treatment. J Neurol 1995; 242: 326–331.

95. Sanchez-Guerrero J, Liang MH, Karlson EW, Hunter DJ, Colditz GA. Postmenopausal estrogen therapy and the risk for developing systemic lupus erythematosus. Ann Intern Med 1995; 122: 430–433.

96. Kreidstein S, Urowitz MB, Gladman DD, Gough J. Hormone replacement therapy in systemic lupus erythematosus. J Rheumatol 1997; 24: 2149–2152.

97. Mok CC, Lau CS, Ho CT, Lee KW, Mok MY, Wong RW. Safety of hormonal replacement therapy in postmenopausal patients with systemic lupus erythematosus. Scand J Rheumatol 1998; 27: 342–346.

98. Sanchez-Guerrero J, Gonzalez-Perez M, Durand-Carbajal M, Lara-Reyes P, Bahina-Amezcua S, Cravioto MC. Effect of hormone replacement therapy (HRT) on disease activity in postmenopausal patients with SLE. A two year follow-up clinical trial. Arthritis Rheum 2001; 44 (Suppl): S263.

99. Walker SE. Treatment of systemic lupus erythematosus with bromocriptine. Lupus 2001; 10: 197–202.

100. Morikawa K, Oseko F, Morikawa S. Immunosuppressive property of bromocriptine on human B lymphocyte function in vitro. Clin Exp Immunol 1993; 93: 200–205.

101. McMurray RW, Allen SH, Braun All, Rodriguez F, Walker SE. Longstanding hyperprolactinemia assoicated with systemic lupus erythematosus: possible hormonal stimulation an autoimmune disease. J Rheumatol 1994; 21: 843–850.

102. McMurray RW, Weidensaul D, Allen SH, Walker SE. Efficacy of bromocriptine in an open label therapeutic trial for systemic lupus erythematosus. J Rheumatol 1995; 22: 2084–2091.

103. Buskila D, Lorber M, Neumann L, Flusser D, Shoenfeld Y. No correlation between prolactin levels and clinical activity in patients with systemic lupus erythematosus. J Rheumatol 1996; 23: 629–632.

104. Jimena P, Aguirre MA, Lopez-Curbelo A, de Andres M, Garcia-Courtay C, Cuadrado MD. Prolactin levels in patients with systemic lupus erythematosus: a case controlled study. Lupus 1998; 7: 383–386.

105. Alvarez-Nemegyei J, Cobarrubias-Cobos A, Escalante-Triay F, Sosa-Munoz J, Miranda JM, Jara LJ. Bromocriptine in systemic lupus erythematosus: a double-blind, randomized, placebo-controlled study. Lupus 1998; 7: 414–419.

106. McMurray RW. Bromocriptine in rheumatic and autoimmune diseases. Semin Arthritis Rheum 2001; 31: 21–32.

107. Van Vollenhoven RF, Engleman EF, McGuire JL. An open study of dehydroepiandrosterone in systemic lupus erythematosus. Arthritis Rheum 1994; 37: 1305–1310.

108. Suzuki T, Suzuki N, Daynes RA, Engleman EG. Dehydroepiandrosterone enhances IL-2 production and cytotoxic effector function of human T cells. Clin Immunol Immunopathol 1991; 61: 202–211.

109. Von Vollenhoven RF, Morabito LM, Engleman EG, McGuire JL. Treatment of systemic lupus erythematosus with dehydroepidandrosterone: 50 patients treated up to 12 months. J Rheumatol 1998; 25: 285–289.

110. Petri MA, Lahita RG, van Vollenhoven RF et al. Systemic lupus erythematosus and autoimmunity effects of prasterone on corticosteroid requirements of women with systemic lupus erythematosus: a double-blind, randomized, placebo-controlled trial. Arthritis Rheum 2002; 46: 1820–1829.

111. Mease PJ, Ginzler EM, Gluck OS et al. Improvement in bone mineral density in steroid-treated SLE patients during treatment with GL701 (prasterone, dehydroepiandrosterone). Arthritis Rheum 2000; 43 (Suppl): S271.

112. Robinzon B, Cutolo M. Should dehydroepiandrosterone replacement therapy be provided with glucocorticoids? Rheumatology 1999; 38: 488–495.

113. Wierzbicki AS. Lipid-lowering drugs in lupus: an unexplored therapeutic intervention. Lupus 2001; 10: 233–236.

127 Treatment – renal involvement

Dimitrios T Boumpas, Gabor G Illei and James E Balow

- Urinalysis is the single most useful test to monitor for renal involvement and relapses after remission

- In moderate to severe proliferative lupus nephritis, neither pulse methylprednisolone of any duration nor short-term pulse cyclophosphamide is as effective as extended courses of pulse cyclophosphamide, with the combination of both being more effective. Plasmapheresis has no benefit when added to standard immunosuppressive therapy

- Combinations of mycophenolate mofetil (MMF) with high doses of corticosteroids are effective in inducing remission in the short term in patients with mild to moderate lupus nephritis, but flares are common when the drug is discontinued

- Patients with mild proliferative disease may benefit from corticosteroids, either alone or in combination with azathioprine

- Patients with membranous disease may benefit from corticosteroids alone or in combination with cyclosporine or cyclophosphamide

- Approximately one-third of lupus patients with moderate to severe proliferative lupus nephritis will relapse after achieving partial or complete remission

- Short courses (3–6 months) of daily or intermittent pulse cyclophosphamide result in responses of limited duration, emphasizing the need for some form of maintenance therapy

- In lupus nephritis aggressive control of blood pressure and dyslipidemia is of paramount importance

INTRODUCTION

Effective treatment in lupus nephritis depends on the recognition of early phases of renal involvement, prior to scarring, atrophy and fibrosis. However, many forms of lupus renal disease, including severe forms of glomerulonephritis, are asymptomatic and insidiously progressive, and clinicians can easily overlook them. The marked heterogeneity among individual patients in terms of pattern and evolution of disease, and response to treatment, presents additional challenges. Yet, notwithstanding the capricious nature of the disease and its intrinsic complexities and subtleties, nephritis is one of the most gratifying aspects of lupus to treat because the majority of patients respond well and eventually reach long-lasting remission.

In this chapter we review selected aspects of the diagnosis and assessment of lupus nephritis, and discuss its treatment based on current evidence from randomized controlled trials. For management issues that have not been adequately studied, we present the experience of investigators in the field and indicate our own preferences.

DIAGNOSIS AND ASSESSMENT OF DISEASE ACTIVITY

Although in published series almost all patients have positive results for antinuclear antibodies (ANA), there are a small number of patients with classic lupus nephritis and either negative or low-positive titers below the laboratory cut-off. At the other end of the spectrum are lupus patients with nephritis but very little evidence of immune complex disease. A careful exclusion of other causes of nephritis should not prevent the physician from establishing the tentative diagnosis of lupus and initiating therapy.

Clinical presentation

In large centers, almost half of the patients present with asymptomatic urine abnormalities such as hematuria and proteinuria. Nocturia and/or foamy urine are common initial complaints but rarely volunteered by the patient unless specifically asked about[1]. Persistent glomerular hematuria is common in lupus nephritis but rarely found without concomitant proteinuria, which is the dominant feature of lupus nephritis. Nephritic syndrome accounts for an additional 30–40% of patients, but rapidly progressive glomerulonephritis is rarer and accounts for less than 10% of initial presentations. Hypocomplementemia (especially C3) and anti-DNA antibodies are commonly found in lupus patients with renal disease. In general, renal involvement tends to appear within the first 2 years of lupus, with its frequency decreasing significantly after the first 5 years.

The clinical presentation does not always predict the underlying histological class of nephritis. This is especially true in patients on therapy that may modify findings. In general, patients with mesangial nephritis have small amounts of proteinuria (<1g/day) with hematuria but typically no cellular casts. Patients with membranous glomerulopathy have proteinuria, often at nephrotic range but otherwise blunt urine sediments. C3 tends to be normal and anti-DNA antibodies, when present, are usually found in low titers. In contrast, patients with proliferative nephritis have hypertension, nephritic urine sediment with various degrees of proteinuria (often at nephritic range), low C3 and typically high titers of anti-DNA antibodies.

In lupus nephritis proteinuria reflects the extent of involvement of peripheral glomerular capillary loops and tends to increase incrementally from mesangial to proliferative to membranous nephropathy. The latter involves all glomerular capillary loops and is characteristically accompanied by heavy proteinuria.

Urinalysis

Urinalysis is the most important and effective method to detect and monitor disease activity in lupus nephritis. In order to ensure its quality, several steps have to be taken. These include expeditious examination of a fresh, early-morning midstream, clean-catch, non-refrigerated specimen; flagging of specimens from patients at substantial risk of developing nephritis; and (ideally) personal review of the urine sediment[1]. Hematuria (usually microscopic, rarely macroscopic) indicates inflammatory glomerular or tubulointerstitial disease. Erythrocytes are fragmented or misshapen (dysmorphic) (Fig. 127.1). Granular and fatty casts reflect proteinuric states, whereas red blood cell, white blood cell and mixed cellular casts reflect nephritic states. Broad and waxy casts

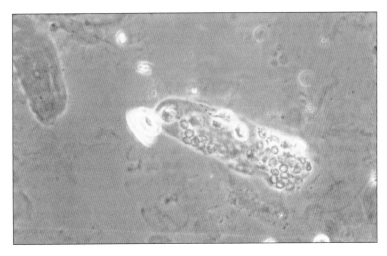

Fig. 127.1 Microscopy of urine. A tubular cast containing red cells, which usually indicates a glomerular origin for concomitant hematuria and in general an active proliferative/infiltrative glomerular disease ($\times$ 400, phase contrast). Courtesy of Dr GB Fogazzi.

TABLE 127.2 ACTIVITY AND CHRONICITY INDICES

Activity index (lesions are scored 0–3+, with maximum score 24 points)

- Hypercellularity: endocapillary proliferation compromising glomerular capillary loops
- Leukocyte exudation: polymorphonuclear leukocytes in glomeruli
- Karyorrhexis/fibrinoid necrosis (weighted ×2): necrotizing changes in glomeruli
- Cellular crescents (weighted ×2): layers of proliferating epithelial cells and monocytes lining Bowman's capsule
- Hyaline deposits: eosinophilic and PAS-positive materials lining (wire loops) or filling (hyaline thrombi) capillary loops
- Interstitial inflammation: infiltration of leukocytes (predominantly mononuclear cells) among tubules

Chronicity index (lesions are scored 0–3+, with maximum score 12 points)

- Glomerular sclerosis: collapse and fibrosis of capillary tufts
- Fibrous crescents: layers of fibrous tissue lining Bowman's capsule
- Tubular atrophy: thickening of tubular basement membranes, tubular epithelial degeneration, with separation of residual tubules
- Interstitial fibrosis: deposition of collagenous connective tissue among tubules

Scored on a scale of 0–3 representing either (a) absent, mild, moderate and severe lesions, or (b) the presence of lesions in none, <25%, 25–50% and 50% of glomeruli, respectively. (Modified from Balow *et al.*[1])

reflect chronic renal failure. In severe proliferative disease, urine sediment containing the full range of cells and casts can be found ('telescopic urine sediment') as a result of severe glomerular and tubular ongoing disease superimposed on chronic renal damage.

Renal biopsy

Renal biopsy rarely helps the diagnosis of lupus, but is the best way of documenting the renal pathology. In addition to the WHO classification (Table 127.1), a semiquantitative analysis (on a scale of 0–3+) of specific histologic features is incorporated into the elements of the activity and chronicity indices (Table 127.2). In several studies of lupus nephritis, type IV nephritis is the most common (approximately 40%), and types III and V follow with an approximate frequency of 25% and 15%, respectively. Transformation from one class to another can occur both spontaneously and as a result of treatment. In the absence of renal abnormalities, renal biopsy has nothing to offer and should not be performed. Standard indications for renal biopsy and general considerations are found in Table 127.3. Practical considerations in evaluating renal biopsy are shown in Table 127.4. Studies have suggested (and ex-

TABLE 127.3 INDICATIONS FOR RENAL BIOPSY IN LUPUS NEPHRITIS

Initial biopsy (before treatment)	Nephritic urine sediment (glomerular hematuria and cellular casts) Glomerural hematuria with proteinuria >0.5–1.0g/day Glomerular hematuria with proteinuria <0.3–0.5g/day and low C3 and/or positive anti-ds DNA Proteinuria >1.0–2.0g/day (especially if C3 is low and/or positive anti-ds DNA)
Repeat biopsy (during or after treatment)	Unexplained worsening proteinuria (e.g. >2g/day increase if non-nephrotic at baseline, or >50% increase if nephrotic) Unexplained worsening of renal function (e.g. reproducible ≥30% increase in serum creatinine) Persistent glomerular hematuria with proteinuria >2g/day or proteinuria >3g/day (especially if C3 is decreased) Nephritic or nephrotic flare

Selected patients with clinical and laboratory evidence of severe lupus nephritis, nephritic or nephrotic syndrome, azotemia and hypertension may not require a renal biopsy prior to treatment with cytotoxic drugs. On the other hand, patients with concomitant serologic abnormalities (i.e. low C3, positive anti-ds DNA) or patients who had previous immunosuppressive treatment may be candidates for renal biopsy even with more subtle findings.

TABLE 127.1 HISTOLOGICAL FEATURES OF THE VARIOUS TYPES OF LUPUS NEPHRITIS

WHO type	
Class I	Normal histology
Class II	Mesangial expansion with cell or matrix; preservation of mostly intact capillary loops. Mesangial immune deposits
Class III	Proliferative, necrotizing or sclerosing lesions affecting less than 50% of glomeruli. Compromised capillary loop lumens by leukocyte infiltration, endocapillary proliferation and endothelial cell swelling and proliferation. Subendothelial immune deposits
Class IV	Same as in class III but affecting more than 50% of glomeruli. Loss of the capillary space is the hallmark
Class V	Widespread basement membrane thickening. Numerous immune deposits early on at epimembranous (subepithelial) and later at intramembranous locations*

* Patients with membranous nephropathy associated with focal or diffuse proliferative lesions are best categorized as class III or IV lesions because prognosis and therapy are dictated by the latter.

perience supports) that both patients and physicians are more willing to make decisions on aggressive therapies when faced with a renal biopsy indicating severe renal involvement[2]. This in turn translates into earlier institution of cytotoxic therapy and better renal outcomes.

Monitoring of lupus nephritis

Renal function

Serum creatinine is a practical but relatively insensitive early indicator of abnormalities in glomerular filtration rate (GFR). Its absolute level is affected by muscle mass and age, as well as GFR. In clinical practice, changes in renal function are more important to detect than absolute

TABLE 127.4 EVALUATION OF RENAL BIOPSY IN LUPUS NEPHRITIS

- Ensure that sample is adequate
- Evaluation of specimens with fewer than 10 glomeruli is suboptimal
- Light microscopy stains
  - Hematoxylin–eosin: best to identify inflammatory cells
  - Trichrome (Masson): best for interstitial fibrosis, glomerulosclerosis
  - Periodic-acid–Schiff (PAS): best for basement membrane abnormalities
- Immunofluorescence studies do not help if diagnosis of lupus is established
- Electron microscopy helps to define distribution (i.e. subendothelial, epithelial, membranous deposits) of immune complexes
- Activity and chronicity indices are useful in organizing renal biopsy report as a complement to WHO classification
- Most important elements to recognize and consider:
  - Activity index: crescents, fibrinoid necrosis
  - Chronicity index: interstitial fibrosis, tubular atrophy, glomerular sclerosis
  - Moderate to high chronicity scores (e.g. >3)

TABLE 127.5 GENERALLY ACCEPTED FACTORS ASSOCIATED WITH ADVERSE PROGNOSIS AND HIGH RISK OF RENAL PROGRESSION IN LUPUS NEPHRITIS

- **Demographic:** Black race; limited access to healthcare (male gender, children)
- **Clinical:** Hypertension; severe extrarenal disease affecting major organ; failure to achieve or marked delay (e.g. >2 years) to renal remission; multiple flares of lupus nephritis; pregnancy
- **Laboratory:** Nephritic urinary sediment; azotemia; anemia; thrombocytopenia; antiphospholipid antibodies; thrombotic microangiopathy; hypocomplementemia (especially falling levels); high anti-DNA (especially rising titers); persistent severe nephrotic syndrome
- **Histologic:** Proliferative glomerulonephritis (WHO class III, IV); mixed membranous (V) and proliferative (III–IV) glomerulonephritis; cellular crescents; fibrinoid necrosis; very high activity index; moderate to high chronicity index[#]; Combinations of active (e.g. cellular crescents) and chronic histologic features (e.g. interstitial fibrosis); extensive subendothelial deposits

Factors with contentious level of impact are shown in parentheses. (Modified from Balow *et al.*[1])

values, and this is best achieved by measuring creatinine clearance. Creatinine clearance is being used only rarely because of several shortcomings, the most important of which is overestimation of true GFR with declining renal function. Serum creatinine measurement is a more practical approach for detecting changes in GFR and is the examination of choice. Significant reproducible changes in serum creatinine (e.g. $\geq$ 20–30% increase) are of concern even if they fall within the normal range, as they indicate significant loss of renal function.

Urine collections

Two or three timed collections of urine to determine 24-hour protein excretion and baseline creatinine clearance is the gold standard. We obtain them before therapy and periodically thereafter, prior to making decisions regarding response and changes to therapy. Collections of urine containing creatinine concentrations that deviate significantly from population averages of 20mg/kg/day (males) or 15mg/kg/day (females) should raise suspicions about the adequacy of the collection. Spot urine protein/creatinine is a simpler method to estimate the severity of proteinuria and could be used in between 24-hour collections (together with serum albumin and cholesterol levels) to provide rough estimates of the response of proteinuria to therapy. In general the numeric ratio approaches the number of grams per day of proteinuria. For example, if the ratio is 2.3 the 24-hour protein excretion is approximately 2.3g/day.

Urinalysis

Resolution of active urine sediment is a feature of renal remission, but to be clinically meaningful has to be sustained for several months. The reappearance of cellular casts with significant proteinuria is an early and reliable predictor of renal relapse, and in most patients usually precedes rises in anti-DNA titers or decreases in C3 by several weeks[3].

Serology

Anti-DNA antibodies and C3 and C4 complement components are useful in monitoring the activity of lupus nephritis and in guiding treatment. In general, changes in anti-DNA titers are more valuable than their absolute values. Patients with rising titers of anti-DNA antibodies warrant close monitoring for evidence of lupus activity. Because C4 deficiency is common in lupus patients; values of C3 and C4 are rarely discordant; and C3 levels correlate best with renal histology on repeat renal biopsies, C3 is the preferred choice for monitoring. Plasma and urinary cytokines or chemokines, or urinary podocytes, may reflect lupus activity, but these tests are not currently used in routine clinical practice.

Assessment of prognosis

Prognosis varies greatly among the many clinical and pathologic forms of lupus nephritis and therefore has important implications for treatment decisions. Numerous demographic and clinical variables can affect prognosis, and individual patients have unique combinations of such risk factors (Table 127.5). Although individual risk factors are extremely heterogeneous and vary in their overall impact, patients with more factors have a worse prognosis and thus need more aggressive treatment. Patient characteristics associated with bad outcomes include black race, azotemia, anemia, failure to respond to initial immunosuppressive therapy, and flares with worsening in renal function. Combinations of severe active (crescents and fibrinoid necrosis) and marked chronic changes (moderate to severe tubulointerstitial fibrosis and tubular atrophy, e.g chronicity index >3) are particularly ominous[4]. The impact of race on determining severity of disease, response to treatment and final outcome is becoming increasingly apparent[4–6]. Significant differences in these risk factors may explain the marked heterogeneity in course, prognosis and treatment responses in randomized controlled studies around the world (see below).

OVERVIEW OF CONTROLLED TRIALS

Of all aspects of lupus, nephritis has been studied most extensively in controlled trials. Still, the total number of patients included thus far is, surprisingly, less than 1000 (approximately 750). Even controlled trials (typically conducted in major referral centers, where patients typically have more severe disease) have been plagued by generic problems, including small numbers of patients, diverse racial mixes and socioeconomic backgrounds, and relatively short follow-up. Because proliferative lupus nephritis has a higher prevalence and worse prognosis most trials have historically involved patients with this type of nephritis.

Corticosteroids and cytotoxic drugs

Controlled studies have established the benefit of cyclophosphamide in combination with corticosteroids in lupus nephritis. Although controlled trials of corticosteroids alone have not been conducted (and in spite of their toxicity), most clinicians feel that their use is warranted at least in the short and medium term, as they have dramatically improved the outcome of lupus nephritis. Short-term ($\leq$6 months) daily oral cyclophosphamide therapy is more efficacious in decreasing disease activity than prednisone alone[7], but it did not protect from renal failure with longer follow-up[8]. This is in contrast to long-term (i.e. until sustained remission is achieved) daily oral cyclophosphamide therapy, which has been shown to reduce the risk of renal failure[9]. Because of the cumulative toxicity of extended courses of daily oral cyclophosphamide this regimen has been abandoned and only short courses are being used. Intermittent pulse cyclophosphamide therapy was shown to be equally effective as daily oral cyclophosphamide but with significantly fewer side effects[9], and the former has become the preferred approach. In the same studies there was no significant difference in outcomes between those treated with corticosteroids, continuous or intermittent cyclophosphamide and azathioprine; however, it could be argued that the small number of patients would preclude the detection of small differences. More notable differences between the various groups became apparent only after the fifth year of the study, emphasizing the importance of long-term follow-up in studies of lupus nephritis[9,10].

Following demonstration of the efficacy of prolonged courses of quarterly pulse cyclophosphamide, subsequent trials were designed to evaluate shorter monthly pulses of cyclophosphamide or methylprednisolone, or longer courses of these agents alone, or the combination of the two. In patients with severe proliferative lupus nephritis (defined as renal impairment or histologic features of very active disease, such as crescents and fibrinoid necrosis in >25% of glomeruli) shorter courses of cyclophosphamide were marginally better than methylprednisolone and less effective than a long course (7 monthly doses followed by quarterly pulses for an additional 2 years) in preventing major flares[11]. In the other study, extended courses (12 months, up to 36 months) of pulse methylprednisolone were not as effective as long courses (3–5 years) of pulse cyclophosphamide[12]. Moreover, the majority of the patients who initially received methylprednisolone eventually required cyclophosphamide for the control of continuous renal disease or renal flares. Extended follow-up (median 11 years) of the study demonstrated greater efficacy of the combination therapy than with cyclophosphamide alone, without a significant increase in toxicity[13]. In another study[14] limited courses (approximately 12 months) of pulse cyclophosphamide or pulse methylprednisolone showed no differences in renal outcomes in the short term.

Plasmapheresis has been studied in several controlled trials of lupus nephritis. All have shown no benefit of adding plasmapheresis to standard immunosuppression with prednisone and cyclophosphamide[15].

Mycophenolate mofetil

Myophenolate mofetil (MMF, 2g/day) was compared to daily oral cyclophosphamide in a controlled trial of 42 patients with mild diffuse proliferative glomerulonephritis. After 6 months, the dose of MMF was decreased to 1g/day. Both groups received azathioprine as maintenance after the first year of the study. There were no differences 2 years later between the two groups in terms of achieving renal remission[16]; however, with longer follow-up there were significantly more relapses in the MMF group. The study was underpowered to prove equivalence of the two drugs.

Conclusions

Neither pulse methylprednisolone of any duration nor short-term pulse cyclophosphamides is as efficacious as extended courses of pulse cyclophosphamide, with the combination of both being more effective. Short courses (3–6 months) of daily or intermittent pulse cyclophosphamide result in responses of limited duration, emphasizing the need for some form of maintenance therapy. There is circumstantial evidence that azathioprine may have a corticosteroid-sparing effect, and that may be marginally better than corticosteroids alone. Studies evaluating azathioprine as maintenance therapy are in progress. Combinations of MMF with high doses of corticosteroids are effective in inducing remission in the short term in patients with mild to moderate lupus nephritis, but flares are common when the drug is discontinued. Plasmapheresis has no benefit when added to standard immunosuppressive therapy.

TREATMENT OPTIONS

Corticosteroids

Most standard immunosuppressive drugs have been used in the management of lupus nephritis. Corticosteroids are effective in inducing rapid control and are included in all treatment regimens. Intravenous pulses of methylprednisolone have become a popular part of initial treatment, following their successful use in transplant rejection in the early 1970s and in Goodpasture syndrome. No formal studies have examined whether they are more efficacious than daily oral corticosteroids or whether there is a significant difference between the two main dosages employed (e.g. 1000mg vs 1g/m²). However, it is the impression of many clinicians that they are more effective to control a rapidly evolving glomerulonephritis, and that when employed in combination with moderate doses of daily corticosteroid, the severity of side effects such as cushingoid appearance, acne and hirsutism may be lessened. Slow infusion over 60 minutes with monitoring of blood pressure and serum glucose (in selected patients), along with a careful search for underlying hidden or low-grade infections (usually in the urinary tract), is essential. Because glucocorticoids inhibit the production of vasodilatory prostaglandins in the kidney, renal perfusion may decrease and serum creatinine may increase for a few days after infusion. Although earlier observations suggested that avascular necrosis of the bone is more common with pulse corticosteroids, subsequent studies have failed to confirm these observations[13]. Recent data suggest that chronic glucocorticoid use induces apoptosis not only in osteoblasts but also in osteocytes, and that these mechanisms may be involved in corticosteroid-induced osteoporosis and osteonecrosis. Bisphosphonates inhibit the apoptosis of these cells and theoretically could prevent osteonecrosis[17]. Early use of corticosteroids in sufficient doses to control acute nephritis, coupled with a regular testing of the feasibility of reducing doses to alternate days by employing additional immunosuppressive drugs is critical, and physicians should not hesitate to use them under these conditions for fear of side effects. Alternate-day prednisone has a modest effect of improving growth in children, in reducing certain infections, and apparently a more powerful benefit in reducing their deleterious effects on the hypothalamopituitary–adrenal axis.

Cytotoxic agents

The use of oral cyclophosphamide for more than 2–3 months is rare in lupus nephritis because of its bladder and other toxicities. Because of their attractive risk/benefit ratio, intermittent pulses of cyclophosphamide have become the cytotoxic agent of choice for moderate to severe disease. Inconvenience related to its administration and the fear of leukopenia, has led groups in Europe to use smaller doses (500mg every 2 weeks) than the NIH protocol (0.75–1g/m² monthly during the induction phase)[18]. Formal testing of the former protocol in a controlled trial is under way (this protocol includes six fortnightly infusions of 500mg IV cyclophosphamide versus eight infusions of 0.75–1g/m² over 1 year) with azathioprine as maintenance therapy[19]. The protocol for the administration of cyclophosphamide that was established at NIH can be found in Table 127.6[1]. Forceful diuresis, the use of antiemetic agents, dose adjustments to keep a safe white blood cell count (WBC) of at least 1500µl and concomitant use of modest doses of corticosteroids (0.5mg/kg/day) have been key elements to its low level of toxicity. In this protocol, when intravenous methylprednisolone is being used in combination with cyclophosphamide it is usually administered just prior to cyclophosphamide because of its antiemetic effects.

Herpes zoster infections are common with pulse cyclophosphamide therapy but are rarely severe or life threatening. Control studies of pulse cyclophosphamide for lupus nephritis have not reported an increased incidence of malignancy, except for an increased incidence of cervical dysplasia, associated in most cases with concurrent human papillo-

TABLE 127.6 NIH PROTOCOL FOR ADMINISTRATION AND MONITORING OF PULSE CYCLOPHOSPHAMIDE THERAPY

- Estimate creatinine clearance by standard methods
- Calculate body surface area (m²): BSA= ⌐Height (cm) × Weight (kg)/3600
- Cyclophosphamide (Cytoxan) (CY) dosing and administration:
  - Initial dose 0.75g/m² (0.5g/m² if creatinine clearance rate is less than one-third of expected normal)
  - Administer CY in 150ml normal saline IV over 30–60min (alternative: equivalent dose of pulse CY may be taken orally in highly motivated and compliant patients)
- WBC at days 10 and 14 after each CY treatment (patient should delay prednisone until after blood tests drawn to avoid transient corticosteroid-induced leukocytosis)
- Adjust subsequent doses of CY to maximum of 1.0g/m² to keep nadir WBC above 1500/l. If WBC nadir falls below 1500/l decrease next dose by 25%
- Repeat CY doses monthly (every 3 weeks in patients with extremely aggressive disease) for 6 months (7 pulses), then quarterly for 1 year after remission is achieved (inactive urine sediment, proteinuria <1g/day, normalization of complement (and ideally anti-DNA), and minimal or no extrarenal lupus activity)
- Protect bladder against CY-induced hemorrhagic cystitis:
  - Diuresis with 5% dextrose and 0.45% saline (e.g. 2 liters at 250ml/h). Frequent voiding; continue high-dose oral fluids for 24h. Patients return to clinic if they cannot sustain an adequate fluid intake
  - Consider Mesna (each dose 20% of total CY dose) intravenously or orally at 0, 2, 4 and 6h after CY dosing. Mesna is especially important to use if sustained diuresis may be difficult to achieve, or if pulse CY is administered in outpatient setting
  - If anticipated difficulty with sustaining diuresis (e.g. severe nephrotic syndrome) or with voiding (e.g. neurogenic bladder) insert a three-way urinary catheter with continuous bladder flushing using standard antibiotic irrigating solution (e.g. 3 liters) or normal saline for 24h to minimize risk of hemorrhagic cystitis
- Antiemetics (usually administered orally):
  - Dexamethasone 10mg single dose plus:
  - Serotonin receptor antagonists: Granisetron 1mg with CY dose (usually repeat dose in 12 hours); ondasetrone 8mg tid for 1–2 days
- Monitor fluid balance during hydration. Use diuresis if patient develops progressive fluid accumulation
- Complications of pulse CY:
  - **Expected**: nausea and vomiting (central effect of CY), mostly controlled by serotonin receptor antagonists; transient hair thinning (rarely severe at CY doses ≤1g/m²)
  - **Common**: significant infection diathesis only if leukopenia not carefully controlled; modest increase in herpes zoster (very low risk of dissemination); infertility (male and female); amenorrhea proportional to age of the patient during treatment and to the cumulative dose of CY. In females at high risk for persistent amenorrhea may consider using leuprolide 3.75mg subcutaneously 2 weeks prior to each dose of cyclophosphamide. In males may use testosterone 100mg intramuscularly every 2 weeks

(Modified from Balow et al.[1])

mavirus (HPV) infections. In view of these reports, vigilance in monitoring for cervical carcinoma is essential.

Of all toxicities associated with cyclophosphamide therapy perhaps the most disturbing is its gonadal toxicity. In women the risk of sustained amenorrhea is dependent on the age of the patient and the cumulative dose. In our series, the rates of amenorrhea after a long course (≥15 pulses) of cyclophosphamide was 17% for women under 25 years of age, 43% for those aged 26–30 years, and 100% in patients over 31 years. Rates of amenorrhea with short courses (≤7 pulses) were 0% for women under 25, 12% for those aged 26–30, and 25% for women older than 31[20]. Recent data suggest that long-acting gonadotropin-releasing hormone agonists (GnRH-a), such as leuprolide 3.75mg (administered as a subcutaneous injection every month 2 weeks prior to pulse cyclophosphamide therapy), reduce the rates of amenorrhea[21]. These agents, after an initial

surge in LH and FSH secretion, downregulate GnRH receptors in the pituitary, suppress FSH and LH production, and ultimately suppress gonadal steroid secretion. Suppression of FSH and LH is thought to prevent accelerated recruitment and depletion of ovarian follicles by cyclophosphamide. In another study[22], depot leuprolide acetate (3.7mg/month) was administered in 18 women under age 40 at least 10 days prior to the cyclophosphamide bolus, together with a transdermal estradiol patch to provide near-physiologic estradiol levels, and depot progestins for contraception and the prevention of endometrial hyperplasia. In this study the odds ratio for ovarian failure after 3 years in untreated versus leuprolide acetate-treated patients was 11. The mechanism for transient or permanent azoospermia observed in men after cyclophosphamide is less clear, but it is implied that cyclophosphamide damages germinal centers with increased mitotic activity. Testosterone (100mg intramuscularly every 15 days) has recently been reported to preserve fertility in patients with nephrotic syndrome treated with a short course of cyclophosphamide[23]. Further clinical trials are needed to better demonstrate the efficacy of these hormonal manipulations and to balance them against their potential side effects (especially, in the case of leuprolide, on bone mineral metabolism).

Azathioprine

Azathioprine in doses of 2–2.5mg/kg/day has been proved to be remarkably safe in the very long term with no significant increase in the risk of infection and probably a marginal risk for malignancy. Leukopenia and hepatotoxicity remain problems in a sizeable number of patients. In addition to its corticosteroid-sparing effects and its acceptable cost, azathioprine is considered as a safe drug during pregnancy, an especially attractive feature for a disease of women of reproductive age. All but two studies have shown that this drug adds marginally to prednisone alone. For this reason, at present azathioprine is used as primary therapy mainly for mild forms of lupus nephritis and in patients strongly opposed to cyclophosphamide. Azathioprine is used in many centers around the world as maintenance therapy after substantial improvements or remission of lupus nephritis[24]; whether is as effective as quarterly pulse cyclophosphamide for maintenance therapy remains to be shown.

Mycophenolate mofetil

Mycophenolate mofetil (MMF) is a reversible inhibitor of the enzyme inosine monophosphate dehydrogenase (IMPDH), a critical rate-limiting enzyme in the de novo synthesis of purines. As lymphocytes require a fully functioning de novo pathway for purine synthesis and proliferation, the drug functions as a relatively selective antimetabolite. Initial dose is 1g/day and can be increased up to 3g/day. This dose, however, is not tolerated well and most patients are usually treated initially with 2g/day. Responses may occur quickly (usually within 6–8 weeks). Its significantly higher cost compared to azathioprine is another important consideration, especially for long-standing maintenance therapy, with some authors recommending switching to azathioprine after the initial 6–12 months of treatment. Adverse effects include leukopenia, nausea, diarrhea and infections. In addition to the controlled study mentioned above, smaller non-RCT studies suggest partial responses in renal function and proteinuria even in patients refractory to pulse cyclophosphamide therapy[25,26]. Although in these patients remissions have rarely been achieved, it is a reasonable choice for patients failing cyclophosphamide. A controlled trial in the USA comparing MMF to pulses of cyclophosphamide is close to completion.

Cyclosporin A

Most reports on treatment of lupus with cyclosporin A (CsA) have evaluated the effects of this drug on the extrarenal manifestations of lupus, with only few patients with active nephritis being treated. There is no permanent nephrotoxicity in patients treated with a low dose

(≤5mg/kg/day) and without an increase in serum creatinine[27]. Serum creatinine should be checked on at least two occasions to obtain a baseline value prior to therapy, and monitored every 2 weeks during the first 3 months and once a month thereafter. Correlation between blood level and clinical effect in autoimmune diseases is suboptimal, so blood level is usually not monitored unless in doses >3mg/day, in which case it is usually done for toxicity purposes. A controlled study of CsA and oral cyclophosphamide in nephrotic children with proliferative lupus nephritis and nephrotic syndrome demonstrated a corticosteroid-sparing effect of CsA[28].

TREATMENT RECOMMENDATIONS

Treatment of lupus nephritis depends on the severity of disease, patient choices and access to medical care. A working classification of the severity of lupus nephritis, although arbitrary, is essential in discussing treatment recommendations (Table 127.7; Figs 127.2–127.5). Patient choice is particular important, with several studies demonstrating an unwillingness of patients to opt for the best therapy (a regimen containing cytotoxic agents) when confronted with the potential side effects. Fertility is an especially emotional issue. Patients at high risk for end-stage renal disease should be thoughtfully counseled not to risk compromising both future health and fertility because of renal failure by rejecting effective therapy for lupus nephritis. At the same time, every effort should be made to accommodate patients' lifestyles by administering cytotoxic drugs on an outpatient basis in specialized units.

Current strategies for the management of lupus nephritis include an initial induction phase aimed at substantially improving disease activity (or even attaining remission), and a maintenance phase whose primary goal is to maximize the therapeutic effect and consolidate the response. During this later phase the balance of benefit between regimens to avoid

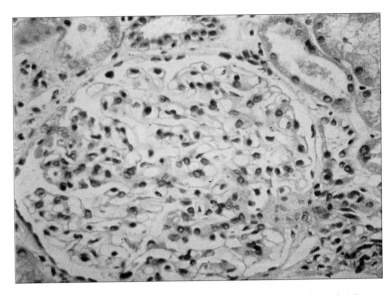

Fig. 127.2 Kidney biopsy showing focal proliferative glomerulonephritis (WHO class III). (Courtesy of Drs Dafna D Gladman and Murray B Urowitz.)

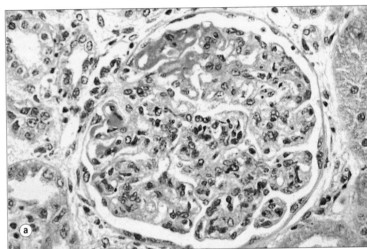

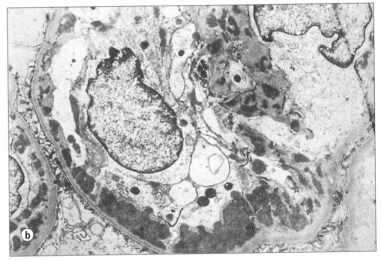

Fig. 127.3 (a) Kidney biopsy showing diffuse proliferative glomerulonephritis (WHO class IV). (b) Electron micrograph of a glomerulus showing subendothelial immune deposits. (Courtesy of Drs Dafna D Gladman and Murray B Urowitz.)

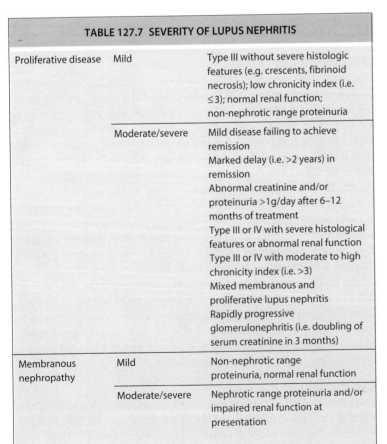

TABLE 127.7 SEVERITY OF LUPUS NEPHRITIS		
Proliferative disease	Mild	Type III without severe histologic features (e.g. crescents, fibrinoid necrosis); low chronicity index (i.e. ≤3); normal renal function; non-nephrotic range proteinuria
	Moderate/severe	Mild disease failing to achieve remission Marked delay (i.e. >2 years) in remission Abnormal creatinine and/or proteinuria >1g/day after 6–12 months of treatment Type III or IV with severe histological features or abnormal renal function Type III or IV with moderate to high chronicity index (i.e. >3) Mixed membranous and proliferative lupus nephritis Rapidly progressive glomerulonephritis (i.e. doubling of serum creatinine in 3 months)
Membranous nephropathy	Mild	Non-nephrotic range proteinuria, normal renal function
	Moderate/severe	Nephrotic range proteinuria and/or impaired renal function at presentation

relapses or smoldering disease activity, and issues such as side effects of the drugs and quality of life, becomes more pressing and difficult to evaluate because of lack of sufficient evidence. Table 127.8 summarizes treatment recommendations for all types of lupus nephritis (see below).

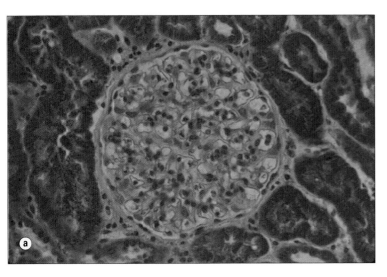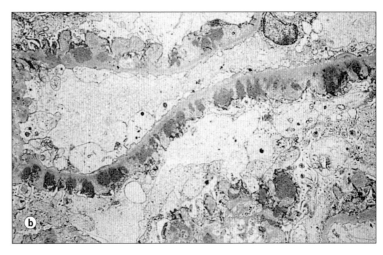

Fig. 127.4 Membranous nephropathy. (a) The capillary walls of the glomerular tuft are prominent and widely patent, resembling 'stiff' structures with decreased compliance. (b) Electron micrograph of a glomerulus showing intramembranous immune deposits. The presence of severe nephrotic-range proteinuria and the absence of significant chronic intersitial changes suggest a moderately severe disease. (Courtesy of Drs Dafna D Gladman and Murray B Urowitz.)

PROLIFERATIVE LUPUS NEPHRITIS

Initial treatment

Mild disease

A limited trial of prednisone (1.0mg/kg/day for up to 8 weeks), gradually tapering to alternate days (~0.25mg/kg) if remission occurs and monitoring for flares, is our preferred approach. If the patient does not achieve complete remission (i.e. clearing of cellular casts and proteinuria, normalization of complement and minimal lupus activity), or if nephritis worsens, we start monthly pulse cyclophosphamide. Delaying cyclophosphamide therapy because of a partial response beyond the 3 or 4 months may have a significant adverse impact on the response to cyto-

toxic therapy (suboptimal response or increase risk of flare). In selected cases the use of three consecutive pulses of methylprednisolone may expedite remission and allow the use of lower doses of corticosteroids (0.5g/kg/day). The addition of alternative immunosuppressive therapy (i.e. azathioprine), either from the beginning or during tapering of corticosteroids, may facilitate tapering or decrease the cumulative dose. Protection against osteoporosis is essential for all patients on chronic (>3 months) corticosteroid use.

Moderate to severe disease

Most authors agree that in addition to high doses of prednisone (0.5–1.0mg/kg/day, tapered after 4 weeks) cytotoxic drugs will have to be added in these patients, at least during the induction period. For the

TABLE 127.8 RECOMMENDED TREATMENT OF LUPUS NEPHRITIS		
	Type of therapy	
Histology/severity	**Induction**	**Maintenance**
Proliferative		
Mild	High-dose corticosteroids (*per os* or bolus); if no remission in 8 weeks, treat as moderate/severe	Low-dose corticosteroids
Moderate/severe	Monthly pulse CY (alone or with MP) (MMF)	Quarterly pulse CY (azathioprine; MMF; ?CsA)
Membranous		
Mild (proteinuria <3g/dl)	High-dose corticosteroids	Low-dose corticosteroids
Moderate/severe	Bimonthly pulse CY (MMF; pulses of MP alternating with oral chlorambucil or CY for 3–6 months; cyclosporin A)	Low-dose corticosteroids (quarterly pulse CY; azathioprine; MMF; CsA)
Mesangial		
Proteinuria >2g/day	Low-dose corticosteroids	Low-dose corticosteroids

See text for dose and further details. Alternative agents are shown in parentheses.
CY, cyclophosphamide; MMF, mycophenolate mofetil; MP, methylprednisone.

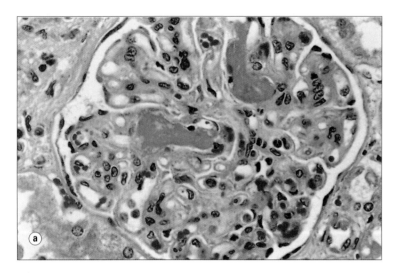
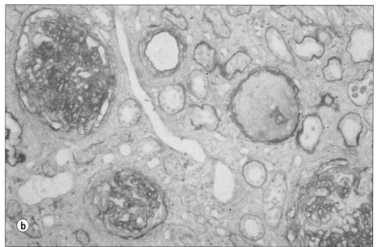

Fig. 127.5 (a) Renal biopsy specimen demonstrating multiple bland thrombi occluding glomerular capillary lumina (hematoxylin & eosin; original magnification × 400) **(Courtesy of Barri J Fessler.)** (b) Kidney biopsy showing advanced sclerosis (WHO class VI). (Courtesy of Drs Dafna D Gladman and Murray B Urowitz.)

induction, we recommend seven monthly pulses of cyclophosphamide, in combination with three initial pulses of methylprednisolone at the start which are continued in patients with more severe disease at monthly intervals (one pulse/month) for the first 6–12 months. Alternative induction therapy for patients strongly opposed to pulses of cyclophosphamide include monthly pulses of methylprednisolone (1.0g/m² daily for three doses) and then at monthly intervals for 6–12 months if there is steady progress to remission; or daily oral mycophenolate mofetil 1g twice a day for 12 months, with an increase to 3g/day if there is no response in 6–8 weeks.

Maintenance therapy

For patients with mild disease low-dose corticosteroids (e.g. 7.5–15mg prednisone on alternate days), azathioprine, mycophenolate mofetil or cyclosporin may be used. For maintenance immunosuppressive therapy in patients with moderate to severe disease, our preferred approach is quarterly pulse cyclophosphamide until 1 year beyond remission. Microscopic hematuria or non-nephrotic proteinuria may not clear for several months, even when most other clinical parameters have remitted. In our experience, in patients with moderate to severe nephritis remission usually occurs at an average of approximately 2 years after therapy. Abandoning pulse cyclophosphamide therapy because remission is not achieved before the completion of at least 2 years of treatment is not justified unless there is definite worsening of the disease (reproducible worsening of renal function, or more than 50% increase in proteinuria in the nephrotic range). Table 127.9 provides general guidelines for the discontinuation of cytotoxic therapy.

MEMBRANOUS LUPUS NEPHROPATHY

Lupus membranous nephropathy with only background mesangial expansion (pure membranous) has a low risk of progression to end-stage renal disease (approximately 20% at 10 years). Persistent nephrotic-range proteinuria, abnormal renal function and, more recently, black race have been implicated as high-risk features. Persistent nephrotic syndrome substantially increases the risk of arteriosclerotic and thromboembolic complications, and may further affect patient survival. Mixed membranous and proliferative histology (especially when diffuse proliferation is present) has a worse prognosis even than pure proliferative disease[1]; these patients should therefore be treated as those with proliferative disease.

TABLE 127.9 GUIDELINES AND CONSIDERATIONS FOR DISCONTINUING CYTOTOXIC THERAPY IN LUPUS NEPHRITIS

Failure to achieve remission

Definite worsening after the first 6–12 months of therapy (e.g. reproducible worsening of renal function or ≥50% increase of proteinuria at the nephrotic range)

Continuous activity after protracted (e.g. 3–4 years) of therapy
 – Renal remission may be delayed more than 2 years

Rule out 'fixed' hematuria or 'proteinuria'. A renal biopsy may be helpful to exclude low-grade renal inflammation

Exclude suboptimal treatment protocols (e.g. lags in treatment intervals, suboptimal doses) and non-lupus related causes of hematuria and worsening renal function (especially drugs and poorly controlled hypertension)

Advanced chronic renal insufficiency
Gradually rising serum creatinine ≥6mg/dl
Inactive urine sediment with broad or waxy casts
Renal biopsy showing only atrophy and fibrosis
Prolonged (≥3 months) dialysis-dependent renal failure with contracted kidney size (<3/4 normal)

Induction and maintenance therapy

Induction therapy

There are no published prospective randomized trials for the treatment of lupus membranous nephropathy. A prospective controlled trial at NIH approaches completion and preliminary results have been presented in Abstract form[29]. In this study alternate-day prednisone alone was compared to treatment regimens with prednisone in combination with pulse cyclophosphamide on alternate months, or with low-dose cyclosporin (≤5mg/kg/day) for 1 year. In a preliminary analysis in a small number of patients at the end of 1 year, 46% of patients treated with pulse cyclophosphamide and a comparable percentage of patients on cyclosporin achieved complete remission (defined as proteinuria <0.3g/day), compared to 13% in the prednisone-only group. Relapses were more frequent after completing cyclosporin (5 of 8 patients) than after cyclophosphamide treatment (1 out of 8 patients). Retrospective analysis of 19 patients from a European center suggested that combination treatment with chlorambucil or oral cyclophosphamide is more effective than prednisone alone[30]. Based on these findings for patients with pure membranous nephropathy with nephrotic-range proteinuria, we recommend alternate-day prednisone (0.5–1mg/kg) for 2 months, tapered to ~0.25mg/kg on alternate days within 3–4 months, with intravenous pulse cyclophosphamide every 2 months (especially if severe) or CsA (≤5mg/kg/day) for 1 year. Alternative treatments for induction therapy include pulse methylprednisolone 1.0g/day for 3 days, followed by 27 days of prednisone (0.5mg/kg/day, alternating with 30 days of chlorambucil 3–6mg/m²/day, three cycles of each therapy over a 6-month period); or oral cyclophosphamide 2mg/kg/day for 3–6 months[30]. Membranous nephropathy with non-nephrotic proteinuria (usually less than 2g/day) does not require therapy but rather careful monitoring for progression to nephrotic syndrome or to mixed membranous and proliferative nephropathy.

Maintenance therapy

Maintenance therapy with azathioprine or lower doses of cyclosporin may help to prevent relapses, although this has not been formally tested.

REMISSION, PARTIAL REMISSION AND RELAPSE

Defining remission and response has implications for the definition of relapse and may facilitate therapeutic decisions. However, there are no universally accepted criteria[31]. We use the term remission when extrarenal disease and urine sediment are inactive (even if small amounts of residual proteinuria, usually below 1g/day is present) and (ideally) complement normalizes for at least 6 months, provided that patients are off immunosuppressive therapy except for low-dose prednisone (<10mg/day). Partial remission ('response') denotes an objective improvement in urine sediment, proteinuria and renal function but persistent abnormalities in urine sediment (i.e. significant glomerular hematuria). Because we have found a high rate of relapse with early discontinuation of cytotoxic drug therapy[32] we do not accept achievement of partial remission as a criterion for discontinuing maintenance therapy unless there are other contraindications to continuing treatment. We therefore continue therapy for several months after remission.

'Fixed proteinuria' or 'hematuria' as a result of severe, irreversible damage to glomerular membranes develop in a small number of patients with inactive disease and can lead to unnecessary overtreatment. In some cases renal biopsy is helpful in defining these fixed abnormalities, as it usually demonstrates marked thickening and lucency of glomerular basement membranes without significant immune deposits. Fixed proteinuria is usually less than 2g/day and the patient has quiescent renal and extrarenal lupus by clinical, serologic and urine sediment criteria.

Approximately one-third to half of patients with moderate to severe proliferative lupus nephritis will relapse after achieving partial or complete remission[32,33]. Nephritic flares with active urine sediment and significant increase of serum creatinine (e.g. a reproducible ≥30% increase) have an adverse effect on renal prognosis, whereas purely proteinuric flares without significant changes in renal function have a more benign prognosis[34]. Patients with substantial loss of renal function (e.g. creatinine >2mg/dl at the time of response), an only partial response to therapy, and high chronicity and activity indices at study entry are more likely to progress to end-stage renal disease after a nephritic flare. These observations argue in support of strategies to minimize the risk of flare. Cyclophosphamide is more effective than corticosteroids alone in preventing renal flares, and our recommendation is to continue quarterly pulse cyclophosphamide for 1 year beyond remission. In our experience flares are more common in African-American patients and patients with undetectable C4 levels[32]. Pre-emptive treatment in the face of a rising

anti-DNA titer without more evidence of clinically active lupus may prevent flares in a few patients, but for the most part these are usually mild and come at the expense of overtreating a much larger number of patients[35]. In selected patients with exquisitely responsive nephritis (remission within 6 months), pulse cyclophosphamide may be stopped earlier in order to maintain fertility while accepting the risk of low-grade lupus nephritis activity. In such patients maintenance with alternate-day prednisone, either alone or with azathioprine, is common practice. Table 127.10 outlines our current approach to the management of renal flares.

COMORBID CONDITIONS

Hypertension

Hypertension is an independent risk factor for progressive renal failure and cardiovascular disease. Target blood pressure is less than 120/75, and in patients with proteinuria >1g/day is ≤110/70[36]. Nephritis contributes to hypertension by producing high renin and angiotensin II states as well as by inducing salt and water retention. Thus, angiotensin-converting enzyme (ACE) inhibitors and diuretics are the initial treatment of choice to control blood pressure in most patients. ACE inhibitors also decrease proteinuria and may be more effective than other antihypertensive agents in reducing the development of end-stage non-diabetic renal disease by mechanisms not necessarily related to the control of blood pressure[37]. Patients on ACE inhibitors or angiotensin receptor antagonists need close monitoring for several weeks after the initiation of therapy for hyperkalemia and worsening renal function. In addition to their antihypertensive effects, these agents may also have beneficial effects in reducing vascular complications and the severity of Raynaud's phenomenon. Calcium channel antagonists may be more effective to control blood pressure than ACE inhibitors in black patients. Occasionally, hypertensive urgencies may develop in patients with acute severe proliferative nephritis requiring the full range of adrenergic antagonists and vasodilators, including minoxidil.

TABLE 127.10 AN APPROACH TO THE MANAGEMENT OF LUPUS NEPHRITIS FLARES

- Confirm flare by looking for extrarenal lupus, active urine sediment, falling levels of C3 or rising titers of anti-ds DNA, or increase in serum creatinine
- Rule out non-lupus-related causes for worsening renal function (e.g. drugs, uncontrolled hypertension, dehydration, contrast agents) or hematuria (e.g. non-glomerular hematuria)
- Nephritic or proteinuric flare?
  - Nephritic flare: active urine sediment, increase in proteinuria, increase in serum creatinine, low C3, rising anti-DNA
  - Nephrotic flare: increase in proteinuria only
- Mild or severe?
  - Mild: active urine sediment with moderate increase in proteinuria (less than twofold increase, or less than 1g/day total) and stable serum creatinine
  - Severe: active urine sediment with either increase in serum creatinine ≥30% from baseline or more than twofold increase in proteinuria to nephrotic range
- Consider renal biopsy
  - Patients with previous biopsy showing proliferative disease with nephritic flare may not need a biopsy
- Treatment:
  - Mild nephritic or proteinuric flare: corticosteroids and/or azathioprine
  - Severe nephritic: corticosteroids with pulse cyclophosphamide

Dyslipidemia and cardiovascular morbidity

It has been suggested that lupus is a significant independent risk factor for atherosclerosis, and most patients with lupus nephritis have multiple cardiovascular risk factors (hypertension, dyslipidemia due to nephrotic syndrome, insulin resistance or hyperglycemia due to corticosteroids, anticardiolipin antibodies and elevated homocysteine levels). Aggressive management of dyslipidemia (LDL-cholesterol target ≤100 for patients with multiple risk factors, and triglycerides <150) is essential. The role of daily aspirin in primary prevention in such patients has not been studied formally but is worth considering. Chronic anemia and hypertension may cause left ventricular hypertrophy (LVH) and heart failure if not managed effectively.

Thrombotic diathesis and renal vasculopathy

Nephrotic syndrome is associated with increased synthesis of clotting factors and loss of fibrinolytic proteins (e.g. proteins S or C) in the urine, and together with antiphospholipid antibodies this is the most important factor for the thrombophilic diathesis in lupus nephritis. The exact role of other factors, such as plasma homocysteine or congenital deficiencies in coagulation proteins, remains ill defined. Patients with nephrotic syndrome (especially those with membranous nephropathy) should be informed about the potential for thrombosis (usually deep vein thrombosis, pulmonary embolism or renal vein thrombosis). Renal vein thrombosis, although it may be asymptomatic, usually manifests itself with flank pain, hematuria and worsening proteinuria.

The role of microvasculopathy in the progression of renal insufficiency in lupus nephritis is perplexing. Extra- and intraglomerular renal vascular lesions, subintimal eosinophilic PAS-positive deposits and intimal hyperplasia are common in lupus, even in the absence of hypertension. Immune complex deposition (with or without necrosis) within arterioles and small arteries is frequent in immunofluorescence studies. The role of antiphospholipid antibodies in microvascular renal injury and other antibodies (e.g. antiendothelial) or inflammatory cytokines has been addressed in several studies. The hypothesis that microthrombi in glomerular capillaries may contribute independently to the progression of renal disease has been put forward, but true microthrombi (thrombotic miroangiopathy) are rare and certainly not more common in patients with antiphospholipid antibodies than in matched antiphospholipid-negative patients[38]. However, antiphospholipid antibody-positive patients have a higher prevalence of fibrous intimal hyperplasia and hypertension. Taking together all available data, we think that antiphospholipid antibodies may be either a surrogate for more severe disease or may contribute (by non-necessarily prothrombotic mechanisms) to disease progression[39]. True thrombotic thrombocytopenic purpura (TTP) – defined as TTP when lupus is inactive, or a TTP-like syndrome in patients with systemic activity – may develop in rare lupus patients; because of their poor prognosis they must be recognized and treated early.

PREGNANCY

Glomerular perfusion increases during pregnancy and the resultant glomerular hyperfiltration decreases serum creatinine levels. As a result of hyperfiltration, women with significant prepregnancy proteinuria (>1g/day) may increase protein excretion (average increase 2–4g/day) between 18 and 36 weeks of gestation, followed by a sharp decrease postpartum[40]. Patients with normal renal function (or near normal, e.g. serum creatinine <1.4mg/dl) at the time of conception have no worsening of renal function, provided there is inactive urine sediment and that proteinuria is less than 1g/day. These women also have a high probability of successful pregnancy. Women with a variety of glomerular diseases and increased serum creatinine at baseline have a 10% risk of developing end-stage renal disease, whereas those with creatinine >2mg/dl have a 35% risk[41]. These patients have also a higher risk of hypertension, worsening proteinuria, prematurity and growth retardation. Falling serum complements and increase in creatinine and uric acid levels during pregnancy should raise the suspicion of lupus nephritis rather than pre-eclampsia. In these patients the presence of nephritic urine sediment is strong evidence for lupus nephritis. Pregnancy in lupus patients with active disease or substantial renal impairment is best managed in consultation with a high-risk obstetrician and a nephrologist. Corticosteroids are safe during pregnancy and are the treatment of choice, with azathioprine added for severe disease or as a corticosteroid-sparing agent.

LUPUS NEPHRITIS IN CHILDREN

Although initial studies suggested that the course of nephritis in children is worse than comparable classes of lupus nephritis in adults, more recent data suggest that this may not be true. As in adults, black race appears to be a high-risk factor in children. Response to treatment does not differ significantly between children and adults[42–44]. Compared to adults, children have a greater capacity to compensate for glomerular damage by compensatory hypertrophy in the less involved glomeruli, thus preserving renal function, although in the long term hyperfiltration may facilitate glomerulosclerosis.

MANAGEMENT OF CHRONIC RENAL INSUFFICIENCY

Similar to other chronic glomerulopathies, progressive renal injury in lupus nephritis involves predominantly non-immune mechanisms. Based on substantial experimental evidence, proteinuria, hypertension and dyslipidemia are often implicated in the deterioration of renal function in animal models. Maladaptive compensatory mechanisms (glomerular hypertrophy, increased blood flow, intraglomerular hypertension etc.) working in cohort with various immunopathogenic processes culminate in a progressive decline of glomerular filtration rate. However, in humans the relative contribution of these maladaptive processes has not been well defined. Experimental evidence and longitudinal clinical studies provide the basis for recommendations for stringent blood pressure and lipemic control, and a low-protein diet in patients with chronic insufficiency[45].

Once chronic renal insufficiency arises in patients with advanced disease several management issues become critical. These include efforts to minimize exposure to nephrotoxic drugs and contrast agents; the correction of anemia by the use of erythropoietin (e.g. 80–100U/kg) administered twice or thrice a week to keep hematocrit about 30% (usually 30–34%); use of calcium carbonate (650mg once to three times a day to decrease intestinal absorption of phosphates and ameliorate metabolic acidosis) and of a low-protein and -potassium diet; and modest salt restriction. If metabolic acidosis is significant (i.e. serum bicarbonate levels <18mEq/l) and does not respond to calcium carbonate, $NaHCO_3$ or bicitra (10–20mEq of base per day) can be used to maintain serum bicarbonate levels above 18mEq/l. In these patients, vitamin D supplementation with active 1,25-dihydroxy vitamin D and multiple vitamins is also prescribed[1].

END-STAGE RENAL DISEASE AND DIALYSIS

Approximately 10–20% of patients with SLE develop end-stage renal disease, but the progression of lupus nephritis to the point of dialysis does not necessarily indicate end-stage renal disease. Approximately 5–10% of lupus patients requiring dialysis recover sufficient function to interrupt dialysis temporarily, or for long periods. Patients with rapid deterioration of renal function are more likely to have a reversible physiologic (e.g. acute tubular necrosis) or pathologic (e.g. crescentic glomerulonephritis) component accounting for their renal failure. In these patients, immunosuppressive therapy (pulse methylprednisolone with pulses of cyclophosphamide $0.4-0.5g/m^2$ administered 8–10 hours before dialysis) may continue during dialysis.

Discontinuation of immunosuppressive therapy is an emotional issue for patients and physicians alike. We generally consider discontinuing therapy in patients with steadily rising creatinine to $\geq 5mg/dl$ with inactive urine sediment, renal biopsy showing exclusively scarring and atrophy, or with contracted renal size (see Table 127.9). Peritoneal dialysis is a reasonable option for lupus patients and offers greater independence.

Most lupus patients with advancing renal disease experience a significant decline in lupus activity. However, up to one half of patients on maintenance hemodialysis continue to experience lupus activity that may be difficult to distinguish from the complications of uremia per se[46]. Lupus activity is more likely to persist on dialysis when renal failure develops rapidly, rather than over a more extended period.

Uremia is a major predisposing factor for infections, and judicious use of corticosteroids and immunosuppressive drug therapy is essential to minimize the high risk of septic death in lupus patients with end-stage renal disease. Cardiovascular and cerebrovascular mortality and morbidity are increased in lupus patients with end-stage renal disease compared to those without[47]. Recent data from the US Renal Data System suggest that, similar to other primary renal diseases, the incidence of end-stage renal disease due to lupus nephritis increased steadily over the period 1982–1995, despite the introduction of efficacious new treatment regimens, an observation that may be related to limited use of these modalities[48].

RENAL TRANSPLANTATION

There are no firm rules for the optimal timing of renal transplantation in lupus nephritis patients. Although some patients with living-related donors proceed directly to transplantation without prior dialysis, a period of at least 3 months on dialysis may allow some patients to recover adequate function for significant periods of time. A recent study in 8481 patients with a variety of renal diseases has suggested that non-use of long-term dialysis improves allograft survival in renal transplants from living donors. Improved immune function after dialysis may have contributed to this effect[49].

Kidney transplantation is a viable alternative for lupus patients, although more recent data suggest an approximately twofold increase in the risk of allograft loss[50]. A recent pediatric study involving 100 renal transplants performed in 94 young lupus patients reported comparable outcomes to those seen in the control group, but an unexplained increase in the incidence of recurrent rejections (four or more) in lupus patients[51]. Recipient mesenchymal cells infiltrate the vascular (neointimal) and interstitial compartments of renal allografts undergoing chronic rejection[52]. Whether mesenchymal cells of lupus patients are more likely to migrate to renal allografts or have a heightened response when present at areas of inflammation in the graft remains to be seen. Recurrence of lupus nephritis in the renal allograft is rare (~2% of transplants) and not an important cause of graft loss. Whether antiphospholipid antibody-related events play an important role, as has been suggested[46], remains to be seen.

FUTURE DIRECTIONS

Unresolved issues

Several issues remain to be addressed in future clinical trials. These include, among others, studies of the comparative benefits of recycling short-term, intense immunosuppressive drug treatment for relapses versus long-term, low intensity maintenance therapies to avert relapses

TABLE 127.11 NOVEL APPROACHES TO TREATMENT OF PROLIFERATIVE LUPUS NEPHRITIS

Approach	Example
Non-specific immunosuppression	
High-dose immunoablative therapy	High-dose cyclophosphamide with HSCT
	High-dose cyclophosphamide without HSCT
Mycophenolate mofetil	
Nucleoside analogs	Fludarabine with cyclophosphamide
Sequential use of IST	Cyclophosphamide induction followed by azathioprine, mycophenolate mofetil or intravenous immunoglobulin
Biologic response modifiers	
Cytokine-directed therapy	Anti-IL-10 antibody, anti IL-6 receptor antibody
Interference with T–B-cell interactions	Anti-CD40 ligand antibodies CTLA4-Ig
B-cell depletion	Anti-CD20 and/or anti-CD22 antibodies
Interference with immune complex formation and deposition	DNAse Anti-idiotypic antibodies and competitive peptides
Induction of tolerance	Toleragen (LJP 394) Co-stimulatory blockade
Potential targets	
Complement components	Anti-C5 monoclonal antibody
BLyS	Anti-BLyS antibodies or soluble receptors
Chemokine modulation	Bindarit
Hormonal agents	Tamoxifen

BLyS, B lymphocyte stimulator; HSCT, hematopoietic stem cell transplantation; IST, immunosuppressive therapy.

and minimize cumulative renal damage in lupus nephritis; studies on the feasibility of corticosteroid-free regimens; and studies to define optimal treatment of lupus membranous nephropathy.

Novel therapies

There are two major approaches to developing novel treatments for lupus nephritis (Table 127.11). The first is to modify existing immunosuppressive therapies by changing the dose or duration of commonly used drugs; to use these drugs in combination or sequentially to reduce adverse events; or to use more recently developed drugs that have been effective in other diseases. The other major approach is to target specific steps in the pathogenesis of lupus nephritis, such as interfering with T- and B-cell activation by blocking co-stimulatory molecules, preventing immune complex formation or deposition, and diverting the autoimmune response by inducing antigen-specific tolerance or by interfering with abnormal cytokine networks.

An example of the first approach is high-dose immunoablative therapy with[53] or without[54] stem cell transplantation, which is currently being evaluated in several trials for the treatment of severe lupus. The goal is to eliminate most pathogenic clones ('reset the immunostat') and allow the reconstituting immune system to develop tolerance to self-antigens. Despite promising early results in some studies, further trials are needed to establish the optimal conditioning and maintenance regimen and to determine whether stem cell replacement provides any benefit over high-dose cyclophosphamide with spontaneous recovery of the hemopoietic and immune systems.

The discovery that a two-stage signaling process is necessary to develop and sustain most antigen-specific immune responses presented new opportunities for targeted immunotherapy. If T lymphocytes are activated through their antigen-specific T-cell receptors in the absence of co-stimulatory 'second' signals mediated by co-stimulatory receptor–ligand pairs, the T-cell receptor–antigen/MHC interaction induces apoptosis, clonal deletion of antigen-specific T cells and, ultimately, anergy or even immune tolerance.

Studies in animal models and in humans have demonstrated the essential role of the co-stimulatory molecule CD40 and its ligand CD40L (CD154) in the production of pathogenic autoantibodies and tissue injury in lupus nephritis. Several groups have reported hyperexpression of CD40L by B and T cells and elevated soluble CD40L levels in the serum of lupus patients. Glomerular and tubular CD40 expression is also markedly upregulated in proliferative lupus nephritis. Anti-CD40L therapy ameliorates renal disease in animal models of SLE and improves survival even when used in animals with established disease. In humans, a short course of treatment with an anti-CD40L antibody in patients with proliferative lupus nephritis reduced anti-dsDNA antibodies, increased C3 levels and decreased hematuria[55]. The aberrancies observed in the peripheral B-cell compartment at baseline normalized with treatment[56] and there was a substantial reduction in the frequency of B cells secreting IgG and IgM anti-DNA antibodies[57]. These in vivo and ex vivo data suggest that the drug has an immunomodulatory effect. Although promising, the clinical potential of this approach is not yet clear as the study had to be stopped prematurely because of an increased number of thromboembolic events in this and other clinical studies using the same antibody[56]. Another study using a different anti CD40L antibody found no clinical benefit in patients with extrarenal lupus.

In animal models, blocking other co-stimulatory pathways (such as CD28 or its ligands) or interfering with several co-stimulatory pathways simultaneously may increase efficacy[58]. CTLA4 is expressed on the surface of T cells after activation and has a high affinity for the B7 antigen (CD80) present on B cells and antigen-presenting cells. CTLA4 binds to CD80 more avidly than CD28 and generates an inhibitory signal in B cells. CTLA4-Ig is a fusion protein derived from the extracellular domain of CTLA4 and the Fc portion of IgG1. CTLA4-Ig prevents the progression of renal disease and prolongs survival in NZB/W mice. In mice with advanced renal disease a combination of CTLA4-Ig and cyclophosphamide improved survival significantly better than either agent alone[59]. CTLA4-Ig has been safely used in patients with psoriasis and rheumatoid arthritis, with initial results suggesting a significant clinical effect as well; a controlled trial of CTLA4-Ig with and without cyclophosphamide is under consideration for lupus nephritis.

Selective depletion of well-defined lymphocyte subsets may lead to better understanding of the pathogenesis and potentially safer therapies. Treating patients with DNAse, or interfering with the complement cascade by blocking C5, or neutralizing pathogenic antibodies by administering specific binding peptides or inducing specific anti-idiotype antibodies may prevent immune complex formation and/or deposition. Breaking the established autoinflammatory circuit may be achieved by blocking important cytokines, such as interleukins 6 and 10, or the action of chemokines.

BLyS (B lymphocyte stimulator; also known as BAFF, zTNF4, TALL-1 and THANK) is a recently described stimulator of B cells. BLyS transgenic mice develop severe B-cell hyperplasia and lupus-like disease, characterized by the presence of autoantibodies against nuclear antigens and immune deposits in the kidney[60,61]. In murine models of SLE there are increased serum levels of BLyS that seem to correlate with disease activity, and treatment with soluble BLyS receptors significantly decreased proteinuria and increased survival in these mice[62]. Elevated levels of BLyS were also found in patients with SLE. The BLyS isolated from these patients was biologically active and was partially associated with elevated anti-dsDNA antibody levels, but not with disease activity[63]. BLyS appears to be an attractive target for therapy in lupus, but further studies are needed to determine its role in human SLE.

REFERENCES

1. Balow JE, Boumpas DT, Austin HA. Systemic lupus erythematosus and the kidney. In: Lahita RG, ed. Systemic erythematosus and the kidney. San Diego: Academic Press, 1999: 657–685.
2. Esdaile JM, MacKenzie T, Kashgarian M et al. The benefit of early treatment with immunosuppressive agents in lupus nephritis. J Rheumatol 1994; 21: 2046.
3. Herbert LA, Dillon JJ, Middendorf DF et al. Relationship between appearance of urinary red blood cell/white blood cell casts and the onset of renal relapse in systemic lupus erythematosus. Am J Kidney Dis 1995; 26: 432–438.
4. Austin HA, Boumpas DT, Vaughan EM et al. High-risk features of lupus nephritis: importance of race and clinical and histological factors in 166 patients. Nephrol Dial Transplant 1995; 10: 1620–1628.
5. Bakir AA, Levy PS, Dunea G. The prognosis of lupus nephritis in African-Americans: a retrospective analysis. Am J Kidney Dis 1994; 24: 159–171.
6. Dooley MA, Hogan S, Jennette C, Falk R. Cyclophosphamide therapy for lupus nephritis: poor renal survival in black Americans. Glomerular Disease Collaborative Network. Kidney Int 1997; 51: 1188–1195.
7. Donadio JVJ, Holley KE, Ferguson RH et al. Treatment of diffuse proliferative lupus nephritis with prednisone and combined prednisone and cyclophosphamide. N Engl J Med 1978; 299: 1151–1155.
8. Donadio JV Jr, Holley KE, Ilstrup DM. Cytotoxic drug treatment of lupus nephritis. Am J Kidney Dis 1982; 2 (Suppl): 178.
9. Austin HA, Klippel JH, Balow JE et al. Therapy of lupus nephritis. Controlled trial of prednisone and cytotoxic drugs. N Engl J Med 1986; 314: 614–619.
10. Steinberg AD, Steinberg SC. Long-term preservation of renal function in patients with lupus nephritis receiving treatment that includes cyclophosphamide versus those treated with prednisone only. Arthritis Rheum 1991; 34: 945–950.
11. Boumpas DT, Austin HA, Vaughn EM et al. Controlled trial of pulse methylprednisolone versus two regimens of pulse cyclophosphamide in severe lupus nephritis. Lancet 1992; 340: 741–745.
12. Gourley MF, Austin HA, Scott D et al. Methylprednisolone and cyclophosphamide, alone or in combination, in patients with lupus nephritis. A randomized, controlled trial. Ann Intern Med 1996; 125: 549–557.
13. Illei GG, Austin HA, Crane M et al. Combination therapy with pulse cyclophosphamide plus pulse methylprednisolone improves long-term renal outcome without adding toxicity in patients with lupus nephritis. Ann Intern Med 2001; 135: 248–257.
14. Sesso R, Monteiro M, Sato E et al. A controlled trial of pulse cyclophosphamide versus pulse methylprednisolone in severe lupus nephritis. Lupus 1994; 3: 107–112.
15. Lewis EJ, Hunsicker LG, Lan SP et al. A controlled trial of plasmapheresis therapy in severe lupus nephritis. The Lupus Nephritis Collaborative Study Group. N Engl J Med 1992; 326: 1373–1379.
16. Chan TM, Li FK, Tang CS et al. Efficacy of mycophenolate mofetil in patients with diffuse proliferative lupus nephritis. Hong Kong–Guangzhou Nephrology Study Group. N Engl J Med 2000; 343: 1156–1162.
17. Weinstein RS, Manolagas SC. Apoptosis and osteoporosis. Am J Med 2000; 108: 153–164.
18. D'Cruz D, Cuadrado MJ, Mujic F et al. Immunosuppressive therapy in lupus nephritis. Clin Exp Rheumatol 1997; 15: 275–282.
19. Houssiau FA, Vasconcelos C, D' Cruz D et al. Comparison of a short-course versus a long-course iv CPM regimen, followed by azathioprine, as treatment of proliferative lupus glomerulonephritis: results of the Euro-Lupus Nephritis Trial, a multicenter randomized study. Arthritis Rheum 2001; 44: S387.
20. Boumpas DT, Austin HA, Vaughan EM et al. Risk for sustained amenorrhea in patients with systemic lupus erythematosus receiving intermittent pulse cyclophosphamide therapy. Ann Intern Med 1993; 119: 366–369.
21. Dooley MA, Patterson CC, Hogan SL et al. Preservation of ovarian function using depot leuprolide acetate during cyclophosphamide therapy for severe lupus nephritis. Arthritis Rheum 2000; 42: S107
22. McCune WJ, Somers EC, Ognenovski V et al. Use of leuprolide acetate for ovarian protection during cyclophosphamide therapy of women with severe SLE: A case control study. Arthritis Rheum 2001; 44: S387.
23. Masala A, Faedda R, Alagna S et al. Use of testosterone to prevent cyclophosphamide-induced azoospermia. Ann Intern Med 1997; 126: 292–295.
24. Berden JH. Lupus nephritis. Kidney Int 1997; 52: 538–558.

25. Dooley MA, Cosio FG, Nachman PH *et al.* Mycophenolate mofetil therapy in lupus nephritis: clinical observations. J Am Soc Nephrol 1999; 10: 833–839.

26. Petri M. Mycophenolate mofetil treatment of systemic lupus erythematosus. Arthritis Rheum 1999; 42: 303.

27. Feutren G, Mihatsch. Risk factors for cyclosporin-induced nephropathy in patients with autoimmune diseases. International kidney biopsy registry of cyclosporin in autoimmune diseases. N Engl J Med 1992; 326: 1654–1660.

28. Fu LW, Yang LY, Chen WP, Lin CY. Clinical efficacy of cyclosporin a in the treatment of paediatric lupus nephritis with heavy proteinuria. Br J Rheumatol 1998; 37: 217–221

29. Austin HA, Vaughan EM, Boumpas DT *et al.* Lupus membranous nephropathy: controlled trial of prednisone, pulse cyclophosphamide, and cyclosporin A (Abstract). J Am Soc Nephrol 1996; 7: 1328.

30. Ponticelli C, Passerini P. Treatment of membranous nephropathy. Nephrol Dial Transplant 2001; 16 (Suppl 5): 8–10.

31. Boumpas Dt, Balow JE. Outcome criteria for lupus nephritis. Lupus 1998; 7: 622–629.

32. Illei GG, Takada K, Parkin P *et al.* Renal flares are common in patients with severe proliferative lupus nephritis treated with pulse immunosuppressive therapy: long-term follow-up of a cohort of 145 patients participating in randomized controlled studies. Arthritis Rheum 2002; 46: 995–1002.

33. Ioannidis JPA, Boki KA, Katsorida ME *et al.* Remission, relapse, and re-remission of proliferative lupus nephritis treated with cyclophosphamide. Kidney Int 2000; 57: 258–264.

34. Moroni G, Quaglini S, Maccario M *et al.* 'Nephritic flares' are predictors of bad long-term renal outcome in lupus nephritis. Kidney Int 1996; 50: 2047–2053.

35. Bootsma H, Spronk P, Derksen R *et al.* Prevention of relapses in systemic lupus erythematosus. Lancet 1995; 345: 1595.

36. Peterson JC, Adler S, Burkart JM *et al.* Blood pressure control, proteinuria, and the progression of renal disease. The modification of diet in renal disease study. Ann Intern Med 1995; 123: 754–762.

37. Giatras I, Lau J, Levey AS. Effect of angiotensin-converting enzyme inhibitors on the progression of non-diabetic renal disease: a meta analysis of randomized trials. Ann Intern Med 1997; 127: 337–345.

38. Vlachoyiannopoulos PG, Kanellopoulos P, Tektonidou MG *et al.* Renal involvement in antiphospholipid syndrome (APS): a controlled study. Arthritis Rheum 2001; 44: S190.

39. Bhandari S, Harnden P, Brownjohn AM, Turney JH. Association of anticardiolipin antibodies with intraglomerular thrombi and renal dysfunction in lupus nephritis. QJ Med 1998; 91: 401–409.

40. Laskin CA, Nadler JN, Clark CA *et al.* Pregnancy-induced hyperfiltration in women with lupus nephritis. Arthritis Rheum 2001; 44: S289.

41. Jones DC, Hayslett JP. Outcome of pregnancy in women with moderate or severe renal insufficiency. N Engl J Med 1996; 355: 226–230.

42. Lehman TJ, Onel K. Intermittent intravenous cyclophosphamide arrests progression of the renal chronicity index in childhood systemic lupus erythematosus. J Pediatr 2000; 136: 243–247.

43. Baqi N, Moazami S, Singh A *et al.* Lupus nephritis in children: a longitudinal study of prognostic factors and therapy. J Am Soc Nephrol 1996; 7: 924–929.

44. Niaudet P. Treatment of lupus nephritis in children. Pediatr Nephrol. 2000; 14: 158–166.

45. Clark WF, Moist LM. Management of chronic renal insufficiency in lupus nephritis: Role of proteinuria, hypertension, and dyslipidemia in the progression of renal disease. Lupus 1998; 7: 649–653.

46. Stone JH. End-stage renal disease in lupus: Disease activity, dialysis, and the outcome of transplantation. Lupus 1988; 7: 654–659.

47. Ward MM. Cardiovascular and cerebrovascular morbidity and mortality among women with end-stage renal disease attributable to lupus nephritis. Am J Kidney Dis 2000; 36: 516–525.

48. Ward MM. Changes in the incidence of end-stage renal disease due to lupus nephritis, 1982–1995. Arch Intern Med 2000; 160: 3136–3140.

49. Mange KC, Joffe MM, Feldman HI. Effect of the use or non-use of long term dialysis on the subsequent survival of renal transplants from living donors. N Engl J Med 2001; 344: 726–730.

50. Ward MM. Outcomes of renal transplantation among patients with end-stage renal disease caused by lupus nephritis. Kidney Int 2000; 57: 2136–2143.

51. Barthosh SM, Fine RN, Sullivan EK. Outcome after transplantation of young patients with systemic lupus erythematosus: a report of the North American Renal Transplant Cooperative Study. Transplantation 2001; 72: 973–978.

52. Grimm PC, Nickerson P, Jeffery J *et al.* Neointimal and tubulointerstitial infiltration by recipient mesenchymal cells in chronic renal-allograft rejection. N Engl J Med 2001; 345: 93–97.

53. Traynor AE, Schroeder J, Rosa RM *et al.* Treatment of severe systemic lupus erythematosus with high-dose chemotherapy and haemopoietic stem-cell transplantation: a phase I study. Lancet 2000; 356: 701–707.

54. Petri M, Jones R, Brodsky R. High dose immunoablative cyclophosphamide (HDIC) open-label trial: complete responders and durability of response. Arthritis Rheum 2000; 44: s387.

55. Boumpas DT, Furie R, Manzi S *et al.* A short course of BG9588 (anti-CD40L) antibody improves serologic activity and decreases hematuria in patients with proliferative lupus glomerulonephritis. Arthritis Rheum 2001; 44: S387.

56. Grammer A C, Shinohara S, Vasquez E, Gur H, Illei G G, Lipsky P E. Normalization of peripheral B cells following treatment of active SLE patients with humanized anti-CD154 Mab(5C8, BG9588). Arthritis Rheum 2001; 44: S282.

57. Davidson A, Budhai L, Reddy B, Vaishnaw A, Furie R. The effect of anti-CD40L antibody on B cells in human SLE. Arthritis Rheum 2000; 43: S271.

58. Daikh DI, Finck BK, Linsley PS, Hollenbaugh D, Wofsy D. Long-term inhibition of murine lupus by brief simultaneous blockade of the B7/CD28 and CD40/gp39 costimulation pathways. J Immunol 1997; 159: 3104–3108.

59. Daikh DI, Wofsy D. Reversal of murine lupus nephritis with CTLA4Ig and cyclophosphamide. J Immunol 2001; 166: 2913–2916.

60. Khare SD, Sarosi I, Xia XZ *et al.* Severe B cell hyperplasia and autoimmune disease in TALL-1 transgenic mice. Proc Natl Acad Sci USA 2000; 97: 3370–3375.

61. Mackay F, Woodcock SA, Lawton P *et al.* Mice transgenic for BAFF develop lymphocytic disorders along with autoimmune manifestations. J Exp Med 1999; 190: 1697–1710.

62. Gross JA, Johnston J, Mudri S *et al.* TACI and BCMA are receptors for a TNF homologue implicated in B-cell autoimmune disease. Nature. 2000; 404: 995–999.

63. Zhang J, Roschke V, Baker KP *et al.* A role for B lymphocyte stimulator in systemic lupus erythematosus. J Immunol 2001; 166: 6–10.

128 Severe lupus

Daniel J Wallace

- Half of patients with SLE have severe lupus, defined as complications that threaten life, organ function or an important bodily function such as sight
- The most common forms of severe lupus, by prevalence, are renal (reviewed elsewhere), cutaneous vasculitis, myocardiopathy, pulmonary vasculitis, autoimmune thrombocytopenia, and central nervous system vasculitis
- Management includes high doses of corticosteroids (usually 1mg/kg/day for at least 6 weeks of prednisone equivalent) and frequently immune-suppressive therapies
- Aggressive management of adjunctive features by a qualified internist to minimize steroid toxicity (e.g. hyperlipidemia, hypertension, hyperglycemia, obesity, bone demineralization), vigilance for fevers and infection, and promotion of healthy lifestyle changes (e.g. diet, exercise) have a significant impact on prognosis

TABLE 128.1 CLINICAL FORMS OF SEVERE LUPUS

Life-threatening (associated with >10% mortality within 3 months)

Myocarditis	Coronary arteritis	Pericardial tamponade
Pancreatitis	Mesenteric vasculitis	Budd–Chiari syndrome
Digital gangrene	Aplastic anemia	TTP
Pulmonary hemorrhage	Pulmonary embolus	Pulmonary hypertension
Central nervous vasculitis	Hemolytic anemia	

Serious lupus (organ-threatening or impairs bodily function but may shorten lifespan)

Libman–Sacks endocarditis	Lupus hepatitis	Biliary cirrhosis
Hyerviscosity	Cryoglobulinemia	Interstitial lung disease
Lupoid sclerosis	Mononeuritis multiplex	Pseudotumor cerebri
Protein enteropathy	Leukopenia	Cutaneous vasculitis
Optic neuritis	Vestibulitis	Proliferative nephritis
Antiphospholipid syndrome		

DEFINITION

Severe lupus is defined as aspects of the disorder associated with a greatly increased morbidity or mortality. Examples are organ-threatening complications that threaten life (e.g. mesenteric vasculitis), organ function (e.g. diffuse proliferative glomerulonephritis, CNS vasculitis), or an important bodily function such as sight (e.g. retinal vasculitis). Approximately half of those with SLE have 'organ-threatening disease' (Table 128.1), and half of these individuals have one of the forms of severe lupus listed below. This section will review several different forms of severe lupus, but some are reviewed elsewhere. Antiphospholipid syndrome is covered in Chapter 131, thrombotic thrombocytopenic purpura in Chapter 122, and nephritis in Chapter 127.

CARDIAC MANIFESTATIONS

Although dynamic echocardiographic evidence for myocardial dysfunction is present in up to 30% of those with SLE, frank inflammatory myocarditis is found in 5–10% of patients during the course of their disease[1] (Table 128.2). About half with lupus myocarditis also have generalized active systemic disease and constitutional symptoms (e.g. fatigue, low-grade fevers, tachycardia, aching) and half have quiescent lupus and develop myocarditis possibly as a consequence of a viral-like process. Most patients report vague chest discomfort not improved with movement or position. An electrocardiogram may reveal non-specific ST-T wave changes, cardiomegaly or infarction, and blood testing

TABLE 128.2 LUPUS AND THE HEART

Pericardial involvement	Painless effusion	Seen in 25% on echocardiogram
	Pericarditis	Common, rarely serious, responds to NSAIDs, steroids
	Pericardial tamponade	Uncommon, life-threatening, diagnosed by 2-D echo
Myocardial involvement	Myocardiopathy	Myocardial dysfunction in 30% on echo, usually no symptoms evident
	Myocarditis	Uncommon, serious, needs steroid therapy
	Coronary arteritis	Very rare, serious, needs steroid therapy
Endocardial involvement	Libman–Sacks	Sterile vegetations can become infected or embolize; serious and mandates a cardiac work-up
Hypertension		In 25% with SLE, associated with steroid use
Atherosclerotic heart disease		Prematurely evident in steroid-treated lupus patients
Costochondritis		More common in SLE, benign
Non-cardiac chest pain		Esophagitis is particularly common in SLE patients
Increased cardiac awareness		In SLE patients with fibromyalgia, mitral valve prolapse, or on steroids, reflects autonomic hypervigilance

demonstrates elevations of muscle enzymes (e.g. creatine phosphokinase, troponins). Skeletal muscle myositis may also be evident. Stress echocardiography shows myocardial dysfunction, and imaging studies ranging from pyrophosphate to indium-111 ([111]I) antimyosin Fab to SPECT scanning suggest inflammation. The diagnosis can be definitively made by myocardial biopsy, but its yield is less than 50%. Pathologically, evidence for a bland lymphocytic inflammatory infiltrate is found along with immune deposits (IgG, IgM, IgA, C3 or fibrinogen) on electron microscopy or immune fluorescence[2]. Lupus myocarditis must be differentiated from gastrointestinal sources of non-cardiac chest pain, costochondritis, atherosclerotic heart disease, pericarditis, autonomically mediated increased cardiac awareness syndromes and infectious myocarditis. Optimal management includes 1mg/kg/day of prednisone for 2–4 weeks, tapering as electrocardiographic improvement is observed, along with laboratory normalization of muscle enzymes. Azathioprine can be a useful steroid-sparing adjunct, but cyclophosphamide is reserved for refractory cases. Most patients with acute lupus myocarditis succumb within weeks if not promptly managed with corticosteroids.

Vasculitis of the coronary arteries is extremely rare and usually associated with generalized active systemic disease. Diagnosed at coronary angiography by its 'beaded' appearance or at myocardial biopsy, **coronary arteritis** is a life-threatening emergency[3]. Approximately half of the reported cases have been found in children, necessitating consideration of Kawasaki's disease. In adults, coronary arteritis can be difficult to distinguish from atherosclerotic heart disease. Coronary arteritis usually responds to high doses of corticosteroids (1mg/kg/day of prednisone equivalent) within days.

At autopsy, 90% of those with SLE have serosal abnormalities and 25% of living patients have incidental pericardial effusions on a 2D echocardiogram. Fortunately, **pericardial tamponade** occurs only in one living case per 100. Life threatening by definition, a scarred pericardium from chronic serositis (e.g. fibrinous or constrictive pericarditis) is an important predisposing factor. Tamponade is diagnosed by equalization of cardiac chamber pressures, pulsus paradoxicus, and most readily by echocardiography. Pericardiocentesis has a high complication rate because of the frequent concurrence of pericarditis with myocarditis. When a flabby myocardium is readily penetrated during the procedure it does not always contract adequately to close a small puncture[4]. The procedure should ideally be performed by a chest surgeon in an operating room with anesthesia back-up. Although pericardial drainage provides temporary relief – and most lupus patients have benefited from drainage followed by fenestration or triamcinolone injections into the pericardium – all need treatment of the underlying disease process and some respond well to pericardiectomy[5].

Sterile vegetations on a heart valve, rings, commissures, chordae tendineae, papillary muscles or mural endocardium characterize Libman–Sacks endocarditis, or atypical verrucous endocarditis. Statistically associated with the presence of antiphospholipid antibodies and prior corticosteroid use, these 1–4mm immune complex desposits are seen on routine echocardiography only 30% of the time, but transesophageal echocardiography identifies them 70% of the time[6,7]. They consist of proliferating and degenerating cells, fibrin, fibrous tissues and hematoxylin bodies. Individuals with these deposits are at high risk for developing superimposed bacterial endocarditis, cerebral embolic events and valvular incompetence. All patients with Libman–Sacks endocarditis should be on a platelet antagonist (e.g. one baby aspirin daily), receive antibiotic prophylaxis prior to dental procedures, and have their cardiac function scrutinized on a regular basis. When clinically appropriate, strong consideration should be given to instituting warfarin therapy.

GASTROINTESTINAL MANIFESTATIONS

Pancreatitis is a serious complication of SLE. Diagnosed by elevations in serum amylase and lipases in a person with severe (usually posterior) abdominal pain and fever, most pancreatitis in lupus patients is due to corticosteroid, azathioprine or sulfa-containing diuretic therapies, as well as to lifestyle decisions (e.g. alcohol abuse). However, at least one-third of all episodes of pancreatitis in SLE result from presumed vasculitis of the pancreatic blood supply[8]. Ascertaining the etiology of pancreatitis is critical, as its management ranges from stopping medication to giving 'pulse' doses of corticosteroids. Solving this etiopathologic conundrum can be assisted by looking for signs of generalized lupus activity (which suggests lupus pancreatitis), and a peritoneal tap if ascites is present or a thoracocentesis if pleural fluid is present. An abdominal CT scan can help in looking for pseudocysts or to rule out more easily reversible etiologies, such as 'gallstone pancreatitis'. Individuals with true lupus pancreatitis are best managed with bed rest, hospitalization, hydration, sparing but supportive use of analgesics, parenteral nutrition, and initially having nothing by mouth. Several hundred milligrams of intravenous methylprednisolone are given daily for the first few days, followed by tapering.

Many individuals with SLE have a mild transaminitis which may reflect disease activity, and in some patients this denotes increased sensitivity to aspirin or non-steroidal anti-inflammatory drugs (NSAIDs). **Autoimmune lupus hepatitis** has been defined as evidence for inflammation, sometimes with vasculitis on liver biopsy in a patient who fulfills the ACR criteria for SLE, and has negative serologies for hepatitis A, B, C and other relevant viruses (Table 128.3)[9]. Although a distinct autoantibody system (e.g. antibodies to the liver–kidney microsomal autoantigen) has been found in 20% of autoimmune hepatitis, another 10% fulfill the ACR criteria for SLE and do not have these autoantibodies. Known as 'lupoid hepatitis with LE cells' prior to the availability of viral serologies, most lupus hepatitis patients present with vague constitutional symptoms, and the diagnosis of autoimmune hepatitis is sought when young women have transaminases in the several hundred range. Those with SLE frequently also have antiribosomal P, smooth muscle and antimitochondrial antibodies. Liver failure is a late complication, and prior to the era of liver transplantation up to half with autoimmune hepatitis succumbed within 5 years. Corticosteroids in combination with azathioprine have been shown to be efficacious in a controlled trial[10]. In the **Budd–Chiari syndrome** occlusion of the hepatic veins and ascites with ensuing cirrhosis and portal hypertension is a complication of antiphospholipid antibodies and occurs in one case of SLE per 1000[11]. A handful of cases of **biliary cirrhosis** have been reported, mostly in individuals with lupus–scleroderma overlap disease[12].

The most feared gastrointestinal complication of SLE is **mesenteric vasculitis**. Carrying a greater than 50% mortality rate, bowel infarction occurs in SLE as a consequence of antiphospholipid syndrome-mediated clots or inflammation of the small- and medium-sized arterioles supplying the mesentery[13] (Fig. 128.1). Patients present with an insidious onset of abdominal pain, nausea, vomiting, diarrhea, ileus and fever, and may initially have dark, bloody stools. MR angiography, indium-111 scanning and technetium scanning may help localize the site or sites of involvement. Gastrografin enemas can reveal classic 'thumbprinting' of the bowel wall. Infections, adhesions, tumors and other causes of obstruction need to be considered. Prompt surgical intervention before peritonitis – and ultimately gangrene – sets in, as well as 1–2mg/kg/day of

---

TABLE 128.3 DEFINITION OF LUPUS HEPATITIS

- Liver biopsy demonstrating autoimmune hepatitis
- Abnormal liver function tests
- Absence of damage from hepatotoxic drugs
- Fulfillment of the ACR criteria for SLE
- Negative hepatitis viral serologies and other infectious etiologies ruled out

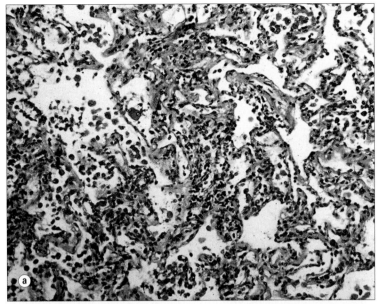

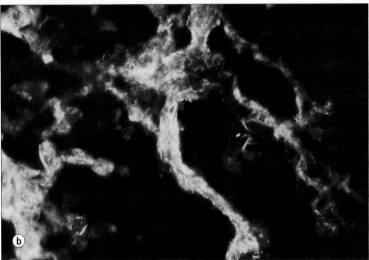

Fig. 128.1 Immunofluorescence of the lung showing immune deposits.

intravenous methylprednisolone, may be life-saving. Mesenteric vasculitis must be distinguished from a more benign form of serositis that occurs in lupus patients and responds to moderate doses of corticosteroids.

Fewer than 100 cases of **protein-losing enteropathy** have been reported[14]. Occurring mostly in children, the presence of severe diarrhea and marked hypoalbuminemia (as low as 0.8g/dl) stimulates the initiation of a malabsorption work-up. Bowel biopsies usually reveal villous atrophy and inflammatory infiltrates, which respond to corticosteroid therapy, and often a gluten-free diet is salutary.

PULMONARY MANIFESTATIONS

Approximately 1–5% of lupus patients experience a sudden onset of shortness of breath, fever, cough and rapid heart rate. As this mimics an acute pulmonary infection, they are often treated with antibiotics or cough suppressants, inhalers or decongestants. **Acute lupus pneumonitis**, however, does not respond to these regimens[15]. Most have active, multisystem SLE. When a chest X-ray is obtained it shows a diffuse interstitial infiltrate. If a bronchoscopy or bronchoalveolar lavage is performed, cultures are negative and evidence for an acute or lymphocytic interstitial pneumonia (LIP) is present, with immune deposits on electron microscopy or immunofluorescence. Acute lupus pneumonitis can be confused with bacterial, fungal, tuberculous and *Pneumocystis carinii*

infections. Time is of the essence, as failure to treat the patient with high doses of corticosteroids (1mg/kg/day or prednisone equivalent) is associated with a 50% mortality rate within weeks.

A chronic process, **interstitial lung disease** is seen in 3% with SLE and is associated with the gradual onset of windedness, dyspnea on exertion and non-productive cough, as well as an increased respiratory rate. Evolving over years, many of these patients will have a lupus overlap with scleroderma, Sjögren's or inflammatory myositis[16]. Chest radiographs demonstrate evidence for a reticulated, diffuse pattern. The process is only worth treating if, by the time it is recognized, the lesions are potentially amenable to anti-inflammatory therapy and are not totally scarred. To this end, pulmonary function testing shows a low diffusing capacity, along with a high-resolution CT scan that documents the diagnosis. However, imaging studies such as indium-111 or gallium scanning may be needed to demonstrate ongoing inflammation, as would tissue obtained at bronchoscopy or lung biopsy. Fortunately, interstitial lung disease rarely leads to pulmonary failure. It is managed with 1mg/kg/day of prednisone daily for 6 weeks, followed by a slow tapering. There is some evidence in the scleroderma literature that this process also responds to 6 months of intravenous cyclophosphamide[17].

In addition to the interstitium, patients with SLE can develop alveolar infiltrates induced by vascular injury, with disruption of the alveolar capillary membranes. Known as **pulmonary hemorrhage**, this rare but serious complication afflicts 1% of lupus patients. Presenting with hemoptysis followed by progressive respiratory failure, pulmonary hemorrhage is usually fatal within weeks even with optimal management[18]. The key to success includes early recognition of the process. Antibiotics do not help, and the degree of anemia present is much greater than that associated with most pneumonias. Chest X-rays reveal a fluffy, bilateral alveolar infiltrate. High-resolution CT scanning demonstrates a 'ground glass' appearance, but bronchoscopic cultures are negative. Instead, IgG and complement deposits of immune material are found in the alveolar septae (Fig. 128.2). Goodpasture's disease can be easily ruled out by obtaining antiglomerular basement membrane antibodies and assessing renal function. If the carer suspects alveolar hemorrhage early on and treats the patient aggressively with pulses of corticosteroids (1g methylprednisolone intravenously for the first few days) along with cyclophosphamide and plasmapheresis, up to half of the patients will survive.

One-third of those with SLE have an antiphospholipid antibody and one-third of these will have a thromboembolic event. Of the 11% with SLE who have sustained this, half have had a **pulmonary embolus**[19].

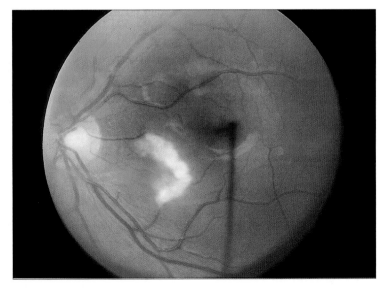

Fig. 128.2 Retinal vasculitis in a 16-year-old girl with multisystem active lupus.

Most have had calf pain and possess additional risk factors, such as oral contraceptive use, or smoking. Ventilation/perfusion scanning of the lungs is usually definitive, as is spiral CT scanning, especially when serum levels of D-dimers are elevated. Patients have sudden onset of focal chest pain, dyspnea, tachycardia and oxygen desaturation. After heparin therapy is administered, lifelong anticoagulation with warfarin is advised.

Pulmonary hypertension is the final serious pulmonary complication of SLE. If caused by recurrent emboli associated with the antiphospholipid syndrome, the process is reversible with chronic anticoagulation. Unfortunately, most pulmonary hypertension in SLE is idiopathic and insidious. The cause is probably related to proliferation of endothelial and smooth muscle cells, angiogenesis, and activation with injury of endothelial cells, producing increased pulmonary vascular resistance[20]. Chest X-rays are often normal and may remain so as late as a few days prior to death. Patients with mixed connective tissue disease and scleroderma overlaps are at increased risk for developing pulmonary hypertension. Many patients deny symptoms, but a careful history will reveal evidence of a sense of breathlessness or being easily winded. On physical examination a tricuspid regurgitation murmur is usually audible. Pulmonary pressures can be estimated by a two-dimensional Doppler echocardiogram of the heart. Many patients with SLE have chronic mild elevations of pulmonary pressure, but the process becomes increasingly progressive when systolic pressures rise above 40mmHg. Of this subgroup, 80% are dead within 5 years. Vasodilating regimens with hydralazine or calcium-channel blockers such as nifedipine are rarely successful but worth a trial. Infusions with a variety of prostacyclin and prostaglandin derivatives are the focus of intense investigation, but these agents are expensive, poorly tolerated, and effective only as long as they are used[21]. Botanseran and sildenafil (Viagra) may be useful adjuncts. This author believes that they should be employed as 'bridge therapy' until a lung transplant can be performed.

TABLE 128.4 DIFFERENTIAL DIAGNOSIS OF CNS VASCULITIS

Entity	Comment
CNS infection	Spinal fluid cultures or serologies or abscess on imaging suggest diagnosis
Organic brain syndrome	Seizures with normal CSF, mental status changes are chronic
Steroid psychosis	Improves within 24 hours of steroid taper and antipsychotic therapy
Aseptic meningitis	Withdraw ibuprofen or related NSAIDs
High-dose antimalarials	Produces manic state with dizziness, ringing in the ears
ITP	Very low platelet counts produce a CNS bleed
TTP	Seen with azotemia, hemolytic anemia, fever, low platelets
Hyperviscosity syndrome	Dizzy, mental fogging with high serum viscosity
Cryoglobulinemia	Dizziness, mental fogging, rash with cryoglobulins
Lupus headache	Migraine with a normal neurologic work-up
Cognitive dysfunction	Normal CSF and MRI; decreased perfusion on SPECT
Fibromyalgia	Tender points with normal neurologic work-up
Cerebral embolic stroke	Related to antiphospholipid antibodies, focal neurologic abnormalities with normal CSF
Cerebrovascular disease	Stroke or TIA associated with hypertension, steroid use, atheroembolic disease; CSF normal

SEVERE LUPUS IN THE NERVOUS SYSTEM

About 10% of lupus patients experience **central nervous system vasculitis** (Table 128.4). This usually occurs early in the course of the disease, the typical patient being a young woman who presents with a flu-like illness followed by fevers, lethargy and headache[22]. Within days she may develop seizures, mental status changes including psychosis, and frank meningismus. Untreated, the process progresses to stupor, coma and death. Infection is usually the first consideration, and indeed it is not uncommon for lupus patients to have true bacterial or viral meningitis or ibuprofen-induced aseptic meningitis. Opportunistic infections as well as corticosteroid or antimalarial drug reactions can mimic some aspects of CNS vasculitis. CNS vasculitis can be mistaken for cognitive dysfunction, organic brain syndrome (where seizures emanate from a scar focus and do not represent an acute inflammatory process), or a clot to the brain related to antiphospholipid antibodies. Any part of the brain can be affected and patients display almost any CNS manifestation, ranging from ataxia to chorea in addition to those listed above. Blood testing is generally unhelpful and may show evidence of active lupus. Cerebral imaging with MR scanning is usually normal, although individuals with thromboembolic disease from antiphospholipid antibodies can show focal infarctions. Cognitive dysfunction (see Chapter 122) without vasculitis is associated with bifrontal and bitemporal hypoperfusion on SPECT scans, but space-occupying lesions (e.g. tumors, AV malformations, abscesses, aneurysms) are better seen on MR images. The definitive diagnosis of CNS vasculitis can be made when spinal fluid demonstrates pleocytosis (seen in 30%), elevated proteins (seen in 40%), or a positive 'multiple sclerosis panel'[23] (Table 128.5). Consisting of IgG synthesis rate, oligoclonal bands and myelin basic protein, these determinations help screen for a coexisting multiple sclerosis (known as **lupoid sclerosis** when confirmatory demyelinating MR images are obtained). These CSF findings are evidence of an immune complex-mediated process (the choroid plexus shows evidence of immune complexes)[24]. The presence of ribosomal P serum antibodies is statistically associated with psychosis but not necessarily vasculitis, and levels are not helpful. Spinal fluid antineuronal antibodies can be elevated in 80% with true CNS vasculitis, but antibodies can also be present in glioblastomas[25]. Because the caliber of vessels involved is small, the yield of an angiogram for CNS vasculitis is only 10%. Brain biopsies and autopsy studies may demonstrate a vasculopathy, with hyalinization, perivascular inflammation, endothelial proliferation, thrombosis, infarction and small vessel vasculitis[26]. However, pathologic findings may not reveal vasculitis in all patients. One assumes that vasculitis is responsible for this diffuse gray and white matter process, but definitive proof for this

TABLE 128.5 DIAGNOSTIC TESTING FOR CNS VASCULITIS

CSF white cells	Increased in 30%
CSF protein	Increased in 40%
CSF IgG synthesis rate	Increased in 50%
CSF oligoclonal bands	Increased in 70%
CSF neuronal antibodies	Increased in 80%
CSF LE cells	Seen on Wright's stain, strongly suggestive of vasculitis
MRI brain with contrast	Normal with acute vasculitis, can show areas of prior activity
SPECT brain	Hypoperfusion to affected areas but not distinguishable from cognitive dysfunction
Angiogram	With or without MR, it has only a 10% yield
Chance of CNS vasculitis if all the above tests are normal: <10%. Brain biopsy can be done in unusual cases	
Not useful: C3, anti-DNA, sedimentation rate, C-reactive protein, antiribosomal P, CBC, chemistry panel.	

particular pathologic process in all patients is lacking. Once the diagnosis is made, pulse dosing of corticosteroids (1g of methylprednisolone intravenously three times daily) should be followed by 1mg/kg/day of prednisone equivalent for several weeks, followed by a slow tapering. This regimen is associated with a 40% relapse rate, which can be reduced to 5% if accompanied by 750mg/m² of cyclophosphamide given intravenously monthly for 6 months[27]. In refractory cases there is some evidence that plasmapheresis is useful as well[28].

Other severe manifestations of severe nervous system lupus include **hyperviscosity syndrome**, where elevated plasma viscosity levels due to high levels of circulating immune complexes induce vascular sludging, dizziness and mental dullness, as does its closely related cousin, **cryoglobulinemia**[29]. These rare complications are managed with anti-inflammatory regimens as well as apheresis. **Lupus myelitis** results from infarction of a spinal artery or inflammation of vessels or nerve tissue in the spinal cord. Paresis, urinary and bowel retention can ensue[30]. Prompt intervention with both pulses of corticosteroids and anticoagulation can be life-saving, as its etiology is rarely ascertained in sufficient time to make a difference in outcome. About one lupus patient in 300 has elevated spinal fluid pressures and headaches, with evidence for **pseudotumor cerebri**, relieved by periodic lumbar punctures[31]. Finally, inflammation of the peripheral nervous system can lead to **mononeuritis multiplex**, which presents with a foot or wrist drop, and burning or tingling. After 3 weeks classic changes are evident on nerve conduction studies, but early on a nerve biopsy may be needed to make the diagnosis[32]. This complication is usually associated with generalized active SLE and responds rapidly to corticosteroid therapy, with the addition of intravenous immune globulin in refractory cases.

HEMATOLOGIC MANIFESTATIONS

Deficiencies of any of the three blood elements can be associated with severe lupus. **Autoimmune hemolytic anemia** (AIHA) is clinically present in 15% of those with SLE at some time during the disease course[33]. Most patients with AIHA have a Coombs' direct positive warm IgG antibody covering red blood cells, which are destroyed prematurely. Hemolysis is induced by active disease, infection and stressful circumstances. The typical symptoms or signs of anemia are manifest in AIHA: fatigue, weakness, dizziness, a pale appearance and lassitude. It is detected by elevations in serum lactic dehydrogenase (LDH), decreases in serum haptoglobin, increased reticulocyte count and evidence of hemolysis on a blood smear (spherocytosis, anisocytosis, macrocytosis). AIHA is among the poorest prognostic subsets of SLE, especially if a hemolytic crisis occurs. Patients in crisis may have nucleated red blood cells, polychromasia, or Howell–Jolly bodies with a hyperplastic bone marrow. Other causes of anemia in SLE, such as B₁₂ deficiency (seen with atrophic gastritis with anti parietal cell antibodies), sickle cell anemia or trait (owing to its prominence in African-Americans), iron deficiency (women predominate in SLE and often have heavy periods), drugs that suppress the bone marrow, renal failure, and the anemia of chronic disease, should be considered. A minority with AIHA are only minimally anemic owing to 'compensated hemolysis', with reticulocyte counts in the range 8–10%. True AIHA is potentially life threatening and appropriate treatments may be delayed by transfusions or erythropoietin therapy. Patients should receive 1–1.5mg/kg/day of prednisone daily for 8–12 weeks, followed by a slow taper. About 50% of the time the addition of a steroid-sparing regimen with azathioprine, cyclophosphamide, danocrine or cyclosporin is needed. The major mistake in managing AIHA is not giving enough corticosteroids for a long enough period of time. **Pure red blood cell aplasia** or **aplastic anemia** due to active disease, with circulating factors inhibiting erythropoiesis and other blood elements, is rare and found in 1 in 1000 lupus patients. Anecdotal reports suggest that cyclosporin therapy is ameliorative[34].

TABLE 128.6 HOW TO MANAGE ITP IN LUPUS PATIENTS

1. For platelets >80 000: manage active lupus if present; no specific therapy for platelets needed

2. For platelets between 50 000 and 80 000: manage active lupus if present. If platelets are the only problem give 1 mg/kg/day of prednisone equivalent for 4–6 weeks then taper by 10% a week.
   - If platelets do not respond obtain hematologic consultation and bone marrow
   - If platelets respond but then fall with tapering, add danocrine 200mg bid as a steroid-sparing drug. If successful, try to taper steroids to less than 10mg of prednisone equivalent a day
   - If danocrine is not tolerated or does not work, add 100–200mg of azathioprine. If successful, try to taper steroids to less than 10 mg of prednisone equivalent a day

3. For platelets between 20 000 and 50 000: manage as in (2). If not successful, evaluate for laparoscopic splenectomy. If not a surgical candidate, or splenectomy has failed, consider cyclophosphamide

4. For platelets <20 000: use intravenous immunoglobulin to raise platelets and then treat as in (2) and (3). If unable to maintain rise in platelet count and splenectomy or cyclophosphamide has failed, consider rituximab

Autoimmune neutropenia is extremely rare and limited to a handful of case reports in SLE. On the other hand, antilymphocyte antibodies, viral infections and disease activity frequently lead to leukopenia as a consequence of **lymphopenia**. White blood cell counts below 2000/mm³ are found in 5% of lupus patients and usually respond to corticosteroids for disease activity, or to antimicrobial therapy[35]. The administration of growth factors such as G-CSF and GM-CSF has been associated with reports of lupus flares and should be used only by experienced practitioners in life-threatening or special circumstances[36].

When platelets are short-lived due to autoantibody formation in the absence of other abnormalities the patient is said to have **idiopathic thrombocytopenic purpura** (ITP) (Table 128.6). Twenty per cent of those with SLE have platelet counts lower than 100 000/mm³ during the course of their disease, but counts of 50 000/mm³ or less are found in only 5%[37]. Most individuals with ITP are asymptomatic. Easy bruisability, spontaneous bleeding, heavy menstrual flow and purpura may be seen in individuals with platelet counts less than 50 000/mm³, and epistaxis, oozing from the gums and petechiae are only found in patients with platelet counts less than 20 000/mm³. ITP usually exists by itself without SLE. The younger a patient with ITP is, the more responsive it is to corticosteroid therapy. Approximately 5–15% of cases of idiopathic ITP ultimately evolve into lupus years later. Patients with ITP usually have a normal physical examination. A large group with ITP and a positive ANA lack lupus symptoms and do not fulfill the ACR criteria for SLE. Among those with SLE, at least half have antiphospholipid antibodies or the circulating lupus anticoagulant. Evans' syndrome, the concurrence of AIHA and ITP, is not uncommon in SLE. ITP can be readily diagnosed when a bone marrow examination shows normal platelet formation in an individual who has low platelet counts. Antiplatelet antibodies are present but difficult to obtain and ascertain clinically. Sometimes, active lupus is associated with lower platelet counts and responds promptly to anti-inflammatory therapy. Our group usually manages ITP with corticosteroids (1mg/kg/day of prednisone equivalent for a few weeks, followed by a rapid taper) when the counts decline below 80 000/mm³. In our pregnant patients we treat counts up to 100 000/mm³ with corticosteroids, especially if they are also using heparin injections for antiphospholipid antibody-mediated previous miscarriages. Steroid-resistant ITP responds to danocrine (200–800mg/day), vincristine, azathioprine, cyclophosphamide and cyclosporin. Case reports of responses to rituximab have appeared[38]. Patients who require chronic immunosuppressive therapy are usually better off undergoing splenectomy, which is successful approximately 70% of the time. Thrombocytopenia due to **thrombotic thrombocytopenic purpura** is discussed in Chapter 122.

SEVERE LUPUS IN THE SKIN AND SENSORY ORGANS

The skin is involved in one form in over 80% of those with SLE. Breakdown of the skin representing severe lupus in the form of **cutaneous vasculitis** is present at some point in 10%[39]. Vasculitic ulceration with skin breakdown occurs rarely, and these lesions can mimic diabetic ulcers, infections, pressure sores and even pyoderma gangrenosum (Fig. 128.3). Most serious cutaneous vasculitis is found in the hands and feet. Infarction can be a complication of Raynaud's phenomenon, as well as cholesterol emboli (especially in nephrotic patients with very high cholesterol levels) or clots related to antiphospholipid antibodies. If not appropriately managed with high doses of corticosteroids and prostaglandin E1 infusions (for vasculitis) with or without anticoagulation, infarction with **digital gangrene** can become a life-threatening complication of the disease[40].

Up to 8% of SLE patients develop inflammation of the retinal artery during the course of their disease. Usually the only symptom is visual impairment. An equal number of patients have infarction of the retinal vasculature owing to the presence of antiphospholipid antibodies. Although both conditions sometimes lead to a 'cottonwool' infarction

pattern visible on ophthalmoscopy or fluorescein angiography (where perivascular exudates and patches of dye leakage along the vessels are seen), the treatment of **retinal vasculitis** consists of 1mg/kg/day of prednisone equivalent for 4–6 weeks, whereas thrombosis is managed with anticoagulation and platelet antagonists[41]. Retinal vasculitis is strongly associated with generalized active systemic disease and usually presents early in the disease process. Retinal infarction can also be seen in bacterial endocarditis ('Roth spots'), sickle cell anemia, diabetes mellitus and atherosclerosis (sometimes caused by prolonged steroid use). Ischemic or **optic neuritis** may also be associated with vasculitis, and the practitioner should consider the possibility of concurrent multiple sclerosis (lupoid sclerosis)[42]. Blurred vision and elevation of eye pressures are almost always a result of patients taking corticosteroids, as opposed to active lupus.

One lupus patient in 500 experiences sudden, usually unilateral, sensorineural hearing impairment, often associated with dizziness due to **autoimmune vestibulitis**[43]. Concurrent therapy with antimalarials, salicylates and non-steroidals mimics this complication, but the symptoms are bilateral. If treated promptly with high-dose corticosteroids, hearing returns to normal within days.

CONCEPTS OF PREVENTIVE MANAGEMENT

Severe lupus usually requires high doses of corticosteroids with or without immunosuppressants, and other innovative, aggressive therapies (e.g. apheresis) (Table 128.7). Survival studies suggest that this group, representing 25% of SLE patients, has only a 50% chance of surviving 15 years. Interestingly, only 25% of the deaths among these individuals are related to disease activity. As very ill patients survive serious inflammatory episodes, the therapies that allowed them to do so predispose to opportunistic infections[44]. Most importantly, the requirement for long-term moderate to high doses of corticosteroids leads to premature atherosclerosis, hyperlipidemia, diabetes mellitus, osteoporosis and cutaneous atrophy, which makes patients vulnerable to complications leading to an early demise. Thus, proactive adjunctive management of

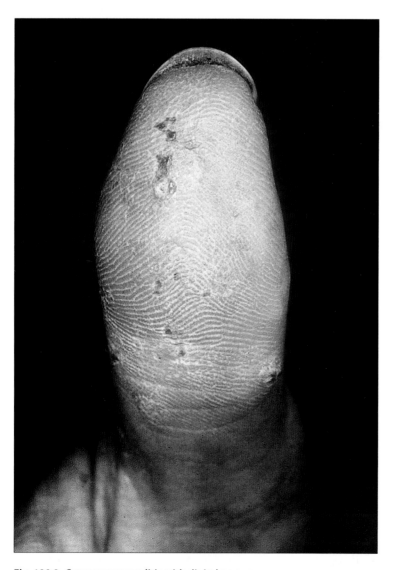

Fig. 128.3 Cutaneous vasculitis with digital gangrene.

TABLE 128.7 NON-STEROIDAL DISEASE-MODIFYING THERAPIES	
Azathioprine	Classic steroid-sparing drug. Controlled studies suggest efficacy for hepatitis, nephritis, interstitial lung disease, multiple sclerosis
Cyclophosphamide	The gold standard for nephritis, pneumonitis, CNS vasculitis
Mycophenolate mofetil	May be useful for nephritis, cutaneous vasculitis, promising for other complications
Cyclosporin	Nephritis, bone marrow hypoplasia
Danocrine	ITP, hemolytic anemia
Surgery	Pericardial tamponade, mesenteric vasculitis, transplant for lung, liver, kidney failure, spinal taps for pseudotumor cerebri, Libman–Sacks
Apheresis	Hyperviscosity, cryoglobulinemia, TTP, refractory pulmonary hemorrhage and CNS vasculitis
Prostaglandins	Digital gangrene, pulmonary hypertension
Anticoagulant/platelet inhibition	Libman–Sacks, Budd–Chiari, pulmonary embolus, certain thromboembolic complications

Not shown to be helpful for severe lupus: methotrexate
Useful in selected circumstances: nitrogen mustard, chlorambucil, 6-mercaptopurine, fludarabine, antilymphocyte globulin, antithymocyte globulin
Potentially useful but not adequately studied: tacrolimus, leflunomide, biologics

TABLE 128.8 SUPPORTIVE MEASURES FOR SEVERE LUPUS

- Visits every 1–3 months with vital signs, physical examination and laboratory tests
- Aggressive proactive management of blood pressure, blood sugars, serum lipids, weight
- Yearly bone densitometry
- Annual electrocardiogram and chest X-rays
- Dietary counseling
- Prompt evaluation of all fevers
- Periodic treadmill or stress testing
- Screening for and prophylactic management of antiphospholipid antibodies

severe lupus is just as important as being vigilant for disease activity. This author's recommendations follow (Table 128.8).

A qualified internist who has experience in managing lupus, such as a rheumatologist, hematologist or nephrologist, should ideally follow all patients with severe lupus. Visits should be scheduled on a regular basis, usually at least every 1–3 months. At these visits, a physical examination with vital signs, followed by laboratory tests including a complete blood count, comprehensive metabolic (chemistry) panel, urinalysis and screening tests for inflammation (e.g. sedimentation rate, C-reactive protein, C3 complement, anti-DNA) appropriate for the patient should be obtained. Blood pressure should be rigorously controlled. More than the usual attention should be paid to reviewing diet, weight and exercise considerations. At least two to three times a year fasting lipid and glucose levels should be obtained. Up to 50% may benefit from intervention with statins. The prevalence of steroid-induced diabetes is high and glycohemoglobin screening or glucose tolerance tests may be indicated. DEXA scanning for bone density should be performed annually. Recent ACR guidelines for glucocorticoid-induced osteoporosis advise intervention with bisphosphonates when starting more than 5mg of prednisone daily for more than 3 months[45]. The author usually performs a complete physical examination and obtains a chest X-ray and electrocardiogram annually. There are no blood tests that screen for heart or lung disease. Patients who have been on moderate-dose corticosteroids for more than 5 years should undergo stress testing (e.g. treadmill) every 2–3 years. The presence of any fever warrants an aggressive work-up to screen for occult infection. Depending on the patients' phospholipid and cardiac profile, platelet antagonists and even warfarin may be advised as prophylaxis against atheroembolic events. It is this writer's belief that attention to the factors listed above can greatly decrease the morbidity and mortality seen in severe SLE patients.

REFERENCES

1. Crozier IG, Li E, Milne MJ et al. Cardiac involvement in systemic lupus erythematosus detected by echocardiography. Am J Cardiol 1990; 1145–1148.
2. Fairfax TJ, Osborn TG, Williams GA et al. Endomyocardial biopsy in patients with systemic lupus erythematosus. J Rheumatol 1988; 15: 593–596.
3. Karrar A, Sequiera W, Block JA. Coronary artery disease in systemic lupus erythematosus: Review of the literature. Semin Arthritis Rheum 2001; 30: 436–443.
4. Berbir N, Allen J, Dubois E. The risk of pericardiocentesis in SLE: case report and literature review. Rev Rhum 1976; 44: 359–362.
5. Kahl LE. The spectrum of pericardial tamponade in systemic lupus erythematosus. Arthritis Rheum 1992; 35: 1343–1349.
6. Bulkey BH, Roberts WC. The heart in systemic lupus erythematosus and the changes induced in it by corticosteroid therapy. A study of 36 necropsy cases. Am J Med 1975; 58: 243–264.
7. Khamashta MA, Cervera R, Asherson RA et al. Association of antibodies against phospholipids with heart valve disease in systemic lupus erythematosus. Lancet 1990; 335: 1541–1544.
8. Saab S, Corr MP, Weisman MH. Corticosteroids and systemic lupus erythematosus pancreatitis: A case series. J Rheumatol 1998; 25: 801–806.
9. Hall S, Czaja AJ, Kaufman Dk et al. How lupoid is lupoid hepatitis? J Rheumatol 1986; 13: 95–98.
10. Hallegua DS, Wallace DJ. Gastrointestinal and hepatic manifestations. In: Wallace DJ, Hahn BH, eds. Dubois' lupus erythematosus, 6th edn. Philadelphia: Lippincott Williams & Wilkins, 2001.
11. Van Streenbergen, Beyls J, Vermylen J et al. Lupus anticoagulant and thrombosis of the hepatic veins (Budd–Chiari syndrome): report of three cases and review of the literature. J Hepatol 1986; 3: 87–94.
12. Nachbar F, Korting HC, Hoffman RM et al. Unusual coexistence of systemic lupus erythematosus and primary biliary cirrhosis. Dermatology 1994; 188: 313–317.
13. Zizic TM, Classen JN, Stevens MB. Acute abdominal complications of systemic lupus erythematosus and polyarteritis nodosa. Am J Med 1982; 73: 525–531.
14. Sunheimer RL, Finck C, Mortazavi S et al. Primary lupus-associated protein-losing enteropathy. Am J Clin Lab Sci 1994; 24: 239–242.
15. Carette S, Macher AM, Nussbaum A, Plotz PH. Severe acute pulmonary disease in patients with SLE: ten years of experience at the National Insitutues of Health. Semin Arthritis Rheum 1984; 14: 52–59.
16. Weinrib L, Sharma OP, Quismorio FP Jr. A long-term study of interstitial lung disease in systemic lupus erythematosus. Semin Arthritis Rheum 1990; 20: 48–56.
17. Varai G, Earle L, Jimenez SA et al. A pilot study of intermittent intravenous cyclophosphamide for the treatment of systemic sclerosis associated lung disease. J Rheumatol 1998; 25: 1325–1329.
18. Schwab EP, Schumacher HR, Freundlich B et al. Pulmonary alveolar hemorrhage in systemic lupus erythematosus. Semin Arthritis Rheum 1993; 23: 8–15.
19. Bick RL, Baker WF. Antiphospholipid syndrome and thrombosis, Semin Thromb Hemost 1999; 25: 333–350.
20. Asherson RA, Higgenbottom TW, Dihn Xuan AT et al. Pulmonary hypertension in a lupus clinic: experience with twenty-four patients. J Rheumatol 1990; 17: 1292–1298.
21. Robins IM, Gaine SP, Schilz R et al. Epoprostenol for treatment of pulmonary hypertension in patients with systemic lupus erythematosus, Chest 2000; 117: 14–18.
22. Tsokos GC, Tsokos M, le Riche NG, Klippel JH. A clinical and pathologic study of cerebrovascular disease in patients with systemic lupus erythematosus. Semin Arthritis Rheum 1986; 16: 70–78.
23. West SG. Systemic lupus erythematosus and the nervous system. in Wallace DJ, Hahn BH, eds. Dubois' lupus erythematosus, 6th edn. Philadelphia: Lippincott Williams & Wilkins, 2001.
24. Hietaharju A, Peltola J, Seppa J et al. The coexistence of systemic lupus erythematosus and multiple sclerosis in a mother and daughter. Scand J Rheumatol 2001; 30: 120–122.
25. Bluestein HG. Antibodies to brain. In: Wallace DJ, Hahn BH, eds. Dubois' lupus erythematosus, 5th edn. Baltimore: Williams & Wilkins, 1997; 517–522.
26. Ellis SG, Verity MA. Central nervous system involvement in systemic lupus erythematosus: review of neuropathologic findings in 57 cases, 1955–1977. Semin Arthritis Rheum 1979; 8: 212–221.
27. Boumpas DT, Yamada H, Patronas NJ et al. Pulse cyclophosphamide for severe neuropsychiatric lupus. QJ Med 1991; 296: 975–984.
28. Neuwelt CM, Lacks S, Kaye BR et al. Role of intravenous cyclophosphamide in the treatment of severe neuropsychiatric systemic lupus erythematosus. Am J Med 1995; 98: 32–41.
29. Garcia-Carrasco M, Ramos-Casals M, Cervera R et al. Cryoglobulinemia in systemic lupus erythematosus: Prevalence and clinical manifestations in a series of 122 patients. Semin Arthritis Rheum 2001; 30: 366–373.
30. Kovacs B, Lafferty TL, Brent LH. Transverse myelopathy in systemic lupus erythematosus: an analysis of 14 cases and review of the literature. Ann Rheum Dis 2000; 59: 120–124.
31. Greeb L, Vinker S, Amital T et al. Pseudotumor cerebri in systemic lupus erythematosus. Semin Arthritis Rheum 1995; 25: 103–108.
32. Omdal R, Mellgren SI, Husby G et al. A controlled study of peripheral neuropathy in systemic lupus erythematosus. Acta Neurol Scand 1993; 88: 41–46.
33. Kokori SI, Ioannidis JP, Voulgarelis M et al. Autoimmune hemolytic anemia in patients with systemic lupus erythematosus. Am J Med 2000; 108: 198–204.
34. Chute JP, Hoffmeister K, Cotelingam J et al. Aplastic anemia as the sole presentation of systemic lupus erythematosus. Am J Hematol 1996; 51: 237–239.
35. Rivero SJ, Diaz-Jouanen E, Alarcon-Segovia D. Lymphopenia in systemic lupus erythematosus. Arthritis Rheum 1978; 21: 295–305.
36. Hellmich B, Schnabel A, Gross WL. Treatment of severe neutropenia due to Felty's syndrome or systemic lupus erythematosus with granulocyte colony-stimulating factor. Semin Arthritis Rheum 1999; 29: 82–99.
37. Hakim AJ, Machin SJ, Isenberg DA. Autoimmune thrombocytopenia in primary antiphospholipid syndrome and systemic lupus erythematosus: Response to splenectomy. Semin Arthritis Rheum 1998; 28: 20–25.
38. Patel K, Berman J, Ferber A et al. Refractory autoimmune thrombocytopenic purpura treatment with rituximab. Am J Hematol 2001; 67: 59–60.
39. Lotti TM, Comacchi C, Ghersetich L. Cutaneous necrotizing vasculitis: relation to systemic disease. Adv Exp Med Biol 1999; 455: 115–125.
40. Langevitz P, Buskila D, Lee P, Urowitz MB. Treatment of refractory ischemic skin ulcers in patients with Raynaud's phenomenon with PgE1 infusions. J Rheumatol 1989; 16: 1433–1435.
41. Ushiyama O, Ushiyama K, Koarada S et al. Retinal disease in patients with systemic lupus erythematosus. Ann Rheum Dis 2000; 59: 705–708.

42. Galindo-Rodriguez G, Avina-Zubeta JA, Pizarro S *et al.* Cyclophosphamide pulse therapy for optic neuritis due to systemic lupus erythematosus: an open trial. Am J Med 1999; 106: 65–69.

43. Andonopoulos AP, Naxikis S, Goumas P *et al.* Sensoneural heating disorders in systemic lupus erythematosus. A controlled study. Clin Exp Rheumatol 1995; 13: 137–141.

44. Urowitz MA, Gladman DD. Prognosis of lupus. In: Wallace DJ, Hahn BH, eds. Dubois' lupus erythematosus, 6th edn. Philadelphia: Lippincott Williams & Wilkins, 2001.

45. American College of Rheumatology Ad Hoc Committee on Glucocorticoid-Induced Osteoporosis. Recommendations for the prevention and treatment of glucocorticoid-induced osteoporosis. Arthritis Rheum 2001; 44: 1496–1503.

129 Pregnancy in SLE

Michelle Petri

- Lupus flares, including renal flares, can occur during pregnancy and postpartum
- Preterm births are frequent in systemic lupus erythematosus pregnancies
- Antiphospholipid antibodies (lupus anticoagulant, anticardiolipin, or both) are associated with pregnancy loss

TYPICAL PATIENT

A 28-year-old woman has had systemic lupus erythematosus (SLE) for 4 years, initially diagnosed on the basis of antinuclear antibody positivity (1:640 titer, speckled pattern), malar rash, nephritis and presence of anti-double-stranded (ds)DNA. Renal biopsy showed World Health Organization Class III focal proliferative glomerulonephritis, which was treated initially with corticosteroids. Corticosteroid treatment proved unsuccessful, and mycophenolate mofetil 2000mg was added. Because of hypertension, an angiotensin-converting enzyme inhibitor was begun. Her current medications are prednisone 10mg, mycophenolate mofetil 2000mg, lisinopril 20mg and hydroxychloroquine 400mg. The most recent laboratory results included: anemia (hemotocrit 28%); urine analysis showing 1+ protein on dipstick testing; 3–5 urine red blood cells per high-powered field; serum creatinine concentration 1.2mg/dl; low C3 concentration (78mg/dl); low C4 concentration (10mg/dl); lupus anticoagulant testing using the modified Russell viper venom time, which showed prolongation and no correction in a mixing study. At a routine follow-up visit, the patient advises the physician that she is 2 months pregnant.

DEFINITION OF THE PROBLEM

The patient described presents with an unplanned pregnancy at a time when there is some evidence of disease activity and when she requires several medications to control her SLE and its complications. In this chapter, contraception, lupus flares during pregnancy, maternal complications and fetal complications are described.

FERTILITY/CONTRACEPTION

Systemic lupus erythematosus is not associated with infertility, unless the woman has been treated with cyclophosphamide, leading to premature ovarian failure. Infertile women with SLE (who do not have ovarian failure) may desire treatment with ovulation induction, with or without *in vitro* fertilization. These treatments confer some risk, in terms of both lupus flares and thrombosis[1]. However, most flares that have been reported were mild[2].

Pregnancies in SLE are associated with important maternal and fetal morbidity. Pregnancies should be planned for a time of good control of maternal disease activity and require adjustment of the medical regimen to avoid drugs with teratogenic potential, and angiotensin-converting enzyme inhibitors. Risk assessment – in terms of checking for anti-phospholipid antibodies (for risk of fetal loss) and for anti-Ro and anti-La antibodies (for risk of neonatal lupus) – should be undertaken before the pregnancy. In many centers, however, planned pregnancies are the exception, rather than the rule. Ideally, patients are counseled to use an effective, but safe means of contraception, to avoid unplanned pregnancies.

Ideally, a woman who has completed her family will choose tubal ligation (or her partner, vasectomy). Barrier contraception (diaphragm, foam, condom) are safe in SLE. The intrauterine device can be used if a woman is in a monogamous relationship and is not receiving major immunosuppression that would predispose to infections. The great majority of premenopausal women with SLE, however, will use progesterone-only contraception, usually depo-provera (the progesterone 'mini-pill' is less favored, because of break-through bleeding, and Norplant is rarely used). Progesterone-only contraception is not associated with SLE flare.

Although estrogen-containing oral contraceptives are the preferred means of contraception in the general population, their use in SLE remains controversial. In the Nurses' Health Study[3], normal women who took oral contraceptives had an increased risk of developing SLE. In one study, women with lupus nephritis had a high flare rate after starting to use oral contraceptives[4]. However, oral contraceptives can also provide benefit in SLE, including control of cyclic disease activity, preservation of fertility in women taking cyclophosphamide and prevention of osteoporosis[5]. The Safety of Estrogen in Lupus: National Assessment (SELENA) study is a randomized double-blind placebo-controlled trial, currently in progress, that aims to address the question of whether oral contraceptives increase the severe flare rate in SLE.

However, the controversy regarding the use of oral contraceptives in SLE extends beyond the issue of disease activity. As many as 50% of patients with SLE make antiphospholipid antibodies (lupus anticoagulant, anticardiolipin, anti-β_2 glycoprotein I) and are therefore at greater risk of thrombosis. The addition of exogenous estrogen would further increase hypercoagulability. In our experience, both oral contraceptives and pregnancy have been inciting factors in the development of the catastrophic form of the antiphospholipid antibody syndrome[6]. Thus, although there may be some gynecologic issues in patients with SLE that require oral contraceptives, such as the management of endometriosis or ovarian cysts, most patients with SLE should be advised to use other forms of contraception. Patients with SLE who have known antiphospholipid antibodies should avoid oral contraceptive pills.

LUPUS FLARES DURING PREGNANCY

An increase in SLE disease activity during pregnancy would be expected, as a result of the increases in estrogen, prolactin and T helper cell 2 cytokines. However, studies of SLE flares in pregnancy show conflicting results (Table 129.1).

Both study design and patient selection likely explain the differing results of SLE flare studies. No one definition of lupus flare is currently accepted. Several studies have used a simple definition based on a 1.0

TABLE 129.1 SLE FLARES DURING PREGNANCY

Study	Design	SLE (pregnant)	SLE (non-pregnant)	Result
Lockshin et al. 1984[7]	Case–control	33	28	No difference
Meehan and Dorsey 1987[8]	Case–control	18	22	No difference
Petri et al. 1991[9]	Prospective, controlled	36	185	0.136 vs 0.054 flares/month
Urowitz et al. 1993[10]	Case–control	61	59	70% vs 80%; no difference
Cabral-Castaneda et al. 1996[11]	Retrospective	84		17.8% flares
Ruiz-Irastorza et al. 1996[12]	Prospective	78	50	65% vs 42% (p=0.0015) Flare rate: 0.082 cf 0.039 (p<0.001)
LeHoung et al. 1997[13]	Prospective	62		27% flares
Johns et al. 1998[14]	Retrospective	28		60.7% flares
Aggarwal et al. 1999[15]	Retrospective	15		2 renal flares
Carmona et al. 1999[16]	Prospective	60		28.3% flares; 0.044 flares/patient per month
Sittiwangkul et al. 1999[17]	Retrospective	48		33% flares
De Bandt et al. 2000[18]	Cohort	59		7 severe flares
Georgiou et al. 2000[19]	Case–control	59	59	13.5% flares

change on a 0–3 Physician's Global Assessment[9], but a more elaborate definition of flare is currently being used in the SELENA study[20]. Patient selection may be the most important variable. There is a general consensus that the ideal patient for pregnancy is one whose disease has been quiescent for 6 months or more; in centers with mostly planned pregnancies, a patient with such a profile is unlikely to experience a disease flare during pregnancy. Other centers, with mostly unplanned pregnancies, more patients taking prednisone, or more patients with recent or current disease activity[9,12] will tend to report greater flare rates.

SLE flares can occur in any trimester, including postpartum. The Hopkins Lupus Pregnancy Center has reported more renal and hematologic flares during pregnancy[21], but this experience is not universal. Patients with SLE flares are more likely to deliver preterm[17,21], but there is not necessarily an increase in fetal loss. Some renal flares have led to irreversible renal deterioration. Renal flares may be difficult to differentiate from pre-eclampsia (and the two conditions may co-exist)[22].

Management of SLE flares must take into account the need both to control disease activity rapidly and to avoid medications with teratogenic effects (Table 129.2).

TABLE 129.2 MANAGEMENT OF SLE FLARES DURING PREGNANCY

Drug	Toxicity concerns
Prednisone (oral)	Metabolized by placenta; increased doses are associated with pre-eclampsia and gestational diabetes
Methylprednisolone (pulse)	
Azathioprine	Crosses placenta; birth defects are rare
Mycophenolate mofetil	Crosses placenta; azathioprine should be substituted
Cyclosporin	Crosses placenta; may be associated with intrauterine growth retardation
Cyclophosphamide	Crosses placenta; major teratogen; used only in late second or third trimester for life-threatening or organ-threatening (renal, central nervous system) flares
Non-steroidal anti-inflammatory drugs	Cross placenta; stopped in first trimester because of adverse effects on ductus arteriosus
Hydroxychloroquine	Crosses placenta, but no eye or ear toxicity in longitudinal or clinical trial experience

Most centers use corticosteroids and azathioprine and cyclosporin, when needed, in SLE pregnancies[23]. Hydroxychloroquine, although it crosses the placenta, has had an excellent safety record[24], including a recent randomized clinical trial[25].

MATERNAL MORBIDITY DURING PREGNANCY

In addition to the obvious morbidity from SLE flares and their treatment, other morbidity is also increased in SLE pregnancy (Table 129. 3). In a case–control study, it was found that urinary tract infections, diabetes mellitus, hypertension, preterm premature rupture of membranes and pre-eclampsia were all increased in SLE[21]. In another case–control study, which used data from the California Health Information for Policy Project, hypertensive complications, renal disease, preterm delivery, non-elective Cesarean section, postpartum hemorrhage and delivery-related deep venous thrombosis occurred more frequently in the 555 women with SLE than in the 600 000 control women (p<0.001)[26].

Pregnancy (and especially the postpartum period) represents an additional thrombotic risk in those patients with SLE who have antiphospholipid antibodies. Patients who are already taking warfarin because of a past venous or arterial thrombotic event are switched to therapeutic

TABLE 129.3 MATERNAL MORBIDITY OF SLE PREGNANCY

- SLE flares
- Urinary tract infections
- Hypertension
- Diabetes mellitus
- Pre-eclampsia
- Preterm rupture of membranes
- Thrombosis

TABLE 129.4 MANAGEMENT OF ANTIPHOSPHOLIPID ANTIBODIES IN PREGNANCY

No past pregnancy morbidity	No treatment or low-dose aspirin (81mg)
One early first-trimester loss	Low-dose aspirin (81mg)
Multiple early losses or one late fetal loss	Prophylactic heparin (either unfractionated or low molecular weight) plus low-dose aspirin (81mg)
Past venous or arterial thrombosis	Therapeutic anticoagulation with heparin, with or without low-dose aspirin (81mg)

doses of heparin (either unfractionated or low molecular weight) as soon as pregnancy is recognized. Patients who have had only fetal losses (or other pregnancy morbidity) from antiphospholipid antibody syndrome are treated with prophylactic doses of heparin and low-dose aspirin (81mg) during subsequent pregnancies. Management of the antiphospholipid antibody syndrome is summarized in Table 129.4. Currently, there is no accepted 'prophylactic' treatment in women with SLE who have antiphospholipid antibodies and no past morbidity, although many would consider the use of low-dose aspirin (81mg), with or without hydroxychloroquine. A retrospective case–control study demonstrated that women with antiphospholipid antibodies who continued to receive low-dose aspirin (81mg) were significantly less likely to suffer a thrombotic event after delivery[27].

Potentially or actually life-threatening complications have occurred, albeit rarely, in the prospective experience of 250 pregnancies at the Hopkins Lupus Pregnancy Center. There have been two maternal deaths, one from a postpartum pulmonary embolus in a patient without antiphospholipid antibodies, and one sudden death postpartum in a patient with lupus myocarditis during pregnancy. Complications of the antiphospholipid antibody syndrome, including pulmonary emboli, strokes in therapeutically anticoagulated patients, and HELLP syndrome (hemolysis, elevated liver enzymes, low platelets), occurred in five others. Another patient suffered a spinal cord hemorrhage on anticoagulation, with permanent pareparesis. Several patients suffered permanent renal impairment requiring later dialysis. One patient, who had a previous Cesarean section, had a uterine rupture during labor.

Because of the maternal morbidity of SLE pregnancy, all SLE pregnancies should be considered high risk and monitored accordingly, by both the obstetrician and rheumatologist.

FETAL MORBIDITY

Fetal loss

Pregnancy losses are significantly increased in SLE compared with control groups[28] (Table 129.5). Fetal loss can occur at any trimester. First trimester losses are associated with antiphospholipid antibodies, but also with markers of lupus activity (such as low complement concentrations and increased anti-dsDNA) and renal disease[29]. Later losses are associated with antiphospholipid antibodies.

The current pregnancy classification criteria for antiphospholipid antibody syndrome were adopted at a consensus conference in Sapporo, Japan[30] and were subsequently validated[31]. The presence of either a lupus anticoagulant or medium- to high-titer anticardiolipin on two occasions, 6 weeks apart, is required, in addition to one of three clinical events: (1) recurrent first trimester losses, (2) one late pregnancy loss or (3) other pregnancy morbidity, such as preterm birth as a result of severe pre-eclampsia, or placental insufficiency. Other antiphospholipid antibodies (anti-β_2 glycoprotein I and anti-phosphatidyl ethanolamine) are also associated with pregnancy loss, but are not yet included in the criteria. Unless the woman has had past arterial or venous thrombosis that requires therapeutic anticoagulation, management of the next pregnancy in a woman with past fetal loss is prophylactic heparin (either unfractionated or low molecular weight) and low-dose aspirin (81mg). A

landmark clinical trial proved that, although both heparin/low-dose aspirin and prednisone/aspirin led to equivalent fetal survival, the heparin/aspirin regimen was associated with less maternal morbidity[32]. Subsequent clinical trials have demonstrated that some pregnancies will be successful with aspirin alone, but that heparin and aspirin together is the best regimen[33].

Some women continue to miscarry in spite of treatment with heparin and aspirin. No set regimen exists for this clinical scenario; some would add intravenous immunoglobulin, which binds antiphospholipid antibodies[34,35], during the next pregnancy or add plasmapheresis[36,37].

Other hypercoaguable states besides antiphospholipid antibody syndrome are also associated with increased fetal loss. Women with SLE with fetal losses who are negative for antiphospholipid antibodies (including lupus anticoagulant, anticardiolipin and anti-β_2 glycoprotein 1) should also be screened for genetic causes of hypercoagulability, such as Factor V Leiden, the prothrombin mutation and hyperhomocysteinemia[16,38].

Preterm birth

Preterm delivery is numerically more of a problem than fetal loss in SLE (Table 129.5)[14,39]. Preterm birth occurs because of pre-eclampsia, premature rupture of the membranes and placental insufficiency. Many centers have documented a greater frequency of preterm birth in patients with SLE than in control pregnancies[15,28]. Preterm premature rupture of membranes is also more common in those with SLE than in non-SLE pregnancies[40]. A greater rate of preterm deliveries, especially pre-eclampsia, is seen with higher doses of prednisone[21,41].

Non-invasive fetal monitoring can help to detect a fetus 'at risk'. Umbilical artery blood flow velocity detects absent or reversed end-diastolic flow velocity, a marker of increased risk of pre-eclampsia, intrauterine growth retardation, Cesarean section and preterm delivery[42].

Intrauterine growth retardation

Intrauterine growth retardation is increased in SLE pregnancies[14,15,41,43]. In the Hopkins Lupus Pregnancy Center there were no clinical or laboratory predictors, but hypocomplementemia was an associated factor in one study[41]. The best ultrasound predictors of intrauterine growth retardation were a fetal abdominal circumference less than 10% and an estimated fetal body weight less than 50%[43].

Neonatal lupus

Neonatal lupus presents as congenital heart block or as lupus rash[44]. It is rare in SLE pregnancies, occurring in 3.5% in one series[29]. It is highly associated with maternal anti-Ro (usually with anti-La also), although the rash can occur with anti-RNP. Because not all anti-Ro/La pregnancies are affected with congenital heart block, prophylactic treatment is not appropriate. Instead, fetal four-chamber cardiac echocardiograms, from the 16th to the 28th week of gestation, are recommended. If heart block (of any degree) is found, dexamethasone 4mg daily is given to the mother, because dexamethasone crosses the placenta. It is unusual for third-degree heart block to be reversible. Rarely, neonatal lupus presents as hepatic or hematologic involvement.

Most babies with congenital heart block can be delivered at term; if there is severe hydrops, early Cesarean section is necessary. In the neonate, pacing is sometimes required[45]. Rarely, children with congenital heart block develop a connective tissue disease in adolescence[46].

Fetal and childhood development

In one case–control study, children of mothers with SLE were shown to have more developmental difficulties, immunorelated disorders and non-righthandedness than controls, especially in male children[47]. Whether this represents preterm delivery, adverse effects of maternal medications or transplacental transfer of maternal autoantibodies is unknown.

TABLE 129.5 FETAL MORBIDITY OF SLE PREGNANCY		
Pregnancy loss	Total	13.1%
	First	6.0%
	Later	7.1%
Preterm birth	≤37 weeks	40.5%
	≤36 weeks	32.1%

CONCLUSION

Because of the risks of SLE pregnancy, safe and effective contraception is important in SLE, and is usually achieved with depo-progesterone or tubal ligation. Maternal risks of pregnancy include SLE flares, urinary tract infections, diabetes mellitus, hypertension, pre-eclampsia and thrombosis. Fetal risks include fetal loss (especially secondary to antiphospholipid antibody syndrome), preterm birth, intrauterine growth retardation and neonatal lupus. Interdisciplinary collaboration in the management of SLE pregnancy by a high-risk obstetrician/rheumatology team, with the help of the ultrasonographer, medical geneticist and perinatologist in selected cases, is important. Even in patients whose disease is stable, monthly rheumatologic visits are urged. Non-invasive fetal monitoring during the late second and third trimesters can help to identify a fetus at risk and help to time delivery. A successful pregnancy outcome is achievable in 90% of SLE pregnancies.

REFERENCES

1. Huong DL, Wechsler B, Piette JC et al. Risks of ovulation-induction therapy in systemic lupus erythematosus. Br J Rheumatol 1996; 35: 1184–1186.
2. Guballa N, Sammaritano L, Schwartzman S et al. Ovulation induction and in vitro fertilization in systemic lupus erythematosus and antiphospholipid syndrome. Arthritis Rheum 2000; 43: 550–556.
3. Sanchez-Guerrero J, Karlson EW, Liang MH et al. Past use of oral contraceptives and the risk of developing systemic lupus erythematosus. Arthritis Rheum 1997; 40: 804–808.
4. Jungers P, Dougados M, Pelissier C et al. Influence of oral contraceptive therapy on the activity of systemic lupus erythematosus. Arthritis Rheum 1982; 25: 618–623.
5. Petri M, Robinson C. Oral contraceptives and systemic lupus erythematosus. Arthritis Rheum 1997; 40: 797–803.
6. Asherson RA, Cervera R, Piette JC et al. Catastrophic antiphospholipid syndrome: clues to the pathogenesis from a series of 80 patients. Medicine (Baltimore) 2001; 80: 355–377.
7. Lockshin MD, Reinitz E, Druzin ML et al. Lupus pregnancy. I. Case–control prospective study demonstrating absence of lupus exacerbation during or after pregnancy. Am J Med 1984; 77: 893–898.
8. Meehan RT, Dorsey JK. Pregnancy among patients with systemic lupus erythematosus receiving immunosuppressive therapy. J Rheumatol 1987; 14: 252–258.
9. Petri M, Howard D, Repke J. Frequency of lupus flare in pregnancy: the Hopkins Lupus Pregnancy Center experience. Arthritis Rheum 1991; 34: 1538–1545.
10. Urowitz MB, Gladman DD, Farewell VT et al. Lupus and pregnancy studies. Arthritis Rheum 1993; 36: 1392–1397.
11. Cabral-Castaneda F, Hernandez-Campos AG, Carballar-Lopez G et al. Systemic lupus erythematosus and pregnancy (analysis of 84 cases). Ginecol Obstet Mex 1996; 64: 363–367.
12. Ruiz-Irastorza G, Lima F, Alves J et al. Increased rate of lupus flare during pregnancy and the puerperium: a prospective study of 78 pregnancies. Br J Rheumatol 1996; 35: 133–138.
13. Le Huong D, Wechsler B, Vauthier-Brouzes D et al. Outcome of planned pregnancies in systemic lupus erythematosus: a prospective study on 62 pregnancies. Br J Rheumatol 1997; 36: 772–777.
14. Johns KR, Morand EF, Littlejohn GO. Pregnancy outcome in systemic lupus erythematosus (SLE): a review of 54 cases. Aust N Z J Med 1998; 28: 18–22.
15. Aggarwal N, Sawhney H, Vasishta K et al. Pregnancy in patients with systemic lupus erythematosus. Aust N Z J Obstet Gynaecol 1999; 39: 28–30.
16. Carmona F, Font J, Cervera R et al. Obstetrical outcome of pregnancy in patients with systemic lupus erythematosus. A study of 60 cases. Eur J Obstet Gynecol Reprod Biol 1999; 83: 137–142.
17. Sittiwangkul S, Louthrenoo W, Vithayasai P, Sukitawut W. Pregnancy outcome in Thai patients with systemic lupus erythematosus. Asian Pac J Allergy Immunol 1999; 17: 77–83.
18. De Bandt M, Palazzo E, Belmatoug N et al. Outcome of pregnancies in lupus: experience at one center. Ann Med Int (Paris) 2000; 151: 87–92.
19. Georgiou PE, Politi EN, Katsimbri P et al. Outcome of lupus pregnancy: a controlled study. Rheumatology (Oxford) 2000; 39: 1014–1019.
20. Kim MY, Buyon JP, Petri M et al. Equivalence trials in SLE research: issues to consider. Lupus 1999; 8: 620–626.
21. Petri M. Hopkins Lupus Pregnancy Center: 1987 to 1996. Rheum Dis Clin North Am 1997; 23: 1–14.
22. Repke JT. Hypertensive disorders of pregnancy. Differentiating preeclampsia from active systemic lupus erythematosus. J Reprod Med 1998; 43: 350–354.
23. Ramsey-Goldman R, Mientus JM, Kutzer JE et al. Pregnancy outcome in women with systemic lupus erythematosus treated with immunosuppressive drugs. J Rheumatol 1993; 20: 1152–1157.
24. Parke A, West B. Hydroxychloroquine in pregnant patients with systemic lupus erythematosus. J Rheumatol 1996; 23: 1715–1718.
25. Levy RA, Vilela VS, Cataldo MJ et al. Hydroxychloroquine (HCQ) in lupus pregnancy: double-blind and placebo-controlled study. Lupus 2001; 10: 401–404.
26. Yasmeen S, Wilkins EE, Field NT et al. Pregnancy outcomes in women with systemic lupus erythematosus. J Matern Fetal Med 2001; 10: 91–96.
27. Erkan D, Merrill JT, Yazici Y et al. High thrombosis rate after fetal loss in antiphospholipid syndrome: effective prophylaxis with aspirin. Arthritis Rheum 2001; 44: 1466–1467.
28. Petri M, Allbritton J. Fetal outcome of lupus pregnancy: a retrospective case–control study of the Hopkins Lupus Cohort. J Rheumatol 1993; 20: 650–656.
29. Rahman P, Gladman DD, Urowitz MB. Clinical predictors of fetal outcome in systemic lupus erythematosus. J Rheumatol 1998; 25: 1526–1530.
30. Wilson WA, Gharavi AE, Koike T et al. International consensus statement on preliminary classification criteria for definite antiphospholipid syndrome: report of an international workshop. Arthritis Rheum 1999; 42: 1309–1311.
31. Lockshin MD, Sammaritano LR, Schwartzman S. Validation of the Sapporo criteria for antiphospholipid syndrome. Arthritis Rheum 2000; 43: 440–443.
32. Cowchock FS, Reece EA, Balaban D et al. Repeated fetal losses associated with antiphospholipid antibodies: a collaborative randomized trial comparing prednisone with low-dose heparin treatment. Am J Obstet Gynecol 1992; 166: 1318–1323.
33. Rai R, Cohen H, Dave M, Regan L. Randomised controlled trial of aspirin and aspirin plus heparin in pregnant women with recurrent miscarriage associated with phospholipid antibodies (or antiphospholipid antibodies). Br Med J 1997; 314: 253–257.
34. Branch DW, Peaceman AM, Druzin M et al. A multicenter, placebo-controlled pilot study of intravenous immune globulin treatment of antiphospholipid syndrome during pregnancy. The Pregnancy Loss Study Group. Am J Obstet Gynecol 2000; 182: 122–127.
35. Gordon C, Kilby MD. Use of intravenous immunoglobulin therapy in pregnancy in systemic lupus erythematosus and antiphospholipid antibody syndrome. Lupus 1998; 7: 429–433.
36. Takeshita Y, Turumi Y, Touma S, Takagi N. Successful delivery in a pregnant woman with lupus anticoagulant positive systemic lupus erythematosus treated with double filtration plasmapheresis. Ther Apher 2001; 5: 22–24.
37. Nakamura Y, Yoshida K, Itoh S et al. Immunoadsorption plasmapheresis as a treatment for pregnancy complicated by systemic lupus erythematosus with positive antiphospholipid antibodies. Am J Reprod Immunol 1999; 41: 307–311.
38. Kupferminc MJ, Eldor A, Steinman N et al. Increased frequency of genetic thrombophilia in women with complications of pregnancy. N Engl J Med 1999; 340: 9–13.
39. Kleinman D, Katz VL, Kuller JA. Perinatal outcomes in women with systemic lupus erythematosus. J Perinatol 1998; 18: 178–182.
40. Johnson MJ, Petri M, Witter FR, Repke JT. Evaluation of preterm delivery in a systemic lupus erythematosus pregnancy clinic. Obstet Gynecol 1995; 86: 396–399.
41. Kobayashi N, Yamada H, Kishida T et al. Hypocomplementemia correlates with intrauterine growth retardation in systemic lupus erythematosus. Am J Reprod Immunol 1999; 42: 153–159.
42. Farine D, Granovsky-Grisaru S, Ryan G et al. Umbilical artery blood flow velocity in pregnancies complicated by systemic lupus erythematosus. J Clin Ultrasound 1998; 26: 379–382.
43. Witter FR, Petri M. Antenatal detection of intrauterine growth restriction in patients with systemic lupus erythematosus. Int J Gynaecol Obstet 2000; 71: 67–68.
44. Tseng CE, Buyon JP. Neonatal lupus syndromes. Rheum Dis Clin North Am 1997; 23: 31–54.
45. Grolleau R, Leclercq F, Guillaumont S, Voisin M. Congenital atrioventricular block. Arch Mal Coeur Vaiss 1999; 92: 47–55.
46. Hubscher O, Carrillo D, Reichlin M. Congenital heart block and subsequent connective tissue disorder in adolescence. Lupus 1997; 6: 283–284.
47. McAllister DL, Kaplan BJ, Edworthy SM et al. The influence of systemic lupus erythematosus on fetal development: cognitive, behavioral, and health trends. J Int Neuropsychol Soc 1997; 3: 370–376.

130 Sjögren's syndrome

Athanasios G Tzioufas and Haralampos M Moutsopoulos

Definition

- A slowly progressive, inflammatory autoimmune disease affecting primarily the exocrine glands
- Lymphocytic infiltrates replace functional epithelium, leading to decreased exocrine secretions (exocrinopathy)
- Characteristic autoantibodies, Ro(SS-A) and La(SS-B), are produced

Clinical features

- Mucosal dryness manifested by keratoconjunctivitis sicca, xerostomia, xerotrachea and vaginal dryness
- Major salivary gland enlargement
- Non-erosive polyarthritis; Raynaud's phenomenon without telangiectasia or digital ulceration
- The periepithelial extraglandular manifestations are the result of lymphocytic invasion in epithelial tissues of lungs, kidneys and liver; they appear early in the disease and have a benign course
- The extraepithelial manifestations, such as skin vasculitis, peripheral neuropathy and glomerulonephritis, with low C4 levels, are associated with increased morbidity and high risk for lymphoma
- Association with other autoimmune diseases (RA, SLE, systemic sclerosis, polymyositis)
- Increased risk of lymphoid malignancy

HISTORY

The various clinical features of keratitis, dry mouth and salivary gland enlargement, were first described in the late 1800s by Hadden, Leber and Mikulicz. However, it was not until the work of Gougerot in France in 1925, and of Sjögren in Sweden in 1933 that association of these findings with polyarthritis and systemic disease was fully appreciated. Sjögren, a Swedish ophthalmologist, wrote the classic monograph on the disease, in which he emphasized that the eye manifestations are local findings of a systemic disorder.[1] In 1953, Morgan and Castleman[2] showed that the intense focal lymphocytic infiltrate of the parotid gland, described in Mikulicz's patient about 60 years earlier, was identical to the characteristic findings in Sjögren's syndrome (Table 130.1). This resolution of nomenclature was followed by an increasing recognition of the diverse clinical spectrum of Sjögren's syndrome and, in the 1960s, by the

TABLE 130.1 SYNONYMS FOR SJÖGREN'S SYNDROME

- Mikulicz's disease
- Gougerot's syndrome
- Sicca syndrome
- Autoimmune exocrinopathy
- Autoimmune epithelitis

discovery of autoantibodies in Sjögren's syndrome patients. Subsequent work has defined a genetic predisposition for the disease marked by specific HLA antigens, and advanced molecular and cellular techniques have dissected the specificity of autoantibodies to cellular components Ro(SS-A) and La(SS-B), the composition and function of the focal lymphocytic infiltrates of the exocrine glands, and the biology of the epithelial cell in the immunopathologic lesion.[3]

EPIDEMIOLOGY

Sjögren's syndrome can occur at all ages, but it affects primarily females during the fourth and fifth decades of life with a female:male ratio of 9:1. Among pediatric presentations, the youngest reported patient was 3 years old, with others being drawn from the full age distribution to the mid-teens.[4]

Studies on geriatric populations revealed that it occurs in approximately 3%.[5] Using a validated questionnaire[6] it was found that the prevalence of definite and probable Sjögren's syndrome in women in a Greek town was 0.6% and 3%, respectively.[7] In another epidemiologic study, performed in Sweden, the calculated prevalence of Sjögren's syndrome in 705 randomly selected women aged 52–72 years was 2.7%.[8] In a cross-sectional population-based survey performed on 1000 adults aged from 18 to 75 years, randomly selected from a population register, it was shown that Sjögren's syndrome affects approximately 3–4% of adults, and in the general population appears to be associated with a clinically significant impairment of the subject's health.[9]

CLINICAL FEATURES

In most patients primary Sjögren's syndrome runs a rather slow and benign course.[10] Initial manifestations can be non-specific, and usually 6 years elapse from the initial symptoms to the full-blown development of the syndrome Table 130.2.[11]

Exocrinopathy (glandular involvement)

Ocular involvement

Diminished tear production leads to the destruction of both corneal and bulbar conjunctival epithelium and a constellation of clinical findings termed keratoconjunctivitis sicca (KCS). Physical signs include dilation of the bulbar conjunctival vessels, pericorneal injection, irregularity of the corneal image and lacrimal gland enlargement. The patient usually complains of a burning, sandy or scratchy sensation under the lids, itchiness, redness and photosensitivity. Sensitive tests are available to detect KCS (Figs 130.1 & 130.2), but these are not specific for Sjögren's syndrome as KCS may occur in a number of other conditions.

Oropharyngeal involvement

Xerostomia, or dry mouth, results from markedly decreased production of saliva by the salivary glands. Patients often report difficulty in swallowing dry food, inability to speak continuously, changes in sense of

TABLE 130.2 CLINICAL MANIFESTATIONS OF PRIMARY SJÖGREN'S SYNDROME AT DIAGNOSIS AND AFTER A 10-YEAR FOLLOW-UP[38]		
	Prevalence at diagnosis (%)	Prevalence at end of follow-up (%)
Glandular disease		
Xerostomia	90	92
Dry eyes	95	95
Parotid gland enlargement	49	53
Extranglandular disease		
Arthralgias/arthritis	70	75
Raynaud's phenomenon	41	48
Pulmonary involvement	23	29
Kidney involvement: Interstitial nephritis	7	9
Glomerulonephritis	0.4	2
Liver involvement	4	4
Peripheral neuropathy	1	2
Myositis	1	1
Central nervous system disease	0	0
Lymphoma	2	4

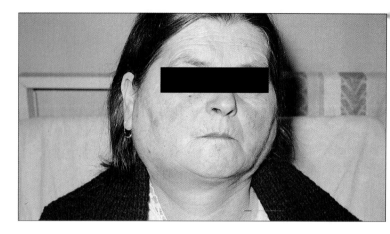

Fig. 130.3 Patient with primary Sjögren's syndrome. Parotid gland enlargement.

taste, a burning sensation in the mouth, an increase in dental caries and problems with wearing complete dentures. Physical examination shows a dry, erythematous sticky oral mucosa, dental caries, scanty and cloudy saliva from the major salivary glands and, on the dorsal tongue, atrophy of the filiform papillae. Parotid or major salivary gland enlargement occurs in 60% of primary Sjögren's syndrome patients. In many patients the salivary gland enlargement occurs episodically, whereas others have chronic, persistent enlargement. The parotid gland swelling may begin unilaterally but often becomes bilateral (Fig. 130.3). Table 130.3 lists con-

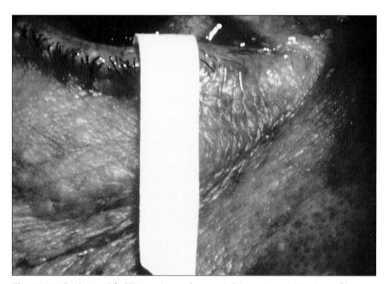

Fig. 130.1 Patient with Sjögren's syndrome. Schirmer's test. Wetting of less than 5 mm/5 min of the filter paper strip is shown.

TABLE 130.3 DIFFERENTIAL DIAGNOSIS OF PAROTID GLAND ENLARGEMENT	
Bilateral	Viral infection (mumps, influenza, Epstein–Barr, Coxsackie A, cytomegalovirus, HIV) Sjögren's syndrome Sarcoidosis Miscellaneous (diabetes mellitus, hyperlipoproteinemia, hepatic, cirrhosis, chronic pancreatitis, acromegaly, gonadal hypofunction) Recurrent parotitis of childhood
Unilateral	Salivary gland neoplasm Bacterial infection Chronic sialadenitis Sialolithiasis

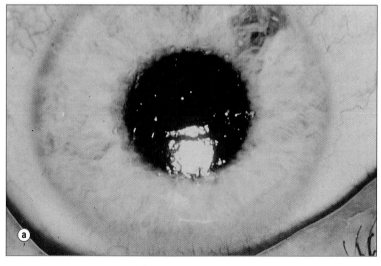
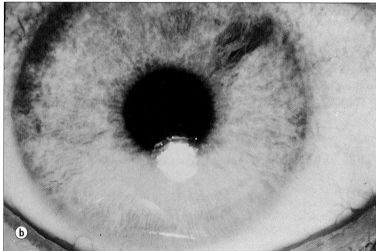

Fig. 130.2 Rose Bengal staining. (a) In a normal volunteer and (b) in a patient with Sjögren's syndrome; retention of the stain in the cornea is apparent.

TABLE 130.4 CAUSES OF XEROSTOMIA	
Psychogenic	
Dehydration	Diabetes mellitus
	Trauma
Drugs	Psychotherapeutic
	Parasympatholytic
	Antihypertensive
Irradiation	
Congenital (absent or malformed glands)	
Viral infection	

TABLE 130.5 FREQUENCY OF EXTRAGLANDULAR MANIFESTATIONS IN PRIMARY SJÖGREN'S SYNDROME	
Clinical manifestation	%
Arthralgia/arthritis (non-erosive)	60–70
Raynaud's phenomenon	35–40
Lymphadenopathy	15–20
Vasculitis	5–10
Lung involvement	10–20
Kidney involvement	10–15
Liver involvement	5–10
Peripheral neuropathy	2–5
Myositis	1–2
Lymphoma	5–8

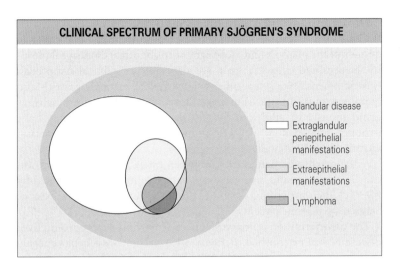

CLINICAL SPECTRUM OF PRIMARY SJÖGREN'S SYNDROME

- Glandular disease
- Extraglandular periepithelial manifestations
- Extraepithelial manifestations
- Lymphoma

Fig.130.4 Clinical spectrum of primary Sjögren's syndrome.

ditions other than Sjögren's syndrome that cause parotid enlargement, and Table 130.4 lists medical conditions that cause xerostomia.

Other glandular involvement

Dryness may affect the upper respiratory tract as well as the oropharynx, and cause hoarseness, recurrent bronchitis and pneumonitis. Loss of exocrine function may also lead to loss of pancreatic function and hypochlorhydria. Patients may also experience dermal dryness and loss of vaginal secretions.

Extraglandular manifestations

Systemic manifestations are seen frequently in primary Sjögren's syndrome patients and may include both general constitutional symptoms, such as easy fatiguability, low-grade fever, myalgias and arthralgias, as well as other organ involvement (Table 130.5). It is now recognized that the extraglandular manifestations in primary Sjögren's syndrome can be divided into two major categories: the periepithelial organ involvement, such as interstitial nephritis, liver involvement and obstructive bronchiolitis, is the result of lymphocytic invasion in the epithelia of organs beyond the exocrine glands. These clinical features appear early in the disease and usually have a benign course. The extraepithelial manifestations – palpable purpura, glomerulonephritis and peripheral neuropathy – are produced from an immune complex deposition as a result of the ongoing B-cell hyperreactivity; they are associated with increased morbidity and risk for lymphoma development (Fig. 130.4; see below).

Arthritis

Of primary Sjögren's syndrome patients, 50% experience episodes of arthritis during the course of their disease. Arthritis may precede overt sicca manifestations. Articular signs and symptoms include arthralgias, morning stiffness, intermittent synovitis and chronic polyarthritis, which may sometimes lead to Jaccoud's arthropathy.[11] In contrast to rheumatoid arthritis (RA), radiographs of the hands usually do not reveal erosive changes.

Skin involvement

Raynaud's phenomenon is the most common skin manifestation, occurring in 35% of primary Sjögren's syndrome patients. It usually precedes sicca manifestations by many years. Primary Sjögren's syndrome patients with Raynaud's phenomenon present with swollen hands but, in contrast to those with scleroderma, they do not develop telangiectasias or digital ulcers. Hand radiographs of these patients may show small tissue calcifications. Non-erosive arthritis has also been shown to be significantly more frequent in patients with Raynaud's phenomenon than in those without.[12] Patients with Raynaud's phenomenon present a higher frequency of non-specific nailfold capillary abnormalities than do patients without.[13] Other skin manifestations include purpura, annular erythema and pernio-like lesions. Flat purpura is usually seen in patients with hypergammaglobulinemia, whereas palpable purpura is a manifestation of dermal vasculitis. Annular erythemas have been described in patients with Sjögren's syndrome from Japan. The erythemas consist of wide elevated erythematous borders with central pallor, located on the face, upper extremities and back. The erythema fades within a few months, leaving no scars or skin pigmentation. Pernio-like lesions (chilblains) were noted in the distal extremities in Japanese patients.[14]

Pulmonary involvement

Manifestations from the trachea to the pleura have been described in patients with Sjögren's syndrome. They are frequent but rarely clinically important. They can present either with dry cough secondary to dryness of the tracheobronchial mucosa (xerotrachea) or dyspnea due to airway obstruction or interstitial lung disease.[15] Interstitial disease in Sjögren's syndrome is rare and is appreciated only after a complete functional and radiologic evaluation of the patient. Papiris et al. used pulmonary function tests to evaluate 61 consecutive non-smoking patients with primary Sjögren's syndrome. Their major finding was small airways obstruction, which was frequently associated with mild hypoxemia. Chest radiography showed mild interstitial-like changes in 27 patients. High-resolution computed tomography (CT) of the lung in patients with abnormal chest radiography revealed wall thickening at the segmental bronchi. Transbronchial and/or endobronchial biopsy specimens in 10 of the 11 sufficient tissue samples disclosed peribronchial and/or peribronchiolar mononuclear inflammation, but interstitial inflammation coexisted in only two patients.[16] Lymphoma should always be suspected when lung nodules or hilar and/or mediastinal lymphadenopathy are present on chest radiographs.

Pleural effusions are usually found in Sjögren's syndrome associated with other rheumatic disorders and not in primary Sjögren's syndrome.[15]

Gastrointestinal and hepatobiliary features

Patients with Sjögren's syndrome often report dysphagia due either to dryness of the pharynx and esophagus or to abnormal esophageal motility. Nausea and epigastric pain are also common clinical symptoms. Gastric mucosa biopsy specimens show chronic atrophic gastritis and lymphocytic infiltrates, similar to those described in minor salivary gland biopsy. In addition, Sjögren's syndrome patients may have hypopepsinogenemia, elevated serum gastrin, low levels of serum vitamin B_{12} and antibodies to parietal cells.

Acute or chronic pancreatitis has been rarely reported. In contrast, subclinical pancreatic involvement is rather common, as illustrated by the fact that hyperamylasemia is found in approximately 25% of Sjögren's syndrome patients.[17]

The association of primary Sjögren's syndrome with chronic liver disease is well established. Patients often present with hepatomegaly (25%) and antimitochondrial antibodies (AMA) (5%). Liver enzymes and alkaline phosphatase are elevated in approximately 70% of patients with Sjögren's syndrome and AMA. In most of these patients liver biopsy discloses a picture of mild intrahepatic bile duct inflammation.[18] There is also a high incidence of secondary Sjögren's syndrome in patients with primary biliary cirrhosis. Sicca manifestations have been described in as many as 50% of primary biliary cirrhosis patients, with 10% being clinically severe.[19]

Renal involvement

Clinically significant renal involvement is observed in approximately 5% of patients with primary Sjögren's syndrome. Patients may present with either interstitial nephritis or glomerulonephritis. Subclinical involvement of the renal tubules can be seen in one-third of patients, as attested by an abnormal urine acidification test. Renal biopsy typically reveals interstitial lymphocytic infiltration. Most of the patients present with hyposthenuria and hypokalemic, hyperchloremic distal renal tubular acidosis, reflecting interstitial infiltration and destruction by lymphocytes. Distal tubular acidosis may be clinically silent, but significant untreated renal tubular acidosis may lead to renal stones, nephrocalcinosis and compromised renal function (Fig. 130.5).[20,21] Such patients may present with recurrent renal colic and/or hypokalemic muscular weakness. Less commonly, Sjögren's syndrome patients have proximal tubular acidosis with Fanconi's syndrome. Membranous or membranoproliferative glomerulonephritis in Sjögren's syndrome has been described in few patients. Cryoglobulinemia, associated with hypocomplementemia, is a consistent serologic finding in these cases. Interstitial nephritis is usually an early feature of the syndrome, whereas glomerulonephritis is a late sequela.[21]

Sjögren's syndrome may also be associated with interstitial cystitis, a non-bacterial disease of the bladder producing constant or intermittent long-lasting symptoms such as nocturia and suprapubic or perineal pain. Bladder biopsy discloses intense inflammation in the mucosa and submucosa, with lymphoid cells and mast cells.[22]

Vasculitis

Vasculitis, found in approximately 5% of Sjögren's syndrome patients, affects small and medium-sized vessels and is manifest most commonly as purpura (Fig. 130.6), recurrent urticaria, skin ulcerations and mononeuritis multiplex. Uncommon cases of systemic vasculitis with visceral involvement affecting the kidneys, lung, gastrointestinal tract, spleen, breast and reproductive tract have been described. Two histopathologic types of vasculitis have been suggested, depending on the type of the infiltrating cell: the mononuclear cell type and the neutrophil type. The neutrophil type is associated with hypergammaglobulinemia, high titers of rheumatoid factor, antibodies to Ro(SS-A) cellular antigen and hypocomplementemia.[23] Another classification of vascular involvement, suggested by Tsokos et al.,[24] has proposed a small

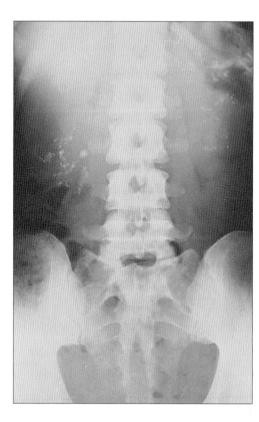

Fig. 130.5 Primary Sjögren's syndrome patient with nephrocalcinosis. Plain abdominal film.

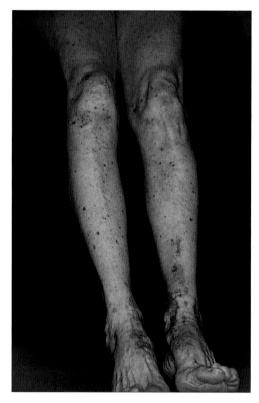

Fig. 130.6 Palpable purpura. Lower extremities of a primary Sjögren's syndrome patient.

vessel vasculitis of the hypersensitivity type, i.e. leukocytoclastic and lymphocytic; a medium vessel vasculitis with acute necrotizing features similar to polyarteritis nodosa but without aneurysm formation; and an endarteritis obliterans seen in Sjögren's syndrome patients with a long-standing history of vasculitis.[24]

Neuromuscular involvement

Neurologic manifestations of Sjögren's syndrome include peripheral sensorimotor neuropathy as a consequence of small vessel vasculitis. Cranial neuropathy, usually affecting single nerves such as the trigeminal or the optic nerve, has been well documented. Central nervous system

(CNS) involvement in Sjögren's syndrome is a matter of considerable controversy. A wide variety of CNS manifestations has been described in Sjögren's patients, including hemiparesis, hemisensory deficits, seizures, movement disorders, transverse myelopathy, and diffuse brain injury expressed as encephalopathy, aseptic meningitis and dementia.[25] Other studies, however, have failed to document severe CNS involvement in patients with primary or secondary Sjögren's syndrome.[26]

Many patients with primary Sjögren's syndrome complain of myalgias, but muscle enzymes are usually normal or only slightly elevated. Polymyositis and inclusion body myositis have been described in Sjögren's syndrome.[27]

Autoimmune thyroid disease

Autoimmune thyroid disease has been described in some cases of primary Sjögren's syndrome patients. In a study by Karsh et al.[28], 50% of Sjögren's syndrome patients presented with antithyroid antibodies and signs of altered thyroid function, as reflected by an elevated basal thyroid-stimulating hormone level. In another study, Ramos-Casals et al.[29] revealed that thyroid disease can be seen in more than one-third of patients with primary SS, but no significant differences were observed when the prevalence of thyroid disease was compared with that in a control group of similar age and gender.

Lymphoproliferative disease

Patients with primary Sjögren's syndrome have a 44 times higher relative risk of developing lymphoma than an age-, sex- and race-matched normal control population. Immunohistologic studies in biopsies of Sjögren's syndrome patients with lymphoma show that these lymphomas are primarily of B-cell origin, expressing usually IgMκ immunoglobulin in their cytoplasm.[30] Immunoglobulin variable region gene analysis disclosed that these lymphomas may frequently develop from B cells producing rheumatoid factor.[31]

High-risk factors for lymphoma development in Sjögren's syndrome patients include persistent unilateral or bilateral parotid gland enlargement, splenomegaly and lymphadenopathy, low C4 complement levels as well as type II mixed monoclonal cryoglobulinemia.[32] The majority of lymphomas are marginal zone B-cell lymphomas, a term which describes the mucosa-associated lymphoid tissue (MALT) and monocytoid B-cell lymphomas. A European multicenter study[33] evaluated the disease characteristics, the clinical course and the evolution in 33 patients with primary Sjögren's syndrome and lymphoma followed up in nine European centers. The majority of patients were in a good clinical performance status and at an early clinical stage. The disease location was mostly extranodal, involving in 55% of cases the salivary glands. In 86% of patients with nodal disease the involved lymph nodes were peripheral (cervical, supraclavicular and/or axillary) and easily accessible for biopsy. Lymphadenopathy, skin vasculitis, peripheral nerve involvement, low-grade fever, anemia, mixed monoclonal cryoglobulinemia and lymphopenia were observed significantly more frequently in Sjögren's syndrome with lymphoma than in general Sjögren's syndrome patients, suggesting that active disease is a risk factor for the development of lymphomas. The survival of these patients was closely associated with the histologic grade of lymphoma. Low-grade lymphomas may remain localized for many years and undergo spontaneous remission without therapy. On the other hand, patients with high and intermediate grades have the worst prognosis.[33]

SECONDARY SJÖGREN'S SYNDROME

The association of Sjögren's syndrome with rheumatoid arthritis (RA) was first described by Sjögren in 1933, but it soon became evident that sicca manifestations can also be found in other autoimmune rheumatic diseases, such as systemic lupus erythematosus (SLE) and progressive

---

TABLE 130.6 ASSOCIATION OF SJÖGREN'S SYNDROME WITH OTHER AUTOIMMUNE RHEUMATIC DISEASES (SECONDARY SJÖGREN'S SYNDROME)

- Rheumatoid arthritis
- Systemic lupus erythematosus
- Scleroderma
- Mixed connective tissue disease
- Primary biliary cirrhosis
- Myositis
- Vasculitis
- Thyroiditis
- Chronic active hepatitis
- Mixed cryoglobulinemia

---

systemic sclerosis. Sjögren's syndrome manifestations have also been described in polymyositis, polyarteritis nodosa and primary biliary cirrhosis (Table 130.6).

The diagnosis of RA usually precedes the diagnosis of Sjögren's syndrome by many years,[34] and Sjögren's syndrome symptoms are primarily KCS. Parotid or other major gland enlargement, as well as extraglandular features of Sjögren's syndrome, including lymphadenopathy and renal involvement, are quite uncommon in Sjögren's syndrome associated with RA.[35]

Such clear differences in the natural history and clinical manifestations of Sjögren's syndrome are not usually found in other associated autoimmune diseases. Systemic lupus erythematosus (SLE) and Sjögren's syndrome have similar disease manifestations, such as arthralgias, rash, peripheral neuropathy and glomerulonephritis.[36] Subjective xerostomia in scleroderma may be due to fibrosis of the exocrine glands. Minor salivary gland biopsies of 44 unselected scleroderma patients showed that 38% had fibrosis, whereas only 22% had lymphocytic infiltration compatible with Sjögren's syndrome.[37]

PROGNOSTIC FACTORS AND OUTCOME

Despite the fact that Sjögren's syndrome is a rather common chronic disease, the prognostic factors of outcome and survival have only recently been determined. Skopouli et al.[38] studied the evolution of the clinical picture and laboratory profile, the incidence and predictors for systemic sequelae, as well as the impact of the disease on overall survival in a prospective cohort study of 261 Greek patients with primary Sjögren's syndrome followed for a 10-year period. The results were compared with the general Greek population, adjusting for age and sex. The glandular manifestations of the syndrome were typically present at the time of diagnosis, and the serological profile of the patients did not change substantially during the follow-up. The extraglandular manifestations can be divided into two different groups with regard to disease outcome. The appearance of arthritis, Raynaud's phenomenon, interstitial nephritis, lung and liver involvement early in the disease process usually has a favorable outcome. Purpura, glomerulonephritis, decreased C4 complement levels and mixed monoclonal cryoglobulinemia were identified as adverse prognostic factors. The overall mortality of patients with primary Sjögren's syndrome compared with that of the general population was increased only in patients with adverse predictors. In another survival study[39] performed in residents of Olmsted County, Minnesota, USA, between 1976 and 1992, 50 cases of primary Sjögren's syndrome and 24 of secondary Sjögren's syndrome were identified. An average of 7.2 years of follow-up was available for patients with primary Sjögren's syndrome and 9.9 years for patients with secondary SS. Increased mortality was found in patients with secondary SS, but not primary SS.

INVESTIGATIONS

Routine laboratory tests reveal a mild anemia of chronic disease in a quarter of patients. Leukopenia is found in 10% of patients, but thrombocytopenia is rather infrequent. Elevated erythrocyte sedimentation rate (ESR) is a very common manifestation of Sjögren's syndrome patients (80–90%), although C-reactive protein levels are normal. Hypergammaglobulinemia is a consistent laboratory finding, found in 80% of primary Sjögren's syndrome patients.[3] Autoantibodies are common and include rheumatoid factors, antinuclear antibodies (ANA), and multiple organ-specific antibodies such as antigastric parietal cell, thyroglobulin thyroid microsomal, mitochondrial, smooth muscle and salivary duct antibodies. Antibodies to Ro(SS-A), La(SS-B) and immune complexes also occur with high frequency.[3] Analyses of the chemical and immunologic parameters of the saliva (sialochemistry) from Sjögren's syndrome patients have been examined extensively, but the results are conflicting and controversial. These analyses offer very little diagnostic value.[44] Numerous tests are available to assess direct exocrine gland secretion and/or the sequelae of decreased secretion.

Schirmer's tear test

Schirmer's tear test is used for the evaluation of tear secretion by the lacrimal glands. The test is performed with strips of filter paper 30mm in length. The strip is slipped beneath the inferior lid, with the remainder of the paper hanging out (Fig. 130.2). After 5 minutes the wetting length of the paper is measured. Wetting of less than 5mm per 5 minutes is a strong indication of diminished secretion. The presence of decreased tear secretion, however, is not diagnostic of KCS.

Rose Bengal staining

The sequela of decreased secretion, KCS, is easily diagnosed using Rose Bengal staining of the corneal epithelium. Rose Bengal is an aniline dye which stains the devitalized or damaged epithelium of both the cornea and the conjunctiva. Slit-lamp examination after Rose Bengal staining shows a punctate or filamentary keratitis (Fig. 130.3).

Determination of tear film break-up

Determination of tear film break-up is another useful clinical assessment. A drop of fluorescein is applied to the eye and the time between the last blink and the appearance of dark, non-fluorescent areas in the tear film is measured. An overly rapid break-up of the tear film indicates either a mucin or a lipid layer abnormality.[40]

Sialometry

Sialometry measures salivary flow rates, with or without stimulation, for the individual parotid or submandibular and sublingual glands, or for total saliva production. Patients with clinically overt Sjögren's syndrome have reduced salivary flow rates. However, flow measurements depend on many factors, such as the age and sex of the patient, drugs taken, and the time of day. Therefore, a wide spectrum of flow rates is found among normal individuals[41] and no single value is diagnostic of Sjögren's syndrome.

Sialography

Sialography is a radiographic method of assessing anatomic changes in the salivary gland duct system. Sialographic studies show an increased incidence of sialectasis in Sjögren's syndrome patients. Sialography is as sensitive and specific as labial minor salivary gland biopsy for the diagnosis of primary Sjögren's syndrome.[42]

Scintigraphy

Scintigraphy provides a functional evaluation of all the salivary glands by observing the rate and density of ^{99m}Tc pertechnetate uptake and time of appearance in the mouth during a 60-minute period after intravenous injection. In patients with Sjögren's syndrome the uptake of the label by the glands and the secretion of labeled saliva in the mouth is delayed or absent. Abnormal scintigraphy correlates with the reduced salivary flow, the sialographic picture and the intensity of minor salivary gland lymphocytic infiltrates. Scintigraphy abnormalities are highly sensitive, but not disease specific.[43]

Minor salivary gland biopsy

Minor salivary gland biopsy serves as a cornerstone for the diagnosis of Sjögren's syndrome. The typical findings are discussed below.

DIFFERENTIAL DIAGNOSIS

Several sets of criteria have been applied for the diagnosis of Sjögren's syndrome by different study groups. The most widely used are those developed and validated from a prospective study involving 26 centers from 12 European countries.[6] They consist of a six-item questionnaire for the determination of dry eyes and mouth – useful for the initial screening for Sjögren's syndrome – and the definition of a new set of diagnostic criteria for SS. An algorithm for the diagnosis of Sjögren's syndrome, using these diagnostic criteria, is presented in Figure 130.7.

Differential diagnosis must include those diseases that may have dry eyes, xerostomia and parotid gland enlargement. Sarcoidosis can mimic

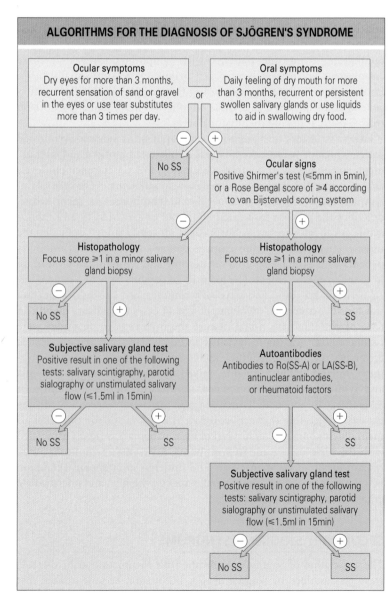

Fig. 130.7 Algorithms for the diagnosis of Sjögren's syndrome (SS).[6]

the clinical picture of Sjögren's syndrome.[45] However, the minor salivary gland biopsy reveals non-caseating granulomas, and autoantibodies to Ro(SS-A) or La(SS-B) antigens are typically absent. Other medical conditions that can mimic Sjögren's syndrome include lipoproteinemias (types II, IV and V), chronic graft-versus-host disease, amyloidosis, and infection with viruses such as human immunodeficiency virus (HIV), human T-lymphocytic virus-I (HTLV-I) and hepatitis C virus (HCV). Patients with HIV infection present with sicca manifestations, parotid gland enlargement, pulmonary involvement and lymphadenopathy (see Chapter 98). These patients had an increased prevalence of HLA-DR5 alloantigen.[46] The two diseases can easily be distinguished, as patients with HIV infection are usually young males, have no autoantibodies to Ro(SS-A) and La(SS-B), and the lymphocytic infiltrates of the salivary glands consist of CD8+ T cells. Hepatitis C virus (HCV) may produce a chronic lymphocytic sialadenitis which mimics Sjögren's syndrome.[47] These patients have a higher mean age, a lower prevalence of parotid gland enlargement and a higher prevalence of liver involvement than patients with primary Sjögren's synrome.[48] On the other hand, Sjögren's syndrome patients do not possess an increased frequency of antibodies to HCV in their sera.[49]

PATHOLOGY

The common feature of all organs affected in Sjögren's syndrome patients is a periepithelial lymphocytic infiltration that causes functional disability and produces various clinical manifestations. Salivary glands are the best-studied organs because they are affected in almost all patients and are readily accessible. The histopathologic characteristics of minor salivary gland biopsy include: focal aggregates of at least 50 lymphocytes, plasma cells and macrophages adjacent to and replacing the normal acini; and the consistent presence of these foci in all or most of the glands in the specimen (Fig. 130.8). Larger foci often exhibit the formation of germinal centers, but epimyoepithelial islands are very uncommon. These pathologic lesions are the characteristic findings of a chronic lymphocytic sialadenitis. However, a minor salivary gland biopsy can be very specific for Sjögren's syndrome if it is obtained through normally appearing mucosa, includes 5–10 glands separated from the surrounding connective tissue, demonstrates focal lymphocytic infiltrates in all or most of the glands in the specimen, and has a focus score above a diagnostic threshold (>1 according to Chilsom).[6,50]

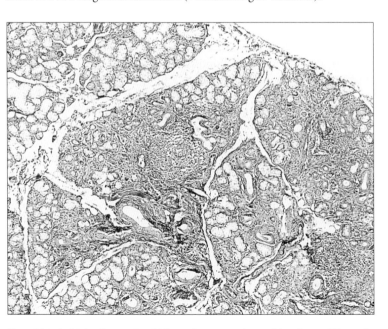

Fig. 130.8 Labial salivary gland biopsy from a patient with primary Sjögren's syndrome. Focal lymphocytic infiltrates are seen. (Hematoxylin and eosin, ×340).

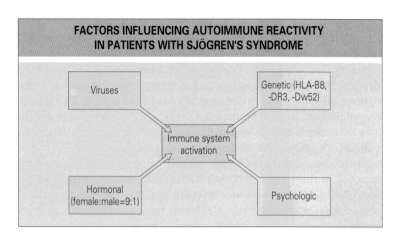

FACTORS INFLUENCING AUTOIMMUNE REACTIVITY IN PATIENTS WITH SJÖGREN'S SYNDROME

Viruses

Genetic (HLA-B8, -DR3, -Dw52)

Immune system activation

Hormonal (female:male=9:1)

Psychologic

Fig. 130.9 Factors influencing autoimmune reactivity in patients with Sjögren's syndrome.

IMMUNOPATHOLOGY

Over the past two decades research on immunopathology, autoantibodies, immunogenetics and viruses has further refined the concepts of pathophysiology and pathogenesis of Sjögren's syndrome (Fig. 130.9). The development of Sjögren's syndrome can be conceptualized in three steps: (1) autoimmunity may be triggered by a given environmental factor which acts on a susceptible genetic background; (2) perpetuation of autoimmune reactivity becomes chronic through normal immune regulatory mechanisms; and (3) tissue lesions occur as a consequence of the ongoing inflammatory process. During recent years clinical and laboratory observations have pointed to the central role of the epithelial cell, and therefore the etiologic name of the disease is proposed to be 'autoimmune epithelitis'.[51]

Environmental triggers of autoimmunity

Autoimmune reactions against virally infected host tissue have been reported in both humans and experimental animals. Despite the fact that viruses have long been suspected of being a major contributory factor in certain autoimmune disorders, no infective agent has so far been discovered.

The concept of viral infection as a cause of primary Sjögren's syndrome has been reinforced during the last few years on the basis of both clinical and experimental observations. First, the epithelial cells of the salivary glands in humans can host a variety of viruses, such as cytomegalovirus (CMV), HIV, HTLV-I and HCV, and create a chronic local immune response with morphologic characteristics similar or even identical to those of the autoimmune sialadenitis of primary Sjögren's syndrome. Studies of minor salivary glands from Sjögren's syndrome patients have shown that the *tax* gene of HTLV-I was present in epithelial cells and that a monoclonal antibody to *tax* protein stained only the epithelial cells.[52] Furthermore, the TCR Vβ gene usage by the infiltrating lymphocytes in the exocrine glands was examined in both primary Sjögren's syndrome and HTLV-I related sialadenitis, using single-strand conformation polymorphism and sequence analysis. T cells expressing TCR with a conserved motif were commonly present in both disease entities.[53] Transgenic mice bearing the *tax* gene develop an autoimmune exocrinopathy resembling Sjögren's syndrome. An initially observed increase and proliferation of the acinar epithelial cells is followed by gradual infiltration by lymphocytes and plasma cells, leading to destruction of the acini. HCV-RNA, as well as HCV core antigen, was detected in the epithelial cells of the salivary gland biopsies from all anti-HCV-positive patients with sialadenitis.[54] Thus, HCV can infect and replicate in the epithelial cells from salivary glands. Two independent lines of transgenic mice carrying the HCV envelope genes have been shown to express the HCV envelope proteins in several organs, including the liver and salivary glands. Despite the fact that no pathological changes were observed in the liver, these animals develop an exocrinopathy involving the salivary and lacrimal glands.[55]

Second, an abundant expression of proto-oncogenes has been described in the immunopathologic lesion of primary Sjögren's sydrome patients. Skopouli *et al.*, utilizing in situ cytohybridization with specific c-*myc* probes, have demonstrated c-*myc* mRNA expression on the acinar epithelial cells in minor salivary glands of Sjögren's syndrome patients. The expression of the proto-oncogene was strongly correlated with the disease duration in the various patients, as well as with the intensity of the T-cell infiltration.[56] Protein expression of p53 and p21 was studied, by immunohistochemistry and Western blot analysis, in minor salivary gland biopsy specimens from patients with primary Sjögren's syndrome and control subjects. The study revealed increased protein expression of p53 and p21 in biopsy specimens from patients compared to controls, and sequence analysis showed that the p53 gene was of the wild type. These findings indicate a probable role for the DNA damage response genes in the pathogenesis of this syndrome.[57] Finally, bcl-2, an apoptosis-inhibitory molecule, is overexpressed in the lymphocytic infiltrates of Sjögren's syndrome patients.[58]

Third, the epithelial cells of the exocrine glands in Sjögren's syndrome have an increased rate of apoptosis.[58] Programmed cell death (apoptosis) can occur after several extrinsic or intrinsic triggering factors, including viral infections. In Sjögren's syndrome, apoptosis of the epithelial cell is mediated through the Fas–Fas ligand interaction and the perforin/granzyme B pathway. The periepithelial lymphocytic infiltrates in the immunopathologic lesion possess cytotoxic properties against the epithelial cells, a finding similar to that observed in the response against virus-infected host cells. Thus, CD8+ T lymphocytes were located around the acinar epithelial cells. The majority of these CD8+ T lymphocytes possess an unique integrin, $\alpha E\beta 7$ (CD103). The acinar epithelial cells adherent to $\alpha E\beta 7$ (CD103)+ CD8+ T lymphocytes were apoptotic.[59] Furthermore, Xanthou *et al.* have demonstrated the existence of a CD4+ cytotoxic cell population that utilizes perforin-mediated cell destruction as they express perforin mRNA.[60]

All the above data suggest a viral etiology for Sjögren's syndrome. Transient or persistent infection of the epithelial cells by a putative virus may lead to neoantigen expression and an increased rate of apoptosis. This initiating event results in the accumulation of helper and/or inducer memory T and B cells, perpetuation of the autoimmune response via autoantigens provided from the apoptotic cells, and ultimately tissue destruction with simultaneous B-cell monoclonal expansion (Fig. 130.10).

Immunogenetics and autoimmunity

Family members of Sjögren's syndrome patients have a higher incidence of SS and a higher incidence of serologic autoimmune abnormalities than do age- and sex-matched controls. Sjögren's syndrome is associated with increased frequencies of HLA-B8, HLA-Dw3 and HLA-DR3.[61] Studies of HLA antigens in primary Sjögren's syndrome patients from various ethnic groups have revealed different associations: HLA-DR5 in Greeks;[62] HLA-DR11, a subtype of HLA-DR5, in Israelis; and HLA-DRw53 in Japanese patients.[63] A DNA-sequence specific oligonucleotide probe typing and a sequence analysis of Israeli Jewish and Greek non-Jewish patients with Sjögren's syndrome have shown that the majority of patients in both groups presented with either DRB1*1101 or DRB1*1104 alleles, which were in linkage disequilibrium with DRB1*0301 and DQA1*0501.[64] Caucasian Americans and black American patients with Sjögren's syndrome also present high frequencies of DQB1*0201 and DQA1*0501.[65] Therefore, the majority of patients with Sjögren's syndrome, independent of racial and ethnic differences, carry the DQA1*0501 allele, suggesting that it may be a determining factor in the predisposition of certain individuals to primary Sjögren's syndrome.

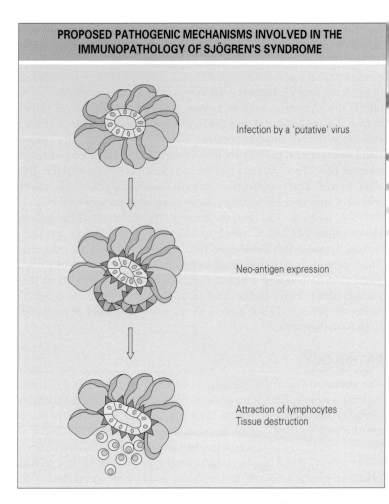

PROPOSED PATHOGENIC MECHANISMS INVOLVED IN THE IMMUNOPATHOLOGY OF SJÖGREN'S SYNDROME

Infection by a 'putative' virus

Neo-antigen expression

Attraction of lymphocytes
Tissue destruction

Fig. 130.10 Proposed pathogenic mechanisms involved in the immunopathology of Sjögren's syndrome.

Perpetuation of autoimmunity: polyclonal hyperreactivity

The most common serologic finding in Sjögren's syndrome is hypergammaglobulinemia. The elevated immunoglobulin levels contain a number of autoantibodies, including rheumatoid factors, antinuclear antibodies, usually with a speckled pattern on immunofluorescence, antibodies to extractable cellular antigens (Ro(SS-A), La(SS-B), RANA), and antibodies to organ-specific antigens found on salivary ductal cells, thyroid gland cells, mitochondria and gastric mucosa.[66] Recently, autoantibodies to α-fordrin,[67] muscarinic receptor 3 (M3),[68] proteasomes[69] and carbonic anhydrase II[70] have been described in Sjögren's syndrome. Their pathogenetic role, if any, and clinical significance remain to be elucidated.

The most common autoantibodies to cellular antigens in Sjögren's syndrome patients are directed against two ribonucleoprotein antigens known as Ro(SS-A) and La(SS-B). Anti-Ro(SS-A) autoantibodies are not specific for Sjögren's syndrome and may be found in other autoimmune diseases, especially SLE and RA. Anti-La(SS-B) autoantibodies are more specific for Sjögren's syndrome. The incidence of anti-Ro(SS-A) antibodies is approximately 40–60% in Sjögren's syndrome and 25–35% in SLE. The anti-La(SS-B) antibody is detected in half of Sjögren's syndrome patients and 10% of SLE patients.[71]

The autoantibodies to Ro(SS-A) recognize a ribonucleoprotein particle composed of hY-RNAs, and protein components of 52 and 60 kDa. These proteins are the main autoimmune targets, as Ro(SS-A) autoimmune sera did not recognize hY-RNA alone. Peptide mapping studies have shown that the 60, the 52 and the 47 kDa La(SS-B) proteins are distinctly different intracellular proteins. Autoantibodies to the 52 kDa component are found in Sjögren's syndrome sera (>80%), whereas antibodies to the 60 kDa component are observed more often in SLE patients' sera.[72]

The La(SS-B) antigen is also a ribonucleoprotein particle associated with all RNA polymerase III transcripts, including the hY-RNAs. Therefore, a subpopulation of La(SS-B) particles may be complexed with Ro(SS-A). La(SS-B) is also associated with several viral transcripts.[71] The human La(SS-B) gene is localized to chromosome 2 and encodes a protein composed of 408 amino acid residues with a calculated molecular weight of 47 kDa. The N-terminal end of the molecule contains an RNA-binding protein consensus motif. Epitope mapping of the autoantigens Ro52Kda, Ro60Kda and La48Kda, performed in several laboratories, disclosed many distinct linear and conformational B-cell antigenic determinants, pointing to the polyclonal nature of the autoimmune response.[73,74] Of particular interest is the sequence 349-364aa of La(SSB), as it presents high specificity and sensitivity for the detection of anti-La(SSB) autoantibodies.[74]

The presence of anti-Ro(SS-A) and/or La(SS-B) autoantibodies is associated with earlier disease onset, longer disease duration, recurrent parotid gland enlargement, splenomegaly, lymphadenopathy and vasculitis in primary Sjögren's syndrome patients. Anti-Ro(SS-A) and/or La(SS-B) autoantibodies correlate with the intensity of the minor salivary gland infiltration (Fig. 130.11) and with multisystem extraglandular disease (Fig. 130.12).

Perpetuation of autoimmunity: oligomonoclonal hyperactivity

Monoclonal immunoglobulins and immunoglobulin light chains have been described in the sera and urine of the majority of primary Sjögren's syndrome patients with lymphoma or extraglandular disease.[75,76] One-third of patients have mixed monoclonal cryoglobulins (type II) containing an IgMκ monoclonal rheumatoid factor.[77] The presence of mixed monoclonal cryoglobulinemia is associated with an increased risk for lymphoma development.[32]

Patients with mixed monoclonal cryoglobulins have κ-positive plasma cell predominance in their minor salivary glands, whereas patients without cryoglobulins or with polyclonal cryoglobulins have almost equal numbers of κ- and μ-positive plasma cells.[78] The above data suggest that very early

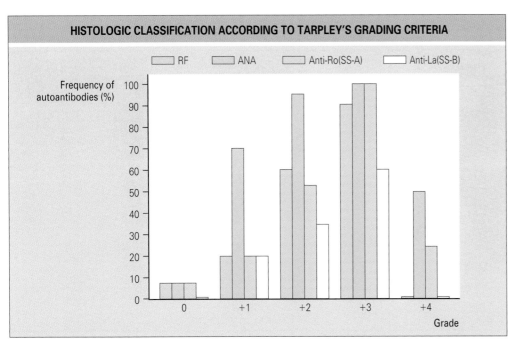

Fig. 130.11 Histologic classification according to Tarpley's grading criteria. Frequency of autoantibodies in patients with primary Sjögren's syndrome according to the grading of the labial minor salivary gland histopathologic lesion (Tarpley's grading system[46]).

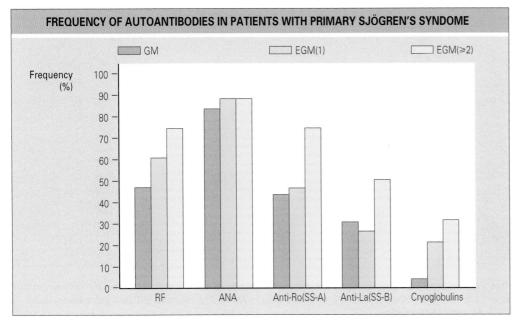

Fig. 130.12 Frequency of autoantibodies in patients with primary Sjögren's syndrome. The patients are grouped according to glandular disease (GM), extraglandular disease with only one manifestation (EGM 1) or more than one extraglandular manifestation (EGM ≥2).

in the disease, patients with Sjögren's syndrome may have both polyclonal B-cell activation and monoclonal B-cell expansion in the salivary glands, with circulating monoclonal immunoglobulins.

Immunogenotypic and immunophenotypic studies have demonstrated oligo- or monoclonal immunoglobulin gene rearrangements in Sjögren's syndrome salivary gland lymphoepithelial lesions.[79] Cloning and sequencing of the variable part (V(H)-D-J(H)) of the immunoglobulin heavy-chain genes expressed in these B cells derived from labial salivary glands and lymph nodes from Sjögren's syndrome patients revealed that a clonal B-cell expansion takes place in the salivary glands of patients with Sjögren's syndrome who do not have histologic evidence of developing lymphoma.[80]

Tapinos et al.[57] performed sequence analysis of the p53 gene on DNA samples obtained from labial salivary glands biopsy samples of seven patients with Sjögren's syndrome and from four patients with Sjögren's syndrome and in situ non-Hodgkin's lymphoma (NHL). It was found that the p53 gene from patients with SS and in situ NHL had two novel mutations in exon 5. These were single-base substitutions and appeared to be functional, as exon 5 is included in the coding region of the p53 gene. These novel mutations implicate dysregulation of this tumor suppressor gene as a possible mechanism for lymphoma development in SS.

Thus, it appears that B-cell activation is the most consistent immunoregulatory aberration in Sjögren's syndrome patients. It begins as polyclonal activation, may evolve to oligoclonal and monoclonal activation, and may end as malignant monoclonal proliferation. Taken together, it is highly likely that the lymphomagenesis in Sjögren's syndrome is a multistep process where the initiating event, which consequently leads to an oligoclonal B-cell expansion, is the chronic ongoing antigenic stimulation that takes place in the immunopathologic lesion of the disease. In a following step, a partial or complete inhibition of the antineoplastic regulatory mechanisms (e.g p53 mutations), could transform the oligoclonal B-cell process into a malignant lymphoma.

Lymphocytes and the immunopathologic lesion

Studies evaluating the immunopathologic lesion of the affected exocrine glands indicate that the majority of the infiltrating lymphocytes are T cells and that the B cells in the lesion are activated (Fig. 130.13).[81] Monocytes, macrophages and natural killer (NK) cells make up less than 5% of the total population. Approximately 60–70% of the T lymphocytes bear the CD4 phenotype, and the majority of them exhibit the memory and/or inducer marker (CD45 RO). Almost all infiltrating T cells express the $\alpha\beta$ T-cell receptor (TCR$\alpha\beta$).[82] Analysis of the TCR

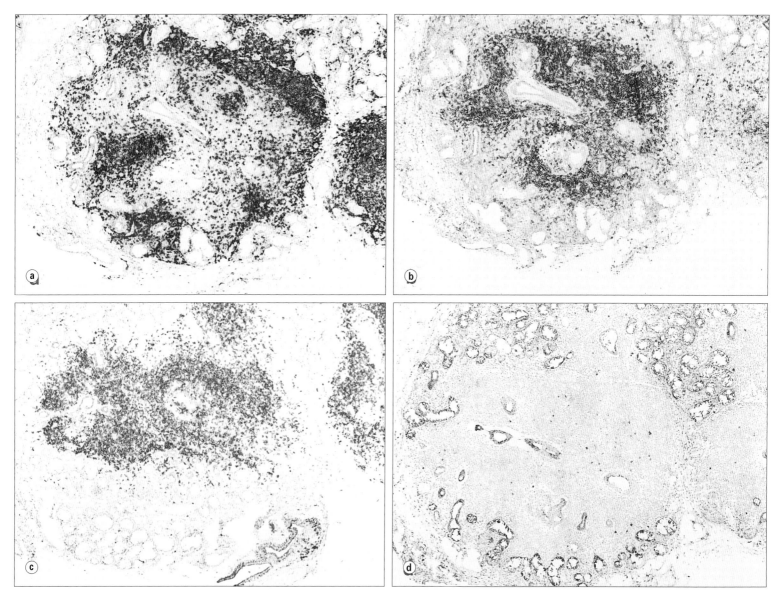

Fig. 130.13 Serial frozen sections from labial minor salivary glands from a patient with primary Sjögren's syndrome. Immunostaining with different monoclonal antibodies. T-cells (Leu4, CD3+) predominate in the lesion and are usually distributed around B cells (a). B cells (L-26) (b). The majority of T-cells are memory cells (UCHL-1+, CD45RO) (c). Very few and scattered Tgd cells (TCR d1+) (d). (Magnification, ×62).

repertoire of the infiltrating T lymphocytes from minor salivary gland biopsies of Sjögren's syndrome patients using quantitative polymerase chain reaction (PCR), revealed that the repertoire of the TCR Vα gene was not restricted.[83] T cells in the lesion are activated, as is attested by the membrane expression of HLA class II molecules, interleukin-2 receptor (IL-2R), lymphocyte function-associated antigen 1 (LFA-1) and interleukin (IL-2) production.[82,84]

Evaluation of the isotypes of intracytoplasmic immunoglobulins of the plasma cells infiltrating the salivary glands of Sjögren's syndrome patients using an immunoperoxidase technique showed that the IgG and IgM isotypes predominate, in contrast to the plasma cells of the normal salivary glands, where the IgA isotype is dominant.[85] Furthermore, B cells in the lesion contain intracytoplasmic immunoglobulins with anti-Ro(SSA) and/or anti-La(SSB) reactivity.[86]

Several studies performed over recent years suggest that the glandular or acinar epithelial cells play a key role in the pathogenesis of the disease. The epithelial cell is activated and possesses properties of an antigen-presenting cell. Histopathologic studies in newly diagnosed cases of Sjögren's syndrome showed that the focal lymphocytic infiltrates start around the ducts. Furthermore, by staining the labial salivary glands with anti-class II HLA monoclonal antibodies, it was shown that the ductal and acinar epithelial cells inappropriately express these molecules. Because γ-interferon (IFN-γ) and tumor necrosis factor (TNF)-α have been shown to induce expression of both histocompatibility antigen classes on the surface of epithelial and other cells, and because these cytokines are produced locally by the activated T cell of the lesion, one is faced with the chicken and egg problem: that is, whether the HLA-DR expression and possible antigen presentation by epithelial cells predates or is a consequence of the lymphocytic infiltration. Subsequent observations, however, suggest that the HLA class II molecule expression by epithelial cells may indicate a specific way of activation of these cells. In this regard, studying proto-oncogene mRNA expression in the minor salivary glands of Sjögren's syndrome patients, it was observed that the c-*myc*, unlike c-*fos* and c-*jun*, was expressed not by the activated lymphocytes, but by the epithelial glandular cells. Because the expression of c-*myc* is so restricted, this phenomenon cannot be attributed to microenvironmental factors.[51] In addition, the salivary gland epithelial cells express B7 molecules.[87] These molecules are expressed on classic antigen-presenting cells and play a critical role in the regulation of immune responses by providing activation or inhibitory signals to T cells through the ligation with CD28 or CTLA4 receptors, respectively. In a recent study, it was shown that B7 molecules expressed in the epithelial cells of primary Sjögren's syndrome patients are functional inducing co-stimulation signal in CD4+ T cells.[88] Furthermore, acinar epithelial cells express autoantigens on their membrane which, in conjunction with class II antigen expression and co-stimulation, may potentially prime an autoimmune response. In fact, translocation and membrane localization of the nuclear antigen La(SS-B) has been observed in conjunctival epithelial cells of Sjögren's syndrome patients.[89] Epithelial cell lines derived from the salivary glands of primary Sjögren's syndrome patients express spontaneously the adhesion molecule ICAM-1, which seems to play an important role in the induction and maintenance of lymphocytic infiltrates of patients.[90] Xanthou *et al.*[91] showed by in situ hybridization and immunohistochemistry that lymphoid chemokines are produced by the epithelial cells in the chronic inflammatory lesions of Sjögren's syndrome patients. Lymphoid chemokines are a newly defined set of chemokines which orchestrate leukocyte microenvironmental homing and contribute to the formation of lymphoid structures. The expression pattern of 'lymphoid' chemokine mRNA points further to the role of epithelial cells in the pathogenesis of SS, and offers new insight into the potential mechanisms that could be involved in leukocyte attraction and in the in-situ formation of secondary lymphoid tissue structures.

Interesting data on cytokine production from the salivary glands of Sjögren's syndrome patients have been reported in the past few years. Almost all proinflammatory (IL-1α, IL-6 and TNF-α) and regulatory cytokines (IFN-γ, IL-4 and TGF-β) are present in the affected salivary glands. Evaluation of IL-1α and IL-6 in labial salivary glands of Sjögren's syndrome patients using oligonucleotide probes, in-situ hybridization and quantitative PCR demonstrated that the mRNA of these cytokines is found in both the infiltrating lymphocytes and the epithelial cells.[84,92] TNF-α is expressed in abundance in almost all the tissues from the salivary glands from Sjögren's syndrome patients. Messenger RNA for IFN-γ is detected in the heavily infiltrated salivary gland tissues and is expressed together with transforming growth factor (TGF)-β, an anti-inflammatory and immunosuppressive cytokine. IL-4, however, is detected in naive cells in the early lesion.[92]

All the above data clearly suggest an in-situ immune response in the exocrine glands of Sjögren's syndrome patients, with the epithelial cell playing the role of an antigen-presenting cell. As a consequence, T cells are attracted and become activated. Cytokines produced by both cell compartments are responsible for inflammatory perpetuation and the stimulation of B lymphocytes.

MANAGEMENT

Sjögren's syndrome is a chronic disease with a wide clinical spectrum. Therefore, patients should be followed regularly for significant functional deterioration, signs of disease complications and significant changes in the course of the disease. Preventive treatment of sicca manifestations is essential.[93]

Dry eyes should be lubricated with artificial tears as often as necessary. A variety of preparations is commercially available, differing primarily in viscosity and preservative content. The thicker, more viscous drops require less frequent application, although they can cause blurring and leave residue on the lashes. Less viscous drops require more frequent application. Patients usually test several different preparations to determine which one is most suitable for their own individual needs. The use of bicarbonate-buffered electrolyte solutions, which mimic the electrolyte composition of human tears, has been shown promising results. Soft contact lenses may help to protect the cornea, especially in the presence of keratitis filamentosa. However, the lenses themselves require wetting, and the patients must be followed very carefully because of an increased risk of infection. Avoidance of windy and/or low-humidity indoor and outdoor environments is helpful. Cigarette smoking and drugs with anticholinergic side effects, such as phenothiazines, tricyclic antidepressants, antispasmodics and antiparkinsonian agents, should be avoided whenever possible. Local stimulators for tear secretion include a cyclic adenosine monophosphate (AMP) derivative, 3-isobutyl-1-methyl-xanthine, which can be administered as eye drops.[94] Local administration of cyclosporin A, 2% in olive oil solution, has been shown to be relatively effective in a placebo-controlled clinical trial. The concominant use of artificial tears alleviates possible local irritation due to cyclosporin A use.[95] In severely dry eyes punctal cauterization should be used. Lateral tarsorrhaphy is indicated to reduce the ocular surface in a case of severe dryness. When corneal perforation occurs, transplantation is recommended.

Treatment of xerostomia is difficult. No single method is consistently effective, and most efforts are aimed only at palliation. Stimulation of salivary flow by sugar-free highly flavored lozenges is rather helpful. In contrast, dry food, heavy smoking and drugs with anticholinergic side effects, which further decrease salivary flow, should be avoided. Most patients carry water, sugarless lemon drops or chewing gum. These must be sugar free because of the risk of rampant dental caries. Adequate oral hygiene after meals is a prerequisite for the prevention of dental disease. Topical treatment with stannous fluoride enhances dental mineralization and retards damage to tooth surfaces. In case of rapidly progressive dental disease the fluoride can be applied directly to the teeth from plastic trays that are used at night. If the salivary hypofunction is severe, pilocarpine hydrochloride, 5mg orally four times daily, may increase the salivary secretion. Pilocarpine hydrochloride stimulates salivary secretion in both normal individuals and patients with impaired salivary function. Pilocarpine is a cholinergic agonist that binds to muscarinic M3 receptors, resulting in smooth muscle contraction. Salivary flow rate increases within 15 minutes of oral administration and is maintained for at least 4 hours.[96] Side effects such as flushing and sweating are usually mild. Newer muscarinic agents, such as cevimeline, have been shown to increase the salivary flow.[97] The recommended dose is 30mg three times daily. Cevimeline should be used with caution in patients with cardiovascular disease.

Vaginal dryness is treated with lubricant jellies and dry skin with moisturizing lotions.

Hydroxychloroquine, 200mg/day, can be effective in a subgroup of patients complaining of arthralgias and myalgias.[93] In a single-center, open-label pilot study, 16 patients with primary Sjögren's syndrome were treated with three infusions, each 3mg/kg, of infliximab, a chimeric human-mouse anti-TNF alpha monoclonal antibody at 0, 2, and 6 weeks. There was statistically significant improvement in all clinical and functional parameters, including patient's global assessment, patient's assessment of pain and fatigue, physician's global assessment, erythrocyte sedimentation rate, salivary flow rate, the Schirmer I test, tender joint count, fatigue score, and dry eyes and dry mouth. This clinical benefit was observed at week 2 and was maintained throughout the study and the 2-month follow-up period. The treatment was well tolerated in all patients, and no significant adverse events were seen.[98]

Systemic corticosteroids (0.5–1mg/kg/day of prednisone) and immunosuppressive drugs such as cyclophosphamide are used for severe extraglandular disease, including diffuse interstitial pneumonitis, glomerulonephritis, vasculitis and peripheral neuropathy. The impact of these agents on the natural course of Sjögren's syndrome is not well established. Treatment of lymphoma depends on the histologic type, the location and the extension. Decisions regarding chemotherapy and/or radiation therapy should be guided by experienced oncologists.

REFERENCES

1. Sjögren H. Auf Kenntnis der Keratoconjunctivitis sicca (Keratitis filiformis bei Hypofunction der Transendrusen). Acta Ophthalmol (Kbh) 1933; 11s(suppl 2): 1–151.
2. Morgan WS, Castleman B. A clinicopathologic study of 'Mikulicz's disease'. Am J Pathol 1953; 29: 471–503.
3. Tapinos NI, Polihronis M, Tzioufas AG, Moutsopoulos HM. Sjögren's syndrome. Autoimune epithelitis. Adv Exp Med Biol 1999; 455: 127–134.
4. Siamopoulou-Mavridou A, Drosos AA, Andonopoulos AP. Sjögren's syndrome in childhood: report of two cases. Eur J Pediatr 1989; 18: 523–524.
5. Drosos AA, Andonopoulos AP, Costopoulos JS et al. Prevalence of primary Sjögren's syndrome in an elderly population. Br J Rheumatol 1988; 27: 123–127.
6. Vitali C, Bombardieri S, Moutsopoulos HM et al. Preliminary criteria for the classification of Sjögren's syndrome. Results of a prospective concerted action supported by the European Community. Arthritis Rheum. 1992; 36: 340–348.
7. Dafni U, Tzioufas AG, Staikos P et al. The prevalence of Sjögren's syndrome in a close rural community. Ann Rheum Dis 1997; 56: 521–525.
8. Jacobsson L, Axell TE, Hansen B et al. Dry eyes or mouth – an epidemiological study in Swedish adults with special reference to primary Sjögren's syndrome. J Autoimmun 1989; 2: 521–527.
9. Thomas E, Hay EM, Hajeer A, Silman AJ. Sjögren's syndrome: a community-based study of prevalence and impact. Br J Rheumatol 1998; 37: 1069–1076.
10. Pavlidis NA, Karsh J, Moutsopoulos HM. The clinical picture of primary Sjögren's syndrome: a retrospective study. J Rheumatol 1982; 9: 685–690.
11. Maini RN. Relationships of Sjögren's syndrome to rheumatoid arthritis. In: Talal N, Moutsopoulos HM, Kassan SS, eds. Sjögren's syndrome: Clinical and immunological aspects. Berlin: Springer-Verlag, 1987; 165–171.
12. Skopouli FN, Talal A, Galanopoulou V et al. Raynaud's phenomenon in primary Sjögren's syndrome. J Rheumatol 1990; 17: 618–620.
13. Tektonidou M, Kaskani E, Skopouli FN, Moutsopoulos HM. Microvascular abnormalities in Sjögren's syndrome: nailfold capillaroscopy. Rheumatology (Oxford) 1999; 38: 826–830.
14. Moutsopoulos HM, Velthuis PJ, De Widde PCM, Kater L. Sjögren's syndrome. In: Kater L, De la Faille HB, eds. Multi-systemic autoimmune diseases. New York: Elsevier, 1995; 173–205.
15. Constantopoulos SH, Moutsopoulos HM. The respiratory system in Sjögren's syndrome. In: Talal N, Moutsopoulos HM, Kassan SS, eds. Sjögren's syndrome: clinical and immunological aspects. Berlin: Springer-Verlag, 1987; 83–89.
16. Papiris SA, Maniati M, Constantopoulos SH et al. Lung involvement in primary Sjögren's syndrome is mainly related to the small airway disease. Ann Rheum Dis 1999; 58: 61–64.
17. Trevino H, Tsianos EB, Schenker S. Gastrointestinal and hepatobiliary features in Sjögren's syndrome. In: Talal N, Moutsopoulos HM, Kassan SS, eds. Sjögren's syndrome: clinical and immunological aspects. Berlin: Springer-Verlag, 1987; 89–95.
18. Skopouli FN, Barbatis C, Moutsopoulos HM. Liver involvement in primary Sjögren's syndrome. Br J Rheumatol 1994; 33: 745–748.
19. Tsianos EB, Hoofnagle JH, Fox PC et al. Sjögren's syndrome in patients with primary biliary cirrhosis. Hepatology 1990; 11: 730–734.
20. Kassan SS, Talal N. Renal disease with Sjögren's syndrome. In: Talal N, Moutsopoulos HM, Kassan SS, eds. Sjögren's syndrome: clinical and immunological aspects. Berlin: Springer-Verlag, 1987; 96–102.
21. Goules A, Masouridi S, Tzioufas AG et al.Clinically significant and biopsy-documented renal involvement in primary Sjögren syndrome. Medicine (Baltimore) 2000; 79: 241–249.
22. Van de Merwe JP, Kamerling R, Arendsen HS et al. Sjögren's syndrome in patients with interstitial cystitis. J Rheumatol 1993; 20: 962–966.
23. Alexander EI. Inflammatory vascular disease in Sjögren's syndrome. In: Talal N, Moutsopoulos HM, Kassan SS, eds. Sjögren's syndrome: clinical and immunological aspects. Berlin: Springer-Verlag, 1987; 102–104.
24. Tsokos M, Lazarou SA, Moutsopoulos HM. Vasculitis in primary Sjögren's syndrome. Histologic classification and clinical presentation. Am J Clin Pathol 1987; 88: 26–31.
25. Alexander EI. Neuromuscular complications of primary Sjögren's syndrome. In: Talal N, Moutsopoulos HM, Kassan SS, eds. Sjögren's syndrome: clinical and immunological aspects. Berlin: Springer-Verlag, 1987; 61–82.
26. Binder A, Snaith ML, Isenberg D. Sjögren's syndrome: a study of its neurological complications. Br J Rheumatol 1988; 27: 275–280.
27. Leroy JP, Drosos AA, Yannopoulos DI et al. Intravenous pulse cyclophosphamide therapy in myositis and Sjögren's syndrome. Arthritis Rheum 1990; 33: 1579–1581.
28. Karsh J, Pavlidis N, Weintraub BD, Moutsopoulos HM. Thyroid disease in Sjögren's syndrome. Arthritis Rheum 1980; 23: 1326–1329.
29. Ramos-Casals M, Garcia-Carrasco M, Cervera R et al. Thyroid disease in primary Sjögren syndrome. Study in a series of 160 patients. Medicine (Baltimore) 2000; 79: 103–108.
30. Tzioufas AG, Moutsopoulos HM, Talal N. Lymphoid malignancy and monoclonal proteins. In: Talal N, Moutsopoulos HM, Kassan SS, eds. Sjögren's syndrome: clinical and immunological aspects. Berlin: Springer-Verlag, 1987; 129–136.
31. Martin T, Weber JC, Levallois H et al. Salivary gland lymphomas in patients with Sjögren's syndrome may frequently develop from rheumatoid factor B cells. Arthritis Rheum 2000; 43: 908–916.
32. Tzioufas AG, Boumba DS, Skopouli FN, Moutsopoulos HM. Mixed monoclonal cryoglobulinemia and monoclonal rheumatoid factor cross-reactive idiotypes as predictive factors for the development of lymphoma in primary Sjögren's syndrome. Arthritis Rheum 1996; 39: 767–772.
33. Voulgarelis M, Dafni UG, Isenberg DA, Moutsopoulos HM. Malignant lymphoma in primary Sjögren's syndrome: a multicenter, retrospective, clinical study by the European Concerted Action on Sjögren's Syndrome. Arthritis Rheum 1999; 42: 1765–1772.
34. Andonopoulos AP, Drosos AA, Skopouli FN et al. Secondary Sjögren's syndrome in rheumatoid arthritis. J Rheumatol. 1987; 1: 1098–1103.
35. Moutsopoulos HM, Webber BL, Vlagopoulos TP et al. Differences in the clinical manifestations of sicca syndrome in the presence and absence of rheumatoid arthritis. Am J Med 1979; 66: 733–736.
36. Kassan SS, Talal N. Sjögren's syndrome with systemic lupus erythematosus mixed connective tissue disease. In: Talal N, Moutsopoulos HM, Kassan SS, eds. Sjögren's syndrome: clinical and immunological aspects. Berlin: Springer-Verlag, 1987; 177–181.
37. Andonopoulos AP, Drosos AA, Skopouli FN, Moutsopoulos HM. Sjögren's syndrome in rheumatoid arthritis and progressive systemic sclerosis. A comparative study. Clin Exp Rheumatol 1989; 7: 203–205.
38. Skopouli FN, Dafni U, Ioannidis JP, Moutsopoulos HM. Clinical evolution, and morbidity and mortality of primary Sjögren's syndrome. Semin Arthritis Rheum 2000; 29: 296–304.

39. Martens PB, Pillemer SR, Jacobsson LT et al. Survivorship in a population based cohort of patients with Sjögren's syndrome, 1976–1992. J Rheumatol 1999; 26: 1296–1300.

40. Kincaid MC. The eye in Sjögren's syndrome. In: Talal N, Moutsopoulos HM, Kassan SS, eds. Sjögren's syndrome: clinical and immunological aspects. Berlin: Springer-Verlag, 1987; 25–34.

41. Skopouli FN, Siouna-Fatourou HI, Ziciadis C, Moutsopoulos HM. Evaluation of unstimulated whole saliva flow rate and stimulated parotid flow as confirmatory tests for xerostomia. Clin Exp Rheumatol 1989; 7: 127–129.

42. Vitali C, Tavoni A, Simi U et al. Parotid sialography and minor salivary gland biopsy in the diagnosis of Sjögren's syndrome: a comparative study of 84 patients. J Rheumatol 1988; 15: 262–267.

43. Parrago G, Rain GD, Bronchierion C, Rocher F. Scintigraphy of the salivary glands in Sjögren's syndrome. J Clin Pathol 1987; 40: 1463–1467.

44. Baum BJ, Fox PC. Chemistry of saliva. In: Talal N, Moutsopoulos HM, Kassan SS, eds. Sjögren's syndrome: clinical and immunological aspects. Berlin: Springer-Verlag, 1987; 25–34.

45. Drosos AA, Constantopoulos SH, Psychos D et al. The forgotten cause of sicca complex; sarcoidosis. J Rheumatol 1989; 16: 1548–1551.

46. Itescu S, Braneato LJ, Buxbaum J et al. A diffuse infiltrative CD8 lymphocytosis syndrome in human immunodeficiency virus (HIV) infection: a host immune response associated with HLA-DR5. Ann Intern Med 1990; 112: 3–10.

47. Haddad J, Deny P, Munz-Gothiel C et al. Lymphocytic sialadenitis of Sjögren's syndrome associated with chronic hepatitis C virus liver disease. Lancet 1992; 339: 321–323.

48. Ramos-Casals M, Garcia-Carrasco M, Cervera R et al. Hepatitis C virus infection mimicking primary Sjögren syndrome. A clinical and immunologic description of 35 cases. Medicine (Baltimore) 2001; 80: 1–8.

49. Vitali C, Sciuto M, Neri R et al. Anti hepatitis C virus antibodies in primary Sjögren's syndrome: false positive results are related to hyper-γ-globulinemia. Clin Exp Rheumatol 1992; 10: 103–104.

50. Daniels TE, Aufdemorte TB, Greenspan JS. Histopathology of Sjögren's syndrome. In: Talal N, Moutsopoulos HM, Kassan SS, eds. Sjögren's syndrome: clinical and immunological aspects. Berlin: Springer-Verlag, 1987; 266–286.

51. Moutsopoulos HM. Sjögren's syndrome autoimmune epithelitis. Clin Immunol Immunopath 1994; 72: 162–165.

52. Papadopoulos GK, Moutsopoulos HM. Slow viruses and the immune system in the pathogenesis of local tissue damage in Sjögren's syndrome. Ann Rheum Dis 1992; 51: 136–138.

53. Sasaki M, Nakamura S, Ohyama Y. Accumulation of common T cell clonotypes in the salivary glands of patients with human T lymphotropic virus type I-associated and idiopathic Sjögren's syndrome. J Immunol 2000; 164: 2823–2831.

54. Arrieta JJ, Rodriguez-Inigo E, Ortiz-Movilla N et al. In situ detection of hepatitis C virus RNA in salivary glands. Am J Pathol 2001; 158: 259–264.

55. Koike K, Moriya K, Ishibashi K. Sialadenitis histologically resembling Sjögren syndrome in mice transgenic for hepatitis C virus envelope genes. Proc Natl Acad Sci USA 1997; 94: 233–236.

56. Skopouli FN, Kousvelari E, Mertz P et al. C-myc mRNA expression in minor salivary glands of patients with Sjögren's syndrome. J Rheumatol 1992; 19: 693–699.

57. Tapinos NI, Polihronis M, Moutsopoulos HM. Lymphoma development in Sjögren's syndrome: novel p53 mutations. Arthritis Rheum 1999; 42: 1466–1472.

58. Polihronis M, Tapinos NI, Theocharis SE et al. Modes of epithelial cell death and repair in Sjögren's syndrome (SS). Clin Exp Immunol 1998; 114: 485–490.

59. Fujihara T, Fujita H, Tsubota K. Preferential localization of CD8+ alpha E beta 7+ T cells around acinar epithelial cells with apoptosis in patients with Sjögren's syndrome. J Immunol 1999; 163: 2226–2235.

60. Xanthou G, Tapinos NI, Polihronis M et al. CD4 cytotoxic and dendritic cells in the immunopathologic lesion of Sjögren's syndrome. Clin Exp Immunol 1999; 118: 154–163.

61. Mann D. Immunogenetics of Sjögren's syndrome. In: Talal N, Moutsopoulos HM, Kassan SS, eds. Sjögren's syndrome: clinical and immunological aspects. Berlin: Springer-Verlag, 1987; 235–243.

62. Papasteriades C, Skopouli FN, Drosos AA et al. HLA-alloantigen associations in Greek patients with Sjögren's syndrome. J Autoimmun 1988; 1: 85–90.

63. Moriuchi J, Ichikawa Y, Takaya M et al. Association between HLA and Sjögren's syndrome in Japanese patients. Arthritis Rheum 1986; 29: 1518–1521.

64. Tambur AR, Friedmann A, Safirmann C et al. Molecular analysis of HLA class II genes in primary Sjögren's syndrome: a study of Israeli and Greek non-Jewish patients. Hum Immunol 1993; 36: 235–242.

65. Reveille JD, Macteod MJ, Whittington K, Arnett FC. Specific amino acid residues n the second hypervariable region of HLA-DQA1 and DQB1 chain genes promote the Ro(SSA)/La(SSB) autoantibody responses. J Immunol 1991; 146: 3871–3875.

66. Harley JB. Autoantibodies in Sjögren's syndrome. In: Talal N, Moutsopoulos HM, Kassan SS, eds. Sjögren's syndrome: clinical and immunological aspects. Berlin: Springer-Verlag, 1987; 218–234.

67. Witte T, Matthias T, Arnett FC et al. IgA and IgG autoantibodies against alpha-fodrin as markers for Sjögren's syndrome. Systemic lupus erythematosus. J Rheumatol 2000; 27: 2617–2620.

68. Bacman S, Sterin-Borda L, Camusso JJ et al. Circulating antibodies against rat parotid gland M3 muscarinic receptors in primary Sjögren's syndrome. Clin Exp Immunol 1996; 104: 454–459.

69. Feist E, Kuckelkorn U, Dorner T et al. Autoantibodies in primary Sjögren's syndrome are directed against proteasomal subunits of the alpha and beta type. Arthritis Rheum 1999; 42: 697–702.

70. Ono M, Watanabe K, Miyashita Y et al. A study of anti-carbonic anhydrase II antibodies in rheumatic autoimmune diseases. J Dermatol Sci 1999; 21: 183–186.

71. Tzioufas AG, Moutsopoulos HM. Clinical significance of antibodies to Ro/SSA and La/SSB. In: Maini R, van Venrooij V, eds. The manual of autoantigens-antibodies. Dordrecht: Kluwer, 1996; 1–14.

72. Ben-Chetrit E, Fox RI, Tan EM. Dissociation of immune responses to the SS-A(Ro) and 52 kd and 60 kd polypeptides in systemic lupus erythematosus and Sjögren's syndrome. Arthritis Rheum 1990; 33: 3449–3555.

73. Scofield RH, Farris AD, Horsfall AC, Harley JB. Fine specificity of the autoimmune response to the Ro/SSA and La/SSB ribonucleoprotein. Arthritis Rheum 1999; 42: 199–209.

74. Moutsopoulos NM, Routsias JG, Vlachoyiannopoulos PG et al. B-cell epitopes of intracellular autoantigens: myth and reality. Mol Med 2000; 6: 141–151.

75. Moutsopoulos HM, Steinberg AD, Fauci AS et al. High incidence of free monoclonal I light chains in the sera of patients with Sjögren's syndrome. J Immunol 1983; 130: 2263–2265.

76. Moutsopoulos HM, Costello R, Drosos AA et al. Demonstration and identification of monoclonal proteins in the urine of patients with Sjögren's syndrome. Ann Rheum Dis 1985; 44: 109–112.

77. Tzioufas AG, Manoussakis MN, Costello R et al. Cryoglobulinemia in autoimmune rheumatic diseases: evidence of circulating monoclonal cryoglobulins in patients with primary Sjögren's syndrome. Arthritis Rheum 1986; 29: 1098–1104.

78. Moutsopoulos HM, Tzioufas AG, Bai AK et al. Serum IgMk monoclonicity in patients with Sjögren's syndrome is associated with an increased proportion of k-positive plasma-cells infiltrating the labial minor salivary glands. Ann Rheum Dis 1990; 49: 929–931.

79. Freinmark B, Fantozzi R, Bone R et al. Detection of clonally expanded salivary gland lymphocytes in Sjögren's syndrome. Arthritis Rheum 1989; 32: 859–869.

80. Gellrich S, Rutz S, Borkowski A et al. Analysis of V(H)-D-J(H) gene transcripts in B cells infiltrating the salivary glands and lymph node tissues of patients with Sjögren's syndrome. Arthritis Rheum 1999; 42: 240–247.

81. Moutsopoulos HM, Manoussakis MN. Immunopathogenesis of Sjögren's syndrome: facts and fancy. Autoimmunity 1989; 5: 17–24.

82. Skopouli FN, Fox PC, Galanopoulou V et al. T-cell subpopulation in the labial minor salivary gland histopathologic lesion of Sjögren's syndrome. J Rheumatol 1991; 18: 210–214.

83. Sumida T, Yonaha F, Maeda T et al. T-cell receptor repertoire of infiltrating T-cells in lips of Sjögren's syndrome patients. J Clin Invest 1992; 89: 681–685.

84. Fox RI, Kang-Ho-II, Ando D et al. Cytokine mRNA expression in salivary biopsies of Sjögren's syndrome. J Immunol 1994; 152: 5532–5539.

85. Bodeuitsch C, de Wilde PCM, Kater L et al. Quantitative immunohistologic criteria are superior to the lymphocytic focus score criterion for the diagnosis of Sjögren's syndrome. Arthritis Rheum 1992; 35: 1075–1087.

86. Tengner P, Halse AK, Haga HJ et al. Detection of anti-Ro/SSA and anti-La/SSB auto-antibody-producing cells in salivary glands from patients with Sjögren's syndrome. Arthritis Rheum 1998; 41: 2238–2248.

87. Manoussakis MN, Dimitriou ID, Kapsogeorgou EK et al. Expression of B7 costimulatory molecules by salivary gland epithelial cells in patients with Sjögren's syndrome. Arthritis Rheum 1999; 42: 229–239.

88. Kapsogeorgou EK, Moutsopoulos HM, Manoussakis MN. Functional expression of a costimulatory B7.2 (CD86) protein on human salivary gland epithelial cells that interacts with the CD28 receptor, but has reduced binding to CTLA4. J Immunol 2001; 166: 3107–3113.

89. Yannopoulos DI, Roncin S, Lamour A et al. Conjunctival epithelial cells from patients with Sjögren's syndrome inappropriately express major histocompatibility complex molecules, La/SSB antigen and heat shock proteins. J Clin Immunol 1992; 12: 259–265.

90. Kapsogeorgou EK, Dimitriou ID, Abu-Helu RF et al. Activation of epithelial and myoepithelial cells in the salivary glands of patients with Sjögren's syndrome: high expression of intercellular adhesion molecule-1 (ICAM.1) in biopsy specimens and cultured cells. Clin Exp Immunol 2001; 124: 126–133.

91. Xanthou G, Polihronis M, Tzioufas AG et al. "Lymphoid" chemokine messenger RNA expression by epithelial cells in the chronic inflammatory lesion of the salivary glands of Sjögren's syndrome patients: possible participation in lymphoid structure formation. Arthritis Rheum 2001; 44: 408–418.

92. Boumba D, Skopouli FN, Moutsopoulos HM. Cytokine mRNA expression in the labial salivary gland tissues from patients with primary Sjögren's syndrome. Br J Rheumatol 1995; 34: 326–333.

93. Moutsopoulos HM, Vlachoyiannopoulos PG. What would I do if I had Sjögren's syndrome? Rheumatol Rev 1993; 2: 17–23.

94. Gilbard JP, Rossi SR, Heyda KG, Dartt DA. Stimulation of tear secretion and treatment of dry eye disease with 3-isobutyl-1-methylxanthine. Arch Ophthalmol 1991; 109: 672–675.

95. Gunduz K, Ozdemir O. Topical cyclosporin treatment of keratoconjunctivitis sicca in secondary Sjögren's syndrome. Acta Ophthalmol (Copenhagen) 1994; 72: 438–442.

96. Vivino FB, Al-Hashimi I, Khan Z et al. Pilocarpine tablets for the treatment of dry mouth and dry eye symptoms in patients with Sjögren syndrome: a randomized, placebo-controlled, fixed-dose, multicenter trial. P92-01 Study Group. Arch Intern Med 1999 25; 159: 174–181.

97. Fox RI, Michelson P. Approaches to the treatment of Sjögren's syndrome. J Rheumatol 2000; 61 (Suppl.): 15–21.

98. Steinfeld SD, Demols P, Salmon I, Kiss R, Appelboom T. Infliximab in patients with primary Sjögren's syndrome: a pilot study. Arthritis Rheum 2001; 44: 2371–5.

131 Antiphospholipid syndrome

E Nigel Harris and Munther A Khamashta

Definition

- A disorder of recurrent vascular thrombosis, and/or pregnancy losses associated with persistently elevated levels of antiphospholipid–protein antibodies

Clinical features

- Complications primarily related to venous or arterial occlusion and recurrent pregnancy losses
- Features of some autoimmune diseases, especially systemic lupus erythematosus, may coexist and even predominate
- Anticoagulation is used to prevent recurrent thrombosis
- Recurrent pregnancy loss may be prevented by treatment with subcutaneous heparin and low-dose aspirin during pregnancy

HISTORY

In 1952 an unusual clotting inhibitor was described in some patients with systemic lupus erythematosus (SLE)[1]. This inhibitor, later named 'lupus anticoagulant', was frequently associated with a biological false positive test for syphilis (BFP-STS).

Initial clinical descriptions of patients with the lupus anticoagulant reported hemorrhage, but it soon became evident that this complication was rare. Indeed, in 1963 Bowie et al[2]. suggested that these patients were paradoxically subject to thrombosis. Thirteen years later, Johannson et al. reported a 'syndrome' of recurrent thrombosis associated with the BFP-STS and lupus anticoagulant[3]. Nilsson et al[4]. first reported that recurrent spontaneous abortion might be associated with the lupus anticoagulant. By the early 1980s, there were many reports of patients with the lupus anticoagulant, thrombosis and recurrent fetal loss[5]. In 1983 Harris and colleagues[6] reasoned that the lupus anticoagulant might be related to the BFP-STS because of a common specificity for the negatively charged phospholipid antigen cardiolipin. They devised a solid-phase anticardiolipin assay that proved to be a sensitive means of detecting patients with this disorder[5]. Subsequent studies have shown that aPL antibodies bind diverse protein antigens, the most prominent of which are β_2 glycoprotein (β_2GP)-1[7,8] and prothrombin[9], as well as negatively charged phospholipids[10]. By the late 1980s, it was evident that aPL antibodies and their associated clinical complications were not confined to patients with SLE and a designation for this 'new' disorder was needed. Of the various suggestions, 'antiphospholipid syndrome' (APS) has acquired the greatest popularity[11]. In 1999, Wilson and an international group of experts [12] developed preliminary classification criteria for APS (Table 131.1).

EPIDEMIOLOGY

A full understanding of the epidemiology of APS awaits more universal agreement about criteria for diagnosis. Its prevalence is unknown. The apparent female predominance may be due to the fact that recurrent

---

TABLE 131.1 PRELIMINARY CRITERIA FOR CLASSIFICATION OF THE ANTIPHOSPHOLIPID SYNDROME

Clinical criteria

- Vascular thrombosis
  One or more clinical episodes of arterial, venous or small vessel thrombosis, in any tissue or organ. Thrombosis must be confirmed by imaging or Doppler studies or histopathology, with the exception of superficial venous thrombosis. For histopathologic confirmation, thrombosis should be present without significant evidence of inflammation in the vessel wall.
- Pregnancy morbidity*
  - One or more unexplained deaths of a morphologically normal fetus at or beyond the 10th week of gestation, with normal fetal morphology documented by ultrasound or by direct examination of the fetus, or
  - One or more premature births of a morphologically normal neonate at or before the 34th week of gestation because of severe pre-eclampsia or eclampsia, or severe placental insufficiency, or
  - Three or more unexplained consecutive spontaneous abortions before the 10th week of gestation, with maternal anatomic or hormonal abnormalities and paternal and maternal chromosomal causes excluded.

In studies of populations of patients who have more than one type of pregnancy morbidity, investigators are strongly encouraged to stratify groups of subjects according to a, b or c above.

Laboratory criteria

- Anticardiolipin antibody of IgG and or IgM isotype in serum, present in medium or high titer, on two or more occasions at least 6 weeks apart, measured by a standardized enzyme-linked immunosorbent assay for β_2 glycoprotein-1 dependent anticardiolipin antibodies.
- Lupus anticoagulant present in plasma on two or more occasions at least 6 weeks apart, detected according to the guidelines of the International Society on Thrombosis and Hemostasis (Scientific Subcommittee on Lupus Anticoagulants/Phospholipid-Dependent Antibodies) in the following steps:
  - Prolonged phospholipid-dependent coagulation demonstrated on a screening test, e.g. activated partial thromboplastin time (aPTT). kaolin clotting time (KCT), dilute Russell's viper venom time (RVTT), dilute prothrombin time (PT) or textarin time (TT).
  - Failure to correct the prolonged coagulation time on the screening test by the addition of excess phospholipid.
  - Exclusion of other coagulopathies, e.g. Factor VIII inhibitor or heparin, as appropriate.

Definite antiphospholipid antibody syndrome is considered to be present if at least one of the clinical criteria and one of the laboratory criteria are met.

* No exclusions other than those contained within the above criteria are needed. However, because of the likelihood that thrombosis may be multifactorial in patients with the antiphospholipid antibody syndrome, the workshop participants recommend that (a) patient populations being studied should be assessed for other contributing causes of thrombosis, and (b) such populations should be stratified according to identifiable or probable risk factors, e.g. age or comorbidities. Specific limits were not placed on the interval between the clinical event and the positive laboratory findings. However, it was the view of many at the workshop that (a) information about such intervals should be assessed when relevant, and that (b) the relatively strict definition of laboratory[1] criteria (including the requirement that results again be positive on repeat tests performed at least 6 weeks after the initial test) would help to exclude antiphospholipid antibody positivity that represents an epiphenomenon to the clinical events.

(Modified from Wilson et al. [12])

pregnancy loss is a prominent feature of the disorder and that early series were often confined to patients with SLE. Although there are several examples of family members having positive anticardiolipin tests, there are few reports of the full syndrome occurring in more than one family member.

In studying the epidemiology of APS, a distinction must be made between patients who have positive anticardiolipin tests alone and those with positive tests and clinical manifestations. Positive tests have been detected in patients with SLE, rheumatoid arthritis (RA) and related systemic autoimmune disorders, as well as in patients with a variety of drug-induced, infectious and other miscellaneous disorders. Patients with syphilis, acquired immunodeficiency syndrome (AIDS) and other infectious disorders, as well as those with drug-induced aPL antibodies, do not usually have clinical features of APS. In other groups, about 30% of patients with the lupus anticoagulant and about 30–50% with high or medium positive IgG anticardiolipin tests have clinical features of APS. Antibody isotype, level, and other yet to be defined characteristics of aPL antibodies, as well as underlying disease, may all be determining features in developing the clinical syndrome.

CLINICAL FEATURES

Overview

Antiphospholipid syndrome is a disorder of recurrent vascular thrombosis and pregnancy losses associated with persistently positive anticardiolipin or lupus anticoagulant tests (Table 131.1)[12]. A variety of abnormalities of the skin, cardiac valves, central nervous system (CNS) and other organ systems, as well as thrombocytopenia, have been described, but the frequency of their occurrence is uncertain. Many patients with APS have clinical and laboratory features found in other autoimmune diseases, particularly SLE. Such patients are defined as having 'secondary' APS to distinguish them from patients with features of APS alone ('primary' APS). However, the clinical and laboratory features of APS appear to be the same in either circumstance[13]. Some patients who present with features of APS alone later develop features

typical of SLE. Conversely, patients with SLE may develop APS some time after the onset of SLE. Clinically, it is important to determine whether a given patient with APS has features of another autoimmune disorder, as complications such as thrombosis or pregnancy losses may be caused by factors other than those related to APS. For example, pregnancy loss in patients with SLE may be related to underlying renal disease, severe systemic disease in the mother, or congenital heart block in the fetus. Similarly, thrombosis may result from a hypercoagulable state induced by the nephrotic syndrome associated with SLE.

Many features of APS are directly related to thrombosis, which may affect large, medium or small vessels. Other features, including thrombocytopenia, Coombs'-positive hemolytic anemia, abnormalities of cardiac valves, non-thrombotic skin lesions and a variety of non-thrombotic CNS abnormalities, are less clearly associated with a specific pathophysiologic mechanism. Whether these features are directly related to the disorder or are part of an associated systemic autoimmune disorder, such as SLE, is uncertain.

Venous thrombosis

All sites in the vascular tree may be subject to thrombosis. Large, medium and small vessels are affected. In the venous circulation the deep and superficial veins of the leg are the most frequently reported sites of thrombosis (Fig. 131.1). Some of these patients have pulmonary emboli. There are rare reports of pulmonary hypertension, due to either recurrent pulmonary emboli or in situ thrombosis. Other reported sites of venous thrombosis include the pelvic, renal, mesenteric, portal, hepatic, axillary and sagittal veins, as well as the inferior vena cava. Venous events usually occur at single sites and these can recur at the same or different sites, months or years apart.

Arterial thrombosis

The arterial circulation is also subject to thrombosis. Stroke and transient ischemic attacks, usually secondary to thrombosis of intracerebral arteries, are most frequently reported (Fig. 131.2). However, cerebral infarction may be silent, and when multiple events occur (Fig. 131.3)

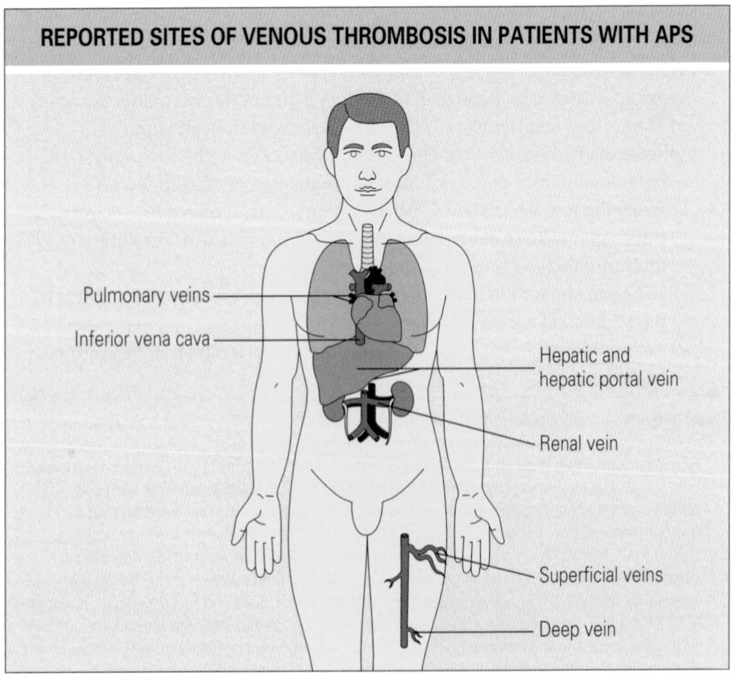

REPORTED SITES OF VENOUS THROMBOSIS IN PATIENTS WITH APS

Pulmonary veins

Inferior vena cava

Hepatic and hepatic portal vein

Renal vein

Superficial veins

Deep vein

Fig. 131.1 Reported sites of venous thrombosis in patients with APS. The deep and superficial veins of the legs are the most frequently reported sites of thrombosis.

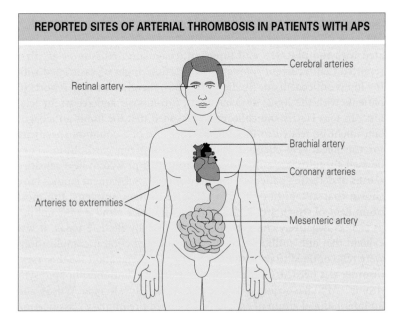

REPORTED SITES OF ARTERIAL THROMBOSIS IN PATIENTS WITH APS

Cerebral arteries

Retinal artery

Brachial artery

Coronary arteries

Arteries to extremities

Mesenteric artery

Fig. 131.2 Reported sites of arterial thrombosis in patients with APS. The intracranial arteries are the most frequently reported sites of thrombosis resulting in stroke and transient ischemic attacks. Myocardial infarction, gangrene of fingers and toes and bowel infarction have all been described and are presumed to be secondary to thrombotic occlusion of arteries supplying these sites. In some instances, occlusion of intracranial arteries may be secondary to emboli from heart valve vegetations.

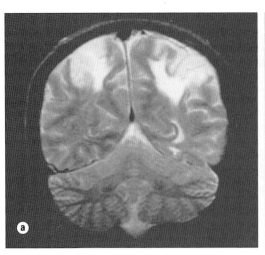 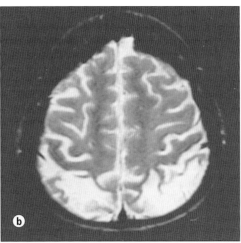

Fig. 131.3 Demonstration by MRI of biparietal infarctions in a 26-year-old woman with antiphospholipid syndrome. This woman also had a right frontal lobe infarct, which is not shown here. She had no risk factors for thrombosis other than the lupus anticoagulant and high positive IgG anticardiolipin antibodies. Her first pregnancy was terminated with intrauterine fetal death at 24 weeks gestation.

patients may first present with symptoms such as seizure or dementia secondary to extensive cerebral damage. Because emboli from heart valve vegetations may be responsible for cerebral infarction it is advisable to perform echocardiograms on patients with APS who present with transient ischemic attacks or stroke.

Other arterial sites, including retinal, coronary, brachial, mesenteric and peripheral arteries, are also subject to thrombosis. The clinical presentation depends on the anatomic site occluded. As with venous thrombosis, arterial events usually occur at single sites and can recur months or years later. A diagnosis of APS should be suspected when patients are young and have no risk factors for atherosclerosis.

Pregnancy complications

Pregnancy losses, fetal distress and premature births are frequent complications in women with APS. Fetal complications may occur at any stage of gestation, although most reports emphasize problems in the third trimester. Thrombotic occlusion of placental vessels and placental infarction are frequently reported. In some instances, however, the extent of placental damage does not appear sufficient to account for the degree of fetal distress. The aborted fetus usually appears normal. Although some babies born to mothers with APS may have positive anticardiolipin tests, complications in neonates due to these antibodies are unusual.

Early impressions suggested that pregnancy losses occurred in up to 85% of females with the lupus anticoagulant, but subsequent investigators have revised these estimates downwards, especially for a first pregnancy. Pregnancy losses occur in more than 50% of women with high or medium IgG anticardiolipin tests and are more likely in women with a history of at least one fetal death. Low positive IgG anticardiolipin, as well as IgM- or IgA-positive tests, seem to be less frequently associated with pregnancy complications.

Nervous system abnormalities

Stroke and transient ischemic attacks (TIA) are the most frequent neurologic complication of APS[14]. They are also the most frequently reported presentation of arterial thrombosis in APS. Angiograms typically demonstrate thrombotic occlusion of intracranial branch or trunk vessels, but in one-third of cases these studies may be normal. In some cases, emboli from cardiac valvular vegetations may account for stroke or TIAs, and echocardiograms are appropriate, particularly where there is no evidence of large vessel occlusion. Without anticoagulant therapy strokes may recur, and patients occasionally present with multi-infarct dementia.

Cerebral venous sinus thrombosis has occasionally been reported in patients with APS. Other causes, such as Factor V Leiden deficiency resulting in activated protein C resistance, should be excluded.

Ocular ischemic events can occur, including anterior ischemic optic neuropathy, central retinal artery occlusion, cilioretinal artery occlusion and amaurosis fugax, as well as occlusion of retinal veins[15]. Sensorineural hearing loss, often presenting as sudden deafness, has also been reported in this disorder[16]. The latter is presumably due to vascular thrombosis, and anticoagulant therapy would be an appropriate treatment choice.

Many other neurologic abnormalities have been reported in APS, but these are not clearly linked to thrombosis. They include transverse myelopathy, chorea, Guillain–Barré syndome, psychosis and migraine headaches[14]. These complications may result from interaction between antiphospholipid antibodies and nervous tissue, or from immune complex deposition in cerebral or spinal cord vessels. Seizures are also reportedly associated with APS, but it would be important to exclude cerebral infarction as a cause.

Cardiac valve abnormalities

Cardiac valvular abnormalities (e.g. Libman–Sacks endocarditis) are observed with Doppler echocardiography in as many as 30–50% of patients with APS[17]. Valvular thickening is most common, but valvular vegetations, stenosis and regurgitation may be present. Any of the four heart valves may be affected, but mitral involvement is most frequent, followed by the aortic valve. Tricuspid and pulmonary valve involvement is uncommon. Mitral regurgitation is the most frequent hemodynamic abnormality, reported in some series to occur in as many as 25% patients, followed by aortic regurgitation, which may be present in 6–10% of patients. Mitral or aortic regurgitation is rarely severe enough to cause symptoms, and requirement for valve replacement is distinctly uncommon. The valvular abnormalities of APS are different from those seen in rheumatic heart disease. In APS valvular thickening is diffuse, whereas in rheumatic heart disease thickening is more localized, present at leaflet tips, and often associated with thickening, fusion and calcification of the chordae tendinae.

The pathogenesis of APS is unclear. Valvular abnormalities are often indistinguishable from those present in patients with SLE who *do not* have aPL antibodies. Hence, these lesions could conceivably be caused by antibodies other than aPL antibodies that may exist in both APS and SLE. Alternatively, circulating autoantibody–antigen complexes might deposit on cardiac valves, resulting in activation of complement, inflammation and heart valve damage. A final possibility is that autoantibodies (aPL or antiendothelial) may interact with valvular antigens directly, resulting in superficial thrombosis, subendocardial mononuclear cell infiltrations and fibrosis.

Skin

The occurrence of leg ulcers was noted in an early description of the antiphospholipid syndrome (APS)[3]. Other skin manifestations reportedly associated with APS include livedo reticularis, leg ulcers, cutaneous necrosis, gangrene of the digits or extremities, thrombophlebitis, necrotizing purpura and nailfold infarcts[18]. These lesions are reported more frequently in dermatologic series, and none are specific to APS. Thrombophlebitis, cutaneous gangrene, gangrene of the extremities and nailfold infarcts are usually consequences of thrombosis of small arteries. Livedo reticularis is the most frequently reported skin manifestation of APS, but its pathogenesis is uncertain. Livedo may occur in a variety of other disorders, including connective tissue diseases, vasculitides, multiple cholesterol emboli syndrome, sepsis, hyperoxaluria, Sneddon's syndrome – where it is associated with stroke – and it may occur in normal individuals. Leg ulcers can be multiple and focal, painful, sharply marginated with a necrotic center or base, non-inflammatory, and form a white atrophic scar on healing. These ulcers tend to occur in the pretibial area and ankle. Occasional patients have single large ulcers that may resemble pyoderma gangrenosum. The latter should also be distinguished from postphlebitic ulcers, which can occur in patients who have had multiple episodes of deep vein thrombosis in the same leg, resulting in chronic edema, characteristic skin changes, skin breakdown and ulceration.

Thrombocytopenia/hemolytic anemia

Thrombocytopenia is a well recognized feature of APS, being present in about one-third patients with the disorder[13]. Platelet levels fluctuate, usually in the range of $100–150 \times 10^9/l$, but are seldom low enough to be associated with hemorrhage ($<50 \times 10^9/l$). Thrombocytopenia may occur in several disorders that may have features similar to APS, including SLE, thrombotic thrombocytopenia pupura (TTP), diffuse intravascular coagulation (DIC), HELLP syndrome (a disorder in late pregnancy characterized by hemolysis, elevate liver enzymes, low platelet counts and severe pre-eclampsia), and heparin-induced thrombocytopenia (which, paradoxically, can be complicated by thrombosis).

The pathogenesis of thrombocytopenia in APS is unclear. Hypotheses include binding of aPL antibodies to platelet membrane phospholipids, β_2GP-1/phospholipid complexes, or coexisting antibodies to platelet membrane glycoproteins. Demonstration that aPL antibodies can activate platelets in the presence of low levels of thrombin or ADP gives credence to the possibility of aPL binding to platelet membranes, which may result in increased platelet uptake and destruction by the reticuloendothelial system.

About 10–20% of patients with APS have a positive Coombs' test, but hemolytic anemia is relatively uncommon. The simultaneous occurrence of hemolytic anemia and thrombocytopenia, referred to as Evans syndrome, is a rare occurrence in series of patients with APS, but in some series positive anticardiolipin tests are frequent[19]. Coombs'-positive tests and hemolytic anemia may result from aPL antibodies binding β_2GP-1/phospholipid complexes on red cell membranes, or might result from the coexistence of antibodies to proteins in red cell membranes.

Catastrophic antiphospholipid syndrome

Catastrophic antiphospholipid syndrome is characterized by thrombosis at multiple organ sites occurring concurrently or over a short period of time in association with positive anticardiolipin antibody or lupus anticoagulant tests. Ischemia of the kidneys, bowels, lungs, heart and/or brain is most frequent, but rarely adrenal, testicular, splenic, pancreatic or skin involvement has been described. Occlusion of small vessels (thrombotic microangiopathy) is characteristic, resulting in symptoms related to dysfunction of the affected organs[20]. Depending on the organs involved, patients may present with hypertension and renal impairment, acute respiratory distress syndrome, alveolar hemorrhage and capillaritis, confusion and disorientation, or abdominal pain and distention secondary to bowel infarction.

Catastrophic antiphospholipid syndrome must be distinguished from thrombotic thrombocytopenic pupura (TTP) or diffuse intravascular

TABLE 131.2 DIFFERENTIAL DIAGNOSIS OF CATASTROPHIC ANTIPHOSPHOLIPID SYNDROME

Laboratory abnormalities	CAPS	TTP*	DIC**
Microangiopathic hemolytic anemia	–	+	+
Thrombocytopenia	+	+	+
Fibrinogen/FDP	Normal/Normal	Normal/Increased	Decreased/Increased
Anticardiolipin antibody	+	–	–
Lupus anticoagulant	+	–	–

DIC, diffuse intravascular coagulation; TTP, thrombotic thrombocytopenia purpura; FDP, fibrinogen degradation products.

coagulation (DIC) (Table 131.2). TTP is characterized by the presence of microangiopathic hemolytic anemia with schistocytes in the peripheral smear; consumptive thrombocytopenia, which can be complicated by hemorrhage; fluctuating neurologic symptoms; fever; and microscopic hematuria/proteinuria, occasionally with renal impairment. DIC is a consumptive coagulopathy characterized by prolonged coagulation tests, increased fibrinogen degradation products, hypofibrinogenemia, thrombocytopenia and schistocytes on peripheral smear.

LABORATORY DIAGNOSIS

Laboratory diagnosis of APS is based on a positive anticardiolipin antibody or lupus anticoagulant test[12]. The anticardiolipin test is positive in about 80% of these patients, the lupus anticoagulant is the only positive test in about 20%, and both are positive in about 60% of cases. It is important that both tests be performed in patients suspected of APS. These assays detect a heterogeneous group of antibodies that bind serum proteins such as β_2GP-1 or prothrombin, cardiolipin and negatively charged phospholipids, and protein/phospholipid complexes.

The anticardiolipin test utilizes an ELISA technique with cardiolipin in the presence of β_2GP-1 as antigen (Fig. 131.4). ELISA plates are coated

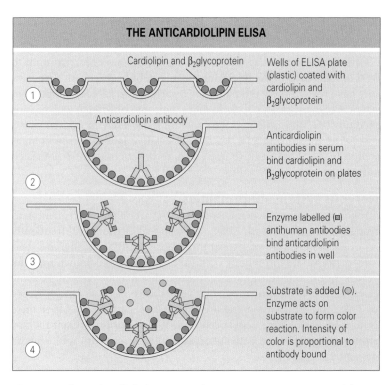

THE ANTICARDIOLIPIN ELISA

① Cardiolipin and β₂glycoprotein — Wells of ELISA plate (plastic) coated with cardiolipin and β₂glycoprotein

② Anticardiolipin antibody — Anticardiolipin antibodies in serum bind cardiolipin and β₂glycoprotein on plates

③ Enzyme labelled (■) antihuman antibodies bind anticardiolipin antibodies in well

④ Substrate is added (○). Enzyme acts on substrate to form color reaction. Intensity of color is proportional to antibody bound

Fig. 131.4 The anticardiolipin ELISA. A diagrammatic representation of the steps involved in the anticardiolipin test.

with cardiolipin and then incubated with bovine or fetal calf serum diluted (10%) in phosphate-buffered saline. The incubation mixture is also used to dilute patient serum samples being tested. The use of fetal calf or bovine serum provides sufficient β_2GP-1 as antigen in the assay. Antibodies bind β_2GP-1, cardiolipin, or some combination of the two. These antibodies cross-react with other negatively charged phospholipids, hence negatively charged phospholipids such as phosphatidylserine can sometimes be used in place of cardiolipin, but to ensure test standardization cardiolipin is preferred.

Anticardiolipin test results are reported according to isotype (IgG, IgM or IgA) and level. Levels of IgG anticardiolipin are reported in GPL (G phospholipid) units, IgM in MPL (M phospholipid) units, or APL (A phospholipid) units, as defined by the First International Workshop on anticardiolipin antibodies[21]. Because absolute levels have a relatively wide error range, the use of semiquantitative measures to report results – normal, *low positive* (10–20 GPL or MPL unit), *moderate positive* (20–80 GPL or MPL units) or *high positive* (above 80 GPL or MPL units) – is preferable. In assessing anticardiolipin test results, a moderate to high positive IgG anticardiolipin test, present on more than one occasion at least 6 weeks apart, is most specific for a diagnosis of APS. However, some patients may have only a positive IgM test, and a few are only IgA positive.

The lupus anticoagulant test is a functional assay which measures the ability of this subset of aPL antibodies to prolong clotting tests such as the partial thromboplastin time (PTT) or the Russell viper venom time (RVVT). These antibodies are inhibitors of clotting in vitro, acting by partially blocking the conversion of prothrombin to thrombin in the presence of a phospholipid template (Fig. 131.5). This inhibitory action delays the formation of fibrin and so prolongs the time to clot formation. The lupus anticoagulant test is performed with patient plasma and requires three basic steps:

1. Prolongation of a phospholipid-dependent coagulation test such as the PTT or RVVT
2. Failure of the test to normalize when patient plasma is mixed with normal plasma – thereby excluding a clotting factor deficiency and demonstrating the presence of a clotting inhibitor
3. Normalization of the test by the addition of a phospholipid preparation (so confirming the 'phospholipid-dependent' characteristic of

these antibodies and excluding other inhibitors such as anti-Factor VIII or antiprothrombin (Factor II))[22].

An unsolved paradox of APS is the ability of this subset of aPL antibodies to act as clotting inhibitors in vitro but to promote clotting in vivo.

Although not part of the laboratory criteria for diagnosis of APS, other assays can be positive in large numbers of these patients. The anti-β_2 GP-1 assay, in which β_2GP-1 is presented on oxidized polystyrene plates (in the absence of phospholipids), is often (but not always) positive in patients with a positive anticardiolipin test[23]. An ELISA kit that utilizes a mixture of negatively charged phospholipids termed the APhL antigen[24] is also nearly as sensitive as the anticardiolipin test. Both anti-β_2GP-1[23] and the APhL ELISA assay[24] have proved more specific for the diagnosis of APS than the anticardiolipin test. A significant minority of patients with APS will have a biologic false positive test for syphilis (BFP-STS), which measures the ability of aPL antibodies to precipitate an antigen (e.g. the VDRL antigen) containing a mixture of cardiolipin, phosphatidylcholine, and cholesterol.

DIFFERENTIAL DIAGNOSIS

Presentations of APS are diverse and the differential diagnosis will vary depending on the particular manifestations of individual patients. Unexplained venous thrombosis is a common presenting feature, and the disease states listed in Table 131.3 should be considered. In patients presenting with clinical features resulting from arterial thrombosis, such as stroke, myocardial infarction, bowel gangrene etc., causes other than APS should be considered (Table 131.4).

In addition to APS, recurrent pregnancy losses may be due to structural abnormalities of the uterus, systemic disease, chronic infections, immunologic dysfunction and environmental factors, including alcohol and drug abuse. Genetic abnormalities of the fetus account for more than half of first trimester and 35% of second trimester pregnancy losses. A careful history, physical examination and appropriate laboratory studies are essential in excluding each of these possibilities.

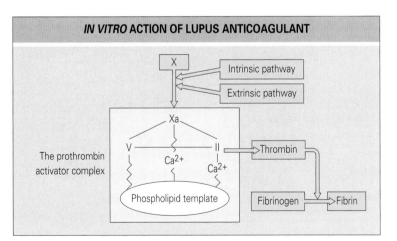

Fig. 131.5 *In vitro* action of lupus anticoagulant. Antiphospholipid antibodies responsible for the lupus anticoagulant test are believed to act at the level of the 'prothrombin activator complex' of the clotting cascade. For prothrombin to be converted to thrombin, a complex of factors Xa, V and prothrombin must be formed on a phospholipid template in the presence of calcium. Antiphospholipid antibodies may bind the prothrombin–phospholipid complex; disrupt the complex and so delay prothrombin-to-thrombin conversion. This will result in a delay of fibrin formation and prolongation of coagulation tests.

TABLE 131.3 DISEASE STATES THAT SHOULD BE CONSIDERED IN PATIENTS WITH UNEXPLAINED VENOUS THROMBOSIS
• Factor V Leiden ('activated protein C resistance')
• Protein C deficiency
• Protein S deficiency
• Antithrombin III deficiency
• Nephrotic syndrome
• Peripartum state
• Estrogen-containing oral contraceptives
• Malignancy (Trousseau's syndrome)
• Behçet's syndrome
• Paroxysmal nocturnal hemoglobinura
• Heparin-induced thrombosis

TABLE 131.4 DISEASE STATES THAT SHOULD BE CONSIDERED IN PATIENTS WITH UNEXPLAINED ARTERIAL THROMBOSIS
• Atherosclerosis
• Vasculitis
• Homocystinuria
• Myeloproliferative disorders
• Protein C, protein S, or antithrombin III deficiency

A diagnosis of APS is more likely when patients have an unequivocally positive lupus anticoagulant test and/or a moderate to high positive IgG anticardiolipin test, in combination with any of the following clinical features: venous or arterial thrombosis without apparent risk factors; involvement of abnormal venous sites (e.g. mesenteric, hepatic, renal, axillary veins); the occurrence of thrombosis in patients less than 45 years old; and multiple unexplained pregnancy losses, particularly in the second or third trimester. In general, patients presenting with combinations of clinical abnormalities characteristic of APS (e.g. arterial and/or venous thrombosis, pregnancy losses, thrombocytopenia) are more likely to have the disorder than those with only one feature. However, patients with SLE may well have a combination of complications, such as recurrent thrombosis, pregnancy losses and thrombocytopenia, that might have explanations other than APS – thus, nephrotic syndrome may account for venous thrombosis, vasculitis for a complication such as stroke, and antiplatelet antibodies (other than aPL) for thrombocytopenia.

PATHOGENESIS

Mechanism of action

The relationship of aPL antibodies to thrombosis and pregnancy loss is unknown. The antibodies may be just 'markers' of the disorder, and thrombosis and pregnancy loss may result from other unknown factors that induce a procoagulant state. Alternatively, the antibodies may contribute directly to a procoagulant state. Even if the antibodies play a direct role, other factors must act in concert to cause thrombosis, as most patients with persistently elevated antibody levels only suffer thrombosis episodically, and others never suffer this complication. The occurrence of placental vessel thrombosis in the absence of systemic disease suggests that local tissue factors within the placenta may favor a procoagulant state. Furthermore, only some subsets of aPL antibodies may be associated with thrombosis, as exemplified by patients with aPL antibodies secondary to infectious or drug-induced disorders who usually do not experience thrombosis.

Induction of thrombosis

Evidence that aPL plays a role in thrombosis is persuasive. Several retrospective and some prospective studies[25] have demonstrated an association of thrombosis with the presence of anticardiolipin antibodies or lupus anticoagulant. Thrombosis is likelier with higher anticardiolipin antibody levels[26]. Numerous studies have shown that mice passively immunized with human polyclonal or monoclonal antibodies have longer and more persistent thrombi, when thrombi are induced by vascular pinch injury[27]. A similar effect on induced thrombus size has also been demonstrated in mice, where antiphospholipid antibodies have been induced by active immunization with β_2GP-1 or human IgG aPL antibodies[28].

Various studies have suggested that aPL antibodies may cause thrombosis by activation of endothelial cells or platelets, or by inhibition of the protein C activation pathway. Several groups of investigators demonstrated that aPL antibodies can cause β_2GP-1 dependent activation of endothelial cells, as evidenced by increased expression of adhesion markers, such as intracellular adhesion molecule-1 (ICAM-1), vascular cell adhesion molecule-1 (VCAM-1) and P-selectin[29]. In separate studies utilizing ICAM-1 knockout or ICAM/P-selectin knockout mice, or monoclonal anti-VCAM-1 antibodies, investigators have demonstrated that each of these molecules is important for aPL-induced thrombosis in vivo[30]. Other investigators have suggested that aPL antibodies may promote tissue factor synthesis by leukocytes[31]. Tissue factor activates Factor VII, which sets in motion the extrinsic coagulation pathway leading to thrombosis.

An alternative route by which aPL antibodies might promote thrombosis is by platelet activation, leading to enhanced platelet adhesion or increased thromboxane synthesis. One group has reported that in the presence of low levels of thrombin or ADP, aPL antibodies can induce platelet activation, as demonstrated by increased expression of platelet GIIb/IIIa[32]. Another group reported increased urinary excretion of the major platelet thromboxane metabolite 11-dehydrothromboxane-α_2 in patients with lupus anticoagulant compared to normal controls[33]. F(ab)$_2$ fractions from lupus anticoagulant-positive patients were also shown to increase thromboxane-α_2 production by washed platelets[33].

A third possibility is that aPL antibodies may inhibit the protein C activation system, which requires a membrane phospholipid catalyst (Fig. 131.6). Activation of the clotting cascade causes the generation of thrombin. Thrombin 'turns off' its own production by binding thrombomodulin in endothelial membranes, and then the thrombin–thrombomodulin complex activates protein C. Activated protein C then inactivates Factors Va and VIIIa, which will 'turn off' the clotting cascade and thrombin formation (Fig. 131.6). Some groups have shown that aPL can inhibit protein C activation[34], and if this occurs it would result in unopposed thrombin generation.

β_2Glycoprotein-1 is a prominent antigen for aPL antibodies and much work has been done to determine how this might relate to thrombus formation. β_2GP-1 is a 50 kDa protein present in human plasma at a concentration of about 200mg/ml. It consists of 326 amino acids organized in five homologous motifs (termed short consensus repeats (SCR)

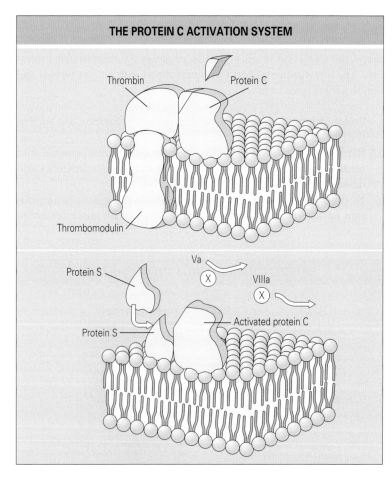

Fig. 131.6 The protein C activation system. This is depicted in two steps. In the first step (top) thrombin binds thrombomodulin, which results in cleavage (and activation) of the protein C molecule. In the second step (bottom), activated protein C in association with protein S (a cofactor) degrades (and so inactivates) protein Va and VIIa. These processes all take place on a phospholipid (membrane) template. Some studies suggest that antiphospholipid antibodies inhibit protein C activation and one study suggests that these antibodies inhibit degradation of factor Va by activated protein C.

or 'sushi' domains) of 60 amino acids each. The protein binds negatively charged molecules, including negatively charged phospholipids. Antiphospholipid antibodies have weak binding affinity for this molecule[35], exhibiting binding when β_2GP-1 is presented on a template of negatively charged phospholipids or irradiated polystyrene plates. The latter surfaces increase antibody binding, either by increasing the density of antigen presented[35] or by altering the conformation of the molecule[23]. Active immunization of mice with β_2GP1 induces aPL antibodies, as well as anti-β_2GP1 antibodies, which promotes thrombus formation[28]. One problem with hypothesizing a role for anti-β_2GP1 in thrombosis is that individuals who have heterozygous or even homozygous deficiencies of β_2GP1 do not appear more susceptible to thrombosis, and β_2GP1 knockout mice also do not appear subject to increased thrombosis.

Pregnancy loss

That aPL antibodies may have a role in pregnancy loss has been demonstrated in several studies of pregnant mice, in which passive immunization with human or mouse polyclonal and monoclonal human antibodies has been shown to cause fetal resorption and decreased litter size[36]. One of the most intriguing hypotheses as to how this might occur relates to aPL displacement of annexin V proteins from trophoblast surfaces[37]. Annexin V belongs to a family of proteins all of which have four domains consisting of 70 amino acids each. Annexin V has potent anticoagulant activity, because it binds negatively charged phospholipids in the presence of calcium and so inhibits binding of coagulation factors to phospholipid catalysts. Annexin V proteins are expressed on the surface of placental trophoblasts, thereby maintaining an anticoagulant trophoblastic surface. Removal of annexin V from trophoblast surfaces by EGTA has been shown to increase coagulation on the surfaces of these cells. One group of investigators has demonstrated that aPL antibodies can reduce annexin V on cultured trophoblasts and endothelial cells, perhaps through competitive binding for phosphatidylserine on the surface of these cells. Displacement of annexin V may make trophoblast surfaces procoagulant and so may account for placental thrombosis and pregnancy loss[37].

MANAGEMENT

Primary thromboprophylaxis of aPL-positive subjects

The controversy concerning whether or not prophylactic treatment is indicated for patients with aPL who have no history of thrombosis remains unresolved. Although low-dose aspirin (75–100mg daily) has been considered to be a logical first option, the Physician Health Study showed that low-dose aspirin (325mg daily) in men with aCL did not protect against deep venous thrombosis or pulmonary embolus[25]. In contrast, hydroxychloroquine may be protective against the development of thrombosis in aPL-positive patients with SLE[38].

A prospective, randomized clinical trial comparing aspirin alone with aspirin plus low-intensity warfarin (INR~1.5) in patients with aPL who have never had thrombosis is currently under way in the United Kingdom. Until these results are available, we suggest that individuals with a persistently positive aCL (moderate/high titers) and/or unequivocally positive lupus anticoagulant tests take low-dose aspirin (75–100mg daily) indefinitely. Cessation of estrogen-containing oral contraceptive use, treatment of hypertension, hyperlipidemia or diabetes if present, and the avoidance of smoking are all additional recommended therapeutic measures. Prophylaxis with heparin administered subcutaneously should certainly be given to cover higher-risk situations, such as surgery and long-haul flights.

Thrombosis

Acute management of venous or arterial thrombosis in patients with APS is no different from that of other patients with similar complications. There is now good evidence from both retrospective[39] and prospective[40] studies that APS patients with thrombosis will be subject to recurrences, and that these can be prevented by long-term anticoagulation. Many patients with APS in whom anticoagulation has been stopped have had major recurrent thrombosis. It is not clear, however, whether prolonged anticoagulation is necessary in APS patients whose first thrombotic episode developed in association with surgery, oral contraceptive use, pregnancy or other circumstantial thrombotic risk factors.

Most patients requiring long-term anticoagulant therapy respond well to warfarin targeted to an international normalized ratio (INR) of 2.0–3.0. However, the optimal intensity of anticoagulation therapy is uncertain for patients with aPL-associated thrombosis. There are reports based on retrospective analyses of observational studies that patients with APS and thrombosis are inadequately protected from recurrent thrombotic episodes if treated at a targeted INR of 2.0–3.0. In the largest retrospective study of 147 aPL-associated thromboses followed up for 10 years, recurrent thrombosis occurred in 69% of patients[39]. High-intensity warfarin (INR >3.0) was the most effective therapeutic option in the secondary prevention of venous and arterial thromboses in these patients. Some dispute this and prefer to advocate an INR of 2.0–3.0 for those with venous thrombosis[40], reserving intensive anticoagulation INR (3.0–4.0) for those with recurrent venous thrombosis or arterial thrombosis.

Oral anticoagulation therapy carries an inevitable risk of serious hemorrhage. In APS, serious bleeding complications may occur but their risk is not higher than that observed in other thrombotic conditions warranting oral anticoagulation.

Concerns exist over the validity of the INR in the control of oral anticoagulant dosing if lupus anticoagulant is present. The inhibitor occasionally increases the prothrombin time and the INR may not reflect the true degree of anticoagulation. This phenomenon seems to be more likely when certain recombinant thromboplastin reagents are used, and can usually be circumvented by careful selection of the thromboplastin to be used for the prothrombin-time test.

The role of steroids and immunosuppressive drugs in the treatment of patients with aPL and thrombosis is uncertain. Such drugs do not always suppress aPL and they have severe side effects when given for prolonged periods. Furthermore, in a large series of patients with APS, corticosteroids and immunosuppressive therapy, prescribed in some patients to control lupus activity, did not prevent further thrombotic events[39]. The use of these drugs is probably justified only in patients with life-threatening conditions with repeated episodes of thrombosis despite adequate anticoagulation therapy, namely catastrophic APS. In this rare but life-threatening condition plasmapheresis and fibrinolytic agents have also been used, with varying success[20].

Recurrent pregnancy loss

The management of pregnancy in women known to have APS is the subject of much debate, and as yet there have been very few randomized controlled trials. Anticoagulation in one form or another is the preferred treatment, rather than steroids (once widely recommended[41,42]). The current choices lie between aspirin, heparin or both. Recently, two prospective trials showed that heparin plus low-dose aspirin is more effective than aspirin alone for achieving live births among women with aPL and first trimester recurrent pregnancy loss[43,44]. A third prospective trial of aPL-positive women with repeated pregnancy loss but no history of thrombosis or SLE, found similar live birth rates (~80%) using either low-dose aspirin or placebo[45], suggesting that treatment may be unnecessary in some women. Although optimal treatment for women with one or more late pregnancy losses (second/third trimester) but no history of thromboembolism is controversial, most obstetricians support the use of heparin therapy in addition to low-dose aspirin[41,42].

Intravenous immunoglobulin (IVIG) has also been used during pregnancy, usually in conjunction with heparin and low-dose aspirin, especially in women with particularly poor past obstetric histories or recurrent pregnancy loss during heparin treatment[46]. However, a randomized controlled pilot study of IVIG treatment during pregnancy in unselected APS cases found no benefit to this expensive therapy compared to heparin and low-dose aspirin[47]. It is currently unclear whether IVIG may play a role in 'refractory' cases. Therefore, it would seem prudent to limit its use to women with APS who have had pregnancy losses despite treatment with aspirin and heparin.

For women with APS on warfarin because of previous thrombosis, who want to become pregnant, it is important to note that there is a warfarin embryopathy, particularly on exposure of the fetus during weeks 6–12 of gestation. Hence, patients should be switched from warfarin to subcutaneous heparin at an early enough time to ensure that there is no fetal exposure during that period. Some physicians prefer to switch before conception is attempted, whereas others do so as soon as pregnancy is determined. Heparin should be initiated at the time of warfarin cessation and should be continued both intrapartum and postpartum until warfarin is reintroduced. Both warfarin and subcutaneous heparin are compatible with breastfeeding.

Pregnancy complicated by APS requires expert care and a team approach by obstetricians and physicians. Close monitoring of both mother and fetus is essential. Ultrasound monitoring of fetal growth and uteroplacental blood flow is crucial. This allows for timely delivery. Some authorities utilize uterine artery waveforms at 20 and 24 weeks' gestation, and those pregnancies with evidence of an early diastolic notch are monitored very closely with 2-weekly growth scans because of the high risk of intrauterine growth restriction. When there are no notches we recommend 4-weekly assessment of growth and amniotic fluid volume. Doppler flow studies of the umbilical artery may be used, as in other pregnancies at high risk of fetal compromise through uteroplacental insufficiency.

Management of other manifestations of APS

Thrombocytopenia is an accompanying problem in 30% of individuals with APS. Generally it is mild, but occasionally severe thrombocytopenia occurs. The treatment of choice is corticosteroids. Anecdotal reports have shown that low-dose aspirin, dapsone, danazol, chloroquine, IVIG and warfarin have improved steroid-resistant thrombocytopenia. Splenectomy has been safely and successfully performed in some patients with APS and refractory thrombocytopenia.

Headache is a common feature in APS and usually responds to conventional treatment. In some patients with APS, headache has been reported to improve remarkably with low-dose aspirin, and in very resistant cases warfarin may be an alternative therapy.

There is a high prevalence of heart valve lesions in patients with aPL. In some cases valvular damage may result in significant hemodynamic compromise requiring surgery. Both biological and mechanical valves have been implanted, with favorable results. Regardless of the valve type used, all patients with APS and valve prosthesis require full anticoagulation.

The outcome of kidney transplantation in patients with SLE and end-stage renal failure appears to be similar to that of patients with renal failure from other causes. However, the presence of aPL seems to be associated with a poorer prognosis[48]. Post-transplant thromboembolic phenomena, the recurrence of thrombotic microangiopathy in the graft despite anticoagulation, and thrombosis of the graft's renal vein, have all been reported.

REFERENCES

1. Conley CL, Hartmann RC. A hemorrhagic disorder caused by circulating anticoagulant in patients with disseminated lupus erythematosus. J Clin Invest 1952; 31: 621–622.
2. Bowie WEF, Thompson JH, Pascuzzi CA, Owen GA. Thrombosis in systemic lupus erythematosus despite circulating anticoagulants. J Clin Invest 1963; 62: 416–430.
3. Johansson EA, Niemi KM, Mustakallio KK. A peripheral vascular syndrome overlapping with systemic lupus erythematosus. Dermatologia 1977; 155: 257–267.
4. Nilsson IM, Astedt B, Hedner V, Berezin D. Intrauterine death and circulating anticoagulant (anti-thromboplastin). Acta Med Scand 1975; 197: 153–159.
5. Carreras LO, Defreyn G, Machin SJ et al. Arterial thrombosis, intrauterine death and lupus anticoagulant: detection of immunoglobulin interfering with prostacyclin formation. Lancet 1981; i: 244–246.
6. Harris EN, Gharavi AE, Boey ML et al. Anticardiolipin antibodies: detection by radioimmunoassay and association with thrombosis in systemic lupus erythematosus. Lancet 1983; ii: 1211–1214.
7. McNeil HP, Simpson RJ, Chesterman CN, Krilis SA. Anti-phospholipid antibodies are directed against a complex antigen that includes a lipid-binding inhibitor of coagulation: β_2 glycoprotein-1 (apolipoprotein H). Proc Natl Acad Sci USA 1990; 87; 4120–4124.
8. Galli M, Comfurius P, Maasen C et al. Anticardiolipin antibodies (ACA) directed not to cardiolipin but to a plasma cofactor. Lancet 1990; 335: 1544–1547.
9. Rao LVM, Hoarg AD, Rapaport SI. Differences in the interaction of lupus anticoagulant. IgG with human prothrombin and bovine prothrombin. Thromb Haemost 1995; 73: 668–674.
10. Pierangeli SS, Dean J, Gharavi AE et al. Studies on the interaction of placental anticoagulant protein (PAP-1), β_2 glycoprotein-1 (β_2 GP1) and antiphospholipid (aPL) antibodies in the prothrombinase reaction and in solid phase anticardiolipin assays. J Lab Clin Med 1996; 128: 194–201.
11. Harris EN. Syndrome of the Black Swan. Br J Rheumatol 1987; 26: 324–327.
12. Wilson WA, Gharavi AE, Koike T et al. International consensus statement on preliminary classification for definite antiphospholipid syndrome. Arthritis Rheum 1999; 42: 1309–1311.
13. Vianna JL, Khamashta MA, Ordi-Ros J et al. Comparison of the primary and secondary antiphospholipid syndrome: a European multicenter study of 114 patients. Am J Med 1994; 96: 3–9.
14. Brey RL. Differential diagnosis of central nervous system manifestations of the antiphospholipid antibody syndrome. J Autoimmun 2000; 15: 133–138.

15. Castanon C, Reyes PA. The eye in the primary antiphospholipid syndrome (Hughes Syndrome). In: Khamashta MA, ed. Hughes Syndrome: antiphospholipid syndrome. London: Springer Verlag, 2000; 89–95.
16. Naarendrop M, Spiera H. Sudden sensorineural hearing loss in patients with systemic lupus erythematosus or lupus-like syndrome and antiphospholipid antibodies. J Rheumatol 1998; 25: 589–592.
17. Nesher G, Ilani J, Rosenman D, Abraham AS. Valvular dysfunction in antiphospholipid syndrome: prevalence, clinical features, and treatment. Semin Arthritis Rheum 1997; 27: 27–35.
18. Alegre VA, Gastineau DA, Winkelmann RK. Skin lesions associated with circulating lupus anticoagulant. Br J Dermatol 1989; 120: 419–429.
19. Deleze M, Oria CV, Alarcon-Segovia DA. Occurrence of both haemolytic anemia and thrombocytopenic purpura (Evans' Syndrome) in systemic lupus erythematosus. Relationship to antiphospholipid antibodies. J Rheumatol 1988; 15: 611–615.
20. Asherson RA, Cervera R, Piette J-C et al. Catastrophic antiphospholipid syndrome. Clinical and laboratory features of 50 patients. Medicine 1998; 77: 195–207.
21. Harris EN, Gharavi AE, Patel S, Hughes GRV. Evaluation of the anti-cardiolipin antibody test: Report of an International Workshop held 4 April 1986. Clin Exp Immunol 1987; 68: 215–222.
22. Brandt JT, Triplett DA, Alving B et al. Criteria for the diagnosis of lupus anticoagulants: an update on behalf of the Subcommittee on Lupus Anticoagulant/Antiphospholipid Antibody of the Scientific and Standardization Committee of the ISTH. Thromb Haemost 1995; 74: 1185–1190.
23. Matsuura E, Igarashi Y, Yasuda T et al. Anticardiolipin antibodies recognize beta(2)-glycoprotein 1 structure altered by interacting with an oxygen modified solid phase surface. J Exp Med 1994; 179: 457–462.
24. Merkel PA, Chong Y, Pierangeli SS, Harris EN, Polisson RP. Comparison between the standard anti-cardiolipin antibody test and a new phospholipid test in patients with a variety of connective tissue diseases. J Rheumatol 1999; 26: 591–596.
25. Ginsburg KS, Liang MH, Newcomer L et al. Anticardiolipin antibodies and the risk for ischemic stroke and venous thrombosis. Ann Intern Med 1992; 997–1002.
26. Levine SR, Salowich-Palm L, Sawaya KL et al. IgG anticardiolipin antibody titer >40GPL and the risk of subsequent thrombo-occlusive events and death: a prospective cohort study. Stroke 1997; 28: 1660–1665.
27. Pierangeli SS, Liu XW, Anderson GH, Barker JH, Harris EN. Induction of thrombosis in a mouse model by IgG, IgM and IgA immunoglobulins from patients with the antiphospholipid syndrome. Thromb Haemost 1995; 74: 1361–1366.

28. Pierangeli SS, Liu XW, Anderson GH, Barker JH, Harris EN. Thrombogenic properties of murine anticardiolipin antibodies induced by β_2 glycoprotein-1 and human immunoglobulin G antiphospholipid antibodies. Circulation 1996; 94: 1746–1751.

29. Del Papa N, Guidali L, Sala A et al. Endothelial cells as target for antiphospholipid antibodies. Human polyclonal and monoclonal anti β_2 glycoprotein-1 induce endothelial cell activation. Arthritis Rheum 1997; 40: 551–561.

30. Pierangeli SS, Espinola RG, Liu XWei, Harris EN. Thrombogenic effects of antiphospholipid antibodies are mediated by intracellular adhesion molecule-1, vascular cell adhesion molecule-1, and P-selectin. Circ Res 2001; 88: 245–250.

31. Reverter JC, Tassies D, Font J et al. Effects of human monoclonal anticardiolipin antibodies on platelet function and on tissue factor expression on monocytes. Arthritis Rheum 1998; 41: 1420–1427.

32. Campbell AL, Pierangeli SS, Wellhausen S, Harris EN. Comparison of the effect of anticardiolipin antibodies from patients with antiphospholipid syndrome and with syphilis on platelet activation and aggregation. Thromb Haemost 1995; 73: 519–524.

33. Lellouche F, Martinuzzo M, Scuid P et al. Imbalance of thromboxane/prostacyclin biosynthesis in patients with lupus anticoagulant. Blood 1991: 78: 2894–2899.

34. Smirnov MD, Triplett DT, Comp PC, Esmon NL, Esmon CT. On the role of phosphatidylethanolamine in the inhibition of activated protein C activity by antiphospholipid antibodies. J Clin Invest 1995; 95: 309–316.

35. Roubey RAS, Eisenberg RA, Harper MF, Winfield JB. 'Anticardiolipin' autoantibodies recognize β_2 glycoprotein-1 in the absence of phospholipid. Importance of Ag density and bivalent binding. J Immunol 1995; 154: 954–960.

36. Blank M, Krause I, Shoenfeld Y. The contribution of experimental models to our understanding of etiology, pathogenesis and novel therapies in the Antiphospholipid Syndrome. In: Khamashta MA, ed. Hughes syndrome: antiphospholipid syndrome. London: Springer Verlag, 2000; 374–388.

37. Rand JH. Antiphospholipid antibody-mediated disruption of the Annexin V antithrombotic shield: a thrombogenic mechanism for the antiphospholipid syndrome. J Autoimmun 2000; 15: 107–111.

38. Petri M. Hydroxychloroquine use in the Baltimore lupus cohort: effects on lipids, glucose, and thrombosis. Lupus 1996; 5(Suppl): 516–522.

39. Khamashta MA, Cuadrado MJ, Mujic F et al. The management of thrombosis in the antiphospholipid–antibody syndrome. N Engl J Med 1995; 332: 993–997.

40. Schulman S, Svenungsson E, Granqvist S and the Duration of Anticoagulation Study Group. Anticardiolipin antibodies predict early recurrence of thromboembolism and death among patients with venous thromboembolism following anticoagulant therapy. Am J Med 1998; 104: 332–338.

41. Esplin MS. Management of antiphospholipid syndrome during pregnancy. Clin Obstet Gynecol 2001; 44: 20–28.

42. Shehata HA, Nelson-Piercy C, Khamashta M. Management of pregnancy in antiphospholipid syndrome. Rheum Dis Clin North Am 2001; 27: 643–659.

43. Kutteh WH. Antiphospholipid antibody-associated recurrent pregnancy loss: treatment with heparin and low-dose aspirin is superior to low-dose aspirin alone. Am J Obstet Gynecol 1996; 174: 1584–1589.

44. Rai R, Cohen H, Dave M, Regan L. Randomised controlled trial of aspirin and aspirin plus heparin in pregnant women with recurrent miscarriage associated with phospholipid antibodies. Br Med J 1997; 314: 253–257.

45. Pattison NS, Chamley LW, Birdsall M et al. Does aspirin have a role in improving pregnancy outcome for women with the antiphospholipid syndrome? A randomized controlled trial. Am J Obstet Gynecol 2000; 183: 1008–1012.

46. Clark AL, Branch DW, Silver RM et al. Pregnancy complicated by the antiphospholipid syndrome: outcome with intravenous immunoglobulin therapy. Obstet Gynecol 1999: 93: 437–441.

47. Branch DW, Peaceman AM, Druzin M et al. A multicenter, placebo-controlled pilot study of intravenous immune globulin treatment of antiphospholipid syndrome during pregnancy. Am J Obstet Gynecol 2000, 182: 122–127.

48. McIntyre JA, Wagenknecht DR. Antiphospholipid antibodies – risk assessments for solid organ, bone marrow and tissue transplantation. Rheum Dis Clin North Am 2001, 27: 611–631.

132 Epidemiology of systemic sclerosis

Virginia D Steen

- Incidence: 20 cases per million population per year

- Prevalence: more than 150 patients per million population

- Race, subtype and antibody predict the course of disease in scleroderma subsets

- African-American patients are younger and typically have diffuse scleroderma, anti-topoisomerase antibody and more severe lung disease

- Limited scleroderma is characterized by anticentromere antibody and increased risk for pulmonary hypertension late in disease

- Anti-RNA polymerase III typifies diffuse scleroderma and is associated with severe skin disease and renal crisis

- Genetics are most closely related to antibodies; twin studies are negative

- Survival has improved in the past decade, but lung involvement is a major cause of death

- There is no conclusive evidence for an occupational cause of scleroderma.

INTRODUCTION

Epidemiology is the study of patterns of disease that help in understanding an illness and give hints to the pathogenesis of the disease. Through such studies we have obtained a better understanding of the natural history of systemic sclerosis and identified a variety of genetic and risk factor studies, which may lead to hypotheses of possible causes of the disease. In this chapter the incidence and prevalence of systemic sclerosis and the survival of affected patients will be reviewed. The features that affect survival, resulting in the differing outcomes, will be discussed. Although autoantibodies do not have a pathogenic role, they are important in determining the outcome for an individual patient and may be closely linked to the genetics of the disease. The clinical subsets, natural history and genetics of this disease will be summarized. Additionally, there have been a number of factors that have been associated with scleroderma-like illnesses. Although no factors have been proven to 'cause' classic scleroderma, these are studies that are helpful in the understanding of the disease.

INCIDENCE AND PREVALENCE

The reported incidence and prevalence of systemic sclerosis are quite variable, depending on the period of time over which the study was done, the definition of disease applied to the cases, and the country in which the study was undertaken. One of the earliest studies in the USA was from Shelby County, Tennessee, from 1947 to 1968 (Table 132.1)[1]. This was a study by Medsger and Masi that looked at patients admitted to hospital with scleroderma. The investigators found rates of 0.6–1.5 new cases per year per million population in the first 10 years, which increased to 4.5 new cases in the 1958–1968 time period. Steen et al.[2],

TABLE 132.1 INCIDENCE AND PREVALENCE OF SYSTEMIC SCLEROSIS

Author	Country	Year	Incidence rate (per million)	Prevalence rate (per million)
Medsger and Masi[1]	Tennessee (USA)	1947–54	0.6	4
		1953–58	1.5	7
		1958–62	4.1	21
		1963–68	4.5	28
Steen et al.[2]	Allegheny County (USA)	1963–72	9.6	
		1973–82	18.7	
Michet et al.[3]	Minnesota	1950–79	13.0	253
Mayes[4]	Detroit	1989–91	18.7	242
Maricq et al.[5]	South Carolina	1985		286 (point prevalence)
Bosmansky and Zitnan[6]	Czechoslovakia	1961–69	7.0	
Silman et al.[7]	England	1980–85	3.7	30.7
Tamaki et al.[8]	Japan	1988		38
Asboe-Hansen[9]	Denmark	1977–79		126
Haustein and Anderegg[10]	Germany	1980–81		100
	Iceland	1975–90	3.8	71
Englert et al.[11]	Austalia (Sydney)	1974–88		45–86
Chandran et al.[12]	Australia (Adelaide)	1993		208 (point prevalence)
Valter et al.[13]	Estonia	1997		2280
Eason et al.[14]	New Zealand	1970–79	6.3	
Arnett et al.[15]	Chocktaw Indians	1990–94		4690

using similar techniques, performed a hospital-based study in Allegheny County in Pennsylvania from 1963 to 1982. In the period during which the years of these studies overlapped, the rates of incidence of systemic sclerosis were similar in Tennessee and Pennsylvania. Over the following 10 years, they increased to 19 new cases per year per million population. Improved diagnosis and recognition were felt to account for most of this increase. However, unlike the women in the study, the men did not show an increase in incidence of the disease. This could mean that at least part of the increase was real. Michet et al.[3] found a similar incidence of 13.0 per million for the years 1950–1979 in Rochester, Minnesota, which already had an excellent record-keeping of disease diagnoses in the community. In a population-based study in Detroit, Michigan, Mayes[16] found a very similar incidence of scleroderma: 18.7 per million, compared with the 19.1 per million value in Allegheny County, even though it was 10 years later.

Prevalence rates are dependent on patient diagnosis and survival: earlier diagnosis and improved survival will increase prevalence. Medsger and Masi's[1] low prevalence calculations in the early time periods of their study may reflect that later diagnosis and earlier death were common in their patients. However, others have reported similar prevalences of around 150 patients per million population. In 1985, Maricq et al.[5] performed the only true community-based survey, using a multiphase survey for the diagnosis of Raynaud's disease in 7000 people randomly selected in South Carolina. Although there were only two definite cases of scleroderma and the investigators used a number of assumptions about people who were not seen, they were still able to calculate that the prevalence of scleroderma patients was 286 patients per million population in South Carolina. The findings of Michet et al.[3] at the Mayo Clinic were similar: 253 prevalent cases per million population. The incidence and prevalence of systemic sclerosis thus seem to have some geographical variation, but there does not appear to be a difference between cold and warm climates within the USA. The greatest prevalence in the USA is among the Choctaw Native American tribe, which will be discussed below.

International studies generally show a decreased incidence and prevalence compared with those reported in studies from the USA (Table 132.1). England[7] and Japan[8] have a significantly lower incidence than Denmark[9] and Germany[10]. The incidence in England[7] was only 3.7 per million population, compared with 10–19 in the USA[2]. The investigators in Iceland[10] found a similar incidence of systemic sclerosis of 3.8 per million, but the prevalence was considerably increased compared with that in England, at 71 per million population. In the mid-1980s, studies in England[7] showed a prevalence of only 30 patients per million population, in contrast to the 150–250 per million in the studies in USA. The Japanese estimate of 7 per million was even smaller[8]. The prevalence of scleroderma was determined in two studies from Australia[11,12]. Techniques and outcomes were quite different. In Sydney, a very thorough search for patients from a variety of hospitals and outpatient physicians, including dermatologists and vascular surgeons, led to identification of 715 cases, which was calculated to be a prevalence of 45–86 per million population in the period 1975–1988[11]. In Adelaide, using primarily outpatient and discharge diagnostic codes from five teaching hospitals, the investigators found 215 cases and calculated a point prevalence of 2080 per million population[12], which is significantly more than that found in Sydney. The study that has provided the greatest amount of data on prevalence was another prospective study, in Estonia[13]. The estimate of the prevalence of disorders in the scleroderma spectrum, based on 13 cases, was 2280 per million population, close to 10 times more than seen in the USA. Although the definition of scleroderma spectrum disorders may have been broader in that study than is commonly used for scleroderma, this does not completely account for the large differences between the Estonia and others countries.

AGE, SEX AND RACIAL FACTORS

Like other connective tissue diseases, systemic sclerosis is also predominant in females: 3–5:1 most commonly, but as high as 14:1 in some populations. The female:male ratio is greatest in the childbearing years, although it is not as dramatic as in systemic lupus erythematosus. Scleroderma in children in general is infrequent but, when present, is also more frequent in girls than boys. In the postmenopausal age range, the female:male ratio is at its lowest, 2.4:1.

Age of onset of scleroderma is most commonly in the range 30–50 years. The mean ages of onset in white men and women are 44 and 42 years. This is similar in patients in both of the two major subsets of scleroderma, limited cutaneous and diffuse cutaneous, although patients with limited scleroderma are not usually diagnosed until 5–10 years later. Systemic sclerosis (as opposed to localized or linear scleroderma) is quite uncommon in children younger than 13 years. One estimate of the incidence of scleroderma in children is 0.1 cases per million population[17]. In comparison with adults, childhood systemic sclerosis is associated with less renal crisis, but more cardiopulmonary problems.

Both male and female African-Americans have an earlier age of disease onset than whites, with a peak in the third decade[2] (Fig. 132.1). The mean ages of onset among African-American men and women are 41 and 38 years, respectively. Female predominance is also present in African-Americans. Elderly African-American males with scleroderma are quite uncommon. The incidence of systemic sclerosis may be slightly greater in African-Americans than in whites. Medsger and Masi[1] showed that the prevalence rate among African-American females was 4.3 per million population, but that in whites was 3.6 (in females); the disparity was even greater in African-American male army veterans: 7.1, compared with 1.9 in whites. Although the overall incidence of scleroderma in African-Americans in the Allegheny County study was not much different than that in whites, African-American females in their 20s had a 10-fold increase[2]. Indeed, in that study there was an increase in the incidence among African-American men and women in several age groups (Fig. 132.1): a two- to threefold increase was present in the 45–55 years age group in African-American women compared to white women, and the overall incidence among African-American men was 9.6 per million, compared with 6.8 in white men, with most of the increase in African-Americans being in the 35–55 years age range.

As with other connective tissue diseases, systemic sclerosis is believed to be more severe in African-Americans. However, the increased severity

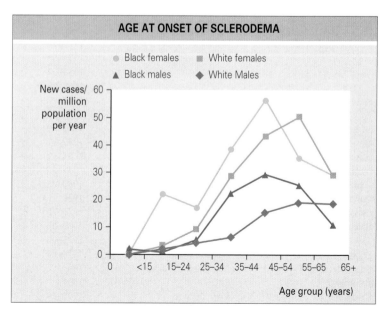

Fig. 132.1 Age at onset of scleroderma. Age at onset of disease among black and white populations in Pennsylvania.

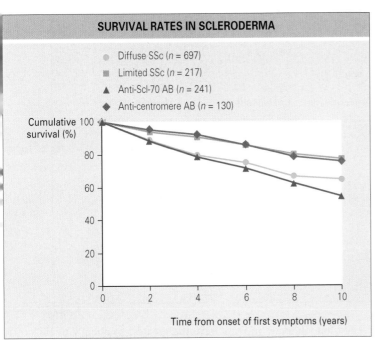

SURVIVAL RATES IN SCLERODERMA

- Diffuse SSc (*n* = 697)
- Limited SSc (*n* = 217)
- Anti-Scl-70 AB (*n* = 241)
- Anti-centromere AB (*n* = 130)

Fig. 132.2 Survival rates in scleroderma. Cumulative survival rates for diffuse and limited systemic sclerosis (SSc) and among those with anti-Scl-70 or anticentromere antibodies (AB).

in scleroderma may be a reflection of the disease subtype, rather than related to socioeconomic factors. Anti-Scl-70 antibody and anti-U3-RNP antibodies are associated with more severe disease and are seen more frequently in African-Americans than is anticentromere antibody, which is associated with milder disease in whites. This may be a major factor contributing to the overall decreased survival of African-American patients with scleroderma (Fig. 132.2). The clinical features of black African patients with scleroderma were very similar to those of African-Americans[18]. Interestingly, there have been no cases reported in Aborigines in Australia, and no formal study has been undertaken in this population.

SCLERODERMA CLASSIFICATION AND SUBSETS

The epidemiology and natural history of scleroderma revolve around the two major scleroderma subsets. The American Rheumatism Association (or now American College of Rheumatology) criteria for the classification (not diagnosis) of scleroderma were established in 1980 and were based on the findings of a large study using patients with primary Raynaud's syndrome or systemic lupus erythematosus as controls[19]. The major criterion is skin thickening proximal to the metacarpophalangeal joints; minor criteria (two of the three minor criteria are required) include sclerodactyly, digital pitting scars and bibasilar pulmonary fibrosis. Patients had to have had symptoms for less than 2 years; this resulted in a smaller number of patients with limited scleroderma, because the early diagnosis of limited scleroderma is infrequent. The criteria were only 69% sensitive for patients with limited scleroderma, because of relatively small numbers of patients in this subgroup.

The CREST syndrome (**c**alcinosis, **R**aynaud's syndrome, **e**sophageal dysmotility, **s**clerodactyly and **t**elangiectasias[20]) was described long ago, and these patients were considered to have an entity distinct from systemic sclerosis. Over the years, there has been controversy and confusion about the use of this term, in that it was used literally, often excluding patients who did not have all five features. Also, patients with long-standing diffuse scleroderma develop many of these features, and were often inappropriately given the diagnosis of CREST. Thus the separation of these patients into two clinically distinct subsets was blurred. With the identification of the scleroderma-specific autoantibodies, particularly anticentromere and antitopoisomerase, it was possible to define further that there were two clinically distinct subsets associated with these antibodies. In 1988, a group of senior scleroderma investigators wrote an editorial describing definitions of these two subsets that were clinically the most meaningful[21]. Patients with limited cutaneous scleroderma have skin thickening limited to the distal extremities and face (Table 132.2). They do not necessarily have all the features of CREST syndrome, although many of them do. The most important features that differentiate these patients from those with diffuse cutaneous scleroderma are the extent of skin thickening and the pace of their disease. The disease onset in patients with limited scleroderma is usually with Raynaud's phenomenon, which is present alone for years before any other manifestations occur; at some time, possibly 5–10 years later, they develop puffy, swollen fingers, digital tip ulcers, telangiectasias or esophageal symptoms that result in the diagnosis of limited scleroderma. In contrast, patients with diffuse cutaneous disease have a much more acute onset of symptoms including Raynaud's phenomenon, swollen hands and legs, carpal tunnel syndrome, arthralgia/arthritis and fatigue, all occurring in a short span of time. Diagnosis of diffuse scleroderma occurs usually after skin thickening becomes evident, 1–12 months after the onset of other symptoms. The pattern of organ system involvement is also different. Both forms commonly have the same type of gastrointestinal disease; interstitial fibrosis occurs in both, but is primarily

TABLE 132.2 CLINICAL DIFFERENCES BETWEEN THE LIMITED AND DIFFUSE CUTANEOUS SCLERODERMA SUBSETS OF SYSTEMIC SCLEROSIS	
Limited scleroderma	**Diffuse scleroderma**
Long duration of Raynaud's phenomenon	Short duration of Raynaud's, often delayed after other symptoms
Puffy fingers, intermittent to persistent	Swollen hands and legs
Mild arthralgias, fatigue, no tendon friction rubs	Acute onset of fatigue, severe arthralgias, carpal tunnel symptoms and tendon friction rubs
Skin thickening late, limited to hands and face	Skin thickening early, moves up extremities and on trunk
Telangiectasias and calcinosis common	Telangiectasias and calcinosis may occur late in disease
Digital tip ischemia	Ischemia of digital tips and dorsum of proximal interphalangeal joints
Esophageal scleroderma	Esophageal scleroderma, some severe intestinal problems
Occasional pulmonary fibrosis	Severe pulmonary fibrosis
Severe pulmonary hypertension	Cardiomyopathy or arrythmias
	Renal crisis
Anticentromere antibodies	Anti-Scl-70
	Anti-RNA-polymerase III

TABLE 132.3 FEATURES SIGNIFICANTLY ASSOCIATED WITH SCLERODERMA-SPECIFIC AUTOANTIBODIES

ACA	Th/To	Pm/Scl	U1-RNP	U3-RNP	RNA pol 3	Scl-70
Fewer males			Younger	Black, young		
Limited	Limited	Limited	Limited	Diffuse	Diffuse	Diffuse
Fewer joints	Fewer joints	Muscles	Muscles, joints	Less inflamed muscle	Tendon rubs less muscle	Tendon rubs
Calcinosis		Calcinosis				
Tuft resorption		Tuft resorption			Less tuft resorption	Tuft resorption
Digital ulcers		Digital ulcers		Digital ulcers		Digital ulcers
	Less GI	Less GI	Less GI			
			Pulmonary fibrosis	Pulmonary fibrosis	Less pulmonary fibrosis	Pulmonary fibrosis
Isolated PHT	Isolated PHT		Isolated PHT	Isolated PHT		
			Heart	Heart		Heart
				Kidney	Kidney	Kidney
5 year CSR 86%	5 year CSR 65%	5 year CSR 92%	5 year CSR 95%	5 year CSR 77%	5 year CSR 90%	5 year CSR 80%

ACA, anticentromere antibody; CSR, cumulative survival rate from diagnosis of scleroderma; GI, gastrointestinal involvement; PHT, pulmonary hypertension; Pm/Scl, Th/To, U3-RNP nucleolar antibodies; RNA pol 3, anti-RNA polymerase III; Scl-70, anti-Scl-70 or topoisomerase.

related to the anti-Scl-70 antibody. Isolated pulmonary hypertension occurs more prominently in limited scleroderma, whereas renal crisis and cardiac disease occur predominately in diffuse scleroderma.

Scleroderma autoantibodies have been shown to be associated with specific patterns of disease consistent with these two major subsets (Table 132.3). Classically, the anticentromere antibody is seen almost exclusively in patients with limited scleroderma, with a greater frequency in women; it is rarely seen in African-Americans. It is seen in 30–90% of patients with limited scleroderma, depending on the definition of limited scleroderma that is applied[22,23]. Antitopoisomerase (or anti-Scl-70) is the other scleroderma antibody for which tests are commercially available. It is associated with classic diffuse scleroderma. However, about 25% of these patients do not have extensive skin, heart or kidney problems, and their disease follows a course similar to that of limited scleroderma. This antibody is seen more frequently in African-Americans. In addition to its association with diffuse cutaneous disease, it is associated with more pulmonary interstitial fibrosis and more vascular problems. However, these patients seem to be protected from the isolated, vasculopathy type of pulmonary hypertension. Frequent cardiac involvement and renal crisis also affect survival in these patients. It is interesting to note that, for unclear reasons, this antibody was seen in low frequencies in both white individuals and African-Americans in a study carried out in Michigan[24]: 18% in both groups. In contrast,

Oklahoma Choctaw Indians have the greatest frequency of this antibody[25].

Anti-RNA polymerase III is another commonly seen scleroderma-specific antibody, which is found almost exclusively in diffuse scleroderma (28%), but assays are not yet commercially available. Patients with this antibody often have very extensive amounts of skin thickening and they have the greatest frequency of renal crisis (25%)[23]. Severe pulmonary fibrosis is uncommon, and the survival of these patients is actually better than that of those with anti-Scl-70, probably because renal crisis is now a more treatable problem than is pulmonary fibrosis.

A nucleolar pattern of antinuclear antibodies is very specific to scleroderma, and three different specific antibodies have been identified. Individually they are not very common, and assays for two are not yet commercially available; however, from an epidemiologic standpoint they are important. One of them, anti-U3-RNP or antifibrillarin, is the most frequent antibody seen in African-Americans. In one study, its frequency in African-American patients with scleroderma was 16%, compared with 5% in whites[26]. It is associated with diffuse cutaneous disease, pulmonary fibrosis and isolated pulmonary hypertension. The other nucleolar antibodies, anti-Th/To and anti-Pm/Scl, are more frequent in white patients with limited scleroderma. Pulmonary hypertension and myositis, respectively, are common features in patients with these anti-

TABLE 132.4 FREQUENCY OF SCLERODERMA AUTOANTIBODIES IN DIFFERENT COUNTRIES

Country	Frequency of limited and diffuse		Frequency of ACA and Scl-70	
	Limited	Diffuse	ACA	Scl-70
USA[22]	50	50	22	26
African-Americans[24]	30	70	14	18.4
Whites[24]	69	31	35	18.6
African-Americans[28]	–	–	4	37
Whites[28]	–	–	36	17
Choctaw Indians[15]	8	92	–	83
Australia[29]				
White Australians	85	15	51	26
Non-white Thais	0	100	2	76
South Africa (blacks)[18]	29	65	0	–
Denmark[30]	–	–	36	14
Italy[31]	90	10	–	–
Greece[32]	49	45	34	34

ACA, anticentromere antibody; anti-Scl-70 or topoisomerase.

bodies. Lastly, anti-U1-RNP antibody, which is the autoantibody associated with the overlap disease, mixed connective tissue disease, is seen with increased frequency in African-Americans with scleroderma and has its own unique constellation of findings.

The most recently described scleroderma-specific autoantibody is an autoantibody to fibrillin-1, a major structural glycoprotein of connective tissue microfibrils. Antifibrillin-1 antibody is seen in high frequencies in Choctaw Indians and Japanese patients, but less commonly in whites and is infrequent in African-Americans[27]. In contrast to other scleroderma-associated autoantibodies, human leukocyte antigen (HLA) class II alleles are not associated with antifibrillin-1 antibodies in patients with scleroderma and, unlike the other scleroderma antibodies, antifibrillin-1 antibodies have no clinical associations.

The etiology of these autoantibodies is not clear. They have not been shown to be pathogenic, but clearly appear to be markers of specific forms of the disease. In general, they are almost always present at the time of first physician evaluation, and rarely disappear. They could be present for years before the onset of symptoms. One possibility is that they represent the body's reaction to different triggers of the disease, perhaps environmental or occupational. However, the varying frequencies of the different antibodies in different countries suggest that ethnicity and genetics are likely to play a larger part. Table 132.4 summarizes the different frequencies of these autoantibodies that are seen in different countries. In general, countries that have a large number of patients with limited scleroderma have a high frequency of anticentromere antibody. This strongly suggests that the antibodies are directly related to the subset of patients, and thus may play a larger part in the pathogenesis than do other factors.

GENETIC FACTORS

Genetic factors have been suggested to have a possible pathogenic role in scleroderma. There have been suggestions that chromosomal breakage rates are greater in patients with scleroderma. This would support the toxic agent theory, but adequate supporting data have not been obtained. More recent data have been based on assessment of variable number tandem repeats, a technique that can show chromosomal abnormalities[33]. The investigators in that study found increased variable number tandem repeat mutations in patients with scleroderma and their offspring compared with a small control group. These mutations did not correlate with a disease subtype or antibodies. The etiology of these alterations is unknown. Another area of a potential pathogenic relationship is the theory of microchimerism, in which the hypothesis is that patients have a reaction to fetal cells from an early pregnancy or from their parents (in order to account for the occurrence in males and nulliparous females)[34], after which the patients develop a graft versus host-like reaction that results in scleroderma. Although the supporting data for this are reasonable, there does not seem to be any relationship with scleroderma subtypes and autoantibodies. Furthermore, although scleroderma is similar to graft versus host disease in some ways, there are primary differences that make it difficult to use this theory as a primary cause of scleroderma.

Early studies of the major histocompatability complex alleles in scleroderma were not correlated with any particular disease pattern. This may have been because of ethnic variability in geographic areas, but most likely because the patients studied had too much clinical heterogeneity. With increasing sophistication of genetic studies, an even greater variety of findings have been seen[35]. A 1987 study showed that C4A-null alleles had the greatest association. DQA2 is associated, and probably represents the old DR3 association. Comparing UK and US findings, it seems that American patients have less frequent B8, DR3 and DQ2 haplotypes. Conversely, the work of Reveille et al.[36] suggests that DQ7 and DQ5 are more common. These are just a few of the many associations, and it

almost appears that these findings are different in every patient group studied. Early on, it was shown that patients with limited scleroderma and anticentromere antibodies were associated with HLA-DR-1, and diffuse scleroderma and antitopoisomerase antibody were associated with HLA-DR-5[22]. Antitopoisomerase antibody is now also associated with DR-2, but these are in linkage disequilibrium with other areas. In an important study, Kuwana et al.[25] studied these autoantibody associations in African-American, white and Japanese populations. HLA-DRB1 alleles differed in Japanese and American Indian patients compared with the others. The findings for anticentromere antibody were only slightly less complex. Although not studied as frequently, anti-U3-RNP has been shown to be associated with alleles HLA-DRB1 and DQB1[26]. Antipolymerase III antibody has also been associated with specific markers[23]. As the genetic analyses have become more complex, even the autoantibody associations that seemed to be the most meaningful have become less clear.

One of the most exciting findings has been the identification of an extremely high prevalence of systemic sclerosis in the Choctaw Native Americans from Oklahoma. The prevalence was calculated to be 4690 per million population, compared to 150 per million population in the remainder of the USA[37]. There was a striking clinical homogeneity among these patients, who had diffuse scleroderma, anti-Scl 70 antibodies and pulmonary fibrosis. The strongest genetic associations in these patients were the haplotypes – HLA-B35, Cw4, DRB181602, DQA1, and DQB1. Interestingly, a Choctaw tribe in another state had the identical associations, but did not have an increased prevalence of scleroderma. Recently, the investigators were able to identify a candidate gene that was different in the two tribes. These studies implicate a 2-cM haplotype, containing the fibrillin 1 gene on chromosome 15, in conferring increased susceptibility to systemic sclerosis[38]. Autoantibodies to fibrillin-1 are commonly seen in patients with scleroderma. African-Americans, Japanese and Choctaw Indians have greater concentrations than do white populations. However, there was no clinical correlation with any scleroderma subsets, antibodies or organ system involvement[27]. Additional studies will focus on what part this gene plays in the pathogenesis of scleroderma. Additionally, advanced techniques have led to the finding that the fibrillin-1 gene is also associated with the tight skin mouse model of scleroderma[39].

Family studies have not shown that there are an excessive number of first-degree relatives who have scleroderma. However, although only 1.6% of patients have a first-degree relative with scleroderma, having a first-degree relative with scleroderma is the strongest risk factor for the disease. The absolute risk factor for an individual family member remains low, at less than 1%[40,41]. Recent twin studies did not show an increase in the disease in identical twins compared with fraternal twins, although positivity for antinuclear antibody was seen more frequently in the identical twins[42]. Previous studies have shown an increased frequency of both antinuclear antibodies and any autoimmune disease in family members of patients with scleroderma.

SURVIVAL

Survival studies in scleroderma are almost as varied as the genetic associations. The patient demographics, clinical subsets and organ system involvement, in addition to the use of different starting times, such as first symptom, diagnosis or first visit, are all important features that lead to difficulty in comparing findings between studies. Most studies agree that old age, male sex, poor socioeconomical status, scleroderma subtype and specific organ involvement all are associated with a decreased survival. Other features, including sedimentation rate and anemia, have been shown to affect survival. Studies have shown that the presence of any major organ involvement is associated with a decreased survival[43,44], but a recent study showed that the decreased survival was primarily associated with severe organ involvement of skin, lung, gastro-intestinal tract, heart and kidney[45]. In patients with severe skin (Rodnan skin score >40), lung (vital capacity <55% predicted), gastrointestinal (malabsorption, pseudo-obstruction), heart (severe arrhythmia or congestive heart failure), or kidney (renal crisis) involvement, the 9-year cumulative survival rate was 38%, whereas in the remainder of the patients, many of whom had mild organ involvement, the survival rate was 72%.

The most dramatic change in survival over time has occurred in those with scleroderma renal crisis. The use of angiotensin-converting enzyme inhibitors is able to control blood pressure, reverse renal failure and, in more than 50% of the cases, avoid or decrease the need for permanent dialysis. The 5-year cumulative survival for patients with scleroderma renal crisis improved from 10% before the advent of angiotensin-converting enzyme inhibitors to 70% after the use of these drugs. In the past 10 years, the patients with renal crisis not requiring dialysis and those who only needed temporary dialysis had a 5-year cumulative survival rate equivalent to that of those patients with diffuse scleroderma who did not have renal crisis: namely, 90% of predicted. Additionally, there was significant improvement in survival, independent of the improved treatment of renal crisis, between the 1970s decade and the 1980s decade[46].

African-Americans have been felt by many to have a decreased survival, because of socioeconomic status[43,44]. However, there is some controversy as to what are the most important risk factors for survival in scleroderma, and particularly in African-Americans. It is possible that autoantibodies are the primary predictors of survival. African-Americans may have a bad outcome because their ethnic and genetic features make them more likely to have high frequencies of anti-Scl-70 and U3-RNP antibodies. These antibodies are associated with bad disease in both races, but are seen more frequently in African-Americans.

In a study from England, a model was developed that was highly predictive of the 5-year survival[47]. Using logistic regression, the investigators identified that proteinuria, an increased sedimentation rate and the presence of antitopoisomerase antibody had a greater than 80% accuracy in predicting mortality.

Worldwide survival studies have recently been carried out in Canada, Hungary, Spain, England, Japan, Denmark, Sweden, Australia, Italy and Greece, and they have similar findings[35]. The variations between these studies primarily relate to the proportions of patients with limited and diffuse scleroderma and the frequency of anticentromere and anti-Scl-70 antibodies.

OCCUPATIONAL AND ENVIRONMENTAL RISK FACTORS

Genetic factors are believed to have some role in the development of systemic sclerosis but, unlike their influence in some of the rheumatic diseases, they do not appear to be the primary factor in scleroderma. There have been occasional clusters of the disease such as that reported by Silman et al.[35], who found a prevalence rate of 150 per million around airports, which was significantly greater than that seen in other areas of England. There have been other clusters in Italy, Detroit and Louisiana, but the most well described is that seen in the Choctaw Indians of Oklahoma, as discussed above. It appears in that last case that genetics is the primary factor that explains the increased prevalence.

Throughout the years, there have been descriptions of relationships of certain environmental or occupational toxins with the development of scleroderma-like illness[48] (Table 132.5). However, one of the oldest associations is that of silica with systemic sclerosis. In 1914, Bramwell[49] reported the occurrence of diffuse scleroderma in stone masons; later, Eramus[50] found a similar increase among gold miners in South Africa, and Rodnan et al.[51] found an increase in scleroderma in the coal miners of Pennsylvania. However, all these studies have some methodological problems, bringing doubts to the findings. In East Germany, there are reports that the relative risk for developing scleroderma is 74%, but others have questioned that figure because of the concern that the use of vibration machines in the uranium mines results in Raynaud's syndrome, which, together with the silica interstitial lung disease, looks like scleroderma. However, in West Germany the frequency of definite scleroderma is 16% in silica-exposed patients[48]. Haustein and Anderegg[10] remain completely convinced that, at least in their area, silica is a definitive causative factor. The silica-induced scleroderma is not a unique entity, and is identical to systemic sclerosis in every way. There does not seem to be any specific associations with disease subtype, autoantibody, duration of exposure or the presence of lung silicosis. There is a lack of any silica exposure in the vast majority of patients. Recent studies from other parts of the world have not been able to confirm that silica plays a definite part in the development of scleroderma.

It has been well established that polyvinyl chloride causes a scleroderma-like illness, but there are no studies that link this compound to more typical systemic sclerosis[48]. Similarly, there are a variety of other chemicals, particularly in the organic solvent family, that have been reported in case reports to cause scleroderm-like illnesses. Nietert et al.[52] showed an increased odds ratio for occupational exposure to trichloroethylene in men with anti-Scl-70 antibody, a fairly small

TABLE 132.5 EXPOSURES THAT HAVE BEEN ASSOCIATED WITH SCLERODERMA-LIKE OR SCLERODERMA ILLNESSES

Study type	Exposure	Type of scleroderma
Cohort studies	Polyvinylchloride (PVC)	Scleroderma-like illness definitely caused by PVC
Individual case reports	*Organic solvents*: trichloroethylene, toluene, polyethylene, hydrocarbons, epoxy resins, etc. *Drugs*: appetite suppressants, carbidopa, bleomycin, pentazocine, cocaine	Individual scleroderma cases, but also many scleroderma like illnesses Individual scleroderma cases
Case–control studies	Silica (in Germany)	Typical scleroderma in every way, supported but not confirmed by studies
Case–control epidemiology studies	Multiple compounds including solvent, silica, implants	No associations with scleroderma except trichloroethylene with Scl-70 positive men
Several cases	Silicone breast implants Toxic oil syndrome, eosinophilic myalgia syndrome (L-tryptophan)	Typical scleroderma, no definite associations Classic scleroderma-like illness definitely caused by these agents

subset of patients. Similar findings were found for the association of anti-Scl-70 antibody with exposure to organic solvents used in hobbies[53].

Drugs have also been reported to be associated with the development of scleroderma, including appetite suppressants, L-5-hydroxy tryptophan, bleomycin, pentazocine and cocaine. However, even if these associations prove to be real, they will only be able to account for a very small number of patients.

Most recently, there has been much controversy as to whether silicone breast implants caused scleroderma. The original article from Japan in the late 1980s suggested that there were a large number of women with implants who developed scleroderma[54]. Since these earliest reports, there have been numerous epidemiological reports, cohort studies, case-control studies and meta-analyses of all the studies[55]. Their conclusion was that there was no significant association of silicon breast implants with systemic sclerosis. These findings were also found by a panel of experts looking at the issues for a Class Action Suit in Alabama and by the Institute of Medicine.

INSTRUMENTS FOR MONITORING DISEASE STATUS

Systemic sclerosis is a multisystem connective tissue disease that affects a wide variety of organs with varying degrees of severity. It is quite difficult to make comparisons between patients, because almost no one patient has similar features to another patient. Measurement of specific organ systems has been the primary means of monitoring these patients. The most frequent of these measurements is the skin score, a semiquantitative measure of the extent and severity of skin thickness. A standardized method of scoring skin thickening, fashioned after Dr Gerald Rodnan's method, the modified Rodnan Skin Score, has been validated both within and between investigators, and is the primary measurement used in clinical trials[56]. A recent study has shown that patients who experience a significant improvement in skin score also have a significant improvement in survival, thus allowing the skin score to be a surrogate for survival[57]. The status of other organs, including lung, heart and kidney, can be monitored reasonably easily by pulmonary function tests, echocardiogram and serum creatinine and blood pressure, but the gastrointestinal tract is much more difficult to evaluate.

The Health Assessment Questionnaire (HAQ) has been used in most of the rheumatic diseases, although most frequently for rheumatoid arthritis. It has been found to be very helpful in documenting changes in disease function over time. This instrument, and several scleroderma-specific visual analog scales, have been validated in scleroderma and collectively termed the Scleroderma HAQ[58]. They definitely correlate with the extent and severity of skin involvement and disability, and the severity with which patients are affected in other organs. This scleroderma-specific HAQ is being used successfully in clinical trials in scleroderma.

For many years, clinical trial and other studies have evaluated and used a variety of instruments to measure disease activity in systemic lupus erythematosus. However, it has been quite difficult to define the 'activity' in scleroderma. A European group is making a valiant attempt to develop a disease activity instrument that can be generally used[59]. Ideally, the use of a self-administered instrument would make disease monitoring more practical but, to date, this has not been established. A disease severity index, which is a set of scales measuring differing degrees of severity of eight different organ systems, has recently been carefully validated[60]. It remains to be seen whether this will become useful in clinical trials or other studies.

REFERENCES

1. Medsger TA Jr, Masi AT. Epidemiology of systemic sclerosis (scleroderma). Ann Intern Med 1971; 74: 714–721.
2. Steen VD, Oddis CV, Conte CG et al. Incidence of systemic sclerosis in Allegheny County, Pennsylvania. A twenty-year study of hospital-diagnosed cases, 1963–1982. Arthritis Rheum 1997; 40: 441–445.
3. Michet CJ Jr, McKenna CH, Elveback LR et al. Epidemiology of systemic lupus erythematosus and other connective tissue diseases in Rochester, Minnesota, 1950 through 1979. Mayo Clin Proc 1985; 60: 105–113.
4. Mayes MD. Classification and epidemiology of scleroderma. Semin Cutan Med Surg 1998; 17: 22–26.
5. Maricq HR, Weinrich MC, Keil JE et al. Prevalence of scleroderma spectrum disorders in the general population of South Carolina. Arthritis Rheum 1989; 32: 998–1006.
6. Bosmansky K, Zitnan D. Screening of collagen diseases in the years 1961–1972 from a selected population sample [in German]. Z Gesamte Inn Med 1976; 31: 979–981.
7. Silman A, Jannini S, Symmons D, Bacon P. An epidemiological study of scleroderma in the West Midlands. Br J Rheumatol 1988; 27: 286–290.
8. Tamaki T, Mori S, Takehara K. Epidemiological study of patients with systemic sclerosis in Tokyo. Arch Dermatol Res 1991; 283: 366–371.
9. Asboe-Hansen G. Scleroderma. J Am Acad Dermatol 1987; 17: 102–108.
10. Haustein UF, Anderegg U. Silica-induced scleroderma – clinical and experimental aspects. J Rheumatol 1998; 25: 1917–1926.
11. Englert H, Small-McMahon J, Davis K et al. Systemic sclerosis prevalence and mortality in Sydney 1974–88. Aust N Z J Med 1999; 29: 42–50.
12. Chandran G, Smith M, Ahern MJ, Roberts-Thomson PJ. A study of scleroderma in South Australia: prevalence, subset characteristics and nailfold capillaroscopy. Aust N Z J Med 1995; 25: 688–694.
13. Valter I, Saretok S, Maricq HR. Prevalence of scleroderma spectrum disorders in the general population of Estonia. Scand J Rheumatol 1997; 26: 419–425.
14. Eason RJ, Tan PL, Gow PJ. Progressive systemic sclerosis in Auckland: a ten year review with emphasis on prognostic features. Aust N Z J Med 1981; 11: 657–662.
15. Arnett FC, Howard RF, Tan F et al. Increased prevalence of systemic sclerosis in a Native American tribe in Oklahoma. Association with an Amerindian HLA haplotype. Arthritis Rheum 1996; 39: 1362–1370.
16. Mayes MD. Scleroderma epidemiology. Rheum Dis Clin North Am 1996; 22: 751–764.
17. Fujikawa S, Okuni M. A nationwide surveillance study of rheumatic diseases among Japanese children. Acta Paediatr Jpn 1997; 39: 242–244.
18. Tager RE, Tikly M. Clinical and laboratory manifestations of systemic sclerosis (scleroderma) in Black South Africans [see comments]. Rheumatology (Oxford) 1999; 38: 397–400.
19. Masi AT, Rodman G, Medsger T et al. Preliminary criteria for the classification of systemic sclerosis (scleroderma). Arthritis Rheum 1980; 23: 581–590.
20. Velayos EE, Masi AT, Stevens MB, Shulman LE. The 'CREST' syndrome. Comparison with systemic sclerosis (scleroderma). Arch Intern Med 1979; 139: 1240–1244.
21. Leroy EC, Black C, Fleischmajer R et al. Scleroderma (systemic sclerosis): classification, subsets and pathogenesis. J Rheumatol 1988; 15: 202–205.
22. Steen VD, Powell DL, Medsger TA Jr. Clinical correlations and prognosis based on serum autoantibodies in patients with systemic sclerosis. Arthritis Rheum 1988; 31: 196–203.
23. Okano Y. Antinuclear antibody in systemic sclerosis (scleroderma). Rheum Dis Clin North Am 1996; 22: 709–735.
24. Laing TJ, Gillespie BW, Toth MB et al. Racial differences in scleroderma among women in Michigan. Arthritis Rheum 1997; 40: 734–742.
25. Kuwana M, Kaburaki J, Arnett FC et al. Influence of ethnic background on clinical and serologic features in patients with systemic sclerosis and anti-DNA topoisomerase I antibody. Arthritis Rheum 1999; 42: 465–474.
26. Arnett FC, Reveille JD, Goldstein R et al. Autoantibodies to fibrillarin in systemic sclerosis (scleroderma). An immunogenetic, serologic, and clinical analysis. Arthritis Rheum 1996; 39: 1151–1160.
27. Tan FK, Arnett FC, Reveille JD et al. Autoantibodies to fibrillin 1 in systemic sclerosis: ethnic differences in antigen recognition and lack of correlation with specific clinical features or HLA alleles [in process citation]. Arthritis Rheum 2000; 43: 2464–2471.
28. Reveille JD, Durban E, Goldstein R et al. Racial differences in the frequencies of scleroderma-related autoantibodies [see comments]. Arthritis Rheum 1992; 35: 216–218.
29. McNeilage LJ, Youngchaiyud U, Whittingham S. Racial differences in antinuclear antibody patterns and clinical manifestations of scleroderma. Arthritis Rheum 1989; 32: 54–60.
30. Jacobsen S, Halberg P, Ullman S et al. Clinical features and serum antinuclear antibodies in 230 Danish patients with systemic sclerosis. Br J Rheumatol 1998; 37: 39–45.
31. Ferri C, Valentini G, Cozzi F et al. Systemic sclerosis: demographic, clinical, and serologic features and survival in 1,012 Italian patients. Medicine (Baltimore) 2002; 81: 139–153.
32. Vlachoyiannopoulos PG, Dafni UG, Pakas I et al. Systemic scleroderma in Greece: low mortality and strong linkage with HLA-DRB1*1104 allele. Ann Rheum Dis 2000; 59: 359–367.
33. Artlett CM, Black CM, Briggs DC et al. DNA allelic alterations within VNTR loci of scleroderma families. Br J Rheumatol 1996; 35: 1216–1222.
34. Evans PC, Lambert N, Maloney S et al. Long-term fetal microchimerism in peripheral blood mononuclear cell subsets in healthy women and women with scleroderma. Blood 1999; 93: 2033–2037.
35. Silman A, Black C, Welsh K. Epidemiology, demographics, genetics. In: Clements P, Furst D, eds. Systemic sclerosis. Baltimore: Williams &Wilkins; 1996: 23–49.

36. Reveille JD, Durban E, MacLeod-St Clair MJ et al. Association of amino acid sequences in the HLA-DQB1 first domain with antitopoisomerase I autoantibody response in scleroderma (progressive systemic sclerosis). J Clin Invest 1992; 90: 973–980.

37. Arnett FC, Howard RF, Tan F et al. Increased prevalence of systemic sclerosis in a Native American tribe in Oklahoma. Association with an Amerindian HLA haplotype. Arthritis Rheum 1996; 39: 1362–1370.

38. Tan FK, Stivers DN, Foster MW et al. Association of microsatellite markers near the fibrillin 1 gene on human chromosome 15q with scleroderma in a Native American population. Arthritis Rheum 1998; 41: 1729–1737.

39. Saito S, Nishimura H, Brumeanu TD et al. Characterization of mutated protein encoded by partially duplicated fibrillin-1 gene in tight skin (TSK) mice. Mol Immunol 1999; 36: 169–176.

40. Englert H, Small-McMahon J, Chambers P et al. Familial risk estimation in systemic sclerosis. Aust N Z J Med 1999; 29: 36–41.

41. Arnett FC, Cho M, Chatterjee S et al. Familial occurrence frequencies and relative risks for systemic sclerosis (scleroderma) in three United States cohorts. Arthritis Rheum 2001; 44: 1359–1362.

42. Kuwana M, Feghali CA, Medsger TA Jr, Wright TM. Autoreactive T cells to topoisomerase I in monozygotic twins discordant for systemic sclerosis. Arthritis Rheum 2001; 44: 1654–1659.

43. Altman RD, Medsger TA Jr, Bloch DA, Michel BA. Predictors of survival in systemic sclerosis (scleroderma). Arthritis Rheum 1991; 34: 403–413.

44. Medsger TA Jr, Masi AT, Rodnan GP et al. Survival with systemic sclerosis (scleroderma). A life-table analysis of clinical and demographic factors in 309 patients. Ann Intern Med 1971; 75: 369–376.

45. Steen VD, Medsger TA. Severe organ involvement in systemic sclerosis with diffuse scleroderma. Arthritis Rheum 2000; 43: 2437–2444.

46. Steen VD, Medsger TA. The survival of patients with systemic sclerosis. Arthritis Rheum 1999; 43: S192.

47. Bryan C, Knight C, Black CM, Silman AJ. Prediction of five-year survival following presentation with scleroderma: development of a simple model using three disease factors at first visit. Arthritis Rheum 1999; 42: 2660–2665.

48. Steen VD. Occupational scleroderma. Curr Opin Rheumatol 1999; 11: 490–494.

49. Bramwell B. Diffuse scleroderma: its frequency, its occurrence in stone masons, its treatment by fibrolysin – elevations of temperature due to fibrolysin injections. Edinburgh Med J 1914; 12: 387.

50. Erasmus LD. Scleroderma in gold miners on the Witzwaterzrand with particular reference to pulmonary manifestations. S Afr J Lab Clin Med 1957; 3: 209–213.

51. Rodnan GP, Benedek TG, Medsger TA Jr, Cammarata RJ. The association of progressive systemic sclerosis (scleroderma) with coal miners' pneumoconiosis and other forms of silicosis. Ann Intern Med 1967; 66: 323–334.

52. Nietert PJ, Sutherland SE, Silver RM et al. Is occupational organic solvent exposure a risk factor for scleroderma? [published erratum appears in Arthritis Rheum 1998; 41: 1512]. Arthritis Rheum 1998; 41: 1111–1118.

53. Nietert PJ, Sutherland SE, Silver RM et al. Solvent oriented hobbies and the risk of systemic sclerosis. J Rheumatol 1999; 26: 2369–2372.

54. Kumagai Y, Shiokawa Y, Medsger TA Jr, Rodnan GP. Clinical spectrum of connective tissue disease after cosmetic surgery. Observations on eighteen patients and a review of the Japanese literature. Arthritis Rheum 1984; 27: 1–12.

55. Janowsky EC, Kupper LL, Hulka BS. Meta-analyses of the relation between silicone breast implants and the risk of connective-tissue diseases. N Engl J Med 2000; 342: 781–790.

56. Clements PJ, Lachenbruch PA, Seibold JR et al. Skin thickness score in systemic sclerosis: an assessment of interobserver variability in 3 independent studies. J Rheumatol 1993; 20: 1892–1896.

57. Steen VD, Medsger TA. Improvement in skin thickening in diffuse scleroderma is associated with improved survival [abstract]. Arthritis Rheum 1999; 42: S309.

58. Steen VD, Medsger TA Jr. The value of the Health Assessment Questionnaire and special patient-generated scales to demonstrate change in systemic sclerosis patients over time. Arthritis Rheum 1997; 40: 1984–1991.

59. Valentini G, Della RA, Bombardieri S et al. European multicentre study to define disease activity criteria for systemic sclerosis. II. Identification of disease activity variables and development of preliminary activity indexes. Ann Rheum Dis 2001; 60: 592–598.

60. Medsger TA Jr, Silman AJ, Steen VD et al. A disease severity scale for systemic sclerosis: development and testing. J Rheumatol 1999; 26: 2159–2167.

133 Clinical features of systemic sclerosis

Fredrick M Wigley and Laura K Hummers

Definition

- A generalized disorder of connective tissue affecting skin and internal organs
- Characterized by fibrotic arteriosclerosis of peripheral and visceral vasculature
- Variable degrees of extracellular matrix accumulation (mainly collagen) occur in both skin and viscera
- Associated with specific autoantibodies, most notably anticentromere and anti-Scl-70 (antitopoisomerase)
- Various subsets of disease with specific clinical features and variable involvement of internal organs

Clinical features

- Raynaud's phenomenon
- Tightening and thickening of skin (scleroderma)
- Involvement of internal organs, including gastrointestinal tract, lungs, heart and kidneys, accounts for increased morbidity and mortality
- Risk of internal organ involvement strongly linked to extent and progression of skin thickening

HISTORY

Although there is evidence in the writings of Galen and Hippocrates of scleroderma, the first convincing description was in 1753 by Carlo Curzio. He described a 17-year-old patient as having 'extensive tension and hardness of skin all over her body'. Curzio managed the case with bloodletting, warm milk and 'small doses of quicksilver'[1]. However, it was only in the mid-19th century that scleroderma was established as a clinical entity and given its current name[2]. In reviewing the described cases to date, Gintrac, in 1847, ascribed the name *sclerodermie*[1]. Maurice Raynaud described Raynaud's phenomenon in 1865[3] and Jonathan Hutchinson reported a case with Raynaud's phenomenon who had definite features of scleroderma in 1883[2]. William Osler referred to the systemic nature of the disease in his 1894 textbook of medicine (patients were 'apt to succumb to pulmonary complaints or to nephritis')[4] and Klemperer, Pollack and Baehr, in 1942, proposed that scleroderma should be considered as a 'systemic disease of the connective tissue'[5]. It was not until 1945, however, that Goetz proposed the term progressive systemic sclerosis to emphasize the degree of visceral disease[6]. In 1964, Winterbauer described the CRST syndrome (now the CREST syndrome of calcinosis, Raynaud's phenomenon, esophageal dysmotility, sclerodactyly and telangiectasia)[7], although it was first described in 1910 and originally termed Thiberge–Weissenbach syndrome after the presenting physicians[8]. In 1969 a major pathologic review delineated the widespread fibrotic and vascular disease of scleroderma[9]. Clinical and pathologic surveys of patients with scleroderma followed, giving new insight into the clinical features, risk factors, pathogenesis of fibrosis and associa-tions of scleroderma with the immune response. In the last decade, there has been remarkable progress in understanding the molecular mechanisms of fibrosis, microvascular injury and the autoimmune process in this rare disease.

EPIDEMIOLOGY

It is estimated that new cases of scleroderma occur at a rate of approximately 18–20 per million of the general population per year[10]. The incidence appears to have increased steadily from the 1940s to the 1970s but according to more recent surveys this trend may have stabilized. The apparent increase in cases may be related to a new awareness of scleroderma created by the introduction of classification criteria in 1980[11]. Surveys that include the full clinical spectrum of scleroderma and the related disorders find the prevalence to be 5–19 times higher than previous reports[12].

The prevalence and severity of scleroderma also vary among different racial and ethnic groups. Estimates of the prevalence in the Japanese suggest 38 per million have scleroderma, while the prevalence is 4690 per million among full-blooded Choctaw Native Americans[13]. A national survey of Iceland reports 71 cases of scleroderma per million, although most of these patients had limited scleroderma[14]. The limited variant of scleroderma is found more commonly in Caucasians[15], while African-American females appear to have an increased risk for diffuse cutaneous scleroderma and a younger age at disease onset[16].

While the incidence of scleroderma is higher in females than in males (3:1), this difference is greater in younger age groups (7:1) and less in patients over 50 years old (2:1)[17]. The average age of onset of disease is approximately 50 years. Scleroderma is uncommon in children. The diagnosis of scleroderma by a physician is often delayed years after symptoms first begin; this is particularly true in patients with the more indolent disease course of the CREST syndrome.

There are several reports suggesting geographic clustering of cases of scleroderma. In some cases environmental etiologies are proposed but definite proof is lacking[18,19]. Typical scleroderma is found among male workers exposed to silica[20] and epidemics of a scleroderma-like illness following exposure to toxins contaminating preparations of tryptophan and rapeseed oil are well described (see Chapter 137).

Familial aggregation and concordance of disease in twin pairs rarely occurs[21]. This suggests that the genetic influence is probably complex, involving multiple genetic susceptibilities. Among twin pairs with at least one twin with scleroderma, there is a strong concordance rate for antinuclear antibody positivity (100% in monozygous pairs). However, none of the healthy twins had scleroderma-specific antibodies and only 6% have concordance for scleroderma[22]. First-degree relatives of patients with scleroderma also have a significantly higher frequency of antinuclear antibody positivity and other autoimmune diseases, but multiplex families of scleroderma are rare[23]. It is very likely that both genetic susceptibility to autoimmune disease and some environmental factors influence the clinical expression of scleroderma.

CLINICAL FEATURES

Systemic sclerosis (scleroderma) is a disfiguring multisystem disease that may alter every aspect of an individual's life. It includes a broad spectrum of disease with varying degrees of organ involvement. Thus subsets of patients exist with unique clinical features and distinct outcomes. Raynaud's phenomenon, the manifestation of perturbation of the terminal arteries of the circulatory system, is almost universal in scleroderma. This outward manifestation of vascular disease is a marker of tissue ischemia that is linked to a progressive fibrosing process in specific target organs: the skin, lung, heart, gastrointestinal tract and kidney. In the diffuse cutaneous variant of scleroderma, fibrosis of the skin and other organs is widespread and potentially life-threatening. In the limited form of scleroderma the skin fibrosis is restricted to the fingers and/or distal limbs with a more benign and indolent disease course. Limited cutaneous scleroderma is less likely to be associated with serious internal organ involvement.

The term scleroderma, therefore, encompasses many unique phenotypic subsets of disease with varying degrees and severity of organ involvement. In many cases the unique clinical subset is associated with specific autoantibodies. For example, the presence of antibody to topoisomerase associates with diffuse cutaneous scleroderma and severe interstitial lung disease (see later).

In addition, patients may have 'overlap' features, in which scleroderma is coupled with another autoimmune diseases such as systemic lupus erythematosus (SLE), polymyositis, Sjögren's syndrome or autoimmune thyroid disease.

Diagnostic criteria

A subcommittee of the American Rheumatism Association (now the American College of Rheumatology) established criteria by consensus for scleroderma in 1980 after initiating a multicenter prospective study of early scleroderma patients and comparing them to patients with other autoimmune diseases (SLE, polymyositis and Raynaud's phenomenon)[11]. Criteria were chosen for their discriminatory value and to assure diagnostic certainty to allow for consistency in research and other comparative purposes. The criteria include proximal skin thickening as the major criteria and evidence of digital ischemia, sclerodactyly and pulmonary fibrosis as minor criteria. These criteria were found to be 97% sensitive and 98% specific for a diagnosis of scleroderma, but they have been criticized for failing to include many patients with signs of limited scleroderma or CREST syndrome. These criteria also do not take into account cases that have subtle features of the disease and specific serological markers known to be associated with scleroderma.

Classification

Patients with scleroderma are classified into subsets of disease by the degree of clinically involved skin (Table 133.1). Attempting to classify or subdivide patients is useful both in terms of uniformity and for prognostic implications. Patients with more diffuse skin disease (i.e. those with higher skin scores) have more severe organ involvement and a worse survival[24]. Several proposals exist defining subsets of scleroderma patients[25–28]. The most popular classification distinguishes between patients with truncal skin involvement (diffuse) and those with limited skin involvement (distal to elbows and knees). The limited group includes patients with CREST syndrome, whose skin findings are limited to the digits and face. Within these two subsets, there are groups of patients who have distinct clinical phenotypes (i.e. patients with limited disease and late-onset pulmonary hypertension).

In addition, there may be mild expressions of scleroderma that do not meet current diagnostic criteria, such as the presence of Raynaud's phenomenon alone with abnormal nailfold capillary loops and

TABLE 133.1 CLASSIFICATION OF SYSTEMIC SCLEROSIS
• **Diffuse scleroderma** – skin thickening present on the trunk in addition to the face, proximal and distal extremities
• **Limited scleroderma** – skin thickening restricted to sites distal to the elbow and knee but also involving the face and neck
– **CREST syndrome** (C, subcutaneous calcinosis; R, Raynaud's phenomenon; E, esophageal dysmotility; S, sclerodactyly; T, telangiectasia)
• *Sine* scleroderma – no clinically apparent skin thickening but with characteristic internal organ changes, vascular and serologic features
• **Overlap syndrome** – criteria fulfilling systemic sclerosis occurring concomitantly with features of SLE, RA or inflammatory muscle disease
• **Undifferentiated connective tissue disease** – Raynaud's phenomenon with clinical and/or laboratory features of systemic sclerosis; these include scleroderma-specific antibodies, abnormal nailfold capillaroscopy, finger edema and ischemic injury

autoantibodies associated with scleroderma. Many of these patients are diagnosed as undifferentiated connective tissue disorder with features of scleroderma. Recently, it has been proposed to include patients with Raynaud's phenomenon and specific scleroderma serologies as definite scleroderma[29]. About 5% of patients may have systemic sclerosis without skin thickening (systemic sclerosis *sine* scleroderma)[30].

Scleroderma patients with definite clinical signs and laboratory parameters of another rheumatic disease such as SLE or polymyositis are considered to have an 'overlap syndrome'. Mixed connective tissue disease is considered to be an overlap syndrome with features of scleroderma, myositis and a polyarthritis. Some consider it a distinct disease entity[31]. Longitudinal studies of patients with mixed connective tissue disease suggest that most eventually meet defined criteria for another rheumatic disease such as scleroderma or SLE[32,33].

Natural history of disease

Other autoimmune illnesses such as SLE are characterized by exacerbations or 'flares,' while the course of scleroderma is predominantly monophasic (Fig. 133.1). A re-flare of the cutaneous disease occurs in

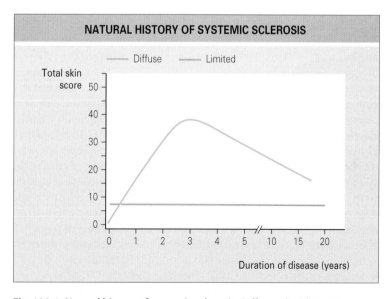

NATURAL HISTORY OF SYSTEMIC SCLEROSIS

Fig. 133.1 Natural history of systemic sclerosis. Diffuse scleroderma is typified by rapid progression of skin involvement in the early years. New internal organ involvement occurs most frequently during the active early phase of disease. Limited disease slowly increases in severity of skin involvement and internal organ involvement is typically delayed until the second decade of disease.

only about 5% of patients. The course of other organ involvement is complex and difficult to define clinically. In general, in the diffuse form of the disease, internal organ involvement tends to progress in concert with cutaneous disease. The clinical course and prognosis vary significantly among the different subsets of disease. Diffuse cutaneous scleroderma has an early rapid phase, usually followed by regression of skin disease after years. In contrast, limited disease has an indolent course, often with years of Raynaud's phenomenon alone before other features of scleroderma become evident.

Diffuse cutaneous scleroderma

In general, patients with diffuse disease have a narrow interval between onset of Raynaud's phenomenon, skin thickening and internal organ involvement. The early stage of scleroderma is usually characterized by inflamed, edematous skin (Fig. 133.2) and significant systemic manifestations such as fatigue, arthralgias, myalgias, diffuse pruritus and an elevated erythrocyte sedimentation rate (ESR). In this initial phase there is early rapid progression of skin thickening over months to years. There is also a significant risk of internal organ involvement, particularly in the first 3 years[34]. The higher the skin score (degree of skin thickening determined by the physician), the greater the risk for renal disease and higher mortality. Approximately 10–20% of patients with diffuse scleroderma will develop severe, life-threatening internal organ disease (heart, renal, pulmonary, gastrointestinal). Further significant internal organ involvement or progression rarely occurs after skin changes have reached a peak or maximal skin score.

The later stages of diffuse cutaneous scleroderma are characterized by gradual softening of the skin[24]. Remission of the skin disease is accompanied by resolution of systemic symptoms and lack of progression (or new development) of internal organ disease. Despite overall improvement in skin thickness, areas of irreversible skin fibrosis, especially in the forearms and hands, often exist. Skin atrophy and deeper tissue fibrosis cause contractures and prolonged disability. A small subset of patients, even in this late stage, will have progressive active disease. Chronic organ dysfunction and failure is also the result of permanent damage caused by prior active disease.

Although patients with scleroderma have a mortality rate four to five times greater than that of the general population, overall mortality for diffuse cutaneous disease has improved over the last 30 years. This is in part because of improved management of scleroderma renal crisis, previously the leading cause of death in scleroderma. Estimates suggest that the 5-year survival has improved from the figure in the 1950s–1970s of 50% to approximately 75% (since 1980)[10,35]. Predictors for higher mortality include higher skin scores (Rodnan score >20), reduced lung diffusion capacity, elevated sedimentation rate and evidence of heart or renal involvement.

Limited scleroderma

The clinical course, survival and clinical features of limited disease are quite different than in the diffuse form (Fig. 133.1). The overall 5-year survival in limited scleroderma is 80–85%, which is significantly better than is seen in diffuse disease[36]. Patients with limited disease often have many years of Raynaud's phenomenon prior to the development of other signs or symptoms of scleroderma. The most common first non-Raynaud's symptom is caused by esophageal dysfunction manifested by dysphagia or gastroesophageal reflux.

The major causes of morbidity and mortality in limited disease are severe Raynaud's phenomenon with occlusive digital vascular disease and pulmonary hypertension. Patients with limited disease, particularly those with anticentromere antibodies, are more likely to have severe digital ischemia and digital loss related to advanced arterial vascular disease (see Figs 133.6–133.8)[37]. Pulmonary hypertension is the leading cause of scleroderma-related mortality among limited disease patients. This complication occurs in approximately 10% of cases with limited scleroderma and often occurs in the absence of interstitial lung disease. In patients who develop pulmonary hypertension, the disease is almost uniformly fatal secondary to progressive right-sided heart failure.

Brief introduction to pathophysiology

The diverse clinical manifestations of scleroderma can be better appreciated by understanding the possible underlying pathophysiological mechanisms involved in this disease (see Chapter 134). The three key pathologic features are:

- a unique vascular disease
- abnormal accumulation of extracellular matrix components (fibrosis)
- autoimmunity.

It is unclear how and when the immune system is involved, but evidence suggests that it is important early in the disease and probably the immune process initiates and propagates the inflammatory process that causes vascular damage and eventual tissue fibrosis. The vasculopathy of scleroderma is fundamental to the other pathological events. It is characterized by arterial vasospasm, smooth muscle hyperactivity, intimal proliferation and eventual vascular occlusion. The vascular disease is manifested clinically by the presence of nailfold capillary changes, telangiectasias, Raynaud's phenomenon and most strikingly by digital and other tissue ischemia. Associated with the vascular disease is tissue fibrosis that varies in degree but occurs in the skin and other targeted organs. Fibrosis is the most characteristic pathologic finding; however, the cause of organ dysfunction is complex and it can be seen in the absence of severe fibrosis. This is particularly true in the gastrointestinal tract, where smooth muscle atrophy is striking and fibrosis is limited.

Raynaud's phenomenon

Raynaud's phenomenon is vasoconstriction of the digital arteries in response to cold. This manifests with color changes in the skin, corresponding to the stage of the vasospastic process. Initially there is sharply demarcated pallor (Fig. 133.3) and/or cyanosis (Fig. 133.4). This is followed by erythema of the skin, a manifestation of the reactive hyperemia that follows the ischemic episode. Raynaud's is caused by vasoconstriction of the muscular digital arteries, precapillary arterioles and arteriovenous (AV) shunts of the skin in response to colder temperature and to neural signals associated with emotional stress.

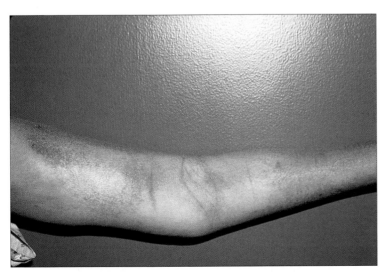

Fig. 133.2 Diffuse scleroderma. Inflamed, indurated skin of the arm in early diffuse scleroderma.

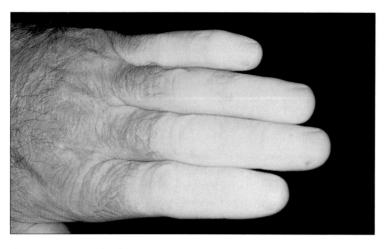

Fig. 133.3 Raynaud's phenomenon. Sharply demarcated pallor of the fingers.

TABLE 133.2 CLINICAL AND LABORATORY FEATURES IN THE DIFFERENTIAL DIAGNOSIS OF RAYNAUD'S PHENOMENON		
Feature	Primary Raynaud's	Systemic sclerosis
Sex	F:M 4:1	F:M 3:1
Age at onset	Puberty	25 years or older
Frequency	Usually <5 per day	>5–10 attacks per day
Precipitants	Cold, emotional stress	Cold
Ischemic injury	Absent	Present
Other vasomotor phenomena	Yes	Yes
Antinuclear antibodies	Absent	90–95%
Anticentromere antibody	Absent	50–60%
Anti-Scl-70 antibody	Absent	20–30%
Abnormal capillaroscopy	Absent	>95%
In vivo platelet activation	Absent	>75%

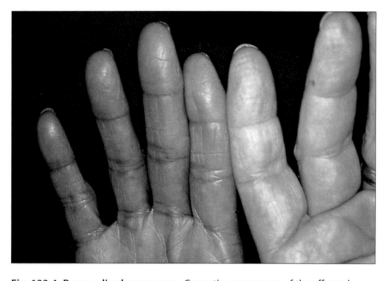

Fig. 133.4 Raynaud's phenomenon. Cyanotic appearance of the affected hand compared with the normal other hand.

Surveys find that 4–15% of the general population have symptoms characteristic of Raynaud's phenomenon[38,39]. In the majority of cases, Raynaud's phenomenon is not associated with either structural vascular changes or ischemic tissue damage (primary Raynaud's phenomenon). Primary Raynaud's typically begins in the teenage years and is more common in women (female:male ratio approximately 4:1). Approximately 30% of the first-degree relatives also have Raynaud's phenomenon. In primary Raynaud's phenomenon, the patients are otherwise healthy, the episodes are symmetric in the fingers and/or toes and they do not lead to tissue ulceration or gangrene. Examination of these patients is unremarkable and laboratory data, including antinuclear antibody and ESR, are normal.

The challenge for the physician is to determine whether the presence of Raynaud's phenomenon is an uncomplicated primary process or the first symptom of a secondary illness such as scleroderma (Table 133.2) or another disease (Table 133.3). Patients who have Raynaud's attacks without digital pitting, ulceration or gangrene and who have normal nailfold capillaries, a normal ESR and a negative antinuclear antibody test, are unlikely to have an underlying disease such as scleroderma[40].

TABLE 133.3 DIFFERENTIAL DIAGNOSIS OF RAYNAUD'S PHENOMENON		
Structural vasculopathies	Large and medium arteries	Thoracic outlet syndrome Brachiocephalic trunk disease (atherosclerosis, Takayasu's arteritis)
	Small artery and arteriolar	Systemic lupus erythematosus Dermatomyositis Overlap syndromes Cold injury Vibration disease Arteriosclerosis (thromboangiitis obliterans) Chemotherapy (bleomycin, vinblastine) Polyvinyl chloride disease
Normal blood vessels	Abnormal blood elements	Cryoglobulinemia Cryofibrinogenemia Paraproteinemia Cold agglutinin disease Polycythemias
	Abnormal vasomotion	Primary (idiopathic) Raynaud's phenomenon Drug-induced (ergots sympathomimetics) Pheochromocytoma Carcinoid syndrome Other vasospastic disorders (migraine, Prinzmetal's angina)

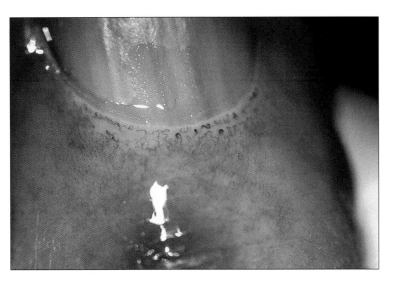

Fig. 133.5 Capillary loop abnormalities. Nailfold capillaroscopy showing the scleroderma pattern with dilated capillary loops and vessel dropout.

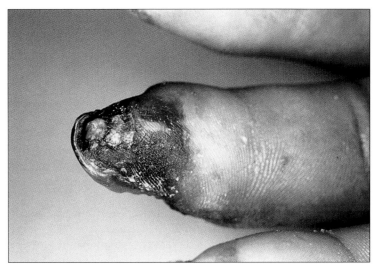

Fig. 133.7 Digital gangrene. Sharply demarcated gangrene of several weeks duration of the fingertip of a woman with CREST syndrome.

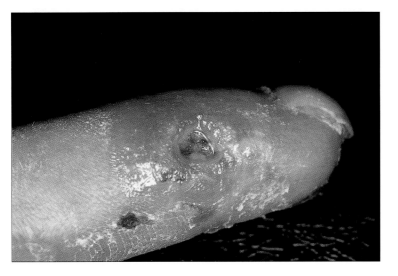

Fig. 133.6 Digital tip ulcer. Typical ulceration of the fingertip in a patient with diffuse scleroderma.

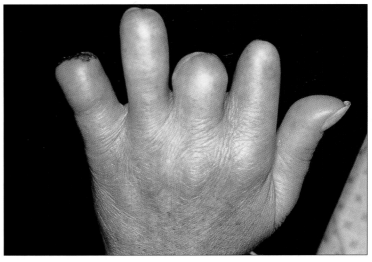

Fig. 133.8 Digital loss. Cumulative loss of multiple digits in a patient with limited scleroderma and anticentromere antibodies.

The presence of nailfold capillaries with enlarged capillary loops and/or the loss of capillaries or avascularity (a scleroderma pattern; Fig. 133.5) suggest that the patient has scleroderma[41,42]. Approximately 13% of patients presenting to a university medical center with Raynaud's phenomenon alone develop a connective tissue disease[43]. Patients with limited scleroderma often have mild or vague symptoms and are initially diagnosed with undifferentiated connective tissue disorder. Predictors of the development of scleroderma among such patients include older age at onset of Raynaud's phenomenon, severe Raynaud's phenomenon, nailfold capillary abnormalities and the presence of antinuclear/scleroderma-specific antibodies[44].

Raynaud's phenomenon and scleroderma

In scleroderma, over 90% of patients have intense Raynaud's phenomenon associated with tissue fibrosis, digital ulceration (Fig. 133.6) and, on occasion, ischemic demarcation and digital amputation (Fig. 133.7). The severity of the Raynaud's attacks is a manifestation of both vasospasm and structural abnormalities of the digital arteries. Compared to normals, scleroderma patients have a more pronounced decrease of both nutritional and thermoregulatory blood flow to the skin in response to cold temperatures. This sensitivity is coupled with long delays in recovery of local blood flow following rewarming and relief of stimulants of vasoconstriction (cold, emotional stress). In addition, reactive hyperemia, which normally follows periods of digital ischemia and is present in patients with primary Raynaud's, is absent in scleroderma, indicating that fixed irreversible structural disease is a significant cause of tissue ischemia[45]. In addition to vasospasm, vascular occlusion occurs secondary to activation of platelets and the intravascular clotting cascade, leading to fibrin deposition and vascular occlusion.

A vascular occlusive event that involves the digital artery or major arteries of the peripheral circulation (palmar arch, ulnar or tibial arteries) can cause deep tissue infarction with gangrene and/or digital amputation (Fig. 133.8). Rarely, major vessel disease may lead to loss of the distal part of a limb. These major vascular events are more likely to occur in patients with limited skin disease who have anticentromere antibody[37].

There is good evidence that a generalized vasospastic disorder exists in scleroderma ('systemic Raynaud's phenomenon') involving the terminal arterial system of the kidney, heart and probably other viscera. The renal crisis of scleroderma is a clear example of reversible vasoconstriction of the cortical blood flow to the kidney[46]. Cold-induced vasospasm of the pulmonary circulation has been more difficult to prove[47,48], in part because irreversible structural changes of the arteries occur very early in the lung. Management of patients with scleroderma must carefully address the systemic vascular disease that is present.

The cutaneous manifestations of scleroderma

The skin disease of scleroderma follows a course characterized by three phases: an inflammatory edematous phase, an indurative phase and an atrophic phase. These stages do not have a distinct beginning and ending and there is a high degree of variability in the duration of inflammatory signs and in the severity and extent of the skin involvement. Evidence also suggests that a subclinical inflammatory process is present even in areas of clinically normal skin.

In the initial edematous stage, the patient experiences puffiness, swelling and a sense of decreased flexibility of the skin, especially in the forearms, hands and digits, as well as in the feet. These symptoms may be accompanied by intense pruritus. The fingers appear puffy (Fig. 133.9) with a moon-like fullness of the fingertip and there is loss of normal digital creases. Reduced sweat and oil production results in drying and scaling of the skin's surface, which may cause small fissures leading to complications such as cellulitis or paronychia. Loss of the finger pad and tapering of the finger due to fingertip ischemia is often seen during this early phase of scleroderma. This inflammatory process may last for months, during which time induration and skin thickening becomes evident.

After the initial intense inflammatory stage has diminished there is a long course of progressive fibrosis of the skin in diffuse cutaneous scleroderma (Fig. 133.10). This is characterized by marked tightening and thickening of the skin that can involve the extremities, chest, neck, face and abdomen. Areas of the midback are usually spared even in severe diffuse disease but the posterior neck and lower flanks of the trunk can have thickened skin. The skin of the abdomen is usually diffusely thickened, or there can be patches of hyperpigmented thick skin that primarily occurs over pressure points such as the belt line. Interestingly, the area around the areola of the breast is spared. In patients with diffuse skin disease, a pulling, tight sensation around the upper chest and shoulder girdle is a common complaint. The anterior neck may develop thick horizontal folds of skin called the scleroderma 'neck sign' (Fig. 133.11). These folds can be present in patients with either limited or diffuse disease.

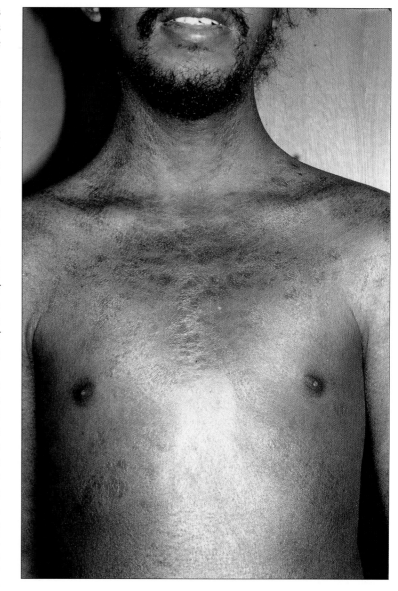

Fig. 133.10 Truncal scleroderma. Skin thickening of the chest and abdomen of a patient with diffuse scleroderma. Both hyperpigmentation and hypopigmentation are demonstrated.

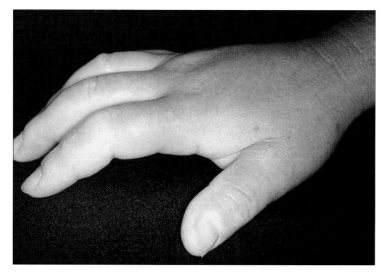

Fig. 133.9 Early puffy scleroderma. Extensive edema of the fingers in a man with several months of preceding Raynaud's phenomenon. Skin was not clinically thickened but became so on follow-up.

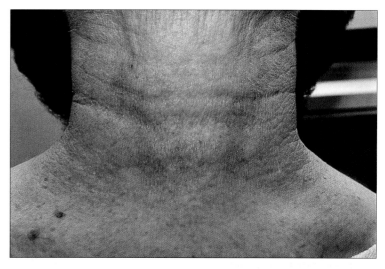

Fig. 133.11 Scleroderma neck sign.

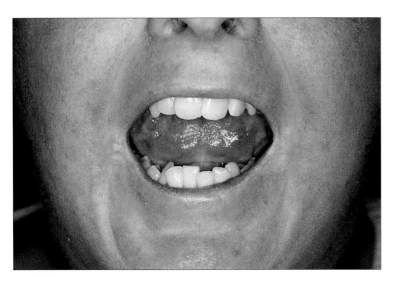

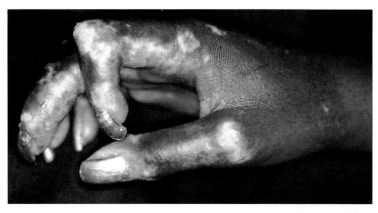

Fig. 133.14 Digital and hand scleroderma. Advanced changes of scleroderma have caused digital contractions and limitation of finger movement.

Fig. 133.12 Facial scleroderma. Taut smooth skin over the face and reduced oral aperture of a woman with long-standing disease. Furrowing is present around the mouth, along with some facial telangiectasias.

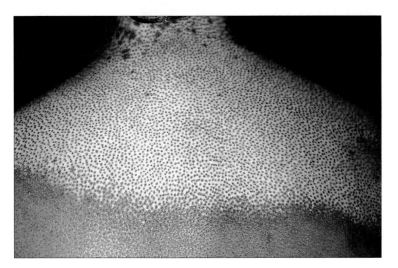

Fig. 133.13 Depigmentation of the skin. 'Salt and pepper' appearance of skin secondary to perifollicular sparing of pigment loss.

The face can appear expressionless because of reduced capacity to smile or move the eyelids or cheeks. The opened mouth becomes circular with a remarkable reduction in the maximum oral aperture. Vertical lines or furrowing of the skin around the lips gives a pursed-lip appearance as though a string had pulled tight the borders of the lips to close the mouth (Fig. 133.12). The tight perioral skin sometimes makes the frontal teeth appear more prominent, especially if there is associated gum retraction caused by local fibrosis and bone resorption. The nose becomes pinched and the facial creases smooth so that the face has a mouse-like appearance (*Mauskopf*).

Pigmentary changes of the skin also occur during the edematous and fibrotic stages of scleroderma but these changes vary in intensity and distribution. Some patients develop areas of depigmentation that is similar to vitiligo, especially in the scalp, eyebrows, upper back and chest and over areas of trauma, such as the dorsum of the hand or shins. This vitiligo pattern gives the skin a 'salt and pepper' appearance because of perifollicular sparing of pigment loss (Fig. 133.13). Some patients develop diffuse tanning of the skin; others have scattered patches of hyperpigmentation, particularly over pressure points. Areas of marked hyperpigmentation can be seen in the skin creases.

On average, after 1–3 years of disease activity, the inflammatory and fibrotic process gradually stops. These areas of the skin begin to thin or remodel and return to clinically normal skin (especially the trunk and proximal limbs). The first signs of improvement may be regrowth of hair on the forearms, a decrease in pruritus and a sense of improved flexibility. In the late stage of scleroderma, the skin becomes atrophic (especially over the fingers, hands and distal limbs) and thinned, with tethering secondary to fibrotic tissue binding to underlying structures. Areas of thinned skin can ulcerate with minor trauma, especially in areas such as the tip of the elbow, the medial or lateral ankle or over sites of a flexion contracture. Flexion contractures of the fingers are very common in the diffuse form of scleroderma (Fig. 133.14). These contractures evolve in the setting of intense deep tissue fibrosis and likely reflect stronger flexors, compared to extensors, of the digits. In severe cases, similar contractures can occur in the wrists, elbows, shoulders, knees, ankles and rarely the hip girdle. Thickened skin and fibrosis of deeper tissue of the palm and hand tendons reduce mobility and cause muscle atrophy and loss of function of the hands.

In patients with limited skin disease, the fibrotic skin changes are usually limited to the fingers (sclerodactyly). Sclerodactyly may present as puffy fingers with thickening only of the very distal digits. Facial changes are much less dramatic in limited disease but perioral furrowing can occur. More prominent in limited disease are small and large mat-like telangiectasias that appear on the face, upper chest, palms, fingertips and mucous membranes (Figs 133.15 & 133.16). These telangiectasias are dilated capillaries, which gradually increase in number. In diffuse cutaneous disease they can appear in the later stages on the face, arms and trunk.

Subcutaneous calcinosis, composed of calcium hydroxyapatite deposits at sites of trauma such as the forearms, elbows or fingers (Fig. 133.17), occurs in all subsets of scleroderma but is more prominent in limited scleroderma and patients with anticentromere antibody. The calcinosis can become superficial, ulcerate the skin and lead to secondary infection. More often the deposits remain bothersome subcutaneous lumps that rarely cause recurrent local inflammation due to the release of crystals of hydroxyapatite into the tissue.

Ulceration of the skin can occur for various reasons in scleroderma. Sudden episodes of ischemic ulceration are common and are seen more frequently during the cold temperatures of the winter months. Digital ischemic ulcerations are located on the fingertips (Fig. 133.18) or distal toes and may be either very small and superficial or deep painful lesions that are 1–2cm in size. They may also occur under the fingernail and appear as a painful hazy area of necrotic debris trapped under the nail. Untreated cutaneous ulcers form a thick eschar of

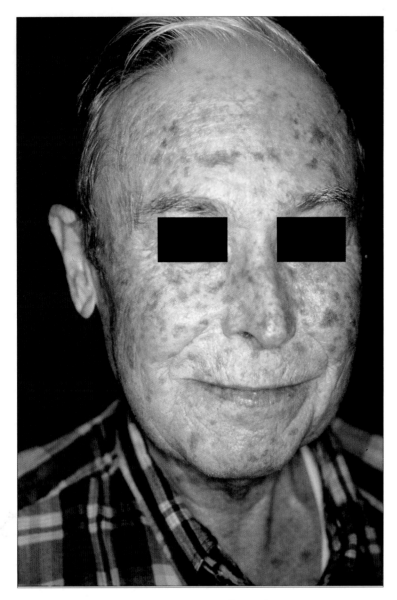

Fig. 133.15 Facial telangiectasias. Extensive facial telangiectasias in a man with CREST syndrome.

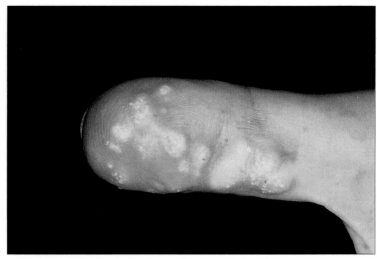

Fig. 133.17 Subcutaneous calcinosis. Calcinosis of the finger tip.

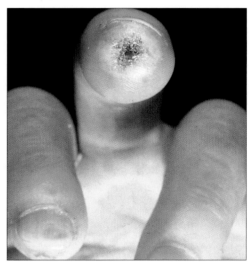

Fig. 133.18 Fingertip ulceration. Large digital infarction in a patient with limited scleroderma.

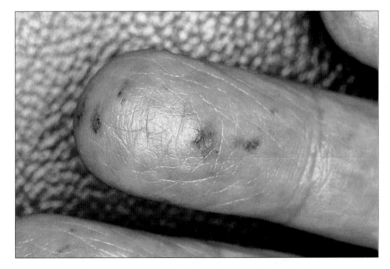

Fig. 133.16 Telangiectasias of the fingers.

debris, which can develop secondary infection with cellulitis. With proper management, healing will occur in 6–9 weeks. After healing of an ulcer, a digital 'pit' remains or there is loss of the pulp of the finger pad. Pitting and digital pad atrophy may occur without definite ulceration.

Traumatic ulceration occurs at sites of flexion contractures or areas of repeated minor trauma such as the pinna of the ear or over the proximal interphalangeal joints of the fingers, a common site of severe flexion contractures. Ankle ulcers are usually traumatic or, rarely, secondary to an associated vasculitis. Vasculitis in scleroderma has been reported to be associated with Sjögren's syndrome[49].

Systemic manifestations of scleroderma
Musculoskeletal features
Non-specific musculoskeletal complaints such as arthralgias and myalgias are one of the earliest symptoms of scleroderma. Synovitis similar to rheumatoid arthritis occurs in a small subset of patients and involves multiple joints, including the fingers, wrists, knees or ankles. These patients represent an overlap syndrome with polyarthritis and scleroderma. This inflammatory arthritis is usually responsive to

typical therapy used for rheumatoid arthritis. The more common situation is that pain and stiffness are generally greater than objective inflammatory signs would predict. Discomfort from joints often extends along tendons and into the muscles of the arms and legs. Pain on motion of the ankle, wrist, knee or elbow may be accompanied by a coarse 'friction' rub caused by fibrinous deposits on the tendon sheath. These rubs are detected in approximately 30% of patients with diffuse scleroderma[50]. The presence of friction rubs can be used as a clinical predictor of worse disease and is associated with higher skin scores, increased frequency of cardiac and renal involvement and increased mortality[50].

The dominant musculoskeletal problem in late scleroderma is muscle atrophy and loss of joint function secondary to restricted motion, usually caused by the abnormal overlying thickened and non-flexible skin. In diffuse scleroderma this can occur over any articulation but is almost universal over the fingers, wrist and elbows. Radiographs of the bones in scleroderma will frequently show osteopenia. Osseous resorption of the digital tuft, secondary to ischemia, and soft tissue calcinosis may also be seen. Joint space narrowing, erosions or bony ankylosis are seen infrequently.

Muscle weakness is a significant problem in scleroderma and often has more than one cause[51]. In diffuse scleroderma, muscle atrophy and weakness can result from deconditioning secondary to restricted mobility and contractures. A myopathy also occurs from a direct extension of the fibrosis process into the muscle itself. These patients present with weakness and fatigue associated with a mild elevation in serum creatine phosphokinase (CPK) and an abnormal electromyogram (EMG)[52]. An 'overlap' syndrome with typical polymyositis or dermatomyositis is seen in a subset of patients with a high CPK, proximal muscle weakness, abnormal EMG and inflammation on muscle biopsy[51,52]. Myopathy secondary to drugs (e.g. corticosteroids, D-penicillamine) used in the treatment of scleroderma can also mimic polymyositis or scleroderma muscle disease. Global weakness and muscle deconditioning are often present in patients with severe disease and multiple organ dysfunction.

Gastrointestinal involvement

Gastrointestinal tract involvement is found in almost every patient with scleroderma and is characterized by abnormal motility secondary to dysfunctions caused by abnormal innervation, smooth muscle atrophy and tissue fibrosis[53]. Every area of the gastrointestinal tract can be involved, including the oropharynx, esophagus, stomach, small and large bowel and rectum. Many scleroderma patients are without significant symptoms despite measurable abnormalities of gastrointestinal function. Unfortunately, severe disease frequently occurs, causing significant morbidity. Patients with both limited and diffuse variants of scleroderma are at equal risk, with gastrointestinal disease being the most common first non-Raynaud's symptom of scleroderma.

The smooth muscle is the major pathologic site of disease in scleroderma gastrointestinal disease. It is not clear, however, whether the smooth muscle abnormality is primary or secondary to abnormal innervation or a defective vascular supply. Although the autonomic nerves of the gastrointestinal tract appear normal by microscopy, functional studies suggest that a neurogenic process precedes muscle dysfunction[54]. The microvascular abnormalities in scleroderma are also seen in the gastrointestinal tract (i.e. intimal proliferation) but clear evidence of ischemic injury is absent. Whatever the primary insult, smooth muscle atrophy and some degree of fibrosis of the submucosal and muscular layers of the gastrointestinal tract becomes the dominant pathology. Irreversible and severe life-threatening bowel dysfunction can result.

Oropharynx

A small oral aperture and dry mucosal membranes with periodontal disease can lead to problems with chewing foods, loss of teeth and failure of good nutrition. Many patients with scleroderma have a sensation of dry eyes and mouth (the sicca complex). Minor salivary gland biopsies usually show fibrosis without the typical lymphocytic aggregates of Sjögren's syndrome. In addition, the majority of scleroderma patients with sicca complaints usually do not have antibodies against Ro/SSA or La/SSB, suggesting that the mechanism of dry membranes in scleroderma is a secondary process different from that seen in Sjögren's syndrome[55].

Upper pharyngeal function is generally considered to be normal in scleroderma unless there is involvement of striated pharyngeal muscles with an inflammatory myositis or a neuromuscular disease. In this case, movement of food from the mouth to the esophagus is abnormal and the patient may complain of coughing upon swallowing, nasal regurgitation of fluids or a sense of inability to swallow.

Esophagus

Esophageal dysfunction affects almost every scleroderma patient, with dysphagia and dyspepsia being the most common symptom. The dysphagia is usually described as solid foods sticking after normal initiation of swallowing. This sensation is relieved by the intake of extra fluids to clear the esophagus. Substernal burning pain may be coupled with a feeling of indigestion or nausea. These reflux symptoms are typically worse after meals, with exercise and after bedtime. Severe esophageal reflux and esophagitis occur equally in patients with either limited or diffuse scleroderma. However, the degree of symptoms does not directly correlate with objective measurements of acid reflux events documented by 24-hour pH monitoring. Patients with motility problems of the esophagus may also present with early satiety, regurgitation of food, progressive weight loss and malnutrition or with emergency impaction of food.

Atypical manifestations of esophageal disease include aspiration, unexplained coughing, hoarseness, a feeling of excess oral secretions, chest pain and localized *Candida* infection.

Low or absent primary and secondary peristalsis of the distal esophagus and low lower esophageal sphincter pressure in the presence of a normal proximal (striated muscle) esophagus are typical manometric findings in scleroderma[56]. Excessive air in the esophagus is commonly detected on routine chest X-ray. Although symptoms are a poor guide to the degree of esophageal disease, patients who are asymptomatic on or off treatment are unlikely to have significant complications. Esophagitis appears to occur only in patients with impaired peristalsis and delayed acid clearance[57].

Untreated or persistent esophagitis can lead to mucosal erosions and occult bleeding, distal esophageal stricture, Barrett's metaplasia or, rarely, adenocarcinoma. Gastrointestinal bleeding occurs from esophagitis, gastritis or gastrointestinal telangiectasias of the stomach, small bowel or colon.

If there is unexplained weight loss with poor caloric intake or other symptoms of esophageal dysfunction, a barium swallow (Fig. 133.19), endoscopic and/or manometric investigation of the esophagus are warranted. A 24-hour pH probe study is a helpful method to quantify the degree and frequency of acid reflux in difficult-to-manage cases.

Stomach and small bowel

Delayed emptying of the stomach with retention of solid foods aggravates reflux and is a frequent cause of bloating, nausea, vomiting, early satiety and poor appetite. Patients frequently reduce their caloric intake to avoid these symptoms and as a consequence lose weight. Gastric

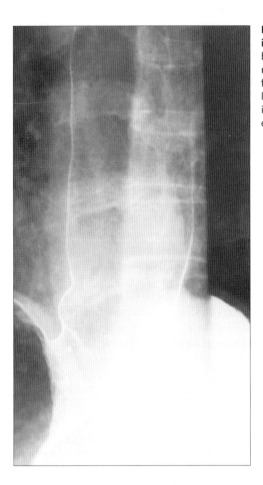

Fig. 133.19 Esophageal involvement. This barium contrast study reveals the characteristic findings of a hypomotile lower esophagus and an incompetent lower esophageal sphincter.

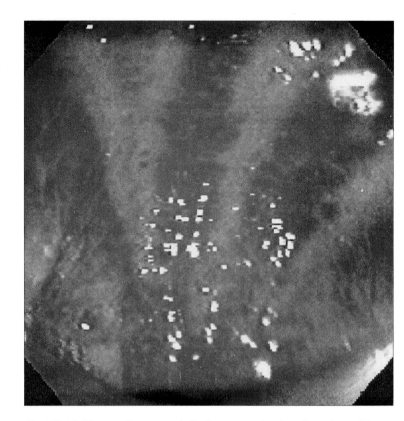

Fig. 133.20 Watermelon stomach. Endoscopy evaluation of a patient with scleroderma with recent gastrointestinal bleeding.

antral vascular ectasia (watermelon stomach) can be a cause of gastrointestinal bleeding in scleroderma patients. Endoscopy of these patients reveals antral gastritis and prominent longitudinal vascular folds that resembles the surface of a watermelon (Fig. 133.20)[58].

Dysmotility of the small intestine may be asymptomatic or it can cause serious intermittent pseudo-obstruction of the intestine presenting with abdominal pain, distention and vomiting that ultimately requires total parenteral nutrition for survival. Motility problems of the small bowel more commonly result in recurrent bouts of mild abdominal pain, diarrhea, weight loss and malnutrition. Malnutrition and diarrhea are usually a consequence of malabsorption caused by bacterial overgrowth in stagnant intestinal fluids. Occasionally, pneumatosis cystoides intestinalis occurs in patients with advanced bowel disease. In this situation, intestinal gas dissects into the bowel wall or, on occasion, into the peritoneal cavity, mimicking a ruptured bowel.

Large bowel

The large intestine and rectum are also affected by scleroderma. Scleroderma patients have decreased distensibility of the colon that does not necessarily correlate with symptoms[59]. Rarely diarrhea, but more frequently constipation, lower abdominal distention or impaction are manifestations of colonic involvement. Because of muscular atrophy of the bowel wall, asymptomatic wide mouthed diverticula unique to scleroderma are commonly found in the transverse and descending colon (Fig. 133.21). Anorectal dysfunction due to reduced capacity, compliance and anal sphincter tone may lead to rectal prolapse and incontinence or alternatively aggravate constipation.

Liver

The liver is rarely involved in scleroderma. An association exists between primary biliary cirrhosis and limited scleroderma[60]. This disease is manifested by cholestatic liver disease with elevations in alkaline phosphatase

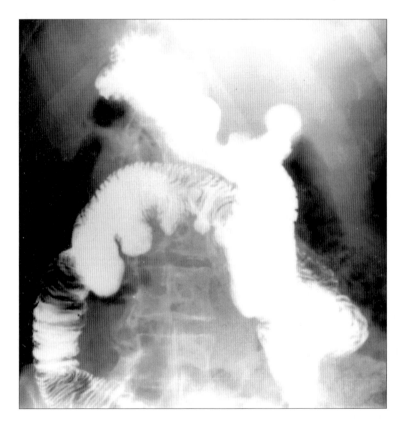

Fig. 133.21 Large bowel involvement. Barium study showing wide-mouthed colonic diverticula.

and jaundice and is associated with antimitochondrial antibodies. Autoimmune hepatitis has been reported in patients with limited scleroderma as well. Transaminase elevations from muscle disease are often mistaken for liver disease in patients with scleroderma.

Pulmonary involvement

Lung involvement in scleroderma is almost universal and now accounts for significant lifetime morbidity and is the leading cause of death. Both interstitial fibrosis and pulmonary arterial vascular disease are present in the lungs of patients with scleroderma but often one pathologic process will be the dominant cause of clinical problems. Pulmonary interstitial fibrosis is more likely to be severe in patients with diffuse skin disease, while pulmonary vascular disease and pulmonary hypertension can be the dominant problem of the lung in patients with the CREST syndrome. Most patients have some degree of both processes and any patient with scleroderma with pulmonary symptoms needs to be evaluated thoroughly for both interstitial lung disease and pulmonary hypertension. Approximately 80% of patients will have abnormal pulmonary function measured by specific and sensitive testing[61]. Yet, the majority of the lung disease will be clinically silent until advanced pulmonary fibrosis or moderate to severe pulmonary arterial hypertension is present.

Patients with interstitial lung disease (ILD) commonly have a rapid decline in pulmonary function that occurs in conjunction with progressive skin disease. Dyspnea on exertion without chest pain is the most common presenting symptom with a dry cough being a late manifestation of ILD. Examination of the patients with ILD reveals 'Velcro-like' crackles at the lung bases in the absence of signs of heart failure. A chest radiograph is relatively insensitive to detect lung disease, but, if abnormal, the fibrosis appears as bilateral reticulonodular changes in the lower lobes of the lung parenchyma (Fig. 133.22).

The most sensitive method for detecting early lung disease in scleroderma is to perform pulmonary function testing. Mild changes in function can be detected before any symptoms develop. The most common changes of pulmonary function testing are either a reduced diffusion capacity (D_LCO) or a reduction in lung volumes (forced vital capacity, FVC) typical of a restrictive ventilatory defect with associated reduction in gas exchange. A high-resolution computed tomography (HRCT) scan of the chest is a very sensitive technique for detecting changes in the lung parenchyma. Findings of ground-glass opacification of the lung bases on HRCT corresponds with active alveolitis and progressive restrictive lung disease.

Bronchoalveolar lavage (BAL) is used to detect inflammation and active alveolitis. BAL demonstrates an increased total number of cells with an increased percentage of neutrophils, eosinophils or CD8+ T cells. Evidence of active alveolitis by either BAL or HRCT predicts progressive lung disease. Therefore, patients with ground-glass findings on HRCT should be studied with a BAL and, if positive, considered for immunosuppressive therapy. When the disease progresses, fibrosis becomes prominent and is irreversible. In this late stage, there is worsening interstitial fibrosis and 'honeycombing' of the lung parenchyma. When lung fibrosis is present, pulmonary function[62,63] testing will show a restrictive ventilatory defect with reduced lung volumes or a low D_LCO.

Pulmonary arterial vascular disease with associated pulmonary hypertension is one of the most difficult clinical problems in scleroderma. The pulmonary vascular process can be indolent and remain clinically undetectable until severe irreversible pulmonary hypertension and signs of right-sided heart failure develop. Significant pulmonary hypertension presents clinically with dyspnea on exertion and fatigue. Physical exam findings include a loud pulmonic component of S2, an S3 gallop and other signs of cor pulmonale such as an elevated jugular venous pulse, hepatomegaly and peripheral edema (Fig. 133.23). Electrocardiography shows evidence of right-sided heart strain with right ventricular hypertrophy and right axis deviation. Pulmonary

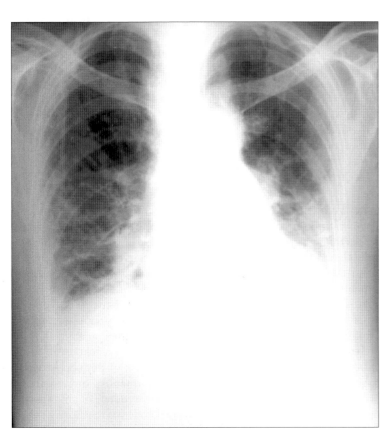

Fig. 133.22 Interstitial lung disease. Chest radiograph in scleroderma showing increased interstitial markings in the lower two-thirds and associated cystic changes.

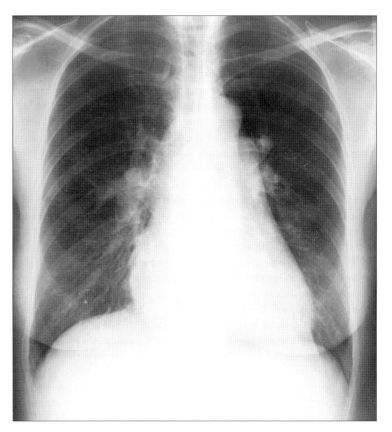

Fig. 133.23 Pulmonary hypertension. This patient had severe pulmonary hypertension documented on right heart catheterization. The lung fields are clear but the left heart border is straightened from elevation of the pulmonary conus and there is enlargement of the pulmonary arteries. This syndrome is most typical of later years of limited scleroderma.

hypertension can be detected early and non-invasively by measuring the pulmonary artery pressure with two-dimensional Doppler echocardiography. Pulmonary function testing often reveals an isolated decrease in diffusion capacity when pulmonary vascular disease is present.

The natural history of the lung disease in scleroderma is highly variable; the majority of patients will have an early but modest decline in function and then follow a stable course or improve[61]. Approximately a third will have a more severe progressive decline in lung function that continues for 4–5 years and then appears to stabilize. Patients with diffuse skin changes tend to have serious lung involvement in the first 5 years of disease, while patients with CREST syndrome usually do not experience clinical symptoms until more than 5 years after diagnosis. Risk factors for serious restrictive lung disease are African-American or Afro-Caribbean race and antitopoisomerase antibodies[64]. A low diffusing capacity (less than 40% predicted)[65] or rapidly declining $D_{L}CO$ and/or lung volumes predict a high mortality rate.

Less common problems of the lung include aspiration pneumonia (secondary to severe esophageal dysfunction), endobronchial telangiectasias, pulmonary hemorrhage, bronchiolitis obliterans organizing pneumonia, pleural reactions and pneumothorax. Studies are inconclusive about the association between pulmonary function impairment and abnormal esophageal function[66]. There is likely an increased risk of lung cancer in patients with ILD[67]. Chest pain is generally not caused by scleroderma lung disease and if present can usually be explained by another process such as musculoskeletal pain, reflux esophagitis, pleurisy or pericarditis.

Cardiac involvement

The clinical manifestations of scleroderma heart disease are quite variable, usually subtle in expression and often not seen until late in the course of the disease. Frequently, when clinical symptoms are absent, sensitive diagnostic testing can detect the presence of cardiac disease. Overt clinical signs of cardiac disease of any type are a poor prognostic sign and predict shortened survival[68].

Symptoms of scleroderma heart involvement include dyspnea on exertion, palpitations and less frequently chest discomfort. Clinical manifestations of pericarditis, congestive heart failure, pulmonary hypertension and arrhythmias are the main categories of cardiac disease reported in both limited and diffuse scleroderma. The evaluation of the heart can be done with a variety of sensitive methods but it must be remembered that many symptoms of cardiac disease are often linked to pulmonary scleroderma. Dyspnea on exertion is more likely to be secondary to scleroderma lung disease than significant heart problems until late in the course of scleroderma. However, palpitations, atypical chest pain or syncope may be secondary to arrhythmia or pericardial disease. A two-dimensional echocardiogram or ambulatory monitoring of the electrocardiogram is helpful in evaluating patients with symptoms suggesting cardiac disease.

Pericardial disease is found frequently by echocardiography and at autopsy but is usually asymptomatic. The most common finding by echocardiography is a pericardial effusion, although pathological specimens at autopsy also reveal fibrinous pericarditis with adhesions and inflammatory infiltrates[69]. Clinically overt pericarditis is uncommon, although hemodynamic compromise and pericardial tamponade can occur that require acute intervention. Uremic pericardial effusions may also occur in renal failure, a consequence of scleroderma renal crisis.

Ischemic chest pain and myocardial infarction are uncommon clinical problems in scleroderma. Thallium perfusion defects reflecting vascular disease of the endomyocardial vessels (not larger coronary arteries) are seen among scleroderma patients both at rest and with exercise. Because of this, the scleroderma patient with angina-like chest pain may need angiographic studies to rule out coronary arteriosclerosis because thallium scans are likely be abnormal as a result of the microvascular disease of scleroderma heart. In fact, cold provocation of Raynaud's phenomenon can temporarily increase the number of thallium scan defects and induce local abnormalities in ventricular wall motion, supporting the notion that reversible vasospasm of the myocardial microcirculation occurs in scleroderma[70]. Thallium scan perfusion defects predict more severe myocardial disease and poor outcome.

Patchy myocardial fibrosis is a fairly common finding at autopsy in scleroderma patients[70]. This finding is thought to occur secondary to ischemia–reperfusion events in the heart microvasculature causing contraction band necrosis of heart muscle. A decline in left ventricular ejection fraction is a late clinical manifestation, primarily in patients with diffuse skin disease. An abnormal left ventricular ejection fraction is demonstrated by radionucleotide scanning during exercise in approximately 40–50% of all patients, and approximately 15% of diffuse scleroderma patients have abnormalities at rest. Echocardiographic studies suggest that both right and left ventricular dysfunction is common in scleroderma and that diastolic left ventricular dysfunction may occur independent of systolic dysfunction. Diastolic dysfunction may be secondary to hypertension (with or without renal disease) or myocardial fibrosis and may manifest with abnormal left ventricular compliance and pulmonary vascular congestion. Unexplained dyspnea on exertion may be the initial clinical manifestation of unappreciated diastolic dysfunction.

Myocarditis can be associated with inflammatory muscle disease and present as sudden onset of congestive heart failure in a patient with scleroderma and myositis. In fact, patients with skeletal myositis are more likely to develop congestive heart failure or sudden cardiac death than patients without skeletal muscle involvement independent of clear evidence of myocarditis[71]. An endomyocardial biopsy may differentiate myocarditis from the muscle fibrosis seen in scleroderma.

Electrocardiography or Holter monitoring often shows conducting system disease or arrhythmias, which are usually clinically silent. Premature ventricular contractions are the most common arrhythmia; frequently they are in couplets or are multifocal. Premature atrial contractions, supraventricular tachycardia, AV or intraventricular conduction disorders are seen less commonly[72]. The prevalence of arrhythmias and conduction defects is greater among patients with diffuse scleroderma than in those with limited disease. The presence of arrhythmias is associated with a worse overall prognosis.

Renal involvement

The most important clinical manifestation of scleroderma kidney is accelerated hypertension and/or rapidly progressive renal failure: the scleroderma renal crisis[73] (see Chapter 135). Surveys suggest that only about 10% of all scleroderma patients develop a crisis. The majority of patients who develop renal crisis have diffuse cutaneous disease and approximately 80% of cases of renal crisis occur within 4 years of disease onset[74]. Risk factors for renal crisis include rapidly progressing diffuse skin disease, tendon friction rubs, new unexplained anemia and the presence of anti-RNA polymerase III antibody. Antecedent use of corticosteroids is also associated with a higher risk of developing renal crisis[75]. Non-malignant hypertension, abnormalities on urinalysis, plasma renin level[76] and the presence of anticentromere or antitopoisomerase antibodies are not predictors of a scleroderma renal crisis.

Patients with renal crisis may present with typical signs of malignant hypertension, including headache, altered vision, signs of heart failure and confusion or neurologic signs such as seizures in the setting of an abnormally high blood pressure (>150/90mmHg). However, there may be no specific symptoms and occasionally a normotensive crisis can occur. Laboratory data show normal or high creatinine, proteinuria and/or microscopic hematuria. A microangiopathic hemolytic anemia and thrombocytopenia can be present, especially in normotensive patients with renal crisis. A poorer outcome is seen in males, patients with an older age of onset and those who present with creatinine levels higher than 3mg/dl (230μmol/l)[77].

The typical vasculopathy of scleroderma is present in the renal vessels of patients with or without renal crisis. This suggests that other factors, such as vasospasm, probably contribute to the development of renal crisis. Scleroderma patients may have a reduced creatinine clearance, proteinuria, microscopic hematuria and non-malignant hypertension, but often another cause for these abnormalities is found. For example, an immune complex process may be the cause for glomerulonephritis in patients with an overlap syndrome of SLE and scleroderma. A reversible proteinuria or even a crescentic glomerulonephritis may occur secondary to treatment with **D**-penicillamine[78].

Other common clinical problems

Nervous system

Although it has been argued that the clinical features of scleroderma could be explained by a diffuse degenerative process in the nervous system, conclusive evidence for a primary nervous system disease is still lacking. Scleroderma spares the central nervous system and therefore signs of central nervous system disease usually have another explanation. The exception is trigeminal neuropathy, which may first present with facial numbness and then later with facial pain. Abnormal neural function, perhaps secondary to microvascular disease, may explain the early manifestation of gastrointestinal disease (see above). Similarly, Raynaud's phenomenon may partially be a manifestation of enhanced adrenergic nerve responses of vascular smooth muscle. Sensitive peripheral nerve testing may disclose abnormal cutaneous sensory thresholds. Entrapment neuropathy occurs from carpal tunnel syndrome or ulnar nerve entrapment at the elbow. A recent survey shows that nearly 50% of patients with scleroderma have symptoms of depression[79]. The severity of depression correlates more with personality traits and the degree of supportive care available than with the severity of the disease. Sexual dysfunction is also common in scleroderma. Impotence among male patients is usually secondary to neurovascular disease, although non-organic dysfunction should be investigated.

Fertility and pregnancy

Investigations thus far do not clarify whether patients with scleroderma have any increased risk for infertility, miscarriage or low-birthweight infants or not. However, it is clear that pregnancy aggravates the gastrointestinal and cardiopulmonary symptoms of scleroderma and adds risk for the patient[80]. There is also evidence that an increased risk for scleroderma renal crisis exists. Therefore, patients should be closely monitored, in conjunction with a high-risk obstetrician, with frequent measurements of blood pressure and urinalyses.

Malignancy in scleroderma

Population-based surveys reveal a higher incidence of malignancy in scleroderma patients[81,82]. The types of cancer reported include lung cancer, non-melanoma skin cancer and liver cancer[81]. Although there has been some controversy over the association of scleroderma with excess breast cancer, there is strong evidence that more lung cancer occurs than would be expected in the general population, probably related to interstitial lung disease[67]. Adenocarcinoma of the esophagus associated with chronic gastroesophageal reflux has also been reported in patients with scleroderma[83].

Endocrinopathy

Hypothyroidism can occur either secondary to thyroid fibrosis or from autoimmune thyroiditis. One study revealed that all patients with hypothyroidism had some degree of fibrosis on microscopic evaluation, although some did have a lymphocytic infiltrate as well[84]. Subclinical thyroid disease was detected in up to 20% of patients by a sensitive evaluation[85]. Other endocrinopathies are no more common in scleroderma patients than in the general population.

INVESTIGATIONS

Measuring disease activity and severity

Ideal clinical and laboratory measurements of disease 'activity' do not exist in scleroderma[86]. The degree of disease activity can be confused with 'severity-damage' or irreversible loss of function of an organ or body system[86]. A variety of laboratory measurements have been proposed as important tools to measure disease, including various cytokines, collagen metabolites, factors signifying vascular perturbation (e.g. von Willebrand factor) and components signifying inflammation or activation of the immune system, although none of these are widely used clinically.

Subjective clinical parameters are also used as measurements of disease activity, although it is unclear what is the best parameter to measure this activity. Popular clinical measurements include skin score, hand extension, oral aperture, finger flexion and global patient and physician assessments of disease activity. Most clinical observations detail the cutaneous manifestations because the skin is directly measurable by observation and palpation. Although the natural course of the skin changes is reasonably well described in diffuse scleroderma, it must be remembered that the cutaneous disease may not be the ideal surrogate for the overall disease activity. For example, significant cardiopulmonary and gastrointestinal disease can emerge later in the course, at a time when the skin may be improving or thinning. In limited scleroderma, the skin fibrosis is minimal and does not parallel the vascular disease such as pulmonary hypertension and digital loss.

Recently, a quantitative measure of disease severity has been developed that documents the degree of severity of involvement of each major organ graded from 0 (normal) to 4 (end-stage)[87] (Table 133.4). This scale has been externally validated on a large group of scleroderma patients and may be helpful in comparing groups of patients in clinical trials and for following disease in individual patients.

Method of measuring skin involvement

Palpation of the skin to detect skin thickening has been shown to be a reliable semiquantitative method that correlates with the weight of a punch biopsy of the skin in the same area[88]. The examiner should attempt to pinch the skin and then assess the thickness of the skinfold between the fingers. Although the thickness is due to an increase in the dermal skin layer, often the skin will be fixed to subdermal tissues. It is important to distinguish thickening of the skin of early disease from 'involved skin' of late disease, which can be thinned (atrophic), tethered or bound down. Late-stage skin is often thinner than normal skin and less flexible.

A simplified total skin score (modified Rodnan skin thickness score) is obtained by the examiner pinching the skin in 17 sites, scoring each area from 0–3 (0 = normal skin; 3 = extreme thickening) and then summing the score of all the palpated sites (Fig. 133.24)[88]. In clinical practice, serial measurements of the skin involvement will help define the stage and course of the skin disease, with higher skin scores suggesting more aggressive internal organ disease.

TABLE 133.4 DISEASE SEVERITY SCALE

System	0 (normal)	1 (mild)	2 (moderate)	3 (severe)	4 (end-stage)
General	Normal	Weight loss of 5.0–9.9kg *or* hematocrit 33.0–36.9	Weight loss of 10.0–14.9kg *or* hematocrit 29.0–32.9	Weight loss of 15.0–19.9kg *or* hematocrit 25.0–28.9	Weight loss of 20+kg *or* hematocrit <25.0
Raynaud's	Normal	Vasodilator-requiring	Digital pitting scars	Active digital pit ulceration	Digital gangrene
Skin score	0	1–14	15–29	30–39	40+
Finger to palm (cm)	<1	1.0–1.9	2.0–3.9	4.0–4.9	5.0+
Proximal weakness	None	Mild	Moderate	Severe	Cannot walk
GI status	Normal	Requires antireflux medication *or* abnormal small bowel series	High dose antireflux medication *or* antibiotics for bacterial overgrowth	Malabsorption syndrome *or* episodes of pseudo-obstruction	TPN required
Lung	Normal	FVC *or* $D_L$co 70–80% predicted *or* rales *or* fibrosis on chest X-ray	FVC *or* $D_L$co 50–69% predicted *or* mild pulmonary hypertension	FVC *or* $D_L$co 50% predicted *or* moderate–severe pulmonary hypertension	Oxygen required
Heart	Normal	ECG conduction defect *or* LVEF 45–49%	Arrhythmia *or* RVE + LVE *or* LVEF 40–44%	LVEF <40%	Congestive heart failure *or* arrhythmia requiring medication
Kidney	Normal	Creatinine 1.3–1.6 *or* uprot 2+	Creatinine 1.7–2.9 *or* uprot 3–4+	Creatinine 3.0+	Requires dialysis

LVE, left ventricular enlargement; LVEF, left ventricular ejection fraction, RVE, right ventricular enlargement; TPN, total parenteral nutrition. (Modified from Medsger *et al.*[87])

CLINICAL ASSESSMENT OF SKIN THICKENING

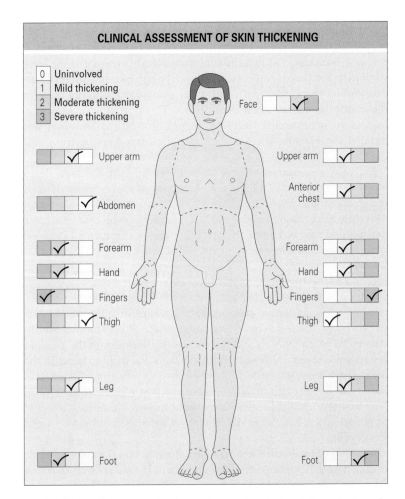

0 Uninvolved
1 Mild thickening
2 Moderate thickening
3 Severe thickening

TABLE 133.5 AUTOANTIBODY ASSOCIATIONS WITH SCLERODERMA

Antibody	Prevalence (%)*	Clinical associations
Anti-topoisomerase 1 (Scl-70)	20–40	Diffuse skin disease Interstitial lung disease Increased mortality Cardiac disease
Anti-centromere	20–40	CREST syndrome Digital loss Pulmonary hypertension Primary biliary cirrhosis
Nucleolar antibodies		
RNA Polymerases	4–20	Renal crisis Cardiac disease Diffuse skin disease Tendon friction rubs Increased mortality
U3snRNP (fibrillarin)	8	African-American males Diffuse skin disease Pulmonary disease
Th	5	Limited skin disease
Nor-90	Rare	Unknown
Pm-Scl	1	Myositis
U1snRNP	5	Mixed connective tissue disease

* Among patients with scleroderma.

Fig. 133.24 Total skin score. Semiquantitative estimates by clinical palpation of the extent and severity of scleroderma skin change. In all cases, the initial areas involved are peripheral and are the most severely affected. The mild skin change on the chest permits classification of this subject as diffuse scleroderma.

Serologic associations

Recent findings suggest that serologic data can help predict clinical features and survival (Table 133.5). Scleroderma patients with anticentromere antibody are more likely to have CREST syndrome and have a relatively good prognosis but may develop pulmonary hypertension, digital amputation or biliary cirrhosis. Patients with anti-RNA polymerase antibody have an increased risk of cardiac or renal disease and a poor prognosis[89], while patients with antitopoisomerase[90] have a higher risk of pulmonary disease. Anti-U3-RNP (antifibrillarin) is seen in approximately 5% of patients, primarily African–American or Afro-Caribbean males with serious pulmonary disease[91]. Anti-PM-Scl and anti-Ku are associated with scleroderma with myositis in Caucasians and Japanese respectively[92].

DIFFERENTIAL DIAGNOSIS

The differential diagnosis of scleroderma includes other disorders associated with Raynaud's phenomenon, toxic exposures, other connective tissue diseases and conditions with cutaneous disease resembling scleroderma (Table 133.6). Silica exposure can cause a disease indistinguishable from idiopathic scleroderma including typical skin changes, Raynaud's phenomenon and antitopoisomerase antibodies in masons, gold and coal miners[93]. Eosinophilia–myalgia syndrome and toxic oil syndrome have skin disease that mimics scleroderma but are distinguished by other manifestations such as cognitive impairment, chronic pain and muscle cramping. Eosinophilic fasciitis causes a widespread deep tissue fibrosis but typically spares the fingers, hands and face. Scleredema also presents with skin thickening, especially in the back, neck and shoulder girdle, and occurs in association with type 1 diabetes and in patients with paraproteinemias. Scleroderma skin changes are seen in a variety of other disorders including chronic graft-versus-host disease, porphyria cutanea tarda, phenylketonuria, progeria-like syndromes, POEMS syndrome, localized lipoatrophies and bleomycin exposure (see also Chapter 137).

TABLE 133.6 DIFFERENTIAL DIAGNOSIS OF SCLERODERMA

Disorders characterized by similar presentations

Systemic lupus erythematosus
Rheumatoid arthritis
Inflammatory myopathy

Disorders characterized by similar visceral features

Primary pulmonary hypertension
Primary biliary cirrhosis
Idiopathic intestinal hypomotility
Collagenous colitis
Idiopathic interstitial pulmonary fibrosis

Disorders characterized by skin thickening

Affecting the fingers
  Diabetic digital sclerosis
  Vinyl chloride disease
  Vibration syndrome
  Bleomycin-induced scleroderma
  Chronic reflex sympathetic dystrophy
  Amyloidosis
  Acrodermatitis
  Scleromyxedema

Sparing the fingers
  Scleredema
  Eosinophilic fasciitis
  Eosinophilia–myalgia syndrome
  Generalized subcutaneous morphea
  Fibrosis associated with augmentative mammoplasty
  Amyloidosis
  Carcinoid syndrome
  Pentazocine-induced scleroderma

REFERENCES

1. Rodnan GP, Benedek TG. An historical account of the study of progressive systemic sclerosis (diffuse scleroderma). Ann Intern Med 1962; 57: 305–319.
2. Barnett AJ. History of scleroderma. In: Clements PJ, Furst DE, eds. Systemic sclerosis. Baltimore, MD: Williams & Wilkins; 1996: 3–22.
3. Raynaud M. On local asphyxia of the extremities, 1864. London: New Sydenham Society; 1888.
4. Osler, W. The principles and practice of medicine. New York: Appleton, 1894: 993.
5. Klemperer P, Pollack AD, Boehr G. Diffuse collagen disease: acute disseminated lupus erythematosus and diffuse scleroderma. JAMA 1942; 119: 331.
6. Goetz RH. Pathology of progressive systemic sclerosis (generalized scleroderma) with special reference to changes in the viscera. Clin Proc (S Afr) 1945; 4: 337–342.
7. Winterbauer RH. Multiple telangiectasia, Raynaud's phenomenon, sclerodactyly, and subcutaneous calcinosis: a syndrome mimicking hereditary hemorrhagic telangiectasia. Bull Johns Hopkins Hosp 1964; 114: 361–383.
8. Meyer O. From Thibierge–Weissenbach syndrome (1910) to anti-centromere antibodies (1980). Clinical and biological features of scleroderma. Ann Med Interne (Paris) 1999; 150: 47–52.
9. D'Angelo WA, Fries JF, Masi AT, Shulman LE. Pathologic observations in systemic sclerosis (scleroderma). A study of fifty-eight autopsy cases and fifty-eight matched controls. Am J Med 1969; 46: 428–440.
10. Medsger TA Jr. Epidemiology of systemic sclerosis. Clin Dermatol 1994; 12: 207–216.
11. Masi AT, Rodnan GP, Medsger TA Jr et al. Preliminary criteria for the classification of systemic sclerosis (scleroderma). Arthritis Rheum 1980; 23: 581–590.
12. Maricq HR, Kel JE, Sith EA et al. Prevalence of scleroderma spectrum disorders in the general population of South Carolina. Arthritis Rheum 1989; 32: 998–1006.
13. Arnett FC, Howard RF, Tan F et al. Increased prevalence of systemic sclerosis in a native American tribe in Oklahoma. Arthritis Rheum 1996; 39: 1362–1370.
14. Geirsson AJ, Steinsson K, Guthmundsson S, Sigurthsson V. Systemic sclerosis in Iceland. A nationwide epidemiological study. Ann Rheum Dis 1994; 53: 502–505.
15. Tan EM, Rodnan GP, Garcia I et al. Diversity of antinuclear antibodies in progressive systemic sclerosis. Anti-centromere antibody and its relationship to CREST syndrome. Arthritis Rheum 1980; 23: 617–615.
16. Laing TL, Gillespie BW, Toth MB et al. Racial differences in scleroderma among women in Michigan. Arthritis Rheum 1997; 40: 734–742.
17. Medsger TA Jr, Masi AT. Epidemiology of systemic sclerosis. Ann Intern Med 1971; 74: 714–721.
18. Silman AJ, Howard Y, Hicklin AJ, Black C. Geographical clustering of scleroderma in south and west London. Br J Rheumatol 1990; 29: 93–96.
19. Maricq HR. Geographic clustering of scleroderma. Br J Rheumatol 1990; 29: 241–243.
20. Haustein UF, Herrmann K. Environmental scleroderma. Clin Dermatol 1994; 12: 467–473.

21. Cook NJ, Silman AJ, Propert J, Cawley MI. Features of systemic sclerosis (scleroderma) in an identical twin pair. Br J Rheumatol 1993; 32: 926–928.

22. Feghali CA, Wright TM. Epidemiologic and clinical study of twins with scleroderma. Arthritis Rheum 1995; 38: S308.

23. Maddison PJ, Stephens C, Briggs D et al. Connective tissue disease and autoantibodies in the kindreds of 63 patients with systemic sclerosis. The United Kingdom Systemic Sclerosis Study Group. Medicine 1993; 72: 103–112.

24. Clements PJ, Hurwitz EL, Wong WK et al. Skin thickness score as a predictor and correlate of outcome in systemic sclerosis. Arthritis Rheum 2000; 43: 2445–2454.

25. Giordano M. Classification of progressive systemic sclerosis (scleroderma). In: Black CM, Myers AR, eds. Systemic sclerosis (scleroderma). New York: Gower; 1985: 21–23.

26. Masi A. Classification of systemic sclerosis (scleroderma). In: Black CM, Myers AR, eds. Systemic sclerosis (scleroderma). New York: Gower; 1985: 7–15.

27. Medsger TA Jr. Classification of systemic sclerosis. In: Jayson MIV, Black CM, eds. Systemic sclerosis: scleroderma. New York: John Wiley & Sons; 1988: 1–6.

28. Barnett AJ. Classification of systemic sclerosis (scleroderma). In: Black CM, Myers AR, eds. Systemic sclerosis (scleroderma). New York: Gower; 1985: 18–20.

29. LeRoy EC, Medsger TA Jr. Criteria for the classification of early systemic sclerosis. J Rheum 2001; 28: 1573–1576.

30. Poormoghim H, Lucas M, Fertig N et al. Systemic sclerosis sine scleroderma: demographic, clinical, and serologic features and survival in forty-eight patients. Arthritis Rheum 2000; 43: 444–451.

31. Alarcon-Segovia D. Mixed connective tissue disease and overlap syndromes. Clin Dermatol 1994; 12: 309–316.

32. Black C, Isenberg DA. Mixed connective tissue disease – goodbye to all that. Br J Rheumatol 1992; 31: 695–700.

33. Van de Hoogen FHJ, Spronk PE, Boerbooms AMT et al. Longterm follow-up of 46 patients with anti-U1snRNP antibodies. Br J Rheumatol 1994; 33: 1117–1120.

34. Steen VD, Medsger TA Jr. Severe organ involvement in systemic sclerosis with diffuse scleroderma. Arthritis Rheum 2000; 43: 2437–2444.

35. Bryan C, Knight C, Black CM et al. Prediction of five-year survival following presentation with scleroderma. Arthritis Rheum 1999; 42: 2660–2665.

36. Jacobsen S, Halberg P, Ullman S. Mortality and causes of death of 344 Danish patients with systemic sclerosis (scleroderma). Br J Rheumatol 1998; 37: 750–755.

37. Wigley FM, Wise RA, Miller R et al. Anti-centromere antibody predicts the ischemic loss of digits in patients with systemic sclerosis. Arthritis Rheum 1992; 35: 688–693.

38. Maricq HR, Carpentier PH, Weinrich MC et al. Geographic variation in the prevalence of Raynaud's phenomenon: Charleston, SC, USA, vs. Tarentaise, Savoie, France. J Rheumatol 1993; 20: 70–76.

39. O'Keeffe ST, Tsapatsaris NP, Beetham WP Jr. Color chart assisted diagnosis of Raynaud's phenomenon in an unselected hospital employee population. J Rheumatol 1992; 19: 1415–1417.

40. LeRoy EC, Medsger TA Jr. Raynaud's phenomenon: a proposal for classification. (Review). Clin Exp Rheumatol 1992; 10: 485–488.

41. Maricq HR, Weinberger AB, LeRoy EC. Early detection of scleroderma-spectrum disorders by in vivo capillary microscopy: a prospective study of patients with Raynaud's phenomenon. J Rheumatol 1982; 9: 289–291.

42. Zufferey P, Depairon M, Chamot AM, Monti M. Prognostic significance of nailfold capillary microscopy in patients with Raynaud's phenomenon and scleroderma-pattern abnormalities. A six-year follow-up study. Clin Rheumatol 1992; 11: 536–541.

43. Spencer-Green G. Outcomes in primary Raynaud phenomenon. Arch Intern Med 1998; 158: 595–600.

44. Kallenberg CG. Early detection of connective tissue disease in patients with Raynaud's phenomenon. Rheum Dis Clin North Am 1990; 16: 11–30.

45. Rodnan GP, Myerowitz RL, Justh GO. Morphologic changes in the digital arteries of patients with progressive systemic sclerosis (scleroderma) and Raynaud phenomenon. Medicine 1980; 59: 393–408.

46. Clements PJ, Lachenbruch PA, Furst DE et al. Abnormalities of renal physiology in systemic sclerosis. A prospective study with 10-year follow-up. Arthritis Rheum 1994; 37: 67–74.

47. Wigley FM, Wise RA, Stevens MB, Newball H. The effect of cold exposure on carbon monoxide diffusing capacity in patients with Raynaud's phenomenon. Chest 1982; 81: 695–698.

48. Shuck JW, Oetgen WJ, Tesar JT. Pulmonary vascular response during Raynaud's phenomenon in progressive systemic sclerosis. Am J Med 1985; 78: 221–227.

49. Oddis CV, Eisenbeis CH, Reidbord HE et al. Vasculitis in systemic sclerosis: association with Sjögren's syndrome and the CREST syndrome variant. J Rheumatol 1987; 14: 942–948.

50. Steen VD, Medsger TA Jr. The palpable tendon friction rub. Arthritis Rheum 1997; 40: 1146–1151.

51. Olsen NJ, King LE, Park JH. Muscle abnormalities in scleroderma. Rheum Dis Clin North Am 1996; 22: 783–796.

52. Clements PJ, Furst DE, Campion DS et al. Muscle disease in progressive systemic sclerosis: diagnostic and therapeutic considerations. Arthritis Rheum 1978; 21: 62–71.

53. Young MA, Rose S, Reynolds JC. Gastrointestinal manifestations of scleroderma. Rheum Dis Clin North Am 1996; 22: 797–823.

54. Cameron AJ, Payne WS. Barrett's esophagus occurring as a complication of scleroderma. Mayo Clin Proc 1978; 53: 612.

55. Clements PJ, Furst DE. Systemic sclerosis. Baltimore, MD: Williams & Wilkins; 1996.

56. Bassotti G, Battaglia E, Debernardi V et al. Esophageal dysfunction in scleroderma. Arthritis Rheum 1997; 40: 2252–2259.

57. Basilisco G, Barbera R, Molgora M et al. Acid clearance and oesophageal sensitivity in patients with progressive systemic sclerosis. Gut 1993; 34: 1487–1491.

58. Watson M, Hally R, McCue P et al. Gastric antral vascular ectasia (watermelon stomach) in patients with systemic sclerosis. Arthritis Rheum 1996; 39: 341–346.

59. Whitehead ME, Taitelbaum G, Wigley FM, Schuster MM. Rectosigmoid motility and myoelectric activity in progressive systemic sclerosis. Gastroenterology 1989; 96: 428–432.

60. Rose S, Young MA, Reynolds JC. Gastrointestinal disorders and systemic disease, Part I. Gastroenterol Clin North Am 1998; 27: 563–594.

61. Schneider P, Hochberg MC, Wise RA, Wigley FM. Serial pulmonary function in patients with systemic sclerosis. Am J Med 1982; 73: 385–394.

62. Steen VD, Conte C, Owens GR, Medsger TA Jr. Severe restrictive lung disease in systemic sclerosis. Arthritis Rheum 1994; 37: 1283–1289.

63. Steen VD. Conte G, Owens GR et al. Isolated diffusing capacity reduction in systemic sclerosis. Arthritis Rheum 1992; 35: 765–770.

64. Greidinger EL, Flaherty KT, White B et al. African-American race and antibodies to topoisomerase I are associated with increased severity of scleroderma lung disease. Chest 1998; 114: 801–807.

65. Peters-Golden M, Wise R, Hochberg M et al. Clinical and demographic predictors of loss of pulmonary function in systemic sclerosis. Medicine 1984; 63: 221–232.

66. Troshinsky MB, Kane GC, Varga J et al. Pulmonary function and gastroesophageal reflux in systemic sclerosis. Ann Intern Med 1994; 121: 6–10.

67. Peters-Golden M, Wise R, Hochberg M et al. Incidence of lung cancer in systemic sclerosis. J Rheumatol 1985; 12: 1136–1139.

68. Clements PJ, Lachenbruch PA, Furst DE et al. Cardiac score. A semiquantitative measure of cardiac involvement that improves prediction of prognosis in systemic sclerosis. Arthritis Rheum 1991; 34: 1371–1380.

69. Byers RJ, Marshall AS, Freemont AJ. Pericardial involvement in systemic sclerosis. Ann Rheum Dis 1997; 56: 393–394.

70. Deswal A, Follansbee WP. Cardiac involvement in scleroderma. Rheum Dis Clin North Am 1996; 22: 841–860.

71. Follansbee WP, Zerbe TR, Medsger TA Jr. Cardiac and skeletal muscle disease in systemic sclerosis (scleroderma): a high risk association. Am Heart J 1993; 125: 194–203.

72. Follansbee WP, Curtiss EI, Rahko PS et al. The electrocardiogram in systemic sclerosis (scleroderma). Study of 102 consecutive cases with functional correlations and review of the literature. Am J Med 1985; 79: 183–192.

73. Steen VD. Renal involvement in systemic sclerosis. Clin Dermatol 1994; 12: 253–258.

74. Traub YM, Shapiro AP, Rodnan GP et al. Hypertension and renal failure (scleroderma) renal crisis) in progressive systemic sclerosis. Review of a 25 year experience with 68 cases. Medicine 1983; 62: 335–352.

75. Steen VD, Medsger TA Jr. Case-control study of corticosteroids and other drugs that either precipitate or protect from the development of scleroderma renal crisis. Arthritis Rheum 1998; 41: 1613–1619.

76. Clements PJ, Lachenbruch PA, Furst DE et al. Abnormalities of renal physiology in systemic sclerosis. A prospective study with 10-year follow-up. Arthritis Rheum 1994; 37: 67–74.

77. Steen VD, Medsger TA Jr. Long-term outcomes of scleroderma renal crisis. Ann Intern Med 2000; 133: 600–603.

78. Garcia-Porrua C, Gonzalez-Gay MA, Bouza P. D-Penicillamine-induced crescentic glomerulonephritis in a patient with scleroderma. Nephron 2000; 84: 101–102.

79. Roca RP, Wigley FM, White B. Depressive symptoms in systemic sclerosis (scleroderma). Arthritis Rheum 1996; 39: 1035–1040.

80. Steen VD. Scleroderma and pregnancy. Rheum Dis Clin North Am 1997; 23: 133–147.

81. Abu-Shakra M, Guillemin F, Lee P. Cancer in systemic sclerosis. Arthritis Rheum 1993; 36: 460–464.

82. Rosenthal AK, McLaughlin JK, Gridley G et al. Incidence of cancer among patients with systemic sclerosis. Cancer 1995; 76: 910–914.

83. Heath EI, Limburg PJ, Hawk ET et al. Adenocarcinoma of the esophagus: risk factors and prevention. Oncology 2000; 14: 507–514.

84. Gordon MB, Klein I, Dekker A et al. Thyroid disease in progressive systemic sclerosis: increased frequency of glandular fibrosis and hypothyroidism. Ann Intern Med 1981; 95: 431–435.

85. Kahl LE, Medsger TA Jr, Klein I. Prospective evaluation of thyroid function in patients with systemic sclerosis (scleroderma). J Rheumatol 1986; 13: 103–107.

86. Clements PJ. Measuring disease activity and severity in scleroderma. Curr Opin Rheum 1995; 7: 517–521.

87. Medsger TA Jr, Silman AJ, Steen VD et al. A disease severity scale for systemic sclerosis: development and testing. J Rheumatol 1999; 26: 2159–2167.

88. Clements P, Lachenbruch P, Seibold J, Wigley FM. Inter- and intra-observer variability of total skin thickness score (modified Rodnan) in systemic sclerosis (SSc). J Rheumatol 1995; 22: 1281–1285.

89. Kuwana M, Kaburaki J, Mimori T et al. Autoantibody reactive with three classes of RNA polymerases in sera from patients with systemic sclerosis. J Clin Invest 1993; 91: 1399–1404.

90. Steen VD, Powell DL, Medsger TA Jr. Clinical correlations and prognosis based on serum autoantibodies in patients with systemic sclerosis. Arthritis Rheum 1988; 31: 196–203.

91. Okano Y, Steen VD, Medsger TA Jr. Autoantibody to U3 nucleolar ribonucleoprotein (fibrillarin) in patients with systemic sclerosis. Arthritis Rheum 1992; 35: 95–100.

92. Reichlin M, Maddison PJ, Targoff I *et al*. Antibodies to a nuclear/nucleolar antigen in patients with polymyositis overlap syndrome. J Clin Immunol 1984; 4: 40–44.

93. Rodnan GP, Benedek TG, Medsger TA Jr *et al*. The association of progressive systemic sclerosis (scleroderma) with coal miners' pneumoconiosis and other forms of silicosis. Ann Intern Med 1967; 66: 323–334.

134 Systemic sclerosis: etiology and pathogenesis

Edwin A Smith

Definition

- Disease characterized by fibrosis and microvascular occlusion

Etiology

- Specific human leukocyte antigen (HLA) types are associated with certain autoantibody specificities, but not with overall disease
- Certain haplotypes containing the fibrillin-1 gene are associated with the disease
- Environmental factors, such as solvent or drug exposure, may be important

Pathogenesis

- Activation of immune system and endothelial cells
- Release of cytokines (transforming growth factor-β, platelet-derived growth factor, interleukin-4 and others) from platelets, macrophages T cells
- Cytokine activation of fibroblasts to increase extracellular matrix production.

INTRODUCTION

Two processes, fibrosis and microvascular occlusion, characterize the pathologic findings seen in all involved organs of patients with systemic sclerosis. Any hypothesis of the pathogenesis of this disease must consider the mechanisms of extracellular matrix accumulation, immune cell activation and its consequences, and vascular endothelial injury. The development of methods to study these phenomena *in situ* in animals, and in cells *in vitro* has allowed a better understanding of these processes in patients with systemic sclerosis.

PATHOLOGY

Dermis

The pathologic hallmark of systemic sclerosis is an excessive accumulation of extracellular matrix in the dermis, which leads to taut skin[1]. Monotonously similar collagen fibers (Fig. 134.1) are present in the reticular dermis and there is thinning of the papillary dermis. There are associated deposits of fibronectin, glycosaminoglycans and tenascin. In the early stages of systemic sclerosis, an infiltration of mononuclear inflammatory cells, predominantly T cells[2], surrounding the dermal blood vessels (Fig. 134.2) is concentrated at the border between the reticular dermis and subcutaneous fat. Thickening of the reticular dermis results from perivascular expansion of collagen surrounding small islands of adipose tissue and encasing the base of hair follicles and cutaneous glands. Obliteration of these fat islands and follicles occurs in the later, atrophic stages of disease.

The vascular lesion shows intimal proliferation with luminal narrowing at the arterial and arteriolar levels. Capillary loss can be seen *in vivo* in the skin by the technique of wide-field nailfold capillaroscopy[3]. There

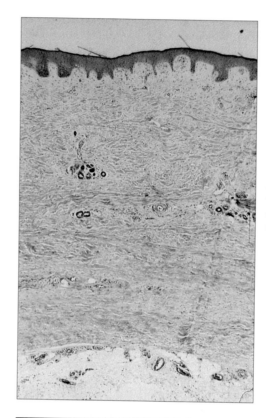

Fig. 134.1 **Excess collagen deposition in the dermis of a patient with systemic sclerosis.** There is marked thickening of the dermis with collagen and some inflammatory infiltrate surrounding vasculature. There is entrapment of cutaneous glands. Although atrophy of the epidermal rete pegs is a frequent finding, it is not evident in this example. (Hematoxylin and eosin.)

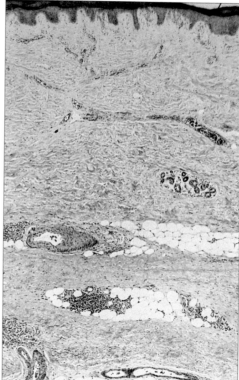

Fig. 134.2 **Inflammatory infiltrate in a dermal systemic sclerosis lesion.** The skin in systemic sclerosis has a mononuclear cell inflammatory infiltrate in the perivascular areas, expansion of the collagenous reticular dermis, encasement of sweat glands and expansion of the collagenous region into the subcutaneous adipose tissue. This biopsy specimen, obtained from a patient with systemic sclerosis of 8 years duration, demonstrates the persistence of the inflammatory infiltrate. (Hematoxylin and eosin.)

is alteration of the very regular, fine forest of dermal capillary loops, with both obliteration of some capillaries and dilatations of others.

One of the vascular hallmarks of systemic sclerosis, of either the limited (subcutaneous **c**alcinosis, **R**aynaud's phenomenon, **e**sophageal dysmotility, **s**clerodactyly, **t**elangiectasia: CREST syndrome) or diffuse form of the disease, is telangiectasia, particularly over the face, hands and anterior chest. These telangiectasias are clumps of dilated dermal capillaries.

Lung

Both fibrotic lesions and vascular lesions are evident in the lungs of patients with systemic sclerosis. Although these often coexist, there is a sizeable group of patients who have one without the other. Dissociation of the two lesions is usually found in patients with limited systemic sclerosis for several decades who develop the isolated vascular lesion. In this setting, marked intimal proliferation with resulting narrowing of the lumen is typically accompanied by medial thickening (Fig. 134.3). The physiologic result is pulmonary hypertension, which may lead to intractable right heart failure with multiple pulmonary emboli found at

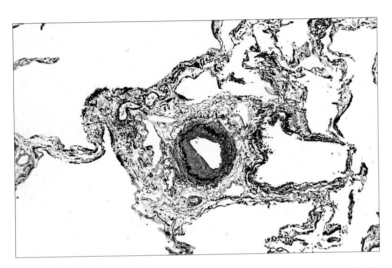

Fig. 134.3 Pulmonary artery intimal fibrosis. This elastin stain (elastin = black) shows the thickening of the intima in a small pulmonary artery in the area on the lumen side of the elastic lamina. There is only mild interstitial fibrosis in this specimen from an individual who died from pulmonary hypertension accompanying limited systemic sclerosis (CREST syndrome).

autopsy. The initial stage of the pulmonary fibrotic lesion is inflammation within alveolar air spaces[4]. In individuals with restrictive pulmonary mechanics, there is an increase in the number of cells obtained by bronchoalveolar lavage compared with the numbers obtained from healthy individuals or from patients with systemic sclerosis without restrictive lung disease. These cells are mostly alveolar macrophages, but there are also more granulocytes (both polymorphonuclear leukocytes and eosinophils).

The histology of fibrotic lung disease is that of expansion of the normally thin alveolar wall interstitial space with the deposition of collagen and other connective tissue components. Progressive collagen accumulation with diminution of the alveolar air space volume, so that ultimately there is more fibrous tissue than air space (Fig. 134.4), causes a gas diffusion blockade, an increase in the alveolar–arterial $P\text{O}_2$ gradient and ventilation–perfusion inequalities. Pulmonary hypertension may develop either as a result of this alveolar fibrosis or because of widespread vascular disease with intimal proliferation and luminal narrowing. The effects on the pulmonic and triscuspid valves and the right atrium and ventricle are those seen in any form of pulmonary hypertension. The pleura can be involved to a minor degree, with inflammatory and fibrotic reactions that are not usually of functional significance.

Heart

Both the pericardium and myocardium can develop lesions. Pericardial disease is characterized by fibrosis with occasional constrictive pericarditis; effusive pericarditis with tamponade is rare. The myocardium shows typical intimal proliferation and luminal narrowing of the small vessels (Fig. 134.5). Surrounding such damaged blood vessels are areas of fibrosis replacing myocardium (Fig. 134.6). The early lesion appears to be the development of contraction band necrosis, similar to that seen early in myocardial infarction. This histologic evidence suggests that the primary insult in the myocardium is ischemic and is the result of structural vascular disease, with superimposed vasospasm.

Gastrointestinal tract

Any part of the gastrointestinal tract with a smooth muscle layer can be affected. Esophageal involvement is most common, but proximal small bowel, stomach and colon are also often affected. There is fibrosis of the lamina propria and submucosa and of the muscular layer, with perivascular collections of inflammatory cells similar to those seen in the dermal lesion. This fibrosis leads to diminished peristalsis. The com-

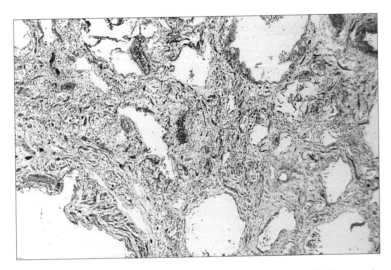

Fig. 134.4 Pulmonary interstitial fibrosis in systemic sclerosis. Thickening of the alveolar septa with connective tissue is evident in this specimen obtained from an individual who died as a result of hypoxemia. An inflammatory component accompanies the increase in matrix substance. (Hematoxylin and eosin.)

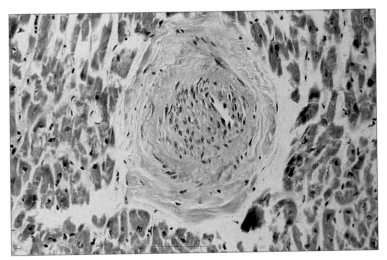

Fig. 134.5 Arterial disease in the myocardium. An intramyocardial artery shows intimal proliferation and consequent narrowing of the vascular lumen, characteristic of arteries throughout the organs involved in systemic sclerosis. There is also some evidence of myocarditis in this specimen, with inflammatory cells located between the myocardial cells. (Hematoxylin and eosin.)

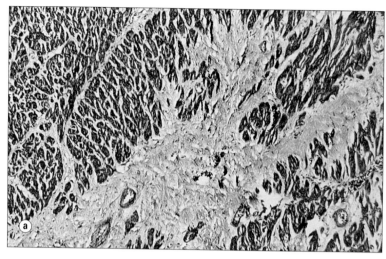 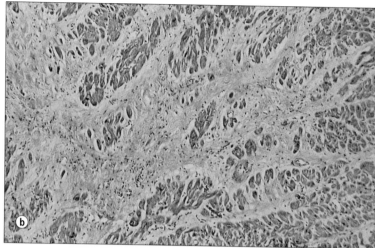

Fig. 134.6 Myocardial fibrosis in systemic sclerosis. (a) There is a remarkable perivascular and perimysial increase in collagen (blue-stained material) in this myocardial specimen (Masson's trichrome). These areas of fibrosis can be quite extensive, resulting in myocardial failure or serving as foci for arrhythmias. (b) Fibrosis can also involve the conducting system, resulting in heart block.

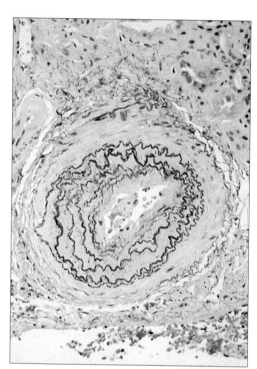

Fig. 134.7 Renal blood vessel in systemic sclerosis. An artery from an individual with renal failure secondary to systemic sclerosis demonstrates the luminal narrowing caused by intimal proliferation. There is evident reduplication of the elastic lamina, as seen in the concentric layering in the media.

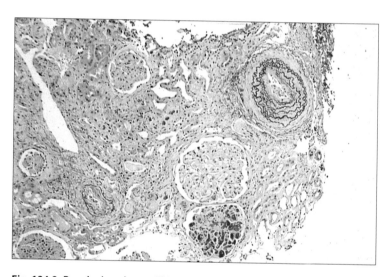

Fig. 134.8 Renal scleroderma. This specimen from a renal biopsy of a patient with renal scleroderma shows the vascular disease in blood vessels (bottom left and upper right), which have narrowed lumina and reduplication of elastic lamina. One glomerulus (top) shows evidence of fibrinoid deposition (darker pink color) as a reflection of thrombosis in the glomerulus.

bined effect of disrupted peristalsis, fibrosis and atrophy of the muscularis results in the development of wide-mouth diverticula in the colon. Recurrent peptic ulcerations in the distal esophagus can result in scarring, with stricture formation. Metaplasia of the lower esophagus (Barrett's esophagus) can develop.

Kidney

Small renal arteries and arterioles are the vessels primarily affected, with intimal proliferation, medial thinning, reduplication of the elastic lamina and, often, fibrinoid necrosis (Fig. 134.7). Duplication of the glomerular basement membrane similar to that in diabetes is seen, but without glomerulonephritis. Shrunken glomeruli, with involvement of individual glomerular capillary tufts, result from local ischemia (Fig. 134.8). Sclerotic glomeruli are characteristic of ischemic cortical infarction and end-stage renal systemic sclerosis. One frequent concomitant renal involvement is microangiopathic hemolysis (Fig. 134.9), resulting from physical disruption of erythrocytes in the severely disordered renal circulation.

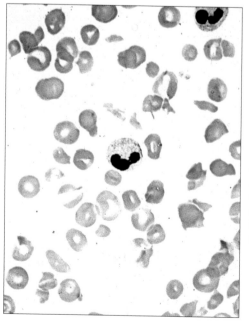

Fig. 134.9 Hemolysis in systemic sclerosis renal disease. A peripheral blood smear from an individual with systemic sclerosis with renal failure shows several fragmented erythrocytes and thrombocytopenia. This change in erythrocyte morphology is the result of thrombosis within arteries and arterioles, with the passage of erythrocytes through fibrin clots resulting in the fragmentation.

Musculoskeletal

Skeletal muscle involvement occurs most commonly as an expansion of the perifascicular fibrous tissue and as disease in the smaller arteries and arterioles, with diminution of the capillary number. This type of skeletal muscle involvement is characterized clinically by only a minimal reduction in strength and a slight increase in serum muscle enzymes. Inflammatory muscle involvement, similar to polymyositis or dermatomyositis with perivascular lymphocytic infiltration, muscle necrosis and degenerating–regenerating muscle fibers, is more rare and associated with clinically significant proximal muscle weakness and major increases in serum concentrations of muscle enzymes.

Tendon sheaths often have deposition of fibrin and collagen, with resultant limitation of movement of tendons, tendon friction rubs and the development of flexion contractures, particularly of the digits. Synovitis may occur occasionally, but erosive arthritis is unusual.

ETIOLOGY

The cause of systemic sclerosis remains unknown. Proposed initiating factors include chemical exposure, mechanical stimuli and viruses. The widespread locations of the pathologic lesions and their structural similarity indicate the systemic nature of systemic sclerosis and that some circulating substance or cell type is important. The cell types involved include microvascular endothelial cells, interstitial fibroblasts, vascular wall smooth muscle cells, T and B lymphocytes, monocytes (macrophages), neutrophils, mast cells and eosinophils. Both cell-to-cell interactions, mediated by direct contact and by interleukins and cytokines, and cell-to-matrix interactions participate in the pathogenesis of systemic sclerosis. Factors influencing disease include both cell-mediated and humoral immunity to vascular structures, enhanced and persistent expression of adhesion molecules on endothelial cells and failure of activated fibroblasts to downregulate matrix production. The last of these is perhaps caused by a defective integrin-dependent signal transduction mechanism or a cytokine-induced change in phenotype.

Genetic factors

Sex strongly influences the risk of developing systemic sclerosis, with the reported female:male ratio ranging from 2:1 to 20:1. The role of female sex hormones in disease pathogenesis is unknown. Systemic sclerosis occurs in more frequently in first-degree relatives of patients with systemic sclerosis than in the general population[5]. Chromosome fragility has been demonstrated in systemic sclerosis and there is reduced telomere (the non-coding ends of chromosomes) length both in patients with systemic sclerosis and in their family members[6]. These may reflect a genetic predisposition to systemic sclerosis or exposure to a common environmental agent.

Studies of major histocompatibility complex (MHC) antigens (human leukocyte antigen, HLA) in patient populations have led to conflicting results. A British study[7] linked Al, B8, DR3 with DR5 and with DRw52 in systemic sclerosis, but an American study showed no link with DR5. In Japan, reports have linked HLA-Bw52, DR2 and DR4. The occurrence of specific autoantibodies is associated with certain MHC class II alleles. Anticentromere antibodies are associated with the *HLA-DQB1*05* allele and less frequently with *DQB1*0301* and *DQB1*0401* or *DQB1*0402*[8]. In contrast, antitopoisomerase I antibodies are associated with *HLA-DQB1*0301* and less strongly with *DQB1*0302* and *DQB1*06* in whites and African-Americans, and with *HLA-DQB1*0601* and *HLA-DQB1*0301* in Japanese patients[9]. All these antitopoisomerase I antibody-associated alleles contain a tyrosine residue at position 30. Antibodies to fibrillarin are associated with *DRB1*1302*, *DQB1*0604*, *DQB1*0301*, *DQB1*0302* and *DQB1*0602*, and are seen in persons with diffuse skin, cardiac and renal involvement, and pulmonary fibrosis[10].

Choctaw Native Americans have a high incidence of systemic sclerosis, and it is likely that Choctaw individuals with systemic sclerosis have a single common ancestor. A 2cM haplotype containing two intragenic markers for the fibrillin-1 (*FBN-1*) gene on chromosome 15q was found to be increased in Choctaw patients with systemic sclerosis[11]. This section of chromosomal DNA was examined because the known genetic defect in the tight skin mouse 1 is in the *FBN* gene. Furthermore, one single nucleotide polymorphism (T to C) in the 5′-untranslated region of the *FBN-1* gene is strongly associated with systemic sclerosis in the Choctaw[12]. This single nucleotide polymorphism is present on two *FBN-1* gene haplotypes found only in the patients with systemic sclerosis. These same two haplotypes are also associated with systemic sclerosis in a cohort of Japanese patients. These data are consistent with the hypothesis that *FBN-1* or a nearby gene on chromosome 15q is involved in susceptibility to systemic sclerosis. The Choctaw, Japanese and African Americans (but not whites) with systemic sclerosis have antibodies to fibrillin-1, but the various ethnic groups recognize different epitopes on the fibrillin-1 protein[13].

No association can be made between systemic sclerosis and types I and III procollagen gene restriction fragment length polymorphisms[14]. There are suggestions of an abnormal fibronectin gene[15] and of a specific restriction fragment length polymorphism in the gene coding for the gamma chain of the T cell receptor[16].

Environmental factors

Several substances have been associated with systemic sclerosis and systemic sclerosis-like conditions (Table 134.1). Although the majority of patients with clear-cut systemic sclerosis can give no history of exposure to such chemicals, exposure-related disease may provide insight into the pathogenesis of idiopathic disease (see Chapters 132 and 137). Among the chemicals most commonly associated with systemic sclerosis-like conditions are organic solvents such as toluene, benzene, trichloroethylene and hexachloroethane. These solvents may induce endothelial damage, with subsequent platelet activation. Whether the immune system is mediating these injury patterns is also unclear. The evidence for a relationship to exposure to organic solvent is most compelling for males who have antibodies to topoisomerase I[17]. Certain alleles of cytochrome P450, important in the metabolism of organic solvents, are associated with systemic sclerosis after exposure to such chemicals[18]. There are specific genotypes, linked to impaired metabolism of organic solvents, that increase susceptibility to systemic sclerosis.

Drugs that cause systemic sclerosis-like illnesses include pentazocine, contaminated L-tryptophan and bleomycin. Bleomycin, when used systemically for treatment of testicular cancer (particularly in combination with *cis*-platinum) may cause Raynaud's phenomenon, lung fibrosis and dermal lesions histologically similar to those seen in idiopathic systemic sclerosis. The development of Raynaud's phenomenon indicates that the

---

TABLE 134.1 ENVIRONMENTAL FACTORS ASSOCIATED WITH SYSTEMIC SCLEROSIS-LIKE CONDITIONS

Chemicals

- Silica
- Vinyl chloride
- Benzene
- Toluene
- Trichloroethylene
- Perchloroethylene

Drugs

- Bleomycin
- Pentazocine
- Spanish toxic oil
- Contaminated L-tryptophan

likely effect of this drug is to damage the endothelium, with resultant sclerosis of the dermis.

Exposure to vinyl chloride leads to the development of Raynaud's phenomenon, acro-osteolysis, sclerotic dermal lesions and pulmonary fibrosis. One study has linked *HLA-DR5* to more severe vinyl chloride disease, along with linkage to the *A1, B8, DR3* autoimmune haplotype[19].

An epidemic of a systemic sclerosis-like illness occurred in Spain as the result of exposure to aniline-adulterated rapeseed cooking oil. The acute illness was characterized by eosinophilia and by constitutional, pulmonary and gastrointestinal symptoms. A chronic phase with myositis, subcutaneous edema, peripheral neuropathy, systemic sclerosis-like dermal lesions and pulmonary hypertension was characterized pathologically by diffuse vasculopathy with early endothelial loss and intimal proliferation.

PATHOGENESIS

Immune system activation

An important role for the immune system in systemic sclerosis pathogenesis is increasingly recognized, as tests for immunologic abnormalities have become more sensitive and specific. There are findings in both the humoral and cell-mediated arms of the system.

Humoral immunity

Non-specific serologic abnormalities including polyclonal hypergammaglobulinemia, cryoglobulinemia, rheumatoid factor and false-positive Veneral Disease Research Laboratory (VDRL) tests occur at frequencies greater than those in a healthy population. The erythrocyte sedimentation rate is variably normal or increased.

About 95% of patients have detectable antinuclear antibodies when proliferating cell lines, such as HEp-2, are used as the detection substrate[20] (Table 134.2) All types of staining patterns may be seen, but nucleolar patterns are more specific than others. Associations exist between the presence of antibodies to certain nuclear antigens and clinical manifestations of systemic sclerosis. Antibodies to centromeres occur in about 40% of patients with limited cutaneous disease, but in only 2–5% of patients with diffuse cutaneous disease. The specific centromeric antigens recognized by sera from patients with the limited cutaneous form have been named CENP-A, CENP-B and CENP-C and are 19, 80 and 140kDa in molecular mass, respectively[21]. The presence of antibodies to these antigens in the sera of patients may account for the high rate of chromosomal breakage and sister chromatid exchange that are seen. In contrast, antibodies to topoisomerase I (Scl-70) are present much more frequently in diffuse cutaneous systemic sclerosis (30–40%). Topoisomerase I is a nuclear enzyme important in the unwinding of DNA for replication and RNA transcription. The presence of antitopoisomerase I antibodies is associated with rapid skin thickening, pul-

monary interstitial fibrosis and renal crisis. T cell help has been shown to be essential for B cell production of antitopoisomerase I antibodies[22].

Antibodies to RNA polymerase types I, II and III are seen frequently in systemic sclerosis, and account for the occurrence of antinucleolar antinuclear antibody (ANA) staining[23]. Antibodies to other extractable nuclear antigens have clinical significance. Antibodies to the antigens Ku and Pm/Scl are seen in some patients with systemic sclerosis with inflammatory myopathy. There are marked racial differences in the occurrence of the various autoantibodies in the clinical subsets of systemic sclerosis, making the regulation of expression of these specific antibodies of interest. Linkage of certain autoantibody types with specific *HLA* loci has been demonstrated (see above).

How antibodies to nuclear materials may be involved in the pathogenesis remains very much a mystery (see Chapter 120). Speculation includes ANA-induced damage to the endothelial cells. Other possibilities include ANA-induced modulation of gene promoter regions, transactivating factors and cell replication. However, how immunoglobulins could cause such effects is unknown. Of course, ANAs may be epiphenomena, occurring as a byproduct of the disease mechanisms but playing no direct part themselves.

One study showed that sera from 19% of patients with systemic sclerosis were able to support antibody-dependent cellular cytotoxicity of human microvascular endothelial cells by peripheral blood mononucleocytes (PBMs) from normal individuals[24]. This phenomenon is mediated by natural killer type lymphocytes, which have Fcγ receptors but lack Tcell receptors for antigen (CD16$^+$, CD3$^-$). The systemic sclerosis sera positive for antibody-dependent cellular cytotoxicity were not cytotoxic in the absence of effector cells, and such effector cells have been found in six of 16 skin biopsies of patients. Antibodies to endothelial cell membranes have been demonstrated in the sera of the majority of patients with systemic sclerosis, particularly those with the lcSSc variant and pulmonary hypertension[25,26]. Such antiendothelial cell antibodies from patients with systemic sclerosis increase adhesion of monocytic cells to endothelial cells by a mechanism dependent on interleukin (IL)-1[27].

Circulating antibodies to connective tissue self proteins also occur in systemic sclerosis. Antibodies to types I, III, IV and VI collagens have been found in patients, particularly early in the disease, and such antibodies, particularly to type IV collagen, have been associated with the severity of interstitial lung disease[28]. Antibodies have also been found that recognize laminin. As both type IV collagen and laminin are important components of subendothelial basement membranes, antibodies to these proteins may have a role in pathogenesis.

Cell-mediated immunity

Lymphocytes

Many studies have analyzed the circulating lymphocyte populations and their function in patients with systemic sclerosis. There is an absolute lymphopenia with a normal ratio of T to B cells, but an increased ratio of T helper-inducer to T suppressor cells. Mononuclear inflammatory cells, almost all of which are activated helper-inducer T cells[2], accumulate in the dermis early in the course of the illness. In the skin of patients with systemic sclerosis, CD4$^+$ T cells predominate, but CD8$^+$ T cells predominate in the lungs. Vδ1$^+$ γ/δ T cells are increased in both the blood and lungs of patients with systemic sclerosis[29].

Circulating lymphocyte populations provide excessive T cell help activity to pokeweed mitogen-driven B cell IgM synthesis. Functional analyses of PBMs, assessed by proliferative responses to non-specific mitogens and by autologous and allogenic mixed lymphocyte reactions, have given conflicting results and add little insight to possible mechanisms of disease. In contrast, Huffstutter *et al*[30]. examined specific stimulation of PBMs in systemic sclerosis and found significant blast transformation in 47% of their patients when the cells were cultured

TABLE 134.2 AUTOANTIBODIES IN SYSTEMIC SCLEROSIS		
Autoantigen recognized	Percentage of patients	SSc type
Nuclei	95	Both
Centromere	10–20	lcSSc
Topoisomerase I (Scl-70)	15–25	dcSSc
RNA polymerase I, II, III	10–25	dcSSc
U3-RNP (fibrillarin)	5–45	dcSSc
Th/To RNP	5	lcSSc
U1-RNP	5–35	lcSSc
Pm/Scl	4	lcSSc with myositis

dcSSc, diffuse cutaneous systemic sclerosis; lcSSc, limited cutaneous systemic sclerosis; SSc, systemic sclerosis.

with laminin, and in 12% when the cells were cultured with type IV collagen. Whether cellular immunity to these endothelial basement membrane antigens is a cause or result of the vascular lesions is unknown.

Despite these limitations, several lines of evidence support a role for T cells in the pathogenesis of systemic sclerosis. Serum concentrations of both IL-2 (a T-cell-derived cytokine) and IL-2 receptors are increased, and correlate with disease severity[31]. IL-2 production by PBMs is augmented by exposure to type I collagen. IL-2 is capable of converting natural killer cells into lymphokine-activated killer cells, which may be important in direct endothelial injury. Studies using more traditional cells for targets have usually shown diminished numbers or function, or both, of natural killer cells[32], but both normal and systemic sclerosis PBMs can be induced to kill endothelial cells equally well when PBMs are preincubated with IL-2[33]. Increased binding of lymphocytes to umbilical vein endothelial cells and a proliferative response of lymphocytes cocultured with endothelial cells have been demonstrated. Chronic graft versus host disease, a model of systemic sclerosis that is manifested, in some bone marrow transplantation recipients, by Raynaud's phenomenon, dermal sclerosis (particularly of the digits) and vascular lesions[34], appears to involve T cells. These findings support the theory that T cells reacting against cellular antigens are likely candidates for a deleterious effector cell involved in systemic sclerosis. Increased concentrations of T cell serine proteases (granzymes) have been found in systemic sclerosis sera and the mRNA for these enzymes is expressed in systemic sclerosis dermis. These enzymes are capable of damaging endothelial cells, and may therefore be an important link between the immune and vascular lesions[35].

Recent research has highlighted a phenomenon known as 'microchimerism'. Circulating fetal immune cells have been demonstrated to persist in previously pregnant women. Because systemic sclerosis has similarities to chronic graft versus host disease occurring after bone marrow transplantation, several investigators have examined patients with systemic sclerosis for this immune cell microchimerism. In one investigation, evidence of Y chromosome material was sought in peripheral blood cells, T lymphocytes and skin biopsies from female patients with systemic sclerosis[36]. Y chromosomal material was found in the peripheral blood cells of 46% of female patients with systemic sclerosis, but only 4% of controls. In three female patients with systemic sclerosis who had male offspring, all had circulating T lymphocytes with Y chromosome sequences. Skin biopsies showed Y chromosome material in 58% of patients with systemic sclerosis. The hypothesis is that lymphocyte microchimerism is one etiologic factor. Systemic sclerosis in males would be explained by microchimerism resulting from transplacental acquisition of maternal lymphocytes.

Mononuclear phagocytes

Macrophages are seen in the dermal mononuclear cell infiltrates of patients with systemic sclerosis[37] and are increased in number in the pulmonary alveoli. These multifunctional cells are important as a source of several secreted products capable of affecting other cell types. Alveolar macrophages are activated and synthesize larger amounts of fibronectin *in vitro* than do similar cells isolated from normal individuals. Activated macrophages are known to be able to produce several other soluble mediators, including transforming growth factor (TGF)-β, platelet-derived growth factor (PDGF), tumor necrosis factor (TNF)-α, IL-1β, IL-6, IL-8, proteases and others, which may be important in the pathogenesis of systemic sclerosis.

Mast cells

Mast cells, which are found closely opposed to the microvessels in systemic sclerosis lesions, contain several very potent substances within their metachromatic granules that can affect endothelial cells and stimulate fibroblasts. Tryptase is a potent endopeptidase capable of injuring endothelial cells and activating TGF-β. Histamine stimulates prolifera-

tion of, and matrix synthesis by, fibroblasts and can cause endothelial cell retraction. Fibroblasts are also capable of engulfing and incorporating mast cell granules into their cytoplasm, a capacity that may make them exquisitely sensitive to signaling by mast cells.

Mast cells are prominent in several *in vivo* fibrotic reactions, including chronic graft versus host disease, interstitial pulmonary fibrosis and the tight skin (TSK/$^+$) mouse model of systemic sclerosis[38]. Mast cells are present in increased numbers in the dermis of lesions. Sera from patients with systemic sclerosis contain four times more eosinophil cationic protein (derived from mast cell granules) than do normal sera[39]. Blockade of mast cell degranulation by either cromolyn sodium or ketotifen in the tight skin mouse diminishes fibrosis.

The fibrotic lesion

The deposition of increased amounts of collagens, fibronectin and glycosaminoglycans in the involved tissues is one of the major clinical hallmarks of systemic sclerosis[40]. The increased deposition of collagen has been confirmed in the dermis, kidney, heart, lung and gastrointestinal tract and is caused by an increased rate of biosynthesis, rather than diminished collagen breakdown, as procollagenase synthesis is increased in the dermis[41]. The occurrence of fine collagen fibrils (about 300Å) with immature cross-banding patterns and the presence of beaded filaments similar to those found in early wound healing reflect this increase in collagen biosynthesis. The beaded structures are the result of materials such as decorin (the core protein of a small dermatan sulfate proteoglycan) attaching to immature collagen fibrils. Fibroblasts isolated from the pulmonary[42] and dermal lesions, particularly fibroblasts from the reticular dermis, continue to synthesize increased amounts of collagen for several generations *in vitro*[43,44]. Thus the accumulation of collagen is the result of increased biosynthesis by the fibroblasts, and the fibrotic lesions in systemic sclerosis can be interpreted to be a result of faulty regulation of collagen synthesis.

Collagens type I and III are increased in systemic sclerosis lesions. In the early dermal lesion there is a preponderance of type III collagen, particularly in the reticular dermis, but this evolves to a more normal ratio in older lesions. Type VI collagen has also been found around the blood vessels. The mRNA for procollagen $\alpha 2(I)$ collagen has been localized predominantly to the areas surrounding dermal blood vessels, suggesting that the fibroblasts in the vicinity of the vessels are activated to collagen biosynthesis. In muscle, myocardium and kidney, the collagen deposition is also initially perivascular.

Biosynthesis of mature fibrillar collagen is a multistep process requiring several enzymatic processes, and is best understood for type I collagen. As for all proteins, the sequence involves mRNA transcription and intron excision. Steady-state mRNA concentrations can be influenced by both message production and decay rates. After ribosomal translation of the message, the procollagen chains are transferred to the rough endoplasmic reticulum, where several unique modifications occur. These modifications include: the removal of signal peptides; hydroxylation of the Y position prolyl residues and of some of the Y position lysine residues; glycosylation of hydroxylysine residues; addition of a mannose-rich polysaccharide to the carboxy-terminal propeptide. The three chains, which form a triple helix through disulfide bonds contained in the globular propeptides that are cleaved, are released from the fibroblasts, amino- and carboxy-terminal propeptides are cleaved, and the helical molecule assembles into collagen fibrils, with the formation of lysine and hydroxylysine-derived cross-links. It remains unknown which steps of the collagen synthetic cascade are dysregulated in systemic sclerosis.

Fibroblast concentrations of procollagen mRNA are increased in systemic sclerosis both *in vivo* and *in vitro*[45]. Increased mRNA concentrations can result from either an increased transcription rate or a decrease in mRNA breakdown. The transcription rate of the gene encoding procollagen $\alpha2(I)$ (*COL1A2*) is increased in systemic sclerosis fibroblasts. The transcription of *COL1A1* has been demonstrated to be increased in systemic sclerosis fibroblasts as a result of DNA sequences in both the promoter region and the first intron[46]. These findings suggest that concentrations or activities of transcription regulatory factors are altered in these cells. As matrix gene mRNA and protein concentrations are coordinately increased in fibroblasts *in vitro*, the regulatory elements in the promoter regions of these genes may be similar in regard to the *trans*-acting protein factors to which they are responsive. Information regarding the promoter region of matrix genes is only currently becoming available, but some evidence for coordinate regulation of two human collagen genes exists[47]. Specifically, *COL1A1* competes effectively with *COL1A2* for fibroblast transcription factors, but not with *COL2A1* (collagen type II is not expressed in fibroblasts). Although there is no striking structural similarity between the promoter regions of *COL1A1* and *COL1A2*, these data suggest that different regulatory sequences may nevertheless bind similar transcription regulatory factors. Thus abnormalities in concentrations or activities of such *trans*-acting factors may account for the phenotype of the systemic sclerosis fibroblast. Competition may be between only one or a small number of *trans*-acting factors, and the critical factors might bind, not directly to the DNA responsive element, but to complexes of other *trans*-acting factors.

Evidence of translational, rather than transcriptional, control of collagen genes is derived from studies demonstrating discrepancies between collagen mRNA concentrations and protein synthetic rates. Fragments of the non-helical amino-terminal region of procollagen are inhibitors of collagen mRNA translation. A synthetic 22-residue peptide analogous to a sequence in the carboxy-terminals of procollagen $\alpha2(I)$ inhibits both collagen and fibronectin synthesis without causing detectable changes in their mRNA concentrations[48]. There is little evidence, however, that systemic sclerosis fibroblasts are hyporesponsive to this negative feedback regulation. Although such a hypothesis is attractive, it does not explain the abnormally high matrix mRNA concentrations seen in systemic sclerosis fibroblasts.

The population of fibroblasts in systemic sclerosis dermis has been shown to be skewed toward cells with a high collagen-producing capacity. This may result from factors (either humoral or cellular) that produce an interstitial environment that gives a high collagen-producing cell population proliferative advantage over those of lower synthetic capacity. Fibroblasts isolated from lesional skin continue to display this altered phenotype for several cell culture propagation passages after removal. Whether this is a result of clonal selection or selective activation is unknown[49].

In addition to the matrix synthesis dysregulation, systemic sclerosis fibroblasts display a subtle alteration of *in vitro* proliferative properties. Systemic sclerosis fibroblasts are not transformed (capable of anchorage independent growth), but rather grow in adherent monolayers in culture. Doubling times and *in vitro* lifespan are comparable to those of normal fibroblasts. However, systemic sclerosis fibroblasts demonstrate persistent proliferation in serum-free conditions and continually express the proliferation-associated proto-oncogene, c-*myc*[50]. They also express increased binding of the PDGF A chain homodimer, PDGF-AA (through the PDGF-α receptor) in response to the cytokine TGF-β, compared with normal fibroblasts. Whether these abnormalities are inherited in individuals who are then more susceptible to the inciting event, or whether they are imprinted on the cells as a result of the local events of the pathogenesis of the disease, is unknown.

The vascular lesion

Endothelial cells

The functions of endothelial cells in healthy microenvironments include separation of blood contents from the interstitial space, prevention of platelet aggregation, inhibition of the coagulation cascade and modulation of the state of smooth muscle contraction (vascular tone). Endothelial cells synthesize and secrete various substances to mediate these multiple functions. Platelet aggregation and platelet interaction with subendothelial connective tissue are inhibited by endothelial production of prostacyclin. If endothelial cells are disrupted, prostacyclin production is diminished and the balance shifted towards platelet activation. Plasma concentrations of factor VIII–von Willebrand factor are increased in systemic sclerosis, indicating endothelial cell activation[51]. Endothelial cells activated in inflammatory lesions by IL-1 and TNF-α express adhesion molecules, which promote leukocyte attachment and trafficking (see Chapter 16). Vascular cell adhesion molecule (VCAM)-1, intercellular adhesion molecule (ICAM)-1, E-selectin and P-selectin (all endothelial cell adhesion molecules) are expressed on endothelial cells of patients with systemic sclerosis. Expression of these molecules early in the disease supports the concept that endothelial activation is important in the developing stages of the lesion[52]. Circulating concentrations of VCAM-1, ICAM-1 and P-selectin are also increased in patients with early, inflammatory-stage systemic sclerosis.

Platelets

Evidence for platelet activation in systemic sclerosis includes an increased number of circulating platelet aggregates and increased plasma concentrations of platelet granule contents (β-thromboglobulin)[53]. Other granule contents include platelet factor 4, thrombospondin, fibroblast-activating factors, TGF-β and PDGF – each with the capacity to profoundly affect endothelial cells, fibroblasts and immune cells. It is likely that the platelet activation is secondary to the disrupted endothelium, rather than a primary defect in platelet function. This secondary platelet activation results in release of the usually sequestered platelet granule contents. The increased vascular permeability allows passage of the platelet-derived substances into the interstitium, where they have significant effects on fibroblasts, generally promoting proliferation, chemotaxis and matrix production.

Cytokines

Increases in IL-2, IL-4, IL-6 and IL-8 in the sera of patients implicate interleukins and cytokines in the pathogenesis of systemic sclerosis (Table 134.3) Increased concentrations of PDGF, TGF-β, TNF-α, IL-8, macrophage-inhibitory protein-1α and RANTES have been demonstrated in the alveolar fluid of patients with systemic sclerosis[54]. Cytokines that directly affect fibroblast proliferation and matrix synthesis are involved in the fibrotic lesions.

Interleukin-1

Interleukin-1 (α and β), a product of macrophages, is capable of stimulating fibroblast proliferation and synthesis of types I and III collagens, but it does not promote chemotaxis[55,56]. Most of the effects of IL-1 on fibroblasts require serum, suggesting an interaction between IL-1 and serum growth factors (largely PDGF and TGF-β), which is poorly understood. Systemic sclerosis fibroblasts from clinically involved dermis produce IL-1α, which is responsible for increases in the production of PDGF A chain and IL-6 by these cells. These observations might link the abnormal production of several cytokines into a pathogenetically meaningful cytokine 'cascade'.

Interleukin-2

Interleukin-2, a product of activated T cells, serves as a T cell growth factor and activates cytolytic lymphokine-activated killer cells. IL-2 and soluble IL-2 receptors (IL-2R) are increased in the sera of patients with systemic sclerosis, and the concentrations of both have been shown to correlate with the rapidity of progression of skin thickening[31]. IL-2 can induce the production of TGF-β by monocytes, providing a link between T cell activation and fibrosis.

TABLE 134.3 CYTOKINES INVOLVED IN THE PATHOGENESIS OF SYSTEMIC SCLEROSIS

Cytokine	Source	Pathophysiologic role
TGF-β	Macrophages Platelets	Induces collagen, fibronectin, IL-1 Inhibits endothelial cells Indirect fibroblast mitogen Attracts fibroblasts, macrophages Primes fibroblasts for PDGF
PDGF	Macrophages Platelets	Fibroblast mitogen Attracts fibroblasts
IL-1	Macrophages	Fibroblast mitogen Induces collagen
IL-2	Lymphocytes	Activates killer cells Increases macrophage TGF-β
IL-4	Lymphocytes	Induces collagen Attracts fibroblasts
IL-6	Macrophages Fibroblasts	Induces collagen
IL-8	Macrophages Neutrophils Fibroblasts	Attracts neutrophils
IL-17	CD4+ T cells	Fibroblast mitogen Induces IL-6 and IL-8
Fibronectin	Macrophages Fibroblasts Hepatocytes	Attracts monocytes, fibroblasts Fibroblast mitogen
Endothelin	Endothelial cells	Vasoconstrictor Increases collagen
TNF-α	Macrophages	Injures endothelial cells Induces IL-1, IL-6 and IL-8
CTGF	Fibroblasts	Fibroblast mitogen

CTGF, connective tissue growth factor.

Each cytokine is presented along with its pathophysiologic role in systemic sclerosis.

Interleukin-4

Interleukin-4, a product of activated T lymphocytes and mast cells, inhibits B and T cells and macrophages, but stimulates extracellular matrix synthesis. IL-4 is a link between inflammation and fibrosis, and has been found in increased amounts in sera of patients with systemic sclerosis.

Interleukin-6

Interleukin-6, a product of macrophages and fibroblasts, has been shown to be produced by systemic sclerosis fibroblasts *in vitro* in concentrations up to 30 times those in normal fibroblasts[57]. Although IL-6 stimulates collagen synthesis only at very high concentrations, it inhibits fibroblast synthesis of the tissue inhibitor of metalloproteinase. Produced locally, IL-6 may therefore promote fibrosis by inhibiting collagenase activity. Studies on circulating IL-6 concentrations in patients with systemic sclerosis have found either increased or normal values. This variation may result from anti-IL-6 antibodies, which have been found in systemic sclerosis and which may interfere with assays for IL-6[58].

Interleukin-8

The chemokine IL-8, a product of macrophages, polymorphonuclear leukocytes and fibroblasts, is a potent attractor and activator of polymorphonuclear leukocytes. Its production is increased by TNF-α. IL-8 is present in bronchoalveolar lavage fluid of patients with systemic sclerosis with alveolitis. It may be extremely important in the early, inflammatory phase of the pulmonary fibrotic lesion[59]. Two polymorphisms of the IL-8 receptor gene, *CXCR-2*, have been associated with systemic sclerosis[60]. *CXCR-2* mediates the transendothelial migration of skin-homing T cells and therefore may be associated with the increased number of dermal T cells in systemic sclerosis.

Interleukin-17

This cytokine, secreted by CD4+ T cells, causes fibroblasts to produce IL-6 and IL-8 and endothelial cells to secrete IL-6. Although IL-17 stimulates fibroblast proliferation, it does not increase collagen synthesis. Systemic sclerosis sera have increased concentrations of IL-17, PBMs from patients with systemic sclerosis make increased IL-17 (but SLE patients do not), and increased IL-17 mRNA is present in the dermis and bronchoalveolar lavage fluid of patients with systemic sclerosis. Increases in IL-17 have been associated with systemic sclerosis of recent onset[61].

Platelet-derived growth factor

The major fibroblast mitogenic factor in serum is PDGF. Originally found in platelet granules, PDGF is also produced by macrophages and fibroblasts. It is most commonly found as a heterodimer of the A and B chains (PDGF-AB), but homodimers (-AA and -BB) are also described. The B chain is coded for by the c-*sis* proto-oncogene. In addition to being a potent mitogen for fibroblasts and smooth muscle cells, PDGF is a chemoattractant important in recruitment of fibroblasts in lesions. Both fibroblast and smooth muscle cells have two types of receptors for PDGF (α and β; β is the predominant form). The intracellular portion of the PDGF-β receptor has a tyrosine kinase domain important in signal transduction and in mechanisms of cellular proliferation.

Potential sources of PDGF in systemic sclerosis lesions include platelets, macrophages and fibroblasts. In patients with systemic sclerosis with pulmonary fibrosis, increased amounts of all three types (AA, BB and AB) are present in bronchoalveolar lavage fluids. Both PDGF B and A chains have been demonstrated by immunohistochemistry in dermal systemic sclerosis lesions. The PDGF-α ligand–receptor system is induced by TGF-β, demonstrating the close relationship of TGF-β and PDGF in the pathogenesis of dermal fibrosis[62]. PDGF-α receptors, which recognize all PDGF isoforms, are increased by TGF-β in systemic sclerosis fibroblasts, but not in normal dermal fibroblasts. That PDGF-AA, which signals only via α receptors, is found in systemic sclerosis lesions makes it likely that this cytokine is important in fibroblast proliferation in systemic sclerosis.

Transforming growth factor-β

Transforming growth factor-β is made by megakaryocytes (and carried in the circulation in the α granules of platelets) and by macrophages, epidermal cells, fibroblasts and T cells; it has several effects on various cell types that are of physiologic significance in systemic sclerosis. TGF-β is the most potent inducer of collagen and fibronectin synthesis by fibroblasts and effectively stimulates formation of extracellular matrix[63]. When TGF-β is injected subcutaneously into animals, there is intense mononuclear cell inflammation, neoangiogenesis and fibrosis within days[64]. TGF-β inhibits growth of epithelial cells, including vascular endothelial cells[65], which may account for endothelial cell damage in systemic sclerosis. Also, TGF-β promotes angiogenesis *in vitro*, enhances the production of type IV collagenase and inhibits the production of tissue inhibitor of metalloproteinase type 2. Because type IV collagen is a prominent component of vascular basement membrane, TGF-β can promote breakdown of the vascular basement membrane, which is probably an important mechanism that enables branching of the vasculature and neovascularization. One might speculate, therefore, that TGF-β is important in the development of telangiectasia in systemic sclerosis.

Additional effects of TGF-β may be important. It is chemotactic for fibroblasts (promoting fibrosis by recruitment of fibroblasts) and induces both monocyte chemotaxis and IL-1 production (augmenting the inflammatory response). TGF-β treatment of fibroblasts *in vitro* increases TGF-β production[66] and expression of PDGF-A and PDGF-α receptors[67]. These effects, in addition to the increased matrix production by fibroblasts, persist after TGF-β has been removed from the culture medium, suggesting that the abnormal phenotype of systemic sclerosis fibroblasts *in vitro* is the result of *in vivo* exposure to this cytokine.

Although no increases in circulating TGF-β are found in the plasma of patients with systemic sclerosis, increased expression of TGF-β1 (but not TGF-β2) has been demonstrated in dermal lesions[68] and in bronchoalveolar lavage fluid[69]. Similarly, some investigators have demonstrated increased fibroblast concentrations of mRNA for TGF-β[70], whereas others have been unable to show increased production of TGF-β or binding of TGF-β by fibroblasts *in vitro*[71]. Attempts to locate mRNA for TGF-β by *in situ* hybridization in skin biopsies have shown variable results[72,73]. A suggestive piece of evidence is the colocalization of TGF-β2 and procollagen αl(I) mRNA in areas surrounding dermal blood vessels[74].

Both types I and II TGF-β receptors are increased on systemic sclerosis dermal fibroblasts[75]. Blockade of TGF-β2 signaling either by antibodies to TGF-β or with antisense oligonucleotide abolishes the increased expression of the collagen gene by scleroderma fibroblasts[76]. Taken together, these results indicate that the increased collagen synthesis seen in systemic sclerosis fibroblasts *in vitro* is dependent on autocrine TGF-β and that controlling signaling by this cytokine is a potential point of treatment for this disease.

An interesting relationship exists between the concentrations of TGF-β1 and TGF-β2 in bronchoalveolar lavage fluid from patients with systemic sclerosis with pulmonary fibrosis[69]. In healthy normal controls, there is very little TGF-β1, whereas TGF-β2 is readily demonstrated. However, in patients with systemic sclerosis the reverse is true, with TGF-β1 concentrations being, on average, six times greater than the very low values seen in healthy controls. TGF-β1 is a mitogen for pulmonary myofibroblasts from patients with systemic sclerosis, increases the proliferative responses of these cells to all three isoforms of PDGF (AA, AB and BB) and induces the expression of the PDGF-α receptor (as it does on dermal fibroblasts).

Connective tissue growth factor (CTGF)

Connective tissue growth factor (CTGF) is directly mitogenic for fibroblasts, and TGF-β has its indirect mitogenic effect on fibroblasts by inducing CTGF. CTGF is persistent in the dermis of patients with systemic sclerosis, and cultured systemic sclerosis fibroblasts express increased amounts of CTGF. Serum concentrations of CTGF are increased in both diffuse cutaneous and limited cutaneous systemic sclerosis, but more so in the fomer. The greatest CTGF concentrations are seen in patients with 1–3 years of disease and in those with pulmonary involvement[77]. TNF-α suppresses TGF-β-induced increases in CTGF production in normal fibroblasts and, to a lesser extent, in systemic sclerosis fibroblasts. However, TNF-α cannot suppress the increased basal concentration of CTGF expression in systemic sclerosis fibroblasts. It is thus suspected that the high level of expression of constitutive CTGF in scleroderma fibroblasts and its inability to respond to negative regulatory cytokines contributes to systemic sclerosis pathogenesis[78].

Fibronectin

This large matrix protein (a dimer of 220kDa subunits) is increased in systemic sclerosis lesions. In addition to its structural role as a matrix protein, fibronectin has effects on cells important in the pathogenesis of systemic sclerosis (Fig. 134.10). It is produced by several cell types, including fibroblasts, endothelial cells, macrophages and hepatocytes. Fibronectin is made up of several functional domains with special roles, such as the binding of matrix components (heparin and collagen). Monocytes and fibroblasts have integrin fibronectin receptors, which are important in cell attachment, spreading, locomotion and response to external stimuli. In addition to serving as an attachment and chemoattractant factor to fibroblasts, fibronectin is a mild growth stimulus and

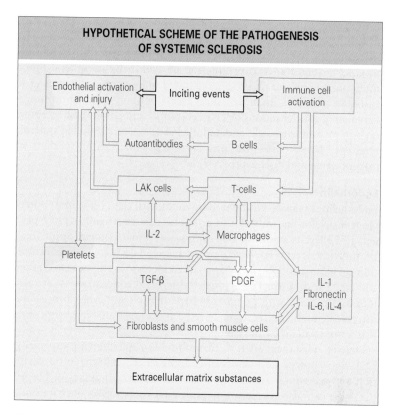

Fig. 134.10 A hypothetical scheme of the pathogenesis of systemic sclerosis. Arrows indicate positive actions of cells, either directly or through the indicated cytokines. IL, interleukin; LAK, lymphokine-activated killer; PDGF, platelet-derived growth factor; TGF, transforming growth factor.

a potent binder of TGF-β. It may, therefore, serve as a reservoir of TGF-β *in vitro*.

Systemic sclerosis fibroblasts synthesize more fibronectin *in vitro* than do normal dermal fibroblasts, and they respond to the matrix-enhancing cytokine, TGF-β, by increasing fibronectin synthesis. Alveolar macrophages synthesize and secrete increased concentrations of fibronectin *in vitro*, and this abnormality has been correlated to the severity of the pulmonary lesion[4]. Whether the fibronectin made by these alveolar macrophages *in vitro* is important, either in activating fibroblasts or in the matrix accumulation itself, is unknown. It may be that the fibronectin is simply a marker of macrophage activation and that other functions of these multipotent cells are more important in the development of the fibrotic lesion.

Tumor necrosis factor-α

Tumor necrosis factor-α is a pleiotropic inflammatory cytokine produced by activated macrophages and other cells and is recognized as a key pathogenic mediator of infectious and inflammatory diseases, including autoimmune disorders. TNF-α has effects on numerous cell types including fibroblasts, macrophages, lymphocytes, endothelial cells and epithelial cells. It induces release of other cytokines such as IL-1, IL-6 and IL-8. Because TNF-α inhibits endothelial cell growth and, in combination with interferon (IFN)-γ, promotes endothelial cytolysis, it seems a likely culprit in endothelial damage. It can also induce endothelial cell adhesion molecules for lymphocytes, thus contributing to vascular damage[79]. TNF-α enhances microvascular permeability and stimulates the expression and signaling of IL-8 responsible for the recruitment of leukocytes to inflammatory sites[80].

The role of TNF-α in systemic sclerosis is uncertain, because it is known to decrease collagen synthesis and to inhibit TGF-β mediated increases in CTGF[78]. However, expression of the *TNF* gene under control of the human surfactant protein SP-C promoter in transgenic mice causes a fibrosing alveolitis resembling systemic sclerosis lung disease[81]. Serum concentrations of TNF-α are increased in patients with systemic sclerosis and are greatest in those with restrictive lung disease[82,83]. Spontaneous production of TNF-α by peripheral blood mononuclear cells has been demonstrated to be significantly greater in systemic sclerosis than in individuals without the condition[84]. Circulating concentrations of TNF receptors I and II and these receptors on skin mononuclear cells and endothelial cells are increased in systemic sclerosis. These concentrations correlate with laboratory signs of inflammation and disease progression[85].

Endothelin

Endothelin, a peptide synthesized by endothelial cells, is the most potent vasoconstrictor known[86]. It also promotes fibroblast synthesis of types I and III collagens and decreases expression of matrix metalloproteinase 1[87]. Individuals with Raynaud's phenomenon have increased concentrations of plasma endothelin and a marked increase in response to cooling compared with normal individuals[88]. Increased concentrations are also found in patients with pulmonary hypertension and lung fibrosis, and increased endothelin receptors have been demonstrated in fibrotic lung tissue from patients with systemic sclerosis[89].

Platelet substances such as thrombin, epinephrine and, especially, TGF-β are potent stimulators of endothelial cell endothelin transcription and secretion[90]. Thus one of the most potent inducers of fibrosis (TGF-β) can also increase a peptide that causes vasoconstriction, a finding which gives an interesting insight into the possible interaction of the fibrotic and vascular lesions in systemic sclerosis.

Interferon-γ

This cytokine, a product of T cells and natural killer cells, is a potent activator of macrophages and is important in the differentiation of T cells into cytolytic cells and in the development of B cells. Thus, as a potent stimulator of the immune system, IFN-γ may be important in the autoimmune phenomenon and macrophage activation that are seen in systemic sclerosis. However, IFN-γ has a strong inhibitory effect on the synthesis of collagen by fibroblasts, including systemic sclerosis fibroblasts[91]. Serum concentrations of IFN-γ are decreased in systemic sclerosis, and *in vitro* stimulation of peripheral blood T cells fails to elicit the increase in its production that is seen in normal T cells. Therefore a defect in T cells of patients with systemic sclerosis that results in an inability to suppress fibrosis may exist.

Vascular endothelial growth factor

Increased concentrations of the angiogenic cytokine, vascular endothelial growth factor, have been correlated with diffuse cutaneous systemic sclerosis and severity of restrictive lung disease[92]. However, angiogenesis may be a reparative process in systemic sclerosis, and the increased concentrations may be a response to the illness.

Non-peptide mediators

Nitric oxide, a gas synthesized by endothelial cells and inflammatory cells, is a potent vasodilator. Inflammatory cytokines (TNF-α and IL-1) increase the endothelial production of nitric oxide by increasing production of the inducible form of nitric oxide synthetase. Production of nitric oxide in systemic sclerosis is increased or decreased, depending on the type of systemic sclerosis and the type of organ involvement. Patients with systemic sclerosis with inflammatory interstitial lung disease exhale more nitric oxide than do those without interstitial lung disease[93]. However, because damaged endothelium is less able to synthesize nitric oxide, patients with pulmonary hypertension exhale less nitric oxide than do those without pulmonary hypertension[94].

Free-radical-induced oxidative stress resulting in lipid peroxidation and tissue damage has been proposed as a potential pathogenic mechanism. Isoprostanes are produced by non-cyclo-oxygenase, free-radical-catalyzed peroxidation of arachidonic acid. Urinary concentrations of isoprostanes are increased in patients with systemic sclerosis[95]. An induction of antioxidant defenses has also been demonstrated in patients with systemic sclerosis who have increased concentrations of plasma superoxide dismutase[96]. This enzyme is important in diminishing oxidative stress.

CONCLUSION

A current theory of the pathogenesis of systemic sclerosis includes several components (Fig. 134.10). Some unknown inciting event triggers endothelial cell injury and immune system activation. The immune system may be the cause of, and almost certainly enhances, endothelial injury. This injury results in release of platelet constituents capable of causing fibroblast proliferation and matrix synthesis. When activated, fibroblasts can also synthesize these materials, leading to a positive feedback loop. Immune cell activation also results in production of materials capable of mesenchymal cell activation. Whether the production of autoantibodies is an epiphenomenon or whether they are important in cellular activation or injury themselves remains an open question.

ACKNOWLEDGMENT

This chapter is dedicated to the memory of Edward Carwile LeRoy MD.

REFERENCES

1. Wigley FM. Scleroderma (systemic sclerosis). In: Goldman L, Bennett JC, eds. Cecil textbook of medicine. Philadelphia: WB Saunders; 2000: 1517–1522.
2. Roumm AD, Whiteside TL, Medsger TA, Rodnan GP. Lymphocytes in the skin of patients with progressive systemic sclerosis. Arthritis Rheum 1984; 27: 645–653.
3. Maricq HR. Widefield capillary microscopy. Technique and rating scale for abnormalities seen in scleroderma and related disorders. Arthritis Rheum 1981; 24: 1159–1166.
4. Kinsella MB, Smith EA, Miller KS et al. Spontaneous production of fibronectin by scleroderma alveolar macrophages. Arthritis Rheum 1989; 32: 577–583.
5. Arnett FC, Cho M, Chatterjee S et al. Familial occurrence frequencies and relative risk for systemic sclerosis (scleroderma) in three United States cohorts. Arthritis Rheum 2001; 44: 1359–1362.
6. Artlett CM, Black CM, Briggs DC et al. Telomere reduction in scleroderma patients: a possible cause for chromosomal instability. Br J Rheumatol 1996; 35: 732–737.
7. Welsh KI, Black CM. Environmental and genetic factors in scleroderma. In: Jayson MIV, Black CM, eds. Systemic sclerosis: scleroderma. New York: Wiley; 1988: 33–48.
8. Reveille JD, Owerbach D, Goldstein R et al. Association of polar amino acids at position 26 of the HLA-DQB1 first domain with the anticentromere autoantibody response in systemic sclerosis (scleroderma). J Clin Invest 1992; 89: 1208–1213.
9. Reveille JD, Durban E, MacLeod-St Clair MJ et al. Association of amino acid sequences in the HLA-DQB1 first domain with the antitopoisomerase I autoantibody response in scleroderma (progressive systemic sclerosis). J Clin Invest 1992; 90: 973–980.
10. Arnett FC, Reveille JD, Goldstein R et al. Autoantibodies to fibrillarin in systemic sclerosis (scleroderma): an immunogenetic, serological and clinical analysis. Arthritis Rheum 1996; 39: 1151–1160.
11. Tan FK, Stivers DN, Foster MW et al. Association of microsatellite markers near the fibrillin 1 gene on human chromosome 15q with scleroderma in a Native American population. Arthritis Rheum 1998; 41: 1729–1737.
12. Tan FK, Wang N, Kuwana M et al. Association of fibrillin-1 single-nucleotide polymorphism haplotypes with systemic sclerosis in Choctaw and Japanese populations. Arthritis Rheum 2001; 44: 893–901.
13. Tan FK, Arnett FC, Reveille JD et al. Autoantibodies to fibrillin-1 in systemic sclerosis. Arthritis Rheum 2000; 43: 2464–2471.
14. Kratz LE, Boughman JA, Needleman BW. Lack of association between scleroderma and types I and III procollagen gene restriction fragment length polymorphisms. Arthritis Rheum 1989; 32: 1597–1600.
15. Verheijen R, Oberye EH, van den Hoogen FHJ, van Venrooij WJ. The mutations in the fibronectin gene described in Japanese patients with systemic sclerosis are not present in Dutch patients. Arthritis Rheum 1991; 34: 490–492.

16. Kratz LE, Broughman JA, Pincus T *et al*. Association of scleroderma with a T cell antigen receptor d gene restriction fragment length polymorphism. Arthritis Rheum 1990; 33: 569–573.
17. Nietert PJ, Sutherland SE, Silver RM *et al*. Is occupational organic solvent exposure a risk factor for scleroderma? Arthritis Rheum 1998; 41: 1111–1118.
18. Povey A, Guppy MJ, Wood M *et al*. Cytochrome P2 polymorphisms and susceptibility to scleroderma following exposure to organic solvents. Arthritis Rheum 2001; 44: 662–665.
19. Black CM, Pereira S, McWhirter A *et al*. Genetic susceptibility to scleroderma-like syndrome in symptomatic and asymptomatic workers exposed to vinyl chloride. J Rheumatol 1986; 13: 1059–1062.
20. Tan EM, Rodnan GP, Garcia I *et al*. Diversity of antinuclear antibodies in progressive systemic sclerosis: anticentromere antibody and its relationship to CREST syndrome. Arthritis Rheum 1980; 23: 617–625.
21. Earnshaw W, Bordwell B, Marino C, Rothfield N. Three human chromosomal autoantigens are recognized by sera from patients with anticentromere antibodies. J Clin Invest 1986; 77: 426–430.
22. Kuwana M, Medsger TA Jr, Wright TM. T and B cell collaboration is essential for the autoantibody response to DNA topoisomerase I in systemic sclerosis. J Immunol 1995; 155: 2703–2714.
23. Hirakata M, Okano Y, Pati U *et al*. Identification of autoantibodies to RNA polymerase II: occurrence in systemic sclerosis and association with autoantibodies to RNA polymerases I and III. J Clin Invest 1993; 91: 2665–2672.
24. Marks RM, Czerniecki M, Andrews BS, Penny R. The effects of scleroderma serum on human vascular endothelial cells: induction of antibody-dependent cellular cytotoxicity. Arthritis Rheum 1988; 31: 1524–1534.
25. Hill MB, Phipps JL, Cartwright RJ *et al*. Antibodies to membranes of endothelial cells and fibroblasts in scleroderma. Clin Exp Immunol 1996; 106: 491–497.
26. Negi VS, Tripathy NK, Misra R, Nityanand S. Antiendothelial cell antibodies in scleroderma correlate with severe digital ischemia and pulmonary hypertension. J Rheumatol 1998; 25: 462–464.
27. Carvalho D, Savage CO, Black CM, Pearson JD. IgG antiendothelial cell autoantibodies from scleroderma patients induce leukocyte adhesion to human vascular endothelial cells in vitro. Induction of adhesion molecule expression and involvement of endothelium-derived cytokines. J Clin Invest 1996; 97: 111–119.
28. Mackel AM, DeLustro F, Harper FE, LeRoy EC. Antibodies to collagen in scleroderma. Arthritis Rheum 1982; 25: 522–531.
29. White B, Yurovsky VV. Oligoclonal expansion of V delta 1+ gamma/delta T-cells in systemic sclerosis patients. Ann NY Acad Sci 1995; 756: 382–391.
30. Huffstutter JE, DeLustro FA, LeRoy EC. Cellular immunity to collagen and laminin in scleroderma. Arthritis Rheum 1985; 28: 775–780.
31. Kahaleh MB, LeRoy EC. Interleukin-2 in scleroderma: correlation of serum level with extent of skin involvement and disease duration. Ann Intern Med 1989; 110: 446–450.
32. Miller EB, Hiserodt JC, Hunt LE *et al*. Reduced natural killer cell activity in patients with systemic sclerosis. Correlation with clinical disease type. Arthritis Rheum 1988; 31: 1515–1523.
33. Silver RM. Lymphokine activated killer (LAK) cell activity in the peripheral blood of lymphocytes of systemic sclerosis (SSc) patients. Clin Exp Rheumatol 1990; 8: 481–486.
34. Jaffee BD, Claman HN. Chronic graft-versus host disease (GVHD) as a model for scleroderma. I. Description of model systems. Cell Immunol 1983; 77: 1–12.
35. Kahaleh MB, Fan PS. Mechanism of serum-mediated endothelial injury in scleroderma: identification of a granular enzyme in scleroderma skin and sera. Clin Immunol Immunopathol 1997; 8332–8340.
36. Artlett CM, Smith JB, Jimenez SA. Identification of fetal DNA and cells in skin lesions from women with systemic sclerosis. N Engl J Med 1998; 338: 1186–1191.
37. Kraling BM, Maul GG, Jimenez SA. Mononuclear cellular infiltrates in clinically involved skin from patients with systemic sclerosis of recent onset predominantly consist of monocytes/macrophages. Pathobiology 1995; 63: 48–56.
38. Walker MA, Harley RA, LeRoy EC. Inhibition of fibrosis in TSK mice by blocking mast cell degranulation. J Rheumatol 1987; 14: 299–301.
39. Gustafsson R, Fredens K, Nettelbladt O, Hallgren R. Eosinophil activation in systemic sclerosis. Arthritis Rheum 1991; 34: 414–422.
40. Rodnan GP, Lipinski E, Luksick J. Skin thickness and collagen content in progressive systemic sclerosis and localized scleroderma. Arthritis Rheum 1979; 22: 130–140.
41. Uitto J, Halme J, Hannuksela M *et al*. Protocollagen proline hydroxylase activity in the skin of normal human subjects and of patients with scleroderma. Scand J Clin Lab Invest 1969; 23: 241–247.
42. Shi-Wen X, Denton CP, McWhirter A *et al*. Scleroderma lung fibroblasts exhibit elevated and dysregulated type I collagen biosynthesis. Arthritis Rheum 1997; 40: 1237–1244.
43. LeRoy EC. Increased collagen synthesis by scleroderma skin fibroblasts in vitro: a possible defect in the regulation or activation of the scleroderma fibroblast. J Clin Invest 1974; 54: 880–889.
44. Uitto J, Bauer EA, Eisen AZ. Scleroderma: increased biosynthesis of triple helical type I and type III procollagens associated with unaltered expression of collagenase by skin fibroblasts in culture. J Clin Invest 1979; 64: 921–930.
45. Jimenez SA, Feldman G, Bashey RL *et al*. Co-ordinate increase in the expression of type I and type III collagen genes in progressive systemic sclerosis fibroblasts. Biochem J 1986; 237: 837–843.
46. Hitraya EG, Jimenez SA. Transcriptional activation on the alpha 1(I) procollagen gene in systemic sclerosis dermal fibroblasts: role of intronic sequences. Arthritis Rheum 1996; 39: 1347–1354.
47. Boast S, Su M-W, Ramirez F *et al*. Functional analysis of cis-acting DNA sequences controlling transcription of the human type I collagen genes. J Biol Chem 1990; 265: 13351–13356.
48. Wiestner M, Krieg T, Hörlein D *et al*. Inhibiting effect of procollagen peptides on collagen biosynthesis in fibroblast cultures. J Biol Chem 1979; 254: 7016–7023.
49. Jelaska A, Arakawa M, Broketa G, Korn JH. Heterogeneity of collagen synthesis in normal and systemic sclerosis skin fibroblasts: increased proportion of high collagen-producing cells in systemic sclerosis fibroblasts. Arthritis Rheum 1996; 39: 1338–1346.
50. Trojanowska M, Wu L, LeRoy EC. Elevated expression of c-myc proto-oncogene in scleroderma fibroblasts. Oncogene 1988; 3: 477–481.
51. Kahaleh MB, Osborn I, LeRoy EC. Increased factor VIII/von Willebrand factor antigen and von Willebrand factor activity in scleroderma and Raynaud's phenomenon. Ann Intern Med 1981; 94: 482–484.
52. Gruschwitz MS, Hornstein OP, von den Driesch P. Correlation of soluble adhesion molecules in the peripheral blood of scleroderma patients with their in situ expression and with disease activity. Arthritis Rheum 1995; 38: 184–189.
53. Kahaleh MB, Osborn I, LeRoy EC. Elevated levels of circulating platelet aggregates and beta-thromboglobulin in scleroderma. Ann Intern Med 1982; 96: 610–613.
54. Bolster MB, Ludwicka A, Sutherland SE *et al*. Cytokine concentrations in bronchoalveolar lavage fluid of patients with systemic sclerosis. Arthritis Rheum 1997; 40: 743–751.
55. Goldring MB, Krane SM. Modulation by recombinant interleukin-l of synthesis of types I and III collagens and associated procollagen mRNA levels in cultured human cells. J Biol Chem 1987; 262: 16724–16729.
56. Postlethwaite AE, Raghow R, Stricklin GP *et al*. Modulation of fibroblast functions by interleukin-l: increased steady-state accumulation of type I procollagen messenger RNAs and stimulation of other functions but not chemotaxis by human recombinant interleukin I α and β. J Cell Biol 1988; 106: 311–318.
57. Feghali CA, Bost KL, Boulware DW, Levy LS. Mechanisms of pathogenesis in scleroderma: I. Overproduction of interleukin 6 by fibroblasts cultured from affected skin of patients with scleroderma. J Rheum 1992; 19: 1202–1211.
58. Suziki H, Takemura H, Yoshizaki K *et al*. IL-6–anti-IL-6 autoantibody complexes with IL-6 activity in sera from some patients with systemic sclerosis. J Immunol 1994; 152: 935–942.
59. Southcott AM, Jones KP, Li D, Majumdar S *et al*. Interleukin-8, differential expression in lone fibrosing alveolitis and systemic sclerosis. Am J Respir Crit Care Med 1995; 151: 1604–1612.
60. Renzoni E, Lympany P, Sestini P *et al*. Distribution of novel polymorphisms of the interleukin-8 and CXC receptor 1 and 2 genes in systemic sclerosis and cryptogenic fibrosing alveolitis. Arthritis Rheum 2000; 43: 1633–1640.
61. Kurasawa K, Hirose K, Sano H *et al*. Increased interleukin-17 production in patients with systemic sclerosis. Arthritis Rheum 2000; 42 : 2455–2463.
62. Yamakage A, Kikucki J, Smith E *et al*. Selective upregulation of platelet-derived growth factor a receptors by transforming growth factor β. J Exp Med 1992; 175: 1227–1234.
63. Ignotz RA, Massague J. Transforming growth factor beta stimulates the expression of fibronectin and collagen and their incorporation into the extracellular matrix. J Biol Chem 1986; 261: 4337–4345.
64. Roberts AB, Sporn MB, Assoian RK *et al*. Transforming growth factor type β: rapid induction of fibrosis and angiogenesis in vivo and stimulation of collagen formation in vitro. Proc Natl Acad Sci USA 1986; 83: 4167–4171.
65. Takehara K, LeRoy EC, Grotendorst GR. TGF-β inhibition of endothelial cell proliferation: alteration of EGF binding and EGF-induced growth regulatory (competence) gene expression. Cell 1987; 49: 415–422.
66. Van Obberghen-Schilling E, Roche NS, Flanders KC *et al*. Transforming growth factor β1 positively regulates its own expression in normal and transformed cells. J Biol Chem 1988; 263: 7741–7746.
67. Ishikawa O, LeRoy EC, Trojanowska M. Mitogenic effect of transforming growth factor β1 on human fibroblasts involves the induction of platelet derived growth factor α receptors. J Cell Physiol 1990; 145: 181–186.
68. Falanga V, Gerhardt CO, Dasch JR *et al*. Skin distribution and differential expression of transforming growth factor β1 and β2. J Dermatol Sci 1992; 3: 131–136.
69. Ludwicka A, Ohba T, Trojanowska M *et al*. Elevated levels of platelet derived growth factor and transforming growth factor-β1 in bronchoalveolar lavage fluid from patients with scleroderma. J Rheumatol 1995; 22: 1876–1883.
70. Vuorio T, Kahari VM, Black C, Vuorio E. Expression of osteonectin, decorin, and transforming growth factor-β1 genes in fibroblasts cultured from patients with systemic sclerosis and morphea. J Rheumatol 1991; 18: 247–251.
71. Needleman BW, Choi J, Burrows-Mezu A, Fontana JA. Secretion and binding of transforming growth factor β by scleroderma and normal dermal fibroblasts. Arthritis Rheum 1990; 33: 650–656.
72. Peltonen J, Kahari L, Jaakola S *et al*. Evaluation of transforming growth factor β and type I procollagen gene expression in fibrotic skin diseases by in situ hybridization. J Invest Dermatol 1990; 94: 365–371.
73. Gruschwitz M, Muller PU, Sepp N *et al*. Transcription and expression of transforming growth factor type beta in the skin of progressive systemic sclerosis: a mediator of fibrosis? J Invest Dermatol 1990; 94: 197–203.
74. Kulozik M, Hogg A, Lankat-Buttgereit B, Krieg T. Co-localization of transforming growth factor β2 with αl(I) procollagen mRNA in tissue section of patients with systemic sclerosis. J Clin Invest 1990; 86: 917–922.
75. Kawakami T, Ihn H, Xu W *et al*. Increased expression of TGF-beta receptors by scleroderma fibroblasts: evidence for contribution of autocrine TGF-beta signaling to scleroderma phenotype. J Invest Dermatol 1998; 110: 47–51.
76. Ihn H, Yamane K, Kubo M, Tamaki K. Blockade of endogenous transforming growth factor beta signaling prevents up-regulated collagen synthesis in scleroderma fibroblasts: association with increased expression of transforming growth factor beta receptors. Arthritis Rheum 2001; 44: 474–480.
77. Sato S, Nagaoka T, Hawesgawa M *et al*. Serum levels of connective tissue growth factor are elevated in patients with systemic sclerosis: association with extent of skin sclerosis and severity of pulmonary fibrosis. J Rheumatol 2000; 27: 149–154.
78. Abraham DJ, Xu S, Black CM *et al*. Tumor necrosis factor alpha suppresses the induction of connective tissue growth factor by transforming growth factor-beta in normal and scleroderma fibroblasts. J Biol Chem 2000; 275: 15220–15225.

79. Kahaleh MB, Smith EA, Soma Y, LeRoy EC. Effect of lymphotoxin and tumor necrosis factor on endothelial and connective tissue cell growth and function. Clin Immunol Immunopathol 1988; 49: 261–272.

80. Pober JC. Effects of tumour necrosis factor and related cytokines on vascular endothelial cells. In: Bock G, Marsh J, eds. Tumour necrosis factor and related cytotoxins. New York: John Wiley; 1987: 70–84.

81. Miyazaki Y, Araki K, Vesin C et al. Expression of a tumor necrosis factor-alpha transgene in murine lung causes lymphocytic and fibrosing alveolitis. A mouse model of progressive pulmonary fibrosis. J Clin Invest 1995; 96: 250–259.

82. Needleman BW, Wigley FM, Stair RW. Interleukin-1, interleukin-2, interleukin-4, interleukin-6, tumor necrosis factor alpha, and interferon-gamma levels in sera from patients with scleroderma. Arthritis Rheum 1992; 35: 67–72.

83. Hasegawa M, Fujimoto M, Kikukuchi K, Takehara K. Elevated serum tumor necrosis factor-alpha levels in patients with systemic sclerosis: association with pulmonary fibrosis. J Rheumatol 1997; 24: 663–665.

84. Kantor TV, Friberg D, Medsger TA Jr et al. Cytokine production and serum levels in systemic sclerosis. Clin Immunol Immunopathol 1992; 65: 278–285.

85. Grushwitz MS, Albrecht M, Vieth G, Haustein UF. In situ expression and serum levels of tumor necrosis factor-alpha receptors in patients with early stages of systemic sclerosis. J Rheumatol 1997; 24: 1936–1943.

86. Yanagisawa M, Kurihara H, Kimura S et al. A novel potent vasoconstrictor peptide produced by vascular endothelial cells. Nature 1988; 332: 411–415.

87. Shi-Wen X, Denton CP, Dashwood MR et al. Fibroblast matrix gene expression and connective tissue remodeling: role of endothelin 1. J Invest Dermatol 2001; 116: 417–425.

88. Kanno K, Hirata Y, Emori T et al. Endothelin and Raynaud's phenomenon. Am J Med 1991; 90: 130–132.

89. Abraham DJ, Vancheeswaran R, Dashwood MR et al. Increased levels of endothelin-1 and differential endothelin-1 and differential endothelin type A and B receptor expression in scleroderma associated fibrotic lung disease. Am J Pathol 1997; 151: 831–841.

90. Kurihara H, Yoshizumi M, Sugiyama T et al. Transforming growth factor β stimulates the expression of endothelin mRNA by vascular endothelial cells. Biochem Biophys Res Commun 1989; 159: 1435–1440.

91. Jimenez SA, Freundlich B, Rosenbloom J. Selective inhibition of human diploid fibroblast collagen synthesis by interferons. J Clin Invest 1984; 74: 1112–1116.

92. Kikuchi K, Kubo M, Kadano T et al. Serum concentrations of vascular endothelial growth factor in collagen diseases. Br J Dermatol 1998; 139: 1049–1051.

93. Rolla G, Colagrande P, Scappaticci E et al. Exhaled nitric oxide in systemic sclerosis: relationships with lung involvement and pulmonary hypertension. J Rheumatol 2000; 27: 1693–1698.

94. Kharitonov SA, Cailes JB, Black CM et al. Decreased nitric oxide in the exhaled air of patients with systemic sclerosis with pulmonary hypertension. Thorax 1997; 52: 1051–1055.

95. Stein CM, Tanner SB, Awad JA et al. Evidence of free radical-mediated injury (isoprostane overproduction) in scleroderma. Arthritis Rheum 1996; 39: 1146–1150.

96. Morita A, Minami H, Sakakibara N et al. Elevated plasma superoxide dismutase activity in patients with systemic sclerosis. J Dermatol Sci 1996; 11: 196–201.

135 Management of systemic sclerosis

Christopher P Denton and Carol M Black

- Effective management of systemic sclerosis requires assessment of the subset, stage and pattern of organ involvement from systemic sclerosis

- No putative antifibrotic or immunosuppressive agents have yet been shown to be of unequivocal benefit in a placebo-controlled clinical trial

- Effective management of organ-based complications is emerging, especially reflux esophagitis, established renal scleroderma crisis and pulmonary arterial hypertension

- High-dose corticosteroids should be used with caution as they may precipitate scleroderma renal crisis

- Systemic sclerosis patients should all undergo regular screening for cardiorespiratory or renal complications, even if asymptomatic. Risk stratification based upon serologic, immunologic or genetic characteristics may be possible in the future so that serial investigation can be individualized

- Better understanding of the key mediators of pathogenesis may allow targeted molecular therapies. Currently, transforming growth factor-β, connective tissue growth factor and endothelin-1 are potential targets under evaluation

INTRODUCTION

The management of the scleroderma spectrum of disorders is a substantial problem but should be approached with a thorough understanding of current concepts of pathogenesis of these disorders, the clinical features, including classification and natural history, and an appreciation that there is much to be offered to patients. In particular, there has been a substantial reduction in disease-related mortality over the past 25 years and this looks set to continue. This has arisen through improvements in the management of organ-based complications of systemic sclerosis, notably renal disease, although these improvements are likely to extend now into other organ-based complications, including pulmonary vascular disease and hopefully also interstitial lung fibrosis. There have also been substantial advances in the treatment of complications such as reflux esophagitis and Raynaud's phenomenon, which have a major impact in terms of morbidity. Other areas of significant recent progress include the establishment and ongoing validation of standardized measures of disease severity and activity, with the development of international consensus scores. On a more negative note, it remains the case that no treatment for systemic sclerosis has been shown in a controlled clinical trial to truly modify mortality or morbidity, based on the extent of cutaneous involvement. There is now, however, an appreciation of what has to be done to demonstrate effectiveness and improvements in clinical trials methodology together with the emergence of a number of attractive candidate molecular therapies that target key pathways or mediators involved in the pathogenesis of systemic sclerosis.

PRINCIPLES OF EFFECTIVE MANAGEMENT

Clinical heterogeneity is a hallmark of the scleroderma spectrum, which includes pre-scleroderma (Raynaud's phenomenon plus systemic-sclerosis-associated autoantibodies) at one end and rapidly progressive diffuse cutaneous systemic sclerosis (dcSSc) at the other[1,2]. The major subsets of systemic sclerosis are described in Table 135.1. Another group comprises patients with overlap syndromes who demonstrate features of

---

TABLE 135.1 CLINICAL FEATURES OF THE MAJOR SYSTEMIC SCLEROSIS SUBSETS

Diffuse cutaneous systemic sclerosis (dcSSc)

33% of patients. Inflammatory features more prominent at onset. Raynaud's may develop later. Skin sclerosis proximal to wrists/elbows and truncal. Prominent pruritus and constitutional symptoms. Tendon friction rubs associated with progressive disease. Significant visceral disease more frequent than in lcSSc. Renal, pulmonary fibrosis (secondary pulmonary hypertension), cardiac, gut. Disease activity appears to remain fairly constant over many years, with prominent vasospastic symptoms.

Limited cutaneous systemic sclerosis (lcSSc)

66% of patients. Long-standing Raynaud's, skin changes hands, face, neck. Compared with dcSSc, renal disease less frequent, isolated pulmonary hypertension, severe gut disease and interstitial lung fibrosis (if anti-topoisomerase-1 present). Florid telangiectasis and calcinosis (especially ACA-positive). Disease activity appears to be maximal in first 3 years from onset then often plateaus and skin involvement may stabilize or improve.

Systemic sclerosis *sine* scleroderma

Less than 2% of patients. Visceral complications without skin sclerosis. Often present with Raynaud's phenomenon and gut, pulmonary or renal complications. Raynaud's generally present; often carries a hallmark systemic sclerosis-associated autoantibody

PREVALENCE OF ORGAN-BASED COMPLICATIONS IN THE MAJOR SYSTEMIC SCLEROSIS SUBSETS*

Clinical feature	lcSSc (%)	dcSSc (%)	Overall (%)
Raynaud's phenomenon	99	98	99
Skeletal myopathy	11	23	15
Esophageal	74	60	69
Other gastrointestinal	7	8	8
Cardiac	9	12	10
Pulmonary fibrosis	26	41	31
Pulmonary hypertension	21	17	20
Renal (overall)	8	18	12
Renal (crisis)	2	10	5

* Data from patients attending the Royal Free Hospital Centre for Rheumatology 1990–2001. ACA, anticentromere antibodies.

other autoimmune rheumatic disorders such as systemic lupus erythematosus, rheumatoid arthritis, polymyositis or Sjögren's syndrome. This group often presents particular management difficulties since there may be differential activity amongst the various disease components. Clearly, not all patients require the same level of investigation or therapeutic intervention.

Optimal management of systemic sclerosis requires:

- accurate diagnosis at the earliest opportunity, notwithstanding the fact that in some cases this may depend upon a period of observation over time
- once the diagnosis is established, patients with scleroderma should be correctly staged and subsetted
- this, together with information obtained by clinical investigation, allows risk-stratification to facilitate stage and subset-appropriate investigation, follow-up and treatment
- screening for important or frequent complications should facilitate effective early treatment of complications
- good patient education and a holistic approach recognizing the impact of the disease on life-style and relationships.

Clinical, serological and genetic markers help to predict particular complications. Thus patients carrying the human leukocyte antigen (HLA)-DR53α genotype or with anti-topoisomerase-1 autoantibodies are at increased risk of developing interstitial lung fibrosis, irrespective of their clinical subset[3]. In contrast, anti-RNA-polymerase (RNApol)-I or -III antibodies are associated with renal involvement, whereas, for limited cutaneous scleroderma, anticentromere antibodies are associated with isolated pulmonary hypertension and with severe gut involvement[4]. Some of these observations are summarized in Table 135.2. These associations offer the possibility of predicting which patients are likely to develop particular complications and may eventually allow frequency

and scope of routine investigations to be tailored on an individual basis. However, associations may differ between ethnic groups[5] and are not absolute, and so at present risk stratification is most useful as an adjunct to routine investigation when interpreting borderline results, and in patient education by allowing reassurance to be given to those at lower risk of internal organ disease.

LINKING THERAPY TO PATHOGENESIS

Systemic sclerosis comprises a heterogeneous group of disorders characterized by fibrosis of the skin or internal organs and vascular abnormalities, notably Raynaud's phenomenon. It sometimes exists in overlap with other autoimmune rheumatic diseases and the diagnosis is essentially clinical. The three underlying pathological processes in systemic sclerosis – vascular damage, immune cell activation and fibrogenesis – may each respond to different therapies. Therefore, combination strategies are more likely to control the disease than single-agent therapies. This may have confounded previous trials, which have generally pursued only single-agent treatments. However, therapies must be matched to disease stage and subset. Thus, for early dcSSc, immunosuppressive treatments may be the most appropriate and studies include the use of immunoablation with peripheral stem cell rescue. At later stages antifibrotic interventions would perhaps be the most important. Throughout the disease course in dcSSc and limited cutaneous systemic sclerosis (lcSSc), vasospasm is a feature and so vascular therapies might be used in combination with these other agents.

The observation that skin fibroblasts from scleroderma, or at least a subset of them, synthesize increased quantities of fibronectin, proteoglycan core proteins and particularly collagens types I and III and to a lesser degree IV and VI was inferred from *ex vivo* studies of skin biopsies but the intriguing finding that this phenotype of matrix overproduction persisted in tissue culture and could be passed on at cell division has provided a paradigm for the mechanisms underlying the development of fibrosis secondary to vascular and immunological perturbation[6]. It has also fueled extensive mechanistic studies to determine the basis for this overproduction and the precise nature of the triggers involved in its initiation. Overproduction of type I collagen is a reflection of increased transcriptional activation of the two pro (I)collagen genes and of increased transcript stability. Transcriptional regulation of collagen genes has itself been a major area of biological study and a number of important *cis*-acting regulatory regions and factors interacting with these regions have been identified. More recent studies have implicated several ubiquitous transcription factors in collagen gene activation in systemic sclerosis fibroblasts, including the Smad proteins and their coactivators[7]. It seems likely that upstream regulators of these factors are disturbed in systemic sclerosis and that this leads to greater levels or more active phosphorylated forms of the transcription factors. Another possibility is that genetic differences in these factors or their regulation contribute to severity or susceptibility to scleroderma, as part of the polygenic background to this disease.

Profibrotic cytokines are likely to be involved in the initiation of fibrosis in scleroderma, and constitutive alterations in the production of some growth factors or responsiveness to their actions has been observed in scleroderma fibroblasts. One of the most potent of these is connective tissue growth factor and there is a body of evidence now suggesting that this could be an important autocrine factor in the maintenance of the scleroderma fibroblast phenotype. Modern molecular genetic methods are now being applied to understanding scleroderma as in other diseases. This includes approaches such as high-density genetic marker maps being used in pedigree and association studies to identify disease-associated loci and especially the application of methods for parallel assessment of protein and gene expression. Different studies have identified various genes, including established candidates already sug-

TABLE 135.2 RISK STRATIFICATION IN SYSTEMIC SCLEROSIS

Serological	Antibody	Clinical association
	Centromere	lcSSc, isolated pulmonary hypertension, bad gut disease
	Topoisomerase-1	Interstitial lung disease, dcSSc, renal crisis
	RNApol I, III	Renal crisis, dcSSc
	Fibrillarin	Pulmonary hypertension, myositis, cardiac disease, poor outcome
	PM-Scl	Myositis
	U1-RNP	Overlap features, cranial neuropathy
Genetic		HLA-DR52a associated with interstitial lung disease. Other severity markers likely to be identified from ongoing genetic association studies
Clinical		Subset classification represents an early example of risk assessment
		DcSSc patients overall more likely to experience a scleroderma renal crisis and systemic-sclerosis-associated lung fibrosis. Pulmonary vascular disease likely to be secondary to fibrosis
		LcSSc patients often manifest more severe peripheral vascular problems and are prone to developing isolated pulmonary hypertension. Presence of anti-RNA-polymerase or anti-topoisomerase autoantibodies appears to increase risk of the associated renal or lung complications observed in dcSSc patients with these reactivities

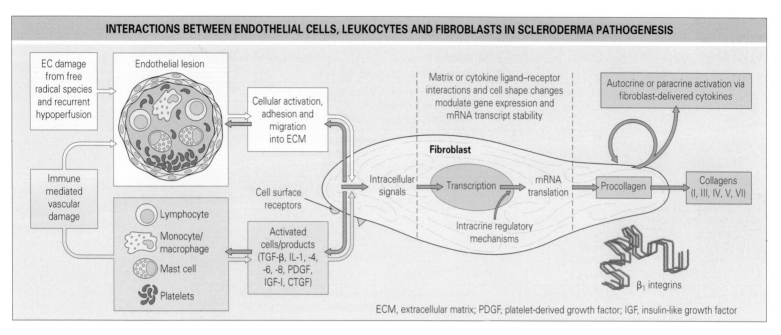

INTERACTIONS BETWEEN ENDOTHELIAL CELLS, LEUKOCYTES AND FIBROBLASTS IN SCLERODERMA PATHOGENESIS

ECM, extracellular matrix; PDGF, platelet-derived growth factor; IGF, insulin-like growth factor

Fig. 135.1 Interactions between endothelial cells (EC), leukocytes and fibroblasts in scleroderma pathogenesis. ECM, extracellular matrix; PDGF, platelet-derived growth factor; IGF, insulin-like growth factor.

gested by linkage studies and novel factors including connective tissue growth factor (CTGF)[8]. Cellular interactions and mediators involved in the pathogenesis of systemic sclerosis are outlined in Figure 135.1.

There is considerable evidence that oxidant stress may play a role in the pathogenesis of systemic sclerosis. It is potentially involved in the fragmentation of autoantigens to expose cryptic epitopes and facilitate the development of antibodies. This has been shown for RNA polymerases and topoisomerase-1 and may be catalyzed by heavy metal ions[9]. There is some data to support an additional association between exposure to heavy metals and the development of autoantibodies[10]. The combination of an appropriate HLA haplotype and exposure to appropriate immunogenic epitopes offers a unifying hypothesis to link different hallmark events in scleroderma. Since tissue hypoxia may occur secondary to Raynaud's phenomenon and the vasculopathy of scleroderma, perhaps in concert with the relative tissue hypoxia of the established lesional tissue, it is possible that oxidant stress may promote disease development. Moreover, there is additional evidence that oxidative modification of proteins may also facilitate the development of scleroderma. Antioxidant strategies for therapy offer an exciting possibility for treatment and are being pursued.

The observation that fetal cells and even naked fetal DNA may persist in the maternal circulation after pregnancy has fueled the hypothesis that some of these fetal cells may become reactivated and that scleroderma could represent a form of graft-versus-host disease[11]. Indeed, it has even been suggested that maternal cells passed to the fetus may persist, allowing an alloreactive process to be implicated in male patients with scleroderma. Although the concept is attractive, there is only weak evidence to support it and recent data have suggested that differences between scleroderma and control levels of foreign DNA are at most quantitative.

ASSESSMENT OF DISEASE

Assessment of disease activity or severity in scleroderma patients is difficult. Rapidly increasing skin sclerosis score or the presence of tendon-friction rubs have been shown to be associated with progression of visceral involvement[12,13] but these are only present in a minority of cases. To provide a more generally applicable assessment tool, modified health assessment questionnaires (HAQs) tailored specifically for systemic sclerosis patients have been developed in the USA and Europe[14].

These will undoubtedly be of considerable use, particularly since constitutional symptoms and functional impairment are among the most troublesome consequences of systemic sclerosis.

For organ-based complications such as pulmonary fibrosis, pulmonary hypertension or renal involvement, objective assessment is easier. There are many investigations that can detect or monitor these manifestations but it is generally important to consider data from several different techniques and to examine changes over time. To provide a more global index of scleroderma severity, a scoring system has recently been reported and is currently being validated[15]. In addition, activity indices are also being developed and tested and may be especially useful for assessing treatment responses in interventional studies[16,17].

Regular follow-up and appropriate assessment is the cornerstone of monitoring scleroderma. Serological markers of disease activity have long been sought and those that may be useful include soluble adhesion molecules such as soluble intercellular adhesion molecule-1, which have been shown to correlate with tissue expression. Other markers of disease activity have also been evaluated, including collagen propeptides, products of the breakdown of collagen type I and serological variables that may reflect immunological activity (e.g. soluble interleukin-2 receptor, neopterin) or vascular activation and damage (soluble E-selectin, thrombomodulin, von Willebrand factor). Some of the markers to assess overall scleroderma severity are listed in Table 135.3.

CLINICAL TRIALS IN SYSTEMIC SCLEROSIS

Difficulties in conducting clinical trials in scleroderma are well recognized[20]. These include clinical heterogeneity, absence of any treatment of proven efficacy to use as an active-control arm and a reluctance of patients with a life-threatening disorder to participate in placebo-controlled studies. To try and improve trials, guidelines for evaluating disease-modifying treatments in systemic sclerosis have been published by the American College of Rheumatology[21].

Although the current climate of evidence-based medicine has encouraged critical appraisal of current treatment approaches for systemic sclerosis, one drawback is that agents may be inadequately evaluated. It is possible that effective therapies risk being discarded because of underpowered studies that give false-negative results. Currently, consortia of clinicians around the world are vigorously improving the infrastructure for multicenter clinical trials, under the auspices of the Scleroderma

TABLE 135.3 MARKERS OF ACTIVITY AND SEVERITY OF SYSTEMIC SCLEROSIS

Skin sclerosis score	Degree of skin involvement graded between 0 (normal) and 3 (severe thickening) at defined sites. Usually 17 or 20 sites assessed. Predicts survival and functional outcome.	
Self-reported disease questionnaires	Disability index of the HAQ	20 activities in eight categories Scored 0 to 3 for analysis Associates with outcome in systemic sclerosis[18]
	SSc-VAS	Self-reported severity scales for symptoms of systemic sclerosis organ-based complications (respiratory, vascular, gastrointestinal, etc.)
	UK Functional Score	Focuses on disability caused by skin tightness in upper limb 11 items – maximum score 33[19]
Organ-based assessments	Renal Cardiac Pulmonary Gastrointestinal Vascular	
Serum markers	Collagen metabolites	Serum carboxy terminal telopeptide of type I collagen Serum amino terminal propeptide (collagen I and III) Urinary pyridinoline cross-link Endostatin (derived from type XVIII collagen)
	Coagulation regulators	Von Willebrand factor propeptide Thrombomodulin
	Adhesion molecules	sVCAM-1, sICAM-1, sE-selectin, sL-selectin, CD44
	Type II pneumocyte products	Surfactant A and D KL-6 glycoprotein
	Cytokines/growth factors	CTGF IL-12 sTNF-α receptor type 1 TGF-β1

CTGF, connective tissue growth factor; IL, interleukin; sICAM, soluble intercellular adhesion molecule; sTNF, soluble tumor necrosis factor; sVCAM, soluble vascular cell adhesion molecule; TGF, transforming growth factor.

Clinical Trials Consortium (SCTC) in the USA and the European Scleroderma Club. Up-to-date information regarding ongoing studies is available at the SCTC website (http://www.sctc-online.org).

One approach to facilitating the recruitment into clinical trials and also to providing demographic and clinical data about systemic sclerosis is through centralized systemic sclerosis clinical databases (or registries). The Michigan (USA) scleroderma registry is now well established and others are being set up in North America and Europe. Such initiatives should increase the number of cases available for studies and also help to standardize treatments.

DISEASE-MODIFYING THERAPIES FOR SYSTEMIC SCLEROSIS

The multifaceted nature of the underlying disease process in systemic sclerosis (scleroderma) makes combination approaches to disease-modifying therapy particularly appropriate. Perturbation of three different components underlies development of systemic sclerosis – the immune system, the vasculature and interstitial connective tissue. Although it is possible that these events occur sequentially, and so targeting, for example, the immune system at a very early stage might prevent other disease events, in practice by the time a diagnosis of systemic sclerosis is confirmed a range of different pathologies are likely to be present, although to different degrees. Modern approaches to disease modifying therapy therefore depend upon a combination of agents which act upon these different aspects of the disease. For early aggressive dcSSc our current approach to therapy is very much in the model of combination chemotherapy, with different parts of the underlying

pathogenic processes being targeted by different therapeutic agents. This is summarized in Figure 135.2. Few of the agents currently used as disease-modifying treatments for scleroderma-spectrum disorders have undergone rigorous placebo-controlled evaluation, and the results for those that have done are disappointing. No agent has been shown to be of unequivocal benefit and, even if such data were available, therapeutic gain must be carefully balanced against toxicity and considered in the context of the natural history of the condition. It may not be justifiable to use treatments with potentially serious side-effects in some scleroderma subsets such as lcSSc, or even in stable late-stage diffuse disease. It is likely that organ-based treatment strategies directed towards complications such as renal disease, pulmonary hypertension or fibrosing alveolitis will have more immediate effect on mortality than the development of generalized disease-modifying strategies. These can be broadly classified as immunosuppressive strategies (Table 135.4) or putative antifibrotic agents (Table 135.5). In addition, the vascular events occurring in systemic sclerosis are likely to have an important role in disease pathogenesis and some of the treatments used for Raynaud's phenomenon can be regarded as potential disease-modifying approaches (Table 135.6). Individual agents are discussed in more detail below.

Immunomodulatory treatments
Cyclophosphamide
Cyclophosphamide is an immunosuppressive drug of proven efficacy in the management of a number of autoimmune rheumatic diseases, especially primary vasculitides and manifestations of systemic lupus

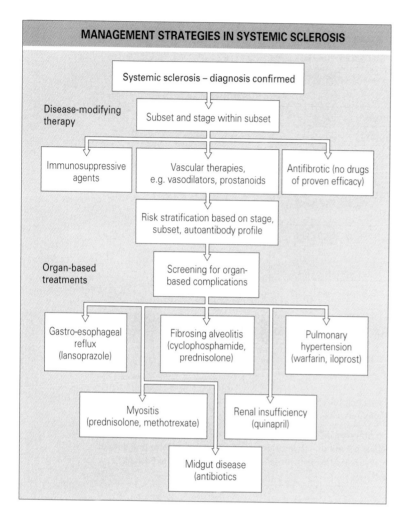

MANAGEMENT STRATEGIES IN SYSTEMIC SCLEROSIS

Systemic sclerosis – diagnosis confirmed

Disease-modifying therapy

Subset and stage within subset

Immunosuppressive agents

Vascular therapies, e.g. vasodilators, prostanoids

Antifibrotic (no drugs of proven efficacy)

Risk stratification based on stage, subset, autoantibody profile

Organ-based treatments

Screening for organ-based complications

Gastro-esophageal reflux (lansoprazole)

Fibrosing alveolitis (cyclophosphamide, prednisolone)

Pulmonary hypertension (warfarin, iloprost)

Myositis (prednisolone, methotrexate)

Renal insufficiency (quinapril)

Midgut disease (antibiotics

Fig. 135.2 Management strategies in systemic sclerosis.

erythematosus such as nephritis. It is also used as treatment for systemic-sclerosis-associated lung fibrosis and a number of retrospective series have suggested efficacy and delineated factors associated with responsiveness. There have also been a number of prospective studies, most recently a small series of five patients treated with intravenous cyclophosphamide[27]. Currently in the UK a major controlled trial is under way to evaluate cyclophosphamide in scleroderma-associated lung fibrosis, and hopefully this will be a crucial step in defining its efficacy. As for other indications, toxicity of cyclophosphamide must be carefully balanced against efficacy. Premature ovarian failure, opportunistic infections and the possibility of late secondary malignancies are important considerations in planning the route, dose and duration of cyclophosphamide administration.

Methotrexate

Methotrexate has been a profoundly effective drug for the treatment of rheumatoid arthritis. There has been reluctance to use it in systemic sclerosis – partly from concern that it can induce eosinophilic pneumonitis and hepatic fibrosis, and so theoretically might be deleterious in a disease having both fibrosis and alveolitis as features. A recent study from The Netherlands[23] included 29 patients and was placebo-controlled – for 24 weeks – followed by a 24-week open-label continuation in those patients who had apparently responded. This trial suggested benefit for skin score and lung function tests. A substantially larger study from North America has recently been reported and failed to confirm clinically significant improvement in skin sclerosis or global disease assessment score[24], although it is likely to have been under powered due to recruitment difficulties. The place of this agent in systemic sclerosis management remains unclear, although it is often effective for overlap syndromes in which arthritis is a prominent feature.

Antithymocyte globulin

The rationale for using antithymocyte globulin as a treatment for systemic sclerosis is based upon its efficacy as an immunosuppressive agent. There were several encouraging case-reports and these have been extended by one larger case series and by a randomized placebo-controlled trial in the UK. The case series of 10 patients from the Mayo Clinic (USA) with early (less than 3 years duration) dcSSc confirmed feasibility and tolerability, but endpoint changes were disappointing[35]. Currently, several centers are using antithymocyte globulin as an induction treatment for diffuse systemic sclerosis according to standardized protocols and hopefully it will be shown to be useful – but perhaps only in carefully selected patients. The short-term (opportunistic infection; hypersensitivity reactions, including serum sickness) and longer-term adverse effects will have to be carefully balanced against any therapeutic benefit. A recent report suggests that antithymocyte globulin in combination with mycophenolate mofetil is a well tolerated treatment in patients with early-stage dcSSc[26].

TABLE 135.4 IMMUNOMODULATORY STRATEGIES FOR DISEASE-MODIFYING TREATMENT OF SYSTEMIC SCLEROSIS

Agent	Clinical trial data	Reference
Cyclosporin A	Open study, 10 patients; improvement in skin score	22
Methotrexate	Placebo-controlled trial, 30 patients; significant improvement in skin score. Larger North American study inconclusive	23, 24
Extracorporeal photopheresis	Recent open study; 6/16 cases showed improvement	25
Antithymocyte globulin	Open study, 13 patients treated with mycophenolate mofetil; skin score improved	26
Cyclophosphamide	Open study, 5 patients; symptomatic improvement	27
Thalidomide	Pilot studies under way	None yet
Rapamycin	Anecdotal benefit	None yet
Oral tolerization to type I collagen	Favorable pilot data; trial ongoing in USA	28
Immunoablation/stem cell transplantation	Ongoing studies USA and Europe	29, 30

TABLE 135.5 ANTIFIBROTIC STRATEGIES FOR DISEASE-MODIFYING TREATMENT OF SYSTEMIC SCLEROSIS

Agent	Clinical trial data	Reference
D-penicillamine	High- vs low-dose study in USA, 134 patients; no apparent benefit	31
Interferon-γ	Open study, 44 patients; showed minor improvements in skin sclerosis	32
Interferon-α	Placebo-controlled trial, 35 patients; better outcome in placebo group	33
Relaxin	Placebo controlled dose-escalation study, 30 patients, stable scleroderma; encouraging. Improved global assessment score. Large phase III study negative. Considered ineffective	34
Halofuginone	Plant alkaloid with *in vitro* and *in vivo* potential to down-regulate collagen (I) gene expression. Little human data available	None yet
Prolylhydroxylase inhibition	Pilot studies under way using topical formulations for skin fibrosis. Systemic administration likely to be toxic	None yet

TABLE 135.6 VASCULAR THERAPIES FOR RAYNAUD'S PHENOMENON

Treatment	Examples	Comments
Simple measures		
Non-drug	Hand warmers; protective clothing	Universally helpful; also useful to minimize cold exposure and ambient temperature changes in work environment
Pharmacological	Evening primrose oil Fish oil capsules Antioxidant vitamins	Evening primrose oil has been shown to be effective in controlled clinical trials Theoretical benefit due to increased synthesis of vasodilator prostanoids Potentially reduce oxidant stress, which may contribute to Raynaud's symptoms and pathology
Oral vasodilators		
Calcium channel blockers	Nifedipine, nicardipine, diltiazem, amlodipine	Variable and differential response to different agents. Slow titration of dose reduced the severity of side-effects. Try each drug for at least 3 weeks if possible
5-HT antagonists	Ketanserin Fluoxetine	5-HT receptor antagonist; limited availability Readily available; fewer vasodilatory side-effects than calcium channel blockers. Depletes platelet 5-HT levels
Angiotensin antagonists	Quinapril, captopril, enalapril Losartan	ACE inhibitors block formation of angiotensin II. Need to observe renal function. Cough may be troublesome Well tolerated, potential remodeling potential by blocking fibrogenic effects of angiotensin II
Parenteral vasodilators	Iloprost, Flolan, prostaglandin E1	Effective at healing ulcers and reducing severity and frequency of Raynaud's attacks. Expensive and limited long-term duration of benefit
Antibiotics	Flucloxacillin, erythromycin	Important adjunct to vasodilator therapy for secondary infection of digital ulcers. Prolonged treatment necessitated by poor tissue perfusion.
Surgical procedures		
Lumbar sympathectomy	Chemical or operative	For severe lower limb Raynaud's
Radical microarteriolysis	Division of adventitia of digital arteries; sometimes termed digital sympathectomy	Useful treatment for individual critically ischemic digits
Debridement, amputation	Surgical or autoamputation	Surgery should be as conservative as possible to allow maximum possibility of spontaneous healing

Cyclosporin A

Cyclosporin A has attractive properties for treating systemic sclerosis, especially for those cases of aggressive dcSSc in which there is marked immunological activation. The main problem has however been toxicity. For scleroderma there are particular risks, especially from nephrotoxicity. One series suggested that the rate of renal systemic sclerosis crisis may be twice that expected for patients with aggressive dcSSc treated using cyclosporin[36]. An open-label study of 48 weeks of administration suggested efficacy, although there was significant toxicity, especially at doses above 3–4mg/kg per day[22]. A recent trial using the related agent FK506 has been reported but, despite its theoretically safer renal side-effect profile, there was still substantial toxicity. However, it is possible that the related agent rapamycin will prove more useful. This is already used in solid-organ transplantation and has attractive antifibrotic properties, in addition to being an effective immunosuppressive drug[37].

Immunoablation with autologous peripheral stem cell rescue
One of the most aggressive approaches to therapy for systemic sclerosis is the use of immunoablation followed by reconstitution using autologous peripheral stem cell rescue. An open phase I/II study of this treatment has been reported[29] and there are additional ongoing programs to evaluate this treatment in Europe and the USA[30]. The rationale for this therapy is similar to that in other autoimmune diseases. Thus, if systemic sclerosis is being driven by an autoimmune process then ablation of self-reactive lymphocyte clones may block pathogenesis. If the immune system is reconstituted in the presence of the neoantigens responsible for autoimmunity then tolerance will be re-established. However, even if such toleration does not occur it is still plausible that the intensive immunosuppression during this treatment will be directly beneficial. A major European multicenter study comparing immunoablation with peripheral stem cell reconstitution against intravenous cyclophosphamide is currently under way (see http://www.astis.org).

Photopheresis for diffuse cutaneous scleroderma
Another immunosuppressive strategy is extracorporeal photopheresis following sensitization of host leukocytes by methylpsoralen. This is of proven value for some cutaneous conditions, notably T cell lymphoma. In view of the presence of an infiltrate of active immune cells in early systemic sclerosis – especially the diffuse cutaneous subset – there was a plausible theoretical basis to using this mode of treatment. It has been undertaken in several centers and a number of uncontrolled studies have reported benefit, although a recent controlled trial was less persuasive[25].

Oral tolerization to type I collagen
In a disease whose pathological hallmark is increased extracellular matrix deposition it is somewhat surprising that oral type I collagen administration is being proposed. The rationale is based upon the observation that oral tolerance to type I collagen can be induced and the hypothesis that there may be an autoimmune reaction to collagen in systemic sclerosis contributing to local production of cytokines[28]. There are some experimental data supporting this and a controlled trial is under way. Oral collagen offers the advantage of being apparently safe and also applicable to established disease, which is otherwise difficult to treat.

Antifibrotic therapy
D-penicillamine
Probably the most widely used agent for treating systemic sclerosis has been D-penicillamine. There have been a large number of studies examining its effect. The pivotal trial, a rigorously designed and carefully executed double-blind controlled clinical trial, has recently been completed and reported, comparing two doses of this drug. Rather disappointingly, this study showed no difference between high (750–1000mg daily) and low (125mg on alternate days) dose regimens, certainly providing no justification for using high doses[31]. Although this study was not positive therapeutically, it has nevertheless provided a large prospectively collected data set documenting the natural history of early dcSSc, which has been instructive about predictors of outcome[18,38]. Penicillamine may still have a place in localized disease, childhood scleroderma or generalized morphea, and in overlap syndromes, when it may also benefit other aspects of the disease such as arthritis, although this is unproven.

Interferons
Interferons (α, β or γ) exert pleiotropic effects on fibroblasts *in vitro* including downregulating extracellular matrix gene expression. This led to the hope that the interferons might have antifibrotic activity *in vivo*. There were a number of encouraging pilot studies and these prompted more extensive evaluation of interferon (IFN)-γ and IFN-α. Following an encouraging open study[39], a placebo-controlled trial of IFN-α for early dcSSc was undertaken in the UK[33]. Unfortunately, a substantial withdrawal rate and mortality was observed – and interim analysis confirmed a greater mortality in the active-treatment arm. Moreover, no benefit for skin sclerosis or pulmonary function, the main study endpoints, was demonstrable. Two studies of IFN-γ have recently been reported, although neither was placebo-controlled. These suggest modest benefit[32], but open studies require cautious interpretation. Overall, it is disappointing that interferons have not fulfilled their early promise; whether they will ultimately have any place in scleroderma treatment remains uncertain. A recent report has suggested that IFN-γ may be useful in treating idiopathic lung fibrosis, and this has rejuvenated interest in this important family of biological mediators[40].

Halofuginone
This plant alkaloid has shown promise as an antifibrotic agent[41] and has been used in small studies in experimental animals with benefit to pathologies including surgical adhesions and postangioplasty stenosis or liver cirrhosis. It appears to selectively downregulate expression of extracellular matrix genes, although its molecular mechanism is poorly defined. It has been used in murine graft-versus-host disease and in tight-skin mice – two animal models of scleroderma[42] – and is currently undergoing preliminary assessment in systemic sclerosis.

Recombinant human relaxin
Another promising agent is recombinant human relaxin. This hormone, normally present in significant amounts only in pregnant woman, appears to have benefit in systemic sclerosis. *In vitro* studies suggest that relaxin reduces synthesis of type I collagen by scleroderma fibroblasts and a dose-escalating placebo-controlled trial has shown benefit, measured by skin score and other endpoints including self-reported health assessment questionnaires[34]. Unfortunately, a large and well-conducted phase III study of relaxin in systemic sclerosis was negative, and so this previously exciting agent is no longer being developed for use in systemic sclerosis.

Minocycline
Another drug that has been tried in a very small study is minocycline. This agent has a number of properties in addition to being an antibiotic. These include an ability to inhibit metalloproteinases – although this would not be helpful in a systemic fibrotic disease. The pilot study of minocycline[43] was widely reported in the lay press and to determine usefulness a larger, formal evaluation is essential. A controlled clinical trial is currently under way to evaluate this treatment and the results are eagerly awaited.

Vascular therapy
The most frequent vascular manifestation of scleroderma is episodic peripheral vasospasm (Raynaud's phenomenon), present in 95% of cases. Although many studies have confirmed the efficacy of oral vasodilators in primary Raynaud's phenomenon, treatment of scleroderma-associated vasospasm is much more difficult. One problem is that side-effects are often dose-limiting and patients with secondary Raynaud's phenomenon may require higher doses than those with the primary form. Responses to individual vasodilators are idiosyncratic, and substantial placebo responses and lack of objective assessment tools confound therapeutic trials.

Intermittent infusion of prostacyclin or its analogs have been shown to be effective[44] but remain inconvenient and costly. In addition to benefiting peripheral vasospasm, one report suggested that iloprost had beneficial effects on renal blood flow, estimated non-invasively. Orally active formulations of prostacyclin or its analogs are an attractive proposition but unfortunately two large studies recently published from Europe and North America have failed to conclusively demonstrate efficacy. In the European study, which followed encouraging results from an earlier investigation of oral iloprost for primary Raynaud's phenomenon, there was some benefit[45] but a parallel North American study was negative.

Other novel therapeutic approaches for Raynaud's phenomenon include probucol, which may exert its effect via its antioxidant properties[46] and low-molecular-weight heparin, which may modulate a number of aspects of the pathogenesis of Raynaud's phenomenon[47]. Some promising preliminary data for losartan, a specific angiotensin receptor antagonist, have also been reported recently[48]. Treatment options for Raynaud's phenomenon are summarized in Table 135.6.

Targeted molecular therapy for systemic sclerosis

Advances in understanding the pathogenic processes that underlie the development and progression of systemic sclerosis raise the possibility of identifying key molecular mediators that are central to the disease and might provide specific targets for therapeutic modulation. Some of these potential targets are listed in Table 135.7. This list is incomplete and rather speculative but illustrates the way in which laboratory studies directed towards understanding disease mechanisms may fuel new approaches to therapy. Some of the novel therapies currently under evaluation are outlined below.

ORGAN-BASED ASSESSMENT AND TREATMENTS

Progress in managing organ-based complications has been made by drawing analogy with other medical disorders such as peptic ulcer disease, idiopathic pulmonary fibrosis and systemic or pulmonary hypertension. As with many other chronic diseases, a multidisciplinary approach to therapy is useful to address the patient's physical, emotional and social requirements as well as their medical problems. Physiotherapy, exercises to maintain finger function, and skin care are all important. Patient education is an integral component of successful management and careful explanation of the disease and its complications is often necessary. Specialist nurse-educators, telephone helplines and patient support organizations all have a valuable place in management.

Cutaneous involvement

Skin sclerosis is present in almost all forms of systemic sclerosis, exceptions being some patients with very early disease and those with the rare subset designated systemic sclerosis *sine* scleroderma, in whom vascular and visceral manifestations occur in the absence of skin involvement. However, treatment of the disease is rarely dictated by its cutaneous manifestations. Visceral involvement is far more important in terms of morbidity and mortality and also even those patients with severe skin sclerosis often demonstrate stabilization and even softening of the skin with time, and overall even the most severe cases of dcSSc show plateauing of skin sclerosis some 2–3 years into the disease. Systemic antihistamine therapy can provide some relief for intractable itching, which is a feature of early dcSSc.

In addition to sclerosis, other cutaneous manifestations include calcinotic nodules, especially in lcSSc. No medical therapy has been shown to be effective but local surgery can be helpful. Another complication is skin ulceration, which can arise through a number of mechanisms – ischaemia from Raynaud's phenomenon, trophic ulcers associated with contractural deformities or underlying calcinosis, and perhaps also large-vessel vasculopathy. Secondary infection should be vigorously treated; poor tissue perfusion may require increased doses or extended courses of antibiotics. Optimizing the circulation using oral or parenteral vasodilators is also important, especially when ulceration is associated with severe peripheral vasospasm. Moisturizing creams, emulsifying ointments and molten wax application help by maintaining skin flexibility and reducing susceptibility to trauma.

Another frequent manifestation of scleroderma is the development of cutaneous dilated loops of small blood vessels (telangiectasias). Although occurring as a prominent feature in lcSSc they are frequently also present in patients with late-stage dcSSc. Indeed they may become more florid in the plateau phase of dcSSc even when the skin sclerosis diminishes. These are distressing for patients and may also cause problems if they are at sites prone to trauma. Hemorrhage from mucosal telangiectasias is also becoming increasingly recognized as a clinical problem and may require local therapy if it is a recurrent problem. Cosmetic camouflage techniques can be very effective for masking facial telangiectasias and appropriate advice should be offered to all patients who might benefit. Recently, the pulsed dye laser has also been used with some success.

Pulmonary disease

With improved survival from renal hypertensive crisis, pulmonary disease (fibrosis and hypertension) is now the most frequent cause of death in systemic sclerosis.

Interstitial pulmonary fibrosis

An algorithm for the investigation and management of pulmonary fibrosis in systemic sclerosis is shown in Figure 135.3. The most common symptoms of respiratory involvement in systemic sclerosis are breathlessness, especially on exertion, and a dry cough. Chest pain is infrequent and frank hemoptysis rare, and if either are present then the presence of additional pathology should be sought. On physical examination the most frequent finding is of bilateral basal crepitations. The classical radiographic features consist of reticulonodular shadowing, usually symmetrical and most marked at the lung bases. However, the chest radiograph is an insensitive indicator of fibrosing alveolitis, and should be used only as an initial screen or to exclude infection or aspiration secondary to esophageal abnormalities. There are many symptomatic patients (often mildly so) with normal chest radiographs despite interstitial lung disease, and lung function tests can be discriminatory. The single-breath diffusion test (D_LCO) is abnormal in over 70% of

TABLE 135.7 CANDIDATE MOLECULAR TARGETS IN SYSTEMIC SCLEROSIS	
Target	**Comments**
Cytokines	
IL-4	Beneficial effect of anti-IL-4 in tight-skin mouse model
IL-6	Anti-IL-6 blocks profibrotic activity of medium conditioned by systemic sclerosis fibroblasts
bFGF	Endothelial-cell-induced activation of fibroblasts blocked by anti-bFGF
TGF-β	Antibody to TGF-β reverses skin fibrosis in the minimal mismatch graft-versus-host disease murine model of scleroderma; anti-TGF-β1 currently being evaluated in early dcSSc
ET-1	Endothelin receptor blockade is effective in treating pulmonary arterial hypertension. Profibrotic and immunostimulatory effects of ET-1 broaden its potential as a therapeutic target.
CTGF	Prototypic member of the CCN family of cytokines. May be important in sustained fibrotic responses.
Adhesion molecules	
ICAM-1	Enhanced lymphocyte-fibroblast interaction for systemic sclerosis cells *in vitro* blocked by anti-ICAM-1
Intracellular signaling	
	Inhibitor of geranylgeranyl transferase specifically downregulates extracellular matrix genes in systemic sclerosis fibroblasts

bFGF, basic fibroblast growth factor; ICAM, intercellular adhesion molecule; IL, interleukin; TGF, transforming growth factor.

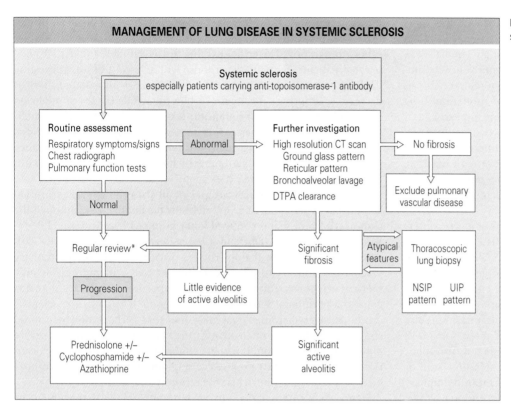

Fig. 135.3 Management of lung disease in systemic sclerosis.

patients with dcSSc (including asymptomatic patients with no complaints and an unremarkable chest radiograph). A reduction in D_LCO is the earliest proven abnormality in patients with systemic sclerosis who develop interstitial lung disease; lung function tests that show normal volumes but reduced transfer of gases in the face of normal imaging are suggestive of pure pulmonary vascular disease (see below).

The application of thin-section (3mm), high-resolution computed tomography (HRCT) scanning of the lungs has been of immense value for definition and assessment of diffuse lung diseases and has revealed the character and distribution of fine structural abnormalities not visible on chest radiographs. Using this technique, the earliest detectable abnormality is usually a narrow, often ill-defined, subpleural crescent of increased density in the posterior segments of the lower lobes. When more extensive, the shadowing often takes on a more characteristic reticulonodular appearance, yet frequently retaining a subpleural distribution. It also becomes associated with fine, honeycomb air spaces and ultimately larger, cystic air spaces an appearance that mirrors the macroscopic appearance.

In predicting the histological pattern, CT, although useful, has not replaced lung biopsy as the 'gold standard' investigation. As yet, patients who appear to have early changes on CT should still be considered for a thoracoscopic biopsy for staging of the disease. Drawing an analogy from studies of idiopathic pulmonary fibrosis (IPF), lung biopsies can be classified as non-specific interstitial pneumonia (NSIP) or usual interstitial pneumonia (UIP; see Chapter 29)[48]. In systemic sclerosis the predominant histological pattern is NSIP whereas in IPF the majority show UIP. Outside the context of systemic sclerosis there is a better long-term outcome for NSIP and this may have important implications for systemic-sclerosis-associated lung disease.

It is not yet possible to distinguish histological subtypes by HRCT and so lung biopsy remains an important clinical and research tool. In the evaluation of diffuse lung disease, bronchoalveolar lavage has now been used for almost 20 years to sample cells and non-cellular material from the lower respiratory tract. The presence of abnormal numbers of granulocytes, particularly neutrophils and eosinophils, is typical for a patient with fibrosing alveolitis occurring alone or in the context of systemic sclerosis. Excess lymphocytes are found in some individuals. In a typical patient with fibrosing alveolitis, bronchoalveolar lavage would produce

an increase in total cell returns of three- to sixfold (up to 6×10^5/ml of fluid return); of these, up to 20% may be neutrophils or eosinophils.

Excess lymphocytes may be found (up to 20% of the total cells) and an increase in mast cells may be observed in a small percentage of patients. The prognostic value of bronchoalveolar lavage has been demonstrated in several studies. Silver et al.[49] reported that patients with scleroderma with persistent alveolitis have greater deterioration in their pulmonary function than alveolitis-negative patients with systemic sclerosis.

The use of diethylenetriaminepenta-acetic acid (DTPA) clearance in the management of systemic sclerosis has been the subject of extensive study and has been shown to be of value. It identifies early disease and also identifies a group of patients whose disease will run a more stable, non-progressive course, i.e. those with normal clearance. The speed of clearance of the isotope is dependent upon the integrity of the epithelial barrier and therefore anything that disrupts this, either inflammation or fibrosis, will increase the rate of clearance. Persistently normal DTPA clearance predicts stable disease and therefore provides a good prognostic index; a study showed significant improvement in pulmonary function tests in 75% of patients whose clearance returned to the normal range whereas similar improvements were not seen in those whose clearance remained normal or abnormally fast[50].

The definition and assessment of lung fibrosis in systemic sclerosis has now reached the stage that the extent, pattern and activity of lung disease can be reliably assessed. Unfortunately, while this provides a number of validated tools to assess outcome, treatments remain unproven. Corticosteroids and cyclophosphamide are the most widely used treatments, while among the studies that have been performed, several suggest benefit. No trial has been prospective, placebo-controlled and of sufficient rigor to confirm efficacy. Fortunately, there are now studies under way in both North America and the UK to assess oral or parenteral cyclophosphamide; the results of these are eagerly awaited.

Pulmonary hypertension

Systemic-sclerosis-related pulmonary vascular disease occurs in several contexts. The most important of these is its manifestation as isolated pulmonary hypertension (PHT), occurring in up to 10% of patients with lcSSc and a smaller proportion of those with dcSSc. There are serological associations for both types, ACA being more common in patients with lcSSc and antifibrillarin (anti-U3RNP) being associated with this complication in diffuse systemic sclerosis. The pathology of isolated PHT in systemic sclerosis is very similar to that of idiopathic or familial PHT and the latter has been used as a treatment paradigm for systemic-sclerosis-associated disease. Patients with associated pulmonary fibrosis may develop secondary PHT, as in other forms of interstitial lung disease, and this may require consideration in managing these cases as it is important to determine the contribution of the two pathologies, which may require different treatment strategies. Other situations in which PHT occurs include associated cardiac disease with diastolic dysfunction. Rare causes include recurrent thromboembolic disease, including that associated with antiphospholipid autoantibodies in the context of systemic sclerosis.

Current treatment and investigation of PHT occurring in the context of systemic sclerosis requires first that the diagnosis is made. The first indication may be from symptoms, which typically include exertional breathlessness and less often chest pain or syncope. In general, patients with systemic sclerosis undergo regular monitoring of pulmonary function, Doppler echocardiography and electrocardiography examination. In the majority of cases the clinical suspicion of pulmonary vascular disease arises because of abnormal tests, as outlined above. Definitive diagnosis requires exclusion of related pathologies such as thromboembolic disease (by ventilation/perfusion lung scan, spiral CT scan or pulmonary angiography) and establishment that the mean pulmonary artery pressure is above 25mmHg at rest or 30mmHg during exercise. Although there is a reasonably good correlation between estimated peak pulmonary artery pressure using Doppler echocardiography and measurements at right heart catheterization at low and high values, this is not always true between 30 and 50mmHg and caution must be used. For this reason, and the additional information which it yields, right heart catheterization has become mandatory for optimal management of these cases. It allows pulmonary venous hypertension to be identified using the pulmonary capillary wedge pressure and the pulmonary vascular resistance, cardiac output (cardiac index) and pulmonary artery pressures to be measured.

All patients with PHT should receive oral anticoagulation and, if appropriate, diuretic therapy (usually spironolactone) and digoxin. If there is evidence of sustained hypoxia (arterial saturation consistently below 90% on air), long-term low-dose oxygen can be helpful by reducing hypoxia-induced pulmonary vasoconstriction. Typically, 2 liters per minute is given, using nasal cannulas.

It has become much more important to detect pulmonary vascular disease now that there are licensed treatments for use both in PHT and in PHT associated with connective tissue disease. The first agent shown to be effective was parenteral prostacyclin in the form of Flolan, in two controlled clinical trials. This is given as a long-term treatment using an ambulatory pump and permanent indwelling central venous line. More recently, other routes of administration have also been shown to improve symptoms, including subcutaneous infusion and inhaled routes.

More exciting still were results of the BREATHE-1 study, which suggest that bosentan, a relatively well tolerated orally active agent, is also an effective treatment for PHT. Bosentan is a broad-spectrum endothelin (ET) receptor antagonist and elevated serum and tissue levels of ET have been clearly demonstrated in systemic sclerosis, providing a rationale for this treatment.

The complex nature of the diagnosis of PHT and of determining its basis, together with the need to diagnose early, when surrogate markers such as $D_L CO$ on pulmonary function testing or evidence of right-sided abnormalities on echocardiography may be equivocal, justifies having a low threshold for right heart catheterization. This allows the diagnosis to be confirmed using pressure measurements at rest and during exercise and also allows cardiac index and pulmonary vascular resistance to be directly measured. These variables often change before significantly elevated pressures can be detected non-invasively, for instance by Doppler echocardiography. Nevertheless, this test is valuable for use in non-selected patients, particularly in those with clinical features suggesting PHT. If on testing pulmonary function there is an isolated marked decrease in diffusing capacity for carbon monoxide (<50% of predicted normal) in the absence of significant restrictive ventilatory abnormalities, then pulmonary hypertension should be strongly suspected. Non-invasive investigative tools such as gated cardiac magnetic resonance imaging and exercise echocardiography hold promise for the future but are not yet widely available.

Pathologically, pulmonary arteries of all sizes show marked intimal and medial hyperplasia; of great interest is the finding that, although the clinical syndrome seems confined to the group with lcSSc, intimal thickening and narrowing, albeit to a lesser degree, occur in patients with dcSSc[51]. In addition to the obstructive vascular lesions, the pulmonary vasculature appears to be abnormally reactive, with significant pulmonary vasoconstriction occurring on exposure to cold, again analogous to a peripheral Raynaud's phenomenon. That systemic sclerosis can be an overwhelmingly vascular disease is perhaps nowhere more convincingly demonstrated than in the subset of patients with severe pulmonary hypertension. It has an extraordinarily poor prognosis; death is usually due to rapidly progressive respiratory insufficiency accompanied by severe right-ventricular hypertrophy and failure.

Figure 135.4 summarizes our current approach to management of systemic-sclerosis-associated pulmonary hypertension.

Renal disease

The most important renal complication is scleroderma renal crisis – typically occurring in the diffuse disease subset within the first 3 years of diagnosis and associated with clinical worsening of skin sclerosis. It has recently been reported that corticosteroid use (more than 20mg prednisolone per day or equivalent) may predispose to the development of scleroderma renal crisis[52]. Patients at risk should be warned to check their blood pressure regularly. At onset this is often elevated markedly, with retinopathy and other signs of end-organ damage, including blood and protein in the urine. Although the widespread early use of angiotensin converting enzyme (ACE) inhibitors, along with other improvements in managing acute renal failure, has undoubtedly improved survival rate[53], the prognosis of established scleroderma renal crisis is still poor, with over 30% of patients progressing to renal replacement therapy. It is nevertheless a significant mark of progress that renal crisis is no longer the most frequent cause of scleroderma-associated death.

Powerful parenteral antihypertensives (e.g. intravenous nitroprusside or labetolol) should be avoided in the management of scleroderma renal crisis since they may exacerbate renal pathology by overdilatation of a vasoconstricted vascular bed, leading to relative hypovolemia and renal hypoperfusion. Similarly, diuretic therapy should also be avoided. Central venous pressure monitoring and an indwelling arterial cannula for systemic arterial pressure measurement should be considered, especially if sclerodermatous involvement of the upper limb causes difficulties in using a sphygmomanometer. It is crucial to avoid administration of potentially nephrotoxic agents such as non-steroidal anti-inflammatory drugs (NSAIDs) and/or X-ray contrast dyes.

Hypertension should be treated using ACE inhibitors. It has been suggested that quinapril may be preferable to other agents, although historically most patients have received either captopril or enalapril, together with calcium channel blockers. Sublingual nifedipine or subcutaneous hydralazine can be used if the patient is vomiting. Intravenous prostacyclin, which may directly benefit the microvascular lesion, is often administered from diagnosis. Regular blood film examination for evidence of red cell fragmentation (including schistocytosis) may provide

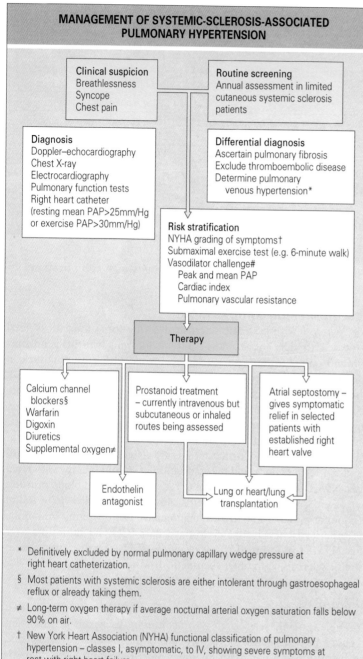

Fig. 135.4 Management of systemic-sclerosis-associated pulmonary hypertension.

* Definitively excluded by normal pulmonary capillary wedge pressure at right heart catheterization. † New York Heart Association (NYHA) functional classification of pulmonary hypertension – classes I, asymptomatic, to IV, showing severe symptoms at rest with right heart failure. ‡ Prostacyclin analog, inhaled nitric oxide or intravenous adenosine may be used. Positive if 20% fall in pulmonary artery pressure (PAP) and pulmonary vascular resistance without fall in cardiac output. § Most patients with systemic sclerosis are either intolerant because of gastroesophageal reflux or are already taking them. ¶ Long-term oxygen therapy if average nocturnal arterial oxygen saturation falls below 90% on air.

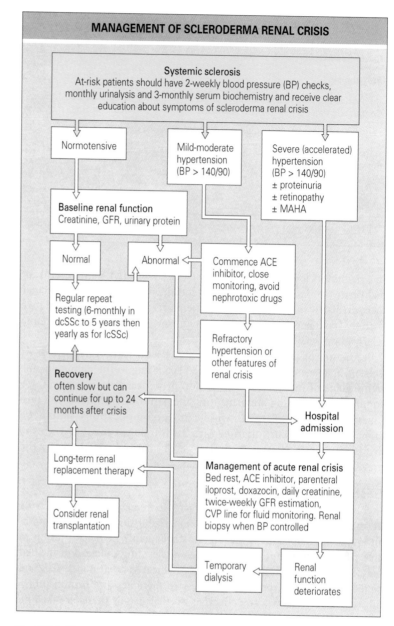

Fig. 135.5 Management of scleroderma renal crisis. CVP, central venous pressure; GFR, glomerular filtration rate; MAHA, microangiopathic hemolytic anemia.

2 years. Therefore decisions regarding renal transplantation should not be made before this time. These management approaches are presented schematically in Fig. 135.5.

Cardiac disease

It is likely that cardiac involvement from scleroderma, although important and life-threatening, is underdiagnosed. This partly reflects the intrinsic difficulties of detection of manifestations such as paroxysmal arrhythmia or cardiac fibrosis. By analogy with advances that have occurred in the other important complications it is likely that cardiac scleroderma management will be facilitated when clinicians are better able to identity the stage, subset and perhaps ethnic groups that are particularly susceptible. Accurate risk stratification will then allow screening resources to be applied in a more focused way. Treatment of cardiac manifestations is currently based on the management of similar clinical events occurring outside the context of systemic sclerosis. Thus antiarrhythmic agents are used for hemodynamically significant dysrhythmias and pacemaker insertion is considered when there is evidence of significant conduction abnormalities. Recent studies suggest that conduction defects are the most frequent electrophysiological disturbances

useful additional information regarding ongoing microangiopathy. Renal function should be monitored until the condition either stabilizes or requires renal replacement therapy. Short-term hemodialysis should be given if necessary and peritoneal dialysis often works well if long-term renal replacement therapy is needed. Considerable recovery in renal function often occurs after an acute crisis, sometimes allowing dialysis to be discontinued, and improvement can continue for up to

TABLE 135.8 MANAGEMENT OF CARDIAC DISEASE IN SYSTEMIC SCLEROSIS

Cardiac disease	Pathology	Frequency	Clinical features	Investigation	Treatment
Arrhythmias	Re-entry mechanism or inflammation	Uncertain	Palpitation, syncope	ECG, especially 24h with symptom diary; stress test	Treat only if hemodynamically significant
Conduction defects	Local fibrosis	10% on ECG	Syncope	ECG	May require pacemaker
Pericardial disease	Inflammation or effusion	10% clinically, 30% at autopsy	Chest pain, dyspnea	ECG, echocardiogram	NSAID, corticosteroids, drainage, fenestration
Myocardial involvement	Myocarditis	Rare	Congestive cardiac failure, arrhythmias	ECG, echocardiogram, MUGA, gated cardiac MRI	Management of heart failure; immunosuppression/ corticosteroids if myocarditis
	Myocardial fibrosis	30–50% dcSSc			

ECG, electrocardiography; MRI, magnetic resonance imaging; MUGA, multiple uptake gated acquisition scan.

in systemic sclerosis, and these may be associated with re-entrant tachyarrhythmias. Some cases of re-entrant monomorphic ventricular tachycardia in systemic sclerosis patients responding to local ablative therapy have been reported. Treatment options for cardiac systemic sclerosis are detailed in Table 135.8.

Predictors of poor cardiac outcome remain to be established. At present, management is individualized according to the hemodynamic significance of myocardial dysfunction or pericardial disease and, for conduction or rhythm abnormalities, the perceived likelihood of a life-threatening event. Patients with cardiac complications should be managed in close consultation with a cardiologist familiar with the disease and an important clinical research goal is to define better the prevalence and natural history of cardiac scleroderma.

Gastrointestinal tract

Involvement of the gastrointestinal tract is extremely frequent in scleroderma. Abnormalities have been demonstrated throughout its length, although the esophagus is the site most frequently involved – in up to 80% of patients. Simple measures such as elevating the head of the bed may be a useful adjunct to more sophisticated treatments. Clinical benefit is obtained from acid-suppressive therapies and proton-pump inhibitors are dramatically effective, so that use of these as first-line treatment is often justified. High doses may be needed to control severe esophagitis. Additional benefit can be obtained from adding cisapride to treat esophageal spasm or dysmotility.

Anal involvement is also common but underdiagnosed, incontinence being the most common complaint. It is important to inquire specifically about anorectal dysfunction so that patients can be offered clear advice to help them cope with this distressing manifestation.

Bacterial overgrowth of the small intestine has been shown to occur frequently in systemic sclerosis and also be associated with more symptoms than in non-systemic-sclerosis cases. This probably reflects changes in small-bowel structure and motility, although the influence of other therapies has also been suggested, notably acid-suppressive treatments. Broad-spectrum antibiotics are helpful in treating bacterial overgrowth and can be dramatically effective in some cases. Sometimes, intermittent single-agent courses are effective but refractory cases may require rotational antibiotics. When this is to be contemplated it is useful to confirm the diagnosis using a hydrogen breath test prior to starting therapy.

Antral venous ectasia has a characteristic appearance at endoscopy, hence the synonym 'watermelon stomach'. It manifests as iron-deficiency anemia due to recurrent or chronic hemorrhage, or as more substantial episodic hematemesis or melena. It is an important diagnosis because it is potentially life-threatening and also because it is amenable to treatment using laser photocoagulation. Such intervention is warranted because chronic hemorrhage from telangiectatic lesions is now recognized as a significant cause of iron deficiency in systemic sclerosis.

Investigation and treatment of gastrointestinal complications of systemic sclerosis is outlined in Table 135.9.

Musculoskeletal complications

Most patients with systemic sclerosis describe some musculoskeletal features. Arthralgia and stiffness are frequent; frank arthritis is uncommon and points towards an overlap syndrome. Other musculoskeletal manifestations include carpal tunnel syndrome, tendinitis (with friction rubs – most often in dcSSc) and the consequences of contractures, especially affecting the hands but also more proximal joints in dcSSc. Regular exercise programs may reduce the development of soft tissue contractures and input from physiotherapists and occupational therapists can be invaluable. Corticosteroids are generally avoided because of their long-term toxicity and the association of steroid therapy with renal crisis. NSAIDs may be detrimental to renal function and blood pressure control and can aggravate esophagitis, although this is likely to be less of an issue for patients who are on maintenance proton-pump inhibitors. The superiority of selective cyclo-oxygenase (COX)-2 inhibitors over other NSAIDs in terms of efficacy or side-effects remains unproven in systemic sclerosis, as in other rheumatic diseases.

SUMMARY

Although systemic sclerosis is an uncommon disease, it is important because it has the highest mortality of any of the rheumatic diseases, and also because it is a paradigm for other more common medical conditions in which immunologically triggered fibrosis occurs, such as liver cirrhosis and idiopathic pulmonary fibrosis. All patients with scleroderma-spectrum disorders should be assessed by physicians familiar with these conditions. In this way the diagnosis is confirmed, patients can be educated about the disease, and follow-up and treatment can be tailored according to stage, subset and activity. Further advances in management will probably depend on collating data from different centers to better define markers of poor prognosis, and will also require interventional studies to confirm efficacy for current treatments and to test novel agents. Management of life-threatening complications should be proactive, with screening of at-risk patients and commencement of therapy at the earliest opportunity. Survival studies strongly suggest that the outcome for scleroderma patients has improved significantly over the past 25 years and scleroderma should now be considered treatable, if not curable. ACE inhibitors appear to have substantially improved survival from renal scleroderma crisis, there is growing evidence that cyclophosphamide is effective in scleroderma-associated fibrosing alveolitis, and prostacyclin analogs are showing promise in patients with pulmonary hypertension. Effective acid-suppressing regimens, notably proton-pump inhibitors, have revolutionized the management of scleroderma-associated esophagitis.

TABLE 135.9 GASTROINTESTINAL TRACT PATHOLOGY IN SYSTEMIC SCLEROSIS

Site	Disorder	Symptom	Investigation	Treatment
Mouth	Tight skin	Cosmetic	None	Facial exercises
	Dental caries	Toothache	Dental radiograph	Dental treatment
	Sicca syndrome	Dry mouth	Salivary gland biopsy	Artificial saliva
Esophagus	Dysmotility/esophageal spasm	Dysphagia	Barium swallow	Proton-pump inhibitors
	Reflux esophagitis	Heartburn	Esophageal scintigraphy	Minimize NSAID and calcium-channel
		Dysphagia	Manometry	blocker use
	Stricture		Endoscopy	Elevate head of bed
				Avoid late meals
Stomach	Gastric paresis	Anorexia	Scintigram	Proton-pump inhibitors
	NSAID-related ulcer	Nausea	Endoscopy	Metoclopramide, domperidone
		Early satiety	Barium meal	
Small bowel	Hypomotility	Weight loss	Barium follow-through	Rotational antibiotics
	Stasis	Postprandial bloating	^{14}C glycocholate or hydrogen breath test	Erythromycin
	Bacterial overgrowth	Malabsorption	Jejunal aspiration	Domperidone, metoclopramide
		Steatorrhea		Octreotide (low dose)
	NSAID enteropathy		Fecal microscopy	Oral nutritional supplements
				Enteral or parenteral nutritional support
	Pseudo-obstruction	Abdominal pain	Plain abdominal radiograph	Conservative management: 'drip and suck'
		Distention		
	Pneumatosis intestinalis	Diarrhea with blood; benign pneumoperitoneum	Plain abdominal radiograph	
Large bowel	Hypomotility	Alternating constipation and diarrhea	Barium enema	Dietary manipulation
				Stool expanders for constipation
				Loperamide for diarrhea
	Colonic pseudodiverticula	Rare perforation	Barium enema	(Resection as a last resort)
	Pseudo-obstruction	Abdominal pain	Plain abdominal radiograph	Conservative management: 'drip and suck'
		Distention		
Anus	Sphincter involvement	Fecal incontinence	Rectal manometry	Protective measures
				Sacral nerve stimulation

However there is much scope for further improvement. The ultimate goal is to develop targeted disease-process-directed treatments in addition to managing organ-based complications. This is only likely to be possible when key events and mediators in pathogenesis are elucidated.

REFERENCES

1. LeRoy EC, Black CM, Fleischmajer R *et al*. Scleroderma (systemic sclerosis): classification, subsets, and pathogenesis. J Rheumatol 1988; 15: 202–205.
2. LeRoy EC, Medsger TA Jr. Criteria for the classification of early systemic sclerosis. J Rheumatol 2001; 28: 1573–1576.
3. Briggs D, Stephens C, Vaughan R et al. A molecular and serologic analysis of the major histocompatibility complex and complement component C4 in systemic sclerosis. Arthritis Rheum 1993; 36: 943–954.
4. Bunn CC, Black CM. Systemic sclerosis: an autoantibody mosaic. Clin Exp Immunol 1999; 117: 207–208.
5. Reveille JD, Fischbach M, McNearney T et al. Systemic sclerosis in 3 US ethnic groups: a comparison of clinical, sociodemographic, serologic, and immunogenetic determinants. Semin Arthritis Rheum 2001; 30: 332–346.
6. LeRoy EC. Increased collagen synthesis by scleroderma skin fibroblasts in vitro. A possible defect in regulation or activation of scleroderma fibroblasts. J Clin Invest 1974; 54: 880–889.
7. Jimenez SA, Saitta B. Alterations in the regulation of expression of the alpha 1(I) collagen gene (COL1A1) in systemic sclerosis (scleroderma). Springer Semin Immunopathol 1999; 21: 397–414.
8. Shi-wen X, Pennington D, Holmes A et al. Autocrine overexpression of CTGF maintains fibrosis: RDA analysis of fibrosis genes in systemic sclerosis. Exp Cell Res 2000; 259: 213–224.
9. Casciola-Rosen L, Wigley F, Rosen A. Scleroderma autoantigens are uniquely fragmented by metal-catalyzed oxidation reactions: implications for pathogenesis. J Exp Med 1997; 185: 71–79.
10. Arnett FC, Fritzler MJ, Ann C, Holian A. Urinary mercury levels in patients with autoantibodies to U3-RNP (fibrillarin). J Rheumatol 2000; 27: 405–410.
11. Artleff CM, Smith JB, Jimenez SA. Identification of fetal DNA and cells in skin lesions from women with systemic sclerosis. N Engl J Med 1998; 338: 1186–1191.
12. Black CM. Measurement of skin involvement in scleroderma. J Rheumatol 1995; 22: 1217–1219.
13. Steen VD, Medsger TA. The palpable tendon friction rub: an important physical examination finding in patients with systemic sclerosis. Arthritis Rheum 1997; 40: 1146–5111.
14. Steen VD, Medsger TA Jr. The value of the Health Assessment Questionnaire and special patient-generated scales to demonstrate change in systemic sclerosis patients over time. Arthritis Rheum 1997; 40: 1984–1991.
15. Medsger TA Jr, Silman AJ, Steen VD et al. A disease severity scale for systemic sclerosis: development and testing. J Rheumatol 1999; 26: 2159–2167.
16. Valentini G, Della Rossa A, Bombardieri S et al. European multicentre study to define disease activity criteria for systemic sclerosis. II. Identification of disease activity variables and development of preliminary activity indexes. Ann Rheum Dis 2001; 60: 592–598.
17. Della Rossa A, Valentini G, Bombardieri S et al. European multicentre study to define disease activity criteria for systemic sclerosis. I. Clinical and epidemiological features of 290 patients from 19 centres. Ann Rheum Dis 2001; 60: 585–591.
18. Clements PJ, Wong WK, Hurwitz EL et al. The Disability Index of the Health Assessment Questionnaire is a predictor and correlate of outcome in the high-dose versus low-dose penicillamine in systemic sclerosis trial. Arthritis Rheum 2001; 44: 653–661.
19. Silman A, Akesson A, Newman J et al. Assessment of functional ability in patients with scleroderma: a proposed new disability assessment instrument. J Rheumatol 1998; 25: 79–83.
20. Pope JE, Bellamy N. Outcome measurements in scleroderma clinical trials. Semin Arthritis Rheum 1993; 23: 22–33.
21. White B, Bauer EA, Goldsmith LA et al. Guidelines for clinical trials in systemic sclerosis (scleroderma). I. Disease-modifying interventions. The American College of Rheumatology Committee on Design and Outcomes in Clinical Trials in Systemic Sclerosis. Arthritis Rheum 1995; 38: 351–360.
22. Clements PJ, Lachenbruch PA, Sterz M et al. Cyclosporine in systemic sclerosis. Results of a forty-eight-week open safety study in ten patients. Arthritis Rheum 1993; 36: 75–83.

23. Van den Hoogen FH, Boerbooms AM, Swank AJ *et al*. Comparison of methotrexate with placebo in the treatment of systemic sclerosis: a 24 week randomized double-blind trial, followed by a 24 week observational trial. Br J Rheumatol 1996; 35: 364–372.

24. Pope JE, Bellamy N, Seibold JR *et al*. A randomized, controlled trial of methotrexate versus placebo in early diffuse scleroderma. Arthritis Rheum 2001; 44: 1351–1358.

25. Krasagakis K, Dippel E, Rameker J *et al*. Management of severe scleroderma with long-term extracorporeal photopheresis. Dermatology 1998; 196: 309–315.

26. Stratton RJ, Wilson H, Black CM. Pilot study of anti-thymocyte globulin plus mycophenolate mofetil in recent-onset diffuse scleroderma. Rheumatology (Oxford) 2001; 40: 84–88.

27. Varai G, Earle L, Jimenez SA *et al*. A pilot study of intermittent intravenous cyclophosphamide for the treatment of systemic sclerosis associated lung disease. J Rheumatol 1998; 25: 1325–1329.

28. McKown KM, Carbone LD, Bustillo J *et al*. Induction of immune tolerance to human type I collagen in patients with systemic sclerosis by oral administration of bovine type I collagen. Arthritis Rheum 2000; 43: 1054–1061.

29. Binks M, Passweg JR, Furst D *et al*. Phase I/II trial of autologous stem cell transplantation in systemic sclerosis: procedure related mortality and impact on skin disease. Ann Rheum Dis 2001; 60: 577–584.

30. Clements PJ, Furst DE. Choosing appropriate patients with systemic sclerosis for treatment by autologous stem cell transplantation. J Rheumatol Suppl 1997; 48: 85–88.

31. Clements PJ, Furst DE, Wong WK *et al*. High-dose versus low-dose D-penicillamine in early diffuse systemic sclerosis: analysis of a two-year, double-blind, randomized, controlled clinical trial. Arthritis Rheum 1999; 42: 1194–1203.

32. Grassegger A, Schuler G, Hessenberger G *et al*. Interferon-gamma in the treatment of systemic sclerosis: a randomized controlled multicentre trial. Br J Dermatol 1998; 139: 639–648.

33. Black CM, Silman AJ, Herrick AI *et al*. Interferon-alpha does not improve outcome at one year in patients with diffuse cutaneous scleroderma: results of a randomized, double-blind, placebo-controlled trial. Arthritis Rheum 1999; 42: 299–305.

34. Seibold JR, Korn JH, Simms R *et al*. Recombinant human relaxin in the treatment of scleroderma. A randomized, double-blind, placebo-controlled trial. Ann Intern Med 2000; 132: 871–879.

35. Matteson EL, Shbeeb MI, McCarthy TG *et al*. Pilot study of antithymocyte globulin in systemic sclerosis. Arthritis Rheum 1996; 39: 1132–1137.

36. Denton CP, Sweny P, Abdulla A, Black CM. Acute renal failure occurring in scleroderma treated with cyclosporin A: a report of three cases. Br J Rheumatol 1994; 33: 90–92.

37. Jam S, Bicknell GR, Whiting PH, Nicholson ML. Rapamycin reduces expression of fibrosis-associated genes in an experimental model of renal ischaemia reperfusion injury. Transplant Proc 2001; 33: 556–668.

38. Clements PJ, Hurwitz EL, Wong WK *et al*. Skin thickness score as a predictor and correlate of outcome in systemic sclerosis: high-dose versus low-dose penicillamine trial. Arthritis Rheum 2000; 43: 2445–2454.

39. Stevens W, Vancheeswaran R, Black CM. Alpha interferon-2a (Roferon-A) in the treatment of diffuse cutaneous systemic sclerosis: a pilot study. UK Systemic Sclerosis Study Group. Br J Rheumatol 1992; 31: 683–689.

40. Ziesche R, Hofbauer E, Wittmann K *et al*. A preliminary study of long-term treatment with interferon gamma-1b and low-dose prednisolone in patients with idiopathic pulmonary fibrosis. N Engl J Med 1999; 341: 1264–1269.

41. Halevy O, Nagler A, Levi-Schaffer F *et al*. Inhibition of collagen type I synthesis by skin fibroblasts of graft versus host disease and scleroderma patients: effect of halofuginone. Biochem Pharmacol 1996; 52: 1057–1063.

42. Levi-Schaffer F, Nagler A, Slavin S *et al*. Inhibition of collagen synthesis and changes in skin morphology in murine graft-versus-host disease and tight skin mice: effect of halofuginone. J Invest Dermatol 1996; 106: 84–88.

43. Le CH, Morales A, Trentham DE. Minocycline in early diffuse scleroderma. Lancet 1998; 352: 1755–1756.

44. Wigley FM, Wise RA, Seibold JR *et al*. Intravenous iloprost infusion in patients with Raynaud phenomenon secondary to systemic sclerosis. A multicenter, placebo-controlled, double-blind study. Ann Intern Med 1994; 120: 199–206.

45. Black CM, Halkier-Sorensen L, Belch JJ *et al*. Oral iloprost in Raynaud's phenomenon secondary to systemic sclerosis: a multicentre, placebo-controlled, dose-comparison study. Br J Rheumatol 1998; 37: 952–960.

46. Denton CP, Howell K, Stratton RJ, Black CM. Long-term low molecular weight heparin therapy for severe Raynaud's phenomenon: a pilot study. Clin Exp Rheumatol 2000; 18: 499–502.

47. Dziadzio M, Denton CP, Smith R *et al*. Losartan therapy for Raynaud's phenomenon and scleroderma: clinical and biochemical findings in a fifteen-week, randomized, parallel-group, controlled trial. Arthritis Rheum 1999; 42: 2646–2655.

48. Veeraraghavan S, Nicholson AG, Wells AU. Lung fibrosis: new classifications and therapy. Curr Opin Rheumatol 2001; 13: 500–504.

49. Silver RM, Miller KS, Kinsella MB *et al*. Evaluation and management of scleroderma lung disease using bronchoalveolar lavage. Am J Med 1990; 88: 470–476.

50. Wells AU, Hansell DM, Harrison NK *et al*. Clearance of inhaled ^{99m}Tc-DTPA predicts the clinical course of fibrosing alveolitis. Eur Respir J 1993 ; 6: 797–802.

51. Follansbee WP, Miller TR, Curtiss EI *et al*. A controlled clinicopathologic study of myocardial fibrosis in systemic sclerosis (scleroderma). J Rheumatol 1990; 17: 656–662.

52. Steen VD, Medsger TA. Case-control study of corticosteroids and other drugs that either precipitate or protect from the development of scleroderma renal crisis. Arthritis Rheum 1998; 41: 1613–1619.

53. Lopez-Ovejero JA, Saal SD, D'Angelo WA *et al*. Reversal of vascular and renal crises of scleroderma by oral angiotensin-converting enzyme blockade. N Engl J Med 1979; 300: 1417–141.

136 Raynaud's phenomenon

Abdul-Wahab Al-Allaf and Jill J F Belch

- Raynaud's phenomenon is an episodic reversible peripheral ischemia provoked by cold or emotion
- Classically, constriction of the digital vessels leads to pallor of the digits, followed by cyanosis secondary to static venous blood
- The recovery phase features reactive hyperemia, with resulting erythema

EPIDEMIOLOGY

The terms 'Raynaud's disease' and 'Raynaud's phenomenon' are often used interchangeably to identify two distinct disorders that initially appear with similar symptoms but then have different sequelae or associated conditions. In the UK, 'Raynaud's phenomenon' is the blanket term usually used to describe any form of cold-related vasospasm, which can be further subdivided into Raynaud's syndrome when there is an associated disorder, and Raynaud's disease when there is not. However, in the USA the terminology most used is 'primary Raynaud's phenomenon' and 'secondary Raynaud's phenomenon'. Thus care must be taken with literature comparisons.

Raynaud's phenomenon may affect as many as 20–30% of young women and have an overall prevalence in the population of approximately 10%, with a female:male ratio of 2:1[1]. By far the largest group of patients presenting to their primary care physician are those with a primary Raynaud's disorder, which typically occurs in young women in their teens and 20s, has a familial predisposition and accounts for the vast majority of all cases of Raynaud's phenomenon. In contrast, more than 50% of the patients referred to hospital will have an associated underlying systemic disease. Recent studies have shown that the Raynaud's syndrome may predate systemic illness by up to two decades.

TABLE 136.1 CONDITIONS ASSOCIATED WITH RAYNAUD'S PHENOMENON

Immune-mediated
- Systemic sclerosis (90%)
- Mixed connective tissue disease (85%)
- Sjögren's syndrome (33%)
- Systemic lupus erythematosus (10–44%)
- Polymyositis/dermatomyositis (29%)
- Rheumatoid arthritis (10–15%)
- Cryoglobulinemia and cryofibrinogenemia (10%)
- Arteritis (e.g. giant cell arteritis, Takayasu arteritis)
- Antiphospholipid syndrome
- Primary biliary cirrhosis

Occupation-related
- Cold injury (e.g. frozen-food packers)
- Polyvinyl chloride exposure
- Vibration exposure
- Ammunition workers (outside work)

Obstructive vascular disease
- Atherosclerosis
- Microemboli
- Thromboangiitis obliterans (50%)
- Thoracic outlet syndrome (e.g. cervical rib)
- Walking-crutch pressure
- Diabetic microangiopathy

Metabolic disorders
- Hypothyroidism
- Carcinoid syndrome
- Pheochromocytoma
- Uremia

Drug-induced
- Antimigraine compounds
- β-blockers (particularly non-selective)
- Cytotoxic drugs
- Cyclosporin
- Bromocriptine
- Sulphasalazine
- Minocycline
- Interferon-α
- Interferon-β
- Ergotamine derivatives

Infections
- Chronic viral liver diseases (hepatitis B and C)
- Cytomegalovirus
- Parvovirus B19
- *Helicobacter pylori*

Miscellaneous
- Arteriovenous fistula
- Artificial acrylic nails
- Carpal tunnel syndrome (60%)
- POEMS syndrome
- Neoplasm
- Complex regional pain syndrome type 1
- Toxic oil syndrome
- Fibromyalgia syndrome
- Polycythemia
- Paraproteinemia
- Myalgic encephalitis (postviral fatigue syndrome)

% values are percentage of patients with disease who have Raynaud's phenomenon.

POEMS, polyneuropathy, organomegaly, endocrinopathy, monoclonal proteins and skin changes

ETIOLOGY

There is a wide spectrum of disease associated with Raynaud's syndrome, including connective tissue disorders, both drug-induced and those associated with thromboangiitis obliterans and with occupational exposure to vibration (Table 136.1).

Raynaud's phenomenon occurs in 90% of patients with systemic sclerosis and 85% of patients with mixed connective tissue disease. Between 10% and 45% of patients with systemic lupus erythematosus, 33% of patients with Sjögren's syndrome and 20% of those with dermatomyositis/polymyositis experience Raynaud's phenomenon. Patients with rheumatoid arthritis have a similar overall prevalence of Raynaud's phenomenon as compared with the general population (10%); however, symptomatology tends to be more severe.

It is estimated that about 50% of all workers using vibrating equipment can develop Raynaud's phenomenon, and it is the most common form of occupational Raynaud's phenomenon. This is now called hand–arm vibration syndrome or HAVS (previously known as vibration white finger syndrome or VWF). β-Blockers are a commonly used group of drugs that can induce Raynaud's phenomenon. More recently, prescribing β-blockers for those suffering from Raynaud's phenomenon has been revolutionized by the development of vasodilating β-blockers. This allows safe prescription of these drugs to patients with Raynaud's phenomenon. In the older age group, obstructive vascular disease is the most common cause of Raynaud's phenomenon and it has been reported that 60% of Raynaud's phenomenon occurring in individuals older than 60 years is atherosclerotic in origin. Many other conditions can be associated with Raynaud's phenomenon and are listed in Table 136.1.

PATHOPHYSIOLOGY

The pathophysiology of the triphasic color changes is well recognized: constriction of the digital vessels leads to pallor of the digits, followed by cyanosis secondary to deoxygenation of static venous blood, and then a reactive hyperemic stage with resulting erythema. There are three pathophysiological mechanisms that may mediate these changes and therefore need to be considered in patients with Raynaud's phenomenon: (1) neurogenic mechanisms; (2) blood and blood vessel wall interactions; (3) abnormalities of the inflammatory and immune responses.

Neurogenic mechanisms

Maurice Raynaud believed that hyper-reactivity of the parasympathetic nervous system caused an increase in vasoconstrictor response to cold. The α-adrenergic receptor and β-presynaptic receptor sensitivity, density, or both, are increased in Raynaud's phenomenon. However, the endothelium possesses at least five different adrenoceptor subtypes (α2A/D, α2C, β1, β2 and β3), which either directly or through the release of nitric oxide, actively participate in the regulation of vascular tone. The central sympathetic system has some role in the pathogenesis of Raynaud's phenomenon, as indicated by the fact that local vibration of one hand induces vasoconstriction of the other, which is abolished by proximal nerve blockade.

In patients with systemic sclerosis, of whom 90% have Raynaud's phenomenon, it has been demonstrated that there is a high incidence of peripheral neuropathy, which supports the neurogenic mechanism for Raynaud's phenomenon. The involvement of nerve terminals reduces the vasodilatory endothelial-dependent or -independent potential of the neuropeptides released by sensory nerve endings. It has also been found that Raynaud's phenomenon is significantly more common in patients with carpal tunnel syndrome, and this could be explained by the presence of autonomic dysfunction, which is evident by swelling of the fingers and dry palms, in addition to the Raynaud's phenomenon.

However, other work does not support the neurogenic concept. Infusions of α- and β-adrenergic agonists in patients with Raynaud's phenomenon do not produce any abnormalities in their response to reflex cooling or indirect heating. Thus, although abnormalities in the nervous system may exist, they are, at present, not clearly defined.

Blood and blood vessel wall interactions

The most important cellular element in Raynaud's phenomenon is the endothelium, which is a functioning organ releasing important mediators, such as prostacyclin (PGI_2), which is a potent antiplatelet agent and vasodilator. It has been found that there are abnormal endothelial responses to both endothelium-dependent and endothelium-independent induced vasodilatation in patients with Raynaud's phenomenon; however, in patients with Raynaud's syndrome secondary to systemic sclerosis, this abnormality is limited to the endothelium-dependent vasodilatation. Here it seems that the disease, perhaps through the injury to the endothelium, jeopardizes the endothelium-dependent vascular control. A reduction in nitric oxide, one of the main endothelial vasodilators, is also involved in the genesis of Raynaud's phenomenon in these patients. It could also be extrapolated from different studies that, in patients with Raynaud's phenomenon, there is possibly a decrease in the synthesis of nitric oxide, rather than impaired sensitivity to it, which could be an important factor in the pathogenesis of Raynaud's phenomenon and may have therapeutic value in the future.

The damaged endothelium in Raynaud's phenomenon can also release factor VIII von Willebrand factor antigen, which can have a prothrombotic effect. Another manifestation of endothelial dysfunction is a defect in the lysis of fibrin. Concentrations of endothelin, another endothelial product that causes vasoconstriction, are increased in Raynaud's phenomenon.

Other blood cellular elements may have a pathological role in Raynaud's phenomenon. The platelets exhibit greater aggregation, releasing increased amounts of the vasoconstrictor and platelet aggregant, thromboxane A_2, and other platelet-release products. The red blood cell appears to be more stiff and rigid, and thus can occlude the microcirculation. An important role has also been claimed for the white blood cell which, when activated, releases prothrombotic free radicals and increases cell aggregation, leading to more reduction in blood flow. Some of the above changes are likely to be a consequence of the Raynaud's phenomenon, rather than a cause, but they may augment the symptoms of vasospasm and their attenuation is a potentially important feature in the drug management of Raynaud's phenomenon.

Abnormalities of the inflammatory and immune responses

Disordered immune and inflammatory processes occur in the majority of severe cases of Raynaud's phenomenon via their association with the connective tissue disorders, but also in HAVS, which has no clear immune/inflammatory basis. Tumor necrosis factor and lymphotoxin, phagocyte/macrophage and T cell derived proteins, along with immune complex deposition in the vessel wall, are likely to be activated in vascular damage seen in Raynaud's phenomenon.

It seems that a combination of the above factors will be involved in the development and propagation of Raynaud's phenomenon.

CLINICAL FEATURES

Detailed history and examination are essential in making the diagnosis, in finding any associated underlying causes, in assessing the likelihood of progression to connective tissue disorder, and in deciding about the most appropriate management plan. A detailed occupational history, particularly in men, allows a diagnosis of HAVS to be made. Drug history is equally important, and it should be noted that even the cardioselective β-blockers produce a degree of peripheral vasoconstriction

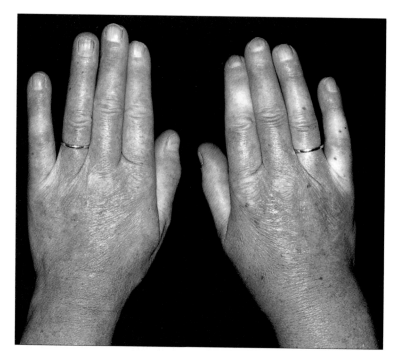

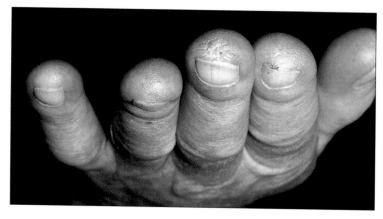

Fig. 136.2 Digital pitting, scarring and sclerodactyly commonly associated with systemic sclerosis. These lesions form two of the three main criteria for systemic sclerosis; the third criterion is pulmonary interstitial fibrosis. A diagnosis of systemic sclerosis requires two of these three findings.

Fig. 136.1 Raynaud's phenomenon in a patient with systemic sclerosis. The white discoloration is an essential clinical finding in Raynaud's phenomenon. The asymmetric involvement and the presence of telangiectasia point to a possibility of a secondary cause for the Raynaud's phenomenon. Digital pitting scarring is one of the main criteria for the diagnosis of systemic sclerosis.

(Table 136.1). Use of the newer vasodilating β-blockers is probably more appropriate in these patients, especially when β-blockade is necessary.

Raynaud's phenomenon is classically manifested by blanching of the affected part (pallor), reflecting vasospasm (Fig. 136.1), followed by cyanosis and then rubor; however, this typical triphasic color change is not necessarily present in all patients. Symptoms associated with Raynaud's phenomenon include numbness, cold and pain, which are secondary to ischemia, which can be severe enough to result in digital ulceration, gangrene and loss of digits. During the reactive hyperemic stage, patients usually experience an unpleasant burning sensation and sweating of the affected parts. The most severely affected patient may experience marked, year-round restrictions in their daily activity. The predictors for the attack rate, severity and pain are the average daily temperature, stress, anxiety, age and sex.

The occurrence of certain clinical features may suggest a greater likelihood of disease progression to connective tissue disorder (Table 136.2). This is important, as we know that, in up to 50% of patients referred to hospital, Raynaud's phenomenon could progress to connective tissue disorder. For instance, sclerodactyly and pitting scars over the finger pulp are associated with later development of connective tissue disorder (Fig. 136.2).

Patients presenting for the first time in their third and fourth decade are at high risk of developing connective tissue disorders, and Raynaud's phenomenon occurring in very young children, although rare, is usually due to an underlying connective tissue disorders. If Raynaud's phenomenon precedes the connective tissue disorder by years, in those who develop systemic sclerosis, the limited form of the disease is more likely to become apparent. Systemic enquiry should concentrate on the presence of migraine (or a family history of migraine), esophageal problems and the presence of vasospastic angina[2].

A full physical examination should be directed to look for any obstructive vascular disease and for signs of associated autoimmune conditions. Simple blood pressure measurement in both arms will help to detect significant occlusive vascular disease above the brachial artery. Looking for evidence of pulmonary hypertension is also important, to point to possible involvement of the pulmonary vascular system. Livedo reticularis could point to cold agglutinin disease or underlying connective tissue disorder. Patients with abnormal nailfold microscopy are more likely to progress to a connective tissue disorder. Patients should also be examined carefully for evidence of carpal tunnel syndrome, as 60% of these patients also have Raynaud's phenomenon.

INVESTIGATIONS

Investigations in patients with Raynaud's phenomenon have three functions: first to confirm the diagnosis of Raynaud's phenomenon, secondly to assess possible disease progression, and thirdly to look for underlying secondary causes or associated conditions[3].

Diagnosis of Raynaud's phenomenon

In the majority of cases the diagnosis of Raynaud's phenomenon can be made from the clinical history. Digital blanching on exposure to cold

---

TABLE 136.2 FEATURES SUGGESTIVE OF PROGRESSION OF RAYNAUD'S PHENOMENON

Clinical

- Older age at onset (>35 years)
- Recurrence of chilblains as adult
- Vasospasm all year round
- Asymmetric attacks (Fig. 136.1)
- Sclerodactyly
- Digital ulceration
- Finger pulp pitting scars

Laboratory

- Increased inflammatory markers
- Detection of autoantibodies
- Increased von Willebrand factor antigen

Nailfold microscopy

- Abnormal vessels

with or without cyanosis or rubor in the absence of clinical evidence of obstructive vascular disease allows the diagnosis of Raynaud's phenomenon to be made. However, in rare situations when the patient is unable to give a clear history, in the presence of occlusive vascular disease when the contribution of vasospasm to the clinical problem needs to be determined, or for medicolegal reasons in HAVS, objective measures of blood flow are needed.

There are many different techniques that can be used to measure blood flow to the digits. However, in clinical practice, measurement of digital systolic blood pressure before and after local cooling of the hands in cool water at a temperature of approximately 15°C is widely used because of its simplicity. A decrease in pressure greater than 30mmHg is usually significant. This technique, however, will give a significant number of false-negative responses unless certain precautions are observed[4]. First, the patient must be warm before the first pressure recordings and, ideally, the starting digital pressure must be as near brachial pressure as can be achieved. Unfortunately, many patients who have cold hands at the start of the tests have been told that they did not have Raynaud's phenomenon when no further pressure decrease was detected after cold challenge. Conversely, on hot days the body itself is too warm, and this will prevent digital vasospasm if digital cooling is used in isolation. Secondly, in premenopausal women, assessment should be avoided in mid-cycle, as poor blood flow before the start of the test can also occur at the time of ovulation. Thirdly, all vasoactive medication should be stopped 24h before the test, as drug-induced vasodilatation can also lead to failure to detect a pressure decrease. For the same reason, the test should be avoided when the patient is in the reactive hyperemic phase. Ideally, patients should not have had a vasospastic attack on the day of the test.

Thermography, radioisotopic clearance and laser Doppler flometry are other methods used to help in the diagnosis of Raynaud's phenomenon. However, these methods have their disadvantages and usually are unnecessary.

Investigations for secondary causes

More than 50% of patients with Raynaud's phenomenon who are referred to hospital will have an associated underlying disease; therefore, once diagnosis of Raynaud's phenomenon is confirmed, it is essential to look carefully for any underlying cause. More importantly, early intervention in these patients could resolve the problem, such as in patients with vibration exposure or those who take vasospastic drugs. Those with an obvious associated disorder will be easily detected, but difficulty arises in diagnosing early connective tissue disorders. Earlier studies had found that progression to connective tissue disorder occurred in 24–50% of patients with Raynaud's phenomenon. However, more recent studies showed that as many as 46–81% of cases of Raynaud's phenomenon have been found to have some underlying secondary condition.

Blood biochemistry, including thyroid function test and full blood count should be carried out. A normochromic, normocytic or microcytic anemia of chronic disease can be found in patients with connective tissue disorders. The inflammatory markers such as erythrocyte sedimentation rate, plasma viscosity or C-reactive protein are usually normal in primary Raynaud's phenomenon, but they may be increased in secondary Raynaud's phenomenon. It should be noted, however, that there might be some impairment of the acute-phase response in patients with systemic sclerosis. Urine analysis will help in detecting early renal disease in patients with connective tissue disorders or diabetes. A chest X-ray will determine whether a bony cervical rib is present, and will show if there is any basal lung fibrosis, which may be seen early in connective tissue disorders. A median nerve conduction study is important in detecting carpal tunnel syndrome when symptoms warrant this.

Immunologic tests will help to detect the immune pathologic origin of the secondary Raynaud's phenomenon. Rheumatoid factor will help in detection of early rheumatoid arthritis, antinuclear antibody and anti-DNA antibodies in systemic lupus erythematosus, anticentromere antibodies for limited systemic sclerosis, and antitopoisomerase antibody (formerly known as scleroderma 70 antibody) for diffuse systemic sclerosis. Anti-La and anti-Ro antibodies may suggest the diagnosis of Sjögren's syndrome. The presence of these antibodies early on in the history of Raynaud's phenomenon suggests that later progression to connective tissue disorder will occur. Increased von Willebrand factor antigen tends to be seen in patients with the secondary Raynaud's phenomenon. Detection of cold-precipitated proteins will help in the diagnosis of cryoglobulinemia and cryofibrinogenemia. Nailfold microscopy may also help to point to Raynaud's phenomenon of rheumatologic origin, especially when associated with positive serum antibodies.

MANAGEMENT

Not all patients experiencing digital vasospasm require drug treatment. The obvious clinical need for medication in patients with digital gangrene and ulceration does not need to be emphasized, but potential prescribers should also be aware that the severity of the pain produced by vasospastic attack and the degree of interruption that a patient may experience in her or his normal daily routine may be profound, and drug treatment should be instituted in these patients.

General measures

Initial treatment in mild disease is conservative, and drug treatment may be avoided. Patients with Raynaud's phenomenon may be apprehensive about their condition and education is important. From our experience, a specialist rheumatology nurse and occupational therapists can provide useful help for the Raynaud's sufferer. It is important to advise patients on protecting themselves from the cold. Electrically heated gloves and socks and chemical hand warmers are the perfect solution for some patients.

Stopping smoking (including exposure to passive smoking) is beneficial. In the case of HAVS, early diagnosis and early discontinuation of vibration exposure resolve the problem. Withdrawal of vasoconstrictor drugs is essential. Although the contraceptive pill has been linked anecdotally to the development of Raynaud's phenomenon, this has never been conclusively proven in epidemiological studies. It is our policy not to discontinue the contraceptive pill or hormone replacement therapy unless it is clearly related to the patient's Raynaud's phenomenon.

In the management of digital ulceration in patients with severe Raynaud's phenomenon, it is essential to treat any infection as soon as possible, and aggressively. Significant infection can be present even in the absence of increased inflammatory markers, formal erythema and pus formation.

Drug treatment of Raynaud's phenomenon

Patients in whom symptoms are severe enough to cause interference with either their social or work lifestyle should be offered drug treatment (Table 136.3).

Calcium channel blockers

Nifedipine has now become the gold standard of Raynaud's treatment. Its mechanism of action is predominantly through vasodilation, but it also has antiplatelet and possibly other antithrombotic effects. The dose in treating Raynaud's phenomenon ranges from 10mg to 20mg two or three times daily, which should be introduced very gradually – for example, 10mg at night for 2 weeks, then twice a day, etc. It has been found to be useful in decreasing the frequency and severity of vasospastic attacks, and improves the objective measures of blood flow after cold exposure. Furthermore, nifedipine is a good alternative to a β-blocker for patients with concomitant hypertension and migraine. Its use, however, is limited by the vasodilatory side effects to which the Raynaud's phenomenon patients appear very susceptible. These effects usually disappear with continued treatment and so, unless they are intolerable, the patient should persevere for at least 2 weeks before a decision is made to discontinue the treatment. The use of the controlled-release preparation is better tolerated than nifedipine itself. If side effects necessitate discontinuation of the treatment, two options are possible. The first is to try another calcium channel antagonist with less vasodilatory effect, such as diltiazem and isradipine. The second option is to use nifedipine capsule (not the Retard tablet) as a rescue medication during a severe spastic attack, the capsule being crushed by the teeth and placed below the tongue.

Other vasodilators

The use of other vasodilators in patients with Raynaud's phenomenon remains controversial, as most studies have been small or uncontrolled. The use of inositol nicotinate and naftidrofuryl has produced encouraging results in mild to moderate Raynaud's phenomenon. Another role of these medications is to use them as adjuncts to calcium channel blockade when adverse effects from calcium antagonists prevent the achievement of high dosage. These drugs may take up to 3 months to produce their effects, suggesting that their action in Raynaud's phenomenon may be through other mechanisms.

Losartan, the angiotensin II receptor antagonist, has been shown in a randomized controlled trial[5] to be effective in treating Raynaud's phenomenon. In a meta-analysis[6], prazosin, an α-blocker, was found to have modest effects. Accordingly, these medications should be considered for those with concomitant hypertension, or as an extra option in those who cannot tolerate the calcium channel blockers. More recently, a pilot study[7] showed that fluoxetine, a selective serotinin reuptake inhibitor, was found to be effective in treating Raynaud's phenomenon.

Prostaglandin treatment

Prostaglandins are the metabolic products of essential fatty acids and both prostacyclin (PGI_2) and alprostadil (PGE_1) have potent vasodila-

tory and antiplatelet properties. Treatments with both PGI_2 and PGE_1, however, require intravenous administration and are very unstable. Thus the use of a more stable analog such as iloprost has been evaluated in a number of studies[8–10].

Iloprost

A number of double-blind placebo controlled studies of iloprost infusion given intravenously have shown benefit in Raynaud's phenomenon[11,12]. In addition to its vasodilatory and antiplatelets effects, iloprost has been shown to downregulate lymphocyte adhesion to the endothelium[13]. When compared with nifedipine, it was found to have the same effect on reducing the frequency of the vasospastic attacks, but was more effective in healing digital ulcers and appeared to produce fewer adverse effects. Accordingly, iloprost is the second-choice treatment for patients with severe Raynaud's phenomenon who have not responded to nifedipine, and the first choice for those who have critical ischemia or digital ulceration, or both. It can be infused through a peripheral vein, and can produce benefit lasting for between 6 weeks and 6 months in most patients.

Alprostadil

A recent study confirmed the efficacy of PGE_1 (alprostadil) in the management of Raynaud's phenomenon secondary to systemic sclerosis. Accordingly, alprostadil could be used in patients who have significant side effects and cannot tolerate iloprost infusion. The effectiveness of using $PGE_1\alpha$–cyclodextrin infusions prophylactically to cover the winter has been proved by a recent study[11].

Oral and transdermal prostaglandins

Studies of orally active prostacyclin analogs have given conflicting results. Cicaprost proved disappointing, whereas oral iloprost has shown clinical benefit in some studies, but this was not confirmed in others[14–17]. A pilot study of oral limaprost, an alprostadil analog, was encouraging[18]. Prostaglandin delivery through the skin has also been studied, but to date no transdermally applied prostaglandin has obtained a license for use in Raynaud's phenomenon.

Role of surgery

Operations to remove part of the terminal phalanx and, occasionally, amputation is necessary for severe ischemia, but this is becoming increasingly infrequent. Patients with peripheral arterial disease and Raynaud's phenomenon of the toes may gain benefit from endovascular intervention. In patients with Raynaud's phenomenon secondary to carpel tunnel syndrome, surgical decompression of the carpal tunnel has been shown to improve the Raynaud's phenomenon symptoms significantly.

Conventional upper limb sympathectomy gives a high relapse rate and poor response in patients with Raynaud's syndrome. However, recent studies show that videoscopic sympathectomy may be successful in a number of patients, despite some untoward effects and partial relapses. Localized digital sympathectomy enjoyed some support initially, as earlier results were encouraging; however, further work is required in this area. Although modified upper limb sympathectomy requires further study, sympathectomy still has an important role in the treatment of Raynaud's phenomenon affecting the feet.

CONCLUSION

Raynaud's phenomenon is a common condition and, until recently, its management was difficult. However, with a careful clinical history and examination and with selection of specific investigations, it is now possible to diagnose correctly both Raynaud's phenomenon and its underlying or associated conditions. When it occurs as a primary phenomenon, it is usually mild, with symmetric involvement and no laboratory

TABLE 136.3 DRUGS COMMONLY USED IN RAYNAUD'S PHENOMENON	
Drug	**Dosage**
Oral	
Nifedipine Retard (or other calcium-channel blocker)	10–20mg two or three times a day
Naftidrofuryl	100–200mg three times a day
Inositol nicotinate	500mg three times, or inositol nicotinate forte 750mg twice a day
Thymoxamine	40–80mg four times a day (initial 2 week trial)
Gamolenic acid	12 capsules a day (3 month trial)
Omega-3 marine triglycerides	10 capsules a day (3 month trial)
Losartan	50mg a day
Fluoxetine	20mg a day
Intravenous infusion	
Iloprost	Start infusion (peripheral line) at 1µg/h, increase by 1µg every 30min until reach maximum tolerable dose (maximum dose should not be greater than 3µg/h) given over 6h each day over 3–7 days on each occasion
Prostaglandin E1	60µg in 250ml physiological infusion over 3h daily for 5–6 days. This could be repeated every 6 weeks to cover the cold weather in severe cases, specially if associated with critical ischemia or digital ulceration

abnormalities, and often needs no drug treatment. Features suggesting secondary Raynaud's syndrome include painful attacks, ischemic digital ulcers, asymmetric attacks, a positive autoantibody test result, and increased inflammatory markers. Vasodilatory treatment is the mainstay of medical management, and calcium channel blockers are usually the drugs of choice. Surgical treatment nowadays is very rarely needed. Lastly, the better evaluation and understanding of the pathophysiology of Raynaud's phenomenon and increasing knowledge on the involvement of vascular adrenoceptors in the condition will contribute to new and better therapeutic approaches. The future of oral and transdermal vasodilators, including prostaglandin analogs, and improvement in the delivery systems still need further study.

ACKNOWLEDGMENT

Professor J J F Belch receives funding from the Raynaud's and Scleroderma Association, UK.

REFERENCES

1. Cooke ED, Nicolaides AN, Porter JM. Raynaud's syndrome. London: Med-Orion Publishing Company; 1991.
2. Belch JJF. Temperature related disorders. In: Tooke J, Lowe GDO, eds. Textbook of vascular medicine. London: Edward Arnold; 1995: 329–352.
3. Bolster MB, Maricq HR, Leff RL. Office evaluation and treatment of Raynaud's phenomenon. Cleve Clin J Med 1995; 62: 51–61.
4. Belch JJF, Zurier RB. Connective tissue diseases, 1E. London: Chapman and Hall Medical; 1995.
5. Dziadzio M, Denton CP, Smith R et al. Losartan therapy for Raynaud's phenomenon and scleroderma: clinical and biochemical findings in a fifteen-week, randomized, parallel-group, controlled trial. Arthritis Rheum 1999; 42: 2646–2655.
6. Pope J, Fenlon D, Thompson A et al. Prazosin for Raynaud's phenomenon in progressive systemic sclerosis. (Cochrane Review). In: The Cochrane Library, Issue 3, 2001. Oxford: Update Software.
7. Coleiro B, Marshall SE, Denton CP et al. Treatment of Raynaud's phenomenon with the selective serotonin reuptake inhibitor fluoxetine. Rheumatology 2001; 40: 1038–1043.
8. Belch JJF, Greer IA, McLaren M et al. The effects of intravenous infusion of ZK36374, a synthetic prostacyclin derivative, on normal volunteers. Prostaglandins 1984; 28: 67–78.
9. Martin MFR, Dowd PM, Ring EFJ et al. Prostaglandin E_1 infusions for vascular insufficiency in progressive systemic sclerosis. Ann Rheum Dis 1981; 40: 350–354.
10. Belch JJF, Drury JK, Capell H et al. Intermittent epoprostenol (prostacyclin) infusion in patients with Raynaud's syndrome – a double-blind controlled trial. Lancet 1983; I: 313–315.
11. Rademaker M, Thomas RHM, Provost G et al. Prolonged increase in digital blood flow following iloprost infusion in patients with systemic sclerosis. Postgrad Med J 1987; 63: 617–620.
12. Wigley FM, Wise RA, Seibold JR et al. Intravenous iloprost infusion in patients with Raynaud phenomenon secondary to systemic sclerosis. Ann Intern Med 1994; 120: 199–206.
13. Della Bella S, Molteni M, Mocellin C et al. Novel mode of action of iloprost: in vitro down-regulation of endothelial cell adhesion molecules. Prostaglandins Other Lipid Mediat 2001; 65: 73–83.
14. Gardinali M, Pozzi MR, Bernareggi M et al. Treatment of Raynaud's phenomenon with intravenous prostaglandin E1alpha-cyclodextrin improves endothelial cell injury in systemic sclerosis. J Rheumatol 2001; 28: 786–794.
15. Lau CS, McLaren M, Saniabadi A et al. The pharmacological effects of cicaprost, an oral prostacyclin analogue, in patients with Raynaud's syndrome secondary to systemic sclerosis – a preliminary study. Clin Exp Rheumatol 1991; 9: 271–273.
16. Pope J, Fenlon D, Thompson A et al. Iloprost and cisaprost for Raynaud's phenomenon in progressive systemic sclerosis. (Cochrane Review). In: The Cochrane Library, Issue 3, 2001. Oxford: Update Software.
17. Belch JJF, Capell HA, Cooke ED et al. Oral iloprost as a treatment for Raynaud's syndrome: a double-blind multi-centre placebo controlled study. Ann Rheum Dis 1995; 54: 197–200.
18. Murai C, Sasaki T, Osaki H et al. Oral limaprost for Raynaud's phenomenon. Lancet 1989; I: 1218.

137

Localized scleroderma and idiopathic and environmentally-induced scleroderma variants

John Varga

Definitions

- Scleroderma variants represent a group of heterogeneous disorders characterized by diffuse or localized skin hardening that may be confused with scleroderma
- In contrast to systemic sclerosis, the scleroderma variants are rarely associated with Raynaud's phenomenon, evidence of systemic involvement or visceral organ damage, or serum autoantibodies
- Some scleroderma variants may be associated with environmental or dietary exposures
- The scleroderma variants generally carry a good prognosis

Clinical points

- Because the natural history, management and prognosis of scleroderma variants differ markedly from those of systemic sclerosis, these two types of conditions associated with skin induration must be differentiated
- When the history and physical examination fail to establish the correct diagnosis, a full-thickness biopsy of the skin is helpful

Numerous disorders are characterized by fibrosis of the skin and subcutaneous tissue. These distinct scleroderma-like diseases occur in sporadic form or as epidemics. The scleroderma variants share similarities that can lead to confusion with scleroderma/systemic sclerosis, but generally show distinct pattern of skin and internal organ involvement and are not associated with Raynaud's phenomenon. Because the complications, prognoses and treatments of the scleroderma variants differ considerably from one another and from those of systemic sclerosis, accurate classification is important. Diagnosis frequently mandates full-thickness skin biopsy and careful histopathological evaluation. The etiology and pathogenesis of most scleroderma variants are unknown. Idiopathic scleroderma-like disorders of skin include the localized forms of scleroderma, as well as scleromyxedema and scleredema (Table 137.1). The epidemic L-tryptophan-induced eosinophilia–myalgia syndrome and the Spanish toxic oil syndrome were associated with eosinophilia, and both clinically and pathologically resembled eosinophilic fasciitis. Ingestion or injection of some drugs may induce scleroderma-like induration, which can also be seen as an infrequent complication of diabetes mellitus and other metabolic diseases. Certain environmental or occupational exposures are associated with a syndrome that is indistinguishable from idiopathic systemic sclerosis/scleroderma.

LOCALIZED FORMS OF SCLERODERMA

Clinical features

In localized scleroderma the skin induration is confined to specific anatomic areas. Localized scleroderma is relatively uncommon, with estimated incidence rates of less than 3/100 000[1]. Women are more often affected than men. In contrast to systemic sclerosis, localized scleroderma is more prevalent in children and adolescents than in adults. Localized scleroderma is subclassified into two closely related but distinct classes: morphea and linear scleroderma (Table 137.2). In morphea, induration of the skin occurs as single or multiple circumscribed small oval plaques. The lesions are 1–10 cm in greatest dimension and tend to have sharply defined margins and a smooth center. The involved skin is firm, thickened and shiny, with an absence of sweat glands and hair. The lesions are distributed in an asymmetric pattern on the trunk, or less commonly on the extremities; the face and fingers are not affected. Guttate morphea is characterized by lesions that are less than 10 mm in diameter. Linear scleroderma most commonly involves the lower limbs in a unilateral fashion. Fibrosis sometimes extends into the subcutaneous tissue, causing atrophy and sclerosis of subjacent fat, fascia and muscle. Occasionally the underlying long bone can be affected[2]. The

TABLE 137.1 SCLERODERMA VARIANTS

Systemic sclerosis	
Localized forms of scleroderma	
Scleredema adultorum of Buschke	
Scleredema diabeticorum	
Scleromyxedema	
Eosinophilic syndrome	Eosinophilia–myalgia syndrome Toxic oil syndrome Eosinophilic fasciitis (diffuse fasciitis with eosinophilia; Shulman's disease)
Chronic graft vs. host disease	
Pseudoscleroderma (local injections of vitamin K, bleomycin, pentazocin)	
Metabolic diseases	Porphyria cutanea tarda Phenylketonuria Werner syndrome Carcinoid syndrome
Polyneuropathy organomegaly endocrinopathy monoclonal gammopathy syndrome (POEMS)	

TABLE 137.2 LOCALIZED FORMS OF SCLERODERMA

Morphea	Morphea en plaque Guttate morphea
Generalized/pansclerotic morphea Linear scleroderma	
	En coup de sabre Progressive hemifacial atrophy

characteristic radiological finding is melorheostosis, a longitudinally distributed cortical hyperostosis of the long bones[3].

Although localized forms of scleroderma are only rarely associated with Raynaud's syndrome or clinically evident internal organ injury, muscle involvement and carpal tunnel syndrome may occur. When the linear lesions cross joints, contractures can develop. In children, disturbed bone growth is a serious concern and may result in substantial leg-length discrepancy. Scleroderma *en coup de sabre* is a form of linear scleroderma involving the face and scalp, and is seen mostly in children. This form of linear scleroderma may be associated with progressive hemifacial atrophy (Parry–Romberg syndrome) and partial alopecia. Seizures, oculomotor nerve palsies and other neurological abnormalities, and uveitis may occur[4–6]. In patients with 'pansclerotic' morphea (seen more frequently in the elderly) there may be generalized involvement of the trunk, extremities and face; the fingers are spared. Localized scleroderma does not evolve into systemic sclerosis, even with widespread skin involvement, and survival is not different from that of the general population[1]. No laboratory test findings are specific for localized scleroderma. Eosinophilia is frequent in the early stage, and correlates with active inflammation[7]. Antinuclear, antimitochondrial and antihistone autoantibodies may be detected in the serum, but do not appear to have diagnostic or prognostic specificity[8,9]. Classic systemic sclerosis-specific autoantibodies are generally not seen in patients with localized scleroderma.

Evaluation and management

In the evaluation of patients with scleroderma-like induration, biopsy of the skin is frequently useful. Full-thickness excisional biopsy involving the dermis, panniculus and subcutaneous fascia is preferred. Perivascular inflammation is prominent in the early lesion. Neutrophils, eosinophils and plasma cells may be seen in the dermis and occasionally the superficial panniculus[10]. With time, there is less inflammation and the dermis becomes progressively more thickened, with swollen and homogenized collagen bundles (Fig. 137.1). Localized scleroderma lesions often show softening or complete resolution even without treatment, generally after 2–4 years. However, therapy may be necessary for patients with widespread or progressive skin induration, joint contractures, or for children with growth retardation. Few controlled treatment trials have been performed, and response to therapy is difficult to evaluate owing to the variable course of localized scleroderma and its tendency for spontaneous resolution. Furthermore, there are no laboratory or clinical markers to reliably assess disease severity and activity.

Localized scleroderma is frequently treated with superpotent topical corticosteroids. Antimalarial agents are also used. Physical therapy can be helpful to reduce joint contractures in linear scleroderma. In patients with extensive localized scleroderma, treatment with D-penicillamine or methotrexate has been shown to result in diminished skin induration after 3–6 months[11,12]. Surgical resection of morphea can be complicated by recurrence in the scar[13]. Phototherapy, with or without psoralens,

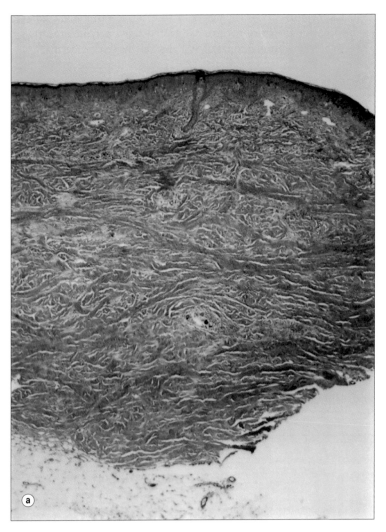
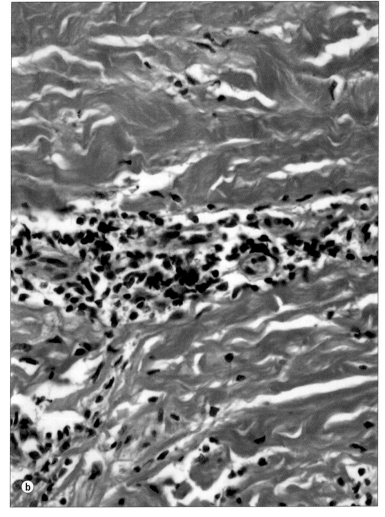

Fig. 137.1 Morphea. Full-thickness skin biopsy from the lower forearm. (a) Low-power view. Marked thickening and acellularity of the dermis. Collagen bundles in the lower dermis are swollen and homogenized. The epidermis is normal. Eccrine glands and hair follicles are absent. (b) High-power view. A focal infiltrate of mononuclear inflammatory cells. (Courtesy of Dr S Takagawa.)

appear to be effective[14,15]. Ultraviolet A irradiation induces local production of collagenase, contributing to enhanced turnover of the extracellular matrix in skin, and regression of tissue fibrosis[16]. Oral 1,25-dihydroxyvitamin D (calcitriol) and intralesional injections of interferon-γ were shown to be moderately effective in reducing the size or inhibiting the development of new lesions[17,18].

Pathogenesis

The etiology of localized scleroderma is not known. A role for local physical injury in triggering the development of cutaneous fibrosis has been suggested based on anecdotal reports[19,20]. Cases of familial pansclerotic morphea have been described[21,22]. Although *Borrelia burgdorferi* has been implicated, the etiological role of this infectious organism remains controversial[23]. The causative relationship between *Borrelia* infection and localized scleroderma is supported by serological, microbiological, immunohistological and DNA-based studies. Interestingly, polymerase chain reaction-based assays for the detection of *Borrelia* mRNA in lesional skin are more often positive in European studies than those from the United States. The extracellular matrix protein fibrillin-1 is implicated in the scleroderma-like skin changes in Tsk mice, a model for human scleroderma[24]. A possible pathogenetic role for fibrillin-1 in localized scleroderma is suggested by the demonstration of serum antibodies directed against fibrillin-1 in many patients[25].

The progenitor cell antigen CD34 identifies a subpopulation of spindle-shaped cells in the skin that are localized in the reticular dermis. The number of CD34-positive dendritic cells is decreased in localized scleroderma, suggesting a role for these unique cells in dermal immunomodulation[26]. Several cytokines and growth factors can initiate and/or sustain elevated production or decreased turnover of the extracellular matrix responsible for dermal fibrosis. Transforming growth factor-β (TGF-β) and inflammatory cell-derived cytokines such as IL-4 are prominent in lesional skin[27,28]. Elevated expression of TGF-β is also seen in periosteal fibroblasts from the melorheostotic bone[29]. In culture, lesional fibroblasts from patients with localized scleroderma display increased expression of the receptor for TGF-β[30]. Connective tissue growth factor (CTGF) is a TGF-β-inducible cytokine that is implicated in the pathogenesis of various forms of tissue fibrosis. The expression of CTGF mRNA is elevated in lesional skin in localized forms of scleroderma[31]. Increased signaling through TGF-β receptors present on lesional fibroblasts at elevated level, and CTGF released by fibroblasts in response to TGF-β together may contribute to an autocrine stimulatory loop that induces and sustains fibroblast proliferation and extracellular matrix production, resulting in fibrosis in localized scleroderma.

SCLEREDEMA

Scleredema adultorum (Buschke's disease) is an uncommon disorder characterized by diffuse cutaneous induration. Scleredema is not infrequently misdiagnosed as scleroderma/systemic sclerosis, although the distribution pattern of skin involvement in these two distinct clinical entities is different[32]. Scleredema frequently follows a febrile illness with upper respiratory symptoms, suggesting an underlying infectious etiology; streptococcal organisms have been implicated[33]. Patients with scleredema of Buschke characteristically present with rapidly evolving brawny induration affecting the nape of the neck, the shoulder girdle and the upper extremities; the scalp and occasionally the trunk may also be involved (Fig. 137.2d). The face may be severely affected and appear mask-like. Mobility of the affected joints is reduced. Whereas the skin induration may be extensive, the hands and feet are generally spared. Furthermore, Raynaud's phenomenon, nailfold capillary abnormalities and visceral organ involvement are not seen. The cutaneous induration is self-limited, regressing in most patients within 2 years. Pathological examination of the lesional skin reveals a thickened dermis with swollen

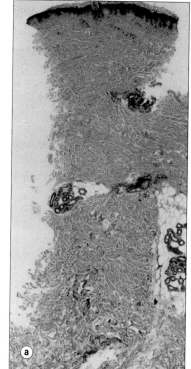
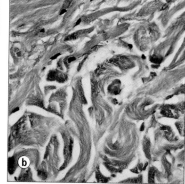
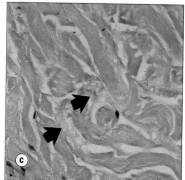
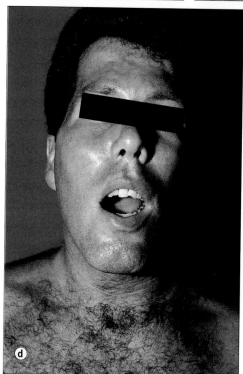

Fig. 137.2 Scleredema. (a–c) Histopathology of the skin. (a) The dermis is markedly thickened without inflammation. (b) Spaces separating collagen bundles in the dermis. (c) Amorphous mucin is identified by Alcian blue in the spaces between collagen bundles. (d) Mask-like appearance of the face.

collagen fibers that are separated by clear spaces (Fig. 137.2a–c). The clear spaces between collagen fibers are filled with amorphous material identified as hyaluronic acid using toluidine blue, Alcian blue, or colloidal iron stains[34,35]. In contrast to the histopathological findings in scleroderma/ systemic sclerosis, the dermal appendages are not obliterated and inflammation is not prominent. Serum monoclonal paraproteins can frequently be detected in adults with scleredema, and may be associated with or even precede multiple myeloma or AL amyloidosis[36,37]. Treatment with corticosteroids or D-penicillamine has been shown anecdotally to have modest benefit in alleviating induration. Photophoresis combined with psoralens may also be effective[38]. Cultured fibroblasts derived from lesional tissue show increased production of collagen and glycosaminoglycans *in vitro*[39].

In contrast to the acute onset characteristic of scleredema of Buschke, insidious evolution of skin induration is seen in scleredema diabeticorum[40]. This relatively frequent complication of long-standing insulin-dependent diabetes mellitus may be associated with carpal tunnel syndrome and Dupuytren's contractures. The appearance of affected skin is similar to that of pansclerotic morphea or scleromyxedema, and the histopathological features of diabetic scleredema are indistinguishable from those of scleredema adultorum of Buschke. With optimal diabetic control the severity of skin induration may improve. Diabetic cheiroarthropathy occurs in the absence of extensive skin involvement. It is characterized by tight skin on the fingers resembling sclerodactyly. However, cheiroarthropathy is not accompanied by nailfold capillary changes, Raynaud's phenomenon or other evidence of systemic sclerosis. Finger joint mobility may be markedly reduced. This complication of diabetes is most frequent in children with insulin-dependent diabetes mellitus. The pathogenesis of diabetic scleredema and cheiroarthropathy is thought to be related to other forms of tissue fibrosis, such as nerve entrapment syndromes and tissue contractures common in diabetes, reflecting non-enzymatic glycosylation and extensive cross-linking of collagen. Furthermore, advanced glycosylation end-products directly stimulate the local production of CTGF, which in turn enhances the deposition of matrix molecules[41].

SCLEROMYXEDEMA

Scleromyxedema or papular mucinosis is characterized by confluent papules causing skin induration. When the lesions are diffuse it may be difficult to distinguish scleromyxedema clinically from systemic sclerosis[42]. The papular lesions are most frequently localized on the upper extremities, face and neck; occasionally the fingers may be affected. Although scleromyxedema is not associated with Raynaud's phenomenon, visceral organ involvement may be prominent[43]. Inflammatory myopathy and esophageal dysmotility are frequent complications, and in some cases contribute to misdiagnosis as systemic sclerosis[44–46]. Monoclonal paraprotein, generally an IgGλ, is frequently detected in the serum and may be associated with multiple myeloma[47]. Some patients develop an erosive arthropathy[48,49]. Neurological abnormalities are frequent. A severe and potentially fatal acute or subacute central nervous system syndrome with fever, convulsions and coma has been reported[50–55]. The cerebrospinal fluid in these patients shows elevated protein, and hyperviscosity may play a role in neurological injury. The syndrome occasionally responds to plasmapheresis.

The etiology of scleromyxedema is unknown. Histopathological examination shows that the affected dermis is filled with amorphous mucin separating the collagen fibers. The mucinous material can be identified with colloidal iron, toluidine blue or Alcian blue stains. The number of fibroblasts appears to be increased. Inflammation in the skin is not prominent, but degranulating mast cells have been described[56,57]. In contrast to the skin, no mucin deposition can be detected in other affected organs, and the pathogenesis of visceral organ involvement in scleromyxedema is unknown[46]. Patients who developed diffuse scleromyxedema-like skin induration associated with hemodialysis treatment have been described[58]. Biopsy of the skin indicated pathological changes indistinguishable from scleromyxedema. The incidence and cause of this newly recognized complication of hemodialysis is unknown.

Unlike the relatively benign and self-limited course characteristic of scleredema of Buschke, scleromyxedema is generally chronic and the cutaneous lesions and internal organ involvement are resistant to therapy. Whereas prednisone is only rarely effective, extracorporeal photophoresis, and in some patients with monoclonal paraproteinemias melphalan, prednisone and plasmapheresis, have been used with success. Sustained cutaneous response in some patients treated with high-dose intravenous immunoglobulin, isotretinoin or interferon-α has been described[59–61].

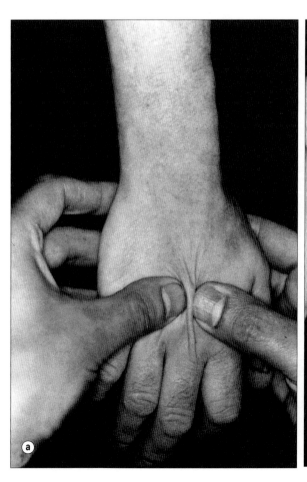 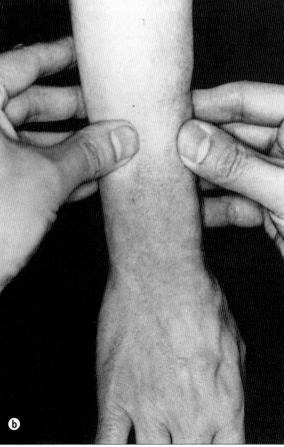

(a) (b)

Fig. 137.3 Characteristic distribution of skin involvement in the eosinophilic fibrosing syndromes. The skin on the hand is unaffected (a), whereas it is indurated and bound to underlying structures on the forearms (b). (Courtesy of Dr S. Jimenez.)

EOSINOPHILIC CUTANEOUS FIBROSES

Three distinct but related scleroderma-like entities are characterized by marked eosinophilia in the blood and/or cutaneous tissues and symmetrical induration of the distal extremities sparing the fingers (Fig. 137.3). These conditions show an acute inflammatory stage, followed by gradual resolution of inflammation but persistence of tissue fibrosis. Eosinophilic fasciitis is a sporadic illness of unknown cause. In contrast, eosinophilia–myalgia syndrome and toxic oil syndrome occurred in discrete epidemic outbreaks and were strongly associated with defined dietary/environmental exposures. The clinical and histopathological features of these three diseases share intriguing similarities.

Eosinophilic fasciitis

Clinical features

Eosinophilic fasciitis was first recognized as a fibrosing skin disorder distinct from scleroderma in the 1970s[62]. Also called diffuse fasciitis with eosinophilia or Shulman's syndrome, eosinophilic fasciitis is relatively uncommon and occurs in sporadic rather than epidemic form. In marked contrast to systemic sclerosis, the onset of eosinophilic fasciitis is typically abrupt and in many cases follows excessive or unusual physical activity. In the acute stage eosinophilic fasciitis is characterized by painful and erythematous swelling of the extremities, accompanied by rapid weight gain, fever and myalgia. Eosinophilia in the peripheral blood, and somewhat less commonly in affected tissue, is prominent at this stage[63,64]. As the disease progresses, edema is replaced by progressive thickening of the skin. Induration is most frequent in the upper extremities, with a symmetrical distribution; less commonly, the lower extremities, neck and trunk may be affected[65]. The absence of skin involvement on the fingers and toes is a helpful clinical clue distinguishing eosinophilic fasciitis from systemic sclerosis/scleroderma. The affected skin is taut and woody, and is firmly bound to the underlying tissue; it often assumes an irregularly puckered *peau d'orange* appearance that is quite distinct from systemic sclerosis/scleroderma. The uplifted arm may display the 'groove' sign, a longitudinal depression in the skin along the course of blood vessels.

Contractures of the underlying joints may develop with long-standing eosinophilic fasciitis. Raynaud's syndrome, and nailfold microvascular abnormalities characteristic of systemic sclerosis/scleroderma, are not seen. Although significant visceral organ involvement is rare, the musculoskeletal system may be affected with arthritis, myopathy, carpal tunnel syndrome and other peripheral neuropathies, compartment syndrome, Dupuytren's contractures and inflammatory arthritis. Non-specific electromyographic abnormalities are common. Autoimmune thyroiditis and diffuse lymphadenopathy have been reported[66,67]. Of greatest concern in patients with eosinophilic fasciitis is the development of hematological abnormalities, including malignant myelodysplastic/lymphoproliferative syndromes. In one series, associated hematological disorders were detected in 10% of patients[65]. In addition to aplastic anemia, thrombocytopenia and hemolytic anemia, lymphoma, chronic lymphocytic leukemia and Hodgkin's disease have been described, suggesting that eosinophilic fasciitis may occur as a paraneoplastic syndrome. The pathogenesis and incidence of these hematological complications are unknown. It may be prudent to perform a bone marrow examination in patients with eosinophilic fasciitis.

In addition to peripheral blood eosinophilia, laboratory investigations reveal hypergammaglobulinemia and elevated erythrocyte sedimentation rate, whereas levels of muscle enzymes are normal, and monoclonal paraproteinemia is rare. The non-specific laboratory findings normalize rapidly in response to glucocorticoid therapy, even when cutaneous manifestations remain unchanged or worsen. Serum antinuclear antibodies have been reported inconsistently, and do not appear to have diagnostic or prognostic utility. The differential diagnosis includes localized forms of scleroderma and other scleroderma variants. Eosinophilic fasciitis must be differentiated from eosinophilia–myalgia syndrome[68] and hypereosinophilic syndromes (Table 137.3). It is important to obtain a careful dietary, drug and occupational exposure history.

Full-thickness wedge biopsy of the clinically involved skin is essential for establishing the accurate diagnosis of eosinophilic fasciitis. Lesional skin demonstrates thickened fascia, which can be recognized even under low-power microscopy (Fig. 137.4). The fascia shows accumulation of lymphocytes, mast cells and plasma cells. The presence of eosinophils or immunohistochemical evidence of eosinophil degranulation in the lesional tissue is variable. Cellular infiltration of the skin is less prominent in established disease, where fibrosis and atrophy of the fascia and often the overlying dermis are characteristic. Inflammation may also be found in the subcutaneous fat, the perimysium and the epimysium. Frank inflammation of the muscle or myocyte degeneration/regeneration are not seen. Magnetic resonance imaging can identify fascial inflammation and fibrosis, and may have a potential role in the non-invasive evaluation of patients with unexplained skin thickening.

Etiology and pathogenesis

The etiology of eosinophilic fasciitis is unknown. In contrast to the eosinophilia–myalgia syndrome associated with L-tryptophan ingestion,

Type of disease	Eosinophilia		Examples
	Tissue	Blood	
Infectious	±	+	Trichinosis, *Schistosoma*, *Toxocara*
Respiratory	+	+	Asthma, Loffler's syndrome, pulmonary infiltrates with eosinophilia (PIE)
Allergic	+	±	Eczema, drug hypersensitivity, atopic dermatitis
Systemic	+	+	Eosinophilia–myalgia syndrome, Churg–Strauss syndrome
Hematologic	+	±	Eosinophilic leukemia, idiopathic hypereosinophilic syndrome

TABLE 137.3 SYNDROMES ASSOCIATED WITH BLOOD OR TISSUE EOSINOPHILIA

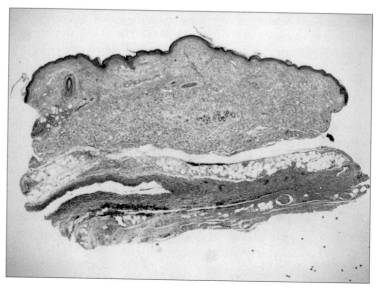

Fig. 137.4 Fascial fibrosis. Low-power view illustrating marked thickening and compact collagen in the subcutaneous fascia in eosinophilic fasciitis.

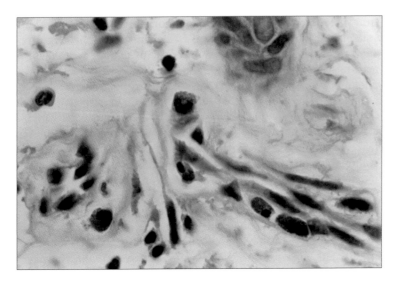

Fig. 137.5 Eosinophil activation in fibrosis. Close topological association between degranulating eosinophils and dermal fibroblasts in area of active collagen production in tissue.

no consistent dietary or environmental exposure history can be elicited. Evidence of infection with *B. burgdorferi* is present in some cases, potentially implicating *Borrelia* in the pathogenesis[69]. Peripheral blood mononuclear cells from patients with eosinophilic fasciitis produce elevated amounts of interleukin-5, which stimulates the production, chemotaxis and survival of eosinophils[70]. Resident fibroblasts secrete increased amounts of collagen in lesional tissue, and display elevated expression of TGF-β_1 and CTGF[28,31]. Because these cytokines stimulate fibroblast proliferation and adhesion, extracellular matrix production and transformation into contractile myofibroblasts, they may be implicated in the intitiation or maintenance of tissue fibrosis.

Eosinophilia is seen in various forms of pathological fibroses (Table 137.3). The association of tissue eosinophil accumulation and/or degranulation with fibrosis, the close topological relationship between degranulating eosinophils and activated resident fibroblasts (Fig. 137.5), and the development of connective tissue fibrosis in animal models of hypereosinophilia suggest a role for eosinophils in the pathogenesis of fibrosis. Numerous mechanisms may account for eosinophil-triggered fibroblast activation. Expression of TGF-β is markedly increased in tissue eosinophils. Furthermore, upon their activation, eosinophils release major basic protein, a strongly cationic protein that stimulates the secretion of interleukin-6 by normal fibroblasts, and directly their transdifferentiation into myofibroblasts. Under culture conditions, fascia-derived fibroblasts show sustained upregulation of collagen, CTGF and TGF-β_1 mRNA expression *in vitro*, suggesting that autocrine stimulatory loops involving TGF-β and CTGF contribute to the pathogenesis of tissue fibrosis.

Treatment

Although the skin induration may improve spontaneously, some patients with eosinophilic fasciitis require therapy. No controlled trials have been reported to date, and thus it is difficult to determine whether any intervention hastens the resolution of fibrosis, prevents the development of hematological complications or modifies the long-term course of the disease. Treatment with daily prednisone at a dose of ~1 mg/kg commonly induces resolution of edema and softening of the skin. A clinical response may be seen within weeks, and is typically preceded by resolution of peripheral blood eosinophilia. Indeed, lack of a marked and rapid decline in the eosinophil count may be evidence of inadequate prednisone dose. The effect of prednisone on the accumulation and degranulation of activated eosinophils in affected tissues is unknown. Cimetidine may be useful in combination with prednisone. Anecdotal reports indicate a beneficial response to plaquenil, methotrexate,

D-penicillamine and psoralen-UVA photochemotherapy. Cyclosporin A and antithymocyte gloubulin have been used in treatment-resistant patients. Severe joint contractures of the wrist, elbow and knee may necessitate surgical fasciectomy. The natural history of eosinophilic fasciitis is unknown. Many patients show partial or full resolution of skin changes within a few years of onset. Recurrence of active disease appears to be rare.

Eosinophilia–myalgia syndrome

In the summer of 1989, a previously unknown eosinophilic fasciitis-like epidemic illness was recognized. The novel syndrome, characterized by marked eosinophilia and widespread myalgia, affected more than 1500 people. Eosinophilia–myalgia syndrome was associated with the ingestion of L-tryptophan, a non-prescription food supplement used widely for insomnia, premenstrual syndrome and other indications. The illness was associated with L-tryptophan originating from a single manufacturer[71]. Analysis of implicated lots of L-tryptophan identified the many contaminants. The best-characterized of these is 1,1'-ethylidenebis (L-tryptophan) (EBT), a tryptophan dimer[72]. Injection of EBT in rodents caused inflammation in the dermis, fascia and perimysium, and EBT stimulates fibroblast proliferation and collagen synthesis *in vitro*. Eosinophilia does not develop in EBT-treated animals, and the precise role of this contaminant in the pathogenesis of eosinophilia–myalgia syndrome remains uncertain. Another contaminant, 3-(phenylamino)-L-alanine, undergoes hepatic biotransformation to 3-(phenylamino)-1,2-propanediol (PAP), which had been previously found in cooking oils implicated in the toxic oil syndrome epidemic in Spain, suggesting that these two clinically similar epidemic diseases, separated by a decade and occurring on separate continents, may have shared a common etiologic agent (Table 137.4)[73].

The majority of patients with eosinophilia–myalgia syndrome are women, reflecting the pattern of L-tryptophan ingestion. The onset of illness was characterized by an abrupt onset of a flu-like syndrome, with fever, myalgia, swelling and skin rashes[74–77]. These symptoms were severe enough to warrant hospitalization in nearly one-third of patients[77]. Laboratory findings in the acute stage included striking eosinophilia, elevated erythrocyte sedimentation rate and non-specific autoantibodies. Curiously, in light of the severe myalgia, serum creatine phosphokinase was low, with elevated aldolase levels. With resolution of the acute phase, more than 50% of patients developed chronic and often progressive symptoms. A prominent late finding was brawny induration of the skin affecting the extremities and trunk but sparing the face, hands and feet, indistinguishable in appearance from eosinophilic fasciitis. Muscle cramps, alopecia and peripheral neuropathy were common delayed and persistent manifestations[78]. Treatment has been empiric,

---

TABLE 137.4 DRUGS, ENVIRONMENTAL AND OCCUPATIONAL EXPOSURES ASSOCIATED WITH SCLERODERMA OR SCLERODERMA VARIANTS

Firm associations

- Rapeseed oil denatured with aniline – toxic oil syndrome (Spain, 1981)
- L-tryptophan manufactured by Showa-Denko – eosinophilia–myalgia syndrome (1989)
- Bleomycin
- Pentazocine
- Vitamin K
- Vinyl chloride
- Trichloroethylene; other organic solvents

Tentative associations

- Silica dust
- Biogenic amines
- Cocaine

and no controlled therapeutic trials have been reported. Glucocorticoids in low to moderate doses were commonly used in the acute stage. Glucocorticoid therapy induced resolution of edema, myalgia and eosinophilia, but did not appear to modify the course of illness or the development of late complications.

Toxic oil syndrome

In spring 1981 an explosive epidemic febrile illness associated with the ingestion of adulterated rapeseed oil broke out in parts of Spain[79]. Toxic oil syndrome affected 20 000 persons, becoming the largest epidemic intoxication on record[80]. Some 12 000 hospitalizations occurred, and more than 300 patients died. With public announcements of the association between the novel illness and the consumption of contaminated oils, the incidence of toxic oil syndrome rapidly declined, and the epidemic abated some 3 months after it broke out[81]. The acute phase of the illness was characterized by fever, cough and dyspnea, edema, myalgia and skin rashes. Peripheral blood eosinophil count was frequently >2000/mm³. The rapeseed oil implicated in the epidemic had been sold illegally as olive oil for cooking, and was found to be denatured with aniline. Toxicoepidemiologic analysis demonstrated the presence of PAP, a trace contaminant also implicated in the eosinophilia–myalgia syndrome. However, PAP failed to reproduce the toxic oil syndrome in experimental animals.

Many patients recovered within 2–4 months of the onset of symptoms, but in more than 50% a chronic illness characterized by progressive woody induration and fibrosis of the skin ensued. Histopathological examination showed eosinophil infiltration and degranulation in the affected dermis and fascia, as well as perimysial and perineurial inflammation indistinguishable from eosinophilia–myalgia syndrome. Joint contractures, muscle atrophy and sensory neuropathy developed in many patients, persisting for as long as 12 years after the outbreak of the epidemic[82]. No recurrence of symptoms has been recorded. In the explosive epidemic phase of toxic oil syndrome, many patients were treated with glucocorticoids. This intervention alleviated the acute respiratory symptoms but did not appear to modify the long-term course of the disease. Although epidemiological investigation firmly implicates aniline-denatured rapeseed oil as the vehicle of the toxic oil syndrome, the precise etiologic agent has not been determined. Attempts to reproduce the illness experimentally have not been successful. The striking similarities in clinical manifestations (abrupt onset, acute eosinophilia, chronic skin induration and neuropathy), the histopathological features of toxic oil syndrome and eosinophilia–myalgia syndrome, and the presence of PAP in implicated vehicles (L-tryptophan and denatured rapeseed oil) raises the possibility that the two diseases may have a shared common etiology and/or pathogenesis.

CHRONIC GRAFT-VERSUS-HOST DISEASE

In the chronic form of graft-versus-host disease following allogeneic bone marrow transplantation, some patients develop scleroderma-like induration of the skin[83]. The face and trunk are most commonly affected. Antinuclear and Scl-70 autoantibodies may develop. Raynaud's syndrome is not seen, but xerostomia may occur. Histopathological examination of lesional skin demonstrates dermal and fascial fibrosis, monocytic/lymphocytic infiltration and mast cell degranulation. A characteristic histopathological finding distinguishing chronic graft-versus-host disease from scleroderma/systemic sclerosis is vacuolization of basal cells in the skin. Experimental bone marrow transplantation in mice resulting in diffuse skin is histologically indistinguishable from human chronic graft-versus-host disease[84]. Study of this animal model has firmly established the crucial roles of monocytes and TGF-β in the development of dermal fibrosis. Thalidomide and photophoresis/photochemotherapy with psoralens may be effective in reducing induration[85,86]. The incidence of scleroderma-like changes in chronic graft-versus-host disease has decreased markedly in the past decade, suggesting that early treatment with glucocorticoids and cyclosporin A may be effective in preventing this late complication of allogeneic bone marrow transplantation[87].

DRUG-ASSOCIATED SCLERODERMA VARIANTS

The antineoplastic/cytotoxic agent bleomycin has been implicated in Raynaud's phenomenon and scleroderma-like induration, in addition to the well-recognized complication of pulmonary fibrosis[88]. The pattern of skin involvement and the histopathological features are identical to those seen in systemic sclerosis/scleroderma. Flexion contractures of the fingers and distal acro-osteolysis develop. The syndrome may resolve with cessation of bleomycin treatment. Repeated subcutaneous injections of pentazocine, a potent analgesic, cause localized brawny induration of the skin resembling morphea. The fibrotic process often involves subcutaneous tissue, including muscle, and soft tissue calcifications may occur. Raynaud's phenomenon and internal organ involvement are not seen[89]. A localized scleroderma-like induration may develop in some patients receiving vitamin K injections[90]. Cocaine abuse has occasionally been linked with systemic sclerosis, but the etiologic relationship remains uncertain[91].

OCCUPATIONAL EXPOSURE-ASSOCIATED SCLERODERMA VARIANTS

Vinyl chloride is a gaseous substance used in the manufacture of polyvinyl chloride (PVC). Several reports have linked occupational PVC monomer exposure with a scleroderma-like syndrome. In one study, the scleroderma-like syndrome developed in 5% of exposed workers[92]. In addition to skin involvement, Raynaud's phenomenon and acro-osteolysis are common. Skin involvement is prominent on the extensor surfaces of the hands and arms, whereas the face and trunk are generally spared. Pulmonary fibrosis and esophageal dysmotility may be seen. Thrombocytopenia and liver fibrosis can be associated, helping to distinguish the syndrome from systemic sclerosis/scleroderma. Trichloroethylene is an organic solvent used extensively to degrease metals and strip paint, and in the dry-cleaning industry. It is readily absorbed both by inhalation and through the skin. Sclerodactyly associated with Raynaud's phenomenon and diffuse morphea have been described in laundry workers, painters and carpenters exposed to trichloroethylene. Scleroderma-like disorder has also been reported in workers engaged in polymerization of epoxy resins, and in those with occupational exposure to biogenic amines[93].

Exposure to silica has been linked with scleroderma-like syndromes. This association is most frequently reported in coalminers, who are exposed to high levels of silica dust. The illness is clinically and pathologically indistinguishable from systemic sclerosis/scleroderma, and is often associated with prominent pulmonary fibrosis[94]. Silica exposure may be considered to be a risk factor for developing systemic sclerosis/scleroderma. Because of their presumed inertness, silicones have been used extensively in medical devices, including breast implants. Fibrosis of the capsular tissue surrounding silicone implants frequently develops, and particles of silicone that had leaked out of the implant can be detected locally or even systemically. Women have been reported who developed scleroderma and morphea several years following silicone breast implants. In some reports, explantation appeared to be associated with clinical improvement. Despite anecdotal reports suggesting a causal relationship between silicone breast implants and systemic sclerosis, presumably owing to leakage of silicone from the implant and activation of a systemic immune reaction, population-based epidemiological surveys and meta-analyses have failed to provide firm support for this association[95,96].

REFERENCES

1. Peterson LS, Nelson AM, Su WP et al. The epidemiology of morphea (localized scleroderma) in Olmsted County 1960–1993. J Rheumatol 1997; 24: 73–80.

2. Moreno Alvarez MJ, Lazaro MA, Espada G et al. Linear scleroderma and melorheostosis: case presentation and literature review. Clin Rheumatol 19; 15: 389–393.

3. Freyschmidt J. Melorheostosis: a review of 23 cases. Eur Radiol 2001; 11: 474–479.

4. Pupillo G, Andermann F, Dubeau F. Linear scleroderma and intractable epilepsy: neuropathologic evidence for a chronic inflammatory process. Ann Neurol 1996; 39: 277–278.

5. Stone J, Franks AJ, Guthrie JA, Johnson MH. Scleroderma "en coup de sabre": pathological evidence of intracerebral inflammation. J Neurol Neurosurg Psychiatry 2001; 70: 382–385.

6. Higashi Y, Kanekura T, Fukumaru K, Kanzaki T. Scleroderma en coup de sabre with central nervous system involvement. J Dermatol 2000; 27: 486–488.

7. Falanga V, Medsger TA Jr, Reichlin M, Rodnan GP. Linear scleroderma. Clinical spectrum, prognosis, and laboratory abnormalities. Ann Intern Med 1986; 104: 849–857.

8. Fujimoto M, Sato S, Ihn H et al. Autoantibodies to mitochondrial 2-oxo-acid dehydrogenase complexes in localized scleroderma. Clin Exp Immunol 1996; 105: 297–301.

9. Parodi A, Drosera M, Barbieri L, Rebora A. Antihistone antibodies in scleroderma. Dermatology 1995; 191: 16–18.

10. Torres JE, Sanchez JL. Histopathologic differentiation between localized and systemic scleroderma. Am J Dermatopathol 1998; 20: 242–245.

11. Uziel Y, Feldman BM, Krafchik BR et al. Methotrexate and corticosteroid therapy for pediatric localized scleroderma. J Pediatr 2000; 136: 91–95.

12. Seyger MM, van den Hoogen FH, van Vlijmen-Willems IM et al. Localized and systemic scleroderma show different histological responses to methotrexate therapy. J Pathol 2001; 193: 511–516.

13. Kamath NV, Usmani A, Pellegrini A. When is surgical treatment not appropriate for morphea? Ann Plast Surg 2000; 45: 199–201.

14. Grundmann-Kollmann M, Ochsendorf F, Zollner TM et al. PUVA-cream photochemotherapy for the treatment of localized scleroderma. J Am Acad Dermatol 2000; 43: 675–678.

15. Karrer S, Abels C, Landthaler M, Szeimies RM. Topical photodynamic therapy for localized scleroderma. Acta Dermatol Venereol 2000; 80: 26–27.

16. Quan T, He T, Voorhees J, Fisher G. Ultraviolet irradiation blocks cellular responses to transforming growth factor-beta by down-regulating its type-II receptor and inducing Smad J Biol Chem published April 24, 2001 as 10.1074/jbc.M010835200

17. Hulshof MM, Bouwes Bavinck JN, Bergman W et al. Double-blind, placebo-controlled study of oral calcitriol for the treatment of localized and systemic scleroderma. J Am Acad Dermatol 2000; 43: 1017–1023.

18. Hunzelmann N, Anders S, Fierlbeck G et al. Double-blind, placebo-controlled study of intralesional interferon gamma for the treatment of localized scleroderma. J Am Acad Dermatol. 1997; 36: 433–435.

19. Komocsi A, Tovari E, Kovacs J, Czirjak L. Physical injury as a provoking factor in three patients with scleroderma. Clin Exp Rheumatol 2000; 18: 622–624.

20. Yamanaka CT, Gibbs NF. Trauma-induced linear scleroderma. Cutis 1999; 63: 29–32.

21. Kornreich HK, King KK, Bernstein BH et al. Scleroderma in childhood. Arthritis Rheum 1977; 20: 343–350.

22. Burge KM, Perry HO, Stickler GB. Familial scleroderma. Arch Dermatol 1969; 99: 681–687.

23. Weide B, Walz T, Garbe C. Is morphoea caused by Borrelia burgdorferi? Br J Dermatol 2000; 142: 636–644.

24. Siracusa LD, McGrath R, Ma Q et al. A tandem duplication within the fibrillin 1 gene is associated with the mouse tight skin mutation. Genome Res 1996; 6: 300–313.

25. Arnett FC, Tan FK, Uziel Y et al. Autoantibodies to the extracellular matrix microfibrillar protein, fibrillin-1, in patients with localized scleroderma. Arthritis Rheum 1999; 42: 2656–2659.

26. Gilmour TK, Wilkinson B, Breit SN, Kossard S. Analysis of dendritic cell populations using a revised histological staging of morphoea. Br J Dermatol 2000; 143: 1183–1192.

27. Higley H, Persichitte K, Chu S et al. Immunocytochemical localization and serologic detection of transforming growth factor beta-1. Association with type I procollagen and inflammatory cell markers in diffuse and limited systemic sclerosis, morphea, and Raynaud's phenomenon. Arthritis Rheum 1994; 37: 278–288.

28. Peltonen J, Kahari L, Jaakkola S et al. Evaluation of transforming growth factor beta and type I procollagen gene expression in fibrotic skin diseases by in situ hybridization. J Invest Dermatol 1990; 94: 365–371.

29. Hoshi K, Amizuka N, Kurokawa T et al. Histopathological characterization of melorheostosis. Orthopedics 2001; 24: 273–277.

30. Kubo M, Ihn H, Yamane K, Tamaki K. Up-regulated expression of transforming growth factor beta receptors in dermal fibroblasts in skin sections from patients with localized scleroderma. Arthritis Rheum 2001; 44: 731–734.

31. Igarashi A, Nashiro K, Kikuchi K et al. Connective tissue growth factor gene expression in tissue sections from localized scleroderma, keloid, and other fibrotic skin disorders. J Invest Dermatol 1996; 106: 729–733.

32. Venencie PY, Powell FC, Su WP, Perry HO. Scleredema: a review of thirty-three cases. J Am Acad Dermatol 1984; 11: 128–134.

33. Cron RQ, Swetter SM. Scleredema revisited. A poststreptococcal complication. Clin Pediatr 1994; 33: 606–610.

34. Cole HG, Winkelmann RK. Acid mucopolysaccharide staining in scleredema. J Cutan Pathol 1990; 17: 211–213.

35. Matsuoka LY, Wortsman J, Carlisle KS et al. The acquired cutaneous mucinoses. Arch Intern Med 1984; 144: 1974–1980.

36. Basarab T, Burrows NP, Munn SE, Russell Jones R. Systemic involvement in scleredema of Buschke associated with IgG-kappa paraproteinaemia. Br J Dermatol 1997; 136: 939–942.

37. Ohta A, Uitto J, Oikarinen AI et al. Paraproteinemia in patients with scleredema. Clinical findings and serum effects on skin fibroblasts in vitro. J Am Acad Dermatol 1987; 16: 96–107.

38. Stables GI, Taylor PC, Highet AS. Scleredema associated with paraproteinaemia treated by extracorporeal photopheresis. Br J Dermatol 2000; 142: 781–783.

39. Varga J, Gotta S, Li L, Sollberg S, Di Leonardo M. Scleredema adultorum: case report and demonstration of abnormal expression of extracellular matrix genes in skin fibroblasts in vivo and in vitro. Br J Dermatol 1995; 132: 992–999.

40. Sattar MA, Diab S, Sugathan TN et al. Scleroedema diabeticorum: a minor but often unrecognized complication of diabetes mellitus. Diabet Med 1988; 5: 465–468.

41. Twigg SM, Chen MM, Joly AH et al. Advanced glycosylation end products up-regulate connective tissue growth factor (insulin-like growth factor-binding protein-related protein 2) in human fibroblasts: a potential mechanism for expansion of extracellular matrix in diabetes mellitus. Endocrinology 2001; 142: 1760–1769.

42. Jablonska S, Blaszczyk M. Scleromyxedema is a scleroderma-like disorder and not a coexistance of scleroderma with papular mucinosis. Eur J Dermatol 1999; 9: 551–554.

43. Gabriel SE, Perry HO, Oleson GB, Bowles CA. Scleromyxedema: a scleroderma-like disorder with systemic manifestations. Medicine (Baltimore) 1988; 67: 58–65.

44. Verity MA, Toop J, McAdam LP, Pearson CM. Scleromyxedema myopathy. Histochemical and electron microscopic observations. Am J Clin Pathol 1978; 69: 446–451.

45. Helfrich DJ, Walker ER, Martinez AJ, Medsger TA Jr. Scleromyxedema myopathy: case report and review of the literature. Arthritis Rheum 1988; 31: 1437–1441.

46. Godby A, Bergstresser PR, Chaker B, Pandya AG. Fatal scleromyxedema: report of a case and review of the literature. J Am Acad Dermatol 1998; 38: 289–294.

47. Kitamura W, Matsuoka Y, Miyagawa S, Sakamoto K. Immunochemical analysis of the monoclonal paraprotein in scleromyxedema. J Invest Dermatol 1978; 70: 305–308.

48. Jamieson TW, De Smet AA, Stechschulte DJ. Erosive arthropathy associated with scleromyxedema. Skeletal Radiol 1985; 14: 286–290.

49. Frayha RA. Papular mucinosis, destructive arthropathy, median neuropathy, and sicca complex. Clin Rheumatol 1983; 2: 277–284.

50. Ochitill HN, Amberson J. Acute cerebral symptomatology, a rare presentation of scleromyxedema. J Clin Psychiatry 1978; 39: 471–475.

51. Reid TL, Spoto DV, Larrabee GJ et al. Monoclonal paraproteinemia with subacute encephalopathy, seizures, and scleromyxedema. Neurology 1987; 37: 1054–1057.

52. Webster GF, Matsuoka LY, Burchmore D. The association of potentially lethal neurologic syndromes with scleromyxedema (papular mucinosis). J Am Acad Dermatol 1993; 28: 105–108.

53. Gonzalez J, Palangio M, Schwartz J et al. Scleromyxedema with dermato-neuro syndrome. J Am Acad Dermatol 2000; 42: 927–928.

54. Nieves DS, Bondi EE, Wallmark J et al. Scleromyxedema: successful treatment of cutaneous and neurologic symptoms. Cutis 2000; 65: 89–92.

55. Johkura K, Susuki K, Hasegawa O et al. Encephalopathy in scleromyxedema. Neurology 1999; 53: 1138–1140.

56. Rongioletti F, Rebora A. Updated classification of papular mucinosis, lichen myxedematosus, and scleromyxedema. J Am Acad Dermatol 2001; 44: 273–281.

57. Varga J, Matsuoka LY, Hashimoto K et al. Papular mucinosis (scleromyxedema) complicating diffuse systemic sclerosis: clinical features and electron microscope observations. Br J Rheumatol 1992; 31: 779–782.

58. Cowper SE, Robin HS, Steinberg SM et al. Scleromyxoedema-like cutaneous diseases in renal-dialysis patients. Lancet 2000; 16; 356: 1000–1001.

59. Tschen JA, Chang JR. Scleromyxedema: treatment with interferon alfa. J Am Acad Dermatol 1999; 40: 303–307.

60. Hisler BM, Savoy LB, Hashimoto K. Improvement of scleromyxedema associated with isotretinoin therapy. J Am Acad Dermatol 1991; 24: 854–857.

61. Milam CP, Cohen LE, Fenske NA, Ling NS. Scleromyxedema: therapeutic response to isotretinoin in three patients. J Am Acad Dermatol 1988; 19: 469–477.

62. Shulman LE. Diffuse fasciitis with hypergammaglobulinemia and eosinophilia: a new syndrome? J Rheumatol 1984; 11: 569–570.

63. Doyle JA, Ginsburg WW. Eosinophilic fasciitis. Med Clin North Am 1989; 73: 1157–1166.

64. Varga J, Griffin R, Newman JH, Jimenez SA. Eosinophilic fasciitis is clinically distinguishable from the eosinophilia–myalgia syndrome and is not associated with L-tryptophan use. J Rheumatol 1991; 18: 259–263.

65. Lakhanpal S, Ginsburg WW, Michet CJ et al. Eosinophilic fasciitis: clinical spectrum and therapeutic response in 52 cases. Semin Arthritis Rheum 1988; 17: 221–231.

66. Farrell AM, Ross JS, Bunker CB. Eosinophilic fasciitis associated with autoimmune thyroid disease and myelodysplasia treated with pulsed methylprednisolone and antihistamines. Br J Dermatol 1999; 140: 1185–1187.

67. Naschitz JE, Misselevich I, Rosner I et al. Lymph-node-based malignant lymphoma and reactive lymphadenopathy in eosinophilic fasciitis. Am J Med Sci 1999; 318: 343–349.

68. Umbert I, Winkelmann RK, Wegener L. Comparison of the pathology of fascia in eosinophilic myalgia syndrome patients and idiopathic eosinophilic fasciitis. Dermatology 1993; 186: 18–22.

69. Granter SR, Barnhill RL, Duray PH. Borrelial fasciitis: diffuse fasciitis and peripheral eosinophilia associated with Borrelia infection. Am J Dermatopathol 1996; 18: 465–473.

70. Viallard JF, Taupin JL, Ranchin V et al. Analysis of leukemia inhibitory factor, type 1 and type 2 cytokine production in patients with eosinophilic fasciitis. J Rheumatol 2001; 28: 75–80.

71. Slutsker L, Hoesly FC, Miller L *et al.* Eosinophilia–myalgia syndrome associated with exposure to tryptophan from a single manufacturer. JAMA 1990; 264: 213–217.

72. Mayeno AN, Lin F, Foote CS *et al.* Characterization of "peak E," a novel amino acid associated with eosinophilia–myalgia syndrome. Science 1990; 250: 1707–1708.

73. Mayeno AN, Belongia EA, Lin F, Lundy SK, Gleich GJ. 3-(Phenylamino)alanine, a novel aniline-derived amino acid associated with the eosinophilia–myalgia syndrome: a link to the toxic oil syndrome? Mayo Clin Proc 1992; 67: 1134–1139.

74. Kaufman LD, Seidman RJ, Gruber BL. L-tryptophan-associated eosinophilic perimyositis, neuritis, and fasciitis. A clinicopathologic and laboratory study of 25 patients. Medicine (Baltimore) 1990; 69: 187–199.

75. Silver RM, Heyes MP, Maize JC *et al.* Scleroderma, fasciitis, and eosinophilia associated with the ingestion of tryptophan. N Engl J Med 1990; 322: 874–881.

76. Martin RW, Duffy J, Engel AG *et al.* The clinical spectrum of the eosinophilia–myalgia syndrome associated with L-tryptophan ingestion. Clinical features in 20 patients and aspects of pathophysiology. Ann Intern Med 1990; 15; 113: 124–134.

77. Varga J, Heiman-Patterson TD, Emery DL *et al.* Clinical spectrum of the systemic manifestations of the eosinophilia–myalgia syndrome. Semin Arthritis Rheum 1990; 19: 313–328.

78. Kaufman LD, Gruber BL, Gregersen PK. Clinical follow-up and immunogenetic studies of 32 patients with eosinophilia–myalgia syndrome. Lancet 1991 4; 337: 1071–1074.

79. Tabuenca JM. Toxic–allergic syndrome caused by ingestion of rapeseed oil denatured with aniline. Lancet 1981; 2: 567–568.

80. Kilbourne EM, Rigau-Perez JG, Heath CW Jr *et al.* Clinical epidemiology of toxic-oil syndrome. Manifestations of a new illness. N Engl J Med 1983; 309: 1408–1414.

81. Rigau-Perez JG, Perez-Alvarez L, Duenas-Castro S *et al.* Epidemiologic investigation of an oil-associated pneumonic paralytic eosinophilic syndrome in Spain. Am J Epidemiol 1984; 119: 250–260.

82. Kaufman LD, Izquierdo Martinez M, Serrano JM, Gomez-Reino JJ. 12-year followup study of epidemic Spanish toxic oil syndrome. J Rheumatol 1995; 22: 282–288.

83. Furst DE, Clements PJ, Graze P *et al.* A syndrome resembling progressive systemic sclerosis after bone marrow transplantation. A model for scleroderma? Arthritis Rheum 1979; 22: 904–910.

84. McCormick LL, Zhang Y, Tootell E, Gilliam AC. Anti-TGF-beta treatment prevents skin and lung fibrosis in murine sclerodermatous graft-versus-host disease: a model for human scleroderma. J Immunol 1999; 163: 5693–5699.

85. Greinix HT, Volc-Platzer B, Rabitsch W *et al.* Successful use of extracorporeal photochemotherapy in the treatment of severe acute and chronic graft-versus-host disease. Blood 1998; 92: 3098–3104.

86. Browne PV, Weisdorf DJ, DeFor T *et al.* Response to thalidomide therapy in refractory chronic graft-versus-host disease. Bone Marrow Transplant 2000; 26: 865–869

87. Siadak M, Sullivan KM. The management of chronic graft-versus-host disease. Blood Rev 1994; 8: 154–160.

88. Kerr LD, Spiera H. Scleroderma in association with the use of bleomycin: a report of 3 cases. J Rheumatol 1992; 19: 294–296.

89. Hertzman A, Toone E, Resnik CS. Pentazocine induced myocutaneous sclerosis. J Rheumatol 1986; 13: 210–214.

90. Sanders MN, Winkelmann RK. Cutaneous reactions to vitamin K. J Am Acad Dermatol 1988; 19 : 699–704.

91. Kerr HD. Cocaine and scleroderma. South Med J 1989; 82: 1275–1276.

92. Black CM, Welsh KI, Walker AE *et al.* Genetic susceptibility to scleroderma-like syndrome induced by vinyl chloride. Lancet 1983; 1: 53–55.

93. Owens GR, Medsger TA. Systemic sclerosis secondary to occupational exposure. Am J Med 1988; 85: 114–116.

94. Haustein UF, Anderegg U. Silica induced scleroderma–clinical and experimental aspects. J Rheumatol 1998; 25: 1917–1926.

95. Hochberg MC, Perlmutter DL, Medsger TA Jr *et al.* Lack of association between augmentation mammaplasty and systemic sclerosis (scleroderma). Arthritis Rheum 1996; 39: 1125–1131.

96. Janowsky EC, Kupper LL, Hulka BS. Meta-analyses of the relation between silicone breast implants and the risk of connective-tissue diseases. N Engl J Med 2000; 342: 781–790

138 Etiology and pathogenesis

Kanneboyina Nagaraju, Paul H Plotz and Frederick W Miller

- The major pathologic findings of myositis consist of focal inflammation, with injury, death and repair of muscle cells (myocytes)
- Differences in the immunopathology of dermatomyositis (perivascular CD4+ T cells, B-cell infiltration, deposition of late complement components and capillary loss) and polymyositis and inclusion body myositis (activated CD8+ T cells and macrophage invasion of myocytes) may reflect different etiologies
- Myositis-specific autoantibodies, which target cytoplasmic molecules involved in protein synthesis, are associated with distinct clinical myositis subsets

INTRODUCTION

An understanding of the mechanisms that produce the clinical signs and symptoms of inflammatory muscle disease requires an understanding of the basic pathology seen in the tissues affected in these autoimmune disorders; the immune abnormalities found in these patients; and the possible environmental and genetic factors associated with the etiology of myositis.

PATHOLOGY

The diagnosis of myositis (inflammatory muscle disease) depends upon a combination of clinical, laboratory and pathologic findings[1]. Although it may seem superfluous to examine muscle tissue directly when everything else points to myositis, a muscle biopsy should be included early in the evaluation of all patients. Even in apparently typical cases another diagnosis may be revealed (see Chapter 141). Inclusion bodies, dystrophic or neuropathic features, amyloidosis, toxic changes, unusual cellular infiltrates, granulomas, arteritis or vacuoles suggesting a metabolic myopathy may be found. All of these findings have major therapeutic implications.

Nevertheless, a muscle biopsy in myositis is not always diagnostic. A non-diagnostic biopsy can be found for several reasons. First, inflammation is not uniformly distributed, either among whole muscle groups or within an individual muscle. It is important to pick an involved muscle (weak but not atrophic) to sample, but even within a weak muscle the damage may be spotty. Sometimes little or no inflammation is visible even if degenerating and regenerating myocytes are present in a section; this is especially a problem if the biopsy has been performed after the institution of therapy, as drug treatment can decrease the degree of inflammation. Second, the inclusions of inclusion body myositis are sometimes not present in a biopsy, so that an early clinical suspicion of the diagnosis may not be confirmed. It is unclear whether this is due to an uneven distribution of the changes or to the fact that they may merely appear later in the pathologic process. The first biopsy in which they appear and establish the diagnosis is usually the last to be performed in a patient, so the point cannot be settled now. Third, many of the changes found in typical cases of myositis are not pathognomonic but also occur in other disorders. For example, inflammation is found in some dystrophies. Fourth, some features characteristic of other disorders can be found in biopsies from typical cases of myositis. For example, small angulated fibers of neuropathic degeneration are sometimes found scattered in myositic muscle.

Muscle pathology

The central pathologic findings of myositis are the injury and death of muscle cells (myocytes) and inflammation. The consequences of the primary process are often evident too: regeneration and hypertrophy of muscle cells, atrophy of muscle cells, and the replacement of muscle by fibrosis and fat. No one of these features alone is diagnostic for myositis, but a combination of characteristics helps separate it from other conditions, and also may distinguish different types of myositis[2].

The pathologic findings are best seen in the hematoxylin and eosin and trichrome stains of an unfixed biopsy specimen taken from a muscle with straight fibers, snap frozen by immersion into isopentane cooled by liquid nitrogen, and then cut frozen after proper orientation. Additional useful information can come from specimens held on stretch by a clamp and then fixed in formalin for light microscopy and in glutaraldehyde for electron microscopy. A portion of the frozen material should be saved for immunologic, metabolic or viral studies. A number of features should be examined: the location of myocytes and cells, the type of inflammatory cells, the interior of individual myocytes.

Location of myocytes and cells

The location of the dying, atrophic and regenerating myocytes, both within the muscle bundle and in relation to one another, and the location of the inflammatory cells need to be established. When for any reason a muscle cell dies, a few inflammatory cells may be found adjacent to it. In myositis, clusters of inflammatory cells may be found not directly in relation to dying myocytes, but between unaffected myocytes (endomysium) and fascicles (perimysium) and surrounding vessels in the interstitial tissue nearby (perivascular) (Fig. 138.1). Furthermore, lymphocytes may be found *within* normal-looking myocytes. Perineural inflammation is not a feature of myositis. If there is abnormal skin overlying a muscle to be biopsied, a full-thickness biopsy should be taken to determine whether fasciitis rather than myositis is responsible for the clinical muscle involvement.

Type of inflammatory cells

Lymphocytes and macrophages predominate in polymyositis and dermatomyositis. A predominance of neutrophils or of eosinophils, or the presence of granulomas, points to another process. With immunologic techniques, the type of lymphocytes found at the various locations can be examined. At the moment, this information is more useful in understanding pathogenesis than in making a diagnosis (see later).

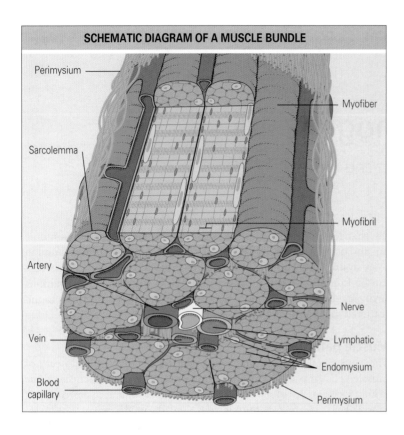

SCHEMATIC DIAGRAM OF A MUSCLE BUNDLE

Fig. 138.1 Schematic diagram of a muscle bundle (fascicle). Individual myofibers (muscle cells or myocytes) are each surrounded by an endomysial membrane. Groups of myocytes are arranged into a bundle or fascicle and surrounded by the perimysium. Muscle fascicles are arranged together as functional units surrounded by a membrane known as the epimysial membrane. The vascular bundle consists of the artery and vein supplying the muscle cells.

Interior of individual myocytes

Vacuoles and inclusions and other tinctorial properties of individual cells with certain stains help distinguish myositis from other entities. Irregular red-rimmed inclusions on the trichrome stain of a frozen specimen are characteristic of the important variant, inclusion body myositis. Recent immunologic studies have shown that the inclusions contain β-amyloid, ubiquitin, phosphorylated τ protein, apolipoprotein E and prion protein, but the role of these proteins in the pathogenesis of the illness has not yet been established[3]. Glycogen (stained red by periodic acid–Schiff (PAS)), fat (identified by the oil red O stain), abnormal mitochondria (the ragged red fiber on trichrome stain) and a variety of other inclusions found in syndromes that can mimic myositis will be revealed in a standard battery of histochemical stains.

High-resolution and special techniques

Because there are few ultrastructural changes specific for the diagnosis of idiopathic inflammatory myopathy, electron microscopy is rarely neces-

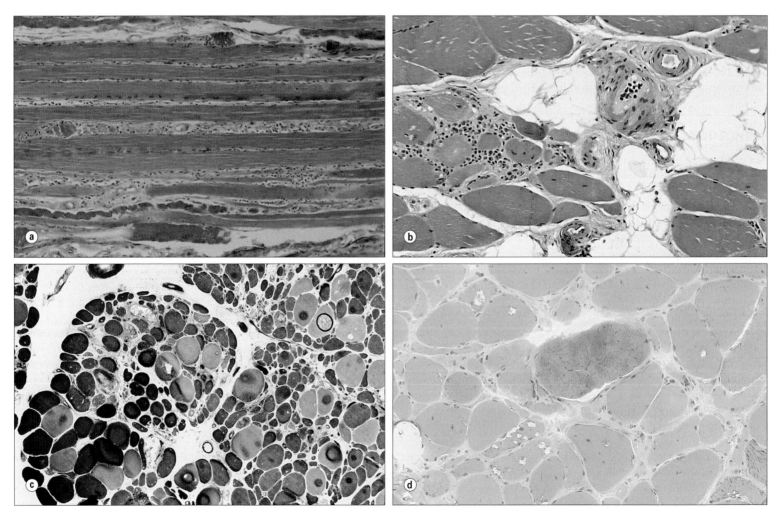

Fig. 138.2 Pathologic changes in myositis by light microscopy. Longitudinal and cross-sectional views of inflammatory myopathy showing variation in cell size, necrosis, regeneration and inflammation (hematoxylin and eosin) (a, b). Perifascicular atrophy in dematomyositis (ATPase) (c). Red-rimmed inclusions, marked cell size variation and relatively sparse inflammation in inclusion body myositis (trichrome) (d). (Courtesy of Dr J Nelson and Dr L Love.)

sary for assessing patients with clinical myositis. Characteristic 15–20 nm diameter nuclear and/or cytoplasmic filaments[4] are one of the proposed criteria for the diagnosis of inclusion body myositis, however, an electron microscopy of muscle should be considered in the evaluation of patients suspected of this diagnosis. The alkaline phosphatase stain is often positive in the interstitium of inflammatory myopathies, and is sometimes useful even if inflammation is not present. Special stains and enzyme assays for rare metabolic conditions are also available and are sometimes essential to avoid the mistake of treating a metabolic disease with immunosuppressive drugs.

Figure 138.2 illustrates myofiber degeneration and regeneration, endomysial and perimysial inflammation with lymphocytes and macrophages, fibrosis, atrophy of residual cells, perifascicular atrophy, perivascular inflammation and the inclusions of inclusion body myositis.

Inflammation is focal

The focal nature of muscle involvement in inflammatory muscle disease is clear clinically, as patients have weakness in only some muscle groups. The focality is both microscopic and macroscopic, and can be demonstrated in a number of ways. Figure 138.3 shows the focal involvement that can occur histologically. The discovery that magnetic resonance imaging (MRI) (see Chapter 141) can detect muscle damage and inflammation may improve the yield of biopsy diagnosis by directing the site of biopsy (Fig. 138.4a)[5]. The reasons for this heterogeneity of muscle involvement are unclear, but it is interesting that the same focal clinical and histologic findings are observed in various models of myositis, including several viral-induced murine models[6].

Sometimes a patient with substantial weakness and the clinical appearance and laboratory tests typical of inflammatory muscle disease will have a normal or near normal biopsy. Weakness then may be due, in part, to metabolic changes in muscle not visible at the resolution of light or even electron microscopy. The information available from magnetic resonance spectroscopy (MRS) may then contribute to understanding the pathogenesis of the weakness. Figure 138.4b illustrates the MRS findings in a normal thigh and in the thigh of a patient with inflammatory muscle disease. In the myositis patient there is a fall in the

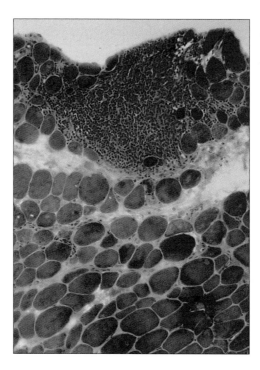

Fig. 138.3 Myositis is focal microscopically. Muscle biopsy showing focal inflammation. (Courtesy of Dr L Love.)

ratio of phosphocreatine to inorganic phosphate, reflecting an abnormality in energy metabolism within the muscle tissue. Whether or not this change can occur in individual cells which are histologically normal, or reflects only changes from visibly damaged cells, is not now known.

Pathologic changes in other organs

Although the clinical picture of dermatomyositis, interstitial lung disease, myocarditis or gastrointestinal disease is usually distinctive enough to make biopsy superfluous, unusual rashes or pulmonary processes may require pathologic study, for example to rule out infection. It is therefore important to recognize the findings that can be attributed to the disease itself (Table 138.1).

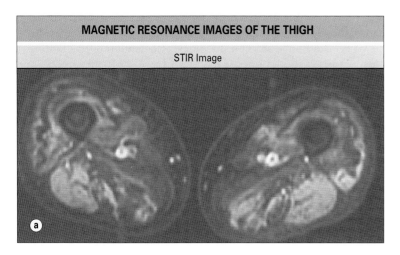

MAGNETIC RESONANCE IMAGES OF THE THIGH

STIR Image

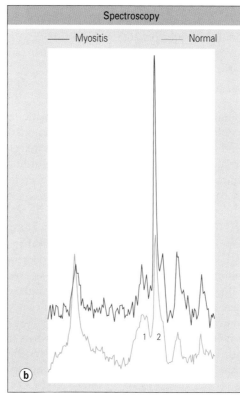

Spectroscopy

Myositis —— Normal

Fig. 138.4 Magnetic resonance images of the thigh. In cross-section using the short tau inversion recover (STIR) technique, atrophy of the anterior muscles is evident. Inflammation shows up as bright areas in the posterior muscles (a). Magnetic resonance spectroscopy of the thigh muscles of a normal person and a patient with myositis. The ratio of the areas under the phosphocreatine (2) and inorganic phosphate (1) peaks is less in the patient with myositis, reflecting abnormal intracellular phosphate metabolism (b). Courtesy of Dr J Frank and Dr D Fraser.

TABLE 138.1 AFFECTED ORGANS AND THEIR EVALUATION IN INFLAMMATORY MUSCLE DISEASE			
Organ system	Modalities of evaluation	Pathologic processes	Findings
Muscle	Biopsy	Myofiber degeneration–regeneration	Myofiber size variation
		Inflammation	Mononuclear cell infiltration
		Fibrosis	Increased interstitium and fatty replacement of muscle
	EMG	Myofiber destruction	Low-amplitude, short, polyphasic potential; spontaneous fibrillations; irritability
	Gallium scan	Inflammation	Increased uptake in affected muscle
	MRI		
	T1 image	Fibrosis	Atrophy of muscle, scarring
	STIR image	Inflammation	Bright signal in inflamed muscle
Heart	ECG, CXR	Myocarditis, fibrosis	Arrhythmias, left ventricular hypertrophy
	Biopsy	Myocarditis, fibrosis	Myofiber size variation, mononuclear cell infiltrates, fibrosis
Lungs	CXR	Inflammation, fibrosis	Interstitial markings
	PFTs	Inflammation, fibrosis	Decreased TLV and $D_{L}CO$
	Radionuclide scan	Inflammation, fibrosis	Ventilation/perfusion mismatches
	BAL	Inflammation, fibrosis	Abnormal leukocyte numbers and differentials
	Biopsy	Inflammation, fibrosis	Mononuclear cell infiltration, destruction of alveolar space and fibrosis
Skin	Biopsy	Inflammation	Vacuolization of the basal layer; mononuclear cell infiltration
Gastrointestinal	Radiographic studies	Inflammation, fibrosis	Reflux and uncoordinated peristalsis

BAL, bronchoalveolar lavage; CXR, chest radiograph; $D_{L}CO$, carbon monoxide diffusion; ECG, electrocardiogram; EMG, electromyogram; PFT, pulmonary function test; TLV, total lung volume.

Skin

In the involved skin of dermatomyositis patients, the non-specific findings of basal layer vacuolopathy, PAS-positive basement membrane thickening, mild mucin deposition and diffuse inflammation are often seen (Fig. 138.5a). Additionally, hyperplasia of the epidermis with acanthosis or papillomatosis, when seen with the above features, may be diagnostic of Gottron's lesions. In an uncommon variant, mucinous deposits predominate. A finding in some patients, especially those with severe juvenile dermatomyositis, is cutaneous calcinosis, which can result in painful or secondarily infected lesions.

Cardiac involvement

Cardiac involvement is common but often clinically asymptomatic in these patients[7]. Both arrhythmias and congestive failure presumed secondary to myocarditis and subsequent fibrosis can be seen, as well as occasional cor pulmonale related to interstitial lung disease. Myocarditis is also a focal process and shows the same pathologic changes as seen in the skeletal muscles of these patients (Figs 138.5b,c).

Pulmonary involvement

In the lung, several different processes may occur, none absolutely diagnostic of myositis. Atelectasis secondary to respiratory muscle weakness is probably the most common and most benign finding. More serious pulmonary pathology results from infectious pneumonitis secondary either to aspiration in patients with dysphagia or to immunodeficiency in those patients on immunosuppressive therapies. The most ominous pulmonary complication is interstitial lung disease, which, when it occurs in association with myositis, is clinically, radiographically and pathologically indistinguishable from the idiopathic variety (Figs 138.5d–f)[8].

Gastrointestinal

Gastrointestinal disease is a common problem in myositis patients, especially at the oropharyngeal, esophageal and gastric levels. Again, the clinical and pathologic findings are neither specific nor treated differently from the dysphagia, abdominal bloating and other symptoms associated with other chronic inflammatory diseases of the gastrointestinal tract. Rarely, the sudden appearance of free peritoneal air and air in the wall of the bowel can mimic an acute abdomen. Recognition of this finding – pneumatosis cystoides intestinalis – can spare a patient unnecessary surgery.

PATHOGENESIS

Unquestionably, study of the pathogenesis of idiopathic inflammatory myopathy must center upon the immunologic abnormalities[9]. There are two principal reasons for this. First, this family of diseases is among those properly designated as autoimmune because of the presence of autoantibodies in the serum of many patients, including some that are specific to myositis[10]. Second, the pathologic processes seen by light microscopy and the alterations of other parameters of immune function implicate the cellular and humoral immune systems[11]. The response to therapy directed at the immune system may be invoked to support an immune pathogenesis, but we know too little of the actions of the anti-inflammatory and cytotoxic drugs to weigh that evidence heavily. Table 138.2 describes the major immunologic abnormalities found in myositis patients.

Cellular immunity

Direct examination of biopsy specimens by immunologic techniques illustrates the role of both the cellular and humoral immune systems in

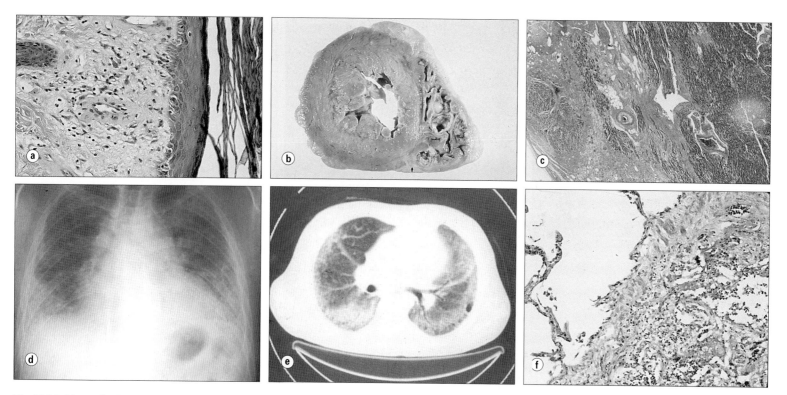

Fig. 138.5 Biopsy findings in extraskeletal muscle. Skin biopsy of a Gottron's lesion in a patient with dermatomyositis. The biopsy demonstrates hyperkeratosis, epidermal thinning, vacuolar degeneration of the basal layer, dilated superficial capillaries with perivascular lymphohistiocytic infiltrates and mild mucin deposition in the dermis. (Courtesy of Dr Maria Turner) (a). Gross autopsy specimen from the heart of a patient with myositis who died from myocarditis showing dilated left ventricle and fibrosis (b). Microscopic sections of the heart shown in (b), demonstrating extensive replacement of the myocardioum with fibrotic tissue (c). The lung in a patient with myositis: standard chest radiograph (d) and CT scan (e) showing typical findings of interstitial lung disease. Microscopic section showing the destructive alveolar changes associated with pulmonary fibrosis and inflammation (f). Courtesy of Dr L Love.

TABLE 138.2 IMMUNOLOGIC ABNORMALITIES IN PATIENTS WITH INFLAMMATORY MYOPATHIES	
Cellular abnormalities	T-cell receptor restriction in inflamed muscle
	Activated T and B lymphocytes expressing co-stimulatory molecules, CD86/CD80; CD28/CTLA4; CD40/CD40L in skeletal muscle
	Increased peripheral mononuclear cell trafficking to muscle
	Increased proportions of peripheral T and B lymphocytes bearing activation markers
	Elevated serum IL-1α, IL-2, soluble IL-2 receptors and soluble CD8 receptors
	Decreased proliferative responses of peripheral mononuclear cells to T-cell mitogens
	Increased proliferative responses of peripheral mononuclear cells to autologous muscle
	Increased expression of cytokines and chemokines in infiltrating mononuclear cells and muscle cells
	Increased MHC class I (HLA-ABC), class II (HLA-DR) and ICAM-1 on skeletal muscle fibers
Humoral abnormalities	Immunoglobulin and complement deposition in muscle vascular endothelium
	Myositis-specific autoantibodies
	Myositis-associated autoantibodies (anti-U1RNP, anti-PM/Scl, anti-Ku)
	Other-autoantibodies (antithyroid, anti-Sm, anti-Ro, anti-La, etc.)
	Hyper-, hypo- and agammaglobulinemia
	Monoclonal gammopathy

muscle damage. The differences between the immunopathologic findings in dermatomyositis, on the one hand, and polymyositis and inclusion body myositis on the other, are of interest and importance in underlining the clinical distinctions among these three groups and may reflect different etiologies.

In idiopathic inflammatory myopathy biopsies there is a tendency for different lymphocytes to accumulate in different regions of the muscle and therefore for several gradients of cell type to be seen[12]. In the perivascular regions there is a predominance of B cells, which decrease in number in the perimysial zone and are least frequent in endomysial sites. Conversely, T cells are most numerous in the endomysial areas and least often found in the perivascular zones. Macrophages seem to be about equally present in all three zones. Different clinical groups, however, show interesting differences in the distribution of lymphocyte subpopulations.

In dermatomyositis B cells are relatively abundant, especially in perivascular regions (Fig. 138.6a). The late components of complement (C5–C9, the membrane attack complex) are found in perivascular areas and within damaged intrafascicular capillaries (Fig. 138.6b)[13]. There are also activated endomysial T cells which are mostly cytotoxic (CD8+). In the perimysial and perivascular regions there is a rising proportion of helper/suppressor (CD4+) T cells. Damage to and dropout of intrafascicular capillaries occurs even before other tissue damage is evident[14].

By contrast, in both polymyositis and inclusion body myositis individual muscle cells which appear otherwise normal may be invaded by T-cytotoxic (Tc) cells, of which a proportion are activated (DR+). The dominant T cells in the inflammatory infiltrate nearby are also CD8+ (Fig. 138.6c). Ultrastructural examination shows that the muscle fibers are honeycombed by cavities filled with both invading macrophages and

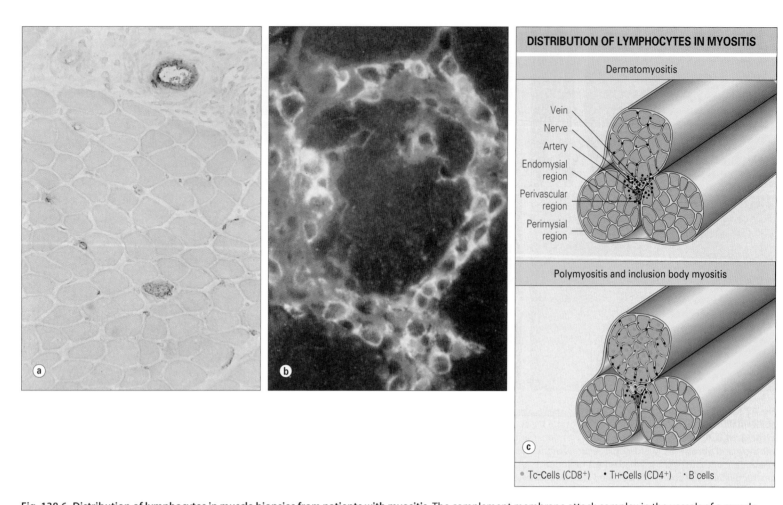

Fig. 138.6 Distribution of lymphocytes in muscle biopsies from patients with myositis. The complement membrane attack complex in the vessels of a muscle from a patient with dermatomyositis. Courtesy of Dr J T Kissel (a). Lymphocytes invading an apparently normal myocyte in a patient with myositis. Double immunofluorescent staining with anti-CD8 (green) and anti-DR (red) antisera. Courtesy of Dr Andrew Engel (b). Distribution of CD4+ and CD8+ lymphocytes in different clinical forms of myositis. Inflammation in dermatomyositis consists predominantly of perivascular B and CD4+ T-cells, and in polymyositis and inclusion body myositis it is mostly endomysial CD8+ T-cells (c). Tc, cytotoxic T cells; TH, helper T cells.

CD8+ cells sending spike-like extensions into the myocytes[15]. In the perimysium and perivascular region the proportion of T-helper (Th) cells rises, but in contrast to dermatomyositis, B cells are not abundant in the lesions. Infiltrating mononuclear cells in both PM and DM show increased expression of costimulatory receptors and ligands such as B7.1, B7.2, CD40, CTLA-4, CD28 and CD40L, suggesting that active interactions among immune cells contribute to the perpetuation of immune inflammation in myositis[16–18]. Natural killer (NK) cells are very uncommon in all three diseases.

Serologic and molecular studies show restricted α-β T-cell receptor (TCR) use by muscle-infiltrating cells. This finding suggests that subpopulations of T cells are selected and expanded in response to as yet uncharacterized antigens, and may explain some of the T cell-mediated pathology seen in these diseases[19]. Different clinical forms of the disease show differences in TCR patterns. In polymyositis and inclusion body myositis oligoclonal patterns of TCR use predominate, whereas in dermatomyositis polyclonal TCR patterns are seen more often.

It is still not possible to determine how much of the inflammatory infiltrate is secondary to muscle cell damage. The inflammation in Duchenne's muscular dystrophy (DMD), though qualitatively similar to that in myositis, is far more sparse, and fewer non-necrotic myofibers are invaded by mononuclear cells. However, there is evidence for both selective T-cell receptor rearrangements and upregulation of inflammatory cell adhesion molecules in DMD[20,21]. In fascioscapulohumeral dys-

trophy, in which inflammation may be significant, mononuclear cells may play a role in muscle damage, but a direct T-cell cytotoxicity appears unlikely[22]. In muscle damaged by excessive exercise, sparse to moderate endomysial and perimysial inflammation occurs, with both macrophages and T cells, but CD4+ cells are the most abundant type[23].

Increased major histocompatibility complex (MHC) class I antigen expression occurs on some necrotic, some non-necrotic, and all regenerating myocytes in a number of diseases, including polymyositis, dermatomyositis and DMD[24]. In myositis, even histologically unaffected cells also have MHC class I on their surface, suggesting that this may be an early event in the pathogenesis of the inflammation. To investigate the role of MHC class I in muscle disease, a conditional transgenic mouse model was recently developed[25]. Overexpression of syngenic MHC class I (H-2K^b) in skeletal muscle led to several features of myositis. The disease is inflammatory, limited to skeletal muscle, self-sustaining, more severe in females, and often accompanied by autoantibodies. The muscle fiber damage appears to occur even in the absence of heavy lymphocyte accumulations. Upregulation of MHC class I in the muscle leads to decreased muscle strength at a very early stage, even before any detectable histological damage in the skeletal muscle of these mice[25]. Similarly, some myositis patients show no detectable inflammatory infiltrate in the muscle biopsy. These patients show increased MHC class I expression on muscle fibers and increased IL-1α expression on capillary endothelial cells, suggesting a potential pathogenic role for these molecules in myositis even in the absence of detectable lymphocyte infiltrates[26,27]. Increased expression of non-classic MHC class I antigen, HLA-G in muscle fibers of various inflammatory myopathies has recently been shown[28]. Although understanding the implications of non-classic MHC class I expression in the pathogenesis of myositis requires further investigation, the distribution of these antigens closely resembles that of classic HLA-A,-B,-C antigens in muscle fibers, infiltrating mononuclear cells and capillaries.

The circulating lymphocytes in patients with active myositis demonstrate many phenotypic abnormalities[29]. Compared to controls, these patients have decreased proportions of cells expressing CD8, but increased proportions of T and B lymphocytes expressing MHC class II antigens (DR). Myositis patients' peripheral lymphocytes also have higher expression of interleukin-2 (IL-2) receptors, and the late T-cell activation markers CD26, a marker of anamnestic responses, and TLiSA1, a marker for cytotoxic differentiation.

As is the case for the quantification of subsets of lymphocytes in the affected muscle, analysis of peripheral mononuclear cells shows that polymyositis and inclusion body myositis are virtually indistinguishable, but differ from dermatomyositis. Dermatomyositis patients have decreased proportions of CD3+DR+ and TLiSA1+ cells, and increased proportions of CD20+ and CD20+DR+ cells compared with patients in the other two groups. Together with the muscle biopsy data, these findings suggest that different mechanisms of systemic immune activation and immunopathology are present in different groups of myositis patients segregated by clinical diagnosis.

Markers of mononuclear cell activation, IL-2 and soluble IL-2 receptors, soluble CD4 and CD8, and IL-1α are also elevated in patients with active myositis and may be useful as indicators of disease activity[30,31].

The factors responsible for attracting inflammatory cells to muscle remain unclear. Abnormal phenotypic changes, including thickening of endothelium in venules and capillaries, are described not only in PM but also in DM and IBM. Capillary endothelial cells in the muscle biopsies express intercellular adhesion molecule (ICAM)-1 and vascular cellular adhesion molecule (VCAM)-1[27]. The ligands of ICAM-1 (leukocyte function-associated molecule, LFA-1α) and VCAM-1 (very-late activating antigen, VLA-4) are also expressed on mononuclear cells, suggesting that ICAM-1/LFA-1α and VCAM-1/VLA-4 pathways are active in recruiting lymphocytes to the inflamed muscle[27,32]. There is evidence for the upregulation of ICAM-1 on both the invading inflammatory cells and the muscle cells in myositis, even on cells that are histologically normal[21,33].

Several pro- and anti-inflammatory cytokines (IL-1α, IL-1β, TNF-α, TGF-β, IFN-γ, IL-2, IL-4, IL-6, IL-10, IL-13 and lymphotoxin) and chemokines (MIP-1α, MIP-1β, MCP-1 and RANTES) may be found in muscle biopsies of myositis patients[34-37]. The majority of these cytokines and chemokines were detected on the infiltrating mononuclear cells, and sometimes on muscle cells and blood vessels. The exact role of cytokines and chemokines in the pathophysiology of myositis remains to be investigated. Recently, it has been shown that the pro-inflammatory cytokine TNF, apart from inducing cell death, can also activate NF-κB, which in turn downregulates Myo-D, a transcription factor critical for the formation of new muscle fibers. Therefore, proinflammatory cytokines such as TNF can cause severe loss in skeletal muscle mass by preventing the formation of new fibers and damaging the existing muscle fibers[38]. The wide variety of cytokines and chemokines in the muscle microenvironment reflects the ongoing immune response, inflammation, cell damage and repair mechanisms in the tissue.

A group of calcium-dependent zinc endoproteinases called matrix metalloproteinases (MMPs) have recently been described in myositis biopsies[39,40]. The proteolytic activity of MMPs is tightly controlled by tissue inhibitors of metalloproteinases (TIMPs). MMPs are involved in the remodelling of the extracellular matrix, and the excess production of these enzymes will lead to degradation, tissue destruction and cell invasion. Excess production of TIMPs leads to fibrosis.

The role of myocytes in initiating the autoimmune response in myositis is not clear. In these diseases myocytes express various cell surface (MHC class I, MHC class II (HLA-DR), ICAM-1, and CD40) and soluble (cytokines and chemokines) molecules involved in antigen presentation. None the less, even in proinflammatory conditions skeletal muscle cells do not express traditional co-stimulatory molecules (CD80/CD86)[16,41]. Therefore, muscle cells may not be very efficient in activating resting naïve T cells. Myocytes may effectively stimulate memory lymphocytes even in the absence of co-stimulatory molecules, and in fact myositis biopsies show increased levels of memory lymphocytes[42], suggesting that muscle cells may be involved in maintaining the autoimmune response by activating memory T cells. On the other hand, infiltrating mononuclear cells may express both MHC and co-stimulatory molecules, suggesting that antigen-presenting cells (dendritic cells) capable of stimulating resting naïve T cells are present locally[16-18]. The muscle microenvironment (e.g. CD40L, GM-CSF) is favorable for the maturation of dendritic cells, and these cells may cross-prime and cross-present muscle autoantigens to resting naïve T cells to initiate the autoimmune response in myositis[43].

Despite the compelling evidence that lymphocytes are involved in the pathogenesis of myositis, their precise role remains to be understood. In dermatomyositis, the early damage to and obliteration of capillaries, antedating muscle weakness, strongly suggests that this vascular injury may be responsible for the later damage to the muscles. Furthermore, the localization of the membrane attack complex of complement to the damaged vessels and the increased proportion of activated B cells peripherally and in the target tissue, suggests that a humoral immune response is involved in the process. So far, however, no humoral antibodies specific to patients with early vascular damage, or even specific to all dermatomyositis patients, have been found. Although the invasion of normal muscle cells by T cells and macrophages does raise the possibility that there are lymphocytes specifically sensitized to muscle cells, data regarding the capacity of lymphocytes to be stimulated by muscle extracts are sparse and not convincing. Although some studies suggest clonal restrictions by muscle-infiltrating T cells in myositis[19], it is not clear that these are due to a primary antigen-driven mechanism or other secondary process[20].

Humoral immunity

Patients with inflammatory muscle disease of any category may have autoantibodies. Not surprisingly, these are most common in patients with an associated connective tissue disease, and least common in those with inclusion body myositis or a cancer-associated myositis. If the analysis is limited to rheumatoid factor, antinuclear antibodies and antibodies to extractable nuclear antigens, there are no significant associations with any particular clinical or pathologic picture. The recent discovery of a family of autoantibodies that appear almost exclusively in patients with myositis (myositis-specific autoantibodies, MSA) has led to a deeper analysis of humoral autoimmunity in this clinically heterogeneous family of diseases[44].

Several outstanding features characterize the MSAs recognized so far. First, they are directed at cell components – proteins and ribonucleoproteins – common to every cell. Second, they are directed at intracellular, usually intracytoplasmic, molecules which are not thought to be expressed on the cell surface. Third, the target molecules (autoantigens) are usually part of the protein synthetic machinery (Fig. 138.7).

In common with many other autoantibodies, MSAs are usually present when the patient first visits the physician, even if that visit is within days of the onset of symptoms, and in at least one case they have been documented to antedate the clinical illness[45]. Also, although they

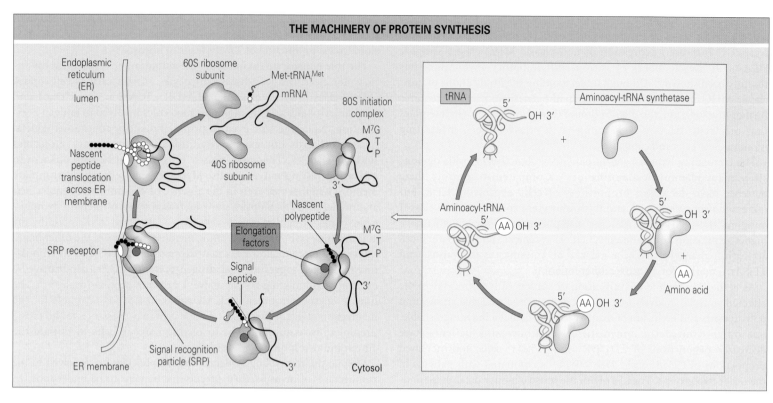

THE MACHINERY OF PROTEIN SYNTHESIS

Fig. 138.7 The machinery of protein synthesis showing some of the targets of myositis-specific autoantibodies.

appear to bind preferentially to the human target autoantigen, they are directed against regions of the molecules which are conserved among species, often quite distant species; and they are apparently directed against the functional site of the molecule, in the sense that they often inhibit the molecule's or particle's recognized function.

Most MSAs are directed at intracytoplasmic components, and thus they are not 'antinuclear' antibodies; a diffuse cytoplasmic staining of target cells is apparent with sera from patients with some MSA. Some patients have both true antinuclear and anticytoplasmic antibodies (Fig. 138.8a). The further analysis of such sera depends upon immuno-diffusion, with a search for lines of identity with well-characterized anti-sera or with the techniques of ribonucleic acid (RNA) and protein immunoprecipitation. Because many of the target antigens are ribo-nucleoproteins (molecular complexes of one or more proteins with one or more molecules of RNA) immunoprecipitation of cytoplasmic extracts and analysis of the precipitated RNA offers the fastest route to a correct characterization of most MSAs (Fig. 138.8b; see also Chapters 20 and 21).

The fact that the target autoantigens of these disease-specific auto-antibodies are both intracellular and common to all cells means that they are unlikely to be the primary pathogenetic agents of muscle damage. If they are agents of muscle cell damage at all, then one must either account for their entry into muscle and not other cells, or explain an event which places the target antigen on a muscle cell surface or other location where the antibody can reach it. For this reason, it is generally hypothesized that these autoantibodies are the footprints of another event, such as a prior viral infection of muscle cells. In this scenario, the infection or other event causes the myositis and also causes the autoantibody synthesis, although the autoantibodies themselves do not participate in damage to the muscles. Considerable research in this area involves a careful analysis of the autoantibody response in the hope that it will yield a clue to the primary agent of muscle cell damage. Recent structural studies of the most common autoantigenic target in myositis, histidyl-tRNA synthetase (Jo-1), have demonstrated that the dominant epitope is a region at the amino terminal end of the molecule whose structure appears to be a pair of side-by-side α helices, the function of which is still unknown[46].

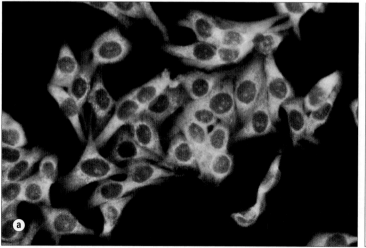

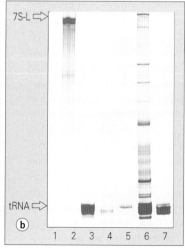

Fig. 138.8 Laboratory demonstration of myositis-specific autoantibodies. Cytoplasmic staining of cultured human cells by immunofluorescence using serum from a patient with antiglycyl-tRNA synthetase antibodies. Courtesy of D. Gracey (a). Immunoprecipitation of cell extract by sera from patients with some myositis-specific autoantibodies. Only the RNA of the protein-RNA immunoprecipitate is shown. 1: normal; 2: anti-SRP; 3: antithreonyl-tRNA synthetase (PL-7); 4: antihistidyl-tRNA synthetase (Jo-1); 5: anti-isoleucyl-tRNA synthetase (OJ), 6: anti-alanyl-tRNA synthetase (PL-12), accompanied by anti-Ro, anti-La and anti-RNP; 7: antiglycyl-tRNA synthetase (EJ). Courtesy of Dr S Cochran (b).

TABLE 138.3 MYOSITIS-SPECIFIC AUTOANTIBODIES AND THEIR ASSOCIATED DISEASE FEATURES

Autoantibody	Autoantigen	Prevalence in IIM (%)	Clinical associations
Antisynthetases			
Anti-Jo-1	HisRS	15–40	Antisynthetase syndrome*
Anti-PL-7	ThrRS	< 5	Antisynthetase syndrome
Anti-PL-12 (1)	AlaRS	< 5	Antisynthetase syndrome
Anti-PL-12 (2)	tRNA-Ala	< 5	Antisynthetase syndrome
Anti-OJ	IleRS	< 5	Antisynthetase syndrome
Anti-EJ	GlyRS	< 5	Antisynthetase syndrome
Anti-SRP	SRP proteins	< 5	Acute, severe polymyositis
Anti-FER	EF1α	< 1	?
Anti-KJ	Unidentified protein	< 1	Interstitial lung disease
Anti-Mi-2	Nuclear helicase	<10	Classic dermatomyositis

* Antisynthetase syndrome is interstitial lung disease, fever, arthritis, Raynaud's phenomenon and 'mechanic's' hands. HisRS/ThrRS/AlaRS/IleRS/GlyRS, histidyl-, threonyl-, alanyl-, isoleucyl- and glycyl-tRNA synthetase respectively; EF1, elongation factor 1; IIM, idiopathic inflammatory myopathy; SRP, signal recognition particle.

For the clinician, and for the clinical investigator exploring new therapies for myositis, the MSAs have another importance. Each of them appears to be connected to a particular *clinical* syndrome, with a group of common clinical features, a predominant human leukocyte antigen (HLA) type, a characteristic onset, and probably a characteristic response to therapy (Table 138.3)[47]. The first hint of this was the recognition that patients with the most commonly recognized MSA, anti-Jo-1, frequently have interstitial lung disease. The target Jo-1 autoantigen is the enzyme histidyl-tRNA synthetase, which joins the tRNA molecules for histidine to the amino acid itself so that it can be incorporated into protein. A startling discovery was that there are a few patients (probably about 5–10% of all myositis patients) who have antibodies to another enzyme of this family (asparaginyl-, glycyl-, threonyl-, isoleucyl- or alanyl-tRNA synthetase), and in addition they usually have interstitial lung disease[47–49]. These same patients also often have fevers, arthritis, Raynaud's phenomenon, and a roughened surface of the lateral and palmar surfaces of their index fingers, termed 'mechanic's hands'. Some of these patients have one of the rashes typical of dermatomyositis, most have HLA-DR3, and almost all have the HLA-DRw52 alloantigen. They often have a rapid onset and an aggressive course, and although they may respond to treatment with corticosteroids they most often require cytotoxic therapy later as corticosteroids are tapered.

A second group of patients has antibodies to Mi-2, (a DNA-dependent nucleosome-stimulated ATPase involved in nucleosome remodeling and histone deacetylase activation) and they almost all have a variant of dermatomyositis, with a rash on the upper chest and back[50,51]. Their HLA type is often DR7, and they respond relatively well to therapy. Recently, PMS1, a DNA mismatch repair enzyme, was identified as a myositis-specific autoantigen. Sera recognizing PMS1 also recognized several other proteins involved in DNA repair and remodeling, including poly (ADP-ribose) polymerase, DNA-dependent protein kinase and Mi-2[52]. The rare patient with antibodies to the intracellular signal recognition particle (SRP) almost always has an extremely rapid and severe disease onset and little extramuscular disease[53]. There are patients with autoantibodies to other cytoplasmic proteins, but the clinical illnesses and the target autoantigens have not yet been so well defined[54]. Nevertheless, the observations in patients with MSAs strongly hint that each of them will form a coherent clinical and immunogenetic group, and that each of these groups may come to be recognized as, in effect, a separate disease – either as a result of a different environmental agent (infection or toxin) for each, or as a result of the same agent having a different effect, depending on the genetic make-up of the individual (Fig. 138.9).

The immunopathogenetic picture of inflammatory muscle disease is thus composed of several elements whose relationship is not currently understood. Patients with dermatomyositis appear to have a primary disease of the small blood vessels of muscle, possibly involving antibodies, as judged by the presence of B cells, Th cells and the late complement components in or near the vessels of affected muscle. Some patients with dermatomyositis have a myositis-specific autoantibody, and some do not. Conversely, the patients with each of the MSAs seem to fall into clinical and genetic groups, but the presence of a dermatomyositis rash, which so clearly marks the histologic events, does not correlate well with the occurrence of particular MSAs. The convergence of studies from these different directions, and from the new direction of identifying the different genetic and environmental risk factors in different subsets of myositis patients, is likely to define groups of patients more clearly[55,56]. In turn, this will focus studies of etiology, therapy and possibly prevention.

Apoptosis

Several groups have investigated apoptotic mechanisms in myositis biopsies and could not detect characteristic apoptotic changes in muscle cells despite the presence of both Fas and Fas ligand in the biopsies. The apparent resistance of muscle cells to apoptosis could be explained by the presence of several antiapoptotic molecules (Fas-associated death domain-like IL-1 converting enzyme-inhibitory protein (FLIP), IAP (inhibitor of apoptosis)-like protein (hILP), Bcl-2, Bcl-XL and cyclin-dependent kinase inhibitory proteins (CdkIs p16 and p57)) in both muscle cells and infiltrating mononuclear cells in myositis biopsies[57–59]. These molecules negatively regulate apoptosis execution by interfering with the caspase machinery which is required for the apoptotic process. Despite the expression of various antiapoptotic molecules, skeletal muscle death and damage occurs in myositis patients, suggesting that alternative mechanisms, such as the granzyme/perforin pathway, may be major players in muscle cell death. In fact, perforin-expressing CD4$^+$ and CD8$^+$ T cells have been shown in the muscle biopsies of both DM and PM patients. Around 43% of CD8$^+$ T cells that contacted a muscle fiber in PM patients showed perforin located vectorially towards the target muscle fiber, suggesting that this pathway may be involved in muscle fiber injury[60].

ETIOLOGY

Infectious agents, drugs and toxins all claim attention as etiologic agents in inflammatory muscle disease (Table 138.4) and, as noted above, there is reason to suppose that the genetic background of the individual may

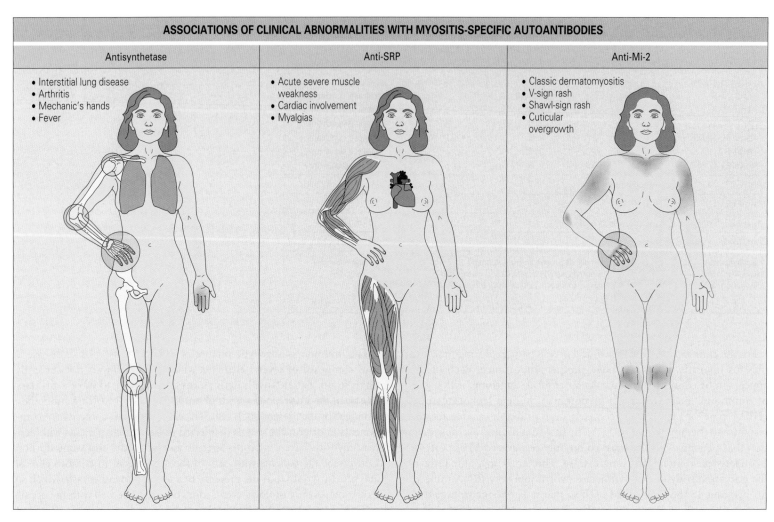

ASSOCIATIONS OF CLINICAL ABNORMALITIES WITH MYOSITIS-SPECIFIC AUTOANTIBODIES

Antisynthetase	Anti-SRP	Anti-Mi-2
• Interstitial lung disease • Arthritis • Mechanic's hands • Fever	• Acute severe muscle weakness • Cardiac involvement • Myalgias	• Classic dermatomyositis • V-sign rash • Shawl-sign rash • Cuticular overgrowth

Fig. 138.9 The anatomic distribution of clinical abnormalities in some groups of patients with myositis.

be important in determining whether a particular agent causes myositis in that person. These claims are based upon direct clinical observation, experimental studies and disease models.

Microchimerism

Chimeric cells of fetal origin have been identified in some autoimmune diseases and these cells have been implicated in their pathogenesis[61,62]. Some patients with graft-versus-host disease develop myositis with cytotoxic T cells around blood vessels and muscle fibers[63]. Recent studies have demonstrated maternal microchimerism in the peripheral circulation and in inflammatory lesions (skin and muscle biopsy samples) of juvenile myositis patients, suggesting a possible role for these cells in the disease process[64,65].

Infectious agents

Bacteria can invade muscle and cause an acute syndrome, with the typical features of an abscess elsewhere. The organism is most often *Staphylococcus aureus*, and the setting is usually the limb of an injured or immunocompromised patient. There is no reason to suppose that this kind of infection is a precursor of dermatomyositis and/or polymyositis or inclusion body myositis. Similarly, a number of parasites directly invade muscle and cause a usually localized myositis. In its acute stages trichinosis, formerly a reasonably common illness in the US, may transiently resemble dermatomyositis and/or polymyositis, but clinical, laboratory and histologic features separate these diseases. There is no connection between the parasitic disease and a later myositis. The same may be said of a number of

other parasites that occasionally invade muscle. The exceptions are *Toxoplasmosis gondii* and *Borrelia burgdorferi*. Although the organisms cannot be cultured from muscle and are not found histologically in the tissues of idiopathic myositis patients, some patients have elevated titers of antibodies against these organisms[66,67]. The reason for this is unknown, but as some patients with myositis do give a history of an antecedent acute inflammatory illness, it remains possible that at least some cases of dermatomyositis and/or polymyositis will prove to be a late consequence of toxoplasma or borrelia infection.

Viral myositis is a well-defined entity for at least three viruses – influenza, coxsackie and echo – and there are individual reports of cases apparently associated with other viruses. The myositis associated with acute influenza and coxsackie infection is well known, usually occurs in children, and is generally self-limited. It is rare in adults. There is a chronic echovirus syndrome closely resembling dermatomyositis that occurs in boys with X-linked agammaglobulinemia, although the virus has rarely been found in the clinically affected muscles[68].

There are, in addition, several reasons to connect viral infection with the idiopathic inflammatory myopathies, dermatomyositis and polymyositis. First, in small and imperfectly controlled observations, some children and adults with idiopathic myositis have been shown to have high titers of antibodies directed against some coxsackie viruses in the early stages of their illness[69,70]. Second, particles resembling picornaviruses have been occasionally observed by ultrastructural examination of myositic muscle[71], although the identity of these is not clearly viral. Third, several less well known picornaviruses (encephalo-

TABLE 138.4 POSSIBLE ETIOLOGIC FACTORS IN ACQUIRED MYOPATHY/MYOSITIS		
Factor	Examples	Comments
Drugs and toxins		
	Cimetidine	
	Chloroquine	Vacuolar myopathy
	Colchicine	Vacuolar myopathy
	Corticosteroids	Type II fiber atrophy
	Emetine	
	Ethanol	Acute rhabdomyolysis and chronic myopathy
	Heroin	
	Penicillamine	Typical polymyositis Mitochondrial myopathy
	Fibrates and statins	Cases of polymyositis, rhabdomyolysis and non-inflammatory myopathies reported
	Zidovudine (AZT) (Many others reported at the case level)	
Infectious agents		
Bacteria	Staphylococci	Most common cause of pyomyositis
	Clostridia	
	Rickettsias	
	Mycobacteria	
Parasites	*Toxoplasma*	
	Trichinella	
	Schistosoma	
	Cysticerca	
	Sarcocystis	
	Trypanosoma	
	Borrelia	
Viruses	Coxsackievirus	Serologic association with juvenile dermatomyositis
	Echovirus	Associated with hypogammaglobulinemia
	Influenza	
	Adenovirus	Cultured from an inclusion body myositis muscle biopsy
	Mumps	
	Hepatitis B	
	HIV	AIDS patients can present with polymyositis
	HTLV-1	High anti-HTLV-1 antibodies in Jamaican myositis patients
Genetic factors		
	HLA DRB1*0301	Other HLA alleles associated with certain myositis-specific autoantibodies and other ethnic groups. Rare familial cases. Other genes probably important
	HLA DQA1*0501	
	TNF2 (−308A)	
	IL1RN A1	

adenovirus was isolated from one case of inclusion body myositis[73]. Mumps virus-specific antisera stained the muscle biopsies from several patients with this disease, but nucleic acid hybridization studies for mumps virus RNA have been negative[74]. Finally, retroviruses, including human immunodeficiency virus (HIV) and human T-cell leukemia/lymphoma virus (HTLV-1), have been associated with myositis in animals[75], individual patients[76] and population studies[77]. However, a highly sensitive search for all of these candidate viruses in the muscle biopsies from patients with myositis failed to demonstrate persistent viral nucleic acid, thereby ruling out continuing viral infection as a cause of the ongoing inflammation[78].

Thus, only circumstantial and indirect evidence points to an infectious initiation of some cases of dermatomyositis and/or polymyositis and inclusion body myositis. Nevertheless, the limited studies to date, and the important implications if infectious agents can be identified as triggers, support the need for further studies in this area of research.

Drugs, toxins and other agents

The list of drugs that can cause an illness that mimics myositis is long[79,80]. In some cases the histology – a vacuolar myopathy for colchicine, a mitochondrial myopathy for AZT – is distinctive enough so that a clear separation is possible. In others, the association between drug and myopathy is clear, but the histology is not distinctive. In still others the myopathy occurs in a patient thought to have an idiopathic myositis, so that the boundaries are difficult to define. The most notable example is the corticosteroid myopathy that complicates the therapy of antecedent myositis. The diagnosis can only be established when strength improves in a patient whose dose of prednisone has been lowered rather than raised when 'unresponsiveness' is recognized.

Statin (lipid lowering agents)-induced myopathy has recently been shown to be the most common side effect in users of this class of drugs. These agents inhibit 3-hydroxy-3-methylglutaryl coenzyme A reductase, the rate-limiting enzyme involved in the conversion of HMG-CoA to mevalonic acid, and hence also prevent the synthesis of bioactive sterol and non-sterol metabolic intermediates in cholesterol biosynthesis. The main adverse effect of statins is a toxic myopathy presenting with muscle pain, CK elevation and occasional rhabdomyolysis. The underlying pathogenetic mechanisms are not yet identified[81,82]. Rare cases of classic biopsy-proven polymyositis or dermatomyositis, however, have been reported following the use of statins.

Other drugs, including D-penicillamine, have also been reported to induce a disease clinically and histologically indistinguishable from an idiopathic inflammatory myopathy such as dermatomyositis or polymyositis. These examples reinforce the possibility that at least some of the apparently idiopathic cases have their origin in an unappreciated environmental exposure[79]. The mechanism of the toxic and drug-related myopathies is not understood, so that it is impossible to do more than guess how such agents might contribute to the idiopathic disease.

Genetic factors

The occasional occurrence of familial idiopathic inflammatory myopathy and the association of specific HLA and non-HLA genes with groups of myositis patients strongly support the role of genetic factors in these conditions[55,83–85]. As is the case with other autoimmune diseases, however, current data imply that multiple genes are involved in the etiology of these complex disorders. Although major histocompatibility genes on chromosome 6, particularly HLA DRB1*0301 and the linked allele DQA1*0501, are the strongest known risk factors for all clinical forms of inflammatory myopathy in Caucasians, it appears that the genetic risk and protective factors for myositis differ considerably among different ethnogeographic groups around the world[86]. Further studies of gene–gene and gene–environment interactions in large, well-

myocarditis virus and mengovirus) which can cause an acute myositis – though only rarely in humans – have been shown to interact with the aminoacyl-tRNA synthetases which are the targets of several myositis-specific autoantibodies[72]. This observation raises the possibility that the virus initiates a viral myositis and autoantibody production. The chronic phase might be due, then, to persistent virus or to self-sustaining cellular or humoral autoimmunity. Fourth, several picornaviruses, including coxsackie and encephalomyocarditis, can cause an acute and sometimes chronic myositis in animals, resembling the human disease. Fifth, defined populations are needed to more fully understand the role of genetics in the myositis syndromes.

The boundary between idiopathic myositis and diseases as superficially different as the genetic dystrophies is not as sharp as their names would suggest. There are, for example, families in which several adults have related neuromyopathic illnesses, not wholly distinct from myositis. In addition, in apparently typical polymyositis, dermatomyositis or inclusion body myositis, neuropathic features may appear on electrophysiologic examination or biopsy.

SUMMARY

A wide range of insults, from drugs and toxins to infectious agents, can result in the clinical and pathologic syndrome of myositis. Although specific environmental agents can be identified in individual cases, in the vast majority the causes are still unclear. New ways of categorizing patients, such as through the use of myositis-specific autoantibodies, should improve our understanding of the complex interactions among the genetic factors, environmental stimuli and immune responses in this heterogeneous group of patients who share chronic muscle inflammation.

REFERENCES

1. Plotz PH, Rider LG, Targoff IN et al. NIH conference. Myositis: immunologic contributions to understanding cause, pathogenesis, and therapy. Ann Intern Med 1995; 122: 715–724.
2. Engel AG, Banker BQ. The polymyositis and dermatomyositis syndromes. In: Engel AG, Banker BQ, eds. Myology. New York: McGraw-Hill, 1986; 1385–1524.
3. Griggs RC, Askanas V, DiMauro S et al. Inclusion body myositis and myopathies. Ann Neurol 1995; 38: 705–713.
4. Mikol J. Inclusion body myositis. In: Engel AG, Banker BQ, eds. Myology. New York: McGraw-Hill, 1986; 1423–1438.
5. Adams EM, Chow CK, Premkumar A, Plotz PH. The idiopathic inflammatory myopathies: spectrum of MR imaging findings. Radiographics 1995; 15: 563–574.
6. Plotz PH, Miller FW. Animal models of myositis. Mt Sinai J Med 1988; 55: 501–505.
7. Askari AD. Cardiac abnormalities. Clin Rheum Dis 1984; 10: 131–149.
8. Tazelaar HD, Viggiano RW, Pickersgill J, Colby TV. Interstitial lung disease in polymyositis and dermatomyositis. Clinical features and prognosis as correlated with histologic findings. Am Rev Respir Dis 1990; 141: 727–733.
9. Hohlfeld R, Engel AG. The immunobiology of muscle. Immunol Today 1994; 15: 269–274.
10. Naparstek Y, Plotz PH. The role of autoantibodies in autoimmune disease. Annu Rev Immunol 1993; 11: 79–104.
11. Engel AG, Arahata K, Emslie-Smith A. Immune effector mechanisms in inflammatory myopathies. Res Publ Assoc Res Nerv Ment Dis 1990; 68: 141–157.
12. Engel AG, Arahata K. Mononuclear cells in myopathies: quantitation of functionally distinct subsets, recognition of antigen-specific cell-mediated cytotoxicity in some diseases, and implications for the pathogenesis of the different inflammatory myopathies. Hum Pathol 1986; 17: 704–721.
13. Kissel JT, Mendell JR, Rammohan KW. Microvascular deposition of complement membrane attack complex in dermatomyositis. N Engl J Med 1986; 31: 329–334.
14. Emslie-Smith AM, Engel AG. Microvascular changes in early and advanced dermatomyositis: a quantitative study. Ann Neurol 1990; 27: 343–356.
15. Arahata K, Engel AG. Monoclonal antibody analysis of mononuclear cells in myopathies III: Immunoelectron microscopy aspects of cell-mediated muscle fiber injury. Ann Neurol 1986; 19: 112–125.
16. Nagaraju K, Raben N, Villalba ML et al. Costimulatory markers in muscle of patients with idiopathic inflammatory myopathies and in cultured muscle cells. Clin Immunol 1999; 92: 161–169.
17. Murata K, Dalakas MC. Expression of the co-stimulatory molecule BB-1, the ligands CTLA-4 and CD28 and their mRNAs in chronic inflammatory demyelinating polyneuropathy. Brain 2000; 123 (Pt 8): 1660–1666.
18. Sugiura T, Kawaguchi Y, Harigai M et al. Increased CD40 expression on muscle cells of polymyositis and dermatomyositis: role of CD40-CD40 ligand interaction in IL-6, IL-8, IL-15, and monocyte chemoattractant protein-1 production. J Immunol 2000; 164: 6593–6600.
19. O'Hanlon TP, Miller FW. T cell-mediated immune mechanisms in myositis. Curr Opin Rheumatol 1995; 7: 503–509.
20. Gussoni E, Pavlath GK, Miller RG et al. Specific T cell receptor gene rearrangements at the site of muscle degeneration in Duchenne muscular dystrophy. J Immunol 1994; 153: 4798–4805.
21. De Bleecker JL, Engel AG. Expression of cell adhesion molecules in inflammatory myopathies and Duchenne dystrophy. J Neuropathol Exp Neurol 1994; 53: 369–376.
22. Arahata K, Ishihara T, Fukunaga H et al. Inflammatory response in facioscapulo-humeral muscular dystrophy (FSHD): immunocytochemical and genetic analyses. Muscle Nerve 1995; 2: S56–S66.
23. Round JM, Jones DA, Cambridge G. Cellular infiltrates in human skeletal muscle: exercise induced damage as a model for inflammatory muscle disease. J Neurol Sci 1987; 82: 1–11.
24. Emslie-Smith AM, Arahata K, Engel AG. Major histocompatibility complex class I antigen expression, immunolocalization of interferon subtypes, and T cell-mediated cytotoxicity in myopathies. Hum Pathol 1989; 20: 224–231.
25. Nagaraju K, Raben N, Loeffler L et al. Conditional up-regulation of MHC class I in skeletal muscle leads to self-sustaining autoimmune myositis and myositis-specific autoantibodies. Proc Natl Acad Sci USA 2000; 97: 9209–9214.
26. Nyberg P, Wikman AL, Nennesmo I, Lundberg I. Increased expression of interleukin 1alpha and MHC class I in muscle tissue of patients with chronic, inactive polymyositis and dermatomyositis. J Rheumatol 2000; 27: 940–948.
27. Lundberg I, Kratz AK, Alexanderson H, Patarroyo M. Decreased expression of interleukin-1alpha, interleukin-1beta, and cell adhesion molecules in muscle tissue following corticosteroid treatment in patients with polymyositis and dermatomyositis. Arthritis Rheum 2000; 43: 336–348.
28. Wiendl H, Behrens L, Maier S et al. Muscle fibers in inflammatory myopathies and cultured myoblasts express the nonclassical major histocompatibility antigen HLA-G . Ann Neurol 2000; 48: 679–684.
29. Miller FW, Love LA, Barbieri SA et al. Lymphocyte activation markers in idiopathic myositis: changes with disease activity and differences among clinical and autoantibody subgroups. Clin Exp Immunol 1990; 81: 373–383.
30. Wolf RE, Baethge BA. Interleukin-1 alpha, interleukin-2, and soluble interleukin-2 receptors in polymyositis. Arthritis Rheum 1990; 33: 1007–1014.
31. Tokano Y, Obara T, Hashimoto H et al. Soluble CD4, CD8 in patients with polymyositis/dermatomyositis. Clin Rheumatol 1993; 12: 368–374.
32. Cid MC, Grau JM, Casademont J et al. Leucocyte/endothelial cell adhesion receptors in muscle biopsies from patients with idiopathic inflammatory myopathies (IIM). Clin Exp Immunol 1996; 104: 467–473.
33. Tews DS, Goebel HH. Expression of cell adhesion molecules in inflammatory myopathies. J Neuroimmunol 1995; 59: 185–194.
34. Lundberg IE: The role of cytokines, chemokines, and adhesion molecules in the pathogenesis of idiopathic inflammatory myopathies. Curr Rheumatol Rep 2000; 2: 216–224.
35. Liang Y, Inukai A, Kuru S et al. The role of lymphotoxin in pathogenesis of polymyositis. Acta Neuropathol (Berlin) 2000; 100: 521–527.
36. Adams EM, Kirkley J, Eidelman G et al. The predominance of beta (CC) chemokine transcripts in idiopathic inflammatory muscle diseases. Proc Assoc Am Phys 1997; 109: 275–285.
37. Confalonieri P, Bernasconi P, Megna P et al. Increased expression of beta-chemokines in muscle of patients with inflammatory myopathies. J Neuropathol Exp Neurol 2000; 59: 164–169.
38. Guttridge DC, Mayo MW, Madrid LV et al. NF-kappaB-induced loss of MyoD messenger RNA: possible role in muscle decay and cachexia. Science 2000; 289: 2363–2366.
39. Choi YC, Dalakas MC. Expression of matrix metalloproteinases in the muscle of patients with inflammatory myopathies. Neurology 2000; 54: 65–71.
40. Kieseier BC, Schneider C, Clements JM et al. Expression of specific matrix metalloproteinases in inflammatory myopathies. Brain 2001; 124: 341–351.
41. Bernasconi P, Confalonieri P, Andreetta F et al. The expression of co-stimulatory and accessory molecules on cultured human muscle cells is not dependent on stimulus by pro-inflammatory cytokines: relevance for the pathogenesis of inflammatory myopathy. J Neuroimmunol 1998; 85: 52–58.
42. De Bleecker JL, Engel AG. Immunocytochemical study of CD45 T cell isoforms in inflammatory myopathies. Am J Pathol 1995; 146: 1178–1187.
43. Heath WR, Carbone FR. Cross-presentation, dendritic cells, tolerance and immunity. Annu Rev Immunol 2001; 19: 47–64.
44. Love LA, Leff RL, Fraser DD et al. A new approach to the classification of idiopathic inflammatory myopathy: Myositis-specific autoantibodies define useful homogeneous patient groups. Medicine 1991; 70: 360–374.
45. Miller FW, Waite KA, Biswas T, Plotz PH. The role of an autoantigen, histidyl-tRNA synthetase, in the induction and maintenance of autoimmunity. Proc Natl Acad Sci USA 1990; 87: 9933–9937.
46. Raben N, Nichols R, Dohlman J et al. A motif in human histidyl-tRNA synthetase which is shared among several aminoacyl-tRNA synthetases is a coiled-coil that is essential for enzymatic activity and contains the major autoantigenic epitope. J Biol Chem 1994; 269: 24277–24283.
47. Miller FW, Twitty SA, Biswas T, Plotz PH. Origin and regulation of a disease-specific autoantibody response: antigenic epitopes, spectrotype stability, and isotype restriction of anti-Jo-1 autoantibodies. J Clin Invest 1990; 85: 468–475.
48. Targoff IN, Arnett FC. Clinical manifestations in patients with antibody to PL-12 antigen (alanyl-tRNA synthetase). Am J Med 1990; 88: 241–251.
49. Hirakata M, Suwa A, Nagai S et al. Anti-KS: identification of autoantibodies to asparaginyl-transfer RNA synthetase associated with interstitial lung disease. J Immunol 1999; 162: 2315–2320.
50. Targoff IN, Reichlin M. The association between Mi-2 antibodies and dermatomyositis. Arthritis Rheum 1985; 28: 796–803.

51. Seelig HP, Renz M, Targoff IN, Ge Q, Frank MB Two forms of the major antigenic protein of the dermatomyositis-specific Mi-2 autoantigen. Arthritis Rheum 1996; 39: 1769–1771.

52. Casciola-Rosen LA, Pluta AF, Plotz PH et al. The DNA mismatch repair enzyme PMS1 is a myositis-specific autoantigen. Arthritis Rheum 2001; 44: 389–396.

53. Targoff IN, Johnson AE, Miller FW. Antibody to signal recognition particle in polymyositis. Arthritis Rheum 1990; 33: 1361–1370.

54. Targoff IN, Arnett FC, Berman L et al. Anti-KJ: a new antibody associated with the syndrome of polymyositis and interstitial lung disease. J Clin Invest 1989; 84: 162–172.

55. Shamim EA, Rider LG, Miller FW. Update on the genetics of the idiopathic inflammatory myopathies. Curr Opin Rheumatol 2000; 12: 482–491.

56. Miller FW, Hess EV, Clauw DJ et al. Approaches for identifying and defining environmentally associated rheumatic disorders. Arthritis Rheum 2000; 43: 243–249.

57. Nagaraju K, Casciola-Rosen L, Rosen A et al. The inhibition of apoptosis in myositis and in normal muscle cells. J Immunol. 2000; 164: 5459–5465.

58. Li M, Dalakas MC. Expression of human IAP-like protein in skeletal muscle: a possible explanation for the rare incidence of muscle fiber apoptosis in T-cell mediated inflammatory myopathies. J Neuroimmunol 2000; 106: 1–5.

59. Vattemi G, Tonin P, Filosto M et al. T-cell anti-apoptotic mechanisms in inflammatory myopathies. J Neuroimmunol 2000; 111: 146–151.

60. Goebels N, Michaelis D, Engelhardt M et al. Differential expression of perforin in muscle-infiltrating T cells in polymyositis and dermatomyositis. J Clin Invest 1996; 97: 2905–2910.

61. Mullinax F. Chimerism in scleroderma. Lancet 1998; 351: 1886.

62. Artlett CM, Smith JB, Jimenez SA. Identification of fetal DNA and cells in skin lesions from women with systemic sclerosis. N Engl J Med 1998; 338: 1186–1191.

63. Parker P, Chao NJ, Ben Ezra J et al. Polymyositis as a manifestation of chronic graft-versus-host disease. Medicine (Baltimore) 1996; 75: 279–285.

64. Artlett CM, Ramos R, Jiminez SA et al. Chimeric cells of maternal origin in juvenile idiopathic inflammatory myopathies. Childhood Myositis Heterogeneity Collaborative Group. Lancet 2000; 356: 2155–2156.

65. Reed AM, Picornell YJ, Harwood A, Kredich DW. Chimerism in children with juvenile dermatomyositis. Lancet 2000; 356: 2156–2157.

66. Magid SK, Kagen LJ. Serologic evidence for acute toxoplasmosis in polymyositis–dermatomyositis. Increased frequency of specific anti-toxoplasmosis IgM antibodies. Am J Med 1983; 75: 313–320.

67. Reimers CD, Pongratz DE, Neubert U et al. Myositis caused by Borrelia burgdorferi: report of four cases. J Neurol Sci 1989; 91: 215–226.

68. Wilfert CM, Buckley RH, Mohanakumar T et al. Persistent and fatal central-nervous-system ECHOvirus infections in patients with agammaglobulinemia. N Engl J Med 1977; 296: 1485–1489.

69. Travers RL, Hughes GRV, Cambridge G, Sewell JR. Coxsackie B neutralization titres in polymyositis/dermatomyositis. Lancet 1977; i: 1268.

70. Christensen ML, Pachman LM, Schneiderman R et al. Prevalence of coxsackie B virus antibodies in patients with juvenile dermatomyositis. Arthritis Rheum 1986; 29: 1365–1370.

71. Pearson CM. Myopathy with viral-like structures. N Engl J Med 1975; 292: 641–642.

72. Mathews MB, Bernstein RM. Myositis autoantibody inhibits histidyl-tRNA synthetase: a model for autoimmunity. Nature 1983; 304: 177–179.

73. Mikol J, Felten-Papaiconomou A, Ferchal F et al. Inclusion-body myositis: clinicopathological studies and isolation of an adenovirus type 2 from muscle biopsy specimen. Ann Neurol 1982; 11: 576–581.

74. Nishino H, Engel AG, Rima BK. Inclusion body myositis: the mumps virus hypothesis. Ann Neurol 1989; 25: 260–264.

75. Dalakas MC, Pezeshkpour GH, Gravell M, Sever JL. Polymyositis associated with AIDS retrovirus. JAMA 1986; 256: 2381–2383.

76. Wrzolek MA, Sher JH, Kozlowski PB, Rao C. Skeletal muscle pathology in AIDS: an autopsy study. Muscle Nerve 1990; 13: 508–515.

77. Morgan OS, Rodgers-Johnson P, Mora C, Char G. HTLV-1 and polymyositis in Jamaica. Lancet 1989; ii: 1184–1187.

78. Leff RL, Love LA, Miller FW et al. Viruses in idiopathic inflammatory myopathies: absence of candidate viral genomes in muscle. Lancet 1992; 339: 1192–1195.

79. Love LA, Miller FW. Noninfectious environmental agents associated with myopathies. Curr Opin Rheumatol 1993; 5: 712–718.

80. Le Quintrec J-S, Le Quintrec J-L. Drug-induced myopathies. Baillière's Clin Rheumatol 1991; 5: 21–38.

81. Sinzinger H, Schmid P, O'Grady J. Two different types of exercise-induced muscle pain without myopathy and CK-elevation during HMG-Co-enzyme-A-reductase inhibitor treatment. Atherosclerosis 1999; 143: 459–460.

82. Argov Z. Drug-induced myopathies. Curr Opin Neurol 2000; 13: 541–545.

83. Pachman LM, Friedman JM, Maryjowski-Sweeney ML et al. Immunogenetic studies of juvenile dermatomyositis. III. Study of antibody to organ-specific and nuclear antigens. Arthritis Rheum 1985; 28: 151–157.

84. Goldstein R, Duvic M, Targoff IN et al. HLA-D region genes associated with autoantibody responses to histidyl-transfer RNA synthetase (Jo-1) and other translation-related factors in myositis. Arthritis Rheum 1990; 33: 1240–1248.

85. Rider LG, Gurley RC, Pandey JP et al. Clinical, serologic, and immunogenetic features of familial idiopathic inflammatory myopathy. Arthritis Rheum 1998; 41: 710–719.

86. Rider LG, Shamim E, Okada S et al. Genetic risk and protective factors for idiopathic inflammatory myopathy in Koreans and American whites: a tale of two loci. Arthritis Rheum 1999; 42: 1285–1290.

139 Inflammatory muscle disease: clinical features

Chester V Oddis and Thomas A Medsger Jr

Definition

- Characterized by chronic inflammation of striated muscle (myositis), distinguishable cutaneous features (rash of dermatomyositis), and a variety of systemic complications
- Cellular and humoral immunologic features including serum autoantibodies that are associated with clinical syndromes with myositis as a major manifestation
- A member of the connective tissue disease family, as indicated by other autoimmune disease associations

Clinical and laboratory features

- Painless symmetric proximal muscle weakness with or without rash
- Increase in serum muscle enzymes, most notably creatine kinase
- Abnormal electromyogram and biopsy showing myositis
- Involvement of other organ systems including the lung, heart, gastrointestinal tract and joints
- Association of dermatomyositis with malignancy in middle-aged and elderly population

HISTORY

The characteristic 'heliotrope' rash of dermatomyositis was recognized before the disease itself in 1875, in a 17-year-old waiter in Paris, France, who presented with fatigue, pain in the extremities and erythema of the eyelids[1]. Eleven years later, in 1886, Wagner coined the term 'polymyositis' to describe a woman presenting with muscle weakness and diffuse muscle and joint pain who developed swelling of the extremities and forearm erythema[2]. In 1888, the first American case of polymyositis documented by muscle biopsy was reported in New York[3]. Because trichinosis was common at that time and could cause periorbital edema and diffuse myalgias, it was necessary that polymyositis or dermatomyositis be a diagnosis of exclusion, requiring an incompatible dietary history and a muscle biopsy lacking *Trichinella spiralis* cysts. In 1891, Unverricht described a 39-year-old pregnant woman with facial erythema and tense, swollen and erythematous legs and thighs, who later delivered a healthy infant. She subsequently developed myalgias with muscle weakness and atrophy and Unverricht introduced the term 'dermatomyositis' to describe her condition[4]. In 1930, Gottron reported on the skin lesions of dermatomyositis that bear his name, describing 'rounded foci of tense atrophy over carpo-metacarpal joints'[5]. The first published cases of dermatomyositis associated with carcinoma were independently reported in 1916[6,7], but Beczny, a Prague dermatologist, suggested a more definitive relationship between dermatomyositis and cancer in 1935[8]. More recently, in 1967, the pathology of inclusion body myositis was described[9], and it was named a short time later, in 1971[10].

EPIDEMIOLOGY

Classification criteria

The purposes of disease classification are to separate the disease of interest from others in order to determine incidence and prevalence, to describe the occurrence of disease in large populations, to compare one patient group with others, and to identify clinically homogeneous subsets of patients. Classification facilitates clinical studies of natural history and response to treatment, in addition to laboratory investigations of pathogenesis and etiology. With no knowledge of cause, and with inadequate understanding of pathogenesis, classifications are necessarily preliminary and must ultimately be revised as appropriate. Classification criteria differ from diagnostic criteria, which pertain to confirming the suspected diagnosis in individual cases[11].

In polymyositis–dermatomyositis, many classification systems have been proposed. For purposes of defining patient groups for clinical research and to aid in the diagnosis of the individual patient, the 1975 Bohan and Peter criteria have served extremely well for more than two decades (Table 139.1)[12]. The essential elements are proximal muscle weakness on physical examination, increased serum muscle enzymes, abnormal electromyogram (EMG), muscle biopsy consistent with myositis and the characteristic rash of dermatomyositis. Definite, probable (most likely diagnosis) and possible (consistent with) disease have been defined. The sensitivity of the Bohan and Peter criteria in a number

---

TABLE 139. 1 BOHAN AND PETER CRITERIA FOR DIAGNOSIS OF POLYMYOSITIS AND DERMATOMYOSITIS

Individual criteria

1. Symmetric proximal muscle weakness
2. Muscle biopsy evidence of myositis
3. Increase in serum skeletal muscle enzymes
4. Characteristic electromyographic pattern
5. Typical rash of dermatomyositis

Diagnostic criteria

Polymyositis:
  Definite: all of 1–4
  Probable: any 3 of 1–4
  Possible: any 2 of 1–4
Dermatomyositis:
  Definite: 5 plus any 3 of 1–4
  Probable: 5 plus any 2 of 1–4
  Possible: 5 plus any 1 of 1–4

(Modified with permission from Bohan and Peter[12].)

TABLE 139.2 INCIDENCE RATES OF POLYMYOSITIS–DERMATOMYOSITIS IN DIFFERENT POPULATIONS

Source	Geographic area	Inclusive dates of study	Annual incidence (per million)	Pertinent features
Rose and Walton (1966)[26]	Northeast England	1954–1964	2.25	
Kurland et al. (1969)[27]	Rochester, MN, USA	1951–1967	6.0	Almost exclusively white population
Findlay et al. (1969)[28]	Transvaal, South Africa	1960–1967	7.5	Includes dermatomyositis only
Medsger et al. (1970)[29]	Memphis and Shelby County, TN, USA	1947–1968	5.0	Hospital-diagnosed cases only; 40% population was African-American
Benbassat et al. (1980)[30]	Israel	1960–1976	2.2	Hospital diagnosed cases only; Bohan and Peter criteria used for diagnosis
Oddis et al. (1990)[31]	Allegheny County, PA, USA	1963–1982	5.5	Hospital diagnosed cases only; predominantly white population (91%); incidence rate 10.2 million during 1978–1982
Weitoft (1997)[32]	Gälveborg, County, Sweden	1984–1993	7.6	Medical center records and biopsy sources
Patrick et al. (1999)[33]	Victoria, Australia	1989–1991	7.4	Hospital diagnosis and muscle biopsy sources

of published studies averaged 70% for definite and 20% for probable myositis. Most probable and possible cases result, not from uncertainty about diagnosis, but instead because one or more of the diagnostic laboratory tests (enzymes, EMG, biopsy) were not performed. The specificity of the Bohan and Peter criteria against 436 patients with systemic lupus erythematosus (SLE) or systemic sclerosis combined was 93%[13]. The addition of myositis-specific serum autoantibodies and magnetic resonance imaging (MRI) to supplement the Bohan and Peter criteria has been recently proposed[14,15]. None of the classification systems mention inclusion body myositis, a more recently recognized entity with distinctive clinical and pathologic features, or amyopathic dermatomyositis, in which patients have the rash of dermatomyositis but no overt muscle weakness.

Association with other disorders

Polymyositis–dermatomyositis frequently occurs in overlap with systemic sclerosis, usually associated with one of several serum autoantibodies, including anti-U1-RNP, anti-PM-Scl or anti-U3-RNP[16,17]. Myositis has been described complicating rheumatoid arthritis[18], SLE[19], Sjögren's syndrome[20], Churg–Strauss vasculitis[21], localized forms of scleroderma[22,23], thrombotic thrombocytopenic purpura[24] and antiphospholipid antibody syndrome[25].

Incidence by age, race and sex

The reported overall annual incidence of polymyositis–dermatomyositis ranges from 2 to 10 new cases per million persons at risk in various populations (Table 139.2)[26–33]. These rates are likely to be underestimates, because not all possible sources of ascertainment were examined. For example, in most instances only hospital-diagnosed cases were sought, and patients with potential misdiagnoses (e.g. muscular dystrophy) were not reviewed. There is a trend towards increasing incidence in several communities over time[29,31], probably because of increased physician awareness, rather than a true increase in disease occurrence. A

nationwide study of inclusion body myositis in The Netherlands revealed a prevalence of 4.9 cases/million per year[34].

Although inflammatory myopathy can occur at any age, the observed pattern of incidence includes childhood and adult peaks and a paucity of patients with onset in the adolescent and young adult years[29,31]. This finding supports the concept of separating childhood from adult forms of the disease. As expected, the mean age of myositis onset is increased when there is an associated malignancy. The overall female: male incidence ratio is 2.5:1. This ratio is lower (nearly 1:1) in childhood disease and with associated malignancy, but is very high (10:1) when there is a coexisting connective tissue disease. Polymyositis–dermatomyositis has a 3–4:1 Afro-American to white ratio of incidence. There is a younger adult-onset peak among Afro-Americans, which is also true of SLE and systemic sclerosis.

The epidemiologic characteristics of the commonly recognized classification subsets are summarized in Table 139.3.

Environmental factors

No striking associations with environmental factors have been identified. Spatial clustering was found in one series[33], but neither spatial nor temporal clustering was detected in another[29]. The relative prevalence of polymyositis–dermatomyositis in Europe increases significantly (sevenfold) with latitude, from the north (Iceland) to the south (Greece), which could have either an environmental or a genetic explanation[35].

Disease onset is more frequent in the winter and spring months, especially in childhood cases, consistent with precipitation by viral and bacterial infections[29]. Serum antibodies to Coxsackie B viruses are more frequent in patients with dermatomyositis in childhood compared with controls with juvenile rheumatoid arthritis[36]. A patient with dermatomyositis and Lyme disease had *Borrelia burgdorferi* organisms detected in his dermatomyositis skin and muscle lesions[37]. Human T cell leukemia/lymphoma virus type-1 infection has been associated with polymyositis, including the identification of viral particles in affected

TABLE 139.3 EPIDEMIOLOGIC CHARACTERISTICS OF POLYMYOSITIS–DERMATOMYOSITIS CLINICAL CLASSIFICATION SUBSETS

	Adult polymyositis	Adult dermatomyositis	Childhood myositis	Myositis/connective tissue disease overlap	Myositis with malignancy	Inclusion body myositis	All patients
Proportion of all patients (%)	50	20	10	10	10	<5	
Mean age at diagnosis (years)	45	40	10	35	60	>65	45
Incidence sex ratio (F:M)	2:1	2:1	1:1	10:1	1:1	1:2	2.5:1
Incidence race ratio (B:W)	5:1	3:1	1:1	3:1	2:1	Unknown	3:1

B:W, black: white; F:M, female:male.

skeletal muscle[38]. Dermatomyositis has occurred in an individual infected with human immunodeficiency virus[39], and polymyositis caused by both a muspiceoid nematode[40] and mycoplasma pneumoniae infection[41] have been reported. In one study, patients with polymyositis–dermatomyositis reported excessive physical exercise and emotional stress antedating the onset of their illness significantly more frequently than did sex-matched unaffected sibling controls[42], but these associations have not been confirmed. Drug-induced myositis occurs with D-penicillamine[43] and the statin agents (see below, section on Drug-induced Myopathy). Despite many case reports, an association between polymyositis–dermatomyositis and bovine collagen injections has not been found in epidemiologic studies[42,44].

Genetic factors

The occurrence of polymyositis–dermatomyositis in monozygotic twins[45] and first-degree relatives of cases[46,47] supports a genetic predisosition, at least in some families. Homozygosity at the human leukocyte antigen *HLA-DQA1* locus has been shown to be associated with familial inflammatory myopathy[48]. Other autoimmune diseases occur four times more frequently in first-degree relatives of patients with polymyositis–dermatomyositis (21.9%) than in first-degree relatives of control probands (4.9%)[49].

The genetics of polymyositis–dermatomyositis has recently been reviewed[50]. Juvenile dermatomyositis has been found to be associated with *HLA-DQA1*0501*[51]. The closely linked *DRB1*0301* allele is also a risk factor for polymyositis–dermatomyositis in white populations[52]. Different *HLA* alleles appear to be important in either conferring risk for or protection from myositis in distinct ethnic, serologic and environmental exposure groups. Certain non-*HLA* genetic risk factors, such as genes regulating cytokines and their receptors – for example, interleukin (IL)-1[53] and tumor necrosis factor α[54] – appear to have a role in the development of myositis.

PRESENTATION

At presentation, the different clinical syndromes vary considerably from patient to patient (Table 139.4). The most frequent problem is insidious, progressive painless symmetric proximal muscle weakness over the course of 3–6 months before the first visit to a physician. Some patients, especially children and young adults with dermatomyositis, have a more acute onset of disease, with muscle pain and weakness developing rapidly over the course of several weeks. In the latter case, constitutional features such as fever and fatigue are more common. A few patients complain only of proximal myalgias. There is also a subset of patients with very slowly evolving weakness over the course of 1–10 years before diagnosis; they are typically older men with weakness of the pelvic girdle and muscles of the distal extremities who have pathologic features of inclusion body myositis on muscle biopsy.

Other presenting features may be attributable to muscle weakness. Several such findings, each occurring in approximately 5% of patients,

TABLE 139.4 TYPES AND FREQUENCIES OF PRESENTING CLINICAL SYNDROMES IN POLYMYOSITIS–DERMATOMYOSITIS

Syndrome	Estimated frequency (%)
Painless proximal weakness (over 3–6 months)	55
Acute or subacute proximal pain and weakness (over weeks to 2 months)	30
Insidious proximal and distal weakness (over 1–10 years)	10
Proximal myalgia alone	5
Dermatomyositis rash alone; extremity edema	<1

are pitting edema of the extremities as a result of lack of muscle tone needed to promote central venous return, hoarseness or dysphagia as a result of bulbar muscle weakness, nasal regurgitation of liquids or aspiration pneumonia, also because of pharyngeal dysphagia, and dyspnea resulting from either ventilatory muscle weakness or interstitial lung disease (ILD).

Presenting features often 'cluster' together, resulting in distinct clinical syndromes. For example, patients with serum anti-aminoacyl tRNA synthetase antibodies such as anti-Jo-1 antibody often have a constellation of findings, including fever, polyarthritis and ILD, in addition to myositis. When polymyositis or dermatomyositis overlap with another connective tissue disease, certain combinations of features tend to occur. When the overlap is with systemic sclerosis, one often finds Raynaud's phenomenon, puffy fingers, sclerodactyly and distal esophageal (smooth muscle) hypomotility. Lupus overlap features include photosensitive and malar rash, alopecia, polyarthralgias, pleurisy and leukopenia. These syndromes are discussed in greater detail below (see section on Clinical Features).

Finally, certain presenting manifestations tend to be mutually exclusive, depending on the patient subset. Of particular note are the rarity of Raynaud's phenomenon and arthralgias in pure (non-synthetase) polymyositis, the absence of calcinosis except in dermatomyositis (typically a late finding) and the unusual condition termed 'amyopathic dermatomyositis' in which the typical dermatomyositis skin rash occurs without objective evidence of myopathy.

CLINICAL FEATURES

Constitutional

Fatigue is a prominent complaint in patients with polymyositis–dermatomyositis and may persist well after adequate treatment with corticosteroids or other immunosuppressive agents. Fever is more commonly observed with childhood dermatomyositis, but adults with the antisynthetase syndrome may have fever accompanying or heralding active disease. Weight loss may occur with any systemic illness, but if it is persistent and severe in a myositis patient, malignancy should be considered. Weight loss also may result from poor caloric intake associated with pharyngeal striated muscle dysfunction or esophageal dysmotility.

Skeletal muscle

Patients complain of difficulty in performing activities requiring normal upper or lower limb strength. Involvement is insidious, bilateral, symmetric, usually painless and proximal greater than distal. An exception is inclusion body myositis, in which asymmetric distal weakness and atrophy are prominent, often accompanied by similar proximal muscle findings. In polymyositis and dermatomyositis, the lower extremity (pelvic girdle) is usually affected initially with difficulty walking up steps or arising from a chair or toilet seat. Walking may become clumsy, with a 'waddling' gait. The patient may fall and be unable to arise without assistance. Upper extremity (shoulder girdle) symptoms follow, with patients experiencing difficulty raising their arms overhead or combing their hair. Neck flexor weakness is manifested by the inability to raise the head from a pillow. Muscle pain may occur and is more common in dermatomyositis, particularly with exercise. Proximal dysphagia, with nasal regurgitation of liquids and pulmonary aspiration reflects pharyngeal striated muscle involvement and is a poor prognostic sign seen with severe disease. Pharyngeal weakness also results in hoarseness or a change in voice, giving it a nasal quality. Ocular or facial muscle weakness is very uncommon[55] in polymyositis–dermatomyositis, and their presence should prompt consideration of another diagnosis.

Physical examination using manual muscle testing is necessary to confirm weakness of individual muscles or groups of muscles, and many such measures are in current use. A standardized grading system for

TABLE 139.5 GRADING OF MUSCLE WEAKNESS IN POLYMYOSITIS–DERMATOMYOSITIS
1. No abnormality on examination
2. No abnormality on examination, but easy fatiguability and decreased exercise tolerance
3. Minimal degree of atrophy of one or more muscle groups, without functional impairment
4. Waddling gait; unable to run, but able to climb stairs without needing arm support
5. Marked waddling gait; accentuated lordosis; unable to climb stairs or rise from a standard chair without arm support
6. Unable to walk without assistance
(Modified with permission of Oxford University Press from Rose and Walton[26].)

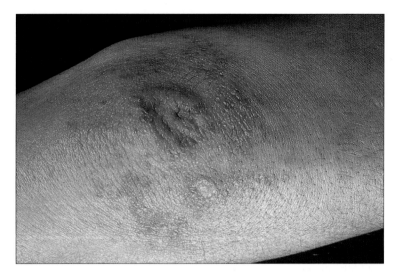

Fig. 139.2 Gottron's sign. Scaling, macular erythema over the extensor surface of the elbow in a patient with dermatomyositis.

muscle weakness has been proposed (Table 139.5). The severity of weakness should be serially assessed and recorded. Quantitative assessment of muscle strength is important, because laboratory tests may not accurately reflect disease activity. However, a more complete assessment should combine muscle strength testing with functional ability. Other means of assessing and quantifying strength include an age- and sex-standardized lower extremity measure[56], a modified sphygmomanometer to quantitate shoulder abductor strength[57] and a hand-held pull gauge to measure isometric strength in different muscle groups[58]. Muscle hypertrophy is seen with muscular dystrophy, not with polymyositis or dermatomyositis. Muscle atrophy and joint contractures are late findings in chronic myositis, as a result of fibrous replacement of muscle or in inclusion body myositis.

Skin

The presence of a characteristic skin rash indicates the clinical subset of dermatomyositis; the rash may precede, develop simultaneously with, or follow muscle symptoms. Gottron's papules and the heliotrope rash are considered pathognomonic cutaneous features of dermatomyositis. Gottron's papules (Fig. 139.1) are scaly, erythematous or violaceous plaques located over bony prominences, particularly the metacarpophalangeal and proximal and distal interphalangeal joints of the hands. Gottron's sign (Fig. 139.2) is a macular erythema that generally occurs in the same distribution, and over other extensor areas such as the elbows, knees and ankles. Either of these rashes is seen in 60–80% of patients

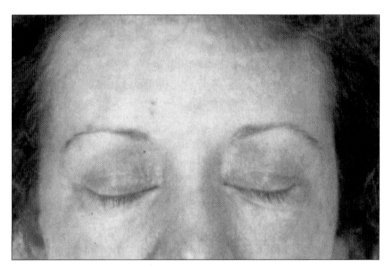

Fig. 139.3 Heliotrope rash of dermatomyositis. The erythematous or violaceous rash over the eyelids of this patient with dermatomyositis and breast cancer is a characteristic cutaneous feature.

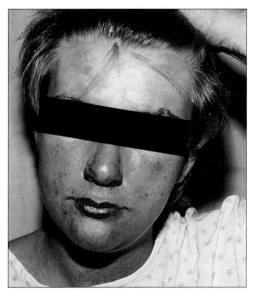

Fig. 139.4 The facial rash of dermatomyositis. Note the malar-like rash of dermatomyositis, which involves the nasolabial area (an area often spared in SLE). Patchy involvement of the forehead and chin is also present.

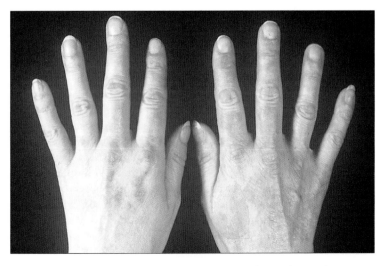

Fig. 139.1 Gottron's papules. This erythematous, scaling rash over the knuckles and dorsum of the hand is a common early sign in dermatomyositis. It can be distinguished from the rash of SLE, which usually affects the phalanges and spares the knuckles.

with dermatomyositis. Later in the disease course, the affected skin lesions may become shiny, atrophic and hypopigmented. The heliotrope rash, seen in fewer than 50% of patients with dermatomyositis, is purplish in color, may be edematous and is located in the periorbital area, especially over the upper eyelids (Fig. 139.3). Cutaneous photosensitivity, with facial erythema (Fig. 139.4) or a 'V sign' over the anterior chest, is more common than reported in dermatomyositis. Pruritus of affected areas is more severe than that seen with the rash of SLE and is particularly common when dermatomyositis involves the scalp (Fig. 139.5)[59]. Another distinguishing feature of the dermatomyositis rash compared with SLE is involvement of the nasolabial area and the forehead with dermatomyositis. The 'shawl sign' refers to a rash located over the upper back and across both shoulders in a shawl-like distribution. Cuticular hypertrophy and hemorrhage with periungual erythema, telangiectasia, infarcts and capillary dilatation are seen in some patients with dermatomyositis and in patients with myositis in overlap with another connective tissue disease. Cracking, fissuring, or both, of the lateral and palmar digital skin pads is termed 'mechanic's hands' (Fig. 139.6), and is most frequently seen in patients with polymyositis who have autoantibodies directed against a tRNA synthetase or the PM-Scl autoantigen[60].

Other cutaneous findings seen in patients with inflammatory myopathy are listed in Table 139.6[61–73]. Panniculitis (with membranocystic changes on biopsy) is being increasingly reported in association with myositis, and may be the presenting feature in some cases[61–65]. In fact, a recent report noted occult MRI abnormalities in the subcutaneous tissue of children with dermatomyositis, indicating active panniculitis, which progressed later to clinically evident calcinosis[65]. 'Centripetal flagellate erythema' consists of non-pruritic linear streaks on the trunk and proximal extremities demonstrating an interface dermatitis on biopsy[66]; it may be a marker of disease activity in dermatomyositis[67]. Hyperkeratotic skin lesions, including pityriasis rubra pilaris, have been reported[68,69].

Some patients may present with the classic biopsy-confirmed rash(es) of dermatomyositis and no muscle weakness, normal muscle enzymes or even a normal EMG. These patients are said to have 'amyopathic dermatomyositis' (ADM) if these findings have been present for 2 years or longer[74]. There are no population-based data that describe the prevalence of adult or childhood ADM, but these patients are more frequently observed in dermatology practices. Many such patients have a favorable outcome, but some may develop malignancy[75,76].

TABLE 139.6 CUTANEOUS FEATURES OF THE IDIOPATHIC INFLAMMATORY MYOPATHIES
Pathognomonic signs in dermatomyositis
Gottron's papules/sign (60–80% of patients)
Heliotrope rash (50% or fewer)
Less specific signs in dermatomyositis
Photosensitivity
'V sign'
Scalp involvement
'Shawl sign'
Nailfold capillary changes with cuticular overgrowth
Other skin findings in polymyositis or dermatomyositis
Calcinosis
'Mechanic's hands'
Panniculitis[61–65]
'Centripetal flagellate erythema' (linear streaks)[66,67]
Pityriasis rubra pilaris (palmar plantar hyperkeratoses)[68,69]
Facial seborrhea[70]
Papular mucinosis (scleromyxedema)[71]
Acquired ichthyosis[72]
Vesiculobullous disorders[73]
Urticarial (lymphocytic) vasculitis
Acanthosis nigricans
Vitiligo
Multifocal lipoatrophy
Poikiloderma

Calcinosis

Soft tissue calcification, which can be a disabling late problem, occurs most commonly in chronic dermatomyositis, especially with onset in childhood, and is uncommon in adult-onset disease. Myositis may be well controlled when calcinosis appears, but patients most often previously have had chronic, active disease or a delay in the initiation of corticosteroid treatment. Recent findings suggest that childhood dermatomyositis may be mediated by activated macrophages, IL-6, IL-1 and tumor necrosis factor, which are found in calcinotic fluid[77]. Calcinosis may be intracutaneous, subcutaneous, fascial or intramuscular in location, with a predilection for sites of repeated microtrauma (elbows, knees, flexor surfaces of fingers and buttocks). Troubling complications of calcinosis include cutaneous ulceration with drainage of calcareous material and secondary infection, and joint contractures that interfere with physical therapy intervention.

Articular

Polyarthralgias or polyarthritis, if they occur, are early in the disease course, rheumatoid-like in distribution and relatively mild. Joint involvement is more common, with overlap syndromes and the antisynthetases, but is frequently encountered in childhood dermatomyositis also[78]. The arthropathy associated with the anti-Jo-1 autoantibody, in addition to other antisynthetases[79], can be chronic and deforming[80], with interphalangeal thumb joint instability ('floppy thumb sign') and erosive[79], with periarticular calcifications[81]. Such 'pseudorheumatoid' changes in a Jo-1-positive patient are depicted radiographically and clinically in Figure 139.7. Other unusual anti-Jo-1 antibody-associated articular features have been described[82,83].

Pulmonary

Lung involvement is common in polymyositis–dermatomyositis (see also Chapter 29), and dyspnea in the patient with myositis warrants an aggressive diagnostic approach (Table 139.7). Pulmonary disease may

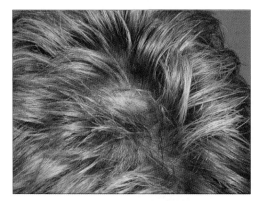

Fig. 139.5 Scalp rash of dermatomyositis. Note the scaling erythema of the scalp in this patient with dermatomyositis.

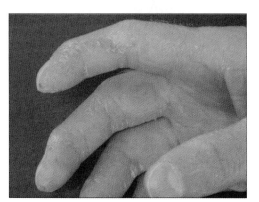

Fig. 139.6 'Mechanic's hands'. Note the hyperkeratotic changes and cracking of the skin on the lateral aspects of the fingers in this patient with the anti-PM-Scl autoantibody.

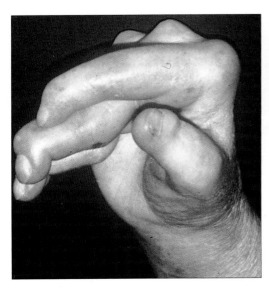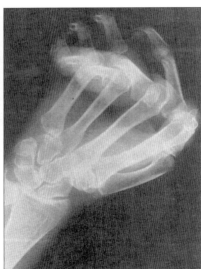

Fig. 139.7 Deforming arthropathy of polymyositis.
(a) Rheumatoid-like deformities of the hand in a patient with the anti-Jo-1 autoantibody. (b) Radiograph of this patient's hand, showing numerous subluxations, but minimal bony erosive changes.

TABLE 139.7 CAUSES OF DYSPNEA IN THE PATIENT WITH IDIOPATHIC INFLAMMATORY MYOPATHY

Non-pulmonary etiology

Respiratory muscle weakness[86–88]
Cardiac involvement (see text)

Pulmonary etiology

Diffuse alveolitis
Adult respiratory distress syndrome[89]
Slowly progressive interstitial lung disease
Pulmonary hypertension
Alveolar hemorrhage[90,91]
Bronchiolitis obliterans organizing pneumonia[92,93]
Pneumomediastinum[94–97]
Pleural effusion
Infection (with or without aspiration due to pharyngeal myopathy)[98,99]
Drug-induced (e.g. methotrexate)

---

overshadow the features of myositis and may be observed in patients without overt myositis or with ADM[84,85]. Dyspnea may result from non-parenchymal problems such as ventilatory (diaphragmatic and intercostal) muscle weakness or cardiac dysfunction (see below). Ventilatory muscle weakness leading to ventilatory failure is uncommon, but four patients have been reported who developed ventilator-dependent respiratory failure with diaphragmatic involvement, and one had myositis of the diaphragm at autopsy[86,87]. Hypercapnia is likely in polymyositis when the vital capacity is less than 55% of predicted normal[88].

In general, the presence of alveolitis with a 'ground glass' appearance on high resolution computed tomography (CT), as opposed to fibrosis characterized by 'honeycombing', indicates a potentially treatment-responsive condition with a more favorable prognosis. Arterial hypoxemia with exercise desaturation is common, and pulmonary function testing reveals restrictive physiology, with a decrease in the diffusion capacity. This type of pulmonary involvement is commonly seen in association with anti-Jo-1 or another antiaminoacyl-tRNA synthetase autoantibody, as part of the 'antisynthetase' syndrome. Interstitial disease may be slowly progressive or even asymptomatic (usually bibasilar) in some patients with polymyositis–dermatomyositis with or without an associated antisynthetase autoantibody. The most ominous intrinsic lung complication is rapidly progressive diffuse alveolitis. This

form of pulmonary involvement may be fatal in weeks to months, often terminating with adult respiratory distress syndrome[89].

Patients with myositis-associated progressive pulmonary fibrosis can develop pulmonary hypertension secondary to pulmonary vasoconstriction as a result of chronic hypoxemia. Diffuse alveolar hemorrhage with pulmonary capillaritis is uncommon[90,91], but bronchiolitis obliterans with organizing pneumonia (BOOP) is increasingly observed as the initial manifestation of polymyositis[92,93]. Pneumomediastinum with subcutaneous emphysema is associated with rapidly progressive ILD and dermatomyositis with cutaneous vasculitis[94–97]. Fulminant *Pneumocystis carinii* pneumonia has been reported in four patients with human immunodeficiency virus-negative dermatomyositis who were lymphopenic before initiation of corticosteroids[98], and *Nocardia* pleural empyema complicated the disease in a Jo-1-positive polymyositis patient during treatment with intravenous immunoglobulin and corticosteroids[99].

Cardiac

Although heart involvement may be common in polymyositis–dermatomyositis, it is seldom symptomatic; the frequency of cardiac abnormalities reported is dependent on the aggressiveness of detection measures[100]. The most common finding is a rhythm disturbance, presumably from inflammatory or fibrotic alteration of the conducting system. More severe forms of cardiac involvement, such as congestive heart failure or pericardial tamponade, may occur on presentation, but are very unusual[101,102]. Congestive heart failure is typically caused by myocarditis or myocardial fibrosis[103,104]. Patients complain of palpitations or dyspnea on exertion and on physical examination have tachycardia and other features of congestive heart failure. Myocardial infarction may result from coronary vasospasm, accelerated atherosclerosis associated with prolonged corticosteroid use or arteritis that may be seen with coronary angiography[105,106].

Gastrointestinal tract

The pharyngeal musculature is striated and thus can become inflamed and weak like striated muscle in other locations. Swallowing problems (upper dysphagia) manifest as difficulty in the initiation of deglutition or nasal regurgitation of liquids, with dysphonia. If severe, aspiration of oral contents leads to chemical pneumonitis, sometimes complicated by secondary bacterial infection. Cricopharyngeal muscle dysfunction also can result in dysphagia, with the complaint of a 'blocking' sensation with swallowing; it is more common in inclusion body myositis[107].

Involvement of the smooth muscle of any portion of the intestinal tract is possible in both overlap disorders or pure polymyositis and dermatomyositis. Patients note a retrosternal 'sticking' sensation on swallowing bread or meat and heartburn (reflux) with esophageal body and gastroesophageal sphincter involvement, respectively. In rare cases, esophageal dysmotility is complicated by megaesophagus or rupture[108]. Postprandial symptoms of bloating, pain and distention (pseudo-obstruction) in addition to watery diarrhea with weight loss (malabsorption syndrome) indicate small bowel involvement. Pneumatosis cystoides intestinalis has been reported[109].

Childhood-onset dermatomyositis is most commonly associated with gastrointestinal ulceration and hemorrhage as a result of vasculitis. Adult-onset dermatomyositis also may have severe gastrointestinal manifestations[110]. Active and quiescent myositis are increasingly reported in conjunction with inflammatory bowel disease[111,112], as are primary biliary cirrhosis, sclerosing cholangitis and celiac disease in adults and children[113–116].

Peripheral vascular system

Raynaud's phenomenon is observed in all subsets of the inflammatory myopathies except for malignancy-associated forms. Systemic vasculitis is common in childhood dermatomyositis, but uncommon in adults[117]. The inflammatory vascular lesions of dermatomyositis include tender dermal and or subcutaneous nodules, periungual infarcts and digital ulcerations.

Kidney

Renal disease is rare in myositis, but an occasional patient has proteinuria and, less commonly, nephrotic syndrome. Patients with overlap syndromes may develop kidney problems from the non-myositis components of their disorders. Polymyositis-induced myoglobuinuric acute renal failure can occur, but is rare[118].

Miscellaneous

Visual complications have been increasingly reported in association with polymyositis–dermatomyositis, including visual blurring and loss as a result of retinopathy or retinal vasculitis[119,120]. Two patients with dermatomyositis developed acute abdominal pain as a result of spontaneous hemorrhage leading to abdominal hematomas[121]. Central nervous system features of polymyositis or dermatomyositis are rare, but progressive multifocal leukoencephalopathy and central nervous system vasculitis have been seen in association with dermatomyositis[122,123].

DIFFERENTIAL DIAGNOSIS

History and physical examination

Among patients with impaired muscle function, only 50% voluntarily complain about 'weakness'. Other frequent symptoms are 'tiredness' and 'fatigue'. The examining physician must differentiate between difficulty in performing a motor task (muscle weakness) or its repetitive performance (fatigue of muscle) and difficulty doing activities of daily living that require more endurance than muscle strength.

Muscle weakness and muscle fatigue imply primary disease of muscle or the neuromuscular unit, whereas inability to perform normal activities may include or be solely caused by cardiovascular, metabolic, endocrine or psychiatric disorders. The patient's complaint of fatigue may refer to a variety of problems that have the common feature of loss of sense of well-being. Fatigue may include indifference to tasks at hand, preoccupation with unimportant activities or difficulty initiating or sustaining an activity. The patient often does not separate physical from mental function. For example, disinclination to interact with one's family members and friends during leisure hours may be termed 'fatigue' by the patient, but be interpreted as a symptoms of depression by the discerning physician. Some of these non-neuromuscular causes of weakness, separated into conditions causing episodic or persistent symptoms, are listed in Table 139.8.

TABLE 139.8 NON-NEUROMUSCULAR CAUSES OF WEAKNESS

Episodic weakness (acute attacks with recurrence)

Hypotension, cardiac arrhythmias
Hypoxia, hypercapnia
Hyperventilation
Hypoglycemia
Cerebrovascular insufficiency
Emotional states (hyperventilation, anxiety)

Persistent weakness

Anemia
Chronic or acute infection
Malignancy
Malnutrition
Advanced organ system failure (lung, heart, liver, kidney)
Metabolic disorders (hyperthyroidism, hyperparathyroidism, hypophosphatemia)

If true muscle weakness is suspected, other medical history features should be elicited because of their usefulness in differential diagnosis. Some complaints are distinctly unusual in polymyositis–dermatomyositis and should suggest alternative diagnoses. A family history of primary myopathy is common in heritable forms of muscle disease. Episodic weakness, especially after exercise or prolonged use of the affected muscles, occurs in myasthenia gravis and metabolic myopathies. Asymmetric or unilateral weakness, muscle cramps and fasciculations suggest a primary neurologic disorder. Facial and ocular muscle weakness rarely occur in myositis, but are frequent in myasthenia gravis. Finally, a list of the patient's medications may uncover an agent recognized to cause skeletal muscle dysfunction.

Non-inflammatory myopathies

The differential diagnosis of adult polymyositis–dermatomyositis is broad and includes numerous conditions capable of affecting skeletal muscle (Table 139.9). History, physical examination and differences in laboratory test results serve as the primary features distinguishing between these conditions. However, even the muscle biopsy may not be diagnostic in some patients with inflammatory myopathy.

Primary diseases of nerve include the spinal muscular atrophies, autosomal recessive disorders leading to slowly progressive degeneration of spinal anterior horn cells (weakness, wasting) and amyotrophic lateral sclerosis, which results in more rapid degeneration of both lower and upper motor neurons (bulbar or pseudobulbar palsy).

Myasthenia gravis is the prototypical disorder of the neuromusclar junction, in which weakness often affects the extraocular and bulbar muscles and becomes worse with prolonged or repetitive use. A similar pattern of activity-increased weakness is found in Eaton–Lambert syndrome. Both of these diseases can cause proximal muscle weakness. They are distinguished from polymyositis–dermatomyositis by their characteristic patterns on the EMG, in addition to absence of increases in serum muscle enzymes, but some patients with myasthenia gravis have been discovered to have myositis on muscle biopsy[124].

The congenital myopathies, including the various forms of muscular dystrophy and nemaline myopathy, are hereditary conditions with onset of symptoms primarily in infancy or childhood, but occasionally in adulthood, with slow but steady progression. Their genetic patterns of occurrence and clinical features have been well described. Some congenital myopathy cases are difficult to differentiate from inflammatory myopathy but have a slowly progressive downhill course unaffected by corticosteroid or immunosuppressive treatment.

Metabolic and mitochondrial myopathies occur because of genetic defects that cause abnormal energy metabolism[125]. Glycogen storage

TABLE 139.9 DIFFERENTIAL DIAGNOSIS OF MUSCLE WEAKNESS

Denervating conditions	Spinal muscular atrophies*, amyotrophic lateral sclerosis*
Neuromuscular junction disorders	Eaton–Lambert syndrome*, myasthenia gravis*
The genetic muscular dystrophies	Duchenne's facioscapulohumeral, limb girdle*, Becker's, Emery–Dreifuss type*, distal, ocular
Myotonic diseases	Dystrophia myotonica*, myotonia congenita
Congenital myopathies	Nemaline, mitochondrial, centronuclear, central core
Glycogen storage diseases	Adult-onset acid maltase deficiency*, McArdle's disease
Lipid storage myopathies	Carnitine deficiency*, carnitine palmityltransferase deficiency*
The periodic paralyses	
Myositis ossificans*	Generalized and local
Endocrine myopoathies*	Hypothyroidism, hyperthyroidism, acromegaly, Cushing's disease, Addison's disease, hyperparathyroidism, hypoparathyroidism, vitamin D deficiency myopathy, hypokalemia, hypocalcemia
Metabolic myopoathies*	Uremia, hepatic failure
Toxic myopathies*	Acute and chronic alcoholism, drugs including penicillamine*, clofibrate*, chloroquine, emetine
Nutritional myopathies	vitamin E deficiency*, malabsorption*
Carcinomatous neuromyopathy*	carcinomatous cachexia
Acute rhabdomyolysis*	
Proximal neuropathies	Guillain–Barré syndrome*, acute intermittent porphyria*, diabetic lower-limb chronic plexopathies*, chronic autoimmune polyneuropathy
Microembolization by atheroma or carcinoma	
Polymyalgia rheumatica*	
Other collagen vascular diseases	Rheumatoid arthritis, scleroderma, systemic lupus erythematosus, polyarteritis nodosa
Infections	Acute viral, including influenza, mononucleosis, rickettsia, coxsackievirus, rubella and rubella vaccination, acute bacterial including typhoid
Parasites	Including *Toxoplasma*, *Trichinella*, *Schistosoma*, *Cysticercus*, *Sarcosporidia*
Septic myositis	Including *Staphylococcus*, *Streptococcus*, *Clostridium perfringens* (*welchii*) and leprosy

* Indicates the conditions that are most commonly confused with muscle weakness.

diseases result from enzyme deficiencies involving the glycolytic pathway. McArdle's disease, or myophosphorylase deficiency, is caused by failure to degrade glycogen for energy under anerobic conditions. It is characterized by acute episodes of pain, weakness and swelling of voluntary muscles, which are contracted frequently or for a prolonged period of time. On occasion, a late proximal myopathy occurs that can simulate polymyositis. Ischemic exercise testing results in failure to produce lactate and muscle biopsy shows glycogen accumulation and absence of myophosphorylase. Acid maltase deficiency, a metabolic disorder known to mimic polymyositis, results in excessive accumulation of glycogen in membrane-bound lysosomes. Progressive proximal weakness, myotonic changes on the EMG and glycogen deposition on muscle biopsy are observed. Carnitine deficiency results in inability to transport long-chain fatty acids into mitochondria for oxidation, leading to lipid accumulation in muscle fibers and a chronic proximal myopathy. The enzyme carnitine palmityltransferase may also be lacking, resulting in a syndrome resembling McArdle's disease, with exertional pain and weakness as a result of inadequte production of adenosine triphosphate from lipids. A similar symptom complex can occur with myoadenylate deaminase deficiency, in which the ischemic exercise test results in the failure to increase ammonia production.

An increasingly recognized form of weakness that occurs in the seriously ill patient includes both 'critical illness polyneuropathy' and 'acute myopathy of intensive care'[126,127]. The latter is associated with the use of high-dose intravenous corticosteroids and non-depolarizing neuromuscular blocking agents, and is a frequent cause of failure to wean tracheally intubated patients from a respirator. Increased serum creatine kinase (CK) concentrations in the first 10 days of the illness, myopathic EMG changes and myofiber necrosis on biopsy are characteristic, and partial or complete recovery is the rule, but may take months[127].

Other causes of non-inflammatory proximal myopathy include vitamin D deficiency, calciphylaxis, adrenal insufficiency, hypophosphatemia, hyperthyroidism, carcinomatous neuropathy and exposures to certain toxic substances.

Other inflammatory myopathies

Infectious agents are capable of producing polymyositis. Viruses reported to cause widespread, but generally mild and self-limited myositis include influenza A and B, hepatitis B, coxsackie, rubella (both natural infection and after immunization with live attenuated virus), echovirus and human immunodeficiency virus. In such cases, the myositis is self-limited and recovery is almost always complete. Echovirus has been associated with myositis in patients with X-linked hypogammaglobulinemia.

Bacterial infection (pyomyositis) caused by staphylococcal or streptococcal organisms is characterized by the insidious onset of fever and myalgias, progressing to acute focal suppuration of skeletal muscle, with abscess formation. Children and young adults or persons with predisposing comorbid conditions such as human immunodeficiency virus infection are most often affected[128]. Although initially reported to occur primarily in persons residing in tropical areas, pyomyositis has been more frequently diagnosed recently in temperate climates. This disorder is potentially fatal if unrecognized, and disabling if foci of osteomyelitis develop.

One parasitic infection capable of causing acute myositis is trichinosis, which also frequently causes conjunctivitis, eosinophilia and increased serum antibody titers. Toxoplasmosis may also cause a polymyositis-like illness in which the organisms are identified in muscle biopsies and an antibody response develops.

Focal nodular myositis, presenting with tumor-like masses and curiously limited to one or several extremities, has been described[129]. Although not an inflammatory condition, diabetic muscle infarction presents with abrupt onset of thigh pain, tenderness, a palpable mass and increased serum CK concentration[130]. Giant cell myositis is rare, but can be encountered in sarcoidosis. Regenerating muscle in other conditions may result in cells having a multinucleate appearance on light microscopy that must be distinguished from true giant cells in a typical granuloma.

Myositis with an eosinophilic inflammatory infiltrate includes a heterogeneous group of rare conditions[131]. A recently proposed classification system divides patients into groups on the basis of whether they have focal eosinophilic myositis, eosinophilic polymyositis (systemic features including myocardial involvement) or eosinophilic perimyositis[132]. These conditions must be distinguished from eosinophilic fasciitis and eosinophilia–myalgia syndrome. In the last two disorders, true myofiber necrosis, with weakness and increased CK are unusual.

Amyloidosis can mimic polymyositis clinically and histologically; the only clue might be other features typical of amyloidosis, failure to respond to corticosteroid treatment and positive Congo red staining of muscle tissue, with immunohistochemical analysis confirming vascular amyloid deposition[133]. For this reason, some recommend routine serum and urine immunoelectrophoresis in all cases of polymyositis–dermatomyositis.

During recent years, a number of patients in France whose symptoms resembled polymyositis or polymyalgia rheumatica have been reported to have subcutaneous and epimysial, perimysial and perifascicular/endomysial infiltration, with large numbers of periodic acid Schiff-positive macrophages[134]. The term 'macrophagic myofasciitis' has been used to describe such patients. Myofibril damage has been minimal, and the symptoms have responded readily to corticosteroid treatment.

Malignancy and myositis

There has been considerable controversy regarding the validity and magnitude of the relationship between malignancy and inflammatory myopathy. Several clinically pertinent questions should be addressed regarding this purported association:

1. Is there an increased risk of cancer in patients with polymyositis–dermatomyositis?
2. If such an association exists, what types of malignancies are increased?
3. Are there clinical findings that identify patients with myositis who are at risk for malignancy?
4. Who should be screened and what is a reasonable screening evaluation for malignancy?
5. What is the pathogenesis of malignancy-associated myositis?

Recent reports strongly support an increased risk of cancer in patients with polymyositis–dermatomyositis. They include consecutive-patient series, hospital-based analyses, national registries and population-based cohort studies of biopsy-proven cases[135–139]. Standardized incidence ratios (SIRs), computed as ratios of observed to expected cases of cancer, have clearly demonstrated the greatest risk of malignancy in patients with dermatomyositis in whom SIR values range from 3.0 to 12.6[136–138]. In a pooled analysis of published national data from Sweden, Denmark and Finland, 618 cases of dermatomyositis were identified, 198 of whom had cancer (SIR 3.0)[137]. Of these, 115 (59%) developed a malignancy after the diagnosis of dermatomyositis was made. Dermatomyositis was strongly associated with ovarian, lung, pancreatic, stomach and colorectal cancer and non-Hodgkin lymphoma. This same study identified a lower but statistically significant increase in cancer associated with polymyositis in 137 of 914 cases (15%), with an increased risk of non-Hodgkin lymphoma and both lung and bladder cancer. In an effort to address several methodologic issues in earlier reports, an Australian study utilizing a cancer registry and a strict definition of myositis based on histologic criteria also demonstrated an increased risk of malignancy in both polymyositis–dermatomyositis and inclusion body myositis (SIR 2.4)[139]. The overall risk of cancer is greatest in the first 3 years after the diagnosis of myositis[139], but a greater risk of malignancy persists through all years of follow-up, emphasizing the importance of continued surveillance[137,139]. Although older individuals with dermatomyositis are at greater risk, the likelihood of malignancy is increased even in dermatomyositis patients younger than 45 years[137].

The sites of origin of malignancy are typical for the age of the patient, but several points are noteworthy. Ovarian cancer is over-represented in some series[137,140], but screening with pelvic examination rarely detects this cancer before the development of metastatic disease. Serum CA-125 screening proved useful in a case–control study of 14 women with dermatomyositis (four of whom subsequently developed ovarian cancer) in which the sensitivity was 50% and specificity 100%[141]. Prospective studies are needed to determine the effect of screening on the stage of ovarian cancer and long-term survival. Asian and Chinese patients with dermatomyositis have a clear increase in nasopharyngeal carcinoma[138,142]. Many other types of cancer occur coincidentally with myositis, including genitourinary malignancies and melanoma.

Clinical and histologic features that may predict the presence of a malignancy in a patient with dermatomyositis include epidermal necrosis, cutaneous leukocytoclastic vasculitis and the presence of amyopathic dermatomyositis[135,143,144]. In a series of 11 patients with adult dermatomyositis, six had malignancy and both clinical and histologic evidence of epidermal necrosis was present in all six, whereas cutaneous necrosis was absent in the five patients with dermatomyositis without cancer[143]. Similarly, in a retrospective study, vasculitis of lesional skin in dermatomyositis predicted concurrent malignancy[144]. Cancer was diagnosed in four of 12 (25%) with ADM followed for an average of 4.3 years after the patient's diagnosis[135]. The presence of pulmonary fibrosis, myositis-associated or specific serum autoantibodies or a clinically confirmed associated connective tissue disease decreases the likelihood of cancer[138].

A cancer evaluation of high-risk patients could reduce mortality. Recommendations vary widely from careful history and physical examination (including gynecologic examination in women) with routine laboratory screening to age-specific studies with extensive invasive investigations. Given the distribution of tumors noted above, it seems prudent also to include chest, abdominal and pelvic CT, along with fecal blood testing and mammography. As the risk of malignant disease continues to be increased long after the development of dermatomyositis, one needs to follow the patient with myositis carefully for a number of years[137].

The etiology of the link between malignancy and the inflammatory myopathies remains obscure. Speculations include the presence of common environmental factors serving as both carcinogens and triggers of inflammation, paraneoplastic phenomena in which tumor antigens generate an inflammatory response against muscle, or the occurrence of malignant transformation by immunosuppressive agents used to treat patients with polymyositis–dermatomyositis. The last of these seems unlikely, given the close temporal association of myositis with malignancy and the lack of increased risk of malignancy in patients with dermatomyositis treated with cytotoxic drugs[145]. The paraneoplastic theory appears most plausible, given the complete resolution of myositis with cancer resection or chemotherapy-induced remission and the recrudescence of muscle symptoms with tumor recurrence. New onset of dermatomyositis in the setting of tumor recurrence also supports this hypothesis.

Drug-induced myopathy

The frequency of toxic myopathy caused by drugs is unknown, but this condition is likely common and certainly under-diagnosed. Many agents

---

TABLE 139.10 DRUGS ASSOCIATED WITH MYOPATHY

Amiodarone	Fibric acid derivatives	Phenylbutazone
Amphetamines	Heroin	Phenytoin
Chloroquine	Hydralazine	Procainamide
Cimetidine	Hydroxychloroquine	Rifampin
Cocaine	Hydroxyurea	Statin drugs
Colchicine	Ipecac (emetine)	Sulfonamides
Corticosteroids	Levodopa	Tiopronin
Cyclosporin	Nicotinic acid	Vecuronium bromide
Danazol	Pancuronium	Vincristine
Epsilon amino-caproic acid	Penicillamine	Zidovudine (AZT)
Ethanol	Pentazocine	

are myotoxic, including both prescription medicines and drugs with high abuse potential. Table 139.10 lists many drugs associated with myotoxicity. The text below describes those most likely to cause myositis-like disorders, including rhabdomyolysis.

All types of cholesterol-decreasing agents have been shown to be toxic to muscles, and the frequency of myopathy increases with combined lipid-decreasing treatment. The hydroxymethyl glutaryl-coenzyme A reductase inhibitors (the statin drugs) utilize the cytochrome P450 (CYP) system (specifically CYP3A4) in their metabolism, and drug inter-actions may result in an increased concentration of the myotoxic statin when agents that inhibit CYP3A4 are administered concomitantly. Inhibitors of CYP3A4 include erythromycin, clarithromycin, fluconazole, cyclosporine, some calcium channel blockers and even grapefruit juice. The resulting toxic myopathy is characterized by severe myalgias, myositis with weakness and increased CK concentrations, or even rhabdomyolysis[146,147]. Pravastatin alone has been associated with a polymyositis-like illness[148] and caused rhabdomyolysis in a patient with mixed connective tissue disease[149]. Lovastatin led to a muscle and cuta-neous syndrome consistent with dermatomyositis[150] and simvastatin to isolated polymyositis and dermatomyositis with lung involvement[151,152]. Cerivastatin has been withdrawn from the US market because of reports of fatal rhabdomyolysis, occurring most frequently with higher doses, in elderly patients or in combination with another lipid-decreasing agent. The fibric acid derivatives (benzofibrate, clofibrate, gemfibrozil) and niacin also cause myopathy and the risk is increased when one of these drugs is used with a statin.

Although muscle symptoms may occur within days of beginning chol-esterol-decreasing drugs, myotoxic reactions have been reported up to 2 years after the commencement of this form of treatment. The frequency of myopathy is dose-dependent and is increased with renal or hepatic impairment, electrolyte disturbances, defective lipid metabolism, hypothyroidism, drugs of abuse and viral infections. Electromyography reveals myopathic changes with prominent spontaneous potentials and muscle biopsy is characterized by necrosis with or without regenerative fibers or myositis. Recognition is crucial, as most syndromes are reversible on discontinuation of the drug. Persistence of myopathy in some patients treated with statins is poorly understood.

Corticosteroid myopathy is the most common drug-induced muscle problem seen in patients with rheumatic disease. It is characterized by slowly progressive, painless proximal weakness that is worse in the hip girdle. Asthmatic individuals may develop diaphragmatic weakness with an excessive dose of inhaled corticosteroids. Steroid myopathy is clearly dose- and duration-dependent and patients who show prominent Cushingoid features seem more prone to its development. The serum CK concentration is normal and the EMG may be normal or only mildly myopathic. The muscle biopsy demonstrates type II myofiber atrophy, without degeneration, regeneration or inflammatory infiltrates. The treatment is withdrawal or tapering of the drug. Colchicine has well-known adverse neuromuscular effects including muscle weakness and polyneuropathy. The CK concentration is often increased and elec-tromyography demonstrates fibrillations, positive sharp waves and polyphasic myopathic potentials. A vacuolar myopathy with accumula-tion of lysosomes and autophagic vacuoles without necrosis is seen on muscle biopsy. Renal impairment increases the risk of myotoxicity. Recently, colchicine-induced rhabdomyolysis has been reported, also in a patient with impaired renal function[153].

First described in 1963, antimalarial neuromyopathy is an uncommon side effect of chloroquine or hydroxychloroquine. Toxicity does not appear to be dose- or duration-dependent. Patients note the insidious onset of painless symmetric muscle weakness predominantly affecting the lower extremities. Cardiomyopathy has been reported. The muscle biopsy has classic changes of a vacuolar myopathy and electron microscopy shows characteristic curvilinear bodies adjacent to large complex secondary lysosomes[154]. In contrast, the myopathy of SLE (for which antimalarial drugs are frequently prescribed) rarely demonstrates vacuolar change and has no curvilinear bodies[154]. In a retrospective chart review of 214 patients begun on antimalarial treatment over a period of 6 years for various rheumatic disorders, three patients with rheumatoid arthritis (all receiving chloroquine) were identified as having a myopa-thy, giving an incidence of 1 per 100 patient-years (95% confidence inter-val 0.2 to 3)[155]. All patients improved within 2 months of discontinuing the drug.

Hydroxyurea is a chemotherapeutic agent that is commonly used in the treatment of myeloproliferative disorders, particularly chronic myel-ogenous leukemia. Cutaneous lesions resembling dermatomyositis without myositis have been reported with this agent up to 7 years after initiation of treatment[156] and the course is usually benign. D-Penicillamine is known to cause an inflammatory myopathy and myas-thenia gravis. Pentazocine, an injectable analgesic agent, causes a fibrous myopathy adjacent to injection sites, but has recently been shown to produce features of polymyositis in a patient after 13 months of treat-ment[157]. Reversible polymyositis occurred during psoralen and ultra-violet A treatment in a patient with vitiligo[158], and other connective tissue diseases have been reported after psoralen and ultraviolet A treat-ment. IL-2[159], interferon-alpha[160] and other cytokines have been used to treat malignancies and are known to be associated with the development of autoantibodies and other immunologic perturbations, including polymyositis. Vinyl chloride, a known carcinogenic agent that is also associated with the development of a systemic sclerosis-like illness, was recently implicated in the development of anti-Jo-1 antibody-positive polymyositis in a middle-aged man[161].

INVESTIGATIONS

General concepts

The assessment of patients with inflammatory myopathy must take into consideration elements of disease activity as opposed to disease damage[162]. Weakness may be the result of myositis, but also of irrepara-ble damage to muscle in the form of atrophy, fatty replacement and fibrosis; the last will not respond to corticosteroids or other immuno-suppressive agents. Similarly, alveolitis in the lung may be reversible but fibrosis, at least today, is not. Polyarthritis, dermatitis and vasculitis are active disease manifestations. Measures of disease activity and damage are currently being developed and validated for the cross-sectional and longitudinal assessment of patients with polymyositis–dermatomyosi-tis[163]. The lack of such indices hampers the practitioner, who must develop an individualized plan to treat his/her patient, and the researcher, who must gauge treatment response in patients enrolled in therapeutic trials.

Routine tests

Low-grade anemia of chronic disease may be found in patients with inflammatory myopathy. However, anemia should always be thoroughly evaluated at diagnosis, particularly in patients with dermatomyositis, in whom an occult malignancy may be present. The erythrocyte sedimen-tation rate is a poor indicator of disease activity, but it and the C-reac-tive protein may be mildly increased (erythrocyte sedimentation rate 30–50mm/h by the Westergren method).

Serum muscle enzymes

Enzymes that leak from injured skeletal muscle into the serum are valu-able aids in detecting active muscle injury. In order of sensitivity, they are CK, aldolase, aspartate and alanine aminotransferases and lactate dehydrogenase. The finding of increased serum transaminases in a patient with fatigue and muscle weakness often leads to an erroneous diagnosis of hepatitis, and an unnecessary liver biopsy.

The serum CK is believed to be the most reliable enzyme test to use in routine patient care. During a flare of disease, the serum CK will usually increase weeks before overt muscle weakness develops. Conversely, with treatment-induced remission, concentrations of this enzyme decrease to normal before objective improvement in strength. The CK is therefore predictive in the management of patients with myositis. However, there are exceptions, as some patients with active biopsy-proven myositis (dermatomyositis > polymyositis and children > adults) have a normal CK and others have circulating inhibitors of CK activity[164]. There is considerable racial variation in CK concentrations, and one cannot apply reference values from white populations to patients of Afro-Caribbean descent, in whom the upper limit of normal CK is increased[165].

Myoglobin is also released from damaged skeletal muscle and cleared by the kidney. Myoglobinemia may be more sensitive than the serum CK concentration in some patients, but the test is cumbersome and not uniformly available; it can be used as an adjunct to routine measurements of serum muscle enzymes in diagnosis and follow-up. Myoglobinuria is less frequent in patients with myositis, but may be followed by acute tubular necrosis of the kidney, with renal failure[166].

Electromyography

Electrical testing is a sensitive but non-specific method of evaluating inflammatory myopathy. Typical findings include irritability of myofibrils on needle insertion and at rest (fibrillation potentials, complex repetitive discharges, positive sharp waves) and short duration, low-amplitude, complex (polyphasic) potentials on contraction. More than 90% of patients with active myositis will have an abnormal EMG, and a normal EMG is a strong point against active disease. Electromyography continues to be helpful in the selection of a muscle for biopsy and it should be performed unilaterally and a contralateral muscle chosen for biopsy, to avoid the confusion of inflammation artifact as a result of injury from the needle itself.

Later in the course of polymyositis–dermatomyositis, EMG examination may be useful for the detection of low-grade disease activity in the setting of chronic damage from fibrosis or fatty infiltration. Unlike biopsy or MRI studies, EMG enables several muscles to be examined.

The EMG may also be useful in the circumstance of normal serum enzyme concentrations and a physical examination of muscle strength that is difficult to interpret. Corticosteroid myopathy causes some electromyographic changes, but the presence of fibrillation potentials suggests another (inflammatory) process.

Muscle biopsy

Biopsy remains the gold standard with which to confirm the diagnosis of inflammatory myopathy. Chronic inflammatory cells in the perivascular and interstitial areas surrounding myofibrils are present in 80% of cases, and lymphocytic invasion of non-necrotic fibers is considered pathognomonic of polymyositis (Fig. 139.8). Besides lymphocytes, other cells – including histiocytes, plasma cells, eosinophils and polymorphonuclear leukocytes – are often present.

More common than inflammatory infiltrates are degeneration and regeneration of myofibrils, with phagocytosis of necrotic fibers and myofibril regeneration (90% of cases). In chronic myositis, fibrous connective tissue or fat replaces necrotic myofibers.

Muscle histopathology is discussed in Chapter 138. There are important differences noted between polymyositis, inclusion body myositis and dermatomyositis. In dermatomyositis, B cells and the late component of complement (C5–C9, membrane attack complex) predominate in the perivascular area. T cells are mostly CD8+ and cytotoxic, but CD4+ cells are found also. Perifascicular myofibril atrophy (Fig. 139.9), endothelial cell hyperplasia of blood vessels, deposition of immune complexes in the vasculature and frank vasculitis are noted. On quantitative morphologic analysis, muscle capillary depletion and dropout are early findings and myofibril damage results from an ischemic microangiopathy. In contrast, polymyositis and inclusion body myositis feature cytotoxic T cell invasion of myofibrils, with relative sparing of the vasculature. T helper cells may also be found in the perivascular and perimysial areas but, unlike the findings in dermatomyositis, B cells are rarely observed.

Eight of 34 patients with polymyositis in one study had increased numbers of eosinophils in their muscle biopsy specimens (>0.3 eosinophils/mm²), but no concomitant blood eosinophilia[167]. These patients had frequent myalgias, myoglobinuria and greater concentrations of serum muscle enzymes, and responded well to corticosteroid treatment, with a relatively benign clinical course compared with the 26 other myositis patients without tissue eosinophilia. These patients did not have the eosinophilia-myalgia syndrome. Whether or not they represent a separate subset of myositis is not yet certain.

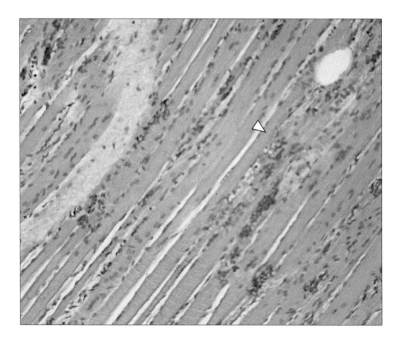

Fig. 139.8 Longitudinal section of fresh-frozen muscle from a patient with polymyositis. Several areas of interstitial involvement, with myofiber destruction, are seen. The arrow indicates an area of degeneration and necrosis of myofibers in association with interstitial lymphocytic and histiocytic cellular infiltration. (Hematoxylin and eosin, medium power.)

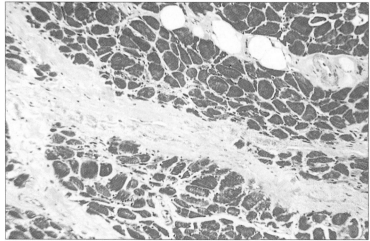

Fig. 139.9 Transverse fresh-frozen section of muscle from a patient with chronic dermatomyositis. Note the atrophic, small fibers in the periphery of the fascicles (perifascicular atrophy) and the increase in fibrous tissue separating bundles of myofibers. (Trichrome stain, low power.)

Despite the characteristic features described above, some patients with active myositis have a normal biopsy, for several reasons. First, the disease is patchy and sampling error precludes 100% sensitivity. Secondly, the wrong muscle may be chosen for biopsy. A weak but not end-stage proximal muscle with EMG abnormalities on the opposite side is the best choice. Open surgical biopsy is the current standard, but percutaneous needle muscle biopsy is a convenient and relatively inexpensive method with a high diagnostic yield in polymyositis–dermatomyositis[168]. Although direct comparison with open techniques is lacking, needle biopsy allows sampling of several muscles with EMG changes, to increase diagnostic sensitivity, and also is useful for detecting other myopathic conditions.

Magnetic resonance imaging

The application of MRI techniques adds an important dimension to our understanding of myositis[169]. MRI is non-invasive and thus has obvious advantages over electromyography and muscle biopsy, particularly in children. Also, large areas of muscle such as both thighs can be visualized, and choosing the most abnormal site can increase the diagnostic yield of biopsy. The T1-weighted image provides excellent anatomic detail, with clear delineation of various muscle groups. Normal tissue is homogeneously dark with a low signal, whereas fat (subcutaneous area and marrow) appears bright, corresponding to a high signal. Muscle is darker on T2-weighted images. Inflammation is bright on both T1 and T2 images. Adding fat suppression in the form of short time inversion recovery (STIR) sequences to the T2 technique improves the detection of muscle inflammation by enhancing the bright signal of inflammation and decreasing the fat signal (dark) (Fig. 139.10). Thus T1-MRI demonstrates damage and chronicity, whereas STIR-MRI shows disease activity. Utilizing these concepts, indications for MRI include (1) documentation of myositis or a disease flare in a patient with a normal CK, EMG or biopsy; (2) confirmation of 'amyopathic dermatomyositis'; (3) distinguishing chronic active from chronic inactive myositis; (4) directing the site of biopsy[170]. Limitations in usefulness remain its expense and focal assessment. Also edema (inflammation on STIR images) is not specific for polymyositis or dermatomyositis, as other inflammatory or even metabolic myopathies may demonstrate similar changes.

Magnetic resonance spectroscopy may provide useful data in conjunction with MRI in children and adults[171]. For example, phosphorus-31 magnetic resonance spectroscopy demonstrated significant differences between patients with amyopathic dermatomyositis and normal controls, indicating inefficient metabolic utilization of ATP and phosphocreatine in the patients dermatomyositis, who had been believed to have no muscle involvement using other objective measures[172].

Other muscle imaging techniques such as ultrasound and CT may have utility in patients with myositis. Ultrasound is commonly available and can image blood flow, but it has a small field of view and cannot provide images deep within muscle. CT provides a larger viewing area and can detect calcification and quantify atrophy, but it cannot detect inflammation in the way that MRI can, and it exposes patients to radiation[169].

Skin

The characteristic cutaneous histopathologic findings of dermatomyositis include focal epidermal atrophy, liquefaction and degeneration of the basal cell layer, and a perivascular or upper dermal mononuclear or lymphocytic infiltrate. Vasculitis or vasculopathy is found in the small vessels of the skin and other organs. Microvascular injury mediated by the terminal components of complement (C_{5b-9}) in the form of the membrane attack complex is well recognized. However, the presence of positive immunofluorescence with immunoglobin or complement staining at the dermal–epidermal junction (i.e. positive lupus band test [LBT]) has been debated. One study noted a positive LBT in only six of 29 patients with dermatomyositis[173], and another found that the presence of a positive LBT correlated strongly with SLE; a negative LBT was seen in dermatomyositis, with a sensitivity of nearly 96%[174]. The latter study emphasized the importance of combining histologic and serologic features to improve sensitivity and specificity; statistically the most powerful predictor of dermatomyositis compared with SLE was the combination of a negative LBT, cutaneous vascular deposition of C_{5b-9} and negative serologic tests for anti-SSA and anti-SSB and anti-U1-RNP antibodies. The variance between the two studies may be the result of the use of different criteria for a positive LBT; lack of standardized criteria will continue to plague interpretation of the literature.

Lung

Reduced ventilatory muscle strength is determined by measuring inspiratory pressures at the mouth. Impaired function results in a weak cough, with an increased risk of aspiration pneumonia. A vital capacity of less than 55% of normal predicts carbon dioxide retention as a result of compromise of the ventilatory musculature. ILD is manifested by restrictive physiology on pulmonary function testing, in addition to reduction in the diffusing capacity for carbon monoxide. The chest radiograph is an insensitive measure of pulmonary interstitial involvement, whereas high-resolution CT can provide greater sensitivity and valuable longitudinal information. High-resolution CT findings include ground-glass opacities (alveolitis), consolidation, subpleural lines or bands, traction bronchiectasis and honeycombing (fibrosis) (Fig. 139.11)[175]. The limiting feature of high-resolution CT is the lack of pathologic correlation in published studies. Radionucleotide gallium scans demonstrate increased radiotracer, and may correlate with active alveolitis and response to treatment, but their sensitivity varies widely among readers.

In an effort to correlate the histologic features of ILD in patients with polymyositis–dermatomyositis with the clinical and radiographic variables, 15 patients with three pathologic patterns were studied: BOOP, interstitial pneumonia and diffuse alveolar damage. Patients with BOOP did well, but all three patients with alveolar damage died[176]. A CD8+ lymphocytic infiltrate is seen in biopsy specimens from patients with ILD who are anti-Jo-1 antibody-positive[177] and CD8+ and DR+ cytotoxic lymphocytes were noted in the bronchoalveolar lavage fluid of eight patients with polymyositis or dermatomyositis and ILD[178].

Other markers are being increasingly reported as indicators of lung involvement in patients with polymyositis–dermatomyositis. Anti-

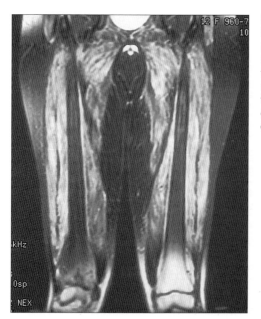

Fig. 139.10
Fat-suppressed MRI. Note the inflammation (white) in the muscles of the thigh in this longitudinal fat-suppressed MRI of a child with active dermatomyositis.

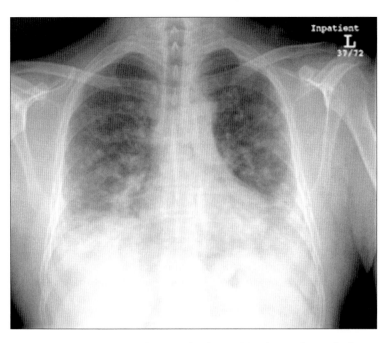

Fig. 139.11 Interstitial lung disease of polymyositis. Chest radiograph of an anti-Jo-1 antibody-positive patient with polymyositis and interstitial lung disease, demonstrating basilar fibrosis and diffuse bilateral interstitial and alveolar infiltrates.

using technitium-99m pyrophosphate or indium-labeled antimyosin may be more sensitive in detecting cardiac abnormalities than electrocardiography or gated blood pool studies[183,184]. The use of endomyocardial biopsy is invasive and subject to sampling error.

The myocardial (MB) fraction of CK (CKMB) is increased in patients with myositis, as a result of the release of this isoenzyme from regenerating myoblasts in damaged skeletal muscle. Search for a more specific enzyme marker of cardiac disease led to the use of cardiac troponin T, but a recent study[185] noted that CKMB was increased in 51% and cardiac troponin T in 41% of patients with myositis who had no clinical evidence of cardiac involvement. Cardiac troponin T has also been shown to be expressed in regenerating skeletal muscle in polymyositis and Duchenne muscular dystrophy, and in normal, non-regenerating skeletal muscle[186]. However, cardiac troponin I was increased in only one of 39 patients with polymyositis or dermatomyositis and now appears to be the most cardiac-specific marker in patients with polymyositis–dermatomyositis[185].

Intestine

In patients with pharyngeal (proximal) dysphagia, the barium swallow shows cricopharyngeal muscle spasm, poorly coordinated motion of the pharyngeal musculature and vallecular pooling of the dye and, occasionally, aspiration of barium into the trachea. Oropharyngeal ultrasound may also aid in serial assessment[187]. Distal dysphagia is most frequently accompanied by esophageal hypomotility demonstrated by cinesophagram or manometry, and may occur in patients with non-overlap myositis. Delayed gastric emptying and small bowel dilatation with hypomotility also are documented by barium studies.

Serum autoantibodies

Serum autoantibodies are commonly found in polymyositis–dermatomyositis and are useful in defining clinically homogeneous subsets of patients. The clinical associations of these autoantibodies are reviewed here, and their relationship to disease pathogenesis is discussed in Chapter 138. Antinuclear autoantibodies or antibodies to cytoplasmic antigens are detected in more than 90% of patients with myositis. Some of these antibodies are termed myositis-specific autoantibodies (MSAs), as they have been previously reported to occur only in patients with features of an inflammatory myopathy. However, the specificity of MSAs is coming under closer scrutiny as more patients without myopathies but having these antibodies are reported[188]. The targets of the MSAs are intracellular antigens (found in all cells) that are commonly involved in protein synthesis, specifically translation. Their role in the pathogenesis of polymyositis–dermatomyositis is unclear; there is no direct evidence that they participate in muscle damage. Autoantibodies typically associated with other connective tissue diseases may also be found in patients with myositis and are termed myositis-associated autoantibodies. Both

endothelial antibodies were found in 20 of 56 patients with myositis and in 10 of 15 with ILD[179]. Their presence did not correlate with antisynthetase antibodies or any particular polymyositis–dermatomyositis subset, but perhaps they relate to pulmonary endothelial damage from a pathogenetic standpoint[179]. KL-6 is a mucinous glycoprotein expressed on type II pneumocytes and bronchiolar epithelial cells. Its concentration is increased non-specifically in the serum of patients with various connective tissue diseases and pneumonitis[180], and decreases over time after treatment for ILD[181]. Cytokeratin 19 fragment (CK19), a cytoskeletal structural protein of bronchial epithelial cells, was measured in 15 patients with myositis, 10 of whom had pulmonary involvement[182]. The CK19 concentrations were significantly greater in individuals with lung disease, and changed as expected with progression or improvement of ILD.

Heart

Cardiac findings are unusual at disease onset in polymyositis–dermatomyositis, but functional heart problems often develop later. Electrocardiographic abnormalities are common, including non-specific ST–T segment changes and various conduction block disturbances. Holter monitoring can detect arrhythmias and cardiac scintigraphy

	Frequency (%)				
Autoantibody	Adult polymyositis	Adult dermatomyositis	Childhood myositis	Overlap	Clinical features
Jo-1	20–30	5	<5	10	Antisynthetase syndrome
PM-Scl	10	<5	5–10	10	Predominantly overlap with systemic sclerosis
U1-RNP	10	5	5–10	30–40	Predominantly overlap with SLE; MCTD
Mi-2		10	5		Classic rash of DM; good response to treatment
SRP	<5		<1%		Severe muscle weakness; no DM rash
PL-7, PL-12, EJ, OJ, KS	<5				Antisynthetase syndrome
PMS-1[194]	8				No unique features
Ku				5	Polymyositis-scleroderma overlap

TABLE 139.11 SERUM AUTOANTIBODIES IN SUBSETS OF PATIENTS WITH POLYMYOSITIS AND DERMATOMYOSITIS

DM, dermatomyositis; MCTD, mixed connective tissue disease.

TABLE 139.12 ANTIAMINOACYL-tRNA SYNTHETASE ANTIBODIES AND THEIR ASSOCIATED ANTIGENS IN POLYMYOSITIS–DERMATOMYOSITIS

Antibody	Antigen	PM–DM patients with antibody (%)
Anti-Jo-1	Histidyl-tRNA synthetase	20
Anti-PL-7	Threonyl-tRNA synthetase	2
Anti-PL-12	Alanyl-tRNA synthetase	1
Anti-OJ	Isoleucyl-tRNA synthetase	1
Anti-EJ	Glycyl-tRNA synthetase	1
Anti-KS	Asparaginyl-tRNA synthetase	<1

PM–DM, polymyositis–dermatomyositis.

MSAs and myositis-associated autoantibodies and their clinical associations are outlined in Table 139.11. Although some patients have more than one autoantibody in their serum, several MSAs are rarely detected in the same patient[189,190]. The frequency of antibody positivity is lower in some myositis subsets such as inclusion body myositis and malignancy-associated myositis, but a negative antinuclear antibody test does not imply that an MSA is absent, as the latter antigens are cytoplasmic in location and the immunoflurorescence staining pattern may be subtle. Testing for serum autoantibodies can both solidify the diagnosis of myositis in patients with atypical clinical features and provide prognostic information regarding the likelihood of future clinical complications.

The MSAs are relatively insensitive markers for myositis. Anti-Jo-1 is the most common MSA and is one of a group of anti-aminoacyl-tRNA synthetases (Table 139.12). Anti-Jo-1 is directed against histidyl-tRNA synthetase, an enzyme that binds histidine to its cognate transfer RNA (tRNA[his]) so that the amino acid can be incorporated into a growing polypeptide chain. The clinical associations of the various antisynthetase antibodies are similar, and have been described previously as comprising the 'antisynthetase syndrome'. The myositis component of antisynthetase antibody-positive patients is often severe with multiple flares, requiring immunosuppressive agents in addition to corticosteroids. Not all patients with an antisynthetase will manifest all features of the syndrome and some will never develop myositis[84]. For example, anti-PL-12 antibody-positive patients are more likely to have ILD without myositis. Other extramuscular features include fever, inflammatory arthritis, Raynaud's phenomenon and mechanic's hands (see earlier sections and Fig. 139.6). The anti-aminocyl-tRNA autoantibody, anti-WS, binds the L-shaped tertiary structure of tRNA and is therefore different from the other antisynthetases, but patients with this antibody also have recurrent fever, polyarthritis and Raynaud's phenomenon without myositis[191], similar to patients with anti-tRNA synthetases. Antibodies against tRNA or tRNA-associated proteins may also be associated with SLE and Sjögren's syndrome[192]

Antibodies to signal recognition particle (anti-SRP) comprise a separate subgroup of MSAs targeting a ribonucleoprotein involved in translocation. To date, all reported patients with this antibody have pure polymyositis, which is generally refractory to treatment, and progressive. There are no pulmonary, articular or systemic manifestations, but the frequency of cardiomyopathy with congestive heart failure is increased. Anti-Mi-2 is an antinuclear antibody directed against a presumed helicase[193], is strongly associated with the rash of dermatomyositis and has been detected in childhood dermatomyositis and in some patients with malignancy. In general, patients positive for anti-Mi-2 have a favorable response to treatment, but the rash can be severe. A recently described antibody to the DNA mismatch repair enzyme, PMS1, was found in 7.5% of a series of 153 myositis sera and has been proposed as a new MSA[194]. No unique or distinguishing clinical features were identified.

Anti-PM-Scl is an antinucleolar antibody that identifies a subset of patients with myositis who also often have features of systemic sclerosis. It has been seen in patients with polymyositis, dermatomyositis or systemic sclerosis alone, and in patients without evidence of either myositis or scleroderma[195]. Anti-U1-RNP antibodies result in a high-titer speckled antinuclear antibody profile and occur in patients with the so-called 'mixed connective tissue disease'; they may have clinical findings of Raynaud's disease, SLE, polymyositis or dermatomyositis or systemic sclerosis, or any combination thereof.

NATURAL HISTORY OF DISEASE

In some patients, dermatomyositis (but seldom polymyositis) is an illness of brief duration followed by remission that does not require continued treatment. The majority of patients, however, have several exacerbations and remissions or persistent disease activity necessitating chronic use of corticosteroids or immunosuppressive drugs. The frequency of clinical and biochemical relapse was found to be 60% in a series of 50 patients with polymyositis, dermatomyositis and overlap syndrome followed closely for a mean of 13 years[196]. The rates of relapse were similar in each of these patient groups and no features predisposing to relapse were identified. Milder, more easily controlled myositis is reported in community studies as compared with series based on medical centers[197].

With each episode of myositis, there is the potential for absolute loss of muscle mass. The rate of progression and amount of muscle loss differ according to clinical classification and serum autoantibody subtype. The best functional outcome occurs in dermatomyositis, whereas the worst is in inclusion body myositis and polymyositis with anti-SRP antibody. Another poor prognostic feature may be an excess of muscle fibers with absent cytochrome oxidase staining and mitochondrial DNA deletions, but clinically these patients resemble individuals with inclusion body myositis[198].

In childhood-onset dermatomyositis, several predictors of chronic active myositis have been identified, including failure to achieve normal muscle strength after 4 months of corticosteroid treatment, continued increased serum muscle enzyme beyond 3 months and increased plasma von-Willebrand factor antigen over 10 months[199]. Anasarca with hypoalbuminemia has been reported to be an indicator of severe disease in this subset of patients[200].

PROGNOSIS

Assessment of prognosis in polymyositis–dermatomyositis is difficult, for several reasons[201]. First, the disease is relatively uncommon. Some studies involve single referral centers reporting retrospectively on small numbers of patients followed for brief periods of time. Secondly, many reports are cross-sectional in design and combine patients with early and late-stage disease. Thirdly, a classification system with disease subsets based on meaningful pathophysiologic and serologic data has not been developed. Finally, objective criteria for improvement (or deterioration) are not standardized. Today, we lack long-term prospective follow-up of well-defined incident cohorts of patients with myositis that have utilized validated outcome measures[201].

Survival

Studies published before the availability of corticosteroids reveal that a high proportion (up to 50%) of untreated patients with polymyositis–dermatomyositis seen at major medical centers died of its complications[201] (Table 139.13). Although there is no double-blind placebo-controlled documentation of their effect, virtually all investigators agree, and mortality rates demonstrate (Table 139.13), that corticosteroids have improved both muscle weakness and survival during the past 30 years[202–213]. Because of this nearly universal acceptance, for ethical

TABLE 139.13 MORTALITY STATISTICS AND PROGNOSTIC FEATURES OF SEVERAL POLYMYOSITIS–DERMATOMYOSITIS SERIES STRATIFIED BY TREATMENT AND DECADE OF PATIENT ENTRY

Author (year)	Dates of patient entry	No. of patients	Mean follow-up from entry (years)	Mortality rate (%)	Comments
Non-corticosteroid-treated patients					
O'Leary and Waisman[202] (1940)	1926–1939	38	Not stated	50	36/38 with dermatomyositis
Sheard[203] (1951)	1927–1950	25	5.0	52	22/25 with dermatomyositis; 5/7 younger than 20 years died
Winkelmann[204] (1968)	Before 1959	122	3.0	29	(See below)
Corticosteroid-treated patients					**Poor prognostic features**
Rose[26] (1966)	1954–1964	89	6.1	30	Malignancy, other connective tissue disease, acute course
Winkelmann et al.[204] (1968)	Before 1959	157	3.0	35	Malignancy, scleroderma, rapid progression
Medsger et al.[205] (1971)	1947–1968	124	2.5 (median)	36	Pulmonary infiltrates, dysphagia, severe weakness, age >50 years, black race
Carpenter et al.[206] (1977)	1947–1971	62	Not stated	45	Dysphagia, severe weakness
Bohan et al.[207] (1977)	1956–1971	153	4.3	14	Malignancy, older age, delayed treatment
Benbassat et al.[208] (1985)	1956–1976	92	1.8	32	Dysphagia, older age, leukocytosis, fever, failure to induce remission, shorter disease remission
Riddoch and Morgan-Hughes[209] (1975)	1960–1970	20	5.0	40	Study excluded children and patients with cancer and connective tissue disease
Henriksson and Sandstedt[210] (1982)	1967–1978	107	5.0	23	Malignancy, older age, delayed treatment, cardiac involvement
Hochberg et al.[211] (1986)	1970–1981	76	Not stated	17	Age >45 years, cardiac involvement
Tymms and Webb[212] (1985)	1970–1982	105	4.0	18	Older age, delayed treatment
Maugars et al.[213] (1996)	1973–1984	69	11.6	33 (at 5 years)	DM: older age, cancer, interstitial lung disease, asthenia-anorexia; PM: older age, failure to improve muscle strength after 1 month of treatment; absence of myalgia at onset

DM, dermatomyositis; PM, polymyositis.
(Modified with permission from Oddis and Medsger[201].)

reasons, corticosteroids cannot be withheld in today's controlled prospective trials.

During the 1960s, three large series described 265 patients followed for 1.8–5.0 years, with mortality rates varying from 14% to 40%[207–209]. A similar three-study composite of 288 patients reported during the 1970s had only 56 (19%) deaths[210–212]. At the present time, the expected mortality in incident cases of polymyositis–dermatomyositis, excluding those associated with malignancy, is less than 10% at 5 years after initial diagnosis. The reasons for improved survival in recent years are unclear, but may include earlier diagnosis, detection of milder cases, better general medical care and more judicious use of immunosuppressive drugs.

Factors associated with poor survival in these reports include older age, malignancy, delayed initiation of corticosteroid treatment, pharyngeal dysphagia with aspiration pneumonia, ILD, myocardial involvement and complications of corticosteroid or immunosuppressive treatment. Additional adverse risk factors for survival among patients with childhood dermatomyositis are gastrointestinal vasculitis and sepsis[214].

The 5-year cumulative survival rate from the time of first physician diagnosis is worst for cancer-associated myositis (55%) and dermatomyositis (80%) and best for connective tissue disease related myositis (85%) and inclusion body myositis (95%). Among the serum autoantibodies, anti-SRP is the worst prognostic marker (5-year survival 30%), followed by the antisynthetase group (65%). The best survival is among patients with anti-PM-Scl (95%) and anti-Mi-2 (95%).

Disability

The determinants of functional status in polymyositis–dermatomyositis are quite different from those of survival. For example, inclusion body myositis has the worst functional outlook, but a good survival because of the lack of visceral involvement. For all types of myositis, each major exacerbation results in a reduction in muscle strength, but treatment almost never improves the patient to the preceding level of total body muscle mass or strength. Fortunately, minor residual atrophy and weakness in one or more muscle groups most often do not translate into functional impairment.

In one 20-year follow-up study of 118 patients, 67% of the 82 survivors had no functional disability[215]. In another report, 87% of 107 patients who improved initially with medical treatment had minimal or no disability after a mean follow-up of 5 years[210]. In a prospective longitudinal study, the patient-completed Health Assessment Questionnaire was used to follow a national cohort of 257 patients with polymyositis–dermatomyositis during years 3–7 after disease diagnosis[216]. Disability (judged by the Health Assessment Questionnaire disability index) increased with disease duration. In individuals with increased disability early in disease, the disability index was highly correlated with the corticosteroid treatment-related complications of osteonecrosis and osteoporotic compression fractures of the lumbar spine.

A childhood Health Assessment Questionnaire for measuring disability in juvenile dermatomyositis has been validated[217]. Children with dermatomyositis have been shown to have decreased calcium absorption, especially while receiving corticosteroids[218], and may thus be at much greater risk for osteoporosis when they become adults. Other disease-related sequelae include calcinosis (especially in juvenile dermatomyositis), arthropathy, Raynaud's phenomenon, respiratory insufficiency as a result of pulmonary interstitial fibrosis or diaphragmatic muscle involvement, and myocardial involvement with congestive heart failure or ventricular arrhythmias.

The contribution of corticosteroid and immunosuppressive drug toxicity to long-term disability has not been adequately addressed, but the frequency of serious adverse reactions has been reported to be 20–40%[12,197,210,212]. The most commonly encountered disabling side effects include osteoporotic bone fractures, osteonecrosis, serious bacterial and fungal infections, and cataracts. Problems that are inconvenient and require frequent physician visits, expensive medications and toxicity monitoring are diabetes mellitus, hypertension and peptic ulcer disease. Early cytopenias, with complications including septicemia, and late hematologic malignancies are serious concerns in patients with myositis requiring immunosuppressive drugs.

REFERENCES

1. Potain. Morve chronique de formed anomale. Bull Soc Méd Paris 1875; 12: 314–318.
2. Wagner EL. Erin Fall von Polymyositis. Dtsch Arch Klin Med 1886; 40: 241–266.
3. Jacoby GW. Subacute progressive polymyositis. J Nerv Ment Dis 1888; 13: 697–726.
4. Unverricht H. Dermatomyositis acuta. Dtsch Med Wochenschr 1891; 17: 41–44.
5. Gottron H. In: Proceedings of the Berlin Dermatologic Society. Dermatol Z 1930; 61: 415–418.
6. Stertz. Polymyositis. Berl Klin Wochenschr 1916; 53: 489.
7. Kankeleit. Über primäre nichteitrige Polymyositis. Dtsch Arch Klin Med 1916; 120: 335–349.
8. Beczeny R. Dermatomyositis. Arch Derm Syph 1935; 171: 242–251.
9. Chou SM. Myxovirus-like structures in a case of human chronic polymyositis. Science 1967; 158: 1453–1455.
10. Yunis EJ, Samaha FJ. Inclusion body myositis. Lab Invest 1971; 25: 240–248.
11. Medsger TA Jr, Oddis CV. Classification and diagnostic criteria for PM and DM [editorial]. J Rheumatol 1995; 22: 581–585.
12. Bohan A, Peter JB. Polymyositis and dermatomyositis. N Engl J Med 1975; 292: 344–347, 403–407.
13. Medsger TA Jr. Polymositis and dermatomyositis. In: Lawrence RC, Shulman LE, eds. Epidemiology of the rheumatic diseases. New York: Gower Medical Publishing; 1984: 176–180.
14. Targoff IN, Miller FW, Medsger TA Jr et al. Classification criteria for the idiopathic inflammatory myopathies. Curr Opin Rheumatol 1997; 9: 527–535.
15. Hausmanowa-Petruseqicz I, Kowalska-Oledzka E, Miller FW et al. Clinical, serologic, and immunogenetic features in Polish patients with idiopathic inflammatory myopathies. Arthritis Rheum 1997; 40: 1257–1266.
16. Okano Y, Steen VD, Medsger TA Jr. Autoantibody to U3 nucleolar ribonucleoprotein (fibrillarin) in patients with systemic sclerosis. Arthritis Rheum 1992; 35: 95–100.
17. Ioannou Y, Sultan S, Isenberg DA. Myositis overlap syndromes. Curr Opin Rheumatol 1999; 11: 468–474.
18. Miro' O, Pedrol EN, Casademont J et al. Muscle involvement in rheumatoid arthritis: clinicopathological study of 21 symptomatic cases. Semin Arthritis Rheum 1996; 25: 421–428.
19. Garton MJ, Isenberg DA. Clinical features of lupus myositis versus idiopathic myositis: a review of 30 cases. Br J Rheumatol 1997; 36: 1067–1074.
20. Gran JT, Myklebust G. The concomitant occurrence of Sjögren's syndrome and polymyositis. Scan J Rheumatol 1992, 21: 150–154.
21. De Vlam K, De Keyser F, Goemaere S et al. Churg–Strauss syndrome presenting as polymyositis. Clin Exp Rheumatol 1995; 13: 505–507.
22. Al Attia HM, Ezzeddin H, Khader T et al. A localised morphoea/idiopathic polymyositis overlap. Clin Rheumatol 1996; 15: 307–309.
23. Dunne JW, Heye N, Edis RH et al. Necrotizing inflammatory myopathy associated with localized scleroderma. Muscle Nerve 1996; 19: 1040–1042.
24. Miyaoka Y, Urano Y, Nameda Y et al. A case of dermatomyositis complicated by thrombotic thrombocytopenic purpura. Dermatology 1997; 194: 68–71.
25. Sherer Y, Livneh A, Levy Y et al. Dermatomyositis and polymyositis associated with the antiphospholipid syndrome – a novel overlap syndrome. Lupus 2000; 9: 42–46.
26. Rose AL, Walton JN. Polymyositis. A survey of 89 cases with particular reference to treatment and prognosis. Brain 1966; 89: 747–768.
27. Kurland LT, Hauser WA, Ferguson RH et al. Epidemiologic features of diffuse connective tissue disorders in Rochester, Minnesota, 1951–1967, with special reference to systemic lupus erythematosus. Mayo Clin Proc 1969; 44: 649–663.
28. Findlay GH, Whiting DA, Simson IW. Dermatomyositis in the Transvaal and its occurrence in the Bantu. S Afr Med J 1969; 43: 694–697.
29. Medsger TA, Dawson WN, Masi AT. The epidemiology of polymyositis. Am J Med 1970; 48: 715–723.
30. Benbassat J, Geffel D, Zlotnick A. Epidemiology of polymyositis–dermatomyositis in Israel, 1960–76. Isr J Med Sci 1980; 16: 197–200.
31. Oddis CV, Conte CG, Steen VD et al. Incidence of PM-DM. A 20-year study of hospital diagnosed cases in Allegheny County, PA 1963–1982. J Rheumatol 1990; 17: 1329–1334.
32. Weitoft T. Occurrence of polymyositis in the country of Gavleborg, Sweden. Scand J Rheumatol 1997; 26: 104–106.
33. Patrick M, Buchbinder R, Jolley D et al. Incidence of inflammatory myopathies in Victoria, Australia, and evidence of spatial clustering. J Rheumatol 1999; 26: 1094–1100.
34. Badrising UA, Maat-Schieman M, van Duninen SG et al. Epidemiology of inclusion body myositis in the Netherlands: a nationwide study. Neurology 2000; 55: 1385–1387.
35. Hengstman GJD, van Venrooij WJ, Vencovsky J et al. The relative prevalence of dermatomyositis and polymyositis in Europe exhibits a latitudinal gradient. Ann Rheum Dis 2000; 59: 141–142.
36. Christensen ML, Pachman LM, Schneiderman R et al. Prevalence of Coxsackie B virus antibodies in patients with juvenile dermatomyositis. Arthritis Rheum 1986; 29: 1365–1370.
37. Hoffman JC, Stichtenoth DO, Zeidler H et al. Lyme disease in a 74-year-old forest owner with symptoms of dermatomyositis. Arthritis Rheum 1995; 38: 1157–1160.
38. Sherman MP, Amin RM, Rodgers-Johnson PEB et al. Identification of human T cell leukemia/lymphoma virus type I antibodies, DNA, and protein in patients with polymyositis. Arthritis Rheum 1995; 38: 690–698.
39. Baguley E, Wolfe C, Hughes GRV. Dermatomyositis in HIV infection [letter]. Br J Rheumatol 1988; 27: 493–494.
40. Dennett X, Siejka SJ, Andrews JRH et al. Polymyositis caused by a new genus of nematode. Med J Aust 1998; 168: 226–227.
41. Perez C, Gurtubay I, Martinez-Ibanex F et al. More on polymyositis associated with mycoplasma pneumoniae infection. Scan J Rheumatol 1999; 28: 125.
42. Lyon ME, Bloch DA, Hollak B et al. Predisposing factors in PM–DM: results of a nationwide survey. J Rheumatol 1989; 16: 1218–1224.
43. Fernandes L, Swinson DR, Hamilton EBD. Dermatomyositis complicating penicillamine treatment. Ann Rheum Dis 1977; 36: 94–95.
44. Hanke CW, Thomas JA, Lee EW-T et al. Risk assessment of polymyositis/dermatomyositis after treatment with injectable bovine collagen implants. J Am Acad Dermatol 1996; 34: 450–454.
45. Harati Y, Niakan E, Bergman EW. Childhood dermatomyositis in monozygotic twins. Neurology 1986; 36: 721–723.
46. Leonhardt T. Familial occurrence of collagen diseases. II. Progressive systemic sclerosis and dermatomyositis. Acta Med Scand 1961; 169: 735–742.
47. Davies MG, Hickling P. Familial adult dermatomyositis. Br J Dermatol 2001; 144: 415–448.
48. Rider LG, Gurley RC, Pandey JP et al. Clinical, serologic, and immunogenetic features of familial idiopathic inflammatory myopathy. Arthritis Rheum 1998; 41: 710–719.
49. Ginn LR, Lin J-P, Plotz PH et al. Familial autoimmunity in pedigrees of idiopathic inflammatory myopathy patients suggests common genetic risk factors for many autoimmune diseases. Arthritis Rheum 1998; 41: 400–405.
50. Shamim EA, Rider LG, Miller FW. Update on the genetics of the idiopathic inflammatory myopathies. Curr Opin Rheum 2000; 12: 482–491.
51. Reed AM, Pachman LM, Hayford J et al. Immunogenetic studies in families of children with juvenile dermatomyositis. J Rheumatol 1998; 25: 1000–1002.
52. West JE, Reed AM. Analysis of HLA-DM polymorphism in juvenile dermatomyositis (JDM) patients. Hum Immunol 1999; 60: 255–258.
53. Rider LG, Artlett CM, Foster CB et al: Polymorphisms in the IL-1 receptor antagonist gene VNTR are possible risk factors for juvenile idiopathic inflammatory myopathies. Clin Exp Immunol 2000; 120: 1–7.
54. Pachman LM, Liotta-Davis M, Hong D, et al. TNF alpha-308A allele in juvenile dermatomyositis: associations with increased production of tumor necrosis factor alpha, disease duration, and pathologic calcifications. Arthritis Rheum 2000; 43: 2368–2377.
55. Bogoussanvsky JE, Perentes E, Regli F, Deruaz JP. Polymyositis with severe facial involvement. J Neurol 1982; 228: 277–281.
56. Csuka ME, McCarty DJ. A rapid method for measurement of lower extremity muscle strength. Am J Med 1985; 78: 77–81.
57. Helewa A, Goldsmith CH, Smythe HA. Patient, observer and instrument variation in the measurement of strength of shoulder abductor muscles in patients with rheumatoid arthritis using a modified sphygmomanometer. J Rheumatol 1986; 6: 1044–1049.
58. Stoll T, Bruehlmann P, Stucki G et al. Muscle strength assessment in polymyositis and dermatomyositis: evaluation of the reliability and clinical use of a new, quantitative, easily applicable method. J Rheumatol 1995; 22: 473–477.
59. Kasteler JS, Callen JP. Scalp involvement in dermatomyositis. JAMA 1994; 272: 1939–1941.
60. Oddis CV, Okano Y, Rudert WA et al. Serum autoantibody to the nucleolar antigen PM-Scl. Arthritis Rheum 1992; 35: 1211–1217.
61. Sabroe RA, Wallington TB, Kennedy CTC. Dermatomyositis treated with high-dose intravenous immunoglobulins and associated with panniculitis. Clin Exp Dermatol 1995; 20: 164–167.
62. Chao Y-Y, Yang L-J. Dermatomyositis presenting as panniculitis. Int J Dermatol 2000; 39: 141–144.
63. Molnar K, Kemeny L, Korom I et al. Panniculitis in dermatomyositis: report of two cases. Br J Dermatol 1998; 139: 161–163.
64. Ishikawa O, Tamura A, Ryuzaki K et al. Membranocystic changes in the panniculitis of dermatomyositis. Br J Dermatol 1996; 134: 773–776.
65. Kimball AB, Summers RM, Turner M et al. Magnetic resonance imaging detection of occult skin and subcutaneous abnormalities in juvenile dermatomyositis. Arthritis Rheum 2000; 43: 1866–1873.
66. Nousari HC, Ha VT, Laman SD et al. 'Centripetal flagellate erythema': a cutaneous manifestation associated with dermatomyositis. J Rheumatol 1999; 26: 692–695.
67. Ferrer M, Herranz P, Manzano R et al. Dermatomyositis with linear lesions. Br J Dermatol 1996; 134: 600–601.

68. Requena L, Grilli R, Soriano L et al. Dermatomyositis with a pityriasis rubra pilaris-like eruption: a little-known distinctive cutaneous manifestation of dermatomyositis. Br J Dermatol 1997; 136: 768–771.

69. See Y, Rooney M, Woo P. Palmar plantar hyperkeratosis – a previously undescribed skin manifestation of juvenile dermatomyositis. Br J Rheumatol 1997; 36: 917–919.

70. Katayama I, Sawada Y, Nishioka K. The seborrhoeic pattern of dermatomyositis. Br J Dermatol 1999; 140: 978–979.

71. Del Pozo J, Almagro M, Martinez W et al. Dermatomyositis and mucinosis. Int J Dermatol 2001; 40: 120–124.

72. Inuzuka M, Tomita K, Tokura Y et al. Acquired ichthyosis associated with dermatomyositis in a patient with hepatocellular carcinoma. Br J Dermatol 2001; 14: 416–417.

73. McCollough ML, Cockrell CJ. Vesiculo-bullous dermatomyositis. Am J Dermatopathol 1998; 20: 170–174.

74. Sontheimer RD. Cutaneous features of classic dermatomyositis and amyopathic dermatomyositis. Cur Opin Rheumatol 1999; 11: 475–482.

75. Osman Y, Narita M, Kishi K et al. Case report: amyopathic dermatomyositis associated with transformed malignant lymphoma. Am J Med Sci 1996; 311: 240–242.

76. Whitmore SE, Watson R, Rosenshein NB et al. Dermatomyositis sine myositis: association with malignancy. J Rheumatol 1996; 23: 1010–1015.

77. Mukamel M, Horev G, Mimouni M. New insight into calcinosis of juvenile dermatomyositis: a study of composition and treatment. J Pediatr 2001; 138: 763–766.

78. Tse S, Lubelsky S, Gordon M et al. The arthritis of inflammatory childhood myositis syndromes. J Rheumatol 2001; 28: 192–197.

79. Wasko MC, Carlson GW, Tomaino MM et al. Dermatomyositis with erosive arthropathy: association with the anti-PL-7 antibody. J Rheumatol 1999; 26: 2693–2694.

80. Oddis CV, Medsger TA Jr, Cooperstein LA. A subluxing arthropathy associated with the anti Jo-1 antibody in polymyositis/dermatomyositis. Arthritis Rheum 1990; 33: 1640–1645.

81. Citera G, Lazaro MA, Cocco JAM et al. Apatite deposition in polymyositis subluxing arthropathy. J Rheumatol 1996; 23: 551–553.

82. Brennan MT, Patronas NJ, Brahim J. Bilateral condylar resorption in dermatomyositis: a case report. Oral Surg Oral Med Oral Pathol 1999; 87: 446–451.

83. Queiro-Silva R, Banegil I, deDios-Jimenez de Aberassturi JR et al. Periarticular calcinosis associated with anti-Jo-1 antibodies sine myositis. Expanding the clinical spectrum of the antisynthetase syndrome. J Rheumatol 2001; 28: 1401–1404.

84. Friedman AW, Targoff IN, Arnett FC. Interstitial lung disease with autoantibodies against aminoacyl-tRNA synthetases in the absence of clinically apparent myositis. Semin Arthritis Rheum 1996; 26: 459–467.

85. Chow SK, Yeap SS. Amyopathic dermatomyositis and pulmonary fibrosis. Clin Rheumatol 2001; 19: 484–485.

86. Selva-O'Callaghan A, Sanchez-Sitjes L, Munoz-Gall X et al. Respiratory failure due to muscle weakness in inflammatory myopathies: maintenance therapy with home mechanical ventilation. Br J Rheumatol 2000; 39: 914–916.

87. Rini BI, Gajewski TF. Polymyositis with respiratory muscle weakness requiring mechanical ventilation in a patient with metastatic thymoma treated with octreotide. Ann Oncol 1999; 10: 913–919.

88. Braun NMT, Aroyan S, Rochester DF. Respiratory muscle and pulmonary function in polymyositis and other proximal myopathies. Thorax 1983; 38: 616–623.

89. Clawson K, Oddis CV. Adult respiratory distress syndrome in polymyositis patients with the anti-Jo-1 antibody. Arthritis Rheum 1995; 38: 1519–1523.

90. Schwarz MI, Sutarik JM, Nick JA et al. Pulmonary capillaritis and diffuse alveolar hemorrhage. A primary manifestation of polymyositis. J Respir Crit Care Med 1995; 151: 2037–2040.

91. Horiki T, Fuyuno G, Ishii M et al. Fatal alveolar hemorrhage in a patient with mixed connective tissue disease presenting polymyositis features. Intern Med 1998; 37: 554–560.

92. Fata F, Rathore R, Schiff C et al. Bronchiolitis obliterans organizing pneumonia as the first manifestation of polymyositis. South Med J 1997; 90: 227–230.

93. Knoell KA, Hook M, Grice DP et al. Dermatomyositis associated with bronchiolitis obliterans organizing pneumonia (BOOP). J Am Acad Dermatol 1999; 40: 328–330.

94. Jansen TLTA, Barrera P, van Engelen BGM et al. Dermatomyositis with subclinical myositis and spontaneous pneumomediastinum with pneumothorax: case report and review of the literature. Clin Exp Rheumatol 1998; 16: 733–735.

95. Yamanishi Y, Maeda H, Konishi F et al. Dermatomyositis associated with rapidly progressive fatal interstitial pneumonitis and pneumomediastinum. Scand J Rheumatol 1999; 28: 58–61.

96. Kono H, Inokuma S, Nakayama H et al. Pneumomediastinum in dermatomyositis: association with cutaneous vasculopathy. Ann Rheum Dis 2000; 59: 372–376.

97. Korkmaz C, Ozkan R, Akay M et al. Pneumomediastinum and subcutaneous emphysema associated with dermatomyositis. Rheumatology 2001; 40: 476–478.

98. Bachelez H, Schremmer B, Cadranel J et al. Fulminant Pneumocystis carinii pneumonia in patients with dermatomyositis. Arch Intern Med 1997; 157: 1501–1503.

99. LaCivita L, Battiloro R, Celano M. Nocardia pleural empyema complicating anti-Jo-1 positive polymyositis during immunoglobulin and steroid therapy. J Rheumatol 2001; 28: 215–216.

100. Gonzalez-Lopez L, Gamez-Nava JI, Sanchez L et al. Cardiac manifestations in dermato–polymyositis. Clin Exp Rheumatol 1996; 14: 373–379.

101. Gordon M-M, Madhok R. Fatal myocardial necrosis. Ann Rheum Dis 1999; 58: 198–199.

102. Chraibi S, Ibnabdeljalil H, Habbal R et al. Pericardial tamponade as the first manifestation of dermatopolymyositis. Ann Med Intern 1998; 149: 464–466.

103. Lie JT. Cardiac manifestations in polymyositis/dermatomyositis: how to get to the heart of the matter. J Rheumatol 1995; 22: 809–811.

104. Anders H-J, Wandes A, Rihl M et al. Myocardial fibrosis in polymyositis. J Rheumatol 1999; 26: 1840–1842.

105. Badui El, Valdespino A, Lepe L et al. Acute myocardial infarction with normal coronary arteries in a patient with dermatomyositis. Angiology 1996; 47: 815–818.

106. Riemekasten G , Optiz C, Audring H et al. Beware of the heart: the multiple picture of cardiac involvement in myositis. Br J Rheumatol 1999; 38: 1153–1157.

107. Shapiro J, DeGirolami U, Martin S et al. Inflammatory myopathy causing pharyngeal dysphagia: a new entity. Ann Otol Rhinol Laryngol 1996; 105: 331–335.

108. Caramaschi P, Biasi D, Carletto A et al. Megaesophagus in a patient affected by dermatomyositis. Clin Rheumatol 1997; 16: 106–107.

109. Kuroda T, Ohfuchi Y, Hirose S et al. Pneumatosis cystoides intestinalis in a patient with polymyositis. Clin Rheumatol 2001; 20: 49–52.

110. Eshraghi N, Farahmand M, Maerz LL et al. Adult-onset dermatomyositis with severe gastrointestinal manifestations: case report and review of the literature. Surgery 1998; 123: 356–358.

111. Braun-Moscovici Y, Schapira D, Balbir-Gurman A et al. Inflammatory bowel disease and myositis. Clin Rheumatol 1999; 18: 261–263.

112. Voigt E, Griga T, Tromm A et al. Polymyositis of the skeletal muscles as an extraintestinal complication in quiescent ulcerative colitis. Int J Colorectal Dis 1999; 14: 304–307.

113. Bondeson J, Veress B, Lindroth Y et al. Polymyositis associated with asymptomatic primary biliary cirrhosis. Clin Exp Rheumatol 1998; 16; 172–174.

114. Seibold F, Klein R, Jakob F. Polymyositis, alopecia universalis, and primary sclerosing cholangitis in a patient with Crohn's disease. J Clin Gastroenterol 1996; 22: 121–124.

115. Russo RAG, Katsicas MM, Davila M et al. Cholestasis in juvenile dermatomyositis. Arthritis Rheum 2001; 44: 1139–1142.

116. Evron E, Abarbanel JM, Branski D et al. Polymyositis, arthritis, and proteinuria in a patient with adult celiac disease. J Rheumatol 1996; 23: 782–783.

117. Oddis CV. Inflammatory diseases of blood vessels. Hoffman GS, Weyand CM, eds. New York: Marcel Dekker, Inc.; 2001: 665–674.

118. Thakur V, DeSalvo J, McGrath J Jr et al. Case report: polymyositis-induced myoglobinuric acute renal failure. Am J Med Sci 1996; 312: 85–87.

119. Yeo LMW, Swaby DSA, Situnayake RD et al. Irreversible visual loss in dermatomyositis. Br J Rheumatol 1995; 34: 1179–1181.

120. Backhouse O, Griffiths B, Henderson T et al. Ophthalmic manifestations of dermatomyositis. Ann Rheum Dis 1998; 57: 447–449.

121. Orrell RW, Johnston HM, Gibson C et al. Spontaneous abdominal hematoma in dermatomyositis. Muscle Nerve 1998; 21: 1800–1803.

122. Tubridy N, Wells C, Lewis D et al. Unsuccessful treatment with cidofovir and cytarabine in progressive multifocal leukoencephalopathy associated with dermatomyositis. J R Soc Med 2000; 93: 374–375.

123. Regan M, Haque U, Pomper M et al. Central nervous system vasculitis as a complication of refractory dermatomyositis. J Rheumatol 2001; 28: 207–211.

124. Aarli JA. Inflammatory myopathy in myasthenia gravis. Curr Opin Neurol 1998; 11: 233–234.

125. Wortmann RL. Metabolic and mitochondrial myopathies. Curr Opin Rheumatol 1999; 11: 462–467.

126. Bolton CF. Critical illness polyneuropathy and myopathy. Crit Care Med 2001; 29: 2388–2390.

127. Lacomis D, Giuliani MJ, Cott AV et al. Acute myopathy of intensive care: clinical, electromyographic, and pathological aspects. Ann Neurol 1996; 40: 645–654.

128. Patel SR, Olenginski TP, Perruquet JL et al. Pyomyositis: clinical features and predisposing conditions. J Rheumatol 1997; 24: 1734–1738.

129. Heffner RR, Armbrustmacher WV, Earle KM. Focal myositis. Cancer 1977; 40: 302–306.

130. Umpierrez GE, Stiles RG, Kleinbart J et al. Diabetic muscle infarction. Am J Med 1996; 101: 245–250.

131. Pickering MC, Walport MJ. Eosinophilic myopathic syndromes. Curr Opin Rheumatol 1998; 10: 504–510.

132. Hall FC, Krausz T, Walport MJ. Idiopathic eosinophilic myositis. Q J Med 1995; 88: 581–586.

133. Mandl LA, Folkerth RD, Pick MA et al. Amyloid myopathy masquerading as polymyositis. J Rheumatol 2000; 27: 949–952.

134. Cherin P, Gherardi RK. Macrophagic myofasciitis. Curr Rheum Reports 2000; 2: 196–200.

135. Whitmore SE, Watson R, Rosenshein NB et al. Dermatomyositis sine myositis: association with malignancy. J Rheumatol 1996; 23: 101–105.

136. Maoz CR, Langevitz P, Livneh A et al. High incidence of malignancies in patients with dermatomyositis and polymyositis: an 11-year analysis. Semin Arthritis Rheum 1998; 27: 319–324.

137. Hill CL, Zhang Y, Sigurgeirsson B et al. Frequency of specific cancer types in dermatomyositis and polymyositis: a population-based study. Lancet 2001; 357: 96–100.

138. Chen Y-J, Wu C-Y, Shen J-L. Predicting factors of malignancy in dermatomyositis and polymyositis: a case–control study. Br J Dermatol 2001; 144: 825–831.

139. Buchbinder R, Forbes A, Hall S et al. Incidence of malignant disease in biopsy-proven inflammatory myopathy. Ann Intern Med 2001; 134: 1087–1095.

140. Whitmore SE, Rosenshein NB, Provost TT. Ovarian cancer in patients with dermatomyositis. Medicine 1994; 73: 153–160.

141. Whitmore SE, Anhalt FJ, Provost TT et al. Serum Ca-125 screening for ovarian cancer in patients with dermatomyositis. Gynecol Oncol 1997; 65: 241–244.

142. Hu W, Chen D, Min H. Study of 45 cases of nasopharyngeal carcinoma with dermatomyositis. Am J Clin Oncol 1996; 19: 35–38.

143. Mautner GH, Grossman ME, Silvers DN et al. Epidermal necrosis as a predictive sign of malignancy in adult dermatomyositis. Cutis 1998; 61: 190–194.

144. Hunger RE, Durr C, Brand CU. Cutaneous leukocytoclastic vasculitis in dermatomyositis suggests malignancy. Dermatology 2001; 202: 123–126.

145. Airio A, Pukkala E, Isomaki H. Elevated cancer incidence in patients with dermatomyositis: a population based study. J Rheumatol 1995; 22: 1300–1303.

146. Lee AJ, Maddix DS. Rhabdomyolysis secondary to a drug interaction between simvastatin and clarithromycin. Ann Pharmacother 2001; 35: 26–31.

147. Renders L, Mayer-Kadner I, Koch C et al. Efficacy and drug interactions of the new HMG-Co-A reductase inhibitors cerivastatin and atorvastatin in CsA-treated renal transplant recipients. Nephrol Dial Transplant 2001; 16: 141–146.

148. Schalke BB, Schmidt B, Toyka K et al. Pravastatin-associated inflammatory myopathy. N Eng J Med 1992; 327: 649–650.

149. Hino I, Akama H, Furuya T et al. Pravastatin-induced rhabdomyolysis in a patient with mixed connective tissue disease. Arthritis Rheum 1996; 39: 1259–1261.

150. Rodriguez-Garcia JL, Serrano Commino M. Lovastatin-associated dermatomyositis. Postgrad Med J 1996; 72: 694.

151. Giordano N, Senesi M, Mattii, G et al. Polymyositis associated with simvastatin. Lancet 1997; 349: 1600–1601.

152. Hill C, Zeitz C, Kirkham B. Dermatomyositis with lung involvement in a patient treated with simvastatin. Aust NZ J Med 1995; 25: 745–746.

153. Dawson TM, Starkebaum G. Colchicine induced rhabdomyolysis. J Rheumatol 1997; 24: 2045–2046.

154. Estes ML, Ewing-Wilson D, Chou SM et al. Chloroquine neuromyotoxicity: clinical and pathologic perspective. Am J Med 1987; 82: 447–455.

155. Avina-Zubieta JA, Johnson ES, Suarez-Almazor ME et al. Incidence of myopathy in patients treated with antimalarials. A report of three cases and a review of the literature. Br J Rheumatol 1995; 34: 166–170.

156. Marie I, Joly P, Levesque H et al. Pseudo-dermatomyositis as a complication of hydroxyurea therapy. Clin Exp Rheumatol 2000; 18: 536–537.

157. Kim HA, Song YW. Polymyositis developing after prolonged injections of pentazocine. J Rheumatol 1996; 2: 1644–1646.

158. Kivanc MT, Klaus MV, Nashel DJ. Reversible polymyositis occurring during psoralen and ultraviolet A (PUVA) therapy. J Rheumatol 2000; 27: 1823–1824.

159. Esteva-Lorenzo FJ, Janik JE, Fenton RG et al. Myositis associated with interleukin-2 therapy in a patient with metastatic renal cell carcinoma. Cancer 1995; 76: 1219–1223.

160. Kalkner K-M, Ronnblom L, Parra AK et al. Antibodies against double-stranded DNA and development of polymyositis during treatment with interferon. Q J Med 1998; 91: 393–399.

161. Serratrice J, Granel B, Pache X et al. A case of polymyositis with anti-histidyl-t-RNA synthetase (Jo-1) antibody syndrome following extensive vinyl chloride exposure. Clin Rheumatol 2001; 20: 379–382.

162. Rider LG. Assessment of disease activity and its sequelae in children and adults with myositis. Curr Opin Rheumatol 1996; 8: 495–506.

163. Miller FW, Rider LG, Churg Y-L et al. Proposed preliminary core set measures for disease outcome assessment in adult and juvenile idiopathic inflammatory myopathies. Rheumatology 2001; 40: 1262–1273.

164. Kagen LJ, Aram S. Creatine kinase activity inhibitor in serum from patients with muscle disease. Arthritis Rheum 1987; 30: 213–217.

165. Johnston JD, Lloyd M, Mathews J et al. Racial variation in serum creatine kinase levels. J Roy Soc Med 1996; 89: 462–464.

166. Rose MR, Kissel JT, Bickley LS et al. Sustained myoglobinuria: the presenting manifestation of dermatomyositis. Neurology 1996; 47: 119–123.

167. Kumamoto T, Ueyama H, Fujimoto S et al. Clinicopathologic characteristics of polymyositis patients with numerous tissue eosinophils. Acta Neurol Scand 1996; 94: 110–114.

168. Campellone JV, Lacomis D, Giuliani MJ et al. Percutaneous needle muscle biopsy in the evaluation of patients with suspected inflammatory myopathy. Arthritis Rheum 1997; 40: 1886–1891.

169. Park JH, Olsen NJ. Utility of magnetic resonance imaging in the evaluation of patients with inflammatory myopathies. Curr Rheum Reports 2001; 3: 334–345.

170. Lampa J, Nennesmo I, Einarsdottir H et al. MRI guided muscle biopsy confirmed polymyositis diagnosis in a patient with interstitial lung disease. Ann Rheum Dis 2001; 60: 423–426.

171. Park JH, Niermann KJ, Ryder NM et al. Muscle abnormalities in juvenile dermatomyositis patients. Arthritis Rheum 2000; 43: 2359–2367.

172. Park JH, Olsen NJ, King LE et al. MRI and P-31 magnetic resonance spectroscopy detect and quantify muscle dysfunction in the amyopathic and myopathic variants of dermatomyositis. Arthritis Rheum 1995; 38: 68–77.

173. Vaughan Jones SA, Black MM. The value of direct immunofluorescence as a diagnostic aid in dermatomyositis – a study of 35 cases. Clin Exp Dermatol 1997; 22: 77–81.

174. Magro CM, Crowson AN. The immunofluorescent profile of dermatomyositis: a comparative study with lupus erythematosus. J Cutan Pathol 1997; 24: 543–552.

175. Akira M, Hara H, Sakatani M. Interstitial lung disease in association with polymyositis-dermatomyositis: long-term follow-up CT evaluation in seven patients. Radiology 1999; 210: 333–338.

176. Tazelaar HD, Viggiano W, Pickersgill J et al. Interstitial lung disease in polymyositis and dermatomyositis. Clinical features and prognosis as correlated with histologic findings. Am Rev Respir Dis 1990; 141: 727–733.

177. Sauty A, Rochat TH, Schoch OD et al. Pulmonary fibrosis with predominant CD8 lymphocytic alveolitis and anti-Jo-1 antibodies. Eur Respir J 1997; 10: 2907–2912.

178. Kourakata H, Takada T, Suzuki E et al. Flow cytomeric analysis of bronchoalveolar lavage fluid cells in polymyositis/dermatomyositis with interstitial pneumonia. Respirology 1999; 4: 223–228.

179. D'Cruz D, Keser G, Khamashta MA et al. Antiendothelial cell antibodies in inflammatory myopathies: distribution among clinical and serologic groups and association with interstitial lung disease. J Rheumatol 2000; 27: 161–164.

180. Nakajima H, Harigai M, Hara M et al. KL-6 as a novel serum marker for interstitial pneumonia associated with collagen diseases. J Rheumatol 2000; 7: 1164–1170.

181. Bandoh S, Fujita J, Ohtsuki Y et al. Sequential changes of KL-6 in sera of patients with interstitial pneumonia associated with polymyositis/dermatomyositis. Ann Rheum Dis 2000; 59: 257–262.

182. Fujita J, Dobashi N, Tokuda M et al. Elevation of cytokeratin 19 fragment in patients with interstitial pneumonia associated with polymyositis/dermatomyositis. J Rheumatol 1999; 26: 2377–2382.

183. Buchpiguel CA, Roizemblatt S, Pastor EH et al. Cardiac and skeletal muscle scintigraphy in dermato- and polymyositis: clinical implications. Eur J Nucl Med 1996; 23: 199–203.

184. Sarda L, Assayag P, Palazzo E et al. Indium antimyosin antibody imaging of primary myocardial involvement in systemic diseases. Ann Rheum Dis 1999; 58: 90–95.

185. Erlacher P, Lercher A, Falkensammer J et al. Cardiac troponin and β-type myosin heavy chain concentrations in patients with polymyositis or dermatomyositis. Clin Chim Acta 2001; 306: 27–33.

186. Bodor GS, Survant L, Voss EM et al. Cardiac troponin T composition in normal and regenerating human skeletal muscle. Clin Chem 1997; 43: 476–484.

187. Sonies BC. Evaluation and treatment of speech and swallowing disorders associated with myopathies. Curr Opin Rheumatol 1997; 9: 486–495.

188. Mierau R, Dick T, Genth E. Less specific myositis autoantibodies? Ann Rheum Dis 2001; 60: 810.

189. Gelpi C, Kanterewicz E, Gratacos J et al. Coexistence of two antisynthetases in a patient with the antisynthetase syndrome. Arthritis Rheum 1996; 39: 692–697.

190. Brouwer R, Hengstman GJD, Vree Eberts W et al. Autoantibody profiles in the sera of European patients with myositis. Ann Rheum Dis 2001; 60: 116–123.

191. Ohosone Y, Matsumura M, Chiba J et al. Anti-transfer RNA antibodies in two patients with pulmonary fibrosis, Raynaud's phenomenon and polyarthritis. Clin Rheumatol 1998; 17: 144–147.

192. Ohosone Y, Ishida M, Takahashi Y et al. Spectrum and clinical significance of auto-antibodies against transfer RNA. Arthritis Rheum 1998; 41: 1625–1631.

193. Seelig HP, Moosbrugger I, Ehrfeld H et al. The major dermatomyositis-specific Mi-2 autoantigen is a presumed helicase involved in transcriptional activation. Arthritis Rheum 1995; 38: 1389–1399.

194. Casciola-Rosen LA, Pluta AF, Plotz PH et al. The DNA mismatch repair enzyme PMS1 is a myositis specific autoantigen. Arthritis Rheum 2001; 44: 389–396.

195. Schnitz W, Taylor-Albert E, Targoff IN et al. Anti-PM/Scl autoantibodies in patients without clinical polymyositis or scleroderma. J Rheumatol 1996; 23: 1729–1733.

196. Phillips BA, Zilko P, Garlepp MJ, Mastaglia FL. Frequency of relapses in patients with polymyositis and dermatomyositis. Muscle Nerve 1998; 21: 1668–1672.

197. Hoffman GS, Franck WA, Raddatz DA, Stallones L. Presentation, treatment and prognosis of idiopathic inflammatory muscle disease in a rural hospital. Am J Med 1983; 75: 433–438.

198. Blume G, Pestronk A, Frank B, Johns DR. Polymyositis with cytochrome oxidase negative muscle fibres: early quadriceps weakness and poor response to immunosuppressive therapy. Brain 1997; 120: 39–45.

199. Huang J-L. Long-term prognosis of patients with juvenile dermatomyositis initially treated with intravenous methylprednisolone pulse therapy. Clin Exp Rheumatol 1999; 17: 621–624.

200. Mitchell JP, Dennis GJ, Rider LG. Juvenile dermatomyositis presenting with anasarca: a possible indicator of severe disease activity. J Pediatr 2001; 138: 942–945.

201. Oddis CV, Medsger TA Jr. Polymyositis–dermatomyositis. In: Bellamy N, ed. Prognosis in the rheumatic diseases. Lancaster: Kluwer Academic Publishers; 1991: 233–249.

202. O'Leary PA, Waisman M. Dermatomyositis. Arch Derm Syph 1940; 41: 1001–1019.

203. Sheard C Jr. Dermatomyositis. Arch Intern Med 1951; 88: 640–658.

204. Winkelmann RK, Mulder DW, Lambert EH. Course of dermatomyositis–polymyositis: comparison of untreated and cortisone-treated patients. Mayo Clin Proc 1968; 43: 545–556.

205. Medsger TA Jr, Robinson H, Masi AT. Factors affecting survivorship in polymyositis: a life-table tudy of 124 patients. Arthritis Rheum 1971; 14: 249–258.

206. Carpenter JR, Bunch TW, Engel AG, O'Brien PC. Survival in polymyositis: corticosteroids and risk factors. J Rheumatol 1977' 4: 208–214.

207. Bohan A, Peter JB, Bowman RI et al. A computer-assisted analysis of 153 patients with polymyositis and dermatomyositis. Medicine 1976; 55: 89–104.

208. Benbassat J, Gefel D, Larholt K et al. Prognostic factors in PM-DM: a computer assisted analysis of 92 cases. Arthritis Rheum 1985; 28: 249–555.

209. Riddoch D, Morgan-Hughes JA. Prognosis in adult polymyositis. J Neurol Sci 1975; 26: 71–80.

210. Henriksson KG, Sandstedt P. Polymyositis – treatment and prognosis: a study of 107 patients. Acta Neurol Scand 1982; 65: 280–300.

211. Hochberg MC, Feldman D, Stevens MB. Adult onset polymyositis/dermatomyositis: an analysis of clinical and laboratory features and survival in 76 patients with a review of the literature. Semin Arthritis Rheum 1986; 15: 168–178.

212. Tymms KE, Webb J. Dermatopolymyositis and other connective tissue diseases. A review of 105 cases. J Rheumatol 1986; 12: 1140–1148.

213. Maugars YM, Berthelot J-MM, Abbas AA et al. Long-term prognosis of 69 patients with dermatomyositis or polymyositis. Clin Exp Rheum 1996; 14: 263–274.

214. Miller LC, Michael AF, Kim Y. Childhood dermatomyositis: clinical course and long-term follow-up. Clin Pediatr 1987; 26: 561–566.

215. DeVere R, Bradley WG. Polymyositis: its presentation, morbidity and mortality. Brain 1975; 98: 637–666.

216. Clarke AE, Bloch DA, Medsger TA Jr, Oddis CV. A longitudinal study of functional disability in a national cohort of polymyositis–dermatomyositis patients. Arthritis Rheum 1995; 38: 1218–1224.

217. Feldman BM, Ayling-Campos A, Luy L et al. Measuring disability in juvenile dermatomyositis: validity of the childhood health assessment questionnaire. J Rheumatol 1995; 22: 326–331.

218. Perez MD, Abrams SA, Koenning G et al. Mineral metabolism in children with dermatomyositis. J Rheumatol 1994; 21: 2364–2369.

140 Management

Luis J Catoggio

- Precise diagnosis is essential and biopsy is mandatory to identify 'non-responding' myopathies such as inclusion body myositis

- Most forms of PM and DM are still approached in a similar manner

- Muscle strength and CPK levels remain the most used measures to monitor disease activity and response to therapy

- Corticosteroids are the main pillar of drug therapy. However, simultaneous use of corticosteroid-sparing drugs may be considered from disease onset

- The main drugs for combined therapy are methotrexate, azathioprine and antimalarials

- Intravenous γ-globulin may have an initial role in some life-threatening cases

- Otherwise, together with plasmapheresis and total body irradiation, they are restricted to refractory cases

GENERAL APPROACH TO MANAGEMENT

As with most rheumatic diseases, the diagnosis of idiopathic inflammatory myopathy must be accurate if therapy is to be adequately planned. In this respect the inflammatory myopathies may prove more difficult to diagnose than other connective tissue diseases because the cardinal signs, proximal weakness and an elevated creatine phosphokinase (CPK), may be due to a variety of conditions (see Chapter 141). Myositis may also occur in the context of, or be associated with, other connective tissue diseases. Therefore, it is important to identify subgroups of the disease. Finally, correct evaluation of muscle biopsies is imperative because some of those myopathies that do not respond as well to treatment, such as inclusion body myositis, can be identified by biopsy.

Although classically considered very similar, recent reports have shown histologic and immunologic differences between polymyositis (PM) and dermatomyositis (DM), suggesting that approaches to treatment and prognosis should be different[1]. Furthermore, there is evidence to suggest that 'myositis-specific' antibody subsets of the disease have different outcomes and may therefore require different approaches to therapy[2]. Although in the future therapies may take into account pathologic findings on muscle biopsy or antibody status, to date controlled studies are lacking to sustain this approach. Therefore, the initial treatment of adult-onset forms of PM and DM remains similar and most commonly guided by the classic Bohan and Peter classification,[3] with the addition of inclusion body myositis (IBM).

Once the correct diagnosis is established and appropriate treatment is under way, lack of response after 4–6 weeks should lead one to consider the possibility of other diagnoses.

Treatment of PM and DM should be tailored to the individual patient, and the initial approach and monitoring of the disease may vary from case to case. There is general agreement that the sooner the condition is treated after onset, the better[1–4]. The degrees of muscle weakness, muscle atrophy or wasting, levels of CPK or functional impairment may lead to different approaches to treatment in individual patients. However, there is general consensus that the different subgroups have the following behaviors (Fig. 140.1):

- Myositis in overlap patients (type V) usually responds to less agressive treatment and rarely relapses. These patients are considered to have the best prognosis.
- Patients with DM (type II) have infrequent relapses and usually respond, recovering with varying degrees of muscle deficit after each treatment period.
- Patients with PM (type I) have more frequent relapses and frequently recover, but with less strength after each bout.
- IBM has the poorest prognosis, with a very variable response to treatment.

Some of these subsets correlate with the presence of myositis-specific or associated antibodies, as shown in Figure 140.1.

The average duration of therapy is around 18–24 months, although some patients will require longer. Malignancy-associated myositis will obviously also depend on the course of the underlying condition.

Although activity and severity may frequently coexist, activity may be present with no severity (damage), and vice versa. The evaluation of both is essential, especially when embarking on treatment of patients who have already received prior therapy and are 'halfway through'.

DRUG THERAPY

An algorithm for the drug management of the inflammatory myopathies is given in Figure 140.2.

Corticosteroids

Corticosteroids continue to be the mainstay of treatment in most cases of PM/DM.

Daily oral corticosteroids

Common practice is to start with doses of prednisone 1–2mg/kg/day or its equivalent. Although single daily doses may succeed in controlling the disease, frequently this is not adequate. The same daily dose given as three or four smaller divided doses may be needed to gain initial control. Once control has been achieved, prednisone is usually reduced to a single morning dose. This dose (in practice usually between 60 and not more than 100mg/day) is maintained until there is substantial clinical improvement and a reduction of CPK levels to normal. The duration of the initial corticosteroid therapy is highly variable but in most responsive cases is between 6 and 8 weeks. Some authors recommend changing to an alternate-day regimen once disease control has been achieved[5]. This may, however, result in relapses if undertaken too early.

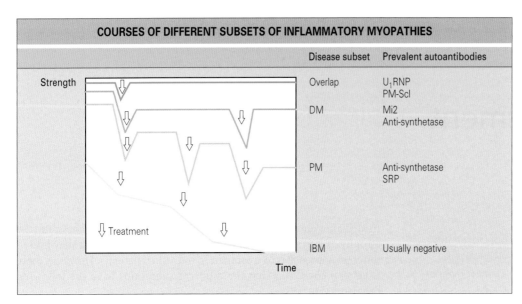

COURSES OF DIFFERENT SUBSETS OF INFLAMMATORY MYOPATHIES

	Disease subset	Prevalent autoantibodies
Strength	Overlap	U₁RNP PM-Scl
	DM	Mi2 Anti-synthetase
	PM	Anti-synthetase SRP
⇩ Treatment	IBM	Usually negative

Time

Fig. 140.1 Courses of different subsets of inflammatory myopathies: correlation with autoantibodies. Patients with overlap myositis may have U₁RNP or PM-Scl antibodies and milder disease that responds relatively well to therapy, with infrequent relapses. Some patients with DM have Mi2 or antisynthetase antibodies, with some relapses after discontinuation of therapy. Patients with PM have even more frequent relapses, with incomplete responses to therapy and antisynthetase or SRP antibodies. IBM usually lacks autoantibodies and shows progression, with poor response to therapy. (Redrawn with permission from Catoggio LJ, Soriano ER, eds. Inflammatory muscle disease: therapeutic aspects. Baillière's Best Practice Clin Rheumatol 2000; 14: 56.)

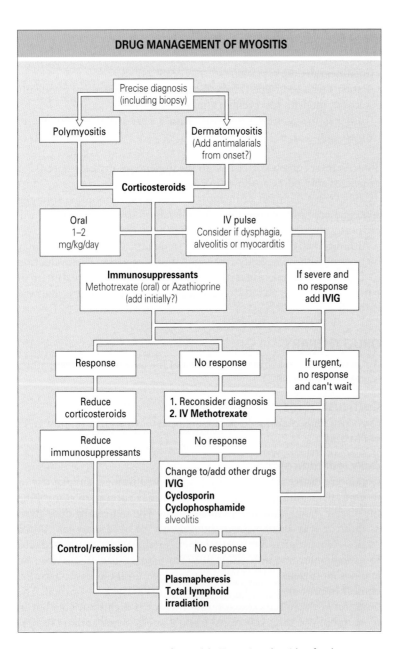

DRUG MANAGEMENT OF MYOSITIS

Fig. 140.2 Drug management of myositis. Tentative algorithm for drug management of polymyositis and dermatomyositis.

Oddis and Medsger have recommended the following regimen to achieve more prolonged control of disease:

- maintain an initial divided dose of prednisone 1mg/kg/day for at least 1 month and until CPK returns to normal; then
- reduce the prednisone dose by 25% monthly to a maintenance dose of 5–10mg/day.

Pulse corticosteroids

Pulse intravenous corticosteroids (1g in total daily for 3 days or methyl-prednisolone 15mg/kg) are increasingly being used in severe, acute myositis, usually followed by high-dose oral corticosteroids. However, whether this results in more rapid control of disease or lower cumulative doses of corticosteroids (and therefore fewer side effects) than do conventional corticosteroid regimens has not been convincingly demonstrated. This approach is probably justified in life-threatening disease such as severe dysphagia, which has a high risk of aspiration, myocardial involvement or active alveolitis[1,2].

Corticosteroid side effects

Probably the most serious side effects of corticosteroids in PM and DM are complications due to osteoporosis, particularly vertebral collapse, and osteonecrosis. In one series the latter was reported in 8.6% of cases[6]. Prescription of calcium supplements and vitamin D is probably warranted, particularly in younger women (see Chapter 199). Recent evidence has shown that bisphosponates are effective in preventing and treating steroid-induced bone loss[7].

Corticosteroid-induced hypertension and heart failure are probably less frequent in clinical practice than has been classically believed. Hyperglycemia may occur, particularly in diabetes-prone patients, and patients with insulin-dependent diabetes who develop myositis are candidates for early use of corticosteroid-sparing agents. Fat redistribution due to iatrogenic Cushing's syndrome is a common and aesthetic problem, particularly in women, as is hirsutism. In our experience, patients prone to the development of Cushing's syndrome even with lower corticosteroid doses tend to be those who also develop osteonecrosis and cataracts.

A propensity for common and uncommon infections in these patients is more frequent and should be kept in mind. Influenza vaccination is indicated in treated patients (WHO recommendations), as is probably pneumoccocal vaccination as well. Prophylactic coverage with isoniazid (300mg/day) is recommended in patients from areas where there is a high incidence of tuberculosis.

Cytotoxic drugs

Reliance on high-dose corticosteroids alone as initial treatment for severe manifestations has been replaced by the early use of cytotoxic drugs combined with corticosteroids. This treatment philosophy is much less well established in myositis; corticosteroids 'alone' continue to be recommended initially. However, the trend in inflammatory myopathies appears to be changing. Earlier combination therapy is being increasingly used both to reduce corticosteroid side effects and because subsets of disease with a poor prognosis can be identified early in the disease course and treated with more aggressive combined therapy[1–3].

The classic approach to the use of cytotoxic drugs in myositis has been to reserve it for patients in whom there is:

- a lack of response to high-dose corticosteroids
- the occurrence of unacceptable corticosteroid side effects, or
- difficulty in reducing high-dose corticosteroids because of flares.

However, although the following is not shared by all, many physicians today add immunosuppressive drugs from the start. The two drugs most used under these circumstances have been methotrexate and azathioprine.

Methotrexate

The clinical experience of methotrexate in myositis is substantial. Many clinicians consider it to be the first choice among immunosuppressive drugs[8–11]. The earliest use of methotrexate was intravenously (i.v.) in doses of 10–15mg/week, increasing to up to 50mg weekly, typically along with corticosteroids. Once control is achieved, the dose is decreased and the interval between injections extended until they are administered once a month. Ideally the aim is to reduce, and if possible discontinue, corticosteroids altogether while maintaining low-dose methotrexate. The rate of dose reduction is highly variable and tailored to the individual patient.

Over the past few years intravenous methotrexate has largely been replaced by oral weekly methotrexate (7.5–15.0mg weekly), similar to regimens used in rheumatoid arthritis (RA). Oral doses of methotrexate may be increased to up to 25mg/week according to tolerance. The ease of use of oral methotrexate and its relative safety has raised the issue of using this drug from the start in combination with corticosteroids, with the goal of reducing the total corticosteroid dose and, at least in theory, potential side effects.

The toxicity of low-dose weekly oral methotrexate in myositis is similar to that in RA and requires careful monitoring via monthly blood counts and transaminase enzymes (SGOT and SGPT)[8–11]. In myositis, problems may arise from the enzyme elevation that results from muscle damage, rather than from liver toxicity. This may not be easy to discern. If the enzymes were normal at onset and then are raised but accompanied by a normal CPK, liver toxicity may be presumed. If CPK is also elevated, the issue may be difficult. In contrast, if SGOT and SGPT are elevated at the initiation of treatment because of myositis, they may decrease after the use of methotrexate. In doubtful situations, suspension or reduction of the dose of methotrexate may be necessary to determine the cause of the rise in enzymes.

Side effects

Serious side effects such as bone marrow suppression may occur more frequently than they do in RA because of the higher doses used. The possibility of methotrexate pneumonitis should be entertained in PM and DM patients with rapidly progressing alveolitis[9]. It has not been determined whether patients with previous lung disease accompanying myositis, or those with the antisynthetase syndrome (more prone to interstitial lung disease), should not be treated with this drug.

Baseline liver biopsy may be warranted only in patients who have a history of prior liver disease or alcohol intake. As in RA, control biopsies are probably not necessary, although until recently this had not been specifically studied in myositis. A recent report suggested that caution is required in patients with myositis and diabetes whose biopsies showed an increased degree of methotrexate-induced fibrosis[11].

Azathioprine

There is considerable experience of azathioprine in myositis. The consensus is that it takes longer to produce an effect than methotrexate[1–3]. The starting dose is usually 1.5–2mg/kg/day, the usual daily dose ranging between 150 and 200mg. Reports have shown that patients treated with this drug in combination with corticosteroids fared better than those with corticosteroids alone, in terms of the degree of disability and total corticosteroid dose required[12]. Optimum regimens have not been determined, but it is suggested that a dose of 150–200mg be maintained until the disease remits and corticosteroids can be decreased to doses below prednisone 15mg/day, at which point the azathioprine dose is reduced.

Cyclophosphamide

Experience of cyclophosphamide in PM and DM is considerably less than is the case for other cytotoxic drugs. Its use has generally been limited to patients who fail other therapies, largely because of concerns about toxicity. Oral doses range from 1 to 2mg/kg/day, usually not exceeding 150mg/day. Cyclophosphamide is more toxic than methotrexate or azathioprine, and reports regarding its benefit are conflicting[1–3,13]. The role of pulse intravenous cyclophosphamide is unclear, although some benefit has been reported in patients with PM or DM, particularly those with overlaps and interstitial lung disease[14,15].

Cyclosporin

There has been increasing experience with cyclosporin in inflammatory myopathies, including the juvenile group[16–19]. Doses used have ranged between 2 and 3.5mg/kg/day; lower doses appear to be less toxic but also less effective. Several recent reports have also shown some success in combination with other drugs, including with intravenous γ-globulin and particularly in patients with myositis and interstitial lung involvement[19]. According to these results, cyclosporin is a useful drug in cases not responding to methotrexate or azathioprine.

Other cytotoxic drugs

Other nitrogen mustard alkylating agents such as chlorambucil have been used in myositis, but experience is limited[20]. A recent paper analysing the use of flutarabine,[21] an adenine analog, showed a partial response in only four of 16 patients enrolled. Mofetil mycophenolate is being increasingly used in connective tissue diseases, and although there are no major trials reported, a recent paper has shown it to be effective as a steroid-sparing agent in four cases of DM[22].

Antimalarials

Antimalarials have been reported to be useful in controlling skin disease in dermatomyositis and in reducing corticosteroid requirements in myositis patients[23,24]. It is generally believed that antimalarials have little or no effect on muscle inflammation *per se*, although this has not been specifically studied. Antimalarials are most commonly recommended early in the course of patients with dermatomyositis, even those with malignancy-associated disease[24]. Antimalarials are often continued when other drugs are stopped, and patients are maintained for prolonged periods on low doses (minimum chloroquine 100mg or hydroxychloroquine 200mg twice weekly).

Skin flares with 'inactive' myositis are also treated with antimalarials, which may control the skin flare without the need to add or increase the dose of corticosteroids. Also, the rare patient with 'dermatomyositis sine myositis' may respond to antimalarials alone, unless they have visceral manifestations warranting other treatment.

Most reports refer to the use of hydroxychloroquine[23]. Whether this is really safer than chloroquine sulfate remains debatable. Most data on the higher retinal toxicity of chloroquine (compared to hydroxychloroquine) involve comparisons of older studies of high-dose chloroquine with more recent studies of hydroxychloroquine[25]. In situations in which drug costs are a major consideration, it is important to recognize that hydroxychloroquine is substantially more expensive than chloroquine sulfate. The usual 'safe' dose of chloroquine is said to be no higher than 4mg/kg/day, and of hydroxychloroquine not over 6.5mg/kg/day.

Side effects

The most serious potential side effect of antimalarials is retinal toxicity. However, this is uncommon with the doses currently used[26]. Whether frequent ophthalmologic monitoring is necessary with current doses is debated by some,[26] although it is generally recommended that funduscopy, together with computed visual fields, should be performed every 6–12 months.

Several side effects of antimalarials can be easily confused with disease manifestations that occur in association with the inflammatory muscle disease. Acute skin eruptions can develop, especially after exposure to sunlight, and may be misinterpreted as dermatomyositis rashes. In addition, progressive muscle weakness from the myopathy induced by antimalarials may similarly be misinterpreted as evidence of ongoing myositis; muscle biopsy may be needed in such patients to determine the cause of the weakness.

OTHER THERAPEUTIC MODALITIES

Intravenous γ-globulin

Recent literature is abundant with case reports on the use of intravenous γ-globulin in the inflammatory myopathies, especially in children. A recent controlled trial reported some benefit for adult patients with dermatomyositis[27]. However, follow-ups of this[28] and other experiences have shown IVIg to be a valuable modality both in refractory patients,[28,29] including children,[30] and in life-threatening cases, especially those with severe esophageal involvement[31].

Total body irradiation

Several reports describe improvements in refractory PM and DM following total body radiation[32]. However, there is little recent experience using this modality, so its use should be limited to exceptional cases.

Plasmapheresis

Although plasmapheresis has been claimed to be benefical in PM and DM, a controlled trial of plasmapheresis and leukapheresis failed to demonstrate any benefits[33]. A more recent article reviewing all patients with PM or DM undergoing plasmapheresis in France was less pessimistic,[34] although its benefits appeared to be limited to patients with early, active disease. Moreover, as plasmapheresis only removes putative immune complexes or pathologic antibodies, it should probably be accompanied by some form of immunosuppression. The substantial cost of the procedure constitutes another limitation.

MONITORING DISEASE ACTIVITY AND RESPONSE TO THERAPY

Careful monitoring of patients with PM or DM is important to evaluate the response to therapy and rehabilitation programs. The two main monitoring tools are muscle strength, at the clinical level, and muscle enzymes at the laboratory level. Although these measures are not useful in all patients because they may not necessarily correlate and others are being evaluated (see below), they remain the two most commonly used in clinical practice.

Muscle strength

An objective evaluation of muscle strength using an instrument such as manual muscle testing (Table 140.1) is important in the initial assessment and follow-up of patients. In addition, quantitative functional evaluations (Table 140.2) provide an assessment of limitations caused by the muscular weakness, and their progress[37,38]. These instruments can be used by physicians or nurse specialists even when rehabilitation expertise may not be widely available.

Muscle weakness may result from inflammation, myofiber damage or, more commonly, a combination of the two. The recovery of muscle strength varies but depends on the extent of damage prior to treatment, the success of treatment and the response to physical therapy. Muscle fibrosis may result in some cases and muscle strength may not fully recover to baseline levels. An incomplete recovery of muscle strength after a reasonable period of treatment, in the presence of other elements suggesting inactive disease, should be a signal to reduce rather than continue or escalate aggressive therapy.

Lack of increase in muscle strength and/or deterioration after prior improvement raises the question: is this activity or relapse of myositis, or is it corticosteroid-induced myopathy (or, rarely, antimalarial-induced myopathy). If it is accompanied by a rise in CPK, then a relapse of myositis is more probable. However, this is not always the case, and distinguishing one condition from the other may be difficult. A biopsy revealing lack of inflammation together with prominent atrophy of

TABLE 140.1 MANUAL MUSCLE STRENGTH TESTING GRADES

0	No muscle contraction
1 (trace)	Palpable contraction, little or no motion
2 (poor)	Motion possible but not against gravity
3 (fair)	Motion against gravity possible
4 (good)	Motion possible against natural resistance
5 (normal)	Motion possible against considerable manual resistance

TABLE 140.2 FUNCTIONAL GRADING SCALE

Activity

1. Transfer from supine to sitting
2. Transfer from sitting to standing
3. Walking
4. Stair climbing
   Ascending
   Descending
5. Care of head and face (e.g. hair, tooth brushing)
6. Dressing
   Donning jacket or buttoned shirt
   Donning pants
7. Lifting objects above shoulder level (elbow extended)
   Light household work
   Heavy household work

Total score

Scoring

Cannot do	0
Requires help from a person	1
Person not needed but does with difficulty (uses aids, e.g. cane, railing, mechanical device)	2
Can do alone without difficulty	3
Maximum score	30

type II muscle fibers may help to suggest corticosteroid myopathy. Nevertheless, this clear-cut situation is not common. A combination of inflammation and atrophy is usually the case, rendering the value of a muscle biopsy relative.

In patients with dermatomyositis, skin disease may run parallel to or be discordant with the course of myositis. Discordance of skin and muscle disease activity is rarely evident at disease onset, and skin flares may be treated 'separately' (usually less aggressively) if muscle disease remains stable.

Muscle enzymes

Creatine phosphokinase and aldolase are the most common laboratory measures used to monitor disease activity, although serum glutamic–oxaloacetic transaminase (SGOT) and serum glutamate pyruvate transaminase (SGPT) may also be indicative of muscle inflammation. Cases with normal CPK and abnormal aldolase have been reported, so it is recommended that CPK, aldolase, SGOT and SGPT are measured initially. How to follow the disease, and with which laboratory test, should be individualized. For instance, we have seen cases where an increase of SGOT or SGPT has heralded a later increase in CPK accompanying a clinical disease flare; the same pattern was observed several times over a 4–5-year period. One should attempt to identify these individual characteristics when possible, because this will improve monitoring of the course of myositis and allow for appropriate changes in drug treatment.

Persistently high CPK values during treatment generally suggest uncontrolled myositis, although 'leakage' of CPK from damaged muscle cells in the absence of muscle inflammation might contribute to the finding in some patients. High values of CPK coinciding with lack of clinical improvement and persisting muscle weakness usually indicate lack of response, and so alternative measures should be considered. Stable or normal CPK values in a patient undergoing corticosteroid treatment who presents with a deterioration of muscle strength should alert the physician to the possibility of corticosteroid myopathy.

In general, the combination of clinical improvement and decrease in CPK is the most commonly used measure to monitor drugs and adapt treatment. Similarly, relapses are usually marked by increased enzymes and clinical deterioration.

Magnetic resonance imaging (MRI)

Recent reports suggest that MRI may be useful in detecting and monitoring disease activity, although not all the data are in agreement[3,35–37] (see Chapter 139). Trained physicians have shown that MRI findings correlate well with muscle strength and enzyme levels. Furthermore, MRI appears to be more sensitive than enzymes in following disease. However, MRI may be normal in patients with abnormal biopsies[3]. Considering its cost, the main indications at present appear to be the evaluation of muscle in patients in whom disease activity is in doubt, orientation of muscle biopsy in difficult cases, and follow-up in patients who have shown disagreement between activity and strength and muscle enzymes.

Myoglobin

Turbidimetric assay of myoglobin has been shown to provide a quick and sensitive method for the assessment of myositis and correlates well with clinical activity[38]. The precise role of the test in clinical practice, however, is still uncertain.

MANAGEMENT OF EXTRAMUSCULAR AND NON-CUTANEOUS MANIFESTATIONS

Cardiac manifestations

Heart involvement is not easy to diagnose in the context of otherwise active disease unless sudden overt cardiac failure or arrythmias appear.

A retrospective analysis showed that only 6% of myositis patients had clinical manifestations, whereas over half had abnormal electrocardiograms (EKG) and almost 40% abnormal diastolic function[39]. A recent report suggests that when the myocardium is affected EKG abnormalities always occur and the muscle–brain (MB) isoenzyme fraction of CPK is elevated[40].

Treatment of these manifestations is the same in principle as for active myositis. Myocarditis may suggest the initial use of pulse corticosteroids and combined therapy. Myocardial involvement also appears to be a feature associated with the antisignal recognition particle (SRP) subset of myositis[2].

Gastrointestinal manifestations

Severe dysphagia with the threat of bronchial aspiration is a serious manifestation of myositis and requires aggressive treatment and other supportive measures. Again, this may be considered an indication for pulse corticosteroids and/or IVIg,[31] especially as some of these patients cannot swallow medication. In extreme cases cricopharyngeal myotomy may be required[41].

Distal involvement of the esophagus, usually in overlap cases and linked to 'sclerodermatous' dysmotility, can be managed with measures tending to improve reflux, including elevation of the head of the bed, antacids, H_2 antagonists or proton pump inhibitors (see Chapter 135). In some cases esophageal dilatation may be required, and occasionally even surgery.

Interstitial lung disease

Interstitial lung disease may be indolent or rapidly progressive, warranting aggressive treatment. The antisynthetase subgroup of patients is more prone to this manifestation, as are those in the overlap group. The alveolitis of the latter may be more responsive to conventional treatment, as is the myositis. The former group may require more aggressive therapy, and it is in this context where pulse cyclophosphamide has been shown to be effective in some patients[14,15]. More recently, cyclosporin has also been shown to be useful in patients not responding to the usual therapies[19]. Bronchoalveolar lavage and/or transbronchial biopsy may be useful in documenting inflammatory changes that may be more responsive to treatment. High-resolution computerized tomography (CT) may also be useful, particularly to monitor response[42].

Calcinosis

Adequate treatment of myositis usually prevents calcinosis, but once this is established therapy does not make it regress. Treatments proposed, including calcium channel blockers[43,44] and vitamin K inhibitors,[45] have provided variable results and all are case reports. A recent paper also describes the disappearance of calcinosis in a child treated with aluminum hydroxide[46].

Surgical procedures may be required to remove calcifications from areas where they are troublesome (e.g. the buttocks). Foci of calcinosis may present flares with inflammation of the surrounding area. It has been proposed that this may be akin to a crystal-related inflammation, and colchicine may be helpful.

MANAGEMENT IN SPECIFIC CLINICAL SITUATIONS

Myositis and infections

Several situations should be considered in the context of infection and myositis.

Muscle infections arising after or during aggressive treatment of myositis

Infectious myositis affecting one or several muscle groups may occur in the context of treated inflammatory myopathies and one should be alert for this, particularly when a limited group of muscles shows a 'flare'. Recent reports describe a case of disseminated muscle tuberculosis (postmortem finding)[47] and pyomyositis occurring in a patient with DM under treatment[48]. Clinical awareness is essential in these cases to permit early diagnosis and institute adequate treatment of the infection[49].

Inflammatory myopathy coexisting with (caused by?) infection

Infections due to uncommon agents may mimic idiopathic PM and DM, and treatment may have to be directed towards both the agent and the myositis. A recent report describes one such case involving *Wuchereria bancroftii* which responded both to treatment of the infectious agent and to corticosteroids[50]. Patients with Lyme disease have been reported to have a clinical picture of myositis very similar to the idiopathic form. A recent report describes one such patient in whom *Borrelia burgdorferi* was implicated as a trigger[51]. Another recent paper shows a patient with AIDS in whom leishmania caused a DM-like rash[52]. Picornaviruses have been implicated in animal models, but search in human biopsies has not rendered evidence of viral infection. Retroviruses, particularly human immunodeficiency virus (HIV), deserve special consideration.

HIV-associated myositis

HIV infection may present as idiopathic myositis (see Chapter 98). Thus, in a newly diagnosed patient with myositis, particularly if he or she belongs to a 'high-risk' group, HIV screening should be requested. Treatment of HIV-associated myositis may be difficult because aggressive therapy for myositis may complicate HIV infection. However, if frank myositis is the main problem, treatment with corticosteroids may be necessary. A further difficulty is that zidovudine may contribute to myopathy[53]. If zidovudine treatment is suspected of causing myopathy and the drug can be reduced or discontinued, this should be attempted. Alternatively, non-steroidal anti-inflammatory drugs (NSAIDs) are recommended and, if unsuccessful, corticosteroids can be added[53].

Inclusion body myositis

Inclusion body myositis requires separate consideration. Prior to its identification it was probably included in the 'non-responding' myositis group. Mandatory muscle biopsies have allowed for a better identification of these patients, who are now known to be more prevalent than previously thought, especially in the older age group. IBM is characterized by a lack of or a slow response, either from the onset of treatment or after a slight improvement. Although it may occur at any age, it should be suspected in an elderly male patient with long-standing weakness, sometimes predominantly distal. Biopsy is essential for diagnosis, but repeat biopsies may be necessary to detect characteristic changes; conversely, an initial biopsy may show the typical findings and a subsequent one may not.

The response to treatment has been considered so poor in these patients that some have recommended that it not be treated at all. Others, however, have reported good results[54,55]. A recent review suggests that patients showing a CPK higher than 1000u/l and whose biopsy shows inflammatory changes are responsive[2] and should merit treatment, as suggested for the other forms of myositis described earlier[54,55]. IVIg, although not impressive, appears to benefit some patients initially, so some recommend its use in severe, rapidly progessive cases[55]. In many cases, weakness progresses regardless of treatment.

PATIENT EDUCATION AND PROGNOSIS

Patient education is essential in order to gain the patient's cooperation and full support in his or her treatment. How much is explained and in what way probably differ around the world, depending on cultural considerations. A description of the different forms of the disease, emphasizing positive aspects, often helps the patient cope. Unless there are elements indicating genuine severity, the approach should be positive as most patients with an accurate diagnosis will respond to treatment, at least initially. Education of the patient's partner and family is also important. An adequate knowledge of the social situation (family and work) is essential so that adequate modifications can be suggested and the best adaptations made possible.

Clinical features suggesting a poor prognosis are: old age, long-standing untreated disease, dysphagia, active heart or lung involvement, previous treatment failures, and malignancy-associated myositis. When these features are present, they should be carefully discussed with the patient and family in order to let them know as much as is considered adequate in each case, without causing needless alarm. Life-threatening aspects should obviously be discussed when present.

Time should be taken to address all of these patient and family education issues. Good patient–physician relations will contribute greatly to successful management of the disease.

PENDING ISSUES

In spite of major research, the IIM are still approached in a similar fashion. Much emphasis has been placed on treating patients according to MRI scans and autoantibody profiles. Controlled studies in these areas should provide us with a better approach to treatment.

Whether pulse steroids lead to fewer corticosteroid side effects in the long term is another issue which has not been addressed, as is the role of antimalarials in sparing steroids, not only in dermatomyositis patients. A more precise role for MRI and IVIg in managing these diseases will probably arise in coming years. Finally, newer drugs already being used in other diseases, such as mofetil mycophenolate and others, may provide help in refractory cases[55].

REHABILITATION IN PATIENTS WITH MYOSITIS

General overview

The classically accepted guidelines were that patients with active disease should refrain from intense physical therapy. Rest was generally recommended in periods of acute inflammation, typically combined with passive range-of-motion exercises to maintain joint motion and avoid contractures. However, this concept has recently been contested with evidence that early rehabilitation is not only not harmful but useful. This argues for the institution of active rehabilitation programs early in the course of myositis, perhaps improving the chances of a faster or more complete muscular recovery[56,57]. As soon as improvement is evident, the patient should begin active exercises, graduated according to muscle improvement.

Experienced physical therapists are extremely valuable in the rehabilitation of myositis patients and are able to devise programs tailored to the patient's needs. However, this service is not always available, and frequently physicians have to instruct patients as to how to proceed gradually with exercises. A recent experience with home exercises has proved successful in improving muscle function in these patients[58].

Specific problems that need to be addressed by the rehabilitation team include muscle weakness, joint limitations (especially in children), fatigue and decreased endurance[59,60].

Muscle weakness

Symmetric proximal weakness is present in 90% of patients. The initial degree of weakness depends on the degree of muscle inflammation present and the time from diagnosis to initiation of treatment. Distal muscle weakness occurs in 15–20% of idiopathic polymyositis, and in up to 50% of patients with inclusion body myositis (IBM). In these cases, hand involvement can interfere significantly with fine motor activities as well as gross grasp. Pharyngeal weakness may be associated with difficulty swallowing.

During treatment, weakness and atrophy of muscle may occur, not only from uncontrolled disease but also as a result of corticosteroid myopathy or fibrosis.

Joint limitations

These occur most frequently in juvenile dermatomyositis with periarticular calcific deposits. These may cause limitation of the elbow and knee joints. Limitations may also be seen in patients with initial incapacity to put their joints through the range of motion, and patients who have been on prolonged bed rest during the acute phase of myositis. This is probably more common in children than in adults, and those on bed rest are particularly prone to shoulder, hip, knee and ankle dorsiflexion contractures.

Fatigue and decreased endurance

Fatigue can be a result of the systemic disease itself, prolonged bed rest, a very low activity level, steroid myopathy, or specific cardiopulmonary involvement from myositis.

Suggested treatment approach[59,60]

Rehabilitation programs need to be tailored to the individual's needs, according to the following:

- Age
- Type of myositis and predicted outcome
- Stage of the disease (acute, recovery or chronic phase)
- Degree of muscle weakness and joint involvement
- Accompanying diseases and/or systemic manifestations
- The patient's work status and lifestyle
- Support systems available to the patient.

With this in mind, different strategies are adopted during the phases of the disease process (Table 140.3). These include plans for the acute phase (Table 140.4), for the early recovery period (Table 140.5) and for the late recovery and chronic phases (Table 140.6)[59].

TABLE 140.3   REHABILITATION IN MYOSITIS

Disease stage	Exercise
Acute	Passive range-of-motion exercises, stretching
Early recovery	Add:
	Muscle re-education, active assisted range-of-motion exercises, isometrics
Late recovery	Add:
	Isotonics (low weight), pool or dry land
Chronic active	Add:
	Aerobic exercise at 60% $\dot{V}O_{2\,max}$ (ergonometer or pool)

TABLE 140.4   AN APPROACH TO REHABILITATION IN ACUTE-PHASE MYOSITIS

- Massage and heat treatment for painful muscles
- Fit with an appropriate collar for neck support
- Use a balanced forearm orthosis on the wheelchair so that some independent feeding is possible
- Support the wrists and ankles with resting splints to prevent flexion contractures
- The patient should go to the rehabilitation department daily to use the tilt table and perform active assisted range-of-motion exercises with gravity eliminated
- Instruct the patient in the use of a long-handled comb and toothbrush, and a sponge to assist with self-care
- Educate the patient about the impact on function of the disease and encourage the patient to understand that function will gradually improve as muscle strength returns
- Regular evaluations and treatment by a speech and language pathologist
- Nurses should be trained in proper bed positioning, the appropriate position to facilitate feeding and prevent aspiration, techniques to facilitate breathing and in bed-to-chair transfers

---

TABLE 140.5   AN APPROACH TO REHABILITATION IN EARLY RECOVERY FROM MYOSITIS

- Begin muscle re-education and strengthening
- Work on improving truncal balance and strength
- Give instruction in active range-of-motion exercise and begin a few isometric contractions to major muscle groups (deltoids, biceps, quadriceps, hip abductors/extensors)
- Work on standing at the parallel bars and begin ambulation training
- Occupational therapy is needed for dressing and bathroom care with appropriate bathroom devices (elevated toilet seat, bars, shower chair, hand-held shower)
- Assess vocational abilities and advise on job retraining if necessary
- Make appropriate recommendations for adaptations in the home setting
- As balance improves and strength becomes good (4/5 range), ambulation with only a straight cane can be done; there may still be some pelvic lurching due to gluteus medius muscle weakness and the gait will be slow; work on negotiating stairs and ramps and practice walking outdoors as well as car transfers
- Work in the kitchen – practice preparing light meals and using the dishwasher, washing machine and dryer
- As enzymes decrease, increase the isometric exercise program to six contractions of each muscle group daily; pool therapy with range-of-motion and stretching exercises is permitted
- Help the patient to incorporate energy conservation strategies into the day

---

TABLE 140.6   AN APPROACH TO LATE RECOVERY AND CHRONIC PHASE MYOSITIS

- Isotonic exercise with low weights (2–4kg) or pool
- Bicycle ergometry without resistance or walking in pool or swimming
- Gradual aerobic exercise (starting at 15min sessions, increasing to 30min sessions, three weekly)

REFERENCES

1. Oddis CV. Current approach to the treatment of polymyositis and dermatomyositis. Curr Opin Rheumatol 2000; 12: 492–497.
2. Targoff IN, Miller FW, Medsger TA, Oddis CV. Classification criteria for the inflammatory myopathies. Curr Opin Rheumatol 1997; 9: 527–532.
3. Rider LG, Miller FW. Idiopathic inflammatory muscle disease: clinical aspects. Baillières Best Pract Res Clin Rheumatol 2000; 14: 37–54.
4. Fafalak RG, Peterson MG, Kagen LJ. The strength in polymyositis and dermatomyositis: best outcome in patients treated early. J Rheumatol 1994; 21: 643–648.
5. Henrikkson KG, Sanstedt P. Polymyositis – treatment and prognosis: a study of 107 patients. Acta Neurol Scand 1982; 65: 280–300.
6. Tymms KE, Webb J. Dermatopolymyositis and other connective tissue diseases: a review of 105 cases. J Rheumatol 1985; 12: 1140–1148.

7. Homik JE, Craney A, Shea B *et al.* A metanalysis on the use of bisphosphonates in corticosteroid induced osteoporosis. J Rheumatol 1999; 26: 1148–1157.
8. Metzger AL, Bohan A, Goldberg LS *et al.* Polymyositis and dermatomyositis: combined methotrexate and corticosteroid therapy. Ann Intern Med 1974; 81: 182–189.
9. Arnett FC, Whelton JC, Zizic TM, Stevens MB. Methotrexate therapy in polymyositis. Ann Rheum Dis 1973; 32: 536–546.
10. Kasteler JS, Callen JP. Low-dose methotrexate administered weekly is an effective corticosteroid-sparing agent for the treatment of the cutaneous manifestations of dermatomyositis. J Am Acad Dermatol 1997; 36: 67–71.
11. Zieglschmid Adams ME, Pandya AG *et al.* Treatment of dermatomyositis with methotrexate. J Am Acad Dermatol 1995; 32: 754–757.
12. Bunch TW. Prednisone and azathioprine for polymyositis: long term follow up. Arthritis Rheum 1981; 24: 45–48.
13. Fries JF, Sharp GC, McDevitt HO, Holman HR. Cyclophosphamide therapy in systemic lupus erythematosus and polymyositis. Arthritis Rheum 1973; 16: 154–162.
14. Yoshida T, Koga H, Saitoh F *et al.* Pulse intravenous cyclophosphamide treatment for steroid-resistant interstitial pneumonitis associated with polymyositis. Intern Med 1999; 38: 733–738.
15. Al Janadi M, Smith CD, Karsh J. Cyclophosphamide treatment of interstitial pulmonary fibrosis in polymyositis/dermatomyositis. J Rheumatol 1989; 16: 1592–1596.
16. Dantzig P. Juvenile dermatomyositis treated with cyclosporin. J Am Acad Dermatol 1990; 22: 310–311.
17. Qushmaq KA, Chalmers A, Esdaile JM. Cyclosporin A in the treatment of refractory adult polymyositis/dermatomyositis: population based experience in 6 patients and literature review. J Rheumatol 2000; 27: 2855–2859.
18. Reiff A, Rawlings DJ, Shaham B *et al.* Preliminary evidence for cyclosporin A as an alternative in the treatment of recalcitrant juvenile rheumatoid arthritis and juvenile dermatomyositis. J Rheumatol 1997; 24: 2436–2443.
19. Nawata Y, Kurasawa K, Takabayashi K *et al.* Corticosteroid resistant interstitial pneumonitis in dermatomyositis/polymyositis: prediction and treatment with cyclosporine. J Rheumatol 1999; 26: 1527–1533.
20. Sinoway PA, Callen JP. Chlorambucil. An effective corticosteroid-sparing agent for patients with recalcitrant dermatomyositis. Arthritis Rheum 1993; 36: 319–324.
21. Adams EM, Pucino F, Yarboro C *et al.* A pilot study: use of flutarabine for refractory polymyositis, dermatomyositis and examination of end point measures. J Rheumatol 1999; 26: 352–360.
22. Gelber AC, Nousari HC, Wigley FM. Mycophenolate mofetil in the treatment of severe skin manifestations of dermatomyositis: a series of 4 cases. J Rheumatol 2000; 27: 1542–1545.
23. Olson NY, Lindsley CB. Adjunctive use of hydroxychloroquine in childhood dermatomyositis. J Rheumatol 1989; 16: 1545–1557.
24. Imamura PM, Catoggio LJ, Soriano ER *et al.* Caracteristicas clinico-serologicas de 34 pacientes argentinos con dermato-polimiositis. Rev Argentina Reumatol 1993; 4: 90–98.
25. Easterbrook M. Ocular effects and safety of antimalarial drugs. Am J Med 1988; 85: 23–29.
26. Spalton DJ, Verdon Roe DM, Hughes GRV. Hydroxychloroquine, dosage parameters and retinopathy. Lupus 1993; 2: 355–358.
27. Dalakas MC, Illa I, Dambrosia JM *et al.* A controlled trial of high-dose intravenous immune globulin infusions as treatment for dermatomyositis. N Engl J Med 1993; 329: 1993–2000.
28. Dalakas MC. Controlled studies with high dose intravenous immunoglobulin in the treatment of dermatomyositis, inclusion body myositis and polymyositis. Neurology 1998; 51: S37–45.
29. Bril V, Allenby K, Midreni G *et al.* IVIG in neurology – evidence and recommendation. Can J Neurol Sci 1999; 26: 139–152.
30. Al-Mayouf SM, Laxer RM, Schneider R *et al.* Intravenous immunoglobulin therapy for juvenile dermatomyositis: efficacy and safety. J Rheumatol 2000; 27: 2498–2503.
31. Marie I, Hachulla E, Levesque H *et al.* Intravenous immunoglobulins as treatment of life threatening esophageal involvement in polymyositis and dermatomyositis. J Rheumatol 1999; 26: 2706–2709.
32. Morgan SH, Bernstein RM, Coppen J *et al.* Total body irradiation and the course of polymyositis. Arthritis Rheum 1985; 28: 831–835.
33. Miller FW, Leitman SF, Cronin ME *et al.* Controlled trial of plasma exchange and leuka-pheresis in polymyositis and dermatomyositis. N Engl J Med 1992; 326: 1380–1386.
34. Cherin P, Auperin I, Bussel A *et al.* Plasma exchange in polymyositis and dermatomyositis. Clin Exp Rheumatol 1995; 13: 270–271.
35. Park JH, Vital TL, Ryder NM *et al.* Magnetic resonance imaging and P-31 magnetic resonance spectroscopy provide unique quantitative data useful in the longitudinal management of patients with dermatomyositis. Arthritis Rheum 1994; 37: 736–746.
36. Schwaitzler ME, Fort J. Cost effectiveness of magnetic resonance imaging in the evaluation of polymyositis . Am J Roentgenol 1995; 165: 1469–1471.
37. Park JH, Niermann KJ, Ryder NM *et al.* Muscle abnormalities in juvenile dermatomyositis patients: P-31 magnetic resonance spectroscopy studies. Arthritis Rheum 2000; 43: 2359–2367.
38. Lovece S, Kagen LJ. Sensitive rapid detection of myoglobin in serum of patients with myopathy by immunoturbidimetric assay. J Rheumatol 1993; 20: 1331–1334.
39. Gonzalez-Lopez L, Gamez-Nava JI, Sanchez L *et al.* Cardiac manifestations in dermatopolymyositis. Clin Exp Rheumatol 1996; 14: 373–379.
40. Cuny C, Eicher JC, Collet E *et al.* Dilated cardiomyopathy disclosing dermatopolymyositis. Manage Ann Cardiol Angio 1993; 42: 155–158.
41. Kagen LJ, Hochman RB, Stron EW. Cricopharyngeal obstruction in inflammatory myopathy (polymyositis/dermatomyositis): report of three cases and review of the literature. Arthritis Rheum 1985; 28: 630–636.
42. Hill C, Romas E, Kirkham B. Use of sequential DTPA clearance and high resolution computerized tomography in monitoring interstitial lung disease in dermatomyositis. Br J Rheumatol 1996; 35: 164–166.
43. Vinen CS, Patel S, Bruckner FE. Regression of calcinosis associated with adult dermatomyositis following diltiazem therapy. Rheumatology (Oxford) 2000; 39: 333–334.
44. Oliveri MB, Palermo R, Mautalen C, Hubscher O. Regression of calcinosis during diltiazem treatment in juvenile dermatomyositis. J Rheumatol 1996; 23: 2152–2155.
45. Matsuoka Y, Miyajima S, Okada N. A case of calcinosis universalis successfully treated with low-dose warfarin. J Dermatol 1998; 25: 716–720.
46. Nakagawa T, Takaiwa T. Calcinosis cutis in juvenile dermatomyositis responsive to aluminum hydroxide treatment. J Dermatol 1993; 20: 558–560.
47. Davidson GS, Voorneveld CR, Krishnan N. Tuberculous infection of skeletal muscle in a case of dermatomyositis. Muscle Nerve 1994; 17: 730–732.
48. Soriano ER, Barcan L, Clara L *et al. Streptococcus pyomyositis* occurring in a patient with dermatomyositis in a country with temperate climate. J Rheumatol 1992; 19: 1305–1307.
49. Bachelez H, Schremmer B, Cadranel J *et al.* Fulminant *Pneumocystis carinii* pneumonia in 4 patients with dermatomyositis. Arch Intern Med 1997; 157: 1501–1503.
50. Poddar SK, Misra S, Singh NK. Acute polymyositis associated with *W. bancrofti.* Acta Neurol Scand 1994; 89: 225–226.
51. Horowitz HW, Sanghera K, Goldberg N *et al.* Dermatomyositis associated with Lyme disease: case report and review of Lyme myositis. Clin Infect Dis 1994; 18: 166–171.
52. Dauden E, Penas PF, Rios L *et al.* Leishmaniasis presenting as a dermatomyositis-like eruption in AIDS. J Am Acad Dermatol 1996; 35: 316–319.
53. Dalakas MC, Illa I, Pezeshkpour GH *et al.* Mitochondrial myopathy caused by long-term zidovudine therapy. N Engl J Med 1990; 322: 1098–1105.
54. Leff RL, Miller FW, Hicks J *et al.* The treatment of inclusion body myositis: a retrospective review and a randomized prospective trial of immunosuppressive therapy. Medicine 1993; 72: 225–235.
55. Dalakas, MC. Progess in inflammatory myopathies: good but not good enough. J Neurol Neurosurg Psychiatry 2001; 70: 569–573.
56. Hicks JE, Miller F, Plotz P *et al.* Isometric exercise increases strength and does not produce sustained creatinine phosphokinase increases in a patient with polymyositis. J Rheumatol 1993; 20: 1399–1401.
57. Wiesinger GF, Quittan M, Graninger M *et al.* Benefit of 6 months long-term physical training in polymyositis/dermatomyositis patients. Br J Rheumatol 1998; 37: 1338–1342.
58. Alexanderson H, Stenstrom CH, Jenner G, Lundberg I. The safety of a resistive home exercise program in patients with recent onset active polymyositis or dermatomyositis. Scand J Rheumatol 2000; 29: 295–301.
59. Hicks JE. Role of rehabilitation in the management of myopathies. Curr Opin Rheumatol 1998; 10: 548–555.
60. Hicks JE. Inflammatory muscle disease: practical problems. In: Klippel JH, Dieppe PA, eds. Rheumatology, 2nd edn. London: Mosby; 1998: 7.16: 9–10.

141 Inflammatory and metabolic myopathies

Robert L Wortmann

Definitions

- The idiopathic inflammatory myopathies are defined by the combination of proximal muscle weakness, increased serum concentrations of enzymes derived from skeletal muscle, myopathic changes on electromyography and inflammation in muscle
- Polymyositis, the prototypic idiopathic inflammatory myopathy, is characterized by cytotoxic T lymphocytic invasion of muscle fibers
- Dermatomyositis, which is differentiated clinically from polymyositis by the presence of a rash, is characterized by perivascular infiltration of helper T cell and B cell lymphocytes
- Inclusion body myositis, which is characterized by rimmed vacuoles in muscle fibers, may be identical to polymyositis, but have neuropathic features also
- Subsets of patients with inflammatory myopathies have circulating myositis-specific autoantibodies, the presence of which tends to predict clinical features in treatment responses
- The differential diagnosis of proximal muscle weakness includes neuropathic, infectious, cancer-related, drug-induced and metabolic disorders, in addition to the inflammatory myopathies
- The primary metabolic myopathies are inherited disorders of muscle glycogen, lipid or mitochondrial metabolism that may cause episodic exercise intolerance, with myoglobinuria or progressive proximal muscle weakness.

INFLAMMATORY DISEASES OF MUSCLE

The idiopathic inflammatory diseases of muscle are a heterogeneous group of conditions characterized by symmetric proximal muscle weakness and non-suppurative inflammation of skeletal muscle (Table 141.1)[1]. In addition, patients with these diseases have increased serum concentrations of enzymes derived from skeletal muscle, myopathic changes demonstrated on the electromyogram (EMG) and inflammatory changes in muscle identified by magnetic resonance imaging. Some patients have circulating myositis-specific autoantibodies.

Patients can be divided into subsets on the basis of their age, coexistence of other disease manifestations, and pathology: (1) primary idiopathic polymyositis, (2) primary idiopathic dermatomyositis, (3) dermatomyositis or polymyositis associated with neoplasia, (4) childhood dermatomyositis (or polymyositis) associated with vasculitis, (5) polymyositis or dermatomyositis with associated collagen vascular disease and (6) inclusion body myositis. The presence or absence of circulating myositis-specific autoantibodies (MSAs) allows further segregation of patients among homogeneous groups with regards to disease manifestations and prognosis[2] (see Chapter 139). A variety of schemes of criteria for the diagnosis of an idiopathic inflammatory myopathy have been proposed. Those proposed in 1975 by Bohan and Peters[3], which are those most commonly used, and those incorporating more recent observations[4–6] are summarized in Tables 141.2–141.5.

Epidemiology

The idiopathic inflammatory myopathies are relatively rare diseases, with estimates of incidence ranging from 0.5 to 8.4 cases per million. The incidence appears to be increasing, although this may simply reflect increased awareness and more accurate diagnosis. The age at onset for the idiopathic inflammatory myopathies has a bimodal distribution, with peaks between ages 10 and 15 years in children and between 45 and 60 years in adults, with the mean ages for specific subsets differing. The age at onset for myositis associated with another collagen vascular disease is similar to that for the associated condition. Myositis associated with malignancy and inclusion body myositis (IBM) are more common after age 50 years. Women are affected more frequently than men, by a 2:1 ratio with the exception of IBM, in which the ratio is reversed. Female predominance is especially great between ages 15 and 45 years, in myositis associated with other collagen vascular diseases, and in blacks populations.

Clinical features

The dominant clinical feature of the idiopathic inflammatory myopathies is symmetric proximal muscle weakness[1,7]. Although strength may be essentially normal at the time of presentation, virtually all patients will develop significant muscle weakness during the course of their illness. The weakness can be accompanied by myalgias and tenderness and, eventually, atrophy and fibrosis. Laboratory investigation reveals increased serum enzyme concentrations of skeletal muscle origin. These include creatine kinase (CK), aldolase, serum glutamic–oxaloacetic transaminase, serum glutamic–pyruvic transaminase, and lactate dehydrogenase. Increased concentrations of these enzymes are found in the inflammatory diseases of muscle, but are not specific for those diagnoses. CK is a dimer and exists in the serum in three isoforms: MM, MB and BB. The MM form predominates in skeletal and cardiac muscle. MB is found primarily

---

TABLE 141.1 CLASSIFICATION OF INFLAMMATORY DISEASES OF MUSCLE

Idiopathic inflammatory myopathies

Polymyositis
Dermatomyositis
Juvenile (childhood) dermatomyositis
Myositis associated with collagen vascular disease
Myositis associated with malignancy
Inclusion body myositis

Other forms of inflammatory myopathy

Localized or focal myositis
Giant cell myositis
Myositis associated with eosinophilia
Myositis ossificans

TABLE 141.2 CRITERIA TO DEFINE POLYMYOSITIS AND DERMATOMYOSITIS PROPOSED BY BOHAN AND PETER[3]

1. Symmetric weakness of limb-girdle muscles and anterior neck flexors, progressing over weeks to months, with or without dysphagia or respiratory muscle involvement
2. Skeletal muscle histology showing evidence of necrosis of type 1 and 2 muscle fibers, phagocytosis, regeneration with basophilia, large sarcolemmal nuclei and prominent nucleoli, atrophy in a perifascicular distribution, variation in fiber size and an inflammatory exudate
3. Increase in serum skeletal muscle enzymes (CK, aldolase, SGOT, SGPT and LDH)
4. Electromyographic triad of: short, small polyphasic motor units; fibrillations, positive waves and insertional irritability; bizarre high-frequency discharges
5. Dermatologic features including a lilac (heliotrope) discoloration of the eyelids with periorbital edema; a scaly, erythematous dermatitis over the dorsa of the hands, especially over the metacarpophalangeal and proximal interphalangeal joints (Gottron's sign); involvement of the knees, elbows, medial malleoli, face, neck and upper torso

CK, creatine kinase; SGOT, serum glutamic–oxaloacetic transaminase; SGPT, serum glutamic–pyruvic transaminase; LDH, lactate dehydrogenase.

TABLE 141.3 DIAGNOSTIC CRITERIA PROPOSED FOR INCLUSION BODY MYOSITIS (IBM)[4]

Pathologic criteria

Electron microscopy
1. Microtubular filaments in the inclusions

Light microscopy
1. Lined vacuoles
2. Intranuclear or intracytoplasmic inclusions, or both

Clinical criteria

1. Proximal muscle weakness (insidious onset)
2. Distal muscle weakness
3. Electromyographic evidence of a generalized myopathy (inflammatory myopathy)
4. Increase in muscle enzyme concentrations (creatine phosphokinase, aldolase, or both)
5. Failure of muscle weakness to improve on a high-dose corticosteroid regimen (at least 40–60mg/day for 3–4 months)

Diagnoses

Definite IBM = Pathologic electron microscopy criterion 1 and cinical criterion 1 plus one other clinical criterion

Probable IBM = Pathologic light microscopy criterion 1 and clinical criterion 1 plus three other clinical criteria

Possible IBM = Pathologic light microscopy criterion 2 plus any three clinical criteria

TABLE 141.4 CLASSIFICATION CRITERIA FOR POLYMYOSITIS/DERMATOMYOSITIS[5]

Classification	Criterion
1	Skin lesions
	(a) Heliotrope rash (red-purple edematous erythema on the upper palpebra)
	(b) Gottron's sign (red-purple keratotic, atrophic erythema, or macules on the extensor surface of finger joints)
	(c) Erythema on the extensor surface of extremity joints; slightly raised red-purple erythema over elbows or knees
2	Proximal muscle weakness (upper or lower extremity and trunk)
3	Increased serum creatine kinase or aldolase concentration
4	Muscle pain on grasping or spontaneous pain
5	Myogenic changes on electromyography (short-duration, polyphasic motor unit potentials with spontaneous fibrillation potentials)
6	Positive anti-Jo-1 (histidyl-tRNA synthetase) antibody
7	Non-destructive arthritis or arthralgias
8	Systemic inflammatory signs (fever >37° C at axilla, increased serum C-reactive protein concentration, or accelerated erythrocyte sedimentation rate of more than 20mm/h by the Westergren method)
9	Pathologic findings compatible with inflammatory myositis (inflammatory infiltration of skeletal muscle with degeneration or necrosis of muscle fibers; active phagocytosis, central nuclei, or evidence of active regeneration may be seen)

Diagnoses

Dermatomyositis	At least one item from criterion 1 and at least four from criteria items 2–9
Polymyositis	At least four from criteria items 2–9

TABLE 141.5 PROPOSED REVISED CRITERIA FOR THE DIAGNOSIS OF IDIOPATHIC INFLAMMATORY MYOSITIS[6]

1. Symmetric proximal muscle weakness
2. Increase in the serum concentrations of enzymes including not only CK concentration, but also aldolase, AST, ALT and lactate dehydrogenase concentrations
3. Abnormal electromyogram with myopathic motor unit potentials, fibrillations, positive sharp waves and increased insertional irritability
4. Muscle biopsy features of inflammatory infiltration and either degeneration/regeneration or perfascicular atrophy
5. Any of one of the myositis-specific autoantibodies (an antisynthetase, anti-Mi-2, or anti-SRP)
6. Typical skin rash of DM that includes Gottron's sign, Gottron's papules, or heliotrope rash

Diagnoses

Possible IIM = any two criteria
Probable IIM = any three criteria
Definite IIM = any four criteria
Patients with IIM who satisfy criterion 6 may be subclassified as having DM. Those who satisfy the proposed criteria for inclusion body myositis may be subclassified as having inclusion body myositis.

Results of magnetic resonance imaging that are consistent with muscle inflammation may be substituted for either criterion 1 or criterion 2.

The application of these criteria assumes that known infectious, toxic, metabolic, dystrophic or endocrine myopathies have been excluded by appropriate evaluations.

ALT, alanine aminotransferase; AST, aspartate aminotransferase; CK, creatine kinase; DM, dermatomyositis; IIM, idiopathic inflammatory myopathy; PM, polymyositis.

in cardiac muscle, composing about 25% of the total CK activity in that tissue; it is a very minor component in skeletal muscle, but is present in that tissue in greater amounts in embryonal and regenerating fibers. BB is the major isoenzyme in brain and smooth muscle. In myositis, most increases are in the MM isoform; however, the MB fraction can occur in myositis with no cardiac involvement and in healthy young women after submaximal eccentric exercise.

The EMG demonstrates myopathic changes that are consistent with, but not specific for, inflammation. The classic electromyographic changes of an idiopathic inflammatory myopathy include the triad of

(1) increased insertional activity, fibrillations and sharp positive waves; (2) spontaneous, bizarre high-frequency discharges; (3) polyphasic motor unit potentials of low amplitude and short duration. However, this complete triad is found in approximately 40% of patients. EMG changes may be limited or localized, and may be completely normal in 10–15% of patients[7].

Histology of skeletal muscle shows changes characteristic of inflammation. These manifestations can occur in a variety of combinations or patterns. Some changes are characteristic and help identify a specific subset of disease, but the changes observed in many biopsies are less helpful. Muscle inflammation may also be apparent using magnetic resonance imaging with T-2 weighting and images, fat-suppression or short time inversion recovery techniques.

Polymyositis in the adult

Polymyositis is perhaps the most characteristic of the idiopathic inflammatory myopathies, as patients with this disease manifest the characteristic features that define the diagnostic criteria[1,7]. Onset is typically insidious over 3–6 months and is not associated with an identifiable precipitating event. The weakness initially affects the muscles of the shoulder and pelvic girdle, with the latter slightly more common. Neck flexor muscle weakness occurs in about 50% of patients. Although mild muscle pain and tenderness are present in about 50% of patients, these findings rarely dominate the clinical picture. Ocular, facial and bulbar muscles are spared.

The inflammatory process is systemic. Accordingly, patients may develop fatigue, morning stiffness, anorexia, weight loss and fever. Periorbital edema may occur. Arthralgias are not uncommon, but frank synovitis is less usual. Pulmonary manifestations may include interstitial fibrosis or pneumonitis[8]. 'Velcro'-like crackles may be heard on chest auscultation. Dysphagia and dysphonia may develop secondary to esophageal dysfunction or cricopharyngeal obstruction. Aspiration pneumonia may complicate the disease course in patients with esophageal dysmotility.

The concentrations of CK and other muscle enzymes are increased at some time during the course of the disease, and in most patients this is a helpful indicator of disease severity. Normal concentrations of CK may be found very early in the disease course, in advanced disease with significant muscle atrophy or, rarely, as a result of circulating inhibitors of CK activity that may be present during active disease.

Although the histopathology of polymyositis is well described, no specific change is pathognomonic, and wide variations in pathologic change can be observed both within the tissue of an individual patient and from individual to individual. Characteristically, necrotic and regenerating fibers are observed, with focal and endomysial infiltration of inflammatory cells. T lymphocytes, especially CD8+ cytotoxic cells, and macrophages are found surrounding and invading the initially non-necrotic fibers. In some cases, the only changes seen are degeneration in the absence of inflammatory cells or type 2 fiber atrophy. Intact fibers may vary in size. As the disease progresses, destroyed fibers are replaced by fibrous connective tissue and fat.

Dermatomyositis in the adult

Patients with dermatomyositis fulfill the criteria for polymyositis and also have cutaneous involvement[9]. Rash may be the presenting complaint, antedating the onset of weakness by more than a year. In some, the severity of the rash and muscle weakness correlate well; in others, the severity of the two problems is unrelated. The rash may change or vary during the course of the disease.

A variety of skin changes can be observed. Gottron's papules, if present, are considered pathognomonic. These are lacy, pink to violaceous, raised or macular areas typically distributed symmetrically on the dorsal aspect of interphalangeal joints, elbows, knees or medial malleoli.

Other characteristic changes include heliotrope or violaceous discoloration of the eyelids, macular erythema of the posterior shoulders and neck (shawl sign), anterior neck and upper chest (V sign), face and forehead. Dystrophic cuticles, periungual telangiectasias, and nailfold capillary changes similar to those observed in patients with scleroderma or SLE can be seen. Darkened or dirty-appearing, horizontal lines may be noted across the lateral and palmar aspects of the fingers. These changes are termed 'mechanic's hands'.

The muscle histopathology of adult dermatomyositis is characteristic. Fiber invasion by inflammatory cells is rare. Instead, the inflammatory infiltration is distributed perivascularly, and is composed of B lymphocytes and CD4+ helper lymphocytes. Other changes include perifascicular atrophy and capillary plugging. Skin histopathology varies according to the stage of the disease and the type of lesion. Epidermal thickening, prominent dermal blood vessels, infiltration of lymphocytes (mostly CD4+), plasma cells and histiocytes, and edema of the superficial layers of the dermis are seen in the earlier erythematous edematous regions. More chronic lesions are characterized by epidermal thinning, inflammatory cell infiltrates in the dermis and increased connective tissue.

The terms 'amyopathic dermatomyositis' and 'dermatomyositis sine myositis' have been used to describe patients with biopsy-confirmed classic cutaneous findings of dermatomyositis but who have no clinical or laboratory evidence of muscle disease. Today, the diagnosis of amyopathic dermatomyositis is applied to patients who have the combination of Gottron's papules or other cutaneous manifestations of dermatomyositis, and no enzymatic or clinical evidence of myopathy. Approximately 33–50% of patients will retain the diagnosis over time, with some attaining partial or complete remission. The remainder progress and develop muscle involvement and weakness. Malignancy has developed in some cases. In making the diagnosis of amyopathic dermatomyositis, one must exclude other causes of similar appearing cutaneous lesions. Trichinosis infection, allergic contact dermatitis and drugs such as hydroxyurea, penicillamine, niflumic acid, diclofenate, tryptophan and practolol can cause cutaneous changes that mimic dermatomyositis.

Juvenile (childhood) dermatomyositis

The general features of juvenile dermatomyositis include rash and weakness similar to those seen in adults. However, the juvenile form differs from that seen in adults because of the coexistence of vasculitis, ectopic calcification and lipodystrophy and arthrtis[10–12]. Classically, children develop cutaneous manifestations, followed by muscle weakness. The rash is typically erythematous and is found on the malar region in addition to the extensor surfaces of the elbows, knuckles and knees. Some lesions scale. Lesions may also become pigmented or depigmented. Weakness, myalgias and stiffness are most severe in the proximal muscles and neck flexors. The involved muscles are often tender on palpation.

Inclusion body myositis

Patients with IBM may present with clinical features identical to those with polymyositis. However, IBM differs from polymyositis with regards to histopathology, treatment, responsiveness and, in some, distribution of muscle weakness[4]. IBM primarily affects older individuals, although a small number of cases have been diagnosed in patients younger than 40 years and, rarely, in childhood.

Onset is typically insidious, and progression is slow. In fact, the disease has often been present for 5 or 6 years before a diagnosis. The clinical picture in some patients differs from that of typical polymyositis in that it may include focal, distal or asymmetric weakness. Dysphagia tends to be a late occurrence, but occasionally is a significant presenting symptom. In some patients, the disease continues a slow, steady progression. In others, it seems to plateau, leaving the individual with fixed weakness, diminished deep tendon reflexes and atrophy of the involved musculature.

Serum CK concentrations are only slightly increased in most patients, are normal in 25% of patients throughout the disease course and are more commonly lower later in the disease. Most patients have myopathic changes on the EMG, with approximately 50% having electromyographic features consistent with neurogenic or mixed neurogenic and myopathic changes.

Histologic changes define the diagnosis. These include necrosis and inflammation consistent with polymyositis that tend to diminish and disappear over time. In addition, 'ragged red' fibers and angulated atrophic fibers may be seen. The characteristic change is the presence of intracellular lined vacuoles. Vacuoles are not specific for IBM, because vacuolar changes are also prominent features in muscle from patients with a wide variety of myopathies. Electron microscopy reveals either intracytoplasmic or intranuclear tubular or filamentous inclusions. These structures are straight and rigid appearing, with periodic transverse and longitudinal striations. Myelin figures and myeloid bodies are membranous whorls that are commonly seen in IBM, but are also not specific.

Myopathies and autoantibodies

The idiopathic inflammatory myopathies can be further defined by the presence or absence of circulating autoantibodies found almost exclusively in patients with polymyositis or dermatomyositis (Table 141.6) [13]. Because of these relationships, they have been termed 'myositis-specific autoantibodies'. The MSAs can be categorized among three types, depending upon the antigen at which the autoantibody is directed: aminoacyl-tRNA synthetases, non-synthetase cytoplasmic antigens, and nuclear antigens (Table 141.7) [2].

The antisynthetases are the most commonly recognized MSAs, and antihistidyl-tRNA synthetase, termed anti-Jo1, is the most common of these. The antisynthetases show immunochemical properties, including the immunoprecipitation of RNA, inhibition of enzyme function and reaction with conformational epitopes that are indicative of autoantibodies. The antisynthetases do not cross-react or occur together. With extremely rare exception, an individual patient will have only one antisynthetase.

Individuals with anti-Jo1 or another antisynthetase may have either polymyositis or dermatomyositis. Patients with these autoantibodies have an increased prevalence of interstitial lung disease, arthritis, Raynaud's phenomenon, fever and mechanic's hands. In fact, perhaps 80% of patients with myositis and interstitial lung disease have circulating antisynthetase syndromes.

In contrast, almost all individuals with anti-SRP antibodies have polymyositis. Anti-SRP may be associated with an acute onset, cardiomyopathy and treatment resistance. Those with anti-Mi-2 antibodies have dermatomyositis and a very good prognosis.

Another group of autoantibodies have been identified in patients with muscle diseases, but are not specific for them. They tend to occur in overlap syndromes or in patients with other autoimmune diseases, such as SLE or scleroderma. Accordingly, they have been termed myositis-associated autoantibodies (Table 141.7).

Localized or focal myositis

Histologic changes identical to those observed in polymyositis occasionally are present in biopsies of focal nodules from patients who have only one muscle or one extremity involved. Characteristically, the nodules are painful, tender and enlarge over a period of weeks. This

TABLE 141.7 MYOSITIS-SPECIFIC AND MYOSITIS-ASSOCIATED AUTOANTIBODIES

Name	Antigen	HLA
Myositis-specific		
Jo1	Histidyl-tRNA synthetase	DR3; DRw52; DRB1*0501
PL-7	Threonyl-tRNA synthetase	DRw52
PL-12	Alanyl-tRNA synthetase	DRw52
EJ	Glycyl-tRNA synthetase	DRw52
OJ	Isoleucyl-tRNA synthetase	DRw52
KS	Asparaginyl-tRNA synthetase	DRw52
SRP	Signal recognition particle	DR5; DRw52
Mi-2	CHO3 and CHO4 helicase components of histone acetylase complexes	DR7; DRw52
Myositis-associated		
56kDa	Components of ribonucleo-protein particle	–
Fer	Elongation factor-1α	–
KJ	Unidentified translocation factor	DRw52
PM-Scl	Unidentified	DR3
Ku	DNA-binding proteins	–
MJ	Unidentified	–
155kDa	Unidentified	–

HLA, human leukocyte antigen.

TABLE 141.6 ADULT AND CHILDHOOD SYNDROMES ASSOCIATED WITH MYOSITIS-SPECIFIC AUTOANTIBODIES

Autoantibody	Clinical features	Treatment response
Anti-Jo1 (and other antisynthetases)	Polymyositis or dermatomyositis with relatively acute onset Interstitial lung disease Fever Arthritis Raynaud's phenomenon 'Mechanic's hands'	Moderate, with disease persistence
Anti-SRP	Polymyositis with very acute onset Severe weakness Cardiomyopathy	Poor
Anti-Mi-2	Dermatomyositis with V sign and shawl sign Cuticular overgrowth	Good

disorder may remit spontaneously, remain focal and confined to one limb for several years, or progress to a distribution of typical polymyositis. These lesions must be differentiated from a skeletal muscle tumor.

Orbital or ocular myositis is a focal myositis limited to extraocular muscles. Patients usually present with orbital or periorbital pain, diplopia, abnormal extraocular motion and proptosis. It can be seen alone or in association with polymyositis. Computed tomography and magnetic resonance imaging are helpful in distinguishing orbital myositis from orbital pseudotumor, cellulitis, cavernous sinus thrombosis or Graves' ophthalmopathy.

Giant cell myositis

Multinucleated giant cells may occur in skeletal muscle in a variety of conditions, including foreign body reactions, tuberculosis, sarcoidosis and giant cell (granulomatous) myositis. Regenerating muscle cells are multinucleated and may closely resemble giant cells. Therefore, the histopathology and overall clinical status of the patient should be reviewed carefully whenever giant cells are found in skeletal muscle.

Eosinophilic myositis

Eosinophilic myositis is a rare disorder characterized by the subacute onset of proximal weakness, myalgias, increased serum concentrations of muscle enzymes, myopathic electromyographic findings and an eosinophilic inflammatory infiltrate in muscle tissue[14]. Eosinophilic myositis can also present as a focal disorder that may relapse or remit spontaneously. It may represent one manifestation of a generalized hypereosinophilic syndrome or can be associated with a predominant overlying eosinophilic fascitis (Shulman's disease). The majority of patients with eosinophilic myositis respond to prednisone.

Myositis ossificans

Myositis ossificans can be localized or widespread. The localized form invariably follows trauma, although the trauma may have seemed trivial or may not be remembered. Initially, a warm, tender swelling of a doughy consistency is noted in the muscle. Soon thereafter, the area takes on the consistency of a mass and becomes firm and hard. At about 1 month, calcifications are seen on radiographs or with computed tomography scanning. Surgical excision is often necessary, and generally leads to a good outcome.

The widespread, progressive form termed 'myositis ossificans progressiva' is inherited in the autosomal dominant pattern, and is first noted during childhood. The warm, tender swellings gradually shrink, become hard and may disappear only to recur. Myositis ossificans progressiva is associated with congenital defects including microdactyly of the great toe and thumb, exostosis, absence of the two upper incisors, hypogenitalism, absence of the ear lobules and deafness.

METABOLIC MYOPATHIES

The term 'metabolic myopathy' represents a heterogenous group of conditions (Table 141.8) that have in common abnormalities in muscle energy metabolism that result in skeletal muscle dysfunction. Some metabolic myopathies should be considered primary and are associated with known or postulated biochemical defects that affect the ability of the muscle fibers to maintain adequate concentrations of ATP[15]. Other metabolic myopathies may be considered secondary and attributed to various endocrine or electrolyte abnormalities.

Primary metabolic myopathies

Disorders of glycogen metabolism

Diseases that have in common an underlying defect in glycogen synthesis, glycogenolysis or glycolysis are termed glycogen storage diseases (GSDs) because the various defects result in an abnormal accumulation of glyco-

gen in skeletal muscle[15–17]. To date, 11 disorders, caused by enzyme deficiencies, are included in this classification (Table 141.8, Fig. 141.1).

The classic clinical manifestation of a GSD is exercise intolerance. This may be attributed to pain, fatigue, stiffness, weakness or intense cramping. Most patients develop some symptoms during childhood, but significant problems such as severe cramping or exercise-induced rhabdomyolysis and myoglobinuria with renal failure may not develop until the teenage years. A subset of patients, however, complain only of easy fatigability, whereas others develop the gradual onset of proximal muscle weakness. The latter presentation often occurs in adulthood, and patients with this presentation may not seek medical attention until middle age.

Affected individuals are generally asymptomatic as long as their muscles do not require carbohydrate for energy production. Accordingly, most afflicted persons are well at rest and can function without difficulty at low levels of activity. Symptoms develop after activities of high intensity or of lesser intensity for longer intervals – times when the majority of energy for muscular work is derived from carbohydrate. Some patients experience a 'second wind' phenomenon. Although they must stop an activity because of exercise-induced symptoms, they are often able to resume the exercise after a brief rest.

Serum CK concentrations are commonly increased, and the EMG shows increased insertional irritability, increased numbers of polyphasic motor unit potentials, fibrillations and positive waves. Muscle biopsy may reveal fiber necrosis and phagocytosis. Thus these nonspecific findings are consistent with the changes seen in inflammatory myopathies.

The diagnosis of GSDs may be suggested by the presence of increased glycogen on muscle biopsy. The finding of excessive glycogen deposition is not specific, however, and may be seen only by electron microscopy. The forearm ischemic exercise test is a useful method of screening for a GSD. Individuals with most GSDs will fail to generate lactate during ischemic exercise. Exceptions include deficiencies of acid maltase, brancher enzyme and phosphorylase b kinase. The putative diagnosis

TABLE 141.8 METABOLIC MYOPATHIES	
Disordered glycogen metabolism	**Endocrine**
Myophosphorylase deficiency (McArdle's disease)	Acromegaly
	Hypothyroidism
Phosphorylase B kinase deficiency	Hyperthyroidism
Phosphofructokinase deficiency	Hyperparathyroidism
Debrancher enzyme deficiency	Cushing's disease
Brancher enzyme deficiency	Addison's disease
Phosphoglycerate kinase deficiency	Hyperaldosteronism
Phosphoglycerate mutase deficiency	Carcinoid syndrome
Lactate dehydrogenase deficiency	
Acid maltase deficiency	**Metabolic–nutritional**
Aldolase deficiency	Uremia
β-Enolase deficiency	Hepatic failure
	Malabsorption
Disordered lipid metabolism and mitochondrial myopathies	Periodic paralysis
Carnitine deficiency	Vitamin D deficiency
• Inherited	Vitamin E deficiency
• Acquired	
Carnitine palmitoyltransferase deficiency	**Electrolyte disorders**
	Hypernatremia
Fatty acid acyl CoA dehydrogenase deficiencies	Hyponatremia
	Hyperkalemia
Coenzyme Q$_{10}$ deficiency	Hypokalemia
Respiratory chain complex deficiencies	Hypercalcemia
	Hypocalcemia
	Hypophosphatemia
	Hypomagnesemia

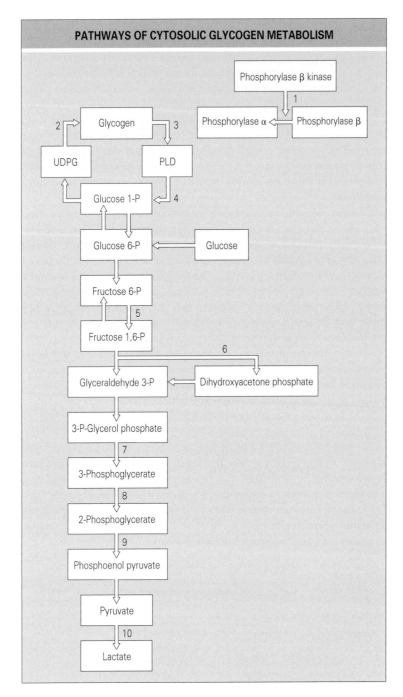

Fig. 141.1 Pathways of cytosolic glycogen metabolism. Deficiencies of numbered enzymes are recognized to cause a glycogen storage disease: 1, phosphorylase b kinase; 2, brancher enzyme; 3, myophosphorylase; 4, debrancher enzyme; 5, phosphofructokinase; 6, aldolase A; 7, phosphoglycerate kinase; 8, phosphoglycerate mutase; 9, β-enolase; 10, lactate dehydrogenase. Note: Acid maltase is not included because it is a lysozomal enzyme. P, phosphate; PLD, phosphorylase limit dextran; UDPG, uridine diphosphate glucose.

should always be confirmed by specific enzyme analysis of muscle tissue whenever it is suspected by histology or ischemic exercise testing.

Like the other GSDs, acid maltase deficiency can present in infantile, childhood or adult forms. The adult form typically presents with proximal muscle weakness beginning after the age of 20 years. Diaphragmatic involvement and respiratory failure develop in 33% of patients. Adult acid maltase deficiency causes characteristic electromyographic changes of intense electrical irritability and myotonic discharges in the absence of clinical myotonia, and the diagnosis can be confirmed by demonstrating deficient α-glucosidase activity in muscle or leukocytes.

The treatment of patients with a GSD includes education regarding physical activity and nutrition. A high-protein diet has helped some. Individuals with myophosphorylase deficiency may also benefit from vitamin B_6 supplementation.

Disorders of lipid metabolism

The disorder of lipid metabolism results from biochemical defects that occur in mitochondria (Table 141.8)[15,17–20]. Those that are caused by defective fatty acid transport or defects in B-oxidation are often referred to as 'lipid storage diseases'. The term 'mitochondrial myopathy' (see below also) is used to represent defects of the respiratory chain and oxidative phosphorylation (Fig. 141.2). Defects in these pathways interfere with energy production in most organs. Therefore, these myopathies may be associated with involvement of other organs. However, some disorders manifest only as skeletal muscle dysfunction.

Carnitine is an amino acid that is required for the transport of long-chain fatty acids into mitochondria. Carnitine deficiency causes abnormal lipid accumulation in skeletal muscle and can result from inherited or acquired causes. Primary carnitine deficiencies can be divided into *systemic* and *muscle* types. *Systemic carnitine deficiency* develops early in life, with episodes of coma and hypoketotic hypoglycemia similar to Reye's syndrome. Patients with *muscle carnitine deficiency* present in later childhood and through the early adult years, with progressive proximal muscle weakness. The process may also involve facial and pharyngeal musculature. Acquired carnitine deficiencies have been reported with pregnancy, renal failure requiring long-term hemodialysis, endstage cirrhosis, myxedema, adrenal insufficiency and treatment with valproate or pivampicillin.

Carnitine deficiency may be confused with polymyositis because serum CK concentrations are increased in more than 50% of patients and electromyography often reveals polyphasic motor unit potentials of small amplitude and short duration. Histochemical analysis by electron microscopy of muscle should demonstrate abnormal deposits of lipid. Almost 50% of patients with carnitine deficiency improve with dietary supplementation with L-carnitine. Treatment with dietary manipulation, prednisone or propranolol may help some patients who are refractory to treatment with L-carnitine.

Carnitine palmitoyltransferase activities are necessary for the transport of the long-chain fatty acid–carnitine complex into mitochondria. Carnitine palmitoyltransferase deficiency is an autosomal recessive disorder that invariably causes attacks of severe myalgia and myoglobinuria. These are typically associated with vigorous physical activity, but may occur with fasting, infection or exposure to cold. Some patients also have exercise intolerance and fatigue. Serum CK concentrations, EMG and muscle histology are normal, except during episodes of rhabdomyolysis. The diagnosis is made by assaying muscle tissue for enzyme activity.

Deficiencies of the three fatty acid acyl-coenzyme A (CoA) dehydrogenase activities have been reported in adults who presented with proximal muscle weakness and neck pain. Further evaluation reveals increased CK concentrations, myopathic changes on EMG and abnormal lipid accumulation in muscle tissue. Treatment with riboflavin, a component of this enzyme, has resulted in normalization of muscle histology and improved strength.

Mitochondrial myopathies

The term 'mitochondrial myopathy' represents a clinically heterogenous group of disorders that have in common morphologic abnormalities in the number, size or structure of mitochondria. The metabolic abnormalities described in these conditions are numerous, and can be attributed to defects in nutrient transport, pyruvate and acetyl-CoA processing, oxidative phosphorylation, the respiratory (electron transport) chain or energy conservation[15,17–20]. It appears that many mitochondrial myopathies are inherited through maternal transmission and are caused by defects in

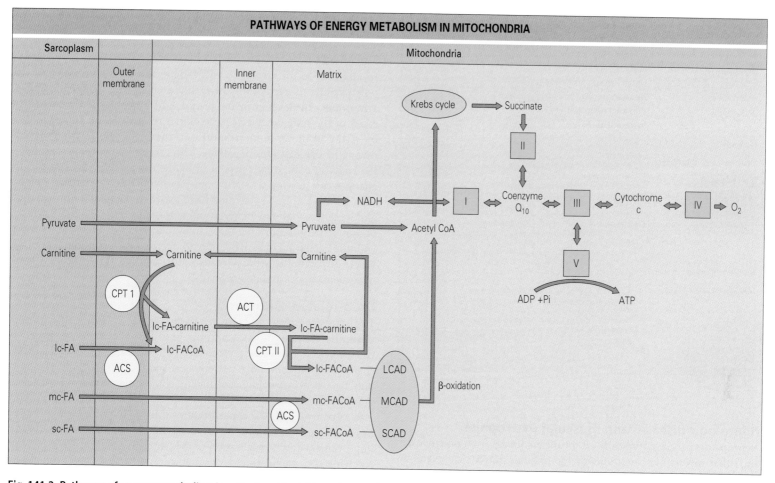

Fig. 141.2 Pathways of energy metabolism in mitochondria. I–IV, respiratory chain complexes; ACS, acyl CoA synthase; ACT, acyl carnitine translocase; CPT, carnitine palmitoyltransferase; LCAD, MCAD, SCAD, long-chain, medium-chain and short-chain fatty acid CoA dehydrogenases; lc-FA, mc-FA, sc-FA, long-chain, medium-chain and short-chain fatty acids; NADH, nicotinamide adenine dinucleotide; Pi, inorganic phosphate.

mitochondrial DNA. The clinical spectrum of these conditions is quite diverse and includes progressive muscular weakness that can be proximal or distal, or both, external ophthalmoplegia with or without proximal myopathy, progressive exercise intolerance and multisystem disease. More than 25 specific enzyme abnormalities have been described, of which at least six may present with exercise intolerance or progressive muscle weakness in adults. Acquired mitochondrial myopathies can develop in patients taking zidovudine and, perhaps, as a consequence of the aging process.

Muscle enzyme and EMG changes are variable and non-specific in the mitochondrial myopathies. Muscle biopsy is required for the specific diagnosis. Non-specific changes such as abnormal lipid or glycogen deposition may be seen with histochemistry and electron microscopy. Electron microscopy may also show mitochondria in increased numbers or with abnormal morphology. The characteristic finding of ragged red fibers can be seen by histology using the Gomori trichrome stain. Identification of the responsible defect requires enzyme analysis of muscle tissue.

Myoadenylate deaminase deficiency

Myoadenylate deaminase deficiency is caused by a nonsense mutation at codon 12 of the adenosine monophosphate deaminase 1 gene. Twenty-two percent of normal individuals and individuals with other recognized neuromuscular diseases are heterozygous for this mutation, 2% are homozygous. This deficiency is not believed to cause myopathy. Almost all patients with myoadenylate deaminase deficiency are asymptomatic. If an individual with this deficiency has muscle weakness, myalgia or fatigue, then another diagnosis should be sought to explain them. Patients with primary myoadenylate deaminase deficiency have normal

serum CK concentrations, normal EMG and normal muscle histology. The forearm ischemic exercise test is, however, abnormal. Myoadenylate deaminase-deficient persons can release lactate into the circulation after ischemic exercise, but fail to generate ammonia.

Secondary metabolic myopathies

Proximal muscle weakness may be a major feature of many endocrine and metabolic disorders (Table 141.8). These include Cushing's syndrome, hypothyroidism, hyperthyroidism and hyperparathyroidism. For reasons that are at present not understood, thyroid and parathyroid diseases may be associated with high concentrations of CK and myopathic changes on the EMG. Disorders that cause abnormal concentrations of sodium, potassium, calcium, magnesium or phosphorus (too much or too little) can cause weakness, fatigue, myalgias or cramps, because normal concentrations of these ions are necessary for the orderly active contraction and relaxation of muscle.

OTHER CAUSES OF MUSCLE WEAKNESS

Myopathic symptoms include fixed muscle weakness, or the inability to perform specific tasks such as climbing stairs or raising the hands above the head, early or premature fatigue and cramping or myalgia after muscular activity. The symptoms of myopathic diseases can range from chronic and mild to acute and fulminant. Some symptoms allow individuals to live comfortably, provided that they sufficiently limit their physical activity; others are severe and are associated with profound disability or rhabdomyolysis, myoglobinuria and renal failure. The list of diseases that cause these symptoms is long (Table 141.9).

TABLE 141.9 CATEGORIES OF DISEASES AND DISORDERS THAT CAN CAUSE MYOPATHIC SYMPTOMS

Neuropathic diseases	Muscular dystrophies	
	Denervating conditions	
	Neuromuscular junction disorders	
	Proximal neuropathies	
	Myotonic diseases	
Neoplasm		
Drug-related conditions		
Infections		
Metabolic	Primary	Glycogen storage diseases
		Mitochondrial myopathies
	Secondary	Nutritional toxic
		Endocrine disorders
		Electrolyte disorders
Rhabdomyolysis		
Miscellaneous causes	Sarcoidosis	
	Atherosclerotic emboli	
	Behçet's disease	
	Fibromyalgia	
	Psychosomatic	

Neurologic diseases and muscular dystrophies

Neuropathic processes typically can be differentiated from polymyositis and other myopathic conditions by the findings on physical examination. Neuropathic conditions typically manifest with asymmetric weakness, distal extremity involvement, altered sensorium or abnormal cranial nerve function. In contrast, the changes in myopathies are limited to proximal and symmetric weakness[21]. Exceptions include some patients with mitochondrial myopathies, IBM, myositis associated with anti-SRP antibodies and myositis with malignancy.

The limb-girdle dystrophies are most easily confused with inflammatory muscle disease. The inheritance is most frequently autosomal recessive. The onset of proximal muscle weakness may occur in the first to third decades of life and is eventually accompanied by muscle wasting. Facioscapulohumeral muscular dystrophy is an autosomal dominant disorder in which the weakness characteristically begins in the facial muscles. Medical attention is usually sought after shoulder weakness develops. Duchenne's muscular dystrophy and Becker's muscular dystrophy are passed by X-linked inheritance. These cause shoulder and pelvic girdle muscle weakness, and usually begin by the age of 5 years. In addition to muscle weakness and wasting, individuals develop winging of the scapulae, a hyperlordotic gait, and pseudohypertrophy of the calf muscles. Patients with Duchenne's muscular dystrophy usually cannot walk after the age of 11 years and die of respiratory failure by the age of 20 years. Becker's muscular dystrophy is similar but generally milder, with patients able to walk beyond the age of 16 years.

The spinal muscle atrophies are generally autosomal recessive disorders that cause degeneration of the spinal anterior horn cells. Onset may occur at any age. These are rarely confused with myositis because the weakness depends on the specific cord segments affected, and accordingly tends to be localized rather than diffuse. Proximal muscle weakness, especially of the upper extremities, may be the dominant clinical feature of myasthenia gravis. The coexistence of extraocular and bulbar muscle involvement, in addition to the marked fatigability helps differentiate it from myositis. Eaton–Lambert syndrome can also be associated with proximal muscle weakness. The syndrome is usually, but not always, associated with neoplastic disease. Proximal neuropathies, including diabetic amyotrophy and plexopathy, Guillain–Barré syndrome and acute intermittent porphyria. These diseases can cause myopathic symptoms and are occasionally confused with polymyositis.

Neoplasia

In addition to the weakness and fatigue that occur in patients with polymyositis or dermatomyositis and a coexisting malignancy, these symptoms can develop in the progress of a neoplastic disease as the result of the systemic effects of cytokines released by the tumor cells or by virtue of the immune response to the malignancy. The proximal myopathy that develops in patients with carcinoid syndrome is probably the result of compounds produced by the cancer cells. Neuromuscular changes can develop as features of paraneoplastic syndrome. Patients with Eaton–Lambert syndrome have excessive fatigability on exertion and weakness that may be profound and exclusively proximal in distribution. Patients report that their strength is reduced at rest but increases with the beginning of activity, only to decrease with continued exercise. Electromyographic studies readily differentiate this diagnosis from myasthenia gravis and polymyositis.

Drug-related conditions

The list of drugs that can cause myopathic changes is long (Table 141.10)[22]. Examples include drugs commonly used in a rheumatology practice. Glucocorticoid can cause proximal muscle weakness and wasting. EMG changes are minimal and, if present, non-specific. Biopsy of muscle shows only type II fiber atrophy. Colchicine, chloroquine and hydroxychloroquine can cause an axonal neuromyopathy. This toxicity is invariably associated with high CK concentrations. Muscle biopsies reveal vacuoles in the tissue. Withdrawal of the drug should rapidly lead to clinical improvement and normalization of the CK concentration. Some patients receiving D-penicillamine develop autoimmune syndromes, including polymyositis and myasthenia gravis.

The exact mechanism by which many drugs cause myopathy is uncertain. Some, such as D-penicillamine, hydralazine and procainamide, are immune-mediated. Some, such as alcohol, may have direct toxic effects. Still others may cause metabolic or electrolyte abnormalities. For example, clofibrate, the hydroxymethyl glutaryl CoA reductase inhibitors (statins) and high-dose niacin probably alter muscle fiber energetics, although simvastatin has been associated with polymyositis. Thiazide diuretics induce hypokalemia, which can cause weakness, myalgias and cramps.

TABLE 141.10 DRUGS THAT CAN CAUSE MYOPATHIC SYMPTOMS OR SYNDROMES*

Alcohol	Fenofibrate	Nicotine acid
Amiodarone	Flecainide	Nalidixic acid
Aspirin	Fluvastatin	Penicillin
Atorvastatin	Gemfibrozil	D-Penicillamine
Bezafibrate	Glucocorticoids	Phenytoin
Chloroquine	Glycyrrhizin	Pivampicillin
Cimetidine	Gold salts	Pravastatin
Clofibrate	Heroin	Propofol
Cocaine	Hydralazine	Ranitidine
Colchicine	Hydroxychloroquine	Rifampin
Cyclosporine	Ipecac	Simvastatin
D-L-Carnitine	Ketoconazole	Sulfonamides
Danazol	Labetalol	L-Tryptophan
Enalapril	Levodopa	Valproic acid
Epsilon aminocaproic acid	Losartan	Vincristine
Etofibrate	Lovastatin	Zidovudine (AZT)

* In addition, any drug or hormone that can increase or decrease serum concentrations of sodium, potassium, calcium, phosphorus or magnesium can induce myopathic symptoms.

TABLE 141.11 INFECTIOUS CAUSES OF MYOSITIS	
Viral	**Bacterial**
Adenovirus 2, 21	*Borrelia burgdorferi* (Lyme spirochete)
Coxsackievirus A9, B1, B2, B3, B4, B5	*Clostridium perfringens*
Cytomegalovirus	*Mycobacterium leprae*
Echovirus A9	*Mycobacterium tuberculosis*
Epstein–Barr virus	*Mycoplasma pneumoniae*
Hepatitis B and C virus	*Rickettsia*
Human immunodeficiency virus	*Staphylococcus*
Human T cell lymphotrophic virus type 1	*Streptococcus*
Influenza A and B viruses	
Mumps virus	**Fungal**
Rubella virus	*Candida*
Varicella zoster virus	*Cryptococcus*
Helminthic	**Parasitic**
Echinococcus	Microsporidia
Trichinella	*Schistosoma*
	Toxoplasma gondii
	Trypanosoma cruzi

TABLE 141.12 CAUSES OF RHABDOMYOLYSIS	
Trauma	Crush injury (with or without coma)
	Excessive exercise (marathon running, military training)
	Electrical shock (lightning, high voltage injury, electroshock therapy)
	Muscle activity (status epilepticus, delirium tremens)
	High temperature (malignant hyperthermia, heat stroke, malignant neuroleptic syndrome, infection)
	Ischemic injury (thromboembolism, sickle-cell trait)
Drugs and toxins	Recreational (alcohol, barbiturates, heroin, cocaine)
	Lipid-decreasing (clofibrate, bezafibrate, gemfibrozil, lovastatin, pravastatin, simvastatin)
	High-dose niacin
	Venoms (rattlesnake, sea snake, hornet, red spider)
Infections	Viral (influenza virus, Coxsackievirus, herpesvirus, echovirus, adenovirus, HIV1)
	Bacterial (*Staphylococcus*, typhoid, *Legionella*, *Clostridium*)
Metabolic causes	Genetic (glycogen storage diseases, CPT deficiency, mitochondrial myopathies)
	Electrolyte imbalance (hypocalcemia, hypernatremia, hypophosphatemia, hyperosmolar non-ketotic states, acidosis)
Collagen vascular diseases	Polymyositis and dermatomyositis
Idiopathic	

CPT, carnitine palmitoyltransferase; HIV1, human immunodeficiency virus 1.

Infections

Numerous infections can cause a myopathy (Table 141.11)[23]. Influenza A and B viral infections can cause severe myalgias, high (up to 15 times normal) CK concentrations, and non-specific myopathic changes, including fiber necrosis and inflammatory cell infiltration on muscle biopsy. A subacute myositis has also been described after rubella infection and after immunization with live attenuated rubella virus.

Weakness is a common finding in patients suffering from acquired immunodeficiency syndrome (AIDS). The possible causes include: the cachexia; central or peripheral nervous system diseases; polymyositis emerging as a consequence of the altered immune function; human immunodeficiency virus, cytomegalovirus, *Mycobacterium avium intracellulare*, *Cryptococcus*, *Trichinella*, and *Toxoplasma* infections; pyomyositis; the toxic effects of antiretroviral treatment. Muscle biopsies from patients with AIDS and the AIDS-related complex may show 'moth-eaten' fibers, type 2 fiber atrophy, endomysial or perimysial or perivascular mononuclear cell infiltrates (or any combination thereof), and vasculitis with perifascicular atrophy. Zidovudine use can cause mitochondrial myopathy.

Pyomyositis is a focal bacterial infection most commonly encountered in tropical zones[17]. Abscesses, most often caused by streptococcal infection, develop in one or more proximal muscles, usually in the lower extremities. Myositis can also be seen in Lyme disease. Among the parasites that cause myositis, *Toxoplasma* is the most common in the USA. Toxoplasmosis can cause an acute or subacute illness resembling polymyositis.

RHABDOMYOLYSIS

Rhabdomyolysis is a syndrome that results from any cause of extensive muscle necrosis (Table 141.12)[24,25]. Clinically, rhabdomyolysis causes intense myalgia with muscle tenderness and swelling. Serum CK concentrations may reach values 2000 times normal. If the cause or offending agent is corrected or removed, the muscle can heal remarkably well. Permanent weakness and atrophy are rare unless the rhabdomyolysis has developed in relation to myositis or vascular insufficiency.

Potential complications of massive muscle necrosis include myoglobinuria, hypocalcemia, hyperkalemia and hyperuricemia. The most threatening complication of rhabdomyolysis is acute renal failure characterized by oliguria, myoglobin-positive urine containing pigmented granular casts, and a high serum creatinine concentration. The risk of this complication increases directly with the serum CK, potassium and phosphorus concentrations, with urine myoglobin concentrations in excess of $1\mu g/ml$, inversely with serum albumin concentrations, and in the presence of dehydration or sepsis as the underlying cause. Treatment is essentially supportive. When myoglobinuria is identified, a diuresis should be established in hopes of preventing renal failure. Alkalinization of the urine is recommended, but has not been proved to alter outcomes. The patient should also be monitored for hyperkalemia, potentially the most life-threatening complication.

Hypocalcemia results from the sequestration of calcium by necrotic muscle, perhaps because the solubility product for calcium phosphate is exceeded locally. The risk of hypocalcemia decreases within the first days after the onset. Serum urate concentrations increase, as a result of the accelerated breakdown of ATP associated with damaged muscle, plus a block in uric acid excretion because of a concomitant acidosis or renal failure.

REFERENCES

1. Oddis C. Idiopathic inflammatory myopathy. In: Wortmann RL, ed. Diseases of skeletal muscles, 1E. Philadelphia: Lippincott Williams & Wilkins; 1999: 45–86.
2. Targoff IN. Autoantibodies. In: Wortmann RL, ed. Diseases of skeletal muscles, 1E. Philadelphia: Lippincott Williams & Wilkins; 1999: 267–292.
3. Bohan A, Peter JB. Polymyositis and dermatomyositis (first of two parts). N Engl J Med 1675; 292: 344–345, 403–407.
4. Calabrese LH, Mitsumoto H, Chou SM. Inclusion body myositis presenting as treatment resistant polymyositis. Arthritis Rheum 1987; 30: 397–403.
5. Tanimoto K, Nakano K, Kano S et al. Classification criteria for polymyositis and dermatomyositis. J Rheumatol 1995; 22: 668–674.
6. Targoff IN, Miller FW, Medsger TA Jr, Oddis CV. Classification criteria for the idiopathic inflammatory myopathies. Curr Opin Rheumatol 1997; 9: 527–535.

7. Bohan A, Peter JB, Bowman BS, Pearson CM. A computer assisted analysis of 153 patients with polymyositis and dermatomyositis. Medicine 1977; 56: 255–286.

8. Marie I, Horton P-Y, Hachulla E et al. Pulmonary involvement in polymyositis and in dermatomyositis. J Rheumatol 1998; 25: 1336–1343.

9. Callen JP. Dermatomyositis. Lancet 2000; 355: 53–57.

10. Pachman LM. Inflammatory myopathy in children: clinical and laboratory indicators of disease activity and chronicity. In: Wortmann RL, ed. Diseases of skeletal muscles, 1E. Philadelphia: Lippincott Williams & Wilkins; 1999: 87–110.

11. Tse S, Lubelsky S, Gordon M et al. The arthritis of inflammatory childhood myositis. J Rheumatol 2001; 28: 192–197.

12. Huemer C, Kitson H, Malleson PN et al. Lipodystrophy in patients with juvenile dermatomyositis – evaluation of clincal and metabolic abnormalities. J Rheumatol 2001; 28: 610–615.

13. Love LA, Leff RL, Fraser DD et al. A new approach to the classification of idiopathic inflammatory myopathy: myositis specific autoantibodies define useful homogeneous patient groups. Medicine 1991; 70: 360–374.

14. Watts RA. Eosinophilia and musculoskeletall disease. Curr Opin Rheumatol 2001; 13: 57–61.

15. Wortmann RL. Metabolic diseases of muscle. In: Wortmann RL, ed. Diseases of skeletal muscles, 1E. Philadelphia: Lippincott Williams & Wilkins; 1999: 157–188.

16. DiMauro S, Lamperti C. Muscle glycogenises. Muscle Nerve 2001; 35: 984–999.

17. Vladutin GD. The molecular diagnosis of the metabolic myopathies. Neurol Clin 2000; 18: 53–104.

18. Simon DK, Johns DR. Mitochondrial disorders: clinical and genetic features. Ann Rev Med 1999; 50: 111–127.

19. Wortmann RL. Metabolic and mitochondrial myopathies. Curr Opin Rheumatol 1999; 11: 462–467.

20. Nardin RA, Johns DR. Mitchondrial dysfunction and meuromuscular disease. Muscle Nerve 2001; 24: 170–191.

21. Lacomis D. Neuropathic disorders and muscular dystrophy. In: Wortmann RL, ed. Diseases of skeletal muscles, 1E. Philadelphia: Lippincott Williams & Wilkins; 1999: 197–220.

22. Pascuzzi RM. Drugs and toxins associated with myopathies. Curr Opin Rheumatol 1998; 10: 511–514.

23. Messner RP. Infections of muscle. In: Wortmann RL, ed. Diseases of skeletal muscles, 1E. Philadelphia: Lippincott Williams & Wilkins; 1999: 129–146.

24. Penn AS. Myoglobulinuria. In: Engel AG, Franzini-Armstrong C, eds. Myology, 2E. New York: McGraw Hill; 1994: 1679–1696.

25. Bolin P. Rhabdomyolysis. In: Wortmann RL, ed. Diseases of skeletal muscles, 1E. Philadelphia: Lippincott Williams & Wilkins; 1999: 245–254.

142

Overlap syndromes

Patrick J W Venables

Definition

- A combination of major features of more than one rheumatic disease present in the same patient and often defined by a specific serologic test

Clinical features

- Raynaud's phenomenon, arthritis and sclerodactyly are common to most overlap syndromes
- Polymyositis and fibrosing alveolitis are frequently the more serious manifestations.

INTRODUCTION

A complete diagnosis of a disease depends on knowledge of its cause. The etiologies of all autoimmune connective tissue diseases are unknown, and diagnosis has had to depend on patterns of symptoms and signs, which now form the basis of internationally accepted diagnostic criteria. Although this approach allows for the selection of reasonably homogeneous patient populations for epidemiologic studies, it is of limited value in individual patients and inadequate for the determination of precise treatment regimens and for assessing prognosis. The problems in rheumatology are heightened by the tendency for one disease type to merge with another. This results in a continuous spectrum of clinical features among the rheumatic diseases, with the traditionally accepted entities such as systemic lupus erythematosus (SLE) or systemic sclerosis occupying only part of the continuum, with the overlap syndromes lying between.

THE DISTINCTIVENESS OF OVERLAP SYNDROMES

To define an overlap syndrome, it is necessary to identify a constellation of distinctive features that constitute a true syndrome. Furthermore, these features should be sufficiently developed to be recognizable as known rheumatic diseases such as myositis, scleroderma or fibrosing alveolitis. Patients with incomplete features (for example a patient with Raynaud's phenomenon, arthralgia and a weak positive antinuclear antibody) are better described as having undifferentiated connective tissue diseases[1]. It is confusing to use the term 'undifferentiated connective tissue disease' interchangeably with overlap syndromes or mixed connective tissue disease (MCTD), as this assumes that overlap syndromes are 'undifferentiated'. Although some cases of MCTD, for example, evolve into systemic sclerosis, many patients with overlap syndromes remain stable for long periods of time. True overlap syndromes can be defined in two ways: on the basis of clinical involvement and by the detection of autoantibodies.

Overlap syndromes defined by clinical features

Raynaud's phenomenon, sclerodactyly and alveolitis are common features of a number of autoimmune rheumatic diseases and cannot be used on their own to define a syndrome. Other features, such as thicken-

ing of the skin proximal to the fingers in scleroderma or the articular erosions in rheumatoid arthritis (RA) are sufficiently disease-specific to suggest that a patient having a combination of both has a true overlap. This may be the basis of the early descriptions of RA/systemic sclerosis overlaps and RA/SLE overlaps or 'rupus'. Before regarding these as distinctive syndromes, it must be remembered that RA is a common disease and could occur by chance in a patient with systemic sclerosis or SLE. Some studies have highlighted a second consideration; namely that erosive arthritis may occur in SLE and systemic sclerosis[2], thus suggesting that RA-like features can, in some patients, be a feature of the disease itself.

Overlap syndromes defined by autoantibodies

A remarkable feature of autoimmune connective tissue diseases is that sera from the majority of patients contain non-organ-specific autoantibodies to DNA, RNA or proteins that bind to them[3]. The antigenic specificity of these antibodies has done much to justify the distinctiveness of the traditionally recognized diseases. For example SLE is associated with the 'markers', anti-double-stranded (ds)DNA or anti-Sm. However, antibody types do not always respect tradition: many coincide with parts of the spectrum in which diseases overlap with each other. The best known examples are antibodies that react mainly with U1-ribonucleoprotein (RNP). These are found in patients with overlapping features of SLE, systemic sclerosis and polymyositis. There are other syndromes that are also associated with myositis and specific antibodies; they include the the rare syndromes closely related to MCTD with antibodies to U2-RNP and U3-RNA, and the polymyositis/fibrosing alveolitis overlaps found in patients with antibodies to Jo-l and the other tRNA synthetases. The polymyositis/scleroderma overlap associated with anti-Pm/Scl is rapidly becoming recognized as an important overlap syndrome that may be underdiagnosed.

Although previously not regarded as markers of an overlap, it is now generally believed that antibodies to the nuclear and cytoplasmic complexes involved in RNA polymerase III transcription, Ro(SS-A) and La(SS-B), occur in patients with Sjögren's syndrome who also have features of SLE – that is, Sjögren's/SLE overlap syndromes. Other antibodies have also been described as markers of overlaps. They include the association of anti-Ro with subacute cutaneous lupus erythematosus and anticardiolipin antibodies with the primary antiphospholipid syndrome. It is arguable that the clinical features of these diseases are not overlapping, more that they represent disease subsets or distinctive syndromes in their own right.

Almost every rheumatic disease has been described as part of an overlap syndrome. In this chapter, the discussion will be restricted to those which combine features of more than one disease and are associated with particular antibody specificities. There are two reasons for emphasizing the importance of the antibodies: first, the antibody provides a reference point with which to compare one study with another and, secondly, the presence of an individual antibody implies, but by no means proves, common etiopathogenic mechanisms, which goes some way towards justifying the term 'diagnosis' in describing these syndromes.

MIXED CONNECTIVE TISSUE DISEASE

Mixed connective tissue disease is an overlap syndrome combining features of SLE, systemic sclerosis and polymyositis, together with the presence of antibodies to U1-RNP (Table 142.1)[3]. Other manifestations, notably trigeminal neuralgia and Sjögren's syndrome (occurring in 25–50% of patients) have also been emphasized[1]. These features are the basis of several sets of diagnostic criteria; those proposed by Alarcon-Segovia and Villanreal are the simplest and likely to be most acceptable (Table 142.2).

History

The evolution of our concept of MCTD has depended on two factors: first, our understanding of the antigen recognized by the antibodies that define the disease and, secondly, by the associated clinical features. A complement fixation test using a saline nuclear extract, termed extractable nuclear antigen, represented the first stage in the development of the serologic test. The assay became refined to a hemagglutination test incorporating enzymatic treatment of the antigen mixture, which led to the definition of MCTD as a diagnostic entity associated

---

TABLE 142.1 CLINICAL FEATURES OF PATIENTS WITH ANTIBODIES TO U1-RNP

Clinical feature	% of patients
Arthritis/arthralgia	95
Raynaud's phenomenon	85
Decreased esophageal motility	67
Impaired pulmonary diffusing capacity	67
Swollen hands	66
Myositis	63
Lymphadenopathy	39
Skin rash	38
Sclerodermatous changes	33
Fever	33
Serositis	27
Splenomegaly	19
Hepatomegaly	15
Renal disease	10
Neurologic abnormalities	10

(Adapted from Sharp et al.[4])

TABLE 142.2 SUGGESTED CRITERIA FOR THE DIAGNOSIS OF MCTD

1. Serologic

Positive anti-RNP at a hemagglutination titer of 1:1600 or higher

2. Clinical

Edema of the hands
Synovitis
Myositis
Raynaud's phenomenon
Acrosclerosis

Requirements for the diagnosis: Serologic criteria plus at least three clinical. (When edema, Raynaud's phenomenon and acrosclerosis are combined, four clinical criteria are required.)

(Adapted from Alarcon-Segovia and reviewed in Von Muhlen and Tan[3].)

---

with antibodies to the ribonuclease (RNase)-sensitive fraction of extractable nuclear antigen[5]. It was claimed that MCTD could be distinguished from SLE on the basis that SLE sera reacted with the RNase-resistant component. Using immunodiffusion[4], the RNase-resistant component was characterized as the previously described Sm antigen and the RNase-sensitive component as a nuclear ribonuclear protein, which was simply termed 'RNP' or 'nRNP'.

Further definition of the RNP and Sm antigens awaited the use of immunoprecipitation of [^{32}P]-labeled cells, which showed, surprisingly, that both Sm and RNP were ribonucleoproteins[6]. The RNP antigen resided on polypeptides bound to the U1 (uridine-rich) RNP complex, whereas the Sm antigen was present on U1, U2, U4, U5 and U6 complexes. Analysis by immunoblotting showed that the major epitopes recognized by MCTD sera were a 68kDa polypeptide bound to U1-RNA, and those for anti-Sm antibodies were a 28kDa doublet and a 16kDa polypeptide. For this reason, the RNP antigen changed its name yet again, to U1-RNP, although Sm has retained its original name.

The clinical features of MCTD, their relationship to antibodies to U1-RNP, and whether they constitute a distinct entity are still debated[1]. In general, almost all reports have confirmed the high frequency of arthritis, Raynaud's phenomenon, myositis and fibrosing alveolitis observed by Sharp and his colleagues[4]. Opinion about the clinical distinctiveness of MCTD has been less harmonious. Arguments against its definition as a separate entity may be summarized as follows:

- If the disease is defined by a serologic reaction (anti-U1-RNP), it is a fallacy to claim that the antibody constitutes a distinctive feature of the disease
- Many patients with anti-U1-RNP have typical features of relatively well-defined diseases such as SLE and can be diagnosed as such[4]
- A substantial proportion of patients with MCTD (75% in one study)[7], evolve into typical cases of SLE or scleroderma after follow-up
- There is no homogeneity in prognosis or in response to treatment
- Some patients with typical features of MCTD have autoantibodies other than anti-U1-RNP. These include those with anti-Jo-1, other tRNA synthetases and some patients with anti-La(SS-B)

Counter to these arguments is that most of the objections listed above are also applicable to accepted entities such as SLE and Sjögren's syndrome. It is particularly noteworthy that serologic reactions are becoming incorporated into diagnostic criteria for these diseases (see Chapters 116, 122 and 130).

Epidemiology and HLA associations

The prevalence of MCTD is unknown. In most studies, the number of patients with clinical and serologic features of the syndrome are about fourfold fewer than patients with SLE, suggesting an overall prevalence in the region of 10/100 000. The female:male ratio is about 9:1 and the disease does not appear to show the relative preponderance of Afro-Caribbeans seen in SLE. No particular environmental agents have been associated with the disease, although it is of interest that occupational exposure to vinyl chloride has been described[8]. Several studies have described an association with DR4, one suggesting that the link could be accounted for by those MCTD patients who had erosive arthritis[9]. A significantly increased frequency of the immunoglobulin allotypes Gm 1.3 and 3 have also been described[9].

Clinical features

Being an overlap syndrome, MCTD lacks any distinctive clinical features. Raynaud's phenomenon is very common, and is often associated with edema of the hands (Fig. 142.1). This feature is often (wrongly) regarded as peculiar to MCTD; swollen hands also occur in early scleroderma, eosinophilic fasciitis and the anti-tRNA (tRNA) synthetase anti-

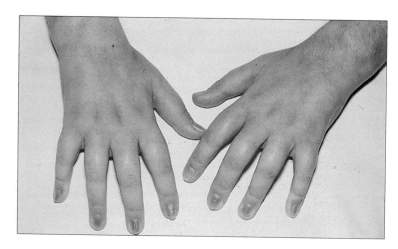

Fig. 142.1 Sausage-shaped fingers in a patient with MCTD. An identical appearance may be found in patients with early scleroderma and eosinopilic fasciitis.

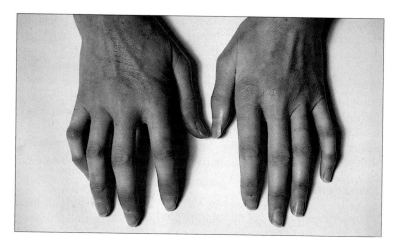

Fig. 142.2 Hands of a patient with MCTD. This shows features of both dermatomyositis (thickening and erythema of the dorsum of the fingers) and scleroderma (sclerodactyly and fixed flexion of the fingers).

body associated overlap syndromes. The appearance of the hands in MCTD may also reflect the overlapping diseases that constitute the syndrome and combine features of scleroderma, SLE and dermatomyositis (Fig. 142.2). Arthritis and arthralgias are also common, but again lack any unique pattern[10]. Joint disease ranging from a relatively mild SLE-like peripheral synovitis through to erosive disease typical of RA, and even arthritis mutilans, has been described[11].

Myositis, fibrosing alveolitis and pulmonary hypertension are the most important common features of the syndrome. There is little evidence to suggest that the pattern of muscle or lung involvement in MCTD differs from that of other diseases, although studies of patients selected purely on the basis of myositis or fibrosing alveolitis suggest that the prognosis in patients with anti-U1-RNP may be marginally better than in those without (Table 142.3)[12]. Nevertheless, both myositis and fibrosing alveolitis are potentially fatal, and pulmonary hypertension, in

particular, is a lethal complication. Some recent studies (reviewed by Hoffman and Greidinger[11]) have suggested that pulmonary hypertension may be associated with coexistent antiphospholipid antibodies. More importantly, the pulmonary artery pressure decreases with prostacycline infusions or treatment with immunosuppressive drugs[11].

Other clinical features of MCTD simply reflect those of the diseases that it overlaps. Skin manifestations include sclerodactyly, scleroderma (usually relatively restricted), calcinosis, telangiectasia, photosensitivity, malar rash and the rash of dermatomyositis. Pleurisy and pericarditis occur in about 60% of patients. Radiologic evidence of esophageal dysmotility has long been recognized as a feature in more than 50% of patients. One recent study has emphasized a high frequency of heartburn (48%) and dysphagia (38%) in patients with MCTD, in addition to more rare gastrointestinal features, including malabsorption syndromes and bowel perforations as a result of vasculitis[13]. Sjögren's syndrome occurs in about 50% of patients with MCTD, although the sicca symptoms are usually less prominent than in those with anti-La(SS-B) antibodies. Trigeminal neuralgia, although a recognized feature of SLE, is a striking feature of MCTD in about 25% of cases.

When first described, MCTD was believed to be characterized by good prognosis and a low frequency of cerebral and renal disease (compared with SLE). This opinion has now been revised, after longer follow-up studies, to the view that the prognosis in MCTD is in fact worse than that in lupus, most of the deaths being attributable to pulmonary hypertension[14]. When renal involvement occurs, it is either membranous nephritis or, less commonly, the renal vasculopathy characteristic of scleroderma, leading to malignant hypertension.

Investigations

The diagnosis of MCTD is critically dependent on the demonstration of high-titer anti-U1-RNP antibodies. In early studies, the hemagglutination assay was most commonly performed, although this test is subject to the criticism that the antigen mixture coating the red cells contained more than one RNase-sensitive antigen. For this reason, it is preferable to demonstrate the antibody by immunodiffusion, either passive double diffusion or counterimmunoelectrophoresis, with the antibody specificity confirmed by a precipitin line of immunologic identity with a reference serum. It is also possible to define the antibody by immunoblotting or immunoprecipitation of [32P]-labeled cell extracts, although these assays suffer from being rather cumbersome and, at best, only semiquantitative. The use of purified or cloned antigens in quantitative enzyme-linked immunosorbent assay are currently the preferred assays in most laboratories. One of the difficulties in serologic diagnosis of MCTD is that most attempts at diagnostic criteria specify a 'high titer'. Although cut-off points of 1:1000 or 1:1600 have been suggested for the hemagglutination test, there has yet to be a defined limit for other assays in more frequent use. The presence of anti-U1-RNP antibodies in the serum means that all MCTD sera will give a speckled nuclear staining pattern on indirect immunofluorescence (Fig. 142.3). Unfortunately, the usefulness of this test is limited by the fact that other autoantibodies, notably anti-Sm and anti-La(SS-B), give very similar staining patterns.

Other investigations show features common to connective tissue diseases in general. The most frequent hematologic findings are leukopenia, thrombocytopenia and a high erythrocyte sedimentation rate. Serum immunoglobulins may be extremely high, with IgG concentrations reaching more than 40g/l in some patients. In contrast to SLE, in MCTD the complement concentrations are usually normal or high. Rheumatoid factors are increased in approximately 70% of patients. Important negative findings are tests for anti-Sm and anti-DNA antibodies. These, if present, in the opinion of Sharp *et al.*[5], represent exclusion criteria for the diagnosis of MCTD, and suggest that the disease lies more firmly in the SLE part of the spectrum.

TABLE 142.3 DEATH DURING A MEAN FOLLOW-UP PERIOD OF 7 YEARS IN PATIENTS PRESENTING WITH ALVEOLITIS AND ITS RELATIONSHIP TO ANTI-U1-RNP		
	Anti-U1-RNP negative	Anti-U1-RNP positive
Polymyositis (n=40)	5/21 (24%)	2/19 (11%)
Fibrosing alveolitis (n=122)	32/107 (30%)	2/15 (13%)
(Adapted from Venables[12].)		

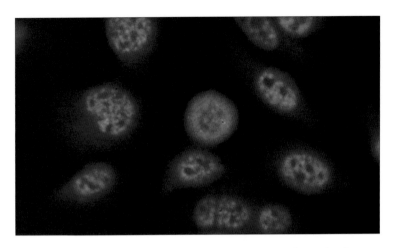

Fig. 142.3 **Indirect immunofluorescence on HEp-2 cells with a patient's serum containing anti-UI-RNP antibody.** This shows speckled nuclear staining, with characteristic sparing of the nucleoli and negative staining of the chromosomes of the cell in early metaphase (center).

Structure and function of the U1-RNP particle

One justification for defining a disease by a serologic test is based on the assumption that anti-U1-RNP and its antigen are intrinsically involved in the pathogenesis of the disease. Although there is no direct evidence to support it, it is a valid hypothesis worthy of investigation.

The U1 RNP particle is one of a series of uridine-rich RNA particles that are involved in the splicing of messenger RNAs (mRNA). It is composed of eight polypeptides linked to RNA, of which two, 68kDa and 33kDa, carry the epitopes recognized by MCTD sera. The other polypeptides, principally 28kDa and 16kDa, react with anti-Sm antibodies (Fig. 142.4). The presence of both U1-RNP and Sm epitopes on the same molecular complex, together with the frequent coexistence of the two antibody specificities, is often taken as evidence for antigen drive by the entire molecular complex. A similar association between the Ro and La antigens (on the hY RNAs) has been proposed as a mechanism for the induction of anti-Ro and anti-La, which also tend to occur together.

Etiology

If the current concept of autoantigen drive is accepted, it is necessary to explain how an intranuclear protein becomes available to the immune system. Such a mechanism could be the expression of intracellular ribonucleoproteins on the cell surface in apoptotic blebs[15]. Tolerance breakdown could then occur as a rsult of post-translational modification

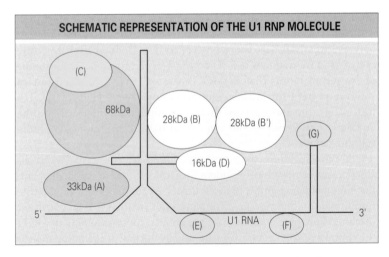

SCHEMATIC REPRESENTATION OF THE U1 RNP MOLECULE

Fig. 142.4 **Schematic diagram of the U1RNP molecule showing the polypeptides bound to U1 RNA.** Those shown in green (68kDa and 33kDa) contain the epitopes for anti-U1-RNP antibodies and those shown in yellow contain the epitopes for anti-Sm antibodies. The letters in parentheses refer to the classification proposed by Lerner and Steitz[6].

TABLE 142.4 U1-RNP AND RETROVIRUS P30 GAG AMINO ACID HOMOLOGY	
U1 RNP	- - R - - - M - - K - - -
	- A - - - - - - M - - - -
Consensus	E T P E E R E E R * R R E T P E E R E E R R
Baboon EV	- - - - - - - A - L I K E Q * - - - - V G E T
Feline LV	- - - - - - - - - L W Q R Q * - - - D K K - H
Murine LV	- - - - - - - - - I - - - - * - - - - - - - -

Homology between the 33kDa U1-RNP polypeptide and the consensus sequence of type C retroviruses and known mammalian retroviruses. EV, endogenous virus; LV, leukemia virus; –, identical or conservative substitutions; *,skipped residue[17].

of the 70kDa molecule[16] or, conceivably, as a result of molecular mimicry with viral antigens. This has been proposed on the basis of sequence similarities between the 33kDa polypeptide of U1-RNP and a consensus sequence common to a number of animal retroviruses (Table 142.4). Infection with a similar exogenous virus or expression of an endogenous retrovirus that is not normally exposed to the immune system could result in the induction of autoantibodies to U1-RNP by molecular mimicry[17]. More recently, James et al.[18] have suggested that sequence similarities between a peptide from Epstein–Barr virus, PPPGRRP, and an immunodominant epitope on the B/B′ component of the splicesosome, PPGMRPP, could be the basis of an etiological role for Epstein–Barr virus in SLE. This hypothesis is supported by epidemiologic studies both in adults and children. Given the clinical and serologic overlap of MCTD with SLE, the virus could be important in MCTD also.

Management

There is no specific treatment for MCTD. One of the original claims in support of MCTD being a 'distinct clinical entity' was its favorable prognosis and unusual responsiveness to treatment with corticosteroids. Like others, this observation has not stood the test of time. It is now agreed that the treatment depends entirely on the pattern of clinical involvement. Mild disease such as arthralgia requires symptomatic treatment only, whereas severe complications such as myositis or fibrosing alveolitis need high-dose corticosteroids, often in combination with immunosuppressive drugs. It should also be borne in mind that MCTD can also differentiate into SLE and that potentially lethal complications, particularly pulmonary hypertension, can be occult at the time of presentation.

Management techniques

All patients with MCTD require careful, long-term follow-up. As in SLE, management is based on clinical assessment and laboratory tests for specific organ involvement. At each visit, every patient's clinical evaluation should include physical examination and blood pressure; laboratory tests should include complete blood count, muscle enzymes and urine analysis for protein. There is no single laboratory test that can be used for monitoring disease activity and progression, although several studies have suggested that an increase in anti-U1-RNP antibodies measured by a quantitative enzyme-linked immunosorbent assay may be helpful in the short term for predicting flares of the disease. In some patients, a decrease in total white cell count (particularly the lymphocyte count) or an increase in erythrocyte sedimentation rate and total immunoglobulin concentrations may be helpful in assessing overall disease activity, although these should never be relied on for dictating treatment options. At intervals, depending on the severity of the disease, a full survey of autoantibodies, including anti-Sm and anti-dsDNA, should be performed as an early warning of those differentiating into SLE.

Pulmonary hypertension, which may or may not be associated with fibrosing alveolitis, is the most frequent cause of death directly attributable to MCTD. This should always be anticipated, by examining patients for basal rales and by performing regular chest radiographs. Because many patients with early pulmonary involvement have no abnormal physical signs and normal radiographs, it is advisable to perform pulmonary function tests and echocardiograms at presentation, and at subsequent intervals to assess progression. If there is evidence of deterioration, bronchial alveolar lavage or biopsy can be used to assess disease activity before treatment.

Drug treatment for MCTD depends on symptoms or the pattern of organ involvement. About 33% of patients have their disease adequately controlled by analgesics or non-steroidal anti-inflammatory drugs. Raynaud's phenomenon can be particularly troublesome, and is characteristically unresponsive to corticosteroids. Most patients derive some benefit from simple conservative treatment with electrically heated gloves, and a minority respond to calcium channel antagonists such as nifedipine. Severe cases respond to infusions of prostaglandin analogs (see also Chapter 136). Arthritis and SLE-like skin involvement is often treated successfully with antimalarial agents such as hydroxychloroquine. There is some anecdotal evidence that patients with MCTD are liable to hypersensitivity to second-line antirheumatic drugs; such drugs should probably be avoided. Low-dose corticosteroids are effective for controlling cutaneous edema, arthritis and pleurisy; high-dose corticosteroids are indicated for the treatment of severe systemic disease such as vasculitis, myositis or fibrosing alveolitis. Myositis is a particularly important complication, requiring the correct use of corticosteroids. Because of the mistaken belief that MCTD is peculiarly corticosteroid-responsive, patients may be given inappropriately low doses. In addition, the apparent lack of an early response may drive the physician into the unnecessary use of cytotoxic drugs. Myositis in MCTD should be treated in the same way as myositis occurring in any other context. High-dose prednisolone (about 1mg/kg per day) should be given for at least 6 weeks before gradual reduction of the dose to a maintenance level.

Immunosuppressive drugs are used in two contexts in MCTD: for the induction of remission or for their corticosteroid-sparing effects. The most common indication for induction of remission is fibrosing alveolitis, although any SLE-like manifestation such as nephritis or systemic vasculitis may also require immunosuppression. The most common drug used in this context is cyclophosphamide, in a daily oral dose of 1–2mg/kg per day in combination with high-dose corticosteroids. Cyclophosphamide may also be given as pulse therapy, either as single intravenous infusions of 500mg to 1g spaced at intervals of 2–4 weeks, depending on the complete blood count, or as weekly oral pulses of 300mg; both regimens to a total dose of 3–6g. Controlled trials comparing these treatments are urgently needed, although the heterogeneity of the clinical expression of MCTD poses considerable problems in designing an appropriate study. Azathioprine is used mainly as a corticosteroid-sparing drug or as maintenance treatment in a dose of 2mg/kg per day after induction of a response with cyclophosphamide. Methotrexate may be effective, although the similarity of one of its side effects to a frequent clinical feature of the disease, pulmonary fibrosis, may pose management problems. Nevertheless, it has been used successfully for the treatment of fibrosing alveolitis in patients with Jo-l antibody[19].

Conclusions

The heat of the argument about the distinctiveness of MCTD as a clinical entity has now largely subsided. Although the original objections to the concept remain valid, MCTD has gained historical respectability and is now a commonly used label for a spectrum of clinical involvement associated with an anti-U1-RNP. The importance of MCTD is not so much in terms of diagnosis, but rather what the antibody tells us about patients. Particularly important is the heterogeneity of the patterns of clinical involvement and the need to tailor treatment accordingly. The clinician must anticipate the potentially lethal complications of myositis fibrosing alveolitis and pulmonary hypertension, and the tendency of the disease to evolve into one of its sister diseases such as SLE or systemic sclerosis. Whether MCTD can be credited with the term 'dia-

gnosis' awaits the demonstration (or otherwise) that anti-U1-RNP antibodies and their associated clinical features are attributable to a single etiologic agent.

tRNA SYNTHETASE ASSOCIATED OVERLAP SYNDROMES

History

The tRNA synthetases are a series of cytoplasmic enzymes that take part in protein synthesis by adding specific amino acids encoded by tRNA during the assembly of polypeptides. A number have been described as autoantigens, although histidyl-tRNA synthetase is by far the most common target for autoimmunity. This antigen, like other soluble cellular antigens, was initially defined as a precipitin reaction obtained with a prototype serum. The antigen, Jo-1, was named after the patient. When first described, anti-Jo-1 was believed to be a marker for myositis, being detected in eight of 26 patients with polymyositis, and rarely in dermatomyositis[20]. Later, it was shown that patients with anti-Jo-1 antibodies had both polymyositis and fibrosing alveolitis; subsequently, other features of systemic connective tissue diseases were described, including Raynaud's phenomenon, arthritis and a number of scleroderma-like features[19]. When it was definitively demonstrated that the Jo-1 antigen was histidyl-tRNA synthetase, other tRNA synthetases, including alanyl and threonyl-tRNA synthetases, were also described as less common autoantigens in polymyositis-associated overlap syndromes.

Clinical features

Several hundred patients with anti-Jo-1 antibodies have now been described in the literature (see also Chapter 139). One of the original large series collected by Marguerie et al.[19] may still be regarded as giving an accurate picture of the widespread patterns of clinical involvement seen in these patients. They found that the clinical features of patients with antibodies to histidyl-tRNA synthetase (Jo-1) were very similar to those with antibodies to other tRNA synthetases; these are therefore presented together in Table 142.5. Overall, the clinical features of patients with anti-tRNA synthetase antibodies are strikingly similar to those with MCTD, such that it would be difficult to predict whether an individual patient with Raynaud's phenomenon, arthritis, myositis and alveolitis would have anti-Jo-1 or anti-U1-RNP antibodies. In contrast, there are differences between the patients analyzed as groups. Patients with anti-Jo-1 antibodies have myositis and fibrosing alveolitis more frequently,

TABLE 142.5 CLINICAL FEATURES OF PATIENTS WITH ANTI-AMINOACYL-tRNA ANTIBODIES	
Clinical feature	% of patients
Raynaud's phenomenon	93
Arthritis/arthralgia	90
Myositis	83
Lung fibrosis	79
Sclerodactyly	72
Sicca	59
Dermatomyositis rash	38
Facial telangiectasia	31
Dysphagia	31
Soft tissue calcification	24
Tendonitis	17
Clubbing	14
(Adapted from Marguerie et al.[19])	

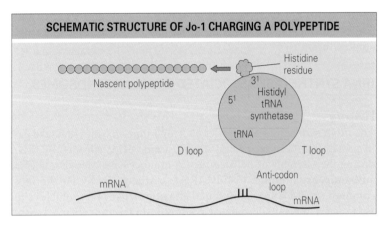

Fig. 142.5 Schematic structure of Jo-1 (histidyl-tRNA synthetase) charging a nascent polypeptide with histidine.

and both are more likely to give rise to the presenting symptoms. In addition, there is some evidence to suggest that the prognosis of the alveolitis is worse in patients with tRNA synthetase antibodies compared with those with anti-U1-RNP. Patients with anti-U1-RNP tend to have more SLE-like features, and may be more likely to differentiate into SLE. It is noteworthy that patients with anti-Jo-1 antibodies may have erosive, deforming arthritis and are often diagnosed as suffering from RA.

Pathogenesis

Evidence that host–virus interactions on the background of genetic susceptibility lead to autoantibody induction is possibly more compelling for the tRNA synthetase antibodies than for any other pattern of autoimmunity in rheumatic disease. Genetic susceptibility is well established, with an almost 100% association between anti-Jo-l antibodies and major histocompatibility complex class II *DR3* alleles. The function of Jo-1 and other tRNA synthetases is shown in Figure 142.5. Histidyl-tRNA synthetase is known to be involved in the aminoacylation of enteroviruses, and it is conceivable that the interaction of host plus virus complex could lead to an anti-host response. Accumulating, but indirect, evidence for the involvement of Coxsackie B viruses in myositis (see Chapter 141) provides a further stimulus for the investigation of induction of anti-tRNA antibodies by a specific etiologic agent. Involvement of the idiotype network in the induction of autoimmunity was proposed in general terms by Plotz[21]. This theory, which suggests that autoantibodies are anti-idiotypes to antiviral antibodies, presupposes that the antiviral antibody reacts with the viral RNA at its site of binding to the host protein, and that the autoantibody (the anti-idiotype) reacts with the host protein at its RNA binding site (Fig. 142.6). Some evidence in support of this hypothesis has been presented on the basis of data from a patient with anti-alanyl-tRNA synthetase antibodies[22].

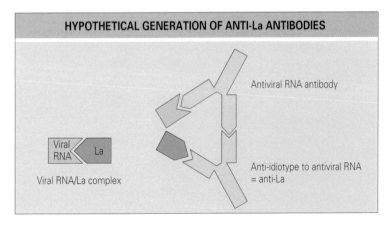

Fig. 142.6 Hypothetical generation of anti-La antibodies. The hypothesis proposed by Plotz applied to the generation of anti-La antibodies.

Diagnosis

One of the major difficulties in diagnosis of the anti-tRNA synthetase-associated overlap syndromes is detecting the antibodies. Since the enzymes involved in aminoacylation by tRNA are cytoplasmic, anti-nuclear antibodies detected by immunofluorescence are often negative. This means that there is no reliable screening test, although cytoplasmic immunofluorescence with a perinuclear distribution may alert the more discriminating diagnostic laboratory to look for antibodies to Jo-1 or one of the related tRNA synthetases. Rabbit thymus extract, the substrate used for detecting antibodies to the so-called extractable nuclear antigens, may give a precipitin reaction that cannot be identified as one of the more common antibody systems such as U1-RNP, Sm, Ro or La, in which case anti-Jo-1 antibodies should be measured. Patients with myositis, fibrosing alveolitis and arthritis should also be tested, although it should be remembered that many patients with Jo-1 antibodies do not have myositis at presentation[19].

Management

The treatment of autoantibody specificity is as for any other multisystem autoimmune disease, except that the relatively poor prognosis of the fibrosing alveolitis should be borne in mind, and should possibly suggest earlier intervention with corticosteroids and immunosuppressive drugs than would be applied in MCTD.

THE PM/SCL ASSOCIATED OVERLAP SYNDROME

Antibodies to Pm/Scl are part of a complex of precipitin reactions originally termed PM-1. Although PM-1 antibody was regarded as a marker antibody for polymyositis occurring in 70% of patients, anti-Pm/Scl was found in about 15%[23] and appeared to be associated with a polymyositis/scleroderma overlap syndrome with clinical features very similar to those of the anti-tRNA-associated overlap syndromes (Table 142.6)[24]. However, there are differences. Myositis and fibrosing alveolitis are described as less frequent, less severe and more likely to respond to treatment with corticosteroids or immunosuppressive drugs. More than 90% of patients are HLA-DR3 positive. It is possible that the Pm/Scl overlap syndrome is as common as the tRNA synthetase syndrome, although it may be underdiagnosed because the serologic assay for it is not widely available. One clue to the presence of anti-Pm/Scl is that serum samples contain antinucleolar antibodies by immunofluorescence, reflecting the nucleolar localization of the antigen.

TABLE 142.6 CLINICAL FEATURES OF PATIENTS WITH ANTI-Pm/Scl ANTIBODIES	
Clinical feature	% of patients
Raynaud's phenomenon	100
Arthritis/arthralgia	97
Myositis	88
Lung fibrosis	78
Sclerodactyly	97
Sjögren's syndrome	34
Dermatomyositis rash	38
Dysphagia	78
Calcinosis	47
(Adapted from Marguerie et al.[24])	

RARE OVERLAP SYNDROMES

Rare syndromes similar to MCTD are found in patients with antibodies to U2-RNP, U3-RNA and Ku. Patients with anti U2-RNP and U3-RNA veer more towards polymyositis/scleroderma overlap syndromes. Patients with anti-Ku antibody may also have overlap syndromes. SLE tends to be the predominant part of the clinical picture, with scleroderma and polymyositis frequently occurring in the same patient[3]. The immunofluorescent staining pattern for antibodies to U2-RNP is the same as for anti-U1-RNP, for U3-RNA, nucleolar and for Ku as 'reticular' nuclear. This suggests that serum samples giving nucleolar immunofluorescence are worth sending to a reference laboratory for both anti-Pm/Scl and anti-U3-RNA testing, if the patient has an overlap syndrome.

THE SLE/SJÖGREN'S SYNDROME OVERLAP DEFINED BY ANTI-LA(SS-B)

History

The antigen La was first reported in 1974 as a cytoplasmic antigen which was a target for autoantibodies in SLE. The Sjögren's syndrome B antigen (SS-B), described 2 years later, suggested properties that were apparently distinct. SS-B was nuclear and anti-(SS-B) antibodies primarily occurred in patients with Sjögren's syndrome. When the two antigens were shown to be identical[5], their different cellular localizations, in addition to the diagnostic associations of their antibodies, suggested a discrepancy, which has subsequently become resolved. The La(SS-B) antigen is known to shuttle between nucleus and cytoplasm and its antibodies occur in both SLE and Sjögren's syndrome, particularly when there are overlapping features of both diseases[25].

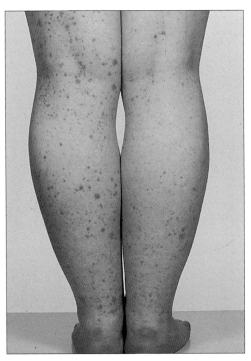

Fig. 142.7 Hypergammaglobulinemic purpura with associated ankle edema in a patient with anti-La antibodies. In this patient there is also a vasculitis accounting for some of the larger, raised lesions.

Clinical features

Patients with anti-La antibodies have Sjögren's syndrome with prominent systemic features (see Chapter 130). Most of the extraglandular features are SLE-like, with a high frequency of arthritis, rashes, Raynaud's phenomenon, leukopenia and thrombocytopenia. Characteristic of the anti-La-associated overlap syndrome is a purpuric hypergammaglobulinemic rash, in about 30% of patients (Fig. 142.7), and a relatively low frequency of nephritis compared with patients with typical SLE. However, renal tubular acidosis (often subclinical) may occur in up to 30% of patients.

Pathogenesis

The La antigen is involved in RNA polymerase III transcription and binds to both host and viral RNAs in infected cells. A clue to a mechanism for the induction of anti-La antibodies may lie in the observations that the La antigen is translocated from the nucleus to the cytoplasm and plasma membrane during virus infection and thus becomes available to the immune system[25]. Its interaction with viral RNA and, possibly, viral proteins could induce anti-La antibodies by tolerance bypass, possibly occurring in the salivary gland itself. In support of this hypothesis is the demonstration that some viruses persist within salivary epithelium, although no one has convincingly demonstrated La antigen presentation within the glands of patients with Sjögren's syndrome.

Management

The treatment of Sjögren's syndrome associated with anti-La is largely symptomatic, with tear and saliva substitutes. Treatment for extraglandular manifestations depends on the pattern of clinical involvement. Hydroxychloroquine, for example, is effective for arthralgia and rashes and will decrease total immunoglobulin concentrations and the erythrocyte sedimentation rate. Anecdotally, it seems to be effective in treating hypergammglobulinemic purpura, although treatment often has to be maintained for more than 6 months before a clinical benefit is observed. Others (personal communications) have also found it helpful for malaise and fatigue, but there are no controlled trial data to substantiate this. Fibrosing alveolitis and myositis both occur in association with anti-La, although less frequently than in MCTD, and may require high-dose corticosteroids and cytotoxic drugs. Similar treatment may be used for systemic vasculitis, which is often manifest as mononeuritis multiplex. A recognized presentation in the elderly is fever, weight loss and lymphadenopathy, sometimes associated with polymyalgia. These patients often do well with a relatively modest dose of corticosteroids.

CONCLUSIONS

The concept of overlap syndromes makes many rheumatologists feel uneasy, although their distinctiveness is no longer the subject of the intense debate that it was in the past. In practice, the diagnosis of an overlap syndrome makes little difference to treatment, although the detection of an autoantibody does help the clinician to anticipate particular complications. The description of overlap syndromes in terms of autoantibodies is based on the assumption that the pattern of autoimmunity reflects the underlying cause for the disease. If this proves to be the case, the definition of disease by an antibody will be justified. Knowledge of disease etiology is the ultimate justification of the use of the term 'diagnosis'.

REFERENCES

1. Mukerji B, Hardin JB. Undifferentiated, overlapping and mixed connective tissue diseases. Am J Med Sci 1993; 305: 114–119.
2. Wild W, Betham WP. Erosive arthropathy in systemic sclerosis. JAMA 1975; 232: 511–512.
3. Von Muhlen CA, Tan EM. Autoantibodies in the diagnosis of systemic rheumatic diseases [review]. Semin Arthritis Rheum 1995; 24: 323–358.
4. Sharp GC, Irwin WS, May CM et al. Association of antibodies to ribonucleoprotein and Sm antigens with mixed connective tissue disease, systemic lupus erythematosus and other rheumatic diseases. N Engl J Med 1976; 29: 1149–1154.
5. Sharp GC, Irwin WS, Tan EM et al. Mixed connective tissue disease: an apparently distinct rheumatic disease syndrome associated with a specific antibody to extractable nuclear antigen. Am J Med 1972; 52: 148–159.

6. Lerner MR, Steitz JA. Antibodies to small nuclear RNAs complexed with proteins are produced by patients with systemic lupus erythematosus. Proc Natl Acad Sci USA 1979; 76: 5495–5499.

7. De Clerk LS, Meijers KA, Cats A. Is MCTD a distinct entity? Comparison of clinical laboratory findings in MCTD, SLE, PSS and RA patients. Clin Rheumatol 1989; 8: 29–36.

8. Kahn MK, Borgeois P, Aeschlimann A, De Truchis P. Mixed connective tissue disease after exposure to vinyl chloride. J Rheumatol 1989; 16: 533–535.

9. Black CM, Maddison PJ, Welsh KI et al. HLA and immunoglobulin allotypes in mixed connective tissue disease. Arthritis Rheum 1988; 31: 131–135.

10. Bennett RM, O'Connel J. The arthritis of mixed connective tissue disease. Ann Rheum Dis 1978; 32: 397–403.

11. Hoffman RW, Greidinger EL. Mixed connective tissue disease [review]. Curr Opin Rheumatol 2000; 12: 386–390.

12 Venables PJW. Antibodies to nucleic acid binding proteins: their clinical and aetiological significance. Cambridge: MD thesis; 1986.

13. Marshall JB, Krertschmar JM, Gerhardt DC et al. Gastrointestinal manifestations of mixed connective tissue disease. Gastroenterology 1990; 98: 1232–1238.

14. Burdt MA, Hoffman RW, Deutscher SL et al. Long-term outcome in mixed connective tissue disease: longitudinal clinical and serologic findings. Arthritis Rheum 1999; 42: 899–909.

15 Casciola-Rosen LA, Anhalt G, Rosen A. Autoantigens targeted in systemic lupus erythematosus are clustered in two populations of surface structures on apoptotic keratinocytes. J Exp Med 1994; 179: 1317–1330.

16. Utz PJ, Anderson P. Posttranslational protein modifications, apoptosis, and the bypass of tolerance to autoantigens [review]. Arthritis Rheum 1998; 41: 1152–1160.

17. Query CC, Keene JD. A human autoimmune protein associated with U1 RNA contains a region of homology that is cross reactive with retroviral p30 gag antigen. Cell 1987; 51: 211–220.

18. James JA, Neas BR, Moser KL et al. Systemic lupus erythematosus in adults is associated with previous Epstein–Barr virus exposure. Arthritis Rheum 2001; 44: 1122–1126.

19 Marguerie C, Bunn CC, Beynon HLC et al. Polymyositis, pulmonary fibrosis and autoantibodies to aminoacyl tRNA synthetases. Q J Med 1990; 77: 1019–1038.

20. Singsen BM, Bernstein HH, Kornreich HK et al. Mixed connective tissue disease in childhood. J Pediatr 1977; 90: 893–900.

21. Plotz PH. Autoantibodies are anti-idiotype antibodies to antiviral antibodies. Lancet 1983; 2: 824–826.

22. Bunn CC, Bernstein RM, Mathews MB. Autoantibodies against alanyl-tRNA synthetase and tRNA coexist and are associated with myositis. J Exp Med 1989; 163: 1281–1291.

23 Reichlin M, Maddison PJ, Targoff I et al. Antibodies to a nuclear/nucleolar antigen in patients with polmyositis overlap syndromes. J Clin Immunol 1984; 4: 40–44.

24 Marguerie C, Bunn CC, Copier J et al. The clinical and immunogenetic features of patients with antibodies to the nucleolar antigen PM-Scl. Medicine 1992; 71: 327–336.

25. Price EJ, Venables PJW. The aetiopathogenesis of Sjögren's syndrome. Semin Arthritis Rheum 1995; 25: 117–133.

THE VASCULITIDES

143 Overview of the inflammatory vascular diseases

Richard A Watts and David G I Scott

- Classification systems currently used are imprecise
- Peak age of incidence is 65–74 years
- Giant cell arteritis is the most common type of vasculitis
- Kawasaki disease and Henoch–Schönlein purpura are the most common types of childhood vasculitis
- Infection must be excluded as far as is practicable before initiation of immunosuppressive treatment
- Urine analysis is the single most important investigation; prognosis is determined by the extent of renal involvement
- Antineutrophil cytoplasmic antibodies should not be used as a substitute for obtaining histology for confirmation of diagnosis
- Biopsies whenever possible should be obtained before treatment
- Treatment should be tailored to the individual patient
- Duration of cyclophosphamide treatment should be kept to a minimum, to reduce toxicity.

INTRODUCTION

Definition

The vasculitides are a heterogeneous group of relatively uncommon diseases characterized by inflammatory cell infiltration and necrosis of blood vessel walls. The severity of vasculitis is related to the size, site and number of vessels affected.

Vasculitis can be isolated to one organ or vessel and be clinically relatively insignificant (e.g. localized cutaneous vasculitis) or may involve many organs and vessels simultaneously and be rapidly life threatening (e.g. polyarteritis nodosa, Churg–Strauss syndrome, Wegener's granulomatosis, microscopic polyangiitis). Muscular arteries may develop focal or segmental lesions. The former can lead to aneurysm formation and possible rupture; segmental lesions (affecting the whole circumference) are more common and may lead to stenosis or occlusion, with distal organ infarction. Hemorrhage or infarction of vital internal organs is the most serious complication of vasculitis and explains the poor prognosis of untreated polyarteritis nodosa[1]. Small vessel vasculitis, particularly when confined to the skin, has a good prognosis and may be self-limiting.

HISTORY

One of the first documented cases of systemic vasculitis (termed periarteritis nodosa) was described in 1866 by Kussmaul and Maier[2], who reported a patient with numerous nodules along the course of small muscular arteries. Earlier reports from the 18th and 19th centuries suggest that vasculitis has been a problem for more than 200 years (reviewed by Matteson[3]). A number of other distinct vasculitic syndromes have been recognized more recently (e.g. Wegener's granulomatosis, Churg–Strauss syndrome), but for many years, especially during the 19th and first three-quarters of the 20th century, 'poly(peri)arteritis nodosa' was used as a generic term for any type of vasculitis. In 1948, Davson et al.[4] described patients with segmental necrotizing glomerulonephritis who also had features of polyarteritis nodosa, with involvement of extrarenal small and medium arteries. He used the term 'microscopic polyarteritis' to describe these patients, in whom the dominant feature was rapidly progressive renal failure. The term 'microscopic polyangiitis' has become widely used since the 1990s for this pattern of disease, emphasizing the difference between it and classical polyarteritis nodosa.

Kawasaki disease (mucocutaneous lymph node syndrome) is an acute vasculitis of unknown etiology that primarily affects infants and young children, and was first described in Japan in 1967 (reviewed by Matteson[5]). Coronary vasculitis is a major cause of morbidity and mortality. Takayasu's arteritis is a chronic granulomatous large vessel arteritis that was described in 1908 by Takayasu, although Savory had described the association between the absence of radial pulses and ocular abnormalities in 1856 (reviewed by Matteson[5]). William Heberden first described a patient with what we would now recognize as Henoch–Schönlein purpura in 1801, and Schönlein initially described acute purpura and arthritis occurring in children in 1837. Subsequently, Henoch described the additional features of colicky abdominal pain and nephritis in 1874 (reviewed by Matteson[5]).

Giant cell arteritis (temporal arteritis) was first described by Hutchinson in 1890 and subsequently in greater detail by Horton in 1932. The systemic nature of the condition was first described by Gilmour in 1941, with the description of an arteritis with infiltration of lymphocytes, plasma cells and formation of multinucleated giant cells (reviewed by Matteson[5]).

CLASSIFICATION

The classification of systemic vasculitis remains confusing and controversial. There is considerable overlap in the clinical expression of the different vasculitic syndromes, and there is evolution of these diseases over time, making a single classification scheme very difficult to use. Even in the presence of infection, the clinical syndrome may be heterogeneous; for example, human immunodeficiency virus (HIV) infection has been associated with polyarteritis nodosa, hypersensitivity vasculitis and large vessel disease[6], in addition to granulomatous angiitis and lymphomatoid granulomatosis.

Zeek[7], in 1952, was the first to classify vasculitis into different groups, mainly on the basis of vessel size, and this has formed the basis of most subsequent classification schemes. She considered necrotizing angiitis to include five separate types of systemic vasculitis: hypersensitivity angiitis, allergic granulomatous angiitis, rheumatic arteritis, periarteritis nodosa and temporal arteritis. She included allergic granulomatous angiitis (now called Churg–Strauss syndrome), but not Wegener's granulomatosis or Takayasu's arteritis, as these conditions were not recognized in the English literature until the late 1950s. Subsequent classification schemes were developed, also based on the histopathological appearances, especially the size of the predominant vessels involved and, more recently, the presence of antineutrophil cytoplasmic antibodies (ANCA).

The classification that we use reflects dominant vessel size and ANCA (Table 143.1, Fig. 143.1)[8]. We place Wegener's granulomatosis, Churg–Strauss syndrome and microscopic polyangiitis in a separate group because they often involve small and sometimes medium-sized arteries, are most frequently associated with ANCA, and are associated with a high risk of glomerulonephritis. The etiology of these diseases is probably unrelated to immune complex formation, in contrast to pure small vessel vasculitis such as Henoch–Schönlein purpura and essential mixed cryoglobulinemia. Our classification also reflects the broad therapeutic approach, with the medium- and small-vessel group responding best to immunosuppression with cyclophosphamide in addition to corticosteroids, whereas the large vessel group require moderate- to high-dose corticosteroids (usually alone), and the small vessel group only sometimes require low-dose corticosteroids (Table 143.2).

Vasculitis may occur secondary to connective tissue disease such as SLE, rheumatoid arthritis or Sjögren's syndrome. Viral infections, in particular hepatitis B virus, hepatitis C virus and HIV are a well-recognized cause of vasculitis (Table 143.3). Bacterial infections, and especially bacterial endocarditis, may mimic systemic vasculitis. Malignancy – classically, hairy cell leukemia – is associated with polyarteritis nodosa and small vessel vasculitis. Vasculitis can be a manifestation of other myeloproliferative diseases and, less commonly, solid malignancies. A wide variety of drugs have been implicated in the precipitation of vasculitis (reviewed by Merkel[10]). The association is strongest with propylthiouracil, hydralazine and allopurinol, which have been associated with high titers of myeloperoxidase (MPO)-ANCA[11]. The leucotriene antagonists have been associated with Churg–Strauss syndrome[12]. A number of recreational drugs have been reported to cause vasculitis, including heroin, cocaine and metamphetamine. They have been particularly associated with cerebral vasculitis.

Classification criteria for individual vasculitic syndromes

The American College of Rheumatology (ACR) addressed the use of classification criteria for vasculitis in 1990[13]. They proposed criteria for classification of seven types of systemic vasculitis: Takayasu's arteritis, giant cell arteritis, Wegener's granulomatosis, polyarteritis nodosa, Churg–Strauss syndrome, hypersensitivity vasculitis and Henoch–Schönlein purpura. The clinical and laboratory features of 807 patients were analysed, criteria being sought that would distinguish one individual disease from another. Thus findings in one group

TABLE 143.1 CLASSIFICATION OF SYSTEMIC VASCULITIS

Dominant vessel	Primary	Secondary
Large arteries	Giant cell arteritis Takayasu's arteritis	Aortitis associated with RA Infection (e.g. syphilis, TB)
Medium arteries	Classical PAN Kawasaki disease	Hepatitis B associated PAN
Small vessels and medium arteries	Wegener's granulomatosis* Churg–Strauss syndrome* Microscopic polyangiitis*	Vasculitis secondary to RA, SLE, Sjögren's syndrome Drugs Infection (e.g. HIV)
Small vessels (leucocytoclastic)	Henoch–Schönlein purpura Cryoglobulinemia Cutaneous leucocytoclastic angiitis	Drugs† Hepatitis C-associated Infection

* Diseases most commonly associated with ANCA (antimyeloperoxidase and antiproteinase 3 antibodies) and a significant risk of renal involvement, and most responsive to immunosuppression with cyclophosphamide.

† For example sulfonamides, penicillins, thiazide diuretics and many others.

PAN, polyarteritis nodosa; RA, rheumatoid arthritis; TB, tuberculosis.

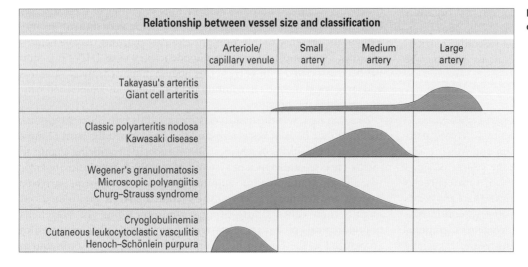

Relationship between vessel size and classification

	Arteriole/ capillary venule	Small artery	Medium artery	Large artery
Takayasu's arteritis Giant cell arteritis				
Classic polyarteritis nodosa Kawasaki disease				
Wegener's granulomatosis Microscopic polyangiitis Churg–Strauss syndrome				
Cryoglobulinemia Cutaneous leukocytoclastic vasculitis Henoch–Schönlein purpura				

Fig. 143.1 Relationship between vessel size and classification.

TABLE 143.2 RELATIONSHIP BETWEEN VESSEL SIZE AND RESPONSE TO TREATMENT

Dominant vessel	Corticosteroids alone	Cyclophosphamide + corticosteroids	Others
Large arteries	+++	–	+
Medium arteries	+	++	++*
Small vessels and medium arteries	+	+++	–
Small vessels	+	–	++

* Includes plasmapheresis, antiviral treatment for Hepatitis B-associated vasculitis, and intravenous immunoglobulin for Kawasaki disease.

(With permission from Scott and Watts[9].)

TABLE 143.3 INFECTION AND VASCULITIS

Vessel involved	Infection	
Large arteries	Bacterial	*Staphylococcus, Salmonella, Mycobacterium, Streptococcus*
	Spirochetal	*Treponema pallidum*
	Fungal	Coccidiomycosis
Medium arteries	Bacterial	Group A *Streptococcus, Mycobacterium*
	Viral	HBV, HCV, HIV, parvovirus B19
Small vessels and medium arteries	Bacterial	*Streptococcus*
	Viral	HBV, HCV, HIV, CMV
Small vessels (leucocytoclastic)	Bacterial	*Staphylococcus, Salmonella, Mycobacterium, Streptococcus, Yersinia, Neisseria*
	Viral	HIV, CMV, herpes zoster, parvovirus B19
	Rickettsiae	

HBV, HCV, hepatitis B and C viruses; CMV, cytomegalovirus.

were compared with those in the remaining groups. The sensitivity and specificity rates varied considerably: from 71.0% to 95.3% for sensitivity and from 78.7% to 99.7% for specificity[14]. The most sensitive and specific criteria were found in Churg–Strauss syndrome, giant cell arteritis and Takayasu's arteritis. Hypersensitivity vasculitis was the least well defined condition and these patients are now usually classified as having Henoch–Schönlein purpura or microscopic polyangiitis. The criteria were not tested against the general population or against patients with other connective tissue diseases or rheumatic conditions. Recently, the criteria have been tested in a cohort of patients with possible vasculitis, and performed poorly in the diagnosis of this group[15].

Definitions for the systemic vasculitides were proposed at an international consensus conference (Chapel Hill Consensus Conference (CHCC))[16]. The objective of this conference was to develop *definitions* for the nomenclature of different systemic vasculitides, based on clinical and laboratory features (Table 143.4). The CHCC produced a clear distinction between classical polyarteritis nodosa and microscopic polyangiitis; the latter condition was not considered by the ACR.

These two developments have now produced clear definitions and classification criteria for the major vasculitides, which should permit studies of more homogeneous groups of patients. However, the two schemes do not necessarily classify individual patients into the same disease category[17]. The most difficult area is the distinction between polyarteritis nodosa, microscopic polyangiitis and Wegener's granulomatosis, with which there is considerable overlap. Recent attempts to improve the CHCC definitions with the use of surrogate parameters showed that they do not work well as diagnostic criteria for Wegener's granulomatosis or microscopic polyangiitis[18].

The ACR and the CHCC did not consider whether ANCA should be used to help classify the vasculitides. Antibodies producing a cytoplasmic staining pattern (cANCA) with specificity against proteinase 3 (PR_3) are predominately found in patients with Wegener's granulomatosis; a perinuclear staining pattern (pANCA), often with specificity for myeloperoxidase, is found in patients with microscopic polyangiitis[19]. ANCA is not associated with large-vessel vasculitis or limited cutaneous small vessel disease, and is rarely found in classical polyarteritis nodosa as defined by the CHCC. ANCA may, however, occur in non-vasculitic conditions, including infection and inflammatory bowel disease[20]. In these circumstances, the target antigens are not PR3 or MPO.

EPIDEMIOLOGY

The systemic vasculitides are all relatively rare conditions, and this has hampered epidemiological studies. The majority of centers with an interest in these diseases are tertiary referral centers with ill-defined catchment populations. In addition, patients seen in such centers may not be representative of those seen in the community. The development of the ACR (1990) criteria[13] and the CHCC definitions[16] has permitted establishment of epidemiological studies using recognized criteria/definitions and, hence, comparison between centers. Interpretation of the older literature is difficult, because of poor and inconsistent classification/diagnosis.

The initial study that estimated the overall incidence of systemic vasculitis came from Bath/Bristol (UK) in the 1970s; the estimated annual incidence was 10 per million[21]. These patients were poorly defined and may have included some cases of hypersensitivity vasculitis. During the period 1988–98, we estimated the annual incidence of the primary systemic

TABLE 143.4 NOMENCLATURE OF SYSTEMIC VASCULITIS*

Large vessel vasculitis

Giant cell (temporal) arteritis	Granulomatous arteritis of the aorta and its major branches, with a predilection for the extracranial branches of the carotid artery. *Often involves the temporal artery. Usually occurs in patients older than 50 years and often is associated with polymyalgia rheumatica*
Takayasu's arteritis	Granulomatous inflammation of the aorta and its major branches. *Usually occurs in patients younger than 50 years.*

Medium-sized vessel vasculitis

Polyarteritis nodosa* (classic polyarteritis nodosa)	Necrotizing inflammation of medium-sized or small arteries without glomerulonephritis or vasculitis in arterioles, capillaries or venules
Kawasaki disease	Arteritis involving large, medium-sized and small arteries, and associated with mucocutaneous lymph node syndrome. *Coronary arteries are often involved. Aorta and veins may be involved. Usually occurs in children*

Small vessel vasculitis

Wegener's granulomatosis[†]	Granulomatous inflammation involving the respiratory tract, and necrotizing vasculitis affecting small to medium-sized vessels (e.g. capillaries, venules, arterioles and arteries). *Necrotizing glomerulonephritis is common*
Churg–Strauss syndrome[†]	Eosinophil-rich and granulomatous inflammation involving the respiratory tract, necrotizing vasculitis affecting small to medium-sized vessels, and associated with asthma and eosinophilia
Microscopic polyangiitis[†] (microscopic polyarteritis)[†]	Necrotizing vasculitis, with few or no immune deposits, affecting small vessels (i.e. capillaries, venules or arterioles). *Necrotizing arteritis involving small and medium-sized arteries may be present. Necrotizing glomerulonephritis is very common. Pulmonary capillaritis often occurs*
Henoch–Schönlein purpura	Vasculitis, with IgA-dominant immune deposits, affecting small vessels (i.e. capillaries, venules or arterioles). *Typically involves skin, gut and glomeruli, and is associated arthralgia or arthritis*
Essential cryoglobulinemic vasculitis	Vasculitis, with cryoglobulin immune deposits, affecting small vessels (i.e. capillaries, venules or arterioles) and associated with cryoglobulins in serum. *Skin and glomeruli are often involved*
Cutaneous leukocytoclastic angiitis	Isolated cutaneous leukocytoclastic angiitis without systemic vasculitis or glomerulonephritis

Large vessel refers to the aorta and the largest branches directed towards the major body regions (e.g. to the extremities and the head and neck); *medium-sized vessel* refers to the main visceral arteries (e.g. renal, hepatic, coronary and mesenteric arteries); *small vessel* refers to venules, capillaries, arterioles and the intraparenchymal distal arterial radicals that connect with arterioles. Some small- and large-vessel vasculitides may involve medium-sized arteries, but large and medium-sized vessel vasculitides do not involve vessels smaller than arteries. Essential components are represented by normal type; *italic type* represents usual, but not essential, components.

* Preferred term. † Strongly associated with antineutrophil cytoplasmic antibodies.

Names and definitions of vasculitides adopted by the CHCC. (With permission from Jeanette *et al.*[16])

---

vasculitides (Wegener's granulomatosis, microscopic polyangiitis, polyarteritis nodosa, Churg–Strauss syndrome) to be 19.8 per million. The peak age at diagnosis was 65–74 years, far older than studies from tertiary referral centers would suggest (Fig. 143.2). There is a preponderance of affected males[22]. This advanced age at onset has been confirmed recently from other centers in Europe (Spain and Scandinavia).

Giant cell arteritis is the most common type of vasculitis seen in North America and Western Europe. There appears to be a distinct racial and geographical distribution of the disease, with a high incidence in Scandinavia compared with Italy and Spain. In Olmstead County, Minnesota, USA, the age- and sex-adjusted incidence was 178 per million adults aged 50 years or more[23] and was significantly greater in women (242 per million). Age-specific incidence rates increased with age, with the greatest incidence in those older than 80 years. The annual incidence rates increased significantly between 1950 and 1954 (73.3 per million) and between 1985 and 1991 (191 per million). The population of Olmstead County contains a high proportion of people of Scandinavian extraction, and this may explain the difference between Olmstead County and the southern USA (Tennessee), where the incidence is approximately 10% that of Olmstead County[24]. The Olmstead county report also noted peaks of incidence at approximately 7-year intervals, suggesting a possible infectious etiology[23].

There are geographical and ethnic differences in the incidence of primary systemic vasculitis. A comparative study in Europe using the same classification criteria in three populations (Lugo, North Western Spain; Norwich, UK; Tromso, Northern Norway) reported that Wegener's granulomatosis appeared to be more common in Norway than in Spain, whereas microscopic polyangiitis had the reverse distribution[25] (Table 143.5). No difference was found in the incidence of systemic vasculitis between the Northern and Southern Germany, or between urban and rural populations[26]. In India and Japan, Wegener's granulomatosis and giant cell arteritis are said to be 'extremely rare', whereas Takayasu's arteritis is 'common', but there is a paucity of data to confirm these assertions.

Two populations with a high incidence of polyarteritis nodosa have been reported. An incidence of 77 per million was reported in a small population of Alaskan Indians among whom hepatitis B infection was endemic[27]. In Kuwait, the incidence of microscopic polyangiitis and polyarteritis nodosa was 45 per million[28]. The reasons for these high incidences is unclear. Classical polyarteritis nodosa as defined by the CHCC is, in our experience, very uncommon.

Andrews and colleagues in Leicester (UK) reported an increase in the annual incidence of Wegener's granulomatosis from 0.7 per million in 1980–86 to 2.8 per million in 1987–89[29]. This was partially attributed to an increase in diagnostic awareness after the introduction of assays for ANCA in 1987. Our data suggest that the incidence was greater in Norwich (10.6 per million) in the 1990s than that in Leicester during the 1980s[25]. Whether this increase is genuine, or reflects changing disease definition or increased physician awareness remains uncertain. However, Koldingsnes and Nossent[30] reported in an increase from 5 per million per year to 12 per million per year over the past 15 years in Tromsø.

Takayasu's arteritis is most common in eastern countries, but occurs worldwide. In most series, however, there appears to be an excess of patients of Asian descent. The peak age of disease onset is in the third decade, and the disease is more common in women. In the USA

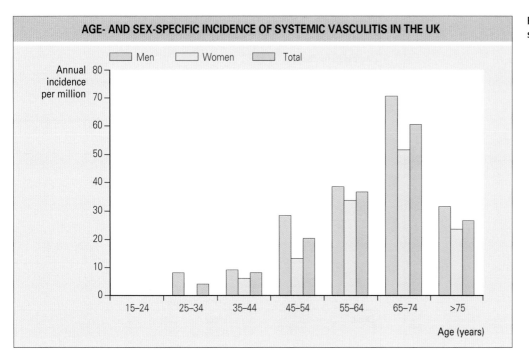

AGE- AND SEX-SPECIFIC INCIDENCE OF SYSTEMIC VASCULITIS IN THE UK

☐ Men ☐ Women ☐ Total

Annual incidence per million

Age (years)

Fig. 143.2 Age- and sex-specific incidence of systemic vasculitis in the UK.

TABLE 143.5 ANNUAL INCIDENCE OF PRIMARY SYSTEMIC VASCULITIS IN THREE REGIONS OF EUROPE

	Incidence (per million)		
	Tromsø	Norwich	Lugo
Wegener's granulomatosis	10.5	10.6	4.9
Churg–Strauss syndrome	0.5	3.1	0.9
Microscopic polyangiitis	2.7	8.4	11.6
Polyarteritis nodosa	0.5	0.0	0.9
Total	13.7	18.9	18.3

Wegener's granulomatosis and Churg–Strauss syndrome classified by the ACR (1990) criteria[13], microscopic polyangiitis and classical polyarteritis nodosa by the CHCC definitions[16].

(Data from Watts et al.[25])

(Olmstead County, Minnesota) three cases were recorded during the period 1971–83, equivalent to an annual incidence of 2.6 per million[31]. The annual incidence in a white population in Sweden during the period 1969–75 was estimated to be 0.8 per million[32]. Since 1988 in Norwich (UK), we have not seen a single new case of Takayasu's arteritis arising in our population of more than 500 000 confirming its relative rarity in the UK.

Childhood vasculitis

The distribution of vasculitis in childhood is different from that seen in adults. The primary systemic vasculitides are all very rare. The annual incidence of Kawasaki disease in 1991–92 in Japan was 900 per million children younger than 5 years. The peak incidence is at age 1 year, and there appears to be a seasonal variation, with more cases occurring in summer than in winter[33]. There have been periodic peaks in incidence in 1979, 1982 and 1986, suggesting an infectious etiology. In the 1990s in the British Isles, the reported annual incidence of Kawasaki disease was 55 per million children younger than 5 years[34]. In Washington State, USA in 1985–86 and 1987–89, the annual incidence was 65 and 152 per million respectively. There are ethnic differences: in 1987–89 in Asian-Americans younger than 5 years, the incidence was 333 per million, compared with 234 per million among African-Americans and 127 per million among whites[35]. This ethnic difference was also documented in the UK series, with Asian children (of Indian subcontinent origin) showing an incidence of 146 per million, compared with 59 per million among those of Afro-Caribbean extraction and 46 per million among whites[34]. It should be noted that, in the UK study, the 'Asians' were from the Indian subcontinent, whereas in the American study they were from South East Asia.

The annual incidence of Henoch–Schönlein purpura in children in the UK is 204 per million[34], but is much lower in adults. The estimated peak annual incidence is age 4–6 years. Afro-Caribbean children have a significantly lower annual incidence than white or Asian children, with a male:female ratio of 1.2:1. In adults, the annual incidence of Henoch–Schönlein purpura is much lower. Applying the ACR (1990) criteria[13] to adults in our population the incidence was 13.0 per million; using the CHCC definition[16] it was 3.4 per million[36].

ETIOLOGY

Infection has long been proposed as one of the most likely triggers for development of vasculitis. Apart from a few specific syndromes associated with hepatitis B and C and HIV, no organism has consistently been identified[37]. HIV-infected patients develop vasculitis, but whether the virus itself or the treatment (e.g. zidovudine) precipitates vasculitis is unclear. Hepatitis C has now been firmly associated with cryoglobulinemia. Giant cell arteritis occurs in cycles, with peaks every 5–7 years[23], and epidemics of Kawasaki disease have been reported, both suggestive of an infectious etiology. In Denmark, peaks of giant cell arteritis occurrence were correlated with occurrence of *Mycoplasma pneumoniae*, *Chlamydia* and parvovirus B19 infection[38].

The predominant respiratory involvement led Duna *et al.*[39] to investigate inhaled agents in Wegener's granulomatosis. They observed an increase in inhaled particulates and fumes in patients with Wegener's granulomatosis in general, but not in those with respiratory disease. A number of other trigger factors have also been reported in association with systemic vasculitis, including silica, solvents, allergy and vaccination.

A case–control study undertaken in Norfolk showed an association between occupations with high exposure to silica and primary systemic vasculitis[40]. In particular, pANCA/MPO-positive patients showed an association, rather than those positive for cANCA/PR3. It is notable that the incidence of microscopic polyangiitis doubled after the Kobe earthquake, in areas where exposure to silica would have been high[41]. Three case–control studies also support the association of silica with

TABLE 143.6 INVESTIGATION OF VASCULITIS

Assessment of inflammation

Blood count and differential (total white cell count, eosinophils)
Acute-phase response (ESR and CRP)
Liver function

Assessment of organ involvement

Urine analysis (proteinuria, hematuria, casts)
Renal function (creatinine clearance, 24-hour protein excretion, biopsy)
Chest radiograph
Liver function
Nervous system (nerve conduction studies, biopsy)
Muscle (EMG, creatine kinase, biopsy)
Cardiac function (ECG, echocardiography)
Gut (angiography)
Skin (biopsy)

Serological tests

ANCA (including proteinase 3 and myeloperoxidase)
Antinuclear antibodies
Rheumatoid factor
Anticardiolipin antibodies
Complement
Cryoglobulins

Differential diagnosis

Blood cultures
Viral serology (HBV, HCV, HIV, CMV)
Echocardiography (two-dimensional, transesophageal, or both)

CRP, C-reactive protein; ECG, electrocardiogram; EMG, electromyogram; ESR, erythrocyte sedimentation rate; HBV, HCV, hepatitis B and C viruses; CMV, cytomegalovirus.

TABLE 143.7 VASCULITIS MIMICS

Multisystem disease	
Infection	Subacute bacterial endocarditis
	Neisseria
	Rickettsiae
Malignancy	Metastatic carcinoma
	Paraneoplastic
Other	Sweet's syndrome
Occlusive vasculopathy	
Embolic	Cholesterol crystals
	Atrial myxoma
	Infection
	Calciphylaxis
Thrombotic	Antiphospholipid syndrome
	Procoagulant states
	Cryofibrinogenemia
Others	Ergot
	Radiation
	Degos syndrome
	Severe Raynaud's
	Acute digital loss
	Buerger's disease
Angiographic	
Aneurysmal	Fibromuscular dysplasia
	Neurofibromatosis
Occlusion	Coarctation

ANCA-positive glomerulonephritis, microscopic polyangiitis and Wegener's granulomatosis[42–44]. Our case–control study also found a significant association of occupational exposure to organic solvents with Wegener's granulomatosis and cANCA-positive vasculitis and also a link with exposure to farming[40].

INVESTIGATION AND DIAGNOSIS OF SYSTEMIC VASCULITIS

Investigation is directed towards: establishing and confirming the diagnosis, assessing the extent of organ involvement, and assessing disease activity (Table 143.6). The initial step in a patient with multisystem disease is to consider that systemic vasculitis might be present. Differentiation must be made from syndromes that may masquerade as primary systemic vasculitis (Table 143.7), infection, malignancy and connective tissue disease. Infection is especially important to exclude, as primary systemic vasculitis is treated with high-dose corticosteroids and immunosuppressive agents.

The single most important investigation is urine analysis. Prognosis is determined mainly by the extent of renal impairment, and renal function can rapidly deteriorate. The detection of proteinuria, hematuria, or both, in a patient with a systemic illness requires immediate further investigation and is a medical emergency.

Assessment of organ involvement
Renal
The extent of renal involvement is assessed by measurement of serum urea and creatinine, urine analysis looking for casts, measurement of glomerular filtration rate and 24-hour urine protein excretion. Renal biopsy will serve to confirm the diagnosis and document the extent of renal inflammation or scarring.

Hematological
A leukocytosis suggests either a primary vasculitis or infection. Leucopenia is a rare presenting feature of vasculitis and, if present, suggests vasculitis secondary to systemic lupus erythematosus or the effects of previous immunosuppressive treatment. A peripheral blood eosinophilia is suggestive of Churg–Strauss syndrome or a drug reaction.

Inflammation
Inflammation may be assessed by measurement of the acute-phase response (erythrocyte sedimentation rate and C-reactive protein). Neither is specific, and may be increased in conditions other than vasculitis. A disproportionate increase in C-reactive protein compared with that in the erythrocyte sedimentation rate should raise the suspicion of infection.

Pulmonary
Chest radiography should be performed in all patients with suspected systemic vasculitis, to assess the presence of infiltrates or granulomata and to exclude infection. High-resolution computed tomography (CT) improves the detection of pulmonary lesions of Wegener's granulomatosis and pulmonary fibrosis, and can be useful in assessing response to treatment. Infection (especially tuberculosis), sarcoidosis and malignancy can mimic the CT appearance of Wegener's granulomatosis. Suspicious lesions should be biopsied to exclude malignancy or infection. High-resolution CT gives a high radiation dose to the patient, and this limits repeat scans.

Ear, nose and throat
Plain sinus films or CT should be obtained to assess the extent of sinus involvement; however, there is difficulty in distinguishing scarring from

active disease. Patients with active ear, nose and throat symptoms should have formal endoscopy by an otolaryngologist, and biopsies should be obtained from areas of inflammation. Histology in active vasculitis is often non-specific, and is difficult to distinguish from chronic infection.

Cardiac

Echocardiography is important to help exclude bacterial endocarditis and atrial myxoma. Myocarditis is especially frequent in Churg–Strauss syndrome, and poor ventricular function can be demonstrated by echocardiography.

Gastrointestinal

Gastrointestinal involvement is associated with a poor prognosis, mainly because of perforation. Visceral angiography (celiac axis, hepatic and renal) will demonstrate the extent of gastrointestinal involvement. Liver function tests may be abnormal, either because of viral infection (e.g. hepatitis B and C) or from non-specific causes.

Neurological

Neurological signs may be subtle, with evidence only of minor sensory impairment. Nerve conduction studies performed on four limbs will demonstrate evidence of mononeuritis multiplex. Cerebrospinal fluid examination in suspected central nervous system vasculitis shows an aseptic meningitis. Vasculitis of the central nervous system is rare. Magnetic resonance imaging (MRI) is the best investigation to assess central nervous system damage, but lacks specificity. The combination of a normal MRI and a normal cerebrospinal fluid examination makes the diagnosis of cerebral vasculitis unlikely, but occasionally biopsy or angiography is required.

Immunology

Antineutrophil cytoplasmic antibodies

Antineutrophil cytoplasmic antibodies were first described by Davis in 1982, but were first associated with Wegener's granulomatosis in 1985[45]. They are antibodies directed against neutrophil granule constituents. Two main patterns of staining are recognized using indirect immunofluorescence: cytoplasmic (cANCA), a coarse granular staining of the cytoplasm, and perinuclear (pANCA), with staining chiefly around the nucleus, leaving the cytoplasm unstained. The main target antigen for cANCA is proteinase 3, whereas pANCA is usually associated with myeloperoxidase. The finding of cANCA in association with proteinase 3 antibodies is highly specific (>90%) for generalized Wegener's granulomatosis[19]. pANCA associated with myeloperoxidase antibodies are typically found in microscopic polyangiitis and Churg–Strauss syndrome. A pANCA pattern may also be associated with other target antigens, including cathepsin-G, elastase and lysozyme. The clinical relevance of these other specificities is less well established.

The ANCA assay may be negative in localized Wegener's granulomatosis, and also in Churg–Strauss syndrome or microscopic polyangiitis. Other forms of vasculitis such as Henoch–Schönlein purpura, giant cell arteritis or Takayasu's arteritis are not associated with ANCA. ANCA without specificity for MPO and PR3 can occur in a number of non-vasculitic disorders, including SLE, rheumatoid arthritis, juvenile idiopathic arthritis, ulcerative colitis and infection, and with drugs. High-titer MPO-ANCA are particularly associated with drug-induced vasculitis[11].

Other autoantibodies

The presence of rheumatoid factors and antinuclear antibodies may indicate vasculitis associated with connective tissue disease. The antiphospholipid syndrome is associated with the presence of anticardiolipin antibodies; it can present with arterial and venous thrombosis, and mimic systemic vasculitis. Antibodies against the cofactor β_2-glycoprotein may correlate better with thrombosis than do anticardiolipin antibodies.

Complement concentrations are low in infection and immune complex mediated vasculitis such as SLE, but high in primary vasculitis. It should be remembered, however, that autoantibodies may occur in conditions other than vasculitis or connective tissue disease.

Confirmation of diagnosis

Tissue biopsy is important, to confirm the diagnosis before treatment with potentially toxic immunosuppressive drugs. The choice of tissue to biopsy is crucial. The old adage of 'go where the money is' usually pays off: biopsy of uninvolved tissue is less likely to yield a positive result. In the acutely sick patient in whom the evidence for vasculitis is strong and infection has been ruled out, then treatment should not be delayed solely to obtain the biopsy. Biopsy may, on occasion, reveal clinically unexpected findings such as cholesterol crystals or myxomatous emboli. It is not usually necessary to biopsy more than one organ to confirm the diagnosis; however, several biopsies may be required to assess the extent of organ involvement and to exclude alternative diagnoses.

Skin lesions (typically purpura or urticaria) are readily biopsied to confirm the presence of vasculitis, but the appearance (usually leukocytoclastic vasculitis) is common to several types of vasculitis. Deposition of IgA demonstrated by immunofluorescence is suggestive of Henoch–Schönlein purpura. It is important to remember that not all purpuric lesions are caused by vasculitis; Wegener's granulomatosis is characterized by the presence of necrotizing granulomata, but their presence is not mandatory for the diagnosis.

Churg–Strauss syndrome is characterized by granulomata and an extravascular eosinophilic infiltrate. In patients with an abnormal urinary sediment, renal biopsy permits confirmation of the diagnosis and estimation of the severity of renal damage. The usual appearance of a focal segmental necrotizing glomerulonephritis is not specific to any one vasculitis syndrome. Sural (or radial) nerve biopsy will confirm the presence of vasculitis of the vasa nervorum causing mononeuritis multiplex. It is often necessary to biopsy pulmonary lesions to exclude malignancy or infection that can mimic vasculitic granulomata.

Giant cell arteritis is ideally diagnosed on temporal artery biopsy. The typical lesion is a panarteritis with fragmentation of the internal elastic lamina and giant cells. The lesions are discontinuous, with skip lesions, thus an adequate length of vessel must be obtained (minimum 2–3cm) and subjected to examination of several sections. The diagnostic yield is greatest before corticosteroids treatment, but treatment should not be delayed to obtain a biopsy. A positive result can be obtained up to 2 weeks after initiation of corticosteroids treatment.

Radiology

Medium- and large-vessel involvement is best assessed by *angiography*. The extent of involvement in Takayasu's arteritis can readily be demonstrated by angiography, the typical long segment rat-tail appearance being confirmatory. In addition, formal angiography permits pressure measurements across stenotic lesions. Medium vessel involvement of visceral organs confirms the diagnosis without need for tissue biopsy. In polyarteritis nodosa, there are typical visceral microaneurysms. Visceral angiography should include the renal, hepatic and mesenteric vessels. Repeat angiography can be used to assess the response to treatment[46].

Magnetic resonance imaging assesses arterial wall thickening and has the advantage over conventional angiography of images in axial, sagittal and coronal planes. The spin echo technique permits differentiation of the arterial lumen from the wall without requiring contrast medium. In large vessel vasculitis, magnetic resonance angiography correlates well with conventional angiography[47]. It has the disadvantage of poor visualization of distal vessels, relatively poor resolution of existing MRI techniques and prolonged scanning time, making it difficult for patients to remain still and hold their breath. These problems may resolve with improved technology. It is, however, non-invasive and does not require ionizing radiation.

Nuclear medicine has several roles in the diagnosis and management of vasculitis – non-specific imaging of ischemic and inflammatory complications of vasculitis, such as ventilation/perfusion lung scanning in patients with medium or large arteries, and brain perfusion imaging in patients with cerebral vasculitis. Specific imaging of inflammation using radioactive agents that specifically target a component of the inflammatory process has the advantages that it helps make a diagnosis in a patient with non-specific symptoms, defines the distribution of inflammatory lesions, and monitors response to treatment (reviewed by Peters[48]).

Fluoro-18 deoxyglucose is an analog of glucose that is taken up by metabolically active cells. Increased glycolysis is seen in inactivated leukocytes and macrophages, and is a feature of vessel inflammation. *Fluoro-18 deoxyglucose positron emission tomography* can demonstrate the extent of vascular involvement in both giant cell arteritis and Takayasu's arteritis.

Labeled leukocyte scintigraphy (using either technetium-99m or indium-111) can be used to image the distribution of inflammation and its response to treatment. This technique will also image pyogenic infection.

High-resolution ultrasonography using a 7.5–10MHz probe has high sensitivity and specificity for stenotic lesions in the carotid vessels. Luminal stenosis and occlusion can be seen, and color *Doppler flow imaging* will permit assessment of flow. *Color duplex ultrasonography* has been used to detect inflammation in temporal vessels in giant cell arteritis, the typical appearance is hypoechoic halo around the perfused lumen of inflamed vessels. This has been reported to disappear with corticosteroid treatment[49].

Other investigations

Blood cultures, viral serology and echocardiography are important to exclude infection and other conditions that may present as systemic multisystem disease and hence mimic vasculitis.

Differential diagnosis

The differential diagnosis of systemic vasculitis is broad and includes infection, malignancy and a number of mimics (Table 143.7). Vasculitis may, of course, be secondary to infection[37] or malignancy[50].

Assessment of disease activity

Modern treatment of the systemic vasculitides has transformed these conditions from acute, fulminating, life-threatening conditions to chronic diseases with considerable morbidity arising either from disease activity or treatment. Several systems have been developed to assess disease activity and damage (reviewed by Carruthers and Bacon[51]). These include the Birmingham Vasculitis Activity Score (BVAS), the Groningen index and the vasculitis activity index. The BVAS is the most widely applicable to different types of necrotizing vasculitis, and has been systematically validated[52]. The BVAS was devised by a group of interested clinicians and pathologists. It is a comprehensive scoring system that includes nine organ systems. Clinical features that are attributable to active vasculitis and that have occurred anew and been present within the previous 4 weeks are recorded. Organ involvement associated with a worse prognosis is given greater weighting. BVAS has also been used to develop definitions of remission and relapse, which are now being used in multicentre trials.

Vasculitis results in organ damage either from the disease itself or as a result of treatment. Damage is defined as an irreversible process that is the result of scars and is not due to acute inflammation or grumbling disease activity. The Vasculitis Damage Index is also an organ-based system and is scored after 3 months. It has been validated[53], is comprehensive, and permits accumulation of damage with time.

The Disease Extent Index is an index specifically developed for use in Wegener's granulomatosis and demonstrates clearly the temporal progression that occurs in this condition. It is an organ-based system that does not specifically study activity or damage alone[54].

The final component of patient assessment is function. The SF-36, which has been validated for use in patients with vasculitis, is included in the Vasculitis Integrated Assessment Log for disease assessment[55].

PROGNOSIS

The natural history of untreated primary systemic vasculitis is of a rapidly progressive, usually fatal, disease. Before the introduction of corticosteroids for the treatment of Wegener's granulomatosis, Walton observed a mean survival of 5 months, with 82% of patients dying within 1 year and more than 90% dying within 2 years[56]. The introduction of corticosteroids resulted in an improvement in survival in polyarteritis nodosa to 50% at 5 years[1]. The median survival in Wegener's granulomatosis was only 12.5 months using corticosteroids alone, with most patients dying of sepsis or uncontrolled disease[57]. The introduction of cyclophosphamide (CYC) combined with prednisolone resulted in a significant improvement in the mortality of WG with a 5-year survival of 82%[58,59], and most modern series report 5-year survival figures of 80–90%.

Overall, however, the prognosis is determined by the extent and number of organs involved. Isolated cutaneous vasculitis has a good prognosis and often does not require any specific treatment. Involvement of other organs such as kidney, gut and nerve is associated with a much poorer outcome. Scoring systems have been developed that give increased weighting to major organ involvement.

The five-factor score was developed in a retrospective study of polyarteritis nodosa and Churg–Strauss syndrome by Guillevin *et al.*[60]. A poor prognosis was associated with age greater than 50 years and the presence of cardiomyopathy, nephropathy (proteinuria >1g/l; creatinine >1.58mg/dl), gastrointestinal tract involvement (bleeding, perforation, infarction or pancreatitis) and central nervous system involvement. A five-factor score of 2 or more is associated with 53% mortality at 6 years, compared with 14% in patients with a score of 0.

The BVAS at presentation is also indicative of prognosis. In a cross-sectional study, patients with a subsequent fatal outcome had a median initial BVAS of 20.5, whereas those with active untreated disease scored 7.5 and those with inactive disease scored 0[52].

TREATMENT

The treatment of vasculitis depends on the size and extent of vessel involvement (Table 143.2). Broadly, patients with large-vessel disease require corticosteroids, possibly with azathioprine or methotrexate. Medium- and small-vessel disease (Wegener's granulomatosis, microscopic polyangiitis, polyarteritis nodosa, Churg–Strauss syndrome) require treatment with cyclophosphamide and corticosteroids. The duration of cyclophosphamide treatment should be kept to a minimum, to reduce toxicity (bladder cancer, hemorrhagic cystitis, infertility, infection); azathioprine or methotrexate should be substituted once remission is achieved. Small-vessel disease may not require any specific treatment. Polyarteritis nodosa associated with hepatitis B or C virus infection should be treated with antiviral medication, in addition to corticosteroids. Intravenous immunoglobulin has a role in Kawasaki disease and also in patients with primary systemic vasculitis resistant to conventional treatment with cyclophosphamide and corticosteroids.

CONCLUSION

The spectrum of vasculitis is broad and presents a challenge to the physician in terms of diagnosis and management. It is important to confirm the diagnosis, if at all possible, with histology before initiating potentially toxic treatment.

REFERENCES

1. Frohnert PP, Sheps SG. Long term follow up of periarteritis nodosa. Am J Med 1967; 43: 8–14.

2. Kussmaul A, Maier R. Uber eine bisher nicht beschriebene eigenthümliche Arterienerkrankung (Periarteritis nodosa), die mit Morbus Brights und rapid fortschreitender allgemeiner Muskellähmung einhergeht. Deutsch Arch Klin Med 1866; 1: 484–514.

3. Matteson EL. A history of early investigation in polyarteritis nodosa. Arthritis Care Res 1999; 12: 294–302.

4. Davson J, Ball J, Platt R. The kidney in periarteritis nodosa. Q J Med 1948; 17: 175–202.

5. Matteson EL. Notes on the history of eponymic idiopathic vasculitis: the diseases of Henoch and Schönlein, Wegener, Churg and Strauss, Horton, Takayasu, Behçet, and Kawasaki. Arthritis Care Res 2000; 13: 237–245.

6. Chetty R. Vasculitides associated with HIV infection. J Clin Pathol 2001; 54: 275–278.

7. Zeek PM. Periarteritis nodosa – a critical review. Am J Clin Pathol 1952; 22: 777–790.

8. Watts RA, Scott DGI. Classification and epidemiology of the vasculitides. Baillière's Clin Rheumatol 1997; 11: 191–217.

9. Scott DGI, Watts RA. Classification and epidemiology of systemic vasculitis. Br J Rheumatol 1994; 33: 897–899.

10. Merkel PA. Drug induced vasculitis. Rheum Dis Clin North Am 27; 2001: 849–862.

11. Choi HK, Merkel PA, Walker AM, Niles JH. Drug associated antineutrophil cytoplasmic antibody-positive vasculitis. Arthritis Rheum 2000; 43: 405–413.

12. Wechsler M, Finn D, Gunawardena D et al. Churg Strauss syndrome in patients receiving montelukast as treatment for asthma. Chest 2000; 117: 708–713.

13. Hunder GG, Arend WP, Bloch DA et al. The American College of Rheumatology 1990 criteria for the classification of vasculitis: introduction. Arthritis Rheum 1990; 33: 1065–1067.

14. Fries JF, Hunder GG, Bloch DA et al. The American College of Rheumatology 1990 criteria for the classification of vasculitis: summary. Arthritis Rheum 1990; 33: 1135–1136.

15. Rao JK, Allen NB, Pincus TD. Limitations of the 1990 American College of Rheumatology classification criteria in the diagnosis of vasculitis. Ann Intern Med 1998; 129: 345–352.

16. Jeanette JC, Falk RJ, Andrassy K et al. Nomenclature of systemic vasculitides. Proposal of an international consensus conference. Arthritis Rheum 1994; 37: 187–192.

17. Watts RA, Jolliffe VA, Carruthers DM et al. Effect of classification on the incidence of polyarteritis nodosa and microscopic polyangiitis. Arthritis Rheum 1996; 39: 1208–1212.

18. Sorensen FA, Slot O, Tvede N, Pedersen J. A prospective study of vasculitis collected in a 5 year period: evaluation of the Chapel Hill nomenclature. Ann Rheum Dis 2000; 59: 478–482.

19. Hagen EC, Andrassy K, Csernok E et al. The diagnostic value of standardised assays for ANCA in idiopathic systemic vasculitis: results of an international collaborative study. Kidney Int 1998; 53: 743–753.

20. Bajema IM, Hagen EC. Evolving concepts about the role of antineutrophil cytoplasmic antibodies in systemic vasculitides. Curr Opin Rheumatol 1999; 11: 34–40.

21. Scott DGI, Bacon PA, Elliott PJ et al. Systemic vasculitis in a district general hospital 1972–80: clinical and laboratory features, classification and prognosis in 80 cases. Q J Med 1982; 203: 292–311.

22. Watts RA, Lane SE, Bentham G, Scott DGI. Epidemiology of systemic vasculitis (SV) – a ten year study. Arthritis Rheum 2000; 43: 422–427.

23. Salvarani C, Gabriel SE, O'Fallon WM, Hunder GG. The incidence of giant cell arteritis in Olmstead County, Minnesota: apparent fluctuations in a cyclic pattern. Ann Intern Med 1995; 123: 192–194.

24. Smith CA, Fidler WJ, Pinals RS. The epidemiology of giant cell arteritis. Report of a ten year study in Shelby County, Tennessee. Arthritis Rheum 1983; 26: 1214–1219.

25. Watts RA, Koldingsnes W, Nossent H et al. Epidemiology of vasculitis in Europe. Ann Rheum Dis 2001; 60: 1156–1157.

26. Reinhold-Keller E, Herlyn K, Wagner-Bastmeyer R et al. No difference in the incidences of vasculitides between north and south Germany: first results of the German vasculitis register. Rheumatology 2002; 41: 540–549.

27. McMahon BJ, Heyward WL, Templin DW et al. Hepatitis B associated polyarteritis nodosa in Alaskan Eskimos: clinical and epidemiological features and long term follow up. Hepatology 1989; 9: 97–101.

28. El-Reshaid K, Kapoor MM, El-Reshaid W et al. The spectrum of renal disease associated with microscopic polyangiitis and classic polyarteritis in Kuwait. Nephrol Dial Transplant 1997; 12: 1874–1882.

29. Andrews M, Edmunds M, Campbell A et al. Systemic vasculitis in the 1980s – is there an increasing incidence of Wegener's granulomatosis and microscopic polyarteritis? J R Coll Physicians Lond 1990; 24: 284–288.

30. Koldingsnes W, Nossent H. Epidemiology of Wegener's granulomatosis in Northern Norway. Arthritis Rheum 2000; 43: 2481–2487.

31. Hall S, Barr W, Lie JT et al. Takayasu arteritis: a study of 32 North American patients. Medicine (Baltimore) 1985; 64: 89–99.

32. Waern AU, Andersson P, Hemmingsson A. Takayasu's arteritis: a hospital-region based study on occurrence, treatment and prognosis. Angiology 1983; 34: 311–320.

33. Yanagawa H, Yashiro M, Nakamura Y et al. Epidemiologic pictures of Kawasaki disease in Japan from the nationwide incidence survey in 1991 and 1992. Paediatrics 1995; 95: 475–479.

34. Gardner-Medwin JM, Dolezalova P, Cummins C et al. Ethnic differences in the incidence of Henoch Schönlein purpura, Kawasaki disease and rare childhood vasculitides in children of different ethnic origins. Lancet 2002; 360: 1197–1202.

35. Davis RL, Waller PL, Mueller BA et al. Kawasaki syndrome in Washington State. Race specific incidence rates and residential proximity to water. Arch Ped Adolescent Med 1995; 149: 66–69.

36. Watts RA, Jolliffe VA, Grattan CEH et al. Cutaneous vasculitis in a defined population – clinical and epidemiological associations. J Rheumatol 1998; 25: 920–924.

37. Somer T, Finegold SM. Vasculitides associated with infections, immunization, and antimicrobial drugs. Clin Infect Dis 1995; 20: 1010–1036.

38. Elling P, Olsson AT, Elling H. Synchronous variations of the incidence of temporal arteritis and polymyalgia rheumatica in different regions of Denmark, association with epidemics of Mycoplasma pneumoniae infection. J Rheumatol 1996; 23: 112–119.

39. Duna GF, Cotch MF, Galperin C et al. Wegener's granulomatosis: role of environmental exposures. Clin Exp Rheumatol 1998; 16: 669–674.

40. Lane SE, Watts RA, Bentham G, Innes NJ, Scott DGI. Are environmental factors important in the aetiology of primary systemic vasculitis (PSV)? Arthritis Rheum 2003; in press.

41. Yashiro M, Muso E, Itoh-Ihara T et al. Significantly high regional morbidity of MPO-ANCA related angiitis and/or nephritis with respiratory tract involvement after the 1995 great earthquake in Kobe (Japan). Am J Kidney Dis 2000; 35: 889–895.

42. Gregorini G, Ferioloi A, Donato F et al. Association between silica exposure and necrotising crescentic glomerulonephritis with p-ANCA and anti-MPO antibodies: a hospital based case control study. Adv Exp Med Biol 1993; 336: 435–40.

43. Nuyts GD, van Vlem, de Vos A et al. Wegener's granulomatosis is associated with exposure to silicon compounds: a case control study. Nephrol Dial Trans 1995; 10: 1162–5.

44. Cohen Tervaert JW, Stegeman CA, Kallenberg CGM. Silicon exposure and vasculitis. Cur Opin Rheumatol 1998; 10: 12–7.

45. Van der Woude FJ, Rasmussen N, Lobatto S et al. Autoantibodies against neutrophils and monocytes: tool for diagnosis and marker of disease activity in Wegener's granulomatosis. Lancet 1985; 1: 425–429.

46. Raza K, Carruthers DM, Exley AR et al. Dramatic aneurysm regression in polyarteritis nodosa following high dose cyclophosphamide therapy. J Rheumatol 2000; 27: 1320–1321.

47. Suwanela N, Piyachon C. Takayasu arteritis in Thailand: clinical and imaging features. Int J Cardiol 1996; 54(suppl): S117–S134.

48. Peters AM. Nuclear medicine in vasculitis. Rheumatology 2000; 39: 463–470.

49. Schimdt WA, Vorpahl K, Volker L et al. Colour duplex ultrasonography in the diagnosis of temporal arteritis. N Engl J Med 1997; 337: 1336–1342.

50. Watts RA, Scott DGI. Secondary vasculitis. In: Isenberg DA, Woo P, Maddison P et al., eds. Oxford textbook of rheumatology, 3E. Oxford: Oxford University Press; (in press).

51. Carruthers D, Bacon P. Activity, damage and outcome in systemic vasculitis. Best Pract Res Clin Rheumatol 2001; 15: 225–238.

52. Luqmani R, Bacon P, Moots R et al. Birmingham vasculitis activity score (BVAS) in systemic necrotising vasculitis. Q J Med 1997; 87: 671–678.

53. Exley A, Bacon P, Luqmani R et al. Development and initial validation of the vasculitis damage index for the standardised clinical assessment of damage in the systemic vasculitides. Arthritis Rheum 1997; 40: 371–380.

54. Reinhold-Keller E, Kekow J, Schnabel A et al. Influence of disease manifestation and antineutrophil cytoplasmic antibody titre on the response to pulse cyclophosphamide therapy in patients with Wegener's granulomatosis. Arthritis Rheum 1994; 37: 919–924.

55. Bacon P, Moots R, Exley A et al. VITAL assessment of vasculitis. Clin Exp Rheumatol 1995; 13: 275–278.

56. Walton EW. Giant cell granuloma of the respiratory tract. BMJ 1958; 2: 265–270.

57. Hollander D, Manning RT. The use of alkylating agents in the treatment of Wegener's granulomatosis. Ann Intern Med 1967; 67: 393–398.

58. Fauci A, Wolff S. Wegener's granulomatosis: studies in 18 patients and a review of the literature. Medicine (Baltimore) 1973; 52: 535–561.

59. Fauci AS, Haynes BF, Katz P, Wolff SM. Wegener's granulomatosis: prospective clinical and therapeutic experience with 85 patients for 21 years. Ann Intern Med 1983; 98: 76–85.

60. Guillevin L, Lhote F, Gayraud M et al. Prognostic factors in polyarteritis nodosa and Churg Strauss syndrome. A prospective study of 342 patients. Medicine (Baltimore) 1996; 75: 17–28.

144 Biology of the vascular endothelium

Ronit Simantov and Roy L Silverstein

- Vascular endothelium has a critical role in the pathogenesis of many rheumatic diseases and inflammatory processes
- The growth and development of new blood vessels involves regulated processes of proliferation, migration and elaboration of proteases
- The endothelium orchestrates trafficking of leukocytes from blood to tissues in a coordinated set of events involving an array of membrane receptors and soluble mediators
- Endothelial functions also include regulation of vascular permeability, hemostasis and thrombosis, and vascular tone.

INTRODUCTION

The endothelium is a single cell layer that forms the continuous lining of the vasculature. The area of this lining is estimated to be several thousand square meters, most of which is found in the microcirculation of the capillary beds. The endothelium is not merely a passive liner; rather it provides a dynamic interface between blood and tissue parenchyma. As long ago as the late 19th century, anatomists recognized the critical role of the endothelium in inflammation. Metchnikoff, in the 1860s, described leukocyte 'paving' on endothelium in inflamed tissue and considered endothelial cells to be second in importance only to leukocytes in the inflammatory response[1]. In the 1970s, with the development by Jaffe et al.[2] and Gimbrone et al.[3] of straightforward methods to maintain, propagate and identify mammalian endothelial cells in culture, interest in the biology of these cells blossomed. In addition to studies following Metchnikoff's legacy on the role of endothelium in inflammation, considerable insight into endothelial cell biology has come from study of the role of endothelium in disease states and the mechanisms by which endothelial cells react to their environment. We now recognize that the vascular endothelium has several critical roles in homeostasis, and that endothelial dysfunction contributes to a great number of pathological processes.

ANATOMY OF THE VASCULAR ENDOTHELIUM

Endothelial cells are heterogeneous, with differences among arterial, venous, sinusoidal, lymphatic and capillary vessels, and among vessels of different organs. In most cases endothelial cells are flat, and continuously attached to each other by numerous intercellular tight junctions. These junctions create a polarity, with phenotypic differences between the apical surface facing the blood and the basal surface facing connective tissue. The most prevalent of the endothelial cell junctions are the adherens junctions, which are mainly localized at the basal side of endothelial cell intercellular contacts. These are formed by homophilic interaction of the extracellular domains of clusters of members of the cadherin family of transmembrane adhesion molecules. The major endothelial cadherin is vascular endothelial cadherin or cadherin-5. Cadherins interact in a dynamic fashion via their cytoplasmic domains

with a network of cytoskeletal proteins, including β-catenin. In addition to its role in cell adhesion and maintaining intercellular connections, the adherens junction is also involved in mediating signal transduction[4]. Regulated and dynamic interactions of vascular endothelial cadherin with cytosolic components are probably important in mediating endothelial cell development and function.

Interendothelial junctions may participate in mediating endothelial cell specialization. Certain endothelial cell–cell contacts, such as in the microcirculation of the brain, are marked by the presence of abundant tight junctions[5]. These are usually localized near the apical side of the lateral cell–cell contact, where they create a high transcellular resistance and thus a barrier to unregulated transport. Tight junction proteins ZO-1 and occludin are heavily and specifically expressed at cell–cell contacts in the microcirculation of the brain. Junctional adhesion molecule 1 also localizes in the brain vasculature and may function in its regulation by interactions with ZO-1 and other junctional proteins[6].

Endothelial ultrastructure was initially described in detail by Weibel and Palade in the 1960s[7]. The presence of surface membrane microdomains (caveolae) and complex intracellular vesicles and channels suggests that considerable transport of macromolecules may occur directly through the cells. The cells also contain numerous unique, electron-dense, membrane-bound organelles, termed Weibel–Palade bodies. These contain a high concentration of high molecular weight multimers of von Willebrand factor and their membranes express the leukocyte adhesion molecule, P-selectin. When endothelial cells are exposed to certain agonists, including thrombin and histamine, the membranes of these organelles fuse with the cell surface membrane and their contents are secreted into the blood. This results in localized high concentration of the more active molecular form of von Willebrand factor and in surface expression of P-selectin. Endothelial heterogeneity is determined in part by differences in embryologic origin, and in part by environmental cues mediating differential gene expression. Current studies using new gene profiling technologies should provide insight into endothelial cell diversity[8].

DEVELOPMENTAL BIOLOGY OF ENDOTHELIAL CELLS

Endothelial cells and hematopoietic cells, which derive from a common precursor, the hemangioblast, aggregate in the developing yolk sac of the embryo to form blood islands. Angioblasts, the precursors of endothelial cells, migrate, proliferate and differentiate to form primary capillary plexi. This process, known as vasculogenesis, is regulated by the vascular endothelial growth factor (VEGF) family of growth factors and receptors. VEGF family members are structurally related to the B chain of platelet-derived growth factor (PDGF) and include VEGFs-A, -B, -C and -D, orf viral VEGF homologs, and placental growth factor[9]. These signal through the receptor tyrosine kinases VEGFR-1 (flt-1), VEGFR-2 (flk or KDR), and VEGFR-3 (flt-4), which are comprised of seven extracellular immunoglobulin homology domains and an intracellular split kinase signaling domain. Murine gene knockout models have provided evidence for the key role of VEGF, VEGFR-1 and VEGFR-2 in early vasculogenic events. Heterozygous gene deletions of VEGF lead to embryonic death at embryonic day 10.5, associated with abnormal blood vessel development in the yolk sac[10]. VEGFR-2 is the first specific marker to appear on primitive endothelial cells, and VEGFR-2 null embryos lack both hematopoietic and endothelial precursors and do not form blood islands[11]. VEGFR-1 knockouts have angioblasts, but do not correctly assemble blood vessels, suggesting a role for VEGFR-1 in later stages of vasculogenesis[12]. VEGFR-3 expression in the adult occurs mainly in the lymphatic endothelium[13]. However, VEGFR-3-deficient embryos die after embryonic day 9.5 because of defects in the remodeling of primary vascular plexus, suggesting a role for the receptor in this process[14]. Overexpression or unregulated expression of VEGF is associated with leaky, hemorrhagic vessels, with an accompanying inflammatory response.

Formation of small and large blood vessels by pruning and growth of blood vessels in the primary capillary plexus is mediated by angiopoietins, which signal through the Tie receptor tyrosine kinases, and by the ephrin ligand/Eph receptor tyrosine kinases. Murine knockout studies have demonstrated that the binding of angiopoietin 1 to endothelial Tie 2 receptors mediates the interaction of endothelial cells with surrounding cells and matrix[15]. In addition, angiopoietin 1 may counteract the effect of VEGF on vascular permeability[16]. Angiopoietin 2 is a Tie 2 antagonist that may have a role in destabilizing blood vessels to initiate remodeling[9]. Vascular development is also mediated by ephrin-B2 and its EphB4 receptor. Ephrin-B2, a transmembrane protein, is expressed in developing arterial blood vessels and binds through direct cell–cell interaction to EphB4 receptors expressed on primordial veins. These findings suggest a role for ephrin-B2/EphB4 in the development and intercalation of arterial and venous capillary beds. There is also evidence that ephrin/Eph signaling is involved in the interactions of endothelial cells with surrounding smooth muscle cells and non-vascular cells[17].

Recent advances in the study of vascular development have been made using the zebrafish, the transparent embryos of which provide an easily visualized vasculature. Angioblast differentiation into the artery and venous structures in the zebrafish have shown to be regulated by a transcriptional repressor protein known as gridlock. Gridlock protein suppresses the development of venous cells, driving angiogblasts to form the aorta. Gridlock expression is induced by the Notch1 receptor signaling pathway, although further studies will need to be done to elucidate the mechanism by the Notch/gridlock pathway acts to determine the fate of angiogblasts[18].

Endothelial cells have been shown to support the development of other organs, even before a functioning vasculature is formed. Early hepatic development was found to be impaired in VEGFR-2-deficient mice, which, as described above, lack angiogblasts and developing endothelial cells. Similarly, hepatic cell growth was inhibited in a liver explant model using VEGFR-2-deficient cells, suggesting that functional endothelial cells were necessary for liver development[19]. Endothelial cells were also shown to participate in the development of the pancreas; lack of functional endothelial cells was associated with impaired pancreatic development, whereas aberrant, increased and insulin-producing cells were found in association with ectopic VEGF in the gastrointestinal tract of a transgenic model[20].

In the adult organism, endothelial cells proliferate at an extremely slow rate; turnover times have been estimated to be as high as decades. Under certain conditions, including ovulation, wound healing, inflammation, tumor growth, diabetic retinopathy and rheumatoid arthritis, new blood vessels can grow rapidly from pre-existing capillaries by a sprouting process similar to embryonic angiogenesis. Folkman and Cotran's observations[21] that growth of malignant tumors beyond 1cm in size required the development of new blood vessels and capillary beds has spawned intense study of the process of angiogenesis. The cellular and molecular mechanisms of angiogenesis are complex, and include at least three pivotal endothelial cell processes: proliferation, migration and elaboration of proteases. Metallo- and serine proteases, such as collagenase and plasminogen activator, degrade extracellular matrix, facilitating cellular migration.

On the basis of *in vitro* assays utilizing cultured capillary endothelial cell monolayers, a number of heparin-binding growth factors have been identified that are capable of eliciting one or more of the activities associated with angiogenesis. These include acidic and basic fibroblast growth factor (FGF), VEGF and hepatocyte growth factor. These growth factors also stimulate angiogenesis in animal model systems such as the rabbit or rodent cornea or the chick chorioallantoic membrane. Figure 144.1a shows an example of a mouse corneal angiogenesis assay, demonstrating robust growth of blood vessels from the limbic vessel towards a pellet containing bFGF. VEGF is now believed to be the most important physiological regulator of angiogenesis, because of its expression in angiogenic tissues, its broad pattern of inducible expression by angiogenic stimuli, and the endothelial cell restricted expression of its receptors. Several chemokines, including interleukin (IL)-8 and neutrophil-activating peptide-2, have angiogenic activity by virtue of their ability to stimulate endothelial cell migration. Other molecules shown to

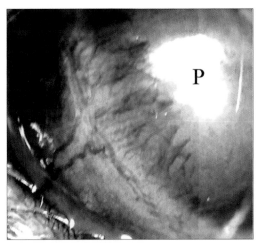
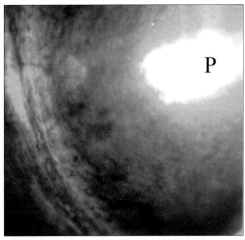
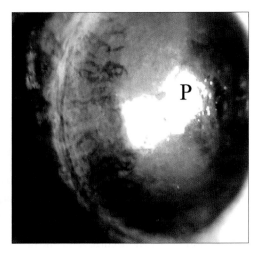

Fig. 144.1 Corneal angiogenesis assay. Hydron/sucralfate pellets containing bFGF or bFGF + thrombospondin-1 were implanted in the corneas of C57Bl/6 mice and photographed after 5 days. (a) Vigorous neovascularization from the limbus towards the pellet (P) induced by bFGF. (b) Inhibition of angiogenesis by thrombospondin-1. (c) No inhibition of neovascularization by thrombospondin-1 in CD36 knockout mice.

have *in vivo* angiogenic activity include PDGF and soluble E-selectin. Interactions of angiogenic endothelial cells with specific extracellular matrix components is also an essential component of the angiogenic response. Expression of $\alpha_v\beta_3$ integrin is increased in angiogenic vessels, and treatment of endothelial cells with inhibitory antibodies or peptides that block the interactions of $\alpha_v\beta_3$ integrin with specific matrix components blocks angiogenesis[22].

Recent attention has focused on angiogenic factors that are selective for specific types of endothelium. An endothelial cell growth factor that is selective for one type of endothelium has been identified. Endocrine-gland-derived vascular endothelial growth factor (EG-VEGF) was found to induce proliferation, migration and fenestration of capillary endothelial cells derived from steroidogenic endocrine gland. EG-VEGF is not structurally related to VEGF, but is functionally similar, in that it is inducible by hypoxia and leads to increased vascular permeability[23]. This suggests that organ-specific angiogenic regulation may be mediated by locally active angiogenic factors.

The regulation of angiogenesis involves both inhibitory and stimulatory influences. Considerable recent attention has focused on matrix-associated molecules as antiangiogenesis factors. These include proteolytic fragments of plasminogen and collagen (endostatin and angiostatin), and thrombospondin-1[24–26]. Angiostatin is a 38kDa internal fragment of plasminogen, which was originally isolated as a tumor product and has been shown to induce apoptosis of endothelial cells. The endothelial cell protein that mediates binding of angiostatin was identified as the $\alpha\beta$ subunits of ATP synthase on the outer membrane of endothelial cells; however, the mechanism by which this inhibits angiogenesis has not been characterized[27]. Endostatin, a fragment of the C-terminal globular domain of collagen XVIII, has also been shown to inhibit endothelial cell proliferation and induce apoptosis.

The most extensively characterized angiogenesis inhibitor is thrombospondin-1, a large molecular weight matrix glycoprotein secreted by endothelial and other vascular cells. Its secretion is regulated by many of the same agonists that control angiogenesis[28]. Thrombospondin-1 and several proteolytic fragments of thrombospondin-1 inhibit endothelial cell migration to angiogenic stimuli and inhibit angiogenesis in animal models[29]. Thrombospondin-1 peptides have been shown to induce endothelial cell apoptosis, and mice null for thrombospondin-1 exhibit increased blood vessel formation in granulation tissue. Although thrombospondin-1 binds to $\alpha_v\beta_3$ integrin and can disrupt focal adhesions, its antiangiogenic activity is mediated by its receptor on capillary endothelial cells, CD36[30]. Antibodies and peptides that block CD36 have been shown to inhibit the effect of thrombospondin-1 on endothelial cell migration, and other CD36 ligands have been shown to have similar antiangiogenic properties . Mice null for CD36, like the thrombospondin-1 null mice, have increased blood vessel formation, and lack an antiangiogenic response to thrombospondin-1[31] (Fig. 144.1b,c). Histidine-rich glycoprotein, a plasma and cellular protein that blocks the binding of thrombospndin-1 to CD36, inhibits the antiangiogenic response to thrombospondin and may serve to modulate the thrombospondin/CD36 antiangiogenic pathway[32].

CIRCULATING ENDOTHELIAL CELLS

Angiogenesis in the adult has long been believed to involve proliferation of endothelial cells derived from the local vasculature. However, recent work has demonstrated that circulating endothelial cell progenitors derived from the bone marrow may participate in this process. Circulating bone marrow-derived endothelial cell progenitors have been identified and characterized in the adult[33,34]. These endothelial precursors, which express VEGFR-2, have been shown to incorporate into new vasculature and proliferate. Recent work has demonstrated that circulating endothelial progenitors are necessary for tumor angiogenesis and are

recruited into the tumor vasculature in association with hematopoietic cells[35].

Differentiated circulating endothelial cells have also been identified in the peripheral blood. Normal adults have approximately circulating endothelial cell concentration of 2.6±1.6/ml blood, and this number is increased in the setting of vascular injury such as sickle-cell disease, myocardial infarction and certain infections. Differentiated circulating endothelial cells differ from circulating progenitors in that they originate from vessel walls rather than from the bone marrow, and have limited proliferative capacity[36].

ENDOTHELIAL CELL ACTIVATION

Central to the critical role of endothelial cells in maintaining homeostasis is their ability to respond to a myriad of environmental signals with specific programmed responses. Included among these signals (summarized in Table 144.1) are biomechanical forces, cytokines, growth factors, bioactive amines, peptides, enzymes, complement components, eicosanoids and nitric oxide. Pathological agents, including bacterial endotoxin, oxidized lipoproteins, viruses and certain antibodies, have also been shown to activate endothelial cells.

Certain endothelial responses are rapid and probably do not require new gene transcription or protein synthesis. These include secretion of Weibel–Palade bodies, activation of eicosanoid and nitric acid metabolic pathways and cytoskeletal/junctional reorganization. Agonists capable of eliciting this type of response include thrombin, histamine and complement components. Many responses, however, are the result of altered transcription of specific endothelial cell gene products. These include the adhesion molecules E-selectin, intercellular adhesion molecules (ICAM)-1 and -2 and vascular cell adhesion molecule (VCAM), proinflammatory cytokines, growth factors, tissue factor procoagulant and plasminogen activator inhibitor (PAI)-1. Perhaps the best described of these endothelial responses is that to the inflammatory mediators IL-1, tumor necrosis factor (TNF)α and bacterial endotoxin. Within a few hours of exposure in culture, the cells begin to express E-selectin and VCAM and increase their expression of ICAM-1. Expression peaks in 4–6 hours and then begins to decrease, reaching baseline at 12–24 hours for E-selectin, and somewhat later for the others. Tissue factor pro-

TABLE 144.1 ENDOTHELIAL CELL AGONISTS

Physiologic agonists	
Biomechanical forces	Shear stress
	Cyclic strains
	Hydrostatic forces
Cytokines	IL-1, IL-4, IL-6, TNFα, interferon-γ
Growth factors	bFGF, aFGF, VEGF, HGF, PDGF
Vasoactive compounds	Histamine, kinins
Enzymes	Thrombin, cathepsin G
Complement components	C5a, C5b-9
Eicosanoids	
Nitric acid	
Pathologic agonists	
Bacterial endotoxin	
DNA viruses	CMV, Herpes simplex
Lipoproteins	Oxidized LDL
Lysophosphatidyl choline	
Antibodies	Antiphospholipid antibodies
Xenoreactive antibodies	

CMV, cytomegalovirus; HGF, hepatocyte growth factor; LDL, low-density lipoprotein; TNF, tumor necrosis factor.

coagulant is also expressed in this setting, along with PAI-1, platelet activating factor (PAF), monocyte chemoattractant protein (MCP)-1, PDGF and IL-1.

Studies have begun to elucidate endothelial cell responses to biomechanical forces, including shear stress, cyclic strain and hydrostatic pressure. Work from the laboratories of Collins and others has identified the essential role of specific nuclear transcription factors in orchestrating the endothelial cell response. In particular, the promoter regions of many of the genes described above contain shear stress response elements and consensus sequences for activation by nuclear factor κB[37]. Transcriptional profiling using cDNA arrays has been used to compare gene expression in cultured endothelial cells under static conditions with those exposed to biomechanical stimulation. These studies have revealed different patterns of gene expression in response to biomechanical activation, and differences in laminar and turbulent shear stresses, although further study will be required to analyze the regulation of the large number of genes in the data generated by these studies.

ENDOTHELIAL CELL FUNCTION

Permeability barrier functions

Regulation of macromolecular and fluid flux between blood and the extravascular space is a critical function of endothelium. Endothelial cells express active transport systems for adenosine, serotonin and low-density lipoprotein (LDL) and may have the capacity to transfer some of these molecules (or their metabolic products) across the cell layer. In certain regions, endothelial cells function to meet highly specialized transport needs, for example as part of the blood–brain barrier, the glomerular filtration system and the pulmonary gas exchange system. Abnormal endothelial barrier function can have considerable untoward effects. Interendothelial gaps can be induced by interferon-γ, other cytokines, kinins, histamine and thrombin, and are associated with changes in endothelial cell shape, cytoskeletal organization and cell junctions. Increased vascular permeability may also play an important part in the pathogenesis of atherosclerosis. Entry of lipoprotein particles, such as LDL and very-low-density lipoprotein, into the subendothelial space in the context of vascular injury places them in a privileged compartment, where they are susceptible to oxidative modification by endothelium- and leukocyte-derived reactive oxygen metabolites[38].

Oxidized lipoproteins can then be taken up by macrophages via 'scavenger' pathways, leading to formation of foam cells and atheromatous plaque. Oxidized LDL and lysophosphatidic lipids can also interact with and activate endothelial cells, smooth muscle cells, leukocytes and platelets, contributing to and augmenting the injury response.

Leukocyte trafficking

Perhaps the most important function of the vascular endothelium with respect to rheumatologic disease is its role in orchestrating the complex trafficking of leukocytes from blood to tissues. Extravasation of leukocytes into inflammatory sites, circulation of naïve lymphocytes and homing of memory/effector lymphocytes require a coordinated set of events involving an array of membrane receptors and soluble mediators. Through this efficient process, up to 10^8 neutrophils per hour can enter a joint afflicted by rheumatoid arthritis, through the flat endothelium of small postcapillary venules. Our current model for leukocyte trafficking, one that is supported by a large amount of elegant experimental cell and molecular biology from many laboratories, involves a multistep cascade of adhesion steps[39]. These steps are mediated by sequential interaction of specific leukocyte adhesion receptors with specific ligands or counter-receptors expressed on the surface of endothelial cells. The multistep adhesion model is summarized in Figure 144.2 and consists of four major steps: (1) tethering of the circulating leukocyte to the endothelial cell, associated with 'rolling' of the leukocyte in certain vascular beds; (2) activation of additional adhesion molecules on the leukocyte surface; (3) firm attachment of leukocyte to endothelial cell; and (4) migration of the leukocyte between adjacent endothelial cells into the subendothelial space.

The initial attachment step is usually mediated by the selectin family of adhesion molecules. These are transmembrane glycoproteins with an amino-terminal C-type lectin carbohydrate recognition domain. P-selectin, stored in the Weibel–Palade bodies, is rapidly expressed in response to inflammatory cytokines and binds preferentially to P-selectin glycoprotein ligand (PSGL)-1, a sulfated sialomucin on the cell surface of neutrophils, monocytes, natural killer cells and some lymphocytes. Endothelial cells also express E-selectin upon stimulation by inflammatory mediators, in a process requiring gene transcription. The major ligands for E-selectin are sialylated fucosylated tetrasaccharides, such as sialyl Lewis[x], and include E-selectin ligand-1 and PSGL-1 on myeloid cells and cutaneous leukocyte antigen (CLA) in lymphocytes.

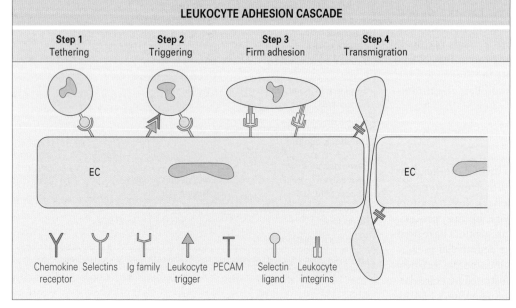

Fig. 144.2 Leukocyte adhesion cascade. Adhesion and transmigration of leukocytes across the endothelial cell layer is a multistep process involving sequential interaction of specific adhesion molecules on the endothelial surface, with counter-receptors on the leukocyte surface. (1) The first step is the tethering or 'rolling' of the leukocyte to selectins expressed on the surface of activated endothelial cells (EC). (2) The second step is a 'triggering' of the tethered leukocyte, which results in activation of leukocyte integrins. Triggering molecules include selectins themselves, platelet activating factor, endothelial cell chemokines and other inflammatory mediators. (3) The third step is firm adhesion and spreading of the leukocyte on the endothelial surface, mediated by interactions of the activated leukocyte integrins with Ig superfamily cell adhesion molecules on the endothelial surface. (4) The final step is transmigration of the leukocyte through the endothelial barrier. This step is mediated by PECAM-dependent homophilic adhesive interactions.

Although *in vitro* cell culture experiments predicted a major role for E-selectin in acute inflammation, murine knockout studies demonstrated that E-selectin null mice had little or no abnormalities[40]. In contrast, P-selectin null mice showed partial inhibition of leukocyte rolling on inflamed mesenteric vessels, blunted delayed-type hypersensitivity and decreased peritoneal recruitment of leukocytes[41]. Interestingly, double E- and P-selectin null mice demonstrated absent rolling, skin infections and poor wound healing, suggesting that the selectins may function cooperatively *in vivo*.

The firm attachment step of the cascade is mediated by the interaction of leukocyte integrins with endothelial cell immunoglobulin gene (Ig) superfamily adhesion molecules. These include the interaction of the β_2 integrins (CD11/CD18) with ICAM-1 and ICAM-2, which are both upregulated on the surface of cytokine-activated endothelial cells. In addition, leukocyte $\alpha_4\beta_1$ integrin interacts with endothelial VCAM-1, which is also expressed by stimulated endothelium. These integrin-mediated interactions are capable of transducing signals to the leukocyte and lead to cytoskeletal reorganization and spreading. In general, the leukocyte integrins are functionally inactive on circulating cells, and a leukocyte triggering or activation step must be interposed between attachment and firm adhesion. Leukocyte triggering is in large part mediated by chemokines, a large family of extracellular signaling molecules that signal through G protein-coupled receptors. These soluble mediators with potent leukocyte chemotactic properties are produced at the site of vascular response. They modulate integrin adhesion by increasing receptor affinity through conformational change of the integrin heterodimer, and by clustering integrins on the cell membrane[42]. Chemokines are classified into two major families containing at least 25 members: the C-X-C family (such as IL-8) and the C-C family (such as MCP-1 and RANTES). Chemokines are produced by activated endothelial cells and may be retained at the endothelial cell surface by heparan sulfate proteoglycans, where they can function on tethered leukocytes in the local microenvironment. Regulation may occur through specificity of chemokines and expression pattern of receptors; for example, IL-8 for neutrophils, MCP-1 for monocytes and RANTES for memory T cells. Order and timing of chemokine activity have also been shown to be important in maintaining the stepwise progression of the leukocyte adhesion cascade: for example, growth-related oncogene α and fractalkine act in initial firm adhesion, whereas MCP-1 is required for leukocyte spreading[43].

Adherent leukocytes transmigrate across the endothelium to the underlying basement membrane by squeezing between the intercellular junctions of adjacent endothelial cells. Work by Muller and colleagues[44] has identified the Ig superfamily molecule, platelet-endothelial cell adhesion molecule (PECAM)-1 (CD31) as necessary for this step. CD31 is expressed on most leukocytes and is also present in high concentration on the endothelial surface, localized to the lateral cell–cell junctions. Leukocyte diapedesis is mediated by homophilic interactions of CD31 on the endothelial cell surface with leukocyte CD31. Blocking CD31 function with specific antibodies or a soluble PECAM-1 molecule significantly inhibits transendothelial migration. Recently, CD99, a 32kDa O-glycosylated transmembrane protein, has been shown to play a part in transendothelial migration of monocytes. Like CD31, CD99 was shown to function through homophilic interactions between leukocytes and endothelial CD99, and mediated diapedesis of monocytes in an *in vitro* model[45].

Naïve lymphocytes migrate into peripheral lymph nodes through the high endothelial cells (HEVs) of postcapillary venules in lymphoid tissues. Tethering and rolling occur through the interaction of lymphocyte L-selectin with its ligands on HEVs, glycosylation-dependent cell adhesion molecule-1 and CD34. The chemokines secondary lymphoid tissue chemokine (SLC, CCL21), Epstein–Barr virus-induced receptor ligand chemokine (ELC, CCL19) and stromal cell derived factor-1α activate the β_2 integrin, lymphocyte function-associated antigen-1, leading to firm adhesion of lymphocytes to endothelial cell ICAM-1[46]. Pioneering studies by Stamper and Woodruff[47] demonstrated that lymphocyte subclasses bound with differing specificities to HEV in thin sections cut from frozen lymphoid tissues: T cells bound preferentially to peripheral node HEV, whereas B cells bound better to Peyer's patch HEV. Subsequent work has revealed that attachment to HEV on Peyer's patches is mediated by an unusual adhesion protein, mucosal addressin cell adhesion molecule (MadCAM), an Ig superfamily member that contains mucin-like domains and thus is capable of binding to both selectins and integrins. MadCAM therefore mediates tethering through interactions with L-selectin and firm attachment through binding of $\alpha_4\beta_7$ integrin. SLC has been shown to activate $\alpha_4\beta_7$ to MadCAM. Lymphocyte transmigration is less well understood, but likely involves regulation of intercellular tight-junction molecules such as members of the junctional adhesion molecule family of junctional proteins[6,48].

Recruitment of memory cells to lymphoid and cutaneous tissues is probably mediated by subtly different pathways. T cells homing to the skin express a unique sialyl Lewis[X] cutaneous lymphoid associated antigen, a modified form of PSGL-1 that mediates tethering to flat cutaneous endothelial cells via E-selectin. Homing of memory lymphocytes to Peyer's patches and postcapillary venules of the gut is mediated through $\alpha_4\beta_7$ binding endothelial MadCAM. Considerable current research is proceeding to identify the precise endothelial 'addressins' and lymphocyte ligands that mediate these myriad and complex trafficking events. Table 144.2 summarizes some of the major adhesion pairs identified to date. The observation that tumor cells may also express specific ligands for endothelial cell adhesion molecules may explain the fairly specific and predictable metastatic patterns of certain cancers.

Hemostatic functions

Under normal conditions endothelial cells present a non-thrombogenic surface to flowing blood and play an active part in maintaining blood fluidity[49] (Fig. 144.3 & Table 144.3). Through the constitutive secretion of low levels of prostacyclin, a potent inhibitor of platelet activation, and expression of CD39, a surface ecto-ADPase[50], endothelial cells prevent inappropriate platelet activation and limit the degree of platelet response to an activating signal. The endothelial surface is also antithrombotic by virtue of constitutive expression of the natural regulators of thrombin generation and fibrin formation. These include tissue factor pathway

TABLE 144.2 FAMILIES OF ENDOTHELIAL CELL ADHESION MOLECULES AND THEIR LEUKOCYTE LIGANDS	
Endothelial cell adhesion molecule	**Leukocyte ligands**
Selectins	
E-selectin	sLe^x, sLe^a, CLA, ESL-1, PSGL-1
P-selectin	sLe^x, sLe^a, PSGL-1
Ig family	
ICAM-1	$\alpha_M\beta_2$, $\alpha_L\beta_2$
ICAM-2	$\alpha_L\beta_2$
VCAM-1	$\alpha_4\beta_1$, $\alpha_4\beta_7$
MadCAM-1	$\alpha_4\beta_7$, L-selectin
PECAM (CD31)	PECAM (CD31)
Mucin-like molecules	
MadCAM-1	$\alpha_4\beta_7$, L-selectin
GlyCAM-1	L-selectin
CD34	L-selectin

CLA, cutaneous leukocyte antigen ; ESL, E-selectin ligand ; sLe, sialyl Lewis.

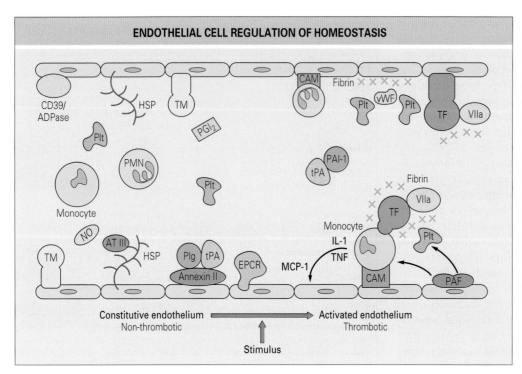

Fig. 144.3 Endothelial cell regulation of homeostasis. The 'resting' endothelium normally expresses a non-thrombotic, non-inflammatory phenotype marked by expression of thrombomodulin (Tm), heparan sulfate proteoglycans (HSP) that serve to bind and activate antithrombin III (AT III), prostacyclin (PGI$_2$), ectoADPase and receptors such as annexin II for plasminogen (Plg) and tissue plasminogen activator (tPA). Upon stimulation (arrow) the cells converts to a prothrombotic, proinflammatory phenotype, marked by loss of Tm and HSP and by induction of expression of cytokines (including IL-1), chemokines (including MCP-1), growth factors (including PDGF), plasminogen activator inhibitor (PAI)-1, platelet activating factor (PAF), von Willebrand Factor (vWF) and cell adhesion molecules (CAM). Leukocytes bound to the CAMs can in turn release cytokines and express tissue factor, amplifying the response. EPCR, endothelial protein C receptor; NO, nitric oxide; Plt, platelets; PMN, polymorphonucleocyte; TF, tissue factor; VIIa, Factor VIIa.

TABLE 144.3 ENDOTHELIAL CELL PRODUCTS INVOLVED IN THE REGULATION OF HEMOSTASIS	
Antithrombotic factors	**Prothrombotic factors**
Thrombomodulin	Tissue factor
tPA/uPA	von Willebrand factor
Annexin II (plasminogen/tPA receptor)	Platelet activating factor
Heparin-like proteoglycans	Plasminogen activator inhibitor-1
Ecto-ADPase	Selectins
Prostacyclin	Ig superfamily cell adhesion molecules
Nitric oxide	Vasoconstrictors
Tissue factor pathway inhibitor	Endothelin, angiotensin
Endothelial protein C receptor	Cytokines
	IL-1, FGF, TGFβ, CSFs
	Chemokines
	MCP-1, IL-8

CSFs, colony-stimulating factors; TGFβ, transforming growth factor β.

inhibitor, the major inhibitor of the coagulation factor VIIa, and antithrombin III, a serine protease inhibitor with specificity for the major vitamin K-dependent proteases of the coagulation cascade. The inhibitory activity of antithrombin III requires the formation of a complex with heparan sulfate proteoglycans expressed on the endothelial surface and within the subendothelial space, thus localizing the inhibitory complexes to areas of vascular injury. The protein C system regulates thrombin generation by proteolytic destruction of the major protein cofactors of the coagulation cascade, factors V and VIII. Protein C is converted to its active form by thrombin-mediated limited proteolytic cleavage. Thrombin gains specificity for protein C only when it is bound on the cell surface to a unique endothelial receptor, thrombomodulin. In addition, endothelial cells express an endothelial cell protein C receptor, which functions to localize and amplify the function of activated protein C. Endothelial cells also constitutively secrete tissue type plasminogen activator (tPA), single chain urinary type plasminogen activator (uPA), and the cellular uPA receptor. Furthermore, annexin II expressed on the endothelial surface functions as a receptor for plas-

minogen and tPA, localizing zymogen and activator to the vessel wall and altering the kinetics of activation to favor plasmin generation. Even though endothelial cells also express PAI-1, evidence suggests that, under normal conditions, the balance favors activators over inhibitors, and that trace amounts of active plasmin are present on the endothelial surface[49].

Although the 'resting' endothelial phenotype is antiplatelet, antithrombin, and profibrinolytic, endothelial cell activation – for example by TNFα or lipopolysaccharide – results in a dramatic change to a prothrombotic phenotype. The molecular basis of this change is complex and includes loss of thrombomodulin and heparan sulfate proteoglycans from the cell surface, decreasing the ability to generate active protein C and functional antithrombin III. PAI-1 secretion also increases, resulting in a net antifibrinolytic state. Thrombin generation is also directly promoted by induced surface expression of tissue factor procoagulant, the most important and efficient initiator of the coagulation cascade. Antiplatelet effects are also downmodulated by the resulting generation of thrombin, a potent platelet agonist, and the concomitant expression of the additional platelet activating agent, PAF. Resting platelets bind to the activated endothelial cell surface through an adhesion cascade that includes PSLG-1 on endothelial cells, the glycoprotein Ib complex on platelets and integrins on both cells. In patients with sickle-cell disease, circulating endothelial cells expressing an activated phenotype have been demonstrated, likely a reflection of a generalized procoagulant, proadhesive vascular endothelium in certain disease states[51]. Many other acquired hypercoagulable states, including cancer, diabetes, the antiphospholipid syndrome and disseminated intravascular coagulation, may be the result of such inappropriate endothelial cell activation[52].

Regulation of vascular tone

Vascular tone is provided primarily by arterial smooth muscle cells under the control of the autonomic nervous system, although endothelium has an important regulatory role. In studies utilizing isolated aortic rings[53], Furchgott and Zawadzki first established that the vasodilatory effect of acetylcholine and histamine required an intact endothelium. The identity of this endothelium-dependent relaxing factor (EDRF) was eventually demonstrated independently by Ignarro et al.[54] to be nitric oxide (NO), consistent with other studies showing that the vasodilatory effect of nitroglycerin-related drugs was due to their metabolism to NO. We now know that NO, by virtue of its ability to activate guanylyl cyclase and generate cGMP, is a potent vasodilator and inhibitor of platelet function. NO is an unstable gas and also binds tightly to hemoglobin and thus has an extraordinarily brief plasma lifespan, limiting its action to the microenvironment in which it is produced. NO is generated from L-arginine by the action of nitric oxide synthetase (NOS), a family of tightly regulated enzymes found in many cells, including in brain, blood vessels and macrophages. Endothelial cells express a constitutive NOS (cNOS) that prevents platelet aggregation and leukocyte adhesion to endothelial cells. Pharmacological inhibitors of cNOS induce an increase in the number of adherent leukocytes, and cNOS knockout mice have an increase in leukocyte rolling and adhesion in postcapillary venules. In addition, endothelial cells may also synthesize a second, inducible form of NOS (iNOS) when exposed to inflammatory cytokines such as TNF. It has been postulated that dysfunction of these systems may contribute to chronic hypertension, atherosclerosis and shock.

Endothelial-dependent relaxation may be lost in the presence of reactive oxygen species, leading to vasoconstriction and vascular injury. Heme oxygenases (HO) are a family of heme-degrading enzymes that catalyze the cleavage of the heme ring to form ferrous iron, carbon monoxide and biliverdin. Synthesis of HO-1 is induced by cytokines, heavy metals and oxidants, and HO-1 has been shown to be expressed by arterial cells in atherosclerosis, angioplasty and hypertension. HO-1 provides a protective effect in the setting of inflammatory injury, by stimulating vascular relaxation in addition to decreasing vascular smooth muscle cell proliferation in models of vascular injury[55].

Endothelial cells constitutively express eicosanoid metabolizing enzymes, including cyclo-oxygenase (COX)-1 and prostacyclin synthase, producing prostacyclin as the major prostaglandin end product[56]. Like NO, this is a potent vasodilator and antiplatelet agent, with an extremely brief plasma half-life. In response to stimulation with thrombin, shear stress and other agonists, phospholipase A_2 and other enzymes are activated, leading to prostacyclin generation. Both platelets and endothelial cells express COX-1, but endothelial cells metabolize its product to prostacyclin and platelets instead form thromboxane as the major prostaglandin metabolite. Inhibition of COX-1 by aspirin or non-steroidal anti-inflammatory agents thus blocks production of both the vasoconstricting, platelet-activating thromboxane, and the vasodilating, antiplatelet prostacyclin. As aspirin inhibits COX-1 irreversibly, and as platelets do not have the capacity to synthesize new proteins, once a platelet is exposed to aspirin, it is permanently paralyzed with respect to thromboxane synthesis. In contrast, endothelial cells have an intact RNA transcriptional and translational system and continue to synthesize new enzymes after a dose of aspirin is metabolized, so that a single low daily dose has very little effect on prostacyclin generation. Perhaps more importantly, endothelial cells also express a second COX isoform (COX-2) that can be induced rapidly in response to TNF and other agonists, increasing the output of prostacyclin after exposure to appropriate stimuli.

Endothelial cells also express vasoconstrictor systems, including angiotensin-converting enzyme, which generates the potent vasoconstrictor, angiotensin II, from its precursor, and endothelin-1, the most potent vasoconstricting substance described to date. Endothelin (ET)-1 is a 21 amino acid peptide formed by enzymatic cleavage of a larger precursor protein and is now known to be a member of a family of peptide hormones related to a family of vasoconstrictor snake venoms. It is secreted basolaterally towards the smooth muscle layer and acts to maintain systemic vascular resistance. Its production and release by endothelial cells is slowly increased in response to epinephrine, thrombin, shear stress and oxidized lipoproteins, suggesting a potential role in the endothelial cell injury response. The biological function of endothelin is mediated by G protein-coupled cellular receptors, ET_A and ET_B. ET_A is expressed predominantly on vascular smooth muscle and mediates the vasoconstrictor effects of ET-1. Binding of ET-1 to ET_B, which is expressed by endothelial cells, causes vasorelaxation in addition to ET-1 clearance.

SUMMARY

This chapter has briefly summarized current concepts of endothelial cell structure and function gained over more than two decades of intense experimentation. It is obvious that the vascular endothelium is a complex organ, precisely regulated to perform many crucial functions, most of which have direct relevance to rheumatic disease. Disordered endothelial function has been implicated in vasculitic syndromes, systemic sclerosis, thrombosis associated with lupus and antiphospholipid syndrome, and rheumatoid synovitis. Antiendothelial cell autoantibodies have been described in many autoimmune diseases, and may be pathogenic in some cases, such as Kawasaki's disease, systemic sclerosis and antiphospholipid syndrome[52]. New therapeutic approaches based on endothelial cell function are being developed for inflammatory disease, thrombotic disease, hypertension, atherosclerosis, cancer, myocardial infarction and the complications of diabetes, and antibody-targeted treatment aimed at specific endothelial antigens is being developed for thrombosis.

REFERENCES

1. Metchnikoff E. In: Lectures on the comparative pathology of inflammation, delivered at the Pasteur Institute in 1891 [translated from the French by Starling FA, Starling EH]. New York: Dover Publications; 1968: 135–137.
2. Jaffe EA, Nachman RL, Becker CG. Culture of human endothelial cells derived from umbilical veins: identification by morphological and immunologic criteria. J Clin Invest 1973; 52: 2745–2758.
3. Gimbrone MA Jr, Cotran RS, Folkman J. Human vascular endothelial cells in culture: growth and DNA synthesis. J Cell Biol 1974; 60: 673–682.
4. Dejana E. Endothelial adherens junctions: implications in the control of vascular permeability and angiogenesis. J Clin Invest 1996; 98: 1949–1953.
5. Bazzoni G, Martinez-Estrada OM, Orsenigo F et al. Interaction of junctional adhesion molecule with the tight junction components ZO-1, cingulin, and occludin. J Biol Chem 2000; 275: 20520–20526.
6. Aurrand-Lions M, Johnson-Leger C, Wong C et al. Heterogeneity of endothelial junctions is reflected by differential expression and specific subcellular localization of the three JAM family members. Blood 2001; 98: 3699–3707.
7. Weibel ER, Palade GE. New cytoplasmic components in arterial endothelial. J Cell Biol 1964; 23: 101–112.
8. Stevens T, Rosenberg R, Aird W et al. NHLBI workshop report: endothelial cell phenotypes in heart, lung, and blood diseases. Am J Physiol Cell Physiol 2001; 281: C1422–C1433.
9. Yancopoulos GD, Davis S, Gale NW et al. Vascular-specific growth factors and blood vessel formation. Nature 2000; 407: 242–248.
10. Carmeliet P, Verreira V, Breier G et al. Abnormal blood vessel development and lethality in embryos lacking a single VEGF allele. Nature 1996; 380: 435–439.
11. Shalaby F, Rossant J, Yamaguchi TP et al. Failure of blood-island formation and vasculogenesis in Flk-1-deficient mice. Nature 1995; 376: 62–66.
12. Fong GH, Rossant J, Gertsenstein M, Breitman ML. Role of the Flt-1 receptor tyrosine kinase in regulating the assembly of vascular endothelium. Nature 1995; 376: 66–70.
13. Partanen TA, Arola J, Saaristo A et al. VEGF-C and VEGF-D expression in neuroendocrine cells and their receptor, VEGFR-3, in fenestrated blood vessels in human tissues. FASEB J 2000; 14: 2087–2096.
14. Dumont DJ, Jussila L, Taipale J et al. Cardiovascular failure in mouse embryos deficient in VEGF receptor-3. Science 1998; 282: 946–949.
15. Suri C, Jones PF, Patan S et al. Requisite role of angiopoietin-1, a ligand for the TIE2 receptor, during embryonic angiogenesis. Cell 1996; 87: 1171–1180.
16. Thurston G, Rudge JS, Ioffe E et al. Angiopoietin-1 protects the adult vasculature against plasma leakage. Nat Med 2000; 6: 460–463.
17. Adams RH, Wilkinson GA, Weiss C et al. Roles of ephrin B ligands and EphB receptors in cardiovascular development: demarcation of arterial/venous domains, vascular morphogenesis, and sprouting angiogenesis. Genes Dev 1999; 13: 295–306.

18. Zhong TP, Childs S, Leu JP, Fishman MC. Gridlock signalling pathway fashions the first embryonic artery. Nature 2001; 414: 216–220.

19. Matsumoto K, Yoshitomi H, Rossant J, Zaret KS. Liver organogenesis promoted by endothelial cells prior to vascular function. Science 2001; 294: 559–563.

20. Lammert E, Cleaver O, Melton D. Induction of pancreatic differentiation by signals from blood vessels. Science 2001; 294: 564–567.

21. Folkman J, Cotran RS. Relation of vascular proliferation to tumor growth. Int Rev Exp Pathol 1976; 16: 207–248.

22. Brooks PC, Montgomery AM, Rosenfeld M et al. Integrin $\alpha_v\beta_3$ antagonists promote tumor regression by inducing apoptosis of angiogenic blood vessels. Cell 1994; 79: 1157–1164.

23. LeCouter J, Kowalski J, Foster J et al. Identification of an angiogenic mitogen selective for endocrine gland endothelium. Nature 2001; 412: 877–884.

24. O'Reilly MS, Boehm T, Shing Y et al. Endostatin: an endogenous inhibitor of angiogenesis and tumor growth. Cell 1997; 88: 277–285.

25. O'Reilly MS, Holmgren L, Shing Y et al. Angiostatin: a novel angiogenesis inhibitor that mediates the suppression of metastases by a Lewis lung carcinoma. Cell 1994; 79: 315–328.

26. Good DJ, Polverini PJ, Rastinejad F et al. A tumor suppressor-dependent inhibitor of angiogenesis is immunologically and functionally indistinguishable from a fragment of thrombospondin. Proc Natl Acad Sci USA 1990; 87: 6624–6628.

27. Moser TL, Stack MS, Asplin I et al. Angiostatin binds ATP synthase on the surface of human endothelial cells. Proc Natl Acad Sci USA 1999; 96: 2811–2816.

28. Bornstein P. The thrombospondins: structure and regulation of expression. FASEB J 1992; 6: 3290–3299.

29. Tolsma S, Volpert OV, Good DJ et al. Peptides derived from two separate domains of the matrix protein thrombospondin-1 have anti-angiogenic activity. J Cell Biol 1993; 122: 497–511.

30. Dawson DW, Pearce SFA, Zhong R et al. CD36 mediates the inhibitory effects of thrombospondin-1 on endothelial cells. J Cell Biol 1997; 138: 707–717.

31. Jimenez B, Volpert OV, Crawford SE et al. Signals leading to apoptosis-dependent inhibition of neovascularization by thrombospondin-1. Nat Med 2000; 6: 41–48.

32. Simantov R, Febbraio M, Crombie R et al. Histidine-rich glycoprotein inhibits the antiangiogenic effect of thrombospondin-1. J Clin Invest 2001; 107: 45–52.

33. Asahara T, Murohara T, Sullivan A et al. Isolation of putative progenitor endothelial cells for angiogenesis. Science 1997; 275: 964–967.

34. Shi Q, Rafii S, Wu MH et al. Evidence for circulating bone marrow-derived endothelial cells. Blood 1998; 92: 362–367.

35. Lyden D, Hattori K, Dias S et al. Impaired recruitment of bone-marrow-derived endothelial and hematopoietic precursor cells blocks tumor angiogenesis and growth. Nat Med 2001; 7: 1194–1201.

36. Lin Y, Weisdorf DJ, Solovey A, Hebbel RP. Origins of circulating endothelial cells and endothelial outgrowth from blood. J Clin Invest 2000; 105: 71–77.

37. Collins T, Palmer J, Whitley Z et al. A common theme in endothelial activation: insights from the structural analysis of the genes for E-selectin and VCAM-1. Trends Cell Biol 1993; 3: 92–97.

38. Ross R. The pathogenesis of atherosclerosis: a perspective for the 1990s. Nature 1993; 362: 801–809.

39. Springer TA. Traffic signals for lymphocytes recirculation and leukocyte emigration: the multistep paradigm. Cell 1994; 76: 301–314.

40. Kontgen F, Stewart CL, McIntyre KW et al. Characterization of E-selectin-deficient mice: demonstration of overlapping function of the endothelial selectins. Immunity 1994; 1: 709–720.

41. Mayadas TN, Johnson RC, Rayburn H et al. Leukocyte rolling and extravasation are severely compromised in P selectin-deficient mice. Cell 1993; 74: 541–554.

42. Worthylake RA, Burridge K. Leukocyte transendothelial migration: orchestrating the underlying molecular machinery. Curr Opin Cell Biol 2001; 13: 569–577.

43. Zernecke A, Weber KS, Erwig LP et al. Combinatorial model of chemokine involvement in glomerular monocyte recruitment: role of CXC chemokine receptor 2 in infiltration during nephrotoxic nephritis. J Immunol 2001; 166: 5755–5762.

44. Muller WA, Weigl SA, Deng X, Phillips DM. PECAM-1 is required for transendothelial migration of leukocytes. J Exp Med 1993; 178: 449–460.

45. Schenkel AR, Mamdouh Z, Chen X et al. CD99 plays a major role in the migration of monocytes through endothelial junctions. Nat Immunol 2002; 3: 143–150.

46. Campbell JJ, Hedrick J, Zlotnik A et al. Chemokines and the arrest of lymphocytes rolling under flow conditions. Science 1998; 279: 381–384.

47. Stamper HB Jr, Woodruff JJ. Lymphocyte homing into lymp nodes: in vitro demonstration of the selective affinity of recirculating lymphocytes for high-endothelial venuls. J Exp Med 1976; 144: 828–834.

48. Martin-Padura I, Lostaglio S, Schneemann M et al. Junctional adhesion molecule, a novel member of the immunoglobulin superfamily that distributes at intercellular junctions and modulates monocyte transmigration. J Cell Biol 1998; 142: 117–127.

49. Nachman RL, Silverstein RL. Hypercoagulable states. Ann Intern Med 1993; 119: 819–827.

50. Marcus AJ, Broekman MJ, Drosopoulos JH et al. The endothelial cell ecto-ADPase responsible for inhibition of platelet function is CD39. J Clin Invest 1997; 99: 1351–1360.

51. Solovey A, Gui L, Key NS, Hebbel RP. Tissue factor expression by endothelial cells in sickle cell anemia. J Clin Invest 1998; 101: 1899–1904.

52. Simantov R, LaSala JM, Lo SK et al. Activation of cultured vascular endothelium by antiphospholipid antibodies. J Clin Invest 1995; 96: 2221–2219.

53. Furchgott RF, Zawadzki JV. The obligatory role of endothelial cells in the relaxation of arterial smooth muscle by acetycholine. Nature 1980; 288: 373–376.

54. Ignarro LJ, Byrns RE, Buga GM, Wood KS. Endothelium-derived relaxing factor (EDRF) released from artery and vein appears to be nitric oxide (NO) or a closely related radical species. Fed Proc 1987; 46: 644.

55. Duckers HJ, Boehm M, True AL et al. Heme oxygenase-1 protects against vascular constriction and proliferation. Nat Med 2001; 7: 693–698.

56. Weksler BB, Marcus AJ, Jaffe EA. Synthesis of prostaglandin 12 (prostacyclin) by cultured human and bovine endothelial cells. Proc Natl Acad Sci USA 1977; 74: 3922–3928.

145 Immunopathogenesis of vasculitis

Wolfgang L Gross

Definition

- The vasculitides are clinicopathologic entities characterized by inflammation and damage to blood vessels
- Most vasculitic syndromes are mediated by immunopathogenic mechanisms ('immune vasculitides')
- Most 'immune vasculitides' are idiopathic (= 'primary' vasculitis) and systemic

Classification

- The 'immune vasculitides' are classified according to their hypersensitivity reaction types:
- Allergic angiitis (I), antineutrophil cytoplasmic antibody (ANCA)-associated vasculitis (AAV) (II), immune-complex vasculitis (ICV) (III), and vasculitis associated with T cell-mediated hypersensitivity (IV)

Immunological features

- Eosinophilia orchestrated by Th2 cells plus elevated IgE in the blood and tissues are characteristic of allergic angiitis and granulomatosis ('Churg–Strauss syndrome' CSS)
- No immune deposits are found *in situ* in AAV ('pauci-immune vasculitis')
- Immune complex deposits, by contrast, are the hallmark of ICV, which is frequently associated with low complement levels
- Inflammatory infiltration induced by Th1 cells distinguishes vasculitis associated with T cell-mediated hypersensitivity (granulomatous arteritis)

INTRODUCTION

The term 'vasculitis' encompasses a heterogeneous group of disorders characterized by inflammatory alteration of the blood vessel wall. Vasculitis can occur as a primary event (primary vasculitis) – e.g. in the ANCA-associated vasculitides (AAV) – or secondary to other established diseases (secondary vasculitis), e.g. in collagen vascular diseases. In both instances the underlying events are thought to be mediated by immunologic mechanisms (immune vasculitis). This inference is based on early clinical observations that serum sickness (induced by large injections of foreign antigen) may be associated with vasculitis, and has since been demonstrated in animal models of immune complex (IC)-mediated disease and in immunologic studies of patients with vasculitis. It is further supported by the response of vasculitis patients to various modes of immunosuppressive therapy. However, it should be in mind that other forms of immune vasculitides exist in which hypersensitivity reactions play little or no part, e.g. those of infectious origin or those closely associated with malignant lymphoma, radiation, transplantation etc. In this chapter we will concentrate on primary immune vasculitides.

Few clues have yet been found regarding the etiology of primary vasculitides: hepatitis B and C virus has been implicated as a causative agent in polyarteritis nodosa (PAN) and essential mixed cryoglobulinemia (EMC), respectively[1]. In AAV there is circumstantial evidence for the causative role of infection:[2] a seasonal variation in the incidence of proteinase 3 autoantibodies (PR3-ANCA) suggests that an infectious agent prevalent in spring or autumn might trigger Wegener's granulomatosis (WG); in addition, PR3-ANCA associated with subacute bacterial endocarditis vanishes after successful antibiotic treatment[3]. Necrotizing glomerulonephritis (GN) and other (ANCA-associated) small vessel vasculitides have been reported as adverse drug reactions to propylthiouracil or hydralazine.

A genetic predisposition is suggested by studies showing a link between small vessel vasculitis and HLA-DQw7, between WG and DR1, and between HLA-Bw52 and giant cell arteritis. More recently, a series of reports have suggested a pivotal role for α_1 antitrypsin (α_1AT) genetic polymorphism, at least in WG, where it appears to be a predictor of disease progression and mortality[4].

NOMENCLATURE

The classification favored by most experts is the one developed in 1992 at the Chapel Hill Conference (CHC). It is based on clinical and histopathological features, on the size of the predominant vessel involved, and on the presence of serological markers and other immune phenomena (e.g. ANCA) in the affected tissue (e.g. immune deposits), as demonstrated by immunohistochemistry[5].

The CHC classification represents a major step forward, as it includes the newer diagnostic tools, e.g. immunological tests for autoantibodies directed against neutrophil cytoplasmic antigens (ANCA), in particular cANCA (mostly induced by PR3-ANCA), which has a 95% specificity for WG, and immunohistochemical studies of tissue biopsies for detection of, for example, the predominantly IgA immune deposits found in the affected small vessels in Henoch–Schönlein purpura (HSP). The framework CHC definition is still based on the main type of vessels involved, as the clinical consequences of vascular inflammation depend on the size, site and number of blood vessels affected. Muscular arteries acquire focal lesions affecting part of the vessel wall and leading to aneurysm formation and possible rupture, or segmental lesions affecting the whole circumference and leading to occlusion and distal infarction. Small vessel vasculitis – arteriole, capillary, venule – if systemic, may be hazardous if sufficient numbers of adjacent vessels are involved, and can lead to necrotizing GN and/or to alveolar hemorrhage syndrome.

IMMUNE-MEDIATED VASCULITIS

Immune mechanisms of vasculitic diseases are traditionally classified using the terminology of Coombs and Gell for the various forms of hypersensitivity reactions (Table 145.1).

TABLE 145.1 IMMUNE PHENOMENA IN SYSTEMIC VASCULITIDES

Name of disease	Coombs & Gell type	Peripheral blood studies	Immunohistochemistry *in situ* (blood vessel)
Churg–Strauss syndrome	I	IgE↑↑, Eos↑↑, ANCA?*	Pauci-immune?* *and* immune deposits?* Eos↑↑
Wegener's granulomatosis	II	PR3-ANCA	Pauci-immune**
Microscopic polyangiitis	II	MPO-ANCA	Pauci-immune**
Kawasaki's disease	II	AECA	?
Polyarteritis nodosa	III	Hepatitis B virus, C'↓	Immune deposits
Henoch-Schönlein purpura	III	IgA↑	IgA dominant immune deposits
Essential cryoglobulinemic vasculitis	III	Hepatitis C virus, C'↓, Cryocrit	IgG/mRF immune deposits
Giant cell arteriitis	IV	CD3+/CD8+↓ activated CD68+↑	CD3+/CD4+↑ activated CD68+↑

* Heterogeneous findings in the literature: ANCA *and* immune deposits have been found.
I, immediate hypersensitivity; II, antibody-mediated hypersensitivity; III, immune complex-mediated hypersensitivity; IV, T-cell mediated hypersensitivity; C↓: complement consumption; Eos↑↑: hypereosinophilia; **pauci-immune: few or no immune deposits in the tissue; CD68, macrophage marker; mR, monoclonal rheumatoid factor; C', complement.
Predominant immune phenomena in systemic vasculitides delineate to the major hypersensitivity reaction type described by Coombs and Gell.

VASCULITIS STRONGLY ASSOCIATED WITH ATOPIC DISORDERS

Type I hypersensitivity reactions occur in atopic individuals. IgE is produced after contact with low levels of innocuous environmental allergens. Mast cells bind IgE via their Fc receptors. On re-exposure to the allergen the IgE becomes cross-linked, inducing degranulation and the release of mediators that produce allergic reactions. Typical examples of allergic reactions are rhinitis and bronchial asthma, which are characteristically found in Churg–Strauss syndrome (CSS, synonyms: allergic granulomatosis and vasculitis). Recently three phases were documented in CSS: a prodromal phase consisting of allergic disease (type I), a second phase characterized by the onset of hypereosinophilia, and a third phase consisting of a life-threatening systemic vasculitis (CSS). In full-blown disease the characteristic pathological findings are blood and tissue eosinophilia, extravascular granulomas and necrotizing vasculitis. Observation of CSS in cases of parasitic disease[6] suggests that immunological stimulation of IgE and eosinophils is involved in the pathogenesis. One key advance was the recognition that eosinophilia is orchestrated by the Th2 subclass of CD4+ T cells. Th2 cells produce interleukins (IL) 4, 5, 9 and 13 and are the immunopathological hallmark of allergic disease. More recently it was demonstrated that the cytokine production pattern of T-cell lines from CSS is that of Th2 cells[7]. In addition, impairment of CD95 ligand-mediated killing of lymphocytes and eosinophils in CSS was recognized as a result of variations in CD95 receptor isoform expression[8]. Drugs that block Th2-cell activity (e.g. interferon-α, IFN-α) have been successfully used in the treatment of CSS.

On the other hand, evidence for a direct role of immediate-type hypersensitivity in the pathogenesis of vasculitis is rather circumstantial and other mechanisms, including IC deposition of IgE-containing circulating IC, have to be considered[9]. Elevated serum levels of circulating IC containing IgE and deposition of various Ig classes and C3 have been observed in renal biopsies.

Urticarial vasculitis (UV), which comprises urticaria-like lesions with histopathological features of leukocytoclastic vasculitis, are divided into two subgroups, those with hypocomplementemia and those with normal complement (C) levels. Hypocomplementemic UV is associated with severe hypocomplementemia (especially of C_{1q}, but also of C4, C2 and C3) and is often accompanied by chronic obstructive pulmonary disease, IC nephritis and central nervous system complications (e.g. pseudotumor cerebri) and cryoglobulinemia. Causes include the binding of IgG antibodies to the collagen-like region of C_{1q}, the presence of a C4 null allele, or a deficiency of C1 inhibitor (either genetic or acquired). In addition, there is usually no response to antihistamines alone, indicating that UV is not caused by mast cell (histamine) mechanisms as is simple urticaria.

VASCULITIS STRONGLY ASSOCIATED WITH AUTOANTIBODIES

Type II hypersensitivity reactions are caused by IgG or IgM (auto-) antibodies directed against cell surface and extracellular matrix antigens. These antibodies can potentially lead to cytotoxic reactions (interactions with complement and a variety of effector cells), or to activation of the target cell (if the antibody binds to the cell receptor, or by engaging the FcγR molecules), or to the activation or inhibition of non-cellular circulating blood molecules such as enzymes, enzyme inhibitors etc.

Antineutrophil cytoplasmic antibodies – ANCA – comprise a heterogeneous group of autoantibodies. ANCA are routinely detected by the indirect immunofluorescence technique, which can distinguish at least three different patterns of fluorescence (Fig. 145.2). These patterns have been assigned the acronyms (cANCA) (classic granular cytoplasmic pattern), pANCA (perinuclear fluorescence pattern), and aANCA (atypical ANCA: more diffuse staining pattern).

cANCA are mostly induced by PR3 autoantibodies (PR3-ANCA), which are highly sensitive and specific for WG. Their sensitivity depends on the extent and activity of disease: it is about 50% for patients in the 'initial phase' of WG (symptoms confined exclusively to granulomatous lesions in the upper and/or lower respiratory tracts without generalized symptoms or clinical signs of vasculitis) and close to 100% for patients with active generalized WG. pANCA directed against myeloperoxidase (MPO), by contrast, is strongly associated with microscopic polyangiitis (MPA). Today the diagnosis of WG and MPA is based on (1) clinical features (often pulmonary renal vasculitis syndrome), (2) immunohistochemical studies ('pauci-immune' vasculitis, or GN with no or few immune deposits) and (3) serological markers (PR3-ANCA or MPO-ANCA, respectively). Biopsies – usually taken from kidneys or lung – typically show a necrotizing vasculitis of the small arteries, capillaries or small veins. In the kidney, necrotizing GN with crescent formation is the most prominent feature. Although it cannot be distinguished from other forms of crescentic GN (e.g. Goodpasture's syndrome or HSP) by light microscopy, immunohistochemistry shows no or only pauci-immune deposits in AAV (Figs 145.1 & 145.2) in contrast to Goodpasture's syndrome (linear IgG deposits along the glomerular basement membrane) and HSP (mesangial immunocomplexes of IgA) (Fig. 145.3)[10].

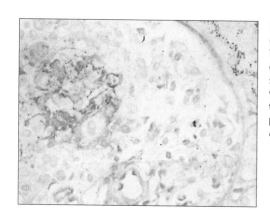

Fig. 145.1 Crescentic glomerulonephritis in Wegener's granulomatosis. There is segmental necrosis within the glomerular tuft (PAS × 1050). (With permission from Gross *et al.*[10])

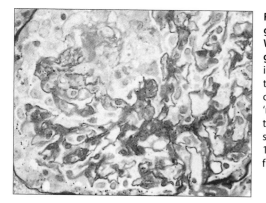

Fig. 145.2 Crescentic glomerulonephritis in Wegener's granulomatosis. Failing immune deposits within the non-necrotic capillaries (although with 'non-specific' IgG trapping in the necrotic segment) (APAP IgG1 × 1050). (With permission from Gross *et al.*[10])

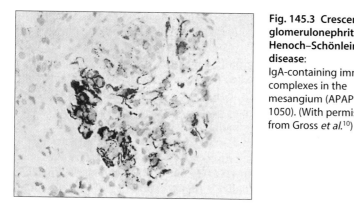

Fig. 145.3 Crescentic glomerulonephritis in Henoch–Schönlein disease: IgA-containing immune complexes in the mesangium (APAP IgA × 1050). (With permission from Gross *et al.*[10])

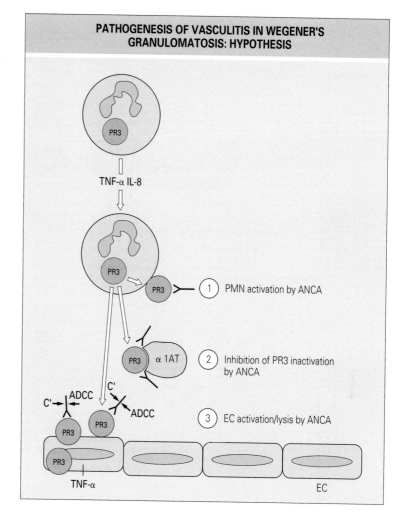

Fig. 145.4 Pathogenesis of vasculitis in Wegener's granulomatosis: hypothesis. In *vitro* models delineating the pathophysiological role of ANCA. 1. PR3- and MPO-ANCA are able to activate primed neutrophils to produce reactive oxygen species and to degranulate via binding PR3 and engaging FcIIR. 2. Products of activated neutrophils (PR3, MPO etc.) induce inflammation which might be potentiated by the interference of ANCA with their natural inhibitor(s), e.g. α_1-antitrypsin (α_1AT). 3. Activated endothelial cells (EC) express PR3 and the subsequent binding of ANCA will be followed by immunopathogenetic pathways ultimately leading to EC lysis. C', complement; ADCC, antibody-dependent cellular cytotoxicity.

PR3 and MPO are stored in the azurophilic granules of human polymorphonuclear leukocytes (PMN) and monocytes; these major ANCA antigens are exposed on the surface of activated or apoptotic PMN[11].

PR3 is a multifunctional protein. In addition to its proteolytic activity, it controls the growth and differentiation of hematopoietic cells, displays microbicidal activity and activates cytokines (transforming growth factor-β, TGF-β) etc.

MPO plays a crucial role in the generation of reactive oxygen species. PR3-ANCA and MPO-ANCA recognize regular conformational epitopes but not linear epitopes[12].

The mechanisms by which ANCA may be involved as a pathogenic factor in the inflammatory processes underlying necrotizing vasculitis are diverse. They include interaction with effector cells (e.g. PMN, monocytes, EC) and interference with the physiological function of the target antigens (e.g. PR3). Several *in vitro* models delineating the pathophysiological role of PR3 and PR3-ANCA interaction have been proposed and are summarized in Figure 145.4. *In vitro*, ANCA can activate primed PMN and can bind to PR3, thereby reducing its proteolytic activity while at the same time preventing complexation and complete inactivation by PR3-α_1-AT[13]. Stimulation of primed PMN and prevention of inactivation of PR3 by α_1-AT may contribute to excessive tissue damage and lead to necrosis and vasculitis[14].

As a unifying concept it was proposed that priming doses of proinflammatory cytokines induce surface expression of ANCA target antigens. Binding of ANCA to these antigens leads to full PMN activation and EC injury, with subsequent vascular damage (for details see Fig. 145.5).

ANCA can activate *primed* (TNF-α pretreated) PMN to produce reactive oxygen species, to release lysosomal enzymes and to cause EC injury[15]. Levels of proinflammatory cytokines and/or their receptors are elevated in the blood of patients with active systemic vasculitis. *In vitro* and *ex vivo* studies revealed that TNF-α and IL-8 act synergistically and induce a translocation of PR3 from the intragranular loci to the cell surface (Fig. 145.5) of PMN[16]. Apart from investigations demonstrating the upregulation of PR3 and the ability of ANCA-positive F(ab)$_2$ preparations to bind to the surface of PMN, to stimulate a respiratory burst, and to modulate PMN migration, recent studies have explored the pathway of full PMN activation in more detail: Murine monoclonal ANCA IgG (but not IgM) binds to PR3 and engages the FcγRIIa to activate the human PMN via a receptor-mediated signal transduction system[17]. Thus, ANCA-mediated neutrophil activation may occur mostly as a consequence of the engagement of FcγRIIa by the Fc region of ANCA and, at least in part, via F(ab)$_2$ binding.

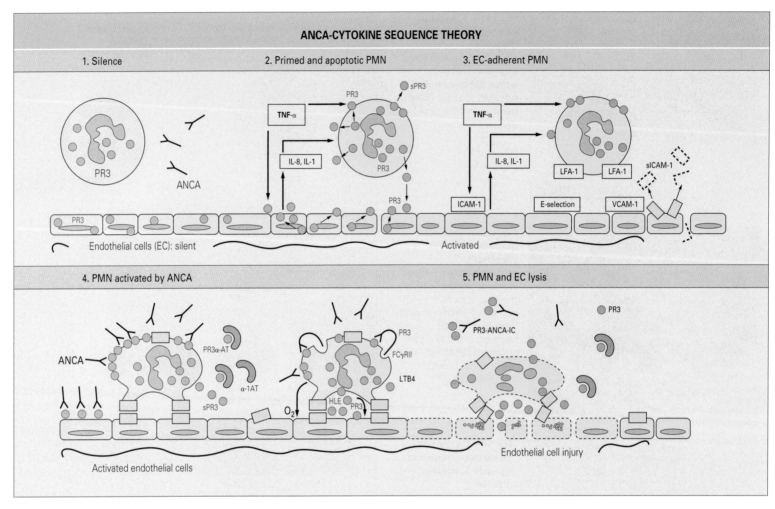

ANCA-CYTOKINE SEQUENCE THEORY

Fig. 145.5 ANCA-cytokine sequence theory. 1. Resting neutrophil-proteinase 3 (PR3) mostly sequestered in azurophil granules. 2. Primed (i.e. by cytokines) and apoptotic PMN. Intracytoplasmic PR3 is translocated to the cell surface and becomes accessible to ANCA: Expression of adhesion molecules. 3. Adhesion of PMN to endothelial cells. 4. Interaction between ANCA and PR3 leads to activation of neutrophils with degranulation, generation of oxygen radicals and endothelial cell injury. 5. This finally results in intravascular lysis of PMN and necrotizing vasculitis.

PR3 exposed on the surface of apoptotic PMN can be equally reached by PR3-ANCA, leading to the opsonization of these cells. It was found that opsonization of the apoptotic neutrophils by PR3-ANCA enhances their recognition and binding by scavenger macrophages, a process which ultimately leads to increased production of proinflammatory mediators[18]. There is an increased rate of apoptosis in WG[19]. Defective apoptosis regulation leads to a persistent presence of inflammatory cells, possibly causing damage to vessel walls[20].

PR3/MPO deposits can be observed in tissue from AAV. Cytokine-induced expression of adhesion molecules (e.g. LFA-1, ICAM-1, ELAM-1) allows close contact between PMN and EC, with consequent shielding from α_1-AT, elafin etc. (Fig. 145.5). Immunohistological studies of vasculitic tissue have demonstrated that both kinds of molecule are upregulated: in active (ANCA-associated) GN-resident cells, EC and infiltrating mononuclear cells express a variety of cytokines (IL-1/3, TNF-α, IL2, IFN-γ, PDGF and TGF-β), cytokine and growth-factor receptors (TNF-R, IL-1R type II, IL-2R, IFN-γR and PDGFβ-R) and the adhesion molecules described above[21]. In renal lesions (of WG) ICAM-1 is abundantly present and the intensity of expression correlates with the presence of glomerular crescents and the number of LFA-1 positive (CD11α) leukocytes; serum levels of soluble adhesion molecules (e.g. sICAM-1) correlate with disease activity and impairment of renal function. Recently, activated PMN and extracellular localization of lysosomal enzymes in renal biopsies were observed. The number of activated PMN in the biopsy correlated with the extent of renal function impairment. Similarly, PR3 and HLE could be found extracellularly in renal tissue.

Apart from PMN, monocytes play a key role in the development of vasculitis, and especially in granuloma formation associated with AAV. Activated monocytes are detected in renal[22] and nasal biopsies from WG[23]. Monocytes can be activated by ANCA enhanced by priming with TNF-α or by ANCA-opsonized PMN and produce chemokines (e.g. monocyte chemoattractant protein-1, MCP-1) or cytokines (e.g. TNF-α) *in vitro*. These mediators participate in the formation of granulomas. Furthermore, monocytes are potent regulators and producers of cytokines, especially when stimulated via endotoxin or Fcγ receptor cross-linking. In this context, recent findings have demonstrated that FcγR cross-linking produces IL-8 in monocytes[24]. These observations might indicate that ANCA binding to PR3 expressed on the surface of monocytes may result in FcγR cross-linking and subsequent IL-8 release. Importantly, IL-8 is released in response to IgG-PR3-ANCA only by TNF-α primed monocytes which express surface PR3, implying that the surface interaction of PR3 with IgG-PR3-ANCA is critical in this disease process.

ANIMAL MODELS FOR AAV

The *in vivo* role of ANCA has been investigated in animal models of systemic vasculitis. However, none of these constitutes an ideal model for human vasculitis. Necrotizing vasculitis can be studied in a number of experimental situations in animal models. Brown Norway rats treated with HgCl develop a number of autoantibodies, including MPO-ANCA, and tissue injury occurs in several organs, with necrotizing vasculitis being especially prevalent in the gut. Despite similarities with human systemic vasculitis, the lack of nephritis in particular is a major weakness of this model.

Five weeks after immunization of brown Norway rats with human MPO, the left kidney was perfused with various injurious agents, including hydrogen peroxidase plus MPO or other products of activated PMN. The rats developed necrotizing crescentic GN and vasculitis. Although MPO, IgG and C3 could be detected along the glomerular basement membrane 24 hours after perfusion, calling into question the 'pauci-immune' character of these renal lesions, the deposits were gone 4 and 10 days after perfusion[25]. In addition, other authors have consistently found immune deposits along the glomerular basement membrane in a similar model based on brown Norway and spontaneously hypertensive rats. Blank et al.[26] immunized BALB/c mice with human ANCA and these animals developed mouse ANCA with specificity both to PR3 and to MPO as well as to antiendothelial autoantibodies (AECA). Moreover, the mice immunized with human ANCA developed perivascular mononuclear cell infiltrates in the lungs that were suggestive of vasculitis. Recently, Jenne et al. identified and characterized murine PR3. Despite the marked similarities between human and murine PR3, PR3-ANCA from WG patients did not recognize the natively folded murine PR3, indicating that the endogenous murine homolog does not present any of the epitopes required to study human ANCA-induced vasculitis in mice. Consequently, it is unlikely that disease observed in mice after immunization with PR3-ANCA is caused by pathogenic antibodies against mouse PR3.[27]

The MRL/lpr strain of mice has been used as an experimental model for the study of systemic lupus erythematosus (SLE) and rheumatoid arthritis. These animals spontaneously develop lymphoproliferation, GN, arteritis and arthritis. Arteritic lesions in these mice are histologically characterized in the early stage of disease by fibrinoid necrosis and neutrophil influx, followed by a chronic infiltration of lymphocytes and granulomatous inflammation. Harper et al. recently demonstrated that 22% of female MRL-lpr mice develop MPO-ANCA. Anti-MPO monoclonal antibodies derived from these mice are polyreactive and react with double-stranded DNA. They bind conformational epitopes on human MPO, which is also expressed by activated human neutrophils. These mice develop a clinical syndrome of vasculitis and GN that is distinct from IC disease. The results suggest that a subset of MRL-lpr mice develops ANCA-related vasculitis rather than SLE and may be used as a spontaneous model for human MPA.[28]

The genetic background, trigger(s) and immune responses of AAV are currently under study.

HLA class II genes are associated with vasculitis and may influence the duration of the associated autoimmune response. Persistence of ANCA is associated with the DQw7 and DR4 haplotypes, whereas end-stage renal disease in WG patients is associated with HLA-DRB1*04.[34]

Several haplotypes on chromosome 6p appear to be strongly associated with PR3-ANCA+ vasculitis[29].

The occurrence of a prodromal 'flu-like' illness in WG and the seasonal variation in its onset further support the hypothesis that this disease is triggered by infection. The Coxsackie B3 virus and parvovirus-B19 infection are possible environmental triggers of ANCA and/or WG. Stegemann and colleagues[30] reported the association of chronic nasal carriage of Staphylococcus aureus with higher relapse rates in WG. Polyclonal B-cell activation, usually seen in chronic infectious diseases, does not appear to play a major role in the induction of ANCA, although V-domain antibody fragments specific for ANCA are known to be present in the normal B-cell repertoire[31]. Furthermore, cANCA have been documented in cases of Entamoeba histolytica infection[32] and in bacterial endocarditis[3].

A growing body of evidence indicates that autoantibody activity in autoimmune diseases might be regulated by idiotype–anti-idiotype

reactions. Observations on the clinical and in vitro effects of pooled human immunoglobulin and interactions with ANCA suggest that a defect in the regulation of the idiotypic network could be involved in the production of these autoantibodies. Furthermore, anti-idiotypic antibodies may prove to be important experimental and therapeutic agents. Our group recently generated a murine monoclonal antibody directed against a human monoclonal anti-PR3 antibody. This anti-idiotypic antibody (type Ab2β, designated 5/7) inhibits the anti-PR3 activity of cANCA in sera from WG patients[33]. These data indicate that idiotypic network regulation may play an important role in the interaction between ANCA and vascular endothelium.

Antibodies reacting with endothelial structures (anti-endothelial cell antibodies: AECA) have been detected in the sera of patients with vasculitis. The association of AECA with clinical manifestations, their ability to recognize EC surface antigen(s) and to display in vitro cytotoxic activity, at least in some sera, provide only indirect evidence that AECA have a role in the induction of vasculitis.

AECA have been observed in sera from many primary (Kawasaki's disease, WG, MPA etc.) and secondary vasculitides (vasculitis associated with rheumatoid arthritis, SLE etc.)[34]. Bound AECA may have the potential to mediate EC injury and lysis via complement fixation with formation of the membrane attack complexes, or via antibody-dependent cellular cytotoxicity, or by inducing more subtle changes in EC function (e.g. leading to enhanced intravascular thrombosis).

In summary, AECA have been demonstrated in several vasculitic disorders. However, because of the lack of assay standardization the incidence of AECA varies widely among investigators and the evidence that AECA may be of pathogenetic significance is only indirect.

VASCULITIS STRONGLY ASSOCIATED WITH IMMUNE COMPLEXES

Some primary vasculitides (e.g. PAN, HSP, essential cryoglobulinemic vasculitis, etc.) and the majority of secondary vasculitides (e.g. in collagen vascular diseases) have an immunopathogenesis that is typical of so-called immune complex vasculitis (ICV). ICV is characterized by the detection of circulating IC using a variety of techniques, the presence of circulating cryoglobulins, by the development of hypocomplementemia and – of major importance – by the immunohistochemical detection of immune deposits consisting of (auto)antibodies, (auto)antigens and complement components in situ, i.e. in the vessel wall (Table 145.2).

Immune complexes are non-covalently bonded molecular arrays of antigens and antibodies whose formation is determined by the law of

---

TABLE 145.2 MECHANISMS IN TYPE III HYPERSENSITIVITY ASSOCIATED WITH IMMUNE COMPLEX VASCULITIS

Immune complexes

1. Interact with the complement system to generate C3a and C5a (anaphylatoxins). C3a and C5a stimulate (a) the release of vasoactive amines (e.g. histamine), (b) the production of chemotactic factors (e.g. for PMN), (c) proinflammatory cytokines (e.g. IL-1, TNF-α), which induce the expression of adhesion molecules, e.g. P- and E-selectin in EC
2. Deposit in blood vessel walls following vasoactive-amine-induced EC retraction
3. Cause increased selectin expression in EC. The attracted PMN exocytose lysosomal enzymes in a frustrated attempt to engulf the deposited immune complex
4. Activate PMN in situ (through Fc binding) to cause inflammation via degranulation, generation of reactive oxygen species, etc.

EC, endothelial cells; PMN, neutrophils.

mass action. With increasing size their solubility decreases until they eventually precipitate. Small IC seldom lead to clinical symptoms, although they remain in the circulation longer than large IC, which tend to precipitate and are therefore more quickly eliminated. The size of IC is determined by the size and valency of the antigens, the class and valency of the antibodies, and the concentration of both (antigen excess, precipitation of gigantic arrays). A well-functioning immune system eradicates IC via complement (which reacts with IC to inhibit immune precipitation, solubilize immune aggregates and promote IC binding to erythrocyte complement receptor (CR) type 1 (CR1), CR (e.g. CR1) and the immunoglobulin Fc, and type 3 and 4 CR-bearing tissue macrophages in the liver and spleen. Inherited deficiencies of C′ proteins (C1, C4 or C2) are associated with impaired defense against microbial infection and with the occurrence of autoimmune disease (e.g. SLE) and vasculitis. A function of the classic pathway may be to remove the self-antigen–antibody complexes that are normally present. In the absence of this pathway these IC accumulate, activate the alternative pathway, become coated with C3d, and are then sufficiently immunogenic to break self-tolerance.

Small IC bind to the Fc-receptors on macrophages in the liver and spleen and are thereby eliminated. In the presence of antigen excess, e.g. in an infection, there is activation of the complement system which results in opsonization of IC by binding of C3b. This causes a reduction in size and a consequent increase in solubility of the IC, which bind via C3b to CR on erythrocytes, are transported rapidly to the liver and spleen, and there transferred to macrophages (RES) which degrade them. Disturbances in this clearing mechanism increase the probability of a vasculitis developing. SLE, for example, is associated with reduced CR1 receptors on erythrocytes, complement deficiencies, and a possible primary or acquired defect in RES function which predisposes to the development of disease by impairing IC clearance. Moreover, pathological IC processing in SLE may result in the persistence of potentially harmful complexes, further systemic and local complement activation, the development of a positive feedback loop stimulating further antigen release and autoantibody production, and finally in tissue damage[35].

ICV therefore represents a hypersensitivity reaction type III IC reaction according to Coombs and Gell (Table 145.2).

Circulating IC are generally recognized to be the cause of ICV. However, circulating IC by themselves do not always cause a vasculitis, and only tissue-bound IC have strong phlogistic potential. The occurrence of IC deposition (as opposed to physiological removal by the reticuloendothelial or mononuclear phagocyte system (RES)) depends on many factors, including flow characteristics within the blood vessel (e.g. turbulence at bifurcations, hydrostatic pressure), quantitative blood supply (e.g. renal glomeruli (=20% cardiac output), open fenestrated endothelium), and the permeability of vascular endothelium (e.g. 'new' antigens induced on the surface, or the appearance of Fc receptors during HSV infection, for example). In addition, the characteristics of IC, such as size, charge etc. (large-latticed IC, cationized antibodies or antigens binding to the glomerular basement membrane with fixed negative charges), facilitate their deposition.

Additional vasoactive factors are required to initiate IC-mediated vessel wall damage, including mast-cell derived histamine (vascular permeabilities), complement-derived anaphylatoxin (C3a, C5a), and mechanical factors such as hydrostatic pressure on the vessel wall and shearing forces (Table 145.2). Whether or not this initial damage results in a clinically manifest vasculitis depends not only on immunological and physicochemical factors, but equally on the effectiveness of repair mechanisms within the vessel wall.

More recently, hepatitis C virus (HCV) was shown to be strongly associated with essential mixed cyroglobulinemia (EMC)[36]. The name cryoglobulin reflects the tendency of these immunoglobulins to precipitate at low temperatures. Cryoglobulinemia has been categorized according to the clonal composition of the Ig into type I (monoclonal only), type II (mixed monoclonal and polyclonal) and type III (polyclonal only). HCV (both antibody and RNA) may be demonstrated in type II cryoprecipitates at a 1000-fold concentration over serum. Chronic HCV infection of lymphocytes triggers a polyclonal B-lymphocyte proliferation, giving rise to a so-called 'benign' lymphoproliferative disease. Different routes of cellular uptake of the HCV have been suggested, such as binding of the HCV envelope protein E2 to CD81 expressed hepatocytes and B cells, or access to the cell via low-density lipoprotein receptor (LDLR)-mediated endocytosis of HCV–very low density lipoprotein (VLDL) complexes. With longer duration of the disease an oligoclonal and – less often – a monoclonal B-lymphocyte proliferation may evolve, sometimes with transition into a malignant lymphoma. Monoclonal IgMk CD5$^+$ B lymphocytes have been detected in liver lymphoid proliferations of patients with type II MC. In contrast, peripheral blood B lymphocytes lack CD5 surface antigen in MC. Various autoantibodies can be detected in HCV-associated CV as a consequence of the polyclonal B-lymphocyte stimulation. The detection of cross-reacting idiotypes on monoclonal IgMk rheumatoid factors, e.g. the WA idiotype, seems to be the consequence of an antigen-independent proliferation of autoreactive B-cell clones. The typical clinical aspects of CV, such as palpable purpura due to cutaneous vasculitis, arthralgia/arthritis, weakness, polyneuropathy, 'cryoglobulinemic' glomerulonephritis and other sequelae, are usually confined to type II MC. Cutaneous vasculitis results from the deposition of complexes of HCV, IgM, RF and IgG. In contrast, demonstration of HCV-related proteins in glomeruli remained difficult, and only recently c22 antigen was found in glomerular lesions[37]. Animal models demonstrated that cutaneous vasculitis developed after the formation of monoclonal RF-containing immune complexes, whereas glomerular lesions were induced by monoclonal RF in the absence of such immune complexes. Complement consumption in the presence of MC shows a typical pattern, with generally low complement C4 and CH50. C3 levels fluctuate with disease activity. Moreover, sCD30 ('Th2 marker') levels correlate with disease activity[38].

Although the etiology of Henoch–Schönlein purpura (HSP) remains unknown, it is clear that IgA plays an important role in its immunopathogenesis. HSP is associated with increased serum IgA (predominant subclass IgA$_1$) concentrations, circulating IC containing IgA, and IgA-rheumatoid factor (IgA-RF).

More recently it has been suggested that abnormal glycosylation of IgA may contribute to glomerular IgA deposition and subsequent damage in HSP. Altered IgA$_1$ O-glycosylation has been reported in HSP with renal involvement.

HSP is characterized by the presence of IgA and fibrinogen in combination with the relative absence of other immunoreactants, a constellation that distinguishes HSP from other forms of IC-mediated vasculitis, which typically have vascular deposits of IgG, IgM and early complement components. This and the finding of C3, properdin and factor B in renal and dermal vascular lesions, suggest that C′ is activated by the alternate pathway. Routine assessment of C′ activation in the blood, i.e. C3, C4 and CH50 assays, usually discloses no abnormality. However, the plasma anaphylatoxins C3a and C4a show a significant correlation with plasma creatinine, and the cytolytic C5b-9 complex (membrane attack complex) was recently colocalized with IgA and C3 in the capillary walls and mesangium of glomeruli of an HSP patient[39].

The immunopathogenetic mechanisms leading to vascular injury in polyarteritis nodosa (PAN) are incompletely understood and probably heterogeneous. PAN is commonly associated with hepatitis B virus infection. Furthermore, an association with other viral infections (e.g. HIV) and with hairy cell leukemia has been described. PAN may also complicate the outcome of several collagen vascular diseases (e.g. Sjögren's syndrome), which calls into question its classification as a 'primary' vasculitis and the commonly held notion that it is an IC-mediated disease. IC deposition with C′ activation and subsequent neutrophil chemotaxis has long been considered a crucial mechanism leading to vascular injury. More recently the phenotype of infiltrating cells in classic PAN lesions showed them to be mainly macrophages and T (CD4⁺ subset) cells. Granulocytes were more abundant in heavily infiltrated vessels than in those with fibrinoid necrosis. In addition to IC-mediated lesions, therefore, an additional T-cell mediated immune mechanism could play a role in the development and perpetuation of PAN lesions[40].

The consequence of C′ activation is the release of anaphylatoxins and chemotactic factors, which induce various cells (basophils, platelets, mast cells) to secrete vasoactive substances (histamine, serotonin, platelet activation factors, PAF) and induce circulating leukocytes and vascular EC to express adhesion molecules (e.g. LFA-1 and ELAM-1). Furthermore, the binding of C3bi to EC allows adhesion of neutrophils via CR3. The intact vessel wall does not normally allow IC precipitation unless the antigen has a particular affinity for the endothelium. An example of this are the DNA anti-ds-DNA antibodies, which have a predilection for the EC membrane. A further factor is a disturbance in permeability which allows the IC to penetrate into the intracellular space. The most important mediators in addition to histamine and serotonin are the proinflammatory cytokine IL-1, PAF and arachidonic acid metabolites.

Deposition of IC in the interstitium activates the mechanisms leading to their elimination. Activated neutrophils adhering to the complement-laden EC penetrate into the vessel wall (diapedesis), phagocytose the precipitates by the Fc and CR, and release lysosomal enzymes (e.g. elastase, collagenase etc.), oxygen radicals and arachidonic acid metabolites. These mediators directly damage the endothelium and result in the generation of other toxic mediators, e.g. eicosanoids such as LTB-4, from arachidonic acid in the cell membrane, the production of inflammatory cytokines (IL-1, TNF-α etc.) from infiltrating lymphocytes, as well as the activation of kallikrein and the components of the extrinsic arm of the coagulation cascade. Many of these factors are chemotactic for leuko-

cytes, thereby promoting further migration of leukocytes and the perpetuation of this process.

If clearing mechanisms predominate, the result is *restitutio ad integrum*. In the presence of perpetuating factors the persistent production of IC in chronic infections (e.g. hepatitis B or C antigenemia) or in autoimmune diseases (e.g. ds-DNA in SLE) results in progressive tissue damage. In animal experiments this IC-mediated damage is limited by depletion of either complement or leukocytes, despite the presence of IC.

VASCULITIS STRONGLY ASSOCIATED WITH T-CELL MEDIATED HYPERSENSITIVITY

The Th1/Th2 model

The discovery of T-helper cell subsets (Th1 and Th2) that differ in their cytokine secretion patterns and effector functions has provided a model for understanding how cytokines regulate pathologic immune and inflammatory responses.

Figure 145.6 summarizes the cell types and cytokines involved in the polarization of T cells and the major differences between Th1 and Th2 cells in terms of cytokine profile and function.

Wegener's granulomatosis

Wegener's granulomatosis (WG) begins with granulomatous changes: the primary granulomas form and develop in connective tissue, but without vascular involvement. Friedrich Wegener wrote: 'The vasculitis that accompanies the granulomatous disease is a secondary feature that represents a later stage'. Thus, it should be possible to obtain insights into the early immunopathogenic mechanisms in WG from studies concentrating on cells in 'pathergic granuloma' or its surroundings (e.g. bronchoalveolar lavage: BAL).

Studies of intercellular interactions that lead to the formation and maintenance of granulomas have now focused on the role of T cells.

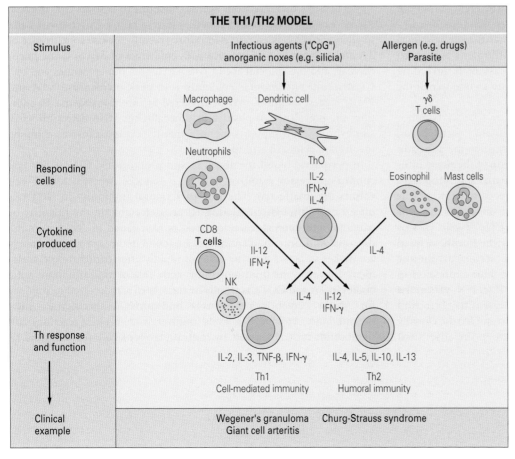

THE TH1/TH2 MODEL

Fig. 145.6 The Th1/Th2 model. This figure summarizes the cell types and cytokines involved in polarization of T cells and the major differences between Th1 and Th2 cells in terms of cytokine profile and function. (Modified with permission from Csernok & Gross[42].)

Because the cellular composition of Wegener's granuloma is diverse (neutrophilic granulocytes, macrophages, epithelioid cells and giant cells, together with lymphocytes and eosinophilic granulocytes), the lesion could equally be induced by Th1 or Th2 cytokines.

The autoimmune phenomena (including ANCA) seen in many patients with WG led to the working hypothesis that generalized WG could be a Th2-associated condition. On the other hand, studies on T cells from peripheral blood have clearly shown that these cells exhibit increased secretion of IFN-γ, thus demonstrating a predominant Th1 response pattern[41].

Recently, the profile of cytokine secretion by T cells was shown to be derived from granulomatous tissue (nasal mucosal biopsy specimens) or from an area close to the site of granulomatous inflammation (BAL). These results demonstrate the existence of a clear-cut Th1 polarization in the granulomatous inflammation seen in WG. Furthermore, immuno-histochemical studies on the presence of CD26 (operational Th1 marker) and CD30 (Th2 marker) indicate that in nasal tissues CD4$^+$/CD26$^+$ T cells may be the main contributors to the polarized Th1 response in the initial phase of WG[23]. The local secretion of high levels of IFN-γ may represent an important amplification loop leading to a tissue-destructive inflammatory response in WG patients. IFN-γ activates local macrophages and granulocytes to produce proinflammatory cytokines and toxic metabolites, which cause damage to the tissue and maintain the inflammation.

Giant cell arteritis

Inflammation of the large arteries is a characteristic feature of granulo-matous giant cell arteritides: giant cell (temporal) arteritis (GCTA) and Takayasu arteritis (TA). The two forms share many clinical and histopathological features but can be differentiated from each other using the definition of the CHC. An increased incidence in women, familial clustering and differences in geographic distribution all support a genetic model for TA. An association with an HLA class I gene, HLA-Bw52, was described in Japanese patients and may be associated with clinically more severe aortic arch syndrome and aortic regurgitation; in North American patients no positive association has been recognized.

Compelling evidence implicates the arterial wall as the site of a local cell-mediated immune response. The cellular infiltrate is composed of T cells, histiocytes and epithelioid cells, occasionally including giant cells and rarely including B cells. It is therefore an example of the hypersensitivity reaction type IV.

A large proportion of the lymphocytes *in situ* are CD4$^+$ T lymphocytes. Plasma cells and neutrophils are scarce or absent. Macrophages, epithelioid cells and giant cells are present and express the adhesion molecules LFA-1, LFA-3 and ICAM-1. Only a fraction of the tissue infiltrating CD4$^+$ T cells but the majority of the accompanying macrophages express HLA-DR antigens and interleukin-2 receptors (IL-2R) as markers of cell activation. Sequencing studies of the T-cell receptor showed that a limited number of idiotypes of the CD4$^+$ T cells (2–5%) undergo clonal expansion and are specifically enriched in the arterial wall compared with the circulating population (localized immune response). RT-PCR technology used to probe cytokine expression in GCTA could show that the T-cell cytokine profile (IL-2, IFN-γ) is of the Th1 type; typically Th1 cells are involved in the hypersensitivity reaction type IV. In GCTA these IFN-γ producing T cells account for the clonally expanded tissue-infiltrating cells; they accumulate in the adventitial

layer, express IL-2, and actively divide. IFN-γ is one of the most potent activators of macrophages. It is thus very likely that the macrophages, which regularly produce proinflammatory cytokines (IL-1β, IL-6 etc.) and TGF-β, are activated by these T cells. Activation of macrophages may precede granuloma formation (Table 145.3). The causative antigen (autoantigen?) is presumed to reside in the internal elastic lamina, as the inflammation seems to be concentrated at this point. Whether or not (abnormal) elastin is the autoantigen remains unclear. Cellular infiltrates in TA tend to be localized in the adventitia and outer part of the media, with marked infiltration of the vasa vasorum. Recent histo-pathologic studies observed perforin-secreting cells in the infiltrate and deposition of perforin on vascular cells and implied that cytotoxic cells, particularly heat-shock protein-recognizing γδ T cells, are responsible for tissue destruction (Table 145.3).

It is possible that infectious agents constitute disease-specific triggers. An increased prevalence of antibodies to respiratory syncytial virus and to adenovirus has been reported. More recently, a close concurrence of TA and polymyalgia rheumatica with epidemics of *Mycoplasma pneumoniae,* and the coincidence of two parvovirus B19 epidemics and one *Clostridium pneumoniae* epidemic with peak incidences of TA and PMR, suggest that both may be triggered by infectious agents. In addition, the prevalence of positive cytomegalovirus DNA detection by *in situ* hybridization supports the idea that the cytomegalovirus could be involved in giant cell arteritis.

In peripheral blood the absolute and proportional CD3$^+$/CD8$^+$ cell count (suppressor cytotoxic T cells) is reduced, whereas total T-cell counts are unaffected. The role of humoral immunity in GCTA is uncertain. Although circulating IC are detectable in the majority of patients, immunohistochemical studies have failed to detect immune deposits. Anticardiolipin antibodies are found in the sera and their levels are higher in active arteritis and fall rapidly after corticosteroid treatment; however, the immunopathogenetic role of anticardiolipin antibodies in TA and GCTA is wholly unclear. Well standardized techniques for ANCA detection only rarely find pANCA specificities. Pro-inflammatory cytokine IL-6 levels (inducer of acute-phase reactions) are significantly raised in serum; by contrast, levels of TNF-α are normal. [42]

TABLE 145.3 PATHOMECHANISMS IN GIANT CELL ARTERITIS

Molecular finding	Suggested pathomechanism
Genetic association with HLA-DRB1 alleles (binding site of the HLA-DR molecule)	Selective binding and presentation of antigens
Activation of circulating monocytes–macrophages resulting in cytokine production	Monocyte–macrophage-activating agent residing outside vasculitic infiltrates
Functional heterogeneity of tissue-infiltrating macrophages	Involvement of distinct macrophage population or distinct functional pathways
In situ clonal expansion of selected CD4 T lymphocytes in inflammatory infiltrates	*In situ* recognition of disease-relevant antigen
Defined profile of *in situ* synthesis of T-cell derived and macrophage-derived cytokine mRNA	*In situ* immune response involving macrophages as antigen-presenting cells and Th1 cells as responding T cells

(With permission from Weyand and Goronzy[43].)

REFERENCES

1. Sundy JS, Haynes BF. Pathogenic mechanisms of vessel damage in vasculitis syndromes. Rheum Dis Clin North Am 1995; 21: 861–881.
2. Jennings JG, Chang L, Savige JA. Anti-proteinase 3 antibodies, their characterization and disease associations. Clin Exp Immunol 1994; 95: 251–256.
3. Choi HK, Lamprecht P, Niles JL et al. Subacute bacterial endocarditis with positive cytoplasmic antineutrophil cytoplasmic antibodies and anti-proteinase 3 antibodies. Arthritis Rheum 2000; 43: 226–231.
4. Elzouki AN, Segelmark M, Wieslander J, Eriksson S. Strong link between the alpha1-antitrypsin PiZ allele and Wegener's granulomatosis. J Intern Med 1994; 236: 543–548.
5. Jennette JC, Falk RJ, Andrassy K et al. Nomenclature of systemic vasculitides. Proposal of an International Consensus Conference. Arthritis Rheum 1994; 37: 187–192.
6. Chauhan A, Scott DGI, Neuberger J et al. Churg–Strauss vasculitis and ascaris infection. Ann Rheum Dis 1990; 49: 320–322.
7. Kiene M, Csernok E, Müller A et al. Elevated interleukin-4 and interleukin-13 production by T cell lines from patients with Churg–Strauss syndrome. Arthritis Rheum 2001; 44: 469–473.
8. Müschen M, Warskulat U, Perniok A et al. Involvement of soluble CD95 in Churg–Strauss syndrome. Am J Pathol 1999; 155: 915–925.
9. Manger BJ, Krapf FE, Gramatzki M et al. IgE-containing circulating immune complexes in Churg–Strauss vasculitis. Scand J Immunol 1985; 21: 369–373.
10. Gross WL, Csernok E, Helmchen U. Antineutrophil cytoplasmic autoantibodies, autoantigens, and systemic vasculitis. APMIS 1995; 103: 81–97.
11. Gilligan HM, Bredy B, Brady HR et al. Antineutrophil cytoplasmic autoantibodies interact with primary granule constituents on the surface of apoptotic neutrophils in the absence of neutrophil priming. J Exp Med 1996; 184: 2231–2241.
12. Chang L, Binos S, Savige J. Epitope mapping of anti-proteinase 3 and anti-myeloperoxidase antibodies. Clin Exp Immunol 1995; 102: 112–119.
13. Dolman KM, Stegemann CA, van de Wiel BA et al. Relevance of classic anti-neutrophil cytoplasmic autoantibody (c-ANCA)-mediated inhibition of proteinase 3-alpha-1-antitrypsin complexation to disease activity in Wegener's granulomatosis. Clin Exp Immunol 1993; 93: 405–410.
14. Gross WL, Csernok E. Antineutrophil cytoplasmic autoantibodies (ANCA). Immuno-diagnostic and pathophysiological aspects. Curr Opin Rheumatol 1995; 7: 11–19.
15. Pall AA, Savage COS. Mechanism of endothelial and injury in vasculitis. Springer Semin Immunpathol 1994; 16: 23–37.
16. Csernok E, Ernst M, Schmitt W et al. Activated neutrophils express proteinase 3 on their plasma membrane in vitro and in vivo. Clin Exp Immunol 1994; 95: 244–250.
17. Porges AJ, Redecha PB, Kimberly WT et al. Antineutrophil cytoplasmic antibodies engage and activate human neutrophils via FcγRIIa. J Immunol 1994; 153: 1271–1280.
18. Moosig F, Csernok E, Kumanovics G, Gross WL. Opsonization of apoptotic neutrophils by anti-neutrophil-cytoplasmic antibodies (ANCA) leads to enhanced uptake by macrophages and increased release of TNFa. Clin Exp Immunol 2000; 122: 499–503.
19. Lorenz HM, Hieronymus T, Grunke M et al. Differential role for IL-2 and IL-15 in the inhibition of apoptosis in short-term activated human lymphocytes. Scand J Immunol 1997; 45: 660–669.
20. Tanigushi Y, Ito MR, Mori S et al. Role of macrophages in the development of arteritis in MRL strains of mice with a deficit in Fas-mediated apoptosis. Clin Exp Immunol 1996; 106: 26–34.
21. Waldherr R, Noronha IL, Niemir Z et al. Expression of cytokines and growth factors in human glomerulonephritides. Pediatr Nephrol 1993; 7: 471–478.
22. Rastaldi MP, Ferrario F, Crippa A et al. Glomerular monocyte–macrophage features in ANCA-positive renal vasculitis and cryoglobulinemic nephritis. J Am Soc Nephrol 2000; 11: 2036–2043.
23. Müller A, Trabandt A, Gloeckner K et al. Localized Wegener's granulomatosis: predominance of CD26 and IFN-γ expression. J Pathol 2000; 192: 113–120.
24. Ralston DR, Marsh CB, Lowe MP, Wewers MD. Antineutrophil cytoplasmic antibodies induce monocyte IL-8 release. J Clin Invest 1997; 100: 1416–1426.
25. Brouwer E, Huitema MG, Klok PA et al. Antimyeloperoxidase-associated proliferative glomerulonephritis: An animal model. J Exp Med 1993; 177: 905–914.
26. Blank M, Tomer Y, Stein M et al. Immunization with anti-neutrophil cytoplasmic antibody (ANCA) induces the production of mouse ANCA and perivascular lymphocyte infiltration. Clin Exp Immunol 1995; 102: 120–130.
27. Jenne DE, Fröhlich L, Hummel AM, Specks U. Cloning and functional expression of the murine homologue of proteinase 3: implications for the design of murine models of vasculitis. FEBS Lett 1997; 408: 187–190.
28. Harper JM, Thiru S, Lockwood CM, Cooke A. Myeloperoxidase autoantibodies distinguish vasculitis mediated by anti-neutrophil cytoplasm antibodies from immune complex disease in MRL/Mp-lpr/lpr mice: a spontaneous model for miscroscopic angiitis. Eur J Immunol 1998; 28: 2217–2226.
29. Gencik M, Meller S, Borgmann S, Fricke H. Proteinase 3 gene polymorphisms and Wegener's granulomatosis. Kidney Int 2000; 58: 2473–2477.
30. Stegemann C, Cohen Tervaert JW, Sluiter WJ et al. Association of chronic nasal carriage of Staphylococcus aureus and higher relapse rates in Wegener's granulomatosis. Ann Intern Med 1994; 120: 12–17.
31. Finnern R, Bye JM, Dolman KM et al. Molecular characteristics of anti-self antibody fragments against neutrophil cytoplasmic antigens from human V gene phage display libraries. Clin Exp Immunol 1995; 102: 566–574.
32. Pudifin D, Duursma J, Gathiram V, Jackson T. Invasive amoebiasis is associated with the development of anti-neutrophil cytoplasmic antibody. Clin Exp Immunol 1994; 97: 48–51.
33. Strunz HP, Csernok E, Gross WL. Incidence and disease associations of a PR3-ANCA idiotype (5/7Id) whose anti-idiotype inhibits PR3-ANCA activity. Arthritis Rheum 1997; 40, 135–142.
34. Meroni PL, D'Cruz D, Khamashta M et al. Anti-endothelial cells antibodies: only for scientists or for clinicians too? Clin Exp Immunol 1996; 104: 199–202.
35. Davies KA. Complement, immune complexes and systemic lupus erythematosus. Br J Rheumatol 1996; 35: 5–23.
36. Wong VS, Egner W, Elsey T et al. Incidence, character and clinical relevance of mixed cryoglobulinaemia in patients with chronic hepatitis C virus infection. Clin Exp Immunol 1996; 104: 25–31.
37. Pasero GP, Bombardieri S, Ferri C. From internal medicine to rheumatology and back: the example of mixed cryoglobulinemia. Clin Exp Rheumatol 1995; 13: 1–5.
38. Lamprecht P, Moosig F, Gause A et al. Immunological and clinical follow-up of hepatitis C virus associated cryoglobulinemic vasculitis. Ann Intern Med 2001; 60: 385–390.
39. Szer IS. Henoch–Schönlein purpura. Curr Opin Rheumatol 1994; 6: 25–31.
40. Cid M-C, Grau JM, Casademont J et al. Immunohistochemical characterization of inflammatory cells and immunologic activation markers in muscle and nerve biopsy specimens from patients with systemic polyarteritis nodosa. Arthritis Rheum 1994; 37: 1055–1061.
41. Csernok E, Gross WL Cytokines and vascular inflammation. In: Hoffman GS, Weyand C, eds. Inflammatory diseases of blood vessels. New York: Marcel Dekker; 2001.
42. Csernok E, Trabandt A, Müller A et al. Cytokine profiles in Wegener's granulomatosis: predominance of type 1 (Th1) in the granulomatous inflammation. Arthritis Rheum 1999; 42: 742–750.
43. Weyand CM, Goronzy JJ. Molecular approaches toward pathologic mechanisms in giant cell arteritis and Takayasu's arteritis. Curr Opin Rheumatol 1995; 7: 30–36.

146 Polyarteritis nodosa and microscopic polyangiitis

Oscar Soto and Doyt L Conn

Definitions

Polyarteritis nodosa

- Polyarteritis nodosa is primarily a vasculitis of medium-sized arteries, causing inflammation of the skin, kidney, peripheral nerves, muscle and gastrointestinal tract

Microscopic polyangiitis

- Microscopic polyangiitis is a systemic necrotizing vasculitis with few or no immune deposits, characterized by involvement of the small vessels (capillaries, venules or arterioles)
- It was initially recognized as a subset of polyarteritis nodosa, with rapid progressive glomerulonephritis and often causing lung hemorrhage

Clinical features

Polyarteritis nodosa

- Constitutional symptoms including, fever, anorexia and weight loss
- Myalgia, arthralgia and arthritis
- Skin involvement, with infarctions and livedo reticularis
- Peripheral neuropathy
- Renal involvement, with mild proteinuria, renal insufficiency and hypertension
- Gut involvement, with abdominal pain, infarction, hemorrhage and liver function abnormalities

Microscopic polyangiitis

- Often, an acute presentation of renal disease, leading to rapid progressive glomerulonephritis
- Pulmonary hemorrhage can be seen
- Lung involvement can accompany renal disease resulting in a pulmonary-renal syndrome
- Skin lesions, most commonly palpable purpura
- Constitutional symptoms, and fever may be present before more definite symptoms appear.

POLYARTERITIS NODOSA

History

Polyarteritis, also called periarteritis and polyarteritis nodosa, is a disease of small and medium-sized arteries. Probably the first description of the disease was in 1842, when Karl von Rokitanski tried to described aneurysm formation of vessels unrelated to trauma[1]. The classic pathologic description of the disease by Kussmaul and Maier was made in 1866, when they reported a case of necrotizing arteritis and called it 'periarteritis nodosa'[2]. Their patient had widespread necrotizing inflammation of small and medium-sized arteries, and in some areas there were focal inflammatory exudations, which gave rise to palpable nodules along the course of the arteries.

Epidemiology

Polyarteritis is an uncommon disease. Estimates of the annual incidence rate for polyarteritis nodosa-type systemic vasculitis in a general population range from 9.0/1 000 000 in Olmsted County, Minnesota, to 77/1 000 000 in a hepatitis B-endemic Alaskan Eskimo population[3], to 19.8/1 000 000 in the UK[4]. These estimates included microscopic polyangiitis, classic polyarteritis nodosa, connective tissue disease-associated polyarteritis and Churg–Strauss syndrome. It is possible that the incidence of polyarteritis has changed as a result of increased diagnostic awareness after the introduction of antineutrophil cytoplasmic autoantibody (ANCA) tests[5]. Watts et al.[6] documented an increased incidence in all systemic vasculitides in a large primary-care population, comparing a 6-year period from 1988 to 1994 against previously determined incidence rates. They reported the mean annual incidence of microscopic polyangiitis to be 2.4 per million (range 0.9–5.3 per million), that of Churg–Strauss syndrome to be 2.4 per million (range 0.9–5.3 per million) and that of systemic rheumatoid vasculitis (secondary polyarteritis) to be 12.5 per million (range 8.5–17.7 per million). Classic polyarteritis nodosa, however, was much less common than previously reported, because of the current more strict definition. None of the 180 patients with systemic vasculitis identified between 1988 and 1994 met current criteria for classic polyarteritis nodosa. This increase in vasculitis generally reflects greater physician awareness and changes in the definition of vasculitis. Classic polyarteritis nodosa affects men more commonly. Microscopic polyangiitis is more common in males, with a reported sex ratio ranging from 1 to 1.8:1[7]. Polyarteritis is observed in children and the elderly, but the average age at onset is about 50 years, ranging from the mid-40s to the mid-60s. It is observed in all racial groups.

Classification

A subcommittee of the American College of Rheumatology (ACR) developed criteria for the classification of seven forms of vasculitis, including polyarteritis, by analysis of data from 1000 cases collected from 48 centers[8]. The gold standard for a patient with one of the forms of vasculitis was the opinion of the committee member. The criteria for each were derived by comparing findings in patients with one form of vasculitis with those from other forms of vasculitis. The criteria selected in these studies were those that both identify each vasculitis and separate it from others (Table 146.1). As a result, the full spectrum of manifestations is not included in all instances, and important but less distinctive clinical features are not recognized and considered irrelevant. Furthermore, each recognized diagnostic criterion is given equal importance, a situation that does not mirror clinical experience. The criteria were developed before the distinction between classic polyarteritis nodosa and microscopic polyangiitis was fully appreciated. The ACR criteria for the classification of polyarteritis nodosa are not particularly

TABLE 146.1 1990 CRITERIA FOR THE CLASSIFICATION OF POLYARTERITIS NODOSA

Criterion	Definition
1. Weight loss >4kg	Loss of 4kg or more body weight since illness began, not due to dieting or other factors
2. Livedo reticularis	Mottled reticular pattern over the skin of portions of the extremities or torso
3. Testicular pain or tenderness	Pain or tenderness of the testicles, not due to infection, trauma or other causes
4. Myalgias, weakness or polyneuropathy	Diffuse myalgias (excluding shoulder and hip girdle) or weakness of muscles or tenderness of leg muscles
5. Mononeuropathy or polyneuropathy	Development of mononeuropathy, multiple mononeuropathies or polyneuropathy
6. Diastolic BP >90mmHg	Development of hypertension with diastolic BP higher than 90mmHg
7. Increased BUN or creatinine	Increase in BUN >40mg/dl (14.3μmol/l) or creatinine >1.5mg/dl (132μmol/l), not due to dehydration or obstruction
8. Hepatitis B virus	Presence of hepatitis B surface antigen or antibody in serum
9. Arteriographic abnormality	Arteriogram showing aneurysms or occlusions of the visceral arteries, not due to arteriosclerosis, fibromuscular dysplasia or other non-inflammatory causes
10. Biopsy of small or medium-sized artery containing PMN	Histologic changes showing the presence of granulocytes or granulocytes and mononuclear leukocytes in the artery wall

BP, blood pressure; BUN, blood urea nitrogen; PMN, polymorphonuclear leukocytes (granulocytes).

The traditional format. For classification purposes, a patient with vasculitis shall be said to have polyarteritis nodosa if at least three of these 10 criteria are present. The presence of any three or more criteria yields a sensitivity of 82.2% and a specificity of 86.6%. (Adapted from Lightfoot et al.[8])

helpful for the clinician to use in the diagnosis of individual patients. However, the criteria do provide a standard way in which to evaluate and describe patients with vasculitis in therapeutic, epidemiologic and other studies, allowing comparisons of results from different centers.

In 1993 a group of physicians from six different countries attempted to standardize and further define the vasculitides, and created the Chapel Hill Consensus Conference on the Nomenclature of Systemic

TABLE 146.2 NAMES AND DEFINITIONS ADOPTED BY THE CHAPEL HILL CONSENSUS CONFERENCE ON SYSTEMIC VASCULITIS NOMENCLATURE

Polyarteritis nodosa (classic polyarteritis nodosa)

Necrotizing inflammation of medium-sized or small arteries without glomerulonephritis or vasculitis in arterioles, capillaries or venules

Microscopic polyangiitis (microscopic polyarteritis)

Essential components
Necrotizing vasculitis, with few or no immune deposits, affecting small vessels (i.e. capillaries, venules or arterioles)

Usual (but not essential components)
Necrotizing arteritis involving small and medium-sized vessels may be present
Necrotizing glomerulonephritis is very common
Pulmonary capillaritis often occurs

(Adapted from Jennette et al.[9])

TABLE 146.3 CLINICAL MANIFESTATIONS OF POLYARTERITIS NODOSA

Organ	Manifestation	Estimated % prevalence Classic PAN	All polyarteritis	MPA
Peripheral nerve	Mononeuritis multiplex	50–70		14–36
Kidney	Focal necrotizing glomerulonephritis			100
	Vascular nephrology	35		
Skin	Palpable purpura, infarctions, livedo		25–60	
Joint	Arthralgias		50	
	Arthritis		20	
Muscle	Achiness		50	
Gut	Abdominal pain, liver function abnormalities		23–70	
Heart	Congestive heart failure, myocardial infarction		low	
Central nervous system	Seizures, cerebrovascular accident		low	
Lung	Interstitial pneumonitis		low	
Eye	Retinal hemorrhage		low	
Testis	Pain		low	
Temporal artery	Jaw claudication		low	

MPA, microscopic polyangiitis; PAN, polyarteritis nodosa.

Vasculitis. From this consensus, microscopic vessel involvement was proposed as a distinguishing feature between polyarteritis nodosa and microscopic polyangiitis. Polyarteritis nodosa was then defined as necrotizing inflammation of medium-sized or small arteries without glomerulonephritis or vasculitis in the arterioles, capillaries or venules (microscopic vessels)[9] (Table 146.2). A practical classification should consider the relationship between primary and secondary vasculitis. The clinician faced with the differential diagnosis of vasculitis must also consider infection, drug, connective tissue disease or malignancy-associated vasculitis.

Clinical features

There is a spectrum of severity from mild, limited disease to progressive disease, which may be fatal. Virtually any organ may eventually be affected (Table 146.3). Typically, the patient experiences constitutional features of fever, malaise, weight loss and diffuse aching, along with manifestations of multisystem involvement such as a skin rash, peripheral neuropathy and an asymmetric polyarthritis. Visceral involvement, such as the kidney or gut, may present coincidentally with these features, or may appear later. In other cases, single organ involvement may be present alone and may remain limited, including isolated involvement of skin, peripheral nerves and visceral organs.

Cutaneous lesions

Cutaneous lesions include palpable purpura, infarctions, ulcerations, livedo vasculitis, subcutaneous nodules and ischemic changes of the distal digits (Figs 146.1 & 146.2). They occur in 25–60% of patients with polyarteritis. Skin lesions may be less common in classic polyarteritis nodosa than in patients with microscopic polyangiitis. Neither category has a particular preferred or distinguishing skin lesion[7].

Musculoskeletal features

Arthralgia or arthritis is present in polyarteritis in as many as 50% of patients. The patient with polyarteritis may present with, or have early in the course of their disease, a polymyalgia rheumatica syndrome. An asymmetric, episodic, non-deforming polyarthritis involving the larger

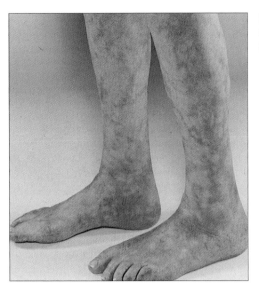

Fig. 146.1 Livedo vasculitis. (With permission from Conn[10].)

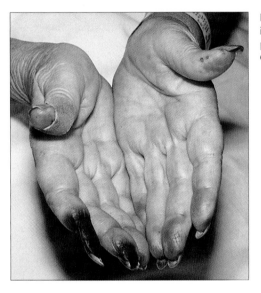

Fig. 146.2 Digital tip infarctions. (With permission from Conn[10].)

involvement. In polyarteritis nodosa, the glomerulus is usually spared. In clinical practice, the distinction is less clear, and there is frequent overlap, with both glomerulonephritis and small and medium-sized artery involvement[13,15].

Polyarteritis nodosa is usually characterized by vascular nephropathy, without glomerulonephritis about 35% of the time[7]. Multiple renal infarctions, the consequence of vascular nephropathy, produce renal failure in classic polyarteritis nodosa. Renal angiography will frequently show several aneurysms and infarcts. Ureteral stenosis and perinephric hematomas (microaneurysm rupture) can complicate classic polyarteritis nodosa. Hypertension develops as a result of renal artery or, less commonly, glomerular involvement. Hypertension, usually mild, occurs in 21–33% of patients with polyarteritis, and is most common in classic polyarteritis nodosa, particularly that associated with hepatitis B infection[7]. Renal infarction and malignant hypertension are commonly found in hepatitis B-associated vasculopathies.

Gastrointestinal involvement

Abdominal pain occurs in 23–70% of patients with polyarteritis[15]. Features of gastrointestinal involvement include abdominal pain, diarrhea, gut hemorrhage and abnormal liver enzyme tests. Hematemesis, melena and hematochezia are caused by vasculitis of the upper or lower gastrointestinal tract, most commonly the small bowel.

The only abnormality reflecting liver involvement may be an increased alkaline phosphatase, without increased bilirubin or transaminase concentrations. Liver involvement is not common clinically, and may be associated with hepatitis B antigen. Hepatitis B-associated vasculitis is more likely to have gastrointestinal and liver manifestations than is polyarteritis without the viral infection.

In cases of severe abdominal pain or distension, mesenteric thrombosis must be considered. The location and extent of vascular involvement on angiography do not correlate with the severity or type of abdominal organ involvement. The hepatic (celiac) and renal circulations are most likely to have microaneurysms, and the presence of microaneurysms predicts clinically severe polyarteritis[16]. A patient may rarely present with localized gallbladder or appendiceal involvement, probably related to a localized Arthus reaction[17]. Polyarteritis should be considered in anyone with cholecystitis and systemic or other organ-specific symptoms, if the symptoms are unexplained by stones or bacterial infection. Endoscopy with biopsy is not very useful in the diagnosis of gut involvement, but may help identify other non-vasculitic causes for abdominal pain.

Cardiac involvement

Cardiac involvement is common pathologically, but is recognized less often clinically. Myocardial infarction, when it occurs, is usually silent. Cardiomegaly occurs in about 20% of patients. Congestive heart failure develops as a result of coronary insufficiency or severe hypertension (or both). Cardiomyopathy is predictive of increased mortality[7,18]. Pericarditis is rare in patients with polyarteritis, except as a complication of uremia.

Pulmonary involvement

Pulmonary involvement is uncommon in polyarteritis nodosa, although pulmonary infiltrates, nodules, cavities or interstitial fibrosis may occur[19]. Pleural effusion occurs in about 5% of classic polyarteritis nodosa, including cases complicated by uremia, congestive heart failure or lung infection[7].

Other features

Diffuse involvement of skeletal muscle arteries may cause ischemic pain and intermittent claudication. Myalgias occur in about 50% of cases of polyarteritis, but generalized myopathy and increased creatine kinase concentrations are unusual[20].

joints of the lower extremity may occur in up to 20% of cases, most commonly early in the disease.

Neuropathy

Peripheral neuropathy may occur in up to 70% of classic polyarteritis nodosa and may be the initial manifestation. The neuropathy affects the lower extremities somewhat more often than the upper extremities. The onset may be sudden, with pain and paresthesias radiating in the distribution of a peripheral nerve, followed in hours or days by a motor deficit of the same peripheral nerve. This may progress asymmetrically to involve other peripheral nerves and produce a mononeuritis multiplex or a multiple mononeuropathy. With additional nerve damage, the final result may be a symmetric polyneuropathy involving all sensory modalities and motor functions. Less commonly, a slowly evolving distal sensory neuropathy or cranial nerve palsy may occur[11]. Clinical manifestations suggestive of central nervous system (CNS) involvement are much less common than those of peripheral nerve involvement, but the two may appear together. CNS involvement includes headache, seizures, cranial nerve dysfunction, cerebral hemorrhage and stroke[12,13]. Between 10% and 20% of patients with polyarteritis (either classic polyarteritis nodosa or microscopic polyangiitis) have some CNS manifestation.

Renal involvement

According to the Chapel Hill criteria, the diagnosis of classic polyarteritis nodosa or microscopic polyangiitis depends on the type of renal

Testicular involvement is manifested by pain, but clinical involvement indicated by swelling or induration occurs only in a small percentage of patients. Orchitis is more common in polyarteritis complicated by gastrointestinal involvement and, in particular, vasculitis associated with hepatitis B.

In the eye, polyarteritis may result in an exudative retinal detachment or toxic retinopathy with retinal hemorrhage or exudates. Ocular, ear, nose and throat complications occur more frequently in microscopic polyangiitis than in classic polyarteritis nodosa[7]. Sore throat, oral ulcers, sinusitis, otitis and hearing loss have all been described.

Temporal artery involvement may infrequently occur in polyarteritis. It may be associated with jaw claudication. The pathologic picture in such cases reveals fibrinoid necrosis without giant cells, and frequently involves smaller muscular branches of the artery.

Secondary polyarteritis nodosa

Polyarteritis may be a manifestation or complication of other diseases. This secondary polyarteritis occurs with rheumatoid arthritis[21], Sjögren's syndrome[22], mixed cryoglobulinemia[23], hairy cell leukemia[24], myelodysplastic syndrome and other hematologic malignancies[25]. Secondary polyarteritis is histopathologically and clinically indistinguishable from the primary forms. However, some forms of secondary polyarteritis have favored clinical presentations. For instance, systemic rheumatoid vasculitis occurs in long-standing rheumatoid arthritis and is most commonly manifest by constitutional symptoms, skin lesions and neuropathy.

Many infectious agents have been associated with vasculitic syndromes[26]. Viruses, including human immunodeficiency virus, are particularly inclined to cause small vessel vasculitis, whereas bacterial infections have been associated with inflammation of all sizes of blood vessels[10]. The clinical picture, including the individual's risk factors for infection, needs to be considered in the evaluation of any vasculitis. As a rule of thumb, secondary vasculitis, particularly that associated with drugs, infections or connective tissue diseases, has prominent cutaneous involvement and is more likely to be associated with hypocomplementemia.

Limited forms of polyarteritis

Isolated polyarteritis of the appendix, gallbladder, uterus or testis is well recognized although uncommon[7]. Vasculitic peripheral neuropathy can occur without other systemic or constitutional symptoms. A cutaneous form of polyarteritis, affecting predominately the lower extremities, is distinguished from systemic polyarteritis by its lack of visceral involvement and benign course[27]. Although the chronic, relapsing, non-lethal nature of the condition has been stressed by some, other investigators have documented the refractory nature of chronic cutaneous vasculitis, and the significant cumulative morbidity related to skin, muscle, joint and nerve involvement[27].

Laboratory tests and angiography

Most tests are non-specific and reflect the systemic inflammatory nature of polyarteritis. An increased erythrocyte sedimentation rate (ESR) and the presence of C-reactive protein, normochromic, normocytic anemia and thrombocytosis, with diminished concentrations of serum albumin are usually present in active polyarteritis. Eosinophilia is not common and is generally associated with pulmonary involvement in Churg–Strauss syndrome.

Rheumatoid factor, other than when present in rheumatoid arthritis, is often associated with cryoglobulins. Low-titer antinuclear antibodies are not seen often. Hypocomplementemia is more common in secondary polyarteritis.

Hepatitis B surface antigen is found in 7–54% of patients with polyarteritis[28,29]. With the widespread use of hepatitis B vaccines, the presence of hepatitis B and hepatitis B-associated vasculitis has significantly

declined. Nevertheless, the evaluation of every patient with polyarteritis should include a study for hepatitis B. Classic polyarteritis nodosa usually manifests within the first 6 months of hepatitis B infection. Hepatitis C infection is associated with polyarteritis, especially in the context of cryoglobulins and hypocomplementemia[30].

Applying the Chapel Hill definition, ANCA occurs rarely in classic polyarteritis nodosa and polyarteritis associated with hepatitis B.

Angiography is useful in patients with suspected polyarteritis, particularly if symptoms and laboratory abnormalities do not direct the choice of biopsy. The angiogram may be the diagnostic procedure of choice in hepatitis B-associated polyarteritis. The typical angiographic appearance includes long segments of smooth arterial stenosis alternating with areas of normal or dilated artery, smooth tapered occlusions, thrombosis and the lack of significant atherosclerosis (Fig. 146.3). The dilated segments include saccular and fusiform aneurysms, which strongly suggest classic polyarteritis nodosa, and aneurysms frequently occur in a more severely affected subset of the disease[16]. It has been suggested that the presence of aneurysms should exclude microscopic polyangiitis as a diagnostic possibility[31]. A number of uncommon conditions can mimic the visceral angiogram appearance of vasculitis, including bacterial endocarditis, atrial myxoma, drug abuse, pancreatitis, abdominal malignancy and disorders of connective tissue.

Pathology

The pathology of polyarteritis consists of focal, necrotizing inflammatory lesions, which extend through the wall of small and medium-sized arteries. The inflammation is characterized by fibrinoid necrosis and pleomorphic cellular infiltration, with predominantly macrophages and lymphocytes, and variable numbers of neutrophils and eosinophils

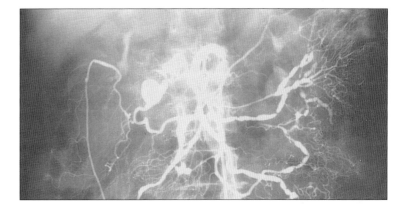

Fig. 146.3 Visceral angiogram in polyarteritis, showing areas of segmental narrowing and aneurysms. (With permission from Conn[10].)

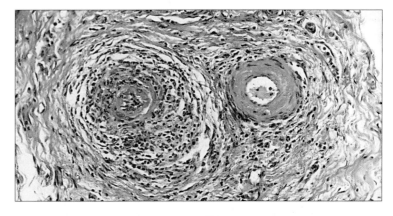

Fig. 146.4 Polyarteritis involving the gallbladder artery, showing pleomorphic inflammatory cell infiltration and fibrinoid necrosis. (With permission from Conn[10].)

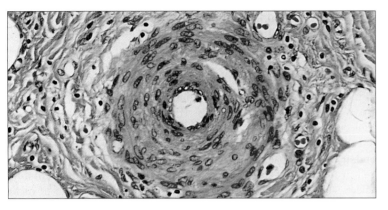

Fig. 146.5 Chronic polyarteritis with intimal proliferation and chronic fibrotic changes. (With permission from Conn[10].)

(Fig. 146.4). The number of neutrophils depends on the presence of fibrinoid necrosis[32]. A significant eosinophilic infiltrate favors the diagnosis of Churg–Strauss syndrome. The normal architecture of the vessel wall, including the elastic laminae, is disrupted. On rare occasions, classic polyarteritis nodosa may appear as granulomatous vasculitis[17]. There may be thrombosis or aneurysmal dilatation at the site of the lesion. Healed areas of arteritis show proliferation of fibrous tissue and endothelial cells, which may lead to vessel occlusion (Fig. 146.5). Lesions at all stages of progression and healing may be seen pathologically if sufficient tissue is available for study. The focal nature of the inflammation increases the risk of a false negative biopsy when the tissue sample is small. The finding of a perivascular inflammation or intimal proliferation without fibrinoid necrosis of the arterial wall suggests, but does not confirm, the diagnosis of polyarteritis.

In autopsy studies of patients with classic polyarteritis nodosa, inflammation in the arcuate and interlobar arteries and arterioles of the kidney is frequently found, along with evidence of infarction.

Arteries of the gastrointestinal tract may be involved in up to 50% of cases studied by autopsy. Vessels of liver and jejunum are the most commonly affected[16]. In the liver, findings include vasculitis along with aneurysms, infarctions and hepatitis. The gallbladder and appendix are affected in 10% of cases with other gut involvement and, rarely, they are the sites of isolated arteritis.

Peripheral nerves may be involved in 50–70% of patients with polyarteritis. The vascular lesions may be widespread and may involve the entire length of an affected nerve. Small arteries, 70–200 μm in diameter, located in the epineurium, are affected. The arterial alterations are similar to those in other organs, and a patient may show a spectrum of pathologic change, from fibrinoid necrosis in acute lesions to intimal proliferation and perivascular fibrosis in more chronic lesions. The axonal degeneration that results depends upon the extent of vascular involvement. The severity of axonal degeneration correlates with the extent of the sensorimotor deficit and the rate of recovery[33]. In some clinically apparent cases, the nerve biopsy may only show severe axonal degeneration. Arterial and peripheral nerve changes in patients with rheumatoid arthritis, Wegener's granulomatosis, and allergic angiitis and granulomatosis are indistinguishable from those changes in microscopic polyangiitis or classic polyarteritis nodosa.

Muscle biopsy is positive in about 50% of patients with polyarteritis who have muscle pain or claudication[20]. The yield on muscle biopsy is lower in asymptomatic cases.

Central nervous system involvement with polyarteritis is uncommon, excluding the CNS morbidity related to hypertension. CNS vasculitis related to polyarteritis is somewhat more likely to result in hemorrhagic stroke than is isolated CNS vasculitis. Inflammation may be found in the vertebral, carotid, meningeal, cerebral and deep arteries within the brain.

The heart is commonly involved in polyarteritis studied at autopsy. These findings include coronary arteritis, myocardial infarction, pericarditis and cardiac hypertrophy. Rarely, cases of isolated coronary arteritis have been described. In the lung, polyarteritis may affect the bronchial arteries[34].

Pathogenesis

Every proposed mechanism for the pathogenesis of vasculitis requires some initial event that primes inflammatory cells and activates endothe-

Fig. 146.6 Vasculitis pathogenesis

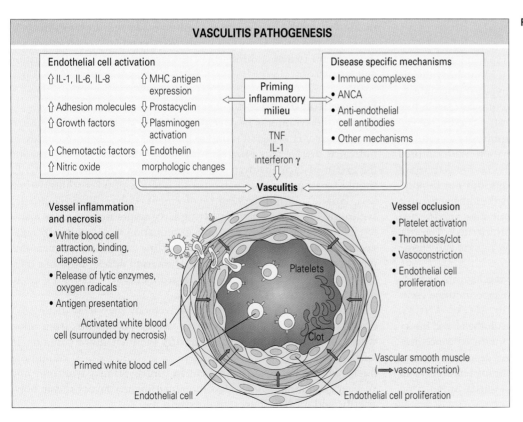

lium with increased concentrations of proinflammatory mediators, locally or systemically. This initial event is not known, but infections, allergic reactions and exposures to other antigen have been suggested. All of the vasculitides, however, share a final common pathway of inflammation, necrosis and occlusion, mediated by primed and activated leukocytes and endothelial cells (Fig. 146.6). The formation of pathogenic immune complexes is one of several proposed specific mechanisms of endothelial cell activation, injury or lysis. Other pathogenic mechanisms proposed include ANCA and neutrophil-mediated endothelial cell damage, antiendothelial cell antibodies (AECA), direct endothelial cell infection, and cellular immune-mediated endothelial cell injury[35]. The location and type of tissue injury depend on the activation and, potentially, the unique properties of different vascular beds[36].

Disease-specific pathogenic mechanisms

Immune complexes

In some vasculitic syndromes, the findings of diminished serum complement, serum immune complexes or cryoglobulins suggest that the arteritis is immune-complex induced. This has been best demonstrated in the vasculitis associated with hepatitis B and C[29,37].

Antineutrophil cytoplasmic autoantibody

Several pathogenic mechanisms for ANCA have been proposed, and each may be contributory. Increasing circulating concentrations of inflammatory cytokines may result from infection or other insults that precede or precipitate the development of vasculitis. Myeloperoxidase and proteinase 3 are expressed on the cell surfaces of cytokine-primed neutrophils. *In vitro* observations document neutrophil activation with the binding of ANCA to these antigens. Activated neutrophils readily bind to cytokine stimulated endothelial cells, degranulate and experience a respiratory burst, releasing toxic oxygen metabolites[38]. Theoretically, proteinase-3 and myeloperoxidase appear on the surface of endothelial cells also. There is *in vitro* evidence for complement-dependent and -independent cytotoxic effects of ANCA directed against stimulated endothelial cells expressing these proteins[45]. Pathogenic theories involving ANCA must take into consideration those patients in clinical remission despite persisting ANCA titers and the small group of patients with microscopic polyangiitis who have persistently negative ANCA.

Antiendothelial cell antibodies

Antiendothelial cell antibodies have been described in many conditions, including HLA matched graft rejection, thrombotic thrombocytopenic purpura, multiple sclerosis, immune-mediated hypoparathyroidism, hemolytic uremic syndrome and many rheumatic diseases, including vasculitis[40]. Antibodies to endothelial cells occur, after endothelial cell activation, as a pathogenic component of the inflammatory cascade, or as a non-pathogenic result of the vascular inflammation. With cultured human umbilical endothelial cells as antigens, antibodies are detected in Kawasaki disease and systemic lupus erythematosus, but not in polyarteritis[40]. When autologous monocytes are used as the antigen because of their antigenic similarity to endothelial cells, antibodies are detected in a variety of vasculitic syndromes, including polyarteritis[41]. The role of AECAs in the pathogenesis of microscopic polyangiitis and classic polyarteritis nodosa is unknown.

There are a number of incompletely understood mechanisms responsible for polyarteritis. The historic focus on pathogenic immune complexes has been augmented by the discovery of AECAs, ANCAs, pathogenic cellular immune responses and direct endothelial cell injury mediated by infection or tumor cell invasion[28,35]. Increased concentrations of S-ICAM, sVCAM-1 and SE-selectin as well as decreased concentrations of L-selectin have been found by a group of researchers in polyarteritis nodosa, suggesting immune and endothelial stimulation during disease activity[42].

Pathogenic mechanisms shared by all vasculitides

Activated endothelial cells can perpetuate and potentiate the inflammatory milieu by producing IL-1, IL-6 and IL-8. IL-1 and TNF-α increase cell expression of ligands, including selectins, leukocyte integrins and other adhesion molecules (ICAM and VCAM)[35]. TNF-α and interferon-γ increase expression of class I major histocompatibility complex (MHC) antigens, and induce class II MHC antigen expression. MHC molecule expression on endothelial cells allows antigen presentation to T cells. IL-8 is a member of the superfamily of cytokines made by endothelial cells that attract leukocytes to the vascular wall[43]. Endothelial cell production of nitric oxide has both anti- and proinflammatory effects. The constitutive, presumably low level, production of nitric oxide maintains the integrity of the vascular endothelium. It inhibits platelet aggregation and platelet and neutrophil adherence to endothelial cells, and reduces microvessel permeability[44]. A high concentration of nitric oxide, induced by IL-1, increases vascular permeability and, combined with superoxide anion released by activated neutrophils, forms peroxynitrite, which may play an important part in tissue injury, thrombosis, vasoreactivity and occlusive vasculopathy.

Occlusive vasculopathy potentially complicates most vasculitis with vasoconstriction, thrombosis and vascular cell proliferation. Coagulation abnormalities in systemic vasculitis are mediated by the endothelial cell[36]. Injured endothelial cells increase the expression of tissue factor that activates the extrinsic clotting pathway. Activated endothelial cells reduce expression of thrombomodulin, decrease active protein C and suppress fibrinolysis with increased synthesis of tissue plasminogen activator inhibitor. Platelet aggregation and adherence to endothelium are enhanced by endothelial cell production of platelet-activating factor. Activated, degranulated platelets adhering to damaged endothelium release preformed thromboxane, promoting vasospasm. Inflammatory mediators released from degranulated platelets also have chemotactic, proliferative, thrombogenic, complement-activating and proteolytic activities that enhance vascular injury. Activated endothelial cells produce growth factors, including granulocyte colony-stimulating factor, granulocyte-macrophage colony-stimulating factor and erythropoietin[43]. These cytokines promote lumen compromise by intimal and medial hypertrophy and proliferation of blood vessel wall cellular elements. However, glucocorticoid inhibition of endothelial cell production of constitutively expressed nitric oxide and prostacyclin could adversely promote endothelin-enhanced vascular constriction and downstream ischemia during the late stages of vascular inflammation and repair[45].

Differential diagnosis

Because the symptoms in polyarteritis are so diverse, the diagnosis is often delayed. However, it is important to make the diagnosis quickly, as untreated disease may progress with time to involve vital organs, and the extent of their involvement determines the outcome. Polyarteritis should be suspected in a patient with findings of fever, chills, weight loss, fatigue and multisystem involvement. Polymyalgia rheumatica syndrome or oligoarthritis involving large joints may be early manifestations of polyarteritis. A careful examination may reveal early cutaneous manifestations, a peripheral neuropathy or renal involvement that might provide clues to the diagnosis. The abrupt development of a multiple mononeuropathy or active renal sediment are important clues to underlying arteritis (Table 146.4).

Determining dominant organ involvement may help distinguish classic polyarteritis nodosa and microscopic polyangiitis from other types of vasculitis. Glomerulonephritis is much more common in microscopic polyangiitis and Wegener's granulomatosis, respiratory tract involvement is most frequent in Churg–Strauss syndrome and Wegener's granulomatosis, and mononeuropathy favors classic polyarteritis nodosa and Churg–Strauss syndrome.

TABLE 146.4 KEY CLINICAL FEATURES SUGGESTIVE OF POLYARTERITIS
Constitutional features (fever, chills, fatigue, weight loss, malaise)
Arthalgia or myalgia
Multiorgan involvement including: • Skin lesions (palpable purpura, livedo reticularis, necrotic lesions, infarcts on digital tips) • Peripheral neuropathy (mononeuritis multiplex) • Renal sediment abnormalities, hypertension • Abdominal pain
(Adapted from Conn[10].)

It is important to be aware of the presence of infectious vasculitis, vasculitis secondary to other systemic illness, and vasculitis mimics[46]. A number of infectious pathogens are associated with small-, medium- and large-vessel vasculitis[26]. Viruses commonly associated with small-vessel vasculitis include human immunodeficiency virus, hepatitis B and C, cytomegalovirus and parvovirus B19. Patients with rheumatoid arthritis, Sjögren's syndrome and other connective tissue diseases may have a complicating polyarteritis[45]. The antiphospholipid syndrome, malignancy, left atrial myxoma or atherosclerosis with peripheral cholesterol embolization may present with features that mimic polyarteritis (Table 146.5)[8,47].

It is important, if possible, to confirm the clinical diagnosis with a tissue biopsy or angiogram to document the vascular involvement objectively. Skin biopsies are easily obtained, and with other appropriate clinical features assist in the diagnosis. Other accessible tissues may include the sural nerve, testes, skeletal muscle and temporal artery. Biopsies of these tissues are useful if symptoms suggest pathologic involvement. In each of these situations, a positive diagnosis is based on the demonstration of small-vessel necrotizing arteritis. Involvement of

TABLE 146.5 DISEASES SIMILAR TO POLYARTERITIS NODOSA	
Disease	**PAN-like features**
Left atrial myxoma	Skin emboli
Cholesterol embolization	Livedo vasculitis of the feet
Infections: staphylococcus gonococcus	Skin emboli
Lyme disease	Peripheral neuropathy
Infective endocarditis	Skin lesions Glomerulitis
Malignancy	Skin lesions Constitutional features
Arterial dissections	Angiographic similarity
Ergotism	Vasospasm

the sural nerve can be verified by electromyography. When the sural nerve biopsy is performed, an entire cross-sectional segment of the nerve must be obtained in order to provide sufficient material for adequate sampling of epineurial arteries. The histopathologic finding of axonal degeneration, without vasculitis, may be sufficient in the appropriate clinical situation[33]. The frequency of a positive muscle biopsy specimen is probably greater when painful or stiff muscles are sampled. There is about a 50% positive yield on directed muscle biopsies[20]. A testicular biopsy should be reserved for those male patients with clinically involved areas of the testis indicated by pain or induration. In patients with microscopic polyangiitis with an abnormal urine analysis, renal biopsy will usually reveal a focal segmental necrotizing glomerulonephritis, the histopathologic equivalent of microscopic polyarteritis. In about 50% of cases, a small-vessel vasculitis may be demonstrated.

Visceral angiography helps diagnose classic polyarteritis nodosa, and may provide information on prognosis. This procedure is most appropriate when involved tissue is not available for biopsy and when there is evidence of hepatitis B infection, intra-abdominal involvement, including liver function abnormalities, or renal sediment abnormalities.

Prognosis

The outcome in polyarteritis is dependent upon the presence and extent of visceral and CNS involvement. Most of the deaths in patients with polyarteritis occur within the first year of disease (Fig. 146.7)[48]. These are usually the result of uncontrolled vasculitis, frequently as a result of delay in the diagnosis of the disease or from infectious complications of treatment. Deaths occurring after 1 year of disease are usually either a result of complications of treatment, such as superimposed infections, or vascular deaths such as a myocardial infarction or stroke. The prognosis of untreated polyarteritis is poor and the 5-year survival is less than 15%. Survival has improved with the use of glucocorticoids, and also with the use of the combination of cyclophosphamide and prednisone in patients with significant major organ involvement. Most studies document a 5-year survival of between 50% and 80%[7]. Lhote and Guillevin[7] have shown that age greater than 50 years at onset, more than 1g/day proteinuria, renal insufficiency at diagnosis, cardiac, gastrointestinal or central nervous system involvement increase the risk of death. Others have confirmed additional mortality risk (relative risk of dying of 2.91 in 5 years) with renal or cardiac involvement[18]. The presence or absence of organs or systems involved has been shown to be associated with

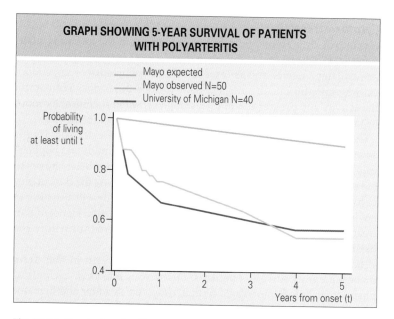

Fig. 146.7 Graph showing 5-year survival of patients with polyarteritis. (Modified with permission from Cohen *et al.*[47] and Sack *et al.*[48])

prognosis of the disease. For example, the presence of neuropathy, including mononeuritis multiplex, does not increase mortality. Comorbid factors, including malignancy, cardiovascular disease, cerebrovascular disease and diabetes mellitus, increase mortality[50]. The five-factor score can be used to predict the survival rate of patients with polyarteritis nodosa. In a prospective study, the following items were identified that predict excess mortality: renal insufficiency (serum creatinine >140µmol/l); proteinuria (>1g/day); visceral involvement (e.g. gastrointestinal); central nervous system involvement; cardiac involvement. When one factor is present, the expected 5-year mortality is 25%; when two factors are present, mortality is 46%. When no factor is found, polyarteritis nodosa is considered to have a good prognosis and the expected mortality is no more than 12%. It has recently been shown that the combination of steroids and cyclophosphamide improves prognosis in patients with a five-factor score of 2 or more, compared with treatment with steroids alone[50].

Relapses are quite common; many patients (perhaps most) are not cured. During a 10-year period of observation, 41% of patients with classic polyarteritis nodosa suffered relapse, with a median time to relapse of 33 months[52]. Classic polyarteritis nodosa is more likely to relapse with a clinical picture similar to its initial presentation. Relapses may be related to the process of tapering off prednisone treatment.

Management

Glucocorticoids

Glucocorticoids are the standard medication used to treat polyarteritis today, their use first having been described in 1951[53]. The initial management of polyarteritis should include high doses of glucocorticoids, most commonly prednisone. Initially, it should be administered in a single daily dose or divided daily doses, ranging from 40 to 60mg a day. Alternate-day doses have no role in the initial management of polyarteritis. Appropriate treatment to prevent steroid-induced osteoporosis should be used in all patients prescribed glucocorticoids.

In the follow-up of patients with polyarteritis, the clinical status and ESR should be monitored. As the clinical status improves and as the ESR returns to normal, tapering of the prednisone can begin. Initially, the decrements can be 5–10mg every 1–2 weeks. As the prednisone dose becomes lower, the decrements should be less. When the total dose of prednisone is down to approximately 15mg a day, the reduction in dose should be 1mg every several weeks. Frequently, the patient must be maintained on a low dose of prednisone for an indefinite period of time.

Cytotoxic treatment

A cytotoxic drug should be added to prednisone in the following situations: (1) On initial evaluation when the vasculitis is rapidly progressing, or involving visceral organs (except isolated gallbladder or appendix); (2) when prednisone in sufficient daily divided doses does not control the activity and progression of disease; and (3) when prednisone cannot be tapered to a tolerable concentration and still control the disease.

Cyclophosphamide is the popular choice when a cytotoxic drug is added to control the disease. The use of cyclophosphamide was popularized by Fauci et al. in 1979[54]. Cyclophosphamide has been shown to reduce mortality in patients with significant disease[51]. As the dose of glucocorticoid is tapered, often the dose of alkylating drug will also have to be decreased, to prevent the development of leukopenia. Concomitant treatment with trimethoprim-sulfa may be considered, to reduce the likelihood of opportunistic infection.

Toxic side effects become one of the major concerns in long-term management of vasculitis patients. Deleterious effects of cyclophosphamide include hemorrhagic cystitis, neoplasia (bladder and hematologic), cytopenias, infection and ovarian failure. Published experience regarding the efficacy of pulse intravenous cyclophosphamide and oral methylprednisolone used every 2 weeks (induction) to 6 months, com-

pared with daily oral methylprednisolone and cyclophosphamide (for first 3–6 months) and azathioprine thereafter, showed no difference in mortality in the first 12 months (85% survival)[52]. There was, however, a reduction in infectious complications in the patients receiving pulse treatment. Renal failure increases the potential morbidity related to high-dose intravenous cyclophosphamide regimens, and necessitates the modification of the dose.

The European Vasculitis Study (EUVAS) Group trials have looked at the use of azathioprine for maintenance therapy in vasculitis. The Cyclophosphamide or Azathioprine as a Remission Therapy for Vasculitis trial[56] demonstrated that, for general vasculitis, azathioprine is as effective as continued cyclophosphamide for maintenance of remission. EUVAS is also supporting a trial in Churg–Strauss syndrome and polyarteritis nodosa, comparing 6 monthly pulses of cyclophosphamide against 12 pulses, classifying patients at diagnosis into groups with good and poor prognosis using the five-factor score. Current trials are also investigating mycophenolate mofetil as an alternative to azathioprine[56]. Antithymocyte globulin is also being studied for refractory vasculitis.

Other treatments

It is unclear whether antiviral treatment such as interferon-α should supersede conventional regimens in patients with hepatitis B-associated vasculitis. There is legitimate concern regarding increased viral replication in some patients receiving conventional treatment using steroids and cyclophosphamide. There is evidence that treating hepatitis B virus-associated vasculitis with antiviral therapy as part of the regimen might be beneficial[57].

Intravenous immunoglobulin treatment has been used successfully in Kawasaki disease to reduce the prevalence of coronary artery aneurysms. In an open-label study of salvage intravenous immunoglobulin treatment for ANCA-associated vasculitis, only six of 15 patients experienced any benefit, which was partial in all cases, and did not improve the nephritis in any[58]. Repeated administration was no more effective than a single course. The use of intravenous immunoglobulin in the treatment of polyarteritis appears to be limited.

When a patient's symptoms progress despite adequate doses of glucocorticoids, the clinician should determine whether glucocorticoid resistant vasculitis, superimposed infection, or progression of occlusive vasculopathy is responsible for the continued symptoms.

It is possible that agents directed towards inhibiting thrombosis, inflammatory cytokines, growth factors and cellular proliferation will be important in the future. There is some anecdotal experience, in addition to current studies with anti-TNF agents in certain types of vasculitis, but not enough experience or formal data to recommend the use of this strategy in this setting.

Vasculopathic complications in vasculitis are the result of the effects of arterial inflammation and glucocorticoid-influenced vascular occlusion and atherosclerosis, and are aggravated by comorbid features of hypertension and diabetes mellitus. Control of blood pressure, cessation of smoking and management of hyperlipidemia and diabetes mellitus are important adjuncts to the management of vasculitis. Proteinuria is an independent risk factor for progression to renal failure. For patients with proteinuria of more than 1g/day, the target blood pressure should be 125/75mmHg[59]. The concomitant use of antiplatelet drugs with glucocorticoid treatment might modify some of these late vascular complications[45].

MICROSCOPIC POLYANGIITIS

History

Microscopic polyangiitis was first described by Wohlwill in 1923[60] and recognized as a different disease in 1948 by Davson et al.[61], as they described a subgroup of patients with polyarteritis nodosa and segmental necrotizing glomerulonephritis. The Chapel Hill international consensus conference distinguished the condition from polyarteritis nodosa by the presence of small-vessel involvement (arterioles, venules or capillaries). The presence of vasculitis in any of these vessels would exclude polyarteritis nodosa[3].

Epidemiology

Microscopic polyangiitis is more common in males, with a reported male:female sex ratio ranging from 1 to 1.8:1[7]. Others have reported a female:male ratio of 1.2:4. The average age at onset seems to be after 50 years, but it can be seen at any age. Further details of the epidemiology of microscopic polyangiitis have been given in the section on polyarteritis nodosa earlier in this chapter.

Classification

In 1994, the Chapel Hill consensus conference on vasculitis nomenclature provided standard definitions for 10 distinct vasculitis entities and grouped them into three familiar groups, based on affected blood vessel size (small, medium and large)[9]. This nomenclature distinguishes classic polyarteritis nodosa from microscopic polyangiitis, with small vessel involvement and glomerulonephritis the definitive differentiating criteria (Table 146.2). Using the Chapel Hill definitions, Scott and Watts[31] were unable to identify even one case of classic polyarteritis nodosa out of 180 recent cases of systemic vasculitis, leading them to suggest that a practical application of the definition should focus on 'dominant vessel involvement'. When distinguishing classic polyarteritis nodosa from microscopic polyangiitis, clinicians must consider the organ systems involved (lung, kidney), and the presence or absence of ANCA, hepatitis infection or angiographic finding of aneurysms. Guillevin and Lhote have assembled histologic and clinical criteria to help distinguish microscopic polyangiitis from polyarteritis nodosa (Table 146.6)[14]. ANCA-positive patients lacking specific features of Wegener's granulomatosis or Churg–Strauss syndrome are described as having microscopic polyangiitis, but in some cases it may be a variant of Wegener's granulomatosis[14].

Clinical features

Renal involvement

Although microscopic polyangiitis has been reported without renal involvement[63], necrotizing, and sometimes rapidly progressive, glomerulonephritis is the major feature of microscopic polyangiitis. Segmental necrosis and crescent formation, together with little or no endocapillary proliferation, are found. Little or no immune deposits and electron-dense deposits are also characteristic. These features can be indistinguishable from the picture seen in Wegener's granulomatosis and idiopathic, rapidly progressive crescentic glomerulonephritis. Proteinuria is common and, rarely, a nephrotic syndrome may develop. There is active urinary sediment, with red cells and red cell casts characteristic of glomerular involvement. Renal insufficiency is frequently noted at presentation, and glomerulonephritis causes oliguric renal failure in 33% of all cases[64]. Dialysis might be necessary in up to 45% of patients[65,66]. The renal angiogram in microscopic polyangiitis is usually normal.

Pulmonary involvement

Pulmonary involvement is common in microscopic polyangiitis, and may vary clinically from dyspnea to massive pulmonary hemorrhage. Pulmonary hemorrhage occurs in up to 29% of patients with microscopic polyangiitis[64], and pleural effusion in about 15%, including cases complicated by uremia, congestive heart failure or lung infection[7]. Nonspecific alveolar infiltrates are found in radiographs. Interstitial fibrosis after recurrent episodes of alveolar hemorrhage has also been reported[67]. Capillaritis is the underlying pathologic feature and, very infrequently, immune deposits are found. Among patients with antiglomerular basement membrane disease (Goodpasture's syndrome), 33% are ANCA-positive[68]; they may have features of systemic vasculitis in addition to rapidly progressive glomerulonephritis and pulmonary disease. Microscopic polyangiitis should be considered in the differential diagnosis of any acute pulmonary–renal syndrome. Pulmonary hemorrhage has recently been found to be a strong independent risk factor for death in patients with microscopic polyangiitis with positive ANCA and glomerulonephritis[69].

Skin involvement

Skin is more commonly involved in microscopic polyangiitis than in polyarteritis nodosa. Palpable purpura is the most common lesion found, although livedo, infarction or ulceration can be present.

Neuropathy

Neuropathy is believed to be less common in microscopic polyangiitis than in classic polyarteritis nodosa[7], and is reported to be present in about 14% of patients. In more recent series, peripheral neuropathy has been found in 57.6% of patients[63].

TABLE 146.6 DISTINGUISHING MICROSCOPIC POLYANGIITIS FROM CLASSIC POLYARTERITIS NODOSA

	Criteria	PAN	MPA
Histology	Type of vasculitis	Necrotizing with mixed cells, rarely granulomatous	Necrotizing with mixed cells, not granulomatous
	Type of vessels involved	Medium- and small-sized muscle arteries, sometimes arterioles	Small vessels (capillaries, venules or arterioles) Small and medium-sized arteries may also be affected
Distribution and localization	Kidney Renal vasculitis with renovascular hypertension, renal infarcts and microaneurysms	Yes	No
	Rapidly progressive glomerulonephritis	No	Very common
	Lung Lung hemorrhage	No	Yes
	Peripheral neuropathy	50–80%	10–30%
Laboratory data	pANCA	Rare <20%	pANCA (80%) and cANCA
	HBV infection	Yes (uncommon)	No
Abnormal angiography	Microaneurysms, smooth tapered vessels, stenosis, poststenotic dilation	Yes (variable)	No

HBV, hepatitis B virus; MPA, microscopic polyangiitis; PAN, polyarteritis nodosa
(Adapted from Guillevin and Lhote[14].)

Laboratory data

As in polyarteritis nodosa, most tests in microscopic polyangiitis are non-specific and reflect the systemic inflammatory nature of polyarteritis. Increased ESR and C-reactive protein, normochromic normocytic anemia, thrombocytosis and diminished concentrations of serum albumin are usually present in active polyarteritis.

In microscopic polyangiitis, rheumatoid factor may be present and not associated with cryoglobulins or low complement concentration[64]. Nearly all patients with microscopic polyangiitis are ANCA-positive; about 50% have cytoplasmic ANCA and the remainder are positive for perinuclear ANCA. The diagnostic usefulness of perinuclear ANCA depends on the prior probability of systemic vasculitis and the antigen specificity for myeloperoxidase[70]. Persistence of ANCA in microscopic polyangiitis after clinical remission does not reflect disease activity, or a risk for mortality[71]. Most patients with microscopic polyangiitis will present with compromised renal function and a nephritic, (red cells, red cell casts) urine sediment[7]. ANCA is a sensitive marker for microscopic polyangiitis and other types of arteritis associated with pauci-immune (few or no immune or complement deposits) glomerulonephritis[72].

Pathology

The distinguishing features of microscopic polyangiitis pathology are found in the lung, with alveolitis leading to capillaritis, and in the kidney, where necrotizing and crescentic glomerulonephritis are essential components[9]. Renal histology is characterized by the presence of focal segmental thrombosing and necrotizing glomerulonephritis. Crescent formation can be seen in almost all the biopsies, and can affect more than 60% of the glomerulus. Biopsy of skin lesions often shows leukocytoclastic vasculitis. (See section on Polyarteritis Nodosa, above, for more details of pathologic features.)

Differential diagnosis

It is important to differentiate both Wegener's granulomatosis and Churg–Strauss syndrome from microscopic polyangiitis. Other small-vessel vasculitis has well-defined immune complex deposits, such as Henoch–Schönlein purpura and cryoglobulinemic vasculitis. Immune complexes will also be found in serum sickness and systemic lupus erythematosus. Isolated cutaneous leukocytoclastic angiitis without systemic vasculitis or glomerulonephritis can occur.

Management

High doses of prednisone should be used, as in polyarteritis nodosa, using the same approach to tapering (see section on Management of polyarteritis nodosa, above). Because renal and pulmonary manifestations are frequent in this disease, treatment with glucocorticoid alone is often not adequate. There are recent data showing that the use of cyclophosphamide along with glucocorticoids to control the disease prevents relapses and decrease mortality[63]. Monitoring of clinical symptoms and laboratory data is important, especially urinary sediment and kidney function. These monitorings should persist after the patient has achieved a stable condition, because relapses are common and difficult to predict. There are no controlled data to support the use of other agents, but there are reports of beneficial use of intravenous immunoglobulin and plasmapheresis, especially in renal involvement[73]. A trial of ANCA-associated vasculitis using plasma exchange is in progress, and results were expected to be available by 2002[48]. Long-term remission in renal vasculitis treated with azathioprine is also being studied[48].

Prognosis

A number of patients with microscopic polyangiitis achieve disease remission with treatment, and relapses have been estimated at about 25–35% in one series[64,74]. Clinical features at relapse differ from those at presentation, and may include organs not previously involved. With microscopic polyangiitis relapse, systemic or constitutional features, or both, and lung or renal involvement are less common, whereas skin lesions and arthralgia more common. In a series of patients with microscopic polyangiitis, the risk of death has been found to be 5.56 times lower in the cyclophosphamide-treated patients than in those treated with corticosteroids alone[69]. The predictors of renal survival in this series were serum creatinine value at the time of the patient's entry to the study ($p = 0.0002$), race (African-Americans having a worse outcome than whites; $p = 0.0008$), and the presence of arterial sclerosis on kidney biopsy ($p = 0.0076$) when control was made for age and ANCA pattern. The relative risk (and 95% confidence interval) of patient death has been estimated to be 8.65 (3.36 to 22.2) times greater in patients who present with pulmonary hemorrhage, and 3.78 (1.22 to 11.70) times greater in patients with cytoplasmic ANCA, compared with those with perinuclear ANCA. The relative risk of pulmonary hemorrhage has been found not to differ with ANCA pattern[69].

REFERENCES

1. Matteson EL. Historical perspective on the classification of vasculitis. Arthritis Care Res 2000; 13: 122–127.
2. Kussmaul A, Maier R. Ueber eine bisher nicht beshriebene eigenthumliche Arterienerkrankung (Periarteritis nodosa), die mit Morbus Brightii und rapid fortschreibtender allgemeiner Muskellahmung einhergeht. Deutsch Arch Klin Med 1866; 1: 484–517.
3. Michet CJ. Epidemiology of vasculitis. In: Conn DL, ed. Rheumatic disease clinics of North America, ch 2. Philadelphia: WB Saunders; 1990: 261–268.
4. Watts RA, Lane SE, Bentham G, Scott DG. Epidemiology of systemic vasculitis. A ten year study in the United Kingdom. Arthritis Rheum 2000; 43: 414–419.
5. Andrews M, Edmunds M, Campbell A et al. Systemic vasculitis in the 1980s – is there an increasing incidence of Wegener's granulomatosis and microscopic polyarteritis? J Roy Coll Phys 1990; 24: 284–288.
6. Watts RA, Carruthers DM, Scott DGI. Epidemiology of systemic vasculitis: changing incidence or definition? Sem Arthritis Rheum 1995; 25: 28–34.
7. Lhote F, Guillevin L. Polyarteritis nodosa, microscopic polyangiitis, and Churg–Strauss syndrome: clinical aspects and treatment. In: Hunder GG, ed. Rheumatic disease clinics of North America, Philadelphia: WB Saunders; 1995; 21: 911–947.
8. Lightfoot RW, Michel BA, Bloch DA et al. The American College of Rheumatology 1990 criteria for the classification of polyarteritis nodosa. Arthritis Rheum 1990; 33: 1088–1093.
9. Jennette JC, Falk RJ, Andrassy K et al. Nomenclature of systemic vasculitis. Arthritis Rheum 1994; 37: 187–192.
10. Conn DL. Polyarteritis. In: Conn AL, ed. Rheumatic Disease clinics of North America, ch 7. Philadelphia: WB Saunders; 1990: 341–362.
11. Davies L. Vasculitic neuropathy. Baillieres Clin Neurol 1994; 3: 193–210.
12. Ford RG, Siekert RG. Central nervous system manifestations of periarteritis nodosa. Neurology 1965; 15: 114–122.
13. Iaconetta G, Benvenuti D, Lamaida E et al. Cerebral hemorrhagic complication in polyarteritis nodosa. Case report and review of the literature. Acta Neurol 1994; 16: 64–69.
14. Guillevin L, Lhote F. Polyarteritis nodosa and microscopic polyangiitis. Clin Exp Immunol 1995; 101(suppl 1): 22–23.
15. Guillevin L, Lhote F, Gallais V et al. Gastrointestinal tract involvement in polyarteritis nodosa and Churg–Strauss syndrome. Ann Med Interne 1995; 146: 260–267.
16. Ewald EA, Griffin D, McCuen WJ. Correlation of angiographic abnormalities with disease manifestations and disease severity in polyarteritis nodosa. J Rheumatol 1987; 14: 952–956.
17. Lie JT. Histopathologic specificity of systemic vasculitis. In: Hunder GG, ed. Rheumatic disease clinics of North America. Philadelphia: WB Saunders; 1995: 883–909.
18. Fortin PR, Larson MG, Watters AK et al. Prognostic factors in systemic necrotizing vasculitis of the polyarteritis nodosa group – a review of 45 cases. J Rheumatol 1995; 22: 78–84.
19. Leatherman JW. The lung in systemic vasculitis. Sem Resp Infect 1988; 3: 274–288.
20. Fort JG, Griffin R, Tahmoush A, Abruzzo JL. Muscle involvement in polyarteritis nodosa: report of a patient presenting clinically as polymyositis and review of the literature. J Rheumatol 1994; 21: 945–948.
21. Luqmani RA, Watts RA, Scott DGI, Bacon PA. Treatment of vasculitis in rheumatoid arthritis. Ann Med Interne 1994; 145: 566–576.
22. Alexander EL, Arnett FC, Provost TT et al. Sjögren's syndrome: association of anti-Ro(SS-A) antibodies with vasculitis, hematologic abnormalities, and serologic hyperreactivity. Ann Intern Med 1983; 98: 155–159.

23. Gorevic PD, Kassab HJ, Levo Y et al. Mixed cryoglobulinemia: clinical aspects and long-term follow-up of 40 patients. Am J Med 1980; 69: 287–308.

24. Gabriel SE, Conn DL, Phyliky RL et al. Vasculitis in hairy cell leukemia: Review of literature and consideration of possible pathogenic mechanisms. J Rheumatol 1986; 13: 1167–1172.

25. Mertz LE, Conn DL. Vasculitis associated with malignancy. Curr Opin Rheumatol 1992; 4: 39–46.

26. Somer T, Finegold SM. Vasculitides associated with infections, immunizations, and antimicrobial drugs. Clin Inf Dis 1995; 20: 1010–1036.

27. Moreland L, Ball GV. Cutaneous polyarteritis nodosa. Am J Med 1990; 88: 426–423.

28. Conn DL, McDuffie FC, Holley KE, Schroeter AL. Immunological mechanism in systemic vasculitis. Mayo Clin Proc 1976; 51: 511–518.

29. Trepo CG, Zuckerman AR, Bird RC et al. The role of circulating hepatitis B antigen/antibody immune complexes in the pathogenesis of vascular and hepatic manifestations in polyarteritis nodosa. J Clin Path 1974; 27: 863–868.

30. Carson CW, Conn DL, Czaja AJ et al. Frequency and significance of antibodies to hepatitis C virus in polyarteritis nodosa. J Rheumatol 1993; 20: 304–309.

31. Scott DGI, Watts RA. Classification and epidemiology of systemic vasculitis. Br J Rheumatol 1994; 33: 897–900.

32. Cid MC, Grau JM, Casademont J et al. Immunohistochemical characterization of inflammatory cells and immunologic activation markers in muscle and nerve biopsy specimens from patients with polyarteritis nodosa. Arthritis Rheum 1994; 37: 1055–1061.

33. Puæchal X, Said G, Hilliquin P et al. Peripheral neuropathy with necrotizing vasculitis in rheumatoid arthritis. Arthritis Rheum 1995; 38: 1618–1629.

34. Travis WD, Colby TV, Lombard C, Carpenter HA. A clinicopathologic study of 34 cases of diffuse pulmonary hemorrhage with lung biopsy confirmation. Am J Surg Path 1990; 14: 1112–1125.

35. Haynes BF. Vasculitis: pathogenic mechanisms of vessel damage. In: Gallin JI, Goldstein IM, Snyderman R, eds. Inflammation: basic principles and clinical correlates, 2E. New York: Raven Press; 1992: 921–941.

36. Savage COS, Cooke SP. The role of endothelium in systemic vasculitis. J Autoimmun 1993; 6: 237–249.

37. Abel G, Zhang QX, Agnello V. Hepatitis C virus infection in type II mixed cryoglobulinemia. Arthritis Rheum 1993; 36: 1341–1349.

38. Jennette JC, Falk RJ. Update on the pathobiology of vasculitis. Monogr Pathol 195; 37: 156–172.

39. Mayet WJ, Schwarting A, Zumbuschenfelde KHM. Cytotoxic effects of antibodies to proteinase 3 (c-ANCA) on human endothelial cells. Clin Exp Immunol 1994; 97: 458–465.

40. Baguley E, Hughes GRV. Antiendothelial cell antibodies. J Rheumatol 1989; 16: 716–717.

41. Brasile L, Kremer JM, Clarke JL et al. Identification of an autoantibody to vascular endothelial cell-specific antigens in patients with systemic vasculitis. Am J Med 1989; 87: 74–80.

42. Coll-Vinet B, Cebrian M, Cid MC et al. Dynamic pattern of endothelial cell expression in muscle and perineural vessels from patients with classic polyarteritis nodosa 1998; 41: 435–444.

43. Introna M, Colotta F, Sozzani S et al. Pro- and anti-inflammatory cytokines: interactions with vascular endothelium. Clin Exp Rheumatol 1994; 12(suppl 10): S19–S23.

44. Moncada S, Palmer RMJ, Higgs EA. Nitric oxide: physiology, pathophysiology, and pharmacology. Pharmacol Rev 1991; 43: 109–142.

45. Conn DL, Tompkins RB, Nichols WL. Glucocorticoids in the management of vasculitis – a double edged sword? J Rheumatol 1988; 15: 1181–1183.

46. Lie JT. Vasculitis simulators and vasculitis look-alikes. Curr Opin Rheumatol 1992; 4: 47–55.

47. Grishman E, Spiera H. Vasculitis in connective tissue diseases, including hypocomplementemic vasculitis. In: Churg A, Churg J, eds. Vasculitis. New York: Igaku-Shoin Medical Publishers; 1991: 273–292.

48. Sack M, Cassidy JT, Bole GG. Prognostic factors in polyarteritis. J Rheumatol 1975; 2: 411–420.

49. Cohen RD, Conn DL, Ilstrup DM. Clinical features, prognosis, and response to treatment in polyarteritis. Mayo Clin Proc 1980; 55: 146–155.

50. Achkar AA, Hall S, Gabriel SE et al. Survival and prognostic factors in polyarteritis nodosa. Arthritis Rheum 1994; 10: S409.

51. Gayraud M, Guillevin L, le Toumelin P et al. Long-term follow up of polyarteritis nodosa, microscopic polyangiitis and Churg–Strauss syndrome. Arthritis Rheum 2001; 44: 666–675.

52. Gordon M, Luqmani RA, Adu D et al. Relapses in patients with a systemic vasculitis. Q J Med 1993; 86: 779–789.

53. Baggenstoss AH, Schick RM, Polley HF. The effect of cortisone on the lesions of periarteritis nodosa. Am J Pathol 1951; 27: 537–559.

54. Fauci AS, Katz P, Haynes BF et al. Cyclophosphamide therapy of severe systemic necrotizing vasculitis. N Engl J Med 1979; 301: 235–238.

55. Bacon PA. Therapy of vasculitis. J Rheumatol 1994; 21: 788–790.

56. Jayne D, on behalf of the European Vasculitis Study Group (EUVAS). Update on the European Vasculitis Study Group trial. Curr Opin Rheumatol 2001; 13: 48–55.

57. Guillevin L, Lhote F, Cohen P et al. Polyarteritis nodosa related to hepatitis B virus. A prospective study with long-term observation of 41 patients. Medicine (Baltimore) 1995; 74: 238–253.

58. Richter C, Schnabel A, Csernok E et al. Treatment of anti-neutrophil cytoplasmic antibody (ANCA)-associated systemic vasculitis with high-dose intravenous immunoglobulin. Clin Exp Immunol 1995; 101: 2–7.

59. Peterson JC et al., for the Modification of Diet in Renal Disease Study Group. Blood pressure control, proteinuria, and the progression of renal disease. Ann Intern Med 1995; 123: 754–762.

60. Wohlwill F. Uber dienur Mikroskopisch erkenbarre Form der Periarititers nodosa. Arch Pathol Anat 1923; 246: 377–411.

61. Davson J, Ball J, Platt R: The kidney in periarteritis nososa. Q J Med 1948; 17: 175.

62. Jennette JC, Falk RJ. Clinical and pathological classification of ANCA-associated vasculitis: what are the controversies? Clin Exp Immunol 1995; 101(suppl 1): 18–22.

63. Guivellin L, Durand-Gasselin B, Cevallos R et al. Microscopic polyangiitis. Clinical and laboratory findings in eighty-five patients. Arthritis Rheum 1999; 42: 421–430.

64. Savage COS, Winearls CG, Evans DJ et al. Microscopic polyarteritis: presentation, pathology, and prognosis. Q J Med 1985; 56: 467–483.

65. Savage COS, Winearls CG, Evans DJ et al. Microscopic polyarteritis: presentation, histopathology and long term outcome. Q J Med 1985; 56: 467–483.

66. Adu D, Howie AJ, Scott DGI et al. Polyarteritis and the kidney. Q J Med 1987; 62: 221–237.

67. Swarchz MI. The nongranulomatous vasculidities of the lung. Semin Respir Crit Care Med 1998; 19: 47.

68. Jayne DR, Marshall PD, Jones SJ, Lockwood CM. Autoantibodies to GBM and neutrophil cytoplasm in rapidly progressive glomerulonephritis. Kidney Int 1990; 37: 965.

69. Hogan SL., Nachman H, Wilkman AS, and the Glomerular Disease Collaborative Network. Prognostic markers in patients with antineutrophil cytoplasmic autoantibody-associated microscopic polyangiitis and glomerulonephritis. J Am Soc Nephrol 1996; 7: 23–32.

70. Jennette JC, Falk RJ. The coming of age of serologic testing for anti-neutrophil cytoplasmic antibodies. Mayo Clin Proc 1994; 69: 908–910.

71. Cohen P, Guillevin L, Baril L et al. Persistence of antineutrophil cytoplasmic antibodies (ANCA) in asymptomatic patients with systemic polyarteritis nodosa or Churg–Strauss syndrome: follow-up of 53 patients. Clin Exp Rheumatol 1995; 13: 193–195.

72. Falk RJ, Jennette JC. Anti-neutrophil cytoplasmic autoantibodies with specificity for myeloperoxidase in patients with systemic vasculitis and idiopathic necrotizing and crescentic glomerulonephritis. N Engl J Med 1988; 318: 1651–1657.

73. Guillevin L, Lhote F, Gayraud M et al. Prognostic factors in polyarteritis nodosa and Churg–Strauss syndrome. A prospective study in 342 patients. Medicine (Baltimore) 1996; 75: 17–28.

74. Nachman PH, Hogan SL, Jennette C, Falk RJ. Treatment response and relapse rate in antineutrophil cytoplasmic autoantibody associated microscopic polyangiitis and glomerulonephritis. J Am Soc Nephrol 1996; 7: 33–39.

147 Polymyalgia rheumatica and giant cell arteritis

Brian L Hazleman

Definitions

Polymyalgia rheumatica

- A clinical syndrome of the middle-aged and elderly, characterized by pain and stiffness in the neck, shoulder and pelvic girdles
- The clinical response to small doses of corticosteroids can be dramatic

Giant cell arteritis

- A vasculitis commonly accompanying polymyalgia rheumatica. Other terms used include temporal arteritis, cranial arteritis and granulomatous arteritis
- Early recognition and treatment can prevent blindness and other complications resulting from occlusion or rupture of involved arteries

Clinical features

Polymyalgia rheumatica

- The musculoskeletal symptoms are usually bilateral and symmetric
- Stiffness is the predominant feature; it is particularly severe after rest and may prevent the patient getting out of bed in the morning
- Muscular pain is often diffuse and is accentuated by movement; pain at night is common
- Corticosteroid treatment is usually required for at least 2 years. Most patients should be able to stop taking corticosteroids after 4–5 years
- Systemic features include low-grade fever, fatigue, weight loss and an increased erythrocyte sedimentation rate

Giant cell arteritis

- There are a wide range of symptoms, but most patients have clinical findings related to involved arteries
- Frequent features include fatigue, headaches, jaw claudication, loss of vision, scalp tenderness, polymyalgia rheumatica and aortic arch syndrome

HISTORY

The earliest description of giant cell arteritis may have been in the 10th century in the *Tadkwat* of Ali Iba Isu, where removal of the temporal artery was recommended as treatment. Dequeker describes two paintings – Jan Van Eyck's work in the Municipal Museum, Bruges, depicting the Holy Virgin with Canon Van der Paele (1436; see Chapter 1) and Pieri di Cosimo's portrait of Francesco Gamberti (1505), now in the Rijksmuseum, Amsterdam[1]. Both show signs of prominent temporal arteries and contemporary accounts document rheumatic pains, difficulty attending morning service with possible stiffness and general ill health.

Recognizable descriptions of polymyalgia rheumatica and giant cell arteritis were recorded throughout the 19th and 20th centuries. Jonathan Hutchinson in 1890 described 'a peculiar form of thrombotic arteritis of the aged, which is sometimes productive of gangrene'[2]. Horton *et al.*[3] described the typical histologic appearances at temporal artery biopsy.

The first description of polymyalgia rheumatica was probably made by Bruce in 1888[4], and Barber[5] suggested the present name in 1957. In 1960, Paulley and Hughes reported on 67 patients, emphasizing the occurrence of 'an arthritic rheumatism' in giant cell arteritis, providing more solid clinical evidence for the relationship between polymyalgia rheumatica and giant cell arteritis[6]. Histologic support came from the work of Alestig and Barr[7], and Hamlin *et al.*[8] confirmed the coexistence of the two conditions.

EPIDEMIOLOGY

Giant cell arteritis affects the white population almost exclusively. Most reports originate from Northern Europe[9] and parts of the northern USA. However, the disease is recognizable worldwide and there have been several reports of its occurrence in American blacks. In Tennessee, there is a lower incidence in the southern white population.

In Europe, studies from Southern Europe (Italy, Spain and France) have consistently reported lower incidence rates than those from Scandinavia. Multiple regression analysis correcting for the effect of increasing incidence with time suggests that there is a significant trend towards increasing incidence with more northerly latitude[10]. O'Brien and Regan[11] proposed that long-term exposure to sunlight (including both infrared and ultraviolet radiation could alter the structure of the internal elastic lamina of superficial arteries, making them antigenic (actinic degeneration). Recently, actinic changes have been demonstrated in the posterior ciliary arteries of patients.

Both polymyalgia rheumatica and giant cell arteritis affect elderly people and are seldom diagnosed in those younger than 50 years. A

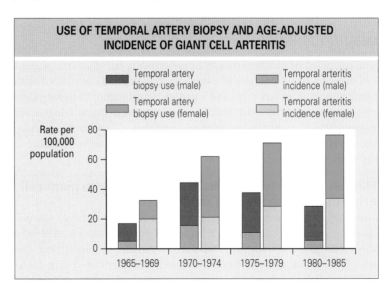

Fig. 147.1 Use of temporal artery biopsy and sex-adjusted incidence of giant cell arteritis. Data for residents of Olmsted County, Minnesota, from 1965 to 1985, per 100 000 population aged 50 years or more. Incidence was also age-adjusted to the 1980 white population of the USA.

study of biopsy-proven giant cell arteritis diagnosed from 1950 through to 1985 in Olmsted County, Minnesota, demonstrated an average annual incidence and prevalence of 17 and 223, respectively, per 100 000 inhabitants aged 50 years or more. The age-adjusted incidence rates were approximately three times greater in women than in men. In addition, the incidence increased in both sexes with old age. The incidence also increased significantly during the period 1950–1985 for females, but decreased in males over the same period (Fig. 147.1)[12]. In Olmsted County, there has been a steady increase of polymyalgia rheumatica, from 7.3 per 100 000 to 19.1 per 100 000 inhabitants aged more than 50 years[13]. The predicted rate of increase was 2.6% every 5 years. Similar increases have been reported from Spain[14] and Scandinavia[15]. The Olmsted County study identified peaks occurring every 7 years, a finding that could be consistent with an infectious etiology[13] (see section on Pathogenesis, below).

The incidence rates reported from Olmsted County are similar to those in Göteborg, Sweden. In a study of 284 biopsy-proven cases of giant cell arteritis collected over a 10-year period (1977–1986) in Göteborg, Nordborg and Bengtsson[16] observed an incidence rate among those aged 50 years or more of 18.3 per 100 000; for women the rate was 25 per 100 000 and for men it was 9.4 per 100 000. The temporal arteries and aorta of all adults who died in Malmö throughout 1 year were examined by Ostberg[17], and although active temporal arteritis was not found, evidence of previous arteritis was found in 1.7% of the 889 cases. It was found that in 75% of these individuals there had been either biopsy evidence or a clinical history suggestive of temporal arteritis.

The epidemiology of polymyalgia rheumatica has been less well defined. Silman and Currey[18] found three cases of polymyalgia among 247 persons older than 65 years who were resident in old peoples' homes and or attending day centers. Only one case had been previously diagnosed. Kyle et al.[19], using a similar questionnaire in 656 patients older than 65 years, found a prevalence of arteritis/polymyalgia of 3300 per 100 000.

Familial aggregation of polymyalgia rheumatica and giant cell arteritis has been reported by several workers. Liang et al. in 1974[20] described four pairs of first-degree relatives, and they noted a further six pairs in the world literature. Clustering of cases in time and space was seen in Liang's study and suggested that, in addition to a genetic predisposition, environmental factors may be important. Rhodes[21] noted that nine of 11 cases seen over 6 years in a practice of 3000 lived in one small part of the same village, and of these, two lived in the same house, two were neighbors and two others were close friends.

IMMUNOGENETICS

The increased prevalence of cases of polymyalgia rheumatica and giant cell arteritis in individuals of European background, compared with other populations, has suggested a genetic relationship. In polymyalgia rheumatica, most genetic studies have involved human leukocyte antigen (HLA) typing using serologic methods. Class I antigens have shown variable results, which suggests that a significant relationship is unlikely.

Human leukocyte antigens in susceptibility to giant cell arteritis and polymyalgia rheumatica

Giant cell arteritis is the best example of an association between vasculitis and genes that lie within the HLA class II region[22]. Most studies have shown an association with *HLA-DRB1*04* alleles[14]. In addition, the severity and risk of visual complications is also associated with *HLA-DRB1*04* alleles.

Polymyalgia rheumatica is associated with *HLA* class II genes, but this varies from one population to another[23]. Relapses of polymyalgia rheumatica, however, have been found to be significantly more common in patients who have the *HLA-DRB1*04* allele, and particularly in those carrying the *HLA-DRB1*0401* allele[14]. A lack of homozygosity of the shared epitope in giant cell arteritis has been reported; this contrasts with observations in rheumatoid arthritis, in which homozygosity of the shared epitope is associated with more severe disease. It has been suggested that the pathology seen in giant cell arteritis may be due to antigenic cross-reactivity after exposure to an infectious agent.

Clonal expansion of T lymphocytes with identical T cell antigen receptor b chains in distinct inflammatory foci within the same temporal artery has been demonstrated in giant cell arteritis, consistent with T-cell activation within the arterial wall in response to disease-specific antigen. This concept gains support by sequence analysis of the *HLA-DRB1* allelic variants, which shows that *DR4*-positive and *DR4*-negative patients share a 'disease associated' sequence of the same four amino acids (DRYF). This 'motif' maps to the second hypervariable region located in the antigen-binding groove of the *HLA-DR* molecule[24]. Patients rarely suffer from both giant cell arteritis and rheumatoid arthritis, consistent with the view that different and distinct domains of the *HLA-DR* molecule are important in determining susceptibility to the two diseases.

Role of tumor necrosis factor in susceptibility to giant cell arteritis and polymyalgia rheumatica

It is likely that other genetic factors may contribute to the susceptibility to these conditions. However, concentrations of tumour necrosis factor (TNF)-α have not been found to be increased in either condition. In Northwestern Spain[25], giant cell arteritis and polymyalgia rheumatica are associated with different TNF microsatellite polymorphisms. Giant cell arteritis is associated with the allele encoding the TNF-α2 microsatellite; this is largely independent of the association of giant cell arteritis with *HLA* class II genes. In contrast, patients with polymyalgia rheumatica have a positive association with TNF-β3, which is also independent of the *HLA* class II genes. Therefore TNF and HLA associations appear to be able to influence susceptibility to these conditions independently of each other[26]. In addition, genetic polymorphisms in endothelial cell adhesion molecules have also been considered to be important candidate susceptibility factors for giant cell arteritis and polymyalgia rheumatica. Recently, Boiardi and colleagues[27] reported a significant association between susceptibility to polymyalgia rheumatica and the interleukin (IL)-1 *RN*2* allele, particularly in the homozygous state.

CLINICAL FEATURES

The mean age at onset of giant cell arteritis and polymyalgia rheumatica is approximately 70 years, with a range of about 50 to more than 90 years of age. Women are twice as likely to be affected as men. The onset of the disease can be dramatic, and some patients can give the date and hour of their first symptom. Equally, the onset can be insidious. In most instances, the symptoms have been present for weeks or months before the diagnosis is established.

Constitutional symptoms, including fever, fatigue, anorexia and weight loss, and depression, are present in the majority of patients. Patients may present with pyrexia/fever of unknown origin and subjected to many investigations. Giant cell arteritis accounts for about 15% of patients older than 65 years presenting with fever of unknown origin. A hidden malignancy can mimic the symptoms of polymyalgia rheumatica. Although, at present, there is no evidence to suggest that malignancy is more common in patients with polymyalgia than in other people, deterioration in health or a poor initial response to corticosteroids must always be taken seriously and a search for an occult neoplasm made. In some cases, onset is associated with recent bereavement.

Polymyalgia rheumatica
Musculoskeletal involvement
Patients usually locate the source of their pain and stiffness to the muscles. The onset is most common in the shoulder region and neck, with eventual

involvement of the shoulder and pelvic girdles and the corresponding proximal muscle groups. Involvement of distal limb muscles is unusual. The symptoms are usually bilateral and symmetric. Stiffness is usually the predominant feature, is particularly severe after rest, and may prevent the patient from getting out of bed in the morning. The muscular pain is often diffuse and movement accentuates the pain; pain at night is common. Muscle strength is usually unimpaired, although the pain makes interpretation of muscle testing difficult. There is tenderness of involved structures, including periarticular structures such as bursae, tendons and joint capsules. In late stages, muscle atrophy may develop, with restriction of shoulder movement that rapidly improves with corticosteroid treatment. Occasionally, the painful arc sign of subacromial bursitis is present; this is important to recognize, as a local injection of corticosteroid will give relief and save the patient from an increase in systemic corticosteroid dosage.

Synovitis

Inflammatory synovitis and effusions have been noted by several authors, the reported incidence varying from 0 to 100% in various series[28]. Synovitis of the knees, wrists and sternoclavicular joints is most common, but involvement is transient and mild. An association between carpal tunnel syndrome and polymyalgia has been noted by several authors. Erosive changes in joints or sclerosis of the sacroiliac joints, or both, have been reported, although they are difficult to demonstrate in the sternoclavicular joints other than by tomography. Abnormal technetium pertechnetate scintigrams have shown widespread uptake over joints, particularly shoulders, knees, wrists and hands.

The synovial tissue shows non-specific inflammatory changes and the synovial fluid has the appearance of a mild inflammatory exudate. The synovitis of polymyalgia differs from that of rheumatoid arthritis in that it does not cause typical juxta-articular osteoporosis and erosions. The discrepancies in frequency of synovitis reported in various studies may be due to differing diagnostic criteria, the definition of synovitis and difficulty in interpretation of scans and radiographs because of coexisting degenerative disease.

Inflammation of synovial cavities and bursae is a common feature of shoulders in polymyalgia rheumatica on histology[29], magnetic resonance imaging and ultrasound assessment[30]. These findings rapidly improve after a few days of corticosteroid treatment. These findings are also seen in patients with symptoms of polymyalgia rheumatica with a normal erythrocyte sedimentation rate (ESR). It has been suggested that this is the basis for the diffuse symptoms in polymyalgia rheumatica. Nevertheless the symptomatology of polymyalgia rheumatica is difficult to explain on the basis of synovitis alone. McGonagle and colleagues[31] have recently demonstrated extracapsular abnormalities in the shoulder of early polymyalgia rheumatica by magnetic resonance imaging. This could explain the diffuse nature of the symptoms.

Salvarani and Hunder[24] have also described peripheral synovitis, distal extremity swelling with pitting edema, and tenosynovitis and carpal tunnel compression in patients with polymyalgia rheumatica and giant cell arteritis.

Kassimos et al.[32] examined the hypothesis that cytidine deaminase may be useful in the differentiation of polymyalgia rheumatica and RA. The mean serum cytidine deaminase concentrations were significantly greater in patients with rheumatoid arthritis compared with those with polymyalgia rheumatica and giant cell arteritis, suggesting that measurement of cytidine deaminase may be a useful laboratory parameter to help distinguish between the two conditions.

Giant cell arteritis

Giant cell arteritis causes a wide range of symptoms, but most patients have clinical features related to affected arteries. Common features include fatigue, headache and tenderness of the scalp, particularly around the temporal and occipital arteries.

Headache

Headache is the most common symptom and is present in 67% or more of patients. It usually begins early in the course of the disease and may be the presenting symptom. The pain is severe and localized to the temple. However, it may be occipital or be less defined and precipitated by brushing the hair. It can be severe even when the arteries are clinically normal and, conversely, may subside even though the disease remains active. The nature of the pain varies; it is described by some patients as shooting and by others as a more steady ache. Scalp tenderness is common, particularly around the temporal and occipital arteries, and may disturb sleep. Tender spots or nodules, or even small skin infarcts, may be present (Fig. 147.2). The vessels are thickened, tender and nodular, with absent or reduced pulsation (Fig. 147.3). Occasionally, they are red and clearly visible.

Ophthalmic features

Visual disturbances have been described in 25–50% of cases of giant cell arteritis. The incidence of visual loss is now regarded as much lower, about 6–10% in most series, probably because of earlier recognition and treatment.

There are a variety of ocular lesions that are essentially caused by occlusion of the various orbital or ocular arteries (Table 147.1 &

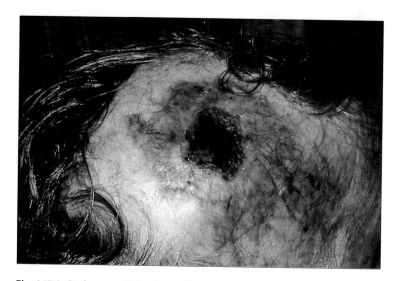

Fig. 147.2 Scalp necrosis in giant cell arteritis.

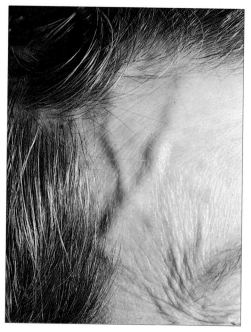

Fig. 147.3 Dilated temporal arteries in a patient with giant cell arteritis.

TABLE 147.1 OCULAR LESIONS IN GIANT CELL ARTERITIS

Lesions	Feature
Optic nerve ischemic lesions:	
Anterior ischemic optic neuropathy	The most common lesion and associated with partial or, more frequently, complete visual loss
Posterior ischemic optic neuropathy	Less common and may cause partial or complete visual loss
Retinal ischemic lesions:	
Central retinal artery occlusion	Leads to severe visual loss
Cilioretinal artery occlusion	Seen occasionally and associated with anterior ischemic optic neuropathy
Choroidal infarcts	Seen rarely
Extraocular motility disorders	Seen rarely and not usually associated with visual loss
Anterior segment ischemic lesions	Seen rarely and not usually associated with visual loss
Pupillary abnormalities	Usually secondary to visual loss
Cerebral ischemic lesions	Associated visual loss is rare

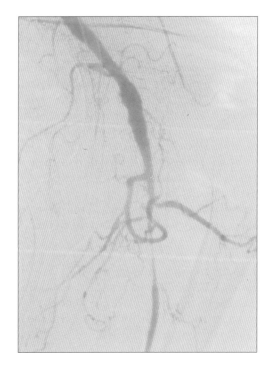

Fig. 147.5 Arteriogram showing narrowing of axillary artery in giant cell arteritis.

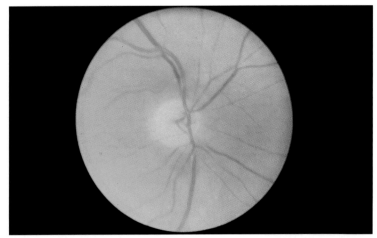

Fig. 147.4 Fundus photograph showing optic atrophy secondary to giant cell arteritis.

Fig. 147.4). Blindness is the most serious and irreversible feature. The visual loss is usually sudden, painless and permanent; it may vary from mistiness of vision, or involvement of a part of the visual field, to complete blindness. There is a risk of the second eye being involved if the patient is not treated aggressively. Blindness may be the initial presentation of giant cell arteritis, but tends to follow other symptoms by several weeks or months[33], premonitory symptoms including blurring of vision or amaurosis fugax or visual hallucinations. Visual symptoms are an ophthalmic emergency; if they are identified and treated urgently, blindness is almost entirely preventable.

The most common ocular lesion resulting from occlusion of orbital or ocular arteries is anterior ischemic optic neuropathy (AION) which usually leads to complete visual loss. In a series of 800 patients with this condition, 12% were found to have the arteritic form[34]. Features suggesting arteritic anterior ischemic optic neuropathy included systemic symptoms, an increased ESR, amaurosis fugax and early visual loss. A chalky white disc was highly suggestive of the arteritic form. Optic disc edema was associated with cilioretinal occlusion and was caused by arteritis. Early non-filling of the choroid on angiography was also associated with arteritis.

Extraocular motility disorders are usually transient and not associated with visual loss. Pupillary abnormalities can be seen secondary to visual

loss. Cerebral ischemic lesions producing visual loss are rare, as are anterior segment ischemic lesions and choroidal infarcts. Retinal ischemic lesions can affect the central retinal artery; this is associated with severe visual loss.

Other symptoms

Pain on chewing, resulting from claudication of the jaw muscles, occurs in up to 67% of patients. Tingling in the tongue, loss of taste, and pain in the mouth and throat can also occur, presumably because of vascular insufficiency.

Less common features of giant cell arteritis include hemiparesis, peripheral neuropathy, deafness, depression and confusion. Involvement of the coronary arteries may lead to myocardial infarction. Aortic regurgitation and congestive cardiac failure may also occur. Abnormalities of thyroid and liver function are well described.

Clinical evidence of large artery involvement is present in 10–15% of cases (Fig. 147.5), and in some instances aortic dissection and rupture occur. Bruits are often present over large arteries and there may be tenderness, particularly over the subclavian artery. An early sign of arteritis

TABLE 147.2 ACR CRITERIA FOR THE CLASSIFICATION OF GIANT CELL ARTERITIS

Criterion	Definition
1. Age at onset >50 years	Development of symptoms or findings beginning aged 50 years or older
2. New headache	New onset of, or new type of, localized pains in the head
3. Temporal artery abnormality	Temporal artery tenderness to palpation or decreased pulsation, unrelated to atherosclerosis of cervical arteries
4. Increased ESR	ESR >50mm/h by Westergren method
5. Abnormal artery biopsy	Biopsy specimen with artery showing vasculitis characterized by a predominance of mononuclear cell infiltration or granulomatous inflammation

A classification of giant cell arteritis requires three of the five criteria.
(From Hunder et al.[35])

is increased sensitivity of the carotid sinus. Light pressure will often lead to transient asystole for two or more beats, so it is advisable for the patient to be lying down when examined.

CLASSIFICATION/DIAGNOSTIC CRITERIA FOR GIANT CELL ARTERITIS/POLYMYALGIA RHEUMATICA

The cause of giant cell arteritis and polymyalgia rheumatic is unknown, and in neither is there a single diagnostic test. As a result, a combination of findings is needed for their diagnosis. The American College of Rheumatology has established criteria for the classification of giant cell arteritis[35] (Table 147.2). Their criteria are best used in research studies involving patients with a diagnosis of vasculitis.

As polymyalgia can mimic a number of different clinical conditions, there should ideally be clear criteria that enable the diagnosis to be made. Currently, there are a number of different criteria sets, all of which differ slightly. The attraction of the criteria proposed by Bird and colleagues[36] (Table 147.3) lies in its practical application in clinical practice. A diagnosis requires three of the seven listed features; the presence of just three features confirms a sensitivity of 92% and a specificity of 80%.

The differential diagnosis between polymyalgia rheumatica and elderly-onset rheumatoid arthritis can be difficult because these conditions may have similar clinical presentations. At present there are no clinical or routine laboratory features allowing early differentiation between polymyalgia rheumatica and rheumatoid arthritis with a polymyalgia rheumatica-like onset. After a 1-year study, 20% of patients presenting with an initial diagnosis of polymyalgia rheumatica developed rheumatoid arthritis[37].

RELATIONSHIP BETWEEN POLYMYALGIA RHEUMATICA AND GIANT CELL ARTERITIS

In recent years, giant cell arteritis and polymyalgia rheumatica have been considered as closely related conditions that form a spectrum of diseases. The conditions may occur independently or may occur in the same patient, either together or separated by time. Certainly, it is difficult to maintain a practical distinction between them by clinical or histologic criteria. Some patients originally suffering from polymyalgia rheumatica have later had symptoms of cranial arteritis, and in a number of patients with typical myalgia and no symptoms from the temporal region, biopsies have shown arteritic changes. Systemic involvement is similar in groups with or without clinical or biopsy evidence of arteritis.

Among patients with polymyalgia rheumatica who have no symptoms or signs of arteritis, positive temporal biopsies are found in 10–15%. There are many similarities between the two conditions. The age and sex distribution is similar, the biopsy findings show an identical pattern and the laboratory features are similar, even though many are non-specific inflammatory changes. In addition, there is similarity in the myalgia, the

associated systemic features and in the response to corticosteroid treatment.

The onset of myalgic symptoms may precede, coincide with or follow that of the arteritic symptoms. No difference has been found between the characteristics of those myalgic patients with a positive biopsy and those with no histologic evidence of arteritis. Mild aching and stiffness may persist for months after other features of giant cell arteritis have remitted. There is little evidence to suggest that the musculoskeletal symptoms are related to vasculitis. Many patients with giant cell arteritis do not have polymyalgia rheumatica, even when large vessels are involved.

MALIGNANCY IN ASSOCIATION WITH POLYMYALGIA RHEUMATICA AND GIANT CELL ARTERITIS

A syndrome resembling giant cell arteritis or polymyalgia rheumatica may occasionally present as a paraneoplastic phenomenon, with a close relationship between the onset of symptoms and the appearance of malignancy. However, several studies have failed to demonstrate that patients with giant cell arteritis or polymyalgia rheumatica appear susceptible to cancer[38]. None of the studies compared the patient population with matched controls, and studies suffered from small numbers and short follow up. Haga and colleagues, who carried out a prospective study using matched controls in the early 1990s[39], showed that patients with a positive biopsy had an increased risk of cancer compared with matched controls. The onset of malignancy was a mean of 6.5 years from diagnosis of giant cell arteritis.

INVESTIGATIONS

The ESR is usually greatly increased in polymyalgia rheumatica/giant cell arteritis and provides a useful means of monitoring treatment, although it must be appreciated that some increase in the ESR may occur in otherwise healthy elderly people. A normal ESR is occasionally found in patients with active biopsy-proven disease[40], and patients with a low ESR at diagnosis had similar clinical characteristics and course of disease as patients with a high ESR at diagnosis[41]. Some investigators have reported varying percentages (7–20%) of patients with polymyalgia rheumatica who had a normal ESR (<40mm/h) at diagnosis.

Anemia, usually of a mild hypochromic type, is common and resolves without specific treatment, but a more marked normochromic anemia occasionally occurs and may be a presenting symptom. Leukocyte and differential counts are generally normal; platelet counts are also usually normal, but may be increased. Protein electrophoresis may show a non-specific increase in α_2-globulin, with less frequent increase in α_1-globulin and gammaglobulin. Quantification of the acute-phase proteins and α_1-antitrypsin, orosomucoid, haptoglobin and C-reactive protein are no more helpful than ESR in the assessment of disease activity[42]. Measurement of α_1-antichymotrypsin concentrations may help in management[43].

Abnormalities of thyroid and liver function have also been well described. In patients with hyperthyroidism, arteritis follows the thyrotoxicosis by intervals of 4–15 years. Individual cases of hypothyroidism have also been reported.

Increased serum values for alkaline phosphatase are commonly found in polymyalgia rheumatica. Sulfobromophthalein retention is also often abnormal and transaminases may be mildly increased. Liver biopsies have shown portal and intralobular inflammation, with focal liver cell necrosis and small epithelioid cell granuloma. Abnormal liver scans may also occur. In patients presenting with non-specific features, the findings of abnormal liver function tests and abnormal scans may be misleading and prompt investigations for malignancy.

A significant number of patients with polymyalgia rheumatica or giant cell arteritis, or both, have increased concentrations of anticardiolipin

TABLE 147.3 BIRD AND COWORKERS' CRITERIA FOR THE DIAGNOSIS OF PMR/GCA[36]
• Age >65 years
• ESR >40mm/h
• Bilateral upper arm tenderness
• Morning stiffness >1 hour
• Onset of illness within 2 weeks
• Depression or weight loss, or both
Diagnosis requires three of the seven listed features. Presence of just three features confirms a sensitivity of 92% and a specificity of 80%.
GCA, giant cell arteritis; PMR, polymyalgia rheumatica.

antibody at presentation[44]. These patients appear to be at increased risk of developing giant cell arteritis or other major vascular complications. It is possible that anticardiolipin may be an independent prognostic marker for future vascular complications with polymyalgia rheumatica or giant cell arteritis. Other studies have shown that anticardiolipin concentrations are greater in patients with active arteritis and decrease rapidly after corticosteroid treatment.

Temporal artery biopsy

Clinicians vary greatly in their approach to temporal artery biopsy. Some emphasize the value of a positive histologic diagnosis, especially months or years later, when side effects of the corticosteroid treatment have developed. Others feel that a high false-negative rate diminishes the value of the procedure. In most instances, the high false-negative rate can be attributed to the focal nature and involvement of the superficial temporal artery by the inflammatory process. A pragmatic policy would include the following:

● Perform biopsy if diagnosis is in doubt, particularly if systemic symptoms predominate
● Biopsy is most useful within 24 hours of starting treatment, but do not delay treatment for sake of biopsy. The artery biopsy will still show inflammatory changes for several days after corticosteroids have been started
● A negative biopsy does not exclude giant cell arteritis
● A positive result helps to prevent later doubts about diagnosis, particularly if treatment causes complications.

A third of patients with signs and symptoms of cranial arteritis may have a negative temporal artery biopsy, which may be the result of localized involvement of arteries in the head and neck. 'Skip' lessons are evident in about 67% of biopsies; some segments showing active disease are as short as 350μm[45]. The rate of false-negative biopsies depends on many variables, including the size of the biopsy, the number of levels examined, whether biopsies were taken from one or both sides of the scalp, and the duration of corticosteroid treatment before the procedure.

Involvement of the temporal arteries occasionally occurs in vasculitides other than giant cell arteritis, among which polyarteritis nodosa appears to be the most common[46]. There have also been sporadic reports of temporal artery involvement in Churg–Strauss syndrome, Wegener's granulomatosis, microscopic polyangiitis, cryoglobulinemia or rheumatoid vasculitis[47].

Occasionally, a temporal artery biopsy reveals small-vessel vasculitis surrounding a spared temporal artery. Esteban and colleagues performed a clinical and histological study of 28 patients with small-vessel vasculitis surrounding a spared temporal artery[48]. The diagnosis of giant cell arteritis can be reasonably established in most of these patients when there is no apparent evidence of additional organ involvement. However, when fibrinoid necrosis is observed or the temporal artery vasa vasorum are not involved, then systemic necrotizing vasculitis must be excluded.

Color Doppler ultrasonography can be used to examine the superficial arteries and is a new, non-invasive method for the diagnosis of giant cell arteritis. Findings include a hypoechoic wall thickening (halo) caused by edema. It disappears within 16 days of corticosteroid treatment in giant cell arteritis[49]. Color Doppler can detect stenosis and occlusion, and is confirmed by simultaneous pulsed-wave Doppler ultrasound. In the cases with abnormal findings, biopsy can be performed to confirm the diagnosis of giant cell arteritis.

Magnetic resonance imaging can demonstrate large-vessel vasculitis in giant cell arteritis, and preliminary positron emission tomography scanning reports support the concept that large-vessel vasculitis may be common in polymyalgia rheumatica[50].

DIFFERENTIAL DIAGNOSIS

The diagnosis of polymyalgia rheumatica is initially one of exclusion. The differential diagnosis (Table 147.4) in an elderly patient with muscle pain, stiffness and a increased ESR is wide, because the prodromal phases of several serious conditions can mimic it. Despite a typical pattern of musculoskeletal symptoms and the presence, in many, of significant systemic features, there is often a considerable delay of several months before diagnosis. Polymyalgia rheumatica can usually be differentiated from late-onset rheumatoid arthritis by the absence of prominent peripheral joint pain and swelling. In patients with polymyositis, the muscular weakness is the predominant factor limiting movement, whereas in polymyalgia rheumatica, pain causes limited function.

The diagnosis of giant cell arteritis should be considered in any patient over the age of 50 years who has recent onset of headache, transient or sudden loss of vision, myalgia, unexplained fever or anemia or an increased ESR. Because the symptoms and signs may vary in severity and be transient, patients must be questioned carefully about recent and current symptoms. The arteries of the head, neck and limbs should be examined for tenderness, enlargement, thrombosis and bruits. Angiography of the temporal arteries is not usually helpful – there is no characteristic abnormality, and false-positives (usually attributable to atheroma) are not uncommon. An angiographic examination of the aortic arch and its branches may prove helpful in patients with symptoms of large-artery involvement. There is usually little difficulty in separating giant cell arteritis from other forms of arteritis, because of the different distribution of lesions, histopathology and organ involvement.

PATHOLOGY

The histologic appearance of giant cell arteritis is one of the most distinctive of vascular disorders. The dense granulomatous inflammatory infiltrates that characterize the acute stages of the disease resemble those of Takayasu's arteritis, but the clinicopathologic features in patients with positive temporal artery biopsies are diagnostic. The arteritis is histologically a panarteritis with giant cell granuloma formation, often in close proximity to a disrupted internal elastic lamina. Large and medium-sized arteries are affected, the involvement is patchy and skip lesions are often found. There is preferential involvement of muscular arteries with well developed internal and external elastic laminae.

The gross features are not characteristic. The vessels are enlarged and nodular and have little or no lumen. Thrombosis often develops at sites of active inflammation. Later, these areas may recanalize. The lumen is narrowed by intimal proliferation (Fig. 147.6). This is a common finding in arteries and may result from advancing age, nearby

TABLE 147.4 DIFFERENTIAL DIAGNOSIS OF POLYMYALGIA RHEUMATICA	
Neoplastic disease	Muscle disease
Joint disease	Polymyositis
Osteoarthritis, particularly of cervical spine	Myopathy
Rheumatoid arthritis	Infections, e.g. bacterial endocarditis
Connective tissue disease	Bone disease, particularly osteomyelitis
Multiple myeloma	Hypothyroidism
Leukemia	Parkinsonism
Lymphoma	Functional

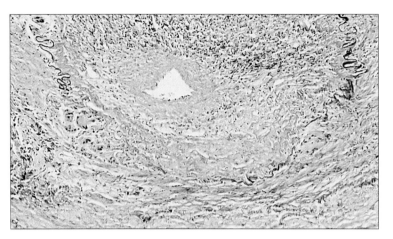

Fig. 147.6 Elastic stain of temporal artery, showing disruption of elastic lamina in giant cell arteritis, and narrowing of the lumen.

chronic inflammation or low blood flow. The adventitia is usually invaded by mononuclear, and occasionally polymorphonuclear, inflammatory cells. There is cuffing of the vasa vasorum and fibrous proliferation is frequent. The changes in the media are dominated by the giant cells, which vary from small cells with two to three nuclei up to masses of 100μm containing many nuclei. There is invasion by mononuclear cells resembling histiocytes. Fibrinoid necrosis is infrequent. Giant cells are not seen in all sections, and therefore are not required for the diagnosis if other features are compatible; however, the more sections that are examined in the area of arteritis, the more likely it is that giant cells will be found.

A progression of changes can be demonstrated, from the active infiltrative phase to the scarred artery with little cellular infiltrate. At first, the most severe changes are centered on the internal elastic lamina, which becomes swollen and fragmented. Fragments of elastic tissue can be demonstrated within giant cells, which are surrounded with plasma cell and lymphocytic infiltration (Fig. 147.7). The findings of electron microscopy studies have suggested that altered or damaged smooth muscle cells are critical in the pathogenesis.

Histologic changes also occur in temporal arteries with advancing age; they differ only in degree with those encountered in giant cell arteritis and it can sometimes be difficult to distinguish between them. However, an inflammatory cell infiltrate does not occur, except in relationship to

large plaques of atherosclerosis. The degree of intimal thickening in arteritis is usually greater, a well-developed smooth muscle layer is seen by the lumen, and loss of the internal elastic lamina is considerable. The histologic changes of healed arteritis include medial chronic inflammation with ingrowth of new blood vessels, focal medial scarring and a bizarre pattern of intimal fibrosis; the last is the most important change. The biopsy finding of healed vasculitis by no means excludes the possibility of active lesions elsewhere. Not infrequently, episodes of vasculitis are recurrent. The widespread nature of the vasculitis has been well documented, and occasionally veins are affected.

Involvement of the aorta and its branches, the abdominal vessels and the coronary arteries have all been described. Giant cell arteritis as a cause of aortic dissection has been recorded rarely at autopsy, and most exceptionally during life. Most patients had a history of hypertension in life or other features of hypertensive disease at autopsy. In addition, the majority of patients described in the literature are women[51].

Although there is a high incidence of involvement of the head and neck vessels in giant cell arteritis, it is interesting that the intracranial vessels are seldom involved. Wilkinson and Russell[52] studied the head and neck vessels and demonstrated a close correlation between susceptibility to arteritis and the amount of elastic tissue present in the arterial wall. The greatest incidence of severe involvement was noted in the superficial temporal arteries, vertebral arteries and ophthalmic and posterior ciliary arteries. The internal carotid, external carotid and central retinal arteries were affected less frequently (Fig. 147.8). In some instances, follow-up biopsy or autopsy surveys showed persistence of mild chronic inflammation even though symptoms had resolved.

There has been little to support a concept of primary muscle disease in polymyalgia rheumatica. Serum aldolase and creatine phosphokinase are normal, and there is no abnormality on electromyography. Muscle biopsy has shown type II atrophy alone and there is no evidence of inflammatory changes[53]. Recently there have been reports of focal changes in muscle ultrastructure and abnormalities of mitochondrial form and function, similar to those associated with inherited mitochondrial myopathies. These abnormalities are not caused by gene deletions or mutations associated with mitochondrial myopathy, and persist even after successful treatment. Arteritis in skeletal muscle appears to be uncommon.

Liver biopsy can show non-specific inflammatory changes or focal liver cell necrosis. There are occasional reports of granulomata and

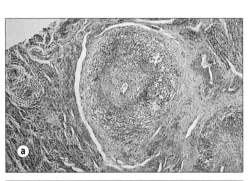
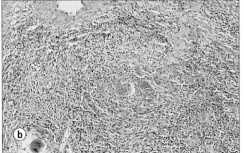

Fig. 147.7 Histology of giant cell arteritis. (a) Low-powered view of arterial wall, showing infiltration by lymphocytes and plasma cells. (b) High-powered view showing giant cells in close relationship to elastic lamina.

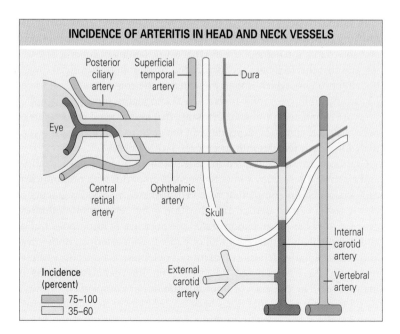

Fig. 147.8 Incidence of arteritis in pathologic study of head and neck vessels.

hepatic arteritis. Synovial biopsy has shown non-specific inflammatory changes with lymphocytic infiltration of knees, sternoclavicular joints and shoulders.

ETIOLOGY AND PATHOGENESIS

At present it is impossible to define the underlying pathologic abnormality in polymyalgia and, indeed, it may well be that there are several different mechanisms responsible for a largely similar pattern of pain. The relative homogeneity of groups of patients and the apparent rapid clinical response to corticosteroids do not exclude this possibility. Although the increasing incidence of giant cell arteritis and polymyalgia rheumatica after the age of 50 years implies a relationship with aging, the significance of this observation is not understood.

A distinct prodromal event resembling influenza or viral pneumonia is often noted by patients. However, viral studies have generally produced negative results. In studies by Bacon et al.[54], hepatitis antigen was not found in any of 12 patients with polymyalgia, although hepatitis B surface antibody was found in nine patients.

Parvovirus B19 infection occurs in epidemic cycles similar to those seen in giant cell arteritis. Salvarani and colleagues[55] have recently used the polymerase chain reaction technique to demonstrate the presence of parvovirus B19 DNA in temporal artery biopsy specimens.

Cimmino and colleagues[56] reported an increase in antibody to respiratory syncytial virus and adenovirus and Duhaut et al.[57] performed a large case–control study suggesting that reinfection with human parainfluenza virus (a virus known to induce human multinucleated giant cells) is associated with the onset of giant cell arteritis, particularly in those with a positive biopsy. No association was seen with other viruses that induce multinucleated giant cells, such as measles, herpes simplex, Epstein–Barr and respiratory syncytial viruses.

In Denmark, peak incidences were correlated with occurrences of Mycoplasma pneumoniae infection[58]. Using a matched case–control method, Russo et al.[59] showed a correlation between infection and onset of giant cell arteritis, but could not identify a specific infection. In addition to cyclic peaks, occasional clusters have been reported; in Jerusalem, Sonnenblick and colleagues[60] observed five cases in a 7-week period when the expected background rate was one case per year. A seasonal pattern of onset has been reported in several studies, but the precise season of maximum occurrence has not been consistent and some studies have failed to document a seasonal effect.

In summary, despite large studies looking for an infectious etiology, no unifying hypothesis has emerged. Cimmino[61] has proposed that infrared and solar radiation damage the internal elastic lamina of superficial arteries, and that this facilitates the localization of an unknown antigen (possibly viral protein), which is then presented in the context of class II major histocompatibility complex molecules. Macrophages and CD4+ lymphocytes are stimulated, producing cytokines that lead to giant cell arteritis or polymyalgia rheumatica, depending on the pattern. This process is accentuated in elderly females with specific HLA-DRB1 alleles.

Giant cell arteritis is limited to vessels with an internal elastic lamina, and electron microscopy shows fragmentation of this with mononuclear cell accumulation compatible with cell-mediated injury. Fragments of elastic tissue can be demonstrated within giant cells. Immunofluorescence studies have also demonstrated the presence of immunoglobulins and complement in the vessel wall of patients with arteritis., Both intra- and extracellularly, deposits of all immunoglobulin classes plus complement (C3) have been noted, adjacent to the internal elastic lamina in many cases. The presence of immunoglobulin or complement within a lesion does not prove that it has been caused by hypersensitivity; rather, it may reflect non-specific immune complex deposition at the site of vascular injury of different cause. Using an immunoperoxidase method, Gallagher and Jones[62] found only intracellular deposits and did not

detect extracellular complement. This pattern of intracytoplasmic staining for immunoglobulins would be anticipated in any chronic inflammatory reaction. It is possible that the changes reflect a non-specific reaction to injury. Immunoglobulin and complement deposition may occur in the synovium in polymyalgia rheumatica, but there are few systematic studies. Dasgupta et al.[63] have reported antibodies against intermediate filaments in 67% of patients at the onset of giant cell arteritis. Antibodies against intermediate filaments are found in viral infections and autoimmune diseases.

Increased numbers of circulating lymphoblasts are seen in patients with active polymyalgia rheumatica, and immunoglobulins are also increased. These observations have led to the suggestion that these diseases may have an immunologic basis, perhaps an age-related autoimmune process directed against arterial wall constituents. The cells from patients with active untreated giant cell arteritis or polymyalgia rheumatica show no difference from normal controls with respect to in vitro lymphocytotoxicity to arterial smooth muscle. The lymphocytes in the arteritic lesions express the T cell phenotype and only a few B cells are found[64].

Lesional T cells are predominately of the CD4 subtype, and produce interferon-γ and IL-2, together with the macrophage products IL-1β, IL-6 and transforming growth factor-β, leading to local and systemic inflammation. They are also the likely source of matrix metalloproteinase 2, and a growth factor for smooth muscle cells, platelet-derived growth factor, which have been implicated in the narrowing and constriction of affected blood vessels[65]. In an animal model of giant cell arteritis in which temporal arteries are implanted onto severe combined immunodeficient mice, arterial T cells are vital to the occurrence of inflammation[66]. T cell clonotypes with identical T cell receptor molecules have been isolated from separate vascular lesions[67]. Immunogenetic studies indicate an association with HLA-DR4[68] and more specifically with HLA DRB*0401[23]. These findings suggest that inflammation in giant cell arteritis is an antigen-driven T-cell-mediated immune process, but the nature of the antigen remains unknown.

Macrophages, epithelioid cells and giant cells are seen in the arterial wall and the majority express HLA-DR antigen, in addition to the adhesion molecules lymphocyte function-associated antigens (LFA)-1 and -3 and intercellular adhesion molecule (ICAM)-1. About 25% of the infiltrating T cells express the HLA-DR antigen and the integrin receptor, vascular leucocyte antigen (VLA)-1, which suggests that these cells are immunologically activated. Further support for a local activation of the T cells is the finding of IL-2 receptors on the lymphocytes from biopsy specimens[69]. The expression of IL-2 receptors on lymphocytes is not as frequent as that of HLA-DR. The reason for this discrepancy is not known, but is seen in other inflammatory lesions. Roche et al.[69] also reported interdigitating reticulum cells in 40% of patients with biopsy-proven giant cell arteritis; these were seen in patients with a shorter disease duration. It has been suggested that interdigitating reticulum cells are seen in lesions in which a local stimulus for an immune response is suspected, but not in diseases caused by immune complexes or degenerative processes. Both IL-2 and interferon-γ are produced by cells located in the inflamed arterial wall. Circulating concentrations of IL-6 are increased, with normal concentrations of TNF-α both in patients with an arteritic presentation of giant cell arteritis and in those presenting with polymyalgia rheumatica. A selective depletion of circulating CD8 T lymphocytes in patients with giant cell arteritis has been observed in most studies. No increase in expression of HLA-DR has been found on circulatory CD4+ T cells; this contrasts with the high incidence on the T lymphocytes in the arterial wall. The surface expression of ICAM-1 by smooth muscle cells within granulomata in the arterial wall in giant cell arteritis might be exposing these cells to LFA-1-mediated macrophage and cytotoxic T cell attack, and suggests that smooth muscle may be an important immune target in giant cell arteritis.

It has been proposed that a serum toxic factor leads to endothelial breakdown and then to disruption of the internal elastic lamina. Elastin fragments are chemotactic to monocytes that have elastolytic potential; this is increased in giant cell arteritis. Also, linear deposits of leukocyte elastase are found along the fragmented internal elastic lamina.

Aging of the immune and neuroendocrine systems may be important factors in the late onset of giant cell arteritis. Breakdown in tolerance, increased susceptibility to infectious triggers or perpetuation of inflammation as a result of relative cortisol deficiency are possible mechanisms. Basal cortisol concentrations are increased in the elderly, but the release of cortisol in response to stress is attenuated.

MANAGEMENT

Corticosteroids are mandatory in the treatment of giant cell arteritis; they reduce the incidence of complications such as blindness and rapidly relieve symptoms. Non-steroidal anti-inflammatory drugs (NSAIDs) will lessen the painful symptoms, but they do not prevent arteritic complications. The response to corticosteroids is usually dramatic, and occurs within days. Corticosteroid treatment has improved the quality of life for patients, although there is no evidence that treatment reduces the duration of the disease. A fear of vascular complications in those patients with a positive biopsy often leads to the use of high doses of corticosteroids. Recent studies have emphasized the importance of adopting a cautious and individual treatment schedule, and have highlighted the efficacy of lower doses of prednisolone.

Initially, the corticosteroids should be given in a dosage sufficient to control the disease; subsequently, they should be maintained at the lowest dose that will control the symptoms and decrease the ESR. In giant cell arteritis, corticosteroids should preferably be given after the diagnosis has been confirmed histologically. However, when giant cell arteritis is strongly suspected, there should be no delay in starting treatment, as the artery biopsy will still show inflammatory changes for several days after corticosteroids have been started, and the result is unlikely to alter therapeutic decisions. If the temporal (or other) artery biopsy shows no arteritis, but the suspicion of disease is strong, corticosteroid treatment should be started. The great danger is delaying treatment, as blindness may occur at any time.

In practice, most studies report using 10–20mg prednisolone daily to treat polymyalgia and 40–60mg for giant cell arteritis, because of the greater risk of arteritic complications in giant cell arteritis. Some ophthalmologists suggest an initial dose of at least 60mg, as they have seen blindness occur in those treated with a lower dose. However, this has to be balanced against the potential complication of high dosage in this older age group. Intravenous corticosteroids are occasionally used if there are visual complications. Patients should be advised that, while they are taking a maintenance dose of corticosteroids, any sudden exacerbation of symptoms, particularly sudden visual deterioration, requires an immediate increase in dose. The initial corticosteroid dose and rate of corticosteroid tapering have been evaluated prospectively by Kyle and Hazleman[70]. They found that patients with polymyalgia relapsed frequently when taking an initial dose of 10mg prednisolone daily, but in those taking 20mg for the first month the disease was well controlled.

Reducing the dosage from 7.5mg to 5mg in the second month was also associated with some relapses. Patients with giant cell arteritis were treated with 40mg for 5 days and then either continued to take 40mg or had their dosage reduced to 20mg for the first month. An initial dose of 40mg controlled symptoms in most cases, whereas giving 20mg and then reducing to 15mg/day after 4 weeks led to more relapses. There is little information on the rate of reduction of corticosteroid dosage once initial symptoms are controlled. Weekly decrements of not more than 5mg have been proposed. The reduction is more gradual when a daily dose of 10mg is reached. It is suggested that 1mg every 2–4 weeks is

sufficient. These dosages are suggestions only, and are not to be interpreted rigidly, as individual cases vary greatly.

Rapid reduction or withdrawal of corticosteroids has been reported to contribute to deaths in patients with giant cell arteritis[71]. Of 17 deaths, 13 were believed to be due to an inadequate dose of corticosteroids or too rapid reduction of the dose. Fortunately, complications are rare, and the activity of the disease seems to decline steadily. Relapses are more likely within 1 year of withdrawal of corticosteroids. There is no reliable method of predicting those most at risk, but arteritic relapses in patients who presented with pure polymyalgia rheumatica are unusual. Temporal artery biopsy does not seem helpful in predicting outcome.

Methylprednisolone has a 20% greater glucocorticoid potency (and a lower mineral corticoid effect) than oral prednisolone. In a prospective study of 60 patients with polymyalgia rheumatica, it has been shown that intramuscular methylprednisolone can confer a remission rate similar to that achieved with oral prednisolone, but with a superior side-effect profile. However, the study excluded patients with giant cell arteritis[72].

Controversy exists as to the expected duration of the disease. Most European studies report that between 33% and 50% of the patients are able to discontinue corticosteroids after 2 years of treatment. Studies from the USA have reported a shorter duration of disease for both polymyalgia rheumatica (75% of patients discontinue corticosteroids by 2 years) and giant cell arteritis (most patients had stopped corticosteroids within 2 years). However, a Mayo Clinic study has substantially confirmed the European view[73]. Both patients with polymyalgia rheumatica and those with giant cell arteritis needed a median duration of treatment of 1.8 years (mean 2.4 years). Most importantly, the median cumulative dose of prednisolone during the treatment period was between 4.5g and 5.4g and with such doses several important side effects were seen. Compared with age matched controls, patients with polymyalgia rheumatica who received corticosteroid treatment were found to have a two to five times greater risk of developing diabetes and vertebral, femoral neck and hip fractures[73]. The consensus view seems to be that stopping treatment is feasible from 2 years onwards.

Dasgupta et al.[74] measured serum T cell subsets before and during treatment in patients with polymyalgia rheumatica and giant cell arteritis, and found a profound and selective reduction of CD8+ suppressor/cytotoxic cells that persisted for up to 1 year, despite satisfactory symptomatic control and a normal ESR and C-reactive protein concentration. After 2 years of treatment, CD8+ cell counts had returned to the values found in normal controls.

Concentrations of IL-6 in combination with the ESR may be of value in determining disease severity and in predicting outcome in subgroups of patients with polymyalgia rheumatica.

Patients who are unable to reduce the dosage of prednisolone because of recurring symptoms, or who develop serious corticosteroid-related side effects, pose particular problems. Azathioprine has been shown to exert a modest corticosteroid-sparing effect. There have been reports of the value of methotrexate in corticosteroid resistant cases of polymyalgia rheumatica or giant cell arteritis, but the overall consensus is that methotrexate, azathioprine and cyclosporin are not effective. Most of the published studies have a relatively small number of patients, with a short duration of follow-up and high numbers withdrawing from treatment.

Relapses

Relapses are most likely in the first 18 months of treatment, but they can occur after apparently successful treatment when corticosteroids have been discontinued. At present, there is no way of predicting those patients most at risk. Diagnosis of relapse should be made on the basis of clinical features, because the ESR and C-reactive protein concentration are often not increased during relapses, or may be increased as a result of other causes. During relapses, the dose of prednisolone should be increased to that given before relapse, or more, depending on the severity of symptoms. The risks of relapse, particularly with arteritic complications, have to be balanced against the risks of corticosteroid-associated side effects.

Complications

Between 20% and 50% of patients may experience serious side effects. Serious side effects are significantly related to high initial doses, maintenance doses, cumulative doses and increased duration of treatment[75]. Side effects can be minimized by using low doses of prednisolone whenever possible, and giving corticosteroid-sparing drugs such as azathioprine and methotrexate when necessary.

Corticosteroid treatment carries the risk of increasing osteoporosis, especially in older patients. It cannot be overly stressed that patients with polymyalgia rheumatica should be given advice and be assessed for the risk of osteoporosis before beginning treatment, and should, as a minimum, be placed on calcium and vitamin D supplements. In this context, deflazacort, or the methyloxazoline derivative of prednisolone, failed to show a significant difference in bone density changes as compared with conventional oral prednisolone[76].

Conclusions

Some conclusions can be drawn (Table 147.5). The overall strategy should be to use an adequate dose of prednisolone for the first month to obtain good symptomatic control, with a decrease in ESR, then to aim for maintenance doses of less than 10mg after 6 months. The exact doses will need to be adjusted to the needs of the individual patient. A possible schedule is 15mg prednisolone/day for polymyalgia rheumatica, reducing the dose to about 7.5–10mg by 6–8 weeks. Patients with giant cell arteritis should be treated with 40mg daily for the first month unless visual symptoms persist, when higher doses (60–80mg) may be needed. A suitable dose reduction would be to 20mg at about 8 weeks. For both conditions, gradual reduction by 1mg every 2–3 months can be attempted, with possible withdrawal of corticosteroids after 2 years. Reduction of doses of prednisolone on alternate days once doses of less than 5mg are reached makes withdrawal easier, and the addition of a non-steroidal anti-inflammatory drug at this stage may reduce some of the minor muscular symptoms that patients develop as corticosteroids are reduced. Some patients, however, find it impossible to stop taking the final 2–3mg, and this level of maintenance dose is probably safe.

Summary

In summary, patients should be warned to expect treatment for at least 2 years, and most should be able to stop taking corticosteroids after 4–5 years. Monitoring for relapse should continue for 6 months to 1 year after discontinuation of corticosteroids; thereafter patients should be asked to report back urgently if arteritic symptoms occur. The risk of this happening is small and unpredictable. A few patients may need low-dose treatment indefinitely. Polymyalgia rheumatica and giant cell arteritis are amongst the more satisfying diseases for clinicians to diagnose and treat, because the unpleasant effects and serious consequences of these conditions can be almost entirely prevented by corticosteroid treatment. Unfortunately, there is no objective means of determining the prognosis in the individual, and decisions concerning duration of treatment remain empirical.

TABLE 147.5 TREATMENT OF POLYMYALGIA RHEUMATICA AND GIANT CELL ARTERITIS	
For polymyalgia rheumatica*	**Initial dosage** Prednisolone 10–20mg initially for 1 month, reduced by 2.5mg every 2–4 weeks to 10mg daily, then 1mg daily every 4–6 weeks (or until symptoms return). **Maintenance dosage** Maintenance dose 5–7mg daily for 6–12 months. Final reduction, 1mg every 6–8 weeks. Most patients require treatment for 3–4 years, but withdrawal after 2 years is worth attempting. **Special points** In patients who cannot reduce prednisolone dosage because of recurring symptoms or who develop serious corticosteroid-related side effects, azathioprine has been shown to have a modest corticosteroid sparing effect, and methotrexate may be more effective. **Main side effects** Weight gain, skin atrophy, edema, increased intraocular pressure, cataracts, gastrointestinal disturbances, diabetes, osteoporosis. **Risk of side effects** Increased risk with high initial doses (>30mg) of prednisolone, maintenance doses of 10mg and high cumulative doses. Maintenance doses of 5mg are relatively safe.
Giant cell arteritis without visual symptoms	Prednisolone 20–40mg daily initially for 8 weeks reduced by 5mg every 3–4 weeks until dose is 10mg daily; then as for polymyalgia rheumatica.
Giant cell arteritis with possible or definite ocular involvement	Prednisolone 40–80mg daily initially for 8 weeks reduced to 20mg daily over next 4 weeks; then as for uncomplicated giant cell arteritis.
*Recurrence of symptoms requires an increase in prednisolone dose.	

REFERENCES

1. Dequeker JV. Polymyalgia rheumatica with temporal arteritis as painted by Jan Van Eyck in 1436. Can Med Assoc J 1981; 124: 1597–1598.
2. Hutchinson J. A peculiar form of neurotic arteritis of the aged which is sometimes productive of gangrene. Arch Surg 1890; 1: 323–327.
3. Horton BT, Magath TB, Brown GE. An undescribed form of arteritis of the temporal vessels. Mayo Clin Proc 1932; 7: 700–701.
4. Bruce W. Senile rheumatic gout. BMJ 1888; 2: 811–813.
5. Barber HS. Myalgic syndrome with constitutional effects. Polymyalgia rheumatica. Ann Rheum Dis 1957; 16: 230–237.
6. Paulley JW, Hughes JP. Giant cell arteritis or arthritis of the aged. BMJ 1960; 2: 1562–1567.
7. Alestig K, Barr J. Giant cell arteritis: biopsy study of polymyalgia rheumatica, including one case of Takayasu's disease. Lancet 1963; i: 1228–1230.
8. Hamlin B, Jonsson N, Landberg T. Involvement of large vessels in polymyalgia arteritica. Lancet 1965; 1: 1193–1196.
9. Gran JT, Myklebust G. The incidence of polymyalgia rheumatica and temporal arteritis in the county of Aust Agder, South Norway: a prospective study 1987–94. J Rheumatol 1997; 24: 1739–1743.
10. Watts RA, Lane S, Bentham G, Scott DGI. Is there a latitudinal variation in the incidence of giant cell arteritis? Proceedings of the American College of Rheumatology, Philadelphia, October 2000. Arthritis Rheum 2000; 43(suppl): S137.
11. O'Brien JP, Regan W. Actinically degenerate elastic tissue: the prime antigen in the giant cell (temporal) arteritis syndrome? New data from the posterior ciliary arteries. Clin Exp Rheumatol 1998; 16: 39–48.
12. Machedo EBV, Michet CJ, Ballard DJ et al. Trends in incidence and clinical presentation of temporal arteritis in Olmsted County, Minnesota 1950–1985. Arthritis Rheum 1988; 31: 745–749.
13. Salvarani C, Gabriel S, O'Fallon W et al. Epidemiology of polymyalgia rheumatica in Olmstead County, Minnesota 1970–1991. Arthritis Rheum 1995; 38: 369–373.
14. González-Gay M, Garcia-Porrua C, Rivas M et al. Epidemiology of biopsy proven giant cell arteritis in North Western Spain: trend over an 18 year period. Ann Rheum Dis 2001; 60: 367–371.
15. Petursdottir V, Johansson H, Nordborg E, Nordborg C. The epidemiology of biopsy-positive giant cell arteritis: special reference to cyclic fluctuations. Rheumatology (Oxford) 1999; 38: 1208–1212.
16. Nordberg E, Bengtsson BA. Epidemiology of biopsy proven giant cell arteritis. J Intern Med 1990; 227: 233–236.
17. Ostberg G. On arteritis with special reference to polymyalgia arteritica. Acta Path Microb Scand 1973; 237(suppl.): 1–59.
18. Silman AJ, Currey HLF. Polymyalgia rheumatica in a defined elderly community. Rheumatol Rehabil 1982; 21: 235–237.
19. Kyle V, Silverman B, Silman A et al. Polymyalgia rheumatica/giant cell arteritis in general practice. BMJ 1985; 13: 385–388.

20. Liang M, Simkin PA, Hunder GG *et al*. Familial aggregation of polymyalgia rheumatica and giant cell arteritis. Arthritis Rheum 1974; 17: 19–24.
21. Rhodes DJ. Giant cell arteritis in general practice. J R Coll Gen Pract 1976; 26: 237–246.
22. Weyand CM, Hunder NH, Hicok K *et al*. HLA-DRB1 alleles in polymyalgia rheumatica, giant cell arteritis and rheumatoid arthritis. Arthritis Rheum 1994; 37: 514–520.
23. Dababneh A, Gonzalez-Gay MA, Garcia-Porrua C *et al*. Giant cell arteritis and polymyalgia rheumatica can be differentiated by distinct patterns of HLA class II association. J Rheumatol 1998; 25: 2140–2145.
24. Salvarani C, Hunder G. Musculoskeletal manifestations in a population-based cohort of patients with giant cell arteritis. Arthritis Rheum 1999; 42: 1259–1266.
25. Gonzalez-Gay M, Garcia-Porrus C, Vazquez-Caruncho M *et al*. The spectrum of polymyalgia rheumatica in Northern Spain: incidence and analysis of variables associated with relapse in ten year study. J Rheumatol 1999; 26: 1326–1332.
26. Matley D, Hajeer A, Dababneh A *et al*. Association of giant cell arteritis and polymyalgia rheumatica with different tumour necrosis factor microsatellite polymorphisms. Arthritis Rheum 2000; 43: 1749–1755.
27. Boiardi L, Salvarani C, Timms J *et al*. Interleukin-1 cluster and tumour necrosis factor-α gene polymorphisms in polymyalgia rheumatica. Clin Exp Rheumatol 2000; 18: 675–681.
28. Meliconi R, Pulsatelli L, Uguccioni M *et al*. Leukocyte infiltration in synovial tissue from the shoulder of patients with polymyalgia rheumatica. Quantitative analysis and influence of corticosteroid treatment. Arthritis Rheum 1996; 39: 1199–1207.
29. Salvarani C, Canitini F, Olivieri I *et al*. Proximal bursitis in active polymyalgia rheumatic. Ann Intern Med 1997; 127: 27–31.
30. Lange V, Teichmann J, Strucke H *et al*. Elderly onset rheumatoid arthritis and polymyalgia rheumatica: ultrasonographic study of the glenohumeral joints. Rheumatol Int 1998; 17: 229–232.
31. McGonagle D, Pease C, Mazo-Ortega H *et al*. Comparison of extracapsular changes by magnetic resonance imaging in patients with rheumatoid arthritis and polymyalgia rheumatica. J Rheumatol 2001; 28: 1837–1840.
32. Kassimos D, Kirwan J, Kyle V *et al*. Cytidine deaminase may be a useful marker in differentiating elderly onset rheumatoid arthritis from polymyalgia rheumatica/giant cell arteritis. Clin Exp Rheumatol 1995; 13: 641–644.
33. Hayreh S, Podhajsky Zimmerman B. Ocular manifestations of giant cell arteritis. Am J Opthalmol 1998; 125: 509–220.
34. Hayreh SS. Anterior ischaemic optic neuropathy. Differentiation of arteritis from non arteritic type and its management. Eye 1990; 4: 25–41.
35. Hunder C, Bloch D, Michel B *et al*. The American College of Rheumatology 1990 criteria for the classification of giant cell (temporal) arteritis. Arthritis Rheum 1990; 33: 1122–1128.
36. Bird HA, Esselinckx W, Dixon AS *et al*. An evaluation of criteria for polymyalgia rheumatica. Ann Rheum Dis 1979; 38: 434–439.
37. Caporali R, Montecncco C, Epis O *et al*. Presenting features of PMR and RA with PMR-like onset: a prospective study. Ann Rheum Dis 2001; 60: 1021–1024.
38. von Knorring J, Somer T. Malignancy in association with polymyalgia rheumatica and temporal arteritis. Scand J Rheumatol 1974; 3: 129–135.
39. Haga H, Eide G, Brun J *et al*. Cancer in association with polymyalgia rheumatica and temporal arteritis. J Rheumatol 1993; 20: 1335–1339.
40. Wise M, Agudelo GA, Chimelewski W, McKnight K. Temporal arteritis with low erythrocyte sedimentation rate: a review of 5 cases. Arthritis Rheum 1991; 34: 1571–1574.
41. Proven A, Gabriel S, O'Fallon W, Hunder G. Polymyalgia rheumatica with low erythrocyte sedimentation rate at diagnosis. J Rheumatol 1999; 26: 1333–1337.
42. Kyle V, Cawston TE, Hazleman BL. ESR and C-reactive protein in the assessment of polymyalgia rheumatica/giant cell arteritis on presentation and during follow up. Ann Rheum Dis 1989; 48: 408–409.
43. Pountain GD, Calvin J, Hazleman BL. α_1-Antichymotrypsin C-reactive protein and erythrocyte sedimentation rate in PMR/GCA. Br J Rheumatol 1994; 33: 550–554.
44. Chakravarty K, Pountain G, Merry P *et al*. A longitudinal study of anticardiolipin antibody in polymyalgia rheumatica and giant cell arteritis. J Rheumatol 1995; 22: 1694–1697.
45. Klein GE, Campbell RJ, Hunder GG, Carney JA. Skip lesions in temporal arteritis. Mayo Clin Proc 1976; 51: 504–508.
46. Généreau T, Lortholary O, Pottier M-A *et al*. Temporal artery biopsy : a diagnostic tool for systemic necrotizing vasculitis. Arthritis Rheum 1999; 42: 2674–2681.
47. Lie JT. When is arteritis of the temporal arteries not temporal arteritis? J Rheumatol 1994; 21: 186–189.
48. Estebann M, Font C, Hernandez-Rodriguez J *et al*. Small-vessel vasculitis surrounding a spared temporal artery. Clinical and pathological findings in a series of 28 patients. Arthritis Rheum 2001; 44: 1387–1395.
49. Schmidt W, Kraft H, Völker L *et al*. Colour Doppler sonography to diagnose temporal arteritis. Lancet 1995; 345: 866.
50. Blockmans D, Maes A, Stoobants S *et al*. New arguments for a vasculitic nature of polymyalgia rheumatica using positron emission tomography. Rheumatology (Oxford) 1999; 38: 444–447.
51. Richardson MP, Lever AML, Fink AM *et al*. Survival after aortic dissection in giant cell arteritis. Ann Rheum Dis 1996; 55: 332–333.
52. Wilkinson IMS, Russell RWR. Arteries of the head and neck in giant cell arteritis. A pathological study to show the pattern of arterial involvement. Arch Neurol 1972; 27: 378–387.
53. Kojima S, Tajagi A, Ida M, Shiozawa R. Muscle pathology in polymyalgia rheumatica: a histochemical and immunohistochemical study. Jpn J Med 1991; 30: 516–523.
54. Bacon PA, Doherty S, Zuckerman AJ. Hepatitis B antibody in polymyalgia rheumatica. Lancet 1975; ii: 476–478.
55. Salvarani C, Casali B, Cantini F *et al*. Detection of parvovirus B19 in temporal arteritis/polymyalgia rheumatic. Arthritis Rheum 2001; 44(suppl): S342.
56. Cimmino M, Grazi G, Balistreri M, Accardo S. Increased prevalence of antibodies to adenovirus and respiratory syncytial virus in polymyalgia rheumatica. Clin Exp Rheumatol 1993; 11: 309–313.
57. Duhaut P, Bosshard S, Calvert A *et al*. Giant cell arteritis, polymyalgia rheumatica, and viral hypothesis: a multicenter, prospective case control study. J Rheumatol 1999; 26: 361–369.
58. Elling P, Olsson AT, Elling H. Synchronous variations of the incidence of temporal arteritis and polymyalgia rheumatica in different regions of Denmark, association with epidemics of *Mycoplasma pneumoniae* infection. J Rheumatol 1996; 23: 112–119.
59. Russo MG, Waxman J, Abdoh AA, Serebro LH. Correlation between infection and the onset of the giant cell arteritis (temporal) arteritis syndrome. Arthritis Rheum 1995; 38: 374–380.
60. Sonnenblick M, Nesher G, Friedlande Y *et al*. Giant cell arteritis in Jerusalem: a 12 year epidemiological study. Br J Rheumatol 1994; 33: 938–941.
61. Cimmino MA. Genetic and environmental factors in polymyalgia rheumatica. Ann Rheum Dis 1997; 56: 576–577.
62. Gallagher PJ, Jones K. Immunohistochemical findings in cranial arteritis. Arthritis Rheum 1982; 25: 75–79.
63. Dasgupta B, Duke O, Kyle V *et al*. Antibodies to intermediate filaments in polymyalgia rheumatica and giant cell arteritis: a sequential study. Ann Rheum Dis 1987; 46: 746–749.
64. Cid MC, Campo E, Ercilla G *et al*. Immunohistochemical analysis of lymphoid and macrophage cell subsets and their immunologic activation markers in temporal arteritis. Influence of corticosteroid treatment. Arthritis Rheum 1989; 32: 884–893.
65. Kaiser M, Weyand C, Bjornsson J, Goronzy J. Platelet derived growth factor, intimal hyperplasia and ischaemic complications in GCA. Arthritis Rheum 1998; 41: 623–633.
66. Brack A, Geisler A, Martinez-Taboada *et al*. Giant cell arteritis is a T cell dependent disease. J Mol Med 1997; 8: 29–55.
67. Weyand CM, Schonberger J, Oppitz U *et al*. Distinct vascular lesions in giant cell arteritis share identical T cell clonotypes. J Exp Med 1994; 179: 951–960.
68. Bignon JD, Ferec C, Barrier J *et al*. HLA class II genes polymorphism in DR4 giant cell arteritis patients. Tissue Antigens 1988; 32: 254–258.
69. Roche N, Fulbright J, Wagner A *et al*. Correlation of interleukin 6 production and disease activity in polymyalgia rheumatica and giant cell arteritis. Arthritis Rheum 1993; 36: 1286–1294.
70. Kyle V, Hazleman BL. Treatment of polymyalgia rheumatica and giant cell arteritis. I. Steroid regimes in the first 2 months. Ann Rheum Dis 1989; 48: 658–661.
71. Nordberg E, Bengtsson BA. Death rates and causes of deaths in 284 consecutive patients with giant cell arteritis confirmed by biopsy. BMJ 1989; 299: 549–550.
72. Dasgupta B, Dolan AL, Panayi GS, Fernandes L. An initially double-blinded controlled 96 week trial of depot methylprednisolone against oral prednisolone in the treatment of PMR. Br J Rheumatol 1998; 37: 189–195.
73. Gabriel S, Sunku J, Salvarani C *et al*. Adverse outcomes of anti-inflammatory therapy among patients with polymyalgia rheumatica. Arthritis Rheum 1997; 40: 1873–1878.
74. Dasgupta B, Duke O, Timms A *et al*. Selective depletion and activation of CD8 lymphocytes from peripheral blood of patients with PMR and GCA. Ann Rheum Dis 1989; 48: 307–311.
75. Kyle V, Hazleman BL. Treatment of polymyalgia rheumatica and giant cell arteritis. II. The relationship between steroid dose and steroid associated side effects. Ann Rheum Dis 1989; 48: 662–666.
76. Krogsgaard M, Thamsborg G, Lund B. Changes in bone mass during low dose corticosteroid treatment in patients with PMR: a double-blind, prospective comparison between prednisolone and deflazocort. Ann Rheum Dis 1996; 55: 143–146.

148

Wegener's granulomatosis and lymphomatoid granulomatosis

John H Stone and Gary S Hoffman

Wegener's granulomatosis

- Wegener's granulomatosis (WG) is a multi-organ system disease of unknown etiology, characterized by granulomatous inflammation, tissue necrosis, and variable degrees of vasculitis in small- and medium-sized blood vessels

- WG has a predilection for causing destructive lesions in upper respiratory tract and lungs. The renal manifestation, a pauci-immune glomerulonephritis, is often associated with rapidly progressive glomerulonephritis

- The majority of WG cases, and particularly those with severe, widespread disease, are associated with anti-neutrophil cytoplasmic antibodies

- Immunosuppressive therapy, which is often life-saving, is effective in the induction of disease remissions. However, WG often flares during or after treatment reduction. Current therapies are associated with substantial morbidity

Lymphomatoid granulomatosis

- Because of its propensity to cause constitutional symptoms, lung nodules, renal dysfunction, and a polymorphic inflammatory infiltrate associated with necrosis, LG may mimic WG clinically. Despite their similar names, however, the two diseases differ substantially in their pathological features

- LG comprises part of a disease continuum, one end of which mimics systemic vasculitis clinically. At the other end of this continuum, the pathological process merges with an aggressive form of diffuse, large B-cell lymphoma

- LG is associated with the transformation of B-lymphocytes by Epstein-Barr virus (EBV)

WEGENER'S GRANULOMATOSIS

Definition

Wegener's granulomatosis (WG) is a multiorgan system disease of unknown etiology characterized by granulomatous inflammation, tissue necrosis, and variable degrees of vasculitis in small- and medium-sized blood vessels. Although WG may affect virtually any organ system, the disease has a predilection for the upper respiratory tract, lungs, and kidneys.

Clinical features

- Destructive inflammation of the nose, sinuses, ears, trachea, bronchi, and lungs
- Glomerulonephritis (GN) with little or no immune complex deposition, typically leading to rapidly progressive renal dysfunction
- Proptosis caused by orbital mass(es) occurring in a retrobulbar location. Other types of ocular inflammation also occur, e.g. scleritis, uveitis and conjunctivitis

- Migratory arthralgias and arthritis are common, but joint destruction is highly atypical
- Immunosuppressive therapy, which is often life saving, is effective in the induction of disease remissions. However, WG often flares during or after treatment reduction. Current therapies are associated with substantial morbidity.

History

In 1931, Heinz Klinger[1] described a 70-year-old physician with constitutional symptoms, joint complaints, proptosis and widespread inflammation of the upper respiratory tract: pansinusitis, bloody nasal crusts and otitis. As his illness evolved, the patient developed a saddle-nose deformity, GN, and pulmonary lesions; he died of an apparent bronchopneumonia. At postmortem, Klinger observed crescentic GN and necrotizing granulomatous vasculitis in both the upper and lower airways. The acute and chronic lesions consisted of a heterogeneous population of cells: neutrophils, lymphocytes, macrophages and multinucleated giant cells. Because of the prominent respiratory tract involvement in this index patient, Klinger speculated that an inhaled agent might have precipitated a 'particular reactivity of the vessels' throughout the involved organs[1]. Several years later, Friedrich Wegener reported three patients with similar findings[2,3]. Because of the striking nasal manifestations in his patients, Wegener entitled his paper 'Rhinogenic granulomatosis with special involvement of the arterial system and kidneys'[3]. Both Klinger and Wegener recognized that these clinicopathological features constituted a unique disease.

Epidemiology

A population-based study from a predominantly Caucasian English county indicated that the annual incidence of WG is at least 8.5 cases per million people[4]. Through examinations of hospital discharge records, the prevalence of WG in the US has been estimated to be at least 30 cases per million[5,6]. Based on US census data from the year 2000, this is equivalent to approximately 8400 prevalent cases. WG afflicts males and females with essentially the same frequency, but has a strong tendency to affect Caucasians, particularly those of northern European origin. However, the disease is known to occur in persons of African-American, Hispanic and Asian descent, and probably occurs in people of all races. Patients are typically in their fourth or fifth decade at the time of diagnosis. WG frequently affects older individuals, but fewer than 15% of cases occur in children.

Organ system involvement

Common individual organ manifestations of WG are depicted in Figure 148.1. Once the full pattern of organ involvement emerges, classic cases of WG may be diagnosed swiftly. For example, the constellation of upper airway complaints, cavitary pulmonary lesions and rapidly progressive GN places WG high on the differential diagnosis. The onset of WG may be acute or insidious. When insidious, evolution to fulminant disease may occur after months or even several years of smoldering symptomatology. All too often, by the time clinicians recognize the pattern of organ dysfunction as suggestive of WG, substantial damage has already occurred.

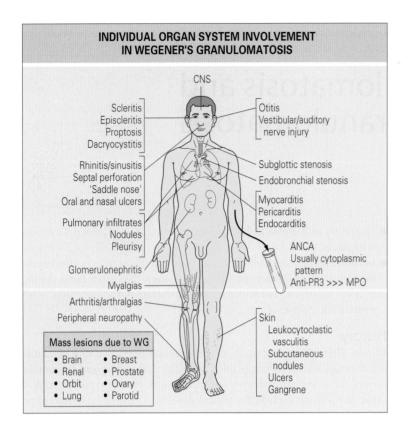

INDIVIDUAL ORGAN SYSTEM INVOLVEMENT IN WEGENER'S GRANULOMATOSIS

CNS

Scleritis
Episcleritis
Proptosis
Dacryocystitis

Otitis
Vestibular/auditory nerve injury

Rhinitis/sinusitis
Septal perforation
'Saddle nose'
Oral and nasal ulcers

Subglottic stenosis
Endobronchial stenosis

Pulmonary infiltrates
Nodules
Pleurisy

Myocarditis
Pericarditis
Endocarditis

ANCA
Usually cytoplasmic pattern
Anti-PR3 >>> MPO

Glomerulonephritis
Myalgias
Arthritis/arthralgias
Peripheral neuropathy

Skin
Leukocytoclastic vasculitis
Subcutaneous nodules
Ulcers
Gangrene

Mass lesions due to WG
- Brain
- Renal
- Orbit
- Lung
- Breast
- Prostate
- Ovary
- Parotid

Fig. 148.1 Individual organ system involvement in Wegener's granulomatosis. (Redrawn with permission from Hoffman GS, Weyand C, eds. Inflammatory Diseases of Blood Vessels. New York: Marcel Dekker, 2002.

Wegener's granulomatosis should be suspected if comparatively mundane problems such as otitis, rhinitis or sinusitis persist for unusual lengths of time; if destructive upper respiratory tract changes occur; or if systemic symptoms or signs develop (e.g. arthralgias, weight loss, or an elevated erythrocyte sedimentation rate). In recent years, testing for antineutrophil cytoplasmic antibodies (ANCA) has facilitated the diagnosis of WG in many cases. As discussed below, these assays have potential shortcomings and must be employed wisely.

Upper respiratory tract and ears

Nasal, sinus, tracheal and/or ear abnormalities comprise the initial symptoms in three-quarters of all patients. More than 90% eventually develop upper airway/ear abnormalities. The nasal symptoms of WG include nasal pain and stuffiness, rhinitis, epistaxis, and crusts that are characteristically brown or bloody. Nasal inflammation may lead to septal erosions, septal perforation and, in many cases, to nasal bridge collapse – the 'saddle-nose deformity' (Fig. 148.2). Any of the bony sinuses (mastoid, maxillary, ethmoid, sphenoid) may be involved. With time, WG may cause erosive disease of the sinuses, but these changes may not be apparent early in the disease course. Because damage to the sinuses heightens susceptibility to infection, the distinction between active WG and/or secondary infections in the sinuses may be challenging.

Two principal categories of ear disease, conductive and sensorineural hearing loss, are typical of WG. 'Mixed' hearing loss – the dual occurrence of both types of auditory lesion – is also common. Conductive hearing loss results from involvement of the middle ear cavity, associated with serous otitis media. Inflammation may compress the seventh cranial nerve as it courses through the middle ear cavity, leading to peripheral facial nerve palsy. Inner ear disease in WG may be associated with sensorineural hearing loss and/or vestibular dysfunction (nausea, vertigo, tinnitus). In contrast to middle ear disease, the mechanism of inner ear problems in WG is poorly understood[7]. Sometimes the cartilaginous structures of the external ears become inflamed, mimicking relapsing polychondritis.

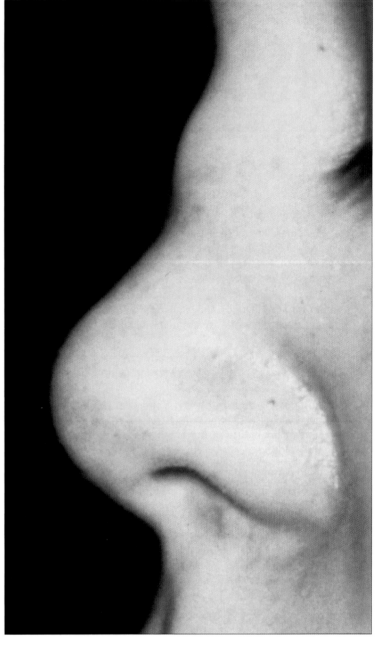

Fig. 148.2 Saddle-nose deformity resulting from collapse of the nasal cartilage in Wegener's granulomatosis.

Trachea

Subglottic stenosis, resulting from tracheal inflammation and scarring below the vocal cords, is a serious and potentially fatal complication of WG. Subglottic involvement is often asymptomatic and may become apparent as hoarseness, pain, cough or wheezing. However, some patients present with the subacute onset of respiratory stridor. With time, airway scarring and profound tracheal narrowing may occur. Severe cases require tracheostomies. Pulmonary function tests (flow–volume loops) may provide a useful, non-invasive means of quantifying both the extent of extrathoracic obstruction and its response to treatment in severe cases. However, flattening of flow–volume loops may only become apparent with advanced stenosis. The most accurate means of assessing tracheal stenosis is by direct laryngoscopy[8].

Eyes

Wegener's granulomatosis has two signature ocular lesions: the orbital mass and necrotizing scleritis. Orbital masses typically occur in a retrobulbar location, causing proptosis (Fig. 148.3). When severe, orbital

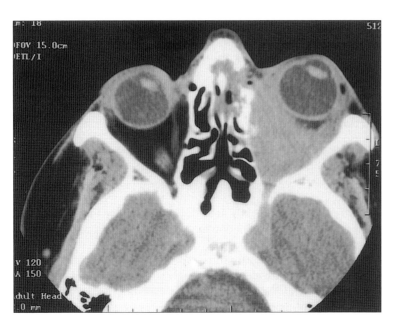

Fig. 148.3 CT scan of a patient with a left orbital mass. This was causing proptosis and visual loss through compression of the optic nerve.

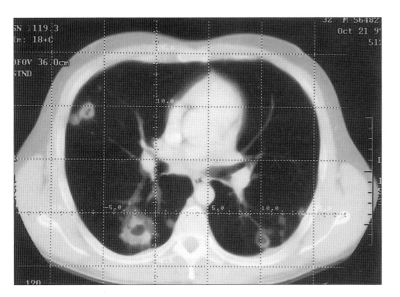

Fig. 148.4 CT scan of the chest in Wegener's granulomatosis. Multiple bilateral pulmonary nodules can be seen, many of which have cavitated.

masses may result in diplopia or visual loss via optic nerve ischemia. Scleritis, which causes eye pain and an angry, purplish discoloration, may lead to scleromalacia perforans and blindness. Other ocular manifestations of WG include conjunctivitis, episcleritis, keratitis, uveitis, nasolacrimal duct obstruction and, occasionally, occlusion of the retinal arteries or veins.

Lungs

The pulmonary manifestions of WG range from asymptomatic lung nodules and fleeting pulmonary infiltrates to fulminant alveolar hemorrhage. The most common radiographic findings are nodules and non-specific infiltrates. The nodules (Fig. 148.4) are usually multiple, bilateral, and often cavitary, leading to confusion with mycobacterial or fungal infections. The infiltrates, which may wax and wane, are often misdiagnosed initially as pneumonia. In one-third of patients with WG, nodules and pulmonary infiltrates are asymptomatic[5]. Pulmonary capillaritis may lead to alveolar hemorrhage, hemoptysis, and rapidly changing alveolar infiltrates (Fig. 148.5). Diffuse alveolar hemorrhage is an

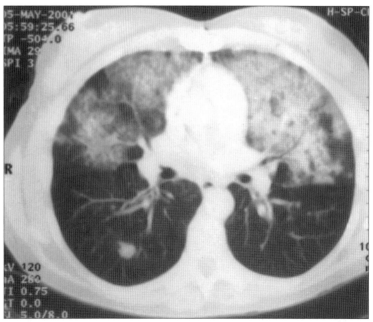

Fig. 148.5 Alveolar hemorrhage in a patient with Wegener's granulomatosis. This has resulted in rapidly changing pulmonary infiltrates. There is also a nodular lesion in the right lung.

immediately life-threatening complication. Hilar and/or mediastinal adenopathy occur rarely in WG, but are reported.

Kidneys

Renal disease is an ominous clinical manifestation of WG. Although fewer than 20% of patients with WG have renal involvement at the time of diagnosis, nearly 80% may develop this complication at some point in their course[5]. The clinical presentation of renal disease in WG is rapidly progressive GN: hematuria, red blood cell casts, proteinuria (usually non-nephrotic), and rising serum creatinine. Without appropriate therapy, irreversible loss of renal function may ensue within days to weeks. Thus, the appearance of active urine sediment or a rise in serum creatinine in WG signals the need for prompt, aggressive treatment.

Other manifestations

Constitutional symptoms, common in WG, serve as important indicators of an active inflammatory process. Prominent musculoskeletal symptoms occur in 60% of patients. Arthralgias are more common than frank arthritis. In addition, cutaneous nodules may occur at sites that are also common locations for rheumatoid nodules. Because approximately one-third of patients with WG are rheumatoid factor positive, rheumatoid arthritis is a common misdiagnosis early in the disease course. Other common constitutional complaints in WG are fever and weight loss. These, however, usually do not occur in isolation.

In addition to the cutaneous extravascular necrotizing granulomas that mimic rheumatoid nodules, skin findings in WG include all of the potential manifestations of cutaneous vasculitis: palpable purpura, vesiculobullous lesions, papules, ulcers, digital infarctions and splinter hemorrhages. Nervous system disease, though present in only a minority of patients at diagnosis, may be severe. Vasculitic neuropathy may lead to a devastating mononeuritis multiplex and/or a disabling sensory polyneuropathy. Central nervous system abnormalities occur in approximately 8% of patients, usually as cranial neuropathies, mass lesions or pachymeningitis. Parenchymal brain involvement by vasculitis is very uncommon in WG, but has been described. Rare neuroendocrine complications of WG include panhypopituitarism[9] and diabetes insipidus[5,10]. WG may also mimic giant cell arteritis, with prominent headaches and symptoms that recall polymyalgia rheumatica.

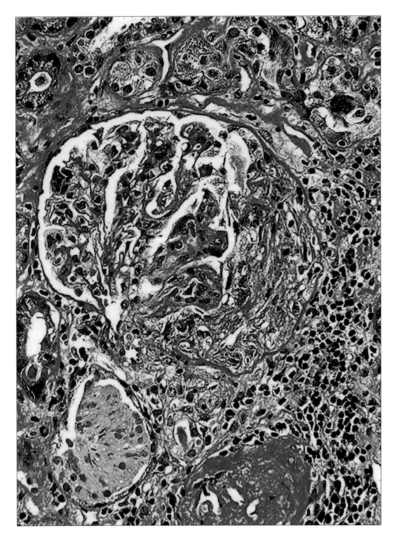

Fig. 148.6 Segmental necrotizing glomerulonephritis with crescent formation, the classic renal histopathology in Wegener's granulomatosis. Immunofluorescence studies in this disease show a paucity of immunoglobulin and complement deposition.

Wegener's granulomatosis rarely affects the heart, gastrointestinal tract, parotid gland, pulmonary artery, breast or genitourinary organs. When these organs do become involved, comorbid processes must be excluded[5,11].

Pathology

The typical renal lesion of WG is a segmental necrotizing GN, often accompanied by crescent formation (Fig. 148.6). Thrombotic changes in the glomerular capillary loops are among the earliest histologic changes. Immunofluorescence studies of renal biopsies demonstrate scant deposition (or complete absence) of immunoglobulin and complement, hence the term 'pauci-immune' GN. This term does not imply the absence of immune-mediated renal injury, but rather the conspicuous absence of immunoglobulin and complement deposition. Although these renal biopsy findings alone are not diagnostic of this disease, the results of renal biopsies often clinch the diagnosis when other clinical, radiologic and serologic data are compatible with WG. The finding of granulomatous inflammation in renal biopsies is unusual.

Wegener's granulomatosis shows its fullest pathologic expression in the lung, where the large amounts of tissue obtained at biopsy (open or thoracoscopic) may capture the entire histologic spectrum of disease[12]. Pulmonary vasculitis in WG may involve arteries, veins and capillaries, with or without granulomatous features. Both the vasculitic and the necrotizing granulomatous features of WG, which do not always coexist,

may be confirmed in lung biopsy specimens. Vascular necrosis begins as clusters of neutrophils within the blood vessel wall, which degenerate and become surrounded by palisading histiocytes. Coalescence of this neutrophilic debris assumes the appearance of microabscesses which, when extensive, are referred to as 'geographic' necrosis (Fig. 148.7). The range of granulomatous inflammation includes scattered giant cells and either palisading or poorly formed granulomas. In addition to the more specific pathological findings, pulmonary WG frequently demonstrates extensive areas of non-specific inflammation, such as bronchiolitis obliterans with organizing pneumonia (BOOP).

In contrast to biopsies of the kidney and lung, tissue samples from involved areas of the upper respiratory tract (nose, sinuses and subglottic region) are frequently non-diagnostic, yielding only non-specific acute and chronic inflammation in up to 50% of biopsies. Upper respiratory tract biopsies demonstrate the full pathologic triad of granulomatous inflammation, vasculitis and necrosis in only about 15% of cases.[13] However, provided that strongly suggestive clinical and radiologic disease manifestations are present, the finding of even only parts of this triad in an upper respiratory tract biopsy (e.g. sterile granulomatous inflammation or isolated vasculitis) may argue compellingly for the diagnosis of WG.

Antineutrophil cytoplasmic antibodies

ANCA, directed against antigens within the primary granules of neutrophils and monocytes, were first reported in 1982[14]. These antibodies were linked to WG in 1985[15]. Two types of assay for these antibodies, immunofluorescence (IF) and enzyme immunoassay (EIA), are now in common use. The current role of ANCA in the diagnosis and management of WG is summarized in Table 148.1.

With IF, three principal patterns of fluorescence are recognized: *cytoplasmic* (c-ANCA), *perinuclear* (p-ANCA), and *atypical* (x-ANCA). In patients with vasculitis, the c-ANCA pattern usually corresponds to the presence of antiproteinase-3 (PR3) antibodies, detected by EIA. The combination of a c-ANCA pattern on immunofluorescence and anti-pr3 antibodies is strongly associated with WG[16]. The p-ANCA pattern, which usually corresponds to the presence of antimyeloperoxidase (MPO) antibodies in vasculitis patients, occurs in approximately 10% of patients with WG but is more typical of microscopic polyangiitis, the Churg–Strauss syndrome, and renal-limited vasculitis. x-ANCA patterns are found in a wide variety of disorders, such as inflammatory bowel disease[17], systemic immune-mediated diseases[18] and infections[19]. These atypical patterns are frequently difficult to distinguish from the p-ANCA

TABLE 148.1 CLINICAL UTILITY OF ANCA TESTING

- Combined testing using IF assays and EIAs for antibodies to PR-3 or MPO is recommended. The most reliable results are positivity by both IF and EIA. However, positive serologies alone are not diagnostic of WG (or any other illness)
- Although the sensitivities of these two techniques are comparable, EIA has a higher specificity than IF
- A host of systemic illnesses (which may mimic WG) including infections, malignancies, and systemic rheumatic conditions may be associated with ANCA
- Despite rigorous serological evaluations, not all patients with WG have ANCA
- Even in patients who are ANCA positive, the titers are unreliable indicators of disease activity. As a rule, predicating treatment decisions on ANCA titers is a mistake.
- The direct role (if any) of ANCA in the pathogenesis of WG remains unclear. Most current evidence suggests that ANCA may amplify inflammation. ANCA enhance the degranulation of cytokine-primed neutrophils *in vitro*, but evidence of a role for these antibodies in the initiation of disease is lacking

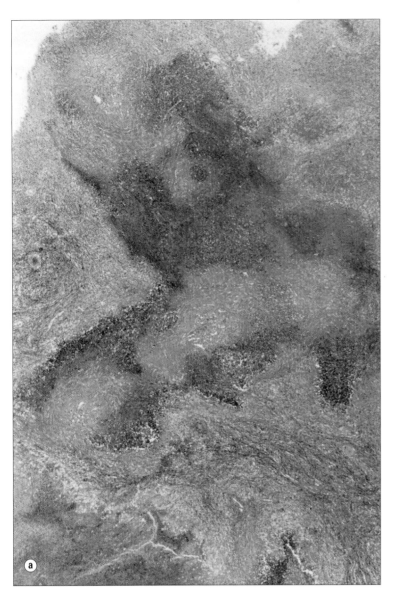
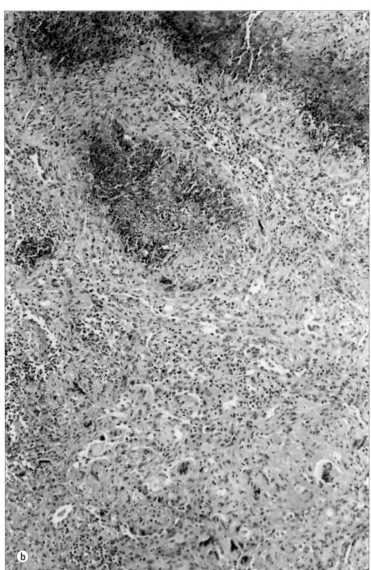

Fig. 148.7 Pulmonary pathology in Wegener's granulomatosis. (a) Extensive coalescent areas of necrosis from a biopsy of a pulmonary nodule. This pathological finding is termed 'geographic' necrosis. (b) Numerous multinucleated giant cells surrounding an ovoid region of necrobiosis.

pattern. Thus, regardless of the IF pattern, positive IF assays should be confirmed by the performance of EIAs for the specific antibodies associated with vasculitis, anti-PR3 and anti-MPO antibodies.

Most series indicate that up to 10–20% of patients with active, untreated WG are ANCA negative[19]. For patients with limited WG, defined as the absence of an immediate threat to either the function of a vital organ or the patient's life[20], 30% or more lack ANCA[19]. Thus, a negative ANCA assay does not preclude the diagnosis of WG.

An additional shortcoming of ANCA is their unreliable correlation with disease activity. Titers of these antibodies tend to decline following the institution of immunosuppressive therapy, but not always: many patients in complete clinical remission remain ANCA positive. Although some of these patients eventually suffer flares of their disease, the period between the rise in ANCA titers and the appearance of renewed disease activity may be a year or more, an interval that calls into question any true association between ANCA elevation and disease flares. In the absence of clinically evident disease, the treatment of patients simply because of rising ANCA titers leads to considerable unnecessary morbidity from heavy-handed immunosuppression.

Despite advances in ANCA testing techniques, the cornerstone of diagnosis in WG remains the combination of typical clinical features and histopathology. When the diagnosis is uncertain, all reasonable attempts to obtain biopsies that confirm the diagnosis should be pursued. On the other hand, appropriate biopsy sites are not always evident. Furthermore, biopsies do not always yield diagnostic findings. In such settings, ANCA assays provide an important adjunct to diagnosis, even though they do not supplant histology in most cases.

Differential diagnosis

In 1954, Godman and Churg noted pathological similarities among three clinically distinct disease entities: WG, microscopic polyangiitis (MPA), and the Churg–Strauss syndrome (CSS)[21]. These observations were insightful, as these conditions are the cardinal forms of vasculitis now recognized to be associated with ANCA in many cases. The typical features of these disorders, which may be difficult to differentiate, are contrasted in Table 148.2.

The 1994 Chapel Hill Consensus Conference on vasculitis nomenclature defined MPA as a process that: 1) involves necrotizing vasculitis with few or no immune deposits (i.e. is pauci-immune); 2) affects the smallest blood vessels (capillaries, venules, and arterioles); 3) may *also* affect medium-sized vessels; and 4) demonstrates tropism for the kidneys (GN) and lungs (pulmonary capillaritis)[22]. The essential difference

TABLE 148.2 COMPARISON OF ANCA-ASSOCIATED VASCULITIDES

	Wegener's granulomatosis	MPA	CSS
ANCA-positive (%)	80–90	75	50
Typical results*	c-ANCA/proteinase 3	p-ANCA/MPO	p-ANCA/MPO
Upper respiratory tract	Nasal septal perforation Saddle-nose deformity Subglottic stenosis	Usually absent or mild	Nasal polyps Allergic rhinitis
Lung	Nodules, infiltrates or cavitary lesions	Alveolar hemorrhage	Asthma Infiltrates
Kidney	NCGN, occasional granulomatous features	NCGN	NCGN
Distinguishing features	Destructive upper airway disease, granulomatous inflammation	No granulomatous inflammation	Asthma, allergy, eosinophilia, granulomatous infiltrates with abundant eosinophils

* These relationships are not absolute. A minority of patients with WG may be p-ANCA/MPO-positive and a minority of patients with MPA or CSS may be c-ANCA/PR3-positive.
The table lists the cardinal features of three vasculitides commonly associated with ANCA.

between WG and MPA is the absence of granulomatous inflammation in MPA. (Because sampling error is impossible to exclude in some tissue biopsies, some patients initially diagnosed with MPA subsequently develop unequivocal features of WG.) Although both MPA and WG may lead to life-threatening alveolar hemorrhage, upper respiratory tract symptoms are not a prominent feature of MPA. Seventy per cent of patients with MPA have ANCA, usually anti-MPO antibodies. These typically produce a p-ANCA pattern on IF testing.

CSS also tends to affect the same organs as WG, albeit often with different manifestations and severity. Asthma and marked eosinophilia typically accompany CSS. More than 90% of CSS patients have histories of asthma, either new-onset or long-standing disease. The finding of peripheral eosinophilia in a patient with features of vasculitis strongly suggests CSS rather than WG. In addition, biopsies from patients with WG sometimes demonstrate mild degrees of eosinophilia, but striking tissue infiltration by eosinophils is atypical. Unlike WG, CSS usually does not produce destructive upper airway disease or cavitary pulmonary nodules.

Henoch–Schönlein purpura (HSP) may mimic WG in its propensity to cause cutaneous vasculitis, arthritis and GN. Although HSP often follows upper respiratory tract infections, these complaints have usually resolved by the time vasculitis appears. This contrasts with the persistent, destructive nasosinus disease process observed in WG. In addition, pulmonary involvement in HSP is exceptional.

Wegener's granulomatosis must be distinguished from pulmonary–renal syndromes such as Goodpasture's disease. In Goodpasture's disease, antiglomerular basement membrane antibodies can be measured in the blood or observed as linear staining in indirect IF studies of lung or kidney tissue. Other characteristic clinical and serologic features distinguish other diseases that may produce pulmonary–renal syndromes, such as systemic lupus erythematosus.

Limited WG may pose a difficult diagnostic problem. The destructive upper airway disease that occurs in limited WG may also be due to infection (mycobacteria, fungi, actinomycosis and syphilis), malignancy (squamous cell carcinoma and extranodal lymphoma), or illicit drug use (intranasal cocaine, or the smoking of crack). Because granulomatous infections of the lung (e.g. mycobacteria or fungi) may also cause vasculitis and necrosis, the diagnosis of WG should not be rendered on lung biopsy specimens until special stains and cultures for infection are negative.

Lymphomatoid granulomatosis, discussed in detail in a later section of this chapter, is an angiocentric immunoproliferative disorder that may mimic WG closely in its presenting features.

Etiology and pathogenesis

Attempts to identify the etiology of WG have centered on the roles of genetics, environmental exposures and microbial pathogens. The striking Caucasian predominance of WG indicates that genes probably do play some role in susceptibility to this disease. However, the rarity of WG in more than one member of the same family suggests that heritable factors alone do not explain the expression of this illness[23]. Attempts to identify links between WG and human leukocyte antigen (HLA) genes have not demonstrated any consistent associations[24]. Large studies employing modern techniques of genetic investigation are now under way.

Environmental exposures – perhaps the proper exposure occurring in a genetically susceptible individual – represent other potential etiologic factors in WG. Granulomas may begin around a nidus of relatively insoluble material derived from inert matter (e.g. asbestos, silica, cement or wood dusts). Many inhaled substances are known to cause inflammatory airway responses, including granuloma formation. Substances such as silica stimulate giant cell formation and simultaneously activate neutrophils. An analysis of the distribution and density of WG cases in New York State revealed several regions of increased prevalence[6]. These data support a potential role for environmental exposures in the etiology of WG. To date, however, studies of known causes of granuloma formation in patients with WG are incomplete. Field studies of disease clusters and their environments are worthy of pursuit. The heterogeneity of WG patients with regard to age, geographic origin and potential environmental exposures casts doubt on any single environmental agent as the cause of WG.

Since the original descriptions of WG by Klinger[1] and Wegener[2,3], microbial pathogens have been regarded as possible precipitants of this disease. Analyses of bronchoalveolar lavage specimens from individuals with active WG who lack overt pulmonary disease indicate that a subclinical neutrophilic alveolitis and ANCA production are present in many[25,26]. In addition, significant abnormalities found on physical examination of the nasal mucosa and radiographic findings in the sinuses have been reported in WG patients who have no clinical symptoms in these organs. This provides further support to the hypothesis that the portal of entry for the putative pathogen(s) is the respiratory tract. Nevertheless, attempts to identify infectious agents in lung tissue using standard pathologic stains, *in situ* hybridization studies and conventional culture techniques for typical and atypical organisms have so far been unrewarding. Modern techniques such as polymerase chain reaction and representational difference analysis are promising approaches to defining the role of infections in WG. These are currently under investigation.

Regardless of the initiating event(s), substantial insights into the pathophysiology of WG have been gained in the past few years. A schematic representation of molecular events involved in the pathogenesis of WG is shown in Figure 148.8. Abnormal regulation of tumor necrosis factor (TNF) and other Th1 cytokines appears to play an important role in this disease. It is known from animal models that antibodies to TNF markedly impair granuloma formation. CD4+ T cells from patients with WG produce elevated levels of TNF, and peripheral blood mononuclear cells secrete increased amounts of interferon-γ, under the direction of interleukin-12[27]. Serum levels of soluble receptors for TNF are elevated in patients with active WG, and normalize with the induction of remission. Finally, *in vitro* priming of activated neutrophils with TNF markedly enhances the ability of ANCA to stimulate neutrophil degranulation, potentially fuelling the vasculitis associated with WG[28]. These insights into the pathogenesis of WG provide the underpinning for current experimental approaches to treating this disease, which include strategies designed to disrupt TNF and to downregulate IL-12.

Treatment

Overview

Current choices for treatment in WG are based on the classification of patients into the categories of either 'severe' or 'limited' disease. This is based upon the clinician's perception of the disease's potential to cause major harm within a short time frame, i.e. days to weeks. Severe WG constitutes an immediate threat to either the function of a vital organ or the patient's life. Conversely, limited WG consists of disease manifestations that do not pose such threats in the short term. Examples of severe disease manifestations that require the most aggressive treat-

ment include rapidly progressive GN, alveolar hemorrhage, intestinal ischemia, necrotizing scleritis and vasculitic neuropathy. Manifestations of limited disease are conductive hearing loss, nasosinus disease, cutaneous lesions, arthritis/arthralgias, and pulmonary nodules or infiltrates that do not significantly compromise lung function.

Data from the 1950s, the period before the availability of effective therapy, indicate that severe WG is generally fatal in the absence of appropriate treatment. In 1958, Walton[29] reported a mean survival of only 5 months (and an 82% mortality at 1 year) in WG. During the 1960s, treatment with corticosteroids appeared to increase mean survival to 12.5 months[30], but the eventual outcome in nearly all patients was death. The possibility of disease remission was realized only in the 1970s, when investigators at the NIH began to employ cyclophosphamide (CYC) to treat WG[31].

Severe disease

Severe WG requires urgent treatment with CYC and high doses of corticosteroids. A longitudinal study from the NIH[5] employed a combination of CYC (2 mg/kg po daily, with doses reduced for patients with renal dysfunction) and corticosteroids (1 mg/kg po daily, tapered over 6 months to a year). This regimen converted a once nearly always fatal disease into one that responded to treatment in more than 90% of cases. In fact, 75% of patients treated in this fashion entered remission. The NIH protocol called for the continuation of daily CYC for 1 full year after the achievement of remission. Although this regimen was effective in controlling WG, patients suffered substantial treatment-related morbidity (see Morbidity and Mortality, below).

Clinical practice regarding the use of either daily or intermittent (e.g. monthly intravenous) CYC varies from center to center. In WG, daily CYC is more likely to result in durable remissions[32,33], but daily administration is also associated with a greater number of side effects (see below). Consequently, meticulous monitoring, particularly of the white blood cell count, is essential. Measuring complete blood counts every 2 weeks is appropriate for patients treated with daily CYC. The induction of neutropenia is *not* required to achieve a therapeutic effect. With daily CYC regimens the avoidance of neutropenia is essential to prevent opportunistic infections. CYC should be withheld temporarily if

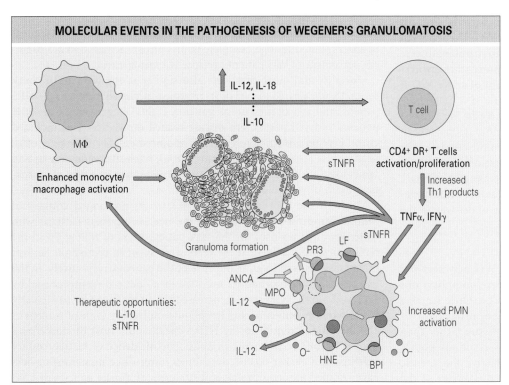

MOLECULAR EVENTS IN THE PATHOGENESIS OF WEGENER'S GRANULOMATOSIS

Fig. 148.8 Molecular events in the pathogenesis of Wegener's granulomatosis. Wegener's granulomatosis is associated with an unbalanced Th1 cytokine pathway, including increased levels of tumor necrosis factor and interferon-γ. These cytokines lead to activation of polymorphonuclear cells and monocyte/macrophages, and to granuloma formation.

the white blood cell count falls below $4.0 \times 10^9/l$. Treatment may be reinstituted at a lower dose after the resolution of neutropenia.

Limited disease

Limited WG may respond to the combination of methotrexate (MTX; up to 25 mg/week) and corticosteroids[5,34,35]. In patients with limited WG, complete remissions are induced in approximately three-quarters of cases (a percentage rivaling that of patients with severe disease treated with CYC). Disease flares during tapers of MTX and prednisone are common, however. MTX is not an appropriate first-line treatment for patients with severe involvement of the kidneys, lungs, peripheral nerves or other vital organs. In addition, because significant renal dysfunction heightens the potential for myelotoxicity, MTX is contraindicated in patients with a serum creatinine of >2.0 mg/dl.

Emergence of a new standard of care

In recent years, a new standard of care has emerged[36]. The greatest current challenge in the management of WG is the absence of a well-tolerated, effective medication for the maintenance of disease remission. To control the disease and yet avoid the side effects of long-term CYC use, many centers now employ shorter courses of induction treatment with CYC (e.g. 3–6 months), followed by longer periods of treatment with either MTX[37] or azathioprine (AZA)[38] to maintain disease remission. The optimal length of treatment with MTX or AZA is not clear, but continuation of these medications for at least 1 year after remission is reasonable in most patients.

Other medical treatments

The use of trimethoprim/sulfamethoxazole (T/S) as a treatment for WG is controversial. A higher rate of disease relapse occurs among patients who have chronic nasal carriage of *Staphylococcus aureus* than in those who do not[39]. In a randomized double-blind trial of relapse prevention, chronic treatment with T/S (one double-strength tablet twice daily) was compared to placebo in 81 WG patients in remission. Relapses occurred less frequently in the T/S group (17%, versus 40% in the placebo group)[39]. However, the reduction in the risk of relapse applied only to the comparatively minor upper respiratory tract disease flares, not to flares involving vital organs. In addition, because of the difficulty in distinguishing secondary bacterial infections from active WG in the sinuses, the reported reduction in upper airway relapses may actually have represented a T/S-induced decrease in secondary bacterial sinusitis which, as noted, may be difficult to distinguish from WG. The results of this study have been used to support the use of T/S to maintain disease remissions in patients with histories of upper respiratory tract involvement. However, the use of T/S alone in the treatment of active WG is not appropriate.

A wide array of other therapies, such as plasmapheresis, intravenous immunoglobulin, mycophenolate mofetil and leflunomide, have been employed in small numbers of patients, but so far insufficient data exist to judge their efficacy. A preliminary study of the use of etanercept, a soluble fusion protein that inhibits TNF, showed encouraging results[40]. Randomized trials of this therapy as a means of facilitating the achievement and maintenance of disease remission are now under way in the United States.

Non-medical interventions

Certain upper respiratory tract complications of WG may respond incompletely to immunosuppressive therapy. These complications include subglottic stenosis (SGS) and nasosinus disease. Once scarring and fibrosis are well established in the subglottic region, airway narrowing may be secondary to the progression of scar tissue rather than to WG-related inflammation. In such cases, SGS responds poorly to immunosuppressive therapy, and the most effective therapeutic approach to this problem is mechanical: surgical dilatations of the airway, augmented by intralesional corticosteroid injections. Serial procedures are often required. If severe SGS precludes a safe dilatation procedure, a patent airway should first be secured by a tracheostomy.

Wegener's granulomatosis often leads to chronic nasosinus dysfunction. This problem results from damage caused by WG itself, superinfections of damaged tissue, the effects of medical therapy, and surgical procedures performed for either diagnosis or treatment. Regardless of disease activity, most patients require daily (or more frequent) saline irrigations to minimize the accumulation of secretions and crusts, and to reduce the incidence of secondary infections. Persistent or recurrent infections may require surgical drainage. Distinguishing between worsening sinus disease caused by active WG and superinfection may be difficult. Both may be present simultaneously. In the absence of a prompt response to antibiotics, surgical drainage and biopsy are often required for a more definitive diagnosis.

Disease assessment

Disease assessment in multiorgan system disorders such as WG is challenging. The Birmingham Vasculitis Activity Score for WG (BVAS/WG) is a validated, WG-specific instrument for the evaluation of disease activity[41]. The one-page evaluation form is shown in Figure 148.9. The BVAS/WG consists of eight groups of organ system-based items, a general category that includes arthritis/arthralgias and fever, and space for the inclusion of other disease manifestations that clinicians attribute to active WG. According to BVAS/WG definitions, remission is the absence of active disease in any organ system[41]. Another recently validated instrument for the assessment of WG is the Disease Extent Index[42]. Currently, there are no disease-specific instruments for the assessment of damage or quality of life in WG.

Morbidity and mortality

Descriptions of two large series of WG patients, the longitudinal NIH cohort ($n = 158$)[5] and a comparably-sized cohort of patients from Lübeck, Germany ($n = 155$)[42], show many similarities with regard to disease course and outcome. Median follow-up times in the two cohorts were comparable: 8 years for the NIH patients, 7 years for those in the Lübeck series. The majority of patients in both series received daily CYC and corticosteroids as treatment. As noted, 75% of patients in the NIH series achieved complete remission, but 50% of these ultimately relapsed (at periods ranging from 3 months to 16 years). Among the Lübeck patients, 54% achieved complete remission but 60% suffered subsequent relapses. Thus, although complete remissions are achieved in a substantial percentage of WG patients, relapse is a major threat.

Mortality and morbidity were also similar in the NIH and Lübeck series. Deaths related to WG or its treatment occurred in 13% of the NIH patients and 12% of the Lübeck patients. Eighty-six per cent of the NIH patients suffered permanent disease-related morbidity. This included chronic renal insufficiency (42%), requirement for dialysis (10%), hearing loss (35%), nasal deformity (28%), tracheal stenosis (13%) and visual loss (8%). Many patients incurred more than one type of permanent morbidity[5].

Much of the morbidity in WG relates to prolonged courses of immunosuppression, particularly the need to re-treat patients who suffer multiple relapses. In the 1229 patient-years of follow-up in the NIH series, only 46% of these years were spent in remission. Serious infections occurred in 46% and 26% of the patients, respectively, in the two series. Other morbidities included drug-induced cystitis caused by CYC (43% in the NIH series), increased risk of malignancy (particularly bladder cancer, leukemia and lymphoma), infertility (57% of women of childbearing potential in the NIH series), and a host of side effects related to the use of corticosteroids. The incidence of bladder injury (cystitis) and cancer has become much lower since numerous centers have adopted induction remission strategies of shorter courses of CYC

BIRMINGHAM VASCULITIS ACTIVITY SCORE FOR WEGENER'S GRANULOMATOSIS EVALUATION FORM

Tick box (□ or ○) only if abnormality is ascribable to the presence of active Wegener's Granulomatosis (chronic damage should be scored separately in the Vasculitis Damage Index, VDI.)

□ Tick box only if the abnormality is **persistent disease activity** since the last assessment and not worse within the previous 28 days.

○ Tick box only if the abnormality is **newly present or worse** within the **previous 28 days**.

△ If no items are present in any section, tick "none".

Major items are in bold and marked with *

All WG-related clinical features need to be documented on this form if they are related to active diseases. Use "OTHER" category as needed.

1. Clinic ID: _ _ _

2. Patient ID: _ _ _

3. Patient name code: _ _ _ _

4. Date form completed: _ _ . _ _ . _ _
   day   month   year

5. Visit ID: _ _ _

	Persistent	New/worse	None
6. GENERAL			△₁
a. arthralgia/arthritis	□₁	○₂	
b. fever (≥ 38.0°C)	□₁	○₂	
7. CUTANEOUS			△₁
a. purpura	□₁	○₂	
b. skin ulcer	□₁	○₂	
c. *gangrene	□₁	○₂	
8. MUCOUS MEMBRANES/EYES			△₁
a. mouth ulcers	□₁	○₂	
b. conjunctivitis/episcleritis	□₁	○₂	
c. retro-orbital mass/proptosis	□₁	○₂	
d. uveitis	□₁	○₂	
e. *scleritis	□₁	○₂	
f. *retinal exudates/hemorrhage	□₁	○₂	
9. EAR, NOSE AND THROAT			△₁
a. bloody nasal discharge/nasal crusting/ulcer	□₁	○₂	
b. sinus involvement	□₁	○₂	
c. swollen salivary gland	□₁	○₂	
d. subglottic inflammation	□₁	○₂	
e. conductive deafness	□₁	○₂	
f. *sensorineural deafness	□₁	○₂	
10. CARDIOVASCULAR			△₁
a. pericarditis	□₁	○₂	
11. GASTROINTESTINAL			△₁
a. *mesenteric ischemia	1	2	
12. PULMONARY			△₁
a. pleurisy	□₁	○₂	
b. nodules or cavities	□₁	○₂	
c. other infiltrate secondary to WG	□₁	○₂	
d. endobronchial involvement	□₁	○₂	
e. *alveolar hemorrhage	□₁	○₂	
f. *respiratory failure	□₁	○₂	

	Persistent	New/worse	None
13. RENAL			△₁
a. hematuria (no RBC casts) (≥ 1+ or ≥ 10 RBC/hpf)	□	○	
b. *RBC casts	□₁	○₂	
b. *rise in creatinine > 30% *or* fall in creatinine clearance > 25%		○₂	

Note: *If both hematuria and RBC casts are present, score only the RBC casts (the major item).*

	Persistent	New/worse	None
14. NERVOUS SYSTEM			△₁
a. *meningitis	□₁	○₂	
b. *cord lesion		○₂	
c. *stroke		○₂	
d. *cranial nerve palsy		○₂	
e. *sensory peripheral neuropathy		○₂	
f. *motor mononeuritis multiplex		○₂	
15. OTHER (describe all items and *items deemed major)			△₁
_____	□₁	○₂	
_____	□₁	○₂	
_____	□₁	○₂	
_____	□₁	○₂	

16. TOTAL NUMBER OF ITEMS:

a.	b.	c.	d.
___	___	___	___
Major New/Worse	Minor New/Worse	Major Persistent	Minor Persistent

DETERMINING DISEASE STATUS

Severe Disease/Flare: ≥ 1 new/worse Major item.
Limited Disease/Flare: ≥ 1 new/worse Minor item.
Persistent Disease: Continued (but not new/worse) activity.
Remission: No active disease, including either new/worse or persistent items.

17. CURRENT DISEASE STATUS (check only one):

Severe Disease/Flare (₁)
Limited Disease/Flare (₂)
Persistent Disease (₃)
Remission (₄)

18. PHYSICIAN'S GLOBAL ASSESSMENT (PGA)
Mark line to indicate the amount of WG disease activity (not including longstanding damage) within the **previous 28 days**:

Remission |—————————————————————| Maximum activity
0   10

19. Value in item No.18: ___ ___ ___ (distance from 0 to tick mark in millimeters)
   mm

20. DATE FORM REVIEWED _ _ . _ _ . _ _
   day   month   year

21. STUDY PHYSICIAN ID: _ _

22. STUDY PHYSICIAN SIGNATURE: _____

23. CLINIC COORDINATOR ID: _ _

24. CLINIC COORDINATOR SIGNATURE: _____

Fig. 148.9 Birmingham Vasculitis Activity Score for Wegener's granulomatosis evaluation form[41]. hpf, high-power field; RBC, red blood cell. (With permission from Stone *et al.*[41]).

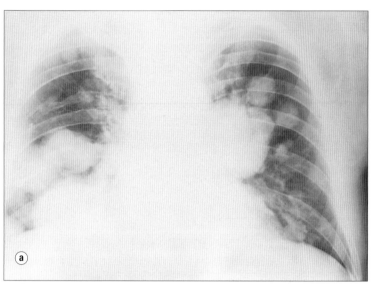
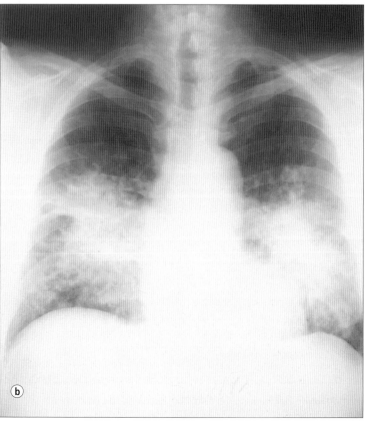
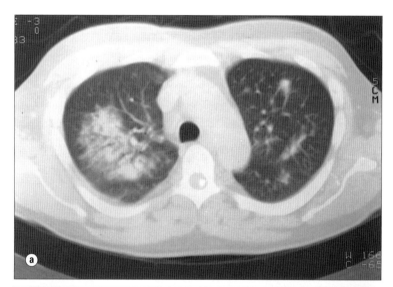
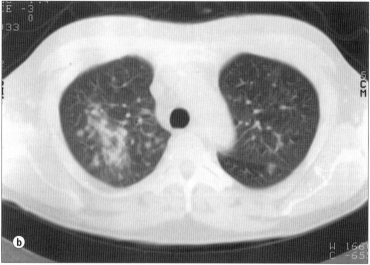

(3–6 months) for patients with severe WG, followed by attempts to maintain remission with MTX or AZA.

Because of the frequency of opportunistic infections with conventional treatment regimens for WG, prophylaxis against *Pneumocystis carinii* pneumonia is an essential component of WG therapy. Either single-strength T/S daily or the double-strength formulation three times a week is suitable. For patients with sulfa allergies, dapsone (100 mg daily) is an appropriate substitute.

All patients who require chronic corticosteroid treatment are at risk for osteoporosis. If bone density studies are normal when treatment begins, calcium and vitamin D supplements should be provided to diminish the risk of osteoporosis. If bone mineral density is already diminished at the time corticosteroids are initiated, bisphosphonate therapy should be added to the treatment regimen.

LYMPHOMATOID GRANULOMATOSIS

Definition

- Lymphomatoid granulomatosis (LG) is an angiocentric and angio-destructive lymphoproliferative disorder associated with the transformation of B lymphoctes by Epstein–Barr virus (EBV).
- Although LG lesions are characterized by angioinvasion of both reactive and atypical lymphocytes, the disorder is not an inflammatory vasculitis in the classic sense. Rather, it comprises part of a disease continuum, one end of which mimics systemic vasculitis clinically. At the other end of this continuum the pathological process merges with an aggressive form of diffuse, large B-cell lymphoma.
- Because of its propensity to cause constitutional symptoms, lung nodules, renal dysfunction, and a polymorphic inflammatory infiltrate

Fig. 148.10 Radiologic studies in lymphomatoid granulomatosis.
(a) Chest radiographs showing bilateral pulmonary nodules of varying sizes.
(b) Cuts from a CT study showing bilateral pulmonary nodules accompanied by interstitial changes. (Courtesy of Fredric B Askin and Stanley S Siegelman.)

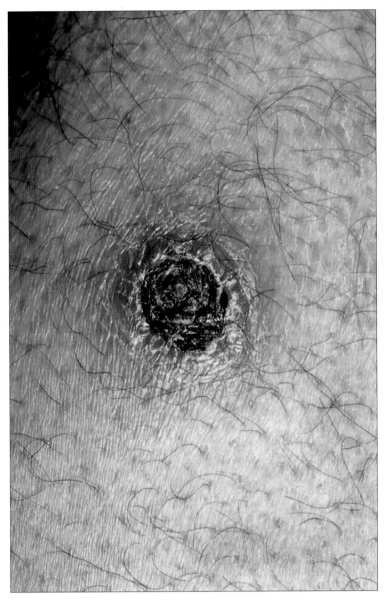

Fig. 148.11 Cutaneous ulcer in a patient with lymphomatoid granulomatosis.

associated with necrosis, LG may mimic WG clinically. Despite their similar names, however, the two diseases differ substantially in their pathological features.

● Complete remissions are possible for all patients within this disease spectrum, including LG and frank angiocentric lymphoma, provided that aggressive treatment is initiated early.

History

Liebow described the pathologic triad of polymorphic lymphoid infiltrate, angiitis and 'granulomatosis' associated with LG in 1972[43]. Because of the disorder's clinical resemblance to WG and the extensive necrosis observed pathologically, 'granulomatosis' was included in the name for this disorder. In fact, LG is a misnomer, as granulomas are not typical of this disease. Although the original name persists in the medical literature, today the term LG is employed most appropriately in settings in which no overt malignancy is evident.

Following its initial description, LG was regarded as an aggressive form of lymphocytic vasculitis. The evolution of many cases into frank lymphoma was soon recognized, however, and in the 1970s and 1980s LG was classified as an 'angiocentric immunoproliferative lesion'[44]. During this period, most studies indicated that LG and related disorders were various stages of peripheral T-cell lymphomas, with a common histology but a propensity to involve a wide variety of organ systems. Thus, 'lethal midline granuloma', 'centrofacial malignant granuloma', 'polymorphic reticulosis', 'midline malignant reticulosis' and LG were all considered to represent essentially the same T-cell disorder.

In most cases, these conditions actually represent distinct disorders of B, NK or T cells. For example, cases of aggressive paranasal sinus disease once identified as 'lethal midline granuloma' are now usually classified as extranodal NK- or T-cell lymphomas[45] and are not considered part of the LG spectrum. In contrast, with rigorous immunohistochemical and molecular analysis, most (or all) cases of LG are now classified as disorders of B cells[46], probably originating from transformation by EBV[47].

Clinical features

LG typically presents in the third to fifth decade of life, and has a male predominance of at least 2:1. Although many cases evolve into lymphoma, adenopathy is unusual at presentation. LG tends to involve extranodal sites such as the lungs, skin, kidney and nervous system (central and peripheral). The involvement of lymph nodes, spleen and bone marrow is a late manifestation of the disease, and usually signals the development of lymphoma.

Most patients with LG have pulmonary involvement. Approximately two-thirds of patients have pulmonary symptoms, which include cough, pleuritic chest pain, deep discomfort within the chest, shortness of breath, and dyspnea on exertion. Pulmonary nodules are the classic manifestation (Fig. 148.10), located bilaterally in the middle and lower lobes. The lesions undergo necrosis and cavitate in 30% of cases.

Skin lesions usually consist of subcutaneous nodules that are painful, erythematous and tender, ranging in size from 1 to 4 cm. These lesions may resemble erythema nodosum, but have a predilection for the trunk. The nodules sometimes erode through the skin, causing ulcers (Fig. 148.11). The renal pathology in LG usually consists of atypical lymphocytic infiltrates within the interstitium, but mild focal GN may occur simultaneously. The clinical manifestations of central nervous system disease derive from mass lesions within the brain or spinal cord, leading to diplopia, ataxia, aphasia, hemiparesis and paresthesia. The cerebrospinal fluid frequently shows abnormal protein concentrations and increased numbers of small T lymphocytes, suggestive of a reactive process. Only rare cases show monoclonal B cells. Peripheral nerve involvement, which mimics vasculitic neuropathy, occurs in approximately 10% of patients.

Pathology

The basic lesion of LG is an angiocentric and angiodestructive infiltrate comprised of atypical lymphoreticular cells. At the malignant end of the disease continuum the disease is essentially a B-cell lymphoma that is rich in T cells. The pleomorphic infiltrate consists of both reactive and atypical cells (lymphocytes, plasma cells, histiocytes and lymphoreticular cells). The degree of atypia varies according to the grade of lesion[44], which correlates with the number of EBV-positive cells[46]. The EBV-transformed cells are large lymphoid cells (immunoblasts) of B-cell origin which show pleomorphic nuclei and prominent nucleoli (Fig. 148.12). In the lesions identified in the lung and other sites, however, most of the infiltrating lymphoid cells are reactive T lymphocytes[44]. In contrast to WG, neutrophils, eosinophils and well-formed granulomas are infrequent or absent.

In LG, the nodular lymphoid infiltrates center on blood vessels. Vascular destruction in this disease is probably multifactorial, involving both angioinvasion by reactive T cells and chemokine-mediated vascular damage. EBV may induce many of the chemokines involved. EBV latent membrane protein is known to cause upregulation of both interferon-inducible protein 10 and the macrophage interferon-γ induced gene (Mig), which can lead to endothelial and vascular damage and fibrinoid necrosis[48]. Vascular obliteration may cause extensive

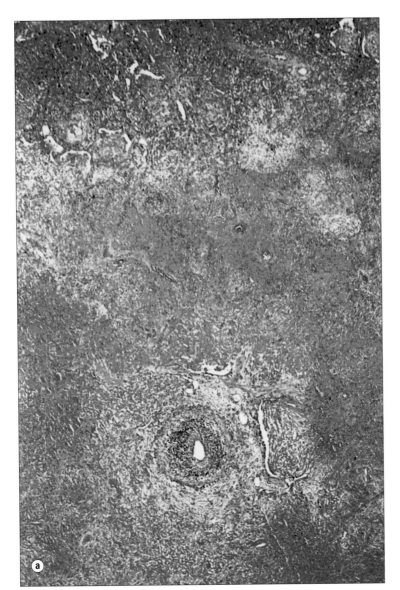
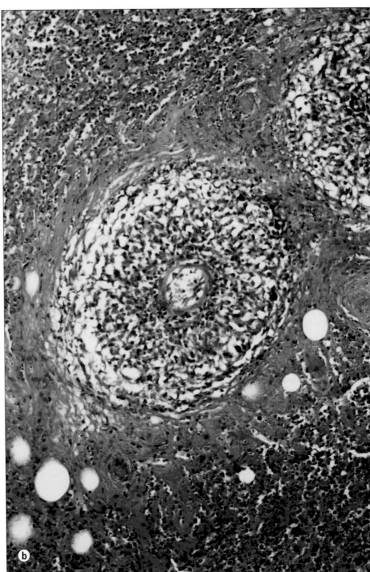

Fig. 148.12 Lung biopsy findings in lymphomatoid granulomatosis. (a) Low-powered view demonstrating extensive areas of necrosis surrounding a blood vessel. (b) Higher-powered view of a pulmonary arteriole, showing fibrinoid necrosis and lymphocytic infiltration. Although lymphomatoid granulomatosis results from the transformation of B lymphocytes, the cellular infiltration is enriched with T lymphocytes.

coagulative necrosis in diseased tissues. The necrotic lesions differ from those of WG in their lack of neutrophils and abundant nuclear debris. As noted, multinucleated giant cells and true granulomas are not a feature of LG.

When carefully evaluated, most patients with LG have defects in cytotoxic T-cell function and diminished levels of CD8+ T-cells[49]. As a consequence, the host response may be ineffective in eradicating the EBV-infected clones.

Treatment and prognosis

Early series reported poor responses to treatment, frequent progression to frank lymphoma, and high mortality[43,50]. In the largest series reported[50] 64% of the patients died, usually within 1 year of diagnosis. Subsequent reports have documented the possibility of complete remission and good long-term survival[44,51]. These series indicate that the single most important prognostic indicator for ultimate survival may be the achievement of complete remission with the initial treatment course. However, because 14–27% of patients experience durable remissions without ever undergoing treatment[50,52], therapy must be individualized in each case.

Up to 25% of patients with LG develop aggressive diffuse large B-cell lymphomas. Rapid disease progression and/or enlarging lymph nodes may herald this. Lymphoma typically occurs later in the disease. At presentation, most patients have low-grade lesions in which reactive cells predominate.

In an NIH series of 15 patients accumulated over a 10-year period, seven of the 13 patients who were treated with both CYC and corticosteroids had complete remissions. The mean duration of treatment with CYC in these patients was long: 37.0 +/– 6.0 months. None of the seven patients who achieved complete remission suffered relapses of LG or developed lymphoma, despite a total follow-up of 5.2 +/– 0.6 years. However, all of the patients who did not achieve complete remission died of lymphoma, despite the subsequent administration of aggressive combination chemotherapy.

Some patients with overt lymphomas have been treated successfully with traditional regimens for these malignancies. Because LG is now regarded as an EBV-associated lymphoproliferative disease, antiviral therapies have been employed. A small number of patients have been treated successfully with interferon-α_{2b}[49]. Because no large experience with this agent is available, however, its use as initial treatment is not appropriate.

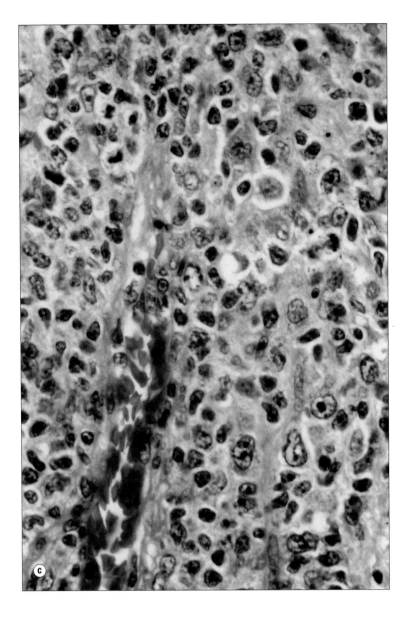

Fig. 148.12 (c) Cellular infiltrate with several large, EBV-transformed B lymphocytes containing pleomorphic nucleoli and prominent nucleoli. (Courtesy of Fredric B Askin.)

REFERENCES

1. Klinger H. Grenzformen der periarteritis nodosa. Frankfurt Z Pathol 1931; 42: 455–480.
2. Wegener F. Über generalisierte, septische Gefasserkrankungen. Verh Dtsch Ges Pathol 1936; 29: 202–210.
3. Wegener F. Über eine eigenartige rhinogene Granulomatose mit besonderer Beteiligung des Arteriensystems und der Nieren. Beitr Pathol Anat Allg Pathol 1939; 36: 36–68.
4. Watts R, Carruthers D, Scott D. Epidemiology of systemic vasculitis: changing incidence or definition? Semin Arthritis Rheum 1995; 25: 28–34.
5. Hoffman G, Kerr G, Leavitt R et al. Wegener's granulomatosis: an analysis of 158 patients. Ann Intern Med 1992; 116: 488–498.
6. Cotch M, Hoffmann G, Yerg D et al. The epidemiology of Wegener's granulomatosis. Estimates of the five-year period prevalence, annual mortality, and geographic distribution from population-based data sources. Arthritis Rheum 1996; 39: 87–92.
7. Stone J, Francis H. Immune-mediated inner ear disease. Curr Opin Rheumatol 2000; 12: 32–40.
8. Langford C, Sneller M, Hallahan C et al. Clinical features and management of subglottic stenosis in patients with Wegener's granulomatosis. Arthritis Rheum 1996; 39: 1754–1760.
9. Roberts G, Erin E, Sinclair H et al. Two cases of Wegener's granulomatosis involving the pituitary. Clin Endocrinol 1995; 323–328.
10. Nishino H, Rubino F, Parisi J. The spectrum of neurologic involvement in Wegener's granulomatosis. Neurology 1993; 43: 1334–1337.
11. Huong D, Papo T, Piette J-C et al. Urogenital manifestations of Wegener's granulomatosis. Medicine 1995; 74: 152–161.
12. Colby T, Specks U. Wegener's granulomatosis in the 1990s – a pulmonary pathologist's perspective (Review). Monogr Pathol 1993; 36: 195–218.
13. Devaney K, Travis W, Hoffman G et al. Interpretation of head and neck biopsies in Wegener's granulomatosis. A pathologic study of 126 biopsies in 70 patients. Am J Surg Pathol 1990; 14: 555.
14. Davies D, Moran J, Niall J et al. Segmental necrotising glomerulonephritis with antineutrophil antibody: Possible arbovirus aetiology. Br Med J 1982; 285: 606.
15. Van der Woude F, Rasmussen N, Lobatto S et al. Autoantibodies against neutrophils and monocytes: Tools for diagnosis and marker of disease activity in Wegener's granulomatosis. Lancet 1985; 1: 425–429.
16. Hagen E, Daha M, Hermans J et al. Diagnostic value of standardized assays for anti-neutrophil cytoplasmic antibodies in idiopathic systemic vasculitis. Kidney Int 1998; 53: 743–753.
17. Mulder A, Broekroelofs J, Horst G et al. Anti-neutrophil cytoplasmic antibodies (ANCA) in inflammatory bowel disease: Characterization and clinical correlates. Clin Exp Immunol 1994; 95: 490–497.
18. Merkel P, Polisson R, Chang Y et al. Prevalence of antineutrophil cytoplasmic antibodies in a large inception cohort of patients with connective tissue disease. Ann Intern Med 1997; 126: 866–873.
19. Hoffman G, Specks U. Antineutrophil cytoplasmic antibodies. Arthritis Rheum 1998; 41: 1521–1537.
20. Hoffman GS, Leavitt RY, Kerr GS et al. The treatment of Wegener's granulomatosis with glucocorticoids and methotrexate. Arthritis Rheum 1992; 35: 1322–1329.
21. Godman G, Churg J. Wegener's granulomatosis: Pathology and review of the literature. Arch Pathol Lab Med 1954; 58: 533–553.
22. Jennette J, Falk R, Andrassy K et al. Nomenclature of systemic vasculitides. Proposal of an international consensus conference. Arthritis Rheum 1994; 37: 187–192.
23. Rottem M, Cotch M, Fauci A et al. Familial vasculitis: report of 2 families. J Rheumatol 1994; 21: 561–563.
24. Cotch M, Fauci A, Hoffman G. HLA typing in patients with Wegener's granulomatosis. Ann Intern Med 1995; 122: 635.
25. Hoffman G, Sechler J, Gallin J et al. Bronchoalveolar lavage analysis in Wegener's granulomatosis. Am Rev Respir Dis 1991; 143: 401–407.

26. Baltaro R, Hoffman G, Sechler J *et al.* Immunoglobulin G antineutrophil cytoplasmic antibodies are produced in the respiratory tract of patients with Wegener's granulomatosis. Am Rev Respir Dis 1991; 143: 275–278.

27. Ludvikkson B, Sneller M, Chua K *et al.* Active Wegener's granulomatosis is associated with HLA-DR+ CD4+ T-cells exhibiting an unbalanced Th1-type T-cell cytokine pattern: reversal with IL-10. J Immunol 1998; 160: 3602–3609.

28. Falk RJ, Terrell RS, Charles LA, Jennette JC. Anti-neutrophil cytoplasmic autoantibodies induce neutrophils to degranulate and produce oxygen radicals *in vitro.* Proc Natl Acad Sci USA 1990; 87: 4115–4119.

29. Walton E. Giant-Cell granuloma of the respiratory tract (Wegener's granulomatosis). Br Med J 1958; 2: 265–270.

30. Hollander D, Manning R. The use of alkylating agents in the treatment of Wegener's granulomatosis. Ann Intern Med 1967; 67: 393–398.

31. Fauci A, Wolff S. Wegener's granulomatosis: studies in eighteen patients and a review of the literature. Medicine 1973; 52: 53–61.

32. Guillevin L, Cordier J-F, Lhote F *et al.* A prospective, multicenter, randomized trial comparing steroids and pulse cyclophosphamide versus steroids and oral cyclophosphamide in the treatment of generalized Wegener's Granulomatosis. Arthritis Rheum 1997; 40: 2187–2198.

33. Hoffman GS. Treatment of Wegener's granulomatosis: time to change the standard of care? Arthritis Rheum 1997; 40: 2099–2104.

34. Sneller MC, Hoffmann GS, Talar-Williams C *et al.* An analysis of forty-two Wegener's granulomatosis patients treated with methotrexate and prednisone. Arthritis Rheum 1995; 38: 608–613.

35. Stone J, Tun W, Hellmann D. Treatment of non-life threatening Wegener's granulomatosis with methotrexate and daily prednisone as the initial therapy of choice. J Rheumatol 1999; 26: 1134–1139.

36. Regan MJ, Hellmann DB, Stone JH. The treatment of Wegener's granulomatosis. Rheum Dis Clin North Am 2001; 27(4): 863–886.

37. Langford C, Talar-Williams C, Barron K *et al.* A staged approach to the treatment of Wegener's granulomatosis: Induction of remission with glucocorticoids and daily cyclophosphamide switching to methotrexate for remission maintenance. Arthritis Rheum 1999; 42: 2666–2673.

38. Jayne D. Update on the European Union Vasculitis Study Group. Curr Opin Rheumatol 2001; 13: 48–55.

39. Stegeman C, Tervaert J, Sluiter W *et al.* Association of chronic nasal carriage of *Staphylococcus aureus* and higher relapse rates in Wegener's granulomatosis. Ann Intern Med 1994; 120: 12–17.

40. Stone J, Uhlfelder M, Hellmann D *et al.* Etanercept combined with conventional treatment in Wegener's granulomatosis: a six month open-label trial to evaluate safety. Arthritis Rheum 2001; 44: 1149–1154.

41. Stone J, Hoffman G, Merkel P *et al.* The Birmingham Vasculitis Activity Score for Wegener's Granulomatosis (BVAS for WG): A disease-specific vasculitis activity index. Arthritis Rheum 2001; 44: 912–920.

42. de Groot K, Gross WL, Herlyn K *et al.* Development and validation of a disease extent index for Wegener's granulomatosis. Clin Nephrol 2000; 55: 31–38.

43. Liebow A, Carrington C, Friedman P. Lymphomatoid granulomatosis. Hum Pathol 1972; 3: 457–558.

44. Lipford E, Margolick J, Longo D *et al.* Angiocentric immunoproliferative lesions: A clinicopathologic spectrum of post-thymic T-cell proliferation. Blood 1988; 72: 1674–1681.

45. Natkunam Y, Warnke R. Angiocentric lymphomas (lymphomatous vasculitis). Semin Diagn Pathol 2001; 18: 67–77.

46. Jaffe E, Wilson W. Lymphomatoid granulomatosis: pathogenesis, pathology, and clinical implications. Cancer Surv 1997; 30: 233–248.

47. Katzenstein A-L, Peiper S. Detection of Epstein–Barr genomes in lymphomatoid granulomatosis: analysis of 29 cases by the polymerase chain reaction. Modern Pathol 1990; 3: 435–441.

48. Sgadari C, Angiolillo A, Cherney B *et al.* Interferon-inducible protein-10 identified as a mediator of tumor necrosis *in vivo.* Proc Natl Acad Sci USA 1996; 93: 13791–13796.

49. Wilson W, Kingma D, Raffeld M *et al.* Association of lymphomatoid granulomatosis with Epstein–Barr viral infection of B lymphocytes and response to interferon-alpha 2b. Blood. 1996; 87: 4531–4537.

50. Katzenstein A, Carrington C, Liebow A. Lymphomatoid granulomatosis: A clinicopathologic study of 152 cases. Cancer 1979; 43: 360–373.

51. Fauci A, Haynes B, Costa J *et al.* Lymphomatoid granulomatosis: Prospective clinical and therapeutic experience over ten years. N Engl J Med 1982; 306: 68–74.

52. James WD, Odom RB, Katzenstein AA. Cutaneous manifestations of lymphomatoid granulomatosis. Arch Dermatol 1981; 117: 196–202.

149 Churg–Strauss syndrome

François Lhote and Loïc Guillevin

Definition

- Pulmonary and systemic antineutrophil cytoplasmic autoantibodies (ANCA)-associated small-vessel vasculitis

Clinical features

- Hypereosinophilic asthma with systemic symptoms (neuropathy, purpura or subcutaneous nodules, arthritis, cardiomyopathy, abdominal pains or nephropathy)

Laboratory results

- Eosinophilia >1000/mm³, antimyeloperoxidase ANCA (70%) and increased IgE concentrations

Treatment

- Corticosteroids form the basis of treatment, sometimes in conjunction with a cytotoxic agent (cyclophosphamide) in the case of nephropathy, cardiomyopathy, gastrointestinal tract and central nervous system involvement
- Relapses occur in 25% of patients
- The 10-year survival rate is 80%.

DEFINITION

The syndrome of allergic granulomatosis and angiitis is a disorder, characterized by pulmonary and systemic small-vessel vasculitis, extravascular granulomas and hypereosinophilia, that occurs in individuals with asthma and allergic rhinitis. It bears the name Churg–Strauss syndrome in honor of the two pathologists, J. Churg and L. Strauss[1], who first described it, in 1951, as a disease entity that is similar to, but clearly distinct from, polyarteritis nodosa. Churg and Strauss established three major histologic criteria based on pathologic examination and postmortem studies: tissue infiltration by eosinophils, necrotizing vasculitis and extravascular granulomas. In fact, these three histologic components rarely coexist temporally or spatially, and are found together in only a minority of cases. Churg–Strauss syndrome is strongly associated with antineutrophil cytoplasmic autoantibody (ANCA), especially antimyeloperoxidase (MPO)-ANCA[2].

EPIDEMIOLOGY

Churg–Strauss syndrome is a rare disease. Since its first description, only small series, including fewer than 400 patients, have been published in the English and French literature[3]. The annual incidence of Churg–Strauss syndrome in Olmstead County, Minnesota (USA), was estimated to be 4 per million inhabitants[4], based on a single case seen during the period 1976–1979. From 1988 to 1998, 14 cases of Churg–Strauss syndrome were diagnosed in the Norwich Health Authority (UK)[5], where the annual incidence of Churg–Strauss syndrome using Lanham's[6] criteria was 3.1 per million inhabitants, much greater than that in Lugo (Spain), where the syndrome is extremely rare, with an annual incidence of 0.9 per million inhabitants[7]. Twelve of the 14 cases of Churg–Strauss syndrome diagnosed at the Norwich Health Authority were living in a rural area, which suggested a role of environmental factors, such as pesticides or pollens.

CLASSIFICATION

Churg–Strauss syndrome was separated from polyarteritis nodosa in 1951, and was characterized by the presence of asthma, eosinophilia and granuloma[1]. It has been considered an autonomous disease, and is now indicated as such in every classification of systemic vasculitides. In 1990, the American College of Rheumatology proposed, six classification criteria for Churg–Strauss syndrome (Table 149.1), with four being necessary for Churg–Strauss syndrome to be diagnosed with 85% sensitivity and 99.7% specificity[8]. In the classification of vasculitides formulated by the Chapel Hill Consensus Conference[9], Churg–Strauss syndrome is included among the group of small-vessel vasculitides. Lanham et al.[6] proposed clinical criteria that are very useful for the diagnosis of Churg–Strauss syndrome: the association of asthma, blood eosinophils count >1500/mm³ and symptoms of systemic vasculitis involving at least two extrapulmonary sites give a sensitivity of 95% and a specificity 95% for the diagnosis. Because of the high frequency of ANCA, it has been suggested that Churg–Strauss syndrome be considered an ANCA-associated vasculitis, like Wegener's granulomatosis and microscopic polyangiitis, and clearly separated from classic polyarteritis nodosa, a disease involving medium-sized arteries and usually not accompanied by ANCA.

TABLE 149.1 1990 AMERICAN COLLEGE OF RHEUMATOLOGY CRITERIA FOR THE CLASSIFICATION OF CHURG–STRAUSS SYNDROME

Criterion	Definition
1. Asthma	History of wheezing or diffuse high-pitched rales on expiration
2. Eosinophilia	Eosinophilia >10% of white blood cell differential count
3. Mononeuropathy or polyneuropathy	Development of mononeuropathy, multiple mononeuropathies or polyneuropathy (i.e. glove/stocking distribution) attributable to vasculitis
4. Pulmonary infiltrates, non-fixed	Migratory or transitory pulmonary infiltrates on radiographs (not including fixed infiltrates), attributable to systemic vasculitis
5. Paranasal sinus abnormality	History of acute or chronic paranasal sinus pain or tenderness or radiographic opacification of the paranasal sinuses
6. Extravascular eosinophils	Biopsy including artery, arteriole or venule, showing accumulations of eosinophils in extravascular areas

For classification purposes, a patient with vasculitis shall be said to have CSS if at least 4 of these 6 criteria are present. The presence of any 4 or more criteria yields a sensitivity of 85% and a specificity of 99.7%.

ACR, American College of Rheumatology; CSS, Churg–Strauss syndrome.

(Adapted from Masi et al.[8])

PATHOGENESIS

Very little information is available concerning the immunopathogenesis of Churg–Strauss syndrome. The immunopathogenetic mechanisms leading to vascular injury in systemic vasculitides are incompletely understood, and are probably heterogeneous. Triggering factors have been identified in Churg–Strauss syndrome, but its etiology has not been elucidated. The development of vascular inflammatory infiltrates in tissue relies on dynamic interactions between polymorphonuclear neutrophils, endothelial cells and extracellular matrix proteins. These interactions, which are mediated by adhesion molecules, are part of the physiologic inflammatory response to injury.

The role of circulating immunoglobulin (Ig)E-containing immune complexes has to be considered. Manger et al.[10] found increased serum concentrations of such complexes in the sera of five patients with Churg–Strauss syndrome, and deposits of various immunoglobulin classes and complement C3 have been observed in renal biopsies[6].

Antineutrophil cytoplasmic autoantibodies might be possible pathogenic factors in the development of endothelial damage in vasculitides, especially in Wegener's granulomatosis, microscopic polyangiitis and Churg–Strauss syndrome[11], as suggested by clinical observations. The ANCA titer may be correlated with disease activity, and patients who are persistently ANCA-positive during remission are prone to developing relapses. In vitro, ANCA activate tumor necrosis factor (TNF)-α-primed neutrophils, leading to the production of reactive oxygen metabolites and the release of lysosomal proteolytic enzymes, including the ANCA antigens themselves. ANCA-mediated activation of neutrophils is also, in part, the result of binding to the low-affinity receptor for the Fc fragment of IgG (FcγRII). Priming results in the expression of ANCA target antigens on the surface of the neutrophils, thereby making these cells accessible for interaction with the antiproteinase 3 and anti-MPO antibodies. ANCA interacts with primed neutrophils when the latter are adherent to endothelium, a process that particularly involves β-integrins. In addition, ANCA can stimulate neutrophil cytotoxicity towards activated endothelial cells in culture. The coexistence of cytokine-primed neutrophils, endothelium and circulating ANCA may permit ANCA to trigger the cascade of events leading to vasculitis[11], especially in small vessels in which neutrophils are in close contact with vessel walls.

Cytokines are potentially involved in the pathogenesis of Churg–Strauss syndrome. Biologically, Churg–Strauss syndrome is characterized by increased serum IgE and eosinophilia that are believed be hallmarks of T helper 2 cell responses. Interleukin (IL)-4 is required for class switching from IgG to IgE, and IL-5, in association with IL-3 and granulocyte–macrophage colony-stimulating factor, is particularly important in regulating the proliferation of eosinophils. Proinflammatory cytokines, such as IL-1β and TNF-α, interact with endothelial cells to induce intercellular adhesion molecules, permitting the egress of eosinophils into inflammatory loci and promoting the expression of adhesion molecules[12]. However, only a few studies have investigated the involvement of cytokines in the pathogenesis of Churg–Strauss syndrome. Grau et al.[13] reported that TNF-α and IL-1β concentrations were increased in the sera of patients with Churg–Strauss syndrome. Tsukadaira et al.[14] obtained similar results, and also showed that IL-5 concentrations were high in the sera of five patients with Churg–Strauss syndrome. Using short-term cultures of polyclonal T cell lines derived from the peripheral blood of patients with Churg–Strauss syndrome, Kiene et al.[15] provided evidence for both a type 1 (characterized by interferon (IFN)-γ) and a type 2 response in Churg–Strauss syndrome. In quantitative terms, the type 2 cytokine pattern (characterized by IL-4, IL-5 and IL-13) appears to predominate.

Patients with Churg–Strauss syndrome often show marked peripheral blood eosinophilia, with various degrees of activation[14], but only a few studies have evaluated the involvement of eosinophils in tissue lesions. Conditions secondary to eosinophilic infiltration of tissues, such as eosinophilic endomyocarditis, are rarely reported[1,16]. Eosinophil granules contain major basic protein, eosinophilic cationic protein and eosinophil-derived neurotoxins. Eosinophilic cationic protein has been found to be increased in serum and bronchoalveolar lavage fluid[17]. Extracellular deposits of eosinophilic cationic protein and major basic protein have also been detected in damaged tissues, at sites of active disease[18,19].

Various precipitating factors have been incriminated in the etiology of some cases of Churg–Strauss syndrome. These putative triggering factors are very diverse, ranging from inhaled antigens to parenterally introduced agents (vaccination or desensitization). It has not been possible to identify any common antigen among them. Suspected precipitating factors were identified in 24 of our patients[20]. Wechsler et al.[21] reported several cases of Churg–Strauss syndrome associated with withdrawal of corticosteroid treatment from asthmatic patients receiving the cysteinyl leukotriene receptor antagonists, zafirlukast or montelukast. The estimated incidences of Churg–Strauss syndrome in the asthmatic population treated with either antagonist are strikingly similar – about 60 per million asthmatics per year. In comparison with the incidence of Churg–Strauss syndrome in the general population, these rates observed in association with leukotriene modifiers appear to represent a large increase. However, analysis of the incidence of Churg–Strauss syndrome[22] in a cohort of patients with asthma who were receiving non-leukotriene-modifying asthma drugs showed a very similar rate (64.4 per million asthmatics per year), suggesting that the Churg–Strauss syndrome was not directly attributable to zafirlukast or montelukast, but rather to an underlying systemic eosinophilic disorder that was chronically masked by systemic or high-dose inhaled corticosteroids prescribed for what was perceived to be severe asthma.

The hypothesis that Churg–Strauss syndrome results from a proliferation of CD4$^+$ T helper 2 cells, triggered by inhaled allergens, vaccinations, desensitization, drugs or infections (parasitic or bacterial), followed by a massive expansion of eosinophils, requires confirmation.

HISTOLOGY

The two lesions characteristic for the diagnosis of Churg–Strauss syndrome[23] are angiitis and extravascular necrotizing granulomas, usually with eosinophilic infiltrates. The vasculitis may be granulomatous or non-granulomatous, and it typically involves both arteries and veins, in addition to pulmonary and systemic vessels. Temporal artery involvement in Churg–Strauss syndrome has been reported anecdotally. Granulomas are typically about 1mm or more in diameter, and are commonly located near small arteries or veins; they are characterized by palisading epithelioid histiocytes arranged around central necrotic zones in which eosinophils are prominent. Necrotizing vasculitis, tissue infiltration by eosinophils and extravascular granulomas rarely coexist temporally or spatially, being found together in only a minority of cases.

In the lungs, the histologic features of Churg–Strauss syndrome combine necrotizing vasculitis and areas resembling eosinophilic pneumonia. Vasculitis affects both arteries and veins. It is characterized by granulomatous inflammation or giant cell infiltration of vessel walls. In some cases, transmural eosinophil and histiocyte infiltrates with fibrinoid necrosis may be seen. Small extravascular granulomas are also common.

Extrapulmonary lesions are more commonly found in the gastrointestinal tract, spleen and heart than in the kidney. Cutaneous and subcutaneous lesions, so-called Churg–Strauss granulomas, lack diagnostic specificity and 50% of such lesions occur in a variety of systemic diseases other than Churg–Strauss syndrome.

CLINICAL FEATURES

Natural history of Churg–Strauss syndrome

Lanham et al.[6] identified three phases of the disease. The prodromal period may last for years (more than 30 years) and consists of asthma and other allergic manifestations (allergic rhinitis and nasal polyposis). A systematic inquiry[20] showed that 63.8% of the patients had a personal history of allergy and 25% had a familial history of allergy[24]. The second phase of the disease is characterized by the onset of peripheral blood and tissue eosinophilia with Löffler's syndrome, chronic eosinophilic pneumonia or eosinophilic gastroenteritis. The eosinophilic infiltrative disease may remit and recur over the years before the systemic vasculitis appears and defines the third phase of the disease. These three phases do not necessarily follow one another in this order. Systemic vasculitis emerges within a mean time of 8.86 ± 10 years after the onset of asthma, and a shorter duration of asthma before the onset of vasculitis is associated with a poorer prognosis. Some authors have proposed a possible relationship between antigenic stimulation (vaccination, desensitization) or inhaled antigens and the onset of vasculitis[12,13], but there is no definitive evidence and coincidence cannot be excluded.

Clinical features of Churg–Strauss syndrome[6,20,24–28] are summarized in Table 149.2. The mean age at the time of diagnosis of Churg–Strauss syndrome is 48.2 ± 14.6 years. The sex ratio is around 1; 53% of the patients were men in our series[20]. General symptoms, such as fever or weight loss, are present in most patients and their development in patients with asthma is suggestive of the diagnosis.

Pulmonary manifestations
Asthma
Asthma is the central feature of Churg–Strauss syndrome and precedes the systemic manifestations in nearly all cases. Unlike common asthma, it appears relatively late, around the age of 35 years[6,20]. The severity and frequency of the asthmatic attacks usually increase until the onset of vasculitis, and 50% of patients requires steroids, at least by spray, and more often orally. Although dramatic remission of asthma may occur when vasculitis emerges, the asthma usually becomes more severe during the weeks preceding vasculitis and becomes corticosteroid-dependent; patients often require admission to hospital to treat asthma attacks or respiratory failure. In one study[24], the severity of asthma justified the use of steroids in 77% of the patients. Upper airway findings can include sinusitis, allergic rhinitis and nasal polyps.

Pulmonary infiltrates
Chest radiographs are often abnormal, and 38–77% of the patients have pulmonary infiltrates. When these are present during the second phase of the disease, and in association with asthma and hypereosinophilia, they may mimic chronic eosinophilic pneumonia. The radiologic features of pulmonary infiltrates are diverse. Transient and patchy infiltrates with an alveolar pattern without lobar or segmental distribution are the most typical radiologic aspect, although a diffuse interstitial infiltrative pattern or massive bilateral nodular infiltrates without cavitation may be seen. The most common finding on computed tomography is non-specific and consists of areas of parenchymal opacification that may be random or peripheral in distribution. Their significance is not univocal: pulmonary eosinophilic infiltration or, more rarely, alveolar hemorrhage can occur.

Pleural effusion
According to recent prospective studies, pleural effusion is rarely present at the time of diagnosis, and was observed in only 3% of patients. The effusion can be unilateral or bilateral and is often asymptomatic. The fluid is an eosinophil-rich exudate and its glucose concentration can be low[3]. Vasculitis and eosinophil infiltration of the pleura can be seen and Churg–Strauss syndrome can, on rare occasions, be diagnosed by pleural biopsy[20].

Neurological involvement
Neuropathy
Peripheral neuropathy, usually mononeuritis multiplex, is found in 64–75% of the patients, and its occurrence is highly suggestive of the diagnosis. Motor and sensory signs are asymmetric and predominantly affect the lower limbs, especially the sciatic nerve and its peroneal and tibial branches; radial, cubital and median nerves are involved less

TABLE 149.2 CLINICAL FEATURES OF CHURG–STRAUSS SYNDROME

Clinical features	Frequency (%)							
Report	Chumbley et al.[25]	Literature review[6]	Lanham et al.[6]	Guillevin et al.[24]	Gaskin et al.[26]*	Haas et al.[27]	Abu-Shakra et al.[28]	Guillevin et al.[20]
No. of patients	30	138	16	43	21	16	12	96
Sex (M/F)	21/9	72/66	12/4	24/19	14/7	12/4	6/6	45/51
Age (years)								
Mean	47	38	38	43.2	46.5	42.5	48	48.2
Range	(15–69)			(7–66)	(23–69)	(17–74)	(28–70)	(17–74)
Asthma	100	100	100	100	100	100	100	100
General symptoms	–	–	–	72	–	100	100	70
Pulmonary infiltrates	27	74	72	77	43	62	58	38
Allergic rhinitis and ENT involvement	70	69	70	21	–	10	83	47
Mononeuritis multiplex	63	64	66	67	70	75	92	78
GI involvement	17	62	59	37	58	56	8	33
CV involvement	16	52	47	49	15	56	42	30
Arthritis, arthralgias	20	46	51	28	43	31	42	41
Myalgias	–	–	68	–	–	43	33	54
Skin involvement	67	–	–	–	50	68	67	51
Purpura	46	48	28	–	25	–	31	
Nodules	27	33	30	21	–	25	–	19
Renal involvement	20	42	49	16	80	31	8	16
Pleural effusion	–	29	29	2.3	–	25	–	–

* Nephrology patients.

ENT, ear, nose and throat; GI, gastrointestinal; CV, cardiovascular; not reported.

Clinical characteristics and frequencies (%) of features of Churg–Strauss syndrome in 372 patients reported in the literature.

frequently. Motor deficit appears abruptly. Sensory signs are responsible for hypo- or hyperesthesia and pain in the area of the motor deficit, which is sometimes present before the sensory loss. Peripheral neuropathy is typically mononeuritis multiplex or multiple mononeuropathy, but can sometimes take on the appearance of bilateral distal sensory neuropathy. Electromyography shows axonal nerve involvement and often detects more extensive involvement than the clinical symptoms would indicate. When performed, neuromuscular biopsies often (63%) showed epineurial vessel involvement[20], and they are good tool for diagnosing vasculitis. Under treatment, mononeuritis multiplex regresses progressively and patients can recover without sequelae. However, when sequelae are present, they are more sensory than motor. Cranial nerve palsy is infrequent, and the most common cranial nerve lesion is ischemic optic neuritis.

Central nervous system involvement

Central nervous system involvement is relatively rare. It occurred in 8.3% of our patients[20]. Clinical manifestations are non-specific – strokes with motor or sensory deficit, meningeal or brain hemorrhage, cognitive dysfunction, or epilepsy – and reflect the presence of brain vasculitis. Computed tomography scans and magnetic resonance images are useful for diagnosis. Central nervous system involvement has been demonstrated to be one of the factors of poor prognosis[29].

Cutaneous lesions

Skin involvement occurs in 40–70% of the patients, and reflects the predilection for small vessels. Purpura is seen in nearly 50% of cases, and subcutaneous nodules in 30%. Skin biopsies show extravascular granulomas. These nodules are the most distinctive skin lesions of Churg–Strauss syndrome, but are not pathognomonic and have been described in other forms of vasculitis, autoimmune diseases and non-Hodgkin's lymphoma. They are red or violaceous and occur primarily on the scalp and the limbs or hands and feet. They are often bilateral and symmetric. Other cutaneous manifestations have been reported, including Raynaud's phenomenon, livedo reticularis (6.2%), urticarial lesions (9.3%), patchy skin necrosis, infiltrated papules, vesicles or bullae, and toe or finger ischemia.

Cardiac involvement

Cardiac involvement is common in Churg–Strauss syndrome and represents the major cause of mortality. Among our patients[20], 22.9% had pericarditis and 13.4% had myocardial involvement. Histologically, granulomatous infiltration of the myocardium and coronary vessel vasculitis are the most common lesions. Endomyocardial fibrosis is very rarely found[1,16]. Congestive heart disease develops rapidly and is often severe; it was responsible for the deaths of five of our 96 patients[20]. Angina pectoris and myocardial infarction are rare, despite frequent coronary vasculitis. Electrocardiograms show abnormalities caused by ischemia or cardiomyopathy. Echocardiography shows diminished contractile parameters that are not specific to vasculitis. Cardiac involvement has been demonstrated to be one of the factors of poor prognosis[29].

Gastrointestinal involvement

Digestive tract symptoms, including abdominal pain, diarrhea and bleeding, occur in 37–62% of patients with Churg–Strauss syndrome. Two different mechanisms of involvement are possible: mesenteric vasculitis is the most common and shares the gastrointestinal location of polyarteritis nodosa, with the risk of bowel perforation; bowel wall infiltration by eosinophils is rare, and may be responsible for obstructive symptoms or diarrhea and bleeding. Bowel perforation is the most severe manifestation and is one of the major causes of death[3,20]. Vasculitis and granulomas can be present throughout the gastrointestinal tract, but are more frequently found in the small intestine or colon.

At endoscopy, the presence of several duodenal and jejunal ulcers may evoke the diagnosis. The sensitivity of angiography to detect microaneurysms appears to be low. The gastrointestinal involvement has been demonstrated to be one of the factors of poor prognosis[29].

Renal involvement

Kidney disease is present in 16–49% of the patients. The glomerular lesion that typifies Churg–Strauss syndrome is focal segmental glomerulonephritis with necrotizing features including crescents, often associated with a perinuclear pattern of ANCA label[26]. Other lesions are possible: vasculitis, eosinophilic interstitial infiltrates and granuloma. Although renal involvement in Churg–Strauss syndrome is generally considered to be mild, seven of the 17 nephrology patients reported by Gaskin et al.[26] had marked renal impairment (creatinine >150µmol/l or 1.7mg/dl), and two required dialysis. Renal involvement has been demonstrated to be one of the factors of poor prognosis[29].

Musculoskeletal involvement

Arthralgias are frequent, and often occur during the first days or weeks. Arthritis with local inflammatory findings is rare, and joint deformity and radiographic erosions do not occur. Although arthralgia can affect all joints, it predominates in the larger articulations. Myalgias are frequent (53–68%)[6,20] and usually regress quickly under treatment. However, sometimes they are so intense that they mimic polymyositis.

Ear, nose and throat and ophthalmologic symptoms

Maxillary sinusitis is frequent in Churg–Strauss syndrome, and 70% of patients have allergic rhinitis or sinus polyposis. A history of chronic sinusitis preceded Churg–Strauss syndrome in 62.5% of our patients[20]. The eye can also be involved, and uveitis, retinal vasculitis, episcleritis and conjunctival nodules have been described[30].

COMPLEMENTARY EXAMINATIONS

Anemia and increased parameters of inflammation, such as erythrocyte sedimentation rate in the first 1 hour and C-reactive protein, are common and were present in 80% of our patients. Eosinophilia is constant and often greater than 1000/mm³ (97%). The absence of eosinophilia may be explained by prior administration of steroids for asthma. The mean eosinophil count in our patients[20] was 7193 ± 6706/mm³, but the eosinophil count can exceed 50 000/mm³. The association of eosinophilia greater than 1000/mm³ with asthma is highly suggestive of the diagnosis of Churg–Strauss syndrome. Corticosteroids promptly reduce the eosinophil count to within the normal range in most patients, and an increase in the eosinophil count usually precedes a relapse of the vasculitis. Serum IgE is increased in 75% of the patients.

Churg–Strauss syndrome is strongly associated with ANCA[2]. ANCA, mostly predominantly anti-MPO, were present in 47.6–85% of the patients (mean 59.2%)[3]. The value of serial ANCA determinations to monitor disease activity in Churg–Strauss syndrome has not been determined. Rheumatoid factor was detected in 53.6% of the patients.

Abdominal and renal angiographies are usually normal.

DIAGNOSIS

Churg–Strauss syndrome is diagnosed on the basis of clinical and pathologic features[3,31]. Patients are usually middle-aged and have a history of asthma that has been present for several years. In addition to asthma, allergic rhinitis and eosinophilia, the appearance of a systemic illness characterized by mononeuritis multiplex, pulmonary infiltrates, cardiomyopathy, calf pain or cramps should lead the physician to consider the diagnosis of Churg–Strauss syndrome. Among the patients with mononeuritis multiplex, asthma and eosinophilia, the prevalence of vasculitis is high. As much as possible, the diagnosis should be substantiated by biopsy of one of the involved tissues. Placing Churg–Strauss syndrome within the spectrum of ANCA-associated vasculitides is based on the frequency of ANCA in patients with this syndrome; however, the contribution of ANCA positivity to the diagnosis of Churg–Strauss syndrome must always be interpreted in light of the patient's clinical condition. For patients with asthma, eosinophilia and mononeuritis multiplex, a positive anti-MPO-ANCA titer is highly indicative of the diagnosis of Churg–Strauss syndrome.

The differential diagnosis of Churg–Strauss syndrome includes polyarteritis nodosa, Wegener's granulomatosis, chronic eosinophilic pneumonia and the idiopathic hypereosinophilic syndrome.

Many similarities exist between polyarteritis nodosa and Churg–Strauss syndrome, and the systemic vasculitis characteristic of the third phase of Churg–Strauss syndrome shares numerous clinical aspects of polyarteritis nodosa, although pulmonary involvement and asthma are usually absent in polyarteritis nodosa. Renal involvement in Churg–Strauss syndrome is characterized by necrotizing glomerulonephritis that is not observed in polyarteritis nodosa. In Churg– Strauss syndrome, the vasculitis involves small vessels, and microaneurysms such as are observed in polyarteritis nodosa are rare. ANCAs are rarely found in polyarteritis nodosa, whereas they are present in 67% of patients with Churg–Strauss syndrome.

Differentiation from Wegener's granulomatosis on clinical grounds is usually not difficult. Asthma and a history of allergy are not prominent features of Wegener's granulomatosis, in which eosinophilia is only an occasional and minor finding. Upper respiratory tract involvement in Churg–Strauss syndrome is not associated with the necrotizing lesions characteristically seen in Wegener's granulomatosis. Renal involvement in Churg–Strauss syndrome is less severe and prominent than in Wegener's granulomatosis. In addition, histopathologic features of the granulomatous lesions of Churg–Strauss syndrome and Wegener's granulomatosis are very different. ANCA are frequently found in both diseases, and may provide another tool for the differential diagnosis: anti-antiproteinase 3 ANCAs are characteristic of Wegener's granulomatosis, whereas most of the ANCAs found in patients with Churg–Strauss syndrome are anti-MPO.

Chronic eosinophilic pneumonia usually affects women and generally does not involve extrapulmonary organs. Granuloma and vasculitis are not among its histologic features.

Hypereosinophilic syndrome is a condition characterized by persistent, marked blood and bone marrow eosinophilia associated with diffuse organ infiltration by eosinophils. Many similarities exist between hypereosinophilic syndrome and Churg–Strauss syndrome. The greater mean peak eosinophil count, typical endomyocardial fibrosis, absence of asthma and history of allergy, absence of vasculitis and granuloma at biopsy, and resistance to steroids observed in the hypereosinophilic syndrome usually make its differentiation from Churg–Strauss syndrome easy.

TREATMENT

Corticosteroids, sometimes in conjunction with cytotoxic agents, are the most effective treatment of Churg–Strauss syndrome. The initial management should include high doses of corticosteroids[32]: 1mg/kg per day of prednisone or its equivalent of methylprednisolone. Treatment should be consolidated into a single morning dose. The administration of methylprednisolone pulses (usually 15mg/kg intravenously over 60min, repeated at 24-hour intervals for 1–3 days) has become widely used at the initiation of treatment for severe systemic vasculitis, because of its rapid action and relative safety, especially in the presence of life-threatening organ involvement or the extension phase of mononeuritis multiplex. The response to corticosteroids is often dramatic; allergic symptoms and eosinophilia regress rapidly and remission of the vasculi-

tis is obtained in most cases. As the patient's clinical status improves and as the erythrocyte sedimentation rate returns to normal, usually within 1 month, tapering of the prednisone dose can begin. However, it is often impossible for the patient to cease taking corticosteroids, because of the residual asthma requiring low doses of prednisone (mean dose 8.85 ± 6.8mg/day in our patients) or inhaled corticosteroids (12% of our patients), or both[20].

The outcome of Churg–Strauss syndrome and other systemic vasculitides is dependent upon the extent of disease dissemination[32]. Therefore, management decisions should also be based on the anatomical distribution, the severity of involvement and the intensity of disease activity. The choice of first-line treatment may be helped by using well-established indicators of severity and prognostic factors. On the basis of a prospective study on 337 patients[29], we determined the clinical, biologic, immunologic and therapeutic factors that are associated with the prognosis of polyarteritis nodosa and Churg–Strauss syndrome. Among all the parameters evaluated, the following five, which had significant prognostic value and were responsible for greater mortality, became the basis of the five-factors score: proteinuria >1g/day, renal insufficiency (creatininemia >140μmol/l or 1.58mg/dl), cardiomyopathy, gastrointestinal tract involvement and central nervous system involvement. Cyclophosphamide is indicated as part of the first-line treatment when one or more factors of poor prognosis are present. The majority of patients with Churg–Strauss syndrome do not have five-factors scores of poor prognosis; thus cyclophosphamide should be prescribed only as second-line treatment, in the case of treatment failure or relapse.

When cyclophosphamide is indicated, an intravenous pulse should be preferred to oral administration. A low dose of cyclophosphamide has conventionally been defined as 2mg/kg per day or less for 1 year and, in combination with corticosteroids, represented the traditional treatment of systemic vasculitides[31,32]. Major side effects associated with daily administration of cyclophosphamide include: hemorrhagic cystitis, bone marrow suppression, ovarian failure, neoplasm (bladder cancer and hematologic malignancies) and severe infections. In an attempt to decrease the morbidity associated with daily cyclophosphamide, pulse cyclophosphamide treatment is now being used increasingly to treat systemic necrotizing vasculitis[32]. In the procedures of the French Vasculitis Study Group, the cyclophosphamide-pulse dose was 0.6g/m², given at 2-week intervals for 1 month, then every month for 6–12 months. Intense hydration and the use of sodium 2-mercaptoethanesulfonate are strongly recommended during pulse treatment. Cyclophosphamide pulses allow a lower cumulative dose to be given and expose the patient to less potential toxicity for shorter periods. Oral cyclophosphamide has been successfully introduced when intravenous administration failed to control disease activity or when a relapse occurred within the first 6 months of treatment[32]. The duration of treatment with corticosteroids and cyclophosphamide should not exceed 1 year.

There is at present no argument to support the systematic prescription of plasma exchanges at the time of Churg–Strauss syndrome diagnosis[33], even for patients with factors of poor prognosis. However, plasma exchanges are a useful tool, as second-line treatment, in Churg–Strauss syndrome refractory to conventional therapy.

Intravenous immunoglobulins, 2g/kg over 2 days, can also be prescribed, as has been done for other ANCA-related vasculitides[33]. This treatment is not recommended as first-line therapy, but may be useful for patients refractory to conventional treatments.

Cyclosporine has been given in anecdotal cases of Churg–Strauss syndrome. One patient who took cyclosporine to prevent cardiac graft rejection suffered a relapse and died[3].

Interferon-α appears to be a promising agent in the treatment of Churg–Strauss syndrome, because it inhibits the degranulation and effector function of eosinophils. High doses of interferon-α (9–63 million units/week) successfully obtained clinical responses in four patients who required this treatment, but most of them suffered relapse at the end of the treatment[34]. Cutaneous lesions have also been successfully treated with interferon-α[35].

OUTCOME

The prognosis of Churg–Strauss syndrome has improved dramatically since the introduction of corticosteroids and, in some cases, cytotoxic drugs. With treatment, remission is rapidly obtained in more than 80% of affected patients (in 88.6% of ours)[20]. During follow-up, relapses occurred in 25.5%, during the first year in half and later in the others, after a mean follow-up of 69.3 months. The clinical symptoms of relapse differed from the initial manifestations of Churg–Strauss syndrome in 50% of the patients, and can be severe and sometimes responsible for death. Some patients experience several relapses.

The 10-year survival rate was 79.4% for our patients[20]. Approximately 75% of the deaths are directly attributable to vasculitis (Table 149.3). Cardiac involvement is the primary cause of death in patients with Churg–Strauss syndrome. Asthma usually persists after recovery from vasculitis. In our patients, 82.2% of the survivors in long-term remission of Churg– Strauss syndrome had persistent asthma and 72.6% of them required maintenance treatment with low doses of prednisone (mean dose 8.85 ± 6.8mg/day) or inhaled corticosteroids (12% of our patients), or both[20]. Permanent morbidity as a result of vasculitis sequelae can be neurologic, such as the consequence of severe peripheral neuropathy or cerebral ischemia. Congestive heart failure is also a major concern in the long term, and some patients may require cardiac transplantation. Renal failure may lead to chronic dialysis.

TABLE 149.3 CAUSE OF DEATH FOR 321 PATIENTS WITH CHURG–STRAUSS SYNDROME

Cause of death	Number							
Report	Churg and Strauss[1]	Chumbley et al.[25]	Literature review[6]	Lanham et al.[6]	Haas et al.[27]	Abu-Shakra et al.[28]	Guillevin et al.[20]	Total
No. of patients	13	30	138	16	16	12	96	321
No. of deaths	11	15	50	1	4	1	23	105
Vasculitis-related	8	7	45	1	2		11	74
Cardiac involvement	3	5	24	1	1		9	43
Renal insufficiency	1	1	9				2	11
GI involvement	1	1	4					9
CNS hemorrhage	3		8		1			11
Iatrogenic complications		2					4	6
Infections		2					2	4
Anticoagulant overdose							2	2
Pulmonary involvement	1	1	5		2		4	13
Respiratory failure			1		1		2	4
Status asthmaticus	1	1	4		1		2	9
Other	1	1				1	3	6
Cancer							2	2
Anaphylaxis							1	1
Pulmonary embolism						1		1
Cachexia	1							1
Miscellaneous			1					1
Unknown	1	4					1	6

GI, gastrointestinal; CNS, central nervous system.

REFERENCES

1. Churg J, Strauss L. Allergic granulomatosis, allergic angiitis and periarteritis nodosa. Am J Pathol 1951; 27: 277–301.
2. Guillevin L, Visser H, Noël LH et al. Antineutrophil cytoplasm antibodies (ANCA) in systemic polyarteritis nodosa with and without hepatitis B virus infection and Churg–Strauss syndrome. 62 patients. J Rheumatol 1993; 20: 1345–1349.
3. Lhote F, Cohen P, Guillevin L. Syndrome de Churg et Strauss. In: Kahn MF, Peltier AP, Meyer O, Piette JC, eds. Maladies et syndromes systémiques ch 22. Paris: Flammarion Médecine-Sciences; 2000: 725–740.
4. Kurland LT, Chuang TY, Hunder G. The epidemiology of systemic arteritis. In: Lawrence RC, Shulman LE, eds. The epidemiology of the rheumatic diseases. New York: Gower; 1984: 196–205.
5. Watts RA, Carruthers DM, Scott DGI. Epidemiology of systemic vasculitis: changing incidence or definition? Semin Arthritis Rheum 1995; 25: 28–34.
6. Lanham JG, Elkon KB, Pusey CD, Hughes GR. Systemic vasculitis with asthma and eosinophilia: a clinical approach to the Churg–Strauss syndrome. Medicine (Baltimore) 1984; 63: 65–81.
7. Watts RA, Gonzalez-Gay MA, Lane SE et al. Geoepidemiology of systemic vasculitis: comparison of the incidences in two regions of Europe. Ann Rheum Dis 2001; 60: 170–172.
8. Masi AT, Hunder GG, Lie JT et al. The American College of Rheumatology 1990 criteria for the classification of Churg–Strauss syndrome (allergic granulomatosis angiitis). Arthritis Rheum 1990; 33: 1094–1100.
9. Jennette JC, Falk RJ, Andrassy K et al. Nomenclature of systemic vasculitides. Proposal of an international consensus conference. Arthritis Rheum 1994; 37: 187–192.
10. Manger BJ, Krapf FE, Gramatzki M et al. IgE-containing circulating immune complexes in Churg–Strauss vasculitis. Scand J Immunol 1985; 21: 369–373.
11. Heeringa P, Jennette JC, Falk RJ. Microscopic polyangiitis: pathogenesis. In: Hoffmann GS, Weyand CM, eds. Inflammatory diseases of blood vessels, ch 23. New-York: Marcel Dekker, Inc.; 2001: 339–353.
12. Rothenberg ME. Eosinophilia. N Engl J Med 1998; 338: 1592–1600.
13. Grau GE, Roux-Lombard P, Gysler C et al. Serum cytokine changes in systemic vasculitis. Immunology 1989; 68: 196–198.
14. Tsukadaira A, Okubo Y, Kitano K et al. Eosinophil active cytokines and surface analysis of eosinophils in Churg–Strauss syndrome. Allergy Asthma Proc 1999; 20: 39–44.
15. Kiene M, Csernok E, Müller A et al. Elevated interleukin-4 and interleukin-13 production by T cell lines from patients with Churg–Strauss syndrome. Arthritis Rheum 2001; 44: 469–473.

16. Ramakrishna G, Connolly HM, Tazelaar HD, Mullany CJ, Midthun DE. Churg–Strauss syndrome complicated by eosinophilic endomyocarditis. Mayo Clin Proc 2000; 75: 631–635.

17. Schnabel A, Csernok E, Braun J, Gross WL. Inflammatory cells and cellular activation in the lower respiratory tract in Churg–Strauss syndrome. Thorax 1999; 54: 771–778.

18. Tai PC, Holt ME, Denny P et al. Deposition of eosinophil cationic protein in granulomas in allergic granulomatosis and vasculitis: the Churg–Strauss syndrome. BMJ 1984; 289: 400–402.

19. Peen E, Hahn P, Lauwers G et al. Churg–Strauss syndrome: localization of eosinophilic major basic protein in damaged tissues. Arthritis Rheum 2000; 43: 1897–1900.

20. Guillevin L, Cohen P, Gayraud M et al. Churg–Strauss syndrome: clinical study and long-term follow-up in 96 patients. Medicine (Baltimore) 1999; 78: 26–37.

21. Wechsler ME, Finn D, Gunawardena D et al. Churg–Strauss syndrome in patients receiving montelukast as treatment for asthma. Chest 2000; 117: 708–713.

22. Martin RM, Wilton LV, Mann RD. Prevalence of Churg–Strauss syndrome, vasculitis, eosinophilia and associated conditions: retrospective analysis of 58 prescription-event monitoring cohort studies. Pharmacoepidemiol Drug Safety 1999; 8: 179–189.

23. Lie JT. Histopathologic specificity of systemic vasculitis. Rheum Dis Clin North Am 1995; 21: 883–909.

24. Guillevin L, Guittard T, Blétry O et al. Systemic necrotizing angiitis with asthma: causes and precipitating factors in 43 cases. Lung 1987; 165: 165–172.

25. Chumbley LC, Harrison EG, De Remee RA. Allergic granulomatosis and angiitis (Churg–Strauss syndrome). Mayo Clin Proc 1977; 52: 477–484.

26. Gaskin G, Clutterbuck EJ, Pusey CD. Renal disease in the Churg–Strauss syndrome. Contrib Nephrol 1991; 94: 58–65.

27. Haas C, Geneau C, Odinot JM et al. L'angéite allergique avec granulomatos : syndrome de Churg et Strauss. Etude rétrospective de 16 observations. Ann Med Interne (Paris) 1991; 142: 335–342.

28. Abu-Shakra M, Smythe H, Lewtas J et al. Outcome of polyarteritis nodosa and Churg–Strauss syndrome. An analysis of twenty-five patients. Arthritis Rheum 1994; 37: 1798–1803.

29. Guillevin L, Lhote F, Casassus P et al. Prognostic factors in polyarteritis nodosa and Churg–Strauss syndrome. A prospective study in 342 patients. Medicine 1996; 75: 17–28.

30. Nissim F, Von der Valde J, Czernobilsky B. A limited form of Churg–Strauss syndrome. Ocular and cutaneous manifestations. Arch Pathol Lab Med 1982; 106: 305–307.

31. Lhote F, Guillevin L. Polyarteritis nodosa, microscopic polyangiitis and Churg–Strauss syndrome. Lupus 1998; 7: 238–258.

32. Guillevin L, Lhote F. Classification and management of systemic vasculitides. Drugs 1997; 53: 805–816.

33. Lhote F, Guillevin L. Indications of plasma exchanges in the treatment of polyarteritis nodosa, Churg–Strauss syndrome and other systemic vasculitides. Transfus Sci 1996; 17: 211–213.

34. Tatsis E, Schnabel A, Gross W. Interferon-α treatment of four patients with the Churg–Strauss syndrome. Ann Intern Med 1998; 129: 370–374.

35. Termeer CC, Simon JC, Schöpf E. Low-dose interferon alpha-2b for the treatment of Churg–Strauss syndrome with prominent skin involvement. Arch Dermatol 2001; 137: 136–138.

150 Takayasu's arteritis

Carol A Langford

Definition
- An inflammatory disease of unknown etiology characterized by granulomatous vasculitis affecting the aorta, its main branches, and the pulmonary arteries
- Occurs most commonly in women of childbearing age

Clinical features
- Examination: absent pulses, bruits, asymmetric blood pressure
- Hypertension is an important contributor to morbidity and mortality
- Common presenting symptoms: claudication, headaches, dizziness, syncope, visual changes, dyspnea, palpitations, vessel tenderness (carotidynia)
- Systemic symptoms may be absent but include: fever, night sweats, fatigue, arthralgias, myalgias

HISTORY

Takayasu's arteritis (TA) is a granulomatous vasculitis of unknown etiology that affects the aorta, its major branches and the pulmonary arteries. The first descriptions of this disease possibly date back to the 1700s and 1800s, when there were several reports of patients with pulselessness and aortic disease. In 1908, at a meeting of the Japanese Society of Ophthalmologists, Mikito Takayasu presented the case of a young woman with a wreathlike arteriovenous anastomosis around the optic disk. Following Takayasu's presentation, Onishi and Kagoshima commented that they had observed similar changes in patients who also lacked radial pulses. Caccamise and Whitman, in 1952, referred to this entity as 'pulseless or Takayasu's disease', and in 1962 Judge and colleagues introduced the term 'Takayasu's arteritis'. Although TA has become the most widely used nomenclature for this disease in the United States, it is known in other countries by different synonyms, including aortic arch syndrome, pulseless disease, middle aortic syndrome, occlusive thromboaortopathy and non-specific aortoarteritis.

EPIDEMIOLOGY

TA has often been characterized as an illness affecting young women of eastern ethnic background. However, descriptions from diverse regions have shown not only that TA occurs throughout the world, but also that it may have a varying clinical spectrum in different populations[1] (Tables 150.1 and 150.2). Whereas Japanese series have demonstrated a female predominance of 9:1, a nearly equal representation among men and women has been reported in Israel and India[2]. Similarly, although TA has been observed to present between the ages of 15 and 25 in Japan, patients from Italy and Sweden have been diagnosed at a mean age of 41 years[2].

TA is believed to be an uncommon disease. In Olmstead County, Minnesota, an incidence of 2.6 cases per million per year was observed, whereas in Sweden the incidence was 1.2 per million per year. In one

Japanese series 100 patients were estimated to develop TA each year, which would suggest a similar incidence[3]. However, it remains possible that geographic differences exist, as detailed data are lacking for many regions where increased prevalence rates have been suggested.

CLINICAL FEATURES

TA has historically been viewed as a triphasic process characterized by an initial systemic phase, a vessel inflammatory phase, and a 'burnt-out' or pulseless phase. Increasing evidence has suggested, however, that such a view is of limited utility as it does not accurately depict the status of blood vessel inflammation and does not follow the course that many patients experience[4].

On physical examination, the most frequent features are bruits, diminished or absent pulses, and asymmetric blood pressure measurements between extremities. Because the subclavian arteries are a frequent site of vessel stenosis, blood pressure measurements in one or both arms may not be representative of aortic root pressure (Fig. 150.1). Hypertension has been reported to occur in 32–93% of TA patients[2,4–10]. It is an important cause of morbidity in TA and contributes to renal, cardiac and cerebral injury. In India, TA is the most common cause of renovascular hypertension, accounting for over 60% of all cases[2].

At the time of diagnosis approximately 20% of patients with TA are clinically asymptomatic, with the disease being detected by abnormal vascular findings on examination[4]. The remaining 80% of patients with TA present as a result of symptoms that are systemic or vascular in nature. Systemic symptoms may be absent in up to 60–80% of patients[6,4] but include fatigue, malaise, weight loss, night sweats, fever, arthralgias or myalgias (Table 150.1).

Vascular symptoms are a direct result of current or previous arteritis. Active inflammation may result in tenderness over the vessel, and

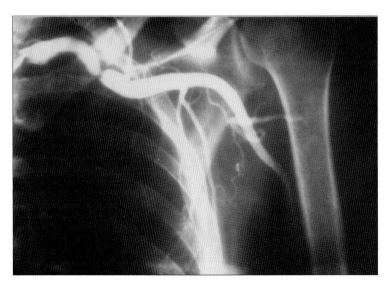

Fig. 150.1 **Tight stenosis of the left subclavian artery seen by arteriography.**

Symptom/sign	Japan[15] (n =52)	India[9] (n =106)	China[7] (n =530)	Korea[12] (n =129)	USA[4] (n =60)	Mexico[8] (n =107)
Fatigue/constitutional	27	–	–	34	43	78
Weight loss	–	9	–	11	20	22
Musculoskeletal	6	5	–	–	53	53
Claudication	13	–	25	21	90	29
Headache	31	44	–	60	42	57
Visual changes	6	12	10	20	30	8
Syncope dizziness	40	26	14	36	35	13
Palpitations	23	19	–	23	10	43
Dyspnea	21	26	11	42	–	72
Carotidynia	21	–	–	2	32	–
Hypertension	33	77	60	40	35	72
Bruit	–	35	58	37	80	94
Decreased pulses	62	–	37	55	60	96
Asymmetric blood pressure	–	–	–	–	47	–

TABLE 150.1 COMMON SYMPTOMS AND SIGNS IN TAKAYASU'S ARTERITIS

carotidynia in particular occurs in 2–32% of patients. Vessel inflammation typically results in either stenosis (Figs 150.1 & 150.2) or aneurysm formation (Fig. 150.3). Arterial stenosis may present with signs or symptoms of diminished blood flow to regions supplied by the affected vessel, and aneurysms can rupture or cause valvular incompetence when affecting the aortic root. The frequencies of common signs and symptoms from different published series are listed in Table 150.1. Decreased circulation to the extremities often presents as intermittent claudication. Cerebral blood flow is supplied by the two carotid and two vertebral arteries. Stenosis or occlusion of these arteries or the vessels proximal to their origin may diminish perfusion and cause injury to the brain and central nervous system. Involvement of these vessels can be completely asymptomatic or present with transient ischemic attacks, stroke, dizziness, syncope, headache or visual changes. Although mesenteric involvement is common in TA, gastrointestinal symptoms such as nausea, diarrhea, vomiting and abdominal pain occur infrequently.

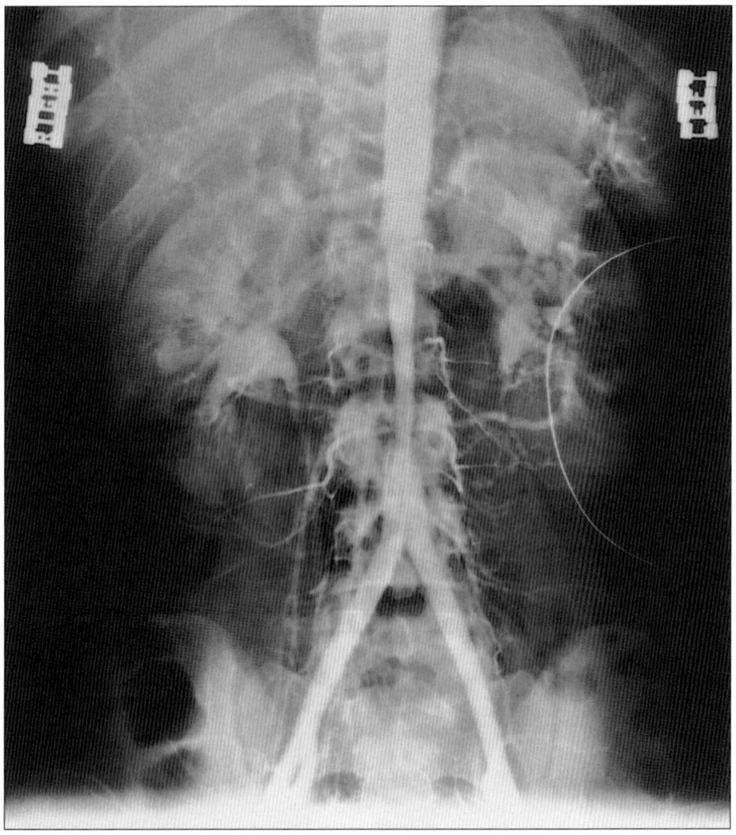

Retinal disease as reported by Takayasu occurs in 14% of patients and results from compromise to the internal carotid circulation with central retinal hypoperfusion[11]. Initially, generalized vasodilation occurs with capillary microaneurysms, but with advancement of the disease arteriovenous anastomosis, capillary dropout and eventual blinding complications may result. Retinopathy may also develop as a direct complication of hypertension.

Cardiac involvement may present with dyspnea, palpitations, angina, myocardial infarction, heart failure or sudden death. Most frequently this is related to aortic valvular regurgitation from dilation of the aortic root, which occurs in 5–55% of patients (Fig. 150.3). Up to 25% of patients may also develop coronary vessel stenosis[12], with other less frequent manifestations including mitral valve regurgitation, cardiomyopathy and myocarditis[1].

By arteriographic studies, pulmonary artery involvement may occur in 50–86% of patients[7,9] (Fig. 150.4). Although this is typically asymptomatic, patients may present with features of pulmonary hypertension, or rarely with hemoptysis. Ventilation/perfusion scans are often abnormal, with pulmonary artery involvement, and such patients may be mistakenly diagnosed with thromboembolic disease.

Cutaneous manifestations occur in 3–28% of patients with TA. The most commonly observed lesions include erythema nodosum, as well as pyoderma gangrenosum, erythema induratum, and papular and ulcerative lesions[13].

Renal involvement in TA is usually characterized by renovascular hypertension. Non-specific glomerular disease from arterial narrowing and hypertension has been observed, as well as occasional reports of other glomerular lesions. Renal amyloidosis has been rarely reported[13].

INVESTIGATIONS

TA is diagnosed by the presence of characteristic arterial lesions in the aorta and its branches, for which other causes of large-vessel abnormalities have been excluded (Table 150.3). The American College of Rheumatology in 1990 proposed classification criteria for the purposes of providing a standard way to describe patients with TA in studies.

Fig. 150.2 Irregularity and stenosis of the abdominal aorta seen by arteriography.

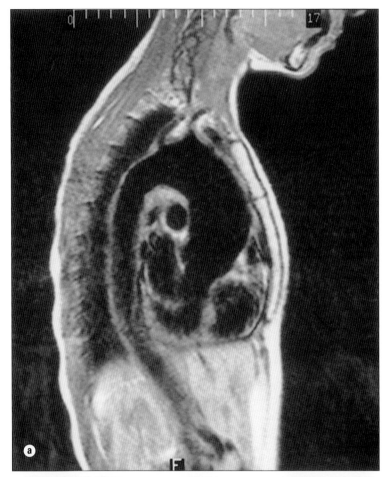

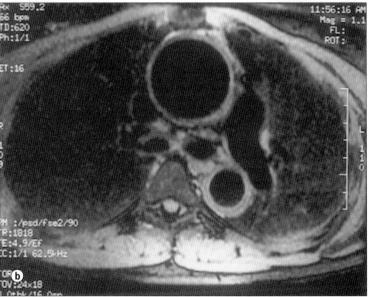

Fig. 150.3 Aneurysm of the aortic root by magnetic resonance imaging (T_1 weighted image). The ascending aorta measures 5.0cm and can be compared against the normal diameter of the descending aorta.

Diagnostic criteria based on patterns of vessel disease and other objective parameters have been studied by investigators from Japan and India[14].

Laboratory and radiographic investigations in TA are initially utilized diagnostically, and thereafter for the purposes of assessing disease activity. The inability to assess disease activity accurately in TA has been a critical limitation in managing the individual patient and in evaluating therapeutic regimens. As no single parameter has proved useful in identifying active disease, one method of assessment has been to examine

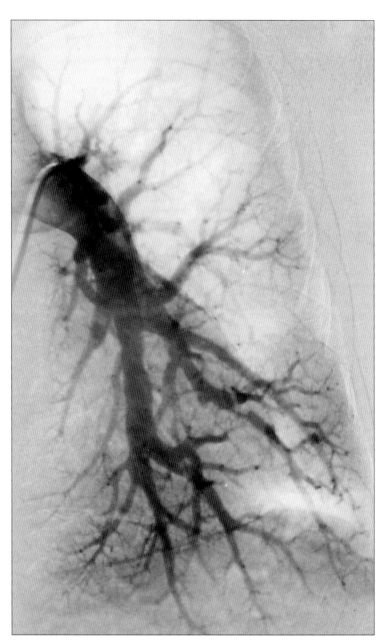

Fig. 150.4 Pulmonary arteriogram in a patient with Takayasu's arteritis. Abrupt termination of a proximal branch to the lingula is seen, as well as a vessel with irregularity and narrowing.

clinical information collectively (Table 150.4). Even using this approach, active arteritis has been observed in 44% of surgical bypass specimens taken from patients judged to be quiescent by current methods[4]. Other studies have similarly demonstrated the presence of ongoing inflammation despite assessment of clinical inactivity.

Laboratory tests

There is no laboratory study that is diagnostic for TA or that correlates consistently with active arteritis. TA is not associated with the presence of antineutrophil cytoplasmic antibodies (ANCA). The most common laboratory findings are reflective of acute inflammation. The complete blood count may reveal a normochromic, normocytic anemia, leukocytosis, and thrombocytosis[8,12,15].

Some series have found the erythrocyte sedimentation rate (ESR) to be a useful marker by which to assess active inflammatory disease[5,16–18], but others have not found it to be uniformly reliable[4,6]. In one series a normal ESR was present in one-third of patients who were felt to have clinically active disease, whereas elevated values were demonstrated in up to 56% of patients in remission[4].

TABLE 150.2 PATTERN OF VESSEL INVOLVEMENT IN TAKAYASU'S ARERITIS

Vessel	Frequency of arteriographic involvement (%)						Symptoms
	Japan[15] (n = 52)	India[9] (n = 106)	China[7] (n = 105)	Korea[12] (n = 129)	USA[4] (n = 60)	Mexico[8] (n = 107)	
Subclavian							
Right	21	28	46	41	8	13	Upper extremity claudication, Raynaud's
Left	56	59	78	61	55	25	
Carotid							
Right	31	7	23	12	7	7	Visual changes, syncope, transient ischemic
Left	40	21	26	32	27	19	attacks, stroke
Vertebral	–	–	13	10	35	19	Visual changes, dizziness
Ascending aorta	46	13	–	1	–	27	
Aortic arch or root	–	19	–	2	35	27	Aortic insufficiency, congestive heart failure
Thoracic aorta	31	26	25	37	17	–	
Abdominal aorta	33	72	55	46	47	67	
Celiac axis	–	3	4	5	18	–	Rarely abdominal pain, nausea, vomiting
Inferior mesenteric	–	8	3	7	–	14	Rarely abdominal pain, nausea, vomiting
Superior mesenteric	–	12	24	16	18	14	Rarely abdominal pain, nausea, vomiting
Renal							
Right	23	53	34	30	17	18	Hypertension, renal failure
Left	15	52	32	33	2	16	
Iliac							
Right	–	15	10	–	2	1	Lower extremity claudication
Left	–	12	8	–	S	6	
Pulmonary	–	49	53	–	–	14	Atypical chest pain, dyspnea
Coronary	–	–	–	23	–	9	Chest pain, myocardial infarction, dyspnea

–, not specified.

TABLE 150.4 CRITERIA FOR ACTIVE DISEASE IN PATIENTS WITH TAKAYASU'S ARTERITIS[4]

- Elevated erythrocyte sedimentation rate
- Systemic symptoms
- New or progressive features of vascular ischemia
- New or progressive arteriographic changes

Active disease said to be defined by the presence of two of the four criteria.

Radiographic studies

Arteriography has remained the gold standard in detecting involved vessels in TA. Unless a strong contraindication exists, diagnostic arteriography should include a complete study of the aorta and its major branches, as the recognition of clinically occult disease may have diagnostic and prognostic importance. The limitations of arteriography, particularly for serial monitoring, are the risks of thromboembolism, and significant contrast and radiation exposure.

The most common arteriographic finding is that of stenosis, which occurs in 85% of patients (Figs 150.1, 150.2). Vessel occlusion or irregularity is also frequently seen. Aneurysms may be saccular or fusiform and typically affect the aorta rather than its branches (Fig. 150.3). Overall, aneurysms occur less frequently than stenosis, but they have been reported as the predominant lesion in some series. Varying patterns of vessel involvement have been observed in different populations, with lesions of the ascending aorta and aortic arch being more common in Japanese patients, whereas involvement of the abdominal aorta and renal arteries is more typical in patients from India[1,19] (Table 150.2). Comparative studies of vessel disease across different regions have been aided by the use of arteriographic classification systems that focus on the distribution of vessel involvement[19] (Fig. 150.5).

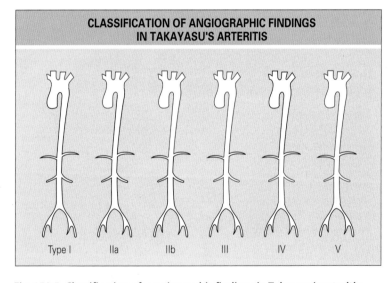

CLASSIFICATION OF ANGIOGRAPHIC FINDINGS IN TAKAYASU'S ARTERITIS

Type I   IIa   IIb   III   IV   V

Fig. 150.5 Classification of arteriographic findings in Takayasu's arteritis. (Redrawn with permission from Hata *et al.*[19])

Interpretation of vessel changes that occur in serial arteriograms is complicated by the fact that progression of vascular disease may result from either active vasculitis or non-inflammatory fibrosis. In one study, although 88% of patients with active disease had new lesions on follow-up arteriography, 61% of patients in clinical remission also had progressive changes[4]. Thus, arteriography demonstrates luminal patency but does not necessarily provide information on the degree of inflammation present in the arterial wall.

Repeat arteriographic studies should be obtained for new or progressive ischemic symptoms. However, in the absence of new symptoms the frequency of obtaining arteriograms must be determined on an individual basis, given the risks of arteriography and the increasing utility of other modalities. Patients with severe lesions affecting cerebral blood flow may warrant closer monitoring, as the availability of collateral circulation may be limited and resultant ischemia potentially catastrophic.

Magnetic resonance (MR) imaging is emerging as a useful adjunctive technique to evaluate vessel disease[20]. Compared with standard arteriography, MR angiography represents a safer and less invasive technique for assessing vessel patency. One series has demonstrated that this technique clearly demonstrates aortic lesions, including stenosis and dilation[21]. However, MR angiography may have limitations in assessment of the aortic branch vessels and may overestimate the severity of vessel narrowing. In contrast to conventional arteriography, MR angiography also cannot provide intravascular pressure measurements. MR using fast spin-echo sequences designed to enhance the detection of vessel wall edema has additionally shown promise in assessing disease activity[22,23]. However, further experience and correlation with vessel pathology are needed to assess this technique fully.

Ultrasonography has been reported to provide useful information about carotid lesions[24]. This technique relies on the skill and interpretation of the operator and will require additional study to determine its general applicability to clinical care.

DIFFERENTIAL DIAGNOSIS

The differential diagnosis of TA includes diseases that affect the aorta, its main branches or the pulmonary arteries (Table 150.3). Although they may appear arteriographically similar to TA, most of these diseases have other clinical manifestations that assist in establishing the diagnosis[25].

PATHOLOGY

In contrast to other vasculitides, tissue biopsies play little to no role in the diagnosis of TA, as histologic examination of the great vessels is

TABLE 150.3 DIFFERENTIAL DIAGNOSIS OF TAKAYASU'S ARTERITIS

Giant cell arteritis
Behçet's syndrome
Cogan's syndrome
Kawasaki's disease
Sarcoidosis
Rheumatoid arthritis
Spondyloarthropathies
Relapsing polychondritis
Systemic lupus erythematous
Reactive arthritis
Buerger's disease
Infections
   Syphilis
   Mycobacterium tuberculosis
   Staphylococcus aureus
   Escherichia coli
   Salmonella
   Rheumatic fever
Atherosclerosis
Thromboembolism
Ehlers–Danlos syndrome
Marfan's syndrome
Neurofibromatosis
Congenital aortic coarctation
Fibromuscular dysplasia
Radiation fibrosis
Traumatic stenosis
Ergotism

usually possible only at the time of vascular procedures or postmortem. TA is a panarteritis that typically occurs as focal 'skip lesions'. During active disease the inflammatory infiltrate is predominantly lymphoplasmacytic, with granuloma formation and giant cells involving the media and adventitia. Later, degeneration of internal elastic lamina of the media, adventitial fibrosis and neovascularization are seen. The characteristic vessel tapering and irregular narrowing are produced by intimal thickening and contraction of the media and adventitia[1,26].

PATHOPHYSIOLOGY

The pathophysiology of TA remains poorly understood and there is no known cause of the disease. In some populations, possible associations between *Mycobacterium tuberculosis* and TA have been reported[8]. However, to date there have been no convincing data linking these two diseases, and treatment with antituberculous therapy has not brought about improvements in TA.

Several lines of reasoning support that TA is immunologically mediated[3]. Defective T-cell regulation has been suggested by one report that demonstrated increased CD4 and decreased CD8 cells in TA patients[27]. In another study, evidence of cell-mediated cytotoxicity was provided by the demonstration of $\gamma\delta$ T lymphocytes, natural killer (NK) cells and cytotoxic T cells in aortic tissue[28]. This study also found that expression of 65 kDa heat-shock protein, intracellular adhesion molecule 1 (ICAM-1), and class I and II human lymphocyte antigens (HLA) was strongly induced in aortic tissue. These factors could facilitate the recognition, adhesion and cytotoxicity of the infiltrating killer cells, particularly $\gamma\delta$ T lymphocytes, and result in vascular cell injury.

A possible role for humoral-mediated mechanisms in the pathogenesis of TA has been questioned, based on the presence of high levels of γ-globulins, rheumatoid factor and circulating immune complexes. Some investigators have demonstrated the presence of antiaortic, antiendothelial[29] and anticardiolipin antibodies in TA patients. However, these have not been found consistently and it remains unclear whether they have a role in disease pathogenesis.

HLA genes have been investigated because of their relevance in regulating immune responses, together with the predilection of the disease for individuals of particular ethnic backgrounds. In studies from Japan and Korea, an association of TA with HLA-Bw52 has been described[3,30]. However, in Indian patients TA is associated with HLA-B5[31], whereas analysis of HLA genes in North America has revealed no association[4]. Because of the clinical differences observed in these populations, some have suggested that HLA play a role in determining the pattern of TA.

MANAGEMENT

General principles

Approximately 80% of patients with TA have features of active disease necessitating treatment. Natural history data would suggest that interruption of active inflammation prior to the development of significant vessel damage improves prognosis. However, this has not been definitively proven and the role of immunosuppressive treatment in lessening morbidity and mortality has been difficult to assess. In addition to limitations in accurately assessing disease activity, treatment is further complicated by the propensity for TA to be a chronic and relapsing disease. In one study, regardless of treatment, 45% of patients were found to experience at least one disease relapse and 23% never achieved a remission[4].

Given these issues, therapeutic decisions are often guided by individual patient variables that include the location and severity of lesions, availability of collateral circulation, nature and intensity of symptoms, and the risks of medication toxicity. Effective management of patients with TA usually includes treatment of not only the active inflammatory disease but also the chronic fixed vascular lesions for which non-medical therapeutic modalities play an important role. Establishing a team of rheumatologists, cardiovascular surgeons and imaging/interventional radiologists early in the course of disease can be helpful in planning overall patient care.

Glucocorticoids

Glucocorticoids are the mainstay of medical treatment in TA, although the data regarding their efficacy have varied. Resolution of systemic symptoms has been reported to occur in 25–100% of glucocorticoid-treated patients[4,5,8,17,18,32]. Objectively, some reports have demonstrated that glucocorticoids have brought about improvement in arteriographic blood flow[33] and a return of previously absent pulses[5,17,18,32].

There have to date been no comparative trials to determine the optimal dose and length of glucocorticoid treatment. Retrospective series have utilized a broad spectrum of initial prednisone doses ranging from 20 to 100mg daily[5,7,17,32–34]. The Systemic Vascular Disorders Research Committee of the Ministry of Health and Welfare of Japan has recommended that patients with evidence of active arteritis be treated initially with prednisolone 30mg daily[32]. In a retrospective analysis of 150 patients who had received glucocorticoids at doses similar to those used in this regimen, 51% had an improved quality of life, 37% experienced no change and 12% worsened, although no definitions of these outcome measures were given[32].

In the largest prospective standardized experience with glucocorticoids in TA, patients initially received prednisone 1mg/kg/day (60mg daily) for the first 1–3 months, with careful observation for adverse effects and response[4,35]. Over the next 2–3 months, when disease activity decreased, the prednisone was tapered to an alternate-day schedule and then decreased further towards discontinuation. In 48 patients with active TA treated with this regimen, first-time therapy resulted in remission in 52% and 60% achieved remission at least once. Although such data support the use of an initial prednisone dose of 1mg/kg/day, a lower starting dose may be considered in selected individuals at high risk for steroid toxicity, provided there is no threat of immediate tissue ischemia.

Cytotoxic therapy

The use of a cytotoxic agent in addition to glucocorticoids is of less proven benefit in TA than in other forms of systemic vasculitis. Cytotoxic therapy in TA is considered primarily in patients who have persistent disease activity despite daily glucocorticoid treatment, or when remission cannot be maintained on alternate-day glucocorticoids. Using these criteria, one study observed that 52% of patients required the addition of a cytotoxic agent during the course of their disease, with 40% of these achieving remission at least once[4].

In considering the choice of cytotoxic agent, the greatest experience has been with the use of methotrexate (MTX), and to a lesser degree cyclophosphamide (CYC). Data regarding the efficacy of other cytotoxic agents in TA is confined solely to case reports[32,36].

MTX has been evaluated in a prospective standardized trial in a glucocorticoid-resistant population[37]. In this regimen, MTX was initiated orally at a dose of 0.3mg/kg (not to exceed 15mg) once a week and increased by 2.5mg every 1–2 weeks, up to a maximum dose of 25mg once a week. This was administered together with prednisone 1mg/kg/day, which was tapered after 1 month to an alternate-day regimen within 3–6 months. If, within 6 months of starting MTX, the symptoms and signs of active disease had resolved and the prednisone dose was able to be reduced, then the MTX was continued for an additional 6 months, after which time it was tapered until discontinuation. Out of 16 patients, this regimen led to remission in 81%, with 25%

experiencing a sustained remission for approximately 1 year in the absence of immunosuppressive medications. However, remission was followed by relapse in 54%, and 19% of patients had progressive disease. Approximately half of the patients who relapsed were reinduced into remission on the same protocol. The therapeutic toxicities in this study included reversible elevated hepatic transaminase levels (28%), nausea (22%), stomatitis (6%), and one episode of *Pneumocystis carinii* pneumonia, which was successfully treated. Other potential side effects of MTX that were not observed in this study include pneumonitis and bone marrow suppression. Although this study has limitations, these data support that MTX may be an effective means of inducing remission and minimizing glucocorticoid toxicity in the difficult to treat TA patient.

CYC was the first studied cytotoxic agent in TA; however, the data regarding its use are limited. In one study, seven patients were treated with daily CYC, all of whom had active arteritis despite 3 months of daily glucocorticoids[35]. In all seven CYC allowed the glucocorticoid dose to be decreased, and cessation of the progression of vascular lesions occurred in four patients, all of whom had experienced progression on prednisone alone. The regimen given in this study was similar to that used for Wegener's granulomatosis, in which prednisone 1mg/kg/day was given together with CYC 2mg/kg/day. The risks of such treatment are an important consideration, as CYC has the potential for serious short- and long-term toxicity that includes bone marrow suppression, infection, permanent infertility, bladder injury, transitional cell carcinoma of the bladder, and myeloproliferative disease.

Given the potential for TA to relapse and the significant side effects of CYC in this predominantly young female population, when a cytotoxic agent is indicated MTX is often considered to be the preferential choice. CYC should be reserved for patients who have clear evidence of active inflammatory disease in which glucocorticoids are effective but cannot be tapered, and where the patient is unresponsive, intolerant, or unable to take MTX.

Other medical therapies

Because of its impact on morbidity and mortality, the treatment of hypertension is important. Renovascular hypertension can be treated either medically or non-medically. In either setting, the level of blood pressure control must be balanced against the risk of worsening ischemia across stenotic sites that require high pressure to maintain blood flow.

Thrombosis of vessels is uncommon in TA and the routine use of anticoagulants is not recommended. Antiplatelet agents such as aspirin and dipyridamole have been used in some retrospective reports, but their potential benefit remains unclear[16,18,32,34].

Surgery and PTCA

Surgical therapy is important in the revascularization of stenosed or occluded vessels that produce significant ischemia. The most frequent indications for surgery include cerebral hypoperfusion, renovascular hypertension, limb claudication, repair of aneurysms, or valvular insufficiency. In carefully selected patients the safety and potential benefits of surgery have been favorable, although the graft patency and complication rates vary greatly[5,16,34,38,39]. Ideally, vascular reconstruction should be deferred until acute inflammation is medically controlled, as aneurysm formation, graft dehiscence or graft occlusion may be more likely in the setting of active arteritis[38]. However, surgery to prevent imminent ischemia of a vital organ should not be delayed because of active inflammation or ongoing immunosuppressive therapy. The role of perioperative glucocorticoids in the clinically quiescent patient remains unclear. Although it is possible that glucocorticoids may have a beneficial role if active arteritis is present, authors caution that this must be tempered against the concern for wound healing, susceptibility to infection, and possible long-term effects on suture line weakening[39].

Percutaneous transluminal angioplasty (PTCA) can be effective to control hypertension related to renal artery stenosis. The ability of PTCA to reduce stenosis has ranged from 56 to 100%[4,40,41] and has improved blood pressure in >85% of patients[40,41]. The durability of results is variable, with the risk of restenosis being highest within the first year[4,41]. Several reports have also found PTCA to be beneficial in treating short stenotic segments of other aortic branches, as well as the aorta[40,42].

OUTCOME

The long-term outcome of patients with TA has varied between studies. Although two North American reports found overall survival to be 94% or greater[4,5], the 5-year mortality rate from other series has ranged from 0 to 35%[7,10,16,43]. Mortality directly related to TA usually occurs from congestive heart failure, cerebrovascular events, myocardial infarction, aneurysm rupture or renal failure[6,7,10,16,34,43]. In two studies, predictors of poor outcome included a progressive disease course and the presence of Takayasu's retinopathy, secondary hypertension, aortic valve insufficiency or aneurysms[16,34]. Even in the absence of life-threatening disease, TA can be associated with substantial morbidity. In one series, 74% of patients were found to have some compromise in activities of daily living and 47% were permanently disabled[4].

PREGNANCY

The safety of pregnancy is an important issue because TA predominantly affects women of childbearing age. Although there remains a limited amount of data, most series have reported favorable maternal and fetal outcomes[4,17,44,45]. Hypertension is the most common cause of complications and must be closely monitored for[44]. Fetal growth retardation has been observed and appears to be influenced by hypertension during pregnancy and maternal vascular disease. Series have varied with regard to whether the presence of TA is associated with any higher rate of fetal death. The induction of labor or cesarean section are not mandatory for women with TA, although advanced planning for the method of delivery is important[44]. For women not on cytotoxic therapy pregnancy is not contraindicated, but careful perinatal care is important in optimizing outcome for both mother and child.

REFERENCES

1. Kerr GS. Takayasu's arteritis. Rheum Dis Clin North Am 1995; 21: 1041–1058.
2. Chugh KS, Sakhuja V. Takayasu's arteritis as a cause of renovascular hypertension in Asian countries. Am J Nephrol 1992; 12: 1–8.
3. Weyand CM, Goronzy JJ. Molecular approaches toward pathologic mechanisms in giant cell arteritis and Takayasu's arteritis. Curr Opin Rheumatol 1995; 7: 30–36.
4. Kerr GS, Hallahan CW, Giordano J et al. Takayasu arteritis. Ann Intern Med 1994; 120: 919–929.
5. Hall S, Barr W, Lie JT et al. Takayasu arteritis. A study of 32 North American patients. Medicine 1985; 64: 89–99.
6. Sharma BK, Sagar S, Singh AP et al. Takayasu arteritis in India. Heart Vessels Suppl 1992; 7: 37–43.
7. Zheng D, Fan D, Liu L. Takayasu arteritis in China: a report of 530 cases. Heart Vessels 1992; 7 (Suppl): 32–36.
8. Lupi-Herrera E, Sanchez-Torres G, Marchushamer J et al. Takayasu's arteritis. Clinical study of 107 cases. Am Heart J 1977; 93: 94–103.
9. Jain S, Kumari S, Ganguly NK et al. Current status of Takayasu arteritis in India. Int J Cardiol 1996; 54 (Suppl): S111–116.
10. Morales E, Pineda C, Martinez-Lavin M. Takayasu's arteritis in children. J Rheumatol 1991; 18: 1081–1084.
11. Chun YS, Park SJ, Park IK et al. The clinical and ocular manifestations of Takayasu arteritis. Retina 2001; 21: 132–140.
12. Park YB, Hong SK, Choi KJ et al. Takayasu arteritis in Korea: clinical and angiographic features. Heart Vessels 1992; 7 (Suppl): 55–59.
13. Sharma BK, Jain S, Sagar S. Systemic manifestations of Takayasu arteritis: the expanding spectrum. Int J Cardiol 1996; 54 (Suppl): S149–154.
14. Sharma BK, Jain S, Suri S et al. Diagnostic criteria for Takayasu arteritis. Int J Cardiol 1996; 54 (Suppl): S141–147.
15. Ueda H, Morooka S, Ito I et al. Clinical observation of 52 cases of aortitis syndrome. Jpn Heart J 1969; 10: 277–288.
16. Ishikawa K, Maetani S. Long-term outcome for 120 Japanese patients with Takayasu's disease. Clinical and statistical analyses of related prognostic factors. Circulation 1994; 90: 1855–1860.
17. Fraga A, Mintz G, Valle L et al. Takayasu's arteritis: Frequency of systemic manifestations (study of 22 patients) and favorable response to maintenance steroid therapy with adrenocorticosteroids (12 patients). Arthritis Rheum 1972; 15: 617–624.
18. Nakao K, Ikeda M, Kimata S-I et al. Takayasu's arteritis. Clinical report of eighty-four cases and immunological studies of seven cases. Circulation 1967; 35: 1141–1155.
19. Hata A, Noda M, Moriwaki R et al. Angiographic findings of Takayasu arteritis: new classification. Int J Cardiol 1996; 54 (Suppl): S155–163.
20. Atalay MK, Bluemke DA. Magnetic resonance imaging of large vessel vasculitis. Curr Opin Rheumatol 2001; 13: 41–47.
21. Yamada I, Nakagawa T, Himeno Y et al. Takayasu arteritis: diagnosis with breath-hold contrast-enhanced three-dimensional MR angiography. J Magn Reson Imaging 2000; 11: 481–487.
22. Flamm SD, White RD, Hoffman GS. The clinical application of 'edema-weighted' magnetic resonance imaging in the assessment of Takayasu's arteritis. Int J Cardiol 1998; 66 (Suppl 1): S151–159.
23. Choe YH, Han BK, Koh EM et al. Takayasu's arteritis: assessment of disease activity with contrast-enhanced MR imaging. AJR Am J Roentgenol 2000; 175: 505–511.
24. Maeda H, Handa N, Matsumoto M et al. Carotid lesions detected by B-mode ultrasonography in Takayasu's arteritis: as an indicator of the disease. Ultrasound Med Biol 1991; 17: 695–701.
25. Hoffman GS. Treatment of resistant Takayasu's arteritis. Rheum Dis Clin North Am 1995; 21: 73–80.
26. Lie JT: Takayasu's arteritis. In: Churg A, Churg J, eds. Systemic vasculitides. New York: Igaku-Shoin, 1991; 159–179.
27. Sagar S, Ganguly NK, Koicha M et al. Immunopathogenesis of Takayasu arteritis. Heart Vessels 1992; 7 (Suppl): 85–90.
28. Seko Y, Minota S, Kawasaki A et al. Perforin-secreting killer cell infiltration and expression of a 65-kD heat-shock protein in aortic tissue of patients with Takayasu's arteritis. J Clin Invest 1994; 93: 750–758.
29. Tripathy NK, Upadhyaya S, Sinha N et al. Complement and cell mediated cytotoxicity by antiendothelial cell antibodies in Takayasu's arteritis. J Rheumatol 2001; 28: 805–808.
30. Dong RP, Kimura A, Numano F et al. HLA-linked susceptibility and resistance to Takayasu arteritis. Heart Vessels 1992; 7 (Suppl): 73–80.
31. Mehra NK, Jaini R, Balamurugan A et al. Immunogenetic analysis of Takayasu arteritis in Indian patients. Int J Cardiol 1998; 66 (Suppl 1): S127–132.
32. Ito I. Medical treatment of Takayasu arteritis. Heart Vessels 1992; 7 (Suppl): 133–137.
33. Ishikawa K. Effects of prednisolone therapy on arterial angiographic features in Takayasu's disease. Am J Cardiol 1991; 68: 410–413.
34. Ishikawa K. Survival and morbidity after diagnosis of occlusive thromboaortopathy (Takayasu's disease). Am J Cardiol 1981; 47: 1026–1032.
35. Shelhamer JH, Volkman DJ, Parillo JE et al. Takayasu's arteritis and its therapy. Ann Intern Med 1985; 103: 121–126.
36. Daina E, Schieppati A, Remuzzi G. Mycophenolate mofetil for the treatment of Takayasu arteritis: report of three cases. Ann Intern Med 1999; 130: 422–426.
37. Hoffman GS, Leavitt RY, Kerr GS et al. Treatment of glucocorticoid-resistant or relapsing Takayasu arteritis with methotrexate. Arthritis Rheum 1994; 37: 578–582.
38. Giordano JM, Leavitt RY, Hoffman GS et al. Experience with surgical treatment for Takayasu's disease. Surgery 1991; 109: 252–258.
39. Tada Y, Sato O, Ohshima A et al. Surgical treatment of Takayasu arteritis. Heart Vessels 1992; 7 (Suppl): 159–167.
40. Khalilullah M, Tyagi S. Percutaneous transluminal angioplasty in Takayasu arteritis. Heart Vessels 1992; 7 (Suppl): 146–153.
41. Tyagi S, Singh B, Kaul UA et al. Balloon angioplasty for renovascular hypertension in Takayasu's arteritis. Am Heart J 1993; 125: 1386–1393.
42. Tyagi S, Khan AA, Kaul UA et al. Percutaneous transluminal angioplasty for stenosis of the aorta due to aortic arteritis in children. Pediatr Cardiol 1999; 20: 404–410.
43. Subramanyan R, Joy J, Balakrishnan KG. Natural history of aortoarteritis (Takayasu's disease). Circulation 1989; 80: 429–437.
44. Wong VCW, Yang RYC, Tse TF. Pregnancy and Takayasu's arteritis. Am J Med 1983; 75: 597–601.
45. Ishikawa K, Matsuura S. Occlusive thromboaortopathy and pregnancy. Am J Cardiol 1982; 50: 1293–1300.

151 Behçet's syndrome

Hasan Yazici, Sebahattin Yurdakul, Vedat Hamuryudan and İzzet Fresko

Definition

- A systemic vasculitis of unknown cause involving veins and arteries of all sizes and having recurrent mucocutaneous and frequent ocular involvement
- A marked geographic distribution along the 'silk route', characterized by greatest prevalence in Turkey, Iran and Japan
- Occurring most commonly in the second or the third decades

Clinical features

- An undulating course that generally abates in intensity with the passage of time
- Males and young patients have a more severe disease course, with increased mortality
- Recurrent oral and genital aphthous ulceration
- Chronic relapsing uveitis with the potential threat of blindness
- A variety of skin manifestations, including the 'pathergy' phenomenon
- Musculoskeletal, neurologic, gastrointestinal and major artery and vein involvement

HISTORY AND EPIDEMIOLOGY

In 1937 Hulusi Behçet from Istanbul described three patients with oral and genital ulceration and hypopyon uveitis. Additional clinical manifestations, including musculoskeletal, neurologic and gastrointestinal involvement, have subsequently been recognized and added to the disease spectrum. The underlying pathology includes an inflammatory process of arteries and veins.

Epidemiologic information is derived mainly from case registries and population surveys conducted in Turkey[1]. The global distribution of reported disease suggests a geographic pattern coincident with the ancient 'silk route'.

CLINICAL FEATURES

The manifestations of Behçet's syndrome (BS) are protean (Table 151.1) and have a tendency to recur. Mucocutaneous lesions constitute the hallmark, whereas uveitis, meningoencephalitis and large vessel disease are the most serious.

Mucocutaneous lesions

Aphthous ulcerations (Fig. 151.1a) are usually the first and most frequently recurrent manifestation of BS. They are usually indistinguishable from ordinary canker sores and usually heal without scarring.

Genital ulcerations (Fig. 151.1b) typically develop on the scrotum and as a rule leave scars. In females the labia are commonly affected, although vaginal and cervical ulcers can also occur.

There are mainly two types of skin lesion. Erythema nodosum-like lesions (Fig. 151.1c) are confined to the lower extremities and heal with residual pigmentation. On histologic sections more elements of vasculitis are observed in these lesions than in erythema nodosum, idiopathic or those due to other causes[2]. Superficial thrombophlebitis, presenting as nodular skin lesions, is also observed in Behçet's and is frequently confused with erythema nodosum. The acne like-lesions are usually indistinguishable from ordinary acne[3]. Papular lesions consistent with cutaneous vasculitis and Sweet's syndrome (neutrophilic dermatosis) can also be associated with BS.

The pathergy reaction

The pathergy reaction (Fig. 151.1d) represents hyperreactivity of the skin to simple trauma, such as a needle prick. Typically, a papule or a pustule forms in 24–48 hours. This is quite specific for Behçet's and represents a general hyperreactivity of tissues to trauma. However, wound healing after biopsy-induced trauma is normal. The prevalence of pathergy is positive on repeated occasions in 60–70% of patients in Turkey or Japan, but is rarely observed in cases reported from northern Europe or the USA.

Eye involvement

Chronic, relapsing bilateral uveitis involving both anterior and posterior uveal tracts is a significant cause of morbidity. Anterior uveitis with hypopyon may be seen in 20% of Mediterranean patients with eye disease and indicates a grave prognosis (Fig. 151.2) Isolated anterior uveitis is infrequent, however, and conjunctivitis is rare.

Posterior uveal inflammation with involvement of the retina can be severe. Retinal lesions consist of exudates, hemorrhages, papilledema and macular disease. Postinflammatory structural changes, including synechiae and retinal scars, are important determinants of the prognosis of eye disease.

Musculoskeletal involvement

Seen in 50% of patients, the typical features of joint involvement include a non-deforming, non-erosive peripheral oligoarthritis that usually lasts a few weeks[4]. Most frequently the knees are involved. Synovial fluid is commonly inflammatory but a good mucin clot is usual. Synovial histology is non-diagnostic. Occasionally, chronic arthritis and osteonecrosis can be seen. Back pain is distinctly uncommon, and properly conducted studies of sacroiliac (SI) joint involvement have not demonstrated an increased prevalence in Behçet's patients.

Patients with BS and arthritis also have more acne lesions[5]. This suggests a link with the reactive arthritides.

Myositis is known to occur in BS. It is usually local, but generalized forms can be seen.

Neurological disease

Neurological involvement is observed in 5% of patients. Most patients have parenchymal involvement, with pyramidal, cerebellar and sensory signs and symptoms, sphincter disturbances and behavioral changes. The remaining have non-parenchymal involvement in the form of intracranial hypertension due to dural sinus thrombosis. Parenchymal

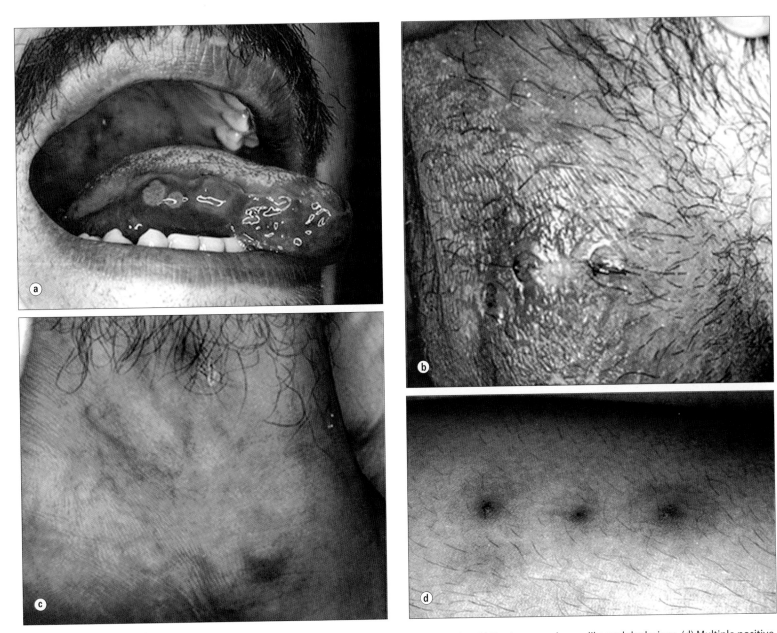

Fig. 151.1 **Mucocutaneous findings in Behçet's syndrome.** (a) Oral apthae. (b) Genital ulceration. (c) Erythema-nodosum-like nodular lesions. (d) Multiple positive pathergy tests.

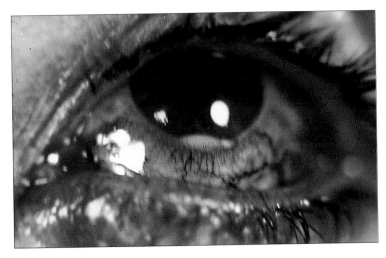

Fig. 151.2 Hypopyon uveitis.

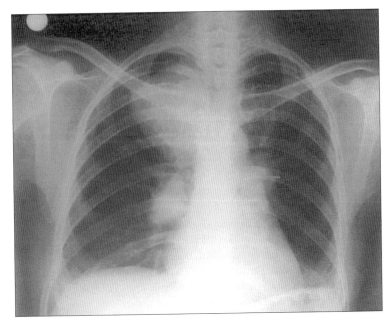

Fig. 151.3 Pulmonary artery aneurysms on chest X ray.

involvement has a more severe course. Peripheral nerve disease is unusual[6].

Cerebrospinal fluid examination reveals non-specific findings, but a high protein or cell count implies a grave prognosis. The most common site of CNS involvement is the brain stem . On the other hand, isolated cerebellar involvement is very uncommon[7].

Venous and arterial lesions

Thrombophlebitis is most frequent in the legs. Thrombosis of the major vessels, such as vena caval obstruction and occlusion of the suprahepatic veins (Budd–Chiari syndrome), is seen less frequently and is more severe in males. Thromboembolism is rarely observed.

The entire arterial tree can be affected by occlusion and/or aneurysm formation[8]. The main pathology is vasculitis of the vasa vasorum.

Pulmonary arterial aneurysms carry a grave prognosis and are usually associated with thrombophlebitis of the large veins[9]. Recurrent hemoptysis is the main manifestation. The aneurysms are seen as non-cavitating shadows on radiographs (Fig. 151.3). The diagnosis can be confirmed by CT scans. Pleural effusions are rare.

Cardiac involvement

There have been sporadic reports of valvular lesions, myocarditis, pericarditis, coronary vasculitis, ventricular aneurysms and intracavitary thrombus formation, but overall cardiac involvement is uncommon in BS.

Gastrointestinal involvement

Mucosal ulcerations, primarily in the ileum and colon, present with colicky abdominal pain and diarrhea. Ileocecal lesions are prone to perforation[10]. Gastrointestinal involvement is seen in about one-third of patients from Japan but is rare among patients from the Mediterranean basin[11].

A slightly enlarged spleen is observed in 20% of male patients.

Other clinical findings

There have been sporadic reports of glomerulonephritis. Amyloidosis of the AA type can accompany Behçet's and presents as nephrotic syndrom[12]. Epididymitis is well recognized and voiding dysfunction due to direct bladder involvement has been reported[13].

PROGNOSIS

Males and younger patients have a more stormy course with increased mortality[14]. The exacerbations in the undulating course become less and less frequent as the patient ages. Complications of chronic uveitis can lead to loss of vision.

Gastrointestinal complications, ruptured peripheral and pulmonary aneurysms and neurologic involvement are the major causes of mortality. Occasionally, the Budd–Chiari syndrome and amyloidosis lead to a fatal outcome.

INVESTIGATIONS

Laboratory findings are non-specific[15]. A moderate anemia of chronic disease and leukocytosis are seen in about 15% of patients. Neither consistently reflects the degree of clinical activity. The erythrocyte sedimentation rate and C-reactive protein may be mildly elevated, but these parameters are not good correlates of disease activity.

Serum immunoglobulins, especially IgA, are occasionally elevated, whereas autoantibodies (rheumatoid factor (RF), antinuclear antibodies (ANA)) are absent. Complement levels may be high. Antineutrophilic cytoplasmic antibodies (ANCA) are not usually positive in BS.

TABLE 151.1 FREQUENCY OF THE CLINICAL MANIFESTATIONS OF BEHÇET'S SYNDROME AND THE INTERNATIONAL STUDY GROUP DIAGNOSTIC CRITERIA

Manifestation	Frequency (%)
Oral ulcers	97–99
Genital ulcers	~85
Skin lesions	
Papulopustular lesions	~85
Erythema nodosum	~50
Pathergy reaction	~60 (Mediterranean countries and Japan)
Uveitis	~50
Arthritis	~50
Subcutaneous thrombophlebitis	25
Deep vein thrombosis	~5
Arterial occlusion/aneurysm	~4
CNS involvement	~5
Epididymitis	~ 15
Gastrointestinal lesions	1–30 (more prevalent in Japan)

In the absence of other clinical explanations, patients must have:
- Recurrent oral ulceration (apthous or herpetiform) observed by the physician or patient recurring at least three times in one 12-month period

and two of the following:
- Recurrent genital ulceration
- Eye lesions: anterior uveitis, posterior uveitis, cells in the vitreous by slit-lamp examination or retinal vasculitis observed by an ophthalmologist
- Skin lesions: erythema nodosum, pseudofolliculitis, papulopustular lesions or acneiform nodules in postadolescent patients not on corticosteroids
- Pathergy read by a physician at 24–48 hours

DIFFERENTIAL DIAGNOSIS

A set of classification criteria has been developed and is in wide use[16] (Table 151.1). Using recurrent aphthous ulceration as a constant feature, these criteria require the presence of two other sets of organ involvement for diagnosis.

Patients with recurrent aphthae and involvement of one other organ system – 'incomplete' forms –present a diagnostic challenge. The diseases that should be considered in the differential diagnosis and their characteristic features are presented in Table 151.2.

TABLE 151.2 DIFFERENTIAL DIAGNOSIS OF BEHÇET'S SYNDROME

Disease	Features not seen in Behçet's syndrome
Reactive arthritis	Urethritis, penile lesions on the glans penis and conjunctivitis
Seronegative arthropathies	Mainly psoriasiform skin lesions, aortic insufficiency, frequent axial involvement
Inflammatory arthropathies	Serological abnormalities
Inflammatory bowel disease	Inflammatory lesions throughout the bowel
Multiple sclerosis	Intranuclear ophthalmoplegia (INO) and optic neuritis
Sarcoidosis	Bilateral hilar adenopathy and parenchymal pulmonary disease
Other systemic vasculitides	Arterial microaneurysms, mononeuritis multiplex, ANCA
Vogt–Koyanagi–Harada syndrome	Peliosis, alopecia and vitiligo
Stevens–Johnson syndrome	Blisters and corneal involvement
Venereal diseases	Glans lesions, specific serologies
Coxsackie and echovirus infections	Subacute course

PATHOGENESIS

Behçet's syndrome is a vasculitis characterized by a heightened inflammatory response. It is believed to be caused by immune dysregulation, but the pathogenesis remains largely unknown.

The syndrome does not have a mendelian inheritance pattern and most cases are sporadic. However, there are a substantial number of familial cases[17], which suggests that genetic factors are also important. Genes in linkage disequilibrium with HLA-B51, such as MHC class I-related gene A (MICA), have been suggested as possible candidates for BS susceptibility, but recent analysis has shown that the genetic marker most strongly related to the syndrome is HLA-B51 itself[18]. The strength of this association is not the same throughout the world[19]. A recent study has proposed that cross-reactivity between self-antigens (retinal S) and an HLA-B51 related peptide (B27PD) may be important[20].

A state of non-specific hyperreactivity, as exemplified by the pathergy test (see Fig. 151.1d), is present in BS. Spontaneous or induced overproduction of proinflammatory Th1-type cytokines from various sources[21] may be another aspect of this non-specific inflammatory state.

Neutrophil hyperreactivity was believed to be central to the pathogenesis of BS[22]. However, this is a matter of debate[23].

T-cell mediated immune responses may also play an important role in pathogenesis. An increase in the proportions of $\gamma\delta^+$ T cells has consistently been reported[24] and a strong Th1 polarization of the immune response during active disease has been shown[25].

Herpes simplex virus (HSV) type I and streptococci (*Streptococcus oralis*) have been implicated in the pathogenesis and BS-like symptoms were produced in ICR mice after inoculation with HSV[26]. The presence of an augmented T- and B-cell response to mycobacterial heat shock proteins and to their human homologs in BS, and the production of uveitis in Lewis rats with some of these proteins, have been proposed as a mechanism of molecular mimicry between bacterial and self-HSP molecules in BS that may trigger the immune response[27]. However, other stigmata of BS are not observed in this animal model, and the hypersensitivity of T cells in BS is not restricted to disease-specific HSP peptides[28].

Some functional abnormalities concerning B cells have been noted; however, the general lack of autoantibodies and the lack of association with Sjögren's syndrome [29] suggest that BS is rather different from classic autoantibody-mediated disorders.

No single coagulation abnormality has been pinpointed in BS despite a propensity towards chronic thrombophlebitis. An increased frequency of factor V Leiden and prothrombin G→A20210 mutations has been demonstrated and increased markers of endothelial activation and injury have been described[30], but their individual contributions to pathogenesis are not clear.

A unifying theory of the pathogenesis of BS should shed light on the mechanisms behind the heightened inflammatory response, including the meaning of the HLA-B51 association that is seen in only a proportion of patients; the effects of gender on the more severe expression of the disease; and the significance of the unique geographic distribution.

MANAGEMENT

Currently, treatment of BS is directed at suppression of inflammation with the aim of preventing the occurrence of irreversible organ damage[31,32]. The presence and severity of symptoms, as well as certain prognostic factors such as male sex and a young age, have an important impact on the selection of therapeutic agents. For example, an elderly female patient with mild disease can be followed up with reassurance and the topical application of steroids and anesthetic creams. However, immunosuppressives (e.g. azathioprine 2.5mg/kg/day) should be considered in a young male patient with similar disease characteristics, as this type of patient is at increased risk for developing systemic complications carrying significant morbidity and mortality[33].

A recent 2-year controlled trial showed that colchicine is more effective than placebo in the treatment of mucocutaneous and joint symptoms, and this effect is especially prominent in females[34]. Thalidomide at a dose of 100mg daily is currently the only agent that can induce prompt and sustained relief from oral and genital ulcers, but symptoms recur after stopping treatment[35]. Furthermore, its side effects, such as teratogenesis and polyneuropathy, also prevent its routine use.

Azathioprine, when used at 2.5mg/kg/day, is effective in maintaining visual acuity and in preventing the emergence of new eye disease[36]. Some data also suggest that the initiation of azathioprine early in the disease course leads to a more favorable outcome in the long term[37]. Cyclosporin A at 5mg/kg/day has been shown to be an effective and rapidly acting drug for the eye involvement[38]. Hypertension, renal impairment and neurotoxicity are the major adverse effects. Neurologic side effects cause a special problem because the toxicity symptoms cannot be easily differentiated from those of CNS involvement of BS. On the other hand, there is the likelihood that the medication itself tends to accelerate the development of CNS system symptoms[39]. Data from uncontrolled trials suggest that interferon-α is a promising drug for various manifestations of BS, including severe eye involvement[40]. Combination of these drugs with steroids, or the combination of azathioprine and cyclosporin A, can be tried in cases resistant to a single agent.

Oral or intravenous cyclophosphamide, either as a single agent or in combination with high doses of steroids, is used on an empirical basis in patients with systemic vasculitis and parenchymal CNS involvement. Similarly, cyclosporin A or azathioprine may be used in the treatment of deep vein thrombosis. The role of anticoagulants or low-dose aspirin with regard to this complication is still not known. The arthritis is usually self-limiting. Azathioprine, sulfasalazine and interferon-α can be used in chronic cases or in cases with frequent recurrences. Gastrointestinal involvement is difficult to manage. Sulfasalazine, thalidomide or azathioprine have been reported to have some value in uncontrolled studies, but wide surgical resections are not infrequently needed and relapses at the anastomosis sites are not rare. Limited experience suggests that TNF-blocking agents may find a place in the treatment of various manifestations of BS in the near future.

With some exceptions, treatment for any serious organ involvement can be stopped after 2 years of remission.

REFERENCES

1. Yurdakul S, Gunaydin I, Tuzun Y *et al*. The prevalence of Behçet's syndrome in a rural area in northern Turkey. J Rheumatol 1988; 15: 820–822.

2. Demirkesen C, Tüzüner N, Mat C *et al*. Clinicopathological evaluation of nodular lesions of Behçet's disease. Am J Clin Pathol 2001; 116: 341–346.

3. Jorizzo JL, Abernethy JL, White WL *et al*. Mucocutaneous criteria for the diagnosis of Behçet's disease: an analysis of clinicopathological data from multiple international centers. J Am Acad Dermatol 1995; 32: 968–976.

4. Yurdakul S, Yazici H, Tüzün Y *et al*. The arthritis of Behçet's disease: a prospective study. Ann Rheum Dis 1983; 42: 505–515.

5. Diri E, Mat C, Hamuryudan V *et al*. Papulopustular skin lesions are seen more frequently in patients with Behçet's syndrome who have arthritis: A controlled and masked study. Ann Rheum Dis 2001; 60: 1074–1076.

6. Akman-Demir G, Serdaroglu P, Tasçi B. Clinical patterns of neurological involvement in Behçet's disease: evaluation of 200 patients. The Neuro-Behçet Study Group. Brain 1999; 122: 2171–2182.

7. Siva A, Kantarci OA, Saip S *et al*. Behçet's disease: diagnostic and prognostic aspects of neurological involvement. J Neurol 2001; 248: 95–103.

8. Koç Y, Güllü I, Akpek G *et al*. Vascular involvement in Behçet's disease. J Rheumatol 1992; 19: 402–410.

9. Hamuryudan V, Yurdakul S, Moral F et al. Pulmonary arterial aneurysms in Behçet's syndrome: a report of 24 cases. Br J Rheumatol 1994; 33: 48–51.

10. Bayraktar Y, Özaslan E, Van Thiel DH. Gastrointestinal manifestations of Behçet's disease. J Clin Gastroenterol 2000; 30: 144–154.

11. Yurdakul S, Tüzüner N, Yurdakul I et al. Gastrointestinal involvement in Behçet's syndrome: a controlled study. Ann Rheum Dis 1996; 55: 208–210.

12. Melikoglu M, Altiparmak MR, Fresko I et al. A reappraisal of amyloidosis in Behçet's syndrome. Rheumatology (Oxford) 2001; 40: 212–215.

13. Cetinel B, Akpinar H, Tufek I et al. Bladder involvement in Behçet's syndrome. J Urol 1999; 161: 52–56.

14. Yazici H, Basaran G, Hamuryudan V et al. The ten-year mortality in Behçet's syndrome. Br J Rheumatol 1996; 35: 139–141.

15. Sakane T, Takeno M, Suzuki N et al. Behçet's disease. N Engl J Med 1999; 341: 1284–1291.

16. International Study Group for Behçet's disease. Criteria for diagnosis of Behçet's disease. Lancet 1990; 335: 1078–1080.

17. Gul A, Inanc M, Ocal L et al. Familial aggregation of Behçet's disease in Turkey. Ann Rheum Dis 2000; 59: 622–625.

18. Mizuki N, Ota M, Yabuki K et al. Localization of the pathogenic gene of Behçet's disease by microsatellite analysis of three different populations. Invest Ophthalmol Vis Sci 2000; 41: 3702–3708.

19. Verity DH, Marr JE, Ohno S. Behçet's disease, the silk road and HLA-B51: historical and geographical perspectives. Tissue Antigens 1999; 54: 213–220.

20. Kurhan-Yavuz S, Direskeneli H, Bozkurt N et al. Anti-MHC autoimmunity in Behçet's disease: T cell responses to an HLA-B-derived peptide cross-reactive with retinal-S antigen in patients with uveitis. Clin Exp Immunol 2000; 120: 62–166.

21. Mege JL, Dilsen N, Sanguedolce V et al. Overproduction of monocyte derived tumor necrosis factor alpha, interleukin (IL) 6, IL-8 and increased neutrophil superoxide generation in Behçet's disease. A comparative study with familial Mediterranean fever and healthy subjects. J Rheumatol. 1993; 20: 1544–1549.

22. Takeno M, Kariyone A, Yamashita N et al. Excessive function of peripheral blood neutrophils from patients with Behçet's disease and from HLA-B51 transgenic mice. Arthritis Rheum 1995; 38: 426–433.

23. Tuzun B, Tuzun Y, Yurdakul S et al. Neutrophil chemotaxis in Behçet's syndrome. Ann Rheum Dis 1999; 58: 658.

24. Freysdottir J, Lau S, Fortune F. Gammadelta T cells in Behçet's disease (BD) and recurrent apthous stomatitis (RAS). Clin Exp Immunol 1999; 118: 451–457.

25. Frassanito MA, Dammacco R, Cafforio P et al. Th1 polarization of the immune response in Behçet's disease: a putative pathogenic role of interleukin-12. Arthritis Rheum 1999; 42: 1967–1974.

26. Sohn S, Lee ES, Bang D et al. Behçet's disease like symptoms induced by the herpes simplex virus in ICR mice. Eur J Dermatol 1998; 8: 21–23.

27. Lehner T. The role of heat shock protein, microbial and autoimmune agents in the aetiology of Behçet's disease. Int Rev Immunol 1997; 14: 21–32.

28. Hirohata S, Hashimoto T. Abnormal T-cell responses to bacterial super-antigens in Behçet's disease. Clin Exp Immunol 1998; 112: 317–324.

29. Gunaydin I, Ustundag C, Kaner G et al. The prevalence of Sjögren's syndrome in Behçet's syndrome. J Rheumatol 1994; 21: 1662–1664.

30. Direskeneli H. Behçet's disease: infectious etiology, new auto-antigens and HLA-B51. Ann Rheum Dis 2001; 60: 996–1002.

31. Kaklamani VG, Kaklamanis PG. Treatment of Behçet's disease – an update. Semin Arthritis Rheum 2001; 30: 299–312.

32. Yazici H, Yurdakul S, Hamuryudan V. The management of Behçet's syndrome. How are we doing? Clin Exp Rheumatol 1999; 17: 145–147.

33. Yazici H, Tuzun Y, Pazarli H et al. Influence of age of onset and patient's sex on the prevalence and severity of manifestations of Behçet's syndrome. Ann Rheum Dis 1984; 43: 783–789.

34. Yurdakul S, Mat C, Ozyazgan Y et al. A double blind trial of colchicine in Behçet's Syndrome. Arthritis Rheum 2001; 44: 2686–2692.

35. Hamuryudan V, Mat C, Saip S et al. Thalidomide in the treatment of the mucocutaneous lesions of the Behçet syndrome. A randomized, double-blind placebo controlled trial. Ann Intern Med 1998; 128: 443–450.

36. Yazici H, Pazarli H, Barnes CG et al. A controlled trial of azathioprine in Behçet's syndrome. N Engl J Med 1990; 322: 281–285.

37. Hamuryudan V, Ozyazgan Y, Hizli N et al. Azathioprine in Behçet's syndrome: effects on long term prognosis. Arthritis Rheum 1997; 40: 769–774.

38. Ozyazgan Y, Yurdakul S, Yazici H et al. Low dose cyclosporin A versus pulsed cyclophosphamide in Behçet's syndrome: a single masked trial. Br J Ophthalmol 1992; 76: 241–243.

39. Kotake S, Higashi K, Yoshikawa K et al. Central nervous system symptoms in patients with Behçet disease receiving cyclosporine therapy. Ophthalmology 1999; 106: 586–589.

40. Kötter I, Eckstein AK, Stubiger N, Zierhut M. Treatment of ocular symptoms of Behçet's disease with interferon alpha 2a: a pilot study. Br J Ophthalmol 1998; 82: 488–494.

152 Kawasaki disease

Tomisaku Kawasaki

Definition

- An acute febrile disease occurring most commonly in infants and children under 5 years of age
- Vasculitis, especially of the coronary arteries, is the most serious and life-threatening complication of the disease

Clinical features

- Fever lasting 5 days or more
- Bilateral conjunctival congestion
- Dry and red lips, inflammation of oral mucous membranes
- Acute non-purulent swelling of cervical lymph nodes
- Polymorphous exanthema of the trunk
- Red palms and soles

HISTORY

The first case of Kawasaki disease was recognized in Japan in 1961 by Dr Tomisaku Kawasaki, who described a syndrome initially named infantile mucocutaneous lymph node syndrome[1]. Cases of sudden death were recognized in 1970, with autopsy findings showing coronary aneurysms and thrombosis[2]. A high frequency of clinical coronary artery involvement has been documented by two-dimensional echocardiography and arteriography[3]. Intravenous γ-globulin was introduced as a treatment for the disease in 1984[4].

EPIDEMIOLOGY

Nationwide surveys of Kawasaki disease (KD) have been carried out in Japan at 2-year intervals since 1970. As of December 1998, the total number of cases reported was 153 803[5]; recurrent cases make up 3–4% of the total. In each survey the peak age of onset has been 1 year of age, with 80–85% of patients being under 5 years of age. The male to female ratio is 1.4:1 and the mortality rate is 0.03–0.14%. As of 1998, the total number of fatal cases was 426 (0.3%). The male to female ratio of patients who have died has been about 3:1. Although cases reported in the United States mostly involve patients from the middle class and above, this has not been observed in Japan, where patients come from many different backgrounds. The annual incidence of KD is 101–111 cases per 100 000 children below 5 years of age, but in epidemic years the number of cases increases about sixfold.

There have been reports of cases of KD from every continent in the world, but the disease is most prevalent in developed countries. In Hawaii, KD is seen in children of all racial backgrounds but particularly affects those of oriental origin, especially children of Japanese ancestry. The lowest rate of occurrence is seen in Caucasian children. The incidence in black children, Hawaiian children and children of mixed ancestry falls midway between these extremes.

CLINICAL FEATURES

Principal symptoms

The typical onset of the disease is with abrupt high fever, with or without prodromal symptoms (Table 152.1). The fever may be remittent or continuous, ranging from 38 to 40°C. In untreated cases it generally lasts 1–2 weeks; fever lasting more than 4 weeks is distinctly unusual and should suggest another disease. Within 2–4 days of onset, bilateral conjunctival congestion (Fig. 152.1) occurs, especially involving the bulbar conjunctivae. Slit-lamp examination may reveal uveitis. Ocular symptoms usually subside within 1 week. Changes in the lips and oral cavity occur 2–5 days after onset. There is dryness, redness and fissuring of the lips, and in some cases bleeding and crust formation (Fig. 152.1). Diffuse reddening of the membranes of the oral cavity and pharynx are seen, without vesicles, aphthae or pseudomembrane formation. The strawberry tongue seen in scarlet fever can also be seen in KD patients. Changes to the mucous membranes subside within 2 weeks, although the reddening of the lips will often continue for several weeks.

Painful cervical lymphadenopathy typically appears 1 day before or simultaneously with the onset of fever. The swelling is firm and non-fluctuant; bilateral swelling is often misdiagnosed as mumps.

Exanthemata can be seen on the trunk and/or extremities (Fig. 152.2) within 1–5 days of onset. They may be morbilliform, urticarial or erythema multiform-like; scarlatiniform exanthemata should be differentiated from scarlet fever. The exanthemata disappear when the fever subsides.

At about the same time as the appearance of the other principal symptoms there is reddening of the palms and soles and indurative edema, which disappear when the fever subsides. Desquamation, beginning in

---

TABLE 152.1 THE SIX PRINCIPAL SYMPTOMS OF KAWASAKI DISEASE

Fever persisting 5 days or more	
Bilateral conjunctival congestion	
Changes in lips and oral cavity	Reddening of lips, strawberry tongue, diffuse injection of oral and pharyngeal mucosa
Acute non-purulent cervical lymphadenopathy	
Polymorphous exanthem	
Changes in peripheral extremities	Reddening of palms and soles, indurative edema in acute phase
Membranous desquamation later	
Diagnosis	
5/6 symptoms present or	
4/6 plus coronary aneurysm visualized by two-dimensional echocardiography or coronary angiography	

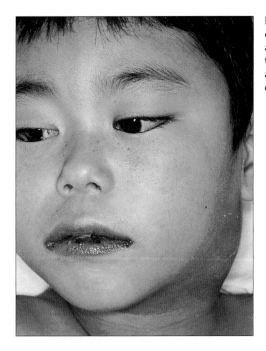

Fig. 152.1 Conjunctival congestion, bleeding and crust formation on the lips and left cervical adenopathy in Kawasaki disease.

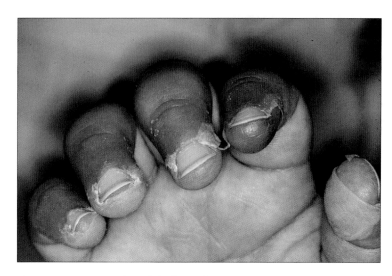

Fig. 152.3 Desquamation of the fingertips.

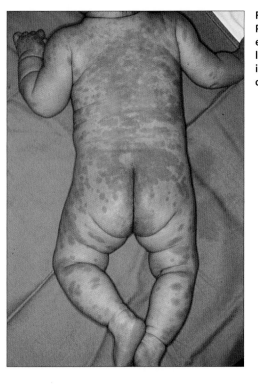

Fig. 152.2 Polymorphous exanthemata on the limbs and trunk of an infant with Kawasaki disease.

the periungual regions of the fingertips (Fig. 152.3) and sometimes extending to the wrists, can be seen 10–15 days from onset.

Other symptoms or findings

The most serious complication of KD is involvement of the cardio-vascular system. In the acute phase more than 80% of cases show signs of carditis, with heart murmurs, gallop rhythms and distant heart sounds on auscultation. On electrocardiogram (ECG) prolonged PR and QT intervals, abnormal Q waves, low voltage, ST-T wave changes and arrythmias may be seen. Cardiomegaly due to myocarditis or peri-carditis can be found on chest radiographs. Coronary artery changes such as dilatation or aneurysms are found on two-dimensional echo-cardiography. In patients with angina pectoris or myocardial infarction, coronary angiography is necessary[6,7] (Fig. 152.4).

Peripheral arteries, such as the axillary, subclavian and iliac, may rarely develop aneurysms. Ischemia, with necrosis of fingers or toes, is distinctly unusual.

Gastrointestinal complications during the acute phase include abdominal pain, vomiting and diarrhea. Mild jaundice may occur from hydrops of the gallbladder. Sometimes there is paralytic ileus and a slight increase in serum transaminase levels due to hepatitis. Neurologic symptoms may be seen in the acute phase, including irritability, facial palsy, limb paralysis and febrile convulsions. Loss of consciousness may occur as a result of encephalitis or encephalopathy.

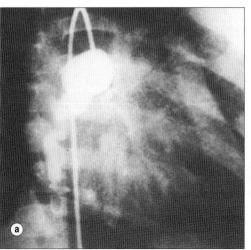
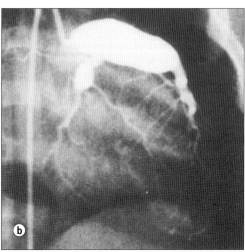

Fig. 152.4 **Coronary angiography.** (a) Right and (b) left coronary artery aneurysms.

Other clinical complications include:

- arthritis in about 20–30% of cases, with involvement of small and large joints
- mild proteinuria and aseptic pyuria
- occasional aseptic small pustules on the elbows, knees and/or buttocks
- upper respiratory signs, such as sneezing and non-productive cough, with normal examination and chest radiograph
- transverse furrows of the fingernails 2–3 months after onset.

INVESTIGATIONS AND DIFFERENTIAL DIAGNOSIS

The differential diagnosis of KD is extensive and includes essentially all febrile illnesses associated with rash in the pediatric population. Laboratory findings suggestive of KD include:

- leukocytosis with left shift of the differential
- increased erythrocyte sedimentation rate (ESR) and C-reactive protein (CRP)
- thrombocytosis; rarely thrombocytopenia
- negative antistreptolysin O (ASO) titers
- negative throat and blood cultures
- pleocytosis in cerebrospinal fluid
- slight increase in serum transaminase activity

PATHOLOGY

The most important pathologic feature of KD is systemic vasculitis, particularly the development of coronary artery changes, including aneurysms[8] (Fig. 152.5). In the acute phase there is vasculitis of medium-sized arteries, such as the main coronary arteries and the interlobular arteries of the kidneys. The angiitis of KD is characterized by an acute inflammation lasting about 7 weeks, with or without fibrinoid necrosis. The course of angiitis may be classified into four stages[9].

In stage I, which occurs during the first 2 weeks following onset, there is perivasculitis of the microvessels (arterioles, capillaries and venules), small arteries and veins. This is followed by inflammation of the intima, adventia and perivascular areas of medium-sized and large arteries, with edema and infiltration with leukocytes and lymphocytes.

The second stage begins around 2 weeks after disease onset and lasts for a period of 2 weeks. It is marked by a decrease in the inflammation of the microvasculature. Aneurysms with thrombi and stenosis occur in the medium-sized arteries, especially the coronary arteries.

During stage three, which lasts from the fourth to the seventh week following onset, there is further reduction of inflammation in the microvasculature and granuloma formation in the medium-sized arteries. Beyond the seventh week there is a fourth stage with scar formation, intimal thickening, aneurysm formation, and thrombotic occlusions and stenosis in the medium-sized arteries. The angiitis can be seen most frequently in the medium-sized and large arteries to the heart and in the iliac arteries.

ETIOLOGY

The etiology of KD is unknown. It is suspected that microorganisms or non-infectious agents may initially act as a trigger for abnormal immunologic activation. Various hypotheses, such as retrovirus,

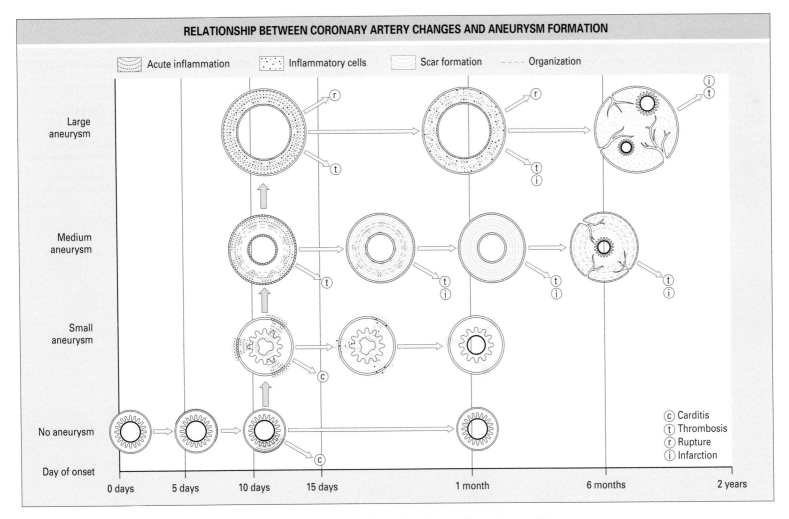

Fig. 152.5 Relationship between coronary artery changes and aneurysm formation. (Adapted from Naoe et al.[8])

superantigens (TSST-1, SPEA,B,C), mercury, mites etc., have been proposed, but none have been confirmed by other investigators.

PATHOGENESIS

The current hypothesis[10] for the development of vasculitis in the acute phase of KD postulates activation of the immune system with the production of cytokines and antibodies. The cytokines, particularly γ-interferon, interleukin-1 and tumor necrosis factor, are thought to interact with endothelial cells, giving rise to neoantigens. It seems to be that antibodies produced against these neoantigens lead to vasculitis and eventual endothelial cell damage. Further investigations as to the role of antibodies in the pathogenesis of Kawasaki disease are needed.

TREATMENT AND MANAGEMENT

Intravenous fluids are often required in KD patients with high fever and inadequate oral intake. Antibiotics are of no value, but may be administered until bacterial infection has been excluded. Coronary artery involvement is assessed by two-dimensional echocardiography performed weekly for the first month following disease onset.

At present the recommended therapy in the acute phase of KD is one infusion of IVIG (2g/kg/8–12h) plus oral aspirin (30–50mg) divided three times daily administered within the first 10 days of illness. After the fever has subsided the aspirin dose can be reduced to 3–5 mg/kg once a day for 6–8 weeks from onset. If coronary artery changes (ectasia or aneurysms) remain, low-dose aspirin (3–5mg/kg/day) should be continued until the changes regress.

The one-dose IVIG therapy with aspirin is very effective to prevent coronary artery abnormalities. Only 2–4% of cases show coronary artery aneurysms[11]. However, persistent or recrudescent fever within 48 hours after initial IVIG therapy is seen in about 10–13% of patients. In half of these cases IVIG with aspirin retreatment (1–2g/kg/8–12h) may reduce the fever. Although coronary artery abnormalities may still be a strong possibility, a third treatment may be either IVIG or pulse methylpredonisolone therapy (20–30mg/kg/day for 1–3 days)[12,13]. If the fever still persists treatment should be aspirin (30–50mg/kg/day) as an anticoagulant measure. In almost all cases fever subsides within 30–40 days. If not, other diseases should be considered.

If large or giant aneurysms are discovered there is an increased risk of stenosis and/or obstruction. In this case, anticoagulants – not only aspirin, but also dipyridamole (5mg/kg), flurbiprofen (4mg/kg), ticlopidin (5mg/kg) and warfarin – should be considered.

Long-term management is necessary in patients with documented coronary artery changes during the acute illness. In addition to two-dimensional echocardiography, coronary angiography should be done and repeated at 1–2-year intervals. In patients with stenotic coronary lesions, exercise ECG and dipyridamole stress myocardial thallium scintigraphy should be considered. In patients with severe coronary artery lesions, coronary bypass surgery may be required.

Patients with Kawasaki disease without clinical coronary artery involvement during the acute illness may develop coronary atherosclerosis. Therefore, long-term follow-up is strongly recommended in all patients.

REFERENCES

1. Kawasaki T, Kosaki F, Okawa S et al. A new infantile acute febrile mucocutaneous lymph node syndrome (MLNS) prevailing in Japan. Pediatrics 1974; 54: 271–276.
2. Kawasaki T. Febrile oculo-oro-cutaneo-acrodesquamatous syndrome: clinical observations of 50 cases. Jpn J Allergy 1967; 16: 178–222.
3. Yoshikawa J, Yanagihara K, Owaki T et al. Cross sectional echocardiographic diagnosis of coronary artery aneurysms in patients with the mucocutaneous lymph node syndrome. Circulation 1979; 59: 133–139.
4. Furusho K, Kamiya T, Nakano H et al. High-dose intravenous gamma globulin for Kawasaki disease. Lancet 1984; 2: 1055–1058.
5. Yanagawa H, Nakamura Y, Yashiro M et al. Incidence survey of Kawasaki disease in 1997 and 1998 in Japan. Pediatrics 2001; 107: e33
6. Kato H, Ichionose E, Kawasaki T. Myocardial infarction in Kawasaki disease: Clinical analysis in 195 cases. J Pediatr 1986; 108: 923–927.
7. Suzuki A, Kamiya T, Kuwahara N et al. Coronary artery lesions of Kawasaki disease: cardiac catheterization findings of 1100 cases. Pediatr Cardiol 1986; 7: 3–9.
8. Naoe S, Shibuya K, Takahashi K et al. Pathological observations concerning the cardiovascular lesions in Kawasaki disease. Cardiol Young 1991; 1: 212–220.
9. Fujiwara H, Hamashima Y. Pathology of the heart in Kawasaki disease. Pediatrics 1978; 61: 100–107.
10. Leung DYM. Immunologic aspects of Kawasaki disease: Implications for pathogenesis and therapy. Clin Cardiol 1991; 14(Suppl.II), II-11–15.
11. Burns JC, Capparelli EV, Brown JA et al. Intravenous gamma-globulin treatment and retreatment in Kawasaki disease. Pediatr Infect Dis J 1998; 17: 1144–1148.
12. Hashino K, Ishii M, Iemura M et al. Retreatment for immune globulin-resistant Kawasaki disease: A comparative study of additional immune globulin and steroid pulse therapy. Pediatrics International. 2001; 43: 211–217.
13. Wright WA, Newburger JW, Baker A et al. Clinical and laboratory observations: Treatment of immune globulin-resistant Kawasaki disease with pulsed doses of corticosteroids. J Pediatr 1996; 128: 146–149.

153 Henoch–Schönlein purpura

Ilona S Szer

Definition

- The most common vasculitis syndrome of childhood
- Generally a benign disorder which follows an intercurrent illness, usually of the upper respiratory tract
- Most children have a self-limited course and systemic involvement or serious sequelae are not frequent

Clinical features

- Purpuric rash, particularly over dependent areas of buttocks and lower extremities
- Arthritis affecting primarily the large joints
- Abdominal cramping with bloody stools
- Microscopic and/or gross hematuria
- The spectrum of the clinical expression of HSP may vary from only minimal petechial rash to severe gastrointestinal (GI), renal, neurologic, pulmonary and joint disease

TABLE 153.1 HENOCH–SCHÖNLEIN PURPURA, CLINICAL MANIFESTATIONS

	% at onset	% during course
Purpura (nl platelet count)	50	100
Subcutaneous edema	10–20	20–50
Arthritis (large joints)	25	60–85
Gastrointestinal	30	85
Renal	?	10–50
Genitourinary (ddx torsion)	?	2–35
Pulmonary (T_LCO)	?	95
Pulmonary hemorrhage	?	Rare, may be fatal
CNS (headache, organic brain syndrome, seizures)	?	Rare, may be fatal

TABLE 153.2 INFLUENCE OF AGE ON CLINICAL MANIFESTATIONS

	< 2 years old (% involved)	> 2 years old (% involved)
Renal	23	43
GI	29	75
Arthritis	56	73
Scalp edema	59	19
Other edema	71	51

(With permission from Allen et al.[10])

HISTORY

The first description of a child with the syndrome that we now know as Henoch–Schönlein purpura was published by Heberden in his 1801 treatise 'On Cutaneous Diseases'[1]. A 5-year-old child with painful subcutaneous edema, abdominal pain, bloody stools and urine, and 'bloody points' over the skin of his legs was described. It was not until 1837 that Schönlein named the association of joint pain and purpura 'purpura rheumatica' and noted 'frequent precipitates in the urine'[2]. Henoch, a student of Schönlein, subsequently highlighted the importance of gastrointestinal and renal involvement[3,4] and thus it is Henoch who is credited with the first place in the Henoch–Schönlein name. In 1915 Frank called the syndrome anaphylactoid purpura, a term no longer used because an allergic etiology has not been substantiated[5].

EPIDEMIOLOGY

Although well described in adults, HSP is much less frequent in adults than in children. In school-aged children the prevalence of HSP is as high as 1.5 per 1000[6]. Interestingly, in children with familial Mediterranean fever (FMF) the prevalence of HSP is 130/1000[7,8]. HSP is a seasonal disorder, occurring more commonly in the spring, winter and fall months and preceded in 50% of the children by an upper respiratory tract infection. Many organisms have been implicated in triggering HSP. Girls and boys are affected equally and the median age of onset is 4 years[6].

CLINICAL FEATURES

The diagnosis of HSP in children requires the presence of palpable purpura and a normal platelet count. Although most children have the classic triad of purpura, colicky abdominal pain and arthritis, up to 50% may present with symptoms other than purpura (Table 153.1), including abdominal pain, arthritis and, importantly, testicular swelling (which must be differentiated from testicular torsion). Numerous manifestations of HSP have been described, including pulmonary hemorrhage which, although exceedingly rare, may be fatal. In a recent study of children with HSP, 95% of those with active disease had decreased carbon monoxide diffusion capacity, which resolved when they recovered from purpura[9].

It is interesting to note that the clinical spectrum differs in younger children from that in older children (Table 153.2): renal disease occurs less often in those under 2 years of age, whereas subcutaneous edema is more common in this age group than in children older than 2[10].

Similar to other rheumatic conditions of childhood, HSP is a syndrome with a varying course. Borrowing from the dermatomyositis disease course, HSP may be thought of as uniphasic in the majority (>80%) of children, polyphasic in 10–20%, and assumes a chronic, continuous course in less than 5%.

Cutaneous manifestations

Palpable non-thrombocytopenic purpura is a prerequisite to the diagnosis and occurs in 100% of patients, but may be a presenting sign in only 50%. Dependent areas of the body, such as the buttocks and the lower extremities, are the most common sites of the rash. Edema of the hands, feet, scalp and ears is a common (20–46%) early finding.

Joint involvement

Arthralgia or arthritis is the second most common symptom of HSP. Acute arthritis, affecting most frequently the knees and the ankles, occurs in 60–84% of patients. Arthritis and arthralgia may precede the rash in 25%. The arthritis is transient and self-limited, but may be painful and may cause the occasional inability to ambulate. There are no permanent sequelae of joint space narrowing and erosions.

Gastrointestinal involvement

Gastrointestinal signs and symptoms have been reported in up to 85% of patients and include colicky pain, nausea, vomiting and gastro-intestinal bleeding. Endoscopic studies commonly reveal hemorrhagic, erosive duodenitis. Less frequently, gastric, jejunal, colonic and rectal erosions have been demonstrated. In a recent study[11] upper GI endo-scopy revealed abnormalities in 6/7 children with HSP, and sigmoid-oscopy revealed abnormalities in one-quarter of the patients. The mucosal changes were more marked in the second part of the duode-num, rather than in the bulb or in the stomach. Endoscopic findings included redness, swelling, petechiae or hemorrhage, as well as erosions and ulceration of the mucosa. Histology of the mucosal biopsy speci-mens revealed non-specific inflammation with positive staining for IgA in the capillaries, but no evidence of vasculitis.

Up to a third of patients with HSP and GI manifestations experience hemoptysis and 50% have occult bleeding, but major hemorrhage occurs in only 5%, and intussusception in 2%. Most cases of abdominal pain are due to submucosal and intramural extravasation of fluid and blood into the intestinal wall, which may lead to localized ulceration of the mucosa and may be associated with diffuse arterial inflammation and fibrinoid necrosis. Radiographic findings are non-specific and may include thickening of bowel wall, blurring of bowel folds due to wall edema, scalloping due to local hemorrhage of bowel wall, filling defects in bowel wall due to vascular occlusion in the submucosa, bleeding into the mesentery, and intussusception. A sudden increase in the intensity of abdominal pain may be secondary to intussusception, bowel infarct, perforation, pancreatitis, or hydrops of the gallbladder. Intussusception is reported in 2% of children with HSP, but other GI complications are extraordinarily rare. The cause of intussusception may be bowel wall edema or a submucosal hematoma. HSP-related intussusception is ileoileal in 65% of cases, compared with idiopathic intussusception which is usually ileocolic. As a result, ultrasonography is more helpful in the diagnosis of intussusception in children with HSP than barium enema, which may miss the ileoileal location. In a recent study[12] of 14 children with HSP and abdominal pain, high-resolution ultra-sonography provided information at three levels:

1. Ultrasound explained the acute abdominal pain by showing in all cases the edematous hemorrhagic infiltration of the intestinal wall, which appeared thickened (3–11 mm): lesions were either diffuse (6 children) or focal (duodenal in 5, jejunal in 2 and ileal in 1).

2. Ultrasound followed the evolution of the disease: extension of lesions in five patients, or resolution in the remaining nine children whose US showed progressive decrease of parietal thickening, re-expansion of the small bowel lumen, and the reappearance of peristalsis.

3. In each case the ultrasound detected surgical complications: ileoileal intussusception in three patients and perforation in one.

Renal involvement

The incidence of renal involvement ranges between 10% and 50%. Children over 9 years of age develop glomerulonephritis more often than their younger peers. Children with bloody stools reportedly have a 7.5-fold increased risk for renal disease compared with children whose stools are hemoccult negative. The overall prognosis for renal disease is favorable, with a 1.1–4.5% incidence of persistent involvement and an approximate <1% progression to end-stage renal failure. Generally, renal involvement occurs within 3 months of onset of the rash. Persistence of rash for 2–3 months is associated with a slightly increased risk of nephropathy.

The clinical expression of nephritis ranges from transient isolated microscopic hematuria to rapidly progressive glomerulonephritis. Hematuria is detected in virtually all children with HSP-associated nephritis. Proteinuria, nephrotic syndrome, hypertension and renal insufficiency are uncommon. If present, the combination of hematuria and proteinuria is associated in 15% of patients with progressive renal insufficiency. Up to 50% of children who present with the nephrotic syndrome and evidence of renal insufficiency develop renal failure within 10 years[13].

Similar to clinical expression, renal histopathology ranges from minimal change to severe crescenteric GN. Electron microscopy may reveal mesangial, subendothelial and subepithelial deposits. Immuno-fluorescence studies reveal diffuse glomerular deposition of IgA, C3, fibrin, IgG, properdin and IgM.

HSP and IgA nephropathy – the latter described almost exclusively in young adults – appear to be related disorders on the same spectrum[13]. It is important to note that 30% of adult patients with IgA nephropathy have rash and joint symptoms similar to HSP. An increased serum IgA level is seen in both disorders and renal biopsy findings are identical. Among important differences, however, is the fact that HSP is a systemic syndrome whereas IgA nephropathy is localized primarily to the kidney. The age of onset is the major difference between these two histologically similar illnesses, and the prognosis remains favorable for HSP and guarded for IgA nephropathy. A question has been asked and remains unanswered: did adults with IgA nephropathy have HSP as children[14]? The natural history of IgA nephropathy suggests that it is not associated with early HSP[15]. In this study, patients with documented IgA nephro-pathy who had presented clinically with hematuria and mild proteinuria were followed for a median of 7 years. During this time over half of the patients progressed to nephrotic syndrome and/or hypertension. Only 14% had complete resolution of renal findings, and the remainder still had hematuria or proteinuria.

Genitourinary involvement

Extrarenal genitourinary involvement has been described in HSP and may precede the rash. Acute scrotal swelling, secondary to inflammation and hemorrhage of the scrotal vessels, has been reported in 2–35% of children. A frequency of 32% was recently reported by Chamberlain and Greenberg[16], who reviewed the medical records of 61 children with HSP and found that 10 had scrotal involvement on physical examination and one patient reported purpuric lesions and scrotal edema 2 days prior to the onset of generalized rash. The differentiation of scrotal edema from acute torsion of the spermatic cord is a challenge in children who have scrotal involvement as the first sign of HSP[17]. In HSP, a normal or increased Doppler and radionuclide flow are expected, whereas in testic-ular torsion both the Doppler flow on the affected side and the uptake of radionuclide are decreased. Therefore, the evaluation of boys with testic-ular swelling should include one or both of the radiographic imaging studies, which may avoid the need for surgical exploration[17]. True testic-ular torsion is rare in HSP, but when it occurs it represents a surgical emergency as vascular insufficiency may lead to infarction and death of the Leydig cells within 10 hours unless blood supply is restored.

Central nervous system involvement

Central nervous system involvement is exceedingly rare but has been described. The most common manifestation is headache followed by subtle encephalopathy with minimal changes in mental status, labile mood, apathy, and hyperactivity. Seizures have been reported. Subdural hematomas, cortical hemorrhage, intraparenchymal bleeding, and infarction have been documented. Peripheral neuropathy has also been reported[18].

Pulmonary involvement

Chaussain[9] documented impairment of lung diffusion capacity in the majority of children with HSP during the active phase of the illness. In a study of 29 children, 28 had a significant decrease of lung transfer for carbon monoxide (56.8% of predicted $T_L\text{CO}$). During the subsequent longitudinal follow-up, $T_L\text{CO}$ normalized in all children who recovered completely but remained abnormal in patients who had evidence of persistent disease activity. The authors concluded that decreased $T_L\text{CO}$ measurement may reflect an alteration of the alveolar capillary membrane secondary to circulating immune complexes, and thus serves as a parameter of disease activity. None of the patients in this study had clinically apparent pulmonary distress. However, massive pulmonary hemorrhage has been reported in HSP. Olson et al.[19] described four children with severe pulmonary bleeding, one of whom died during the initial massive pulmonary hemorrhage. Although no autopsy was performed, previous reports of postmortem pulmonary specimens revealed periarteriolar infiltrates and fibrinoid necrosis of the lungs.

INVESTIGATIONS

The diagnosis of HSP is based on clinical signs and symptoms. Skin biopsy, if obtained, shows leukocytoclastic vasculitis with neutrophils within vessel walls, necrosis of vessel walls, and deposits of pink amorphous fibrin within and around the walls of small vessels. Immunofluorescence studies may show IgA and C3 along the small vessels of the skin and in the renal glomeruli. Routine laboratory studies are usually normal and abnormalities reflect particular organ involvement or bleeding. There are no diagnostic studies, although an elevated serum level of IgA is suggestive of HSP. Laboratory evaluation is aimed at excluding other disorders and assessing the extent of organ involvement.

DIFFERENTIAL DIAGNOSIS

An entity known as acute hemorrhagic edema (AHE) of childhood, described almost exclusively in the European literature in children under 24 months of age, may or may not represent HSP in infants[20]. The manifestations of AHE are edema and ecchymotic, targetlike purpura on the limbs and face. Most patients have a history of either a recent illness, drug exposure or immunizations. Systemic symptoms such as bloody stools or renal involvement seem to occur less frequently in AHE than in HSP, although these symptoms are also uncommon in infants and toddlers thought to have HSP. Spontaneous and complete resolution occurs within 1–3 weeks, but one to three recurrences are frequent. Leukocytoclastic vasculitis is seen when a skin biopsy is obtained. It is not known whether or not AHE is an IgA-related vasculitis.

Recently, a subcommittee of the American College of Rheumatology (ACR) defined criteria for the classification of several forms of vasculitis in adults, including hypersensitivity vasculitis (HV; Table 153.3) and Henoch–Schönlein purpura (Table 153.4)[21]. Because the two entities share many clinicopathologic features and HSP is often considered a type of HV, Michel et al. compared the characteristics of HV and HSP as separate and definable clinical syndromes, using the ACR study database[22]. Both disorders share the common feature of leukocytoclastic vasculitis of small vessels, with prominent skin involvement. Major differences with respect to frequency and type of organ involvement were found, suggesting that these are indeed distinct entities which carry varying prognoses. Although hematuria and proteinuria were more often seen in HSP, elevated BUN and creatinine as factors reflecting functional renal impairment (and likely to reflect worse prognosis) were

TABLE 153.3 1990 CRITERIA FOR THE CLASSIFICATION OF HYPERSENSITIVITY VASCULITIS

Criterion	Definition
Age at disease onset >16 years	Development of symptoms after age 16
Medication at disease onset	Medication was taken at the onset of symptoms that may have been a precipitating factor
Palpable purpura	Slightly elevated purpuric rash over one or more areas of the skin; does not blanch with pressure and is not related to thrombocytopenia
Maculopapular rash	Flat and raised lesions of various sizes over one or more areas of the skin
Biopsy including arteriole and venule	Histologic changes showing granulocytes in a perivascular or extravascular location

For purposes of classification, a patient shall be said to have hypersensitivity vasculitis if at least three of the five criteria are present. The presence of any three or more criteria yields a sensitivity of 71% and a specificity of 83.9%.

(With permission from Calabrese et al.[21])

TABLE 153.4 CRITERIA FOR DIFFERENTIATING HENOCH–SCHÖNLEIN PURPURA FROM HYPERSENSITIVITY VASCULITIS

Criterion	Definition
Palpable purpura	Slightly elevated purpuric rash over one or more areas of the skin not related to thrombocytopenia
Bowel angina	Diffuse abdominal pain worse after meals, or bowel ischemia, usually including bloody diarrhea
GI bleeding	GI bleeding, including melena, hematochezia or positive test for occult blood in the stool
Hematuria	Gross hematuria or microhematuria (>1/hpf)
Age at onset <20	Development of first symptoms at age 20 or less
No medications	Absence of any medication at onset of disease which may have been a precipitating factor

The presence of any three or more of the six criteria yields a correct classification of HSP cases of 87.1%. The presence of two or fewer criteria yields a correct classification of HV cases in 74.2%.

(With permission from Calabrese et al.[21])

significantly more frequent in HV. Generally, important organ involvement was found more often in HV (pleuritis, pericarditis, congestive heart failure, and more extensive involvement of skin, mucosa and muscle). Similarly, tests which classically reveal active inflammatory processes, i.e. ESR and C4 levels, were more frequently abnormal in patients with HV than those with HSP. Frank arthritis was significantly more common in HSP, whereas arthralgia was reported more frequently in HV. HSP in adults tended to affect organs more extensively and the prognosis appeared to be worse with regard to renal disease than in children and adolescents with HSP. In summary, this study corroborates the concept that HV and HSP are distinct clinical disorders within the broader group of small vessel vasculitis with prominent skin involvement.

BASIC SCIENCE

Etiology

The etiology of HSP remains unknown. Controversy exists regarding seasonal increases in its occurrence, with reports of peaks in the spring, fall and winter months. In addition, at least 50% of children have had a preceding upper respiratory tract infection. Numerous organisms have been implicated in triggering HSP, including streptococci, *Mycoplasma pneumoniae, Yersinia, Legionella*, Epstein–Barr virus, hepatitis B, varicella, adenovirus, cytomegalovirus and parvovirus B19. Several case reports link vaccinations against typhoid, paratyphoid A and B, measles, cholera and yellow fever with the subsequent development of HSP. This suggests that more than one infectious agent may trigger the expression of the disease. In addition, allergens such as drugs (penicillin, ampicillin, erythromycin, quinine and quinidine), as well as foods, exposure to cold and insect bites, have been implicated as potential triggers[23].

Pathogenesis

HSP is believed to be an immune complex-mediated small vessel vasculitis. Serologic studies document elevated levels of IgA in 50% and activation of the alternate pathway of the complement system. IgA levels become elevated because of either increased production or decreased clearance. It is hypothesized that an unknown antigen(s) stimulates IgA production, activating pathways leading to necrotizing vasculitis. Levels of C3 and C4 complement components are normal. Histopathology of the skin and other affected organs reveals polymorphonuclear cells in vessel walls, with IgA, C3 and immune complexes seen in venules, arterioles and capillaries[10].

In HSP, complement fixing immune complexes (IC) are present in the circulation and deposited on the interior of blood vessels of the skin. IC are capable of activating complement, leading to the formation of chemotactic factors such as C5a, which in turn recruit PMN leukocytes at the site of deposition. Release of lysosomal enzymes follows the ingestion of immune complexes by PMN, resulting in vessel damage. The C5b-9 complex, also known as membrane attack complex (MAC), was recently colocalized with IgA and C3 on vessel walls of the skin and on capillary walls and mesangium of the glomeruli in patients with HSP-related nephritis. Kawana and Nishiyama[24] assessed the degree of *in vivo* terminal activation by measuring serum concentrations of the terminal complement complex (TCC). The results show that vascular endothelial cells in each MAC-positive case were injured, even in papillary dermal vessels in which no PMNs could be detected but C5b-9 deposition was seen. This suggests that not only leukocytes but also MAC are necessary for endothelial cells to incur damage. Using the C5b-9 enzyme immunoassay, the serum concentration of C5b-9 was shown to be significantly increased in most HSP patients. Complement activation leading to terminal complement sequence is thus shown to occur in the circulation as well as the skin of patients with HSP. Immune complexes may possibly contribute to this terminal complement activation. TCC increased significantly at the time of disease flare-up, but dropped to the normal range during remission and showed close correlation with disease activity during its course. The authors conclude that the assay for TCC should prove useful in monitoring the activity of HSP. Routine assessment of complement activation, i.e. C3, C4 and CH50, showed no abnormality. However, the measurement of plasma anaphylatoxins C3a and C4a in 46 patients with HSP and IgA nephropathy showed a significant correlation with plasma creatinine and urea levels[25]. In addition, an association between C3a and creatinine was reported. These observations suggest a role for anaphylatoxin determination as a sensitive indicator of complement activation and a useful tool in monitoring the activity of disease in affected patients. Similar to this study, a group of investigators from Heidelberg, Germany[26], investigated the possibility that the local inflammatory and thrombotic process may be regulated by increased biosynthesis of vasoactive prostanoids, including thromboxane A_2 (TxA$_2$), a potent vasoconstrictor and platelet agonist; prostacyclin, a vasodilator and platelet antagonist; and prostaglandin E_2, a mediator of inflammation. The results of their study of 14 children with HSP revealed that both thromboxane A_2 and prostacyclin were significantly increased during the acute phase of the disease, and again during

subsequent recurrences of HSP. Of note, both patients with nephrotic syndrome had the highest concentrations of renal thromboxane A_2. The enhanced TxA2 formation is consistent with phasic platelet activation in HSP. The increased prostacyclin biosynthesis probably reflects endothelial cell damage and may be a response of the vascular endothelium to modulate platelet–vessel wall and leukocyte–vessel wall interactions.

That serum IgA levels are elevated in children with HSP is well known. To investigate the mechanism(s) leading to this finding, Kondo et al.[27] studied 12 children with HSP and found that serum IgA levels were significantly elevated within 2 weeks (5–14 days) of onset, whereas serum levels of both IgG and IgM were normal. Although the percentage of surface IgA-bearing cells was not increased in the children, the numbers of IgA-secreting cells were significantly increased within 2 weeks of onset. In Northern blotting experiments the secreted αs-chain gene was well expressed compared with the membrane-bound αm-chain gene, within 2 weeks of onset of HSP. These data provide strong evidence for a selective triggering of differentiation of IgA-secreting cells which appears to correlate with disease activity. Yang et al.[28] report elevated levels of IgA anticardiolipin antibodies as well as TGF-β secreting T cells in the blood of 26 Chinese children only during the active phase of HSP. The abnormalities resolved during convalescence. This is interesting because TGF-β is important in class switching to IgA. These observations were further expanded by two reports of rare thrombotic complications of HSP: one child had a brain infarct and another developed thrombosis of the spermatic cord[29,30]. Both cases suggest that some signs and symptoms of HSP might be explained by differing pathologic mechanisms in individual patients. Ault et al.[31] have reported a significant association of C4B deficiency in a subset of patients with HSP-related glomerulonephritis (19% of children with glomerulonephritis had C4B deficiency vs. 3% of controls). Because the complement system plays a crucial role in the solubilization and clearance of immune complexes, deficiency of C4B complement component may predispose to renal disease. Using radial immunodiffusion and ELISA, Saulsbury[32] investigated the heavy- and light-chain composition of serum IgA and IgA rheumatoid factors in 34 children with HSP. As expected, serum IgA concentrations were elevated in children with HSP compared with controls. The predominant subclass was IgA$_1$, whereas levels of IgA$_2$ remained normal. The majority of the patients (19/34) had circulating rheumatoid factors composed primarily of IgA$_1$. There were no IgG or IgM rheumatoid factors. Determination of the light-chain composition of serum IgA$_1$ was similar in both patients and controls. However, the IgA$_1$ rheumatoid factors were enriched in κ light chains. The predominance of IgA$_1$ is not surprising, as 80–90% of serum IgA is the IgA$_1$ subclass. A similar finding was reported in patients with IgA nephropathy, highlighting the similarity between the disorders.

During the last several years there has been a profusion of articles characterizing the spectrum of antineutrophil cytoplasmic antibodies (ANCA) associated with systemic vasculitis syndromes and a variety of inflammatory disorders. It is now apparent that ANCA are a family of related but distinct autoantibodies. Their putative role in the pathogenesis of both HSP and IgA nephropathy was suggested by one group of investigators who detected IgA ANCA in 55% of patients with HSP and 15% of patients with Berger's nephropathy[33]. However, in a study by O'Donoghue et al.[34] this finding was not confirmed. Indeed, of the 30 children with early HSP none had ANCA. Similarly, of the 100 adult patients with IgA nephropathy only two were found to have ANCA. Both of these patients had IgG antimyeloperoxidase antibodies (p-ANCA), and even though both had persistent microscopic hematuria with slowly progressive renal failure, neither had glomerular crescents nor focal necrosis, which are classically associated with p-ANCA. It appears therefore that IgA ANCA are not involved in the pathogenesis of HSP or in the pathogenesis of glomerular injury in IgA nephropathy, even in patients who develop rapidly progressive renal insufficiency. The detection of IgG antimyeloperoxidase antibodies in a small minority of patients raised the possibility that a small subset of IgA-related renal disorders shares the immunopathogenic mechanisms with other systemic vasculitides classically associated with ANCA. O'Donaghue et al. further studied the relationship of specific IgG autoantibodies directed against glomerular antigens in the serum of patients with active HSP: 61% of children with HSP complicated by nephritis had IgG antiglomerular antibodies, compared with 1/6 children without overt renal involvement[35]. The finding that IgG antibodies were not detected during remission or in patients without renal manifestations further supports the hypothesis that IgG antibodies may play a direct role in renal injury.

MANAGEMENT

Treatment of HSP is largely supportive and includes adequate hydration and monitoring of vital signs. Non-steroidal anti-inflammatory drugs (NSAIDs) help with joint pain and do not worsen the purpura. However, it may be prudent to avoid NSAIDs in the setting of renal insufficiency, particularly in older patients. Steroids are helpful in the management of painful edema but there is no clear indication for this. Consensus regarding the treatment of children with HSP includes the use of analgesics and/or NSAIDs for the control of joint pain and inflammation, and steroids for painful cutaneous edema[10]. Most physicians agree that these interventions achieve their intended outcome.

Corticosteroids are still used, particularly in children with severe abdominal pain, but the efficacy of the treatment has not been proven.

Should steroids be used in treatment of abdominal pain in HSP?

In a retrospective analysis, Rosenblum and Winter[36] evaluated the effect of corticosteroids on the duration of abdominal pain in 43 children with HSP and abdominal pain. Twenty-five patients received oral prednisone at a dose of 2mg/kg/day and 18 children served as controls. Results showed that during the first 24 hours abdominal pain resolved in 44% of children who received steroids, compared with spontaneous resolution in only 14% of children who were not treated ($P = 0.02$). Over the next 24 hours, respectively 65% vs 45% no longer had abdominal pain. After 72 hours three-quarters of patients in both groups were well. It is this experience that has influenced many physicians to treat abdominal pain with corticosteroids. In addition, similar observations by Allen[10] included the finding that painful edema and arthritis resolved either with or without steroids within 24–48 hours after onset, and that steroids had no effect on either purpura or renal disease. Notably, none of the patients with abdominal pain who received steroids developed intussusception.

To further address this issue, Glasier et al.[37] designed another retrospective study of 22 children admitted to hospital with abdominal pain. Their findings agreed with Rosenblum and Allen: 20/22 (91%) children recovered with or without steroids. Numerous case reports suggest improvement of abdominal pain, melena and massive hemorrhage with the use of steroids. This is supported by many physicians who have 'successfully' treated children with abdominal pain admitted to hospital using steroids. However, to date there has been no placebo-controlled study and we are left with experience and reason but not a proven fact on which to base the recommendation to treat.

The treatment of nephritis is highly controversial[38]. Treatment modalities have included daily, alternate-day and pulse corticosteroids, cyclophosphamide, plasmapheresis, anticoagulation, cyclosporin and azathioprine. The results of these different treatments are difficult to interpret, as most patients were not randomized and many may recover without treatment.

Should steroids be used to prevent the onset of delayed HSP nephritis?

To answer this question, Buchanec et al.[39] designed a retrospective study of 32 children with HSP and no evidence of renal involvement. Twenty-three patients received corticosteroids at 2mg/kg/day and 10 did not. Of the treated children only one (5%) developed nephritis, whereas in the untreated group five patients (50%) developed renal manifestations. These authors concluded that immediate treatment with steroids prevented renal disease in a significant proportion of patients. Mollica et al.[40] continued the study in a modified prospective but open and non-randomized design in which 84 children received corticosteroids and 84 did not receive any intervention. The results, which included 2 years of follow-up, showed no renal involvement in any of the treated children, whereas in the non-intervention group 10 children developed hematuria ($P < 0.001$) and, of those, four still had hematuria 12 months later and two developed renal insufficiency 18 months after onset[40]. This study was immediately followed by the retrospective observations of Saulsbury, who similarly treated 20 children without renal disease with steroids while observing 30 who had no intervention. In both groups there was a 20% frequency of subsequent renal involvement within 3 months of initial presentation, suggesting that pretreatment with steroids did not prevent the onset of delayed nephritis in children with HSP[41].

The seemingly confusing results regarding the prevention of delayed onset of renal disease are difficult to interpret. One explanation may be an inherent flaw in the design of each study: neither was placebo controlled nor randomized and two of three were retrospective observations. There were also inconsistencies regarding the timing of corticosteroid administration between the studies, further contributing to difficulty in interpreting the results.

Poor prognostic signs

The controversy regarding management of HSP nephritis is centered primarily on children whose disease is associated with a high risk for

---

TABLE 153.5 CORRELATIONS BETWEEN INITIAL CLINICAL MANIFESTATIONS AND RENAL OUTCOME AFTER 1 YEAR OF FOLLOW-UP

Manifestation	n	Clinical remission	Minimal urinary abnormalities	Persistent nephropathy	Renal failure
Hematuria	2	2	0	0	0
Proteinuria (<1g/day)	16	7	6	3	0
Proteinuria (>1g/day)	42	17	10	9	6
Nephrotic syndrome	64	32	14	10	8
Nephrotic syndrome and renal failure	27	8	2	2	15
Total	151	66	32	24	29

(With permission from Niaudet et al.[13])

TABLE 153.6 CORRELATIONS BETWEEN INITIAL CLINICAL MANIFESTATIONS AND RENAL OUTCOME AFTER 1 YEAR OF FOLLOW-UP

Biopsy finding	n	Clinical remission	Minimal urinary abnormalities	Persistent nephropathy	Renal failure
Mesangiopathic GN	2	2	0	0	0
Focal segmental GN	47	26	15	4	2
Proliferative endocapillary GN	13	8	3	1	1
Endocapillary and extracapillary GN					
crescents <50%	21	11	3	6	1
crescents >50%	68	19	11	13	25
Total	151	66	32	24	29

Only children whose initial renal biopsy results were available are included.

(With permission from Niaudet et al. [13])

renal insufficiency and/or failure. For the majority of children with HSP renal involvement is transient, but for the 1–5% who develop chronic renal disease and up to 1% who may go on to renal failure, the management that would prevent this sequela is not known[42].

To examine which patients are at highest risk, the study by Allen[10] provides multiple insights. A retrospective review of 74 children revealed that 40 had no renal findings, 24 presented with hematuria only, and 10 had hematuria and proteinuria. One year later, 80% of the children who had no renal involvement at onset and 71% of mildly affected children remained well. In contrast, only 40% of those who presented with severe involvement were free of renal findings[8]. In a similar study by Niaudet et al.[11] none of the children with mild initial renal findings (hematuria only, or proteinuria of <1g/day) developed renal disease more than 1 year later. However, of the patients who presented with either nephrotic syndrome, renal insufficiency and/or renal failure, a significant number went on to chronic renal failure (Table 153.5). The same authors then correlated biopsy findings with clinical renal manifestations and reported a significant association between proliferative glomerulonephritis with >50% crescents and the development of future renal failure (Table 153.6).

Attempts have been made to identify other reliable predictors of severe renal disease. Muller et al.[43], in a prospective study, measured urinary excretion of two tubular proteins: N-acetyl-β-D-glucosamine (NAG) and α_1 microglobulin (α_1MG). The results show that elevated urinary levels of both proteins correlated with renal disease at 1, 6 and 12 months after onset of HSP. Absence of both markers had a strong negative predicting power. If confirmed, these findings may allow the physician to identify patients at risk for more aggressive renal disease.

In summary, the presence of hematuria with nephrotic-range proteinuria confers a 15% risk of renal failure, whereas nephrosis with renal insufficiency and documentation of >50% crescenteric glomerulonephritis may lead to renal failure in up to 50% of patients with renal HSP after a 10-year course. Aggressive treatment should therefore be attempted to prevent late sequelae. Children with nephrotic-range proteinuria, nephrotic syndrome and signs of renal insufficiency should undergo renal biopsy to determine the extent of renal involvement.

How should children with severe HSP nephritis be treated?

Several studies have recommended various treatment modalities for children with severe renal involvement, including pulse or oral corticosteroids, either alone or in combination with immunosuppressive agents such as azathioprine, cyclophosphamide or cyclosporin; plasmaphere-

sis; high-dose IVIG; danazol; and fish oil[40–50]. The studies suffer from small numbers of subjects, retrospective analysis of data, and lack of placebo-controlled groups. In addition, renal biopsy findings are inconsistently available and interventions are given at different times in the course of the illness. It is therefore difficult to draw meaningful conclusions from these reports[51].

Although the value of renal therapy is being debated, three uncontrolled trials suggest that early aggressive treatment may change the natural history of severe nephritis. Oner et al.[47] treated 12 children with HSP and biopsy-proven rapidly progressive crescenteric glomerulonephritis with a combination of methylprednisolone at 30mg/kg/day for 3 consecutive days, followed by oral corticosteroids at 2mg/kg/day, cyclophosphamide at 2mg/kg/day for 2 months and dipyridamole at 5mg/kg/day for 6 months. At the 3-month evaluation, GFR had normalized in 11/12 children, nephrosis resolved in 8/12, and hematuria was no longer detectable in 9/12. Furthermore, at 30 months after the treatment only one patient had persistent nephrotic syndrome and one child had developed renal failure (Table 153.7). In addition, both Iijima et al.[49] and Foster et al.[50] evaluated the efficacy of prednisone in combination with azathioprine and found an improved outcome in their patients compared with historical controls. The merit of combination therapies will not be fully documented until multicenter prospective trials are completed. Until such time, we will continue to treat individual patients based on limited information[51].

TABLE 153.7 RENAL OUTCOME IN HENOCH–SCHÖNLEIN PURPURA: CONCLUSIONS FROM LITERATURE REVIEW

Reference	Conclusion (study design)
Levy et al.[44]	Improved with steroids (pilot)
Counahan et al.[45]	No improvement with steroids (retrospective analysis)
Mollica et al.[40]	Steroids prevent delayed renal disease (open, non-randomized, controlled prospective trial)
Saulsbury[41]	Steroids do not prevent delayed renal disease (retrospective analysis)
Rostoker et al.[46]	High-dose IgG stabilizes poor renal function in HSP/IgA nephropathy (open prospective cohort study)
Oner et al.[47]	Triple therapy may be effective in severe HSP nephritis (see text, pilot)
Rostoker et al.[48]	Low-dose IgG slows progression of renal disease (open, uncontrolled, prospective trial)

REFERENCES

1. Heberden W. Commertarii de Marlbaun. Historia et curatione, London: Payne; 1801.
2. Schonlein JL. Allgemeine und specielle Pathologie und Therapie, 3rd edn. Wurzburg: Herisau; 1837.
3. Henoch EHH. Ubereine eigenthumliche form von Purpura. Klin Wochenschr 1874; 11: 641.
4. Henoch EHH. Vorlesungen uber Kinderkrankheiten. In: Hirschward A, ed. Vohlesunger uber Kinderkrankheiten. Berlin: Aufl. 1899.
5. Frank E. Die essentielle Thrombopenie. Berl Wochenschr 1915; 52: 454.
6. Robson WLM, Leung AKC. Henoch–Schönlein purpura. Adv Pediatr 1994; 41: 163–194.
7. Schlessinger et al. HSP an FMF. Israel J Med Soc 1985; 21: 83–85.
8. Flautau E, Kohn D, Schiller D et al. Schonlein–Henoch syndrome in patients with familial Mediterranean fever. Arthritis Rheum 1982; 25: 42–47.
9. Chaussain M, De Boissieu D, Kalifa G et al. Impairment of lung diffusion capacity in HSP. J Pediatr 1992; 121: 12–16.
10. Allen DM, Diamond LK, Howell DA. Anaphylactoid purpura in children (Henoch–Schönlein syndrome). Am J Dis Child 1960; 99: 147–168.
11. Kato S, Shibuya H, Neganuma H, Nekagawa H. Gastrointestinal endoscopy in Henoch–Schönlein purpura. Eur J Pediatr 1992; 151: 482–484.
12. Couture A, Veyrac C, Baud C et al. Evaluation of abdominal pain in Henoch–Schönlein syndrome by high frequency ultrasound. Pediatr Radiol 1992; 22: 12–17.
13. Niaudet P, Murcia I, Beaufils H et al. Primary IgA nephropathies in children: Prognosis and treatment. Adv Nephrol 1993; 2: 121–140.
14. Nakamoto Y et al. Primary IgA glomerulonephritis and Schonlein–Henoch purpura nephritis: clinico-pathological and immuno-histochemical characteristics. Q J Med 1978; 47: 495–516.
15. Szeto CC, Lai FM, To KF et al. The natural history of immunoglobulin a nephropathy among patients with hematuria and minimal proteinuria. Am J Med 2001; 110: 434–437.
16. Chamberlain RS, Greenberg LW. Scrotal involvement in Henoch–Schönlein purpura: A case report and review of the literature. Pediatr Emerg Care 1992; 8: 213–215.
17. Singer JI, Kissoon N, Gloor J. Acute testicular pain: Henoch–Schönlein purpura versus testicular torsion. Pediatr Emerg Care 1992; 8: 51–53.
18. Belman AL, Eicher CR, Moshe SL, Mezey AP. Neurologic manifestations of Schonlein–Henoch Purpura: Report of three cases and review of the literature. Pediatrics 1985; 75: 687–692.
19. Olson JC, Kelly KJ, Pan CG, Wortmann DW. Pulmonary disease with hemorrhage in Henoch–Schönlein purpura. Pediatrics 1992; 89: 1177–1181.
20. Ince E, Mumcu Y, Suskan E et al. Infantile acute hemorrhagic edema: a variant of leucocytoclastic vasculitis. Pediatr Dermatol 1995; 12: 224–227.
21. Calabrese LH, Michel BA, Bloch DA et al. The ACR 1990 criteria for the classification of hypersensitivity vasculitis. Arthritis Rheum 1990; 33: 1108–1113.
22. Michel BA, Hunder GG, Bloch DA, Calabrese LH. Hypersensitivity vasculitis and Henoch–Schönlein purpura: A comparison between the 2 disorders. J Rheumatol 1992; 19: 721–728.
23. Szer IS. Henoch–Schönlein purpura. Current science. Curr Opin Rheumatol 1994; 6: 25–31.
24. Kawana S, Nishiyama S. Serum SC5b-9 (Terminal complement complex) level, a sensitive indicator of disease activity in patients with Henoch–Schönlein purpura. Dermatology 1992; 184: 171–176.
25. Abou-Ragheb HHA, Williams AJ, Brown CB, Milford-Ward A. Plasma levels of the anaphylatoxins C3a and C4a in patients with IgA nephropathy/Henoch–Schönlein nephritis. Nephron 1992; 62: 22–26.
26. Tonshoff B, Momper R, Schweer H et al. Increased biosynthesis of vasoactive prostanoids in Schonlein–Henoch purpura. Pediatr Res 1992; 32: 137–140.
27. Kondo N, Kasahara K, Shinoda S, Orii T. Accelerated expression of secreted alpha-chain gene in anaphylactoid purpura. J Clin Immunol 1992; 12: 193–196.
28. Yang YH, Huang MT, Lin YT. Increased transforming growth factor beta secreting T cells and IgA anti-cardiolipin antibody levels during acute stage of childhood HSP. Clin Exp Immunol 2000; 122: 285–290.
29. Sokol DK, McIntyre JA, Short RA et al. HSP and stroke: antiphosphatidyl-ethanolamine antibody in CF and Serum. Neurology 2000; 55; 1379–1381.
30. Diana A, Gaze H, Laubscher B et al. A case of pediatric HSP and thrombosis of spermatic veins. J Pediatr Surg 2000; 35: 1843.
31. Ault BH, Stapleton FB, Rivas ML et al. Association of Henoch–Schönlein purpura glomerulonephritis with C4B deficiency. J Pediatr 1990; 117: 753–755.
32. Saulsbury FT. Heavy and light chain composition of serum IgA rheumatoid factor in Henoch–Schönlein purpura. Arthritis Rheum 1992; 35: 1377–1380.
33. Shaw G, Ronda N, Bevan JS et al. Antineutrophil cytoplasmic antibodies (ANCA) of IgA class correlate with disease activity in adult Henoch–Schönlein purpura. Nephrol Dial Transplant 1992; 7: 1238–1241.
34. O'Donoghue DJ, Nusbaum P, Noel LH et al. Antineutrophil cytoplasmic antibodies in IgA nephropathy and Henoch–Schönlein purpura. Nephrol Dial Transplant 1992; 7: 534–538.
35. O'Donoghue DJ, Jewkes F, Postlethwaite RJ, Ballardie FW. Autoimmunity to glomerular antigens in Henoch–Schönlein nephritis. Clin Sci 1992; 83: 281–287.
36. Rosenblum ND, Winter HS. Steroid effects on the course of abdominal pain in children with HSP. Pediatrics 1987; 79: 1018–1021.
37. Glasier CM, Siegel MJ, McAlister WH et al. Henoch–Schönlein syndrome in children: gastrointestinal manifestations. AJR (Am J Roentgenol) 1981; 136: 1081–1085.
38. Szer IS. Gastrointestinal and renal involvement in vasculitis: management strategies in HSP. Cleveland Clin J Med 1999; 86; 312–317.
39. Buchanec J, Galanda V, Belakova S et al. Incidence of renal complications in Schonlein–Henoch purpura syndrome in dependence of early administration of steroids. Int J Nephrol 1988; 20: 409–412.
40. Mollica F, Li Volti S, Garozzo R, Russo G. Effectiveness of early prednisone treatment in preventing the development of nephropathy in anaphylactoid purpura. Eur J Pediatr 1982; 151: 140–144.
41. Saulsbury FT. Corticosteroid therapy does not prevent nephritis in Henoch–Schönlein purpura. Pediatr Nephrol 1993; 7: 69–71.
42. Scharer K, Kramar R, Querfel U et al. clinical outcome of HSP nephritis. Pediatr Nephrol 1999; 13: 816–823.
43. Muller D, Greve D, Eggert D. Early tubular proteinuria and the development of nephritis in HSP. Pediatr Nephrol 2000; 15; 85–89.
44. Levy M, Broyer M, Arsan A et al. Anaphylactoid purpura nephritis in childhood: Natural history and immunopathology. Adv Nephrol 1976; 6: 183–189.
45. Counahan R, Winterborn MH, White RHR et al. Prognosis of Henoch–Schönlein nephritis in children. Br Med J 1977; 2: 11–14.
46. Rostoker G, Desvaux-Belghiti D, Pilatte Y et al. High-dose immunoglobulin therapy for severe IgA nephropathy and Henoch–Schönlein purpura. Ann Intern Med 1994; 120: 476–484.
47. Oner A, Tinaztepe K, Erdogan O. The effect of triple therapy on rapidly progressive type of Henoch–Schönlein nephritis. Pediatr Nephrol 1995; 9: 6–10.
48. Rostoker G, Desvaux-Belghiti D, Pilatte Y et al. Immunomodulation with low-dose immunoglobulins for moderate IgA nephropathy and Henoch–Schönlein purpura. Nephron 1995; 69: 327–334.
49. Iigima K, Ito-Kariya S, Nakamura H et al. Multiple combined therapy for severe HSP nephritis in children. Pediatr Nephrol 1998; 12: 244–248
50. Foster BJ, Bernard C, Drummond K, Sharma AK. Effective therapy for severe HSP nephritis with prednisone and azathioprine: a clinical and histopathologic study. J Pediatr 2000; 136; 370–375.
51. Szer IS. HSP: When to treat and how. J Rheumatol 1996: 23; 1661–1665.

154 Panniculitis

Jeffrey P Callen

Definition

- Panniculitis (inflammation within adipose tissue) most commonly affects the subcutaneous fat
- A variety of associated systemic diseases and clinical syndromes exist
- These are classified histopathologically into septal, lobular or mixed forms

Clinical features

- Subcutaneous, tender nodules
- Associated manifestations and course of the disease are dependent on the clinical syndromes

HISTORY AND CLASSIFICATION

The panniculitides are divided into four categories based on histopathologic criteria: septal panniculitis, lobular panniculitis, mixed, with septal and lobular components, or panniculitis with vasculitis (Table 154.1).

The term erythema nodosum (EN) was first introduced by Willan in 1798; Erasmus Wilson clearly described the clinical features of EN in 1842. The classic modern description of the disease ascribes EN to a reactive process secondary to a variety of underlying disorders, most commonly infections and drugs[1].

Weber–Christian disease (WCD) was first described by Pfeifer in 1892 in the German literature, and by Gilchrist and Kenton in the English literature. In the 1920s, Weber and Christian described similar patients and the eponym Weber–Christian disease was first used in 1936 by Brill in a series of papers dedicated to Henry A. Christian. The modern description by Panush et al.[2] suggests that this disease is less specific and is essentially a reactive process, occasionally associated with enzymatic abnormalities or with factitial disease. The most recent study by White and Winkelmann has suggested that with careful study and follow-up most patients with Weber–Christian disease can be reclassified as one of the more classic panniculitides[3].

TABLE 154.1 CLASSIFICATION OF THE PANNICULITIDES

Septal panniculitis	Erythema nodosum Vilanova's disease – subacute nodular migratory panniculitis

Lobular panniculitis	Weber–Christian – relapsing febrile nodular nonsuppurative panniculitis
	Rottiman–Maka syndrome – lipogranulomatosis subcutanea
	Subcutaneous fat necrosis of the newborn
	Poststeroid panniculitis
	Calcifying panniculitis
	Enzymatic panniculitis
	    Pancreatic
	    α1-antitrypsin deficiency
	Physical or factitial panniculitis
	Histiocytic cytophagic panniculitis
	Lipodystrophy syndromes
	Connective tissue panniculitis – scleroderma or rnyositis
	Sclerosing panniculitis – lipodermalosclerosis

Mixed panniculitis	Lupus profundus – lupus erythematosus panniculitis Erythema nodosum-like lesions of Behçet's
Panniculitis with vasculitis	Small-vessel vasculitis (postcapillary venule), leukocytoclastic vasculitis Medium-sized-vessel vasculitis (arterioles or small arteries) Polyarteritis nodosa Erythema induratum

EPIDEMIOLOGY

The panniculitides can affect all ages, including children. The peak age for EN is varied but WCD and lupus erythematosus panniculitis (LEP) tend to occur in young adults. Most panniculitides are more prevalent in women, although the reasons for this are unclear. No racial or genetic associations have been clearly identified (Table 154.2).

TABLE 154.2 EPIDEMIOLOGY OF THE MAJOR PANNICULITIDES

	Erythema nodosum	Weber–Christian disease	Lupus erythematosus panniculitis
Peak age (years)	25–40	37	27
Sex distribution (M:F)	1:4	3:7	1:9
Prevalence (/100 000)	<1	<1	<1
Annual incidence (/100 000)	2–3	<1	<1
Racial predilection	None	None	None
Genetic associations	HLA-B8	Unknown	Unknown

CLINICAL FEATURES

Panniculitis is a dynamic process that progresses through inflammation with neutrophils to lymphocytes and then to histiocytes, ending with fibrosis[4,5]. In the histiocytic phase it can become granulomatous. The exact nature of the infiltrate depends on the timing of the biopsy in relation to the age of the lesion. Frequently, the panniculitides are associated with systemic disease, and often the separation of one syndrome from another is made only after a period of observation.

Erythema nodosum

A relatively common process, EN is usually acute and self-limited. The typical clinical presentation is the sudden onset of one or more tender, erythematous nodules on the anterior legs that are more easily palpated than visualized (Fig. 154.1). The eruption is often preceded by a prodrome of fever, malaise and/or arthralgias. As the lesions age they may develop an ecchymotic appearance. Over a 4–6 week period they eventually heal without scar formation. Ulceration of the primary process is rare. Although EN is usually an acute process, patients with chronic or recurrent disease have been described using terms such as chronic EN, EN migrans, subacute nodular migratory panniculitis (Vilanova's

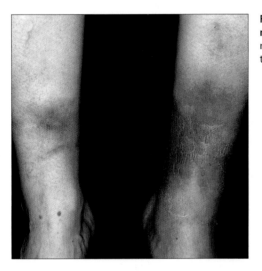

Fig. 154.1 Erythema nodosum. Tender, red nodules on the anterior tibial surface.

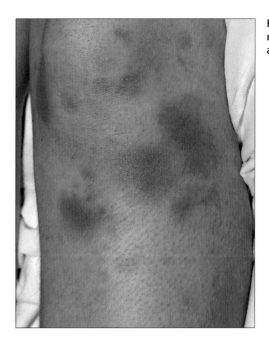

Fig. 154.2 Erythema nodosum secondary to acute sarcoidosis.

disease) or septal granulomatous panniculitis. Chronic or recurrent EN most commonly occurs in middle-aged women. The disease is often present for several years, and is most common on the legs.

Etiologic or associated conditions are present in about 50% of patients with EN. The associated conditions can be divided into three broad categories: infections, drugs or systemic diseases (usually inflammatory disorders). A partial list of the known associations is given in Table 154.3. Garcia-Porrua et al.[6] and Psychos et al.[7] reported that sarcoidosis accounted for 20 and 28% of the cases, an infection for 34 and 18% of the patients, usually in the upper respiratory tract and often β-hemolytic streptococcal infection, and the cause was unknown in roughly 35% of patients. A few patients in each study were noted to have Sweet's syndrome, Behçet's disease, pregnancy, drugs or inflammatory bowel disease as associated processes/causes. The infectious agents associated with EN tend to primarily affect the respiratory or gastrointestinal tract and are most often bacterial or fungal in origin. The most common drugs are antibiotics and oral contraceptives. Pregnancy, particularly in its second trimester, is a known association, and the EN will recur with subsequent pregnancies or with the administration of oral contraceptives. EN-like lesions may occur in Behçet's disease and are accompanied by oral and genital ulcerations, pathergy, uveitis, and/or central nervous system (CNS) disease or other systemic manifestations[8]. A specific variant of sarcoidosis associated with EN is known as Löfgren's syndrome[9] (Fig. 154.2). This is an acute, self-resolving process in which EN occurs with bilateral hilar lymphadenopathy, arthritis and anterior uveitis. Granulomatous colitis (Crohn's disease), regional enteritis and ulcerative colitis have been associated with EN. In patients with inflammatory bowel disease, it appears that the EN parallels the activity of the bowel disease. At least half of the cases of EN are not found to have an associated or underlying process.

Weber–Christian disease

The existence of Weber–Christian disease has often been questioned. Traditionally, Weber–Christian disease is characterized by multiple recurrent subcutaneous nodules with accompanying fever (Fig. 154.3). Biopsy of the nodules reveals a lobular panniculitis with an early neutrophilic infiltrate with fat degeneration, foamy histiocytes and giant cell formation. Eventually fibrosis occurs and this, plus the destruction of fat, results in the clinical finding of an atrophic scar. Other clinical features that commonly occur are arthralgias and myalgias. Some patients also have recurrent abdominal pain. In addition to the skin lesions, any area of the body containing fat can be affected by WCD. Several cases of

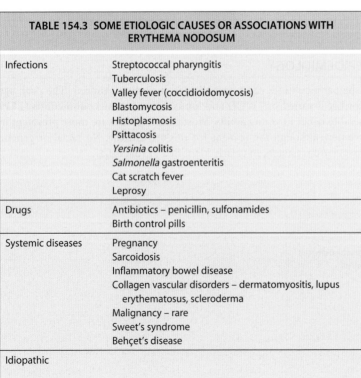

TABLE 154.3 SOME ETIOLOGIC CAUSES OR ASSOCIATIONS WITH ERYTHEMA NODOSUM	
Infections	Streptococcal pharyngitis
	Tuberculosis
	Valley fever (coccidioidomycosis)
	Blastomycosis
	Histoplasmosis
	Psittacosis
	Yersinia colitis
	Salmonella gastroenteritis
	Cat scratch fever
	Leprosy
Drugs	Antibiotics – penicillin, sulfonamides
	Birth control pills
Systemic diseases	Pregnancy
	Sarcoidosis
	Inflammatory bowel disease
	Collagen vascular disorders – dermatomyositis, lupus erythematosus, scleroderma
	Malignancy – rare
	Sweet's syndrome
	Behçet's disease
Idiopathic	

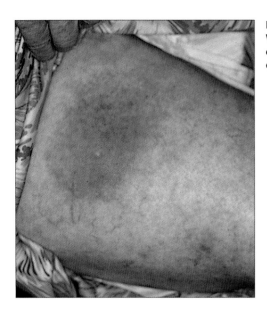

Fig. 154.3 **Weber–Christian disease.** Tender, deep erythematous nodules.

mesenteric panniculitis have been reported, and involvement of the heart, lungs, liver and/or kidneys has also been reported. The disease is chronic but can result in death in 10–15% of cases. White and Winkelmann[3] retrospectively studied 30 cases diagnosed as Weber–Christian panniculitis and found that 26 could be classified as another form of panniculitis, including erythema nodosum (12), post-phlebitic syndrome (6), factitial panniculitis (5), and one case each of cytophagic panniculitis, lymphoma or leukemia. This report suggests that when followed and studied closely most of the patients with Weber–Christian disease have another panniculitic syndrome.

The laboratory abnormalities associated with WCD include an elevated sedimentation rate, anemia, leukopenia or leukocytosis, depression of complement components and evidence of circulating immune complexes.

α_1-antitrypsin deficiency

Patients with a lobular, septal or mixed panniculitis have been found to have a deficiency of α_1-antitrypsin. In a study of 96 patients with panniculitis, Smith et al.[10] found 15 patients with α_1-antitrypsin deficiency. Such patients were more likely to have ulceration and drainage, and correspondingly had greater amounts of fat necrosis and elastic tissue destruction. It was suggested that induction of lesions by trauma was more likely in the antitrypsin-deficient group. The recognition of these patients is important for several reasons. First, debridement of the lesion should be avoided; secondly, in patients felt to have factitial panniculitis, α_1-antitrypsin deficiency should be considered; thirdly, these patients

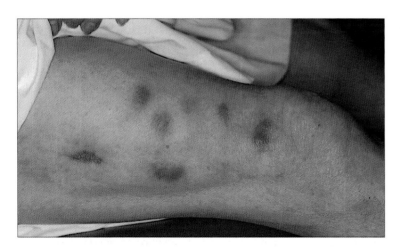

Fig. 154.4 **Pancreatic panniculitis.**

should be evaluated for pulmonary disease and should be counseled to avoid smoking; and lastly, therapy with α_1-proteinase inhibitor concentrate may be helpful.

Pancreatic panniculitis

Patients with pancreatic diseases may develop subcutaneous fat necrosis (lobular panniculitis) (Fig. 154.4) with accompanying polyarthritis and osseous intramedullary fat necrosis. A variety of pancreatic pathologic changes have been implicated in the development of this process, including pancreatitis, pancreatic carcinoma (acinar cell), pancreatitis secondary to cholelithiasis, post-traumatic lesions, pancreatic ischemia, pancreatic pseudocyst and pancreas divisum (a congenital pancreatic abnormality)[11]. It is not clear whether the elevated lipase in the circulation is primarily involved in the pathogenesis of the fat necrosis, or whether its presence follows the fat necrosis. Histopathologically, there is extensive fat necrosis with a basophilic alteration of lipocytes. Ghost cells with absent nuclei are also common.

Calcifying panniculitis of renal failure

Patients with renal failure often have abnormal calcium–phosphorus metabolism. These patients may develop acute, erythematous, tender indurated nodules as a manifestation of calciphylaxis[12]. The panniculitic lesions can progress to necrosis and ulceration. The prognosis is poor, and treatment should consist of attempts to correct the calcium–phosphorus imbalance. Parathyroidectomy with or without renal transplantation may be helpful.

Post-steroid panniculitis

Panniculitis following withdrawal of corticosteroid therapy is a rare entity which seems to be limited to children[13]. Patients reported have been treated with corticosteroids for a wide array of problems, including leukemia, nephrotic syndrome, rheumatic carditis and encephalopathy. Interestingly, the panniculitis may clear upon readministration of the corticosteroids. The pathogenesis of this rare complication is not understood.

Lipoatrophic panniculitis

Several conditions have been described in children that often result in lipoatrophy following the inflammatory reaction. There exists a spectrum that perhaps includes Rothman–Makai syndrome (lipogranulomatosis subcutanea), lipoatrophic panniculitis, lipophagic panniculitis of childhood and localized lipoatrophy (atrophic connective tissue disease panniculitis)[14]. These children tend to have multiple erythematous lesions, most commonly on the extremities, that resolve with subcutaneous atrophy. The patients often also manifest fever. They may have associated 'autoimmune' phenomena, such as juvenile rheumatoid arthritis, Hashimoto's thyroiditis or diabetes mellitus. There is no known effective therapy, although some patients have responded to oral corticosteroids, oral antimalarials or oral dapsone.

Histiocytic cytophagic panniculitis

Histiocytic cytophagic panniculitis was described by Crotty and Winkelmann[15] as a chronic histiocytic disease of the subcutaneous fat, with accompanying inflammatory panniculitis, fever, serositis and 'reticuloendotheliomegaly'. Recently Craig et al.[16] have suggested that there are two, perhaps distinct, patterns of disease, one that is benign and is termed cytophagic histiocytic panniculitis, and one that is malignant and is termed subcutaneous T-cell lymphoma. In both instances the hemophagocytic syndrome may occur, but in cytophagic histiocytic panniculitis there is often a response to prednisone and/or cyclosporin. Some of these patients perhaps have EB virus within their lesions. The diagnosis of subcutaneous T-cell lymphoma is at times very difficult to confirm[17] (Bush and Callen, personal communication). Aggressive therapy with cytotoxic agents used early in this process may be helpful[18].

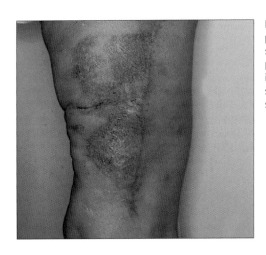

Fig. 154.5 Factitial panniculitis. Multiple scars are present in this patient, who was injecting a foreign substance into her subcutaneous tissue.

Factitial panniculitis

Factitial panniculitis due to external trauma or from the injection of foreign substances is not common, but should be considered in patients with unusual clinical or histopathologic features of panniculitis (Fig. 154.5). In traumatic lesions there may be an organizing hematoma demonstrated histologically; whereas with injections one encounters refractile bodies or a 'Swiss cheese' effect. Occasionally, spectroscopic and/or chromatographic techniques are necessary to identify the causative injected material.

Lupus erythematosus panniculitis (lupus profundus)

Lupus erythematosus panniculitis (LEP) is a rare cutaneous manifestation of lupus erythematosus occurring in 1–3% of patients with LE[19]. The lesions are tender, red–blue subcutaneous nodules that may eventually ulcerate. They tend to occur on the face, upper arms, thighs and/or buttocks. The lesions may underlie a typical lesion of discoid LE. Histopathologic changes include a panniculitis that is both lobular and septal. When the overlying epidermis and/or dermis demonstrate changes of LE, the diagnosis of LEP can be histologically confirmed. The activity of the panniculitic lesion does not seem to follow the course of the systemic disease.

Sclerosing panniculitis

Jorizzo et al. coined the term sclerosing panniculitis to describe a group of patients with well-circumscribed, indurated inflammatory plaques of the lower extremity[20]. These lesions most frequently occur in women and are often accompanied by signs of venous insufficiency. Histopathologically this disorder is characterized by fat necrosis, sclerosis and a lobular panniculitis. Fat microcysts with foci of membranous fat necrosis are also commonly observed in the later stages of the disease. Sclerosing panniculitis is probably a manifestation of venous insufficiency, and thus therapy should include support stockings, elevation and rest. Measures for the prevention of phlebitis are also warranted. Low-dose aspirin or other non-steroidal anti-inflammatory drugs (NSAIDs) may be helpful. Intralesional injection of triamcinolone acetonide may also be helpful.

Panniculitis with vasculitis

Nodular vasculitis, polyarteritis nodosa (both cutaneous and systemic varieties) and small vessel vasculitis may involve subcutaneous vessels and result in inflammatory or ischemic changes in the subcutaneous fat. Erythema induratum is a form of nodular vasculitis felt to be due to tuberculosis.

INVESTIGATIONS

The evaluation of the patient with panniculitis should include a careful history and physical examination. The possibility of infection of the upper respiratory tract should be considered, and a throat swab for a rapid streptococcal screen, skin tests for tuberculosis and a chest radiograph should be obtained. In general, neither inflammatory bowel disease nor infectious enteritis is asymptomatic and thus it is not necessary to perform endoscopic or radiographic procedures in these patients. Tests for enzymatic abnormalities, such as amylase, lipase or α_1-antitrypsin deficiency should be ordered. The possibility of a coexistent collagen vascular disease should also be considered.

DIFFERENTIAL DIAGNOSIS

The differential diagnosis of EN involves distinguishing it from (1) other forms of panniculitis (all of which may present with tender subcutaneous nodules), (2) insect bites, (3) thrombophlebitis or (4) cellulitis. Insect bites may be tender, red, infiltrated lesions. The distribution is dependent upon the type of bite, and in general the patient is otherwise asymptomatic. Often there is a puncture site within the lesion. Cellulitis rarely manifests as subcutaneous nodules. When the diagnosis is in question a wedge biopsy or deep punch biopsy which includes subcutaneous fat will be helpful.

The differential diagnosis of WCD includes other lobular panniculitides, EN and LEP (lupus profundus). EN can be separated on clinical and histopathologic grounds. Lupus profundus occurs in conjunction with typical LE skin lesions or in patients with SLE. This latter group may be difficult to distinguish from WCD, particularly in view of the reports of WCD in some patients with SLE.

MANAGEMENT

The treatment of EN and other panniculitides first involves assessment of a causative disease and its treatment. In the absence of a treatable disorder, therapy is symptomatic. Acute EN is often self-limited, thus nontoxic therapies are advised. Bed rest and leg elevation are very helpful in controlling symptoms. In patients who need to continue to be ambulatory, support stockings or tights may be helpful. Aspirin or other NSAIDs may be helpful. Sometimes, however, treatment with aspirin does not produce results prior to toxicity, and oral indomethacin (25–75mg/day) is therefore recommended.

In patients with chronic EN or frequent recurrences, oral potassium iodide 300–900mg/day has been useful in open clinical trials. When the drug is stopped or the dose is lowered the disease often relapses, only to respond again with reinstitution of therapy. Other therapies that may be considered include oral corticosteroids, colchicine, hydroxychloroquine or an immunosuppressive agent. Cyclosporin has been used successfully in some patients. One adjunctive therapy that can be helpful is intralesionally injected triamcinolone acetonide.

There is no specific therapy for WCD. Reports have centered on the use of anti-inflammatory agents including aspirin, NSAIDs, oral corticosteroids, antimalarials and immunosuppressives, including cyclophosphamide and cyclosporin. In addition, colchicine, dapsone and potassium iodide may be effective in some individual cases.

Patients with cytophagic histiocytic panniculitis should be aggressively treated with corticosteroids and/or immunosuppressive agents. Despite this treatment, many patients develop the hematophagocytic syndrome, and multiple deaths have been reported in this seemingly benign inflammatory process.

Patients with LEP may respond to antimalarials or to intralesional injections of triamcinolone. Corticosteroids and/or immunosuppressives are rarely necessary for LEP.

SUMMARY

Panniculitides form a wide array of syndromes which perhaps can be best separated on the basis of clinical features, associated disorders and/or histopathologic findings. Unfortunately, several of the syndromes seem to have overlapping features, the pathogenesis is not understood for most, and therapeutic options are similar for all. The differential diagnosis often depends on an adequate specimen for histopathologic investigation. Thus a fusiform incisional biopsy or a wedge biopsy should be performed. Furthermore, the youngest lesion should be biopsied. Sections should be serially cut to identify the pattern of the panniculitis: lobular, septal, vasculitis or mixed. Evaluation for the underlying process should be performed and includes ingestants, infections, malignancy and autoimmune disorders. Treatment, in the absence of an underlying disease, is aimed at control of the inflammatory reaction with agents such as NSAIDs, corticosteroids, dapsone, potassium iodide, antimalarials, colchicine or cytotoxic/immunosuppressive agents.

REFERENCES

1. Weinstein L. Erythema nodosum. Disease-A-Month 1969; June: 1–30.
2. Panush RS, Vonker RA, Diesk A *et al.* Weber–Christian disease. Medicine 1985; 64: 181–190.
3. White JW, Winkelmann RK. Weber–Christian panniculitis: a review of 30 cases with this diagnosis. J Am Acad Dermatol 1998; 39, 56–62.
4. Black MM. Panniculitis: problems with diagnosis. Aust J Dermatol 1988; 29: 79–84.
5. Patterson JW. Panniculitis: New findings in the third compartment. Arch Dermatol 1987; 123: 1615.
6. Garcia-Porrua C, Gonzalez-Gay MA, Vazquez-Caruncho M *et al.* Erythema nodosum: etiologic and predictive factors in a defined population. Arthritis Rheum 2000; 43: 584–592.
7. Psychos DN, Voulgari PV, Skopouli FN *et al.* Erythema nodosum: the underlying conditions. Clin Rheumatol 2000; 19: 212–216.
8. Chun SI, Su WPD, Lee S, Rogers RS III. Erythema nodosum-like lesions in Behçet's syndrome: a histopathologic study of 30 cases. J Cutan Pathol 1989; 16: 259–265.
9. Mana J, Gomez-Vaquero C, Montero A *et al.* Lofgren's syndrome revisited: a study of 186 patients. Am J Med 1999; 107: 240–245.
10. Smith KC, Su WPD, Pittelkow MR, Winkelmann RK. Clinical and pathologic correlations with 96 patients with panniculitis, including 15 patients with deficient levels of alpha-1-antitrypsin. J Am Acad Dermatol 1989; 21: 1192–1196.
11. Dahl PR, Su WPD, Cullimore KC, Dicken CH. Pancreatic panniculitis. J Am Acad Dermatol 1995; 33: 413–417.
12. Ivker RA, Woosley J, Briggaman RA. Calciphylaxis in three patients with end-stage renal disease. Arch Dermatol 1995; 131: 63–68.
13. Roenigk HH, Haserick JR, Arundell FD. Post steroid panniculitis. Report of a case and review of the literature. Arch Dermatol 1964; 90: 387–391.
14. Winkelmann RK, McEvoy MT, Peters MS. Lipophagic panniculitis of childhood. J Am Acad Dermatol 1989; 21: 971–978.
15. Crotty C, Winkelmann R. Cytophagic histiocytic panniculitis with fever, cytopenia, liver failure, and terminal hemorrhagic diathesis. J Am Acad Dermatol 1981; 4: 181–194.
16. Craig A J, Cualing H, Thomas G *et al.* Cytophagic histiocytic panniculitis – a syndrome associated with benign and malignant panniculitis: case comparison and review of the literature. J Am Acad Dermatol 1998; 39; 721–736.
17. Weenig RH, Ng CS, Perniciaro C. Subcutaneous panniculitis-like T-cell lymphoma. An elusive case presenting as lipomembranous panniculitis an a review of 72 cases in the literature. Am J Dermatopathol 2001; 23; 206–215.
18. Perniciaro C, Winkelmann RK, Ehrhardt DR. Fatal systemic cytophagic histiocytic panniculitis: a histopathological and immunohistochemical study of multiple organ sites. J Am Acad Dermatol 1994; 31: 901–905.
19. Martens PB, Moder KG, Ahmed I. Lupus panniculitis: clinical perspectives from a case series. J Rheumatol 1999; 26; 68–72.
20. Jorizzo JL, White WL, Zanolli MD *et al.* Sclerosing panniculitis: a clinicopathologic assessment. Arch Dermatol 1991; 127: 544–548.

155 Cutaneous vasculitis

Jeffrey P Callen

Definition

- Polymorphonuclear inflammation of the vessel wall of small to medium-sized vessels that supply nutrients to the skin
- Circulating immune complexes are involved in the pathogenesis, but a complex interaction of cytokines and vasoactive amines with endothelial cells is necessary for disease expression

Clinical features

- Cutaneous involvement: palpable purpura or urticaria-like lesions are most common; less common are livedo reticularis, ulcerations or necrosis
- Systemic involvement: arthritis, glomerulonephritis, gastrointestinal hemorrhage or colic are most common
- The acute variant is often self-limiting
- Prognosis is dependent upon the organ systems involved and the severity of involvement

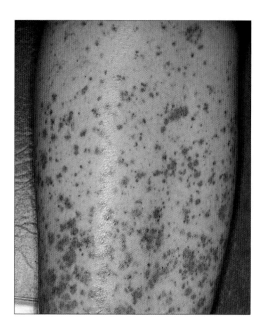

Fig. 155.1 Palpable purpura representing a leukocytoclastic vasculitis.

CLINICAL FEATURES

Cutaneous vasculitis refers to a neutrophilic inflammation within the small to medium-sized vessels that supply nutrients to the skin. Cutaneous vasculitic syndromes may be classified o the basis of the size of the vessel involved (Table 155.1)[1–3]. There are several classification schemes; however, none of those proposed satisfactorily predicts prognosis. There have been many recent papers that separate hypersensitivity vasculitis from Henoch–Schönlein purpura; however, in my opinion their separation remains somewhat arbitrary[4,5]. Most forms of cutaneous vasculitis represent a systemic disorder that may or may not have recognizable abnormalities in other organ systems. Vessel disease is caused by circulating immune complexes and usually begins as a 'leukocytoclastic' vasculitis. With repair mechanisms, a mononuclear cell infiltrate may develop and become demonstrable when the biopsy is taken late in the course of the individual lesion. In leukocytoclastic vasculitis (LCV), there is fibrinoid necrosis of the vessel walls, with infiltration of polymorphonuclear leukocytes, some of which are disrupted, resulting in the presence of nuclear debris with the tissue[6].

The lesions observed in patients with cutaneous vasculitis can vary from transient urticaria-like lesions to necrosis of wide areas of skin[3].

The type of lesion, in general, reflects the size of the vessel involved and thus varies somewhat with the specific vasculitic syndrome. The most common cutaneous finding is palpable purpura (Fig. 155.1) followed by urticaria-like lesions.

Palpable purpura

Sams et al.[6] suggested that the development of the clinical lesion is in some manner dynamic, often beginning as non-palpable purpura that eventually becomes palpable. Furthermore, they suggested that in 'later stages, some lesions become nodular, bullous, infarctive and ulcerative'. Most often, the patient has only one type of lesion, which fades as reparative processes begin. There are patients who will have nodules, bullae, ulcers, necrosis or livedo reticularis, either in combination with palpable purpura or as the sole manifestation of LCV.

Purpuric lesions are most frequent on dependent surfaces, in particular the legs or buttocks. Palpable purpura is characterized by smooth, discrete papules with relatively uniform lesional hemorrhage. Piette and Stone[7] attempted to distinguish IgA-related palpable purpura from other forms of LCV. They described a distinct pattern for IgA-associated cutaneous vasculitis, in which the lesions were superficial plaques (palpable purpuric plaques) with multifocal areas of hemorrhage and necrosis, arranged in a retiform pattern (Fig. 155.2). The lesions of vasculitis can, on occasion, become generalized, and this often suggests more severe internal involvement.

Urticarial lesions

Urticarial lesions of vasculitis are the second most common cutaneous manifestation (Fig. 155.3). These lesions differ from urticaria in the following characteristics: the individual lesions are most often long-lived, lasting between 6 and 72 hours; the lesions may resolve with some

TABLE 155.1 CUTANEOUS CLASSIFICATION OF VASCULITIS
1. Vasculitis of the postcapillary venule
2. Vasculitis of the small mid-dermal arterioles
3. Vasculitis of the arterioles within the panniculus
4. Vasculitis of the medium-sized arteries

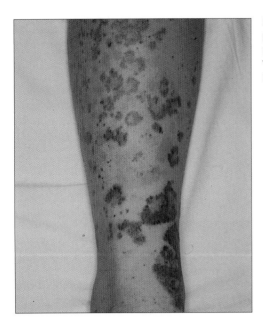

Fig. 155.2 Retiform purpuric plaques are present in this patient with Henoch–Schönlein purpura.

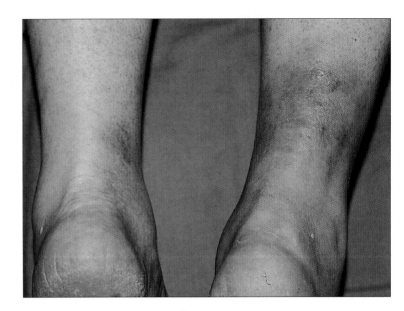

Fig. 155.5 Nodular lesions of leukocytoclastic vasculitis.

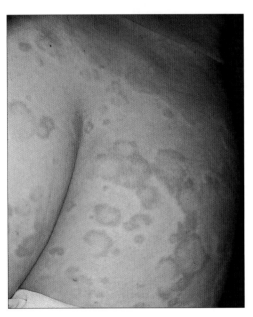

Fig. 155.3 Urticarial vasculitis.

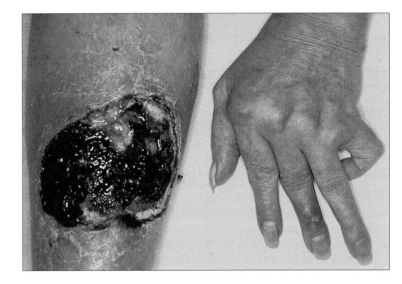

Fig. 155.6 Leukocytoclastic vasculitis with ulceration in a patient with rheumatoid arthritis.

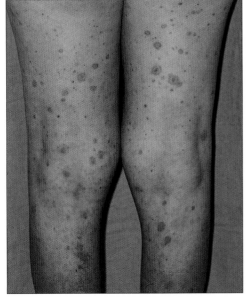

Fig. 155.4 Erythema multiforme-like lesions of leukocytoclastic vasculitis.

residual pigmentation or ecchymosis; the lesions are often characterized by pain or burning rather than pruritus; the patients tend to have symptoms or signs of multisystem disease such as arthralgias, fever, gastrointestinal pain, lymphadenopathy or abnormal urine sediment[8]. The lesions of urticarial vasculitis are usually generalized. Demonstration of the long-lived nature of these lesions can be achieved by encircling several lesions and evaluating them for the onset of resolution.

Other cutaneous lesions

A wide array of other cutaneous lesions can also occur and include erythematous plaques, erythema multiforme-like lesions (Fig. 155.4), nodules (Fig. 155.5), ulcerations (Fig. 155.6), necrosis and livedo reticularis. Table 155.2 demonstrates the varying, yet overlapping, cutaneous manifestations that occur in the traditional vasculitic syndromes. The occurrence of palpable purpura, the hallmark of LCV, in all syndromes except large-vessel vasculitis has resulted in some of the controversy surrounding the classification.

Systemic manifestations

The systemic manifestations correlate with the syndrome and the size of the vessel involved (Table 155.3). This section will focus on LCV and its full spectrum; Henoch–Schölein purpura is considered in Chapter 153, and polyarteritis nodosa, Wegener's granulomatosis and Churg–Strauss syndrome are covered in more detail in Chapters 146, 148 and 149, respectively.

The most common manifestation of vasculitis is involvement of organs with a rich vascular supply, such as the gut, the kidneys, the lungs and the musculoskeletal system (Table 155.4). In a study of 82 patients selected for cutaneous LCV, only about 50% had any systemic manifestations that were clinically evident, and in general this group of patients had involvement that was not life-threatening[9]. Similarly, Blanco et al.[10] found that a majority of patients with cutaneous vasculitis had a relatively benign course. However, their data for adults differed from that of children. Of the 172 adults in their study, 23 had the cutaneous disease as a manifestation of a systemic necrotizing vasculitis. They also noted that cutaneous vasculitis was a manifestation of a connective tissue disease in 20 patients, essential mixed cryoglobulinemia in 11 patients, bacterial endocarditis in four and malignancy in four.

Vasculitic syndromes

Acute hemorrhagic edema of infancy

Acute hemorrhagic edema of infancy is a rare condition that occurs in infants younger than 2 years[11]. It has an acute onset, often following an upper respiratory tract infection or drug ingestion. The rash begins as urticarial plaques, but rapidly becomes intensely purpuric. Fever and generalized edema are common. Acute hemorrhagic edema of infancy has been separated from Henoch–Schönlein purpura by clinical and

TABLE.155.2 RELATIONSHIP BETWEEN THE DIFFERENT VASCULITIC SYNDROMES AND THE CUTANEOUS MANIFESTATION	
Clinical syndrome	Gross cutaneous morphology
Leukocytoclastic vasculitis (dermal vasculitis, hypersensitivity angiitis)	Palpable purpura, urticarial lesions, erosion, hemorrhagic bullae, livedo reticularis, cutaneous infarcts, nodules, ulcerations
Henoch–Schönlein purpura	Retiform purpuric plaques
Wegener's granulomatosis	Ulcerative nodules, palpable purpura, peripheral gangrene
Polyarteritis nodosa	Subcutaneous nodules, livedo reticularis, ulcerations, peripheral gangrene

TABLE 155.3 SYSTEMIC DISEASES ASSOCIATED WITH LEUKOCYTOCLASTIC VASCULITIS
Other vasculitic syndromes: Wegener's granulomatosis, polyarteritis nodosa, polyangiitis syndromes
Rheumatic disorders: Systemic lupus erythematosus, RA, dermatomyositis, Sjögren's syndrome
Infections: Hepatitis B infection, HIV disease, streptococci, subacute bacterial endocarditis
Paraproteins: Cryoglobulinemia, macroglobulinemia, hyperglobulinemia, cryofibrinogenemia
Other: Inflammatory bowel disease, neoplasia, cystic fibrosis, bowel bypass syndrome, C2 deficiency, a_1-antitrypsin deficiency

TABLE 155.4 SYSTEMIC INVOLVEMENT IN VASCULITIS
Musculoskeletal: Arthralgias, myalgias, arthritis, myositis
Renal: Hematuria, proteinuria, azotemia, hypertension
Gastrointestinal: Colic, hemorrhage, ulceration, perforation
Pulmonary: Infiltrates, pleuritis, nodules, asthma
Neurologic: Neuropathy, cephalagic stroke
Other: pancreatitis, pericarditis, myocarditis

immunologic differences. For example, patients with the former have IgM within the dermal vessels, whereas those with Henoch–Schönlein purpura have IgA. The process of acute hemorrhagic edema of infancy is basically benign and self-limiting; therefore supportive treatment is all that is necessary.

Urticarial vasculitis

McDuffie et al.[12] first described urticarial vasculitis when they reported four patients with recurrent attacks of erythematous urticarial and hemorrhagic skin lesions associated with synovitis and, sometimes, abdominal distress. Their patients did not have lupus erythematosus or paraproteinemia, but did have hypocomplementemia; two had nephritis. In 1977 Soter[13], demonstrated that necrotizing vasculitis (LCV) could occur in patients with chronic urticaria, and this pathologic finding correlated with complement activation as manifested by hypocomplementemia. Monroe et al.[8] demonstrated that LCV could be observed in chronic-like lesions, and that this correlated with long duration of an individual lesion (more than 24 hours), the presence of immunoglobulin in the biopsy specimen, and an increased erythrocyte sedimentation rate. The correlation was present, but imperfect, and there was little correlation with the presence of arthralgias.

Urticarial lesions may also be an early clinical manifestation of lesions that become typical palpable purpura. The spectrum of 'urticarial vasculitis' has also grown, in recent years, to include the presence of lung disease characterized by 'asthma' or obstructive lung disease[14]. Patients with obstructive disease may have hypocomplementemia. Many patients, however, have primarily chronic urticaria, with little or no systemic involvement.

Lastly, a syndrome of chronic urticaria with macroglobulinemia has been described, known as Schnitzler's syndrome[15]. Other etiologies or associated diseases in patients with urticarial vasculitis have included lupus erythematosus, viral hepatitis, infectious mononucleosis, serum sickness, Sjögren's syndrome and other paraproteinemias. Thus urticarial vasculitis can manifest many of the features and associations typical of other forms of LCV, and is only distinguishable on the basis of the clinical skin lesion.

Vasculitis associated with paraproteinemia

Almost any clinical lesion, from urticarial through palpable purpura to necrosis and ulceration, can occur in patients with an abnormal circulating protein. Patients with cryoglobulins may have a predilection for acral disease, otherwise there are few clinical clues that suggest a paraprotein. There are therapeutic implications of paraproteinemia, and

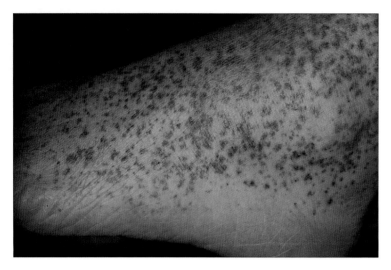

Fig. 155.7 Non-palpable purpura of hyperglobulinemic purpura of Waldenström.

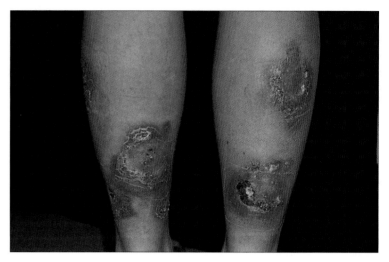

Fig. 155.8 This patient with Crohn's disease also has cutaneous polyarteritis.

thus almost all patients with chronic or recurrent cutaneous vasculitis should be evaluated for a paraprotein, including cryoglobulins. In many of the patients with mixed cryoglobulinemia, a link with hepatitis C virus infection has been noted[16]. These patients may have non-inflammatory occlusive disease or a small-vessel vasculitis. Treatment with interferon alfa-2α or ribavirin, or both, has led to disease control in many of these patients[17].

In some reports, hyperglobulinemic purpura has been separated from other vasculitides[18]. Perhaps this is because some of the lesions of hyperglobulinemic purpura are non-palpable (Fig. 155.7) and do not reveal LCV on biopsy. This may indicate that these lesions are early or late manifestations, and in my experience, if timed appropriately, the skin biopsy usually reveals LCV. Hyperglobulinemic purpura has recently been associated with Sjögren's syndrome and lupus erythematosus. These patients commonly demonstrate the anti-Ro(SS-A) antibody.

Paraneoplastic vasculitis

Cutaneous or systemic vasculitis, or both, has been reported on several occasions in patients who have or have had malignancies. Sanchez-Guerrero *et al.*[19] reported that 11 of 222 patients had what they termed 'paraneoplastic vasculitis'. In most of these patients (nine of the 11), the vasculitis was limited to the small cutaneous vessels and was histologically characterized as LCV. In three patients, the vasculitis was the presenting manifestation of neoplasia (squamous cell carcinoma of the esophagus, T cell lymphoma and myeloblastic leukemia).

The mechanisms underlying 'paraneoplastic' vasculitis are unknown. The vasculitis can at times be directly related to tumor treatment, but in many cases the occurrence appears to be coincidental. The exact incidence of neoplasia with vasculitis is not known, and thus extensive evaluation of malignancy cannot be recommended; unexplained symptoms, however, should be evaluated. Lymphoreticular malignancies, in particular hairy cell leukemia, have been the most frequently reported type of neoplasia, but also a wide variety of solid tumors have occurred in patients with vasculitis.

Cutaneous polyarteritis nodosa

Cutaneous polyarteritis nodosa is characterized clinically by nodules, livedo reticularis, ulcerations or a combination of these lesions (Fig. 155.8)[20]. Histopathologically, the lesions are characterized by LCV of the arterioles, often in the subcutaneous tissue, with a surrounding panniculitis. The nodular lesions must be differentiated from erythema nodosum or other panniculitides. Livedo reticularis can occur with thrombotic disorders of several causes. Cutaneous polyarteritis nodosa is generally associated with a good prognosis, but patients with ulcerations tend to have neuropathy more frequently[20]. Patients with cutaneous polyarteritis nodosa have been reported with a variety of systemic disease associations, including inflammatory bowel disease, rheumatoid arthritis and paraproteinemia. Recently, the cutaneous and systemic forms of polyarteritis nodosa have been linked to long-term treatment of acne vulgaris with minocycline[21,22]. Systemic polyarteritis nodosa may manifest skin lesions similar to those of the cutaneous form, but has disease involving muscular arteries in other organs. A more detailed discussion of polyarteritis nodosa is given in Chapter 146.

Erythema elevatum diutinum

Erythema elevatum diutinum is a rare form of LCV having its major manifestation in the skin[23,24]. The lesions begin as red–purple or yellow papules that coalesce to form plaques. The most prominent involvement occurs on the extensor surfaces such as the knees, elbows and dorsal hands (Fig. 155.9). The only systemic manifestation a arthralgia, which occurs in 20–40% of patients. Some of the patients with erythema elevatum diutinum are found to have an IgA paraprotein.

Cutaneous vasculitis in patients with rheumatic diseases

Cutaneous vasculitis, as manifest by palpable purpura, urticarial lesions or ulcerations, is commonly observed in systemic lupus erythematosus, rheumatoid arthritis and Sjögren's syndrome. The appearance of cutaneous vasculitis is usually associated with active systemic disease.

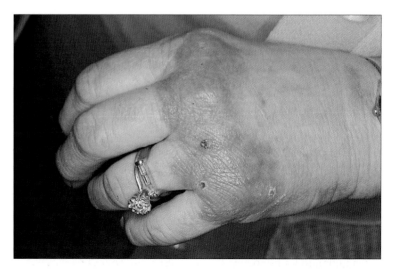

Fig. 155.9 Erythema elevatum diutinum.

INVESTIGATIONS

Patients who present with palpable purpura, urticarial lesions or other cutaneous lesions that represent LCV have been classified within several schemas. The basic premise of evaluation is first to find an etiologic association, and second to assess the presence, and severity, of systemic involvement[10]. Table 155.5 presents the basic work-up that is recommended for patients with vasculitis. In patients with acute disease, in whom there is an obvious etiology such as a drug or infection, the evaluation is streamlined and need not assess all possible causes. Skin biopsy of an early lesion is necessary to confirm the presence of LCV, but is often not performed in children with typical lesions[10].

In patients with chronic disease, or in whom there is not an obvious etiology, the work-up is more extensive. An assessment for paraproteins is necessary in this group of patients, but evalution for malignancy is probably not necessary unless there are other symptoms or signs. Cutaneous immunofluorescence biopsy can be useful when Henoch–Schönlein purpura is considered.

DIFFERENTIAL DIAGNOSIS

The differential diagnosis of cutaneous vasculitis differs with each clinical lesion. Palpable purpura must be differentiated from traumatic purpura, insect bites, embolic phenomena and a variety of infections. Infectious agents that cause purpuric lesions similar to vasculitis can do so by embolizing material that occludes the vessels or by the formation of immune complexes. At times, both processes may be operative, particularly in patients with subacute bacterial endocarditis. Other embolic processes that can mimic vasculitis include atheromatous emboli or emboli from a left atrial myxoma. In addition, endocarditis may mimic cutaneous vasculitis[10].

Urticarial lesions must be differentiated from 'garden-variety' urticaria, bites, erythema multiforme and drug eruptions. Ulcerations can occur from non-inflammatory vessel occlusion such as atherosclerosis, malignant processes or bites, or from non-vessel-based inflammatory conditions such as pyoderma gangrenosum. Livedo reticularis usually occurs with involvement of medium-sized vessels and occurs secondary to atherosclerosis, emboli or occlusive vasculopathy associated with the antiphospholipid antibody syndrome.

PATHOGENESIS

Current evidence suggests that LCV, whether of the small or medium-sized vessels, is related to immune complexes[25]. It is presumed that antibodies are formed to an antigen that binds and forms circulating immune complexes. Most vasculitides are related to IgG or IgM immune complexes, although Henoch–Schönlein purpura is related to IgA immune complexes.

Soluble immune complexes that are not removed by the mononuclear–phagocyte system can become lodged between the endothelial cells of the vessel wall. This process can be exacerbated by vasoactive amines (specifically, histamine) that can dilate the vessel, creating spaces between endothelial cells (this observation can be used clinically to reproduce lesions). Once lodged, the circulating immune complexes will activate complement via the classic pathway, resulting in the release of chemotactic factors, in particular C5a, and the formation of the membrane attack complex that may damage the endothelial cells directly[26]. In addition, the complement component C5a specifically attracts polymorphonuclear leukocytes, which release lysosomal enzymes and cause tissue destruction, with resultant edema and hemorrhage. Mononuclear cells eventually clear the destroyed tissue. Thus polymorphonuclear leukocytes precede the mononuclear cells in the dynamic process. This is demonstrated schematically in Figure 155.10.

In addition to immunologic factors, several non-immunologic factors are involved in disease expression. Increased hydrostatic pressure predis-

TABLE 155.5 EVALUATION OF THE PATIENT WITH CUTANEOUS VASCULITIS
1 History:
Infections? Drug ingestion? Prior history of one of the 'associated' disorders? Are there systemic symptoms?
2. Physical examination:
General appearance Type of skin lesion
3. Skin biopsy:
Immunofluorescence is optional, perhaps useful when considering IgA disease
4. Laboratory studies:
Necessary: Complete blood count Urine analysis, test of renal function Chest radiograph Test for collagen vascular diseases – ANA, anti-Ro(SS-A), rheumatoid factor, etc. Hepatitis B surface antigen, hepatitis C antibody Tests for paraproteins, cryoglobulins, cryofibrinogens, etc. When appropriate or under special circumstances: Total hemolytic complement Circulating immune complexes Sedimentation rate Anticardiolipin antibody Blood cultures

poses certain areas of involvement, explaining the observation that vasculitis is more common on the legs and buttocks. Fibrinolytic activity may also be abnormal in some patients, and the result is a non-healing ulceration, or stellate scars. This process is evident in cryofibrinogenemia, and perhaps in the histologically bland lesions of 'livedoid vasculitis' or atrophie blanche.

There is well-documented experimental evidence in animals suggesting that LCV is a dynamic process[27]. Gower et al.[28] evaluated the histopathologic and immunopathologic findings in experimentally induced lesions over time. The infiltrate varied, but it is not clear whether or not the characteristics of the infiltrate changed with time. In a single case of naturally occurring LCV studied by Zax et al.[29], repeated biopsies suggested that the infiltrate changed from polymorphonuclear predominance to mononuclear predominance. This is in contrast to data from Soter et al.[30] and Alexander and Provost[31], who have suggested that two distinct subgroups of inflammatory vasculopathy exist – those with neutrophil predominance and others with mononuclear inflammatory disease[31]. Furthermore, these investigators have suggested that associated phenomena such as serologic reactivity, hypocomplementemia and central nervous system involvement correlate with the presence of a neutrophilic infiltrate. Although their patients have undergone repeated biopsies, none has had serial biopsies of their lesions. Despite these contradictory studies, experimental evidence in both humans and animals does suggest that the process is dynamic.

In recent years, it has become evident that the pathogenesis of vasculitis is more complex than can be explained by immune complex disease alone. It appears that there may be cellular immune and inflammatory interactions of neutrophils, eosinophils, monocytes, lymphocytes and endothelial cells. It is likely that soluble mediators such as cytokines, prostaglandins and products of the coagulation or fibrinolytic pathways, or both, are involved in disease expression. Lastly, expression of the disease may be linked to abnormalities of the cell adhesion molecules.

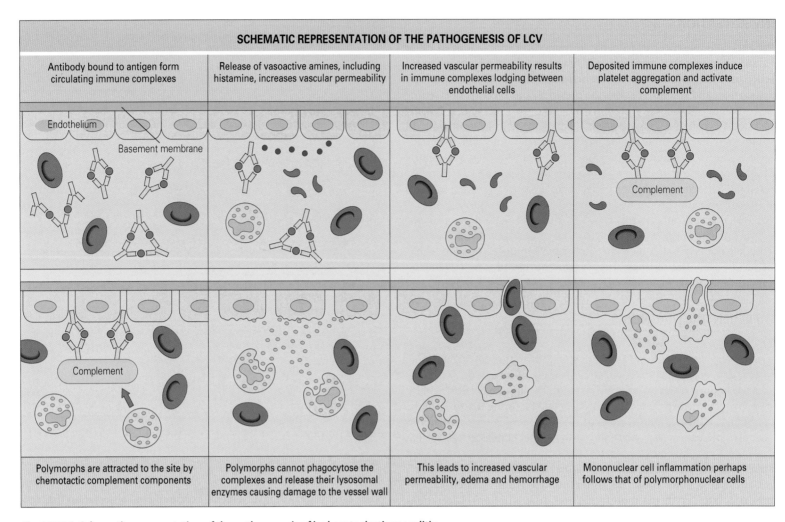

Fig. 155.10 Schematic representation of the pathogenesis of leukocytoclastic vasculitis.

Syndrome	First choice	Alternate choices	Comments
Hypersensitivity vasculitis	Identify and remove antigen	Colchicine, dapsone, immunosuppressive agent, corticosteroids	A thorough evaluation is needed to exclude other vasculitic syndromes that may manifest as palpable purpura
Henoch–Schönlein purpura	Observation	Corticosteroids or an immunosuppressive agent, or both	There are no data that demonstrates that treatment alters the course. Often this condition is self-limiting
Urticarial vasculitis – normocomplementemic	Antihistamines	Colchicine, dapsone, corticosteroids, immunosuppressive agents, intravenous immune globulin	Chronic urticaria, particularly when associated with vasculitis, is probably an immune-mediated disorder
Urticarial vasculitis – hypocomplementemic	Corticosteroids or immunosuppressives	Intravenous immune globulin	This disorder is difficult to treat. Associated pulmonary disease may occur and there is no known effective treatment
Vasculitis associated with hepatitis C	Interferon with or without ribavirin		Suppression of the viral load may decrease the vasculitis
Livedo vasculitis	Smoking cessation	Pentoxyfylline, anabolic steroids	This process is often not a true vasculitis, but rather an occlusive process that may be related to a coagulopathy
Cutaneous polyarteritis nodosa	Corticosteroids or immunosuppressives	Intravenous immune globulin	Although there is a primary focus on the skin, patients may develop ulcers or may have associated inflammatory bowel disease or arthritis
Erythema elevatum diutinum	Dapsone	Corticosteroids	–

TABLE 155.6 TREATMENT OF CUTANEOUS VASCULITIS, BASED ON SYNDROME

MANAGEMENT

The treatment of cutaneous vasculitis depends on whether or not there is clinical evidence of systemic disease, or on the severity of the cutaneous disease. Table 155.6 highlights some of the treatments that might be considered for various cutaneous vasculitic syndromes. The patient with severe systemic necrotizing vasculitis should be treated rapidly and aggressively with systemic corticosteroids and an immunosuppressive agent. Pulsed treatment with either methylprednisolone or cyclophosphamide can result in a rapid control of the disease. However, in the patient with chronic cutaneous vasculitis without clinically apparent systemic involvement, treatments associated with less toxicity should be considered. Each therapeutic agent should be evaluated for the possible risks versus the benefits.

Patients with chronic cutaneous vasculitis tend to be frustrated, and frequently desire treatment for symptomatic relief or for cosmetic reasons. In some cases, small recurrent purpuric lesions with superficial ulceration can compromise the patient's ability to work, and in this instance effective treatment that can allow the patient to become functional is warranted. In patients with acute disease such as Henoch–Schönlein purpura, it may not be necessary to treat other than with agents for symptomatic relief.

It is important to identify and remove any offending antigen that may be present. In addition, underlying diseases that have specific treatments should also be treated. Some examples are the identification of an ingestant such as a drug, food or food additive that can be removed. Lunardi et al.[32] described five patients with chronic cutaneous vasculitis in whom dietary factors were found to be causative. Some patients with 'paraneoplastic' vasculitis whose tumors are removed will resolve their vasculitis. Two patients in the author's experience, one with an adenocarcinoma and one with a pheochromocytoma, had resolution of their cutaneous vasculitis with tumor resection. Patients with paraproteinemia may be good candidates for treatment with an immunosuppressive agent to suppress the formation of the abnormal protein, or, in the case of hepatitis C virus-associated cryoglobulinemic purpura, interferon alpha-2α with or without ribavirin has been useful[17]. Patients with erythema elevatum diutinum seem to respond extremely well to oral dapsone. Finally, patients with a cyrofibrinogen may respond to thrombolytic agents such as stanazolol (V Falanga, personal communication, 1991).

Patients without an identifiable cause or associated phenomenon who require therapy can be treated with a variety of agents. A therapeutic ladder can be designed from which treatment can be sequentially selected until an appropriate and effective agent is located. Because the postulated mechanism for cutaneous vasculitis involves immune complex-mediated disease, complement activation, chemotaxis of polymorphonuclear leukocytes, lysosomal release and resultant cell destruction, modulated by vasoactive substances, agents that interfere with any of these processes may be beneficial. Agents such as antihistamines, nonsteroidal anti-inflammatory agents, antimalarials and sulfones have been reported to be therapeutic in individual cases, but they have not been uniformly effective. Corticosteroids, if given in a sufficiently high dosage, are almost always effective. In open-label trials colchicine was effective for 75–80% of patients with cutaneous vasculitis[33]; however, in the only published double-blind, placebo-controlled trial, colchicine failed to demonstrate efficacy[34]. In my view, that trial was compromised by biases that favored a response in the placebo group. Immunosuppressive agents such as azathioprine, cyclophosphamide, methotrexate, mycophenolate mofetil or cyclosporin are also often effective.

The burning or itching of the lesions most often irritates patients with urticarial vasculitis. The patient should be first treated with antihistamines. Histamine 1 receptor (H_1) antagonists can be combined with H_2 antagonists, but the doses required often result in drowsiness. In some cases, the use of doxepin hydrochloride, which has effects on both H_1 and H_2 receptors, is effective. Lastly, the newer, less sedating agent, cetirizine, or non-sedating agents such as fexofenadine or loratadine, or can be used during waking hours and a soporific agent before retiring.

Colchicine

In patients with chronic cutaneous vasculitis of unknown cause, oral colchicine given at a dose of 0.6mg twice daily has been reported to be useful for the cutaneous and joint manifestations[33].. The only double-blind, placebo-controlled study of this agent failed to demonstrate its efficacy[34]. However, this study included patients with urticarial vasculitis, patients with hepatitis C-associated vasculitis and patients who had failed to respond to other non-steroidal treatment, such as dapsone. This study was small, and the inclusion of patients from the above categories may well have altered the results. Colchicine is an alkaloid that is known to inhibit polymorphonuclear leukocyte chemotaxis, block lysosomal formation and stabilize lysosomal membranes. These factors are believed to be involved in the pathogenesis of the clinical lesion. In open-label trials, about 80% of patients treated with colchicine will respond, as judged by the disappearance of existing lesions and lack of appearance of new ones. In most patients in whom a response occurs, if the colchicine is stopped the disease returns, and with reinstitution of the treatment the clinical signs are again suppressed. The onset of action is rapid, usually occurring within the first 4–7 days; if no response is noted by 2 weeks, the treatment should be considered a failure.

In addition to the cutaneous benefits, arthralgias or arthritis may respond to colchine. However, no changes are noted in circulating immune complex concentrations or abnormalities of proteins. This treatment is reserved for those patients who lack severe systemic involvement. Colchicine is generally well tolerated and can be used over long periods of time.

Toxicity is most frequently gastrointestinal, but long-term use should not be undertaken in potentially pregnant women; blood counts should be monitored periodically.

Immunosuppressive agents

Corticosteroids can be used to stop progress of disease when it is acute, or for severe systemic involvement, but their use in chronic, non-life-threatening cutaneous small-vessel vasculitis is often complicated by several side effects. For this reason, immunosuppressive agents can be used. Cyclophosphamide has been selected in many cases as the agent of choice, especially for severe necrotizing vasculitis or Wegener's granulomatosis[35]. Jorizzo et al.[36] have reported the use of low-dose methotrexate as a corticosteroid-sparing agent for cutaneous polyarteritis nodosa. In three patients, 7.5–15mg methotrexate given orally once weekly led to control of disease and cessation of oral corticosteroids. Finally, azathioprine has been reported to be effective in patients with a variety of vasculitic syndromes, including those with chronic recalcitrant cutaneous LCV[37].

REFERENCES

1. Fan PT, Davis JA, Somer J et al. A clinical approach to systemic vasculitis. Semin Arthritis Rheum 1980; 9: 248–304.

2. Jennette CJ, Falk RJ. Small-vessel vasculitis. N Engl J Med 1997; 337: 1512–1523.

3. Stone JH, Nousari HC. 'Essential' cutaneous vasculitis: what every rheumatologist should know about vasculitis of the skin. Curr Opin Rheumatol 2001; 1 3: 23–34.

4. Callen JP. Are Henoch–Schönlein purpura and hypersensitivity vasculitis in adults truly distinct entities? A dermatologist's perspective. Clin Exp Rheumatol 2000; 18: 659–660.

5. Garcia-Porrua C, Gonzalez-Gay MA. Comparative clinical and epidemiological study of hypersensitivity vasculitis versus Henoch–Schönlein purpura in adults. Semin Arth Rheum 1999; 28: 404–412.

6. Sams WM Jr, Thorne EG, Small P *et al.* Leukocytoclastic vasculitis. Arch Dermatol 1976; 112: 219–226.

7. Piette WN, Stone MS. A cutaneous sign of IgA-associated small dermal vessel leukocytoclastic vasculitis in adults (Henoch–Schönlein purpura). Arch Dermatol 1989; 125: 53–56.

8. Monroe EW, Schulz CI, Maize JC *et al.* Vasculitis in chronic urticaria: an immunopathologic study. J Invest Dermatol 1981; 76: 103–107.

9. af Ekenstam E, Callen JP. Cutaneous leukocytoclastic vasculitis: clinical and laboratory features of 82 patients seen in private practice. Arch Dermatol 1984; 120: 484–489.

10. Blanco R, Martinez-Toboada VM, Rodriguez-Valerde V, Garcia-Fuentes M. Cutaneous vasculitis in children and adults: associated diseases and etilologic factors in 303 patients. Medicine (Baltimore) 1998; 77: 403–418.

11. Saraclar Y, Tinaltepe K, Adalioguin G *et al.* Acute hemorrhagic edema of infancy (AHEI). A variant of Henoch–Schönlein purpura or a distinct clinical entity? J Allergy Clin Immunol 1990; 86: 473–483.

12. McDuffie FC, Sams WM Jr, Maldonado JE *et al.* Hypocomplementemia with cutaneous vasculitis and arthritis. Possible immune complex syndrome. Mayo Clin Proc 1973; 48: 340–348.

13. Soter NA. Chronic urticaria as a manifestation of necrotizing vasculitis. N Engl J Med 1977; 296: 1440–1442.

14. Wisneski JJ, Baer AN, Christensen J *et al.* Hypocomplementemic urticarial vasculitis syndrome. Medicine 1995; 74: 24–41.

15. Lipsker D, Veran Y, Grunenberger F *et al.* The Schnitzler Syndrome: four new cases and review of the literature. Medicine (Baltimore) 2001; 80: 37–44.

16. Levey JM, Bjornsson B, Banner B *et al.* Mixed cryoglobulinemia in hepatitis C infection. Medicine 1994; 73: 53–67.

17. Misiani R, Bellavita P, Fenili D *et al.* Interferon alfa-2a therapy in cryoglobulinemia associated with hepatitis C virus. N Engl J Med 1994; 330: 751–756.

18. Hudson CP, Callen JP. Cutaneous leukocytoclastic vasculitis with hyperglobulinemia and splenomegaly. Arch Dermatol 1984; 120: 1224–1226.

19. Sanchez-Guerrero J, Satierrez-Urena S, Vidaller A *et al.* Vasculitis as a paraneoplastic syndrome. Report of 11 cases and review of the literature. J Rheumatol 1990; 17: 1458–1462.

20. Daoud MD, Hutton KP, Gibson LE. Cutaneous periarteritis nodosa: a clinicopathological study of 79 cases. Br J Dermatol 1997; 136: 706–713.

21. Schaffer JV, Davidson DM, McNiff JM, Bolognia JL. Perinuclear antinuetrophilic cytoplasmic antibody-positive cutaneous polyarteritis nodosa associated with minocycline therapy for acne vulgaris. J Am Acad Dermatol 2001; 44: 198–206.

22. Schrodt BJ, Callen JP. Polyarteritis nodosa attributable to minocycline treatment for acne vulgaris. Pediatrics 1999; 103: 503–504.

23. Katz SI, Gallin JI, Hertz KL *et al.* Erythema elevatum diutinum. Skin and systemic manifestations, immunologic studies and successful treatment with dapsone. Medicine (Baltimore) 1972; 56: 443–455.

24. Grabbe J, Haas N, Moller A, Henz BM. Erythema elevatum diutinum – evidence for disease dependent leucocyte alterations and response to dapsone. Br J Dermatol 2000; 143: 415–420.

25. Mackel SE, Jordon RE. Leukocytoclastic vasculitis. A cutaneous expression of immune complex disease. Arch Dermatol 1982; 118: 296–301.

26. Boom BW, Out-Leiting CJ, Baldwin WM *et al.* Membrane attack complex of complement in leukocytoclastic vasculitis of the skin. Arch Dermatol 1987; 123: 1192–1195.

27. Cream JJ, Bryceson AD, Ryder G. Disappearance of immunoglobulin and complement from the Arthus reaction and its relevance to studies of vasculitis in man. Br J Dermatol 1971; 84: 106–109.

28. Gower RG, Sams WM Jr, Thorne EG *et al.* Leukocytoclastic vasculitis. Sequential appearance of immuno-reactants and cellular changes in serial biopsies. J Invest Dermatol 1977; 69: 477–484.

29. Zax RH, Hodge SJ, Callen JP. Cutaneous leukocytoclastic vasculitis: serial histopathologic evaluation demonstrates the dynamic nature of the infiltrate. Arch Dermatol 1990; 126: 69–72.

30. Soter NA, Mihm MC Jr, Gigli I *et al.* Two distinct cellular patterns in cutaneous necrotizing angiitis. J Invest Dermatol 1976; 66: 344–350.

31. Alexander E, Provost IT. Sjögren's syndrome: association of cutaneous vasculitis with central nervous system disease. Arch Dermatol 1987; 123: 801–810.

32. Lunardi C, Bambara LM, Biasi D *et al.* Elimination diet in the treatment of selected patients with hypersensitivity vasculitis. Clin Exp Rheumatol 1992; 10: 131–135.

33. Callen JP. Colchicine is effective in controlling chronic cutaneous leukocytoclastic vasculitis. J Am Acad Dermatol 1985; 13: 193–200.

34. Sais G, Vidaller A, Jucgla A *et al.* Colchicine in the treatment of cutaneous leukocytoclastic vasculitis: results of a prospective, randomized trial. Arch Dermatol 1995; 131: 1399–1402.

35. Fauci AS, Katz P, Haynes BF *et al.* Cyclophosphamide therapy in severe systemic necrotizing vasculitis. N Engl J Med 1979; 301: 235–238.

36. Jorizzo JL, White WL, Wise CM *et al.* Low-dose weekly methotrexate for unusual neutrophilic vascular reactions: cutaneous polyarteritis nodosa and Behçet's disease. J Am Acad Dermatol 1991; 24: 973–978.

37. Callen JP, Spencer LV, Burruss JB *et al.* Azathioprine: an effective, corticosteroid sparing therapy for patients with recalcitrant cutaneous lupus erythematosus or with recalcitrant cutaneous leukocytoclastic vasculitis. Arch Dermatol 1991; 127: 515–522.

156 Cryoglobulinemia

Alessandra Della Rossa, Antonio Tavoni and Stefano Bombardieri

Definition

- Cryoglobulinemia is characterized by the presence in serum of one or more immunoglobulins, which precipitate at temperatures below 37°C and redissolve on rewarming (cryoglobulins)

- Three types of cryoglobulin are recognized according to the Brouet classification. Type I are composed of an isolated monoclonal immunoglobulin with rheumatoid factor (RF) activity. Types II and III (mixed cryoglobulins) are composed of an IgG and an anti-IgG RF, either an IgM of monoclonal origin (type II) or an IgM of polyclonal origin (type III)

Clinical features

- A disease which predominantly affects middle-aged persons
- Females affected more often than males: F/M ratio 3:1
- HCV positivity in more than 90% of cases
- Histologically: small vessel leukocytoclastic vasculitis
- Clinically: dependent purpura, appears in almost all patients. Other common features: weakness, arthralgias, liver involvement, Raynaud's phenomenon and multiplex mononeuritis

HISTORY

The term cryoglobulinemia refers to the presence in the serum of one or more immunoglobulins which precipitate at temperatures below 37°C and redissolve on rewarming. This phenomenon was first described in 1933 by Wintrobe and Buell in a case of multiple myeloma. Table 156.1 summarizes the history of the disease. Lerner and Watson, in 1947, first referred to the cryoprecipitable molecules as cryoglobulins and described them in association with purpura, glomerulonephritis and urticaria. The presence of cryoglobulins had by then been reported in a wide array of disorders, ranging from neoplastic to inflammatory and infective conditions.

According to Brouet et al. the cryoglobulins can be subdivided into three subgroups: type I contains an isolated monoclonal immuno-globulin; type II are generally comprised of IgG and an IgM rheumatoid factor of monoclonal origin; and type III are comprised of IgG and a polyclonal IgM rheumatoid factor.

Type I cryoglobulins are frequently of the IgG isotype; less frequently they may be comprised of IgG, IgA or light chains. They are present in high concentrations (up to 8 g/l), rarely have rheumatoid factor activity and do not interfere with complement-mediated functions in vitro. They precipitate promptly at low temperatures and this feature is not affected by warming to 56°C or by cycles of freezing and thawing. An explanation on a molecular level of this temperature-dependent solubility is still lacking, but it is probably linked to an excess of hydrophobic aminoacidic residuals[1]. Type I cryoglobulinemia is frequently associated with immunoproliferative disorders.

Mixed cryoglobulins (types II and III) are comprised of IgG plus an IgM (rarely of either IgA or IgG) with RF activity. They represent up to 80% of all cryoglobulins and are generally present in lower concentrations than monoclonal cryoglobulins; they precipitate after a longer period of exposure to low temperatures (from 24 h to over 1 week at 4°C); they have strong anticomplement activity and, unlike monoclonal cryoglobulins, repeated freezing and thawing cycles reduce or abolish their cryoprecipitability. Mixed cryoglobulinemia (MC) has been described in association with chronic infections and autoimmune disorders[2].

In 1966 Meltzer and Franklin described for the first time a syndrome characterized clinically by the triad of weakness, arthralgias and Raynaud's phenomenon, and by the presence of mixed cryoglobulins without any known precipitating factor; this condition was termed 'essential mixed cryoglobulinemia'[1].

However, the frequent finding of liver involvement in MC patients, which is much less common in other immune complex-mediated diseases, suggested the hypothesis that an environmental factor, possibly a hepatotropic virus, might be the actual trigger for the disease. An association with the hepatitis B virus (HBV) was suggested, but this was not confirmed by subsequent studies in which HBV antigenemia was only occasionally detected in subjects with antibodies against the HBV surface antigen. At the same time, analysis of large groups of MC patients made it possible to define more clearly the organ involvement associated with the disease. The main clinical features are purpura, arthralgias, and renal and liver involvement, together with a benign lymphoproliferative disorder taking the form of lymphoid aggregates in the spleen and bone marrow[3]. Studies in the 1990s on large series of MC patients definitively eliminated HBV as a causative agent in most cases of mixed cryoglobulinemia, and the hypothesis of a hepatotropic virus became less convincing[4].

Subsequently, however, the identification of HCV as the main causative agent of non-A, non-B hepatitis[5] provided fresh support for this hypothesis. Because HCV is a hepatotropic virus which can cause chronic infection with liver involvement, its prevalence was evaluated in a small series of MC patients. Using first-generation tests, antibodies against HCV were initially demonstrated in 30–54% of all MC patients. With the introduction of second-generation ELISA and RIBA tests, the

TABLE 156.1 THE HISTORY OF MIXED CRYOGLOBULINEMIA	
Date	Discovery
1933	Cryoprecipitable molecule in a case of multiple myeloma
1947	Cryoglobulins
1962	Mixed cryoglobulins with rheumatoid factor activity
1966	Clinical picture of essential mixed cryoglobulinemia
1974	Classification of cryoglobulins
1977	Association with HBV antigenemia
1990–1991	Association of HCV infection with mixed cryoglobulinemia

prevalence was found to be even higher, ranging from 70 to 100%; there was a comparable prevalence of HCV viremia in the same subjects. Increasing evidence suggested that this association also has pathogenetic significance[6–8]. In particular, the demonstration of the specific concentration of HCV in type II cryoglobulins, immunohistochemical evidence of HCV-associated antigens in vasculitic skin biopsy specimens, the presence of HCV RNA in serum and plasma samples and of HCV infection in the peripheral mononuclear cells (PBMC) of MC patients, all lend support to the etiopathogenetic role of HCV in MC[1,9].

EPIDEMIOLOGY

The prevalence of mixed cryoglobulinemia varies widely from country to country; it is more frequent in southern Europe than in northern Europe or North America. On the whole, this disease is considered to be relatively rare, but its frequency may be underestimated because of its clinical polymorphism. The geographic distribution of mixed cryoglobulinemia seems to be closely related to the endemic presence of HCV infection. Genotype 2a has been described to be more frequent in mixed cryoglobulinemia patients than in chronic HCV carriers without MC. Table 156.2 shows the main epidemiological findings in mixed cryoglobulinemia patients[9].

TABLE 156.2 EPIDEMIOLOGY OF MIXED CRYOGLOBULINEMIA	
Peak age (years)	42–52
Sex distribution (F:M)	3:1
Geography	Southern Europe
Genetic association	Controversial

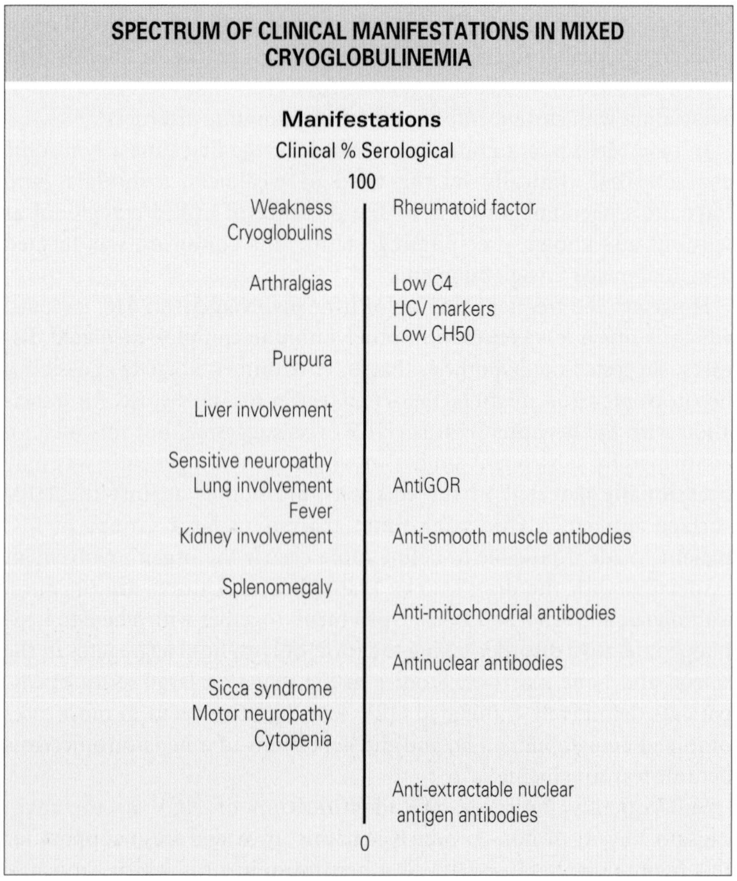

SPECTRUM OF CLINICAL MANIFESTATIONS IN MIXED CRYOGLOBULINEMIA

Manifestations
Clinical % Serological
100

Weakness	Rheumatoid factor
Cryoglobulins	
Arthralgias	Low C4
	HCV markers
	Low CH50
Purpura	
Liver involvement	
Sensitive neuropathy	
Lung involvement	AntiGOR
Fever	
Kidney involvement	Anti-smooth muscle antibodies
Splenomegaly	
	Anti-mitochondrial antibodies
	Antinuclear antibodies
Sicca syndrome	
Motor neuropathy	
Cytopenia	
	Anti-extractable nuclear antigen antibodies

0

Fig. 156.1 Spectrum of clinical manifestations in mixed cryoglobulinemia. RF, rheumatoid factor; ASMA, antismooth muscle antibodies; AMA, antimitochondrial antibodies; ANA, antinuclear antibodies; ENA, antiextractable nuclear antigen antibodies.

CLINICAL FEATURES

Mixed cryoglobulinemia is a virus-triggered immune complex-mediated disease which generally shows a slow progression with periods of exacerbation and remission and rare acute flares. Figure 156.1 shows the spectrum of disease manifestations that characterize mixed cryoglobulinemia[1].

Purpura

Purpura almost always occurs in MC patients, most commonly as the presenting feature. It is characteristically non-pruritic, intermittent, and typically involves the lower extremities, as venous stasis favors the precipitation of cryoglobulins (Fig. 156.2). Histologically it is characterized by dermal vasculitis with a variable degree of involvement of the subcutaneous interstitium. Leg ulcers associated with purpura are the presenting symptoms in approximately one-quarter of patients[3]. Immunohistochemical evidence of HCV-associated antigens in vasculitic skin biopsy specimens suggest that HCV-containing circulating immune complexes (CIC) play a major role in the pathogenesis of cryoglobulinemic purpura[1].

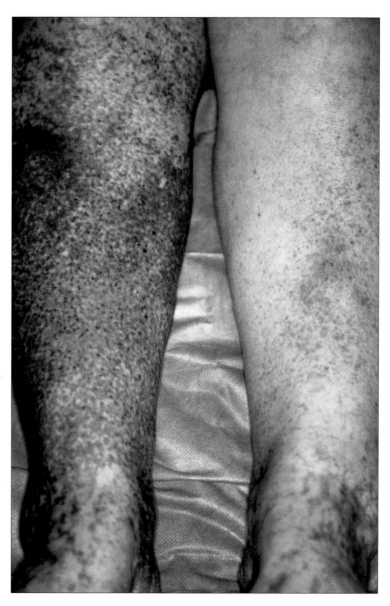

Fig. 156.2 Patient with cryoglobulinemic purpura involving the lower limbs. The right limb is more involved than the left, as venous stasis favors the precipitation of cryoglobulins (the patient had venous insufficiency on the right side).

Raynaud's phenomenon

Raynaud's phenomenon is another feature of MC, being present in one-quarter of patients at diagnosis. Symptoms are mild, involve all of the extremities, and are not usually associated with trophic derangement.

Arthralgias/arthritis

Arthralgias are present in the majority of cases and usually recur intermittently during the course of the disease. The most frequently involved joints are the hands, knees, ankles and elbows. Occasionally, the same joints show the presence of frank non-erosive arthritis[3].

Renal involvement

Renal involvement is one of the most serious complications of MC and affects approximately one-third of patients. Histologically it almost invariably takes the form of a membranoproliferative glomerulonephritis with a varying degree of interstitial and vascular damage. Clinically, renal involvement ranges from isolated proteinuria to nephritic syndrome. The disease course is generally characterized by periods of remission and exacerbation and, if not adequately treated, may eventually lead to renal failure[10].

Peripheral nerve involvement

Another common feature in MC patients is peripheral neuropathy. However, the real frequency of this manifestation is often underestimated, owing to its smouldering clinical course. In MC this manifestation generally seems to take the form of an impairment of the sensory fibers. Subjective symptoms suggesting peripheral neuropathy were present in the majority (91%) of our MC patients, and objective manifestations as well as sensory motor conduction velocity abnormalities were detected in half. The finding of pure motor neuropathy is a rarer (about 5%) but disabling condition. Electrophysiologic variables are altered in more than 80% of patients.

The nerve injury may be caused by immunologically mediated demyelinization, vasculitis or occlusion of the vasa nervorum by cryoglobulin precipitation. Histological studies have shown inflammatory vessel damage with axonal degeneration. The correlation found between serum cryoglobulin levels and various neurologic findings suggest that an immune complex-mediated mechanism might be responsible for this nerve damage[1,9,11].

Liver involvement

Liver involvement is present in over two-thirds of MC patients. Clinically, it is generally asymptomatic and the laboratory evidence of cell damage is usually mild or absent. However, the correlation between clinical liver disease and histology is low, for the latter shows in all instances various degree of periportal inflammation, with fibrosis, architectural derangement and evidence of cirrhosis in one-third of cases[1,3].

Lymphoproliferative disorders

Mixed cryoglobulinemia is frequently associated with a benign lymphoproliferative disorder taking the form of distinct lymphoid infiltrates with B cells bearing surface monoclonal rheumatoid factor (IgMk) in the portal tracts, spleen and bone marrow. This disorder, which is responsible for the monoclonal rheumatoid factor in type II cryoglobulins, can evolve in a limited number of subjects to a frank non-Hodgkin's B-cell lymphoma. The frequency of malignant lymphoma in MC patients may be as high as 40%. The malignancy appears 1–11 years after disease onset and the histologic type is generally immunocytoma.

Hepatitis C virus has been detected in the peripheral blood mononuclear cells (PBM) and marrow cells, and more interestingly, in the lymphomatous cells of patients with type II MC or chronic hepatitis C evolving to non-Hodgkin's lymphoma (NHL). These observations suggest a possible role of HCV in some lymphoproliferative disorders, a hypothesis that is further strengthened by the finding of a high frequency of HCV infection among unselected patients affected by idiopathic NHL[9,12].

Hyperviscosity syndrome

Although increased blood viscosity and reduced blood filtration can be demonstrated in a high percentage of MC patients, a patent hyperviscosity syndrome is relatively uncommon. Indeed, the trend towards an increase in blood viscosity is compensated for by a parallel decrease in the hematocrit in MC patients[13].

Other manifestations

Other manifestations are dryness of eyes and mouth, bilateral parotid swelling, generalized lymphadenopathy, recurrent abdominal pain and CNS involvement[3]. In some patients with acute abdomen, laparoscopy will disclose a vasculitis of the small mesenteric vessels. Lung involvement has been frequently observed by us, particularly at the level of small airways and the pulmonary interstitial spaces. Possibly related to immune complex deposition, this involvement is generally mild[14].

INVESTIGATIONS

The laboratory hallmark of mixed cryoglobulinemia is the presence of type II or type III cryoglobulins with rheumatoid factor (RF) activity. High levels of circulating immune complexes and low levels of complement (primarily via activation of the classic pathway) are characteristic findings. Patients with MC may have a monoclonal component in their serum, usually an IgM of the κ type; this reflects the presence of clones of lymphoid cells in the portal tracts of the liver, spleen and bone. It has already been demonstrated that HCV participates in the production of both cryoglobulins and immune complexes, and probably plays a major role in the pathogenesis of MC (Fig. 156.3). In particular, the demonstration of the concentration of HCV specifically in type II cryoglobulins and the presence of HCV RNA in serum and plasma samples[1,6–9] point to the relevance of HCV in the pathogenesis of MC.

The key laboratory parameters for the diagnosis of MC, as specified in the GISC diagnostic criteria[15] (Table 156.3), are: (i) cryoglobulins; (ii) rheumatoid factor; (iii) C4 and or CH50; and (iv) anti-HCV antibodies and HCV RNA in the patient's serum.

Detection of cryoglobulins

A 20 ml blood sample should be stored at 37°C until completely coagulated, centrifuged at 37°C at 2500 rpm for 5 minutes, and then stored at 4°C for 1 week. A white precipitate in the bottom of the tube indicates the presence of cryoglobulins. When the tube is rewarmed to 37°C the precipitate will dissolve.

To quantify the amount of cryoglobulins present in the serum sample a cryocrit should be performed. Briefly, the serum is centrifuged in a graduated tube at 4°C and 2500 rpm, and the percentage of cryoglobulins is calculated.

To characterize the cryoglobulins a variety of immunological methods can be used, although immunofixation and immunoblotting are the methods of choice for the typing of cryoglobulins and for the accurate assessment of clonality. Combining the two procedures may be particularly helpful in determining the oligoclonality of each component of the complex[16].

Detection of rheumatoid factor

Rheumatoid factor may be detected either by means of a latex fixation test or by laser nephelometry.

Detection of complement

Antigenic analysis of complement proteins makes use of several immune precipitation techniques. Single radial immunodiffusion according to

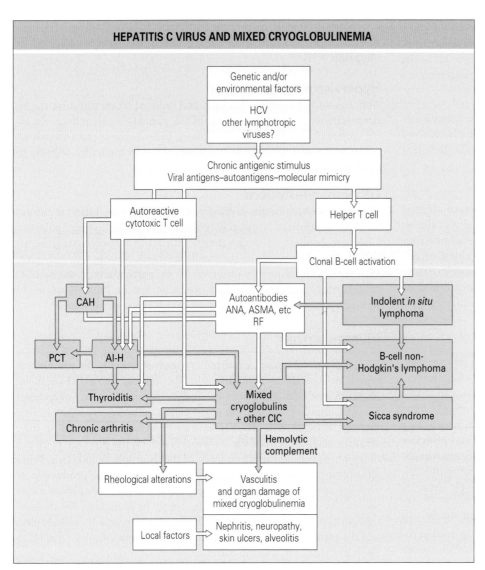

HEPATITIS C VIRUS AND MIXED CRYOGLOBULINEMIA

Fig. 156.3 Hepatitis C virus (HCV) and mixed cryoglobulinemia. The flowchart illustrates the etiopathogenetic role of HCV in mixed cryoglobulinemia and HCV-related disorders. AIH, autoimmune hepatitis; ANA, ASMA, antinuclear, anti-smooth-muscle antibodies; CAH, chronic active hepatitis; CIC, circulating immune complexes; PCT, porphyria cutanea tarda; RF, rheumatoid factor. (With permission from Ferri C, Zignego AL. Relation between infection and autoimmunity in mixed cryopglobulinemia. Curr Opin Rheumatol 2000;12: 53–60. © 2000 Lippincott Williams & Wilkins.)

TABLE 156.3 GISC CLASSIFICATION CRITERIA

- 6 months duration of symptomatic cryoglobulinemia
- plus the presence of at least two of the following symptoms:
  - Purpura
  - Arthralgias
  - Weakness
  - Detection of high RF activity and/or low complement factor (C4)
- **Exclusion criteria**: coexistence of autoimmune, lymphoproliferative or other infectious disease except HCV infection

---

either Fahey or Mancini is the most commonly employed method for quantifying protein. In both methods antigen is added to wells in a gel that contains antibody, and rings of precipitation are formed. Mancini's procedure, which is both sensitive and accurate, employs a relatively simple endpoint methodology with antibody excess in the gel (most commercial firms use the Mancini method in the preparation of immunodiffusion plates).

The CH50 titer is the reciprocal of the dilution of the patient's serum yielding 50% lysis of sheep erythrocytes sensitized with an optimal amount of rabbit anti-Forssman antibody. Immune hemolysis is the result of a complex series of reactions that occur on the cell surface. Photometric measurements indicate the proportion of cells lysed by this series of reactions[17].

Detection of HCV

Anti-HCV antibodies can be detected in the sera of cryoglobulinemia patients by means of commonly employed ELISA or immunoblotting methods. The presence of HCV antigens and HCV genotypes should be detected using polymerase chain reaction tests[18].

DIFFERENTIAL DIAGNOSIS

Systemic vasculitides

HCV infection may be associated with different types of systemic vasculitides. Polyarteritis nodosa (PAN), although most frequently associated with hepatitis B infection, can in a limited number of cases be associated with hepatitis C virus. However, as the prevalence of this infection among PAN patients is low (5–10%), the significance of the association remains a matter of debate[19]. Moreover, in a small number of patients with polyarteritis nodosa cryoglobulins are also detectable, and this makes the differential diagnosis even more difficult. Patients with polyarteritis nodosa present more often with life-threatening systemic vasculitis, malignant hypertension, cerebral angiitis and ischemic abdominal pain than do patients with mixed cryoglobulinemia. Moreover, kidney and liver microaneurysms involving the medium-sized vessels are a hallmark of PAN, compared to the small vessel involvement in mixed cryoglobulinemia. Finally, peripheral nerve involvement almost always takes the form of a severe multifocal sensorimotor neuropathy in PAN, compared to the more frequent distal moderate sensory neuropathy of mixed cryoglobulinemia[20].

Leukocytoclastic vasculitis has been claimed to be associated with hepatitis C virus infection. Whether this condition is a separate entity or represents an incomplete form of cryoglobulinemia is an unresolved issue. However, the presence of HCV infection in a patient affected by leukocytoclastic vasculitis renders mandatory the search for cryoglobulins[19].

Sjögren's syndrome

Mixed cryoglobulinemia and Sjögren's syndrome (SS) share a number of clinical and serological features (Table 156.4). Moreover, chronic HCV infection, even in the absence of cryoglobulins, may mimic the main clinical, histological and immunological features of primary Sjögren's syndrome. This renders the differential diagnosis very difficult in some instances. Another intriguing similarity between MC and SS is the increased frequency in both diseases of lymphoproliferative disease. The prevalence of HCV infection among European patients with Sjögren's syndrome ranges from 5 to 19% and the frequency of the HCV seems to be analogous. A small number of patients with MC have anti-Ro/SSA and anti-La/SSB antibodies. Therefore, in at least some instances a true overlap between the two conditions may exist. In the other cases, differentiating between the two conditions can be unusually difficult. Distinguishing features might include a lower prevalence of symptoms of dryness, a significant increase in the prevalence of liver involvement, a lower prevalence of anti-Ro/SSA and anti-La/SSB autoantibodies and a milder expression of lymphocytic infiltrates on the salivary glands in HCV-positive patients (Table 156.4)[21,22].

ETIOPATHOGENESIS

MC is a complex disorder with a broad spectrum of clinical manifestations, representing an intersection between autoimmune disorders, immune complex-mediated disorders and lymphoproliferative processes. It is now clear that HCV plays a central role in the etiopathogenesis of MC: the immediate pathogenesis arises from autoantibody production through molecular mimicry (i.e. GOR, LKM1) or

TABLE 156.4 FEATURES OF PRIMARY SJÖGREN'S SYNDROME AND MIXED CRYOGLOBULINEMIA

	Primary Sjögren's syndrome	Mixed cryoglobulinemia
Sex ratio (M/F)	1/10	1/3
Keratoconjunctivitis sicca	+++	+
Xerostomia	+++	+
Arthralgia	++	++
Raynaud's phenomenon	+	+
Renal involvement	Interstitial	Glomerular
Lung interstitial involvement	+	++
Liver involvement	+	+++
Purpura	+	++
Peripheral neuropathy	+	+
Lymphoproliferative disorder	+	+
Antinuclear antibodies	+++	+
Anti Ro/La antibodies	++	-
Rheumatoid factor	+++	+++
Hypergammaglobulinemia	+++	+++
Reduced C4 level	+	+++
Circulating immune complexes	++	++
Cryoglobulins	+	+++
Monoclonal gammopathy	+	++
HLA association	++	-

Comparison of the demographic, clinical and laboratory features of primary Sjögren's syndrome and mixed cryoglobulinemia (With permission from Vitali C, Bombardieri S. Sjögren's syndrome, mixed cryoglobulinaemia and the monoclonal gammopathies. Clin Exp Rheumatol 1996; 14 (Suppl. 14) S59–S63.)

from the deposition of HCV-containing immune complexes in the vascular system and tissues. The immune complex behavior depends on many variables. The antigen/antibody ratio; the action of rheumatoid factor, which constantly modifies complement-mediated functions; and the heterogeneity of the immunocomplex types, some of which are cryoprecipitable, all influence the pathogenicity and precipitability of CIC[1,9].

Similarly to other RNA viruses, HCV is characterized by a high degree of genetic heterogeneity and may occur either spontaneously or as a result of host immune pressure. Mutation of the HCV genome during replication in a single infected individual results in a quasispecies genotype distribution with a master sequence and a large series of related variants, and the accumulation of mutations during the evolution of the virus has led to the emergence of several viral genotypes.

It is not clear why some individuals infected with HCV develop an autoimmune disorder: although a specific HLA association has not been demonstrated in MC patients, genetic susceptibility probably plays an important role. In this regard, recently differing immune reactivities to a non-structural protein of HCV (NS4) were demonstrated among different disorders associated with HCV infection. Antibodies reactive against a recombinant peptide from NS4 were detected in 64% of sera from patients with autoimmune hepatitis (AIH), 51% of chronic hepatitis C (CHC) sera, and 22% of mixed cryoglobulinemia sera. Thus, the differing expression of the immune repertoire among different individuals, a factor which is genetically determined, probably influences the response to HCV and the appearance of autoimmunity.

This hypothesis is further strengthened by the demonstration that the majority of monoclonal IgM rheumatoid factor in type II cryoglobulinemia in HCV-infected patients bear the WA idiotype, a public idiotype frequently found on monoclonal rheumatoid factor. However, the mechanisms leading to the disorders associated with HCV infection are still unknown, as are the single steps leading to the spectrum of manifestations of MC. HCV lymphotropism is probably responsible for the viral persistence and the chronic stimulation of the immune system that, together with the direct action of the microrganism, contribute to the persistent derangement of immune regulation and, eventually, lymphomagenesis. HCV seems to be directly involved in this process, possibly through the activation of oncogenes.

Recently, a high frequency of t(14;18) translocation has been described in MC patients. During this translocation the *bcl-2* gene normally located on chromosome 18 is transferred to chromosome 14, and an overexpression of the gene is the result. As *bcl-2* is an antiapoptotic gene, there is an inhibition of apoptosis. *bcl-2* rearrangement was demonstrated not only in patients with chronic HCV infection and MC, but also in one-third of patients with HCV-related chronic liver disease without cryoglobulinemia. Because *bcl-2* rearrangement characterizes the majority of follicular B-cell lymphomas, it could be hypothesized that this gene contributes to the promotion of lymphomagenesis in patients with MC and chronic hepatitis C through the selection of a clone protected against apoptosis.

The possible ethiopathogenesis of MC may be summarized as follows. Among the different possible noxious agents, HCV, either alone or in combination with other still unknown factors, plays an important role. Autoimmunity may be a virus-triggered epiphenomenon perpetuated by a variety of factors, including genetic susceptibility, environmental factors, and host and viral factors (genotype, superinfection with unrelated strains, escape from the immunological system etc.). The viral persistence represents a continuous challenge for the host, and the chronic stimulation of the immune system on the one hand triggers the appearence of autoantibodies through molecular mimicry or other unidentified mechanisms, and on the other hand favors the emergence of clones protected against apoptosis, possibly maintaining in this way through a vicious circle the pathway of autoimmunity[1,9,12]. In this regard, the discovery of the close association of MC with a virus should not rule out other potential etiopathogenetic factors, such as autoimmunity and organ-specific autoantibodies.

For instance, several years ago autoantibodies reactive against a 50 kDa antigen were isolated from a glomerular extract from patients with mixed cryoglobulinemia. Through sequencing this molecule was identified as α enolase. The frequency of these autoantibodies was higher in a group of patients with active renal involvement, and in a follow-up study their amount fluctuated either spontaneously or in response to therapy. It was then hypothesized that these antibodies could contribute to the induction of glomerulonephritis in MC through the formation of *in situ* immune complexes. Further studies have demonstrated that anti-α enolase can frequently be detected in other systemic autoimmune disorders. In SLE and MC they are associated with nephritis and in SSc they are associated with severe endothelial damage. α Enolase is ubiquitous, but it is highly expressed in the kidney and also on the membrane of several cell types, including endothelial cells. Thus, antibodies against α enolase could contribute to renal injury not only through the local formation of immune complexes, but also by direct damage to endothelial cells[23].

The vascular deposition of immunocomplexes composed of cryoglobulins, with the involvement of viral markers and autoantigens, is responsible for the organ damage observed in mixed cryoglobulinemia and in the vasculitis associated with HCV infection. HCV imposes a chronic stimulus on the immune system, and infects blood mononuclear cells. Monoclonal or polyclonal B-cell expansion is the most important consequence of this process. Autoantibody production is another result. The activation of oncogenes leads to the emergence of clones protected against apoptosis. This, as previously mentioned, possibly favours the persistence of autoreactive clones and the promotion of lymphoproliferative disorders[1,9,12].

MANAGEMENT

Mixed cryoglobulinemia has a multifactorial origin and the tissue damage results from various mechanisms. The most important are the deposition of (HCV-containing) immune complexes, chronic stimulation by HCV infection, and the presence of a benign smoldering lymphoproliferative process. The spectrum of disease manifestations is characterized by a broad polymorphism, and the clinical picture may vary from very mild symptoms (such as weakness and arthralgias) to life-threatening conditions (including rapidly progressive glomerulonephritis). Furthermore, the clinical course is characterized by alternating periods of remission and exacerbation.

Another feature of MC is that serological parameters cannot be used as guides to therapy, as none of these correlates with clinical activity or disease severity. Therefore, treatment should not focus on lowering the levels of cryoglobulins or normalizing the complement values, but rather on controlling the prevailing symptoms. Moreover, the treatment chosen is often based on the results of uncontrolled studies or experience gained during clinical practice at single tertiary care centres.

Recently light has been shed on the triggers of the disease. In particular, the close association between MC and HCV infection has induced clinicians to reconsider their previous approach to the disease. In fact, the aggressive use of cytotoxic drugs should be ceased, because of the risk of progression of HCV infection. Table 156.5 summarizes the main therapeutic modalities in MC. Non-steroidal anti-inflammatory drugs can help to relieve non-erosive polyarthritis or some of the diffuse arthralgias and should be used symptomatically. Medium to low doses of cortico-

TABLE 156.5 PRINCIPAL THERAPEUTIC MODALITIES AND THEIR CLINICAL INDICATIONS IN MIXED CRYOGLOBULINEMIA

Manifestation	Drug/ therapeutic modality
Arthralgias	Low-dose steroids
	Non-steroidal anti-inflammatory drugs
Glomerulonephritis	High-dose steroids
Severe hypertension	Plasmapheresis
Motor neuropathy	Cytotoxic agents
Systemic vasculitis	
Liver involvement	Low antigen content diet
	Low dose steroids
	Interferon-α
	Ribavirin

steroids (0.1–0.3 mg/kg/day) are usually sufficient to control most of the minor symptoms of MC, such as purpura, arthralgias, arthritis and weakness. Larger doses (0.5–1.5 mg/kg/day) are necessary for the management of renal involvement, peripheral neuropathy and serositis.

A low antigenic diet has been proposed as a potentially effective supportive measure for the management of MC. This diet is based on the hypothesis that the ICC compete with other inputs to the mononuclear phagocytic system. Under normal conditions these inputs consist primarily of blood-borne constituents and high molecular weight exogenous substances which cross the mucosal barrier of the gut and enter the circulation through the lymph and portal vein. A low antigen content diet which reduces the levels of these components could help to restore a saturated mononuclear phagocytic system, freeing it to remove the immune complexes. A short-term placebo-controlled study demonstrated a beneficial effect in MC patients in terms of both clinical and laboratory parameters. However, because of the difficulties of maintaining this diet long-term studies have not been conducted and its long-term effects are uncertain.

Aggressive therapies, such as plasma exchange, are to be used in cases of life-threatening or disabling conditions. Plasma exchange, with or without immunosuppressive drugs, has been successfully employed to treat rapidly progressive glomerulonephritis, motor neuropathy and hyperviscosity syndrome. Double filtration plasmapheresis seems to be as effective as conventional apheresis but reduces the need for the substitution of proteins and fluids.

In 1986 the first pilot study on interferon in the treatment of MC was performed. Subsequently, a strong association between MC and HCV infection was demonstrated. Given the antiviral, immunomodulatory and antiproliferative effects of interferon, the use of this agent in the treatment of MC has been advocated and several studies on its long-term effects in MC patients have been performed. Clinical and biological remissions have been reported in a high proportion of patients. However, the initial enthusiasm for this drug was soon dampened by the high relapse rate observed after the cessation of therapy. To ensure a higher proportion of long-term responders, the administration schedule or the dosage might be adjusted, or alternatively combination therapy could be tried. At present, the main indication for the administration of interferon therapy in MC remains the presence of active liver involvement. Several recent studies indicate that interferon–ribavirin combination therapy may have beneficial effects in patients with symptomatic cryoglobulinemia who are unresponsive to interferon, and in particular in those with liver disease[24,25].

REFERENCES

1. Della Rossa A, Ferri C, Bombardieri S. From essential mixed cryoglobulinemia to virus induced autoimmnunity: ten years of research in mixed cryoglobulinemia. In: Shoenfeld Y, ed. The decade of autoimmunity. Amsterdam: Elsevier Science, 1999; 235–243.

2. Winfield JB. Cryoglobulinemia. Hum Pathol 1983; 14: 350–354.

3. Gorevich PD, Kassab HJ, LevoY et al. Mixed cryoglobulinemia: clinical aspects and long term follow up of 40 patients. Am J Med 1980; 69: 287–308.

4. Galli M, Monti G, Invernizzi F et al. and the Italian Group for the Study of Cryoglobulinemia (GISC). Hepatitis B virus-related markers in secondary and essential mixed cryoglobulinemias: a multicentre study of 596 cases. Ann It Med Int 1992; 7: 209–214.

5. Choo QL, Kuo G, Weiner AJ et al. Isolation of a c-DNA clone derived from a blood borne non-A, non-B viral hepatitis genome. Science 1989; 244: 359–362.

6. Ferri C, Greco F, Longombardo G et al. Antibodies to hepatitis C virus in patients with mixed cryoglobulinemia. Arthritis Rheum 1991; 34: 1606–10.

7. Ferri C, Greco F, Longombardo G et al. Association between hepatitis C virus and mixed cryoglobulinemia. Clin Exp Rheumatol 1991; 9: 621–624.

8. Agnello V, Chung RT, Kaplan LM. A role for hepatitis C virus infection in type II cryoglobulinemia. N Engl J Med 1992; 327: 1490–1495.

9. Ferri C, La Civita L, Longombardo G et al. Mixed cryoglobulinemia: a cross road between autoimmune and lymphoproliferative disorders. Lupus 1998; 7: 275–279.

10. Tarantino A, Campise M, Banfi G et al. Long-term predictors of survival in essential mixed cryoglobulinemic glomerulonephritis. Kidney Int 1995; 47: 618–623.

11. Caniatti LM, Tugnoli V, Eleopra R et al. Cryoglobulinemic neuropathy related to hepatitis C virus infection. Clinical, laboratory and neurophysiological study. J Periph Nerv Syst 1996; 1: 131–138.

12. Ramos Casals M, Treyo O, Garcia-Carrasco M et al. Mixed cryoglobulinemia: new concepts. Lupus 2000; 9: 83–91.

13. Ferri C, Mannini L, Bartoli V et al. Blood viscosity and filtration abnormalities in MC patients. Clin Exp Rheumatol 1990; 8: 271–281.

14. Bombardieri S, Paoletti P, Ferri C et al. Lung involvement in essential mixed cryoglobulinemia. Am J Med 1979; 66: 748–756.

15. Lamprecht P, Moosig F, Gause A et al. Immunological and clinical follow-up of hepatitis C virus associated cryoglobulinaemic vasculitis. Ann Rheum Dis 2001; 60: 385–390.

16. Kallemuchikkal U, Gorevich PD. Evaluation of cryoglobulins. Arch Pathol Lab Med 1999; 123: 119–125.

17. Wasiuddin AK, Delbert RV, Michael MF. Complement and chinins mediators of inflammation. In: Henry JB, ed. Clinical diagnosis and management by laboratory methods, 19th edn. Philadelphia: WB Saunders, 1996; 928–946.

18. Erensoy S. Diagnosis of hepatitis C virus (HCV) infection and laboratory monitoring of its therapy. J Clin Virol 2001; 21: 271–281.

19. Wener MH, Johnson RJ, Sasso EH. Hepatitis C virus and rheumatic disease. J Rheumatol 1996; 23: 953–959.

20. Cacoub P, Maisonobe T, Thibault V et al. Systemic vasculitis in patients with hepatitis C. J Rheumatol 2001; 28: 109–118.

21. Vitali C, Bombardieri S. Sjögren's syndrome, mixed cryoglobulinaemia and the monoclonal gammoapathies. Clin Exp Rheumatol 1996; 14(Suppl.14): 59–63.

22. Ramos-Casals M, Garcia Carrasco M, Cervera R, Font J. Sjögren's syndrome and hepatitis C virus. Clin Rheumatol 1999; 18: 93–100.

23. Pratesi F, Moscato S, Sabbatini A et al. Autoantibodies specific for alpha-enolase in systemic autoimmune disorders. J Rheumatol 2000; 27: 109–115.

24. Lunel F, Cacoub P. Treatment of autoimmune and extrahepatic manifestations of HCV infection. Ann Med Interne (Paris) 2000; 151: 58–64.

25. Tavoni A, Mosca M, Ferri C et al. Guidelines for the management of essential mixed cryoglobulinemia. Clin Exp Rheumatol 1995; 13(suppl. 13): S191–S195.

157 Primary angiitis of the central nervous system

Leonard H Calabrese

Definition

- Vasculitis limited to the brain spinal cord and overlying leptomeninges
- Clinically heterogeneous, with several recognized clinical subsets

Clinical features

- Confirmed by either biopsy of tissues within the central nervous system or cerebral angiography
- Confirmed only after meticulous exclusion of all conditions capable of producing vasculitis within the central nervous system, or those conditions capable of mimicking the angiographic findings seen in vasculitis

HISTORY

The modern era of primary angiitis of the central nervous system (PACNS) began in the late 1950s with the elegant description of several patients with a progressive and fatal form vasculitis limited to the CNS characterized by a rich granulomatous pathology. The disease was named granulomatous angiitis of the CNS (GACNS) and remained a diagnosis of extreme rarity, with fewer than 40 cases reported over the next 25 years[1]. The 1970s and 1980s witnessed an increased use of cerebral angiography and an increase in reported cases; however, many of these newly reported cases lacked histologic confirmation. The next major change in the approach to PACNS came in the early 1980s with successful reports of therapy utilizing a combination of cyclophosphamide and glucocorticoids, which served to increase the enthusiasm for diagnosing the disorder. This combination of increased diagnosis by angiography combined with a decreasing frequency of biopsy confirmation, led to increasing numbers of patients being treated with prolonged and intensive immunosuppressive regimens based on the belief that each (i.e. angiographically and histologically undocumented, as well as antemortem biopsy proven) case represented a progressive and fatal form of granulomatous arteritis.

In the 1990s we and others[2,3] began to question whether all cases of PACNS diagnosed solely on the basis of cerebral angiography were indeed equivalent to those diagnosed by antemortem biopsy. It was at this time suggested that within the spectrum of angiographically diagnosed PACNS existed a subset of patients with a predictably more benign outcome requiring far less intensive therapy. This subset was named benign angiopathy of the central nervous system (BACNS), emphasizing the term *angiopathy* as opposed to *angiitis* to indicate the uncertainty as to the nature of the underlying vascular pathology. The last several years have witnessed an increasing appreciation of the complexity of PACNS and the need for a multidisciplinary approach[4].

DIAGNOSTIC CRITERIA

In 1988 Calabrese and Mallek[1] proposed three working criteria for the diagnosis of PACNS. Although imperfect and not validated by con-

TABLE 157.1 CONDITIONS RESEMBLING PACNS EXCLUDED BY THE PRELIMINARY DIAGNOSTIC CRITERIA

Systemic vasculitides	Polyarteritis nodosa Allergic granulomatosis Hypersensitivity vasculitis group disorders Vasculitis with connective tissue disease Wegener's granulomatosis Temporal arteritis Takayasu's arteritis Behçet's disease Lymphomatoid granulomatosis Cogan's syndrome
Infections	Viral, bacterial, fungal, spirochetes, rickettsial
Neoplasm	Primary CNS lyphoma Angioimmunoproliferative disorders Carcinomatous meningitis Infiltrating glioma Malignant angioendotheliomatosis
Drug use	Amphetamines Ephedrine Phenylpropanolamine Cocaine Ergotamine
Vasospastic disorders	Postpartum angiopathy Eclampsia Pheochromocytoma Subarachnoid hemorrhage Migraine and exertional headache
Other vasculopathies and mimicking conditions	Atherosclerosis Fibromuscular dysplasia Moyamoya disease Thrombotic thrombocytopenic purpura Sickle cell anemia Neurofibromatosis Demyelinating disease Sarcoidosis Emboli (i.e. SBE, cardiac myxoma, paradoxical emboli) Hypercoagulable states, including antiphospholipid antibody syndrome Acute posterior placoid pigment epitheliopathy and cerebral vasculitis CADASIL (cerebral autosomal dominant arteriopathy with subcortical infarcts and leukoencephalopathy) MELAS syndrome (myopathy, encephalopathy, lactic acidosis and stroke-like episodes Retinocochleocerebral vasculopathy (Susac syndrome)

trolled investigation, these criteria have been useful for both the clinical management of suspected patients as well as assisting in nosologic classification. The criteria proposed are:

1. A history of an unexplained neurologic deficit that remains after a vigorous diagnostic work-up, including lumbar puncture and neuroimaging
2. Either classic angiographic evidence (high probability) of vasculitis or histopathologic demonstration of vasculitis within the CNS
3. No evidence of systemic vasculitis or any other condition to which the angiographic or pathologic evidence can be attributed. These conditions include but are not limited to those in Table 157.1.

Following the diagnosis of PACNS all attempts should be made to categorize the patient into one of the recognized subsets or clinical variants as described below. These subsets appear to have varyingly important prognostic and therapeutic implications.

CLINICAL SUBSETS

Granulomatous angiitis of the central nervous system

Granulomatous angiitis of the central nervous system, or GACNS, represents approximately 20% of all patients fulfilling the diagnostic criteria for PACNS (Fig. 157.1). The epidemiology of the disease is poorly understood, but it does appear to be male predominant and occurs at virtually any age. It is most often characterized by a long prodromal period of frequently 6 months or more. Examples of acute onset have been reported, but it is far more commonly subacute or chronic in its presentation. The most common clinical manifestations of GACNS are headache and mental status changes. In addition to these features the majority of patients develop additional neurologic symptoms and signs during the course of their illness, including mental status changes, transient ischemic episodes, varying degrees of paresis, seizures, ataxia, visual changes, aphasia, and rarely even coma. It is the combination of evolving focal and diffuse neurologic dysfunction that is the hallmark of GACNS.

In a review of 136 reported cases of GACNS, Younger and colleagues[5] identified a number of associated conditions, including lymphoproliferative diseases, varicella zoster infection, amyloidosis, sarcoidosis and several others. Whether such cases are equivalent to GACNS occurring in isolation is unknown, and further analysis is needed to determine whether such confounded cases need to be approached differently. Several of these disorders are discussed below under Clinical variants.

A number of less common clinical manifestations of GACNS have also been reported, including a presentation as an acute or subacute encephalopathy or, rarely, as a pure dementia. It is far more common, however, to experience fluctuating levels of consciousness during the course of the illness. A pseudo multiple sclerosis-like presentation has

also been described. Of note is the fact that signs of symptoms of systemic vasculitis, such as peripheral neuropathies, fever, weight loss and rash, are rarely if ever part of GACNS. Wasting and low-grade fever may occasionally be observed, but this is generally believed to be due to disability secondary to neurologic dysfunction, and not part of the primary disorder.

Diagnosis and treatment

The most critical elements in securing the diagnosis of GACNS, apart from brain biopsy, are the lumbar puncture and neuroradiographic studies, in particular magnetic resonance imaging (MRI). Examination of the cerebral spinal fluid is essential, given that it is abnormal in approximately 90% of patients with GACNS, and thus a totally normal lumbar puncture weighs heavily against this as a probable diagnosis[2,6]. In addition, the lumbar puncture is essential for ruling out malignancies and infection, which may mimic the disease. The characteristic findings of the lumbar puncture in GACNS are those of aseptic meningitis. The white count is rarely over 250 cells/mm³ and the protein rarely exceeds 500mg%[2]. Because the disease is chronic, the lumbar puncture remains abnormal in the untreated patient over many weeks to months and thus presents within the differential diagnosis of chronic meningitis.

Neuroimaging studies are vital in the diagnostic work-up, and in general MRI is the investigation of choice[7]. There is no specific MRI finding that is diagnostic of GACNS, but the most suspicious findings are those of multifocal cerebral ischemic lesions occurring over time. These lesions are generally multiple and bilateral and located within the cortex, deep white matter or leptomeninges. Rarely is the disease confined to the white matter, and gray–white matter lesions are generally more suspicious for vasculitis. Enhancement, particularly in the leptomeninges, may occasionally be observed and serves to increase the sensitivity of a biopsy guided to the affected area. Collectively, abnormalities of the MRI or CSF analysis are noted in close to 100% of patients, and thus when normal make the diagnosis of GACNS unlikely. Angiography has a limited role in the diagnosis of GACNS. The literature has suggested that angiography may be normal in up to 40% of GACNS[2], but in our recent experience only 10–20% of such patients have abnormal studies. Although the specificity of angiography is extremely low in securing the diagnosis of PACNS[8], a high-probability angiogram in the setting of a chronic meningitis formula is highly suspicious for vasculitis if infection can be soundly ruled out. Unfortunately this is not always possible, and thus biopsy is frequently warranted.

The gold standard for the diagnosis of GACNS is biopsy of the CNS. The histology of GACNS has been well described[9], and the gross findings consist of multiple small foci of infarction or hemorrhage, with occasional larger areas being observed. At the microscopic level GACNS is characterized by segmental necrotizing granulomatous inflammation of small and medium-sized arteries affecting predominantly the leptomeninges and underlying cortical blood vessels. Veins are affected in about half the cases. The majority of the inflammatory infiltrate is composed of small lymphocytes, with an admixture of epithelioid cells, plasma cells, macrophages and giant cells of both of the Langerhans and foreign body types (Fig. 157.2). Clearly not all features are present in every patient, including the presence of giant cells. Unfortunately, from the diagnostic perspective the lesions are distributed in a patchy manner throughout the CNS, leading to the possibility of skipped lesions and false negative biopsies. Frank well-formed granulomas may rarely be seen, but more commonly there is loose granuloma formation. Lastly, lymphocytic-predominant lesions without prominent granulomas can be seen in up to 20% of biopsy-proven cases of PACNS, and it is unclear whether these cases, which are similar to GACNS in every other respect, are clinically equivalent or whether they represent a distinct nosologic entity. These will be discussed later under Atypical forms.

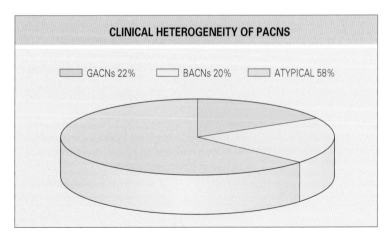

CLINICAL HETEROGENEITY OF PACNS

GACNs 22%   BACNs 20%   ATYPICAL 58%

Fig. 157.1 Clinical heterogeneity of PACNS. Frequency of distribution of nosologic subsets of PACNS at the Cleveland Clinic Foundation (*n* = 65).

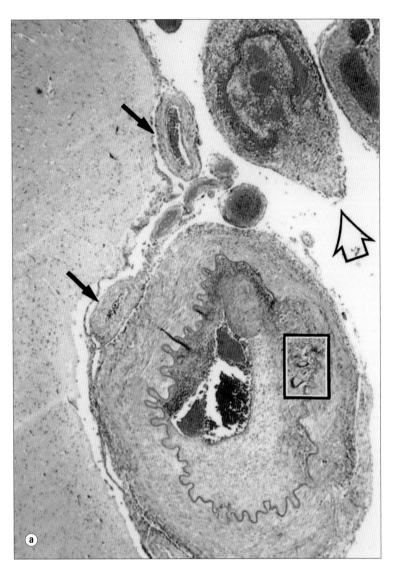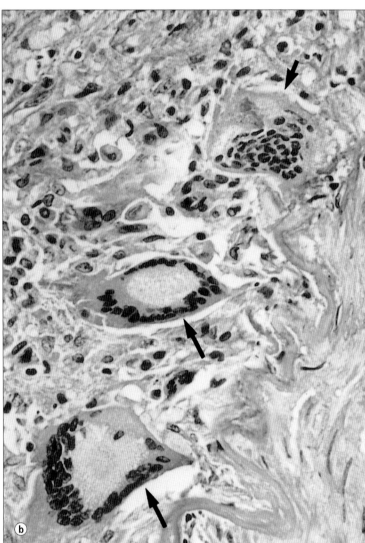

Fig. 157.2 Granulomatous vasculitis. (a) Brain biopsy findings of granulomatous vasculitis side by side with a polyarteritis-type necrotizing arteritis (open arrow). (b) Close-up view of (a) showing foreign body (short arrow) and foreign body (long arrow) giant cells in granulomatous vasculitis. Hematoxylin and eosin, × 64 and 400 respectively. (With permission from Calabrese *et al.*[4])

The differential diagnosis of GACNS primarily includes those conditions considered within the differential diagnosis of chronic meningitis[10]. Infections are the most important category of illness to rule out in this setting. Infections of particular importance, which may be overlooked, include HIV, *Borrelia burgdorferi* and varicella zoster virus (VZV). As discussed later, VZV may confound the diagnosis of GACNS, as CNS vasculitis may occur in the wake of clinical VZV infection as well as be detected within vasculitic lesions, even in the absence of clinical infection[11]. In general, given the gravity of the diagnosis as well as the profound nature of the therapy, we favor CNS biopsy as the preferred diagnostic technique. It should be remembered that the importance of the biopsy is not only to secure the diagnosis of GACNS but also to rule out the many mimicking conditions noted in Table 157.1[12].

Based on the historical literature there is little doubt that GACNS is a progressive and highly fatal disorder. Although there are no controlled clinical therapeutic trials in GACNS, informal therapeutic guidelines have been proposed based on the assumption of its progressive and fatal nature. In general, the majority of patients with documented GACNS should be treated with a combination regimen consisting of oral cyclophosphamide and glucocorticoids. Originally it was felt that oral cyclophosphamide needed to be continued for approximately 1 year after the patient was in clinical remission, but more recently – and similar to the treatment of ANCA-associated vasculitis – the patient's

exposure to alkylating agents should ideally be limited. It is now our practice to treat with oral cyclophosphamide for 3–6 months, and once the patient is in clinical remission to switch to an antimetabolite such as azathioprine or methotrexate for the duration of therapy[13]. Oral glucocorticoids are used similar to their application in treating Wegener's granulomatosis, starting with 1mg/kg of oral prednisone and gradually tapering to a small daily dose over 8–12 weeks. Given the debilitating nature of the disease and the intensity of the immunosuppressive regimen, we also advocate antimicrobial prophylaxis with trimethoprim sulfamethoxazole to prevent *Pneumocystis carinii* pneumonia[13].

One of the most critical problems in the management of GACNS is following disease activity. Clinical symptoms and signs of neurologic damage are slow to change, similar to any other ischemic event in the brain. MRI changes should improve but are likely to leave residual scars, and thus are difficult to interpret. In our experience improvement in CSF abnormalities serves as a useful indicator of decreased disease activity and should be documented after 8–12 weeks of therapy. Following clinical stability, which generally includes lessening or the absence of headaches in the absence of new neurologic signs and symptoms, serial MRI examinations at 3–4-month intervals should be performed during the first year. These are not performed primarily to look for radiographic resolution but rather to search for silent progression (i.e. new ischemic lesions) during the tapering of the immunosuppressive regimen. Similar to the treatment of other forms of systemic necrotizing vasculitis with high intensity immunosuppressive regimens, PACNS patients treated with cyclophosphamide and prednisone need to be carefully monitored to reduce and prevent treatment-related morbidity from infections, osteoporosis and other complications[13].

Benign angiopathy of the central nervous system (BACNS)

Clinical features

Growing evidence now suggests that some cases of PACNS diagnosed based solely on classic or high-probability angiograms represent a distinct nosologic subset, clearly distinguishable from GACNS based on their clinical features, prognosis and recommended therapy. Evidence supporting this hypothesis includes numerous case reports and clinical series of patients diagnosed on the basis of angiography alone with far more benign outcomes than that described for GACNS[4]. Retrospective analyses of angiographically and histologically documented cases have revealed significant clinical and laboratory differences as well[14]. Based upon such observations the term BACNS has been used to describe a discrete entity with specific clinical features (Table 157.2). Patients presenting with BACNS in its fully developed form are not difficult to recognize and contrast sharply with GACNS patients, with their long prodrome and progression of focal and non-focal neurologic dysfunction. Alternatively, BACNS patients generally present with an acute onset of a headache or neurologic event and display a clinical course that is relatively brief and monophasic. Unfortunately, at times the presentation may be profound and heralded by such complications as stroke with or without cerebral hemorrhage, leading to catastrophic sequelae. Thus not all cases of BACNS are truly benign, but the term has been applied to distinguish the overall better prognosis, distinctive clinical features and less intense therapeutic requirements for this subset of PACNS.

Hajj-Ali and colleagues[15] have recently described a large series of patients with BACNS. In their cohort of 16 patients, the mean age was 40 years with a female to male ratio of 4.3:1. Headache was the most common presenting symptom, observed in 88% of cases, followed by focal symptoms in 63% and diffuse symptoms in 44%. All patients had highly abnormal cerebral angiography and MRI abnormalities were present in 77%. Severe CSF abnormalities were present in only a single patient. Interestingly and importantly, 12 of their patients underwent follow-up cerebral angiography over a period ranging from 4 weeks to 8 months, revealing total or near total resolution of their changes (Fig. 157.3). These investigators proposed that follow-up angiography is essential to secure the diagnosis of BACNS. Also reported in this study was a prospective evaluation of long-term follow-up utilizing a standardized index specifically designed to assess post-stroke morbidity, demonstrating that 94% of the patients experienced significant recovery, with 71% showing no evidence of long-term disability. Only a single patient relapsed in this group.

TABLE 157.2 ESSENTIAL FEATURES OF BENIGN ANGIOPATHY OF THE CENTRAL NERVOUS SYSTEM		
Clinical	Most common in young women
	Acute onset (hours to days)
	Severe headache and or focal neurologic event
	Normal or near normal CSF analysis
Radiographic	High-probability angiogram for vasculitis (segmental narrowing, ectasia or beading in multiple vascular beds)
	Reversibility of angiographic abnormalities after therapy
Exclusions	Diseases and conditions in Table 157.1

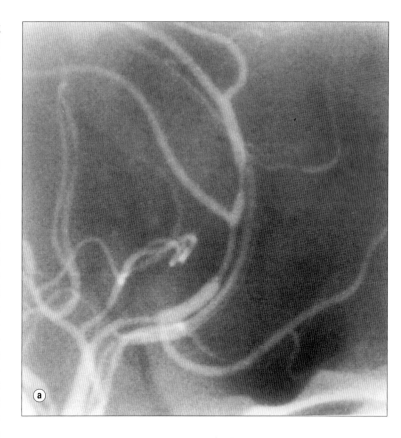

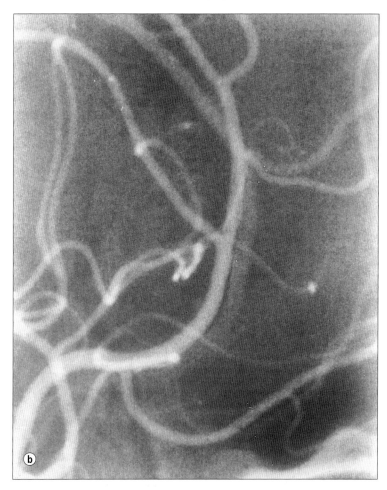

Fig. 157.3 Angiographic findings in a patient with BACNS. (a) Prior to therapy, demonstrating alternating areas of stenosis in branches of the middle cerebral artery. (b) Angiographic findings in the same patient approximately 4 weeks into therapy, demonstrating total resolution. (With permission from Hajj-Ali *et al.*[15])

BACNS is described as an *angiopathy,* implying the uncertainty of what is actually happening within the vessel wall, rather than an *angiitis,* which implies true vascular inflammation. This is because by definition the disease is angiographically defined, and in the few patients who have been subject to biopsy the procedure has been unrevealing. Given the pathophysiologic uncertainty, it has been proposed that many or even most patients with BACNS may be experiencing a form of reversible vasoconstriction or spasm rather than true arteritis[4,16]. In support of this contention is the fact that the clinical and angiographic picture of patients with BACNS is often identical to the cerebral vascular syndromes seen after exposure to sympathomimetic drugs, that found in the setting of complex headaches, with pheochromocytoma, and rarely in the postpartum period[4,16]. In all of these settings reversible vasoconstriction appears likely, but in the absence of definitive pathophysiologic investigations the underlying vascular pathology remains unknown. It is also possible that some patients presenting with the diagnostic criteria for BACNS have true angiitis, but limited numbers of biopsies performed in such patients have always been unrevealing.

Diagnosis and treatment

As opposed to GACNS, the diagnostic procedure of choice in patients presenting with a BACNS-like presentation is cerebral angiography. The angiographic features are illustrated in Figure 157.3 and classically include alternating areas of stenosis or ectasia in vessels in more than a single vascular bed. At times the vessels may appear beaded or, alternatively, display long areas of smooth tapering or areas of cutoff. It is important to appreciate that the cerebral angiogram is incapable of differentiating cerebral vasospasm from vasculitis, and thus only the rapid dynamic change can support its reversible and probably vasoconstrictive basis. Cerebral spinal fluid analysis is also vital in such patients, as by definition it must be normal or near normal. The presence of high numbers of cells or markedly elevated protein should warrant other diagnostic considerations. In all patients presenting with this clinical and/or angiographic picture a diligent search for sympathomimetic drug use, including over-the-counter agents such as phenylpropanolamine, as well as herbal products that contain ephedrine or ephedrine-based compounds, should be undertaken. In patients with unexplained hypertension screening for pheochromocytoma is essential. Although the cerebral angiogram is by definition normal in patients suffering from migraine headaches, there are rare reported cases of complex headaches, generally exertional in nature, associated with a similar angiographic picture[16]. Whether such patients should be viewed as having a distinct disorder or whether they represent mere clinical variants is currently unknown. The postpartum state is a setting for BACNS, and most cases of so-called postpartum angiitis no doubt represent a BACNS-like illness.

In our experience there is often a strong history of cigarette smoking and multiple risk factors, although these data are anecdotal. Other conditions that must be considered in the differential diagnosis of the acute onset of headache and angiographic abnormalities include emboli and hypercoagulable states.

There are no controlled therapeutic studies in patients with BACNS, although in general patients suspected of this clinical subset require far less intense therapy than those with GACNS. In the experience of Hajj-Ali et al.[15], no patient was treated with more than 6 months of oral glucocorticoids and the majority were treated with adjunctive calcium channel blockers. In our experience, we generally initiate therapy with prednisone 1mg/kg/day given in divided doses, and in addition start verapamil 240mg/day. If symptoms are not controlled, especially headaches, the dose of verapamil is increased as needed. In patients presenting with more catastrophic clinical manifestations, such as stroke, hemorrhagic stroke or marked focal neurologic deficits, intravenous methylprednisolone pulse therapy is initiated. The rationale for the use of high-dose glucocorticoids is based not only on their anti-inflammatory properties but also their application in the treatment of experimentally induced vasoconstriction in animal models. As noted above, it is essential that when clinical signs and symptoms have abated repeat cerebral angiography be performed to document total or near total resolution of the underlying abnormalities. We believe that this can be done as early as 4 weeks, but we generally perform this between 6 and 12 weeks, depending upon the clinical situation. Failure to improve – or, even worse, when there is angiographic progression – should warrant complete diagnostic re-evaluation. In particular, the absence of dynamic angiographic change on therapy suggests either atherosclerotic disease, embolic disease, a hypercoagulable state, and only rarely the possibility that this is an aggressive form of true angiitis which is being undertreated. Finally, it should be noted that not all investigators agree as to the benign nature of patients presenting in such fashion. We believe, however, that the inclusion of the requirement for angiographic reversibility will more clearly define the group requiring the least intense therapy.

Atypical PACNS

As demonstrated in Figure 157.1, a majority of patients (60%) with either angiographically or histopathologically documented PACNS do not fall neatly within the diagnostic categories of GACNS or BACNS and thus are considered atypical. Given our limited knowledge of the spectrum of PACNS disease, it is quite possible that further subclassifications will be developed in the future. Most patients falling within this category have either clinical features that preclude them from a ready diagnosis of BACNS, such as abnormal spinal fluid, or a more subacute to chronic presentation than one generally sees. Also represented are those rare cases of patients presenting with a BACNS-like presentation who upon repeat angiography fail to show dynamic improvement. As stated previously, we believe that most of these patients have non-arteritic forms of disease, but we cannot preclude that some have refractory forms of CNS vasculitis requiring more aggressive therapy. Other atypical cases would include those patients presenting with a GACNS-like presentation but whose biopsies reveal non-granulomatous pathology. Alternative patterns of histopathology include a predominantly lymphocytic angiitis (Fig. 157.4), or occasionally eosinophilic or even leukocytoclastic variants. It is unclear how patients who are characteristic in all other facets of the syndrome of GACNS should be so classified if their histology fails to show typical granulomatous changes.

Also included within the atypical category are those patients with unusual anatomic presentations. Spinal cord involvement is uncommon in PACNS but has been well documented[4]. Spinal cord involvement may or may not coincide with cortical involvement and when isolated poses a formidable diagnostic challenge. The vast majority of cases of spinal cord involvement reported in the literature have been diagnosed postmortem, with only rare examples of antemortem diagnosis described. The presentation of spinal cord variant PACNS is non-specific and similar to any other vascular and/or inflammatory myelopathy. Most commonly progressive paraparesis is observed, whereas acute transverse myelitis is rare. Several unusual variants of spinal cord involvement have been reported, including the presence of multiple aneurysms leading to acute spinal subdural hemorrhage. Several cases have also been described in association with lymphoproliferative diseases. There are no specific findings for spinal cord arteritis on neuroimaging, but a few cases have described enhancement within the cord and have suggested an infiltrating appearance[17]. Most cases of spinal cord vasculitis are associated with granulomatous pathology. There is no way of diagnosing PACNS within the spinal cord without biopsy, and thus surgical exploration for tissue confirmation is essential. Treatment is similar to that for GACNS.

Another poorly appreciated variant of PACNS are those cases presenting with mass lesions. This has been observed in about 15% of our

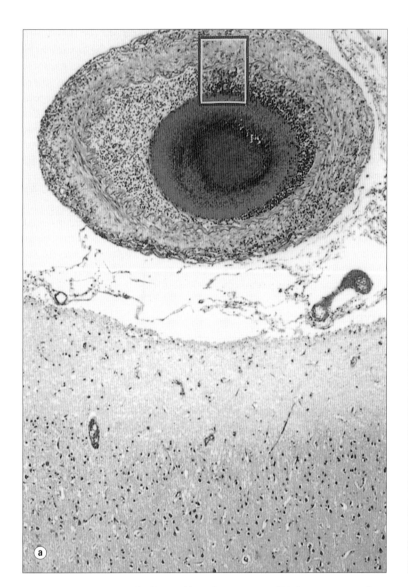
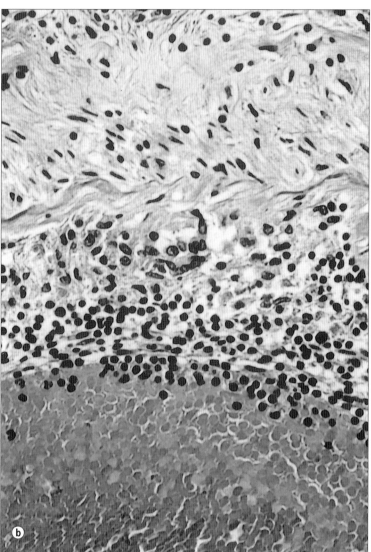

Fig. 157.4 Brain biopsy findings of lymphocytic vasculitis in a patient with PACNS with thrombosis. (b) Close-up view of the area in (a), demonstrating lyphocytic infiltrate in vessel wall. Hematoxylin and eosin, ×64 and 400 respectively. (With permission from Calabrese *et al.*[4])

cases. As always, a patient presenting with a mass lesion, demonstrated by neuroimaging techniques, should be suspected of having an infection or neoplasm until proven otherwise. Most all cases of PACNS with mass lesion presentations are diagnosed only at biopsy. Angiograms are generally normal save for demonstrating a mass effect if the lesion has achieved critical size. Neuroimaging of these types of mass lesions by CT or MRI has demonstrated variable degrees of enhancement, and thus there are no specific features to suspect the diagnosis. In our experience, a mass lesion presentation is the sole indication for stereotactic biopsy, which has been successful in diagnosing PACNS on rare occasions. A sizable percentage of such lesions display non-granulomatous lesions, often with leukocytoclastic features[4]. The optimal therapy for such patients is unknown, but rare reports of excisional cure have been documented. We generally treat patients with high-dose glucocorticoids, following them frequently with neuroimaging and adding cyclophosphamide only if the condition fails to respond. As always, it is essential to provide adequate tissue for special analysis, such as for clonality, particularly when there is a lymphocyte-predominant infiltrate.

The principles of diagnosis outlined for GACNS and BACNS apply equally to patients presenting with these atypical presentations. In patients displaying a chronic meningitis cerebral spinal fluid formula, the differential diagnosis is largely chronic infections, neoplasms and other inflammatory diseases[10]. In general, brain biopsy is the preferred technique in patients with inflammatory spinal fluid formulas suspected of CNS vasculitis.

In patients presenting more acutely with unexplained stroke-like syndromes angiography is generally the preferred diagnostic technique. If, however, patients present with an acute stroke syndrome associated with abnormal spinal fluid or evidence of systemic inflammation, then the decision whether to perform angiography and/or biopsy may be dictated by the availability of technical support, including a willing neurosurgeon. As discussed below, a team approach is clearly the best strategy when approaching suspected CNS angiitis.

With regard to the treatment of patients with atypical PACNS, there are no clinical trials to guide therapy. In general, in the absence of histopathologically documented GACNS, most cases of PACNS in the atypical category can be initially treated with glucocorticoids alone. If the presentation is fulminant and there are clear signs of rapid progression, then combined glucocorticoid and cyclophosphamide therapy, similar to that for GACNS, is recommended. For those patients with acute presentations and features which may suggest a reversible vasoconstrictive component, the addition of a calcium channel blocker is warranted.

Variants of PACNS

PACNS associated with varicella zoster infection (VZV)

It would seem that PACNS associated with an infection with VZV would most likely be considered a form of secondary CNS vasculitis; however, the relationship between VZV and cerebral vasculitis is highly complex and often subtle. The association of VZV infection with CNS vascular disease has been well described[18,19] and there is a broad range of CNS vascular pathology described in the literature. VZV causes chicken pox, usually in childhood, with most children manifesting no or only minimal neurologic sequelae. After chicken pox resolves, the virus becomes latent in the neurons and the spinal ganglia of nearly all infected individuals. In immunocompetent patients with reactivated virus the most common spread is a centrifugal pattern, manifesting as the dermatomal rash of shingles. Less commonly the spread from the ganglia is centripetal, with migration towards the spinal cord or brain, resulting in a variety of neurologic signs and symptoms. The virus may spread to the proximal nerve routes, including the cranial nerves, or even more centrally to the spinal cord and its meninges. Alternatively, the virus may also spread to the large vessels at the base of the brain, causing one of several distinct syndromes.

The best-described neurovascular syndrome associated with VZV follows infection of the trigeminal nerve, particularly when it involves its ophthalmic division[11]. In this syndrome, several weeks to months following VZV infection the patient suffers an ischemic event secondary to vasculitis of the middle cerebral artery, several of its branches, and occasionally the internal carotid artery. The mechanism appears to be due to retrograde spread of VZV to the cerebral circulation via anastomotic branches of the gasserian ganglion[19]. In general the disease remains anatomically localized (i.e. angiographically) and monophasic in course, but the mortality in such patients may approach 25%. We do not consider patients with this typical monophasic illness limited to the ipsilateral side of brain to the infection to have true PACNS, as they are readily differentiated on clinical and/or angiographic grounds. A more complex VZV-associated vascular syndrome of the CNS has been described in patients who are frequently elderly or who have other alterations in their host defenses. In this instance the syndrome may become indistinguishable from classic GACNS[20]. Interestingly, this disease may evolve either in the setting of VZV infection of the trigeminal nerve or a somatic dermatome, or even in the absence of clinical VZV infection (i.e. zoster sine herpete). In each of these vascular syndromes VZV has been occasionally isolated in inflamed vascular tissues. Anatomically it has been found in the outer layers of the vessel, as opposed to the endothelium. It has also been occasionally isolated in the CSF by polymerase chain reaction[19], though its presence in CSF may be only transient. Pathologically a spectrum of vascular involvement exists, ranging from frank necrotizing vasculitis to moderate vascular inflammation, to thrombosis without inflammation, or rarely an intimal proliferative lesion indistinguishable from atherosclerosis. Given that the clinical suspicion for VZV infection has traditionally been low in suspected cases of PACNS, without outward evidence of VZV infection, an unanswered question is how many patients may have clinically unrecognized VZV disease? The treatment of such cases is problematic but probably requires a combination of prolonged antiviral therapy and varying degrees of immunosuppression, as well as antiplatelet and/or anticoagulant therapy. There are no controlled therapeutic trials in this disease.

CNS sarcoid vasculitis

Another complex subgroup of patients are those with sarcoidosis and a clinical and histologic picture indistinguishable from that of GACNS[5,21]. As shown in Figure 157.5, GACNS at times may display well-formed non-necrotizing perivascular granulomas indistinguishable from sarcoid. In several of these cases, including the one illustrated, there was no evidence of any sign of sarcoidosis outside the central nervous system. Classification of such patients is problematic. Similar pathology in a patient with well-documented systemic sarcoidosis would clearly warrant the diagnosis of CNS vascular sarcoid. In the absence of such systemic disease such patients would probably best be classified as GACNS. Therapy of such patients is similar to that outlined under GACNS.

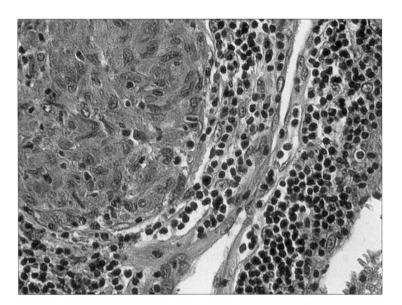

Fig. 157.5 Marked mononuclear inflammatory infiltrate in a cortical vessel with a well-formed paravascular granuloma. Magnification ×200. (With permission from Calabrese LH. Vasculitis of the cental nervous system. Rheum Dis Clin North Am 1995; 21: 1059–1076.)

PACNS and amyloidosis

There are growing numbers of case reports of patients with cerebral amyloid and features of PACNS, generally similar to GACNS. In their review, Younger and colleagues[5] expressed the belief that such patients were clinically and pathologically inseparable from others with GACNS. Clinically, headache, mental status changes, multifocal cerebral signs and gait disturbances were noted in 70% of patients and progressive neurologic dysfunction was common. Postmortem findings revealed an admixture of diffuse granulomatous angiitis of the CNS combined with cerebral amyloid angiopathy.

From a pathophysiologic perspective, the question has been raised as to whether these conditions are linked or merely coincidental. In a recent detailed report by Anders and colleagues[22] describing six patients with GACNS and cerebral amyloid, these authors pointed out that the inflammatory infiltrate in their series was somewhat atypical for GACNS. They noted that mononuclear cells were only found in the outer portion of the vessels and surrounding brain parenchyma, and not generally in a transmural distribution. These authors also demonstrated the presence of β/A4 peptide deposition in the thickened media of amyloid-damaged vessels and within the cytoplasm of multinucleated giant cells. These authors proposed that the granulomatous angiitis most likely represented a foreign body response to amyloid proteins, with a secondary destruction of the vessel wall. Optimal therapy of this variant is unclear, but the condition has been rarely reported to respond to aggressive therapy similar to that for GACNS.

DIAGNOSTIC APPROACH

As can be seen from Table 157.1, the differential diagnosis of PACNS is extensive and complex and there is no single subspecialty which has sufficient expertise in all of these conditions to be highly competent in their diagnosis and treatment. Thus we strongly believe that the optimal approach to PACNS requires a well-constructed team. This should include a rheumatologist or immunologist interested in vascular inflammatory disease and competent in the use of immunosuppressive drugs. It also should include a neurologist subspecializing in cerebrovascular disease with expertise in the broad differential of non-inflammatory acquired CNS vascular disorders. A capable neurosurgeon who is willing to tailor biopsy of CNS tissues is essential, as is a neuroradiologist who understands the use and limitations of neurodiagnostic techniques, especially angiography. Finally, a neuropathologist with experience and an interest in such unusual cases is essential.

The approach to suspected PACNS is not uniform, and from the descriptions of the clinical subsets described above varies depending upon the presentation and the clinical setting. For patients presenting with chronic meningitis, the differential diagnosis of infections, neoplasms and inflammatory diseases requires extensive laboratory testing, sampling of cerebral spinal fluid, and ultimately a biopsy of CNS tissues to confirm the diagnosis of PACNS. When brain biopsy is indicated in this setting, the preferred technique is an open biopsy of the temporal tip of the non-dominant hemisphere, including both leptomeninges and underlying cortex[23]. Sampling of the basilar meninges is important when attempting to exclude certain indolent infections or sarcoidosis. In the presence of leptomeningeal enhancement, a directed biopsy to involved areas is the preferred approach. Sterotactic biopsy is probably not indicated unless approaching a mass lesion. Regardless of the technique, tissue samples should be stained and cultured for microorganisms, with an effort being made to preserve frozen tissues for further investigations (i.e. immunohistochemistry, molecular analysis etc.) as needed. In general temporal artery biopsy has no role in the diagnosis of PACNS.

In patients presenting acutely, such as described for those with BACNS, an exhaustive search for emboli and hypercoagulability is essential. If none is found, cerebral angiography is generally the next logical step. Magnetic resonance angiography (MRA) is a poor substitute for high-quality cerebral angiography even though it is easier to perform and associated with less risk. Critical in the interpretation of cerebral angiography is the appreciation that virtually no findings, regardless of how 'classic', can alone secure the diagnosis of cerebral arteritis. Cerebral vasospasm, intravascular tumor, clot or atheromas and vascular inflammation secondary to infection may at times be indistinguishable from the findings in idiopathic PACNS. Thus, as with all diagnostic tests, this diagnostic test must be interpreted in the context of the clinical situation. Even in a highly biased referral population for suspected CNS vasculitis, Duna and colleagues[8] found that the specificity of cerebral angiography was only in the region of 26%. These data emphasize that the greatest pitfall in the diagnosis of CNS angiitis is overreliance on the specificity of neuroradiographic studies.

Neuroimaging studies such as CT and MRI are important in the diagnosis of PACNS in its varying subsets[24]. It can be stated that MRI is more sensitive than CT and is the preferred diagnostic imaging technique when CNS vasculitis is suspected. Common MRI findings in PACNS include multiple and often bilateral infarcts, including lesions in the cortex, deep white matter and/or leptomeninges. Occasionally such lesions demonstrate increased signal intensity with contrast enhancement, but this is a non-specific finding. Contrast enhancement in the leptomeninges provides an ideal place for biopsy and may increase the yield of this technique, but it is not specific for arteritis. Atypical neuroradiographic presentations of PACNS have been reported, including white matter disease mimicking multiple sclerosis. More advanced neuroradiographic techniques, such as SPECT and PET scanning, merely increase the sensitivity for detecting abnormalities of cerebral vascular flow while limiting specificity even further. The diagnosis of CNS vasculitis should never be made on the basis of nonvascular neuroimaging studies.

The relationship between MRI and cerebral angiography has been studied by several groups and most recently and extensively by Pomper et al.[25] In this investigation they studied 18 patients with varying forms of CNS angiitis, the majority of whom had PACNS. Each patient underwent both MRI and cerebral angiography. The authors observed that MRI was abnormal in 100%, but interestingly there was only a modest correlation between MRI abnormalities and lesions noted on angio-

graphy, and they concluded that the two procedures are complementary and necessary in the evaluation of suspected CNS angiitis.

Perhaps the most important admonition in the diagnostic process for suspected CNS vasculitis is the fact that most patients will have a disease other than arteritis. Although in this day and age of aggressive neuro-diagnostics patients are still too frequently left without a definite diagnosis, such diagnostic uncertainty should not in itself lead to a conclusive diagnosis of CNS arteritis. A thoughtful differential diagnosis, accompanied by the appropriate use of cerebral angiography and/or biopsy, with appropriate exclusionary diagnosis, remains the gold standard.

DISEASE ACTIVITY IN PACNS

Regardless of the clinical subset or the specific therapy applied to a given patient with PACNS, a major problem for the clinician is how to monitor such therapy from the perspective of disease activity. The CNS, once injured, is slow to regenerate (if it ever does) and thus improvement in signs or symptoms due to fixed tissue ischemia and necrosis is problematic. Other signs or symptoms due to transient ischemia and/or inflammation, such as headache, or transient ischemic attacks, seizures and weakness, are only crude and non-specific markers of activity. Furthermore, we have found that many patients with PACNS will long complain of new and occasionally severe headaches that persist after the acute phase of the illness has been treated, and these may not be true indicators of disease activity. In our experience, calcium channel blockers are often extremely helpful in treating this associated symptom.

Even serial MRI examinations may not be helpful, as signs of tissue necrosis are slow to resolve. Alternatively, serial MRIs are extremely valuable in identifying silent progression of ischemia, particularly during periods of tapering immunosuppressives, even when the patient is stable. The appearance of new infarctive lesions is strong evidence of increased disease activity even in the absence of symptoms or signs. For patients with GACNS, ensuring that CSF inflammation is subsiding is reassuring that treatment is effective. We generally perform repeat lumbar punctures after approximately 2–3 months of therapy to ensure declining cell counts and protein.

For patients with abnormal cerebral angiograms repeating this study is an option to assure oneself that there is improvement. In patients with BACNS, who by definition have abnormal angiograms, assuring angiographic reversibility is essential, not only to assure the adequacy of therapy but, as previously discussed, to verify the underlying diagnosis[15]. Failure to reverse suggests an alternative diagnosis. The precise timing of repeat angiography is uncertain, but in general we wait 6–12 weeks. Non-invasive assessments of cerebral blood flow, such as transcranial Doppler ultrasound and SPECT scanning, may also be useful, but at present there are no data regarding this application.

SECONDARY FORMS OF CNS VASCULITIS

Infection

In evaluating CNS vasculitis it is essential to search for infections, as the clinical and angiographic presentations of infection-related cerebral arteritis may mimic those of PACNS. Complicating this evaluation is the fact that infection may be occult when neurovascular complications arise. Table 157.3 lists those pathogens that have been described in association with either focal or diffuse cerebral vasculitis[4]. The search for a specific pathogen begins with an assessment of the epidemiologic features and individual risk factors in the suspected patient. Among viral pathogens that have been implicated in the development of CNS vasculitis, VZV has already been discussed in detail. HIV has been incriminated in a number of cases of CNS vasculitis, though the

TABLE 157.3 INFECTIOUS ETIOLOGIES OF CNS VASCULITIS
• Viruses (HIV-1, varicella-zoster virus, hepatitis C virus, others)
• Syphilis
• *Borrelia burgdorferi*
• *Bartonella*
• *Mycobacterium tuberculosis*
• Fungi (*Aspergillus, Coccidioides,* others)
• Bacteria (multiple)
• Ricketsiae

precise mechanism of its involvement is as yet unclear. More recently, hepatitis C virus has been associated with several cases both with and without the presence of associated cryoglobulinemia[26]. Ruling out infectious causes is particularly important in patients presenting with inflammatory changes in their spinal fluid. Certain pathogens, such as *Mycobacterium tuberculosis,* are notoriously difficult to identify and may take long periods of time to culture. Advances in molecular detection have minimized but not eliminated this problem. At times empiric therapy for both infectious agents and cerebral arteritis is required concomitantly.

Drugs

The relationship between drug use and CNS vasculitis is complex and has recently been reviewed[27,28]. The most commonly implicated drugs in the development of CNS vasculitis are oral and intravenous amphetamines, cocaine, ephedrine, phenylpropanolamine and heroin. It should be noted that most reported cases of 'drug-induced CNS vasculitis' have been defined by cerebral angiography in the absence of pathologic confirmation. Because most of the implicated drugs are capable of inducing vasospasm, some of these cases may have conceivably represented CNS angiopathy due to reversible vasoconstriction, rather than true angiitis. Despite this suggestion, well documented cases of drug-associated vasculitis have been reported, with pathology ranging from perivascular cuffing to frank vasculitis with or without vascular necrosis.

A high index of suspicion leading to prompt withdrawal of the offending drug is clearly the cornerstone of treatment. In addition to removing of the offending agent, we recommend the use of a calcium channel blocker and a short course of glucocorticoids in most cases where the drug is a sympathomimetic. The use of long-term glucocorticoid therapy and/or the addition of cytotoxic drugs should be reserved for those patients with biopsy-proven disease or those with progressive clinical findings.

Malignancy-associated CNS vasculitis

Central nervous system vasculitis has been reported in association with Hodgkin's lymphoma, non-Hodgkin's lymphoma and angioimmuno-lymphoproliferative lesions (AIL)[4]. It is of interest to note that the lymphoproliferative disease has been identified both outside and within the CNS. Clinical features of CNS vasculitis in association with lymphoproliferative disease are similar to those found in idiopathic PACNS, with mass lesions, spinal cord involvement and CNS hemorrhage all being reported. In other cases the clinical presentation and pathology may be indistinguishable from GACNS. In most cases therapy should be directed at the underlying lymphoproliferative disease and may consist of combination chemotherapy and/or radiotherapy. Favorable neurologic responses have been reported.

In view of the recent data incriminating VZV as a possible etiologic agent in cases of widespread CNS vasculitis in compromised hosts, we believe all cases of CNS vasculitis occurring in the setting of lymphoproliferative disease should be carefully screened for VZV.

Systemic vasculitides

CNS vasculitis may occur with any of the systemic vasculitides, but it is most commonly reported in polyarteritis nodosa, Behçet's syndrome, and in the ANCA-associated vasculitides[29]. The true prevalence of CNS vasculitis in the systemic vasculitides is problematic to estimate, as the diagnosis is frequently presumptive. In the setting of the systemic vasculitis, the new onset of neurologic signs or symptoms should raise the possibility of arteritic involvement of the CNS but also should raise the possibility of intercurrent complications, such as opportunistic infections, or the sequelae of uncontrolled hypertension or other comorbidities. Treatment of CNS disease is generally directed at the underlying systemic vasculitis and generally consists of high doses of glucocorticoids in combination with a cytotoxic drug, particularly cyclophosphamide.

Central nervous system complications of giant cell arteritis (GCA) deserve special consideration. In general CNS vasculitis is an uncommon complication of GCA, and when CNS signs or symptoms arise in the setting of GCA it is more likely to be due to either atherosclerosis in the elderly than the rarely encountered large vessel arteritis at the base of the brain. Extracranial vascular involvement, particularly of the carotid artery, is not uncommon. Rarely the proximal intracranial segments of both the carotids and vertebrals may be affected[30,31]. Among pathologically documented cases of GCA with intracranial involvement, inflammation has been generally limited to the proximal segments of the major arteries to the brain, and in a single example of a branch of the circle of Willis[30]. Small vessel involvement in the setting of true GCA is distinctly uncommon.

Miscellaneous and mimicking conditions

As described in Table 157.1, there are numerous conditions capable of mimicking either the clinical and/or the angiographic characteristics of CNS vasculitis. Perhaps one of the most common and difficult to differentiate is cerebral atherosclerosis. Because of the ability of atherosclerosis to mimic the angiographic findings of vasculitis, the use of angiography as the sole diagnostic modality in elderly patients or those with multiple cardiovascular risk factors is particularly problematic. Another condition which may at times be difficult to differentiate is demyelinating disease. The MRI appearance of demyelinating plaques, particularly when large, may be difficult to discriminate from that secondary to ischemic lesions[32,33]. The anatomic configuration of these lesions, as well as their confinement to white matter and characteristic CSF findings, is helpful in strongly suspecting demyelinating disease, but equivocal cases may require biopsy.

The antiphospholipid antibody (APL) syndrome may be at times difficult to distinguish from CNS arteritis, as it is clearly associated with CNS ischemic events related to arterial thrombosis. An angiographic study of a series of APL patients revealed that 59% had solely intracranial lesions, of which 60% were solitary arterial occlusions and 40% were suggestive of vasculitis[34]. This is potentially misleading, as the occurrence of true vasculitis in the APL syndrome is distinctly unusual.

Other conditions that may pose problems in differentiation include intravascular neoplasms, such as malignant angioendotheliomatosis, a neoplasm of B-cell origin which may be confined to the CNS and associated with both inflammatory CSF and angiographic abnormalities[35]. Carcinomatous meningitis may present as chronic meningitis and may be problematic to identify. Multiple lumbar punctures with high-volume CSF analysis may be required to secure this diagnosis. Radiation vasculitis may also be problematic to differentiate unless a careful history reveals an exposure to therapeutic irradiation in the appropriate anatomic areas[36].

REFERENCES

1. Calabrese LH, Mallek JA. Primary angiitis of the central nervous system: Report of eight new cases, review of the literature and proposal for diagnostic criteria. Medicine 1988; 67: 20–40.
2. Calabrese LH, Furlan AJ, Gragg LA et al. Primary angiitis of the central nervous system: Diagnostic criteria and clinical approach. Cleveland Clin J Med 1992; 59: 293–306.
3. Hankey GJ. Isolated angiitis/angiopathy of the central nervous system. Cerebrovasc Dis 1991; 1: 2–15.
4. Calabrese LH, Duna GF, Lie JT. Vasculitis in the central nervous system. Arthritis Rheum 1997; 40: 1189–1201.
5. Younger DS, Calabrese LH, Hays AP. Granulomatous angiitis of the nervous system. Neurol Clin 1997; 15: 821–834.
6. Stone JH, Pomper MG, Roubenoff R et al. Sensitivities of noninvasive tests for central nervous system vasculitis: a comparison of lumbar puncture, computed tomography, and magnetic resonance imaging. J Rheumatol 1994; 21: 1277–1285.
7. Wynne PJ, Younger DS, Khandji A, Silver AJ. Radiographic features of central nervous system vasculitis. Neurol Clin 1997; 15: 779–804.
8. Duna G, Calabrese L. Limitations in the diagnostic modalities in the diagnosis of primary angiitis of the central nervous system (PACNS). J Rheumatol 1995; 22: 662–669.
9. Lie JT. Primary (granulomatous) angiitis of the central nervous system: a clinicopathologic analysis of 15 new cases and a review of the literature. Hum Pathol 1992; 23: 164–171.
10. Gripshover BM, Ellner JJ. Chronic meningitis. In: Mandell GL, Bennett JE, Dolin R, eds. Principles and practice of infectious diseases, 4th edn. Philadelphia: Churchill Livingstone; 1998.
11. Gilden DH, Kleinschmidt-DeMasters BK, LaGuardia JJ et al. Neurologic complications of the reactivation of varicella zoster virus. N Engl J Med 2000; 342: 635–645.
12. Moore PM. Vasculitis of the central nervous system. Semin Neurol 1994; 14: 307–312.
13. Calabrese LH. Therapy of systemic vasculitis. Neurol Clin 1997; 15: 973–992.
14. Calabrese L, Gragg LA, Furlan AJ. Benign angiopathy: a distinct subset of angiographically defined primary angiitis of the central nervous system. J Rheumatol 1993; 20: 2046–2050.
15. Hajj-Ali, Hajj-Ali R, Furlan A et al. Benign angiopathy of the central nervous system (BACNS): cohort of 16 patients with clinical course and long term follow up. Arthritis Care Res (in press).
16. Solomon S, Lipton RB, Harris PY. Arterial stenosis in migraine: spasm or arteriopathy. Headache 1990; 30: 52–61.
17. Giovanini MA, Eskin TA, Mukherji SK, Mickle JP. Granulomatous angiitis of the spinal cord: a case report. Neurosurgery 1994; 34: 540–542.
18. Martin JR, Mitchell WJ, Henken DB. Neurotropic herpes viruses, neural mechanisms and arteritis. Brain Pathol 1990; 1: 6–13.
19. Gilden DH, Kleinschmidt-DeMasters, La Guardia JJ et al. Neurologic complications of the reactivation of Varicella-Zoster virus. N Engl J Med 2001; 342: 635–644.
20. Lie JT. Primary (granulomatous) angiitis of the central nervous system: a clinical pathologic analysis of 15 new cases and a review of the literature. Hum Pathol 1992; 23: 164–171.
21. Ulrich H. Neurosarcoidosis or granulomatous angiitis: a problem of definition. Mount Sinai J Med 1977; 44: 718–725.
22. Anders KH, Wang ZZ, Kornfeld M et al. Giant cell arteritis with cerebral amyloid angiopathy: immunohistochemical and molecular studies. Hum Pathol 1997; 28, 1237–1246.
23. Parisi JE, Moore PM. The role of biopsy in vasculitis of the central nervous system. Semin Neurol 1994; 14: 341–348.
24. Wynne PJ, Younger DS, Khandji A, Silver AJ. Radiographic features of central nervous system vasculitis. Neurol Clin 1997; 15: 779–804.
25. Pomper MG, Miller TJ, Stone JH et al. CNS vasculitis in autoimmune disease: Magnetic resonance imaging findings and correlation with angiography. Am J Neuroradiol 1999; 20: 75–85.
26. Petty GW, Duffy J, Huston J. Cerebral ischemia in patients with hepatitis C virus infection and mixed cryoglobulinemia. Mayo Clin Proc 1996; 71: 671–678.
27. Calabrese LH, Duna GF. Drug-induced vasculitis. Curr Opin Rheumatol 1996; 8: 34–40.
28. Buxton N. Amphetamine abuse and intracranial hemorrhage. J Roy Soc Med 2000; 93: 472–477.
29. Moore P, Calabrese LH. Neurologic manifestations of systemic vasculitides. Semin Neurol 1994; 14: 300–306.
30. Caselli R J, Hunder GG. Neurologic aspects of giant cell (temporal) arteritis. Rheum Dis Clin North Am 1993; 19: 941–953.
31. Rhodes R H, Madelaire C, Petrelli M et al. Primary angiitis and angiopathy of the central nervous system and their relationship to giant cell arteritis. Arch Pathol Lab Med 1995; 119, 334–349.
32. Trizulzi F, Scotti F. Differential diagnosis of multiple sclerosis: contribution of magnetic resonance imaging techniques. J Neurol Neurosurg Psychiatry 1998; 64(Suppl): S6–S14.
33. Finelli PF, Onyiuke HC, Uphoff DF. Idiopathic granulomatous angiitis of the CNS manifesting as diffuse white matter disease. Neurology 1997; 49: 1696–1699.
34. Provenzale JM, Barboriak DP, Allen NB, Ortel TL. Antiphospholipid antibodies: findings at arteriography. Am J Neuroradiol 1998; 19: 611–616.
35. Lie JT. Malignant angioendotheliomatosis (intravascular lymphomatosis) clinically simulating primary angiitis of the central nervous system. Arthritis Rheum 1992; 35: 831–834.
36. Alfonso ER, De Gregorio MA, Mateo P et al. Radiation myelopathy in over-irradiated patients: MR imaging findings. Eur Radiol 1997; 7: 400–404

OTHER SYSTEMIC ILLNESSES

158 The hereditary periodic fevers

Daniel L Kastner

Definition

- The hereditary periodic fevers are a group of inherited systemic illnesses characterized by episodes of fever with localized inflammation, often affecting serosal membranes, joints and skin

- There are two recessively inherited periodic fevers, familial Mediterranean fever (FMF) and the hyperimmunoglobulinemia D with periodic fever syndrome (HIDS). There are three dominantly inherited periodic fevers, the TNF-receptor-associated periodic syndrome (TRAPS), Muckle–Wells syndrome (MWS) and familial cold autoinflammatory syndrome (FCAS)

- FMF, MWS and FCAS are all caused by mutations in the pyrin family of proteins, which appear to be important in the regulation of apoptosis, NFκB activation and cytokine production. TRAPS is caused by mutations in the 55kDa TNF-α receptor, while HIDS is caused by mutations in mevalonate kinase, a key enzyme in the synthesis of cholesterol and non-sterol isoprenes

Clinical features

- Episodes of fever and localized inflammation, the duration and details of which vary with the specific disorder, but can include abdominal pain, pleuritic chest pain, arthritis or arthralgia, myalgia, rash and conjunctivitis

- In FMF, TRAPS, MWS and rarely FCAS, an increased risk of systemic AA amyloidosis

Treatment

- Colchicine prevents the attacks and amyloidosis of FMF

- Experience to date indicates that etanercept may reduce the frequency and severity of attacks in TRAPS

- There is no consensus on the optimal treatment for HIDS, MWS or FCAS

INTRODUCTION

The hereditary periodic fevers (Table 158.1) are a group of inherited systemic disorders characterized by episodes of fever with a variety of localized inflammatory manifestations, often including arthralgia or arthritis. A subset of patients also develop secondary AA amyloidosis. The hereditary periodic fevers can be thought of as inborn errors of inflammation.

Familial Mediterranean fever (FMF), a recessively inherited condition, is perhaps the prototype of this family of diseases, both because of its prevalence in certain populations and the degree to which it has been studied. The other hereditary periodic fevers include the recessively inherited hyperimmunoglobulinemia D with periodic fever syndrome (HIDS) and three dominantly inherited illnesses: the tumor necrosis factor (TNF)-receptor-associated periodic syndrome (TRAPS), Muckle–Wells syndrome (MWS) and familial cold autoinflammatory syndrome (FCAS; formerly familial cold urticaria or FCU). Although the adjective 'periodic' suggests that patients with these conditions experience relatively regular attacks, this is frequently not the case, and in some patients the febrile episodes are quite unpredictable. Antigen-specific T cells and high-titer autoantibodies appear not to play a major role in the pathogenesis of these illnesses, and thus they are sometimes termed autoinflammatory diseases[1,2]. Since these diseases often present in childhood, the differential diagnosis includes juvenile chronic arthritis and the syndrome of periodic fever with aphthous stomatitis, pharyngitis and cervical adenopathy (PFAPA).

Based on their often dramatic clinical presentation, the hereditary periodic fevers have long been viewed as potential keys to understanding how inflammation and innate immunity are regulated. Each of these conditions segregates as a single-gene disorder in families, but until the 1990s the nature of the proteins encoded by these genes was purely a matter of conjecture. With the advent of the Human Genome Project and positional cloning techniques, it became feasible to search systematically for these genes. In 1992 the FMF gene, designated *MEFV*, was mapped to the short arm of chromosome 16 (Ref. 3) and within the ensuing 10 years the genes underlying all five illnesses were identified. *MEFV*, the first of these genes to be cloned[4,5], encodes a previously unknown protein called pyrin (or marenostrin) that is predominantly expressed in leukocytes. The N-terminal 92 amino acids (aa) of this protein form a novel 6-helix homotypic interaction motif (the pyrin domain)[6] that defines a family of over 20 proteins involved in the regulation of inflammation and apoptosis. Mutations in one of these proteins, cryopyrin, have recently been found to cause both MWS and FCAS[7]. In 1999 a group of somewhat heterogeneous families with dominantly inherited periodic fevers were found to harbor mutations in *TNFRSF1A*, which encodes the 55kDa TNF-α receptor[1]. This permitted a major reclassification of these conditions into a single entity, TRAPS. Shortly thereafter two independent groups reported that HIDS is caused by mutations in a key enzyme in cholesterol biosynthesis[8,9], underscoring the fact that very divergent molecular lesions can sometimes lead to a similar phenotype.

The impact of these discoveries on the practice of clinical medicine is still evolving. Genetic tests are now available for all five of the hereditary periodic fevers discussed here, permitting a re-examination of the clinical and geographic bounds of these illnesses. Indications for genetic testing, as well as the sensitivity and specificity of various laboratory methods, are still being worked out and there is lively debate over the use of clinical versus genetic criteria in the diagnosis of these conditions. Mutational analysis of the known periodic fever genes does not account for all of the cases with clinical disease, raising the possibility that there may be yet more of these genes to be identified. In the case of TRAPS, the recognition that this condition is caused by mutations in the 55kDa TNF-α receptor has provided the conceptual underpinnings for the use of TNF-α inhibitors in this illness.

The discoveries of the last 10 years lay the foundation for the challenges and opportunities of the next decade. At the basic science level, these will include deepening our understanding of the function of the periodic fever genes, learning the molecular basis for how mutations cause disease and defining the relevant biochemical pathways. Such insights may well suggest new candidate genes for mutational screening

TABLE 158.1   THE HEREDITARY PERIODIC FEVERS

	Familial Mediterranean fever	TNF-receptor-associated periodic syndrome	Hyper-IgD syndrome	Muckle–Wells syndrome	Familial cold autoinflammatory syndrome
OMIM number	249 100	142 680	260 920	191 100	120 100
Inheritance	Autosomal recessive	Autosomal dominant	Autosomal recessive	Autosomal dominant	Autosomal dominant
Ethnic distribution	Jewish, Arab, Armenian, Turkish, Italian	Broad ethnic distribution; originally Irish/Scottish	Dutch, French	Northern European	Primarily European
Gene (chromosome)	*MEFV* (16p13.3)	*TNFRSF1A* (12p13)	*MVK* (12q24)	*CIAS1* (1q44)	*CIAS1* (1q44)
Protein	Pyrin (marenostrin)	55kDa TNF-α receptor	Mevalonate kinase	Cryopyrin (PYPAF1, NALP3)	Cryopyrin (PYPAF1, NALP3)
Typical attack length	1–3 days	>7 days	3–7 days	1–2 days	30min–72h
Serosal manifestations	Mild abdominal pain to peritonitis; pleurisy; pericardial involvement usually asymptomatic; acute scrotum	Mild abdominal pain to peritonitis; pleurisy; pericarditis; scrotal pain	Abdominal pain, but peritonitis uncommon; pleurisy rare	Abdominal pain; pleurisy rare	Absent
Musculoskeletal manifestations	Exercise-induced myalgia; protracted febrile myalgia (rare); monoarticular arthritis; chronic arthritis of hip; sacroiliitis	Migratory myalgia; arthralgia more common than arthritis; when present, arthritis is monoarticular or pauciarticular	Myalgia uncommon; self-limited symmetric polyarticular non-destructive arthritis	Myalgia, arthralgia common; large joint oligoarticular arthritis	Polyarthralgia, myalgia
Cutaneous manifestations	Erysipelas-like erythema (ELE); Henoch–Schönlein purpura in 5% of children	Migratory erythema often accompanying myalgia	Erythematous macules and papules most common; aphthous ulcers of mouth, vagina	Urticarial rash (granulocytes predominate)	Urticarial rash (granulocytes predominate)
Lymphadenopathy	Uncommon	Sometimes found	Cervical adenopathy common during attacks	Can occur	Absent
Neurosensory	Aseptic meningitis (rare)	Conjunctivitis, uveitis, periorbital edema	Uncommon	Sensorineural deafness; conjunctivitis, episcleriitis; elevation of optic disc	Headache, conjunctivitis
Amyloidosis risk	Varies according to genotype, environment	~14% of cases	None reported	~25% of cases	Infrequent (~2%)
Genotype–phenotype associations	M694V/M694V associated with amyloidosis, arthritis, ELE, possibly other severe manifestations; E148Q low penetrance	Cysteine mutations associated with increased penetrance, amyloidosis; R92Q, P46L are low penetrance mutations	Nearly all cases have at least one copy of V377I; HIDS-associated mutations distributed throughout the gene	None to date	None to date
Treatment	Daily oral colchicine	Prednisone, etanercept	No established treatment; NSAID for fever; statins investigational	In some cases, colchicine or high-dose steroids	NSAID for fever, arthralgia; long-term steroids effective, but limited by toxicity

Regularly updated lists of mutations in the respective genes can be found on the Internet at http://fmf.igh.cnrs.fr/infevers/.

(OMIM = online Mendelian inheritance in man, available on the Internet at http://www.ncbi.nlm.nih.gov/omim).

in patients with currently unexplained autoinflammatory diseases. Moreover, the known periodic fever genes and their biochemical partners may also have a role in the more prevalent inflammatory diseases, just as mutations in *CARD15/NOD2* cause both Blau syndrome (a rare granulomatous disorder) and the much more common Crohn's disease[10–12]. The following pages will summarize the current state of knowledge for each of the hereditary periodic fevers and highlight the questions yet to be answered in this rapidly moving field.

FAMILIAL MEDITERRANEAN FEVER

Background, basic genetics and epidemiology

Although the earliest recognizable description of FMF appeared in the medical literature in 1908[13], the first series of cases was not reported until 1945[14]. Shortly thereafter, detailed descriptions were published by clinicians in France and Israel, and the current name, familial Mediterranean fever, was proposed[15–17]. Other synonymous terms are still occasionally found in the literature, including recurrent polyserositis, recurrent hereditary polyserositis, familial paroxysmal polyserositis and periodic peritonitis.

Familial Mediterranean fever is generally thought of as a recessively inherited disorder most frequent in individuals of non-Ashkenazi Jewish, Armenian, Arab and Turkish ancestry. The availability of genetic testing has led to the realization that FMF is also relatively common among individuals of Ashkenazi (east European) Jewish and Italian ancestry[18,19], often with less severe clinical manifestations than in the populations where it has been more extensively described. DNA analysis has also confirmed the presence of FMF in individuals with no known Mediterranean or Middle Eastern ancestry. The recessive mode of inheritance means that it is possible that neither parent of an affected individual will have FMF (although one or both parents may be affected), but both parents must at least be carriers. As in other recessive conditions, a history of consanguinity is sometimes elicited. The expected frequency of offspring born to two parents who are FMF carriers is 25%; for the offspring of an affected individual and a carrier, it is 50%; and for the offspring of two affected individuals, it is 100%. Particularly in countries where smaller families predominate, it is not at all uncommon for there to be no family history of FMF in individuals with clinically typical, genetically confirmed disease. DNA studies have raised the possibility that at least for certain relatively rare *MEFV* mutations, dominant inheritance is possible[20].

Based on large case series reported before the cloning of *MEFV*, approximately 90% of patients with FMF exhibit their first symptoms by the age of 20[17,21] and thus the diagnosis is most frequently made by pediatricians or pediatric rheumatologists[22]. Increasingly, though, genetic testing has allowed the recognition of relatively mild disease in adults, who on close questioning often give a history dating back to childhood. There is an excess of male cases over females (usually with an M:F ratio of about 1.5–2.0:1), which may be due to a number of factors, including the misdiagnosis of FMF abdominal attacks as gynecological disease, possible hormonal effects on FMF symptoms (in some women symptoms begin at menarche, and pregnancy may be associated with an amelioration or remission of febrile attacks[17,21]) and/or underreporting by females for social/cultural reasons. Despite the possibility of underdiagnosis, the incidence of FMF has been found to be as high as 1:248 in the Libyan Jewish population[23], implying a carrier frequency of at least 1:8.

Clinical features and laboratory findings

Acute attacks

The acute attacks of FMF are typically characterized by fever and either serositis, synovitis or skin rash. The duration of attacks is usually 24–72 hours, although arthritic attacks sometimes last up to 1 week. The attacks can occur as often as once a week or as infrequently as once every few years, and even for a given patient the frequency may vary greatly over time, for no apparent reason. Physical exertion, emotional stress and menses have all been associated with attacks in some patients, but in many cases there is no obvious provocation. Some patients experience a prodromal sensation for several hours before the onset of the attack and chills often herald the onset of fever.

The magnitude of temperature elevation can vary greatly among individuals and even from one episode to the next in a given individual. Fevers are generally higher in children than in adults and, especially in infants and toddlers, fever may be the only finding[22]. During an episode, antipyretics may ameliorate the fever and help prevent febrile seizures in infants, but, untreated, the temperature generally stays elevated throughout the episode.

Abdominal pain is the second most common manifestation of FMF and occurs at some time in over 90% of patients. At its worst, the abdominal pain of FMF mimics an acute surgical abdomen, with absence of bowel sounds, board-like rigidity and rebound tenderness. Many patients who present in this way early in their disease undergo one or more exploratory laparotomies, which usually reveal sterile peritonitis and sometimes unexplained adhesions, but no evidence of appendicitis. After the attack subsides, upper GI series, barium enema and endoscopic investigations are normal unless amyloidosis is present. CT scanning of the abdomen performed during an acute attack may reveal a small amount of free fluid in the peritoneum, probably representing the inflammatory exudate. Patients who remain undiagnosed after several attacks frequently avoid medical attention in subsequent episodes out of frustration; these patients often give a history of staying at home in bed for the duration of their attacks. It should, however, be emphasized that even those patients who experience attacks of the severity described above sometimes have milder abdominal episodes that do not preclude work or school activities.

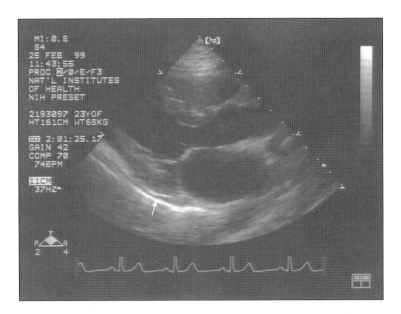

Fig. 158.1 Small posterior pericardial effusion (arrow) in a young woman with FMF. Two-dimensional echocardiogram, parasternal long-axis view.

Pleural attacks are also common in FMF, either alone or in combination with abdominal attacks. Pleurisy may be more frequent among Armenians than in other populations[21]. Pleural attacks are usually unilateral, with sharp, stabbing chest pain on inspiration or coughing, and sometimes with shoulder pain referred from the diaphragm. A pleural effusion may be present and thoracentesis reveals an exudative fluid rich in neutrophils, but frequently no effusion is detectable on upright or lateral decubitus films.

Symptomatic non-uremic pericarditis is relatively rare in FMF, although it has been reported, even with tamponade[24,25]. Nevertheless, small pericardial effusions with mild or no symptoms can sometimes be detected by echocardiography, as illustrated in Figure 158.1.

The incidence of arthritis in FMF[26] varies considerably among ethnic groups. Individuals carrying two copies of the M694V mutation have been shown to be at increased risk for arthritis[27–30] and the incidence of arthritis roughly parallels the population frequency of this mutation. In the North African Jewish population, where this mutation is very common, as many as 75% of FMF patients experience synovial attacks at some point in their illness[17,26]. FMF arthritis often first presents in childhood. The most frequent presentation is monoarticular, commonly affecting the knee or ankle, followed by symmetric two-joint arthritis; other patterns, such as polyarticular symmetric arthritis and oligoarticular asymmetric arthritis, are less frequent[22]. During the acute arthritic attacks of FMF, there may be large sterile synovial effusions with neutrophil counts of the magnitude seen in septic arthritis. Despite this, the natural history of the acute arthritis of FMF is usually complete resolution with no radiographic residua. In patients not treated with colchicine, chronic monoarticular arthritis can develop and, when located in the hip, this can eventually necessitate joint replacement[26,31]. FMF patients may also be at increased risk of sacroiliitis, irrespective of HLA-B27 status or colchicine prophylaxis[32].

The most characteristic skin lesion of FMF, which is considered pathognomonic by some, is a tender erythematous plaque on the dorsum of the foot, ankle or lower leg that is termed erysipelas-like erythema (ELE). An early case report of the histology of this lesion described a perivascular infiltrate that was primarily polymorphonuclear[33], consistent with the composition of serosal and synovial fluids from FMF patients. A larger, more recent study showed a more mixed cellular infiltrate[34], as is seen in Figure 158.2; possibly, colchicine prophylaxis alters the histology. Deposits of C3 can be demonstrated in vessel

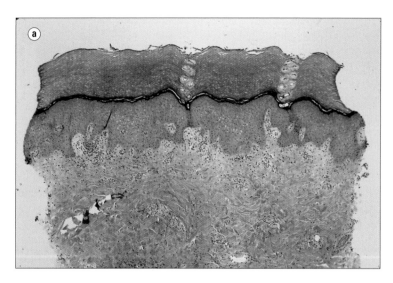

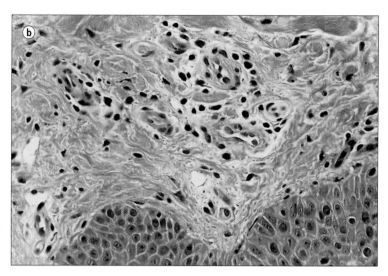

Fig. 158.2 (a) Skin biopsy specimen taken from the site of erysipelas-like erythema (ELE) in a young man with FMF. Note the predominantly perivascular distribution of the inflammatory infiltrate (hematoxylin and eosin staining, magnification ×40). (b) Higher magnification of the biopsy shown in panel (a), demonstrating a mixed, predominantly mononuclear infiltrate (×1000).

walls, but vasculitis is not observed. A number of other rashes, most notably Henoch–Schönlein purpura[17], can present as non-specific manifestations of FMF.

Attacks of FMF can involve other anatomic compartments. Exertional myalgia of the lower extremities, usually without fever and lasting from a few hours to 2–3 days, occurs in about 20% of patients, and a shorter-lasting, mild myalgia can sometimes occur without strenuous exercise[22]. In a small percentage of patients, there can be prolonged (up to 6 weeks) episodes of severe, debilitating myalgia of the extremities, with fever, accelerated erythrocyte sedimentation rate (ESR) and a normal creatine kinase (CK)[35]. This 'protracted febrile myalgia' is thought to be due to vasculitis. A small percentage of boys with FMF develop acute scrotal pain resulting from inflammation of the tunica vaginalis, an embryologic remnant of the peritoneal membrane[36]. There have also been isolated reports of aseptic meningitis in FMF[37].

Laboratory investigations

Laboratory studies performed during FMF attacks show a non-specific acute phase response, including leukocytosis, an accelerated ESR and elevations in the C-reactive protein (CRP), serum amyloid A (SAA), fibrinogen and haptoglobin[38]. Patients may have moderate hypergammaglobulinemia irrespective of whether they are in an attack, and serum IgD levels can be moderately elevated, especially in patients homozygous for the M694V mutation[39]. As noted previously, autoantibodies, including the antinuclear antibody (ANA), rheumatoid factor (RF), anticardiolipin antibodies (ACA) and antineutrophil cytoplasmic antibody (ANCA) are usually negative, or present only in low titer.

Between their attacks FMF patients have no residual symptoms. Nevertheless, the majority of FMF patients show persistent elevations of their acute phase reactants, especially the CRP and SAA, even when they are between attacks[40]. Moreover, obligate carriers of FMF mutations have also been shown to have increased acute phase reactants, relative to non-carriers[40]. Taken together, these data suggest that the acute attacks of FMF probably represent the tip of the inflammatory iceberg.

Associated disorders

Several other inflammatory/rheumatologic disorders have been observed in association with FMF. As noted above, the protracted febrile myalgia of FMF is thought to be due to vasculitis, and two other vasculitides, Henoch–Schönlein purpura[17] and polyarteritis nodosum[41], are seen

more frequently in FMF patients than in the general population. There are also data that non-amyloid glomerulitis may present at an increased frequency in FMF patients. In addition, fibromyalgia, while not an inflammatory disease in its own right, is seen in association with FMF, just as it is seen in the setting of other inflammatory diseases.

Systemic amyloidosis

Systemic amyloidosis is an extremely serious manifestation of FMF[17]. It is caused by the deposition of a degradation product of SAA, an acute phase reactant made by the liver, in a number of different organs. The most common sites of amyloid deposition in FMF are the kidneys, liver, spleen, gastrointestinal tract, testes, thyroid and adrenals. Before the advent of colchicine prophylaxis, amyloidosis was a frequent cause of kidney failure and death in FMF patients. Amyloid deposits in FMF seldom occur in the heart, peripheral nerves or joints (except in the setting of chronic hemodialysis). Amyloidosis usually occurs in patients who are already experiencing the acute febrile episodes of FMF (phenotype I), but rarely occurs as the first manifestation of FMF (phenotype II).

There are a number of factors that determine the risk of amyloidosis for a given patient. The older literature notes ethnic differences in the risk of amyloidosis, with North African Jews having a higher risk than Iraqi Jews, who in turn have a higher risk than Ashkenazi Jews[42]. With the cloning of *MEFV*, most series indicate an increased risk of amyloidosis in patients who are homozygous for the M694V mutation[27–30,43–46]. The differences in amyloid risk among Jewish subpopulations roughly parallel the M694V mutation frequencies. Although there are less data, the M694I mutation may also confer increased amyloid risk[45]. These mutations tend to associate with other more severe manifestations of FMF, suggesting a connection between disease severity and amyloidosis. There is an excess of M694V homozygotes even among the phenotype II patients, suggesting that phenotype II may be explained by asymptomatic episodes of severe 'biochemical inflammation'. However, it should be emphasized that even among patients with milder, relatively low risk *MEFV* mutations such as E148Q, amyloidosis has been observed[18,47].

Over and above the effect of specific *MEFV* mutations, a positive family history of amyloidosis confers increased amyloid risk. Recent data on Armenian FMF patients indicate that the SAA1 α/α genotype may account for at least part of this risk and male gender has also been associated with increased risk of amyloidosis in FMF[48]. An excess of amyloidosis among untreated Armenian FMF patients in Armenia, relative to Armenian–Americans before the use of colchicine, suggests an additional role for environmental factors.

All FMF patients should be regularly screened for amyloidosis by urinalysis. Patients who have significant proteinuria on repeated urinalyses performed between febrile attacks may require tissue diagnosis. Renal biopsy has the highest sensitivity, with rectal biopsy a slightly less sensitive but also less invasive alternative[49]. Bone marrow biopsy is less often undertaken, but also has a high sensitivity. Aspiration of the abdominal fat pad, while less invasive, is not a sensitive test for amyloidosis in FMF[50]. If not treated, the natural history of amyloidosis in FMF is progression to renal failure usually within 3–5 years of diagnosis. In those patients who undergo dialysis or renal transplantation who are not adequately treated, amyloid deposition will continue in the transplanted kidney and other organs, leading to amyloid goiter, malabsorption and diarrhea due to gastrointestinal deposition, and occasionally cardiac involvement.

Molecular genetics

The FMF gene, *MEFV*, was mapped to the short arm of chromosome 16 in 1992[3] and was identified by positional cloning by two independent groups in 1997[4,5]. It is a 10-exon gene spanning approximately 15 kb of genomic DNA and it encodes a 781-aa protein product that has been named pyrin, to connote its relationship to fever, or marenostrin, after the Latin name for the Mediterranean sea (*mare nostrum,* our sea), by the two teams. Four missense mutations in exon 10 – the substitution of isoleucine for methionine at codon 680 (M680I), the substitution of valine for methionine at position 694 (M694V), the substitution of isoleucine for methionine at codon 694 (M694I) and the substitution of alanine for valine at position 726 (V726A) – were found in absolute association with disease in two large panels of families. Moreover, M694V and V726A were found in several populations, each associated with a unique haplotype (essentially a genetic fingerprint), suggesting that present-day carriers of these two mutations are respectively descended from two different common ancestors. Based on the histories of the populations involved, the ancestral mutations probably arose 2500 or more years ago. Similar findings have subsequently been reported for the E148Q mutation[19] in exon 2.

Pyrin is expressed predominantly in neutrophils, eosinophils and cytokine-activated monocytes, but not at significant levels in lymphocytes[51]. Although initial computational analyses of the coding sequence suggested that pyrin might be a transcription factor, transfected full-length pyrin is cytoplasmic when examined by fluorescence microscopy[52]. The product of a relatively non-abundant alternative splice form lacking exon 2 does enter the nucleus[53], but the physiologic significance of this isoform is still uncertain. Full-length pyrin associates with microtubules[52], suggesting a possible mechanism by which colchicine exerts its therapeutic effect in FMF.

Since the positional cloning of *MEFV*, a number of other proteins have been identified that are homologous to the N-terminal ~92 aa of pyrin[6,54], encoded by exon 1. Although this domain has not yet been crystallized, computational secondary structure analysis and studies of circular dichroism predict that this domain is the fourth member of a superfamily that includes death domains, death effector domains and caspase recruitment domains (CARD). Each has a six α-helix configuration that promotes homotypic interactions: death domains associate with death domains, pyrin domains with pyrin domains, etc.

Recognition of the pyrin domain (PYD) is the basis for the current working hypothesis on pyrin function (Fig. 158.3). Pyrin has been shown to bind an adaptor protein called ASC (apoptosis-associated speck-like protein with a caspase recruitment domain)[55] that consists of an N-terminal PYD and a C-terminal CARD. The PYD of pyrin binds the PYD of ASC, and the CARD of ASC is then free to bind other CARD proteins, which are known to regulate apoptosis, NFκB activation and cytokine production. Alternatively, pyrin may associate directly with other PYD-containing proteins, which have similarly been implicated in these three cellular processes. If normal wild-type pyrin acts to promote leukocyte apoptosis or to suppress cytokine production, then loss-of-function mutations might lead to the persistence of leukocytes that would ordinarily undergo apoptosis, and/or the increased production of proinflammatory cytokines, thus permitting the amplification of otherwise innocuous stimuli[54].

A recent review summarized a total of 29 known *MEFV* mutations associated with FMF[56]. Of these 29 mutations, 18 are in exon 10 and six are in exon 2. Twenty-six represent single aa substitutions, two are single

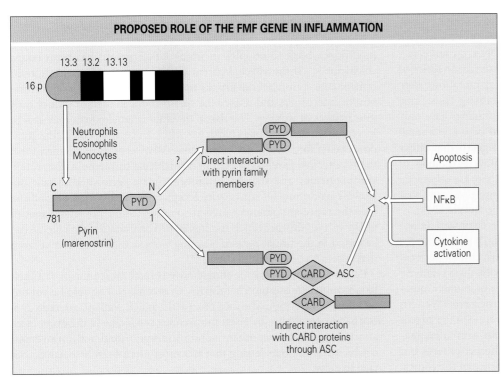

Fig. 158.3 Proposed role of the FMF gene in inflammation. Pyrin, the FMF protein, associates with other proteins through its interactions with the adaptor protein ASC (apoptosis-associated specklike protein with a caspase recruitment domain) at the N-terminal pyrin domain (PYD). ASC has a caspase recruitment domain (CARD) which in turn can bind other inflammatory proteins. Alternatively, it is hypothesized that pyrin may also interact directly with other PYD proteins. Either pathway may lead to the regulation of apoptosis, NFκB or cytokine activation.

aa in-frame deletions and only one is a truncation (at codon 688). Three mutations have been described at each of the codons 680 and 694 and two at codon 148. The preponderance of missense mutations may explain the episodic nature of FMF, since these mutations may lead to subtle functional changes and a delicate equilibrium state[4]. As previously noted, M694V homozygotes have an increased risk of amyloidosis[27–30,43–46], and some studies additionally associate this genotype with an earlier age of onset, greater frequency of attacks, arthritis and ELE[27–30]. M694I and M680I may also confer a more severe phenotype. There is evidence that the deletion mutation at codon 694 is dominantly inherited[20]. The E148Q substitution is generally regarded as a less penetrant, milder mutation, that is usually found in FMF patients who are compound heterozygotes for E148Q and an exon 10 mutation. E148Q can also be seen as a complex allele in *cis* with an exon 10 mutation[19,57]. The relative frequencies of various *MEFV* mutations, especially M694V and E148Q, may explain some of the differences in FMF severity among ethnic groups.

Identification of *MEFV* has permitted the direct enumeration of FMF carriers in high-risk populations and has produced estimates of FMF carrier frequencies as high as 1:3 to 1:5 in certain ethnic groups[19,56,58]. To put these figures in perspective, the carrier frequency for cystic fibrosis, the most common lethal recessive disorder in North American Caucasians, is only about 1:20. Such high FMF carrier rates strongly suggest a selective advantage, perhaps resistance to one or more infectious agents, for heterozygous carriers of *MEFV* mutations. Since the number of affected individuals predicted by these figures exceeds the population-based estimates, it is likely that there are significant numbers of non-penetrant/undiagnosed individuals carrying two *MEFV* mutations who do not carry the diagnosis of FMF[19,59]. Certain mutations in *MEFV* may also increase an individual's risk of other inflammatory disorders, including Behçet's disease[60], inflammatory bowel disease[61] and secondary amyloidosis[62].

Diagnosis

At the time *MEFV* was cloned, many expected that FMF would become purely a genetic diagnosis, particularly in light of the high frequency of just four mutations in the initial panels of families. However, as experience has broadened, it has become clear that the diagnosis of FMF cannot be made or refuted on the basis of genetic testing alone. Because of the aforementioned issue of non-penetrance, the identification of two *MEFV* mutations in the absence of clinical information is of limited value. Conversely, it is widely recognized that current methods of mutation detection, usually based on sequencing of genomic DNA, do not detect all of the mutations that 'should' be present. In one recent series of 90 patients with clinically diagnosed FMF[19], only 142 mutations were identified, accounting for 79% of the expected 180 mutations. Thus, some patients with FMF diagnosed on the basis of clinical findings have only one demonstrable mutation (rather than the expected two) and a small number will have no identifiable mutations. This suggests that either current methods do not identify a substantial percentage of the pool of *MEFV* mutations in the populations studied or that there are other loci, perhaps encoding pyrin homologs or proteins in the same pathway, that may interact with *MEFV* to produce the signs and symptoms of FMF.

The most frequently employed clinical criteria for FMF were established at the Tel-Hashomer Medical Center in Israel[63] and include a schema of major, minor and supportive criteria. These criteria perform well in a number of Middle Eastern populations, with their relatively high pretest probability of FMF and restricted number of founder mutations, but they are still under evaluation in more heterogeneous Western European and North American populations. Moreover, with the advent of DNA testing for *MEFV* mutations, there are patients with inflammatory episodes that do not conform with the Tel Hashomer criteria, but who have two mutant alleles at *MEFV*. These cases broaden the clinical spectrum of *MEFV*-associated illness[18,64] and may eventually lead to a somewhat revised set of clinical criteria.

For patients from high-risk populations with typical clinical manifestations of FMF, the diagnosis can still be made with confidence without the use of DNA studies. Genetic testing, however, can play an important adjunctive role in more heterogeneous populations, particularly for physicians with little experience with this disorder. The finding of two *MEFV* mutations may add certainty to the diagnosis in such a setting, while the absence of any mutations may help refute the diagnosis in a dubious case. However, particularly in those circumstances where only one mutation is found by genetic testing, clinical judgment will continue to have an important place in the diagnosis of FMF.

Treatment

The mainstay of treatment for FMF is daily oral prophylactic colchicine. There is solid evidence that 1–2mg per day of colchicine both prevents the acute inflammatory attacks of FMF[65–67] and the development of systemic amyloidosis[68]. Intermittent dosing at the time of attacks is not nearly as effective in controlling symptoms and there is no evidence that such a regimen prevents amyloidosis. The major limiting toxicities of colchicine are gastrointestinal – diarrhea, cramping and bloating. These side effects can be minimized by starting at a low dose and gradually advancing the dose as tolerated, by dividing the daily dose, by using simethicone for flatulence and by treating the lactose intolerance that can develop. With attention to these details, most adults can tolerate 1.2mg per day and many can tolerate 1.8mg/d. Dosages above 2mg per day are rarely tolerated for prolonged periods. Young children may require lower dosages, but children over the age of 5 years often require the same dose as adults. Colchicine induces a near cessation of FMF attacks in about 70% of patients and provides at least some relief in over 90%.

Rarer side effects of colchicine include bone marrow suppression and a myoneuropathy that is most often seen in elderly adults with renal insufficiency[69]. This latter condition often presents with proximal muscle weakness, an elevated CK and electromyographic changes consistent with polymyositis, and for this reason may initially be misdiagnosed. There are anecdotal reports of male infertility due to colchicine[70], but most men with FMF are able to father children without discontinuing the drug. It should also be noted that there are no controlled studies of sperm count or function before and after starting colchicine and that the amyloidosis of FMF may itself cause testicular dysfunction[71].

There is a slight increase in the risk of trisomy 21 (Down's syndrome) in children born to couples in which either parent has been taking colchicine[72,73]. If the affected parent discontinues the drug through the time of conception, febrile attacks may ensue that diminish opportunities for intercourse and reduce the sperm count in men or induce early miscarriages in women. The risk of developing amyloidosis may also be increased while not taking colchicine. After conception, colchicine at the doses taken for FMF is not teratogenic. Many centers recommend that the prospective parent(s) remain on colchicine throughout conception and pregnancy and that an amniocentesis be performed to rule out Down's syndrome. Of course, the acceptability of this plan depends on how the expectant parents would act on the possible prenatal diagnosis of Down's syndrome, which is a highly personal matter. Colchicine can be found in the breast milk of lactating women with FMF, but at levels that appear to be safe for the infant[74].

Patients taking colchicine should have regular measurements of their blood counts and serum chemistries. Oral colchicine should be continued if possible even in the face of an FMF attack. Patients on daily oral colchicine should not be given intravenous colchicine in the event of an attack, since the concomitant administration of oral and intravenous colchicine is the one setting that has most often been associated with fatal toxicity[75–77].

In FMF patients who already have amyloidosis, intensive treatment with at least 1.5mg of colchicine per day may arrest the progression of amyloid nephropathy[78]. Regardless of the colchicine dose, the prognosis is much worse in patients who already have renal insufficiency. Recent data indicate that the total amyloid burden may be reduced in patients in whom the circulating SAA levels are lowered to normal[79]. In patients who progress to renal failure, renal transplantation confers a better prognosis than chronic hemodialysis. At least 1.5mg of colchicine per day should be given to minimize the risk of amyloid deposition either in the transplanted kidney or other organs[78]. Because colchicine and cyclosporin are metabolized by the same enzyme system in the liver, the concomitant administration of the two drugs raises the risk of toxicity from either one[73].

In patients who have an unsatisfactory response to colchicine or are unable to tolerate the drug, there are unfortunately few alternatives. Corticosteroids are ineffective in either treating or preventing the acute attacks of FMF and there are anecdotal data that they may even accelerate the amyloidosis of FMF. Interferon-α 2B, at a dose of 3 million units subcutaneously, may abort FMF attacks if given at the first sensation of an attack[80]. However, any beneficial effect must be weighed against the transient fever and flu-like syndrome induced by interferon. Moreover, there are no data on the efficacy of interferon in preventing amyloidosis and therefore if interferon is given, it should be used in conjunction with, but not instead of, colchicine.

It should also be noted that certain manifestations or complications of FMF require treatments other than colchicine. Most notably, the protracted febrile myalgia of FMF[35], as well as Henoch–Schönlein purpura, require the use of corticosteroids, and polyarteritis nodosum often requires both corticosteroids and cyclophosphamide.

TNF-RECEPTOR-ASSOCIATED PERIODIC SYNDROME

Background

The TNF receptor-associated periodic syndrome (TRAPS) subsumes those dominantly inherited periodic fevers that are caused by mutations in *TNFRSF1A,* the gene encoding the 55kDa receptor for TNF-α. In contrast with FMF, where there is an evolving relationship between clinical criteria and *MEFV* mutational status, TRAPS was first proposed as a genetic diagnosis. Thus, only those patients with demonstrable TNF-α receptor mutations should be included as cases of TRAPS.

Before this terminology was proposed, there had been a number of case descriptions of dominantly inherited periodic fever in families of diverse ethnic backgrounds. Perhaps the best characterized of these was a large pedigree of Irish-Scottish ancestry first described by Williamson and colleagues in 1982[81] and termed familial Hibernian (Irish) fever (FHF). The inflammatory attacks observed in this family resembled FMF in some respects, including the presence of abdominal pain, pleurisy, joint pain, an accelerated ESR and neutrophilia. However, there were important differences[81,82], including a much longer duration of attacks, migratory areas of erythema, swelling and myalgia, conjunctivitis and periorbital edema, a dominant pattern of inheritance, poor response to colchicine and a relatively prompt response to corticosteroids.

There were a number of other reports of families with similar, although not identical, dominantly inherited periodic fevers. They included a large Australian family of Scottish ancestry denoted benign autosomal dominant familial periodic fever (FPF)[83], as well as smaller families of Swedish, Spanish, German, Finnish, Dutch, Austrian and mixed Irish/English/German ancestry. Although each of these families exhibited dominant inheritance and attacks generally lasting longer than 7 days, there were a number of differences, including ethnicity, the type of skin rash and the presence or absence of systemic amyloidosis. Therefore, it was not clear whether these cases represented a single disease with varying severity and manifestations or completely different disorders.

There were two key breakthroughs that led to the emergence of TRAPS as a unique diagnostic entity. The first was the discovery in 1998 that both FHF and FPF map to the same region of the short arm of chromosome 12 (Refs 83, 84), thus suggesting that mutations at a common locus might account for FHF, FPF and perhaps even some of the other dominant families and laying to rest any possibility that either FHF or FPF is caused by mutations in *MEFV*. Based on this linkage information, genes from the pertinent region of chromosome 12 were screened for disease-associated mutations. Among the possibilities on the transcript map was *TNFRSF1A*, the gene encoding the 55kDa receptor for TNF-α. It was an attractive candidate both because of the central role of TNF-α in inflammation and because of the observation of abnormal levels of soluble 55kDa receptor in patients' blood. Remarkably, in seven families of varied ethnic background, an international team found six different mutations in *TNFRSF1A* that segregated with disease[1]. This second advance led to the proposal of a common nomenclature for families with *TNFRSF1A* mutations. Although historical names such as FHF might still be used to denote individual variants, it seemed likely that perpetuating a classification scheme based on ethnicity might delay appropriate genetic studies for some patients.

The subsequent 3 years have vindicated the concept of TRAPS as a distinct clinical entity with a broad ethnic distribution[85]. Mutations have been reported among patients of African–American, Puerto-Rican, French, Belgian, Dutch, Portuguese, Italian, Arabic, Czech, Mexican, Jewish, German and Finnish background. With these reports, the clinical spectrum of TRAPS has broadened, but a number of common themes have endured.

Clinical features and laboratory findings

Acute attacks

As noted above, an attack duration of greater than 7 days was a common feature of the first families identified with TRAPS. As more cases have been diagnosed and the inventory of mutations has grown from six to 19 at this writing, the usual duration of episodes in TRAPS remains substantially longer than for the other hereditary periodic fevers. However, shorter attacks can occur in TRAPS and the occasional patient may only experience episodes lasting less than 7 days. The interval between attacks in TRAPS, as in FMF, is highly variable between patients and over time in any given patient. Although episodes sometimes develop with no apparent provocation, physical or emotional stress, physical trauma and menses are sometimes associated with attacks; pregnancy may be associated with an amelioration of symptoms. A small minority of patients, most notably with the R92Q mutation, experience waxing and waning symptoms on a nearly daily basis. Fever usually heralds the onset of inflammatory episodes and is sometimes the sole manifestation of TRAPS, especially in children. The median age of onset of TRAPS attacks is 3 years[85].

Pleuritic chest pain and severe abdominal pain, with or without peritoneal signs, occur in TRAPS, as they do in FMF. Early in their disease patients may undergo exploratory laparotomy and it is not unusual for patients to develop peritoneal adhesions, presumably the sequelae of recurrent peritoneal inflammation. Also similar to FMF, symptomatic pericardial involvement is much less common than peritoneal or pleural inflammation. Scrotal pain, presumably due to inflammation of the tunica vaginalis, is another uncommon feature of both illnesses. Arthralgia is more frequent than arthritis in TRAPS. When present, arthritis is usually non-erosive and monoarticular, most frequently involving the hips, knees or ankles. Chronic arthritis of the type seen in FMF has not been observed in TRAPS.

Among the features that distinguish TRAPS from FMF are the characteristic migratory myalgia and rash that are seen at some time in nearly all TRAPS patients. Typically, this occurs as a localized area of cramping muscle pain, often with warmth and tenderness to palpation, and an overlying erythematous, blanchable rash (Fig. 158.4), usually on the torso or the extremities. When it occurs on the limbs, the area of inflammation migrates centrifugally over the course of several days and is often associated with synovitis and effusion as it crosses a joint. Muscle enzymes are not elevated and magnetic resonance imaging demonstrates edema in discrete muscular compartments and intramuscular septa (Fig. 158.5).

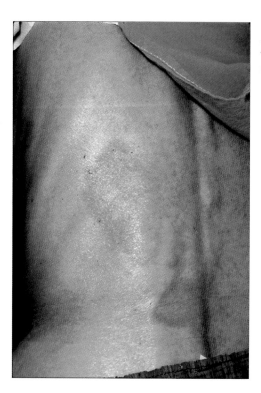

Fig. 158.4 Migratory erythematous lesion on the trunk of a TRAPS patient.

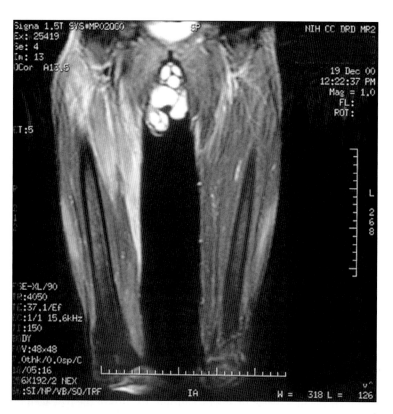

Fig. 158.5 Sagittal view of the proximal thighs of a TRAPS patient using STIR magnetic resonance imaging. The scan demonstrates edematous changes within muscle compartments, intraseptal regions and extending to the skin.

Consistent with the normal muscle enzymes, a recently reported full-thickness biopsy demonstrated predominantly panniculitis, fasciitis and perivascular inflammation, but not involvement of the myofibrils themselves[86]. In the skin there is a superficial and deep perivascular and interstitial infiltrate of lymphocytes and monocytes[87]. It is possible that the centrifugal migration represents propagation along fascial planes.

Ocular involvement is another feature that distinguishes TRAPS from FMF[85]. Approximately 80% of patients experience conjunctivitis, periorbital edema or periorbital pain. Much less commonly, patients may develop iritis or uveitis.

Laboratory investigations

As is the case for FMF, the acute attacks of TRAPS are associated with a neutrophilia and thrombocytosis (particularly in children) and a global acute phase response, including an accelerated ESR and an elevated CRP, SAA, haptoglobin and fibrinogen. Although these parameters may fluctuate with attacks, they often remain elevated even between attacks. Many patients exhibit an anemia of chronic disease, polyclonal hypergammaglobulinemia and low titer IgM and IgG anti-cardiolipin antibodies. The ANA, RF and ANCA are usually negative. When measured, soluble 55kDa TNF-α receptor levels tend to be subnormal between attacks and, in contrast to other inflammatory disorders, increase only modestly during active disease[1].

Systemic amyloidosis

As noted above, systemic amyloidosis was one of the features that was observed in only a subset of the families in the initial description of TRAPS. Amyloidosis was common among the families with the C30R, C52F and C88Y mutations, but was rare or not observed in the families with C33Y, T50M and C88R mutations. A recent analysis of cases followed at the US National Institutes of Health or compiled from the literature found that 14 of 100 patients with TRAPS had evidence of systemic amyloidosis[88]. The series was almost evenly divided between patients with nine different mutations involving cysteine residues and seven non-cysteine mutations, yet 13 of the 14 patients with amyloidosis had cysteine mutations.

As is the case for FMF, the amyloidosis of TRAPS is secondary to the deposition of a presumed cleavage product of SAA (Fig. 158.6) and the tissue distribution of amyloid deposits is similar in the two diseases.

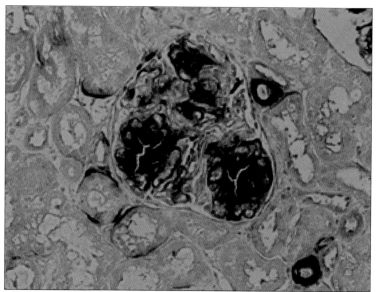

Fig 158.6 Glomerular and vascular amyloid deposition in a renal biopsy specimen from a TRAPS patient. The specimen has been stained with an enzyme-conjugated monoclonal antibody against AA amyloid (×400). Kindly provided by Drs Charles Alpers and James E Balow.

The most frequent complication of TRAPS amyloidosis is renal failure, although hepatic failure has also been observed. All TRAPS patients, but particularly those with cysteine mutations, should undergo regular urinalyses to monitor for albuminuria, an early sign of renal amyloidosis.

Molecular genetics

There are two receptors for the proinflammatory cytokine TNF-α, a 55kDa molecule (p55) encoded by *TNFRSF1A* on chromosome 12p, and a 75kDa receptor (p75) encoded by *TNFRSF1B* on chromosome 1p. The p55 receptor is expressed on most cell types, while expression of the p75 receptor is restricted to leukocytes and endothelial cells. TRAPS is caused by mutations in the p55 receptor; to date there are no known periodic fever patients with mutations in the p75 receptor.

Both TNF-α receptors belong to a family of membrane proteins with repeating cysteine-rich extracellular motifs. By X-ray crystallography, each cysteine-rich domain (CRD) is comprised of a loop structure constrained by three disulfide bonds[89] (Fig. 158.7). The p55 receptor has four of these extracellular CRDs, a transmembrane segment and an intracellular carboxy-terminal death domain (similar in structure to the pyrin domain) that is actually a homotypic interaction motif. All of the 19 currently known mutations[1,88,90–95] in TRAPS are found in the first two CRD, at the amino-terminus of the protein.

Of the first six TRAPS mutations described, five involved substitutions at cysteines involved in disulfide bonds: the substitution of arginine for cysteine at codon 30 (C30R), the substitution of tyrosine

for cysteine at codon 33 (C33Y), the substitution of phenylalanine for cysteine at codon 52 (C52F) and the substitution of either arginine or tyrosine for cysteine at codon 88 (C88R, C88Y). All five of these mutations would disrupt the disulfide bonding of the extracellular portion of p55. The sixth mutation was a substitution of methionine for threonine at codon 50 (T50M), which would disrupt a conserved hydrogen bond in CRD1 (Fig. 158.7).

Figure 158.7 depicts the 19 TRAPS mutations published at the time of this writing. Ten of these mutations are in CRD1 and eight are in CRD2. The nineteenth known mutation is a splicing defect causing a 4 aa insertion in the second loop (L2) of CRD1. Altogether, 11 of the 19 known mutations involve cysteine substitutions, seven are non-cysteine substitutions and one is the aforementioned insertion. As noted above, systemic amyloidosis in TRAPS is seen more frequently in the patients with cysteine substitutions than the other mutations.

Two of these mutations, R92Q (glutamine for arginine at codon 92) and P46L (leucine for proline at codon 46) are seen in about 1% of control chromosomes[88,95], but are found at even higher frequencies among TRAPS patients. Since the frequency of TRAPS does not approach 1% of the population, the penetrance of these mutations (i.e., the probability of having disease if an individual has the mutation) must be low. Overall, the non-cysteine substitutions have a lower penetrance than the cysteine mutations. Patients with R92Q have a wider spectrum of clinical manifestations than other TRAPS patients[85] and this mutation has been observed at increased frequency in a non-TRAPS early arthritis clinic[88], suggesting that R92Q may have a more general role in inflammatory disease.

The dominant inheritance of TRAPS is probably a consequence of the fact that p55 receptors trimerize on the cell surface. Even though patients with TRAPS inherit one normal copy of *TNFRSF1A* and one abnormal copy, assuming that both gene products are found at equal concentrations, 1/8 trimers on the cell surface will comprise only normal p55 molecules, and 7/8 trimers will include at least 1 abnormal p55. If in fact one abnormal receptor is enough to affect the function of the trimer, most of the trimers in a heterozygote would be dysfunctional.

The mechanism by which p55 mutations cause a hyperinflammatory phenotype is still under investigation. At least one probable mechanism is depicted in Figure 158.8. In normal individuals (top), stimulation through TNF-α receptors leads both to the activation of inflammatory cellular pathways and to the metalloprotease-mediated cleavage of the receptors from the cell surface. This is thought to have a negative homeostatic effect on inflammation, both because receptor clearance reduces the chances of repeated stimulation and because shed receptors can bind soluble ligand and thereby act as competitive antagonists. In patients with the C52F *TNFRSF1A* mutation, activation-induced receptor cleavage is markedly diminished, leading to higher levels of membrane p55, lower levels of soluble p55, and impaired homeostasis[1]. This phenomenon has been demonstrated for some but not all TRAPS mutations[2,88], suggesting that additional as yet unknown mechanisms must be operative.

Diagnosis

The diagnosis of TRAPS is established by identifying a mutation in *TNFRSF1A* in a patient with unexplained periodic fever. Because of the large and still-growing number of TRAPS mutations, the preferred method is genomic DNA sequencing. To date all of the TRAPS-associated mutations have been in CRD1 and CRD2, encoded by exons 2–5. Genetic analysis should be considered in patients with unexplained periodic fevers even if there is no family history, because of the phenomenon of reduced penetrance. In fact, at this writing the most common mutation found in newly diagnosed TRAPS patients is R92Q, which is known to have a low penetrance.

It should also be emphasized that TRAPS has been found in many ethnic groups, including those with a high frequency of FMF[88,95].

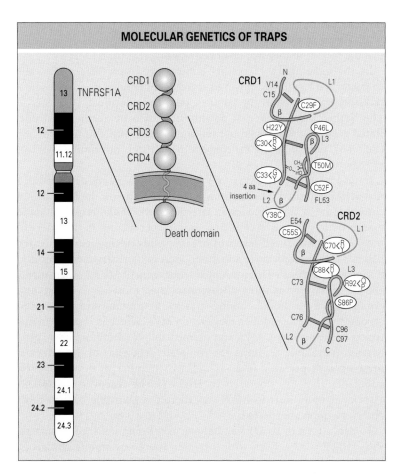

Fig 158.7 Molecular genetics of TRAPS. *TNFRSF1A*, the gene encoding the p55 TNF-α receptor, is located on the distal short arm of chromosome 12. Currently known TRAPS-associated mutations are in the first two (N-terminal) cysteine-rich domains (CRDs). The crystallographically determined structure of the protein is shown on the right. Disulfide bonds are indicated as thick blue lines, and structurally conserved regions of the CRD are represented by thicker lines. Mutations are shown as circled amino acids. Looped domains are denoted as L1–L3, β turns are indicated by β. A regularly updated tabulation of TRAPS mutations can be found on the Internet at http://fmf.igh.cnrs.fr/infevers.

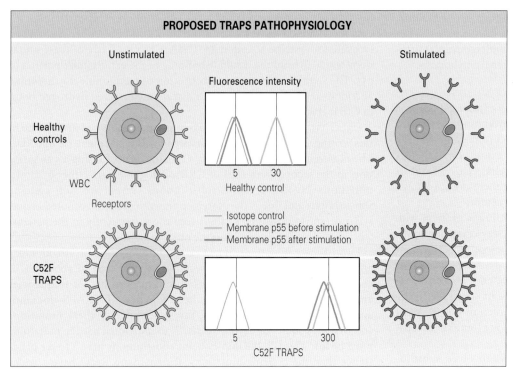

Fig 158.8 Proposed TRAPS pathophysiology. In healthy control individuals (upper panel), p55 TNF-α receptors are shed from the cell surface upon cellular activation. The box in the middle depicts p55 cell surface staining, by flow cytometry, before and after stimulation. In TRAPS patients with the C52F mutation (lower panel), there is an impairment of activation-induced p55 shedding, leading to higher p55 receptor densities on the cell membrane. Flow cytometric analysis shows a minimal left-shift of staining after stimulation. Adapted from Ref. 1.

Although it may be cost-effective to screen periodic fever patients of Mediterranean ancestry for FMF first, those patients who test negative for *MEFV* mutations should be considered for *TNFRSF1A* screening. Some centers perform an initial screen for subnormal soluble p55 levels in the serum. The sensitivity and specificity of this approach, relative to mutational screening, especially for the more recently identified mutations, has not been established.

Treatment

As previously noted, colchicine is ineffective in preventing the febrile attacks of TRAPS and recent data suggest that it does not prevent the development of systemic amyloidosis, either. Corticosteroids can be used to treat the attacks of TRAPS, but patients frequently require escalating dosages with time, often with diminishing efficacy and serious toxicity. Azathioprine, cyclosporin, thalidomide, cyclophosphamide, chlorambucil, intravenous immunoglobulin, dapsone and methotrexate have all been tried empirically but have not been found effective.

Preliminary experience with etanercept, the p75:Fc fusion protein, has been favorable in reducing the frequency and severity of TRAPS attacks[2,85] and a larger dose-escalation study is nearing completion. The efficacy of etanercept in preventing amyloidosis in TRAPS is still under investigation. One patient with the C33Y mutation and amyloidosis was found to have a marked reduction in proteinuria and regression of amyloid as demonstrated on serum amyloid P scanning[96]. However, a different patient with the C52F mutation experienced the new onset of proteinuria, with amyloid on renal biopsy, while taking etanercept[97]. In TRAPS patients at high risk for amyloidosis, it may be appropriate to use SAA levels in the serum to guide therapy.

HYPERIMMUNOGLOBULINEMIA D WITH PERIODIC FEVER SYNDROME

Background

The hyperimmunoglobulinemia D with periodic fever syndrome (HIDS) is a recessively inherited disorder first described in six Dutch patients in 1984[98]. Although these patients manifested some findings that were consistent with FMF, their abdominal pain was less severe than that usually seen in FMF and they had much more significant lymphadenopathy. In addition, they had constant elevations in serum IgD and large numbers of IgD+ plasma cells in the bone marrow, findings not usually seen in FMF. For these reasons van der Meer and colleagues correctly proposed that the condition they had described was different from FMF.

In the ensuing 15 years this clinical syndrome was extensively characterized[99] and was shown to segregate in families as an autosomal recessive trait. Most of the families identified continued to cluster in The Netherlands, France or neighboring areas of northern Europe. Initial genetic studies ruled out linkage to *MEFV* on chromosome 16p (Ref. 100), substantiating the concept that HIDS is not simply a variant of FMF.

In 1999 two independent groups from The Netherlands demonstrated that HIDS is caused by mutations in *MVK*, a gene on the long arm of chromosome 12 that encodes an enzyme in the cholesterol/isoprenoid biosynthetic pathway[8,9]. The first group, specializing in disorders of metabolism, measured levels of organic acids in the urine of Dutch patients with periodic fever and found increased urinary mevalonic acid during febrile crises[8]. This prompted sequencing of *MVK* in the patients and the discovery of three disease-associated mutations. The second group used a positional cloning strategy, first establishing linkage to chromosome 12q24 and then focusing on *MVK*, which is encoded in this region of the genome[9]. *MVK* was deemed an interesting candidate gene because mevalonic aciduria, the complete deficiency of this enzyme, presents with periodic fever as well as a number of developmental anomalies that are not seen in HIDS[101]. The discovery of HIDS-associated mutations in *MVK* was therefore plausible but, to most observers, quite unexpected.

To date a total of 20 *MVK* mutations have been published in patients with HIDS[8,9,102–104]. Even with a greater awareness among clinicians, HIDS remains a relatively rare condition, with a total of 170 patients tabulated in a registry maintained in The Netherlands[105]. In general, elevations in serum IgD and mutations in *MVK* correlate well. However, there are occasional patients with periodic fevers and HIDS-associated *MVK* mutations who have normal IgD levels[8,106] and, conversely, there are somewhat larger numbers of patients with periodic fever and elevated serum IgD and no demonstrable *MVK* mutations (variant-type HIDS)[104,107]. These observations suggest a somewhat more complicated picture than would be predicted by a simple equivalence of HIDS with specific *MVK* mutations[108], raising the possibility that one or more additional HIDS genes or modifiers will eventually be found.

Clinical features and laboratory findings

Acute attacks

Typically, HIDS presents very early in life, with a median age of onset of 6 months[99]. It is not unusual for childhood vaccinations to precipitate febrile episodes. Other provocative factors include infections, emotional stress, trauma and surgery, but in many instances there is no obvious trigger. Patients frequently report some type of premonitory symptoms and the usual attacks of HIDS last approximately 3–7 days, intermediate in length between the typical attacks of FMF and TRAPS. Headache is a frequent but non-specific concomitant of HIDS attacks. As with the other periodic fever syndromes, the attacks are usually not truly periodic, but rather episodic, and the inter-attack interval can vary greatly both between patients and over time for any given patient. With increasing age there is a tendency for the attacks to become less frequent and less severe[99].

Although the abdominal attacks reported in the initial description of HIDS were somewhat less dramatic than those often seen in FMF, the majority of HIDS patients have attacks of abdominal pain, sometimes severe enough to warrant exploratory laparotomy. Unexplained adhesions are sometimes found, consistent with a history of peritoneal inflammation[99]. In contrast with FMF, diarrhea is often seen with HIDS attacks, usually towards the end of the episode. Vomiting is also common. Pleurisy and pericardial involvement are rare in HIDS.

Arthralgia is very common with HIDS episodes and arthritis was documented in nearly 70% of patients in one series[99], with children more frequently affected than adults. Large joints, especially the knees and ankles, tend to be most commonly involved and, in contrast to FMF, HIDS arthritis is often polyarticular, sometimes accompanying abdominal pain. Synovial fluid leukocyte counts are high, with a predominance of granulocytes, but cultures are sterile.

Mucocutaneous lesions are common during HIDS attacks[99,109]. Crops of erythematous macules, ranging from 0.5–2cm in diameter and sometimes affecting the palms and soles, are the most frequent skin manifestation of HIDS (Fig. 158.9). Other dermatologic findings include

erythematous papules and nodules, urticaria, annular erythema and purpura. A large series of HIDS skin biopsies reported swelling of endothelial cells, perivascular edema and mixed cellular perivascular infiltrates[109]. Painful aphthous ulcers of the mouth or vagina are also sometimes seen in HIDS[105].

Diffuse lymphadenopathy is one of the clinical features that is much more common in HIDS than the other hereditary periodic fevers[99,105]. Swelling of the cervical nodes fluctuates with attacks; inguinal, axillary and mesenteric adenopathy may also be present. Histologic examination shows non-specific reactive lymphadenitis. Splenomegaly is also frequently found in children with HIDS.

Laboratory investigations

During their febrile episodes HIDS patients manifest the same vigorous but non-specific acute phase response seen in the other hereditary periodic fevers. This includes acceleration of the ESR and elevation of the CRP, SAA, haptoglobin and fibrinogen. There is also a leukocytosis with left shift. Several cytokines, including interferon-γ, TNF-α and IL-6, are increased in the serum during attacks[110,111]. Urinary neopterin, a marker for cellular immune activation, is also increased during febrile attacks[111]. Urinary mevalonate levels correlate well with HIDS attacks (Fig. 158.10). Autoantibodies are generally not found in HIDS.

Prior to the identification of the underlying gene, measurement of elevated serum IgD (>100IU/ml or >14.1mg/dl) on more than one occasion at least 1 month apart was required for the diagnosis of HIDS[99]. Levels do not fluctuate with attacks, nor do they correlate with overall disease severity between individuals or in a given individual over time. IgA levels (primarily of the IgA1 subclass) are also increased in over 80% of patients with HIDS.

Systemic amyloidosis

In contrast with the other hereditary periodic fevers, amyloidosis has not been reported in HIDS patients[105]. It is not known whether this dichotomy represents some fundamental difference in the pathogenesis of HIDS, reflects a difference in severity of inflammation integrated over time or is simply the result of coincidental differences in amyloid-related environmental or genetic factors stratified in the populations in which HIDS is usually found.

Molecular genetics

There is now abundant evidence that HIDS is caused by recessively inherited mutations in *MVK*, the gene for mevalonate kinase

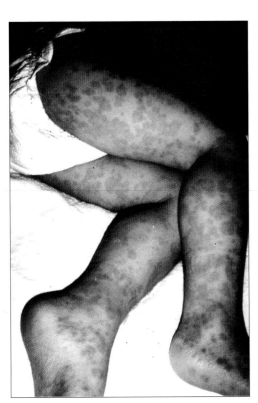

Fig 158.9
Diffuse erythematous maculopapular rash in a young child with HIDS.

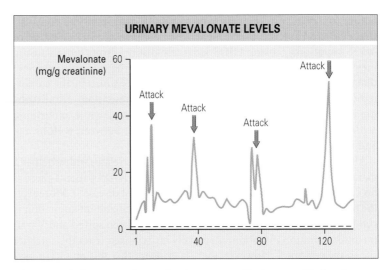

URINARY MEVALONATE LEVELS

Fig 158.10 Urinary mevalonate levels, measured by isotope dilution, in a patient with HIDS, demonstrating a close correlation with clinical symptoms. Kindly provided by Dr Richard I Kelley.

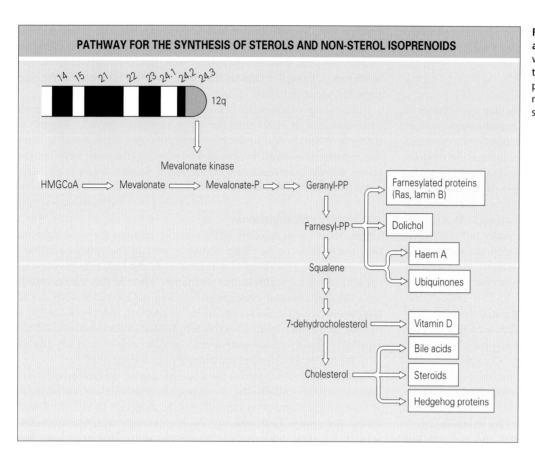

PATHWAY FOR THE SYNTHESIS OF STEROLS AND NON-STEROL ISOPRENOIDS

Fig 158.11 Pathway for the synthesis of sterols and non-sterol isoprenoids. Mevalonate kinase, which is encoded on chromosome 12q, catalyzes the conversion of mevalonate to mevalonate phosphate. In HIDS, activity of this enzyme is reduced. In mevalonic aciduria, which is more severe, enzyme activity is almost absent.

(MK)[8,9,102–104], which catalyzes the conversion of mevalonic acid to 5-phosphomevalonic acid (Fig. 158.11). The first papers reporting the HIDS gene enumerated a total of four missense mutations, one deletion and one null allele. At this writing, a total of 20 HIDS-associated *MVK* mutations, most of them missense substitutions, have been reported in the literature. Nearly all mutation-positive HIDS patients harbor at least one copy of the substitution of isoleucine for valine at codon 377 (V377I)[102,103], and the substitution of threonine for isoleucine at position 268 (I268T) is the second most common mutation[103].

Lymphocytes and fibroblasts from HIDS patients exhibit reduced but not absent MK enzymatic activity. In contrast, patients with the much more severe mevalonic aciduria have almost no residual enzymatic activity. These latter patients experience many of the inflammatory manifestations of HIDS, but also develop dysmorphic facies, cataracts, cerebellar ataxia, cerebral atrophy, mental retardation, hypotonia and failure to thrive[101,112]. Their urinary mevalonic acid levels are constitutively elevated at levels much higher than are seen in HIDS. The set of *MVK* mutations causing HIDS is largely distinct from those causing mevalonic aciduria, although there is some overlap owing to the fact that an individual's MK enzymatic activity is determined by the combination of two mutant alleles. HIDS-associated mutations are distributed throughout the coding region of the gene, while mevalonic aciduria-associated mutations are concentrated between codons 243 and 334[103].

Although the residual MK enzymatic activity correlates with whether a patient has HIDS or mevalonic aciduria, among HIDS patients there is no correlation between MK activity and severity of disease[107]. Moreover, the biochemical connection between MK mutations and inflammation is still unclear. The crystal structure of rat MK has been solved and V377I, the most common mutation, is spatially far removed from the catalytic site of the enzyme[113]. However, there is evidence that this mutation may destabilize the protein and thereby lead to reduced enzyme activity[8]. Cholesterol levels in HIDS patients are usually in the low-normal range, suggesting that unavailability of cholesterol is not the mechanism of

inflammatory episodes[112]. Another unproven possibility is that HIDS mutations decrease the post-translational prenylation of signaling molecules involved in inflammation.

It is unlikely that elevations in IgD itself are the cause of fever and inflammation. Besides the fact that the frequency and severity of attacks do not correlate with IgD levels, there are a number of other conditions, including diabetes mellitus, pregnancy and cigarette smoking, in which IgD levels are modestly increased[99] but there are no symptoms compatible with HIDS.

Diagnosis

Before the discovery of *MVK* mutations, the diagnosis of HIDS was established by the reproducible demonstration of elevated serum IgD in a patient with compatible clinical findings. Based on the genetics and biochemistry of *MVK*, additional approaches are possible: mutational screening, quantitation of urinary mevalonic acid and measurement of MK activity in cultured fibroblasts or leukocytes.

The genomic structure of *MVK* was recently published, which facilitates use of genomic DNA for mutation detection, rather than relying on technically more demanding cDNA assays. Since a large percentage of HIDS patients have at least one copy of either the V377I or I268T mutation, it is cost-effective to screen for these mutations first before undertaking a more comprehensive sequencing effort.

Urinary mevalonate levels can be measured by routine gas chromatography/mass spectroscopy or by isotope dilution methods[106,112]. The former approach is usually sensitive enough to detect the elevations in urinary mevalonate that occur during HIDS attacks. The latter method detects the elevations that are present in HIDS patients between their attacks, but is only available in specialized centers. Enzymatic assay in cultured cells is probably the most technically demanding of these approaches.

In the majority of patients, all of these assays, if performed, would be in agreement. However, as noted above, there are a small number of patients who have *MVK* mutations but normal IgD levels[8,106] and there are a somewhat larger numbers with 'variant-type HIDS' who have increased serum IgD but no *MVK* mutations[104,107,108]. Patients with variant-type HIDS tend to have a negative family history, lower IgD levels, fewer symptoms and lower ESR; it is currently not known if these patients have some other defect in cholesterol/isoprenoid synthesis. Further complicating matters, there can be modest elevations in the serum IgD in a minority of patients with FMF[39,114] and TRAPS[82], as well as some patients with the syndrome of periodic fever, aphthous stomatitis, pharyngitis and cervical adenopathy (PFAPA)[115].

When confronted with a patient with unexplained periodic fever in whom FMF and TRAPS are unlikely or have been ruled out, it is advisable to test the serum IgD in conjunction with either *MVK* mutational analysis or one of the biochemical assays. Patients with definite IgD elevations but normal mutational screens could be classed as variant-type HIDS. There is currently no agreement on a term for patients with *MVK* mutations but normal IgD levels, although some have advocated the term 'Dutch type periodic fever (DPF)' for patients with periodic fever and reduced MK activity, irrespective of the IgD[108]. Patients with elevated IgD levels and evidence for *MVK* mutations and/or MK dysfunction are sometimes called 'classic-type HIDS'[107] and the designation DPF would also apply.

Treatment

There is currently no proven treatment for HIDS. Non-steroidal anti-inflammatory drugs may help control fever and arthralgia. Corticosteroids may help to control attacks in some patients, but long-term toxicity is a major concern, especially in children. There have been mixed results with colchicine, intravenous gamma globulin and cyclosporin[105]. A recent small double-blind crossover trial of thalidomide demonstrated modest decreases in acute phase reactants, without an effect on the attack rate[116]. There is anecdotal evidence that etanercept may be useful in some patients and a trial of 3-hydroxy-3-methylglutaryl (HMG)-coenzyme A reductase inhibitors (statins) is under way[105].

MUCKLE–WELLS SYNDROME

Background

In 1962 two English physicians described a large Derbyshire family in which several members were affected with an apparently new syndrome consisting of episodes of rigors, malaise, limb pains and an urticaria-like skin rash[117]. These 'aguey bouts' were relatively brief, usually lasting 36 hours at most, and were not ameliorated by antihistamines or low doses of corticosteroids. Several members of the family developed nephropathy, with renal amyloidosis proven at autopsy in two, and sensorineural hearing loss developed in association with nephropathy in five members of the family. Although there was some variability in the constellation of findings manifested in individual family members, there was a clear four-generation dominant pattern of inheritance. Over time a number of other similar kindreds, as well as a few sporadic cases, were described with what came to be known as Muckle–Wells syndrome, in recognition of the original describers.

In 1999 a large collaborative group reported the results of a genome-wide search for linkage in a panel of three large families with MWS[118]. The results clearly excluded linkage to chromosomes 16p13, 12p13 or 12q24, where the genes for FMF, TRAPS and HIDS had already been respectively identified. Instead, the causative locus was mapped to a relatively broad region on the distal part of the long arm of chromosome 1. The following year Hoffman and colleagues[119] mapped another dominantly inherited periodic fever, familial cold autoinflammatory syndrome (FCAS, also known as familial cold urticaria) to the same region of chromosome 1, and about 1 year later this group found that both MWS and FCAS are caused by mutations in the same gene[7]. This gene, which they denoted *CIAS1* (cold-induced autoinflammatory syndrome 1), was

screened for mutations in part because it encodes a protein with an N-terminal pyrin domain, as does the FMF protein. The MWS/FCAS protein has been named 'cryopyrin,' to connote its relationship both to cold exposure and to fever, although two other names, PYPAF1 and NALP3, are also found in the literature and sequence databases.

Clinical features and laboratory findings

Acute attacks

Muckle–Wells syndrome attacks have a variable age of onset, ranging from infancy to adolescence, and last from about 12–48 h[117,120]. Some patients give a history that temperature change (cold for some patients, heat for others), fatigue or emotion exacerbates attacks. Besides chills, fever and malaise, attacks are comprised of urticaria-like skin rash (Fig. 158.12), arthralgia, arthritis, aching limb pain and sometimes abdominal pain, conjunctivitis or episcleritis. Lymphadenopathy may also be present.

The rash of MWS is comprised of erythematous geographical plaques ranging from 1–7cm in diameter. They are described as 'aching' but are usually not pruritic. There have only been a few reports of skin biopsies taken from MWS patients, with the histology showing sparse perivascular infiltrates of neutrophils or lymphocytes[121].

Arthralgia is more common than arthritis, but some patients develop transient synovitis with their attacks and, less commonly, persistent neutrophil-rich effusions[122]. Knees and ankles are most frequently involved.

As with the other periodic fevers, there is an acute phase response during febrile episodes, but many patients have evidence of ongoing inflammation, with an accelerated ESR, even between attacks. Persistent hypergammaglobulinemia is also common. Fluctuations in serum IL-6 levels with attacks have been documented in one patient[123].

Sensorineural hearing loss

In a compilation of 78 cases of MWS, 55 (70%) had progressive sensorineural hearing loss[120]. Audiography demonstrates a downsloping curve when the hearing level is plotted against tonal frequency, with the air and bone conduction giving nearly identical results (Fig. 158.13). Postmortem examinations in the original MWS family showed absence of the organ of Corti and vestibular sensory epithelium, atrophy of the cochlear nerve and ossification of the basilar membrane, but no amyloidosis in the inner ear[117].

Amyloidosis

Systemic amyloidosis has been observed in about one quarter of cases of MWS and is not required for the diagnosis[120]. Most cases develop in

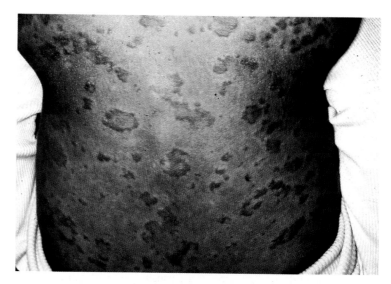

Fig 158.12 Urticarial skin rash in a patient with Muckle–Wells syndrome.

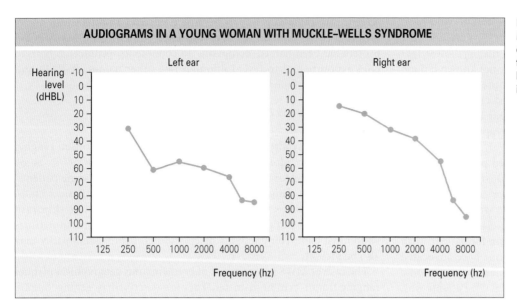

AUDIOGRAMS IN A YOUNG WOMAN WITH MUCKLE–WELLS SYNDROME

Fig 158.13 Audiograms in a young woman with Muckle–Wells syndrome, demonstrating markedly downsloping hearing levels with increasing frequency. Consistent with sensorineural hearing loss, air conduction and bone conduction are nearly identical.

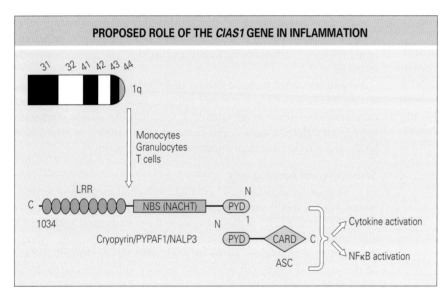

PROPOSED ROLE OF THE *CIAS1* GENE IN INFLAMMATION

Fig 158.14 Proposed role of the *CIAS1* gene in inflammation. *CIAS1*, the gene for both Muckle–Wells syndrome and familial cold autoinflammatory syndrome, is encoded on chromosome 1q. It encodes cryopyrin, a 1034 aa protein with an N-terminal pyrin domain (PYD) as well as a nucleotide binding site domain (NBS, NACHT subtype) and a leucine-rich repeat domain (LRR). Cryopyrin binds ASC through homotypic interactions at their PYD, leading to NFκB activation.

middle age. Deposits occur in the kidneys, adrenals, spleen and testes and, consistent with this distribution, the deposits are comprised of AA fibrils.

Molecular genetics

CIAS1, the gene that is mutated in both MWS and FCAS, is encoded on chromosome 1q44 and expressed in monocytes, granulocytes and T cells[7,124]. The protein product, variously named cryopyrin, PYPAF1 and NALP3, has a number of alternative splice forms, the largest of which consists of 1034 aa with a predicted size of 118kDa without post-translational modifications. Cryopyrin has three distinct motifs: an N-terminal pyrin domain (PYD), a nucleotide-binding site (NBS, NACHT subfamily) and a leucine-rich repeat (LRR) region. Cryopyrin is one of over 20 newly discovered PYD proteins, which have been implicated in regulating the activation of NFκB, cytokine processing and apoptosis. Recent functional studies indicate that cryopyrin binds the adaptor protein ASC through homotypic PYD interactions, leading to activation of NFκB and cytokines (Fig. 158.14)[124].

Diagnosis

Until late 2001, the diagnosis of MWS was purely clinical, based on the presence of typical febrile episodes. The presence of sensorineural hearing loss, while not required, greatly increases diagnostic confidence.

The identification of *CIAS1* now raises the possibility of genetic diagnosis. At this writing it is still too early to know whether most patients with clinical MWS will have *CIAS1* mutations or whether *CIAS1* mutations may also be found in patients with unexplained arthritis, rash, hearing loss or amyloidosis, who would not completely fit the clinical diagnosis of MWS.

Treatment

In some patients colchicine[118] or high dose corticosteroids may attenuate MWS attacks. It is unknown whether these agents prevent either the hearing loss or amyloidosis associated with this disorder.

FAMILIAL COLD AUTOINFLAMMATORY SYNDROME

Background

In 1940 Kile and Rusk reported a 47 member pedigree, 23 of whom exhibited a dominantly inherited form of cold urticaria[125]. Typically, in cold weather the affected members of this family developed urticaria within 30 min to 1 hour of going outdoors. Other concomitant symptoms included fever, chills, headache and joint stiffness. The duration of attacks ranged from 6–8 hours to 48 hours, depending on the degree of cold exposure. In the propositus case, experimental immersion of the arm in a 50°F (10°C) water bath caused pain and erythema within 2 minutes, with urticaria appearing 4 hours later.

About 20 families have been reported in the literature with similar findings and the disorder has variously been called familial cold urticaria, familial polymorphous cold eruption, cold hypersensitivity, cold pathergy and cold-specific vasomotor neuropathy. The nomenclature used here, FCAS, was proposed by the group that mapped and cloned the underlying gene[7,126]. This term recognizes the fact that the rash is not true urticaria (mast cells are not part of the dermal infiltrate and tissue histamine levels are normal) and emphasizes the systemic autoinflammatory nature of the illness. In 95% of patients, the age of onset is within the first 6 months of life[126].

As noted in the MWS section, *CIAS1* is mutated in both FCAS and MWS. Early in a genome-wide scan for the FCAS susceptibility locus, Hoffman and colleagues established linkage to chromosome 1q44, the same region that had already been implicated in MWS[119]. The following year, this group identified *CIAS1* by positional cloning and demonstrated that the gene encodes a new member of the pyrin family of proteins[7].

Clinical features and laboratory findings
Acute attacks
A recent analysis of six American FCAS families, comprised of 45 affected and 68 unaffected members, found that rash was the most common feature of acute episodes, occurring in 100% of affected individuals[126]. Other findings included arthralgia (96%), fever and chills (93%), conjunctivitis (84%), profuse sweating (78%), drowsiness (67%), headache (58%), extreme thirst (53%) and nausea (51%).

In this study the average duration of cold exposure required to provoke an attack was 52 minutes, although at colder temperatures shorter exposures were required, and the severity of symptoms was proportionate to the length and degree of cold exposure. The delay of symptoms after cold exposure averaged 2.5 hours and the mean duration of attacks was 12 hours, with a range of up to 72 hours. Symptoms tended to be worse in the evening, often with resolution by the morning. Patients had a diurnal variation in minor symptoms nearly every day, with superimposed cold-induced exacerbations. Neither consumption of cold beverages nor localized exposure to cold (such as holding an ice cube to the skin) provokes attacks.

The rash of FCAS usually begins on the extremities or face and generalizes to the remainder of the body over the course of the episode. It should be emphasized that the rash occurs both on cold-exposed areas and areas of the skin that are covered by clothing. Skin biopsy during an attack demonstrates an intense polymorphonuclear leukocyte infiltrate, with moderate edema in the upper dermis. The infiltrate includes neutrophils, eosinophils and lymphocytes and is concentrated around the walls of dilated capillaries. Vasculitis is not present.

Polyarthralgia is often severe, most commonly affecting the hands (88%), knees (68%) and ankles (54%). Frank arthritis is rare, but myalgia may occur. Ocular findings include red eyes, increased watering, blurred vision and pain. Periorbital edema appears to be uncommon.

Hearing loss, amyloidosis
Hearing loss is not a feature of FCAS. Systemic amyloidosis is rare, but has been reported, in FCAS. Several members of a large Indian family with an MWS/FCAS overlap have developed amyloidosis; the susceptibility locus in this family also maps to chromosome 1q44, and recently a missense mutation in *CIAS1* was identified in affected members of the family[127].

Laboratory findings
During their attacks FCAS patients often have a marked polymorphonuclear leukocytosis, with white counts sometimes exceeding 30 000/mm³. The ESR is accelerated and the CRP, haptoglobin and other acute phase reactants are also elevated. Serum IL-6 and granulocyte colony-stimulating factor levels are reportedly elevated during attacks. Kinins, histamine and other mast-cell mediator levels are normal and neither cold agglutinins nor cryoglobulins are present.

Molecular genetics
Mutations in *CIAS1*, which is encoded on chromosome 1q44 and expressed in monocytes, granulocytes and T cells, cause both MWS and FCAS[7]. Of the four reported missense mutations in this gene, three segregate in families with FCAS. Additional details on this gene and its protein product are summarized in the MWS section above.

Diagnosis
Clinical criteria for FCAS have recently been proposed[126] and include:

- recurrent intermittent episodes of fever and rash following generalized cold exposure
- autosomal dominant pattern of inheritance

TABLE 158.2 COMPARISON OF FAMILIAL COLD AUTOINFLAMMATORY SYNDROME WITH ACQUIRED COLD URTICARIA

	Familial cold autoinflammatory syndrome	Acquired cold urticaria
Inheritance	Autosomal dominant	Sporadic
Age of onset	Infancy, early childhood	Usually adulthood
Prognosis	Lifelong episodes	Spontaneous resolution in months to years
Type of cold exposure required to provoke an attack	Generalized cold exposure	Localized (ice cube diagnostic test)
Delay of symptoms after cold exposure	~2.5h	Minutes
Duration of symptoms	30min–72h	Minutes to several hours
Rash	Maculopapular rash with perivascular infiltrate of polymorphonuclear leukocytes	Urticaria, with mast cells present
Other symptoms during attacks	Fever, arthralgia, conjunctivitis	Angioedema, wheezing, hypotension
Laboratory findings	Polymorphonuclear leukocytosis	Increased serum histidine

Adapted from Ref. 126.

- age of onset <6 months
- duration of attacks <24 hours
- conjunctivitis associated with attacks
- absence of deafness, periorbital edema, lymphadenopathy and serositis.

Besides the other hereditary periodic fevers, the major diagnostic consideration is acquired cold urticaria (ACU). Features that distinguish FCAS from ACU are summarized in Table 158.2.

With the discovery of *CIAS1* mutations in FCAS, molecular diagnosis is also possible. At this writing genetic testing has been available for too short a time to compare clinical and genetic diagnosis of FCAS. At least some *CIAS1* mutations appear to be associated with more than one clinical entity[128–130].

Treatment

There is currently no consistently effective treatment for FCAS[126]. Non-steroidal anti-inflammatory drugs have a modest effect, particularly on arthralgia. High dose corticosteroids are effective in some patients, but carry with them side effects that many find unacceptable. Gold salts and anabolic steroids have been beneficial in some patients, but colchicine appears not to be effective in preventing the attacks of FCAS.

Note added in proof

Recently two independent groups have found *CIAS1* mutations in patients with a third autoinflammatory disorder that is variously called chronic infantile neurologic cutaneous and articular (CINCA) syndrome or neonatal onset multisystem inflammatory disease (NOMID)[129,130].

REFERENCES

1. McDermott MF, Aksentijevich I, Galon J et al. Germline mutations in the extracellular domains of the 55kDa TNF receptor, TNFR1, define a family of dominantly inherited autoinflammatory syndromes. Cell 1999; 97: 133–144.
2. Galon J, Aksentijevich I, McDermott MF et al. TNFRSF1A mutations and autoinflammatory syndromes. Curr Opin Immunol 2000; 12: 479–486.
3. Pras E, Aksentijevich I, Gruberg L et al. Mapping of a gene causing familial Mediterranean fever to the short arm of chromosome 16. N Engl J Med 1992; 326: 1509–1513.
4. International FMF Consortium. Ancient missense mutations in a new member of the RoRet gene family are likely to cause familial Mediterranean fever. Cell 1997; 90: 797–807.
5. French FMF Consortium. A candidate gene for familial Mediterranean fever. Nature Genet 1997; 17: 25–31.
6. Fairbrother WJ, Gordon NC, Humke EW et al. The PYRIN domain: a member of the death domain-fold superfamily. Protein Sci 2001; 10: 1911–1918.
7. Hoffman HM, Mueller JL, Broide DH et al. Mutation of a new gene encoding a putative pyrin-like protein causes familial cold autoinflammatory syndrome and Muckle–Wells syndrome. Nature Genet 2001; 29: 301–305.
8. Houten SM, Kuis W, Duran M et al. Mutations in MVK, encoding mevalonate kinase, cause hyperimmunoglobulinaemia D and periodic fever syndrome. Nature Genet 1999; 22: 175–177.
9. Drenth JPH, Cuisset L, Grateau G et al. Mutations in the gene encoding mevalonate kinase cause hyper-IgD and periodic fever syndrome. Nature Genet 1999; 22: 178–181.
10. Hugot J-P, Chamaillard M, Zouali H et al. Association of NOD2 leucine-rich repeat variants with susceptibility to Crohn's disease. Nature 2001; 411: 599–603.
11. Ogura Y, Bonen DK, Inohara N et al. A frameshift mutation in NOD2 associated with susceptibility to Crohn's disease. Nature 2001; 411: 603–606.
12. Miceli-Richard C, Lesage S, Rybojad M et al. CARD15 mutations in Blau syndrome. Nature Genet 2001; 29: 19–20.
13. Janeway TC, Mosenthal HO. An unusual paroxysmal syndrome, probably allied to recurrent vomiting, with a study of the nitrogen metabolism. Trans Assoc Am Phys 1908; 23: 504–518.
14. Siegal S. Benign paroxysmal peritonitis. Ann Intern Med 1945; 23: 1–21.
15. Mamou H, Cattan R. La maladie périodique (sur 14 cas personnels dont 8 compliqués de néphropathies). Semin Hop Paris 1952; 28: 1062–1070.
16. Heller H, Sohar E, Sherf L. Familial Mediterranean fever. Arch Int Med 1958; 102: 50–71.
17. Sohar E, Gafni J, Pras M, Heller H. Familial Mediterranean fever. A survey of 470 cases and review of the literature. Am J Med 1967; 43: 227–253.
18. Samuels J, Aksentijevich I, Torosyan Y et al. Familial Mediterranean fever at the millennium: clinical spectrum, ancient mutations, and a survey of 100 American referrals to the National Institutes of Health. Medicine (Baltimore) 1998; 77: 268–297.
19. Aksentijevich I, Torosyan Y, Samuels et al. Mutation and haplotype studies of familial Mediterranean fever reveal new ancestral relationships and evidence for a high carrier frequency with reduced penetrance in the Ashkenazi Jewish population. Am J Hum Genet 1999; 64: 949–962.
20. Booth DR, Gillmore JD, Lachmann HJ et al. The genetic basis of autosomal dominant familial Mediterranean fever. QJM 2000; 93: 217–221.
21. Schwabe AD, Peters RS. Familial Mediterranean fever in Armenians. Analysis of 100 cases. Medicine (Baltimore) 1974; 53: 453–462.
22. Majeed HA, Rawashdeh M, el-Shanti H et al. Familial Mediterranean fever in children: the expanded clinical profile. QJM 1999; 92: 309–318.
23. Yuval Y, Hemo-Zisser M, Zemer D et al. Dominant inheritance in two families with familial Mediterranean fever (FMF). Am J Med Genet 1995; 57: 455–457.
24. Zimand S, Tauber T, Hegesch T, Aladjem M. Familial Mediterranean fever presenting with massive cardiac tamponade. Clin Exp Rheumatol 1994; 12: 67–69.
25. Kees S, Langevitz P, Zemer D et al. Attacks of pericarditis as a manifestation of familial Mediterranean fever (FMF). QJM 1997; 90: 643–647.
26. Heller H, Gafni J, Michaeli D et al. The arthritis of familial Mediterranean fever (FMF). Arthritis Rheum 1966; 9: 1–17.
27. Pras E, Langevitz P, Livneh A et al. Genotype-phenotype correlation in familial Mediterranean fever (a preliminary report). In: Sohar E, Gafni J, Pras M, eds. Familial Mediterranean fever. First international conference. London: Freund; 1997: 260–264.
28. Dewalle M, Domingo C, Rozenbaum M et al. Phenotype-genotype correlation in Jewish patients suffering from familial Mediterranean fever (FMF). Eur J Hum Genet 1998; 6: 95–97.
29. Brik R, Shinawi M, Kepten I et al. Familial Mediterranean fever: clinical and genetic characterization in a mixed pediatric population of Jewish and Arab patients. Pediatrics 1999; 103: 70.
30. Cazeneuve C, Sarkisian T, Pêcheux C et al. MEFV-gene analysis in Armenian patients with familial Mediterranean fever: diagnostic value and unfavorable renal prognosis of the M694V homozygous genotype – genetic and therapeutic implications. Am J Hum Genet 1999; 65: 88–97.
31. Sneh E, Pras M, Michaeli D et al. Protracted arthritis in familial Mediterranean fever. Rheumatol Rehabil 1977; 16: 102–106.
32. Langevitz P, Livneh A, Zemer D et al. Seronegative spondyloarthropathy in familial Mediterranean fever. Semin Arthritis Rheum 1997; 27: 67–72.
33. Azizi E, Fisher BK. Cutaneous manifestations of familial Mediterranean fever. Arch Dermatol 1976; 112: 364–366.
34. Barzilai A, Langevitz P, Goldberg I et al. Erysipelas-like erythema of familial Mediterranean fever: clinicopathologic correlation. J Am Acad Dermatol 2000; 42: 791–795.
35. Langevitz P, Zemer D, Livneh A et al. Protracted febrile myalgia in patients with familial Mediterranean fever. J Rheumatol 1994; 21: 1708–1709.
36. Livneh A, Madgar I, Langevitz P, Zemer D. Recurrent episodes of acute scrotum with ischemic testicular necrosis in a patient with familial Mediterranean fever. J Urol 1994; 151: 431–432.
37. Gedalia A, Zamir S. Neurologic manifestations in familial Mediterranean fever. Pediatr Neurol 1993; 9: 301–302.
38. Eliakim M, Levy M, Ehrenfeld M. Recurrent polyserositis (familial Mediterranean fever, periodic disease). Amsterdam: Elsevier North-Holland; 1981: 87–95.
39. Medlej-Hashim M, Petit I, Adib S et al. Familial Mediterranean fever: association of elevated IgD plasma levels with specific MEFV mutations. Eur J Hum Genet 2001; 9: 849–854.
40. Tunca M, Kirkali G, Soytürk M et al. Acute phase response and evolution of familial Mediterranean fever. Lancet 1999; 353: 1415.
41. Ozen S, Ben-Chetrit E, Bakkaloglu A et al. Polyarteritis nodosa in patients with familial Mediterranean fever (FMF): a concomitant disease or a feature of FMF? Semin Arthritis Rheum 2001; 30: 281–187.
42. Pras M, Bronshpigel N, Zemer D, Gafni J. Variable incidence of amyloidosis in familial Mediterranean fever among different ethnic groups. Johns Hopkins Med J 1982; 150: 22–26.
43. Shohat M, Magal N, Shohat T et al. Phenotype–genotype correlation in familial Mediterranean fever: evidence for an association between Met694Val and amyloidosis. Eur J Hum Genet 1999; 7: 287–292.
44. Livneh A, Langevitz P, Shinar Y et al. MEFV mutation analysis in patients suffering from amyloidosis of familial Mediterranean fever. Amyloid 1999; 6: 1–6.
45. Ben-Chetrit E, Backenroth R. Amyloidosis induced, end stage renal disease in patients with familial Mediterranean fever is highly associated with point mutations in the MEFV gene. Ann Rheum Dis 2001; 60: 146–149.
46. Grateau G. The relation between familial Mediterranean fever and amyloidosis. Curr Opin Rheumatol 2000; 12: 61–64.
47. Akar N, Akar E, Yalçinkaya F. E148Q of the MEFV gene causes amyloidosis in familial Mediterranean fever patients. Pediatrics 2001; 108: 215.
48. Cazeneuve C, Ajrapetyan H, Papin S et al. Identification of MEFV-independent modifying genetic factors for familial Mediterranean fever. Am J Hum Genet 2000; 67: 1136–1143.
49. Blum A, Sohar E. The diagnosis of amyloidosis. Ancillary procedures. Lancet 1962; 1: 721–724.
50. Tishler M, Pras M, Yaron M. Abdominal fat tissue aspirate in amyloidosis of familial Mediterranean fever. Clin Exp Rheumatol 1988; 6: 395–397.

51. Centola M, Wood G, Frucht DM *et al.* The gene for familial Mediterranean fever, *MEFV*, is expressed in early leukocyte development and is regulated in response to inflammatory mediators. Blood 2000; 95: 3223–3231.
52. Mansfield E, Chae JJ, Komarow HD *et al.* The familial Mediterranean fever protein, pyrin, associates with microtubules and colocalizes with actin filaments. Blood 2001; 98: 851–859.
53. Papin S, Duquesnoy P, Cazeneuve C *et al.* Alternative splicing at the MEFV locus involved in familial Mediterranean fever regulates translocation of the marenostrin/pyrin protein to the nucleus. Hum Mol Genet 2000; 9: 3001–3009.
54. Kastner DL, O'Shea JJ. A fever gene comes in from the cold. Nature Genet 2001; 29: 241–242.
55. Richards N, Schaner P, Diaz A *et al.* Interaction between pyrin and the apoptotic speck protein (ASC) modulates ASC-induced apoptosis. J Biol Chem 2001; 276: 39320–39329.
56. Touitou I. The spectrum of familial Mediterranean fever (FMF) mutations. Eur J Hum Genet 2001; 9: 473–483.
57. Bernot A, da Silva C, Petit J-L *et al.* Non-founder mutations in the *MEFV* gene establish this gene as the cause of familial Mediterranean fever (FMF). Hum Mol Genet 1998; 7: 1317–1325.
58. Stoffman N, Magal N, Shohat T *et al.* Higher than expected carrier rates for familial Mediterranean fever in various Jewish ethnic groups. Eur J Hum Genet 2000; 8: 307–310.
59. Kogan A, Shinar Y, Lidar M *et al.* Common *MEFV* mutations among Jewish ethnic groups in Israel: high frequency of carrier and phenotype III states and absence of a perceptible biological advantage for the carrier state. Am J Med Genet 2001; 102: 272–276.
60. Touitou I, Magne X, Molinari N *et al.* MEFV mutations in Behçet's disease. Hum Mutat 2000; 16: 271–272.
61. Cattan D, Notarnicola C, Molinari N, Touitou I. Inflammatory bowel disease in non-Ashkenazi Jews with familial Mediterrranean fever. Lancet 2000; 355: 378–379.
62. Booth DR, Lachmann HJ, Gillmore JD *et al.* Prevalence and significance of the familial Mediterranean fever gene mutation encoding pyrin Q148. QJM 2001; 94: 527–531.
63. Livneh A, Langevitz P, Zemer D *et al.* Criteria for the diagnosis of familial Mediterranean fever. Arthritis Rheum 1997; 40: 1879–1885.
64. Grateau G, Pêcheux C, Cazeneuve C *et al.* Clinical versus genetic diagnosis of familial Mediterranean fever. QJM 2000; 93: 223–229.
65. Zemer D, Revach M, Pras M *et al.* A controlled trial of colchicine in preventing attacks of familial Mediterranean fever. N Engl J Med 1974; 291: 932–934.
66. Dinarello CA, Wolff SM, Goldfinger SE *et al.* Colchicine therapy for familial Mediterranean fever. A double-blind trial. N Engl J Med 1974; 291: 934–937.
67. Goldstein RC, Schwabe AD. Prophylactic colchicine therapy for familial Mediterranean fever. A controlled, double-blind study. Ann Intern Med 1974; 81: 792–794.
68. Zemer D, Pras M, Sohar E *et al.* Colchicine in the prevention and treatment of the amyloidosis of familial Mediterrranean fever. N Engl J Med 1986; 314: 1001–1005.
69. Kuncl RW, Duncan G, Watson D *et al.* Colchicine myopathy and neuropathy. N Engl J Med 1987; 316: 1562–1568.
70. Ehrenfeld M, Levy M, Margalioth EJ, Eliakim M. The effects of long-term colchicine therapy on male fertility in patients with familial Mediterranean fever. Andrologia 1986; 18: 420–426.
71. Ben-Chetrit E, Backenroth R, Haimov-Kochman R, Pizov G. Azoospermia in familial Mediterranean fever patients: the role of colchicine and amyloidosis. Ann Rheum Dis 1998; 57: 259–260.
72. Ferreira NR, Buoniconti A. Trisomy after colchicine therapy. Lancet 1968; 2: 1304.
73. Ben-Chetrit E, Levy M. Colchicine: 1998 update. Semin Arthritis Rheum 1998; 28: 48–59.
74. Ben-Chetrit E, Scherrmann J-M, Levy M. Colchicine in breast milk of patients with familial Mediterranean fever. Arthritis Rheum 1996; 39: 1213–1217.
75. Putterman C, Ben-Chetrit E, Caraco Y, Levy M. Colchicine intoxication: clinical pharmacology, risk factors, features, and management. Semin Arthritis Rheum 1991; 21: 143–155.
76. Simons RJ, Kingma DW. Fatal colchicine toxicity. Am J Med 1989; 86: 356–357.
77. Wallace SL, Singer JZ. Review: systemic toxicity associated with the intravenous administration of colchicine. Guidelines for use. J Rheumatol 1988; 15: 495–499.
78. Livneh A, Zemer D, Langevitz P *et al.* Colchicine treatment of AA amyloidosis of familial Mediterranean fever. An analysis of factors affecting outcome. Arthritis Rheum 1994; 37: 1804–1811.
79. Gillmore JD, Lovat LB, Persey MR *et al.* Amyloid load and clinical outcome in AA amyloidosis in relation to circulating concentration of serum amyloid A protein. Lancet 2001; 358: 24–29.
80. Tunca M, Tankurt E, Akbaylar Akpinar H *et al.* The efficacy of interferon alpha on colchicine-resistant familial Mediterranean fever attacks: a pilot study. Br J Rheumatol 1997; 36: 1005–1008.
81. Williamson LM, Hull D, Mehta R *et al.* Familial Hibernian fever. QJM 1982; 51: 469–480.
82. McDermott EM, Smillie DM, Powell RJ. Clinical spectrum of familial Hibernian fever: a 14-year follow-up study of the index case and extended family. Mayo Clin Proc 1997; 72: 806–817.
83. Mulley J, Saar K, Hewitt G *et al.* Gene localization for an autosomal dominant familial periodic fever to 12p13. Am J Hum Genet 1998; 62: 884–889.
84. McDermott MF, Ogunkolade BW, McDermott EM *et al.* Linkage of familial Hibernian fever to chromosome 12p13. Am J Hum Genet 1998; 62: 1446–1451.
85. Hull KM, Drewe E, Aksentijevich I *et al.* TNF receptor-associated periodic syndrome: emerging concepts of an autoinflammatory disorder. Medicine 2002; 81: 349–368.
86. Hull KM, Wong K, Wood GM *et al.* Monocytic fasciitis: a new clinical feature of TNF receptor dysfunction. Arthritis Rheum 2002; 46: 2189–2194.
87. Toro JR, Aksentijevich I, Hull K *et al.* Tumor necrosis factor receptor-associated periodic syndrome: a novel syndrome with cutaneous manifestations. Arch Dermatol 2000; 136: 1487–1494.
88. Aksentijevich I, Galon J, Soares M *et al.* The tumor-necrosis-factor receptor-associated periodic syndrome: new mutations in *TNFRSF1A*, ancestral origins, genotype-phenotype studies, and evidence for further genetic heterogeneity of periodic fevers. Am J Hum Genet 2001; 69: 301–314.
89. Banner DW, D'Arcy A, Janes W *et al.* Crystal structure of the soluble human 55 kD TNF receptor-human TNFβ complex: implications for TNF receptor activation. Cell 1993; 73: 431–445.
90. Dodé C, Papo T, Fieschi C *et al.* A novel missense mutation (C30S) in the gene encoding tumor necrosis factor receptor 1 linked to autosomal dominant recurrent fever with localized myositis in a French family. Arthritis Rheum 2000; 43: 1535–1542.
91. Aganna E, Aksentijevich I, Hitman GA *et al.* Tumor necrosis factor receptor-associated periodic syndrome (TRAPS) in a Dutch family: evidence for a *TNFRSF1A* mutation with reduced penetrance. Eur J Hum Genet 2001; 9: 63–66.
92. Jadoul M, Dodé C, Cosyns J-P *et al.* Autosomal-dominant periodic fever with AA amyloidosis: novel mutation in tumor necrosis factor receptor 1 gene. Kidney Int 2001; 59: 1677–1682.
93. Simon A, Dodé C, van der Meer JWM, Drenth JPH. Familial periodic fever and amyloidosis due to a new mutation in the *TNFRSF1A* gene. Am J Med 2001; 110: 313–316.
94. Simon A, van Deuren M, Tighe PJ *et al.* Genetic analysis as a valuable key to diagnosis and treatment of periodic fever. Arch Intern Med 2001; 161: 2491–2493.
95. Aganna E, Zeharia A, Hitman GA *et al.* An Israeli Arab patient with a de novo *TNFRSF1A* mutation causing tumor necrosis factor receptor-associated periodic syndrome. Arthritis Rheum 2002; 46: 245–249.
96. Drewe E, McDermott EM, Powell RJ. Treatment of the nephrotic syndrome with etanercept in patients with the tumor necrosis factor receptor-associated periodic syndrome. N Engl J Med 2000; 343: 1044–1045.
97. Hull KM, Kastner DL, Balow JE. Hereditary periodic fever. N Engl J Med 2002; 346: 1415.
98. van der Meer JWM, Vossen JM, Radl J *et al.* Hyperimmunoglobulinaemia D and periodic fever: a new syndrome. Lancet 1984; 1: 1087–1090.
99. Drenth JPH, Haagsma CJ, van der Meer JWM. International Hyper-IgD Study Group. Hyperimmunoglobulinemia D and periodic fever syndrome. The clinical spectrum in a series of 50 patients. Medicine (Baltimore) 1994; 73: 133–144.
100. Drenth JPH, Mariman ECM, van der Velde-Visser SD *et al.* Hyper-IgD Study Group. Location of the gene causing hyperimmunoglobulinemia D and periodic fever syndrome differs from that for familial Mediterranean fever. Human Genet 1994; 94: 616–620.
101. Hoffmann G, Gibson KM, Brandt IK *et al.* Mevalonic aciduria – an inborn error of cholesterol and nonsterol isoprene biosynthesis. N Engl J Med 1986;314: 1610–1614.
102. Houten SM, Koster J, Romeijn G-J *et al.* Organization of the mevalonate kinase (*MVK*) gene and identification of novel mutations causing mevalonic aciduria and hyperimmunoglobulinaemia D and periodic fever syndrome. Eur J Hum Genet 2001; 9: 253–259.
103. Cuisset L, Drenth JPH, Simon A *et al.* Molecular analysis of *MVK* mutations and enzymatic activity in hyper-IgD and periodic fever syndrome. Eur J Hum Genet 2001; 9: 260–266.
104. Frenkel J, Houten SM, Waterham HR *et al.* Clinical and molecular variability in childhood periodic fever with hyperimmunoglobulinaemia D. Rheumatology 2001; 40: 579–584.
105. Drenth JPH, van der Meer JWM. Hereditary periodic fever. N Engl J Med 2001; 345: 1748–1757.
106. Kelley RI, Takada K, Aksentijevich I. Hereditary periodic fever. N Engl J Med 2002; 346: 1416.
107. Simon A, Cuisset L, Vincent M-F *et al.* for the International HIDS Study Group. Molecular analysis of the mevalonate kinase gene in a cohort of patients with the hyper-IgD and periodic fever syndrome: its application as a diagnostic tool. Ann Intern Med 2001; 135: 338–343.
108. Frenkel J, Houten SM, Waterham HR *et al.* Mevalonate kinase deficiency and Dutch type periodic fever. Clin Exp Rheumatol 2000; 18: 525–532.
109. Drenth JPH, Boom BW, Toonstra J, van der Meer JWM and the International Hyper IgD Study Group. Cutaneous manifestations and histologic findings in the hyperimmunoglobulinemia D syndrome. Arch Dermatol 1994; 130: 59–65.
110. Drenth JPH, van Deuren M, van der Ven-Jongekrijg J *et al.* Cytokine activation during attacks of the hyperimmunoglobulinemia D and periodic fever syndrome. Blood 1995; 85: 3586–3593.
111. Drenth JPH, Powell RJ, Brown NS, van der Meer JWM. Interferon-γ and urine neopterin in attacks of the hyperimmunoglobulinemia D and periodic fever syndrome. Eur J Clin Invest 1995; 25: 683–686.
112. Kelley RI. Inborn errors of cholesterol biosynthesis. Adv Pediatr 2000; 47: 1–53.
113. Fu Z, Wang M, Potter D *et al.* The structure of a binary complex between a mammalian mevalonate kinase and ATP: insights into the reaction mechanism and human inherited disease. J Biol Chem 2002; 277: 18134–18142.
114. Livneh A, Drenth JPH, Klasen IS *et al.* Familial Mediterranean fever and hyperimmunoglobulinemia D syndrome: two diseases with distinct clinical, serologic, and genetic features. J Rheumatol 1997; 24: 1558–1563.
115. Padeh S, Brezniak N, Zemer D *et al.* Periodic fever, aphthous stomatitis, pharyngitis, and adenopathy syndrome: clinical characteristics and outcome. J Pediatr 1999; 135: 98–101.
116. Drenth JPH, Vonk AG, Simon A *et al.* Limited efficacy of thalidomide in the treatment of febrile attacks of the hyper-IgD and periodic fever syndrome: a randomized, double-blind, placebo-controlled trial. J Pharmacol Exp Ther 2001; 298: 1221–1226.
117. Muckle TJ, Wells M. Urticaria, deafness, and amyloidosis: a new heredo-familial syndrome. QJM 1962; 31: 235–248.
118. Cuisset L, Drenth JPH, Berthelot J-M *et al.* Genetic linkage of the Muckle–Wells syndrome to chromosome 1q44. Am J Hum Genet 1999; 65: 1054–1059.
119. Hoffman HM, Wright FA, Broide DH *et al.* Identification of a locus on chromosome 1q44 for familial cold urticaria. Am J Hum Genet 2000; 66: 1693–1698.
120. Muckle TJ. The 'Muckle–Wells' syndrome. Br J Dermatol 1979; 100: 87–92.

121. Lieberman A, Grossman ME, Silvers DN. Muckle–Wells syndrome: case report and review of cutaneous pathology. J Am Acad Dermatol 1998; 39: 290–291.

122. Watts RA, Nicholls A, Scott DGI. The arthropathy of the Muckle–Wellls syndrome. Br J Rheumatol 1994; 33: 1184–1187.

123. Gerbig AW, Dahinden CA, Mullis P, Hunziker T. Circadian elevation of IL-6 levels in Muckle–Wells syndrome: a disorder of the neuro-immune axis? QJM 1998; 91: 489–492.

124. Manji GA, Wang L, Geddes BJ et al. PYPAF1, a PYRIN-containing Apaf1-like protein that assembles with ASC and regulates activation of NF-κB. J Biol Chem 2002; 277: 11570–11575.

125. Kile RL, Rusk HA. A case of cold urticaria with an unusual family history. J Am Med Assoc 1940; 114: 1067–1068.

126. Hoffman HM, Wanderer AA, Broide DH. Familial cold autoinflammatory syndrome: phenotype and genotype of an autosomal dominant periodic fever. J Allergy Clin Immunol 2001; 108: 615–620.

127. Aganne E, Martinon F, Hawkins PN et al. Association of mutations in the NALP3/CIAS1/PYPAF1 gene with a broad phenotype including recurrent fever, cold sensitivity, sensorineural deafness, and AA amyloidosis. Arthritis Rheum 2002; 46: 2445–2452.

128. Dodé C, Le Dû N, Cuisset L et al. New mutations of CIAS1 that are responsible for Muckle-Wells syndrome and familial cold urticaria: a novel mutation underlies both syndromes. Am J Hum Genet 2002; 70: 1498–1506.

129. Feldmann J, Prieur A-M, Quartier P et al. Chronic infantile neurological cutaneous and articular syndrome is caused by mutations in CIAS1, a gene highly expressed in polymorphonuclear cells and chondrocytes. Am J Hum Genet 2002; 1: 198–203.

130. Aksentijevich I, Nowak M, Mallah M et al. De novo CIAS1 mutations, cytokine activation, and evidence for generic heterogeneity in patients with neonatal-onset multisystem inflammatory disease (NOMID): a new member of the expanding family of pyrin-associated autoinflammatory diseases. Arthritis Rheum 2002; 46: 3340–3348.

OTHER SYSTEMIC ILLNESSES

159 Sarcoidosis

Sterling G West and Brian L Kotzin

Definition

- A systemic disorder of unknown etiology characterized by non-caseating, granulomatous inflammation that can affect virtually any organ

Clinical features

- Acute and chronic forms of polyarthritis, particularly involving the knees and ankles
- Cystic bone lesions that may produce dactylitis or rarely involve the skull, vertebrae, ribs or pelvis
- Muscle involvement is usually asymptomatic but may cause acute or chronic myopathies or nodular masses
- Non-musculoskeletal features are common and include bilateral hilar adenopathy, pulmonary infiltrates, uveitis, cardiac and neurologic involvement, and skin lesions such as erythema nodosum and lupus pernio

HISTORY

Sarcoidosis derives from Greek *sarco* meaning flesh, *eidos,* meaning like, and *osis,* meaning condition[1]. In 1880, Dr Jonathan Hutchinson described the first case at King's College Hospital in London. Dr Ernest Besnier in 1889 described lupus pernio, the cutaneous hallmark of chronic sarcoidosis. Later, Dr Caesar Boeck advanced the description of sarcoidosis by emphasizing the granulomatous inflammation characteristic of this disease. With the introduction of skeletal radiography in the late 1890s, bone involvement by sarcoidosis was soon recognized. In 1903, Dr Karl Kreibich found the classic pattern of radiolucencies in the distal ends of the second phalanges of a patient with sarcoidosis. Later, he associated these bony lesions with lupus pernio and concluded that sarcoidosis represented a distinct granulomatous process not related to tuberculosis. Drs Kuznitzky and Bittorf in 1915 emphasized internal organ involvement, and in 1935 the Kveim–Siltzbach skin test for diagnosis was introduced. One year later, Drs Burman and Mayer described chronic sarcoid arthropathy. In 1953, Dr Sven Löfgren described the acute sarcoidosis syndrome of bilateral hilar adenopathy and erythema nodosum, frequently associated with arthritis, fever and uveitis. Over the past century, sarcoidosis has become recognized as a multisystem granulomatous disorder with protean manifestations that may affect any organ[2].

EPIDEMIOLOGY

Sarcoidosis occurs worldwide. In most series it affects females slightly more often than males. People of all ages can be involved, but it particularly occurs in young adults 20–40 years old. Sarcoidosis has been reported in all races and ethnic groups, but with marked variations. Prevalence estimates range from less than 1 per 100 000 (Spain, Portugal, Italy, Saudi Arabia, and India) to 20–40 per 100 000 (US Puerto Ricans/ Hispanics) to over 50 per 100 000 (Sweden, Denmark, and US African-Americans). In the United States the annual incidence rates are three times higher for African-Americans than for Caucasians, with a lifetime risk of sarcoidosis for US blacks of 2.4% and for US whites of 0.85%[3].

Clinical evidence indicates that the presentation and severity of sarcoidosis varies according to race and ethnicity. Caucasians are more likely to have erythema nodosum, less extrapulmonary involvement and less age-adjusted mortality than other racial groups. The Japanese may have more cardiac involvement, and African-Americans have the most severe disease with higher mortality rates.

CLINICAL FEATURES

Sarcoidosis is a systemic inflammatory disorder. The clinical spectrum is protean, ranging from an abnormal chest radiograph in an asymptomatic individual to severe multiorgan involvement[2]. Because there is no specific test for sarcoidosis, the diagnosis is established when well recognized clinical and radiographic findings are supported by histologic evidence of widespread epithelioid granulomata in more than one organ system[4,5]. Other granulomatous diseases caused by mycobacterial infection, fungal infection, berylliosis, and local reaction to tumors or lymphoma must be excluded. The presenting manifestations and cumulative organ involvement in sarcoidosis patients are shown in Table 159.1.

Respiratory tract

The entire respiratory tract from sinuses (2–18%) to lungs can be involved in sarcoidosis. Pulmonary involvement is the most common visceral manifestation, occurring in 95% of patients[6]. The clinical spectrum ranges from asymptomatic hilar adenopathy to an interstitial lung disease with alveolitis. Pleural effusions are rare. Endobronchial involvement is found on biopsy in 50% and may lead to airway stenosis (10%).

TABLE 159.1 CLINICAL FEATURES OF SARCOIDOSIS		
Manifestation	**Presenting (%)**	**Cumulative (%)**
Pulmonary	25	95
Constitutional	24	33–70
Adenopathy	20	90
Joint disease	14	≤ 38
Uveitis	7	25–50
Hepatosplenomegaly	4	5–10*
Cutaneous	3	25–30
Other	4	–
Heart	< 1	5–10*
Neurologic	< 1	5–10
Muscle	< 1	5*
Bone	< 1	3–13

* At autopsy, 20–67% have heart involvement; on biopsy, 50–80% have muscle and liver involvement.

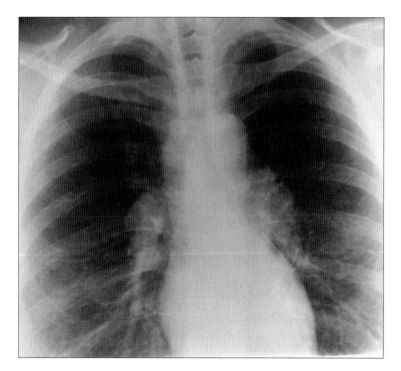

Fig. 159.1 Pulmonary sarcoidosis. Chest radiograph demonstrating bilateral hilar adenopathy.

Symptoms of lung disease include dry cough (30%), dyspnea (28%) and chest pain (15%). Hemoptysis is rare and occurs primarily in patients with fibrosis and cavitation filled with aspergillomas. For chest radiographs the modified Scadding staging system is used: Stage 0 – normal; Stage I – bilateral hilar adenopathy; Stage II – adenopathy with pulmonary infiltrates; Stage III – pulmonary infiltrates only; and Stage IV – end-stage pulmonary fibrosis (Fig. 159.1). Notably, the stages are not chronologic. High-resolution computerized tomography (HRCT) scans of the lungs may show abnormalities when chest radiographs are normal (Fig. 159.2). Pulmonary function testing shows restricted lung volumes and loss of diffusing capacity. Obstruction of large and small airways can also be seen, indicating endobronchial granulomas and/or bronchiolitis, and is a poor prognostic sign suggesting extensive and progressive disease. Bronchoalveolar lavage (BAL) fluid shows an elevated lymphocyte percentage with predominantly $CD4^+$ T cells. Transbronchial biopsy usually consists of six specimens from the upper and lower lobes. With an abnormal chest radiograph the diagnostic yield is over 90%.

Ophthalmologic

The eye is involved in 25–50% of patients[7]. Because it may be asymptomatic, all patients with sarcoidosis should have a baseline eye examination. Any area of the eye may be involved, but acute anterior uveitis manifested by blurred vision, photophobia and excessive lacrimation is the most common presentation. Involvement is frequently bilateral, which distinguishes it from the unilateral uveitis seen in HLA-B27 associated spondyloarthropathies. Other ophthalmologic manifestations include interstitial keratitis, posterior uveitis, scleral plaques, lacrimal gland enlargement, and corneal/conjunctival nodules. Approximately 20% of patients with uveitis will suffer some visual loss.

Cutaneous

Skin involvement occurs in up to 30% of cases, can be of a variety of morphologies, and may be present at disease onset[8]. Hyperpigmented maculopapular lesions commonly occur on the face, nape of the neck and upper back, whereas nodules occur more frequently on the torso and extremities. Skin plaques and annular lesions are associated with

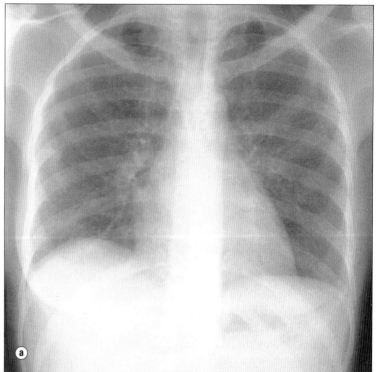

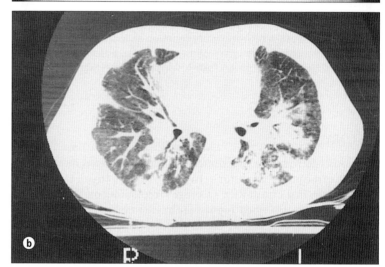

Fig. 159.2 Pulmonary sarcoidosis. (a) Radiograph of patient with pulmonary sarcoidosis showing minimal changes. (b) CT scan of the chest done at the same time shows extensive changes.

chronic disease and a poor prognosis when they occur on the head and neck. Scars and tattoos can become infiltrated with sarcoidosis. Subcutaneous sarcoidosis of Darier and Roussy presents with nodules deep in the dermis and subcutaneous tissue and can remit spontaneously. Lupus pernio has a predilection for black women and is the most characteristic skin manifestation of sarcoidosis (Fig. 159.3). Lesions are indurated and violaceous, occurring primarily on the nose, cheeks, ears, lips and fingers. They tend to be slowly progressive and can be disfiguring. Lupus pernio has a significant association with chronic upper respiratory tract involvement, pulmonary fibrosis, and bony lesions of the phalanges. Conversely, erythema nodosum occurs more commonly in young Caucasian and Puerto Rican females and usually is associated with an acute presentation and benign course. A variety of atypical lesions ranging from ulcers to ichthyosis can also be seen.

Cardiac

Symptomatic cardiac involvement occurs in 5% of sarcoidosis patients but is considerably more common at autopsy (20% in US to 67% in

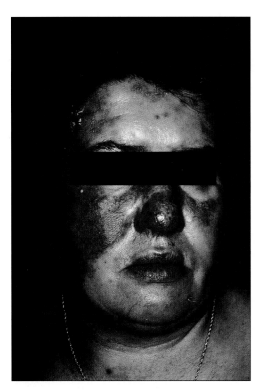

Fig. 159.3 Lupus pernio. Violaceous nodular and plaque-like eruptions on the nose, cheeks and forehead in a patient with chronic sarcoidosis.

Japan)[9,10]. Sarcoidosis may affect any part of the heart except the valves. Manifestations include sudden death, conduction disturbances, papillary muscle dysfunction, infiltrative cardiomyopathy with congestive heart failure, and pericarditis.

Cor pulmonale can also develop as a consequence of severe restrictive lung disease. Over 50% of sarcoidosis patients with cardiac involvement will have electrocardiographic abnormalities. Echocardiography can show granulomatous inflammation in the myocardium, manifesting as a 'snowstorm' pattern. A similar pattern may be observed in cardiac AA amyloid deposition, which may also occur as a complication of chronic sarcoidosis. Other findings include left ventricular hypertrophy and dysfunction, papillary muscle involvement, and asymptomatic pericardial effusions (20%) which are usually associated with myocardial involvement. Myocardial scintigraphy with thallium-201 can show areas of decreased uptake at rest, corresponding to granulomatous/fibrous infiltration. These areas decrease in size with stress imaging (i.e. reverse distribution, separating it from ischemic coronary artery disease)[11]. Magnetic resonance imaging (MRI) with gadolinium enhancement and gallium-67 scans can show increased uptake, which may predict a response to immunosuppressive therapy. Endomyocardial biopsies are often negative, as cardiac sarcoid lesions tend to be heterogeneous and have a predilection for the left ventricular free wall. Cardiac sarcoidosis is more common in patients with neurosarcoidosis and is indicative of severe disease.

Nervous system

Symptomatic involvement of the central or peripheral nervous systems occurs in approximately 5% of patients, although it is three times more common at autopsy[9,12]. Neurosarcoidosis has a predilection for the base of the brain and can occur without pulmonary or systemic features of sarcoidosis. Unilateral cranial nerve palsy, most frequently of the seventh nerve, is the most common (50%) presentation. Heerfordt's syndrome is the combination of fever, parotid enlargement, uveitis and facial nerve palsy, and usually has a poor prognosis. Other features of neurosarcoidosis include leptomeningeal involvement (25%), other cranial neuropathies, hypothalamic and pituitary lesions, localized mass lesion, seizures, and psychiatric and cognitive dysfunction, as well as other less common manifestations. Peripheral neuropathy occurs in 8.5–24% of patients with neurosarcoidosis[13]. Chronic sensorimotor polyneuropathy is the most common presentation, although mononeuritis multiplex, pure sensory neuropathy, intercostal neuritis and acute Guillain–Barré syndrome can be seen.

MRI with gadolinium enhancement is the best imaging technique to evaluate sarcoid involvement of brain parenchyma, meninges or spinal cord, as well as response to therapy. Positron emission tomography (PET) scans may be useful to identify areas of activity to biopsy. Cerebrospinal fluid (CSF) analysis can show elevated protein (70%) and lymphocytic pleocytosis (50%), high IgG index and oligoclonal bands (≤ 50%). The CSF can have an elevated angiotensin-converting enzyme (ACE) level, mostly due to secretion by central nervous system granulomas. Brain biopsies are invasive and may not reveal definitive pathologic changes. The prognosis of neurosarcoidosis is guarded, and symptoms can be chronic or relapsing. Mortality can be as high as 10%.

Musculoskeletal
Joints

Joint manifestations, including arthritis and periarthritis, occur in 14–38% of patients. Arthralgias are considerably more common (70%). Rheumatic involvement is generally divided into acute and chronic types. The most common form of joint involvement is an acute polyarthropathy/periarthritis. The arthritis may be migratory, resembling rheumatic fever; intermittent, resembling palindromic rheumatism; or additive, resembling rheumatoid arthritis, and can precede other manifestations of sarcoidosis by several months. More commonly, however, it is non-migratory and accompanied by other features of acute sarcoidosis. In patients with acute sarcoidosis presenting with bilateral hilar adenopathy and erythema nodosum (Löfgren's syndrome) 70% will have this form of poly/periarthritis, often associated with fever and uveitis (Fig. 159.4)[14]. This presentation most commonly occurs in young Caucasian women and is rare in blacks. Large joints, especially the ankles and knees, are most frequently affected, although other peripheral large and small joints may also be involved. Joint manifestations may be painless, whereas palpation elicits severe tenderness, indicating that this process is more a periarthritis. Joint radiographs show soft tissue swelling without bony changes. Arthrocentesis reveals no or only minimal synovial fluid, which is mildly inflammatory with a lymphocyte

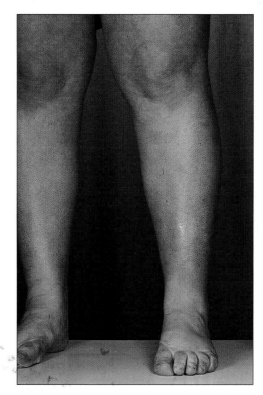

Fig. 159.4 Lofgren's syndrome. Patient presenting with knee arthritis, erythema nodosum and bilateral hilar adenopathy on chest radiograph.

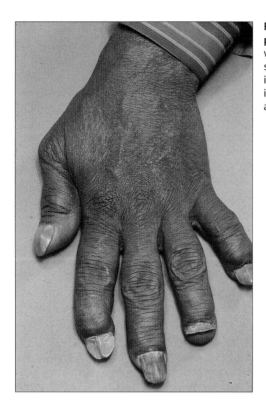

Fig. 159.5 Chronic polyarthritis. Patient with long-standing sarcoidosis and involvement of the interphalangeal joints and nails.

usually a non-destructive oligoarthritis or monoarthritis involving the shoulders, wrists, knees, ankles and/or small joints of the hands and feet. A chronic polyarthritis resembling rheumatoid arthritis, or sacroiliitis mimicking a spondyloarthropathy or mycobacterial infection are uncommon presentations. Radiographs show soft tissue swelling, but bony destruction is uncommon. Arthrocentesis reveals a mildly inflammatory fluid with a mononuclear cell predominance. In contrast to acute sarcoid arthritis, synovial biopsies in chronic sarcoid arthropathy characteristically show granulomatous inflammation. Tenosynovitis of the wrist, ankle, patella or Achilles tendons can also occur (5–13%).

Bone

The frequency of bone involvement ranges from 3 to 13%[16]. Bone changes may be present at disease onset, but are more frequently seen in patients with chronic and established disease. Women are affected more than men (2:1) and blacks more than other racial groups. Bone lesions occur frequently in patients with lupus pernio and/or other granulomatous skin lesions and predict a poor prognosis with excessive mortality. There is a predilection for the phalanges of the hands and feet. Other bones, particularly the nasal bones in patients with lupus pernio (Fig. 159.6) and the calcaneus, causing heel pain mimicking a spondyloarthropathy, can be involved. The skull, vertebrae, ribs, pelvis, sternum and the distal ends of long bones are rarely affected.

Bone lesions of the phalanges can be lytic, permeative and/or destructive, and tend to be bilateral in distribution. Lytic lesions are rounded, 'punched-out' bone defects on radiographs and are most frequently located at the ends of the proximal and middle phalanges (Fig. 159.7). Permeative lesions reflect granulomatous involvement of cortex and trabeculae of the phalangeal shafts, resulting in a reticular, lace-like appearance on radiographs. This may result in the phalangeal shafts becoming tubular. In advanced cases sclerosis or fractures may develop, or joints may be affected owing to subchondral bony involvement and collapse. Notably, sarcoid bone lesions are not associated radiographically with periostitis and rarely sequestra, helping to separate sarcoidosis from chronic osteomyelitis. Bone scans with technetium-99 diphosphonate can help detect osseous involvement in sarcoidosis.

The reason that sarcoidosis has a predilection for the phalanges is unknown. Pathologically, granulomatous infiltration into the marrow results in rarefaction of the trabeculae. In the cortical bone there is irregular resorption, with enlargement of Haversian canals containing granulomas. Occasionally, granulomatous inflammation can extend into surrounding tissues, causing infiltration of tendon sheaths. MRI can distinguish soft tissue involvement from bony lesions. Granulomatous

predominance. Synovial biopsies show mild, non-specific synovitis without granuloma formation.

Patients presenting with acute polyarthropathy have or will develop erythema nodosum in 50–75% of cases. Bilateral hilar adenopathy is present in over 90% of these individuals at disease onset, but in some patients will not develop for several weeks, making the diagnosis of sarcoidosis difficult. The acute form of joint involvement is usually associated with a benign course. Joint pain may resolve within weeks or persist for several months (average 3 months); however, 10–15% will have several recurrences or persistently active joint disease. Patients with a normal serum ACE level at diagnosis are most likely to completely resolve their disease without recurrences.

Chronic polyarthritis without involvement of adjacent bone is most likely to occur in black patients (Fig. 159.5)[15]. This less common type of joint involvement is caused by synovitis and usually accompanies the slower-onset, more chronic and systemic form of sarcoidosis. The arthritis may be mild and transient, recurrent or protracted. There is

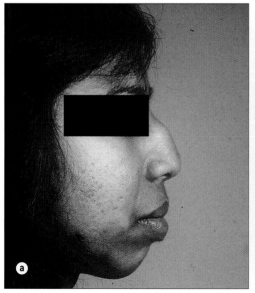
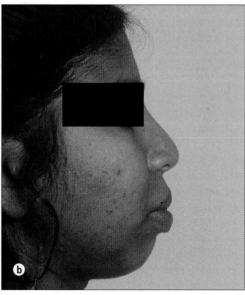

Fig. 159.6 Sarcoidosis involving the nasal bones. (a) Stage I nasal involvement in a patient with sarcoidosis and lupus pernio. (b) The same patient shown after treatment with oral prednisolone for 1 year.

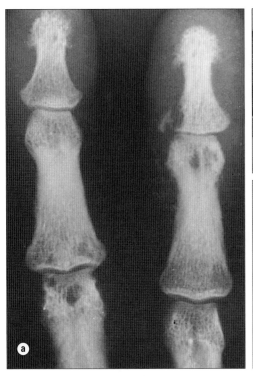

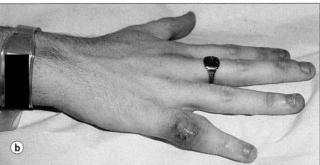

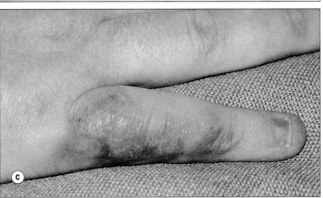

Fig. 159.7 Bone cysts and sarcoid dactylitis. (a) Radiograph of small bones of the hand showing bone cysts in an asymptomatic patient with bilateral hilar adenopathy. (b) Dactylitis with underlying bone cyst. (c) Resolution of dactylitis after treatment with oral prednisolone.

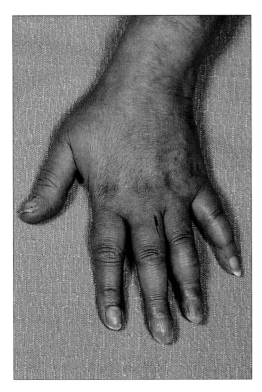

Fig. 159.8 Sarcoid dactylitis. Soft tissue swelling of the digits in a patient with long-standing sarcoidosis.

involvement of tendon sheaths can result in sarcoid dactylitis, with swelling over the affected digits associated with pain and stiffness (Fig. 159.8). The overlying skin can be erythematous, and when the terminal phalanges are involved the nails may become thickened and dystrophic.

Osteopenia and osteoporosis due to dysregulated calcium metabolism and medications used in therapy can occur in up to two-thirds of patients. All sarcoidosis patients on corticosteroids or who are postmenopausal should have bone density measurements.

Muscle

Asymptomatic muscle involvement is common (20–80%), whereas symptomatic involvement occurs in less than 5% of patients. A random muscle biopsy in a sarcoidosis patient without myopathic symptoms will show granulomas in up to 80% of cases and can be used for tissue diagnosis. The most common form of symptomatic muscle disease is a chronic myopathy[17]. This evolves slowly over several years, resulting in symmetric proximal muscle weakness and wasting, similar to muscular dystrophy. Neurogenic atrophy due to granulomatous infiltration of nerves can occur. In patients with muscle involvement electromyography shows myopathic changes, but muscle enzymes are frequently normal or only minimally elevated.

Acute myopathy and muscle nodules are rare manifestations of sarcoidosis. Acute sarcoid myopathy has been reported in fewer than 20 cases[18], mostly in black females. Patients present similarly to polymyositis with myalgias, proximal muscle weakness, muscle tenderness, high levels of muscle enzymes, and muscle necrosis/inflammation on biopsy. Many patients have fever at the time of presentation. Palpable granulomatous nodules and mass or tumor-like lesions may cause pain, stiffness and cramping of the involved muscle[19].

The response of acute myopathy to treatment with corticosteroids is good, and the course is usually benign. However, in chronic myopathy and nodular disease the response to therapy is unpredictable, with variable remissions and exacerbations requiring continued suppression and adjustments of the corticosteroid dose.

An association of myasthenia gravis (MG) with sarcoidosis has been reported in rare patients. Sarcoidosis has developed during remission of MG in some patients and during recurrences in others. Regression of MG and sarcoidosis after thymectomy has been reported, whereas in other patients the MG improves but the sarcoidosis does not.

Other organ systems

Constitutional symptoms of fever, fatigue, weight loss, and/or malaise occur in over a third of patients. Peripheral lymphadenopathy is common and usually non-tender. Sarcoid granulomas have been reported to involve virtually any organ. The oral, pharyngeal and nasal mucosae can be involved, leading to obstruction and sometimes disfigurement. Parotid and minor salivary gland enlargement occurs in 6% and can cause sicca symptoms, mimicking Sjögren's syndrome[20]. The thyroid can be infiltrated, and antithyroid antibodies have been reported. The liver and spleen show granulomas on biopsy in 50–80% of patients[21]. Alkaline phosphatase is frequently elevated (33%), but significant liver dysfunction is unusual. Cholestasis can result from granulomatous cholangitis or hepatic hilar adenopathy. Hepatosplenomegaly can occur and is associated with progressive fibrotic disease in other organs. Portal hypertension has been reported as a result of granulomatous phlebitis of hepatic or portal veins. Sarcoidosis can cause granulomatous ulcers or masses in the gastrointestinal tract. Pancreatic sarcoidosis is rare. Renal involvement is also rare, but overproduction of 1,25-dihydroxyvitamin D can lead to increased intestinal absorption of calcium, causing hypercalciuria (40–60%), nephrocalcinosis, nephrolithiasis (10%) and renal insufficiency. The risk of nephrolithiasis is 20% greater than in the general population. Interstitial nephritis, glomerulonephritis and amyloidosis may also occur. All areas of the male and female genitourinary tract have been reported to be involved in case series. Sarcoidosis has been rarely associated with vasculitis, and all sizes of blood vessels can be involved[22]. African-American and Asian children are more likely to have large vessel involvement.

CHILDHOOD SARCOIDOSIS

Children of both sexes can develop sarcoidosis. The characteristic presentation is in a child less than 5 years old who presents with mild constitutional symptoms; painless, boggy and effusive large joint polyarthritis and tenosynovitis; skin lesions; uveitis; and lymphadenopathy/splenomegaly without typical lung disease[23]. This presentation must be differentiated from the rare autosomal dominant familial granulomatous disorder, Blau's syndrome. Children with sarcoidosis usually have a spontaneous resolution of disease, but some suffer residual complications. Corticosteroids with or without methotrexate are the treatment of choice for children with severely symptomatic or progressive disease.

PREGNANCY

Sarcoidosis may improve in some women during pregnancy, possibly owing to physiologic increases in corticosteroids. Occasionally sarcoidosis may relapse in the postpartum period, especially in patients who have had their corticosteroid therapy tapered during pregnancy. Overall, sarcoidosis has no adverse effect on pregnancy or fetal outcome.

SARCOIDOSIS ASSOCIATIONS

A variety of autoimmune disorders that may occur in association with sarcoidosis have been described in case reports[24]. These include rheumatoid arthritis, scleroderma, systemic lupus erythematosus, Sjögren's syndrome, spondyloarthropathies, primary biliary cirrhosis and other autoimmune liver diseases, autoimmune cytopenias, autoimmune thyroiditis alone or as part of polyglandular autoimmune syndrome type III, polymyositis, insulin-dependent diabetes mellitus, dermatitis herpetiformis, vitiligo, and pernicious anemia. Sarcoidosis has also been associated with common variable immunodeficiency and has been reported to occur before or simultaneously with various malignancies or following chemotherapy[25]. Malignant lymphoma, lung cancer, testicular cancer and lymphoproliferative disorders have been reported most often. Medication-induced sarcoidosis has been described following interferon-α therapy for various diseases.

INVESTIGATIONS

The diagnosis of sarcoidosis is made by the combination of clinical, radiologic and laboratory findings and confirmed by characteristic histology[4,5]. Patients with a classic presentation such as Löfgren's syndrome may not need tissue biopsy. However, in all doubtful cases and in cases where immunosuppressive treatment is likely to be needed, histologic confirmation or, much less commonly, Kveim testing is essential.

Laboratory

Laboratory evaluation of patients with sarcoidosis shows many abnormalities[26]. Most patients will have anemia of chronic disease and lymphopenia. Some may have eosinophilia. Leukocyte and platelet counts are normal unless there is significant bone marrow involvement, hypersplenism or another associated autoimmune disease. Chemistries are obtained to rule out diabetes insipidus due to pituitary involvement or renal insufficiency due to nephrocalcinosis. Hypercalciuria occurs in up to 17% of cases owing to non-suppressible alveolar macrophage secretion of 1,25-dihydroxyvitamin D_3[27]. Notably, patients with normal serum calcium levels may have elevated 1,25-dihydroxyvitamin D levels, which can cause increased calcium absorption from the gastrointestinal tract and hypercalciuria, placing the patient at risk for nephrolithiasis and renal insufficiency. Liver-associated enzymes may be abnormal in up to one-third of patients, showing elevations in alkaline phosphatase and γ-glutamyl transferase (GGT) more often than elevated aminotransferase levels.

Serologic abnormalities, including elevations of erythrocyte sedimentation rate, C-reactive protein and hypergammaglobulinemia, are common during active sarcoidosis. Low-titer rheumatoid factor is seen in up to 38% of patients, depending on the method used, and is more likely in those with chronic lung disease. A positive antinuclear antibody test with a speckled pattern of immunofluorescence in low titer is seen in up to 34% of patients. Antibodies against specific nuclear antigens are typically negative, although an occasional patient (6%) has been reported to have elevated antibodies against double-stranded DNA[28].

Angiotensin-converting enzyme (ACE) levels are elevated in 40–90% of sarcoidosis patients. Elevations correlate with active pulmonary disease and will normalize with successful therapy. This enzyme is produced by epithelioid cells and alveolar macrophages at the periphery of granuloma in response to an ACE-inducing factor released by T lymphocytes. ACE may contribute to the formation of granulomas by producing angiotensin II locally, which is chemotactic for macrophages and enhances phagocytosis. Elevated ACE levels are not specific for sarcoidosis and may be due to other diseases, such as hyperthyroidism, Gaucher's disease, diabetes mellitus, leprosy, α_1 antitrypsin deficiency, Kaposi's sarcoma in HIV patients, silicosis, hypersensitivity pneumonitis, cirrhosis, histoplasmosis and asbestosis. Therefore, an elevated ACE level may be supportive, but not diagnostic, of sarcoidosis.

Radiology

Chest radiographs are abnormal in 90–95% of patients. The radiographic staging system has been previously described (see Respiratory Tract). In the majority of patients hilar node enlargement is bilateral, but unilateral hilar (usually right-sided) and/or unilateral paratracheal adenopathy is present in up to 4% of patients. The HRCT scan is more sensitive than the chest radiograph and may show mediastinal node involvement and/or unexpected parenchymal disease in patients with normal chest radiographs[29]. Moreover, HRCT scan changes may match pulmonary function abnormalities more closely than a plain chest radiograph.

Gallium-67 citrate scanning may reveal a characteristic pattern of uptake in sarcoidosis (Fig. 159.9)[30]. The panda sign is the image of a panda bear produced by parotid and lacrimal gland uptake by sarcoid granulomas. The lambda sign is absorption by paratracheal and bilateral hilar lymph nodes, forming the Greek letter lambda (λ). It is important to note that gallium-67 is also taken up by tissues in other inflammatory and malignant diseases, including fungal infection, tuberculosis and lymphomas.

Other radiographic tests have been used, including MRI with gadolinium enhancement for brain involvement, myocardial disease, muscle disease and bone involvement. Myocardial scintigraphy with thallium-201 and technetium-99 pertechnetate reveals defects but is not specific

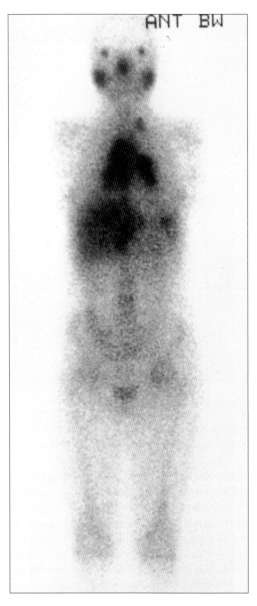

Fig. 159.9 **Abnormal gallium scan in sarcoidosis.** The scan shows uptake in the lacrimal, parotid and salivary glands (panda sign) as well as mediastinal lymph nodes (lambda sign) and lungs.

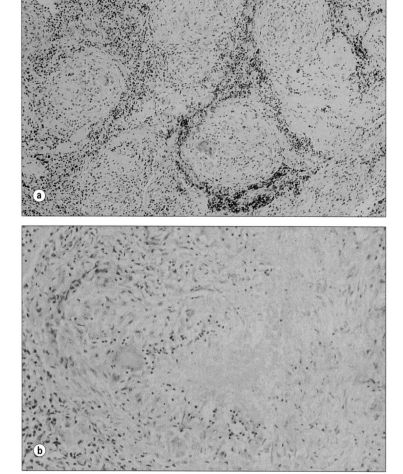

Fig 159.10 **Sarcoid granulomas.** Histology of lymph node showing non-caseating epithelioid and giant cell granulomas (a). Histology from patient with acute sarcoidosis showing non-caseating granulomas with central eosinophilic necrosis of collagen (b). There was subsequent natural resolution without treatment in this case.

for sarcoidosis. Technetium-99 diphosphonate scanning can be used to detect bone lesions.

Physiologic testing

Pulmonary function tests typically show a restrictive pattern, with a reduction in vital capacity, residual volume and total lung capacity[4,5]. The loss of diffusing capacity is the most common abnormality. Obstruction of large and small airways may occur because of endobronchial granulomas or bronchiolitis. Two-dimensional and M-mode echocardiography in patients with cardiac sarcoidosis can show pericardial effusions, concentric left ventricular hypertrophy with 'snow-storm' pattern due to granulomatous infiltration of myocardium, restrictive cardiomyopathy, ventricular dyskinesis, and valvular incompetence due to papillary muscle dysfunction.

Biopsy

Tissue biopsy is the gold standard to confirm a clinicoradiographic diagnosis of sarcoidosis.

Tissue biopsy should be performed on any patient with an atypical presentation, or if therapy is being considered, in order to exclude infection or malignant disease. Transbronchial, lymph node and skin biopsies are the most common, but a specimen can be obtained from any clinically involved organ. The diagnostic yield is as follows: transbronchial lung biopsy with normal chest radiograph, 30–50%; transbronchial lung biopsy with abnormal chest radiograph, >90%;

lymph node, > 90%; minor salivary gland, 36%; parotid, 93%; muscle, 50–80%; liver, 50–80%; synovium in chronic arthropathy, 80%; conjunctival and lacrimal gland, 10–55%; and skin, > 90%. The characteristic histologic finding is that of well-circumscribed non-caseating granulomas of the epithelioid type (Fig. 159.10). However, the presence of noncaseating granulomas are not diagnostic of sarcoidosis until other granulomatous diseases are excluded (see Differential Diagnosis).

The Kveim–Siltzbach skin test is rarely used[31]. This test consists of an intradermal injection (0.2ml) of a 10% saline suspension of lymph node or spleen homogenate from a known sarcoid patient into the skin of a patient being evaluated for sarcoidosis. If the patient has sarcoidosis, biopsy of a papule 4–6 weeks after the injection shows characteristic non-caseating granulomas. The test is positive in 50–70% of patients, particularly with early disease. The test, however, is not well standardized, not widely available, and has a 5% false positive rate.

Additional tests

Bronchoalveolar lavage (BAL) abnormalities are common. Although not diagnostic, a characteristic BAL fluid cell differential shows greater than 30–50% lymphocytosis with a CD4/CD8 T-cell ratio greater than 3.5 (94% specific, 52% sensitive)[32]. The lymphocytes are in an activated state (HLA-DR positive, IL-2R positive and CD45RO positive). Tuberculin and anergy skin testing show that many patients with active disease are anergic. Two tests which should be done as a baseline in all patients are an electrocardiogram and ophthalmologic examination with slit-lamp examination to rule out asymptomatic abnormalities. Electrocardiographic abnormalities can occur in 20–30% of patients with various dysrhythmias, conduction disturbances and non-specific ST- and T-wave changes. A 24-hour Holter monitor should be done in patients with arrhythmias or palpitations. Fluorescein angiography is helpful to document posterior uveitis.

DIFFERENTIAL DIAGNOSIS

Several diseases can result in similar clinical presentations and granulomas on biopsies, resembling sarcoidosis. Acute histoplasmosis can simulate Lofgren's syndrome and must be excluded by serologies and cultures. Acute arthritis with erythema nodosum, but without hilar adenopathy, can occur in inflammatory bowel disease, coccidiomycosis, histoplasmosis, psittacosis, and reactions to various medications. The pattern of arthritis in these patients is also similar to that seen in sarcoidosis. In patients with more insidious presentations other diseases need to be considered, depending on the organ involved. Patients with pulmonary disease should have chronic berylliosis excluded by clinical history of exposure and a beryllium lymphocyte proliferation test. Hypersensitivity pneumonitis is ruled out by a history of occupational and environmental exposure and results of serologic precipitins. Other inorganic agents, such as metals, silica and talc, are excluded by a good history. Fungal serologies or stains/cultures for organisms rule out fungal and mycobacterial disease. Wegener's granulomatosis is excluded by the absence of a positive antineutrophil cytoplasmic antibody (c-ANCA) test and the absence of vasculitis on biopsy. Churg–Strauss syndrome patients have a history of asthma and prominent eosinophilia. Tissue biopsy will exclude lymphoma. Patients with cutaneous granulomatous lesions should have treponemal infections, leprosy, tularemia and leishmaniasis excluded by serologies and/or cultures. Granuloma annulare and granulomatous rosacea are ruled out clinically by lack of systemic involvement. Lupus vulgaris due to mycobacterial infection may mimic cutaneous plaques of sarcoidosis. Primary biliary cirrhosis can cause liver granulomas but is associated with antimitochondrial antibodies. Fungal or mycobacterial infections and brucellosis should be considered in patients with monoarticular axial or peripheral arthritis. Fungal infections, leprosy, brucellosis, syphilis, Wegener's granulomatosis, eosinophilic granuloma, multiple myeloma and lymphoma can cause bony lesions similar to those due to sarcoidosis. Toxoplasmosis can mimic acute and chronic sarcoid myopathy, and various neoplasms and infections need to be excluded in patients with a muscle mass.

ETIOLOGY

The cause of sarcoidosis is unknown. Several reports of community outbreaks, increased work-related risk for nurses and firefighters, seasonal clustering of cases in the winter and early spring months, case contact studies, and cases transmitted by cardiac and bone marrow transplantation suggest that environmental and/or transmissible factors are involved in the pathogenesis of sarcoidosis[33]. Inorganic and organic pollutants as well as many infectious agents have been reported to be isolated from sarcoid granulomas (Table 159.2). Three organisms have received particular attention. Human herpesvirus 8 DNA sequences have reportedly been isolated from sarcoidosis tissue, but serologic evidence of infection has not been consistently found. *Propionibacterium* species genomic DNA has also been found by polymerase chain reaction in lymph node biopsies from sarcoidosis patients. Finally, cell wall-deficient forms (L-forms) of mycobacteria have been isolated from the blood of the majority of sarcoidosis patients but not from controls. However, the inability of any of these agents to cause sarcoidosis in animal models, the diversity of tissues involved in sarcoidosis which are not typically involved by some of these organisms, the lack of response to antibiotics but improvement with immunosuppressive agents, and

TABLE 159.2 REPORTED ETIOLOGIC FACTORS IN SARCOIDOSIS	
Environmental	**Genetic**
Pollutants	• HLA Class I
• Beryllium	• HLA Class II
• Zirconium	• Factor B
• Pine pollen	• Tumor necrosis factor alpha
• Peanut dust	• Interleukin-1 alpha
• Clay	• Interferon regulatory factor
Viruses	• C-C chemokine receptor
• Epstein–Barr	• Angiotensin-converting enzyme
• Human herpesvirus 8	• Angiotensin II type 1 receptor
• Adenovirus	
• Others	
Mycobacteria	
• *M. tuberculosis*	
• Atypical mycobacteria	
• Cell wall-deficient mycobacteria	
• Phage-transformed mycobacteria	
Other bacteria	
• *Mycoplasma pneumoniae*	
• Nocardia species	
• Corynebacterium species	
• Propionibacterium acnes	
• *Borrelia burgdorferi*	

(Adapted from James and Zurnia[33].)

the failure to decrease the prevalence of sarcoidosis in countries where BCG vaccination is used, are all evidence against a single infectious agent causing sarcoidosis.

Other environmental factors may also influence the development or expression of sarcoidosis. The possibility of a non-infectious environmental agent is suggested by a comparison of sarcoidosis to chronic beryllium disease. This histologically identical process is caused by exposure to beryllium metal or alloy in the workplace. An example of an environmental factor that decreases the probability of developing sarcoidosis is cigarette smoke. It is postulated that the acrolein (breakdown product of cyclophosphamide) in cigarette smoke is cytotoxic to lymphocytes trying to enter the lungs, accounting for the decreased prevalence of sarcoidosis in cigarette smokers.

Genetic factors also play a role in the racial and ethnic variations in prevalence, clinical presentations and severity of sarcoidosis[34]. Reports of several hundred families with two or more affected members are considered the strongest evidence for a genetic component to this disease. Familial aggregation has been reported to occur in 19% of affected African-American families and 5% of Caucasian families. Additionally, the concordance rate is two to four times higher in monozygotic than in dizygotic twins, further supporting a genetic basis for this disease.

The intraracial heterogeneity of clinical manifestations and prognoses makes it unlikely that a single gene is responsible for sarcoidosis. Studies have shown that the HLA-A1, B8, DR3 haplotype and HLA-DR17 (a subset of DR3) are associated with an increased risk of developing sarcoidosis in Caucasians. In contrast, HLA-DR5 was associated with chronic disease. HLA-DRw52 was reported to be associated with sarcoidosis in Japanese patients, and the DPB1*0201 allele was increased in African-Americans and some Caucasian ethnicities. Other candidate genes suggested to be associated with disease in specific ethnic groups of sarcoidosis patients include certain alleles of factor B (F allele), TNF-α (308*2 allele), interleukin-1α, interferon regulatory factor protein (IRF-4), C-C chemokine receptor 2 for macrophage chemotactic protein-1 (MCP-1), angiotensin-converting enzyme (DD genotype), and angiotensin II type 1 receptor.

Several large studies are presently ongoing that will further our understanding of the causes of sarcoidosis. A multicenter case control study of the pathogenesis of sarcoidosis is being conducted by the National Institutes of Health (NIH) to address environmental and other factors. This research group is developing common definitions and assessments of organ involvement to better delineate the multiple clinical variations of this disorder[35]. These studies will help verify which genetic factors are associated with disease in patients with carefully defined clinical manifestations within different ethnic populations. Recently, two large registries of familial sarcoid have been established, one of African-Americans in the United States and one of Caucasians in Germany. Whole genome scans of genetic material from these patient samples may enable researchers to map genetic loci linked to sarcoidosis.

IMMUNOPATHOGENESIS

The non-caseating epithelioid granuloma is the histologic hallmark of sarcoidosis and is formed by a stepwise series of events[36,37].

Step 1: lymphocytic alveolitis

The initial event in sarcoidosis is thought to be the uptake and processing of a triggering antigen by antigen-presenting cells (type II alveolar epithelial cells, alveolar macrophages and dendritic cells) bearing HLA class II molecules in the lower respiratory tract. The recognition of antigen by $CD4^+$ T cells is considered to be a critical event in the development of disease. The alveolar macrophage secretion of interleukins (IL)-8, -12, -15 and RANTES, and the alveolar epithelial cell secretion of IL-16, increases the recruitment of inflammatory cells and lymphocytes. Additionally, the upregulation of endothelial cell adhesion molecules (ICAM-1, VCAM-1, LFA-3 and selectins) caused by lymphocyte and macrophage-derived cytokines, including TNF-α, interferon-γ (IFN-γ), IL-1 and IL-15, is central to the marked accumulation of inflammatory cells in the lung alveoli. Studies indicate that inflammatory alveolitis precedes granuloma formation and is composed primarily of $CD4^+$ T lymphocytes and mononuclear phagocytes. In patients with established disease the accumulation of $CD4^+$ T cells in the lung (and BAL fluid) includes oligoclonal expansions of T cells bearing particular T-cell receptors, indicative of expansion by antigen.

Step 2: granuloma formation

The accumulation and activation of antigen-specific T-helper 1 (Th1) lymphocytes is a critical event in the development of granulomatous inflammation. The alveolar macrophage/dendritic cell cytokine IL-12 is critical to the differentiation of naïve $CD4^+$ T lymphocytes into Th1 cells. The Th1 cells secrete the Th1 cytokines IL-2 and IFN-γ. IL-2 acts synergistically with IL-15 and TNF-α from macrophages to stimulate further T-lymphocyte proliferation and differentiation. Other T-lymphocyte cytokines stimulate macrophage recruitment, activation and proliferation (GM-CSF and MCP-1) as well as B-cell growth and differentiation (IL-2, BCGF and BCDF). The Th1 cytokine IFN-γ amplifies the immune response through its effects on multiple target cells and is critical to granuloma formation.

The sarcoid granuloma is well circumscribed, round or oval, non-caseating, and made up of compact, radially arranged epithelioid cells with pale nuclei. The typical giant cell is of the Langerhans type, in which the nuclei are arranged in an arc or circular pattern around a central granular zone. Stellate asteroid (entrapped collagen) and blue Schaumann inclusion bodies (altered lysosomes in giant cells) are occasionally observed. The center of the granuloma is composed of macrophage-derived cells and $CD4^+$ Th1 lymphocytes, whereas the outer zone contains many CD4 and $CD8^+$ T lymphocytes, fibroblasts, and interdigitating antigen-presenting cells entwined in bands of collagen. The initial events leading to this granuloma formation involve the local proliferation of the Th1 T-cell subset and reciprocal suppression of the Th2 subset. Macrophage-derived IL-1β, IL-12 and IL-15 promote Th1 proliferation. IL-12, in turn, specifically upregulates IFN-γ from Th1

lymphocytes, which enhances macrophage function. Both IL-1β and IFN-γ are important in the early recruitment stage of granuloma formation, and TNF-α may be particularly important in the later maintenance of granuloma formation and perpetuation of inflammation. Many other macrophage-derived cytokines also contribute to granuloma formation and tissue damage, including the CXC chemokine, IFN-γ inducible protein (IP-10), which is produced by epithelioid cells and macrophages within granulomas and is a powerful stimulus to the direct migration of activated T cells to the periphery of granulomas.

Step 3: granuloma resolution

The immunologic factors that determine the ultimate fate of sarcoid granulomas are poorly understood. If the granuloma does not resolve spontaneously or with therapy, it becomes converted into fibrotic scar. The alveolar macrophages and mast cells probably contribute to this fibrotic process by releasing profibrotic growth factors. Macrophages promote fibroblast recruitment through the secretion of TNF-α. Once attracted to this site, fibroblasts proliferate in response to several macrophage-derived cytokines, including TGF-β, basic fibroblast growth factor, insulin-like growth factor 1, platelet-derived growth factor, and prostaglandin E. Additionally, IL-8, leukotriene B_4 and other macrophage-derived chemokines recruit neutrophils from the blood, which may participate in fibrosis by producing superoxide radicals and proteases. This is reflected in the association of lung fibrosis with neutrophilia in BAL fluid.

NATURAL HISTORY AND PROGNOSIS

The natural history of untreated sarcoidosis is difficult to predict in an individual patient[38]. Most patients (60%) undergo spontaneous remission, with an additional 10–20% resolving with corticosteroid therapy. However, in 10–30% the course is chronic. Of those having a chronic course, half will have progressive pulmonary disease and half will display involvement of critical extrapulmonary organs, such as the eye, brain and heart. The probability of a spontaneous remission can be predicted by the patient's clinical and radiologic presentation. Up to 80% of patients presenting with hilar adenopathy alone (radiographic Stage I disease) have a spontaneous resolution, and patients with Löfgren's syndrome have the best overall prognosis for full remission within 2 years. Fifty to sixty per cent of patients with radiographic Stage II disease experience remission, in contrast to fewer than 30% of those with Stage III disease. The mortality rate of patients with pulmonary fibrosis (radiographic Stage IV with vital capacity less than 1.5 l) is 25–40%. Although the overall prognosis for sarcoidosis is good, at least 50% of patients have some degree of permanent organ dysfunction. In addition, there is a 5% mortality rate, with progressive pulmonary disease accounting for half and cardiac/neurologic disease causing the other half of all deaths from sarcoidosis. Of patients with cardiac or neurologic manifestations, up to 10% will die from organ failure. In Japan, patients die of cardiac complications, whereas in the United States pulmonary disease causes most of the deaths. In general, the more severe the involvement and the more organ systems involved at the time of diagnosis, the worse the prognosis. Cutaneous sarcoidosis is a poor prognostic sign, as is black race, disease onset after 40 years of age, and symptoms lasting longer than 6 months[2,39].

MANAGEMENT

Because the cause of sarcoidosis is unknown, therapy is empiric. Whenever possible, patients with good prognostic signs should be observed for the first 3–6 months without immunosuppressive therapy because of the potential for spontaneous resolution. In patients with progressive disease the recommended doses of corticosteroids and adjunctive therapies vary, depending on the organ system involved.

There have been few controlled, randomized trials to establish the appropriate dose and duration of any therapy for sarcoidosis. Despite a lack of well-controlled clinical trials proving that corticosteroids improve long-term outcome, oral corticosteroids are used as first-line treatment for symptomatic and progressive lung disease (a decrease in forced vital capacity of 10% or more, or 20% or greater decrease in lung diffusion of carbon monoxide), Stage II and III pulmonary disease, malignant hypercalcemia, and severe ocular, neurologic, cardiac, skin and musculoskeletal involvement.

Pulmonary

Two prospective randomized studies showed short-term benefit of corticosteroid therapy for patients with deteriorating lung function or serious extrapulmonary disease[40,41]. For the 15% of patients who develop progressive lung involvement, current guidelines suggest the use of 40–60mg (1mg/kg/day) of prednisone daily for 8–12 weeks, with a gradual tapering of the dose to 30mg every other day by 6 months, 20mg every other day by 9 months, and 10mg every other day by 12 months. Other regimens have been published[42,43]. More than 70% of patients respond favorably, but relapses occur in 25–50% after tapering or discontinuation of corticosteroids. Some patients need 10–20mg every other day indefinitely to prevent relapses.

A variety of other medications have been tried to reduce oral corticosteroid dependence and in patients who do not respond or have intolerable side effects[44]. Two double-blind randomized studies failed to demonstrate that inhaled corticosteroids were more efficacious than placebo for preventing pulmonary deterioration. A randomized trial of chloroquine (750mg/day, tapering by 250mg every 2 months) showed benefit in 23 patients with symptomatic advanced pulmonary disease[45]. In a randomized controlled trial, methotrexate showed a steroid-sparing effect in patients with acute sarcoidosis[46]. In an uncontrolled report, 70% of 50 patients with chronic sarcoidosis treated with methotrexate were able to reduce their prednisone use after 6 months. However, relapses were frequent after methotrexate was discontinued. Experience with other immunosuppressive medications, including azathioprine, cyclophosphamide, chlorambucil and cyclosporin, has been limited to small, uncontrolled trials and anecdotal case reports. Of these, azathioprine is used most often. The therapeutic effectiveness of cyclosporin in pulmonary sarcoidosis has generally been disappointing. In patients for whom corticosteroids and immunosuppressive drugs have failed, mechanical dilatation of bronchial stenosis can be effective but often needs to be repeated. In patients with end-stage pulmonary fibrotic disease lung transplantation offers a potential cure, although higher than normal rates of rejection and recurrence of sarcoidosis in the allograft have been observed[47].

Ophthalmic

Eye manifestations are treated with topical, injectable and systemic corticosteroids. Topical steroids and cycloplegics are usually sufficient for anterior uveitis, although granulomatous involvement of ocular structures and posterior segment inflammation require oral corticosteroid or periocular steroid injections. Azathioprine and methotrexate have been effective for steroid-refractory chronic uveitis[7].

Cutaneous

Topical corticosteroids and monthly intralesional injections of triamcinolone are often effective therapy for small sarcoid papules or plaques. Larger, disfiguring skin lesions require systemic corticosteroid therapy (30mg every day to every other day). Several small studies have found chloroquine (500mg/day for 2 weeks, then 250mg/day) and hydroxychloroquine (200–400mg/day) to be useful in the treatment of skin disease, with an overall 35% response rate. Mucosal lesions of the upper respiratory tract have also been reported to respond to antimalarial therapy. Methotrexate has been reported to be an effective steroid-

sparing agent for severe cutaneous sarcoid. Thalidomide, allopurinol, minocycline, PUVA and retinoids have been anecdotally successful in a few patients with refractory sarcoid skin lesions[8].

Cardiovascular

Cardiac and neurologic sarcoid are uncommon but are important causes of mortality. Large doses of prednisone (60mg/day or greater) should be initiated in patients with ventricular arrhythmias or cardiomyopathy[10]. Antiarrhythmic agents and medications for heart failure should be used as adjunctive therapies. Magnetic resonance imaging of the heart and myocardial scintigraphy may be useful in monitoring the response to therapy. In patients with severe or refractory disease, high-dose pulse methylprednisolone, azathioprine, methotrexate, chlorambucil and cyclophosphamide have been used with some success. Implantable pacemakers and heart transplantation have been used for patients in whom medical management failed. Sarcoid vasculitis is uncommon and may require treatment with immunosuppressive drugs.

Neurologic

Neurologic sarcoidosis is treated with oral prednisone 40–80mg/day[12]. Antiseizure medications are used as adjunctive therapy in patients with seizures. Patients with severe and refractory disease have been treated with immunosuppressive therapy, similar to cardiac sarcoidosis. Uncontrolled reports have also suggested that antimalarials, methotrexate, azathioprine, cyclophosphamide (oral and monthly pulse), cyclosporin and cranial radiation may be effective[48]. Surgical intervention is necessary for hydrocephalus and mass lesions that are expanding or causing increased intracranial pressure. Because of the possibility of devastating sequelae and the reactivation of neurosarcoidosis, most patients are maintained on low-dose prednisone and a second immunomodulatory medication for life.

Arthritis

Acute sarcoidosis with arthritis/periarthritis (Löfgren's syndrome) requires no specific therapy other than analgesics or non-steroidal anti-inflammatory drugs (NSAIDs) such as indomethacin, as spontaneous resolution is the most likely outcome. Colchicine appears to shorten attacks in some patients. For chronic synovitis, low-dose corticosteroids may be helpful if NSAIDs or analgesics fail. Chloroquine, hydroxychloroquine, azathioprine and methotrexate (7.5–20mg/week) have been used successfully in patients with severe musculoskeletal manifestations refractory to corticosteroids[49].

Bone and muscle

Osteosarcoidosis responds poorly to therapy. Corticosteroids will decrease swelling, but will not completely normalize bony destruction[10]. Hydroxychloroquine, chloroquine and methotrexate have been reported anecdotally to be helpful adjunctive therapies. Acute sarcoid myositis responds well to corticosteroids, but chronic myopathy and mass lesions respond much less well. Bisphosphonates are beneficial to prevent osteoporosis.

Renal

Hypercalciuria usually responds rapidly to 10–20mg/day of prednisone. Chloroquine and ketoconazole act more slowly but produce a more sustained lowering of calcium after cessation of therapy[27]. A low-calcium diet, avoidance of vitamin D supplements and limited exposure to sunlight are helpful adjunctive measures. Patients should keep well hydrated to help prevent nephrolithiasis.

FUTURE THERAPY

New therapies for sarcoidosis will depend on a better understanding of its cause and immunopathogenesis[50]. TNF-α, IL-12 and other cytokines involved in the Th1 response have been shown to be increased in active sarcoidosis. Pentoxifylline (400mg three times daily) inhibits the synthesis of TNF-α and has been reported to reverse the loss of pulmonary function. Other TNF-α inhibitors, including monoclonal antibodies and TNF-α receptors currently used to treat rheumatoid arthritis and inflammatory bowel disease, may be useful in sarcoidosis. Clinical trials using these agents are in progress. Finally, IL-4 and IL-10, which are potent suppressors of Th1 activity and granuloma formation, may be useful as future therapies.

MONITORING THERAPY

Many tests have been used to determine disease activity and response to therapy. However, no serologic test, including the ACE level, has proved to be a reliable marker[51]. The best assessment is through longitudinal observation of symptoms, chest radiographs, HRCT scans and measurement of pulmonary function tests and other parameters reflecting internal organ involvement. Gallium scans and MRI with gadolinium may be useful in assessing activity in some organs that are difficult to access, such as heart, brain and bone. The ongoing NIH-sponsored multicenter case–control study should help better define the course and outcome of treated and untreated sarcoidosis.

ACKNOWLEDGMENT

The authors wish to thank Dr Donald N. Mitchell for his contributions and figures from the last edition used in this chapter. We also thank Nancy Hoffmann for her expert editorial assistance in manuscript preparation.

REFERENCES

1. James DG. Historical background. In: James DG, ed. Sarcoidosis and other granulomatous disorders: lung biology in health and disease. New York: Marcel Dekker; 1994: 1–18.
2. Newman LS, Rose CS, Maier LA. Medical progress: sarcoidosis. N Engl J Med 1997; 336: 1224–1234.
3. Rybicki BA, Malariak MJ, Major M et al. Epidemiology, demographics, and genetics of sarcoidosis. Semin Respir Infect 1998; 13: 166–173.
4. Huninghake G, Costabel U, Ando M et al. Statement on sarcoidosis. Sarcoidosis Vasc Diffuse Lung Dis 1999; 16: 149–173.
5. ATS Statement. Sarcoidosis. Am J Respir Crit Care Med 1999; 160: 736–755.
6. Lynch JP III, Kazerooni EA, Gay SE. Pulmonary sarcoidosis. Clin Chest Med 1997; 18: 755–785.
7. Smith JA, Foster CS. Sarcoidosis and its ocular manifestations. Int Ophthalmol Clin 1996; 36: 109–125.
8. English JC, Patel PJ, Greer KE. Sarcoidosis. J Am Acad Dermatol 2001; 44: 725–743.
9. Lynch JP III, Sharma OP, Baughman RP. Extrapulmonary sarcoidosis. Semin Respir Infect 1998; 13: 229–254.
10. Sekiguchi M, Yazaki Y, Isobe M, Hiroe M. Cardiac sarcoidosis: diagnostic, prognostic, and therapeutic considerations. Cardiovasc Drugs Ther 1996; 10: 495–510.
11. Mana J. Nuclear imaging. Clin Chest Med 1997; 18: 799–811.
12. Zajicek JP, Scolding NJ, Foster O et al. Central nervous system sarcoidosis: diagnosis and management. Q J Med 1999; 92: 103–117.
13. Zuniga G, Ropper AH, Frank J. Sarcoid peripheral neuropathy. Neurology 1991; 41: 1558–1561.
14. Mana J, Gomez-Vaquero C, Montero A et al. Lofgren's syndrome revisited: a study of 186 patients. Am J Med 1999; 107: 240–245.
15. Spilberg I, Siltzbach LE, McEwen C. The arthritis of sarcoidosis. Arthritis Rheum 1969; 12: 126–137.
16. Wilcox A, Bharadwaj P, Sharma OP. Bone sarcoidosis. Curr Opin Rheumatol 2000; 12: 321–330.
17. Wolfe SM, Pinals RS, Aelion JA, Goodman RE. Myopathy in sarcoidosis: clinical and pathologic study of four cases and review of the literature. Semin Arthritis Rheum 1987; 16: 300–306.
18. Ost D, Yeldani A, Cugell D. Acute sarcoid myositis with respiratory muscle involvement. Case report and review of the literature. Chest 1995; 107: 879–882.
19. Zisman DA, Biermann JS, Martinez FJ et al. Sarcoidosis presenting as a tumorlike muscular lesion. Medicine (Baltimore) 1999; 78: 112–122.
20. Drosos AA, Constantopoulos SH, Psychos D et al. The forgotten cause of sicca complex: sarcoidosis. J Rheumatol 1998; 16: 1548–1551.
21. Ishak KG. Sarcoidosis of the liver and bile ducts. Mayo Clinic Proc 1998; 73: 467–472.
22. Fernandes SRM, Singsen BH, Hoffman GS. Sarcoidosis and systemic vasculitis. Semin Arthritis Rheum 2000; 30: 33–46.
23. Pattishall EN, Kendig EL. Sarcoidosis in children. Pediatr Pulmonol 1996; 22: 195–203.
24. Enzenauer R, West S. Sarcoidosis in autoimmune disease. Semin Arthritis Rheum 1992; 22: 1–17.
25. Askling J, Grunewald J, Eklund A et al. Increased risk for cancer following sarcoidosis. Am J Respir Crit Care Med 2000; 160: 1668–1672.
26. Costabel U, Teschler H. Biochemical changes in sarcoidosis. Clin Chest Med 1997; 18: 827–842.
27. Sharma OP. Vitamin D, calcium, and sarcoidosis. Chest 1996; 109: 535–539.
28. Weinberg I, Vasiliev L, Gotsman I. Anti-dsDNA antibodies in sarcoidosis. Semin Arthritis Rheum 2000; 29: 328–331.
29. Putman CE, Rothman SL, Littner MR. Computerized tomography in pulmonary sarcoidosis. Comput Tomogr 1977; 1: 197–209.
30. Sulavik SB, Spencer RP, Palestro CJ et al. Specificity and sensitivity of distinctive chest radiographic and/or 67Ga images in the noninvasive diagnosis of sarcoidosis. Chest 1993; 103: 403–409.
31. Munro C, Mitchell D. The Kveim test: still useful, still a puzzle. Thorax 1987; 44: 371–372.
32. Winterbauer RH, Lammert J, Selland M et al. Bronchoalveolar lavage cell populations in the diagnosis of sarcoidosis. Chest 1993; 104: 352–361.
33. James DG, Zumla A, eds. The granulomatous disorders. Cambridge: Cambridge University Press; 1999.
34. Luisetti M, Beretta A, Casali L. Genetic aspects of sarcoidosis. Eur Respir J 2000; 16: 768–780.
35. Judson MA, Baughman RP, Teirstein AS et al. Defining organ involvement in sarcoidosis: the ACCESS proposed instrument. Sarcoidosis Vasc Diffuse Lung Dis 1999; 16: 75–86.
36. Conron M, DuBois RM. Immunological mechanisms in sarcoidosis. Clin Exper Allergy 2001; 31: 543–554.
37. Agostini C, Basso U, Semenzato G. Cells and molecules involved in the development of sarcoid granuloma. J Clin Immunol 1998; 18: 184–192.
38. Gideon NM, Mannino DM. Sarcoidosis mortality in the United States 1979–1991: an analysis of multiple-cause mortality data. Am J Med 1996; 100: 423–427.
39. Mana J, Salazar A, Manresa F. Clinical factors predicting persistence of activity in sarcoidosis: a multivariate analysis of 193 cases. Respiration 1994; 61: 219–225.
40. Gibson GJ, Prescott RJ, Muers MF et al. British Thoracic Society sarcoidosis study: effects of long-term corticosteroid treatment. Thorax 1996; 51: 238–247.
41. Huninghake GW, Gilbert S, Pueringer R et al. Outcome of the treatment of sarcoidosis. Am J Respir Crit Care Med 1994; 149: 893–898.
42. Judson MA. An approach to the treatment of pulmonary sarcoidosis with corticosteroids: the six phases of treatment. Chest 1999; 115: 1158–1165.
43. Jones CJ, Michele TM. The clinical management of sarcoidosis. A 50-year experience at the Johns Hopkins Hospital. Medicine (Baltimore) 1999; 78: 65–111.
44. Baughman RP, Lower EE. Steroid-sparing alternative treatments for sarcoidosis. Clin Chest Med 1987; 18: 853–864.
45. Baltzan M, Mehta S, Kirkham TH et al. Randomized trial of prolonged chloroquine therapy in advanced pulmonary sarcoidosis. Am J Respir Crit Care Med 2000; 160: 192–197.
46. Baughman RP, Winget DB, Lower EE. Methotrexate is steroid sparing in acute sarcoidosis: results of a double blind, randomized trial. Sarcoidosis Vasc Diffuse Lung Dis 2000; 17: 60–66.
47. Judson MA. Lung transplantation for pulmonary sarcoidosis. Eur Respir J 1998; 11: 738–744.
48. Sharma OP. Effectiveness of chloroquine and hydroxychloroquine in treating selected patients with sarcoidosis with neurological involvement. Arch Neurol 1998; 55: 1248–1254.
49. Kaye O, Palazzo E, Grossin M et al. Low-dose methotrexate: an effective corticosteroid-sparing agent in the musculoskeletal manifestations of sarcoidosis. Br J Rheumatol 1995; 34: 642–644.
50. Semenzato G. Chemotactic cytokines: from the molecular level to clinical use. Sarcoidosis Vasc Diffuse Lung Dis 1998; 15: 131–133.
51. Muller-Quernheim J. Serum markers for the staging of disease activity of sarcoidosis and other interstitial lung diseases of unknown etiology. Sarcoidosis Vasc Diffuse Lung Dis 1998; 15: 22–37.

OTHER SYSTEMIC ILLNESSES

160 Relapsing polychondritis

Harvinder S Luthra

Definition

- A rare autoimmune disease of unknown etiology with episodic but potentially progressive inflammatory manifestations
- Cartilaginous structures throughout the body are primarily involved, including the ears, nose, eyes, laryngobronchial and costal cartilage and joints, in a heterogeneous pattern and sequence
- May be associated with other autoimmune and the myelodysplastic syndrome diseases

Clinical features

- Chondritis of the auricular, nasal, laryngotracheal, costal and articular cartilage
- Ocular and inner ear inflammation
- An associated systemic vasculitis, or glomerulonephritis may contribute significant morbidity and premature mortality
- Extremely varied in its manifestations, course and response to therapy

TABLE 160.1 CONDITIONS ASSOCIATED WITH RELAPSING POLYCHONDRITIS

- Rheumatoid arthritis
- Systemic lupus erythematosus
- Scleroderma
- Sjögren's syndrome
- Overlap connective tissue disease
- Ankylosing spondylitis and sacroiliitis
- Psoriatic arthritis
- Reactive arthritis
- Wegener's granulomatosis
- Polyarteritis nodosa
- Churg–Strauss vasculitis
- Behçet's disease
- Myelodysplastic syndromes
- Lymphoma
- Inflammatory bowel disease
- Primary biliary cirrhosis

HISTORY

Relapsing polychondritis is a rare disease of unknown etiology. The first clinical description of it is attributed to Jaksch-Wartenhorst[1], who called it 'polychondropathia' and considered it to be a degenerative disorder. Pearson et al.[2] reported in the English literature the case of a 32-year-old brewer with fever, asymmetric polyarthritis, pain in and swelling of his external ears, and collapse of his nose bridge. This patient went on to develop external auditory canal stenosis and diminished hearing. A biopsy of the nasal septum showed a hyperplastic mucous membrane and the absence of any cartilage. Pearson et al. first coined the term 'relapsing polychondritis', which is the currently accepted name.

EPIDEMIOLOGY

Relapsing polychondritis (RP) is a rare disease, as demonstrated by the estimated annual incidence rate of 3.5/million in Rochester, Minnesota (personal communication, C. J. Michet). The peak age at onset is between 40 and 50 years, but cases have been observed in children and in the very elderly (over the age of 80 years). It occurs with equal frequency in both sexes and all racial groups. Over 30% of the cases are associated with an existing autoimmune or hematologic disease (Table 160.1), the chondritis usually occurring after the onset of the other condition. One transplacental case has been observed, but there are no documented reports of familial RP. The life expectancy of RP patients is reduced, with an estimated 5-year survival of 74% in one large series. In the subgroup of patients with systemic vasculitis the estimated survival is similar to that of patients with polyarteritis – 45% at 5 years. Infection and respiratory involvement are frequent and contribute to reduced survival[3].

CLINICAL FEATURES

Otorhinolaryngeal disease

The classic clinical manifestation of RP is acute unilateral or bilateral auricular chondritis. The onset is characteristic, with redness or violaceous discoloration, warmth and swelling involving the cartilaginous portion of the pinna, sparing the lobe (Fig. 160.1a). The episode lasts days to weeks and resolves with or without treatment. Over time and

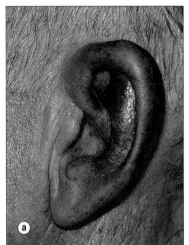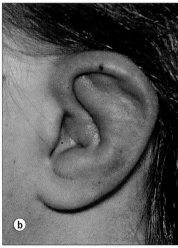

Fig. 160.1 **Otorhinolaryngeal disease in relapsing polychondritis.** (a) The pinna of the ear becomes inflamed: note the sparing of the non-cartilaginous portion of the ear. (b) Recurrent attacks cause loss of cartilage, with the ear flopping over.

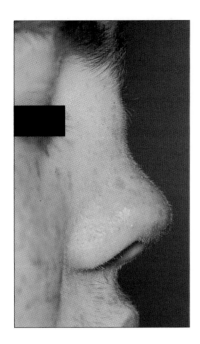

Fig. 160.2 Otorhinolaryngeal disease in relapsing polychondritis. The saddle nose deformity is caused by damage to the nasal bridge.

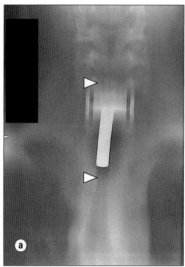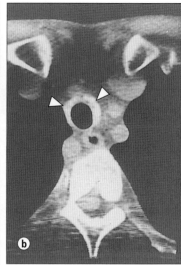

Fig. 160.3 Localized tracheobronchial obstruction due to relapsing polychondritis. (a) The radiograph shows narrowing in both the larynx above the tracheostomy tube and the tracheal stenosis below. (b) CT scan of the trachea shows the thickening of the tracheal wall due to inflammatory changes.

with repeated attacks, the pinna loses its firmness and becomes soft and flops over (Fig. 160.1b) or assumes a knobbly, cauliflower appearance. In our series[3] of 112 patients at the Mayo Medical School this was the presenting feature in 39%, ultimately developing in up to 85% of the patients. Damage to the nasal bridge causes the saddle nose deformity (Fig. 160.2). Swelling of the external auditory canal causes conductive deafness. Vasculitis of the internal auditory artery, or its cochlear or vestibular branches, results in auditory and/or vestibular impairment leading to varying degrees of vertigo and/or neurosensory hearing loss. This may occur in up to 30% of patients (Table 160.2)[4].

Respiratory disease

Respiratory symptoms are common and can be potentially lethal. At onset, 25% of patients present with these, although ultimately 50% develop them. Tenderness of the thyroid cartilage and the anterior trachea, hoarseness, persistent cough, choking spells, and wheezing and dyspnea on exertion can occur. Inflammation of the tracheobronchial tree leads to varying degrees of localized (Fig. 160.3) or diffuse obstruction, and damage to the cartilaginous rings can cause a dynamic obstruction leading to respiratory difficulty in inspiration and during anesthesia. Strictures usually form in the subglottic region, causing

TABLE 160.2 CLINICAL MANIFESTATIONS OF RELAPSING POLYCHONDRITIS		
	Frequency (%)	
Clinical manifestations	**Initial**	**Total**
Auricular chondritis	39	85
Saddle nose deformity	18	29
Hearing loss	9	30
Arthritis	36	52
Costochondral	2	2
Nasal cartilage	24	54
Ocular	19	51
Scleritis/episcleritis	19	47
Laryngotracheal–bronchial	26	48
Laryngotracheal stricture	15	23
Systemic vasculitis	3	10
Valvular dysfunction	0	6
Cutaneous	7	28

(Modified from Izaak et al.[4])

increased susceptibility to secondary infections. The reported mortality from respiratory complications varies from 10 to 50% – the lower figure is probably more realistic[3–8].

Musculoskeletal symptoms

The arthritis of RP is episodic, seronegative, asymmetric oligo- or polyarticular. It can occur before, during or after the diagnosis is established, and is the presenting feature in 30% of cases, ultimately developing in 75%. The episodes may last weeks to months, but the arthritis is non-deforming and non-erosive. Its activity does not correlate with the activity of RP. The joints most commonly involved are the ankles, followed by the wrists, proximal interphalangeal and metacarpophalangeal joints, elbows and metatarsophalangeal joints. The hips, knees and sacroiliac joints are involved less frequently, and inflammation of the costochondral cartilages may lead to a pectus deformity. Because RP can be accompanied by another connective tissue disease, the patient may have the musculoskeletal manifestations of the associated disease[2–5,9].

Cardiovascular disease

The cardiovascular system is involved in less than 10% of cases. The spectrum of vasculitis is broad, with small-vessel disease presenting as cutaneous leukocytoclastic vasculitis and large-vessel disease presenting as Takayasu's arteritis. Aneurysms of the thoracic and abdominal aorta can occur. Systemic polyarteritis nodosa has been observed in 9% of cases; the underlying disease dictates the prognosis. Aortitis causes thinning of the media and leads to dilatation of the root of the aorta and leakage of the aortic valve. Aortic and mitral valves can be sites of inflammation, with incompetence of the valve developing because of aortic root dilation, valvulitis or papillary muscle dysfunction. Conduction abnormalities causing arrhythmias, heart block and supraventricular tachycardia, owing to myocarditis and involvement of the conduction system, occur rarely. Myocarditis and pericarditis are infrequent. Recurrent aneurysms and valvular function abnormalities can occur in spite of treatment[10].

Ocular symptoms

The eye is a frequent site of involvement. Initially, 19% of patients have eye symptoms but eventually about 50% are affected. The extraocular involvement includes periorbital edema, tarsitis, chemosis and proptosis. Extraocular muscle palsy can occur. Episcleritis – local or diffuse –

and scleritis, both anterior and posterior, can occur at onset or during the course of this disease. Keratitis, thinning of the cornea and corneal melt have been reported but are rare. Iridocyclitis, chorioretinitis, retinal hemorrhages and retinal vasculitis have been observed[4].

Renal disease

In RP, although up to 26% of patients may have abnormal urinalysis, creatinine is elevated in only 10%[11]. A few patients have had renal biopsies showing segmental proliferative glomerulonephritis with crescent formation. Immunoglobulins (IgG or IgM) and C3 component of complement, deposited in a granular pattern or as subendothelial and mesangial deposits, have been observed on electron microscopy. Renal involvement by the associated autoimmune disease, for example systemic vasculitis, Wegener's granulomatosis or systemic lupus erythematosus, has also been observed.

Dermatologic disease

The skin manifestations are variable. They can be seen as the initial manifestation in 15% of patients, although ultimately in up to 35%. These include skin changes of associated underlying disease. The presence of skin changes does not have any prognostic significance[4,12]. The presence of palpable purpura, urticaria and angioedema has been observed. Livedo reticularis, migratory superficial thrombophlebitis, erythema nodosum, erythema multiforme and panniculitis are rare but known.

Neurologic disease

Vasculitis involving the central and peripheral nervous system is seen in some patients who develop cranial neuropathies, headaches, encephalopathy, aseptic meningitis, hemiplegia and ataxia. Transverse myelitis, mononeuritis multiplex and temporal artery non-granulomatous vasculitis have been observed[13].

Miscellaneous

Several cases of RP associated with the myelodysplastic syndrome have been described[14]. Fever has been observed in 22% of the patients at presentation and up to 44% during the course of the illness. The pattern is variable and a few patients have presented as fever of unknown origin. The coexistence of RP with Behçet's syndrome (MAGIC syndrome) has been reported in a few cases. This is an interesting presentation of two rare diseases occuring together, suggesting shared pathogenic mechanisms. Elastin has been suggested as a common antigen[15].

DIAGNOSIS AND INVESTIGATIONS

Although the diagnosis of RP is relatively easy, many conditions can mimic the initial changes, or an associated disease may confuse the clinical picture. McAdam et al.[16] used the following criteria, requiring three or more of the clinical features to confirm the diagnosis:

- bilateral auricular chondritis
- non-erosive, seronegative inflammatory polyarthritis
- nasal chondritis
- ocular inflammation (conjunctivitis, keratitis, scleritis and/or episcleritis, uveitis)
- respiratory tract chondritis (laryngeal and/or tracheal cartilages)
- cochlear and/or vestibular dysfunction (neurosensory hearing loss, tinnitus and/or vertigo)
- cartilage biopsy confirmation of a compatible histologic picture.

Biopsy of auricular chondritis is performed to confirm the diagnosis of polychondritis (Fig. 160.4). In patients where the presentation is very characteristic, such as simultaneous chondritis in both auricles or chon-

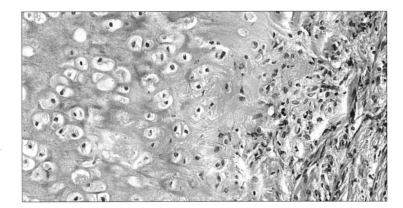

Fig. 160.4 Biopsy of auricular chondritis. Biopsy of the ear shows perichondritis with presence of mononuclear cells and occasional polymorphonuclear leukocytes at the fibrochondral junction. Hematoxylin and eosin, original magnification × 200. (Courtesy of Dr Lester E Wold.)

dritis in multiple sites, a biopsy is frequently not necessary. In others, if there is early disease or another underlying disease, it may be required.

All patients should be evaluated for laryngotracheal disease because of the potential for serious airway involvement (Fig. 160.3a). Pulmonary function tests, such as inspiratory and expiratory flow–volume curves, as well as a radiologic assessment by tomography or computed tomography (CT) scanning each are necessary, as either test alone may not reveal the full functional impact on the airway[6–8]. Combinations of intra- and extrathoracic airway involvement with expiratory and inspiratory obstruction occur. Laryngotracheal biopsy should be considered with caution as it may be hazardous, leading to acute respiratory distress in cases with stenotic or collapsing airways.

The usual findings on CT of the trachea include wall thickening by edema or granulation tissue (Fig. 160.3b), collapse of the lumen by edema or granulation tissue, fibrosis and calcification of the tracheal wall. An examination of the respiratory cycle by cine CT may demonstrate flaccidity of the airway, with dynamic collapse during breathing.

Renal status should always be investigated to exclude the possibility of an accompanying glomerulonephritis[11]. Echocardiography may be indicated to evaluate the valves and CT/MRA for large vessel involvement. Non-specific parameters of inflammation are often observed, including an elevated erythrocyte sedimentation rate (ESR), anemia of chronic disease, leukocytosis, thrombocytosis and hypergammaglobulinemia. If macrocytic anemia is present, the possibility of a rare associated early myelodysplastic syndrome should be considered.

Positive serologic tests, such as rheumatoid factor and antinuclear antibodies, are observed in the setting of RP associated with rheumatoid arthritis or other connective tissue disease. Complement levels are usually normal in RP. The arthropathy of polychondritis is radiographically characterized by a non-erosive process resulting in juxta-articular osteoporosis and uniform joint-space narrowing. The antineutrophil cytoplasmic antibody (ANCA) has been reported with RP; however, because Wegener's granulomatosis or renal 'microscopic' polyarteritis nodosa are occasionally accompanied by RP, it is possible that this reflects underlying associated disease. Few cases of both c-ANCA and p-ANCA positivity in low titers have been reported to be present with active RP. The significance of this is unclear. Anti-type II collagen antibody tests are not routinely available, and when they are undertaken antibodies are not observed in all cases. Currently, however, no reliable laboratory marker for ongoing cartilage damage is clinically available.

DIFFERENTIAL DIAGNOSIS

Although the clinical manifestations of this disease are characteristic, there are circumstances when the diagnosis may be difficult. The pinna of the ear is readily exposed to injury by trauma, chemicals, frostbite and so on. The trachea is similarly liable to be injured during prolonged endotracheal intubation. Acute streptococcal infection, fungal infection, syphilis and leprosy all may lead to perichondritis that may be easily mistaken for RP. Although the sparing of the ear lobe is characteristic, sometimes the only way to make a definite diagnosis is to perform a biopsy. Nasal damage can occur as a result of several different conditions, including local infections from fungi, tuberculosis, syphilis and leprosy, or granulomatous lesions, such as Wegener's granulomatosis, lymphomatoid granulomatosis and lethal midline granuloma. Eye involvement by RP or the associated disease can be difficult to separate. Necrotizing scleritis and keratitis can occur with rheumatoid arthritis, Wegener's granulomatosis, polyarteritis nodosa, Behçet's syndrome or Cogan's syndrome. Other features of these associated diseases aid differential diagnosis. Systemic vasculitis with pulmonary, renal, central nervous system (CNS) and other organ involvement can occur. Involvement of the root of the aorta by other diseases should be considered, especially Ehlers–Danlos syndrome, Marfan's syndrome, idiopathic medial cystic necrosis or associated ankylosing spondylitis.

STRUCTURE AND PATHOGENESIS

Cartilage is an avascular structure made up of chondrocytes, type II collagen, proteoglycan aggregates and non-collagenous matrix proteins. It is immunologically protected and thus tolerance does not develop to these antigens. This is also the reason that it is likely to be a target for an autoimmune response. Because of the association of RP with autoimmune disease, the finding of immune-mediated changes in sites of damage and humoral and cell-mediated immunity to cartilage components, and the recent observation of similar changes in rats and mice, this disease should be classified as an autoimmune disorder.

Over the past 10 years there have been several reports of cartilage antigens functioning as autoantigens and possibly leading to disease. That this may be involved in the pathogenesis of RP is suggested by several lines of evidence. The pathology of the lesion shows collections of lymphocytes and few plasma cells. The presence of immunoglobulins and C3 component of complement locally at the fibrocartilaginous junction suggests local complement activation[17]. Antibodies to type II collagen have been reported, and cell-mediated immunity to cartilage antigens has been observed in patients with RP. Recently, investigators have observed chondritis in rats immunized with native type II collagen, and fawn-hooded rats developing it spontaneously. In addition, doubly transgenic mice for human HLA-DQ6 and HLA-DQ8 have recently been observed to develop chondritis and arthritis following type II collagen immunization[18], and another group have demonstrated relapsing polychondritis developing following cartilage martix protein-matrilin-1 injections in mice[19]. A recent study from France reported an increase of HLA DR4 (56.1%) in patients with RP compared to controls (25.5%). However, when these investigators performed oligonucleotide-based genotyping, no significant subtype was found to be increased[20].

These observations reconfirm that autoimmune mechanisms are probably important in the pathogenesis of RP. The role of enzymatic destruction is probably just as important, and local release of proteinases and oxygen metabolites contribute to the damage. Whether the immune damage initiates the process that is perpetuated by the enzymatic damage, or whether enzymatic damage exposes the privileged antigens that can activate the immune system, thus allowing the disease to appear, is not known.

MANAGEMENT

The initial management of acute RP is well established. In situations of mild auricular and/or nasal chondritis or arthritis, initial treatment is with non-steroidal anti-inflammatory drugs and low-dose prednisone. For cases with serious manifestations, such as laryngotracheal or ocular symptoms, inner ear inflammation, severe auricular or nasal chondritis, systemic vasculitis, aortitis or glomerulonephritis, prednisone at a dose of 1mg/kg is indicated. In most instances the acute inflammation responds well and the corticosteroids can be gradually tapered off. However, if relapses occur with dose reduction, patients require maintenance doses of prednisone to control the disease. Strategies for refractory disease or frequent relapses during tapering are less certain.

As RP is so rare, controlled therapeutic trials have not been carried out. The literature is replete with successful anecdotes of therapies ranging from dapsone and colchicine to immunosuppressants. Generally, the former two may be useful in milder disease as corticosteroid-sparing agents, whereas immunosuppressants are reserved for those with manifestations refractory to moderate to high-dose steroids. Plasmapheresis, azathioprine, cyclophosphamide, chlorambucil and cyclosporin have all been reported to be beneficial, but patients may not respond reliably to any of these. Treatment with some of the new agents, e.g. lefunomide, etanercept and infliximab, has not been reported but personal use in some difficult cases has not been productive. Further experience is needed to evaluate these. Treatment is monitored by clinical response.

The ESR may be useful in some cases. Urinary glycosaminoglycans, serum anticollagen antibodies and antibodies to 148 kDa non-collagenous cartilage matrix protein have all been proposed as potential laboratory markers for disease activity, but their roles in monitoring RP have not been satisfactorily established.

In the situation of an initial presentation with unilateral auricular chondritis alone, the differential diagnosis and initial treatment must include the possibility of a bacterial external otitis, cellulitis and/or perichondritis. A biopsy with culture may be necessary in this setting, as well as concurrent treatment with an antibiotic until culture results are known.

Laryngotracheal involvement presents special management issues in following the activity of the disease and dealing with the consequences of a structurally impaired airway. Indirect laryngoscopy and serial CT scanning of the trachea can be used to monitor disease activity, although experience with this radiographic procedure in RP is limited. Once airway damage has occurred, tracheostomy is necessary to treat a symptomatic subglottic stenosis. If diffuse airway involvement with flaccid collapse has occurred, effective therapies are limited. Recurrent pulmonary infections require antibiotic and respiratory care treatment. Experience with successful tracheal stents is limited. Nasal continuous positive airway pressure can be tried at night to assist the patient in keeping the airway open while recumbent and asleep. Surgical correction of subglottic stenosis and collapsed nasal cartilage can be performed once the disease is quiescent.

Heart valve replacement and aortic graft surgery have been successful. Owing to the nature of the disease, surgical failure has been observed: continued annular inflammation leading to perivalvular leaks, as well as recurrent aortitis adjacent to grafts. Successful pregnancies have been accomplished[21].

REFERENCES

1. Jaksch-Wartenhorst R. Polychondropathia. Wien Arch F Inn Med 1923; 6: 93–100.
2. Pearson CM, Kline HM, Newcomer VD. Relapsing polychondritis. N Engl J Med 1960; 263: 51–58.
3. Michet CJ Jr, McKenna CH, Luthra HS, O'Fallon WW. Relapsing polychondritis; survival and predictive role of early disease manifestations. Ann Intern Med 1986; 104: 74–78.
4. Isaak BL, Liesegang TJ, Michet CJ Jr. Ocular and systemic findings in relapsing polychondritis. Ophthalmology 1986; 93: 681–689.
5. Trentham DE, Le CH. Relapsing polychondritis. Ann Intern Med 1998; 129: 114–122.
6. Krell WS, Staats BA, Hyatt RE. Pulmonary function in relapsing polychondritis. Am Rev Respir Dis 1986; 133: 1120–1123.
7. Adliff M, Ngato D, Keshavjee S et al. Treatment of diffuse tracheomalacia secondary to relapsing polychondritis with continuous positive airway pressure. Chest 1997; 112: 1701–1704.
8. Booth A, Dieppe PA, Goddard PL, Watt I. The radiological manifestations of relapsing polychondritis. Clin Radiol 1989; 40: 147–149.
9. O'Hanlon M, McAdam LP, Bluestone R, Pearson CM. The arthropathy of relapsing polychondritis. Arthritis Rheum 1976; 19: 191–194.
10. Delrosso A, Petix NR, Pratesi M et al. Cardiovascular involvement in relapsing polychondritis. Semin Arthritis Rheum 1997; 26: 840–844.
11. Chang-Miller A, Okamura M, Torres VE et al. Renal involvement in relapsing polychondritis. Medicine. 1987; 66: 202–217.
12. Frances C., El Rassi R, Laporte JL et al. Dermatologic manifestations of relapsing polychondritis. A study of 200 cases at a single center. Medicine 2001; 173–179.
13. Stewart SS, Ashizawa T, Dudley AW Jr et al. Cerebral vasculitis in relapsing polychondritis. Neurology 1988; 38: 150–152.
14. Myers B, Gould J, Dolan G. Relapsing polychondritis and myelodysplasia: a report of two cases and review of the literature. Clin Lab Haematol 2000; 22: 45–48.
15. Firestein GS, Gruber HE, Weisman MH et al. Mouth and genital ulcers with inflamed cartilage: MAGIC syndrome. Am J Med 1985; 79: 65–72.
16. McAdam LP, O'Hanlon MA, Bluestone R, Pearson CM. Relapsing polychondritis: prospective study of 23 patients and a review of the literature. Medicine 1976; 55: 193–215.
17. Homma S, Matsumoto T, Abe H et al. Relapsing polychondritis: pathological and immunological findings in an autopsy case. Acta Pathol Jpn 1984; 34: 1137–1146.
18. Bradley DS, Das P, Griffiths MM et al. HLA-DQ6/8 double transgenic mice develop auricular chondritis following type II collagen immunization: a model for human relapsing polychondritis. J Immunol 1998; 161: 5046–5053.
19. Hansson AS, Heinegard D, Holmdahl R. A new animal model for relapsing polychondritis, induced by cartilage matrix protein (matrilin-1). J Clin Inv 1999; 104: 589–598.
20. Lang B, Rothenfusser A, Lanchbury JS et al. Susceptibility to relapsing polychondritis is associated with HLA-DR4. Arthritis Rheum 1993; 36: 660–664.
21. Papo T, Wechsler B, Bletry O et al. Pregnancy in relapsing polychondritis: twenty-five pregnancies in eleven patients. Arthritis Rheum 1997; 40: 1245–1249.

161 Miscellaneous arthropathies

Daniel A Albert and H Ralph Schumacher

- Miscellaneous conditions include a variety of disorders that mimic conventional rheumatic diseases
- Localized arthritis can be caused by metastatic disease, cartilagenous tumors, foreign body synovitis, synovial osteochondromatosis, pigmented villonodular synovitis, synovial sarcomas and occasionally palindromic rheumatism
- Polyarthritis can be caused by carcinomatous polyarthritis, bypass arthritis, hypertrophic osteoarthopathy, intermittent hydroarthrosis, multicentric reticulohistiocytosis, SAPHO syndrome and Whipple's disease
- Systemic syndromes can be associated with angioimmunoblastic lymphadenopathy, Castleman's disease and leukemia

ANGIOIMMUNOBLASTIC LYMPHADENOPATHY

Angioimmunoblastic lymphadenopathy is a lymphoproliferative syndrome[1] which is frequently mistaken for an autoimmune disease because of lymphadenopathy, hepatosplenomegaly, fever, and constitutional symptoms[2]. Occasionally there is a maculopapular or urticarial rash with polyarthritis and serologic abnormalities[3]. Polyclonal hypergammaglobulinemia, Coombs-positive hemolytic anemia and less commonly other autoantibodies have been reported. The diagnosis is based on the characteristic pathologic appearance of small arborizing vessels within the lymph nodes with an inflammatory infiltrate that includes lymphocytes, immunoblasts and plasma cells. The infiltrate is oligoclonal with rearrangements of the T cell receptor and abnormal cytogenetic studies demonstrating trisomy 3 and 5. It is now thought to be premalignant or a low grade malignancy, with up to 20% of patients developing high grade non-Hodgkin's lymphoma[4].

BYPASS ARTHRITIS

Patients who underwent a jejunal ileal (but not gastric) bypass for weight reduction frequently suffered from an intermittent polyarthritis with constitutional symptoms[5]. This procedure is now rarely done because of these complications. Occasionally papular skin lesions would accompany attacks and were thought to result from blood borne dissemination of bacterial debris or immune complexes from the blind loop created by the surgery. Both the joint and the skin lesions were exquisitely painful and were reminiscent of gonococcal arthritis. Patients could develop symptoms of immune complex disease[6] with polyserositis and mild glomerulonephritis. Skin biopsies showed immune complexes and leukocytoclastic vasculitis, but laboratory studies were unrevealing. Synovial fluid was usually inflammatory and antibiotic treatment for blind loop is often helpful. In spite of this some patients needed reversal of the bypass because of persistent articular and dermatologic symptoms.

CANCER-RELATED ARTHROPATHIES

Cancer associations

An association of malignancy and autoimmune disease is clearly demonstrated for several rheumatologic disorders and hypothesized for others[7,8]. The clearest association is between adult onset polymyositis and adult onset dermatomyositis. A full description of the details of this association is beyond the scope of this chapter; however, in individuals beyond the age of 50 years there is a significant increase in malignancies, particularly solid tumors that are common in this age group. For example, in women there is an association with breast and ovarian carcinoma. In men there is an association of prostate carcinoma and in both genders there is an association with lung and gastrointestinal cancer. In addition, there are case reports of the myopathy resolving after curative resection of the malignancy. An evaluation for underlying malignancy is indicated for these patients but the extent of the workup is not well defined.

Another clear association is between lymphoproliferative diseases and both rheumatoid arthritis and Sjögren's syndrome (primary and secondary). In these conditions a two- or more fold increase in primarily B cell lymphomas is found. In Sjögren's syndrome there is a suggestion that the lymphoproliferative feature of the disease becomes more and more oligoclonal as the disease progresses toward malignancy. These associations are clouded by a probable increased risk of lymphoma conferred by some of the drugs such as azathioprine, methotrexate, cyclosporine and cyclophosphamide used to treat the disease[9]. There are emerging data on associations of systemic lupus and lymphoid malignancies and cervical carcinoma again clouded by a probable cyclophosphamide effect. There is an increase in osteogenic sarcoma in patients with Paget's disease, primarily in involved long bones. Lastly, there may be a small increase in risk of cancer in scleroderma (particularly Scl-70-positive patients) which includes the rare alveolar cell carcinoma and ovarian carcinoma[10]. Another association that is clearly recognized is relapsing polychondritis and myeloproliferative disorders, especially myelodysplasia. Likewise Sweet's syndrome is also associated with myelodysplastic syndromes and occasionally other cancers, as is multicentric reticulohistiocytosis. Lastly, gout can complicate any hyperproliferative disorder and is especially common in leukemia and aggressively treated malignancies with or without tumor lysis syndrome.

Metastatic disease

Metastatic disease from lung or breast carcinoma and rarely from kidney or prostate can present with swelling in or around a joint due to metastasis in the proximal or distal end of long bones (Fig. 161.1). This is typically around the knee but many regions are involved and even the small joints of the hands are reported. Very rarely there are multiple lesions reported resulting from disseminated carcinoma. Metastasis to the synovium is virtually unreported. Involvement of the synovium with cutaneous tumors is rare[9].

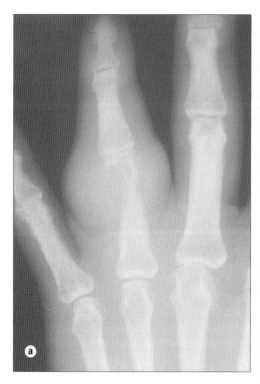

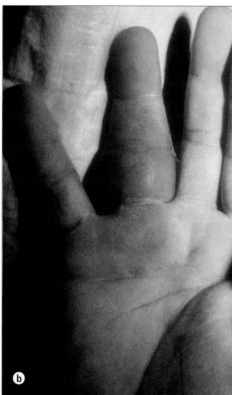

Fig. 161.1 Metastatic cancer of lung. (a) Radiograph of digit showing destructive changes. (b) Finger with inflammatory appearance.

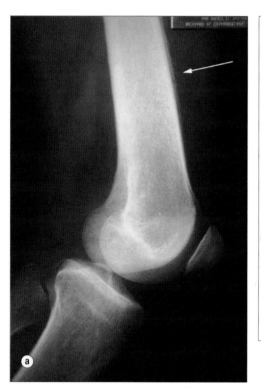

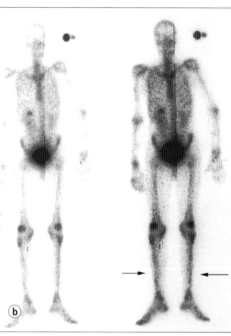

Fig. 161.2 Hypertrophic osteoarthropathy. (a) Radiograph of knee showing periosteal new bone formation along the shaft of the femur. (b) Technetium bone scan with arrows indicating increased uptake in the tibias.

Carcinomatous polyarthritis

Solid tumours particularly of the breast and lung are rarely accompanied by an asymmetric inflammatory polyarthritis of the large and small joints. This is a nonerosive seronegative condition which frequently remits upon treatment of the underlying disorder and otherwise can be treated with nonsteroidal anti-inflammatory medications. Very rarely it can be an early diagnostic clue to the presence of an occult malignancy. A different syndrome seen with pancreatitis and occasionally pancreatic carcinoma[11–13] results in arthritis involving large joints, especially the ankles, with subcutaneous nodules that resemble erythema nodosum,

however they may ulcerate and drain. Biopsies of these nodules, which are often several centimeters and intensely inflamed, reveal septal panniculitis similar to erythema nodosum but accompanied by fat necrosis, presumably from release of lipase from the pancreas. Synovial or bursal fluid can be milky in appearance because of large numbers of fat droplets from necrosis of the fatty synovium.

Hypertrophic osteoarthropathy

Hypertrophic osteoarthropathy (Figs 161.2 & 161.3) is present in two distinct syndromes (see also Chapter 162). One is a rare inherited disorder

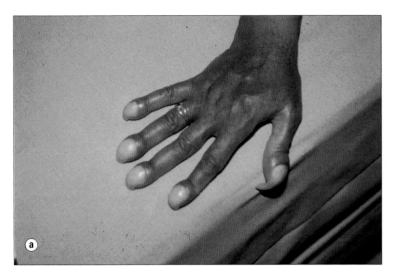
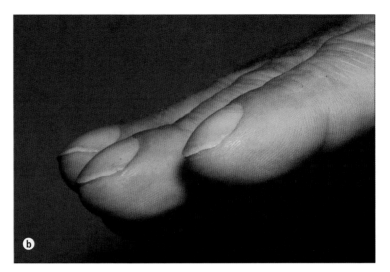

Fig. 161.3 Clubbing. (a) Hereditary clubbing without skin changes of pachydermoperiostitis. (b) Acquired clubbing showing loss of the angle at the base of the nail.

alternatively known as pachydermoperiostitis[14] in which the musculo-skeletal changes are associated with characteristic thickened furrowed skin. There is usually a family history often suggesting an autosomal dominant mode of transmission. The musculoskeletal changes are radiographically demonstrable periostitis with involvement in adjacent joints. The joints themselves are swollen and tender with bland effusions. Characteristic findings are seen on radionucleotide (technetium) bone scans with increased uptake at the distal end of long bones.

When these findings are acquired and present in the absence of skin changes, the syndrome is secondary and often associated with malignancy especially lung carcinoma[15]. Rarely, it can be seen in nonmalignant disorders such as chronic liver disease, inflammatory bowel disease, cyanotic heart disease, and other forms of shunts (e.g. cavernous hemangiomas and arteriovenous fistula)[16]. If the underlying disease is correctable the musculoskeletal manifestations may resolve suggesting a humoral factor[17]. The sedimentation rate is frequently elevated because of the underlying malignancy thus mimicking an inflammatory rheumatic disease. This condition usually responds to nonsteroid antiinflammatory agents.

Palmar fasciitis syndrome

In 1982 two reports of the association of palmar fasciitis (Fig. 161.4) and ovarian carcinoma appeared[18,19]. These reports and subsequent series described a syndrome present in a variety of neoplastic diseases primarily ovarian[20,21], but also breast, gastric[22], lung and pancreatic[21] carcinoma and others[23]. Subsequently case reports of patients with Hodgkin's disease[21], chronic myelogenous leukemia[21] and even some non-neoplastic diseases such as tuberculosis and thyroid disease have appeared. The syndrome is difficult to distinguish from reflex sympathetic dystrophy (RSD) but generally spares the shoulders and by contrast with RSD palmar fasciitis is frequently associated with inflammatory synovitis. However, the reports vary in the differentiation from features of RSD and some authors consider it a variant of RSD.

Biopsy of palmar fasciitis reveals nodules or whorls of fibroblasts surrounded by dense connective tissue with fibrous septae. Some studies suggest an autoimmune etiology based on the depositions of immunoglobulin[7].

Palmar fasciitis may improve with chemotherapy or surgery for the underlying malignancy but patients often have widespread metastatic disease at the time of presentation[7].

Malignant conditions that mimic rheumatic disease

The most difficult condition that mimics a rheumatic disease is childhood leukemia (acute lymphoblastic leukemia) which can be misdiagnosed as systemic onset juvenile rheumatoid arthritis[24]. Bone pain which is difficult to distinguish from joint pain often in a distribution that suggests juvenile rheumatoid arthritis, fever, constitutional symptoms and occasionally rash and hematologic changes are common to both. If any concern arises then a bone marrow examination is mandatory. Suggestions that it might be leukemia are severe night pain, bone tenderness to palpation, unresponsiveness to non-steroidals and leukopenia rather than leukocytosis. Radiolucent lines near the epiphyses can be present and suggest the diagnosis[25]. Similarly, both leukemia and lymphoma can mimic adult onset Still's disease, but more frequently they present with bone pain and lytic lesions.

Occasionally, neoplasias may mimic dermato or polymyositis presenting as an asymmetric neuromyopathy. Both electromyography and muscle biopsy tend to show atypical features. Also polyarthralgias, constitutional symptoms and positive antinuclear antibody and/or positive rheumatoid factor occasionally cause confusion. Lastly, pulmonary nodules that may cavitate can occur with lung cancer and mimic Wegener's granulomatosis. Hairy cell leukemia, a rare B cell lymphoproliferative condition, usually presents with massive splenomegaly and pancytopenia. However, a small number of patients have a cutaneous small vessel vasculitis[26,27]. Other solid tumors have been associated with cutaneous leukocytoclastic vasculitis especially lung, prostate, colon and breast[10]. Likewise, antiphospholipid syndrome with or without vasculitis can accompany many different types of malignancies. Generalized aching, constitutional symptoms and an elevated sedimentation rate can occur with a variety of cancers, mimicking polymyalgia rheumatica, which itself probably has a very weak if positive association with malignancy.

Myeloma

Multiple myeloma can present primarily in the elderly with a variety of musculoskeletal problems including bone pain, pathologic fractures, elevated sedimentation rate, amyloidosis (usually presenting as carpal tunnel syndrome and/or cardiomyopathy with or without macroglossia and/or shoulder pad sign), gout, hyperviscosity syndrome (especially in Waldenström's macroglobulinemia), hypercalcemia, cryoglobulinemia, polyneuropathy and the rare POEMS syndrome. Radiographs showing lytic lesions and bone marrow examination showing an increased number of plasma cells is usually sufficient for the diagnosis. POEMS (polyneuropathy, organomegaly, endocrinopathy, M spike and skin changes) has sclerotic bone lesions, a slowly progressive demyelinating polyneuropathy, organomegaly, skin changes and a variety of endocrinologic features including diabetes and hypogonadism[28–32]. This syndrome may be, in part, cytokine mediated[33] and may mimic rheumatic disease[33,34]. Improvement has been noted in one patient treated with all *trans*-retinoic acid[35].

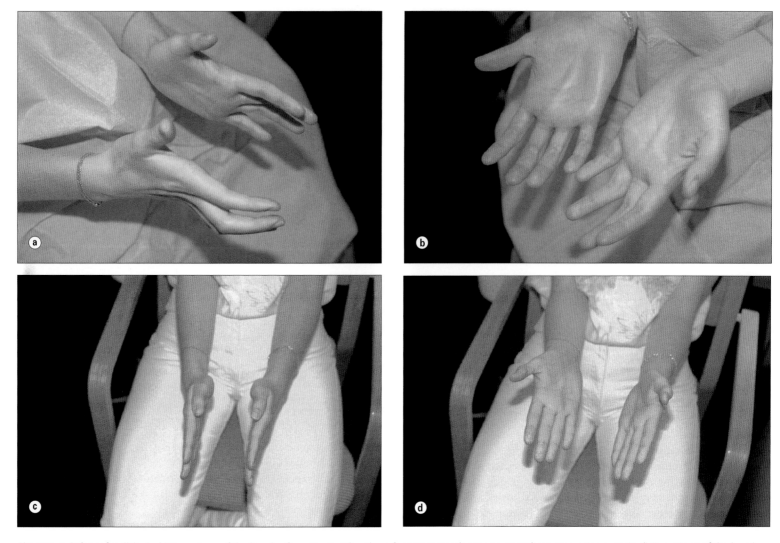

Fig. 161.4 Palmar fasciitis. (a, b) Two views of the hands of a patient with palmar fasciitis secondary to a nonmalignant ovarian cyst. (c, d) Two views of the hands of the same patient after removal of the ovarian cyst demonstrating resolution of the findings.

CARTILAGINOUS TUMORS

Based on radiologic appearance cartilaginous tumors are divided into two types. Endophytic lesions grow into the medullary cavity of the appendicular or the axial skeleton. They are frequently associated with or at the site of the epiphyseal growth plate. Exophytic lesions arise from the cortical surface of the bone. These tumors are further divided into benign and malignant conditions, with the benign much more commonly encountered, especially as incidental radiographic findings. Their location is often juxta-articular and they may present with pain in the adjacent joint.

Enchondroma

Enchondroma is an endophytic lesion that is the most common cartilaginous tumor and almost always found incidentally on hand radiographs done for other purposes. Rarely enchondromas may present as a pathologic fracture or may undergo malignant transformation. The mass arises in the central portion of the medullary cavity and shows a well defined lobulated eroded contour with or without dystrophic calcification. An inherited form of multiple enchondromas appearing early in life is known as Ollier's disease, which has a 20% rate of transformation to a malignancy. If it is accompanied by soft tissue hemangiomas it is called Maffucci's disease. If enchondromas are symptomatic they can be treated with operative curetting and bone grafting.

Chondroblastoma

This rare endophytic malignant tumor is usually found in a juxta-articular location especially around the knee, where it presents with joint pain and often an effusion. Chondroblastomas are slow growing but may metastasize to the lung.

Osteochondroma

The most common exophytic tumor arises from the junction of the epiphyseal plate and the cortex of the bone. It presents as slowly growing masses either pedunculated or sessile on the surface of the bone with a cartilaginous cap. Large and more proximal lesions are at higher risk for malignant transformation and the appearance of a malignant lesion often includes large irregular calcifications.

Chondrosarcoma

These tumors are either exophytic or endophytic and may arise within one of the benign tumors. They can occur at any age; however, if they present in childhood they are often aggressive and similar in course to osteogenic sarcomas. In adults they have an unpredictable course[36]. Radiographically, they are usually rapidly growing destructive lesions, with a variable amount of matrix calcification. Altogether, chondrosarcomas represent 10% of bone tumors[37]. Treatment is surgical with poor response to radiation.

CASTLEMAN'S DISEASE

Castleman's disease, described in 1956 (also known as giant lymph node hyperplasia), is an unusual syndrome of adults with diffuse lymphadenopathy and a variety of systemic symptoms[38,39]. The pathology reveals two different types, a hyaline vascular subtype (90%) and a plasma cell subtype (10%)[40]. The later, if multicentric, is often accompanied by autoimmune serology mimicking a systemic autoimmune disease such as systemic lupus or Sjögren's syndrome. Amongst the autoimmune features that have been described are polyclonal hyper-gammaglobulinemia, cold agglutinins, elevated erythrocyte sedimentation rate (ESR), thrombocytopenia, myelofibrosis, lupus anticoagulant[41], sensory motor polyneuropathy, and glomerulonephritis. There is an overlap of this syndrome and the POEMS syndrome, with some patients having the clinical features of POEMS and the pathological features of Castleman's. It can also be confused with angio-immunoblastic lymphadenopathy[42]. Interestingly, recent reports suggest that the germinal centers of the affected lymph nodes produce a large quantity of IL-6[43] and that monoclonal antibodies to IL-6 can ameliorate or reverse the disease process[44], although the mortality rate is high due to progressive disease, opportunistic infection, malignancy, especially lymphoma and Kaposi's sarcoma, or renal failure. Corticosteroids, chemotherapy and radiation have all been used[45] with variable success.

FOREIGN BODY SYNOVITIS

This unusual form of arthropathy has been described primarily as a monarticular arthritis as a consequence of a penetrating injury from a foreign object[46,47]. Objects fall into two categories: organic objects, usually plant thorns[48] or spines from sea urchins[49] or pieces of seashells; and inorganic material, both of natural and manufactured origin. A special case of the latter is fragments from prosthetic joints which predominantly are silicone, polyethylene and metallic. Occasionally cement used in arthroplasties, usually methylmethacrylate, has been described. Table 161.1 gives the reported associations. Typical patients with organic foreign bodies are young males engaged in one of the vocations or avocations which put them at risk for penetrating injury, such as farming, gardening, and marine activities.

The joints involved include those that are most susceptible to penetrating injuries and predominately the hands and knees. The presentation is generally an acute or subacute monarticular arthritis, but inflammation may be episodic. Synovial fluid is inflammatory with between 5000 and 50 000 white blood cells, typically with a polymorphonuclear leukocyte predominance suggesting the possibility of a septic joint. Cultures are frequently negative although on rare occasions the introduced material may be contaminated and cause a coexisting septic arthritis. The inflammatory condition in the non-septic foreign body synovitis is typically granulomatous. Synovial biopsy, either closed or open, shows a nonspecific granulomatous reaction. This could be mistaken for a variety of granulomatous diseases such as sarcoidosis. When

a foreign body is suspected, the patient's pathologic material may be examined using polarizing microscopy and this often reveals a birefringent structure suggestive of a plant material. Radiographs are sometimes helpful; usually they show just soft tissue swelling but erosive changes have been noted. If the material is radio opaque it can be seen on X-ray, but the vast majority of vegetable material is radiolucent and thus not visible on standard radiographs. The appropriate treatment is an excisional biopsy.

SILICONE SYNOVITIS

Prosthetic joints that contain silicone often fracture, generating wear particles. These wear particles are ingested by macrophages and generate an inflammatory reaction. This reaction is severe and can be debilitating, and requires removal of the prosthesis[50]. Many of the plastics used in prosthetic joints have been implicated, including Teflon, the original coating of total hip replacement, polyethylene[51], the current most common plastic used in prosthetic joints, and silicone, used primarily for metacarpophalangeal replacements. Aside from removal of the prosthetics this inflammatory problem has been largely treated symptomatically.

INTERMITTENT HYDRARTHROSIS

Intermittent hydrarthrosis is a rare syndrome of women that is characterized by symmetrical swollen joints, particularly the knees, that occurs periodically, often monthly, at or around the menses. The pathogenic mechanism is not understood. The patients are symptomatic with mild to moderate joint pain and stiffness. On examination there are effusions but the joint fluid is bland or mildly inflammatory. No satisfactory therapy exists but the process is nondestructive.

MULTICENTRIC RETICULOHISTIOCYTOSIS

Multicentric reticulohistiocytosis (Fig. 161.5) is a rare disorder characterized by the insidious onset of polyarthritis that often evolves into a severe erosive deforming arthritis and characteristic skin lesions composed of nodules and plaques containing lipid-laden (periodic-acid–Schiff-positive) histiocytes and multinucleated giant cells[52]. The syndrome is found predominantly, but not exclusively, in adults, females more than males and can be mistaken for rheumatoid arthritis, gout, leprosy or psoriatic arthritis. Biopsy of the skin lesions or the synovium can lead to diagnostic confirmation. The mechanism of disease is unknown but abnormal regulation of several cytokines including increased tumor necrosis factor (TNF)-α, interleukin (IL)-1β and IL-12 have been described[53,54].

Skin lesions are pleomorphic, may be pruritic and are often around the joints[55]. The most characteristic lesions are in a 'string of pearls' or 'coral bead' pattern at the base of the nails. Joint involvement is symmetrical and is similar in distribution to rheumatoid arthritis, except that distal interphalangeal joints are frequently involved. If untreated it is very destructive. There are no characteristic laboratory patterns although most patients have mild anemia and 30% have a serum lipid abnormality and almost 50% are tuberculin-positive. Interestingly, occasional patients have an autoimmune disease but 25% have an associated malignancy including carcinoma of the breast, stomach, cervix, ovary, colon and lung. Recent reports emphasize the efficacy of treatment with disease-modifying antirheumatic drugs (DMARDs), especially methotrexate and cyclophosphamide[56,57].

PALINDROMIC RHEUMATISM

A palindrome is a word or phrase that is symmetrical about an axis. The most famous is the sentence said to be uttered by Napoleon, 'able was I ere I saw Elba'. Palindromic rheumatism is an intermittent inflammatory condition that affects one or at most a few joints in an

TABLE 161.1 REPORTED ASSOCIATIONS OF FOREIGN BODY SYNOVITIS	
Organic	**Inorganic**
Plant	**Natural**
Date palm	Stone
Sentinal palm	Gravel
Blackthorn	
Rose	**Manmade**
Cactus	Glass
Citrus	Rubber
Mesquite	Fiberglass
Toxic	Plastic
Wood splints	
	Iatrogenic
Animal	Starch
Sea urchin spine	Talc
Fish bone	Methylmethacrylate
Sea shell	Silicone
Bee stinger	Teflon
	Metal

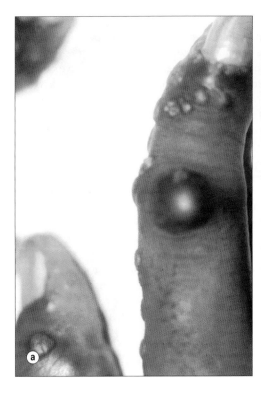

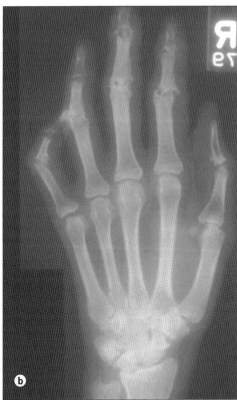

Fig. 161.5 Multicentric reticulohistiocytosis.
(a) Finger with glistening pearly white nodules – 'string of pearls sign'. (b) Radiographic appearance of digits showing destructive arthropathy.

unpredictable pattern lasting hours to a few days at most[58]. In between attacks the affected joints are normal and the attacks never result in joint damage. Swelling, heat, erythema, and tenderness with inflammatory joint fluid is found at the affected joints[59]. The condition may affect the same or different joints with repeated attacks. Acute phase reactants may be elevated during attacks but not in the intercurrent period. The attacks may persist or spontaneously resolve but approximately one third of patients (especially those who are rheumatoid factor positive) go on to develop conventional rheumatoid arthritis[60,61]. Non-steroidals and glucocorticoids may be used during attacks but do not shorten their duration. Hydroxychloroquine and other DMARDs have been used to prevent attacks but have not been systematically evaluated. Crystal arthropathies and other intermittent disorders such as familial Mediterranean fever need to be considered in the differential diagnosis.

PIGMENTED VILLONODULAR SYNOVITIS

Pigmented villonodular synovitis (PVNS) (Fig. 161.6) is a benign proliferation of synovial tissue that usually presents as an indolent progressive monoarticular arthritis or tenosynovitis. Clinically it is divided into three forms:

● an isolated tenosynovitis often in the hand[62]
● a diffuse form commonly found in the knee[63]
● a pedunculated form that floats freely in the joint cavity often causing the clinical picture of a loose body.

This disorder is seen throughout the age spectrum and is approximately equally found in men and women. One study suggested a prevalence of 9.2 cases per million population.

Pigmented villonodular tenosynovitis usually presents as an enlarging mass adherent to a tendon usually in adults and is more common in women than men. Excision is generally curative and recurrences are rare. Tendon and adjacent bone damage can occur but is usually not excessive or disabling. It is similar in presentation to a ganglion and never becomes malignant.

The diffuse form of PVNS presents as a slowly developing painful single joint swelling. The knee is most commonly affected, followed by the hip and ankle. Rarely it can occur in the hand, shoulder, wrist or vertebrae. In joints with a tight capsule such as the hip and the vertebral column, the lesion is destructive often generating the hallmark radiologic appearance of scalloped erosions, usually with a sclerotic margin thought to be a consequence of pressure or direct invasion from the mass. Joint effusions can be brown or hemorrhagic. The least common form of PVNS is the localized pedunculated nodule that is a villous like projection into the synovial cavity.

Plain radiographs do not show the lesion[63,64] but it is visible on magnetic resonance imaging (MRI) as a soft tissue mass, often with altered signal secondary to hemosiderin deposition resulting in a black appearance on T2-weighted images[65].

The etiology is unknown but all three types are thought to have a common pathogenesis since the histology of all three types is identical. Microscopically there is a proliferation[66] of sheets of pale staining synovial cells, foam cells which contain lipid and hemosiderin and multinucleated giant cells resulting in a hypertrophic red brown and occasionally yellow hued tissue[67]. Hemophilia, hemosiderosis from recurrent hemarthroses, and hemochromatosis can also produce iron pigmented tissue. Thus, not all brown stained proliferative synovitis is PVNS. All in all this appearance is more consistent with a benign proliferative and inflammatory process than a neoplastic one, which is borne out by the lack of examples of PVNS that degenerated to a malignancy. It might be thought of as analogous to pannus in rheumatoid arthritis. Some investigators propose that hemorrhage into the joint plays a role in the pathogenesis of the lesion. Attempts to reproduce the lesion with injections of blood into the joint cavity of animals results in an inflammatory synovitis that most closely resembles the arthropathy that accompanies hemophilia than PVNS.

The management of patients with PVNS is through surgical excision. This is usually curative with PVN tenosynovitis and the pedunculated form, but it is substantially less effective and less satisfactory for the diffuse form. In this instance the location of the lesion is critical since wide excisions are possible in the knee but are less successful elsewhere.

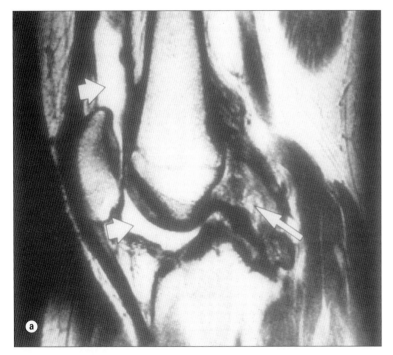

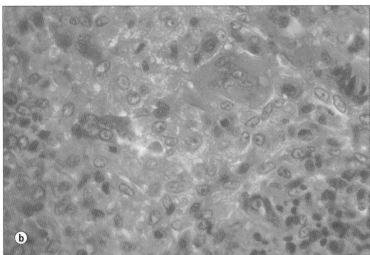

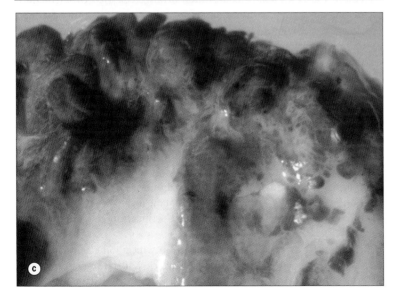

Fig. 161.6 Pigmented villonodular synovitis. (a) MRI of knee with fat arrows indicating joint effusion in suprapatellar pouch and a lobulated mass with typical dark image on T2-weighted scans in the popliteal fossa just below the thin arrow. (b) Histology of PVNS showing clusters of cells with large pale nuclei and foamy cytoplasm, giant cells, and hemosiderin in the right lower corner. (c) Gross appearance of PVNS synovium with pigmented nodules.

It is particularly difficult to perform a curative resection in the vertebral column. There is a long history of attempts to use radiotherapy for non-resectable and recurrent disease[68]. Both yttrium-90 silicate and dysprosium-65 ferric hydroxide macroaggregate have been used with some success often in combination with extensive surgical debridement. External radiation is not commonly used. Arthroscopic resection alone is inadequate therapy for these lesion. In the knee and hip there is considerable difficulty achieving an adequate resection and this combined with the bony destruction makes prosthetic joint replacement the most common approach. Total knee replacement and total hip replacement combined with a total synovectomy has a very low recurrence rate[69].

SAPHO SYNDROME

The SAPHO syndrome is an acronym that is applied to a clinical constellation which contains some or all of the following items: synovitis; acne; pustulosis; hyperostosis; ostitis[70]. This uncommon disorder of young adults has been observed in all age groups including children and the elderly and has been known under a variety of acronyms and appellations including recurrent multifocal osteomyelitis and acne induced arthritis[71]. However, the term SAPHO was coined in 1987 and refers to a heterogeneous patient population whose hallmarks include osteosclerotic bone lesions with sterile osteomyelitis and skin lesions that are heterogeneous and include both pustulosis and acne.

The typical skin involvement with the syndrome is palmoplantar pustulosis[72,73] which affects approximately half the patients. The other half have a variety of different skin manifestations including psoriasis, hidradenitis suppurativa[74], severe acne, and, rarely, Sweet's syndrome.

The typical bone lesion is osteosclerotic hyperostosis, often of the acromioclavicular and sternoclavicular joints. These sclerotic bone lesions have increased uptake on technetium scan but are sterile if the bone is biopsied and cultured with the exception that a small number are positive for *P. acne*. Other typical sites for the lesions include the anterior chest wall, sternum, clavicle, symphysis pubis, thoracic and cervical spine as well as the mandible. If the bone lesions are adjacent to a joint an inflammatory synovitis can develop which is sterile but is erosive. Approximately 13% of patients are positive for the HLA-B27 gene and many of these patients have sacroiliitis or spondylitis[75].

Approximately 8% of patients have inflammatory bowel disease with the predominance of Crohn's rather than ulcerative colitis.

The mainstay of treatment is nonsteroidal anti-inflammatory agents, which help approximately two thirds of the patients. In those failing nonsteroidals, corticosteroids will help in the majority. A few patients have progressive disease and will either need methotrexate or sulfasalazine. Patients have been tried on doxycycline for prolonged periods for the presumption of an infectious agent, even when biopsy is unrevealing[76]. This treatment is associated with improvement in a small minority of patients. A few patients appear to respond to colchicines.

Patients are likely to remain symptomatic, however this disease does not appear to be overwhelmingly disabling. This disease is often characterized by sporadic outbreaks or attacks that acquire new osteosclerotic bone lesions. The skin tends to be more persistent and less responsive to therapy. It is not known if aggressive treatment of the skin disease ameliorates the bone disorder. Acquisition of various manifestations may take prolonged periods of time and individual attacks are characterized by one or more organ system involvement[77].

SYNOVIAL OSTEOCHONDROMATOSIS

Synovial osteochondromatosis (Fig. 161.7) is an uncommon condition resulting from metaplasia of synovial tissue into cartilage which can subsequently calcify or ossify giving rise to the typical radiographic

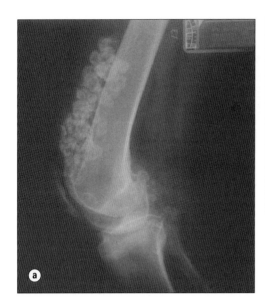

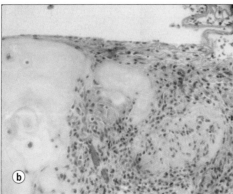

Fig. 161.7 Synovial osteochondromatosis.
(a) Radiograph of knee with typical 'popcorn'-shaped calcification. (b) Hematoxylin and eosin stain of synovial biopsy showing osteochondrometaplasia on the left.

appearance of 'popcorn' within the joint cavity. The disorder is arbitrarily divided into primary and secondary depending on the presence or absence of degenerative disease[78]. However, it is not clear what factors precipitate this condition since osteoarthritis is so rarely associated with it and the primary form has no obvious precipitating factors[79].

Clinically, the condition presents as joint pain, swelling and tenderness primarily in a monoarticular distribution. Over half of the cases are in the knee and the most common other joints are hip and elbow, but many joints have been described. Although it has been described in children the majority of patients are older and average around 50 years. There is no striking gender predominance but overall males are more commonly affected than females.

Radiographs show the characteristic appearance if the lesions are calcified. If they are not calcified, they should be visible on MRI[80]. There are no detailed analyses of synovial fluid, but CPPD crystals have been described.

The differential diagnosis includes loose bodies from trauma and tumoral calcinosis.

The pathogenesis is unknown but the synovium is strikingly hypertrophied with numerous villi. Cartilaginous nodules are seen within the synovium and free within the synovial cavity. Interestingly, although these represent metaplastic tissue, there are no descriptions of this disorder degenerating to a malignancy.

Conservative management usually involves nonsteroidal anti-inflammatory drugs. Operative management usually involves an open arthrotomy with removal of loose bodies as well as a synovectomy. In principle this could be done with an arthroscope[81].

SYNOVIAL SARCOMA

Synovial sarcoma is a rare tumor with a poor prognosis that arises from tissue adjacent to the joint but rarely if ever from the synovium[82]. Thus it is a misnomer. It is generally a mass lesion around large joints of the extremities, lower (especially around the knee) greater than upper, which is only mildly to moderately painful[83]. It presents in children and adolescents[84]. These tumors are adherent to the structures they encroach upon and the symptoms are a consequence of local invasion. They can present as painless superficial or deep structures or painful rapidly growing lesions. The average time from onset to diagnosis is months to years and they are often misdiagnosed as benign growths before histologic analysis.

Radiographs reveal a soft tissue mass that may appear well circumscribed and frequently has calcium within it or at the margin, but about half of the time the radiographs are normal[85]. Occasionally periosteal

reaction and even invasion of the bone is noted. Bone scans and computed tomography scans are abnormal and show the extent of the lesion and a bony reaction. Angiograms show typical neovascularization and tumor blush but the imaging procedure of choice is the MRI which shows the full extent of the lesion and degree of involvement of all the other soft tissue structures in the area such as vessels and nerves. In addition, the MRI can help localize the optimal site for biopsy, which should include the tumor and its margin if possible[86].

The gross pathology of the tumor is that of a circumscribed mass adherent to the underlying tissue and to adjacent tissue structures. It is usually solid but cystic changes are noted on occasion. The histologic evaluation of the tissue is difficult and expertise should be sought for. Diagnoses are not infrequently changed on rereview of the tissue slides. Other tumors confused with synovial sarcoma are epithelioid sarcomas, clear cell sarcomas, and fibrosarcoma. The typical histologic pattern is biphasic with two distinct cell types, a fibrosarcoma like spindle shaped cell and epithelial cell. The spindle cells are usually the predominant cell type and have a characteristic swirling orientation with large nuclei, scant cytoplasm and a monotonous appearance. These swirls appear to make clefts and the epithelial cells are often arranged at the border of these clefts. The more frequent mitotic figures that are seen the more dedifferentiated the tumor and poorer prognosis as is vascular invasion. The epithelial component is occasionally scarce but can be visualized by silver stains that identify reticulin in the cytoplasm. By contrast the fibroblast cells have keratin which can be identified by immunohistochemistry. Occasionally a single cell type (most often spindle cells) is seen, leading to difficulties in diagnosis. If the cell type is poorly differentiated there is a poorer prognosis.

Overall the prognosis is very poor. At the time of presentation the tumor has frequently metastasized, often widely through a hematologic distribution, most often to the lungs and less frequently locally through the lymphatics[87]. The 5-year survival is about 50% with better outlook for younger patients, tumors less than 5cm, localized disease and the histologic features we discussed above. Calcification connotes a better prognosis[86].

Treatment is primarily surgical resection with good results for small localized tumors with good histologic features. Radical resection with or without amputation is done for larger less well differentiated tumors. All too frequently, distant metastases are subsequently found. Radiation therapy (5000–7000rad) is frequently given with evidence of better survival and decreased relapse rates over surgery alone[88,89]. Combination chemotherapy is often given in addition to surgery and radiation and also appears to improve overall prognosis and lengthens the time of disease free interval[90].

WHIPPLE'S DISEASE

In 1907 George Hoyt Whipple, Nobel laureate in medicine and physiology, described a patient who was a 36-year-old physician. He had been working as a medical missionary in Constantinople and developed cough, shortness of breath and periodic arthritis[91]. His joints were hot, swollen and tender and the episodes lasted for 6–8 hours. Many different joints were affected and the patient gradually lost weight, and developed chronic diarrhea with fat malabsorption. Later he developed a swollen abdomen and dark skin, with probable ascites. Radiographs of joints revealed only soft tissue swelling. In spite of force-feeding the patient (including four raw eggs a day), he lost weight and died. On autopsy a peculiar 'intestinal lipodystrophy' was seen and these findings characterize a rare disease, which was found in 1961 to be caused by a fastidious organism[92] that stained positively with periodic-acid–Schiff (PAS) stain named *Tropheryma whippelii*[93]. Later reports document molecular diagnosis by polymerase chain reaction (PCR)[94] or electron microscopy[95], even in PAS-negative individuals. This rare disorder (less than 1000 cases reported) primarily afflicts middle-aged Caucasian males and may be more common in those with renal disease or immunodeficiency syndromes and individuals with a farming occupation. In addition to the migratory arthritis reports have emerged of other manifestations including uveitis[96], cardiac[97], and a characteristic central nervous system manifestation known as 'oculomasticatory myorhythmia'[98]. A staging system has been proposed that delineates the extent of disease. Late manifestations include dementia, and cerebellar dysfunction. Some patients develop a spondyloarthropathy and are found to be HLA-B27-positive. Most patients have anemia and an elevated sedimentation rate. Lymphadenopathy is shown on examination and by imaging. Upper gastrointestinal studies reveal thickened duodenal folds which, when biopsied, demonstrate that the intestinal mucosa contains PAS-positive diastase resistant macrophages. The organisms can be seen on electron microscopy, but PCR testing can be done if the diagnosis is equivocal. Celiac disease and tuberculosis should be ruled out. Most patients do well with antibiotic treatment although the response time is variable and the optimal antibiotic regimen is unknown. Initial treatment is often penicillin and streptomycin followed by trimethoprim/sulfamethoxazole or tetracycline given for 1 year[99,100].

REFERENCES

1. Frizzera G, Moran EM, Rappaport H. Angio-immunoblastic lymphadenopathy. Diagnosis and clinical course. Am J Med 1975; 59: 803.
2. Steinberg AD, Seldin MF, Jaffe ES et al. NIH conference. Angioimmunoblastic lymphadenopathy with dysproteinemia. Ann Intern Med 1988; 108: 575–584.
3. Boumpas DT, Wheby MS, Jaffe ES et al. Synovitis in angioimmunoblastic lymphadenopathy with dysproteinemia simulating rheumatoid arthritis. Arthritis Rheum 1990; 33: 578–582.
4. Gravallese EM, Winalski CS, Longtine J, Helfgott SM. Polyarthritis in a 78-year-old-woman (rheumatology grand rounds). Arthritis Rheum 1994; 37: 1087–1095
5. Stein HB, Schlappner OL, Boyko W et al. The intestinal bypass: arthritis–dermatitis syndrome. Arthritis Rheum 1981; 24: 684–690.
6. Rose E, Espinoza LR, Osterland CK. Intestinal bypass arthritis: association with circulating immune complexes and HLA B27. J Rheumatol 1977; 4: 129–134.
7. Naschitz JE, Rosner I, Rozenbaum M et al. Rheumatic syndromes: clues to occult neoplasia. Semin Arthritis Rheum 1999; 29: 43–55.
8. Naschitz JE. Cancer-associated rheumatic disorders: clues to occult neoplasias. Sem Arthritis Rheum 1995; 24: 231–241.
9. Beauparlant P, Papp K, Haraoui B. The incidence of cancer associated with the treatment of rheumatoid arthritis. Semin Arthritis Rheum 1999; 29: 148–158.
10. Abu-Shakra M, Guillemin F, Lee P. Cancer in systemic sclerosis. Arthritis Rheum 1993; 36: 460–464.
11. Gibson TJ, Schumacher HR, Pascual E and Brighton C. et al. Arthropathy, skin and bone lesions in pancreatic disease. J Rheumatol 1975; 2: 7–13.
12. Halla JT, Schumacher HR Jr, Trotter ME. Bursal fat necrosis as the presenting manifestation of pancreatic disease: light and electron microscopic studies. J Rheumatol 1985; 12: 359–364.
13. Smukler NM, Schumacher HR, Pascual E et al. Synovial fat necrosis associated with ischemic pancreatic disease. Arthritis Rheum 1979; 22: 547–553.
14. Matucci-Cerinic M, Lotti T, Jajic I et al. The clinical spectrum of pachydermoperiostosis (primary hypertrophic osteoarthropathy). Medicine (Baltimore) 1991; 70: 208–214.
15. Schumacher HR Jr. Articular manifestations of hypertrophic pulmonary osteoarthropathy in bronchogenic carcinoma. Arthritis Rheum 1976; 19: 629–636.
16. Schumacher HR Jr. Hypertrophic osteoarthropathy: rheumatologic manifestations. Clin Exp Rheumatol 1992; 10(suppl. 7): 35–40.
17. Padula SJ, Broketa G, Sampieri A et al. Increased collagen synthesis in skin fibroblasts from patients with primary hypertrophic osteoarthropathy. Evidence for trans-activational regulation of collagen transcription. Arthritis Rheum 1994; 37: 1386–1394.
18. Medsger TA, Dixon JA, Garwood VF. Palmar fasciitis and polyarthritis associated with ovarian carcinoma. Ann Intern Med 1982; 96: 424–431.
19. Irigoyen-Uyarzabal MV, Patino Ruiz E, Tinture-Eguren T. The fasciilitis–polyarthritis syndrome. Rev Clin Esp 1992; 191: 27–29.
20. Vinker S, Dgani R, Lifschitz-Mercer B et al. Palmar fasciitis and polyarthritis associated with ovarian carcinoma in a young patient. A case report and review of the literature. Clin Rheumatol 1996; 15: 495–497.
21. Pfinsgraff J, Buckingham RB, Killian PJ et al. Palmar fasciitis and arthritis with malignant neoplasms: a paraneoplastic syndrome. Semin Arthritis Rheum 1986; 16: 118–125.
22. Enomoto M, Takemura H, Suzuki M et al. Palmar fasciitis and polyarthritis associated with gastric carcinoma: complete resolution after total gastrectomy. Intern Med 2000; 39: 754–757.
23. Grados F, Houvenagel E, Cayrolle G et al. Two new cancer locations accompanied with palmar fasciitis and polyarthritis. Rev Rheum Engl Ed 1998; 65: 212–214.
24. Evans TI, Nercessian BM, Sanders KM. Leukemic arthritis. Semin Arthritis Rheum 1994; 24: 48–56.
25. Weinberger A, Schumacher HR, Schimmer BM et al. Arthritis in acute leukemia. Clinical and histopathological observations. Arch Intern Med 1981; 141: 1183–1187.
26. Westbrook CA, Golde DW. Autoimmune disease in hairy-cell leukaemia: clinical syndromes and treatment. Br J Haematol 1985; 61: 349–356.
27. Gabriel SE, Conn DL, Phyliky RL et al. Vasculitis in hairy cell leukemia: review of literature and consideration of possible pathogenic mechanisms. J Rheumatol 1986; 13: 1167–1172.
28. Bardwick PA, Zvaifler NJ, Gill GN et al. Plasma cell dyscrasia with polyneuropathy, organomegaly, endocrinopathy, M protein, and skin changes: the POEMS syndrome. Report on two cases and a review of the literature. Medicine (Baltimore) 1980; 59: 311–322.
29. Soubrier MJ, Dubost JJ, Sauvezie BJ. POEMS syndrome: a study of 25 cases and a review of the literature. French Study Group on POEMS Syndrome. Am J Med 1994; 97: 543–553.
30. Miralles GD, O'Fallon JR, Talley NJ. Plasma-cell dyscrasia with polyneuropathy. The spectrum of POEMS syndrome. N Engl J Med 1992; 327: 1919–1923.
31. Imawari M, Akatsuka N, Ishibashi M et al. Syndrome of plasma cell dyscrasia, polyneuropathy, and endocrine disturbances. Report of a case. Ann Intern Med 1974; 81: 490–493.
32. Waldenstrom JG, Adner A, Gydell K, Zettervall O. Osteosclerotic 'plasmacytoma' with polyneuropathy, hypertrichosis and diabetes. Acta Med Scand 1978; 203: 297–303.
33. Rose C, Zandecki M, Copin MC et al. POEMS syndrome: report on six patients with unusual clinical signs, elevated levels of cytokines, macrophage involvement and chromosomal aberrations of bone marrow plasma cells. Leukemia 1997; 11: 1318–1323.
34. Murphy N, Schumacher HR Jr. POEMS syndrome in systemic lupus erythematosus. J Rheumatol 1992; 19: 796–799.
35. Authier FJ, Belec L, Levy Y et al. All-trans-retinoic acid in POEMS syndrome. Therapeutic effect associated with decreased circulating levels of proinflammatory cytokines. Arthritis Rheum 1996; 39: 1423–1426.
36. Henderson SE. Chondrosarcoma of bone – a study of two hundred and eighty eight cases. J Bone Joint Surg 1963; 45A: 1450.
37. Larsson SE, Lorentzon R. The incidence of malignant primary bone tumours in relation to age, sex and site. A study of osteogenic sarcoma, chondrosarcoma and Ewing's sarcoma diagnosed in Sweden from 1958 to 1968. J Bone Joint Surg 1974; 56B: 534–540.
38. Peterson BA, Frizzera G. Multicentric Castleman's disease. Semin Oncol 1993; 20: 636–647.
39. Frizzera G, Banks PM, Massarelli G, Rosai J. A systemic lymphoproliferative disorder with morphologic features of Castleman's disease. Pathological findings in 15 patients. Am J Surg Pathol 1983; 7: 211–231.
40. Shahidi H, Myers JL, Kvale PA. Castleman's disease. Mayo Clin Proc 1995; 70: 969–977.
41. Yebra M, Vargas JA, Menendez MJ et al. Gastric Castleman's disease with a lupus-like circulating anticoagulant. Am J Gastroenterol 1989; 84: 566–570.
42. Kessler E, Beer R. Multicentric giant lymph node hyperplasia clinically simulating angioimmunoblastic lymphadenopathy. Associated Kaposi's sarcoma in two of three cases. Isr J Med Sci 1983; 19: 230–234.
43. Hsu SM, Waldron JA, Xie SS, Barlogie B. Expression of interleukin-6 in Castleman's disease. Hum Pathol 1993; 24: 833–839.
44. Beck JT, Hsu SM, Wijdenes J et al. Brief report: alleviation of systemic manifestations of Castleman's disease by monoclonal anti-interleukin-6 antibody. N Engl J Med 1994; 330: 602–605.
45. Castleman B, Iverson L, Menendez VP. Localized mediastinal lymph-node hyperplasia resembling thymona. Cancer 1956; July–August: 822–830.

46. Reginato AJ, Ferreiro JL, O'Connor CR *et al*. Clinical and pathologic studies of twenty-six patients with penetrating foreign body injury to the joints, bursae, and tendon sheaths. Arthritis Rheum 1990; 33: 1753–1762.

47. Sugarman M, Stobie DG, Quismorio FP *et al*. Plant thorn synovitis. Arthritis Rheum 1977; 20: 1125–1128.

48. Olenginski TP, Bush DC, Harrington TM. Plant thorn synovitis: an uncommon cause of monoarthritis. Semin Arthritis Rheum 1991; 21: 40–46.

49. Cracchiolo A III, Goldberg L. Local and systemic reactions to puncture injuries by the sea urchin spine and the date palm thorn. Arthritis Rheum 1977; 20: 1206–1212.

50. Khoo CT. Silicone synovitis. The current role of silicone elastomer implants in joint reconstruction. J Hand Surg Br 1993; 18: 679–686.

51. Gelb H, Schumacher HR, Cuckler J *et al*. In vivo inflammatory response to polymethylmethacrylate particulate debris: effect of size, morphology, and surface area. J Orthop Res 1994; 12: 83–92.

52. Levin RW, Schumacher HR. Multicentric reticulohistiocytosis. Int Med Specialist 1989; 10: 148–157.

53. Gorman JD, Danning C, Schumacher HR *et al*. Multicentric reticulohistiocytosis: case report with immunohistochemical analysis and literature review. Arthritis Rheum 2000; 43: 930–938.

54. Samaan SS, Schumacher HR Jr, Villanueva T *et al*. Unusual immunocytochemical and ultrastructural features of synovial fluid cells in multicentric reticulohistiocytosis. A case report. Acta Cytol 1994; 38: 582–588.

55. Conaghan P, Miller M, Dowling JP *et al*. A unique presentation of multicentric reticulohistiocytosis in pregnancy. Arthritis Rheum 1993; 36: 269–272.

56. Ginsburg WW, O'Duffy JD, Morris JL, Huston KA. Multicentric reticulohistiocytosis: response to alkylating agents in six patients. Ann Intern Med 1989; 111: 384–388.

57. Liang GC, Granston AS. Complete remission of multicentric reticulohistiocytosis with combination therapy of steroid, cyclophosphamide, and low-dose pulse methotrexate. Case report, review of the literature, and proposal for treatment. Arthritis Rheum 1996; 39: 171–174.

58. Mattingly S. Palindromic rheumatism. Ann Rheum Dis 1966; 25: 307–317.

59. Schumacher HR. Palindromic onset of rheumatoid arthritis. Clinical, synovial fluid, and biopsy studies. Arthritis Rheum 1982; 25: 361–369.

60. Guerne PA, Weisman MH. Palindromic rheumatism: part of or apart from the spectrum of rheumatoid arthritis. Am J Med 1992; 93: 451–460.

61. Schreiber S, Schumacher HR, Cherian PV. Palindromic rheumatism with rheumatoid nodules: a case report with ultrastructural studies. Ann Rheum Dis 1986; 45: 78–81.

62. Jones FE, Soule EH, Coventry MB. Fibrous xanthoma of synovium (giant-cell tumor of tendon sheath, pigmented nodular synovitis). A study of one hundred and eighteen cases. J Bone Joint Surg 1969; 51A: 76–86.

63. Flandry F, Hughston JC, McCann SB, Kurtz DM. Diagnostic features of diffuse pigmented villonodular synovitis of the knee. Clin Orthop 1994; 298: 212–220.

64. Flandry F, McCann SB, Hughston JC, Kurtz DM. Roentgenographic findings in pigmented villonodular synovitis of the knee. Clin Orthop 1989; 247: 208–219.

65. Hughes TH, Sartoris DJ, Schweitzer ME, Resnick DL. Pigmented villonodular synovitis: MRI characteristics. Skeletal Radiol 1995; 24: 7–12.

66. Myers BW, Masi AT. Pigmented villonodular synovitis and tenosynovitis: a clinical epidemiologic study of 166 cases and literature review. Medicine (Baltimore) 1980; 59: 223–238.

67. Schumacher HR, Lotke P, Athreya B, Rothfuss S. Pigmented villonodular synovitis: light and electron microscopic studies. Semin Arthritis Rheum 1982; 12: 32–43.

68. O'Sullivan B, Cummings B, Catton C *et al*. Outcome following radiation treatment for high-risk pigmented villonodular synovitis. Int J Radiat Oncol Biol Phys 1995; 32: 777–786.

69. Hamlin BR, Duffy GP, Trousdale RT, Morrey BF. Total knee arthroplasty in patients who have pigmented villonodular synovitis. J Bone Joint Surg 1998; 80A: 76–82.

70. Kahn MF, Chamot AM. SAPHO syndrome. Rheum Dis Clin North Am 1992; 18: 225–246.

71. Knitzer RH, Needleman BW. Musculoskeletal syndromes associated with acne. Semin Arthritis Rheum 1991; 20: 247–255.

72. Sonosaki H, Kawashima M, Hongo O *et al*. Incidence of arthroosteitis in patients with pustulosis palmaris and plantaris. Ann Rheum Dis 1981; 40: 554–557.

73. Sonozaki H, Mitsui H, Miyanaga Y *et al*. Clinical features of 53 cases with pustulotic arthro-osteitis. Ann Rheum Dis 1981; 40: 547–553.

74. Rosner IA, Richter DE, Huettner TL *et al*. Spondyloarthropathy associated with hidradenitis suppurativa and acne conglobata. Ann Intern Med 1982; 97: 520–525.

75. Maugars Y, Berthelot JM, Ducloux JM, Prost A. SAPHO syndrome: a followup study of 19 cases with special emphasis on enthesis involvement. J Rheumatol 1995; 22: 2135–2141.

76. Ballara SC, Siraj QH, Maini RN, Venables PJ. Sustained response to doxycycline therapy in two patients with SAPHO syndrome. Arthritis Rheum 1999; 42: 819–821.

77. Hayem G, Bouchaud-Chabot A, Benali K *et al*. SAPHO syndrome: a long-term follow-up study of 120 cases. Semin Arthritis Rheum 1999; 29: 159–171.

78. Milgram JW. Synovial osteochondromatosis: a histopathological study of thirty cases. J Bone Joint Surg 1977; 59A: 792–801.

79. Jones HT. Loose body formation in synovial osteochondromatosis with special reference to etiology and pathology. J Bone Joint Surg 1924; 6A: 407–458.

80. Sundaram M, McGuire MH, Shields JB. Magnetic resonance imaging of lesions of synovial orgins. Skeletal Radiol 1986; 15: 110–116.

81. Dorfmann H, De Bie B, Bonvarlet JP, Boyer T. Arthroscopic treatment of synovial chondromatosis of the knee. Arthroscopy 1989; 5: 48–51.

82. Cadman NL, Soule EH, Kelly PJ. Synovial sarcoma: an analysis of 134 tumors. Cancer 1965; 18: 613–627.

83. Ariel IM, Pack GT. Synovial sarcoma review of 25 cases. N Engl J Med 1963; 268: 1273.

84. Andrassy RJ, Okcu MF, Despa S, Raney RB. Synovial sarcoma in children: surgical lessons from a single institution and review of the literature. J Am Coll Surg 2001; 192: 305–313.

85. Horowitz AL, Resnick D, Watson RC. The roentgen features of synovial sarcomas. Clin Radiol 1973; 24: 481–484.

86. Wetzel LH, Levine E. Soft-tissue tumors of the foot: value of MR imaging for specific diagnosis. AJR 1990; 155: 1025–1030.

87. Ryan JR, Baker LH, Benjamin RS. The natural history of metastatic synovial sarcoma: experience of the Southwest Oncology group. Clin Orthop 1982; 164: 257–260.

88. Suit HD, Proppe KH, Mankin HJ, Wood WC. Preoperative radiation therapy for sarcoma of soft tissue. Cancer 1981; 47: 2269–2274.

89. Leibel SA, Tranbaugh RF, Wara WM *et al*. Soft tissue sarcomas of the extremities: survival and patterns of failure with conservative surgery and postoperative irradiation compared to surgery alone. Cancer 1982; 50: 1076–1083.

90. Pezzi CM, Pollock RE, Evans HL *et al*. Preoperative chemotherapy for soft-tissue sarcomas of the extremities. Ann Surg 1990; 211: 476–481.

91. Whipple GH. A hitherto undescribed disease characterized anatomically by deposits of fat and fatty acids in the intestinal and mesenteric lymphatic tissues. Johns Hopkins Hosp Bull 1907; 198: 382.

92. Raoult D, Birg ML, La Scola B *et al*. Cultivation of the bacillus of Whipple's disease. N Engl J Med 2000; 342: 620–625.

93. Relman DA, Schmidt TM, Macdermott RP, Falkow S. Identification of the uncultured bacillus of Whipple's disease. N Engl J Med 1992; 327: 293–301.

94. O'Duffy JD, Griffing WL, Li CY *et al*. Whipple's arthritis: direct detection of *Tropheryma whippelii* in synovial fluid and tissue. Arthritis Rheum 1999; 42: 812–817.

95. Wilcox GM, Tronic BS, Schecter DJ *et al*. Periodic acid-Schiff-negative granulomatous lymphadenopathy in patients with Whipple's disease. Localization of the Whipple bacillus to noncaseating granulomas by electron microscopy. Am J Med 1987; 83: 165–170.

96. Rickman LS, Freeman WR, Green WR *et al*. Brief report: uveitis caused by *Tropheryma whippelii* (Whipple's bacillus). N Engl J Med 1995; 332: 363–366.

97. Silvestry FE, Kim B, Pollack BJ *et al*. Cardiac Whipple disease: identification of Whipple bacillus by electron microscopy of a patient before death. Ann Intern Med 1997; 126: 214–216.

98. Adler CH, Galetta SL. Oculo-facial-skeletal myorhythmia in Whipple disease: treatment with ceftriaxone. Ann Intern Med 1990; 112: 467–469.

99. Durand DV, Lecomte C, Cathebras P *et al*. Whipple disease. Clinical review of 52 cases. The SNFMI Research Group on Whipple Disease. Société Nationale Française de Medecine Interne. Medicine (Baltimore) 1997; 76: 170–184.

100. Caples SM, Petrovic LM, Ryu JH. Successful treatment of Whipple disease diagnosed 36 years after symptom onset. Mayo Clin Proc 2001; 76: 1063–1066.

162 Hypertrophic osteoarthropathy

Manuel Martínez-Lavín and Carlos Pineda

Definition

- Hypertrophic osteoarthropathy (HOA) is a syndrome characterized by abnormal proliferation of the skin and osseous tissues at the distal parts of the extremities

Clinical features

- Three features are typically present: a peculiar bulbous deformity of the tips of the digits conventionally described as 'clubbing', periostosis of the tubular bones and synovial effusions

HISTORY

Digital clubbing is perhaps the oldest clinical sign in medicine. Its original recognition has been attributed to Hippocrates (circa 450 BC)[1]. Marie in 1890[2] and Bamberger in 1891[3] described the fully developed syndrome. Marie distinguished it from acromegaly and suggested the term pulmonary hypertrophic osteoarthropathy (HOA). Paleopathologic studies have demonstrated changes consistent with HOA in human skeletal remains from pre-Hispanic Mesoamerica[1].

EPIDEMIOLOGY

There are no systematic studies of the prevalence of digital clubbing in either the general population or hospital inpatients. The deformity is associated with a variety of internal illnesses, so that most clinicians, regardless of their specialty, have frequent encounters with patients that display this abnormality.

The veterinary literature contains reports of this illness in different species of mammals, in which the syndrome appears in response to the same illnesses as those reported for humans. HOA has been artificially produced in dogs by surgically caused right-to-left shunts of blood or by chemically induced lung cancer. Nevertheless, a stable animal model of the syndrome, accessible for systematic studies, has not been developed[4].

CLASSIFICATION

Classification of HOA is outlined in Figure 162.1. There is now evidence to sustain the belief that clubbing and HOA represent different stages of the same disease process[5]. In the overwhelming majority of cases, the finger deformity is the first manifestation and, as the syndrome progresses, periostosis becomes evident. The degree of association of clubbing with the diverse illnesses varies from it being a constant finding, as in cases with cyanotic heart diseases, to being a rare manifestation, as in patients with cancer of the lung, liver cirrhosis or Graves' disease.

Synonyms for the deformity, besides clubbing, include drumstick, pendulum and hippocratic fingers. Primary HOA is also known as pachydermoperiostosis. The term 'acropachy' is etymologically the most appropriate, and has been used to describe either clubbing or the fully developed syndrome.

CLINICAL FEATURES

In HOA there is a spectrum of symptoms. At one extreme, patients may be asymptomatic and unaware of the deformity of their digits. Other patients, in particular those with malignant lung tumors, may notice a burning sensation of the fingertips and may also suffer incapacitating bone pain. Characteristically, this pain is deep-seated, more prominent in the lower extremities and is aggravated by dependency of the limbs.

Physical examination is of foremost importance in diagnosis, because the bulbous deformity of the fingertips is unique (Fig. 162.2). The nail becomes convex (watch-crystal nail), and the skin overlying its base becomes thin and shiny, with disappearance of the normal creases. The edema and increased soft tissue produce rocking of the nail bed on

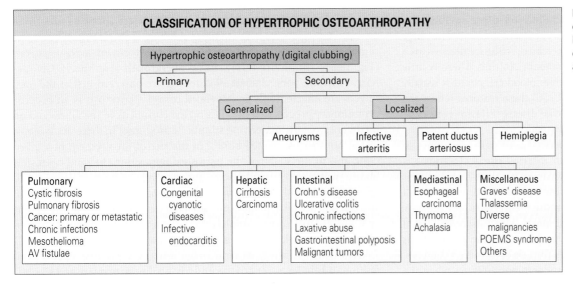

Fig. 162.1 Classification of hypertrophic osteoarthropathy. AV, arteriovenous; POEMS, polyneuropathy, organomegaly, endocrinopathy, monoclonal proteins and skin changes.

CLASSIFICATION OF HYPERTROPHIC OSTEOARTHROPATHY

Hypertrophic osteoarthropathy (digital clubbing)
- Primary
- Secondary
  - Generalized
  - Localized
    - Aneurysms
    - Infective arteritis
    - Patent ductus arteriosus
    - Hemiplegia

Pulmonary	Cardiac	Hepatic	Intestinal	Mediastinal	Miscellaneous
Cystic fibrosis	Congenital	Cirrhosis	Crohn's disease	Esophageal	Graves' disease
Pulmonary fibrosis	cyanotic	Carcinoma	Ulcerative colitis	carcinoma	Thalassemia
Cancer: primary or metastatic	diseases		Chronic infections	Thymoma	Diverse
Chronic infections	Infective		Laxative abuse	Achalasia	malignancies
Mesothelioma	endocarditis		Gastrointestinal polyposis		POEMS syndrome
AV fistulae			Malignant tumors		Others

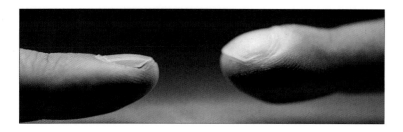

Fig. 162.2 Clubbing deformity. The finger on the right is clubbed compared with the normal finger shape on the left.

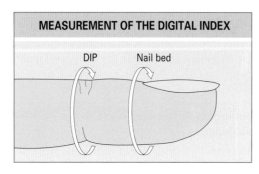

MEASUREMENT OF THE DIGITAL INDEX

DIP   Nail bed

Fig. 162.3 The Digital Index. The perimeter of each of the 10 fingers is measured at the nail bed (NB) and at the distal interphalangeal joint (DIP). If the sum of the 10 NB:DIP ratios is more than 10, clubbing is probably present.

palpation. Toes are also affected, but early changes are more difficult to discern here, because of the splaying of the normal toe tip.

The Digital Index provides a practical method to measure clubbing (Fig. 162.3). Using a non-elastic string, the perimeter of each finger is measured at the distal interphalangeal joint (DIP) and at the nail bed (NB). If the sum of the 10 NB:DIP ratios is more than 10, clubbing is probably present. There is variation in the prominence of clubbing, and the Digital Index serves to assess the severity of the deformity, or to compare groups of patients or responses to treatment[6]. The most advanced stages, with a Digital Index greater than 11, are seen predominantly among patients with cyanotic heart diseases or primary HOA.

It is worth noting that, in the majority of cases, clubbing is the only manifestation of the syndrome. When the complete features of HOA are present, however, skin hypertrophy may be evident at other levels: with coarsening of the facial features, or non-pitting cylindrical soft tissue swelling at the ankles ('elephant legs'). Thickening of the tubular bones may be evident in areas of the extremities not covered by muscles, as in the case of the ankles and wrists.

Periostosis may be accompanied by tenderness on palpation of the involved area, but in some instances gives no symptoms whatsoever. Effusions into the large joints are frequently observed and are more easily detected in the knees and wrists. At the ankle, they are more difficult to detect because of the surrounding soft tissue swelling. On palpation, there is no hypertrophy of the synovial membrane. The range of motion of the joints may be slightly decreased. Arthrocentesis yields a very thick fluid with tendency to spontaneous clotting. There is little inflammatory cell exudation, and the white blood cell count is usually less than 500/mm³ in the synovial fluid[7]. All these features reflect the fact that HOA is not a proliferative synovial disease. Effusions are most likely a sympathetic reaction to the nearby periostosis.

There are other clinical findings associated with particular types of HOA that echo the involvement of an internal organ. Cyanosis is prominent in heart malformations associated with right-to-left shunts of blood. These patients present the prototype of HOA, as almost all have life-long presence of clubbing, and more than 33% display the fully developed syndrome[8]. No other internal illness is so closely associated with HOA. A lesser degree of cyanosis is seen when the acropachy is associated with cystic fibrosis, pulmonary fibrosis or chronic infections. Jaundice, ascites and palmar erythema are common findings when the

syndrome is secondary to liver cirrhosis. Chronic diarrhea is a constant finding in intestinal HOA.

Thyroid acropachy is a rare manifestation of Graves' disease and is independent of the state of thyroid function. Clubbing usually coexists with exophthalmos and pretibial myxedema. The myxedema bears resemblance to the elephant legs described in other types of HOA. Thyroid acropachy is characterized by an exuberant periosteal proliferation, located mostly at the small tubular bones of the hands and feet[9]. Patients with the POEMS syndrome (**p**olyneuropathy, **o**rganomegaly, **e**ndocrinopathy, **m**onoclonal proteins and **s**kin changes) often display features of HOA, such as digital clubbing, skin thickening and hyperhidrosis[10].

Forms of HOA localized to one or two limbs may be seen. Most of them occur as a result of a prominent endothelial injury of that particular limb, such as in cases of arterial aneurysms or endothelial infections. A growing number of cases with localized HOA secondary to infection of an arterial graft have been reported. These are characterized by painful swelling of the affected limb, associated with radiographic periostosis; clubbing has been reported in a minority of such cases[11]. Another form of localized HOA is secondary to patent ductus arteriosus complicated by pulmonary hypertension. In these instances, clubbing and sometimes periostosis are limited to the cyanotic limbs[12].

Primary HOA is characterized by a clear-cut hereditary predisposition, with 33% of cases having a close relative with the same illness. The male:female ratio is 9:1. Primary cases are prone to display a more disseminated skin hypertrophy, hence the term 'pachydermoperiostosis'. This overgrowth roughens the facial features and it can reach the extreme of cutis verticis gyrata, the most advanced stage of cutaneous hypertrophy. In such cases, the scalp takes on a cerebroid appearance. Another cutaneous alteration more frequently seen in idiopathic cases is glandular dysfunction manifested as hyperhidrosis, seborrhea or acne, or combinations thereof. A variety of associated abnormalities have been described in primary HOA: cranial suture defects, males with female escutcheon, and hypertrophic gastropathy[13]. In primary HOA, the activity of the illness is usually limited to the growth period, adults becoming asymptomatic. Nevertheless, there are instances of primary HOA that show an enigmatic clinical paradox. HOA will occur as late complications in disease entities that are also well recognized causes of secondary HOA, such as persistent ductus arteriosus, Crohn's disease or myelofibrosis.

INVESTIGATIONS

At the present time there are no useful serologic tests for HOA. An array of biochemical abnormalities, however, may be found, reflecting the underlying illness.

Of utmost importance for the correct assessment of HOA are plain radiographs of the extremities, which may detect abnormalities in an asymptomatic patient: long-standing clubbing is characterized by a bone remodeling process that usually takes the form of acro-osteolysis (Fig. 162.4) and, more rarely, tuftal overgrowth (Fig. 162.5). Characteristically, the bone changes of clubbing are observed first at the toes; fingers are affected only in advanced cases[14]. Periostosis is an orderly, evolutionary process that depends on the chronicity of the illness and on the intensity of the underlying stimuli. It progresses in three dimensions: in the number of affected bones, in the site of involvement of a given bone and in the shape of the periosteal apposition. In mild cases, few bones are affected (usually tibias and fibulas), periostosis is limited to the diaphysis and it has a monolayer configuration (Fig. 162.6). In advanced cases, all tubular bones are affected: in addition to the diaphysis, the metaphysis and epiphysis are also involved and the periostosis takes on an irregular configuration (Fig. 164.4).

Periostosis has a symmetric distribution and evolves in a centripetal fashion. It is independent of the underlying illness; primary and second-

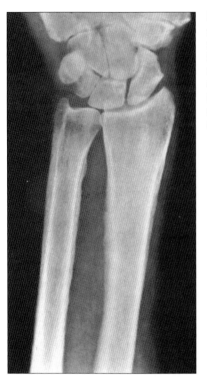

Fig. 162.4 Hypertrophic osteoarthropathy. Wrist radiograph showing periostosis at the distal ends of the radius and ulna. The coarse, layered appearance is most evident along the diaphyses. The relative sparing of the radial epiphyses is characteristic.

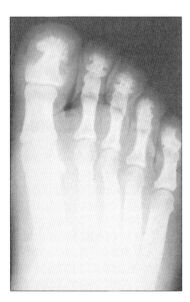

Fig. 162.5 Clubbing and hypertrophic changes. Anteroposterior view of the foot of a 34-year-old male with primary HOA, demonstrating marked clubbing and hypertrophic changes, with 'mushrooming' of the tufts.

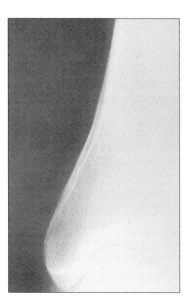

Fig. 162.6 Monolayer periostosis. Typical location of the early periosteal changes of HOA. A monolayer type of periostosis is seen in this anteroposterior view of the ankle of a 20-year-old woman with Fallot's tetralogy.

ary cases feature similar changes[14]. Typical of HOA is preservation of joint space and the absence of erosions or para-articular osteopenia.

Radionuclide bone scanning is a sensitive method for demonstrating periosteal involvement. There is hyperconcentration of the bone-seeking tracer at the periosteum. Using this method, the diagnosis of HOA is sometimes made serendipitously in patients with known malignant disease who develop bone pain, the study being requested in the evaluation of metastatic cancer.

DIFFERENTIAL DIAGNOSIS

When HOA is fully expressed, the drumstick fingers are so unique that its recognition poses no dilemma. Nonetheless, there are borderline cases in which neither a careful examination nor the Digital Index would clarify the situation. The most appropriate approach for such cases is to assume the presence of clubbing and to search for an underlying illness.

Diagnostic criteria for HOA are the combined presence of clubbing and radiographic evidence of periostosis of the tubular bones. Synovial effusion is not essential for the diagnosis. Nevertheless, it should be emphasized that in some patients – particularly those with malignant lung tumors – painful arthropathy may be the presenting manifestation of the syndrome, in advance of clubbing. Such cases could be misdiagnosed as suffering from an inflammatory type of arthritis[15]. Here, important clinical features in the differential diagnosis are the location of pain – in HOA not only the joint is involved, but also the adjacent bone – plus the fact that rheumatoid factor is usually absent and synovial fluid is 'non-inflammatory' in nature.

Some patients with HOA have an exuberant skin hypertrophy that may resemble acromegaly. The presence of clubbing and periostosis, plus the absence of prognathism, enlarged sella turcica or abnormal circulating concentrations of growth hormone should lead to the correct diagnosis. A patient should be classified as having the primary form of the syndrome only after a careful scrutiny fails to reveal an underlying illness.

The importance of recognizing HOA cannot be overstated. If, in a previously healthy individual, any of the manifestations of the syndrome become evident, a thorough search for an underlying illness should be undertaken. Special attention must be directed to the chest, because nowadays the most frequent cause of an 'acute' onset of HOA in adults is malignant lung tumor, either primary or metastatic. Conversely, if a patient previously diagnosed with any of the chronic illnesses outlined in Figure 162..1 develops clubbing, this is by itself an unfavorable prognostic sign, indicating that the disease has reached an advanced stage.

In some clinical situations, the presence of acropachy signals a serious but treatable complication. If clubbing appears in a patient with known rheumatic heart disease, infective endocarditis should be strongly suspected. A similar consideration applies to patients with prior history of prosthetic vascular surgery who develop periostosis of a limb.

STRUCTURE

The bulbous deformity of the digits is secondary to excessive laying down of collagen fibers and interstitial edema. There is also vascular hyperplasia and thickening of the vessels walls, with a perivascular infiltrate of lymphocytes.

Electron microscopic studies have confirmed the structural vessel damage demonstrated by the presence of Weibel–Palade bodies and the prominence of Golgi complexes[16]. Similar changes have been observed in the bones. At this level, excessive connective tissue elevates the periosteum and new osteoid matrix is deposited beneath.

Histologic studies of the joints have found minimal synovial cell proliferation but a prominent artery wall thickening, with intravascular deposition of electron dense material[7].

ETIOLOGY AND PATHOGENESIS

Significant advances in the understanding of HOA have been made in recent years. Any valid theory attempting to unravel its pathogenesis must explain the peculiarities of the syndrome, namely how such different illnesses can induce so unique a deformity. It must also explain the reason for the acropachy – why the syndrome begins at the most distal parts of the extremities, evolving in a centripetal fashion. Lastly, it must also account for the pathologic features of edema, localized endothelial hyperplasia and excessive collagen deposition. Several hypotheses that have been proposed to explain these peculiarities are now supported by experimental data[5,17].

The majority of illnesses associated with HOA have in common alteration of lung function. Such an alteration may be the result of exclusion of this organ from part of the circulation – a phenomenon evident in cyanotic heart diseases but also present to a lesser degree in some cases of cancer of the lung – by intestinal polyposis or in the hepatopulmonary syndrome of liver cirrhosis. In the last condition there is an 'intrapulmonary' shunting of blood[18]. A particularly strong argument in favor of the key role of lung bypass in the development of HOA is the existence of patients with patent ductus arteriosus complicated by pulmonary hypertension in whom the acropachy is limited to the cyanotic

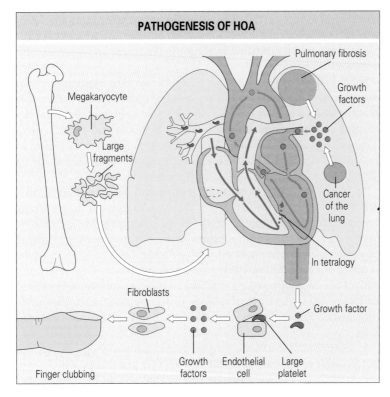

PATHOGENESIS OF HOA

Megakaryocyte

Large fragments

Pulmonary fibrosis

Growth factors

Cancer of the lung

In tetralogy

Fibroblasts

Growth factor

Finger clubbing

Growth factors | Endothelial cell | Large platelet

Fig. 162.7 Theoretical hypertrophic osteoarthropathy. Megakaryocytes emerge from the bone marrow and, in normal circumstances, are fragmented in the lung microvasculature. In individuals with cyanotic heart disease (in this case Fallot's tetralogy), the large fragments would not enter the pulmonary circulation; instead they would directly enter the systemic circulation, reach its most distal sites, release growth factors, activate endothelial cells and thus inducing finger clubbing. In individuals with lung cancer, a growth factor derived from abnormal tissue would enter the systemic circulation and induce clubbing.

limbs[12]. Another form of alteration of lung function results from a direct injury to the lung parenchyma, from an assortment of diffuse interstitial illnesses listed in Figure 162.1.

The lack of inflammatory and autoimmune phenomena by conventional serology, in addition to the excessive collagen deposition evident in histologic studies, led to a proposal that a fibroblast growth factor could be at the epicenter of the syndrome[5]. This factor would normally be present in the central venous circulation and removed in the lung. A platelet-derived growth factor was chosen on the basis of a mathematical model suggesting that, in normal circumstances, large platelets are fragmented in the pulmonary circulation. It was suggested that, in the patients with right-to-left shunts of blood, large thrombocytes that escaped fragmentation in the lung would enter the systemic circulation and reach its most distal parts on axial streams, there releasing growth factors and inducing acropachy[17].

Studies of patients with HOA associated with cyanotic heart diseases are consistent with these explanations. It has been found that these patients have a bizarre platelet population, characterized by the presence of macrothrombocytes with aberrant volume-distribution curves[19]. Such cyanotic patients also display alterations in another distal part of the circulation; the renal glomeruli. Histologic studies have disclosed glomerular enlargement, with trapped megakaryocyte nuclei inside[20]. These features concur with the theory of platelet fragmentation in the lung. Furthermore, it has also been demonstrated that these cyanotic patients, and patients with primary HOA, have increased circulating concentrations of von Willebrand factor antigen, an abnormality that reflects activation of the platelet/endothelial cell[21]. There are theoretical grounds to suggest that similar mechanisms may be operative in other illnesses associated with acropachy. Endothelial cell activation is a prominent feature of endarteritis and endocarditis of infective etiology.

These data suggest that localized activation of the platelet/endothelial cells, with the subsequent release of growth factor(s), has a key role in the development of HOA (Fig. 162.7). Vascular endothelial growth factor (VEGF) may also be involved in the pathogenesis of HOA. It is an angiogenic agent produced by malignant tumors as mechanism of cancer growth. It is also one of the cytokines released during platelet activation, with important effects on the development of endothelial hyperplasia. Furthermore VEGF is a hypoxia-induced agent. Thus the action of this cytokine theoretically explains how different neoplastic or hypoxic illnesses may induce HOA. It may also explain the histologic abnormalities of HOA (vascular hyperplasia, endothelial cell activation and edema). Plasma concentrations of VEGF are significantly greater in patients with primary HOA and with HOA associated with lung cancer, compared with those in normal controls[22].

All this new information awaits assessment by independent investigators.

MANAGEMENT

Apart from its unsightliness, clubbing is usually asymptomatic and does not require treatment. For patients with painful osteoarthropathy, nonsteroidal anti-inflammatory drugs are effective in alleviating pain in most patients. Removal of a lung tumor, correction of a heart malformation or successful treatment of infective endocarditis is followed by a dramatic regression of all features of the syndrome.

REFERENCES

1. Martínez-Lavín M, Mansilla J, Pineda C, Pijoán C. Evidence of hypertrophic osteoarthropathy in human skeletal remains from prehispanic Mesoamerica. Ann Intern Med 1994; 12: 238–241.
2. Marie P. De l'ostéo-arthropie hypertrophiante pneumique. Rev Med 1890; 10: 1–36.
3. Bamberger E. Uber knochenveränderugen bei chronishen lungen und herzkrankheiten. Z Klin Med 1891; 18: 193–217.
4. García A, Martínez-Lavín M. La osteoartropatía hipertrófica de los animales. Rev Mex Reumatol 1989; 4: 146–148.
5. Martínez-Lavín M. Digital clubbing and hypertrophic osteoarthropathy: a unifying hypothesis. J Rheumatol 1987; 14: 6–8.
6. Vazquez-Abad D, Pineda C, Martínez-Lavín M. Digital clubbing: a numerical assessment of the deformity. J Rheumatol 1989; 16: 518–520.

7. Schumacher R. Articular manifestations of hypertrophic pulmonary osteoarthropathy in bronchogenic carcinoma. Arthritis Rheum 1976; 19: 629–635.

8. Martínez-Lavín M, Bobadilla M, Casanova J et al. Hypertrophic osteoarthropathy in cyanotic congenital heart disease. Arthritis Rheum 1982; 25: 1186–1193.

9. Kinsella R, Back D. Thyroid acropachy. Med Clin North Am 1968; 52: 393–398.

10. Martínez-Lavín M, Vargas AS, Cabré J et al. Features of hypertrophic osteoarthropathy in patients with POEMS syndrome. A metaanalysis. J Rheumatol 1997; 24: 2268–2269.

11. Stiles R, Resnick D, Sartoris D, Savoia M. Unilateral lower extremity hypertrophic osteoarthropathy associated with aortic graft infection. South Med J 1988; 81: 788–791.

12. Martínez-Lavín M. Elucidation of digital clubbing may help in understanding the pathogenesis of pulmonary hypertension associated with congenital heart defects. Cardiol Young 1994; 4: 228–231.

13. Martínez-Lavín M, Pineda C, Valdez T et al. Primary hypertrophic osteoarthropathy. Semin Arthritis Rheum 1988; 17: 156–162.

14. Pineda C, Fonseca C, Martínez-Lavín M. The spectrum of soft tissue and skeletal abnormalities of hypertrophic osteoarthropathy. J Rheumatol 1990; 17: 626–632.

15. Segal A, Mackenzie A. Hypertrophic osteoarthropathy: a 10-year retrospective analysis. Semin Arthritis Rheum 1982; 12: 220–232.

16. Padula S, Broketa G, Sampieri A et al. Increased collagen synthesis in skin fibroblasts from patients with primary hypertrophic osteoarthropathy. Arthritis Rheum 1994; 37: 1386–1394.

17. Dickinson CJ, Martin JF. Megakaryocytes and platelet clumps as the cause of finger clubbing. Lancet 1987; ii: 1434–1435.

18. Stoller J, Moodie D, Schiavone W et al. Reduction of intrapulmonary shunt and resolution of digital clubbing associated with primary biliary cirrhosis after liver transplantation. Hepatology 1990; 11: 54–58.

19. Vazquez-Abad D, Martínez-Lavín M. Macro-thrombocytes in the peripheral circulation of patients with cardiogenic hypertrophic osteoarthropathy. Clin Exp Rheumatol 1991; 9: 59–62.

20. Perloff JK, Latta H, Barsotti P. Pathogenesis of the glomerular abnormality in cyanotic congenital heart disease. Am J Cardiol 2000; 86: 1198–1204.

21. Matucci-Cerinic, Martínez-Lavín M, Rojo F et al. Von Willebrand factor antigen in hypertrophic osteoarthropathy. J Rheumatol 1992; 19: 765–767.

22. Silveira LH, Martínez-Lavín M, Pineda C et al. Vascular endothelial growth factor and hypertrophic osteoarthropathy. Clin Exp Rheumatol 2000; 18: 57–62.

OTHER SYSTEMIC ILLNESSES

163 Cogan's syndrome

E William St Clair and Rex McCallum

Definition

- Cogan's syndrome is a rare, chronic inflammatory disease of unknown cause affecting the eye and inner ear

Clinical features

- The hallmarks of Cogan's syndrome are interstitial keratitis and recurrent Ménière's-like episodes often leading quickly to deafness
- Cogan's syndrome may also be accompanied by systemic vasculitis
- The differential diagnosis of Cogan's syndrome includes a variety of infectious and inflammatory diseases with ocular and inner ear manifestations
- Auditory outcomes may benefit from prompt initiation of corticosteroid therapy

HISTORY

In 1945, David Cogan, an ophthalmologist, described four patients with non-syphilitic interstitial keratitis and vestibuloauditory symptoms[1]. The ocular and inner ear symptoms had begun in each case within a few days to weeks of each other. Cogan had discovered an earlier report describing a young man with similar eye and inner ear manifestations characterized by interstitial keratitis, iritis and Ménière's-like attacks[2]. Three of Cogan's cases were young women with severe vestibuloauditory symptoms whose course was marked by rapidly progressive, bilateral deafness. The other case, a man, had relatively mild vestibuloauditory symptoms and transient hearing loss. All of the patients had bilateral eye redness, photophobia and reduced vision. Cogan's examination revealed a yellowish-white nodular patchy infiltrate in the deep corneal stroma, with a paucity of inflammatory reaction in the anterior chamber and no abnormality of the iris. Each of the cases exhibited a 'nerve type' hearing loss with hypoactive or absent vestibular function. Serological studies for syphilis were uniformly negative. The only laboratory abnormality was mild leukocytosis.

Cogan distinguished this new syndrome from the interstitial keratitis and hearing loss of congenital and tertiary syphilis. In syphilis, Cogan explained, the cornea has a ground-glass or opalescent opacity, often associated with iridocyclitis; the disease begins abruptly, peaks within 1–2 weeks, and then vascularizes with corneal thickening, followed by gradual improvement. In contrast, the eye disease in Cogan's cases began slowly and the cornea showed little change in appearance even after months of follow-up. Cogan also stressed that deafness from syphilis usually occurs with severe interstitial keratitis and a dearth of vestibular symptoms; it 'comes on slowly, and does not begin for months or years after the ocular signs'[1].

Shortly thereafter, Cogan and colleagues described nine more cases with the same features and chronicled the long-term follow-up of these new cases plus the original four[3,4]. The clinical picture consisted of recurrent and chronic corneal involvement of both eyes and rapidly fluctuating, profound hearing loss. Bilateral, severe visual loss developed in only one of the surviving 11 patients. All but two of the 13 patients had marked hearing loss or deafness. Two of the patients died during follow-up. One death was attributed to rheumatic fever, an enlarged heart, and aortic insufficiency. In retrospect, the aortic valvular disease may have been due to aortitis, a now-recognized feature of Cogan's syndrome. Cogan also speculated that three of the patients in this series had 'polyarteritis', but tissue biopsies were never done to confirm the diagnoses.

In 1953, Oliner and coworkers[5] described a 21-year-old woman with interstitial keratitis, abrupt onset of vertigo and total bilateral deafness who later in the course developed nodular scleritis and a biopsy-proven, systemic necrotizing vasculitis. Several case reports then followed that established a link between Cogan's syndrome and systemic vasculitis[6,7]. In 1980, Haynes and his colleagues[8] described 13 new cases of Cogan's syndrome seen at the National Institutes of Health (NIH), and reviewed the literature up to this point. This contribution afforded new insights into the clinical manifestations of Cogan's syndrome and for the first time provided a conceptual framework for effective management. In this review, the authors divided Cogan's syndrome into 'typical' and 'atypical' forms. The syndrome was deemed 'atypical' if the latency between the eye and inner ear manifestations exceeded 2 years, or if interstitial keratitis was accompanied by serious inflammatory eye disease, such as scleritis, posterior uveitis, or retinal vascular disease. This distinction arose from observations suggesting that systemic vasculitis occurred more often with 'atypical' than 'typical' forms. In 1986, Vollertsen et al.[9] described 18 additional cases of Cogan's syndrome from the Mayo Clinic. The division of Cogan's syndrome into two forms no longer appears valid because many examples are now available documenting systemic vasculitis in cases of typical Cogan's syndrome.

EPIDEMIOLOGY

Cogan's syndrome occurs primarily in young adults, with no gender predisposition. The mean age of onset was 22 years for the NIH[8] and Mayo Clinic[9] series. At Duke, 47 patients with Cogan's syndrome (which includes the 13 patients from the NIH series) had a mean age of onset of 29 years[10]. Cogan's syndrome has been infrequently described in children[11] and the elderly[12]. There have been no population studies of the incidence or prevalence of Cogan's syndrome, but this diagnosis is made rarely even at tertiary medical centers.

PATHOPHYSIOLOGY

Eye disease

The defining ocular manifestation of Cogan's syndrome is interstitial keratitis, a corneal inflammatory disease. The cornea is a dome-like structure on the anterior surface of the eye. Ordinarily it is transparent and non-vascular, acting as the primary refractive structure of the eye. The cornea is composed of five layers: epithelium (external) and basement membrane, Bowman's layer, stroma, Descemet's membrane, and endothelium. Innervation of the cornea comes from the trigeminal nerve. In Cogan's syndrome, the inflammatory process in the cornea initially involves the superficial and middle layers and then affects the deeper layers. Histopathological studies of this lesion are limited. Corneal tissue from a single autopsy specimen has shown focal thickening of the epithelium, destruction of Bowman's membrane, a lymphocytic stromal infiltrate and neovascularization[7].

Hearing loss and vestibular dysfunction

Cogan's syndrome damages the inner ear structures, causing sensorineural hearing loss and vestibular dysfunction. The inner ear is embedded in the temporal bone and consists of the osseous labyrinth, membranous labyrinth, and the endolymphatic duct and sac. The endolymphatic sac and duct communicate with both the cochlea and the vestibular apparatus. The osseous labyrinth houses the cochlea and its organ of Corti, the semicircular canals, and the saccule and utricle. The membranous labyrinth forms an interconnected network of spaces bathed in potassium-rich endolymph. This fluid provides a suitable metabolic environment for normal inner ear function. The endolymph is produced by the stria vascularis, the richly vascularized epithelial lining of the cochlear wall.

The cochlea is a prime target in Cogan's syndrome. Auditory function requires an intact cochlea, which is a coiled duct with nerve fibers and specialized cells. Sound reaches the cochlea via mechanical transmission through the external auditory canal, the tympanic membrane and the ossicles (malleous, incus and stapes) of the middle ear. The ossicular chain vibrates the oval window and displaces the endolymphatic fluid of the cochlear duct. The fluid displacement moves the hair cells of the organ of Corti, which in turn converts the mechanical energy into neural stimulation. The nerve impulses are conveyed to the brain stem through the afferent cochlear nerve fibers of cranial nerve VIII and then relayed to the speech centers of the brain.

The semicircular canals, the maculae of the utricle and the sacculae are affected in Cogan's syndrome. These structures detect angular and linear acceleration of the body, delivering nerve impulses through the cochlear branch of cranial nerve VIII to the ipsilateral and contralateral vestibular nuclei of the brain stem. These nuclei also receive major neural input from the muscles of the truck and extremities, the cerebellum and the visual cortex to maintain the body's balance and equilibrium and coordinate the eyes in such a way to keep images focused on the retina. Dyscoordinated inputs from the inner ear can provoke vertigo, oscillopsia (perception of objects jiggling back and forth) and nystagmus, typical features of Cogan's syndrome. The vestibular system has the ability to repair itself through the reorganization of synaptic contacts to preserve the symmetry of input required for equilibrium, a process termed vestibular compensation. After an acute inflammatory episode, vestibular function usually improves because of this compensatory mechanism.

Histopathological analysis of the inner ear has been limited to temporal bone specimens from autopsies of four patients who died with Cogan's syndrome. In these cases, inner ear pathology has shown lymphocytic and plasma cell infiltration of the spiral ligament, endolymphatic hydrops, degenerative changes in the organ of Corti, neoosteogenesis, and demyelination and atrophy of the vestibular and cochlear branches of cranial nerve VIII[7,13–15]. New bone formation appears to be a late finding. No trace of vasculitis has been found.

Vasculitis

In Cogan's syndrome the vascular involvement resembles that seen with polyarteritis nodosa and Takayasu's arteritis. The walls of affected medium-sized muscular arteries show typical histopathologic changes of polyarteritis, including infiltration with lymphocytes and plasma cells, intimal thickening and fibrosis, and aneurysmal dilatation[8,16] (Fig. 163.1). The inflammatory process may also involve veins in a manner similar to microscopic polyangiitis[7]. Large artery involvement takes the form of a Takayasu's-like arteritis and is characterized by infiltration of the walls with polymorphonuclear cells, mononuclear cells and multinucleated giant cells, intimal proliferation, fibrinoid necrosis, and disruption of the elastic lamina[17,18].

The aorta can be affected in up to 10% of patients with Cogan's syndrome. Proximal aortitis may cause enlargement of the ascending aorta. The inflammatory process can extend to the coronary ostia and aortic valve, leading to coronary stenosis and valvular regurgitation[7,18,19]

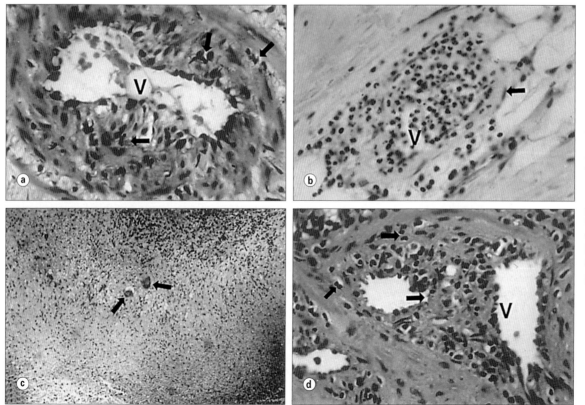

Fig. 163.1 Histology of vascular and splenic inflammation in a patient with Cogan's syndrome. (a) Inflammatory cells infiltrating and surrounding the wall of a medium-sized vessel in the dermis (arrow). V, vessel lumen (hematoxylin and eosin). (b) Inflammatory infiltrate in the lumen (V) as well as infiltrating and surrounding the wall of an artery in the gastric serosa (hematoxylin and eosin). (c) Giant cells (arrows) within the granulomatous inflammatory infiltrate in the spleen (hematoxylin and eosin). (d) A splenic muscular artery with inflammatory cells infiltrating the vessel wall and within the intraluminal thrombus (arrows) (hematoxylin and eosin). (With permission from Allen et al.[18])

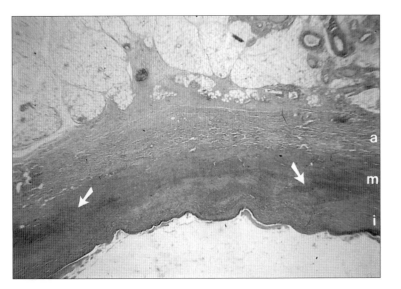

Fig. 163.2 Cogan's syndrome and aortitis. Low-power view of the histopathology of the aorta. The inflammatory response is characterized by intimal proliferation and an acute inflammatory infiltrate. a, adventitia; m, media; i, intima. Hematoxylin and eosin.

(Fig. 163.2) Defective aortic valves removed from patients with Cogan's syndrome have shown cusp detachments, outpouchings, fenestrations, thinning, thickening and retraction[16,17,19,20]. Histopathological analysis of the valve leaflets has revealed patchy infiltration with mononuclear cells, fibrinoid necrosis, myxomatous degeneration, and irregular thickening of the endocardium[16,17,19–21]. Two patients with Cogan's syndrome have been reported with aneurysmal dilatation of the descending thoracic and abdominal aorta[22]. Histopathology of the aorta from one of these cases showed a dense lymphocytic infiltrate of the media and adventitia, with marked destruction of the medial elastic lamina.

ETIOLOGY

Infection has long been suspected as a trigger for Cogan's syndrome, but proof of a microbial etiology has been elusive. The resemblance of this disorder to the ocular and vestibuloauditory manifestations of congenital and tertiary syphilis has stimulated ongoing interest in a possible infectious cause, starting with its first description more than five decades ago. Several attempts have been made to link Cogan's syndrome with a variety of infectious agents, including *Borrelia burgdorferi* and various chlamydial species, but with inconsistent and largely negative results.

Because *Chlamydia trachomatis* causes a chronic eye infection, evidence of this pathogen has been frequently sought in Cogan's syndrome. For example, IgM and IgG antibodies to *C. trachomatis* were detected at the NIH in sera from 4 of 13 and 9 of 13 patients with Cogan's syndrome[8]. Other studies have found positive and negative serological evidence of chlamydial infection in this disease population. There have been repeated failures to directly isolate the organisms from affected eyes. However, an interesting case of a 15-year-old girl has been described with sudden onset of interstitial keratitis, sensorineural hearing loss, aortic valve thickening and coronary vasculitis in which *C. psittaci* was isolated from the conjunctiva[23]. At present, no evidence supports a direct link between infection and Cogan's syndrome.

IMMUNOLOGIC MECHANISMS

Immune mechanisms probably play an important role in the pathogenesis of Cogan's syndrome. Once considered immunologically privileged sites, the cornea and the inner ear are both capable of mounting an immune response. Ordinarily, the cornea and anterior chamber of the eye produce factors that suppress delayed-type hypersensitivity, a

TABLE 163.1 IMMUNOLOGIC MECHANISMS OF THE INNER EAR

- Endolymphatic sac contains antigen-presenting cells, T cells, B cells, IgM, IgG and IgA
- IL-1, IL-2 and transforming growth factor-β produced with immune response
- Spiral modular vein acquires morphology of high endothelial venules and expresses intracellular adhesion molecule (ICAM)-1 and vascular cell adhesion molecule-1 (VCAM-1) during immune response, leading to recruitment of leukocytes
- Transfer of T-cell lines reactive with heterologous preparation of inner ear antigen produces experimental labyrinthitis in rat model

process termed anterior chamber-associated immune deviation. However, infection, trauma or toxins can set in motion a robust inflammatory response. For example, herpes simplex keratitis and corneal allograft rejection, widely studied immune disorders of the cornea, are characterized by an influx of CD4 and CD8 T cells and activated Langerhans' cells (antigen-presenting cells of the eye) and secretion of IL-1 and TNF-α[24]. An experimental model of autoimmune keratitis has been developed in the rat[25]. In this model, transfer of corneal-specific activated T cells into irradiated rats produces a severe keratitis, with T-cell and macrophage infiltration of the cornea.

The inner ear can also generate a vigorous immune response to an array of insults[26] (Table 163.1). This appears to depend on the integrity of the endolymphatic sac. During periods of quiescence the endolymphatic sac contains antigen-presenting cells, T cells and B cells, as well as IgM, IgG and IgA. IL-1, IL-2 and transforming growth factor-β are produced during an immune response. The spiral modular vein is important for trafficking leukocytes to sites of inflammation[27]. It acquires the morphology of high endothelial venules (HEV), which function to recruit leukocytes into inflamed tissue. In experimental models, antigenic challenges upregulate the expression of intracellular adhesion molecule (ICAM)-1 and vascular cell adhesion molecule (VCAM)-1 on the surface of the spiral modular vein[28]. In a rat model, labyrinthitis can be induced by transfer of T-cell lines reactive with a heterologous preparation of inner ear antigens[29]. These studies suggest that autoreactive T cells can mediate vestibuloauditory inflammation. Regardless of the insult, however, animal studies show that immunologic reactions culminate in rapid accumulation of dense extracellular matrix. The inner ear is incapable of clearing this matrix, leading to endosteal cell activation, neosteogenesis and irreversible injury.

Relatively little evidence can be found to substantiate a role for organ-specific autoimmunity in the pathogenesis of Cogan's syndrome. Although serum IgG antibodies to corneal antigens have been associated with Cogan's syndrome[30–33], these studies have been difficult to interpret because of the small numbers of patients in these studies, the absence of controls, and the poorly characterized antigen preparations. Investigators have also searched for serum antibodies to inner ear antigens. Moscocki *et al.*[34] found serum antibodies to a 68 kDa inner ear protein in 42 (58%) of 72 patients with idiopathic, progressive bilateral sensorineural hearing loss. However, these autoantibodies were absent in sera from all eight patients with Cogan's syndrome used as controls in this study.

CLINICAL FEATURES

Ocular manifestations

Cogan's syndrome is commonly heralded by ocular signs and symptoms (Table 163.2). Although ocular pain, redness and photophobia are the dominant complaints, blurry vision, tearing, diplopia, foreign-body sensation and visual field defects have also been described at

TABLE 163.2 MAJOR CLINICAL FEATURES OF COGAN'S SYNDROME

Manifestations		Proportion of cases (%)
Inflammatory eye disease		100
	Interstitial keratitis	70
	Conjunctivitis	35
	Iridocyclitis	30
	Episcleritis/scleritis	30
	Papillitis	5
	Posterior uveitis	5
	Retinal vasculitis	5
	Vitritis	5
	Exophthalmos	<5
Vestibuloauditory dysfunction		100
	Hearing loss	95
	Vertigo	90
	Tinnitus	75
	Nausea and vomiting	65
	Ataxia	45
	Nystagmus	30
	Oscillopsia	15
Systemic vasculitis		15
	Aortitis with or without aortic insufficiency	10
	Large vessel vasculitis	10
	Medium vessel vasculitis	<5

(With permission from McCallum et al.[35])

presentation[8–10,30]. In the Duke series, the ocular diagnoses were varied and included interstitial keratitis (72%) (Fig. 163.3), conjunctivitis (34%), iridocyclitis (32%), scleritis/episclerits (20%) (Fig. 163.4), corneal ulceration (4%), vitritis, choroiditis and subretinal neovascular membrane (2%), pars planitis (2%), orbital pseudotumor (2%) and cottonwool spots (2%)[10]. The ocular manifestations may be fleeting and repetitive eye examinations may be required to document ocular inflammatory disease, particularly interstitial keratitis[9,36,37].

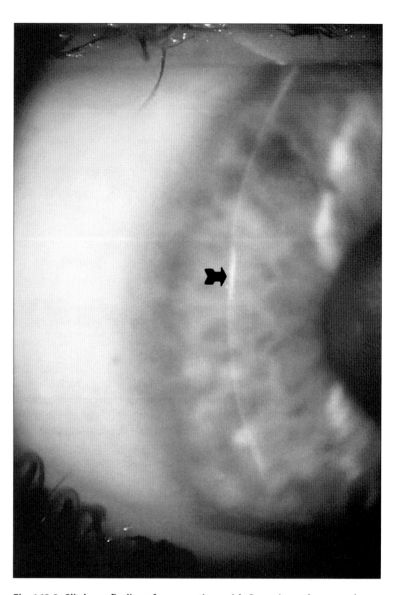

Fig. 163.3 Slit-lamp findings from a patient with Cogan's syndrome and interstitial keratitis. Subtle stroma infiltrate (arrow) typical of early interstitial keratitis is demonstrated in the narrow band of light. (With permission from McCallum et al.[35])

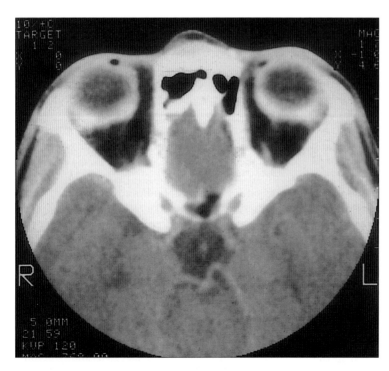

Fig. 163.4 Severe posterior scleritis in a patient with Cogan's syndrome. CT scan of the orbits reveals thickening of the posterior sclerae, compatible with posterior scleritis. (With permission from McCallum et al.[35])

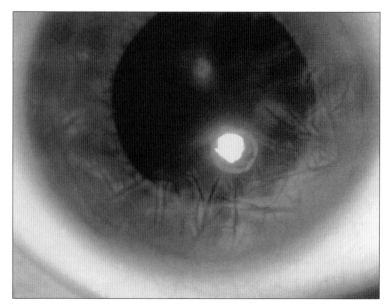

Fig. 163.5 Cornea from the right eye of a patient with a 29-year history of Cogan's syndrome. Note the formation of ghost vessels, remnants of neovascularization. (With permission from Haynes et al.[8])

The earliest corneal findings in patients with Cogan's syndrome and interstitial keratitis are 'faint cornea infiltrates, measuring 0.5–1.0mm in diameter. They mimic the lesions seen in adenoviral or chlamydial keratitis[37]. For this reason, the initial diagnosis may be viral keratitis, particularly in the absence of vestibuloauditory symptoms. These early corneal lesions resolve promptly with topical or systemic corticosteroid therapy. Approximately 15% of patients acquire faint subepithelial scars and fewer than 5% of patients develop corneal erosions[37]. Later, these early findings evolve into the classic 'granular type of corneal infiltrates', with progressive neovascularization (Fig. 163.5)[3,36]. Scarring and vascularization opacify the cornea and reduce visual acuity, but these complications are unusual for patients appropriately treated with topical or systemic corticosteroids[1,37].

Conjunctivitis and anterior uveitis may occur with or without interstitial keratitis in Cogan's syndrome[9,10,37]. Other types of eye disease have been associated with Cogan's syndrome and include posterior uveitis, vitritis, retinochoroiditis, papillitis, vitreous hemorrhage, conjunctival nodule, central venous occlusion and retinal arterial disease[8–10].

Vestibuloauditory manifestations

Vestibuloauditory dysfunction develops abruptly in Cogan's syndrome, with Ménière's-like attacks of vertigo, nausea, emesis, tinnitus and hearing loss[8–10,38]. Vestibuloauditory manifestations include Ménière's-like attacks with hearing loss (92%), nystagmus (32%) and oscillopsia (15%), Ménière's-like attacks without hearing loss (4%), and hearing loss only (4%)[10]. Disease exacerbations can produce down-fluctuations in hearing and eventually deafness in many cases. The sudden Ménière's-like attacks are incapacitating and require hospitalization for acute management.

Vasculitis

Vasculitis occurs in 15% of patients with Cogan's syndrome[8–10]. It can be divided into three categories: aortitis, large vessel vasculitis involving the aorta and great vessels (Takayasu's-like), and medium-sized arteritis (polyarteritis-like) or other vasculitic syndrome[39].

Aortitis develops in 10% of patients with Cogan's syndrome, typically within weeks to a few years of disease onset. Proximal aortic inflammation can dilate the aortic ring and damage the heart valves, producing aortic regurgitation. The symptoms of aortitis range from an asymptomatic murmur to exertional dyspnea, chest pain and congestive heart failure, with severe aortic regurgitation[9,16,18,40–43]. Associated findings include coronary arteritis[18,42], myocardial infarction[3], pericarditis[43,44], left ventricular hypertrophy[9] and arrhythmias[9].

Large vessel vasculitis (Takayasu's-like) is the most common type of vasculitis in Cogan's syndrome (Fig. 163.6). The presenting manifestations of large vessel vasculitis are diverse and reflect the ischemic territory of the affected vessel. Angiograms have shown occlusive disease of the major branches of the aorta[10,18]. Varied clinical presentations have resulted from mesenteric insufficiency[7,45], spontaneous rupture of a renal artery[7] or renal artery stenosis[46] (Fig. 163.6). Medium-sized vasculitis has manifested as gastrointestinal bleeding[47], proteinuria and microscopic hematuria[9,10], ischemic loss of limb[7], coronary arteritis[18,42] (Fig. 163.6), muscle involvement[6] and testicular pain[7]. Neurologic involvement is relatively uncommon in Cogan's syndrome, but it can result in meningismus, encephalitis, psychosis, seizures, cerebral infarction, cavernous sinus thrombosis and trigeminal neuralgia[7–10,48]. Cutaneous vasculitis may present as palpable purpura, urticaria or nodules[8–10,48].

Other systemic features

Patients with Cogan's syndrome often develop non-specific systemic symptoms (Table 163.3), including fever, weight loss, fatigue, headache, arthralgia and myalgia[8–10,49]. One of the authors has seen a patient with Cogan's syndrome and persistent oligoarthritis. Also, Crohn's disease[8,46],

ulcerative colitis[50], sarcoidosis[8], hypothyroidism[8] and interstitial nephritis[51] have occurred in association with Cogan's syndrome.

INVESTIGATIONS

Blood and cerebrospinal fluid

Patients with Cogan's syndrome frequently have abnormal hematological parameters (Table 163.4). Leukocytosis is the most common finding. The

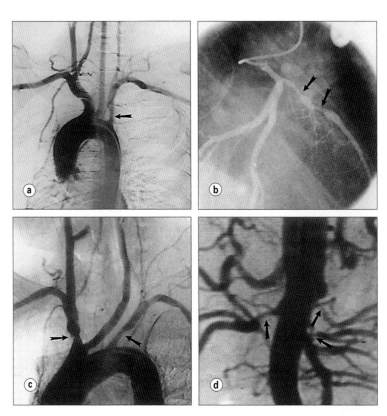

Fig. 163.6 Large vessel vasculitis in Cogan's syndrome. (a) Stenotic lesion of the left subclavian artery (arrow). (b) Stenotic lesions in the left anterior descending coronary artery (arrows) with post-stenotic dilatation. (c) Stenotic lesions in the right innominate artery (left arrow) and the left subclavian artery (right arrow). (d) Multiple lesions in the single right and duplicated left renal arteries (arrows). (With permission from Allen *et al.*[18])

TABLE 163.3 SYSTEMIC MANIFESTATIONS OF COGAN'S SYNDROME

Manifestations	% of cases
Fever	25
Fatigue	20
Arthralgias/myalgias	15
Arthritis	15
Weight loss	15
Abdominal pain	10
Gastrointestinal bleeding	10
Lymphadenopathy	10
Hepatomegaly	10
Splenomegaly	10
Central nervous system findings	5
Cutaneous nodules	5
Pleuritis	5
Rash	5
Peripheral nervous system findings	<5
Polychondritis	<5

(With permission from McCallum and Haynes[51].)

TABLE 163.4 LABORATORY ABNORMALITIES IN COGAN'S SYNDROME

Laboratory study	Abnormal studies (%)	Mean	Range
White blood cell count	75	13 700/mm^3	1600–47 000/mm^3
Neutrophilia	50		
Relative lymphopenia	25		
Eosinophilia (mild)	17		
Leukocytosis > 24 000 cells/ml	10		
Erythrocyte sedimentation rate > 20mm/h	75	40mm/h	3–128mm/h
Hemoglobin/hematocrit (anemia)	33		
Platelet count (thrombocytosis)	30		
Cerebrospinal fluid	25		
Cryoglobulins	17–23		
Decreased C3	21		
Decreased total hemolytic complement	17		
Decreased C4	17		
Antinuclear antibodies (low titer)	17		
Rheumatoid factor (low titer)	14		

(With permission from McCallum *et al.*[35])

erythrocyte sedimentation rate is elevated above 20mm/h in 75% of patients[9]. Cogan's syndrome has been associated with abnormalities of serum protein electrophoresis compatible with a chronic inflammatory response[8,9]. Low titers of serum rheumatoid factor and antinuclear antibodies have been reported in 14% and 17%, respectively, of patients with Cogan's syndrome[8,9]. Some patients have false positive tests for syphilis[8,9]. Cryoglobulins were detected in three (23%) of 13 patients at the NIH[8] and one (6%) of 16 patients at the Mayo Clinic[9]. Total hemolytic complement was diminished in two (17%) of 12 patients at the Mayo Clinic, with a low C3 component in three (21%) of 14 patients and low C4 component in two (17%) of 12 patients[9]. Direct Coombs' tests and assays for serum anti-DNA antibodies, anti-smooth muscle antibodies, anti-Ro antibodies, anti-La antibodies and hepatitis B surface antigen have been uniformly negative in Cogan's syndrome[8,9]. Approximately 25% of patients with Cogan's syndrome show abnormalities of cerebrospinal fluid, including pleocytosis[8,9,49], elevated protein[51] and increased γ-globulins[8,9].

Ocular procedures

Slit-lamp examinations are routinely performed to evaluate the corneal and anterior segment of the eye. Changes in the cornea and other diseased segments may be documented during follow-up using ophthalmic photography[36]. Fluorescein angiography is useful for diagnosing and monitoring patients with retinal vasculitis or retinochoroiditis[53].

Audiometry

More than 95% of patients with Cogan's syndrome have an abnormal audiogram[8–10,49]. Hearing loss is most pronounced at the highest and lowest frequencies, with relative sparing of the mid-range (Fig. 163.7), a pattern similar to that of Ménière's syndrome. Cochlear damage causes abnormalities in brainstem auditory evoked potentials. Vestibular injury results in absent or abnormal caloric responses[9].

Brain imaging

In some patients with Cogan's syndrome, brain magnetic resonance imaging (MRI) and computed tomography (CT) have shown soft tissue and calcified obliteration of vestibular and cochlear structures[54,55]. MRI scans with gadolinium have revealed enhancement of vestibular and cochlear structures, implying disruption of the blood–labyrinthine barrier[39].

Cardiovascular procedures

Echocardiographic abnormalities have been described in patients with Cogan's syndrome and aortic regurgitation, including 'fluttering' of the anterior mitral valve leaflet[9], thickening of the valve cusps[9,56], paradoxical movement of the ascending aorta during systole[18] and left ventricular enlargement[9,18,56]. Cardiac catheterization has been useful for diagnosing aortic valvular disease and evaluating hemodynamics[17,18,36]. Coronary angiography has shown ostial coronary stenosis[16,43] as well as distal coronary arteritis[30]. Visceral angiography has revealed the typical lesions of Takayasu's-like or polyarteritis-like vasculitis[9,17,18,56,57].

APPROACH TO THE PATIENT

Diagnosis

The care of patients with Cogan's syndrome requires close coordination between ophthalmologists, otolaryngologists, audiologists and rheumatologists. The rheumatologist often organizes the care. The ophthalmologist is instrumental for evaluating the cornea, other parts of the anterior segment, and the vitreous, choroid and retinal vasculature. Localizing the site of the vestibuloauditory lesion benefits from the input of a skilled otolaryngologist, and sometimes a neurologist. Hearing loss is quantified using pure tone audiograms. An MRI scan is typically done to exclude the possibility of an acoustic neuroma or other brainstem lesion.

The laboratory studies are directed toward identifying sites of systemic involvement and excluding other diagnoses. They include a complete blood count and urinalysis and measurement of serum electrolytes, creatinine, liver transaminases and erythrocyte sedimentation rate. Serologic tests are routinely performed to exclude syphilis and Lyme disease. Because of the prevalence of aortitis in Cogan's syndrome, 2D echocardiography should be done at the time of diagnosis to evaluate for aortic valvular dysfunction. Cardiac catheterization may be indicated for hemodynamically significant valvular disease. When performing cardiac catheterization for this reason, coronary angiography should also be done to identify coronary ostial lesions or more distal artery involvement. Coronary angiography is also warranted if there are signs or symptoms of ischemic heart disease. Patients with suspected vasculitis elsewhere should undergo the appropriate angiographic studies or tissue biopsy for diagnostic purposes.

The differential diagnosis of Cogan's syndrome is broad and varies depending on clinical presentation. Several disorders produce ocular inflammation and vestibuloauditory dysfunction similar to Cogan's syndrome (Table 163.5) Examples include syphilis, Lyme disease, Vogt–Koyanagi–Harada (VKH) syndrome, toxic exposures and

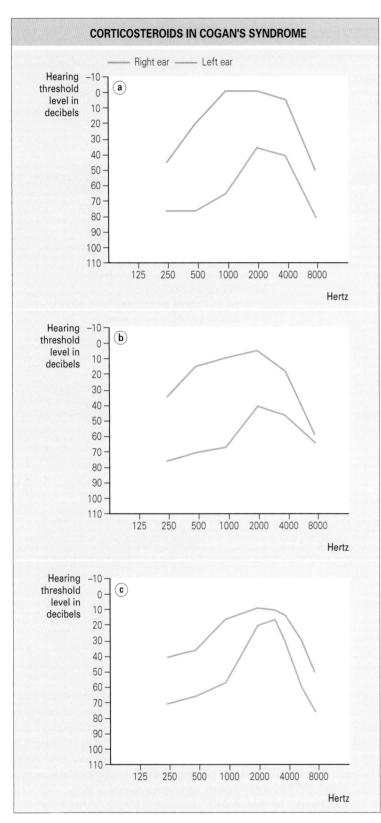

CORTICOSTEROIDS IN COGAN'S SYNDROME

Fig. 163.7 **Corticosteroids in Cogan's syndrome.** Serial pure tone audiograms over an 8-year period. Note the higher hearing thresholds at the upper and lower frequencies. (a) 2 months after onset of CS while on daily corticosteroid therapy. (b) 4.5 years later on alternate-day corticosteroid therapy. (c) 3 years later, demonstrating stable to improved hearing over the period of the tests. (O—O, right ear; X—X, left ear). (With permission from Haynes *et al.*[8])

Mèniére's disease. VKH syndrome causes panuveitis, vitiligo, poliosis, aseptic meningitis and, in 75% of cases, hearing loss. Although interstitial keratitis may occur in VKH syndrome, ocular inflammation predominates at other sites and is vision-threatening[44].

MANAGEMENT

Eye

Interstitial keratitis and iridocyclitis are treated with topical ocular corticosteroids and mydriatics to control inflammation and prevent synechiae[58]. Low-potency topical corticosteroids are often adequate for treating interstitial keratitis. Systemic corticosteroids are not generally indicated for the treatment of interstitial keratitis or iridocyclitis. However, they may be utilized in these settings for the rare case failing topical therapy[8,58]. If interstitial keratitis does not improve with topical corticosteroid therapy, then chlamydial infection should be considered as a possible cause of the inflammation and consideration given to treatment with a tetracycline antibiotic[59]. In Cogan's syndrome the ocular signs and symptoms of interstitial keratitis usually respond within 3–7 days of starting therapy[8,9]. Only rarely is the course complicated by the development of corneal opacity and visual loss[60]. Cataracts may develop secondary to chronic inflammation or corticosteroid therapy. Surgical extraction of the cataracts and lens implantation may be needed to restore satisfactory vision. Vision is particularly important for deaf individuals who must rely on lip reading and sign language for communication.

Conjunctivitis, scleritis and episcleritis are also treated with topical corticosteroids. Alternatively, episcleritis and scleritis can be managed with topical or systemic non-steroidal anti-inflammatory therapy[58]. Nodular scleritis warrants more aggressive therapy with systemic corticosteroids or other potent immunosuppressive drug[61] (Fig. 163.8). Posterior segment ocular inflammation calls for systemic corticosteroid therapy if the inflammation is progressive, persistent, or interferes with vision[8,58]. Progression of posterior ocular inflammation despite systemic corticosteroids may require the addition of methotrexate, azathioprine, cyclophosphamide or cyclosporin[18,58].

Vestibuloauditory

A trial of systemic corticosteroid therapy is indicated for a patient newly diagnosed with Cogan's syndrome and hearing loss[8,10,58,62]. The severity of hearing loss should be quantified using audiometry (Fig. 163.9). After establishing the degree of auditory dysfunction systemic corticosteroids are initiated at a dose of 1–2mg/kg/day of prednisone (or its equivalent)[8,58]. Corticosteroids are usually begun in divided doses for the first 3–7 days, with subsequent consolidation to a single morning dose[58]. If adequate improvement occurs over 10–14 days, then prednisone is continued at that dose for 2–4 weeks. Every effort should be made to taper the prednisone therapy to an alternate-day regimen within 6–8 weeks. The dose can then be tapered to discontinuation over the next 3–4 months, provided auditory acuity remains stable. Certain patients with recurrent episodes of hearing loss may require long-term daily corticosteroid therapy to maintain auditory function[10]. If possible, the dose of prednisone should be kept to 10mg/day or less in these cases.

Some patients may fail to improve following a 14-day course of prednisone 1–2mg/kg/day. In these instances the dose should be rapidly tapered to discontinuation and the patient considered a treatment failure. Anecdotal evidence suggests that other immunosuppressive drugs may be effective for treating corticosteroid-resistant hearing loss[58]. Cyclophosphamide 1–2mg/kg/day has been utilized most often in this situation. The length of treatment and threshold for response should be predefined to avoid a prolonged course of immunosuppression with low likelihood of benefit. For example, an adequate response to cyclophosphamide therapy might be defined as a minimum of 10dB improvement in hearing after 8 weeks of treatment.

Some patients with Cogan's syndrome may not be able to reduce the prednisone dose below 10mg/day without experiencing a disease flare. If so, then an empiric trial of another immunosuppressive agent should be considered for steroid-sparing effects[58]. Methotrexate, azathioprine and

TABLE 163.5 DIFFERENTIAL DIAGNOSIS OF COGAN'S SYNDROME

Disorder	Eye manifestations	Ear manifestations	Other features
Chlamydia infection	Conjunctivitis, IK	Otitis media, CHL	Respiratory tract symptoms
Lyme disease	Conjunctivitis, episcleritis, uveitis, IK, choroiditis, retinitis, optic neuritis		Erythema migraines, meningitis, carditis, arthritis
Congenital syphilis	IK	SNHL	+FTA-ABS
Whipple's disease	Uveitis, vitritis	SNHL	Diarrhea, weight loss, fever, arthritis, skin hyperpigmentation
Sarcoidosis	Conjunctivitis, IK anterior uveitis, retinitis, keratoconjunctivitis sicca	SNHL	Hilar adenopathy, pulmonary fibrosis, CNS involvement, skin lesions, parotid gland enlargement
Vogt–Koyanagi–Harada	Panuveitis, iridocyclitis	Vertigo, SNHL	Aseptic meningitis, vitiligo, alopecia, poliosis
KID syndrome (congenital)	Keratoconjunctivitis, corneal vascularization	SNHL	Ichthyosis
Sjogren's syndrome	Keratoconjunctivitis sicca	SNHL	Xerostomia, parotid gland enlargement, serum ANA
Rheumatoid arthritis	Episcleritis, scleritis	SNHL	Arthritis, serum rheumatoid factor
SLE	Retinitis, optic atrophy	SNHL (mild)	Skin rash, arthritis, pleurisy, glomerulonephritis, cytopenias, serum ANA
APA	Retinal vascular occlusion	SNHL	Deep vein thrombosis, pulmonary emboli, arterial thrombosis, thrombocytopenia, serum APA
Polyarteritis nodosa	Retinal vasculitis	SNHL	Renal failure, hypertension, arthritis, skin lesions, neuropathy, CNS involvement, elevated ESR
Wegener's granulomatosis	Conjunctivitis, episcleritis scleritis, uveitis, retinitis	Otitis media (CHL), SNHL	Sinusitis, pulmonary infiltrates, glomerulonephritis, serum ANCA
Relapsing polychondritis	Conjunctivitis, IK, scleritis uveitis	SNHL	Auricular, nasal, and laryngotracheal chondritis, systemic vasculitis
Behçet's syndrome	Anterior uveitis, episcleritis, IK, retinal vasculitis, chorioretinitis	Vertigo, SNHL	Oral and genital ulcers, CNS involvement, arthritis, skin lesions
Ulcerative colitis	Anterior uveitis	SNHL	Colitis
Crohn's disease	Anterior uveitis	SNHL	Enterocolitis
CNS lymphoma	Corneal, anterior chamber and vitreous opacities, sub-RPE infiltrates	SNHL	Cerebellopontine mass
CLL	Optic neuropathy	Otitis media, SNHL	CNS involvement, CSF lymphocytosis
Retinocochleocerebral vasculopathy	Retinal arteriolar occlusions	SNHL	CNS microangiopathy

ANA, antinuclear antibodies; ANCA antineutrophil cytoplasmic antibodies; APA, antiphospholipid antibody; CHL, conductive hearing loss; CLL, chronic lymphocytic leukemia; CNS, central nervous system; CSF, cerebrospinal fluid; FTA-ABS, fluorescent treponemal antibody absorption; IK, interstitial keratitis; KID, keratitis, ichthyosis, and deafness; RPE, retinal pigment epithelial; SLE, systemic lupus erythematosus; SNHL sensorineural hearing loss.
(With permission from McCallum *et al.*[35])

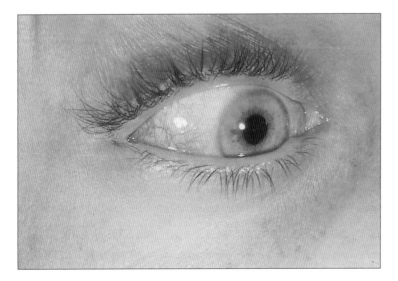

Fig. 163.8 Nodular scleritis seen laterally in a patient with CS. Note nodule under the light reflex. This finding is an indication for aggressive therapy of eye inflammation.

cyclophosphamide have been successfully used under these circumstances[39]. The use of cyclophosphamide therapy for more than 1 year increases the risk for bladder cancer and hematopoietic malignancy, and should be avoided if possible[63]. The relative efficacy of corticosteroids and other immunosuppressive drugs in Cogan's syndrome is unclear. However, in the Duke series a hearing threshold of <60dB was noted in 16 of 22 (73%) patients treated with corticosteroids alone, and in 9 of 11 (81%) patients treated with corticosteroid plus other immunosuppressive therapy[10].

Persistent or recurrent inner ear disease may lead to cochlear hydrops[8,64]. Cochlear hydrops produces short-lived hearing fluctuations ranging in duration from hours to 3–5 days. Such down-fluctuation may be associated with the menstrual cycle in women, eating salty foods, allergies, or upper respiratory illnesses. Cochlear hydrops cannot reliably be distinguished from a bout of inner ear inflammation. However, an inflammatory process can be suspected, with concomitant ocular inflammation, vestibular symptoms, or elevation in sedimentation rate. Hearing fluctuations due to cochlear hydrops may be observed or treated with a diuretic[58]. If the hearing fails to improve within 3–5 days of a down-fluctuation, then consideration should be given to an empiric

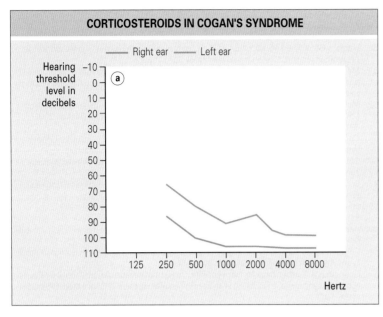

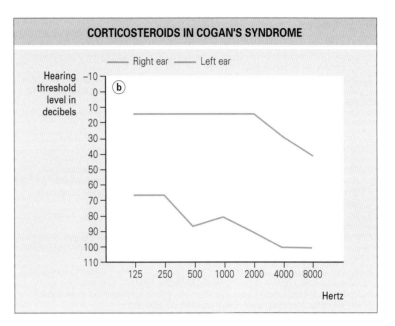

Fig. 163.9 Corticosteroids in Cogan's syndrome. Audiometry demonstrating response to therapy with corticosteroids in a patient with CS. (a) Hearing thresholds prior to therapy. (b) Hearing thresholds after therapy for active CS. (O—O, right ear; X—X, left ear). (With permission from McCallum *et al.*[35])

trial of prednisone therapy or an increase in prednisone dose. Finally, permanent deafness can be treated with cochlear implants[39].

Cardiovascular

The presence of aortic insufficiency implies aortitis and should be treated with high doses of corticosteroids in a manner similar to a systemic vasculitis[18]. If aortic insufficiency develops or worsens during corticosteroid therapy, then other immunosuppressive agents should be added to the treatment regimen[18]. For example, cyclophosphamide 2mg/kg/day has been useful for treating potentially serious or life-threatening cases of vasculitis[58]. Patients with Cogan's syndrome have successfully undergone aortic valve replacement soon after the discovery of aortic insufficiency[8,9,49]. Aortic insufficiency may also stabilize with aggressive medical therapy[18].

Systemic vasculitis is treated with prednisone 1mg/kg/day, either alone or in combination with another immunosuppressive agent. Among the other immunosuppressants, cyclosporin 3.5–5mg/kg/day has been the most effective for the treatment of large vessel vasculitis[18,58], and cyclophosphamide 2mg/kg/day has produced beneficial results for patients with polyarteritis-like disorders[8,43]. When using prednisone in combination with another immunosuppressive agent, the prednisone dose should be converted from a daily to an alternate schedule within 3 months to minimize toxicity. With disease control, the prednisone dose may then be gradually tapered to discontinuation. Typically, cyclosporin A or cyclophosphamide are administered for 1 year after the onset of complete remission[18,58]. Surgery may be indicated for bypass of obstructed vessels. Vascular stenoses can produce ischemic symptoms or threaten viability of an organ or tissue. Ideally, surgical procedures are carried out when the disease is under control.

PROGNOSIS

Ocular outcomes in patients with Cogan's syndrome are excellent. In the Duke series only 6% of patients had a visual acuity of less than 20/30 in either eye, the worst being 20/60[10]. At the Mayo Clinic, blindness occurred in 5% of eyes[9]. In a literature review, severe visual loss was described in only 4% of patients with Cogan's syndrome and ocular inflammation beyond the anterior segment[8].

Deafness is a frequent outcome in Cogan's syndrome, occurring in 25–50% of cases[8–10]. Hearing loss is the major debilitating sequela of CS. Bilateral deafness developed in 12 of 18 (67%) patients from the Mayo Clinic[9]. In the Duke series, 26 (70%) of 37 patients with Cogan's syndrome had a pure tone audiometry threshold of less than 60dB (severe hearing loss) after a median follow-up of 72 months[10]. A retrospective analysis of patients with Cogan's syndrome at Duke suggests that corticosteroid therapy may improve auditory outcomes. Auditory acuity was less than 60dB in one (17%) of six patients without corticosteroid therapy and 25 (81%) of 31 patients who received systemic corticosteroid therapy[8]. Vestibular manifestations improve for most patients with Cogan's syndrome. However, in the Duke series 15% of patients had persistent oscillopsia[9].

Systemic vasculitis has been successfully treated in four of five patients from the Duke series[10]. A large vessel vasculitis developed in a patient who was receiving cyclosporin A therapy but was later successfully treated with cyclophosphamide[10]. Another patient has been described with persistent vasculitis who died despite aggressive therapy with several different immunosuppressive agents[65].

CONCLUSION

The diagnosis of Cogan's syndrome depends on the presence of interstitial keratitis and vestibuloauditory neuronitis, usually occurring for the first time within a few weeks to months of each other. Some patients with Cogan's syndrome can develop more serious inflammatory eye disease or systemic vasculitis. Thus, ophthalmologists, otolaryngologists and rheumatologists must be alert for this constellation of clinical features. The cause of this disease is unknown, but its pathogenesis appears to involve immunological mechanisms. Although controlled studies are lacking, experience suggests that prompt initiation of corticosteroid therapy offers the best opportunity to restore acute hearing deficits. Cochlear implants can improve auditory function and quality of life for those patients with permanent and severe hearing loss.

REFERENCES

1. Cogan DG. Syndrome of nonsyphilitis interstitial keratitis and vestibuloauditory symptoms. Arch Ophthalmol 1945; 33: 144–149.

2. Morgan RF, Baumgartner CJ. Ménière's disease complicated by recurrent interstitial keratitis: excellent results following cervical ganglionectomy. West J Surg 1934; 42: 628–631.

3. Cogan DG. Nonsyphilitic interstitial keratitis with vestibuloauditory symptoms. Report of four additional cases. Arch Ophthalmol 1949; 42: 42–49.

4. Norton EWD, Cogan DG. Syndrome of nonsyphilitic interstitial keratitis and vestibuloauditory symptoms. A long-term follow-up. Arch Ophthalmol 1959; 61: 695–697.

5. Oliner L, Taubenhaus M, Shapira TM et al. Nonsyphilitic interstitial keratitis and bilateral deafness (Cogan's syndrome) associated with essential polyangiitis (periarteritis nodosa). A review of the syndrome with consideration of a possible pathogenic mechanism. N Engl J Med 1953; 248: 1001–1008.

6. Crawford WJ. Cogan's syndrome associated with polyarteritis nodosa. A report of three cases. Penn Med J 1957; 60: 835–838.

7. Fisher ER, Hellstrom HR. Cogan's syndrome and systemic vascular disease. Analysis of pathologic features with reference to its relationship to thromboangiitis obliterans (Buerger). Arch Pathol 1961; 72: 572–592.

8. Haynes BF, Kaiser-Kupfer MI, Mason P et al. Studies in thirteen patients, long-term follow-up, and a review of the literature. Medicine 1980; 59: 426–441.

9. Vollertsen RS, McDonald TJ, Younge BR et al. Cogan's syndrome: 18 cases and a review of the literature. Mayo Clin Proc 1986; 61: 344–361.

10. McCallum RM, Allen NB, Cobo LM et al. Cogan's syndrome: clinical features and outcomes(abstract). Arthritis Rheum 1992; 35(Suppl): S51.

11. Podder S, Shepherd RC. Cogan's syndrome: a rare systemic vasculitis. Arch Dis Child 1994; 71: 163–164.

12. Fidler H, Jones NS. Late onset Cogan's syndrome. J Laryngol 1989; 103: 512–514.

13. Wolff D, Bernhard WG, Tsutsumi S et al. The pathology of Cogan's syndrome causing profound deafness. Ann Otol Rhino Laryngol 1965; 74: 507–520.

14. Rarey KE, Bicknell JM, Davis LE. Intralabyrinthine osteogenesis in Cogan's syndrome. Am J Otolaryngol 1986; 4: 387–390.

15. Schuknecht HF, Nadol JB. Temporal bone pathology in a case of Cogan's syndrome. Laryngoscope 1994; 104: 1135–1142.

16. Gelfand ML, Kantor T, Gorstein F. Cogan's syndrome with cardiovascular involvement: aortic insufficiency. Bull NY Acad Med 1972; 48: 647–660.

17. Cochrane AD, Tatoulis J. Cogan's syndrome with aortitis, aortic regurgitation, and aortic arch vessel stenosis. Ann Thorac Surg 1991; 52: 1166–1167.

18. Allen NB, Cox CC, Cobo M et al. Use of immunosuppressive agents in the treatment of severe ocular and vascular manifestations of Cogan's syndrome. Am J Med 1990; 88: 296–301.

19. Livingston JZ, Casale AS, Hutchins GM et al. Coronary involvement in Cogan's syndrome. Am Heart J 1992; 123: 528–530.

20. Eisenstein B, Taubenhaus M. Nonsyphilitic interstitial keratitis and bilateral deafness (Cogan's syndrome) associated with cardiovascular disease. N Engl J Med 1958; 22: 1074–1079.

21. Pinals RS. Cogan's syndrome with arthritis and aortic insufficiency. J Rheumatol 1978; 5: 294–298.

22. Tseng JF, Cambira RP, Aretz T et al. Thoracoabdominal aortic aneurysm in Cogan's syndrome. J Vasc Surg 1999; 30: 565–568.

23. Darougar S, John AC, Viswalingam et al. Isolation of Chlamydia psittaci from a patient with interstitial keratitis and uveitis association with otological and cardiovascular lesions. Br J Opthalmol 1978; 62: 709–714.

24. Dana MR, Qian Y, Hamrah P. Twenty-five year panorama of corneal immunology. Cornea 2000; 19: 625–643.

25. Verhagan C, Mor F, Kipp JBA et al. Experimental autoimmune keratitis induced in rats by anti-cornea T-cell lines. Invest Ophthalmol Vis Sci 1999; 40: 2191–2198.

26. Harris JP, Heydt J, Keithley EM et al. Immunopathology of the inner ear: an update. Ann NY Acad Sci 1997; 830: 166–178.

27. Harris JP, Fukuda S, Keithley EM. Spiral modular vein: Its importance in inner ear inflammation. Acta Otoloaryngol (Stockh) 1990; 110: 357–365.

28. Zhang C, Huang W, Song H. Expression of vascular cell adhesion molecule-1, α_4-integrin and L-selectin during inner ear immunity reaction. Acta Otolaryngol 2000; 120: 607–614.

29. Gloddek B, Gloddek J, Arnold W. A rat T-cell line that mediates autoimmune disease of the inner ear in the Lewis rat. ORL J Otorhinolaryngol Relat Spec 1999; 61: 181–187.

30. Arnold W, Gebbers J-O. Serum-antikörper gegen kornea- und innenohrgewebe beim Cogan-syndrom. Laryng Rhinol Otol 1984; 63: 428–432.

31. Arnold W, Pfaltz R, Altermatt H-J. Evidence of serum antibodies against inner ear tissues in the blood of patients with certain sensorineural hearing disorders. Acta Otolaryngol (Stockh) 1985; 99: 437–444.

32. Majoor MHJM, Albers FWJ, van der Gaag R et al. Corneal autoimmunity in Cogan's syndrome? Report of two cases. Ann Otol Rhinol Laryngol 1992; 101: 679–684.

33. Hughes GB, Kinney SE, Barna BP et al. Autoimmune reactivity in Cogan's syndrome: a preliminary report. Otolaryngol Head Neck Surg 1983; 91: 24–32.

34. Moscicki RA, San Martin JE, Qunitero CH et al. Serum antibody to inner ear proteins in patients with progressive hearing loss. Correlation with disease activity and response to corticosteroid treatment. JAMA 1994; 272: 611–616.

35. McCallum RM, St. Clair EW, Haynes BF. Cogan's syndrome. In: Hoffman GS, Weyand CM, eds. Inflammatory diseases of blood vessels. New York: Marcel Dekker; 2002: 491–509.

36. Cogan DG, Dickerson GR. Nonsyphilitic interstitial keratitis with vestibuloauditory symptoms: A case with fatal aortitis. Arch Ophthalmol 1964; 71: 172–175.

37. Cobo LM, Haynes BF. Early corneal findings in Cogan's syndrome. Ophthalmology 1984; 91: 903–907.

38. Benitez JT: Evidence of central vestibulo-auditory dysfunction in atypical Cogan's syndrome: A case report. Am J Otol 1990; 11: 131–134.

39. St. Clair EW, McCallum RM. Cogan's syndrome. Curr Opin Rheumatol 1999; 11: 47–52.

40. Hammer M, Witte T, Mugge A et al. Complicated Cogan's syndrome with aortic insufficiency and coronary stenosis. J Rheumatol 1994; 21: 552–555.

41. Cogan DG. Corneoscleral lesions in periarteritis nodosa and Wegener's granulomatosis. Trans Am Ophthalmol Soc 1955; 53: 321–344.

42. Eisenstein B, Taubenhaus M. Nonsyphilitic interstitial keratitis and bilateral deafness (Cogan's syndrome) associated with cardiovascular disease. N Engl J Med 1958; 258: 1074–1079.

43. Livingston JZ, Hutchins GM, Shapiro EP. Coronary involvement in Cogan's syndrome. Am Heart J 1992; 123: 528–530.

44. Nussenblattt RB, Palestine AG. The Vogt–Kayanagi–Harada syndrome. In: Nussenblattt RB, Palestine AG, eds. Uveitis: fundamentals and practice. Chicago: Year Book Medical Publishers; 1989: 274–290.

45. LaRaja RD. Cogan syndrome associated with mesenteric vascular insufficiency. Arch Surg 1976; 111: 1028–1031.

46. Thomas HG. Case report: clinical and radiological features of Cogan's syndrome – non-syphilitic interstitial keratitis, audiovestibular symptoms and systemic manifestations. Clin Radiol 1997; 45: 418–421.

47. Cheson BD, Bluming AZ, Alroy J. Cogan's syndrome: A systemic vasculitis. Am J Med 1976; 60: 549–555.

48. Ochonisky S et al. Cogan's syndrome: An unusual etiology of urticarial vasculitis. Dermatologica 1991; 183: 218–220.

49. Bielory L, Conti J, Frohman L. Cogan's syndrome. J Allergy Clin Immunol 1990; 85: 808–815.

50. Jacob A, Ledingham MB, Kerr AIG et al. Ulcerative colitis and giant cell arteritis associated with sensorineural deafness. J Laryngol Otol 1990; 104: 889–890.

51. McCallum RM, Haynes BF. Cogan syndrome. In: Pepose JS, Holland GN, Wilhelmus KR, eds. Ocular infection and immunity. St. Louis: Mosby-Year Book Inc; 1996: 446–459.

52. Djupesland G, Flottorp G, Hansen e Sjaastad O. Cogan syndrome: The audiological picture. Arch Otolaryngol 1974; 99: 218–225.

53. Mandava N, Guyer DR, Yannuzzi LA. Ancilllary Test – Fluorescence Angiography. In: Yanof FM, Duker JS, eds. Ophthalmology. St Louis, Mosby, Inc; 1999.

54. Majoor MHJM, Albers FWJ, Casselman JW. Clinical relevance of magnetic resonance imaging and computed tomography in Cogan's syndrome. Acta Otolaryngol (Stockh) 1993; 113: 625–631.

55. Casselman JW, Majoor MHJM, Albers FW. MR of the inner ear in patients with Cogan's syndrome. AJNR Am J Neuroradiol 1994; 15: 131–138.

56. Kundell SP, Ochs HD. Cogan syndrome in childhood. J Pediatr 1980; 97: 96–98.

57. Char DH, Cogan DG, Sullivan WR. Immunologic study of nonsyphilitic interstitial keratitis with vestibuloauditory symptoms. Am J Ophthalmol 1975; 80: 491–494.

58. McCallum RM. Cogan's syndrome. In Franunfelder FT, Roy FH, eds. Current ocular therapy, 5th edn. Philadelphia: WB Saunders; 2000; 161–163.

59. Whitcher JP. Chlamydial diseases. In: Smolin G, Thoft RA, eds. The cornea: scientific foundations and clinical practice. Boston: Little, Brown; 1983; 210–221.

60. Cogan DG, Kuwabara T. Late corneal opacities in the syndrome of interstitial keratitis and vestibulo-auditory symptoms. Acta Ophthalmol 1989; 67: 182–187.

61. Foster CS. Immunosuppressive therapy for external ocular inflammatory disease. Ophthalmology 1980; 87: 140–150.

62. Haynes BF, Pikus A, Kaiser-Kupfer M, Fauci AS. Successful treatment of sudden hearing loss in Cogan's syndrome with corticosteroids. Arthritis Rheum 1981; 24: 501–503.

63. Kovarsky J. Clinical pharmacology and toxicology of cyclophosphamide: emphasis of use in rheumatic diseases. Semin Arthritis Rheum 1983; 12: 359–372.

64. Paparella MM, Da Costa SS, Fox R, Yoon TH. Ménière's disease and other labyrinthine diseases. In: Papatella MM, Shumrick DA, Gluckman JL, Meyerhoff WL, eds. Otolaryngology: otology and neurotology. Philadelphia: WB Saunders; 1991; 1689–1714.

OSTEOARTHRITIS AND RELATED DISORDERS

164 Osteoarthritis: epidemiology and classification

Elaine Dennison and Cyrus Cooper

- Osteoarthritis (OA) is the most common joint disorder in the world
- A variety of different systems of classification have been proposed, because of the heterogeneity of the condition
- Studies suggest that the prevalence of radiographic OA rises steeply with age at all joint sites
- Risk factors influencing a generalized predisposition to OA include heredity, obesity, reproductive variables, hypermobility and cigarette smoking
- Local biomechanical factors influencing the risk of OA at specific joint sites include joint shape, trauma, occupation and physical activity
- The natural history of knee, hip and hand OA is heterogeneous

INTRODUCTION

Osteoarthritis (OA) is the most common joint disorder in the world. It has been found in skeletal remains from as far back as Neolithic times[1]. Archeological studies suggest that the relative frequencies of OA at certain joints within and between ethnic groups have changed with time[2]; in Western populations, radiographic evidence of OA occurs in the majority of people by 65 years of age and in about 80% of those aged over 75 years. In the USA, it is second only to ischemic heart disease as a cause of work disability in men over 50 years of age, and accounts for more hospitalizations than rheumatoid arthritis (RA) each year. Despite this public health impact, OA remains an enigmatic condition to the epidemiologist. Consensus has only recently emerged as to its definition; the etiology, clinical features and natural history remain the subject of intense investigation and the generation of effective preventive strategies appears a more attainable goal. This chapter reviews four aspects of the epidemiology of OA:

- approaches to the definition and classification of OA
- the prevalence and incidence of OA
- the individual risk factors for development of OA
- the natural history of OA.

DEFINITION AND CLASSIFICATION

Definition

The subdivision of arthritic conditions into discrete pathological entities is a relatively recent phenomenon in the history of medicine. Earlier this century, pathologists differentiated between two broad groups of arthritis: atrophic and hypertrophic[3–5]. Atrophic disorders were characterized by synovial inflammation with erosion of cartilage and bone, and came to include RA and septic arthritis. The hypertrophic group were never subdivided, however, and gradually became synonymous with what is now termed OA[6]. The term thus encompasses a large and heterogeneous spectrum of idiopathic joint disorders.

Any working definition of OA entails consideration of pathologic, radiologic and clinical components. The key pathological features of the disorder have been recognized for many decades and include focal destruction of articular cartilage, followed by changes in subchondral bone. Initial autopsy studies[7,8] recognized the occurrence of soft tissue changes but emphasis was still placed on age-related degeneration of cartilage as the central feature. Subsequent pathologic and anatomic studies, mainly but not exclusively involving the hip joint, led to a more complex and dynamic concept of OA. Lloyd-Roberts, for example, highlighted the importance of capsular changes in hip OA[9], and Byers and colleagues[10] obtained indirect evidence that cartilage damage was not necessarily progressive. Bullough[11] stressed the importance of joint anatomy in controlling focal loss of cartilage, and Sokoloff and others[12] also pointed out that much of the pathology of an OA joint represents real or attempted repair, rather than degeneration. The concept that OA can largely be explained as a natural reaction of synovial joints to injury and is a product of normal remodeling or repair processes in joints stems from the work of Trueta and others[13] and has gained considerable support from recent literature. Two other facets of the OA process have also been documented in pathological studies: synovial inflammation and crystal deposition. However, the role of these factors in disease pathogenesis remains controversial.

Taken together, these studies have led to an altered concept of OA that has developed over the last two decades and is enshrined in current approaches to definition of the disorder[14]. It is now widely viewed as an age-related dynamic reaction pattern of a joint in response to insult or injury. All tissues of the joint are involved, although the loss of articular cartilage and changes in adjacent bone remain the most striking features. In this regard, OA represents failure of the joint as an organ, analogous to renal or cardiac failure, and the pathological observations in advance to disease are as much a product of attempted repair as of the primary insult or damage that contributed to initiation of the process. Hence, the American College of Rheumatology (ACR) currently defines the disorder as: 'a heterogeneous group of conditions that lead to joint symptoms and signs which are associated with defective integrity of articular cartilage, in addition to related changes in the underlying bone at the joint margins'[15]. A more comprehensive definition summarizing the clinical, pathophysiological, biochemical and biomechanical changes that occur in OA was developed in 1986[16] and is summarized in Table 164.1.

By contrast, another recent definition underscores the concept that OA may not represent a single disease entity, and is summarized as follows:

Osteoarthritis is a group of overlapping distinct diseases, which may have different etiologies but with similar biologic, morphologic, and clinical outcomes. The disease processes not only affect the articular cartilage, but involve the entire joint, including the subchondral bone, ligaments, capsule, synovial membrane and periarticular muscles. Ultimately, the articular cartilage degenerates with fibrillation, fissures, ulceration, and full thickness loss of the joint space[17].

TABLE 164.1   FEATURES OF OA

Clinical	Joint pain
	Joint tenderness
	Limitation of movement
	Crepitus
	Occasional effusion
	Variable local inflammation without systemic side-effects
Pathological	Irregular loss of cartilage, especially in areas of increased load
	Sclerosis of subchondral bone
	Subchondral cysts
	Marginal osteophytes
	Increased metaphyseal blood flow
	Variable synovial inflammation
Histological	Fragmentation of cartilage surface
	Cloning of chondrocytes
	Vertical clefts in the cartilage
	Variable crystal deposition
	Remodeling and violation of the tidemark by blood vessels
	Osteophytes
	Loss of cartilage
	Sclerosis of subchondral bone
	Focal osteonecrosis of subchondral bone
Biomechanical	Alteration in tensile, compressive and shear properties
	Altered cartilage hydraulic permeability
	Excessive cartilage swelling
	Increased stiffness of subchondral bone
Biochemical	Reduction in proteoglycan concentration
	Possible alteration in size and aggregation of proteoglycans
	Alteration in collagen fibril size and weave
	Increased synthesis and degradation of matrix macromolecules

TABLE 164.2   RADIOGRAPHIC GRADING SYSTEM FOR OA

Grade	Classification	Description
0	Normal	No features of OA
1	Doubtful	Minute osteophyte, doubtful significance
2	Minimal	Definite osteocyte, unimpaired joint space
3	Moderate	Moderate diminution of joint space
4	Severe	Joint space greatly impaired with sclerosis of subchondral bone

(Adapted from the Atlas of Standard Radiographs. Oxford: Blackwell Scientific.)

Radiography

The radiographic features conventionally used to define OA include joint space narrowing, osteophyte formation, subchondral sclerosis, subchondral cysts and abnormalities of bone contour. These features were originally selected to measure various aspects of cartilage loss and subchondral bone reaction. Although several radiographic grading systems have been proposed, most epidemiologic studies have used the Empire Rheumatism Council system, first described over three decades ago by Kellgren and Lawrence[18]. This system assigns one of five grades (0–4) to OA at various joint sites: knee, hip, hand and spine. Grading is performed by comparing the index radiograph with reproductions in a radiographic atlas. The criteria for increasing severity of OA are shown in Table 164.2 and relate to the assumed sequential appearance of osteophytes, joint space loss, sclerosis and cyst.

Epidemiologic studies support the notion that any radiographic grading system should be joint-specific. The age- and sex-specific prevalence of OA, the individual risk factors for the disorder and the rela-

tionship between radiographic change and symptoms are all known to differ according to joint site.

There are, however, two important caveats to the use of this overall grading system[19]. First, inconsistencies in the descriptions of radiographic features of OA by Kellgren and Lawrence themselves have led to studies being performed using criteria that are discordant. Second, the prominence awarded to the osteophyte at all joint sites remains controversial. To address these issues, recent studies have broken up this overall radiographic grading system into its component features, quantified each feature more precisely and assessed the reproducibility and clinical correlates of each. These studies have been attempted for OA at the knee, hip and hand. For the knee, each of joint space narrowing, osteophyte and the overall Kellgren/Lawrence grade show good within-observer reproducibility, but the scoring of osteophyte is most closely associated with knee pain[20]. At the hip, comparison of joint space narrowing, osteophyte, sclerosis and an overall grading system suggest that measurement of joint space was more reproducible than that of osteophyte, sclerosis or the composite score, and was most closely associated with reported hip pain[21]. Finally, in the hand, joint space narrowing, osteophyte and overall Kellgren/Lawrence grade can all be assessed reproducibly, but osteophyte appears to be more closely associated with pain[22]. Recent atlases of standard radiographs have helped to ensure a more consistent approach to the grading of these individual features and permit greater extrapolation between the results of different studies[23,24].

Radiographic measures also remain a cornerstone in the assessment of the progression of OA. A consensus meeting of the American Academy of Orthopedic Surgeons, the National Institutes of Health and the World Health Organization has recently produced recommendations for the use of radiographic measures for this purpose[25]. Careful attention must be paid to patient positioning and to the inclusion of views that permit assessment of different compartments of a joint (see Chapter 168). Thus, assessment of the knee requires a weight-bearing view to assess the tibiofemoral joint, as well as views to include the patellofemoral compartment. For the knee, the narrowest point of the tibiofemoral joint space can be measured in millimeters and both joint space narrowing and osteophyte can be graded 0–3 in all compartments. For the hip joint, progression should be recorded for joint space narrowing, both by millimeter measurements of the interbone distance and by visual grading (0–3 according to a standardized atlas). Femoral osteophytes are also graded 0–3 and features such as cyst, sclerosis, attrition and migration pattern can be recorded as present or absent. Radiographic features of knee disease should be recorded separately for the medial, lateral and patellofemoral compartments. Although advanced techniques can be used to assist assessment of the radiographs (e.g. digitization of the images with computerized methods for the assessment of interbone distance or osteophyte), these techniques remain research tools and have not yet superseded radiographic assessment by eye.

In recent years, other techniques have emerged in the assessment of OA. These include radionuclide scintigraphy, whose main role is to detect the activity of different types of process in a joint, and magnetic resonance imaging, which produces high-contrast soft tissue images in any spatial plane. In addition, there is increasing interest in the use of biochemical marker assays (such as type II collagen degradation and synthesis products) to study the disease process in OA, although at present none of the available markers can be specifically recommended as providing a measure of disease progression.

Clinical correlates

Two broad clinical areas are relevant to any definition or classification of OA: the symptoms associated with the condition and the degree of disability constituting its longer-term sequelae. Joint pain is the dominant symptom of OA. The prevalence of joint pain rises markedly with age in the general population. However, the association between joint pain and

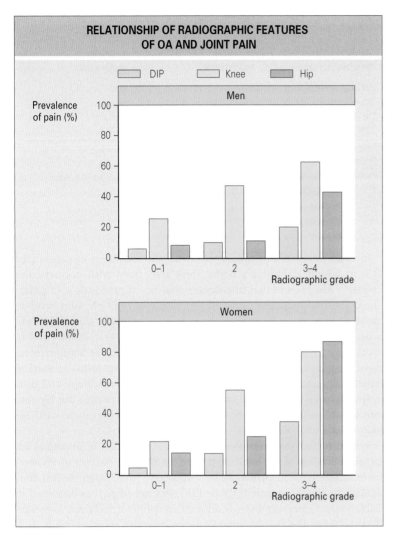

RELATIONSHIP OF RADIOGRAPHIC FEATURES OF OA AND JOINT PAIN

Fig. 164.1 Relationship of radiographic features of OA and joint pain. (Data from Lawrence[26].)

TABLE 164.3 ACR CRITERIA FOR OA OF THE HIP, KNEE AND HAND

	Items required for presence of OA
Hand	
Clinical	
1. Hand pain, aching or stiffness for most days of prior month	1, 2, 3, 4 or 1, 2, 3, 5
2. Hard tissue enlargement of ≥ 2 of 10 selected hand joints*	
3. MCP swelling in ≤ 2 joints	
4. Hard tissue enlargement of ≥ 2 DIP joints	
5. Deformity of ≥ 1 of 10 selected hand joints*	
Hip	
Clinical and radiographic	
1. Hip pain for most days of the prior month	1, 2, 3 or 1, 2, 4 or 1, 3, 4
2. ESR ≤ 20mm/h (laboratory)	
3. Radiograph femoral and/or acetabular osteophytes	
4. Radiograph hip joint-space narrowing	
Knee	
Clinical	
1. Knee pain for most days of prior month	1, 2, 3, 4 or 1, 2, 5 or 1, 4, 5
2. Crepitus on active joint motion	
3. Morning stiffness ≤ 30min in duration	
4. Age ≥ 38 years	
5. Bony enlargement of the knee on examination	
Clinical and radiographic	
1. Knee pain for most days of prior month	1, 2 or 1, 3, 5, 6 or 1, 4, 5, 6
2. Osteophytes at joint margins (radiograph)	
3. Synovial fluid typical of OA (laboratory)	
4. Age ≥ 40 years	
5. Morning stiffness ≤ 30min	
6. Crepitus on active joint motion	

* 10 selected hand joints include bilateral 2nd and 3rd proximal interphalangeal joints, 2nd and 3rd distal interphalangeal (DIP) joints and 1st carpometacarpal joints

ESR, erythrocyte sedimentation rate; MCP, metacarpophalangeal.

the radiographic features of OA is not constant. In studies performed during the 1950s in the north of England (Fig. 164.1), the relationship between pain and radiographic evidence of OA was considerably stronger for the hip and knee than for distal interphalangeal (DIP) joint involvement[26]. In a more recent study of 400 women aged 45–65 years living in Chingford, Essex, UK, Hart *et al.*[27] noted that the prevalence of symptomatic knee OA was only 2.3% compared to 17% for radiologically defined knee OA.

Diagnostic criteria

The heterogeneity of OA has led to attempts to establish diagnostic criteria for the disorder at various joint sites. The most widely used such criteria were developed by the American College of Rheumatology[15,28,29]. These criteria sets identify subjects or patients with clinical OA, the major inclusion parameter being joint pain for most days of the prior month. This contrasts with the use of radiographic changes alone as many, if not most, subjects do not report joint pain. The algorithms for classification were developed by comparing patients with clinically diagnosed OA and controls with site-specific joint pain due to other arthritic or musculoskeletal diseases. The sensitivity, specificity and accuracy of the whole range of clinical and radiographic measures in discriminating between these two groups were assessed. Table 164.3 illustrates the criteria for hand, knee and hip.

The method whereby the criteria sets were derived will influence their usefulness in different settings. For clinical studies and randomized controlled trials of new interventions, selection based on the ACR criteria

enhances comparison between studies. The use of the ACR criteria in population-based research is less clearly defined and prevalence estimates using the ACR case definitions are likely to be substantially lower than those based on traditional radiographic criteria. Thus, the prevalence of symptomatic knee OA among women aged 45–65 years in one study was only 2.3%, in contrast with an estimate of 17% for radiographically defined disease[27].

Classification

Two major systems have been proposed for the classification of OA: etiologic and articular. The recognition that pathologic and radiologic features of OA could follow almost any established joint disorder led to the suggestion that OA could be classified as primary (idiopathic) or secondary[30]. Several disorders are recognized as causes of secondary OA. They can be divided into four main categories (Table 164.4):

● metabolic disorders such as ochronosis, which lead to joint damage that can be indistinguishable from OA
● anatomic derangements such as a slipped epiphysis, which can lead to OA of the one affected joint only
● major trauma or surgery to a joint, such as a meniscectomy
● a previous inflammatory arthropathy, such as RA, resulting in a secondary OA process in some of the affected joints.

TABLE 164.4   CLASSIFICATION OF OA

Classification by the joints involved

- Monoarticular, oligoarticular or polyarticular (generalized)
- Chief joint site (index joint site) and localization within the joint:
  - Hip (superior pole, medial pole or concentric)
  - Knee (medial, lateral, patellofemoral compartments)
  - Hand (interphalangeal joints and/or thumb base)
  - Spine (apophyseal joints or intervertebral disc disease)
  - Others

Classification into primary and secondary forms of OA

- Primary = idiopathic
- Secondary indicates that a likely cause can be identified
  Causes of secondary OA:
  1. **Metabolic:** examples include
     Ochronosis
     Acromegaly
     Hemochromatosis
     Calcium crystal deposition
  2. **Anatomic:** examples include
     Slipped femoral epiphysis
     Epiphyseal dysplasias
     Blount's disease
     Legg–Perthes disease
     Congenital dislocation of the hip
     Leg-length inequality
     Hypermobility syndromes
  3. **Traumatic:** examples include
     Major joint trauma
     Fracture through a joint or osteonecrosis
     Joint surgery (e.g. meniscectomy)
     Chronic injury (occupational arthropathies)
  4. **Inflammatory:** examples include
     Any inflammatory arthropathy
     Septic arthritis

Classification by the presence of specific features

- Inflammatory OA
- Erosive OA
- Atrophic or destructive OA
- OA with chondrocalcinosis

TABLE 164.5   ASSOCIATION BETWEEN DIFFERENT JOINT GROUPS IN OA

Radiographic definition of OA	Grade 2+ (odds ratio)	Grade 3+ (odds ratio)
DIP–DIP (row)	5.0	10.0
PIP–PIP(row)	3.7	3.1
DIP–PIP (ray)	3.7	5.9
CMC–IP	1.4	1.3

CMC, carpometacarpal (1st); DIP, distal interphalangeal; IP, interphalangeal; PIP, proximal interphalangeal.

Clustering of hand joint involvement among perimenopausal women. The odds ratios indicate the hierarchies of association between different joint groups. (Data from Egger et al.[34])

However, the distinction between primary and secondary OA is not always clear. For example, it has been shown that after meniscectomy 20–25% of people will develop premature OA in the operated knee joint some 20 years later[31]. However, there is also evidence that the 20% who do get secondary OA have some generalized predisposition to the disorder. Furthermore, in an individual patient it can be difficult to judge whether or not an abnormality reported many years previously is of significance for their current OA.

The second basis for subclassifying OA relates to the number and distribution of joint sites expected. Just as there is great heterogeneity in the effects and manifestations of OA at one joint, there is variation in the pattern of joint distribution in different individuals. The condition shows a particular predilection for the DIP joints of the hand, the thumb base, the knee, hip and intravertebral facet joint. Involvement of more than one joint is common, and many population surveys have reported that subjects with OA in one joint have a greater frequency in other joints that cannot be explained by chance or age alone. Furthermore, there appear to be differences in the degree of association between OA at different joint sites. There is a stronger association between hand and knee OA than between hip and knee disease in Caucasian populations[32]. These differences justify the contention that OA at different sites should be treated as separate conditions.

In 1952, Kellgren and Moore described the condition of generalized OA, in which Heberden's nodes were associated with polyarticular disease[33]. They found that first-degree relatives of probands with generalized OA had twice the expected prevalence of multiple joint involvement. They went on to confirm the hereditary nature of this diathesis in a twin study. This subgroup of OA has been better characterized in recent years[34,35]. It shows a predilection for polyarticular hand involvement (particularly the interphalangeal and thumb base joints), a marked female preponderance, early inflammatory symptomatology and pronounced node formation. When large joints, for example the hip, are affected there is a tendency to diffuse (bilateral and concentric) cartilage loss.

Symmetry of joint involvement in this disorder is pronounced. Detailed studies of the hand joints suggest that the pattern of involvement is determined primarily by symmetry, with much weaker tendencies to cluster by row (DIP or PIP) and ray (digit), as displayed in Table 164.5. Generalized OA is difficult to define: it has been suggested that it means the involvement of three or more joint sites but such definitions depend upon the age of subjects, the radiographic severity adopted for definition, the number of joint sites included in any survey and the degree of certainty required regarding coincident involvement of joints on the basis of chance alone.

Several other features of OA have been used in attempts to subset the disorder. For example, the term *inflammatory OA* is sometimes used for patients with obvious inflammation and multiple joint involvement[36]. However, the joints appear to pass through phases in which this inflammation is more or less prominent, and no clear differences between patients with and without extensive inflammatory features of OA have been delineated. Some patients develop erosions of their interphalangeal joints, leading to the classification of the subset of erosive OA[37]. This disorder tends to occur in middle-aged women, presents acutely with features of inflammation and subsides over a period of months to years, leaving joint deformity and occasional ankylosis. Recent controlled data suggest that erosions in OA may simply be an aggressive form of joint destruction in a joint that is already at risk[38]. Similarly, atrophic and destructive forms of OA probably represent ends of the spectrum of disease rather than separate entities. Finally, insights into OA are provided by a variety of rare or geographically localized diseases that are associated with the development of premature disease. Examples include dysplastic conditions such as Blount's disease[39].

MORBIDITY

Prevalence

Attempts have been made to assess the prevalence of pathologic features of OA in systematic autopsy studies. In a series of 1000 cases in 1926, Heine[7] documented almost universal evidence of cartilage damage in people aged over 65 years. More recent studies report that cartilage

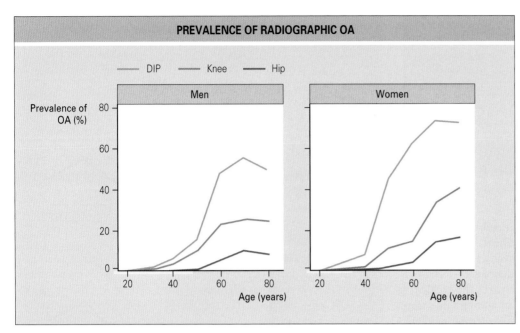

PREVALENCE OF RADIOGRAPHIC OA

— DIP — Knee — Hip

Men

Women

Prevalence of OA (%)

Age (years)

Fig. 164.2 Prevalence of radiographic OA. Estimates for the prevalence of radiographic OA affecting the DIP joint, knee and hip in a large Dutch population sample.

erosions, subchondral reaction and osteophyte are present in the knees of 60% of men and 70% of women who die in the seventh and eighth decades of life. Prevalence estimates from such studies tend to be higher than those from radiographic surveys, partly because relatively mild pathologic change is not apparent on radiographs and also because pathologic studies examine the whole joint surface.

Radiographic surveys of prevalence

Most currently available information on the epidemiology of OA comes from population-based radiographic surveys. In the earliest such studies, attention was focused on OA of the hand joints, or on generalized (polyarticular) OA. More recent studies from Europe and the USA present prevalence data for individual joints, which permit comparison between studies. The two most comprehensive surveys are those from the US National Health Survey[40] and the Zoetermeer Community Survey in The Netherlands[41].

The prevalence of radiographic OA rises steeply with age at all joint sites. The Netherlands study[41] included 6585 inhabitants randomly selected from the population of a Dutch village. A total of 75% of women aged 60–70 years had OA of their DIP joints (Fig. 164.2) and, even by 40 years of age, 10–20% of subjects had evidence of severe radiographic disease of their hands or feet. Knee disease appears less frequent than hand and foot involvement. Population-based studies in the USA suggest comparable prevalence rates to those in Europe (Table 164.6), rising from less than 1% for severe radiographic disease among people aged 25–34 to 30% in those aged 75 years and above. Both hand and knee disease appear to be more frequent among women than men, although the female-to-male ratio varies among studies from 1.5 to 4.0. Hip OA is less common than knee OA, and prevalence rates for OA at this site in men and women appear more similar. Some, but not all, studies have reported a male preponderance in hip OA.

Geographic variation in prevalence

Although OA is worldwide in its distribution, geographic differences in prevalence have been reported. These are often difficult to interpret because of differences in sampling procedure and radiographic consistency. European and American data do not appear to differ markedly for hand and knee disease[42]. However, hand involvement appears to be particularly frequent in Pima and Blackfoot Indian populations within the USA. African-American females have a higher age-adjusted prevalence of knee OA than Caucasian females but are less likely to have Heberden's nodes on physical examination[43–45]. Studies among African

TABLE 164.6		PREVALENCE OF OA BY AGE AND SEX IN THE USA			
		Grades 2–4		Grades 3 and 4	
Site	Ages (years)	Males	Females	Males	Females
Hands	25–34	4.8	2.1	0.1	–
	35–44	17.5	11.3	0.6	1.1
	45–54	39.0	34.0	1.8	5.5
	55–64	56.6	68.8	12.6	21.5
	65–74	71.0	77.1	22.4	37.0
Knees	25–34	–	0.1	–	0.0
	35–44	1.7	1.5	0.1	0.5
	45–54	2.3	3.6	0.2	0.5
	55–64	4.1	7.3	1.0	0.9
	65–74	8.3	18.0	2.0	6.6
Hips	25–34	0.4	–	0.2	–
	35–44	0.1	–	–	–
	45–54	0.7	–	0.1	–
	50–54	–	0.8	–	0.1
	55–64	2.6	2.8	0.7	1.6
	65–74	4.6	2.7	2.3	1.2

Prevalence per 100 of radiologic changes of OA in hands, knees and hips by age and sex in the US National Health Survey.

blacks in Nigeria and Liberia, as well as Jamaican blacks confirm the lower prevalence of Heberden's nodes[26]. Greater variation has been found in the distribution of hip OA, with low or similar rates reported among African blacks[44,46,47], Asian Indians[48] and Hong Kong Chinese[49] and, most recently, Chinese men and women living in Beijing[50,51]. These differences have been attributed to a lower rate of developmental hip disorders among these populations, as well as the common use of the squatting posture, which forces the hip joint through an extreme range of motion. By contrast, knee OA is common in the Beijing elderly. In a recent survey, despite being thinner, Chinese women had a much higher prevalence of knee OA than their US Caucasian counterparts, whereas Chinese men had lower levels of radiographically defined OA than their American counterparts[50].

Incidence

Few studies have examined the incidence of OA and most available data have been obtained in the USA (Table 164.7). Such studies typically rely on ascertainment of new cases that develop between duplicate

TABLE 164.7 EPIDEMIOLOGICAL STUDIES OF OA INCIDENCE				
Study	Date	Site	Sex	Incidence rate (per 100 000)
Wilson et al.[52]	1990	Hip	M + F	47.3
		Knee	M + F	163.8
Kallman et al.[53]	1990	Hand	M	100
Oliveria et al.[54]	1995	Hip	M + F	88
		Knee	M + F	240
		Hand	M + F	100

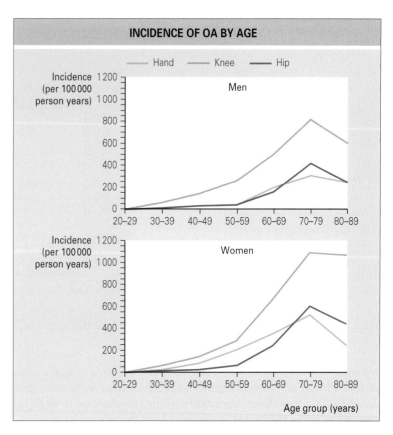

Fig. 164.3 Incidence of OA by age. Incidence of symptomatic OA of the hand, knee and hip. (Data from the Fallon Community Health Plan[54].)

cross-sectional surveys. Kallman et al.[22] examined hand radiographs of around 200 men in the Baltimore Longitudinal Study of Aging who had undergone radiography on at least four occasions over a 20-year follow-up period. They reported an incidence of OA, defined by Kellgren/Lawrence or individual features scales, of 4% per year. The incidence rate rose steeply with age and reached 10% each year among subjects in the oldest age group. Incidence estimates were even higher for hand OA among female participants of the Tecumseh Community Health Study[55]. In a population-based incidence study of hip and knee OA using the medical record linkage section of the Mayo Clinic, age- and sex-adjusted rates for OA of the hip and knee were found to be 47.3/100 000 person-years (95% confidence interval, CI 27.8–66.8) and 163.8/100 000 person-years (95% CI 127.1–200.6), respectively[52]. Age-adjusted rates for OA of the hip and knee were similar for men and women. In men, the results point to a steadily increasing rate with age. In women, there was a plateau in incidence after the menopause.

The most recent data to characterize the incidence of symptomatic hand, hip and knee OA were obtained from the Fallon Community Health Plan, a health maintenance organization located in the northeast USA[54]. In this study, the age- and sex-standardized incidence rate of hand OA was 100/100 000 person-years (95% CI 86–115), for hip OA 88/100 000 person-years (95% CI 75–101) and for knee OA 240/100 000 person-years (95% CI 218–262). The incidence of hand, hip and knee disease increased with age and women had higher rates than men, especially after the age of 50 years (Fig. 164.3). A leveling off occurred for both groups at all joint sites around the age of 80 years. By the age of 70–89 years, the incidence of symptomatic knee OA among women approached 1% per year. Comparison of these data with age- and sex-adjusted arthroplasty rates in the northern USA suggests that the rate of surgery is beginning to match the incidence rate of severe hip disease but that a considerable shortfall exists between surgical treatment and disease incidence for knee OA.

INDIVIDUAL RISK FACTORS

The individual risk factors for OA may be conveniently viewed as acting through two major pathogenetic mechanisms:

- factors influencing or marking a generalized predisposition to the condition
- factors resulting in abnormal biomechanical loading at specific joint sites (Fig. 164.4).

Generalized susceptibility

Heredity
A hereditary component in the etiology of OA is most likely for the polyarticular form. Both twin and family studies have pointed to a strong hereditary predisposition to generalized OA. In studies by Stecher[56], a twofold excess of Heberden's nodes was found among mothers of probands, and a threefold excess among sisters, when com-

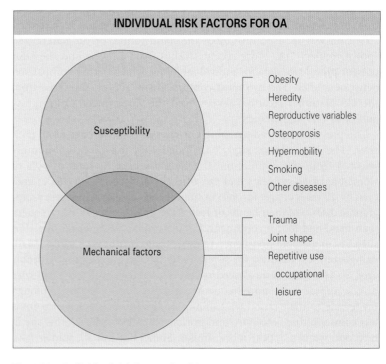

Fig. 164.4 Individual risk factors for OA.

pared with age-expected values. Subsequent analyses of the mode of inheritance suggested an autosomal dominant pattern consistent with a single gene model. Further studies of the genetic factors conducted in the UK suggested a striking familial aggregation of Heberden's nodes with a 4.5-fold excess among female relatives of female probands and an 8.5-fold excess among female relatives of male probands[26]. A recent British twin study confirmed greater concordance of OA among monozygous than dizygous twin pairs[57]. More recently, attention has focused upon abnormalities in the genes coding for collagen synthesis, with reports that certain defects segregate with disease in multi-case families. (See Chapter 167 for further details on this subject.)

Obesity

Adiposity is clearly associated with the development of knee OA in both sexes. Population-based studies suggest that the increase in risk of knee OA between the highest and lowest fifths of the distribution of body mass index is between four- and sevenfold and there appears to be a linear dose–response relationship[58]. Furthermore, obesity is more strongly associated with bilateral than unilateral knee OA and the strength of the association is not diminished by adjustment for potential confounding variables, including age, race, blood pressure, serum cholesterol, serum uric acid, body fat distribution or history of diabetes[59].

Until recently, it was not clear whether obesity preceded (and perhaps caused) OA, or whether obesity resulted from the sedentary lifestyle of patients with OA. Longitudinal studies now suggest that the former assertion is correct. First, analysis from the Framingham study in the US has revealed that body mass index measured at onset (between 1948 and 1951) predicted the presence of radiographic knee OA 36 years later. Other longitudinal studies to evaluate the association between obesity and OA include the Chingford Study[60], the Baltimore Longitudinal Study of Aging[61], the Matsudai Precursors Study[62], the Johns Hopkins Precursors Study[63] and a longitudinal study conducted in Bristol, UK[64]. It therefore seems likely that prevention of weight gain that results in obesity may be an important part of primary preventive strategies against knee OA. Data are conflicting regarding whether joint symptoms may be alleviated with weight loss[65,66] but, in the Framingham study, weight loss was associated with a reduced risk of knee OA at baseline and, in the prospective study, a reduced risk of developing OA compared with individuals whose weight remained stable.

The association of obesity with hand OA remains controversial. Studies based on the US Health Examination Survey and the Baltimore Longitudinal Study of Aging have failed to demonstrate statistically significant associations among men or women[67]. However, the trends in several studies point consistently towards an association that is simply less marked than that observed for knee OA. Prospective data, analyzed from the Tecumseh Community Health Study, found that baseline obesity was a significant independent predictor of both the incidence and severity of hand OA[68]. By contrast, an analysis of data from the Baltimore Longitudinal Study of Aging did not find an association between increased body weight and incidence and progression of hand OA in men[69]. The gradient of risk between obesity and hip OA appears intermediate between those for hand and knee disease[70–72].

The reason for the association between obesity and OA remains speculative. Although mechanical loading appears to be an attractive mechanism at first sight, it does not explain the differential effects of adiposity at the hip and knee. Some studies point toward a stronger association of OA and obesity among women than men, suggesting that metabolic, rather than mechanical, factors may explain the link.

The effect of loading of body weight through the knee joint may be influenced by joint alignment. Hence, a recent longitudinal study of 237 subjects with primary knee OA has demonstrated that having malalignment of greater than 5° in both knees at baseline was associated with significantly greater functional deterioration during the 18 months of follow-up than having malalignment of less than 5°, after adjusting for age, sex, body mass index and pain; in this study, varus alignment predicted increased risk of medial compartment progression and valgus alignment increased the risk of lateral compartment progression[73]. It has been similarly proposed that dysplasia of the femoral condyles alters the biomechanical stability of the knee joint and predisposes to OA.

Reproductive variables

The marked female predominance of polyarticular OA has led many commentators to suggest that this clinical subgroup is hormonally mediated[74]. The disorder appears to increase in prevalence after the menopause in women, and OA has been associated with previous hysterectomy[75]. Epidemiological studies suggest that the use of postmenopausal hormone replacement therapy (HRT) may retard the development of knee OA[76]. A systematic review of observational studies of the relationship between HRT use and OA supported a protective association[77], and recent prospective studies have reported non-significant reductions in radiographic knee OA in women who were current HRT users[78,79]. However, recent work has also suggested that women using HRT had a greater risk of developing symptomatic arthritis than those who did not[80] and Sandmark et al.[81] noted that postmenopausal women who underwent total knee replacement were more likely to have taken HRT. Results from randomized placebo-controlled trials are hence eagerly awaited.

Osteoporosis

Osteoarthritis at particular sites also appears to have an inverse association with osteoporosis[82]. The strongest evidence for this lies at the hip joint, where studies consistently observe that elderly patients with hip OA have high levels of bone mineral density[83]. In patients with hand OA and polyarticular disease, studies of bone density have produced inconsistent results[84]. The association is stronger in patients with hypertrophic OA characterized by osteophytes rather than atrophic OA characterized by joint space narrowing. The OA–osteoporosis relationship supports the view that abnormal mechanical behavior of subchondral bone underlies accelerated cartilage damage. Certainly, in rare inherited bone diseases such as osteopetrosis, where the skeleton is diffusely sclerotic, there is a high incidence of premature polyarticular OA.

Hypermobility

The range of motion of any joint has a normal distribution in the population. Generalized ligamentous laxity is therefore seen in a small proportion of healthy people. Hypermobility diminishes rapidly throughout childhood and then more slowly during later life. Women are more mobile than men, and Chinese/Japanese more mobile than Caucasians. Generalized joint laxity is a feature of several rare inherited disorders of collagen, such as Ehlers–Danlos syndrome. Hypermobility in the absence of identifiable collagen gene abnormalities may result in a wide variety of overuse lesions, as well as OA. The strength of the association with OA, as well as its precise mechanism, remain subjects for further study (see also Chapter 207).

Cigarette smoking

Analysis of some, but not all, population-based data sets suggests that cigarette smoking has a protective influence on the development of OA[84]. This effect remains after adjustment for potential confounding variables such as body weight, and may reflect an influence of smoking on hepatic metabolism of female sex hormones.

Other diseases

Associations have been documented between OA and diabetes mellitus, hypertension and hyperuricemia that are independent of obesity[84]. The association with diabetes may have particular etiological significance through the increased prevalence of diffuse idiopathic skeletal hyperostosis (Forestier's disease) in this condition.

Mechanical factors

Trauma

Major injury is a common cause of knee OA. Two specific types of injury are associated with a knee OA: cruciate ligament damage and meniscal tears. Follow-up studies of patients with cruciate rupture (particularly when bilateral) have reported cartilage loss, even in young patients. Following meniscectomy, most studies have reported an increased frequency of subsequent OA[85]. The risk rises with advancing age, presence of a generalized predisposition to OA (as evidenced by Heberden's nodes) and time since meniscectomy. Major injury, particularly fracture, may alter mechanical function and predispose to OA at other sites. Most notable among these are fractures of the femoral shaft (hip OA), tibia (ankle OA), humerus (shoulder OA) and scaphoid (wrist OA). The association between lower limb injury during young adulthood and an increased risk for knee OA has recently been confirmed in a longitudinal study of male physicians[86].

Joint shape

The sites at which joint shape has been most closely linked with later development of OA are the hip and knee. It is well established that childhood hip disorders such as Perthes disease, slipped capital epiphysis and congenital dislocation of the hip lead to premature hip OA. It is also likely that milder degrees of acetabular dysplasia account for a proportion of hip OA even among older subjects[87].

Occupation

Occupational physical activity exemplifies stereotyped repetitive use of particular joint groups. The association of hand OA with handedness, and the relatively infrequent involvement of paretic limbs by the condition, point to a role for repetitive activity in the etiology of OA. Several observational studies comparing the prevalence of symptomatic or radiographic knee OA in different occupational groups have reported a higher prevalence of disease among manual workers[88]. Thus, knee OA has been shown to be more frequent among miners, dock workers, concrete workers and shipyard workers than among clerical or office staff. These observations have been extended in cohort studies from the USA and Sweden.

Perhaps the most compelling evidence linking knee OA with occupational knee use comes from population-based surveys relating risk to particular types of activity. These studies suggest significant increases in the risk of symptomatic knee OA among men and women who engage in prolonged kneeling or prolonged squatting and who have jobs associated with high physical demands[89]. A systematic review and meta-analysis of the relationship between occupational physical activity and lower limb OA was published by Maetzel and colleagues[90].

Epidemiological studies from the USA, Sweden and the UK suggest that hip OA occurs more frequently than expected among agricultural laborers. These observations are consistent, and the increase in risk varies between two- and eightfold[70,71]. The precise reasons for the increased risk among this occupational group remain uncertain but are most likely related to regular lifting of very heavy loads and walking over rough ground. Elegant studies have suggested that the localization of hand OA to particular joint groups in the hands of cotton workers is also related to specific activities performed in the workplace.

Sports and leisure physical activity

Sporting activity combines the risks of major joint damage with those of repetitive use. In a case-control study reported from Hong Kong[91], women who performed gymnastics regularly were at a sixfold increased risk of hip OA and those who performed kung fu had an odds ratio of 22 for OA of the knee. In a study of incident knee OA in Framingham, USA, heavy physical activity was associated with an increased risk of knee OA in both sexes; adjustment for body mass index, weight loss, knee injury, health status, calorie intake and smoking strengthened the association[92]. A cross-sectional study of participants in the Study of Osteoporotic Fractures[71] found that the risk of moderate to severe radiographic hip OA in older age was modestly increased in women who had performed more physical activity as teenagers.

PROGRESSION

Knee osteoarthritis

The knee is a complex joint with three major compartments: the medial and lateral tibiofemoral joints and the patellofemoral joint. Each of these areas can be affected by OA separately, or in any combination. Isolated medial compartment or medial plus patellofemoral disease are the most common combinations[93]. Table 164.8 lists the studies that have examined the natural history of knee OA.

Disease evolution is slow, usually taking many years. However, there is evidence that, once established, the condition can remain relatively stable, both clinically and radiologically, for a further period of several years. The correlation between the clinical outcome of knee OA and its radiographic course is not strong. In a large study, Dougados et al.[95] demonstrated that, although radiographic improvement was rare, overall clinical improvement at 1 year follow-up was common. Longer-term studies confirmed that radiographic deterioration occurs in between one-third and two-thirds of patients and that radiographic improvement is unusual. A Swedish study documented that, among patients with struc-

TABLE 164.8 STUDIES OF THE NATURAL HISTORY OF KNEE OA					
Study	Year	No. of subjects	Measure	Follow-up (years)	% deteriorated
Hernborg[100]	1977	84 knees	C	15	55
			R	15	56
Danielsson[112]	1970	106 knees	R	15	33
Massardo et al.[94]	1989	31	R	8	62
Dougados et al.[95]	1991	353	C	1	28
			R	1	29
Schouten[96]	1991	142	R	12	34
Spector et al.[97]	1991	63	R	11	33
Spector et al.[60]	1994	58	R	2	22
Ledingham et al.[98]	1995	350 knees	R	2	72
McAlindon[92]	1998	470	R	4	11*
Cooper et al.[64]	2000	354	R	5	22
Pavelka et al.[99]	2000	139	R	5	25

* Incident OA.

C, clinical; R; radiographic.

tural change, for example tibial or femoral sclerosis, the majority experienced radiographic and symptomatic deterioration over 15 years[100]. Of those subjects with only osteophyte on baseline radiography, a much smaller proportion suffered deterioration. This is broadly in accord with an American study[101] in which joint space narrowing was judged to be a more important determinant of progression in knee OA than was the presence of osteophyte. However, when variables were considered in combination, this study reported that a score based on joint space narrowing, osteophyte and sclerosis was reasonably reproducible and a better predictor of progression than any other combination.

Recent British studies[97,102] have also examined the progression of knee OA, both among subjects attending hospital outpatient departments and in the general population. In an 11-year follow-up study of 63 subjects who had baseline knee radiographs, the majority of knees did not show a worsening of overall grade of OA, with only 33% deteriorating in Kellgren/Lawrence score over the time period[97]. When a more sensitive global scoring system was used on paired films, the proportion showing a slight deterioration increased to 50%, and 10% showed improvement. The latter estimate is within the limits imposed by imprecision in radiographic grading. The visual analogue pain scores remained stable over the time period, but it was reported that those with knee pain at baseline had a greater chance of progressing, as did those with existing OA in the contralateral knee.

A similar follow-up study was performed in 58 women aged 45–64 from the general population, in whom unilateral knee OA (Kellgren/Lawrence grade 2 or higher) was present at baseline[60]. Follow-up radiographs at 24 months revealed that 34% of the women developed disease in the contralateral knee and that 22% progressed radiologically in the index joint. Table 164.9 shows the change in radiographic score of knee OA during a 5-year follow-up period in 354 British men and women, aged 55 years or over, who participated in a longitudinal study conducted by Cooper et al.; rates of incidence and progression were 2.5% and 3.6% per year respectively[64].

Despite these studies, several questions remain about the natural history of knee OA. Some studies have excluded from follow-up subjects whose symptoms were severe enough for them to need surgery. In other studies, many of the patients initially seen were subsequently lost to follow-up. This loss could have occurred because the patients had surgery, or because their knee symptoms had remitted and they felt no need to return. Studies of the natural history of knee OA are shown in Table 164.8, and include a cohort of 500 clinically diagnosed patients with lower limb arthritis, the majority of whom reported a worsening of their condition with an increase in disability and use of walking aids[102].

Hip osteoarthritis

As with knee OA, it remains uncertain whether the anatomically recognized subsets of hip OA represent part of a spectrum or discrete pathophysiological entities. These anatomical subtypes are best classified by the pattern of cartilage loss apparent on hip radiography. The most frequent pattern is superolateral, estimated to occur in some 60% of patients with hip OA. The other two patterns are medial and concentric cartilage loss occurring in 25% and 15% of patients respectively.

The natural history of hip OA is very variable. Many cases that come to surgery have a relatively short history of severe symptoms, suggesting that a progressive phase lasting between 3 months and 3 years often precedes the advanced stages of OA.

There are fewer prospective studies of hip OA than of knee OA. In a Danish follow-up study of 121 hips, the majority (65%) showed radiographic deterioration over a ten year follow-up period[103]. Symptomatic improvement in this series was surprisingly common, occurring in the majority of patients. This is at variance with the results of another longitudinal study which documented frequent deterioration in the clinical course of hip OA patients[104]. In a Dutch study of patients identified from the general population who had established OA in one or both hips, 29% of the subjects showed a worsening of their radiographic scores over a 12-year follow-up period[105]. Nonetheless, unlike knee OA, a few patients with hip OA can experience clear cut radiologic and symptomatic recovery[106]. This appears to occur most often among patients who have marked osteophytosis and in those with concentric disease.

Osteonecrosis is the major complication of hip OA and tends to occur late in the natural history. Rapidly progressive OA can lead to an unusual appearance, with extensive bone destruction and a wide interbone distance. This appearance was initially observed among patients who ingested anti-inflammatory drugs and was termed analgesic hip[107,108]. However, it is now recognized to occur in groups of subjects who ingest few or no such agents. Studies of the natural history of hip OA are shown in Table 164.10 and include data from a study of 136 hospital-referred patients with hip OA[109] and French data from a cohort of 508 patients with hip OA[110].

Hand osteoarthritis

Osteoarthritis principally affects the DIP, PIP and thumb base in the hand. The evolution of hand OA is usually complete after a period of a few years. It has been studied both clinically and radiographically. The condition usually starts with aching in the affected joints and tends to have a remitting and relapsing course over the initial years. There is often clear evidence of inflammatory phases in which individual joints become warm and tender. Bony swelling develops during this phase and cysts may form. After a variable time period, often lasting several years, these flares and the pain tend to subside. The swellings become firm and fixed and joint movement becomes progressively reduced. The condition then appears to enter a stable phase during the seventh and eighth decades of life. Imaging studies show this evolution of change to be accompanied by sequential changes in joint anatomy and physiology.

Kallman and colleagues reported that, among men with DIP joint OA, more than 50% experienced progression of radiographic disease over 10 years[53]. The progression was fastest in the DIP joints and was slower in PIP joints and the thumb base. The presence of narrowing at baseline increased the risk that subjects would develop subsequent osteophytes, and joints with severe radiographic changes at baseline had slower progression rates than joints with milder radiographic changes. The rates of OA progression in individual subjects paralleled the rate of progression hinted at by cross-sectional studies, in which subjects are studied at different ages. Similarly, Harris et al. reported a study of 59 subjects with paired hand radiographs over a 10-year period[111]. Radiographs were scored in three areas: DIP, PIP and carpometacarpal joints using the methods of Kellgren and Lawrence and for osteophytes and narrowing. Virtually all subjects (97%)

TABLE 164.9 PROGRESSION OF OA

Baseline Kellgren/Lawrence score	Follow-up Kellgren/Lawrence score					
	0	1	2	3	4	All
0	148	14	16	–	–	178
1	3	32	27	2	–	64
2	–	–	59	16	1	76
3	–	–	–	28	3	31
4	–	–	–	–	5	5
All	151	46	102	46	9	354

Change in radiographic score of knee OA during 5-year follow-up in men and women aged 55 years or over. The analysis was based on the worst-affected knee at baseline and follow-up. (Data derived from Cooper et al.[64])

TABLE 164.10   STUDIES OF THE NATURAL HISTORY OF HIP OA

Study	Year	No. of subjects	Measure	Follow-up (years)	% deteriorated
Danielsson[103]	1964	121 hips	C	10.0	19
			R	10.0	65
Seifert et al.[104]	1969	83 hips	C	5.0	83
Van Saase et al.[105]	1989	86	R	12.0	29
Ledingham et al.[109]	1993	136	C	2.3	66
			R	2.3	47
Dougados et al.[110]	1996	508	R	1	22

TABLE 164.11   DETERMINANTS OF PROGRESSION OF HIP AND KNEE OA

	Strength of association	
	Knee	Hip
Generalized OA diathesis	++	+
Obesity	++	+
Joint injury	++	+
Crystal deposition	+	
Neuromuscular dysfunction	+	
Physical activity	++	++

deteriorated when the total scores of all joints were calculated, with new osteophytes appearing in 48% of DIP joints over the follow-up period.

In conclusion, OA is firmly established as a public health problem. Recent advances in defining the disorder, and in its measurement clinically and radiographically have allowed epidemiological studies designed to collect data on the incidence and progression of OA. It is clear that these figures are joint-specific, and that there may be disease subsets at each site in which progression depends on different groups of factors (Table 164.11). The challenge of identifying subjects at risk of rapid progression is currently the subject of intensive research.

REFERENCES

1. Rogers J, Dieppe P, Watt I. Arthritis in Saxon and medieval skeletons. Br Med J 1981; 283: 668–671.
2. Inoue K, Hukuda S, Fardellon P et al. Prevalence of large-joint osteoarthritis in Asian and Caucasian skeletal populations. Rheumatology 2001; 40: 70–73.
3. Goldthwaite JW. The treatment of disabled joints resulting from the so-called rheumatoid diseases. Boston Med Surg J 1987; 136: 79–84.
4. Nichols EH, Richardson FL. Arthritis deformans. J Med Res 1909; 21: 149–223.
5. Adams R. A treatise on rheumatic gout, or chronic rheumatic arthritis of all the joints. London: John Churchill; 1857.
6. Garrod AE. Rheumatoid arthritis, osteoarthritis and arthritis deformans. In: Allbitt TC, Rolleston HD, eds. A system of medicine. London: Macmillan; 1907: 3–43.
7. Heine J. Uber die arthritis deformans. Virchows Archiv 1926; 260: 521–563.
8. Collins DH. Osteoarthritis. J Bone Joint Surg 1953; 35B: 518–520.
9. Lloyd-Roberts GC. The role of capsular changes in osteoarthritis of the hip joint. J Bone Joint Surg 1953; 35B: 627–642.
10. Byers PD, Contepomi CA, Farkas TA. A post-mortem study of the hip joint. Ann Rheum Dis 1970; 29: 15–31.
11. Bullough PG. The geometry of diarthrodial joints, its physiologic maintenance and the possible significance of age-related changes in geometry to loan distribution and the development of arthritis. Clin Orthop Rel Res 1981; 156: 61–66.
12. Sokoloff L. The biology of degenerative joint disease. Chicago: Chicago University Press; 1969.
13. Trueta J. Studies of the development and decay of the human frame. New York: Heinemann; 1968.
14. Hutton C. Osteoarthritis: the cause not result of joint failure? Ann Rheum Dis 1989; 48: 958–961.
15. Altman R, Asch E, Bloch D et al. The American College of Rheumatology criteria for the classification and reporting of osteoarthritis of the knee. Arthritis Rheum 1986; 29: 1039–1049.
16. Brandt KD, Mankin HJ, Shulman LE eds. Workshop on etiopathogenesis of osteoarthritis. J Rheumatol 1986; 13: 1126–1160.
17. Keuttner K, Goldberg VM eds. Osteoarthritic disorders. Rosemont, IL: American Academy of Orthopedic Surgeons, 1995: xxi–xxv.
18. Kellgren JK, Lawrence JS. Radiological assessment of osteoarthritis. Ann Rheum Dis 1957; 15: 494–501.
19. Spector TD, Cooper C. Radiographic assessment of osteoarthritis in population studies: Whither Kellgren and Lawrence? Osteoarthritis Cartilage 1993; 1: 203–206.
20. Spector TD, Hart DJ, Byrne J et al. Definition of osteoarthritis of the knee for epidemiological studies. Ann Rheum Dis 1993; 52: 790–794.
21. Croft P, Cooper C, Wickham C, Coggon D. Defining osteoarthritis of the hip for epidemiologic studies. Am J Epidemiol 1990; 132: 514–522.
22. Kallman DA, Wigley FM, Scott WW Jr et al. New radiographic grading scales for osteoarthritis of the hand: reliability for determining prevalence and progression. Arthritis Rheum 1989; 32: 1584–1591.
23. Altman RD, Hochberg M, Murphy WA et al. Atlas of individual radiographic features in osteoarthritis. Osteoarthritis Cartilage 1995; 3(suppl A): 3–70.
24. Burnett S, Hart DJ, Cooper C, Spector TD. A radiographic atlas of osteoarthritis. London: Springer-Verlag, 1994: 1–45.
25. Dieppe DA. Recommended methodology for assessing the progression of osteoarthritis of the hip and knee joints. Osteoarthritis Cartilage 1995; 3: 73–77.
26. Lawrence JS. Rheumatism in populations. London: William Heinemann; 1977.
27. Hart DJ, Leedham-Green M, Spector TD. The prevalence of knee osteoarthritis in the general population using different clinical criteria: the Chingford Study. Br J Rheum 1991; 30: 72.
28. Altman R, Alarcon G, Appelrough D et al. The American College of Rheumatology criteria for the classification and reporting of osteoarthritis of the hand. Arthritis Rheum 1990; 33: 1601–10.
29. Altman R, Alarcon G, Appelrough D et al. The American College of Rheumatology criteria for the classification and reporting of osteoarthritis of the hip. Arthritis Rheum 1990; 34: 505–514.
30. Mankin HJ, Brandt KD, Shulman LE. Workshop on etiopathogenesis of osteoarthritis: proceedings and recommendations. J Rheumatol 1986; 13: 1130–1160.
31. Doherty M, Watt I, Dieppe P. Influence of primary generalised osteoarthritis on the development of secondary osteoarthritis. Lancet 1983; 2: 8–11.
32. Cushnagan J, Dieppe P. Study of 500 patients with limb joint osteoarthritis. I. Analysis by age, sex and distribution of symptomatic joint sites. Ann Rheum Dis 1991; 50: 8–13.
33. Kellgren JH, Moore R. Generalized osteoarthritis and Heberden's nodes. Br Med J 1962; 1: 181–187.
34. Egger P, Cooper C, Hart DJ et al. Patterns of joint involvement in osteoarthritis of the hand: the Chingford study. J Rheumatol 1995; 22: 1509–1513.
35. Cooper C, Egger P, Coggon D et al. Generalised osteoarthritis in women: pattern of joint involvement and approaches to definition for epidemiological studies. J Rheumatol 1996; 23: 1938–1942.
36. Ehrlich GE. Inflammatory osteoarthritis. I. The clinical syndrome. J Chronic Dis 1972; 25: 317–328.
37. Utsinger P, Resnick D, Shapiro RF et al. Roentgenologic, immunologic and therapeutic study of erosive (inflammatory) osteoarthritis. Arch Intern Med 1978; 18: 683–697.
38. Cobby M, Cushnaghan J, Creamer P et al. Erosive osteoarthritis: is it a separate disease entity? Clin Radiol 1990; 42: 258–263.
39. Zayer M. Osteoarthritis following Blount's disease. Inst Orthop 1980; 4: 63–66.
40. Lawrence RC, Helmick CG, Arnett FC et al. Estimates of the prevalence of arthritis and selected musculoskeletal disorders in the United States. Arthritis Rheum 1998; 41: 778–799.
41. Van Saase JLCM, Van Romunde LKJ, Cats A et al. Epidemiology of osteoarthritis: Zoertermeer survey. Comparison of radiologic osteoarthritis in a Dutch population with than in 10 other populations. Ann Rheum Dis 1989; 48: 271–280.

42. Lawrence JS, Sebo M. The geography of osteoarthritis. In: Nuki G, ed. The etiopathogenesis of osteoarthritis. Baltimore, MD: University Park Press, 1980: 155–183.

43. Anderson JJ, Felson DT. Factors associated with osteoarthritis of the knee in the First National Health and Nutrition Examination Survey (HANES-1): evidence for an association with overweight, race, and physical demands of work. Am J Epidemiol 1988; 128: 179–189.

44. Hochberg MC, Lawrence RC, Everett DF, Cornoni-Huntley J. Epidemiologic associations of pain in osteoarthritis of the knee: data from the National Health and Nutrition Examination Survey and the National Health and Nutrition Examination – I Epidemiologic follow-up survey. Semin Arthritis Rheum 1989; 18(suppl 2): 4–9.

45. Sowers M, Lachance L, Hochberg M, Jamander D. Radiographically defined osteoarthritis of the hand and knee in young and middle-aged African American and Caucasian women. Osteoarthritis Cart 2000; 8: 69–77.

46. Solomon L, Beighton P, Lawrence JS. Osteoarthritis in a rural South African negro population. Ann Rheum Dis 1976; 35: 274–278.

47. Jordan JM, Linder GF, Renner JB, Fryer JG. The impact of arthritis in rural populations. Arthritis Care Res 1995; 8: 242–250.

48. Mukhopadhaya B, Barooah B. Osteoarthritis of the hip in Indians: an anatomical and clinical study. Indian J Orthop 1967; 1: 55–63.

49. Hoaglund FT. Osteoarthritis of the hip and other joints in the Southern Chinese in Hong Kong. J Bone Joint Surg 1973; 55: 245–257.

50. Nevitt M, Xu L, Zhang Y et al. Very low prevalence of hip osteoarthritis among Chinese elderly in Beijing, China, compared with whites in the United States: The Beijing Osteoarthritis Study. Arthritis Rheum 2002; 46: 1773–1779.

51. Felson D, Nevitt M, Zhang Y et al. High prevalence of lateral knee osteoarthritis in Beijing Chinese compared with Framingham caucasian subjects. Arthritis Rheum 2002; 46: 1217–1222.

52. Wilson MG, Michet CJ, Ilstrup DM, Melton LJ. Idiopathic symptomatic osteoarthritis of the hip and knee: a population based incidence study. Mayo Clin Proc 1990; 65: 1214–1221.

53. Kallman DA, Wigley FM, Scott WW et al. The longitudinal course of hand osteoarthritis in a male population. Arthritis Rheum 1990; 33: 1323–1332.

54. Oliveria SA, Felson DT, Reed JI et al. Incidence of symptomatic hand, hip and knee osteoarthritis among patients in a health maintenance organization. Arthritis Rheum 1995; 38: 1134–1141.

55. Sowers M, Zobel D, Weissfeld L et al. Progression of osteoarthritis of the hand and metacarpal bone loss: a twenty-year following of incident cases. Arthritis Rheum 1991; 34: 36–42.

56. Stecher RM. Heberden's nodes: heredity in hypertrophic arthritis of the finger joints. Am J Med Sci 1941; 210: 801–809.

57. Spector TD, Cicuttini F, Baker J et al. Genetic influences on osteoarthritis in women: a twin study. Br Med J 1996; 312: 940–944.

58. Felson DT, Anderson JJ, Naimark A et al. Obesity and knee osteoarthritis: the Framingham study. Ann Intern Med 1988; 109: 18–24.

59. Davis MS, Ettinger WH, Neuhaus JM, Mallon KP. Knee osteoarthritis and physical functioning: evidence from the NHANES-1. Epidemiologic follow-up survey. J Rheumatol 1991; 18: 591–598.

60. Spector TD, Hart DJ, Doyle DV. Incidence and progression of osteoarthritis in women with unilateral knee disease in the general population: the effect of obesity. Ann Rheum Dis 1994; 53: 565–568.

61. Lethbridge-Cejku M, Creamer P, Wilson PD et al. Risk factors for incident knee osteoarthritis: data from the Baltimore Longitudinal Study on ageing. Arthritis Rheum 1998; 419: S182.

62. Shiozaki H, Koga Y, Omori G et al. Obesity and osteoarthritis of the knee in women: results from the Matsudai Knee Osteoarthritis Survey. Knee 1999; 6: 189–192.

63. Gelber AC, Hochberg MC, Mead LA et al. Body mass index and the risk of subsequent knee and hip osteoarthritis. Am J Med 1999; 107: 542–548.

64. Cooper C, Snow S, McAlindon TE et al. Risk factors for the incidence and progression of radiographic knee osteoarthritis. Arthritis Rheum 2000; 43: 995–1000.

65. Schouten JSAG, van den Ouweland FA, Valkenburg HA. A twelve year follow-up study in the general population on prognostic factors of cartilage loss in osteoarthritis of the knee. Ann Rheum Dis 1992; 51: 932–937.

66. Felsen DT, Zhang Y, Anthony JM et al. Weight loss reduces the risk for symptomatic knee osteoarthritis in women: the Framingham study. Ann Intern Med 1992; 116: 535–539.

67. Hochberg MC, Lethbridge-Cejku M, Scott WW Jr et al. Obesity and osteoarthritis of the hands in women. Osteoarthritis Cart 1993; 1: 129–135.

68. Carman WJ, Sowers M, Hawthorne VM, Weissfield LA. Obesity as a risk for osteoarthritis of the hand and wrist: a prospective study. Am J Epidemiol 1994; 139: 119–29.

69. Hochberg MC, Lethbridge M, Wigley F et al. Factors predicting progression of hand osteoarthritis in males: data from the Baltimore Longitudinal Study of Aging. Arthritis Rheum 1991; 34(Suppl 9): S34.

70. Croft P, Cooper C, Wickham C, Coggon D. Osteoarthritis of the hip and occupational activity. Scand J Work Env Health 1992; 18: 59–63.

71. Lane NE, Hochberg MC, Pressman A et al. Recreational physical activity and the risk of osteoarthritis of the hip in elderly women. J Rheumatol 1999; 26: 849–854.

72. Croft P, Coggon D, Cruddas M, Cooper C. Osteoarthritis of the hip: an occupational disease in farmers. Br Med J 1992; 304: 1269–1272.

73. Sharma L, Song J, Felson DT et al. The role of knee alignment in disease progression and functional decline in knee osteoarthritis. JAMA 2001; 286: 188–195.

74. Spector TD, Campion GD. Generalized osteoarthritis: a hormonally mediated disease. Ann Rheum Dis 1989; 48: 523–527.

75. Spector TD, Brown GC, Silman A. Increased rates of previous hysterectomy and gynaecological operations in women with osteoarthritis. Br Med J 1988; 297: 899–900.

76. Hannan MT, Felson DT, Anderson JJ et al. Estrogen use and radiographic osteoarthritis of the knee in women. Arthritis Rheum 1990; 33: 525–532.

77. Nevitt MC, Felson DT. Sex hormones and the risk of osteoarthritis in women: epidemiological evidence. Ann Rheum Dis 1996; 55: 673–676.

78. Zhang Y, McAlindon TE, Hannan MT et al. Estrogen replacement therapy and worsening of radiographic knee osteoarthritis: the Framingham study. Arthritis Rheum 1998; 41: 1867–1873.

79. Hart DJ, Doyle DV, Spector TD. Incidence and risk factors for radiographic knee osteoarthritis in middleaged women: the Chingford Study. Arthritis Rheum 1999; 42: 17–24.

80. Sayhoun N, Brett KM, Hochberg MC, Pamuk ER. Estrogen replacement therapy and incidence of self-reported physician-diagnosed arthritis. Prev Med 1999; 28: 458–464.

81. Sandmark H, Hogstedt C, Lewold S, Vingard E. Osteoarthritis of the knee in men and women in association with overweight, smoking, and hormone therapy. Ann Rheum Dis 1999; 58: 151–155.

82. Nevitt MC, Cummings SR, Lane NE et al. Association of estrogen replacement therapy with the risk of osteoarthritis of the hip in elderly white women. Arch Intern Med 1996; 156: 2073–2080.

83. Stewart A, Black AJ. Bone mineral density in osteoarthritis. Curr Opin Rheumatol 2000; 12: 464–467.

84. Hochberg MC. Osteoarthritis. In: Silman AS, Hochberg MC, eds . Epidemiology of rheumatic diseases. Oxford: Oxford University Press; 2001.

85. Rangger C, Kathrein A, Klestil T, Glotzer W. Partial meniscectomy and osteoarthritis. Implications for treatment of athletes. Sports Med 1997; 23: 61–68.

86. Gelber AC, Hochberg MC, Mead LA et al. Joint injury in young adults and risk for subsequent knee and hip osteoarthritis. Ann Intern Med 2000; 133: 321–328.

87. Lane NE, Lin P, Christiansen L et al. Association of mild acetabular dysplasia with an increased risk of incident hip osteoarthritis in elderly white women: the study of osteoporotic fractures. Arthritis Rheum 2000; 43: 400–404.

88. Cooper C. Occupational activity and the risk of osteoarthritis. J Rheumatol 1995; 22(suppl 43): 10–12.

89. Cooper C, McAlindon T, Egger P et al. Occupational activity and osteoarthritis of the knee. Ann Rheum Dis 1994; 53: 90–93.

90. Maetzel A, Makela M, Hawker G, Bombardier C. Osteoarthritis of the hip and knee and mechanical occupational exposure; a systematic review of the evidence. J Rheumatol 1997; 24: 1599–1607.

91. Lau EC, Cooper C, Dam D et al. Factors associated with osteoarthritis of the hip and knee in Hong Kong Chinese: obesity, joint injury and occupational activities. Am J Epidemiol 2000; 152: 855–862.

92. McAlindon TE, Wilson PWF, Aliabadi P et al. Level of physical activity and the risk of radiographic and symptomatic knee osteoarthritis in the elderly: the Framingham study. Am J Med 1999; 106: 151–157.

93. McAlindon TE, Snow S, Cooper C, Dieppe P. Radiographic patterns of knee osteoarthritis in the community: the importance of the patellofemoral joint. Ann Rheum Dis 1992; 51: 844–849.

94. Massardo L, Watt I, Cushnaghan J et al. Osteoarthritis of the knee joint: an eight year prospective study. Ann Rheum Dis 1989; 48: 893–897.

95. Dougados M, Gueguen A, Nguyen M et al. Longitudinal radiologic evaluation of osteoarthritis of the knee. J Rheumatol 1992; 19: 378–383.

96. Schouten J. A twelve year follow up study of osteoarthritis of the knee in the general population. PhD thesis, Erasmus University, The Netherlands: 1991.

97. Spector TD, Dacre JE, Harris PA, Huskisson EC. The radiological progression of osteoarthritis: an eleven year follow up study of the knee. Ann Rheum Dis 1992; 51: 1107–1110.

98. Ledingham J, Regan M, Jones A, Doherty M. Factors affecting radiographic progression of knee osteoarthritis. Ann Rheum Dis 1995; 54: 53–58.

99. Pavelka K, Gatterova J, Altman RD. Radiographic progression of knee osteoarthritis in a Czech cohort. Clin Exp Rheumatol 2000; 18: 473–477.

100. Hernborg JS, Nilsson BE. The natural course of untreated osteoarthritis of the knee. Clin Orthop 1977; 123: 130–137.

101. Altman RD, Fries JF, Bloch DA et al. Radiographic assessment of progression in osteoarthritis. Arthritis Rheum 1987; 30: 1214–1225.

102. Dieppe P, Cushnaghan J, Tucker M et al. The Bristol OA500 Study: progression and impact of the disease after 8 years. Osteoarthritis Cartilage 2000; 8: 63–68.

103. Danielsson LG. Incidence and prognosis of coxarthrosis Acta Orthop Scand 1964; 66(suppl): 1–87.

104. Seifert MH, Whiteside CG, Savage O. A five year follow up of 50 cases of idiopathic osteoarthritis of the hip (abstract). Ann Rheum Dis 1969; 28: 325–326.

105. Van Saase JLCM. Osteoarthrosis in the general population: a follow up study of osteoarthrosis of the hip. PhD thesis, Leiden State University, The Netherlands; 1990.

106. Bland JH, Cooper SM. Osteoarthritis: a review of the cell biology involved and evidence for reversibility. Semin Arthritis Rheum 1984; 14: 106–133.

107. Newman NM, Ling RSM. Acetabular bone destruction related to non-steroidal anti-inflammatory drugs. Lancet 1985; 2: 11–14.

108. Rashad S, Revell P, Hemingway A et al. The effect of non-steroidal anti-inflammatory drugs on the course of osteoarthritis. Lancet 1989; 2: 519–522.

109. Ledingham JM, Dawson S, Preston B, Doherty M. Radiographic progression of hospital referred hip osteoarthritis. Ann Rheum Dis 1993; 52: 263–267.

110. Dougados M, Gueguen A, Nguyen M et al. Radiographic features predictive of radiographic progression of hip osteoarthritis. Rev Rheum Engl Ed 1997; 64: 795–803.

111. Harris PA, Hart DJ, Dacre JE et al. The progression of radiological hand osteoarthritis over 10 years: a clinical follow-up study. Osteoarthritis Cartilage 1994; 2: 247–252.

112. Danielsson L, Hernborg J. Clinical and roentgenologic study of knee joints with osteophytes. Clin Orthop 1970; 69: 224–226.

1791

165 Clinical features

Roy D Altman and Carlos J Lozada

- Osteoarthritis is the most common articular disease
- About 50% of those with radiographic osteoarthritis have symptoms
- Pain is the most common reason the patient consults the physician
- Pain in osteoarthritis has many potential sources. There is no direct pain from cartilage, synovial fluid or the inner two-thirds of menisci. Pain fibers are present in the remaining tissues surrounding the joint
- A variety of other symptoms can result from osteoarthritis that impact on function and quality of life
- Signs of osteoarthritis can be absent, subtle or severe
- Although osteoarthritis can involve virtually any joint in the body, the most commonly involved joints are hands and feet, hips and knees

INTRODUCTION

Osteoarthritis (OA) is the most common form of arthritis, accounting for 30% of physician visits[1]. It may be defined as a 'heterogeneous group of conditions that lead to joint symptoms and signs which are associated with defective integrity of articular cartilage, in addition to related changes in the underlying bone and at the joint margins'[2]. It is usually classified as either primary (idiopathic) or secondary (associated with a known condition). Although OA is present by histologic or radiographic criteria in nearly 80% of people by the age of 80 years, only half have symptoms[3], and these are often variable and intermittent. It affects as many as 12% in the US population between the ages of 25 and 74 years[4]. There is a modest correlation between the presence of symptoms and the severity of anatomic changes.

Although variable in its presentation and course, OA often carries significant morbidity. In addition to the effects on the individual, the cost of OA to society is significant[1], related to its high prevalence, the reduced ability of those affected to perform both occupational and non-occupational activities, the occasional loss of a patient's ability to undertake self-care, and the related drain on health-care resources[5].

Osteoarthritis is no longer considered a 'degenerative' or 'wear and tear' arthritis, but rather involves dynamic biomechanical, biochemical and cellular processes[6]. Indeed, the joint damage that occurs in OA is, at least in part, the result of active remodeling involving all the joint structures. Although articular cartilage is at the center of change, OA is currently viewed as a disease of the entire joint and, therefore, the failure of the joint as an organ[7].

Although symptoms are often unilateral, evidence of OA is almost always present bilaterally. However, even when symptoms are bilateral, there is a tendency for one side to be more symptomatic than the other. The symptomatic side may also alternate over time. Unilateral disease may suggest OA secondary to trauma. However, despite the presence of continuing trauma, progression is more common with bilateral disease. In contrast to systemic inflammatory arthritides, OA lacks constitutional symptoms.

TABLE 165.1 SYMPTOMS AND SIGNS OF OSTEOARTHRITIS

Symptoms	Signs
Pain	Altered gait
Stiffness	Tenderness
Swelling	Enlargement
Altered function	Crepitus
Weakness	Limitation of motion
Deformity	Deformity
Grinding or clicking	Instability
Instability	

When OA is symptomatic, the most prominent complaint is pain. It remains unclear why fewer than 50% of persons with severe radiographic OA (Kellgren and Lawrence grade III and IV[8]) report pain[9]. Most often, the onset of OA symptomatology is insidious. Symptoms and signs of OA are listed in Table 165.1.

SYMPTOMS

Pain

Pain is most often the reason a patient with OA seeks the help of a physician[10]. When pain is present, its cause is often not clear, as the stimulus for pain in OA has many potential mechanisms (Table 165.2)[11]. Pain can be difficult to localize to an area within the joint. In knee OA, patients will commonly describe their pain as involving the entire joint. In one study, medial knee pain was reported in 34% of patients with OA of the knee, as compared with 52% reporting 'generalized' knee pain[12]. Joint pain may be referred proximally, but is more commonly referred distally, for example hip pain referred into the thigh and knee pain referred to the anterior or medial upper tibia. Anterior knee pain may represent patellofemoral (anterior compartment) OA. Patients often ascribe increasing pain and stiffness to changes in weather. Investigation in this area has been inconclusive. Some have suggested that changes in any two of temperature, humidity and barometric pressure may lead to changes in OA symptomatology.

The severity of pain should be noted and, ideally, measured at each visit. The two most commonly used pain scales are the five-point Likert scale (0 = none; 1 = mild; 2 = moderate; 3 = severe; 4 = very severe) or a 100mm visual analog scale (from 0mm = no pain to 100mm = the most pain possible). An alternative to the visual analog scale is a 10-point Numerical Rating Scale (from 0 = no pain to 10 = the most pain possible).

Pain can also be quantified through standardized testing. The Western Ontario McMaster Universities (WOMAC) Osteoarthritis Index pain subscale quantifies five measures of pain. It also measures stiffness and function in separate subscales. The algofunctional scale of Lequesne is

TABLE 165.2 RELATIONSHIP BETWEEN ANATOMIC SITE AND POSSIBLE PHYSIOLOGIC MECHANISM FOR PAIN IN OA

Anatomic site	Mechanism
Cartilage (defective or loss)	*Synovial:* inflammation induced by cartilage 'char' fragments, cartilage crystal shedding, cartilage release of cytokines (e.g. interleukin-1), enzymes (e.g. metalloproteinases). *Subchondral bone:* mechanical stress (see below) *Instability:* stress on capsule
Menisci	Tear or degeneration: stretch at insertion to the joint capsule, catch between surfaces
Synovial cavity	Stretch of joint capsule, transport of inflammatory mediators between synovium and cartilage
Synovium	Inflammation
Subchondral bone	Ischemia with increased pressure, decreased oxygen tension and increased pH. Avascular necrosis. Regeneration or repair of infarcted bone
Osteophytes	Periosteal elevation. Neural impingement
Joint capsule	Stretch from joint distention. Stress at insertion to periosteum and bone
Ligaments	Stress at insertion to periosteum and bone
Bursae	Inflammation, with or without calcification
Muscle	Spasm. Nocturnal myoclonus
Central nervous system	Dysthymia, cyclothymia, fibromyalgia. Ethnic, cultural, coping skills

that usually occurs across smooth cartilage surfaces. Movement across uneven surfaces results in a grinding or clicking sensation to the patient and crepitus on examination. These sensations can be accompanied by pain.

When damaged cartilage 'char' fragments are released into the synovial cavity, an attempt is made at clearing them, precipitating an inflammatory synovial response. Other microscopic and submicroscopic particulate material released from damaged articular cartilage – such as collagen, proteoglycans, crystals, proteolytic enzymes and cytokines – trigger a synovial inflammatory response to varying degrees. Although inflammation of the synovium in joints affected by OA is most often less severe than in the traditional 'inflammatory' arthritides (e.g. rheumatoid arthritis and gout), activation of inflammatory responses always occurs in OA joints, at both the synoviocyte and chondrocyte level (justifying the terminology 'osteo*arthritis*')[15,16].

Abnormal cartilage may contain a variety of calcium crystals, including calcium pyrophosphate dihydrate, hydroxyapatite and basic calcium phosphate. Surface disruption may allow 'crystal shedding' into the joint cavity, stimulating varying degrees of inflammation[17]. In cases in which cartilage is fissured and the subchondral bone is exposed, hydroxyapatite crystals from bone or cartilage may leach or be sheared into the synovial cavity. These crystals stimulate intracellular mechanisms of inflammation. In addition, the absence of articular cartilage allows loosening and instability of the joint, with resultant changes in the periarticular structures.

Other loose bodies in the joint, such as 'joint mice' or osteochondromatosis are potential indirect causes of pain. The disrupted portion of torn *menisci* can be displaced and inserted between normally smooth, gliding articular surfaces, stretching the joint capsule. Pain can sometimes be elicited on examination when the torn meniscus is stressed at its outer one-third or when partially torn menisci 'catch' between cartilage surfaces. Horizontal fissures do not usually cause symptoms, but fragments of the defective menisci may elicit an inflammatory response or act as loose bodies in the joint cavity.

also a reliable and validated instrument that combines pain and function (see Chapter 170 for further discussion of these and other disease-specific instruments for clinical assessment in OA).

The quality of the pain may hint as to its pathological origin. Pain that occurs after exercise is often caused by subchondral ischemia – so called 'bone angina'. This pain is often aching and deep seated. Pain along the joint margin, with tenderness at the site may indicate periosteal pain from stretching of the capsule or ligaments or overgrowing osteophytes. The sudden onset of pain with a catching sensation of the knee may be associated with a torn meniscus.

A thorough history and physical examination may help direct symptomatic treatment by revealing the source of the pain, which may be categorized by anatomic site (Table 165.2). This then allows the physician to target his therapeutic intervention. The contribution of the different tissues to pain are discussed below.

Articular cartilage

Damage to *articular cartilage* is the hallmark of osteoarthritis, yet articular cartilage is not a direct source of pain, because it lacks nerve endings[13,14]. *Menisci*, similarly, do not contain nerves in their weight-bearing surfaces (i.e. the inner two-thirds), and cannot directly account for pain. Teleologically, it makes evolutionary sense that compressive or shear forces on cartilage would not elicit pain, as pain would make ambulation problematic. Nevertheless, abnormalities in *articular cartilage*, *menisci*, and even *synovial fluid* can indirectly cause pain in OA.

Damaged *articular cartilage* causes symptoms that derive from loss of its structural integrity, cartilage debris and absence of cartilage. Structurally damaged cartilage loses the ability to allow the even gliding

Synovium

Synovial fluid can indirectly cause pain by serving as a transport medium, distending the joint capsule or limiting joint function. The synovial fluid shuttles inflammatory mediators between cartilage and synovium. Synovial fluid also serves as a reservoir for inflammatory cytokines, cells and crystals. Furthermore, synovial fluid distends the joint, potentially compressing synovial blood vessels and stimulating pressure receptors in the capsule[18-20]. A distended joint compromises the normal transport of nutrition and gases by synovial fluid between cartilage and synovium. The residual waste products linger in the synovial space and perpetuate inflammation.

The *synovium* contains nerve fibers. These include Aβ (large myelinated mechanoreceptors), Aδ (small myelinated nociceptors) and C (small non-myelinated nociceptors). The latter nociceptors can release both substance P and calcitonin gene-related peptide. Substance P stimulates both the pain response and inflammation[21]. These pain receptors may also be activated through peripheral mechanical, thermal and noxious stimuli. These noxious stimuli include bradykinin, histamine, prostaglandins and leukotrienes[22].

Bone

The *subchondral bone* is directly related to pain in OA[23]. When subchondral ischemia or increased venous pressure occur, peptides such as substance P and calcitonin gene-related peptide are released from the nerve endings in bone[24]. The pain of ischemic bone is aching and deep-seated. When bone death occurs (osteonecrosis), there is a pain-free period. Pain recurs with bone repair and remodeling. In OA, subchondral cysts and sclerosis are the eventual radiographic evidence that localized osteonecrosis has taken place. Providing relief from the pain of ischemic bone has not been specifically studied. It is uncertain whether there is a neurogenic pain component to the bone pain of OA.

Osteophytes are the most consistent pathologic and radiographic finding associated with the presence of pain[25]. The mechanisms are not clear, but osteophytes may cause pain directly by distending the periosteum; pain can sometimes be elicited by applying pressure over an osteophyte of knee or hand. Pain from osteophytes may be due to concomitant inflammation. Osteophytes in the spinal facets are often an indirect cause of pain and other symptoms by compressing nerves as they traverse the spinal foramina (e.g. cervical, lumbar lateral recess) or within the spinal canal (e.g. lumbar spinal stenosis).

Capsule and related tissues

The *joint capsule* and periarticular *ligaments* are stretched by synovial effusions or instability, and may cause pain through mechanoreceptors and nociceptors. Stress at the ligamentous insertion on the *periosteum* stimulates nociceptors. When the joint periarticular tissues are distorted, the ligaments may be abnormally stressed or may be understressed (e.g. varus deformity of the knee stresses the lateral ligaments and fully relaxes the medial ligaments). These phenomena, labeled 'stress enhancement' and 'stress deprivation'[26], result in contractures of the capsule and ligaments. Contractures result in decreasing function and increasing pain from stress at ligamentous insertions, and periarticular muscle spasm.

Periarticular *bursae* may become inflamed and, hence, be a source of pain. Bursal inflammation is sometimes associated with calcium formation (e.g. calcific bursitis).

Muscle

Muscle spasm is probably a common source of pain in OA. Muscle spasm may occur in the form of nocturnal myoclonus, altering sleep patterns and resulting in fibromyalgia-like symptoms[27]. In a study of 429 patients older than 65 years with OA of the knee, there were problems with sleep onset (31%), sleep maintenance (81%) and early morning awakening (51%)[28]. This was influenced by additional psychosocial and medical comorbidities. Muscle spasm of the lower extremities must be differentiated from pain of vascular (e.g. night cramps) or spinal radicular origin. Joint contractures in OA can cause pain upon stretching of the periarticular muscles.

Psychological factors and pain

Joint pain is modulated by the individuals' perception of pain and unique ethnic, cultural and personal circumstances. It tends to be more severe in evenings, at weekends and early in the work week[29]. Pain is complicated by the presence of dysthymia, other forms of depression, cyclothymia and secondary gains. Psychologic evaluation may be needed to determine the overlying psychologic and coping influences on the pain response. In knee OA, a passive coping style that led to resting was found to predict a higher level of disability within 36 weeks[30]. Self-efficacy beliefs appear to relate to functional decline when associated with lower extremity muscular weakness[31].

Stiffness

Stiffness may be defined as a sensation of a 'gelling' or tightening of the involved joint that usually occurs after inactivity, such as in the morning or when arising after sitting for a prolonged period. In contrast to inflammatory arthritides (e.g. rheumatoid arthritis), stiffness in OA usually lasts only a few minutes, almost always less than 30 minutes. However, the duration of stiffness has been found to be of less use than the character of the stiffness, in distinguishing OA from rheumatoid arthritis (Silman A, personal communication). In contrast to the diffuse stiffness of rheumatoid arthritis, that of OA is usually confined to the involved joints.

Other symptoms

The patient may have a sensation of fullness and swelling about the joint. There may be associated warmth and loss of function.

Weight-bearing joints that are inflamed or contracted, or both, are associated with gait disturbance, increased muscle spasm and reduced quality of life. A contracted knee or hip can produce a prominent limp (see below). Aids to ambulation may reduce the severity of altered function.

Impaired function of a weight-bearing joint places stress on the contralateral weight-bearing joints. It is not uncommon for the patient with impaired right knee function (perhaps with pain) to have difficulty with the left hip.

Hypertrophic bone formation in interphalangeal joint OA may contribute to reduced dexterity and difficulty performing fine movements, such as knitting, sewing or playing a musical instrument. OA of the 1st carpometacarpal (CMC) joint may make it difficult to hold a pen.

Inactivity secondary to pain may lead to significant weakness, and can be compounded by periarticular muscle atrophy.

Patients may complain of enlargement of the joints of the hands or knee. They may also complain of increasing deformity of the knees, such as 'knock knees' (valgus) or 'bowing' (varus).

Patients may complain of a click or grinding sensation with joint motion. The grinding may be associated with pain.

Finally, the sensation of instability may cause the patient to seek assistance in ambulation, such as a cane or crutch. In the knee, instability is often associated with a feeling that the knee is 'giving out.'

SIGNS

Gait

Osteoarthritis of weight-bearing joints leads to altered gait patterns, mostly by a conscious or subconscious attempt to protect the joint. Hip, knee, ankle and foot arthritis provide distinctive gait patterns. One should note the patient's gait pattern and make appropriate use of aids to ambulation.

Tenderness

There may be tenderness of soft tissues (e.g. synovium, capsule, bursae, periarticular muscles) or periosteum at the insertion of capsule or ligaments.

Joint swelling

There may be enlargement of the joint from synovitis, synovial effusion, bony enlargement, joint mice or osteochondromatosis. Effusions are usually cool or slightly warm to palpation. The distal interphalangeal joint (DIP) swelling may present as a cystic herniation (Fig. 165.1); aspiration often reveals a jelly-like material reminiscent of a ganglion cyst. Swelling of the joint from an effusion frequently leads to loss of extension. This is in contrast to a periarticular bursitis or tendinitis, in which the joint is splinted, often in full extension.

Crepitus

Crepitus over a joint with OA may be of soft tissue or bony origin. It may be localized (e.g. chondromalacia patella and anterior compartment crepitus of the knee). Grinding, crunching or cracking may be present over a joint with OA. This represents uneven surfaces moving across each other. Although present with passive joint motion, it is most often best demonstrated with active motion of the joint. This should be contrasted with the benign 'cracking' of the metacarpophalangeal (MCP) joints that occurs when smooth cartilage surfaces are separated, creating a vacuum sound.

Needle arthroscopy has been used to define the origin of crepitus of the knee[32]. Transmitted bony crepitus was a specific finding for bone-

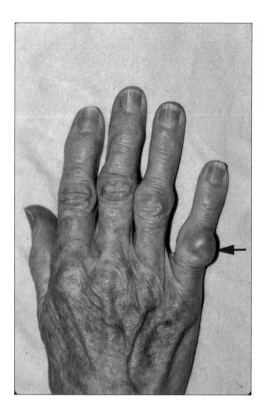

Fig. 165.1 Interphalangeal osteoarthritis of the hand, with cystic herniation of the 5th proximal interphalangeal joint.

on-bone in the compartment being assessed. Added tibiofemoral stress was 65% sensitive and 94% specific for cartilage disruption in the compartment assessed.

Limitation of motion

There may be loss of function with reduced motion as a result of synovitis/effusion or periarticular soft tissue contractures. When there is limitation of motion of a weight-bearing joint, it places additional stress on ipsilateral and contralateral weight-bearing joints.

As above, performance measures can be assessed on examination[32]. The WOMAC physical function subscale score correlates with several performance measures such as walking, stair climb, rising from a chair and range of motion in OA of the knee and hip[33].

Deformity

Deformity may be present in any of the peripheral joints with OA. However, it is most notable in the interphalangeal joints with enlarge-

ment and subluxation, the 1st CMC joint, the knees (varus/valgus) or the hips (shortened extremity). Bony enlargement is a form of deformity. Deformity may be associated with joint fusion or instability.

Instability

Taking joints through their arc of movement may reveal instability in various planes of motion. For example, instability of the knee may be demonstrated in anterior-posterior planes (cruciate ligament laxity or deficiency) or in mediolateral planes (collateral ligament laxity, loss of medial compartment bony stock).

CLINICAL PRESENTATIONS

Osteoarthritis may involve virtually any joint in the body. As it usually has an insidious onset of symptoms, an acute presentation suggests a concomitant inflammatory component (e.g. crystalline synovitis). OA is most often monarticular in presentation, slowly evolving to the contralateral side.

There are patterns to joint involvement. In general, OA of the knees and of the hips occur in different patient populations. OA of the hands and feet are generally present in the same individual, to varying degrees. There appears to be a subset of patients that have osteoarthritis of both central and peripheral joints, which is known as 'generalized' OA[34]. The characteristics of OA at individual sites are discussed below.

Shoulder

Shoulder pain is sometimes related to glenohumeral OA. Pain is typically aching in nature, and associated with the extremes of motion or after activity of the shoulder. There is not usually much loss of function, but crepitus can be found on examination. OA of the shoulder usually coexists with, and is difficult to differentiate from, other abnormalities of the shoulder, e.g. rotator cuff abnormalities, adhesive capsulitis, bursitis.

A peculiar destructive arthropathy (Milwaukee shoulder) is associated with persistent shoulder pain, large synovial effusions and demonstration of a variety of calcium crystals (Fig. 165.2) (see Chapter 180).

Acromioclavicular joint OA can produce pain that can be aggravated by weight bearing or other stressful activities. Painless enlargement of the acromioclavicular joint is common and may be associated with reduced shoulder motion.

Hands

Patients often present for unsightly enlargement of digits or pain at the base of the thumb. Examination demonstrates bony enlargement and

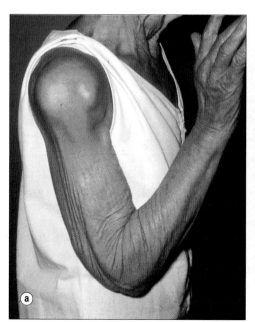

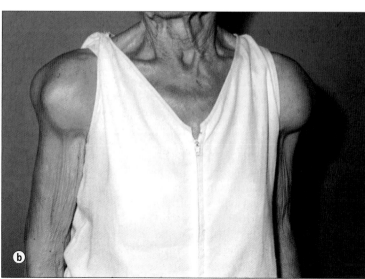

Fig. 165.2 Destructive arthropathy (Milwaukee) of the shoulder. A large synovial effusion is apparent (a) over the lateral aspect of the humerus or (b) anteriorly in front of the glenohumeral joint.

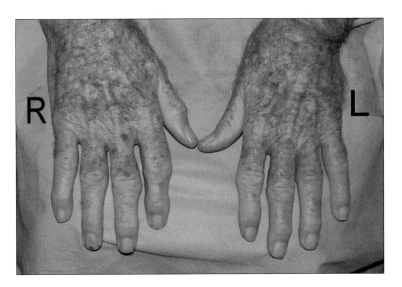

Fig. 165.3 Interphalangeal osteoarthritis of the hands. Knobby, hard tissue changes of the DIP joints. Hard and soft tissue changes of the proximal interphalangeal joints, with deformity. The MCP joints and wrists are spared. There is knobby deformity at the base of the left thumb, reflecting radial subluxation of the 1st proximal metacarpal at the 1st CMC joint.

deformities of the interphalangeal joints. There may be tenderness, and occasionally other signs of inflammation. There is often a partial loss of range of motion.

Distal interphalangeal joints are typically involved, with slow bony enlargement over a period of years (Heberden's nodes) (Fig. 165.3). These nodes are more common in women, and are often present in more than one family member. They often appear around the time of the menopause, but a clear relation to reduced estrogen concentrations

has not been established. The enlargement is not confined to any one aspect of the joint, although there is a predilection for the radio- and ulnodorsal aspects of the joints. Involvement of the 2nd and 3rd DIPs is particularly common. Enlargements are often more severe in the dominant hand. There is often associated deformity, with radial, ulnar or palmar deviations; these are unsightly rather than painful. A predominant palmar subluxation may have the appearance of a 'mallet' finger. There may be some loss of dexterity. OA of the DIPs may result in vertical ridges on the adjacent fingernails. There may be an acute swelling of the DIP, with cystic herniation of the capsule (Fig. 165.1). Aspiration of these cysts yields a jelly-like material. Microscopic examination reveals large polymorphonuclear leukocytes, with several refractile inclusion cysts that stain for fat (reminiscent of the fluid extracted from a wrist ganglion).

There are often associated hard or soft tissue changes in the proximal interphalangeal (PIP) joints (Bouchard's nodes) and erosive changes radiographically. Deformities of the PIPs are particularly common (Fig. 165.3). The 2nd and 3rd PIPs are most commonly involved. Involvement of the MCP joints is uncommon.

The 1st CMC (trapezioscaphoid) joints are commonly involved, particularly in women with hypermobility[35]. There is a tendency for osteophytes to develop on the distal ulnar surface of the trapezoid, associated with subluxation and radial deviation of the proximal head of the 1st metacarpal. This gives the base of the thumb a 'knobby' clinical appearance (Fig. 165.3). In contrast to PIP and DIP involvement, this deviation is commonly associated not only with pain, but also with disability.

Although the course is usually insidious and not very inflammatory, in a subset of these patients the disease may have an aggressive and destructive course. This has suggested classification into a nodal (noninflammatory) and non-nodal (inflammatory) or erosive interphalangeal OA. On occasion, the evolution of interphalangeal OA may be

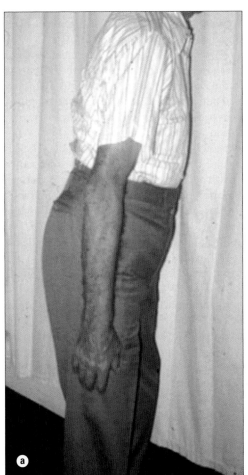

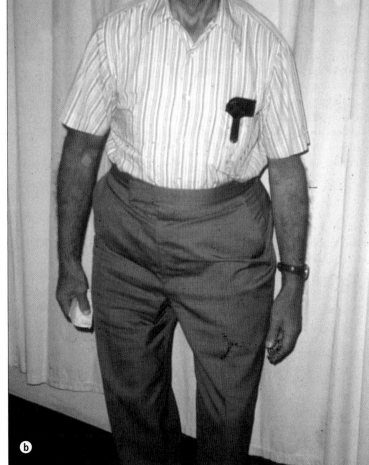

Fig. 165.4 Osteoarthritis of the hips. Severe osteoarthritis secondary to pelvic Paget's disease causes medial migration of the femoral heads into the acetabuli, resulting in hip flexion contractures. The patient stands with a bent forward posture apparent from a lateral (a) or anterior (b) view.

indistinguishable from early-onset rheumatoid arthritis or a spondyloarthropathy, particularly psoriatic arthritis.

Hips

Patients most often present with groin or anterior hip pain that radiates into the thigh. Pain is associated with weight bearing and is relieved by rest. Examination most often reveals difficulty rising from a seated position, altered gait favoring the arthritic hip and reduced range of motion on examination, with pain on motion.

Hip OA is most commonly associated with an insidious onset of pain (*malum coxae senilis*, coxarthropathy). Pain is noted on weight-bearing activity and must be distinguished from referred lumbar pain. In contrast to hip pain, low back pain is most often aggravated by prolonged sitting and improves with ambulation. Both lumbar and hip OA may be painful when the patient rises from a seated or reclined position and during early ambulation. Pain from lumbar stenosis often has its onset after ambulating for a distance, and is more suggestive of claudication (pseudoclaudication). More symptomatic hip OA may be painful at all times, even at rest. Pain is usually localized to the groin or medial thigh, but may be lateral, suggesting (and associated with) trochanteric bursitis. Hip pain may also be referred posteriorly or toward the knee.

Hip OA is associated with a particular gait – one in which the patient overshifts their weight while walking, to reduce the pain (antalgic gait). There is loss of extension that often goes unnoticed. Loss of hip flexion/rotation is noticed by the patient, because of difficulty while attempting to put on socks or shoes. When severe, flexion contracture is associated with a prominent limp (Fig. 165.4). Significant OA of the hip is associated with a loss of internal rotation (less than 15°) on examination[36]. The severely involved hip is flexed, externally rotated and adducted. The Trendelenburg sign may be present – standing on the involved extremity leads to a drop in the contralateral hip from weakening of the ipsilateral hip abductors. Another late sign is shortening of the extremity as the femoral head migrates into the acetabulum, in association with a flexion contracture of the hip.

Most hip OA is slowly progressive. However, there is a subset of patients with a rapidly progressive form of hip OA, evolving over a few months. Unfortunately, at this time, there is no particular clinical characteristic or set of characteristics that can separate those with rapidly progressive OA from the less aggressive forms.

Hip pain must be distinguished from referred lumbar spine pain, trochanteric bursitis, avascular necrosis, and hip fractures that can be difficult to detect on routine radiography. Additional differential considerations include transient osteoporosis of the hip, non-displaced fracture (e.g. femoral neck or intertrochanteric) and osteonecrosis.

Knee

Patients often present with an insidious onset of pain about the knee, particularly with weight bearing and climbing stairs. They may have noticed enlargement, swelling, varus/valgus deformity. Examination sometimes reveals swelling with loss of the usual crease in the skin over the inner (null) facet between the patella and the condyle, in addition to a bulging suprapatellar sac. When present, the effusions are usually cool to palpation. There may be tenderness, but redness is uncommon. Reduced function may be seen with a flexion contracture (unable to extend to 0°) and sometimes an extension contracture (unable to flex to 115°). There is often tenderness of the anserine bursa and crepitus on active motion of the knee.

Knee OA is also associated with pain on weight bearing (gonarthritis). There is often pain when rising from a seated position. It may be aggravated with climbing stairs or bending. The most common form of symptomatic OA of the knee is from medial tibiofemoral compartment involvement. Pain is often along the medial joint margin and associated

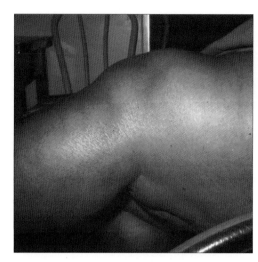

Fig. 165.5
Osteoarthritis of the knee. This morbidly obese woman has an enlarged knee with a flexion contracture. Lack of mobility is reflected by her use of a wheelchair. Synovial effusion of the knee is difficult to detect by inspection or palpation in a knee distal to a thigh of this size.

with tenderness, and may radiate along the upper medial leg. Pain may also be felt distally along the anterior proximal tibia. A knee limp may be present. The knee may be unsteady on weight bearing, causing the patient to complain of a feeling that the knee is buckling or 'giving out.' A flexion contracture may be demonstrated (Fig. 165.5).

There is often crepitus on motion that is best detected on active joint motion. A usually cool, palpable effusion may be present. Occasional distention of the popliteal semitendinosus bursa (Baker's cyst) may be present. There may also be herniation or rupture of the bursa into the thigh or leg (herniated or ruptured popliteal cyst), reminiscent of thrombophlebitis (pseudothrombophlebitis syndrome). Marginal osteophytes, intrasynovial loose bodies (joint mice) or moveable bodies (osteochondromas) may be palpable. There may be a loss of full extension, aggravating the limp. Medial joint space narrowing may lead to a varus deformity, whereas lateral joint space narrowing may lead to a valgus deformity. Varus deformity with valgus deformity of the contralateral knee gives the patient a 'wind-swept' appearance. There is often associated quadriceps weakness and atrophy.

Knee OA may be associated with pain at the distal medial joint margin (anserine bursitis at the insertion on the pes anserinus of the tibia). This is particularly common in the elderly with significant varus deformity. Both varus alignment and standing balance correlate with the severity of knee OA[37]. Thus knee OA has been associated with quadriceps weakness, reduced knee proprioception and increased postural sway[38]. When present, reduced proprioception was present in the contralateral knee[39]. It was felt that both pain and muscle weakness influenced postural sway. Although quadriceps strength was significantly lower in patients with OA of the medial compartment of the knee, the hip adductor muscles were actually stronger, perhaps compensating for the varus deformity[40].

Meniscal tears may be difficult to determine on physical examination of patients with knee OA. A positive McMurray test is the only true predictor of an unstable meniscal tear[41]. A history of swelling and synovial effusion are not helpful.

Patellofemoral OA is not commonly symptomatic, except in young women (chondromalacia patella). Anterior compartment pain is aggravated by sitting in low chairs (e.g. movie theaters) and can be precipitated by pressure and mediolateral movement of the patella in the intercondylar groove. Symptoms from patellofemoral OA are usually self-limiting, resolving in a period of several months.

Osteoarthritis of the knee may be associated with varying degrees of subchondral osteonecrosis. This is suspected in patients with a rather abrupt onset of particularly severe pain refractory to the usual therapy. In early phases, it is best detected by magnetic resonance imaging. Uncommonly, there is a destructive arthropathy associated with a variety of calcium crystals.

Ankle

Talonavicular and subtalar joint osteoarthritis is often secondary, for example to trauma with or without ligamentous damage. Patients complain of ankle pain on weight bearing. Examination reveals synovitis of the ankle that must be distinguished from a variety of conditions, such as Achilles bursitis, plantar fasciitis, talocalcaneal coalition, post-traumatic osteoarthritis (e.g. after calcaneal fracture), painful os trigonum, talonavicular osteoarthritis, posterior tibial tendinitis and pedal edema.

Feet

Patients most often present with pain and enlargement of the 1st metatarsophalangeal (MTP) joint, particularly with walking. Examination commonly reveals an enlarged joint, with medial subluxation and lateral deviation of the big toe. There are sometimes signs of inflammation over the involved joint, with tenderness and loss of dorsiflexion. There are commonly abnormalities of additional toes.

The same processes that occur in the hands can occur concomitantly in the feet. Different members of the same family may have predominant hands or feet involvement.

The typical pattern of involvement of the feet includes the 1st MTP joint, commonly called the 'bunion' joint (hallux valgus) (Fig. 165.6). The joint enlarges medially, with a lateral drift of the 1st toe.

There may be loss of function of the 1st MTP (hallux rigidus), usually occurring without drifting of the great toe, but limiting 'toe off' with ambulation. In this condition, the enlargement is usually dorsal.

There is often painful and tender swelling of foot joints. Associated contractures of additional (cock-up) toes with loss of plantar fat pads are often seen. Disabling painful ambulation may ensue. Pes planus, with relaxation of the transtarsal ligament and a pronator forefoot deformity, aggravates the symptoms. The patient may find it difficult to wear certain types of shoes, particularly those with high heels.

Temporomandibular

Temporomandibular OA is often associated with hyperextensibility, perhaps with recurrent subluxations. However, most temporomandibular OA is associated with meniscal tears or malalignment between mandible and maxilla.

EVALUATION

Laboratory tests

There are no laboratory tests that are diagnostic of OA. Low-grade inflammation in OA can be detected by measurement of serum acute-phase reactants. Increases in erythrocyte sedimentation rate are more often attributable to age rather that to OA. Subtle, but definite increases in C-reactive protein are present in patients with active OA, and appear to predict disease progression[42].

Synovial fluid and serum markers of OA are being investigated as tools to detect the presence of OA or to predict disease progression. To date, no individual marker has accomplished either of these goals, and a combination of markers may be needed.

Synovial fluid from patients with OA is usually clear and colorless, and the polymorphonuclear leukocyte content is less than 2000/ml. More inflammatory synovitis in OA may demonstrate inflammatory synovial effusions, particularly in the presence of calcium crystals. Synovial fluid from a DIP cyst is often jelly-like and contains large polymorphonuclear leukocytes with several refractile inclusion cysts. Synovial fluid from a joint with osteochondromatosis is often very viscous and relatively acellular.

Crystals may be present in as many as 70% of synovial fluid specimens from patients with OA[43]. Although all calcium crystals have been shown to precipitate inflammation, the relationship between hydroxyapatite and several forms of basic calcium phosphate to the synovitis that is present in patients is not well established.

Imaging

A detailed description of the imaging characteristics of OA is given in Chapter 168.

SUMMARY

Symptomatic OA of the extremities is common, and affects a large segment of the population, particularly those older than 50 years. Although OA can affect nearly any joint in the body, OA of the weight-bearing joints leads to the most disabling symptoms. Hip and knee OA can cause significant morbidity, disability and impairment. Pain is the most common complaint that brings the patient to seek a physician's assistance. Examination often reveals loss of function and may reveal signs of inflammation. The findings on careful history and physical examination should lead to the formulation of an individualized program of therapy.

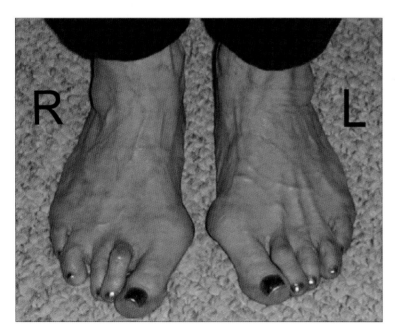

Fig. 165.6 MTP and interphalangeal osteoarthritis of the feet. There is bilateral enlargement of the 1st MTP joint, with medial subluxation of the phalanx. Flexion contraction of toes (particularly of the right 2nd digit) with subluxation of the MTP, has an associated callus over the dorsum of the PIP joint. The right 3rd digit is subluxed under the 2nd digit. There is relaxation of the transtarsal ligament, with medial subluxation of the MTP and bony enlargement of the 5th MTP joints (Tailor bunion, bunionette).

REFERENCES

1. Kramer JS, Yelin EH, Epstein WV. Social and economic impacts of four musculoskeletal conditions: a study using national community-based data. J Rheumatol 1983; 26: 901–907.

2. Altman RD, Asch E, Bloch D et al. Development of criteria for the classification and reporting of osteoarthritis: classification of osteoarthritis of the knee. Arthritis Rheum 1986; 29: 1039–1049.

3. Hochberg MC, Lawrence RC, Everett DF, Cornoni-Huntley J. Epidemiologic associations of pain in osteoarthritis of the knee: data from the National Health and Nutrition Examination Survey and the National Health and Nutrituion Examination. I: epidemiologic follow-up survey. Semin Arthritis Rheum 1989; 18(suppl 2): 4–9.

4. Lawrence RC, Hochberg MC, Kelsey JL et al. Estimates of the prevalence of selected arthritic and musculoskeletal diseases in the United States. J Rheumatol 1989; 16: 427–441.

5. Levy E, Ferme A, Perocheau D, Bono I. Socioeconomic costs of osteoarthritis in France. Rev Rhum 1993; 60: 63S–67S.

6. Kuettner KE, Goldberg VM. Introduction. In: Kuettner KE, Goldberg VM, eds. Osteoartritic disorders. Rosemont, IL: American Academy of Orthopaedic Surgeons; 1995: xxi–xxv.

7. Lozada CJ, Altman RD. Chondroprotection in osteoarthritis. Bull Rheum Dis 1997; 46: 5–7.

8. Kellgren JH, Lawrence RC. Radiological assessment of osteoarthrosis. Ann Rheum Dis 1957; 16: 494–501.

9. Lethbridge-Cejku M, Scott WW, Reichle R et al. Association of radiographic features of osteoarthritis of the knee with knee pain: data from the Baltimore Longitudinal Study of Aging. Arthritis Care Res 1995; 8: 182–188.

10. Brandt KD. Pain, synovitis, and articular cartilage changes in osteoarthritis. Semin Arthritis Rheum 1989; 18(suppl 2): 77–80.

11. Altman R, Dean D. Introduction and overview: pain in osteoarthritis. Semin Arthritis Rheum 1989; 18(suppl 2): 1–3.

12. Creamer P, Lethbridge-Cejku M, Hochberg MC. Where does it hurt? Pain localization in osteoarthritis of the knee. Osteoarthritis Cartilage 1998; 6: 318–323.

13. Harkness IAL, Higgs ER, Dieppe PA. Osteoarthritis. In Wall PD, Melzadk R, eds. Textbook of pain. London: Churchill Livingstone; 1984: 215–224.

14. Wyke B. The neurology of joints: a review of general principles. Clin Rheum Dis 1981; 7: 223–239.

15. Lindblad S, Hedfors E. Arthroscopic and immunohistologic characterization of knee joint synovitis in osteoarthritis. Arthritis Rheum 1987; 30: 1081–1088.

16. Lindblad S, Hedfors E. Arthroscopic and synovial correlates of pain in osteoarthritis. Semin Arthritis Rheum 1989; 18(suppl 2): 91–93.

17. Schumacher HR. The role of inflammation and crystals in the pain of osteoarthritis. Semin Arthritis Rheum 1989; 18(suppl 2): 81–85.

18. Schaible H-G, Schmidt RF. Effects of an experimental arthritis on the sensory properties of fine articular afferent units. J Neurophysiol 1985; 54: 1109–1122.

19. Grigg P, Schaible H-G, Schmidt RF. Mechanical sensitivity of group III and IV afferents from posterior articular nerve in normal and inflamed cat knee. J Neurophysiol 1986; 55: 635–643.

20. Schaible H-G, Neugebauer V, Schmidt RF. Osteoarthritis and pain. Semin Arthritis Rheum 1989; 18: 30–34.

21. Kolasinski SL, Haines KA, Siegel EL et al. Neuropeptides and inflammation. A somatostatin analog as a selective antagonist of neutrophil activation by substance P. Arthritis Rheum 1992; 35: 369–375.

22. Kantor TG. Concepts in pain control. Semin Arthritis Rheum 1989; 18(suppl 2): 94–99.

23. Badalamente MA, Cherney SB. Periosteal and vascular innervation of the human patella in degenerative joint disease. Semin Arthritis Rheum 1989; 18(suppl 2): 61–66.

24. Kiaer T, Gronlund J, Sorensen KH. Intraosseous pressure and partial pressures of oxygen and carbon dioxide in osteoarthritis. Semin Arthritis Rheum 1989; 18(suppl 2): 57–60.

25. Altman RD, Asch E, Bloch D et al. Development of criteria for the classification and reporting of osteoarthritis: classification of osteoarthritis of the knee. Arthritis Rheum 1986; 29: 1039–1049.

26. Akeson WH, Garfin S, Amiel D et al. Para-articular connective tissue in osteoarthritis. Semin Arthritis Rheum 1989; 18(suppl 2): 41–50.

27. Moldofsky H. Sleep influences on regional and diffuse pain syndromes associated with osteoarthritis. Semin Arthritis Rheum 1989; 18(suppl 2): 18–21.

28. Wilcox S, Brenes GA, Levine D et al. Factors related to sleep disturbance in older adults experiencing knee pain or knee pain with radiographic evidence of knee osteoarthritis. J Am Geriatr Soc 2000; 10: 1241–1251.

29. Bellamy N, Sothern RB, Campbell J et al. Circadian and circaseptan variation in pain perception in osteoarthritis of the knee. J Rheumatol 1990; 17: 364–372.

30. Steultjens MP, Dekker J, Bijlsma JW. Coping, pain, and disability in osteoarthritis: a longitudinal study. J Rheumatol 2001; 28: 1068–1072.

31. Rejeski WJ, Miller ME, Foy C et al. Self-efficacy and the progression of functional limitations and self-reported disability in older adults with knee pain. J Gerontol B Psychol Sci Soc Sci 2001; 56: S261–265.

32. Ike R, O'Rourke KS. Compartment-directed physical examination of the knee can predict articular abnormalities disclosed by needle arthroscopy. Arthritis Rheum 1995; 38: 917–925.

33. Lin YC, Davey RC, Cochrane T. Tests for physical function of the elderly with knee and hip osteoarthritis. Scand J Med Sci Sports 2001; 11: 280–286.

34. Kellgren JH, Moore R. Generalized osteoarthritis and Heberden's nodes. BMJ 1952; 1: 181–187.

35. Jonsson H, Valtysdottir ST. Hypermobility features in patients with hand osteoarthritis. Osteoarthritis Cartilage 1995; 3: 1–5.

36. Altman RD, Chairman, for the ACR Subcommittee on Classification Criteria of Osteoarthritis. The American College of Rheumatology criteria for the classification and reporting of osteoarthritis of the hip. Arthritis Rheum 1991; 34: 505–514.

37. Birmingham TB, Kramer JF, Kirkley A et al. Arch Phys Med Rehabil 2001; 82: 1115–1118.

38. Hassan BS, Mockett S, Doherty M. Static postural sway, proprioception, and maximal voluntary quadriceps contraction in patients with knee osteoarthritis and normal control subjects. Ann Rheum Dis 2001; 60: 612–618.

39. Koralewixz LM, Engh GA. Comparison of proprioception in arthritic and age-matched normal knees. J Bone Joint Surg Am 2000; 82A: 1582–1588.

40. Yamada H, Koshino T, Sakai N, Saito T. Hip adductor muscle strength in patients with varus deformed knee. Clin Orthop 2001; 386: 179–185.

41. Dervin GF, Stiell IG, Wells GA et al. Physician's accuracy and interrator reliability for the diagnosis of unstable meniscal tears in patients having osteoarthritis of the knee. Can J Surg 2001; 44: 267–274.

42. Spector TD, Hart DJ, Nandra D et al. Low-level increases in serum C-reactive protein are present in early osteoarthritis of the knee and predict progressive disease. Arthritis Rheum 1997; 40: 723–727.

43. Olmez N, Schumacher HR Jr. Crystal deposition and osteoarthritis. Curr Rheumatol Rep 1999; 1: 107–111.

166 Pathogenesis of osteoarthritis

Frank A Wollheim

- Osteoarthritis (OA) may be defined as joint failure, and cartilage destruction is the most constant and best studied feature. However, OA involves all parts of the joint, including synovial tissue and bone

- OA is accompanied by chondrocyte senescence but is different from normal aging

- Chondrocyte function and extracellular matrix biology are regulated by cytokines and growth factors. Interleukin-1 is the major cytokine involved. Fibronectin fragments are mediators of catabolic signals to chondrocytes. Crystals deposited in cartilage may constitute other important endogenous mediators of catabolic changes in OA

- Inflammation is present, but in limited form in many cases of OA, and may influence the course of disease. There is evidence that markers of inflammation indicate a poor prognosis

- Induced and spontaneous OA in animals remain useful investigative tools, and gene manipulation is of value to create new models and to test pathogenetic mechanisms

- Mechanical factors are involved in the pathogenesis of OA. These are generated by joint incongruity, laxity, muscle weakness and impaired proprioception in addition to trauma and heavy physical load

- Local cartilage-related resistance factors have been found that may explain differences in prevalence of OA between different joints, e.g. knee and ankle

- Gene analysis is an emerging investigative tool. It has helped to define differences between early and late stages of cartilage changes in OA

INTRODUCTION

Osteoarthrosis or osteoarthritis (OA) was traditionally defined as a degenerative condition in the elderly, accelerated by certain external factors such as trauma and obesity. Conventional radiography combined with clinical characteristics have been the dominating if not the only diagnostic tools in practice as in science. Therapy was far from exciting and consisted mostly of pain killers and physiotherapy, until joint replacement and other orthopedic procedures became available. This conferred an air of dullness to OA[1]. The situation is now changing, stimulated by an explosive expansion of information regarding matrix composition and cell biology of cartilage and bone. Emerging claims of disease-modifying remedies for OA have also created wider interest among patients to seek help from non-operating physicians. This chapter presents some current knowledge of the pathogenesis of OA, as interpreted by a clinician for clinicians. Wherever possible, putative targets for therapy will be addressed.

JOINT CARTILAGE IN FOCUS

Although OA is a disease of all joint tissues, it is appropriate first to focus on cartilage, since much of the research has dealt with cartilage

pathology. In previous editions of this textbook, this chapter was solely devoted to cartilage[2]. Better knowledge of the life cycle of chondrocytes in embryonic and adult life will lead to new understanding of disease processes and eventually new treatment strategies for OA and other diseases[3].

Adult cartilage consists of chondrocytes dispersed in abundant extracellular matrix containing 65–80% water and 20–35% solids. Approximately 5–6% of the tissue is inorganic, mostly hydroxyapatite. The water content is critically balanced, mainly by restraint from the scaffolding collagen framework and the attraction by negatively charged proteoglycan side chains. Even slight alterations in content or quality of the organic components of cartilage extracellular matrix will affect water content and cartilage function.

Formation and turnover of cartilage

In the embryo, chondrogenesis starts from mesenchymal precursor cells under the influence of extracellular growth and differentiation factors, which include bone morphogenic proteins, fibroblast growth factors (FGF), parathyroid-hormone-related peptide (PTHrP), and members of the hedgehog and Wnt families. Members of the Sox family play a leading role in the process. These are highly conserved molecules containing a high mobility group (HMG) DNA binding box. Sox9 is highly expressed in embryonic chondrogenic cells and mutations of Sox9 have been identified as the congenital defect in campomelic dysplasia[4]. These individuals suffer from skeletal anomalies related to widespread hypoplasia of enchondral bone formation. They also have other defects, such as XY sex reversal and heart and kidney malformations. This indicates different functions for Sox9. Two other members of the Sox family, L-Sox5 and Sox6, are linked to chondrocyte maturation and matrix formation[5]. Knock-out experiments in mice indicate that these two transcription factors are largely redundant. They have been shown to directly activate type II collagen genes distinguishing the chondrocyte phenotype. Sox9 also inhibits transition of proliferating chondrocytes into hypertrophic chondrocytes and thus plays a role in the prevention of chondrocyte apoptosis. Fibroblast growth factor and PTHrP formed in periarticular perichondrium and Indian hedgehog co-operate to delay the transformation of proliferating chondrocytes into hypertrophic collagen-X-producing chondrocytes. A transcription factor, core binding factor $(Cbf)\alpha_1$, on the other hand, promotes this process and is important for both enchondral bone formation and osteoblast differentiation[6]. Some features of this chondrocyte regulation are depicted in Figure 166.1.

Joint cartilage matrix

Hyaline joint cartilage consists of 1% or less chondrocytes, which live in an abundance of extracellular matrix. The chondrocytes both secrete the building blocks of and produce substances that degrade the matrix, from which they also derive their nutrition. Different zones (Fig. 166.2) and compartments (Fig. 166.3) are characteristic of hyaline joint cartilage. They differ in composition and in the orientation of the fibrillar

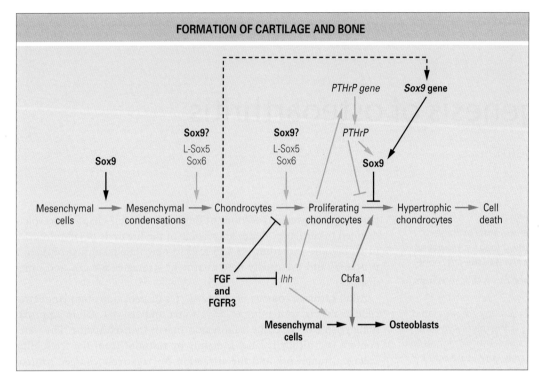

FORMATION OF CARTILAGE AND BONE

Fig 166.1 Formation of cartilage and bone. Diagram of the transcription factors that control the chondrocyte and osteoblast differentiation pathways. (Redrawn with permission from De Crombrugghe *et al.*[5])

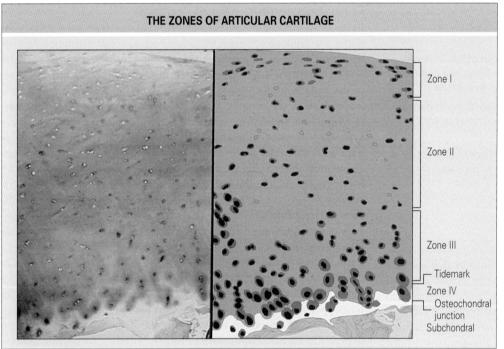

THE ZONES OF ARTICULAR CARTILAGE

Fig 166.2 The zones of articular cartilage. Light micrograph of human articular cartilage from the medial tibial plateau of a 66-year-old woman. Weigert's acid iron chloride hematoxylin, safranin O and fast green stain (proteoglycans: red; collagen: green; calcified cartilage: yellow). Cartilage thickness: 1.8mm. The corresponding computer-enhanced schematic illustration of the different layers of articular cartilage from the surface to the subchondral bone is shown on the right. Zone I: tangential zone; zone II: transitional zone; zone III: radial zone, followed by the tidemark that separates the non-calcified cartilage from the calcified zone (zone IV). The osteochondral junction links the subchondral bone with the cartilage.

network. The chondrocyte has the capacity to synthesize both the matrix components and regulators of its metabolism. Figure 166.4 shows the different types of collagen produced by chondrocytes. Type II collagen is the main component of the collagen fibrils, which also incorporate type XI and, on the surface, type IX.

Formation and maintenance of the extracellular matrix in articular cartilage is essential for normal joint function. This matrix is a microcosm of collagens, aggrecan and other non-collagenous macromolecules that interact to form a scaffold of fibrils and a highly charged, water-binding, resilient matrix. Cell-surface–protein interactions and protein–protein interactions are involved (Fig. 166.5). Some of the matrix constituents, such as type II collagen and aggrecan, exist mainly in cartilage, whereas others are generally distributed in several tissues; fibronectin is one example. All are, however, produced locally. Figure 166.5 depicts some of the identified macromolecules and their cellular, territorial and interterritorial interactions. It can be seen that the collagen fibrils consist of type II–XI collagen fibers held together by decorin, type IX collagen and cartilage oligomeric matrix protein (COMP). Integrins and chondroadherin anchor some fibrils to the chondrocyte. Knowledge of normal cartilage matrix is obviously essential in order to understand the pathology of OA.

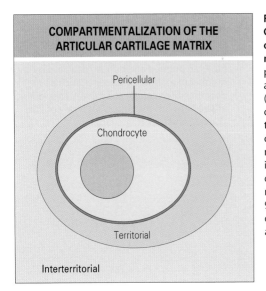

COMPARTMENTALIZATION OF THE ARTICULAR CARTILAGE MATRIX

Fig 166.3 Compartmentalization of the articular cartilage matrix. The thin rim of pericellular matrix (red) and the territorial matrix (light blue) form the cell-associated matrix, the metabolically active compartment. The metabolically 'inert' interterritorial matrix compartment (dark blue) makes up more than 90% of the total volume of the matrix in human adult articular cartilage.

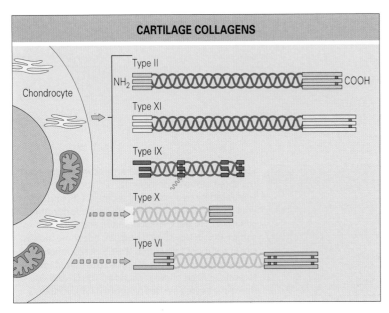

CARTILAGE COLLAGENS

Fig.166.4 Cartilage collagens. The different collagen types synthesized by chondrocytes. The chondrocyte, depicted on the left side of the figure, constitutively produces three collagen types: type II, type XI and type IX. These three collagens, shown inside the bracket, are incorporated into the same collagen fibril. The proportions of these collagens in the fibrils changes with age. The other two collagen types, type X and type VI (marked with dashed arrows), are not made by all chondrocytes. Type X collagen is synthesized only by the hypertrophic chondrocytes in growth-plate cartilage or in articular cartilage near the tidemark and through the calcified cartilage. Type VI collagen is not synthesized in embryonic cartilage but appears in mature cartilage. The levels of both type X and type VI collagen in articular cartilage appear to increase in osteoarthritis. All the cartilage collagens are synthesized as molecules containing at least two different kinds of domains, triple helical and non-helical. The helical regions are depicted as three-chained coils and the non-helical regions are contiguous small boxes. In some collagen types (II and XI) the non-helical regions (yellow) are removed as fibrils are formed. The other collagen types (IX, X and VI) retain their non-helical regions and are shown as one solid color through the entire molecule. Type IX collagen is also a proteoglycan and contains one glycosaminoglycan chain (small orange kinked chain). Disulfide bonds between two collagen chains are shown as red boxes. All the molecules and their domains are drawn approximately to scale as a linear representation of their respective molecular weights.

Polymeric collagen constitutes two-thirds of adult joint cartilage. In addition to the main fibrillar collagen constituents, types II, XI and IX, types III, VI, X, XII and XIV are also normal constituents, although less abundant. Type III collagen synthesis is a feature of clustering chondrocytes as seen in OA cartilage. Mutations affecting the *COLII*, *COLIX* or *COLXI* genes result in chondrodysplasia and an accelerated form of OA[7], proving their critical structural function. Collagen type X is only synthesized by hypertrophic chondrocytes and is normally restricted to a rim of calcified cartilage covering the subchondral bone.

The 40 or more non-collagenous macromolecules belong to several chemical families and have both structural and cell-regulating functions[8]. Aggrecan is the most studied and abundant proteoglycan (Fig. 166.6). Genetic defects of aggrecan core protein result in brachymorphism in mice, nanomelia in chickens and matrix deficiency in mice. Aggrecan depletion is an early feature in experimental arthritis. Aggrecan and the related versican share structural features. Both have an N-terminal globular G_1 domain and a C-terminal G_3 domain. Aggrecan has an additional G_2 domain, which shares features of the G_1 domain but lacks the ability to attach to hyaluronan[9]. The production and folding of the aggrecan core protein with its globular domains and the side chain sulfation is the result of complex intracellular processing and trafficking and chaperone interactions[10]. The folding of the nascent core protein chains is protected by chaperones such as calreticulin/calnexin. Failure to form the G_3 domain results in retention in the endoreticulum and the lethal anomaly nanomelia. Impaired sulfation of the aggrecan side-chains is associated with diastrophic dysplasia, achondrogenesis and atelosteogenesis[8].

In human cartilage the N-terminal region undergoes progressive loss of the G_3 domain with age, and cartilage from 65-year-old individuals contains 92% less than that from newborn children[11]. The G_3 domain can ligate with a number of bipolar proteins, such as tenascins, fibulins and fibrillin[12]. The metabolism of the N-terminal hyaluronan-binding part of aggrecan is much slower than that of the remaining aggrecan monomers, with half-lives of 25 and 3.4 years respectively[13]. Changes in the carbohydrate composition also occur, such as accumulation of advanced glycation end-products[14].

Decorin and biglycan belong to the growing family of small leucine-rich repeat proteins, which have important functions. Like fibromodulin and lumican they can bind type II collagen on the collagen fibrils, whereas biglycan locates at some distance from these[9]. Other molecules that are located to distinct regions, and presumably have distinct functions, are cartilage intermediate layer protein (CILP)[15,16] and cartilage superficial layer protein (SZP)[17,18]. SZP is synthesized by chondrocytes close to the cartilage surface and is concentrated in synovial fluid, where it has a strong lubricating effect. CILP is present in increased amounts in OA and in old age.

Cartilage oligomeric matrix protein was initially described as a cartilage-specific macromolecule[19]; this was later found to be not strictly true[20,21]. COMP is of paramount functional importance both in embryonic and adult cartilage, as shown by numerous examples of pseudo-achondroplasia related to COMP mutations[22]. COMP is a member of the thrombospondin family and a pentamer (Fig. 166.7)[19,23]. It has gained particular attention as an investigative tool in arthritis and OA, since its serum concentration relates to development of progressive OA[24–27]. COMP is also emerging as a valuable tool for monitoring experimental joint damage[28].

SPONTANEOUS AND EXPERIMENTALLY INDUCED OSTEOARTHRITIS IN ANIMALS

Osteoarthritis models have been used widely in attempts to understand the pathogenesis of the disorder and derive therapeutic strategies for its management. Initially, drastic measures such as injections of noxious substances and mechanical destruction of parts of joints were used. Later, Pond and Nuki[29] refined the model of Paatsama[30] of trans-section of the anterior cruciate ligament in the dog, which has been extensively

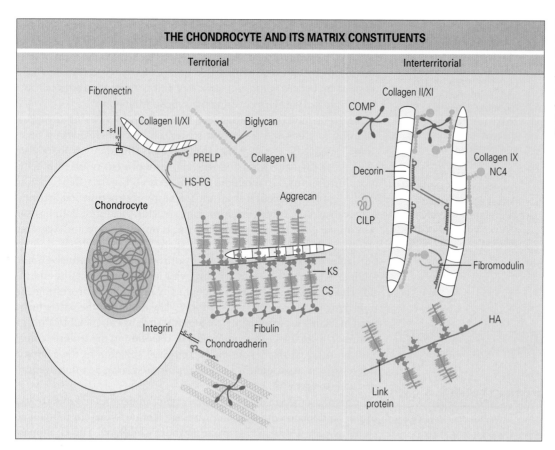

THE CHONDROCYTE AND ITS MATRIX CONSTITUENTS

Territorial | Interterritorial

Fig 166.5 Chondrocyte and its matrix constituents. The chondrocyte communicates with the matrix with integrins, receptors and hyaluronan chains. Collagen fibrils are formed and tightly regulated by a number of matrix components, such as decorin, fibromodulin and COMP. They differ in size between the zones. (Courtesy of Pilar Lorenzo and Dick Heinegård.)

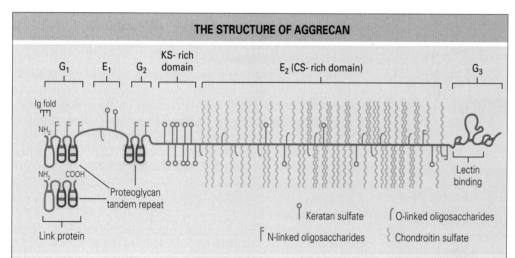

THE STRUCTURE OF AGGRECAN

Fig. 166.6 The structure of aggrecan. In aggrecan the three globular domains (G_1, G_2 and G_3) are separated by two extended segments (E_1 and E_2), which carry the glycosaminoglycans chondroitin sulfate (CS, in the CS-rich domain) and keratan sulfate (KS, in the KS-rich domain, but some also in the E_1 segment and within the CS-rich domain). Furthermore, the core protein is substituted with N- and O-linked oligosaccharides. The G_1 and G_2 domains, as well as the link protein (LP), contain a double loop structure (proteoglycan tandem repeat, PTR). In addition, both G_1 and LP show an additional loop structure (immunoglobulin fold, Ig fold) which can selectively interact with HA to form aggregates. The G_3 domain contains a lectin-binding region.

studied up to recent times. Basically, most of the older models induce injury and study attempted repair[31]. The models in Table 166.1 are based on induced instability or induction of abnormal loading. Other methods target cells by injection of toxic substances such as colchicine and osmic acid, which cause synovial inflammation, or iodoacetamide, which penetrates cartilage and affects chondrocytes. Inflammation is often induced in these experiments and the relevance for human OA can be questioned. However they have been important tools for the study of cartilage injury and repair[32].

More relevant but harder to study are the spontaneous forms of OA in rats, guinea pigs, dogs, horses, Rhesus monkeys and other species. Some mouse strains develop 'spontaneous' OA and in one such strain, STR/1N, evidence of attempted repair, chondrocyte hypertrophy and increased bone formation has been studied[33]. Another strain, STN/ort, was derived from STR/1N after a period of outbreeding and in this strain

85% of male animals develop OA by week 35. This model has many features of human OA and allows precise monitoring of the process on magnetic resonance imaging (MRI), scanning electron microscopy and by biomarkers such as COMP[34]. The medial knee joint is generally affected whereas the lateral parts are spared. Ankle deformities are not unusual but it is unclear whether this represents real OA or is a manifestation of joint laxity. Patellar subluxation was originally believed to be of pathogenetic importance but the correlation is not strong. Soft tissue calcifications are also a feature in the STR/ort strain. Net cartilage matrix proteoglycan depletion and metalloproteinase and aggrecanase expression occur just like in human OA. Increased chondrocyte apoptosis is present. Inflammation is not prominent in STR/ort disease. A recent study looked at gene expression of aggrecan and type II, X and XI collagen in non-OA prone CBA mice in comparison with STR/ort mice[35]. All genes were expressed in both young and old mice of both species.

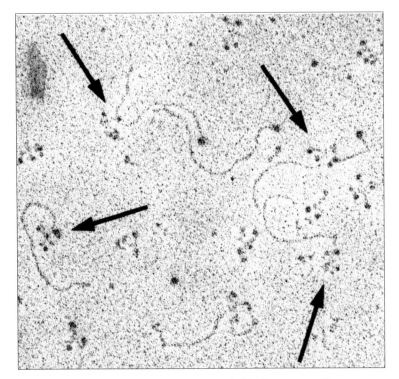

Fig. 166.7 Cartilage oligomeric matrix protein binding to procollagen visualized by electron microscopy. COMP was incubated with procollagen II, at the molar ratio 1:8, and dialyzed overnight against 0.2mol/l ammonium formate, pH .4, with 1mmol/l zinc for glycerol spraying/rotary shadowing. COMP binds via a globular end to the collagen filament and often bridges between different collagens. To identify the polarity of collagen, procollagen II was used as its C terminus, seen as a globular domain (arrows). The bars represent 100nm. (Modified with permission from Rosenberg et al.[23])

TABLE 166.1 SOME EARLY INDUCED ANIMAL MODELS OF OSTEOARTHRITIS	
	Features
Mono-articular	
Bennett–Baurer (1932)	Patellar displacement in dog
Bruce–Walmsley (1942)	Patellectomy in dog
Paatsama–Pond–Nuki (1952, 1973)	Anterior cruciate ligament transection in dog
Moskowitz (1973)	Partial meniscectomy in rabbit
Reimann (1973)	Osteotomy in rabbit
Arsever–Bole (1986)	Tenotomy in guinea pig
Johnson–Poole (1988)	Osteotomy in dog
Polyarticular	
Radin et al. (1978)	Repetitive impulsive knee-loading in rabbit
Radin (1984)	Exercise on cement in sheep

These models are based on creating joint instability and/or destroying joint structures. For references see Brandt[36].

However all four genes were inactive adjacent to OA lesions. Thus it is unlikely that OA development is caused by failure to synthesize the proteins but, once the lesions are manifest, synthesis may be down-regulated. The molecular basis of this interesting model needs further investigation.

A comprehensive review of spontaneous, chemically and physically induced animal models emphasize that the only way to validate a model

is to show that it is responsive to measures proved to be effective in human OA[36]. Instability is a well established route to OA in the Pond–Nuki model. Neurogenic acceleration, influence of immobilization and muscle weakness and evidence against a primary role of subchondral bone stiffening have all been convincingly documented. Therapeutic studies were also reviewed. Cyclo-oxygenase (COX) inhibitors are without effect on joint damage. Doxycycline has a striking inhibiting effect in the Pond–Nuki model, possibly through matrix metalloproteinase (MMP) inhibition. Co-administration of pentosan sulfate and insulin-like growth factor (IGF)-1 is also protective, presumably by lowering MMPs and increasing tissue inhibitor of metalloproteinase (TIMP).

An exiting new generation of animal models has been created by means of gene manipulation. Targeted deletions directed at components of the structural collagen network that predispose animals to premature OA confirm their importance for cartilage function. An example is the transgenic Del1 mouse which carries a deletion in exon 7 and intron 7 of the COL2α gene, resulting in early OA[28]. A transient upregulation of the COMP gene compared to non-transgenic control C57B1×DBA mice at the border to the calcified cartilage and a shift from interterritorial to pericellular location closely mimics similar changes in human OA and testifies to the relevance of the model. In the same model, expression of the Sox9 gene and deposition of embryonic collagen type IIA characteristic of early chondrogenesis were found in some areas indicative of repair.

Metalloproteinase and inhibitor expression has also been explored. MMP-13 and TIMP-1 were absent in degrading cartilage but were found to be upregulated in hyperplastic synovial tissue, subchondral bone and calcified cartilage[37,38]. Neoepitopes of aggrecan resulting from MMP-13 catabolism were found in the same location. The interpretation of these experiments is that MMP-13 is not a primary mediator of the OA-like process.

Such models thus have great potential for the study of initial and later phases of the OA process, for identifying candidate genes, for the identification of biomarkers and in the end for investigating therapeutic interventions.

NORMAL AGING IS DIFFERENT FROM OSTEOARTHRITIS

Age is the strongest risk factor for OA, and it is not far-fetched to consider OA as a form of premature aging. However, prevalence of clinical OA does not increase after the age of 75, and degenerative cartilage changes are prevalent starting at age 15[39]. Normal aging must be distinguished from OA. Table 166.2 depicts some of the differences. Matrix swelling due to increased water content is seen in OA and is caused by breaks in the restraining collagen meshwork. Chondrocyte proliferation and increased metabolism are other features seen only in OA. Subchondral bone sclerosis is not seen in normal aging. Chondrocytes, like other cells, have a limited life span and a limited capacity for division, which decreases with age. Responsiveness to growth factors platelet-derived growth factor (PDGF), IGF-1 and transforming growth

TABLE 166.2 OSTEOARTHRITIS VS AGING	
Osteoarthritis	**Aging**
↑ cartilage hydration	↓ cartilage hydration
↓ proteoglycan concentration	↔ proteoglycan concentration
↓ collagen concentration	↔ collagen concentration
↑ chondrocyte proliferation	↔ or ↓ chondrocyte proliferation
↑ metabolic activity	↔ metabolic activity
↑ subchondral bone thickness	Normal subchondral bone

Cartilage changes in aging differ from those in OA. (Adapted with permission from Loeser[39].)

factor (TGF)-β is reduced in chondrocytes obtained at knee replacement. Telomere length is reduced as is synthetic capacity in chondrocytes derived from old persons[40,41]. The telomerase defect can now be reversed *in vitro* by retroviral transfection with telomerase[42]. This is exciting progress but does not answer the question of what distinguishes normal aging chondrocytes from OA chondrocytes.

CYTOKINES AND INFLAMMATION

Traditionally, OA has been looked at as a 'degenerative' and non-inflammatory condition and it was often termed 'osteoarthrosis'. Classical signs of inflammation are absent but synovial swelling and tenderness and joint effusion, clinical indications of inflammation, are common albeit transient events in the course of OA. They could be a secondary response to tissue injury and not a primary pathogenetic event. Moderate macroscopic and histologic evidence of synovial inflammation was found in 55% of patients with knee OA and normal radiographs by arthroscopy[43]. Modest increases of the sensitive acute-phase proteins SAA and CRP have been observed in several studies of OA as well as in post-traumatic joint disease[44,45]. Increased levels of CRP in serum and synovial fluid have been related to rapid progression of OA[46,47].

Inflammatory components in the pathogenesis of OA have been suggested for more than a decade[48]. Developing knowledge of cell biology with molecular definition of cytokines, nitric oxide (NO) and other mediators of inflammation has transformed the question of whether or not inflammation is involved in OA into one of semantics[49]. It may be argued that the chondrocyte in OA releases mediators very similar to activated macrophages (Fig. 166.8). The chondrocyte diameter is seven times that of the average macrophage. According to this view, the osteoarthritic joint can be described as a chronic but localized inflammation. Analysis in a number of laboratories of human OA cartilage has shown up-regulation of mRNA by real time polymerase chain reaction (PCR) for several proinflammatory cytokines as well as increased 'spontaneous' synthesis in OA compared to normal cartilage (Fig. 166.9). Furthermore, gene chip analysis has shown increased expression of genes for several MMPs, COX-2, IL-8 but also for TGF-β (Fig. 166.9). Little is known of which mediators are causing these changes. IL-17 has been suggested in one report[50] but there are many other candidates. Regulators and mediators of inflammation have therefore moved into the forefront of putative targets for intervention in many laboratories. A simplified cartoon shows the influences of some important cytokines on chondrocyte function (Fig. 166.10).

PROTEASES AND MATRIX CONTROL

The mechanism of the proteolytic attack on the main components of cartilage, aggrecan and type II collagen, has been and is the subject of intense research efforts. Aggrecan has an average turnover in adult cartilage of a few years, compared to several decades for collagen[2]. Aggrecan depletion is an early event in the development of OA[51]. *In vitro* MMPs, for instance collagenase 3 (MMP-13) can be shown to degrade aggrecan at the Asn[341]-Phe[342] site of the aggrecan core chain in the region between G_1 and G_2. However analysis of aggrecan fragments in synovial fluid from patients with OA showed fragments with a cleavage site at Glu[373]-Ala[374], indicating involvement of a novel proteinase[52]. This was called aggrecanase and was later identified as a member of the ADAM-TS family and cloned[53,54]. ADAM-TS is a descriptive name and stands for 'a disintegrin and metalloprotease with thrombospondin motifs'. Aggrecanase cleavage products have also been confirmed in *in vitro* experiments in which chondrocyte cultures are exposed to IL-1 or retionoids[55]. It appears that ADAM-TS4 and ADAM-TS5, also called aggrecanase-1 and -2, are both involved in this degradation and that synthetic inhibitors specific for these enzymes can protect cartilage *in vitro*[56]. It has also been shown that the thrombospondin motif is essential for enzyme function by binding to the GAG chains of aggrecan[57]. The *ADAM-TD4* gene is expressed more in RA synovial fibroblast-like cells than in OA, in contrast to *ADAM-TS5*, which is constitutively expressed in both conditions; it can be up-regulated by IL-1, tumor necrosis factor (TNF)-α and TGF-β[58]. This new information has a clear bearing on early and later catabolic events in cartilage in OA and may help to develop new remedies.

The discovery of collagenase by Gross and Lapiere was a landmark event[59]. At present more than 25 MMPs have been identified[60]. One can distinguish between, for example, collagenases (MMP-1, -8 and -13), gelatinases (MMP-2 and -9), stromelysins (MMP-3, -10 and -11), and membrane-type MMPs, of which at least six are known. The enzymes exist in inactive proforms and must undergo a series of activation steps. Thus presence of MMP as such does not prove a pathogenetic role in disease. Redundancy must also be considered. In OA cartilage, MMP-1, -3, -8, -9 and -13 have been detected[61]. The different MMPs are in part found in different zones of the cartilage, indicating different roles. The membrane bound proteases, TM-MMPs, participate in activation of MMPs but may also have a direct matrix-degrading function.

The same cells that produce MMPs also produce inhibitors, TIMPs. In rheumatoid arthritis (RA) and OA there is an imbalance, leading to relative dominance of MMPs over TIMPs. In general, proinflamma-

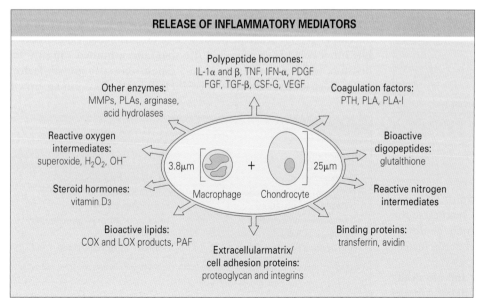

RELEASE OF INFLAMMATORY MEDIATORS

Polypeptide hormones:
IL-1α and β, TNF, IFN-α, PDGF
FGF, TGF-β, CSF-G, VEGF

Other enzymes:
MMPs, PLAs, arginase, acid hydrolases

Coagulation factors:
PTH, PLA, PLA-I

Reactive oxygen intermediates:
superoxide, H_2O_2, OH⁻

Bioactive digopeptides:
glutalthione

3.8μm   +   25μm

Macrophage   Chondrocyte

Steroid hormones:
vitamin D3

Reactive nitrogen intermediates

Bioactive lipids:
COX and LOX products, PAF

Binding proteins:
transferrin, avidin

Extracellularmatrix/
cell adhesion proteins:
proteoglycan and integrins

Fig.166.8 Release of inflammatory mediators. Common inflammatory mediators that are released by activated macrophages and OA-affected chondrocytes. CSF, colony stimulating factor; PAF, platelet activation factors; PLA, phospholipase A; PTH, parathyroid hormone; TNF, tumor necrosis factor; VEGF, vascular endothelial growth factor. (Redrawn with permission from Attur *et al.*[48])

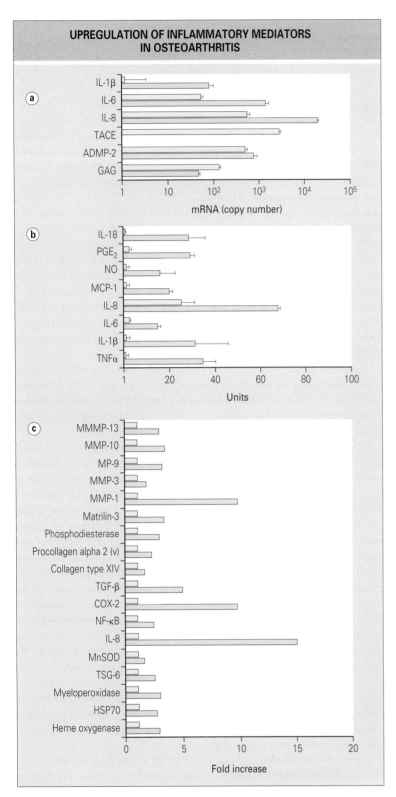

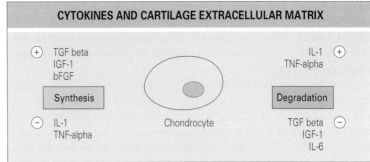

Fig 166.10 Cytokines and cartilage extracellular matrix. Some cytokines influencing cartilage matrix synthesis and degradation.

Fig. 166.9 Up-regulation of inflammatory mediators in osteoarthritis. Normal human cartilage is represented by the red bars and OA-affected cartilage by the blue bars. (a) Real time PCR of mRNA transcripts in normal and OA-affected cartilage. (b) Spontaneous production of inflammatory mediators by normal and OA-affected cartilage *in vitro*. (c) Gene chip analysis of selected proinflammatory mediators and stress genes in normal and OA-affected cartilage. The human Affymetrix U95 gene chip was probed with a pool (*n* = 10) of normal and OA-affected cartilage RNAs. (Redrawn with permission from Attur *et al.*[48])

tory signals increase MMP gene expression and reduce TIMP gene expression.

Gene manipulation of MMPs in animals has generated confusing results. MMP-3-deficient mice have a normal phenoptype[61]. Over-expression of MMP-13 in mice, however, produces OA-like defects[62]. Targeting MMPs in animal models such as the STR/ort has produced promising results[63]. However no clinically useful MMP inhibitor for therapy of OA is presently available.

NITRIC OXIDE AND OSTEOARTHRITIS

Nitric oxide is produced by three distinct synthases (NOS), indicating the diverse and important physiologic functions of this molecule. Two calcium-dependent constitutively expressed enzymes – endothelial and neuronal NOS, eNOS and nNOS – produce pico- or nanomolar amounts of NO with important functions for normal microcirculation. In contrast, the inducible iNOS manufactures micromolar concentrations of NO. Human chondrocytes obtained from OA patients undergoing joint replacement express iNOS and produce micromolar amounts of NO in culture[64]. This lasts for 5–7 days, indicating upregulation due to factors present in cartilage. In normal chondrocyte cultures iNOS expression requires *in vitro* stimulation.

The mechanisms by which NO could contribute to OA pathogenesis are in part hypothetical. NO inhibits actin polymerization, which affects cell adhesion, signaling from extracellular matrix and phagocytosis[65]. Furthermore, NO can inhibit matrix synthesis and promote apoptosis of chondrocytes[66,67]. OA chondrocytes in culture exposed to NO pregulated COX-2 and produced prostaglandin E₂. It is possible, but not proved, that this is mediated by iNOS. NO has been reported both to inhibit and stimulate prostaglandin E production, perhaps depending on the cell type or COX isotype[68].

A possible role for iNOS in OA receives support from observations in animal models. Selective inhibition of iNOS with *N*-iminoethyl-L-lysine (L-NIL) reduces destruction in the Pond–Nuki model[69]. Selective iNOS inhibitors are in development as putative therapeutic agents in human disease. A beneficial effect in the Pond–Nuki model by tetracycline may in part be explained by its iNOS inhibition[70]. Finally, a dual inhibitor of COX and lipoxygenase (licofelone ML-3000), which is in clinical development, inhibits chondrocyte apoptosis and iNOS expression[71].

APOPTOSIS

Evidence of reduced cellularity in OA cartilage and inability to heal lesions are obvious factors which raise suspicion that cell death may be involved in the pathogenesis of OA. The likely role of NO was discussed in the previous section. NO in micromolar concentrations is known to increase apoptosis[66]. NO alone does not induce apoptosis but requires additional exposure to reactive oxygen[72]. However, it is evident that chondrocytes in adult cartilage must have strong inherent resistance to apoptosis. The tissue is avascular and thus there is no access for mesenchymal stem cells. Mitoses are unusual in healthy cartilage. Cell–cell contact, which in other tissues generates protection against apoptosis, does not occur, which puts the burden on the cell itself and its contact with the surrounding extracellular matrix. It has been shown that chondrocytes in monolayer culture are more vulnerable to apoptosis than when they are grown in three-dimensional gel, showing the importance of extracellular factors[73].

Direct observations of apoptosis in OA cartilage have yielded conflicting results. Whereas some authors find widespread apoptosis in OA cartilage and correlation with the severity of damage, others have not been able to confirm this[73]. In a careful study of normal cartilage obtained at autopsy, 'early' OA cartilage obtained from arthroscopy and advanced OA cartilage obtained at joint replacement procedures, little evidence of apoptosis or reactive cell proliferation could be detected[74]. Indeed, clustering could only be seen in superficial parts of specimens from far advanced OA. In this careful investigation no mitoses were seen among more than 100 000 cells examined under the microscope. The sensitive cell surface proliferation marker Ki-67 was detected in the upper and middle zones of only six of 18 OA specimens. Furthermore, examination of histologically empty-appearing lacunae showed strong in situ staining for rRNA and mRNA, indicating the presence of living cells. Likewise, the TUNEL technique disclosed only occasional positive cells in seven of 18 OA specimens and in none of the control non-calcified cartilage areas examined. In contrast, half of the empty lacunae in the calcified cartilage of all three groups were empty by the RNA method. The proportion of TUNEL positive cells in this zone constituted less than 1% of all cells. There are technical difficulties with the TUNEL method, which can result in false-positive results that are not always realized and that may have caused overestimation of the role of apoptosis in earlier studies. The role of apoptosis may therefore be overestimated in discussions of OA pathogenesis.

SYNOVITIS

Whereas much interest has focused on the importance of inflammation in general, and proinflammatory cytokines in particular, relatively little attention has been given to a possible role of the synovium in human OA. In the Pond–Nuki and other animal models, signs of synovitis are the rule rather than the exception[32,36]. Periarticular tissues and synovium are a likely source of pain and stiffness in OA patients. An early study found a high prevalence of intact and degranulated mast cells in OA synovium, indicating a role of the synovium in the disease[75]. Another study focused on granzymes A and B, markers of cytotoxic T lymphocytes and natural killer (NK) cells. Such cells were found in the synovium from 60% of patients with RA but also in 40% of OA synovial biopsies; 75% of the positive cells carried NK cell markers[76]. Using the rabbit partial meniscectomy model, cartilage and synovial tissue were obtained at various intervals after surgery. Histologic signs of synovitis were present at 4 weeks but not later[77]. MMP-3 (stromelysin) was elevated in culture supernatants, in particular in the early phases, whereas the inhibitor TIMP was decreased at this stage[77]. Signs of synovitis were found in areas close to the cartilage but not at other locations in knee joints of patients with early destructive probable OA[78].

A large and systematic Australian study leaves no doubt about the presence of synovitis in early OA[79]. The study involved both arthroscopic biopsies and material obtained at the time of joint replacement. Varying degrees of synovitis were seen, notably with some overlap with normal control synovium. The inflammatory signs were most pronounced in the surgical specimens, where lymphocyte infiltrates were seen in one-third. Immunohistology showed presence of IL-1α, IL-1β and TNF-α, which correlated to the cellularity. In the most pronounced cases the changes were not too different from those seen in RA. Thus it is established that synovitis is present in OA, although more discrete and episodic than in RA. What remains to be elucidated is whether synovitis is primary or secondary to the initial event in OA. The latter appears more likely in view of the variable etiologies of OA. Prospective studies

are needed to establish if early signs of inflammation are a predictor in OA. One such study indicated that elevated inception C-reactive protein (CRP) levels in a population-based cohort of knee pain, correlated with later development of knee-joint OA[80].

CRYSTAL DEPOSITION

It is well established that articular deposition of crystals is a common finding in OA and this raises several questions. Is it an epiphenomenon, is it a consequence of OA or do crystals cause OA or exacerbate the disease?

Basic calcium phosphate or calcium hydroxyapatite (BCP) and calcium pyrophosphate dihydrate (CPPD) are common findings in advanced OA[81]. CPPD is easily detected on routine radiography. In a population-based study from Catalonia, patients with deposits had a relative risk of between 3 and 4 of developing knee or hand OA[81]. Although this was not a strict epidemiologic study and the size was small, it is safe to conclude that it confirms several earlier studies indicating that CPPD is common among the elderly and is associated with increased risk of developing clinical OA. Monosodium urate crystal deposition is associated with Heberden's nodes. Such associations do not necessarily indicate a pathogenetic role for crystals; they could also be a consequence of preferential deposition in diseased tissue[81].

In several studies, the prevalence of crystal occurrence relates to duration and severity of OA. Crystal deposition does not locate to typical OA joints but is often seen in shoulders, wrists and elbows, where OA is uncommon[81]. No close relation has been found between signs of synovial inflammation and finding of crystals in joint tissue.

Crystals could participate in joint tissue damage in several ways. Injection of CPPD into joints in the partial meniscectomy model in rabbits accelerated joint damage;[82] however, injection of crystals in normal rabbit joints did not cause any harm[83]. This indicates a modifying rather than an initiating role for crystals. One speculation is that crystals, by virtue of their hardness, could damage cartilage mechanically. More likely are biologic effects of crystals on cell signaling and metabolic cellular events. Thus it has been shown that BCP crystals in vitro in concentrations commonly present in OA joints act like growth factors on fibroblasts, synovial cells and chondrocytes. This results in mitogenesis and increased production of prostaglandins, proto-oncogenes c-fos and c-myc, and secretion of several MMPs, including MMP-1, -3, -8 and -13[84]. Signal transduction in fibroblasts uses the calcium-dependent protein kinase (PK)C-α pathway as well as the independent p44/42 MAPK pathway[84]. The emerging evidence thus favors a signaling pathway depicted in Figure 166.11. A similar study also identified a three- to fourfold increase in MMP-1 and MMP-13 secretion induced by BCP crystals in vitro and, interestingly, showed synergism with added TNF-α or IL-1β. It had been previously shown that the crystals could induce secretion of these cytokines[85].

These studies not only indicate a role for BCP, and perhaps other crystals, in the pathogenesis of OA but also point to putative therapeutic strategies for the future.

Some drugs in clinical use may act as inhibitors of MMPs. This has been shown for tetracycline and may relate to the binding of tetracycline to BCP[81]. Antimalarial drugs have inhibiting effect on the synthesis of MMP in vitro but no clinical trials in OA have been reported. Probenecid may have yet another way to reduce crystal-induced pathology. It has been shown to inhibit the formation by TGF-β of CPPD crystals in chondrocytes[81].

SUBCHONDRAL BONE AND OSTEOPHYTES

In contrast to RA, OA is usually accompanied by signs of new bone formation, so called subchondral sclerosis and osteophyte formation. Traditionally, the latter has been considered secondary to altered joint stability and a sign of attempted healing, and for many years the former

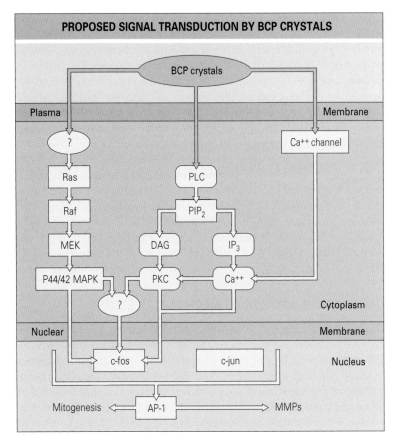

PROPOSED SIGNAL TRANSDUCTION BY BCP CRYSTALS

Fig.166.11 Proposed signal transduction by BCP crystals. Proposed model of BCP crystal-induced signal transduction in human fibroblasts. The p44/42 MAPK and PKC signal transduction pathways activated upon BCP crystal stimulation initially function independently, ultimately leading to an increase in mitogenesis and MMP synthesis. The pathways may converge downstream of p44/42 MAPK and PKC to mediate BCP-crystal-induced cellular responses. A question mark (?) indicates that this component of the signal transduction pathway is currently unknown. (Redrawn with permission from Reuben *et al.*[84])

has been either neglected or alternatively considered to impose a damaging influence on the joint cartilage by means of its hardness. Does OA start in the cartilage or in the bone or elsewhere? It has also been taught that osteoporosis and OA are mutually exclusive conditions. It is necessary to examine the validity of these dogmas in the light of newer evidence.

In the canine OA model of anterior cruciate ligament transection, cartilage swelling and disturbance of proteoglycan metabolism are the initial events, although later subchondral and other bone changes are prominent[36]. In human OA it is feasible that the process starts simultaneously in cartilage and bone. Indirect evidence was provided by a Swedish study using biomarkers for cartilage and bone in a population-based cohort of knee pain. Both markers increased concomitantly in ultra-early stages of what later developed into regular radiographic OA[86].

However, abnormal bony growth has for a long time been a suggested initiating pathogenetic factor in OA[87]. In a spontaneous form of OA in primate adult *Cynomolgus* macaques, early bone changes rather than cartilage abnormalities support such a view[88]. Human data regarding occurrence of osteoporosis and OA are conflicting. In a majority of older reports, published in the 1980s and 1990s, an inverse relation was stressed[89–91]. Increased levels of growth factors IGF-1, IGF-2 and TGF-β have been identified in OA but not in osteoporotic patients and were proposed as a possible mechanism protecting OA patients from fractures[92]. More recent studies are either in conflict with[93–94] or support[95] the inverse relation concept. One study examined the subchondral bone thickness and density in 100 knee joint preparations from 72 patients using high-resolution radiography and correlated the results with gross cartilage damage and body mass index. The specimens were obtained

from a tissue bank and may not have been representative of the average aging population. An age-related increase in cartilage damage correlated inversely with subchondral bone thickness in the lateral tibial region but not in any of the other sites examined. Cartilage damage in the tibial or femoral region did not correlate with subchondral bone thickness or quality. This indicates that the subchondral bone changes observed in OA may be more related to age than to OA[96]. What seems clear, however, is that OA patients are not protected entirely from acquiring osteoporosis and that some as yet unidentified confounding factors may exist. Indeed, the use of the antiresorptive bisphosphonates have been suggested as therapy in OA and a promising pilot study has been performed[97].

Significant advances have been made in the understanding of osteophyte formation. Osteophyte formation in experimental OA typically starts at sites of joint stress with a growth-plate-like formation, chondrocyte formation and later calcification. Growth factors can be shown to stimulate this process. TGF-β_1 concentration is increased in OA joint fluid and repeated intra-articular injection of TGF-β_1 can induce proteoglycan synthesis in cartilage, synovial inflammation and formation of typical osteophytes[98]. More recently, these investigators confirmed the results by administering a TGF-β_1 gene with an adenovirus vector, and showed inhibition of osteophyte formation with clodronate. Synovial inflammation is also involved in the osteophyte formation.

But TGF-β_1 seems to have a dual role, insofar as it promotes aggrecan synthesis and preservation/healing of cartilage and counteracts the catabolic effects induced by IL-1β. Endogenous TGF-β can be blocked by soluble receptor TGF-β-RII. In a model of papain-induced OA, administration of this blocking agent completely inhibited osteophyte formation but also resulted in cartilage matrix depletion and thinning. This was probably mediated by upregulation of MMP-3 and -13 but not ADAM-TS4/5[99].

Another growth factor that has been studied experimentally is IGF-1. IGF-1 serum levels did not correlate with incident or progressive OA in the Framingham study but it has been found to be expressed in a collagenase-induced murine OA model[100]. Chondrocytes in OA, in contrast to normal chondrocytes, are unresponsive to this important growth factor. Their reactivity can be restored *in vitro* by anti-IL-1 reagents.

A further insight in osteophyte formation was a study looking at NO, expression of vascular endothelial growth factor (VEGF) and apoptosis in a rabbit OA model[101]. It was shown that hypertrophic chondrocytes express this angiogenic factor and later express NO and undergo apoptosis. Other investigations have shown expression of type X collagen. All these features can be interpreted as a kind of distorted enchondral bone formation. The interest in all this for the clinician is connected with the observation that many of the symptoms of OA, in particular pain, are generated in or near osteophytes.

ROLES OF LOADING IN THE DEVELOPMENT OF OSTEOARTHRITIS

Osteoarthritis has often been characterized as a mechanically triggered joint failure mediated by biochemical reactions. It is well established by *in vitro* experiments that normal chondrocyte function is dependent on intermittent loading, without which matrix synthesis stops. Therefore it is in the best interests of joint cartilage health to use the joints, and repetitive low-impact exercises do not normally result in increased risk of developing OA. High-impact exercises involving torsion forces and risk of injury are, however, recognized accelerators of OA in the affected joints. Low-impact in contrast to high-impact exercises are not osteogenic[102].

Occupations involving demanding physical activity are known to increase the risk to develop OA in hips[103] or knee joints[104], indicating that OA at times could be considered an occupational disease. In the Framingham study, the amount of heavy physical activity was related to the risk of incident radiographic knee OA[105]. A significant odds ratio of

1.3 per hour of daily activity was found, and adjustment for a number of risk factors such as body mass index, weight loss, smoking and knee injury failed to eliminate the association.

Joint loading is a plausible causative factor in these occupational as well as in overweight and joint-instability-related OA. Gait analysis has established a correlation between loading and radiographic signs of OA in the knee joint. Loading can be measured by adduction moment and has been found to be associated with severity of medial compartment OA in the knee[106]. Another study found a significantly higher than normal peak external knee adduction during walking in a group of OA patients[107]. Increased adduction moment during gait may be an important cause of pain during walking. For many years wedge osteotomy of the knee, which redistributes the load to more lateral parts of the joint, was a popular procedure in knee OA. Wedged shoes have also been used for this purpose, but with uncertain success. Wearing of shoes with high heels leads to a 23% increase in femoropatellar force and may contribute to the development of OA in predisposed individuals.

A large number of studies have investigated congenital acetabular dysplasia as a risk factor for development of OA of the hip, but not all have found a correlation. A prospective study adjusting for age and weight found a relative risk of 3 in individuals with mild asymptomatic dysplasia, indicating the importance of anatomic factors in the pathogenesis of hip OA[108].

It is remarkable how resistant joints are to loading. Normal walking involves impacts on knee joints amounting to three to four times the body weight, and in squatting it may reach 10 times. Controlled deceleration reduces the impact substantially in normal and athletic activities. It has been postulated, but never proven, that impaired muscular control, sometimes called 'microklutziness'[109], contributes to impact-related joint damage in the pathogenesis of OA. Neuromuscular reflexes need time to get activated. Therefore unexpected minor missteps may result in a high impact and cause damage by imposing an excessive load.

Increased bone mineral density is a common finding in individuals with progressive hip and knee OA[103]. This could add to the load damage by increased stiffness of subchondral bone[110].

In summary, joint load is an established accelerating factor in OA, regardless of whether the cause is excessive physical activity, overweight, increased bony stiffness or altered anatomy.

NEUROMUSCULAR FUNCTION AND PROPRIOCEPTION

Decreased muscle function in OA was usually considered to be a consequence of OA and OA-related pain and other symptoms. Improvement in muscle function has been a long-time goal of rehabilitation efforts in OA and it was considered to be symptomatic treatment of one of the consequences of OA. However, evidence has emerged to indicate that it could in addition be implicated in the pathogenesis. Thus, weakness of the quadriceps muscle in patients with knee OA is often present at the start of symptoms. In a population-based study that included asymptomatic individuals with radiographic signs of OA, quadriceps weakness was a strong predictor of radiographic changes[111]. Knee extensor strength was 18% lower in individuals who later developed OA. Another study also found quadriceps weakness at onset of knee OA[112]. However, neither study found a relation between stable or progressive OA and quadriceps weakness. This indicates that muscle control may have a preventive influence on the occurrence of symptomatic or subclinical OA. Interference with innervation through induced spinal lesions has been documented to augment the onset and severity of arthritis in the Pond–Nuki model[36]. These important observations indicate the value of physical activity, in particular in patients at risk of developing OA. The elderly is one such risk group.

Proprioception is the ability to perceive limb position in space. It is generated from receptors in the muscle spindles and in the ligaments, mainly close to their insertion. Signaling through the proprioceptive sensory nerves results eventually in activation of corresponding motor nerves. Intact proprioception is necessary for appropriate joint stability and it can be measured with some degree of accuracy. As expected, it is impaired in patients with anterior cruciate ligament injuries. Several cross-sectional studies have shown impairment in proprioception in patients with OA compared to age-matched controls[113]. In one study, overweight, reduced quadriceps strength and impaired proprioception, combined with increased postural sway, were all associated with knee OA[114]. Impaired proprioception could be a pathogenetic factor or a consequence of OA or a combination of both. In the absence of a prospective study one cannot at present distinguish between these alternatives. In patients with joint laxity, impaired proprioception has been documented[113]. It is very likely that this is a factor increasing the risk to develop OA in this population. Several reports have shown that knee orthoses can improve proprioception. A recent study compared a standard elastic bandage with a looser bandage, and showed reduced pain and improved postural sway control with the latter, although it did not influence proprioception[115]. Use of the standard bandage worsened proprioception.

CARTILAGE RESPONSE TO MECHANICAL STRESS

During normal locomotion and other physical activity, joint surfaces are exposed to forces amounting to several multiples of the body weight, and cartilage must be able to adapt to this load stress, and still maintain its shape and keep its surface smooth and low friction. The compressive stiffness of chondrocytes is several orders of magnitude lower than that of the surrounding matrix. Therefore, chondrocytes will undergo deformation when cartilage is compressed during load. Enhanced flow of tissue fluid will potentially allow exposure of the cells to high concentrations of cytokines and growth factors. This will critically influence chondrocyte biology, and knowledge in this area may be crucial in order to understand the pathogenesis of OA. Proteoglycan content is normally high in areas exposed to high load but the synthetic activity may not be increased[116]. This could indicate reduced breakdown of matrix.

Normal chondrocytes can be studied in explant cultures, which can be exposed to regulated loading conditions. Such studies using explants from normal joints have shown that intermittent loading stimulates whereas static load inhibits matrix synthesis, and indicates that chondrocyte phenotypic variation is load-dependent[117]. Strenuous exposure of dogs to load for 1 year increased proteoglycan content. Triathletes have a larger weight-bearing knee joint surface, indicating another adaptive mechanism towards mechanical stress[118]. This group found no or only marginal correlation between cartilage volume and body weight or body height, but stronger correlation with leg muscle volume as measured on MRI.

Normal human chondrocytes exposed to intermittent loading increase mRNA for aggrecan and decrease mRNA for MMP-3 via an integrin-dependent IL-4 autocrine/paracrine loop. OA chondrocytes do not show this anabolic type of response. The integrin $\alpha_5\beta_1$ serves as the mechanoreceptor in both OA and normal chondrocytes but downstream signaling appears abnormal in OA[119]. Understanding the pathogenesis of OA has taken another significant step forward.

CARTILAGE METABOLISM IN ANKLE AND KNEE JOINTS

It is well known that OA has a strong preference for some joints while sparing others unless exposed to non-physiologic stress. Circus performers who earn their livelihood by walking upside down develop osteophytes and symptoms of OA in the elbows. Whereas hip and knee joints are prone to develop OA, the ankle joints are usually spared. Histologically, ankle joints often show cartilage fissures but rarely full-blown cartilage destruction. Normal ankle joint cartilage is only 1mm thick. This could indicate local resistance factors in the ankle joint. Cartilage explant cultures, and other techniques[120], have been used to explore whether metabolic chondrocyte-related differences could explain the relative susceptibility or resistance to the development of OA[116,121].

Paired knee and ankle cartilage explants were obtained within 24 hours post-mortem. The initial macroscopic and histologic examination showed that, even though none of the patients had had a diagnosis of OA, only 37% of the knee specimens and 54% of the ankle specimens were completely normal. Explant cultures from paired ankle and knee joints with normal histology detected consistently higher matrix synthesis in the ankle preparations. Static pressure suppressed synthesis more in the ankle than in the knee explant. Matrix synthesis was stimulated by intermittent (dynamic) pressure in the ankle joint but this was not tested in knee explants. Interestingly, knee explants were six times more sensitive to inhibition of synthesis by IL-1 and recovered more slowly after exposure. This could possibly be explained by differences in IL-1 receptors on the chondrocyte surface. It had been shown previously that an amino-terminal thrombin-generated 29kDa fragment of fibronectin inhibits matrix synthesis after intra-articular injection into rabbit joints[122]. The inhibition can be abrogated by antisense peptides to α_5 integrin[123]. Such fragments from normal matrix constituents have been postulated to have a regulatory role in matrix homeostasis (Fig. 166.12). Knee cartilage showed 30–50% inhibition from day 7 to day 28 or longer in culture, while ankle joint cartilage was unaffected throughout by fibronectin fragments.

These interesting results show that intrinsic biochemical chondrocyte differences may in part explain why some joints are more prone to develop OA and others more resistant.

GENE EXPRESSION IN DIFFERENT STAGES OF OSTEOARTHRITIC CARTILAGE

Gene expression can be studied by three different techniques. The cDNA gene array technique requires large amounts of RNA but allows screening for a large number of identified genes simultaneously. Quantitative PCR determination of individual genes can be applied to minute amounts of tissue using *ex vivo* material. Finally, differential display technology can be used to detect new genes[124,125]. This approach has yielded a wealth of data, some of which are unexpected and need confirmation.

Chondrocytes occur in different phenotypes distinguished by synthesis of different collagens. Adult chondrocytes produce mainly type IIB collagen. Type I and III collagen is secreted by dedifferentiated chon-

drocytes. Type IIA collagen is made by progenitor chondrocytes, and type X collagen by hypertrophic chondrocytes. Type IIA collagen is alternatively spliced and contains a cysteine-rich segment in exon 2 that is not present in adult type IIB collagen. Evidence of type III collagen gene expression was present in middle zones of OA cartilage, whereas type IIA and type X mRNA was seen in deeper layers, where apoptosis could be observed. These results indicate reversion to immature phenotypes and are not surprising. A new collagen type XVI was identified and, interestingly, tenascin, which is absent in normal chondrocytes[124].

Early results comparing normal, early and late OA cartilage show mRNA expression of aggrecan and decorin in all three groups of cartilage, indicating active synthesis. In contrast biglycan, type II and type III collagen mRNA was only detected in advanced OA (Fig. 166.13). MMP-3 was only present in early OA whereas MMP-2, MMP-11 and

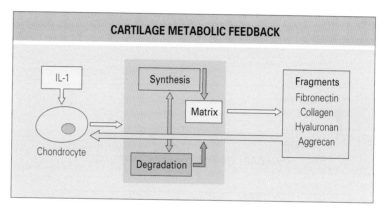

Fig.166.12 Cartilage metabolic feedback. Chondrocytes respond to IL-1 through their receptors by shifting the maintenance of homeostasis through a decrease in matrix synthesis and increase in matrix loss. Matrix loss occurs as the components become proteolytically degraded. The fragments generated through degradation appear to generate an endogenous metabolic feedback that will generate a response from the chondrocytes. The effect of the fragments on the chondrocytes may result in greater matrix damage than IL-1 itself, apparently by acting through the cell-surface receptors, activating degradative pathways and further potentiating the process of matrix destruction. (Adapted with permission from Cole and Kuettner[121].)

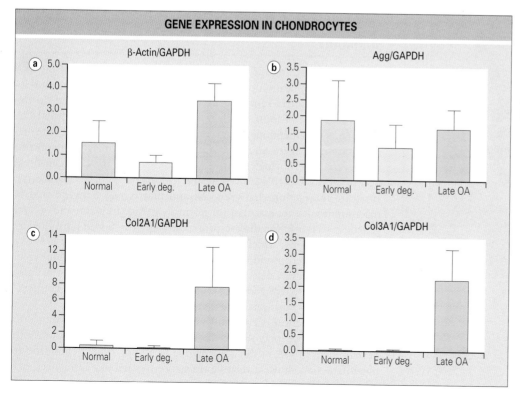

Fig. 166.13 Gene expression in chondrocytes. Quantitative PCR analysis of expression levels of (a) housekeeping gene *β-actin* and (b–d) matrix proteins (normalized to *GAPDH*) in normal (*n* = 9), early degenerative OA (*n* = 6), and late-stage OA (*n* = 6) cartilage. Bars show the mean and SD. Agg, aggrecan; deg, degenerative. (Redrawn with permission from Aigner *et al.*[125])

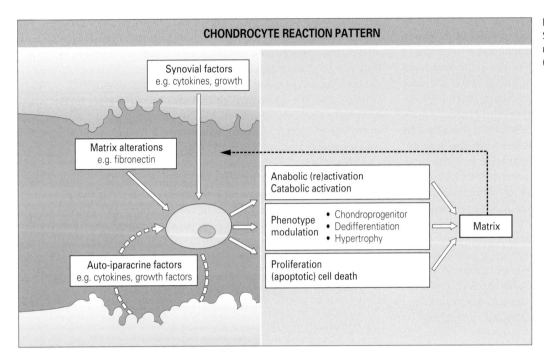

CHONDROCYTE REACTION PATTERN

Synovial factors
e.g. cytokines, growth

Matrix alterations
e.g. fibronectin

Auto-iparacrine factors
e.g. cytokines, growth factors

Anabolic (re)activation
Catabolic activation

Phenotype modulation
• Chondroprogenitor
• Dedifferentiation
• Hypertrophy

Proliferation
(apoptotic) cell death

Matrix

Fig. 166.14 Chondrocyte reaction pattern. Schematic representation of basic chondrocyte reaction pattern and main factors influencing it. (Redrawn with permission from Aigner[128].)

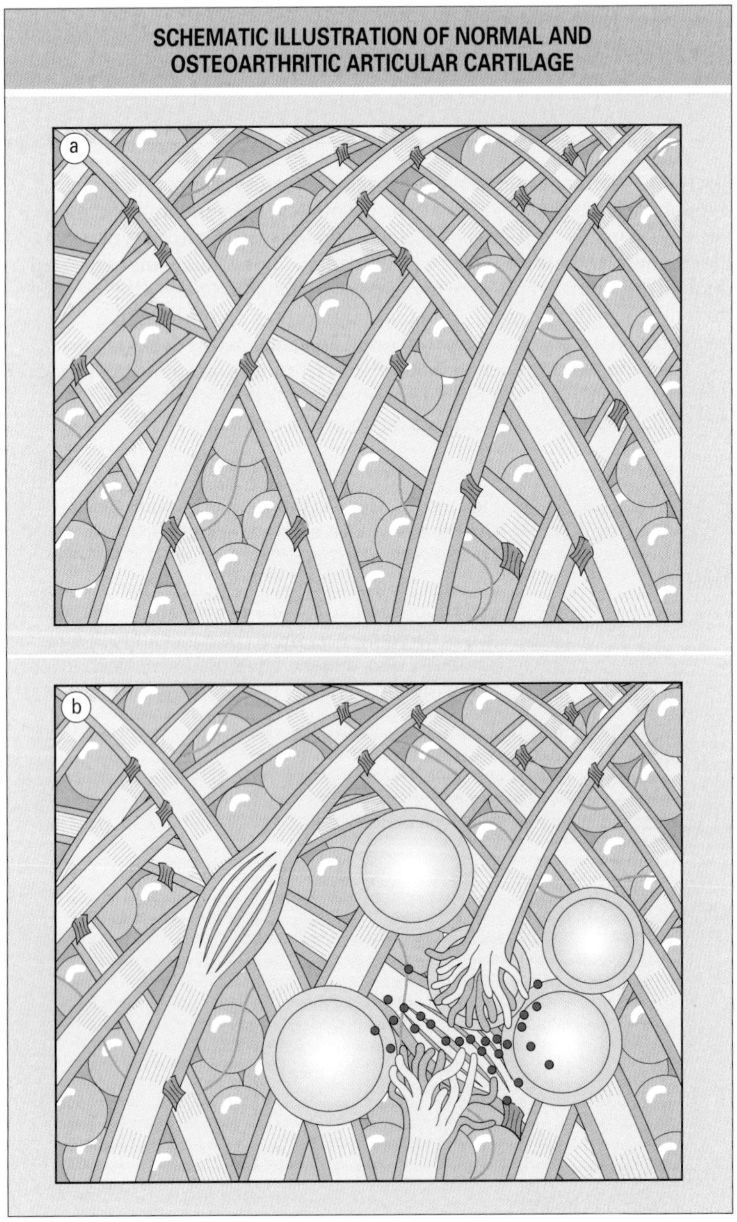

SCHEMATIC ILLUSTRATION OF NORMAL AND OSTEOARTHRITIC ARTICULAR CARTILAGE

a

b

Fig.166.15 Schematic illustration of normal and osteoarthritic articular cartilage. (a) The blue balls denote hydrated but compressed aggrecan monomers that bind non-covalently to hyaluronate (green), thus forming large supramolecular proteoglycan aggregates. The swelling pressure generated by these compressed molecules is counterbalanced by the tight collagen network (orange–brown) which is strengthened by the intercollagen crosslinks (red). This unique composite structure allows healthy articular cartilage to resist major pressure and shear forces. (b) In the early stages of OA, loss of aggrecan molecules allows the remaining proteoglycan molecules to swell and become 'decompressed'. The cartilage becomes softer and the pressure, as well as shear resistance, is diminished, leading to further damage to the collagen network.

MMP-13 were found in late OA. Surprisingly, no MMP-1 and MMP-8 mRNA was detected. As the authors point out, variability was a feature in these experiments and they should not be overinterpreted[125].

SUMMARY

Knowledge regarding the pathogenesis of OA is rapidly increasing as a result of the application of new methodology. The chondrocyte and its surrounding matrix remain a main target of research, based on the prominent role of joint cartilage damage in human and animal OA (Fig. 166.14). As mentioned, aggrecan metabolism is rapid under normal conditions and aggrecan repair is possible. Type II collagen in contrast has a very slow normal turnover, and damage of the collagen fibril network leads to cartilage swelling and irreversible damage (Fig. 166.15). Intricate interactions between cell and matrix and between matrix macromolecules are essential for normal cartilage function and several genetic defects result in disease-prone cartilage. This is well illustrated by COMP mutations, which have been linked to a number of OA-like conditions called pseudoachondrodysplasia and multiple epiphyseal dysplasia. However, deletion of COMP by gene manipulation in mice produced a normal phenotype[126]. This indicates that unknown compensatory measures may wait to be discovered.

Solid information is emerging regarding variations in resistance to OA. Osteoporosis may not exclude affliction with OA. Resistance to development of OA in the ankle is due to a joint-related chondrocyte phenotype that shows a relative resistance to catabolic influences and enhanced response to anabolic signals as provided by OP-1[116,121,127]. The resistance of normal chondrocytes to cell death and the role of apoptosis in human OA are still not fully understood[128]. Improved experimental models, in part based on gene manipulation, and expanding knowledge of the cell biology of joint tissue in particular cartilage have brought cartilage repair a long way from science fiction to clinical reality[129]. Ultimately, however, new insights into the pathogenesis of OA should point to effective strategies for prevention.

REFERENCES

1. Dieppe P. Osteoarthritis. In: Dieppe P, Wollheim FA, Schumacher HR Jr, eds. Classic papers in rheumatology. London: Martin Dunitz; 2002: 256–273.
2. Kuettner KE, Thonar EJ-MA. Cartilage integrity and homeostasis. In: Klippel JH, Dieppe PA. Rheumatology, 2nd ed. London: Mosby; 1998: 8.6.1–8.6.15.
3. Shum L, Nuckolls G. The life cycle of chondrocytes in the developing skeleton. Arthritis Res 2002; 4: 94–106.
4. Kwok C, Weller PA, Guioli S et al. Mutations in SOX9, the gene responsible for Campomelic dysplasia and autosomal sex reversal. Am J Hum Genet 1995; 57: 1028–1036.
5. De Crombrugghe B, Lefebvre V, Nakashima K. Regulatory mechanisms in the pathways of cartilage and bone formation. Curr Opin Cell Biol 2001; 13: 721–727.
6. Takeda S, Bonnamy JP, Owen MJ et al. Continuous expression of Cbfa1 in nonhypertrophic chondrocytes uncovers its ability to induce hypertrophic chondrocyte differentiation and partially rescues Cbfa1-deficient mice. Genes Dev 2001; 15: 467–481.
7. Eyre D. Collagen of articular cartilage. Arthritis Res 2002; 4: 30–35.
8. Roughley PJ. Articular cartilage and changes in arthritis: noncollagenous proteins and proteoglycans in the extracellular matrix of cartilage. Arthritis Res 2001; 3: 342–347.
9. Heinegård D, Lorenzo P, Saxne T. Matrix glycoproteins, proteoglycans, and cartilage. In: Ruddy S, Harris ED Jr, Sledge CB, eds. Kelley's textbook of rheumatology, 6th ed. Philadelphia, PA: WB Saunders; 2001: 41–53.
10. Chen TL, Wang PY, Luo W et al. Aggrecan domains expected to traffic through the exocytic pathway are misdirected to the nucleus. Exp Cell Res 2001; 263: 224–235.
11. Bolton MC, Dudhia J, Bayliss MT. Quantification of aggrecan and link-protein mRNA in human articular cartilage of different ages by competitive reverse transcriptase-PCR. Biochem J 1996; 319: 489–498.
12. Olin AI, Morgelin M, Sasaki T et al. The proteoglycans aggrecan and Versican form networks with fibulin-2 through their lectin domain binding. J Biol Chem 2001; 276: 1253–1261.
13. Maroudas A, Bayliss MT, Uchitel-Kaushansky N, et al. Aggrecan turnover in human articular cartilage: use of aspartic acid racemization as a marker of molecular age. Arch Biochem Biophys 1998; 350: 61–71.
14. Verzijl N, DeGroot J, Bank RA et al. Age-related accumulation of the advanced glycation endproduct pentosidine in human articular cartilage aggrecan: the use of pentosidine levels as a quantitative measure of protein turnover. Matrix Biol 2001; 20: 409–417.
15. Lorenzo P, Bayliss MT, Heinegard D. A novel cartilage protein (CILP) present in the mid-zone of human articular cartilage increases with age. J Biol Chem 1998; 273: 23463–23468.
16. Lorenzo P, Aman P, Sommarin Y, Heinegard D. The human CILP gene: exon/intron organization and chromosomal mapping. Matrix Biol 1999; 18: 445–454.
17. Flannery CR, Hughes CE, Schumacher BL et al. Articular cartilage superficial zone protein (SZP) is homologous to megakaryocyte stimulating factor precursor and Is a multifunctional proteoglycan with potential growth-promoting, cytoprotective, and lubricating properties in cartilage metabolism. Biochem Biophys Res Commun 1999; 254: 535–541.
18. Su JL, Schumacher BL, Lindley KM et al. Detection of superficial zone protein in human and animal body fluids by cross-species monoclonal antibodies specific to superficial zone protein. Hybridoma 2001; 20: 149–157.
19. Oldberg A, Antonsson P, Lindblom K, Heinegard D. COMP (cartilage oligomeric matrix protein) is structurally related to the thrombospondins. J Biol Chem 1992; 267: 22346–22350.
20. DiCesare P, Hauser N, Lehman D et al. Cartilage oligomeric matrix protein (COMP) is an abundant component of tendon. FEBS Lett 1994; 354: 237–240.
21. Smith RK, Zunino L, Webbon PM, Heinegard D. The distribution of cartilage oligomeric matrix protein (COMP) in tendon and its variation with tendon site, age and load. Matrix Biol 1997; 16: 255–271.
22. Briggs MD, Chapman KL. Pseudoachondroplasia and multiple epiphyseal dysplasia: mutation review, molecular interactions, and genotype to phenotype correlations. Hum Mutat 2002; 19: 465–478.
23. Rosenberg K, Olsson H, Morgelin M, Heinegard D. Cartilage oligomeric matrix protein shows high affinity zinc-dependent interaction with triple helical collagen. J Biol Chem 1998; 273: 20397–20403.
24. Sharif M, Saxne T, Shepstone L et al. Relationship between serum cartilage oligomeric matrix protein levels and disease progression in osteoarthritis of the knee joint. Br J Rheumatol 1995; 34: 306–310.
25. Petersson IF, Sandqvist L, Svensson B, Saxne T. Cartilage markers in synovial fluid in symptomatic knee osteoarthritis. Ann Rheum Dis 1997; 56: 64–67.
26. Conrozier T, Saxne T, Fan CS et al. Serum concentrations of cartilage oligomeric matrix protein and bone sialoprotein in hip osteoarthritis: a one year prospective study. Ann Rheum Dis 1998; 57: 527–532.
27. Clark AG, Jordan JM, Vilim V et al. Serum cartilage oligomeric matrix protein reflects osteoarthritis presence and severity: the Johnston County Osteoarthritis Project. Arthritis Rheum 1999; 42: 2356–2364.
28. Salminen H, Perala M, Lorenzo P et al. Up-regulation of cartilage oligomeric matrix protein at the onset of articular cartilage degeneration in a transgenic mouse model of osteoarthritis. Arthritis Rheum 2000; 43: 1742–1748.
29. Pond MJ, Nuki G. Experimentally-induced osteoarthritis in the dog. Ann Rheum Dis 1973; 32: 387–388.
30. Paatsama S Ligament injuries in the canine stifle joint. A clinical and experimental study. Thesis, Helsinki, 1952.
31. Pritzker KP. Animal models for osteoarthritis: processes, problems and prospects. Ann Rheum Dis 1994; 53: 406–420.
32. Brandt KD, Myers SL, Burr D, Albrecht M. Osteoarthritic changes in canine articular cartilage, subchondral bone, and synovium fifty-four months after transection of the anterior cruciate ligament. Arthritis Rheum 1991; 34: 1560–1570.
33. Benske J, Schunke M, Tillmann B. Subchondral bone formation in arthrosis. Polychrome labeling studies in mice. Acta Orthop Scand 1988; 59: 536–541.
34. Mason RM, Chambers MG, Flannelly J et al. The STR/ort mouse and its use as a model of osteoarthritis. Osteoarthritis Cartilage 2001; 9: 85–91.
35. Chambers MG, Kuffner T, Cowan SK et al. Expression of collagen and aggrecan genes in normal and osteoarthritic murine knee joints. Osteoarthritis Cartilage 2002; 10: 51–61.
36. Brandt KD. Animal models of osteoarthritis. Biorheology 2002; 39: 221–235.
37. Salminen H, Vuorio E, Samaanen AH. Expression of Sox9 and type IIA procollagen during attempted repair of articular cartilage damage in a transgenic mouse model of osteoarthritis. Arthritis Rheum 2001; 44: 947–955.
38. Salminen HJ, Saamanen AM, Vankemmelbeke MN et al. Expression of collagen and aggrecan genes in normal and osteoarthritic murine knee joints. Ann Rheum Dis 2002; 61: 591–597.
39. Loeser RF Jr. Aging and the etiopathogenesis and treatment of osteoarthritis. Rheum Dis Clin North Am 2000; 26: 547–567.
40. Guerne PA, Blanco F, Kaelin A et al. Growth factor responsiveness of human articular chondrocytes in aging and development. Arthritis Rheum 1995; 38: 960–968.
41. Martin JA, Buckwalter JA. Telomere erosion and senescence in human articular cartilage chondrocytes. J Gerontol A Biol Sci Med Sci 2001; 56: B172–B179.
42. Piera-Velazquez S, Jimenez SA, Stokes D. Increased life span of human osteoarthritic chondrocytes by exogenous expression of telomerase. Arthritis Rheum 2002; 46: 683–693.
43. Myers SL, Brandt KD, Ehlich JW et al. J Synovial inflammation in patients with early osteoarthritis of the knee. Rheumatol 1990; 17: 1662–1669.
44. Sukenik S, Henkin J, Zimlichman S et al. Serum and synovial fluid levels of serum amyloid A protein and C-reactive protein in inflammatory and noninflammatory arthritis. J Rheumatol 1988; 15: 942–945.
45. Spector TD, Hart DJ, Nandra D et al. Low-level increases in serum C-reactive protein are present in early osteoarthritis of the knee and predict progressive disease. Arthritis Rheum 1997; 40: 723–727.
46. Wolfe F. The C-reactive protein but not erythrocyte sedimentation rate is associated with clinical severity in patients with osteoarthritis of the knee or hip. J Rheumatol 1997; 24: 1486–1488.
47. Conrozier T, Chappuis-Cellier C, Richard M et al. Increased serum C-reactive protein levels by immunonephelometry in patients with rapidly destructive hip osteoarthritis. Rev Rhum Engl Ed 1998; 65: 759–765.
48. Attur MG, Dave M, Akamatsu M et al. Osteoarthritis or osteoarthrosis: the definition of inflammation becomes a semantic issue in the genomic era of molecular medicine. Osteoarthritis Cartilage 2002; 10: 1–4.
49. Pelletier JP, Roughley PJ, DiBattista JA et al. Are cytokines involved in osteoarthritic pathophysiology? Semin Arthritis Rheum 1991; 20(suppl 2): 12–25.
50. Benderdour M, Tardif G, Pelletier JP et al. Interleukin 17 (IL-17) induces collagenase-3 production in human osteoarthritic chondrocytes via AP-1 dependent activation: differential activation of AP-1 members by IL-17 and IL-1β. J Rheumatol 2002; 29: 1262–1272.
51. Caterson B, Flannery CR, Hughes CE, Little CB. Mechanisms involved in cartilage proteoglycan catabolism. Matrix Biol 2000; 19: 333–344.
52. Sandy JD, Flannery CR, Neame PJ, Lohmander LS. The structure of aggrecan fragments in human synovial fluid. Evidence for the involvement in osteoarthritis of a novel proteinase which cleaves the Glu 373–Ala 374 bond of the interglobular domain. J Clin Invest 1992; 89: 1512–1516.
53. Tortorella MD, Burn TC, Pratta MA et al. Purification and cloning of aggrecanase-1: a member of the ADAMTS family of proteins. Science 1999 4; 284: 1664–1666.
54. Abbaszade I, Liu RQ, Yang F et al. Cloning and characterization of ADAMTS11, an aggrecanase from the ADAMTS family. J Biol Chem 1999 Aug 13; 274: 23443–23450.
55. Sztrolovics R, White RJ, Roughley PJ, Mort JS. The mechanism of aggrecan release from cartilage differs with tissue origin and the agent used to stimulate catabolism. Biochem J 2002 1; 362: 465–472.
56. Tortorella MD, Malfait AM, Deccico C, Arner E. The role of ADAM-TS4 (aggrecanase-1) and ADAM-TS5 (aggrecanase-2) in a model of cartilage degradation. Osteoarthritis Cartilage 2001; 9: 539–552.

57. Malfait AM, Liu RQ, Ijiri K *et al*. Inhibition of ADAM-TS4 and ADAM-TS5 prevents aggrecan degradation in osteoarthritic cartilage. J Biol Chem 2002 21; 277: 22201–22208.
58. Yamanishi Y, Boyle DL, Clark M *et al*. Expression and regulation of aggrecanase in arthritis: the role of TGF-beta. J Immunol 2002 1; 168: 1405–1412.
59. Gross J, Lapiere CM. Collagenolytic activity in amphibian tissues: a tissue culture assay. Proc Natl Acad Sci U S A 1962; 48: 1014–1022.
60. Brinckerhoff CE, Matrisian LM. Matrix metalloproteinases: a tail of a frog that became a prince. Nat Rev Mol Cell Biol 2002; 3: 207–214.
61. Mengshol JA, Mix KS, Brinckerhoff CE. Matrix metalloproteinases as therapeutic targets in arthritic diseases: bull's-eye or missing the mark? Arthritis Rheum 2002; 46: 13–20.
62. Neuhold LA, Killar L, Zhao W *et al*. Postnatal expression in hyaline cartilage of constitutively active human collagenase-3 (MMP-13) induces osteoarthritis in mice. J Clin Invest 2001; 107: 35–44.
63. Brewster M, Lewis EJ, Wilson KL *et al*. Ro 32–3555, an orally active collagenase selective inhibitor, prevents structural damage in the STR/ORT mouse model of osteoarthritis. Arthritis Rheum 1998; 41: 1639–1644.
64. Amin AR, Di Cesare PE, Vyas P *et al*. The expression and regulation of nitric oxide synthase in human osteoarthritis-affected chondrocytes: evidence for up-regulated neuronal nitric oxide synthase. J Exp Med 1995 Dec 1; 182: 2097–2102.
65. Clancy RM, Rediske J, Tang X *et al*. Outside-in signaling in the chondrocyte. Nitric oxide disrupts fibronectin-induced assembly of a subplasmalemmal actin/rho A/focal adhesion kinase signaling complex. J Clin Invest 1997; 100: 1789–1796.
66. Van 't Hof RJ, Hocking L, Wright PK, Ralston SH. Nitric oxide is a mediator of apoptosis in the rheumatoid joint. Rheumatology (Oxford) 2000; 39: 1004–1008.
67. Kobayashi K, Mishima H, Hashimoto S *et al*. Chondrocyte apoptosis and regional differential expression of nitric oxide in the medial meniscus following partial meniscectomy. J Orthop Res 2001; 19: 802–808.
68. Clancy R, Varenika B, Huang W *et al*. Nitric oxide synthase/COX cross-talk: nitric oxide activates COX-1 but inhibits COX-2-derived prostaglandin production. J Immunol 2000; 165: 1582–1587.
69. Pelletier JP, Jovanovic DV, Lascau-Coman V *et al*. Selective inhibition of inducible nitric oxide synthase reduces progression of experimental osteoarthritis in vivo: possible link with the reduction in chondrocyte apoptosis and caspase 3 level. Arthritis Rheum 2000; 43: 1290–1299.
70. Amin AR, Attur MG, Thakker GD *et al*. A novel mechanism of action of tetracyclines: effects on nitric oxide synthases. Proc Natl Acad Sci U S A 1996; 93: 14014–14019.
71. Boileau C, Martel-Pelletier J, Jouzeau JY *et al*. Licofelone (ML-3000), a dual inhibitor of 5-lipoxygenase and cyclooxygenase, reduces the level of cartilage chondrocyte death in vivo in experimental dog osteoarthritis: inhibition of pro-apoptotic factors. J Rheumatol 2002; 29: 1446–1453.
72. Del Carlo M Jr, Loeser RF. Nitric oxide-mediated chondrocyte cell death requires the generation of additional reactive oxygen species. Arthritis Rheum 2002; 46: 394–403.
73. Lotz M, Hashimoto S, Kühn K. Mechanisms of chondrocyte apoptosis. Osteoarthritis Cartilage 1999; 7: 389–389.
74. Aigner T, Hemmel M, Neureiter D *et al*. Apoptotic cell death is not a widespread phenomenon in normal aging and osteoarthritis human articular knee cartilage: a study of proliferation, programmed cell death (apoptosis), and viability of chondrocytes in normal and osteoarthritic human knee cartilage. Arthritis Rheum 2001; 44: 1304–1312.
75. Dean G, Hoyland JA, Denton J *et al*. Mast cells in the synovium and synovial fluid in osteoarthritis. Br J Rheumatol 1993; 32: 671–675.
76. Kummer JA, Tak PP, Brinkman BM *et al*. Expression of granzymes A and B in synovial tissue from patients with rheumatoid arthritis and osteoarthritis. Clin Immunol Immunopathol 1994; 73: 88–95.
77. Mehraban F, Lark MW, Ahmed FN *et al*. Increased secretion and activity of matrix metalloproteinase-3 in synovial tissues and chondrocytes from experimental osteoarthritis. Osteoarthritis Cartilage 1998; 6: 286–294.
78. Lindblad S, Hedfors E. Arthroscopic and immunohistologic characterization of knee joint synovitis in osteoarthritis. Arthritis Rheum 1987; 30: 1081–1088.
79. Smith MD, Triantafillou S, Parker A *et al*. Synovial membrane inflammation and cytokine production in patients with early osteoarthritis. J Rheumatol 1997; 24: 365–371.
80. Lindell M, Månsson B, Petersson IF, Saxne T. Serum C-reactive protein and COMP in knee joint osteoarthritis. Arthritis Rheum 2000; 43(suppl): S339.
81. Olmez N, Schumacher HR Jr. Crystal deposition and osteoarthritis. Curr Rheumatol Rep 1999; 1: 107–111.
82. Sanmarti R, Kanterewicz E, Pladevall M *et al*. Analysis of the association between chondrocalcinosis and osteoarthritis: a community based study. Ann Rheum Dis 1996; 55: 30–33.
83. Fam AG, Morava-Protzner I, Purcell C *et al*. Acceleration of experimental lapine osteoarthritis by calcium pyrophosphate microcrystalline synovitis. Arthritis Rheum 1995; 38: 201–210.
84. Reuben PM, Brogley MA, Sun Y, Cheung HS. Molecular mechanism of the induction of metalloproteinases 1 and 3 in human fibroblasts by basic calcium phosphate crystals. Role of calcium-dependent protein kinase C alpha. J Biol Chem 2002; 277: 15190–15198.
85. McCarthy GM, Westfall PR, Masuda I *et al*. Basic calcium phosphate crystals activate human osteoarthritic synovial fibroblasts and induce matrix metalloproteinase-13 (collagenase-3) in adult porcine articular chondrocytes. Ann Rheum Dis 2001; 60: 399–406.
86. Petersson IF, Boegard T, Svensson B *et al*. Changes in cartilage and bone metabolism identified by serum markers in early osteoarthritis of the knee joint. Br J Rheumatol 1998; 37: 46–50.
87. Hulth A. Does osteoarthrosis depend on growth of the mineralized layer of cartilage? Clin Orthop 1993: 19–24.
88. Carlson CS, Loeser RF, Purser CB *et al*. Osteoarthritis in cynomolgus macaques. III: Effects of age, gender, and subchondral bone thickness on the severity of disease. J Bone Miner Res 1996; 11: 1209–1217.
89. Astrom J, Beertema J. Reduced risk of hip fracture in the mothers of patients with osteoarthritis of the hip. J Bone Joint Surg 1992; 74B: 270–271.
90. Hannan MT, Anderson JJ, Zhang Y *et al*. Bone mineral density and knee osteoarthritis in elderly men and women. The Framingham Study. Arthritis Rheum 1993; 36: 1671–1680.
91. Dequeker J. Inverse relationship of interface between osteoporosis and osteoarthritis. J Rheumatol 1997; 24: 795–8.
92. Dequeker J, Mohan S, Finkelman RD *et al*. Generalized osteoarthritis associated with increased insulin-like growth factor types I and II and transforming growth factor beta in cortical bone from the iliac crest. Possible mechanism of increased bone density and protection against osteoporosis. Arthritis Rheum 1993; 36: 1702–1708.
93. Schneider DL, Barrett-Connor E, Morton DJ, Weisman M. One mineral density and clinical hand osteoarthritis in elderly men and women: the Rancho Bernardo study. J Rheumatol 2002; 29: 1467–1472.
94. Karvonen RL, Miller PR, Nelson DA *et al*. Periarticular osteoporosis in osteoarthritis of the knee. J Rheumatol 1998; 25: 2187–2194.
95. Stewart A, Black A, Robins SP, Reid DM. Bone density and bone turnover in patients with osteoarthritis and osteoporosis. J Rheumatol 1999; 26: 622–626.
96. Yamada K, Healey R, Amiel D *et al*. Subchondral bone of the human knee joint in aging and osteoarthritis. Osteoarthritis Cartilage 2002; 10: 360–369.
97. Cocco R, Tofi C, Fioravanti A *et al*. Effects of clodronate on synovial fluid levels of some inflammatory mediators, after intra-articular administration to patients with synovitis secondary to knee osteoarthritis. Boll Soc Ital Biol Sper 1999; 75: 71–76.
98. Van Beuningen HM, van der Kraan PM, Arntz OJ, van den Berg WB. Transforming growth factor-beta 1 stimulates articular chondrocyte proteoglycan synthesis and induces osteophyte formation in the murine knee joint. Lab Invest 1994; 71: 279–290.
99. Scharstuhl A, Glansbeek HL, Van Beuningen HM *et al*. Inhibition of endogenous TGF-β during experimental osteoarthritis prevents osteophyte formation and impairs cartilage repair. J Immunol 2002; 169: 507–514.
100. Okazaki K, Jingushi S, Ikenoue T *et al*. Expression of insulin-like growth factor I messenger ribonucleic acid in developing osteophytes in murine experimental osteoarthritis and in rats inoculated with growth hormone-secreting tumor. Endocrinology 1999; 140: 4821–4830.
101. Hashimoto S, Creighton-Achermann L, Takahashi K *et al*. Development and regulation of osteophyte formation during experimental osteoarthritis. Osteoarthritis Cartilage 2002; 10: 180–187.
102. Vuori IM. Dose-response of physical activity and low back pain, osteoarthritis, and osteoporosis. Med Sci Sports Exerc 2001; 33(suppl): S551–S586.
103. Hurwitz DE, Sumner DR, Block JA. Bone density, dynamic joint loading and joint degeneration. A review. Cells Tissues Organs 2001; 169: 201–209.
104. Felson DT, Hannan MT, Naimark A *et al*. Occupational physical demands, knee bending, and knee osteoarthritis: results from the Framingham Study. J Rheumatol 1991; 18: 1587–1592.
105. McAlindon TE, Wilson PW, Aliabadi P *et al*. Level of physical activity and the risk of radiographic and symptomatic knee osteoarthritis in the elderly: the Framingham study. Am J Med 1999; 106: 151–157.
106. Sharma L, Hurwitz DE, Thonar EJ *et al*. Knee adduction moment, serum hyaluronan level, and disease severity in medial tibiofemoral osteoarthritis. Arthritis Rheum 1998; 41: 1233–1240.
107. Baliunas AJ, Hurwitz DE, Ryals AB *et al*. Increased knee joint loads during walking are present in subjects with knee osteoarthritis. Osteoarthritis Cartilage 2002; 10: 573–579.
108. Lane NE, Lin P, Christiansen L *et al*. Association of mild acetabular dysplasia with an increased risk of incident hip osteoarthritis in elderly white women: the study of osteoporotic fractures. Arthritis Rheum 2000; 43: 400–404.
109. Radin EL, Burr DB, Caterson B *et al*. Mechanical determinants of osteoarthrosis. Semin Arthritis Rheum 1991; 21(suppl 2): 12–21.9.
110. Burr DB. The importance of subchondral bone in osteoarthrosis. Curr Opin Rheumatol 1998; 10: 256–262.
111. Slemenda C, Brandt KD, Heilman DK *et al*. Quadriceps weakness and osteoarthritis of the knee. Ann Intern Med 1997 15; 127: 97–104.
112. Sharma L, Song J, Felson DT *et al*. The role of knee alignment in disease progression and functional decline in knee osteoarthritis. JAMA 2001; 286: 188–195.
113. Sharma L, Pai YC. Impaired proprioception and osteoarthritis. Curr Opin Rheumatol 1997; 9: 253–258.
114. Hassan BS, Mockett S, Doherty M. Static postural sway, proprioception, and maximal voluntary quadriceps contraction in patients with knee osteoarthritis and normal control subjects. Ann Rheum Dis 2001; 60: 612–618.
115. Hassan BS, Mockett S, Doherty M. Influence of elastic bandage on knee pain, proprioception, and postural sway in subjects with knee osteoarthritis. Ann Rheum Dis 2002; 61: 24–28.
116. Kerin A, Patwari P, Kuettner K *et al*. Molecular basis of osteoarthritis: biomechanical aspects. Cell Mol Life Sci 2002; 59: 27–35.
117. Little CB, Ghosh P. Variation in proteoglycan metabolism by articular chondrocytes in different joint regions is determined by post-natal mechanical loading. Osteoarthritis Cartilage 1997; 5: 49–62.
118. Eckstein F, Faber S, Muhlbauer R *et al*. Functional adaptation of human joints to mechanical stimuli. Osteoarthritis Cartilage 2002; 10: 44–50.
119. Salter DM, Millward-Sadler SJ, Nuki G, Wright MO. Differential responses of chondrocytes from normal and osteoarthritic human articular cartilage to mechanical.
120. Häuselmann HJ, Masuda K, Hunziker EB *et al*. Adult human chondrocytes cultured in alginate form a matrix similar to native human articular cartilage. Am J Physiol 1996; 271: C742–52.121.

121. Cole AA, Kuettner KE. Molecular basis for differences between human joints. Cell Mol Life Sci 2002; 59: 19–26.
122. Homandberg GA, Kang Y, Zhang J et al. A single injection of fibronectin fragments into rabbit knee joints enhances catabolism in the articular cartilage followed by reparative responses but also induces systemic effects in the non-injected knee joints. Osteoarthritis Cartilage 2001; 9: 673–683.
123. Homandberg GA, Costa V, Ummadi V, Pichika R. Antisense oligonucleotides to the integrin receptor subunit alpha decrease fibronectin fragment mediated cartilage chondrolysis. Osteoarthritis Cartilage 2002; 10: 381–393.
124. Aigner T, McKenna L. Molecular pathology and pathobiology of osteoarthritic cartilage. Cell Mol Life Sci 2002; 59: 5–18.
125. Aigner T, Zien A, Gehrsitz A et al. Anabolic and catabolic gene expression pattern analysis in normal versus osteoarthritic cartilage using complementary DNA-array technology. Arthritis Rheum 2001; 44: 2777–2789.
126. Svensson L, Aszodi A, Heinegard D et al. Cartilage oligomeric matrix protein-deficient mice have normal skeletal development. Mol Cell Biol 2002; 22: 4366–4371.
127. Eger W, Schumacher BL, Mollenhauer J et al. Human knee and ankle cartilage explants: catabolic differences. J Orthop Res 2002; 20: 526–534.
128. Aigner T, Kim HA. Apoptosis and cellular vitality. Issues in osteoarthritic cartilage degeneration. Arthritis Rheum 2002; 46: 1986–1996.
129. Hunziker EB. Articular cartilage repair: basic science and clinical progress. A review of the current status and prospects. Osteoarthritis Cartilage 2002; 10: 432–463.

167 The genetics of osteoarthritis

Nisha J Manek, Flavia M Cicuttini and Timothy D Spector

- Evidence suggests that genetic factors play a major role in osteoarthritis (OA).

- This genetic influence has now been estimated to be of the order of 50–65% and first-degree relatives have a two- to threefold increased risk of disease

- The nature of the genetic influence in OA is speculative and may involve either a structural defect (i.e. collagen) or alterations in cartilage or bone metabolism

- Mutations in collagen genes have been identified in some rare familial forms of OA that segregate as a simple mendelian genetic trait; however, the genetic basis of the common forms of OA is currently unknown. Finding the genes involved is likely to lead to important therapeutic and diagnostic advances in this most common disabling rheumatic disease

INTRODUCTION

The multifactorial nature of osteoarthritis (OA) is well recognized, with a number of environmental risk factors such as obesity[1], previous injury and meniscectomy[2] being strongly associated with its development. The role of genetic factors in the development of OA has been poorly understood but has recently received considerable attention, aided by our rapidly expanding knowledge of molecular biology. This chapter will review the data that support the role of genetic variation in the common as well as the rare forms of OA.

EVIDENCE FOR INHERITANCE OF OA

For over 50 years a strong genetic component to certain forms of OA has been believed to be present and several clinical studies have been conducted (Table 167.1). In 1941 Stecher[3] demonstrated that Heberden's nodes of the fingers were three times as common in the sisters of 64 affected subjects as in the general population. Subsequently, in 1944 Stecher et al. concluded that these lesions were inherited as a single autosomal dominant gene with a strong female predominance[4].

The most common form of inherited OA is primary generalized OA, which was first described as a clinical entity by Kellgren and Moore in 1952[5]. This form is characterized by the presence of Heberden's and Bouchard's nodes and premature degeneration of articular cartilage, often in a concentric pattern in many joints. Family studies performed in the early 1960s in the UK of 20 male and 32 female probands with generalized OA, based on the presence of five radiologically affected joint groups, suggested that first-degree relatives were twice as likely to have radiographic generalized disease as well[6]. Subsequent studies provided additional evidence for the familial occurrence of Heberden's and Bouchard's nodes and of osteoarthritis involving multiple joints[6]. In a study of 391 cases of OA, 120 patients, largely middle-aged women, were identified as having a polyarthritis characterized by signs of inflammation and acute onset of symptoms. Of these patients, 20% gave a family history of similar joint disease[5]. This and other studies suggested a polygenic form of inheritance rather than a single gene defect to primary generalized OA[5,6].

These earlier studies therefore suggested that specific forms of common OA cluster within families. Lindberg[7] further supported this observation in a retrospective radiographic analysis of hip OA in which siblings of patients who had undergone total hip replacement were noted to have twice the incidence of radiographic hip OA than that of age- and gender-matched controls. Similarly, two other studies found an overall increase in the rate of joint replacement among the patients' siblings compared with their spouses[8,9]. These studies demonstrate that relatives of affected individuals have higher rates of OA than the general population. Clustering within families may either be explained by closely related affected individuals inheriting the same OA-predisposing DNA variants or alleles from their parents, or that they share similar environmental influences.

TABLE 167.1 CLINICAL STUDIES EXAMINING THE INHERITANCE OF OA		
Study	Subjects	Conclusions
Stecher[4]	Hand OA (64 cases)	Frequency of Heberden's nodes 3 times greater in sisters of cases compared with general population
Kellgren and Moore[5]	Generalized OA (391 cases)	20% family history of OA
Keligren et al.[6]	Generalized OA (20 men + 32 women)	First degree relatives 2-fold increased risk of generalized radiologic OA
Lawrence[9]	Radiologic OA (10 twin pairs)	Increased concordance in identical pairs at a number of joint sites
Spector et al.[10]	500 normal female twins (age 45–70 years)	Heritability of radiologic knee and hand OA 39–65%

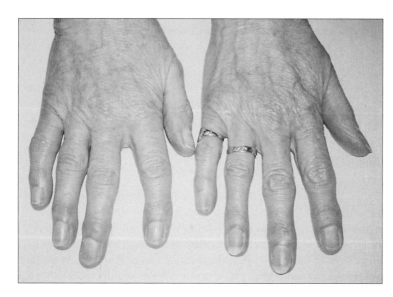

Fig. 167.1 The right hands of a pair of identical twins: note the similarities in Heberden's and Bouchard's nodes

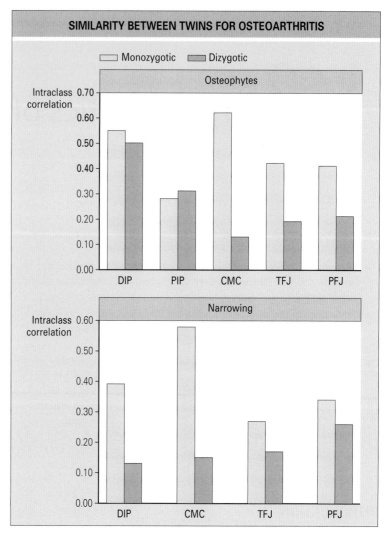

Fig. 167.2 Similarity between twins for osteoarthritis. Correlations between 130 identical (MZ) and 120 non-identical (DZ) female twin pairs for the presence of osteophytes and narrowing at different joint sites. CMC, first carpometacarpal; DIP, distal interphalangeal; PFJ, patellofemoral joint; PIP, proximal interphalangeal; TFJ, tibiofemoral. (From Spector *et al.*[13])

Several studies have examined the inheritance of genetic markers in individuals with primary generalized OA and in their relatives with no disease. A genetic predisposition to primary generalized OA has also been suggested by the association with HLA haplotypes and with α_1 antitrypsin isoform[10]. However, not all studies have found this association[11] and whether there is a true relationship remains unclear.

TWIN AND FAMILY STUDIES

The relative contribution of genetic and environmental factors to common forms of OA affecting the hands and knees remains unclear. A classic twin study is a very useful design to determine the extent to which genetic factors determine variation in the radiographic measures of OA, as twins are uniquely matched for age and for many known or unknown environmental factors. Because monozygotic twins are completely concordant for germline genetic factors, any intrapair variation is assumed to be due to environmental factors, whereas because dizygotic twins share on average half their genes, any intrapair variation is due to both environmental and genetic factors. Thus a comparison of the similarities in monozygotic and dizygotic twins allows us to estimate the extent to which genetic factors determine variation in the measures of OA (Fig. 167.1).

Lawrence[12] briefly reported data from a study of 10 twin pairs that suggested increased concordance in identical pairs at a number of joint sites. Using a cohort of 130 monozygotic and 120 dizygotic female twin pairs, Spector and colleagues[13] observed higher intraclass correlations among monozygotic twins than in dizygotic twins for several clinical and radiographic features of hand and knee OA (Fig. 167.2). The influence of genetic factors was estimated to be between 39% and 65%, independent of known environmental or demographic confounders. This genetic effect was consistent whichever radiographic diagnosis of OA was used (i.e. osteophyte or narrowing) and was also found using a clinical definition based on knee pain or Heberden's nodes. There was a genetic influence at both the tibiofemoral and patellofemoral joints of the knee, though not at the proximal interphalangeal joints of the hands. A similar effect of inheritance was seen when the analyses were limited to osteophytes or narrowing scores separately or to the knee joint alone. The same group carried out a similar study on radiographic hip OA in female twins and found familial clustering attributable to genetic factors for joint space narrowing. The numbers of pairs concordant for definite osteophytes in the sample was too low to assess this feature. A significant heritability of 64% for joint space narrowing and a

heritability of 58% for OA overall at the hip joint was calculated[14]. Acetabular dysplasia has been shown to be associated with a modestly increased risk of incident hip OA[15]. A subsequent twin study has also shown that genetic factors account for most of the variation in acetabular anatomy at the hip joint[16]. This genetic variation was found to be largely due to unique factors with only a small proportion being shared with genetic factors underlying acetabular shape.

These results demonstrate a clear genetic effect for primary OA of the hand and knee in women, with a heritability of up to 65%, independent of environmental or demographic confounders (Fig. 167.2). However, there was no clear evidence to support generalized OA as a separate genetic entity, as the genetic effect for Heberden's nodes, a postulated marker for generalized OA, was similar to that for tibiofemoral and patellofemoral OA.

Large population-based family studies have now confirmed the findings of the twin study with similar heritability estimates for all forms of common OA. Investigators of the Rotterdam study[17] found a strong genetic effect for hand OA and degenerative disc disease in enrolled sibling pairs. The estimated heritabilities were 0.56 for hand OA and 0.75 for disc degeneration. Hirsch and colleagues[18] found a significant correlation for OA with regard to joint location and number of affected joints as well as severity when they examined sibling pairs in the Baltimore Longitudinal Study of Aging cohort. Although no direct esti-

TABLE 167.2 HEREDITARY FORMS OF OA

Primary OA	
Secondary familial	Familial calcium pyrophosphate deposition disease
	Familial hydroxyapatite deposition disease
	Hereditary arthroophthalmopathy (Stickler's syndrome)
	Chondrodysplasias, e.g. achondroplasia
	Spondyloepiphyseal dysplasias
	Multiple epiphyseal dysplasias
	Kniest's dysplasia
	Blount's disease

mation of heritability was done, the risk was estimated at between 0.33 to 0.81. Analysis of the Framingham cohort by Felson and associates[19] suggested a major genetic component for generalized OA incidence that best fit a mendelian recessive model with a multifactorial component (either polygenic or environmental factors), although others have interpreted the data differently[20].

FAMILIAL DISORDERS ASSOCIATED WITH OA

A number of rare subtypes of OA have a genetic basis and have been described as secondary familial forms of OA (Table 167.2).

Familial calcium pyrophosphate deposition disease

Familial calcium pyrophosphate deposition disease (CPPD) is characterized by the deposition of calcium-containing crystals in and around hyaline articulate cartilage and fibrocartilage, leading to arthritis-like symptoms. Early-onset CPPD has been described in several large families in which the disease progresses to severe OA[21]. In these families an autosomal dominant mode of inheritance is observed, with an age at onset between the second and fifth decades[21]. An autosomal recessive CPPD leading to precocious OA has also been described in 13 pedigrees[22]. Genetic linkage analysis has been undertaken to map the disease gene(s) for familial CPPD. A study conducted on a British family with the phenotype of primary chondrocalcinosis and childhood seizures demonstrated genetic linkage to a region of chromosome 5p[23]. A study of a large family from Maine, USA, excluded linkage to the COL2A1 locus; in this family, genetic linkage was demonstrated between CPPD and chromosome 8q[24]. The arthropathy of CPPD has a distinct distribution: it occurs in sites less commonly involved in the usual form of generalized OA, such as the metacarpophalangeal, radioscaphoid, and

patellofemoral joint articulations[25]. For further details on this syndrome, see Chapter 179.

Hydroxyapatite arthritis

Another form of inherited crystal deposition disease is associated with the deposition of hydroxyapatite crystals in articular cartilage. The clinical features and pathologic manifestations of this disease are similar to those of CPPD, except for the nature of the crystals deposited. From the published pedigrees it is clear that this disease also has an autosomal-dominant inherited pattern with full penetrance[26]. This disorder results in periarticular disease in the form of tendinitis or bursitis, and less frequently true articular disease[27,28]. Genetic linkage analyses in families with hydroxyapatite deposition disease have been more limited. A linkage study of a Argentinian family with hydroxyapatite arthritis associated with spondyloepiphyseal dysplasia (SED) excluded several candidate genes, including types II and X collagens[29].

Stickler's syndrome

The classic form of Stickler syndrome was originally described in 1965 by Gunnar Stickler and was termed hereditary progressive arthroophthalmopathy[30]. It is characterized by prominent ocular involvement and severe OA which develops most frequently in the third or fourth decades. This syndrome is a relatively common autosomal-dominant disorder with a prevalence of approximately 1 in 10 000 births. Associated clinical symptoms include myopia, progressive sensorineural hearing loss, cleft palate and mandibular hypoplasia, and epiphyseal dysplasia.

Stickler syndrome is increasingly classified into clinical subtypes that generally reflect the disorder's underlying genetic basis. COL2A1 was a likely candidate gene in early studies of the molecular defect in Stickler syndrome because of its expression in both articular cartilage and the vitreous of the eye. Linkage analysis of several Stickler syndrome kindreds showed that the disease is linked to COL2A1 in some, but not all, affected families[31-33]. Patients with Stickler syndrome who lack eye involvement have mutations in the COL11A2 gene, consistent with this gene's lack of expression in the vitreous of the eye[34]. Furthermore, Stickler syndrome patients with more severe hearing impairment tend to have COL11A1 or COL11A2 mutations rather than COL2A1 mutations[35,36].

Chondrodysplasias

The chondrodysplasias are a group of clinically heterogeneous hereditary disorders characterized by abnormalities in the growth and development of articular and growth plate cartilages. The most common is

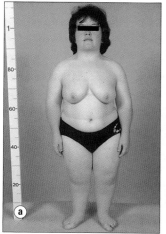
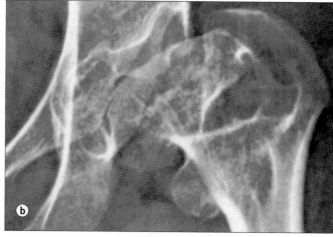
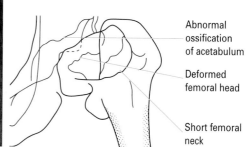

Abnormal ossification of acetabulum

Deformed femoral head

Short femoral neck

Fig.167.3 Epiphyseal dysplasia. (a) A 24-year-old woman with multiple epiphyseal dysplasia who is developing premature OA of the hips. (b) Hip radiograph from another patient with epiphyseal dysplasia showing severe deformation of the acetabulum and femoral head.

achondroplasia, which has a frequency of 1 in 50 000 births and represents the classic form of 'short-limb' dwarfism. Although this often occurs sporadically, it may also be inherited as an autosomal-dominant trait. Mutations have recently been found in the fibroblast growth factor gene[37]. Many laboratories have examined a variety of chondrodysplasias in attempts to link their phenotype with an abnormal genetic locus. Linkage to COL2A1, the gene for type II procollagen, has been demonstrated in some cases but excluded in others[38].

Spondyloepiphyseal dysplasias (SEDs)

The SEDs comprise a heterogeneous group of disorders characterized by abnormal development of the axial skeleton and severe alterations of the epiphyses of the long bones, often resulting in dwarfism. This group of disorders includes autosomal-recessive, autosomal-dominant and X-linked patterns of inheritance. The epiphyseal abnormalities often result in severe, disabling OA in both weightbearing and non-weightbearing joints at a very early age (Fig. 167.3).

Genetic studies reported in 1989 and 1990 showed a linkage between the phenotype of precocious OA/late-onset SED and a mutation in the COL 2A1 gene[39,40]. The first report of a COL2A1 mutation in a kindred with SED was a heterozygous Arg519→Cys base substitution[41]. Four additional families with an identical mutation have now been identified[42].

A second dominant Arg→Cys base substitution at position 75 of the type II collagen triple helix has been identified in another kindred with precocious OA and mild SED[43].

Multiple epiphyseal dysplasias (MEDs)

The MEDs are a heterogeneous group of disorders characterized by alterations in epiphyseal growth that causes irregularity and fragmentation of the epiphyses of long bones. There is minimal or no spinal involvement. The epiphyseal abnormalities result in precocious, crippling OA of both weightbearing and non-weightbearing joints. Multiple joints are usually involved in a symmetrical fashion, particularly involving the knees, hips, hands, wrists and shoulders. Affected individuals typically present in childhood with pain and stiffness in multiple joints and an abnormal gait. The symptoms progress and evolve into severe osteoarthritis. There are no ocular or retinal abnormalities. MED is inherited in an autosomal dominant pattern with high penetrance.

Linkage analysis of some families with MED excluded the genes for collagen types II and VI[44]. However, close linkage to the pericentromeric region of chromosome 19 was observed in some families[45]. Subsequent studies identified mutations in the gene encoding the cartilage oligomeric protein (COMP) in three patients affected with MED and clinically related pseudo achondroplasia[46]. There is now evidence from linkage analysis that a mutation in COL9A1 gene causes MED[47]. This group also found that the phenotypic heterogeneity of MED may be due to locus heterogeneity; the study of four MED families showed recombination between the candidate genes COL9A1, COL9A2, COL9A3 and COMP and the MED phenotype.

Kneist's dysplasia

Kneist's dysplasia is an extremely rare disorder characterized by shortening of the trunk and limbs, flattening of the face and bridge of the nose, protuberance of the eye globes and severe joint abnormalities. This condition has an autosomal dominant pattern of inheritance. The joints are usually very large at birth and continue to enlarge during childhood and early adolescence. The majority of affected individuals develop severe premature osteoarthritis, particularly involving the knees and hips. The articular cartilage is soft and has decreased resilience. Histologically the articular cartilage has large cystic lesions, giving an appearance that has been compared to Swiss cheese. It has been suggested that this disease may result from abnormalities in the processing of type II procollagen, as large inclusions, containing the carboxyl propeptide of type II procol-

lagen, have been found in the dilated rough endoplasmic reticulum[48]. Most of the cases of Kniest dysplasia studied to date demonstrate mutations in the type II procollagen gene[49,50].

Blount's disease

Blount's disease is a rare disorder of the knee joint seen mostly in African and Arab children. Also known as tibia vara or osteochondrosis deformans tibiae, it occurs in two forms: an infantile form which is usually bilateral and develops during the first 3 years of life, and an adolescent form, often unilateral, that develops between the ages of 8 and 15 years. There is local disturbance of growth of the medial aspect of the proximal tibial epiphysis, thought to be due to a combination of growth arrest and trauma and resulting in severe deformities (Fig. 167.4). Although early walking and obesity have been blamed for causing damage to the epiphysis, Siebert and Bray[51] provided evidence for a probable dominant inheritance with variable penetrance.

Blount's disease predisposes to OA of the knees[52]. Classic Blount's disease is both an obvious and a rare cause of OA. However, it is of interest that it has been suggested that more minor forms of local dysplasias of the knee or hip could be a common cause of OA in these joints[53].

Alkaptonuria

Ochronosis (alkaptonuria) is described fully in Chapter 190. It is one of the classic 'inborn errors of metabolism' and is inherited as an autosomal recessive disorder. It leads to the deposition of homogentisic acid pigment in the connective tissues[54]. One of the effects of this is premature OA with an unusual joint distribution, which includes many sites rarely affected by idiopathic OA, including the shoulders and the lateral compartments of the knees.

THE NATURE OF THE GENETIC INFLUENCE IN OA: A ROLE FOR TYPE II PROCOLLAGEN

The nature of the genetic influence in the rarer subtypes of OA discussed above confirms the importance of the integrity of collagen and cartilage as well as bone metabolism in normal healthy joints. Alterations in the structure and function of these tissues undoubtedly predispose to OA, which is often severe. The abnormal bone and joint anatomy characteristic of these disorders (epi- and metaphyseal dysplasia, genu varum and valgum, coxa vara and valga) predisposes to the biomechanical overload of some joints. The cartilage and subchondral bone are often defective, especially as a result of mutations in the collagen genes, particularly COL2A1[55,56]. Several other factors are considered which suggest that the failure of the collagenous component of articular cartilage may be responsible for the degeneration of joint tissue in OA:

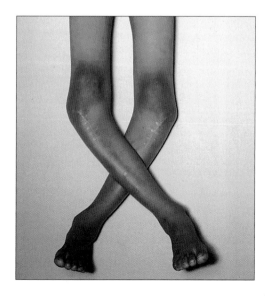

Fig. 167.4 Blount's disease: note the marked varus deformity of the knee joints due to underdevelopment of the medial tibial condyle.

- Collagen plays an important role in the maintenance of the biomechanical properties of cartilage.
- The normal assembly of cartilage collagen serves as a mechanical constraint to prevent the expansion of the highly hydrated proteoglycans into the large hydrodynamic domains that are characteristic of proteoglycans free in solution.
- Articular cartilage contains a remarkable degree of molecular complexity with regard to the number of biochemical species of collagen.
- A failure of normal assembly of cartilage collagen, the main component of the organic matrix of articular cartilage, would result in increased hydration of the tissue, softening of the matrix and cartilage degradation.

OTHER CANDIDATE GENES

New genetic and molecular biological research might enable a better understanding of some forms of idiopathic OA. Although the available studies provide conclusive evidence that mutations in COL2A1 are present in affected individuals from some families who display the phenotype of primary generalized OA and mild spondyloepiphyseal dysplasia, other studies have shown that COL2A1 is not the disease locus in other families with OA[55]. Primary generalized OA may be a heterogeneous disease at the genetic level, and mutations in genes other than COL2A1 are likely to be responsible for this phenotype. For example, yet to be fully explored is the role of mutations in the genes encoding the minor collagen types (e.g. types IX, X, XI). Transgenic mouse models with a central deletion in the α_1 chain of the type IX collagen gene suggest that this gene may be important, as heterozygous mice develop OA with no signs of chondrodysplasia[57]. Also, the role of genes influencing the other extracellular matrix proteins, such as aggrecan, decorin and the link protein, will need to be investigated.

One of the most consistent candidates for OA from association studies has been the vitamin D receptor gene (a well recognized candidate gene for osteoporosis), although results differed when subjects were defined by osteophytes or joint space[58,59] or site of OA[60]. Another potential candidate related to bone is transforming growth factor (TGF)-β, which has been found to have a small effect on bone density[61] and an association with disk degeneration[62]. Lumbar disc degeneration has also been associated with mutations in the gene for collagen type IX in the Finnish population[63]. Other candidate genes include estrogen receptor genes, aggrecan, CRT, tumor necrosis factor (TNF) and interleukin (IL)-1.

EVIDENCE FOR GENETIC ABNORMALITIES IN COMMON FORMS OF OA

There is currently little evidence that the common forms of OA are due to collagen mutations. Ritvaniemi and colleagues[56] evaluated COL2A1 in 45 patients with familial OA and found a single putative mutation. This result suggests that among patients with common OA the incidence of COL2A1 mutations is low, probably below 2%.

A recent study used gene-specific highly polymorphic markers and affected sibling pair analyses to investigate genetic linkage between generalized OA (GOA) and three cartilage matrix genes: COL2A1, which encodes type II collagen; CRTL1, which encodes the cartilage link protein; and CRTM, which encodes the cartilage matrix protein[64]. The analyses showed no linkage between GOA and the three genes in the 38 sibling pairs examined. These results suggest that COL2A1, CRTL1 and CRTM are not major susceptibility loci for GOA, although the power of the study to detect more modest effects was low.

THE HETEROGENEITY OF OA

Previous chapters have stressed the heterogeneity of the expression of OA. In this context it is interesting to note that rare genetic causes, such as families with a defect of COL2A1, or those with alkaptonuria, develop a different disorder from that commonly seen in idiopathic OA. The distribution of joints affected is different (with early involvement of the shoulders and predominant lateral tibiofemoral disease at the knee, for example), and the condition starts much earlier in life than in the majority of sporadic cases. This has led to the suggestion that there are three distinct forms of OA:

- Where trauma to a single site is the major cause, resulting in premature disease of a single site;
- Where a genetic defect is the major cause, resulting in a generalized condition at a number of sites; and
- Sporadic disease of the elderly, which is age-related and in which distribution is determined by evolutionary aspects of the development of our musculoskeletal system[65]. In fact all three 'subtypes' are likely still to be determined by both genetic and environmental influences, although the genes are likely to be different and may also be site specific. In any case, the genetic predisposition to common age-related sporadic forms of OA is likely to be quite different from the genetic (often monogenic) defects described in the rare premature familial cases.

SUMMARY

The improvement in genetic techniques in the past 10 years has enabled us to identify a number of genes that can cause OA associated with skeletal disease. There have been tremendous efforts directed to finding genes that confer risk for both rare and common forms of OA. The study of the genetics of OA is likely to be beneficial in several ways. First, the study of OA associated with simple mendelian genetic disease phenotypes will help confirm the role of a gene or protein whose importance has been suspected. Second, the study of these heritable disorders will help identify new genes, proteins and biologic pathways that are essential to normal skeletal growth and function.

Third, genetic studies will identify patients and families at highest risk for the development of OA because they segregate a disease predisposing allele. Because of clinical homogeneity, these individuals with disease predisposing mutations can facilitate the evaluation of new biologic markers that are being developed as measures of disease status. Validating the usefulness of a biologic marker in a well-defined population at highest risk of developing OA may hasten the marker's application among individuals at low or moderate risk of development of common OA. The presymptomatic diagnosis of individuals at high risk of developing OA has practical importance with respect to genetic and occupational counseling. Lastly, uncovering genes for OA is likely to lead to discoveries of novel pathways that might provide new therapeutic tools for preventing or treating OA. The next decade will provide genomic tools, such as rapid cheap genotyping on a large scale, that facilitate our ability to study complex skeletal diseases such as common OA, in which the phenotype may be subtle, the number of contributing genes large and the pattern of inheritance unclear.

REFERENCES

1. Anderson JJ, Felson DT. Factors associated with osteoarthritis of the knee in the first national health and nutrition examination survey (NHANES I). Am J Epidemiol 1988; 128: 179–189.
2. Cooper C, McAlindon T, Snow S et al. Mechanical and constitutional factors for symptomatic knee osteoarthritis: differences between medial tibiofemoral and patellofemoral disease. J Rheumatol 1994; 21: 307–313.
3. Stecher RM. Heberden's nodes. Heredity in hypertrophic arthritis of the finger joints. Am J Med Sci 1941; 201: 801–812.
4. Stecher RM, Hersh AH, Hauser H. Heberden's nodes; the mechanisms of inheritance in hypertrophic arthritis of the fingers. J Clin Invest 1944; 23: 699–704.
5. Kellgren JH, Moore R. Generalized osteoarthritis and Heberden's nodes. Br J Med 1952; 1: 181–187.
6. Kellgren JH, Lawrence JS, Bier F. Genetic factors in generalised osteoarthritis. Ann Rheum Dis 1963; 22: 237–255.
7. Lindberg H. Prevalence of primary coxarthrosis in siblings of patients with primary coxarthrosis. Clin Orthop 1986; 203: 273–275.
8. Chitnavis J, Sinsheimer JS, Clipsham K et al. Genetic influences in end-stage osteoarthritis – sibling risks of hip and knee replacement for idiopathic osteoarthritis. J Bone Joint Surg [Br] 1997; 79: 660–664.
9. Lanyon P, Muir K, Doherty S, Doherty M. Assessment of a genetic contribution to osteoarthritis of the hip: sibling study. Br Med J 2000; 321: 1179–1183.
10. Pattrick M, Manhire A, Ward M, Doherty M. HLA-A, B antigens and alpha-1-antitrypsin phenotypes in nodal and generalized osteoarthritis and erosive osteoarthritis. Ann Rheum Dis 1989; 48: 470–475.
11. Ercilla MG, Brancos MA, Breysse G et al. HLA antigens in Forestier's disease, ankylosing spondylitis, and polyarthrosis of the hands. J Rheumatol 1977; 4(Suppl 3): 89–93.
12. Lawrence JS. Rheumatism in populations. London: Heinemann; 1977; 144–155.
13. Spector TD, Cicuttini F, Baker J, Hart DJ. Genetic influences on osteoarthritis in women: a twin study. Br Med J 1996; 312; 940–944.
14. MacGregor AJ, Antoniades L, Matson M et al. The genetic contribution to radiographic hip osteoarthritis in women. Results of a classic twin study. Arthritis Rheum 2000; 43: 2410–2416.
15. Lane NE, Lin P, Christiansen L et al. Association of mild acetabular dysplasia with and increased risk of incident hip osteoarthritis in elderly white women: the study of osteoporotic fractures. Arthritis Rheum 2000; 43: 400–404.
16. Antoniades L, Spector TD, MacGregor AJ. The genetic contribution to hip morphometry and relationship to hip cartilage thickness. Osteoarthritis Cartilage 2001; 9: 593–595.
17. Bijkerk C, Houwing-Duisterman JJ, Valkenburg HA et al. Heritabilities of radiologic osteoarthritis in peripheral joints and of disc degeneration of the spine. Arthritis Rheum 1999; 42: 1729–1735.
18. Hirsch R, Lethbridge-Cejku M, Hanson R et al. Familial aggregation of osteoarthritis: data from the Baltimore Longitudinal Study on Aging. Arthritis Rheum 1998; 41: 1227–1232.
19. Felson DT, Couropmitree NN, Chaisson CE et al. Evidence for a Mendelian gene in a segregation analysis of generalized radiographic osteoarthritis: the Framingham Study. Arthritis Rheum 1998; 41: 1064–1071.
20. Spector TD, Snieder H, Keen R et al. Interpreting the results of a segregation analysis of generalised radiographic osteoarthritis: comment on the article by Felson et al. Arthritis Rheum 1999; 42: 1068–1070.
21. Ryan LM, McCarty DJ. Calcium pyrophosphate crystal deposition disease: pseudo-gout; articular chondrocalcinosis. In: McCarty DJ, Koopman WJ, eds. Arthritis and allied conditions, 12th edn. Philadelphia: Lea & Febiger; 1993; 1835–1855.
22. Rodriguez-Valverde V, Zuniga M, Casanueva B et al. Hereditary articular chondrocalcinosis. Clinical and genetic features in 13 pedigrees. Am J Med 1988; 84: 101–106.
23. Hughes AE, McGibbon D, Woodward E et al. Localisation of a gene for chondrocalcinosis to chromosome 5p. Hum Mol Genet 1995; 4: 1225–1228.
24. Baldwin CT, Farrer LA, Adair R et al. Linkage of early onset osteoarthritis and chondrocalcinosis to human chromosome 8q. Am J Hum Genet 1995; 56: 692–697.
25. Riestra JL, Sanchez A, Rodriguez-Valverde V et al. Radiographic features of hereditary articular chondrocalcinosis. A comparative study with the sporadic type. Clin Exp Rheumatol 1988; 6: 369–372.
26. Hajiroussou VJ, Webley M. Familial calcific periarthritis. Ann Rheum Dis 1986; 42: 469–470.
27. Dieppe PA, Huskisson EC, Crocker P, Willoughby DA. Apatite deposition disease: a new arthropathy. Lancet 1976; 1: 266–269.
28. Ferri S, Zanardim M, Barozzi L et al. Familial apatite deposition disease (FADD) in a Northern-Italian kindred. Arthritis Rheum 1994; 37: S413.
29. Marcos JC, Arturi AS, Babini C et al. Familial hydroxyapatite chondrocalcinosis with spondyloepiphyseal dysplasia: Clinical course and absence of genetic linkage to the type II procollagen gene. J Clin Rheumatol 1995; 1: 171–178.
30. Stickler GB, Belau PG, Farrell FJ et al. Hereditary progressive arthro-ophthalmopathy. Mayo Clin Proc 1965; 40: 433–455.
31. Francomano CA, Liberfarb RM, Hirose T et al. The Stickler syndrome: evidence for close linkage to the structural gene for type II collagen. Genomics 1987; 1: 293–296.
32. Knowlton RG, Weaver EJ, Struyk AF et al. Genetic linkage analysis of hereditary arthro-ophthalmopathy (Stickler syndrome) and the type II procollagen gene. Am J Hum Genet 1989; 45: 681–688.
33. Bonaventure J, Philippe C, Plessie G et al. Linkage study in a large pedigree with Stickler syndrome: exclusion of COL2A1 as the mutant gene. Hum Genet 1992; 90: 164–168.
34. Vikkula M, Mariman ECM, Lui VCH et al. Autosomal dominant and recessive osteochondrodysplasia associated with the (COL11A2) locus. Cell 1995; 80: 431–437.
35. Annunen S, Korkko J, Czarny M et al. Splicing mutations of 54-bp exons in the COL11A1 gene cause Marshall syndrome, but other mutations cause overlapping Marshall/Stickler phenotypes. Am J Hum Genet 1999; 65: 974–983.
36. Melkoniemi M, Brunner HG, Manouvrer S et al. Autosomal recessive disorder otospondylomegaepiphyseal dysplasia is associated with loss-of-function mutations in the COLL11A2 gene. Am J Hum Genet 2000; 66: 368–377.
37. Shiang R, Thompson LM, Zhu Y-Z et al. Mutations in the transmembrane domain of FGFR3 cause the most common genetic form of dwarfism, achondroplasia. Cell 1994; 78: 335–342.
38. Wordsworth P, Ogilvie P, Priestley L et al. Structural and segregational analysis of the type II collagen gene (COL2A1) in some heritable chondrodysplasias. J Med Genet 1988; 25: 521–527.
39. Palotie A, Vaisanen P, Ott J et al. Predisposition to familial osteoarthritis linked to type II collagen gene. Lancet 1989; i: 924–927.
40. Knowlton RG, Katzenstein PL, Moskowitz RW et al. Genetic linkage of a polymorphism in the type II collagen gene (COL2A1) to primary osteoarthritis associated with a mild chondrodysplasia. N Engl J Med 1990; 322: 526–530.
41. Alla-Kokko L, Baldwin CT, Moskowitz RW, Prockop DJ. A single base mutation in the type II procollagen gene (COL2A1) as cause of primary osteoarthritis associated with a mild chondrodysplasia. Proc Natl Acad Sci USA 1990; 87: 6565–6568.
42. Bleasel JF, Holderbaum D, Brancolini V et al. Five families with Arg 519 to cysteine mutation in COL2A1: evidence for three distinct founders. Hum Mut 1998; 12: 172–176.
43. Williams CJ, Rock M, Considine E et al. Three new point mutations in type II procollagen (COL2A1) and identification of a fourth family with the COL2A1 Arg519 to Cys base substitution using conformation sensitive gel electrophoresis. Hum Mol Genet 1995; 4: 309–312.
44. Weaver EJ, Summerville GP, Yeh G et al. Exclusion of type II and type IV procollagen gene mutations in a five-generation family with multiple epiphyseal dysplasia. Am J Med Genet 1993; 45: 345–352.
45. Oehlman R, Summerville GP, Yeh G et al. Genetic linkage mapping of multiple epiphyseal dysplasia to the pericentric region of chromosome 19. Am J Hum Genet 1994; 54: 3–10.
46. Briggs MD, Hoffinan SMG, King LM et al. Pseudo achondroplasia and multiple epiphyseal dysplasia due to mutations in the cartilage oligomeric matrix protein gene. Nature Genet 1995; 10: 330–336.
47. Czarny-Ratajczak M, Lohiniva J, Rogala P et al. A mutation in COL9A1 cause multiple epiphyseal dysplasia. Further evidence for locus heterogeneity in MED. (in press).
48. Poole AR, Pidoux I, Reine A et al. Kniest dysplasia is characterized by an apparent abnormal processing of the C-propeptide of type II cartilage collagen resulting in imperfect fibril assembly. J Clin Invest 1988; 81: 579–589.
49. Bogaert R, Wilkin DJ, Wilcox WR et al. Expression in cartilage of a seven amino acid deletion in type II collagen from two unrelated individuals with Kniest dysplasia. Am J Hum Genet 1994; 55: 1128–1136.
50. Winterpacht A, Hilbert M, Schwarze U et al. Kniest and Stickler dysplasia phenotypes caused by collagen type II gene (COL2A1) defects. Nature Genet 1993; 3: 323–326.
51. Siebert JR, Bray PT. Probable dominant inheritance of Blount's disease. Clin Genet 1977; 11: 394–401.
52. Zayer M. Osteoarthritis following Blount's disease. Int Orthop 1980; 4: 63–66.
53. Cooke D, Saidamore A, Li J et al. Axial lower-limb alignment: comparison of knee geometry in normal volunteers and osteoarthritis patients. Osteoarthritis Cartilage 1997; 5: 39–48.
54. Hamdi N, Cooke TD, Hassan B. Ochronotic arthropathy: case report and review of the literature. Int Orthop 1999; 23: 122–125.
55. Williams CJ, Jimenez SA. Heritable diseases of cartilage caused by mutations in collagen genes. J Rheumatol 1995; 22(Suppl 43): 28–33.
56. Ritvaniemi P, Korkko I, Bonaventure et al. Identification of COL2A1 gene mutations with chondrodysplasias and familial osteoarthritis. Arthritis Rheum 1995; 38: 999–1004.
57. Nakata K, Ono K, Miyazaki J et al. Osteoarthritis associated with mild chondrodysplasia in transgenic mice expressing αI(IX) collagen chains with a central deletion. Proc Natl Acad Sci USA 1993; 90: 2870–2874.
58. Keen RW, Hart DJ, Lanchbury JS, Spector TD. Association of early osteoarthritis of the knee with a Taq I polymorphism of the vitamin D receptor gene. Arthritis Rheum 1997; 40: 1444–1449.
59. Uitterlinden AG, Burger H, Huang Q et al. Vitamin D receptor genotype is associated with radiographic osteoarthritis at the knee. J Clin Invest 1997; 100: 259–263.
60. Jones G, White C, Sambrook P, Eisman J. Allelic variation in the vitamin D receptor, lifestyle factors and lumbar spinal degenerative disease. Ann Rheum Dis 1998; 57: 94–99.
61. Keen RW, Snieder H, Molloy H et al. Evidence of association and linkage disequilibrium between a novel polymorphism in the transforming growth factor beta 1 gene and hip bone mineral density: a study of female twins. Rheumatology (Oxford) 2001; 40: 48–54.
62. Yamada Y, Okuizumi H, Miyauchi A et al. Association of transforming growth factor beta1 genotype with spinal osteophytosis in Japanese women. Arthritis Rheum 2000; 43: 452–460.
63. Paassilta P, Lohiniva J, Goring HH et al. Identification of a novel common genetic risk factor for lumbar disk disease. JAMA 2001; 285: 1843–1849.
64. Loughlin J, Irven C, Fergusson C, Sykes B. Sibling pair analysis shows no linkage of generalized osteoarthritis to the loci encoding type II collagen, cartilage link protein or cartilage metrix protein. Br J Rheumatol 1994; 33: 1103–1106.
65. Dieppe PA. Therapeutic targets on osteoarthritis. J Rheumatol 1995; 22(Suppl 43): 136–139.

OSTEOARTHRITIS AND RELATED DISORDERS

168 Imaging

Christopher Buckland-Wright

- Plain radiography is the most reliable method of imaging in clinical practice, for diagnosis and grading severity, and in assessing disease progression in osteoarthritis
- Ultrasonography is used for evaluating synovial hypertrophy, tendons and other soft tissue changes
- Arthroscopy visualizes changes to the surface of the articular cartilage and other intra-articular structures
- Radionucleotide scintigraphy can be used to assess disease activity in soft tissues and bone, particularly osteophytosis and subchondral sclerosis
- Magnetic resonance imaging provides anatomical imaging of all tissues and can provide quantification of lesions and assessment of biochemical changes in the tissue

INTRODUCTION

The osteoarthritic diseases are a group of disorders which, despite different causes, result in anatomical changes to the synovial joint, leading to the characteristic pathologic features of osteoarthritis (OA) (Fig. 168.1). The emphasis that many authors place on loss of articular cartilage thickness underscores its significance as a principal component within the disease process. However, OA is a condition affecting the synovial joint, and in particular the osteochondral junction, and changes in the cartilage are inseparable from those in bone. There are two principal modalities used to image the changes in OA joints and which form the basis of this chapter. They are:

- Anatomical imaging, such as radiography, ultrasonography and arthroscopy, which detects structural alterations that have already occurred in the joint.
- Physiological imaging of radionucleotide scans and magnetic resonance imaging (MRI), which provide an assessment of the dynamic disease processes that cause these changes.

ANATOMICAL IMAGING

Plain radiographs

Plain radiographs are the most important imaging method in OA. They are widely available, inexpensive and readily understood. The radiograph examinations have three purposes: (1) to establish the diagnosis or severity of OA, (2) to monitor disease activity, progression and possible therapeutic responses and (3) to look for complications of the disorder or of treatment.

Good quality radiography is essential to achieve these aims, because this determines whether small anatomical changes, characteristic of the disease process, are detected[1,2]. Radiographic image quality is influenced by the sensitivity of the imaging system and the radiographic view. The latter is the most important of these, because it must be constant both within and between patient examinations. Failure to standardize the radioanatomic positioning of the joint between examinations will lead to distortion in the features recorded in the radiograph[1–3]. For example variation in joint flexion will affect the assessment of the joint space width (Fig. 168.2), and joint rotation can result in osteophytes appearing either larger or smaller at successive examinations[3]. The recommended methods for radiography of the different joints are described below.

Radiographic features of osteoarthritis

X-ray features of OA in the early stages of the disease must be distinguished from age-related changes in joint anatomy. These include a degree of subchondral trabecular condensation, the presence of small hard spurs at the joint margin and in the knee, spiking of the tibial spines. Such features do not, however, alter greatly over time. In contrast, in OA, subchondral sclerosis and osteophytosis are generally the earliest radiographic features. They increase with time in both extent and size[4,5], and precede articular cartilage loss, which is detected radiographically as joint space narrowing[5,6] (Fig. 168.3). The temporal separation in the appearance of these features is primarily due to the rich blood supply of the bone, which permits bone to make an early response to the altered conditions in the joint. By contrast, the detection of joint space narrowing requires the physical loss of the articular cartilage, which occurs at a later stage of the disease[4,5,6]. Importantly, it is the range of anatomical changes, rather than the presence of any one single item, that assists in the confirmation of a diagnosis.

Osteophytosis

Osteophyte formation occurs as outgrowths at sites where mechanical load is minimal[8]. It thus appears at articular margins, capsular insertions and at central articular regions in the unloaded region of joints[9] (Fig. 168.3). Localized osteopenia at the periarticular region occurs immediately adjacent to sites of osteophyte formation[9], from an increased vascular supply associated with new bone formation. The degree of bony changes seen in OA may vary between patients, from 'hypertrophic' to 'atrophic' (Fig. 168.4).

Subchondral bone sclerosis

Increased subchondral cortical plate thickness and subjacent trabecular sclerosis are also among the earliest changes of OA. Sclerosis is greater at concave than at convex articular surfaces, and increases in extent and density with disease progression[6,7]. Reduced bone mineral density has been detected in the subarticular region in the knee below the trabecular sclerosis[10], which appeared osteoporotic (Fig. 168.3).

Joint space narrowing

The 'interbone distance' reflects articular cartilage thickness in load-bearing views of the joint[1,2]. Joint space narrowing is focal and not uniform, reflecting compression of the biomechanically weakened articular cartilage in joints with early to moderately advanced disease[1,5,6].

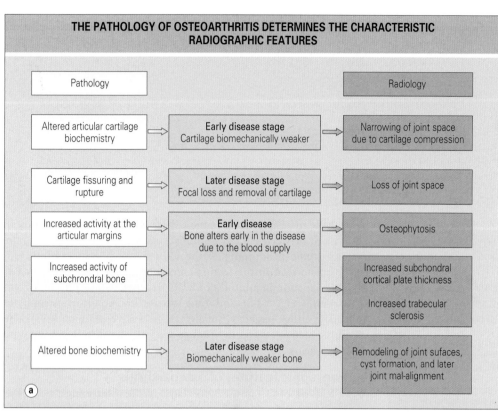

THE PATHOLOGY OF OSTEOARTHRITIS DETERMINES THE CHARACTERISTIC RADIOGRAPHIC FEATURES

Pathology		Radiology
Altered articular cartilage biochemistry	**Early disease stage** Cartilage biomechanically weaker	Narrowing of joint space due to cartilage compression
Cartilage fissuring and rupture	**Later disease stage** Focal loss and removal of cartilage	Loss of joint space
Increased activity at the articular margins	**Early disease** Bone alters early in the disease due to the blood supply	Osteophytosis
Increased activity of subchrondral bone		Increased subchondral cortical plate thickness Increased trabecular sclerosis
Altered bone biochemistry	**Later disease stage** Biomechanically weaker bone	Remodeling of joint sufaces, cyst formation, and later joint mal-alignment

Fig. 168.1 **The pathology of OA determines the characteristic radiographic features.** (a) identifies those features that are visualized in the plain radiograph of joints with early and late stage disease. OA is a disease affecting the osteochondral junction which leads to the appearance in the radiograph of subchondral sclerosis and osteophyte formation. Loss of articular cartilage appears later as a narrowing of the interbone distance on a radiograph. (b) is a radiograph of a healthy knee with normal anatomy and (c) with late disease showing most of the features listed in (a).

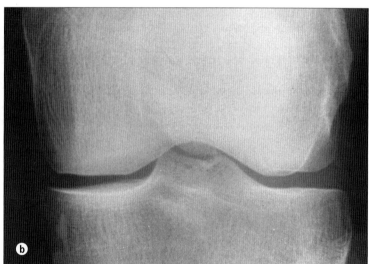

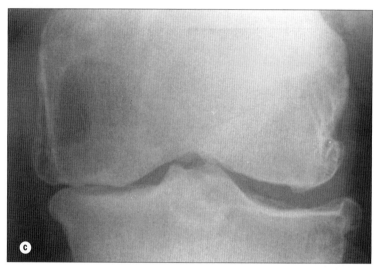

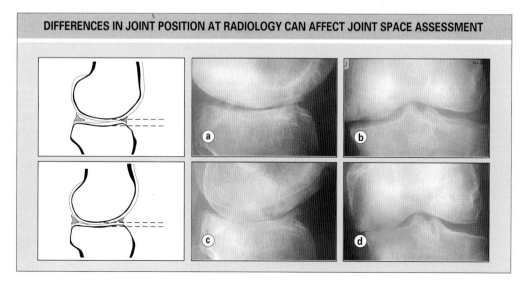

DIFFERENCES IN JOINT POSITION AT RADIOLOGY CAN AFFECT JOINT SPACE ASSESSMENT

Fig. 168.2 **Differences in joint position at radiography can affect joint space assessment.** The illustration shows focal cartilage loss occurring at the central and posterior surfaces of the femur and tibia. With the knee extended (top row), radiography does not reveal joint space narrowing, but in the semiflexed position (bottom row) joint space narrowing is detected. With advanced disease, when no cartilage is left, lateral radiographs in the standing extended knee view (a) show that the femoral condyle sits forward on the anterior rim of the tibial plateau, producing a gap visible as a joint space in the anteroposterior view (b). Conversely, in the same knee radiographed at the same visit in the semi-flexed view, the femoral condyle occupies the central region of the tibial plateau (c) where there is no cartilage present, and consequently no joint space is visible in the anteroposterior view (d). Articular cartilage thickness is not reliably assessed in the extended knee view. (b) A small subchondral cyst is visible in the medial femoral condyle.

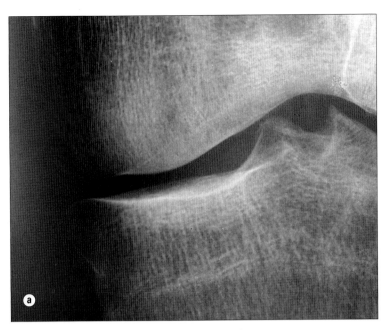
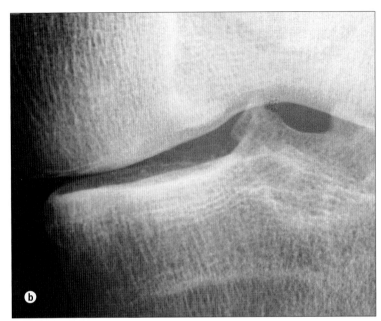

Fig. 168.3 Radiographic progression in the anatomical features of OA. Part of macroradiographs (reduced) showing the medial compartment in osteoarthritic knees. (a) Early disease: joint space width >3mm. (b) Definite disease: joint space width <3mm. With progressive joint space loss, there is an increase in the thickness of the subchondral cortical plate and subjacent horizontal trabeculae, resulting in a ladder-like appearance. Periarticular osteopenia in (a) is present adjacent to the developing marginal osteophyte; the osteopenia is not visible in (b), as osteophytic growth appears to have halted. Osteophyte formation at the tibial spine appears as an irregular outgrowth in (a) and as a clearly defined feature in (b). A marginal osteophyte at the posterior rim of the tibia is also visible in (b).

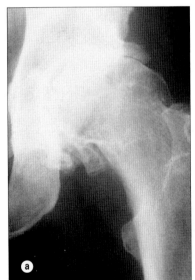
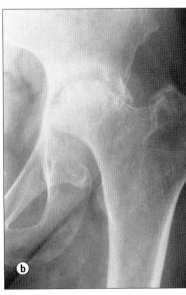
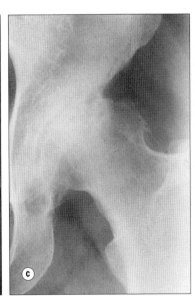
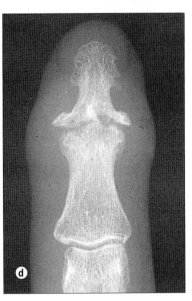

Fig. 168.4 The range of radiographic changes seen in OA. (a) In 'hypertrophic' OA of the hip there is concentric narrowing of the joint space, with extensive osteophytosis and subchondral bone sclerosis characteristic of the marked bony reaction at this end of the spectrum of OA changes. (b) 'Atrophic' or destructive OA of the hip: the other end of the spectrum of changes in OA. Some joints show destruction of subchondral bone, with a relative paucity of osteophyte formation in association with joint space narrowing. (c) 'Secondary' OA of the hip. Here the cause of the OA is a dysplastic hip, with a shallow acetabulum and uncovering of the head of the femur, resulting in OA of the upper pole of the joint, with joint space narrowing, subchondral sclerosis of bone, cysts and osteophytosis. (d) 'Erosive' OA at this distal interphalangeal joint shows that, apart from the joint space narrowing, subchondral sclerosis and osteophytosis, there is loss of the cortical margin, central erosions and marked soft tissue swelling.

Marked joint space narrowing, attributed to tissue loss, is more typical of later stages of the disease[4,5,6] (Figs 168.2 & 168.3b).

Subchondral radiolucencies

Radiolucencies in the subchondral bone are a frequent finding, and fall into two main categories: (1) juxta-articular radiolucencies, similar to erosions, which are associated with a low-grade inflammation[4], and (2) cysts, which occur in more advanced OA at sites of increased mechanical load and frequently communicate with the articular surface (Fig. 168.2d).

Remodeling and attrition of the bone

Subchondral bone in OA patients is less stiff and dense and is mechanically 'weaker' than in those with non-arthritic joints[11]. It is detected radiographically as a flattening and increased congruity between the articular elements (Fig. 168.5). With cartilage loss in the load-bearing compartment, tongue-in-groove corrugation may appear as a manifestation of the variable pattern of weakness of the bone. With complete loss of cartilage, the weakened subchondral bone is further flattened, acquiring greater articular congruence (Fig. 168.5b). Ultimately, the surfaces

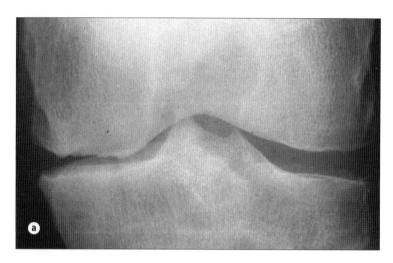 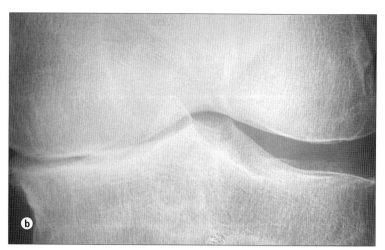

Fig. 168.5 Articular bone distortion and flattening in OA, caused by weaker bone. (a) OA knee radiographed in the standing extended view with a medial compartment joint space width >2mm, clearly showing marked subchondral sclerosis with tongue-in-groove corrugations on the femoral and tibial articular surfaces of the medial compartment. (b) The same knee radiographed in the same view 21 months later, showing flattening of the articular surfaces. The corrugations visible in (a) are now reduced or absent, resulting in greater articular congruence.

become distorted and deformed, with the collapse of the bone leading to altered limb alignment and deformity. These later stages can be assessed by use of long leg films (Fig. 168.6).

RADIOGRAPHIC PROCEDURES

The absence of standardization, either in personnel or in radiographic method, leads to errors in the assessment of the severity and progression of the OA[1-3]. The implementation of validated procedures for the radiographic assessment of OA joints has largely overcome these difficulties.

Standardized radiographic procedures are based on minimizing any distortion in the radiographic image of the joint. This is achieved by positioning the joint so that the central ray of the X-ray beam passes between the margins of the joint space, with the result that the margins and the space are optimally defined when the joint is in a position consistent with weight-bearing, as during normal activity[1,2,3] (Fig. 168.7).

Knee radiography

Tibiofemoral compartment

The most reliable and reproducible method for imaging this compartment is the standing semiflexed view. Comparative studies[12] have shown that the non-fluoroscopic standing semiflexed view of the knee (Fig. 168.8a) is the most accurate method for positioning the joint, and the most reproducible method for repositioning the joint at successive examinations and for measuring joint space width. A major advantage is that correction for radiographic magnification is not required between repeat examinations when changes in joint space width are measured.

An alternative reproducible method, which ensures that the center of the X-ray beam is parallel to the tibial plateau, is to screen the joint into the correct radioanatomical position, using fluoroscopy, before obtaining the radiograph[1,2,13,14] (Fig. 168.8b).

Patellofemoral compartment

The axial or 'skyline' view is more precise than the lateral view of the joint at localizing changes in the medial and lateral facets of the patellofemoral joint[1,2,13]. This view is obtained with the patient standing and the knee flexed to 30° from the vertical[1,2,13] (Fig. 168.9).

Hip radiography

Joint space width is more reliably assessed with the patient standing with the feet internally rotated (15–20° angle between the feet)[1,2,15], rather than

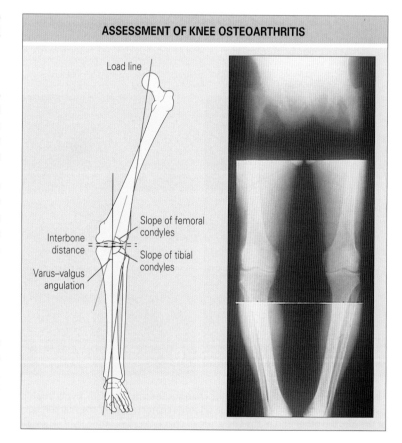

Fig. 168.6 Assessment of knee OA with long leg films. The diagram indicates the measurements that can be made which might indicate dysplasia of the knee, and the assessment of the load line and varus–valgus angulations from the long leg film. This is a particularly important investigation before surgery. The long leg films shown illustrate a case of varus angulation of the knee joints caused by dysplasia, with an oversized lateral femoral condyle resulting in an abnormal alignment of the knee joints and secondary varus deformity of the tibiae.

lying down. Furthermore, image distortion is minimized when the X-ray beam is centered on each joint. Lateral oblique views of the hip help detect OA at the posterior articular surface, not visible in the anteroposterior view.

PLANE FOR MEASUREMENT OF MINIMUM JOINT WIDTH

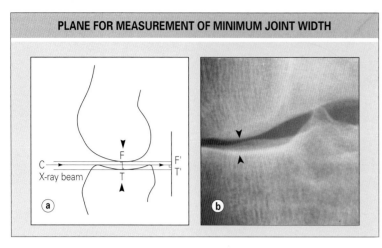

Fig. 168.7 Plane of measurement for minimum JSW measurement. (a) The illustration defines the plane for minimum JSW measurement in the tibiofemoral compartment which is taken in the middle of the joint, coinsident with load transmission (arrows), perpendicular to the central ray (C) of the X-ray beam and parallel to the film. Arrowheads also identify the corresponding site in the anteroposterior radiograph of an OA knee. F, femur; T, tibia; F' and T' their projection onto the X-ray film.

Hand radiography

The optimal position for joint assessment is obtained with the fingers held together and in line with the wrist and forearm when laid flat on the X-ray film holder[1,2].

RADIOGRAPHIC ASSESSMENT OF DISEASE SEVERITY AND MEASUREMENT OF DISEASE PROGRESSION

Grading systems

Semiquantitative grading systems based on global score of the radiographic features, such as that of Kellgren and Lawrence[16], although widely used to assess disease severity and progression, are based upon the following assumptions that may be incorrect:

- the change in any one radiographic feature is linear and constant during the course of the disease
- the relationship between the radiographic features is constant
- progression of radiographic features is similar in different joints.

Consequently, a number of investigators have developed alternative methods for scoring individual radiographic features for the separate joints and their compartments[17]. Methods of scoring are susceptible to fairly high levels of observer variability.

Quantitative methods

Direct measurement of the joint space width is recommended as the outcome measure in clinical drug trials[1,2,18]. The sensitivity of this measurement as a surrogate for articular cartilage thickness is determined by the parameters described below[1–3].

Radioanatomic plane of measurement

The plane of measurement is determined by the radiographic view of the joint as described above (Figs 168.8 & 168.9). Reproducible repositioning of the limb can be achieved by foot maps, which the patient stands in at subsequent examinations[1–3,13,14].

Methods of measurement

Although the simplest tool of measurement is the ruler with millimeter divisions, it is inaccurate, and does not reliably measure joint space width[3]. More accurate methods are either those using a graduated

EVALUATION OF KNEE OA

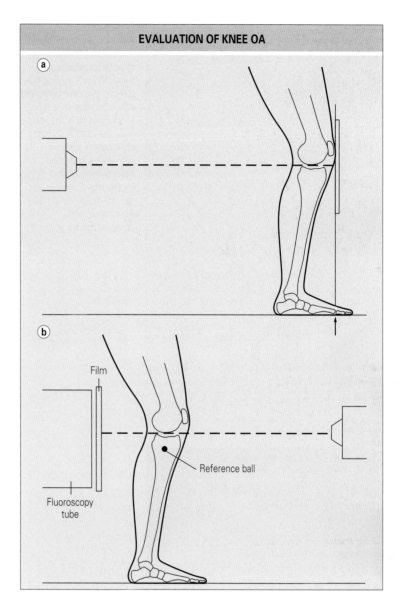

Fig. 168.8 Evaluation of knee OA. Reproducible radiographic methods for reliable evaluation. (a) The patient stands in the semi-flexed position, both knees are bent and in contact with the film cassette, and the feet are slightly externally rotated (about 15°). The first metatarsophalangeal joint of each foot (arrow) is positioned immediately below and in line with the front edge of the film cassette. The X-ray beam is directed midway between the knees and the tube's positioning light is aligned with the horizontal plane of the joint. (b) The semi-flexed view of the knee can be positioned with greater reproducibility by using fluoroscopy to position the tibial plateau horizontally and parallel to the X-ray beam. A metallic reference ball is used to correct for radiographic magnification.

magnifying lens placed on the film across the joint space[3,14], or other digitization methods using calipers or cross-wire cursors linked to digitization tablets[3]. Computerized methods of joint space width measurement from digitized radiographs[14,15] overcome the limitations of observer variability, providing a reproducible and accurate method of measurement[14].

Which measure of joint space width?

The accuracy and precision of measurement of the joint space width at its narrowest site (minimum joint space width) has been validated[18] as a method for detecting progression of OA in the knee, hip and hand. This measure has been recommended for all manual and computerized methods of measurement[1–3,18]. The alternatives of joint space width area and mean joint space width area measurements require computerized methods[15]. Their limitation is that focal loss of articular cartilage in OA

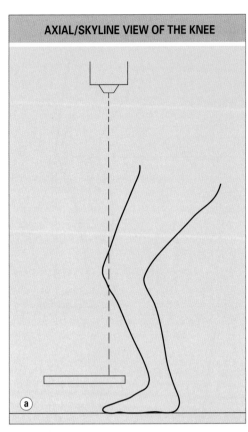

AXIAL/SKYLINE VIEW OF THE KNEE

(a)

Fig. 168.9
Axial or skyline view of the knee. (a) The illustration shows the method for X-raying the patello-femoral joint. The film is placed on a step. In this position the joint is under load. (b) This view of the joint provides a reliable assessment of the interbone distances at the medial and lateral patellofemoral compartments.

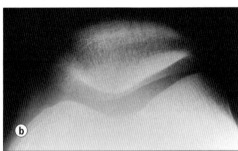

(b)

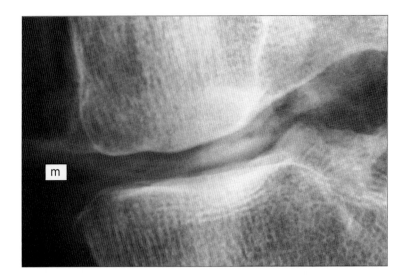

Fig. 168.10 Double-contrast arthrogram of the knee. View of the medial compartment showing focal cartilage loss and surface irregularities. The meniscus (m) is extruded.

can lead to the joint space widening within the same compartment, rendering this measure less sensitive to detecting changes in joint space width.

Effect of radiographic magnification

Radiographic magnification in large joints can lead to imprecise measurements of the joint space width[1,2,13,14]. Use of a sized metal ball placed at the side of the joint can correct radiographic magnification[13,14] (Fig. 168.8b).

OTHER ANATOMICAL IMAGING TECHNIQUES

Magnification radiography

Magnification techniques such as microfocal radiography[4–7] are characterized by a micron-sized X-ray (15–50μm) source, which produces enlarged radiographic images ($\times$4 to $\times$8) with high spatial resolution (200 lines/cm, equivalent to an object size of 25μm). The size and quality of these images permit direct measurements to be made of the dimensions of the radiographic features[4–7]. This has provided valuable additional information on early radiographic features of OA[4–7] (Fig. 168.3) and in quantifying the effect of drug treatment[1,2,5]. Because of the need for dedicated equipment, this method will not be of

routine use, but does provide value in research and in longitudinal studies.

Computerized image analysis

Increasingly, computer programs are being used to measure joint space width from digitally stored images of OA joints – procedures that are necessary in clinical trials, because they avoid the limitations of observer variability. The reproducibility of measurements obtained with these systems is excellent[14,15]. Digital image analysis has also been used to assess the fractal signature of the trabecular pattern of subchondral bone, a technique that may provide a very sensitive way of assessing change in osteoarthritis[7].

Arthrograms

The introduction of a positive (radiopaque) or negative (radiolucent) contrast medium, or both, into a joint can be valuable. A double-contrast arthrogram can also be used as an alternative to arthroscopy to assess cartilage or meniscal damage, highlighting focal lesions and allowing more accurate measurement of cartilage thickness[1,2] (Fig. 168.10). However, arthrography has the disadvantages of being time consuming and invasive, and has largely been replaced by MRI.

Dual energy X-ray absorptiometry

Dual energy X-ray absorptiometry provides a reproducible assessment of bone mineral density of the subchondral and periarticular regions affected by OA. The extensive region of osteoporosis in the subarticular bone (Fig. 168.3) has been quantified[10]. The lower than normal bone mineral density in knee OA appeared to be related to the radiographic changes at the joint[10]. Increasingly, this method is being used to follow changes in bone that occur as OA progresses, or as a consequence of the altered weight bearing of joints[19].

Ultrasonography

This modality is increasingly being used in the assessment of soft tissue involvement. It is widely available, and provides real-time imaging, with no radiation hazard. Its disadvantages are that it is highly operator-dependent, it lacks standardized diagnostic criteria and reproducibility is difficult.

Ultrasonography can depict synovial hypertrophy, tendon sheath widening, tendon degenerative changes and tears, in addition to visualizing joint effusions at inaccessible sites such as the hip. Furthermore, Baker's cysts and joint ruptures can be detected[20] (Fig. 168.11). Hyaline

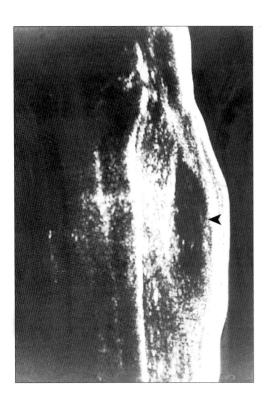

Fig. 168.11 Ultrasound of the knee joint, showing a popliteal cyst (arrow).

cartilage can also be visualized at some sites, and focal defects and generalized thinning have been recorded. Ultrasonography makes intra-articular treatment easier and safer, allowing the inserted needle to be guided until the tip is seen within the selected target area.

Arthroscopy

This method offers the most direct way of visualizing and imaging the cartilage defects of OA and evaluating the structural integrity and mechanical stability of the menisci and intra-articular ligaments. This method has been used as a means of detecting and quantifying cartilage lesions and following the progression of OA[21]. It has the limitation of being invasive, and in only visualizing the surface of articular cartilage; deep chondral abnormalities are invisible with this technique. The arthroscope is used most frequently in OA as a tool with which to deliver surgical treatment. It also has an important role in patients with knee pain for whom OA is part of the differential diagnosis, as in the following settings[22]:

- painful swollen knees with normal radiographs and non-inflammatory fluid
- OA of a joint with pain out of proportion to radiographic findings and refractory to conventional treatment
- chronic stable OA with profound worsening of symptoms
- OA with predominant 'mechanical' symptoms
- OA with unexpected synovial fluid characteristics.

PHYSIOLOGICAL IMAGING

Radionucleotide scintigraphy

One method of scintigraphy involves the use of [99m]technetium-labeled methylene or hydroxymethylene diphosphonate and a conventional gamma camera with a suitable collimator, with imaging immediately after the intravenous injection and a delayed acquisition 3–4 hours later. This gives information on blood flow within bone and soft tissues, perivascular edema and protein leakage, and overall bone mineral turnover and activity. Spatial resolution is not as good as that obtained with radiography, and correlation with plain films may be difficult.

Scintigraphy is extremely sensitive, but non-specific because it will detect any cause of local pathology. Quantification of the image is also difficult.

Evidence to suggest that changes in bone occur early in the development of OA came from bone scans. In hand OA, the increase in isotope concentration identified joints with OA before the onset of radiographic changes and was predictive of subsequent radiographic abnormalities of joint space loss and osteophytosis[23,24]. In addition, hand joints showed variable levels of disease activity, switching between an active and a quiescent phase[23,24] (Fig. 168.12). Increased isotope uptake was found to be associated with osteophyte growth and remodeling and, in later stages, with increased subchondral sclerosis.

Radioisotope studies in OA of the knee confirmed the earlier work in OA of the hand[23,24] on the predictive nature of this methodology in identifying joints likely to show progression. In the tibiofemoral compartment, three main categories of abnormality can be detected[25]:

- Generalized activity: this correlates best with pain and with evidence of effusions on plain radiographs. This type of activity can be suppressed by intra-articular injection of corticosteroid and presumably reflects inflammation, protein binding and leakage, rather than increased subchondral blood flow (Fig. 168.13)
- 'Tramline' activity along the joint margins: this correlates well with subchondral bone sclerosis, and may also reflect active osteophytic growth
- 'Extended' activity in the subchondral bone: this shows some correlation with clinical and radiographic evidence of severe disease, and may indicate progressive disease.

In any one patient, a number of the above patterns may be present, both within the entire knee or in any one compartment. Inactivity of any type of bone scan activity is a strong negative predictor of subsequent radiographic progression, irrespective of the severity of the initial structural change, emphasizing the fact that the disease process often stabilizes.

Magnetic resonance imaging

Magnetic resonance imaging combines multiplanar tomography with unparalleled soft tissue contrast, allowing all components of the joint to be examined simultaneously. Whole-organ joint evaluation is particularly useful in OA, in view of the interest in understanding this heterogeneous group of disorders, which involve several components of the synovial joint, including muscle and nerve.

Anatomical data

Compared with radiography, MRI is more sensitive at detecting marginal and, especially, central osteophytes in OA[26] (Fig. 168.14), but poor at delineating the sclerotic regions below the subchondral cortex, because of the low signal intensity of bone. MRI has the unique capability for evaluating joint effusions, hypertrophic synovial tissue, the integrity of the menisci, and the cruciate and collateral ligaments of the knee. In addition, subarticular bone marrow edema, which has recently been shown to be strongly associated with the presence of pain in knee OA[27], is saliently depicted with MRI (Fig. 168.15). These lesions generally reflect increased blood or other fluid inside bone, which may be associated with intraosseous hypertension as a result of poor venous drainage from the marrow[27]. MRI has been shown to detect arthroscopically demonstrable cartilage defects in the knee with high sensitivity and specificity[28,29] (Fig. 168.16). Techniques have also been developed for accurately quantifying cartilage volume and for mapping the cartilage thickness[30,31] (Fig. 168.17). In addition, MRI is already the investigation of choice in the evaluation of a number of pathologies seen in association with OA, including:

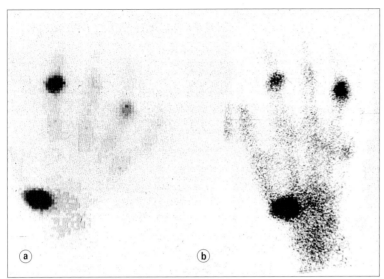
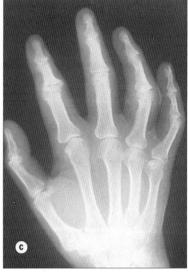
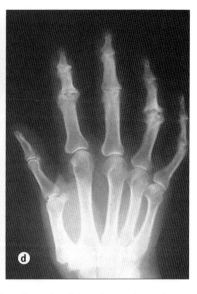

Fig. 168.12 Scintigraphy indicates the 'phasic' nature of OA and can predict subsequent radiographic changes. These films show the plain radiographs and late-phase scans of the same patient, taken 2 years apart. The initial radiograph (c) shows early OA of some of the interphalangeal joints, whereas on the scan (a), the thumb base and index proximal interphalangeal joint (PIP) are most active. Two years later, the radiograph (d) shows progression of changes at the 'hot' interphalangeal joint, and the appearance of changes at the thumb base. The second scan (b) shows that the activity in the index PIP is now subsiding, but the ring finger PIP is now becoming more active.

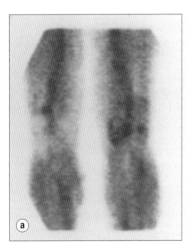
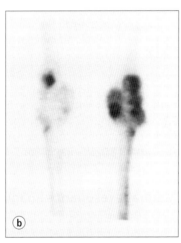

Fig. 168.13 Detecting inflammation in knee OA using scintigraphy. The left knee shows generalized increased uptake both in the perfusion-phase (a) and the late-phase (b) scans. The inflammatory component is documented by the increased vascularity. In the right knee, some tracer uptake is seen at the patellofemoral joint.

- osteonecrosis of bone and marrow
- internal joint derangement
- some periarticular pathologies, such as rotator cuff lesions.

Physiological data

Magnetic resonance imaging is also capable of measuring a variety of compositional parameters relevant to the osteoarthritic process. The concentration of water proton provides the basis for the MRI signal in hyaline cartilage. Cartilage matrix modifies the signal behavior of these water protons, so that cartilage has a slightly greater signal intensity than water on T1-weighted images and a markedly lower signal intensity than water on T2-weighted images (Fig. 168.18). Disruption or loss of the normal collagen–proteoglycan matrix in OA increases the water content (and therefore the proton density) and decreases T1-relaxation and T2-relaxation. This can be associated with a striking increase in signal intensity in morphologically normal-appearing cartilage on T2-weighted images (Fig. 168.19). Although these patterns of signal alteration in degenerating cartilage are well documented, their longitudinal behavior has not been carefully defined. Nevertheless, it is anticipated that T1-weighting, T2-weighting and proton density will prove to be

Fig. 168.14 Delineating osteophytes with MRI. (a) Coronal T1-weighted MRI of the knee delineates large marginal osteophytes. (b) Sagittal image of a different knee shows a central osteophyte (arrow) in the trochlear groove of the femur.

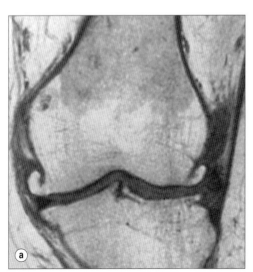
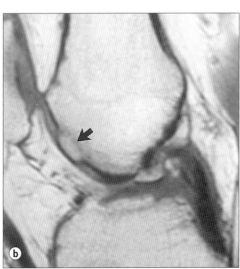

useful parameters for tracking early degenerative changes in articular cartilage in patients with established OA and, even more importantly, for identifying patients who are at risk of developing OA (e.g. obese women with a family history of OA).

Using specialized phase-sensitive pulse sequences, MRI is also able to quantify the diffusion coefficient of water in cartilage[32]. This parameter increases with proteoglycan loss, and may prove to be a valuable indicator for early OA, although more work is needed to make this parameter attainable *in vivo*. MRI contrast media such as the anionic gadolinium-diethylene triamino-pentacetic acid or the cationic agents, such as Mn^{2+}, can assist in detecting changes in the biochemical status of the cartilage.

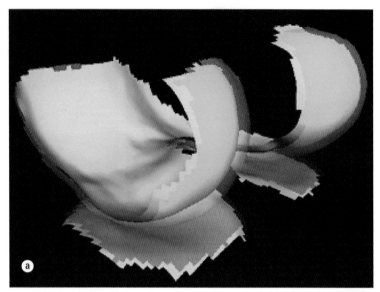

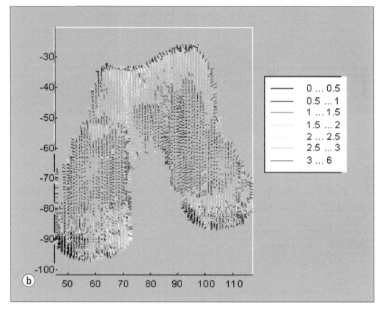

Fig. 168.17 **Quantitative assessment of cartilage volume in OA knee using MRI.** (a) Three-dimensional rendering of the femoral and tibial cartilages in the knee of a patient, obtained from serial high-resolution three-dimensional acquisitions with fat-suppression MRI. (b) Summing the voxels within each of these cartilage images determines their precise volumes, which are then displayed as normalized femoral and tibial volume maps (scale in mm), showing here patterns of cartilage loss in the medial and lateral femoral condyles. (With permission of ArthroVision, Montreal, Quebec, Canada.)

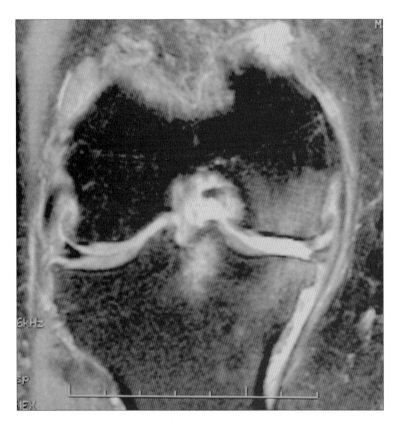

Fig. 168.15 **Subchondral bone marrow edema in OA revealed with MRI.** Coronal fat-suppressed T2-weighted MRI of the knee, showing water signal in the normally fatty bone marrow of the medial femoral condyle and tibial plateau adjacent to the area of articular cartilage loss. Scale in millimeters. (Courtesy of Dr Curtis W Hayes, University of Michigan, Ann Arbor, MI.)

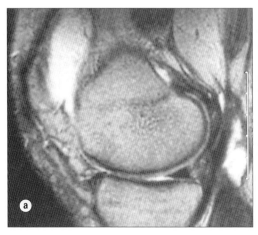
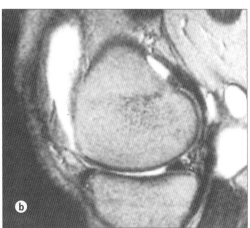

Fig. 168.16 **Monitoring cartilage loss with MRI.** (a) Sagittal T2-weighted MRI of the knee of a patient with a meniscal tear shows intact articular cartilage in the medial femorotibial joint at the time of initial presentation. (b) Repeat MRI 16 months later shows extensive loss of cartilage in the same compartment. Note the large Baker's cyst on both images.

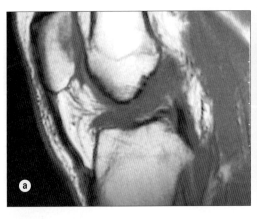 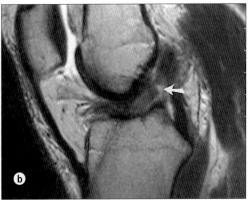

Fig. 168.18 MRI signal behavior of articular tissues. (a) Sagittal T1-weighted image of the knee, showing high signal intensity in marrow fat and adipose tissue, intermediate signal intensity in cartilage and muscle, low signal intensity in synovial fluid, tendons, ligaments and menisci, and signal void in cortical and trabecular bone. (b) T2-weighted image showing high signal intensity in synovial fluid, intermediate signal intensity in fat, and low signal intensity in muscle and cartilage. Fibrous structures and cortical and trabecular bone show signal void. Discontinuity of the anterior cruciate ligament on the T2-weighted image is indicative of tear (arrow).

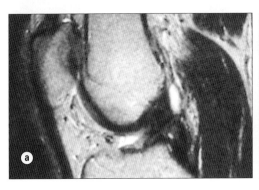 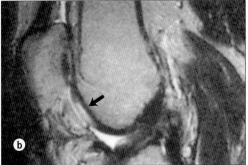

Fig. 168.19 Detection of early cartilage degeneration with MRI. (a) Sagittal T2-weighted magnetic resonance image of the knee in a patient with acute anterior cruciate ligament tear, showing normal low signal in the intact femoral cartilage. (b) A repeat MRI 14 months after repair of the cruciate ligament shows increased signal within the cartilage (arrow), indicative of loss of matrix.

SUMMARY

The plain radiograph remains the most popular technique for epidemiologic studies and everyday assessments of the OA joint, but care must be taken with obtaining, interpreting and, particularly, measuring features recorded in the image. Other imaging modalities, in particular MRI, have an undoubted role in the detection of local pathology, and in research into the disease process.

REFERENCES

1. Buckland-Wright JC. Quantitation of radiographic changes. In: Brandt KD, Lohmander S, Doherty M, eds. Osteoarthritis. Oxford: University Press; 1998: 459–472.
2. Buckland-Wright JC. Protocols for radiography. In: Brandt KD, Lohmander S, Doherty M, eds. Osteoarthritis. Oxford: University Press; 1998: 578–580.
3. Buckland-Wright JC. Radiographic assessment of osteoarthritis: comparison between existing methodologies. Osteoarthritis Cart 1999; 7: 430–433.
4. Buckland-Wright JC, Macfarlane DG, Lynch JA, Clark B. Quantitative microfocal radiographic assessment of progression in osteoarthritis of the hand. Arthritis Rheum 1990; 33: 57–65.
5. Buckland-Wright JC, Macfarlane DG, Lynch JA, Jasani MK. Quantitative microfocal radiography detects changes in OA knee joint space width in patients in placebo-controlled trial of NSAID therapy. J Rheumatol 1995; 22: 937–943.
6. Buckland-Wright JC, Macfarlane DG, Jasani MK, Lynch JA. Quantitative microfocal radiographic assessment of osteoarthritis of the knee using weight-bearing tunnel and semi-flexed standing views. J Rheumatol 1994; 21: 1734–1741.
7. Buckland-Wright C, Lynch J, Macfarlane D. Fractal signature analysis measures cancellous bone organisation in macroradiographs of patients with knee osteoarthritis. Ann Rheum Dis 1996; 55: 749–755.
8. Alexander CJ. Osteoarthritis: a review of old myths and current concepts. Skeletal Radiol 1990; 19: 327–333.
9. Resnick D, Niwayama G. Degenerative disease of extraspinal locations. In: Resnick D, Niwayama G, eds. Diagnosis of bone and joint disorders, 2E. Philadelphia: WB Saunders; 1988: 1365–1479.
10. Karvonen RL, Miller PR, Nelson DA et al. Periarticular osteoporosis in osteoarthritis of the knee. J Rheumatol 1998; 25: 187–194.
11. Li B, Aspden RM. Mechanical and material properties of the subchondral bone plate from the femoral head of patients with osteoarthritis or osteoporosis. Ann Rheum Dis 1997; 56: 247–254.
12. Buckland-Wright JC, Wolfe F, Ward RJ et al. Substantial superiority of semiflexed (MTP) views in knee osteoarthritis: a comparative radiographic study, without fluoroscopy, of standing extended, semiflexed (MTP), and schuss views. J Rheumatol 1999; 26: 2664–2674.
13. Buckland-Wright C. Protocols for precise radio-anatomical positioning of the tibio-femoral and patello-femoral compartments of the knee. Osteoarthritis Cart 1995; 3(suppl A): 71–80.

14. Buckland-Wright JC, Macfarlane DG, Williams SA, Ward RJ. Accuracy and precision of joint space width measurements in standard and macro-radiographs of osteoarthritic knees. Ann Rheum Dis 1995; 54: 872–880.
15. Conrozier T, Lequesne M, Tron AM et al. The effects of position on the radiographic joint space in osteoarthritis of the hip. Osteoarthritis Cart 1997; 5: 17–22.
16. Kellgren JH, Lawrence JS. Radiological assessment of osteoarthritis. Ann Rheum Dis 1957; 16: 494–501.
17. Altman M, Hochberg M, Murphy WA et al. Atlas of individual radiographic features in osteoarthritis. Osteoarthritis Cart 1995; 3(suppl A): 3–70.
18. Altman R, Brandt K, Hochberg M, Moskowitz R. Design and conduct of clinical trials in patients with osteoarthritis. Osteoarthritis Cart 1996; 4: 217–243.
19. Madsen OR, Schaadt O, Bleddal H et al. Bone mineral distribution of the proximal tibia in gonarthrosis assessed in vivo by photon absorption. Osteoarthritis Cart 1994; 2: 141–146.
20. Richardson ML, Selby B, Montana MA, Mack LA. Ultrasonography of the knee. Radiol Clin North Am 1988; 26: 63–75.
21. Ayral X, Dougados M, Listrat V et al. Chondroscopy: a new method for scoring chondropathy. Semin Arthritis Rheum 1993; 22: 289–297.
22. Ike RW. The role of arthroscopy in the differential diagnosis of osteoarthritis of the knee. Rheum Dis Clin N Am 1993; 19: 673–696.
23. Hutton CW, Higgs ER, Jackson PC et al. 99mTc-HMDP bone scanning in generalised nodal osteoarthritis. I. Comparison of the standard radiograph and four hour bone scan image of the hand. Ann Rheum Dis 1986; 45: 617–621.
24. Hutton CW, Higgs ER, Jackson PC et al. 99mTc-HMDP bone scanning in generalised nodal osteoarthritis. II. The four hour bone scan image predicts radiographic change. Ann Rheum Dis 1986; 45: 622–626.
25. McCrae F, Shoels J, Dieppe P, Watt I. Scintigraphic assessment of osteoarthritis of the knee joint. Ann Rheum Dis 1992; 51: 938–942.
26. Chan WP, Lang P, Stevens MP et al. Osteoarthritis of the knee: comparison of radiography, CT, and MR imaging to assess extent and severity. Am J Radiology 1991; 157: 799–806.
27. Felson DT, Chaisson CE, Hill CL et al. The association of bone marrow lesions with pain in knee osteoarthritis. Ann Intern Med 2001; 134: 541–549.
28. Recht MP, Pirraino DW, Paletta GA et al. Accuracy of fat-suppressed three dimensional spoiled gradient echo FLASH MR imaging in the detection of patellofemoral articular cartilage abnormalities. Radiology 1996; 198: 209–212.

29. Disler DG, McCauley TR, Kelman CG *et al*. Fat-suppressed three-dimensional spoiled gradient-echo MR imaging of hyaline cartilage defects in the knee: comparison with standard MR imaging and arthroscopy. Am J Radiology 1996; 167: 127–132.

30. Peterfy CG, van Dijke CF, Janzen DL *et al*. Quantification of articular cartilage in the knee by pulsed saturation transfer and fat-suppressed MRI: optimization and validation. Radiology 1994; 192: 485–491.

31. Peterfy CG, Genant HK. Emerging applications of magnetic resonance imaging for evaluating the articular cartilage. Radiol Clin North Am 1996; 34: 195–213.

32. Burstein D, Gray ML, Hartman AL *et al*. Diffusion of small solutes in cartilage as measured by nuclear magnetic resonance (NMR) spectroscopy and imaging. J Orthop Res 1993; 11: 465–478.

169 Pathology of osteoarthritis

Peter G Bullough

- The function of a joint is to provide for movement and stability while withstanding the applied loads.

- The function is fulfilled through the architecture of the joint and the mechanical properties of the matrices of the connective tissues of which the joint is constructed. The geometry of the articulating surfaces is particularly important and an intact neuromuscular system essential.

- Osteoarthritis is a dysfunction of the joint resulting from a failure in the materials, an alteration in the geometry or ligamentous injury.

- Malfunction of the neuromuscular system frequently results in amplification of joint dysfunction.

- In most instances the etiology of osteoarthritis is multifactorial.

- The pathogenesis follows a course of injury, repair, repetitive injury and chronic repair. Injury may affect primarily the tissues or the architectural structure, but eventually both will be affected. Repair, to be effective, must include repair of the structure.

- The disease process may stabilize without treatment and is not necessarily relentless in its clinical course. In some case there may be morphologic and/or clinical improvement.

THE NORMAL JOINT

Arthritis (i.e. joint dysfunction) can be understood only when the process of normal function has been comprehended. Discussions of the pathology of arthritis which deal only with the morbid anatomy of the diseased joint do not by themselves help our understanding[1].

Osteoarthritis is a functional disorder of joints characterized by altered anatomy, especially a change in shape of the articular surfaces and a loss of articular cartilage. Unlike many other forms of arthritis (rheumatoid, psoriatic or infectious) it is not obviously inflammatory, although it must be stressed that all types of injury, even mechanical, result in an inflammatory response.

Osteoarthritis does not have a single cause but is the result of a number of different pathophysiologic pathways.

Function and anatomy

Normal joint function can be characterized by three properties: first, the freedom of the opposed articular surfaces to move painlessly over each other within the required range of motion; second, by the correct distribution of load across joint tissues, which might otherwise be altered either by mechanical overloading resulting in damage, or habitual underloading[2,3] resulting in disuse atrophy; and third, by the maintenance of stability. These three interdependent aspects of joint function further depend on three features of joint design.

First, the geometry of its opposed articulating surfaces is the most obvious feature of a joint. In general one articular surface is convex, whereas the other is concave. These complementary shapes are necessary to permit the range of motion required, to provide stability and to

ensure the most equitable loading during use. It was long thought that precise fit or congruence was a normal feature of a joint[4]; however, as many joints are multiaxial, if they were to remain congruent in all positions then the opposed surfaces would have to be perfectly spherical. As they are not[5,6], no joint can be congruent in all positions, though it may be more congruent in one position than in others (Figs 169.1, 169.2).

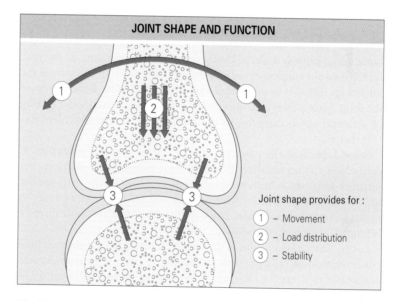

JOINT SHAPE AND FUNCTION

Joint shape provides for :
1. – Movement
2. – Load distribution
3. – Stability

Fig. 169.1 Joint shape and function.

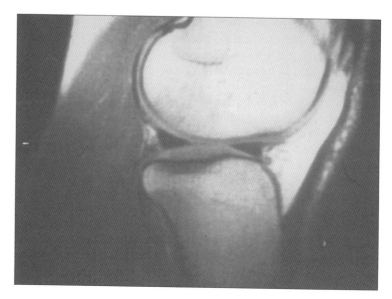

Fig. 169.2 Sagittal magnetic resonance image (MRI) of a normal knee. This shows the gross incongruity of the cartilaginous surfaces, partially corrected by the interposed meniscus which acts as a load-bearing structure

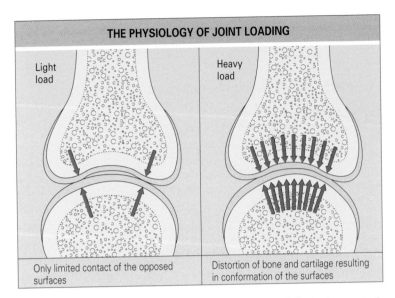

Fig. 169.3 The physiology of joint loading. Light load: only limited contact of the opposed surfaces. Heavy load: distortion of bone and cartilage resulting in conformation of the surfaces

The tissues of the joint surface, particularly the cartilage, but also the bone, when loaded, undergo elastic deformation. Therefore, as the load is increased the surfaces come into increasing contact. In this way, as the load is increased it is more equitably distributed. The deformation of the joint space under load also provides for the circulation and mixing of synovial fluid, essential to the metabolism of the chondrocytes (Fig. 169.3).

Second, because the physicochemical and mechanical properties of connective tissues are determined by their extracellular matrices, the intrinsic cells which both synthesize and break down the extracellular matrix must be subject to highly sensitive feedback systems in order to maintain matrix equilibrium. These feedback systems have only recently begun to be studied (see below).

Lastly, any consideration of functional joint anatomy must include consideration of both the role of ligaments and the neuromuscular control of motion. As recognized by Charcot in the 19th century, a breakdown of neuromuscular coordination can lead to profound arthritis[7].

Tissue heterogeneity

Heterogeneity of the articular cartilage matrix, including biochemical, structural and biomechanical variations, is observed within different regions of a normal weightbearing joint. Thus, Maroudas et al.[8] observed topographical variations in proteoglycan content in the cartilage of the femoral head. Kempson et al.[9] further observed that the variation in stiffness seen in different areas of the femoral head was related to proteoglycan content and to the amount of water held by the tissue.

An example of normal geographic variation can be readily observed in the tibial plateau, of humans as well as of other animals, where there are distinct differences between the articular cartilage which is covered by the meniscus and that which is not. These differences consist of a rough surface and soft matrix in the uncovered area, compared to the smooth, firm matrix found in those areas covered by the meniscus. Bennet et al.[10] reported that all individuals over 16 years showed focal roughening of the uncovered cartilage on the tibial plateau. The author, in an examination of both adult human and dog knee joints at autopsy, found that articular cartilage not covered by meniscus always showed matrix softening and superficial fibrillation (Fig. 169.4)[11]. Naturally occurring variations in both matrix structure and mechanical properties may relate to the patterns of joint loading experienced in normal everyday use[12]. In the normally functioning knee, load is transmitted through

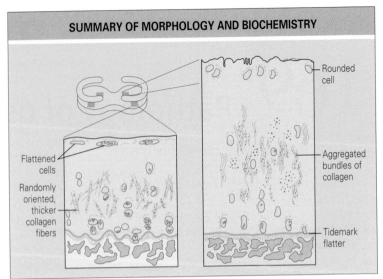

Fig. 169.4 Summary of morphology and biochemistry. Left: In the covered area the surface is smooth, there is an amorphous electron-dense layer and cells are flattened. With respect to lipid, there is an increased intracellular accumulation in all three layers, there is an increased extracellular accumulation at the surface and there are increased numbers of extracellular matrix vesicles in the deep zone. Collagen appears in randomly oriented fibers with thicker mean diameters, there is regular binding or proteoglycan and the concentration per wet weight is increased. Proteoglycan shows an increased concentration per wet weight. The tidemark is irregular. Right: In the uncovered area, the surface is irregular, there is a detached electron-dense layer and cells are rounded. The concentration of water per unit volume is increased. Collagen appears in wavy aggregated bundles with thinner mean diameters (small range), and binding of proteoglycan is ill defined. An increased amount of proteoglycan can be extracted. The tidemark is smooth. In both the covered and the uncovered areas, the cell size is the same histologically and there is the same amount of DNA per dry weight of cartilage tissue. (Adapted from Bullough et al.[11])

the meniscus and on to the underlying tibial cartilage, whereas the exposed tibial cartilage, i.e. that which is not covered by the meniscus, remains relatively underloaded[13].

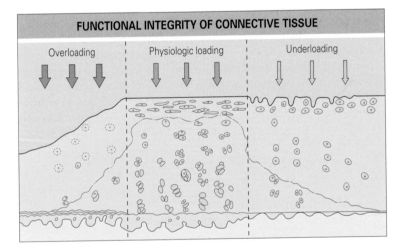

Fig. 169.5 Functional integrity of connective tissue. The continued optimal functional integrity of connective tissue depends on balanced rates of matrix production and breakdown by the cells. Healthy tissue (center) results from a physiologic range of stress that maintains optimal cell activity and matrix production. If this range of stress is exceeded (left), the result is cell injury and eventual necrosis (in cartilage this is called chondrolysis). If the stress is inadequate (right), disuse atrophy, i.e. lack of adequate matrix production by the cells, may occur. In cartilage this is associated with increased water content, superficial fibrillation of the collagen, altered organization of collagen fibrils and increased ease of dissociation of proteoglycan from the collagen framework.

Other similar areas of possible disuse atrophy demonstrating 'chondromalacia and fibrillation' have been described around the rim of the radial head[14]. in the roof of the acetabulum and on the perifoveal and inferomedial aspects of the femoral head[15]. All these joints (the knee, the hip and the elbow) in later life frequently show morphologic, though not necessarily clinical, evidence of osteoarthritis.

Both *in vivo* and *in vitro* studies have demonstrated that changes in the loading of the joint may lead to alterations in the composition and mechanical properties of the cartilage matrix[11,16–18]. In general it seems that low levels of mechanical stress (i.e. below the physiologic range) are associated with enhanced catabolic activity, whereas stress within the physiologic range is associated with anabolic activity[19–22]. Under conditions of supraphysiologic stress, the chondrocytes are unable to adapt. In other words, there is a window of physiologic loading above or below which the chondrocytes cannot synthesize or maintain an adequate functional matrix (Fig. 169.5)[23–25].

Joint modeling

Wolff's hypothesis states that both bone density and the spatial distribution of bone tissue correlate with the magnitude and direction of the applied loads. It follows therefore that the articular end of a bone, in particular the subchondral bone trabeculae, must undergo continuous modeling which is self-regulated to maintain a joint shape capable of optimal load distribution (Fig. 169.6)[26–29]. The joint shape as seen on a radiologic image depends on the subchondral bone endplate and the calcification front (or tidemark) at the base of the articular cartilage that covers it. An advance of the calcification front or the subchondral bone endplate will result in a change in the shape of the articular surface.

Chondroyctes close to the calcification front produce substances that promote mineralization. Extracellular matrix vesicles around these chondrocytes may provide sites for many such factors, including hydroxyapatite deposition[30], enzymes that increase local calcium and phosphate concentration[31–33], phosphoproteins[34], glycoproteins[35], proteolipids[36] and calcium phospholipid complexes[37]. On the other hand, other factors may inhibit or limit the extent of calcification. These inhibitory substances include proteoglycans[38], nucleotide triphosphate and pyrophosphate[39].

It is hypothesized that cellular control of shape, through the regulation of calcification, is related to patterns of joint use and loading. An advance of the calcification front would be expected to result in thinning of the overlying viable cartilage and thickening of the calcified cartilage. However, this does not happen because the additional calcified cartilage is remodeled into bone through the mechanism of endochondral ossification, and the extracellular matrix and chondrocytes of the viable cartilage are continuously being replaced throughout life.

THE ARTHRITIC JOINT, WITH PARTICULAR EMPHASIS ON OSTEOARTHRITIS

Although this chapter is mainly concerned with the pathology of osteoarthritis, a number of features, both clinical and anatomic, are common to all cases of arthritis whatever their etiology.

Arthritis is a clinical term which describes the consequences of a breakdown in the joint's normal function. These dysfunctions include loss of capacity of the articulating surfaces to move over one another easily, loss of joint stability and, almost always, pain.

The loss of freedom of motion, with its associated pain and instability, can be related to several morphologic features:

- a change in the joint shape, which in turn may result in severe non-physiologic incongruities
- a change in both the quantitative and qualitative composition of the extracellular matrices of the tissues that make up the joint, especially the articular cartilage, which in turn will affect their mechanical properties
- alterations in either ligamentous integrity and/or neuromuscular control which affect stability, movement and loading.

It follows therefore that malfunction of a joint may result from either acute or chronic injuries that produce either:

- anatomic alterations in the shape of articulating surfaces (which may result from a subarticular or transarticular fracture; or a metabolic disturbance affecting bone modeling)
- loss of integrity of the support structures around the joint (for example an inflammatory or traumatic destruction of ligaments, tendons or capsular tissue)
- alterations in the mechanical properties of the tissue matrices making up the joint, owing to disturbances affecting:
  - matrix synthesis (e.g. ochronosis)[40]
  - enzymatic degradation of the connective tissue matrices resulting from an inflammatory condition (e.g. rheumatoid arthritis).

There are certain common morphologic features (macroscopic and microscopic) which occur in an arthritic joint, whatever its cause, and these will be discussed next.

Macroscopic changes

A change in joint shape resulting from cartilage and bone loss is common to most forms of arthritis. Sometimes these changes are characteristic of a particular form of arthritis, for example the concentric loss of cartilage and bone that occurs in the inflammatory arthritides, the collapse of the joint surface that occurs in the late stage of osteonecrosis or acutely in subchondral fracture in elderly osteoporotic females[41], and the gross deformities of a Charcot's joint or advanced Paget's disease. However, in the osteoarthritic process, although bone and cartilage loss plays an important part, it is the addition of new bone and cartilage in the form of osteophytes, particularly at the joint periphery and sometimes beneath the articular surface, that forms one of its most characteristic features[42].

Microscopic cellular and tissue changes

Regardless of the etiology, microscopic evidence of bone and cartilage injury is characterized by alterations in both the cells and the extracellular matrix. Generally there is both macroscopic and microscopic evidence of degeneration and of repair[43].

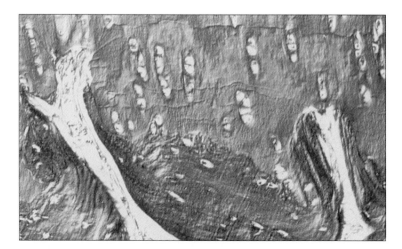

Fig. 169.6 Photomicrograph demonstrating vascular invasion with subsequent bone formation in the calcified region of normal articular cartilage. Through this regulated mechanism of endochondral ossification the articular bone end is remodeled. Hematoxylin and eosin × 10.

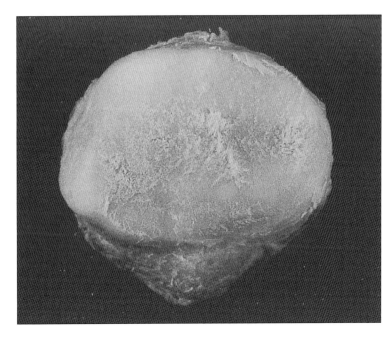

Fig. 169.7 Fibrillation of the superficial cartilage. Photograph of the articular surface of a patella obtained from a young individual at autopsy. Photographed using ultraviolet light.

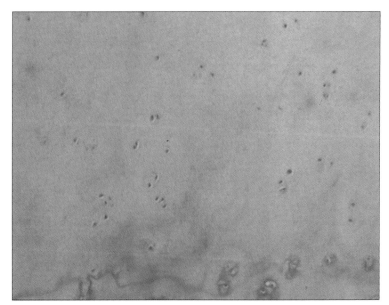

Fig. 169.8 Photomicrograph showing areas of cartilage with no chondrocytes, a consequence of focal cell necrosis. Hematoxylin and eosin × 10.

The alterations seen in the extracellular matrix of the connective tissues may result from a number of phenomena, including direct physical injury, alterations in the cellular synthesis of the matrix, or enzymatic breakdown of the matrix constituents. In any individual case of arthritis all these factors may be expected to contribute; however, their relative importance will vary depending on the etiology. The etiology of any observed matrix degradation or injury usually cannot be determined from the microscopic appearance.

Cartilage injury

Macroscopic evidence of injury to cartilage is evident only in its extracellular matrix. One of the earliest findings is a disruption of the surface collagen which, instead of having the smooth appearance of normal articular cartilage, becomes rough and/or eroded (Fig. 169.7)[44]. Three patterns of macroscopic alteration can be identified involving the cartilage surface, and to a variable degree the underlying tissue: fibrillation, erosion (ulceration) and cracking[45].

In considering the pathogenesis of these three histologic types of cartilage matrix damage it is important to recognize that in the early stages of osteoarthritis the damage may affect only one of the opposed articular surfaces. For this reason, fibrillation and other cartilage alterations cannot solely be ascribed, as they usually are, to wear and tear as the opposed articular surfaces move over each other.

Softening of the cartilage (chondromalacia) results from an increase in the ratio of water to the proteoglycan in the cartilage matrix[46]. Chondromalacia and fibrillation usually occur together, but the former may be present before there is any evidence of the latter.

Cellular injury is recognizable only under a microscope. Cell necrosis, a common finding in arthritis, can be identified when only the ghost outlines of the chondrocytes remain. This ghosting is usually focal in distribution (Fig. 169.8); less often, all of the chondrocytes are seen to be necrotic. Sublethal cell injury needs special techniques such as electron microscopy for its recognition.

CARTILAGE REGENERATION

The chondrocytes are intimately involved in both the breakdown and synthesis of cartilage matrix, and a wide range of growth factors and cytokines are involved in these processes, both as part of the regulation of normal matrix and in the processes involved in the repair of osteoarthritic cartilage. The enzymes that break down collagen and proteoglycan, the metalloproteinases, are themselves regulated by proinflammatory cytokines such as tumor necrosis factor (TNF) and interleukin-1 (IL-1). Three main groups of metalloproteinases, the stromelysins, gelatinases and collagenases, have been identified. The stromelysins degrade the proteoglycans and basement membranes and the collagenases the fibrillar proteins. It is probably important to realize that whereas the proteoglycans are broken down and replaced rapidly, replacement of the fibrillar collagen is very slow. It might therefore be useful therapeutically to block collagenase activity in the early stages of the arthritic process.

In a damaged joint, repair of the hyaline cartilage takes the form of cell proliferation and synthesis of new matrix. It may be initiated from either or both of two possible sites[47]. It may come from the damaged cartilage itself, in which case the process can be thought of as 'intrinsic' repair. Extrinsic repair of cartilage may develop from the subchondral bone or from the joint margin.

Intrinsic repair

In intrinsic repair there is microscopic evidence of focal cell proliferation and clumps, or clones, of chondrocytes 'within' the damaged cartilage matrix (Fig. 169.9). When the tissue is stained with methylene blue

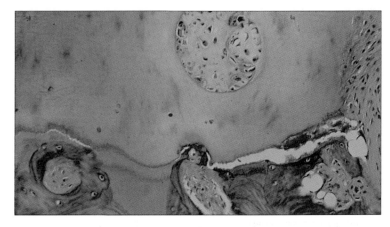

Fig. 169.9 Photomicrograph of a portion of degenerate cartilage which demonstrates a large nest of proliferating chondrocytes in the deep zone. Hematoxylin and eosin × 10.

there is often intense metachromasia around the proliferating chondrocytes, which indicates an increased synthesis of sulfated glycosaminoglycans[48].

Using a combination of immunohistochemical, biochemical and *in situ* hybridization techniques Von der Mark et al. identified three types of chondrocytes in osteoarthritic cartilage[49]. Normal chondrocytes were observed secreting type II collagen; clusters, or clones, of chondrocytes, having undergone focal dedifferentiation, were found secreting type I and type III collagen; in the middle and deep zones, particularly in areas with a deeply fibrillated surface, hypertrophic chondrocytes were seen producing increased amounts of type X collagen, a non-fibrillar collagen related to vascularization. This latter finding is probably related to the increased number of tidemarks and the underlying increased vascular remodeling of the calcified cartilage that is a feature of osteoarthritic cartilage.

Caterson et al.[50] have used specific monoclonal antibodies directed against different proteoglycan epitopes to detect subtle changes in chondroitin sulfate in the early stages of osteoarthritis. Altered proteoglycans may identify a change in the phenotypic expression of chondrocytes with the onset of disease.

Extrinsic repair

Extrinsic repair which arises from the joint margin may be seen as a cellular layer of cartilage extending over, and sometimes dissecting into, the existing cartilage. This extrinsically repaired cartilage is usually much more cellular than the pre-existing articular cartilage, and the chondrocytes are evenly distributed throughout the matrix. On microscopic examination of an H&E-stained section this type of repair cartilage can easily be overlooked. However, examination under polarized light will clearly demonstrate the discontinuity between the collagen network of the repaired cartilage and that of the pre-existing cartilage (Fig. 169.10).

In arthritic joints in which loss of the articular cartilage has denuded the underlying bone, especially in cases of osteoarthritis, there are frequently small pits in the bone surface from which protrude small nodules of firm white tissue. On microscopic examination these nodules have the appearance of fibrocartilage and they appear to arise in the marrow spaces of the subchondral bone. They may eventually extend over the previously denuded surface to form a more or less continuous layer of repair tissue[51].

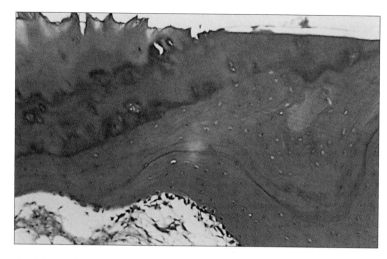

Fig. 169.11 Photomicrograph showing increased osteoblastic activity and trabecular thickening underlying an area of cartilage erosion. Section taken from the edge of a denuded and eburnated area. Hematoxylin and eosin × 10.

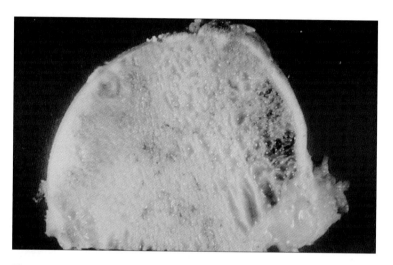

Fig. 169.12 A portion of the eburnated surface of an osteoarthritic joint. This demonstrates focal superficial bone and bone marrow necrosis, which is seen macroscopically as an opaque yellow area.

Bone injury and repair

Osteoarthritis is a disease that affects not only the articular cartilage but also the underlying bone and the structures around the joint. In subarticular bone that has been denuded there is usually a proliferation of osteoblasts, with the formation of new bone to buttress and strengthen the existing bone trabeculae (Fig. 169.11). This process results in the bony sclerosis seen on radiographic images[52]. A further result of the increased local stress in denuded sclerotic bone is focal pressure necrosis, which is seen in both bone and bone marrow. This superficial necrosis interferes with the development of extrinsic cartilage repair from the underlying bone (Fig. 169.12)[53].

In those cases of arthritis where there is significant inflammation, or where the patient has been treated with steroids or with non-steroidal anti-inflammatory drugs (NSAIDs), the reparative response in the subchondral bone may be significantly reduced, resulting in a progression of bone destruction.

Rapidly destructive arthrosis (RDA) of the hip joint, first reported by Postel and Kerboull in 1970[54], is a relatively uncommon form of arthritis of the hip seen mostly in elderly women. A normal joint space is the typical initial finding on radiography, followed within a few months by rapid disappearance of the femoral head. The majority of cases are unilateral (Fig. 169.13).

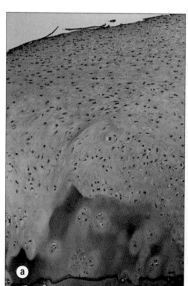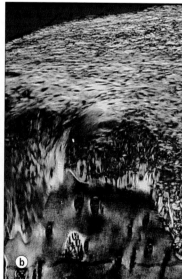

Fig. 169.10 Cartilage repair. (a) Photomicrograph of a section through the articular surface of an arthritic joint demonstrating extensive fibrocartilaginous repair overlying residual hyaline cartilage. Hematoxylin and eosin × 4. (b) The same field photographed with polarized light.

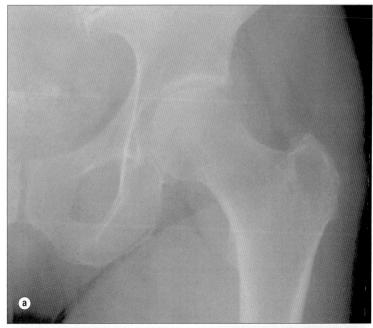

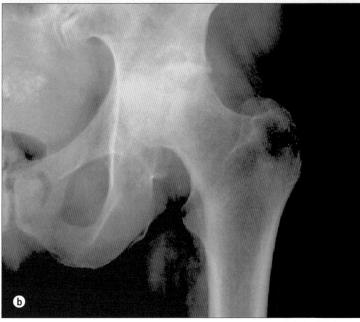

Fig. 169.13 An 80-year-old woman presented with severe pain in the hip joint. (a) A radiograph showed no obvious abnormality. (b) Three months later a radiograph of the hip showed loss of the joint space and collapse of the femoral head. This pattern of destruction is typical in cases of rapid destructive arthritis.

Various etiologies have been suggested in the literature, including idiopathic chondrolysis, apatite crystal deposition, drug toxicity or abnormal immunoreaction; however, the condition is generally considered to be idiopathic. Recently, we described a number of cases that had been diagnosed both clinically and by imaging as osteonecrosis, but were found histopathologically to have had subchondral insufficiency fracture of the femoral head (SIF)[41] (Fig. 169.14). In our experience this condition appears to be relatively common in the elderly osteoporotic population. Some of our cases of SIF have shown rapid disappearance of the joint space[55]. The relationship between the two entities, RDA and SIF, is suggested by the presence of a unique granulomatous lesion in the marrow space, which had been previously observed only in advanced cases of RDA[56]. We consider such lesions to be the result of the rapid rate of bone destruction, which does not allow for resorption of the resulting detritus in the usual way (Fig. 169.15). Being overweight

increases the risks for both SIF and subsequent joint destruction. Many factors may play an important role in the pathogenesis of rapid joint destruction, including increased levels of bone-resorptive enzymes[57] as well use of anti-inflammatory drugs or corticosteroid injection into the joint after the insufficiency fracture has occurred.

Subarticular cysts are usually seen only where the overlying cartilage is absent. They are believed to result from transmission of intra-articular pressure through defects in the articulating bony surface into the marrow spaces of the subchondral bone[58,59]. The cysts increase in size until the pressure within them is equal to the intra-articular pressure (Fig. 169.16).

Separated fragments of bone and cartilage from a damaged joint surface may remain free as loose bodies in the joint cavity or become incorporated into the synovial membrane and, depending on their size and rate of production, be digested (Fig. 169.17). Under certain circumstances proliferation of cartilage cells occurs at the surface of these loose bodies, which consequently grow larger[60].

Ligamentous injury and repair

In the ligamentous and capsular tissue around an arthritic joint, microscopic evidence of both lacerations and repair by scar tissue is common. Whether the lacerations precede the arthritic process or whether they are a consequence of it cannot usually be determined by tissue examination; however, there is abundant evidence from clinical studies that severe ligamentous injury is a significant cause of osteoarthritis, especially in athletes.

Synovial inflammation

Even when cases of inflammatory arthritis, where the disease process is primarily in the synovium, are excluded, microscopic examination generally demonstrates some degree of chronic synovitis. The injury and breakdown of cartilage and bone, such as occurs in osteoarthritis, results in increased amounts of bone and cartilage debris within the joint cavity. The debris is subsequently removed from the synovial fluid by the phagocytic cells of the synovial membrane. In consequence, the membrane becomes both hypertrophic and hyperplastic. In addition, the phagocytosed breakdown products themselves evoke an inflammatory response. It is for these reasons that some degree of chronic inflammation can be expected in the synovial membrane of the osteoarthritic joint, even when the injury has been purely mechanical (Fig. 169.18)[61,62]. Histologic studies have shown that there may be a similarity between the degree of inflammatory response as seen in some cases of severe osteoarthritis and that of rheumatoid arthritis[63].

Inflammation is especially prominent where there has been rapid breakdown of the articular components, as evidenced by the presence in the synovium of abundant bone and cartilage detritus. This is likely to occur in Charcot joints as well as in elderly osteoporotic patients with subchondral fractures. The use of anti-inflammatory drugs that inhibit matrix synthesis will exacerbate this process.

Extension of the hyperplastic synovium on to the articular surface of the joint (i.e. pannus) is a common finding even in osteoarthritis, particularly in the hip. However, the extent and the aggressiveness of this pannus with respect to underlying cartilage destruction is much less marked in osteoarthritis than in rheumatoid arthritis.

Osteophytosis

The most significant morphologic features of an osteoarthritic joint are a change in shape, an increase in size, damage to the articular cartilage and bony sclerosis. In the weightbearing areas of the joint the cartilage may be entirely absent, and the exposed subchondral bone may have a dense, polished appearance like that of marble (eburnation).

When the affected joint is sectioned, in the areas without cartilage the subarticular bone usually is markedly thickened (sclerotic). Adjacent to the surface, cystic defects filled with loose fibromyxoid tissue (or sometimes a thick fluid) may be found. The superficial bone in the eburnated

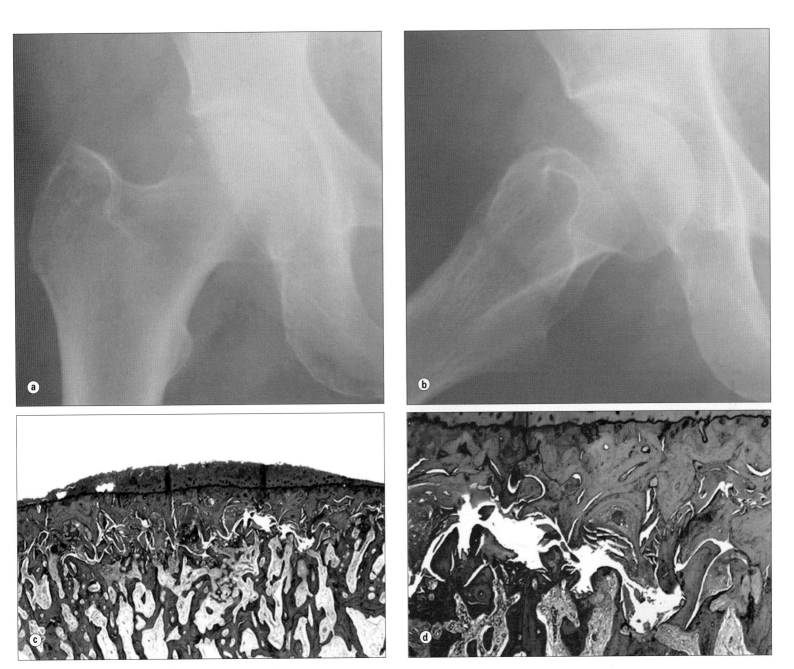

Fig. 169.14 A 68-year-old woman presented with severe acute onset pain in the hip joint. (a+b) Radiographs of the hip showed no abnormality. Magnetic resonance images (not shown) were interpreted as showing osteonecrosis and an isotope study showed increased uptake. (c & d) A total hip replacement was performed and no evidence of osteonecrosis was present in the resected femoral head. However, there was a subchondral fracture involving approximately 20% of the articular surface and located on the superolateral aspect. Hematoxylin and eosin × 4.

areas may be focally necrotic[64]. In areas of the joint that do not bear weight, and around its margins, bony and cartilaginous overgrowths, or osteophytes, develop.

For each joint the location of the osteophytes associated with osteoarthritis is characteristic. In the distal interphalangeal (DIP) joints the osteophytes (Heberden's nodes) are prominent on the dorsal and palmar aspects of both articulating surfaces. In the metatarsophalangeal (MTP) joint of the big toe, the osteophyte is on the medial joint margin (hallux valgus). In the hip joint, although osteophytes are usually present around the entire joint margin, there is characteristically a large flat osteophyte on the medial articular surface of the femoral head, extending to the fovea (Fig. 169.19). The shape and position of the osteophyte depends on the amount of instability and the extent of subluxation of the joint in question. Despite the loss of bone and cartilage in some parts of the joint, which is assumed to be the late result of overloading and mechanical abrasion, in cases of osteoarthritis the net effect of the osteophytes is an overall increase in joint size.

Osteophytes form through the process of endochondral ossification in one of two ways. The first involves vascular penetration into existing cartilage. In the base of this type of osteophyte there are often remnants of the original tidemark and calcified cartilage. In some cases these remnants themselves undergo secondary ossification, not only from the region of the original subchondral bone but also from the osteophyte itself (Fig. 169.20).

Secondary osteophytes may form from foci of cartilaginous metaplasia at the capsular and ligamentous insertions at the joint margins, and may be the result of traction injuries[65]. In this type of osteophyte the cartilage overlying the bone overgrowth is usually hypercellular, and histologically the process resembles the epiphyseal growth plate of a child.

Examination of the residual cartilage remaining on the joint surface reveals many clefts in its substance, most but by no means all of which are vertically oriented. Proteoglycan staining of the matrix is usually diminished[66], although, as discussed previously, there is evidence from

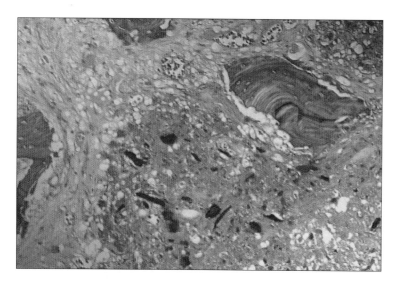

Fig. 169.15 Photomicrograph to demonstrate the granulomatous lesion made up of fibrin, bony detritus and found within the subarticular marrow space, which typifies cases of rapid destructive arthritis. Hematoxylin and eosin × 10.

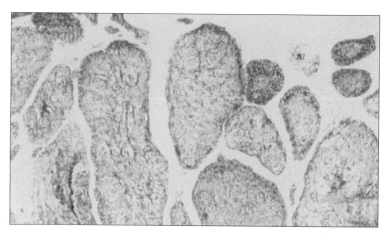

Fig. 169.18 Photomicrograph of the synovial membrane in a patient with osteoarthritis. The villous pattern of the synovium and hyperplasia of the synovial lining cells are evident. In this patient, as with many patients with osteoarthritis, one may also note a mild chronic inflammatory infiltrate in the synovial tissue (this inflammation can be quite severe in some individuals). Hematoxylin and eosin × 10.

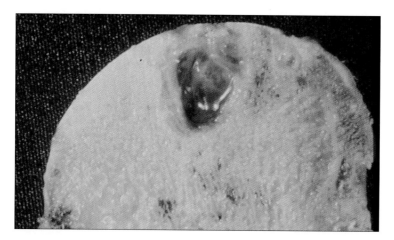

Fig. 169.16 An area of cystic degeneration in the subchondral bone of the superior surface of a femoral head. Such cysts are usually seen only in the absence of the overlying articular cartilage. Note the large flat osteophyte on the medial surface.

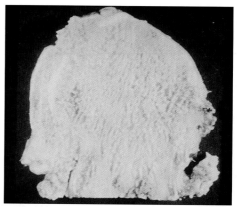

Fig. 169.19 Osteophytosis (on the left hand side of this photograph). A large, flat medial osteophyte associated with subluxation of the femoral head in a patient with osteoarthritis of the hip. The osteophyte extends from the joint margin to the region of the fovea. The residual cartilage of the medial surface of the femoral head can still be seen.

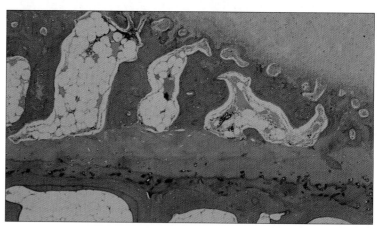

Fig. 169.20 Photomicrograph of a section through a marginal osteophyte. This shows a wedge of bone formation dissecting into the cartilage. The cartilage on the articular side of the osteophyte is cellular, and there is more active endochondral ossification on this surface than on the lower surface that faces the bone. Hematoxylin and eosin × 4.

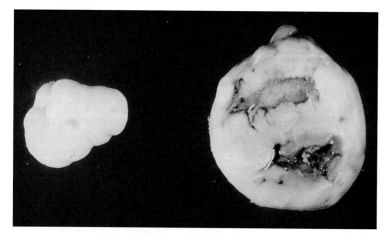

Fig. 169.17 Traumatic arthritis of the elbow. A loose body (left) has arisen from the portion of the articular surface that is missing from the radial head (right).

radioactively labeled sulfate uptake studies that the amount of proteoglycan produced by the chondrocytes in osteoarthritis may be increased. This paradox may be explained by increased leakage of proteoglycan into the synovial fluid and by decreased binding of those proteoglycans

being produced to the surrounding collagen fibrils. The chondrocytes away from the areas of eburnation may show considerable evidence of cell replication, with the formation of prominent cell nests. However, these cell nests are not usually seen in the cartilage immediately adjacent to eburnated areas.

In areas of residual cartilage there is often marked duplication and irregularity of the tidemark. Histologic evidence of increased endochondral ossification, which expands the subchondral bone periphery

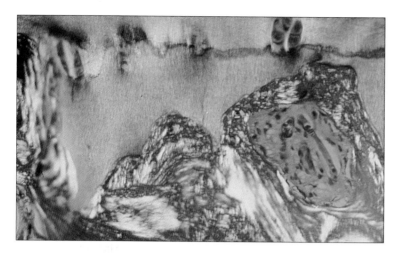

Fig. 169.21 Photomicrograph taken with polarized light showing woven bone formation in the subchondral region. This is an indication of an accelerated rate of replacement of cartilage by bone and hence an increased rate of modeling in a case of osteoarthritis. × 25.

without actually forming an osteophyte, is seen as increased irregularity of the bone cartilage interface, increased vascular penetration of the calcified cartilage, and deposition of woven (immature) bone at the bone–cartilage interface (Fig. 169.21). Again, the net result of this process is to enlarge the end of the bone.

PATHOGENESIS OF OSTEOARTHRITIS

This review has highlighted a number of questions concerning the pathogenesis of osteoarthritis. Is osteoarthritis a single disorder or a family of disorders? What are the roles of acute and chronic trauma in pathogenesis? Is osteoarthritis an inevitable consequence of aging? How do the anatomic, physiologic and biochemical alterations, as well as changes in the mechanical properties of the matrix, interrelate in the pathogenesis of osteoarthritis? What roles do extracartilaginous structures play in osteoarthritis? Under what circumstances does inflammation develop in osteoarthritis, and what role does it play in the perpetuation of disease? Does articular cartilage undergo repair in osteoarthritis?

Osteoarthritis appears to comprise a family of disorders. In about one-fifth of patients it is evident to the clinician that an antecedent condition is causally related to the osteoarthritis (e.g. childhood dysplasia, Perthes' disease, sickle cell disease, hemophilia, Paget's disease, acromegaly etc.). Such cases are often referred to as secondary osteoarthritis and are likely to present clinically at a younger age than those with idiopathic osteoarthritis, who are often over 60 years of age.

The pathogenesis of osteoarthritis can be understood only in terms of the interdependence of anatomy, physiology, biochemistry and mechanical function. All components of the joint have a role in both the etiology and the pathogenesis of the disease: it is not just a disease of the cartilage. Tissue breakdown results in inflammation, which must play a role in the perpetuation of disease processes. Both acute and chronic trauma play a role both in the pathogenesis as well as in the etiology of osteoarthritis. Finally, articular cartilage does undergo repair in osteoarthritis.

When the changes of injury and repair within cartilage, bone and synovium are considered it is clear that joint function depends on the anatomy of the entire joint structure[67]. If the repair processes observed in the various tissues are not directed towards the eventual restoration of the shape of the joint, its stability and an equitable loading pattern over the joint surfaces, then such processes may serve no useful purpose.

The most easily recognized evidence of the attempt at functional restoration is the production of new bone, in the form of osteophytes, at various sites along the joint surface, particularly at the joint margins. Such remodeling may occur early in the degenerative process[68] and the extent can be considerable. The presence of osteophytes, as seen in radiographs of the knee and hip, by no means always heralds the development of progressive symptomatic osteoarthritis. Radiographic studies of large populations of non-symptomatic subjects have shown that even when followed up for as long as 17 years, two-thirds of knees that exhibit evidence of osteophyte formation do not develop other degenerative changes[69].

A number of autopsy studies have demonstrated the prevalence of OA in various joints, as well as its progression from mild to severe disease[70]. The availability of a large volume of tissue specimens from hip replacement arthroplasty, together with the availability of these patients' clinical radiographs and case histories, has enabled us to gain further insights into the natural history of osteoarthritis of the hip[71]. Not all cases are progressive but some – albeit few – show radiographic improvement, with restoration of joint space and a decrease in bone sclerosis and subchondral cysts.

SUMMARY

Osteoarthritis is not necessarily the consequence of aging *per se*, as certain joints in most people remain essentially normal even into extreme old age[72].

In 1909 Nichols and Richardson[73], on the basis of anatomic features, distinguished the two major categories of chronic arthritis by separating inflammatory arthritis from degenerative arthritis. They stated that 'these joint lesions can be divided with great definiteness into two pathological groups:

- those which arise from primary proliferative changes in the joints, chiefly in the synovial membrane and in the perichondrium
- those which arise primarily as a degeneration of the joint cartilage.

These two pathological groups are characterized by distinct gross and histological differences'. Nichols and Richardson went on to say that 'the earliest change to be observed in hypertrophic arthritis is a roughening of the cartilage, which begins near the center of the articular surface, i.e. at the point where pressure and friction between the ends of the bones is greatest.'

Since the time of that report most investigators have concluded that the earliest changes are found in those areas in which it is assumed that weightbearing is pre-eminently concentrated, and which therefore are the most severely subjected to shearing and twisting types of stress[74].

The 'wear-and-tear' theory of the causation has had a stultifying effect on medical opinion with regard to its views concerning the prevention and treatment of osteoarthritis. It would seem more helpful to regard clinical disease not as a result of an inevitable wearing out of the joint but rather as the consequence of a breakdown of the normal functional and physiologic pathways. Such a breakdown is frequently the result of mechanical trauma. Thus the etiology of arthritis can be defined in general terms as any condition that changes the shape of the articulating surface, changes the joint support or alters the tissue matrices.

For example, a fracture through the subarticular bone will alter the geometry of a joint. Such a fracture may occur in young people because of severe injury, or in elderly people as a result of minor trauma in the presence of severe osteoporosis. Another condition that leads to altered joint shape is excessive or altered modeling at the bone–cartilage interface such as occurs (dramatically) in Paget's disease and various endocrinopathies, especially acromegaly[75]. If, as happens in ochronosis as a result of an alteration in collagen tissue structure the cartilage is rendered stiffer and more brittle, with use the cartilage disintegrates and arthritis ensues.

As has already been emphasized, the joints that often develop osteoarthritis may be those that show evidence of cartilage degeneration in early adulthood. The knee is a good example of this. Contrary to previously expressed views that particular areas in the knee and other joints degenerate because of excessive loading, we and others have taken the view that these areas degenerate because of underuse rather than overuse[76]. It is possible that the alteration in joint modeling, which occurs as a normal result of aging and which may be subtly affected by various endocrinopathies, has a contributory role in accelerating cartilage breakdown in areas of previously disused or underused cartilage as the patterns of loading change.

Osteoarthritis is not an inevitable disease resulting from wearing out of the joint by long use. Rather, it is a syndrome of multiple etiologies and the search for a single all-encompassing cause is fruitless[75,77,78]. Rational therapy can only proceed from understanding the pathology. As far as possible treatment should be prophylactic and be directed towards the reasonable avoidance of injury; the early treatment of acute injury, inhibiting continuing injury of the matrix and cells; and promoting repair.

Although dysfunction may begin in any of the structures that make up the joint, by the time the disease comes to the attention of a clinician most of the joint is involved. Because of this overall involvement it is usually impossible for the pathologist to determine the etiology in a given case of arthritis; this is especially true in later stages of the disease. Only continuing autopsy studies in presumably symptomless individuals, with clinical and imaging correlation and the application of new technologies, will fill in the essential background necessary to a full understanding of this common disease state.

ACKNOWLEDGMENT

I am extremely grateful to Philip Rusli for all his invaluable help in the preparation of this manuscript.

REFERENCES

1. Byers PD, Contepomi CA, Farkas TA. A post-mortem study of the hip joint. Ann Rheum Dis 1970; 29: 15–31.
2. Palmoski MJ, Colyer RA, Brandt KD. Joint motion in the absence of normal loading does not maintain normal articular cartilage. Arthritis Rheum 1980; 23: 325–334.
3. Bullough PG. The geometry of diarthrodial joints, its physiological maintenance and the possible significance of age-related changes in geometry to load distribution and the development of osteoarthritis. Clin Orthop 1981; 156: 61–66.
4. Hammond BT, Charnley J. The sphericity of the femoral head. J Med Biol Eng 1967; 5: 445.
5. Walmsley T. The articular mechanism of the diarthroses. J Bone Joint Surg 1928; 10A: 40–45.
6. MacConaill MA. The movements of bones and joints. J Bone Joint Surg 1950; 32B: 244–252.
7. Connor BL, Palmoski MJ, Brandt KD. Neurogenic acceleration of degenerative joint lesions. J Bone Joint Surg 1985; 67A: 562–572; 1976; 58B: 176–183.
8. Maroudas A, Evans H, Almeida L. Cartilage of the hip joint; topographical variation of glycosaminoglycan content in normal and fibrillated tissue. Ann Rheum Dis 1973; 32: 1–9.
9. Kempson GE, Muir H, Swanson A, Freeman MAR. Correlates between stiffness and the chemical constituents of cartilage of the human femoral head. Biochim Biophys Acta 1970; 215: 70–77.
10. Bennett GA, Waine H, Bauer W. Changes in the knee joint at various ages, with particular reference to the nature and development of degenerative joint disease. New York: The Commonwealth Fund, 1942.
11. Bullough PG, Yawitz PS, Tafra L et al. Topographic variations in the morphology and biochemistry of adult canine tibial plateau articular cartilage. J Orthop Res 1985; 3: 1–16.
12. Tammi M, Paukkonen K, Kiviranta I et al. Joint loading-induced alterations in articular cartilage. In: Joint loading. Bristol: Wright, 1987; 64–88.
13. Bullough PG, Walker PS. The distribution of load through the knee joint and its possible significance to the observed patterns of articular cartilage breakdown. Bull Hosp Jt Dis 1977; 37: 110–132.
14. Goodfellow JW, Bullough PG. The pattern of ageing of the articular cartilage of the elbow joint. J Bone Joint Surg 1967; 49B: 175–181.
15. Bullough PG, Goodfellow J, O'Connor JJ. The relationship between degenerative changes and local bearing in the human hip. J Bone Joint Surg 1973; 55B: 746–758.
16. Thompson RC Jr, Basset CAL. Histological observations on experimentally induced degeneration of articular cartilage. J Bone Joint Surg 1970; 52A: 435–443.
17. Caterson B, Lowther DA. Changes in the metabolism of the proteoglycans from sheep articular cartilage in response to mechanical stress. Biochim Biophys Acta 1978; 540: 412–422.
18. Palmoski MJ, Perricone E, Brandt KD. Development and reversal of a proteoglycan aggregation defect in normal canine knee cartilage after immobilization. Arthritis Rheum 1979; 22: 508–517.
19. Veldhuijzen JP, Bourret LA, Rodan GA. In vitro studies of the effect of intermittent compressive forces on cartilage cell proliferation. J Cell Physiol 1979; 98: 299–306.
20. Jones IL, Klamfeldt A, Sandstrom T. The effect of continuous mechanical pressure upon the turnover of articular cartilage proteoglycans in vitro. Clin Orthop 1982; 165: 283–289.
21. Palmoski MJ, Brandt KD. Effects of static and cyclic compressive loading on articular cartilage plugs in vitro. Arthritis Rheum 1984; 27: 675–681.
22. DeWitt MT, Handley CJ, Oakes BW, Lowther DA. In vitro response of chondrocytes to mechanical loading. The effect of short term mechanical tension. Connect Tissue Res 1984; 12: 97–109.
23. Lippiello L, Kaye C, Neumata T, Mankin HJ. In vitro metabolic response of articular cartilage segments to low levels of hydrostatic pressure. Connect Tissue Res 1985; 13: 99–107.
24. Dingle JT, Knight G. The role of the chondrocyte microenvironment in the degradation of cartilage matrix. In: Verbruggen G, Veys EM, eds. Degenerative joints, Vol. 2. Amsterdam: Elsevier, 1985.
25. Van Kampen GPJ, Vledjuijzen JP, Kuijer R et al. Cartilage response to mechanical force in high density chondrocyte cultures. Arthritis Rheum 1985; 28: 419–424.
26. Ogston A. On articular cartilage. J Anat 1876; 10: 49–74.
27. Johnson LC. Morphologic analysis in pathology: The kinetics of disease and general biology of bone. In: Frost HM, ed. Bone biodynamics. Boston: Little, Brown, 1964; 543–654.
28. Green WT Jr, Martin GN, Eanes ED, Sokoloff L. Microradiographic study of the calcified layer of articular cartilage. Arch Pathol 1970; 90: 151–158.
29. Bullough PG, Jagannath A. The morphology of the calcification front in articular cartilage. J Bone Joint Surg 1983; 65B: 72–78.
30. Ali SY, Anderson HC, Sajdera SW. Enzymatic and electromicroscopic analysis of extracellular matrix vesicles associated with calcification in cartilage. Biochem J 1971: 122: 56.
31. Matsuzawa T, Anderson HC. Phosphatases of epiphyseal cartilage studied by electron microscopic cytochemical methods. J Histochem Cytochem 1971; 19: 801–808.
32. Felix R, Fleisch H. Pyrophosphatase and ATPase of isolated cartilage matrix vesicles. Calcif Tissue Int 1976; 22: 1–7.
33. Fortuna T, Anderson HC, Carty RP, Sajdera SW. Enzymatic characterization of the chondrocytic alkaline phosphatase isolated from bovine fetal epiphyseal cartilage. Biochim Biophys Acta 1979; 570: 291–302.
34. Leaver AG, Triffitt JT, Holbrook IB. Newer knowledge of non-collagenous protein in dentin and cortical bone matrix. Clin Orthop 1975; 110: 269–292.
35. Termine JD, Belcourt AB, Conn KM, Kleinman HK. Mineral and collagen-binding proteins of fetal calf bone. J Biol Chem 1981; 256: 10403–10408.
36. Boyan-Salyers BD. Proteolipid and calcification of cartilage. Trans Orthop Res Soc 1980; 5: 9–13.
37. Boskey AL. The role of Ca-PL-PO$_4$ complexes in tissue mineralization. Metab Bone Dis 1978; 1: 137–148.
38. Blumenthal NC, Posner AS, Silverman LD, Rosenberg LC. The effect of proteoglycans on in vitro hydroxyapatite formation. Calcif Tissue Int 1979; 27: 75–82.
39. Blumenthal NC, Betts F, Posner AS. Stabilization of amorphous calcium phosphate by Mg and ATP. Calcif Tissue Int 1977; 23: 245–250.
40. Lagier R. The concept of osteoarthritic remodeling as illustrated by ochronotic arthropathy of the hip: An anatomico-radiological approach. Virchows Arch 1980; 385: 293–298.
41. Yamamoto T, Bullough PG. Subchondral insufficiency fracture of the femoral head: a differential diagnosis in acute onset of coxarthrosis in the elderly. Arthritis Rheum 1999; 42: 2719-2723.
42. Jeffery AK. Osteophytes and the osteoarthritis femoral head. J Bone Joint Surg 1975; 57B: 314–324.
43. Weiss C. Ultrastructural characteristics of osteoarthritis. Fed Proc 1973; 32: 1459–1466.
44. Meachim G. Light microscopy of Indian ink preparations of fibrillated cartilage. Ann Rheum Dis 1972; 31: 457–464.
45. Cutignola L, Bullough PG. Photographic reproduction of anatomical specimens using ultraviolet illumination. Am J Surg Pathol 1991; 15: 1096–1099.
46. Mankin HJ, Thrasher AZ. Water content and binding in normal and osteoarthritic human cartilage. J Bone Joint Surg 1975; 57A: 76–80.
47. Nakata K, Bullough PG. The injury and repair of human articular cartilage: A morphological study of 192 cases of osteoarthritis. J Jpn Orthop Assoc 1986; 60: 763–775.
48. Meachim G, Collins DH. Cell counts of normal and osteoarthritic articular cartilage in relation to the uptake of sulphate ($^{35}SO_4$) in vitro. Ann Rheum Dis 1962; 21: 45–50.

49. Von der Mark K, Kirsch T, Aigner T *et al.* The fate of chondrocytes in OA cartilage. Regeneration, dedifferentiation or hypertrophy. In: Kuetnerr K *et al.*, eds. Articular cartilage and osteoarthritis. New York: Raven Press, 1992; 221–234.

50. Caterson B, Hughes CE, Johnstone B, Mort JS. Immunological markers of cartilage proteoglycan metabolism in animal and human OA. In: Kuettner K *et al.*, eds. Articular cartilage and osteoarthritis. New York: Raven Press, 1992; 415–428.

51. Storey GO, Landells JW. Restoration of the femoral head after collapse in osteoarthritis. Ann Rheum Dis 1971; 30: 406–412.

52. Christensen SB. Osteoarthritis: Changes in bone, cartilage and synovial membrane in relation to bone scintigraphy. Acta Orthop Scand 1985; 214(Suppl.): 1–43.

53. Milgram JW. Morphologic alterations in the subchondral bone in advanced degenerative arthritis. Clin Orthop 1983; 173: 293–312.

54. Poste M, Kerboull M. Total prosthetic replacement in rapidly destructive arthrosis of the hip joint. Clin Orthop 1970; 72: 138–144.

55. Yamamoto T, Bullough PG. The role of subchondral insufficiency fracture in rapid destruction of the hip joint. A preliminary report. Arthritis Rheum 2000; 43: 2423–2427.

56. Mitovic DR, Riera H. Synovial, articular cartilage and bone changes in rapidly destructive arthropathy (osteoarthritis) of the hip. Rheumatol Int 1992; 12: 17–22.

57. Komiya S, Inoue A, Sasaguri Y *et al.* Rapidly destructive arthropathy of the hip: studies on bone resorptive factors in joint fluid with a theory of pathogenesis. Clin Orthop 1992; 284: 273–282.

58. Landells JW. The bone cysts of osteoarthritis. J Bone Joint Surg 1953; 35B: 643–649.

59. Rhaney K, Lamb DW. The cysts of osteoarthritis of the hip. A radiological and pathological study. J Bone Joint Surg 1955; 37B: 663–675.

60. Villacin AB, Brigham LN, Bullough PG. Primary and secondary synovial chondrometaplasia. Hum Pathol 1979; 10: 439.

61. Goldenberg DL, Egan MS, Cohen AS. Inflammatory synovitis in degenerative joint disease. J Rheumatol 1982; 9: 204–209.

62. Gordon GV, Villanueva C, Schumacher HR, Gohel V. Autopsy study correlating degree of osteoarthritis, synovitis and evidence of articular calcification. J Rheumatol 1984; 11: 681–686.

63. Ito S, Bullough PG. Synovial and osseous inflammation in degenerative joint disease and rheumatoid arthritis of the hip. Histometric study. In: Proceedings of the 25th Annual Meeting or the ORS, 1979: 199.

64. Yamamoto T, Yamaguchi T, Lee KB, Bullough PG. A clinicopathologic study of osteonecrosis in the osteoarthritic hip. Osteoarthritis Cartilage 2000; 8: 303–308.

65. Moskowitz RW, Goldberg VM. Studies of osteophyte pathogenesis in experimentally induced osteoarthritis. J Rheumatol 1987; 14: 311–320.

66. Christensen SB, Reimann I. Differential histochemical staining of glycosaminoglycans in the matrix of osteoarthritic cartilage. Acta Pathol Microbiol Scand 1980; 88: 61–68.

67. Radin EL, Burr DB. Hypothesis: Joints can heal. Semin Arthritis Rheum 1984; 13: 293–302.

68. Gilbertson EMM. Development of periarticular osteophytes in experimentally induced osteoarthritis in the dog. Ann Rheum Dis 1975; 34: 12–25.

69. Lawrence JS, Brenner JM, Bier F. Osteoarthrosis: Prevalence in population and relationship between symptoms and x-ray changes. Ann Rheum Dis 1966; 25: 1–24.

70. Heine J. Uber die Arthritis Deformans. Virchows Arch 1926; 260: 521–663.

71. Macys JR, Bullough PG, Wilson PD Jr. Coxarthrosis: A study of the natural history based on a correlation of clinical, radiographic and pathologic findings. Semin Arthritis Rheum 1980; 10: 66–80.

72. Collins DH. The pathology of osteoarthritis. Br J Rheumatol 1938; 14: 253.

73. Nichols EH, Richardson FL. Arthritis deformans. Med Res 1909; 21: 149.

74. Bennett GA, Waine H, Bauer W. Changes in the knee joint at various ages. New York: Commonwealth Fund, 1942.

75. Johanson NA. Endocrine arthropathies. Clin Rheum Dis 1985; 11: 297–323.

76. Harrison MHM, Schajowicz F, Trueta J. Osteoarthritis of the hip: a study of the nature and evolution of the disease. J Bone Joint Surg 1953; 35B: 598–626.

77. Sokoloff L. Endemic forms of osteoarthritis. Clin Rheum Dis 1985; 11: 187–202.

78. Solomon L. Patterns of osteoarthritis of the hip. J Bone Joint Surg 1976; 58B: 176–183

170 Clinical assessment in osteoarthritis

Nicholas Bellamy

- In clinical practice, the need to perform quantitative assessments is driven by the need to establish current clinical status, detect change in clinical status, and quantify response to treatment
- The establishment of current clinical status is a useful goal, particularly when assessing new patients, or those not seen for some time. It provides a quantification of an individual's disease burden, and serves to more closely describe the consequence of their disease
- The detection of change in status provides evidence for worsening or improvement over time
- The quantification of response to therapy facilitates decision making as to whether the therapeutic objective has been achieved, and whether further intervention is required

This chapter concerns assessment of the clinical severity and consequence of osteoarthritis (OA), rather than issues involved in establishing the diagnosis, or determining the severity of structural damage. Readers interested in reviewing the general theory that underpins the measurement process in rheumatology should consult Chapter 4.

FUNDAMENTAL DIFFERENCES BETWEEN MEASUREMENT IN CLINICAL PRACTICE AND CLINICAL RESEARCH ENVIRONMENTS

In general the clinimetric issues surrounding assessment of health status in clinical practice are similar to those in clinical research. In both environments health status measures are required to be valid, reliable and responsive. There are, however, several important differences; these differences are outlined in Table 170.1.

Each of these differences has potential impact on the transfer of evaluation techniques originally developed for clinical research purposes into clinical practice environments.

Measurement in clinical practice

Measurement of osteoarthritis (OA) in clinical practice may be difficult, complex and vary in purpose, during the course of a disorder that can last several decades. In two postal surveys conducted in Australia and Canada[1,2], it was noted that approximately 50% of rheumatologists did not longitudinally follow their OA patients over time. Furthermore, while clinical assessments were made, standardized health status measures, including those specifically developed for OA patients, were rarely used[1,2]. A very recent re-evaluation in Australia (unpublished data) suggests that 5 years later this situation has not changed. It appears from these studies that clinicians require not only measures that are valid, reliable and responsive, but also measures that they perceive as brief, simple, and easy to score. While those who develop instruments and routinely use them in clinical research may be of the opinion that existing measures fulfill these requirements, it is clear that the uptake of these instruments in clinical practice has been gener-

ally poor. This may be due to a number of reasons, such as lack of familiarity, or because the value of routinely performing standardized quantitative assessment has not been conclusively demonstrated to the satisfaction of clinicians or those agencies that might under appropriate circumstances require the collection, application, archiving and availability of such data for patient management and quality audit purposes.

Clinical-based assessment

The skill, knowledge and ability to conduct a thorough interview and physical assessment are generic requirements in the musculoskeletal disciplines. Through a combination of verbal, tactile and visual cues, an impression is gained regarding the nature, severity and consequence of the condition. In particular it is important for the clinician to appreciate the distribution of OA, noting which joints are involved, and which are symptomatic. Often one or two joints are the main problem, even

---

TABLE 170.1 ASSESSMENT ISSUES IN CLINICAL PRACTICE THAT DIFFER FROM CLINICAL RESEARCH ENVIRONMENTS

1 PURPOSE: The purpose of the assessment process is to optimize the outcome for each individual patient
2 FOCUS: The focus is on individual patients rather than groups of patients
3 SELECTION: Patients are not included or excluded from clinical care by virtue of protocol-driven selection criteria
4 CENSORING: The degree of left and right censoring depends on the clinical environment (population-based versus general practice versus rheumatologist versus orthopedic surgery)
5 STRUCTURE: The approach to health status assessment is less structured with respect to domain and instrument selection, and time frame and timing
6 RESOURCES: Resource requirements may be challenging
7 CULTURE: The use of standardized health status questionnaires is neither routine nor ubiquitous
8 EFFECTIVENESS: The effectiveness of the use of quantitative measurement in routine clinical care in OA may not have been adequately demonstrated
9 COST-EFFECTIVENESS: The cost-effectiveness of the use of quantitative measurement in routine clinical care in OA may not have been adequately demonstrated
10 OBLIGATION: There is no obligation or requirement currently to collect data using standardized HSM in routine clinical care
11 ANALYSIS AND INTERPRETATION: The analysis and interpretation of health status data at an individual level has received relatively little attention, compared to statistical methods for group data that are quite routine
12 EXPECTATION: Patients do not generally expect or demand quantitative information
13 EVOLUTION: Some patients are followed over much longer periods of time during which joint involvement may evolve
14 CO-MORBIDITY: Some patients are followed over much longer periods of time during which comorbidities develop
15 FOLLOW-UP: Some patients may be seen on a single occasion or be discharged from longitudinal follow-up
16 SCHEDULING: Clinic attendances and hospitalizations may be unscheduled and the intervals between highly variable

though many may be involved. Based on a detailed examination, fully-trained rheumatologists are able, in general, to agree on which joints are involved in an individual patient[3], even without the aid of radiographic information[4]. Subclinical disease, of course, will not be evident, but symptomatic OA is more readily appreciable.

The distribution of OA can be recorded on a homunculus indicating, for example, involvement of the distal interphalangeal (DIP), proximal interphalangeal (PIP), first carpometacarpal (CMC), hip or knee joints. This simple descriptive exercise provides a basis for tracking the disorder's evolution.

The following features should be assessed: bony enlargement, tenderness on palpation, pain on motion, presence of erythema and effusion or soft-tissue swelling. Erythema (unusual except in DIP and PIP joints), and effusion (unusual except in the knee joints), suggest active inflammation. The exact cause of joint line tenderness is less certain. Evidence of inflammation may provide added support for a management strategy including the use of anti-inflammatory agents.

The detection of joint instability or malalignment indicates a biomechanical abnormality that may require physical forms of therapy or a definitive surgical solution.

Performance-based assessment

Although the 50 foot walk time and to a lesser extent ascent time have been used previously in clinical research studies they are not generally useful in routine clinical practice. In particular suitable conditions for performing the assessment may not be available, and the testing environment may not adequately capture the complexities of comparable 'real world' activities.

Joint goniometry is attended by some degree of intra-observer variability, while plurimetry is a less familiar method of assessing the excursion of joint movement. Nevertheless, quantifying joint range of movement in specific joints is useful for following treatment response, especially to physical and surgical forms of therapy. It is less applicable for assessing the response to analgesic, anti-inflammatory and injectable (hyaluronic acid and corticosteroid-based) forms of treatment. Similar limitations apply to the use of measures such as intercondylar distance and intermalleolar straddle. The usefulness of joint goniometry is restricted because it is the patient's functioning in everyday living, rather than performance on a clinical test, that is important in determining health-related quality of life.

Like measures of joint range of movement, grip strength and pinch grip are easy to conduct in a clinic setting. Issues of intra-observer variability apply, as do issues of clinical consequence. These measures are probably more popular in clinical practice than clinical research settings. Applicable only to hand involvement, they can provide useful information in following response to physical and surgical forms of treatment.

Health Status Questionnaire (HSQ)-based assessment

There is no doubt that in the clinical research environment the use of standardized HSQ is being widely recommended[5,6,7]. Orthopedic associations such as the American Academy of Orthopedic Surgeons and the Hip and Knee Society are ahead of their colleagues in rheumatology in actively promoting the use of HSQ for tracking patient outcomes in routine clinical practice. The measures being recommended are not being used routinely in rheumatology practice. It appears therefore that the problem is in part cultural and the solution is in part within the provenance of professional societies. This raises question as to whether there is compelling evidence to support the benefits of performing quantitative measurement in routine clinical care. A relevant literature search of this area neither highlights the demand by patients for such information, nor evidence for the effectiveness of providing such information to clinicians in improving patient out-

comes. Nevertheless, there are several excellent reasons to perform standardized quantitative measurements:

- Pain is an entirely subjective sensation[8], and has several components that are not readily appreciated by asking a single global pain question. A patient may experience pain in one setting (e.g. while walking), but not in another (e.g. at night). Knowledge of the severity of pain in different settings can be helpful in planning a management program.
- The disability experience differs considerably between patients, and knowledge of the patient's individual profile can be useful in management planning.

Given that (1) pain and disability are the two key symptoms of OA, (2) valid reliable and responsive standardized measures of pain and disability are currently available, and (3) knowledge of the profile and severity of pain and function are useful in management planning, it seems reasonable to conclude that the routine use of quantitative measurement procedures adds value to the management process.

The global approach to questioning, which seems to be used frequently in clinical practice, lacks standardization, and the process by which patients review their symptom experience, select weight and aggregate information is poorly understood. An excessive reliance on global questioning may at times provide an incomplete appreciation of the clinical situation.

Standardized methods of health status assessment provide enhanced opportunities for within-patient comparisons during longitudinal follow-up. They also provide an opportunity for between-patient comparisons when estimating the probability of response to therapy.

Standardized forms of HSQ-based measurement provide data that are immediately available in the clinic, can be given to the patient, and can be used to assist clinical decision making.

Measurement during routine clinical care

The selection of measurement tools depends on the measurement objective. Measurement may be conducted at the level of an individual joint (e.g. left knee) or anatomic region (e.g. hand or hands), the disease in its entirety (e.g. overall OA) or the person as a whole (e.g. health related quality of life). Furthermore, one or more aspects of the condition may be the focus of assessment (e.g. pain and/or function and/or strength and/or range of movement). It is important to tailor the measurement process to the specific clinical requirements. In general different types of measure are mutually complementary, and a battery of measures, used in combination, often represents a robust approach. A few general points are worth considering:

- The general measures of health-related quality of life provide an excellent appreciation of an individual's overall condition. However, these measures lack the necessary content and attribution to understand the specific status of the musculoskeletal condition, since HRQOL scores are often influenced by comorbidities.
- General arthritis measures provide an excellent overview of the musculoskeletal condition but do not have the necessary content and attributions to clearly define the status of individual joints.
- Disease-specific measures, when appropriately worded are capable of defining the condition of individual joints or joint areas, but do not provide the information provided by HRQOL or general arthritis measures.
- The more generalized the OA and the greater the comorbidity, the greater the difference in the type of information being provided by the three different types of measures.
- Measures of strength and joint range of movement provide information about impairment but not about ability/disability or handicap/participation. The consequence to the individual of impaired strength

TABLE 170.2 ASSESSMENT METHODS (ALTERNATIVES SHOWN IN BRACKETS) FOR EVALUATING THE DIFFERENT ASPECTS OF HEALTH

| Joints | Quantitative measurement tools | | | | |
	HRQOL	GAM	DSM	Strength	Motion
Hip	SF36 (EUROQOL)	HAQ (AIMS2)	WOMAC (ICS)	–	ICD/IMS/GON
Knee	SF36 (EUROQOL)	HAQ (AIMS2)	WOMAC (ICS)	–	GON
Hand	SF36 (EUROQOL)	HAQ (AIMS2)	AUSCAN (Cochin/FIHOA)	Grip/pinch	GON

HRQOL, health-related quality of life; GAM, general arthritis measure; DSM, disease specific measure; Strength, muscle strength; Motion, joint range of motion; SF-36, short form 36; HAQ, Health Assessment Questionnaire; WOMAC, Western Ontario and McMaster Universities Osteoarthritis Index; EuroQol, Eurpoean Quality of Life Measure; AIMS2, Arthritis Impact Measurement Scales2; ICS, Indices of Clinical Severity; AUSCAN, Australian/Canadian Osteoarthritis Hand Index; Cochin, Cochin Hand Index; FIHOA, Functional Index of Hand Osteoarthritis; ICD, intercondylar dIstance; IMS, intermalleolar straddle; GON, goniometry (or plurimetry).

or range of movement is not described by such measures, which therefore need supplementing with other functional status measures. Furthermore these types of measures are subject to intra-observer variation and circadian variation

Clinicians, while frequently using global-type questions, should be cautious when interpreting responses, in that global responses are reductionist, and may conceal important information.

The quantitative assessment tools needed to perform such measurements are readily available. Table 170.2 provides a list of suggested assessment methods (alternatives shown in brackets) suitable for evaluating the different aspects of health. It should be noted that the different instruments do not all contain the same dimensions (e.g. the AUSCAN contains pain, stiffness and function while the Cochin and FIHOA [Dreiser Index] only contain function). More detailed information on these measurement techniques can be found in Chapter 4 and in Tables 170.3 and 170.4[9–18]. Though the general item content of several OA specific measures is shown in Tables 170.3 and 170.4, the tables do not provide the exact wording, but simply identify the domains and the areas of enquiry. It is recommended that users contact the index developers prior to using these measures in order to obtain authentic versions of the questionnaires and instructions on administration and scoring.

The measurement battery identified in Table 170.2 is based on the same or similar instruments proposed in Osteoarthritis Society International (OARSI) guidelines documents for the conduct of clinical research in hip, knee and hand OA[5,6]. The advantages from using the same instruments in clinical research and clinical practice are self-evident, but include continuity, familiarity and efficiency.

DATA MANAGEMENT

At the present time clinicians will most often store information in paper form within the patient's clinical file or chart. However, as familiarity with computer systems increases, and computer-based measurement procedures are developed and validated, the opportunity to integrate health status measurement within an electronic medical record will improve. Recent experience using mouse-driven and touch screen navigation in self-completion of the WOMAC Osteoarthritis Index has been positive. Further advances in improving the efficiency of data acquisition, reducing human resource requirements, and immediately providing graphic and tabular information in a user-friendly format can be anticipated within a short period of time. Computer-based systems for

TABLE 170.3 GENERAL ITEM AREAS FOR WOMAC AND ICS INDICES

WOMAC (hip and knee)	Lequesne hip (ICS)	Lequesne knee (ICS)
How much pain Walking on flat Stairs While in bed Sitting/lying Standing **Stiffness** After first wakening Later in day **Degree of difficulty** Descending stairs Ascending stairs Rising from sitting Standing Bending to floor Walking on flat surface Getting in/out of car/bus Shopping Putting on socks/stockings Rising from bed Taking off socks/stockings Lying in bed Getting in/out bath Sitting Getting on/off toilet Performing heavy domestic duties Performing light domestic duties	**Pain or discomfort** During nocturnal bedrest Morning stiffness/regressive pain after rising After standing for 30 min While ambulating Getting up from sitting without using arms **Maximum distance walked** **Activities of daily living** Put on socks by bending forward Pick up an object from the floor Climb up and down a flight of stairs Get into/out of car	**Pain or discomfort** During nocturnal bedrest Morning stiffness/regressive pain after rising After standing for 30 min While ambulating Getting up from sitting without using arms **Maximum distance walked** **Activities of daily living** Climb up standard flight of stairs Climb down standard flight of stairs Squat or bend on knees Walk on uneven ground

TABLE 170.4 GENERAL ITEM AREAS FOR AUSCAN, COCHIN AND FIHOA INDICES

AUSCAN	Cochin	Dreiser/FIHOA
How much pain	**In the kitchen**	Turn key
At rest	Hold bowl	Cut meat
Gripping	Seize full bottle	Cut cloth/paper
Lifting	Hold full plate	Lift full bottle
Turning	Pour liquid	Clench fist
Squeezing	Unscrew lid	Tie knot
How much stiffness	Cut meat	Sew (women)/use screwdriver (men)
After first wakening	Prick things	Fasten buttons
How much difficulty	Peel fruit	Write for long period
Taps	**Dressing**	Accept handshake
Doorknobs	Button shirt	
Buttons	Open/close zipper	
Jewellery	**Hygiene**	
Opening jar	Squeeze tube	
Carrying full pot	Hold toothbrush	
Peeling vegetables/fruits	**At the office**	
Picking up large/ heavy objects	Write short sentence	
Wringing out cloths	Write letter	
	Other	
	Turn door knob	
	Cut paper	
	Pick up coins	
	Turn key	

storing, retrieving, analyzing and displaying data have been developed, but their use to date has not been widespread. Data volume increases in part as a function of time, the number of patients evaluated and followed longitudinally, and the information obtained at each visit. It is important therefore, for the clinical practitioner to recognize the logistic demands that attend progressively increasing data volume.

Data interpretation in clinical practice

Changes in clinical status based on dichotomous data are relatively simple to interpret. A joint is either tender or not tender, effused or not effused, and erythematous or not erythematous, compared to some prior assessment. In contrast, continuous data are more difficult to interpret because some judgment is required regarding the clinical importance of the change which has been observed. The recent publication of the OARSI responder criteria has improved the capability to make such judgments[19]. However, the criteria are joint and class specific, developed around measures of pain, function and patient global assessment and based on data acquired using specific measurement tools. Furthermore, the criteria require a certain minimum score prior to intervention, otherwise it is impossible for the patient to improve sufficiently to be designated a responder, even if improvement occurs.

Differentiating real change from change occurring due to measurement error can be difficult. For this reason several different definitions of change have emerged. More detailed information concerning this issue is provided in Chapter 4.

In general change is important if it is appreciable to the patient, and also results in a meaningful change for better or worse in their health status. It should be noted that patients may reevaluate and reprioritize their treatment goals with continuing experience of OA, and that these processes may influence the interpretation of health status information. In particular the value of recent health gains may be diminished and new health priorities established.

Finally it should be appreciated that a number of factors including social and emotional status, coping, helplessness and fatigue can modulate pain and disability, creating complex and often dynamic bi-directional inter-relationships that may be difficult to interpret.

CONCLUSION

In clinical practice there is a trade off between the benefits and resource costs of acquiring, storing and using quantitative information. Understanding the patient's goals, the musculoskeletal condition and factors mediating and modulating health outcomes is paramount. Measurement procedures should be conducted purposefully, with well identified objectives. Osteoarthritis is a dynamic condition symptomatically and patients may shift their health priorities over the course of this common chronic condition. Nevertheless, there are many excellent valid, reliable and responsive measurement tools for assessing various aspects of the condition. Many are familiar to specialist rheumatologists, and are closely linked to basic skills in interviewing and musculoskeletal examination. Others, in particular generic health-related quality of life measures, general arthritis measures and disease-specific measures, are very familiar to clinical researchers, and their more widespread use in clinical practice is strongly encouraged.

REFERENCES

1. Bellamy N, Kaloni S, Pope J et al. A survey of outcome measurement procedures used in routine rheumatology outpatient practice by Canadian rheumatologists. J Rheumatol 1998; 25: 852–858.
2. Bellamy N, Muirden KD, Brooks P et al. A survey of outcome measurement procedures used in routine rheumatology outpatient practice by Australian rheumatologists. J Rheumatol 1999; 26: 1593–1599.
3. Bellamy N, Klestov A, Muirden K et al. Perceptual variation in categorizing individual peripheral joints for the presence or absence of osteoarthritis using a standard homunculus: observations based on an Australian twin registry study of osteoarthritis. Inflammopharmacology 1999; 7: 37–46.
4. Bellamy N, Klestov A, Muirden K et al. Perceptual variation in categorizing individuals according to American College of Rheumatology classification criteria for hand, knee and hip osteoarthritis: observations based on an Australian twin registry study of osteoarthritis. J Rheumatol 1999; 26: 2654–2658.
5. Osteoarthritis Research Society (OARS) Task Force Report. Design and conduct of clinical trials of patients with osteoarthritis: recommendations from a task

force of the Osteoarthritis Research Society. Osteoarthritis Cart 1996; 4: 217–243.

6. Bellamy N, Kirwan J, Boers M *et al*. Recommendation for a core set of outcome measures for future phase III clinical trials in knee, hip and hand osteoarthritis – consensus development at OMERACT III. J Rheumatol 1997: 24, 799–802.

7. Poss R, Clark CR and Heckman JD. A concise format for reporting the longer-term follow-up status of patients managed with total hip arthroplasty. Editorial, J Bone Joint Surg Am 2001; 83.

8. Wall PD. Introduction. In: Textbook of pain, 2nd edn. Eds. Wall PD and Melzack R. Edinburgh: Churchill Livingstone; 1989.

9. Ware JE Jr, Sherbourne CD. The MOS 36-item Short-Form Health Status survey (SF-36): 1. Conceptual framework and item selection. Med Care 1992; 30: 473–483.

10. Fries JF, Spitz P, Kraines RG, Holman HR. Measurement of patient outcome in arthritis. Arthritis Rheum 1980; 23: 137–145.

11. Bellamy N, Buchanan WW, Goldsmith CH *et al*. Validation study of WOMAC: a health status instrument for measuring clinically important patient relevant outcomes to antirheumatic drug therapy in patients with osteoarthritis of the hip or knee. J Rheumatol. 1988; 15: 1833–1840.

12. Economic and Health Outcomes Research Group: Hurst NP, Jobanputra P, Hunter M *et al*. Validity of Euroqol – a generic health status instrument – in patients with rheumatoid arthritis. Br J Rheumatol 1994; 33: 655–662.

13. Meenan RF, Mason JH, Anderson JJ *et al*. AIMS2 – the content and properties of a revised and expanded arthritis impact measurement scales health status questionnaire. Arthritis Rheum 1992; 35: 1–10.

14. Lequesne MG, Mery C. Samson M, Gerard P. Indexes of severity for osteoarthritis of the hip and knee: validation-value in comparison with other assessment tests. Scand J Rheumatol 1987; 65(suppl): 85–89.

15. Bellamy N, Campbell J, Haraoui B *et al*. Clinimetric properties of the AUSCAN Osteoarthritis Hand Index: an evaluation of reliability validity and responsiveness Osteoarthritis Cart 2002 (In Press).

16. Poiraudeau S, Chevalier X, Conrozier T *et al*. Reliability, validity and sensitivity to change of the Cochin hand functional disability scale in hand osteoarthritis. Osteoarthritis Cart 2001; 9: 570–577.

17. Drieser RL, Maheu E, Guillou GB *et al*. Validation of an algofunctional index for osteoarthritis of the hand. Rev Rhum 1995; 62(suppl): 43S–53S.

18. Bellamy N. Musculoskeletal clinical metrology. Dordrecht: Kluwer Academic; 1993: 1–367.

19. Dougados M, LeClaire P, van der Heijde D *et al*. Special article: response criteria for clinical trials on osteoarthritis of the knee and hip: a report of the Osteoarthritis Research Society International Standing Committee for Clinical Trials Response Criteria Initiative. Osteoarthritis Cart 2000; 8: 395–403.

OSTEOARTHRITIS AND RELATED DISORDERS

171 Management of limb joint osteoarthritis

Carlos J Lozada and Roy D Altman

- Osteoarthritis (OA) is the most common form of arthritis and pain is the patient's major symptom
- Distinguishing articular from periarticular sources of pain is important in designing an appropriate therapeutic intervention
- Currently, the aims of treatment are to reduce pain and minimize disability
- The management of OA should be individualized and should include both non-pharmacologic and pharmacologic intervention
- Patient education, weight control and exercise are the cornerstones of the successful management of OA
- Systemic pharmacologic therapies often effectively relieve pain and include non-steroidal anti-inflammatory drugs, cyclo-oxygenase-2 specific inhibitors, non-opioid analgesics and opioid analgesics
- Intra-articular agents include corticosteroids and hyaluronate products, which may be useful in the symptomatic treatment of knee joint OA
- The adverse event profile of the therapeutic plan should be minimized whenever possible
- Pharmacologic structure-modifying interventions are currently under active investigation
- Surgical interventions are available for those that fail to respond to the non-pharmacologic and pharmacologic interventions

INTRODUCTION

Osteoarthritis (OA) is the most common articular rheumatologic disorder[1]. It is characterized by articular cartilage deterioration, subchondral bone remodeling and osteophyte formation. Risk factors include (among others) increasing age, weight, genetic factors and prior trauma. Traditionally, OA has been viewed as an inevitable degenerative condition of the cartilage. It is now viewed as a biomechanical and biochemical inflammatory disease of the entire joint[2]. New insights into pathogenesis have revealed a role for inflammatory pathways in the natural history of the disease[3]. This understanding of inflammation in OA has led to a new focus on the potential for structure modification[4]. Some new investigational approaches include: enzyme inhibitors, cytokines/cytokine blockers and nutritional supplements[5].

The goals of therapy for OA of the perieral joints are summarized in Table 171.1. The patient must know and understand their disease. Because there is no single program that is effective for everyone, the program needs to be individualized. Although alteration of the course of OA is desirable, present programs improve function and reduce disability by treating symptoms. It is felt that the future will identify and prove that it is possible to alter the course of OA with disease/structure modification.

Therapeutic approaches are generally geared to symptom relief and include non-pharmacologic therapy (e.g. exercise and weight loss), pharmacologic therapies (e.g. topical preparations, intra-articular drugs,

systemic pharmacologic agents) and surgery (Table 171.2)[6]. Guidelines for the management of OA at specific sites have been developed and reported by such bodies as the American College of Rheumatology (ACR)[7] and the European League of Associations of Rheumatology[8].

TABLE 171.1 GOALS IN MANAGEMENT OF OA

- Patient education
- Individualize therapeutic regimen (patient specific morbidities)
- Treat symptoms (e.g. reduce pain)
- Minimize disability
- Slow structural change/disease progression

TABLE 171.2 THERAPEUTIC MODALITIES FOR OA

Non-pharmacologic

Patient education
Disease process and prognosis
Management issues
Patient geared literature
Support groups

Psychosocial measures
Identify and treat depression
Identify and treat sleep disturbances
Weight management (if overweight)

Physical modalities
Thermal modalities
Exercise: isotonic, isometric
- range of motion
- passive
- active
Exercise: aerobic
Supportive devices
- canes
- orthotics
Modifications in activities of daily living

Pharmacologic (drug based) therapy

Topical agents
Intra-articular agents
Oral (systemic) agents
Adjunct therapies
Nutraceuticals
Investigational therapies

Surgical interventions

OA involves both axial and peripheral joints. Peripheral limb joint involvement is common, particularly the proximal interphalangeal (PIP), distal interphalangeal (DIP) and first carpometacarpal (CMC) joints of the hand, and the hip and knee.

Pain is the most frequent symptom of OA and is the symptom that most often brings the patient to see the physician. Pain has multiple potential causes, and a careful assessment of the patient may reveal the source of pain, helping to tailor a therapeutic plan. Potential sources include raised intraosseous pressure, peri-articular muscle and ligament strain, capsular stretching, periosteal elevation at joint margins and synovitis[9]. 'Gelling' of involved joints after prolonged immobility is characteristic. Morning stiffness with OA is rarely more than 30 minutes.

Psychosocial factors, like social isolation, anxiety and depression, contribute to the experience of pain and degree of disability in patients with OA[10,11]. The variety of factors influencing the pain experience in OA emphasize the need for careful assessment and determination of appropriate therapy on an individual basis.

Until a structure (disease) modifying agent is available, the objectives in managing the patient with OA are: reducing/eliminating pain and optimizing function, hence minimizing disability. Fortunately, new basic and clinical research suggests a variety of agents that may alter the course of OA, making the potential for disease (or structure) modification more of a reality (Table 171.3).

Guidelines for the conduct of clinical trials in OA have been developed[12,13]. The principal variable for evaluating the efficacy of symptom modifying therapy is pain relief, usually measured with a visual analog scale (VAS). Other tools for measuring symptomatic relief in OA include the Lequesne 'algofunctional index' and the Western Ontario and McMaster Universities (WOMAC) Osteoarthritis Index. For studies of structure modifying drugs the primary outcome measure has been the radiographic joint space assessment in semiflexed, AP radiographs of the knee and weight-bearing views of the hip. It is expected that magnetic resonance imaging (MRI) will be validated in prospective trials and may replace the radiograph as the surrogate for progression. Biochemical markers and arthroscopy are other potential tools for measuring disease modification in OA[14].

NON-PHARMACOLOGIC THERAPIES

Optimal use of non-pharmacologic modalities improves patient outcomes. Non-pharmacologic approaches include: patient education, psychosocial measures, exercise, support devices, thermal modalities and others and should constitute the base on which all other therapeutic interventions are added. Non-pharmacologic therapies also include potentially disease modifying interventions such as weight loss.

Patient education

Patients should be educated on their diagnosis. Misconceptions often exist about OA. Patients are concerned about possible rapid progression to disability. There should be an emphasis on the natural history of OA and its typically slow progression. Therapeutic options need to be discussed that emphasize lifestyle changes such as exercise and weight control that might be helpful. Lifestyle changes should be individualized, minimizing limitations in activities of daily living.

'Alternative' or 'unproven' therapies and remedies should be openly and objectively discussed. There is a tendency for patients to not advise their physician about 'alternative' pharmaceuticals and nutraceuticals, creating a suboptimal management environment. Educational pamphlets, for example available in the USA through the Arthritis Foundation, may help.

Psychosocial measures

Older age, ethnic background, gender, lower educational level, lower income and unmarried status have been linked to the tendency to become disabled in patients with musculoskeletal complaints[15]. In addition there are a variety of psychosocial factors that modulate the perception of pain and associated disability, including family relationships and secondary gains. Depression needs to be identified and treated; the overall therapeutic program will rarely be effective if depression is not addressed. Continuing emotional support is important, but need not be achieved through frequent doctor visits. Telephone contact with the patient between visits, even by non-professionals, may improve outcomes[16].

Reassurance, counseling and education may minimize the influence of psychosocial factors. Patients must participate in their care, understand their disease and take responsibility for their therapeutic program[17,18]. With a variety of techniques aimed at coping, education and psychosocial factors, one can better achieve patient acceptance, adaptation, compliance and an improved outcome.

A potential application of psychosocial intervention is with the obese patient; weight loss 'groups' and a stable social support system are more effective than simple instructions to diet.

Weight management

There is an epidemiological association between obesity and OA, which is strongest in women with OA of the knee[19–22]. A link between weight and OA of the hands has been proposed as well[23,24]. The mechanisms have not been clearly elucidated and may include increase in body mass, altered biodynamics of gait[25], genetic predisposition (genetically obese mice get more OA), and/or altered metabolism (e.g. estrogens). Pharmacologic approaches to achieving weight loss have been traditionally difficult to achieve. By contrast, through a combination of nutritional consultation, exercise and general lifestyle modifications, patients may be able to succeed. Modest weight loss has been accompanied by a decrease in joint symptoms[26], and perhaps reduced radiographic progression. It may be that a reduction in percentage of body fat, rather than weight itself, may be significant in reducing pain from OA of the knee[27].

Physical measures

There are a variety of physical modalities available for the relief of pain, reducing stiffness, and limiting muscle spasm. These include strengthening the peri-articular structures to provide improved joint support and improve balance. Physical measures make up an integral part of any successful therapeutic program for OA. They can be subdivided into exercise, supportive devices, alterations in activities of daily living, and thermal modalities.

Exercise

Patients with OA should exercise in order to maintain good muscle tone and to help in weight control[28]. Exercise programs have been linked to reduced pain and improved function in OA[29]. In theory, improved muscle support of the joint may retard the progression of OA through improved biomechanics. Care should be taken to choose exercises that maximize muscle strengthening while minimizing stress on the affected

TABLE 171.3 POSSIBLE STRUCTURE/DISEASE MODIFYING AGENTS IN OA*
Glucosamine
Degradative enzyme inhibitors, e.g. tetracyclines, specific metalloproteinase inhibitors
Bisphosphonates
Diacerein
Cytokine inhibitors
Cartilage repair
*Agents in which clinical trials have been initiated

joints. In general, the onset of pain in the involved joint indicates that exercise tolerance has been reached. Peri-articular strengthening exercises can also be recommended depending on the joints involved. An example of this is quadriceps strengthening exercise in managing OA of the knee. Clinically, quadriceps strengthening appears to help with joint stability and provide symptomatic relief. However, in patients with significant varus or valgus deformity, quadriceps strength may accelerate disease progression[30].

Low impact aerobic exercise such as walking or swimming should be recommended in most patients, unless contraindicated because of concurrent illness. Swimming is particularly effective in that it exercises multiple muscle groups and is useful in nearly all forms of OA. In most instances, exercises can be performed by the patient after basic instruction. Some particular sports or activities, however, may need to be curtailed. There are exceptions where specific exercises may actually worsen symptoms: e.g. chondromalacia patella may be worsened by bicycle riding.

A supervised program of fitness walking and education improves functional status without worsening OA of the knee[31]. The intensity of the exercise program should be graded. If the regimen is advanced too quickly, symptoms may worsen. The patient should be advised that worsening pain during exercise is a warning sign that exercise tolerance has been reached and the exercise should be discontinued.

There should be a commitment from the patient to continue an exercise program. If a program is discontinued, benefit is lost. The benefits of a formal exercise program can be lost 9 months after discontinuation[32].

Support devices

Supportive devices can significantly unload a joint and reduce pain from OA[33]. They include canes (walking sticks), crutches, walking frames, and orthotics for shoes. These various supports are intended to improve patient activity, increase compliance, and allow the patient to retain functional independence.

Canes, when properly used, can increase the base of support, decrease loading, and demands on the lower limb and its joints[34]. A cane can unload an affected hip by as much as 60%[33]. They should be used in the contralateral hand and moved together with the limb with the affected joint(s) and height measured to produce about 20 degrees of flexion at the elbow. The total length of a properly measured cane should be equal to the distance between the upper border of the greater trochanter of the femur and the bottom of the heel of the shoe. In general, a single posted cane is preferred unless there is neurologic impairment. The healthier limb should precede the affected limb when climbing up stairs. However, when climbing down stairs, the cane and the affected limb should be advanced first.

Proper footwear is often of great potential value. An orthotic device, or shoe insert, may help the patient with subluxed metatarsophalangeal joints[35]. Trainers may mitigate pain of walking in firm leather shoes. Trainers are generally lighter than leather shoes and have good arch support. A running trainer has a slightly higher heel than a walking trainer and may be of additional help with forefoot abnormalities. Walking ability and pain from medial compartment OA of the knee may be lessened by the use of a lateral heel wedged insole[36,37]. Athletic shoes can be helpful if attention is paid to selecting ones that have good mediolateral support, good medial arch, and calcaneal cushion.

A knee cage or brace may be of use in patients with tibiofemoral disease, especially those with lateral instability or those with a tendency for the knee to 'give out'[38,39]. The knee cage is not helpful and may worsen symptoms when significant valgus or varus deformity is present. Medial taping of the patella has been advocated by some in order to relieve the symptoms of OA of the knee and particularly in those with chondromalacia patella[40].

The use of the devices should be monitored to insure proper use. For example, cane/crutch tips should be changed when worn, in order to avoid slipping on smooth or wet surfaces.

Thermal modalities

Heat or cold applications are potentially helpful to patients with OA. The use of heat, cold, or alternating heat and cold are based on patient preference and not on any scientific superiority[41]. For chronic pain, most patients prefer the symptomatic relief obtained from heat applications to that obtained from cold. Traditionally, the more acute the process, the more likely cold applications will be of benefit (reduction in blood flow and reduction in pain). Sources of heat include: warm packs, heating pads, paraffin baths, ultrasound and others. The use of heat can be subdivided into superficial and deep, with no proven advantage of one over the other. The therapeutic value of applying heat includes decreasing joint stiffness, alleviating pain, relieving muscle spasm, and preventing contractures. Because of the risk of burns, heat modalities should be used with caution in anesthetized, somnolent or obtunded patients. The use of heat is contraindicated over tissues with inadequate vascular supply, bleeding, or cancer. Heat should also be avoided in areas close to the testicles or near developing fetuses. The range of temperatures used is from 40–45°C (104–113°F)[42] for 3–30 minutes. Dehydration is a risk from prolonged hot baths, particularly in the elderly. Cold is mostly applied through cold packs. Cold can relieve muscle spasm, decrease swelling in acute trauma, and relieve pain from inflammation. There have been no studies demonstrating superiority of spas over home applications in providing heat/cold applications.

Activities of daily living

Alteration in activities of daily living may improve symptoms. For example, raising the height of a chair or toilet seat can be helpful since the hip and knee are subjected to the highest pressures during the initial phase of rising from the seated position.

Miscellaneous

There are several miscellaneous physical modalities that may warrant additional study, such as massage, yoga therapy, acupressure, magnets, pulsed electromagnetic fields and transcutaneous neural stimulation (TENS). In a meta-analysis of seven published trials of OA of the knee acupuncture reduced pain but did not alter function[43].

PHARMACOLOGIC MODALITIES

Since no one agent is uniformly effective in treating the symptoms of OA, there are many pharmacologic agents that are presently in use (Table 171.4). Pharmacologic modalities could potentially be divided into topical, intra-articular and oral (systemic) agents. Furthermore, systemic therapies can be divided into those that relieve symptoms and agents that have the potential of structure (disease) modification[44]. Furthermore, those that relieve symptoms may have a rapid or slow onset of effect.

Topical agents

Capsaicin ointments applied to the skin without rubbing have been formally tested in OA of hand joints[45,46]. Clinically, they are potentially helpful in relieving pain in other joints such as the knees. Capsaicin products are derived from the common hot pepper plant and are usually in concentrations of 0.025 or 0.075%. Capsaicin is also available in a 'roll on' form. The proposed mechanism of action is depletion of the neurotransmitter substance P[47].

The patient feels heat in the area where these are applied. If the patient uses them regularly (e.g. 3–4 times a day), the heat sensation lessens and there is persistent relief of pain. Care should be taken to avoid contact with the eyes as capsaicin can be quite irritating.

TABLE 171.4 PHARMACOLOGIC THERAPY FOR OA

Topical agents

Capsaicin preparations
Salicylate preparations
Topical non-steroidal anti-inflammatory agents

Intra-articular agents

Corticosteroids
Hyaluronan

Systemic agents – rapid onset of effect

Non-narcotic analgesics
Acetaminophen
Opioid related analgesics
Tramadol
Propoxyphene
Codeine
Opioid analgesics (may be topical)
Non-steroidal anti-inflammatory drugs
Non-selective inhibitors
COX-2 specific inhibitors

Systemic agents – slow onset of effect

e.g. glucosamine, chondroitin sulfate, unsoponafiable oils, diacerein

Adjuvants

Antidepressants
Muscle relaxants

There are a variety of non-steroidal anti-inflammatory drug (NSAID) preparations that are available for topical application. Most, but not all, published trials have shown superiority over placebo[48,49].

Intra-articular therapy

Depot corticosteroids have been widely used as intra-articular agents for treatment of peripheral joints with OA[50]. Depot corticosteroids presumably relieve symptoms through an anti-inflammatory effect. The duration of effect of intra-articular depot corticosteroids is usually for more than 1 month and is not related to several risk factors examined[51]. This therapy can be particularly helpful in allowing a patient to participate in physical therapy. There may be a benefit in reducing the reaccumulation of joint effusions. The patient should be warned, however, not to overuse the joint as this may result in paradoxical increase in symptoms. Depot corticosteroids may also be useful in the management of periarticular disease, such as anserine bursitis, that commonly accompanies OA. Because of concerns over deleterious effects on cartilage[52], it is generally not recommended that a joint be injected with depocorticosteroids more than four times per year[53].

The amount of depot corticosteroid injected varies depending on the joint and the volume to be injected. Infection is the major risk of intra-articular depocorticosteroids injections, though this is fortunately uncommon. In addition, depot corticosteroids are prepared as crystals for their prolonged effect; they may induce a crystalline synovitis[54]. This 'flare' typically occurs within hours of the injection. This is in contrast to infection, which most often happens 24–72 hours after the procedure. The application of cold compresses often reduces the pain of a crystalline flare until symptoms resolve spontaneously within several hours. There is no role for systemic corticosteroids in the management of OA.

Intra-articular hyaluronate (HA) may reduce the symptoms of OA of the knee. HA is administered as 3–5 intra-articular weekly injections[55].

HA is a normal component of synovial joints[56]. Preparations vary widely in molecular weight from 0.5 to over 6 million kDa, with no proven advantage of size or viscosity. Because of a limited half life in the joint, intra-articular HA exerts a short term lubricant and biomechanical effect. The HA long term effects may be due to an anti-inflammatory effect, reduced neuroreceptor activity, altered cartilage metabolism, and/or altering synoviocyte behavior. HA preparations may reduce pain for prolonged periods of time and potentially improve mobility[57]. A problem in studying these and other intra-articular compounds for OA has been a high placebo group response rate[58]. An intra-articular HA (Hyalgan®) derivative was compared to oral naproxen or placebo in a 14 week double blind study. Pain relief was prolonged with the HA, and at 6 months over 60% of the completers had at least a 20% reduction of pain, with half of that group pain free. Even though 40% of the placebo group improved, there was significant improvement in the HA injected group when compared to placebo. The benefit compared favorably to naproxen with significantly fewer adverse effects (fewer gastrointestinal complaints). In another study, three weekly intra-articular injections of HA (Synvisc®) were compared to their combination with an NSAID, and to the NSAID alone. At week 12 and a telephone follow up after 26 weeks, the groups receiving the HA were better in terms of rest pain and lateral joint tenderness[59]. The major adverse effect is a local transient painful reaction in the joint or at the injection site.

Formal use for knee OA has been approved in the USA and trials are underway studying use in other joints such as the shoulders, ankles and hips.

Oral (systemic) pharmacologic agents
Symptom modifying agents
This group of agents includes analgesics such as non-opioid analgesics [e.g. acetaminophen (paracetamol) and tramadol] and opioid analgesics, or anti-inflammatory agents such as NSAIDs. Analgesia may be potentiated by adjuvant agents, such as agents intended to reduce muscle spasm and low dose antidepressant medications, particularly tricyclic antidepressants.

Non-opioid analgesics
For many patients with OA, relief of mild to moderate joint pain can be achieved with acetaminophen (paracetamol). Oral acetaminophen 1g four times daily has a benefit equivalent to ibuprofen 2.4g/day in treating the pain of OA by most measured parameters[60]. However, in several trials, NSAIDs have been more efficacious, particularly in those with moderate to severe symptoms from their OA[61,62]. The revised ACR recommendations for the medical management of OA allow for selection of an NSAID or a COX-2 selective inhibitor as initial therapy in those with more symptomatic OA[63].

There is concern for hepatotoxicity with acetaminophen when taken at doses above the recommended maximum (4g/day). Care should be taken to avoid other acetaminophen containing compounds, such as cold remedies, if the patient is already consuming full OA doses of acetaminophen.

Opioid analgesics
Although there is limited published clinical research, weak opioid analgesics such as propoxyphene and codeine have been commonly administered for OA.

Tramadol has a dual mechanism of action: inhibition of the μ opioid receptor and inhibition of serotonin uptake. It does not have significant addiction potential[64]. Starting doses of less than 50mg daily minimize nausea and other central nervous system adverse effects. High doses have been associated with seizures and allergic reactions[65]. The dose can be titrated to a maximum of 100mg four times daily. Tramadol can be added to medication regimens that use NSAIDs as base therapy and may have NSAID-sparing properties[66]. Tramadol can also be combined with acetaminophen for an added analgesic effect[67].

Stronger narcotics or narcotic derivatives are also useful in selected patients with OA. The World Health Organization stepladder guidelines for the use of narcotic analgesics should be followed. Additional guidelines have been published[68]. Dependence is always of concern, but is less common in patients with OA. Narcotics are used most often as rescue medications for severe pain. Constipation should be anticipated as it is an often encountered adverse effect. Although tablet forms are most often prescribed, alternative dosing regimens such as slow release patches are available.

Non-steroidal anti-inflammatory drugs

Non-steroidal anti-inflammatory drugs continue to be the most commonly used agents in the therapy of OA. NSAIDs are available in both prescription and over-the-counter dose forms. NSAIDs are analgesic, anti-inflammatory and antipyretic, exerting their therapeutic effect by blocking cyclooxygenase (COX) at sites of pain and/or inflammation. Their effects are mostly at peripheral sites of inflammation, but have some central analgesic effects.

Even though non-selective NSAIDs are effective in OA, potential adverse events, particularly gastrointestinal, are of concern. These include gastroduodenal ulcers that can result in pain, bleeding, perforation or obstruction. Some estimates are that, in the USA, NSAID use is linked to 16 000 deaths and over 100 000 hospitalizations a year from gastrointestinal bleeding. Although most major gastrointestinal events occur without warning, there are risk factors that predispose patients to these events. They include: older age, higher dose of NSAIDs, prior history of peptic ulcer disease or of gastrointestinal bleeding, comorbid conditions such as heart disease and concurrent use of systemic corticosteroids and oral anticoagulants.

Various strategies have been utilized to reduce this risk of NSAID-associated gastrointestinal toxicity. The addition of a proton pump inhibitor to the medication regimen has been proven to reduce the incidence of endoscopic peptic ulcers in those on NSAIDs[69]. Misoprostol, a prostaglandin analog, reduces the incidence of clinical GI adverse events when used at a dose of $200\mu g$ four times daily[70]. Diarrhea is a potential side effect. Over the counter doses of H-2 blockers and antacids have not been shown to reduce either endoscopic or clinical gastrointestinal events.

Two distinct cyclooxygenase isoenzymes, COX-1 and COX-2, have been identified. COX-1 is constitutive and appears to protect the gastric mucosa from the acidic environment of the stomach. In contrast, COX-2 is mostly inducible and commonly expressed at sites of inflammation such as joints.

COX-2 selective inhibitors have been developed for use in OA[71]. Although no more effective than aspirin or non-selective NSAIDs, there is considerable evidence that they have less gastrointestinal toxicity[72,73]. Platelet aggregation and bleeding time are not significantly affected by COX-2 selective inhibition[74]. The use of daily aspirin for cardiovascular or cerebrovascular prophylaxis reduces, but does not eliminate, COX-2 selective inhibitor derived gastrointestinal protection. The various issues of aspirin/NSAID-COX-2 interactions remain an active area of investigation[75]. Like non-selective NSAIDs, some patients will have increased hypertension and/or peripheral edema with COX-2 selective inhibitors. Both COX-1 and COX-2 are present in the kidney and COX-2 selective inhibitors can precipitate renal insufficiency. As with traditional NSAIDs, they should be used with caution in the presence of even mild renal insufficiency.

Celecoxib, rofecoxib, and valdecoxib are the first available COX-2-selective inhibitors. Recent trials have attempted to compare their efficacy, and that of acetaminophen, in OA[76]. Meloxicam has COX-2 selective inhibition at the recommended doses[77]. More highly selective COX-2 agents are under development (e.g. etoricoxib); the increased selectivity has uncertain additional clinical benefit at this time[78].

Adjunct therapies

Any analgesic program can be supplemented with tricyclic antidepressant medication[79,80]; the antidepressants appear to potentiate the analgesic effects of the other agents. In addition, they may exert part of their benefit by improving sleep patterns altered by nocturnal myoclonus and fibromyalgia-like complaints.

Oral *anti-spasmodics* are purported to reduce muscle pain and spasm in OA[81]. The value of oral medications in relieving the pain of muscle spasm is controversial. However, centrally acting agents may be helpful for improving sleep patterns through their sedating qualities and potential for disrupting neurologic transmission of the pain sensation. Pain associated with muscle spasm may be reduced with a local injection of lidocaine with or without a depot corticosteroid.

'Nutraceuticals'

'Nutraceuticals' are nutritional supplements that appear to have medicinal properties[82]. For a variety of reasons nutraceuticals have gained in popularity. There are increasing attempts to subject nutraceuticals to rigorous clinical research. Some are being tested in double-blind, randomized clinical trials.

Glucosamine sulfate 1500mg/day, has been tested in several clinical trials comparing it to placebo and other NSAIDs. In small European trials it has shown pain relief comparable to that of ibuprofen 1200mg/day in OA of the knee but with a slower onset of action (3–4 weeks)[83,84]. Structure modification with reduced progression of joint space narrowing of the knee was demonstrated in two 3-year, double blind, randomized trials when compared to placebo[85,86]. Serial radiographs of the knee (in full extension) assessed joint space width. Very small joint space benefit has been seen favoring the glucosamine groups.

Oral *chondroitin sulfate*, a glycosaminoglycan with a molecular mass of around 14 000, is composed of repeating units of N-acetyl galactosamine and glucuronic acid. Chondroitin sulfate 800–1600mg/day reduced pain in OA of the knee[87]. There is a relatively slow onset of benefit; NSAIDs have more rapid pain relief.

There is little information on the combination of glucosamine and chondroitin.

A National Institutes of Health sponsored study is currently examining glucosamine hydrochloride, chondroitin sulfate, the combination, a COX-2 selective inhibitor, and placebo in patients with knee OA.

S-adenosylmethionine (SAM-e), a methyl group donor and oxygen radical scavenger, has been used by intravenous loading and oral maintenance[88]. Limited information is available.

MSM (methylsulfonylmethane) has been touted as a 'sulfate donor' (especially through the internet). This 'natural' product is actually chemically manufactured. It is related to DMSO, a solvent that has also been proposed as a remedy for several different conditions. There is minimal information on MSM's efficacy and/or toxicity available in the peer-reviewed scientific literature.

A ginger extract was recently reported to be superior to placebo in a randomized clinical trial of OA of the knee[89].

Other nutraceuticals are entrenched in popular culture. These include compounds such as 'cat's claw' and shark cartilage that are being used with increasing frequency and being sold over the counter in pharmacies and health food stores. There are no carefully performed trials to support their use.

Miscellaneous agents

Although research continues into symptom-modifying medications for OA, there is a new emphasis on the development of structure modifying agents. Structure modifying medications are intended to retard, prevent or reverse the progression of OA.

Since there is no direct measure of progression of OA, imaging studies are used as a surrogate measure of structure modification by measuring the joint space[90]. Several groups of agents are under investigation, mostly directed at cartilage repair:

- growth factors and cytokines
- sulfated and non-sulfated sugars
- hormones and other steroids
- enzyme inhibitors
- chondrocyte/stem cell transplantation.

Tetracyclines, apart from any antimicrobial effect, are inhibitors of tissue metalloproteinases[91] and may have effects on nitric oxide synthase[92]. Doxycycline has reduced the severity of OA in canine models[93] and is currently being evaluated in a multi-center, double blind, placebo controlled trial for 'structure-modification' in obese women with OA of the knee.

Specific metalloproteinase inhibitors are also under investigation for structure modification in OA.

Diacerein[94] and its active metabolite rhein are anthraquinones related to senna compounds. They inhibit the synthesis of interleukin-1 (IL-1) beta in human OA synovium in vitro as well as the expression of IL-1 receptors on chondrocytes[95]. No effects have been reported on TNF or its receptors. Collagenase production and articular damage have been reduced in animal models[96–98]. Early human clinical trials have shown improved pain scores as compared to placebo and comparable efficacy to NSAIDs but slower onset of action[99]. Diarrhea is the main adverse effect[100]. It is usually self-limited. One trial suggested disease/structure modification in OA of the hip joint. Unfortunately, the study had a dropout rate that approached 50%[100]. Furthermore, symptomatic benefit couldn't be confirmed. On the strength of these trials, diacerein has been proposed as a slow acting symptom-modifying and perhaps disease/structure modifying drug for OA.

Oral preparations of *avocado and soya unsaponifiables* (ASU) have been studied in OA of the knee and hand. The unsaponifiable residues of avocado and soya oils are mixed in a 1:2 ratio. *In vitro* studies on cultured chondrocyte have shown partial reversal of IL-1β effects. IL-1β roles in OA are thought to include inhibition of prostaglandin synthesis by chondrocytes and stimulation of MMP and nitric oxide (NO) production. Metalloproteinases and nitric oxide can degrade cartilage matrix and cause chondrocyte apoptosis. Use of ASU also results in inhibited production of IL-6, IL-8, matrix metalloproteases and stimulation of collagen synthesis. The mechanism through which these effects occur is unknown as is the active ingredient in ASU[101]. Symptomatic benefit in double-blind human trials in OA of the hip and knee has also been reported[102]. Some abstract presentations have suggested structure/disease modification in human hip OA[103].

MANAGEMENT OF OA AT SPECIFIC SITES

The hand

Hand joints commonly affected in OA include the first carpometacarpal (CMC) joints, distal interphalangeal joints (DIP) and proximal interphalangeal (PIP) joints. Topical agents such as capsaicin have been tested in OA of these joints and are helpful. Involvement of the CMC joint at the base of the thumb can be particularly disabling. The patient often benefits from intra-articular injection of a corticosteroid preparation. Orthoses, such as a thumb splint, can help a patient that is having difficulty with vocational or avocational chores. Surgery may be needed if the patient cannot be helped with conservative interventions[104].

The knee

Knee crepitus, pain on activity and gelling after prolonged inactivity are characteristic. In some, effusions are evident. A careful assessment as to the cause of the pain should be made. Tendinitis/bursitis components, particularly anserine bursitis should be identified.

Quadriceps strengthening exercises should be taught and the patient should perform them at least every other day. General exercise, such as walking or swimming will help and will also contribute to limb strength. High impact activities such as stair climbing and jogging should be discouraged. When exercising, if pain ensues in the affected joint, it is an indication that exercise tolerance has been reached and the patient should rest. Weight loss is important in overweight individuals but is very difficult to achieve.

In more severe cases, a cane may help unload the joint. It should be held in the contralateral hand and may not only reduce pain, but perhaps increase exercise tolerance. Heel and forefoot wedges may help those with varus deformities[105]. Medial taping of the patella can be useful in those with patellofemoral OA.

Topical agents and systemic therapies such as acetaminophen, NSAIDs or COX-2 selective inhibitors are often used in these patients. Joint aspiration and infiltration with depot corticosteroids or hyaluronate preparations may be helpful in relieving the symptoms of those with knee OA[106]. Tidal lavage with 0.5–1 liter of saline has been tried with some success[107].

Surgical intervention is effective in those refractory to more conservative management. There are no firm guidelines for surgery; however, surgery may be indicated for joint pain due to the OA that is not relieved with the other interventions; particularly if it interferes with the patient's ability to perform his daily activities. Arthroscopic intervention should be limited to patients in whom an additional diagnosis of internal derangement is suspected. Surgical arthroscopy is useful for repair and for partial removal of damaged menisci in some patients; benefit decreases with increasing age. The value of synovectomy and debridement has not been established in OA. Abrasion chondroplasty leads to partial cartilage repair and provides the same symptomatic improvement as irrigation and debridement alone[108]. Arthroscopic lavage has also been tried, with some success. Large-bore needle lavage with saline may be of value in selected patients[109]. It has been shown to be effective in the relief of pain in OA of the knees for up to 6 months[110].

Osteotomies and arthroplasties appear cost effective when the improved quality of life and the alternatives are considered. Osteotomies may serve as alternatives to arthroplasty, in younger, overweight patients, and in unicompartmental disease of the knee. This may delay progression of disease (hence the need for total joint replacement). However, only 50% of patients with knee osteotomies have satisfactory results at 10 years[111].

Total knee arthroplasties have improved the morbidity and probably the indirect mortality of OA. Most series report good to excellent long-term results in over 90% of patients undergoing knee replacement. Overweight patients, along with those with marked varus or valgus deformities and those with flexion contractures offer particular challenges to the orthopedic surgeon. Knee fusions are not recommended because of the poor resulting function. They are only employed in those who have failed arthroplasty.

A particular presentation in younger adults with patellar (anterior knee) pain is chondromalacia patellae. In chondromalacia, there is damage to the patellar cartilage and pain is most notable when walking uphill or upstairs. Avoidance of these activities and quadriceps strengthening exercises should be recommended.

The hip

Symptomatic hip OA is usually insidious in onset. Diminished internal rotation, a limp and groin pain are characteristic. Complaints of pain in

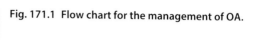

FLOW CHART FOR THE MANAGEMENT OF OA

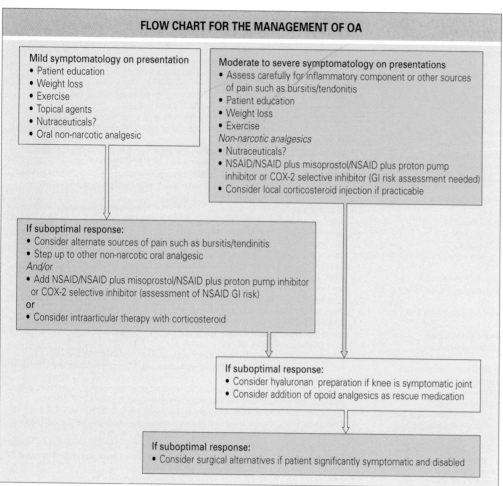

Mild symptomatology on presentation
- Patient education
- Weight loss
- Exercise
- Topical agents
- Nutraceuticals?
- Oral non-narcotic analgesic

Moderate to severe symptomatology on presentations
- Assess carefully for inflammatory component or other sources of pain such as bursitis/tendonitis
- Patient education
- Weight loss
- Exercise
Non-narcotic analgesics
- Nutraceuticals?
- NSAID/NSAID plus misoprostol/NSAID plus proton pump inhibitor or COX-2 selective inhibitor (GI risk assessment needed)
- Consider local corticosteroid injection if practicable

If suboptimal response:
- Consider alternate sources of pain such as bursitis/tendinitis
- Step up to other non-narcotic oral analgesic
And/or
- Add NSAID/NSAID plus misoprostol/NSAID plus proton pump inhibitor or COX-2 selective inhibitor (assessment of NSAID GI risk)
or
- Consider intraarticular therapy with corticosteroid

If suboptimal response:
- Consider hyaluronan preparation if knee is symptomatic joint
- Consider addition of opoid analgesics as rescue medication

If suboptimal response:
- Consider surgical alternatives if patient significantly symptomatic and disabled

Fig. 171.1 Flow chart for the management of OA.

the buttocks, sciatic region or even knee are not uncommon. Pain in the lateral aspect of the upper thigh that is reproducible on palpation most often represents trochanteric bursitis. Local depocorticosteroid infiltration is particularly effective in managing the bursitis.

The initial management is similar to that for knee OA. Weight loss and exercise are important. Both range of motion and strengthening exercises are important. Formal referral for physical therapy may be necessary in some, particularly in older, debilitated patients. Unloading with a cane should be recommended to significantly symptomatic patients. Use of a cane can reduce stress on the joint by about 20–30%[23].

Systemic pharmacologic therapy is often needed if pain interferes with adequate ambulation. Acetaminophen, NSAIDs or COX-2 selective inhibitors can be used. Opioid analgesics should be used with caution but may be necessary in some and can delay the need for operative therapy. Intra-articular corticosteroid infiltration is not generally advisable but, if performed, fluoroscopic guidance is often needed.

Osteotomy and arthroplasty are the surgical methods employed in those with more severe involvement. The choice of procedure generally depends on the patient's circumstances. Osteotomies are less useful than for knee OA. Arthroplasty provides excellent pain relief and superior function. The need for revision arthroplasty later on in life because of heavier loading, greater duration of usage, and prosthesis deterioration and/or loosening is of concern in younger patients. There has

been an 85% success rates at 20 years followup of the Charnley total hip prosthesis.

Materials used for prostheses include polyethylene and stainless steel. The polyethylene components can 'wear' with time. Loosening of either the acetabular or femoral component is another potential clinical issue. There has been some controversy regarding the use of cemented (polymethylmethacrylate) versus uncemented prostheses and the rates of complications such as loosening. A combination used widely is an uncemented acetabular component with a cemented femoral component. Some have tended to try uncemented femoral components in younger, more active patients. Hip fusion provides more restricted function and is mostly used for failed arthroplasties.

SUMMARY

The therapy of OA involves establishing the diagnosis of OA and trying to determine the cause of the patients symptoms and signs. An algorithm is proposed (Fig. 171.1) that includes a combination of non-pharmacologic therapy, pharmacologic therapy and surgery. As with any chronic disease, therapy is not curative and a stepwise approach is needed that is guided by the severity and impact of OA on the patient. The future therapies of OA will involve attempts at altering the course of OA, either by prevention, stabilization or reversal of the pathogenic mechanisms involved.

REFERENCES

1. Kramer JS, Yelin EH, Epstein WV. Social and economic impacts of four musculoskeletal conditions: a study using national community-based data. J Rheumatol 1983; 26: 901–907.

2. Liang MH, Fortin P. Management of osteoarthritis of the hip and knee. Editorial. N Eng J Med 1991; 325: 125–127.

3. Poole AR, Howell DS. Etiopathogenesis of osteoarthritis. In: Moskowitz R, Howell D, Altman R *et al.*, eds. Osteoarthritis: diagnosis and management, 3rd edn. Saunders: Philadelphia; 2001: 29–47.

4. Lozada CJ and Altman RD. Chondroprotection in osteoarthritis. Bull Rheum Dis 1997; 46: 5–7.

5. Lozada CJ and Altman RD. New and investigational therapies for osteoarthritis. In: Moskowitz R, Howell D, Altman R et al., eds. Osteoarthritis: diagnosis and management, 3rd edn. Saunders: Philadelphia; 2001: 447–448.

6. Lozada CJ and Altman RD. Osteoarthritis: A comprehensive approach to management. J Musculoskeletal Med 1997; 14: 26–38.

7. ACR Subcommittee on osteoarthritis guidelines. Recommendations for the medical management of osteoarthritris of the hip and knee: 2000 update. Arthritis Rheum 2000; 43: 1905–1915.

8. Pendleton A, Arden N, Dougados M et al. EULAR recommendations for the management of knee osteoarthritis. Ann Rheum Dis. 2000; 59: 936–944.

9. Felson DT, Chaisson CE, Hill CL, Totterman SMS et al. The association of bone marrow lesions and pain in knee osteoarthritis. Ann Intern Med 2001; 134: 541–549.

10. Summers MN, Haley WE, Reveille JE, Alarcon GS. Radiographic assessment and psychological variables as predictors of pain and functional impairment in osteoarthritis of the hip or knee. Arthritis Rheum 1988; 31: 204–209.

11. Salaffi F, Cavalieri F, Nolli M et al. Analysis of disability in knee osteoarthritis: relationship with age and psychological variables but not with radiographic score. J Rheumatol 1991; 18: 1581–1586.

12. Altman R, Brandt K., Hochberg M. et al. Design and conduct of clinical trials in patients with osteoarthritis: recommendations from a task force of the Osteoarthritis Research Society. Osteoarthritis Cart 1996; 4: 217–243.

13. Lequesne M, Brandt K, Bellamy N et al. Guidelines for testing slow acting drugs in osteoarthritis. J Rheumatol 1994; 21(suppl 41): 65–73.

14. Altman R. and Lozada CJ. Laboratory findings in osteoarthritis. In: Moskowitz R, Howell D, Altman R et al., eds. Osteoarthritis: diagnosis and management, 3rd edn. Saunders: Philadelphia; 2001: 273–91.

15. Cunningham,LS and Kelsy, JL. Epidemiology of musculoskeletal impairments and associated disability. AJPH 1984; 74: 574–579.

16. Weinberger M, Tierney WM, Cowper PA et al. Cost-effectiveness of increased telephone contact for patients with osteoarthrits. Arthritis Rheum 1993; 36: 243–246.

17. Lorig KR, Mazonson PD, Holman HR. Evidence suggesting that health education for self-management in patients with chronic arthritis has sustained health benefits while reducing health care costs. Arthritis Rheum 1993; 36: 439–446.

18. Hampson SE, Glasgow RE, Zeiss AM et al. Self-management of osteoarthritis. Arthritis Care Res 1993; 6: 17–22.

19. Felson DT. The epidemiology of knee osteoarthritis: results from the Framingham Osteoarthritis Study. Semin Arthritis Rheum 1990; 20: 42–50.

20. Hubert HB, Bloch DA, Fries JF. Risk factors for physical disability in an aging cohort: The NHANES 1 epidemiologic followup study. J Rheumatol 1993; 20: 480–488.

21. Hochberg MC, Lethbridge-Cejku M, Scott WW Jr et al. The association of body weight, body fatness and body fat distribution with osteoarthritis of the knee: data from the Baltimore Longitudinal Study of Aging. J Rheumatol 1995; 22: 488–493.

22. Spector TD, Hart DJ. Incidence and progression of osteoarthritis in women with unilateral knee disease in the general population: the effect of obesity. Ann Rheum Dis 1994; 53: 565–568.

23. Oliveira SA, Felson DT, Cirillo PA, Reed JI. Body weight, body mass index, and incident symptomatic osteoarthritis of the hand, hip, and knee. Epidemiology 1999; 10: 161–166.

24. Carman WJ, Sowers M, Hawthorne VM, Weissfeld LA. Obesity as a risk factor for osteoarthritis of the hand and wrist: a prospective study. Am Med J Epidemiol 1994; 139: 119–129.

25. Leach RE, Baumgard S, Broom J. Obesity: its relationship to osteoarthritis of the knee. Clin Orthop 1973; 93: 271–273.

26. Felson DT., Zhang Y, Anthony JM et al. Weight loss reduces the risk for symptomatic knee osteoarthritis in women. Ann Intern Med 1992; 116: 535–539.

27. Toda Y, Toda T, Takemura S et al. Change in body fat, but not body weight or metabolic correlates of obesity, is related to symptomatic relief of obese patients with knee osteoarthritis after a weight control program. J Rheumatol 1998; 25: 2181–2186.

28. Minor MA. Exercise in the management of osteoarthritis of the knee and hip. Arthritis Care Res. 1994; 7: 198–204.

29. van Baar ME, Dekker J, Oostendorp RA, Bijl D. The effectiveness of exercise therapy in patients with osteoarthritis of the hip or knee: a randomized clinical trial. J Rheumatol 1998; 25: 2432–2439.

30. Sharma L, Song J, Felson DT et al. The role of knee alignment in disease progression and functional decline in knee osteoarthritis. J Am Med Assoc 2001; 286: 188–195.

31. Kovar PA, Allegrante JP, Mackenzie R et al. Supervised fitness walking in patients with osteoarthritis of the knee. Ann Intern Med 1992; 16: 529–534.

32. van Baar ME, Dekker J, Oostendorp RAB et al. Effectiveness of exercise in patients with osteoarthritis of hip or knee: nine months' followup. Ann Rh Dis 2001; 60: 1123–1130.

33. Brand SA, Crowinshield RD. The effect of cane use on hip contact force. Clin Orthop 1980; 147: 181–184.

34. Blount WP. Don't throw away the cane. J Bone Joint Surg 1956; 38-A: 695–708.

35. Thompson JA, Jennings MB, Hodge W. Orthotic therapy in the management of osteoarthritis. J Am Podiatr. Med Assoc 1992; 82: 136–139.

36. Keating EM, Faris PM, Ritter MA, Kane J. Use of lateral heel and sole wedges in the treatment of medial osteoarthritis of the knee. Orthop Rev 1993; 22: 921–924.

37. Sasaki T, Yasuda K. Clinical evaluation and treatment of osteoarthritis of the knee using designed wedge insoles. Clin Orthop 1987; 221: 181–187.

38. Rubin G, Dixon M, and Danisi M. prescription procedures for knee orthosis and knee–ankle–foot orthosis. Orthot Prosthet 1977; 31: 15–25.

39. Marks R, Quinney AH, Wessel J. Reliability and validity of the measurement of position sense in women with ostearthritis of the knee. J Rheumatol 1993; 20: 1919–1924.

40. Cushnagan J, McCarthy C, Dieppe PA. Taping the patella medially: a new treatment for osteoarthritis of the knee joint? Br Med J 1988; 308: 753–755.

41. Swezey RL. Essentials of physical management and rehabilitation in arthritis. Semin Arthritis Rheum 1974; 3: 349–368.

42. Basford JR. Physical agents and biofeedback. In: DeLisa JA et al. eds. Rehabilitation medicine – principles and practice. Philadelphia: Lippincott; 1988: 257–275.

43. Ezzo J, Hadhazy V, Birch S et al. Acupuncture for osteoarthritis of the knee: a systematic review. Arthritis Rheum 2001; 44: 819–825.44.

44. Dougados M, Devougelaer MP, Annerfeldt M et al. Recommendations for the registration of drugs used in the treatment of osteoarthritis. Ann Rheum Dis 1996; 55: 552–557.

45. McCarthy GM, McCarthy DJ. Effect of topical capsaicin in the therapy of painful osteoarthritis of the hands. J Rheumatol 1992; 19: 604–607.

46. Altman RD, Aven A, Holmburg CE et al. Efficacy of topical capsaicin cream 0.025% as monotherapy in patients with osteoarthritis: a double-blind study. Sem Arthrit Rheum 1994; 23(suppl 3): 25–33.

47. Virus RM, Gebhart GF. Pharmacologic actions of capsaicin: apparent involvement of substance P and serotonin. Life Science 1979; 25: 1273–1284.

48. Moore RA, Tramer MR, Carroll D et al. Quantitative systematic review of topically applied non-steroidal anti-inflammatory drugs. Brit Med J 1998; 316: 333–338.49.

49. Ottilinger B, Gomort B, Michel A et al. Efficacy and safety of eltenac gel in the treatment of knee osteoarthritis. Osteoarthritis Cartilage 2001; 9: 273–280.

50. Miller JH, White J, Norton TH. he value of intra-articular injections in osteoarthritis of the knee. J. Bone Joint Surg 1958; 40A: 636–643.

51. Jones A, Doherty M. Intra-articular corticosteroids are effective in osteoarthritis but there are no clinical predictors of response. Ann Rh Dis 1996; 55: 829.52.

52. Wada J, Koshino T, Morii T, Sugimoto K. Natural course of osteoarthritis of the knee treated with or without intraarticular corticosteroid injections. Bulletin – Hospital for Joint Diseases 1993; 53: 45–48.

53. Schnitzer TJ. Osteoarthritis treatment update. Postgrad Med 1993; 93: 89–93.

54. Altman RD. Osteoarthritis: aggravating factors and therapeutic measures. Postgrad Med 1986; 80: 150–163.

55. Lohmander L, Dalen N, Englund G et al. Intra-articular hyaluronan injections in the treatment of osteoarthritis of the knee: a randomized double-blind, placebo controlled multicentre trial. Ann Rheum Dis 1996; 55: 424–431.

56. Peyron JG. Intraarticular hyaluronan injections in the treatment of osteoarthritis: state-of-the art review. J Rheumatol 1993; 20(suppl 39): 10–15.

57. Dougados M, Nguyen M, Listrat V, Amor B. High molecular weight sodium hyaluronate (hyalectin) in osteoarthritis of the knee: a 1 year placebo-controlled trial. Osteoarthritis and Cartilage 1993; 1: 97–103.

58. Altman RD, Moskowitz R. Intraarticular sodium hyaluronate (Hyalgan) in the treatment of osteoarthritis of the knee: a randomized clinical trial. Hyalgan Study Group. J Rheumatol 1998; 25: 2203–2212.

59. Adams MF, Atkinson M, Lussler AJ et al. Comparison of intra-articular Hyalgan G-F (Synvisc), a viscoelastic derivative of hyaluronan and continuous NSAID therapy in patients with osteoarthritis of the knee. Arthritis Rheum 1993; 37: S165.

60. Bradley JD, Brandt KD, Katz BP et al. Comparison of an antiinflammatory dose of ibuprofen, an analgesic dose of ibuprofen, and acetaminophen in the treatment of patients with osteoarthritis of the knee. N Eng J Med 1991; 325: 87–91.

61. Pincus T, Koch GG, Sokka T et al. A randomized, double-blind crossover clinical trial of diclofenac plus misoprostol versus acetaminophen in paients with osteoarthritis of the hip or knee. Arthritis Rheum 2001; 44: 1587–1598.

62. Altman, RD and the IAP Study Group: Ibuprofen, acetaminophen and placebo in osteoarthritis of the knee: a six-day double-blind study. Arthritis Rheum 1999; 42(suppl): S403.

63. ACR Subcommittee on osteoarthritis guidelines. Recommendations for the medical management of osteoarthritris of the hip and knee: 2000 update. Arthritis Rheum 2000; 43: 1905–1915.

64. Raffa, RB, Friederichs E, Reimann W et al. Opioid and non opioid components independently contribute to the mechanism of action of tramadol, an 'atypical' opioid analgesic. J Pharmacol Exp Ther 1992; 260: 275–285.

65. Goeringer KE, Logan BK, Christian GD. Identification of tramadol and its metabolites in blood from drug-related deaths and drug-impaired drivers. J Anal Toxicol 1997; 21: 529–537.

66. Schnitzer TJ, Kamin M, Olson WH. Tramadol allows reduction of naproxen dose among patients with naproxen-responsive osteoarthritis pain: a randomized, double-blind, placebo-controlled study. Arthritis Rheum 1999; 42: 1370–1377.

67. Mullican WS, Lacy JR Tramadol/acetaminophen combination tablets and codeine/acetaminophen combination capsules for the management of chronic pain: a comparative trial. Clin Ther 2001; 23: 1429–1445.

68. AGS Panel on Chronic Pain in Older Persons. The management of chronic pain in older persons. J Amer Geriatric Soc 1998; 46: 635–651.

69. Hawkey CJ, Karrasch JA, Szczepanski L et al. Omeprazole compared with misoprostol for ulcers associated with nonsteroidal antiinflammatory drugs. Omeprazole versus misoprostol for NSAID-induced ulcer management (OMINUM) study group. N Engl J Med 1998; 338: 727–734.

70. Graham DY, Agrawal NM, Roth SH. Prevention of NSAID-induced gastric ulcer with misoprostol: multicenter, double-blind, placebo-controlled trial. Lancet. 1988; 2: 1277–1280.

71. Schnitzer TJ, Hochberg MC. Cox-2 selective inhibitors in the treatment of arthritis. Cleve Clin J Med 2002; 69(suppl 1): SI 30–30.

72. Silvestein FE, Faich G, Goldstein JL et al. Gastrointestinal toxicity with celecoxib vs. nonsteroidal antiinflammatory drugs for osteoarthritis and rheumatoid arthritis: the CLASS study: a randomized controlled trial. Celecoxib Long-term Arthritis Safety Study. J Am Med Assoc 2000; 284: 1247–1255.

73. Bombardier C, Laine L, Reicin A *et al.* Comparison of upper gastrointestinal toxicity of rofecoxib and naproxen in patients with rheumatoid arthritis. VIGOR Study Group. N Engl J Med. 2000; 343: 1520–1528.

74. Leese PT, Hubbard RC, Karim A *et al.* Effects of celecoxib, a novel cyclooxygenase-2 inhibitor, on platelet function in healthy adults: a randomized, controlled trial. J Clin Pharmacol 2000; 40: 124–132.

75. Ouellet M, Riendeau D, Percival MD. A high level of cyclooxygenase-2 inhibitor selectivity is associated with a reduced interference of platelet cyclooxygenase-1 inactivation by aspirin. Proc Natl Acad Sci USA 2001; 98: 14583–14588.

76. Geba GP, Weaver AL, Polis AB *et al.* Vioxx, acetaminophen, celecoxib trial (VACT) Group. Efficacy of rofecoxib, celecoxib, and acetaminophen in osteoarthritis of the knee: a randomized trial. J Am Med Assoc 2002; 287: 64–71.

77. Yocum D, Fleischmann R, Dalgin P *et al.* Safety and efficacy of meloxicam in the treatment of osteoarthritis: a 12-week, double-blind, multiple-dose, placebo-controlled trial. Arch Intern Med 2000; 23: 2947–2954.

78. Camu F, Beecher T, Recker DP, Verburg KM. Valdecoxib, a COX-2-specific inhibitor, is an efficacious, opioid-sparing analgesic in patients undergoing hip arthroplasty. Am J Ther 2002 ; 9: 43–51.

79. Riendeau D, Percival MD, Brideau C *et al.* Etoricoxib (MK-0663): preclinical profile and comparison with other agents that selectively inhibit cyclooxygenase-2. J Pharmacol Exp Ther 2001; 296: 558–566.

80. Kantor TG. The pharmacological control of musculoskeletal pain. Can J Physiol Pharmacol 1991; 69: 713–718.

81. Curatolo M, Bogduk N. Pharmacologic pain treatment of musculoskeletal disorders: current perspectives and future prospects. Clin J Pain 2001; 17: 25–32.

82. Deal CL, Moskowitz RW. Nutraceuticals as therapeutic agents in osteoarthritis. The role of glucosamine, chondroitin sulfate, and collagen hydrolysate. Rheum Dis Clin North Am 1999; 25: 379–395.

83. Qiu GX, Gao SN, Giacovelli G, Rovati L. Efficacy and safety of glucosamine sulfate versus ibuprofen in patients with knee osteoarthritis. Arzneimittelforschung 1998; 48: 469–474.

84. Muller-Fabender H, Bach GL, Haase W *et al.* Glucosamine sulfate compared to ibuprofen in osteoarthritis of the knee. Osteoarthritis and Cartilage 1994; 2: 61–69.

85. Reginster J-Y, Deroisy R, Rovati LC *et al.* Long term effects of glucosamine sulphate on osteoarthritis progression: a randomized, placebo-controlled clinical trial. Lancet 2001; 357: 251–256.

86. Pavelka K, Gatterova J, Olejarova M *et al.* Glucosamine sulfate decreases progression of knee osteoarthritis in a long-term, randomized, placebo-controlled, independent, confirmatory trial. Arthritis Rheum 2000; 43(suppl): S384.

87. Leeb BF, Schweitzer H, Montag K, Smolen JS. A metaanalysis of chondroitin sulfate in the treatment of osteoarthritis. Rheum 2000; 27: 205–211.

88. Bradley JD, Flusser D, Katz BP *et al.* A randomized, double blind, placebo controlled trial of intravenous loading with S-adenosylmethionine (SAM) followed by oral SAM therapy in patients with knee osteoarthritis. J Rheumatology 1994; 21: 905–911.

89. Altman RD, Marcussen KK. Effects of a ginger extract on knee pain in patients with osteoarthritis. Arthritis Rheum 2000; 44: 2531–2538.

90. Lozada CJ and Altman RD. Chondroprotection in osteoarthritis. Bull Rheum Dis 1997; 46: 5–7.

91. Yu LP Jr., Smith GN Jr, Hasty KA, Brandt KD. Doxycycline inhibits type XI collagenolytic activity of extracts from human osteoarthritic cartilage and of gelatinase. J Rheumatol 1991; 18: 1450–1452.

92. Amin AR, Attur MG, Thakker GD *et al.* A novel mechanism of action of tetracyclines: Effects on nitric oxide synthases. Proc Natl Acad Sci USA 1996; 93: 14014–14019.

93. Brandt KD, Yu LP, Amith G *et al.* Therapeutic effect of doxycycline (doxy) in canine osteoarthritis (OA). Osteoarthritis and Cartilage 1993; 1: 14.

94. Spencer CM and Wilde MI. Diacerein. Drugs 1997: 53: 98–108.

95. Martel-Pelletier J, Mineau F, Jolicoeur FC *et al.* In vitro effects of diacerhein and rhein on interleukin 1 and tumor necrosis factor-alpha systems in human osteoarthritic synovium and chondrocytes. J Rheumatol 1998; 25: 753–762.

96. Carney SL, Hicks CA, Tree B, Broadmore RJ. An in vivo investigation of the effect of anthraquinones on the turnover of aggrecans in spontaneous osteoarthritis in the guinea pig. Inflamm Res 1995; 44: 182–186.

97. Brun PH. Effect of diacetylrhein on the development of experimental osteoarthritis. A biochemical investigation (letter). Osteoarthritis Cartilage 1997; 5: 289–291.

98. Brandt K, Smith G, Kang SY *et al.* Effects of diacerhein in an accelerated canine model of osteoarthritis. Osteoarthritis Cartilage 1997; 5: 438–449.

99. Pelletier JP, Yaron M, Haraoui B *et al.* Efficacy and safety of diacerein in osteoarthritis of the knee. Arthritis Rheum 2000; 43: 2339–2348.

100. Dougados M, Nguyen M, Berdah L *et al.* Evaluation of the structure-modifying effects of diacerein in hip osteoarthritis: ECHODIAH, a three-year, placebo-controlled trial. Evaluation of the chondromodulating effect of diacerein in OA of the hip. Arthritis Rheum 2001; 44: 2539–2547.

101. Henroitin YE, Labasse AH, Jaspar JM *et al.* Effects of three avocado/soybean unsaponifiable mixtures on metalloproteinases, cytokines and prostaglandin E2 production by human articular chondrocytes. Clin Rheumatol 1998; 17: 31–39.

102. Maheu E, Mazieres B, Valat JP *et al.* Symptomatic efficacy of avocado/soybean unsaponifiables in the treatment of osteoarthritis of the knee and hip. A prospective, randomized, double-blind, placebo-controlled, multicenter clinical trial with six-month treatment period and two-month followup demonstrating a persistent effect. Arthritis Rheum 1998; 41: 81–91.

103. Lequesne M, Maheu E, Cadet C *et al.* Effect of avocado/soya unsaponifiables (ASU) on joint space loss in hip osteoarthritis (HOA) over 2 years. A placebo controlled trial. Arthritis Rheum 1996; 39(suppl 9): S227.

104. Pellegrini VD. Osteoarthritis at the base of the thumb. Orthop Clin N Am 1992; 23: 83–102.

105. Keating EM, Faris PM, Ritter MA, Kane J. Use of lateral heel and sole wedges in the treatment of medial osteoarthritis of the knee. Orthop Rev 1993; 22: 921–924.

106. Gaffney K, Ledingham J, Perry J. Intra-articular triamcinolone hexacetonide in knee osteoarthritis: factors influencing the clinical response. Ann Rheum Dis 1995; 54: 379–381.

107. Chang RW, Falconer J, Stulberg SD *et al.* Randomized controlled trial of arthroscopic surgery versus closed needle joint lavage for patients with osteoarthritis of the knee. Arthritis Rheum 1993; 36: 289–296.

108. Gibson JNA, White MD, Chapman VM *et al.* Arthroscopic lavage and debridement for osteoarthritis of the knee. J Bone Joint Surg 1992; 74-b: 534–537.

109. Liveseley PJ, Doherty M, Needoff M *et al.* Arthroscopic lavage of osteoarthritic knees. J Bone Joint Surg 1991; 73-B: 922–926.

110. Ravaud P, Moulinier L, Giraudeau B *et al.* Effects of joint lavage and steroid injection in patients with osteoarthritis of the knee. Arthritis Rheum 1999; 42: 475–482.

111. Oldenbring S, Egund N, Knutson K *et al.* Revision after osteotomy for gonarthrosis: a 10–19 year follow-up of 314 cases. Acta Orthop Scand 1990; 61: 128–130.

172 Diffuse idiopathic skeletal hyperostosis

Geoffrey Littlejohn

Definition

- A chronic, age-related condition, with characteristic new bone growth especially at entheses

Clinical features

- Characteristic radiologic findings
- Hyperostosis, increase in bone mass generally
- Few symptoms related to diagnostic changes in thoracic spine
- Risk of important cervical and lumbar arthropathy and enthesopathy
- Stiffening peripheral arthropathy
- Associations with obesity, diabetes, gout, dyslipidemia, hypertension, hyperinsulinemia
- Growth factors, particularly insulin, implicated in pathogenesis

HISTORY

Diffuse idiopathic skeletal hyperostosis (DISH), also known as ankylosing hyperostosis or Forestier's disease, is a ubiquitous skeletal condition, affecting many species and most human populations studied. Thus, hyperostosis of the spine, typical of that seen in DISH, has been observed in dinosaurs, prehistoric reptiles, current day cetaceans (whales, dolphins) as well as dogs, horses, monkeys and bears. Paleopathologic studies have identified DISH in Egyptian mummies[1], Roman Britons and Saxons[2] and medieval and postmedieval skeletons[3].

In 1824, Wenzel[4] described irregular bony outgrowths 'immobilizing' two or more adjacent vertebrae in elderly subject's spines, with similar findings, subsequently reported by others. Over a century later, Forestier and Rotés-Querol[10] presented comprehensive anatomic, radiologic and clinical data on the disorder, which was then termed ankylosing hyperostosis. The condition was thus seen as a well-defined syndrome with both axial and peripheral manifestations, and expressed from head (hyperostosis frontalis) to foot (calcaneal spurs). The diffuse nature of the condition later led to the terminology DISH[11] (Table 172.1).

EPIDEMIOLOGY

There is a 2:1 reported male predominance in DISH with the prevalence in both sexes rising with age and weight[12,13] (Fig. 172.1), the condition being very uncommon before the age of 45 years[14].

TABLE 172.1 HISTORY OF DISH TERMINOLOGY		
Wenzel[4]	1824	Spinal bony outgrowths
Rokitansky[5]	1856	Pathologic spinal variants
Bechterew[6]	1899	Pathologic spinal variants
Meyer and Forster[7]	1938	Hyperostose moniliforme du flanc droit de la colonne dorsale
Oppenheimer[8]	1942	Spondylitis ossificans ligamentosa
Lacapère[9]	1948	Vertebral melorheostosis
Forestier and Rotés-Querol[10]	1950	Senile ankylosing hyperostosis of spine
Resnick et al.[11]	1975	Diffuse idiopathic skeletal hyperostosis

Summary of principal terminology used to describe DISH.

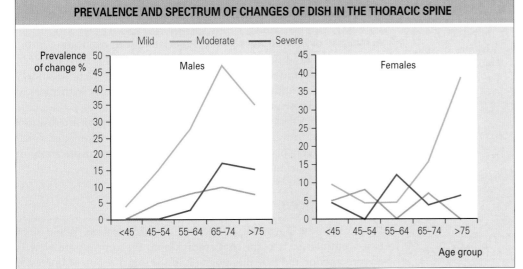

PREVALENCE AND SPECTRUM OF CHANGES OF DISH IN THE THORACIC SPINE

— Mild — Moderate — Severe

Males

Females

Prevalence of change %

Age group

Fig. 172.1 Prevalence and spectrum of changes of DISH in the thoracic spine. Data from 296 subjects at autopsy[13]. Mild: entheseal new bone present at at least two levels; moderate: continuous new bone spanning less than 4 levels; and severe: continuous new bone spanning ≥ 4 levels (typical DISH).

Although diagnostic criteria vary, population surveys indicate that this is a common condition. In Scandinavia the annual cumulative incidence is estimated to be 7/1000 in males and 4/1000 in females beyond the age of 30[15]. Prevalence rates vary in different populations but are consistent with these findings[16]. Approximately 10–15% of males and 5–10% of females over the age of 65 will have DISH, although some populations have increased predisposition for the disorder (Table 172.2). It is thus not only perhaps the oldest known rheumatic disorder but also one of the most common.

CRITERIA AND CHARACTERISITC DESCRIPTION

Criteria

Criteria for diagnosis of DISH rely principally on radiologic appearances in the thoracic spine. These typically require the new bone formation to bridge four contiguous vertebral bodies (see Fig. 172.1) in the absence of degenerative disc disease and the absence of inflammatory sacroiliac or facet changes[19]. As the acronym DISH implies, the condition is characterized by widespread new bone formation, with an increase in the amount of normal bone, heterotopic bone formation and, specifically, the presence of new bone growth into the entheseal regions. The enthesis is that region where tendon, ligament, joint capsule or annulus fibrosis fibers insert into bone[20]. The prominent new bone growth in the anterolateral entheseal regions along the thoracic spine first brought attention to this condition.

DISH may affect any skeletal structure but it varies in severity to the degree that the underlying unity may not be appreciated.

It is most characteristic in the relatively non-mobile parts of the thoracic spine, where uninterrupted new bone may 'flow' from one vertebra to another. It is more prominent on the right side of the thoracic vertebrae, thought to be a consequence of the pressure effect of the left-sided aorta. The presence of the anterior longitudinal ligament over the anterior two thirds of the vertebral bodies dictates the distribution of the new bone formation. The new bone is typically much thicker than the normal anterior ligament, implying ligamentous overgrowth prior to ossification. There is often a gap in the new bone adjacent to the intervertebral disc or between the new bone and the intact original cortex. When disc changes are absent, the new bone formation may be applied quite closely to the vertebral bodies and can, at times, mimic an inflammatory spondylitis. In DISH the original cortex remains under the ossified ligament, while in spondylitis the erosion of the cortex is characteristic particularly at the corners, with underlying sclerosis when the inflammation is active. In some instances DISH may coexist with such a spondylitis. As the condition is more prominent with increased age, it commonly coexists with intervertebral disc change. In such situations the bulging of disc material anteriorly may give rise to spectacular anterior spinal hyperostosis.

In the more mobile cervical and lumbar spine, spondylotic changes are more characteristic than bland bridging, and syndromes of spinal stenosis may result.

TABLE 172.2 PREVALENCE OF DISH

Caucasian populations (various studies)[14–16]	Males 10%
	Females 8%
Pima Indians[17]	Males 54%
	Females 14%
Males with gout[18]	58%

The table gives the prevalence of DISH at age 65 years or over (selected studies [17,18]). Diagnostic criteria vary slightly.

There is a spectrum of spinal new bone formation with increasing amounts laid down with increasing duration[13]. The well-defined condition occurs over several years, but regression of new bone growth over a short period of time has been noted in the context of the pressure effect from an enlarging aortic aneurysm[21]. It is apparent that the new bone formation is a dynamic process with deposition and remodeling occurring as in other areas of the skeleton. Peripheral new bone formation is also most prominent in the entheseal areas, particularly around heels, knees and elbows, among other regions. Such changes also occur on a spectrum ranging from minor through to quite marked hyperostosis[22]. Pronounced peripheral hyperostosis may precede the spinal changes diagnostic of DISH.

The 'diffuse hyperostosis' of DISH includes increased bone formation as demonstrated by phalangeal tufting, increased cortical thickness of tubular bones of the hand and increase in the size of the sesamoid bones[23]. In addition, there is increase in bone mineral density[24] indicating lowered risk of osteoporosis.

Reports have indicated an increased incidence of heterotopic new bone formation after surgical procedures, such as total hip replacement, in patients with DISH[25].

DISH may coexist with inflammatory joint diseases such as rheumatoid arthritis, psoriatic arthritis, other spondyloarthropathies or gout. It has been shown to modify the radiologic reaction to rheumatoid arthritis with less destructive bone disease and a tendency to heal erosions more quickly if the disease remits (RADISH)[26]. There is an increased prevalence of DISH in patients with gout and Paget's disease[18,27]. It can influence the radiologic expression of those diseases, with more exuberant new bone formation being the characteristic observation.

CLINICAL FEATURES

The deposition of new bone in DISH is usually asymptomatic, apart from increased stiffness in the neck, back or peripheral joints[28,29]. Uncommonly, fractures through bony bridges may occur which are difficult to diagnose and treat.

In peripheral joints, a stiffening arthropathy due to thickening and shortening of ligaments can be seen long before the characteristic spinal changes, and identified by the association with hyperinsulinemia[28]. Clinically, there is painless reduction of internal rotation of shoulders and hips, and reduced flexion of fingers and knees. The process may change the biomechanics of joint action and lead to osteoarthritis[30].

Pain may be present in some patients with peripheral enthesopathy, e.g. from a calcaneal spur, this likely being due to abnormal biomechanical stress causing injury to the enthesis. However, while the majority of such extraspinal entheseal changes are asymptomatic adequate controlled studies are lacking.

Important clinical features arise when new bone growth obstructs or impinges on other tissues. In the cervical spine DISH may give rise to dysphagia[31] or cervical myelopathy. Association with ossification of the posterior longitudinal ligament[32] can result in myelopathy and even quadriplegia. In the lumbar spine, spinal stenosis may occur secondary to posterior osteophytic ridges and facet arthropathy with marked hyperostosis. These problems are not common.

DISH is associated with a particular type of degenerative hip disease[33] and increased prevalence of Heberden nodes[34]. The elongated tibial spines common in obesity-related knee osteoarthritis are ossifications of the entheseal attachments of the cruciate ligaments[22].

INVESTIGATIONS

DISH cannot be diagnosed without radiologic evaluation. While often first identified on a plain chest radiograph, the appropriate view is posteroanterior and lateral radiograph of the spinal region of interest[35].

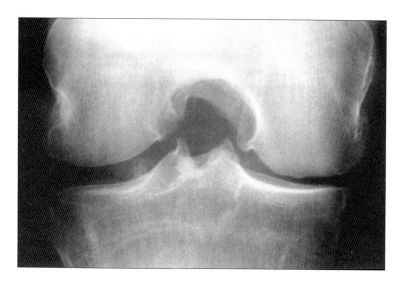

Fig. 172.2 Peripheral arthropathy of DISH in the right knee. Ossification of the insertions of the cruciate ligaments reflect thickening and shortening of these structures. There is narrowing of medial compartment space, while lateral compartment space is preserved. Ossification of the margin of the articular cartilage of the medial femoral condyle is seen adjacent to the femoral notch.

Computed tomography will provide more spectacular images, but is not necessary unless the presence of conditions such as spinal stenosis are being sought. Magnetic resonance imaging shows the ligamentous thickening that precedes ossification. Plain films of peripheral areas will show variable degrees of peripheral enthesopathy (Fig. 172.2). Bone scans show no change in the involved areas, but may help identify an associated process, such as osteoarthritis, spinal fracture or mechanically induced inflammatory entheseal changes.

Routine biochemical studies and the erythrocyte sedimentation rate are normal. Abnormalities associated with hyperinsulinemia may be present which, in addition to the clinical findings of hypertension and obesity, include results compatible with maturity-onset diabetes, dyslipidemias and gout[36,37].

DIFFERENTIAL DIAGNOSIS

The most important differential is that of ankylosing spondylitis. The new bone formation may be smooth and tightly fused to the underlying cortex, and thus difficult to differentiate from ankylosing spondylitis. Usually, however, the exuberant and bumpy bony change within the anterior longitudinal ligament, with preservation of the original cortex, is characteristic of DISH. This problem is occasionally compounded by anterior osteophytosis of the sacroiliac joints which may lead to a change falsely interpreted as post-inflammatory 'fusion' of the joints.

Degenerative disc disease (osteochondrosis) of the thoracic or lumbar spine characteristically give disc space narrowing with horizontal osteophytes, prominent anteriorly. Facet joint hypertrophic changes are commonly seen as age progresses and may narrow the neural foramina as well as the spinal canal. The hyperostotic peripheral joint changes of DISH resemble primary osteoarthritis in distribution, as well as osteophytosis, but is distinguished by early stiffening, with relative preservation of joint space in the early stages[23,28].

Peripheral enthesopathy of DISH shows well defined and often quite prominent new bone growth usually, but not always, connected to the subjacent bony mass. It lacks the erosions or periosteal proliferation seen in the B-27 related inflammatory arthropathies, and is distinct from the linear calcifications that may be seen in calcium pyrophosphate crystal deposition disease[38].

Acromegaly is also characterized by new bone formation, but in addition subcutaneous soft tissue and cartilage thickening are prominent (see Chapter 182). In early acromegaly, there is hypermobility in striking contrast to the stiffening characteristic of DISH. The bony spurs and hyperostosis of DISH may at times be identical to those seen in acromegaly and both conditions associate with hyperostosis frontalis interna[39]. There is no increase in joint space in DISH nor in soft tissue thickness[23]. Repetitive trauma, fluorosis, hypervitaminosis A or retinoid therapy may all produce enthesopathy, which may require differentiation from DISH.

ETIOLOGY AND PATHOGENESIS

The principal changes in DISH occur at the enthesis (Fig. 172.3). The earliest change, preceding ossification, is connective tissue proliferation,

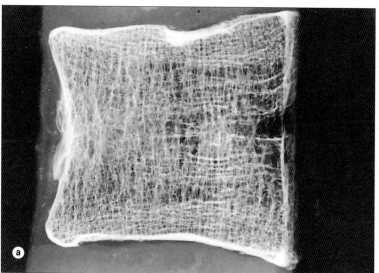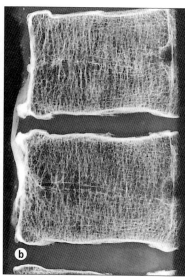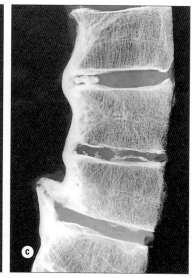

Fig. 172.3 Progressive spinal entheseal changes in DISH. The earliest change is shown in (a), with ossification at the site of attachment of the anterior longitudinal ligament to the middle of the vertebral body, well away from the annulus. Note the separation of the ossification from the intact cortex, except at the site of attachment. Moderately advanced changes are seen in (b), with ossification bridging the disc space, but still firmly attached to cortex at the middle of the vertebral body. Advanced changes are shown in (c), with smooth attachment of the new bone to the original cortex. The ossified ligament is much thickened and interrupted at the lower level.

relatively rich in matrix and cellularity, separating randomly oriented collagen bundles. There are islands of fibrocartilaginous metaplasia with a further increase in cellularity. Chondrocytes are found in recognizable lacunae and there is an increase in the proteoglycan content with a decrease in collagen. The ossification develops within the cartilage, with an irregular mineralization front, or tide mark, at the interface between calcified and uncalcified cartilagenous tissue at the enthesis (Fig. 172.3). Later, vascular invasion occurs from the adjacent cortical haversian canals. Preferential ossification occurs at, or close to, the enthesis which eventually leads to the characteristic radiologic appearance of DISH[13,40]. These features may subside with age, and be least impressive when the ossification is most mature.

DISH is, however, a diffuse systemic condition whose expression is modified by local mechanical factors acting on entheses in particular locations. It is likely that the propensity to deposit new bone has an underlying metabolic cause.

Since the early reports of Forestier, an association between obesity and DISH has been noted[10]. Subsequently a link was observed with impaired glucose tolerance and related adult-onset diabetes[36,41]. The prevalence of these abnormalities in patients with DISH reportedly ranges from 17–60% and thus is much higher than in the general population. Conversely, the prevalence of DISH in patients with adult-onset diabetes ranges between 13 and 50%, these findings being greatly in excess of non-diabetic controls. Glucose intolerance and obesity seem to act as independent factors in their association with DISH, although there is no relationship between the degree of hyperglycemia and the severity of the bony change. No patients with juvenile-onset (i.e. type 1 or insulin deficient) diabetes have been found to have DISH.

As indicated previously, patients with acromegaly have many radiologic features in common with DISH. The level of growth hormone and non-suppressible insulin-like activity, including somatomedin, has been found to be similar in patients with DISH and in controls. This is true both in the resting and stimulated state. In contrast, insulin has been found to be significantly higher in DISH subjects compared to controls, both in the resting and stimulated state (Fig. 172.4)[42]. In such studies

patients were carefully matched for body mass index to exclude the effect of obesity *per se* on insulin secretion. Insulin has a growth factor-like activity and may well be involved in the new bone deposition in this condition. Other studies have shown increased bone density in patients with hyperinsulinemia compared to those with low serum insulin levels[28]. This possibility is further supported by the finding of the extremely high prevalence of obesity, hypertension, adult-onset diabetes and associated hyperinsulinemia in groups such as the Pima Indians who also have a very high prevalence of DISH[17]. Male gouty patients also have this association. Furthermore, hyperinsulinemia has been associated with hyperostosis frontalis interna.

Chronic vitamin A toxicity in animals will produce DISH-like changes[43]. Studies of vitamin A and metabolites in stimulated states indicate an increased level of these retinoids in patients with DISH when compared to controls[44] but the significance of this remains speculative.

In summary it seems likely that a systemic metabolic factor, probably hyperinsulinemia causes the new bone growth through action on entheseal growth plates and osteoblasts. The effect of this bony change is then influenced by mechanical forces acting at entheseal regions, particularly in the spine, heel and elbow areas. The resultant changes occurring over several years lead to a well-characterized syndrome (Table 172.1), i.e. DISH, but clearly variants and early forms of this condition are more common. The hyperinsulinemia also relates to the documented associations between DISH, upper-body obesity, hypertension, lipid abnormalities and increased risk of vascular disease[45].

MANAGEMENT

Prevention

A high risk of DISH may be anticipated in large-boned, large muscled subjects with upper abdominal obesity, especially those with gout, hypertension, peripheral enthesopathies, limited internal rotation of hips or shoulders or large stiff fingers. Laboratory screening may show a characteristic lipid profile; with elevated triglycerides, low high-density lipoprotein–cholesterol and high low-density lipoprotein–cholesterol. Glucose abnormalities are not usual at this stage, but hyperinsulinemia may be found in fasting samples, or more convincingly with a glucose tolerance test[28]. The best therapy at this stage is weight reduction, ideally with a fitness program.

Specific interventions

There is no specific medical therapy of value for the established condition apart from treatment of factors contributing to hyperinsulinemia, for instance, ideal body weight should be attained. Physical therapy can be of value in maintaining range of motion and muscle strength and help relieve symptoms, although there is little published literature to confirm its benefits.

Surgical interventions may be needed for complications such as osteophytic dysphagia or spinal stenosis.

Peripheral entheseal pain may be helped by using carefully placed local anesthetic/corticosteroid injections followed by 5 days without weight-bearing.

The risk of heterotopic bone formation following hip arthroplasty, although uncommon, may be reduced by use of low-dose radiation or nonsteroidal anti-inflammatory medications[46]. Radiation has been associated with an increased risk of nonunion of the greater trochanter.

Peripheral osteoarthropathy is often preceded by striking asymmetric acceleration of capsular thickening and new bone formation around the joint with stiffening further increasing crushing forces through the joint[31]. Anecdotally, local corticosteroid injections may increase range of movement and relieve pain.

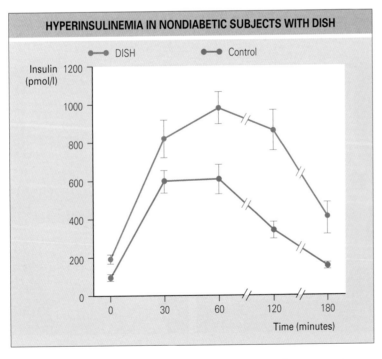

HYPERINSULINEMIA IN NONDIABETIC SUBJECTS WITH DISH

● DISH ● Control

Fig. 172.4 Hyperinsulinemia during a standard glucose tolerance test in nondiabetic subjects with DISH, as compared with controls matched for age, gender and body mass index[42]. Values are mean ± standard error in pmol/l.

REFERENCES

1. Moodie RL. Paleopathology: an introduction to the study of ancient evidence of disease. Urbana: University of Illinois Press; 1923: 403–404.
2. Rogers J, Watt I, Dieppe P. Arthritis in Saxon and mediaeval skeletons. Br Med J 1981; 283: 1668–1671.
3. Rogers J, Watt I, Dieppe P. Paleopathology of spinal osteophytosis, vertebral ankylosis, ankylosing spondylitis and vertebral hyperostosis. Ann Rheum Dis 1985; 44: 113–120.
4. Wenzel G. Ueber die krankheiten an ruckgrathe. Wesche: Bamber; 1824.
5. Rokitansky C. Lehrbuch der pathologische anatomie, vol 1, 3rd edn. Wien: Braumuller; 1856: 99–102.
6. Bechterew W von. Neue beobachtungen und pathologisch-anatomische untersuchungen über steifigheit der wirbelsaule. Deutsch Z Nervenheilk 1899; 15: 45–50.
7. Meyer M, Forster E. Considérations pathogéniques sur 'l'hyperostose moniliforme du flanc droit de la colonne dorsale'. Rev Rhum 1938; 5: 286–293.
8. Oppenheimer A. Calcification and ossification of vertebral ligaments (spondylitis ossificans ligamentosa). Roentgen study of pathogenesis and clinical significance. Radiology 1942; 38: 160–164.
9. Lacapère J. Etude de l'osteophytose vertebrale. Acta Physiother Rheumatol Belg. 1948; 48: 145–158.
10. Forestier J, Rotés-Querol J. Senile ankylosing hyperostosis of the spine. Ann Rheum Dis. 1950; 9: 321–330.
11. Resnick D, Shaul SR, Robins JM. Diffuse idiopathic skeletal hyperostosis (DISH): Forestier's disease with extra spinal manifestations. Radiology 1975; 115: 513–524.
12. Utsinger PD. Diffuse idiopathic skeletal hyperostosis. Clin Rheum Dis 1985; 11: 325–351.
13. Fornasier VL, Littlejohn GO, Urowitz MB et al. Spinal entheseal new bone formation: the early changes of diffuse idiopathic skeletal hyperostosis. J Rheum. 1983; 10: 939–947.
14. Sèze De S, Claisse MR. Hyperostose vertébrale lombaire juvenile. Rev Rhum 1960; 27: 219–225.
15. Julkunen H, Heinonen OP, Knekt P, Maatela J. The epidemiology of hyperostosis of the spine together with its symptoms and related mortality in a general population. Scand J Rheumatol 1973; 40: 581–591.
16. Boachie-Adjei O, Bullough PG. Incidence of ankylosing hyperostosis of the spine (Forestier's disease) at autopsy. Spine 1987; 12: 739–743.
17. Henrard JC, Bennett PH. Etude epidemiologique de l'hyperostose vertébrale. Enquête dans une population adulte d'indiens d'amérique. Rev Rhum Mal Osteoartic 1973; 40: 581–591.
18. Littlejohn GO, Hall S. Diffuse idiopathic skeletal hyperostosis and new bone formation in male gouty subjects. Rheum Int 1982; 2: 83–86.
19. Littlejohn GO. More emphasis on the enthesis. J Rheumatol 1989; 16: 1020–1021.
20. Resnick D, Niwayama G. Radiographic and pathologic features of spinal involvement in diffuse idiopathic skeletal hyperostosis (DISH). Radiology 1976; 119: 559–568.
21. Chaiton A, Fam A, Charles B. Disappearing lumbar hyperostosis in a patient with Forestier's disease: an ominous sign. Arthritis Rheum 1979; 22: 799–802.
22. Littlejohn GO, Urowitz MB. Peripheral enthesopathy in diffuse idiopathic skeletal hyperostosis (DISH): a radiological study. J Rheumatol 1982; 9: 568–572.
23. Littlejohn GO, Urowitz MB, Smythe HA, Keystone EC. Radiographic features of the hand in diffuse idiopathic skeletal hyperostosis (DISH): a comparative study with normals and acromegalics. Radiology 1981; 140: 623–629.
24. Di Franco M, Mauceri MT, Sili-Scavalli A et al. Study of peripheral bone mineral density in patients with diffuse idiopathic skeletal hyperostosis. Clin Rheumatol 2000; 19: 188–192.
25. Resnick D, Linovitz RL, Feingold ML. Post operative heterotopic ossification in patients with ankylosing hyperostosis of the spine (Forestier's disease). J Rheum 1976; 3: 313–320.
26. Resnick D, Curd J, Shapiro RF et al. Radiographic abnormalities of rheumatoid arthritis in patients with diffuse idiopathic skeletal hyperostosis. Arthritis Rheum 1978; 21: 1–5.
27. Mazières B, Jung-Rozenfarb M, Arlet J. Rapports de la maladie de Paget avec l'hyperostose vertébrale ankylosante et l'hyperostose frontale interne. Sem Hop Paris 1978; 54: 521–525.
28. Smythe HA. Osteoarthritis, insulin and bone density. J Rheumatol 1987; 14(suppl 14): 91–93.
29. Mata S, Fortin PR, Fitzcharles MA et al. A controlled study of diffuse idiopathic skeletal hyperostosis. Clinical features and functional status. Medicine (Baltimore) 1997; 76: 104–117.
30. Smythe HA. The mechanical pathogenesis of generalised osteoarthritis. J Rheumatol 1983; 10(suppl 9): 11–12.
31. Akhtar S, O'Flynn PE, Kelly A, Valentine PM. The management of dysphagia in skeletal hyperostosis. J Laryngol Otol 2000; 114: 154–157.
32. Epstein NE. Simultaneous cervical diffuse idiopathic skeletal hyperostosis and ossification of the posterior longitudinal ligament resulting in dysphagia or myelopathy in two geriatric North Americans. Surg Neurol 2000; 53: 427–431.
33. Arlet J, Jacqueline F, Depeyre M et al. Le hanche dans l'hyperostose vertébrale. Rev Rhum Mal Osteoartic 1978; 45: 17–26.
34. Schlapbach P, Beyeler C, Gerber NJ et al. The prevalence of palpable finger joint nodules in diffuse idiopathic hyperostosis (DISH). A controlled study. Br J Rheumatol 1992; 31: 531–534.
35. Mata S, Hill RO, Joseph L et al. Chest radiographs as a screening test for diffuse idiopathic skeletal hyperostosis. J Rheumatol 1993; 20: 1905–1910.
36. Littlejohn GO. Insulin and new bone formation in diffuse idiopathic skeletal hyperostosis. Clin Rheumatol 1985; 4: 294–300.
37. Reaven GM, Lithell H, Landsberg L. Mechanisms of disease: hypertension and associated metabolic abnormalities – the role of insulin resistance and the sympathoadrenal system. New Engl J Med 1996; 334: 374–381.
38. Resnick D, Niwagama G. Entheses and enthesopathy. Radiology 1983; 146: 1–9.
39. Littlejohn G, Hall S, Brand C, Davidson A. New bone formation in acromegaly: pathogenetic implications for diffuse idiopathic skeletal hyperostosis. Clin Exp Rheum 1986; 4: 99–104.
40. Ono K, Yonenobu K, Miyamoto S, Okada K. Pathology of ossification of the posterior longitudinal ligament and ligamentum flavum. Clin Orthop 1999; 359: 18–26.
41. Forgacs SS. Diabetes mellitus and rheumatic disease. Clin Rheum Dis 1986; 12: 729–753.
42. Littlejohn GO, Smythe HA. Marked hyperinsulinemia after glucose challenge in patients with diffuse idiopathic skeletal hyperostosis. J Rheumatol 1981; 8: 965–968.
43. Seawright A, English P, Gartner R. Hypervitaminosis A and hyperostosis of the cat. Nature 1965; 206: 1171–1172.
44. Abiteboul M, Arlet J, Sarrabay MA et al. Etude du métabolism de la vitamine A au cours de la maladie hyperostatique, de Forestier et Rotés-Querol. Rev Rhum 1986; 53: 143–145.
45. DeFronzo RA, Ferrannini E. Insulin resistance: a multifaceted syndrome responsible fo NIDDM, obesity, hypertension, dyslipidemia, and atherosclerotic cardiovascular disease. Diabetes Care 1991; 14: 173–194.
46. Nilsson OS, Persson PE. Heterotopic bone formation after joint replacement. Curr Opin Rheumatol 1999; 11: 127–131.

173 Neuropathic arthropathy

Dimitrios G Kassimos and Paul Creamer

Definition

- Progressive destructive joint disease associated with sensory loss
- Characterized by relative lack of pain and by atrophic changes on plain radiography

Clinical features

- Relatively painless due to sensory neuropathy
- Bony swelling and soft tissue enlargement, effusion, laxity, instability, deformity
- Common sites of joint involvement are the mid-foot, ankle and knee and, less commonly, the hip, spine, shoulder and wrist

Radiologic features

- Joint destruction, subluxation, heterotopic new bone formation and recurrent or persistent joint effusion

HISTORY

Neuropathic joint disease was first described by the French neurologist Jean-Martin Charcot (1825–1893)[1,2]. As chief physician of l'Hospice de la Salpêtrière, an ancient hospital with 5000 chronically ill inmates, he described in 1868 severe osteoarthritic changes associated with tabes dorsalis in a soldier subjected to long periods of marching. He believed that 'spontaneous fractures' were due purely to degeneration of certain nerves, with resultant bone atrophy. Although the condition was named after Charcot by Sir James Paget in 1882, earlier descriptions of neuropathic arthropathy exist. William Musgrave of Exeter (1657–1721) described arthritis due to tertiary syphilis. Charcot himself recognized the reports of the American physician J. K. Mitchell of Philadelphia, who in 1831 described arthropathy in a patient with paraplegia due to spinal tuberculosis. The Germans Volkmann and Virchow proposed the mechanical theory for neuropathic arthritis in 1886. They believed that the changes occur mechanically as a result of loss of normal proprioceptive reflexes via posterior roots of the spinal cord. In 1873, Laborde reported a case of poliomyelitis complicated by neurogenic arthropathy, and in 1892 both Sokoloff and Sverdleff reported cases of 'syringomyelic osteoarthropathies'. In 1917 Eloesser assessed the role of trauma in the development of neuropathic joints by cutting the posterior roots of the spinal cord in cats, resulting in analgesia, anesthesia and ataxia. His work was used to support the neurotraumatic theory of pathogenesis. In 1936 Jordan gave the initial description of neuroarthropathy associated with diabetes.

Since that time neuropathic arthropathy has been described in a variety of other conditions[3], including leprosy[4], syringomyelia[5], multiple sclerosis, spinal bifida with meningomyelocele, amyloidosis, congenital insensitivity to pain[6], spinal cord tumors[7], spinal cord trauma, arachnoiditis after spinal anesthesia or meningitis, repeated intra-articular corticosteroid injections, familial dysautonomia (Riley–Day syndrome), familial and other polyneuropathies[8,9], peroneal muscular atrophy (Charcot–Marie–Tooth disease), neurofibromatosis[10] and idiopathic disease[11].

EPIDEMIOLOGY

Neuropathic arthropathy can complicate a variety of neurologic disorders, all having in common a sensory neuropathy[12], although no neurological disorder is found in up to 30%. Neuropathic arthropathy occurs in 0.1–0.5% of diabetic patients, with an approximately equal sex ratio[14]. Causes other than diabetes are relatively rare and epidemiologic data are therefore scarce. However, neuropathic arthropathy is said to occur in 5–10% of patients with tabes dorsalis[13], 14% of patients with leprosy[4] and 20–25% of patients with syringomyelia[5]. In childhood the most common cause of neuropathic arthropathy is spina bifida[7].

CLINICAL FEATURES

The distribution of joint involvement depends on the underlying neuropathy (Table 173.1). In general, tabes dorsalis and leprosy involve the large joints of the lower limbs, syringomyelia the large joints of the upper limbs, with the shoulder being affected in 80% of cases (Fig. 173.1), and diabetes mellitus the joints of the foot. Mono- or oligoarticular involvement is most common, but polyarticular forms do occur.

When the knee is involved the onset of neuropathic arthropathy is usually gradual, though it may be subacute or even acute, occurring within a few hours ('pseudoinflammatory'). The knee becomes warm and swollen, with signs of joint effusion. Because there is relatively little pain and functional disability patients often do not seek medical consultation until progressive deterioration has occurred. The knee may become permanently symptomatic and swollen, with instability leading to valgus, varus or recurvatum deformities, and enlargement of the articular bones and periarticular tissues. Although abnormalities are gross and the clinical picture even alarming, the joint may be painless. The patient is able to walk, although with a limp.

A similar clinical picture is seen in other major limb joints. When the hip is affected (Fig. 173.2) there is often extensive joint destruction,

TABLE 173.1 JOINT INVOLVEMENT IN NEUROPATHIC ARTHROPATHY

Disease	Site of involvement
Diabetes mellitus	Metatarsophalangeal, tarsometatarsal, intertarsal
Syringomyelia	Shoulder, elbow, wrist
Amyloidosis	Knee, ankle
Congenital sensory neuropathy	Knee, ankle, intertarsal, metatarsophalangeal
Tabes dorsalis	Knee, hip, ankle
Leprosy	Tarsal, tarsometatarsal

shortening of the leg, severe loss of function and a limp[7,15]. When the shoulder is involved joint destruction may be rapid and associated with swelling and tenderness.

The hindfoot, tarsometatarsal joints and the toes are most commonly affected regions in the foot (Fig. 173.3). Mediotarsal joint involvement is often associated with edema of the ankle and dorsal foot extending to the plantar arch, which is often collapsed. Tarsometatarsal joint involvement is associated with edema of the dorsum of the foot and bony deformities, with dorsal prominence or plantar protrusion. Downward collapse of the tarsal bones may produce abnormal convexity of the plantar surface. On examination the range of motion is usually subnormal, but may even be excessive as result of a laxity and subluxation (Fig. 173.4). Instability becomes permanent and deteriorates with time. Localization of neuropathic arthropathy in the metatarsophalangeal joints may result in swelling and other signs of inflammation. The articular disorder is frequently accompanied by trophic skin lesions and ulcers on the sole of the foot. The ulcers have well-defined edges. Infection of ulcers is a major problem and effective eradication of bacteria is often impossible.

The hand is rarely involved and the manifestations in general are less severe. They include vasomotor problems, digital ulcers, thickening of

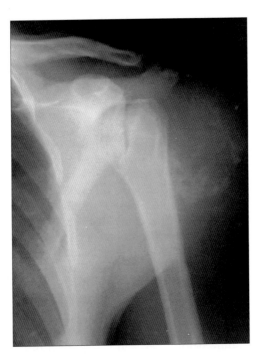

Fig. 173.1 Syringomyelia with neuropathic disease of the shoulder, showing atrophic changes and soft tissue calcification. (Courtesy of Dr I Watt.)

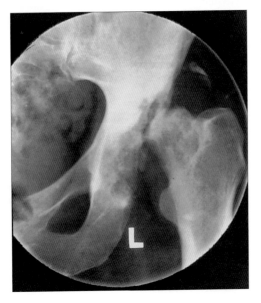

Fig. 173.2 Neuropathic hip secondary to tabes dorsalis. (Courtesy of Dr I Watt.)

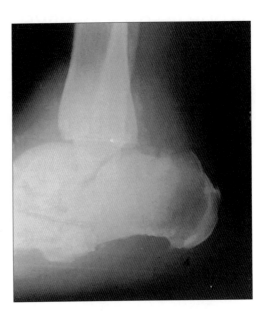

Fig. 173.3 Diabetic neuropathy of the hindfoot. Destruction of the joint with collapse and fragmentation.

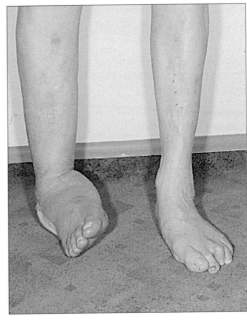

Fig. 173.4 Neuropathic ankle. Marked instability of the subtalar and midtarsal joints are seen with collapse on weightbearing.

the fingers and painless subluxation of the finger joints. In the spine localization is most frequent in the lumbar region, although the cervical and dorsal spine may also be involved. Severe deformity (kyphosis, scoliosis) may result despite normal mobility and relative absence of pain. Because of this paucity of symptoms, the condition is often first discovered during routine examination. Occasionally, signs of nerve root compression are present.

The belief that neuropathic joints are relatively painless is probably untrue. Arthralgia is well documented in up to 50% of patients[12], though the symptoms are usually less than expected from the degree of joint destruction.

INVESTIGATIONS

Plain radiography

Neuropathic arthropathy is usually diagnosable by conventional radiographic techniques (Fig. 173.5). In the early stages, radiographic findings may be normal or show only soft tissue swelling. Other early features include periosteal calcification and joint effusion. The presence of an enlarging and persistent effusion, minimal subluxation, fracture and fragmentation suggests the possibility of neuroarthropathy. After a

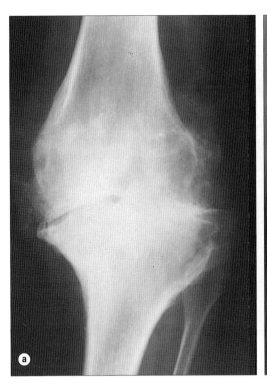
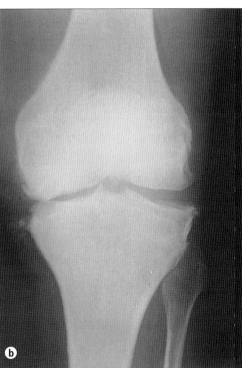

Fig. 173.5 Neuropathic disease of the left knee (tabes dorsalis). (a) Advanced form of the disease in the knee. (b) The same knee 13 years previously showing partial fracture of the tibial epiphysis.

few weeks the calcification becomes more dense and the bone margin less well defined. Ultimately, the radiographic picture is that of a disorganized joint, characterized by bone resorption and formation occurring simultaneously. Fractures may occur and free fragments of bone may be seen in the joint cavity. The degree of sclerosis, osteophytosis and fragmentation in this articular disorder is greater than that in any other process. However, the bone fragments and irregular articular surfaces resulting from the osseous destruction and collapse accompanying this disease are generally well defined and sharp. Poorly marginated, ill-defined bone contours, as occur in septic arthritis, are not evident unless infection has become superimposed on the neuropathic process. This latter complication, however, is not infrequent, especially in diabetic patients and in the more superficial joints (e.g. metatarsophalangeal).

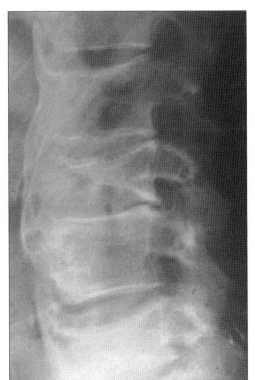

Fig. 173.6 Neuropathic disease of the lumbar spine (tabes dorsalis). Lateral radiograph of the lumbar vertebra showing partial destruction of L2 and diffuse exuberant osteophytes.

Intra-articular bony fusion is an uncommon manifestation of neuroarthropathy at any site, with the exception of the spine[3] (Fig. 173.6).

Progression from the early stage can be very rapid, suggesting that microfractures exist that evolve quickly into gross fragmentation, with complete destruction of the articulation within a few weeks.

Other imaging techniques

Bone scintigraphy (late phase) appears to allow detection before radiographs become abnormal[16–18]. The role of magnetic resonance imaging (MRI) and computed tomography (CT) in the early detection of neuropathic disease remains to be established. Both allow the extent of the soft tissue lesions to be defined, but may not differentiate from infection of bone or joint[19]. Low signal intensity areas on MRI have been reported in the medullary cavity of the bone on both T_1- and T_2-weighted spin-echo images in syringomyelia even before the actual resorptive process[20].

Laboratory investigations and histology

The synovial fluid may be serous, serosanguinous or frankly hemorrhagic, and lipid crystals secondary to subchondral bone lesions may be seen. Biopsy of the synovial membrane usually shows nonspecific changes; however, bone biopsy may sometimes be useful to exclude other diagnoses, such as osteosarcoma, metastatic carcinoma or osteomyelitis. The most common histologic findings are fibrosis with cartilaginous and bony metaplasia and embedded fragments of necrotic or viable bone ('detritic synovitis'). The histopathologic findings in most of the cases reported have been of synovium and not of the underlying bone. Necrotic and reactive cartilage and rice body-like articular fibrinous material have also been described in the joint. Laboratory evidence of an acute-phase response or systemic disturbance is lacking[12].

DIFFERENTIAL DIAGNOSIS

In a typical case the differential diagnosis is not a problem, but if a neurologic disorder is not readily apparent or if the clinical or radiographic appearances are unusual, then the diagnosis may be more difficult. The characteristic combination of joint disease with gross clinical manifestations in the presence of relative lack of pain and good functional capacity, together with a typical radiographic picture, makes the diagnosis simple. A careful neurologic examination should be carried out, as this may identify the neuropathy responsible, which should have a sensory component. Greater diagnostic difficulty exists in the mild and moderate stages of neuropathic joint disease. In the spine, joint space loss, sclerosis and fragmentation in the early stages of neuroarthropathy can resemble the changes of osteoarthritis. Destructive arthropathy associated with hydroxyapatite crystal or calcium pyrophosphate deposition may cause a similar picture[21], the latter being described as causing 'pseudoneuropathic arthropathy'[22]. Diagnosis is made by the identification of crystals in synovial fluid. Bony fragmentation and collapse are also manifestations of osteonecrosis, which may occur after corticosteroid therapy, excessive alcohol intake, or spontaneously in diseases such as systemic lupus erythematosus (SLE) (see Chapter 174). Similar appearances have been reported in post-traumatic osteoarthritis, after intra-articular corticosteroid injections, tumor and alkaptonuria. The important differential of septic arthritis has been described above, and if there is any clinical doubt one should aspirate the involved joint and send synovial fluid for microscopy and culture.

In the spine, early findings of neuroarthropathy, such as intervertebral disc space narrowing and vertebral sclerosis, resemble those of intervertebral osteochondrosis, infection, Paget's disease or alkaptonuria. With the appearance of significant fragmentation, sclerosis and osteophytosis, the diagnosis of axial neuropathy is not difficult. Finally, the differential diagnosis of an acutely swollen neuropathic joint is that of any other monoarthritis including, as indicated above, septic arthritis or crystal arthritis[23].

ETIOLOGY

Tabes dorsalis

Of patients with tertiary syphilis, 5–10% develop neuroarthropathy. It is still the classic model for neuropathic joint disease despite its decreasing incidence. Both sexes are equally affected. The onset is usually in adulthood, as well as in the advanced stages of tabes. The lower limb joints are affected in 60–75% of cases, with involvement of knee, hip, ankle, shoulder, elbow in descending order of frequency (Fig. 173.7). Other joints involved are the forefoot, midfoot, vertebral column and sternoclavicular. Monoarticular involvement predominates, but is not universal. Diagnosis requires identification of specific antitreponemal antibodies in blood and cerebrospinal fluid (VDRL, FTA-ABS, TPI).

Syringomyelia

It has been estimated that 20–25% of patients with syringomyelia develop neuroarthropathy. The disease is more common in men than in women, with onset between the ages of 20 and 40 years, and it usually progresses slowly. It is common in the joints of the upper extremity, especially the glenohumeral, elbow, wrist (Fig. 173.8b,c), fingers and, more rarely, the cervical spine. Approximately 75–80% of syringomyelia patients with neuroarthropathy demonstrate abnormalities in one or more of these sites. Bilateral and symmetric involvement is less frequent in syringomyelia than in tabes dorsalis. Neurologic manifestations due to spinal cord damage include loss of pain and temperature sensation, although tactile and postural sensitivity is preserved; wasting of the intrinsic muscles of the hand (Fig. 173.8a); and amyotrophic paralysis in the upper limb. Myelography, CT and MRI (Fig. 173.9) can demonstrate spinal cord enlargement[24], especially in the cervical region, and laboratory analysis can indicate increases in cerebrospinal fluid pressure and protein content.

Leprosy

Leprotic patients develop peripheral neuropathy with a variety of secondary changes in the feet. Neuroarthropathy can result from long-standing neuropathy, with little evidence of active leprosy[4,25]. The disease alters the shape of the hands and feet owing to subluxation of individual joints. In the feet the changes usually start in the medial arch and later

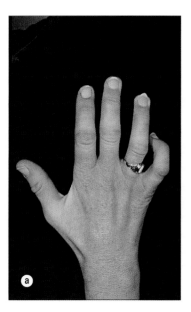
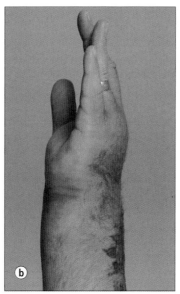
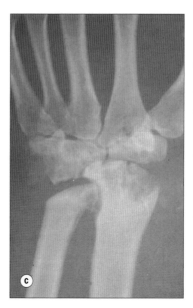

Fig. 173.7 Syphilitic Charcot knee joints showing gross destructive changes.

Fig. 173.8 Syringomyelia. (a) Wasting of the intrinsic muscles of the hand and 'claw' deformity. (b) A neuropathic wrist joint in a patient with mild syringomyelia. Note the swelling and deformity of the joint. (c) Radiograph showing the gross destruction of the proximal carpal row with attrition and simplification of the bony margins. Residual fragments of bone and considerable soft tissue swelling can also be seen.

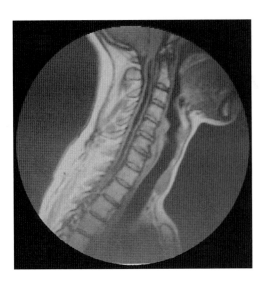

Fig. 173.9 MRI of cervical spine in syringomyelia, showing the fluid-filled syrinx in the center of the spinal cord.

involve the lateral arch, talus and calcaneus. In extreme cases, dissolution of the midfoot results in separation of the forefoot and the hindfoot, and the tibia is driven downward to become weightbearing. The pathogenesis in this type seems to be mainly direct trauma to the forefoot.

Diabetes mellitus

Sensory diabetic neuropathy complicates long-standing (poorly controlled) type I or type II diabetes mellitus; it has become the major cause of neuropathic arthropathy.

Congenital indifference to pain

This group includes congenital insensitivity to pain and hereditary sensory neuropathies types I to IV. The pathogenesis appears to be the same as that in other causes of Charcot's joints. Often, there is marked disproportion between the severity of the disease process and the clinical symptoms[6].

Meningomyelocele (spinal dysraphism)

Neuropathic changes in childhood raise the possibility of congenital indifference to pain or meningomyelocele. Principally the ankle and the tarsal articulations are affected. In active children changes may appear in the first 3 years of life and include osteoporosis, diaphyseal and metaphyseal fractures, injuries of the growth plate, epiphyseal separations, persistent effusions, articular destruction and soft tissue ulcerations.

PATHOGENESIS

The pathogenesis of neuropathic arthropathy remains controversial. Although sensory impairment, overuse and trauma are recognized as predisposing factors these are neither necessary nor sufficient to account for the observed clinical and pathologic features. Any theory of pathogenesis must attempt to explain the facts that only a small minority of patients with severe peripheral sensory neuropathy develop Charcot's joints, and the chances of developing a Charcot joint do not appear to relate either to the severity of neuropathy or the degree of physical activity[27]. The reason for the bizarre local response with marked destructive changes and loss of bone seen in early atrophic lesions and the overgrowth of bone seen in some hypertrophic Charcot's joints is also unclear.

Two main theories have been proposed. The first or 'neurotraumatic' theory suggests that somatic muscular reflexes that normally protect the joint from exceeding certain 'safe' limits in range of movement are lost in the presence of neuropathy, leading to repeated trauma and ultimately joint destruction. Volkmann and Virchow described the changes as resulting from 'a multiplicity of subclinical traumas which are unperceived because of the insensitivity of the affected joints'. The second or 'neurovascular' theory states that a Charcot's joint develops when the sensory deficit disrupts the normal neurovascular reflexes around the joint, resulting in hyperemia and active resorption of bone[12].

Implicit in both these theories is the notion that peripheral sensory nerves actively prevent development of Charcot's arthropathy in normal joints, and disruption of these nerves should lead inevitably with normal use to a Charcot's joint. In fact, there is surprisingly little evidence that this is the case. Attempts to create Charcot's joints in cats, rabbits and dogs have met with variable success. It is unknown whether these differences reflect species-specific responses to the same basic experimental protocol, whether neuropathic arthropathy develops because of subclinical microtrauma during day-to-day activities, or whether gross trauma is necessary to initiate the process. It is clear that even extensive deafferentation of a joint does not necessarily lead to joint pathology in the absence of trauma or infection. In a series of important experiments the effect of denervation at the dorsal root ganglion on the development of osteoarthritis (OA) has been studied in the canine anterior cruciate ligament (ACL) transection model. It was found that whereas ACL section inevitably led to OA in active dogs, denervation of the limb alone did not lead to OA or Charcot's joints even if the dogs were allowed to remain active[28]. However, the combination of ACL section and denervation led to more severe OA than ACL section alone[27,29]. These results suggest that intact peripheral nerves are not important in preventing joint destruction in stable knees, but may have a protective role in preventing the unstable joint from destruction[30]. Analysis of the gait pattern of denervated dogs showed abnormality, with an increased range of knee extension, but in the absence of instability knee OA did not occur[31]. Finally, if dorsal root ganglion section is delayed until 52 weeks after ACL section, the resulting OA is no worse than that seen with ACL section alone, suggesting that over time the central nervous system may acquire the ability to protect the unstable joint[32]. The model of accelerated OA above differs from the conventional ACL section model in the neurologically intact dog in a number of ways: osteophytes are more prominent, a detritic synovitis is present[30], and periosteal new bone formation is seen[33]. This suggests that interruption of sensory input from the limb may affect the regulation of osteogenesis in the mechanically unstable joint.

Although these experiments strictly examined the role of nerve section in the development of OA rather than neuropathic arthritis, the conclusions are likely to be relevant, particularly as some forms of OA, such as those associated with apatite deposition[21], bear a marked clinical and radiographic resemblance to neuropathic joints.

These experiments refute the theory that neuropathic joints result from a peripheral sensory neuropathy in the presence of normal activity, although they would explain the development of joint destruction in the presence of neuropathy and instability. The role of joint instability in the development of human neuropathic joints is currently unknown.

On current evidence, neuropathic joints are best explained by the neurovascular theory with a neurally initiated vascular reflex leading to active bone resorption by osteoblasts[12]. This is supported by the finding of increased blood flow to affected joints seen on bone scans and angiography, and by histologic evidence of hypervascularity of bone, osteoclastic activity and dilatation of Haversian canals. There may or may not be a secondary pathologic fracture and subsequent productive repair[12]. This depends upon whether the joint is insensitive or whether it is subjected to continued weightbearing. If the latter, then the neurotraumatic mechanism comes into play, but only secondarily.

MANAGEMENT

Despite progress in our understanding of the disease, curative treatment of established neuropathic arthropathy remains impossible. The most important part of management is early diagnosis and the prevention of further deterioration. Treatment of the neurologic disorder, such as surgical repair of syringomyelia, is indicated when possible but will not reverse established arthropathy.

The treatment of the neuropathic joint depends on the joint involved and the stage of the disease. The key to successful conservative treatment is early recognition in order to prevent joint destruction. If activity is resumed too early, further breakdown of the joint may occur[21]. Immobilization of the joint is important and should be done as soon as possible. In cases where the lower limb is involved, cessation of weight-bearing is important. This is mandatory during periods of apparent flare in activity. Joint immobilization and rest should last for between several weeks and 3 months, and can lead to stabilization of the joint and improvement in the osteoarticular lesion. Orthotic devices such as plaster casts, crutches, stabilizing splints or braces are used as required to permit limited mobilization, though a balance has to be struck between restricting mobility and allowing a return to weightbearing ambulation. A Charcot Restraint Orthotic Walker (CROW) has been developed to provide the prolonged protection required in the diabetic neuroarthropathic patient[34]. The CROW is a rigid, custom-built, full-foot enclosure ankle–foot orthosis used after an initial period of cast immobilization.

Ulcers require rigorous hygiene: disinfection, sterile bandaging and antibiotic treatment of any superimposed infection.

Recently the bisphosphonate pamidronate has been used in an attempt to halt the underlying bone resorption in neuroarthropathy[35]. There was a significant reduction in bone turnover as judged by alkaline phosphatase activity, and this may be an area for increased therapeutic intervention, especially with newer, more potent bisphosphonates.

Indications for surgery in neuropathic arthropathy include ulceration and unacceptable deformity. In these situations healing time is pro-longed and the risk of further bony breakdown is increased. The surgical treatment of the neuropathic knee is generally arthrodesis. The relatively small numbers in each series make definitive conclusions impossible, but it is agreed that the major problem with this treatment is non-union[36,37]. Successful arthrodesis may be improved by attention to particular procedural details[36], including rigorous removal of all cartilage and debris; removal of sclerotic bone down to bleeding, well vascularized tissue; careful fashioning of congruent bone surfaces for apposition; firm fixation of the bones, either by an intramedullary rod or other device; and debridement of all synovial tissue and scarred capsule. Neuropathic knees can be treated by total joint arthroplasty[38,39] if severe bone loss is corrected by either bone grafting or a custom-augmented prosthesis, and if ligamentous balancing is adequately secured. Unfortunately, the combination of marked joint destruction and, not infrequently, superimposed infection makes amputation the only viable option. In cases of neuropathic disease of the lumbar vertebrae leading to nerve root compression, laminectomy has given satisfactory results. Spinal arthrodesis has also reportedly been successful.

SUMMARY

Neuropathic joint disease is a chronic form of arthropathy associated with reduced sensory innervation of the joints. Apart from an association with diabetes the condition is rare, but important as early recognition and treatment may significantly alter the prognosis. It should be considered in any patient presenting with a monoarthritis, and in an appropriate clinical setting should prompt a careful neurologic examination. The mechanism by which sensory changes result in such gross destructive arthritis is unclear. The disease bears a marked resemblance to certain forms of atrophic OA: this, combined with recent animal experiments, raises the intriguing possibility that neurologic factors may play a role in OA.

REFERENCES

1. Charcot JM. On arthropathies of cerebral or spine origin (Reprint). Clin Orthop Rel Res 1993; 296: 4–7.
2. Gupta R. A short history of neuropathic arthropathy. Clin Orthop Rel Res 1993; 296: 43–49.
3. Resnick D. Neuroarthropathy. In: Resnick D, Niwayama G. Diagnosis of bone and joint disorders. Philadelphia: WB Saunders; 1988; 3154–3185.
4. Horibe S, Tada K, Nagano J. Neuroarthropathy of the foot in leprosy. J Bone Joint Surg 1988; 70B: 481–485.
5. Barnett JHM, Foster JB, Hudgson P. Syringomyelia. Philadelphia: WB Saunders; 1973; 3–7.
6. Piazza RM, Bassett SG, Bunnell PW. Neuropathic spinal arthropathy in congenital insensitivity to pain. Clin Orthop Rel Res 1988; 236: 175–179.
7. Martinet P, MBappe P, Lebreton C et al. Neuropathic arthropathy: a forgotten diagnosis? Two recent cases involving the hip. Rev Rheum Eng Ed 1999; 66: 284–287.
8. Guille JT, Forlin E, Bowen JR, Delaware W. Charcot joint disease of the shoulders in a patient who had familial sensory neuropathy with anhidrosis. J Bone Joint Surg 1992; 74A: 1415–1417.
9. Chappel R, Willems J, Martin JJ. Charcot joint in idiopathic sensorimotor neuropathy. Clin Rheumatol 2000; 19: 153–155.
10. McCann P, Herbert J, Feldman F, Kelly MA. Neuropathic arthropathy associated with neurofibromatosis. J Bone Joint Surg 1992; 74A: 1411–1414.
11. Blanford AT, Keane SP, McCarty DJ, Albers JW. Idiopathic Charcot joint of the elbow. Arthritis Rheum 1978; 21: 723–726.
12. Brower AC, Allman RM. Pathogenesis of the neuropathic joint: neurotraumatic vs neurovascular. Radiology 1981; 139: 349–354.
13. Jaffe HL. Metabolic, degenerative and inflammatory diseases of bones and joints. Philadelphia: Lea & Febiger; 1972: 847–866.
14. Gray RG, Gottlieb NL. Rheumatic disorders associated with diabetes mellitus: literature review. Semin Arthritis Rheum 1976; 6: 19–34.
15. Regan M, Jones JKL, Snape J. Destructive large joint arthritis. Ann Rheum Dis 1995; 54: 626–627.
16. Sakarelles JC, Swift TR. Shoulder enlargement as the presenting sign in syringomyelia. A report of two cases and a review of the literature. JAMA 1976; 236: 2878–2879.
17. Hatzis N, Kaar TK, Wirth MA et al. Neuropathic arthropathy of the shoulder. J Bone Joint Surg Am 1998; 80: 1314–1319.
18. Nigrisoli M, Moscato M, Padovani G. Syringomyelic arthropathy: a description of two cases and a review of the literature. Chir Organi Mov 1991; 76: 237–244.
19. Kapila A, Lines M. Neuropathic spinal arthropathy: CT and MR findings. J Comput Assist Tomogr 1987; 1: 736–739.
20. Rawat B, Bell RS. Case report: rapidly progressive neuropathic arthropathy in syringohydromyelia. Radiographic and magnetic resonance imaging findings. Clin Radiol 1994; 49: 504–507.
21. Dieppe PA, Doherty M, MacFarlande DG et al. Apatite associated destructive arthritis. Br J Rheumatol 1984; 23: 84–91.
22. Menkes CJ, Simon F, Delrieu F et al. Destructive arthritis in chondrocalcinosis articularis. Arthritis Rheum 1976; 19: 329–348.
23. Johnson JTH. Neuropathic fractures and joint injuries. Pathogenesis and rationale of prevention and treatment. J Bone Joint Surg Am 1967; 49A: 1–30.
24. Pojunas K, Williams AL, Daniels DL, Haughton VM. Syringomyelia and hydromyelia: Magnetic resonance evaluation. Radiology 1984; 153: 679–683.
25. Horibe S, Tada K, Nagano J. Neuroarthropathy of the foot in leprosy. J Bone Joint Surg Br 1988; 70B: 481–485.
26. Salo PT, Theriault E, Wiley RG. Selective ablation of rat knee joint innervation with injected immunotoxin: a potentia the study of neuropathic arthritis. J Orthop Res 1997; 15: 622–628.
27. O'Connor BL, Brandt KD. Neurogenic factors in the aetiopathogenesis of osteoarthritis (Review). Rheum Dis Clin North Am 1993; 19: 581–605.
28. O'Connor BL, Palmoski MJ, Brandt KD. Neurogenic acceleration of degenerative joint lesions. J Bone Joint Surg Am 1985; 67A: 563–572.
29. O'Connor, Visko DM, Brandt KD et al. Neurogenic acceleration of osteoarthrosis. J Bone Joint Surg Am 1992; 74A: 367–376.
30. Myers SL, Brandt KD, O'Connor BL et al. Synovitis and osteoarthritis changes in canine articular cartilage after anterior cruciate ligament transection. Effect of surgical haemostasis. Arthritis Rheum 1990; 33: 1406–1415.
31. Vilensky JA, O'Connor BL, Brandt KD et al. Serial kinematic analysis of the canine knee after L4–S1 dorsal root ganglionectomy: implications for the cruciate deficiency model of osteoarthritis. J Rheumatol 1994; 21: 2113–2117.
32. O'Connor BL, Visko DM, Brandt KD et al. Sensory nerves only temporarily protect the unstable canine knee joint from osteoarthritis. Evidence that sensory nerves reprogramme the central nervous system after cruciate ligament transection. Arthritis Rheum 1993; 36: 1154–1163.

33. Myers SL, Brandt KD, O'Connor B *et al*. Periosteal new bone formation in canine neuropathic model of osteoarthritis. Arthritis Rheum 1997; 40: 1756–1759.

34. Morgan JM, Biehl WII, Wagner FW. Management of neuropathic arthropathy with the Charcot Restraint Orthotic Walker. Clin Orthop Rel Res 1993; 296: 58–63.

35. Selby PL, Young MJ, Boulton AJM. Bisphosphonates: A new treatment for diabetic Charcot neuroarthropathy? Diabetic Med 1994; 11: 28–31.

36. Drennan DB, Fahey JJ, Maylahd DJ. Important factors in achieving arthrodesis of the Charcot knee. J Bone Joint Surg 1971; 53A: 1180–1193.

37. Sticha RS, Frascone ST, Wertheimer SJ. Major arthrodeses in patients with neuropathic arthropathy. J Foot Ankle Surg 1996; 35: 560–566.

38. Soudry M, Binazzi R, Johanson NA *et al*. Total knee arthroplasty in Charcot and Charcot-like joints. Clin Orthop Rel Res 1985; 208: 199–204.

39. Yoshino S, Fujimoro J, Kajino A *et al*. Total knee arthroplasty in Charcot's joint. J Arthroplasty 1993; 8: 335–340.

OSTEOARTHRITIS AND RELATED DISORDERS

174 Osteonecrosis

Bernard Mazières

Definition

- Osteonecrosis is cell death in components of bone: hematopoietic fat marrow and mineralized tissue

- Osteonecrosis is not a specific disease entity. It is the final common pathway of a number of conditions, most of which lead to impairment of the blood supply to the femoral head; this explains the frequently used terms of 'avascular necrosis' or 'aseptic necrosis'

Clinical features

- Radiologic changes are typical at the late stages of the disease, but radiographs can be normal at early stages. Magnetic resonance imaging is especially useful in these stages

- Predisposing factors (mainly corticosteroids and alcoholism) should be carefully sought

- The femoral head is the most common and severely affected site of osteonecrosis. However, it may also develop in other locations (including the distal femur[1], humeral head and small bones of the wrist and foot)

CLINICAL DISEASE

History

As early as 1794, James Russell published his book on necrosis of bone[2]. In the 19th century Jean Cruveilhier, a French anatomist, described gross deformation of the femoral head as a late complication of trauma presumably resulting from vascular impairment. The distinction between septic and aseptic necrosis was not recognized until 1888, by Axhausen and Koenig. In the 1930s and 1940s, Phemister and his associates wrote a series of articles on the etiology, pathogenesis and treatment of this condition that remain classics[3,4].

The modern history of osteonecrosis began in the 1960s with the cases reported by Mankin and Brower[5], the concept of 'creeping substitution' proposed by Glimcher and Kenzora[6] and the first cases of preradiologic, pathologically proven osteonecrosis described by Ficat and Arlet[7]. During the 1970s more data became available on its natural history: contralateral hip involvement is present in 30–70% of cases at the time of the first examination, and anatomic and functional deterioration leads to a surgical procedure in more than 50% of cases within 3 years of diagnosis[8–11]. In the 1990s, a reappraisal of the necrotic area on radiographs and magnetic resonance imaging (MRI) has led to the conclusion that both extent and location of this area are important in predicting the evolution toward collapse[12].

Epidemiology

Although there are no reliable data on incidence, it has been estimated that approximately 15 000 new cases occur annually in the USA[13]. Osteonecrosis is thought to account for over 10% of the more than 500 000 total hip arthroplasties performed each year in the USA[14].

A Japanese survey of bone necrosis estimated that non-traumatic osteonecrosis of the femoral head occurred in 2500–3300 adults during 1988; 35% of cases were due to corticosteroid treatment, 22% to alcohol abuse and 37% were considered idiopathic[15].

The disease occurs far more frequently in men than in women, the overall male to female ratio being in the range of 8:1[17]. The age distribution is wide. The vast majority of cases, however, are younger than 50 years. The average age of osteonecrosis is 36 years[18]. The average age of female cases exceeds that of males by almost 10 years[17]. The first case of idiopathic osteonecrosis of the hip in twins was reported recently[19].

Clinical features

The femoral head is the most common location of osteonecrosis but it may also develop in other locations, including the distal femur, humeral head and small bones of the wrist and foot (Fig. 174.1). Approximately 3% of the total population with osteonecrosis have multifocal disease. The distribution of joints affected by multifocal osteonecrosis is hip (91%), knee (87%), shoulder (72%) and ankle (35%). There is a high index of suspicion of multifocal osteonecrosis in patients treated with steroids; indeed, 91% of recognized cases have been treated with steroids[16].

Symptoms associated with osteonecrosis of the femoral head are non-specific. In many instances, the patient may remain entirely asymptomatic, and the condition is often diagnosed from X-ray films, taken because of symptoms in the opposite hip (Marcus's 'silent hip'[12]). In other instances, the patient may develop pain that persists for weeks to months before radiographs show any changes.

When pain does develop, it is most often located in the groin but may also be in the buttock, the thigh or even the knee. It is usually exacerbated by weight-bearing but it is often present at rest. Later, the patient may notice a limp and, still later, decreased range of motion.

Physical findings are also non-specific. Examination of the hip in many cases is within normal limits, even after radiographic films show advanced disease. Once the femoral head has begun to collapse, the range of motion will be limited, with pain at its extremes. Only after extensive femoral head collapse is shortening apparent[13].

Investigations

Radiographic changes

In the earliest stages of the disease, plain radiographs will be normal. During these stages, the pathologic process can be detected by other techniques[7], particularly MRI. Early radiographic changes include, within the femoral head, diffuse osteopenia, a central area of radiolucency with a sclerotic border and linear sclerosis. None of these changes are specific to osteonecrosis. Anteroposterior (AP) in extension, AP in flexion of 30° (Fig. 174.2), and lateral views (Fig. 174. 3) of the hips must be obtained to determine whether the shape of the head is still spherical without subchondral radiolucency. Later in the disease process, a subchondral radiolucency (the 'crescent sign') may appear, indicating a subchondral fracture (Fig. 174.4). This picture is almost

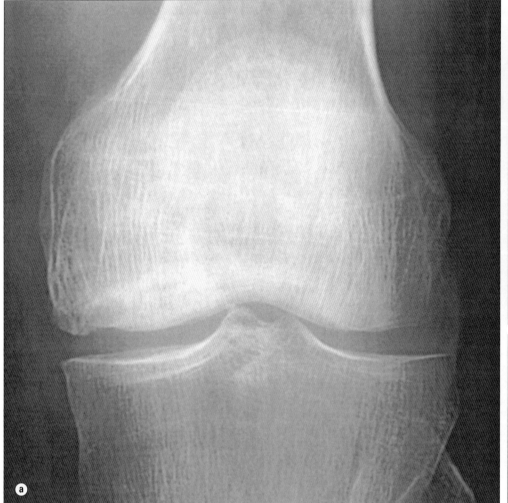

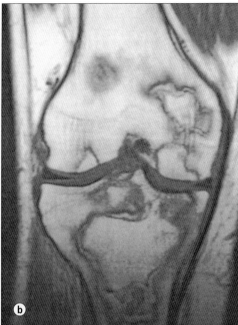

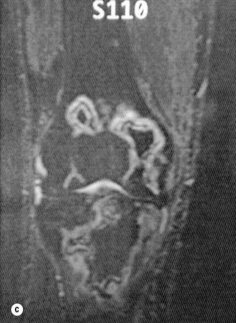

Fig. 174.1 Osteonecrosis of the left medial femoral condyle. (a) Plain radiograph of the knee of a 45-year-old man with hepatic grafting 8 months ago shows flattening and collapse of the medial femoral condyle. Both T1-weighted (b) and T2-weighted (c) MRI scans show multiple characteristic wavy margins delineating the areas of osteonecrotic bone.

pathognomonic of osteonecrosis, as are the changes that appear later – flattening and often gross collapse (Fig. 174.5) of the femoral head. The sphericity of the femoral head is lost, then a triangular zone of sclerotic bone is observed in the weight-bearing area. The joint space and the acetabulum are still normal.

Eventually, secondary osteoarthritic changes occur, with joint-space narrowing and sclerotic and cystic changes of the acetabulum. Sometimes, total destruction of the femoral head is noted.

Radionuclide bone scan

Conventional bone scan using a bone-imaging agent (methylene bisphosphonate labeled with technetium-99m) has been used for more than 30 years in investigation of osteonecrosis. It usually shows increased uptake, either due to new bone formation or simply as a result of metabolic activity around the necrotic area. The technique is very helpful because increased uptake may be observed even in early stages of the disease, when radiographs are normal or nearly normal. However, the technique does have limitations:

- it is non-specific except when a characteristic but rare decreased uptake is observed in the center of an uptake area within the femoral head ('cold in hot' image; Fig. 174.6)
- it can be judged only by comparison with the contralateral hip and so it is often of little use in bilateral involvement

- it is relatively insensitive in the precollapse stages, where it gives a positive result in only 70% of cases[20].

Computed tomography

Considerable progress in imaging of osteonecrosis came with the introduction of computed tomography (CT)[21]. CT images display early sclerosis in the central part of the femoral head ('asterisk sign'[22]) and give a better evaluation of the size of the sequestrum. Above all, CT shows well the anterior part, which is preferentially involved in osteonecrosis of the femoral head, and slight anterior collapse is in some cases visible only on CT images (Fig. 174.7).

Magnetic resonance imaging

Magnetic resonance imaging with axial and coronal T1- and T2-weighted images in early osteonecrosis displays an area of low-intensity signal in the medial aspect of the femoral head, especially in the subchondral zone (Fig. 174.8). This focal defect involving the anterosuperior aspect of the femoral head, but sometimes extending to the metaphysis, is the most frequent abnormality observed (96% of cases). In some cases, early changes

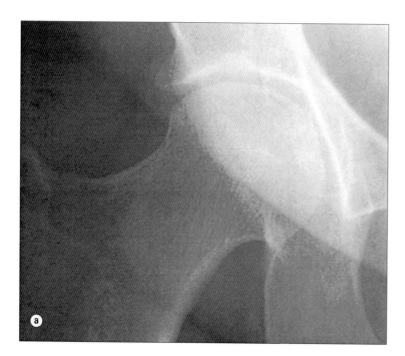
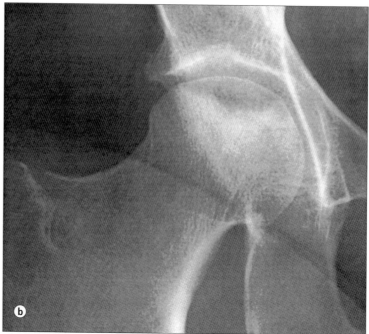

Fig. 174.2 Radiographic assessment of the femoral head in osteonecrosis. Both extended and semi-flexed AP views are necessary to ensure that the femoral head is normal. This 23-year-old woman complained of right hip pain 3 months post-partum. The extended AP radiograph (a) was normal, but the 30° flexion view (b) displayed a radiolucent area of the superior aspect of the femoral head, which already showed stage 2 disease.

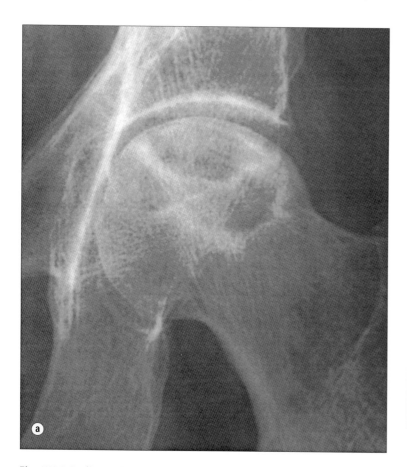
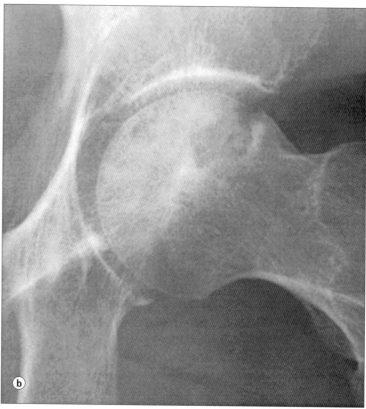

Fig. 174.3 Radiographic assessment of the femoral head in osteonecrosis. This 52-year-old woman, alcoholic and treated with steroids for asthma, had complained of left hip pain for 13 months. (a) The AP view shows an extensive radiolucent area delineated by a sclerotic band without flattening of the femoral head. (b) The lateral view depicts a fracture of subchondral bone (stage 4).

depicted in fat suppression images will precede the classic band pattern[23]. As there is excellent agreement between full and screening MRI, a shorter technique may be useful and enable time (< 4min) and potential cost reduction[24].

The most characteristic image is a margin of low signal on T1- and T2-weighted images. It is observed in 60–80% of cases[25–27]. According to Mitchell *et al.*[26], the central region delineated by the line of low signal may give a high or a low signal on T1- as on T2-weighted images, leading

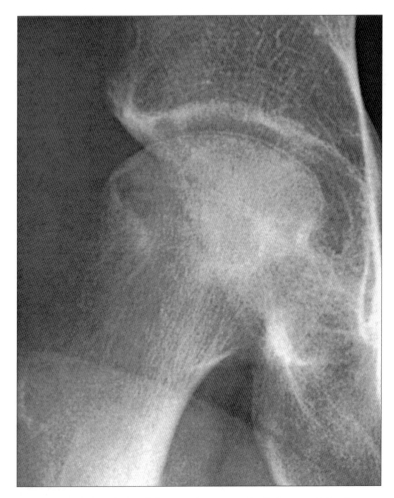

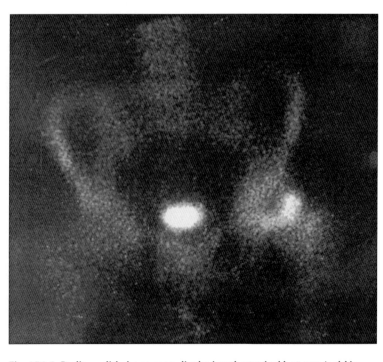

Fig. 174.6 Radionuclide bone scan displaying the typical but rare 'cold in hot' image in the left hip. This patient had had a renal transplant 2 years previously and presented with pain in the left buttock only. X-rays were normal. MRI confirmed osteonecrosis.

Fig. 174.4 Subchondral radiolucency ('crescent sign') characteristic of osteonecrosis. More often detected on lateral than on AP views, this signals a subchondral fracture (stage 3).

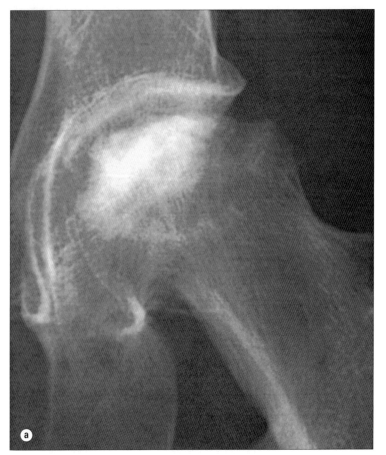

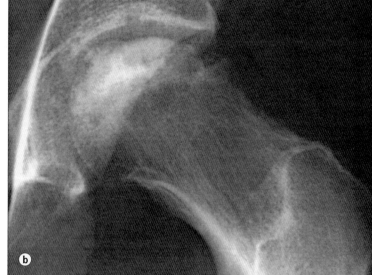

Fig. 174.5 Collapse of the femoral head due to osteonecrosis. This systemic lupus erythematosus patient was treated with 12mg of prednisone (prednisolone) for 4 years and complained of pain in the left buttock over a period of 12 months. On radiography, the gross collapse was detectable, on both AP (a) and lateral views (b). Note the sclerotic margin within the femoral head, which delineates the area of the necrotic zone (stage 4).

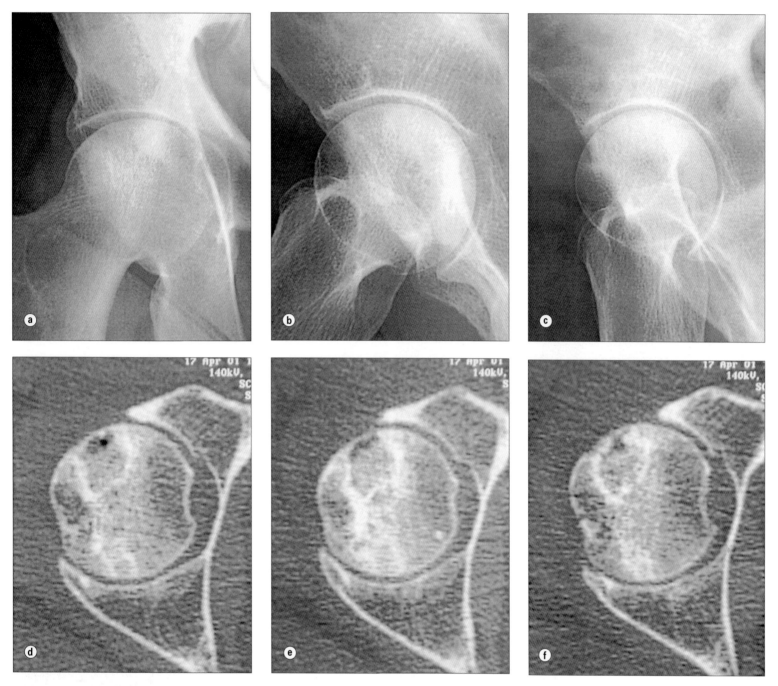

Fig. 174.7 Radiographs and CT of stage 4 osteonecrosis. AP (a), lateral (b) and profile (c) views are nearly normal except for a slight condensation of the upper part of the femoral head. CT scans (d–f) allow evaluation of the size of the sequestrum in the anterior aspect of the right femoral head and the subchondral fracture that identifies stage 4. (The patient was a 41-year-old fireman without any etiological factor for osteonecrosis except a direct contusion – a fall from a truck – on the right trochanteric area 11 months before.)

to a classification in four classes, A–D. On T1-weighted images the majority of precollapsed osteonecrosis cases display a high signal (classes A or B), while the majority of collapsed osteonecrosis cases display a low signal (classes C or D). Injection of gadolinium or fat-suppression sequences enhance profiles of the marrow spaces and are more sensitive for the diagnosis of osteonecrosis[28].

Joint fluid is shown well as an intense signal on T2-weighted images. In osteonecrosis, this fluid is more frequently present and more extensive after collapse has occurred[29].

Magnetic resonance imaging is highly sensitive; indeed, all cases of collapse of the femoral head display an identical image on MRI. At early stages, even before collapse, MRI has the best sensitivity and the best accuracy (75–100%) compared with other modes of investigation[30–35].

However, true osteonecrosis cases with negative MRI have been reported[36].

Other investigations

Functional bone exploration (including bone-marrow pressure, stress test with injection of saline and intramedullary venography) demonstrates the decreased bone blood flow with increased bone marrow pressure that occurs even at the early stages in all cases of osteonecrosis[7]. These explorations are very sensitive but not specific and may be abnormal in osteoarthritis of the hip, transient osteoporosis of the hip and pagetic hip arthropathy. Superselective angiography, which discloses interruption of the superior retinacular arteries, has also been used.

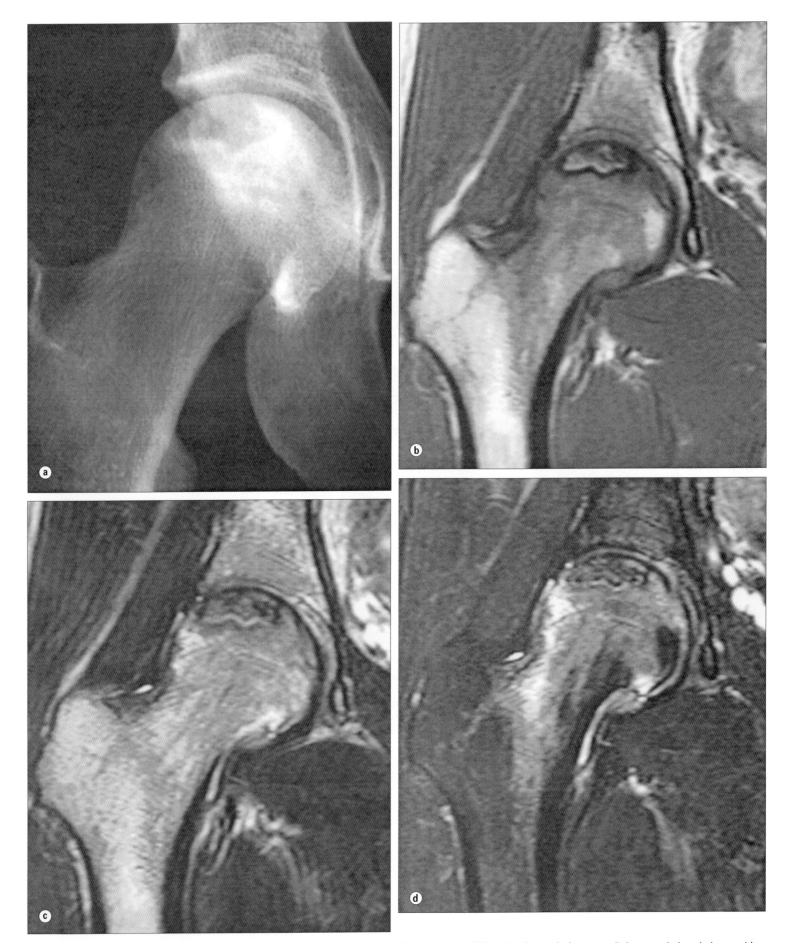

Fig. 174.8 MRI of stage 2 osteonecrosis. A 37-year-old man treated with corticosteroids for asthma. (a) The AP radiograph shows a radiolucent subchondral area with normal contour of the femoral head (i.e. stage 2, confirmed on lateral view and CT scan, not shown). (b) The T1-weighted MRI image shows a subarticular lesion in the femoral head delimited by a characteristic wavy, low-signal margin. This pattern is virtually pathognomonic for osteonecrosis. A more diffuse pattern of low signal extends down the right femoral neck. On the T2-weighted image (c) and overall on the fat saturation image (d), the diffuse pattern in the femoral neck exhibits high signal intensity consistent with marrow edema[95]. The osteonecrotic region in the femoral head does not contain any high signal to indicate acute edema or liquefaction. A small, high-signal-intensity joint effusion is visible beneath the femoral head and the neck.

TABLE 174.1 STAGING OF OSTEONECROSIS		
Stage	Findings	Techniques
0	All techniques normal or non diagnostic, necrosis on biopsy	Biopsy and histology
1	X-rays and CT scan normal Positive result from at least one of the techniques opposite	Radionuclide scan MRI
2	X-ray abnormalities without collapse (sclerosis, cysts, osteopenia)	MRI
3	Crescent sign	X-rays
4	Flattening or evident collapse	CT scan initially
5	As for stage 4, with narrowing of joint space	X-rays only
6	As for stage 5, with destruction of the joint	

However, these invasive techniques have been eclipsed by MRI, except for pathogenic investigations[36].

STAGING SYSTEMS FOR OSTEONECROSIS

The sequence of changes seen by radiography and other investigation techniques have formed the basis of several proposed staging systems[7,35,37,38]. Recently, the Subcommittee of Nomenclature of the International Association on Bone Circulation and Bone Necrosis (ARCO: Association Research Circulation Osseous), has reassembled the results of these classifications to establish an internationally accepted system of classification of the various stages of osteonecrosis (Table 174.1). It is believed by the committee that a uniform system is necessary in order to be able to carry out comparative epidemiologic studies, as well as to be able to compare and contrast the results of different methods of treatment.

Stage 0

All diagnostic examinations are normal and the patient is asymptomatic. The diagnosis is made purely on the basis of histology that demonstrates osteonecrosis. In one sense, stage 0 is a theoretical stage, but it is useful for autopsy studies or to define the silent osteonecrosis that might be diagnosed at the time of intervention for the opposite hip. Acceptance of this stage is recognition that osteonecrosis can exist histologically without any associated clinical signs or symptoms.

Stage 1

The radiographs, both AP and lateral views, and the CT scan are normal but the pathologic condition is suspected from other procedures, including standard technetium bone scan, angioscintigraphy, MRI and functional exploration of bone. Stage 1 is defined by one of these being abnormal. However, the only confirmation of stage 1 is by histology (biopsy) or by MRI, when a low-signal-intensity band on T1- and T2-weighted images is visible or a cold spot is observed on the radionuclide scan. The patient may or may not be symptomatic at this stage.

Stage 2

A variety of radiologic abnormalities that are the early signs of eventual bone death are evident within the femoral head. These may include areas of linear sclerosis, focal bead mineralization or cysts in the femoral head or neck. However, the femoral head is perfectly spherical, as seen on both AP and lateral radiographs and on the CT scan. There is no subchondral radiolucency. Because stage 2 covers a wide range of radio-graphic abnormalities, a subclassification according to the area of radiologic involvement is included: A, less than 15% of the head involved, as detected on radiographs or MRI; B, 15–30%; C, more than 30%.

Stage 3

In stage 3 the femoral head has begun to fail mechanically. The hallmark of this stage is a radiolucent 'crescent sign' appearing just beneath the subchondral endplate and indicating collapse of the subchondral cancellous trabeculae. The spherical configuration of the articular surface remains intact. This crescent sign does not always develop as the femoral head progresses from earlier to later stages of involvement. Because the head remains spherical, it is at least theoretically possible to preserve its integrity by surgical procedures that allow the necrotic and collapsed bone to be replaced by viable tissue. The extent of involvement is divided as follows: A, crescent beneath less than 15% of the articular surface; B, crescent beneath 15–30%; C, crescent beneath more than 30%.

Stage 4

Any evidence of flattening or eccentric joint-space increase is the first sign of stage 4 and has important therapeutic implications because the hip has now progressed to the point at which the changes are irreversible. This collapse usually occurs in the anterolateral or superior weight-bearing region. The differentiation between stage 2 and stage 4 can best be shown by CT scan, which is more sensitive than plain radiographs. Stage 4 is divided into three subsets to quantify the lesion: A, less than 15% of the surface has collapsed and depression is less than 2mm; B, 15–30% collapsed or 2–4mm depression; C, more than 30% collapsed or more than 4mm depression.

Stage 5

Any or all of the preceding radiographic changes may be evident and in addition there is a decrease in the joint space. In this case, there is osteoarthritis secondary to the mechanical collapse of the femoral head, with sclerosis, cysts of the acetabulum and occasionally marginal osteophytes.

Stage 6

Extensive destruction of the femoral head occurs, following the degenerative process.

DIFFERENTIAL DIAGNOSIS

At stages 3 and 4, radiographs are specific and no differential problem occurs. When late stage 5 and stage 6 are observed for the first time, unless an early radiograph is available it is quite impossible to diagnose osteonecrosis as the cause of the destruction of the hip. However, the question is not of practical relevance, since the only therapeutic possibility is total hip replacement.

The difficult differential diagnoses concern stages 1 and 2. In stage 1, all the diseases of the hip affecting bone, cartilage or synovial tissue may be considered. An algorithm that may be useful in diagnosis in the patient at risk of osteonecrosis is given in Figure 174.9. Arthrography of the hip allows identification of chondromatosis, synovitis or synovial tumors, labrum tear or local thinning of cartilage in the weight-bearing area, which signals early osteoarthritic change.

In stage 2, non-specific bone lesions on radiographs prompt radionuclide scan or MRI if patients are thought to be at risk of osteonecrosis. The most difficult differential diagnosis is transient osteoporosis of the hip or hip algodystrophy, in which the same osteopenia of the femoral head can be observed on radiographs, with the same radionuclide uptake and possibly the same low-signal area on T1-weighted MRI. The only difference is on the T2-weighted image, in which algodystrophy displays a high signal as opposed to the low signal seen in osteonecrosis[39]. Subchondral

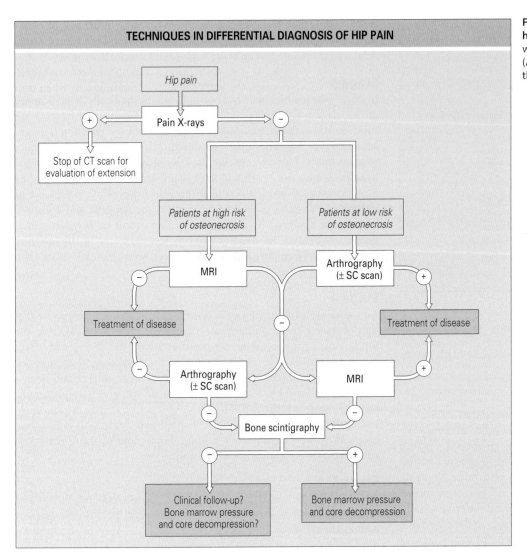

TECHNIQUES IN DIFFERENTIAL DIAGNOSIS OF HIP PAIN

Fig. 174.9 Techniques in differential diagnosis of hip pain. This approach may be especially useful when radiographs are normal or nearly normal. (Adapted from Beltran *et al.*[34] with permission from the Radiological Society of North America.)

stress fracture is also difficult to diagnose even on MRI. Chondroblastoma of the femoral head is a very rare condition.

Diagnostic criteria

In a multicenter study including 122 hips with osteonecrosis and 155 hips with other diseases, a set of four diagnostic criteria of osteonecrosis was proposed[40], using histology as gold standard with 100% sensitivity and 100% specificity (Table 174.2). The sensitivity and specificity of these criteria are given in Table 174.3.

NATURAL HISTORY AND EVOLUTION

Contralateral silent hip involvement is present in 30–70% of cases at the time of the first examination.

Evidence suggests that the rate of progression is high, particularly in symptomatic patients. At least 68–80% of femoral heads with osteonecrosis will collapse within 4 years[35,41]. There is no correlation between underlying etiology and the time to collapse. In the later stages of the disease, after subchondral collapse and loss of joint congruity, progressive osteoarthritis is considered to be inevitable. Anatomic and functional deterioration leads to a surgical procedure in more than 50% of the cases within 3 years of diagnosis[8–10].

However, both extent and location of the necrotic area are important to predict the evolution of collapse. Good prognostic signs with minimal risk of evolution to collapse are involvement of less than one-fourth of the diameter of the head, necrosis of less than one-third of the weight-bearing area and involvement of less than 30% of the femoral head[11,42].

TABLE 174.2 DIAGNOSTIC CRITERIA FOR OSTEONECROSIS[40]

	Tool	Criterion
1	X-rays	Collapse of the femoral head (depression or crescent sign)
2	X-rays	Demarcating sclerosis in the femoral head
3	Bone scan	'Cold in hot' spot
4	MRI	Low-intensity band on T1-weighted images (band pattern)

To fulfill criteria 1 and 2, there must be no joint-space narrowing and no acetabular abnormality.

TABLE 174.3 SENSITIVITY AND SPECIFICITY OF COMBINATIONS OF THE CRITERIA LISTED IN TABLE 174.2[40]

Criteria combinations	Sensitivity (%)	Specificity (%)
One positive criterion	100	94
Two positive criteria	91	99
Three positive criteria	79	100

According to the Japanese classification[35], mainly based on the location of the lesion, medial lesions rarely progress (only 9%), lateral involvement has the worst prognosis and central osteonecrosis has intermediate severity[43].

However, a complete review of the literature on the natural history of osteonecrosis shows that only 31–35% of precollapse osteonecrosis had a satisfactory clinical result without an operative procedure[18]. Non-progressive medial lesions do not exceed 12% of total cases and the vast majority of patients should undergo a surgical procedure to avoid collapse as far as possible.

In prospective studies of the relative usefulness of scintigraphy and MRI as screening tests for groups at high-risk for osteonecrosis (e.g. patients with systemic lupus erythematosus, allograft recipients, patients under steroids for autoimmune disorders), the condition was diagnosed in about 15% of the cases, mainly during the first 6 months of follow-up[44]. Interestingly, some patients have unilateral decreased scintigraphy uptake (photopenia) on one or more bone scans that is transient and normalizes on subsequent scans without any other subsequent evidence of osteonecrosis[45]. Similar transient images on MRI have been reported[46], including low-signal-intensity areas that do not lead to osteonecrosis, but when the area is band-like the predictive value for osteonecrosis is nearly 70%[47].

BASIC SCIENCE

Pathology

As the etiology and pathogenesis of the disease are not known, pathology is so far the gold standard for diagnosis of osteonecrosis. Osteonecrosis involves the cells of the two tissues of bone: osteocytes and marrow cells. Necrosis of the marrow is easier to observe. The only sign of necrosis of bone tissue is disappearance of the osteocytes, the cavities of which are empty and often enlarged. At least partial necrosis, 50% or more empty osteocyte-lacunas of the trabecular bone, must be found. Following the stages of the disease, several pictures may be described.

In advanced stages, as observed in femoral heads removed at the time of total hip replacement (Fig. 174.10), the triangular sequestrum is made

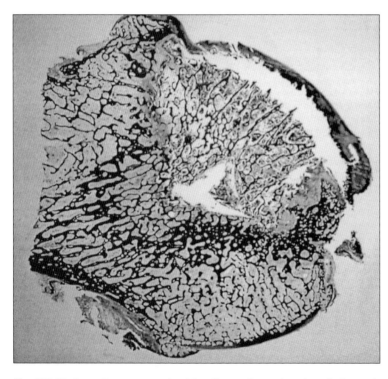

Fig. 174.10 Stage 5 osteonecrosis with collapse. Coronal section of a femoral head retrieved during total hip replacement. The cartilage above the sequestrum is of irregular height and osteophytes of the superior and inferior aspects of the femoral head are observed. Note the sclerotic border delineating the sequestrum. The trabecular architecture is preserved and lesions of the bone marrow tissue are suspected (blue-stained zones are fibrous or necrotic tissues). (Masson's stain, original magnification × 0.5.)

up of dead trabeculae without osteocytes but with preserved architecture. The bone marrow tissue becomes a magma characterized by the disappearance of the stem cells, adipocyte nucleolysis and membrane loss, sometimes replaced by eosinophilic debris with no recognizable cell remnants. In some cases, the adipocytes are mummified, as when only shadows of fat cells are found, without nuclei and with discontinuous outlines resulting from the persistence of pericellular reticulin[48]. This necrotic area is located under the subchondral plate. Its size is variable, sometimes very limited, sometimes extending well into the metaphysis. The subchondral fracture at the origin of the collapse is usually located in the subchondral dead bone, typically more or less parallel with the edges of the epiphysis that produces the radiological 'crescent sign'. The dead tissue of the sequestrum is usually in continuity with the concave zone of 'repair' (Phemister's creeping substitution[3]), including fibrovascular proliferation, and below active bone resorption and new living bone apposition on the remains of old, dead trabeculae. Osteonecrosis is due to a single event and it appears that an increase in size of the necrotic area is extremely rare (0.3%)[49].

More interesting are the lesions observed either before collapse, as described on specimens taken in core biopsies, or when the collapsed area of the femoral head is removed from within the metaphysis, far from the sequestrum area[50]. The earlier marrow lesions are edema or stasis, hemorrhages, fibrilloreticulosis, hypocellularity, necrosis of the hematopoietic cells, and disorganization and reticular eosinophilic atrophy of the lipocytes. These lesions are at first localized, then diffuse. Several authors maintain that bone marrow lesions precede the osteocytic ones[51–53]. Bone marrow necrosis can be found alone in osteonecrosis but lacks specificity[54]. The study of biopsies obtained from core decompression may have two potential pitfalls: a false-negative result due to the biopsy not containing the necrotic area, and a false-positive result because of artificial necrosis on the edges of the sample due to mechanical or thermal artifacts (more frequent with motorized drillings)[50,55].

Unfortunately, the histologic criteria used for diagnosis of osteonecrosis are not always detailed in the literature and their inappropriate use has sometimes led to confusion and minimization of the diagnostic value of histology, especially when new data obtained using other techniques such as MRI[56] are discussed.

Osteonecrosis pathology is complex because one is usually dealing with chronic incomplete ischemia in which truly ischemic lesions, secondary reactive lesions and reconstruction phenomena may be both sequential and simultaneous, depending upon time and area. Arlet and Durroux proposed a classification into four types of pathologic changes[53] (Table 174.4). Electron microscopy displays the necrosis of the various components of bone (Fig. 174.14).

TABLE 174.4 PATHOLOGICAL CLASSIFICATION OF OSTEONECROTIC LESIONS[53]	
Type	**Description**
Type I	The predominant lesions are clearly prenecrotic and confined to bone marrow, although occasionally both foam cells and small areas of eosinophilic reticular necrosis of the fatty marrow are seen. The most common lesion is interstitial edema or plasmostasis (Fig. 174.11).
Type II	The most characteristic finding is that all the medullary spaces are filled with necrotic tissue, resulting in eosinophilic reticular necrosis extending one to several centimeters in the specimen (Fig. 174.12).
Type III	Marrow necrosis is associated with clear trabecular necrosis, with 50–100% of the lacunae empty.
Type IV	The previous lesions (type III) are present, but foci of marrow fibrosis are also encountered, and the dead trabeculae are increased in number and surrounded by living, newly formed bone (Fig. 174.13).

TABLE 174.5 ETIOLOGICAL FACTORS IN OSTEONECROSIS[40]

Osteonecrosis of known etiology
Traumatic
    Fracture of the femoral neck
    Dislocation or fracture-dislocation of the hip
Non-traumatic
    Caisson and divers' diseases
    Gaucher's disease
    Sickle-cell anemia
    Radiotherapy
Osteonecrosis with probable etiologic relationships
Traumatic
    Minor trauma
Non traumatic
    Arteriosclerosis and other occlusive vascular disorders
    Carbon tetrachloride poisoning
    Corticosteroid administration
    Cushing's disease
    Diabetes mellitus
    Disturbances of lipid metabolism
    Dysplasia of the acetabulum
    Excessive alcohol intake
    Fatty liver
    Hyperuricemia and gout
    Osteomalacia
    Pancreatitis and Weber-Christian disease
    Pregnancy
    Transplantations (renal, hepatic,…)
    SLE and other connective tissue disorders
    Thrombophlebitis disorders
    Tumors

Etiology

Osteonecrosis is often seen in association with a number of different conditions (Table 174.5).

Trauma with fracture of the femoral neck, especially in the subcapital region, interrupts the major part of the blood supply to the head and may lead to osteonecrosis. The risk has been reported to be as high as 10–43% after a displaced femoral neck fracture. The perfusion and viability of the femoral head are critical for successful fracture healing and may be predicted by arteriography, radionuclide scintigraphy or, easily, by dynamic MRI (which is a non-invasive technique and whose sensitivity and specificity seem good – 81% and 100% respectively)[57]. Dislocation and fracture–dislocation are much less common than hip fracture but the incidence of osteonecrosis may be as high as 40% if reduction is delayed more than 12 hours after dislocation[58].

Corticosteroids and alcoholism are the two main predisposing factors other than trauma. The risk of osteonecrosis with corticosteroid therapy is dose-related. Low dose therapy (average daily dosage 8mg) does not, however, protect patients against the development of osteonecrosis. Thus in rheumatoid arthritis 12% of femoral heads removed for total hip arthroplasties were affected by classical osteonecrosis (6%) or demonstrated osteonecrosis in association with degenerative changes (6%). In all, 81% and 68% respectively of patients on steroid therapy demonstrated these two types of osteonecrosis, whereas only 33% of patients who had not received steroids had osteonecrosis[59]. Few cases of osteonecrosis after long-term topical steroid application have been reported[60].

Some risk factors have been postulated based on temporal association or increased incidence in groups of patients exhibiting particular characteristics. For example, an association has been suggested[61] between

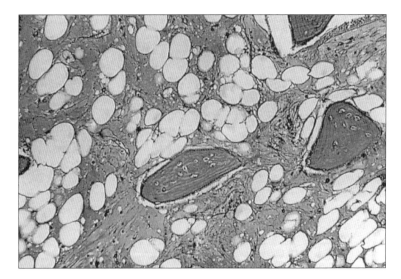

Fig. 174.11 Type I osteonecrosis. Interstitial edema or plasmostasis with lipocytes that are still normal, and living trabecular bone. (Hematoxylin and eosin stain, original magnification × 200.)

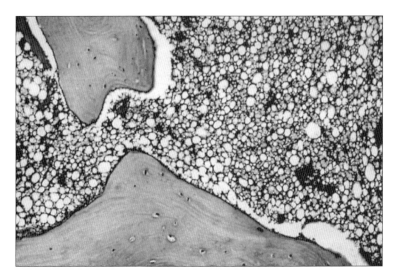

Fig. 174.12 Type II osteonecrosis. Surrounding two normal trabeculae, the bone marrow fat is disorganized and atrophied with fat drops of various diameter, displaying the typical eosinophilic reticular necrosis. (Hematoxylin and eosin stain, original magnification × 100.)

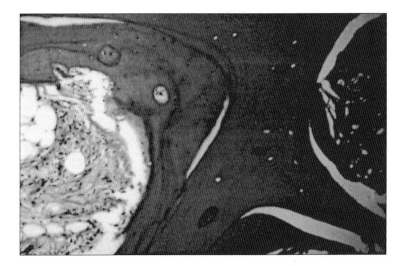

Fig. 174.13 Type IV osteonecrosis. A new living bone trabecula is laid down on the left side of an old necrotic trabecula with empty lacunas; a dense fibrosis is observed at the right side of the necrotic trabecula. (Hematoxylin and eosin stain, original magnification × 200.)

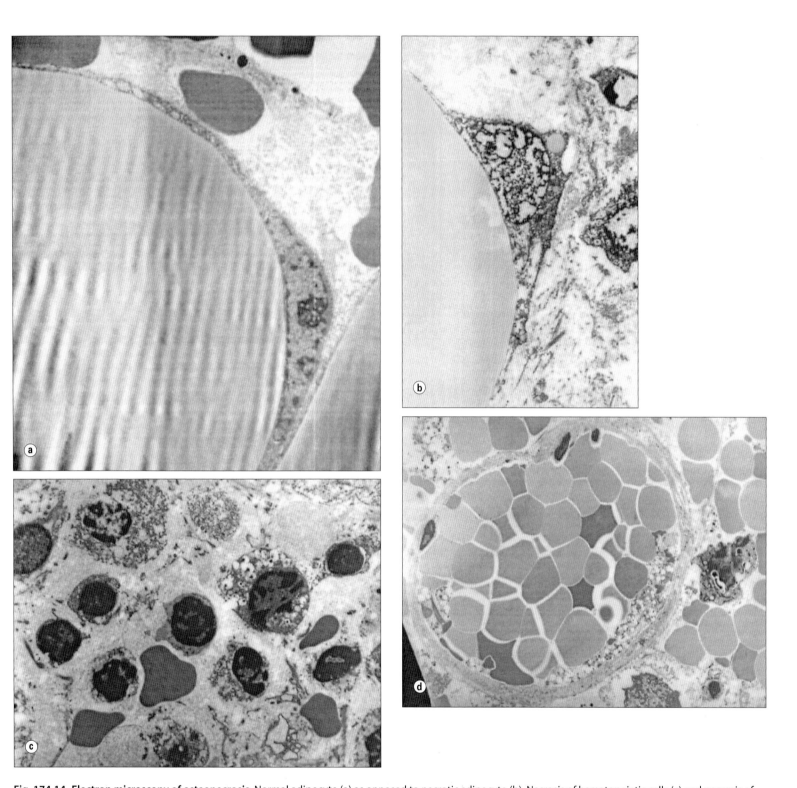

Fig. 174.14 Electron microscopy of osteonecrosis. Normal adipocyte (a) as opposed to necrotic adipocyte (b). Necrosis of hematopoietic cells (c) and necrosis of the wall of a vessel (d). (Original magnification × 3000.)

elevated serum cholesterol levels and idiopathic osteonecrosis of the femoral head.

In many of these instances, the pathophysiologic relationship between the causal agent and the subsequent necrosis is either poorly understood or under dispute. Osteonecrosis has been reported in human immuno-deficiency virus (HIV)-positive patients but the condition is more likely to be explained by other well-known concomitant etiological factors[62], mainly steroids[63]. Several cases of osteonecrosis occurring in pregnancy have been reported[64].

Caisson disease, sickle-cell disease, Gaucher's disease and radiotherapy for malignancies represent causes of osteonecrosis in a small percentage

of cases, although sickle-cell disease is the main cause in some African countries.

Pathogenesis

A mechanical interruption to the circulation of the femoral head is common to most of the conditions associated with osteonecrosis. In the case of a displaced fracture or a dislocation, gross disruption of the vessels occurs. In Caisson disease and sickle-cell disease, osteonecrosis is commonly attributed to an engorgement of sinusoidal circulation by either nitrogen bubbles or rigid sickle cells. However, the mechanism of ischemia and/or necrosis is still in question for most other non-traumatic forms of osteonecrosis[65]. Several hypotheses can be summarized, as follows.

Microfractures and osteoporosis

Frost[66] supposed that repeated microfractures in the weight-bearing area would induce microvascular lesions, then ischemia in fragile bone. Laurent et al.[67] found osteopenia in 20 and osteomalacia in seven out of 35 iliac crest biopsy specimens from patients with osteonecrosis. However, osteonecrosis does not seem to be a complication of post-menopausal osteoporosis.

Vascular problems

Primary vascular problems in the arterial, venous or capillary part of the vascular network may make osteonecrosis a 'coronary disease of the hip'[68]. Recent arteriographic studies have given a new impulse to this old hypothesis[69]. Histopathologic study of the vessels of the osteonecrosis femoral head show increased thrombosis, presence of lipid droplets in the small bone vessels and thickening of arterial vessel walls compared with osteoarthritic femoral heads or controls[70]. Furthermore, corticosteroids favor the development of hypertension and coronary arteriosclerosis, and the background of osteonecrosis patients is very similar to that of diabetic, arteritic and alcoholic patients, with hyperlipidemia and blood hyperviscosity[71].

Experimental interruption of venous drainage of bone in animals induces osteonecrosis but this factor is not proved in human disease. Venous drainage is in fact decreased, as demonstrated by intramedullary phlebography, but this is just a reflection of the slowing of the whole bone vascular network. Finally, the 'compartment syndrome' theory[7,68] suggests compression of bone microvasculature in the rigid trabecular network by increased medullary pressure and blood viscosity[71] as causes, but it is not known whether these increases are primary or secondary. Recently, with gadolinium-enhanced MRI and MR hydrogen-1 spectroscopy for marrow composition study, it was demonstrated that femoral head perfusion was greater in corticosteroid-treated systemic lupus erythematosus patients than in controls[72]. These data do not therefore support the role of a compartment syndrome mechanism with impaired perfusion that results from lipocyte hypertrophy in the development of osteonecrosis in this condition.

In spite of case reports, antiphospholipid antibodies are not more frequent in osteonecrosis patients than in age- and sex-matched controls[73].

Fat embolism

Jones showed lung- and kidney-fat embolism from fatty liver, and induced experimental osteonecrosis by intra-arterial injection of lipiodol[37]. However, it has not been proved that the lipid droplets observed in the subchondral vessels of the necrotic femoral head are from the fatty liver. Jones proposed three possible origins for the fat emboli: fatty liver, destabilization and coalescence of plasma lipoproteins, and disruption of fatty bone marrow.

Hypertrophy of fat cells

Experimentally, corticosteroids have been shown to induce enlargement of marrow fat cells and marrow volume, to increase intramedullary pressure and reduce bone blood flow[74]. However, the relevance of these findings to corticosteroid-induced osteonecrosis is unclear.

MANAGEMENT

Introduction

When the subchondral shell is intact, there is a possibility of healing; following collapse, healing is obviously impossible. By contrast, the evolution of osteonecrosis in the contralateral hip, which progresses to collapse in more than 50% of cases, is an important issue in management.

Prevention

When the risk of osteonecrosis is high, and when an etiologic factor is reversible, prevention is the best approach.

- Most decompression accidents can be avoided if all decompressions follow the established rules (slow resurfacing with staged decompression).
- Hyperlipidemia and diabetes should be treated and alcohol intake minimized.
- Each time corticosteroid treatment is undertaken in moderate or high doses, particularly more than 20mg of prednisone (prednisolone) or equivalent daily for more than a month, the risk of bone necrosis must be recognized and weighed against the benefits to be derived from this therapy. Corticosteroid use should be kept as low as possible. Statins – agents that dramatically reduce cholesterol levels in blood and tissues – may offer some protection against the development of osteonecrosis when steroid treatment is necessary. Indeed there is only a 1% incidence of osteonecrosis in statin-plus-steroid-treated patients versus the 3–20% usually reported for patients receiving high-dose steroids[75].

Medical treatment

- Weight-bearing on the affected hip should be restricted for at least 4–8 weeks. Use of crutches is classically proposed but the only conditions for which this might be effective are osteonecrosis with involvement of the medial aspect of the femoral head, an extension of less than one-fourth of the diameter of the head or necrotic volume of less than 20% on MRI with minimal risk of evolution to collapse.
- Vasoactive drugs may play a role in treating early cases of osteonecrosis, although it is difficult to prove the efficacy of so-called peripheral vasodilators such as naftidrofuryl oxalate, dihydroergotamine or vincamine. These drugs are extensively used in Africa in the treatment of sickle-cell crises. They seem to reduce bone marrow pressure[76].
- Promising results have been reported using pulsing electromagnetic fields applied externally[77]. This technique is still being evaluated and developed.

Surgical treatment

Osteonecrosis involves ischemic events followed by death of bone and marrow elements. A process of repair is then initiated but, unless the lesion is small, involving less than 15% of the femoral head, or medially located, this repair weakens subchondral bone with subsequent collapse of the articular surface. The results of hip arthroplasty in patients with osteonecrosis are, however, relatively poor, with failure rates ranging from 10% to 50% at an average follow-up of 5 years. Thus emphasis has been placed on modalities aimed at femoral head preservation. The surgical alternatives may include core decompression, osteotomies, non-vascularized and vascularized bone grafting, all of which might be enhanced with the use of growth and differentiation factors[41].

Core decompression decreases the intramedullary pressure within the femoral head and neck and as a consequence has been postulated to improve circulation to the femoral head. The results of this technique are still controversial: 34–95% of good results are obtained in the early stages[78,79] but they are always better than discontinuing weight-bearing.

Bone grafting using cortical or cancellous bone, grafts with an attached muscle pedicle or with microvascular anastomosis, with intra- and extra-articular techniques, also provides decompression of the femoral head[65,82–84]. The probability of total hip replacement rescue within 5 years after the procedure is statistically lower in precollapse stages compared with the other groups[82,84]. Future approaches may also include the use of specific cytokines (such as bone morphogenetic protein) or medullary stem cells that promote bone healing[80,81].

Numerous osteotomies have been performed in various planes[85–90]. The stated goal is to remove the diseased section of the femoral head from the region of major weight-bearing and to replace it with a normal portion of the femoral head. Here also, the absence of collapse is associated with a good clinical result and a collapse of 2mm or more leads to clinical failure[86]. There are two radiological factors reported to correlate with the results of transtrochanteric rotational osteotomy:

- the extent of the intact articular surface of the femoral head under the weight-bearing portion of the acetabulum on the postoperative AP film
- the extent of the intact femoral articular surface of either the anterior or posterior area on the preoperative, true lateral radiograph (preoperative lateral intact area)[89].

The best postoperative results are usually obtained in young, active patients with unilateral involvement and necrotic angle less than 200° in whom the osteotomy is performed before collapse. The results obtained in 50 hips from 40 patients (six stage 2 (Arlet–Ficat) and 44 stage 3) were strongly dependent on the amplitude of the necrotic (Kerboul) angle ($p < 0.01$), the preoperative mobility of the hip ($p < 0.01$), and age[90]. In cases of extensive necrosis in which the necrotic area occupies two-thirds or more of the weight-bearing zone of the femoral head, both transtrochanteric rotational osteotomy of the femoral head and vascularized pedicle iliac bone graft may be performed if age makes total hip replacement undesirable[84].

Cup arthroplasty, surface replacement arthroplasty and femoral endoprosthetic replacement were almost completely abandoned once the effectiveness of total hip replacement was established. But the results of total hip replacement in osteonecrosis patients have generally been poorer, with a higher revision rate compared with age-matched patients with other diagnoses[91]. Furthermore, the success of this surgery is related to the etiology of osteonecrosis: good or excellent results are seen in 92% of idiopathic cases, 87% of alcohol-induced cases, 78% of renal transplant cases and 62.5% of systemic lupus erythematosus cases[92]. The results are also poor in osteonecrosis due to sickle cell disease[93], leading some authors to treat the collapse by injecting acrylic cement into the necrotic area until the collapse is corrected[94].

A number of problems confront attempts to determine the efficacy of surgical procedures used to treat osteonecrosis. The existence of several staging systems makes it difficult to compare the results of many studies. The multifactorial etiology of osteonecrosis makes it hard to be certain that every center is treating the same disease. Results are difficult to evaluate if there are technical differences in the way a procedure has been applied. Finally, uniformly accepted criteria for success need to be established.

However, it is possible to indicate the main procedures that can be proposed according to disease stage. It is of prognostic significance to determine the integrity of the subchondral plate using the most accurate method available. In precollapse stages, core decompression with or without bone grafting may be an effective procedure; in later stages with evident collapse, total hip replacement may be the most reasonable technique. In cases of crescent sign or slight flattening, especially in young patients, the decision is more difficult: bone graft or osteotomy may be the best alternatives.

REFERENCES

1. Mont MA, Baumgarten KM, Rifai A et al. Atraumatic osteonecrosis of the knee. J Bone Joint Surg 2000, 82A: 1279–1290.
2. Russell J. An essay on necrosis: section I. General remarks and description of appearances. Clin Orthop Rel Res 1978; 130: 5–7.
3. Phemister DB. Lesions of bones and joint arising from interruption of the circulation. J Mt Sinai Hosp 1948; 15: 55–63.
4. Phemister DB. Treatment of the necrotic head of the femur in adults. J Bone Joint Surg 1949; 31A: 55–66.
5. Mankin HJ, Brower TB. Bilateral idiopathic aseptic necrosis of the femur in adults: 'Chandler's disease'. Bull Hosp Joint Dis 1962; 23: 42–57.
6. Glimcher MJ, Kenzora JE. The biology of osteonecrosis of the human femoral head and its clinical implications: an abridged communication. Clin Orthop Rel Res 1978; 130: 47–50.
7. Ficat RP, Arlet J. Ischemia and necroses of bone. Baltimore, MD: Williams & Wilkins; 1980.
8. Jacobs B. Epidemiology of traumatic and nontraumatic osteonecrosis. Clin Orthop Rel Res 1978; 130: 51–67.
9. Renier JC, Bregeon C, Boasson M et al. Contribution à la connaissance de l'évolution de l'ostéonécrose primitive de la tête fémorale. Rev Rheum Mal Ostéo-Articul 1972; 39: 697–708.
10. Bradway JK, Morrey BF. The natural history of the silent hip in bilateral atraumatic necrosis of the femoral head. J Arthroplasty 1993; 8: 383–387.
11. Shimizu K, Moriya H, Akita T et al. Prediction of collapse with magnetic resonance imaging of avascular necrosis of the femoral head. J Bone Joint Surg 1994; 76A: 215–223.
12. Marcus ND, Enneking WF, Massam RA. The silent hip in idiopathic aseptic necrosis. J Bone Joint Surg 1973; 55A: 1351–1366.
13. Steinberg ME, Steinberg DR. Avascular necrosis of the femoral head. In: Steinberg ME, ed. The hip and its disorders. Philadelphia, PA: WB Saunders; 1991: 623–647.
14. Mankin HJ. Nontraumatic necrosis of bone (osteonecrosis). N Engl J Med 1992, 326: 1473–1479.
15. Ninomiya S. An epidemiological survey of idiopathic avascular necrosis of the femoral head in Japan. Annual Report of Japanese Investigation Committee for Intractable Disease. Osaka: University Publisher; 1989.
16. Collaborative Osteonecrosis Group. Symptomatic multifocal osteonecrosis. Clin Orthop Rel Res 1999; 369: 312–326.
17. Calandriello B, Grassi G. Idiopathic osteonecrosis of the femoral head. Epidemiological and aetiological factors. Ital J Orthop Trauma 1982; 8(suppl): 9–18.
18. Mont MA, Hungerford DS. Current concepts review : nontraumatic avascular necrosis of the femoral head. J Bone Joint Surg 1995; 77A: 459–474.
19. Nobillot R, Le Parc JM, Benoit J et al. Idiopathic osteonecrosis of the hip in twins. Ann Rheum Dis 1994; 53: 702.
20. Mazières B, Arlet J, Boussaton M et al. Assessment of intramedullary pressure versus bone scintigraphy in the diagnosis of osteonecrosis of femoral head. In: Arlet J, Mazières B, eds. Bone circulation and bone necroses. Berlin: Springer-Verlag; 1990: 264–266.
21. Masuda T. Computed tomography and bone scintigraphy in avascular necrosis of the femoral head. Monthly Book Orthop 1988; 8: 4–50.
22. Dihlmann W. CT analysis of the upper end of the femur: the asterisk sign and ischæmic bone necrosis of the femoral head. Skeletal Radiol 1982; 8: 251–228.
23. Fujioka M, Kubo T, Nakamura F et al. Initial changes of non-traumatic osteonecrosis of the femoral head in fat suppression images: bone marrow edema was not found before the appearance of band patterns. Magn Reson Imaging 2001; 19: 985–991.
24. Khanna AJ, Yoon TR, Mont MA et al. Femoral head osteonecrosis : detection and grading by using a rapid MR imaging protocol. Radiology 2000; 217: 188–192.
25. Gires F, Leroy-Willig A, Chevrot A et al. L'ostéonécrose de la tête fémorale. Etude par IRM de 60 cas. J Radiol (Paris) 1987; 68: 503–510.
26. Mitchell DG, Rao VM, Dalinka MD et al. Femoral head avascular osteonecrosis: correlation of MR imaging, radiographic staging, radionuclide imaging and clinical findings. Radiology 1987; 162: 709–715.
27. Sarrat P, Aquaviva PC, Lafforgue P et al. Ostéonécrose aseptique de la tête fémorale. Apports de l'imagerie par résonance magnétique (IRM). Ann Radiol (Paris) 1988; 31: 133–139.
28. Nadel SN, Debatin JF, Richardson WJ et al. Detection of acute avascular necrosis of the femoral head in dogs: dynamic contrast-enhanced MR imaging vs spin-echo and STIR sequences. AJR 1992; 159: 1255–1261.
29. Mitchell DG, Rao VM, Dalinka MD et al. MRI of joint fluid in the normal and ischemic hip. AJR 1986; 146: 1215–1218.
30. Mazières B, Mignonat H, Rousseau H et al. Femoral head osteonecrosis: MR imaging and correlations with scintigraphy, CT scan, and bone marrow pressure (abstract A48). Arthritis Rheum 1989; 32(suppl 2): 20.
31. Coleman BG, Kressel HY, Dalinka MD et al. Radiographically negative avascular necrosis: detection with MR imaging. Radiology 1988; 168: 525–528.
32. Robinson HJ, Hartleben PD, Lund G et al. Evaluation of magnetic resonance imaging in the diagnosis of osteonecrosis of the femoral head. Accuracy compared with radiographs, core biopsy and intraosseous pressure measurements. J Bone Joint Surg 1989; 71A: 650–663.
33. Stulberg BN, Levine M, Bauer TW et al. Multimodular approach to osteonecrosis of the femoral head. Clin Orthop Rel Res 1989; 240: 181–193.
34. Beltran J, Herman LJ, Burk JM et al. Femoral head avascular necrosis: MR imaging with clinical–pathologic and radionuclide correlation. Radiology 1988; 166: 215–220.
35. Ohzono K, Saito M, Takaoka K. Natural history of nontraumatic avascular necrosis of the femoral head. J Bone Joint Surg, 1991; 73-B: 68–75.

36. Koo KH, Kim R, Cho SH *et al*. Angiography, scintigraphy, intraosseous pressure and histologic findings in high-risk osteonecrotic femoral heads with negative magnetic resonance images. Clin Orthop 1994; 308: 127–138.

37. Jones JP Jr. Osteonecrosis. In: McCarty DJ, ed. Arthritis and allied conditions. Philadelphia, PA: Lea & Febiger; 1989: 1545–1562.

38. Steinberg ME, Hayken GD, Steinberg DR. A quantitative system for staging avascular necrosis. J Bone Joint Surg 1995; 77B: 34–41.

39. Guerra JJ, Steinberg ME. Distinguishing transient osteoporosis from avascular necrosis of the hip. J Bone Joint Surg 1995; 77A: 616–624.

40. Sugano N, Kubo T, Takaoka K *et al*. Diagnostic criteria for non-traumatic osteonecrosis of the femoral head. A multicentre study. J Bone Joint Surg 1999; 81B: 590–595.

41. Mont MA, Jones LC, Einhorn TA *et al*. Osteonecrosis of the femoral head. Potential treatment with growth and differentiation factors. Clin Orthop 1998; 355S: S314–S335.

42. Mazières B, Marin F, Chiron P *et al*. Influence of the volume of osteonecrosis on the outcome of core decompression of the femoral head. Ann Rheum Dis 1997; 56: 747–750.

43. Ohzono K, Saito M, Sugano N *et al*. The fate of nontraumatic avascular necrosis of the femoral head. A radiologic classification to formulate prognosis. Clin Orthop 1992; 277: 73–78.

44. Sakamoto M, Shimizu K, Iida S *et al*. Osteonecrosis of the femoral head. A prospective study with MRI. J Bone Joint Surg 1997; 79B: 213–219.

45. Halland AM, Klemp P, Botes D *et al*. Avascular necrosis of the hip in systemic lupus erythematosus : the role of magnetic resonance imaging. Br J Rheumatol 1993; 32: 972–976.

46. Siddiqui AR, Kopecky KK, Wellman HN *et al*. Prospective study of magnetic resonance imaging and SPECT bone scans in renal allograft recipients: evidence for a self-limited subclinical abnormality of the hip. J Nucl Med 1993; 34: 381–386.

47. Kokubo T, Takatori Y, Ninomiya S *et al*. Magnetic resonance imaging and scintigraphy of avascular necrosis of the femoral head. Clin Orthop 1992; 277: 54–60.

48. Hauzeur JP, Sintzoff SA Jr, de Maertelaer V *et al*. Relationship between magnetic resonance imaging and histologic findings by bone biopsy in non traumatic osteonecrosis of the femoral head. J Rheumatol 1992; 19: 385–392.

49. Yamamoto T, DiCarlo EF, Bullough PG. The prevalence and clinicopathological appearance of extension of osteonecrosis in the femoral head. J Bone Joint Surg 1999; 81-B: 328–332.

50. Hauzeur JP, Pasteels JL. Pathology of bone marrow distant from the sequestrum in non traumatic aseptic necrosis of the femoral head. In: Arlet J, Mazières B, eds. Bone circulation and bone necrosis. Berlin: Springer-Verlag; 1989: 73–76.

51. Rutishauser E, Taillard W. L'ischémie articulaire en pathologie humaine et expérimentale. Rev Chir Orthop 1966; 52: 197–202.

52. Kenzora JC, Steele RE, Yosipovitch ZH, Glimcher MJ. Experimental osteonecrosis of the femoral head in adult rabbits. Clin Orthop Rel Res 1978; 130: 8–46.

53. Arlet J, Durroux R. Diagnostic histologique précoce de l'ostéonécrose aseptique de la tête fémorale par le forage-biopsie. In: Ficat P, Arlet J. Compte rendu du 1° symposium international sur la circulation osseuse. Paris: Editions INSERM; 1973: 293–302.

54. Solomon L. Bone marrow oedema syndrome. J Bone Joint Surg 1993; 75B: 175–176.

55. Bauer TW, Stulberg BN. The histology of osteonecrosis and its distinction from histologic artefacts. In: Schoutens A, Arlet J, Gardeniers JWN, Hughes SPF, eds. Bone circulation and vascularization in normal and pathological conditions. New York: Plenum Press; 1993: 283–292.

56. Vandeberg BC, Malghem J, Goffin EJ *et al*. Transient epiphyseal lesions in renal transient recipients: presumed insufficiency stress fractures. Radiology 1994; 191: 403–407.

57. Hirata T, Konishiike T, Kawai A *et al*. Dynamic magnetic resonance imaging of femoral head perfusion in femoral neck fracture. Clin Orthop 2001; 393: 294–301.

58. Rodriguez-Merchan EC. Osteonecrosis of the femoral head after traumatic hip dislocation in the adult. Clin Orthop 2000; 377: 68–77.

59. Zabinski SJ, Sculco TP, Dicarlo EF *et al*. Osteonecrosis in the rheumatoid femoral head J Rheumatol 1998; 25: 1674–1680.

60. Kubo T, Kojima A, Yamazoe S *et al*. Osteonecrosis of the femoral head that developed after long-term topical steroid application. J Orthop Sci 2001; 6: 92–94.

61. Moskal JT, Topping RE, Franklin LL. Hypercholesterolemia: an association with osteonecrosis of the femoral head. Am J Orthop 1997; 26: 609–612.

62. Scribner AN, Troia-Cancio PV, Cox BA *et al*. Osteonecrosis in HIV: a case-control study. J AIDS 2000; 25: 19–25.

63. Glesby MJ, Hoover DR, Vaamonde CM. Osteonecrosis in patients infected with human immunodeficiency virus: a case-control study. J Infect Dis 2001; 184: 519–253.

64. Montella BJ, Nunley JA, Urbaniak JR. Osteonecrosis of the femoral head associated with pregnancy. A preliminary report. J Bone Joint Surg 1999; 81A: 790–798.

65. Sotereanos DG, Plakseychuk AY, Rubash HE. Free vascularized fibula grafting for the treatment of osteonecrosis of the femoral head. Clin Orthop 1997; 344: 243–256.

66. Frost HM. The etiodynamics of aseptic necrosis associated with hypercorticism. Mayo Clin Proc 1969; 44: 255–258.

67. Laurent J, Meunier P, Courpron P *et al*. Recherches sur la pathogénie des nécroses aseptiques de la hanche. Nouv Presse Méd 1973; 2: 1755–1757.

68. Hungerford DS, Zizic TM. Pathogenesis of ischemic necrosis of the femoral head. In: Hungerford DS, ed. The hip. Proceedings of the Eleventh Open Scientific Meeting of the Hip Society. St Louis:, MO CV Mosby; 1983: 249–56.

69. Atsumi T, Kuroki Y, Yamamo K. A microangiographic study of idiopathic osteonecrosis of the femoral head. Clin Orthop Rel Res 1989; 246: 186–194.

70. Cheras PA, Freemont AJ, Sikorski JM. Intraosseous thrombosis in ischemic necrosis of bone and osteoarthritis. Osteoarthritis Cartilage 1993; 1: 219–232.

71. Arlet J, Pradère J, Tabarly A *et al*. La viscosité sanguine dans les ostéonécroses de la tête fémorale. Rev Rheum Mal Ostéoarticul 1986; 53: 595–599.

72. Bluemke DA, Petri M, Zerhouni EA. Femoral head perfusion and composition: MR imaging and spectroscopic evaluation of patients with systemic lupus erythematosus and at risk for avascular necrosis. Radiology 1995; 197: 433–438.

73. Dromer C, Marc V, Laroche M *et al*. No link between avascular necrosis of the femoral head and antiphospholipid antibodies. Rev Rhum (Engl Ed) 1997; 64 : 382–385.

74. Wang GJ, Sweet DE, Reger SI *et al*. Fat-cell changes as a mechanism of avascular necrosis of the femoral head in cortisone treated rabbits. J Bone Joint Surg 1977; 59A: 729–735.

75. Pritchett JW. Statin therapy decreases the risk of osteonecrosis in patients receiving steroids. Clin Orthop 2001; 386: 173–178.

76. Arlet J, Mazières B, Thiéchart M *et al*. The effect of IV injection of naftidrofuryl (praxilène) on intramedullary pressure in patients with osteonecrosis of the femoral head. In: Arlet J, Mazières B, eds. Bone circulation and bone necrosis. Berlin: Springer-Verlag; 1990: 405–406.

77. Aaron RK, Lennox DW, Bunce GE *et al*. The conservative treatment of osteonecrosis of the femoral head: a comparison of core decompression and pulsing electromagnetic fields. Clin Orthop 1989; 249: 209–218.

78. Ficat RP. Idiopathic bone necrosis of the femoral head. J Bone Joint Surg 1985; 67B: 3–9.

79. Stulberg BN, Bauer TW, Belhobek GH. Making core decompression work. Clin Orthop 1990; 261: 186–195.

80. Mazières B, Chiron P, Aziza R *et al*. Bone morphogenetic protein (BMP) used in core decompression surgical technique of the hip in pig model. Pathological findings (abstract #32). Rev Rhum Mal Ostéo-Articul 1994; 61: 590.

81. Hernigou P. Autologous bone marrow grafting of avascular osteonecrosis before collapse (abstract no. 44). Rev Rhum Mal Ostéo-Articul (Engl Ed) 1995; 62: 650.

82. Urbaniak JR, Coogan PG, Gunneson EB *et al*. Treatment of osteonecrosis of the femoral head with free vascularized fibular grafting: a long-term follow-up of one hundred and three hips. J Bone Joint Surg 1995; 77A: 681–694.

83. Pavlovcic V, Dolinar D, Arnez Z. Femoral head necrosis treated with vascularized iliac crest graft. Int Orthop (SICOT) 1999; 23: 150–153.

84. Noguchi M, Kawakami T, Yamamoto H. Use of vascularized pedicle iliac bone graft in the treatment of avascular necrosis of the femoral head. Arch Orthop Trauma Surg 2001; 121: 437–442.

85. Sugioka Y, Katsuki I, Hotokebuchi T. Transtrochanteric rotational osteotomy of the femoral head for the treatment of osteonecrosis. Follow-up statistics. Clin Orthop Rel Res 1982; 169: 115–126.

86. Matsuda T, Matsuno T, Hasegawa I *et al*. Results of transtrochanteric rotational osteotomy for nontraumatic osteonecrosis of the femoral head. Clin Orthop 1988; 228 : 69–74.

87. Scher MA, Jakim I. Intertrochanteric osteotomy and autogenous bone-grafting for avascular necrosis of the femoral head. J Bone Joint Surg 1993; 75A: 1119–1133.

88. Barbos P, Balbo C, Rossi P. Middle and long-term results of flexion osteotomy for avascular necrosis of the femoral head. J Orthop Traumatol 1992; 18: 53–61.

89. Miyanishi K, Noguchi Y, Yamamoto T *et al*. Prediction of the outcome of transtrochanteric rotational osteotomy for osteonecrosis of the femoral head. J Bone Joint Surg 2000; 82B: 512–516.

90. Dinulescu I, Stanculescu D, Nicolescu M *et al*. Long-term follow-up after intertrochanteric osteotomies for avascular necrosis of the femoral head. Bull Hosp Joint Dis 1998; 57: 84–87.

91. Ortiguera CJ, Pulliam IT, Cabanela ME. Total hip arthroplasty for osteonecrosis : matched-pair analysis of 188 hips with long-term follow-up. J Arthroplasty 1999; 14 : 21–28.

92. Brinker MR, Rosenberg AG, Kull L *et al*. Primary total hip arthroplasty using noncemented porous-coated femoral components in patients with osteonecrosis of the femoral head. J Arthroplasty 1994; 9: 457–468.

93. Moran MC. Osteonecrosis of the hip in sickle cell hemoglobinopathy. Am J Orthop 1995; 24: 18–24.

94. Hernigou P, Bachir D, Galacteros F. Avascular necrosis of the femoral head in sickle-cell disease. Treatment of collapse by the injection of acrylic cement. J Bone Joint Surg 1993; 75B: 875–880.

95. Turner DA, Templeton AC, Selzer PM *et al*. Femoral capital osteonecrosis: MR finding of diffuse marrow abnormalities without focal lesions. Radiology 1989; 171: 135–140.

CRYSTAL-RELATED ARTHROPATHIES

175 History, classification and epidemiology of crystal-related arthropathies

Gyula Poór and Mila Mituszova

- The crystal-related arthropathies represent a heterogenous group of disorders in which minerals are deposited in musculoskeletal tissue, resulting in further pathologic alterations. Intra-articular crystals may be inert but can cause acute and chronic inflammation and joint damage via biomechanical as well as biochemical pathways.

- Synovial fluids can contain a number of crystals and other particulate substances. Some of these, particularly monosodium urate monohydrate (MSUM), calcium pyrophosphate dihydrate (CPPD) and basic calcium phosphates (BCP), such as hydroxyapatite (HA), are pathogenic; others including cholesterol and various other particles are of doubtful significance[1]. Table 175.1 lists the main forms of particulate substances that have been identified in synovial fluids.

- The most common crystal-related arthropathies are gout, calcium pyrophosphate dihydrate disease or 'pseudogout', and calcific periarthritis/tendinitis. In terms of its prevalence and clinical significance gout is considered the most important condition among crystal-related arthropathies.

GOUT

Definition

Gout is a clinical syndrome caused by an inflammatory response to MSUM crystals formed in humans with elevated serum urate concentration (hyperuricemia).

Acute and chronic forms of gout are known. The acute form usually appears as relapsing, self-limiting severe inflammatory arthritis. In the chronic form, aggregates of MSUM crystals (tophi) are deposited chiefly in and around joints which sometimes lead to bone and joint destruction. Gout is commonly associated with obesity, heavy alcohol intake, hypertension, renal impairment involving glomerular, tubular, and interstitial tissues and blood vessels, and diuretic use. Hyperuricemia alone, even when complicated by uric acid urolithiasis, should not be called gout.

History

The description of gout dates back to the time of Babylon. Evidence of the disease has been found in several early skeletal remains. However, the best early description can be found in the works of Hippocrates. The familial nature of gout was mentioned by Seneca in the 1st century AD, while Galen described the tophi (3rd century AD).

TABLE 175.1 INTRINSIC AND EXTRINSIC CRYSTALS AND PARTICLES DETECTED IN SYNOVIAL FLUID

Extrinsic crystals or particles (introduced from outside)		Intrinsic crystals or particles (formed within the joint)	
Pathogenic	Nonpathogenic	Pathogenic	Nonpathogenic
Corticosteroid can cause short lived inflammatory episode	From air-dust, fungal spores, (lens) tissue fibres, etc.; many are birefringent	MSUM – vely birefrigent needles 1–20 μm. Can form in 'beachball' array	Fibrin. Hair-like strands under HP 1000×. Found in many SF
	Storage artefacts – Brushite, +vely birefringent rods 10 μm+ in 'star-bursts'	CPPD + vely birefringent rods/ rhomboids. 1–20 μm. Can form 'beachballs'	Non-birefringent 1–20 μm 'broken glass' cartilage in all SF
			Larger (100 μm+) birefringent 'silk-sheen' cartilage in damaged/arthritic joints
	'Drying-out' SF gives spectacular birefringent particles resembling MSUM, CPPD, etc.	BCP – submicroscopic, very weakly birefringent. Aggregates 2–80 μm visible if stained.	Meniscal fragments = silksheen + fibrillar appearance.
	Ovoid starch granules from gloves, 10–100 μm+ birefringent weak 'Maltese cross'	NB Mixed crystal populations are common	Fragments many contain CPPD/MSUM Fragments of fibrillar cruciate ligament – joint injury
	Corticosteroids (all strongly birefringent crystals 1–40 μm)	CPPD + BCP (often)	Fragments of synovium – villi + birefringent fibrous core
	Lederspan (1–10 μm) resembles CPPD	MSUM + CPPD	Rice bodies – aggregates of synovial tissue in RA SF
		MSUM + cholesterol, etc.	Lipid crystals, 1–30 μm ovoids. Birefringent. Bright 'Maltese cross'
			Cholesterol 5–40 μm + vely birefringent notched plates. Lipid globules – non-birefringent (resemble air bubbles)

SF, synovial fluid; MSUM, monosodium urate monohydrate; CPPD, calcium pyrophosphate dihydrate; RA, rheumatoid arthritis.

The term gout, derived from the Latin *gutta* (drop), was introduced in the 13th century AD, and points to the belief that a poison falling drop by drop into the joint causes the disease. Van Leeuwenhoek (1679) was the first who identified crystals microscopically in a tophus (without knowing anything about their chemical composition). Important milestones in the history of gout were (1) the description of the classic symptoms of acute attack (Sydenham, 1683); (2) the discovery of uric acid by Scheele (1776); (3) the demonstration of uric acid in tophi by Wollaston (1797); and (4) the 'thread' test of Garrod (1859) showing that the amount of uric acid is increased in the blood of gouty patients. This called attention to the association between gout and elevated serum levels of urate. The first radiologic description of gout was reported by Huber (1896). In understanding the pathomechanism of gout, the demonstration that uric acid is a urine compound was also an important step (Fischer, 1898).

Concerning the modern history of gout it is worth mentioning the observations of His and Freudweiler (1899) showing that injected synthetic MSUM crystals induce inflammatory responses in man. From the clinical point of view, the measurement of serum urate concentration (Folin and Denis, 1913), the efficacious use of colchicine in the treatment of gout (1936), and the demonstration of uricosuric effect of probenecid (Talbot, Gutman and Yu, 1950) are also important. The constant presence of MSUM crystals in gouty joint fluid was first reported by McCarty and Hollander (1961) rediscovering their pathogenetic role. The detection of allopurinol as a clinically applicable xanthine oxidase inhibitor by Hitchings and Elion (1963) is also an important landmark in the modern history of gout.

Finally it has to be mentioned that the description of hypoxanthine-guanine phosphoribosyltransferase (HGPRT) deficiency in gouty patients (Seegmiller, Rosenbloom and Kelley, 1967) as well as the finding that phosphorybosil pyrophosphate (PRPP) synthetase overactivity can be the cause of urate overproduction (Sperling *et al.*, 1972) were extremely helpful to clarify the biochemical background of uric acid disturbance. We have also to emphasize that Schumacher (1979) demonstrated urate crystals in some uninvolved joints of patients with gout.

Diagnostic and classification criteria for gout

The key diagnostic features, reflected in the classification criteria, are recurrent attacks of acute monoarthritis of the first metatarsophalangeal or tarsal joints with maximal inflammation, producing redness over the involved joint, developing within one day, and the presence of tophus.

TABLE 175.2 ROME AND NEW YORK CRITERIA FOR DIAGNOSIS OF GOUT

Rome criteria for diagnosis of gout

- Serum urate concentration ≥7mg/100ml in males, ≥6mg/100ml in females
- Painful joint swelling, with abrupt onset, clearing in 1–2 weeks initially
- Presence of urate crystals in synovial fluid
- Presence of a tophus

New York criteria for diagnosis of gout

- Chemical or microscopic demonstration of urate crystals in the synovial fluid or in the tissues; or
- Presence of two or more of the following criteria
- Two attacks of painful limb joint swelling with abrupt onset, remitting in 1–2 weeks initially
- A single such attack involving the great toe
- Response to colchicine, with major decrease in inflammation in 48 hours.
- Presence of a tophus

Several diagnostic criteria for gout have been proposed (Table 175.2). In 1963, the Council for International Organizations of Medical Sciences (CIOMS), under the joint auspices of UNESCO and WHO, set forth requirements that two or more of the Rome criteria be met to establish the diagnosis[2]. In 1968 the CIOMS, with support from the National Institute of Arthritis and Metabolic Diseases and the American Rheumatism Association, proposed the New York diagnostic criteria[3]. Neither set of criteria proved satisfactory. For example, in a population study of gout sufferers, the author found eight subjects who satisfied the Rome criteria only, four who satisfied the New York criteria only, and ten who satisfied both[4]. An advantage of the Rome criteria was the epidemiologic definition of hyperuricemia, however better established parameters were necessary for clinical and research purposes. The New York criteria emphasized the demonstration of synovial urate crystals as an absolute criterion; however, they lacked the radiological abnormalities and the hyperuricemia.

In 1975 the American Rheumatism Association subcommittee on classification criteria for the acute arthritis of gout analysed data from more than 700 patients with gout, pseudogout, rheumatoid arthritis, or septic arthritis[5]. Fifty-three variables were evaluated statistically; of

---

TABLE 175.3 ARA CRITERIA FOR ACUTE ARTHRITIS OF PRIMARY GOUT

Clinical setting	Survey setting
1. More than one attack of acute arthritis	1. More than one attack of acute arthritis
2. Maximum inflammation developed within 1 day	2. Maximum inflammation developed within 1 day
3. Monoarthritis attack	3. Oligoarthritis attack
4. Redness observed over joints	4. Redness observed over joints
5. First MTP joint painful or swollen	5. First MTP joint painful or swollen
6. Unilateral first MTP joint attack	6. Unilateral first MTP joint attack
7. Unilateral tarsal joint attack	7. Unilateral tarsal joint attack
8. Tophus (proven or suspected)	8. Tophus (proven or suspected)
9. Hyperuricemia	9. Hyperuricemia
10. Asymmetric swelling within a joint on X-ray*	10. Asymmetric swelling within a joint on X-ray*
11. Subcortical cysts without erosions on X-ray	11. Complete termination of an attack
12. Monosodium urate monohydrate microcrystals in joint fluid during attack	
13. Joint fluid culture negative for organisms during attack	

*This criterion could logically be found on examination as well as on X-ray. However, the protocol did not request this information in regard to examination.
MTP, metatarsophalangeal.

the 30 which significantly discriminated primary gout from the other diseases, 13 were selected that could be used on a patient's first visit (Table 175.3). The preliminary criteria performed best when the following diagnostic rules were used:

- the presence of characteristic urate crystals in the joint fluid (item 12 in Table 175.3)
- a tophus proved to contain urate crystals by chemical or polarized light microscopic means (item 8 in Table 175.3)
- the presence of six out of 12 clinical, laboratory and radiographic features (excluding items 12 and 8 in Table 175.3).

The combined criteria were both sensitive (98%) and specific (98%) compared with rheumatoid arthritis of greater than 2 years' duration and 89% compared with pseudogout and septic arthritis. Presence of urate crystals in synovial leukocytes or a proven tophus establish the diagnosis irrespective of the other positive findings. This set of criteria was modified for epidemiologic purposes since synovial fluid is rarely obtained in population studies. Information ascertained by removing criteria 12 and 13 had a sensitivity for gout of 85% and a specificity of at least 93% in differentiating gout from other rheumatic diseases (Table 175.3).

There are no agreed criteria for assessing disease severity or measuring outcome in gout. All clinical trials use their own guidelines.

Reliability of synovial fluid examination

There are a large number of techniques that can be used to identify crystals that can be found in synovial fluid, nearly all of which rely on microscopy of one sort or another because of the small size of the individual particles. They range from the very simple, like Garrod's famous 'string test' to the furiously complex, such as laser microscopy or atomic force microscopy. In clinical practice we need a relatively simple, affordable technique with a reasonable degree of sensitivity and specificity. Polarized light microscopy remains the only possibility that comes anywhere near fulfilling these needs: it is available in most hospitals and is relatively inexpensive.

Unfortunately, in practice, three problems interfere with the usefulness of synovial fluid examination. First, obtaining fluid can be difficult. The high reported success rates (>90%) of aspiration from the first metatarsophalangeal joint are not matched in general practice. Second, tiny amounts of synovial fluid are sufficient for crystal identification but one needs to be able to examine the fluid promptly. Delay or discarding the needle used for aspiration (to minimize risk of needlestick) can lead to failure despite a potentially diagnostic aspirate. Third, synovial fluid examination for crystals is not highly reliable in clinical practice. Errors in the identification of urate crystals are not uncommon, and the error rate is even higher for CPPD crystals[1].

Classification criteria for hyperuricemia and gout

The biochemical hallmark and prerequisite of gout is hyperuricemia. The concentration of uric acid in body fluids is determined by the balance between rates of production and elimination of urate. Within the disease cluster of gout, subsets may be identified using classification criteria. Hyperuricemia and gout may be classified as primary or secondary (Table 175.4). Primary hyperuricemia or gout refers to those cases that are neither secondary to another acquired disorder nor a subordinate manifestation of an inborn error that leads to a major disease other than gout. Although some cases of primary gout will have a genetic basis, others do not. Secondary hyperuricemia or gout includes those cases that develop in the course of another disease or as a consequence of drug treatment. The designation 'idiopathic' gout is used when a more precise classification cannot be assigned. Further subdivisions within each major category are based on the identification of

TABLE 175.4 CLASSIFICATION OF HYPERURICEMIA AND GOUT

Type	Inheritance
Primary	
Overproduction (10% of primary gout)	Polygenic
Specific enzyme mutations	
Increased activity of PP-ribose-P synthetase	X-linked
Partial deficiency of hypoxanthine-guanine phosphoribosyltransferase	X-linked
Underexcretion (90% of primary gout)	Polygenic?
Mutations in enzymes involved in renal handling of urate causing inhibited tubular secretion or increased distal reabsorption	
Secondary	
Overproduction	
Specific enzyme mutations	X-linked
Virtually complete deficiency of hypoxanthine-guanine phosphoribosyltransferase (Lesch-Nyhan syndrome)	
Increased nucleic acid turnover or ATP degradation	Most not familial
Lympho- and myeloproliferative disorders, tumors	
High purine, fructose or alcohol intake	
Heavy exercise	
Obesity and hypertriglyceridemia	
Underexcretion	
Severe renal diseases inhibiting glomerular filtration or tubular secretion of urate	Most not familial
Drugs (eg. thiazide diuretics, low-dose salicylate, cyclosporin, PZA) and alcohol intake	
Metabolites (lactate, ketones, etc.)	
Hypertension	
Overproduction plus underexcretion	
Glucose-6-phosphatase deficiency or absence (glycogen storage disease, von Gierke)	Autosomal recessive
Fructose-1-phosphate aldolase deficiency (juvenile familial nephropathy)	Autosomal recessive

overproduction or underexcretion of uric acid as responsible for the hyperuricemia.

A proportion of primary gouty patients, probably no more than 10%, will have overproduction of uric acid and, in a minority of these, abnormal purine enzyme activity can be identified. The enzyme abnormalities associated with uric acid overproduction are: hypoxanthine-guanine phosphoribosyl transferase (HGPRT) deficiency, phosphoribosyl-pyrophospate (PRPP) synthetase overactivity, glucose-6-phosphatase deficiency, and fructose-1-phosphate aldolase deficiency[6–10]. The first of these are rare, but heterozygosity for fructose-1-phosphate aldolase deficiency has a prevalence of at least 1 in 250, of whom one-third may develop gout; hence, this enzyme abnormality may be a relatively common cause of familial gout. If an enzyme defect is suspected and high 24h urinary urate excretion is confirmed, then specific enzyme assays can be performed on erythrocytes or lymphocytes.

In the majority (up to 90%) of patients with primary gout uric acid excretion by the kidneys is decreased compared with that in healthy persons with comparable serum urate levels .

Epidemiology of hyperuricemia and gout
Hyperuricemia

The biochemical hallmark of gout is not apparent at the time of the acute attack in all patients with gout but it is manifested in about 98% of individuals with gout. Hyperuricemia may be defined either in statistical terms from epidemiological studies of normal and gouty populations or from the physicochemical properties of urate.

Epidemiological surveys have resulted in an arbitrary definition of hyperuricemia as a serum urate level greater than 7.0mg/dl for males and 6.0mg/dl for females. However, it should be realized that this definition of hyperuricemia results in considerable overlap between the normal and gouty populations. This is due in part to the nonGaussian distribution of serum urate values in the normal population with a skewing toward the higher values. In addition, the normal range of values is dependent upon the population under study, since the serum urate has been reported to vary with age, sex, environmental, ethnic and anthropomorphic differences.

Hyperuricemia has been described in 2.3–17.6% of the populations studied. In adults, serum urate levels correlate strongly with serum creatinine and urea nitrogen levels, body weight, height, blood pressure and alcohol intake. Serum urate values show positive correlation with weight and with body surface area in people of widely differing races and cultures[11–14].

The urate level of adult ethnic males in Oceania is higher than in most other populations studied. All three ethnic groups in Malaysia, Malays, Tamil and Chinese show higher mean urate levels compared with most Caucasian populations, whereas black Africans, Japanese and American Indians have generally lower values than Caucasian populations. Acculturation has led to higher urate levels in Filipinos and Malayo–Mongoloids, Tokelauans and Polynesians and Chinese[15].

Gout

For more than a century, elevated serum urate levels have been known to be a risk factor for gout. The precise magnitude of that risk remains unclear. Only a few epidemiological studies have attempted to quantify the risk of gouty arthritis in relation to prior urate levels. The Sudbury study found occurrence of acute gout confined to those whose serum urate levels were above the 90th percentile[16]. The most widely cited study is the one from Framingham, describing cumulative incidence of acute gout over 12 years of 36% for those with urate level of 8mg/dl or more. A widely quoted figure from that study was the 90% frequency of gout in males with a urate concentration of more than 9mg/dl; however, this was based on only 10 subjects at risk[12]. The survey of Campion et al. presents the results of a prospective, longitudinal study over 15 years of asymptomatic hyperuricemia with 30.15 human years of follow up. It found the incidence of gout to be remarkably low[17]. For men with a serum urate level of 9mg/dl or more, the incidence rate of new gouty arthritis is 4.9%/year. The cumulative incidence of gout in these hyperuricemic men is 22% after 5 years. The two studies can be reconciled quite well once incidence and prevalence are clearly distinguished and once temporal trends in serum urate levels are considered.

In 1992 the prevalence of gout was estimated in the USA by using self-reported data as opposed to rates derived from physician evaluations. Overall prevalence in respondents of all ages, both sexes and all races combined was 8.4 cases per 1000 persons. This corresponds to an estimated 2.1 million persons with gout: 1.56 million men and 550 000 women. Prevalence was higher at all ages in men than in women and higher in blacks aged 45 and older than in whites in the same age group[18,19].

The determination of the precise incidence rate of gout is not easy because of the remitting and relapsing nature of the disease and the frequent misdiagnosis. One has to consider that due to alterations in lifestyle, drugs, weather conditions and seasonal changes, and increasing span of life the epidemiology of gout (e.g. the ratio of males to females) is changing. The ratio of males to females (which was formerly 20:1) is now 2–7:1, the prevalence rate (/1000) in males 5–28, and 1–6 in females. The annual incidence shows also a characteristic sex difference: 1–3/1000 in males and 0.2 in females. Concerning the geographical distribution of the disease, the regional differences may mirror genetic disorders (inherited enzyme abnormalities, inherited urate underexcretion), environmental factors (such as diet, drugs, toxins), moreover racial inclination[20–22].

Racial differences in the incidence of gout were found in two cohorts of male medical students followed up by Hochberg et al.[23]. Over a mean period of 28 years, the cumulative incidence of gout was 10.9% in blacks and 5.8% in whites. Systolic blood pressure in the black cohort was the only baseline characteristic predictive of the development of gout. The development of hypertension during the period of observation was an independent risk factor for the development of gout in both cohorts. Thiazide diuretic use could have been a major factor in the association of hypertension and gout.

Gout has generally been considered to be rare in African blacks. However, Cassim et al. reported on a series of 107 patients with gout seen in an urban South African hospital over a 5-year period[24]. This report was the largest series of gout ever reported in black Africans and seems to reflect a trend of increased reporting of gout in this population. Although this increase may result from a greater awareness of the disease, the authors speculate that a high prevalence of hypertension and diuretic therapy may be important factors as well. An increased frequency of HLA-B14 (26 versus 6% in controls) was found in patients with primary gout[24]. Further studies will be needed to confirm the significance of this finding, because no association with HLA antigens was reported in any previous studies of gout[25].

There is no convincing evidence that the prevalence of gout is increasing overall, although a study from New Zealand suggested that this was the case in both Maori and European men[26].

Some cases with gout have been attributed to chronic lead intoxication especially as occupational exposure. Saturnine gout that accounts for less than 5% of all causes of gout is mostly resulted from damaged renal tubular or glomerular function caused by lead intoxication[27].

The problem of transplant hyperuricemia was explored by Marcen et al. In one of the several studies, Lin et al. found that 7% of patients treated with cyclosporine developed gout posttransplant and 80% were hyperuricemic[28]. Thus, improvement of immune modulation via cyclosporine has brought with it a minor epidemic of gouty arthritis.

CALCIUM PYROPHOSPHATE DIHYDRATE DEPOSITION DISEASE

Definition

The hallmark of calcium pyrophosphate dihydrate deposition disease is the formation of CPPD crystals in articular hyaline and fibro-cartilage. These crystals can produce an inflammatory arthritis known as *pseudogout,* and even more commonly are associated with severe, atypically distributed form of structural joint damage called *pyrophosphate arthropathy.* Chondrocalcinosis is a term reserved for pathologically or radiologically evident cartilage calcification.

History

Adams (1857) was the first who described that articular cartilage calcification is a common phenomenon occurring either alone or in association with arthritis. In 1903, Bennet reported the autopsy of patients with polyarticular chondrocalcinosis owing to crystalline chalk containing tiny rhomboidal crystals. Two types of meniscal calcification were differentiated in 1927 by Mandel. A primary type predominating in the aged, occurred without antecedent trauma and was frequently asymptomatic and bilateral. Microscopically, punctate deposits of granular calcific material of the involved cartilage were noted. A secondary type found in younger adults was symptomatic and unilateral, this type usually followed trauma to the joint. A well documented case reported by Werwath in 1928 contained the first roentgenogram showing the characteristic pattern of calcification; he correlated this pattern with the pathological findings at meniscectomy. In 1929, Tobler examined menisci from cadavers and found degenerative changes in 75% and calcification in 25% of menisci. Subsequently, studies by Bennett and colleagues (1941), as well as other investigators, described small deposits of granular material in semilunar cartilages showing interstitial matrix markedly altered by degenerative changes[29].

In 1958 Zitnan and Sitaj described the clinical and roentgenological features of what they called chondrocalcinosis articularis (familiaris). They presented 27 patients with chondrocalcinosis, 21 of whom were members of five different families of Hungarian origin, suggesting the hereditary nature of the disease[30]. In 1962 McCarty et al. identified previously unrecognized square rod-like, or rhomboid nonurate crystals. These crystals which could be distinguished from sodium urate crystals by their optical properties when examined with compensated polarized light microscopy, subsequently were identified as calcium pyrophosphate dihydrate by their X-ray diffraction powder pattern. Clinical similarity to gout promoted the term pseudogout for this new 'crystal-induced arthropathy'[31]. It was soon realized that chondrocalcinosis polyarticularis was also caused by CPPD. In 1970, Martel reported the first characteristic radiographic features in prospective study[32]. The clinical presentations of CPPD crystal deposition disease are highly variable and mimic of the common rheumatic syndromes. McCarty (1976) described clinical patterns of joint involvement[33].

The finding of metabolic disease associations and varying forms of familial predisposition further reinforced the analogy to urate crystals in gout and led to division into hereditary, disease-associated or sporadic/idiopathic forms of chondrocalcinosis. Genetic factors, which are becoming more commonly recognized in many diseases, are clearly important in some CPPD-associated diseases. Familial cases have now been reported from countries around the world. Two clinical forms of familial CPPD crystal deposition have been observed. A relatively benign, early-onset form is characterized by polyarticular distribution, recurrent episodes of crystal-positive acute pseudogout and chondrocalcinosis without chronic deforming arthropathy. The second form is a more destructive, late-onset oligoarthritis, with deforming progressive osteoarthritis. The inheritance pattern is consistent with autosomal dominant transmission. Early-onset osteoarthritis and chondrocalcinosis are linked to chromosome 8q[34]. A syndrome of chondrocalcinosis associated with recurrent childhood seizures is linked to chromosome 5p[35].

Identification of gene defects in families with inherited CPPD crystal deposition disease and understanding of the gene product will contribute to the understanding of molecular events involved in cartilage function[36].

Diagnostic and classification criteria

It was suggested that cases of CPPD crystal deposition disease be identified as possible, probable or definite, depending on the presence or absence of certain clinical, radiological or crystal criteria[37]. For example synovial fluid crystal identification or roentgenographic calcification of the cartilage alone represents a probable diagnosis (Table 175.5). The presence of both criteria is necessary for the diagnosis of definite disease. Chemical, electron or X-ray diffraction identification of crystals as CPPD alone represent a definite diagnosis. We have no information on either the specificity or the sensitivity of these criteria.

One should accept the diagnosis when the CPPD crystals are demonstrated in synovial fluid or articular tissues using compensated polarized light microscopy. Although radiologic patterns, especially chondrocalcinosis, are suggestive, they are not of themselves diagnostic.

Classification

CPPD deposition disease can be subclassified as hereditary, secondary, chiefly associated with metabolic disease, or sporadic according to the presence or absence of recognized predisposing factors. A tentative classification is given in Table 175.6.

TABLE 175.5 DIAGNOSTIC CRITERIA FOR CALCIUM PYROPHOSPHATE DEPOSITION DISEASE

Criteria

I. Definitive identification of CPPD crystals obtained by joint aspiration or biopsy by X-ray or electron diffraction, intrared spectroscopy or chemical analysis

IIa. Identification of monoclinic or triclinic crystals showing no birefringence or a weakly positive elongation by compensated polarized light microscopy

IIb. Presence of typical calcifications of fibrocartilage and hyalin cartilage on X-rays

IIIa. Acute arthritis attacks, especially knees, wrists

IIIb. Subacute or chronic arthritis, with or without acute episodes

Categories

A. Definite diagnosis: Criterion I, or IIa plus IIb

B. Probable diagnosis: Criterion IIa or IIb

C. Possible diagnosis: Criterion IIIa or IIIb in any combination

---

TABLE 175.6 CLASSIFICATION OF CALCIUM PYROPHOSPHATE DEPOSITION DISEASE

I. Hereditary

(e.g. Slovakian, Chilean, Dutch, Canadian, Spanish, French, Israeli, Japanese, Swedish, Mexican types)

II. Secondary

A. High probability
Primary hyperparathyroidism
Hemochromatosis
Familial hypocalciuric hypercalcemia
Hemosiderosis
Hypophosphatasia
Hypomagnesemia
Bartter syndrome
Gitelman syndrome
Gout
Neuropathic osteoarthropathy
Amyloidosis
Hypermobility syndrome
Long-term corticosteroid therapy
Aging

B. Modest probability
Osteoarthritis
Hypothyroidism
Nephrolithiasis
Diffuse idiopathic skeletal hyperostosis
Ochronosis
Wilson's disease
Hemophilia arthritis

C. Low probability
Diabetes mellitus
Paget's disease
Acromegaly
Hypertension
Azotemia
Inflammatory bowel disease
Rheumatoid arthritis

III. Sporadic (idiopathic)

According to the clinical manifestation and course three classifications were elaborated and proposed for clinical use. McCarty has classified CPPD deposition disease into six clinical patterns[33]. These are: pseudogout (type A), pseudorheumatoid arthritis (type B), pseudo-osteoarthritis, with acute attacks (type C), and without inflammation (type D), lanthanic or asymptomatic (type E) and pseudoneurotrophic (type F). Doherty and Dieppe (1986) classified only two groups of the disease, as acute CPPD induced synovitis (pseudogout) and chronic CPPD arthropathy[38]. Fallet (1989) distinguished acute mono- or oligoarthritis (pseudogout), relapsing inflammatory polyarthropathy, chronic arthralgia and destructive mono-, oligo- or polyarticular arthropathy[39]. During the course of the disease the knees are the most frequently involved joints.

Epidemiology

Intra-articular calcification is a common finding in older individuals and may occur as an asymptomatic, incidental finding, or may be associated with arthritis.

The largest epidemiological survey of the prevalence of articular chondrocalcinosis in the general population was carried out in the American population of Framingham[40]. In this study, radiological knee chondrocalcinosis was found in 8% of subjects in the age range 63–93 and ranging from 3% in those aged < 70, to 27% in those > 85 years. Data reported in this study are in good agreement with those of other authors in that articular chondrocalcinosis is an age-related disorder, and its occurrence increases dramatically with age. Analysing the prevalence in both sexes in each five year age group also described a higher frequency in women in each group but a similar prevalence of articular chondrocalcinosis in men and women aged over 80 years was noted[38,41,42].

Chondrocalcinosis is reported from several countries and different ethnic groups. The pattern of inheritance varies, though autosomal dominance is usual. Two clinical phenotypes have been emphasized, the first characterized by early-onset, florid, polyarticular chondrocalcinosis and the second by late-onset oligoarticular with arthritis resembling sporadic pyrophospate arthropathy. A familial study from Madrid, consisting of 21 kindreds with definite CPPD, that were collected from a systematic familial study of 'sporadic cases', revealed a familial aggregation of up to 38% for chondrocalcinosis, compared with 0% in 15 kindreds of patients with other rheumatic disease, which were used as controls. This was the first controlled study showing a prevalence of about 18 percent pyrophospate arthropathy in kindreds with CPPD compared with 0% observed in the some control group[43].

An association with a variety of endocrine and metabolic conditions is well accepted[44]. In most instances, the nature and significance of such associations cannot be assessed, and the combination of CPPD crystal deposition disease and another disorder merely may represent the chance occurrence of two diseases. The following diseases have been reported in association with CPPD crystal deposition disease (Table 175.6). The strongest evidence relates to hyperparathyroidism and hemochromatosis, in which the independent effect from aging has been demonstrated. Hemochromatosis is the one metabolic disease that causes structural arthropathy rather than just chondrocalcinosis and pseudogout attacks.

BASIC CALCIUM PHOSPHATE (HYDROXYAPATITE) CRYSTAL DEPOSITION DISEASE

The terms basic calcium phosphate and hydroxyapatite are used synonymously though apatite is not the only form of BCP. BCP describes a mixture of partially carbonate substituted HA, octacalcium phosphate, and sometimes tricalcium phosphate that is found in clinical specimens.

Definition

Deposition of HA and other related BCP crystals in and around the joints have very different clinical manifestations, ranging from asymptomatic *periarticular* deposits to acute calcific periarthritis, from acute *intra-articular* hydroxyapatite arthritis to apatite-associated destructive arthropathy, including 'Milwaukee shoulder–knee' syndrome.

History

The scapulohumeral form of calcific periarthritis was described in 1870 and radiographically first demonstrated in 1907. In addition to this form, three decades later, periarticular calcifications at other sites were also recognized. In 1966 McCarty and Gatter described that the calcific material consisted of hydroxyapatite[45]. In 1976 Dieppe *et al.* described aggregates of apatite in knee synovial fluids from patients with osteoarthritis and suggested that these may contribute to the inflammatory exacerbations[46]. In 1979 Fam and associates demonstrated HA crystals by scanning and transmission electronmicroscopy in synovial fluid in a variety of joint diseases[47]. Later, by using ultrastructural and physical microanalysis techniques the aggregates of apatite-like crystals as well as their various chemical compositions have been further defined[48,49].

In 1981 McCarty *et al.* drew attention to a new entity, when they reported a group of patients with 'Milwaukee shoulder–knee' syndrome and emphasized the presence of BCP crystals, particulate collagens, and proteolytic enzymes in joint effusions[50]. A variety of other terms have been used to describe the disorder 'apatite-associated destructive arthropathy' (AADA)[51] and 'idiopathic destructive arthropathies' (IDA)[52]. Historical or clinical findings in some patients with HA crystal deposition, such as familial occurrence, particular age range, polyarticular distribution, and increased prevalence of certain histocompatibility antigens suggest that a metabolic rather than a local degenerative process may be operative.

Diagnostic criteria and classification

BCP crystal deposition disease is diagnosed on the basis of roentgenography and synovial fluid analysis.

Specific identification of BCP crystals in synovial fluid by light microscopy is difficult, owing to their small size. Demonstration of the crystals and definite diagnosis of the disease requires the use of techniques including electron probe or transmission electronmicroscopy. The radiographic demonstration of periarticular calcifications is highly diagnostic, however, the radiography is generally both insensitive and nonspecific. Computed tomography or magnetic resonance imaging may be helpful in revealing small calcific deposits. Definitive identification of HA and other related BCP crystals[53] often requires the use of one or more specialized techniques (Table 175.7).

Due to the heterogenous nature of BCP crystal deposition disease, its classification is difficult. Our suggestion is summarized in Table 175.8.

Epidemiology

No comparable epidemiologic data have been reported subsequently, although a number of smaller pathologic or radiographic studies have

TABLE 175.7 SPECIALIZED TECHNIQUES USED IN THE DIAGNOSTICS OF BASIC CALCIUM PHOSPHATE CRYSTAL DEPOSITION DISEASE

Imaging	X-ray
	Computed tomography
	Magnetic resonance imaging
Crystal identification in synovial fluids and tissues	Polarized light microscopy
	Transmission electron microscopy
	Scanning electron microscopy
	Fourier transform infrared spectroscopy
	Alizarin red S calcium stain
	Raman microscopy
	Atomic force microscopy
	Energy-dispersive X-ray microbe elemental analysis

TABLE 175.8 SUGGESTED CLASSIFICATION OF BASIC CALCIUM PHOSPHATE CRYSTAL DEPOSITION DISEASE
I. Localization
A. Periarticular BCP crystal deposition
Asymptomatic periarticular deposits or acute calcific periarthritis (tendinitis, bursitis, enthesopathies)
B. Intra-articular BCP crystal deposition
Acute hydroxyapatite arthritis or apatite-associated destructive arthritis including Milwaukee shoulder–knee syndrome
II. Conditions associated with BCP crystal deposition
A. Hereditary
Familial bursitis, tendinitis, arthritis or destructive arthropathies reported from different countries (United States, England, France, Spain, Italy, Argentina, etc.)
Enthesopathy in X-linked hypophosphatemia
Epiphyseal dysplasia
Fibrodysplasia ossificans progressiva
B. Secondary
Chronic renal failure managed with long-term dialysis
Connective tissue disease (scleroderma, dermatomyositis, polymyositis, SLE)
Hypercalcemia due to primary hyperparathyroidism, hypervitaminosis D or sarcoidosis
Heterotrophic calcification associated to neurologic diseases (hemiplegia, paraplegia, coma, etc.)
Intra-articular corticosteroid injections
C. Sporadic (idiopathic)
Unifocal (including hydroxyapatite pseudopodagra) or multifocal depositions

documented the relatively high frequency of periarticular calcification. Asymptomatic periarticular calcification affects both sexes equally and is particularly common between the ages of 40–70 years. Prevalence of shoulder deposits occur in about 2.7–7.5% of adults. The shoulder is the most common site (60%); this is followed by the hip (15%), knee, elbow, wrist and ankle joints[54,55,56].

The prevalence of intra-articular apatite deposition has not been established. Intra-articular BCP crystals are detected in synovial effusions of 26–52.5% of OA joints[57] but the prevalence in normal joints at different ages is not known. The 'Milwaukee shoulder–knee' syndrome tends to occur in elderly patients and is of unknown prevalence.

Large, periarticular tumoral tophus-like deposits containing masses of HA and other BCP crystals are rare. This may occur as an idiopathic condition or in association with chronic renal failure, hyperparathyroidism, scleroderma, or systemic lupus erythematosus[53]. Uremic tumoral calcinosis occurs in about 1–7% of patients with end-stage renal disease undergoing chronic hemodialysis[58].

OTHER CRYSTALS

Other types of crystal depositions, such as oxalate, cholesterol, cryoglobulin and corticosteroid crystals, occur relatively frequently. Damage induced by such crystals may change the mechanical properties of tissues and sometimes initiate arthritis, while in other cases they may act as an 'amplification loop'. These crystals are found less often than MSUM, CPPD, and HA, but sometimes may be confused with them. The identification of such crystals in synovial fluid can be very important in the diagnosis of a systemic disease, e.g. in the case of cryoglobulinemia[59].

Oxalate crystals

Oxalate crystals in joint fluids were first reported in 1982 by Hoffman *et al.* in joints of patients in overt renal failure[60]. Oxalate deposition disease is a rare metabolic disorder that may be a result of familial enzymatic defects leading to increased oxalate production or end-stage renal disease requiring long-term dialysis. Acute and chronic arthritis resulting from oxalate deposition can occur in a variety of joints (knees, hands, ankles, feet, tendons and bursae) and often have been confused with MSUM, CPPD, and HA depositions. Oxalates may also involve intervertebral discs and contribute to disc destruction in dialysis patients. Oxalosis can cause vascular insufficiency with gangrene, cardiomegaly, heart block, milliary skin deposits, peripheral neuropathy and aplastic anemia. Synovial fluid aspiration and examination for crystals, or biopsy of joints, bones or other tissues are essential to definitive diagnosis[61].

Cholesterol crystals

In 1964, Zuckner and his colleagues described a number of cases of rheumatoid arthritis in whom synovial fluid cholesterol crystals were seen and positively identified by infrared spectrophotometry. Cholesterol crystals are occasionally detected in rheumatoid arthritis joints, pleural and pericardial fluid, bursal effusions, or tumoral calcinosis in patients with dermatomyositis, systemic lupus erythematosus, chronic tophaceous gout, osteoarthritis, and in a variety of other chronic effusions[59]. Their inflammatory capacity has not been established; the clinical presentations of the small number of inflammatory cells, and the lack of crystal phagocytosis from aspirates suggest a minor inflammatory role at most. The crystals may be an incidental finding in joint disease of little clinical significance.

An alternative viewpont has been put forward in 1981 by Fam *et al.* who suggested that cholesterol crystals are potent causes of fibrosis, capable of making an important contribution to synovial pathology[62]. Patients with subcutaneous cholesterol crystal nodules have been described, and no associations have been found with lipid disorders or arthritis[63]. A syndrome that is interesting even though it has not been related to any type of arthritis or to the presence of subcutaneous nodules is the gastrointestinal blood loss due to cholesterol crystal embolization. Clinical signs involved in this syndrome are blue toes, renal insufficiency, and eosinophilia; it occurs in elderly patients with atherosclerosis. In 1995, this syndrome was reviewed by Moolenaar and Lamers[64].

The cholesterol crystal depositions can be classified according to the site of crystal deposition[59]:

- skin (xanthomas, cholesterol tophus, MSUM tophus, rheumatoid nodules)
- joints, burses, tendons (rheumatoid arthritis, SLE, SPA, degenerative osteoarthritis, chronic tophaceous gout, hyperbetalipoproteinemia)
- bones (unicameral bone cysts, bone granulomatosis)
- pleura/pericardial effusions; arteries (atheromas, cholesterol emboli).

CRYOGLOBULIN CRYSTALS

It has long been recognized that paraproteins produced in the course of plasma cell dyscrasias may crystallize. The spontaneous crystallization of paraproteins at low temperatures first described by von Bonsdorf in 1938 and subsequently termed cryocrystalglobulinemia. In this disorder, crystals have been seen within the bone marrow, cornea, synovium, liver, spleen and kidneys. Symptomatic cryocrystalglobulinemia is rare and has been considered a paraneoplastic syndrome associated with multiple myeloma[65]. Patients have symptoms and signs of systemic necrotizing vasculitis with progressive renal failure, arthritis, cutaneous purpura and mucosal ulcerations. Cryoglobulin crystals have been reemphasized as causes of both destructive arthritis and vasculopathy. Serum and synovial fluid studies showed large paraprotein crystals with very different shapes and a strongly positive or a strongly negative birefringence. Monoclonal antibodies detected in joint effusions can provide specific identification[66]. Spontaneous formation of immunoglobulin crystals is often asymptomatic and is sometimes noted only in blood samples *in vitro*.

CORTICOSTEROID CRYSTALS

Intra-articular injection of steroids was pioneered in 1951 by Hollander and is widely used. The use of intrasynovial corticosteroid therapy was accompanied inconstantly by local exacerbations of symptoms in the treated joint. The inflammatory reaction, called 'the post injection flare' usually began several hours following injection, and subsided spontaneously in 24–72 h. The incidence of post-injection flares is variable and

was found by Hollander in 2% of patients. McCarty and Hogan (1964) demonstrated a subclinical leukocyte response in synovial fluid after injection of hydrocortisone acetate[67]. The crystals might remain inside joints for weeks and months and can be confused with CPPD or MSUM crystals. The appearance of corticosteroid crystals in synovial fluid has been described by Kahn and colleagues in 1970[68]. Depot corticosteroid crystal-induced inflammation appears to be more common with triamcinolone hexacetonide than other preparations. Diagnosis can be supported by aspiration and identification of pleomorphic crystals that include irregular shaped rods and squares with intense positive or negative birefringence. McCarty described radiographic evidence of the appearance of calcification around joints after injection with depot corticosteroids[69].

REFERENCES

1. Dieppe PA, Swan A. Identification of crystals in synovial fluid. Ann Rheum Dis 1999; 58: 261–263.
2. CIOMS Criteria, Rome. Appendix I: Proposed diagnostic criteria for use in population studies. In: Kellgren JH, Jeffrey MR and Ball J, eds. Epidemiology of chronic rheumatism. Oxford: Blackwell Scientific; 1963: 327.
3. CIOMS Criteria, New York. Recommendations. In: Bennett PH and Wood PHN, eds. Population studies of the rheumatic diseases. Amsterdam: Excerpta Medica; 1968: 457.
4. O'Sullivan JB. Gout in a New England town. A prevalence study in Sudburry, Massachusetts. Ann Rheum Dis 1972; 31: 166–169.
5. Wallace SL, Robinson H, Masi AT et al. Preliminary criteria for the classification of the acute arthritis of primary gout. Arthritis Rheum 1977; 20: 895–900.
6. Seegmiller JE, Rosenbloom EM, Kelley WN. An enzyme defect associated with sex-linked neurological disorder and excessive purine synthesis. Science 1967; 155: 561–567.
7. Kelley WN, Rosenbloom EM, Henderson JF et al. A specific enzyme defect in gout associated with overproduction of uric acid. Proc Nat Acad Sci 1967; 57: 1735–1740.
8. Kelley WN, Fox IH, Palella TD. Gout and related disorders of purine metabolism. In: Kelley WN, Harris ED, Ruddy S, Sledge CB, eds. Textbook of rheumatology, 3rd edn. Philadelphia: Saunders; 1989: 1395–1448.
9. Seegmiller JE, McAlindon T, Dieppe P et al. An aberration of fructose metabolism in familial gout identified by ^{31}P magnetic resonance spectroscopy. Clin Res 1990; 38: 309.
10. Simmonds HA, Duley JA, Fairbanks LD et al. When to investigate for purine and pyrimidine disorders. Introduction and review of clinical and laboratory indications. J Inher Metab Dis 1997; 29: 214–226.
11. Mikkelsen WM, Dodge HJ, Valkenburg H et al. The distribution of serum uric acid values in a population unselected as to gout or hyperuricemia. Am J Med 1965; 39: 242–251.
12. Hall AP, Barry PE, Dawlen TR et al. Epidemiology of gout and hyperuricemia. Am J Med 1967; 42: 27–37.
13. Pauls HE, Contts A, Calabro JJ et al. Clinical significance of hyperuricemia in routinely screened hospitalized men. JAMA 1970; 211: 277–279.
14. Duff IF, Mikkelsen WM, Dodge HJ et al. Comparison of uric acid levels in some Oriental and Caucasian groups unselected as to gout or hyperuricemia. Arthritis Rheum 1968; 11: 184–190.
15. Darmawan J, Lutalo SK. Gout and hyperuricemia. Baillière's Clin Rheumatol 1995; 9: 83–94.
16. O'Sullivan JB. The incidence of gout and related uric acid levels in Sudbury, Massachusetts. In: Bennett P, Wood P, eds. Population studies of the rheumatic diseases. New York: Excerpta Medica; 1968: 371–376.
17. Campion EW, Glynn RJ, Delabry MA. Asymptomatic hyperuricemia. Am J Med 1987; 82: 422–426.
18. Benson V, Marano MA. Current estimates from the National Health Interview Survey, United States, 1992. Vital Health Stat 1994; 10: 189.
19. Lawrence RC, Helmick CG, Arnett FC et al. Estimates of the prevalence of arthritis and selected musculoskeletal disorders in the United States. Arthritis Rheum 1998; 41: 778–799.
20. Yu TF. Some unusual features of gouty arthritis in females. Semin Arthritis Rheum 1977; 6: 247–255.
21. Roubenoff R. Gout and hyperuricemia. Rheum Dis Clin North Am 1990; 16: 539–550.
22. Harris CM, Lloyd DC, Lewis J. The prevalence and prophylaxis of gout in England. J Clin Epidemiol 1995; 48: 1153–1158.
23. Hochberg MC, Thomas J, Thomas DJ et al. Racial differences in the incidence of gout. Arthritis Rheum 1995; 38: 628–632.
24. Cassim B, Mody GH, Deenadayalu VK et al. Gout in black South Africans: a clinical and genetic study. Ann Rheum Dis 1994; 53: 759–762.
25. Mituszova M, Judák A, Poór G. Clinical and family studies in Hungarian patients with gout. Rheumatol Int 1992; 12: 165–168.
26. Klamp P, Stansheld SA, Castle B et al. Gout is on the increase in New Zealand. Ann Rheum Dis 1997; 56: 22–26.
27. Poór Gy, Mituszova M. Saturnine gout. Baillière's Clin Rheumatol 1989; 3: 51–61.
28. Lin HY, Rocher LL, McQuillan MA et al. Cyclosporine-induced hyperuricemia and gout. N Eng J Med 1989; 321: 287–292.
29. Dieppe PA, Doherty M. The first description of chondrocalcinosis. Arthritis Rheum 1989; 32: 139–140.
30. Zitnan D, Sitaj S. Chondrocalcinosis articularis. Ann Rheum Dis 1963; 22: 142–152.
31. Kohn NN, Huges RE, McCarty DJ et al. The significance of calcium pyrophosphate crystals in the synovial fluid of arthritic patients: The 'pseudogout syndrome'. II. Identification of crystals. Ann Intern Med 1962; 56: 738–745.
32. Martel W, Champion CK, Thompson GR et al. A roentgenologically distinctive arthropathy in some patients with the pseudogout syndrome. An J Roentgenol 1970; 109: 587–605.
33. McCarty DJ. Calcium pyrophosphate dihydrate crystal deposition disease – 1975. Arthritis Rheum 1976; 19(suppl): 275–286.
34. Baldwin CT, Farrer LA, Adain R et al. Linkage of early-onset osteoarthritis and chondrocalcinosis to human chromosome 8q. Am J Hum Genet 1995; 56: 692–697.
35. Huges A, McGibbon P, Woodward E et al. Localisation of a gene for chondrocalcinosis to chromosome 5p. Hum Mol Genet 1995; 4: 1225–1228.
36. Andrev LJ, Brancolini V, de la Pena LS et al. Refinement of the chromosoma 5p locus for familial calcium pyrophosphate dihydrate deposition disease. Am J Hum Genet 1999; 64: 136–145.
37. McCarty DJ. Crystal and arthritis. Dis Mon 1994; 6: 253–300.
38. Doherty M, Dieppe P. Crystal deposition disease in the elderly. Clin Rheum Dis 1986; 12: 97–116.
39. Fallet GH. Chondrokalzinose. In: Fehr K, Miehle W, Schattenkirchner M et al., eds. Rheumatologie in Praxis und Klinik. Stuttgart: Thieme Verlag; 1989: 919–929.
40. Felson DT, Anderson JJ, Naimark A et al. The prevalence of chondrocalcinosis in the elderly and its association with knee osteoarthritis: the Framingham Study. J Rheumatol 1989; 16: 1241–1245.
41. Wilkins E, Dieppe P, Maddison P. Osteoarthritis and articular chondrocalcinosis in the elderly. Ann Rheum Dis 1983; 42: 280–284.
42. Sanmarti R, Panella D, Broncos MA et al. Prevalence of articular chondrocalcinosis in elderly subjects in a rural area of Catalonia. Ann Rheum Dis 1993; 53: 418–422.
43. Fernandez Dapica MP, Reginato AJ. Familial chondrocalcinosis in Spain. Arthritis Rheum 1992; 35: 45.
44. Jones AC, Chuck AJ, Arie EA et al. Diseases assiciated with calcium pyrophospate deposition disease. Semin Arthritis Rheum 1992; 22: 188–202.
45. McCarty DJ, Gatter RA. Recurrent acute inflammation associated with local apatite crystal deposition. Arthritis Rheum 1966; 9: 804–819.
46. Dieppe PA, Huskisson EC, Crocken P et al. Apatite deposition disease: a new arthropathy. Lancet 1976; 1: 266–269.
47. Fam AG, Pritzker JL, Stein JB. Apatite associated arthropathy: a clinical study of 14 cases and of 2 patients with calcific bursitis. J Rheumatol 1979; 6: 461–471.
48. McCarty DJ, Lehr JR, Halverson PB. Crystal populations in human synovial fluid. Identification of apatite, octacalcium phosphate and tricalcium phosphate. Arthritis Rheum 1983; 26: 1220–1224.
49. Swan AJ, Chapman B, Heap P et al. Submicroscopic crystals in osteoarthritic synovial fluids. Ann Rheum Dis 1994; 53: 467–470.
50. McCarty DJ, Halverson PB, Carrera GF et al. 'Milwaukee shoulder' – association of microspheroids containing hydroxyapatite crystals, active collagenase, and neutral protease with rotator cuff defects. I. Clinical aspects. Arthritis Rheum 1981; 24: 464–473.
51. Dieppe PA, Doherty M, Macfarlane DG et al. Apatite associated destructive arthritis. Br J Rheumatol 1984; 23: 84–91.
52. Zakaoui L, Schumacher HR, Rothfuss S et al. Idiopathic destructive arthropathies: clinical light and electron microscopic studies. J Clin Rheumatol 1996; 2: 9–17.
53. Fam AG. Basic calcium phosphate (calcium apatite) crystal deposition diseases. In: Smyth CJ, Holers VM, eds. Gout, hyperuricemia and other crystal-associated arthropaties. New York: Marcel Dekker; 1999: 333–358.
54. Sandstrom C. Peritendinitis calcarea. A common disease of middle life. Its diagnosis, pathology and treatment. Am J Roentgen 1938; 40: 1–21.
55. Resnick D. Calcium hydroxyapatite crystal deposition disease. In: Resnick D, ed. Diagnosis of bone and joint disorders, 3rd edn. Philadelphia: Saunders; 1995: 1615–1648.
56. Chow HY, Recht MP, Schils J et al. Acute calcific tendinitis of the hip: case report with magnetic resonance imaging findings. Arthritis Rheum 1997; 40: 974–977.

57. Gibilisco PA, Schumacher HR, Hollander JL *et al.* Synovial fluid crystals in osteoarthritis. Arthritis Rheum 1985; 28: 511–515.

58. Cogan F, Garcia S, Combalia A *et al.* Uraemic tumoral calcinosis in patients receiving long-term hemodialysis therapy. J Rheumatol 1999; 26: 379–385.

59. Reginato AJ, Falasca GF. Calcium oxalate and other miscellaneous crystal related arthropathies. In: Smyth CJ, Holers VM, eds. Gout, hyperuricemia and other crystal-associated arthropathies. New York: Marcel Dekker; 1999: 369–393.

60. Hoffman GS, Schumacher HR, Paul H *et al.* Calcium oxalate microcrystalline associated arthritis in end stage renal disease. Ann Intern Med 1982; 97: 36–42.

61. Reginato AJ, Kurnik BRC. Calcium oxalate and other crystals associated with kidney diseases and arthritis. Semin Arthritis Rheum 1989; 18: 198–224.

62. Fam AG, Pritzker KPH, Cheng PT *et al.* Cholesterol crystals in osteoarthritic joint effusions. J Rheumatol 1981; 8: 273–280.

63. Gun M, Ehrenfeld M. The benign long term effect of cholesterol crystal synovial cysts. Clin Rheumatol 1994; 13: 537–542.

64. Moolenar W, Lamers CBHW. Gastrointestinal blood loss due to cholesterol crystal embolization. J Clin Gastroenterol 1995; 21: 220–223.

65. Ball JF. Crystalglobulinemia syndrome: a manifestation of multiple myeloma. Cancer 1993; 71: 1231–1234.

66. Podell DN, Packmann CH, Maniloff J *et al.* Characterization of monoclonal IgG cryoglobulins: fine structural and morphological analysis. Blood 1987; 69: 677–681.

67. McCarty DJ, Hogan JM. Inflammatory reaction after intrasynovial injection of microcrystalline adrenocorticosteroid esters. Arthritis Rheum 1964; 7: 359–367.

68. Kahn GB, Hollander JL, Schumacher HR. Corticoid crystals in synovial fluid. J Am Med Assoc 1970; 211: 807–809.

69. McCarty DJ. Treatment of rheumatoid joint inflammation with triamcinolone hexacetonide. Arthritis Rheum 1972; 15: 157–173.

176 The pathogenesis of gout

Lachy McLean

Key points

- Acute gout is a severe arthritis caused by the inflammatory response to urate crystals
- Gout is the most common inflammatory arthritis in men
- Hyperuricemia is the central biochemical precursor for gout
- Defects in purine metabolic enzymes are a well characterized cause but account for less than 1% of gout cases
- In most patients the main problem is renal under-excretion of uric acid, exacerbated by a purine rich diet, diuretics, and/or alcohol
- In addition to conventional phagocytosis, urate crystal surfaces can interact directly with signaling proteins and membranes to cause cell activation and lysis
- While chemokine activated neutrophils predominate in the synovial fluid, it is likely that the acute gout attack is initiated by resident synovial cells including phagocytes and mast cells
- The molecular and genetic basis of the renal defect underlying most patients' gout remains poorly understood
- Alcohol, the treatment of heart failure, calcineurin antagonists and Filipino or Polynesian ethnicity are associated with difficult gout

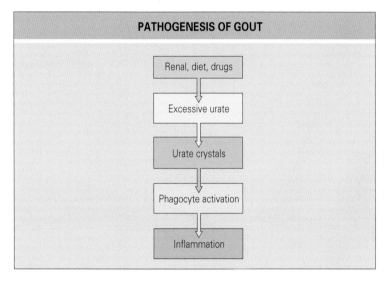

PATHOGENESIS OF GOUT

Fig. 176.1 Pathogenesis of gout. Simplified version; many hyperuricemic subjects do not form crystals, and phagocytes can ingest urate crystals without necessarily triggering inflammation.

TABLE 176.1 PHYSIOLOGICAL FUNCTIONS OF PURINES

- Antioxidant (urate)
- Co-enzymes (co-enzyme-A, FAD, NAD)
- Elementary building blocks for nucleic acids DNA and RNA
- Extracellular messengers (adenosine, ATP)
- High-energy reactions (ATP)
- Intracellular second messengers (G-protein-coupled receptors)
- Metabolic regulators (cyclic AMP; phosphorylation by ATP)
- Neurotransmitters

Acute gout is one of the most painful conditions that rheumatologists encounter, with a pain intensity to rival that of childbirth and long bone fractures. Gout is also one of the best understood of the rheumatic disorders (Fig. 176.1), and is one of the few for which we have effective and reasonably safe long-term disease-modifying therapy. Yet patients who fail medical treatment are common and anecdotes of medical mismanagement abound. Certain groups of patients continue to pose difficult management problems: allograft recipients, patients with severe heart failure, patients with renal failure including those with tubulo-interstitial renal disease, and patients with Filipino or Polynesian ethnicity.

NORMAL PURINE FUNCTIONS

Purines take part in a range of important physiological activities (Table 176.1). All cells utilize purines and pyrimidines for the synthesis of nucleic acids and coenzymes, and purines act as important extracellular and intracellular messengers.

The main purine structures are shown (Figs 176.2 & 176.3). The generic purine structure is a 6-atom pyrimidine ring coupled to an imidazole. Uric acid is a weak acid. The acidic proton (position 9) has a pKa of around 5.75, so that at physiological pH almost all uric acid exists in the ionized form as the urate ion. The solubility of urate falls with reducing pH, although changes within the usual physiological range do not have a great impact. In the extracellular locale most of the salt is formed with

sodium, as the most abundant cation. Uric acid and monosodium urate (MSU) have similar solubility in aqueous solutions. For simplicity both MSU and the hydrated salt found in the crystal lattice (monosodium urate monohydrate) are often referred to simply as 'urate.'

Uric acid is the end-product of purine degradation in man, but may itself have an important physiological role. Humans have higher concentrations of uric acid than most other mammals. With increasing age many of us teeter on the brink of urate supersaturation. Uric acid can act as an anti-oxidant, removing damaging reactive oxygen metabolites[1], and on a molecule-for-molecule basis is as effective an antioxidant as ascorbate (vitamin C). Correlations have been noted between hyperuricemia and longevity, intelligence, and social achievement[2]. It has been suggested that our higher urate levels help humans compensate for losing the ability to make our own ascorbate.

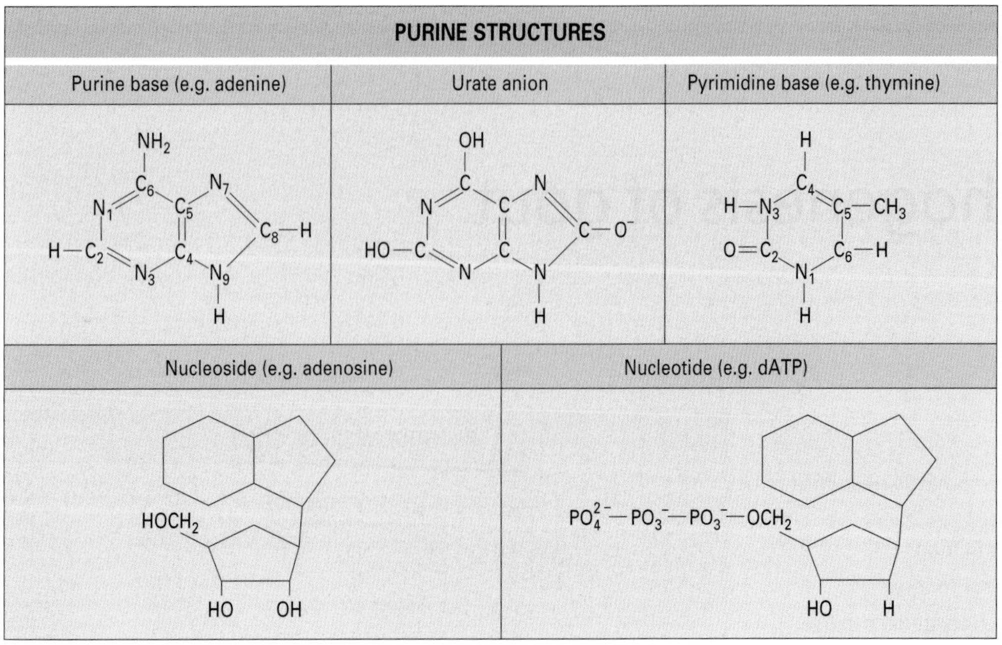

PURINE STRUCTURES

Purine base (e.g. adenine)	Urate anion	Pyrimidine base (e.g. thymine)

Nucleoside (e.g. adenosine)	Nucleotide (e.g. dATP)

Fig. 176.2 Purine structures. Positions in the base rings are numbered 1–9 (purine) or 1–6 (pyrimidine); pentose sugar positions are numbered 1' (attached to the base at N-9) to 5'. The –OH group at the 2' carbon of the ribose sugar is replaced by –H in deoxyribose. Nucleoside: purine or pyrimidine base linked to a ribose or deoxyribose sugar. Nucleotide: phosphate ester of the nucleoside (AMP, ATP, dAMP etc.). One, two, or three phosphate groups are attached via the 5' carbon of the sugar. Nucleotidase: removes the phosphate group. Phosphorylase: removes the phosphate group and the sugar. Kinase: transfers a high energy phosphate group (e.g. to convert ATP). The nucleoside of hypoxanthine is known as inosine, and its nucleotide is IMP.

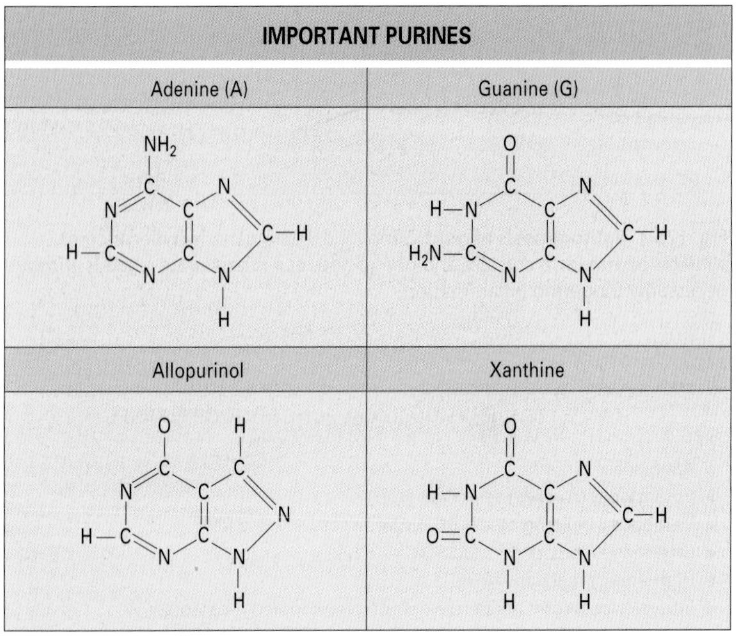

IMPORTANT PURINES

Adenine (A)	Guanine (G)
Allopurinol	Xanthine

Fig. 176.3 Important purines. Allopurinol is an analogue of hypoxanthine, with the N and C atoms at positions 7 and 8 interchanged. Xanthine oxidase hydrolyzes allopurinol to the active metabolite oxypurinol. Oxypurinol binds tightly to the active site of XO.

TABLE 176.2 DIETARY FACTORS AFFECTING PURINE DISPOSITION

Chemical composition	Total caloric intake (obesity, leptin)
	Triglycerides
	Carbohydrates (insulin)
	Protein (aspartate, glutamine, glycine)
	DNA (cellularity, nucleus/cytoplasm ratio)
	RNA (transcriptional activity, messengers)
Specific food examples	Bacon
	Beer
	Legumes
	Liver
	Shellfish
	Thymus, pancreas
	Yeast extracts

In addition to the direct contributions of dietary purines and protein as uric acid precursors, diet can adversely influence renal urate excretion. The renal actions of insulin and leptin may mediate some of these effects.

HYPERURICEMIA

An elevated urate level is the key biochemical precursor of gout and is the strongest prospective risk factor. The higher a person's urate level, the greater the chance of gout[3,4]. Hyperuricemia can be defined as a serum or plasma urate concentration greater than 7.0mg/dl (0.42mmol/l) in males and 6.0mg/dl (0.36mmol/l) in females. The risk of supersaturation in physiological fluids rises with urate concentration. While increasing hyperuricemia favors crystal formation *in vitro* (typically above 6.8mg/dl in serum) the relationship is not linear. In plasma, synovial fluid and tissue fluids urate can be considerably more soluble than in water. The solubility of urate varies according to the other constituents in biological fluids. This accounts for some of the difference in the threshold for gout associated with a given elevation in urate level.

The amount of urate in the body depends on the balance between purine nucleotide synthesis, breakdown and recycling, and excretion. At a basic biochemical level, hyperuricemia may result from the overproduction of urate or the underexcretion of urate, and is often a combination of the two. In overproduction of urate, the purine precursors may be of endogenous (cell turnover and metabolism) or exogenous (dietary) origin. More than one factor may be involved in the etiology of hyperuricemia in an individual patient. An excessive ingestion of purines and primary renal underexcretion of urate are the most common combination. The normal physiology of each of the components of normal purine metabolism will be reviewed prior to examples of abnormalities associated with hyperuricemia and gout.

Purine intake

Purine availability can be altered by several dietary factors (Table 176.2). Purines can be derived by synthesis from small molecular precursors or directly from the diet. The dietary intake of DNA and ribonucleotides has a significant impact on how much uric acid the body must dispose of. The complete elimination of purines from the diet reduces urate excretion by up to 5mg/kg per day and after ten days can reduce the serum urate level by 25%. This indicates a substantial dietary contribution to the purine load[5], and affirms the potential of dietary manipulation in the management of gout. Unfortunately, reductions of this magnitude are seldom obtained in clinical practice.

Uric acid itself is not a normal component of food, and if present is poorly absorbed. Unless the bowel has been sterilized, urate from the diet or which has been excreted into the gut is degraded to allantoin by uricase-positive colonic bacteria. This process of intestinal uricolysis accounts for around a third of purine excretion. A proportion of ingested dietary purines are also catabolized directly within the gut rather than entering the body's recycling purine pool.

The purine content of particular foods (Table 176.2) depends on their relative cellularity (hence their content of nuclei) and on the transcriptional and metabolic activity of the cells present. Purine precursors are digested in several steps. Pancreatic ribonuclease and deoxyribonucleases hydrolyze nucleic acids into oligo- and mononucleotides, and phosphodiesterases then break oligonucleotides into simple nucleotides. Pancreatic and mucosal enzymes remove most of the phosphate and sugar groups. The resulting digestion products can be absorbed either as nucleosides or as free bases, with around 50% of the purines from dietary RNA and 25% of those from DNA being eventually absorbed. A diet rich in protein also adds to the pool of purine precursors. The amino acids aspartic acid, glutamine, and glycine each contribute molecular groups to the purine chemical backbone (Fig. 176.4).

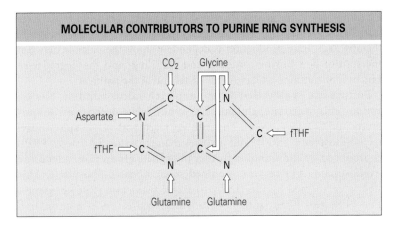

MOLECULAR CONTRIBUTORS TO PURINE RING SYNTHESIS

Fig. 176.4 Molecular contributors to purine ring synthesis. The purine ring atoms are derived from amino acids, carbon dioxide, and formyl groups. fTHF: N^{10}-formyl-tetrahydrofolate.

Purine biosynthesis and salvage

The pathways of production of uric acid are outlined in Figure 176.5 and are covered well in standard biochemistry texts[6]. Several stages in the synthesis and salvage of purines are worthy of further attention as they have been implicated in the pathogenesis of gout. In addition to *de novo* synthesis, purine bases derived from tissue nucleic acids are re-utilized. These salvaged purines arise from physiological cell turnover.

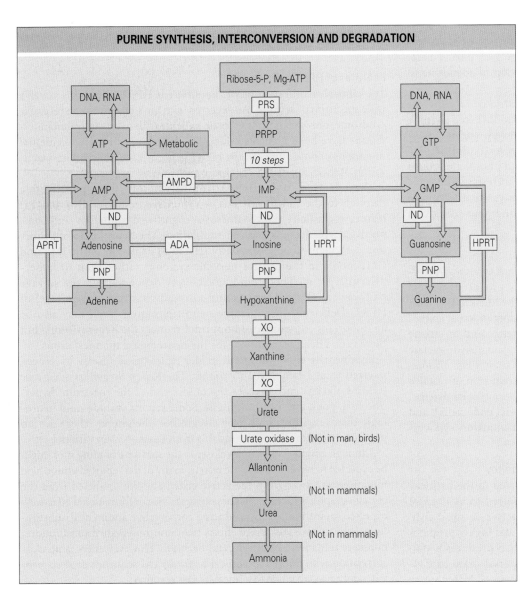

PURINE SYNTHESIS, INTERCONVERSION AND DEGRADATION

Fig. 176.5 Purine synthesis, interconversion and degradation. The gene for urate oxidase has been inactivated in man and higher primates. Intermediates and enzymes not implicated in hyperuricemia and gout have been omitted for simplicity. AMPD, AMP deaminase/adenylate deaminase; GMP, guanosine monophosphate; ND, 5′-nucleotidase; XMP, xanthosine monophosphate; XO: xanthine oxidoreductase. For other abbreviations see text.

The amounts can be greatly increased in inflammatory and proliferative disorders, particularly hematologic malignancies, and by cytotoxic therapy. Net urate production is dependent upon the balance between the sum of new purine synthesis and recycling, and the degradative function of xanthine oxidase at the distal end of the pathway.

Purines are synthesized from simple chemical building blocks: amino acids (aspartate, glutamine, glycine), folate derivatives, ammonium, and CO_2 (Fig. 176.4). The pathway starts with 5'-phosphoribosyl 1-pyrophosphate (PRPP) and involves many intermediate steps. PRPP is produced by addition of a further phosphate group from adenosine triphosphate (ATP) to the modified sugar ribose-5-phosphate. This step is performed by the family of *PRPP synthetase* (PRS) enzymes. The PRS1 and PRS2 isoforms are widely expressed in mammalian cells. This step and several others later in the pathway are subject to feedback inhibition by purines.

Purine interconversion and salvage reactions

The next step (and the first committed step for the *de novo* purine pathway) is the reaction of PRPP with glutamine to add an amine. This is followed by a further nine enzymatic reactions, finishing with closure of the purine ring (Fig. 176.2) to produce inosine monophosphate (IMP; also known as inosinic acid or inosinate; Fig. 176.3). The different purine bases are closely related chemically and can be interconverted in simple enzymatic steps (Fig. 176.5). IMP is converted to the adenine and guanine nucleotides, respectively adenosine monophosphate (AMP, adenylate) and guanosine monophosphate (GMP, guanylate). Nucleotidases and phosphatases convert the nucleotides AMP, IMP and GMP into the corresponding nucleosides and bases. *Purine nucleotide phosphorylase* (PNP) catalyses the reversible reaction to remove the sugar group from the purine nucleosides, yielding the free purine base. *Adenosine deaminase* (ADA) catalyses the conversion of adenosine to inosine, and *AMP deaminase* converts AMP to IMP.

The enzyme *hypoxanthine-guanine phosphoribosyl transferase* (HPRT; formerly HGPRT) salvages hypoxanthine to IMP and guanine to GMP (Fig. 176.5). In an analogous salvage pathway, *adenine phosphoribosyl transferase* (APRT) converts adenine to AMP. Both HPRT and APRT use PRPP as the donor of the ribose and phosphate groups needed to convert the purine base back into the corresponding ribonucleotide. Abnormalities in these salvage pathways are uncommon but well characterized causes of hyperuricemia and gout (discussed below).

Purine catabolism

Xanthine oxidase (XO) is a flavoprotein enzyme which catalyses the formation of hypoxanthine from inosine, then in turn produces uric acid from hypoxanthine. The final degradation to urate by XO is irreversible. This enzyme is widespread in human tissues including mucosal epithelia, vascular smooth muscle cells and endothelia, and in tissue macrophages. It can be converted to an NAD-dependent dehydrogenase form; the two are sometimes referred to together as *xanthine oxidoreductase*. XO also plays an important role in the production of reactive oxygen species (ROS)[7], which can contribute to antimicrobial defense. XO has also been demonstrated in inflamed synovial endothelia[8], and ROS have been implicated in the aggravation of inflammatory synovitis during ischemic perfusion cycles[9].

Urate oxidase, a species-wide metabolic 'deficiency'

Unfortunately for gout patients, XO is the final step in the pathway for humans. The enzyme *urate oxidase* (also referred to as *uricase*) degrades urate to allantoin. Urate oxidase is active in most fish, amphibians, and non-primate mammals. In man and higher primates the gene (*UOX*) is inactivated by a mutation which produces a stop codon in the fifth of the eight exons[10]. This universal urate oxidase 'deficiency' [on-line Mendelian inheritance in man (OMIM) entry 191540; www3.ncbi.nlm.nih.gov/omim/] sets the scene for gout in humans. The evolutionary gain from this is unclear, but might include the increased antioxidant effect. Uricase is in therapeutic use[11,12]. Further steps in the pathway, degrading allantoin to urea and ammonia, were lost at an early stage in mammalian evolution.

Abnormalities in purine metabolism

HPRT deficiency

Defects in HPRT (OMIM 308000) are the most extensively studied purine enzyme abnormality leading to hyperuricemia and gout[13,14]. This enzyme is a crucial step in recycling hypoxanthine and guanine back into the pool of nucleotides available for nucleic acid synthesis (Fig. 176.5). The HPRT gene comprises nine exons, eight introns and a putative promoter region, and is located on the X chromosome. Over 200 different mutations have been described[15]. Single base substitutions (including CpG transitions) account for the majority (63%), followed by deletions (24%) and a lesser number of insertions and base duplications. Half of the described deletions are of an entire exon or more. Disease-associated mutations have been reported throughout the HPRT gene, although there are a few mutation 'hot spots'. These include the CpG motifs, prone to mutation of the cytosine (C) to a thymine (T) base through methylation then deamination.

Hypoxanthine cannot be reutilized without HPRT, and can only be degraded to urate. The underutilization of PRPP by the salvage pathway in HPRT and APRT deficient patients further contributes to hyperuricemia, as an elevated concentration of PRPP drives the *de novo* biosynthetic pathway to a markedly increased level. The decrease in IMP and GMP levels also contribute to hyperuricemia by reducing feedback inhibition on *de novo* purine synthesis.

Features of HPRT deficiency

The clinical manifestations of the different HPRT mutations cover a wide spectrum of severity. As expected with an X chromosome recessive syndrome, only a handful of female patients with overt clinical manifestations have been identified. These patients either have coincidental mutations of both copies of the HPRT gene, or have nonrandom inactivation of their 'normal' X chromosome[15].

The effects in males range from asymptomatic hyperuricemia through to the full-blown *Lesch–Nyhan syndrome* (OMIM 300322) featuring spasticity, choreoathetosis, cognitive dysfunction, and compulsive aggressiveness and self-mutilation. The neurological dysfunction is thought to be particularly related to depletion of the IMP and GMP pools in the central nervous system[16] rather than to hyperuricemia *per se*. The brain appears very dependent on the salvage pathway for GMP synthesis and normally has a very high level of HPRT. Deficiency in dopamine neurotransmitter levels may also be an important component. Allopurinol reduces the hyperuricemia but there is no effective treatment for the neurological manifestations.

Intermediate conditions with milder neurological disease have been referred to as Lesch–Nyhan *variants*. The *Kelley–Seegmiller syndrome* (OMIM 300323) encompasses the milder end of the spectrum: hyperuricemia, gout, and nephrolithiasis. Some reports include mild neurologic disease within the Kelley–Seegmiller phenotype. There are no precise criteria for distinguishing this from Lesch–Nyhan variants.

Although amino acid changes closer to the substrate binding sites might be expected to have more drastic effects, many of the reported amino acid mutations are away from the active enzymatic site predicted from the crystallographic structure[17,18]. These may act via conformational effects. As expected, point mutations producing conservative amino acid substitutions tend to have less severe effects than nonconservative substitutions, nonsense mutations, insertions and deletions. However, there is no clear correlation with particular clinical features, and sequence analysis provides only a rough guide to clinical disease severity.

On the other hand the level of residual HPRT enzymatic activity expressed *in vitro* with different mutations shows a reasonable inverse correlation with the severity of the clinical phenotype. In general, gout is likely to develop with HPRT activity between 2% and 20% of normal, and severe neurologic manifestations only if the functional activity of the enzyme is less than 2% of normal.

Genetic deficiency in APRT (OMIM 102600) tends to present with renal stones rather than gout. It is rare in Caucasians but more common among Japanese, who have a gene frequency of over 1%. The APRT mutations reported are far less diverse than those found in HPRT[19].

PRS superactivity

Mutations in the PRPP synthetase genes can result in overactivity of the pathway and excessive production of urate[20]. PRS overactivity is an uncommon disorder and is inherited as an X-linked dominant trait. The molecular defects reported to lead to PRS overactivity are diverse, and the basis for excessive transcription of PRS in these patients is unknown but may lie in trans-acting genes[21].

Fructose intolerance

Patients homozygous for a recessively inherited defect of the enzyme aldolase B (causing congenital fructose intolerance) may also develop hyperuricemia due to excessive degradation of adenine nucleotides[22]. Around 1% of Caucasians are heterozygous for aldolase B deficiency. Heterozygotes with gout have been reported. Urinary urate excretion can appear normal until a fructose load is administered.

Severe hyperuricemia also occurs in patients with the glucose-6-phosphatase deficiency. In part this is due to overproduction of urate, secondary to increased purine synthesis. However, the persistently elevated serum lactate levels that usually occur in this disease further contribute to the hyperuricemia by competing for renal tubular excretion of urate (see below).

Allopurinol, XO substrate and inhibitor

Allopurinol, an isomer of hypoxanthine (Fig. 176.3), was originally developed as a cancer chemotherapeutic drug. It is both a substrate and a potent inhibitor of xanthine oxidase. Fortunately the build-up of purine metabolites at the proximal stages in the pathway when XO is inhibited therapeutically does not seem to have significant adverse consequences. Severe genetic deficiency of XO can cause xanthinuria, with an increase in both hypoxanthine and xanthine. XO activity is also reduced in animal models of chronic renal impairment[23], a factor which may ameliorate the degree of hyperuricemia occurring with renal failure.

The degradative products hypoxanthine and xanthine are freely filtered at the glomerulus and do not undergo significant net tubular re-absorption. Occasional XO deficient patients have a metabolic arthropathy, myopathy, or xanthine renal stones. The majority are asymptomatic. On the other hand, inhibition of azathioprine or mercaptopurine degradation by allopurinol can have disastrous consequences with agranulocytosis and aplastic anemia despite careful dose reduction.

Interconversion enzymes

Leucocytes are particularly prone to the effects of high concentrations of accumulated purine nucleotides. Although both ADA and PNP are widely expressed in mammalian tissues[24] the main clinical manifestation of genetic deficiency of either enzyme is a severe combined immune deficiency (SCID). A similar effect can be obtained with therapeutic inhibition of PNP, providing a novel approach to immunosuppression[25]. Methotrexate inhibits the folate-dependent enzyme 5-amino-4-imidazole carboxamide ribonucleotide (AICAR) transformylase, the penultimate step in IMP biosynthesis. The increased concentration of AICAR inhibits both ADA and AMP-deaminase. The accumulating adenosine translocates to the extracellular space immediately surrounding the leucocyte, and delivers an inhibitory signal via the membrane A2a, A2b and A3 G-protein coupled receptors (GPCR) for adenosine. This is believed to be an important mechanism for the activity of low dose methotrexate in inflammatory synovitis[26].

RENAL ELIMINATION OF URIC ACID

As in other primates, uric acid disposal in humans is mainly via the kidneys. Enteric excretion contributes almost all of the nonrenal urate disposal, about a third of the daily total in healthy subjects[27], and increases in the face of hyperuricemia and impaired renal excretion. The majority of patients with gout and hyperuricemia demonstrate urate underexcretion[28] (urate clearance of less than 6ml/min or a urate-to-creatinine clearance ratio of less than 6%), with no other demonstrable abnormality of renal function. The renal excretion of urate in these patients does increase in response to a higher serum urate level, but still lags behind the excretion rate needed to clear the higher circulating load.

Renal urate excretion is exquisitely sensitive to volume status and hemodynamic changes, to competition with other organic anions including endogenous metabolites such as lactate, and to certain drugs. Hyperuricemia is disproportionately severe with drugs and diseases which affect tubulointerstitial function.

Stages of renal urate excretion

Renal urate handling can be considered in four physiological compartments: glomerular filtration, tubular re-absorption, tubular secretion, and post-secretory absorption. Only a small proportion of plasma urate binds to plasma proteins, including a urate binding globulin, and this interaction is weak. Over 95% of the urate entering the kidney in plasma is freely ultrafiltered at the glomerulus. However, almost all of this filtered urate load is re-absorbed by the early proximal tubule (Fig. 176.6). The physiological advantages of this and the later re-absorptive step are not clear[29,30].

On ultrastructural grounds the proximal tubule can be subdivided into three segments S1, S2 and S3. The stages of bi-directional urate movement have been defined functionally. While the correlation between urate movement and these anatomic sites is not definite, most of the initial pre-secretory reabsorption probably occurs in the S1 and S2 segments. Urate absorption is likely to involve counter-transport with other anions: hydroxyl or bicarbonate on the luminal side of proximal tubule epithelial cell (the cell's apical membrane), and the entry of chloride on the basal side towards the peri-tubular capillary network. As with absorption of other anions, active sodium/hydrogen ion exchange on the basal aspect provides the pH gradient that drives the system. Most gout patients have tubular function that is normal apart from net urate underexcretion, arguing against defects in transporter systems shared by other major ions.

Net urate excretion is mainly determined by the balance between the next two steps: active tubular secretion of around 50% of the re-absorbed urate (mainly S2), followed by a second post-secretory absorptive phase (S3 and early distal tubule) which removes all but 10% of the filtered urate load. Clearly, abnormalities at either the tubular secretion or the final postsecretory re-absorption steps could have a profound effect on net urate excretion.

Urate transport systems

Despite these uncertainties, significant progress has been made in our understanding of renal tubular ion transport. As with urate reabsorption, urate movement into the lumen is probably in exchange for reabsorption of another abundant anion (e.g. chloride) through an associated membrane channel. Organic acids such as lactate, β-hydroxybutyrate, acetoacetate and salicylate, together with the antituberculous

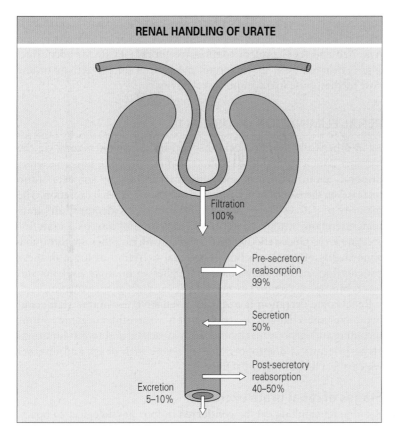

Fig. 176.6 Renal handling of urate. Renal urate movement can be divided into four physiological compartments. The existence of a discrete fourth compartment (postsecretory reabsorption) is controversial, and the anatomical correlations are not certain. Urate ion movement involves counter-transport with other anions, and is driven in part by a pH gradient produced by active sodium/hydrogen ion exchange. Selective urate transporter molecules (hUAT1, hUAT2) and a transporter shared with other organic anions (hOAT3) have been identified. The molecular basis of the defect in tubular urate handling in gout is unknown.

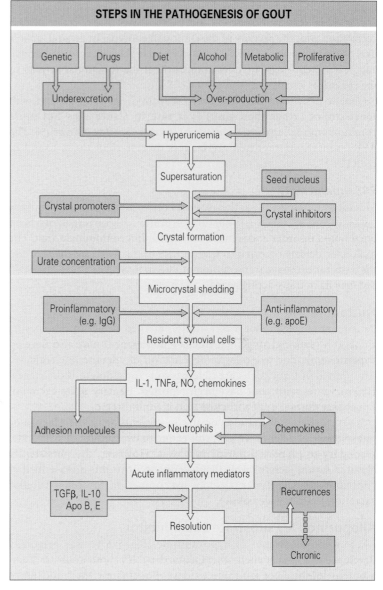

Fig. 176.7 Steps in the pathogenesis of gout. Many signals impact at the critical points in this pathway. Hyperuricemic patients do not necessarily form urate crystals, and crystals ingested by phagocytes sometimes elicit remarkably little inflammation. The factors leading to the spontaneous termination of the acute gout attack are unclear. Inflammation is usually low grade in chronic gout.

agent pyrazinamide, decrease urate excretion by inhibiting tubular secretion of urate. This suggests that they share the same anion channel.

Urate is not a significant substrate for the human renal organic anion transporters (hOAT) described initially[31]. However, the recently characterized channel hOAT3 is expressed on the basolateral membranes of proximal tubular epithelia and mediates sodium-dependent urate transport[32]. hOAT3 also interacts with other relevant compounds including estradiol, NSAID, and diuretics.

The highly selective urate transporter membrane channels hUAT1 (galectin 9) and hUAT2 were recently identified in man, and characterized at a functional and molecular level[33]. They are integral membrane proteins with multiple transmembrane domains. The hUAT were initially identified through structural similarities with parts of the urate oxidase molecule. UAT are also expressed in the gut. It will be useful to define their ultrastructural distribution and polymorphisms.

The contribution of hUAT1, hUAT2 and hOAT3 to the different physiological stages of urate excretion has not been explored and defective function of these and other ion channels in gout patients is open to speculation. The molecular basis for the relative renal underexcretion of urate that underlies gout in most patients remains unknown.

PROGRESSION TO GOUT: URATE CRYSTAL FORMATION

There are a number of factors that determine whether hyperuricemia leads to urate crystal formation, and in turn whether these crystals trigger acute inflammation (Fig. 176.7 & Table 176.3).

Factors influencing urate crystal formation

A critical step in the pathogenesis of gout is whether the hyperuricemic patient forms urate crystals. The main factors are the concentration of urate and cations at the site of crystal formation; the local temperature; the presence or absence of substances maintaining urate in solution, particularly proteoglycans; and the presence or absence of inhibitors and promoters of crystal nucleation and growth[34–36]. Gradual diffusion of water out of a joint, leaving behind progressively increasing concentrations of uric acid and crystallization promoters, has been postulated to aid crystallization[37], and this may contribute to the diurnal variation in gout onset.

The initial stage of crystal nucleation in a fluid phase generally occurs around a solid particle, and proceeds best if there is a surface on which the urate molecules can accumulate. Small fragments of cartilage or synovial debris may provide such a seed nucleus. This may account for some of the predilection that tophi have for Heberden's nodes.

In addition to their opsonic role (see below), immunologically specific urate crystal antibodies may also promote crystal formation by stabilizing the growing surfaces[38–40]. The identities and mechanisms of action of

TABLE 176.3 GOUT PROMOTERS AND INHIBITORS	
Crystal formation	Seed nucleus (particulate)
	Specific antibody?
	Phagocytes
	Low temperature
	Low pH
	Cation concentration
	Intra-articular dehydration
	Unknown macromolecules
Triggering the acute flare	Rapid change in urate level
	Microcrystal release
	IgG coat (apolipoproteins B, E inhibitory)
	Adhesion molecule activation
	Local trauma?
	Susceptible phagocytes, mast cells

A diverse array of mediators have been identified on the surfaces of urate crystals. In addition to their proinflammatory effect through opsonizing existing crystals, antibodies may promote crystal formation by providing a stable molecular platform for crystal nucleation and growth. Apolipoproteins are the best characterized of the anti-inflammatory molecules that coat crystals. The differentiation stage of the phagocyte encountering the crystals may be crucial.

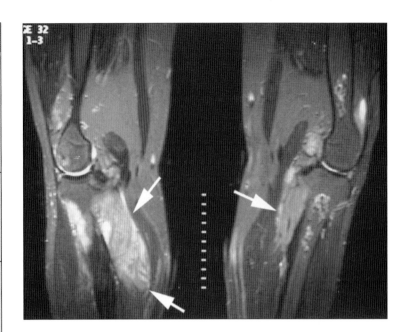

Fig. 176.8 Giant tophaceous pseudotumors. Coronal MRI, distal thigh to proximal calves, 33-year-old Polynesian man with tubulointerstitial disease and severe polyarticular tophaceous gout who presented with gradual bilateral calf swelling. Massive tophaceous deposits, with maximum dimensions of 8 × 12cm on the right, and together estimated at over 1kg of monosodium urate. Markers: 1cm. Large tophi often elicit very little inflammatory response. (Courtesy of Drs Peter Gow and Sunil Kumar.)

the other crystal promoters and inhibitors are unknown. There is some evidence that tissue macrophages may play an active role in the deposition of urate in their microenvironment[41].

With decreasing temperatures the solubilities of both uric acid and monosodium urate decrease. The saturation limit of 6.4mg/dl in physiological saline at body core temperature falls to 4.5mg/dl at 30ºC. The predilection of gout to affect exposed peripheral joints such as the first metatarsophalangeal and the distal interphalangeal joints has been attributed to the lower temperature of these joints. The seasonal variation in acute gout attacks has been cited as further support for the role of locally decreased temperature, with the onset of colder weather helping to precipitate acute attacks[42]. However two recent studies noted gout to be more common in the spring than in fall or winter, and found no correlation with mean monthly temperature or humidity[43,44]. Seasonal dietary changes could also confound the interpretation of this variation.

Synovial fluid pH, which normally approximates that in blood, has also been invoked as a factor. Synovial fluid acidosis has been described in RA and relates to the degree of joint damage[45]. There is no information about changes in synovial fluid pH preceding an attack of gout.

THE INFLAMMATORY RESPONSE TO URATE CRYSTALS

An acute attack of gout occurs when urate crystals trigger a marked inflammatory response. Some evidence suggests that this is associated with the shedding of microcrystals from a small, preformed synovial tophus rather than the formation of new crystals *in situ*. Whereas calcium pyrophosphate crystals mainly occur in the cartilage and menisci, urate crystals and microtophi are found in the synovial membrane.

Although dermal and subcutaneous tophi are generally regarded as features of long-standing gout, microtophi have been demonstrated in superficial areas of the synovium at an early phase in the acute attack[46]. The presence of synovial microtophi at the first attack suggests that urate crystals have been accumulating for some time without triggering inflammation. At later stages of the disease numerous microtophi may be present on the synovial membrane and can be demonstrated during arthroscopy.

In acute gout the predominant synovial fluid cell is the neutrophil, and it is activation of the neutrophil that is thought to contribute the bulk of the proinflammatory stimulus. Healthy joints do not contain a resident population of neutrophils. Urate crystals instead have their initial interaction with physiological synovial cell types. These include

cells of the monocyte-macrophage lineage (type A synoviocyte), fibroblast-like (type B) synoviocytes, and possibly mast cells. In the first acute attack of gout, synovial proliferation with phagocytosis of urate crystals has been demonstrated[47]. This is associated with vascular congestion and an inflammatory infiltrate.

Crystal phagocytosis

As discussed above, part of the reason that many persistently hyperuricemic people do not get gout may lie in the individual's propensity for forming crystals. This depends on seed nuclei, the balance between promoters and inhibitors, crystal-stabilizing antibodies, joint trauma or osteoarthritis, and peripheral temperature.

Despite their potent proinflammatory potential, the presence of urate crystals does not necessarily trigger acute inflammation. Patients may have urate crystals in clinically uninvolved joints[48,49], and heavily crystal-laden fluid can be found in relatively uninflamed bursae and joints[50]. Tophi comprise dense masses of urate crystals but can reach massive dimensions (Fig. 176.8) with surprisingly little inflammatory response. When in unusual axial or visceral sites, tophi can enlarge progressively until they eventually cause symptoms by acting as a space-occupying lesion. Similarly, patients with chronic gout may have prolonged periods with absent or relatively low grade synovitis.

Some crystals may simply be too large to stimulate the necessary inflammatory response. Initiation of the acute attack depends on the macrophage phagocytic response to urate microcrystals, which may form afresh or be released either from larger crystals or from tophi (Fig. 176.9). This is consistent with the long-standing clinical observation that gout flares are associated more closely with rapid changes in urate concentration than with the absolute level of urate. Overly vigorous hypouricemic therapy is more likely to precipitate acute flares than a slow lowering in urate level. This may be because reducing the urate concentration in the microenvironment around a large urate mass to below the saturation level partially re-dissolves the urate at the margins of the deposit, releasing fresh microcrystals.

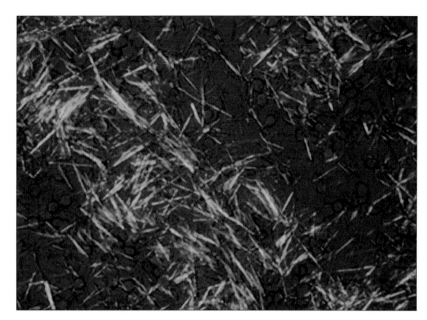

Fig. 176.9 Urate crystals. Crystals aspirated from a subcutaneous tophus. The patient was still hyperuricemic but had not had an acute gout attack for several months and had no local inflammatory symptoms associated with the tophus. One factor in the failure of some crystals to trigger acute gout may be their size. These relatively large (20μm+) crystals are eliciting a minimal inflammatory response. The protein coat surrounding the crystal and the condition of the responding phagocyte are other crucial factors. Polarized transmission white (halogen) light; 90° extinction filter; 530nm first order compensator.

Proteins binding to urate crystals

Urate crystals are composed of a highly ordered, regular array of urate, sodium, and hydrogen ions, and water molecules. Although the surface has a net negative charge, some positive charges are also exposed. Urate crystal surfaces bind immunoglobulin G (IgG), both through charge interactions and with hydrogen bonding. This induces a conformational change in IgG analogous to that produced by antigen binding or immunoglobulin aggregation. This encourages phagocytosis by cells with Fcγ receptors.

Crystal-bound IgG can also activate complement. The surfaces of urate microcrystals are highly reactive with a range of other protein molecules in addition to IgG, and they can directly activate complement even in the absence of bound immunoglobulin[51,52]. This provides further opsonization via C3b on the crystal exterior, and additional neutrophil chemoattraction from the soluble split products C3a and C5a.

A coating of apolipoproteins can counter the opsonic effects of IgG Fc and decrease the attractiveness of urate crystals to phagocytes. In particular, ApoB is a major component of the serum low density lipoprotein (LDL) fraction. It can coat crystals and inhibit the stimulation of neutrophils[53]. ApoE has similar effects[54] and can be made locally by synovial macrophages. A wide range of proteins have been detected on urate crystals from *in vivo* sources, including other complement activation products, lysosomal enzymes, and TGFβ. Their relative inflammatory potential may reflect the balance between pro- and anti-inflammatory elements of this coating.

Phagocyte responsiveness

The interaction between phagocytes and crystals is a key factor in triggering the acute gout flare. Despite this it is well established that synovial fluid phagocytes from non-inflamed joints may contain urate crystals[55]. One study found intracellular crystals in synovial fluid cells from all of 43 intercritical gout patients not on treatment with hypouricemic drugs[56]. Clearly there are additional factors which determine whether the intra-articular phagocytosis of urate crystals precipitates acute inflammation (Table 176.3 & Fig. 176.10). The protein coat acquired by the crystals may be one such factor, important not only in promoting or inhibiting phagocytosis[57], but influencing whether the crystals provide an appropriate stimulus to trigger an acute inflammatory response once phagocytosed.

Alternatively, the type of cell initially interacting with the crystals may be a crucial determinant. Most phagocytes containing crystals in non-inflamed joints are macrophages rather than neutrophils[58]. With advancing degrees of differentiation, murine macrophage cell lines can effectively phagocytose urate microcrystals *in vitro* without triggering an inflammatory cascade[59]. Similarly, human monocytes isolated fresh from the blood mount a vigorous response to urate crystals, whereas

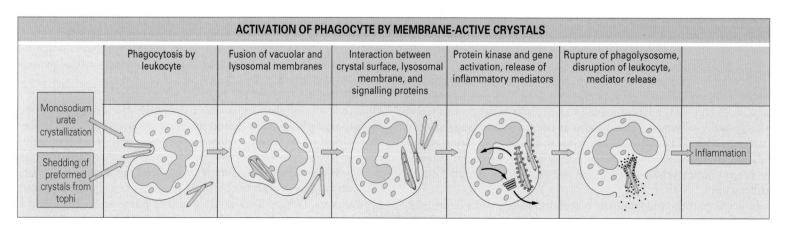

Fig. 176.10 Activation of phagocyte by membrane-active crystals. Protein kinase and gene activation, release of inflammatory mediators. Urate and other crystals interact with lipid membranes. They also bind to cytosolic and membrane-bound proteins and cross-link them, acting directly at important control steps in proinflammatory signaling.

macrophages differentiated *in vitro* for 7 days show a greatly reduced proinflammatory mediator response despite internalizing the crystals equally well[60]. Mature phagocytes resident in human synovium may be able to interact with crystals without triggering acute synovitis, whereas the entry of fresh monocytes or neutrophils into the joint contributes to the triggering of an acute gout attack.

GOUT, RHEUMATOID ARTHRITIS AND RENAL FAILURE

There is a strong negative association between gout and rheumatoid arthritis[61,62]. In most case reports of gout and RA occurring in the same patient, the gouty arthritis preceded the onset of the RA. This apparent protective effect of RA has generally been ascribed to alterations in the protein constituents of the synovial fluid that inhibit crystal formation or phagocytosis. Rheumatoid factor may inhibit the interaction between phagocytes and the exposed Fc portions of crystal-bound IgG[63].

Alternatively this could reflect differences in the phagocyte population resident in the rheumatoid synovial membrane and fluid. RA patients do not show a reduced inflammatory response to urate crystals injected intradermally[64], arguing against a more generalized alteration in phagocyte function. Other indirect evidence for the crucial role of phagocyte responsiveness comes from the observation that acute gout is relatively rare in end stage renal disease considering the degree of hyperuricemia in many renal patients. Monocytes from patients with renal failure produce lower levels of the cytokines interleukin (IL)-1, IL-6 and TNF after stimulation *in vitro* with urate crystals[65].

THE ACUTE ATTACK OF GOUT

Urate crystals are a highly potent inflammatory stimulus. Crystals interact with phagocytes through two broad mechanisms, depending on their concentration and surface reactivity. First, they can activate the cell through the conventional route as opsonized and phagocytosed particles, analogous to the response seen with phagocytosed microorganisms. This elicits the stereotypical phagocyte response of lysosomal fusion, respiratory burst, and the release of inflammatory mediators. The other mechanism involves the particular properties of the urate crystal surface, and its interactions through direct contact with lipid membranes and proteins.

This strong surface reactivity enables the crystals to cross-link membrane glycoproteins and directly activate proinflammatory signaling pathways at any of several levels within the phagocyte. Urate microcrystals interact with signaling glycoproteins in the cell membrane, including integrins and FcRγ[66,67]. Signal transduction from receptors on the phagocyte surface usually requires tyrosine kinase phosphorylation, but urate crystals can bypass the normal membrane receptor routes and directly activate second messenger systems including membrane-associated and cytosolic kinases[68].

Phospholipases and GPCRs, including chemokine receptors in the phagocyte membrane, are also cross-linked and activated. Monocyte activation by urate crystals *in vitro* is reduced by inhibitors of the p38 mitogen activated protein (MAP) kinase[69], a key regulatory point for many of the cytokines implicated in this and other forms of inflammatory arthritis. Both urate and calcium pyrophosphate crystals activate the kinases JNK, ERK-1 and ERK-2, and induce binding of the NF-κB and AP-1 nuclear factors to the CXCL8 (IL-8) promoter in monocytic cells[70].

Acute inflammatory mediators

Activation of resident cells by urate microcrystals leads to the production of IL-1, IL-6, chemokines including CXCL8, granulocyte-macrophage colony stimulating factor (GM–CSF) and tumor necrosis factor alpha (TNFα)[71-74]. The early effects of these cytokines include increased expression on nearby vascular endothelial cells of E-selectin[75]. An alternative model is primary recruitment of immature blood monocytes in response to endothelial changes (e.g. trauma, sepsis)[60].

Chemokines

Chemokines of the CXC family are important for attracting and activating the neutrophils so prominent in acute gout, and are major cytokines in the synovial fluid from acute gout patients. Mice with a targeted disruption ('knockout') in the gene for the chemokine receptor CXCR2 lack the normal neutrophil component of the response to urate crystals[76], suggesting a dominant role for chemokines in recruiting neutrophils among the diverse array of proinflammatory mediators in gouty synovial fluid (Figs 176.10 & 176.11 & Table 176.4). In addition to CXCL-8, CXCL-1 (Gro-α), CXCL -2 (MIP-2α, Gro-β) and CXCL-3 (MIP-2β, Gro-γ) have been implicated.

The chemokine family is large, with over 40 distinct chemokines, 18 chemokine receptors, and substantial overlap between the various chemokines binding a given receptor[77]. While all leucocytes and many connective tissue cell types can be persuaded to produce a chemokine such as CXCL-8 *in vitro*, the expression *in vivo* is more restricted. The relative importance of the individual chemokines in human gout has not been established.

Urate crystals also induce the *de novo* synthesis of the inducible form of cyclo-oxygenase (COX-2) and of phospholipase-A2, producing the inflammatory prostanoids prostaglandin-E_2 and thromboxane-A_2 in phagocytes[69]. PG-E_2 causes vasodilatation, edema, and further leukocyte immigration. In addition to providing prostanoid precursors, the phospholipase A_2 induced in the activated phagocyte produces lysophosphatidylcholine (LPC), which acts via the G2A GPCR[78] to modulate the chemotaxis and activation of inflammatory cells.

Reactive nitrogen metabolites

Urate crystals incite nitric oxide (NO) production by human monocytes and synovial fibroblasts[79]. NO synthesis by the inducible isoform of nitric oxide synthetase (NOS2; also known as *iNOS*) has been demonstrated in macrophages, fibroblasts, chondrocytes, and endothelia in many species. NOS2 has been implicated in RA and osteoarthritis, and

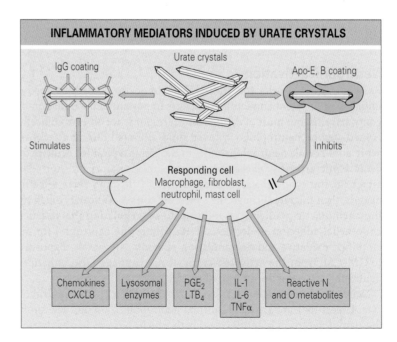

Fig. 176.11 Inflammatory mediators induced by urate crystals. Urate crystals can stimulate a variety of cells to produce a diverse array of inflammatory mediators, depending on the coating of the crystal and the receptiveness of the cell.

TABLE 176.4 INFLAMMATORY EVENTS IN THE ACUTE GOUT ATTACK

Sequence of cellular events

1. Release of urate microcrystals, proinflammatory coating
2. Initial interaction with monocytes ± fibroblasts, mast cells
3. Release of cytokines, especially IL-1, TNF-α, CXCL8
4. Activation of endothelial cell adhesion molecules
5. Emigration, attraction and activation of neutrophils
6. Aggressive phagocytosis of crystals by neutrophils
7. Delayed phagocyte apoptosis
8. Cross-linking of inflammatory signaling proteins
9. Membrane perturbation, phagolysosome rupture
10. Neutrophil death, massive enzyme and mediator release
11. Resolution – cytokines (TGFβ), mature macrophages

Soluble mediators

Prostaglandins	Leukotrienes
Reactive oxygen species	Reactive nitrogen species
Chemokines, particularly CXCL family	Proteases
IL-1	IL-6
TNF-α	Complement split products

Urate crystals can activate many cell types and trigger the release of a diverse array of proinflammatory mediators. Some have been detected both after *in vitro* stimulation of phagocytes and in gout patients' synovial fluid. The clinical efficacy of the inhibition of prostanoids has established their role beyond doubt. Intervention *in vivo* with selective inhibitors of other mediators to 'prove' their role in man has not been practical. Most of the numerous chemokines and cytokines have not been examined in gout, either in clinical specimens or using *in vitro* phagocyte stimulation models.

in inflammatory disorders affecting other organ systems. The human NOS2 gene has cytokine-inducible NF-κB promoter elements in common with rodent NOS2, although the promoter organization and phagocyte cytokine responses are different[80].

NO can have toxic, regulatory, and either pro- or anti-apoptotic effects, and depending on its concentration can either inhibit or enhance neutrophil activation. Although a role in the acute inflammation of gout seems likely there are no published data on NOS-2 activation by urate crystals *in vivo*, nor on NO or its metabolites in gout. On the other hand, uric acid may actually counteract some of the effects of reactive nitrogen species via its oxidative radical scavenging activity [81].

Neutrophil activation

Resident synovial cells and trafficking monocytes contribute to the initial burst of proinflammatory mediators important in the initiation of gouty arthritis, but most of the full-blown response we observe clinically is mediated by neutrophils. Synovial fluid aspirated during attacks of acute gout reveals neutrophil counts in the range typical for acute pyogenic septic arthritis. These classic acute inflammatory effector cells attach to the synovial vascular endothelium through their selectin ligands, then migrate through the synovium to the joint cavity aided by the chemotactic gradient. In addition to up-regulating the vascular endothelial adhesion molecules, TNFα primes the neutrophil for an amplified oxidative and degranulation response to crystals. Exposure to GM-CSF from the activated synovial macrophages also enhances neutrophil activation by opsonized crystals[82].

Neutrophils have a shorter half-life than any other circulating leukocyte. Unless they are activated, normal neutrophils soon die. The short lifespan of neutrophils and the ease with which they are activated artefactually during *in vitro* study makes the neutrophil a difficult cell to study, both in gout and in other inflammatory arthropathies. Inflammatory mediators, particularly colony stimulating factors, IL-1, IL-6, chemokines, and prostaglandins, prolong neutrophil survival by inhibit-

ing their usual spontaneous apoptosis[83]; there is conflicting data on the effects of TNF on neutrophil apoptosis.

Neutrophils within the synovial fluid avidly engulf urate crystals. Lysosomal enzymes then start to remove the protein coating the crystal has acquired in the synovial cavity. Restored to their naked state, the crystals have increased reactivity with proteins and membranes. Neutrophil activation is marked both by activation of phospholipases[87] and by inositol triphosphate production leading to a cytoplasmic calcium flux[88]. Urate crystals also induce leukotriene (LT) production[89].

Depending on their concentration and coating the crystals can then directly initiate lysis of the phagolysosomal membrane, spilling toxic lysosomal contents into the neutrophil cytoplasm[90,91]. The detailed molecular mechanisms for the interaction between the urate crystal surfaces and membranes have yet to be determined, but as discussed above include direct actions on lysosomal membrane lipids and glycoproteins[92].

Membrane lysis causes death of the neutrophil and releases the lysosomal contents and newly synthesized acute inflammatory mediators into the local microenvironment. Depending on the intensity of the response and on the size and number of joints affected, cytokines including IL-1, IL-6 and TNFα are produced in sufficient quantity to spill over into the circulation in sufficient amounts to stimulate a systemic acute phase response. Patients with acute gout are often systemically unwell, with fever and leucocytosis. The symptomatic response to COX-2 inhibitors suggests that prostanoids are prominent mediators of the extreme pain so characteristic of acute gout. Other pain mediators may include kinins, neuropeptides such as substance P, and mast cell products.

Major mediators of inflammation

This intense activation of both resident synoviocytes and immigrant phagocytes produces an imposing array of overlapping mediators, as detected in synovial fluids from acute gout and as mimicked following *in vitro* stimulation with urate microcrystals. Just as the majority of chemokines have yet to be fully examined for their potential role in gout, there are many other cytokines and nonprotein mediators whose known actions suggest they could play a role in aspects of gout. It is difficult to categorically ascribe elements of the acute gout flare syndrome to particular molecules unless selective inhibitors are exploited, analogous to confirming the key roles of prostanoids, IL-1 and TNFα in aspects of rheumatoid arthritis.

INTERCRITICAL AND CHRONIC GOUT

Termination of the acute attack

Even without medical intervention, acute gout is self-limiting. The classic attack resolves spontaneously within a week or two. The increase in vascular permeability once acute synovitis has begun allows increased entry of large molecules from plasma into the synovial compartment. The binding of Apo B to the crystals remaining in the joint may help terminate the attack[53,73]. Together with TGFβ and IL-10, induction of the nuclear hormone receptor PPARg and its ligand 15deoxy-PG12 by urate crystals helps reduce inflammation[93]. Other endogenous anti-inflammatory molecules have yet to be examined. Resolution of the acute attack may be aided by progressively more differentiated macrophages, in response to the cytokine milieu and as the neutrophils present undergo apoptosis and are themselves phagocytosed by mature macrophages[60].

Recurrent gout

The majority of patients with an episode of acute gout will have a further attack within a year, and 78% within 2 years. Other than the serum urate level, the risk factors for recurrence during this intercritical phase have not been studied in detail, but are likely to be the same as for the initial gout incidence. Hyperuricemia, synovial membrane microtophi and synovial fluid crystals persist in a large proportion of these patients. Despite their potent reactivity, urate crystals can be tolerated remarkably well within the synovial compartment for many months, without exciting an inflammatory response until other factors (see above) come into play.

Chronic gout

There is little information on the microscopic or molecular pathology of chronic gout, where clinically there is ongoing but often relatively low grade inflammation. Persistent nests of crystals are surrounded by a granuloma-like chronic inflammatory response, with fibrous tissue, macrophages, and giant cells. These macrophages show a relatively mature phenotype[41]. There may be a balance with anti-inflammatory mediators and a predominance of phagocytes with a less inflammatory phenotype.

MECHANISMS OF CLINICAL ASSOCIATIONS WITH GOUT

Many medical conditions have been associated with hyperuricemia and gout, with varying certainty as to the strength and mechanism of the association (Table 176.5). From a practical point of view the acquired 'lifestyle' conditions are particularly important, due to their potential for prevention or reversibility[94–98]. In most cases the link is via hyperuricemia rather than by modulating the thresholds for crystal formation or for triggering an inflammatory response from phagocytes. Many of these conditions contribute through both an enhanced production and a decreased excretion of urate.

A multiple regression analysis of the serum levels of leptin (the *ob* gene product elevated in obese subjects) in normal and diabetic individuals showed an independent association with urate levels[99], and it is possible that leptin also mediates an effect on renal urate handling. Some authors have included hyperuricemia as a manifestation of the metabolic Syndrome X of insulin resistance, obesity, hypertension, hyperlipidemia, and atherosclerosis. Hyperlipidemia, particularly with elevated triglycerides, is common in patients with gout. Triglyceride and cholesterol levels have been independently correlated with serum urate level[100–102], although it is difficult to fully separate their contributions from those of total caloric intake and obesity.

Hypertension

The association of hypertension with hyperuricemia and gout remains controversial. Uric acid concentrations increase with age, vascular disease, and obesity, diuretic and alcohol use. Hypertension reduces the renal excretion of urate[100,103] and increases adenine nucleotide turnover. Similarly, pre-eclampsia raises urate levels through both increased adenosine production and an effective reduction in blood volume, but in pregnant women the resulting hyperuricemia is not associated with gout.

It is uncertain whether hyperuricemia itself contributes to hypertension. Hyperuricemia *per se* is no longer believed to cause renal damage. Extreme hyperuricemia can lead to chronic urate nephropathy, with urate crystal deposition and microtophus formation in the medullary interstitium causing significant effects from inflammation, a giant cell reaction, and fibrosis[104,105]. Chronic urate nephropathy is now rare. Hyperuricemia has complex associations with glucose intolerance and cardiovascular disease[106–112].

Malignancy

Malignant hemopoietic cells can have a greatly increased rate of cell turnover and metabolic activity. The increased nucleic acid catabolism yields a marked increase in purines, and can lead to hyperuricemia and gout. In the tumor lysis syndrome aggressive cytotoxic chemotherapy regimens cause massive death of the malignant cells. The abrupt release of purines can cause sudden severe hyperuricemia. Uric acid crystals can form in the renal tubules and distal collecting system, causing an acute obstructive nephropathy. Acute elevations in potassium, phosphate, and lactate also contribute[113].

Drug influences

Many drugs reduce net renal urate excretion (Tables 176.6 & 176.7). The urate retention caused by diuretics is related both to dysfunction of tubular ion transport and to effective volume depletion. A reduction in effective blood volume enhances proximal tubular urate reabsorption[114,115], to the extent that urate clearance and serum urate level

---

TABLE 176.5 CONDITIONS ASSOCIATED WITH HYPERURICEMIA AND GOUT

Age

Male gender or postmenopausal

Direct causal link

- Bartter's and Gitelman's syndromes
- Glycogen storage diseases
- Hemolytic disorders
- Hemopoietic malignancies
- Lactic or keto acidosis
- Lead nephropathy, chronic low level lead exposure
- Pre-eclampsia*
- Renal impairment†
- Systemic inflammatory conditions (including psoriasis, RA‡)
- Vasopressin resistant diabetes insipidus

Associated disorders§

- Diabetes mellitus
- Hyperlipidemia
- Hyperparathyroidism
- Hypertension
- Hypothyroidism
- Obesity

Common precipitants of the acute attack

- Aggressive introduction of hypouricemic therapy
- Alcohol or shellfish binges
- Sepsis, myocardial infarction, other acute severe illness
- Sudden cessation of hypouricemic therapy
- Trauma, surgery, dehydration

* Hyperuricemia is a sensitive indicator both of effective volume status and of tubular dysfunction. † Uremia appears to blunt the inflammatory response to urate crystals, so that gout is less common that might be expected for a given degree of hyperuricemia. ‡ RA is associated with hyperuricemia but not gout. § A causal relationship has not been established with many of the associated disorders.

TABLE 176.6 DRUGS THAT WORSEN OR PRECIPITATE GOUT

- Aspirin (low dose)
- Cyclosporin
- Chemotherapeutic cytotoxics
- Diuretics (especially thiazides)
- Ethambutol
- Ethanol
- Levodopa
- Nicotinic acid
- Pyrazinamide
- Tacrolimus

TABLE 176.7 ROLE OF ALCOHOL IN GOUT

- Lactate competition for tubular transport
- Direct renal tubular effect?
- Hypertension
- Adenosine triphosphate turnover
- Guanosine content (beer)
- Poor hypouricemic compliance

are sensitive markers of volume status in clinical settings such as dehydration and pre-eclampsia.

By contrast some of the specific antagonists of the angiotensin II receptor (ATR) have modest uricosuric effects. This has been studied most with losartan, and is mainly mediated by direct inhibition of the renal tubular urate-anion exchange rather than being secondary to improved renal haemodynamics[116]. This is not a class effect common to all ATR antagonists, and in hypertensive patients the effect on serum uric acid levels is unlikely to be clinically significant in the face of gout[117]. Calcium channel antagonists have also been reported to augment renal excretion of uric acid in the post-allograft setting, but it is unclear whether this is because of a specific tubular action rather than improved renal blood flow[118]. Again the net effect is small.

Low-dose aspirin is well established as a contributor to decreased renal urate excretion. This effect is most marked in elderly patients with low circulating albumin levels. This same group of patients is often treated with thiazide diuretics.

Gout in transplant recipients

Gout is common and particularly difficult to manage in allograft recipients. The major factor is treatment with the calcineurin antagonists cyclosporin and tacrolimus. Up to 80% of cyclosporin treated patients become hyperuricemic. Around one in ten develop gout, although in one case series 28% were affected[119]. Allograft-associated gout is more likely to be tophaceous and extra-articular, as the steroid component of the immunosuppressive regimen delays overt inflammatory presentations until a large urate load has accumulated[115]. Most studies of calcineurin antagonists have implicated their effects on renal tubular handling of uric acid. As with thiazide diuretics there is disagreement on the contribution from tubular dysfunction. Other work has implicated reduced glomerular filtration and hemodynamic effects as the dominant factors at lower cyclosporin levels[114]. Similar problems have not been reported with sirolimus.

Transplant recipients pose many additional difficulties. Both renal and cardiac transplant patients are often treated with diuretics. The threshold for hypouricemic therapy might be accordingly lower in allograft recipients, and the case could be made for treatment of significant hyperuricemia before overt gout occurs. But the potential for adverse outcomes is high. Allopurinol inhibits the degradation of the purine drug azathioprine commonly used as part of the rejection prophylaxis regimen, and fatal bone marrow suppression has been reported despite careful reductions in azathioprine dose. Mycophenolate mofetil inhibits *de novo* purine synthesis and its metabolism is not affected by allopurinol. Cost considerations have worked against its more widespread use as an alternative to azathioprine.

Lead ingestion

Although classical lead-induced (*saturnine*) gout is now rare, chronic low-level exposure to lead has been studied as a potential risk factor for 'primary' gout. Chronic lead nephropathy should be considered when the degree of hyperuricemia is disproportionate to the reduction in

glomerular filtration, and is again related mainly to tubulointerstitial damage. A recent study of Chinese patients with chronic renal disease and gout demonstrated a marked improvement in urate clearance after four weeks of lead chelation with intravenous calcium-EDTA[120]. In most communities the levels involved are insufficient to have an impact on hyperuricemia and gout[121]. Nevertheless, careful enquiry will occasionally reveal a relevant domestic hobby or occupational exposure to lead.

MODELS FOR GOUT

Rodents, usually the most convenient source of arthritis animal models, do not suffer spontaneous gout. Mice with a homozygous targeted uric oxidase gene disruption have severe hyperuricemia. Half die before four weeks of age from renal failure due to intra-renal uric acid deposition[122] and the rest develop severe nephrogenic diabetes insipidus. Gouty synovitis is not a reported feature of the model.

HPRT-deficient mice have a normal phenotype. It was postulated that this is because rodents rely more on APRT than on HPRT for purine salvage. However, interbreeding HPRT and APRT knockout lines to produce mice completely deficient in both pathways (in an attempt to generate a model for Lesch–Nyhan syndrome) yielded animals with normal urate excretion rates and no overt behavioral changes[123].

Non-rodent animal models

Other species with spontaneous hyperuricemia have not provided good models for gout. One reason is that visceral urate deposition is more common than articular deposition with acute gout attacks in these animals. Genetically gout-prone strains of chicken have been reported[124], and have a selective defect in tubular urate excretion[125]. As in humans, the transport of urate across the tubular epithelium of gouty chickens utilizes an ion channel distinct from that for p-aminohippurate (PAH).

In Dalmatian dogs, urate deposition most commonly manifests as renal stone formation. As in man and in the uricase knockout mouse, renal impairment may suppress the inflammatory response to articular urate crystal deposition in this and other hyperuricemic animals. Crocodiles have been noted to suffer a spontaneous gouty arthritis of peripheral joints, especially with cooler environments, but have not had wide acceptance as a laboratory model.

Urate crystal injection

Uric acid crystals have been injected locally in several species, including rodents, pigs and man, and provoke a transient dose-dependent acute inflammatory response[64,75,76,126]. The 10–20mg doses of urate crystals used in earlier *in vivo* human experiments were sufficient to provoke severe inflammation with marked pain and a systemic acute phase response[127]. The intradermal injection of a more moderate dose of urate microcrystals (2.5mg or less) provokes a local acute inflammatory response, providing a safe and reasonably predictable model to study aspects of cell trafficking, inflammatory regulation and mediator release under controlled circumstances *in vivo*[128].

THE GENETICS OF GOUT

Gout is a disease of great antiquity. It is almost two millennia since Seneca first noted the familial nature. A positive family history has been reported in as few as 10% or as many as 80% of gout patients. This wide range suggests differences in the populations studied, the definitions used, or both. Obviously this depends on how vigorously such a history is pursued, and estimates from two large series were around 40%.

Gout is a genetically complex disease, with environmental factors required to exacerbate an underlying genetic predisposition. Assessing the relative contributions of genes and environment is difficult. There are many potential environmental contributors to hyperuricemia and gout that are hard to stratify for in family studies. For example, dietary habits are a strongly familial but non-genetic variable that may affect the intake of purine precursors, clinical expression of the metabolic syndrome, and renal tubular function. Nevertheless it has been possible to estimate that the heritable component of the serum uric acid level is around 40%, after adjusting for alcohol intake and body mass index[129]. By comparison with other common rheumatic diseases, the heritability of gout is at least as strong as that of RA, broadly in line with nodal osteoarthritis, but less marked than ankylosing spondylitis.

The genetic contribution to gout

It is likely that there is a polygenic component in most patients, although a predominant contribution from a single gene (for example a putative renal urate transporter mutation) cannot be eliminated[129]. Monozygotic twins show a tighter concordance than dizygotic for renal fractional urate clearance[130], consistent with a genetic contribution to the renal under-excretion component of hyperuricemia. There are many potential contributors to the genetics of gout (Table 176.8). Multi-case pedigrees are common, especially in ethnic groups with a high incidence of severe, young onset, hard-to-treat gout[131–137].

The genetic component of gout is mainly mediated through hyperuricemia, as the obvious biochemical precursor. Apart from the rare purine metabolic enzyme defects outlined above, the molecular basis of genetic hyperuricemia has not been delineated. The defective UOX gene is located at chromosome 1p22[138] but is not usually considered a 'disease gene' as the same lesion is common to all humans.

Polymorphism in metabolic genes

Although the predominant defect in most gout patients is at the level of renal urate excretion, part of the genetic influence may be through minor alterations in the activity of metabolic enzymes due to otherwise innocent polymorphisms. For example, genes involved in the metabolic syndrome may contribute to the genetic load for hyperuricemia and gout. The

Trp64Arg mutation in the β3 adrenergic receptor has been associated with central obesity, insulin resistance, and hypertension. In hyperuricemic Japanese patients this was no more frequent than in controls[139], whereas in a recent Italian study there was a significant association with this genotype[140]. A variety of glycolytic pathway polymorphisms have been implicated in a small groups of patients.

X chromosome genes

With the strong male predominance of gout it is tempting to speculate that a defective gene or genes on the X chromosome might be involved. As with HPRT mutations males, lacking the back-up 'normal' copy on the other X chromosome as in females, would bear the full brunt of such defects[141]. The increase in the incidence of gout in women after the menopause is in part due to increased diuretic use, but is also consistent with hormonal influences rather than a direct effect of an X chromosome gene. Urate clearance in women is up to 20% higher than in men, and exogenous estrogens given to transgender males raised the urate clearance by 20–30%.

A study of 61 postmenopausal Japanese women noted a significant reduction in serum urate levels with hormone replacement therapy[142], adding further support to the hormonal hypothesis. A recent analysis of urate levels in 196 families (obese but otherwise well, and stratified for body mass index) found no segregation of microsatellite markers with plasma urate levels[143]. At present there is no positive evidence for a direct role for X chromosome genes in most cases of gout.

Genes influencing crystals and inflammation

An individual's genetic propensity for gout at a given urate level could also be mediated by genetic factors influencing crystal formation or inflammatory trigger thresholds. For example, ApoE polymorphisms could influence the ability of the apolipoprotein to provide an anti-inflammatory coating for urate crystals. One study found no association between apolipoprotein phenotypes and gout overall[144]. The apo-E4 allele has been correlated with cholesterol and triglyceride levels in Japanese gout patients[145].

Numerous polymorphisms have been identified in the genes for inflammatory cytokines and their receptors[146], and one or more of these might modulate the inflammatory response to urate crystals. Many of these have been examined in RA and other chronic inflammatory conditions, but not yet studied in the context of gout.

Familial juvenile hyperuricemic nephropathy

Familial juvenile hyperuricemic or gouty nephropathy (FJHN, FJGN; OMIM 162 000) features an early onset of hyperuricemia followed by gout. Some authors regard the phenotype as an extreme form of classical gout. There is a reduced fractional clearance of uric acid, which precedes a more general decline in renal function[147]. In the later stages tubulointerstitial damage supervenes, although this does not seem to be due directly to intra-renal urate deposition. Progressive renal impairment develops by middle age. The pathogenesis remains unclear. Possible mechanisms include hyperuricemia as the underlying cause of the nephropathy; hyperuricemia consequent on impaired renal hemodynamics; or the most likely option, a primary defect in luminal anion exchange[148–150].

Although classically regarded as an autosomal dominant disorder, genetic heterogeneity and variable penetrance have been noted in FJHN. It is possible that a milder lesion in the same gene could contribute to the renal urate underexcretion common in primary gout. A locus for the FJHN gene was identified on chromosome 16p11.2–12[151–152]. Sequencing of candidate genes in patients from multicase families revealed that mutations in the gene coding for uromodulin (UMOD) were responsible both for type 2 autosomal dominant medullary cystic kidney disease and for FJHN[153].

TABLE 176.8 POSSIBLE GENETIC FACTORS IN GOUT

Genetic influence mainly via hyperuricemia	Purine metabolic enzymes Renal excretion
Crystallization seeds, promoters, inhibitors	Inflammation threshold Phagocyte activation Endogenous anti-inflammatory mediators
Well characterized examples	Abnormalities in APRT, HPRT, PRS enzyme genes
Associated syndromes with genetic component	Obesity Insulin resistance Tubulointerstitial disorders
Candidate genes and loci	16p11.2–12/uromodulin Apolipoprotein polymorphisms Cytokine and cytokine receptor polymorphisms hUAT1, hUAT2, hOAT3 transporter genes Metabolic (purine and glycolytic) enzyme polymorphisms Other (unknown) renal organic anion transporters?

The strong familial nature of gout has been recognized since the 1st century AD. Despite the obvious contributions of environmental factors such as diet and alcohol, heredity is thought to contribute substantially (40%) to urate levels. The defect in renal urate handling that underlies gout in most patients may have a genetic basis, perhaps in the gene coding for a tubular urate transporter.

SUMMARY

Acute gouty arthritis results from the inflammatory response to urate microcrystals, which have formed on a background of hyperuricemia and urate supersaturation. Major steps in the pathogenesis are the accumulation of excessive urate, the formation of urate microcrystals, and the attraction and activation of susceptible phagocytes.

Mutations in purine metabolic enzymes such as HPRT are a rare but well characterized cause of an excessive urate load. The more common situation is a dietary excess of purine precursors on a background of inadequate renal tubular urate excretion. Associated disorders are frequent in industrialized societies and contribute to both purine supply and renal under-excretion. Most of the drugs causing hyperuricemia do so by reducing renal urate excretion.

Urate microcrystals are potent stimulators of acute inflammation response, although this depends on the coat of the crystal and state of the responding cell. Macrophages and possibly mast cells are stimulated first followed by the influx and activation of neutrophils, leading to a diverse array of potent proinflammatory mediators. Intradermal urate crystal injection provides a useful *in vivo* human inflammatory model.

The genetic contribution to gout is thought to be mainly through hyperuricemia, but genes affecting the inflammatory threshold may also play a role. Although there has been great progress towards unraveling the pathogenesis of gout there are still many unresolved issues (Table 176.9). In clinical practice this 'easy' disease often proves difficult.

TABLE 176.9 SOME ISSUES IN THE PATHOGENESIS OF GOUT, 2003

- Causal component of the association with ischemic heart disease?
- Endogenous anti-inflammatory responses?
- Genetic basis of gout: Oligo- or polygenic?
  Which gene(s)?
  Same in Polynesians and Filipino gout?
- How much do the renal effects of insulin and leptin contribute?
- Importance of the anti-oxidant role of uric acid?
- Inhibitors and promoters of crystal formation and of crystal phagocytosis?
- Molecular characterization of renal urate transport
- Relative contributions of the hemodynamic and direct tubular effects of drugs affecting urate excretion
- What are the dominant cytokines, chemokine(s), other mediators?
- Why are renal impairment and rheumatoid arthritis 'protective'?
- Why is acute gout so painful?
- How does acute gout resolve spontaneously?

REFERENCES

1. Ames BN, Cathcart R, Schiviers E, Hochstein P. Uric acid provides an anti-oxidant defense in humans against oxidant and radicals causing aging and cancer: a hypothesis. Proc Natl Acad Sci USA 1981; 78: 6858–6862.
2. Dunn JP, Brooks GW, Mausner J et al. Social class gradient of serum uric acid levels in males. JAMA 1963; 185: 431–436.
3. Campion EW, Glynn RJ, De Labry LO. Asymptomatic hyperuricemia. Am J Med 1987; 82: 421–426.
4. Lin KC, Lin HY, Chou P. The interaction between uric acid level and other risk factors on the development of gout among asymptomatic hyperuricemic men in a prospective study. J Rheumatol 2000; 27: 1501–1505.
5. Coe FL, Moran E, Kavalich AG. The contribution of dietary purine over-consumption to hyperuricosuria in calcium oxalate stone formers. J Chron Dis 1976; 29: 793–800.
6. Stryer L. Biochemistry. New York: Freeman; 1995.
7. Chambers DE, Parks DA, Patterson G et al. Xanthine oxidase as a source of free radical damage in myocardial ischemia. J Mol Cell Cardiol 1985; 17: 145–152.
8. Stevens CR, Benboubetra M, Harrison R et al. Localisation of xanthine oxidase to synovial endothelium. Ann Rheum Dis 1991; 50: 760–762.
9. Blake DR, Merry P, Unsworth J et al. Hypoxic–reperfusion injury in the inflamed human joint. Lancet 1989; 1: 289–293.
10. Wu X, Lee CC, Muzny DM, Caskey CT. Urate oxidase: primary structure and evolutionary implications. Proc Natl Acad Sci USA 1989; 86: 9412–9416.
11. Goldman SC, Holcenberg JS, Finklestein JZ et al. A randomized comparison between rasburicase and allopurinol in children with lymphoma or leukemia at high risk for tumor lysis. Blood 2001; 97: 2998–3003.
12. Davis S, Park Y, Abuchowwski A, Davis F. Hypouricaemic effect of polyethyleneglycol modified urate oxidase. Lancet 1981; 1.
13. Seegmiller JE, Rosenbloom RM, Kelley WN. An enzyme defect associated with a sex-linked human neurologic disorder and excessive purine synthesis. Science 1967; 155: 1682–1684.
14. Kelley WN, Rosenbloom EM, Henderson JF, Seegmiller JE. A specific enzyme defect in gout associated with overproduction of uric acid. Proc Natl Acad Sci USA 1967; 57: 1735–1739.
15. Jinnah HA, De Gregorio L, Harris JC et al. The spectrum of inherited mutations causing HPRT deficiency: 75 new cases and a review of 196 previously reported cases. Mut Res 2000; 463: 309–326.
16. Curto R, Voit EO, Cascante M. Analysis of abnormalities in purine metabolism leading to gout and to neurological dysfunctions in man. Biochem J 1998; 329: 477–487.
17. Eads JC, Scapin G, Xu Y, Grubmeyer C, Sacchettini JC. The crystal structure of human hypoxanthine–guanine phosphoribosyltransferase with bound GMP. Cell 1994; 78: 325–334.
18. Balendiran GK, Molina JA, Xu Y et al. Ternary complex structure of human HGPRTase, PRPP, Mg²⁺, and the inhibitor HPP reveals the involvement of the flexible loop in substrate binding. Prot Sci 1999; 8: 1023–1031.
19. Kamatani N, Hakoda M, Otsuka S et al. Only three mutations account for almost all defective alleles causing adenine phosphoribosyltransferase deficiency in Japanese patients. J Clin Invest 1992; 90: 130–135.
20. Sperling O, Eilam G, Persky-Brosh S, De Vries A. Accelerated erythrocyte 5-phosphoribosyl-1-pyrophosphate synthesis. A familial abnormality associated with excessive uric acid production and gout. Biochem Med 1972; 6: 310–316.
21. Ahmed M, Taylor W, Smith PR, Becker MA. Accelerated transcription of PRPS1 in X-linked overactivity of normal human phosphoribosylphosphate synthetase. J Biol Chem 1999; 274: 7482–7488.
22. Seegmiller JE, Dixon RM, Kemp GJ. Fructose-induced aberration of metabolism in familial gout identified by 31P magnetic resonance spectroscopy. Proc Natl Acad Sci USA 1990; 87: 8326–8330.
23. Vaziri ND, Freel RW, Hatch M. Effect of chronic experimental renal insufficiency on urate metabolism. J Am Soc Nephrol 1995; 64: 1313–1317.
24. Moriwaki Y, Yamamoto T, Higashino K. Enzymes involved in purine metabolism – a review of histochemical localization and functional implications. Histol Histopathol 1999; 14: 1321–1340.
25. Bantia S, Miller PJ, Parker CD, Ananth SL. Purine nucleoside phosphorylase inhibitor BXC-1777 (Immucillin-H): a novel potent and orally active immunosuppressive agent. Internat Immunopharmacol 2001; 1: 1199–1210.
26. Montesinos MC, Desai A, Delano D et al. Adenosine A2A or A3 receptors are required for inhibition of inflammation by methotrexate or its analog MX-68. Arthrit Rheum 2003; 48: 240–247.
27. Sorenson LB, Levinson DJ. Origin and extrarenal elimination of uric acid in man. Nephron 1975; 14: 7–20.
28. Simkin PA. When, why, and how should we quantify the excretion rate of urinary uric acid? J Rheumatol 2001; 28: 1207–1210.
29. Levinson DJ, Sorensen LB. Renal handling of uric acid in normal and gouty subjects: evidence for a 4-component system. Ann Rheum Dis 1980; 39: 173–179.
30. Maesaka JK, Fishbane S. Regulation of renal urate excretion: a critical review. Am J Kid Dis 1998; 32: 917–933.
31. Race JE, Grassl SM, Williams WJ, Holtzman EJ. Molecular cloning and characterization of two novel human renal organic anion transporters (hOAT1 and hOAT3). Biochem Biophys Res Comm 1999; 255: 508–514.
32. Cha SH, Sekine T, Fukushima JI et al. Identification and characterization of human organic anion transporter 3 expressing predominantly in the kidney. Mol Pharmacol 2001; 59: 1277–1286.
33. Lipkowitz MS, Leal-Pinto E, Rappoport JZ, Najfeld V, Abramson RG. Functional reconstitution, membrane targeting, genomic structure, and chromosomal localization of a human urate transporter. J Clin Investig 2001; 107: 1103–1115.
34. Wilcox WR, Khalef A. Nucleation of monosodium urate crystals. Ann Rheum Dis 1975; 34: 332–339.
35. Dieppe PA, Doherty M. The role of particles in the pathogenesis of joint disease. Curr Topic Pathol 1982; 71: 199–233.
36. McGill NW, Dieppe PA. Evidence for a promoter of urate crystal formation in gouty synovial fluid. Ann Rheum Dis 1991; 50: 558–561.
37. Simkin PA, Pizzorno JE. Transynovial exchange of small molecules in normal human subjects. J Appl Physiol 1974; 36: 581–587.
38. Kam M, Perl-Treves D, Caspi D. Antibodies against crystals. FASEB J 1992; 6: 2608–2613.
39. Gross M. Crystallographic antibodies. Nature 1995; 373: 105–106.
40. Perl-Treves D, Kam M, Addadi L. Interaction between antibodies and crystal surfaces. Mol Cryst Liq Cryst 1996; 278: 1–15.
41. Palmer DG, Highton J, Hessian PA. Development of the gout tophus. Am J Clin Pathol 1989; 91: 190–195.
42. McLeod J. Gout and fibrositis in cold weather. Med J Aust 1972; 1: 943.

43. Schlesinger N, Gowin KM, Baker DG *et al*. Acute gouty arthritis is seasonal. 1998; 25: 342–344.

44. Gallerani M, Govoni M, Mucinelli M *et al*. Seasonal variation in the onset of acute microcrystalline arthritis. Rheumatology 1999; 38: 1003–1006.

45. Geborek P, Saxne T, Petterson H, Wollheim FA. Synovial fluid acidosis correlates with radiological joint destruction in rheumatoid arthritis knee joints. J Rheumatol 1989; 16: 468–472.

46. Agudelo C, Schumacher HR. The synovitis of acute gouty arthritis. Hum Pathol 1973; 4: 265–279.

47. Schumacher HR. Pathology of crystal deposition disease. Rheum Dis Clin North Am 1988; 14: 269–288.

48. Weinberger A, Schumacher HR, Agudelo CA. Urate crystals in asymptomatic metatarsophalangeal joints. Ann Intern Med 1979; 91: 56–57.

49. Bomalaski JJ, Lluberas G, Schumacher HR. Monosodium urate crystals in the knee joints of patients with asymptomatic nontophaceous gout. Arthrit Rheum 1986; 39: 1480–1484.

50. Horowitz MD, Abbey L, Sirota DK. Intraarticular noninflammatory free urate suspension (urate milk) in three patients with painful joints. J Rheumatol 1990; 17: 712–714.

51. Terkeltaub R, Tenner AJ, Kozin F. Plasma protein binding by monosodium urate crystals: analysis by two-dimensional gel electropheresis. Arthrit Rheum 1983; 26: 775–783.

52. Doherty M, Whicher JT, Dieppe PA. Activation of the alternative pathway of complement by monosodium urate monohydrate crystals and other inflammatory particles. Ann Rheum Dis 1983; 42: 285–291.

53. Terkeltaub R, Martin J, Curtiss L. Apoliproprotein B mediates the capacity of low density lipoprotein to suppress neutrophil stimulation by particulates. J Biol Chem 1986; 261: 15662–15667.

54. Terkeltaub R, Dyer C, Martin J. Apolipoprotein E (apo E) inhibits the capacity of monosodium urate crystals to stimulate neutrophils: characterization of intraarticular aop E and demonstration of apo E binding to urate crystals *in vivo*. J Clin Invest 1991; 87: 20–26.

55. Gordon TP, Bertouch JV, Walsh BR, Brooks PM. Monosodium urate crystals in asymptomatic knee joints. J Rheumatol 1982; 9: 967–969.

56. Pascual E, Batlle Gualda E, Martinez A *et al*. Synovial fluid analysis for diagnosis of intercritical gout. Ann Inter Med 1999; 131: 756–759.

57. Ortiz-Bravo E, Sieck MS, Schumacher HR. Changes in the proteins coating monosodium urate crystals during active and subsiding inflammation. Immunogold studies of synovial fluid from patients with gout and of fluid obtained using the rat subcutaneous air pouch model. Arthrit Rheum 1993; 36: 1274–1285.

58. Pascual E, Jovani V. A quantitative study of the phagocytosis of urate crystals in the synovial fluid of asymptomatic joints of patients with gout. Brit J Rheumatol 1995; 34: 724–726.

59. Yagnik DR, Hillyer P, Marshall D *et al*. Noninflammatory phagocytosis of monosodium urate monohydrate crystals by mouse macrophages. Implications for the control of joint inflammation in gout. Arthrit Rheum 2000; 43: 1779–1789.

60. Haskard DO, Landis RC. Interactions between leukocytes and endothelial cells in gout: lessons from a self-limiting inflammatory disease. Arthritis Res 2002; 4 (suppl 3): 91–97.

61. Rizzoli AJ, Trujeque L, Bankhurst AD. The coexistence of gout and rheumatoid arthritis. J Rheumatol 1980; 7: 316–324.

62. Atdjian M, Fernandez-Madrid F. Coexistence of chronic tophaceous gout and rheumatoid arthritis. J Rheumatol 1981; 8: 989–992.

63. Gordon TP, Ahern MJ, Reid C, Roberts-Thomson PJ. Studies on the interaction of rheumatoid factor with monosodium urate crystals and case report of coexistent tophaceous gout and rheumatoid arthritis. Ann Rheum Dis 1985; 44: 384–389.

64. Dieppe PA, Doherty M, Papadimitriou GM. Inflammatory responses to intradermal crystals in healthy volunteers and patients with rheumatic diseases. Rheumatol Int 1982; 2: 55–58.

65. Schreiner O, Wandel E, Himmelsbach F *et al*. Reduced secretion of proinflammatory cytokines of monosodium urate crystal-stimulated monocytes in chronic renal failure: an explanation for infrequent gout episodes in chronic renal failure patients? Nephrol, Dial, Transplant 2000; 15: 644–649.

66. Barabe F, Gilbert C, Liao N. Crystal-induced neutrophil activation VI: involvement of Fc gamma RIII PMN (CD16) and CD11b in response to inflammatory microcrystals. FASEB J. 1998; 12: 209–220.

67. Gaudry M, Gilbert C, Barabe F *et al*. Activation of *lyn* is a common element of the stimulation of human neutrophils by soluble and particulate agonists. Blood 1995; 86: 3567–3574.

68. Burt HM, Jackson JK, Salari H. Inhibition of crystal-induced neutrophil activation by a protein tyrosine kinase inhibitor. J Leuk Biol 1994; 55: 112–119.

69. Pouliot M, James MJ, McColl SR *et al*. Monosodium urate microcrystals induce cyclooxygenase-2 in human monocytes. Blood 1998; 91: 1769–1776.

70. Liu R, O'Connell M, Johnson K *et al*. Extracellular signal-regulated kinase-1/extracellular signal-regulated kinase-2 mitogen-activated protein kinase signaling and activation of activator protein-1 and nuclear factor kB transcription factors play central roles in interleukin-8 expression stimulated by monosodium urate monohydrate and calcium pyrophosphate crystals in monocytic cells. Arthrit Rheum 2000; 43: 1145–1155.

71. Di Giovine FS, Malawista SE, Nuki G. Interleukin-1 (IL-1) as a mediator of crystal arthritis: stimulation of T cell and synovial fibroblast mitogenesis by urate crystal-induced IL-1. J Immunol 1987; 138: 3213–3218.

72. Guerne PA, Terkeltaub R, Zuraw B, Lotz M. Inflammatory microcrystals stimulate interleukin-6 production and secretion by human monocytes and synoviocytes. Arthrit Rheum 1989; 32: 1443–1452.

73. Terkeltaub R, Zachariae C, Santoro D *et al*. Monocyte-derived neutrophil chemotactic factor/IL-8 is a potential mediator of crystal-induced inflammation. Arthrit Rheum 1991; 34: 894–903.

74. Di Giovine FS, Malawista SE, Thornton E, Duff GW. Urate crystals stimulate production of tumor necrosis factor alpha from human blood monocytes and synovial cells. J Clin Invest 1991; 78: 1375–1381.

75. Chapman PT, Jamar F, Harrison AA *et al*. Characterisation of E-selectin expression, leucocyte traffic and clinical sequelae in urate crystal-induced inflammation: an insight into gout. Rheumatology 1996; 35: 323–334.

76. Terkeltaub R, Baird S, Sears P *et al*. The murine homolog of the interleukin-8 receptor CXCR-2 is essential for the occurrence of neutrophilic inflammation in the air pouch model of acute urate crystal-induced gouty synovitis. Arthrit Rheum 1998; 41: 900–909.

77. Murphy PM, Baggiolini M, Charo IF *et al*. International Union of Pharmacology. XXII. Nomenclature for chemokine receptors. Pharmacol Rev 2000; 52: 145–176.

78. Kabarowski JHS, Zhu K, Le LQ *et al*. Lysophosphatidylcholine as a ligand for the immunoregulatory receptor G2A. Science 2001; 293: 702–704.

79. Oliviero F, Schiltz C, Champy R *et al*. Effect of monosodium urate crystals on nitric oxide pathway. Arthrit Rheum 2001; 44: S129.

80. Ganster RW, Taylor BS, Shao L, Geller DA. Complex regulation of human inducible nitric oxide synthase gene transcription by Stat 1 and NF-kB. Proc Natl Acad Sci USA 2001; 98: 8638–8643.

81. Squadrito GL, Cueto R, Splenser AE *et al*. Reaction of uric acid with peroxynitrite and implications for the mechanism of neuroprotection by uric acid. Arch Biochem Biophys 2000; 376: 333–337.

82. Burt HM, Jackson JK. The priming action of tumour necrosis factor-alpha (TNF-a) and granulocyte–macrophage colony-stimulating factor (GM–CSF) on neutrophils activated by inflammatory microcrystals. Clin Exp Immunol 1997; 108: 432–437.

83. Coletta F, Re F, Pollentarutti N *et al*. Modulation of granulocyte survival and programmed cell death by cytokines and bacterial products. Blood 1992; 80: 2012–2020.

84. Akahoshi T, Nagaoka T, Namai R *et al*. Prevention of neutrophil apoptosis by monosodium urate crystals. Rheumatol Int 1997; 16: 231–235.

85. Tudan C, Fong D, Duronio V *et al*. The inhibition of spontaneous and tumor necrosis factor-alpha induced neutrophil apoptosis by crystals of calcium pyrophosphate dihydrate and monosodium urate monohydrate. J Rheumatol 2000; 27: 2463–2472.

86. Hamilton JA, McCarthey G, Whitty G. Inflammatory microcrystals induce murine macrophage survival and DNA synthesis. Arthritis Research 2001; 3: 242–246.

87. Bomalaski JS, Baker DG, Brophy LM, Clark MA. Monosodium urate crystals stimulate phospholipase A2 enzyme avtivities and the synthesis of a phospholipase A2-activating protein. J Immunol 1990; 145: 3391–3397.

88. Onello E, Traynor-Kaplan A, Sklar L, Terkeltaub R. Mechanism of neutrophil activation by an unopsonized inflammatory particulate: monosodium urate crystals induce pertussis toxin-insensitive hydrolysis of phosphatidylinositol 4,5-biphosphate. J Immunol 1991; 146: 4289–4299.

89. Serhan CN, Lundberg U, Weissman G, Samuelsson B. Formation of leukotrienes and hydroxy acids by human neutrophils and platelets exposed to monosodium urate. Prostaglandins 1984; 27: 563.

90. Schumacher HR, Phelps P. Sequential changes in human polymorphonuclear leukocytes after urate crystal phagocytosis. Arthrit Rheum 1971; 14: 513–526.

91. Shirahama T, Cohen AS. Ultra-structural evidence for leakage of lysosomal contents after phagocytosis of monosodium urate crystals. Am J Pathol 1974; 76: 501–520.

92. Burt HM, Jackson JK. Role of membrane proteins in monosodium urate crystal-membrane interactions. II. Effect of pretreatments of erythrocyte membranes with membrane permeable and impermeable protein crosslinking agents. J Rheumatol 1990; 17: 1359–1363.

93. Akahoshi T, Namai R, Murakami Y *et al*. Rapid induction of peroxisome proliferator-activated receptor g expression in human monocytes by monosodium urate monohydrate crystals. Arthrit Rheum 2003; 48: 231–239.

94. Wingrove CS, Walton C, Stevenson JC. The effect of menopause on serum uric acid levels in non-obese healthy women. Metabol Clin Exper 1998; 47: 435–438.

95. Faller F, Fox IH. Ethanol-induced hyperuricemia: evidence for increased urate production by activation of adenine nucleotide turnover. N Engl J Med 1982; 307: 1598–1602.

96. Emmerson BT. Alteration of urate metabolism by weight reduction. Aust NZ J Med 1973; 3: 410–412.

97. Yamashita S, Matsuzawa Y, Tokunaga K *et al*. Studies on the impaired metabolism of uric acid in obese subjects: marked reduction of renal urate excretion and its improvement by a low-calorie diet. Int J Obesity 1986; 10: 255–264.

98. Ter Maaten JC, Voorburg A, Heine RJ *et al*. Renal handling of urate and sodium during acute physiological hyperinsulinaemia in healthy subjects. Clin Sci 1997; 92: 51–58.

99. Fruehwald Schultes B, Peters A, Kern W *et al*. Serum leptin is associated with serum uric acid concentrations in humans. Metabol Clin Exper 1999; 48: 677–680.

100. Emmerson BT. Abnormal urate excretion associated with renal and systemic disorders, drugs, toxins. In: Weiner IM, ed. Uric acid (Handbook Exp Pharm, vol 51). Berlin: Springer Verlag, 1978: 287–324.

101. Nakanishi N, Suzuki K, Kawashimo H *et al*. Serum uric acid: correlation with biological, clinical and behavioral factors in Japanese men. J Epidemiol 1999; 9: 99–106.

102. Chu NF, Wang DJ, Liou SH, Shieh SM. Relationship between hyperuricemia and other cardiovascular disease risk factors among adult males in Taiwan. Eur J Epidemiol 2000; 16: 13–7.

103. Messerli FH, Frohlich ED, Dreslinski GR *et al*. Serum uric acid in essential hypertension: an indication of renal vascular involvement. Ann Intern Med 1980; 93: 817–821.

104. Johnson RJ, Kivlign SD, Kim YG *et al*. Reappraisal of the pathogenesis and consequences of hyperuricemia in hypertension, cardiovascular disease, and renal disease. Am J Kid Dis 1999; 33: 225–234.

105. Tarng D-C, Lin H-Y, Shong M-L *et al*. Renal function in gout patients. Am J Nephrol 1995; 15: 31–37.

106. Fang J, Alderman MH. Serum uric acid acid and cardiovascular mortality. The NHANES I epidemiologic follow-up study, 1971–1992. J Am Med Assoc 2000; 283: 2404–2410.

107. Culleton BF, Larson MG, Kannel WB, Levy D. Serum uric acid and risk for cardiovascular disease and death: the Framingham Heart Study. Ann Intern Med 1999; 131: 7–13.

108. Herman JB, Goldbourt U. Uric acid and diabetes: observations in a population study. Lancet 1982; 2: 240–241.

109. Chou P, Lin K-C, Lin H-Y, Tsai S-T. Gender differences in the relationships of serum uric acid with fasting serum insulin and plasma glucose in patients without diabetes. J Rheumatol 2001; 28: 571–576.

110. Facchini F, Chen Y-D, Hollenbeck CB, Reaven GM. Relationship between resistance to insulin-mediated glucose uptake, urinary uric acid clearance, and uric acid concentration. J Am Med Assoc 1991; 266: 3008–3011.

111. Rathmann W, Funkhauser E, Dyer C, Roseman JM. Relations of hyperuricemia and the various components of the insulin resistance syndrome in young black and white adults: the CARDIA study. Coronary artery risk development in young adults. Ann Epidemiol 1998; 8: 250–261.

112. Clausen JO, Borch-Johnsen K, Ibsen H, Pedersen O. Analysis of the relationship between fasting serum uric acid and the insulin sensitivity index in a population-based sample of 380 young healthy Caucasians. Eur J Epidemiol 1998; 138: 63–69.

113. Andreoli SP, Clark JH, McGuire WA, Bergstein JM. Purine excretion during tumor lysis in children with acute lymphoblastic leukemia receiving allopurinol: relationship to acute renal failure. J Paediat 1986; 109: 292–298.

114. Hansen JM, Fogh-Andersen N, Leyssac PF, Strandgaard S. Glomerular and tubular function in renal transplant patients treated with and without ciclosporin A. Nephron 1998; 80: 450–457.

115. Clive DM. Renal transplant-associated hyperuricemia and gout. J Am Soc Nephrol 2000; 11: 974–979.

116. Edwards RM, Trizna W, Stack E, Weinstock J. Interaction of nonpeptide angiotensin II receptor antagonists with the urate transporter in rat renal brush–border membranes. J Pharmacol Exp Ther 1996; 276: 125–129.

117. Puig JG, Mateos FA, Buno A et al. Effect of eprosartan and losarten on uric acid metabolism in patients with essential hypertension. J Hypertens 1999; 17: 1033–1039.

118. Zawadzki J, Grenda R, Januszewicz P. Effect of nifedipine on tubular handling of uric acid in transplanted kidney on cyclosporine A treatment. Nephron 1995; 70: 77–82.

119. Delaney V, Sumrani N, Daskalakis P et al. Hyperuricemia and gout in renal allograft recipients. Transplant Proc 1992; 24: 1773–1774.

120. Lin J-L, Yu C-C, Lin-Tan D-T, Ho H-H. Lead chelation therapy and urate excretion in patients with chronic renal diseases and gout. Kidney Int 2001; 60: 266–271.

121. Shadick NA, Kim R, Weiss S et al. Effect of low level lead exposure on hyperuricemia and gout among middle aged and elderly men: the normative aging study. J Rheumatol 2000; 27: 1708–1712.

122. Wu X, Wakamiya M, Geske R et al. Hyperuricemia and urate nephropathy in urate oxidase-deficient mice. Proc Natl Acad Sci USA 1994; 91: 742–746.

123. Engle SJ, Womer DE, Davies PM et al. HPRT–APRT-deficient mice are not a model for Lesch–Nyhan syndrome. Hum Mol Genet 1996; 5: 1607–1610.

124. Peterson DW, Hamilton WH, Lilyblade AL. Hereditary susceptibility to dietary induction of gout in selected lines of chickens. J Nutr 1971; 101: 347–354.

125. Zmuda MJ, Quebbemann AJ. Localization of renal tubular uric acid transport defect in gouty chickens. Am J Physiol 1975; 229: 820–825.

126. Faires JS, McCarty DJ. Acute arthritis in man and dog after intrasynovial injection of sodium urate crystals. Lancet 1962; 2: 682–685.

127. Hutton CW, Collins AJ, Chambers RE et al. Systemic response to local crystal induced inflammation in man: a possible model to study the acute phase response. Ann Rheum Dis 1985; 44: 533–536.

128. Pickering MC, Haskard DO. Behcet's syndrome. J R Coll Phys Lond 2000; 34: 169–177.

129. Wilk JB, Djousse L, Borecki I et al. Segregation analysis of serum uric acid in the NHLBI family heart study. Hum Genet 2000; 106: 355–359.

130. Emmerson BT, Nagal SL, Duffy DL, Martin NG. Genetic control of the renal clearance of urate: a study of twins. Ann Rheum Dis 1992; 51: 375–377.

131. Gibson T, Waterworth R, Hatfield P et al. Hyperuricaemia, gout and kidney function in New Zealand Maori men. Brit J Rheumatol 1984; 23: 276–282.

132. Prior IAM, Welby TJ, Ostbye T et al. Migration and gout: the Tokelau Island migration study. Brit Med J 1987; 295: 457–461.

133. Klemp P, Stansfield SA, Castle B, Robertson MC. Gout is on the increase in New Zealand. Ann Rheum Dis 1997; 56: 22–26.

134. Chang SJ, Ko YC, Wang TN et al. High prevalence of gout and related risk factors in Taiwan's aborigines. J Rheumatol 1997; 24: 1364–1369.

135. Healey LA. The epidemiology of Filipino hyperuricaemia. In: Holers VM, ed. Gout, hyperuricaemia, and other crystal-associated arthropathies. New York: Marcel Dekker, 1999; 121–126.

136. Chou TC, Chao PM. Lipid abnormalities in Taiwan aborigines with gout. Metabolism 1999; 48: 131–133.

137. McKinney K, Abu-Maree M, Dalbeth N et al. Genes for gout in New Zealand Maori and Pacific people. NZ Med J 2001; 114: 319.

138. Yeldandi AV, Patel YD, Liao M et al. Localization of the human urate oxidase gene (UOX) to 1p22. Cytogenet Cell Genet 1992; 61: 121–122.

139. Hayashi H, Nagasaka S, Ishikawa S-E et al. Contribution of a missense mutation (Trp64Arg) in b3-adrenergic receptor gene to the multiple risk factors in Japanese men with hyperuricemia. Endo J 1998; 45: 779–784.

140. Strazzullo P, Iacone R, Siani A et al. Relationship of the Trp64Arg polymorphism of the beta3-adrenoceptor gene to central adiposity and high blood pressure: interaction with age. Cross-sectional and longitudinal findings of the Olivetti prospective heart study. J Hypertens 2001; 19: 399–406.

141. Chang SJ, Chang JG, Chen CJ et al. Identification of a new single nucleotide substitution on the hypoxanthine-guanine phosphoribosyltransferase gene (HPRT Tsou) from a Taiwanese aboriginal family with severe gout. J Rheumatol 1999; 26: 1802–1807.

142. Sumino H, Ichikawa S, Kanda T et al. Reduction of serum uric acid by hormone replacement therapy in postmenopausal women with hyperuricaemia. Lancet 1999; 354: 650.

143. Reed DR, Price RA. X-linkage does not account for the absence of father–son similarity in plasma uric acid concentrations. Am J Med Genet 2000; 92: 142–146.

144. Moriwaki Y, Yamamoto T, Takahashi S et al. Apolipoprotein E phenotypes in patients with gout: relation with hypertriglyceridaemia. Ann Rheum Dis 1995; 54: 351–354.

145. Takahashi S, Yamamoto T, Moriwaki Y et al. Increased concentrations of serum Lp(a) lipoprotein in patients with primary gout. Ann Rheum Dis 1995; 54: 90–93.

146. Bidwell J, Keen L, Gallagher G et al. Cytokine gene polymorphism in human disease: on-line databases (suppl 1). Gene Immun 2001; 2: 61–70.

147. Moro F, Ogg CS, Simmonds HA et al. Familial juvenile gouty nephropathy with renal urate hypoexcretion preceding renal disease. Clin Nephrol 1991; 35: 263–269.

148. Puig JG, Miranda ME, Mateos FA et al. Hereditary nephropathy associated with hyperuricemia and gout. Arch Intern Med 1993; 153: 357–365.

149. McBride MB, Rigden S, Haycock GB et al. Presymptomatic detection of familial juvenile hyperuricaemic nephropathy in children. Pediatr Nephrol 1998; 12: 357–364.

150. Lhotta K, Gruber J, Sgonc R et al. Apoptosis of tubular epithelial cells in familial juvenile gouty nephropathy. Nephron 1998; 79: 340–344.

151. Stiburkova B, Majewski J, Sebesta I et al. Familial juvenile hyperuricemic nephropathy: localization of the gene on chromosome 16p11.2 and evidence for genetic heterogeneity. Am J Hum Genet 2000; 66: 1989–1994.

152. Kamatani N, Moritani M, Yamanaka H et al. Localization of a gene for familial juvenile hyperuricemic nephropathy causing underexcretion-type gout to 16p12 by genome-wide linkage analysis of a large family. Arthrit Rheum 2000; 43: 925–929.

153. Hart TC, Gorry MC, Hart PS et al. Mutations of the UMOD gene are responsible for medullary cystic disease 2 and familial juvenile hyperuricaemic nephropathy. J Med Genet 2002; 39: 882–892.

177 Clinical features of gout

Terry Gibson

Clinical features

- Abrupt initial onset involving, most commonly, big toe, ankle or other joints of foot
- Upper limbs are affected in chronic tophaceous or recurrent acute gout, especially the distal interphalangeal joint
- Men in middle life who are obese and drink alcohol regularly are the most susceptible
- Women when affected are most commonly on diuretics or heavy alcohol drinkers
- There are associations with hypertension, hypertriglyceridemia and mild renal impairment
- HPRT deficiency, PRPP synthetase overactivity or hereditable renal disease should be suspected in children, adolescents or young adults with gout

HISTORICAL BACKGROUND

The common concept of gout comprises an image of a stout, portly gentleman of substance with his foot elevated on a stool and a glass of alcoholic beverage and a table heavy with food near at hand. In 19th century England, this image of 'aldermanic' gout was perpetuated by satirical and political illustrators who wished to lampoon royalty and politicians. The picture of male predominance and an indirect association with excess of wine was recognized much earlier by Hippocrates in his aphorisms. The nature of gout and tophi was discussed in the first and second centuries by Celsus, Galen and Aretaeus the Cappadocian. Pliny and Seneca noted the absence of gout in the early period of the Roman republic, viewing it as a sign of decadence and debauchery in the empire of the first century. A succession of authorities over several subsequent centuries attested to the consistent pattern of the arthritis and its association with plenty. Sydenham himself was a sufferer and added a commentary on the distinctive nature of gout and a first-hand description of tophaceous material.

The picture of unmistakable classical tophaceous gout was described vividly in 16th century Spanish manuscripts. However, the separate recognition of chronic gout from rheumatoid arthritis and other forms of rheumatism was a discussion point until the early 19th century, when Landre Beavais and then Heberden in his commentaries, clarified that gout was indeed a separate condition. The clinical distinction of gout was further emphasized by Sir Alfred Garrod in the same century and to a much smaller extent by his son Sir Archibald at the close of the century.

A galaxy of 20th century clinicians, including Talbott, Scott and Emmerson, wrote extensively on the clinical and biochemical features of gout. The role of the kidney in the pathogenesis of gout and its sequential impairment were pursued relentlessly by Guttman and Yu.

The underlying purine metabolic defects of gout and their clinical expression received impetus from yet more 20th century figures of stature such as Seegmiller, Kelley, Holmes, Simmonds and Wyngaarden.

Meanwhile, the importance of the monosodium urate to the initiation of acute gout was confirmed and consolidated by McCarty, Phelps and Schumacher. By contrast to acute gout the clinical picture of the chronic disease is still poorly appreciated. Even less well remarked upon are the acute and chronic manifestations affecting the axial skeleton, the bizarre displays of subcutaneous tophi, the compressive effects of tophi on nerves, spinal column and bone and the associated non-articular features of hypertension, renal dysfunction, alcoholism and hypertriglyceridemia. This chapter attempts to extend the clinical spectrum beyond the stereotypical image and also to describe the rare causes of juvenile gout and the clinical picture associated with women and older people.

ACUTE GOUT

Risk factors

The archetypical patient is male, age 40–50, overweight and with a proclivity for regular alcohol consumption. No race or social class is excluded. There are plentiful exceptions to this picture and these are also described in this chapter. A family history of gout may be evident. Acute episodes seem to occur more commonly in the spring but this does not seem to be associated with variations of serum uric acid levels or with diet[1,2]. An episode of acute gout is more likely to occur during an infectious or other illness or during a period of hospital in-patient care or following trauma. Withdrawal from alcohol during such an illness may cause a consequent fall in serum uric acid level[3] and disturbance of urate homeostasis. This may in turn induce any microtophi within the joint to fragment, releasing urate crystals which excite local inflammation. There may be other explanations for the relationship between incidental illness, hospital admission and precipitation of gout but these are unknown.

Clinical features

The sudden onset of pain and swelling is often preceded by a period of irritability or the premonition of an attack. The first indication of pain is

TABLE 177.1 DISTRIBUTION OF INDIVIDUAL ACUTE AND CHRONIC JOINT INVOLVEMENT IN 354 PATIENTS WITH RECURRENT ACUTE GOUT

Joint	Cumulative frequency (%)
Big toe	76
Ankle or foot	50
Knee	32
Finger	25
Elbow	10
Wrist	10
Other joint	4
Bursitis	3
More than one site simultaneously	11

Half the patients had experienced gout for more than 10 years[5].

often at night. Usually a single joint is affected and the initial episode involves the first metatarsophalangeal joint (podagra) in most cases. Next in frequency are the mid tarsal and hind foot joints including the ankle. The foot is involved in nearly all cases at some time and if not affected in the first episode, is very likely to become so in subsequent acute events. The susceptibility of the foot and its pre-eminence in gout has no known explanation. With the passage of time, recurrent acute arthritis may involve multiple sites including the knee and the joints of the upper limbs. The shoulders are usually spared but may be involved. Not only does acute gout seem to spread upward from the feet with the cumulative frequency of episodes but the number of joints involved is also increased so that polyarticular acute gout tends to be a later feature, thus departing from the classical monarticular description and expanding the differential diagnosis. Acute gout affecting more than four sites simultaneously is an uncommon initial presentation but two to three joints may be affected during the first episode in a third of cases[4]. Involvement of the wrist and elbow has a clear relationship to disease duration[5]. Bursae which are near to or communicate with joints may also be the site of acute inflammation. Olecranon and pre-patellar bursitis are the most common of these[6].

The pain of acute gout is often extreme, especially in the first few episodes. This regularly interrupts sleep, prevents walking and interferes with work and leisure. The severity of disability ranges from complete prostration to a slight limp. The experience of recurrent acute episodes and the development of chronic tophaceous gout are associated with increased tolerance of the symptoms. Patients adapt in other ways. They may amend their footwear by cutting holes in shoes or wear slippers or sandals in inappropriate circumstances, visible evidence of their diagnosis and their desperation (Fig. 177.1). The involved joint becomes red, shiny and very tender especially when the big toe is affected. There may be surrounding cellulitis especially when the ankle or a bursa is involved. This may be extensive and suggestive of local infection. These symptoms and signs develop over a period of hours. The intense inflammation is often accompanied by fever which when associated with a neutrophilia and a pronounced acute phase response is highly suggestive of septic arthritis or infective cellulitis of surrounding soft tissues. Fever is more common in polyarticular acute gout[7] but the degree of fever and of leukocytosis does not correlate with the number of affected joints[4]. The natural history of acute gout is of resolution over a period of several days or when multiple joints are affected simultaneously, over a few weeks. As the inflammation recedes, the red apple shine is replaced by a purple plum hue associated with exfoliation of overlying skin.

Some patients experience a single isolated episode without recurrence. For some of those who do not receive appropriate advice and prophylaxis, there may be recurrent sporadic episodes of acute pain and swelling affecting one or more joints at variable intervals.

Differential diagnosis

Alternatives to the diagnosis of acute gout need to be considered in all situations except a recurring, painful swelling of the big toe in a middle age, overweight male. The likelihood of an alternative diagnosis in this context is improbable. Any history of acute, intermittent painful swelling and discoloration of the foot in males should be considered to be gout until proved otherwise. When a joint or joints other than the ankle or foot is inflamed and when multiple sites are involved, the diagnostic options are increased. When acute arthritis affects one or a few joints the possible diagnoses include pseudogout, septic arthritis and reactive arthritis. This is especially problematic when a knee joint is inexplicably hot and swollen without a preceding history of articular symptoms. A likely clinical diagnosis in an elderly, slender woman not receiving diuretics is probably that of pseudogout but in an obese male who drinks a lot of beer, gout is the more likely. A patient with quiescent rheumatoid arthritis, an infected leg ulcer and an acute hot swollen knee very likely has septic arthritis. In a slender young man or woman with a recent history of diarrhea or urethritis, reactive arthritis is probable. The presence of fever does not distinguish between them. The ruddy facial flush of alcohol excess, the clinical features of alcoholic liver disease or of alcoholic peripheral neuropathy and the presence of chalk like tophi on the ears or fingers and tophaceous nodules on the elbows, knees or Achilles tendons may provide corroborative evidence of gout (Figs 177.2 & 177.3). A prosthetic joint which becomes hot and swollen is most likely due to sepsis but gout, especially when a previous history is noted, could be the cause[8]. Patients with systemic lupus erythematosus (SLE) with worsening joint pain, especially in the context of renal failure and when the fingers and toes are affected may have gout rather than lupus arthri-

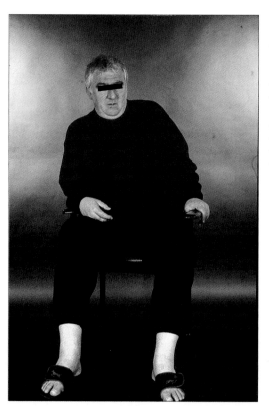

Fig. 177.1 This patient presented complaining of painful big toes. His body habitus and the shoes he was wearing on a cold morning suggested a diagnosis of gout. This was supported by the tophi visible on his fingers.

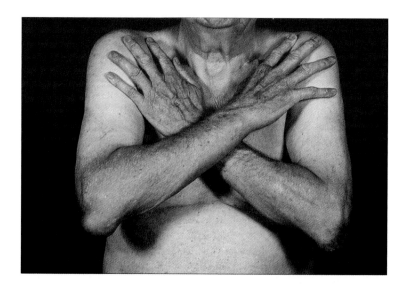

Fig. 177.2 Tophi on the elbows in a patient with chronic polyarthritis affecting the fingers. He was thought to have nodular rheumatoid arthritis and was treated with sodium aurothiomalate injections despite a negative test for rheumatoid factor.

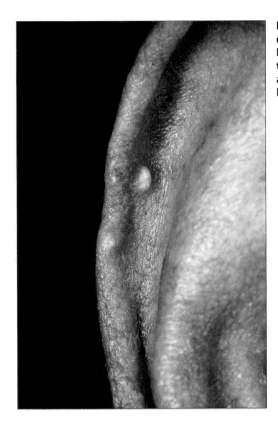

Fig. 177.3 The true diagnosis of gout became evident when the patient developed a chalk-like tophus on his right ear.

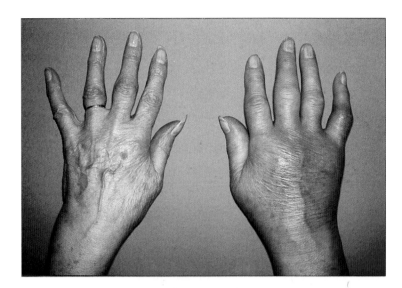

Fig. 177.4 Chronic tophaceous gout affecting the small joint of the fingers reminiscent of rheumatoid arthritis.

tis. In some of the described cases, large tophi have developed over the fingers and toes helping to simplify the diagnosis[9,10]. The chronic renal failure of SLE together with the prescription of diuretics in this illness explain the occasional concurrence with tophaceous gout. The co-existence of gout and other chronic peripheral joint diseases has been rarely documented but may be under estimated. Gout arising in a patient with rheumatoid arthritis has been described[11]. The theoretical risk of hyperuricemia and gout co-existing with rheumatoid arthritis is increased among those receiving cyclosporine as a disease modifying agent. The crucial investigation to discriminate between these possibilities is the examination of synovial fluid or nodules for the presence of monosodium urate crystals. Even when the clinical diagnosis of gout seems secure, the immediate satisfaction of diagnostic confirmation by synovial fluid analysis and the documented diagnostic clarification make it worthwhile.

CHRONIC TOPHACEOUS GOUT

When recurrent acute gout and hyperuricemia go untreated and when there is a failure to eradicate causative factors such as alcohol excess, obesity or diuretic therapy, the condition may evolve from a picture of sporadic acute mono and oligoarthritis through recurrent polyarthritis to persistent low grade joint inflammation, joint deformity and deposition of urate crystals to form visible tophi. Tophaceous deposits develop within the same joints affected by acute gout and especially the first metatarsophalangeal joint. The relatively mild discomfort of chronic gout may be punctuated by episodes of acute arthritis. About one third of chronic gout patients develop visible tophi[12]. Within the joints, tophi contribute to the development of bone erosions especially in the big toe but also elsewhere. Tophi are classically found on the pinnae, the elbows and Achilles tendons but they may be distributed more widely, occurring within and around the finger joints, in the finger tip pulp, around the knee and within olecranon and pre-patellar bursae. Swelling and deformity become the characteristic signs, but without the intense inflammation (Fig. 177.4) associated with acute gout. No diarthrodial joint is immune to this process and although the joints of the feet are

notoriously involved in the acute illness it is the hands where evidence of chronic gout is more evident. Swelling of the distal, and proximal interphalangeal and metacarpophalangeal joints are often due to articular and periarticular tophi. Swan neck, Boutonniere and flexion deformities may develop resembling rheumatoid arthritis. The diagnosis is sometimes suggested by the pallor of tophaceous material beneath the skin which is stretched over an involved joint. Toes, ankles, elbows and wrists may all be similarly affected. Careful inspection of tophi may reveal a white subcutaneous granular appearance due to the accumulation of monosodium urate crystals. Tophi may emerge at unexpected sites becoming suddenly visible and discharging uric acid crystals as a paste or pus like material, especially during hypouricemic treatment.

Differential diagnosis

The swelling and deformity of fingers and toes may affect the metacarpophalangeal and proximal interphalangeal joints symmetrically. Typical rheumatoid-like deformities may add to the confusion and when tophi are confined to the elbows they may be so suggestive of rheumatoid nodules that the diagnosis is followed by antirheumatoid treatment. This clinical pitfall may be compounded by radiological joint erosions reminiscent of rheumatoid arthritis. A perceptive clinician would seek further information if such a patient had negative tests for rheumatoid factor since positive tests would be the normal expectation in a patient with nodular rheumatoid disease. Involvement of the distal interphalangeal joints and fusiform swelling of fingers indicative of dactylitis may suggest psoriatic arthritis or chronic reactive arthritis (Fig. 177.5). Only the diligent search for tophi or the examination of synovial aspirates for urate crystals may establish the true diagnosis. Widespread, visible tophi over the fingers, especially when these ulcerate, can resemble the calcium hydroxyapatite deposits of scleroderma. The converse is also true. The radiolucency of tophi and the demonstration of urate crystals in aspirate or exudate will resolve this dilemma. Localized subcutaneous or dermal tophi may also suggest infection with pus formation. Many tophi which discharge their contents are treated mistakenly with antibiotics (Fig. 177.6).

Atypical clinical features

In acute gout, unusual presentations departing from the classical description are on close inspection usually atypical episodes of established but sporadic gout. Recognition of acute gout affecting the manubriosternal, acromioclavicular and cervical spine joints is usually on a background of previous more typical and sometimes forgotten gouty arthritis affecting

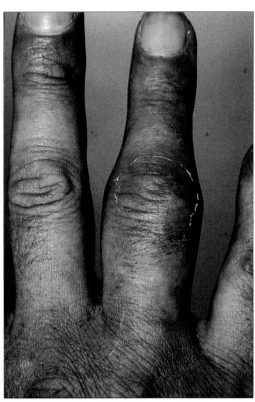

Fig. 177.5 Gouty dactylitis of a finger. This appearance is indistinguishable from other rheumatic diseases such as psoriatic or reactive arthritis. Cutaneous exfoliation indicates the resolving of a recent episode of acute gout affecting the interphalangeal joint.

the foot[13,14,15]. Acute involvement of the knee may be associated with popliteal cyst formation, leakage of synovial fluid and lower limb cellulitis or swelling simulating a deep vein thrombosis[16].

It is chronic tophaceous gout which provides more opportunity for anecdotal reports of uncommon manifestations. Tophi within the flexor tendons of the hand and wrist may cause discrete palmar or extensor swelling and carpal tunnel syndrome[17]. These tumorous swellings may also compress the spinal cord as well as peripheral nerves. Tophi and acute gout within the cervical and lumbar spine have been well documented causing acute and chronic spinal pain, cord compression and paralysis. Fever, a raised acute phase response and suggestive X-ray or MRI scans may confuse these complications with an infective discitis or an epidural abscess[18,19]. Spinal involvement may occur without visible tophi and reportedly as an initial manifestation of gout[20]. In addition to subcutaneous tophi which arise within or around the joints, the skin itself may contain intradermal deposits which may appear as widespread pustules mainly on the legs and forearms[21,22]. These are seen in severe tophaceous gout, often in association with renal failure and diuretic treatment.

INVESTIGATIONS

The concurrence of hyperuricemia with acute or chronic joint symptoms and signs is not sufficient to establish a diagnosis of gout. Both musculoskeletal pain and unrelated hyperuricemia are common in all communities and for a variety of environmental reasons. Furthermore, acute gout may occur in the presence of normouricemia and although the presumption is that such patients have been hyperuricemic in the past, an anecdotal case has been made for gout developing despite consistently normal blood uric acid levels[23].

Demonstration of urate crystals

Metatarsophalangeal joint aspiration is rarely justifiable in a patient with podagra and obvious susceptibility features. The certain diagnosis of both acute and chronic gout, however, requires the demonstration of monosodium urate crystals in samples of synovial fluid, tophaceous material, synovial or other tissue. It is most often required when an isolated joint and especially a knee is hot and swollen without previous history or other diagnostic distinguishing features. The synovial fluid is usually turbid because of large numbers of polymorphs. It may be sufficiently purulent to suggest sepsis and is occasionally milky in appearance[24]. So called 'urate milk' tends to contain few leukocytes and comprises a dense sediment of monosodium urate crystals presumably from intra-articular or bursal tophi[23]. In the acute synovitis of gout the urate crystals can usually be identified lying within phagocytic cells

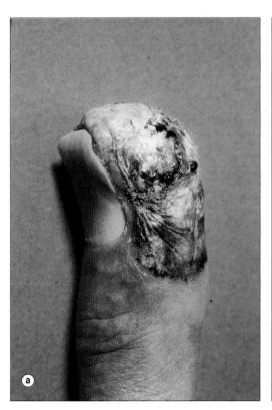
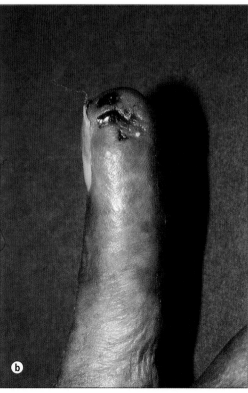

Fig. 177.6 Tophus on a finger tip. (a) During antibiotic treatment for a presumed mistaken diagnosis of local infection; (b) after treatment with allopurinol for 6 months.

which often contain several crystals of different sizes. Visualization and morphological recognition of these slender often pointed crystals is easily achievable with an ordinary light microscope but compensated polarizing microscopy is useful in distinguishing monosodium urate from calcium pyrophosphate dihydrate crystals on the basis of their birefringent properties as well as allowing an esthetic appreciation of their appearance. Urate crystals tend to be more numerous than calcium pyrophosphate crystals and are much brighter under polarizing microscopy. Their number is not related to the severity of the arthritis but they do diminish in both number and size as the attack recedes. It is important to recognize that occasionally gout and sepsis or pseudogout may co-exist so bacteriological examination is a pre-requisite for every turbid sample[26,27]. When gout is suspected but a joint effusion is not detectable, needle aspiration is still worth attempting because a drop of aspirate may contain crystals even when it appears to be blood. In effusions which persist after the signs of inflammation have resolved, the clinical picture of so called inter-critical gout, urate crystals may still be apparent[27]. This can be helpful confirmation of the diagnosis in patients who have an arthritis of unknown cause and whose most recent episode of pain appears to have resolved. By contrast there are occasions when crystals are not demonstrable in synovial fluid. Such fluid is probably from sympathetic joint effusions which have arisen adjacent to periarticular inflammation due to gouty bursitis[28]. Diagnostic scraping or needle probing of tophi or biopsy of synovium and suspect lumps, may yield sheets of monosodium crystals sometimes serendipitously. These specimens are often dramatic under compensated polarizing microscopy but contain no cells.

Blood tests and urine

As stated above, the reliance on a high serum uric acid level for the diagnosis of acute gout is misplaced. A period of sustained hyperuricemia is required before accretions of uric acid accumulate on the cartilage and synovial surfaces but the blood level may normalize before crystals are liberated into the joint cavity. It is a fall in serum uric acid which so often precipitates acute episodes by encouraging tophus dissolution. It has been estimated that about one third of patients are normouricemic during episodes of acute gout and the majority of such cases are not taking hypouricemic drugs[29]. However, hyperuricemia is the most common biochemical abnormality in acute and chronic gout and the higher the level, the more predictive of gout does it become, either as a diagnostic aid or a guide to the future development of gout[30].

There is no requirement to estimate urine uric acid excretion as a routine practice except in children and young adults with gout who are not taking diuretics, low dose aspirin, pyrazinamide or cyclosporine. All of these agents will cause hyperuricemia by reducing uric acid renal clearance. In the rare and exceptional cases of juvenile gout a high excretion of uric acid may denote deficiency of the hypoxanthine-guanine phosphoribosyltransferase (HPRT) or an increase in activity of the phosphoribosylpyrophosphate synthetase (PP-rib-P) enzyme. A very low urate clearance, in a young woman especially, may be evidence of familial nephropathy with hyperuricemia[31]. The overwhelming majority of patients with gout have impaired urate clearance[32].

During an acute episode of gout a modest neutrophilia is common but usually does not exceed 15.0×10^{-9}/l. A rise of erythrocyte sedimentation rate (ESR) and c-reactive protein (CRP) is usual in both acute and chronic gout but in the former, the acute phase response is striking, the ESR frequently exceeding 50mm/h. This often leads investigators to consider more sinister pathology including malignancy and sepsis. An ESR of more than 80mm/h would not be exceptional in the context of acute gout and the search for myeloma or polymyalgia rheumatica is predictably fruitless in such cases.

In chronic gout, a fall in hemoglobin to levels as low as 9.0g/dl reflects chronic low grade inflammation although use of non-steroidal anti-inflammatory drugs (NSAIDs) may contribute an element of iron deficiency. The etiology of gout in an individual case is often suggested by the macrocytosis of alcohol abuse. Sometimes this is accompanied by alcohol induced thrombocytopenia or neutropenia. Alcoholic liver dysfunction is a common accompaniment with elevation of serum transaminases, alkaline phosphatase or bilirubin.

Imaging

Standard radiology contributes little to the diagnosis of acute gout in the absence of an antecedent history. Plain films may simply confirm soft tissue swelling. However, radiographs of the feet may occasionally show evidence of first metatarsophalangeal joint erosion despite the absence of previous symptoms, attestation of tophaceous development within the joint over a period (Fig. 177.7). The appearance of bone erosions due to tophi is characterized by well demarcated round or oval shaped deficits with sclerotic margins, sometimes with an overhanging margin of bone (Fig. 177.8). The erosions and cysts in the big toe may precede any clinical evidence of tophaceous deposits and in chronic gout, radiographic evidence may be apparent in almost half of those without visible tophi[12,33]. More extensive erosive damage resembling rheumatoid and psoriatic arthritis may develop in the toes, ankles, fingers, wrists and elsewhere in chronic tophaceous gout.

On MR scanning, tophi appear of intermediate signal intensity on T1-weighted images and as heterogeneous signal intensity on T2-weighted images. These views may demonstrate spread of tophaceous material along fascial planes and show early bone damage not visible on standard radiographs[34,35].

DISORDERS ASSOCIATED WITH GOUT

In primary gout there is often a constellation of other health problems including obesity, alcohol abuse, hypertension, renal dysfunction and hypertriglyceridemia. Their cause and effect relationships are complex. In diverse populations there is a striking positive correlation between blood uric acid levels and both body weight and alcohol consumption[36,30]. These traits are even more striking among those with gout. The rise in serum urate following alcohol consumption is higher in gouty compared with normouricemic subjects[37]. Almost half of gout patients

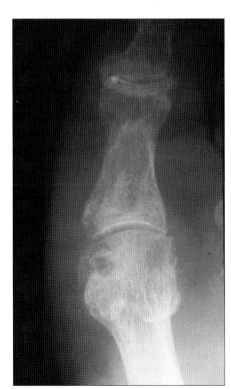

Fig. 177.7 X-ray of big toe showing round erosions due to tophi in the first metatarsophalangeal joint.

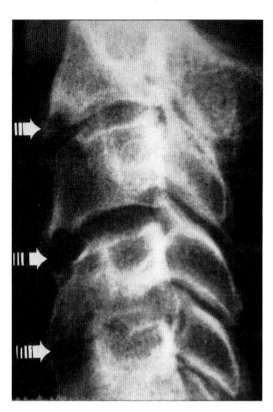

Fig. 177.8 Radiograph of cervical spine showing probable gouty erosions of vertebral bodies (arrows). The patient had severe, disabling tophaceous gout with episodes of neck pain associated with episodic acute peripheral gout.

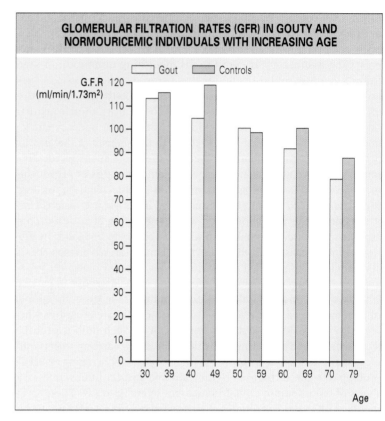

Fig. 177.9 Glomerular filtration rates (GFR) in gouty and normouricemic individuals with increasing age. There is a steady decline in both groups but the GFR in the gouty patient is always less than that of the control population.

drink 60g of alcohol or more a day[38]. Such a heavy intake is inevitably associated with an increased prevalence of alcohol dependence, liver dysfunction, depression and the central and peripheral nerve sequelae of alcoholism. Alcohol may cause a rise in blood pressure and together with obesity accounts for some of the increased prevalence of hypertension in gout. This has been reported in as many as 50% of cases in one series[5]. Among hypertensive patients there is a similar frequency of hyperuricemia[39]. Whether it is principally the adverse impact of hypertension on renal function or whether it is an effect of impaired kidneys on blood pressure, the association is real and the cause and effect mechanisms may operate in both directions. Hypertensive patients with gout do have renal dysfunction and lower urate clearance than normal people. The possibility that the renal impairment is the primary phenomenon and causes both the hyperuricemia and the hypertension has been suggested[40]. However, the demographic data strongly implicate environmental factors as well as a relative reduced urate clearance in the development of gout and it is likely that in most patients, hypertension and renal failure are partly if not wholly co-morbid features. Among Polynesian peoples, a relative impairment of urate clearance accounts for their susceptibility to hyperuricemia and in general, they do not develop renal failure although renal function may show a modest decline among those who develop gout[41]. Among Caucasians with gout there is a reduction of glomerular filtration rates, urine concentrating ability and renal disposal of hydrogen ion at all ages[32] (Fig. 177.9).

The question of whether gout itself can cause renal failure is moot. Hyperuricemia in a non-gouty population does not seem deleterious to the kidneys but prior to the availability of effective treatments, there were plentiful descriptions of renal failure, death and urate deposits within the renal parenchyma[42]. This is now a rare event but persistent hyperuricemia among those with gout does seem to cause a slow decline of kidney function[43]. Improvements in renal function have been recorded after treatment of hyperuricemia in gout but this may be partly an effect of a reduced requirement for NSAIDs[44]. Renal failure, whatever the etiology, will cause hyperuricemia but there is no convincing evidence beyond anecdote that the presence of uremia suppresses the acute inflammation of gout and reduces its incidence in chronic renal failure. Some patterns of renal disease, particularly that of familial inter-stitial nephritis may cause pronounced hyperuricemia and precocious gout as a first manifestation[45]. Other renal disorders preferentially involving tubular function and urate clearance include Bartter's syndrome, Alport's syndrome and saturnine gout due to chronic lead ingestion. These may all cause acute and chronic gout in advance of renal failure. The overproduction and increased excretion of uric acid in HPRT or PP-rib-P synthetase abnormalities tend to produce gout, kidney stones and renal failure whereas the sudden, massive rise in urine uric acid seen during treatment of some malignant disorders is more likely to precipitate acute renal failure due to crystal obstructive nephropathy than gout.

Allied to obesity and alcohol excess is dyslipidemia. This is mostly due to raised serum triglyceride levels which correlate with degrees of obesity[46]. The levels are even higher among those who drink a lot of alcohol. Both serum uric acid and triglyceride can be lowered independently by reducing body weight or alcohol intake[3,47]. There are conflicting reports about a link between high serum cholesterol levels and gout but a strong association has not been demonstrated[48]. Of those with both gout and hypertriglyceridemia, almost three quarters have impaired glucose tolerance and about ten per cent of gouty individuals have or will develop non-insulin-dependent diabetes mellitus[49,50]. The common factor is obesity. It is surprising that cardiovascular disease does not feature more prominently in surveys of gout given the frequency of obesity, hypertension and impaired glucose tolerance. There are population data which support an indirect relationship between hyperuricemia and the risk of coronary artery disease[51,52] but in clinical practice this translates into a recognition that gout may signal the presence of additional health problems.

GOUT IN YOUNG PEOPLE

The possibility of gout needs to be considered in all children, adolescents and young adults of either gender who develop spontaneous pain and swelling of the first metatarsophalangeal joint, the hind foot or the ankle and for which no other explanation is apparent. None of the classical predisposing factors such as obesity, diuretic therapy and alcohol is likely to be present. A family history of gout or renal failure should arouse curiosity and prompt measurement of the blood uric acid level, but no such clues may be available. Such instances are rare and many rheumatologists will not encounter a case of juvenile or adolescent gout within their professional lives.

Diagnosis

If a diagnosis of gout is proven by demonstration of monosodium urate crystals in a joint or by persistent hyperuricemia then further investigation must include an estimate of renal function including creatinine or clearance especially if the serum creatinine and urea are normal or only slightly elevated. The next essential investigation is measurement of 24 hour urine uric acid excretion and calculation of the urate clearance and its expression as a percentage of glomerular filtration (fractional urate clearance). Further investigation of purine metabolism may need to be undertaken if the patient is found to be excreting increased amounts of uric acid. These can be performed at several well known world centres and include measurement of the excretion of other purines and assay of purine enzymes using skin fibroblasts, lymphocytes or red cells. A diagnosis may then be pursued and confirmed by genetic mutation detection techniques.

The diagnosis may be suggested by other features including a personal or family history of renal failure, kidney stones, gout itself or neurological abnormalities.

Purine enzyme abnormalities

There are two purine enzyme abnormalities which result in overproduction of uric acid, precocious gout and increased uric acid excretion in the urine. This results in tubular obstruction by urate crystals, the formation of renal interstitial tophi and uric acid urolithiasis.

HRPT Deficiency

One of the enzyme aberrations is a deficiency of hypoxanthine guanine phosphoribosyl transferase (HPRT), a vital enzyme in the purine salvage pathway. The HPRT gene resides on the X chromosome and of the almost 300 reported cases, only five have been female. The defect in females arises as a result of mutations in the maternal or paternal allele with non-random inactivation of the other allele[53]. A spectrum of disease is seen depending on the severity of enzyme deficiency. In the devastating childhood disease known as Lesch–Nyhan syndrome, the enzyme is entirely absent. This is a syndrome of severe neurological illness with cognitive impairment, spasticity, extra-pyramidal motor dysfunction and a propensity to self mutilation by biting. These features are allied to hyperuricosuria and kidney failure. Gout and tophi may develop depending on survival and the duration of disease. The illness usually causes death within the first decade of life. Lesser deficiencies of the enzyme are associated with a longer life expectation and may cause gout, renal dysfunction and varying degrees of pyramidal and extrapyramidal disease but without self-mutilation. The mildest phenotype may be associated with gout and kidney stones only. Cases with residual enzyme activity are sometimes referred to as the Kelley–Seegmiller syndrome. The gene for HPRT possesses nine exons. The many described mutations associated with HPRT deficiency are spread throughout the gene and neither specific locations nor particular base substitutions and deletions can predict the phenotype except in a very limited fashion.

PP-rib-P synthetase superactivity

The second enzyme aberration involves superactivity of phosphoribosylpyrophosphate synthetase (PP-rib-P synthetase). This is a substrate for nucleotide synthesis and like the HPRT gene, it is found on the X chromosome. Gout may occur mainly in male children and young adults but two major phenotypes have been described. When the more serious of these affects heterozygous males, there is neurological impairment, severe sensorineural deafness and death in childhood. In heterozygous females the disease expression of this phenotype is milder but they may also have deafness as well as overproduction of uric acid and gout[54,55]. The other phenotype is not associated with deafness and presents in adolescence or adulthood as gout or urolithiasis. The PP-rib-P synthetase genes (PRPS1 and PRPS2) map to different regions of the X chromosome. Both contain seven exons. The genetic basis of the illness appears to be due to point mutations of the PRPS1 gene.

Familial juvenile hyperuricemic nephropathy

In patients with the rare disorder, familial juvenile hyperuricemic nephropathy there may be a childhood presentation with pain in the big toe due to gout[31]. There is not always a family history of either gout or kidney failure but in affected patients there is usually early evidence of renal impairment as measured by glomerular filtration and tubular function studies. In some families, females are more susceptible. Reduced urate clearance is more pronounced than is anticipated from the degree of renal impairment. The disease is characterized by gout, progressive renal dysfunction, hypertension, reduced kidney size and the histopathological changes of tubulointerstitial nephritis and ischemic damage, fibrosis and tubular atrophy. There is still a debate about whether the hyperuricemia has a renal pathogenetic role but the same familial clinical and pathological picture may occur in the absence of hyperuricemia indicating that the renal disease causes the gout and not vice versa. The condition is transmitted as an autosomal dominant gene which has been localized on chromosome 16p11.2. There is evidence of heterogeneity and reduced penetrance[56,57]. Another pattern of interstitial nephropathy associated with precocious gout and hyperuricemia is autosomal dominant medullary cystic kidney disease (ADMCKD). This typically causes a defect of urine concentrating ability and has clinical and pathological similarity to the recessive disorder, inherited juvenile nephronophthisis which is another renal cystic disease. However, their genetic loci appear to be different. Two loci have been inferred for ADMCKD. One of these is on chromosome 16p12[58].

Glycogen storage diseases

Hyperuricemia is also a feature of some glycogen storage diseases. These are largely autosomal recessive hereditary disorders of glycogen metabolism comprising hepatic and muscular forms of illness. In type 1A (von Gierke's disease) children are short in stature and have large livers. This hepatic form of disease is further characterized by multiple xanthomata, fasting hypoglycemia, elevated serum triglyceride and hyperuricemia leading in adolescence to acute and chronic gout. Liver biopsy reveals deficient glucose-6-phosphatase. There is accelerated ATP turnover causing increased degradation of adenine nucleotides to inosine, hypoxanthine, xanthine and uric acid. Other hepatic forms are not consistently associated with hyperuricemia. Of the muscular forms of glycogen storage disease it is type V (McCardle's disease) and type VII which have been both firmly associated with gout. In type V disease, a deficiency of muscle phosphorylase may be detected on muscle biopsy but the mechanism of the muscle breakdown and fatigue remain uncertain[59]. Patients may remain asymptomatic until adolescence when fatigue and muscle cramps occur after exercise, sometimes followed by myoglobinuria and rhabdomyolysis with renal failure. Exercise may not be followed by the normal rise of venous serum lactate. However, there is a demonstrable increase in blood levels of hypoxanthine, xanthine and uric acid after exercise accounting for the sporadic reports of associated gout[60]. In the type VII disease the clinical picture is similar to type V except that there is associated hemolysis. The disease is caused by muscle phosphofructokinase deficiency. These observations suggest that the hyperuricemia is caused by an increase of purine nucleotide turnover.

Treatment

In all of the disorders which can cause hyperuricemia and gout in young people, allopurinol is effective at reducing the level of blood uric acid. In the two enzyme abnormalities, HPRT deficiency and PP-rib-P synthetase overactivity, the impact of uric acid overproduction on renal function may be obviated but successful treatment does not influence the neurological features of these disorders. In the interstitial kidney diseases associated with precocious gout hypouricemic treatment has no influence on the progression of the renal disease, management of which usually entails dialysis and kidney transplantation in the course of time. Gout associated with glycogen storage disease can also be treated by conventional hypouricemic drugs.

GOUT IN WOMEN

Population surveys have consistently demonstrated higher serum uric acid levels in men than in women. Although female values rise around the menopause and approximate those of males, a disparity persists[61,62,63]. This phenomenon may not be the result of the menopause *per se* since pre and post menopausal subjects of the same age have similar serum uric acid levels[64]. The prevalence of hyperuricemia among females varies between 1–15% depending on the survey population and the definition of hyperuricemia[65]. It is therefore not surprising that of large series of gout patients, women represent a quarter or less of the total[5,66]. As anticipated, most women who develop gout are post-menopausal and a majority are receiving diuretics. The relationship of gout with obesity and alcohol excess is not as apparent in women. There is a stronger association in women of gout with hypertension and renal dysfunction[67]. A growing number of females with gout are renal transplant recipients treated with cyclosporine[68]. A rare familial juvenile hyperuricemic nephropathy may in some families afflict only the females, presenting in childhood or more likely young adulthood as gout or renal failure[31,45]. The pattern of acute and chronic arthritis in women is similar to that of men. Podagra is the most common initial manifestation but polyarticular features are more common than in men at the time of presentation. A predilection for Heberden and Bouchard nodes to be affected by acute and chronic gouty arthritis and as sites for the development of tophaceous deposits are features described mainly in women on diuretics[69,70] (Fig. 177.10). Whether this is due to their older age at presentation and the greater frequency of nodal osteoarthritis among women of this age group is not clear but it is the one clinical characteristic that tends to distinguish women from men with gout

although not exclusively. The presence of previous cartilage damage may predispose the osteoarthritic finger joints to urate crystal deposition. The same mechanism has been proposed to explain the susceptibility of the first metatarsophalangeal joint in podagra[71].

GOUT IN OLDER PEOPLE

There is a widely held view that when gout presents in old age, acute arthritis is less common than a polyarticular, deforming arthritis. This impression is partly due to the cumulative impact of chronic gout on the joints with aging and time. The description of elderly women on diuretics with tophaceous deposits over the fingers and elsewhere is firmly established and many of these appear to have no history of acute symptoms[72]. This syndrome is not confined to women but the gender distribution of gout in the elderly approximates parity. Large tophi especially at atypical sites and a chronic polyarthritis in the absence of any history of acute mono- or oligoarticular arthritis can be puzzling. The tophi within joints can cause considerable malformation[73].

Co-morbidity is common and the high percentage of diuretic induced gout and the small contribution of low dose aspirin to the hyperuricemia in this age group reflect the frequency of heart disease. Other concurrent diseases may include hypertension, renal failure and diabetes mellitus. The accentuated risks of gastrointestinal (GI) bleeding and of acute renal failure in the elderly together with the occasional need for anticoagulation in this age group, prohibit the standard NSAIDs traditionally used in acute gout. It is far better to prescribe a short course of oral corticosteroids in reducing dose over 10 days than take the risk of using NSAID in gouty patients over the age of 75 years. Alternatively, joint aspiration and intra-articular injection or intra-muscular injection of a long acting corticosteroid are effective. When NSAIDs are the preferred option of clinicians and their patients, selective Cox II inhibitors will lessen the risk of GI bleeding but not of renal impairment. Colchicine for acute episodes is not recommended because it is reportedly poorly tolerated in the elderly[74]. It retains its value when used in small doses in the early phase of hypouricemic drug treatment as a prophylaxis against recurrent acute gout. The choice of blood uric acid lowering agent in the elderly is allopurinol. Relative kidney impairment which is so common at this age lessens the effectiveness of uricosuric drugs. By the same token, renal impairment reduces the elimination of allopurinol metabolites and increases the risk of associated side effects such as rash and serious vasculitis[75]. Doses of 50–100mg daily are safer and usually adequate.

ASYMPTOMATIC HYPERURICEMIA

Within large population samples the prevalence of hyperuricemia varies depending on the definition of hyperuricemia and the population itself. In a survey of English people the frequency was about 4% in men and in women 0.4% before and about 2% after the menopause[61]. Multiple studies have corroborated the correlation of serum uric acid levels with body weight[63,76] and it is therefore likely that in many areas of the world, the frequency of hyperuricemia is increasing. Average blood uric acid levels vary between populations and are higher in native Taiwanese[77] and most famously among Polynesian people[41]. The gender difference and the association of hyperuricemia with obesity and alcohol excess still pertain to these communities and have been consistently observed over several decades and in all ethnic groups.

The fact that primates convert purines to uric acid and eliminate it through the kidneys is almost unique among mammals. Given the evolutionary standing of the human animal it could be assumed that there is a developmental advantage in the absence of uricase in human tissue and the apparent preference for urate rather than urea excretion. Historically, gout and hyperuricemia have been associated with the

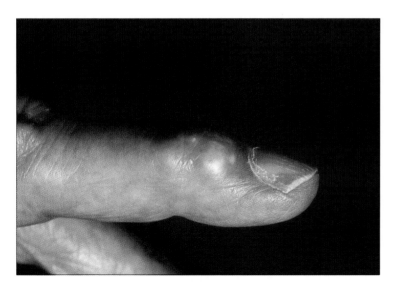

Fig. 177.10 Tophus overlying a Heberden's node in a woman on a diuretic.

upper echelons of society. This observation together with a social class gradient of blood uric acid levels and the recording of gout among worthy and intellectually profound men such as Goethe, Darwin and Newton led to the hypothesis that gout is a correlate of intelligence. As recently as 1963, the documentation of higher blood uric acid levels among executives compared with craftsmen gave support to this notion[78]. The explanation is probably more prosaic. The financial rewards of talent and endeavor together with inherited affluence were until recent times the best guarantees of plentiful food and drink. Hyperuricemia is a condition of affluence and gout does not occur among the malnourished. In western cultures, obesity was until recently a measure of prosperity. The widespread availability of inexpensive food and a decline in levels of physical activity have seen a reversal in the social scale of fatness. No contemporary population data exist but in all likelihood, western affluence and egalitarianism have dissipated the socioeconomic clustering of hyperuricemia and make untenable the always improbable correlation of hyperuricemia with intellectual capacity. This removes the only evolutionary advantage so far proposed for the essential human need to synthesize and excrete uric acid rather than urea and water as the end products of purine turnover.

If hyperuricemia is not to the good in what way is it to the bad? The occurrence of gout is the main risk of asymptomatic hyperuricemia and over a five year period there was a cumulative incidence of gout in 18% of one series of subjects[30]. However, within a given population, the majority with hyperuricemia will not develop gout and a small number of normouricemic individuals will do so[79]. Treating hyperuricemia to prevent gout is not justifiable. The demonstration of hyperuricemia in individuals may be an important health indicator of serious pathology such as alcoholism and hypertension[36,30]. There are no data which support a deleterious affect of hyperuricemia on kidney function despite the association of gout with mild renal impairment[80,81]. Hyperuricemia in chronic renal failure is common and is an effect rather than the cause of the kidney impairment. In renal, liver and cardiac transplant patients receiving cyclosporine, hyperuricemia is a regular finding because of the reduction of urate clearance caused by this agent.

Hyperuricemia has been associated with a panoply of disorders, some real, some contested and others dubious[82]. The serious hyperuricosuria and occasional mild hyperuricemia which occur with myeloproliferative diseases and myelomatosis are accentuated by their treatment unless deflected by allopurinol. The transient impairment of renal urate secretion in diabetic ketoacidosis and starvation will cause a rise of blood uric acid as will renal failure. Gout will not be precipitated by these events alone. Psoriasis has been linked to hyperuricemia in some studies[83] but not in others[84,85]. The evidence so far linking hyperuricemia directly with hypothyroidism, Paget's disease, hyperparathyroidism, sickle cell disease and sarcoidosis is not impressive and is reliant on small series of subjects and anecdotal reports.

There is no convincing evidence that hyperuricemia is by itself an independent risk factor for cardiovascular disease[51,86] although it is associated with an increased relative risk of death from all causes including coronary heart disease, stroke and hepatic disease[52]. It is likely that any association of hyperuricemia with the risk of ischemic heart disease is mediated mainly through the impact of obesity[87]. In any population survey this is compounded by the common prescription of low dose aspirin and diuretics in heart disease. Both drugs may cause hyperuricemia by reducing renal urate clearance. An association of non-diuretic-induced hyperuricemia with both right and left heart failure has been observed but the cause and effect relationships await explanation[88]. There are no benefits from treating asymptomatic hyperuricemia by drugs alone. Incidental reduction of blood uric acid levels consequent on weight reduction and alcohol restriction may be associated with less risk of liver and cardiovascular disease. Hypouricemic drugs do not improve renal impairment which may coincidentally accompany asymptomatic hyperuricemia.

REFERENCES

1. Schlesinger N, Gowin K, Baker DG, Bentler A. Acute gouty arthritic is seasonal. J Rheumatol 1998; 25: 342–344.
2. Gallerani M, Govoni M, Mucinelli M et al. Seasonal variation in the onset of acute microcrystalline arthritis. Rheumatology 1999; 38: 1003–1006.
3. Gibson T, Kilbourn K, Horner I, Simmonds HA. Mechanism and treatment of hypertriglyceridaemia in gout. Ann Rheum Dis 1979; 38: 31–35.
4. Hadler NM, Franck WA, Bress NM, Robinson DR. Acute polyarticular gout. Am J Med 1974; 56: 717–719.
5. Grahame R, Scott JT. Clinical survey of 354 patients with gout. Ann Rheum Dis 1970; 29: 461–468.
6. Dawn B, Williams JK, Walker SE. Prepatellar bursitis: a unique presentation of tophaceous gout in a normouricemic patient. J Rheumatol 1999; 24: 976–978.
7. Ho G, De Nuccio M. Gout and pseudogout in hospitalized patients. Arch Int Med 1993; 153: 2787–9270.
8. Beutler AM, Epstein AL, Policastro D. Acute gouty arthritis involving a prosthetic knee joint. J Clin Rheumatol 2000; 6: 291–293.
9. Helliwell M, Crisp AJ, Grahame R. Co-existent tophaceous gout and systemic lupus erythematosus. Rheum Rehab 1982; 21: 161–163.
10. Veerapen K, Schumacher HR, van Linthoudt D et al. Tophaceous gout in young patients with systemic lupus erythematosus. J Rheumatol 1993; 20: 721–724.
11. Owen DS, Toone E, Irby R. Co-existent rheumatoid arthritis and chronic tophaceous gout. J Am Med Assoc 1966; 197: 953–956.
12. Nakayama DY, Barthelemy C, Carrera G et al. Tophaceous gout: a clinical and radiographic assessment. Arthritis Rheum 1984; 27: 468–470.
13. Kernodle GW, Allen NB. Acute gout presenting in the manubrio-sternal joint. Arthritis Rheum 1986; 29: 570–572.
14. Musgrave DS, Ziran BH. Monarticular acromioclavicular joint gout: a case report. Am J Orthop 2000; 29: 544–547.
15. Sabharwal S, Gibson T. Cervical gout. Br J Rheumatol 1988; 27: 412–413.
16. Nelson C, Haines JD, Harper CA. Gout presenting as a popliteal cyst. A case of pseudothrombophlebitis. Postgrad Med 1987; 82: 73–74.
17. Chen CK, Chung CB, Yeh L et al. Carpal tunnel syndrome caused by tophaceous gout: CT and MR imaging features in 20 patients. Am J Roentgenol 2000; 175: 655–659.
18. St George E, Hillier CE, Hatfield R. Spinal cord compression: an unusual neurological complication of gout. Rheumatology 2001; 40: 712–714.
19. Barett K, Miller ML, Wilson JT. Tophaceous gout of the spine mimicking epidural infection: case report and review of the literature. Neurosurgery 2001; 48: 1170–1173.
20. Varga J, Gianpolo C, Goldenberg DL. Tophaceous gout of the spine in a patient with no peripheral tophi: case report and review of the literature. Arthritis Rheum 1985; 28: 1312–1315.
21. Fam AG, Assaad D. Intradermal urate tophi. J Rheumatol 1997; 24: 1126–1131.
22. Vazquez-Mellado J, Cuan A, Magana M et al. Intradermal tophi in gout: a case-control study. J Rheumatol 1999; 26: 136–140.
23. McCarty DJ. Gout without hyperuricemia. J Am Med Assoc 1994; 271: 302–303.
24. Horowitz M, Abbey L, Sirota DK, Spiera H. Intra-articular non-inflammatory free urate suspension (urate milk) in three patients with painful joints. J Rheumatol 1990; 17: 712–714.
25. Fam AG, Reis MD, Szalai JP. Acute gouty synovitis associated with urate milk. J Rheumatol 1998; 25: 2285–2286.
26. Hamilton ME, Parris TM, Gibson RS, Davis JS. Simultaneous gout and pyarthrosis. Arch Intern Med 1980; 140: 917–919.
27. Pascual E, Batlle-Gualda E, Martinez A et al. Synovial fluid analysis for diagnosis of intercritical gout. Ann Intern Med 1999; 131: 756–759.
28. Schumacher HR, Jimenez SA, Gibson T et al. Acute gouty arthritis without urate crystals identified on initial examination of synovial fluid. Arthritis Rheum 1975; 18: 603–612.
29. Snaith ML, Coomes EN. Gout with normal serum urate concentration. Brit Med J 1977; 1: 685–686.
30. Lin KC, Lin HY, Chou P. The interaction between uric acid level and other risk factors on the development of gout among asymptomatic hyperuricemic men in a prospective study. J Rheumatol 2000; 27: 1501–1505.
31. Warren DJ, Simmonds HA, Gibson T, Naik RB. Familial gout and renal failure. Arch Dis Child 1981; 56: 699–704.
32. Gibson T, Highton J, Potter C, Simmonds HA. Renal impairment and gout. Ann Rheum Dis 1980; 39: 417–423.
33. Barthelemy CR, Nakayama DA, Carrera GF et al. Gouty arthritis: a prospective radiographic evaluation of sixty patients. Skeletal Radiol 1984; 11: 1–8.
34. Popp JD, Bridgood WD, Edwards NL. Magnetic resonance imaging of tophaceous gout in the hands and wrists. Sem Arthritis Rheum 1996; 25: 282–289.

35. Yu JS, Chung C, Recht M et al. MR Imaging of tophaceous gout. Am J Roentgenol 1997; 168: 523–527.

36. Yano K, Rhoads GG, Kagan A. Epidemiology of serum uric acid among 8000 Japanese–American men in Hawaii. J Chron Dis 1977; 30: 171–184.

37. Gibson T, Rodgers AV, Simmonds HA, Toseland P. Beer drinking and its effect on uric acid. Br J Rheumatol 1984; 23: 203–209.

38. Gibson T, Rodgers AV, Simmonds HA et al. A controlled study of diet in patients with gout. Ann Rheum Dis 1983; 42: 123–127.

39. Garrick R, Bauer GE, Ewan CE, Neale FC. Serum uric acid in normal and hypertensive Australian subjects. Aust NZ J Med 1972; 4: 351–356.

40. Gibson T, Highton J, Simmonds HA, Potter CF. Hypertension, renal function and gout. Postgrad Med J 1979; 55(suppl. 3): 21–25.

41. Gibson T, Waterworth R, Hatfield P et al. Hyperuricaemia, gout and kidney function in New Zealand Maori men. Br J Rheumatol 1984; 23: 276–282.

42. Brown J, Mallory GK. Renal changes in gout. N Engl J Med 1950; 243: 325–329.

43. Gibson T, Rodgers V, Potter C, Simmonds HA. Allopurinol treatment and its effect on renal function in gout: a controlled study. Ann Rheum Dis 1982; 41: 59–65.

44. Perez-Ruiz F, Calabozo M, Herrero-Beites AM et al. Improvement of renal function in patients with chronic gout after proper control of hyperuricaemia and gouty bouts. Nephron 2000; 86: 287–291.

45. Puig JG, Miranda ME, Mateos FA et al. Hereditary nephropathy associated with hyperuricemia and gout. Arch Intern Med 1993; 153: 357–365.

46. Gibson T, Grahame R. Gout and hyperlipidemia. Ann Rheum Dis 1974; 33: 298–303.

47. Dessein PH, Shipton EA, Stanwix AE et al. Beneficial effects of weight loss associated with moderate calorie/carbohydrate restriction, and increased proportional intake of protein and unsaturated fat on serum urate and lipoprotein levels in gout: a pilot study. Ann Rheum Dis 2000; 59: 539–543.

48. Darlington LG, Scott JT. Plasma lipid levels in gout. Ann Rheum Dis 1972; 31: 487–489.

49. Berkowitz D. Gout, hyperlipidemia and diabetes inter-relationships. J Am Med Assoc 1966; 197: 117–120.

50. Whitehouse FW, Cleary WJ. Diabetes mellitus in patients with gout. J Am Med Assoc 1966; 197: 113–116.

51. The Coronary Drug Project Research Group. Serum uric acid: its association with other risk factors and with mortality in coronary heart disease. J Chronic Dis 1976; 29: 557–569.

52. Tomita M, Mizuno S, Yamanaka H et al. Does hyperuricemia affect mortality? A prospective cohort study of Japanese male workers. J Epidemiol 2000; 10: 403–409.

53. Jinnah HA, De Gregorio L, Harris JC et al. The spectrum of inherited mutations causing HPRT deficiency: 75 new cases and a review of 196 previously reported cases. Mut Res 2000; 463: 309–336.

54. Simmonds HA, Webster D, Wilson J, Lingham S. An X-linked syndrome characterised by hyperuricemia, deafness and neurodevelopmental abnormalities. Lancet 1982; 2: 68–70.

55. Becker MA, Mateos FA, Jimenez ML et al. Inherited superactivity of phosphoribosyl pyrophosphate synthetase: association of uric acid overproduction and sensorineural deafness. Am J Med 1988; 85: 383–390.

56. Stiburkova B, Majewski J, Sebesta I et al. Familial juvenile hyperuricemic nephropathy: localization of the gene on chromosome 16p11.2 and evidence for genetic heterogeneity. Am J Hum Genet 2000; 66: 1989–1994.

57. Kamatani N, Moritani M, Yamanaka H et al. Localization of a gene for familial juvenile hyperuricemic nephropathy causing underexcretion-type gout to 16p12 by genome-wide linkage analysis of a large family. Arthritis Rheum 2000; 43: 925–929.

58. Kroiss S, Huck K, Berthold S et al. Evidence of further genetic heterogeneity in autosomal dominant medullary cystic kidney disease. Nephrol Dial Transplant 2000; 15: 818–821.

59. DiMauro S, Lamperti C. Muscle glycogenoses. Muscle Nerve 2001; 24: 984–999.

60. Jinnai K, Kono N, Yamamato Y et al. Glycogenosis type V (McCardle's disease) with hyperuricemia: report and clinical investigation. Eur Neurol 1993; 33: 204–207.

61. Popert AJ, Hewitt JV. Gout and hyperuricemia in renal and urban populations. Ann Rheum Dis 1962; 21: 154–163.

62. Mikkelsen WM, Dodge HJ, Valkenburg H. The distribution of serum uric acid values in a population unselected as to gout or hyperuricemia. Am J Med 1965; 39: 242–251.

63. Munan L, Kelly A, Petitclerc C. Population serum urate levels and their correlates. The Sherbrooke regional study. Am J Epidemiol 1976; 103: 369–382.

64. Bengtsson C, Tibblin E. Serum uric acid levels in women. Acta Med Scand 1974; 196: 93–102.

65. Lin KC, Lin HY, Chou P. Community based epidemiological study on hyperuricemia and gout in Kn Hu, Kinmen. J Rheumatol 2000; 27: 1045–1050.

66. Kuzell WC, Schaffarzick RW, Naugler WE et al. Some observations on 520 gouty patients. J Chron Dis 1955; 2: 645–669.

67. Lally EV, Ho G, Kaplan SR. The clinical spectrum of gouty arthritis in women. Arch Intern Med 1986; 146: 2221–2225.

68. Park YB, Park YS, Song J et al. Clinical manifestations of Korean female gouty patients. Clin Rheumatol 2000; 19: 142–146.

69. Macfarlane D, Dieppe PA. Diuretic induced gout in elderly women. Br J Rheumatol 1985; 24: 155–157.

70. Simkin PA, Campbell PM, Larsen EB. Gout in Heberden's nodes. Arthritis Rheum 1983; 26: 94–97.

71. Simkin PA. The pathogenesis of podagra. Ann Intern Med 1977; 86: 230–233.

72. Doherty M, Dieppe PA. Crystal deposition disease in the elderly. Clin Rheum Dis 1986; 12: 97–116.

73. van der Klooster, Peters R, Burgmans JP, Grootendorst AF. Chronic tophaceous gout in the elderly. Neth J Med 1998; 53: 69–75.

74. Fam AG. Gout in the elderly. Clinical presentation and treatment. Drugs and Aging 1998; 13: 229–243.

75. Dieppe PA. Investigation and management of gout in the young and elderly. Ann Rheum Dis 1991; 50: 263–266.

76. Gertler MM, Garn SM, Levine SA. Serum uric acid in relation to age and physique in health and coronary heart disease. Ann Intern Med 1951; 34: 1421–1431.

77. Chou CT, Lai JS. The epidemiology of hyperuricaemia and gout in Taiwan Aborigines. Br J Rheumatol 1998; 37: 258–262.

78. Dunn JP, Brooks GW, Mausner J et al. Social class gradient of serum uric acid levels in males. J Am Med Assoc 1963; 185: 431–436.

79. Rigby A, Wood PH. Serum uric acid levels and gout: what does this herald for the population? Clin Exp Rheumatol 1994; 12: 395–400.

80. Fessel WJ, Siegelaub AB, Johnson ES. Correlates and consequences of asymptomatic hyperuricemia. Arch Intern Med 1973; 132: 44–54.

81. Campion EW, Glynn RJ, DeLabry LO. Asymptomatic hyperuricemia: risks and consequences in the normative aging study. Am J Med 1987; 82: 421–426.

82. Smyth CJ. Disorders associated with hyperuricemia. Arthritis Rheum 1975; 18: 713–719.

83. Goldman M. Uric acid in the etiology of psoriasis. Am J Dermatopathol 1981; 3: 397–404.

84. Scott JT, Stodell MA. Serum uric acid levels in psoriasis. Adv Exp Med Biol 1984; 165: 283–285.

85. Lambert JR, Wright V. Serum uric acid levels in psoriatic arthritis. Ann Rheum Dis 1977; 264–267.

86. Myers AR, Epstein FH, Dodge HJ, Mikkelsen WM. The relationship of serum uric acid to risk factors in coronary heart disease. Am J Med 1968; 45: 520–528.

87. Klein R, Klein BE, Cornoni JC et al. Serum uric acid. Its relationship to coronary heart disease risk factors and cardiovascular disease, Evans County, Georgia. Arch Intern Med 1973; 132: 401–410.

88. Hoeper MM, Hohlfeld JM, Fabel H. Hyperuricaemia in patients with right or left heart failure. Eur Respir J 1999; 13: 682–685.

178 The management of gout

Bryan T Emmerson

Principal goals of treatment

- Treating acute attacks early and effectively
- In some cases, correcting hyperuricemia either by determining a correctable cause or by using drugs

Acute gout

- Choose either non-steroidal anti-inflammatory agents (NSAID), colchicine or corticosteroids
- Use colchicine prophylaxis between attacks

Prevention and correction of hyperuricemia

- Seek and correct factors contributing to hyperuricemia, e.g. regular alcohol, high purine intake, obesity, diuretic therapy, suboptimal urine flow, hypertension, or
- Use a urate lowering drug regularly and permanently.

Therapy in gout is directed primarily towards the treatment of acute attacks and secondarily towards the correction of the hyperuricemia, which is the basic cause of these attacks (Fig. 178.1). Treatment should also aim to reverse any complications that may have arisen and attention should also be given to any concomitant or etiologically related conditions such as renal impairment, hypertension or factors promoting vascular disease.

When considering therapy for gout, it is important to distinguish clearly between therapy for reducing inflammation in acute gout and that for managing hyperuricemia. Rarely does any agent offer clinically useful control of both factors. Indeed, the inappropriate use of antihyperuricemic agents during acute gout can cause severe exacerbations of the joint inflammation. An outline of the general principles used in the management of gouty arthritis is given in Table 178.1.

ACUTE GOUT

The management of the acute attack of gout is the same, whatever its underlying cause. There are three effective treatments, the particular

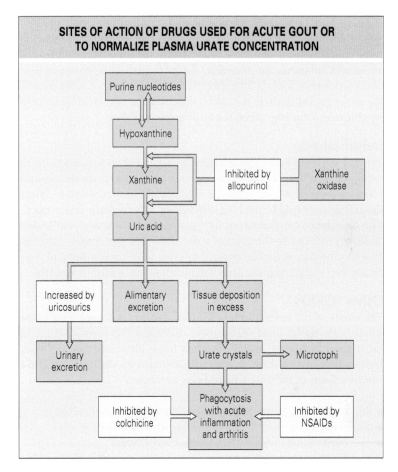

Fig. 178.1 **Sites of action of drugs used for acute gout or to normalize plasma urate concentration.**

choice depending upon what other diseases are affecting the patient or to which the patient is predisposed. These are colchicine[1,2], (ii) non-steroidal anti-inflammatory drugs (NSAIDs)[3,4] and corticosteroids. NSAIDs are superior to colchicine in terms of speed of onset of action but are relatively contraindicated in some patients, particularly those with renal insufficiency, hypertension, peptic ulceration or congestive heart failure. Despite having been used for centuries, colchicine is now usually reserved for those patients in whom NSAIDs are contraindicated. Corticosteroids, often administered as an intra-articular injection, are usually effective and, indeed, joint aspiration alone will often ease the pain. Oral corticosteroids may be chosen if colchicine or NSAIDs are not desired, and parenteral corticosteroids may be used if the gastrointestinal route is not feasible. Whichever drug is chosen in acute gout, the earlier the therapy is instituted the quicker the resolution of the attack. Patients who have had previous attacks of gout should be advised, and soon learn, to have therapy readily available and to take it at the first indication of an attack. Taken so early, only one or two doses may be sufficient to abort an attack of gout.

TABLE 178.1 GENERAL APPROACHES TO THE MANAGEMENT OF GOUT	
Acute gout	Nonsteroidal anti-inflammatory drugs Colchicine Corticosteroids Do not attempt to modify plasma urate concentrations
Recurrent gout or chronic gout	Reverse factors promoting hyperuricemia Maintain urine output . 1400ml/day When asymptomatic, add agent to lower plasma urate concentration (e.g. probenecid or allopurinol) Continue prophylactic doses of colchicine for at least 12 months after normalization of the plasma urate concentration

Among the various NSAIDs, indomethacin has been the most widely used but most other NSAIDs, if they are used in appropriate doses, have been shown to be effective in the treatment of an acute attack of gout[5]. The newer COX-2 selective inhibitors, celecoxib and rofecoxib, have not yet been assessed in the management of an intense inflammatory arthritis such as occurs in gout, but it is likely that they would be effective if given in appropriate anti-inflammatory dosage[6].

Numerous regimens exist for the use of these drugs in the acute attack and these recommendations provide a guide which may be altered depending upon the severity of the attack and the response to therapy. Nonetheless, it must be noted that the commonest cause of difficulty in controlling an attack is the simultaneous administration (or withdrawal) of drugs that alter the plasma urate concentration. Both increases and decreases in the plasma urate concentration may precipitate or prolong an attack of gout. Therefore, therapy aimed at reducing urate concentrations should be delayed until the complete resolution of all signs of inflammation. However, should the patient be stabilized on a constant dose of a urate-lowering drug at the time of an acute attack, the urate-lowering drug should be continued at the same dose until specific treatment has caused the acute gout to subside.

Indomethacin

Patients will often notice that the pain has begun to ease within 2 hours of taking the first dose. Generally, 50mg four times a day is an average and effective dose schedule, although mild attacks may respond to lower doses. This dose may be doubled with benefit in particularly severe cases[7]. The dose should be maintained for 2 days or until the severe pain settles, and then reduced to three times a day. Provided the attack continues to settle, the dose is further reduced to 25mg three times a day and continued for 1–2 days after the acute inflammation has settled completely.

Other NSAIDs

The doses of the several other NSAIDs used to treat gout tend to be towards the upper limit of, or above, the usual therapeutic range. In most cases, a higher initial dose has been advocated and, as with indomethacin, the dose is generally reduced as the inflammation resolves. Some of the dose schedules are as follows:

- ibuprofen 800mg every 8 hours reducing to 400mg every 6 hours[8]
- diclofenac 50mg every 8 hours reducing to 25mg every 8 hours
- naproxen 750mg initially, then 250mg every 8 hours
- piroxicam 40mg daily for 5 days[9]
- sulindac 200mg initially, then 100mg every 6 hours[10].

Several of the NSAID available in suppository or injectable form may be useful in patients unable to take oral medications.

Corticosteroids

Intra-articular administration of corticosteroids is a particularly effective means of terminating an attack of gout[11]. Resolution is typically complete within 12–24 hours. This form of treatment is of particular value in some patients with monoarticular gout associated with renal impairment and other conditions where the use of full doses of other drugs may be relatively contraindicated. A good response without rebound has been reported with either oral prednisone 30–50mg/day tapering over 7–9 days, with intramuscular adrenocorticotropic hormone (ACTH) (40IU)[12] or triamcinolone acetonide (60mg)[13] or betamethasone (7mg), or with intravenous methylprednisolone (125mg)[14].

Colchicine

Colchicine is an alkaloid derived from the autumn crocus, *Colchicum autumnale*. It has an anti-inflammatory action in acute attacks of gout and a prophylactic effect against recurrent attacks. It has no effect on the serum urate concentration or on urate metabolism[15].

TABLE 178.2 MECHANISMS OF ACTION OF COLCHICINE

- Inhibits phagocytosis by the formation of a tubulin–colchicine dimer which caps the assembly ends of the microtubules

- Alters the motility and adhesion of the neutrophil leukocyte by an effect on the membrane

- Reduces the release of the eicosanoids PGE_2 and LTB_4 by monocytes and neutrophil leukocytes by inhibiting phospholipase A_2

- Affects chemotaxis

The effect of colchicine is principally mediated by changes to the neutrophil leukocyte population. Its effects on this cell are multiple and there is controversy as to which effect is the dominant one determining its effectiveness in the treatment of gout[16]. However, by a combination of these mechanisms, colchicine interrupts the inflammatory response to the tissue deposition of urate crystals (Table 178.2).

Pharmacokinetics

Because of its lipid solubility, colchicine rapidly passes into all tissues of the body. After intravenous (i.v.) administration, it has a half-life in plasma of less than 1 hour and is distributed throughout a volume greater than the extracellular water. After oral administration, it is absorbed through the upper small bowel, has a peak plasma concentration in 1–2 hours[17] and a half-life of about 4 hours. It is not bound to plasma protein and does not displace protein-bound drugs. However the drug persists in leukocytes, where it may be detected for up to 10 days following administration. It also appears to be concentrated in the liver, kidney, spleen and intestine. It is extensively metabolized within the liver and is excreted principally in the bile and intestinal secretions. There may be some enterohepatic recirculation. A total of 20% is excreted unchanged in the urine, so that, during chronic administration, the dose should be reduced in the presence of pre-existing renal disease. Traces of the drug can still be found in the urine 10 days after its last administration.

Dosage

Colchicine is usually available in 0.5mg tablets and is most effective in acute gouty arthritis if given early in the acute attack. The therapeutic dose, however, is close to the toxic dose, so that when given orally the dose needs to be graduated to the individual response. The initial dose is usually given as 1mg, with 0.5mg being repeated every 2 hours until the patient develops diarrhea or vomiting, the gout begins to settle or the maximum dose is reached. This maximum dose can range up to 6mg, and caution and close supervision need to be exercised in the use of doses larger than this. Acute gouty arthritis usually subsides within 24 hours of administration of an effective dose of colchicine. The tablets are sensitive to light and may deteriorate.

In some countries, an intravenous preparation is available. If so, it can be given in a dose of 1–2mg initially, with a further 1mg dose in 6 hours if there has been no relief. However, the total dose should not exceed 4mg and this should be reduced in the presence of hepatic or renal disease, in an older patient or if there has been previous dosing with colchicine[18]. The intravenous route has fewer gastrointestinal side effects but it may take 6 hours to be fully effective and the potential for serious systemic toxicity is much greater than by the oral route, particularly in patients with renal insufficiency, volume depletion and underlying cytopenia. It should be administered by intravenous line, well diluted with considerable care to avoid extravasation.

Colchicine is often thought to be specific for gout, and certainly three-quarters of patients with uncomplicated acute gout will respond to a course of colchicine. However, it is not completely specific to gout and will also cause subsidence of sarcoid and psoriatic arthritis and some crystal arthropathies due to hydroxyapatite or pyrophosphate crystals.

Adverse reactions

Most of the adverse effects of colchicine are dose-related and will disappear if a sufficiently low dose is taken. The principal adverse effects are gastrointestinal and usually consist of diarrhea or vomiting. Prolonged high dosage can lead to a malabsorption syndrome and, if sufficiently severe, a hemorrhagic gastroenteritis. Although it is recognized to have an antimitotic effect, bone marrow suppression has been extremely rare. Ovarian and testicular function have generally remained normal during prolonged prophylactic treatment.

More importantly, however, a myoneuropathy has been reported in some patients taking a prophylactic dose of colchicine who were suffering from minor degrees of renal insufficiency[19,20]. Most of these patients presented with proximal muscle weakness or showed elevation of the serum creatine kinase concentrations. An axonal polyneuropathy could be demonstrated, together with disruption of the cytoskeleton in the muscle cells. This report suggests that the prophylactic dose should not exceed 0.5mg per day in the presence of renal insufficiency[21]. Poisoning from colchicine, usually with suicidal intent, causes severe damage to most tissues and presents clinically with severe diarrhea and vomiting with dehydration, hyponatremia, shock and disseminated intravascular coagulation. It has been treated successfully with colchicine-specific Fab fragments[22] but these are not readily available.

Drug prophylaxis of acute gout

Whatever the serum urate concentration, acute attacks of gout may be inhibited by small regular doses of either colchicine or NSAID. Such drug prophylaxis is particularly important because of the increased risk of acute attacks of gout both prior to and during the introduction of urate-lowering drugs and other therapy designed to correct hyperuricemia, at which time there may be considerable fluctuations in the serum urate concentration. Colchicine prophylaxis was totally effective in 82% of such patients and satisfactory in a further 12%[23].

The prophylactic dose of colchicine is usually 0.5mg twice a day but some patients will tolerate only 0.5mg once daily. The prophylactic dose should be adjusted so as not to produce any gastrointestinal symptoms and it should be continued until the patient has been normouricemic and has had no attacks of gout for 1–2 years[23]. The lowest dose should be used in the presence of hepatic or renal disease.

Practical prescribing tips

- Colchicine prophylaxis is of special value in patients with recurrent attacks of gout in whom acute attacks are precipitated by drugs or procedures to normalize the plasma urate concentration.
- Colchicine prophylaxis should be continued until the patient has had no symptoms of gout for about 12 months and the serum urate concentration has remained normal for that time.
- An acute attack of gout in a patient on prophylactic colchicine is usually best treated with an NSAID, although there is no specific reason why a course of oral colchicine should not be used if not contraindicated.
- No controlled comparison between the prophylactic efficacy of low doses of colchicine and NSAID has been carried out. However, their side-effect profile would suggest that colchicine is the preferable agent and should be used on a regular basis, with NSAID being added if colchicine alone is inadequate[24].
- The prophylactic use of these drugs over many years should be undertaken in association with measures to optimize urate concentrations.

TABLE 178.3 CORRECTABLE FACTORS CONTRIBUTING TO HYPERURICEMIA

- Obesity
- Hypertriglyceridemia
- Regular alcohol consumption
- Diuretic therapy
- Inadequately controlled hypertension
- High dietary purine consumption
- Suboptimal urine flow (<1ml/min)

CORRECTION OF THE CAUSES OF HYPERURICEMIA

Prevention of gout is directed at restoring the plasma urate concentration to normal (Fig. 175.1). Many factors contributing to an elevation of the urate concentration have been recognized and a number of these factors can be identified in individual patients with gout. In addition, some of these may be correctable leading to a fall in the serum urate level[25]. Sometimes the resultant plasma urate concentration may be sufficiently low that it is no longer associated with gout. Thus, long-term drug treatment may be avoided and other complications secondary to these contributing factors may not occur (Table 178.3).

Factors already identified as contributing to hyperuricemia include the syndrome of obesity, hypertriglyceridemia, hypertension and insulin resistance, which is an increasing public health and nutritional problem in western societies[26]. Correction of obesity can cause a remission of hyperuricemia[27,28] and even a moderate loss of weight can facilitate the renal excretion of urate. However, the necessary changes in lifestyle and diet are rarely maintained long term, although increasing community recognition of the need to maintain a healthy lifestyle may help this in the future. In addition, diuretic therapy or inadequately treated hypertension will contribute to hyperuricemia[29,30].

A high purine intake will also contribute. Whereas high purine foods are well-recognized contributors, it is less commonly appreciated that a large helping of a food with a medium concentration of purines may provide a much larger purine load than a small helping of a food high in purines. A low purine diet is not a practical solution in the management of hyperuricemia, but rather that moderation of purine intake and avoidance of high purine foods is desirable in most patients with gout, particularly if there is any difficulty in achieving a normal plasma urate. A urine flow rate of less than 1ml/min is also suboptimal for renal elimination of urate[31].

Dietary restriction of purines rarely causes a fall in the plasma urate concentration of more than 1.0mg/dl (0.06mmol/l) unless the diet has had a large purine content. Moreover, such dietary restriction can rarely be sustained for long and is only occasionally clinically useful.

In contrast, alcohol restriction can have a much greater effect on the plasma urate concentration, depending upon the amount previously consumed[32]. Consequently, permanent modification of excessive alcohol consumption should contribute significantly to lowering the plasma urate concentration. Maintaining a urine volume of at least 1400ml/day will also facilitate urate excretion, although this will in itself have only a small impact on plasma urate concentrations.

Effective management of gout requires the patient to understand the nature of his underlying disease and the factors which contribute to it. Such an education needs to be provided by the physician and reinforced by printed material providing a guide to management and prevention[33].

CORRECTION OF HYPERURICEMIA BY DRUG THERAPY

The decision to introduce drugs to normalize hyperuricemia depends in part on the number of previous attacks of acute gout, the degree of hyperuricemia, the presence of reversible factors and the presence of tophi. Urate-lowering drugs will not normally be used after only a single attack of gout but should be considered after the second or third attacks. They should always be used for tophaceous gout. The patient needs to be aware that the decision to commence antihyperuricemic therapy usually implies life-long treatment and the patient, as well as the physician, needs to be committed to this policy.

The goal should be a sustained level of plasma urate of less than 6mg/dl (0.36mmol/l). Lower levels are necessary for the resorption of tophi[34]. This can occur from their surface when an adequately reduced plasma urate concentration [desirably below 5mg/dl (0.30mmol/l)] is maintained for many years. Once a satisfactory urate level is achieved, regular monitoring is desirable to ensure it continues to be maintained.

Antihyperuricemic drugs must not be commenced until an acute attack of gout has settled completely, since this may delay subsidence of the inflammation. In addition, prophylactic doses of colchicine (usually 0.5mg twice daily) should be administered concomitantly to minimize the risk of inducing an attack of acute gout.

Choice of drug

Drugs to correct hyperuricemia act either by promoting the renal excretion of urate (uricosuric agents) or by decreasing urate production by inhibiting xanthine oxidase (allopurinol) (Table 178.4). Although it would be logical to use a uricosuric agent when there is primary urate underexcretion and a xanthine oxidase inhibitor when there is urate overproduction, many patients show features of both overproduction and underexcretion of urate. Thus, the choice between uricosuric agents and allopurinol for an individual with hyperuricemia will depend more upon associated diseases. A uricosuric would be less favored if there had been a history of renal colic or there was coexistent renal disease (creatinine clearance less than 60ml/min), whereas allopurinol would be less favored if there was a history of drug sensitivity. Similarly, a high urine urate excretion would favor the use of allopurinol and a low urinary urate excretion would favor the use of a uricosuric agent (Table 178.5).

Uricosuric agents

A uricosuric agent is one which lowers the serum urate concentration by increasing the excretion of uric acid by the kidney (Fig. 178.2). This will be associated with an increase in the uric acid concentration in the urine

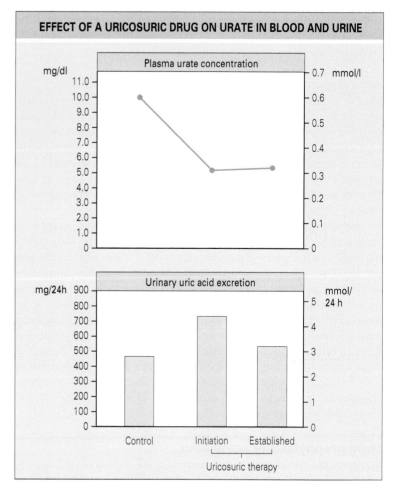

EFFECT OF A URICOSURIC DRUG ON URATE IN BLOOD AND URINE

Fig. 178.2 Effect of a uricosuric drug on urate in blood and urine.

unless there is a corresponding increase in the urine flow rate. The tendency for uric acid crystal formation would also be reduced by alkalinization of the urine. Like uric acid, most uricosuric agents are weak organic acids.

Pharmacokinetics and pharmacodynamics

Aspirin or salicylate in high dosage (5g/24h) is uricosuric, whereas low dosage (1–2g/24h) may retain urate. The uricosuric effect depends upon the concentration of salicylate in the tubular fluid, which can be increased by alkalinization of the urine. Thus, a daily dose of 5g of aspirin and 5g of sodium bicarbonate functions as an effective uricosuric agent. However, such doses are not a practical option for long-term therapy. Diflunisal is a fluorinated salicylate which retains the uricosuric effect, and which can usefully lower the serum urate concentration during long-term therapy[35]. Azapropazone is another NSAID with a uricosuric action that can result in modest serum urate-lowering effects[36].

Probenecid was the first modern drug able to produce lowering of the serum urate by a uricosuric action[37]. The drug is well absorbed from the gastrointestinal tract and has a half-life of 6–12 hours, the actual value being dose dependent. It is moderately protein bound (90%) and is thus confined to extracellular fluid. Its metabolism is rapid, with its major metabolite being an acylmonoglucuronide, in which form 40% of the drug is excreted within 48 hours[38]. There are several other active metabolites. Availability of particular uricosuric drugs may vary from country to country.

Sulfinpyrazone, a derivative of phenylbutazone, is a more potent uricosuric agent. It is rapidly absorbed, reaching a peak within an hour and is strongly (98%) bound to plasma proteins. Its metabolites are also actively uricosuric and are rapidly excreted with 20–40% of the drug being excreted unchanged within 24 hours[39].

TABLE 178.4 DRUG MECHANISMS TO NORMALIZE HYPERURICEMIA
Uricosuric drugs
Facilitate urate excretion by the kidney with an increase in the urate clearance and the fractional excretion of filtered urate. Especially useful in urate underexcretion.
Xanthine oxidase inhibiting drugs
Reduce urate production by inhibiting the final enzyme in its pathway. Especially useful in patients with urate overproduction, both primary and secondary.

TABLE 178.5 INDICATIONS FOR ALLOPURINOL WHEN AN ANTIHYPERURICEMIC AGENT IS REQUIRED
Urate overproduction, primary or secondary
Acute uric acid nephropathy
— tumor lysis syndrome
Nephrolithiasis of any type
Renal impairment (dose 100mg/day per 30ml/min glomerular filtration rate)
Low urine volume
24 hour urinary uric acid > 0.42g (2.5mmol) (an arbitrary value on a low purine diet)
Intolerance or allergy to uricosuric agents

Benzbromarone is also an active uricosuric agent. It is not as readily available as probenecid or sulfinpyrazone and has no special benefit except its potency.

Indications and clinical use
Uricosuric drugs are indicated to correct hyperuricemia and gout when there is defective renal excretion of urate and the patient is persuaded that long-term drug therapy is necessary. These drugs are contraindicated if there is a history of renal calculi or if there is a poor urine volume (< 1ml/min). They are relatively ineffective in the presence of renal disease with a glomerular filtration rate (GFR) of less than 60ml/min.

Initial doses should be small with gradual increments to minimize side effects, particularly any potential adverse effects from the increased urinary concentration of uric acid which results. Because of the increased amount of uric acid excreted in the urine during the first few weeks of treatment or after a dose increment, the urine should be alkalinized during this time to minimize the risk of uric acid crystal deposition in the renal tubules and collecting ducts of the kidney. When drug dosage is stable, the alkalinization could be stopped but a good urine volume (always greater than 1500ml/day) should be maintained permanently.

Probenecid in a dose of 1–3g/day in two to three divided doses is usually well tolerated. The starting dose should not be greater than 0.5g/day in order to minimize the risk of a flare-up of acute gout. The usual dose is 0.5g two or three times a day.

Sulfinpyrazone is three to six times as potent as probenecid on a weight for weight basis and more effective than probenecid in patients with renal disease. The initial dose should be 50mg twice a day, increasing to 100mg, then 200mg twice daily. Occasionally, up to 800mg/day may be used.

Efficacy and variability in response
The ultimate effectiveness of these drugs is judged by the degree of fall in the serum urate concentration. This may be affected by many other non-drug factors such as alcohol consumption, diet and hypertension. Despite this, up to 75% of patients receiving 1.5g probenecid daily will develop a serum urate of less than 6.7mg/dl (0.4mmol/l). If the initial fall in the serum urate is inadequate, the dose should be increased to the maximum but should not be increased beyond this until all other factors promoting hyperuricemia have been corrected. The uricosuric response is reduced when there is any impairment of glomerular function.

Adverse reactions
Probenecid blocks the tubular excretion of salicylate, the penicillins and some other uricosuric agents. Its uricosuric effect is blocked by concomitant administration of salicylate. It has numerous effects upon membrane transport, particularly within the kidney. It increases the serum furosemide concentration and augments its diuretic effect[40]. It reduces the renal excretion of indomethacin[41] and dapsone, and prolongs the metabolism of heparin. It is still used to prolong the effects of many other drugs excreted by the kidney, particularly the penicillins and zidovudine.

Fluctuations in the serum urate concentration, whether resulting in an increase or a reduction in the concentration, will often induce a flare-up of an acute attack of gout. Thus, any drug treatment which lowers the serum urate may precipitate an acute attack of gout. This is minimized by starting with a low dose and increasing to full dosage very gradually. Probenecid can cause upper gastrointestinal side effects in 3–8% of patients and a hypersensitivity rash in 2–5% of patients. Nonetheless, serious side effects are rare and the drug is acceptable in 95% of patients.

An important potential complication from all uricosuric agents is uric acid crystalluria in either the renal tubules or the urinary tract. This is a particular risk in the early stages of uricosuric treatment when the urinary urate concentration is high[42]. During this time it is important to alkalinize the urine and keep the urine dilute by means of water diuresis. Once the initial uricosuria has passed and the serum urate has fallen, the increase in urinary urate excretion will be relatively small and the risk of urate crystal formation within the renal tract reduced (see Fig. 178.2).

Sulfinpyrazone is also well tolerated and, although its uricosuric effect is also neutralized by concurrent salicylates, it has an additional specific effect of reducing platelet adhesiveness. It also prolongs platelet survival and reduces the tendency to thrombosis in arteriovenous (AV) shunts and mechanical intravascular devices.

Practical prescribing tips
When instituting uricosuric therapy it is important to:

- use concurrent colchicine prophylaxis (0.5mg once or twice daily)
- use an initial low dose and increase the dose gradually to an effective level over several weeks
- maintain an alkaline diuresis by water loading and the addition of oral sodium bicarbonate 0.5g four times a day (or more) to achieve an alkaline urine
- not use uricosuric agents in patients whose urine volume is less than 1400ml/24h
- ensure the patient always maintains a good urine volume whenever uricosuric agents are being taken. This must be continued even through hot weather when the urine volume may fall despite the maintenance of a usually adequate fluid intake.

The biggest problem in any therapy to lower the serum urate in a gouty patient is the patient's realization that the treatment must be continued even throughout the asymptomatic years. To achieve this it is important that urate-lowering therapy is not started too early, that is before the patient is persuaded of the need to take life-long therapy. If a uricosuric agent is to be used to lower the serum urate concentration in a patient with significant renal disease, the most potent uricosuric agent will probably be needed.

Allopurinol
Allopurinol, a hydroxypyrazolopyrimidine, is an isomer of hypoxanthine which lowers the urate concentration by inhibition of xanthine

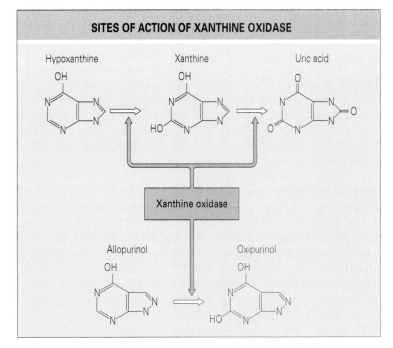

Fig. 178.3 Sites of action of xanthine oxidase.

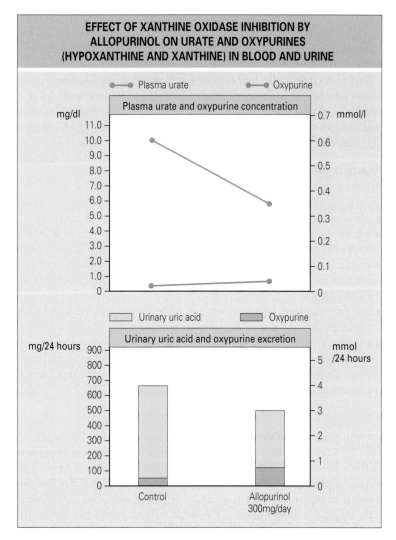

Fig. 178.4 Effect of xanthine oxidase inhibition by allopurinol on urate and oxypurines (hypoxanthine and xanthine) in blood and urine.

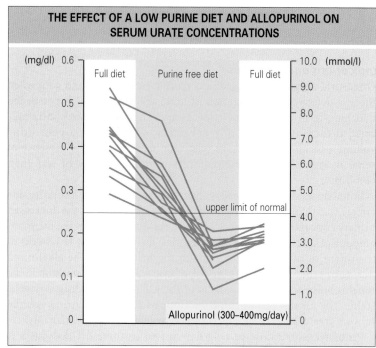

Fig. 178.5 The effect of a low purine diet and allopurinol on serum urate concentrations. There is a consistent but usually small fall in serum urate concentrations with low purine diet alone. The addition of allopurinol reliably normalizes the serum urate concentrations an effect which is largely maintained when the patients return to a full diet. (Adapted from Emmerson BT. Aust Ann Med 1969; 16: 205–214.)

oxidase (Fig. 178.3). It reduces the concentration of urate in blood and urine and increases the concentration of the urate precursors xanthine and hypoxanthine[43] (see Fig. 178.4). Except in patients with hypoxanthine phosphoribosyltransferase (HGPRT) enzyme deficiency, allopurinol also reduces total purine production. This is probably because allopurinol utilizes the high energy phosphate compound, phosphoribosyl pyrophosphate (PRPP), which is also necessary for *de novo* purine synthesis. This reaction requires the HGPRT enzyme. Although the increased amount of xanthine produced is less soluble than urate, problems do not arise because the purine excretion is spread among three substances, which reduces the risk of crystallization of any one of these. Allopurinol is itself metabolized by xanthine oxidase to oxypurinol, which is responsible for most of its effects on urate and purine metabolism.

Pharmacokinetics

Allopurinol has a short half-life of about 40 minutes, although this can sometimes be extended to a couple of hours. Most allopurinol, however, is rapidly converted into its principal metabolite, oxypurinol, with small amounts being converted into the ribonucleoside and ribonucleotide of allopurinol. Oxypurinol has a half-life of 14–28 hours and is largely excreted by the kidney, although small amounts are converted into the ribonucleoside. It is oxypurinol, therefore, which is principally responsible for the clinical effect of inhibition of xanthine oxidase. Allopurinol is well absorbed from the alimentary tract but oxypurinol in ordinary tablet form is poorly absorbed, which is why oxypurinol is not a useful therapeutic agent. However, a rapid release preparation of oxypurinol sodium

is available in some countries and appears to be clinically effective[44]. It is noteworthy that uricosuric drugs increase the excretion of oxypurinol whereas renal insufficiency reduces the excretion of oxypurinol. Both allopurinol and oxypurinol are distributed throughout body water and neither is significantly bound to the plasma protein.

Pharmacodynamics

Allopurinol and its metabolite oxypurinol are responsible for the fall in the concentration of urate in serum and urine (Fig. 178.5). The maximum effect is seen between 4–14 days and results in a stable fall of the serum urate. These two compounds deplete cells of PRPP, which is most readily observed with red cell PRPP concentrations. The increased concentrations of hypoxanthine and xanthine in serum and urine rarely cause problems because they are usually well below their solubility limits. After the drug is withdrawn, its effect on urate metabolism mostly disappears in 3–4 days, although some of the more complex metabolic effects may last considerably longer. The concentration of oxypurinol needed to completely inhibit xanthine oxidase activity is well within the therapeutic range usually achieved in clinical practice[45].

Interactions

The main interaction is with 6-mercaptopurine and azathioprine, or with any other drug whose oxidation is inhibited by allopurinol. Their co-administration with allopurinol greatly potentiates all their effects, both beneficial and toxic, and necessitates a reduction in their dose to 25% of normal. The co-administration of ampicillin with allopurinol results in a three-fold increase in the risk of a skin rash. Allopurinol also potentiates the toxic effects of cyclophosphamide, although the mechanism is not clear. It also inhibits several hepatic drug metabolizing enzymes but there is little resultant implication for therapy.

Dosage

Allopurinol is available in 100mg and 300mg tablets. The requisite dose needs to be given once daily and should be adjusted to bring the serum urate concentration to less than 6.0mg/dl (0.36mmol/l). Usually, 300mg per day will be necessary to achieve this, but occasionally 200mg, 400mg or even 600mg per day may be needed. However, should a dose of 400mg not restore the serum urate to this level, it is wise to seek and correct additional factors promoting the hyperuricemia rather than increase the dose further. Since oxypurinol is excreted principally by the kidney, the dose should be reduced in the presence of renal insufficiency. Whereas the dose might be 300mg per day for a GFR or creatinine clearance of 100ml/minute, the dose should be reduced to 200mg/day when the creatinine clearance is 50–60ml/min and to 100mg per day when the GFR is 20–30ml/min[46].

Indications

Allopurinol is immediately indicated in the presence of urate overproduction, either of endogenous origin or of dietary origin, or because of increased marrow cell turnover due to myeloproliferative disorders (so-called secondary gout). It is also used prophylactically against the tumor lysis syndrome when a large initial loading dose should be used to produce a rapid effect. It is effective in HGPRT deficiency and in other varieties of acute uric acid nephropathy. It is also of special value in the presence of renal calculi, either of uric acid or of calcium oxalate[47].

When given in combination with uricosuric agents, such as probenecid, allopurinol prolongs the half-life of the uricosuric agent and the uricosuric agent promotes excretion of oxypurinol, thereby reducing the inhibitory effect on xanthine oxidase. It is therefore better to avoid the simultaneous use of uricosuric agents and allopurinol if possible.

Variability in response and efficacy

There appears to be a moderate degree of variability in the effect of a 300mg dose of allopurinol on the serum urate in different individuals. However, some of this variability may be due to differences of body size and metabolism. Plasma oxypurinol concentrations are of considerable value when patients remain hyperuricemic despite the usual doses of allopurinol. Plasma oxypurinol concentrations between 0.46–1.52mg/dl (30–100μmol/l) are usually effective in maintaining a normal serum urate concentration[46]. However, these readily increase in renal insufficiency unless the dose of allopurinol is reduced in proportion to renal function. Because of inhibition of xanthine oxidase, plasma xanthine concentrations rise significantly, which provides an index of the metabolic effect.

Adverse reactions

Up to 5% of patients are unable to tolerate allopurinol because of adverse reactions. Minor gastrointestinal intolerance is common but can usually be minimized by administering the tablets with food. The major adverse effect is a sensitivity reaction which may range from an erythematous skin rash through to a life-endangering illness which requires corticosteroid therapy. Most commonly it is seen after 3 weeks of therapy. If the reaction is confined to the skin, the rash usually settles after withdrawal of the allopurinol, but may require local or systemic steroids. The more serious allopurinol hypersensitivity reaction involves fever and rash with systemic features of eosinophilia, acute interstitial nephritis[48] (including renal insufficiency) and hepatitis. The severity ranges through an acute interstitial nephritis to a Stevens-Johnson syndrome, to a toxic epidermal necrolysis requiring prolonged steroid therapy and intensive care. There is a 25% mortality. The risk of allopurinol hypersensitivity increases considerably in the presence of renal insufficiency and sometimes appears to be related to the use of higher doses of allopurinol than are indicated. It is therefore important that the dose of allopurinol be lowered in proportion to the GFR and that the three-fold increased risk of sensitivity in the presence of renal insufficiency be avoided.

In some of the less severe cases where the only manifestation of allopurinol sensitivity is cutaneous, slow oral desensitization has been pos-

sible with doses of allopurinol beginning at 50μg and increasing very gradually over a 4 week period to 100 mg/day or sometimes more[49, 50, 51]. In a recent study[52], over 70% of such patients were able to continue to take allopurinol, although sometimes late adjustment of the dose was needed. Even relatively small doses of allopurinol may be very effective in controlling hyperuricemia in some patients with gout and renal disease who do not respond to uricosurics. There is some evidence that the lymphocyte response in these patients is a reaction to oxypurinol rather than to allopurinol itself[53, 54].

Practical prescribing tips

- Allopurinol therapy should be initiated only after the acute attack of gout has entirely resolved. Administration to a patient with subsiding gout can cause severe exacerbation of the gout.
- It is wise to increase the dose of allopurinol slowly so that the full proposed dosage is reached only after 2–4 weeks. This considerably minimizes the risk of an acute exacerbation of gout.
- Concurrent colchicine prophylaxis (0.5mg twice daily) is also of value in preventing acute flare-ups during the institution of urate-lowering therapy. The dose should be adjusted in the presence of renal insufficiency in proportion.
- If no adequate fall occurs in the serum urate concentration, seek an alternative factor which might be maintaining the hyperuricemia. If none can be found and if the patient is still hyperuricemic despite an apparently adequate dose of allopurinol, it would be wise to measure plasma oxypurinol concentrations[46].

Hyperuricemia not responding to drugs

Associated conditions such as renal insufficiency, hypertension, abdominal obesity, hyperlipidemia and regular increased alcohol intake are commonly seen in patients with gout. Each of these conditions needs to be managed at the same time as the hyperuricemia and together they are often more threatening to longevity. In occasional patients, full dosage of allopurinol (300–400mg/day) will not cause the urate concentration to be reduced sufficiently and, in such a case, another factor (e.g. regular alcohol consumption or diuretic therapy) is usually operating[55]. Rarely, patients may need to be treated with the combination of a uricosuric drug and a xanthine oxidase inhibitor but this should be avoided if at all possible because the uricosuric agents alter the pharmacokinetics of oxypurinol. Another uncommon situation is the patient who has a history of renal calculi as well as being intolerant of allopurinol. If urate-lowering therapy is required in such a patient, a uricosuric agent may be cautiously begun with strict attention to maintaining an alkaline urine and a high urine volume. In extreme situations other therapy, including parenteral uricase, may be considered[56].

Asymptomatic hyperuricemia

Whereas the treatment of hyperuricemia is certainly of value in patients with recurrent attacks of gout, there is currently no evidence of benefit to be obtained from treating sustained asymptomatic hyperuricemia unless this is severe [urate > 12mg/dl (0.7mmol/l)] or in situations where there may be acute urate overproduction (as with tumor lysis). Although, as documented earlier, hyperuricemia is associated with a significant risk for the development of gout and a smaller risk of nephrolithiasis and possible renal impairment, it is usually many years between the detection or the development of hyperuricemia and the presentation of any of these problems, if they arise at all[57]. Only when acute severe overproduction of urate can be anticipated should prophylactic therapy with a xanthine oxidase inhibitor be considered. In patients with asymptomatic hyperuricemia, long-term urate-lowering drug therapy cannot be justified either in terms of the risks of drug complications or cost effectiveness.

GOUT IN THE ELDERLY

Gout may develop in the elderly with prolonged hyperuricemia such as that due to diuretics, hypertension or renal insufficiency[58]. Acute attacks may be few, but they may be polyarticular and involve the upper limbs and tophi may develop at a relatively early stage[59]. Although the same principles of management apply, there is a greater frequency of side effects from therapy and NSAID and colchicine are often poorly tolerated. Steroids may be useful for acute attacks. Therapy to normalize the serum urate may need to be considered and this follows the choices as enumerated. One must be particularly alert to the increased risk of side effects, particularly sensitivity to allopurinol. With the age dependent decline in renal function, the renal elimination of the allopurinol metabolite oxypurinol is reduced and its dose needs to be reduced in proportion to renal glomerular function (see previous page). The lowest dose possible to achieve the desired effect on the plasma urate should be used[60].

SURGERY

Surgery is rarely indicated for tophi except in unusual presentations where tophi exert pressure on an important structure (e.g. spinal cord). In other less vital situations, control of the hyperuricemia will cause resorption of the tophi provided there is no urgency to have them removed. Infected tophi can usually be managed with antibiotics and local measures, but debridement may be needed, particularly when there is associated vascular disease.

REFERENCES

1. Ahern MJ, Reid C, Gordon TP et al. Does colchicine work? The results of the first controlled study in acute gout. Aust NZ J Med 1987; 17: 301–304.
2. Roberts WN, Liang MH, Stern SH. Colchicine in acute gout: reassessment of risks and benefits. J Am Med Assoc 1987; 257: 1920–1922.
3. Griffin MR, Piper JM, Daugherty JR et al. Nonsteroidal anti-inflammatory drug use and increased risk for peptic ulcer disease in elderly persons. Ann Intern Med 1991; 114: 257–263.
4. Unsworth J, Sturman S, Lunec J, Blake DR. Renal impairment associated with non-steroidal anti-inflammatory drugs. Ann Rheum Dis 1987; 46: 233–236.
5. Arnold MH, Preston SJ, Buchanan WW. Comparison of the natural history of untreated acute gouty arthritis vs acute gouty arthritis treated with non-steroidal anti-inflammatory drugs. Br J Clin Pharmacol 1988; 26: 488–489.
6. Boutsen Y, Esselinckx W. Novel nonsteroidal anti-inflammatory drugs. Acta Gastroenterol Belg 1999; 62: 421–424.
7. Emmerson BT. Regimen of indomethacin therapy in acute gouty arthritis. Br Med J 1967; 2: 272–274.
8. Schweitz MC, Nashel DJ, Alepa FP. Ibuprofen in the treatment of acute gouty arthritis. J Am Med Assoc 1978; 239: 34–35.
9. Widmark PH. Piroxicam: its safety and efficacy in the treatment of acute gout. Am J Med 1982; 72: 63–65.
10. Calabro JJ, Khoury MI, Symth CJ. Clinoril in acute gout. Acta Reuma Port 1974; 8: 163–166.
11. Gray RG, Tenenbaum J, Gottlieb NL. Local corticosteroid injection treatment in rheumatic disorders. Semin Arthritis Rheum 1981; 10: 231–254.
12. Axelrod D, Preston S. Comparison of parenteral adrenocorticotropic hormone with oral indomethacin in the treatment of acute gout. Arthritis Rheum 1988; 31: 803–805.
13. Alloway JA, Moriarty MJ, Hoogland YT, Nashel DJ. Comparison of triamcinolone acetonide with indomethacin in the treatment of acute gouty arthritis. J Rheumatol 1993; 20: 111–113.
14. Werlen D, Gabay C, Vischer TL. Corticosteroid therapy for the treatment of acute attacks of crystal-induced arthritis: an effective alternative to nonsteroidal antiinflammatory drugs. Rev Rhum Engl Ed 1996; 63: 248–254.
15. Wallace SL. Colchicine. Semin Arthritis Rheum 1974; 3: 369–381.
16. Spilberg I, Mandell B, Mehta J et al. Mechanism of action of colchicine in acute urate crystal-induced arthritis. J Clin Invest 1979; 64: 775–780.
17. Ferron GM, Rochdi M, Jusko WJ, Scherrmann JM. Oral absorption characteristics and pharmacokinetics of colchicine in healthy volunteers after single and multiple doses. J Clin Pharmacol 1996; 36: 874–883.
18. Wallace SL, Singer JZ. Review: systemic toxicity associated with the intravenous administration of colchicine – guidelines for use. J Rheumatol 1988; 15: 495–499.
19. Kuncl RW, Duncan G, Watson D et al. Colchicine myopathy and neuropathy. N Engl J Med 1987; 316: 1562–1568.
20. Tapal MF. Colchicine myopathy. Scand J Rheumatol 1996; 25: 105–106.
21. Wallace SL, Singer JZ, Duncan GJ et al. Renal function predicts colchicine toxicity: guidelines for the prophylactic use of colchicine in gout. J Rheumatol 1991; 18: 264–269.
22. Baud FJ, Sabouraud A et al. Brief report: treatment of severe colchicine overdose with colchicine-specific Fab fragments. N Engl J Med 1995; 332: 642–645.
23. Yu TF. The efficacy of colchicine prophylaxis in articular gout – a reappraisal after 20 years. Semin Arthritis Rheum 1982; 12: 256–263.
24. Kot TV, Day RO, Brooks PM. Preventing acute gout when starting allopurinol therapy. Colchicine or NSAID? Med J Aust 1993; 159: 182–184.
25. Emmerson BT. Identification of the causes of persistent hyperuricaemia. Lancet 1991; 337: 1461–1463.
26. Emmerson, BT. Hyperlipidaemia in hyperuricaemia and gout. Ann Rheum Dis 1998; 57: 509–510.
27. Facchini F, Chen Y-DI, Hollenbeck CB, Reaven GM. Relationship between resistance to insulin-mediated glucose uptake, urinary uric acid clearance and plasma uric acid concentration. J Am Med Assoc 1991; 266: 3008–3011.
28. Yamashita S, Matsuzawa Y, Tokunaga K et al. Studies on the impaired metabolism of uric acid in obese subjects: marked reduction of renal urate excretion and its improvement by a low-calorie diet. Int J Obesity 1986; 10: 255–264.
29. Macfarlane DG, Dieppe PA. Diuretic induced gout in elderly women. Br J Rheumatol 1985; 24: 155–157.
30. Scott JT, Higgens CS. Diuretic induced gout: a multifactorial condition. Ann Rheum Dis 1992; 51: 259–261.
31. Brøchner-Mortensen K. Uric acid in blood and urine. Acta Med Scand 1937; 84(suppl): 127–153.
32. Eastmond CJ, Garton M, Robins S, Riddoch S. The effects of alcoholic beverages on urate metabolism in gout sufferers. Br J Rheumatol 1995; 34: 756–759.
33. Emmerson BT. Getting rid of gout – a guide to management and prevention. Melbourne: Oxford University Press; 1996.
34. McCarthy GM, Barthelemy CR, Veum JA, Wortmann RL. Influence of antihyperuricemic therapy on the clinical and radiographic progression of gout. Arthritis Rheum 1991; 34: 1489–1494.
35. Emmerson BT, Hazelton RA, Whyte IM. Comparison of the urate lowering effect of allopurinol and diflunisal. J Rheumatol 1987; 14: 335–337.
36. Gibson T, Simmonds HA, Armstrong RD et al. Azapropazone – a treatment for hyperuricaemia and gout? Br J Rheumatol 1984; 23: 44–51.
37. Bishop C, Rand R, Talbot JH. Effect of benemid (p-[di-n-propyl sulfanyl]-benzoic acid) on uric acid metabolism in one normal and one gouty subject. J Clin Invest 1951; 30: 889–905.
38. Dayton PG, Perel JM. The metabolism of probenecid in man. Ann NY Acad Sci 1971; 179: 399–402.
39. Dieterle W, Faigle JW, Mory H et al. Biotransformation and pharmacokinetics of sulfinpyrazone (Anturan) in man. Eur J Clin Pharmacol 1975; 9: 135–145.
40. Chennavasin P, Seiwell R, Brater DC, Liang WM. Pharmacodynamic analysis of the furosemide–probenecid interaction in man. Kidney Int 1979; 16: 187–195.
41. Brooks PM, Bell MA, Sturrock RD et al. The clinical significance of indomethacin–probenecid interaction. Br J Clin Pharmacol 1974; 1: 287–290.
42. Kovalchik MT. Sulfinpyrazone induced uric acid urolithiasis with acute renal failure. Connecticut Med 1981; 45: 423–424.
43. Rundles RW, Metz EN, Silberman HR. Allopurinol in the treatment of gout. Ann Intern Med 1966; 64: 229–258.
44. Walter-Sack I, de Vries JX et al. Disposition and uric acid lowering effect of oxipurinol: comparison of different oxipurinol formulations and allopurinol in healthy individuals. Eur J Clin Pharmacol 1995; 49: 215–220.
45. Graham S, Day RO et al. Pharmacodynamics of oxypurinol after administration of allopurinol to healthy subjects. Br J Clin Pharmacol 1996; 41: 299–304.
46. Emmerson BT, Gordon RB, Cross M, Thomson DB. Plasma oxipurinol concentrations during allopurinol therapy. Br J Rheumatol 1987; 26: 445–449.
47. Ettinger B, Tang A, Citron JT et al. Randomized trial of allopurinol in the prevention of calcium oxalate calculi. N Engl J Med 1986; 315: 1386–1389.
48. Hande KR, Noone RM, Stone WJ. Severe allopurinol toxicity – description and guidelines for prevention in patients with renal insufficiency. Am J Med 1984; 76: 47–56.
49. Meyrier A. Desensitization in a patient with chronic renal disease and severe allergy to allopurinol. Br Med J 1976; 2: 458.
50. Fam AG, Lewtas J et al. Desensitization to allopurinol in patients with gout and cutaneous reactions. Am J Med 1992; 93: 299–307.
51. Kelso JM, Keating RM. Successful desensitization for treatment of a fixed drug eruption to allopurinol. J Allergy Clin Immunol 1996; 97: 1171–1172.
52. Fam AG, Dunne SM et al. Efficacy and safety of desensitization to allopurinol following cutaneous reactions. Arthritis Rheum 2001; 44: 231–238.
53. Emmerson BT, Hazelton RA, Frazer IH. Some adverse reactions to allopurinol may be mediated by lymphocyte reactivity to oxypurinol. Arthritis Rheum 1988; 31: 436–440.
54. Hamanaka H, Mizutani H et al. Allopurinol hypersensitivity syndrome: hypersensitivity to oxypurinol but not allopurinol. Clin Exp Dermatol 1998; 23: 32–34.
55. Emmerson BT. The management of gout. N Engl J Med 1996; 334: 445–451.
56. Rozenberg S, Roche B, Koeger AC et al. Repeated administration of urate oxidase: treatment for heart transplant gouty arthritis. Arthritis Rheum 1994; 37(suppl): 414.
57. Campion EW, Glynn RJ, De Labry LO. Asymptomatic hyperuricemia: risks and consequences in the normative ageing study. Am J Med 1987; 82: 421–426.
58. Scott JT, Higgins CS. Diuretic induced gout – a multifactorial condition. Ann Rheum Dis 1992; 51: 259–261.
59. Fam AG. Gout in the elderly. Clinical presentation and treatment. Drugs and Aging 1998; 13: 229–243.
60. Turnheim K, Krivanek P, Oberbauer R. Pharmacokinetics and pharmacodynamics of allopurinol in elderly and young subjects. Br J Clin Pharmacol 1999; 48: 501–509.

179 Calcium pyrophosphate dihydrate crystal-associated arthropathy

Michael Doherty

Definition

- Arthropathy and other locomotor disease associated with calcium pyrophosphate dihydrate (CPPD) crystal deposition
- Sporadic, familial and metabolic disease-associated forms recognized

Clinical features

- Predominantly a disease of the elderly
- Acute self-limiting synovitis ('pseudogout')
- Chronic arthropathy showing association and overlap with osteoarthritis
- Target joints – knees, wrists, shoulders and hips

HISTORY

Adams (1857) is credited with the first description of articular cartilage calcification (chondrocalcinosis) in pathological specimens. With the advent of skeletal radiography it soon became apparent that chondrocalcinosis is a common phenomenon, occurring either alone or in association with arthritis. Mandl (1927) was the first to emphasize the clinical and pathologic diversity of chondrocalcinosis at the knee, distinguishing primary (asymptomatic, bilateral, no cartilage damage) from secondary chondrocalcinosis (symptomatic, localized, often post-traumatic, with cartilage fibrillation). In 1957 Sitaj and Zitnan utilized chondrocalcinosis as a diagnostic feature for arthritis in five Czech families – 'chondrocalcinosis polyarticularis'. The observation that chondrocalcinosis often preceded the development of radiographic damage in these families reinforced previous contentions (Werwath, 1928; Harman, 1944) that chondrocalcinosis was a cause of arthritis. Undoubtedly a major milestone, however, was when, in 1961, McCarty and Hollander introduced compensated polarized microscopy as a technique to identify urate crystals in gout. Within a year McCarty and colleagues discovered non-urate crystals, identified by x-ray diffraction as calcium pyrophosphate dihydrate ($Ca_2P_2O_7.2H_2O$) (CPPD) in knee fluids from patients with acute synovitis and chondrocalcinosis. The clinical similarity to gout prompted the term pseudogout for this new 'crystal-induced arthropathy'[1]. It was soon realized that chondrocalcinosis polyarticularis was also caused by CPPD. Cadaveric studies subsequently established CPPD as the most common – but not the exclusive – cause of knee chondrocalcinosis, resulting in the term chondrocalcinosis often being used synonymously with CPPD. The perspective of CPPD crystals as primary, causal agents in joint disease was readily supported by the demonstration of CPPD crystals in acute arthritis, the *in vitro* evidence that CPPD crystals are potent inflammatory agents, and the induction of synovitis by injection of CPPD into normal canine or human joints. The finding of metabolic disease associations and varying forms of familial predisposition further reinforced the analogy to urate crystals in gout. Consequently, CPPD arthropathy was separated into hereditary, metabolic disease-associated or sporadic/idiopathic forms.

Following initial descriptions of pseudogout, however, a variety of other clinical settings for CPPD deposition were reported. Many presentations appeared to mimic other forms of arthritis, encouraging the proliferation of numerous 'pseudo' syndromes and a complex clinical classification of 'pseudogout' (type A), 'pseudorheumatoid arthritis' (type B), 'pseudo-osteoarthritis' (with acute attacks, type C; without inflammation, type D), 'lanthanic or asymptomatic' (type E) and 'pseudoneurotrophic' (type F), to which other forms were later added[2]. In an attempt to simplify matters the term 'CPPD crystal deposition disease' was introduced to incorporate all instances of CPPD crystal deposition, the term pyrophosphate arthropathy later being used, particularly in Europe, for cases with accompanying arthritis.

Although knowledge of CPPD has increased in recent years, the relationship between CPPD crystals and arthritis remains unclear. The paradox of asymptomatic deposition of inflammatory crystals, the wide spectrum of clinical presentation and the lack of disease specificity have challenged recognition of CPPD deposition as a discrete 'crystal deposition disease'. The strong overlap with osteoarthritis (OA) has led many to consider pyrophosphate arthropathy more as a 'subset' of OA, with CPPD deposition being a 'process' marker for certain cartilage changes that occur in OA[3].

The confusing nomenclature in crystal-associated locomotor disease is currently under review. For clarity, the following definitions are used:

- chondrocalcinosis – calcification of articular fibro- or hyaline cartilage
- pyrophosphate arthropathy – structural abnormality of cartilage and bone (cartilage loss, osteophyte, cysts) associated with intra-articular CPPD deposition
- pseudogout – the clinical syndrome of acute synovitis associated with intra-articular CPPD deposition.

EPIDEMIOLOGY

Data on chondrocalcinosis, derived from radiographic and pathologic surveys, are sparse and largely confined to the knee[2–5] (Table 179.1). All studies, however, suggest a female preponderance and a striking association with aging, the prevalence for radiographic chondrocalcinosis being low under age 50 but rising from 10–15% in those aged 65–75 to 30–60%

TABLE 179.1 EPIDEMIOLOGY OF PYROPHOSPHATE ARTHROPATHY

Peak age (years)	6–75
Sex distribution (F:M)	2–7:1
Prevalence rate (/100,000)	8100 (CC only, age range 63–93)
Annual incidence (/1000)	Unknown
Geography	Appears ubiquitous
Genetic associations	Genes on chromosomes 5p (1 UK and 1 French family) and 8q (1 American family)

in those over 85[2,3]. The only large population-based radiographic survey is the Framingham study[5], which in the age range 63–93 showed an overall prevalence rate of 8%, ranging from 3% in those aged <70 to 27% in those over 85. This study also confirmed a female preponderance (age-adjusted relative risk 1.3), though less pronounced than that derived from patient series[2,3].

Chondrocalcinosis is reported from most countries and racial groups, but there are insufficient data to confirm a racial predisposition. Familial predisposition, however, is well reported from several countries and different ethnic groups, including the former Czechoslovakia, Chile, Holland, France, Canada, Germany, Sweden, United States, Spain, Japan, Israel, Tunisia and the United Kingdom[2,3,6–9]. The pattern of inheritance varies, though autosomal dominance is usual. Two clinical phenotypes have been emphasized, the first characterized by early onset in the third to fourth decades, florid polyarticular chondrocalcinosis, and variable severity of arthropathy ranging from mild to destructive[6,7,9], and the second characterized by late onset in the sixth to seventh decades, oligoarticular chondrocalcinosis mainly confined to the knees, and arthritis resembling sporadic pyrophosphate arthropathy[8,9]. The latter familial form may be more common than is recognized, the late onset of disease expression and geographic dispersal of families posing difficulties in this respect. An association with benign childhood fits appears unique to one UK family with early-onset polyarticular chondrocalcinosis[9], the responsible gene – chondrocalcinosis gene 2 (CCAL2) being located to chromosome 5p15[10]. The gene in two other kindreds from France and Argentina have also been localized to the same region of 5p15[11]. The other reported locus (CCAL1), in an American family with premature OA and associated CPPD deposition, is on chromosome 8q[12].

No epidemiologic data exist for pyrophosphate arthropathy. Most patient series report a mean age at presentation of between 65 and 75 years[2,3], with a female predominance (2–3:1). Associated metabolic disease (see Fig. 179.12; after Jones et al.[13]) and familial predisposition are rarely identified, though each may be associated with a younger age of presentation (<55 years) and florid, polyarticular chondrocalcinosis. Although numerous metabolic associations have been suggested, many reflect a chance concurrence of common age-related conditions, as suggested by controlled studies for diabetes, uremia and Paget's disease[13]. The strongest evidence relates to hyperparathyroidism and hemochromatosis. With rare conditions, evidence is based on the occurrence of premature chondrocalcinosis in just a few cases, as reported for hypophosphatasia and hypomagnesemia[13]. Hemochromatosis is the one metabolic disease that causes structural arthropathy rather than just chondrocalcinosis and pseudogout attacks.

CLINICAL FEATURES

Chondrocalcinosis can be an incidental finding, but the two common presentations are acute synovitis and chronic arthritis[2,3,14,15]. Other presentations are rare.

Acute synovitis ('pseudogout')

This classic presentation is the most common cause of acute monoarthritis in the elderly. Acute attacks may be the only manifestation of otherwise asymptomatic chondrocalcinosis or pyrophosphate arthropathy; in older, mainly female patients, however, they often superimpose upon chronic symptomatic arthropathy. Any joint may be involved, including the first metatarsophalangeal ('pseudopodagra'), but the knee is by far the commonest site (Fig. 179.1), followed by the wrist, shoulder, ankle and elbow. Concurrent attacks in more than one joint are unusual[1] (<10% of cases) and polyarticular attacks rare. The typical attack develops rapidly, with severe pain, stiffness and swelling, maximal within just 6–24 hours of onset. As with gout, the patient may

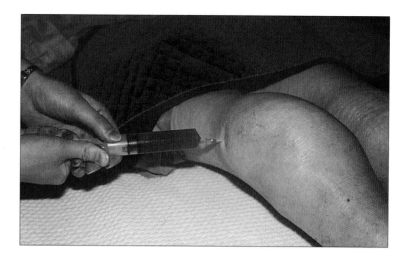

Fig. 179.1 Pseudogout affecting the knee. Seen here in an elderly woman with background chronic pyrophosphate arthropathy. Bloodstaining of synovial fluid is common in this situation.

TABLE 179.2 SITUATIONS THAT MAY TRIGGER ACUTE PSEUDOGOUT
• Direct trauma to joint
• Intercurrent medical illness (e.g. chest infection, myocardial infarction)
• Surgery (especially parathyroidectomy)
• Blood transfusion, parenteral fluid administration
• Institution of thyroxine replacement therapy
• Joint lavage
Most cases of pseudogout develop spontaneously

describe pain as the 'worst ever' and be unable to tolerate even light pressure from clothing or bedding. Overlying erythema is common and examination reveals a tender joint, with signs of marked synovitis – increased warmth, a large or tense effusion, joint line tenderness, and restricted movement with stress pain. Fever is common and occasionally marked. Elderly patients may appear unwell and mildly confused, especially with knee or multiple joint involvement.

Acute attacks are self-limiting and usually resolve within 1–3 weeks. Transient, less severe 'petit' attacks are probably common but difficult to confirm. Most pseudogout develops spontaneously but several provoking factors are recognized which may precede the attack by 1–3 days (Table 179.2), the commonest being stress response to intercurrent illness or surgery.

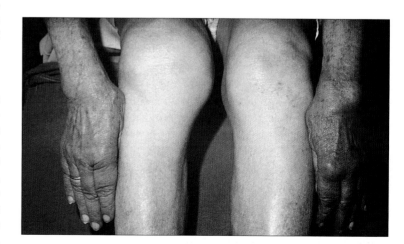

Fig. 179.2 Chronic pyrophosphate arthropathy.

Chronic pyrophosphate arthropathy

Symptomatic patients with this common condition are mainly elderly and female. Like pseudogout it principally targets large and medium-sized joints, the knees being the most common and severely affected sites, followed by wrists, shoulders, elbows, hips and midtarsal joints (Figs 179.2 & 179.3). In the hand, the metacarpophalangeal joints (particularly the second and third) are the commonest most severely affected site. Presentation is with chronic pain, early morning and inactivity stiffness, limitation of movement and functional impairment: acute attacks may be superimposed upon this chronic history. Symptoms are often restricted to just a few joints, though single or multiple joint involvement also occurs.

Affected joints usually reveals signs of OA – bony swelling, crepitus, restricted movement – with varying degrees of synovitis. Synovitis, represented by increased warmth, joint line and/or capsular tenderness, stress pain, effusion and soft tissue thickening, may be marked, and is usually most evident clinically at the knee, radiocarpal or glenohumeral joints. Knees typically show bi- or tricompartmental disease, with marked or predominant patellofemoral involvement. In severe cases fixed flexion with either valgus or varus deformity may occur. Other deformities, such as recurvatum or posterior tibial subluxation, are less common.

Examination, particularly of elderly women, often reveals more widespread but asymptomatic arthropathy. Generalized OA with Heberden's nodes, for example, is a common accompaniment, but pyrophosphate arthropathy may be clinically distinguished from non-crystal associated OA by: (1) the pattern of involvement (wrists, shoulder, ankles and elbows are uncommonly affected in OA; knee involvement usually predominates in the medial compartment); (2) the often marked inflammatory component; and (3) the superimposition of acute attacks.

The natural history of chronic pyrophosphate arthropathy is poorly documented. However, despite often severe symptoms and structural change at presentation, one 5-year hospital-based study[16] suggests that most patients run a benign course, particularly in respect of small and medium-sized joint involvement. As expected, most symptom progression in this study occurred in large lower limb joints, but even in severely affected knees (the usual site of presentation) 60% showed stabilization or improvement of symptoms. However, in a second hospital-based prospective study of 350 OA knees, the presence of synovial fluid CPPD crystals or chondrocalcinosis was associated with radiographic progression, especially bone attrition (odds ratio 3.44, 95% CI 1.97–6.02) and clinical deterioration[17], suggesting that CPPD is a marker for poor prognosis in knee OA. In keeping with this is the occasional development of rapidly progressive arthropathy, particularly at the knee, shoulder or hip. Such 'destructive pyrophosphate arthropathy' ('pseudoneuropathic joint'[2]) is virtually confined to elderly women, usually accompanied by severe night and rest pain, and associated with a poor outcome[18]. Some such patients have problematic recurrent hemarthrosis, particularly of the shoulder and knee; joint leakage may cause extensive bleeding, swelling and bruising of adjacent tissues. Interestingly, the occurrence of rapidly destructive apatite-associated arthritis at the hip (without CPPD) appears more common in patients with chondrocalcinosis or pyrophosphate arthropathy at other sites, though the mechanism for this is obscure[3]. Again, such rapidly progressive arthropathy is virtually confined to elderly women (see Chapter 180).

Incidental finding

Because isolated chondrocalcinosis is a common age-associated phenomenon it is often observed as an incidental radiographic finding in elderly subjects. Though less well documented, it is likely that asymptomatic pyrophosphate arthropathy is also common in the eighth and ninth decades[4,5]. Therefore, as with OA, clinical or radiographic evidence of pyrophosphate arthropathy or chondrocalcinosis may be a confounding factor; only a thorough history and examination can elucidate their relevance to symptom causation.

Uncommon presentations
Atypical arthropathic and axial presentations

Marked proximal stiffness accompanying glenohumeral and polyarticular involvement may rarely suggest polymyalgia rheumatica. Severe spinal stiffness, particularly in Czech, Chilean and other familial forms, may cause 'pseudoankylosing spondylitis'; indeed, spinal ankylosis may occur in Chilean families[7]. The putative association with diffuse idiopathic skeletal hyperostosis (DISH)[19] may further complicate this issue. Acute attacks in axial joints are difficult to confirm, and some self-limiting spinal syndromes, described in relation to the periodontoid ('crowned dens' syndrome), cervical and lumbar regions, may reflect pseudogout attacks. Certainly in elderly subjects acute self-limiting meningitic episodes may occur in relation to CPPD deposition in degenerative ligamenta flava and cervical discs; such deposits rarely associate with chronic myeloradiculopathy. Preferential deposition of CPPD in ligamenta flava at C3–C6 remains unexplained but corresponds to the level of greatest mobility.

Tendinitis and tenosynovitis

Acute inflammatory episodes relating to CPPD deposition in tendons are described for triceps, flexor digitorum and Achilles tendons, and tenosynovitis is reported for hand flexors and extensors[20]. Tendinitis

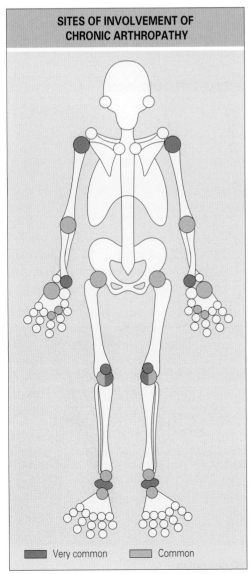

SITES OF INVOLVEMENT OF CHRONIC ARTHROPATHY

Very common ▪ Common ▪

Fig. 179.3 Chronic arthropathy. Common sites of involvement of chronic pyrophosphate arthropathy.

and tenosynovitis usually, but not inevitably, occur in patients with accompanying chondrocalcinosis or pyrophosphate arthropathy. Flexor tendon involvement may associate with carpal tunnel syndrome, and less frequently with combined median and ulnar nerve entrapment at the wrist[20,21], the entrapment appearing to relate more to soft tissue factors than structural arthropathy. Tendon rupture (hand extensors, Achilles) is a rare complication.

Bursitis

Olecranon, infrapatellar and retrocalcaneal bursitis is a rare clinical manifestation, again predominating in patients with widespread pyrophosphate arthropathy. It is thought most likely that CPPD crystals migrate to bursal tissues from adjacent cartilage and capsule of tendon rather than deposit *de novo* in soft tissues.

Tophaceous CPPD deposition

Tophaceous ('tumoral') CPPD deposition is rare, but reported in intra- or periarticular sites that include the elbow, finger, jaw, acromioclavicular joint and hip[22]. Lesions are solitary and usually develop in areas of chondroid metaplasia without predisposing metabolic abnormality or evidence of CPPD deposition elsewhere. Malignancy is often suspected and the diagnosis follows the examination of excised material.

INVESTIGATIONS

Central investigations for diagnosis are (1) fluid and tissue analysis (primarily synovial fluid, rarely bursal or tenosynovial aspirate, biopsy material) for the presence of CPPD crystals; and (2) plain radiographs. Other investigations may be undertaken to exclude alternative or coexisting arthropathy, and once the diagnosis is confirmed further investigation for predisposing metabolic disease may be indicated.

CPPD crystal identification

In pseudogout, aspirated fluid is often turbid or bloodstained, with diminished viscosity and greatly elevated cell count (usually >90% neutrophils). Macroscopic appearance, viscosity and cell counts in chronic arthropathy are more variable and range from 'inflammatory' to 'non-inflammatory'. The CPPD crystals are poorly visualized by plain light microscopy, but compensated polarized light microscopy (× 400) will reveal predominantly intracellular CPPD crystals (Fig. 179.4), recognized by their morphology (usually rhomboids or rods, occasionally acicular, ~2–10μm long), weak positive birefringence and inclined extinction (15–20°): 'twinning' of crystals, leaving a chip at one corner, is occasionally seen. Crystals of CPPD are less readily identified and often less numerous than urate crystals, and can often be missed. A careful search in areas of cellular debris and fibrin, and examination of a spun deposit may both increase detection. Although the crystals are robust, early examination of fresh fluid avoids problems of dissolution and post-

aspiration artifact. For histologic samples, tissue preparation in neutral buffers and stains should be used to avoid dissolution: crystals may readily be lost during decalcification (often done for tissue submitted with bone).

As with other synovial fluid particles, identification by polarized light microscopy is associated with both false positives and false negatives, and identification using more definitive analytical means (e.g. infrared spectrophotometry, electron microscopic methods, x-ray diffraction) is ideal. However, such methods often require a high crystal load for analysis, are expensive and take time. Therefore, for routine clinical purposes polarized microscopy of fresh fluid represents a convenient, rapid and adequate compromise.

Plain radiographic features

Radiographic aspects relate both to the calcification and the arthropathy associated with CPPD deposition[3,23].

Calcification

This may affect several joint tissues (Fig. 179.5). Chondrocalcinosis most commonly affects fibrocartilage (particularly knee menisci, wrist triangular cartilage, symphysis pubis), but also occurs in hyaline cartilage (particularly knee, glenohumeral joint, hip) as thick linear deposits, parallel to and separate from subchondral bone (Fig. 179.6). Although occasionally localized to a single joint, such as one knee, chondrocalcinosis usually affects several joints: if absent from knees, wrists or symphysis pubis it is unlikely to be present elsewhere. Capsular and synovial calcification is less common than chondrocalcinosis and is usually most obvious at metacarpophalangeal joints (Fig. 179.7) and the knee. Florid synovial calcification occasionally stimulates synovial osteochondromatosis. Deposition in tendon insertions particularly favors the

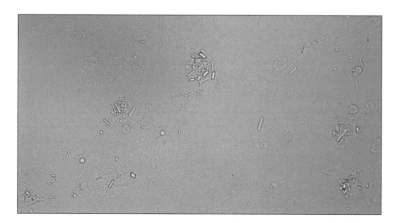

Fig. 179.4 Synovial fluid CPPD crystals.

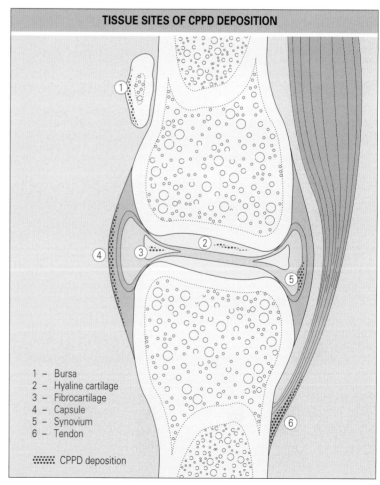

TISSUE SITES OF CPPD DEPOSITION

1 – Bursa
2 – Hyaline cartilage
3 – Fibrocartilage
4 – Capsule
5 – Synovium
6 – Tendon

▓▓▓▓ CPPD deposition

Fig. 179.5 Tissue sites of CPPD deposition.

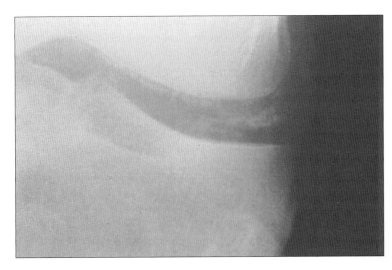

Fig. 179.6 Knee radiograph showing chondrocalcinosis of both fibrocartilage (meniscus) and hyaline cartilage.

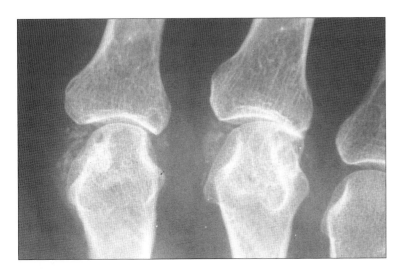

Fig. 179.7 Calcification affecting metacarpophalangeal joints.

Achilles (Fig. 179.8), triceps and obturators, and is typically linear and extensive compared to the discrete nummular calcification of apatite. Diffuse calcification of bursae (subacromial, olecranon, retrocalcaneal) is an occasional finding. Both chondrocalcinosis and calcification are dynamic and may increase or decrease with time. Chondrocalcinosis may become less evident, particularly if cartilage thickness is lost or if crystals are 'shed' from cartilage during acute or recurrent inflammatory episodes[16,24].

Chondrocalcinosis and calcification may be readily visible on standard radiographs, though meticulous technique using optimal resolution undoubtedly enhances detection. Plain radiographs, tomography and CT imaging are relatively insensitive and detect only sizable CPPD deposits. The presence of detectable calcification is not a prerequisite for diagnosis of CPPD-associated syndromes.

Structural changes

The changes of pyrophosphate arthropathy are those of OA, namely cartilage loss, sclerosis, cysts and osteophytes[3,23]. Characteristics purported to aid distinction, however, include:

- Joint distribution and involvement within articulations that are atypical of OA. For example, glenohumeral, metacarpophalangeal, ankle or elbow disease; isolated or predominant involvement of patellofemoral compartment, radiocarpal joint (sometimes with characteristic scapholunate dissociation), or talocalcaneonavicular articulation; and
- Often prominent, exuberant osteophyte and cyst formation (particularly at the knee and wrist).

Such combined features may present a distinctive 'hypertropic' appearance and distribution that suggest CPPD even in the absence of chondrocalcinosis (Figs 179.9 & 179.10). Many cases of pyrophosphate arthropathy, however, appear not dissimilar to 'uncomplicated' OA as regards structural change (and vice versa). Furthermore, because nodal generalized OA often coexists in such patients it is common to find otherwise typical OA changes in some joints, with more distinctive changes of pyrophosphate arthropathy in others. One study of 300 OA

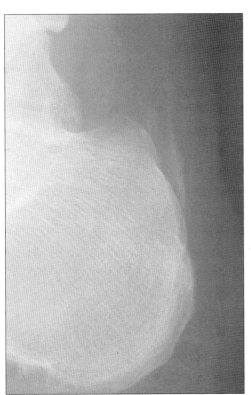

Fig. 179.8 Achilles tendon calcification.

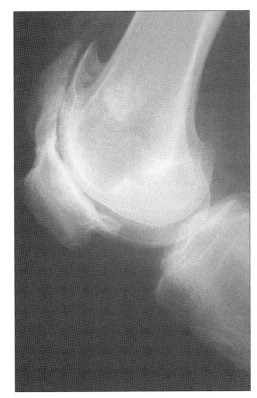

Fig. 179.9 Knee radiograph showing hypertrophic OA features. Note prominent patellofemoral involvement, typical of pyrophosphate arthropathy.

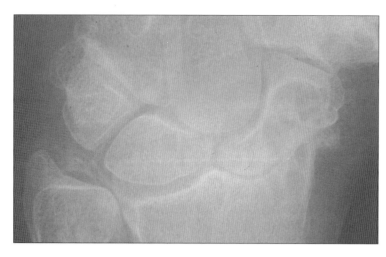

Fig. 179.10 Hand radiograph showing typical radiocarpal involvement. Note prominent cyst formation, chondrocalcinosis of the triangular ligament and 'pressure erosion' of the distal radius.

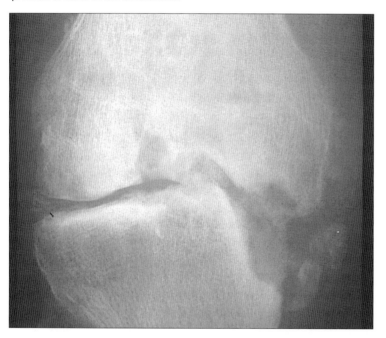

Fig. 179.11 Rapidly destructive knee arthropathy in an elderly woman. Note marked bone attrition, bony 'loose bodies' and chondrocalcinosis.

knees, importantly including asymptomatic as well as symptomatic joints, showed no association between synovial fluid CPPD and specific radiographic features at this site[25]. The presence of CPPD, however, did associate both with extent (tri- and bicompartmental OA) and overall severity of radiographic OA. Sequential radiographic changes are variable. The few patients with destructive arthropathy show marked attrition of cartilage and bone, with occasional fragmentation and loose osseous bodies that may resemble the 'disorganization' of a Charcot joint; such cases may show rapid, progressive change (Fig. 179.11).

Marginal erosions (non-proliferative or proliferative) are not a feature of pyrophosphate arthropathy, though smooth 'pressure' erosions (reflecting chronic effusions or bone 'wear') are not infrequent, particularly on the anterior distal femur and around distal inferior radioulnar and radiocarpal joints. In patients with coexistent RA and CPPD ('pseudorheumatoid arthritis') a modified radiographic appearance may occur (Fig. 179.12), characterized by retained bone density, prominent osteophytes, prominent well-corticated cysts and paucity of erosion – in other words, predominance of reparative OA rather than atrophic destructive change[26].

Additional investigations

In pseudogout, Gram stain and culture should always be performed on aspirated fluid. Septic arthritis is the principal differential diagnosis, and concurrence with pseudogout occasionally occurs. Other synovial fluid investigations are of little diagnostic value in this situation. Lactate levels, for example, are often in the range seen in sepsis. Pseudogout commonly triggers a moderate acute-phase response, with elevation of plasma viscosity, erythrocyte sedimentation rate (ESR), acute-phase reactants (e.g. C-reactive protein) and peripheral white cell count predominantly neutrophils). Such changes are occasionally impressive, particularly with pseudogout affecting multiple large joints and in patients with triggering intercurrent illness.

In chronic arthropathy, mild anemia with a modest elevation of plasma viscosity and acute-phase reactants (including ferritin) is not uncommon. The frequency of other biochemical and serologic abnormalities, however, is no different from that in other subjects of the same age.

Screening for predisposing metabolic disease

Metabolic predisposition is rare and routine screening of all CPPD patients is unrewarding. Nevertheless, chondrocalcinosis and arthritis

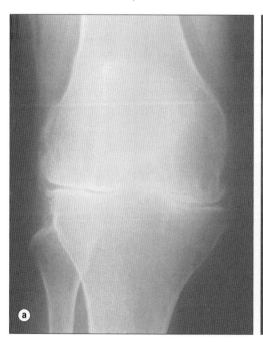
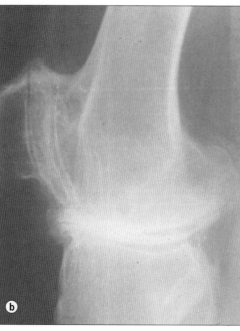

Fig. 179.12 Knee radiograph of patient with coexistent rheumatoid arthritis (RA) and CPPD deposition. On the anteroposterior view (a) there is widespread cartilage loss, but the lateral view (b) shows marked new bone formation atypical of RA.

TABLE 179.3 METABOLIC DISEASES PREDISPOSING TO CPPD DEPOSITION

	CC	Pseudogout	Chronic PA
Hemochromatosis	Yes	Yes	Yes
Hyperparathyroidism	Yes	Yes	No
Hypophosphatasia	Yes	Yes	No
Hypomagnesemia	Yes	Yes	No
Hypothyroidism	Probably	No	No
Gout	Possibly	Possibly	No
Acromegaly	Possibly	No	No
Familial hypocalciuric hypercalcemia	Possibly	No	No
X-linked hypophosphatemic rickets	Possibly	Possibly	Possibly

CC, chondrocalcinosis; PA, pyrophosphate arthropathy.

may be the presenting feature of metabolic disease (Table 179.3), and a search is warranted in the following circumstances:

- early-onset arthritis (<55 years)
- florid polyarticular, as opposed to pauciarticular, chondrocalcinosis
- recurrent acute attacks more than chronic arthropathy
- the presence of additional clinical or radiographic clues that suggest the diagnosis.

A 'blanket' screen for young-onset, polyarticular chondrocalcinosis includes serum calcium, alkaline phosphatase, magnesium, ferritin and liver function, but investigation may be more focused if additional clues suggest specific conditions. Hemochromatosis may present radiographic changes similar to those of sporadic pyrophosphate arthropathy, although possible differentiating features include more widespread metacarpophalangeal involvement, the absence of scapholunate dissociation, multiple 'ring cysts' in large joints, and subchondral bone fragmentation at the hip[23,27]. In older patients with typical pauciarticular disease and no added features, further tests other than calcium studies (performed for additional reasons in this age group) are probably unwarranted.

DIFFERENTIAL DIAGNOSIS

Acute pseudogout

The occurrence of acute synovitis in one or a few joints, overlying erythema, pyrexia, systemic upset and purulent joint fluid (particularly in the setting of preceding surgery, trauma or infective illness) should always lead to the consideration and exclusion of sepsis. Because sepsis may coexist with crystal synovitis, Gram stain and culture of joint fluid should always be undertaken (culture of blood and other body fluids may also be appropriate), even once CPPD crystals are identified or radiographic chondrocalcinosis demonstrated. Gout is the other principal condition to consider, diagnosis again resting on synovial fluid analysis. Occasionally heavy bloodstaining of joint fluid may lead to consideration of other causes of hemarthrosis, especially bleeding disorder (low vitamin C levels in the elderly may encourage hemarthrosis) or subchondral fracture (particularly with preceding, provoking trauma). However, if CPPD crystals are identified, the clotting screen is normal, there is no lipid in the aspirated fluid and no radiographic fracture, the diagnosis of pseudogout alone can be accepted. If localized tenderness and pain on weightbearing persist following resolution of synovitis, repeat radiographs (± subsequent bone scan) may be justified to detect missed fracture.

Chronic pyrophosphate arthropathy

In most cases the characteristic distribution, radiographic features and joint fluid findings permit a ready diagnosis. In older patients, however,

a marked inflammatory component, polyarthritis with metacarpophalangeal involvement and modest elevation of ESR may lead to consideration of RA (pseudorheumatoid arthritis[2]), particularly as large joint involvement may predominate in elderly patients with RA. Nevertheless, with pyrophosphate arthropathy the following considerations usually permit distinction: infrequency of metatarsophalangeal arthropathy; infrequency of tenosynovitis; infrequency of severe systemic upset; absence of extra-articular features; lack of juxta-articular osteopenia and erosions; lack of strong seropositivity for rheumatoid factor; and positive joint fluid and radiographic findings for pyrophosphate arthropathy.

Patients with marked proximal stiffness and elevated ESR are differentiated from those with polymyalgia rheumatica mainly by careful locomotor examination, and by positive joint fluid and radiographic findings. Oral corticosteroids often improve symptoms in such patients but rarely give the rapid 'cure' of polymyalgia: response to local intra-articular corticosteroid may be more impressive.

Differentiation from uncomplicated OA is often by the different pattern of distribution between and within articulations; the more florid inflammatory component; the presence of superimposed acute attacks; radiographic findings of atypical distribution for OA, chondrocalcinosis, prominent osteophyte and cyst formation; and synovial fluid CPPD crystals.

Although destructive pyrophosphate arthropathy may radiographically resemble a neuropathic joint (shoulder involvement suggesting syringomyelia, knee involvement tabes) such joints are severely symptomatic and arise in the absence of overt neurologic or serologic abnormality.

Although the description of clinical presentations by the addition of 'pseudo' to other diagnostic labels suggests the close mimicry of other joint disease, the diagnosis is usually suspected on clinical grounds alone, and confirmed by the synovial fluid and radiographic findings. However, CPPD deposition commonly coexists or is superimposed upon other recognizable joint disease, making the prefix 'pseudo-' clearly inappropriate[3]. The commonest associated condition is OA (generalized, pauciarticular or post-traumatic) affecting the same or distant joints, though coexistent gout, sepsis, rheumatoid, apatite-associated destructive arthropathy or true Charcot arthropathy may all occur. In such cases the diagnostic label should reflect both conditions, though the relative contribution of each may vary at different sites in the same individual.

Although rare, tophaceous CPPD should be considered with malignancy, tophaceous gout and tumoral calcinosis in the differential diagnosis of calcified lesions involving periarticular soft tissues. Examination of biopsy material is inevitably required for correct diagnosis[22].

STRUCTURE AND FUNCTION

Pyrophosphate metabolism

Inorganic pyrophosphate (PPi) is produced as a byproduct of multiple intracellular biosynthetic reactions throughout the body[28]. Despite very high turnover (estimated in kg/day) both intra- and extracellular concentrations are maintained at a generally low level by ubiquitous pyrophosphatases which metabolize PPi (complexed to magnesium) to orthophosphate. Despite its high-energy phosphoester bond (implicated in the biochemical origin of life), PPi is not known to be an energy source in mammals, nor it is known to be synthesized de novo.

Numerous biological roles for PPi are now recognized, including participation in intracellular Ca^{2+} traffic, mediation of nucleotide and iron transport, modulation of enzyme systems, storage of molecules in cellular granules and effects on mitogenesis[28]. In locomotor tissues, however, an important role derived from the study of matrix vesicles is

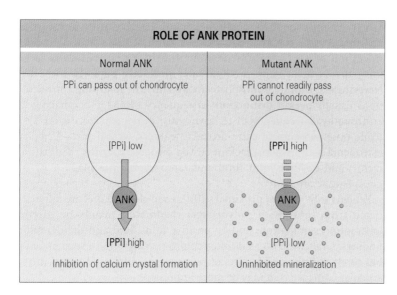

ROLE OF ANK PROTEIN

Normal ANK	Mutant ANK
PPi can pass out of chondrocyte	PPi cannot readily pass out of chondrocyte
[PPi] low	[PPi] high
ANK	ANK
[PPi] high	[PPi] low
Inhibition of calcium crystal formation	Uninhibited mineralization

Fig. 179.13 Role of ANK protein. The role of ANK protein in regulating the exit of pyrophosphate from cells with subsequent inhibition of apatite mineralization.

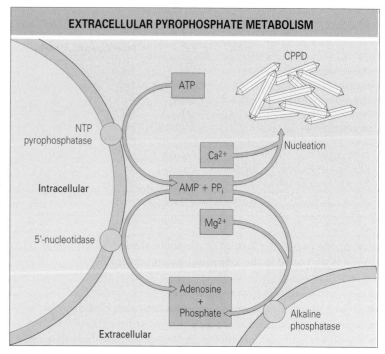

EXTRACELLULAR PYROPHOSPHATE METABOLISM

Fig. 179.14 Extracellular pyrophosphate metabolism. Outline of main factors relating to extracellular pyrophosphate metabolism. AMP, adenosine monophosphate; for other abbreviations, see text.

modulation of apatite mineralization[29]. A certain level of PPi is required for the initial nucleation of apatite from amorphous calcium phosphate and for subsequent crystal growth. Paradoxically, higher levels of PPi inhibit these processes by preventing nucleation and by adsorbing to the surface of apatite crystals, preventing further crystal growth and acting as a crystal poison. Alkaline phosphatase is the principal pyrophosphatase at the extracellular site of mineralization, and its effect on PPi levels alone could theoretically control apatite formation and growth.

The source of extracellular PPi remains uncertain. As the substrates for its formation are nucleoside triphosphates (NTP), the majority of PPi derived from NTP-dependent biosynthetic reactions probably originates intracellularly. As a phosphate ester, however, PPi cannot passively cross membranes. A transport system exchanges PPi for adenosine diphosphate (ADP) at the mitochondrial level, but until recently no active or facilitative transport mechanism for PPi was recognized at the cell surface. The multipass membrane-transporter protein ANK, however, is now known to regulate the passage of PPi to the exterior of the cell[30]. Defects in the ANK protein can result in high intracellular but low extracellular levels of PPi (Fig. 179.13). The subsequent low extracellular PPi levels and reduced inhibition of apatite formation and growth may then result in abnormal mineralization of locomotor tissues. Such extensive calcification in and around joints results in the 'ankylosis' mouse phenotype from which the protein and its gene were first determined[30]. It has not yet been confirmed, however, whether defects in the ANK gene and ANK protein relate to chondrocalcinosis or calcific periarthritis in humans.

The family of phosphodiesterase nucleotide pyrophosphatase (PDNP) enzymes includes plasma cell membrane glycoprotein 1 (PC1, located on the membrane of cells and matrix vesicles), autotaxin (secreted from cells) and PDNP3 (intracellular). All these PDNP enzymes hydrolyze the phosphodiesterase 1 bond of purine and pyrimidine NTPs and thus have NTP pyrophosphohydrolase (NTPPPH) activity[31]. The ectoenzyme PC1 appears particularly important in generating PPi from extracellular NTP at sites of CPPD formation in cartilage[31]. The activity of surface 5′-nucleotidase may influence this reaction in favor of PPi production (Fig. 179.14). The principal extracellular NTP substrate for PC1 is adenosine triphosphate (ATP). ATP is released from chondrocytes, particularly following mechanical loading[32], during increased cell activity, cell division and injury, and possibly during vesicular extrusion of matrix components and other products[28]. Extracellular ATP may have cell signaling functions, activating P2 purinoceptors of chondrocytes to raise

intracellular calcium levels, and also directly activate pain fibers. The level of extracellular ATP, however, together with PC1 activity, is also important in determining extracellular PPi levels and hence possible CPPD crystal formation[28,33].

Extracellular PPi, complexed with magnesium, is normally rapidly processed by surface alkaline phosphatase to orthophosphate, which can readily cross membranes. In organ culture adult hyaline and fibrocartilage, but not synovium or bone, elaborate extracellular PPi. Increased production of PPi is observed in growth cartilage and human OA cartilage. The addition of ATP to cultured articular cartilage encourages CPPD crystal formation, particularly around articular chondrocyte vesicles (ACVs)[33]. These vesicles, analogous to matrix vesicles of growing cartilage, are trilaminar, phospholipid membrane-limited structures adjacent to chondrocytes. They avidly bind calcium and are rich in all the enzymes that generate PPi and orthophosphate. Cultured ACVs mineralize in the presence of calcium and ATP[34]. Depending on the ratio of PPi to orthophosphate (excess ATP producing a high, and restricted ATP a low, ratio), ACVs produce either CPPD, basic calcium phosphate or both[34]. However, factors other than ATP concentration can influence extracellular PPi elaboration in cartilage. For example, transforming growth factor-β, (TGF-β) stimulates PPi elaboration from hyaline cartilage, fibrocartilage and ligament (but not synovium) whereas insulin-like growth factor (IGF)-1 inhibits this effect[35,36]. Aging also influences the elaboration of extracellular PPi by chondrocytes. For example, TFG-β increases PPi levels to a greater extent in chondrocytes from older subjects, whereas the stimulus to cell proliferation from IGF is attenuated in such cells[37]. Several cell signaling pathways may be of relevance in moderating such responses – protein kinase C activation stimulates and adenyl cyclase stimulation diminishes PPi elaboration[38].

Compared to normal knees, elevated synovial fluid concentrations of PPi are reported both in chronic pyrophosphate arthropathy and uncomplicated OA[28,39], the normal plasma and urinary concentrations in such cases supporting increased intra-articular production. Less impressive synovial fluid elevations are seen in pseudogout, with subnormal levels in RA[28,39], these lower levels perhaps reflecting increased clearance of PPi in inflamed states. Extracellular ATP, the major substrate for PPi,

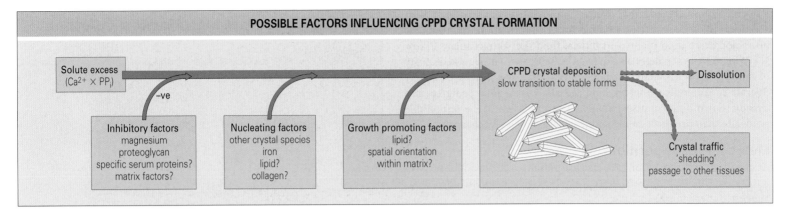

Fig. 179.15 Possible factors influencing CPPD crystal formation.

has been confirmed in synovial fluid, with higher levels in pyrophosphate arthropathy than in OA or RA[28]. However, correlation between PPi levels and NTPPPH, alkaline phosphatase and 5′-nucleotidase activities is inconsistent, and no clear-cut pattern of altered enzyme activity has emerged.

CPPD crystal formation

Factors likely to affect the formation, growth and dissolution of CPPD crystals are outlined in Figure 179.15. The formation of CPPD appears restricted principally to fibro- and hyaline cartilage (less commonly capsule, tendon) with only two of 12 known crystallographic forms occurring – the triclinic (t-CPPD) and monoclinic (m-CPPD) dimorphs[40]. Unlike monosodium urate (MSUM), CPPD crystals require exacting physicochemical conditions for formation, and crystals resembling those occurring *in vivo* are very difficult to manufacture from solution systems. To date no animal model has been developed, and most knowledge derives from model systems employing gels (nonbiologic, gelatin or native collagen gels) in various study designs. From these the following generalities appear true:

- In addition to the product ($Ca^{2+} \times PPi$), local magnesium concentration importantly influences CPPD deposition by inhibiting nucleation and growth, and by enhancing dissolution. Orthophosphates, chondroitin sulfate and proteoglycan are also inhibitory to nucleation and growth. With proteoglycan this effect depends on the spatial arrangement of carboxylate ligands, which may operate via calcium binding or spatial regulation of Mg^{2+}, phosphate or unidentified small molecular weight promoters and inhibitors.
- Conversely, nucleating and growth-promoting factors include iron ($Fe^{3+}>Fe^{2+}$) and seeded MSUM crystals. Interestingly, seeded apatite has little epitaxial effect but efficiently traps PPi, leading to more stable CPPD growth. A possible promoting role for collagen and acidic phospholipid has been suggested.
- Formation of m-CPPD and t-CPPD is slow, occurring via intermediate crystal species, with t-CPPD being the final, most stable form. Such formation–dissolution–reformation facilitates a localized ionic concentrating process.

Histologic studies suggest that CPPD crystals form extracellularly in pericellular sites, usually the collagenous matrix outside the lacunar area, in the midzone of fibro- and hyaline cartilage[41]. A close association is reported with hypertropic or metaplastic chondrocytes containing Sudan-positive lipid granules[41], and similar lipid may occur around CPPD crystals, the involved matrix often being proteoglycan deplete and degenerate. Such findings support the importance of tissue ('soil') factors, implying that reduction of inhibitors (e.g. proteoglycan) and an increase in promoters (e.g. lipid) combine to copromote CPPD forma-

tion. Conversely, elevation of synovial fluid PPi, perhaps released from hypertrophic and metabolically active chondrocytes, argues in favor of 'seed' components. The relative importance of these multiple factors may vary in different clinical settings. With respect to dissolution, CPPD crystals are extremely insoluble but can, however, be dissolved by alkaline phosphatase[42]. Magnesium enhances dissolution via both enzyme stimulation and enhanced release of PPi ions from the crystal surface, whereas calcium slows dissolution via enzyme inhibition.

ETIOLOGY

Although several associations are described (Table 179.4), the linking mechanisms are poorly understood.

Aging

This appears to be a major predisposing factor. Levels of PPi in synovial fluid from normal knees show no increase with age[43], suggesting that age-related alteration in matrix factors may be more important than alteration in PPi metabolism. A role for senile amyloid, which avidly binds calcium and PPi, has been suggested, although histologic investigation shows no correlation, chondrocalcinosis and amyloid predominating at different locations within cartilage[44]. An indirect association could come from the positive correlation with OA, but chondrocalcinosis commonly occurs in otherwise normal cartilage and this association remains unexplained.

Familial predisposition

A primary cartilage abnormality is suggested from histologic studies of Swedish and Japanese cases, the former demonstrating proteoglycan depletion, which may precede crystal formation[6], and the latter showing similar hypertrophic lipid-laden chondrocytes to those identified in sporadic chondrocalcinosis[41]. Conversely, a generalized abnormality of PPi metabolism is suggested by two reports[28] of increased intracellular PPi concentration (skin fibroblasts or transformed lymphoblasts) in French and American kindreds with familial chondrocalcinosis. Both studies,

TABLE 179.4 ASSOCIATIONS OF CPPD CRYSTAL DEPOSITION	
Positive	Aging
	Familial predisposition
	Metabolic disease
	Joint insult, osteoarthritis
	(DISH)
Negative	Rheumatoid arthritis

however, found considerable overlap with controls (and patients with sporadic CPPD[28]), and these findings await confirmation. Interestingly, no major overt abnormality of synovial fluid (i.e. extracellular) PPi or NTPPPH activity was detectable in five UK kindreds[9]. The clinical diversity of familial chondrocalcinosis suggests that different mechanisms may operate in different pedigrees. Linkage analysis in four pedigrees has already shown different associations[10–12], and isolation of the responsible genes and their products should shortly elucidate these mechanisms.

Metabolic predisposition

Associations with metabolic disease are rationalized through putative effects on PPi metabolism, extrapolated largely from *in vitro* data. Suggested mechanisms include:

- reduced breakdown of PPi by alkaline phosphatase, due to:
  - reduced levels (hypophosphatasia)
  - the presence of inhibitory ions (calcium, iron or copper in hyperparathyroidism, hemachromatosis, Wilson's disease, respectively)
  - impaired complexing with magnesium (hypomagnesemia)
- enhanced nucleation of CPPD crystals by increased iron (hemachromatosis) or copper (Wilson's disease)
- increased calcium concentration (hyperparathyroidism)
- increased PPi production through parathyroid hormone (PTH) stimulation of adenylate cyclase (hyperparathyroidism).

Effects on PPi metabolism are supported by the finding of elevated synovial fluid PPi in asymptomatic, structurally normal knees of patients with untreated hyperparathyroidism, hemochromatosis or hypomagnesemia[45] and elevated urinary and blood levels in hypophosphatasia[46]. Such differences may represent the clinical counterpart of matrix vesicle and ACV studies where a modest increase in PPi (mild hypophosphatasia) stimulates apatite but a great elevation (classic hypophosphatasia) is inhibitory to apatite but effectively predisposes to CPPD.

Mechanisms other than effects on PPi metabolism may also operate. Bone and cartilage changes may be marked in these disorders, and in those with frequent subchondral bone change and arthropathy (particularly hemochromatosis and Wilson's disease) CPPD deposition may be secondary to joint damage mediated via alterations in cartilage matrix factors.

Osteoarthritis and joint insult

The precise relationship between OA and CPPD remains unclear. Although both frequently coexist, each can occur without the other and both associate with age. Nevertheless, convincing evidence for a strong positive association, at least at the knee, comes from histologic[4,44] and epidemiologic[5] studies. The Framingham study, for example, confirmed an increased rate of radiographic OA in those with chondrocalcinosis (age-adjusted relative risk 1.52) and a similar link between chondrocalcinosis and severe OA (relative risk 1.52). Such data accord with many clinical surveys noting a high frequency and greater severity of OA in patients with associated CPPD.

Several observations support a relationship between preceding joint insult and the subsequent development of chondrocalcinosis[3], for example the high frequency of chondrocalcinosis (often localized, premature) in knees that have undergone surgery for osteochondritis dissecans or total meniscectomy; the frequency of CPPD in lumbar disc fibrocartilage removed at revision surgery; and reports of localized pyrophosphate arthropathy as a late complication of juvenile chronic arthritis, joint instability or trauma[3]. However, although CPPD commonly occurs with OA, controlled radiographic and synovial fluid surveys suggest a negative correlation between CPPD deposition and RA[26]. Furthermore, the occurrence of atypical osteoarthritic radiographic features in patients with coexistent disease suggests that the

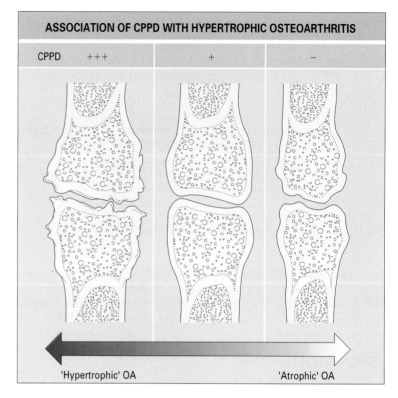

Fig. 179.16 Association of CPPD with hypertrophic osteoarthritis.

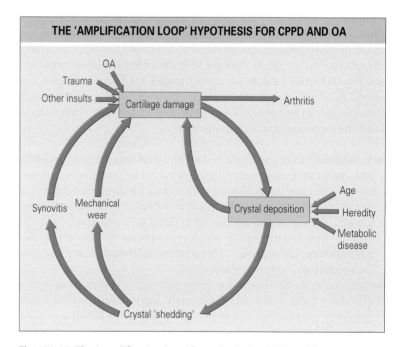

Fig. 179.17 The 'amplification loop' hypothesis for CPPD and OA.

primary association of CPPD is with hypertrophic tissue response and/or OA, rather than joint insult *per se* (Fig. 179.16). The increasing prevalence of knee synovial fluid CPPD crystals the more extensive and severe the radiographic OA[25] further supports this view. CPPD in the context of OA would therefore seem to reflect more a joint process (accompanying changes in cartilage) than a specific disease entity.

Another hypothesis to explain the variable interrelationship between OA and CPPD is the 'amplification loop' hypothesis (Fig. 179.17). This suggests that CPPD deposition may be enhanced by the tissue changes that accompany OA, and that, once formed, the CPPD crystals hasten further joint damage via inflammatory and mechanical effects[3]. Moderation of CPPD deposition by aging, familial factors and metabolic disease can influence the crystal load, and fissuring of cartilage increases the tendency to crystal shedding and superimposed acute attacks.

Factors accompanying joint damage and repair that explain positive and negative associations with CPPD are unknown, though alterations in both PPi and matrix factors could be relevant. For example, synovial fluid PPi levels are elevated in uncomplicated OA but reduced in RA[39], this difference perhaps reflecting chondrocyte activity and division rather than increased clearance by hypervascular synovium. Also, differential alterations in matrix-promoting or -inhibiting factors might influence crystal formation and growth. In this respect the strong negative correlation between RA and gout is of interest, suggesting that the presence of non-specific crystal inhibitors, or the absence of promoters, may be a characteristic of rheumatoid tissues.

The characteristic distribution of chronic pyrophosphate arthropathy, compared with OA, remains unexplained. Aging and gender, however, could be important confounders in that the prevalence both of OA at different joint sites and of CPPD deposition varies markedly according to these factors. The glenohumeral joint, for example, may appear a target site for pyrophosphate arthropathy because it only becomes a common site for OA in elderly women. Correction for age and gender may greatly reduce this often emphasized disparity in distribution between OA and chronic pyrophosphate arthropathy.

Diffuse idiopathic skeletal hyperostosis

This putative association[19] awaits confirmation. Interestingly, spinal hyperostosis in mild hypophosphatasia appears identical[46].

PATHOGENESIS

Crystal-associated inflammation

Crystals of CPPD, as with MSUM, have been studied mainly in respect of acute inflammation[47]. In general, laboratory-prepared CPPD crystals are markedly phlogistic particles in a wide variety of *in vitro* and *in vivo* systems, though less so on an equal-weight comparison, than MSUM.

Effects on humoral mediators, cell-derived mediators and cell membranes have all been demonstrated[47]. For example, CPPD crystals activate complement *in vitro* via effects on both classic and alternative pathways, and greatly elevated synovial fluid complement breakdown products (C3dg) occur in pseudogout, though interestingly not in chronic pyrophosphate arthropathy despite the presence of often marked clinical inflammation. Hageman factor is also activated *in vitro*, leading to the generation of kallikrein, bradykinin, plasmin and other soluble mediators. A dramatic effect of CPPD is marked perturbation of plasma membranes which causes membranolysis (lysosomes, red cells, neutrophils) as well as non-lytic platelet and neutrophil secretory responses. Crystals of CPPD induce superoxide production by neutrophils and the release of lysosomal enzymes, chemotactic factor and lipoxygenase-derived products of arachidonic acid, including leukotriene B$_4$, following phagocytosis. Other CPPD–cell interactions include the secretion of interleukin-1 (IL-1) and tumor necrosis factor by monocytes, and the release of newly synthesized IL-6 from synoviocytes and monocytes (in accord with the high synovial fluid IL-6 levels demonstrated in pseudogout).

Many of these effects result from direct crystal contact, though some (e.g. classic pathway complement activation) may be enhanced or mediated via IgG adsorbed on to the crystal surface (Fig. 179.18). In biological systems CPPD crystals avidly attract both anionic and cationic proteins, with some preferential selection for immunoglobulin, especially IgG. Although the altered stereochemical configuration of adsorbed IgG may be proinflammatory, other protein binding may be inhibitory. Of most interest in this respect are apo B-containing low-density and high-density lipoproteins, binding with which, for example, inhibits CPPD-induced cytolysis of neutrophils.

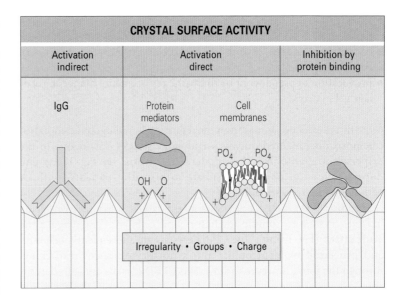

Fig. 179.18 Crystal surface activity. Potential interactions and blocking at the crystal surface.

Certain physical characteristics of CPPD and other crystals appear to relate to inflammatory potential. In general, smaller crystals are more inflammatory than large ones; this may result from mechanical effects (e.g. greater ease of phagocytosis) or merely reflect the greater surface area/weight presented for protein or membrane interaction. 'Roughness' and net negative surface charge are also important. Crystal surfaces of inflammatory membranolytic crystals (MSUM, CPPD) are irregular and possess a high density of charged groups that give a high negative δ potential, whereas surfaces of non-inflammatory crystals (diamond, stishovite) are smooth, with low or zero δ potential; brushite and apatite are intermediate in these respects and are associated with more modest inflammatory effects.

Less is known of chronic CPPD-induced tissue damage, though postulated mechanisms included persistent synovial inflammation and altered cell metabolism. Intradermal injection of CPPD causes a chronic 'granulomatous' reaction lasting several weeks; unlike acute inflammation, CPPD is more potent that MSUM in this respect. Stimulation of collagen production by fibroblasts is well studied with respect to other crystals (asbestos, silica) and may occur without much overt inflammation.

There are few data on the possible mechanical effects of crystals in joints. Deposition of hard CPPD crystals within the cartilage matrix might theoretically be disadvantageous for cartilage, but equally might facilitate impact force transmission, depending on the shape, size, extent and orientation of the crystals[48]. However, the occurrence of free crystals at the cartilage–cartilage interface is likely to be damaging through their effects as 'wear' (abrasive) particles[49]. Although usually quickly cleared from synovial fluid, the presence of even small amounts of CPPD crystals may thus be more harmful than very much larger deposits within cartilage.

Crystal shedding

Given the difficult physicochemical requirements of *in vitro* manufacture, nucleation and growth of CPPD crystals in synovial fluid would seem unlikely, and the preferred mechanism to explain the occurrence of CPPD within synovial fluid is 'shedding' from preformed deposits within cartilage[24]. This could be accomplished by a reduction in crystal size, fissuring of cartilage or alteration in cartilage matrix that allows the easier escape of crystals. Circumstantial evidence to support each of these includes:

- provocation of pseudogout by joint lavage with crystal solubilizing agents, or by situations (acute stress response, parathyroidectomy) associating with reduction in ionized calcium (reduced crystal size)

- provocation of pseudogout by trauma (microfissuring, 'shaking loose')
- concurrence of pseudogout and sepsis ('enzymatic strip mining' of crystals)
- provocation of pseudogout by thyroxine replacement (change in cartilage gel matrix).

More direct evidence comes from the reduction in radiographic chondrocalcinosis documented during pseudogout attacks (analogous to the dispersal of apatite in acute calcific periarthritis; see Fig. 179.17 and during follow-up of pyrophosphate arthropathy patients, with or without associated cartilage loss[16,24].

Shedding from cartilage deposits might expose previously protected 'naked' crystals to soluble mediators and cells and thus trigger the acute attack (Fig. 179.19). The CPPD crystals are subsequently taken up and processed by neutrophils and synoviocytes; such 'trafficking' through the joint, however, is slow, and CPPD crystals are still identifiable in synovial fluid as the attack settles. What 'turns off' the attack and permits inflammatory crystals to reside in synovial fluid during non-inflamed intercritical periods remains unexplained. Nevertheless, coating by inhibitory proteins (some acute-phase reactants?) appears more plausible than altered responsiveness or changes in the physical properties of CPPD.

PATHOLOGY

Unlike MSUM, CPPD crystals do not deposit in all connective tissues but are virtually confined to locomotor structures. Pathologic data largely support primary deposition in cartilage (less commonly, capsule, tendon) with secondary release and uptake by synovium, tenosynovium or bursae.

Microscopy of cartilage usually shows rounded, sharply demarcated crystal deposits within a granular matrix in the midzone[4,41,44]. The earliest lesions are perilacunar, but with widespread chondrocalcinosis superficial cartilage may be involved, with tophus-like deposits predominating in the midzone. Electron microscopy studies may dislodge CPPD crystals, and those visualized often appear vacuolated and 'foamy' (artefactual) with a bumpy contour, perhaps representing adsorbed protein. Surrounding cartilage may appear normal or show loss of metachromasia, chondrocyte cloning or fibrillation; occurrences of associated lipid-laden hypertrophic metaplastic chondrocytes have particularly been emphasized[41]. With severe cartilage changes subchondral bone may show thickened trabeculae with multiple cysts; cyst fracture occasionally results in bone fragmentation and collapse. In synovium, CPPD crystals usually occur superficially in the interstitial space and synoviocyte vacuoles, often surrounded by fibrocytes and connective tissue; neutrophil and lymphocyte infiltrates may be present, but the prominent response is lining cell hyperplasia. Tophus-like deposits, surrounding giant cell reactions and osteochondral bodies, are occasional findings. In advanced disease, masses of CPPD crystals may virtually replace ischemic-appearing villi. Changes in bursae and tendon sheaths resemble those in synovium.

Additional findings may occur with predisposing disease. In hemochromatosis iron is present in chondrocytes and synovium, appearing most abundant in synthetic synovial lining cells rather than in deeper cells and macrophages (as seen with repeated bleeds). Ochronosis is also readily identified by the grossly black, microscopically golden brown pigmentation in cartilage or in cartilage fragments in synovium.

MANAGEMENT

Acute synovitis

The aims of management for pseudogout are to reduce symptoms; identify and treat triggering illness; and rapidly mobilize as inflammation settles.

Rapid mobilization is particularly important, as many patients are elderly and especially prone to complications due to prolonged immobility. Many also have coexisting medical problems and are especially at risk from drug side effects and interactions. In general, therefore, local rather than systemic therapy is preferred, particularly as pseudogout affects usually only one or a few joints.

Aspiration, injection

In most cases aspiration alone greatly relieves symptoms and may be the only treatment required. Fluid reaccumulation, however, is common, particularly early in the attack. Therefore, for florid pseudogout intra-articular corticosteroid injection is appropriate, either at the time of initial aspiration or as a second procedure following reaccumulation (some prefer the reassurance of a negative Gram stain and/or culture before injecting). Joint lavage (normal saline, room temperature) can help settle attacks but is reserved for troublesome relapsing or prolonged episodes unresponsive to corticosteroid injection.

Oral drugs

Simple analgesic and non-steroidal drugs may give additional benefit, but these must be used with caution in elderly or medically unfit patients. Oral colchicine is effective but rarely warranted. For severe polyarticular attacks unresponsive to aspiration and injection of the largest affected joints, oral corticosteroid may be considered, though its efficacy is anecdotal.

Additional measures

Identification of triggering illness that requires specific treatment (e.g. chest infection) is by appropriate patient enquiry and examination.

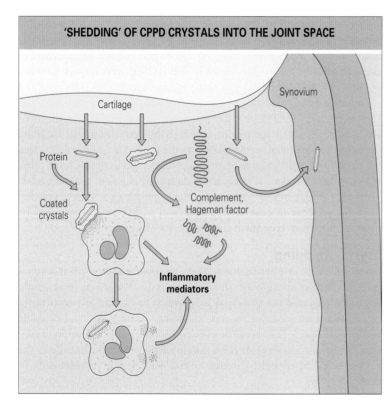

Fig. 179.19 'Shedding' of CPPD crystals into the joint space. The preformed CPPD crystals initiate an acute attack but then become protein coated and processed by synoviocytes and inflammatory cells.

Once the synovitis is settling, increasing mobilization with attention to muscle training exercises should be undertaken.

Chronic pyrophosphate arthropathy

Unlike gout there is no specific therapy, and treatment of any underlying metabolic disease (e.g. hyperparathyroidism, hemochromatosis) does not influence locomotor outcome. The aims of management are the same as those for OA: to educate and advise the patient, to reduce and control symptoms, and to retain or improve function. The choice of interventions is also the same as for OA and a variety of strategies may be beneficial (see Chapter 171). Whether the presence of chondrocalcinosis or synovial fluid CPPD crystals is a predictor of response to individual treatments for OA, however, has not been formally examined in clinical trials.

General principles

All patients should receive:

- Education concerning the nature of their arthritis
- A prescription of exercise – both local strengthening and aerobic/ fitness exercise
- Reduction of adverse mechanical factors – for example, reduction of obesity, 'pacing' of activities through the day, use of a cane or other walking aid, appropriate footwear
- Simple analgesia – paracetamol is the oral drug of first choice; topical NSAIDs and capsaicin cream are also both safe and often effective, especially for knee and hand involvement.

In discussion with the patient, a variety of other options may then be selected according to individual patient beliefs and requirements, disease severity, and the coexistence of any comorbidity and chronic therapy. Recognition and management of depression and the use of coping strategies are as applicable to elderly patients with pyrophosphate arthropathy as to young patients with RA.

Control of chronic synovitis

Despite the presence of often marked structural abnormality, intra-articular corticosteroid injection often greatly improves symptoms. Though often temporary, this may improve the patient's optimism, encourage adherence in other aspects of treatment, and provide a useful interval for effective physiotherapy or enjoyment of an important life event (e.g. holiday).

Intra-articular radiocolloid (yttrium-90) may be considered in patients with troublesome knee (or shoulder) synovitis who show definite, but temporary, improvement following corticosteroid injection. Prolonged symptomatic benefit may be obtained with such treatment, even in cases with gross structural change[3]. If synovitis recurs (again corticosteroid responsive), single repeat treatment may be considered. Radiosynovectomy is also useful for recurrent hemarthrosis, presumably by induction of synovial fibrosis.

Other symptomatic drugs

Stronger analgesics, such as opioids, NSAIDs, coxibs, nefopam and tramadol, may be required but carry an appreciable incidence of side effects and drug interactions. As for pseudogout, such symptomatic drugs are used with caution in the elderly. The patient should be clearly informed regarding optimal usage, the requirement for oral drugs should be regularly reviewed, and 'repeat' prescribing avoided. One 6-month placebo-controlled study of oral magnesium supplementation, given to enhance solubility and inhibit the formation of CPPD, showed limited symptomatic benefit without alteration in radiographic chondrocalcinosis[3]. Such treatment was well tolerated and further long-term studies seem warranted.

Surgery

Patients with progressive or destructive large joint arthropathy who require replacement appear to derive benefit equal to those with uncomplicated OA, without any increased risk of prosthetic failure.

REFERENCES

1. Kohn NN, Hughes RE, McCarty DJ, Faires JS. The significance of calcium pyrophospate crystals in the synovial fluid of arthritic patients: The 'pseudogout syndrome'. II. Identification of crystals. Ann Intern Med 1962; 56: 738–745.
2. McCarty DJ. Calcium pyrophosphate dihydrate crystal deposition disease – 1975. Arthritis Rheum 1976; 19(suppl); 275–286.
3. Doherty M, Dieppe PA. Clinical aspects of calcium pyrophosphate dihydrate crystal deposition. Rheum Dis Clin North Am 1988; 14: 395–414.
4. Mitrovic DR, Stankovic A, Iriarte-Borda O et al. The prevalences of chondrocalcinosis in the human knee joint. An autopsy survey. J Rheumatol 1988; 15: 633–641.
5. Felson DT, Anderson JJ, Naimark A et al. Recently fitted. The prevalence of chondrocalcinosis in the elderly and its association with knee osteoarthritis: the Framingham study. J Rheumatol 1989; 16: 1241–1245.
6. Bjelle AO. Morphological study of articular cartilage in pyrophosphate arthropathy. (Chondrocalcinosis articularis or calcium pyrophosphate dihydrate crystal deposition disease). Ann Rheum Dis 1972; 31: 449–456.
7. Reginato AJ. Articular chondrocalcinosis in the Chiloe Islanders. Arthritis Rheum 1976; 19: 395–404.
8. Riestra JL, Sanchez A, Rodriguez-Valverde V, Alonson JL. Radiographic features of hereditary articular chondrocalcinosis. A comparative study with the sporadic type. Clin Exp Rheumatol 1988; 6: 369–372.
9. Doherty M, Hamilton E, Henderson J et al. Familial chondrocalcinosis due to calcium pyrophosphate dihydrate crystal deposition in English families. Br J Rheumatol 1991; 30: 10–15.
10. Hughes A, McGibbon D, Woodward E et al. Localisation of a gene for chondrocalcinosis to chromosome 5p. Hum Mol Genet 1995; 4: 1225–1228.
11. Andrew LJ, Brancolini V, Serrano de la Pena L et al. Refinement of the chromosome 5p locus for familial calcium pyrophosphate dihydrate deposition disease. Am J Hum Genet 1999; 64: 136–145.
12. Baldwin CT, Farrer LA, Adair R et al. Linkage of early-onset osteoarthritis and chondrocalcinosis to human chromosome 8q. Am J Hum Genet 1995; 56: 692–697.
13. Jones AC, Chuck AJ, Arie EA et al. Diseases associated with calcium pyrophosphate deposition disease. Semin Arthritis Rheum 1992; 22: 188–202.
14. Dieppe PA, Alexander GM, Jones H et al. Pyrophosphate arthropathy: a clinical and radiological study of 105 cases. Ann Rheum Dis 1982; 41: 371–376.
15. Doherty M. Pyrophosphate arthropathy – a clinical study. MD thesis, Cambridge University, 1987.
16. Doherty M, Dieppe PA, Watt I. Pyrophosphate arthropathy: a prospective study. Br J Rheumatol 1993; 32: 189–196.
17. Ledingham J, Regan M, Jones A, Doherty M. Factors affecting radiographic progression of knee osteoarthritis. Ann Rheum Dis 1995; 54: 53–58.
18. Menkes CJ, Simon F, Delrieu F et al. Destructive arthropathy in chondrocalcinosis articularis. Arthritis Rheum 1976; 19: 329–348.
19. Okazaki T, Saito T, Mitommo Y, Sicta Y. Pseudogout: clinical observations and chemical analyses of deposits. Arthritis Rheum 1976; 19: 293–305.
20. Gerster JC, Lagier R. Upper limb pyrophosphate tenosynovitis outside the carpal tunnel. Ann Rheum Dis 1989; 48: 689–691.
21. Pattrick M, Watt I, Dieppe PA, Doherty M. Peripheral nerve entrapment at the wrist in pyrophosphate arthropathy. J Rheumatol 1988; 15: 1254–1257.
22. Sissons HA, Steiner GC, Bonar F et al. Tumoral calcium pyrophosphate deposition disease. Skeletal Radiol 1989; 18: 79–87.
23. Resnick D, Niwayama G. Calcium pyrophosphate dihydrate (CPPD) crystal deposition disease. In: Resnick D, Niwayama G. Diagnosis of bone and joint disorders. Philadelphia: WB Saunders, 1981; 1520–1574.
24. Doherty M, Dieppe PA. Acute pseudogout: 'Crystal shedding' or acute crystallisation? Arthritis Rheum 1981; 24: 954–957.
25. Pattrick M, Hamilton E, Wilson R et al. Association of radiographic changes of osteoarthritis, symptoms and synovial fluid particles in 300 knees. Ann Rheum. Dis 1993; 52: 97–103.
26. Doherty M, Dieppe PA, Watt I. Low incidence of calcium pyrophosphate dihydrate crystal deposition in rheumatoid arthritis with modification of radiographic features in coexistent disease. Arthritis Rheum 1984; 27: 1002–1009.
27. Adamson TC, Resnik CS, Guerra J et al. Hand and wrist arthropathies of haemochromatosis and calcium pyrophosphate deposition disease: distinct radiographic features. Radiology 1983; 147: 377–381.
28. Rachow JW, Ryan LM. Inorganic pyrophosphate metabolism in arthritis. Rheum Dis Clin North Am 1988; 14: 289–302.
29. Einhorn Tenancy Agreement, Gordon SL, Siegel SA, Hummel CF et al. Matrix vesicle enzymes in human osteoarthritis. J Orthop Res 1985; 3: 160–169.
30. Ho AM, Johnson MD, Kingsley DM. Role of the mouse ank gene in control of tissue calcification and arthritis. Science 2000; 289: 265–270.
31. Johnson K. Hashimoto S, Lotz M et al. Up-regulated expression of the phosphodiesterase nucleotide pyrophosphatase family member PC-1 is a marker

and pathogenic factor for knee meniscal cartilage matrix calcification. Arthritis Rheum 2001; 44: 1071–1081.

32. Graff RD, Lazarowski ER, Banes AJ, Lee GM. ATP release by mechanically loaded porcine chondrons in pellet culture. Arthritis Rheum 2000; 43: 1571–1579.

33. Ryan LM. Kurup IV, Derfus BA, Kushnaryov VM. ATP-induced chondrocalcinosis. Arthritis Rheum 1992; 35: 1520–1525.

34. Derfus BA, Rachow JW, Mandel NS et al. Articular cartilage vesicles generate calcium pyrophosphate dihydrate-like crystals in vitro. Arthritis Rheum 1992; 35: 231–240.

35. Olmez U, Ryan LM, Kurup IV, Rosenthal A. Insulin-like growth factor-1 suppresses pyrophosphate elaboration by transforming growth factor beta1-stimulated chondrocytes and cartilage. Osteoarthritis Cartilage 1994; 2: 149–154.

36. Rosenthal AK, McCarty BA, Cheung HS, Ryan LM. A comparison of the effect of transforming growth factor β1 on pyrophosphate elaboration from various articular tissues. Arthritis Rheum 1993; 36: 539–542.

37. Rosen F, McCabe G, Quach J et al. Differential effects of aging on human chondrocyte responses to transforming growth factor β. Arthritis Rheum 1997; 40: 1275–1281.

38. Ryan LM, Kurup IV, Cheung HS. Transduction mechanisms of porcine chondrocyte inorganic pyrophosphate elaboration. Arthritis Rheum 1999; 42: 555–560.

39. Pattrick M, Hamilton E, Hornby J, Doherty M. Synovial fluid pyrophosphate and nucleoside triphosphates pyrophosphatase: comparison between normal and diseased and between inflamed and non-inflamed joints. Ann Rheum Dis 1991; 50: 214–218.

40. Mandel N, Mandel G. Calcium pyrophosphate crystal deposition in model systems. Rheum Dis Clin North Am 1988; 14: 21–40.

41. Ishikawa K, Masuda I, Ohira T, Yokoyama M. A histological study of calcium pyrophosphate dihydrate crystal-deposition disease. J Bone Joint Surg 1989; 71A: 875–876.

42. Xu Y, Pritzker KPH, Cruz TF. Characterisation of chondrocyte alkaline phosphatase as a potential mediator in the dissolution of calcium pyrophosphate dihydrate crystals. J Rheumatol 1994; 21: 912–919.

43. Hamilton E, Pattrick M, Doherty M. Inorganic pyrophosphate, nucleoside triphosphates pyrophosphatase, and cartilage fragments in normal human synovial fluid. Br J Rheumatol 1991; 30: 260–264.

44. Sokoloff L, Varma AA. Chondrocalcinosis in surgically resected joints. Arthritis Rheum 1988; 31: 750–756.

45. Doherty M, Chuck A, Hosking D, Hamilton E. Inorganic pyrophosphate in metabolic diseases predisposing to calcium pyrophosphate dihydrate crystal deposition. Arthritis Rheum 1991; 34: 1297–1303.

46. Chuck AJ, Pattrick MG, Hamilton E et al. Crystal deposition in hypophosphatasia: a reappraisal. Ann Rheum Dis 1989; 48: 571–576.

47. Terkeltaub RA, Ginsberg MH. The inflammatory reaction to crystals. Rheum Dis Clin North Am 1988; 14: 353–364.

48. Clift SE, Harris B, Dieppe PA. Load concentrations around crystal aggregates in articular cartilage under short-term loading. J Eng Med 1993; 207: 35–40.

49. Hayes A, Harris B, Dieppe PA, Clift SE. Wear of articular cartilage: the effects of crystals. Proc IME 1993; 207: 41–58.

180

Basic calcium phosphate crystal deposition disease

Geraldine M McCarthy

Definition

Calcific periarthritis

- Periarticular deposits of calcific material (hydroxyapatite)
- May result in calcific periarthritis, tendinitis or bursitis

Intra-articular deposition

- Intra-articular deposits of basic calcium phosphate (BCP) crystals may be found in joint fluid as well as in articular cartilage and synovium

Clinical features

Calcific periarthritis

- The shoulder is the main site affected but deposits have been described near many other joints
- Deposits are often inert and asymptomatic
- Deposits can rupture, causing a local acute, crystal-induced inflammation
- Deposits may also be associated with local chronic pain and functional impairment

Intra-articular deposition

- Deposits are often inert and asymptomatic
- Deposits often occur in patients with osteoarthritis
- Crystals can occasionally be shed into the joint, resulting in an acute synovitis resembling gout
- BCP crystals are also found in abundance in the joints of older patients with large joint destructive arthropathies, such as the 'Milwaukee shoulder' syndrome

HISTORY

Calcific periarthritis

Calcific scapulohumeral periarthritis was first described in 1870 and radiographic demonstration of periarticular shoulder calcifications was accomplished by 1907[1]. These calcifications were initially regarded as having arisen in the subdeltoid bursa but were subsequently demonstrated to occur chiefly in the supraspinatus tendon or the shoulder joint capsule. Thirty years later, renewed interest in periarthritis of the shoulder led to further descriptions of the phenomenon and also the recognition of periarticular calcifications at other sites[2]. After another 30 years, it was recognized that the calcific material consisted of hydroxyapatite[3], and the pathophysiologic theory of primary tendon necrosis leading to secondary calcification followed[4]. Subsequently, aggregates of basic calcium phosphate (BCP) crystals with their various crystalline structures and chemical compositions have been further defined using ultrastructural and physical microanalysis techniques, including analytical electron microscopy, X-ray diffraction and Fourier transformation

infrared spectroscopy[5]. The term BCP includes crystals of partially carbonate substituted hydroxyapatite, octacalcium phosphate, and rarely found tricalcium phosphate.

Intra-articular BCP crystal deposition

The earliest description of the pathoanatomical features of the consequences of intra-articular BCP crystal deposition appears to have been by Robert Adams in 1857 and called 'chronic rheumatic arthritis of the shoulder'[6]. In his 1934 monograph, Codman reported the case of a 51-year-old woman who had what he called subacromial space hygroma. He described recurrent swelling of the shoulder, absent rotator cuff, cartilaginous bodies attached to the synovial tissue and severe destructive glenohumeral arthritis[7]. These clinical descriptions were made without the benefit of modern diagnostic tests. The condition has subsequently been known by many different names. In the French literature, the terms 'les caries séniles hémorragique de l'épaule' and 'l'arthropathie destructrice rapide de l'épaule' have been used[8], and in the English literature terms such as 'cuff-tear arthropathy' appear[9]. All early descriptions stress the involvement of older females and the localization to the shoulder joint[10].

The association of intra-articular deposits of BCP crystals with joint disease is much more recent. The presence of solid deposits of BCP crystals in the menisci of postmortem knees was noted in 1966[11], but it was not until 1976 that the first description of BCP crystals in degenerative joint diseases was recorded. Clumps of BCP crystals were discovered in the synovial fluid of patients with osteoarthritis (OA) using analytical electron microscopy[12], a finding which was confirmed by others[13,14]. In 1981, McCarty's group described a similar large joint destructive arthropathy, seen most commonly in the shoulder joints of elderly women, called it 'Milwaukee shoulder', and noted the presence of large quantities of BCP crystals associated with collagenase in the synovial fluid. They hypothesized that the BCP crystals caused the associated joint destruction[15]. Subsequently, others noted that many large joints could be involved, and terms such as 'apatite-associated destructive arthritis' and 'idiopathic destructive arthritis of the shoulder' were added to the list of names. BCP crystals were also described in the joint fluids of a few patients with acute synovitis and other forms of arthropathy[14].

EPIDEMIOLOGY

Calcific periarthritis

There have been very few systematic studies of the incidence or prevalence of juxta-articular deposits of BCP crystals. These deposits are often asymptomatic and are most commonly noted by chance on a radiograph taken for other reasons (Fig. 180.1). In a unique, very large study of office workers published in 1941, a 2.7% prevalence of shoulder deposits was noted in a North American, predominantly Caucasian population, 34–45% of which were associated with clinical problems[16]. Females were affected more commonly than males and the prevalence was highest in those aged between 31 and 40 years (19.5%). No comparable

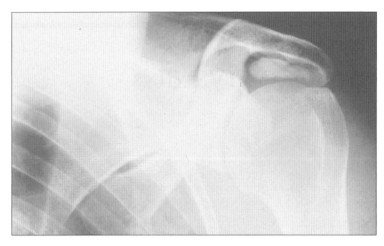

Fig. 180.1 Anteroposterior radiograph of the shoulder joint showing a large calcific deposit in the supraspinatus tendon. The deposit is dense, homogenous and well defined, findings characteristic of inert periarticular deposits of calcific material.

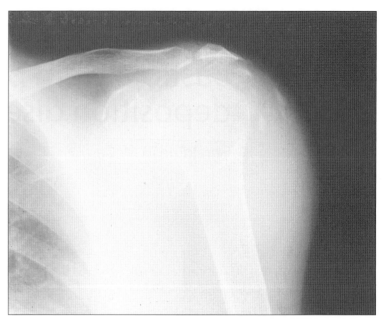

Fig. 180.2 Anteroposterior radiograph of the shoulder during an attack of severe acute calcific periarthritis. The deposit has become indistinct and ill defined as the crystals are shed into the surrounding tissues. In this elderly patient the communication between the shoulder joint and the subacromial bursa led to a large effusion of the glenohumoral joint and a huge extension of the bursa into the upper arm, as shown by the soft tissue swelling seen in the radiograph.

epidemiologic data have been reported subsequently, although a number of smaller pathologic or radiographic studies have documented the relatively high frequency of periarticular calcification. Calcific periarthritis has been reported in children as young as 3 years old, but appears to be relatively uncommon in the elderly. This suggests that many of the deposits seen in young adults must disappear spontaneously.

Articular calcification

The prevalence of intra-articular BCP crystal deposition has not been established. Apatite crystals are found in up to 60% of synovial fluid samples from patients with knee OA[17,18]. The prevalence of BCP crystals in approximately 50% of 53 preoperative OA knees has been noted recently[19]. The prevalence in normal joints at different ages is not known. The 'Milwaukee shoulder' syndrome and related BCP crystal-associated destructive arthropathies are uncommon, tend to occur in elderly individuals and are of unknown prevalence.

CLINICAL FEATURES

Calcific periarthritis

Periarticular calcific deposits are often asymptomatic. However, they are also associated with a number of clinical syndromes (Table 180.1). The most striking clinical presentation is acute calcific periarthritis, which

most commonly involves the shoulder but can occur in association with almost any joint. The episode may be preceded by mild trauma or overuse, but most cases present with a spontaneous onset.

Patients present with sudden onset of severe pain, and within hours the affected part is usually swollen, with redness and warmth of the overlying skin. There is extreme local tenderness and associated loss of function. At the shoulder the pain is most marked around the subacromial region, radiating down the outside of the arm. Glenohumoral movement is usually severely restricted. Severe pain may last for several days, but symptoms then usually resolve slowly over a period of 2–3 weeks. A 'frozen shoulder' may result.

Calcific periarthritis is thought to result from rupture of a calcific deposit into an adjacent soft tissue space or bursa, initiating an acute inflammatory reaction. In the shoulder the crystals may induce intense inflammation in the subacromial bursa (Fig. 180.2). Radiographically, calcium deposits appear dense, with well-defined borders, prior to an attack. With the onset of an attack, however, these calcific deposits appear fluffy, with poorly defined margins. Ultimately, there is a reduction in the size of the deposit seen radiographically, and it may disappear completely.

Calcific deposits in the periarticular tissues are also associated with chronic pain syndromes. However, in the shoulder it is difficult to define what contribution, if any, the deposits themselves make to the clinical findings. This is for two reasons: both chronic shoulder pain and calcification are common; and prior damage to tendons may predispose to the calcification. Moderate to severe pain is described, with varying degrees of tenderness and restriction of motion. Pain usually radiates to the insertion of the deltoid and sometimes beyond, to the forearm. Lying on the affected shoulder is painful and may interfere with sleep. In some patients recurrent acute attacks around the shoulder, separated by pain-free periods of months or years, are followed by the development of chronic pain. Damage to the tendons and muscles of the rotator cuff may result and may lead to total disruption of the cuff apparatus.

The shoulder is the most commonly affected site, followed by the hip, knee, elbow, wrist and ankle joints. The joints of the feet and toes are

TABLE 180.1 SYNDROMES ASSOCIATED WITH BCP CRYSTALS

Subcutaneous deposits (e.g. calcification of hands in scleroderma)	Asymptomatic chance finding Acute and chronic inflammation Skin ulceration Secondary infection Pressing necrosis of surrounding tissues Mechanical interference with function
Periarticular deposits (e.g. calcification of supraspinatus tendon)	Asymptomatic chance finding Acute calcific periarthritis Chronic periarticular pain and/or dysfunction
Intra-articular deposits (e.g. synovial and cartilage deposits in damaged joints)	Asymptomatic chance finding Acute synovitis Severe osteoarthritis Destructive arthropathies of older people

Clinical syndromes that can be associated with the deposition of BCP crystals in and around joints.

less commonly involved (less than 1% of all reported cases), as are those of the hands and fingers[20]. Hydroxyapatite pseudopodagra is a term used to describe acute calcific arthritis at the first metatarsal phalangeal joint, usually in young women[21]. Acute neck pain attributed to calcifications surrounding the odontoid process has been described and called the 'crowned dens' syndrome. Calcifications appear to be composed of apatite or calcium pyrophosphate dihydrate, or a combination of both[22].

Some patients with multifocal deposits develop symptoms at several sites, suggesting a more generalized condition rather than a chance localized process with resultant calcification. This manifestation can cause diagnostic confusion and may even mimic a seronegative polyarthritis. Several reports describe familial occurrences of calcific periarthritis[23].

INTRA-ARTICULAR BCP CRYSTALS

Our understanding of the exact relationship between intra-articular BCP crystals and joint pathology is incomplete, especially as special techniques are required to identify the crystals. None the less, current data support the pathogenic role of BCP crystals in articular tissue degeneration (Fig. 180.3). BCP crystals have been linked with several different diseases.

Acute synovitis

Acute attacks of arthritis associated with intra-articular BCP crystals in relatively young individuals have been described in the knee as well as other sites. Pain, swelling and erythema resembled gout[24]. These attacks appear to be rare and the diagnosis is difficult to establish. Occasionally, crystals from a periarticular deposit can rupture into the joint itself, causing acute synovitis. This can occur in some older individuals who have a direct communication between the subacromial bursa and the glenohumeral joint.

Chronic monoarthritis, with or without erosions

A chronic, sometimes erosive monoarthritis has been linked with intra-articular BCP crystals. BCP crystals have been particularly implicated in finger joint arthropathies, including erosive or inflammatory forms of OA[25]. However, this also appears to be a rare phenomenon and the direct contribution of BCP crystals to the observed pathology remains to be established.

Osteoarthritis

The concurrence of BCP crystals and OA is well established. It has been suggested that many OA joint fluids contain clusters of BCP crystals, which are too small or too few in number to be identified by conventional techniques[26]. Ample data support the role of BCP crystals in cartilage degeneration, as their presence correlates strongly with the severity of radiographic OA[27], and larger joint effusions are seen in affected knee joints when compared with joint fluid from OA knees without crystals[28]. Although the basis of cartilage damage by BCP crystals has been the subject of numerous investigations, there are ongoing controversies concerning the direction of the relationship between calcium-containing crystals and OA, i.e. do the crystals cause cartilage damage or are they present as a result of joint damage?

Large joint destructive arthropathies

A distinctive type of destructive arthropathy has been described in elderly individuals and is associated with rotator cuff defects and numerous aggregates of BCP crystals in the fluids of affected joints[15].

The clinical picture is characteristic (Fig. 180.4a). Patients are nearly always over 70 years old, and approximately 90% are females. They usually present with a history (months or years) of increasing pain, swelling and loss of function of the affected joint, usually the shoulder. The dominant side is usually involved initially, although 60% have bilateral involvement[29]. The pain may be mild but is usually most apparent at night and on joint use. Examination reflects extensive damage to the periarticular soft tissues as well as to cartilage and subchondral bone on both sides of the joint. There is a reduced active range of motion in all affected joints, sometimes associated with pronounced joint instability. Crepitation and pain may be noted, especially when the humerus is grated passively against the glenoid. The rotator cuff is generally

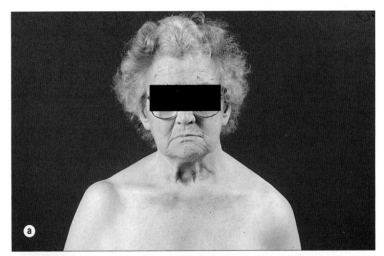

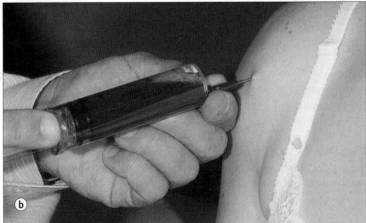

Fig. 180.4 BCP crystal-associated destructive arthritis ('Milwaukee shoulder'). (a) This elderly patient has visible swellings of both shoulders. (b) Aspiration revealed a large amount of bloodstained fluid which contained numerous particles of basic calcium phosphates.

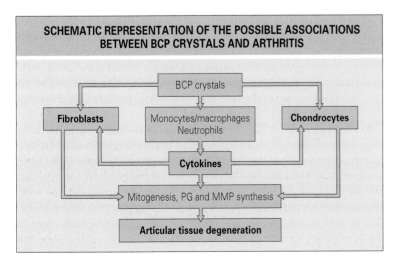

Fig. 180.3 Schematic representation of the possible associations between BCP crystals and arthritis. PG, prostaglandins; MMP, matrix metalloproteases.

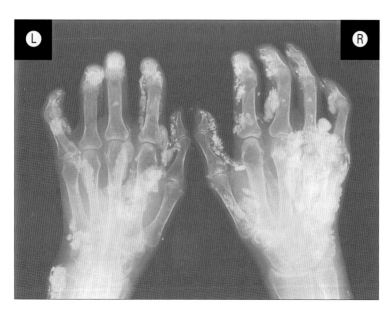

Fig. 180.5 **Anteroposterior radiograph of the hands of a patient with severe subcutaneous calcification associated with mild scleroderma.**

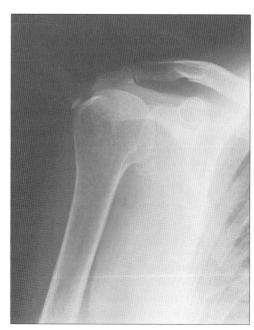

Fig. 180.6 **Anteroposterior radiograph of the shoulder joint showing a small periarticular calcific deposit.** Other views may be needed to identify small deposits and the site of deposition.

completely destroyed. Joint effusion is typically present and may be massive, extending into the subdeltoid region. Aspiration of affected shoulder joints routinely yields blood-tinged synovial fluid that has a low, predominantly mononuclear, cell count (Fig. 180.4b). Rupture of the effusion can lead to a massive extravasation of blood and synovial fluid into the surrounding tissues[30]. Although the shoulder predominates, knees, hips, elbows and other joints may be involved[31].

The natural history of the condition is unclear, but many cases seem to stabilize after a year or two, with reduction of symptoms, joint effusions and no further radiographic changes.

ASSOCIATED DISEASES AND OTHER CLINICAL PRESENTATIONS

A number of secondary forms of BCP crystal-associated arthropathies have been described. BCP crystal deposits have been reported in the joints and periarticular tissues of renal failure patients, mostly when undergoing dialysis. Renal failure also predisposes to calcium oxalate, monosodium urate, calcium pyrophosphate dihydrate (CPPD) and aluminum phosphate crystal deposition[32]. Intra-articular injection of triamcinolone hexacetonide has been associated with the formation of periarticular calcifications along the injection tract, which may become apparent months after the injection. Such calcification may gradually be resorbed over a period of months to years. Occasionally, severe neurologic damage has been followed by heterotopic ossification in periarticular tissues that may mimic arthritis.

BCP deposition is also associated with the connective tissue diseases, particularly scleroderma and dermatomyositis. Following dermatomyositis in childhood, massive sheets of fascial calcification can occur. In scleroderma the deposits are usually subcutaneous. They are associated with the CREST syndrome, but in some patients there is extensive calcification with very little in the way of other features of the disease (calcinosis cutis) (Fig. 180.5). Occasionally the hand calcification occurs on its own. 'Tumoral calcinosis' is a rare condition in which calcification of bursae, such as the olecranon bursa, occurs in the absence of other problems.

INVESTIGATIONS

Imaging

The plain radiograph is the easiest method with which to detect and describe the calcific material of calcific periarthritis (Fig. 180.6).

Anteroposterior and lateral radiographs are usually sufficient, but special views, with internal or external rotation of the shoulder, may be necessary to visualize retrohumeral deposits. The deposits are usually visualized in the rotator cuff, particularly the supraspinatus tendon a few centimeters from its insertion, but may also be seen in the subacromial bursa. Various appearances have been described, with size varying from a few millimeters to several centimeters across. Other imaging investigations are rarely helpful in calcific periarthritis, although arthrography can be used to confirm cuff rupture, and techniques such as computed tomography (CT) or magnetic resonance imaging (MRI) may help demonstrate small deposits or other changes in the tissues around the lesion. Because bilateral calcification is common, a radiograph of the contralateral side (usually the shoulder) may be warranted. Radiographs of other sites (pelvis, knees, wrists and hands), even if asymptomatic, will sometimes reveal multiple deposits. During acute attacks of periarthritis the deposits may change and disappear, only to reappear subsequently.

Calcification around joints is sometimes mistaken for ossification, although the presence of trabeculae in the latter should permit differentiation. The only other differential diagnosis on the images is with the very rare formation of periarticular deposits of CPPD. These occasionally occur in periarticular tendons but, as in joints, they usually appear as linear rather than nummular shadows.

Intra-articular BCP deposits are rarely visible with any of the conventional imaging procedures. Occasionally, articular calcifications of a nummular sort are seen, contrasting with the linear deposits of chondrocalcinosis due to CPPD crystals. However, pathologic studies indicate that individual aggregates of crystals in cartilage synovium or synovial fluid are generally tiny and well below the size that gives any chance of their being visible on a radiograph.

Radiographs in Milwaukee shoulder syndrome are striking (Fig. 180.7), showing upward subluxation of the humeral head or arthrographic evidence of rotator cuff defects in the majority of patients. Other findings may include cystic degeneration of the humeral tuberosities, erosions of cortical bone at the site of insertion of the rotator cuff, degenerative changes of the humeral head and/or glenoid of the scapula, degenerative changes of the acromioclavicular joint and calcification of the tendinous rotator cuff. Pseudarthrosis formation between the humeral head and the acromion and clavicle is common.

MRI can be used to further define the anatomical changes associated with Milwaukee shoulder syndrome, including loss of cartilage, peri-

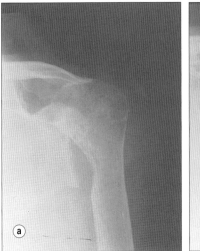
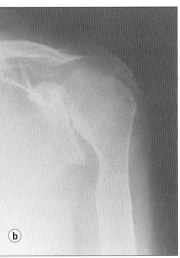

Fig. 180.7 Anteroposterior radiographs of a shoulder joint affected by BCP crystal-associated destructive arthritis ('Milwaukee shoulder'). The extensive destruction of periarticular tissues, including the rotator cuff, has led to instability of the shoulder. The upward subluxation (a) of the humerus can be overcome by traction on the shoulder (b). Note the extensive atrophic destruction and loss of bone of both the acromion and the glenohumeral joint.

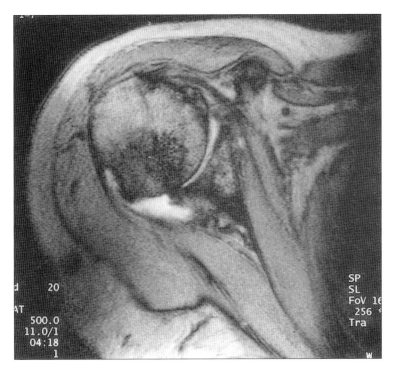

Fig. 180.8 Axial T2-weighted MRI scan of a shoulder joint affected by BCP crystal-associated destructive arthritis ('Milwaukee shoulder'). There is advanced glenohumeral joint degeneration with loss of articular cartilage, truncation of the anterior and posterior labrum, narrowing of the joint space, osteophyte formation, muscle atrophy and joint effusion.

articular bone marrow edema, rupture of the rotator cuff, synovial hypertrophy and joint effusion (Fig. 180.8).

Metabolic

Apatite deposition usually occurs in the absence of any detectable metabolic abnormality. However, if multiple deposits are detected, or if the deposits are unusually large or in unusual sites, the calcium and phosphate levels, as well as renal function, should be checked. High serum phosphate levels seem more likely to predispose to deposition than abnormalities of calcium alone.

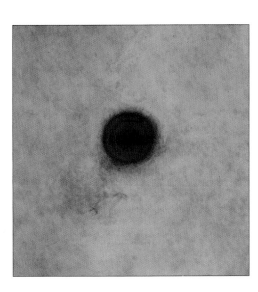

Fig. 180.9 Alizarin red S stain of a BCP particle isolated from the synovial fluid of a patient with osteoarthritis.

Synovial or bursal fluid

In acute calcific periarthritis it is sometimes possible to aspirate a mixture of calcium deposits and inflammatory matter from the bursa or periarticular tissues. This may look like toothpaste, or be a creamy fluid obviously full of 'chalk'. In cases of intra-articular BCP deposition the synovial fluid findings vary. Usually the fluids that contain BCP have a low cell count, are viscous, and are very much the same as fluids from any patient with OA. In the destructive arthropathies of the elderly there is frequent bloodstaining of the fluid. In addition, there may be numerous cartilage fragments and other debris, although the cell count is low.

Identification and characterization of BCP crystals

The study of BCP crystal-associated arthritis has been relatively difficult because of the lack of a simple, easily accessible, reliable diagnostic test[5]. BCP crystals are not birefringent[33]. Therefore, polarized light microscopy is not useful for their detection. This is because individual BCP crystals, which are usually needle-shaped and less than 0.1 μm long, cannot be resolved by light microscopy and are randomly oriented in the much larger aggregates (2–19 μm) in which they are usually found. Plain and polarized light microscopy of samples containing apatite may show globular clumps of crystals, which can look like shiny coins, but the usual appearance of these crystals is non-descript.

Calcium stains such as Alizarin red S have been used by some investigators to identify BCP crystals. Clumps of crystals show up with a 'halo' of stain (Fig. 180.9). Alizarin red S is highly sensitive, but frequent false positive results suggest that it lacks sufficient specificity to qualify for the routine identification of BCP crystals without some other type of confirmatory testing.

A semiquantitative binding assay for BCP crystals has been described which uses [¹⁴C]ethane-1-hydroxy-1,1-diphosphonate (EHDP)[13]. Diphosphonates are analogs of inorganic pyrophosphate that adsorb to the surface of BCP crystals but not to monosodium urate, CPPD, cartilage fragments or any other known particulates in joint fluid. This method is performed on a synovial fluid pellet resuspended in phosphate-buffered saline and the results are expressed as μg/ml of hydroxyapatite standard. The limit of sensitivity is approximately 2 μg/ml standard hydroxyapatite.

Electron microscopy can be used to visualize the crystals in synovial fluid pellets, and if elemental analysis or electron diffraction is possible their identity can be confirmed (Fig. 180.10). If sufficient material is available, for example from surgical specimens, other analytical techniques, such as X-ray powder diffraction or Fourier transformation infrared spectroscopy (FTIR), can be used to identify the material. The latter has shown that BCP crystal deposits consist of mixtures of

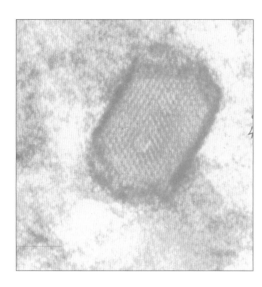

Fig. 180.10 High magnification transmission electron micrographs of BCP crystals. The crystal lattice structure as well as the morphology of the crystals is apparent.

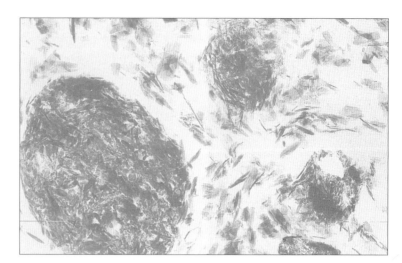

Fig. 180.11 Transmission electron micrograph of BCP crystals from a tendon deposit. This shows the clumps of crystals, dense globular structures of various sizes, and isolated crystals.

hydroxyapatite, octacalcium phosphate and, rarely, tricalcium phosphate crystals. Combinations of BCP and CPPD are not infrequent.

Atomic force microscopy has been applied recently to the identification of synovial fluid microcrystals. This technique is capable of achieving subnanometer resolution of crystal surface topology and measurement of lattice unit cell dimensions[34].

The ability to identify apatite is less crucial from a clinical perspective than the identification of monosodium urate or calcium pyrophosphate dihydrate crystals, as no drug has as yet been identified that specifically inhibits the pathologic effects of BCP crystals *in vivo*.

DIFFERENTIAL DIAGNOSIS

Acute calcific periarthritis
The differential diagnosis of acute calcific periarthritis should include gout, pseudogout and sepsis. However, the distribution of the lesions and the acute onset are often characteristic. Radiographs showing the evolution of the calcific deposit are virtually pathognomonic. The diagnosis can be confirmed if material can be aspirated from the area.

Chronic periarticular syndromes
The usual features are those of a tendonitis, and the only way of implicating crystal deposition in the diagnosis is through visualizing the deposit on the radiograph. Other causes of tendonitis, such as trauma, impingement and inflammatory arthritis, are possible differential diagnoses.

Acute and chronic arthritis
Acute inflammatory arthritis which may mimic gout, pseudogout or other systemic inflammatory rheumatic disease has been attributed to BCP crystals[12,24]. BCP crystals are often detected in osteoarthritic joints and appear to promote the degenerative process, as their presence is associated with more advanced radiographic change and larger joint effusions than in joints without BCP crystals[27,28]. Erosive arthritis with recurrent episodes of pain and swelling involving the wrists and the finger joints has been associated with BCP crystal deposition[25].

Destructive arthropathies of the elderly
The main differential diagnoses include neuropathic or Charcot joints, chronic sepsis, advanced rheumatoid disease, osteonecrosis and CPPD deposition disease. Radiographic involvement of both sides of the joint helps differentiate this condition from osteonecrosis. The absence of any neurologic deficit distinguishes it from Charcot's arthropathy. Synovial fluid examination and culture will aid the differentiation from CPPD deposition disease and sepsis.

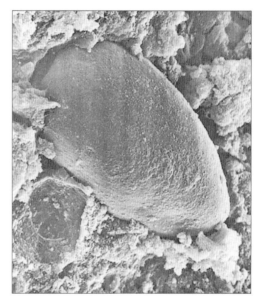

Fig. 180.12 Scanning electron micrograph of a calcific deposit isolated from a tendon.

STRUCTURE AND FUNCTION

Nature of the crystals
Hydroxypatite is a form of calcium phosphate represented by the formula $Ca_5(PO_4)_3OH2H_2O$ and is usually found in partially substituted carbonated form. In periarticular calcific deposits, light microscopy usually shows multifocal aggregates of crystals separated by fibrocollagenous tissue. On transmission electron microscopy the deposits appear as rounded aggregates with isolated crystals in a matrix of fragmented collagen fibers (Fig. 180.11). On scanning electron microscopy they look like rocky bulks embedded in mortar (Fig. 180.12). The crystals are very heterogeneous, both within the sample and in different patients. Typically, they include compounds of varying crystallinities, ranging from amorphous BCP to well-structured stable elements similar to those of bone and tooth, but with a larger crystal size than most of those seen in bone. In bone, poorly crystalline partially carbonated crystals of hydroxyapatite, each of about 500 Å in length, are the main mineral phase. The crystals of periarticular deposits are often more carbonated than bone crystals, and high-resolution electron microscopy suggests that some of them are coated with electron-dense material.

In synovial fluid samples mixed populations of BCP crystals have been reported, including partially carbonate-substituted hydroxyapatite, octacalcium phosphate ($Ca_8H_2(PO_4)_6 \cdot 5H_2O$) and, rarely, tricalcium phosphate ($Ca_3(PO_4)_2$). They frequently coexist with CPPD crystals and are associated with particulate collagens[35]. One recent report suggested that crystals extracted from the synovial fluid were more like those found in periarticular calcific deposits than in bone crystals, suggesting that they were derived from newly formed deposits and not from subchondral bone[36].

Another form of BCP, magnesium whitlockite, has been identified in the superficial region of articular cartilage. Recent studies suggest that it may be a frequent finding in normal as well as diseased hyaline cartilage[37]. This observation, coupled with the identification of some hydroxyapatite crystals in normal cartilage, has led to speculation that some BCP minerals may have a physiologic, rather than a pathologic, role in cartilage homeostasis. However, whitlockite crystals elicit biologic cellular responses, including mitogenesis and matrix metalloprotease production *in vitro* which suggest potential pathogenicity in arthritis[38].

ETIOLOGY

The mechanism of periarticular calcification is largely unknown, although periarticular intratendinous deposits have been thought to be due to ectopic calcification of damaged tendons. In most patients no obvious local, metabolic or genetic cause for the calcification is found. The frequent occurrence of bilateral and multifocal deposits suggests the operation of a generalized predisposition as well as local factors. This is supported by the fact that the sites of deposition in sporadic cases of calcific periarthritis are the same as those associated with a known systemic predisposition, such as diabetes mellitus, hyperthyroidism or parathyroid disorders. The classic description of a relationship between repetitive shoulder use and the formation of calcific deposits has not been established. There is no known relationship with any HLA specificity or other genetic marker, in spite of the known occurrence of familial cases.

PATHOGENESIS

Calcific periarthritis

Pathologic assessments have shown that the calcific deposits are located in tendons, peritendinous tissues, bursae or ligaments. Original studies suggested that 'dystrophic' tendon calcification occurs as a consequence of local trauma, ischemia and necrosis of tendons. Calcific periarthritis frequently localizes to the supraspinatus tendon in a poorly vascularized area of the tendon sheath known as the 'critical zone', at a distance of a few millimeters from the bone insertion. Similarly, calcification in other tendons seems to occur preferentially in hypovascular segments, suggesting local necrosis followed by ectopic calcification.

Some evidence has indicated that calcifying tendinitis is an active cell-mediated process in which local vascular and mechanical changes result in focal transformation of tendinous tissues into fibrocartilaginous material containing chondrocytes. This is followed by local deposition of hydroxyapatite crystals within extracellular matrix vesicle-like structures derived from these chondrocytes[39].

No good animal or *in vitro* model is available to study the formation of periarticular or intra-articular deposits. Aging and the degeneration of collagen fibers do not seem to be sufficient explanation for the phenomenon.

The frequent tolerance of deposits without any apparent inflammation or other response is difficult to explain. The absence of any phagocytic cells in the calcified area may be significant, although the formation of granuloma-like reactions has been reported.

Acute calcific periarthritis appears to be induced by rupture of the deposit and the shedding of crystals into more cellular vascular areas. BCP crystals have been shown to be intrinsically phlogistic. They are phagocytosed *in vitro*, resulting in the release of inflammatory media-

tors[40]. Similarly, *in vivo* models of inflammation show a brisk inflammatory reaction to apatite, and injection into the tissues of human volunteers results in an inflammatory response[41]. Phagocytosis may be one of the main ways in which the crystals are removed.

There is evidence that coating of the crystals, which have highly adsorptive surfaces, can either stimulate or suppress the inflammatory response, depending on the nature of the proteins that attach to the crystals[42]. Immunoglobulins, for example, may activate inflammatory responses, whereas coating of apolipoproteins on the crystal surfaces will suppress it.

RELATIONSHIP WITH OSTEOARTHRITIS AND DESTRUCTIVE ARTHROPATHIES

Crystals of BCP are frequently found in OA cartilage, synovium and synovial fluid. Evidence suggests that human articular cartilage contains matrix vesicles which are capable of progressive mineralization and can generate either BCP or CPPD *in vitro*[43]. However, more than one source of formation is likely. For example, the ANK gene product, a cell membrane protein which regulates extracellular inorganic pyrophosphate (ePPi), has recently been identified. ePPi is an important inhibitor of the nucleation and growth of BCP. This investigation has led to the concept of ANK-mediated control of ePPi levels as a possible mechanism of regulation of tissue calcification[44].

The degree of damage that can occur in apatite-associated destructive arthropathies is marked (Fig. 180.13). The basis of cartilage damage by calcium-containing crystals is still somewhat speculative. Theoretically, crystals in cartilage may directly injure chondrocytes. However, in pathologic specimens crystals are rarely seen in immediate contact with chondrocytes, and even less frequently found engulfed by chondrocytes.

It is more likely that cartilage damage ultimately results from the effects of the crystals on synovial lining. *In vitro* properties of BCP crystals have been observed which emphasize their pathogenic potential. The first is their ability to induce mitogenesis, a characteristic which presumably leads to synovial proliferation, characteristic of both 'Milwaukee shoulder' syndrome and apatite-associated OA[45,46]. Increased cell numbers in the synovial lining enhance the capacity for secretion of cytokines, which may promote chondrolysis. The second is their ability to induce the secretion of proteolytic enzymes, leading to degradation of intra-articular collagenous structures, an observation which correlates with the detection of collagenase and neutral protease activities in synovial fluid from patients with Milwaukee shoulder syndrome[47]. BCP crystals induce production of collagenase 1, stromelysin and 92 kDa gelatinase from human fibroblasts and collagenases 1 and 3 from porcine chondrocytes[46]. Lastly, BCP crystals induce cyclo-oxygenases-1 and -2, followed by increased prostaglandin E_2 in human fibroblasts[48].

Despite the association of BCP crystals with OA and joint destruction and the biological effects noted *in vitro*, the specific role of the crystals in joint degeneration is controversial. Some hypothesize that BCP crystal aggregates found in association with destructive arthropathies actually originate from damaged subchondral bone and are merely an epiphenomenon. More studies will be necessary to further differentiate between crystals as a cause of cartilage damage and crystals as a result of cartilage damage. An improved understanding of the biological effects of BCP crystals is essential to the ultimate prevention or reversal of the consequences of deposition.

MANAGEMENT

Calcific periarthritis

Asymptomatic deposits require no treatment. Acute attacks of calcific periarthritis have been treated successfully with immobilization and

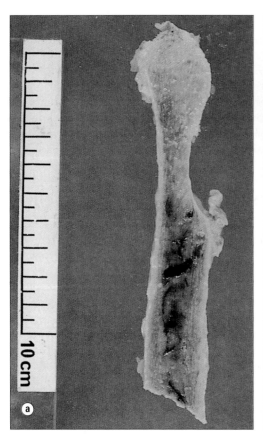
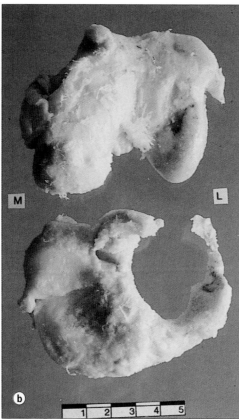

Fig. 180.13 Bones from a patient with advanced BCP crystal-associated destructive arthritis. (a) The humerus shows extensive bony attrition characteristic of this condition. (b) The tibial condyles show the characteristic destruction of the lateral tibiofemoral joint, with extensive loss of subchondral bone.

a variety of non-steroidal anti-inflammatory drugs (NSAIDs) or colchicine. Most patients have markedly reduced symptoms within 5 days and virtual complete resolution within 1–3 weeks. Untreated attacks may last several weeks. Needle aspiration of the paste-like calcific deposits, with or without irrigation, may be helpful. The use of corticosteroids is controversial: local corticosteroid injections will help the acute attacks to resolve but may possibly make further calcification and recurrent attacks more likely.

For patients with chronic periarticular syndromes the treatment is in general much the same as it would be whether the deposit was there or not. There is no known medical way of dispersing or dissolving the deposit. In chronic calcific tendinitis ultrasound treatment helps resolve calcifications and is associated with short-term clinical improvement[49].

If the problem persists and large calcific deposits are present, other treatments can be considered. Local corticosteroid therapy should be used with caution because of the risk of disrupting the deposit or seeding further calcification. Needle aspiration is usually difficult in chronic cases, but arthroscopic or surgical removal may provide permanent symptomatic relief in refractory cases.

Articular BCP crystals
Currently, patients with OA complicated by BCP crystal deposition should be treated in the same manner as if they had simple OA.

Hopefully, ongoing research endeavors will ultimately lead to the development of more specific treatment for apatite deposition. For example, phosphocitrate, a potent inhibitor of hydroxyapatite crystal formation and a relatively non-toxic compound, inhibits BCP crystal-induced cell activation *in vitro*[50,51]. This compound may ultimately prove useful in protecting articular tissues from the harmful biological effects of BCP crystals.

At the time of diagnosis of BCP crystal-associated destructive arthropathies, such as Milwaukee shoulder syndrome, advanced destructive changes are usually present and may even be asymptomatic. The treatment of symptomatic disease is generally unsatisfactory. A conservative approach, including analgesics and NSAIDs, repeated shoulder aspirations and decreased joint use, has sometimes controlled symptoms satisfactorily. Surgical therapy is sometimes successful for the relief of pain and restoration of function, but may be difficult because of the extent of damage to the joint and periarticular tissues. Surgical procedures include arthroscopic lavage and/or debridement, humeral tuberoplasty, arthrodesis, arthroplasty or hemiarthroplasty[7]. Some patients have responded to closed needle tidal-joint irrigation followed by the injection of methylprednisolone acetate (40 mg) and tranexamic acid (0.5g)[52]. Other pain-relieving measures, such as suprascapular nerve blocks for shoulder disease, or transcutaneous nerve stimulation, have been used with some success. Pain may subside with time alone.

REFERENCES

1. Painter CF. Subdeltoid bursitis. Boston Med Surg J 1907; 156: 345–349.
2. Sandstrom C. Peritendinitis calcarea. A common disease of middle life: Its diagnosis, pathology and treatment. Am J Radiol 1938; 40: 1–21.
3. McCarty DJ, Gatter RA. Recurrent acute inflammation associated with focal apatite crystal deposition. Arthritis Rheum 1966; 9: 804–819.
4. Uhthoff HK, Sarker K, Maynard JA. Calcifying tendonitis. A new concept of its pathogenesis. Clin Orthop 1976; 118: 164–168.
5. Rosenthal A, Mandel N. Identification of crystals in synovial fluids and joint tissues. Curr Rheumatol Rep 2001; 3: 11–16.
6. McCarty DJ. Robert Adams' rheumatic arthritis of the shoulder: "Milwaukee Shoulder" revisited. J Rheumatol 1989; 16: 668–670.
7. Jensen K, Williams G, Russell I, Rockwood C. Rotator cuff tear arthropathy. J Bone Joint Surg Am 1999; 81–A(9): 1312–1324.
8. Lequesne M, Fallut M, Couloumb R. L'arthropathie destructice rapide de l'epaule. Rev Rhum 1982; 49: 427–437.
9. Neer CS, Craig EV, Fakuda H. Cuff-tear arthropathy. J Bone Joint Surg 1983; 65A: 1232–1244.
10. Campion GV, McCrae F, Alwan W et al. Idiopathic destructive arthritis of the shoulder. Semin Arthritis Rheum 1988; 17: 232–245.
11. McCarty DJ, Hogan JM, Gatter RA, Grossman M. Studies on pathological calcifications in human cartilage. J Bone Joint Surg 1966; 48: 309–325.

12. Dieppe PA, Huskisson EC, Crocker P, Willoughby DA. Apatite deposition disease: a new arthropathy. Lancet 1976; 1: 266–269.
13. Halverson PB, McCarty DJ. Identification of hydroxyapatite crystals in synovial fluid. Arthritis Rheum 1979; 22: 389–395.
14. Schumacher HR, Cherian PV, Reginato AJ et al. Intra-articular apatite crystal deposition. Ann Rheum Dis 1983; 42(Suppl 1): 54–59.
15. McCarty DJ, Halverson PB, Carrera GF et al. Milwaukee shoulder: association of microspheroids containing hydroxyapatite crystals, active collagenase, and neutral protease with rotator cuff defects. i: Clinical aspects. Arthritis Rheum 1981; 24: 464–473.
16. Bosworth BM. Calcium deposits in the shoulder and subacromial bursitis. A survey of 12,222 shoulders. JAMA 1941; 116: 2477–2482.
17. Dieppe PA, Crocker PR, Corke CF et al. Synovial fluid crystals. Q J Med 1979; 192: 533–553.
18. Gibilisco PA, Schumacher HR, Hollander JL, Soper KA. Synovial fluid crystals in osteoarthritis. Arthritis Rheum 1985; 28: 511–515.
19. Kurian J, Daft L, Carrera G, Derfus B. The high prevalence of pathologic calcium crystals in pre-operative joints. Arthritis Rheum 1999; 42: S145.
20. McCarthy GM, Carrera GF, Ryan LM. Acute calcific periarthritis of the finger joints: a syndrome of women. J Rheumatol 1993; 20: 1077–1080.
21. Fam AG, Rubenstein J. Hydroxyapatite pseudopodagra. A syndrome of young women. Arthritis Rheum 1989; 32: 741–747.
22. Bouvet J-P, le Parc J-M, Michalski B et al. Acute neck pain due to calcifications surrounding the odontoid process: the crowned dens syndrome. Arthritis Rheum 1985; 28: 1417–1420.
23. Hajeroussan VJ, Short CL. Familial calcific periarthritis. Ann Rheum Dis 1983; 42: 469–470.
24. Schumacher HR, Smolyo AP, Tse RL, Maurer K. Arthritis associated with apatite crystals. Ann Intern Med 1977; 87: 411–416.
25. Schumacher HR, Miller JL, Ludivico C, Jessar RA. Erosive arthritis associated with apatite crystal deposition. Arthritis Rheum 1981; 24: 31–37.
26. Swan A, Chapman B, Heap P et al. Submicroscopic crystals in osteoarthritic synovial fluids. Ann Rheum Dis 1994; 53: 467–470.
27. Halverson PB, McCarty DJ. Patterns of radiographic abnormalities associated with basic calcium phosphate and calcium pyrophosphate crystal deposition in the knee. Ann Rheum Dis 1986; 45: 603–605.
28. Carroll GJ, Stuart RA, Armstrong JA et al. Hydroxyapatite crystals are a frequent finding in osteoarthritic synovial fluid, but are not related to increased concentrations of keratan sulfate or interleukin 1b. J Rheumatol 1991; 18: 861–866.
29. Halverson PB, Carrera GF, McCarty DJ. Milwaukee shoulder syndrome: Fifteen additional cases and a description of contributing factors. Arch Intern Med 1990; 150: 677–682.
30. McCarty D, Swanson A, Ehrhart R. Hemorrhagic rupture of the shoulder. J Rheumatol 1994; 21: 1134–1137.
31. Dieppe PA, Doherty M, Macfarlane DG et al. Apatite associated destructive arthritis. Br J Rheumatol 1984; 23: 84–91.
32. Halverson PB. Arthropathies associated with basic calcium phosphate crystals. Scanning Microscopy 1992; 6: 791–797.
33. Paul H, Reginato AJ, Schumacher HR. Alizarin red S staining as a screening test to detect calcium compounds in synovial fluid. Arthritis Rheum 1983; 26: 191–200.
34. Blair JM, Sorensen LB, Arnsdorf MF, Ratneshwar L. The application of atomic force microscopy for the detection of microcrystals in synovial fluid from patients with recurrent synovitis. Semin Arthritis Rheum 1995; 24: 259–269.
35. McCarty DJ, Lehr JR, Halverson PB. Crystal populations in human synovial fluid. Identification of apatite, octacalcium phosphate and tricalcium phosphate. Arthritis Rheum 1983; 26: 247–251.
36. Heywood BR, Swan A, Dieppe PA. Chemical, structural and morphological analyses of mineral deposits in synovial fluid. Br J Rheumatol 1991; 30(Suppl 2): 129.
37. Scotchford CA, Ali SY. Magnesium whitlockite deposition in articular cartilage: a study of 80 specimens from 70 patients. Ann Rheum Dis 1995; 54: 339–344.
38. Ryan L, Cheung H, LeGeros R et al. Cellular responses to whitlockite. Calcif Tiss Int 1999; 65: 374–377.
39. Sarker K, Uhthoff HK. Ultrastructural localization of calcium in calcifying tendinitis. Arch Pathol Lab Med 1978; 102: 266–269.
40. Dayer J-M, Evequoz V, Zavadil-Grob C et al. Effect of synthetic calcium pyrophosphate and hydroxyapatite crystals on the interaction of human blood mononuclear cells with chondrocytes, synovial cels and fibroblasts. Arthritis Rheum 1987; 30: 1372–1381.
41. Dieppe P, Doherty M, Papadimitriou GM. Inflammatory responses to intradermal crystals in healthy volunteers and patients with rheumatic diseases. Rheumatol Int 1982; 2: 55–58.
42. Terkeltaub RA, Ginsberg MH. The inflammatory reaction to crystals. Rheum Dis Clin North Am 1988; 14: 353–364.
43. Kranendonk S, Ryan L, Buday M et al. Human osteoarthritic vesicles generate both monoclinic calcium pyrophosphate dihydrate and apatite crystals in vitro. J Bone Joint Surg 1994; 18: 502–503.
44. Ho A, Johnson M, Kingsley D. Role of the mouse ank gene in control of tissue calcification and arthritis. Science 2000; 289: 265–269.
45. Cheung HS, Story MT, McCarty DJ. Mitogenic effects of hydroxyapatite and calcium pyrophosphate dihydrate crystals on cultured mammalian cells. Arthritis Rheum 1984; 27: 668–674.
46. McCarthy G, Westfall P, Masuda I et al. Basic calcium phosphate crystals activate human osteoarthritis synovial fibroblasts and induce matrix metalloproteinase-13 (collagenase-3) in adult porcine articular chondrocytes. Ann Rheum Dis 2001; 60: 399–406.
47. McCarthy GM, Mitchell PG, Struve JS, Cheung HS. Basic calcium phosphate crystals cause co-ordinate induction and secretion of collagenase and stromelysin. J Cell Physiol 1992; 153: 140–146.
48. Morgan M, Fitzgerald D, McCarthy C, McCarthy G. Basic calcium phosphate crystals cause increased production of prostaglandin E2 by induction of both cyclooxygenase-1 and cyclooxygenase-2 in human fibroblasts. Arthritis Rheum 2000; 43: S281.
49. Ebenbichler G, Erdogmus C, Resch K et al. Ultrasound therapy for calcific tendinitis of the shoulder. N Engl J Med 1999; 340: 1533–1538.
50. Cheung H, Sallis J, Mitchell P, Struve J. Inhibition of basic calcium phosphate crystal-induced mitogenesis by phosphocitrate. Biochem Biophys Res Commun 1990; 171: 20–25.
51. Cheung H, Sallis J, Struve J. Specific inhibition of basic calcium phosphate and calcium pyrophosphate crystal-induction of metalloproteinase synthesis by phosphocitrate. Biochim Biophys Acta 1996; 1315: 105–111.
52. Caporali R, Rossi S, Montecucco C. Tidal irrigation in Milwaukee shoulder syndrome. J. Rheumatol 1994; 21: 1781–1782.

181 Other crystals

H Ralph Schumacher Jr

Clinical features

- The clinical significance of joint crystals other than monosodium urate monohydrate (MSUM), calcium pyrophosphate dihydrate (CPPD) and hydroxyapatite varies widely depending on the crystal
- Oxalate and depot corticosteroid crystals have established pathogenic potential
- Other crystalline material with possible pathogenic implications include liquid lipid crystals, cholesterol, other lipids, hematoidin, immunoglobulins, Charcot–Leyden crystals and foreign bodies

HISTORY

The identification of infrequently found joint, bursal or subcutaneous crystals is a recent and still evolving topic. This has largely been motivated by techniques of polarized light microscopy introduced by Hollander and McCarty in the early 1960s, and by the expanded use of microscopic examination of joint fluids as part of the routine diagnostic evaluation of arthritis. Oxalate crystals in joint fluids were first reported in 1982[1] and depot corticosteroids have, since their introduction in 1951, been known to be able to cause occasional inflammation[2].

In this chapter the suggestive clinical features and appropriate investigations will be described for these and several less common crystals.

CRYSTAL TYPES

Oxalate crystals

To date, oxalate crystals have only been described in the joints of patients with renal failure[1,3] and should be considered primarily in this setting. Oxalate deposition has also been noted complicating amyloid-induced renal failure in patients with rheumatoid arthritis (RA)[4]. Acute or chronic arthritis resulting from oxalate deposition can occur in a variety of joints, with the sites most frequently involved being the knees and hands. There are also reports of involvement of wrists, ankles, feet, tendon sheaths and bursae. Synovial fluid total leukocyte and differential counts have varied, but there are generally less than 2000/mm³.

Inflammatory reactions in tissue may be absent or there may be a granulomatous response around the crystals. Oxalates may also be found in intervertebral discs and contribute to disc destruction in dialysis patients[5]. Because oxalosis is also generalized in many of these patients, crystal deposition may also occur at other sites. Oxalosis can thus cause vascular insufficiency, with gangrene[6], cardiomegaly, heart block, miliary skin deposits, peripheral neuropathy and aplastic anemia[3]. Oxalosis can occur as a primary disease with stone formation, but to date, bone and articular oxalosis has only been diagnosed after renal failure is established. Thus although oxalosis can occur with small bowel resection or intestinal disease, oxalate arthritis has not yet been reported as a complication of these. Birefringent oxalate crystals have been

described in a foot infected with *Aspergillus niger*[7] in a patient with normal serum oxalate levels.

Definitive diagnosis is by crystal identification in joint fluid or by biopsy of joints, bones or other tissues. Synovial fluid crystals can be pleomorphic, but characteristically include at least some with bipyramidal or envelope-like shapes (Fig. 181.1). Sizes range from 5 to 30 μm. Most crystals are strongly birefringent, though some of the smaller rod-like ones can have positive elongation that could cause confusion with CPPD. Most also stain brightly with calcium stains such as alizarin red S, which might cause further confusion with the various apatite-like crystals or CPPD. It is important to search carefully for those with the classic bipyramidal shape. Under electron microscopy oxalates are electron dense and foamy and are thus indistinguishable from CPPD without elemental analysis, which shows that the oxalates contain calcium but no phosphorus. X-ray or electron diffraction, infrared spectroscopy with Fourier transformation or Raman spectroscopy can be helpful in diagnosis when available and used by experienced staff.

Radiographs of joints can be helpful in suggesting a diagnosis of oxalosis. However, the opacification of articular structures seen from oxalates can be in cartilage or soft tissue and can mimic either CPPD or apatite-associated diseases. Some patients with articular oxalates will have no calcification visible on radiographs. Oxalate-infiltrated bones show varying patterns, including sclerosis and demineralization.

Depot corticosteroid-induced iatrogenic inflammation

The obvious clinical clue to this phenomenon is known or suspected recent intra-articular or bursal injection[8]. If an inflammatory reaction is to occur it is most frequent during the first 8 hours following injection. This tends to help distinguish this phenomenon from an infection, which generally develops considerably more slowly. Depot corticosteroid crystal-induced inflammation appears to be more common with

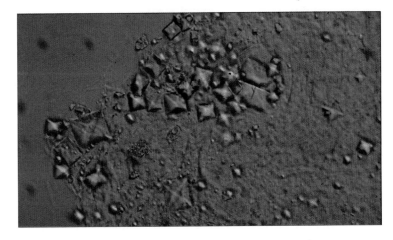

Fig. 181.1 Oxalate crystals from synovial fluid seen with regular, unpolarized light. Note that some crystals have the characteristic bipyramidal shape, × 400.

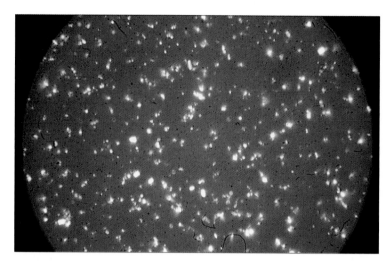

Fig. 181.2 Bright irregular depot corticosteroid crystals. Crystal morphology can vary widely with preparation, batch and duration of storage. Compensated polarized light, × 400.

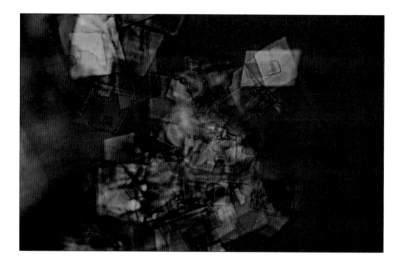

Fig. 181.3 Classic cholesterol plates with overlapping and some corner notching. Compensated polarized light, × 400.

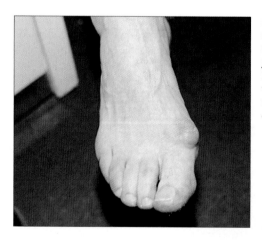

Fig. 181.4 Red tender swelling at first metatarsophalangeal joint in a patient with RA from which fluid with large numbers of massive cholesterol crystals was aspirated.

triamcinolone hexacetonide than with other preparations. This preparation is also less soluble, which may increase the chance of producing acute inflammation. The inflammation may be transient because the steroid suppresses the inflammation as it dissolves in the joint. Even osteoarthritis (OA) joints that are dramatically improved promptly after corticosteroid injection may transiently show depot corticosteroid

crystal phagocytosis and mildly increased synovial fluid leukocyte counts[9]. Diagnosis can be supported by aspiration and identification of pleomorphic crystals that include irregular shapes, rods and squares with intense positive or negative birefringence (Fig. 181.2). Radiographs are not helpful, although it may be necessary to perform a Gram stain and obtain cultures to exclude infection.

Lipid crystals: cholesterol, lipid liquid crystals and others

Lipids, as pathogenic or potentially confusing factors in rheumatic diseases, should be considered in several clinical settings. Cholesterol crystals (Fig. 181.3) are seen most commonly as a complication of joint effusions resulting from RA (Fig. 181.4) as well as other known causes of arthritis, including OA. They are also found in sites such as olecranon bursae. Cholesterol crystals are most often seen as broad plates with a notched corner. Needle-shaped crystals with negative elongation (which are not MSUM crystals) may also be seen in cholesterol-laden fluids[10]. Such fluids may have a glossy golden appearance. Cholesterol crystals may develop in rheumatoid nodules, in gouty tophi, and have been found in rheumatoid pericarditis. There is some debate that, although they are often too large to be phagocytosed, they may contribute in some way to perpetuation of inflammation. For example, injection of cholesterol crystals subcutaneously has stimulated inflammation[11], and injection into guinea pig gallbladders caused increases in interleukin (IL)-1, myeloperoxidase, prostaglandin (PG)E$_2$ and PGF in luminal fluid[12]. Cholesterol-containing subcutaneous tophi or ganglion-like nodules have also been described[13], and because of the sites involved some may be related to repeated local microtrauma. Recent hemarthrosis or trauma followed by joint inflammation is another clinical setting in which lipids might be considered.

Lipid liquid crystals are caused by lipid states with characteristics of both liquids and solids forming layered arrays which appear as birefringent microspherules[14,15]. These form from phospholipids released from red blood cells or other cells. Trauma has not been evident in all cases, so that other sources of these lipid spherules, such as other antecedent inflammatory exudation, should be considered. When present in large numbers, lipid liquid crystals resembling Maltese crosses may be phagocytosed and associated with acute joint symptoms. Most patients have a monoarthritis. The knees are most frequently involved, but cases with wrist involvement and even polyarthritis, with possibly similar mechanisms, have been reported. Synovial fluids have been inflammatory and contain 10 000–40 000 leukocytes/mm³ with intracellular 'Maltese crosses' identified in many samples. Polymorphonuclear leukocytes or macrophages are the predominant cells.

Lipid liquid crystals are readily identified under compensated polarized light as 2–20 μm Maltese Cross-like spherules with the two blue parts of the cross lined up parallel to the axis of slow vibration of the compensator (positive elongation) (Fig. 181.5). Rare Maltese crosses are not clinically significant, but when they are frequent and intracellular

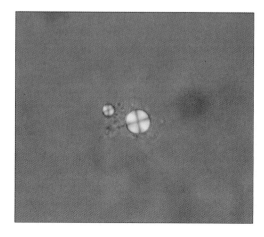

Fig. 181.5 Positively birefringent Maltese cross-like lipid microspherules from the synovial fluid of a patient with otherwise unexplained acute arthritis. Compensated polarized light, × 1000.

they should be considered as possible causes of arthritis if no other explanation is evident. Lipid liquid crystals need to be distinguished from starch from gloves, which has a more polygonal outline, and from rare urate microspherules that have negative birefringence.

There is interest in whether lipid crystals can explain some of the arthritis and tenosynovitis reported to complicate types II and IV hyperlipoproteinemias. Incompletely characterized brightly positively birefringent rod-like crystals have been described in a tendon of a hypercholesterolemic man with Achilles tendinitis[16], but most hyperlipidemic patients do not have lipid crystals. Non-birefringent droplets composed largely of neutral lipids are common after trauma, lymphatic obstruction, in pancreatic disease, and occasionally in type IV hyperlipoproteinemia. Needle-shaped crystals with negative elongation can precipitate in these droplets, especially during storage, and can be a source of confusion with urates. Uricase digestion can be used to see if urate crystals are present, although this may be difficult to interpret if only rare urates are mixed with lipid crystals. Crystalline lipids generally do not stain with fat stains as do neutral fat droplets.

Protein crystals

There is an interesting case report of one patient who had chronic polyarthritis that appeared to be due to massive intra-articular crystalline precipitates of an IgG cryoprecipitable paraprotein[17]. This patient had an erosive arthritis with inflammatory synovial fluid (30 000 leukocytes/mm³, 90% polymorphonuclear neutrophil leukocytes) and chronic inflammation in the synovium surrounding deposits of crystals. Other patients with cryoglobulinemia may have arthritis without synovial fluid crystals. In vessels, crystallized cryoglobulin or myeloma proteins can cause vascular obliteration. Cryoglobulin crystals have been emphasized as causes of both destructive arthritis and vasculopathy[18]. A mouse model for IgG3 cryo crystal globulinemia has been reported with deposits in kidneys[19].

Immunoglobulin crystals are pleomorphic and may be over 60 µm in size. However, they can also appear as smaller squares, hexagons, rhomboids or rods, and be potentially confused with known pathogenic crystals. Because they are proteins they will stain with methylene blue (Fig. 181.6). Some crystals are negatively birefringent. Monoclonal antibodies can provide specific identification. Other protein crystals described in synovial fluid include Charcot–Leyden crystals[20,21], felt to be composed of lysophospholipase in eosinophil-laden fluids, hemoglobin and hematoidin. Charcot–Leyden crystals have a characteristic spindle shape and are weakly birefringent, with positive or negative elongation. Hematoidin crystals, derived from the breakdown of hemoglobin, are rhomboids very similar to CPPD, except for their golden color on regular light microscopy. Other golden debris and stellate arrays are rarely seen but have been identified as hematoidin at other sites[22,23]. Their identification and possible modes of formation have been reviewed[22,24]. As hematoidin and Charcot–Leyden crystals can be phagocytosed they may have phlogistic potential. Hemoglobin has also rarely been noted to crystallize out as rods in dried smears containing red cells[23].

Crystalline foreign bodies

Foreign bodies can cause acute or recurrent arthritis that is usually monoarticular. The penetrating injury may not be recalled. Most foreign bodies become embedded or sequestered in synovial tissue and so are not seen in synovial fluid. Thus, arthroscopy or arthrotomy may be required for diagnosis. Plant thorns can show dramatic packing of cells and cellulose that is accentuated with polarized light. Calcium carbonate from sea urchin spines is birefringent and irregular; fiberglass birefringent fibrils, or polyethylene and methacrylate in patients with replacement joints, have also been described in joints. Aluminum crystals have been reported in joints in systemic aluminium toxicity. Most foreign bodies are not radio-opaque and magnetic resonance imaging (MRI) may help identify some of these.

INVESTIGATIONS AND DIFFERENTIAL DIAGNOSIS

Methods for investigation and differential diagnosis span the variety of techniques in use for the more commonly recognized crystal-associated syndromes. These can include regular and polarized light microscopy, electron microscopy, elemental analysis, X-ray or electron diffraction, Fourier transformed infrared analysis and atomic force microscopy. In addition, monoclonal antibodies can be used to stain immunoglobulin crystals and the Fouchet stain can probably help identify hematoidin[22]. To exclude the more common diseases, uricase or pyrophosphatase digestion may be attempted. Artifacts seen on wet preparations with regular or polarized light have frequently been a source of diagnostic confusion (Table 181.1). Figures 181.7–181.10 illustrate some of the artifacts found.

ETIOLOGY AND PATHOGENESIS

As each new crystal of suspected pathogenic significance has been suggested, new techniques have been used by investigators to help establish their identity and to test their phlogistic potential. Crystals can be tested for inflammatory properties by intra-articular injection, injection into the pleural space, or into air pouches on the dorsum of the rat

---

TABLE 181.1 CRYSTAL-LIKE ARTIFACTS SEEN IN SYNOVIAL FLUID WET PREPARATIONS[23]

- Depot corticosteroid crystals
- Glass fragments
- Nail polish from sealed cover slip edges
- Wood fragments from sticks used in transport
- Starch from gloves
- Anticoagulant crystals – sodium oxalate, lithium, heparin
- Precipitates from storage – calcium phosphates, oxalates, hemoglobin, hematoidin, lipids, unidentified material
- Dust
- Lens paper fibrils

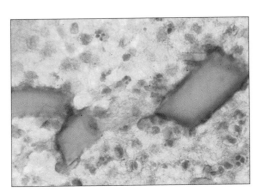

Fig. 181.6 Purple stained cryoglobulin crystals from synovial fluid of patient. Wright–Giemsa stain containing methylene blue, × 400.

Fig. 181.7 Slivers of glass from cover slips can be needle shaped and mimic MSUM crystals even to the point of having faint negative elongation in compensated polarized light, × 400.

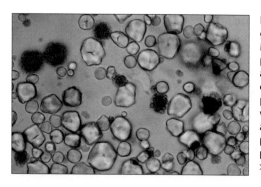

Fig. 181.8 Starch from gloves produces Maltese cross-like particles that are more angular than liquid lipid crystals. Calcium phosphates stained here with alizarin red S are also present in some powders. Compensated polarized light, × 400.

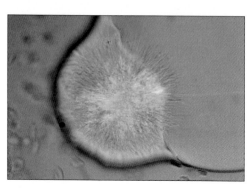

Fig. 181.9 Negatively birefringent needles precipitate in synovial fat droplets during storage. When these are released into the joint fluid they can mimic MSUM crystals. Polarized light, × 400.

Fig. 181.10 As fluid dries birefringent salts precipitate. Compensated polarized light, × 100.

that produce a synovial-like space[25]. *In vitro* incubation with various cells and chemotactic assays are also used. Some crystals may not produce acute readily detectable inflammation but may interact with chronic inflammatory cells and still have a long-term impact. Studies may well be worth extending to better define any important roles of crystals such as cholesterol, the lipid liquid crystals and hematoidin, and also to investigate prosthetic wear particles and polymethyl-methacrylate (PMMA) cement that may produce inflammation in ways similar to crystals[25]. Injection of PMMA into rat air pouches[25] does produce inflammation. Cholesterol crystals can activate complement[26], suggesting a process that might be involved in atherosclerotic plaques as well as in joints or bursae. Surface charge and binding properties, which are being most actively investigated with MSUM crystals, can also be studied with other crystal or crystal-like particles. An organic matrix is associated with oxalate stones, and proteins may well also bind to oxalates in joints.

The reasons why only very few individuals have deposits of the crystals discussed above despite apparent similar risks are also potential areas for investigation. Some investigations suggest a direct mechanism. Thus lipid liquid crystals were shown to result from hemarthrosis, after blood was injected into joints and Maltese cross-like particles developed[27].

MANAGEMENT

Treatment of inflammatory episodes related to these less common crystals has not been studied systematically. Non-steroidal anti-inflammatory drugs are generally used when the clinical situation permits for oxalate-associated inflammation or to temporarily help with depot corticosteroid-induced bouts. Rarely, depot corticosteroid crystals have to be aspirated in unusually prolonged iatrogenic cortico-steroid crystal-induced inflammation. Measures to deplete the crystals discussed here are not known. Oxalate accumulation in hemodialysis patients may be slowed by avoiding the use of vitamin C, which is metabolized to oxalate. Foreign bodies, of course, are best managed by removal.

REFERENCES

1. Hoffman GS, Schumacher HR, Paul H *et al*. Calcium oxalate microcrystalline associated arthritis in end stage renal disease. Ann Intern Med 1982; 97: 36–42.
2. Hollander JL. Hydrocortisone and cortisone injected into arthritis joints. JAMA 1951; 147: 1629–1635.
3. Reginato AJ, Kurnik BRC. Calcium oxalate and other crystals associated with kidney diseases and arthritis. Semin Arthritis Rheum 1989; 18: 198–224.
4. Schumacher HR, Reginato AJ, Pullman S. Synovial oxalate deposition complicating rheumatoid arthritis with amyloidosis and renal failure. J Rheumatol 1987; 14: 361–366.
5. Kaplan P, Resnick D, Murphey M *et al*. Destructive non-infectious spondyloarthropathy in hemodialysis patients. A report of 4 cases. Musculoskel Radiol 1987; 162: 241–244.
6. Baethye BA, Sanusi ID, Landreneau M *et al*. Livedo recticularis and peripheral gangrene with primary hyperaoxaluria. Arthritis Rheum 1988; 31: 1199–1203.
7. Louthrenoo W, Park YS, Phillipe L, Schumacher HR. Localized peripheral calcium oxalate crystal deposition caused by *Aspergillus niger* infection. J Rheumatol 1990; 17: 407–412.
8. McCarty DJ, Hogan JM. Inflammatory reaction after intrasynovial injection of microcrystalline adrenocorticosteroid esters. Arthritis Rheum 1964; 7: 359–367.
9. Gordon GV, Schumacher HR. Electron microscopic study of depot corticosteroid crystals with clinical studies after intra-articular injections. J Rheumatol 1979; 6: 7–14.
10. Nye WHR, Terry R, Rosenbaum DL. Two forms of crystalline lipids in cholesterol effusions. Am J Clin Pathol 1968; 49: 718–727.
11. Zucker J, Uddin J, Gantner GE, Dorner R. Cholesterol crystals in synovial fluid. Ann Intern Med 1964; 60: 436–446.
12. Prystowsky JB, Rege RV. The inflammatory effects of crystalline cholesterol monohydrate in the guinea pig gall bladder *in vivo*. Surgery 1998; 123: 258–263.
13. Selvi E, Hammoud M, DeStefano R *et al*. A cholesterol 'ganglion'. J Rheumatol 2001; 28: 1112–1113.
14. Trostle DC, Schumacher HR, Medsger RA, Kapoor WN. Microspherule associated acute arthritis. Arthritis Rheum 1986; 29: 1166–1169.

15. Rivest C, Hazeltine M, Gariepy G, de Medicis R. Acute polyarthritis associated with birefringent lipid microspherules occurring in a patient with longstanding rheumatoid arthritis. J Rheumatol 1992; 19: 617–620.
16. Schumacher HR, Michael R. Recurrent tendonitis and Achilles tendon nodule with positively birefringent crystals in a patient with hyperlipoproteinemia. J Rheumatol 1989; 16: 1387–1389.
17. Langlands DR, Dawkins RL, Matz LR *et al*. Arthritis associated with crystallizing cryo-precipitate IgG paraprotein. Am J Med 1980; 68: 461–465.
18. Papo T, Musset L, Bardino T *et al*. Cryocrystalglobulinemia as a cause of systemic vasculopathy and widespread erosive arthropathy. Arthritis Rheum 1996; 39: 335–340.
19. Rengers JU, Touchard G, Decourt C *et al*. Heavy and light chain primary structures control IgG3 nephritogenicity in an experimental model for cryocrystalglobulinemia. Blood 2000; 95: 3467–3472.
20. Dougados M. Benhanou L, Amor B. Charcot–Leyden crystals in synovial fluid. Arthritis Rheum 1983; 26: 1416.
21. Brown JP, Rola-Pleszoynski M, Menard H. Eosinophilic synovitis: clinical observations on a newly recognized subset of patients with dermatographism. Arthritis Rheum 1986; 29: 1147–1151.
22. Schumacher HR, Reginato AJ. In: Atlas of synovial fluid analysis and crystal identification. Philadelphia: Lea & Febiger, 1991.
23. Tate GA, Schumacher HR, Reginato AJ *et al*. Synovial fluid crystals derived from erythrocyte degradation products. J Rheumatol 1992; 19: 1111–1114.
24. Brenner DS, Drachenberg CB, Papadimitriou JC. Structural similarities between hematoidin crystals and asteroid bodies: evidence of lipid composition. Exp Mol Pathol 2001; 70: 37–42.
25. Nagase M, Baker DG, Schumacher HR. Prolonged inflammatory reactions induced by artificial ceramics in the rat air pouch model. J Rheumatol 1988; 15: 1334–1338.
26. Vogt W, Von Zabern I, Damerau B *et al*. Mechanisms of complement activation by crystalline cholesterol. Mol Immunol 1985: 22: 101–106.
27. Choi SJ, Schumacher HR, Clayburne G. Experimental haemarthrosis produces mild inflammation associated with Maltese crosses. Ann Rheum Dis 1986; 45: 1025–1028.

ENDOCRINE AND HEMOGLOBIN-RELATED ARTHRITIS AND STORAGE DISEASES

182 Acromegaly

Sándor S Forgács

Definition

- Acromegaly is a disease caused by overproduction of growth hormone, usually as a result of a pituitary tumor. This has a significant effect on connective tissue causing characteristic changes in the bones and joints (acromegalic arthropathy)

Clinical features

- Characteristic changes in the external appearance of the facial features and enlargement of the hands and feet
- Soft tissue thickening, hirsutism and excessive sweating
- Premature osteoarthritis, cartilage overgrowth, kyphosis and entrapment neuropathy

HISTORY

One of the first descriptions of acromegaly was published by Pierre Marie in 1886[1]. In 1931, Erdheim[2] directed attention towards the relationship between pituitary tumors and degenerative joint changes and, in the 1960s, Silberberg[3] demonstrated the effect of growth hormone on joints in animal experiments. Since then, a number of authors have documented the clinical and radiographic features of acromegalic arthropathy.

CLINICAL FEATURES

Acromegaly

When acromegaly manifests itself in the prepubertal period it results in gigantism. Typically, this is proportional gigantism, although it is not infrequent that hypogonadotropic hypogonadism coexists, resulting in eunuchoid body proportions. The disease usually develops during the ages of 20–40 years and is more frequent in females. However, there is no significant difference between the sexes.

In adults, the disease progresses slowly and includes characteristic changes in the external appearance of the patient's head and face (Fig. 182.1). Enlargement of the hands and feet is also characteristic. Thickening of the skin is often associated with increased follicular function, which manifests as hirsutism and sweating in 75% of patients. Moderate darkening of the skin and small sessile fibrous skin tags are also common. In addition, the tongue and internal organs enlarge, especially the heart, liver and kidneys. Diabetes secondary to glucose intolerance develops in 25% of cases. Due to pressure on the optic chiasma, the enlarging pituitary tumor will cause characteristic scotomas and symptoms of elevated brain pressure, particularly headache.

The disease is often diagnosed in this stage, although the rheumatologic symptoms may remain unnoticed. Nevertheless, in the majority of acromegalic patients, osteoarticular symptoms will develop in the initial stage of the disease although they will not become clinically evident until the later phases.

Musculoskeletal features

Backache

Approximately 50% of acromegalic patients suffer backache, particularly in the lower spine. This symptom may be associated with local tenderness and a normal or increased range of spinal and hip motion. Painful kyphosis of the thoracic spine may also be observed.

Limb arthropathy

Peripheral arthropathy is most common in the large joints (knees, shoulders and hips). In the early stages, coarse crepitus with little or no pain and full range of joint motion are characteristic. In later stages, secondary degenerative changes, particularly in the knees and shoulders, may produce pain, limitation of motion, deformity and angulation. In this stage, the leading symptom is arthralgia which affects 70–90% of patients. Palpable thickening of the synovial bursae, such as the prepatellar, olecranon or subacromial regions, may also be involved. Marked effusions are rare.

In the hands, the first carpometacarpal joints are usually involved and enlarged distal interphalangeal joints show a wide range of pain-free movement. Coarse thickened skin is also a characteristic clinical symptom.

Neuropathy

Several forms of neuropathy are associated with acromegaly:

- compression neuropathy where thickening of connective tissues and bony overgrowths produce signs of compression
- ischemic neuropathy secondary to the proliferation of endoneural and perineural tissues
- possible metabolic effects on the neuron related to growth hormone.

Carpal tunnel syndrome is particularly characteristic, occurring in about 30–50% of acromegalic patients, frequently with a bilateral distribution. Compression and hypertrophy of the median nerve are the most important factors in the pathogenesis of the syndrome. Typically treatment of the pituitary lesion results in complete recovery. In some patients, palpable enlargement of the ulnar and popliteal nerves with paresthesia and decreased or absent deep tendon reflexes have been observed. In other cases, spinal cord compression or cauda equina compression have been seen.

Myopathy

Proximal myopathy will develop in up to 50% of acromegalic patients with long-standing disease. The clinical symptoms are usually mild. The main symptoms are proximal muscle weakness and decreased exercise tolerance. The muscle weakness is often out of proportion to the increased muscle mass. Less frequently, myalgia may occur.

Radiologic features

Acromegaly causes characteristic alterations in the osteoarticular system. These radiologic changes correlate well with the pathologic picture (Table 182.1).

TABLE 182.1 PATHOLOGIC–RADIOGRAPHIC CORRELATION IN ACROMEGALY

Pathology	Radiology
Hypophysis adenoma	Sella turcica enlargement
Connective tissue hyperplasia	Increased thickness of skin and heel pad
Cartilage hypertrophy	Widening of articular spaces and intervertebral spaces
Cartilaginous degeneration (fragmentation, ulceration)	Narrowing of articular and intervertebral spaces
Periosteal new bone formation	Thickening of cranial vault Mandibular enlargement Prominence of facial bones Cortical thickening of tubular bones Enlargement of phalangeal tufts
Marginal and subligamentous new bone formation	Large bridging osteophytosis Calcification of anterior longitudinal ligament of the spine Excrescenses on patella, tuberosities, trochanters, etc. Calcaneal spurs
Capsular calcification	Periarticular calcifications
Bone resorption	Intracortical striation Medullary widening Vertebral scalloping Overtubulation of metatarsals and other tubular bones

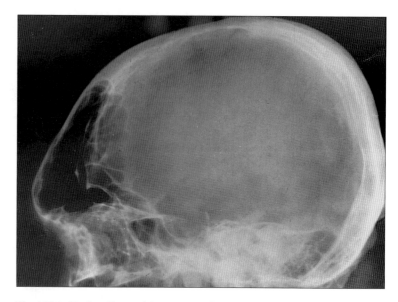

Fig. 182.2 Skull radiograph in acromegaly: showing the usual features of expanded pituitary fossa and enlarged paranasal sinuses.

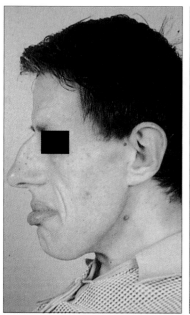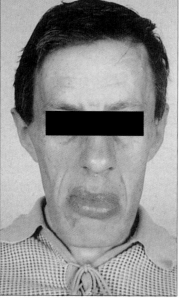

Fig. 182.1 Characteristic facial appearance in acromegaly.

Abnormalities of the skull

These include enlargement of the pituitary fossa which may be very marked. Alterations of the pituitary fossa may be detected in 98–99% of acromegalic patients. Recently, computerized tomography (CT) and magnetic resonance imaging (MRI) examination of the sellar region have become indispensable. Hyperostosis frontalis interna and/or hyperostosis calvariae diffusa can be seen causing thickening of the cranial vault. In addition, there may be enlargement and excessive pneumatization of paranasal sinuses (particularly frontal sinuses) and mastoids; enlargement of facial bones (mandible, zygomatic bones); and prominence of supraorbital ridges and occipital protuberance (Fig. 182.2).

Abnormalities of the vertebral column

An increased intervertebral disc space is usually seen, particularly in the lumbar region as a result of stimulation of endochondral bone formation (Fig. 182.3). This abnormality, as well as the loose ligaments, are responsible for hypermobility. However, the height of the discs will decrease because of degenerative processes in advanced stages of the disease.

Elongation and widening of the vertebral bodies are more frequent in the thoracic region and less common in the cervical spine. There is also increased dorsal kyphosis. Scalloping of the posterior margins of the vertebral bodies is also a frequently observed abnormality, particularly in the lumbar spine region. Steinbach et al.[4] postulated that these changes could be secondary to pressure erosions from enlarged soft tissues, or could be related to resorption and modeling as a direct effect of growth hormone. However, this radiologic sign is not pathognomonic of acromegaly, being found in a variety of other disease processes.

Because of soft tissue and bony overgrowth, myelography and CT scan can reveal characteristic findings, including extradural defects[5]. Anterior and lateral osteophytes may be extensive[6,7]. In advanced stages, a continuous ligamentous calcification can develop resembling the changes seen in diffuse idiopathic skeletal hyperostosis (DISH) syndrome. On the basis of this symptom, and other hyperostotic alterations in acromegaly, it is assumed that growth hormone may also have a role in the development of the DISH syndrome[8].

Osteoporosis in acromegaly

Active acromegaly is not associated with osteoporosis[9]. However, osteoporosis is often a misdiagnosis in active acromegaly because of the thickened bone trabeculae which resembles hypertrophic atrophy. In the majority of cases, however, genuine osteoporosis will develop as the disease progresses as a result of hypogonadism. Diamond et al.[10] measured the mineral bone content in acromegalic patients and found that the forearm and vertebral mineral measurements were different. The forearm bone mineral content of patients with active disease, regardless of gonadal status, was significantly higher than that of normal subjects. Vertebral bone densities were lower in acromegalic patients and were also associated with the gonadal status of the patients. Therefore, the gonadal status should always be taken into consideration in the examination of osteoporosis in acromegalic patients[11].

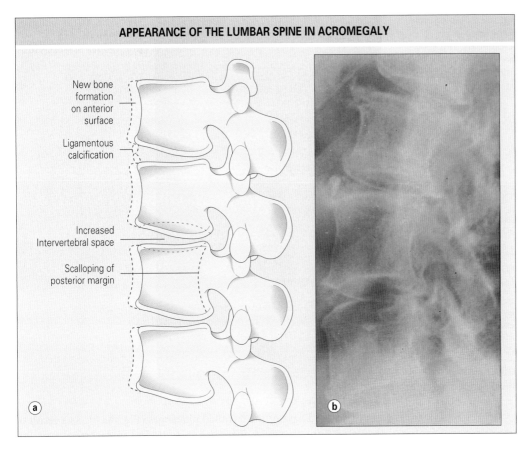

APPEARANCE OF THE LUMBAR SPINE IN ACROMEGALY

New bone formation on anterior surface

Ligamentous calcification

Increased Intervertebral space

Scalloping of posterior margin

(a)

(b)

Fig. 182.3 The appearance of the lumbar spine in acromegaly. (a) Typical changes including scalloping of the posterior margin of the vertebrae, new bone formation on the anterior surfaces and increased intervertebral space. (b) Radiograph of the lumbar spine showing the decrease in disc height due to late degenerative disease.

In growth hormone-deficient adult patients, hormone substitution can result in increasing bone mass[12]. On these grounds, attempts have been made to use growth hormone in the treatment of osteoporosis.

Changes in skin thickness

Thickening of the skin is a manifestation of the effect of growth hormone on collagen tissue. The thickness of the skin can be measured by radiologic and ultrasound methods with the measurement of the thickness of the heel pad being of particular importance (Fig. 182.4). The thickness of the heel pad shows wide individual variation and is also dependent on body weight. Values greater than 23mm in men and 21.5mm in women are suggestive of acromegaly; values greater than 25mm in men and 23mm in women are highly diagnostic of this disease if local causes of skin thickening are excluded. The heel pad thickness is related to the severity of the disease and correlates well with the serum level of growth hormone. The variation in heel pad thickness is reversible and is a simple measure of disease activity.

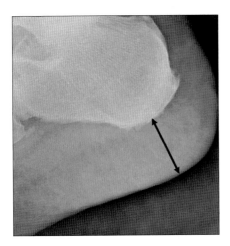

Fig. 182.4 Heel pad thickening in acromegaly. This lateral radiograph illustrates the increased thickness of the heel pad which is a useful confirmatory sign in diagnosis.

Articular abnormalities

Acromegalic arthropathy causes characteristic alterations in both the large joints (especially the knees and shoulders) and in the small joints. These articular symptoms are partly pathognomonic for acromegaly. Most authors categorize these abnormalities into two groups:

- cartilage hypertrophy
- cartilaginous and osseous degeneration.

These forms of abnormality, however, represent two main stages in the onset of acromegalic arthropathy rather than two different types of disease.

Cartilage hypertrophy

Acromegaly is the only disease where genuine diffuse cartilage thickening occurs. Radiologically this is seen as widening of the articular joint space. It can be measured exactly by ultrasonography[13]. This finding may be combined with soft tissue and synovial hypertrophy. Widening of the joint is most frequently observed in the knees (Fig. 182.5), in the metacarpophalangeal joints and interphalangeal joints. Softening and thickening of the capsular and ligamentous structures produces joint laxity which can be observed on clinical examination, as well contributing to the prominence of the joint cavity. The thickened cartilage will form impressions on the articular surfaces. The epiphyses may undergo deformation, with their regular rounded shape becoming squarer; this is enhanced by the appearance of small osteophytes on the edges of the articular surfaces. This symptom may be seen particularly clearly in the metacarpophalangeal joints.

Cartilaginous and osseous degeneration

The thickened cartilage is liable to early degeneration. One of the first symptoms of this may be the 'vacuum' sign in knee joints (see Fig. 182.5). Initially, small osteophytes are seen, which in combination with a normal or widened joint space are suggestive of acromegaly. In later stages of the disease, articular space narrowing, cyst formation, sclerosis and progres-

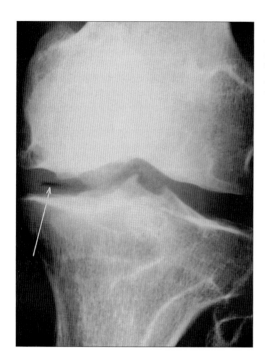

Fig. 182.5 Radiograph of the knee in acromegaly. This shows the widening of the articular joint space and 'vacuum' sign.

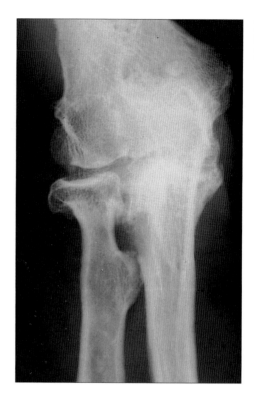

Fig. 182.6 Deformation of the epiphysis and progressive osteophytosis.

sive osteophytosis are seen (Fig. 182.6). In this stage, limitation of motion becomes apparent, particularly in the shoulders. Clinical and radiographic pictures may resemble those of the primary degenerative disease[14,15] and severe osteophytosis may develop.

Although detectable on histologic section, intra- and periarticular calcifications are rarely observed on radiography; tuberosity and thickening of osteal ends can be seen frequently. Periosteal appositions may develop, and the muscular and tendinous insertions will become sclerosed, as in the DISH syndrome.

The thickening of the sesamoid bones of the hand is a measurable parameter in acromegaly (sesamoid index), although opinions vary as to its value[16,17]. A characteristic feature of acromegaly is the enlargement

of the tuft and base of the terminal phalanges (Fig. 182.7). As a result of increased bone turnover, marginal erosions and intracortical striation develop in the short tubular bones[18].

Cortical thickening is sometimes associated with a decrease in the spongioid substance. This may result in tubulation or overconstriction. This symptom is sometimes referred to as hypostosis, and occurs mostly in the metatarsal bones, in the upper pubic bone region and in the phalanges. Accordingly, examination of the hands is of primary importance in acromegaly (Fig. 182.7). The following changes can often be seen:

APPEARANCE OF THE HAND IN ACROMEGALY

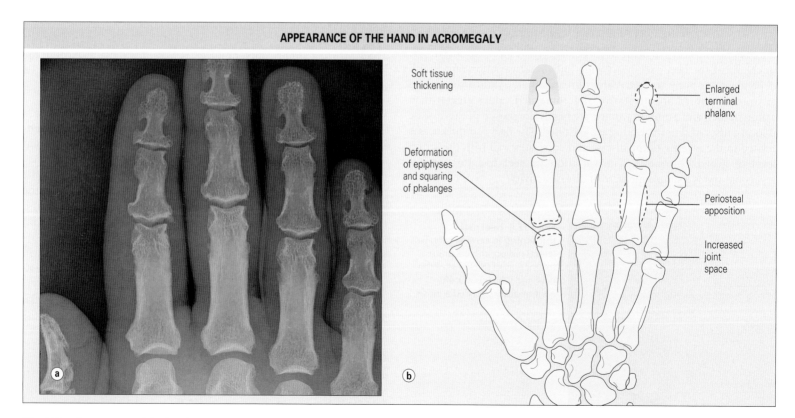

Fig. 182.7 Appearance of the hand in acromegaly. (a) Apart from the soft tissue thickening of the hand, this radiograph also shows the increased joint space and enlargement and tufting of the terminal phalanges. (b) Examination of the hand is important for the diagnosis of acromegaly.

- thickening of the soft parts of the hand
- widening of articular spaces
- deformation of metacarpal heads and later the epiphyses
- rough thickening of terminal phalanges
- periosteal appositions on tubular bones
- rare symptoms – hypostosis, chondrocalcinosis
- intracortical striation can be detected by a special technique (micro-radioscopy), indicating increased bone turnover.

In bone scintigraphy radionuclide uptake is increased[19], but no significant difference is seen in any area between the active and non-active acromegalic patients[20].

ETIOLOGY AND PATHOGENESIS

Acromegaly is usually caused by a benign pituitary tumor (acidophilic adenoma) which results in overproduction of growth hormone. Rarely, hyperplasia of the anterior pituitary lobe may be the cause. Other rare causes include adenomas which develop in the pharynx and the sphenoidal sinus, and bronchial adenomas, pancreatic islet cell tumors or carcinoid tumors which produce growth hormone. On hematoxylin–eosin staining, these tumors are often acidophilic. These are slow-growing, benign tumors, whereas the fast-growing, intracranially expanding tumors show mixed (chromophobic and eosinophilic) histologic pictures.

Effects of growth hormone in acromegaly

Growth hormone (GH) consists of biologically active and inactive components and serum levels may show daily and even hourly fluctuations. This should be taken into account when assessing average serum GH levels. In normal individuals, the GH level is suppressed when there is a rise in circulating glucose. However, in acromegaly this effect is absent and the hormone level may even increase following a glucose load.

Growth hormone stimulates the growth of all tissues and affects metabolic processes at several levels. Its major metabolic effect is the enhancement of protein synthesis, which is the basis of its effect on the skeleton. This is exerted mainly by stimulating the proliferation of epiphyseal chondrocytes. In adults, where the epiphyses are closed, GH will reactivate chondral proliferation and the potentially osteogenic and chondrogenic foci may resume activity. At the biochemical level, the effect is mainly due to increased sulfate incorporation into chondroitin sulfate and to increased collagen synthesis. This can be measured by the procollagen III propeptide level (PIIIP), which may show changes proportional to the activity of disease. In addition, alkaline phosphatase concentrations can be used as a measure of disease activity[21].

According to experimental studies, GH has a direct effect on bone and cartilage tissue. However, an indirect effect via somatomedin stimulation is probably more significant. The somatomedin hypothesis has been verified by the finding that insulin-like growth factor-I (IGF-I) produced by the liver stimulates target cells in specific cartilage plates. Based on a positive correlation between bone growth and levels of IGF-I, it has been suggested that locally produced IGF-I plays a more significant role in the regulation of skeletal growth than does circulating IGF-I[22]. Experimental studies suggest that the effect of GH is unavoidable in all phases of bone formation. Therefore, the hormone will accelerate the aging process and will increase the occurrence and severity of osteoarthritis (OA). This observation agrees well with the clinical findings that severe OA develops in young acromegalic patients. In addition, GH levels in primary OA are significantly higher than in osteoporotic controls[23]. The low prevalence of OA in patients with GH deficiency also suggests that GH is an important factor in the development of osteoarthritis[24].

DIFFERENTIAL DIAGNOSIS

A combination of clinical and radiographic findings is sufficiently characteristic of acromegaly that accurate diagnosis is not difficult. However, the later stages of acromegalic joint disease include findings which are similar to the abnormalities of primary degenerative joint diseases and differentiation may be more difficult. Generally, in acromegaly, unlike OA, the non-weight-bearing joints such as the shoulders and elbows are also involved.

In the early stages of acromegaly, osteophytosis without joint space narrowing and, in the later stages, extreme osteophytosis are characteristic of the disorder. However, the hyperostotic changes may resemble DISH syndrome. Scalloped vertebrae are not pathognomonic for acromegaly as they are also seen in a variety of other diseases.

An acromegaly-like syndrome has been associated with pachydermoperiostosis[25]. However, in this disease there is no sellar enlargement or articular space abnormalities.

MANAGEMENT

The fate of the patient is decisively determined by the growth of the tumor in the skull. Untreated, the disease is characterized by a prognosis of variable rate, with the mortality rate being two-fold that of the normal population. In addition, the slow-growing forms of the tumor must also be treated. Irradiation, neurosurgery and medication have all been used in treatment.

Radiotherapy is a classic method. However, damage to the optic, and often to other cranial nerves and to the hypothalamus, can occur. Therefore, a surgical solution is the most widespread method at present, with good results being seen from transsphenoidal hypophysectomy. Medication also seems to show promising results. The most common drug currently being used is the dopamine agonist, bromocriptine. Recently, a long-acting somatostatin analog has been administered to patients, which is dependent upon the dose required to suppress maximally growth hormone somatomedin C level.

However, the question facing rheumatologists is how the osteoarticular symptoms can be improved by surgery or by chemically decreasing the GH level. In general, soft tissue malformations are reversible; the thickness of the heel pad can decrease and the clinical symptoms of carpal tunnel syndrome can be improved. The degenerative hyperostotic changes are, however, naturally irreversible, but the remission of acromegalic symptoms (e.g. crepitus) has been observed at a high rate even in these cases[26–28]. Following treatment of the underlying disease, the late degenerative processes should be treated, as for primary OA. Sometimes, surgical removal of large osteophytes which limit motion can also be considered.

REFERENCES

1. Marie P. Sur deux cas d'acromegalie: hypertrophic singuliere noncongenitale des extremites superieures, inferieures et cephalique. Rev Med 1886; 6: 297.
2. Erdheim J. Uber wirbelsaulenveranderungen bei akromegalie. Virchows Arch (Pathol Anat) 1931; 281: 197.
3. Silberberg M, Silberberg R. Modifications of degenerative foint disease of mice by somatotrophin (STH). Endocrinology 1960; 67: 540–546.
4. Steinbach H, Feldman R, Goldberg M. Acromegaly. Radiology 1959; 72: 535–549.
5. Efird T, Genant H, Wilson C. Pituitary gigantism with cervical spinal stenosis. Am J Roentgenol 1980; 134; 171–173.
6. Podgorsky M, Robinson B, Weissberger A et al. Articular manifestations of acromegaly. Aust NZ J Med 1988; 18: 28–35.
7. Woo C. Radiological features and diagnosis of acromegaly. J Manipulation Physiol Ther 1988; 11: 206–213.
8. Forgács S, Gacs G. Growth hormone level in diabetes with hyperostotic spondylosis. IRCS Med Sci 1974; 1: 13–73.

9. Bolanowski M, Wielgus W, Milewicz A, Marciniak R. Axial bone mineral density in patients with acromegaly. Acad Radiol 2000; 7: 592–594.

10. Diamond T, Mery L, Posen S. Spinal and peripheral bone mineral densities in acromegaly: the effect of excess growth hormone and hypogonadism. Ann Intern Med 1989; 111: 567–573.

11. Lesse G, Fraser W, Farquharson R et al. Gonadal status an important determinant of bone density in acromegaly. Clin Endocrinol 1988; 48: 59–65.

12. Kann P, Piepkorn B, Schehler B et al. Effect of long term treatment with GH on bone metabolism, bone mineral density and bone elasticity in GH-deficient adults. Clin Endocrinol 1988; 48: 561–568.

13. Colao A, Marzullo P, Vallone A et al. Reversibility of joint thickening in acromegalic patients: an ultrasonographic study. J Clin Endocr Metab 1998; 83: 2121–2125.

14. Perpignano G, Cacace E, Beccaris A et al. L'artropatia acromegalica.Clin Ter 1993; 143: 3–9.

15. Lieberman S, Bjorkengren A, Hoffman A. Rheumatologic and skeletal changes in acromegaly. Endocrinol Metab Clin N Am1992; 21: 615–631.

16. Anton H. Hand measurements in acromegaly. Clin Radiol 1972; 2: 445–450.

17. Duncan T. Validity of the sesamoid index in the diagnosis of acromegaly. Radiology 1975; 115: 617–619.

18. Fischer E. Zeichen an der tuberositas phalangis distalis der finger bei der akromegalie (high bone turnover). ROFO 1990; 153: 456–460.

19. Pounds T, Hattner R, Helms C, Chang S. Skeletal scintigraphic findings in acromegaly. Clin Nucl Med 1994; 19: 461–462.

20. Peretianu D, Grigorie D, Popescu F, Zaharescu J.Bone scintigraphy in acromegaly. Endocrinologie 1990; 28: 199–205.

21. Hampel R, Rose H, Jahreis G et al. Alkalische knochenphosphatase als aktivitatsparameter der akromegalie. Dtsch Med Wschr 1990; 115: 363–366.

22. Rappaport R. New aspects of growth: its neuro-endo-paracrine regulation triangle. Clin Endocrinol 1989; 28: 57–67.

23. Dequeker J, Burssens A, Bouillon R. Dynamics of growth hormone secretion in patients with osteoporosis and in patients with osteoarthrosis. Horm Res 1982; 16: 353–356.

24. Bagge E, Eden S, Rosen T, Bengtsson B. The prevelance of radiographic osteoarthritis is low in elderly patients with growth hormone deficiency. Acta Endocrinol Copenh 1993; 129: 296–300.

25. Harbison J, Nice C Jr. Familial pachidermoperiostosis presenting as acromegaly-like syndrome. AJR 1971; 112: 532–536.

26. Layton M, Fudman E, Barkan A et al. Acromegalic arthropathy. Arthritis Rheum 1988; 31: 1022–1027.

27. Lacks S, Jacobs R. Acromegalic arthropathy: a reversible rheumatic disease. J Rheumatol 1986; 13: 634–636.

28. Dons R, Resselet P, Pastakia B et al. Arthropathy in acromegalic patients before and after treatment: a long-term follow-up study. Clin Endocrinol 1988; 28: 515–524.

183 Bone and joint abnormalities in thyroid diseases

Robert Igwe and Michael Kleerekoper

Definition

- Musculoskeletal abnormalities are seen in patients with hyperthyroidism as well as hypothyroidism. They are most commonly seen in the elderly and postmenopausal women

Clinical features

- Long silent/asymptomatic period
- Osteoporotic fractures at the spine and hip
- Thyroid acropachy: clubbing, periostitis
- Proximal muscle weakness
- Arthralgia and arthritis
- Hypercalcemia

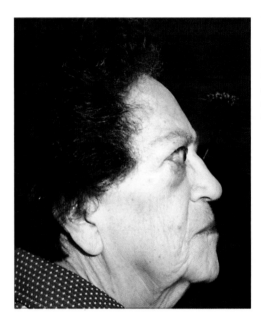

Fig. 183.1 Hyperthyroidsim. Profile of a patient with hyperthyroidism who developed thyroid acropachy, demonstrating the exophthalmus that was present.

INTRODUCTION

Bone disease and myopathies can occur both in hyper- and hypothyroidism. They may be manifest at presentation with thyroid disease or, less commonly, result from therapy (e.g. thyroid acropachy following the treatment of hyperthyroidism). Disturbances in bone and mineral metabolism secondary to hyperthyroidism were reported as early as in 1891 when von Recklinghausen described decalcification with 'worm-eaten' appearance of the long bones of a young woman who died from hyperthyroidism[1]. It is likely that one of his original cases of 'hyperparathyroidism' was in fact suffering from hyperthyroidism instead.

Effects of hypothyroidism on the skeleton can be seen in cretins, who are congenitally deficient in thyroid hormone. They have been shown to have stunted growth and other skeletal abnormalities including epiphyseal dysgenesis and delayed dental development. Joint abnormalities are rare in primary thyroid disease. However, chronic rheumatic disorders including rheumatoid arthritis (RA), Sjögren's syndrome, systemic lupus erythematosus (SLE) and scleroderma have been reported in association with thyroid abnormalities. In part this is probably because many thyroid diseases also have an immune etiology.

CLINICAL FEATURES

Hyperthyroidism

Thyroid hormone excess leads to a reduction in the amount of cancellous bone, increased cortical porosity in all ages and reduced cortical thickness in elderly females[2]. However clinically detectable skeletal manifestations are uncommon, being most apparent in older patients (in whom thyroid disease may be extremely difficult to detect clinically because of the absence of a goiter and limited peripheral signs) (Fig. 183.1). A particular problem occurs in patients (mainly postmenopausal women) treated with excessive doses of exogenous thyroid hormone. Although the patients do not develop signs or symptoms of overt hyperthyroidism, the doses of thyroid hormone are sufficient to produce a decreased bone mass. When clinically apparent, the skeletal complications of hyperthyroidism include back pain and increased dorsal kyphosis from pathologic fractures of the vertebral bodies. Fractures of the femoral neck, other long bones and metacarpals may also be seen[3].

Apathetic hyperthyroidism

In elderly patients the typical hyperactive features of hyperthyroidism may be replaced by a syndrome of blunted affect, muscle weakness and wasting, and marked immobility. This has been termed apathetic hyperthyroidism and is quite uncommon. The diagnosis is often missed because it is so antithetical of what is expected. The etiology of this form of hyperthyroidism is not known but it is felt by some to simply be a manifestation of a very profound thyroid myopathy.

Hypothyroidism

The most significant effects of hypothyroidism are seen in infants and children who manifest growth retardation, delayed skeletal maturation and slow dental development. A gibbus deformity can occur due to deformities of the twelfth thoracic and first lumbar vertebral bodies. Other conditions that may be associated with hypothyroidism include slipped capital femoral epiphysis, epiphyseal dysgenesis, osteonecrosis, gout and/or pseudogout, and erosive osteoarthritis[4,5].

Thyroid acropachy

Thyroid acropachy is an uncommon condition that occurs at any age after years of hyperthyroidism. Since it is usually seen in the setting of exophthalmos and pretibial myxedema, acropachy is regarded as one of the immune manifestations of hyperthyroidism seen only in Graves' disease. Thyroid acropachy is a painless soft tissue swelling of fingers and toes, clubbing and periostitis[6]. Bone changes usually occur in the peripheral skeleton, most often in the hands. It occurs in equal frequency in males and females and tends to develop years after the patient has been treated for hyperthyroidism.

Myopathy

Proximal muscle weakness, usually painless, may be seen both in hyper- and hypothyroidism. Stiffness, cramps and muscle pains increasing with activity are common in hypothyroidism, particularly stiffness[7].

Carpal tunnel syndrome

Myxedematous deposits in the wrist sufficient to compress the median nerve result in a carpal tunnel syndrome, and may be seen in as many as 10% of hypothyroid patients[8]. Hypothyroidism should be considered in all patients with carpal tunnel syndrome, and serum thyroxine and/or thyroid-stimulating hormone should be measured in each such patient (Fig. 183.2).

Osteoporosis

Osteoporosis[9] has already been alluded to above, but is of sufficient importance to repeat. All patients with newly diagnosed osteoporosis should be carefully examined clinically for evidence of hyperthyroidism. Even if the history and examination is not suggestive of hyperthyroidism, screening blood studies should be performed on every newly diagnosed osteoporotic subject. Conversely, patients on therapy for hypothyroidism should have the dose of thyroid replacement carefully monitored, mainly to avoid the deleterious effects of thyroxine on the skeleton. Other consequences of overmedication such as palpitations, irritability, diarrhea, weight loss and so on may be more profound and lead to dose reduction without close monitoring of blood levels. However, the progressive bone loss is clinically silent and can only be avoided by close monitoring of thyroxine or thyrotropin levels.

INVESTIGATIONS

Radiographic investigations

Radiologic examinations are the most useful tools in detecting bony abnormalities of thyroid disorders. Newer biochemical tests are becoming increasingly helpful. Bone biopsy is rarely indicated and it may be difficult to clearly distinguish the increased resorption and formation of hyperthyroidism from that of hyperparathyroidism.

Hyperthyroidism

Thyroid acropachy is the only skeletal abnormality unique to hyperthyroidism, specifically Graves' disease. It is characterized by periostitis with periosteal new bone formation and overlying soft tissue swelling;

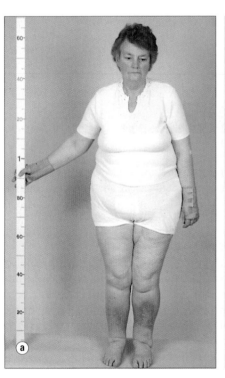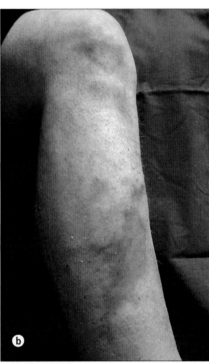

Fig. 183.2 Hypothyroidism. A patient who presented with carpal tunnel syndrome (note the wrist splints) and typical facial and other features of (a) hypothyroidism and (b) pretibial myxedema.

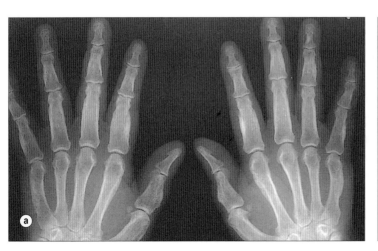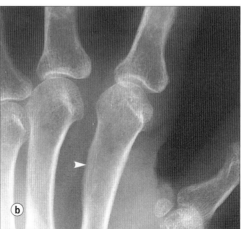

Fig. 183.3 Thyroid acropachy. Arrows show (a) periosteal new bone formation and (b) longitudinal striation within the cortex.

the hand is the most common site (Fig. 183.3a) for this (uncommon) skeletal manifestation of hyperthyroidism. As noted, the lesion may not become apparent until long after the patient has been rendered euthyroid by therapy. More commonly in hyperthyroidism there is radiolucency of the phalanges with longitudinal striation within the cortex (Fig. 183.3b). In the spine there may be compressed or wedged vertebral bodies, and widely spaced trabeculae associated with distorted contour of vertebrae, especially in the lumbar and thoracic area[10]. In the skull, the radiolucency is more focal and may appear microcystic. Joint radiographs tend to be normal unless there is an association with other rheumatic disorders. In children with hyperthyroidism, radiographs reveal an acceleration of bone maturation. Bone mineral density measured by quantitative radiographic techniques such as dual-energy X-ray absorptiometry (DEXA) may show low values at any measurement site; DEXA detects changes far earlier than conventional plane radiographs.

Hypothyroidism

Thyroid hormone deficiency may lead to soft tissue calcifications due to altered calcium metabolism. In children deficient in thyroid hormones since birth – cretins – there is delay in ossification of epiphyseal centers, with irregular patterns of multiple foci of ossifications. When these foci coalesce, the resultant 'stippled' appearance is known as epiphyseal dysgenesis[11].

Biochemical investigations

Thyroid hormone is one of the known regulators of bone remodeling or turnover, leading to activation of the remodeling cycle. Changes in the levels of various biochemical markers of bone remodeling reflect the effects of thyroid hormones on bone. Serum alkaline phosphatase and osteocalcin levels are increased in hyperthyroidism and normal or low in hypothyroidism[12]. Similarly urine excretion of the several markers of bone resorption (hydroxyproline, pyridinoline cross-links of collagen, N- and C-terminal telopeptides of these cross-links) is increased in hyperthyroidism and normal or low in hypothyroidism[13,14]. In hyperthyroidism there is often mild hypercalcemia. This can be distinguished from hyperparathyroidism in most cases because the serum inorganic phosphate is not low (and may in fact be slightly elevated) and the serum parathyroid hormone is suppressed[15]. In hypothyroid patients with articular involvement, joint aspiration usually yields highly viscous joint fluid with elevated hyaluronic acid concentration and a low white cell count (< 1000 cells/mm^3). Hyperthyroid patients with proximal muscle weakness usually have normal serum muscle enzymes; muscle biopsy shows the absence of inflammatory changes. Muscle enzymes, however, are elevated in hypothyroid patients with myopathy, with histology showing focal necrosis, regeneration and mucinous deposits.

DIFFERENTIAL DIAGNOSIS

In all patients with decreased bone mass, with or without fragility fractures, hyperthyroidism has to be excluded. Hypothyroidism must be considered in all cases of growth retardation and delayed epiphyseal closure. The other musculoskeletal manifestations in hyper- and hypothyroidism appear indistinguishable from those seen in many other conditions. The exception to this is of course thyroid acropachy, described earlier. Since this lesion may occur long after the patient has been treated for Graves' disease, the connection between the two conditions may not be readily apparent. Fortunately acropachy is quite uncommon and is almost invariably seen in patients who also have ophthalmopathy[16]. Muscle weakness, usually proximal and usually painless, may occur in both hyper- and hypothyroidism. Muscle weakness occurs in hypokalemic familial periodic paralysis, which may be associated with both hypothyroidism and thyrotoxicosis. Stiffness may be a dominant feature in many patients with hypothyroidism, causing confusion with many other rheumatologic disorders. Usually the patient will have sufficient additional clinical features of hypothyroidism for the correct diagnosis to be made.

Etiology and pathogenesis

In the physiologic state, bone remodeling is the result of equal rates of bone resorption and formation, thereby maintaining a constant total bone mass. Bone remodeling proceeds in a sequence of activation, resorption and osteoblastic bone formation. The product of this process is called the bone structural unit. Thyroid hormone increases the frequency of activation of these units. Thus in hyperthyroidism, there is an increased bone turnover with bone resorption being more predominant. The actions of thyroid hormone on osteoclastic bone resorption leads to elevation in serum calcium, with a feedback suppression of parathyroid hormone secretion and reduced conversion of 25-hydroxyvitamin D into 1,25-dihydroxyvitamin D. Lower levels of active vitamin D leads to decreased absorption of calcium from the intestine. There are direct correlations between the severity and duration of thyrotoxicosis and the induction of bone disease. However, bone changes are more frequently seen in patients at risk for osteoporosis, especially those with a low peak bone mass and postmenopausal women. In children, deficiency of thyroid hormone causes retardation of growth and development[17]. There is little cartilage cell proliferation in the growth plates of the long bones. In adults with hypothyroidism, bone abnormalities are infrequent. There is reduction in the frequency of activation of the bone units with marked prolongation of the remodeling cycle. This results from a reduction in osteoblastic as well as osteoclastic activity. Occasionally the bone may be more compact. In thyroid acropachy, elevated plasma concentrations of long-acting thyroid stimulating (LATS) hormone are detected.

The pathogenesis of proximal myopathy in thyrotoxicosis and hypothyroidism is not well understood. The excess of thyroid disease in patients with autoimmune rheumatic disease has led some to postulate a common genetic link between these two groups of disorders. Family studies show that non-HLA, non-Gm linked genes are likely to be involved in the genetic predisposition common to the two diseases[18]. Others have postulated that the muscle membranes are 'leaky' in hypothyroidism and that this is in some way responsible for elevated serum levels of muscle enzymes, usually to a greater degree than anticipated from the clinical symptoms of muscle involvement.

MANAGEMENT

Appropriate treatment of endogenous hyperthyroidism will prevent skeletal lesions in most patients. Usually the disease is clinically apparent before irreversible skeletal disease has occurred. The exception to this is thyroid acropachy which is apparent only several years after the patient has been rendered euthyroid and for which there is no recognized effective therapy. In patients with exogenous hyperthyroidism the skeletal disease may be the only clinical manifestation and irreversible bone loss may have already occurred.

While specific therapy for osteoporosis (estrogen in postmenopausal women, calcitonin, bisphosphonates, selective estrogen receptor modulators) may be of benefit, it is essential to first try and reduce the dose of thyroxine therapy such that the patient is no longer hyperthyroid. A euthyroid state should be maintained for at least 6 months before considering therapy with drugs that inhibit bone resorption such as those mentioned above[19,20]. Biochemical indices of bone remodeling should have been reduced considerably by that time[14], with a concomitant increase in bone mass.

REFERENCES

1. Ross DS. Hyperthyroidism; thyroid hormone therapy and bone. Thyroid 1994; 4: 319–326.
2. Meema HE, Meema S. Comparison of microradioscopic and morphometric findings in the hand bones with densitometric findings in the proximal radius in thyrotoxicosis and renal osteodystrophy. Invest Radiol 1972; 7: 88–96.
3. Cummings SR, Nevitt MC, Browner WS et al. The study of osteoporotic fractures. Risk factors of hip fracture in white women. N Engl J Med 1995: 332; 767–73.
4. McLean RM, Podell DN. Bone and joint manifestations of hypothyroidism. Semin Arthritis Rheum 1995; 24: 282–290.
5. Dorwatt BB, Schumacher HR. Joint effusions, chondrocalcinosis and other rheumatic manifestations in hypothyroidism. A clinicopathologic study. Am J Med 1975; 59: 780–790.
6. Kinsella RA, Back DK. Thyroid acropachy. Med Clin North Am 1968; 52: 393–398.
7. Bland JH, Frymoyer JW. Rheumatic syndromes of myxedema. N Engl J Med 1970; 282: 1171–1174.
8. Frymoyer JW, Bland JH. Carpal tunnel syndrome in patients with myxedematous arthropathy. J Bone Joint Surg 1973; 55A: 78–82.
9. Poa HL, Knockover MR. Thyroid-induced osteoporosis. Curr Opin Orthop 1995; 6; 39–44.
10. Wartofsky L. Bone disease in thyrotoxicosis. Hos Prac 1994; 15: 69–80.
11. McLean RM, Podell DN. Bone and joint manifestations of hypothyroidism. Semin Arthritis Rheum 1995; 24: 282–290.
12. Cooper DS, Kaplan MM, Ridgway CC et al. Alkaline phosphatase isoenzyme patterns in hyperthyroidism. Ann Intern Med 1979: 90; 164–168.
13. Krakauer JC, Kleerekoper M. Borderline low serum thyrotropin level is correlated with increased fasting urinary hydroxyproline excretion. Arch Intern Med 1992: 152; 360–364.
14. Garnero P, Vassy V, Bertholin A et al. Markers of bone turnover in hyperthyroidism and the effect of treatment. J Clin Endocrinol Metab 1994: 78; 955–959.
15. Mosekilde L, Eriksen EF, Charles P. Effects of thyroid hormone on bone and mineral metabolism. Endocr Metab Clin North Am 1990; 19: 35–63.
16. Fatourechi V, Pajouhi M, Fransway AF. Dermopathy of Graves disease (pretibial myxedema). Review of 150 cases. Medicine 1994; 73: 1–7.
17. Weber G, Mora S, Bellini A et al. Bone mineral metabolism and thyroid replacement therapy in congenital hypothyroid infants and young children. J Endocrinol Invest 1995; 18: 277–282.
18. Sanders PA, Grennan DM, Dyer PA et al. Immunogentic studies in families with rheumatoid arthritis and auto-immune thyroid disease. J Med Genet 1985; 22: 451–456.
19. Franklyn JA, Betteridge J, Holder R, Sheppard MC. Effect of estrogen replacement therapy upon bone mineral density in thyroxine-treated postmenopausal women with a past history of thyrotoxicosis. Thyroid 1995: 5: 359–363.
20. Kung AW, Yeung SSC. Prevention of bone loss induced by thyroxine suppressive therapy in postmenopausal women: The effect of calcium and calctonin. J Clin Endocrinol Metab 1996; 81: 1232–1236.

184 Diabetes mellitus

Sándor S Forgács

Definition

- Diabetes mellitus is a syndrome characterized by chronic hyperglycemia which is accompanied by protein and lipid metabolic disorders
- It is important from the rheumatologic standpoint to distinguish between the two main types of diabetes mellitus:
  - type I: Juvenile-onset, insulin-dependent diabetes
  - type II: Maturity-onset, non-insulin-dependent diabetes

Clinical features

- A variety of rheumatologic disorders occur in patients with diabetes including diabetic osteoarthropathy, stiff hands syndrome, neuropathic joints and calcific periarthritis

INTRODUCTION

Diabetes mellitus affects the connective tissue in a variety of ways and it is not surprising that the complex metabolic disturbances in diabetes cause a variety of alterations in the musculoskeletal system (Table 184.1). These appear not only as independent disease processes (e.g. diabetic osteoarthropathy), but also as modifications in the frequency and course of common rheumatic conditions. Experimental data prove that bone could be structurally altered in diabetes[1].

The incidence of diabetes is about 1.5–2.5% of the general population, and as a result of the rising number of diabetic patients and their increased life expectancy, musculoskeletal symptoms in diabetes are being encountered more frequently by rheumatologists.

TABLE 184.1 BONE AND JOINT ALTERATIONS IN DIABETES MELLITUS

Osteoporosis	Subclinical in most cases
Hyperostosis	DISH syndrome occurs frequently, particularly in type II diabetes
Osteoarthritis	Frequent in diabetes?
Diabetic osteoarthropathy	Destructive bone changes which are severe late complications of type I diabetes
Diabetic hand syndrome	Diabetic alterations of soft tissues of hands
Dupuytren's contracture and shoulder periarthritis	Frequent in diabetes
Rheumatoid arthritis	Immunologic connections between rheumatoid arthritis and diabetes mellitus

OSTEOPOROSIS AND DIABETES MELLITUS

From the preinsulin era to the 1950s, diabetes was considered to predispose an outward form of diabetic osteopathy. Modern radiologic and biochemical methods, however, have allowed us to re-evaluate the relationship between diabetes and osteoporosis in recent decades.

Diabetes was previously considered to predispose patients to osteoporosis as it occurred in about half of adult patients with diabetes. Numerous factors were presumed to be the cause, the most important of which was prolonged negative nitrogen balance leading to a decrease in the protein matrix of the bones. However, numerous observations have since called into question the connection between diabetes and osteoporosis[2]. Recently photon absorptiometry has been used to measure bone mineral content in diabetics. Although bone loss can be detected in type I diabetes, bone mass in type II diabetes may be greater than that in controls[3].

Diabetes during pregnancy does not alter whole body mineral content in infants[4] but a 10–20% reduction of mineral content has been observed at the onset of type I diabetes which progresses in relation to the duration of diabetes and the control of metabolic disturbance. Various metabolic abnormalities have been detected which could be related to low bone mass in insulin-dependent diabetes. Clinical and experimental studies have reported elevated alkaline phosphatase levels, decreased vitamin D_3, parathyroid hormone (PTH) and osteocalcin levels, impaired intestinal calcium absorption, and increased urinary excretion of hydroxyproline[5–6]. Insulin stimulates collagen synthesis and the uptake of amino acids into bone. Reduced production or activity of insulin-like growth factor (IGF-1) and probably IGF-2 may be contributing factors in the development of a diabetic osteoporosis.

Insulin promotes calcification in bone, explaining the phenomenon that in type II maturity-onset diabetes, when there is usually hyperinsulinemia, no osteoporosis develops; indeed, bone mass is increased. There is general consensus that insulin deficiency induces osteoporosis either by the impairment of bone formation[7] or by increasing bone loss[8].

Bone loss in type I diabetes is subclinical in most cases, and is detectable only by special measurements. In a series of 230 diabetics over the age of 60, spontaneous vertebral compression was found in only 19 cases (8.3%), no more than in the non-diabetic population of similar age[9]. Careful control of diabetes is thought to be important in the prevention of bone loss. Recent studies indicate that diabetes is a risk factor for fractures[10].

HYPEROSTOSIS AND DIABETES MELLITUS

The pathology of hyperostosis is essentially metaplastic calcification and ossification of the anterior longitudinal ligaments of the spine, most readily diagnosed on lateral view spinal radiographs. Calcification of spinal ligaments is frequently accompanied by a generalized ossification of ligaments and tendons and may be the first manifestation of the syndrome. These changes are summarized under the name diffuse idiopathic skeletal hyperostosis (DISH syndrome). DISH syndrome has characteristic radiologic signs although the clinical symptoms are often milder than would be expected from the severity of the radiologic changes (see Chapter 172).

Hyperostotic spondylosis occurs in 1.6–13.0% of the normal population[9]. However, among diabetics the prevalence is 13–49%[11]. In addition, in patients with hyperostotic spondylosis, 12–80% were found to have diabetes or impaired glucose tolerance, depending on the criteria used. In a separate study[12], among 500 non-selected diabetic patients over 40 years old, hyperostosis was detected in 118 (26%), whereas this rate was only 3.1% in an age-matched control group.

DISH is a disease which occurs in the elderly; it is rare in the young. In diabetics, however, hyperostosis develops earlier, and is also more frequent in each subsequent age group than in the non-diabetic population (Fig. 184.1). The common occurrence of hyperostosis and type II diabetes is characteristic. Almost three times as many patients with hyperostosis had type II diabetes rather than type I diabetes[9]. However, there were no clear correlations between hyperostosis and duration of diabetes. Bone abnormalities are often detected in newly diagnosed diabetics, although hyperostosis is often detected prior to diagnosis of the diabetes. This is clinically important as diabetes should be excluded in patients presenting with radiologic signs of hyperostosis.

Insulin (or insulin-like growth factor) at prolonged and high level may thus promote new bone growth, particularly in the region of the entheses. This hypothesis would explain why hyperostosis is more frequent in type II diabetes in which there is prolonged hyperinsulinemia. Furthermore, hyperostosis is nearly three times more frequent among diabetics with hyperlipoproteinemia than among those without lipid changes. Hyperostotic alterations have many features in common with acromegaly (see Chapter 182). However, levels of growth hormone in diabetics with hyperostotic spondylitis would appear to be normal[12].

In conclusion, DISH syndrome is not a specific diabetic complication and hyperostosis is not a direct consequence of diabetes. There is, however, a frequent common occurrence of hyperostosis in diabetic patients. The exact causes of the hyperostosis in diabetes have not been clearly established. Disturbance of carbohydrate, lipid and urate metabolism, as well as hyperinsulinemia and perhaps growth hormone overproduction, may all play a role[9].

OSTEOARTHRITIS AND DIABETES

Several studies have reported an association of early onset osteoarthritis (OA) in diabetes. In type II diabetes the frequency of OA of both small and large joints have been reported to be increased. Any association with OA, however, cannot be regarded as unambiguous since OA of weight-bearing joints may be related to obesity rather than to diabetes itself. In a large osteoarthritic patient study, the mean fasting glucose concentration was significantly higher than in controls. However, long-term diabetes occurred in only 5.5%[13].

DIABETIC OSTEOARTHROPATHY

The term diabetic osteoarthropathy applies to destructive lytic bone changes which are severe late complications of diabetes and occur mainly in the pedal bones.

Diabetic osteoarthropathy occurs in 0.1–1.4% of diabetic patients[14], a sizable number considering the prevalence of diabetes. The age and sex distribution from 299 reported cases in the literature are shown in Table 184.2. Changes are most frequent in the age group 50–69 years. No differences in the sex distribution of diabetic osteoarthropathy are apparent.

Clinical features

Bone abnormalities increase with the duration of diabetes (Table 184.3). Changes are especially frequent in those patients in whom attempted control with oral hypoglycemic agents in the month before development of bone lesions has failed, and insulin is required. The localization of joints (or groups of joints) affected by osteoarthropathy in 372 cases

TABLE 184.2 SEX AND AGE DISTRIBUTION OF PATIENTS WITH DIABETIC OSTEOARTHROPATHY

Age group (years)	Reported cases in the literature [11]		Results from Sinha et al. [15]	Total
	Males	Females		
Under 20	–	1	–	1
20–29	9	7	7	23
30–39	8	9	16	33
40–49	19	14	16	49
50–59	29	33	35	97
60–69	24	27	25	76
70–79	8	10	2	20
Total	97	101	101	299

TABLE 184.3 DURATION OF DIABETES IN DIABETIC OSTEOARTHROPATHY

Duration of diabetes (years)	Number of reported cases (%)
0–5	27 (9.4)
6–10	50 (17.5)
11–20	153 (53.5)
Over 21	56 (19.6)
Total	286 (100)

Relationship between duration of diabetes and incidence of diabetic osteorthropathy.

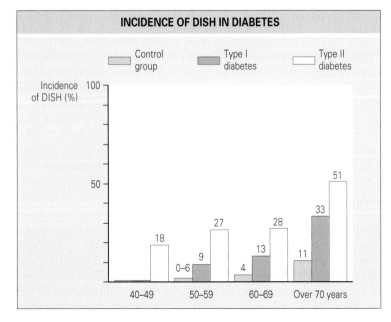

INCIDENCE OF DISH IN DIABETES

Control group • Type I diabetes • Type II diabetes

Fig. 184.1 Incidence of DISH in diabetes.

TABLE 184.4 LOCALIZATION OF DIABETIC OSTEOARTHROPATHY	
Joints	Number of reported cases (%)
Ankle	38 (10.2)
Tarsus	81 (21.8)
Tarsometatarsal joints	102 (27.4)
Metatarsophalangeal joints	117 (31.5)
Interphalangeal joints	34 (9.1)
Total	372 (100)

reported in the literature is summarized in Table 184.4. The metatarsophalangeal (MTP) joints are most commonly involved.

In diabetic osteoarthropathy, the clinical symptoms are much milder than would be expected on the basis of radiologic findings. This explains why diabetic osteoarthropathy is often revealed only after severe irreversible bone changes have developed. The clinical symptoms and soft tissue changes have been classified into four groups[15]:

- Neurologic symptoms. The signs of peripheral neuropathy are present in every case and at each stage of diabetic osteoarthropathy. The majority of patients have paresthesias and often diminished reflexes. An early and permanent sign is the loss of sensation to vibration.
- Skin involvement, soft tissue ulcer. Skin involvement is closely related to neurologic and circulatory disorders. Four types of skin lesions can occur: (1) erythema (with or without necrosis); (2) purpura or pigmentation; (3) yellow nails and (4) skin atrophy. Diabetes is the most frequent cause of neuropathic plantar ulcers, which often become secondarily infected. In most cases, a painless, sharply outlined, slightly oozing ulcer is visible (Fig. 184.2). Ulcer and bone destruction often develop simultaneously and at the same site; a typical example is when the metatarsal head above the ulcer is affected (Fig. 184.3).

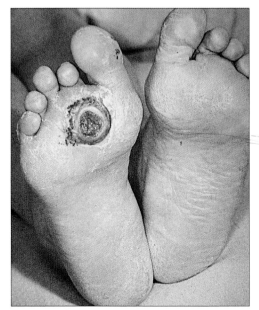

Fig. 184.2 Neuropathic plantar ulcer in diabetic osteoarthropathy.

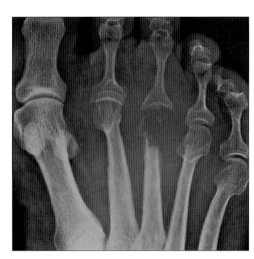

Fig. 184.3 Osteolysis in diabetic osteoarthropathy. This is a radiograph of the foot of the patient in Figure 184.2, showing subluxation of the second MTP joint (first stage) and osteolysis of the third metatarsal head with periosteal reaction towards the diaphysis (second stage).

- Loose joints, articular swelling. These symptoms include the loosening of the articular capsule and ligaments, and pathologic mobility of the joint. Owing to the appearance of loose joints and to the diabetic innervation disorder of the long flexor and extensor muscles, a simultaneous contraction develops, resulting in dorsal flexion and subluxation of the MTP joints. In other cases, the soft tissue surrounding the joint is swollen. Painless articular swelling is a characteristic sign of diabetic osteoarthropathy.
- Deformities. In advanced stages the soft tissues, deprived of their supporting structures, undergo contraction, resulting in structural changes in the shape of the foot and deformities. Because of destruction of the tarsometatarsal joints, the foot shortens, the medial contour becomes smooth and the arch of the foot collapses (so-called 'cubic foot' or 'rockerbottom sole').

Stages and radiologic symptoms of diabetic osteoarthropathy

Diabetic osteoarthropathy can be diagnosed only by X-ray examination[16]. The modern imaging methods have an important role in the diagnosis. Computerized tomography (CT) examination, an accurate method of demonstrating the extent of the disease, bone scintigraphy and especially magnetic resonance imaging (MRI) are valuable adjuncts in the evaluation of diabetic osteoarthropathy[17,18].

Based on the characteristic radiologic signs, three stages can be distinguished (see Table 184.5).

Stage I: Initial symptoms
- Circumscribed porosis. Osteoporosis is often subchondral and gradually turns into osteolysis.

TABLE 184.5 RADIOLOGIC SIGNS OF DIABETIC OSTEOARTHROPATHY	
1st stage: Initial symptoms	Circumscribed porosis Cortical defects Subluxation
2nd stage: Progression	Osteolysis Fragmentation Fractures Periosteal reactions
3rd stage: Healing	Filling of cortical defect Pointed bones Development of arthrosis deformans Ankylosis Total restitution

- Cortical defects. This starts as a juxta-articular cortical defect, or multiple defects, in bones of normal density. These lesions have a good prognosis. Rupture of the cortical border with osteolysis may occur.
- Subluxation, dislocation. This develops in the otherwise intact joint. It is an extremely important sign as it warns about the risk of later osteolysis (Fig. 184.3).

Stage II: Progression

- Osteolysis. This is the most important symptom of diabetic osteoarthropathy and includes two basic types: destructive and mutilating forms. The radiograph of osteolysis is variable, depending on the localization of the lesion (Figs 184.4 & 184.5). The articular surfaces are progressively destroyed and a marked fragmentation is characteristic (Fig. 184.4a).
- Fractures with or without dislocation. Due to the relative insensitivity to pain, so-called spontaneous fractures are relatively frequent in diabetic osteoarthropathy, particularly in the circumscribed porotic areas.
- Periosteal reaction. This may appear simultaneously with extensive osteolysis (Fig. 184.5). In the advanced stage of the process, the periosteal reaction transforms into a thick periosteal calcification.

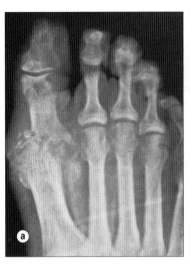 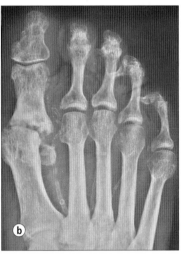

Fig. 184.4 Diabetic osteoarthropathy. (a) Fragmentation and severe osteolysis on the articular surfaces of the first MTP joint. (b) The process has healed with moderate deformation of the articular surfaces.

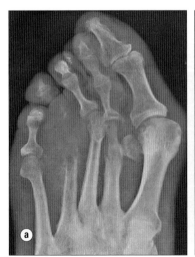 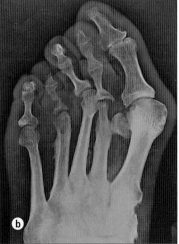

Fig. 184.5 Osteolysis. (a) Severe osteolysis of the fourth toe and metatarsal bone with signs of healed osteoarthropathy in the second MTP joint. (b) After conservative treatment, a significant remodeling can be seen.

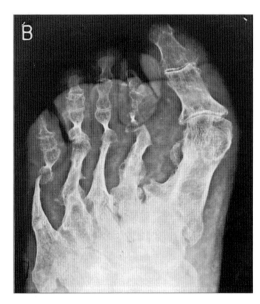

Fig. 184.6 End stage diabetic osteoarthropathy. Deformed, widened diabetic foot with pointed metatarsals after long-standing mutilating arthropathy and spontaneous fractures.

Stage III: Healing

Degeneration of all articular components can be found. The radiographic signs of healing include filling of cortical defects; 'pointed bones' (Fig. 184.6), development of arthrosis deformans, ankylosis, and complete restitution.

The process has no characteristic histologic features. Degeneration of all articular components can be found.

Differential diagnosis

In differential diagnosis, diabetic osteoarthropathy must be distinguished from inflammatory, tumorous, degenerative processes and neurogenic arthropathies of other origin. The disease is often misdiagnosed as osteomyelitis. Recently, MRI has become the most important method in the evaluation of an infectious process[17–20].

Pathogenesis of diabetic osteoarthropathy

Diabetic peripheral neuropathy plays the greatest role in the development of diabetic osteoarthropathy (Table 184.6). Evidence supporting the role of neuropathy is summarized as follows:

- The clinical signs of diabetic neuropathy are detectable in all diabetic osteoarthropathy cases.
- Increased protein levels in the cerebrospinal fluid, which is a frequent symptom of diabetic neuropathy, are found in diabetic osteoarthropathy cases.

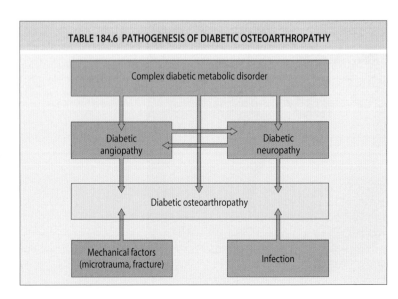

TABLE 184.6 PATHOGENESIS OF DIABETIC OSTEOARTHROPATHY

- Diabetic osteoarthropathy is often accompanied by neuropathic plantar ulcers.
- The clinical, radiographic and histologic manifestations of diabetic osteoarthropathy display many similarities with other bone abnormalities of possible neurogenic origin.
- Histologic findings of nerve biopsies performed in diabetic osteoarthropathy display signs of diabetic neuropathy.

Infection, vascular factors[21] (diabetic micro- and macroangiopathy) and joint traumas[22] also play a role in the pathogenesis.

Prognosis

In a number of cases, the prognosis is remarkably good. In addition, lesions may heal very quickly. Even if the disease is not initially treated, or insufficiently treated, the osteolytic course may stop at a certain stage and recovery will start.

Management

Clinical management is determined by evaluation of each pathogenic factor. Conservative treatment is indicated in most cases when the dominating factor is neuropathy. Healing may be ensured even in severe bone destruction (Fig. 184.5b). The most important task is to ensure good diabetic control, which often means changing from oral hypoglycemic agents to insulin therapy. Bed rest and protection of the foot from weight bearing are also important. The lesions are inclined to recur and residual symptoms are often encountered by the rheumatologist. The foot undergoes deformation and radiographic changes characteristic of stage III development (Fig. 184.6).

Even extensive bone destruction is not an indication for surgical treatment, and caution is especially necessary before deciding on amputation. In cases of non-healing plantar ulcers, and especially for the maintenance of remission after recovery, resection of destroyed capitulum and/or the base of the phalanx is recommended[23]. Empiric broad-spectrum antibiotic regimens are generally preferred because of the polymicrobial nature of most pedal infection. Care should be taken not to overestimate the extent of possible infection: severe osteolysis often results not from inflammatory but from neurogenic processes.

Amputation is only indicated if the process is accompanied by severe macroangiopathy or gangrene. Examinations of the leg always form an important part of diabetic management. Good diabetic control and foot hygiene are fundamentally important in the prevention of diabetic osteoarthropathy.

DIABETIC CHEIROARTHROPATHY (DIABETIC HAND SYNDROME)

The stiff hands syndrome of juvenile diabetes is characterized by thick, tight, waxy skin, joint restriction and sclerosis of tendon sheaths reminiscent of scleroderma. These clinical features have been termed 'diabetic hand syndrome' or 'diabetic cheiroarthropathy (Fig. 184.7).

Diabetic hand syndrome occurs in 8–50% of type I diabetic patients. In the typical case, the symptoms develop after a long duration of diabetic metabolic disturbance. Most cases were originally observed in type I diabetic children. Subsequently, it has been reported to occur in adults and even in type II diabetics, also involving small and large joints[24,25]. In the early phase, paresthesias and slight pain develop. The symptoms increase very slowly and greater pain, aggravated by movement of the hands, may supervene. On histologic examination, more or less pronounced loss of elastic fibers in the corium is observed. In addition, larger joints such as wrists, elbows and ankles are occasionally involved.

The association of diabetic cheiroarthropathy with other diabetic complications, in particular retinopathy and nephropathy, has been described. The relationship between limited joint mobility and frozen shoulder has also been established.

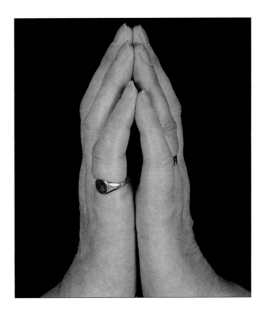

Fig. 184.7 Diabetic hand syndrome. The patient is unable to press both hands together.

The cause of limited joint mobility is probably multifactorial. Diabetic microangiopathy could be the main factor in the pathogenesis. In diabetic microangiopathy, the basic abnormality is thickening of the basement membrane. In addition, the direct metabolic changes in the skin and connective tissue may either be the cause or the effect of diabetic microangiopathy. It is not yet known whether the capillary changes occur first and predispose to ischemia and fibrosis of connective tissue or whether the collagen changes occur first and cause small vessel disease as a secondary phenomenon. It is also possible that diabetes mellitus predisposes to both microangiopathy and cheiroarthropathy independently, in a susceptible population. Diabetic neuropathy (which is closely connected with microangiopathy) may also play a role in the pathogenesis.

Specific management of diabetic cheiroarthropathy is not known. Good diabetic control is considered to be important in preventing progression. In addition, vasodilator drugs and symptomatic treatment are recommended.

DUPUYTREN'S CONTRACTURE AND DIABETES

It is estimated that up to two-thirds of diabetics have symptoms of Dupuytren's disease[8] Conversely, among patients with Dupuytren's contracture, 8–47% are diabetic. Contracture occurs more frequently in long-standing diabetes although the severity of diabetes does not modify the frequency or clinical pattern of contractures. The contractures are generally mild and rarely require surgery.

PERIARTHRITIS OF THE SHOULDER AND DIABETES

Numerous reports have confirmed the association between periarthritis of the shoulder and diabetes mellitus[12,26]. Periarthritis occurs in younger patients who can develop marked loss of shoulder movement and it is more difficult to influence therapeutically. Pain may be less marked than in non-diabetics. Calcifications around shoulder joints occur frequently in diabetics although they are often asymptomatic[12].

RHEUMATOID ARTHRITIS AND DIABETES

Associations with HLA-DR3 and/or DR4, as well as decreases in C4 serum levels, have been detected in both RA and type I diabetes. In RA and type I diabetes, islet cell antibodies and numerous other systemic and organ-specific antibodies have been detected in similar numbers[26,27]. Familial clustering of the two diseases has also been verified.

A question arises of how the pathologic process of RA is modified by concomitant diabetes. In type I diabetes, an unfavorable effect has been reported[11]. Rapidly progressing, mutilating articular processes also involving the large joints are not infrequent. Presumably a role is attributable to diabetic neuropathy which frequently occurs in these cases and which is a predisposing factor in itself to the development of destructive processes.

REFERENCES

1. Balint E, Szabo P, Marshall C, Sprague S. Glucose induced inhibition *in vitro* bone mineralization. Bone 2001; 28: 21–28.
2. Forgács S, Rosinger A, Vértes L. Diabetes mellitus and osteoporosis. Endocrinologie 1976; 67: 343–350.
3. Christiansen J, Svendsen O. Bone mineral in pre- and postmenopausal women with insulin dependent and non-insulin dependent diabetes mellitus. Osteoporosis Int 1999; 10: 307–311.
4. Lapillone A, Guerin S, Braillon P *et al*. Diabetes during pregnancy does not alter whole body mineral content in infants. J Clin Endopcrinol Metab 1997; 82: 3993–3997.
5. Selby P, Shearing P, Marschall S. Hydroxyprolin excretion is increased in diabetes mellitus and related to the presence of microalbuminuria. Diab Med I995; 12: 240–243.
6. Campos Pastor MM, Lopez-Ibarra PJ, Escobar-Jimenez F *et al*. Intensive insulin therapy and bone mineral density in type 1 diabetes mellitus: a prospective study. Osteoporos Int 2000; 11: 455–459.
7. Kermik S, Hermus A, Swinkels L *et al*. Osteopenia in insulin dependent diabetes mellitus, prevalence and aspects of pathophysiology. J Endocrinol Invest 2000; 23.295–303.
8. Tuominen J, Impivaara O, Puukka P, Rönnemaa T. Bone mineral density in patients with type 1 and type 2 diabetes. Diabetes Care 1999; 22: 1196–1200.
9. Forgács S. Diabetes mellitus and rheumatic disease. Clin Rheum Dis 1986; 12: 729–753.
10. Schwartz A, Sellmeyer D, Ensrud K *et al*. Older women with diabetes have an increased risk of fracture. A prospective study. J Clin Endocr Metab 2001; 86: 32–38.
11. Forgács S. Hyperostotische knochenverenderungen bei diabetikern. Der Radiologe 1973; 13: 167–173.
12. Forgács S. Bones and joints in diabetes mellitus. The Hague: Martinus Nijhoff/Akademia Press; 1982.
13. Cimmino M, Cutulo M. Plasma glucose concentration in symptomatic osteoarthritis: a clinical and epidemiological survey. Clin Exp Rheumatol 1990; 39: 477–482.
14. Smith R, Barnes B, Sands A *et al*. Prevalence of radiographic foot abnormalities in patients with diabetes. Foot Ankle Int 1997; 18: 342–346.
15. Forgács S. Clinical picture of diabetic osteoarthropathy. Acta Diabetol Lat 1976; 13: 111–129.
16. Forgács S. Stages and roentgenological picture of diabetic osteoarthropathy. ROFO 1977; 126: 36–42.
17. Enderle M, Coerper S, Schweizer H *et al*. Correlation of imaging techniques to histopathology in patients with diabetic foot syndrome and clinical suspicion of chronic osteomyelits. The role of high resolutional ultrasound. Diabetes Care 1999; 22: 294–299.
18. Vesco L, Boulahdour H, Hamissa S *et al*. The value of combined radionuclide and magnetic resonance imaging in the diagnosis and conservative management of minimal or localized osteomyelitis of the foot in diabetic patients. Metabolism 1999; 48:922–927.
19. Craig J, Amin M, Wu K *et al*. Osteomyelitis of the diabetic foot : MR imaging–pathologic correlation. Radiology 1997; 203: 849–855
20. Lipsky B. Osteomyelitis of the foot in diabetic patients. Clin Infect Dis 1997; 25: 1318–1326.
21. Hill S, Holzman G, Buse R. The effect of peripheral vascular disease with osteomyelitis in the diabetic foot. Am J Surg 1999; 177: 282–286.
22. Young M, Marshall A, Adams J *et al*. Osteopenia, neurological dysfunction, and the development of Charcot neuroarthriopathy. Diabetes Care 1995; 18: 34–38.
23. Hintermann B. Operative behandlungsmöglichkeiten des diabetischen fusses. Schweit Rundsch Med Prax 1999; 88: 1191–1195.
24. Clarke C, Pisowicz A, Spathis G. Limited joint mobility in children and adolescents with insulin-dependent diabetes mellitus. Ann Rheum Dis 1990; 49: 236–237.
25. Renard E, Jacques D, Chammas M *et al*. Increased prevalence of soft tissue hand lesions in type 1 and 2 diabetes mellitus: various entities and associated significance. Diabetes Metab 1994; 20: 513–521.
26. Thomas J, Young A, Gossuch A. Evidence for an association between rheumatoid arthritis and autoimmune endocrine disease. Ann Rheum Dis 1983; 42: 297–300.
27. Gerthner E, Sukerik S, Gladman D *et al*. HLA antigens and nailfold capillary microscopy studies in patients with insulin-dependent and noninsulin-dependent diabetes mellitus and limited joint mobility. J Rheumatol 1990; 17: 1375–1379.

185 Dialysis arthropathy

Thomas Bardin and Daniel Kuntz

Definition

- Musculoskeletal disorders that develop in patients with end-stage renal failure treated by long-term intermittent dialysis

Clinical features

- Crystal-related arthritides due to apatite or, more rarely, calcium oxalate crystal deposition
- Amyloid carpal tunnel syndrome and chronic arthropathy
- Destructive arthropathies of the spine and/or peripheral joints

HISTORY

Hemodialysis was introduced into clinical medicine in the early 1960s and rheumatologic complications were promptly recognized. In Seattle, Caner and Decker[1] reported acute attacks of arthritis or periarthritis which were subsequently found to be related to apatite crystal deposition. The frequency of the attacks was observed to decrease with more efficient treatment of hyperphosphatemia.

Carpal tunnel syndrome was described as a complication of dialysis treatment around 1975, and its association with amyloid was recognized by Assenat et al[2]. Chronic arthropathies were first thought to be due to secondary hyperparathyroidism, but were subsequently recognized as being most frequently caused by β_2 microglobulin.

EPIDEMIOLOGY

Periarticular calcifications suggestive of apatite deposition disease are found in 15–50% of patients treated with chronic hemodialysis or peritoneal dialysis[3]. Histologic evidence of β_2 microglobulin amyloidosis can be found before or soon after the initiation of dialysis. The frequency of carpal tunnel syndrome and amyloid arthropathy varies with the duration of dialysis. These complications are found in less than 5% of patients in the first 5 years, in 65% after 10 years, and in 75–100% after 15 years. Their frequency also increases with patient age.

CLINICAL FEATURES

Crystal-related arthritis

Gout, which is common in renal failure patients before dialysis, is seldom observed in hemodialysis patients. Hemodialysis effectively clears uric acid from serum[4]. Calcium pyrophosphate dihydrate crystal deposition disease is also rare (Fig. 185.1). Calcium oxalate deposition can be a source of chondrocalcinosis, synovial, cutaneous and periarticular calcifications, and acute, inflammatory or chronic, paucicellular joint effusions[3,5]. Involvement of flexor tendons results in flexion contracture of the fingers (Fig. 185.2).

Calcium phosphate – mainly apatite – crystals are the main component of most para-articular calcium deposits in dialysis patients (Fig. 185.3). Deposits vary in size from small flecks of juxta-articular calcium to large pseudotumoral masses that may impair joint motion. Although most frequently asymptomatic, these para-articular calcifications may lead to episodes of acute periarthritic inflammation[3]. Apatite deposition disease in dialysis patients can also be responsible for acute episodes of microcrystalline arthritis, the definitive diagnosis of which requires electron microscopy. Apatite crystals can also be observed in the clinical setting of destructive arthropathies (see below).

Carpal tunnel syndrome

Carpal tunnel syndrome is a well-established complication of long-term hemodialysis and peritoneal dialysis. Males and females are affected roughly equally. Median nerve compression is usually bilateral and severe.

Chronic arthropathy

A chronic arthropathy frequently develops in association with carpal tunnel syndrome in long-term dialysis patients and is associated with articular and periarticular amyloid[6–8] (see below). Arthralgias are a prominent feature; they predominantly involve the shoulders, are usually bilateral, and often worsen during dialysis sessions. Ultrasonography or MRI can demonstrate thickening of the rotator cuff tendons, which can lead to an impingement syndrome. Synovial hypertrophy may occur. Loss of joint mobility is frequent, particularly in the shoulders, wrists and fingers. A chronic tenosynovitis of the finger flexors can lead to progressive loss of extension of the involved fingers, frequently associated with trigger finger phenomena. Joint swelling,

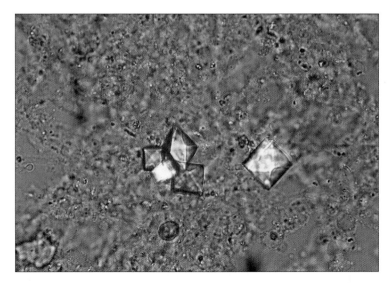

Fig. 185.1 Calcium oxalate dihydrate (weddelite) crystal viewed by polarized light microscopy in a synovial fluid aspirate.

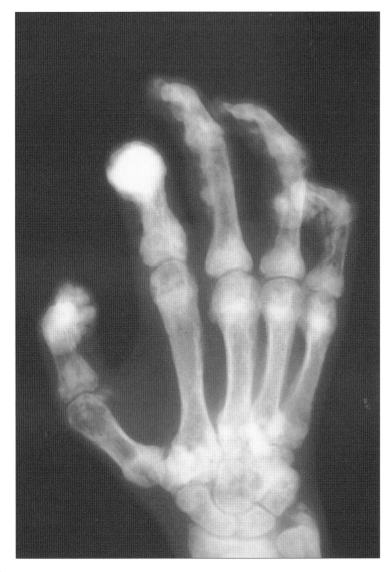

Fig. 185.2 **Hand radiograph showing extensive subcutaneous and flexor tendon deposits of calcium oxalate in a patient on hemodialysis, with characteristic finger flexion contracture.**

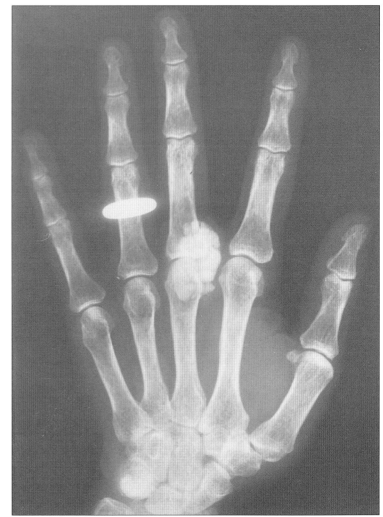

Fig. 185.3 **Periarticular calcium deposit involving the third metacarpophalangeal joint.**

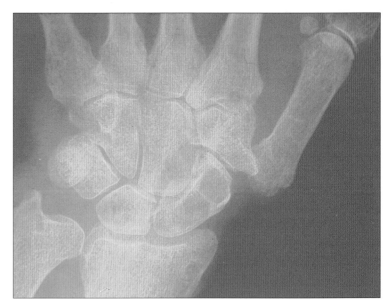

Fig. 185.4 **Amyloid cysts in carpal bones.** Note the trapezometacarpal involvement.

pauciarticular effusions and recurrent hemarthroses may also be observed. Subchondral bone erosions (Fig 185.4) are a characteristic feature and may cause pathological fractures of the femoral neck.

Destructive arthropathies

Destructive arthropathies can develop in long-term dialysis patients. Destructive spondylarthropathies involve mainly the cervical spine and are frequently multiple[9]. Characteristically, disc-space narrowing is associated with erosions of the adjacent endplates. There is no osteophytosis. Lesions may be rapidly progressive. Interapophyseal joints can be affected, causing severe spondylolisthesis (Fig. 185.5) and neurologic compression. Bone lucencies may be observed in the posterior arch, in particular by CT scan. No or very little local increase of isotope uptake may be discernible by bone scan. MRI usually shows a low signal intensity of the involved disk in T1- and T2-weighted sequences. Most frequently, these radiologic lesions are asymptomatic or mildly painful, although they may cause severe neurologic complications. The atlantoaxial joint can also be affected by β_2 microglobulin amyloid deposition (Fig. 185.6). This involvement can result in an erosion of the base of the odontoid process, which leads to an increase risk of fracture. As a consequence, cervical spine radiographs are required before intubation[12].

Destructive arthropathies of large peripheral joints are also frequently multiple and affect the hip, knee, shoulder and wrist. Cartilage narrowing is preceded by subchondral bone lucencies and/or erosions and is usually rapid, being complete within 3–12 months[10]. At a later stage, osteosclerosis, but no osteophytosis, can be observed.

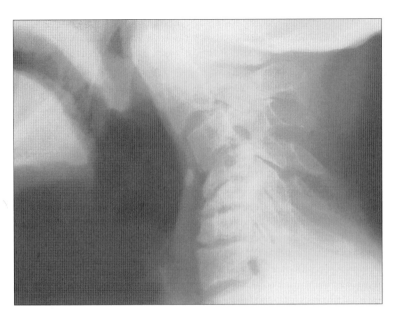

Fig. 185.5 Destructive spondylarthropathy of the cervical spine. Note the multiple involvement and the spondylolisthesis.

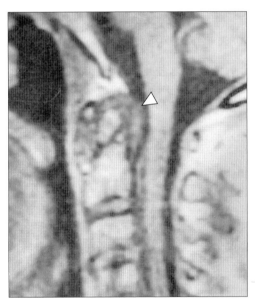

Fig. 185.6 MRI of the cervical spine. T1 sequence: periodontoidal mass.

Interphalangeal joints may be the site of severely erosive or lytic arthropathies which may develop early in the course of dialysis therapy and are not associated with local amyloid deposition. Erosive arthropathy of the trapeziometacarpal joint can also develop and be responsible for a superior and anterior luxation of the first metacarpal bone (Fig. 185.3).

INVESTIGATIONS

The diagnosis of β_2 microglobulin amyloid currently relies on radiologic and pathologic criteria. Thickening of soft tissues of the hip or shoulder, as shown by ultrasonography[11], and subchondral bone erosions on radiographs are valuable diagnostic features of β_2 microglobulin amyloid[6,8]. These erosions are usually multiple and have a roughly symmetric distribution. They are seen exclusively in the vicinity of synovial joints and involve sites of capsular and ligament attachment and/or areas of synovial reflexion. Lesions are evolutive and serial radiographs may show an increase in their size and number. The hips, wrists (Fig. 185.4) and shoulders are predominantly affected.

Dialysis amyloid can be sought in synovial fluid aspirates, surgical samples, particularly from the carpal tunnel, or in synovial biopsies. It has a high Congo red affinity (Fig. 185.4) that is sensitive to potassium permanganate treatment. β_2 microglobulin can be characterized in deposits by immunoperoxidase or immunofluorescence techniques. Scintigraphy using radiolabeled serum amyloid P component or β_2 microglobulin has recently been used to demonstrate amyloid deposits in dialysis patients[8].

Serum β_2 microglobulin level is constantly elevated, but this elevation does not correlate with the occurrence of dialysis arthropathy or carpal tunnel syndrome.

DIFFERENTIAL DIAGNOSIS

Septic arthritides have a much higher frequency in dialysis patients than in the general population. They are frequently polyarticular and may be due to unusual microorganisms, especially in patients treated with desferrioxamine. Diagnosis requires joint fluid aspiration to perform white cell count and careful bacteriologic studies. The cell content of amyloid synovial fluids is characteristically low. High white blood cell (WBC) counts suggest apatite-induced or septic arthritis. Infectious diskitis is similarly an important differential diagnosis of the destructive spondyloarthropathies of dialysis patients.

Renal osteodystrophy can be a source of pain mimicking arthritis. Severe secondary hyperparathyroidism is a source of skeletal pain, bone erosions and painful enthesis involvement, which can lead to tendinous ruptures. Aluminum overload caused limb root pain that could be confounded with amyloid arthropathy.

Finally, any rheumatic disease can develop in patients treated by hemodialysis, and these should not be mistaken for amyloid arthropathy. The diagnosis of these non-related conditions may be difficult in dialysis patients, given the high frequencies of both amyloid arthropathies and non-specific elevations of the erythrocyte sedimentation rate (ESR) in this particular context.

ETIOLOGICAL FACTORS OF DIALYSIS AMYLOIDOSIS

β_2 microglobulin

Hemodialysis-related amyloidosis is composed of β_2 microglobulin, a 118kDa molecule with a β-pleated sheet configuration that is non-covalently associated with the heavy chain of HLA class I antigens[4]. It is normally filtered by the glomerulus and metabolized by the kidney tubules. In long-term hemodialysis patients serum β_2 microglobulin levels are up to 60 times the normal value, and the chronic accumulation of the molecule appears to play a key role in the pathophysiology of the disease. High serum levels in dialysis patients result from loss of renal function, inability to filter β_2 microglobulin through the dialysis membrane and, possibly, increased production due to dialysis procedures employing bioincompatible membranes[13]. β_2 microglobulin modified with advanced glycation products has been identified in deposits and shown to stimulate monocyte chemotaxis and macrophage secretion of tumor necrosis factor and interleukin-1[14]. The amyloid associated with hemodialysis mainly involves articular and para-articular tissues, although symptomatic systemic deposits can rarely develop in long-term dialysis patients and lead to life-threatening complications. The reason for such predilection could be the high affinity of this type of amyloid for articular constituents, including glycosaminoglycans and type II collagen modified by end glycation products.

Apatite crystals

Apatite is the most stable form of calcium phosphate and constitutes the main mineral phase of bone. Its extraskeletal deposition in dialysis patients is favored by hyperphosphatemia that leads to the elevation of serum calcium–phosphorus product over the saturation point.

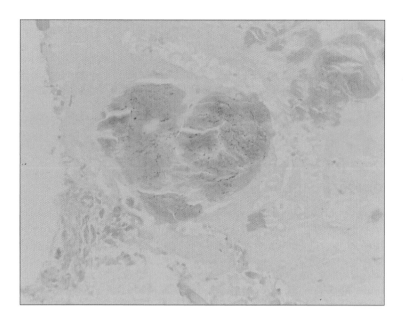

Fig. 185.7 Discal specimen, stained by Congo red, demonstrating amyloid deposit.

Calcium oxalate deposits

Oxalate is a terminal product of several amino acids and is excreted in the urine. Oxalosis can therefore develop in renal failure patients treated by hemodialysis when this technique does not allow sufficient removal of oxalate, and is favored by the ingestion of oxalate precursors such as vitamin C (Figs 185.6 and 185.7) .

PATHOGENESIS

The role of microcrystalline inflammation in most of the acute peri-articular episodes is well recognized. However, a number of joint effusions remain unexplained even when apatite crystals are searched for by electron microscopy.

Local deposition of β_2 microglobulin amyloid appears as a prominent finding in long-term dialysis patients requiring surgery for carpal tunnel syndrome. Vascular factors and edema on the side of the fistula can also be the etiological factors of medial nerve compression, especially when the condition develops early in the course of treatment. Vitamin B_6 deficiency is another potential factor.

Survival on dialysis for long periods is usually necessary for the development of chronic dialysis arthropathy. Aging is another important factor, as the prevalence of this arthropathy in patients treated by long-term dialysis correlates with age. A great number of pathologic reports are in favor of the amyloid nature of this condition.

The pathophysiology of destructive arthropathies is probably multifactorial. Massive amyloid deposits have been repeatedly observed in destructive arthropathies of large peripheral joints and of the spine, but these are not common features of the other articular amyloids. Premature aging, mechanical factors, crystal deposition, aluminum, iron or silicon overloads and secondary hyperparathyroidism are potential factors. Apatite crystals have been identified in disc biopsies of destructive spondyloarthropathy and in a few destructive arthropathies of peripheral joints.

MANAGEMENT

Symptomatic treatments

Standard analgesics are useful in the symptomatic management of chronic dialysis arthropathy. Non-steroidal anti-inflammatory drugs expose dialysis patients to an increased risk of gastroduodenal ulcerations and bleeding. Their prescription should be limited to short courses aimed at the relief of crystal-induced acute inflammation. The use of coxibs is uncomfortable in hemodialysis patients, who experience a high rate of atherosclerosis. Long-term treatment with colchicine (1mg/day) can dramatically lower the frequency of recurrent crystal-induced episodes. Corticosteroid injections carry an important risk of infection and should be avoided. Low-dose corticosteroid therapy (i.e. prednisone 0.1mg/kg/day) usually leads to dramatic relief of chronic arthropathy but its use should be restricted to severe involvements, given its potential risks of osteopenia, accelerated atherosclerosis and immunosuppression[15].

Surgery should be performed early in the course of carpal tunnel syndrome, before the appearance of neurologic defects that do not always recover after nerve decompression. Resection of the acromioclavicular ligament can be proposed in painful shoulders, associated with marked thickening of rotator cuff tendons. Total arthroplasties of the hip and/or the knee are indicated in severely disabling destructive arthropathies. Neurologic compressions can be improved by surgical fusion of the affected, unstable segment.

The use of highly permeable and biocompatible membranes has been reported to improve dialysis arthropathy. Kidney transplant usually dramatically improves dialysis arthropathy when joint pain is not associated with destructive changes[16].

Preventive treatment

Strict control of serum calcium–phosphorus product, and particularly of phosphatemia, allows reduction of both the extent of apatite crystal deposition and the frequency of crystal-induced episodes. Dialysis technique could influence the extent of β_2 microglobulin accumulation and delay the onset of symptomatic amyloid[8,13]. However, dialysis arthropathy has been described in patients treated with all currently available techniques of artificial kidney replacement. The frequency and severity of amyloid arthropathy in long-term dialysis patients leads to the promotion of early kidney transplantation in terminal renal failure patients with a life expectancy exceeding 10 years.

REFERENCES

1. Caner JEZ, Decker JL. Recurrent acute (gouty?) arthritis in chronic renal failure treated with periodic hemodialysis. Am J Med 1964; 36: 571–582.
2. Assenat H, Calemard E, Charra B et al. Hémodialyse, syndrome du canal carpien et substance amyloïde (letter). Nouv Presse Méd 1980; 9: 1715.
3. Bardin T, Bucki B, Voisin L, Ortiz-Bravo E. Calcium microcrystals and dialysis associated arthropathy. Rev Rhum (Engl Ed) 1994; 49S–54S.
4. Chou CT, Wasserstein A, Schumacher HR, Fernandez P. Musculoskeletal manifestations in hemodialysis patients. J Rheumatol 1985; 12: 1149–1153.
5. Reginato AJ, Seoane JLF, Alvarez CB et al. Arthropathy and cutaneous calcinosis in hemodialysis oxalosis. Arthritis Rheum 1986; 29: 1387–1396.
6. Kay J, Bardin T. Osteoarticular disorders of renal origin: disease-related and iatrogenic. Baillière's Clin Rheumatol 2000; 14: 285–305.
7. Munoz-Gomez J, Gomez-Perez R, Llopart-Buisan E, Solé-Arqués M. Clinical picture of the amyloid arthropathy in patients maintained on haemodialysis using cellulose membranes. Ann Rheum Dis 1987; 46: 573–579.
8. Van Ypersele de Strihou C, Drüeke T. Dialysis amyloid. Oxford: Oxford University Press, 1996.
9. Kuntz D, Naveau B, Bardin T et al. Destructive spondylarthropathies in hemodialysed patients. Arthritis Rheum 1984: 27; 369–375.
10. Bardin T, Zingraff J, Shirahama T et al. Hemodialysis associated amyloidosis and beta-2 microglobulin: a clinical and immunohistochemical study. Am J Med 1987; 83: 419–424.
11. Kay J, Benson CB, Lester S et al. Utility of high resolution ultrasound for the diagnosis of dialysis-related amyloidosis. Arthritis Rheum 1992; 35: 926–932.
12. Rousselin B, Henelon O, Zingraff J et al. Pseudotumor of the craniocervical junction during long-term hemodialysis. Arthritis Rheum 1990; 33: 1567–1573.
13. Bardin T, Zingraff J, Kuntz D, Drüeke T. Dialysis related amyloidosis. Nephrol Dial Transplant 1986; 1: 151–154.
14. Miyata T, Inagi R, Lida Y et al. Involvement of β_2-microglobulin modified with advanced glycation end products in the pathogenesis of hemodialysis-associated amyloidosis. J Clin Invest 1994; 93: 521–528.
15. Bardin T. Low-dose prednisone in dialysis related amyloid arthropathy. Rev Rhum (Engl Ed) 1994; 97S–100S.
16. Bardin T, Lebail-Darné JL, Zingraff J et al. Dialysis arthropathy: outcome after renal transplantation. Am J Med 1995; 99: 243–248.

186 Primary hyperlipidemias and xanthomatosis

Thomas Bardin and Daniel Kuntz

Definition

- Primary hyperlipidemias (hyperlipoproteinemias) result from abnormal metabolism of lipoproteins with an increase in their blood levels
- There are six types of hyperlipoprotein, which differ based on lipoprotein profiles and musculoskeletal manifestations
- Tendon xanthomas comprise lipid infiltrates, which result in irregular thickening of the involved tendon
- They can be observed in types IIa and III hyperlipoproteinemia and be associated with or preceded by episodes of acute tendinitis, particularly in type IIa

Clinical features

- Arthralgias and/or arthritis can be a feature of type IIa and type IV hyperlipoproteinemia
- Tendon xanthomas are observed in types IIa and III and may be associated with acute tendinitis, particularly in type IIa
- Osseous xanthomas, aggregates of spumous macrophages, are rare and have been reported mainly in type III hyperlipoproteinemia
- Hyperuricemia and gout can be associated with the hypertriglyceridemia of types I, IV and V
- Sicca-like syndromes, probably due to fatty infiltration of lacrimal and salivary glands, with subsequent enlargement of parotids, can develop in patients suffering from types II, IV and V hyperlipoproteinemia

EPIDEMIOLOGY

The prevalence of the various types of primary hyperlipidemias (Table 186.1) which are associated with tendinous xanthomas is diverse. Homozygous familial hypercholesterolemia is a rare disease estimated to involve 1 per 10^6 of the Caucasian population. However, the heterozygous disease is much more common, its prevalence being estimated at 1 per 500[1]; the prevalence of type III hyperlipoproteinemia is in the same range. More than half of the patients suffering from these two disorders develop tendinous xanthomas, so that this cannot be considered exceptional. However, most xanthomas are asymptomatic and patients are only rarely referred to rheumatologists.

Arthritis associated with primary hyperlipidemia is certainly very rare. In his original report, Khachadurian[2] noted that episodes of arthritis affected 10 out of the 18 homozygous children he examined. In the heterozygotes, figures for articular involvement usually ranged from 5 to 10%, and some studies even failed to show an increased frequency of rheumatic features compared to a control population. Currently, there are fewer than 10 patients with type IV hyperlipoproteinemia reported to suffer from arthritis.

CLINICAL FEATURES

Familial hypercholesterolemia (type IIa hyperlipoproteinemia)

Tendinous xanthomas are a prominent feature of familial hypercholesterolemia (type IIa), but are virtually absent in type IIb

TABLE 186.1 RHEUMATIC FEATURES OF HYPERLIPOPROTEINEMIAS					
Type	Increased lipoprotein	Result of lipoprotein electrophoresis	Serum cholesterol	Serum triglyceride	Rheumatic feature
I	Chylomicrons	↑ Chylomicrons	↑	↑↑↑	Gout
IIa	LDL	↑ β-lipoprotein	↑↑↑	Normal	Tendinous xanthomas Arthritis Sicca syndrome
IIb	LDL VLDL	↑ β-lipoprotein ↑ Pre-β-lipoprotein	↑↑↑	↑	–
III	LDL (remnant VLDL)	Abnormal β-lipoprotein	↑↑	↑↑	Tendinous and osseous xanthomas
IV	VLDL	↑ Pre-β-lipoprotein	N	↑↑	Gout Sicca syndrome Arthritis
V	VLDL and chylomicrons	↑ Chylomicrons ↑ Pre-β-lipoprotein	↑↑	↑↑↑	Gout Sicca syndrome

WHO classification.

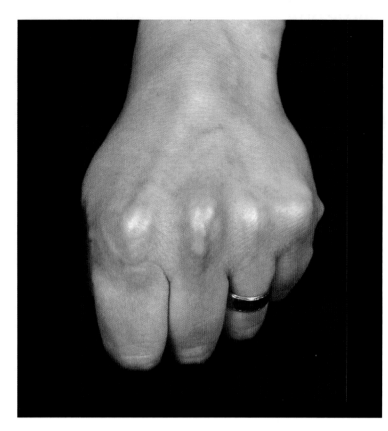

Fig. 186.1 Xanthomatosis of finger extensors.

hyperlipoproteinemia. Familial hypercholesterolemia homozygotes inevitably develop tendon xanthomas in childhood. Heterozygotes develop tendinous xanthomas at the end of the second decade. By the third decade, tendon xanthomas are present in roughly 50% of heterozygotes, and by the time of death 80% have them.

Tendinous xanthomas are usually bilateral and symmetric, and are mainly seen over the finger extensors in the dorsum of the hands (Fig. 186.1) and, less frequently, over the Achilles tendons, near their insertion at the calcanei (Fig. 186.2). They can also develop in insertions of the triceps at the olecranon and of the quadriceps tendon at the tibial tuberosity. The extensor tendons of the toes are more rarely involved. The plantar fascia is occasionally infiltrated. Subperiosteal xanthomas may affect the olecranon process and/or the tibial tuberosity in both homozygotes and heterozygotes. Calcifications in tendinous xanthomas

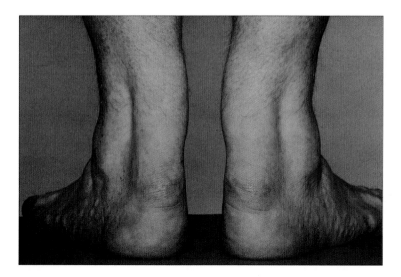

Fig. 186.2 Xanthomatosis of the Achilles tendon. (Courtesy of Professor AF Lant.)

can be observed radiographically, along with well-defined periarticular cortical erosions which result from long-standing pressure applied by adjacent tendon masses. The small bones of the hands are most frequently affected by these secondary erosions[3].

Tendon involvement is usually asymptomatic, the non-tender masses being of only cosmetic concern. It can also be a source of pain, however, through tendinitis or tenosynovitis episodes, or due to irritation of Achilles tendon xanthomas by the shoe. In homozygous children tendinitis can develop, especially in the Achilles tendon, before xanthomas become noticeable. Spontaneous rupture of the tendon may occur in rare cases. Painful episodes are usually self-limited.

Acute migratory polyarthritis was first reported in homozygous children with familial hypercholesterolemia[1]. An atheromatous involvement of the cardiac valves may make the differential diagnosis with rheumatic fever even more difficult (see Chapter 86). The erythrocyte sedimentation rate and levels of plasma fibrinogen may be elevated even in the absence of joint symptoms in homozygotes. Acute mono- or oligoarthritides can also be observed in familial hypercholesterolemia patients, most frequently involving the knee or the ankle[4,5]. Symptoms last for a few days, and the affected joint always returns to normal function. Recurrences are frequent. Synovial biopsy may demonstrate infiltration of the synovium by foam cells. Arthralgias have also been reported[5].

Familial dysbetalipoproteinemia (type III hyperlipoproteinemia)

Tendinous xanthomas (particularly in the Achilles tendon) develop in approximately 10–25% of patients suffering from familial dysbetalipoproteinemia[6]. Intraosseous xanthomas may affect the medullary canal of one or more bones and appear in radiographs as multiple, well-defined, small round or oval-shaped radiolucencies. The small bones of the hands are frequently involved, but xanthomas can also involve the skull, spine, pelvis and long bones. The latter locations can lead to pathologic fractures.

Type IV hyperlipoproteinemia

Patients with type IV hyperlipoproteinemia very rarely develop a chronic oligoarticular involvement characterized by synovial thickening, paucicellular, occasionally lactescent joint effusions. On radiographs subchondral lucencies may be seen. Foam cells may be detected on synovial biopsy[7,8].

Tendinous xanthomas in normocholesterolemic disorders

Tendon involvement is a feature of cerebrotendinous xanthomatosis[9], a rare autosomal recessive disorder characterized by deposition of cholestanol and cholesterol in the brain, lungs and tendons. It is associated with normal or low levels of serum cholesterol, and believed to be due to a lack of hepatic mitochondrial 26-hydroxylase. This disorder is also associated with osteoporosis and an increased rate of fractures[10]. Tendinous xanthomas can also be seen in phytosteroluria, an even rarer inherited sterol storage disease. These two rare diseases must be suspected in young patients developing tendon xanthomas associated with normal, or only slightly elevated, serum cholesterol.

INVESTIGATIONS AND DIFFERENTIAL DIAGNOSIS

The diagnosis of hyperlipidemia requires measurement of the serum fasting levels of triglyceride and cholesterol; a lactescent serum strongly suggests hypertriglyceridemia. Levels of the high-density lipoprotein (HDL) cholesterol fraction will provide information about vascular risk. Lipoprotein electrophoresis may be useful to determine precisely the type of dyslipidemia, especially when both cholesterol and triglyceride are elevated. Ultrasonography may help in diagnosing intratendinous xanthomas, especially in the Achilles tendon[11]. Virtually no other tendon disorder can be mistaken for xanthomas, because of their very progressive growth, their multiplicity and their rough symmetry. Furthermore, other clinical features of hyperlipidemia, i.e. cutaneous xanthomas and arcus cornae, are frequently associated. Occasionally xanthomas can be confused with giant cell tumors of the tendon sheath, but the latter are solitary and not associated with other features of dyslipidemia.

The arthritis associated with hyperlipoproteinemia may be a source of diagnostic problems, particularly the migratory polyarthritis that can affect children suffering from familial hypercholesterolemia. However, the presence of xanthomas and a familial history, together with the lack of signs of streptococcal infection, usually allow the exclusion of rheumatic fever. The other types of arthritis are non-specific and can easily be confused with numerous inflammatory diseases of the synovium. Great care should therefore be taken in excluding other musculoskeletal disorders which can coexist with serum lipid abnormalities. Gout attacks should be excluded when facing acute episodes, as the frequency of gout is increased in hypertriglyceridemic patients.

Etiology

Familial hypercholesterolemia

Familial hypercholesterolemia is a hereditary autosomal dominant disease characterized by a defect in the gene coding for the cellular receptor for plasma low density lipoprotein (LDL). This results in a decline in the rate of removal of LDL from plasma. Plasma LDL levels rise and LDL deposits in connective tissues and scavenger cells, producing xanthomas and atheromas[3]. Familial hypercholesterolemia heterozygotes have a twofold elevation in plasma cholesterol from birth and suffer from premature atherosclerosis and coronary heart disease. Homozygotes have a severe hypercholesterolemia, and frequently die from coronary heart disease before the age of 30.

Familial dysbetalipoproteinemia

The primary molecular defect of familial dysbetalipoproteinemia is the presence of a mutant form of apolipoprotein E (apoE). The mutant differs from normal apoE by a single amino acid substitution, and as a consequence does not bind normally to lipoprotein receptors. This results in the accumulation in plasma of chylomicrons and very low-density lipoprotein (VLDL) remnants (β VLDL), which are taken up by macrophages in peripheral tissues, producing atheromas and xanthomas.

Type IV hyperlipoproteinemia

Type IV hyperlipoproteinemia is characterized by high levels of triglycerides. The molecular basis for this form of hyperlipoproteinemia has not been elucidated. The most consistent feature is an increased production of VLDL by the liver.

PATHOGENESIS

The pathophysiology of tendinous xanthomas is still poorly understood. Tendons are mainly infiltrated by foam cells, which seem to result from excessive endocytosis of circulating lipoproteins (LDL in familial hypercholesterolemia, VLDL remnants in type III hyperlipoproteinemia) by macrophages, with subsequent lysosomal processing and accumulation of intracellular cholesterol. Areas of deposition of cholesterol crystals, surrounded by granulomatous reaction, are less common. Foam cell death could be the source of these extracellular crystals.

The cause of the articular episodes is unknown. Synovial biopsy demonstrates the infiltration of synovium by foam cells, which are believed to be lipid-laden macrophages. Cholesterol crystals are not usually observed in the synovial fluid in this clinical setting, so these do not appear to be responsible for the acute episodes. Apatite crystals have been observed in the mitochondria of synovial cells[5], a finding that could either be considered a non-specific consequence of cellular degeneration or hypothesized to be the source of the acute episodes.

MANAGEMENT

The painful episodes related to dyslipidemias are usually self-limited or promptly relieved by non-steroidal anti-inflammatory drugs. Lowering of serum cholesterol can lead to regression of the size of tendon xanthomas[12], and surgical excision has been performed in a few patients resulting in long-lasting relief, although this can be followed by recurrences[13]. Lowering of the serum lipid levels can similarly improve the arthritis of types IIa and IV hyperlipoproteinemia, but such improvements are very inconsistent. Lipid-lowering drugs can lead to muscular or tendinous side effects[14,15], which should not be confused with musculoskeletal symptoms of the treated dyslipidemia.

REFERENCES

1. Goldstein JL, Brown MS. Familial hypercholesterolemia. In: Scriver CR, Beaud et al, Sly WS, Valle D, eds. The metabolic basis of inherited disease, 6th edn. New York: McGraw-Hill; 1989; 1215–1250.
2. Khachadurian AK. Migratory polyarthritis in familial hypercholesterolemia (type II hyperlipoproteinemia). Arthritis Rheum 1968; 11: 385–393.
3. Yaghami I. Intra- and extraosseous xanthomata associated with hyperlipidemia. Radiology 1978; 128: 49–54.
4. Mathon G, Gagné C, Brun D et al. Articular manifestations of familial hypercholesterolemia. Ann Rheum Dis 1985; 44: 599–602.
5. Menkès CJ, Paris MN, Laoussadi S, de Gennes JL. Le rhumatisme de l'hypercholestérolémie de type IIa. Rev Rhum 1986; 53: 231–236.
6. Mahley RW, Rall SC. Type III hyperlipoproteinemia (dysbetalipoproteinemia): the role of apolipoprotein E in normal and abnormal lipoprotein metabolism. In: Scriver CR, Beaud et AL, Sly WS, Valle D, eds. The metabolic basis of inherited diseases, 6th edn. New York: McGraw-Hill, 1989; 1195–1213.
7. Buckingham RB, Bole GG, Basset DR. Polyarthritis associated with type IV hyperlipidemia. Arch Intern Med 1975; 135: 286–290.
8. Menkès CJ, Laoussadi S, Auvert L, Charrier J. Oligo-arthrite associée à une hyperlipoprotéinémie de type IV. Presse Méd 1987; 16: 1414–1418.
9. Burnstein M, Buckwalter KH, Marten W, McClatchey KD, Quint D. Case report 427. Skel Radiol 1987; 16: 346–349.
10. Berginer WV, Shany S, Alkalay D et al. Osteoporosis and increased bone fractures in cerebrotendinous xanthomatosis. Metabolism 1993; 42: 69–74.
11. Budo RO, Adler RS, Bassett DR et al. Heterozygous familial hypercholesterolemia: detection of xanthomas in the Achilles tendon with US. Radiology 1993; 188: 567–571.
12. Klemp P, Halland AM, Majoos FL, Steyn K. Muscoloskeletal manifestations in hyperlipemia: a controlled study. Ann Rheum Dis 1993; 52: 44–48.
13. Fahey JJ, Stark HH, Donovan WF, Drennan DB. Xanthoma of the Achilles tendon. Seven cases with familial hyperbetalipoproteinemia. J Bone Joint Surg 1973; 55A: 197–211.
14. Chazerain P, Hayem G, Hamza S et al. Four cases of tendinopathy in patients with statin therapy. Joint Bone Spine 2001; 68: 430–433.
15. Victor M, Sieb JP. Myopathies due to drugs, toxin and nutritional deficiency. In: Engel AG, Franzini-Arnstrong C, eds. Myology. Basic and clinical, 2nd edn. New York: McGraw-Hill; 1994; 1697–1725.

187 Hemophilia

John R York

Definition

- A sex-linked inherited disorder of blood coagulation producing a deficiency of factor VIII (hemophilia A) or IX (hemophilia B)
- Its most frequent complication is musculoskeletal hemorrhage

Clinical features

- Widespread hemorrhage, either spontaneously or with minor trauma
- Recurrent hemarthroses with subsequent progressive arthropathy
- High incidence of human immunodeficiency virus-1 (HIV-1) and other viral infections, including hepatitis B and C associated with the use of human donor blood products until the introduction of effective screening techniques

HISTORY

The term hemophilia[1] (Gk: love of blood) is attributed to Schönlein in 1818, although his pupil Hopf first referred it to in a dissertation. The disease was well recognized and documented by Jewish religious writers in the 5th century AD because of the hazards of circumcision in hemophilic babies. Firm rules were laid down to prohibit circumcision in certain circumstances because of an observed bleeding disorder affecting males and transmitted by females. Albucasis, who documented the deaths of men and boys in a certain Spanish village from uncontrollable hemorrhage after trivial wounds and bleeding, recorded the first published medical recognition of the disorder some 500 years later.

Joint disease due to chronic intra-articular bleeding was increasingly noted from the early 19th century onwards, with major contributions to the literature being made by König[2], Legg[3], and Bulloch and Fildes[4]. The appearance of hemophilia in the British royal family in Queen Victoria's offspring, and its transmission to several of the royal families of Europe during the late 19th and early 20th centuries, spurred on research. The young Tsarovich Alexei's severe hemophilia and the resultant established chronic joint disease distracted his parents and almost certainly significantly altered the course of history in Russia leading up to the revolution of 1917. The elucidation of the underlying coagulation defect and the advent of effective clotting factor replacement during the 20th century revolutionized the management of hemophilia in general and allowed the potential prevention of joint disease and the surgical correction of established deformity. Early therapeutic optimism was unfortunately diminished by the high incidence of HIV-1 infection in patients treated with blood products between 1980 and 1985. The advent of synthetic factor VIII and IX concentrates, together with donor screening and heat treatment of naturally obtained concentrates, has almost completely prevented this problem, but the synthetic products are still very expensive and not available in most developing countries.

EPIDEMIOLOGY

Hemophilia A has an incidence of 1/5000 male births and hemophilia B 1:30 000. The distribution is generally uniform in the world and there are no obvious HLA associations[1]. The likelihood of hemophilia occurring in females is infinitely small, but Sir Frederick Treves reported such a case in 1856 resulting from a consanguineous marriage between a man with hemophilia and a female carrier[1].

CLINICAL FEATURES

Mild, moderate and severe forms of the hemophilias are defined by plasma coagulation factor levels corresponding to 6–30%, 2–5% and 1% or less of normal, respectively. Musculoskeletal bleeding, although not as dramatic as life-threatening bleeding episodes such as intracerebral hemorrhage, is the most common complication of hemophilia. Bleeding into muscle occurs with about one-tenth the frequency of joint bleeds.

Acute hemarthrosis

This is the initiating event in hemophilic arthropathy, frequently occurring spontaneously or in response to minor trauma in severe or moderate disease. It is manifested by prodromal stiffness, acute pain, warmth and swelling. The rising intra-articular pressure eventually terminates bleeding and resolution occurs slowly, accompanied by bruising. Milder bleeding episodes may present less dramatically and be limited to the subsynovium, or be unrecognized as is apparently the case when established arthritis develops in a joint where there has been no history of bleeding.

The age of onset and frequency of acute hemarthroses depend mainly on the severity of the factor deficiency. Levels of 5% of normal or less are almost invariably associated with recurrent hemarthroses, and established arthritis may less frequently occur with levels up to 20%[5]. Weightbearing joints on the dominant side are more commonly affected, coinciding with the child's beginning to walk. The shape and stability of the joint are also relevant, and the knee, elbow and ankle are the joints most frequently involved. Avascular necrosis of the femoral head due to hemorrhage into the hip joint may also occur, with clinical and radiological features resembling Perthes' disease.

Muscle hemorrhage in specific sites may be potentially crippling, such as bleeding into the psoas muscle leading to hip contractures and femoral nerve palsy, and into the forearm causing acute compartment syndromes and subsequent ischemic muscle atrophy and nerve damage. At times large hemocysts develop within muscle (Fig. 187.1).

Subacute arthropathy

This usually follows repeated hemarthroses and often targets one or several joints, in which bleeding is more frequent. A persistent 'boggy synovitis' with synovial thickening, chronic joint effusion and variable levels of pain in the absence of recent hemorrhage indicate the onset of this stage. Muscle weakness and joint laxity contribute to further bleeding from the friable thickened synovium, causing continuing damage.

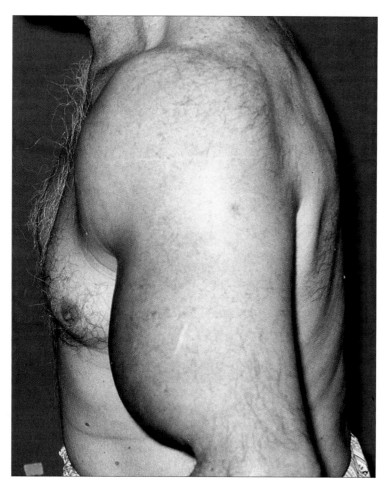

Fig. 187.1 Hemocyst – left upper arm.

The hyaline articular cartilage is progressively eroded by the inflammation associated with iron deposition. In addition, there is the production of lysosomal enzymes and catabolic cytokines, especially monokines, resulting ultimately in deep pits filled with friable blood clot and surviving plateaux of less damaged articular cartilage. Subarticular cyst formation is common and cartilage collapse may result in large bony defects.

Chronic arthropathy

The end result after periods ranging from several months to years is a disorganized joint exhibiting bony thickening, deformity, loss of movement and coarse crepitus due to loss of articular cartilage and sclerosis of subchondral bone. Joint contracture due to fibrosis or ankylosis is common. Soft tissue swelling and effusions are rare at this stage, and pain is fluctuating and variable, but at times severe[6].

Hemophilic pseudotumours

Hemophilic pseudotumors[7] may develop in bone, causing locally destructive lesions sometimes associated with pathological fractures, skin ulceration and infection, and compromised vascular and nerve function. The majority of pseudotumours that occur in the long bones of adults are due to repeated hemorrhage, either subperiosteally or into adjacent muscle, with subsequent encapsulation and calcification of the hematoma and progressive enlargement. These events are postulated to be due to osmotic gradients across the fibrous capsule of the lesion. In children they tend to be distally situated and result from trauma. Surgery on these lesions is hazardous and reserved for life-threatening complications.

IMAGING

Conventional radiology, ultrasound examination and, more recently, magnetic resonance imaging (MRI) have provided increasing detail about the degree and progression of joint damage.

Characteristic radiological changes described in hemophilic arthropathy include the following (many are not specific and occur in other arthropathies, especially those of childhood, most notably in juvenile chronic arthritis).

- Early
  - Periarticular soft tissue swelling
  - Periarticular demineralization
  - Increased radiodensity of thickened synovium* (Fig. 187.2)
- Intermediate
  - Harris (growth arrest) lines
  - Epiphysial widening and/or premature fusion
  - Widening of femoral and humeral intercondylar notches*
  - Squaring of inferior border of patella – lateral view (see Fig. 187.5)

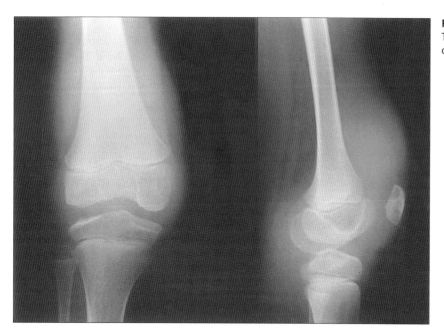

Fig. 187.2 Radiograph showing subacute hemophilic arthropathy. There is synovial thickening and radiologic density due to iron deposition.

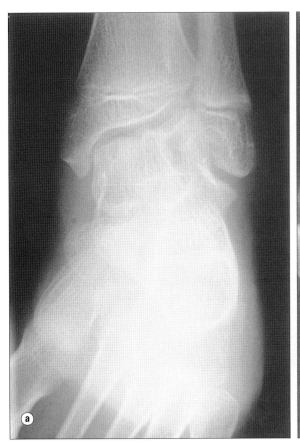
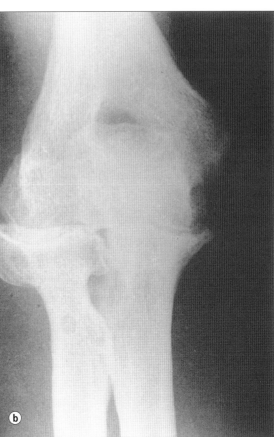

Fig. 187.3 Hemophilic arthropathy. (a) Radiograph of ankle showing tibiotalar slant. (b) Radiograph of elbow showing enlarged radial head.

– Ankle deformities – tibiotalar slant (Fig. 187.3a)
– Flattening of talus
– Proximal radial head enlargement* (Fig. 187.3b)
● Late
  – Cartilage irregularity and narrowing, central and marginal erosions
  – Incongruity of joint surfaces
  – Subarticular sclerosis and osteophyte formation
  – Subarticular bone cysts
  – Subluxations, joint disorganization
  – Bony ankylosis

(* considered to be specific for hemophilic arthropathy).

The most widely used classification of the radiological changes in hemophilic arthropathy is that of Pettersson et al.[8] and subsequent classifications have also included clinical criteria[6]. Where surgery is contemplated in patients with pseudotumours, CT scans to determine the extent of bone and soft tissue involvement, and regional angiography to define the vascular supply to the lesion, are indicated (Fig. 187.4).

Ultrasound examination is a useful and non-invasive technique to demonstrate the degree of synovial hypertrophy in a joint and the anatomy of soft tissue lesions such as muscle hematomata.

MRI has the capacity to not only confirm the presence of blood within the joint cavity or subsynovium but also to detect early hyaline cartilage changes not apparent on conventional radiographs and to assess the degree of synovial hypertrophy. The changes in the articular cartilage in the MRI (Fig. 187.5) were not apparent on plain X-ray. It is important to request specific cartilage sequences using a surface coil that adds extra definition, as these are not always routinely done. The expense of the procedure and lack of availability in many less affluent countries limits its potential usefulness at present.

Radionuclide bone scanning may be helpful in assessing the number of joints involved[9], whereas *in vivo* radiolabeling of red blood cells has a limited place in detecting further bleeding in already damaged joints[10].

ETIOLOGY

Conventional theories of blood coagulation until recently described an intrinsic and an extrinsic pathway, with hemophilias A and B being attributed to the effect of a deficiency of factors VIII or IX, respectively, on the midphase of the process. Roberts et al.[11] have developed an *in vitro* model of the clotting pathway recognizing the critical importance of tissue factor (TF) VIIa in the initiation of coagulation by activating factors IX and X through the TF VIIa pathway. In addition, its role in the interactions involving factors VIII and IX appears to result in a burst of thrombin generation on the platelet surface and effective blood clotting. This proposed model closely mimics *in vivo* conditions and has led to a revision of previous theories of blood coagulation. It does away with the concept of intrinsic and extrinsic pathways, although it is apparent that other inadequately effective routes of thrombin generation may coexist in situations of deficient clotting factors.

Haemophilia is inherited as a recessive trait and occurs in two forms, hemophilia A (factor VIII deficiency) and hemophilia B or Christmas disease (factor IX deficiency), the ratio of A to B being approximately 6 : 1. Deficiencies of other clotting factors are very rare, as is an acquired form of hemophilia A.

The cloning and characterization of the factor IX gene and subsequently the gene for factor VIII in the first half of the 1980s led to increased understanding of the molecular basis of the hemophilias and increased accuracy in carrier detection and prenatal diagnosis within families. The availability of phenotypic and genotypic carrier identification has made genetic counseling more accurate[12]. Also, fetoscopy and chorionic villous sampling, available in several highly specialized centers, have enabled prenatal detection of hemophilia, thus providing the

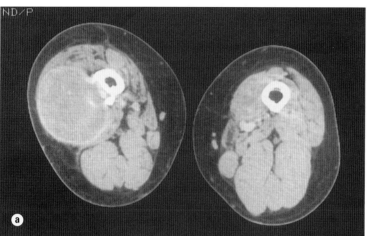

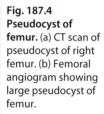

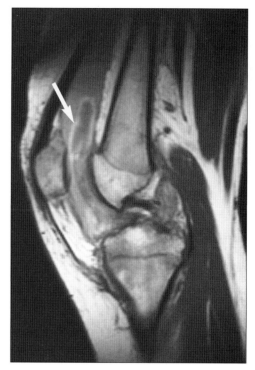

Fig. 187.5 Hemophilic arthropathy. T1-weighted MRI of the knee showing a bloody effusion containing high-signal-intensity methemoglobin (arrow). There is 'squaring' of the inferior pole of the patella. (Courtesy of Professor RD Duthie.)

Fig. 187.4 Pseudocyst of femur. (a) CT scan of pseudocyst of right femur. (b) Femoral angiogram showing large pseudocyst of femur.

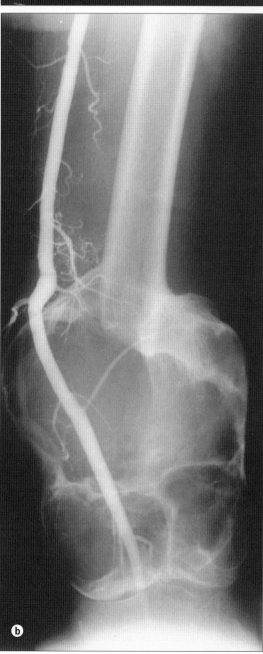

lates stabilized by a non-covalent association with von Willebrand factor.

Gene deletions, gene insertions, missense mutations and gene rearrangements have all been implicated in the chromosomal abnormalities resulting in hemophilia A. The most frequent abnormality is a translocation occurring within intron 22 resulting in the so-called 'flip-tip' abnormality, causing hemophilia A in 40–50% of severe cases throughout the world. By contrast, 90% of mothers of hemophilia patients with no family history of the disease carry this genetic defect, and the patient's normal grandfather supplies almost exclusively the affected gametes. This would suggest that the mutation resulting in Queen Victoria's carrier status could be traced back to her father Edward, the Duke of Kent, son of George III.

The factor IX gene[14] is also situated on the long arm of the X chromosome at band Xq27, and spans 34 kb with eight exons. Genetic screening in hemophilia B has been more straightforward owing to the gene's smaller size; also, because of its earlier sequencing and the smaller number of patients it has also allowed more detailed investigation. Missense and nonsense types account for 80% of the mutations in hemophilia B, and there is no factor IX equivalent of the common factor VIII inversion. Gene deletions and gene rearrangements only account for about 3% of the total mutations but correlate strongly with inhibitor formation.

In both forms of the disease the propensity to inhibitor formation has at least two genetic components, one related to the type of clotting factor gene mutation and one or more involving immune function.

PATHOGENESIS

The evidence increasingly points towards iron deposition being critical in the production of the synovitis[15] (Fig. 187.6). Mechanisms of damage include ferritin-induced production of superoxide anions and OH radicals, damaging cell membranes, and in synovial fluid the demonstrated presence of latent collagenases and other proteolytic enzymes and prostaglandins. Elevated levels of lymphokines and monokines, such as tumour necrosis factor-α (TNF-α) and interleukins IL-1 and IL-6, are found in the synovial fluid from hemophilic joints but in smaller concentrations than in rheumatoid arthritic synovial fluids. The tissue disruption caused by repeated hemorrhage, coupled with the chemical

option of termination if acceptable to the parents. However, a high rate of spontaneous mutation (up to 25%) results in many *de novo* cases[6].

The factor VIII gene[13] is situated on the long arm of the X chromosome at band Xq28 and is 168 kilobases (kb) in length, with six exons and 25 introns. Factor VIII is a large plasma glycoprotein which circu-

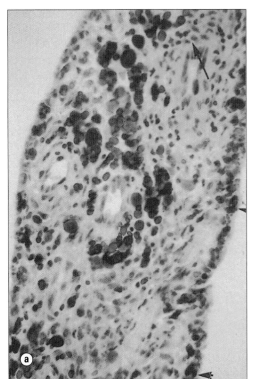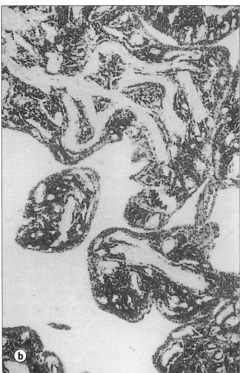

Fig. 187.6 Hemophilic synovitis. (a) Synovial hypertrophy, monocyte infiltration (arrow), heavy synovial and subsynovial deposition of hemosiderin (arrow), and new vessel formation. (H&E, original magnification × 100). (b) Iron deposition (Prussian blue, original magnification × 100).

damage to synovium and cartilage, ultimately leads to dense fibrosis of the joint.

MANAGEMENT

The concept of the hemophilia center providing multidisciplinary expertise has been a major advance in hemophilia care. Such centers provide a wide spectrum of medical, surgical and allied health professional skills, and the key contact person is usually the hemophilia nursing sister.

Prompt and adequate treatment of acute hemarthroses is vital. Factor replacement with consistently potent and safe concentrates is now possible with high-purity heat-treated concentrates, and more recently with synthetic factor VIII and IX produced by recombinant DNA techniques. Replacement protocols are summarized in Table 187.1. Acute hemophilic arthropathy is usually easily identified in previously diagnosed patients, the clinical features having been described earlier. Occasionally musculoskeletal haemorrhage is the first indication of the underlying condition which, if not recognized, can result in major morbidity or mortality. In this event the differential diagnoses include other causes of hemarthrosis, such as joint trauma including intra-articular fractures, bleeding disorders such as platelet deficiencies or anticoagulant therapy, other blood dyscrasias, villonodular synovitis, acute inflammatory arthritides such as pyrophosphate arthropathy in older patients, and rarely, joint neoplasms.

A deficiency or dysfunction of the adhesive glycoprotein von Willebrand factor causes the more common von Willebrand disease, which occurs in males and females with a frequency of 1 : 1000, but although acute joint bleeding does occur in this condition chronic arthropathy is rarely seen.

Some female carriers of the hemophilia genes have relatively low factor levels and may have problems during menstruation and with hemostasis during surgery and dental extractions, but bleeding into the joints is exceptionally uncommon.

As blood is an excellent culture medium associated bacterial infection must be considered and, if in doubt, aspiration and culture of the synovial fluid must be undertaken.

A coagulation screen, including bleeding time, platelet count, prothrombin time, partial thromboplastin time and factor VIII and IX levels, will confirm the diagnosis of hemophilia. It is important that intramuscular injections and aspirin and other drugs affecting platelet function are withheld. If parenteral therapy of any type is necessary it should be administered by intravenous injection until hemophilia has been excluded. In previously undiagnosed cases joint aspiration will almost certainly have been necessary to confirm the presence of blood,

TABLE 187.1 REPLACEMENT PROTOCOLS			
Indication for treatment	Factor VIII or IX elevation (units/100ml)	Frequency/day	Duration of therapy (days)
Hemarthrosis	30	1	1–2
Hematoma	30	1	1–2
Surgery	100	3	2–3
	50	2	3–4
	30	1	2–3
	or by continuous infusion		
Prophylaxis	>10	3/week	Indefinitely
(Adapted from York[1].)			

or where the diagnosis of hemophilia has already been confirmed, if aspiration of the joint is indicated it should immediately be followed by appropriate factor replacement.

Universal precautions to prevent the transmission of viral or other pathogenic agents should be observed, and although the procedure is a 'clean' rather than a sterile one, gloves should be worn, no-touch techniques observed and eye protection used. Should needlestick injury occur, appropriate initial treatment, counseling and follow-up are mandatory. If bacterial infection is suspected synovial fluid should be plated out and also collected directly into blood culture media, and blood cultures taken. HIV-1 positive patients have a significantly increased risk of infection in damaged joints, particularly if their CD4 count is low[16], but sepsis is also more common in joints damaged from any cause and a high index of suspicion should be maintained.

Although aspiration of all the blood from the affected joint would seem logical given the role of iron in the pathophysiology of hemophilic synovitis and cartilage damage, it is often impracticable. Many patients have already received home-based prophylactic or demand factor replacement, and aspiration may be difficult and for young patients quite traumatic. Conservative treatment is usually adequate and aspiration only indicated if the joint is very distended or if infection is suspected.

Local treatment initially, with rest, ice packs and analgesics, followed by graduated physiotherapy, local ultrasound and short-term factor replacement for 48 hours, is usually effective. Isometric exercises should be commenced the next day and graduated active physiotherapy should be encouraged after the first 24 hours, with prophylactic factor replacement if necessary, and the patient or carers instructed in a regular program to be followed. Short-term use of both oral and intra-articular corticosteroids may confer some additional benefit, but repeated use may result in significant side effects. For many families the spectre of the transmission of HIV-1 in human blood products between 1980 and 1985 and the subsequent high mortality among infected individuals has resulted in resistance to treatment. The advent of recombinant factor VIII and IX and virally screened factor concentrates has virtually eliminated that risk, the risk of hepatitis B, and more recently that of hepatitis C. Current concerns about prion transmission are still being evaluated[17]. In developed countries such as Australia newly diagnosed boys who have not received any human plasma products previously are provided with recombinant factor VIII or IX. This favorable situation is unfortunately not realized for up to 80% of the world's hemophilia patients who do not receive adequate treatment.

The subacute stage of the disease, with the development of a 'boggy synovitis' and characteristic radiographic changes, indicates potential permanent joint damage and necessitates carefully planned management. Prompt treatment of joint bleeding is again vital, and where target joints are emerging, prophylactic factor replacement three times weekly, elevating factor VIII or IX levels to 20% for 6–8 weeks, may be effective in controlling bleeding while muscle strength is improved. The excellent results of early prophylactic treatment[18] as soon as possible after diagnosis and before joint damage has occurred have been well documented for many years, and only limited by inadequate clotting factor availability or the development of inhibitors.

Physiotherapy to maintain strong muscles around joints is an important component of treatment to minimize bleeding, and where necessary splinting may be used in an attempt to prevent or correct deformity. Non-steroidal anti-inflammatory agents are not of proven value, and there is insufficient evidence to recommend the use of so-called second-line antirheumatic drugs such as D-penicillamine[1]. Intra-articular and short courses of oral corticosteroid agents have only produced short-lived benefit, but where total joint replacement surgery is not available repeated intra-articular injections have proved a useful compromise[19]. Intra-articular chemical or radioactive agents producing synoviorthesis reduce the frequency of intra-articular bleeding in the knee, elbow and ankle, and fears about the hazards of irradiation in young subjects have proved

unfounded[20]. Intra-articular sclerosants have been widely used in countries where radiocolloids are not available, including rifampin (rifampicin)[21], ethamolin and tetracyclines. Arthroscopy and lavage of the joint contents with appropriate factor cover is sometimes beneficial. Surgical synovectomy in the knee, either arthroscopically or by open operation, may also reduce the frequency of bleeding but is associated with significant postoperative problems. Synovectomy of the elbow and excision or trimming of the often enlarged radial head is an established procedure.

Chronic arthropathy represents a failure of conservative treatment, but unfortunately it has not been entirely preventable even with meticulous care. Aspirin should be avoided, but other non-steroidal anti-inflammatory drugs, preferably COX-2 specific agents, are often helpful in pain relief, but surgery is frequently the only treatment option. Patellectomy has been carried out in patients who had marked problems with retropatellar pain, crepitus, poor extensor function and instability. The results of this procedure have been unpredictable and it may compromise knee function and lead to the need for secondary reconstructive surgery. When pain, fixed deformities and disabilities interfere with the patient's life and work, joint stabilization or total joint replacement should be considered. Arthrodesis of the knee in the hemophilia patient remains a sound procedure with predictable lasting results and few complications. Total knee replacement has been used successfully for this problem (Fig. 187.7), particularly in patients with severe bony changes; but it is a technically difficult operation because of soft tissue contractures, subchondral bone loss and deformity. Furthermore, joint replacement in patients with hemophilia has a high rate of complications, including infection and loosening. For these reasons this treatment should normally be deferred for as long as possible, although in HIV-1 positive individuals short-term comfort and mobility while they are still comparatively active are important priorities. Should the hip be severely affected, total joint arthroplasty may again be indicated, and has given good results. As in all types of chronic joint disease total ankle arthroplasty has not proved to be a long-term solution, and ankle fusion is an effective option for advanced chronic hemophilic arthropathy.

MANAGEMENT PROBLEMS

It is essential that orthopedic surgery in hemophilia patients be performed in major hemophilia centers by operators experienced in the surgery of the condition and with the full back-up of expert hematological support, adequate laboratory facilities and secure supplies of appropriate factor replacement.

Open surgical synovectomy is rarely performed now, and arthroscopic synovectomy has largely been replaced by radioactive or chemical synoviorthesis, which is effective in controlling recurrent bleeding as well as shrinking the thickened synovium.

In the knee joint major preoperative joint deformity and lack of movement, and the young age of many of the hemophilic candidates for joint replacement surgery, mean that the postoperative complications, range of movement and the necessity for subsequent revision will be less favorable. The range of movement following total knee replacement is generally not significantly altered, but a reduction in the almost invariable preoperative fixed flexion deformity shifts the arc of movement into a more functionally useful range. Although the overall results in hemophilia patients by orthopedic standards are less impressive than those following this procedure in other arthritic disorders, the relief of pain and enhanced ability to walk are considered worth the risks, despite the fact that the long-term outcome cannot be assured, and subsequent revision may be difficult and hazardous[22]. Surgery in HIV-1 positive patients is ideally performed when they are on stable antiviral therapy and generally well. However, if their CD4 count is at or below 200/μl prophylaxis against opportunistic infection should be given as well as standard antibiotic cover for the procedure. Individual preference and clinical judgment determine the choice of pros-

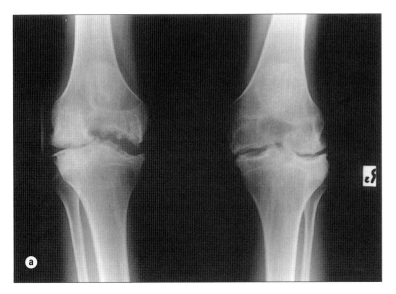 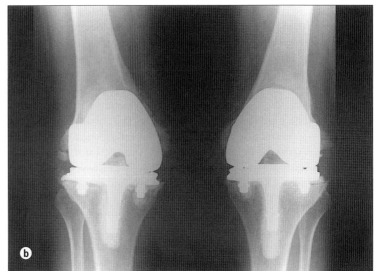

Fig. 187.7 Chronic hemophilic arthropathy. Radiographs showing chronic hemophilic arthropathy and joint destruction of the knee (a) and the consequent arthroplasties (b).

thesis, the use of cemented or non-cemented components and whether the patella should be resurfaced or not. Continuous passive mobilization is generally commenced postoperatively. Continuous intravenous infusion of factor VII or IX during and after surgery has resulted in economy of clotting factor usage, with at least equal and perhaps improved effectiveness.

Surgery in hemophilia B prior to the availability of synthetic factor IX was regarded as more hazardous than in classic hemophilia because of possible postoperative thromboembolic disease resulting from some factor IX concentrates. However, highly purified concentrates and rFactor IX minimize the risk of this very rare occurrence of a disseminated intravascular coagulation syndrome. These new agents have unfortunately not eliminated anaphylactic reactions,which can be life-threatening.

The ankle joint is rapidly overtaking the knee joint as a source of disability in hemophilia because unlike in the knee joint, arthroplasty has not been technically successful. Early radiographic changes in the ankle joint may not be associated with significant symptoms. The development of tibiotalar slant (Fig. 187.3a) alters the alignment of the joint surfaces, and advanced radiologic changes and severe symptoms almost invariably supervene, often despite few documented episodes of intra-articular bleeding. Sudden deterioration in function may occur after variable periods of time, even many years later, attributed to the collapse of surviving islands of articular cartilage and underlying subchondral bone. The use of shock-absorbing insoles or heel pads and suitable footwear, the avoidance of high foot-impacting sports and other activities, and splinting, are often beneficial, but ultimately ankle fusion may be necessary. The range of motion in the ankle at this stage is frequently limited to a few degrees of painful movement, so that pain relief at the cost of little increased disability is a boon. However, if the subtaloid joints are involved surgery is more extensive and recovery slower. Wound healing is slow in this area, so that surgical techniques with limited exposure have been developed[23].

The role of the physiotherapist at all stages of the management of hemophilic arthropathy is critical to minimize joint contractures. Knee flexion deformities and ankle equinus due to joint and muscle disease severely limit mobility, and elbow limitation and forearm muscle contractures interfere with many activities of daily living. Similarly, intensive postoperative physiotherapy is an important determinant of a successful result following joint and soft tissue surgery, especially after joint replacement. The documentation of ranges of joint mobility and related functional limitation is the basis of continuing studies currently being undertaken.

Although periarticular demineralization is a radiological feature of hemophilic joints generalized osteoporosis as a result of chronic hemo-

philic arthropathy has recently been reported (unpublished work, 6th Musculoskeletal Congress of the World Federation of Haemophilia, Lahore, 2001). Fortunately, new and effective therapeutic agents for the prevention and treatment of this condition are available.

Pain control in chronic hemophilic arthropathy is often a significant problem. Pain can be severe and persistent, and narcotic addiction in severely affected hemophiliacs is not uncommon and is best managed in a consultative situation. The cooperative efforts of the pain clinic, liaison psychiatrist, social worker, family members, and most essentially the patient, are essential. The recognition of the severity of the pain by the staff members and the development of positive strategies of non-pharmacological management, as well as the use of appropriate analgesic and antidepressant drugs, including opiates when necessary, are all important considerations.

The hazards of the transmission of infective agents via blood products are well known. HIV-1 infection was a devastating and lethal complication of treatment prior to blood donor HIV-1 screening and heat treatment of factor concentrates. The hepatitis viruses and other viral agents are responsible for a high prevalence of morbidity, and new synthetic factor replacements should prevent these and other more rare infective complications. Meanwhile, the problems of reduced stamina, liver cirrhosis in up to 20% of cases, and the increased incidence of hepatocellular carcinoma continue to bedevil chronic hemophilia A and B sufferers. A legacy of HIV-1 infection has been an increased risk of septic arthritis[16], in addition to the other results of immune dysfunction, resulting in tumors such as Kaposi's sarcoma and non-Hodgkin's lymphoma.

Coagulation factor inhibitors occur in 5–15% of hemophiliacs overall but they are less commonly found in hemophilia B. They are a particular problem in so-called high responders who develop an anamnestic response on re-exposure to clotting factors. In such patients, replacement therapy and surgical treatment have been restricted to life-threatening situations. Previous treatments have included the use of heterologous products such as porcine factor VIII, prothrombin complex materials and activated prothrombin complex materials. The induction of immune tolerance using large doses of factor replacement with immunosuppression using oral corticosteroids and in some protocols cyclophosphamide has been used for over 20 years, with impressive quoted success rates. The use of the technique has been limited because of cost and some doubts about long-term efficacy. Recombinant factor VIIa (rF VIIa) has been available for use in hemophilia A and B patients with inhibitors for bleeding episodes or if undergoing surgery over the last 5 years, but this treatment is very expensive.

The ideal treatment for hemophilia would involve the *in vivo* synthesis of adequate amounts of factor VIII or IX. Genetic engineering resulting in gene insertion therapy, whereby suitable cells containing the appropriate portion of the normal X chromosome are introduced into the body, is technically feasible but still elusive despite recent optimism. In animal studies therapeutic levels of factor VIII and IX have been achieved in mice, dogs and monkeys, inducing factor VIII production and factor IX in hemophilia B dogs using either mammalian cell lines or viruses as vectors to introduce appropriate genetic material[24]. Encouraging early results have recently been reported in severe hemophilia A patients using autologous dermal fibroblasts obtained at skin biopsy, transfected with plasmid-containing sequences of the gene encoding factor VIII and reimplanted laparoscopically into the patient's omentum[25].

At present the available products, such as high-purity viral screened human donor-derived coagulation factors and synthetic factor VIII and IX, avoid the known infective hazards, and initial concerns about increased antigenicity with the latter appear unfounded. However, the products still need to be given by intravenous infusion, with the small but definite risk associated with repeated venepuncture.

Currently replacement therapy is given by intermittent venepuncture, most frequently administered by the patient or a relative. In some centers implanted central venous catheters with a subcutaneous port, such as the Port-A-Cath, have been used for convenience and ease of access, especially in the very young. The most frequent complication is bacteremia, and to minimize this risk meticulous implantation techniques and handling protocols are essential. There is still considerable debate about their long-term safety and effectiveness and prospective data are not yet available.

The inconvenience and hazards of repeated i.v. infusion mean that any non-invasive method of delivery would be a major advantage. The search for alternative non-venous routes of access for coagulation proteins has a long history, but so far novel techniques such as the oral administration of factor VIII trapped in liposomes[1] have not proved therapeutically effective, and subcutaneous bolus injections have similarly been ineffective.

The prevalence of severe hemophilic arthropathy has been reduced by the tragic mortality due to HIV-1 infection. At the same time the incidence of acute hemarthroses and consequent chronic joint disease has been reduced in the developed countries because of the availability of safe, effective factor replacement therapy and expert medical care from an early age.

This chapter has been written from the perspective of the treatment available in affluent largely western societies, and paints a very favorable prognosis for the young hemophilia patient in that situation.

Hemophilia is ubiquitously distributed and the reality of the situation is that probably 80% of those with the condition worldwide do not receive adequate treatment, if any, even if the diagnosis has been made. The suffering so engendered is obvious but must not be allowed to obscure the fact that within the lifetime of this author, and in that of many of the authors quoted, hemophilia care in their countries was underdeveloped and relatively primitive by present standards. The challenge is to not be daunted by the task but to set achievable goals of care in collaboration with government agencies, the World Health Organization, blood transfusion services, medical and allied health professionals, local hemophilia associations and patients and carers.

The World Federation of Hemophilia is the vital coordinating body in these programs to achieve the feasible rather than the unattainable ideal in the management of hemophilia.

ACKNOWLEDGMENT

I would like to thank Professor RD Duthie for his contribution to the second edition, which has been incorporated into this chapter.

REFERENCES

1. York JR. Musculoskeletal disorders in the haemophilias. In: Sturrock RD, ed. Hematological disorders and rheumatic disease. Baillière's Clin Rheumatol – Int Pract Res 1991; 5: 197–220.
2. König F. Die gelenkerkrankungen bet blutern mit besonderer berucksichtigungder diagnose. Klin Vortrage 1892; 36: 233–240. (Translation in Clin. Orthop 1967; 52: 5–11.)
3. Legg JW. A treatise on haemophilia: sometimes called the hereditary haemorrhagic diathesis. London: HK Lewis, 1872.
4. Bulloch W, Fildes P. Hemophilia. In: Pearson K, ed. The treasure of human inheritance, eugenics laboratory memoirs. London: Dulau, 1912; 1: 169–253.
5. Steven MM, Yogarajah S, Madhok R, Forbes CD, Sturrock RD. Hemophilic arthritis. Q J Med 1986; 58: 181–197.
6. Arnold WD, Hilgartner MW. Hemophilic arthropathy. Current concepts of pathogenesis and management. J Bone Joint Surg 1977; 59A: 287–305.
7. Gilbert MS. Surgical management of the adult haemophilic blood cyst (pseudotumour). In: Rodriguez-Merchan EC, Goddard NJ, Lee CA, eds. Musculoskeletal aspects of haemophilia. Oxford: Blackwell Science, 2000: 92–96.
8. Pettersson H, Ahlberg A, Nilsson IM. A radiological classification of hemophilic arthropathy. Clin Orthop 1980; 233: 149–183.
9. Steven MM, Lewis D, Madhok R et al. Radioisotopic joint scans in hemophilic arthropathy. Br J Rheumatol 1985; 24: 263–268.
10. Green D, Spies SM, Rana NA, Milgram JW, Mintzer R. Hemophilic bleeding evaluated by blood pool scanning. Thromb Haemost (Stuttgart) 1981; 45: 208–210.
11. Roberts HR, Monroe DM, Oliver JA et al. Newer concepts of blood coagulation. Haemophilia 1998; 4: 331–334.
12. Goodeve AC. Advances in carrier detection in haemophilia. Haemophilia 1998; 4: 358–364.
13. Peake I. The molecular basis of haemophilia A. Haemophilia 1998; 4: 346–349.
14. Lillicrap D. The molecular basis of haemophilia B. Haemophilia 1998; 4: 350–357.
15. Rosendaal G, Mauser-Bunschoten EP, De Kleijn P et al. Synovium in haemophilic arthropathy. Haemophilia 1998; 4: 619–627.
16. Ragni MV, Handley EN. Septic arthritis in hemophilic patients and infection with human immunodeficiency virus. Ann Intern Med 1989; 110: 69–170.
17. Aguzzi A, Weissmann C. Prion diseases. Haemophilia 1998; 4: 619–627.
18. Ljung RC. Prophylactic treatment in Sweden – overtreatment or the optimal model? Haemophilia 1998; 4: 409–412.
19. Rodriguez-Merchan EC, Villar A, Quintana M et al. Intra-articular corticosteroid therapy for haemophilic synovitis of the knee. In: Rodriguez-Merchan EC, Goddard NJ Lee CA, eds. Musculoskeletal aspects of haemophilia. Oxford: Blackwell Science, 2000; 57–60.
20. Fernandez-Palazzi F. Treatment of acute and chronic synovitis by non-surgical means. Haemophilia 1998; 4: 518–523.
21. Caviglia H, Galatro G, Duhald C et al. Haemophilic synovitis: is rifampicin an alternative? Haemophilia 1998; 4: 514–517.
22. Rodriguez-Merchan EC, Wiedel JD. Total knee arthroplasty. In: Rodriguez-Merchan EC, Goddard NJ Lee CA, eds. Musculoskeletal aspects of haemophilia. Oxford: Blackwell Science, 2000; 78–84.
23. Rodriguez-Merchan EC, Goddard NJ. Joint debridement, alignment osteotomy and arthrodesis. In: Rodriguez-Merchan EC, Goddard NJ Lee CA, eds. Musculoskeletal aspects of haemophilia. Oxford: Blackwell Science, 2000; 66–70.
24. Connelly S, Kaleko M. Haemophilia A gene therapy. Haemophilia 1998; 4: 380–388.
25. Roth DA, Tawa NE, O'Brien JM et al. Nonviral transfer of the gene encoding coagulation factor VIII in patients with severe hemophilia A. N Engl J Med 2001; 344: 1735–1742 (also review article and editorial in same issue).

FURTHER READING

Sohail MT, Heijnen L. Comprehensive haemophilia care in developing countries with emphasis on musculoskeletal aspects. Lahore: Ferozsons; 2001.

Buzzard B, Beeton K. Physiotherapy management of haemophilia. Oxford: Blackwell Science; 2000.

188 Joint and bone lesions in hemoglobinopathies

Sharon Cordner and Karel De Ceulaer

Definition

- Hemoglobinopathies result from a defect in synthesis and structure of hemoglobin
- Rheumatic manifestations occur in homozygous sickle cell disease (SS), Hb SC disease, S-β-thalassemia
- Sickle cell trait does not cause rheumatic disease

Clinical features

- Hemolytic anemia as well as systemic and rheumatologic manifestations
- Specific bone and joint lesions include painful crisis, dactylitis and osteonecrosis
- Other features include osteomyelitis and gout

INTRODUCTION

Specific rheumatic complaints are mostly caused by sickle hemoglobinopathies. Other hemoglobinopathies (e.g. α thalassemia, Hb CC) will rarely cause joint disease, mainly through hemochromatosis. Sickle cell disease results from a single nucleotide substitution in the beta-globin gene (the normal codon GAG at position $β^6$ has been replaced by GUG); this results in the substitution of valine for glutamic acid. In hypoxic conditions the hemoglobin S forms liquid crystals, deforming the erythrocytes into rigid sickle shaped cells. Vaso-occlusion of the microvasculature due to sickled red blood cells may lead to a variety of joint and bone abnormalities of which painful crisis, dactylitis and osteonecrosis are the most common. Other major complications include osteomyelitis and gout. Although most frequent in homozygous sickle cell disease, all these complications may also occur in the milder sickle hemoglobinopathies, such as S-$β^+$-thalassemia. Osteonecrosis is as common in sickle cell hemoglobin C (SC) disease as in homozygous sickle cell (SS) disease.

In sickle cell trait, red cell sickling only occurs in non-physiologic conditions. Therefore rheumatic complaints should never be ascribed to the presence of the sickle cell trait. Many patients with fibromyalgia or connective tissue diseases believe that their sickle cell trait, discovered during routine blood checks, is the cause of their symptoms. Media reports on the frequency of sickle cell traits in various populations have contributed to this false impression.

It is a common misconception that the sickle hemoglobin only occurs in people of African ethnicity; it is also found in people from Southern Italy, Northern Greece, Southern Turkey, Saudi Arabia and Central and Southern India. In cases of unexplained bone pains and avascular necrosis, screening with the sickle cell test should be performed on a wide variety of patients. If positive this should be followed up with a hemoglobin electrophoresis.

CLINICAL FEATURES

Painful crisis

The painful crisis is the most characteristic musculo-skeletal complication of sickle cell hemoglobinopathies[1]. The event is caused by vaso-occlusion in the bone marrow. The pains occur most frequently in the juxta-articular areas of the long bones, but also in the back, ribs and occasionally the abdomen. Acute low back pain may be the only feature. Often multiple sites are involved, sometimes in a symmetrical fashion; the pain may spread from one area to another in an additive or migratory pattern. Localized swelling may be very pronounced, especially at the tibial epiphysis. Rib involvement causes a pleuritic chest pain. During the painful crisis one or more joints may become inflamed[2]. The duration of the painful crisis varies from 10 minutes to several weeks, but persistence of pains beyond 2 weeks is rare in uncomplicated painful crises.

A severe painful crisis usually consists of four distinct clinical phases. During the prodromal phase, the patient becomes restless and experiences vague feelings of being unwell. The second phase (initial phase) is characterized by increased jaundice and a sudden pain of increasing intensity, which reaches its maximum during the established phase. During the resolving phase the pains gradually decrease and by 2 weeks the steady state is restored in most of the patients.

Factors precipitating painful crises include dehydration, infections, exposure to cold, pregnancy, emotional stress and traveling at high

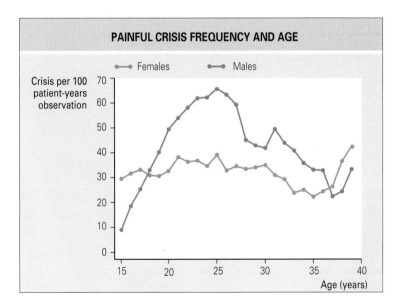

Fig. 188.1 Painful crisis frequency and age. The figure shows the incidence of painful crises according to age in male patients and non-pregnant female patients. In female patients there is little age-related change, whereas in male patients the incidence increases dramatically between 15 and 25 years and falls again after the age of 32 years. Adapted from Baum *et al.* Arch Intern Med 1987; 147: 1231–1234.

altitude. Painful crises are less frequent in female than in male patients; in the latter, a strikingly steep increase in incidence is seen between the ages of 15 and 25 years (Fig. 188.1). Pain frequency correlates with high total hemoglobin levels and low fetal hemoglobin[3]. SS patients over 20 years of age with a high frequency of painful crises show a higher mortality than SS patients with a fewer number of painful episodes[3]. Occasionally myonecrosis and myofibrosis have been observed.

Dactylitis

In young children, the vaso-occlusions frequently occur in the bones of hands and feet, leading to dactylitis (also called hand-foot syndrome). This complication typically occurs between 6 months and 2 years, but cases have been described up to 7 years of age. Clinical examination reveals an acute, painful and non-pitting swelling of hands and feet. Symptoms may improve after 1 week, but recurrences are common. Dactylitis usually heals without sequelae, but occasionally the necrosis of the central part of the epiphysis may lead to premature fusion and shortened digits (Fig. 188.2). This results in disruption of the continuity of alignment of the metacarpophalangeal joints.

Osteonecrosis

Osteonecrosis of the femoral head occurs in up to 20% of patients with sickle cell disease and has been diagnosed at as early as 5 years of age. At onset the pains are indistinguishable from a painful crisis, but the symptoms do not disappear after 2 weeks and usually get worse on walking and at night. With continued weight-bearing the pain increases, due to the progressive collapse of the femoral head. The final outcome is related to the age of the patient: children may retain normal hip function despite flattening of the femoral head, while adults show a progressive deterioration of joint function. However, not infrequently, hips affected by osteonecrosis remain asymptomatic. Osteonecrosis of the femoral head due to hemoglobinopathy is virtually absent in patients with Hb SC disease and S-β-thalassemia who are under the age of 15 years[4]. In contrast the rate of osteonecrosis in Hb SC disease in older patients (over 35 years) is striking. Osteonecrosis can occur in other joints, especially the shoulder. Pain and limitation of abduction and rotation occur, but the condition is less symptomatic because of the absence of weight bearing.

Osteomyelitis and septic arthritis

Osteomyelitis, when it occurs, usually follows an episode of painful crisis. It should be suspected if there are marked signs of inflammation, a sharp rise in temperature, a corrected white blood cell count >28 000. It also is a prime consideration if the crisis lasts longer than 2 weeks. Multiple sites of involvement may occur and may present with a symmetrical pattern. Soft tissue swelling and persistent pyrexia are frequently noted. Osteomyelitis may be complicated by osteonecrosis of the adjacent joint, adhesive capsulitis of the shoulder and pathologic fractures. The development of chronic osteomyelitis significantly increases the morbidity of affected patients. *Salmonella* remains the commonest organism causing osteomyelitis in SS disease[5]. The second most frequently seen organism is Staphylococcus aureus, with gram-negative enteric bacilli being third. One center in the USA however reported the detection of *Staphylococcus aureus* infection in eight out of 15 patients with sickle osteomyelitis[6]. It is possible that chronic sickling of the intestine's vasculature predisposes the devitalized bowel to invasion by enteric bacteria.

Septic arthritis is uncommon in sickle cell disease. It may occur in the presence of acute osteomyelitis, but more commonly it occurs secondary to hematogenous spread. Gram-negative infections predominate, especially *Salmonella*. Because of the usually associated bone pains and general ill feeling, septic arthritis may proceed for days without being attended to, despite marked joint swelling and tenderness.

Patients with known osteonecrosis of the hip who experience a sudden increase of hip pains and disability should be investigated for superimposed infection[7].

Gout

Gouty arthritis is rare in sickle cell disease[8], despite the fact that hyperuricemia occurs in over 40% of these patients. In contrast with primary gout, the involvement of the big toe is less frequently seen than arthritis of knees, wrists and small finger joints. Tophaceous gout is extremely uncommon.

Miscellaneous

A chronic arthritis with rapid chondrolysis of the hip may be related to the increased phagocytic activity in some sickle cell patients[9].

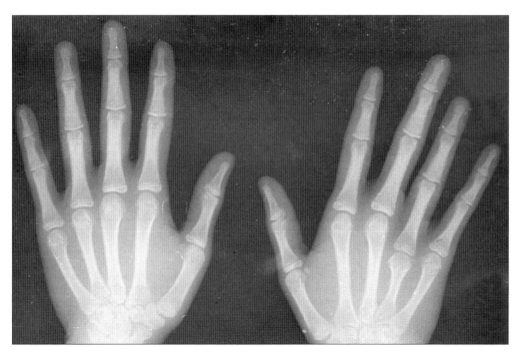

Fig. 188.2 Shortened fingers due to premature fusion of the epiphyses of two metacarpal bones. Careful examination of the position of the metacarpophalangeal joints will reveal which bone is affected.

Occasionally chronic synovitis with pronounced lymphocytic and plasma cell infiltration of the synovium and early cartilage destruction has been described[10]. Bilateral protrusio acetabuli may result from osteoporosis due to the expanded marrow. Arthritis of the ankle may develop in association with an ischemic ulcer at the medial or lateral malleolus[2]. The arthritis tends to occur at the early stages of impending leg ulceration, when the skin surface is still intact, but the tissues look shriveled and hyperpigmented. The ankle suddenly becomes stiff and tender with impaired gait; non-steroidal anti-inflammatory drugs result in a fast improvement of function. When left untreated, the pains and dysfunction of the ankle lessen when the leg ulceration develops, but persistent limitation is common as long as the ulcer persists.

Patients with SS disease rarely develop rheumatoid arthritis, but it is not clear if this is caused by early mortality or ischemic factors preventing synovium proliferation. SS patients may develop a chronic asymmetrical seronegative oligoarthritis, which needs to be defined. The coexistence of SS disease and SLE is not frequent enough to allow speculation about complement abnormalities in SS disease leading to the development of SLE.

INVESTIGATIONS

The hemoglobin and reticulocyte count should be checked with every painful crisis, because of possible associated aplastic crisis. An aplastic

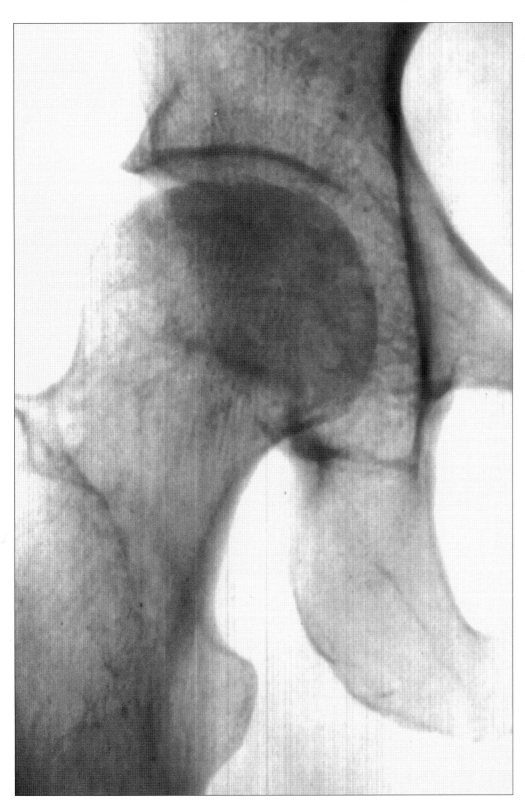

Fig. 188.3 Very early osteonecrosis of the femoral head (Steinberg stage 2). The femoral head shows sclerotic and radiolucent areas.

crisis can be caused by concomitant parvovirus infection. Determining white blood cell counts by Coulter counter methods can be misleading as immature nucleated red blood cells are detected and read as leukocytes. Therefore a corrected white cell count should be obtained. An increasing ESR and leukocytosis with left differential shift might suggest osteomyelitis. In uncomplicated SS patients the erythrocyte sedimentation rate (ESR) is usually low, due to the unique rheology of sickled red blood cells. However it rises during the resolving phase of the painful crisis and to a greater extent if infection is present. Plasma viscosity and C-reactive protein (CRP) determinations are more reliable than the ESR when monitoring an inflammatory process.

Radiographs of affected bones are not helpful at the early stages of osteomyelitis, as even periosteal reaction can be seen in uncomplicated painful crisis. Blood cultures should be performed if the patient's temperature exceeds 38°C. Joint aspiration is necessary in painful crisis with associated arthritis. In uncomplicated arthritis, the synovial fluid is non-inflammatory, straw-colored and sterile. Blood cultures are always indicated in dactylitis, as Salmonella infections have been documented in this complication[11].

Patients with osteonecrosis of the femoral head can be radiographically staged by the Steinberg classification system[12]. At the early stages plain radiographs are normal, but the hip is symptomatic with groin or thigh pain, which is worse at night (Steinberg stage 1). However at this stage MRI can detect abnormalities, even where bone scans fail. The overall reported sensitivity is 91%. Therefore MRI should be performed if avascular necrosis is suspected. Stage 2 hips show sclerosis and radiolucent areas on X-rays (Fig 188.3), while the patient has similar symptoms as in stage 1. In stage 3 there is on plain films a lucent subchondral line, followed by a cortical discontinuity (crescent sign) (Fig. 188.4); it appears only after several weeks of illness. At this stage the pains and limitation have increased and ambulation may only be possible with a cane. In stage 4, there is segmental flattening of the femoral head without radiological evidence of acetabular involvement (Fig. 188.5). Stage 5 shows progressive destruction of the hip joint with joint space narrowing, cysts sclerosis and osteophytes (Fig. 188.6). Stage 6 includes advanced degenerative joint disease with extreme narrowing or obliteration of the joint space. It is important to recognize that the correlation

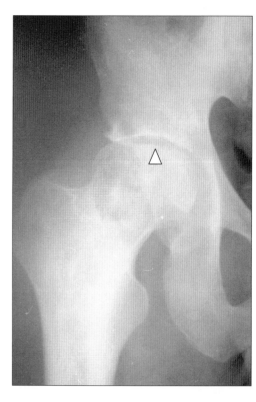

Fig. 188.5 Osteonecrosis of the femoral head (Steinberg stage 4). Mild flattening of the superolateral part of the femoral head despite long-standing disease.

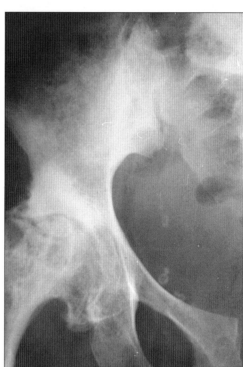

Fig. 188.6 Advanced osteonecrosis of the femoral head (Steinberg stages 5–6). Gross destruction and remodeling of the femoral head. There are significant osteoarthritic changes.

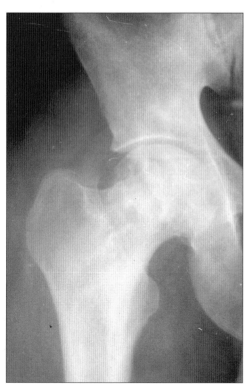

Fig. 188.4 Early osteonecrosis of the femoral head (Steinberg stage 3). There is a short break in the cortical line of the superolateral segment of the femoral head.

between the clinical symptoms and radiologic features of osteonecrosis is poor.

Osteomyelitis should be suspected if the patient's temperature exceeds 38°C or if the painful crisis lasts longer than 2 weeks. *Salmonella* and *Staphylococcus aureus* are the commonest organisms. Radiographic changes are only apparent after weeks of illness. Plain radiographs and bone scans are unable to differentiate between painful crisis and osteomyelitis. At present soft tissue ultrasound and gadolinium enhanced MRI are the best imaging techniques to suggest bone infection, although the exact specificity of these investigations is not yet clear. With ultrasound, a finding of a 4mm depth or more of subperiosteal fluid is highly suggestive of osteomyelitis[13]. On gadolinium enhanced MRI acute infarcts demonstrate thin, linear rim enhancement, while osteomyelitis shows a more geographic and irregular marrow enhancement[14].

The diagnosis of gouty arthritis should only be made after identification of urate crystals in the joint fluid. Indeed, hyperuricemia is common in uncomplicated sickle cell disease and therefore cannot be used as a criterion for the presence of gouty arthritis. Also, intermittent joint swelling may be only a part of a painful crisis, rather than of a gouty attack.

DIFFERENTIAL DIAGNOSIS

The painful crisis can mimic attacks of rheumatic fever, which typically starts as a migratory polyarthritis. In both diseases, cardiac murmurs are extremely common (SS patients often have left ventricular hypertrophy) and mild antistreptolysin O elevations are frequently seen. Of note these conditions may also coexist, especially in developing countries where rheumatic fever is not uncommon.

Infectious processes of joints and bones should be considered in each case, as patients with hemoglobinopathies are more susceptible to infections, especially with *Haemophilus influenzae*, *Streptococcus pneumoniae* and *Salmonella*. This is compounded by their susceptibility to encapsulated organisms due to their functional asplenia.

A chronic destructive synovitis has been described in sickle cell disease and needs to be differentiated from rheumatoid arthritis.

Although there is no evidence for an increased frequency of SLE in SS disease, SS patients may be frequently positive for low titer ANA and antiphospholipid antibodies. It needs to be established if the latter antibodies are contributing to the acute chest syndrome, stroke and recurrent miscarriages which are common complications of SS disease.

PATHOGENESIS

The occlusion of the small blood vessels of the active bone marrow by sickled erythrocytes is the cause of many complications such as the painful crisis, dactylitis and osteonecrosis. Factors disrupting the microcirculation leading to a painful crisis include polymerization of hemoglobin S in a deoxygenated state, which leads to decreased red blood cell deformability[15]. The polymerization of HbS is influenced by various factors including the intracellular concentration of Hb S and the concentrations of Hb F and C. Others are the oxygen saturation of the blood, the pH, the ionic strength, temperature and 2,3-DPG. Once a sufficient number of rigid sickled cells with polymerized hemoglobin are created microvascular occlusion will occur. Subsequent hypoxia of the tissues supplied causes tissue damage. After the initial ischemia, a secondary inflammatory reaction mediated by K^+, H^+, histamine, bradykinin and prostaglandins occurs causing increased intramedullary pressure and bone pains.

The increased incidence of salmonella osteomyelitis in sickle cell disease remains unexplained. Bone damage due to vaso-occlusion seems to be a necessary condition. The blockage of the reticuloendothelial system by erythrocyte fragments, the iron overload and a defect in the alternative pathway of complement, have been implicated in the increased susceptibility[16].

Hyperuricemia and gout are caused by a decreased renal tubular excretion of urate, rather than urate overproduction secondary to increased purine turnover[17]. Hyperuricemia may contribute to the decreased renal function observed in sickle cell patients over 40 years of age.

MANAGEMENT

The management of the acute painful crisis depends on the patient's response to analgesics during previous crises, the severity and extent of the painful episode and the presence of complications such as acute chest syndrome and paralytic ileus[18].

Because of the associated dehydration the treatment of painful crises starts with the administration of large amounts of fluids. Intravenous administration of 3–4 liters/24h with unlimited amounts orally has been the standard. However it has been shown that the majority of uncomplicated painful crises can be effectively managed by oral hydration and analgesia alone. Mild painful crises respond to simple analgesics, such as acetaminophen (paracetamol), but in the case of severe crisis, narcotic analgesics (pethidine, pentazocine, hydromorphone) are necessary. In the presence of normal gastrointestinal motility, oral, controlled-release morphine is a reliable, non-invasive alternative[19]. Narcotic analgesics should be prescribed in the full therapeutic doses at regular 2–4 hour dosing intervals to relieve pains, and not restricted to an 'as needed' basis. Smaller additional doses should be prescribed for breakthrough pains. The pain severity and its response to treatment should be reassessed frequently. Non-steroidal anti-inflammatory drugs, sedatives and anti-histamines may reduce the amount of narcotics needed in the treatment of a painful crisis and can be used in combination with narcotics. Tramadol, a centrally acting analgesic that is administered orally, induces minimal respiratory depression and is useful in the outpatient management of vaso-occlusive crises. Anti-sickling agents and pentoxyfilline have shown disappointing results, once the pains have set in.

Because of the recurrent nature of the pains, sickle cell patients are at risk of addiction and drug dependence. Paranoia about this issue has often led to the sub-optimal treatment of sickle cell painful crises with unnecessary suffering by the patients. Reluctance of hospital staff to prescribe and administer narcotic analgesia is seen by the patients as a sign of indifference, and perpetuates a lack of confidence in the care.

While in the past most patients with moderate or severe painful crisis were treated as in-patients in hospital, recent studies have shown that day-care centers may provide an adequate alternative way of treating patients with SS crisis[20]. Hospitalization has been suggested because of concern for undetected infection and sickle cell related complications. In addition there is the perception that adequate pain relief rarely can be obtained on an out-patient basis. However a specialized day-care unit will be able to assess patients more rapidly, titrate the analgesia to individual needs and may avoid the sub-optimal treatment, which commonly occurs on hospital wards. However when systemic infections are suspected, the patient should be admitted for IV antibiotic treatment, in addition to the analgesic medication. Another indication for hospitalization is extensive associated chest syndrome, where early exchange transfusion could be life-saving.

Attention should be paid to prevention of painful crises. These include life-style changes (avoidance of stress, alcohol, over-exertion, swimming, getting caught in the rain, high altitudes) and medications. Hydroxyurea increases the haemoglobin F concentration, with a moderated reduction of neutrophils, reticulocytes and young, low density SS red cells. Clinically hydroxyurea has shown to reduce the frequency of painful crises in adult SS patients and is cost-effective[21]. Magnesium pidolate supplements prevent erythrocyte dehydration and hence reduce sickling[22].

If osteonecrosis of the femoral head is documented, the patient should be on complete bed rest and totally avoid weight bearing. In children this can be achieved by casting, immobilizing the knee at a 30° angle. Only when the femoral head is severely damaged (Steinberg stage 5 or 6), is a total hip replacement indicated. Indeed the results of total hip replacement in SS patients are much less favorable than in patients with osteoarthritis. Apart from peri-operative complications, prosthesis loosening and infection cause poor long-term replacement outcome, compared to primary degenerative hip disease[23,24]. Therefore attention should be directed to the detection of osteonecrosis at an early stage and prevention of progression with conservative treatment or core decompression. The latter however is only superior to conservative treatment in early osteonecrosis (Steinberg stage I)[25].

When osteomyelitis is suspected, traditional treatment tended to include the use of ampicillin or trimethoprim/sulphamethoxazole, as *Salmonella* is the main cause of this complication. However emerging resistance is decreasing its potential efficacy. Newer β lactams and third generation cephalosporins may be suitable alternatives. Quinolones are relatively contraindicated in children because of their potential for chondrotoxicity, arthropathy and tendon rupture. Resistance to ciprofloxacillin has already been described[26]. In established osteomyelitis, antibiotic therapy is usually continued for at least for 3 months.

Septic arthritis needs early surgical drainage, debridement and splinting in order to prevent ankylosis. This complication carries a poor prognosis[27].

Recurrent gouty arthritis is treated with non-steroidal anti-inflammatory drugs and allopurinol. Patients with SS disease and gout are likely to have renal impairment and a challenged liver function. Therefore 4-monthly checks of renal and liver function are indicated.

When SS disease is associated with rheumatoid arthritis, anti-malarials and sulphasalazine may be used together with non-steroidal anti-inflammatory drugs. Caution is exercised when using corticosteroids. Patients on doses of Prednisone of 10mg or more have been observed to develop prolonged painful crises lasting over many weeks. This may be due to the increased blood viscosity caused by corticosteriods. There is concern with the use of weekly methotrexate, as many SS patients are already folate depleted, which might lead to a sudden drop in hemoglobin Likewise leflunomide may prove toxic to an already overburdened liver. However treatment with disease modifying drugs may be beneficial by reducing the anemia of chronic disease superimposed on the hemolytic anemia.

REFERENCES

1. Serjeant GR. The painful crisis. In: Serjeant GR, ed. Sickle cell disease. Oxford: Oxford University Press; 1985: 196–205.
2. De Ceulaer K, Forbes M, Roper D, Serjeant GR. Non-gouty arthritis in sickle cell disease: report of 37 consecutive cases. Ann Rheum Dis 1984; 43: 599–603.
3. Platt OS, Thorington BD, Brambilla DJ *et al*. Pain in sickle cell disease. N Engl J Med 1991; 325: 11–16.
4. Milner PF, Kraus AP, Sebes JI *et al*. Sickle cell disease as a cause of osteonecrosis of the femoral head. N Engl J Med 1991; 325: 1476–1481.
5. Chambers JB, Forsythe DA, Bertrand SL *et al*. Retrospective review of osteoarticular infections in a pediatric sickle cell age group. J Pediatr Orthop 2000; 20: 682–685.
6. Epps CH, Bryant DD, Coles MJM, Castro O. Osteomyelitis in patients who have sickle cell disease. J Bone Joint Surg 1991; 73A: 1281–1294.
7. Phillips FM, Pottenger LA. Acute septic arthritis in chronic osteonecrosis of the hip. J Rheumatol 1988; 15: 1713–1716.
8. Reynolds MD. Gout and hyperuricemia associated with sickle cell anemia. Semin Arthritis Rheum 1983; 12: 404–413.
9. Schumacher HR, Van Lindthoudt, Manno CS *et al*. Diffuse chondrolytic arthritis in sickle cell disease. J Rheumatol 1993; 20: 385.
10. Schumacher HR, Dorwart BB, Bond J *et al*. Chronic synovitis with early cartilage destruction in sickle cell disease. Ann Rheum Dis 1977; 36: 413–419.
11. Noonan WJ. Salmonella osteomyelitis presenting as 'hand-foot syndrome' in sickle cell disease. Br Med J 1982; 248: 1464–1465.
12. Steinberg ME, Hayken GD, Steinberg DR. A quantitave system for staging avascular necrosis. J Bone Joint Surg 1995; 77B: 34–41.
13. William RR, Hussein SS, Jeans WD *et al*. A prospective study of soft-tissue ultrasonography in sickle cell disease patients with suspected osteomyelitis. Clin Radiol 2000; 55: 307–310.
14. Umans H, Haramati N, Flusser G. The diagnostic role of gadolinium enhanced MRI in distinguishing between acute medullary bone infarct and osteomyelitis. Magn Reson Imaging 2000; 18: 255–262.
15. Ballas SK, Mohandas N. Sickle cell disease. Pathophysiology of vaso-occlusion. Hematol/Oncol Clin North Am 1996; 10: 1221–1239.
16. Johnston RB, Newman SL, Struth AG. An abnormality of the alternate pathway of complement activation in sickle cell disease. N Engl J Med 1973; 288: 803–808.
17. Diamond HS, Meisel AD, Holden D. The natural history of urate overproduction in sickle cell anemia. Ann Intern Med 1979; 90: 752–757.
18. Ballas SK. Sickle cell disease: clinical management. Baillière's Clin Haematol 1998; 11: 185–214.
19. Jacobson SJ, Kopecky EA, Joshi P, Babul N. Randomised trial of oral morphine for painful episodes of sickle-cell disease in children. Lancet 1997; 350: 1358–1361.
20. Ware MA, Hambleton I, Ochaya I, Serjeant GR. Day-care management of sickle cell painful crisis in Jamaica: a model applicable elsewhere? Br J Haematol 1999; 104, 93–96.
21. Moore RD, Charache S, Terrin ML *et al*. Cost-effectiveness of hydroxyurea in sickle cell anemia. Am J Hematol 2000; 64: 26–31.
22. De Franceschi L, Bachir D, Galacteros F *et al*. Oral magnesium pidolate: effects of long-term administration in patients with sickle cell disease. Br J Haematol 2000; 108: 284–289.
23. Vichinsky EP, Neumayr LD, Haberkern C *et al*. The perioperative complication rate of orthopedic surgery in sickle cell disease: report of the National Sickle Cell Surgery Study Group. Am J Hematol 1999; 62: 129–138.
24. Bishop AR, Roberson JR, Eckman JR, Fleming LL. Total hip arthroplasty in patients who have sickle-cell hemoglobinopathy. J Bone Joint Surg Am 1988; 70: 853–855.
25. Castro FP, Barrack RL. Core decompression and conservative treatment for avascular necrosis of the femoral head: a meta-analysis. Am J Orthop 2000; 29: 187–194.
26. Workman MR, Philpott-Howard J, Bragman S *et al*. Emergence of ciprofloxacin resistance during treatment of Salmonella osteomyelitis in three patients with sickle cell disease. J Infect 1996; 32: 27–32.
27. Anand AJ, Glatt AE. Salmonella osteomyelitis and arthritis in sickle cell disease. Sem Arthritis Rheum 1994; 24: 211–221.

189 Hemochromatosis

K Sigvard Olsson

Definition

- Hemochromatosis is a genetically inherited disease with iron loading of tissues caused by increased iron absorption
- The detection of the mutant gene, *HFE*, has greatly simplified diagnosis
- Early recognition and treatment can prevent organ damage

Clinical features

- The severity of the disease is variable
- Liver disease and symmetric arthropathy in middle-aged patients is the most common presentation
- The classic clinical picture is only found in a small fraction of homozygotes

HISTORY

The term hemochromatosis was first used by von Recklinghausen in 1889, although similar cases had been described earlier under the names of pigment cirrhosis and bronze diabetes.

In 1927 Sheldon suggested that the disease was the result of an inborn error of metabolism. At this time, most cases were not diagnosed until autopsy[1]. By 1955 a better understanding of the disease had been acquired when Finch and Finch published their review showing that classic hemochromatosis represented the end result of a prolonged period of iron loading caused by abnormal iron absorption from a normal diet[2]. An invariable finding was an iron saturated transferrin. The excess iron can be removed by phlebotomy, a procedure that has been in use since 1946.

In 1972 the serum ferritin method was introduced as a convenient measure of iron stores. In 1975 Simon *et al.* showed that the hemochromatosis gene should be found on chromosome 6 close to HLA locus[3]. These breakthroughs meant that individuals with the genetic defect could be diagnosed early, before the appearance of clinical symptoms and signs. A major breakthrough came in 1996 when Feder *et al.*[4] identified a gene, *HFE*, that was mutated in hemochromatosis. A new diagnostic test using modern DNA technology was thus available, replacing liver biopsy for the diagnosis of hemochromatosis, simplifying family studies and screenings of populations. The prevalence of the *HFE* mutation is higher than was originally thought, making hemochromatosis one of the most common hereditary disorders in populations of northern European origin. However, it is still considered a rare disorder.

GENETICS AND EPIDEMIOLOGY

Epidemiologic data for hemochromatosis is shown in Table 189.1. Simon *et al.*[3] discovered that the putative gene was inherited together with human leukocyte antigen (HLA) genes on the short arm of chromosome 6. They postulated that the founder of the mutation was of northern European origin and carrying HLA A3. An ancestral haplotype carrying HLA A3 and the hemochromatosis gene was constructed and attracted intensive positional cloning studies.

In 1996 Feder *et al.*[4] identified a gene, *HFE*, that was mutated in 85% of patients with hereditary hemochromatosis. One mutation resulted in a cysteine to tyrosine substitution at amino acid 282, C282Y, another in a histidine to aspartic acid substitution at position 63, H63D. Subsequent studies confirmed that more than 90% of hereditary hemochromatosis patients in northern Europe were C282Y/C282Y and 5% C282Y/H63D[1]. These compound heterozygotes were more mildly affected. In southern Europe hereditary hemochromatosis families have been found without *HFE* mutations[1].

The age of the C282Y mutation has been estimated to about 60–70 generations or 2000 years[5]. It did occur in a founder living in the north-west of Europe carrying HLA A3, supporting the hypothesis of Simon *et al.*[3] Figure 189.1 shows the ancestor's haplotype on chromosome 6 extending over a physical distance of 5Mb. Approximately half the hemochromatosis chromosomes of today still carry the same long DNA fragment as that of the founder, resistant against recombinations. Half carry different HLA marker haplotypes resulting from recombinations. The pedigree given in Figure 189.2 is an illustration. The C282Y mutation reaches its highest prevalence in Ireland, Brittany, the UK, Norway, Denmark and Sweden[7], countries that came into contact with the Vikings. The prevalence declines as one travels south and east across Europe and is absent from the original populations of Australia, Asia, etc. A prevalence of C282Y homozygosity of 30–80/10 000 means that hereditary hemochromatosis is one of the most common hereditary disorders in whites[1]. Positive selection might explain the high prevalence in these northern European countries in which iron deficiency was common in the past[2]. There is no reproductive disadvantage and heterozygosity might prevent iron deficiency in women and thus confer a reproductive advantage.

Those with only the genetic predisposition for hereditary hemochromatosis (individuals carrying C282Y/C282Y and C282Y/H63D) should be separated from those with a phenotypic or clinical expression,

TABLE 189.1 EPIDEMIOLOGY OF HEMOCHROMATOSIS

Peak age (years)	40–60
Sex distribution (F:M)	1:4
Prevalence	20–80/10 000
Annual incidence	2–4/100 000
Geographical distribution	Most prevalent in northern European populations
Genetic associations	Related to a point mutation, C282Y, of the *HFE* gene on chromosome 6
Relative risk (RR)	HLA-A3–B14 (RR 23)

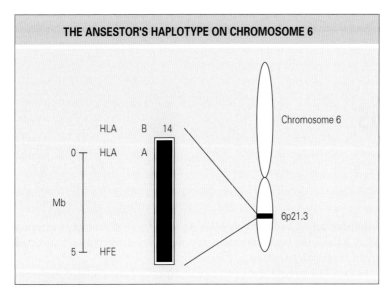

Fig. 189.1 The ancestor's haplotype on chromosome 6. The ancestor's haplotype starts centromeric of the HLA A3 locus and extends telomerically for more than 5Mb, including *HFE* and its mutation C282Y.

CLINICAL FEATURES

Hereditary hemochromatosis is a genetic disease with iron loading of the parenchymal cells of the body and resultant tissue injury. Hemochromatosis can also be caused by multiple blood transfusions and portacaval anastomosis. These secondary forms of iron overload will not be discussed further here.

The concept of hemochromatosis was originally associated with liver cirrhosis, skin pigmentation and diabetes. This classic picture of 'bronze diabetes' also included hypogonadism and cardiac insufficiency as organ manifestations of severe, widespread iron overload. However, this is not a representative description of clinical iron overload seen today; instead it has to be considered as a diagnostic failure. The arthropathy associated with hemochromatosis[9] is a much more common manifestation than diabetes, hypogonadism or cardiomyopathy[8,10] and this can be the first signal of the iron loading process. Screenings of families and populations using phenotypic tests have shown that mildly affected patients are common[1,6]. Even if recent population studies using genotype tests have shown that not all homozygotic carriers express clinical iron overload[8], there remain 1 in 300–400 of northern European populations who express the disease. These findings mean that physicians serving relevant populations will meet these patients and have to keep a diagnostic awareness of the disease. If an early diagnosis is made, effective treatment can be instituted.

because 25% do not seem to develop iron overload[8]. Those who develop a phenotypic expression present a very variable degree of iron overload and the fraction of homozygotes who ultimately develop severe clinical disease is unknown.

CLINICAL MANIFESTATIONS

Clinical manifestations usually appear between the ages of 40 and 60 years (Fig. 189.3). However, the severity of the disease is very

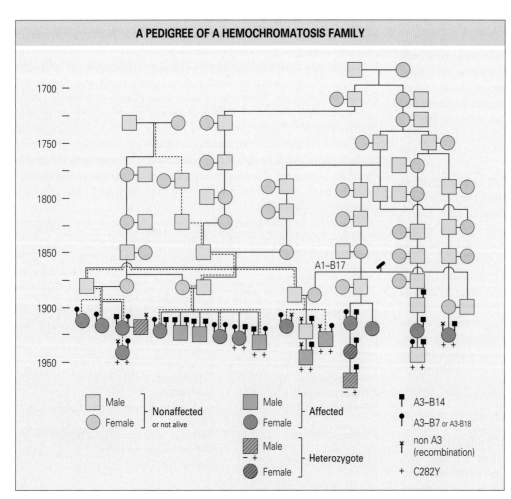

Fig. 189.2 A pedigree of a hemochromatosis family. Six 'unrelated' hereditary hemochromatosis families were found to have the ancestor's HLA marker A3–B14 in common. A family investigation had fortunately been done, revealing that all the patients could be traced to common ancestors in the late 17th century. Recent studies have confirmed the presence of the *HFE* mutation C282Y (marked with +) in members of all six families. The marked A1B17 haplotype was the result of a recombination. (Adapted from Ritter *et al*.[6] and Raha-Chowdhury and Gruen[7].)

variable. A rare fraction express a more 'malignant' form, developing the full-blown clinical picture at 20 years of age. This juvenile form is not *HFE*-related and is caused by a defect gene on chromosome 1q[11]. A neonatal form has been described, not genetically related to hereditary hemochromatosis.

It is useful to consider hemochromatosis as an 'a' disorder, with asthenia, arthropathy and alanine aminotransferase (ALT) elevations as the most common manifestations[10].

Asthenia, in the form of chronic fatigue, weakness, increased sleep requirement and lassitude, may lead to diagnosis in a paradoxical way, iron tests being taken because of suspected iron deficiency.

Liver abnormalities with chronic ALT elevations are probably the most constant manifestation, most often presented accidentally at health checks, sometimes with symptoms of abdominal pain and discomfort. All patients with 'transaminitis' should be investigated for iron overload, instead of being regarded as alcoholics, enabling early diagnosis before the establishment of liver cirrhosis[12]. Treatment started in the precirrhotic stage often means an excellent prognosis. Those with established cirrhosis run a 200-fold increased risk of developing hepatocellular carcinoma despite therapy[13].

The skin pigmentation is seldom diagnostic, is most often a slate-gray color rather than brownish and is caused by melanin rather than iron. Diabetes is a late manifestation and occurs most often when liver cirrhosis is already present. Myocardial involvement is not particularly common, but arrhythmia can be an early manifestation of a cardiomyopathy caused by iron. Hypogonadism with decreased libido, impotence, amenorrhea and sparse body hair is caused by gonadotrophic insufficiency and is usually a late manifestation of iron overload.

ARTHROPATHY

Arthropathy associated with hemochromatosis is a common symptom, present in 24–81%[8,14–19]. The highest figures are probably influenced by biased ascertainment. A population-based study reported arthritis in 6/16 homozygotes (37%)[8] and a study free of ascertainment bias found arthropathy in 33% of homozygous males over 40 years old[18].

It is surprising that this common manifestation was not appreciated until 1964[9]. Arthropathy can be the first manifestation of the iron-loading process (Fig. 189.4)[15,17,19], although more often it occurs later, even following treatment[9]. A German study reported a diagnostic delay of up to 15 years in 11 patients referred to rheumatologists. Ten had already established cirrhosis and one had been treated for 8 years for arthritis when he was found to have hepatocellular carcinoma caused by iron overload[15]. Most joints can be affected but osteoarthritis-like changes of the metacarpophalangeal (MCP) joints of the second and third fingers are the most common (Fig. 189.4). The disease can also affect proximal interphalangeal (PIP) joints, wrists, knees, hips, ankles and shoulders[19,20]. In rare cases, a progressive destructive osteoarthritis can be seen.

It is therefore important that the primary care physician who sees a patient who has trouble gripping and holding on to things and difficulty in unscrewing jar lids, turning the ignition key, changing gear, etc. considers the diagnosis of iron overload. These patients also report stiffness and pain, sometimes when shaking hands or after excessive use. Slight bony swellings and inability to extend and flex the second and third MCP joints may be seen. The tenderness is mild and there is no erythema or increased warmth. The sedimentation rate is often normal and rheumatoid arthritis serology is negative. Some hereditary hemochromatosis sufferers who have had arthropathy for several years have reported being reassured that 'this is not rheumatoid arthritis' when they were referred to a rheumatologist. However, the correct diagnosis was not considered.

Radiographs may show cystic lesions with sclerotic walls, joint space narrowing, sclerosis, osteophytes and osteoporosis (Fig. 189.5)[19].

Sometimes acute episodes of inflammatory arthritis occur, due to deposition of calcium pyrophosphate dehydrate (CPPD). These may involve the cartilage of the knee, wrist, intervertebral disk and symphysis pubis[19,21].

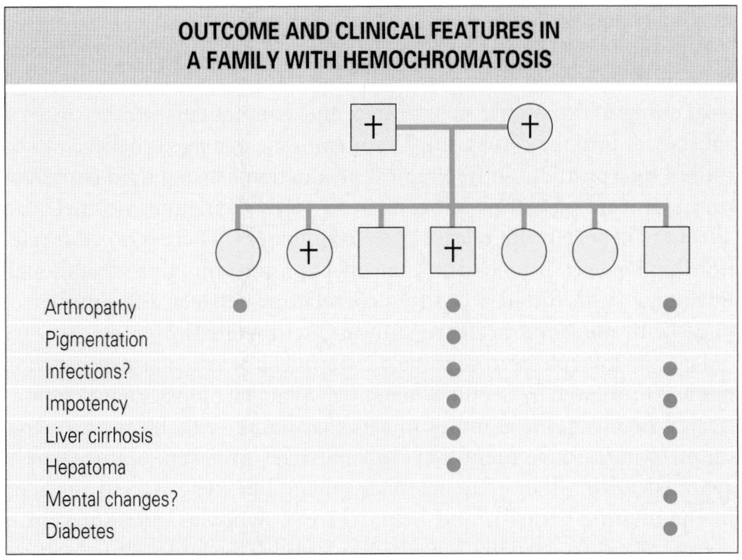

OUTCOME AND CLINICAL FEATURES IN A FAMILY WITH HEMOCHROMATOSIS

Fig. 189.3 Outcome and clinical features in a family with hemochromatosis. A record from 1936 showed that the father had suffered from 'polyarthritis' from age 48. He died at age 49 from 'diabetes bronze and myocarditis' proven by autopsy. Fifty years later his eldest daughter developed arthropathy and underwent total hip replacement. Child no. 4, a son, died from a hepatoma. Child no. 7, the youngest son, has had arthropathy from age 26, abdominal pains from age 30, a diagnosis of 'seronegative polyarthritis' at age 39, hypogonadism at age 44 and the diagnosis hemochromatosis with cirrhosis at age 46. Nos 3, 5 and 6 are mainly free of symptoms, despite being homozygous. Homozygosity for C282Y was confirmed in available members. (Adapted from Ritter *et al.*[6])

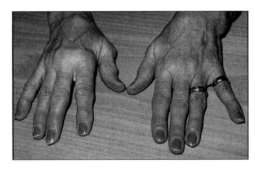

Fig. 189.4 The hands of a patient with hemochromatosis. The bony swelling of the MCP joints is apparent.

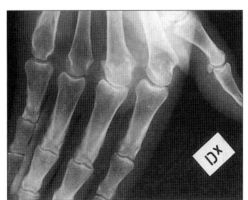

Fig. 189.5 Radiograph of the hands of a 45-year-old man with hemochromatosis. There are cystic lesions of the metacarpal heads, joint space narrowing and osteophytes at the second and third MCP joint.

Even if the arthropathy is most often of a mild, non-inflammatory nature, it is a prominent clinical factor affecting quality of life in hemochromatosis[14].

INVESTIGATIONS

Diagnosis of hereditary hemochromatosis is not difficult providing that it is considered. The simple screening tests are transferrin saturation, expressed as serum iron × 100/total iron binding capacity, which is elevated (>45%), in combination with increased serum ferritin concentration (>200µg/l in males; >100µg/l in females). If an inflammatory condition is superimposed in patients with hemochromatosis, the percentage transferrin saturation drops (Fig. 189.6), which should be kept in mind during a screening using transferrin saturation. If the screening tests are abnormal, they should be followed by the *HFE* genotype test. A finding of homozygosity for C282Y or compound heterozygosity for the two mutations C282Y/H63D confirms the diagnosis. These findings mean that a liver biopsy is no longer needed for the diagnosis, which today can be established by the local doctor from a simple blood sample sent to a laboratory. Only if the liver tests are abnormal and serum ferritin signals severe iron overload (>1000) is a liver biopsy recommended for prognostic purposes (fibrosis, cirrhosis)[1].

Once the diagnosis is established, all first-degree relatives should be screened with genotype and iron tests[1].

A general screening of northern European populations using genotype tests has been proposed. Strong arguments have been raised against such screening because of uncertain penetrance of the genotype and its very variable clinical expression[1].

DIFFERENTIAL DIAGNOSIS

Secondary iron overload, which sometimes produces arthropathy, is excluded by a patient history that does not include blood transfusions, parenteral iron administration and anemia (β-thalassemia, sideroblastic anemia). Porphyria cutanea tarda also presents with elevated percentage transferrin saturation, increased serum ferritin concentration and abnormal liver tests. However, these patients have more intense pigmentation, skin fragility, blisters and hirsutism and are diagnosed by increased urinary excretion of uroporphyrins[1]. Interestingly, the C282Y mutation has been found to be involved in the pathogenesis of 40% of cases of porphyria cutanea tarda[22].

Alcoholic liver disease might be associated with increased serum ferritin concentration and elevated transferrin saturation. Abstinence often results in a rapid drop of these parameters.

PATHOGENESIS

In hemochromatosis there is an increased absorption of iron from the diet. As iron excretion is minimal, the result is progressive iron loading of parenchymal tissues, particularly the liver[1]. Two major cell types are involved in the disturbed iron metabolism of hereditary hemochromatosis; the intestinal epithelial cell regulating absorption and the macrophage responsible for the iron released into plasma from red cell destruction. The macrophage seems to suffer from iron incontinence in hereditary hemochromatosis[23] and cannot store iron, which leaks to plasma and saturates the transferrin. Transferrin molecules that have both binding sites occupied by iron are preferentially taken up by the transferrin receptors of cells. Since the detection of the *HFE* mutation a number of new components of the iron pathway have been found and have recently been reviewed[1].

The HFE protein, a HLA class I protein, interferes with cellular iron uptake by binding to the transferrin receptor on the cell surface. The defective C282Y protein cannot be fully expressed on the cell surface, with reduced control of cellular iron uptake.

The intestinal epithelial cell uses a divalent metal transporter, DMT-1, for uptake of iron through the luminal cell membrane. Upregulation of DMT-1 increasing the transfer of iron has been seen in hereditary hemochromatosis patients lacking normal HFE protein[1].

There is experimental evidence that gene therapy with normal *HFE* can cure the iron incontinence of the macrophage in hereditary hemochromatosis[23].

Within the cell, extra iron is stored in lysosomes as ferritin and hemosiderin. It has been proposed that iron causes cell damage through weakening of lysosomal membranes and consequent leakage of toxic substances into the cytoplasm. The membrane damage is believed to be caused by iron-induced free radical production causing lipid peroxidation. An iron load of no more than 3g (only four times normal) can affect the liver cell with release of transaminases[12]. There is no clear relationship between iron load and the effect on the synovium[17,19], although Pavlotsky *et al.* found a positive correlation between the number of joints with subchondral arthropathy and serum ferritin[21].

The possible role of iron in the development of articular degeneration has been reviewed by Schumacher *et al.*[24] Synovial biopsies have demonstrated hemosiderin granules in synovial lining cells. Electron microscopic studies have identified iron particles preferentially in type B synovial cells rather than in macrophage-like type A cells, as seen in rheumatoid arthritis and hemarthrosis. Synovial inflammation is scarce[9]. Ferritin particles have been identified in intact chondrocytes together with CPPD crystals in the cartilage. However, the CPPD deposits were not spatially related to the iron[24]. Similarities between the osteoarticular changes of hyperparathyroidism and hemochromatosis (both conditions described by von Recklinghausen) was noted by Pavlotsky *et al.*[21]. These authors found a correlation between the serum concentration of the midregion 44–68 of parathyroid hormone and osteoarticular changes. Osteoporosis associated with hemochromatosis is a late manifestation, most pronounced in patients who have developed hypogonadism. A recent review of the arthropathy in hereditary hemochromatosis has been presented by von Kempis[25].

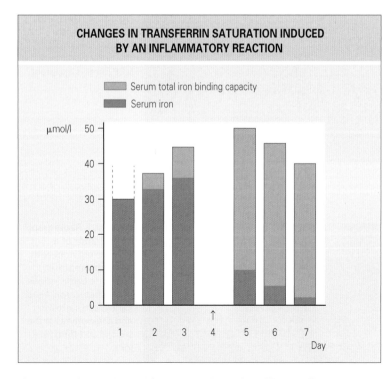

Fig. 189.6 Changes in transferrin saturation induced by an inflammatory reaction. The patient, aged 69, suffered a myocardial infarction on day 4 (arrow), while in hospital because of hemochromatosis.

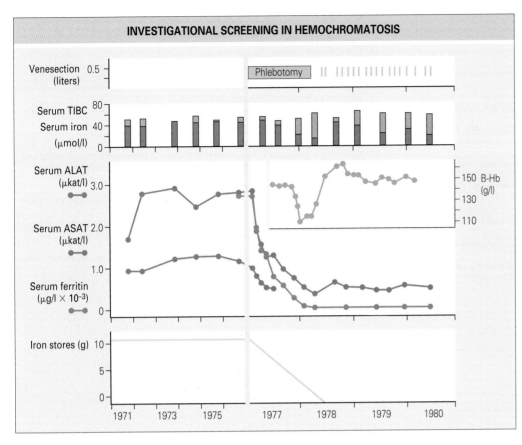

INVESTIGATIONAL SCREENING IN HEMOCHROMATOSIS

Fig. 189.7 Investigational screening in hemochromatosis. Findings from a broad biochemical laboratory profile show constantly abnormal transferrin saturation and elevated transaminases in a 44-year-old man with pseudogout as the presenting symptom. Liver biopsy confirmed the diagnosis of hemochromatosis in the cirrhotic stage. The effect of phlebotomy is obvious. ALAT, alanine-aminotransferase; ASAT, aspartate aminotransferase.

ENVIRONMENTAL FACTORS

Several factors other than age can influence the phenotypic expression of the disease. In women, menstrual blood loss and a lower food intake delay the rate of iron accumulation. Environmental factors, such as a poor diet and different drinking habits (milk instead of wine?) may explain why hereditary hemochromatosis patients in Scandinavia are less iron-loaded than their genetic relatives living in Germany, Australia or other more fertile areas[13,15,17]. Fortification of food with iron and excessive alcohol intake have an additive influence on the liver damage induced by iron.

The highly variable phenotypic expression in homozygotes might be explained by genetic modifiers. Those carrying the ancestor's haplotype with HLA A3 have been reported to have a more severe phenotypic expression than those with recombinations and different HLA marker haplotypes[1].

MANAGEMENT

Excess iron is removed from the body by weekly phlebotomy, a procedure that has been in use for decades. Each unit of blood (450cm[3]) contains 200–250mg of iron. This quantity is mobilized from stores and transported to the bone marrow for incorporation into newly formed hemoglobin. Blood letting is well tolerated and substitution of the plasma loss is not necessary. Serum iron, transferrin saturation and serum ferritin can be checked at monthly intervals. Serum alanine-

aminotransferase levels can also be regularly followed because the falling curve might encourage the patient to continue heavy phlebotomy (Fig. 189.7). After iron depletion, maintenance phlebotomy, three to six times a year, is required to keep the transferrin saturation normal. No dietary restrictions are recommended. The diagnosis and institution of treatment may be a relief to the patient, who may often have been considered to be an alcoholic because of abnormal liver tests. Liver function improves during phlebotomy (Fig. 189.7), abdominal pains disappear and there is a general increase in wellbeing. Even the cardiomyopathy is reversible if treatment is instituted soon enough and for the necessary length of time. However, diabetes and hypogonadism are usually not affected by iron removal.

Arthropathy does not usually improve with phlebotomy and the damage to the synovial membrane and cartilage seems to be irreversible. In a study by Schumacher *et al.*, 32% of the patients reported no effect, 40% became worse and 27% improved with iron removal[20]. Treatment of these symptoms with non-steroidal anti-inflammatory drugs is helpful in the majority of patients. With time, many hereditary hemochromatosis patients need surgical arthroplasties. The prevalence of such arthropathy compared to age-matched controls has not been studied.

Generally, outcome is excellent if treatment is started early in the course of the disease[13]. Patients detected in the cirrhotic stage run a 200-fold increased risk of hepatoma, even after phlebotomy[13]. It is thus of considerable importance to detect and treat these patients as early as possible.

REFERENCES

1. Powell LW, Subramaniam VN, Yapp TR. Haemochromatosis in the new millennium. J Hepatol 2000; 32: 48–62.
2. Finch SC, Finch CA. Idiopathic haemochromatosis, an iron storage disease. A. Iron metabolism in hemochromatosis. Medicine (Baltimore) 1955; 34: 381–430.
3. Simon M, Bourel M, Fauchet R, Genetet B. Association of HLA-A3 and HLA-B14 antigens with idiopathic haemochromatosis. Gut 1976; I7: 332–334.
4. Feder JN, Gnirke A, Thomas W et al. A novel MHC class I like gene is mutated in patients with hereditary hemochromatosis. Nat Genet 1996; 13: 399–408.

5. Ajioka RS, Jorde LB, Gruen JR *et al*. Haplotype analysis of hemochromatosis: evaluation of different linkage-disequilibrium approaches and evolution of disease chromosomes. Am J Hum Genet 1997; 60: 1439–1447.

6. Ritter B, Safwenberg J, Olsson KS. HLA as a marker of the hemochromatosis gene in Sweden. Hum Genet 1984; 68: 626.

7. Raha-Chowdhury R, Gruen JR. Localization, allelic heterogeneity and origins of the hemochromatosis gene. In: Barton JC, Edwards CQ, eds. Hemochromatosis. Cambridge: Cambridge University Press 2000: 75–90.

8. Merryweather-Clarke AT, Pointon JJ, Jouanolle AM *et al*. Geography of *HFE* C282Y and H63D mutations. Genet Test 2000; 4: 183–198.

9. Schumacher HR. Hemochromatosis and arthritis. Arthritis Rheum 1964; 7: 41–50.

10. Brissot P, Guyader D, Loreal O *et al*. Clinical aspects of hemochromatosis. Transfus Sci 2000: 23: 193–200.

11. Roetto A, Totaro A, Cazzola M *et al*. Juvenile hemochromatosis locus maps to chromosome 1q. Am J Hum Genet 1999; 64: 1388–1393.

12. Olsson KS, Ritter B, Lundin PM. Liver affection in iron overload studied with serum ferritin and serum aminotransferases. Acta Med Scand 1985; 217: 79–84.

13. Niederau C, Fischer R, Sonnenberg A *et al*. Survival and causes of death in cirrhotic and noncirrhotic patients with primary hemochromatosis. N Engl J Med 1985; 313: 1256–1262.

14. Adams PC, Speechley M. The effect of arthritis on the quality of life in hereditary hemochromatosis. J Rheumatol 1996; 23: 707–710.

15. Gottschalk R, Neeck G, Wigand R *et al*. Hemochromatotic arthropathy – an early manifestation of genetic hemochromatosis [In German]. Z Rheumatol 1997; 56: 156–162.

16. Sinigaglia L, Fargion S, Fracanzani AL *et al*. Bone and joint involvement in genetic hemochromatosis: role of cirrhosis and iron overload. J Rheumatol 1997; 24: 1809–1813.

17. Bell H, Berg JP, Undlien DE *et al*. The clinical expression of hemochromatosis in Oslo, Norway. Excessive oral iron intake may lead to secondary hemochromatosis even in *HFE* C282Y mutation negative subjects. Scand J Gastroenterol 2000; 35: 1301–1307.

18. Bulaj ZJ, Ajioka RS, Phillips JD *et al*. Disease-related conditions in relatives of patients with hemochromatosis. N Engl J Med 2000; 343: 1529–1535.

19. Faraawi R, Harth M, Kertesz A, Bell D. Arthritis in hemochromatosis. J Rheumat 1993; 20: 448–452.

20. Schumacher HR, Straka PC, Krikker MA, Dudley AT. The arthropathy of hemochromatosis. Ann NY Acad Sci 1988; 526: 224–233.

21. Pawlotsky Y, Le Dantec P, Moirand R *et al*. Elevated parathyroid hormone 44–68 and osteoarticular changes in patients with genetic hemochromatosis. Arthritis Rheum 1999; 42: 799–806.

22. Roberts AG, Whatley SD, Morgan RR *et al*. Increased frequency of the haemochromatosis Cys282Tyr mutation in sporadic porphyria cutanea tarda. Lancet 1997; 349: 321–323.

23. Montosi G, Paglia P, Garuti C *et al*. Wild-type HFE protein normalizes transferrin iron accumulation in macrophages from subjects with hereditary hemochromatosis. Blood 2000; 96: 1125–1129.

24. Schumacher HR. Haemochromatosis. Baillière's Best Pract Res Clin Rheumatol 2000; 14: 277–84.

25. Von Kempis J. Arthropathy in hereditary hemochromatosis. Curr Opin Rheumatol 2001; 13: 80–83.

190 Ochronosis

Daniel Kuntz and Thomas Bardin

Definition

- A feature of alkaptonuria, a rare autosomal recessive disorder resulting from a constitutional lack of homogentisic acid oxidase and the subsequent accumulation of its substrate
- This metabolic defect is evidently the cause of ochronosis and ochronotic arthritis but the pathophysiology remains unknown

Clinical features

- Homogentisic aciduria, pigmentation of cartilages and other connective tissues and, in later years, osteoarthritis

HISTORY

In 1859 Boedeker was the first to recognize alkaptonuria in a patient suffering from lumbar pain[1]. This patient's urine had reducing properties unlike those of a diabetic's urine, and turned dark when alkali was added. Boedeker named the constituent responsible for this 'alkapton'. In 1866 Virchow described the pigmentation that gradually develops in alkaptonuria in the connective tissue of a 67-year-old man. Microscopically, the pigment was ochre in color and for this reason Virchow named the condition ochronosis.

The chemical structure of alkapton was established in 1891 by Wolkow and Baumann[3], who named it homogentisic acid because of its close structural relationship to gentisic acid. With the aromatic structure of homogentisic acid thus established, tyrosine and phenylalanine, as the known aromatic amino acids, were considered to be the source of this abnormal urinary component. Wolkow and Baumann demonstrated that the urine of alkaptonuric patients fed extra tyrosine contained greatly increased amounts of homogentisic acid, and this important observation initiated determination of the metabolic pathway by which tyrosine and phenylalanine are metabolized to homogentisic acid. In 1928 Neubauer suggested a preliminary scheme, based on feeding experiments with alkaptonuric patients[4]. This has remained essentially unchanged for the past 70 years.

Garrod's hypothesis of 1908[5], that a specific enzyme is lacking in alkaptonuria, was confirmed in 1958 by direct biochemical assay of alkaptonuric liver homogenates[6].

Epidemiology

The inheritance of alkaptonuria was first described in 1902 by Garrod, who presented evidence that this condition is congenital and familial and that it occurs more often in families in which there are consanguineous marriages. He suggested that alkaptonuria might be transmitted as a single recessive mendelian trait. In 1932 Hogben et al. carefully studied all the known cases of alkaptonuria reported up to that time[7]. They confirmed the recessive character of the disease in nearly all the families, and they observed that at least half of the affected individuals were the offspring of consanguineous matings. At the present time, most if not all cases appear to represent the inheritance of a single autosomal recessive gene. This is supported by the fact that a single enzyme system is inactive in this condition and that only one clinical form of alkaptonuria is known.

An unusually high incidence of alkaptonuria has been observed in an area of Germany near the border of the Czech Republic. More than 100 alkaptonuric individuals have been identified among the 16 000 inhabitants of this area. Genetic analyses of the affected families show a concentration of alkaptonuric patients within specific localities, presumably as a result of inbreeding within the isolated hamlets of this region.

While the possibility that a dominant type of alkaptonuria exists cannot be absolutely excluded, no convincing evidence for it has yet been presented. Furthermore, the chromosomal location of the gene defect related to alkaptonuria has not been identified.

CLINICAL FEATURES

Ochronosis

The pigmentation of the sclera or the ear is rarely seen before an alkaptonuric patient is 20–30 years old. This is one cause of the generally late diagnosis of ochronosis[8]. However, the pigmentation observed in the tissues of an elderly patient is always striking. For example, the costal, laryngeal and tracheal cartilages are densely pigmented, appearing coal black in some areas. Although the pigment is presumably a polymer derived from homogentisic acid, its precise chemical structure has yet to be determined.

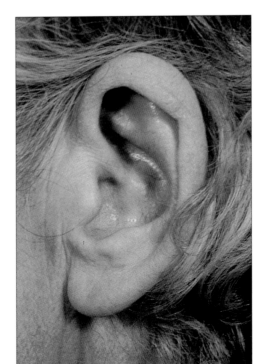

Fig. 190.1 Black-gray pigmentation of the ear cartilage can be seen in this ochronotic patient.

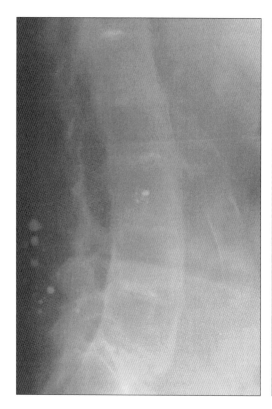
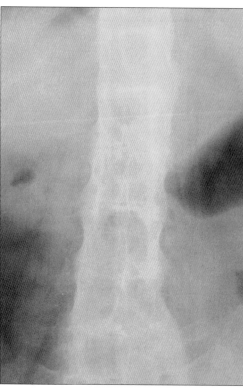

Fig. 190.2 Radiographs of the spine showing narrowing and calcification of the intervertebral discs.

The deposition of ochronotic pigment in the eye is usually visible at the insertion of the rectus muscle but it may be more diffuse, involving the conjunctiva and cornea. Pigmentation of the ear cartilage is first seen in the concha, antihelix and later the tragus, giving a slate-blue or gray coloration (Fig. 190.1). The pigment appears in perspiration; clothing near the axillary regions may be stained, and the skin too may have a brownish discoloration in the axillary and genital regions.

Light microscopic studies disclose ochronotic cartilage embedded in synovium, hemosiderin and ochronotic pigment in macrophages, ochronotic interstitial collagen, occasional multinucleated giant cells around ochronotic shards of cartilage, and focal inflammatory infiltrates of lymphocytes and plasma cells. The ochronotic pigment has a yellow-brown color on staining with hematoxylin and eosin. Synovial lining cell hyperplasia and increased vascularity have been observed in some cases.

Ochronotic arthritis

The earliest symptom of ochronotic arthritis is usually some degree of limitation of motion of the hips, knees or, less frequently, the shoulders. Episodes of acute inflammation of these joints can occur. Later there is usually rather marked limitation of motion of the lumbar spine. The radiographic features in the lumbar spine are almost pathognomonic of ochronotic spondyloarthropathy (Fig. 190.2). Typical wafer-like calcifications are seen in the intervertebral discs, with narrowing of disc spaces and osteoporotic rarefaction of the vertebral bodies. Similar changes may be observed in the thoracic and cervical spine. In rare cases the sacroiliac joints and the symphysis pubis show narrowing of the joint spaces and subchondral bone sclerosis.

The radiographic changes in the large peripheral joints, such as the knee, glenohumeral and, to a lesser extent, the hip joints, are generally observed about 10 years after spinal changes. Narrowing of the joint space, a marked subchondral sclerosis and small osteophytes are frequently noted (Fig. 190.3). Multiple intra-articular radiopaque loose bodies can be seen in the knees and may cause locking episodes. The small joints in the hands, wrists, feet, elbows and ankles are rarely affected[9].

In about 50% of patients joint effusions form in the knee, as a result of fragmentation of damaged cartilage with subsequent inflammation

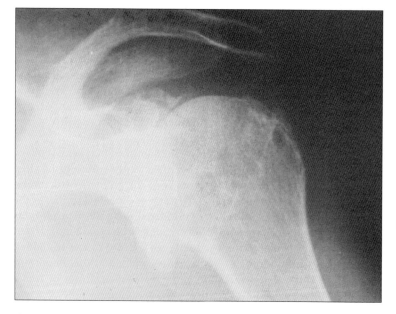

Fig. 190.3 Ochronotic arthritis of the shoulder.

of synovium. The synovial fluid is characteristically non-inflammatory, containing 100–700 cells/mm^3, most of which are mononuclear cells. Both pyrophosphate deposition disease and apatite crystals have been described in association with ochronosis[8].

The high prevalence of osteoarthritis in the general population and the long period before the joint lesion becomes symptomatic in alkaptonuric patients are further factors in the late diagnosis of ochronotic arthropathy. However, in the elderly the joint lesions are often severe and painful and may lead to a marked disability.

Urinary changes

According to the classic description, alkaptonuric patients have dark urine, or urine that turns dark when left standing. However, many patients have never noted any abnormality in the color of their urine

TABLE 190.1 PERIPHERAL OCHRONOTIC ARTHROPATHY VERSUS OSTEOARTHRITIS

	Joint involved	Narrowing of the joint space	Osteophytosis
Ochronosis	Knees, shoulders +++ Hips ++ Sacroiliac joints ±	Symmetric or asymmetric	Absent or sparse
Osteoarthritis	Hips +++ Knees +++ Hands +++	Symmetric or asymmetric	Present

TABLE 190.2 OCHRONOTIC SPONDYLOARTHROPATHY VERSUS ANKYLOSING SPONDYLITIS (RADIOGRAPHIC FEATURES)

	Ochronosis	Ankylosing spondylitis
Calcification of intervertebral discs	++	±
Syndesmophytes	±	+++
Ossification of ligaments	+++	+
Erosion and fusion of sacroiliac joints	±	+++
Osteoporotic vertebral bodies	++	+

during childhood, and the diagnosis has been made only once arthritis has occurred during their later years. In some cases diagnosis has followed discovery of the characteristic radiographic changes in the spine.

Alkaptonuric urine turns dark because it contains an abnormal constituent: homogentisic acid. It has been reported that an alkaptonuric patient excretes about 5–8g of homogentisic acid per day. Its ease of oxidation results in the gradual darkening of the urine downwards from the surface until the entire sample is dark brown. Diagnosis of alcaptonuria is now possible using rapid analysis of homogentisic acid in urine and plasma by high-performance liquid chromatography[10].

DIFFERENTIAL DIAGNOSIS

Osteoarthritis and ankylosing spondylitis are the disorders most likely to be confused with ochronotic arthritis, but calcium pyrophosphate deposition disease must also be kept in mind.

The main differences between peripheral ochronotic arthropathy and osteoarthritis, and between ochronotic spondyloarthropathy and ankylosing spondylitis, are summarized in Tables 190.1 & 190.2.

SYNTHESIS AND DEGRADATION OF HOMOGENTISIC ACID

Biosynthesis

In mammals most of the dietary phenylalanine and tyrosine is oxidized to acetoacetic acid by an enzyme system localized primarily in the liver and kidney (Fig. 190.4). La Du et al.[6] have shown that, in preparations of human liver, homogentisic acid accumulates quantitatively from tyrosine or p-hydroxyphenylpyruvic acid in the presence of an inhibitor of homogentisic acid oxidase. This enzyme is widely distributed in nature and where it is located it is associated with the other enzymes involved in the metabolism of tyrosine and phenylalanine to acetoacetic acid.

Homogentisic acid oxidase catalyzes the oxidative cleavage of the ring of homogentisic acid. In 1951 Suda and Takeda described 'homogentisicase', an enzyme extracted from a strain of Pseudomonas adapted to tyrosine, which catalyzed the degradation of homogentisic acid. They then studied the properties of a similar enzyme from rabbit liver[11]. Homogentisicase has been purified to some degree in several laboratories and many of its

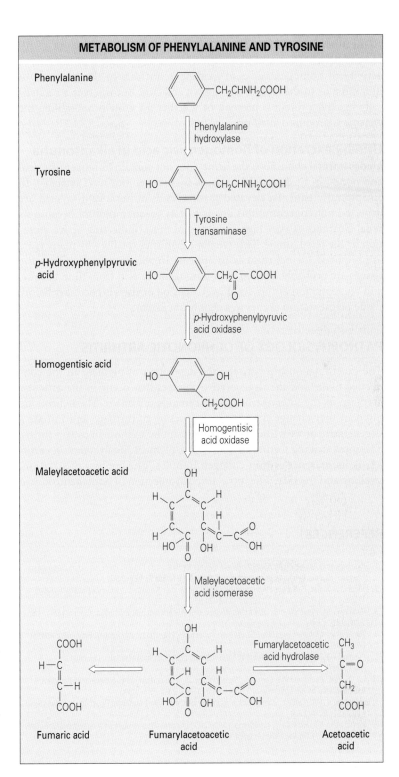

METABOLISM OF PHENYLALANINE AND TYROSINE

Fig. 190.4 Steps in the oxidation of phenylalanine and tyrosine to acetoacetic acid.

properties have been described. The optimal pH for this enzyme is about 7.0. It contains essential sulfhydryl groups and requires ferrous iron, as do several of the other oxygenases involved in ring cleavage reactions. The only function that has been demonstrated for ascorbic acid in this enzymatic reaction is to maintain iron in the reduced form. The requirement for ferrous iron is specific, since other bivalent metals cannot replace it. Homogentisic acid oxidase is inhibited by sulfhydryl-binding agents and by metal-chelating agents that react with ferrous iron. The highest homogentisic acid oxidase activity is found in the soluble fraction of liver and no significant activity has been found in any of the other tissues so far examined, such as blood, salivary glands and muscle.

By a careful analysis of the enzymes involved in tyrosine metabolism in normal and alkaptonuric human liver, La Du et al.[6] demonstrated that only homogentisic acid oxidase is missing in this disorder and that all the other enzymes have about the same activity in normal and alkaptonuric tissue. They also obtained evidence suggesting that the lack of activity of homogentisic acid oxidase is not due to the presence of inhibitors or to the lack of any known cofactor. But whether a catalytically inactive protein is present, or whether no protein resembling the enzyme is produced at all remains unknown.

Urinary excretion of homogentisic acid in alkaptonuria

Under normal conditions the urine does not contain homogentisic acid and none can be detected in plasma by the methods now available. In alkaptonuric patients, elevated plasma levels of homogentisic acid are expected but concentrations are as low as 50–400mmol/ml because its renal clearance is very high (400–500ml/min), indicating active secretion by the renal tubule. This renal mechanism explains why many years are required for ochronosis to appear. In alkaptonuric patients the tissues are probably flooded with homogentisic acid from time to time, and the repetition of this event over a period of years is necessary before tissue pigmentation occurs to a significant extent.

PATHOPHYSIOLOGY OF OCHRONOTIC ARTHRITIS

The exact relationship between the deposition of pigment in the connective tissue and the degenerative changes that occur in the articular cartilage or the intervertebral discs remains unknown. The ochronotic pigment may change the chemical structure of cartilage and initiate a degenerative process leading to changes similar to those in osteoarthritis. The most striking feature of ochronotic pigment involvement in cartilage is its presence within collagen bundles, causing loss of striation, swelling and fracture. The intra-articular injection of homogentisic acid into the knees of rabbits produces local lesions in cartilage resembling those seen in ochronosis. Another hypothesis is that either the ochronotic pigment or homogentisic acid itself inhibits some of the enzymes involved in cartilage metabolism; inhibition of chick embryo lysyl hydroxylase by homogentisic acid has been demonstrated. This enzymatic inhibition is probably important, since it would reduce the amount of hydroxylysine and the number of cross-linkage bonds, which are essential for the tensile strength of collagen fibers. The actual inhibitory agent may be a product of the oxidation of homogentisic acid, such as benzoquinone acetic acid[12]. Human skin and cartilage contain an enzyme called homogentisic acid polyphenol oxidase, which catalyzes the oxidation of homogentisic acid to an ochronotic-like pigment. Benzoquinone acetic acid has been identified as an intermediary metabolite in this oxidation. Chemical reactions between a polymer of benzoquinone acetic acid and the connective tissues may lead to ochronosis and ochronotic arthritis.

Kirkpatrick et al. studied the effects on articular chondrocytes of homogentisic acid at concentrations of 5mg/ml or above[13] which was found to be cytotoxic to rabbit adult articular chondrocytes. A similar effect on fetal articular chondrocytes was observed at concentrations of 1mg/ml. Angeles et al.[14] showed that growth of rabbit, and human, cartilage chondrocytes in monolayer culture was inhibited by homogentisic acid and decreased proportionally to increasing concentrations of homogentisic acid (0.001–1.0mol/l). Substantial chondrocyte morphologic abnormalities were observed when the concentration of homogentisic acid was similar to that found in the plasma of alkaptonuric patients (0.005mol/l). It is of interest that ascorbic acid reduced this inhibition of growth and prevented the morphologic changes. It has also been shown that free radicals may have an important etiologic role in ochronotic arthritis.

MANAGEMENT

Some data suggest that, by protecting lysyl hydroxylase from inhibition, prolonged maintenance of relatively high tissue concentrations of ascorbic acid might delay and possibly reduce the degree of pathologic change in the connective tissues. However, because it is not possible to treat the underlying enzymatic defect, treatment is based on symptomatic measures such as non-steroidal anti-inflammatory drugs, physical therapy, joint overuse and weight loss. Intra-articular injections of glucocorticoids are useful, especially in the knee joint when synovitis is severe. Arthroplasty of the knee or hip is required in the most severe cases of ochronotic arthropathy.

REFERENCES

1. Boedeker C. Ueber das Alcapton; ein neuer Beitrag zur Frage: welche Stoff des Harns können Kupferreduction bewirken? Z Rat Med 1859; 7: 127–155.
2. Virchow R. Ein Fall von allgemeiner Ochronose der Knorpel und knorpelähnlichen Theile. Arch Patol Anat 1866; 37: 212–218.
3. Wolkow M, Baumann E. Uber das Wesen der Alkaptonurie. Z Physiol Chem 1891; 15: 228–285.
4. Neubauer O. Intermediärer Eiweisstoffwechsel. Handb Norm Pathol Physiol 1928; 5: 671–676.
5. Garrod AE. The Croonian lectures on inborn errors of metabolism. Lecture II. Alkaptonuria. Lancet 1908; 2: 73–79.
6. La Du BN, Zannoni VG, Laster L, Seegmiller JE. The nature of the defect in tyrosine metabolism in alkaptonuria. J Biol Chem 1958; 230: 251–260.
7. Hogben L, Worrall RL, Zieve I. The genetic basis of alkaptonuria. Proc R Soc Edin (Biol) 1932; 52: 264–270.
8. Konttinen YT, Hoikka V, Landtman M et al. Ochronosis: a report of a case and a review of literature. Clin Exp Rheumatol 1989; 7: 435–444.
9. Selvi E, Manganelli S, Mannoni A et al. Chronic ochronotic arthritis : clinical, arthroscopic, and pathologic findings. J Rheumatol 2000; 27: 2272–2274.
10. Bory C, Boulieu R, Chantin C, Mathieu M. Diagnosis of alcaptonuria: rapid analysis of homogentisic acid by HPLC. Clin Chim Acta 1990; 189: 7–11.
11. Suda M, Takeda Y. Metabolism of tyrosine. II. Homogentisicase. J Biochem (Tokyo) 1950; 37: 381–387.
12. La Du BN. Alkaptonuria. In: Scriver CR, Beaudet AL, Sly WS, Valle D. The metabolic basis of inherited disease, 6th ed. New York: McGraw Hill; 1989: 1371–1386.
13. Kirkpatrick CJ, Mohr W, Mutschler W. Experimental studies on the pathogenesis of ochronotic arthropathy. The effects of homogentisic acid on adult and fetal articular chondrocyte morphology, proliferative capacity and synthesis of proteoglycans in vitro. Virchows Arch B (Cell Pathol) 1984; 47: 347–360.
14. Angeles AP, Badger R, Gruber HE, Seegmiller JE. Chondrocyte growth inhibition induced by homogentisic acid and its partial prevention with ascorbic acid. J Rheumatol 1989; 16: 512–517.

191 The amyloidoses

Joel Buxbaum

Definition

- The amyloidoses are disorders of secondary protein structure in which the affected precursor molecules become insoluble and form fibrillar deposits that compromise organ function

- The systemic amyloidoses are characterized by the extracellular deposition of fibrils, usually derived from a circulating soluble precursor. In some local forms aggregates can be detected intracellularly

- The amyloid nature of the deposits is defined pathologically by three features: binding of Congo red with green–yellow birefringence under polarized light; a characteristic fibrillar ultrastructure; demonstration of the presence of the serum amyloid P-component immunologically

- At least 23 different proteins (Table. 191.1) form amyloid *in vivo* in humans

Clinical features

- There are systemic and localized forms of deposition

- In the AA, AL and $A\beta_2$-microglobulin amyloidoses, the tissue dysfunction produced by the amyloid adds to that produced by the primary disorder (infection and/or inflammation, multiple myeloma and renal failure, respectively)

- Mutations in the amyloid precursors transthyretin, gelsolin, cystatin, lysozyme, fibrinogen, $A\beta PP$, apolipoprotein A1 and apolipoprotein A2 are the proximal causes of autosomal dominant disorders in which the deposition is the sole pathology

- The formation of some amyloids is associated with aging.

- The manifestations of the amyloidoses are determined by the site, extent and rate of formation of the deposits and the nature of the underlying primary disorder.

- Clinical presentations include renal disease (AA, AL, AApoA1, AApoA2, lysozyme, fibrinogen), heart disease, primarily in AL and ATTR; peripheral and autonomic neuropathy (AL and ATTR); and intracutaneous, intramuscular, gastrointestinal or CNS hemorrhage secondary to amyloid infiltration of blood vessels.

HISTORY

The long, early phase of amyloid investigation (1842–1959) was largely descriptive and nosologic. Clinical (e.g. primary, secondary, familial) and pathologic classifications (e.g. perireticular versus pericollagenous) were proposed, none of which could accommodate all the available observations. The finding that the histologically amorphous deposits had a defined ultrastructure, which could serve as a parameter of identification for candidate molecules, was critical when a method for extraction and isolation of tissue amyloid was developed. The discovery that fibrils from fresh or frozen infiltrated organs could be released, in a physical state amenable to chemical analysis, by extraction with distilled water enabled the modern study of amyloidosis. From this followed the detection and characterization of the discrete precursor proteins and molecular classification of the pathologic entities (Table 191.1).

Clinical knowledge of the amyloidoses was initially dominated by the identification of amyloid deposits in a multitude of disease states. The recognition that Congo red binding with position birefringence was virtually pathognomonic for amyloid allowed the division of homogeneous, eosinophilic material noted in clinical samples into Congophilic and non-Congophilic deposits. High-yield tissue sampling techniques such as rectal biopsy and subcutaneous fat aspiration made diagnosis possible with little risk to the patient.

In addition to the inflammation-associated deposition of AA amyloid, systemic deposition was found to be associated with malignancies (AL and AA amyloidoses) and iatrogenic interventions ($A\beta_2$-microglobulin amyloidosis in dialysis patients). Systemic or tissue-specific amyloids were found in autosomal dominant genetic disorders (ATTR, AApoA1, AapoA2, AGel, ACys, ALys, AFib). Amyloids localized to the central nervous system (CNS) or cerebral vessels (APrP, $A\beta PP$, ACys) were identified as critical in the pathogenesis of Creutzfeldt–Jakob disease, Alzheimer's disease and cerebral angiopathy. Chemical analyses of fibrils extracted from local deposits not associated with systemic amyloidoses revealed a set of distinct single-tissue amyloidoses (AIAPP, ACal, AANF).

Identification of precursors and the use of reagents capable of immunohistochemically distinguishing different amyloids, along with safer techniques for sampling tissues have simplified diagnosis and clarified the nature of the syndromes associated with each precursor.

Progress in treatment has lagged behind diagnosis, but principles of therapy, dependent on the molecular nature of the amyloid precursor and a greater understanding of the process of fibrillogenesis, have been established. Elimination of the infectious or inflammatory stimulus (AA), antineoplastic treatment (AL) and organ transplantation as either replacement (AL, AA) or gene therapy (familial amyloidotic polyneuropathy) have been salutary but not curative. Improved supportive measures have prolonged survival and enhanced the quality of life for patients. Current investigation is based on insights into pathogenesis gained in the last decade and is focused on the development of molecules designed to interfere with the processes of aggregation, fibril formation and deposition.

EPIDEMIOLOGY AND RISK FACTORS

Each of the amyloidoses has its own epidemiology. The relative frequencies of AL, AA and ATTR in amyloid-positive tissues in different countries is shown in Table 191.2. Amyloid formation represents a final common pathway reached from a variety of etiologic starting points. It is not clear if there is a generic risk for amyloid formation *per se*. In autopsy studies the incidence of more than one amyloid, derived from different precursors, in the same individual increases with age[1]. This observation may reflect multiple independent processes influenced by the passage of time or the disruption of a single age-sensitive pathway

TABLE 191.1 CHEMICAL CLASSIFICATION OF HUMAN AMYLOID

Amyloid protein	Precursor	Mechanism of amyloidogenesis	Clinical syndromes
AA	ApoSAA	Increased production; cleavage of amyloidogenic isoform	Chronic infection/inflammation; familial Mediterranean fever; familial amyloid nephropathy with urticaria and deafness; tumors (Muckle–Wells syndrome)
AL	Ig light chain, κ or λ	Primary structure; deletion; proteolysis	Primary myeloma-associated
AH	Ig heavy chain	Deletion	Primary
ATTR	Transthyretin	Mutation ? cleavage	Familial amyloidotic polyneurocardiomyopathy; senile systemic (cardiac) amyloid
AApoAI	Apolipoprotein A_1	Mutation	Familial amyloidotic polyneuropathy; senile systemic (cardiac) amyloid
AApoA2	Apolipoprotein A_2	Mutation	Familial nephropathy
AGel	Gelsolin	Mutation-altered cleavage	Finnish corneal lattice dystrophy with cranial neuropathy
ACys	Cystatin	Mutation	Hereditary cerebral hemorrhage with amyloid
AβPP	β-protein precursor	Mutation; altered secretion and/or cleavage?	Alzheimer's disease
$Aβ_2M$	$β_2$-microglobulin	Diminished excretion, polymerization, glycosylation, cleavage?; increased production	Dialysis amyloid
APrP	Prion protein	Mutation conformational change	Creutzfeldt–Jakob, Gerstmann's, Straüssler–Scheinker disease, fatal familial insomnia
ABri	Bri(2)	Mutation	Familial neurodegeneration
ACal	Procalcitonin	Local overproduction	Medullary thyroid carcinoma
AANF	Atrial natriuretic factor	Local overproduction	Atrial amyloid of aging
AIAPP	Islet amyloid polypeptide	Local overproduction	Senile amyloid of the pancreas
ALys	Lysozyme	Mutation	Ostertag renal amyloid
AFib	A-Fibrogen	Mutation	Hereditary renal amyloid
APin	?	Local overproduction	Odontogenic tumor
Ack Pending	Cytokeratins	Local overproduction	Cutaneous
Apro	Prolactin	Wild-type	Aging pituitary
AIns	Insulin	Wild-type	Local deposition
ALac	Lactoferrin	Wild-type	Corneal deposition
Amedin	Lactadherin	Fragment	Aortic media deposits

From Westermark P *et al*. Nomenclature of amyloid fibril proteins. Report from the meeting of the International Nomenclature Committee on Amyloidosis, July 19, 20, 2001, in Amyloid: Protein Folding Disord 2002; 9: 197–200.

TABLE 191.2 TYPES OF SYSTEMIC AMYLOID WORLDWIDE

Country	Time period	No.	Tissues	AA (%)	AL (%)	ATTR (%)
Japan	1987–89	140	Autopsy	56	32	4
India	1968–86	104	Autopsy + biopsy	84	12	–
Netherlands	1964–86	162	Autopsy + biopsy	64	36	–
UK	1973–82	131	Autopsy + biopsy	58	42	–
UK	1976–88	17	Renal biopsy	65	35	–
UK	1990–99	46	Biopsy	35	65	-
Spain	1974–86	48	Renal biopsy	77	23	–
Germany	1975–90	225	Renal biopsy	64	36	–
Malaysia*	1978–83	186	Biopsy	3	6	-
Sweden	1952–79	148	Autopsy	83	17	–
Sweden	1974–84	150	Subcutaneous fat aspirate	76	21	–
USA (Mayo)[†]	1981–92	1315	Autopsy + biopsy	3	70	–
USA (BU)[†]	1981–85	83	Autopsy + biopsy	21	63	–
USA (BU)[†]	1990–99	728	Subcutaneous fat aspirate	3	83	13
USA (LA County)	1952–85	431	Autopsy	18	50	32[‡]
Caucasian		170		30	24	46
Hispanic		191		11	86	3
African-American		70		4	17	79

* Very high frequency of atrial and local forms of amyloid. † Referral centers. ‡ Late-onset cardiac amyloid.

These figures were derived from a variety of published studies performed in various countries. Time periods of the studies are indicated as are the sources of tissue for the analysis.

for maintaining *in vivo* protein solubility in the face of various forms of non-enzymic modification.

The pathogenic properties of the protein product in AL, a monoclonal disorder of the B-cell lineage, may be greater than the prolifera-tive potential of the involved clone[2]. It is the most common form of systemic amyloidosis seen in the USA. Since AL is generally fatal, autopsy estimates of prevalence are reliable if the demographics of the reporting institution do not change and the proportion of individuals autopsied is high. Such data, from Olmstead County (MN, USA), between 1950 and 1989, suggest that approximately 1 in 100 000 (0.001%) will develop AL amyloidosis[3]. Death certificate data, which are less reliable, indicate a prevalence of 1:75 000 in The Netherlands[4].

About 20% of people with multiple myeloma are found to have AL amyloidosis. Among AL cases identified at the Mayo Clinic, 18% had myeloma while a similar number (16%) was classified as having monoclonal gammopathies of undetermined significance prior to the diagnosis of amyloidosis.

The most common form of systemic amyloidosis worldwide is the AA type. The fibril is derived from the acute-phase protein serum amyloid A (SAA), a molecule found to be elevated in a variety of diseases, that plays a role in cholesterol transport during inflammation. The protein exists as three isoforms, SAA1, 2 and 4. They are encoded by three homologous genes[5]. SAA1 has five alleles (Table 191.3). SAA2 has two. SAA 1 and 2 have been identified as amyloid components. SAA4 has not. Particular alleles have been associated with a predisposition to amyloid formation in inflammatory diseases in specific populations, for example SAA1γ in Japanese with rheumatoid arthritis, SAA1α in Caucasians with juvenile chronic arthritis and in individuals with familial Mediterranean fever[6,7]. While a prolonged and substantial elevation of SAA is required for AA deposition, there are many instances in which there is a chronic moderate increase without apparent AA formation. This has recently been identified in individuals with active coronary artery disease and has been cited as evidence for the inflammatory nature of atherosclerosis[8].

The disorders associated with clinically significant AA amyloidosis are identified in Table 191.4. In industrialized countries non-infectious inflammatory conditions are most common, while in countries with endemic chronic infectious diseases, particularly tuberculosis and leprosy, AA is associated with infection.

In the USA the distribution of various amyloidoses varies with the reporting institution. The proportions of AL and AA are different in referral centers from those in a hospital providing general health services for a socioeconomically defined population. In the latter it may be possible to discern ethnic differences in prevalence, since environmental influences on the various populations are minimized. Thus, in mid-20th century Los Angeles, AL was more common in individuals of Mexican–Hispanic origin than in either whites or African–Americans[9]. African–Americans had the lowest prevalence of AL and AA but the highest incidence of isolated late-onset cardiac amyloidosis derived from transthyretin (see Table 191.2). The relationship between AL and AA prevalence in the entire population was closer to that in USA referral centers than in other countries. These observations suggest that, if environmental agents play a role in the pathogenesis of the amyloidoses, hereditary factors must also be involved in susceptibility.

The incidence of amyloidosis in the spectrum of inflammatory arthropathies varies with both the country and the means of diagnosis. The data for rheumatoid arthritis (RA) are shown in Table 191.5. They suggest that biopsy sampling of a single tissue site gives lower prevalence estimates than autopsy series in the same population. However, it may be that patients with RA coming to autopsy have had more severe disease and it is the chronicity and severity that have led to more extensive amyloidosis. While amyloid prevalence at autopsy seems to be comparable in most countries, results obtained by tissue sampling and clinical assessment vary.

There is considerable geographic variation in the incidence of amyloidosis in patients with ankylosing spondylitis and juvenile chronic arthritis (JCA) (Table 191.6). Some discrepancies may reflect statistical distributions in small samples; others represent actual population differences in susceptibility. It is clear that AA is more common in JCA with systemic rather then articular presentation. AA appears to be associated with inflammatory disease more frequently in Europe than in the USA. The reasons are uncertain and may reflect the natural history of the inflammatory disease in different populations either on a genetic or an environmental basis. More likely is that, in the past, less aggressive anti-inflammatory therapy has allowed a longer period of persistent SAA elevation. It is possible that other, unsuspected, factors also play some role.

Familial Mediterranean fever (see Chapter 158) demonstrates how interaction between different genetic elements can influence the incidence of renal AA. The M694V mutation in the pyrin gene is more highly associated with AA amyloidosis than other mutations in the same gene. Rather than the mutation being a specific amyloidogenic risk factor, clinical studies suggest that the inflammatory disease is more severe with homozygous M694V and in individuals homozygous for complex (two substitutions on the same allele) mutations. In both instances the incidence of amyloidosis is increased in the presence of

TABLE 191.3 HUMAN SAA GENES AND PROTEINS

SAA1.1	(SAA1α)	V52A	A57V	G73D
SAA1.2	(SAA1β)	V52A	A57V	
SAA1.3	(SAA1γ)	V52A	A57V	D60N
SAA1.4	(SAA1δ)	V52A	A57V	
SAA1.5	(SAA1β)	V52A	A57V	
SAA2.1	(SAA2α)	V52A	A57V	D60N	F69L	G70T	N84K	G90R
SAA2.2	(SAA2β)	V52A	A57V	D60N	F69L	H72R	N84K	G90R

Amino acid sequences are identical except for positions noted: A, alanine; D, aspartic acid; F, phenylalanine; G, glycine; H, histidine; K, lysine; L, leucine; N, asparagines; R, arginine; T, threonine; V, valine.

TABLE 191.4 DISEASES ASSOCIATED WITH AA WORLDWIDE

Country	No.	Tissue	RA (%)	Other inflammatory diseases* (%)	Tuberculosis (%)	Other infectious diseases† (%)	Tumor (%)
Japan	68**	Autopsy	68	–	4	29	20
Sweden	123	Autopsy	46	6	15	19	9
India	87	Autopsy & biopsy	–	–	72	–	–
UK	76	Autopsy & biopsy	62	16	11	8	3
USA (Mayo)	64	Autopsy & biopsy	48	30	–	17	3
Netherlands	104	Autopsy & biopsy	60	13	3	14	5
Spain	37	Renal biopsy	8	43	14	30	–
Germany	144	Renal biopsy	41	30	8	13	2

* Including ankylosing spondylitis, inflammatory bowel disease, juvenile chronic arthritis, familial Mediterranean fever. † Other chronic infections, including pyelonephritis, osteomyelitis, bronchiectasis
** In some instances individual AA cases had more than one category of underlying disease, either of which could have stimulated AA deposition, hence the total is greater than 100%. Where percentages do not add up to 100% quantitatively minor forms were not included.

TABLE 191.5 AA IN RA

Country	Year	Tissue	No.	%
UK	1956	Autopsy	181	14
UK	1963	Rectal biopsy	115	5
USA	1960	Consecutive autopsy	42	26
USA	1965	Gingival biopsy	192	5
Sweden	1974	Rectal biopsy + subcutaneous fat aspiration	47	4
Israel	1972	Autopsy + biopsy	54	17
Japan	1991	Autopsy	81	21
Japan	1991	Gastroduodenal biopsy	107	13
Estonia	1993	Subcutaneous fat aspiration	47	23
Egypt	2001	Subcutaneous fat aspiration	112	7
Hungary	1992	Consecutive autopsy	215	17
Hungary	2001	Consecutive autopsy	161	21

TABLE 191.6 AA PREVALENCE IN SELECTED INFLAMMATORY AND INFECTIOUS DISEASES

Disease	Country	Prevalence (%)	Comments
JCA	USA (1977)	0.14	1946 study 1.8%
	Denmark	4	
	Russia	5.1	
	Poland	11	
	UK	7.4	Incidence reduced by chlorambucil administration
	Germany	3.1	
	Sweden	9	
	France	16.7	Small series
Ankylosing spondylitis	USA	3	Small series
	UK	6	Autopsies
	West Germany	4	
	Former Yugoslavia	8.6	
	Finland	13	Decreased 1979–93
Inflammatory bowel disease	USA	0.7	Crohn's disease, ileocolitis
		0.1	Ulcerative colitis
Behçet's syndrome	Turkey	0.4	
Osteomyelitis	Nigeria	10	
Subcutaneous drug abuse	USA (New York)	5	1981–83; secondary to skin abscesses
SLE			Case reports only

homozygosity for the $\alpha 1$ allele of the SAA 1.1 gene (Table 191.3). M694V is more common in populations that have a very high incidence of renal AA amyloidosis accompanying familial Mediterranean fever, but it is the combination of the two gene products that appears to be responsible[10].

The clinical penetrance, as familial amyloidotic polyneuropathy, of the most common mutation (TTR V30M) in transthyretin (TTR), a normal serum protein which carries retinol-binding protein charged with retinol and 25% of serum thyroxine, varies in the different countries in which it is found. It is higher and of earlier onset in Portugal and Japan than it is in Sweden. In addition differences in penetrance have been seen within and among Portuguese families. Haplotype analysis indicates more than one founder for the mutation. The epidemiologic observations suggest that, while the TTR mutations generally follow an autosomal dominant mode of inheritance, environmental or other presently unknown genetic elements influence clinical expression.

Dialysis amyloidosis ($A\beta_2$-microglobulin) becomes clinically evident in some patients after 5–7 years on dialysis[11]. Within 10 years 25–50% are affected, and by 15 years virtually all patients have deposits. Cellulose-based cuprophan dialysis membranes appear to be associated with a higher incidence of amyloid formation than do acrylonitrile or polysulfone membranes, perhaps related to the copper content. The incidence

is lower in patients undergoing peritoneal dialysis and, rarely, individuals with renal failure develop $A\beta_2$-microglobulin deposits before beginning dialysis. There are data suggesting that individuals carrying the Apolipoprotein E4 allele develop this form earlier in the course of dialysis than those carrying other apo E alleles.

CLINICAL FEATURES

Synovial and periarticular amyloid infiltration occur in a small percentage of patients with AL[12]. This may involve small or large joints either symmetrically or asymmetrically. Stiffness is more characteristic than pain. Shoulder involvement may be particularly striking with the joints creating the appearance of an American football player in shoulder pads (see Fig. 191.1). The synovial fluid is non-inflammatory and may contain fibrils which have the tinctorial and ultrastructural features of amyloidosis.

$A\beta_2$-microglobulin (dialysis-associated) amyloidosis always involves the musculoskeletal system with infiltration of the carpal ligaments, bone cyst formation, frequently in apposition to joints, scapulohumeral periarthritis, painful stiff fingers and destructive cervical spondyloarthropathy with cyst formation and occasional odontoid fracture[11,13]. Cervical disease usually shows vertebral end-plate erosion without

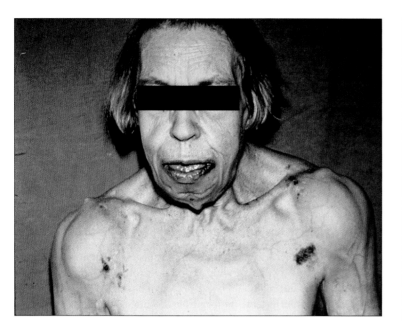

Fig. 191.1 Shoulder pad arthropathy. Reproduced with permission from the American College of Rheumatology clinical slide collection.

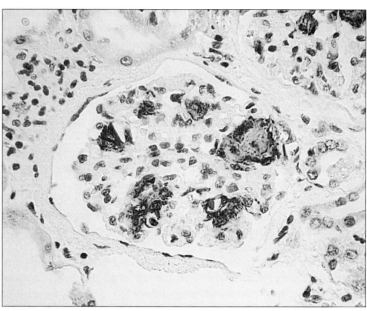

Fig. 191.2 AA amyloid in the kidney. Glomerulus stained with anti-SAA antibody coupled to peroxidase (PAP).

osteophyte formation. Ultrasonography of the wrist is useful for defining thickening of the carpal ligament[14]. Sonograms of the shoulder can distinguish amyloidosis from other forms of shoulder disease. Renal transplantation halts disease progression but does not relieve the symptoms caused by the existing lesions. Pain relief cannot be achieved with surgery, but functional improvement may be obtained in joints that are accessible by arthroscopy.

In familial Mediterranean fever, arthritis is associated with febrile episodes, while Muckle–Wells syndrome patients and those with familial cold urticaria have arthralgias accompanying urticaria. Both develop renal AA amyloidosis.

Joint involvement is not a major feature of the TTR amyloidoses although erosive arthritis has been reported in patients with both Met 30 and Tyr 77 mutations[15]. The severe neuropathy can result in Charcot's joints secondary to trauma. Carpal tunnel syndrome is a common manifestation of familial amyloidotic polyneuropathies and has also been noted with localized normal-sequence TTR amyloid deposition[16].

Renal disease is the dominant clinical manifestation of systemic AA and AL deposition. It is the primary manifestation of the hereditary amyloidoses related to fibrinogen, apolipoprotein A1, apolipoprotein A2 and lysozyme mutations and a late event in some families with familial amyloidotic polyneuropathies associated with TTR mutations. When renal disease is suspected on clinical grounds, AA amyloidosis has been diagnosed in 10–15% (USA), 22% (Japan) and 30% (Finland) of RA patients undergoing renal biopsy[17]. In Finland, however, mesangial glomerulonephritis was a more common form of renal pathology than AA in RA.

The usual presentation is proteinuria, frequently within nephrotic range (> 3g), with a progressive course leading ultimately to renal failure. The proteinuric phase may be brief or not observed until the patient presents with acute or subacute renal insufficiency. Tissue examination has indicated that glomerular deposition (Figs 191.2 & 191.3) is responsible for the proteinuria and that renal failure occurs early when the major site of deposition is interstitial[18]. Serum creatinine above 2mg/dl (152.5mmol/l) at the time of presentation is a poor prognostic sign. Unless another cause of renal failure can be identified the prospects for renal salvage are poor. Renal tubular abnormalities, most commonly

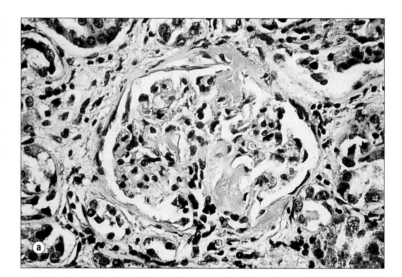

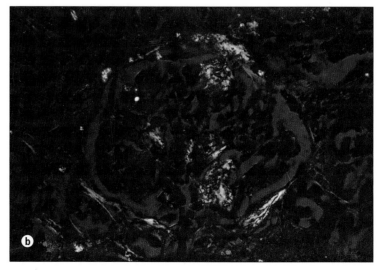

Fig. 191.3 Renal amyloidosis. Glomerulus stained with Congo red viewed under (a) normal and (b) polarized light. The Congo red-stained section shows the characteristic apple-green birefringence for amyloid.

renal tubular acidosis, have been seen during the proteinuric phase. Renal vein thrombosis is increased in nephrotic patients regardless of the cause, but there may be a greater risk among amyloidosis patients[19]. Hematuria reflects amyloid deposition anywhere in the genitourinary tract. There does not seem to be a distinction between the renal disease produced by AA and that by AL.

Heart disease is the major manifestation in 20% of AL patients[2]. Clinical cardiac involvement is rare in AA ($<$ 10%), but has been associated with myopathic and coronary vascular syndromes, sometimes involving only the intramyocardial vessels. Cardiomyopathy is prominent in the TTR amyloidoses. The heart is the primary site for deposition with many of the TTR mutations (familial amyloidotic cardiomyopathy) and a significant secondary site in some of those with primary neurologic involvement (familial amyloidotic polyneuropathy). Mutant and normal sequence forms of TTR are associated with isolated late-onset cardiomyopathy[20,21].

The pathophysiologic features of the infiltrative process are the same regardless of the precursor. However, the rate of AL deposition is more rapid than that seen in the TTR-related disorders. To date, the earliest observed echocardiographic abnormality is loss of isovolumic relaxation with a change in the flow velocity during ventricular filling. This can be detected during Doppler echocardiography as reversal of the early atrial (E/A) flow velocities[22]. This precedes the stage of restrictive cardiomyopathy in which cardiac filling is compromised but a good ejection fraction is retained. The latter is diminished late in the course or in the presence of other heart disease. Arrhythmias may occur at any time, depending on the site rather than the amount of cardiac amyloid deposition. In the familial amyloidoses, involvement of autonomic fibers to the heart may affect beat-to-beat intervals and predispose to 'standstill' syndromes. Similar severe autonomic dysfunction has recently been reported to be common in AL cardiomyopathy.

Peripheral nerve disease is the presenting manifestation in 10–20% of AL patients and most familial amyloidotic polyneuropathy kindreds. The peripheral neuropathy is sensorimotor with both distal and proximal involvement[2]. The dysesthesia may be difficult to manage. Sural nerve biopsy is useful. However, in some cases the lesion is proximal to the sural nerve. Only non-specific degenerative changes are seen and the Congo red stain is negative when the tissue is examined[23]. Biopsies of other sites, particularly the contralateral sural nerve, may be positive. In many patients with familial amyloidotic polyneuropathy, autonomic neuropathy dominates the clinical picture with diarrhea and urinary incontinence the major manifestations. Orthostatic hypotension occurs in both familial amyloidotic polyneuropathy and AL. Neuropathy is not seen in AA amyloidosis. Isolated peripheral neuropathy, in the absence of other suggestive history or signs, is rarely, if ever, the only manifestation of systemic amyloidosis.

Amyloid deposits of all systemic types are found in the gastrointestinal tract, either in the bowel wall or in vessels in almost every region of the gut from the tongue and gingiva to the rectum[24]. Macroglossia, most common in AL, is rarely seen in other amyloidoses. It can prevent adequate food intake and interfere with articulate speech. Laser surgery may be required.

Bleeding from amyloid lesions within the gut is amplified by the non-compliant nature of amyloidotic blood vessels. The clotting disorders sometimes seen in AL make this complication even more problematic. Extensive infiltration of the bowel may result in malabsorption, intestinal obstruction or pseudo-obstruction. In the familial amyloidotic polyneuropathies, autonomic nerve plus bowel wall involvement can produce diarrhea, constipation, nausea and vomiting. Weight loss is almost universal.

Hepatosplenomegaly is a feature of both AA and AL and in some patients with AApoA1. Severe cholestasis has been associated with AL deposition. Clotting abnormalities are relatively common in AL. The most severe of these is an acquired factor X deficiency, which is probably related to binding of the factor to some amyloid fibrils, although other factors may play a role[25]. In cases in which infiltrative splenomegaly is associated with bleeding, splenectomy may be life saving. Untreated, all systemic amyloidoses have a fatal outcome. In the past AL was the most rapidly lethal, with a 2–14 month life expectancy. Familial amyloidotic polyneuropathy patients could expect to survive for 7–15 years after diagnosis. Survival for patients with disease associated with AA was shortened by renal failure consequent to amyloid deposition. Life expectancy has improved for all forms of systemic amyloidosis, in part because of earlier diagnosis, but primarily because of improved supportive measures.

INVESTIGATIONS

Certain clinical signs and symptoms should suggest a diagnosis of one of the amyloidoses. Any patient with significant proteinuria and hypogammaglobulinemic serum should be suspected of having AL, particularly in the presence of peripheral neuropathy or congestive heart failure. A patient with long-standing, active inflammatory joint disease, especially RA, who develops proteinuria must be investigated for AA deposition. Patients on hemodialysis or those in chronic renal failure and not on dialysis who exhibit carpal tunnel syndrome are likely to have β_2-microglobulin amyloidosis. Patients with cardiac or neurologic symptoms and a family history suggestive of hereditary neuropathy or cardiomyopathy with geographic origins in countries with known familial amyloidotic polyneuropathy kindreds warrant investigation for the presence of mutant amyloid precursors.

No blood or urine test is specifically diagnostic for amyloidosis. Studies confirming the presence of chronic inflammatory disease, e.g. erythrocyte sedimentation rate (ESR), C-reactive protein (CRP), serum SAA level, etc., are not discriminant since most patients with chronic inflammation do not develop amyloidosis.

Studies of serum proteins, particularly albumin and immunoglobulins, may be helpful in that hypoalbuminemia in the presence of proteinuria supports the diagnosis of nephrotic syndrome. Hypogammaglobulinemia in the presence of proteinuria suggests AL or its non-fibrillar analog light chain deposition disease (LCDD) or light and heavy chain deposition disease (LHCDD)[26]. AL, AH, LCDD and LHCDD can be grouped as the monoclonal immunoglobulin deposition diseases (MIDD). Serum and urine electrophoresis and immunoelectrophoresis may reveal a monoclonal immunoglobulin in the serum and/or urine and the generalized proteinuria characteristic of the nephrotic syndrome. The absence of a monoclonal protein does not eliminate the possible diagnosis of AL since a monoclonal serum or urine protein is not detectable in 15–20% of AL patients, and some patients with other amyloidoses have a coincidental monoclonal serum protein. Bone marrow biopsy with immunophenotyping by immunofluorescent, immunohistologic or immuno-electron microscopic staining for light chain class will demonstrate a monoclonal population of plasma cells, with excess light chain production, even in patients with no identifiable serum or urine monoclonal protein. The clonal population in the marrow can be followed during therapy[27]. The biopsy can also be examined for the presence and type of amyloid.

Non-invasive techniques

Many non-invasive techniques are useful for assessing organ involvement but do not establish whether the findings are related to amyloid. Renal sonography may reveal normal size (34%), small (54%) or large (11%) kidneys[19]. In patients with AL kidney enlargement may be more common (42% versus 4% with small kidneys). Intravenous pyelography should not be performed if AL is suspected, since there is a risk of precipitating acute renal failure.

The echocardiographic findings in amyloid heart disease are suggestive rather than diagnostic[22]. Changes in diastolic filling, detected by Doppler ultrasound, occur early but are not specific. Thickening of the posterior interventricular septum (>15mm) has been noted, as has 'sparkling' of the myocardial echoes. Neither has a high degree of sensitivity or specificity. In advanced disease, ventricular voltage measured in the precordial leads is low relative to ventricular mass.

A number of reports have indicated that technetium-99 is concentrated in soft tissues infiltrated with amyloid, particularly the heart. This is not a consistent finding, but is useful when present.

Several laboratories have been developing more specific non-invasive assays both to determine the presence of tissue amyloid and to measure the extent of deposition. One set of assays are based on the binding of serum amyloid P-component (SAP) to amyloid fibrils *in vivo*. Radio-iodinated purified SAP is administered intravenously to patients with various forms of amyloid who are then scanned with a gamma camera[28,29]. The results have been impressive in AA, AL and ATTR, less so in $A\beta_2$-microglobulin. The reduction in deposition after successful therapy is striking as are the increases associated with treatment failure. The technique visualizes the liver, spleen, adrenals, kidneys and joints very well, but has not proved useful in assessing cardiac, peripheral nerve or brain disease. A similar procedure using technetium tagged aprotinin has been reported to be more discriminant in defining cardiac amyloidosis, but needs further investigation at other centers, as does scanning with Tc99 3,3-diphosphono-1,2-propanodicarboxic acid (DPD)[30].

Biopsy

The definitive diagnostic test is biopsy of either easily accessible tissues expected to contain amyloid or clinically affected organs. Rectal biopsy (Fig. 191.4) and subcutaneous fat aspiration (Fig. 191.5) are the procedures of choice. The diagnostic yield from published studies which utilize a variety of sampling procedures in the three major forms of systemic amyloidosis is shown in Table 191.7. In AA patients subcutaneous fat aspiration and rectal biopsy were found to have sensitivities of 0.97 and 0.82 respectively[31]. In AL patients the sensitivities were 0.62 and 0.72 with bone marrow biopsy being somewhat less sensitive (0.50)[32]. With Congo red staining as the indicator, specificity is 99%, with false positives due only to Congo red overstaining. Sampling procedures are less risky than specific organ biopsy, since they can be carried out under direct vision with hemostatic control which is not possible during needle puncture of internal organs. If results are negative, or there is a reason to believe that clinical organ involvement is not due to amyloid, then more invasive procedures such as renal, liver or endomyocardial biopsy can be performed. The yield of positive biopsies from amyloid-compromised organs is above 90%.

Samples obtained from any of these procedures are stained with hematoxylin eosin, Congo red (with polarized light) or thioflavine T or S to demonstrate the characteristic metachromasia, antibodies against SAP (positive with all amyloids) and all available precursor specific antibodies (anti-kappa and -lambda light chains, anti-AA, anti-TTR, anti-β_2-microglobulin and if appropriate anti-α-fibrinogen, antilysozyme, anti-procalcitonin, anti-ANF)[33]. They can also be prepared for electron

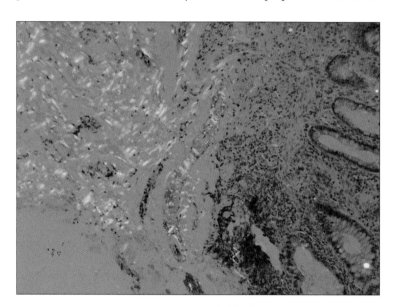

Fig. 191.4 Rectal biopsy positive for amyloidosis. The tissue has been stained with Congo red and examined by polarized light. Note the apple-green birefringence.

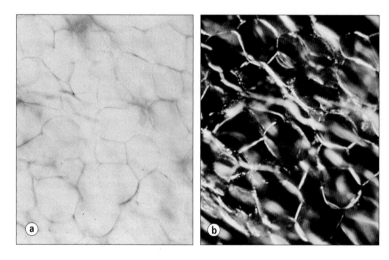

Fig. 191.5 Amyloidosis in subcutaneous fat. Subcutaneous abdominal fat is obtained by needle aspiration. Regular light microscopy (a) is compared with polarized microscopy (b) after staining with Congo red. (Reproduced with permission from the American College of Rheumatology teaching slide collection.)

TABLE 191.7 DIAGNOSTIC YIELD OF TISSUE SAMPLING PROCEDURES IN THE MAJOR AMYLOIDOSES			
Tissue	**AL**	**AA**	**ATTR**
Subcutaneous fat aspiration*	541/689 (79%)	56/91[†] (62%)	58/71(82%)
Rectal biopsy*	146/194 (75%)	54/65 (85%)	
Bone marrow biopsy	221/394 (56%)	12/26 (46%)	
Stomach and small bowel biopsy	19/23 (83%)	15/16 (94%)	
Labial salivary gland biopsy	13/16 (81%)	13/14 (93%)	

* Neither subcutaneous fat aspiration nor rectal biopsy is useful in $A\beta_2$-microglobulin. [†] The results of subcutaneous fat aspiration in AA amyloid do not include patients with familial Mediterranean fever, who are generally not positive from this site.

microscopy and immuno-electron microscopy. The assays detect amyloid and identify the precursor, thereby defining the therapeutic options.

ETIOLOGY AND PATHOGENESIS

Amyloid formation reflects a conformational disorder of the precursor protein and represents a final common pathway of disease reached from a variety of etiologic starting points. It is not clear if there is a generic risk for amyloid formation *per se*. In autopsy studies occurrence of more than one amyloid, derived from different precursors, in the same individual increases with age[1]. The observation may reflect multiple independent processes influenced by the passage of time, or disruption of a single age-sensitive pathway for maintaining *in vivo* protein solubility in the face of various forms of non-enzymic modification.

The amyloid precursors shown in Table 191.1 do not share any region of amino acid sequence. With the exceptions of PRP, lysozyme and SAA, they all have considerable β-pleated sheet secondary structure in the soluble state. However, when PRP undergoes fibrillogenesis it fully adapts the β-structure. The deposited fibrils are antiparallel β-sheet. Proteins with the same primary structure (amino acid sequence) can exist in more than one conformation. If amyloid precursors have fibrillogenic and non-fibrillogenic conformations, amyloidogenesis must involve an increase in the proportion of molecules assuming the amyloidogenic conformation. The factors responsible for controlling the relative proportions of the two conformers are not known. One important element is precursor structure. All are relatively small proteins. In some, a smaller 'core peptide' sequence, which possesses all the *in vitro* fibrillogenic capacity of the whole protein, has been identified. It is possible that *in vivo* the native intramolecular environment surrounding the core peptide maintains it in the non-fibrillar conformation; when that environment is disturbed fibrillogenesis is initiated.

Changes in primary protein structure produced by germline mutations are responsible for the hereditary amyloidoses. While normal TTR has intrinsic amyloidogenicity, demonstrated *in vivo* by the occurrence of normal sequence TTR amyloid deposits in the heart and carpal tunnel in the elderly, single mutations changing more than 50 of 127 amino acids in TTR are associated with various forms of familial amyloidotic polyneuropathies and familial amyloidotic cardiomyopathy due to amyloid formation earlier in life[34,35]. In vitro assays have demonstrated that the fibrillogenic potential of mutant molecules is greater than that of native TTR.

In AL, lambda light chains are more amyloidogenic than kappa chains and the V lambda$_{VI}$ subclass is more so than any of the others[26]. Furthermore, amino acid substitutions which are unusual in non-fibrillogenic light-chain v regions are enriched among amyloid proteins[36]. There is also early evidence suggesting that the L-chain subgroup determines where the major site of tissue deposition will be. Biosynthetic studies have shown that unusually sized (larger and smaller) light-chain synthetic products can be found in bone marrow cells of some patients with AL[37,38]. The smaller molecules may represent the products of genes containing deletions or intact chains which have undergone rapid limited postsynthetic proteolysis. The larger chains appear to be glycosylated. Either may increase amyloidogenicity.

Carbohydrate analyses of AL fibrils have indicated that 35% of the light chains are glycosylated[26]. Since only 15% of normal human light chains have sugar side chains, it is possible that glycosylation enhances light-chain fibrillogenicity.

Non-enzymic glycosylation has also been implicated in the amyloidogenicity of Aβ_2-microglobulin. However, in this circumstance and in Alzheimer's disease it has been suggested that, rather than acting through their effect on primary structure, the molecules interact with receptors for advanced glycation end products (AGE) on macrophages and glial cells to stimulate an inflammatory response which produces cytotoxicity[39].

Since the marrow cells from only a fraction of AL patients have been shown to produce short light chains and most deposits consist largely of truncated light-chain proteins beginning with an intact v region and extending for some distance into the c region, proteolysis has been identified as a participant in the process of amyloidogenesis. Limited proteolysis of amyloidogenic light chains will produce Congo red binding fibrils *in vitro*. Thus, there is circumstantial evidence that digestion plays a role in AL fibrillogenesis.

The protein SAA has a molecular size of 12 500Da. AA isolated from fibrils varies between 3500 and 7000Da[40]. Proteolysis, which may be tissue specific, is responsible for the truncation. Neutrophil elastase, monocyte proteases and some cathepsins have been shown to be capable of digesting SAA. The question remains: what is the active protease *in vivo*? There seems to be polymorphism in the monocyte ectoproteases, in that cells from some individuals digest SAA to small peptides while others digest it to a size approximating that of AA[41]. One proposed scheme of pathogenesis of AA has the increased amounts of intact amyloidogenic isomorph of SAA produced during inflammation released from the circulating SAA–apolipoprotein complex, binding to tissue and being digested *in situ* to form the fibrils. Tissue culture studies have shown the generation of Congophilic material by murine peritoneal macrophages incubated with soluble SAA[42].

It has also been suggested that proteolysis accounts for the presence of fragments, as well as intact precursor, in both TTR and β_2-microglobulin deposits. Whether the fragments are epiphenomena or intrinsic to the process of amyloidogenesis is unknown.

Increased production of precursor is a factor in AA disease associated with inflammation. SAA gene transcription in the liver is stimulated by the cytokine interleukin (IL)-6 produced by inflammatory cells. Also, IL-1 and tumor necrosis factor (TNF) may influence SAA production but it is uncertain whether their effects are direct or via stimulation of IL-6 synthesis.

Clonal expansion results in increased production of amyloidogenic light chains in AL disease. It is also likely that the local amyloids (AIAPP, ACal and AANF) are the result of local overproduction, either because of clonal expansion (medullary carcinoma of the thyroid) or persistent stimulation (AANF, AIAPP). Aβ_2-microglobulin appears to be related to the failure of some dialysis membranes to clear the normal quantity of β_2-microglobulin produced daily. An alternative hypothesis suggests that the membranes have the capacity to increase the synthesis of β_2-microglobulin by inflammatory cells. It may be that both contribute to the enlarged precursor pool that ultimately leads to deposition.

Precursor synthesis in ATTR is no greater than normal and clearance experiments indicate that mutant TTR leave the serum more rapidly than the normal molecule, observations consistent with either more rapid catabolism or sequestration of the subunits into deposits. The data are not conclusive enough to define the role of precursor catabolism in amyloidogenesis.

Other components of amyloid deposits

Analyses of amyloid deposits have shown that other components (in addition to the fibril) are present. Three molecules which appear to be constituents of all amyloid deposits are the serum amyloid P-component (SAP), apolipoprotein E (ApoE) and the several heparan sulfate proteoglycans (HSPG) including perlecan, glypican and several syndecans. Of these, only ApoE has any intrinsic fibrillogenic potential; however, it is not extracted with the fibrils. It is possible that other accessory molecules will be discovered.

Serum amyloid P is a normal human serum protein that belongs to the same molecular family as CRP (pentraxins) and behaves like an acute phase reactant in the mouse but not in humans. Antibodies to SAP also react with some normal basement membranes. However, the molecular basis of the immunologic reactivity is not yet clear. Mice, in which the SAP gene has been inactivated by targeted disruption, have higher levels of circulating DNA and anti-DNA antibodies suggesting that the normal function of the protein is to bind free DNA[43]. Current data suggest that the P-component binds to the fibril after deposition and stabilizes it against digestion or resolubilization. In the non-fibrillar light-chain deposits of LCDD, P-component is not incorporated into the deposits. In patients who have both amyloid and non-amyloid light-chain deposits, only the amyloid contains P-component. Hence, staining of Congo red-positive tissue with anti-P-component serum is a confirmatory assay for the amyloid nature of the deposits.

The role of the HSPG, perlecan, is unclear. It binds to all amyloid fibrils and ultrastructural studies indicate that the relationship is intimate[44]. Recent data provide evidence that anionic small molecular HSPG analogs can inhibit experimental AA amyloid formation in mice[45]. The absence of other good, readily available, *in vivo* amyloid models has delayed the assessment of the effects of these molecules on other forms of amyloid, but the association of HSPG with the deposits has been established.

Other non-fibril precursor molecules have been found in some forms of amyloid, but not in others. Laminin and other basement membrane molecules have been isolated from some AA deposits. α_1-antichymotrypsin and α-synuclein have been found in Alzheimer's plaques. An 85kDa protein, of uncertain function, has been found in Aβ_2-microglobulin deposits.

Any attempt to integrate current knowledge into a general scheme of amyloidogenesis must account for a general failure to find fibrils in the cell synthesizing the precursor and that most precursors interact with other ligands while in the circulation. It must also consider a role for accessory molecules in either deposition or fibril stabilization. It could also be hypothesized that precursor molecules are always in an equilibrium state between amyloidogenic and non-amyloidogenic conformers and that equilibrium is influenced by synthetic (including secretory) and catabolic rates and interactions with other molecules, most of which function to prevent what happens to the precursors in the test tube from happening *in vivo* (Fig. 191.6).

It is not clear whether organ dysfunction is produced by toxicity to normal cells, replacement of normal structures by fibrils, a combination of both or other mechanisms yet to be elucidated.

MANAGEMENT

The therapeutic approach to AA consists of treatment of the primary infectious or inflammatory process. Chemotherapy for tuberculosis has resulted in a decrease in the incidence of AA and some reports of resolution. The use of chlorambucil for the treatment of JCA has reduced the frequency of AA in that disorder, although with a risk of subsequent leukemia[46]. It may be assumed that effective control of the inflammatory process with any other disease-modifying agent (e.g. methotrexate) would have a similar impact. Similarly, the discovery that colchicine reduced the frequency of inflammatory episodes in patients with Familial Mediterranean Fever with a reduction in the incidence of renal AA deposition was a powerful demonstration of prophylaxis by reducing inflammation (see Chapter 158). It is still uncertain whether the institution of colchicine treatment after the appearance of AA disease is effective. There have been sporadic reports of resolution of AA associated with other disorders during the administration of colchicine. Colchicine has not shown efficacy in any amyloid other than AA and the basis for its effect is likely to be related to its capacity to suppress some forms of inflammation by altering expression of cell surface molecules required for neutrophil–endothelial cell interactions. It appears that reduction of the SAA level to less than 10 mg/l allows resorption of the deposits and prevents further accumulation.

Two studies have shown increased survival in AL patients treated with a regimen similar to that used for multiple myeloma, i.e. melphalan and prednisone every 6 weeks[47,48]. The rationale is reduction of the number of cells producing the amyloid precursor with an accompanying reduction in protein product and fibril formation. In terms of survival, patients with cardiac disease are the least responsive. Colchicine did not add to the efficacy of the melphalan–prednisone regimen. An extension of this approach has been the use of intensive alkylating agent treatment followed by autologous stem cell transplantation. Long-term studies of this modality are in progress in myeloma and some centers are using similar protocols in AL[49,50]. Although no randomized prospective control studies have been done, survival of AL patients has been prolonged relative to historic controls. The danger with this interpretation

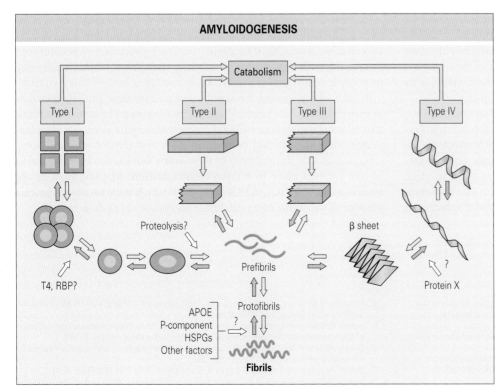

AMYLOIDOGENESIS

Fig. 191.6 In vivo amyloidogenesis is a function of the quality and quantity of the precursor protein. Quality is defined in terms of precursor conformation, i.e. whether conformation closer to the protofibrillar state than the native protein. The amount of precursor molecule in that conformation is determined by the absolute concentration of the native protein, subject to its rate of synthesis and degradation, and the nature of the equilibrium between amyloidogenic and non-amyloidogenic conformations. The four types of amyloid depicted here reflect different pathways of generating the amyloidogenic precursor. Type I typified by transthyretin is dependent on a population of potentially misfolded monomers arising from the tetramer. It may also be seen in some instances of AL. Type II results from cleavage of a non-amyloidogenic parent molecule, releasing an amyloidogenic fragment. This is seen in the generation of Aβ from AβPP in Alzheimer's disease or in the gelsolin diseases, where a mutation generates a new cleavage site in the parent molecule. Type III is represented by AA, in which the apparently physiologic cleavage of SAA to small peptides is incomplete, yielding the amyloidogenic AA fragment. Type IV is the least well understood, the precursor going from a soluble to protofibrillar conformation, in an apparently templated fashion, without any form of modification. This appears to be the case in the prion disorders.

is that the patients offered the procedure are highly selected for features that may be associated with good outcome even without high intensity chemotherapy. Individuals with reduced ventricular ejection fractions have been uniformly eliminated as candidates because of severe, sometimes fatal complications surrounding the procedure. The role of the procedure should become clarified over the next year or two.

Attempts to treat TTR amyloidosis have also focused on reducing the production of the amyloidogenic precursor. A number of familial amyloidotic polyneuropathy and cardiomyopathy patients have undergone liver transplantation in an effort to replace the organ expressing the gene encoding the amyloidogenic protein with one bearing two normal alleles[28]. Early outcomes suggest that the procedure will be successful if it is performed before the patient becomes malnourished secondary to autonomic involvement of the gut. The first therapeutic responses were in symptoms related to the autonomic neuropathy, with reductions in diarrhea. In general it appears that progression of the neurologic disease is arrested, with improvement in some patients. There is some evidence that cardiac disease, in patients other than those having the val30met transthyretin mutation, progresses despite a successful transplant. The combination of liver and heart transplantation has been performed in some patients. It is still too early to evaluate the full impact of the procedure.

Although there is no direct treatment for $A\beta_2$-microglobulin, dialysis centers are moving from cuprophan membranes to other membranes which seem to remove β_2-microglobulin more effectively. In addition, methods are being developed for removal of the molecule during dialysis. It is too early to assess the impact of these measures on the frequency or severity of this form of amyloidosis.

There is no therapeutic measure currently available which acts on the processes of fibrillogenesis and deposition. Dimethyl sulfoxide (DMSO) has been proposed as a therapeutic agent which may solubilize deposits and a number of patients with both AA and AL have received the material in uncontrolled trials. There appeared to be salutary effects in some patients with AA, but the accompanying body odor made it unacceptable. It is now only used topically in individuals with extensive cutaneous amyloidosis.

Supportive therapy for patients with the amyloidoses has improved considerably. The availability of antibiotics to treat symptoms of bacterial overgrowth, urinary tract infections occurring secondary to neurogenic bladder and infections occurring while on antineoplastic or immunosuppressive agents have all added to survival and quality of life.

Ephedrine compounds can be used to treat orthostatic hypotension in the course of either AL or familial amyloidotic polyneuropathy. Octreotide, a peptide homolog of somatostatin, has been effective in reducing diarrhea in some patients with amyloid enteropathy.

Patients with amyloid heart disease present major therapeutic problems. Loop diuretics are the main therapeutic agents for the management of fluid overload. However, maintaining a balance between edema and intravascular contraction can be difficult. In patients with reaccumulating pleural effusions with severe dyspnea, it is possible to place a pleuroabdominal shunt so that the fluid drains into the abdomen where it may be better tolerated. In patients who have substantial hepatosplenomegaly this is not an option. Digitalis glycosides and calcium channel blockers should be avoided in patients with cardiac involvement. Both have been reported to increase heart failure[51,52]. Digoxin has also been associated with arrhythmias. Although the poor outcomes were reported with nifedipine and verapamil, it is reasonable to assume that the effect is generic and will also be seen with newer members of this family of drugs. The mechanism of toxicity appears to be related to the fibrils' capacity to bind the drugs, effectively increasing their concentration in the myocardium. Binding has been demonstrated *in vitro* but not *in vivo*; increased myocardial concentrations have not been documented.

Transplants have proved successful for patients with organ failure. In AA, particularly if the primary inflammatory process can be modified or aborted, renal transplant is reasonable. A number of patients with AL or AA and renal failure have undergone renal transplantation[53]. Some of them have died of other manifestations of their disease. Others have accumulated amyloid in the transplanted organ within 4 years after transplantation. In the latter group of patients it is not clear whether their initial therapy stopped the production of the amyloidogenic light chain. If that were the case, amyloid might not recur in the new kidney unless the same clone re-emerged.

Current approaches to treatment have involved the development of small molecules which interfere with the processes of fibrillogenesis and deposition. One compound with such potential (4-iodo-4-doxirubicin) was identified serendipitously during the course of a clinical trial for multiple myeloma[54]. The drug has been shown to reduce deposits in both animal models and humans. However responses are not uniform. A recent trial involving three centers showed some effect in 15% of the patients. It may be a useful agent in some patients, probably in conjunction with other treatment.

Two other trials are in early stages. One is testing an anionic sulfonate which inhibits AA deposition in animals, presumably by interfering with the interaction between the fibril and perlecan[45]; the other is evaluating a compound that blocks the binding of SAP to fibrils *in vitro*.

Laboratory studies suggested that sulfite might inhibit formation of the transthyretin fibril precursor in TTR amyloidosis. A more systematic approach based on ligand binding studies have suggested that a variety of molecules can stabilize the ttr tetramer and reduce fibril formation *in vitro*[55].

Current thinking suggests that a variety of agents targeting various steps in the pathway of amyloidogenesis will be required to achieve consistent clinical results, thus agents reducing precursor concentration, interfering with aggregation, inhibiting tissue deposition or allowing proteolytic removal may all have a role sometime in the clinical course.

In each case potential therapeutic compounds were initially tested in *in vitro* fibrillogenesis assays. While the *in vitro* assays have provided substantial information concerning the structural requirements for fibril formation, they are generally performed under non-physiologic conditions. Compounds that show activity in these assays will have to be evaluated in *in vivo* systems prior to human administration. At present there are animal models for AA, ATTR and ABPP which may be useful for this purpose as well as for more detailed investigations of pathogenesis.

REFERENCES

1. Wright MD, Calkins E, Breen W *et al*. Relationship of amyloid to aging. Review of the literature and systematic study of 83 patients derived from a general hospital population. Medicine 1969; 48: 39–60.
2. Kyle RA, Gertz MA. Primary systemic amyloidosis: clinical and laboratory features in 474 cases. Sem Hemat 1995; 32: 45–59.
3. Kyle RA, Linos A, Beard CM *et al*. Incidence and natural history of primary systemic amyloidosis in Olmsted County, Minnesota, 1950 through 1989. Blood 1992; 79: 1817–1822.
4. Hazenberg BPC, van Rijswijk MH. Clinical and therapeutic aspects of AA amyloidosis. Baillière's Clin Rheumatol 1994; 8: 661–690.
5. Sipe J. Revised nomenclature for serum amyloid A (SAA). Nomenclature Committee of the International Society of Amyloidosis. Part 2. Amyloid 1999; 6: 67–70.
6. Booth DR, Booth SE, Gillmore JD *et al*. SAA1 alleles as risk factors in reactive systemic AA amyloidosis. Amyloid 1998; 5: 262–265.
7. Baba S, Masago SA, Takahashi T *et al*. A novel allelic variant of serum amyloid A, SAA1 γ: genomic evidence, evolution, frequency and implication as a risk factor for

reactive systemic AA-amyloidosis. Hum Molec Genet 1995; 4: 1083–1087.

8. Danesh J, Muir J, Wong YK et al. Risk factors for coronary heart disease and acute-phase proteins. A population-based study. Euro Heart J 1999; Jul 1920: 954–959.

9. Buck FS, Koss MN, Sherrod AE et al. Ethnic distribution of amyloidosis: an autopsy study. Mod Pathol 1989; 2: 372–377.

10. Gershoni-Baruch R, Brik R, Shinawi M et al. SAA1 gene polymorphism as a risk factor for the development of amyloidosis of FMF. IXth International Symposium on Amyloidosis, Budapest, 17 July 2001.

11. Schaffer J, Floege J, Koch KM. Clinical aspects of dialysis-related amyloidosis. Contrib Nephrol 1995; 112: 90–96.

12. Pras M, Itzchaki M, Prelli F et al. Amyloid arthropathy: characterization of the amyloid protein. Clin Exp Rheumatol 1985; 3: 327–331.

13. Westmark KD, Weissman BN. Complications of axial arthropathies. Orthoped Clin North Am 1990; 21: 423–435.

14. Ikegaya N, Hishida A, Sawada K et al. Ultrasonographic evaluation of the carpal tunnel syndrome in hemodialysis patients. Clin Nephrol 1995; 44: 231–237.

15. Eyanson S, Benson MD. Erosive arthritis in hereditary amyloidosis. Arth Rheum 1983; 26: 1145–1149.

16. Kyle RA, Gertz MA, Linke RP. Amyloid localized to tenosynovium at carpal tunnel release. Immunohistochemical identification of amyloid type. Am J Clin Pathol 1992; 97: 250–253.

17. Helin HJ, Korpela MM, Mustonen JT et al. Renal biopsy findings and clinicopathologic correlations in rheumatoid arthritis. Arth Rheum 1995; 38: 242–247.

18. Bohle A, Wehrmann M, Eissele R et al. The long-term prognosis of AA and AL renal amyloidosis and the pathogenesis of chronic renal failure in renal amyloidosis. Pathol Res Practice 1993; 189: 316–331.

19. Ekelund L. Radiologic findings in renal amyloidosis. Am J Roentgen 1977; 129: 851–853.

20. Jacobson DR, Gorevic PD, Buxbaum JN. A homozygous transthyretin variant associated with senile systemic amyloidosis: evidence for a late-onset disease of genetic etiology. Am J Hum Genet 1990; 47: 127–136.

21. Christmansson L, Betsholtz C, Gustavsson Å et al. The transthyretin cDNA sequence is normal in transthyretin-derived senile systemic amyloidosis. FEBS Lett 1991; 281: 177–180.

22. Simons M, Isner JM. Assessment of relative sensitivities of noninvasive tests for cardiac amyloidosis in documented cardiac amyloidosis. Am J Cardiol 1992; 68: 425–427.

23. Simmons Z, Blaivas M, Aguilera AJ et al. Low diagnostic yield of sural nerve biopsy in patients with peripheral neuropathy and primary amyloidosis. J Neurol Sci 1993; 120: 60–63.

24. Lee JG, Wilson JAP, Gottfried MR. Gastrointestinal manifestations of amyloidosis. Southern Med J 1994; 87: 243–247.

25. Mumford AD, O'Donnell J, Gillmore JD et al. Bleeding symptoms and coagulation abnormalities in 337 patients with AL-amyloidosis. Brit J Haematol 2000; 110: 454–460.

26. Buxbaum JN. Mechanisms of disease: monoclonal immunoglobulin deposition. Hematol Oncol Clin N Am 1993; 6: 323–346.

27. Gertz MA, Greipp PR, Kyle RA. Classification of amyloidosis by the detection of clonal excess of plasma cells in the bone marrow. J Lab Clin Med 1991; 118: 33–99.

28. Holmgren G, Ericzon BG, Groth CG et al. Clinical improvement and amyloid regression after liver transplantation in hereditary transthyretin amyloidosis. Lancet 1993; 341: 1113–1116.

29. Hawkins PN, Cavender JP, Pepys MB. Evaluation of systemic amyloidosis by scintigraphy with ^{125}I-labeled serum amyloid P component. N Engl J Med 1990; 323: 508–513.

30. Aprile C, Marinone G, Saponaro R et al. Cardiac and pleuropulmonary AL amyloid imaging with technetium-99m labelled aprotinin. Eur J Nucl Med 1995; Dec 1922: 1393–1401.

31. Klemi PJ, Sorsa S, Happonen RP. Fine-needle aspiration biopsy from subcutaneous fat. An easy way to diagnose secondary amyloidosis. Scand J Rheumatol 1987; 16: 429–431.

32. Gertz MA, Li CY, Shirahama T et al. Utility of subcutaneous fat aspiration for the diagnosis of systemic amyloidosis (immunoglobulin light chain). Arch Intern Med 1988; 148: 929–933.

33. Gallo GR, Feiner HD, Chuba JV et al. Characterization of tissue amyloid by immunofluorescence microscopy. Clin Immunol Immunopathol 1986; 39: 479–490.

34. McCutchen SL, Lai Z, Miroy GJ et al. Comparison of lethal and nonlethal transthyretin variants and their relationship to amyloid disease. Biochemistry 1995; 34: 13527–13536.

35. Benson MD, Uemichi T. Transthyretin amyloidosis. Amyloid. Internat J Experiment Clin Invest 1996; 3: 44–56.

36. Stevens FJ, Myatt EA, Chang CH et al. A molecular model for self-assembly of amyloid fibrils: immunoglobulin light chains. Biochemistry 1995; 34: 10697–106702.

37. Buxbaum J. Aberrant immunoglobulin synthesis in light chain amyloidosis. Free light chain and light chain fragment production by human bone marrow cells in short-term tissue culture. J Clin Inv 1986; 78: 798–806.

38. Preud'homme JL, Ganeval D, Grunfeld JP. Immunoglobulin synthesis in primary and myeloma amyloidosis. Clin Exp Immunol 1988; 73: 389–396.

39. Miyata T, Inagi R, Lida Y et al. Involvement of beta$_2$ microglobulin with advanced glycation end products in the pathogenesis of hemodialysis-associated amyloidosis. J Clin Invest 1994; 93: 521–528.

40. Sipe JD. Amyloidosis. Ann Rev Biochem 1992; 61: 947–975.

41. Lavie G, Zucker-Franklin D, Franklin EC. Degradation of serum amyloid A protein by surface-associated enzymes of human blood monocytes. J Exp Med 1978; 148: 1020–1031.

42. Kluve-Beckerman B, Manaloor J, Liepnieks JJ et al. SAA is processed intracellularly by macrophages prior to deposition as amyloid. IXth International Symposium on Amyloidosis, Budapest, 17 July 2001.

43. Botto M, Hawkins PN, Bickerstaff MC et al. Amyloid deposition is delayed in mice with targeted deletion of the serum amyloid P component gene. Nat Med 1997; 3: 855–859.

44. Inoue S, Kuroiwa M, Saraiva MJ et al. Ultrastructure of familial amyloid polyneuropathy amyloid fibrils: examination with high-resolution electron microscopy. J Struct Biol 1998; 124: 1–12.

45. Kisilevsky R, Lemieux LJ, Fraser PE et al. Arresting amyloidosis in vivo using small-molecule anionic sulphonates or sulphates: implications for Alzheimer's disease. Nat Med 1995; 1: 143–148.

46. David J, Vouyiouka O, Ansell BM et al. Amyloidosis in juvenile chronic arthritis: a morbidity and mortality study. Clin Exp Rheumatol 1993; 11: 85–90.

47. Kyle RA, Gertz MA, Garton JP et al. Primary systemic amyloidosis (AL): randomized trial of colchicine vs. melphalan and prednisone vs. melphalan, prednisone, and colchicine. In: Kisilevsky R, Benson MD, Frangione B et al., eds. Amyloid and amyloidosis 1993. New York: Parthenon; 1994: 648–650.

48. Skinner M, Anderson J, Simms R et al. Treatment of 100 patients with primary amyloidosis: a randomized trial of melphalan, prednisone, and colchicine versus colchicine only. Am J Med 1996; 100: 290–298.

49. Dember LM, Sanchorawala V, Seldin DC et al. Effect of dose-intensive intravenous melphalan and autologous blood stem-cell transplantation on al amyloidosis-associated renal disease. Ann Intern Med 2001; 134: 746–753.

50. Dispenzieri A, Lacy MQ, Kyle RA et al. Eligibility for hematopoietic stem-cell transplantation for primary systemic amyloidosis is a favorable prognostic factor for survival. J Clin Oncol 2001; 1919: 3350–3356.

51. Gertz MA, Skinner M, Connors LG et al. Selective binding of nifedipine to amyloid fibrils. Am J Cardiol 1985; 55: 1646.

52. Rubinow A, Skinner M, Cohen AS. Digoxin sensitivity in amyloid cardiomyopathy. Circulation 1981; 63: 1285–1288.

53. Pasternack A, Ahonen J, Kuhlback B. Renal transplantation in 45 patients with amyloidosis. Transplantation 1986; 42: 598–601.

54. Merlini G, Anesi E, Garini P et al. Treatment of AL amyloidosis with 4'-Iodo-4'-deoxydoxorubicin: an update. Blood 1999; 93: 1112–1113.

55. Klabunde T, Petrassi HM, Oza VB et al. Rational design of potent human transthyretin amyloid disease inhibitors. Nat Struct Biol 2000; 7: 312–321.

SECTION
16

METABOLIC BONE DISEASES

192 Bone structure and function

Nancy Lane, Jan Dequeker and Gregory R Mundy

- The unique physical and chemical properties of bone relate to its three main functions: the provision of support and protection, and calcium homeostasis
- Macroscopically, there are two types of bone: dense cortical bone and spongy cancellous bone
- Bone turnover is mediated by coupling of the bone-forming cellular activity of osteoblasts and the bone-resorbing osteoclasts
- The bone matrix consists of type I collagen fibers and the mineral apatite
- Proteoglycans, Gla-containing proteins and glycoproteins, such as osteocalcin and bone sialoprotein, are unique to the osteogenic phenotype and play key functional roles
- Polypeptide growth factors such as IGF-I and IGF-II play an important role in the growth, development and homeostasis of skeletal tissues
- Bone remodeling and repair are mediated by systemic hormones and local factors

The skeleton occupies about 9% of the body by bulk and about 17% by weight. The stability and immutability of dry bones and their persistence for centuries, and even millions of years, after the soft tissues have turned to dust give us a false idea of bone during life. Its fixity after death is in sharp contrast to its ceaseless activity in life. (Cooke 1955)[1]

BONE AS AN ORGAN

Functional structure

The unique physical and chemical attributes of bone mirror the diversity of its functions. The most obvious function is its supportive role: strong, hard bones make useful limbs. A second important function is the protection of vital soft tissues such as the brain, spinal cord, heart and bone marrow. Thirdly, bone is involved in calcium homeostasis. Bone also plays an important role as a trap for a variety of bloodborne ions, such as lead, fluoride and strontium, which may exchange with calcium ions or otherwise become incorporated within the apatite crystal lattice or bound to the organic matrix of bone.

Bone is an ideal supporting material by virtue of its remarkable strength. It is a two-phase material, consisting of two contrasting substances: fibrous protein collagen (which is strong in tension) and the mineral apatite (which is strong in compression). The crystallites of apatite (or calcium phosphates) are exceedingly small and are aligned along the collagen fibrils. The way in which these two substances are actually bound together is still not properly understood. If the mineral matter is removed by acids (e.g. ethylenediaminetetraacetic acid, EDTA), the result is a rubbery bone which is very flexible. If only the organic matter is destroyed, a brittle bone results. In some way the mineral matter locks in the protein to form an organic material that is

able to survive for millions of years. Presumably, the close packing of the crystals seals off the organic matter from naturally destructive agents.

The internal architecture must be appropriate for the function it has to perform. For a given volume of material to support a certain weight, it is more efficient that this material is organized in the form of a hollow cylinder rather than as a solid block, as seen in the long bones of the limbs.

Macroscopic organization of bone

The outer cortex of the midshafts is the solid, compact part of limb bones. At the ends, where they approach the joints, the bones have a loose, spongy texture. When examined closely, this spongy-looking tissue is, in fact, well organized, showing a delicate internal architecture. There is a series of narrow beams, or trabeculae, joined by minor cross struts, which together form an intricate three-dimensional scaffolding. The main trabeculae line up along the major axes of force to which the bone is subjected during development. When the weight of the body is transmitted from one bone to another, as at the knee or hip joints during walking, for example, the forces are distributed through the trabeculae to the compact cortex of the outer parts of the shafts. This complexity at the ends of the bones is necessary because both movement and weight have to be transmitted with the bones in different positions. In whatever manner the limbs are positioned, within reason, the forces can still be effectively distributed through the trabeculae[2].

At the macroscopic level there are thus two major types of bone: compact or cortical bone and trabecular or cancellous bone (Fig. 192.1). Cortical bone is located in the diaphyses of long bones and on the surfaces of flat bones. There is also a thin cortical shell at the epiphyses

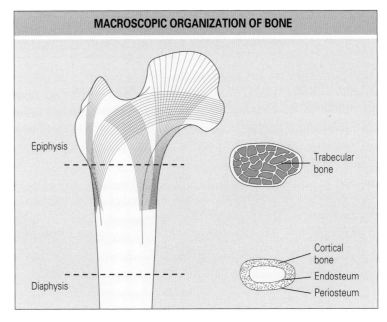

MACROSCOPIC ORGANIZATION OF BONE

Epiphysis

Trabecular bone

Cortical bone

Endosteum

Periosteum

Diaphysis

Fig. 192.1 Macroscopic organization of bone.

and metaphyses of long bones. Trabecular bone is limited to the epiphyseal and metaphyseal regions of long bones and is present within the cortical coverings in the smaller flat and short bones. Consequently, there are two bone surfaces. Where the bone is in contact with the soft tissues is an external surface (periosteal) and where the bone is in contact with the bone marrow there is an internal surface (endosteal). These surfaces are lined with osteogenic cells organized in layers termed the periosteum and endosteum, respectively.

The difference between cortical bone and trabecular bone is both structural and functional. They are, however, constituted of the same cells and the same matrix elements. The structural differences are essentially quantitative: 80–90% of the volume of compact bone is calcified, versus 15–25% in trabecular bone (the remaining volume is occupied by the bone marrow), but 70–85% of the interface with soft tissues is at the endosteal bone surface. The functional differences are a consequence of these structural differences, and vice versa. Cortical bone fulfils mainly (but not exclusively) a mechanical and protective function and the trabecular bone a metabolic and mechanical function[3].

Cortical bone
Macroscopically, cortical bone appears dense and is histologically characterized as haversian bone. The haversian systems, or secondary osteons, are approximate cylindric structures with concentric lamellae. The osteons in the diaphyses of the long bones are oriented in the direction of the long axis of the bone. Figure 192.2 is a schematic representation of cortical bone tissue. However, when bone is formed very rapidly (e.g. during histogenesis, fracture healing, tumors or metabolic bone diseases) there is no preferential organization of collagen fibers. They are then found in more or less randomly oriented bundles. This type is called woven bone, as opposed to lamellar.

An osteon is a packet of bone formed in the haversian system. The degree of mineralization of neighboring osteons varies considerably. The bone in young osteons is less dense, as revealed by microradiography, and the density or mineral content increases with age. This end phase of mineralization may take weeks, months or even years to be completed. This less dense bone may often undergo resorption before achieving complete mineralization.

Cancellous bone
Cancellous bone is structurally a three-dimensional lattice composed of bone plates and bone column within the cortical shell. The mechanical properties and the role in mineral metabolism of both types of bone architecture are critical to the skeleton's strength.

BONE AS A TISSUE

Microscopic organization
Bone matrix and mineral
Bone is formed by collagen fibers (type I – 90% of total proteins), usually oriented in a preferential direction, and ground substance. Spindle-shaped crystals of hydroxyapatite ($Ca_{10}(PO_4)_6(OH)_2$) are found on the collagen fibers, within them and in the ground substance. They are generally oriented in the same preferential direction as the collagen fibers. The ground substance is essentially composed of glycoproteins and proteoglycans. These highly anionic complexes have a very high ion-binding capacity and are thought to play an important role in the calcification process and the fixation of hydroxyapatite crystals to the collagen fibers.

Cellular organization within the bone matrix: osteocytes
The calcified bone matrix is not metabolically inert and cells (osteocytes) are found embedded deep within the bone in small osteocytic lacunae (25 000/mm³ of bone). They were originally bone-forming cells (osteoblasts) but have been trapped by their own production of bone matrix which later became calcified. These cells have numerous, long cell processes, rich in microfilaments, which are in contact with cell processes from other osteocytes (frequent gap junctions), or with processes from the cells lining the bone surface (osteoblasts or flat lining cells in the endosteum or periosteum). These processes are organized during the formation of the matrix and before its calcification; they form a network of thin canaliculi within the entire bone matrix (Fig. 192.3). There is a space between the osteocyte plasma membrane and the bone matrix itself, both in the lacunae and in the canaliculi, termed the periosteocytic space, which is filled with extracellular fluid (bone ECF).

Whether osteocytes are able to synthesize new bone matrix or resorb it at the surface of the osteocytic lacunae is still questionable. On the other hand, osteocytes may be the primary cells in bone which respond to the mechanical loading by sending signals through the canaliculi to the cell surface. The fate of the osteocytes is to be phagocytosed or to apoptose and be digested, together with the other components of bone, during

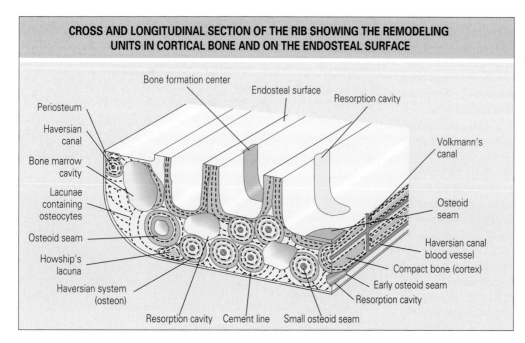

CROSS AND LONGITUDINAL SECTION OF THE RIB SHOWING THE REMODELING UNITS IN CORTICAL BONE AND ON THE ENDOSTEAL SURFACE

Labels: Bone formation center; Endosteal surface; Resorption cavity; Periosteum; Haversian canal; Bone marrow cavity; Volkmann's canal; Lacunae containing osteocytes; Osteoid seam; Howship's lacuna; Osteoid seam; Haversian canal blood vessel; Compact bone (cortex); Haversian system (osteon); Early osteoid seam; Resorption cavity; Resorption cavity; Cement line; Small osteoid seam

Fig. 192.2 Cross and longitudinal sections of the rib showing the remodeling units in cortical bone and on the endosteal surface. Three-dimensional view of the gross and microscopic structure of adult human bone. (Adapted from Jaworsky[3].)

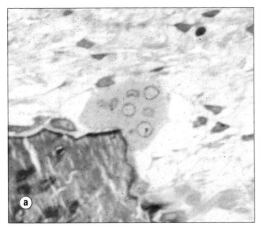

SCHEMATIC REPRESENTATION OF BONE CELL TYPES, ORIGIN AND MARKERS

Fig. 192.3 Schematic representation of bone cell types, origin and markers. ALP, alkaline phosphatase; CZ, clear zone; TRAP, tartrate-resistant acid phosphatase.

deformation is critical even to the survival of these cells. In addition, with disuse the osteocytes express collagenase, suggesting that this cell has the ability to regulate the recruitment of bone forming and resorbing cells, as well as modulate its own local microenvironment.

Cells of the bone surface

Mesenchymal cells line the bone surfaces. These cells line the external endosteal surfaces of both cortical and trabecular bone and the internal endosteal surfaces of haversian bone. The periosteal surface of all bones is covered by a much more extensive cellular layer of mesenchymal cells and fibroblasts.

The osteoblast and bone formation

The osteoblast is the bone-lining cell responsible for the production of the matrix constituents (collagen and ground substance). It also plays an important part in the calcification process. It originates from a local mesenchymal stem cell (bone marrow stromal stem cell or connective tissue mesenchymal cell). The presence of the nuclear factor, CBFA1, designates differentiation of mesenchymal stem cells into the osteo-blastic lineage. These precursors, following the correct stimulation, undergo proliferation and differentiate into preosteoblasts and the mature osteoblasts. Osteoblasts never appear or function individually but are always found in clusters of cuboidal cells along the bone surface (approximately 100–400 cells per bone-forming site).

At the light microscopic level the osteoblast is characterized by a round nucleus at the base of the cell. Osteoblasts are always found lining a layer of bone matrix which they are producing which is not yet calci-fied (osteoid tissue). The presence of the osteoid is due to a time lag between matrix formation and its subsequent calcification: the osteoid maturation period takes about 10 days. Behind the osteoblast are usually found one or two layers of activated mesenchymal cells and pre-osteoblasts. The plasma membrane of the osteoblast is characteristically

osteoclastic bone resorption. Osteocytes may also play a role in the local regulation of bone turnover. Recent evidence that mechanical strain actually reduces the rate of osteocyte apoptosis, suggests that matrix

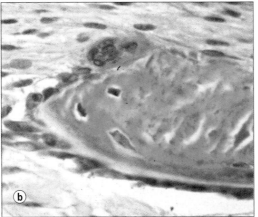

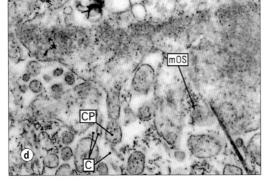

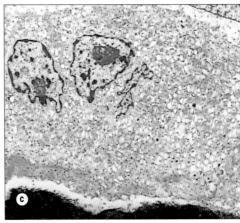

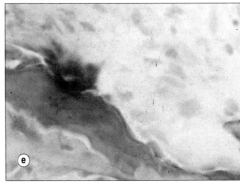

Fig. 192.4 Osteoclasts. Osteoclasts are large cells, irregularly delimited, with prolongations of their abundant basophilic cytoplasm. The size and number of nuclei are variable. Osteoclasts are thought to be derived from blood monocytes but it is not known whether they form from repeated nuclear divisions in the cell or from fusion of a number of cells. Osteoclasts are mostly found on the bone surface at sites of active bone resorption, where they erode into the bone. These resorption sites are called Howship's lacunae. (a) Micrograph of a toluidine blue-stained epoxy resin section showing an osteoclast with six nuclei on the bone surface. (b) Micrograph of a gold-stained acrylic resin section of bone showing active osteoblast deposition of new osteoid as well as active resorption by a multinucleate osteoclast lying in a Howship's lacuna. (c) Electron micrograph of an osteoblast showing a ruffled border on the osteoclast interface with bone. Many Golgi, lysosomes, secretory vesicles and abundant mitochondria can be observed. (d) High-power electron micrograph of the ruffled border showing numerous fine cytoplasmic processes extending into the osteoid, with some fragments of mineralized osteoid between the processes. (e) Micrograph of a frozen section of bone showing abundant acid phosphatase activity in an osteoclast. (Reproduced with permission from Stevens and Lowe[4].)

rich in alkaline phosphatase, whose presence in the serum alkaline phosphatase is used as an index of bone formation. The membrane has also been shown to have receptors for parathyroid hormone (PTH), though not for calcitonin. Osteoblasts also express estrogen receptors in their nuclei. Towards the end of the secreting period the osteoblasts suffer one of a number of fates, including apoptosis (50%), becoming a flat lining cell or an osteocyte. The lifespan of the osteoblast varies from 15 days to 8 weeks. Glucocorticoid use reduces the lifespan of osteoblasts by increasing the rate of programmed cell death, or apoptosis, and this may account for some of the reduction in bone formation with glucocorticoid use.

The osteoclast and bone resorption

The osteoclast is the bone-lining cell responsible for bone resorption. Osteoclast precursors arise from hematopoietic stem cells in the bone marrow. Osteoclast precursor cells arise from the macrophage lineage through M-CSF stimulation, which is necessary for the differentiation, proliferation and survival of the cells of the macrophage lineage. The further progression into a functional osteoclast (presence of calcitonin receptor and carbonic anhydrase expression) requires other local factors, including the presence of bone stromal or osteoblast cells. A protein from the osteoblastic cell-receptor activator of NK (natural killer)-κB ligand (RANKL) functions as a receptor and interacts with receptor activator of NK-κB (RANK) receptor on the precursor osteoclast cells and stimulates osteoclastogenesis. Interestingly, a decoy receptor, osteoprotegerin (OPG), is found on osteoblastic cells and this controls the amount of osteoclastogenesis[7–9].

The osteoclast is a giant multinucleated cell (4–20 nuclei) usually found in contact with a calcified bone surface and within a lacuna (Howship's lacuna) which is the result of its own resorptive activity (Fig. 192.4). It is possible to find up to four or five osteoclasts in the same resorptive site, but there usually are only one or two per site. The contact zone with the bone is characterized by the presence of a ruffled border and of dense patches on each side of it, called the sealing zone (clear zone). The sealing zone separates the ruffled border from the extracellular space and may function to isolate the space in which the cellular activity resulting in dissolution of bone by the osteoclast takes place. The characteristic enzymatic marker of the osteoclast is tartrate-resistant acid phosphatase (TRAP).

Lysosomal enzymes are actively synthesized by the osteoclast and are found in the endoplasmic reticulum, Golgi, and many transport vesicles. These lysosomal enzymes are secreted, via the ruffled border, into the extracellular bone resorbing compartment where they achieve high extracellular concentrations because the compartment is sealed off. The transport and targeting of these enzymes for secretion at the apical pole of the osteoclast involves mannose-6-phosphate receptors.

The extracellular bone resorbing compartment is therefore the functional equivalent of a secondary lysosome with (i) a low pH, (ii) lysosomal enzymes, and (iii) the substrate. The low pH dissolves the crystals, exposing the matrix; the enzymes, now at optimal pH, degrade the matrix components. The residues from this extracellular digestion are either internalized, transported across the cell (transcytosis) and released at the basolateral domain, or released during periods of relapse of the sealing zone.

Chronologically, the crystals are mobilized by digestion of their links to collagen (non-collagenous proteins) and dissolved by the acid environment; the residual collagen fibers are digested by either the activation of latent collagenase or the action of cathepsins at low pH. Clinically, this explains why bone resorption may affect Ca and inorganic phosphate (P_i) levels in the plasma, and why hydroxyproline concentration in the urine is used as an indirect measurement of bone resorption in humans (collagen type I is highly enriched in hydroxyproline).

Coupling bone formation–bone resorption

The activity of these bone cells along the surfaces of bone results in bone remodeling. This is the process by which bone grows and is turned over. Bone formation and resorption do not, however, occur along the bone surface at random: they are part of the turnover mechanism replacing old bone with new. In the normal adult skeleton, bone formation occurs only where bone resorption has previously occurred. The sequence of events at the remodeling site is therefore activation–resorption–formation (Fig. 192.5). During the intermediate phase between resorption and formation (reversal phase) osteoclasts undergo apoptosis[5] and a cement line, marking the limit of resorption and 'cementing' together the old

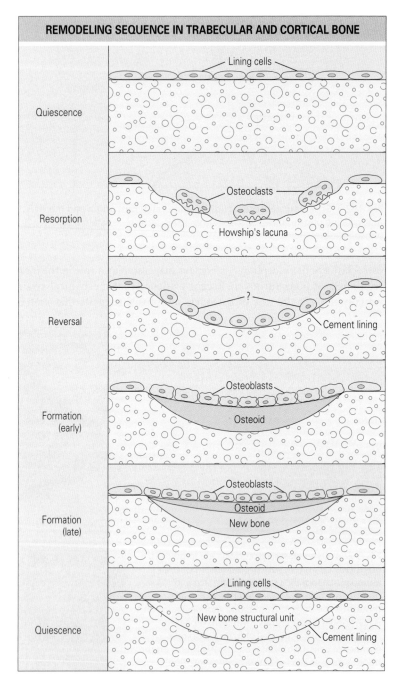

REMODELING SEQUENCE IN TRABECULAR AND CORTICAL BONE

Quiescence — Lining cells

Resorption — Osteoclasts — Howship's lacuna

Reversal — ? — Cement lining

Formation (early) — Osteoblasts — Osteoid

Formation (late) — Osteoblasts — Osteoid — New bone

Quiescence — Lining cells — New bone structural unit — Cement lining

Fig. 192.5 Remodeling sequence in trabecular and cortical bone. The remodeling sequence of bone is initiated by osteoclastic resorption followed by the absence of osteoclasts or osteoblasts (the reversal phase). Subsequently, osteoblasts appear within the resorption bay (Howship's lacuna) and synthesize matrix (the formative phase) until a new packet of bone (the osteon) is produced. In non-growing young adults the amounts of matrix resorbed and synthesized are in equilibrium. In older individuals, on the other hand, the amount of new bone is less than the amount removed, resulting in a net decrease in skeletal mass.

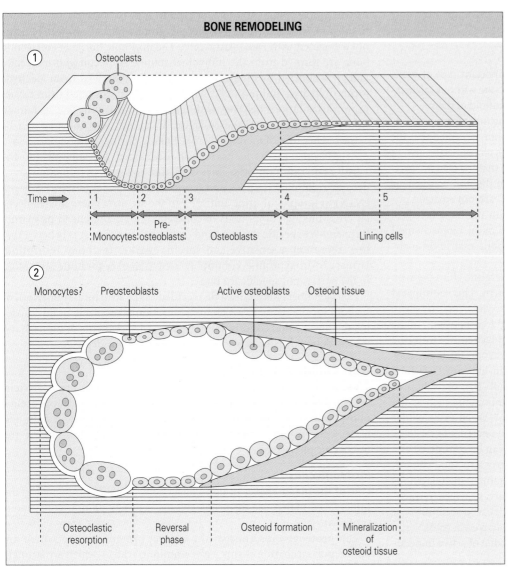

BONE REMODELING

Fig. 192.6 Bone remodeling. Three-dimensional illustration of remodeling through a trabecular plate. (1) Osteoclasts resorb the bone to form a Howship's lacuna. Preosteoblasts divide and become osteoblasts, which form osteoid. After a certain time the osteoid is mineralized and the osteoblasts dedifferentiate to flat lining cells. (2) Bone remodeling unit in the haversian envelope. This shows a cutting cone with osteoclastic resorption and a closing cone with lamellar bone formation. (Adapted from Eriksen[6].)

and the new bone, is formed (Fig. 192.6). At present, the exact coupling mechanism between bone formation and bone resorption is not yet elucidated. However, it is thought that locally produced cytokines (e.g. growth factors) may play a crucial role in the process[7–9].

THE CONSTITUENTS OF BONE

Bone is a complex tissue containing more than one type of component. The predominant component is the mineral (i.e. crystalline hydroxyapatite). The major macromolecule of bone is type I collagen forming the frame for the deposition of the crystals. A number of non-collagenous molecules bound in the mineral phase have recently been discovered and are all probably important for the regulation of bone.

Mineral chemistry

Bone mineral is a highly complex and insoluble particulate material which has a relatively long biological half-life and which fulfils morphologic and mechanical functions in the skeleton that are complementary to those of collagen. However, it is the mineral portion of the skeleton that is involved in the unique role played by bone tissue in maintaining mineral metabolism and homeostasis. Because no comparable physiologic function is ascribed to the components of the organic matrix of bone, it would appear that from a biological point of view the mineral is actually the least inert fraction of all the structural constituents of bone tissue[10].

Chemically, the mineral portion of bone is composed of calcium, phosphate salts, which contain a small but significant amount of carbonate (4–6% by weight), and very small amounts (less than 1%) of other ions such as sodium, potassium, magnesium, fluoride and chloride. Interestingly, about half of the body's magnesium is in the skeleton. This mineral is essential for life. It is an activator of enzymes, some of which are found mainly in the skeleton, such as the alkaline phosphatases and pyrophosphatases, and is the fourth most abundant cation in the skeleton.

Bone apatite is distinct from the geological apatites in that it is smaller in size (10–40nm) and less perfect in atomic arrangement and stoichiometry, making it a more reactive and soluble mineral. The chemical character of bone mineral is no longer believed to be a mixture of an X-ray amorphous tricalcium phosphate and hydroxyapatite, but a poorly crystalline carbonate containing an analog of hydroxyapatite for which the empirical formula is $Ca_{10}(PO_4)_6(OH)_2$. Because of its small crystalline size and large surface per unit weight, a high proportion of bone mineral particles are available for exchange and reaction with body fluids. Ions of similar size and charge to the component Ca^{2+}, PO_4^{2-} and OH ions readily substitute for these ions on the surface and within the growing crystal. Hence, bone has the ability to incorporate such bone-seeking ions as magnesium, strontium and the lanthanides from the body fluid. In general, the uptake of such ions makes the mineral crystals more imperfect and more soluble. In contrast, fluoride, by substituting for OH in the apatite structure, produces larger, less soluble bone mineral crystals. This effect is in great part the basis for the development of fluoride treatment, both to retard caries formation and to stabilize rapidly remodeling mineral crystals, reducing bone loss in osteoporotic patients.

Bone matrix

'The organic matrix (Eastoe, 1968[11]) is the most important part of bone, because, although it is possible to have histological bone without calcification, it is not possible to have bone at all without a scaffold of matrix'[12].

The extracellular matrix of bone is a composite structure whose predominant component (85–90%) is type I collagen. It is now accepted that the backbone of the gene for type I collagen is identical in all connective tissues throughout the body. Therefore, it is most probable that the genetic specificity of the bone extracellular matrix resides within the non-collagenous constituents of the tissue. These proteins, however, are not spatially isolated within bone but are intimately associated with the bone collagen, forming a composite structure fulfilling all the biochemical, biomechanical and homeostatic requirements demanded of the bone matrix throughout life.

The formation of mineralized bone tissue is a synergistic effort between the secretory cells (osteoblasts) and the vascular system. This coordinated action results in the building of a functional extracellular matrix where the involvement of these two tissues is reflected by the composition of the matrix. Macromolecular components derived endogeneously from the tissue-specific cell(s), such as collagen, osteocalcin, osteonectin, bone sialoprotein(s), bone growth-promoting proteins (insulin-like growth factor I (IGF-I), IGF-II, transforming growth factor-β (TGF-β)), phosphoproteins, proteoglycans and from the circulation components such as the plasma proteins, can be found as part of the mineralized extracellular matrix. This is illustrated in Figure 192.7, with special reference to the location of events. In this dynamic scheme the osteoid can be considered as a zone of mineralization inhibition in which the matrix structural components are assembled. Collagen, proteoglycans and some non-collagenous proteins are secreted at the osteoblast–osteoid interface. Conversely, osteocalcin, and perhaps other macromolecules which appear to accumulate at the mineralization front or in the mineral phase, arrive via osteoblastic processes and are secreted directly at the front, the zone of active mineralization.

Collagen

The collagen in bone is type I, which is the same in skin and tendon. Except for collagen V, no other forms of collagen are found in the bone

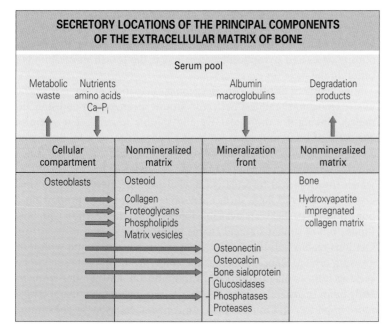

SECRETORY LOCATIONS OF THE PRINCIPAL COMPONENTS OF THE EXTRACELLULAR MATRIX OF BONE

Fig. 192.7 The probable secretory locations of the principal components of the extracellular matrix of bone.

matrix proper. Small amounts of type III and IV collagen are confined to the bone vasculature or to adherent, unmineralized connective tissue not associated with osteoblastic cells. The insoluble fibrils of collagen in bone are formed from the individual soluble tropocollagen molecules and are stabilized by intermolecular cross-links derived from aldehyde forms of hydroxylysine and lysine. Bone collagen extracted from tissues in various solutions behaves, with maturity, in the same way as human skin, tendon and cartilage collagen. With age, less collagen can be extracted because of increasing cross-linking during the aging process[12].

At present, methods have been developed for analysis of the 3-hydroxypyridinium cross-links of mature collagen, pyridinoline (pyr), deoxypyridinoline (D-pyr), and serum N-telopeptides of type I collagen (NTX) in samples of urine and NTX in the serum[13]. These intermolecular cross-linking compounds of collagen are only present in its mature form and are specific for bone and cartilage. Therefore, it is believed that they represent a sensitive and specific marker for bone resorption. Urinary hydroxyproline, commonly used as marker for bone resorption in the past, is not specific for bone.

Collagen fibers may at least be regarded as the structural framework or scaffold for the tissue in which mineralization takes place. In this capacity, the fibers could conceivably serve as passive elements of support and merely define the spaces into which mineral may be deposited.

Non-collagenous proteins

The major non-collagenous proteins of bone are proteoglycans, γ-carboxyglutamic acid (Gla)-containing proteins, glycoproteins, phosphoproteins and plasma proteins. The proteins osteocalcin and bone sialoprotein appear to represent unique expressions of the osteogenic phenotype.

Proteoglycans

One of the major classes of non-collagenous protein represented in the mineralized matrix are the proteoglycans ($\pm 10\%$ of all non-collagenous proteins).

The proteoglycans consist of a central protein core to which are bound polysaccharide chains – glycosaminoglycans – which are strongly polyanionic due to carboxyl and sulfate groups. Some proteoglycans are able to bind non-covalently to chains of the non-protein bound glycosaminoglycan hyaluronate with the aid of link proteins, thus forming very large molecular complexes. Two small proteoglycans have been identified in bone: PG-I (now termed 'biglycan', as two side chains are attached) and PG-II ('decorin', as it seems to decorate collagen fibers)[14]. Although no definite function for any of the proteoglycans found in developing or mature bone is known, many studies *in vitro* and histochemical localization *in situ* showed that proteoglycans are found in close association with collagen fibers and that they affect both the rate of fiber growth and the diameter of collagen fibers; it is possible that they influence the collagen scaffolding[15].

Bone Gla-containing proteins (BGP) – osteocalcin

One low molecular weight protein that has received considerable attention is bone Gla protein or osteocalcin. Among the principal non-collagenous proteins of bone matrix, osteocalcin stands as the numerically most abundant and the most thoroughly characterized molecular species.

The name osteocalcin derives from the abundance of this protein in osseous tissue (10–20% of the non-collagenous protein), and its affinity for Ca^{2+}. Osteocalcin has also been called 'the vitamin K-dependent protein of bone'. The biochemical function of this molecule remains to be established. Osteocalcin is distinguished by its small size (molecular weight 5.2–5.9 kDa, depending on species) and its content of two or three residues of Gla. Although vitamin K is known to be required for the formation of Gla residues in osteocalcin, no obvious changes in bone histology and mineral metabolism occur in experimental situations of vitamin K antagonism using dicoumarol or warfarin[16].

Circulating levels of osteocalcin have been studied clinically to establish their significance as diagnostic parameters in disorders of bone and calcium metabolism. Serum osteocalcin increases in situations where the bone formation rate is elevated or where bone turnover is increased. Osteocalcin binds tightly to hydroxyapatite. The protein is believed to have a function in the assembly of mineralized bone, perhaps by participating in the regulation of hydroxyapatite crystal growth. The synthesis of osteocalcin is stimulated severalfold when 1,25-dihydroxyvitamin D_3 is added in osteoblast culture or *in vivo*[17].

Analogous proteins containing γ-carboxyglutamic acid have also been found in bone as well as in cartilage. They have been named matrix Gla proteins[18].

Glycoproteins

Many glycoproteins are found in bone. Principal among these are bone sialoprotein, osteopontin, osteonectin, alkaline phosphatase and the bone growth factors such as bone morphogenetic protein (BMP) and IGF. Only a few glycosylated non-collagenous proteins have been isolated and characterized to any degree.

Sialoproteins

Bone sialoprotein was one of the first non-collagenous proteins identified by Herring[19], who did pioneering work in the field of bone matrix proteins. Sialoproteins constitute 61% of the non-collagenous proteins.

Two sialoproteins, osteopontin and bone sialoprotein (BSP), previously called sialoproteins I and II, are both cell adhesion molecules, mediating cell attachment of a number of cell types *in vitro*, including bone cells. The presence of an Arg–Gly–Asp (RGD) sequence confers to bone protein cell-binding properties of both sialic acid-rich proteins. In addition, the sialoprotein binds strongly to hydroxyapatite. Both proteins, however, behave differently *in vitro* and probably have a different function *in vivo*. The synthesis of BSP is inhibited by 1,25-dihydroxyvitamin D_3, whereas it is stimulated by dexamethasone added to the cultured osteoblasts[20]. In contrast, the synthesis of osteopontin by osteoblasts is stimulated by 1,25-dihydroxyvitamin D_2. Oldberg *et al.*[19] suggested that sialoprotein I be named osteopontin, denoting that it is a product of cells in the osteoid matrix and that it can form a bridge (pons) between cells and the mineral in the matrix.

Heinegard and Oldberg[18], using an immunogold technique, have demonstrated that osteopontin is located at the clear zone of osteoclasts binding to mineral, whereas it is not present in the ruffled border region. In view of this information, together with the fact that 1,25-dihydroxy-vitamin D_3 stimulates osteopontin formation and mobilization of calcium from the skeleton, they have postulated that osteopontin has a role in recruiting osteoclast precursor cells and in binding them to the mineralized matrix of bone (Fig. 192.8). In support of this hypothesis, osteoclasts express large amounts of an adhesion (integrin) receptor identical, or closely related to, the vitronectin receptor. They propose that this integrin is the receptor for osteopontin. In contrast to osteopontin, BSP may not be specific to bone tissue although bone cells are believed to be the major source of BSP message production. Other tissues, such as cartilage, decidua and placenta, also contain small amounts of message for BSP.

Osteonectin and other attachment glycoproteins

Osteonectin, osteopontin, bone sialoprotein and many other glycoproteins of bone may be considered to be attachment glycoproteins (like fibronectin, laminin and chondronectin in other tissues), which bind to collagen, proteoglycan and cell surface receptors, creating an ordered supramolecular complex. These glycoconjugates not only maintain the structure of the extracellular matrix but also help to regulate the functions of the resident cells. These so-called attachment proteins have various biological activities, including mediating cell attachment and spreading and stimulating cell growth, migration and differentiation. The attachment glycoproteins from one tissue can also suppress the growth of cells from other tissue, presumably as a mechanism to maintain the segregation of different cell types. Alterations in the interaction of cells with the extracellular matrix occur in inflammation and in other diseases and may lead to the loss of tissue structure and function.

Alkaline phosphatases

The classic vertebrate alkaline phosphatases are a group of isozymic membrane-bound glycoproteins with molecular weights of 100–200kDa. The wide organ and tissue distribution of alkaline phosphatase activity suggests some type of generalized function. That this glycoprotein is primarily located in the plasma membrane implies either a carrier or a signal transducer function. Several possible actions of alkaline phosphatase in biomineralization have been proposed:

- increasing local concentrations of inorganic phosphate (P_i);
- local destruction of mineral crystal growth inhibitors via expression of phosphohydrolase activity;
- acting as a P_i-transporter;
- acting as a Ca-binding protein;
- acting as a Ca-pump (Ca^{2+}-ATPase) in cells or vesicle membranes; and
- acting as a regulator of cellular division or differentiation, by acting as a tyrosine-specific phosphoprotein phosphatase.

Although there are supportive data for each, no singular function appears to be the principal action of the enzyme.

Growth factors in bone matrix

Polypeptide growth factors play an important role in the development and growth of osseous tissue. Bone is unique because of its abundant mineralized extracellular matrix, which sequesters growth factors and modulates their biological action through complex modes of release and presentation to responding cells. It has now been demonstrated that most of the growth regulatory peptides for bone cells are produced by

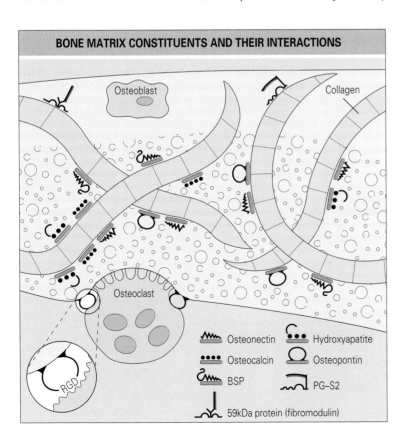

Fig. 192.8 Bone matrix constituents and their interactions. (Adapted from Heinegard and Oldberg[20].)

TABLE 192.1 BONE GROWTH FACTORS

Factor	kDa	Relative abundance		Actions on osteoblasts	
		Bone	Bone cell conditioned medium	Proliferation	Differentiation
SGF/IGF-II	7.5	++++	++++	↑	↑
IGF-I	7.7	+	+	↑	↑
TGF-b	25	+++	++	↑↓	↑
FGF (basic)	16	+	?	↑	?
FGF (acidic)	17	+	?	↑	?
PDGF	32	+	+/?	↑	↑
BMP-1	?	+	?	?	?
BMP-2A	16	+	?	?	?
BMP-3	18	+	?	?	?
OIF	20–30	+	?	?	↑
Osteogenin	28–43	+	?	↑	↑
IL-1	17.5	?	+	+	↑
IL-3	28	?	+	?	?
IL-6	23_30	?	+	?	?
G-CSF	18–22	?	+	?	?
GM-CSF	14–35	?	+	↑	↑

+, present; ↑, increase; ↓, decrease; ?, not known.
Data from Mohan and Baylink[22,29]. SGF, skeletal growth factor. PDGF, platelet-derived growth factor, OIF, osteoinductive factor, G–CSF, granulocyte colony-stimulating factor, GM–CSF, granulocyte-macrophage colony-stimulating factor.

osteoblasts as they differentiate. These growth factors are then laid down in the bone matrix, together with the structural proteins of bone, such as type I collagen.

Polypeptide growth factor effects on bone are necessarily divided into two areas of study: exogenously produced endocrine factors, which act on specific bone target cells, and endogenously produced 'local' factors with possible autocrine or paracrine action.

Many growth factors have been shown to modulate bone cell function (Table 192.1). The difficulty now is to distinguish between the useful and the irrelevant. At present it is clear that single factors do not control cell functions: cell behavior is the result of a concerted action of several growth and differentiation factors on several points of control. These points of control can be at transcription, translation or post-translational gene expression, at release of factors or at the activity of the secreted molecules, e.g. modulating receptor number and affinity. The existence of natural inhibitors of growth factors and cytokines is only just being elucidated. It is still not clear whether circulating levels are relevant, or how highly localized production or action of growth factors and cytokines can be achieved.

Insulin-like growth factors (IGF-I and IGF-II)

Insulin-like growth factors are peptides with a high degree of structural homology to proinsulin, with important effects on all metabolism (insulin-like effects) and on cell growth, differentiation and mitosis. Two main forms are known to exist: IGF-I (synonymous with somatomedin C) and IGF-II (synonymous with skeletal growth factor). Recently, a number of IGF-binding proteins (IGF-BP) have been discovered. The actions of IGF can be modulated at the local level by the presence of these IGF-BP. The presence of multiple IGF-BP forms and evidence for their local modulation suggest that these proteins could function throughout the body to provide tissue specificity for the actions of the IGFs. Tissue specificity would seem to be essential, given the diverse actions of the IGFs in different tissues and the fact that the IGFs function as hormones as well as local factors. The precise role of the IGF-BPs is not understood. They may prolong the half-life of IGF, neutralize or enhance its biological activity, or be involved in the transport of IGF to its target cells.

Based on findings that IGF-II is present in bone, is produced by bone cells and acts on bone cells, it has been proposed that IGF-II is an

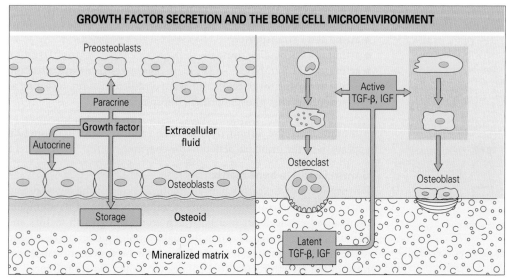

GROWTH FACTOR SECRETION AND THE BONE CELL MICROENVIRONMENT

Fig. 192.9 Growth factor secretion and the bone cell microenvironment. Model illustrating growth factor secretion towards matrix and extracellular fluid.

important local regulator of bone cell metabolism. A model of how IGF-II may act in the bone cell microenvironment is shown in Figure 192.9. This model can also be applied to other bone growth factors, for example TGF-β, which is also produced by osteoblasts. According to this model, bone cells secrete IGF-II, which is either incorporated into bone matrix or diffuses to the extracellular fluid. Recent findings suggest that the IGF-II is fixed into the matrix by means of an IGF-II BP that has strong affinity for hydroxyapatite. IGF-II stored in bone would act only after being released in an active form from bone via bone resorption. IGF-II secreted into extracellular fluid will have an acute action on osteoblast-like cells. In this regard, IGF-II can act on the same cell that produces it in an autocrine manner, or it can act on cells that are in the near vicinity in a paracrine manner.

Bone morphogenetic protein (BMP)

Currently, the BMPs are under intensive investigation. The BMPs are members of the TGF-β superfamily and have powerful stimulatory effects on bone formation. Various methods of purifying BMP have been attempted since Urist[23] experimented with bone induction in demineralized bone in 1965. Purification is difficult because BMP is present in a much smaller amount than other non-collagenous proteins and is insoluble in many solvents. *In vivo* it has been shown that BMP is involved in the differentiation of progenitor mesenchymal-type cells into cartilage, and that the subsequent process of endochondral bone differentiation may be synergized by other growth factors. Spectacular results can be obtained when purified BMP is implanted in a muscle pouch, subcutaneous space or diffusion chamber. It may induce differentiation of cartilage and woven bone within 10 days, of lamellar bone within 20 days and of an ossicle containing bone marrow within 30 days. However, when infused or injected locally over a normal bone surface, it causes bone formation without a cartilaginous phase. It has been demonstrated that the BMPs comprise a mixture of possibly 10–14 molecules. It seems quite likely that the BMP activity derived from bovine bone matrix represents the combined action of multiple factors acting at specific points during bone development[16].

Fibroblast growth factors

Recently, it has been shown that members of the heparin-binding fibroblast growth factor (FGF) family are important in normal skeletal development. Point mutations and receptors for several members of this family result in various disorders of skeletal development, such as achondroplasia. Moreover, when added to bone surfaces *in vivo* or injected or infused systematically into rodents, both basic and acidic FGF (FGF-II and FGF-I) result in profound increases in new bone formation systematically. Like the other growth regulatory factors in the bone matrix, the FGFs are expressed and secreted by osteoblasts during osteoblast proliferation and differentiation. They act in an autocrine and a paracrine manner on osteoblasts. Their major effect *in vitro* is to increase osteoblast proliferation, presumably increasing the pool of committed osteoblasts which could later differentiate to more mature bone-forming cells[22,24].

Plasma proteins

Mineralized tissue contains serum proteins. A number of plasma proteins have been identified and quantified. Some of them have been found to be highly concentrated in bone by factors of about 15 for α_2-HS glycoprotein, 11–19 for α_2-acid glycoprotein and 306–515 for IgE[25].

SKELETAL DEVELOPMENT: GROWTH AND MODELING

Endochondral ossification

Tubular bones develop predominantly (but not exclusively) by endochondral ossification. Transformation of cartilage to bone initially occurs at ossification centers within the cartilaginous model and at the

perichondrium. As longitudinal growth occurs the physis (growth plate) forms, consisting of four anatomically distinct zones. The zone of resting cartilage is firmly adherent to the overlying epiphyseal bone. The proliferating zone is characterized by vertical columns of chondrocytes, which expand the plate interstitially until they enter the hypertrophic zone, where they enlarge and polarize. It is in this zone that oxygen tension is lowest and cellular metabolism entirely anaerobic. Alkaline phosphatase is produced by the hypertrophic cells closest to the metaphysis, presumably promoting formation of the zone of calcified cartilage.

The formation of mineralized cartilage is a pivotal step in endochondral growth, as this calcified matrix serves as a lattice for deposition of bone in the primary spongiosa (Fig. 192.10)[26]. This complex of mineralized cartilage and woven bone is eventually resorbed and replaced by lamellar bone, forming the secondary spongiosa or metaphyseal trabeculae. Therefore, while the physis is expanded by interstitial growth of the proliferative zone it is replaced by bone on the metaphyseal side, resulting in elongation of the shaft.

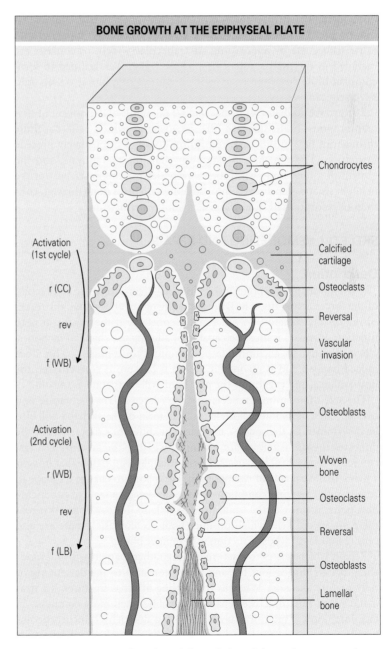

BONE GROWTH AT THE EPIPHYSEAL PLATE

Chondrocytes

Activation (1st cycle)

r (CC)

rev

f (WB)

Activation (2nd cycle)

r (WB)

rev

f (LB)

Calcified cartilage

Osteoclasts

Reversal

Vascular invasion

Osteoblasts

Woven bone

Osteoclasts

Reversal

Osteoblasts

Lamellar bone

Fig. 192.10 Bone growth at the epiphyseal plate. Schematic representation of the cellular events occurring at the growth plate in long bones. r, resorption; rev, reversal; f, formation; CC, calcified cartilage; WB, woven bone; LB, lamellar bone.

As the bone grows longitudinally it becomes necessary to expand and shape it to adult proportions. This is called modeling. Structural modeling is accomplished by intramembranous ossification, involving apposition and resorption at appropriate locations on the subperiosteal and endosteal surfaces. Growth and modeling occur only in the developing skeleton and cease with growth plate closure. Because skeletal development requires matrix formation at some surfaces and resorption at others, growth and modeling are characterized by an anatomic disassociation of the activities of osteoblasts and osteoclasts (see Figs 192.5 and 192.6).

Intramembranous ossification

Intramembranous ossification, the process responsible for development of the major part of the axial skeleton, differs from its endochondral counterpart in that no cartilage is formed. Because bone cannot grow interstitially, intramembranous bone develops only by apposition.

The process originates with mesenchymal cells clustering together in centers of ossification. These cells differentiate into large osteoblasts, which in turn produce a collagen matrix and ground substance. Coincidentally with the secretion of alkaline phosphatase, mineralization occurs. This initial trabeculum lined by osteoblasts branches into other trabeculae by apposition. As trabeculae widen, osteoblasts are included in the matrix osteocytes. Those trabeculae destined to form compact bone continue to expand, incorporating blood vessels into haversian canals.

The growth in diameter of the shaft is the result of deposition of new membranous bone beneath the periosteum which will continue throughout life. In this case, resorption does not immediately precede formation. The midshaft is narrower than the metaphysis, and the growth of a long bone will progressively destroy the lower part of the metaphysis and transform it into a diaphysis. This is done through continuous resorption by osteoclasts beneath the periosteum.

SKELETAL REMODELING AND REPAIR

Description

The overall shape of a bone and its internal architecture are a reflection of the forces acting upon it. During the life of any individual, the forces acting on the skeleton do not remain constant. If the organism is to function properly, it must be capable of altering the shape of its bones, albeit slightly, to accommodate changing requirements. This does indeed happen and is obvious if a limb is broken. If correctly set, the limb will heal and eventually the new bone will be as good as the old.

The size of an animal reflects to a very large extent the nature and overall shape of its internal skeleton. The form of the skeleton will also be determined by the species' lifestyle. The different proportions of the bones of the limbs tell us, for example, whether the creature is a fast runner or a powerful burrower. These examples emphasize that bone is a living tissue capable of regeneration. For a bone to change its shape in response to changing conditions, as well as being capable of producing new bone, it must at the same time be able to destroy bone. Whereas there are special cells which produce bone (osteoblasts), there are also cells (osteoclasts) whose function is to remove bone.

Repair, which relates to fracture healing rather than growth and modeling, occurs throughout life and is not confined to the developing or fully mature skeleton. Whereas the healing of gross fractures is a dramatic event, microfracture repair is probably much more common. In fact, inhibition of microfracture repair by agents such as glucocorticoids is thought by some to underlie many of the skeletal complications of steroid-induced bone disease, such as osteonecrosis. Remodeling, like repair, is a lifelong event. It is the skeletal process intimately related to mineral homeostasis and probably serves to remove and replace effete bone. Unlike growth, modeling and repair, remodeling is characterized by an anatomic coupling or tethering of the activities of osteoclasts and osteoblasts. The process, which occurs dysynchronously at thousands of sites in the human skeleton at all times, is initiated by recruitment of osteoclasts to a target site on the bone surface. Because of its high surface-to-volume ratio, many more remodeling sites are to be found per unit volume of trabecular than of cortical bone. Thus, disorders of remodeling, such as renal osteodystrophy, disuse, glucocorticoid-induced bone loss or postmenopausal osteoporosis, are more likely to become manifest in cancellous rather than cortical bone.

Once in contact with matrix the osteoclast resorbs a packet of bone, resulting in a 'Howship's lacuna' or 'resorption bay' approximately 50mm deep. Osteoclasts then depart, ultimately to be replaced by osteoblasts which in young individuals fill the resorption bay with new bone in amounts equal to that initially removed. In the normal state the remodeling that occurs is imperceptible: bone is constantly being resorbed and renewed. In adult life there is a delicate equilibrium between these two processes which only begins to break down in old age or in diseases such as hyperthyroidism, when the rate of resorption is greater than the rate of redeposition[6]. The bones become more porous, resulting in osteoporosis (Fig. 192.11). They are then less able to withstand the strains normally placed on them and become more liable to fracture. It is this net deficit of bone, occurring in many thousands of remodeling sites throughout the skeleton, that leads to the universal bone loss associated with aging (Fig. 192.12). Moreover, the coupling of matrix resorbing and synthesizing activities of bone cells is in large part responsible for the challenge in attempting to cure osteoporosis. Specifically, bone-seeking hormones tend to either accelerate or suppress remodeling. In so doing, they generally have similar effects on both matrix resorptive and synthesizing cells and hence may not alter net bone mass. Clearly, a major goal for treating osteoporosis is the development of agents able to disassociate the activities of osteoblasts and osteoclasts, and recently there has been substantial progress made in this area.

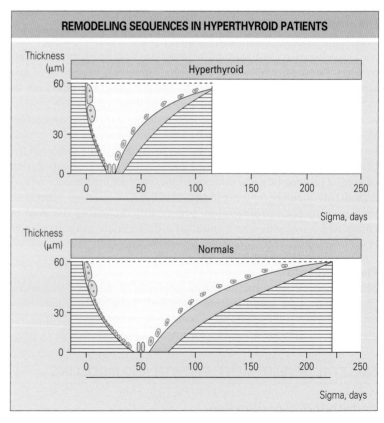

Fig. 192.11 Remodeling sequences in hyperthyroid patients. The sequences are compared with age- and sex-matched normals. (Adapted from Melsen and Mosekilde[27].)

BONE TURNOVER, BALANCE, AND BONE LOSS

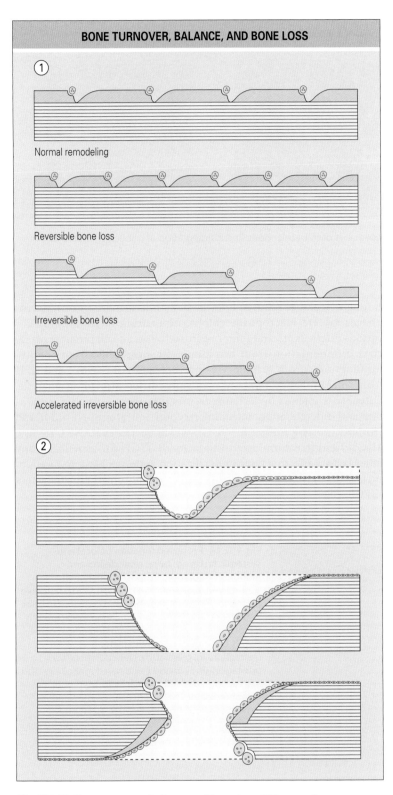

Normal remodeling

Reversible bone loss

Irreversible bone loss

Accelerated irreversible bone loss

Fig. 192.12 Bone turnover, balance and bone loss. (1) In every bone remodeling unit there is a temporary bone loss caused by osteoclastic resorption, which is reversible as long as bone formation fully compensates. If the frequency of remodeling increases there is an associated increase in bone loss, which will be irreversible if this is not fully compensated by new bone formation. (2) Perforation of a bone plate can occur through resorption.

Aging and the architectural consequences of remodeling

Non-load-bearing trabecular bone in younger individuals is constructed of uniform trabecular plates forming a honeycomb structure which combines maximum strength with minimum bone mass. The architecture of load-bearing trabecular bone is characterized by thick plates and columns orientated in the direction of the compressive forces, sustained by thinner trabecular struts in the non-load-bearing plane (anisotrophy). The trabecular elements in the young are completely interconnected, giving maximum support. However, with age this trabecular framework changes. The thick load-bearing plates are successively perforated during remodeling processes and converted into columns, and the thinner non-load-bearing trabeculae are disconnected and often disappear. The biomechanical consequences of this loss of continuity in the three-dimensional lattice are pronounced (Fig. 192.13).

During adulthood the skeleton shows a generalized tendency towards slow appositional growth, leading to an increased diameter of tubular bones and an expansion of the marrow cavity due to a positive balance at the periosteal envelope and a negative balance on the endosteal envelope. Similar changes have been observed in irregular weight-bearing bones, where they might to some extent reduce the effect on bone strength by the reduction in trabecular bone mass with age[27].

Mediators of bone remodeling and repair

Bone remodeling is regulated by systemic hormones and by local factors which affect cells of the osteoclast and osteoblast lineages. The regulation of bone metabolism by hormones has been studied extensively, but it is now clear that local non-systemic factors play a direct and important role in bone remodeling.

Circulating hormones may act on skeletal cells, either directly or indirectly, modulating the synthesis or effects of a local growth factor, which in turn stimulates or inhibits bone formation or bone resorption. The function of local factors is currently not entirely clear: it is conceivable that circulatory hormones provide a non-specific environment to maintain normal tissue function, whereas the precise regulation of tissue growth is provided by local growth factors. These factors may play a critical role in the coupling of bone formation to bone resorption, and possibly in pathologic processes. Bone remodeling is regulated by polypeptide, steroid and thyroid hormones and by local factors outlined in Table 192.2.

TABLE 192.2 HORMONAL AND LOCAL REGULATORS OF BONE REMODELING		
Hormones		
Polypeptide hormones	Parathyroid hormone (PTH) Calcitonin Insulin Growth hormone	
Steroid hormones	1,25-dihydroxyvitamin D_3 [1,25(OH)$_2D_3$] Glucocorticoids Sex steroids	
Thyroid hormones		
Local factors		
Synthesized (or presumably synthesized) by bone cells	IGF-I and IGF-II β_2-microglobulin TGF-β BMPs FGFs PDGF	
Synthesized by bone-related tissue	Cartilage-derived	IGF-I FGFs (basic) TGF-β
	Blood-cell-derived	IL-1 TNF
Other factors	Prostaglandins Binding proteins	

LOSS OF CONTINUITY OF TRABECULAR BONE

Fig. 192.13 Loss of continuity of trabecular bone. Different stages in the age-dependent loss of trabecular bone and disintegration of trabecular structure. (Adapted from Melsen and Mosekilde[27].)

Although the local regulatory mechanisms of normal bone remodeling are not fully understood, much information on bone cell interactions has been derived from studies of bone cells *in vitro*. The mechanism of bone turnover is complicated, entailing communication between several cell types which respond to systemic hormones and locally released factors. The sequential activation of bone cells is initiated by recruitment of bone resorbing osteoclasts to the remodeling site. The resorption phase is followed by the arrival of osteoblasts, which replace the bone excavated by the osteoclasts. Mononuclear cells of the monocyte– macrophage lineage may be involved in the coordination of the two phases. The rates of bone resorption and formation are closely related, and this tight 'coupling' is conserved under many pathologic conditions. Osteoclasts and osteoblasts communicate

through cytokines released into the bone microenvironment. Macrophages secrete macrophage colony-stimulating factor – M-CSF – various interleukins, and tumor necrosis factor, and all promote osteoclast differentiation from hematopoietic stem cells, from colony-forming units from granulocyte–macrophages (CFU-GM), and CFU from macrophages (CFU-M) to fully differentiated osteoclasts. Osteoblasts interact by secreting factors that affect osteoclast maturation and differentiation, including receptor activator of NF-$\kappa\beta$ ligand (RANKL), osteoprotegerin (ODG), which decreases RANKL release, M-CSF, and transforming growth factor-β (TGF-β), as well as many other factors affecting bone mineralization and osteoblast maturation, such as insulin-like growth factors (IGFs) and fibroblast growth factors (αFGF, βFGF)[8,9].

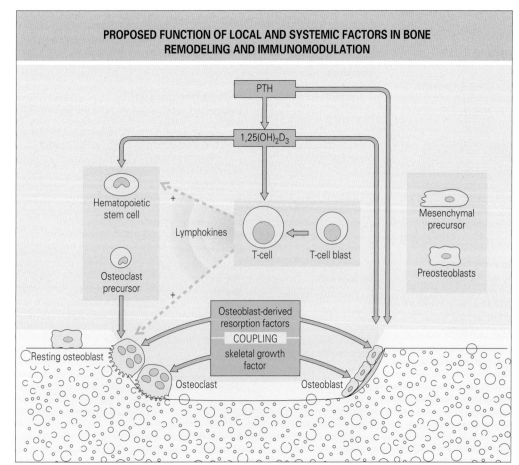

PROPOSED FUNCTION OF LOCAL AND SYSTEMIC FACTORS IN BONE REMODELING AND IMMUNOMODULATION

Fig. 192.14 Proposed function of local and systemic factors in bone remodeling and immunomodulation. Proposed function of 1,25-dihydroxyvitamin D$_3$ [1,25(OH)$_2$D$_3$], parathyroid hormone (PTH), lymphokines, and cytokines in bone remodeling and immunomodulation. Local growth factors: skeletal cell-derived somatomedin C or IGF-I, TGF-β, bone-derived growth factor or β_2 microglobulin, platelet-derived growth factor, prostaglandin E$_2$, blood cell-derived monokines (IL-1, macrophage-derived growth factor), lymphokines (lymphotoxin or TNF, interferon), prostaglandins. Systemic factors: hormones (PTH, 1,25(OH)$_2$D$_3$, calcitonin, corticosteroids, sex hormones, thyroxine, growth hormone).

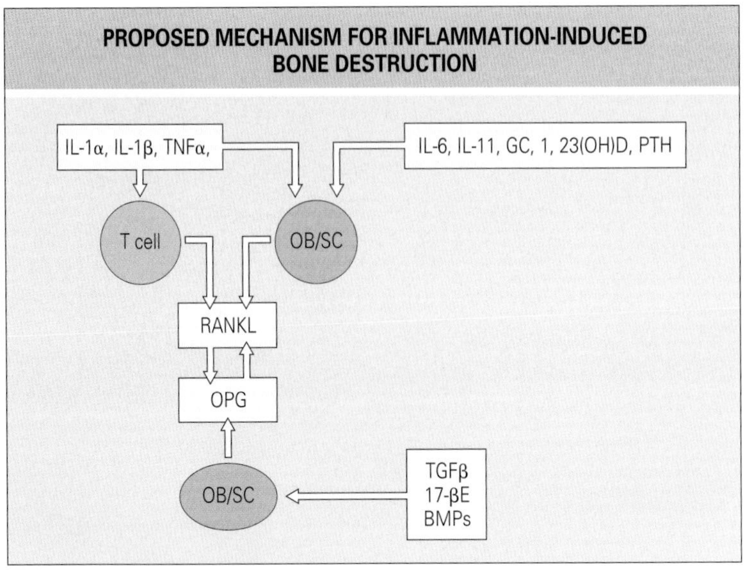

PROPOSED MECHANISM FOR INFLAMMATION-INDUCED BONE DESTRUCTION

Fig. 192.15 Proposed mechanism for inflammatory induced bone destruction. Many proinflammatory and anti-inflammatory cytokines interact with RANKL-OPG and the net result determines the differentiation, activation and survival of osteoclasts. Osteoclast activity then directly influences the amount of bone loss in inflammatory arthritis. 1,25(OH)2D, 1,25 dihydroxyvitamin D; 17βE, 17-β estrogen; BMP, bone morphogenetic protein; GC, glucocorticoids; OB/SC, osteoblast/stromal cell; OPG, osteoprotegerin; PTH, parathyroid hormone; RANKL, receptor activator of nuclear factor-κB ligand; TGF, transforming growth factor; TNF, tumor necrosis factor. (Adapted with permission from Rehman and Lane[29].)

Coupling of the catabolic and anabolic phases of bone remodeling may also explain the ability of the major bone resorbing hormones (PTH and 1,25-dihydroxyvitamin D_3) to stimulate bone formation.

Clearly, the concept of bone cell coupling is important for the interpretation of inflammatory tissue reactions in bone.

In addition to direct cell contact, interactions of the osteoblast and osteoclast lineages may entail the release of messenger molecules. Bone surface-lining cells may generate signals governing the recruitment of osteoclasts. This hypothesis is strengthened by the observation that osteoblasts, but not osteoclasts, express receptors for the bone-resorbing hormones PTH and 1,25-dihydroxyvitamin D_3[3]. However, osteoclasts express receptors for the bone resorption inhibitor calcitonin. Moreover, matrix constituents are potent chemoattractants for bone-resorbing cells, and osteoblasts may 'uncover' the resorption site by hormonally regulated release of matrix degrading enzymes. Similarly, the recruitment and proliferation of osteoblasts following resorption may depend on autocrine or paracrine growth factors positioned in the bone matrix, or released locally by osteoblasts or mononuclear cells[7]. Figure 192.14 illustrates the proposed functions of 1,25-dihydroxyvitamin D_3, lymphokines and cytokine receptors in bone remodeling and immunomodulation.

Inflammatory arthritides are commonly characterized by localized and generalized bone loss. Localized bone loss in the form of joint erosions and periarticular osteopenia is the hallmark of rheumatoid arthritis. Recent studies have highlighted the importance of RANKL-dependent osteoclast activation by inflammatory cells and subsequent bone loss. Adjuvant-induced arthritis (AIA) is an animal model of T lymphocyte-mediated inflammatory arthritis characterized by destruction of bone and cartilage similar to that in RA. In this model, activated T cells express RANKL protein on their surface, and through binding of RANKL to RANK on preosteoclasts these cells promote osteoclastogenesis and subsequent bone loss. Treatment of these AIA animals with OPG resulted in a decrease in osteoclast number and preservation of bone and joint structure, whereas control animals had both bone destruction and an increased number of osteoclasts. Various combinations of inflammatory and anti-inflammatory cytokines converge on RANKL-OPG, and the net balance determines bone loss in inflammatory arthritis (Fig. 192.15)[28,29].

REFERENCES

1. Cooke AM. Osteoporosis. Lancet 1955; 1: 878–82; 929–937.
2. Halstead B, Middleton J. Bare bones, an explanation in art and science. Edinburgh: Oliver and Boyd; 1972.
3. Jaworski ZGF. Proceedings of the first workshop on bone morphometry. Ottawa: University of Ottawa Press; 1973: 3–7.
4. Stevens A, Lowe J. Histology. London: Mosby; 1992.
5. Parfitt AM, Mundy GR, Roodman GD et al. Local control of bone resorption, with particular reference to the effects of bisphosphonates. J Bone Miner Res 1996; 11: 150–159.
6. Eriksen EF. Normal and pathological remodeling of human trabecular bone: three-dimensional reconstruction of the remodeling sequence in normals and in metabolic bone diseases. Endocrinol Rev 1986; 7: 379–408.
7. Mundy GR. Local control of bone formation by osteoblasts. Clin Orthop Rel Res 1995; 313: 19–26.
8. Rubin CT, Rubin JE. Biology, physiology and morphology of bone. In: Ruddy S, Harris ED, Sledge CB, eds. Textbook of rheumatology, 6th edn. Philadelphia: W B Saunders; 2001; 1611–1634.
9. Hofbauer LC, Khosla S, Dunstan CR, Lacey DL, Boyle WJ, Riggs BL. The roles of osteoprotegerin and osteoprotegerin ligand in the paracrine regulation of bone resorption. J Bone Miner Res 2000; 15: 2–12.
10. Termine JD. Bone matrix proteins and the mineralization process. In: Favers MJ, ed. Primer on the metabolic bone diseases and disorders of mineral metabolism. Kelseyville: American Society of Bone and Mineral Research; 1990; 6–18.
11. Eastoe JE. Chemical aspects of the matrix concept in calcified tissue organization. Calcif Tissue Res 1968; 2: 1–6.
12. Dequeker J, Merlevede W. Collagen content and collagen extractability pattern of adult human trabecular bone according to age, sex, and amount of bone mass. Biochim Biophys Acta 1971; 244: 410–420.
13. Black D, Duncan A, Robins SP. Quantitative analysis of the pyridinium crosslinks of collagen in urine using ion-paired reversed phase high-performance liquid chromatography. Anal Biochem 1988; 169: 197–203.
14. Fisher LW, Hawkins GR, Tuross N, Termine JD. Purification and partial characterization of small proteoglycans I and II, bone sialoproteins I and II, and osteonectin from the mineral compartment of developing human bone. J Biol Chem 1987; 262: 9702–9708.
15. Gehron Robey P. The biochemistry of bone. Endocrinol Metabol Clin North Am 1989; 18: 859–902.
16. Hauschka PV, Reid ML. Vitamin K-dependence of a calcium binding protein containing gamma carboxyglutamic acid in developing chick bone. J Biol Chem 1978; 253: 9063–9068.
17. Geusens P, Vanderschueren D, Verstraeten A et al. Short-term course of 1,25(OH)$_2$D$_3$ stimulates osteoblasts but not osteoclasts in osteoporosis and osteoarthritis. Calcif Tissue Int 1991; 49: 168–173.
18. Price PA. Vitamin K-dependent bone proteins. In: Cohn HV et al., eds. Calcium regulation and bone metabolism: basic and clinical aspects. Vol. 9. Amsterdam: Elsevier Science; 1987; 419–425.
19. Herring GM. Studies on the protein-bound chondroitin sulphate of bovine cortical bone. Biochem J 1968; 107: 41–49.
20. Heinegard D, Oldberg A. Structure and biology of cartilage and bone matrix noncollagenous macromolecules. FASEB J 1989; 3: 2042–2051.
21. Oldberg A, Franzen A, Heinegärd D. Cloning and sequence analysis of rat bone sialoprotein (osteopontin) in DNA reveals an Arg–Gly–Asp cell-binding sequence. Proc Natl Acad Sci USA 1986; 83: 8819–8823.
22. Mohan S, Baylink D. Bone growth factors. Clin Orthop Rel Res 1991; 263: 30–48.
23. Urist MR. Bone: formation by induction. Science 1965; 150: 893–899.
24. Wronski TJ, Ratkus AM, Thomsen JS et al. Sequential treatment with basic fibroblast growth factor and parathyroid hormone restores lost cancellous bone mass and strength in the proximal tibia of aged ovariectomized rats. J Bone Miner Res 2001; 16: 1399–1407.
25. Mbuyi JM, Dequeker J, Bloemmen F, Stevens E. Plasma proteins in human cortical bone: Enrichment of alpha$_2$ HS-glycoprotein, alpha$_1$ acid-glycoprotein and IgE. Calcif Tissue Int 1982; 34: 229–231.
26. Baron R. Anatomy and ultrastructure of bone. In: Favers MJ, ed. Primer on the metabolic bone diseases and disorders of mineral metabolism. Kelseyville: American Society of Bone and Mineral Research; 1990; 3–7.
27. Melsen F, Mosekilde L. Calcified tissues: cellular dynamics. In: Nordin BEC, ed. Calcium in human biology. London: Springer Verlag; 1988; 181–208.
28. Dequeker J, Geusens P. Osteoporosis and arthritis. Ann Rheum Dis 1990; 49: 276–280.
29. Rehman Q, Lane NE. Bone loss. Therapeutic approaches for preventing bone loss in inflammatory arthritis. Arthritis Res 2001; 3: 221–227.

193

Investigation of bone: biochemical markers

Patrick Garnero and Pierre D Delmas

INTRODUCTION

Bone turnover is characterized by two opposite activities, the formation of new bone by osteoblasts and the resorption of old bone by osteoclasts. The rate of formation or degradation of bone matrix can be assessed either by measuring an enzymatic activity of the bone-forming or -resorbing cells – such as alkaline and acid phosphatase – or by measuring bone matrix components released into the circulation during formation or resorption (Table 193.1). These have been separated into markers of formation and resorption, but it should be borne in mind that in disease states where both events are coupled and change in the same direction, such as osteoporosis, any marker will reflect the overall rate of bone turnover. Bone markers cannot discriminate between turnover changes in a specific skeletal envelope, i.e. trabecular versus cortical, but reflect whole body net changes. Although bone markers might be useful in the management of a variety of metabolic bone diseases, most studies have focused on their potential use in postmenopausal osteoporosis. Bone turnover markers may be used to predict the rate of postmenopausal bone loss, and the occurrence of osteoporotic fractures. In addition, they may have a role in monitoring the efficacy of treatment, especially antiresorptive agents (hormone replacement therapy, bisphosphonates and calcitonin), but also more recently anabolic treatment such as parathyroid hormone. The suggestion that measurement of bone turnover before treatment might be useful to select the type of therapy (antiresorptive or bone-stimulating agent) has not been substantiated by adequate prospective studies. In this chapter we will review the recent development in bone marker technology and then discuss the use of these markers for the management of osteoporosis and Paget's disease of bone.

BIOCHEMICAL MARKERS OF BONE FORMATION

Serum alkaline phosphatase

Skeletal alkaline phosphatase (ALP) is an enzyme localized in the membrane of osteoblasts which is released into the circulation by an unclear mechanism. Among the several tissues containing alkaline phosphatase, the liver and bone isoenzymes are the major contributors to the serum level. The intestinal isoenzyme can also account for part of the circulating levels in some non-fasting patients, and placental alkaline phosphatase circulates during pregnancy. In serum, bone alkaline phosphatase (bone ALP) exists in three different isoforms: B/I (70% of bone and 30% of intestinal ALP), B1 and B2. The major forms are B1 and B2, which can be differentiated by high-performance liquid chromatography (HPLC)[1]. Trabecular bone has higher total (B1+B2) ALP activity than cortical bone. In addition, the distribution of the two isoforms also differs between the bone compartments. Cortical bone has about twofold higher activity of B1 than B2, whereas trabecular bone has twofold higher activity of B2 than B1, suggesting that measurements of specific bone ALP activity may provide information on bone metabolism within specific bone envelopes[2]. Serum total alkaline phosphatase (total ALP) activity was until recently the most commonly used marker of bone formation, but for the above reasons it lacks sensitivity and specificity. In an attempt to improve the specificity and the sensitivity of serum alkaline phosphatase measurement, techniques have been developed to differentiate the bone and the liver isoenzymes, which differ only by post-translational modifications as they are coded by a single gene. These techniques rely on the use of differentially effective activators and inhibitors (heat, phenylalanine and urea), separation by electrophoresis, and indirect separation by liver-specific antibodies[3–5]. In general, these assays have slightly enhanced the sensitivity of this marker, but most of them are indirect and/or technically cumbersome. A real improvement has been achieved by using monoclonal antibodies that preferentially recognize the bone isoenzyme. These direct immunoassays have been shown to exhibit a low cross-reactivity with the circulating liver isoenzyme (15–20%) and to be more sensitive than the total ALP activity to detect the increase in bone turnover following menopause[6,7]. More recently, an automated immunoassay for serum bone ALP with improved precision over manual immunoassay and high throughput has been developed.

TABLE 193.1 BIOCHEMICAL MARKERS FOR BONE REMODELING

Formation

Serum
- **Osteocalcin (OC)**
- Total and **bone alkaline phosphatase (bone ALP)**
- Procollagen type I C- and N-propeptides (PICP and **PINP**)

Resorption

Plasma/serum
- Tartrate-resistant acid phosphatase (TRACP)
- Free pyridinoline (free PYD) and deoxypyridinoline (free DPD)
- C-terminal cross-linking telopeptide of type I collagen generated by MMPs (CTX-MMP)
- N-terminal (S-NTX) and C-terminal (**S-CTX**) cross-linking telopeptide of type I collagen
- Bone sialoprotein (BSP)

Urine
- **Free pyridinoline (PYD) and deoxypyridinoline (DPD)**
- **N-terminal (U-NTX) and C-terminal (U-CTX) crosslinking telopeptide of type I collagen**
- Calcium
- Hydroxyproline (Hyp)
- Galactosylhydroxylysine
- Helicoidal peptide 620-633

The markers with the best performance characteristics in osteoporosis are in bold type.

Serum osteocalcin or bone Gla protein

Osteocalcin (OC) is a small non-collagenous protein which is specific for bone tissue and dentine. Its precise function remains unknown[8], although data in osteocalcin-deficient mice suggest that OC could limit *in vivo* bone formation[9]. OC is predominantly synthesized by osteoblasts and is incorporated into the extracellular bone matrix, but a fraction of newly synthesized osteocalcin is released into the circulation where it can be measured by radioimmunoassay[10–13]. OC mRNA has been detected in bone marrow megakaryocytes and peripheral blood platelets, but the protein itself was undetectable in human platelets[14], suggesting that platelet osteocalcin is unlikely to contribute significantly to either serum or plasma levels. Circulating OC has a short half-life and is rapidly cleared by the kidney[11,15]. Serum OC concentrations correlate with skeletal growth at the time of puberty, and are increased in a variety of conditions characterized by increased bone turnover, such as primary and secondary hyperparathyroidism, hyperthyroidism, Paget's disease and acromegaly. Conversely, they are decreased in hypothyroidism, hypoparathyroidism, in glucocorticoid-treated patients, and in some patients with multiple myeloma and malignant hypercalcemia (reviewed in [16]). Comparisons of serum OC levels with iliac crest histomorphometry and calcium kinetic data have shown that under most conditions serum osteocalcin is a valid marker of bone turnover when resorption and formation are coupled, and is a specific marker of bone formation whenever formation and resorption are uncoupled[17–21].

Using a battery of monoclonal antibodies directed against various epitopes of the human osteocalcin molecule, we found that the intact molecule represents about one-third of the immunoreactivity in the adult serum (or plasma). One-third is represented by several small fragments and another third by a large N-terminal–midmolecule fragment (N–mid fragment)[22]. This latter large fragment (about 43 amino acids, compared to 49 for the intact molecule) is generated *in vitro* by osteoblastic cells in culture and circulates *in vivo*. Recent preliminary *in vitro* studies using purified rat osteoclasts cultured on bovine bone slices have, however, suggested that both intact and fragmented osteocalcin could also be released from bone matrix during the process of bone resorption[23]. However, the relative contribution of osteoclast- versus osteoblast-generated OC to the total circulating level is unknown. We have shown that short-term treatment with a potent bisphosphonate did not decrease either intact or the major circulating N–mid fragment[22], despite dramatic decrease of bone resorption, suggesting that *in vivo*, serum OC mainly reflects bone formation. The possibility cannot be excluded, however, that some specific osteocalcin fragments could actually reflect bone resorption. After a few hours of incubation of serum samples at room temperature, a significant fraction of plasma intact OC is rapidly converted into the large N–mid fragment, resulting in a significant loss of immunoreactivity with intact OC assay and with most polyclonal antibodies because they recognize the C-terminal end of the molecule. The heterogeneity of circulating OC forms, together with the lability of the intact molecule, probably accounts for most of the discrepancies reported in the literature[24] and for the surprisingly very wide scatter of individual values observed in several studies, and stresses the importance of standardization. From a practical point of view, however, it is recommended to use assays measuring both the intact molecule and the N–mid fragment, which results in a more robust and sensitive assay. In addition, such an assay reduces by 50% the long-term precision error when osteocalcin measurement is repeated over months in a single patient.

Procollagen type I propeptides

During the extracellular processing of type I collagen, there is cleavage of the amino terminal (PINP) and carboxy terminal (PICP) extension peptides prior to fibril formation. These peptides circulate in blood, where they might represent useful markers of bone formation as collagen is by far the most abundant organic component of bone matrix. Serum PICP levels correlate modestly with histological bone formation in patients with vertebral osteoporosis ($r = 0.36–0.50$)[25]. The menopause induces a significant but marginal (+20%) increase in serum PICP concentration which is not correlated with the subsequent rate of bone loss measured by densitometry[26]. In contrast to significant increases in both serum bone ALP and OC concentration in osteoporotic patients treated with fluoride, serum PICP levels decreased under therapy[27]. Conversely, the decrease of serum PICP in osteoporotic patients treated with estrogen is consistent with the decrease of serum bone ALP and OC[28].

In contrast to serum PICP, which is a single glomerular protein with a size of the authentic propeptide[29], immunoreactive PINP circulates as different forms. These include the intact PINP corresponding to the authentic trimeric *in vivo* cleaved propeptide, a low molecular weight form[30], and fragments. Recently it has been shown that the low molecular weight form represents monomers of intact α chains of type I collagen propeptide[31]. The trimeric structure is unstable at 37°C and can be transformed to the stable monomeric forms. The first assays developed for serum PINP, using as immunogen synthetic peptides from the α_1 chain of type I collagen propeptide, recognized both trimeric and monomeric forms and PINP fragments[32] and, as serum PICP, have been disappointing in osteoporosis[33,34]. In contrast, the assay recognizing specifically the intact trimeric form of PINP[30] has been shown to be more sensitive than PICP, and to be as valuable as OC and bone ALP to detect the increase in bone turnover following menopause[35] and for monitoring the response to antiresorptive therapy[35–38]. Serum PINP, together with bone ALP, has also recently been shown to be the most sensitive marker to assess disease activity and monitor the efficacy of bisphosphonate treatment in patients with Paget's disease of bone[39,40].

The reasons for the different sensitivities of PICP and PINP are not clear, but could be related to the contribution of tissues other than bone for PICP[32] and/or to their metabolism. Both propeptides are not cleared by the kidney because they are either too large (PICP) or have an elongated shape (PINP). The propeptides are actively taken up and metabolized by the endothelial cells of the liver, via the mannose receptor for PICP[41] and the scavenger receptor for the PINP[42]. These two clearance systems are independent of each other and also seem to be regulated separately by hormones such as thyroid hormones or IGF-I[43].

BIOCHEMICAL MARKERS OF BONE RESORPTION

Fasting urinary calcium, hydroxyproline and hydroxylysine glycosides

Fasting urinary calcium measured on a morning sample and corrected for creatinine excretion is the cheapest assay of bone resorption. It is useful in detecting a marked increase of bone resorption, but lacks sensitivity. Fasting urinary calcium reflects the amount of calcium released during resorption, but also the renal handling of calcium that is influenced by calcium-regulating hormones and by estrogens. Hydroxyproline (Hyp) is found mainly in collagen and represents about 13% of the amino acid content of the molecule[44]. Hyp is derived from proline by a post-translational hydroxylation occurring within the peptide chain. Because free Hyp released during degradation of collagen cannot be reutilized in collagen synthesis, most of the endogenous Hyp present in biologic fluids is derived from the degradation of various forms of collagen[45]. Because half of human collagen resides in bone, where its turnover is probably faster than in soft tissues, excretion of Hyp in urine is regarded as a marker of bone resorption. The C1q fraction of complement, however, contains significant amounts of Hyp and could account for up to 40% of urinary Hyp[46]. About 90% of the Hyp released by the breakdown of collagen in the tissues, especially during bone resorption, is degraded to the free amino acid that circulates in plasma, is filtered, and is almost entirely reabsorbed by the kidney. It is eventually completely oxidized in the liver and is degraded to carbon dioxide and urea[47,48]. About 10% of the Hyp released by the breakdown of collagen circulates in a peptide-bound form, and these peptides are filtered and excreted in urine without any further metabolism. Thus, the urinary total Hyp represents only about 10% of total collagen catabolism. Colorimetric assay of Hyp is usually performed on a hydrolyzed urine sample and therefore reflects the total excretion of the amino acid. As a consequence of its tissue origin and metabolism pattern, urinary Hyp is poorly correlated with bone resorption assessed by calcium kinetics or bone histomorphometry[16].

Hydroxylysine is also an amino acid unique to collagen or proteins containing collagen-like sequences. Like hydroxyproline, hydroxylysine is not reutilized for collagen biosynthesis, and although it is much less abundant than hydroxyproline it is a potential marker of collagen degradation. Hydroxylysine is present in part as galactosyl hydroxylysine and in part as glucosyl-galactosyl hydroxylysine. The relative proportion and total content of galactosyl hydroxylysine and glucosyl-galactosyl hydroxylysine varies in bone and soft tissues, with a higher content of galactosyl hydroylysine in bone, suggesting that its urinary excretion might be a more sensitive marker of bone resorption than urinary hydroxyproline. Urinary galactosyl hydroxylysine increases with aging[49]. Recently a serum assay for free galactosyl hydroxylysine has been reported[50]. Using this assay, increased levels were found in patients with Paget's disease, and levels decreased after treatment with the bisphosphonate etidronate with a magnitude similar to that of urinary galactosyl hydroxylysine. Finally it has been reported that urinary excretion of galactosyl hydroxylysine is increased in women with a history of fracture compared to controls, despite similar levels of bone resorption between the two groups, as assessed by the urinary excretion of total deoxypyridinoline[51]. These data suggest that increased levels of galactosyl hydroxylysine may reflect overglycosylation of hydroxylysine in bone matrix that may be associated with changes in bone collagen quality and increased susceptibility to fracture, an intriguing hypothesis that needs to be confirmed by prospective studies.

Plasma tartrate-resistant acid phosphatase

Acid phosphatase is a lysosomal enzyme that is present primarily in bone, prostate, platelets, erythrocytes and spleen. Bone acid phosphatase is resistant to L(+)-tartrate, whereas the prostatic isoenzyme is inhibited[52]. The structure and functions of tartrate-resistant acid phosphatase (TRACP) have recently been reviewed[53]. Mice with a heterozygous null mutation into the TRACP gene showed evidence of mild osteopetrosis, and homozygous mice also exhibit abnormal ossification, suggesting that TRACP is required for normal mineralization of developing bone as well as for the resorption of adult bone[54]. Additional experiments using transgenic mice in which tissue-specific overexpression of TRACP gene was observed in several cell lineages – including osteoclasts – resulted in mild osteoporosis with decreased density of trabecular bone. The increase in osteoclast activity was, however, partly compensated by an increase in bone formation rate[55].

Acid phosphatase circulates in blood and shows higher activity in serum than in plasma because of the release of platelet phosphatase activity during the clotting process. In normal plasma TRACP corresponds to plasma isoenzyme 5, which originates partly from bone, as osteoclasts contain TRACP that is released into the circulation[56]. Isoenzyme 5 is represented by two subforms, 5a and 5b, and recent data indicate that TRACP 5b is more specific for osteoclasts[57]. Usefully, total plasma TRACP activity is measured by colorimetric assays. However, the lack of specificity of plasma TRACP activity for the osteoclast, its instability in frozen samples, and the presence of enzyme inhibitors in serum are potential drawbacks that will limit the development of clinically useful enzymatic TRACP assays in osteoporosis. Part of the instability of TRACP in plasma is explained by this enzyme forming complexes with α_2 macroglobulin[58]. These complexes can be only partly disrupted by acidification and/or calcium chelators such as EDTA[59]. To overcome these limitations, antibodies have been developed against TRACP isolated from spleens of patients with hairy cell leukemia[60], human cordon[61] or, more recently, recombinant human TRACP or purified bone TRAP[62,63] to develop immunoassays for TRACP 5b.

Plasma TRACP activity measured by conventional colorimetric assays is increased in a variety of metabolic bone disorders with increased bone turnover[64], and is elevated after oophorectomy[65] and in vertebral osteoporosis[66], but it is not clear whether this marker is actually more sensitive than urinary hydroxyproline[65]. When measured by recent specific immunoassays, serum TRACP 5b isoenzyme has been shown to increase by about 30–40% after the menopause[62,67], with a larger increase (+70–80%) in patients with Paget's disease and breast cancer with bone metastases[67]. In a small group of postmenopausal women treated with estrogens, the decrease of TRACP 5b was higher than that of total TRACP activity[63], suggesting that this marker may be a useful indicator of the effect of antiresorptive therapy on bone resorption, although additional studies comparing its performance with collagen-related markers would be useful.

Collagen pyridinium cross-links and associated type I collagen peptides

Pyridinoline (PYD) and deoxypyridinoline (DPD), also called respectively hydroxylysylpyridinoline (HP) and lysylpyridinoline (LP), are two non-reducible pyridinium cross-links present in the mature form of collagen. This post-translational covalent cross-linking generated from lysine and hydroxylysine residues is unique to collagen and elastin molecules. It creates interchain bonds which stabilize the molecule within the extracellular matrix. The highest concentration of PYD (expressed in mol/mol of collagen) is found in articular cartilage, whereas DPD is present in minute amounts in this tissue[68]. PYD and DPD are present in tendon and aorta but absent from the skin, an abundant source of type I collagen[68]. As both cross-links result from a post-translational modification of collagen molecules, they cannot be reutilized during collagen synthesis. PYD and DPD are released into the circulation after resorption of bone matrix and then excreted in urine, where they are found as free and peptide-bound forms (Fig. 193.1). Studies performed with osteoclastic cells cultured on human bone particles indicated that peptide-bound but not free cross-links are generated directly at the bone resorption site[69]. It has also been shown that the proportion of free cross-links is about two times lower in serum than in urine (16–20% vs. 40%) and that the renal clearance is about four times higher for free than for peptide-bound cross-links[70], suggesting a cleavage of peptide-bound cross-links to free forms in the liver and/or kidney. If this conversion of peptide-bound to free cross-links is saturable, this could explain part of the inverse relationship between increased bone turnover and decreased free cross-link fraction in urine[71]. The total amount of PYD cross-links can be measured by fluorimetry after reversed-phase HPLC of a cellulose-bound extract of hydrolyzed urine[72,73]. In patients with vertebral osteoporosis, the urinary cross-link levels, especially of DPD, are correlated with bone turnover measured by calcium kinetics[74] and bone histomorphometry[75], contrasting with poor correlation obtained with urinary Hyp.

Immunoassays for the PYD cross-links and related telopeptide fragments which substitute advantageously for the HPLC measurement of the total excretion are now available and represent currently the best indices of bone resorption. These comprise measurement of urinary free PYD (free PYD) and DPD (free DPD)[76,77] and of related peptides in urine, and more recently in serum. These peptides include the C-terminal cross-linking telopeptide of type I collagen generated by matrix metalloproteases (MMPs) (S-CTX-MMP, also called ICTP)[78], the C-terminal

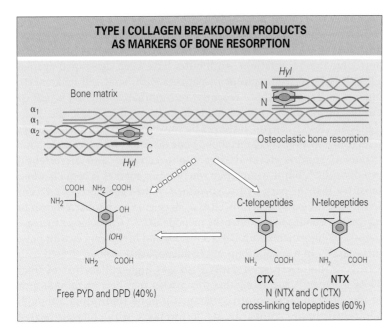

Fig. 193.1 Type I collagen breakdown products as markers of bone resorption. Type I collagen molecules in bone matrix are linked by pyridinoline cross-links (pyridinoline or deoxypyridinoline) in the region of N- and C-telopeptides. Pyridinoline (PYD) differs from deoxypyridinoline (DPD) by the presence of a hydroxyl residue shown in italic. During osteoclastic bone resorption pyridinoline cross-links are released into the circulation mainly as peptide-bound cross-links, i.e. attached to fragments of C-terminal (CTX) or N-terminal (NTX) telopeptides. Parts of the peptide-bound cross-links are further degraded in the kidney in free cross-links. Immunoassays are available that detect specifically free PYD, free DPD, CTX and NTX in serum or urine.

cross-linking telopeptide of type I collagen in serum (S-CTX)[79] and in urine (U-CTX)[80] and the N-terminal cross-linking telopeptide of type I collagen in serum (S-NTX)[81] and in urine (U-NTX)[82]. Most of these type I collagen-related resorption markers can be measured either manually or by automated systems with improved precision and high throughput (Table 193.2). The first peptide assay was a radioimmunoassay for the S-CTX-MMP in serum[78]. The antibody was raised against a cross-link-containing collagen peptide (Mw 8.5 kDa) isolated by trypsin digestion of human bone collagen. The antigenic determinant requires a trivalent cross-link, including two phenylalanine-rich domains of the telopeptide region of the α_1 chain of type I collagen. The tissue specificity and the clinical significance of S-CTX-MMP levels are, however, unclear. In particular, S-CTX-MMP levels increase after treatment with anabolic steroids, which are believed to decrease bone resorption and to

stimulate collagen synthesis[83], which contrasts with the absence of change in S-CTX[84]. Nevertheless, and in contrast to its poor sensitivity in osteoporosis[85], CTX-MMP appears to be a useful bone resorption marker in patients with multiple myeloma[86] or bone metastases[87-91]. The different sensitivities of this marker in these two clinical situations is unclear. One hypothesis could relate to differences in the pattern of type I collagen degradation between osteoporosis and bone metastases because of changes in the relative contributions of the various collagenolytic enzymes, namely the cysteine proteases and MMPs. It has been shown recently that the epitope of CTX-MMP is destroyed by cathepsin K activity[92], an osteoclast-specific cysteine protease which is the key enzyme responsible for bone collagen degradation in normal physiological conditions[93,94], whereas it is generated by MMPs whose activity has been suggested to play an important role in collagen degradation associated with cancer (Fig. 193.2). In contrast, CTX and NTX epitopes are highly efficiently generated by cathepsin K and poorly by MMPs[95]. The degradation of CTX-MMP epitope by cathepsin K explains the absence of increase of this marker in postmenopausal women and its paradoxical increase in patients with pycnodosystosis, a disease characterized by a mutation in the cathepsin K gene, contrasting with the expected decrease of CTX and NTX in this condition[96]. Currently, available

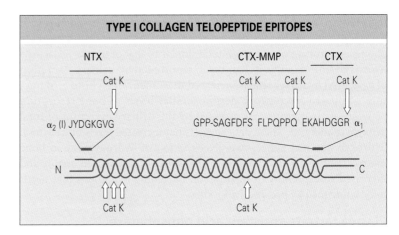

Fig. 193.2 Type I collagen telopeptide epitopes. Schematic representation of the different type I collagen telopeptide epitopes used as markers of bone resorption and sites of cleavage by cathepsin K (Cat K) on type I collagen. The NTX epitope and CTX epitopes in the N and C telopeptide regions, respectively, are efficiently generated by Cat K, the main enzyme responsible for type I collagen degradation in physiological conditions, but not by matrix metalloproteases (MMP)[94,95], which have been proposed to participate in bone resorption in physiological conditions, but also in metastatic processes. In contrast, CTX-MMP epitope is destroyed by the action of Cat K and is generated by MMPs[92,95].

TABLE 193.2 TYPE I COLLAGEN-RELATED BONE RESORPTION MARKERS AND RESPECTIVE ASSAYS

Marker	Serum/urine	Commercial denomination (manufacturer)	Type of assay
CTX	S	Serum Crosslaps One Step (Osteomer Biotech)	Manual ELISA
CTX	S	β-Crosslaps/serum (Roche Diagnostics)	Automated (Elecsys)
CTX	U	Crosslaps ELISA (Osteometer Biotech)	Manual ELISA
α-CTX	U	α-Crosslaps RIA (Osteometer Biotech)	Manual RIA
NTX	S	Osteomark NTx Serum (Ostex)	Manual ELISA
NTX	U	Osteomark Assay (Ostex)	Manual ELISA
NTX	U	Vitros NTX (Ortho-Clinical Diagnostics)	Automated (Vitros Eci)
CTX-MMP	S	ICTP (Orion Diagnostica)	Manual ELISA
Free DPD	U	Pyrilinks D (Metra Biosystems)	Manual ELISA/RIA
Free DPD	U	Pyrilinks D (DPC)	Automated (ACS 180)
Free DPD	U	Pyrilinks D (Chiron)	Automated (Immulite)

markers of type I collagen degradation are based on the measurement of either pyridinoline cross-links or associated cross-linked C or N telopeptides, both originating from the telopeptide region. Recently, a type I collagen-specific peptide corresponding to residues 620–633 of the helicoidal region of the α_1 chain has been isolated from the urine of patients with Paget's disease of bone. Although the enzymatic processes involved in the generation of this peptide are currently unknown, they may reflect different aspects of bone resorption than the telopeptide-derived fragments. We recently found that the urinary excretion of that helicoidal peptide increased markedly after the menopause and it was as sensitive as urinary CTX measurements to assess the antiresorptive effects of bisphosphonate and estrogens[97], suggesting that it may be useful for the investigation of patients with osteoporosis, although additional studies are required to fully evaluate its clinical utility.

Post-translation modifications of type I collagen other than PYD cross-links occur in bone matrix and some of them may be of clinical relevance for the investigation of metabolic bone diseases. Probably one of the most interesting of these modifications is the racemization and β isomerization of the Asp–Gly sequence [1209]AHDGGR[1214] of the C-telopeptide of type I collagen[112,113] generating four isomers: the native form (αL) and three age-related forms: an isomerized (βL), a racemized (αD) and an isomerized/racemized (βD) form (Fig. 193.3). The relative rates at which the age-related CTX-isoforms are generated in bone matrix have been shown to be βL > βD > αD[113]. Thus, αL-CTX reflects the resorption of newly synthesized bone, whereas βL-, βD- and αD-CTX reflect the degradation of aged bone, old bone and very old bone, respectively. Histological studies have shown a decreased degree of isomerization/racemization within the woven pagetic bone, reflected by increased urinary αL/βL and αL/αD ratios[114,115]. These results suggest

that the newly synthesized collagen fibers found in the woven pagetic bone are characterized by a marked decrease of the degree of isomerization. The urinary ratio αCTX/βCTX returned within the normal range in most patients within weeks of treatment with bisphosphonate[115]. Because patients with bone metastases from prostate cancer are also characterized by a marked increase of bone turnover in localized area of the skeleton, with the replacement of lamellar by woven bone, one could expect a higher increase of U-αL CTX compared to U-βL CTX and U-αD CTX, leading to increased αL/βL and αL/αD ratios in these patients. In a recent study involving 39 patients with prostate cancer and bone metastases[116], although the αL/βL ratio was normal, the ratio between the urinary degradation products of the newly formed (αL) and the oldest (αD) forms of collagen was increased twofold compared to controls. These data suggest that the pattern of type I collagen isomerization/racemization is indeed altered in sclerotic metastases, and that the urinary αL/αD ratio may represent a useful index to assess abnormalities of bone matrix in that situation. More recently, in a prospective study of postmenopausal women (OFELY study) we found that racemization/isomerization of type I collagen was also significantly decreased in the 65 women who sustained incident fractures compared to the 343 women of the same cohort who did not fracture during an average follow-up of 6 years. An increased urinary ratio between native and age-related forms of type I collagen CTX was associated with increased fracture risk independently of the level of BMD of the hip and of bone turnover rate[117]. These data suggest that a decreased degree of type I collagen isomerization/racemization could be associated with alterations in bone strength properties. This hypothesis needs to be confirmed by studies correlating the degree of type I collagen racemization/isomerization with the mechanical properties of bone

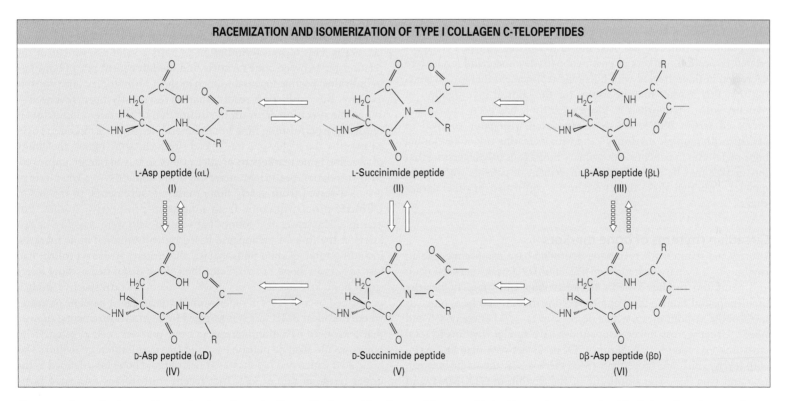

RACEMIZATION AND ISOMERIZATION OF TYPE I COLLAGEN C-TELOPEPTIDES

L-Asp peptide (αL) (I) L-Succinimide peptide (II) Lβ-Asp peptide (βL) (III)

D-Asp peptide (αD) (IV) D-Succinimide peptide (V) Dβ-Asp peptide (βD) (VI)

Fig. 193.3 Racemization and isomerization of type I collagen C-telopeptides. An attack by a peptide backbone nitrogen on the side chain carbonyl group of an adjacent aspartyl residue can result in the formation of a succinimide ring (I→II). The succinimide ring is prone to hydrolysis and racemization, producing peptides and β-aspartyl peptides in both the D and L configurations. Racemization is thought to proceed primarily through the succinimide pathway (II→V), but other pathways such as direct proton abstraction (I↔IV and III↔VI) may also contribute to the formation of D-aspartyl. Throughout the figure, the peptide backbone is shown as a bold line. The four types of C-telopeptide are present in bone matrix: the native form (αL) and three age-related forms: an isomerized (βL), a racemized (αD) and an isomerized/racemized (βD) form. With increasing age of type I collagen molecules, the proportion of β-isomerized and D-racemized forms within bone matrix increases. Degradation products of these four CTX forms of type I collagen can be measured in urine independently by immunoassays using specific conformational monoclonal antibodies. (With permission from Cloos and Fledelius[113].)

specimens. Clearly these findings open new perspectives for the clinical use of bone markers, not only to measure quantitative changes in bone turnover, but also to assess changes of bone quality.

Bone sialoprotein (BSP)

BSP is a phosphorylated glycoprotein with an apparent MW of 70–80 kDa and accounts for 5–10% of the non-collageneous matrix of bone[118]. The protein has been shown to be a major synthetic product of active osteoblasts and odontoblasts, but was also found in osteoclast-like and malignant cell lines[119–121]. Compared to other non-collagenous protein, the tissue distribution of BSP is quite restricted and mRNA has been detected in dentine and in bone with higher BSP concentration in the osteocartilaginous interfaces[122] that are involved early in joint diseases such as osteoarthritis and rheumatoid arthritis. However, BSP immunoreactivity has also been detected in platelets[123]. BSP contains an Arg–Gly–Asp (RGD) integrin recognition sequence and binds preferentially to the α_2 chain of collagen[124]. It nucleates hydroxyapatite crystal formation in vitro[125] and appears to enhance osteoclast-mediated bone resorption[126], suggesting that this protein may play an important role in the local regulation of bone remodeling and in the organization of the extracellular matrix of mineralized tissues.

Several immunoassays based on polyclonal antibodies raised against bovine or human BSP have been developed[123,127,128]. However, little is known about the exact nature of the respective epitopes recognized by these antibodies. Whether the assays recognize the intact newly synthesized molecule or fragments released during resorption of bone matrix and/or by proteolytic degradation of the protein in the circulation remains to be established. Increased serum BSP has been reported in patients with different metabolic bone diseases, including Paget's disease, primary hyperparathyroidism and women with postmenopausal osteoporosis[129,130]. Based on these clinical data and the rapid decrease in serum BSP levels following intravenous bisphosphonate treatment, it is likely that serum BSP reflects processes mainly related to bone resorption[129]. Serum BSP has been shown to correlate to type I collagen-related resorption markers in postmenopausal women, and levels were decreased in those treated with hormone replacement therapy, suggesting that this marker may be useful for the clinical investigation of patients with osteoporosis[131]. More recently it has been shown that increased serum BSP levels were associated with poor survival in patients with multiple myeloma[132] and with increasing risk of developing bone metastases in patients with primary breast cancer[133], suggesting that this marker may be useful in the management of patients with malignancies, although these data need to be confirmed in other larger studies.

Circadian rhythms of bone markers

Urinary and serum markers of bone resorption have significant circadian rhythms[98–111]. Urinary excretion of PYD and DPD peaks between 0200 and 0800 and reaches a nadir between 1400 and 2300. In healthy premenopausal women the magnitude of the rhythm may be as much as 100% of the 24-hour mean, with a decrease of 25–35% between 0800 and 1100[105]. Urinary cross-linked telopeptides have similar rhythms to total cross-link excretion[99,100,104]. Serum CTX peaks between 0130 and 0430, with levels which are more than twice the levels at the nadir between 1100 and 1500[102,110]. The amplitude of the rhythm of CTX-MMP and S-NTX is only 15–20% of the 24-hour mean[101,108], suggesting that the different type I collagen peptides may indeed have different bone specificities and/or reflect different aspects of bone resorption. Circadian rhythms of markers of bone resorption may be attenuated by several factors. Evening calcium supplementation may diminish the rhythmicity of markers of bone resorption, but this effect may depend on whether it is given over a period of weeks or as a single dose[99,106]. Bisphosphonate

therapy reduces the amplitude of the circadian rhythm of urinary NTX although the pattern is maintained[107,108]. In recent studies, fasting has been shown to result in a diminution in the amplitude of the circadian rhythm of urinary – and more markedly – of serum CTX[109–111]. This effect remains to be investigated for the other resorption markers, including the total urinary excretion of pyridinoline cross-links, but if confirmed could give new insights into the pathophysiology and treatment of osteoporosis. In summary, although the amplitude of the circadian rhythm differs according to the markers, its effect is substantial for most of them and indicates the importance of standardizing the time of sampling and the fasting condition of the patient.

CLINICAL USES OF BONE TURNOVER MARKERS IN OSTEOPOROSIS

Bone markers and rate of bone loss

Several cross-sectional studies suggest that bone turnover increases rapidly after the menopause. It has been shown recently that this increase in both bone formation and bone resorption is sustained long after the menopause, for up to 40 years[134]. BMD measured at various skeletal sites is inversely correlated with bone turnover assessed by various markers in postmenopausal women. We have shown that the correlation between bone markers and BMD becomes much stronger with advancing age, so that in women more than 30 years after the menopause bone turnover accounts for 40–50% of the variance of bone mineral density of the whole skeleton[134]. These cross-sectional data suggest that a sustained increase of bone turnover in postmenopausal women induces a more rapid rate of bone loss and therefore an increased risk of osteoporosis. Longitudinal studies are required to confirm this hypothesis. When the rate of bone loss is assessed by annual measurement of bone mineral density at the spine, hip or radius over only 2–4 years, the amount of loss is of the same order of the magnitude of the precision error of repeated measurements in a single individual, i.e. 3–4%. This technical limitation impairs a valid assessment of the relationship between bone turnover and the subsequent rate of bone loss in individual postmenopausal women in short-term studies, and probably explains the conflicting results that have recently been reviewed[135]. When the precision error on the estimation of the rate of bone loss is reduced by performing nine bone mineral density measurements over 24 months at a highly precise skeletal site such as the radius, the ability of baseline bone markers to predict rate of loss is markedly improved, with correlation coefficient increasing from about 0.2–0.4 when rate of loss is assessed from yearly bone mass measurements, to 0.7–0.8[136]. Ultimate proof will come from long-term prospective studies. For example, Hansen et al.[137] found that women who were classified as fast losers at the time of menopause based on conventional bone markers, including total alkaline phosphatase and urinary hydroxyproline, had lost 50% more bone 12 years later than those diagnosed as slow losers (total bone loss 26.6% versus 16.6%, $P<0.001$) A retrospective study[138] performed over 13 years in older women (mean age at baseline 62 years) where calcaneal BMD loss was assessed by eight measurements, showed that 1 standard deviation increase in bone markers such as osteocalcin, bone-specific alkaline phosphatase and free pyridinoline cross-links was associated with a twofold increased risk of rapid bone loss, defined as the upper tertile of rate of loss. In a recent study of 305 untreated postmenopausal women[139] we found that baseline values of serum OC, serum PINP, serum CTX[139,140], urinary CTX and urinary NTX were inversely correlated with the rate of bone loss at the forearm over the next 4 years, with correlation coefficient of the order of 0.4–0.5. However, when correlation coefficients were corrected for the precision error in individual rate of bone loss and bone marker levels, r values increased and reached 0.7–0.9. These data strongly suggest that assays

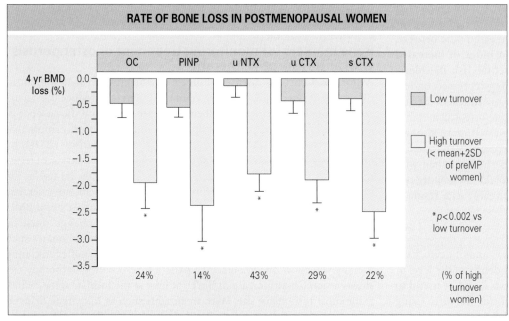

Fig. 193.4 Rate of bone loss in postmenopausal women. The rate of bone loss is shown with high and low bone turnover. Bone loss at the forearm was evaluated by measuring BMD by DXA on four occasions over a 4-year period in 305 post-menopausal women (mean age 64 years), as described in the legend to Table 193.2. For each bone marker each woman was placed in a low and high bone turnover using as a cut-off the mean value +2SD of 134 premenopausal women. The figure shows the percentage of bone loss from baseline during the study period in low and high bone turnover groups. Women whose baseline marker values indicated high bone remodeling lost bone two to six times faster over the next 4 years than those whose marker values were normal. (With permission from Garnero *et al.*[139])

that reduce the short- and long-term variability of bone markers are likely to improve the ability of bone markers to predict the rate of bone mass change. At present, however, it appears that it would be difficult to predict absolute rate of bone loss in individual women using a measurement of bone markers. Nevertheless, the measurement of bone markers may be useful to identify women at a higher risk of being fast bone losers in the following years. Interestingly, we found that women whose marker levels exceeded mean values in premenopausal women by more than 2 SD lost bone two to six times faster than those whose marker levels were normal (Fig. 193.4).

Bone markers and the risk of fragility fractures

With the emergence of effective (but rather expensive) treatments it is essential to detect those women at higher risk of fracture. Several prospective studies have shown that a standard deviation (SD) decrease in bone mineral density (BMD) measured by dual X-ray absorptiometry (DXA) or heel ultrasound is associated with a two- to fourfold increase in relative fracture risk, including the hip, spine and forearm. In this context the question arises to what extent bone markers could add to bone mass measurement in order to improve the assessment of fracture risk.

Relating baseline bone turnover levels with the subsequent risk of osteoporotic fractures is the only valid methodology to assess their clinical utility, as it is difficult from retrospective studies to determine whether differences in bone turnover levels between patients with fractures and controls are related to the underlying rate of bone turnover leading to fracture, or to changes of bone turnover occurring after the fracture.

Prospective studies relating levels of bone formation markers to the risk of fracture have yielded conflicting results. Indeed, either a decrease, no difference or an increase[141,144] in bone formation markers has been reported to be associated with increased fracture risk. The difference between studies may be related to the type of fracture, the populations studied or the duration of follow-up. Thus, whether bone formation marker levels are related to fracture risk remains unclear. In contrast to bone formation markers, data on the relationship between bone resorption markers and fracture risk are very consistent, as reviewed recently[145]. Riis *et al.*[146] reported that women within 3 years of menopause classified as 'fast bone losers' had a twofold higher risk of sustaining vertebral and peripheral fractures during a 15-year follow-up than women classified as 'normal' or 'slow' losers. Interestingly, bone

mineral density (BMD) and rate of bone loss predispose to fractures to the same extent, with odds ratio of about 2. Women with both a low BMD and a fast rate of bone loss after the menopause had a higher risk of subsequently sustaining fractures than women with only one of the two risk factors. Concordant results have been obtained in three large prospective studies (EPIDOS, Rotterdam and OFELY), indicating that increased levels of bone resorption markers are associated with increased risk of hip, vertebral and non-hip and non-vertebral fractures over follow-up periods ranging from 1.8 to 5 years[141,144,147]. This predictive value is consistently of the order of a twofold increase in the risk of fracture for levels above the upper limit of the premenopausal range.

Pyridinium cross-links

Increased levels of both serum and urinary CTX and of free DPD have been shown to be associated with a higher risk of hip, vertebral and other non-vertebral fractures. Increased bone resorption is associated with increased risk of fracture only for values that exceed a threshold, suggesting that bone resorption becomes deleterious for bone strength only when it exceeds the normal physiological range. As the level of bone resorption predicts fracture independently of BMD, these data suggest that increased bone resorption can lead to increased skeletal fragility in two ways. First, a prolonged increase in bone turnover will lead after several years to a lower BMD, which is a major determinant of reduced bone strength. Second, increased bone resorption above the upper limit of the normal range may induce microarchitectural deterioration of bone tissue, such as perforation of trabeculae, a major component of bone strength.

Osteocalcin

OC contains three residues of γ-carboxyglutamic acid (Gla), a vitamin K-dependent amino acid. It was postulated that impaired γ-carboxylation of osteocalcin could be an index of both vitamin D and vitamin K deficiency in elderly populations. Vitamin K status may be involved in the maintenance of skeletal integrity, and recently it has been shown that vitamin K_2 treatment in postmenopausal women with osteoporosis decreases serum levels of undercarboxylated osteocalcin (ucOC), increases spine BMD and reduces the risk of fragility fractures[148]. In two prospective studies performed in a cohort of elderly institutionalized women followed for 3 years[149,150], and in a population of healthy elderly women (EPIDOS study)[151], levels of ucOC over the premenopausal range were associated with a two- to threefold increase in the risk of hip fracture, although total osteocalcin was not predictive. Like markers of bone resorption, the prediction was still significant after adjusting for hip BMD. More recently, it was reported that a decreased ratio between carboxylated and total osteocalcin – which is an index of increased ucOC – was also associated with increased fracture risk in elderly women living at home[152]. The mechanisms relating increased under-carboxylation of osteocalcin and fracture risk are unclear. Serum ucOC[153] and the ratio between carboxylated and total osteocalcin[154], but not total osteocalcin, have been found to be associated more strongly with ultrasonic transmitted velocity (which has been suggested to reflect in part changes in bone structure) at the os calcis and tibia than with BMD[153], suggesting that poor bone quality may explain the fracture risk associated with undercarboxylated osteocalcin, possibly as a result of inadequate vitamin K status.

Using combination data

Because increased levels of bone resorption markers and of ucOC have been shown to predict the risk of fracture independently of the level of BMD, the combination of these two diagnostic tests could be useful to improve the identification of women at high risk for fracture. Using the database of the EPIDOS study, it was shown that combining a bone resorption marker (ucOC) and hip BMD measurement can detect elderly women at very high risk of hip fracture. Indeed, elderly women with both osteoporosis (total hip BMD T-score below –2.5) and high bone resorption had a four- to fivefold higher risk of hip fracture than the general population. This has been confirmed for vertebral and non-vertebral and non-hip fractures in younger postmenopausal women[143]. In addition, using such combinations the specificity of hip fracture prediction is increased without a loss of sensitivity[155]. As recently discussed by Kanis et al.[156], the use of odds ratios is not ideal for clinical decision making, as the risk may decrease or remain stable with age, whereas absolute risk increases. Thus calculating absolute risks such as 10-year probabilities – which depend on knowledge of the fracture and death hazards – is probably more appropriate. Based on the probability of hip fracture in the Swedish population and on the marker data of the EPIDOS study it was found that combining urinary CTX with BMD or history of previous fracture results in a 10-year probability of hip fracture that was about 70–100% higher than that associated with low BMD alone (Table 193.3)[156]. Similar findings also apply for the prediction of all fractures in the younger postmenopausal woman from the OFELY study[156]. Thus, the use of multiple risk factors such as BMD, biochemical markers and other important risk factors, such as personal history of previous fracture, is clearly likely to perform better than the use of BMD alone. Such a combined strategy

has been found to be powerful to identify individuals at high risk for cardiovascular disease[157].

Bone markers for monitoring treatment of osteoporosis with anti-resorptive therapy

As for most chronic diseases, monitoring the efficacy of treatment of osteoporosis is a challenge. The goal of treatment is to reduce the occurrence of fragility fractures, but their incidence is low and the absence of events during the first year(s) of therapy does not necessarily imply that treatment is effective. Measurement of bone mineral density (BMD) by dual-energy X-ray absorptiometry (DXA) is a surrogate marker of treatment efficacy that has been widely used in clinical trials. Its use in the monitoring of treatment efficacy in the individual patient, however, has not been validated. Given a short-term precision error of 1–1.5% of BMD measurement at the spine and hip, the individual change must be greater than 3–5% to be seen as significant. With bisphosphonates such as alendronate and risechonate, repeating BMD 2 years after initiating therapy will allow one to detect if a patient is responding to therapy, i.e. shows a significant increase in BMD, at least at the lumbar spine, which is the most responsive site. With treatments such as raloxifene or nasal calcitonin that induce much smaller increases in BMD, DXA is not appropriate to monitor therapy, and with any treatment DXA does not permit the identification of all responders within the first year of therapy. Failure to respond may be due to non-compliance – probably the most important single factor – to poor intestinal absorption (especially with bisphosphonates), to other factors contributing to bone loss, or to other unidentified factors. Monitoring may improve compliance, although this has not been proven for osteoporosis treatment.

Several randomized placebo-controlled studies found that antiresorptive therapy was associated with a prompt decrease of bone resorption markers that can be seen as early as 2 weeks, with a plateau being reached within 3–6 months. The decrease of bone formation markers is delayed, reflecting the physiological coupling of formation to resorption, and a plateau is usually achieved within 6–12 months (Fig. 193.5)[158]. The decrease of bone turnover markers under antiresorptive therapy, usually expressed as a percentage of the initial value, is correlated to a varying degree with the increase in BMD. All published studies of HRT in the past 10 years[159–165] except one[166] have shown that the short-term (3–6 months) decrease in bone turnover markers is significantly correlated with the long-term (1–2 years) increase in BMD at the spine, radius and hip (Fig. 193.6). A marked decrease of markers is associated with a positive subsequent BMD response, whereas non responders show little or no changes of bone markers, suggesting that bone markers, especially new sensitive and specific ones, could be used to monitor HRT. Similarly,

TABLE 193.3 RISK FACTORS FOR HIP FRACTURE

Risk factor	Threshold value	Prevalence (%)	Odds ratio	Relative risk*	10-year probability (%)
Average	–	100		1.0	18.0
Low BMD	T-score <–2.5	56	2.8	1.40	23.6
Prior fracture	Yes	39	3.5	1.77	28.8
High CTX	Above premenopausal values	23	2.4	1.82	29.5
Low BMD + prior fracture	As above	23	4.1	2.39	36.3
Low BMD + high CTX	As above	16	4.1	2.74	40.1
Prior fracture + high CTX	As above	12	5.3	3.50	47.3
All of the above	As above	7	5.8	4.43	54.5

* Adjusted for the prevalence of the risk factor in the population.

The effect of risk factors alone or in combination on the relative risk of hip fracture in women at the age of 80 years. The right-hand column gives the probability of hip fracture within the next 10 years. From Kanis et al.[17]

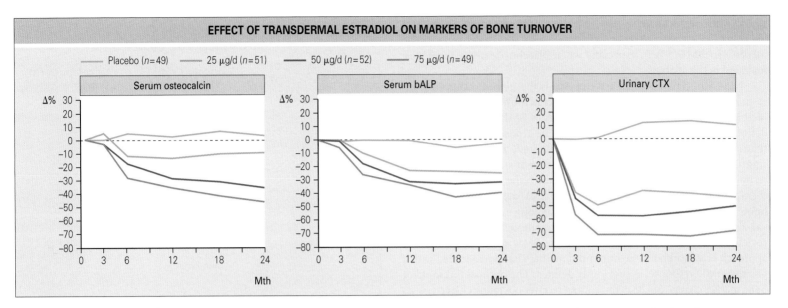

Fig. 193.5 Effect of transdermal estradiol on markers of bone turnover. In this study, 201 postmenopausal women aged 40–60 years with a time since menopause shorter than 6 years were given either a placebo or a new matrix delivery transdermal 17β estradiol in a dosage of 25, 50 or 75 μg twice a week for 28 days. The decrease of bone formation markers (osteocalcin and bALP) is delayed compared to that of bone resorption (urinary CTX), reflecting the coupling mechanism. This delayed decrease of bone formation is amplified by the transdermal route of administration of estradiol. (With permission from Cooper et al.[158])

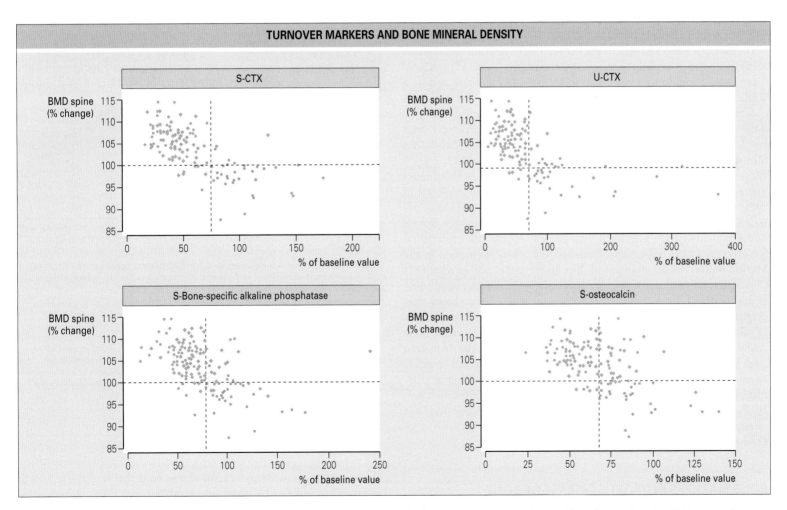

Fig. 193.6 Turnover markers and bone mineral density. Relationships between early changes in turnover markers and late changes in spine BMD assessed by DXA in postmenopausal women treated by estradiol 1 mg/day (orange diamonds), estradiol 2 mg/day (orange circles) or placebo (purple circles). The optimum cut-offs of biochemical markers of bone turnover, i.e. the best trade-off between sensitivity and specificity, were derived from ROC analyses and were used to calculate the accuracy of the marker changes after 6 months of treatment to predict the long-term changes in spine BMD after 3 years. For example a 37% decrease in serum CTX (S-CTX) at 6 months provided a sensitivity of 86.9%, a specificity of 88.6%, a positive predictive value of 95.6% and a negative predictive value of 70.5%. (With permission from Bjarnason and Christiansen[163].)

studies with alendronate suggest that the magnitude of the short-term decrease in bone turnover is correlated with the magnitude of the increase in BMD[85,166,170], especially when placebo-treated patients are included in the analysis.

For the clinician, the primary concern is the identification of non-responders, i.e. patients who will fail to demonstrate a significant increase in BMD after 2 years of treatment. A BMD response has been defined either as a positive BMD change or a positive change greater than the precision error in a single individual, also called the least significant change. Several methods have been suggested to identify responders/non-responders according to the bone marker response to therapy. One approach is to consider the least significant change of a bone marker based on the short term or long term within-subject variability in untreated women; this method has been recently reviewed[171] (Table 193.4), regardless of the BMD response[161]. Another approach is to search for the minimum marker change associated with a positive BMD response, as previously defined. The optimal threshold of bone marker change can be defined using receiver operating characteristics analysis, or by using logistic regression models[162,167,168]. The percentage change and/or the absolute value of the marker under treatment can be used[169], and cut-off values can be obtained with a prespecified sensitivity or specificity[162,169]. Retrospective analyses of several clinical trials using HRT or alendronate suggest that, for a given marker of resorption or formation, a cut-off value under treatment can be defined that provides an adequate predictive value of the subsequent 2-year BMD response in a single patient[172] (Table 193.5). These cut-off values should be tested in other cohorts using the same therapeutic regimens in order to strengthen their clinical utility.

The value of BMD changes to predict the risk of fracture under treatment is debated, especially because some treatments – such as raloxifene – can induce a 30 to 50% reduction in vertebral fracture rate despite a small 2 to 3% increase of BMD at all skeletal sites. Thus, BMD changes may not be an adequate surrogate endpoint to analyze the ability of bone markers to predict fracture risk. Unfortunately, there have been few attempts to correlate bone marker changes with fracture risk. In a retrospective analysis of a small placebo controlled trial of HRT, Riggs[173] suggested that changes in bone turnover (assessed by histomorphometry) predict change in vertebral fracture risk as well as change in BMD in osteoporotic women. Interestingly, it was found that the short-term changes of serum osteocalcin and serum bone alkaline phosphatase under raloxifene were associated with the subsequent risk of vertebral fractures in a large subgroup of osteoporotic women enrolled in the MORE study, while changes in hip BMD were not predictive[174] (Fig. 193.7). More recently, in postmenopausal women with osteoporosis treated with oral risedronate (VERT study) it has been shown that changes of urinary CTX and NTX after 3 to 6 months predicted the risk of subsequent incident vertebral fractures after both 1 and 3 years, these changes accounting for 66–67% of the vertebral fracture risk reduction over 3 years.[175] Clearly, such analyses should be performed in other ongoing and recently completed large clinical trials performed in postmenopausal women with osteoporosis treated with bisphosphonates, HRT, or SERMs and cut-off values to predict responders and non responders to therapy should be defined using incident fractures as an endpoint.

BONE MARKERS IN PAGET'S DISEASE OF BONE

Introduction

Paget's disease of bone is a localized disorder characterized by a marked increase of bone turnover, leading to the overproduction of poor-quality bone responsible for hypertrophy, osteosclerosis and bone fragility[176]. The architecture of the lamellar texture of pagetic bone matrix is dis-

TABLE 193.4 WITHIN-SUBJECT VARIABILITY (CV%) OF BONE MARKERS IN POSTMENOPAUSAL WOMEN

	Short-term CV (%) (1–5 weeks)	Long-term CV (%) (3 months–3 years)
Bone formation		
Serum		
OC	7–13	8–27*
Bone ALP	7–13	9
PINP	–	7.5
PICP	10.6	8.6
Bone resorption		
Serum		
NTX	6.3	7.5
CTX	8 (fasting)	9–13
	14 (non-fasting)	
Urine		
Total DPD (HPLC)	12–24	17–63
Free DPD (ELISA)	12	9–13
CTX	–	18–24
NTX	10–18	16–25

* The figure of 27% was obtained using a conventional bovine-based radioimmunoassay recognizing mainly intact osteocalcin and highly sensitive to sampling procedures.

(With permission from Hannon and Eastell[171].)

TABLE 193.5 EARLY CHANGES IN BONE REMODELING MARKERS TO PREDICT THE EFFICACY OF ESTROGEN REPLACEMENT THERAPY WITH A 90% SPECIFICITY IN INDIVIDUAL PATIENTS

Marker	Cut-off value for the bone marker decrease after 3 or 6 months (%)	Sensitivity* (%)	Likelihood of a positive response† (%)
Serum OC (6 months)	–21	51	89
Serum bone ALP (6 months)	–20	49	89
Serum CTX (3 months)	–33	68	87
Urinary CTX (3 months)	–45	60	88

* Proportion of women whose bone marker value decrease at 3 to 6 months into therapy was equal to or greater than the cut-off, among those with a greater than 2.26% BMD increase 2 years into therapy.

† Proportion of women with a greater than 2.26% BMD increase 2 years into therapy, among those whose bone marker value decrease at 3 to 6 months into therapy was equal to or greater than the cut-off.

In this study, 569 postmenopausal women aged 40–60 years with a time since menopause shorter than 6 years were given either a placebo or transdermal estrogen in a dosage of 25, 50 or 75µg twice a week for 28 days (continuous treatment) or 50, 75 or 100µg twice a week for 25 days per cycle (cyclic therapy). Bone mineral density (BMD) at the spine was measured at baseline and after 2 years using dual-energy X-ray absorptiometry (DXA). Women with a BMD increase versus baseline greater than 2.26% (i.e. twice the short-term coefficient of variation for DXA) were classified as treatment responders and women with a BMD decrease versus baseline of more than 2.26% as non-responders. The table shows the sensitivity and the likelihood of a positive response obtained using a 3 to 6 month bone marker decrease cut-off associated with 90% specificity. (From Delmas *et al.*[162])

organized, with a predominance of woven bone that is characterized by an irregular and patchy arrangement of collagen fibers. Biochemical markers of bone turnover are routinely used for assessing the disease activity and for monitoring the efficacy of bisphosphonate therapy. Because of the marked increased in bone turnover, serum total alkaline phosphatase activity is the most commonly used bone marker in Paget's disease of bone for both applications. The level of this marker has been shown to be correlated with the extent of the disease ($r = 0.66$) assessed

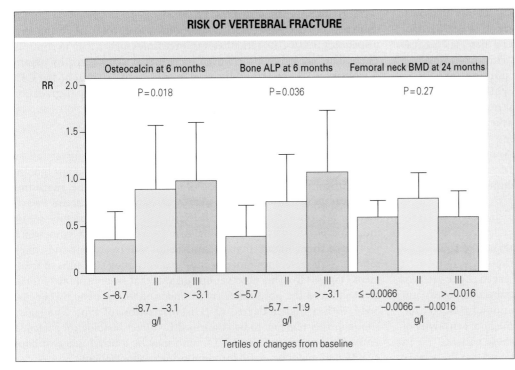

Fig. 193.7 Risk of vertebral fracture. The relative risk of new vertebral fracture at 3 years (raloxifene vs placebo) by tertile of change in serum osteocalcin, serum bone alkaline phosphatase (bone ALP) after 6 months and in femoral neck BMD after 24 months. Postmenopausal women with osteoporosis participating in the MORE study were treated by raloxifene (60 or 120mg/day) or placebo for 3 years. Note that there was a significant relationship between the magnitude of changes in bone markers at 6 months and the relative risk of new vertebral fracture at 3 years, whereas changes in femoral neck BMD at 24 months were not predictive. The P values are for interaction and indicate the presence of a differential antifracture efficacy across tertile of changes for a model including tertile of change, therapy and tertile therapy. $n = 2413$, 2403 and 6745 for osteocalcin, bone ALP and femoral neck BMD, respectively. (With permission from Bjarnason et al.[174])

TABLE 193.6 SENSITIVITY OF BONE MARKERS IN PAGET'S DISEASE OF BONE

Bone marker	Polyostotic disease (n = 27) (increase over control values)	Monostotic disease (n = 16) (increase over control values)
Formation		
Total alkaline phosphatase	× 5.2	× 2.1
Bone alkaline phosphatase	× 8.1	× 3.5
Intact PINP	× 8.9	× 2.7
PICP	× 1.8	× 1.4
Osteocalcin	× 2.4	× 1.5
Bone resorption		
Urinary hydroxyproline	× 3.9	× 1.7
Urinary NTX	× 31	× 7.2
Serum TRACP	× 1.5	× 1.1
Serum CTX-MMP	× 2.0	× 1.3
Urinary DPD	× 3.2	× 1.4
Urinary β-CTX	× 3.1	× 1.2

Data are expressed in -fold increase over control values: From Alvarez et al.[39]

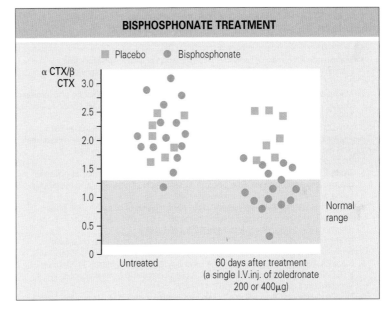

Fig. 193.8 Bisphosphate treatment. Effect of bisphosphonate treatment on the urinary ratio of non-isomerized to β-isomerized C-telopeptide breakdown products (αCTX/βCTX) in Paget's disease. A total of 28 patients with active Paget's disease of bone were studied before and 2 months after a single injection of the bisphosphonate zoledronate (200 or 400μg) or placebo. Before treatment most patients (93%) were characterized by elevated urinary αCTX/βCTX ratio with a mean 2.7-fold increase compared to controls (2.1 vs 0.8). Two months after treatment, the αCTX/βCTX was decreased by 50% in zoledronate-treated patients and returned within the normal range (gray area: mean±2SD) in 65% patients. No significant change was observed in the placebo-treated group. (With permission from Garnero et al.[115])

by bone scanning[177]. Although serum total alkaline phosphatase is adequate to monitor most patients with an active disease, this marker may lack sensitivity in two clinical presentations: in patients with monostotic disease affecting a small bone, and in patients with purely osteolytic lesions.

New markers

To overcome these limitations, the new specific markers described above and validated in osteoporosis have been studied in patients with Paget's disease of bone. However, because a given marker may not perform equally well in different metabolic bone diseases, they must be tested independently in pagetic patients. A study comparing a panel of different markers of bone formation and bone resorption in 43 patients with Paget's disease, including 16 with monostotic lesions and 27 with poly-

ostotic disease showed that bone ALP and PINP were the most sensitive bone formation markers for assessing disease activity[39] (Table 193.6). These two markers might be particularly interesting in patients with monostotic disease. Interestingly, both markers also demonstrated a more pronounced decrease than total alkaline phosphate activity after treatment with the bisphosphonates pamidronate[6] and tiludronate[40]. Although osteocalcin is one of the most sensitive markers in osteoporosis, it lacks sensitivity in Paget's disease[178]. The reasons for this are unknown, but it has been postulated that the fraction of newly synthesized osteocalcin that is incorporated into bone matrix might be increased because of the high mineral content of the woven bone. This may result in a decrease in the fraction of osteocalcin released into the circulation. Alternatively, a dysregulation of osteocalcin synthesis by pagetic osteoblasts could also be involved, although this has not been tested. For bone resorption, the type I collagen-related markers have replaced urinary hydroxyproline. Among these, urinary NTX and urinary non-isomerized α CTX (see below) currently appear to be the most sensitive bone resorption markers both for assessing disease activity and for monitoring efficacy of bisphosphonate therapy[39,40,115] (Table 193.6).

As discussed above, the pagetic bone matrix is characterized by an impaired degree of β isomerization of type I collagen molecules[114] (see Fig. 193.3). We have shown by direct immunoassay of collagenase digest of human bone specimens that the proportion of β-isomerized type I collagen molecules was indeed decreased in pagetic bone (40% of β CTX) compared to normal bone taken from trabecular (68%) and cortical compartments (71%)[114]. This lower proportion of β-isomerized type I collagen in pagetic bone probably explains the poor sensitivity of urinary β CTX for assessing disease activity in these patients[39,114]. In 26 patients with active Paget's disease of bone, we found that the urinary

excretion of non-isomerised α CTX was markedly increased (13.5fold vs controls) compared to β CTX (3.5-fold vs controls), resulting in a urinary α CTX/β CTX ratio that was three times higher than in controls. These data suggest that the woven bone matrix synthesized by pagetic osteoblasts is characterized by an altered β isomerization of the CTX which can be detected *in vivo* by measuring the urinary degradation products arising from bone collagen resorption.

Use of bone markers in monitoring treatment

Bisphosphonates induce a marked decrease of bone turnover rate in pagetic patients, and histological studies have shown that a few months of treatment induce the formation of normal lamellar bone, suggesting that treatment restores bone quality[179]. In patients with active Paget's disease we found that a single injection of zoledronate 200–400μg induces a significant decrease of the urinary α CTX/β CTX ratio, which was three times higher than in controls before treatment and which returns to the reference range in most patients after 2 months of treatment (Fig. 193.8). This observation suggests that bisphosphonate treatment induced the progressive replacement of woven bone by lamellar bone with a higher degree of β isomerization of type I collagen, although this remains to be confirmed by direct histological evidence. Thus, the urinary α CTX/β CTX ratio may be a novel index of bone quality that might be useful for monitoring pagetic patients.

REFERENCES

1. Magnusson P, Lofman O, Larsson L. Determination of alkaline phosphatase isoenzymes in serum by high performance liquid chromatography with post-column reaction detection. J Chromatogr 1992; 576: 79–86.
2. Magnusson P, Larsson L, Magnusson M et al. Isoforms of bone alkaline phosphatase: characterization and origin in human trabecular and cortical bone. J Bone Miner Res 1999; 14: 1926–1933.
3. Moss DW. Alkaline phosphatase isoenzymes. Clin Chem 1982; 28: 2007–2016.
4. Farley JR, Chestnut CJ, Baylink DJ. Improved method for quantitative determination in serum alkaline phosphatase of skeletal origin. Clin Chem 1981; 27: 2002–2007.
5. Duda RJ, O'Brien JF, Katzmann JA et al. Concurrent assays of circulating bone gla-protein and bone alkaline phosphatase: Effects of sex, age, and metabolic bone disease. J Clin Endocrinol Metab 1988; 66: 951–957.
6. Garnero P, Delmas PD. Assessment of the serum levels of bone alkaline phosphatase with a new immunoradiometric assay in patients with metabolic bone disease. J Clin Endocrinol Metab 1993; 77: 1046–1053.
7. Gomez B, Ardakanis S, Ju J et al. Monoclonal antibody assay for measuring bone-specific alkaline phosphatase in serum. Clin Chem 1995; 41: 1560–1566.
8. Price PA. Vitamin K-dependent bone proteins. In: Cohn DV, Martin TJ, Meunier PJ, eds. Calcium regulation and bone metabolism: basic and clinical aspects. Vol. 9. Amsterdam: Elsevier Science, 1987; 419–426.
9. Ducy P, Desbois C, Boyce B et al. Increased bone formation in osteocalcin-deficient mice. Nature 1996; 382: 448–452.
10. Price PA, Parthemore JG, Deftos LJ. New biochemical marker for bone metabolism. J Clin Invest 1980; 66: 878–883.
11. Price PA, Williamson MK, Lothringer JW. Origin of vitamin K-dependent bone protein found in plasma and its clearance by kidney and bone. J Biol Chem 1981; 256: 12760–12766.
12. Lian JB, Gundberg CM. Osteocalcin. Biochemical considerations and clinical applications. Clin Orthop Rel Res 1988; 226: 267–291.
13. Delmas PD, Stenner D, Wahner HW et al. Serum bone gla-protein increases with aging in normal women: Implications for the mechanism of age-related bone loss. J Clin Invest 1983; 71: 1316–1321.
14. Thiede MA, Smock SL, Petersen DN et al. Presence of messenger of ribonucleic acid encoding osteocalcin, a marker of bone turnover, in bone marrow megakaryocytes and peripheral blood platelets. Endocrinology 1994; 135: 929–937.
15. Delmas PD, Wilson DM, Mann KG et al. Effect of renal function on plasma levels of bone gla-protein. J Clin Endocrinol Metab 1983; 57: 1028–1030.
16. Delmas PD. Biochemical markers of bone turnover for the clinical assessment of metabolic disease. Endocrinol Metab Clin North Am 1990; 19: 1–18.
17. Brown JP, Delmas PD, Malaval L et al. Serum bone Gla-protein: A specific marker for bone formation in postmenopausal osteoporosis. Lancet 1984; 1: 1091–1093.
18. Charles P, Poser JW, Mosekilde L, Jensen FT. Estimation of bone turnover evaluated by 47 calcium kinetics. Efficiency of serum bone gamma-carboxyglutamic acid containing protein, serum alkaline phosphatase and urinary hydroxyproline excretion. J Clin Invest 1985; 76: 2254–2258.
19. Delmas PD, Malaval L, Arlot ME, Meunier PJ. Serum bone gla-protein compared to bone histomorphometry in endocrine diseases. Bone 1985; 6: 329–341.

20. Delmas PD, Demiaux B, Malaval L et al. Serum bone gla-protein (osteocalcin) in primary hyperparathyroidism and in malignant hypercalcemia. Comparison with bone histomorphometry. J Clin Invest 1986; 77: 985–991.
21. Bataille R, Delmas PD, Sany J. Serum bone gla-protein in multiple myeloma. Cancer 1987; 59: 329–334.
22. Garnero P, Grimaux M, Seguin P, Delmas PD. Characterization of immunoreactive forms of human osteocalcin generated *in vivo* and *in vitro*. J Bone Miner Res 1994; 9: 255–264.
23. Ivaska KK, Heino TJ, Hentunen TA, Väänänen. Osteocalcin released during resorption *in vitro*. J Bone Miner Res 2001; 16 (suppl 1) : S329.
24. Delmas PD, Christiansen C, Mann KG, Price PA. Bone gla-protein (osteocalcin) assay standardization report. J Bone Miner Res 1990; 1: 5–11.
25. Parfitt AM, Simon LS, Villanueva AR et al. Procollagen type I carboxy-terminal extension peptide in serum as a marker of collagen biosynthesis in bone. Correlation with iliac bone formation rates and comparison with total alkaline phosphatase. J Bone Miner Res 1987; 2: 427–436.
26. Hassager C, Fabbri-Mabelli G, Christiansen C. The effect of the menopause and hormone replacement therapy on serum carboxyterminal propeptide of type I collagen. Osteoporosis Int 1993; 3: 50–52.
27. Ebeling PR, Peterson JM, Riggs BL. Utility of type I procollagen propeptide assays for assessing abnormalities in metabolic bone diseases. J Bone Miner Res 1992; 7: 1243–1250.
28. Hasling C, Eriksen EF, Melkko J et al. Effects of a combined estrogengestagen regimen on serum levels of the carboxy-terminal propeptide of human type I procollagen in osteoporosis. J Bone Miner Res 1991; 6 : 1295–1300.
29. Melkko J, Niemi S, Risteli L, Risteli J. Radioimmunoassay of the carboxyterminal propeptide of human type I procollagen. Clin Chem 1990; 40: 1328–1332.
30. Melkko J, Kauppila S, Niemi S et al. Immunoassay for intact amino-terminal propetide of human type I procollagen. Clin Chem 1996; 42: 947–954.
31. Brandt J, Kroch T, Jensen CH et al. Thermal instability of the trimeric structure of the N-terminal propeptide of human procollagen type I in relation to assay technology. Clin Chem 1999; 45: 47–53.
32. Risteli J, Risteli L. Products of bone collagen metabolism. In: Seibel MJ, Robins SP, Bilezikian JP, eds Dynamics of bone and cartilage metabolism. San Diego: Academic Press, 1999; 275–287.
33. Ebeling PR, Peterson JM, Riggs BL. Utility of type I procollagen propeptide assays for assessing abnormalities in metabolic bone diseases. J Bone Miner Res 1992; 7: 1243–1250.
34. Linkhart SG, Linkhart TA, Taylor AK et al. Synthetic peptide-based immunoassay for amino-terminal propeptide of type I procollagen: Application for evaluation of bone formation. Clin Chem 1993; 39: 2254–2258.
35. Garnero P, Vergnaud P, Delmas PD. Amino terminal propeptide of type I collagen (PINP) is a more sensitive marker of bone turnover than C-terminal propeptide in osteoporosis. J Bone Miner Res 1997; 12: s497.
36. Cabrera, CD Henriquez M, Traba ML et al. Biochemical markers of bone formation in the study of postmenopausal osteoporosis. Osteoporos Int 1998; 8: 147–151.
37. Hannon R, Blumsohn A, Naylor K, Eastell R. Response of biochemical markers of bone turnover to hormone replacement therapy: impact of biological variability. J Bone Miner Res 1998 ; 13: 1124–1133.

38. Garnero P, Tsouderos Y, Marton I *et al.* Effects of intranasal 17 β estradiol on bone turnover and serum insulin like growth factor I in postmenopausal women. J Clin Endocrinol Metab 1999; 84: 2390–2397.

39. Alvarez L, Peris P, Pons F *et al.* Relationships between biochemical markers of bone turnover and bone scintigraphy indices in assessment of Paget's disease activity. Arthritis Rheum 1997; 40: 461–468.

40. Alvarez L, Guanabens N, Peris P *et al.* Usefulness of biochemical markers of bone turnover in assessing response to treatment of Paget's disease. Bone 2001; 29: 447–452.

41. Smedsrod B, Melkko J, Risteli L, Risteli J. Circulating C-terminal propeptide of type I procollagen is cleared mainly via the mannose receptor in liver endothelial cells. Biochem J 1990; 271: 345–350.

42. Melko J, Hellevick T, Risteli L *et al.* Clearance of NH$_2$ terminal propetide of types I and III procollagen is a physiological function of the scavenger receptor in liver endothelial cells. J Exp Med 1994; 179: 405–412.

43. Toivonen J, Tahtela R, Laitinen K *et al.* Markers of bone turnover in patients with differentiated thyroid cancer on and off thyroxine suppressive therapy. Eur J Endocrinol 1994; 138: 667–673.

44. Prockop OJ, Kivirikko KI. Hydroxyproline and the metabolism of collagen. In: Gould BS, ed. Treatise on collagen. New York: Academic Press, 1968; 215–246.

45. Prockop OJ, Kivirikko KI, Tuderman K *et al.* The biosynthesis of collagen and its disorders. N Engl J Med 1979; 301: 13–23.

46. Krane SM, Kantrowitz FG, Byrne M *et al.* Urinary excretion of hydroxylysine and its glycosides as an index of collagen degradation. J Clin Invest 1977; 59: 819–827.

47. Kivirikko KI. Excretion of urinary hydroxyproline peptide in the assessment of bone collagen deposition and resorption. In: Frame B, Potts JT, eds. Clinical disorders of bone and mineral metabolism. Amsterdam: Excerpta Medica, 1983; 105–107.

48. Lowry M, Hall DE, Brosnan JJ. Hydroxyproline metabolism by the rat kidney: Distribution of renal enzymes of hydroxyproline catabolism and renal conversion of hydroxyproline to glycine and serine. Metabolism 1985; 39: 955.

49. Moro L, Mucelli RSP, Gazzarrini C *et al.* Urinary b-1-galactosyl-O-hydroxylysine (GH) as a marker of collagen turnover of bone. Calcif Tissue Int 1988; 42; 87–90.

50. Al-Dehaimi AW, Blumsohn A, Eastell R. Serum galactosyl hydroxylysine as a biochemical marker of bone resorption. Clin Chem 1999; 45: 676–681.

51. Lo Cascio V, Bertoldo F, Gambaro G *et al.* Urinary excretion of galactosyl-hydroxylysine in postmenopausal osteoporotic women: a potential marker of bone fragility. J Bone Miner Res 1999; 14: 1420–1424.

52. Li CY, Chuda RA, Lam WKW *et al.*, Acid phosphatase in human plasma. J Lab Clin Med 1973; 82: 446–460.

53. Oddie GW, Schenk G, Angel N *et al.* Structure, function and regulation of tartrate-resistant acid phosphatase. Bone 2000; 27: 575–584.

54. Hayman AR, Jones SJ, Boyde A *et al.* Mice lacking tartrate-resistant acid phosphatase (Acp5) have disrupted endochondral ossification and mild osteopetrosis. Development 1996; 122: 3151–3162.

55. Angel NZ, Walsh N, Forwood MR *et al.* Transgenic mice overexpressing tartrate-resistant acid phosphatase exhibit an increased rate of bone turnover. J Bone Miner Res 2000; 15: 103–110.

56. Minkin C. Bone acid phosphatase: tartrate-resistant acid phosphatase as a marker of osteoclast function. Calcif Tissue Int 1982; 34: 285–290.

57. Hayman AR, Bune AJ, Bradley *et al.* Osteoclastic tartrate-resistant acid phosphatase (Acp 5). Its localization to dendritic cells and diverse murine tissues. Histochem Cytochem 2000; 48: 219–228.

58. Brehme CS, Roman S, Shaffer J, Wolfert R. Tartrate resistant acid phosphatase forms complexes with a 2 macroglobulin in serum. J Bone Miner Res 1999; 14: 311–318.

59. Hallen JM, Hentunen TA, Karp M *et al.* Characterization of serum tartrate-resistant acid phosphatase and development of a direct two-site immunoassay. J Bone Miner Res 1988 ; 13: 683–687.

60. Kraenzlin ME, Lau KH, Liang L *et al.* Development of an immunoassay for human serum osteoclastic tartrate-resistant acid phosphatase. J Clin Endocrinol Metab 1990; 71: 442–451.

61. Cheung C, Panesar N, Haines C *et al.* Immunoassay of a tartrate-resistant acid phosphatase in serum. Clin Chem 1995; 41: 679–686.

62. Hallen JM, Karp M, Viloma S *et al.* Two-site immunoassays for osteoclastic tartrate-resistant acid phosphatase based on characterization of six monoclonal antibodies. Bone Miner Res 1999; 14: 464–469.

63. Hallen JS, Alatalo SL, Suominen H *et al.* Tartrate-resistant acid phosphatase 5b: a novel serum marker of bone resorption. J Bone Miner Res 2000; 15: 1337–1345.

64. Stepan JJ, Silinkova-Malkova E, Havrenek T *et al.* Relationship of plasma tartrate-resistant acid phosphatase to the bone isoenzyme of serum alkaline phosphatase in hyperparathyroidism. Clin Chim Acta 1983; 133: 189–200.

65. Stepan JJ, Pospichal J, Presl J *et al.* Bone loss and biochemical indices of bone remodeling in surgically induced postmenopausal women. Bone 1987; 8: 279–284.

66. Piedra C, Torres R, Rapado A *et al.* Serum tartrate resistant acid phosphatase and bone mineral content in postmenopausal osteoporosis. Calcif Tissue Int 1989; 45: 58–60.

67. Hallen JM, Alatalo SL, Janckila AJ *et al.* Serum tartrate-resistant acide phosphatase 5b is a specific and sensitive marker of bone resorption. Clin Chem 2001; 47: 597–600.

68. Eyre DR, Koob TJ, Van Ness KP. Quantitation of hydroxypyridinium crosslinks in collagen by high-performance liquid chromatography. Anal Bioche 1984; 137: 380–388.

69. Apone S, Lee MY, Eyre DR. Osteoclasts generate crosslinked collagen N-telopeptides (NTx) but not free pyridinolines when cultured on human bone. Bone 1997; 21: 129–136.

70. Colwell A, Eastell R. Renal clearance of free and conjugated pyridinium crosslinks of collagen. J Bone Miner Res 1996; 11: 1976–1980.

71. Garnero P, Gineyts E, Arbault P *et al.* Different effects of bisphosphonate and estrogen therapy on free and peptide-bound crosslinks excretion. J Bone Miner Res 1995; 10: 641–649.

72. Eyre DR, Koob TJ, Van Ness KP. Quantitation of hydroxypyridinium crosslinks in collagen by high-performance liquid chromatography. Anal Biochem 1984; 137: 380–388.

73. Black D, Duncan A, Robins SP. Quantitative analysis of the pyridinium crosslinks of collagen in urine using ion-paired reversed-phase high-performance liquid chromatography. Anal Biochem 1988; 169: 197–203.

74. Eastell R, Colwell A, Hampton L, Reeve J. Biochemical markers of bone resorption compared with estimates of bone resorption from radiotracer kinetic studies in osteoporosis. J Bone Miner Res 1997; 12: 59–65.

75. Delmas PD, Schlemmer A, Gineyts E *et al.* Urinary excretion of pyridinoline crosslinks correlates with bone turnover measured on iliac crest biopsy in patients with vertebral osteoporosis. J Bone Miner Res 1991; 6: 639–644.

76. Seyedin S, Zuk R, Kung V *et al.* An immunoassay to urinary pyridinoline: the new marker of bone resorption. J Bone Miner Res 1993; 8: 635–642.

77. Robins SP, Woitge H, Hesley R *et al.* Direct, enzyme-linked immunoassay for urinary deoxypyridinoline as a specific marker for measuring bone resorption. J Bone Miner Res 1994; 9: 1643–1649.

78. Risteli J, Elomaa I, Niemi S *et al.* Radioimmunoassay for the pyridinoline cross-linked carboxy-terminal telopeptide of type I collagen: a new serum marker of bone collagen degradation. Clin Chem 1993; 39: 635–640.

79. Rosenquist C, Fledelius C, Christgau S *et al.* Serum crosslaps one step ELISA. First application of monoclonal antibodies for measurement in serum of bone-related degradation products from C-terminal telopeptides of type I collagen. Clin Chem 1998; 44: 2281–2289.

80. Bonde B, Qvist P, Fledelius C *et al.* Immunoassay for quantifying type I collagen degradation products in urine evaluated. Clin Chem 1994; 40: 2022–2025.

81. Clemens JD, Herrick MV, Singer FR, Eyre DR. Evidence that serum NTX (collagen I N-telopeptides) can act as an immunochemical marker of bone resorption. Clin Chem 1997; 43: 2058–2063.

82. Hanson DA, Weiss MAE, Bollen AM *et al.* A specific immunoassay for monitoring human bone resorption: Quantitation of type I collagen cross-linked N-telopeptides in urine. J Bone Miner Res 1992; 7: 1251–1258.

83. Hassager C, Jensen LT, Podenphant J *et al.* The carboxy-terminal pyridinoline cross-linked telopeptide of type I collagen in serum as a marker of bone resorption: the effect of nandrolone decanoate and hormone replacement therapy. Calcif Tissue Int 1994; 54: 30–33.

84. Qvist P, Lovejoy JC. Serum Crosslaps is a biochemical marker of bone resorption and is not influenced by anabolic steroid-induced increase in soft tissue turnover. J Bone Miner Res 2001; 16 (Suppl 1); S465.

85. Garnero P, Shih WJ, Gineyts E. Comparison of new biochemical markers of bone turnover in late postmenopausal osteoporotic women in response to alendronate. J Clin Endocrinol Metab 1994; 79: 1693–1700.

86. Elomaa I, Virkkunen P, Risteli L, Risteli J. Serum concentration of the cross-linked carboxy terminal telopeptide of type I collagen is a useful prognostic marker in multiple myeloma. Br J Cancer 1992; 66: 337–341.

87. Ulrich U, Rhiem K, Schmolling J *et al.* Cross-linked type I collagen C- and N-telopeptides in women with bone metastases from breast cancer. Arch Gynecol Obstet 2001; 264: 186–190.

88. Aruga A, Koizumi M, Hotta R *et al.* Usefulness of bone metabolic markers in the diagnosis and follow-up of bone metastasis from lung cancer. Br J Cancer 1997; 76: 760–764.

89. Blomqvist C, Risteli L, Risteli J *et al.* Markers of type I collage degradation and synthesis in the monitoring of treatment responses in bone metastases from breast cancer. Br J Cancer 1996; 73: 1074–1079.

90. Kylmala T, Tammela TLJ, Risteli L *et al.* Type I collagen degradation product (ICTP) gives information about the nature of bone metastases and has prognostic value in prostate cancer. Br J Cancer 1995; 71: 1061–1064.

91. Garnero P. Markers of bone turnover in prostate cancer. Cancer Treat Rev 2001; 27: 187–192.

92. Sassi M-L, Eriksen H, Risteli L *et al.* Immunochemical characterization of assay for carboxyterminal telopeptide of human type I collagen: Loss of antigenicity by treatment with cathepsin K. Bone 2000; 26: 367–373.

93. Saftig P, Hunziker E, Wehmeyer O *et al.* Impaired osteoclastic bone resorption leads to osteopetrosis in cathepsin K deficient mice. Proc Natl Acad Sci USA 1998; 95: 13453–13458.

94. Garnero P, Borel O, Byrjalsen I *et al.* The collagenolytic activity of cathepsin K is unique amongst mammalian proteinases. J Biol Chem 1998; 273: 32347–32352.

95. Karsdal MA, Garnero P, Ferreras M *et al.* The type I collagen fragments ICTP and CTX reveal distinct enzymatic pathways of bone collagen degradation. J Bone Miner Res 2001; 16 (Suppl 1): S195.

96. Nishi Y, Atley L, Eyre DR *et al.* Determination of bone markers in pycnodysostosis: effects of cathepsin K deficiency on bone matrix degradation. J Bone Miner Res 1999; 14: 1902–1908.

97. Garnero P, Delmas PD. A new immunoassay for type I collagen alpha 1 helicoidal peptide 620-633 as a marker of bone resorption in osteoporosis. J Bone Miner Res 2001; 16 (Suppl 1): S346.

98. Eastell R, Calvo MS, Burritt MF *et al.* Abnormalities in circadian patterns of bone resorption and renal calcium conservation in type I osteoporosis. J Clin Endocrinol Metab 1992; 74: 487–94.

99. Blumsohn A, Herrington K, Hannon RA *et al.* The effect of calcium supplementation on the circadian rhythm of bone resorption. J Clin Endocrinol Metab 1994; 79: 730–735.

100. Greenspan SL, Dresner-Pollak R, Parker RA *et al.* Diurnal variation of bone mineral turnover in elderly men and women. Calcif Tissue Int 1997; 60: 419–423.

101. Hassager C, Risteli J, Risteli L *et al.* Diurnal variation in serum markers of type I collagen synthesis and degradation in healthy premenopausal women. J Bone Miner Res 1992; 7: 1307–1311.

102. Wichers M, Schmidt E, Bidlingmaier F, Klingmuller D. Diurnal rhythm of CrossLaps in human serum. Clin Chem 1999; 45: 1858–1860.

103. Schlemmer A, Hassager C, Jensen SB, Christiansen C. Marked diurnal variation in urinary excretion of pyridinium cross-links in premenopausal women. J Clin Endocrinol Metab 1992; 74: 476–480.

104. Aoshima H, Kushida K, Takahashi M *et al.* Circadian variation of urinary type I collagen crosslinked C-telopeptide and free and peptide-bound forms of pyridinium crosslinks. Bone 1998; 22: 73–78.

105. Schlemmer A, Hassager C, Pedersen BJ, Christiansen C. Posture, age, menopause, and osteopenia do not influence the circadian variation in the urinary excretion of pyridinium crosslinks. J Bone Miner Res 1994; 9: 1883–1888.

106. Sairanen S, Tahtela R, Laitinen K *et al.* Nocturnal rise in markers of bone resorption is not abolished by bedtime calcium or calcitonin. Calcif Tissue Int 1994; 55: 349–352.

107. Sairanen S, Tahtela R, Laitinen K *et al.* Effects of short-term treatment with clodronate on parameters of bone metabolism and their diurnal variation. Calcif Tissue Int 1997; 60: 160–163.

108. Gertz BJ, Clemens JD, Holland SD *et al.* Application of a new serum assay for type I collagen cross-linked N- telopeptides: assessment of diurnal changes in bone turnover with and without alendronate treatment. Calcif Tissue Int 1998; 63: 102–106.

109. Schlemmer A, Hassager C. Acute fasting diminishes the circadian rhythm of biochemical markers of bone resorption. Eur J Endocrinol 1999; 140: 332–337.

110. Christgau S, Jensen OB, Bjarnason NH *et al.* Serum CrossLaps provides a rapid assessment of therapy response compared to BMD measurements. Bone 2000; 26: 505–511.

111. Christgau S. Circadian variation in serum Crosslaps concentration is reduced in fasting individuals. Clin Chem 2000; 46: 431.

112. Fledelius C, Johnsen AH, Cloos PAC *et al.* Characterization of urinary degradation products derived from Type I collagen. J Biol Chem 1997; 272: 9755–9763.

113. Cloos PAC, Fledelius C. Collagen fragments in urine derived from bone resorption are highly racemized and isomerized: a biological clock of protein aging with clinical potential. Biochem J 2000; 345: 473–480.

114. Garnero P, Fledelius C, Gineyts E *et al.* Decreased β isomerisation of C-telopeptides of type I collagen in Paget's disease of bone. J Bone Miner Res 1997; 12: 1407–1415.

115. Garnero P, Gineyts E, Shaffer AV *et al.* Measurement of urinary excretion of nonisomerized and β-isomerized forms of type I collagen breakdown products to monitor the effects of the bisphosphonate zoledronate in Paget's disease. Arthritis Rheum 1998; 41: 354–360.

116. Garnero P, Buchs J, Zekri J *et al.* Bone turnover markers for the management of patients with bone metastases from prostate cancer. Br J Cancer 2000; 82: 858–864.

117. Garnero P, Cloos P, Sornay-Rendu E *et al.* Type I collagen racemization and isomerization and the risk of fracture in postmenopausal women: The OFELY prospective study. J Bone Miner Res (in press).

118. Fisher LW, Whitson SW, Avioli LW, Termine JD. Matrix sialoprotein of developing bone. J Biol Chem 1983; 258: 12723–12727.

119. Chen J, Shapiro HS, Wrana JL *et al.* Localization of bone sialoprotein (BSP) expression to sites of mineral tissue formation in fetal rat tissue by *in situ* hybridization. Matrix 1991; 11: 133–143.

120. Shapiro HS, Chen J, Wrana JL *et al.* Characterization of porcine bone sialoprotein: primary structure and cellular expression. Matrix 1993; 13: 431–444.

121. Bianco P, Fisher LW, Young MF *et al.* Expression of bone sialoprotein (BSP) in developing human tissues. Calcif Tissue Int 1991; 49: 421–426.

122. Debri E, Reinholt FP, Heinegard D *et al.* Bone sialoprotein and osteopontin distribution at the osteocartilaginous interface. Clin Orthop 1996; 330: 251–260.

123. Chenu C, Delmas PD. Platelets contribute to circulating levels of bone sialoprotein in humans. J Bone Miner Res 1992; 7: 47–54.

124. Fujisawa R, Nodasaka Y, Kuboki Y. Further characterization of interaction between bone sialoprotein (BSP) and collagen. Calcif Tissue Int 1995; 56: 140–144.

125. Hunter GK, Goldberg HA. Modulation of crystal formation by bone phosphoproteins: Role of glutamic acid-rich sequences in the nucleation of hydroxyapatite by bone sialoprotein. Biochem J 1994; 302: 175–179.

126. Raynal C, Delmas PD, Chenu C. Bone sialoprotein stimulates *in vitro* bone resorption. Endocrinology 1996; 137: 2347–2354.

127. Saxne T, Zunino L, Heinegard D. Increased release of bone sialoprotein into synovial fluid reflects tissue destruction in rheumatoid arthritis. Arthritis Rheum 1995; 1: 82–90.

128. Karmatschek M, Woitge HW, Armbruster FP *et al.* Improved purification of human bone sialoprotein and development of a homologous radioimmunoassay. Clin Chem 1997; 43: 2076–2082.

129. Seibel MJ, Woitge HW, Pecherstorfer M *et al.* Serum immunoreactive bone sialoprotein as a new marker of bone turnover in metabolic and malignant bone disease. J Clin Endocrinol Metab 1996; 81: 3289–3294.

130. Woitge HW, Pecherstorfer M, Li Y *et al.* Novel markers of bone resorption and comparison with established urinary indices. J Bone Miner Res 2000; 14: 792–801.

131. Fall PM, Kennedy D, Smith JA *et al.* Comparison of serum and urine assays for biochemical markers of bone resorption in postmenopausal women with and without hormone replacement therapy. Osteoporosis Int 2000; 11: 481–485.

132. Pecherstorfer M, Horn E, Keck A-V *et al.* Serum bone sialoprotein as a marker of tumour burden and neoplastic bone involvement and as a prognostic factor in multiple myeloma. Br J Cancer 2001; 83: 344–351.

133. Diel IJ, Solomayer E-F, Seubel MJ *et al.* Serum bone sioloprotien in patients with primary breast cancer is a prognostic marker for subsequent bone metastases. Clin Cancer Res 1999; 5: 3914–3919.

134. Garnero P, Sornay-Rendu E, Chapuy MC, Delmas PD. Increased bone turnover in late postmenopausal women is a major determinant of osteoporosis. J Bone Miner Res 1996; 11: 337–349.

135. Stepan JJ. Prediction of bone loss in postmenopausal women. Osteoporosis Int 2000; 11 (Suppl 6): S45–S54.

136. Uebelhart D, Schlemmer A, Johansen J *et al.* Effect of menopause and hormone replacement therapy on the urinary excretion of pyridinium crosslinks. J Clin Endocrinol Metab 1991; 72: 367–373.

137. Hansen MA, Kirsten O, Riss BJ, Christiansen C. Role of peak bone mass and bone loss in postmenopausal osteoporosis: 12 years study. Br Med J 303: 961–964.

138. Ross PD, Knowlton W. Rapid bone loss is associated with increased levels of biochemical markers. J Bone Miner Res 1998; 13: 297–302.

139. Garnero P, Sornay-Rendu E, Duboeuf F, Delmas PD. Markers of bone turnover predict postmenopausal forearm bone loss over 4 years: The OFELY Study. J Bone Miner Res 1999; 14 : 1614–1621.

140. Garnero P, Borel O, Delmas PD. Evaluation of a fully automated serum assay for C-terminal crosslinking telopeptide of type I collagen in osteoporosis. Clin Chem 2001; 47: 694–702.

141. Van Daele PLA, Seibel MJ, Burger H *et al.* Case–control analysis of bone resorption markers, disability, and hip fracture risk: The Rotterdam study. Br Med J 1996; 312: 482–483.

142. Garnero P, Hausher E, Chapuy MC *et al.* Markers of bone resorption predict hip fracture in elderly women: The Epidos prospective study. J Bone Miner Res 1996; 11: 1531–1538.

143. Garnero P, Sornay-Rendu E, Claustrat B, Delmas PD. Biochemical markers of bone turnover, endogenous hormones and the risk of fractures in postmenopausal women : The OFELY study. J Bone Miner Res 2000; 15: 1526–1536.

144. Ross PD, Kress BC, Parson RE *et al.* Serum bone alkaline phosphatase and calcaneus bone density predict fractures: A prospective study. Osteoporosis Int 2000; 11: 76–82.

145. Garnero P. Markers of bone turnover for the prediction of fracture risk. Osteoporosis Int 2000; 11 (Suppl. 6): S55–S65.

146. Riis SBJ, Hansen AM, Jensen K *et al.* Low bone mass and fast rate of bone loss at menopause – equal risk factors for future fracture. A 15 year follow-up study. Bone 1996; 19: 9–12.

147. Chapurlat RD, Garnero P, Brèart G *et al.* Afternoon sampled serum type I collagen breakdown product (serum CTX) predicts hip fracture in elderly women: Results of the Epidos study. Bone 2000; 27: 283–286.

148. Shiraki M, Shiraki Y, Aoki C, Miura M. Vitamin K2 (menatetrenone) effectively prevents fractures and sustains lumbar spine bone mineral density in osteoporosis. J Bone Miner Res 2000 ; 15: 515–521.

149. Szulc P, Chapuy MC, Meunier PJ, Delmas PD. Serum undercarboxylated osteocalcin is a marker of the risk of hip fracture in elderly women. J Clin Invest 1993 ; 91: 1769–1774.

150. Szulc P, Chapuy MC, Meunier PJ, Delmas PD. Serum undercarboxylated osteocalcin is a marker of the risk of hip fracture: a three year follow-up study. Bone 1996; 5: 487–488.

151. Vergnaud P, Garnero P, Meunier PJ *et al.* Undercarboxylated osteocalcin measured with a specific immunoassay predicts hip fracture in elderly women: the EPIDOS study. J Clin Endocrinol Metab 1997; 82: 719–724.

152. Luukinen H, Kakonen SM, Pettersson K *et al.* Strong prediction of fractures among older adults by the ratio of carboxylated to total serum osteocalcin. J Bone Miner Res 2000; 15: 2473–2478.

153. Liu G, Peacock M. Age-related changes in serum undercarboxylated osteocalcin and its relationships with bone density, bone quality, and hip fracture. Calcif Tissue Int 1998; 62: 286–289.

154. Sugiyama T, Kawai S. Carboxylation of osteocalcin may be related to bone quality: a possible mechanism of bone fracture prevention by vitamin K. J Bone Miner Metab 2001; 19: 146–149.

155. Garnero P, Dargent-Molina P, Hans D *et al.* Do markers of bone resorption add to bone mineral density and ultrasonographic heel measurement for the prediction of hip fracture in elderly women? The EPIDOS prospective study. Osteoporosis Int 1998; 8: 563–569.

156. Johnell O, Oden A, De Laet C, Garnero P, Delmas PD, Kanis JA. Biochemical markers and the assessment of fracture probability. Osteoporosis Int (in press).

157. Ulrich S, Hingorani AD, Martin J, Vallance P. What is the optimal age for starting lipid lowering treatment. A mathematical model. Br Med J 2000; 320: 1134–1140.

158. Cooper C, Stakkestad JA, Radowicki S *et al.* Matrix delivery transdermal 17 β estradiol for the prevention of bone loss in postmenopausal women. Osteoporosis Int 1999; 9: 358–366.

159. Johansen JS, Riis BJ, Delmas PD *et al.* Plasma BGP: an indicator of spontaneous bone loss and effect of estrogen treatment in postmenopausal women. Eur J Clin Invest 1988; 18: 191–195.

160. Rosen CJ, Chesnut CH III, Mallinak NJS. The predictive value of biochemical markers of bone turnover for bone mineral density in early postmenopausal women treated with hormone replacement or calcium supplementation. J Clin Endocrinol Metab 1997; 82: 1904–1910.

161. Hannon R, Blumsohn A, Naylor K, Eastell R. Response of biochemical markers of bone turnover to hormone replacement therapy: impact of biological variability. J Bone Miner Res 1998; 13: 1124–1133.

162. Delmas PD, Hardy P, Garnero P, Dain MP. Monitoring individual response to hormone replacement therapy with bone markers. Bone 2000; 26: 553–560.

163. Bjarnason NH, Christiansen C. Early response in biochemical markers predicts long-term response in bone mass during hormone replacement therapy. Bone 2000; 26: 561–569.

164. Chailurkit L, Ongphiphadhanakul B, Piaseu N *et al.* Biochemical markers of bone turnover and response of bone mineral density to intervention in early postmenopausal women: An experience in a clinical laboratory. Clin Chem 2001; 47: 1083–1088.

165. Marcus R, Holloway L, Wells B *et al.* The relationship of biochemical markers of bone turnover to bone density changes in postmenopausal women: results from the postmenopausal estrogen/progestin interventions (PEPI) trial. J Bone Miner Res 1999; 14: 1583–1595.

166. Greenspan SL, Parker RH, Fergusson L *et al.* Early changes in biochemical markers of bone turnover predict the long term response to alendronate therapy in representative elderly women: a randomized clinical trial. J Bone Miner Res 1998; 13: 1431–1438.

167. Ravn P, Clemmesen B, Christiansen C. Biochemical markers can predict the response in bone mass during alendronate treatment in early postmenopausal women. Bone 1999; 24: 237–244.

168. Ravn P, Hosking D, Thompson GC *et al.* Monitoring of alendronate treatment and prediction of effect on bone mass by biochemical markers in early postmenopausal intervention cohort of study. J Clin Endocrinol Metab 1999; 84: 2363–2368.

169. Garnero P, Darte C, Delmas PD. A model to monitor the efficacy of alendronate treatment in women with osteoporosis using a biochemical markers of bone turnover. Bone 1999; 24: 603–609.

170. Watts NB, Jenkins DK, Viosr JM *et al.* Comparison of bone and total alkaline phosphatase and bone mineral density in postmenopausal women treated with alendronate. Osteoporosis Int 2001; 12: 279–288.

171. Hannon R, Eastell R. Preanalytical variability of biochemical markers of bone turnover. Osteoporosis Int 2000; 11(Suppl 6): S30–S44.

172. Riggs BL, Melton LJ III, O'Fallon WM. Drug therapy for vertebral fractures in osteoporosis: evidence that decreases in bone turnover and increases in bone mass both determine antifracture efficacy. Bone 1996; 18(Suppl 3): 197S–201S.

173. Delmas PD, Eastell R, Garnero P *et al.* The use of biochemical markers of bone turnover in osteoporosis. Osteoporosis Int 2000; 11(Suppl 6): S2–S17.

174. Bjarnason NH, Christiansen C, Sarkar S *et al.* for the MORE Study Group. 6 months changes in biochemical markers predict 3-year response in vertebral fracture rate in postmenopausal, osteoporotic women : results from the MORE study. Osteoporosis Int (in press).

175. Eastell T, Barton I, Hannon RA *et al.* Antifracture efficacy of risedronate: prediction by change in bone resorption markers. J Bone Miner Res 2001; 16 (Suppl 1): S163.

176. Delmas PD, Meunier PJ. The managment of Paget's disease of bone. N Engl J Med 1997; 336: 558–566.

177. Meunier PJ, Salson C, Mathieu L *et al.* Skeletal distribution and biochemical parameters of Paget's disease. Clin Orthop 1986; 217: 37–44.

178. Delmas PD, Demiaux B, Malval L *et al.* Serum bone gla-protein is not as sensitive marker of bone turnover in Paget's disease of bone. Calcif Tissue Int 1986; 38: 60–61.

179. Delmas PD, Chapuy MC, Vignon E *et al.* Long term effects of dichloromethylene diphosphonate in Paget's disease of bone. J Clin Endocrinol Metab 1982; 54: 837–844.

194 Epidemiology and classification

L Joseph Melton, III and B Lawrence Riggs

- Osteoporosis is a syndrome divided into primary (idiopathic and involutional) and secondary forms

- Most populations of aging women and men lose bone, although patterns of loss differ by skeletal site

- As defined by the World Health Organization (bone mineral density ≥2.5 standard deviations below the young normal mean), about 20% of postmenopausal white women have osteoporosis at the femoral neck, with lower proportions among women of other races and men

- Risk factors for low bone mineral density relate either to inadequate bone formation during growth or to excessive bone loss thereafter, but the underlying pathogenesis remains somewhat obscure

- Fractures, the clinical manifestation of osteoporosis, increase dramatically with aging and are more frequent in women than men and in Caucasians than in other races

- Hip fractures are most devastating in terms of mortality, morbidity and cost but other types of fracture contribute substantially to the social burden of osteoporosis

- Although all are related to bone density, hip and forearm fractures are usually precipitated by a fall, whereas vertebral fractures commonly result from excessive spinal loads imposed by everyday activities

- Because of the dramatic growth of the elderly population worldwide, the number of osteoporotic fractures will increase substantially in future years unless cost-effective control programs can be implemented

INTRODUCTION

Osteoporosis is the most common metabolic bone disease. It affects both sexes and all races, although to different degrees. A variety of pathophysiologic mechanisms contribute to a decline in bone density (a pathogenic trait), which causes a disproportionate decrease in bone strength (asymptomatic disease) and leads to an increase in fractures (symptomatic disease), the clinical manifestation of osteoporosis. These fractures are not only extremely common but also devastating, both to the affected patients and to the societies that must bear the enormous costs of fracture treatment and subsequent disability. Although mainly a concern in Western Europe and North America so far, osteoporosis is a global problem which will increase in significance with the growing elderly population. Every clinician will encounter patients with osteoporosis in his or her practice. At present, however, many of them go unrecognized and untreated. Some understanding of the risk factors for bone loss and fractures may foster enhanced efforts to identify and manage this important problem.

HISTORY

Osteoporosis is a disease of antiquity. Skeletons with evidence of spinal osteoporosis have been found that date from 4000 years ago. However, it was only in 1820 that a French pathologist, Jean G.C.F.M. Lobstein, coined the term 'osteoporosis', based on the appearance of affected tissue (= porous bone) under the microscope. Around the same time, Sir Astley Cooper, an English surgeon, called attention to the age-related degeneration of bone tissue associated with skeletal fragility and fractures. From these early days, then, the main elements were present that comprise the current consensus definition of osteoporosis, i.e., 'a systematic skeletal disease characterized by low bone mass and microarchitectural deterioration of bone tissue, with a consequent increase in bone fragility and susceptibility to fractures.'[1] However, the condition was accorded little clinical or scientific significance until the 1940s, when Harvard endocrinologist Fuller Albright defined the clinical syndrome of osteoporosis. Albright showed that the disease was due to bone loss in the central skeleton, leading to vertebral fractures. Because these were found mainly in postmenopausal women, he attributed causation to estrogen deficiency and then showed that estrogen therapy reversed the negative calcium balance that was present prior to treatment. In the absence of a convenient and reliable test for osteoporosis, however, most of the patients who came to clinical attention in subsequent years were women who experienced a vertebral fracture in the early post-menopausal period. Indeed, vertebral fractures and osteoporosis are still synonymous in the minds of many. It was only with the advent of bone densitometry in the early 1960s (see Chapter 195) that the influence of osteoporosis on other types of fracture, in men as well as women, began to be recognized and the scope of the public health problem posed by osteoporosis became apparent. This, in turn, prompted the development of many new therapeutic options for osteoporosis prevention and treatment (see Chapter 198).

CLASSIFICATION OF OSTEOPOROSIS

Bone loss may have many causes and take several clinical forms, and so osteoporosis should be considered a syndrome. A traditional classification of generalized osteoporosis is provided in Table 194.1. In this scheme, osteoporosis is categorized as primary or secondary by the absence or presence of associated medical diseases, surgical procedures, or medications known to be associated with accelerated bone loss[2]. Although this categorization is a useful guide to evaluation and treatment, it is somewhat misleading because it suggests that the primary and secondary causes are independent when they may, in fact, be additive. Thus, vertebral fractures are more likely to occur in postmenopausal women taking corticosteroids than in premenopausal women on the same regimen. Primary osteoporosis is usually divided, in turn, into idiopathic (the uncommon forms of primary osteoporosis found in children and young adults) and involutional (the common form of osteoporosis that begins in midlife and becomes increasingly more frequent with advancing age). The term 'idiopathic' is appropriate for the forms of osteoporosis that occur in children and young adults, the pathogenesis of which remains unclear. However, it is not always obvious why some but not other postmenopausal women develop osteoporosis, nor are the

TABLE 194.1 CLASSIFICATION OF GENERALIZED OSTEOPOROSIS		
Primary	Idiopathic juvenile osteoporosis	
	Idiopathic osteoporosis in young adults	
	Involutional osteoporosis	Type I ('postmenopausal' osteoporosis)
		Type II ('senile' osteoporosis)
Secondary (partial listing)	Hypercortisolism	
	Hypogonadism	
	Hyperthyroidism	
	Hyperparathyroidism	
	Seizure disorder (anticonvulsants)	
	Malabsorption syndrome	
	Rheumatoid arthritis	
	Connective tissue disease	
	Chronic neurological disease	
	Chronic obstructive lung disease	
	Malignancy	
From Khosla et al.[3]		

exact mechanisms by which aging produces bone loss entirely understood. Thus, involutional osteoporosis is also partially 'idiopathic'.

The pathophysiology of involutional osteoporosis is complex (see Chapter 196), but heterogeneity in the age- and sex-specific patterns of bone loss and fracture risk suggest the existence of several subtypes. The syndromes that Albright called 'postmenopausal' and 'senile' osteoporosis have been refined and relabeled by the authors as types I and II osteoporosis[4]. As summarized in Table 194.2, type I is characterized by the occurrence of fractures at skeletal sites that contain relatively large amounts of cancellous bone, such as the vertebrae, and typically affects women within 15–20 years after the menopause. Type II osteoporosis can occur at any age but is the predominant form of the disease in women and men over 70 years of age. The fractures associated with type II osteoporosis occur at sites that contain both cancellous and cortical bone and are more frequent in women than men. Type I osteoporosis is associated with an exaggeration or prolongation of the rapid phase of bone loss at the menopause. This undue responsiveness of bone to estrogen deficiency leads to greatly increased bone turnover, with excessive bone resorption that results in a compensatory suppression of parathyroid hormone levels. In type II osteoporosis, estrogen deficiency results in impairments of calcium absorption and conservation that lead to secondary hyperparathyroidism, although impaired function of bone-forming osteoblasts may also play a role. These estrogen-related effects may also account for type II osteoporosis in men[5].

EPIDEMIOLOGY OF OSTEOPOROSIS

As noted above, the real magnitude of the osteoporosis problem only became apparent with the introduction of non-invasive techniques to measure bone mass (see Chapter 195). Although bone mineral density (BMD) assessed *in vivo* is not completely synonymous with the changes in bone architecture that are responsible for skeletal fragility, there is nonetheless a strong correlation between BMD and the breaking strength of bone *in vitro*. Moreover, it has been shown conclusively that BMD is predictive of future fracture risk, and the relationship is at least as strong as that between blood pressure measurements and the risk of stroke[6]. Thus, it is important to evaluate the changes in bone density that occur over life and to identify the factors associated with excessive bone loss.

Patterns of bone loss

The bone that a person has later in life, and consequently their risk of fracture, depends on the amount formed during growth (peak bone

TABLE 194.2 CHARACTERIZATION OF THE TWO MAIN TYPES OF INVOLUTIONAL OSTEOPOROSIS		
	Type I	Type II
Age (yr)	51–75	> 70
Sex ratio (F:M)	6:1	2:1
Type of bone loss	Mainly cancellous	Cancellous and cortical
Rate of bone loss	Accelerated	Not accelerated
Fracture sites	Vertebrae (crush) and distal radius	Vertebrae (multiple wedge) and hip
Parathyroid function	Decreased	Increased
Calcium absorption	Decreased	Decreased
Estrogen effects	Mainly skeletal	Mainly extraskeletal
Main causes	Menopause plus individual predisposing factor(s)	Factors related to aging including late effects of estrogen deficiency
Modified from Riggs et al.[4]		

mass) and the amount lost subsequently. During the linear growth spurt there is a rapid and massive increase in bone mass which ceases by age 20. Bone mass may continue to increase for a time at some skeletal sites ('consolidation'), but at some point the bone formed in each remodeling cycle is less than that which was resorbed, and net bone loss ensues (see Chapter 197). Most populations of aging women and men lose bone, although patterns appear to differ by skeletal site[7]. At the femoral neck, for example, bone loss over life is approximately linear in men and women of all races and begins before the age of 20 (Fig. 194.1). By contrast, when lumbar spine BMD is assessed in the customary AP projection, women do not appear to lose significant bone until around the time of menopause, and men exhibit no decline in AP lumbar spine BMD. This is an artifact of age-related increases in aortic calcification and vertebral osteophytosis, as bone loss is clearly evident in both sexes when the vertebral bodies are isolated on lateral scans. In the appendicular skeleton, bone loss begins around the time of menopause in women and at a comparable age in men, but trends can be difficult to interpret owing to systematic changes in bone size. Thus, age-related increases in bone diameter cause BMD measurements to decline, as bone area increases more than bone mineral content, but the redistribution of bone tissue to a more peripheral location helps maintain skeletal strength[8]. It is important to bear in mind, however, that low BMD in an older individual may not be due to excessive bone loss but rather to inadequate peak bone mass development[9].

Prevalence of osteoporosis

Although age-related bone loss is more or less universal, determining the prevalence of osteoporosis requires the selection of a cut-off level to define abnormal bone density. Because the relationship between bone density and fracture risk is continuous, like that between blood pressure and stroke, this choice is necessarily somewhat arbitrary. Initially, 'osteopenia' was taken to be BMD more than 2 standard deviations (SD) below the young normal mean, and osteoporosis was not considered present until a characteristic fracture had occurred. This ignored the damage to bone structure that had originally defined osteoporosis, which by this definition was absent one day and present the next when a fracture was diagnosed. Alternatively, abnormality was defined as a 'fracture threshold' (e.g. the 90th percentile of BMD in fracture patients), but this value was also about 2 SD below the young normal mean. In 1994, the World Health Organization defined osteoporosis operationally as a femoral neck BMD value 2.5 SD or more below the young normal mean for white women, or a *t*-score of −2.5[11]. For consistency with the older definition, patients with BMD *t*-scores below −2.5 who also have fractures are said to have severe or 'established' osteoporosis. Somewhat confusingly, perhaps, 'osteopenia' is now defined as a BMD value more than 1 SD but less than 2.5 SD below the young normal mean.

Using the World Health Organization definition, it is now possible to assess osteoporosis prevalence in different populations. In the Third National Health and Nutrition Examination Survey (NHANES III), a large probability sample of the United States population, 20% of post-menopausal white women had osteoporosis at the femoral neck[12]. The prevalence would be greater if additional assessments had been made, as BMD values at different skeletal sites are not always closely correlated. If normative data for white women are used also to define the condition for non-white women, the prevalence of osteoporosis at the femoral neck appears to be about 10% in Hispanic women and only 5% in black women. However, greater areal BMD (g/cm²) in black than in white women, and in white than in Asian women, results from differences in bone size, and race-specific differences are reduced when size is adjusted for by assessing volumetric BMD (g/cm³). Using the same absolute cut-off level for defining osteoporosis in men as in women (0.56g/cm² for femoral neck BMD), the prevalence among white, Hispanic and black

men age 50 years and over was 4%, 2% and 3%, respectively, in the NHANES study[12]. The lower prevalence of osteoporosis in men than in women also results partly from the fact that standard areal BMD is over-estimated in those with larger skeletons, i.e. men.

Risk factors for bone loss

The pathophysiology of osteoporosis is delineated in Chapter 196. From the epidemiologic perspective, however, the risk factors for low BMD relate either to inadequate peak bone mass development or to excessive bone loss. Whereas this is clear conceptually, a bewildering array of risk factors has been identified in different studies. Many of these are highly intercorrelated, and quirks in the data allow weight, for example, to be a predominant risk factor for bone loss in one study, whereas the next identifies body mass index as the stronger predictor and still another claims that weight loss is the most important variable. Adding to the confusion is the fact that different investigators assess different sets of potential risk factors. In the most comprehensive study to date, the Study of Osteoporotic Fractures, a cohort of over 9500 elderly white women, the determinants of bone density were assessed cross-sectionally (Table 194.3). Later age at menopause, estrogen or thiazide use, non-insulin-dependent diabetes, and greater height, weight, strength and dietary calcium intake were all positively associated with bone mass at the distal radius, whereas greater age, cigarette smoking, caffeine intake, prior gastric surgery and maternal history of fracture were negatively associated[13]. Greater height and weight, older age at menopause, a history of arthritis, greater physical activity, use of alcoholic beverages, diuretic treatment and current estrogen replacement therapy were associated with higher lumbar spine BMD, whereas later age at menarche and a maternal history of fracture were associated with lower levels. Increasing age was positively correlated with spinal BMD in these elderly women, probably because of the hypertrophic changes noted previously. Femoral neck BMD was positively associated with most of the same protective factors, along with quadriceps strength, calcium intake, and a history of non-insulin-dependent diabetes. A maternal history of fracture and a personal history of prior wrist fracture were correlated with low femoral neck BMD. Greater age was a risk factor for low femoral neck BMD, as it was for low BMD of the radius.

Although risk factors like these may be of clinical interest, the underlying mechanisms that account for their effects are often obscure. In addition, conditions that may have a devastating effect on the individual patient, but which are uncommon (e.g. Cushing's disease), rarely appear among the independent risk factors identified in large epidemiologic

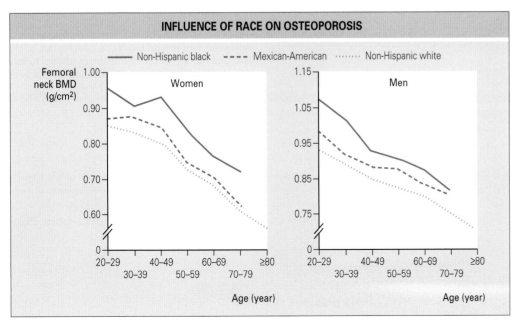

Fig. 194.1 Influence of race on development of osteoporosis. Age-related patterns of bone loss from the proximal femur among women and men of different races. (Redrawn with permission from Looker *et al*.[10])

TABLE 194.3 RISK FACTORS FOR OSTEOPOROSIS

Variable	Lumbar spine	Femoral neck	Distal radius
Age		−	−
Weight	+++	+++	+++
Height	++	++	++
Fracture in mother	−	−	−
Age at menopause	+	+	++
Estrogen use	+++	+++	+++
Quadriceps strength		++	
Grip strength			+++
Thiazide use	+++	++	+++
Non-thiazide diuretic use	++		
Current smoker			− −
Number of alcoholic drinks in lifetime	+		
Dietary calcium intake		++	+
Lifetime caffeine intake			−
Non-insulin-dependent diabetes		+++	+++
Gastric surgery			− −
Recent or past physical activity	+	+	

The strength of correlations from multivariate analyses is indicated by the number of symbols: Three symbols indicate ≥3% change in bone density per unit change in the variable; two symbols a 1–3% change; and one symbol a change of < 1%.

Risk factors (−) and protective factors (+) for axial and appendicular bone density among elderly white women. (From Orwoll et al.[13])

studies. Moreover, the relative importance of specific risk factors may vary from one individual to another. Consequently, it has proved difficult to identify patients at high risk for osteoporosis on the basis of clinical risk factors alone. Despite the large number of potential risk factors assessed in the Study of Osteoporotic Fractures, models incorporating all of the independent predictors together explained only 20–34% of the variance in bone density at the different skeletal sites[13]. This indicates that clinically important risk factors remain to be elucidated. One potential candidate that has recently emerged is low serum bioavailable estrogen levels, which are strongly associated with bone loss in men as well as in women[5].

Epidemiology of fractures

Osteoporosis is of clinical concern because of the associated fractures. Hip and spine fractures are associated with increased mortality, and all fractures may lead to disability and a reduced quality of life[14]. Although fractures are common among adolescents, these typically involve the long bones and result from significant trauma, in boys more often than girls. By contrast, osteoporotic fractures increase dramatically with aging and are more frequent in women than in men. They typically result from moderate trauma (defined by convention as equivalent to a fall from standing height or less) and more often involve the proximal femur (hip), the thoracic or lumbar vertebral bodies (spine), or the distal radius and/or ulna (wrist). Indeed, osteoporotic fractures have often been defined on the basis of these epidemiologic characteristics. However, large epidemiologic studies have shown convincingly that most fractures in older women and men are due, at least in part, to the skeletal fragility associated with age-related bone loss[15,16]. Nevertheless, this review focuses on fractures of the hip, spine and distal forearm, the skeletal sites traditionally associated with osteoporosis.

Hip fractures

Because of their disproportionate impact on morbidity, mortality and cost[14], hip fractures have been studied more extensively than other osteoporotic fractures. Hip fracture incidence rates increase exponentially with age in most populations, reaching annual rates of about 3% among white women and 2% among white men ≥ 85 years of age in the United States (Fig. 194.2). This is due not only to increased skeletal fragility but also to an age-related increase in the falls that are responsible for most hip fractures in the elderly[17]. Indeed, the likelihood of falling at least once annually rises between ages 50 and 85 years from 24% to 48% in women and from 16% to 35% in men[18]. As men experience less bone loss and fewer falls, hip fracture incidence in men is about half that in women at any age. Only in some lesser developed countries are sex-specific incidence rates comparable, but hip fractures are uncommon in those regions and more often associated with severe trauma[14]. Because women live longer, the lifetime risk of hip fracture from age 50 years onward has been estimated at 17% for white women but only 6% for white men in the United States. Lifetime risk in both sexes will increase as life expectancy continues to improve[19].

An estimated 1.7 million hip fractures occurred worldwide in 1990, about 1 197 000 in women and another 463 000 or so in men[14]. However, hip fracture incidence varies substantially from one population to another, and is much lower among non-white than white women and men (Fig. 194.3). The explanation is obscure but may relate to a lower risk of falling, as bone density measurements are similar in white and non-white women and men after correction for differences in bone size. It is important to note that incidence rates are increasing rapidly in

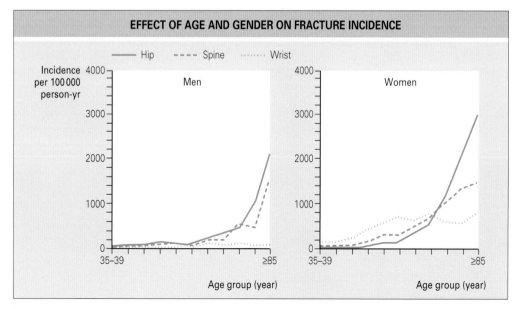

EFFECT OF AGE AND GENDER ON FRACTURE INCIDENCE

— Hip   - - - Spine   ⋯⋯ Wrist

Fig. 194.2 Effect of age and gender on fracture incidence. Age-specific incidence rates for hip, vertebral (spine), and distal forearm (wrist) fractures in Rochester, Minnesota, men and women. (Redrawn with permission from Cooper and Melton[20].)

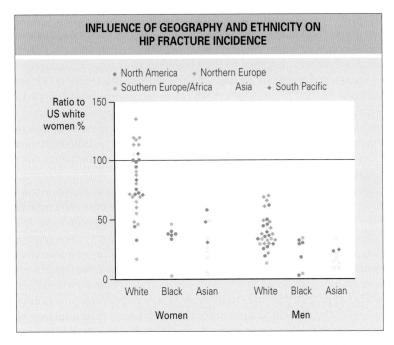

INFLUENCE OF GEOGRAPHY AND ETHNICITY ON HIP FRACTURE INCIDENCE

- North America
- Northern Europe
- Southern Europe/Africa
- Asia
- South Pacific

Ratio to US white women %

Fig. 194.3 Influence of geography and ethnicity on hip fracture incidence. Hip fracture incidence around the world as a ratio of the rates observed in each population to those expected for US white women of the same age (=100). Each point corresponds to a published report. (Redrawn with permission from Melton[13].)

some of these other populations[21]. It is also unclear why hip fracture incidence varies substantially within populations of a given race and gender[14]. Thus, age-adjusted rates are higher among white women in Scandinavia than among comparable women in North America, whereas hip fracture incidence differs more than sevenfold among countries within Europe, and a similar variation is seen even within countries. In an analysis of county-level data in the United States, hip fracture incidence in elderly white women was negatively associated with latitude (higher in the south), water hardness and January sunlight, and positively associated with poverty, the proportion of the land in farms, and fluoridated water supplies. Regional differences were not accounted for by variation in activity levels, obesity, cigarette smoking, alcohol consumption or Scandinavian heritage[22].

Important clinical risk factors for hip fractures have been described, although some of them remain unexplained mechanistically. An exhaustive set of potential risk factors was evaluated among elderly women in the Study of Osteoporotic Fracture, and the independent predictors of hip fracture are delineated in Table 194.4. Hip fracture incidence was 17 times greater among 15% of the women who had five or more of these risk factors, exclusive of bone density, than in the 47% of the women who had two risk factors or fewer[24]. However, the women with five or more risk factors had an even higher risk of hip fracture if their bone density was in the lowest tertile for age. Men have not been studied as intensively, but various diseases associated with secondary osteoporosis and falling seem to be more important in them[25]. It is important to point out, however, that the multifactorial nature of hip fracture pathogenesis resembles that for other common chronic diseases (e.g. atherosclerosis, osteoarthritis) that share the pattern of exponentially increasing incidence with age. Termed 'gompertzian' (after the British actuary Benjamin Gompertz, who discovered that mortality increases exponentially with aging), they share a number of fundamental characteristics in common: almost everyone is at risk of these disorders, which begin early in life and progress silently for decades, until some individuals develop clinical manifestations late in life. The rate of progression depends on the interplay of numerous risk factors, and many people never experience the ultimate clinical expression of the disease. This helps explain why no single factor (e.g. BMD) can completely account for hip fracture occurrence.

Spine fractures

Compared to hip fractures the epidemiology of vertebral fractures is poorly known, mainly because there is no universally accepted definition and because a substantial proportion of these fractures remain asymptomatic. Indeed, the number of people said to have a vertebral fracture depends to a large extent on the criteria or definition used for diagnosis (Fig. 194.4). By assessing the anterior, middle and posterior

	Relative risk (95% CI)	
TABLE 194.4 RISK FACTORS FOR HIP FRACTURE		
Variable	**Base model**	**Add fractures and bone density**
Age (per 5 years)	1.5 (1.3–1.7)	1.4 (1.2–1.6)
History of maternal hip fracture (vs none)	2.0 (1.4–2.9)	1.8 (1.2–2.7)
Increase in weight since age 25 (per 20%)	0.6 (0.5–0.7)	0.8 (0.6–0.9)
Height at age 25 (per 6cm)	1.2 (1.1–1.4)	1.3 (1.1–1.5)
Self-rated health (per 1-point decrease)	1.7 (1.3–2.2)	1.6 (1.2–2.1)
Previous hyperthyroidism (vs none)	1.8 (1.2–2.6)	1.7 (1.2–2.5)
Current use of long-acting benzodiazepines (vs not)	1.6 (1.1–2.4)	1.6 (1.1–2.4)
Current use of anticonvulsant drugs (vs not)	2.8 (1.2–6.3)	2.0 (0.8–4.9)
Current caffeine intake (per 190mg/day)	1.3 (1.0–1.5)	1.2 (1.0–1.5)
Walking for exercise (vs not)	0.7 (0.5–0.9)	0.7 (0.5–1.0)
On feet ≤ 4h/day (vs >4h/day)	1.7 (1.2–2.4)	1.7 (1.2–2.4)
Inability to rise from chair (vs no inability)	2.1 (1.3–3.2)	1.7 (1.1–2.7)
Lowest quartile for depth perception (vs other three)	1.5 (1.1–2.0)	1.4 (1.0–1.9)
Low-frequency contrast sensitivity (per 1SD decrease)	1.2 (1.0–1.5)	1.2 (1.0–1.5)
Resting pulse rate > 80bpm (vs ≤ 80 bpm)	1.8 (1.3–2.5)	1.7 (1.2–2.4)
Any fracture since age of 50 (vs none)	–	1.5 (1.1–2.0)
Calcaneal bone density (per 1SD decrease)	–	1.6 (1.3–1.9)

The table lists risk factors with and without adjustment for prior fractures and calcaneal bone density among elderly white women. (From Cummings et al.[24])

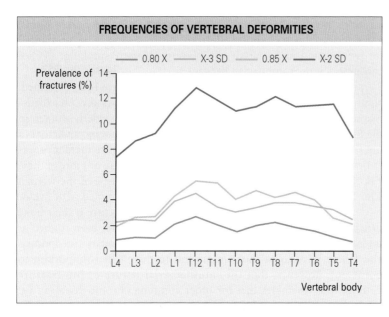

FREQUENCIES OF VERTEBRAL DEFORMITIES

Fig. 194.4 Frequencies of vertebral deformities. Frequency of any vertebral deformity at each vertebral level in elderly white women using different cut-off criteria. Overall, i.e. across all levels combined, prevalence varies from a high of 63% when the vertebral height ratio is more than 2 standard deviations below the mean ($\bar{x}$ –2SD) down to 25% when a 3 standard deviation cut-off is used ($\bar{x}$ –3SD) compared to 28% when the height ratio is reduced by 15% (0.85$\bar{x}$) and to only 12% when the ratio is reduced by 20% or more (0.80$\bar{x}$). (Redrawn with permission from Black *et al.*[28])

heights of the thoracic and lumbar vertebrae in comparison with population norms (vertebral morphometry), the overall prevalence of vertebral deformities among postmenopausal white women is generally estimated at 20–25%. The prevalence of the more severe vertebral deformities is about 10%. The latter are the ones that are more likely to produce chronic symptoms and account for the majority of vertebral fractures that come to clinical attention[26]. Thus, the annual incidence of clinically diagnosed vertebral fractures among postmenopausal white women (5 per 1000) is only a third of the total estimated incidence (18 per 1000) as judged by vertebral morphometry[27]. Fewer than 10% of all vertebral fractures necessitate hospitalization.

Despite these methodological problems, it is clear that the incidence of vertebral fracture increases with age (see Fig. 194.2). About a quarter can be attributed to the age-related increase in falls, but most vertebral frac-

tures are associated with the remarkably large compressive loads, easily capable of fracturing a vertebral body weakened by bone loss, that can result from seemingly benign everyday activities such as opening a stuck window[29]. Because vertebral fracture incidence rates are generally greater in women and women live longer, the lifetime risk of a clinically evident vertebral fracture is about 16% in white women, compared to just 5% in white men. Nonetheless, recent population-based studies have documented a prevalence of vertebral fractures in men as great as that seen in women[30]. The relatively high prevalence in young and middle-aged men suggests that a substantial fraction of these deformities are attributable to causes unrelated to osteoporosis (e.g. trauma).

Despite their lower hip fracture rates, the prevalence of vertebral fractures among Asians is as high as that in whites[31]. Few data are available for other ethnic groups, although vertebral fractures appear to be less common among black and Hispanic men and women[14]. The explanation for these differences is unclear at present. Among white women, vertebral fractures are strongly associated with lumbar spine BMD[6] and, after adjusting for bone density, with elevated rates of bone turnover[32]. It is also apparent that the occurrence of a vertebral fracture greatly increases the likelihood of additional ones[33]. Other than a history of previous vertebral fractures, it has not been possible to identify a consistent set of clinical factors that are strongly predictive of vertebral fracture risk. The risk factors found in different studies of women have included late menarche, early menopause, short duration of fertility, low consumption of cheese and yogurt, decreased height, low physical activity and family history of hip fracture, whereas oral contraceptive use and alcohol consumption were protective[14]. Other risk factors have been suggested, but they do not discriminate well between women who do and do not have a vertebral fracture (Table 194.5). Some of them (e.g. corticosteroid use) may only be associated with severe vertebral crush fractures[34]. In men, age, cigarette smoking, use of alcoholic beverages and secondary osteoporosis (particularly corticosteroid use, gastrectomy and hypogonadism), as well as a history of trauma, tuberculosis or peptic ulcer were risk factors for vertebral fracture, but obesity was protective. It has been proposed that patient-reported risk factors (history of vertebral fracture, history of non-vertebral fracture, age, height loss and prior diagnosis of osteoporosis) could serve clinically to screen for the presence of undetected vertebral fractures[35], but the circularity here seems evident.

Wrist fractures

Unlike hip fractures, which usually result from falling backwards or to the side, forearm fractures almost always follow a fall on the out-

TABLE 194.5 RISK FACTOR PREVALENCE AND RELATIVE RISK OF SPINE FRACTURES AMONG JAPANESE-AMERICAN WOMEN			
Variable	Prevalence	Relative risk	*p* value
Premature menopause (≤ age 40)	4.7%	1.6	NS
Family history (vs none)	1.7%	2.7	NS
Short stature (height ≤1.57m/62in)	87.2%	1.6	NS
Leanness (body mass index ≤19.7)	14.7%	1.7	NS
Calcium deficiency (≤500mg/day)	83.9%	1.2	NS
Physical activity (score ≤26.9)	7.8%	2.5	NS
Nulliparity (vs not)	5.7%	1.6	NS
Smoking (vs none)	16.8%	1.2	NS
Alcohol consumption (≥2g/day)	4.8%	1.7	NS
Asian ancestry (vs not)	100.0%	–	–
Caffeine intake (≥300mg/day)	29.6%	2.1	NS
Chronic gastrointestinal disease (vs none)	4.1%	1.0	NS
(Modified from Wasnich *et al.*[36])			

TYPICAL PATTERNS OF FALLING

Hip fracture

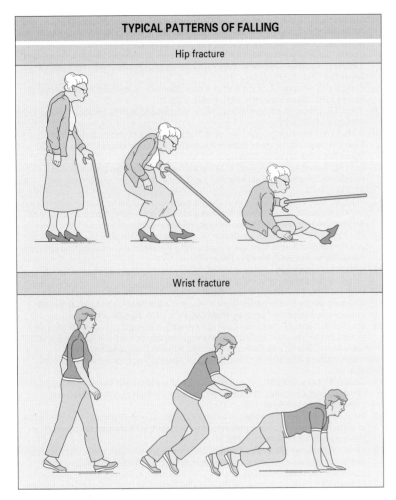

Wrist fracture

Fig. 194.5 Typical patterns of falling. Falling directly on the hip leads to a hip fracture (top) and on the outstretched forearm to a wrist fracture (bottom). (Redrawn with permission from Schwartz et al.[17])

TABLE 194.6 RISK FACTORS FOR DISTAL FOREARM FRACTURE AMONG ELDERLY WHITE WOMEN

Variable	Relative risk (95% CI)
Age (per 5 years)	0.87 (0.74–1.02)
Distal radius bone density (per 0.1g/cm² increase)	0.55 (0.43–0.69)
Fracture since age 50 years (vs none)	1.26 (0.91–1.73)
Blocks walked per week (per 100 blocks)	1.18 (1.00–1.41)
Visual acuity score (per 10 letters correctly identified)	0.83 (0.69–1.01)
Fall in previous year (vs not)	1.31 (0.95–1.81)
Estrogen replacement therapy (per 5 years use)	0.86 (0.74–1.01)
Weight (per 10kg increase)	1.02 (0.90–1.17)
Age at menopause (per 5 years)	0.87 (0.78–0.98)

(Modified from Kelsey et al.[39])

showed that a history of falls or fractures and the distance walked each week were linked to an increased risk of forearm fractures among women, whereas greater age, higher bone density, better vision and estrogen replacement therapy were protective (Table 194.6). Some of these factors were no longer statistically significant in a multivariate analysis, and none of them were particularly powerful except for bone density[39]. Other epidemiological studies have additionally identified low calcium intake, chronic anticonvulsant use and height loss as increasing the risk of a forearm fracture[40,41]. Despite these somewhat equivocal results, wrist fractures are clearly associated with osteoporosis[42]. More importantly, perhaps, forearm fractures are associated with a doubling in the risk of subsequent osteoporotic fractures[33]. Because they occur, on average, about 15 years before hip fractures do, wrist fractures may represent a sentinel event indicating a need for osteoporosis evaluation and therapy.

CONCLUSIONS

Because of the large number of people affected and the extensive and protracted care often required, the cost of fractures is enormous. In the United States alone, direct medical expenditures for osteoporotic fractures were estimated at $13.8 billion in 1995 (17 billion in 2001 dollars)[43]. These costs are likely to rise in the future as the number of elderly people increases. Worldwide, the 323 million individuals aged 65 years and over in 1990 will grow to an estimated 1555 million by 2050, and this demographic change alone could cause the number of hip fractures worldwide to increase from the estimated 1.7 million in 1990 to a projected 6.3 million in 2050[14]. If, in addition, hip fracture incidence rates increase by 1% annually, the projected number of fractures in 2050 could be 8.2 million; if incidence rates stabilize in Europe and North America but increase by 3% annually in the other regions, the total number of hip fractures in the world each year could exceed 21 million by 2050[44]. If the impact of these fractures is to be reduced, increased attention must be given to the design and implementation of effective control programs. The issue is how to accomplish this at a socially acceptable cost[45].

stretched arm (Fig. 194.5). This may explain the different incidence pattern compared to hip or vertebral fractures (see Fig. 194.2). In most studies, rates in women increase linearly to around age 65 years and then stabilize, possibly owing to the fact that elderly women with slower gait and impaired neuromuscular coordination are more likely to fall on their hip than on their wrist[37]. Indeed, the women who experience forearm fractures seem relatively healthy. Compared to hip fractures, which mostly occur indoors, a greater proportion of wrist fractures occur outdoors, and a winter peak in incidence has been associated with periods of icy weather[38]. In men, the incidence of forearm fractures is low and increases little with aging, so that the majority of such fractures occur in women. Although the female to male ratio of 4:1 is more marked than for hip or vertebral fractures, the incidence of wrist fracture varies from one geographic area to another generally in parallel with hip fracture rates[14]. Also, like most other osteoporotic fractures, forearm fracture incidence is lower in non-white than in white populations.

It has been difficult to identify important clinical risk factors for wrist fractures. An analysis of data from the Study of Osteoporotic Fractures

REFERENCES

1. Kanis JA, Glüer CC. An update on the diagnosis and assessment of osteoporosis with densitometry. Osteoporosis Int 2000; 11: 192–202.
2. Khosla S, Melton LJ III. Secondary osteoporosis. In: Riggs BL, Melton LJ III, eds. Osteoporosis: etiology, diagnosis, and management, 2nd edn. Philadelphia: Lippincott-Raven, 1995; 183–204.
3. Khosla S, Riggs BL, Melton LJ III. Clinical spectrum. In: Riggs BL, Melton LJ III, eds. Osteoporosis: etiology, diagnosis, and management, 2nd edn. Philadelphia: Lippincott-Raven, 1995; 205–223.
4. Riggs BL, Khosla S, Melton LJ III. The Type I/Type II model for involutional osteoporosis: update and modification based on new observations. In: Marcus R, Feldman D,

Kelsey J, eds. Osteoporosis, 2nd edn. Vol. 2. San Diego: Academic Press, 2001; 49–58.

5. Riggs BL, Khosla S, Melton LJ III. Sex steroids and the construction and conservation of the adult skeleton. Endocr Rev 2002; 23: 279–302.

6. Marshall D, Johnell O, Wedel H. Meta-analysis of how well measures of bone mineral density predict occurrence of osteoporotic fractures. Br Med J 1996; 312: 1254–1259.

7. Melton LJ III, Khosla S, Atkinson EJ et al. Cross-sectional versus longitudinal evaluation of bone loss in men and women. Osteoporosis Int 2000; 11: 592–599.

8. Beck TJ, Looker AC, Ruff CB et al. Structural trends in the aging femoral neck and proximal shaft: analysis of the Third National Health and Nutrition Examination Survey dual-energy X-ray absorptiometry data. J Bone Miner Res 2000; 15: 2297–2304.

9. Heaney RP, Abrams S, Dawson-Hughes B et al. Peak bone mass. Osteoporosis Int 2000; 11: 985–1009.

10. Looker AC, Wahner HW, Dunn WL et al. Proximal femur bone mineral levels of US adults. Osteoporosis Int 1995; 5: 389–409.

11. Kanis JA, Melton LJ III, Christiansen C et al. Perspective: the diagnosis of osteoporosis. J Bone Miner Res 1994; 9: 1137–1141.

12. Looker AC, Orwoll ES, Johnston CC Jr et al. Prevalence of low femoral bone density in older U.S. adults from NHANES III. J Bone Miner Res 1997; 12: 1761–1768.

13. Orwoll ES, Bauer DC, Vogt TM et al. Axial bone mass in older women. Study of Osteoporotic Fractures Research Group. Ann Intern Med 1996; 124: 187–196.

14. Melton LJ III, Cooper C. Magnitude and impact of osteoporosis and fractures. In: Marcus R, Feldman D, Kelsey J, eds. Osteoporosis, 2nd edn. Vol. 1. San Diego: Academic Press, 2001; 557–567.

15. Seeley DG, Browner WS, Nevitt MC et al. Which fractures are associated with low appendicular bone mass in elderly women? The Study of Osteoporotic Fractures Research Group. Ann Intern Med 1991; 115: 837–842.

16. Nguyen TV, Eisman JA, Kelly PJ et al. Risk factors for osteoporotic fractures in elderly men. Am J Epidemiol 1996; 144: 255–263.

17. Schwartz AV, Capezuti E, Grisso JA. Falls as risk factors for fractures. In: Marcus R, Feldman D, Kelsey J, eds. Osteoporosis, 2nd edn. Vol. 1. San Diego: Academic Press, 2001; 795–807.

18. Winner SJ, Morgan CA, Evans JG. Perimenopausal risk of falling and incidence of distal forearm fracture. Br Med J 1989; 298: 1486–1488.

19. Oden A, Dawson A, Dere W et al. Lifetime risk of hip fractures is underestimated. Osteoporosis Int 1998; 8: 599–603.

20. Cooper C, Melton LJ III. Epidemiology of osteoporosis. Trends Endocrinol Metab 1992; 3: 224–229.

21. Lau EMC, Cooper C. The epidemiology of osteoporosis. The Oriental perspective in a world context. Clin Orthop 1996; 323: 65–74.

22. Jacobsen SJ, Goldberg J, Miles TP et al. Regional variation in the incidence of hip fracture: US white women aged 65 years and older. JAMA 1990; 264: 500–502.

23. Melton LJ III. Differing patterns of osteoporosis across the world. In: Chesnut CH III, ed. New dimensions in osteoporosis in the 1990s. Asia Pacific Congress Series 125. Hong Kong: Excerpta Medica, 1991; 13–18.

24. Cummings SR, Nevitt MC, Browner WS et al. Risk factors for hip fracture in white women. The Study of Osteoporotic Fractures Research Group. N Engl J Med 1995; 332: 767–773.

25. Poór G, Atkinson EJ, O'Fallon MW et al. Predictors of hip fractures in elderly men. J Bone Miner Res 1995; 10: 1900–1907.

26. Ettinger B, Black DM, Nevitt MC et al. Contribution of vertebral deformities to chronic back pain and disability. The Study of Osteoporotic Fractures Research Group. J Bone Miner Res 1992; 7: 449–456.

27. Cooper C, Atkinson EJ, O'Fallon MW et al. Incidence of clinically diagnosed vertebral fractures: A population-based study in Rochester, Minnesota, 1985–1989. J Bone Miner Res 1992; 7: 221–227.

28. Black DJ, Cummings SR, Stone K et al. A new approach to defining normal vertebral dimensions. J Bone Miner Res 1991; 6: 883–892.

29. Myers ER, Wilson SE. Biomechanics of osteoporosis and vertebral fracture. Spine 1997; 22(Suppl 24): 25S–31S.

30. O'Neill TW, Felsenberg D, Varlow J et al. The prevalence of vertebral deformity in European men and women: The European Vertebral Osteoporosis Study. J Bone Miner Res 1996; 11: 1010–1018.

31. Ross PD, Fujiwara S, Huang C et al. Vertebral fracture prevalence in women in Hiroshima compared to Caucasians or Japanese in the US. Int J Epidemiol 1995; 24: 1171–1177.

32. Riggs BL, Melton LJ III, O'Fallon WM. Drug therapy for vertebral fractures in osteoporosis: Evidence that decreases in bone turnover and increases in bone mass both determine antifracture efficacy. Bone 1996; 18(Suppl 3): 197S–201S.

33. Klotzbuecher CM, Ross PD, Landsman PB et al. Patients with prior fractures have an increased risk of future fractures: a summary of the literature and statistical synthesis. J Bone Miner Res 2000; 15: 721–739.

34. Melton LJ III, Atkinson EJ, Khosla S et al. Secondary osteoporosis and the risk of vertebral deformities in women. Bone 1999; 24: 49–55.

35. Vogt TM, Ross PD, Palermo L et al. Vertebral fracture prevalence among women screened for the Fracture Intervention Trial and a simple clinical tool to screen for undiagnosed vertebral fractures. Mayo Clin Proc 2000; 75: 888–896.

36. Wasnich RD, Ross PD, MacLean CJ et al. The relative strengths of osteoporotic risk factors in a prospective study of postmenopausal osteoporosis. In: Christiansen C, Johansen JS, Riis BJ, eds. Osteoporosis 1987, Volume 1. Proceedings of the International Symposium on Osteoporosis, Copenhagen: Osteopress ApS, 1987; 394–395.

37. Nevitt MC, Cummings SR. Type of fall and risk of hip and wrist fractures: the study of osteoporotic fractures. The Study of Osteoporotic Fractures Research Group. J Am Geriatr Soc 1993; 41: 1226–1234.

38. Jacobsen SJ, Sargent DJ, Atkinson EJ et al. Contribution of weather to the seasonality of distal forearm fractures: A population-based study in Rochester, Minnesota. Osteoporosis Int 1999; 9: 254–259.

39. Kelsey JL, Browner WS, Seeley DG et al. Risk factors for fractures of the distal forearm and proximal humerus. Study of Osteoporotic Fractures Research Group. Am J Epidemiol 1992; 135: 477–489.

40. Nguyen TV, Center JR, Sambrook PN et al. Risk factors for proximal humerus, forearm, and wrist fractures in elderly men and women. The Dubbo Osteoporosis Epidemiology Study. Am J Epidemiol 2001; 153: 587–595.

41. Melton LJ III, Achenbach SJ, Khosla S et al. Secondary osteoporosis and the risk of distal forearm fractures in men and women. Bone 2002; 31: 119–125.

42. Eastell R. Forearm fracture. Bone 1996; 18(Suppl 3): 203S–207S.

43. Ray NF, Chan JK, Thamer M et al. Medical expenditures for the treatment of osteoporotic fractures in the United States in 1995: Report from the National Osteoporosis Foundation. J Bone Miner Res 197; 12: 24–35.

44. Gullberg B, Johnell O, Kanis JA. World-wide projections for hip fracture. Osteoporosis Int 1997; 7: 407–413.

45. Eddy D, Johnston CC, Cummings SR et al. Osteoporosis: Review of the evidence for prevention, diagnosis, and treatment and cost-effectiveness analysis. Osteoporosis Int 1998; 8(Suppl 4): 1–88.

195

Investigations of bone: densitometry

Kenneth G Faulkner

- There are several different options for bone density assessment, including dual X-ray absorptiometry (DXA), quantitative computed tomography (QCT) and quantitative ultrasound (QUS)
- For the assessment of osteoporosis, estimation of fracture risk, and monitoring of skeletal changes, DXA measurements of the spine and proximal femur are preferred
- Appropriate subjects for bone density testing include all women over 65, postmenopausal women with risk factors, men and women with low trauma fractures, and men and women currently taking medications known to influence bone (such as glucocorticoids)
- The most clinically important value from a bone density examination is the T-score, which compares the measured bone density to the young adult average

DENSITOMETRY TECHNIQUES

Radiographic techniques

Before the development of bone densitometers, bone mineral density (BMD) was estimated from conventional X-rays by comparing the brightness of the skeleton to the surrounding tissues. Dense bone appears relatively white on a standard X-ray, while demineralized bone has an appearance closer to soft tissue. However, this technique is qualitative and does not provide an accurate measure of BMD. It has been suggested that bone mineral losses of at least 30% are required before they may be visually detected on a conventional X-ray[1].

Because of the insensitivity of X-ray images to bone density changes, several techniques have been developed to improve the accuracy and precision of conventional radiographs for bone mass assessment. Many of these techniques were based on measurements of the hand and forearm, because of easy access for measurement. The primary advantage of these methods is equipment cost, as all medical institutions have standard X-ray units. The disadvantages, however, include alternations

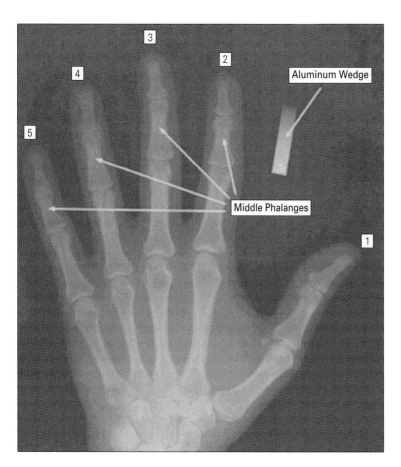
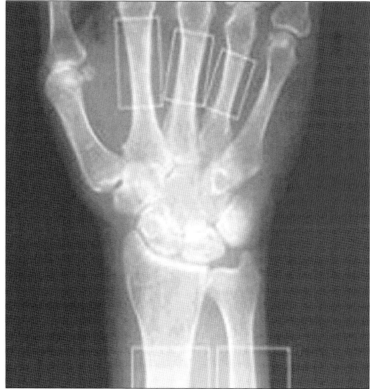

Fig. 195.1 Bone density measurements obtained from radiographs of the hand.

in imaging technique, most notably X-ray energy and type of X-ray film, both of which can cause apparent changes in bone density. To adjust for differences in imaging technique, a calibration wedge is often used during image acquisition as a BMD reference (Fig. 195.1).

To analyze the radiographs and produce a BMD value, some techniques require centralized analysis of the radiographs by a third party[2]. Recent improvements include systems that permit local analysis of hand and forearm radiographs, eliminating the need for shipment to a central analysis facility. Results are obtained using custom analysis software for evaluating the digitized images to produce BMD values. Despite these improvements, X-rays are still primarily qualitative images and are not specifically intended for measuring bone density. This has led to the development of devices specifically designed to quantify bone density at various skeletal sites using X-ray and ultrasound technology.

Single-energy densitometry

Because of the problems and inaccuracies of using radiographs for measuring bone mass, researchers developed the first dedicated bone densitometer in the 1960s[3]. This device passed a beam of radiation through the forearm and determined the difference between the incoming and the outgoing radiation, called the attenuation. The higher the bone mineral content, the greater the attenuation. With the introduction of these devices, physicians were now able to precisely measure bone density at a very low radiation dose. For the first time, it was possible to accurately and precisely monitor changes in bone density that might occur as the result of aging or treatment.

Single-energy densitometry has important limitations. The technique is limited to measuring peripheral bones such as the heel and forearm, as the measurement site must be immersed in water. Placing the measurement site in water cancels the effect of the overlying soft tissues, so that only the differential attenuation of the bone can be measured. This approach is reasonable for the measurement of the peripheral skeleton, but it is not practical to immerse the entire body in water to obtain measurements of the spine or the hip. Today, virtually all manufacturers of single-energy densitometers have switched to producing dual-energy systems.

Dual-energy densitometry

As stated above, the primary limitation of single-energy densitometry is an inability to directly measure the spine and hip. The challenge was to devise a method that eliminated the need for a water bath so that any skeletal site could be measured. Researchers found that if a dual-energy radiation source was used, the influence of soft tissue could be eliminated without the need for a water bath to equalize soft tissue attenuation. With this technique, it is possible to measure the central skeleton, specifically the lumbar spine and proximal femur. Today, dual X-ray absorptiometry, or DXA (sometimes referred to as DEXA), represents the clinical technique of choice for measuring BMD.

Several different types of DXA systems are available, but they all operate on similar principles. A radiation source is aimed at a radiation detector placed directly opposite the site to be measured. The patient is placed on a table in the path of the radiation beam. The source/detector assembly is then scanned across the measurement region. The attenuation of the radiation beam is determined and is related to the BMD[4].

Dual X-ray absorptiometry technology can measure virtually any skeletal site, but clinical use has been concentrated on the lumbar spine, proximal femur, forearm, and total body. DXA systems are available as either full table systems (capable of multiple skeletal measurements, including the spine and hip) or as peripheral systems (limited to measuring the peripheral skeleton). Because of their versatility, and the ability to measure the skeletal sites of greatest clinical interest, full table DXA systems are the current clinical choice for osteoporosis assessment (Fig. 195.2). Peripheral DXA systems, portable and less expensive than

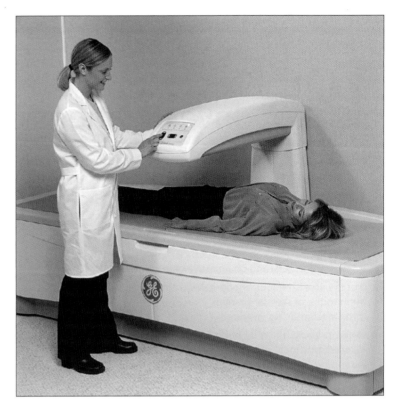

Fig. 195.2 Full table dual X-ray absorptiometry system.

full table systems, are more frequently used as screening and early risk assessment tools.

Spine and proximal femur scans represent the majority of the clinical measurements performed using DXA. Most full table DXA systems are able to perform additional studies, including lateral spine BMD measurements, evaluation of vertebral fractures, assessment of bone around prosthetic implants, measurements of children and infants, small-animal studies and measurements of excised bone specimens.

Early DXA systems used a pencil beam geometry and a single detector, which was scanned across the measurement region. Modern full table DXA scanners use a fan-beam source and multiple detectors, which are swept across the measurement region. Fan beam provides the advantage of decreased scan times compared to single-beam systems, but these machines typically cost more because of the need for multiple X-ray detectors. Fan-beam systems use either a single-view or multiview mode to image the skeleton.

Magnification error

Single-view systems measure the skeleton with a single pass of the X-ray source and detector across the measurement site. However, single-view fan-beam systems introduce a magnification error to the measurement that depends on the position of the object between the X-ray source and the detectors. By measuring the skeleton from only one angle, the location of the object between the source and detector cannot be determined. This is similar to trying to visually judge the distance of an object when one eye is covered – depth perception is lost when only one view is available. Fortunately, BMD measurements are not significantly affected by this magnification error, so in clinical use, single-view fan beam systems yield accurate BMD results[5,6].

When using a single-view fan beam, area and bone content values must either be corrected for body size or object height, or reported as 'estimated' to allow for some variation in the position of the patient between the source and detector[6,7]. For accurate assessment of bone area and content, multiview fan beam systems have been developed. By using overlapping images from different measurement angles, the object plane

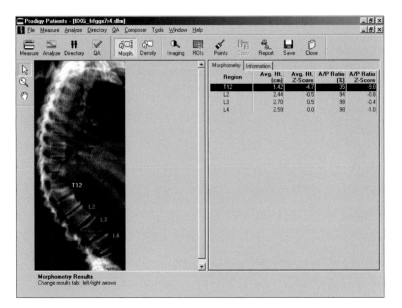

Fig. 195.3 Vertebral fracture assessment from a dual x-ray absorptiometry image of the spine. Use of dual energy images facilitates the visualization of the lumbar and thoracic spine in a single image. In this example, a fracture has been identified at T12.

can be accurately determined. This allows multiview fan beam systems to accurately determine bone area, content and geometry. This is of particular importance for evaluating follow-up BMD measurements, where consistency in area can be used as a gauge of positioning precision. In addition, geometric measurements, such as hip axis length (discussed below), require highly accurate and precise length measurements to be clinically useful.

Vertebral fracture assessment

For assessing vertebral heights (also called vertebral morphometry), special software is used to determine vertebral body dimensions[8,9]. The computer (with the help of the technologist) places points on the superior and inferior endplates of each vertebra. The vertebral heights are calculated and compared to each other as well as to the expected normal dimensions. With the advent of higher-resolution DXA systems, visual assessment of fractures is also possible from DXA-based lateral spine images (Fig. 195.3). In this situation, the DXA system essentially functions as a digital X-ray imaging device. Visual assessment is performed from a computer monitor or high-resolution printout. To optimize the assessment, the use of high-definition dual-energy images has been recommended[10].

Using a DXA system for assessing vertebral fracture status has several advantages. The evaluation of spine fractures can be performed without a conventional lateral spine X-ray. This can be done at the same time and at the same place as the BMD measurement, with much less radiation than a conventional spine X-ray. Despite the apparent advantages, the future of vertebral fracture assessment using DXA remains unclear.

Skeletal radiologists have criticized the technique for being insensitive and inaccurate for detecting vertebral fractures. A DXA image is of lower

resolution than a conventional X-ray and might fail to identify other potential problems or diseases that would be apparent on a spine film. At this time, DXA devices are not generally accepted as a surrogate for spinal X-rays, though they may provide a useful screening tool in higher-risk patients when spinal X-rays are unavailable. For example, individuals over 65, subjects reporting significant height loss or patients on long term glucocorticoid therapy who have not had previous vertebral fractures or spinal radiographs could benefit from a vertebral fracture assessment.

Femoral dual X-ray absorptiometry

Newer applications of DXA include sequential measurement of both femurs as well as geometric measurements incorporated into the DXA scanning software. Several studies have shown that left and right femur measurements are highly correlated[11,12]. Yet, for clinical purposes, the relevant question is how often a difference between the left and right femur will change either the diagnosis or the management of an individual patient.

Studies have confirmed that the average BMD difference between left and right femurs is negligible[11,12]. However, the standard error between

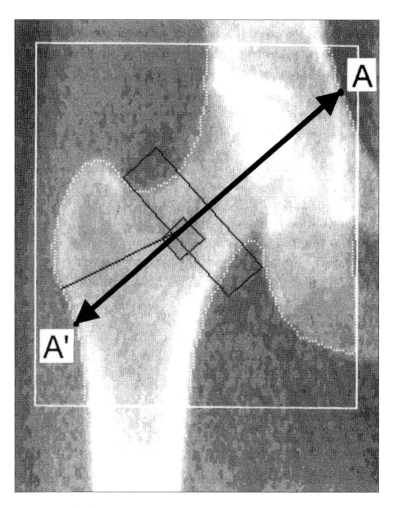

Fig. 195.4 The hip-axis length, defined as the length along the femoral neck axis from the base of the greater trochanter to the inner pelvic brim.

TABLE 195.1 POTENTIAL FOR MISSED DIAGNOSIS OF OSTEOPOROSIS IF ONLY A SINGLE HIP IS MEASURED													
T-score of first hip	0.0	−0.5	−1.0	−1.5	−1.6	−1.7	−1.8	−1.9	−2.0	−2.1	−2.2	−2.3	−2.4
% with second hip at −2.0 or less	0.0	0.1	2.3	15.9	21.2	27.4	34.5	42.1					
% with second hip at −2.5 or less	0.0	0.0	0.1	2.3	3.6	5.5	8.1	11.5	15.9	21.2	27.4	34.5	42.1

In situations where the first hip is within a half of a T-score of a diagnostic or therapeutic criterion, measurement of the second hip is recommended.

the left and right measurements is 0.05g/cm^2, both at the total hip and the femoral neck. Thus, if only one hip is measured, the other hip will differ by an average of ±0.05g/cm^2, equivalent to half a T-score. For patients with T-scores approaching the threshold for osteoporosis, the potential for misclassification becomes significant (Table 195.1). For example, if the left femoral neck has a T-score of –1.8, there is a 34% chance that the opposite femoral neck will be –2.0 or less and an 8% chance that it will be –2.5 or less. Thus the use of the second hip measurement can have an impact on patient management. In addition, the use of both hips greatly reduces precision error and facilitates the evaluation of skeletal response at the femur.

The hip axis length (Fig. 195.4) has been identified as an independent indicator of hip fracture risk[13–19]. This measurement can be obtained from a standard DXA scan of the proximal femur, although on some systems an increased scan field may be required. Each centimeter (10%) increase in hip-axis length doubles the risk for hip fracture. For short-term prediction of hip fracture (within 2 years), hip-axis length was shown to predict hip fractures independent of BMD.

While hip-axis length cannot be viewed as a stand-alone clinical predictor, it can potentially provide utility in conjunction with BMD to identify high-risk patients. Based on the available data, elderly Caucasian women with height- and weight-adjusted hip axis length more than 1cm above normal have twice the risk of hip fracture than those with an average hip-axis length. The use of hip-axis length in younger women, men and non-Caucasians has not yet been studied. However, for those with low BMD, hip-axis length can be considered as another factor to help identify those at increased risk for hip fracture.

Quantitative computed tomography

Before the advent of DXA, several researchers reported using computed tomography (CT) scanners to obtain bone density measurements[20–22]. This technique is called quantitative CT (QCT) to differentiate it from imaging CT. QCT is the only non-invasive three-dimensional bone mass measurement technique available. QCT reports a volumetric density (in milligrams per cubic centimeter) as opposed to the area density (in grams per square centimeter) obtained using other techniques. Initially, QCT was performed without any special equipment (other than the CT system) by measuring the average CT number of the vertebral body. More advanced procedures have been developed to improve the accuracy and precision of the measurement.

Quantitative computed tomography is used clinically to measure the bone density of the spine. It has the advantage of measuring the central bone of the vertebral body, which is a more sensitive site for detecting bone mineral changes than most other skeletal sites[23]. QCT can be performed on most commercial CT systems with the addition of a bone mineral standard for calibration of the CT measurement (Fig. 195.5). Several different types of calibration system are commercially available from CT manufacturers and third-party vendors.

In the standard QCT protocol, three or four lumbar vertebral bodies are measured using a single 8–10mm slice through the center of each vertebra[24]. The calibration standard must also be measured, either at the same time or immediately after the patient is measured. Low-dose settings are used to reduce radiation exposure to well below that of a standard CT examination but still well above other types of bone density measurement (such as DXA). From the CT images, the average attenuation of the vertebral body bone is determined as well as the attenuation of the calibration standard. Using the known density of each of the standards and the measured CT values of the bone mineral standard, the vertebral CT value is converted to a physical density.

While most QCT studies are limited to the lumbar spine, specialized QCT systems (called peripheral QCT, or pQCT) have been introduced for measuring the forearm. This technique offers the advantages of measuring the volumetric density of the forearm as well as providing

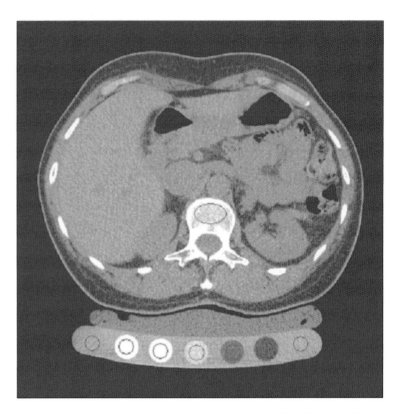

Fig. 195.5 Quantitative computed tomography study of the lumbar spine.

measures of trabecular, cortical and integral (trabecular plus cortical) bone. These scanners are limited to the forearm and can cost as much as full table DXA devices capable of density measurements at multiple skeletal sites.

When properly performed, QCT can be a useful clinical tool. The measurement of a purely trabecular bone sample may have some utility for the diagnosis of osteoporosis, assessing fracture risk and monitoring bone changes. There have been relatively few published prospective studies regarding the use of QCT for predicting fracture. The vast majority of prospective studies have been with DXA. For predicting hip fracture, it is generally agreed that a direct femoral measurement using DXA is the best choice. QCT may offer some advantage in elderly subjects by avoiding artifact introduced in DXA by the degenerative changes typically seen at the spine. On the other hand, it is conceivable that the ability of DXA to measure both cortical and trabecular bone provides some advantage for predicting fracture compared to QCT. Bone strength is influenced by both cortical and trabecular bone, so that measurement of both components by DXA might provide an advantage.

Quantitative computed tomography shows twice to three times the change in BMD seen with DXA, either due to aging or response to therapy. Yet QCT is typically less precise than DXA. Precision errors with QCT are reported to be twice to three times as great as for DXA, because of difficulties with patient positioning, consistent slice location, system stability and consistent placement of the region of interest. Thus, any increased sensitivity of QCT is offset by the increased precision error of the technique, resulting in no significant advantage for monitoring changes.

As with DXA, it is essential to use proper quality control when monitoring changes with QCT. As CT instruments are designed for imaging and not for quantitative assessment, it is essential that the stability of the system is monitored frequently. Acquisition protocols (tube voltage and current) must be consistent from one examination to another. Daily quality control measures must be maintained to guard against drifts in either the X-ray tube or detectors that might influence the BMD

TABLE 195.2 EFFECTIVE DOSES IN DENSITOMETRY COMPARED TO OTHER COMMON RADIATION SOURCES	
Radiation source	Effective dose (µSv)
Single X-ray absorptiometry	1
Dual X-ray absorptiometry	1–5
Quantitative computed tomography	60
Lateral spine film	700
Natural background (per day)	5–8
Round trip (8–10h) airplane flight	60

(Data from Kalender.[25])

result. All QCT manufacturers provide tools for monitoring system performance that should be followed to ensure consistent results.

An additional consideration with repeated use of QCT is radiation dose (Table 195.2). Compared to most radiological examination techniques, QCT has a very low dose, equivalent to that of a mammogram. Yet a single QCT examination has an effective dose equivalent to 50–100 times that of a DXA examination[25]. Improperly performed scans (using imaging protocols rather than BMD protocols) can increase this dose by another factor of 10. As with all radiological examinations, QCT should be performed only at appropriate intervals to avoid excess or unnecessary exposure.

In addition to the clinical and technical considerations, there are a few practical issues regarding the use of QCT. Foremost is the need for a CT scanner. This limits the use of the technique to radiology facilities with the proper equipment and available scanner time. Often, the lack of scanner time can be the most significant barrier to performing QCT. Daily quality assurance procedures require 15 minutes each day to monitor the QCT system. The examination itself takes 15–30 minutes to perform, including time for patient preparation and scan acquisition. With competing pressures for scanner time in many radiology departments, it can be difficult to find time to schedule patients for measurement of bone density.

Quantitative ultrasound

Ultrasound has been used for many years to investigate the mechanical properties of various engineering materials. Several commercial ultrasound devices have been introduced for investigating bone status, primarily of the heel (Fig. 195.6). This technique is termed quantitative ultrasound (QUS) to distinguish it from the more commonly known imaging ultrasound techniques. Clinical QUS looks at the transmission of high-frequency sound through bone, whereas pure imaging ultrasound devices employ sound reflection to produce their image. More advanced QUS devices do provide an image, but it is used to identify the measurement region, in much the same way as an image from a DXA system is used (Fig. 196.6).

Quantitative ultrasound offers the advantages of small equipment size, relatively quick and simple measurements, and no need for ionizing radiation. QUS is most easily performed at skeletal sites with minimal and consistent soft tissue covering, such as the calcaneus, radius, tibia, patella and phalanges. QUS is markedly different from X-ray-based techniques in employing mechanical vibration, rather than electromagnetic waves, to interrogate the bone tissue. The interaction of high-frequency sound with bone, as with any material, uses completely different mechanisms from X-rays.

When measuring the skeleton using QUS, two primary measurements are obtained – the speed of sound and the broadband ultrasound attenuation in the site being measured. Most QUS devices define these parameters in a unique way. In addition, QUS is not standardized in terms of sound frequencies, coupling to the measurement site (water, gel or a combination) and methods for signal processing and analysis. Yet, despite these inconsistencies in instrumentation and physical differences

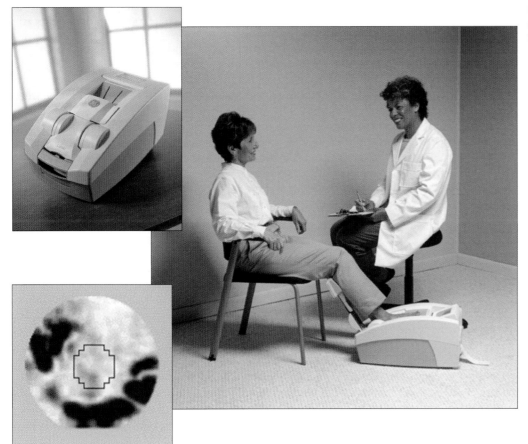

Fig. 195.6 Quantitative ultrasound device for measuring the heel, which incorporates a real-time image for more accurate assessment.

from X-ray-based systems, QUS yields a measurement that is reasonably well correlated with X-ray BMD values at the same skeletal site, particularly at the calcaneus[26]. However, the correlation of calcaneal QUS with density measurements at other skeletal sites is less strong[27]. Much of this discrepancy is due to simple discordance between different skeletal sites and is not related to technical differences between QUS and X-ray technology[28].

Data from several prospective studies using different QUS devices have shown BUA to be predictive of hip fracture[29–32]. Furthermore, the predictive ability of QUS appears to be at least partially independent of X-ray-based BMD measurements[31]. This has fueled interest in QUS as a measure of bone quality as well as density. While the future of QUS appears promising, there are still some questions that remain to be answered. For example, researchers are still not certain exactly which parameters of the bone are being measured with QUS.

Comparisons with other BMD techniques indicate that QUS is measuring a combination of bone density and some other property of the bone. It has been speculated that QUS may be measuring a parameter related to bone structure, such as trabecular size and spacing. If this is true, then a QUS measurement would be valuable in combination with bone density to get a better measure of the bone status. It also remains to be determined how QUS can be used to monitor skeletal response to different therapies. However, the compact size and non-radiation-based qualities of QUS make it an attractive choice for population-based screening programs.

CLINICAL USE OF MEASUREMENTS OF BONE MINERAL DENSITY

For BMD measurements to be clinically useful, they must be compared with established normative ranges. All BMD manufacturers provide normative databases for this purpose. These databases are derived from measurements of large groups of men or women of different ages and races. Comparisons are expressed either as a percentage of the expected normal value or as the number of standard deviations (SD) from the expected normal value. The T-score is the most important comparison. The T-score is the number of SD by which the measured BMD differs from the gender-matched young normal (YN) value.

For the diagnosis of osteoporosis, the World Health Organization has defined the following criteria for the assessment of osteoporosis based on the T-score[33,34]:

- **Normal:** A BMD not more than 1SD below YN (T-score ≥ –1)
- **Osteopenia (low bone mass):** A BMD between 1 and 2.5SD below YN (T-score between –1 and –2.5)
- **Osteoporosis:** A BMD 2.5 or more SD below YN (T-score ≤ –2.5)
- **Severe osteoporosis:** A BMD 2.5 or more SD below YN (T-score ≤ –2.5) and the presence of one or more fragility fractures.

The WHO definitions were not intended to be used in diagnosis of osteoporosis in individuals. They have nevertheless become commonly used for this purpose in clinical practice. Several researchers have pointed out the shortcomings of using T-scores and the WHO criteria for individual diagnosis[28,35].

Figure 195.7 shows a comparison of the age-related decline in T-scores with different BMD measurements. The central skeleton, particularly the spine, shows the largest T-score decline with age. However, there is considerable variation in the T-scores at different skeletal sites. The normative data crosses the –2.5SD level at age 60 with QCT compared to age 77 for DXA spine measurements. At age 60, the prevalence of osteoporosis using the WHO definition is 50% using QCT compared to 14% with spinal DXA.

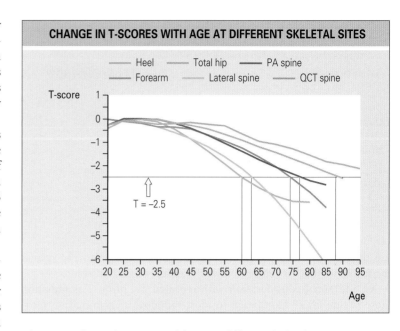

CHANGE IN T-SCORES WITH AGE AT DIFFERENT SKELETAL SITES

Fig. 195.7 Change in T-scores with age at different skeletal sites.

It is clear from Figure 195.7 that some techniques, such as spinal QCT and lateral DXA, produce T-scores that are significantly different than with other measurements. This is predominantly because of differences in the normal data from which the T-scores are derived, resulting in a smaller relative SD for QCT compared to DXA[28]. For this reason, it is now acknowledged that a single T-score criterion cannot be universally applied to all BMD measurements. Specifically, use of the WHO guidelines with lateral DXA or QCT will result in an overestimation of osteoporosis and fracture risk. For the diagnosis of osteoporosis, it is recommended that the lowest T-score from a DXA measurement of the lumbar spine, proximal femur or total hip be used.

WHO SHOULD RECEIVE A BONE MINERAL DENSITY TEST?

In 1998, the National Osteoporosis Foundation (NOF) in the USA, in collaboration with 10 other professional societies, created a set of guidelines for the use and interpretation of BMD measurements[36]. They recommend BMD measurements for postmenopausal Caucasian women who:

- are under the age of 65 and have one or more additional risk factors for osteoporosis (besides menopause)
- are aged 65 and older regardless of additional risk factors
- present with fractures
- are considering therapy for osteoporosis, if BMD testing would facilitate the decision
- have been on hormone replacement therapy for prolonged periods.

At present, the NOF recommendations are limited to Caucasian women because only limited data are available for other populations. However, many physicians are applying these guidelines to postmenopausal women of other races as well. In addition to the NOF recommendations, other high-risk populations should be considered for measurement. The most evident risk population includes both men and women presenting with low-trauma fracture. BMD should be assessed to confirm the diagnosis of osteoporosis. In addition, individuals on long term glucocorticoid therapy should have BMD assessed based on recommendations from the American College of Rheumatology.[37] Patients taking 5mg/day of prednisone (prednisolone) or its equivalent for more than 3 months should receive a BMD test and be considered for antiresorptive therapy to reduce bone loss associated with steroid therapy. In addition, men 65 and older, particularly those with risk factors such as alcoholism or hypogonadism or with radiographic evidence of bone loss, as well as men and women taking drugs known to influence bone density, should be considered for BMD testing.

USE OF BONE MINERAL DENSITY TESTING TO GUIDE TREATMENT

Treatment guidelines were typically developed for use with central DXA measurements[36]. When applied to peripheral measurements, particularly in those under 65 years of age, skeletal discordance can cause significant variation in T-scores between sites. Because of differences in skeletal aging and normative data at the different skeletal sites, variations of a full T-score or more can be expected. Usually, it is the central skeleton that will show the first signs of age-related bone loss, so it is recommended that treatment decisions are based on the lowest T-score at the spine, femoral neck or total hip measured by DXA. In patients with low peripheral T-scores and several additional risk factors, such as age over 70, the risk may be sufficient to warrant treatment based on this information alone[36].

If peripheral densitometry is used for screening, the concern is that a normal T-score at the heel, hand or forearm cannot guarantee that the score at the spine and/or hip would not be low[38,39]. To guard against this situation, a conservative screening approach should be used. If the peripheral skeleton yields a T-score of −1.0 or greater, the patient can be considered to be at low risk. If the T-score at the peripheral skeleton is −2.0 or lower, the central skeleton will typically be as low, if not lower, and the patient should be considered at high risk. For peripheral T-scores between −1.0 and −2.0, additional measurements should be considered, including central densitometry. However, additional risk factors, particularly age and previous fracture history, should be incorporated in any screening program. It is also important to recognize that there is no single BMD measurement, peripheral or central, that will proper identify all patients at risk for fracture.

SUMMARY

While all BMD techniques have clinical utility, differences in versatility, specifically the ability to measure both the spine and hip, favor DXA over other methods. As a result, DXA has become the densitometry technique of choice in many clinical departments. While other methods are still used in some clinics, there is a continued shift to DXA as the clinical standard. DXA has the primary disadvantage of cost, as commercial units typically cost significantly more than pDXA or QUS devices. Because of the advantages of low cost and portability, peripheral densitometry is often used for screening programs or in clinics where central densitometry cannot be accommodated.

The proper clinical use of densitometry requires an understanding of the available techniques, their appropriate application and the potential sources of measurement error. Clinical guidelines recommend that all women over the age of 65 and all postmenopausal women with risk factors should have their bone density assessed. In addition, BMD measurements should be considered in men 65 years of age and older, individuals with low trauma fractures and individuals on long-term glucocorticoid therapy.

With the advent of smaller, portable devices, bone density measurements are now widely available. In particular, ultrasound techniques, which do not use radiation, have particular promise for widespread screening applications. Peripheral densitometry alone cannot adequately address all clinical questions, particularly the question of monitoring subtle changes in bone density. Also, although one skeletal site may be found to have normal BMD, it is possible that the density at other skeletal site(s) could be low. In individuals with multiple risk factors, a moderately low BMD assessment in the peripheral skeleton should be verified by scanning another skeletal site, preferably the spine or hip. For any bone density measurement to be clinically useful, it must be performed with careful attention to detail, particularly with regard to instrument calibration, patient positioning, measurement analysis and interpretation.

REFERENCES

1. Resnick D. Osteoporosis: radiographic-pathologic correlation. In: Genant HK, ed. Osteoporosis update 1987. San Francisco, CA: Radiology Research and Education Foundation, University of California; 1987: 31–39.
2. Cosman F, Herrington B, Himmelstein S et al. Radiographic absorptiometry: a simple method for determination of bone mass. Osteoporosis Int 1991; 2: 34–38.
3. Cameron JR, Sorenson G. Measurements of bone mineral in vivo: an improved method. Science 1963; 142: 230–232.
4. Nord RH. Technical considerations in DPA. In: Genant HK, ed. Osteoporosis update 1987. San Francisco, CA: Radiology Research and Education Foundation, University of California; 1987: 203–212.
5. Faulkner KG, Gluer CC, Estilo M, Genant HK. Cross-calibration of DXA equipment: upgrading from a Hologic QDR 1000/w to a QDR 2000. Calcif Tissue Int 1993; 52: 79–84.
6. Mazess RB, Barden HS. Evaluation of differences between fan-beam and pencil-beam densitometers. Calcif Tissue Int 2000; 67: 291–296.
7. Young JT, Carter KA, Marion MS, Greendale GA. A simple method for computing hip axis length using fan-beam densitometry and anthropometric measurements. J Clin Densitometry 2000; 3: 325–331.
8. Steiger P, Cummings SR, Genant HK, Weiss H. Morphometric X-ray absorptiometry of the spine: correlation in vivo with morphometric radiography. Osteoporosis Int 1994; 4: 238–244.
9. Genant HK, Jiao L, Wu CY, Shepherd JA. Vertebral fractures in osteoporosis: a new method for clinical assessment. J Clin Densitometry 2000; 3: 281–290.
10. Rea JA, Steiger P, Blake GM, Fogelman I. Optimizing data acquisition and analysis of morphometric X-ray absorptiometry. Osteoporosis Int 1998; 8: 177–183.
11. Faulkner KG, Genant HK, McClung M. Bilateral comparison of femoral bone density and hip axis length from single and fan beam DXA scans. Calcif Tissue Int 1995; 56: 26–31.
12. Bonnick SL, Nichols DL, Sanborn CF et al. Right and left proximal femur analyses; is there a need to do both? Calcif Tissue Int 1996; 57: 340–343.
13. Faulkner KG, Cummings SR, Black D et al. Simple measurement of femoral geometry predicts hip fracture: the study of osteoporotic fractures. J Bone Miner Res 1993; 8: 1211–1217.
14. Faulkner KG, McClung M, Cummings SR. Automated evaluation of hip axis length for predicting hip fracture. J Bone Miner Res 1994; 9: 1065–1070.
15. Glüer CC, Cummings SR, Pressman A et al. Prediction of hip fractures from pelvic radiographs: the study of osteoporotic fractures. J Bone Min Res 1994; 9: 671–677.
16. Boonen S, Koutri R, Dequeker J et al. Measurement of femoral geometry in type I and type II osteoporosis: differences in hip axis length consistent with heterogeneity in the pathogenesis of osteoporotic fractures. J Bone Miner Res 1995; 10: 1908–1912.
17. Peacock M, Turner CH, Liu G et al. Better discrimination of hip fracture using bone density, geometry and architecture. Osteoporosis Int 1995; 5: 167–173.
18. Rosso R, Minisola S. Hip axis length in an Italian osteoporotic population. Br J Radiol 2000; 73: 969–972.
19. Frisoli A, Paula AP, Szejnfeld V et al. Comparison between hip axis length of elderly osteoporotic Brazilian women with and without hip fracture. J Bone Min Res 2000; 15: S538.
20. Ruegsegger P, Elsasser U, Anliker M et al. Quantification of bone mineralisation using computed tomography. Radiology 1976; 121: 93–97.
21. Cann CE, Genant HK. Precise measurement of vertebral mineral content using computed tomography. J Comput Assist Tomogr 1980; 4: 493–500.
22. Genant HK, Cann CE, Ettinger B, Gorday GS. Quantitative computed tomography of vertebral spongiosa: a sensitive method for detecting early bone loss after oophorectomy. Ann Intern Med 1982; 97: 699–705.
23. Faulkner KG. Bone densitometry: choosing the proper skeletal site to measure. J Clinical Densitometry 1998; 1: 279–285.
24. Steiger P, Block J, Steiger S et al. Spinal bone mineral density measured with quantitative CT: effect of region of interest, vertebral level, and technique. Radiology 1990; 175: 537–543.
25. Kalender WA. Effective dose values in bone mineral measurements by photon absorptiometry and computed tomography. Osteoporosis Int 1992; 2: 82–87.

26. Glüer CC, Vahlensieck M, Faulkner KG *et al.* Site-matched calcaneal measurements of broadband ultrasound attenuation and single X-ray absorptiometry: do they measure different skeletal properties? J Bone Miner Res 1992; 7: 1071–1079.

27. Faulkner KG, McClung MR, Coleman LJ, Kingston-Sandahl E. Quantitative ultrasound of the heel: correlation with densitometric measurements at different skeletal sites. Osteoporosis Int 1994; 4: 42–47.

28. Faulkner KG, von Stetten E, Miller P. Discordance in patient classification using T-scores. J Clinical Densitometry 1999; 2: 343–350.

29. Bauer D, Glüer C, Cauley J *et al.* Bone ultrasound predicts fractures strongly and independently of densitometry in older women: a prospective study. Arch Intern Med 1997; 157: 629–634.

30. Porter R, Miller C, Grainger D, Palmer S. Prediction of hip fracture in elderly women: a prospective study. Br Med J 1990; 301: 638–641.

31. Hans D, Dargent-Molina P, Schott A *et al.* Ultrasonic heel measurements to predict hip fracture in elderly women: the EPIDOS prospective study. Lancet 1996; 348: 511–514.

32. Marshall D, Johnell O, Wedel H. Meta-analysis of how well measures of bone mineral density predict occurrence of osteoporotic fractures. Br Med J 1996; 312: 1254–1259.

33. The WHO Study Group (1994) Assessment of fracture risk and its application to screening for postmenopausal osteoporosis. Geneva: World Health Organization.

34. Kanis JA. Assessment of fracture risk and is application to screening for postmenopausal osteoporosis: synopsis of a WHO report. Osteoporosis Int 1994; 4: 368–381.

35. Greenspan SL, Maitland-Ramsey L, Myers E. Classification of osteoporosis in the elderly is dependent on site-specific analysis. Calcif Tissue Int 1996; 58: 409–414.

36. National Osteoporosis Foundation. Physician's guide to prevention and treatment of osteoporosis. Washington, DC: National Osteoporosis Foundation; 1998.

37. American College of Rheumatology Ad Hoc Committee on Glucocorticoid-induced Osteoporosis. Recommendations for the prevention and treatment of glucocorticoid-induced osteoporosis: 2001 update. Arthritis Rheum 2001; 44: 1496–1503. Available on the Internet at www.rheumatology.org

38. Baran DT, Faulkner KG, Genant HK *et al.* Diagnosis and management of osteoporosis: Guidelines for the utilization of bone densitometry. Calcif Tissue Int 1997; 61: 433–440.

39. Miller PD, Bonnick SL, Johnston CC *et al.* The challenges of peripheral bone density testing: Which patients need additional central density skeletal measurements? J Clinical Densitometry 1998; 1: 211–217.

196 Pathogenesis of osteoporosis

Graham Russell

- The pathogenesis of osteoporosis reflects the complex interplay among genetic, metabolic and environmental factors that determine:
  - bone growth
  - peak bone mass
  - calcium homeostasis
  - bone loss
- These factors are influenced by:
  - aging
  - physical inactivity
  - sex hormone deficiency
  - nutritional status

INTRODUCTION

Osteoporosis is the most common clinical disorder of bone metabolism. Its pathophysiological basis includes a genetic predisposition to low peak bone mass, and subtle alterations in bone remodeling, due to changes in systemic and local hormones, coupled with environmental influences.

The remarkable advances in the study of osteoporosis and its treatment have occurred mainly since the early 1990s. The published literature is vast, and this chapter can only deal with highlights. Readers are referred to recent reviews for further information[1–4].

THE FEATURES OF OSTEOPOROSIS

Osteoporosis literally means 'holes in bones'. Tunnels created by bone resorption but not refilled with new bone characteristically occur in cortical bone, while in trabecular bone there is thinning of the bony plates so that they eventually perforate.

These changes occur progressively and are present in almost everyone in later decades of life. Fractures are the clinical endpoint of this loss of bone. There are therefore analogies between the decline in bone mass and the occurrence of fractures in osteoporosis with the relationships that exist between risk factors and other diseases, such as elevated serum cholesterol and myocardial infarction, and hypertension and stroke. In fact the relationship between bone mass, measured as bone mineral density (BMD), and fractures is the strongest of these three examples.

There are therefore problems in defining osteoporosis in a precise manner. A definition that relies solely on the presence of fracture impedes the clinical identification of individuals at high risk whose bones have not yet fractured. Conversely a definition based on bone mass will include individuals who never experience fractures and exclude patients who sustain fractures despite having a bone mass above the defined threshold.

The single most important advance that has allowed the spectacular progress in this field over the past decade has been the development of reproducible and accurate methods of measuring bone mass by non-invasive techniques. The technical advances in bone densitometry based in particular on dual energy X-ray absorptiometry (DXA) were key to this.

In 1994, the World Health Organization (WHO) produced a definition of osteoporosis based on low BMD. Osteoporosis was defined by a BMD of 2.5SD or more below the mean for young adults (i.e. a T score of less than −2.5). Severe osteoporosis was defined by a T score of less than −2.5 plus one or more fracture. Individuals with T scores between −1.0 and −2.5 were defined as having osteopenia. These definitions are important because they have, perhaps unintentionally, become related to thresholds for therapeutic intervention, since entry to drug trials is usually based on these values. They are also important in discussions of pathogenesis, where causative associations are identified from epidemiological studies based on T score definitions of osteoporosis.

It is increasingly appreciated that better predictors of fracture risk than BMD alone are needed. BMD is only one of several factors that predict fractures. Moreover, changes in BMD only partially account for responses to treatment. The definition of osteoporosis and risk of fracture needs to evolve to include not only the traditional measures of bone quantity, such as mass, but also measures of bone quality, which contributes to bone strength.

The most recent definition of osteoporosis issued by a Consensus Development Conference[5] sponsored by the National Institutes of Health now refers to decreased bone strength instead of just low BMD, and is worded as follows: 'Osteoporosis is a skeletal disorder characterized by compromised bone strength predisposing a person to an increased risk of fracture.'

The pathogenesis of fracture: bone fragility and falls

Fractures occur when bones are too fragile to resist relatively minor degrees of trauma, which should not normally result in fracture. The conventional definition of osteoporotic fracture in terms of being 'non-traumatic' poses problems of defining the degree of trauma. Practically, the occurrence of any fracture in an elderly person is often considered to be osteoporotic, especially if it was related to a fall from no more than a standing height, or if there was little or no recognized trauma.

While not the focus of this chapter, one must remember that an increased susceptibility to falls contributes to increased risk of fracture, and reducing falls might be expected to reduce fractures in the elderly[6]. The wearing of hip-protecting devices has been shown to reduce rates of fracture in controlled trials[7].

Usually, osteoporotic fractures heal quite normally, unlike fractures associated with other pathological conditions such as bone metastases.

THE PATHOGENESIS OF OSTEOPOROSIS AND FRACTURES

The pathogenesis of osteoporosis involves many different factors. It results from a complex interaction among genetic, hormonal and environmental influences. Factors that contribute to osteoporosis and fractures that have been identified from epidemiological[8] and other studies are listed in Table 196.1.

TABLE 196.1 FACTORS ASSOCIATED WITH OSTEOPOROSIS (LOW BONE MINERAL DENSITY) IN EPIDEMIOLOGIC STUDIES

- Sex (women > men)
- Age
- Ethnicity (especially Caucasian and Asian)
- Low body weight and body mass index
- High bone turnover
- Maternal history of fracture
- Sex hormone deficiency (especially estrogen)
- Early menopause, ovariectomy, amenorrhea
- Previous low-trauma fracture
- Physical inactivity
- Drugs, especially glucocorticosteroids, anticonvulsants
- Endocrine disorders (hyperthyroidism)
- Neoplastic disorders (multiple myeloma)
- Gastrointestinal disease (celiac disease, etc.)
- Rheumatoid arthritis, ankylosing spondylitis
- Vitamin D deficiency
- Cigarette smoking
- Excessive alcohol consumption

Bone is metabolically active throughout life. Growth *in utero* can influence bone mass in later life[9]. After skeletal growth is complete, remodeling of both cortical and trabecular bone continues. The remodeling of both cortical and trabecular bone requires the sequential and co-ordinated actions of osteoclasts to remove bone and osteoblasts to replace it (Fig. 196.1). These processes may be monitored by histological means. Cortical bone is replaced at a lower rate (~2% per annum) than trabecular bone (~10% per annum).

The purpose of remodeling is to allow the bone to adapt to changes in distribution of mechanical forces and to repair microdamage, which can occur in response to repeated loading[10]. The amount of bone made under normal conditions corresponds very closely to the amount removed, so that, in any remodeling cycle within bone, the total amount of bone tends to remain constant.

Bone loss in osteoporosis results from an imbalance between the two components of the bone renewal process – bone resorption and bone formation[11]. This is the fundamental basis of osteoporosis. Specifically, the numbers of sites of bone remodeling increase, the extent of resorption may be greater and the amount of bone replaced smaller[12] (Fig. 196.2).

In cortical bone incomplete replacement of osteons creates tunnels, which may coalesce to create points of weakness[13].

Peak bone mineral mass and bone loss in later life

Peak bone mass is defined as the amount of bone that can be accumulated by early to mid adult life, when it is greater than at other times of life.

Peak bone mass is determined by many factors, only some of which are alterable. Inherited factors are probably the most important and may set the potential upper limit attainable. A wide variety of lifestyle, nutritional, environmental and medical factors modify this genetic potential.

Bone mass at any time in later life is the net sum of this peak achieved in earlier life and subsequent loss, particularly after the menopause in women (Fig. 196.3).

Postmenopausal bone loss is the single most important cause of bone loss. The rate of loss is greatest early after the menopause. Age-related bone loss starts before the menopause and continues from 30–50 years of age onwards in both men and women. Loss from different bone sites occurs at different ages and at different rates.

Changes in bone mass and effects of age on fracture risk

Bone mass declines with age and this is a major contributor to the susceptibility to fracture. The relationship between BMD and fracture is such that fracture rates approximately double for every SD reduction in BMD.

Changes in bone mass are measured as decreases in BMD (see Chapter 195). Although this is very useful in clinical practice, BMD is calculated in two dimensions, so that the important effects on strength of bone size

It is helpful to define the contributory processes at multiple biological levels as well as in terms of known risk factors, and to identify their functional inter-relationships.

The biological levels include molecular, biochemical and cellular changes, and their effects on bone as a tissue, and on the altered physiology of mineral metabolism in osteoporosis. The relevant biological processes are considered below.

Bone growth and development: modeling and remodeling

A consideration of the normal process of bone modeling and remodeling is fundamental to the understanding of the pathogenesis of osteoporosis. During growth, the skeleton enlarges in size. In long bones this is achieved by the epiphysial growth plates, which produce increases in length, while increases in diameter result from deposition of new bone on the periosteal surfaces, accompanied by resorption from the endosteal surfaces.

During development and growth, bone is produced by two main processes – intramembranous ossification, as occurs in skull bones, and endochondral ossification involving the growth plate, as occurs in limb bones. Modeling is the process that results in bones achieving their characteristic shape and overall structure.

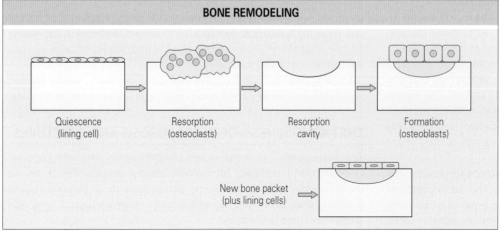

BONE REMODELING

Quiescence (lining cell) → Resorption (osteoclasts) → Resorption cavity → Formation (osteoblasts)

New bone packet (plus lining cells) →

Fig. 196.1 Bone remodeling. The remodeling cycle within bone involves a similar sequence of cellular activity at both cortical and trabecular sites. Trabecular surfaces are shown here. An initial phase of osteoclastic resorption is followed by a more prolonged phase of bone formation mediated by osteoblasts. Under normal conditions the amount of bone removed during resorption is replaced completely.

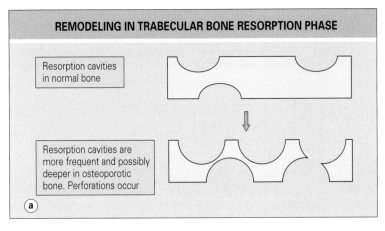

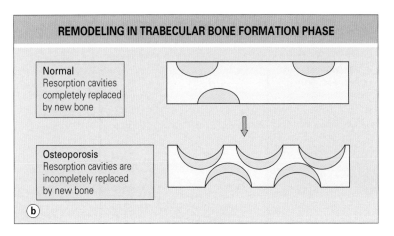

Fig. 196.2 Remodeling in trabecular bone. These figures show remodeling under normal conditions and in osteoporosis. (a) Resorption phase. (b) Formation phase. There may be subtle differences between the sexes, with bone thinning predominating in men because of reduced bone formation. Loss of connectivity and complete trabeculae predominates in women.

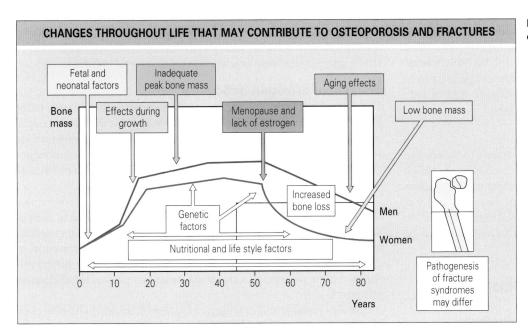

Fig. 196.3 Changes throughout life that may contribute to osteoporosis and fractures.

and dimensions are not assessed. Age itself is a very important risk factor for osteoporotic fractures that is independent of but obviously closely related to low BMD (Fig. 196.4)[14].

Age may also be a surrogate measure for falls. In common with other structures, the tissues of the musculoskeletal system undergo many changes with aging. In addition to the changes in bone that lead to osteoporosis and fractures, muscle changes (sarcopenia) contribute to frailty.

THE CELLULAR BASIS OF OSTEOPOROSIS

Osteoblasts[15] within trabecular bone differentiate from stromal cell precursors in bone marrow and manufacture a complex extracellular matrix, which subsequently mineralizes (see Chapter 192). The older concept that the bone matrix is entirely normal in osteoporosis is undergoing revision as knowledge increases. For example, there may be subtle but significant changes in the type I collagen matrix due to the Sp1 polymorphism (see below), and also in cross-linking within collagen.

Many growth factors affect bone formation. These include insulin-like growth factors (IGFs), fibroblast growth factors (FGFs), and especially members of the transforming growth factor (TGF)-β family, particu-

larly the bone morphogenetic proteins (BMPs). Many of these factors are produced by bone cells themselves and can be deposited in bone matrix. Changes in the production and action of these many regulatory factors are clearly potentially important in the pathogenesis of osteoporosis but detailed knowledge is very limited at present.

Osteoclasts are the major cells involved in bone resorption[16]. Osteoclasts differentiate from hematopoietic stem cell precursors under the direction of factors that include cytokines such as the RANK/RANK-ligand system, colony stimulating factors (CSFs, especially m-CSF), interleukins (e.g. IL-1, IL-11) and other factors. Prostaglandins and nitric oxide (NO) are other endogenous mediators that have complex effects on osteoclast function.

Bone loss is a feature of several inflammatory diseases. This loss may be systemic, leading to fractures, as in rheumatoid arthritis, while local erosive lesions occur in bone in osteomyelitis, rheumatoid arthritis and periodontal disease. The pathogenic mechanisms probably involve proinflammatory cytokines such as IL-1, TNF and IL-6, and aberrant expression of RANK-ligand.

Apoptosis (programmed cell death) is emerging as a major means of regulating the life span of bone cells of all lineages, osteoclasts, osteoblasts and osteocytes[17]. This may contribute to changes in bone

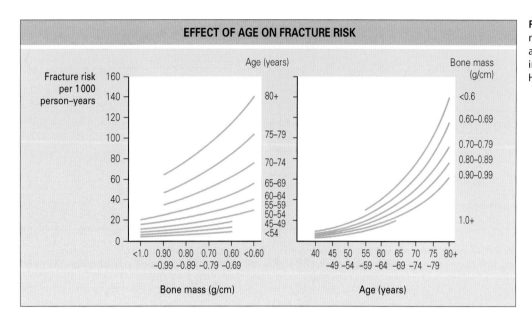

Fig. 196.4 Effect of age on fracture risk. Fracture risk increases with age independent of bone density and also increases with declining bone density irrespective of age. (Adapted with permission from Hui *et al.*[14])

turnover under physiological and pathological conditions. Drugs with adverse effects on bone such as glucocorticoids induce osteoblast and osteocyte apoptosis, while therapeutic agents that inhibit bone resorption, including estrogens and bisphosphonates, shorten the lifespan of osteoclasts. Increased apoptosis of osteocytes is a feature seen in fractures of the femoral neck in patients with osteonecrosis.

Rates of bone turnover and bone loss

There is increasing use of biochemical measurements to assess and monitor rates of bone resorption and formation (see Chapter 193). High rates of bone turnover predict fractures independently of other factors such as BMD. There is evidence that rates of bone loss vary, and that patients defined as 'fast' losers based on biochemical measurements do lose more bone mass than 'slow' losers. Responses to treatment may be greater in those with high turnover[18].

THE PHYSIOLOGICAL BASIS OF OSTEOPOROSIS

Physiological regulation of calcium metabolism

The physiological regulation of calcium homeostasis involves three main organs: the gut, the kidney and the skeleton. The fluxes of calcium and phosphate through these organs contribute to the integration of calcium metabolism throughout growth and adult life.

The physiological control of calcium metabolism and of skeletal remodeling is under the regulation of systemic hormones, especially the calcium regulating hormones, parathyroid hormone (PTH), 1,25-dihydroxy vitamin D (calcitriol) and calcitonin, acting in concert with other hormones and local mediators. Many hormones, including thyroid and pituitary hormones and adrenal and gonadal steroids, have major effects on the skeleton, as seen in clinical disorders in which their secretion is abnormally high or low.

The set-point for plasma calcium concentrations is determined mainly by the renal tubular reabsorption of calcium and the effects of PTH on this process.

Intestinal absorption of calcium is enhanced by calcitriol but the efficiency of absorption may be lowered with age. Production of calcitriol may be impaired, particularly if renal function is reduced. PTH values rise with age, possibly in response to impaired intestinal absorption of calcium, and this may contribute to bone loss.

Interestingly the challenges of pregnancy and lactation seem to have no lasting adverse effects on bone. Examples of osteoporosis associated with pregnancy are exceedingly rare.

In women the loss of estrogen at the menopause is the major change leading to loss of bone but many other factors contribute, and there is a strong interplay between genetic and environmental influences.

The role of estrogen deficiency

The effects of estrogen in bone are of particular interest in relation to the loss of bone after the menopause in women and the therapeutic use of estrogen to prevent this. Estrogen receptors (α and β isoforms) are widely distributed in the body and there are many ways that estrogens can exert their effects on their various target tissues. Some effects of estrogens are mediated by non-genomic means.

The bone loss associated with estrogen deficiency is accompanied by increased bone resorption. Part of this may be due to loss of direct effects on osteoclasts and their precursors, but indirect actions on the immune system may also be involved. The production of cytokines such as IL-1, TNF-α and IL-6, all of which can potentially enhance bone resorption, can be suppressed by physiological doses of estrogen[19].

It is also possible that estrogens have significant anabolic effects on bone by stimulating osteoblasts or their precursors.

The pathogenesis of osteoporosis in men is less well studied than in women but is clinically important, with secondary causes, e.g. hypogonadism, being common. It is now thought that estrogens derived by metabolism from androgens play an important role in protecting against bone loss in men[20,21].

THE GENETIC BASIS OF OSTEOPOROSIS

The many genetic factors that regulate skeletal development and function are rapidly being identified, and recent examples include the *CBFA1* gene for osteoblast differentiation and the RANK/RANK-ligand system for osteoclasts.

Osteoporosis is common and there are strong genetic contributors to skeletal size and composition. Comparisons of identical and non-identical twins have led to estimates that more than 50% of peak bone mass is determined by genetic factors.

Overall physique affects susceptibility to osteoporosis and may underlie racial differences in prevalence. Hip fractures typically occur in the thin and frail rather than the fat and robust, and low body weight is a risk factor. Hip axis length is a quantifiable geometric measure related to fracture risk.

Rarely, osteoporosis or unusually high bone mass can occur as the result of mutations in a single gene. Thus inactivating mutations in the lipoprotein receptor-related protein 5 gene are the cause of the osteoporosis–pseudoglioma syndrome, whereas the high bone mass syndrome is caused by activating mutations of the same gene[22]. In the various forms of osteogenesis imperfecta (brittle bone disease) defects in the synthesis or structure of type I collagen occur due to a range of different mutations in type I collagen genes (see Chapter 204).

In the commoner forms of osteoporosis, genetic factors play an important role in regulating skeletal size and geometry, BMD, ultrasound properties of bone, and bone turnover, as well as contributing to the pathogenesis of osteoporotic fracture[23]. These phenotypes are determined by the combined effects of several genes and environmental influences. Genome-wide linkage studies in man have identified loci on chromosomes 1p36, 1q21, 2p21, 5q33–35, 6p11–12 and 11q12–13 that show definite or probable linkage to BMD but so far the causative genes remain to be identified. Linkage studies in mice have similarly identified several loci that regulate BMD.

Most research has so far been done on candidate genes. Among the best studied are the vitamin D receptor and the collagen type I α1 gene. Polymorphisms of vitamin D receptor have been associated with bone mass in several studies, and there is evidence to suggest that this association may be modified by dietary calcium and vitamin D intake. A functional polymorphism affecting an Sp1 binding site has been identified in the collagen type I α1 gene that predicts osteoporotic fractures independently of bone mass by influencing collagen gene regulation and bone quality[24]. An important problem with most candidate gene studies is small sample size, and this has led to inconsistent results in different populations. This is also complicated by the multiple clinical endpoints (BMD, fracture, rates of bone loss, etc.) to which genetic factors may contribute in different ways.

There is evidence that genetic variants in various hormones and cytokines and their receptors that are involved in bone remodeling may also contribute to the development of osteoporosis.

NUTRITIONAL FACTORS AND OSTEOPOROSIS

Dietary calcium is obviously a potentially important factor in osteoporosis. Calcium restriction in experimental animals results in osteopenia. In humans, calcium deficiency in childhood leads to rickets. Although low calcium intake might be expected to be associated with osteoporosis, the nature of the relationship between calcium intake and osteoporosis remains controversial.

Results from calcium balance studies suggest that premenopausal women require calcium intakes in excess of about 800mg per day to avoid net bone loss, whereas postmenopausal women may require as much as 1500mg per day, perhaps less if receiving sex hormone replacement therapy.

Calcium supplementation in many trials in patients with osteoporosis results in gains in bone mass but to a lesser extent than can be achieved when antiresorptive drugs are given as well.

Dietary calcium intake during growth may play a role in the development and maintenance of peak BMD. It is likely that various other environmental and lifestyle factors, particularly exercise, may modulate this effect. Calcium supplementation in growing children produces small increases in BMD, which tend not to be maintained, and may represent increased mineralization of existing osteons rather than true and sustained increases in bone mass.

Poor nutrition in pregnancy may affect bone in postnatal life, since low birth weight is associated with low bone mass in later life.

Calcium is not the only component of diet that may affect bone; magnesium also may be important. Vitamin D is vital for optimal absorption of calcium from the diet. In many countries vitamin D is added to food stuffs; otherwise adequate skin exposure to ultraviolet light is necessary to maintain vitamin D levels from endogenous synthesis.

There is little evidence that micronutrients such as zinc, copper and boron have major effects on bone health. Some diets, particularly those rich in soy protein, can provide significant sources of estrogens. Excessive salt and caffeine intake may have adverse effects on bone, perhaps by increasing urinary calcium excretion directly and thus contributing to a negative calcium balance. However, these effects are probably relatively minor. Alcohol is another dietary component that may be quite important, with adverse effects in excess but perhaps beneficial effects at moderate levels of intake.

PHYSICAL ACTIVITY, MECHANICAL LOADING AND OSTEOPOROSIS

Mechanical forces exert strong influences on bone shape and modeling. At a cellular level, the osteocytes, which lie embedded within individual lacunae in mineralized bone, are believed to be the cellular system that responds to mechanical deformation and loading. Osteocytes connect with each other via the canalicular system and thus form a cellular network, much like a neural network. Early biochemical responses to mechanical loading may include induction of prostaglandin synthesis, increased nitric oxide production and later increases in IGFs, changes in amino acid transporters and eventually increases in new bone formation. There may be a 'mechanostat', so far hypothetical only, that senses and responds to loading. Estrogens may affect the set-point at which bone responds[25].

Immobilization, for example following major injury and illness, can be associated with rapid bone loss. If sustained, as in patients with paraplegia or hemiplegia, fractures can occur.

The excessive bone resorption associated with immobility can also result in 'immobilization hypercalcemia', particularly in the presence of renal impairment.

Bone loss associated with microgravity may be a limiting factor for long-term space flight.

The positive effects of mechanical loading on bone mass can be seen in weight lifters and other athletes. Sometimes the increased bone density is localized to the loaded side, for example in tennis players' arms.

Physical inactivity correlates with low BMD and fractures in epidemiological studies. However the potential beneficial effects of exercise programs may only produce limited changes in bone mass and have not yet been shown to reduce fractures.

DRUGS AND OSTEOPOROSIS

Several drugs have adverse effects on the skeleton and thereby reduce bone mass and increase the risk of fracture. Glucocorticoids are among the most important of these and are an important cause of bone loss and fractures. They are discussed in detail in Chapter 199.

Anticonvulsant drugs such as phenytoin and various barbiturates have long been thought to modify vitamin D metabolism but their contribution to osteoporosis is probably not major. Heparin is another agent that reduces bone mass.

Since deficiency of estrogen and testosterone both contribute to bone loss, drugs that reduce sex hormone levels cause bone loss. Androgen deprivation therapy with agonists of gonadotropin releasing hormone is now frequently used in the treatment of recurrent and metastatic prostate cancer because it induces medical castration, which renders these men hypogonadal. This is becoming an important iatrogenic cause of osteoporosis.

The use of tamoxifen appears to cause bone loss by antagonizing estrogen in premenopausal women with breast cancer, whereas it has a weak protective effect against bone loss in postmenopausal women. Depot medroxyprogesterone used as a contraceptive in premenopausal women can result in bone loss.

Epidemiological studies show that tobacco smoking is a risk factor for osteoporotic fracture. The mechanisms are uncertain but may include direct adverse effects on bone, induction of early menopause, changes in acid–base status and increased falling secondary to cerebrovascular disease.

In contrast, several drugs may increase bone mass and reduce fractures. Thus, thiazide diuretics decrease urinary calcium excretion and have been associated with increased BMD and reduced hip fracture rates.

There has also been much recent interest in the statins. These drugs are used to reduce cholesterol and have been shown experimentally to induce BMP-2 and increase bone mass in rats. A variety of epidemiological studies suggest that statin users have lower rates of hip fracture than non-users but it has proved difficult to demonstrate large effects on bone mass and turnover in prospective clinical trials.

Of course, those drugs actually used in the therapy of osteoporosis increase bone mass. They include sex hormone replacement therapy with estrogens, calcitonin, selective estrogen receptor modulators and the bisphosphonates (see Chapters 198 and 199), all of which reduce bone resorption and decrease the rate of incident vertebral fractures. Only estrogen and the nitrogen-containing bisphosphonates have been shown to reduce the risk of non-vertebral fractures in postmenopausal women. Anabolic agents, such as intermittent PTH given as a daily subcutaneous injection, increase bone formation and reduce fracture risk.

SUMMARY

Osteoporosis is clearly a multifactorial disorder and much has been learnt in recent years about the many pathogenic processes that contribute to bone loss and fragility. Drug treatments are now available to prevent bone loss and reduce fracture, and there are prospects for modifying some of the pathogenic processes themselves.

REFERENCES

1. Seeman E. Pathogenesis of bone fragility in women and men. Lancet 2002; 359: 1841–1850.
2. Melton LJ III, Cooper C. Magnitude and impact of osteoporosis and fractures. In: Marcus R, Feldman D, Kelsey J, eds. Osteoporosis, 2nd ed (vol 1). San Diego, CA: Academic Press, 2001: 557–567.
3. Delmas PD. Treatment of postmenopausal osteoporosis. Lancet 2002; 359: 2018–2026.
4. Favus MJ, ed. Primer of the metabolic bone diseases and disorders of mineral metabolism, 4th ed. Philadelphia, PA: Lippincott Williams & Wilkins; 1999.
5. Consensus Development Conference. JAMA 2001; 285: 785–795.
6. Francis RM. Falls and fractures. Age Ageing 2001; 30(suppl 4): 25–28.
7. Royal College of Physicians. Osteoporosis: clinical guidelines for prevention and treatment. Including supplement on resource database of randomised controlled trials in osteoporosis. London: Royal College of Physicians of London; 1999, 2000.
8. Cummings SR, Melton LJ. Epidemiology and outcomes of osteoporotic fractures. Lancet 2002; 359: 1761–1767.
9. Javaid MK, Cooper C. Prenatal and childhood influences on osteoporosis. Best Pract Res Clin Endocrinol Metab 2002, 16: 349–367.
10. Burr DB, Robling AG, Turner CH. Effects of biomechanical stress on bones in animals. Bone 2002; 30: 781–786.
11. Parfitt AM. Skeletal heterogeneity and the purposes of bone remodelling: implications for the understanding of osteoporosis. In: Marcus R, Zfeldman D, Kelsey J, eds. Osteoporosis. San Diego, CA: Academic Press; 2001: 433–444.
12. Lips P, Courpron P, Meunier PJ. Mean wall thickness of trabecular bone packets in the human iliac crest: changes with age. Calcif Tissue Res 1978; 10: 13–17.
13. Jordan GR, Loveridge N, Bell KL et al. Spatial clustering of remodeling osteons in the femoral neck cortex: a cause of weakness in hip fracture? Bone 2000; 26: 305–313.
14. Hui S, Slemeda C, Johnston C. Age and bone mass as predictors of fracture in a prospective study. J Clin Invest 1988; 81: 1804–1809.
15. Ducy P, Schinke T, Karsenty G. The osteoblast: a sophisticated fibroblast under central surveillance. Science 2000; 289: 1501–1504.
16. Teitelbaum SL. Bone resorption by osteoclasts. Science 2000; 289: 1504–1508.
17. Manolagas SC. Birth and death of bone cells: basic regulatory mechanisms and implications for the pathogenesis and treatment of osteoporosis. Endocr Rev 2000; 21: 115–137.
18. Bjarnason NH, Christiansen C. Early response in biochemical markers predicts long-term response in bone mass during hormone replacement therapy in early postmenopausal women. Bone 2000 26: 561–569.
19. Pfeilschifter J, Köditz R, Pfohl M, Schatz H. Changes in proinflammatory cytokine activity after menopause. Endocr Rev 2002; 23 : 90–119.
20. Riggs BL, Kholsa S, Melton LJ III. A unitary model for involutional osteoporosis: estrogen deficiency causes both type 1 and type 2 osteoporosis in postmenopausal women and contributes to bone loss in aging men. J Bone Miner Res 1998; 13: 763–773.
21. Szulc P, Munoz F, Claustrat B et al. Bioavailable estradiol may be an important determinant of osteoporosis in men: the MINOS study. J Clin Endocrinol Metab 2001; 86: 192–199.
22. Gong Y, Slee RB, Fukai N et al. LDL receptor-related protein 5 (LRP5) affects bone accrual and eye development. Cell 2001; 107: 513–523.
23. Ralston SH. Genetic control of susceptibility to osteoporosis. J Clin Endocrinol Metab 2002; 87: 2460–2466.
24. Mann V, Hobson EE, Li B et al. A COL1A1 Sp1 binding site polymorphism predisposes to osteoporotic fracture by affecting bone density and quality. J Clin Invest 2001; 107: 899–907.
25. Lanyon L, Skerry T. Postmenopausal osteoporosis as a failure of bone's adaptation to functional loading: a hypothesis. J Bone Miner Res 2001; 16: 1937–1947.

197

Osteoporosis: clinical features

Piet Geusens

- Osteoporosis is the most common disease that affects bone, and is associated with increased risk of fragility fractures
- The most frequent osteoporotic fractures are those in the spine, hip, and wrist, but fractures related to osteoporosis also occur at many other skeletal sites
- Short- and long-term consequences of osteoporosis fractures include increased mortality, pain, physical impairment, increased costs of medical care, decreased quality of life, and increased risk for new fractures
- Osteoporosis is a multifactorial disease. Clinical features evident before the first fracture has occurred include a number of clinical risk factors, many of which can be readily recognized clinically (e.g. age, gender, low body weight, history of fracture, familial history of fracture, immobilization, and use of glucocorticoids)
- Osteoporosis is more common in women than in men, but the problem in men is by no means insignificant

INTRODUCTION

Osteoporosis is a disease characterized by decreased bone mass and a deterioration of bone architecture. These changes result in weaker, more fragile bone and, therefore, a higher risk of fractures. For the purpose of determining the prevalence of disease, osteoporosis has been defined as having a bone density T-score lower than −2.5. The condition is considered to be severe (symptomatic) if a fragility fracture is present in addition to low bone density[1].

In this chapter we will review the clinical features of osteoporosis. These features include the clinical consequences of fractures (clinical outcome) (Table 197.1) and the clinical predisposition (clinical risk factors) for osteoporosis and fractures (Table 197.2, Fig. 197.1). The clinical features of osteoporosis in men will be discussed separately from those in women.

Osteoporosis increases the risk of fractures, just as hypertension increases the risk of stroke. The estimated lifetime risk of fracture is 40% in 50-year-old white women and 13% in 50-year-old men

TABLE 197.2 RISK FACTORS FOR HIP FRACTURE

Bone		Falls
Bone mass	Age	**Neuromuscular function**
	Gender	**Cognitive functions**
	Hyperthyroidism	**Vision**
Architecture	Genetics	**Medication**
Micro	**Familial fractures**	Fall mechanisms
Macro	**Previous fracture**	Energy absorption
Secondary mineralization	Length	**Balance**
Bone turnover	Weight	**Gait**
	Smoking	
	Mobility	
	Glucocorticoids	
	General health	
	Calcium intake	
	Vitamin D	

Risk factors that can be directly evaluated by clinical examination are indicated in bold[94,108,109].

TABLE 197.1 CLINICAL CONSEQUENCES OF HIP, VERTEBRAL AND WRIST FRACTURES

	Hip	Vertebrae		Wrist
		Clinical	Radiographic	
Excess mortality	++	+	+	−
Increased fracture risk	+	+	+	+
Pain				
Acute	+	+	+ or −	+
Chronic	−	+	+ or −	+
Functional decline				
short-term	+++	+	+	+
long-term	++	+	+	+
Psychosocial decline	++	+	+	−
Quality of life	+++	++	+	+

+, Yes; −, No.

OSTEOPOROSIS: VISCIOUS CIRCLES AFTER FRACTURE

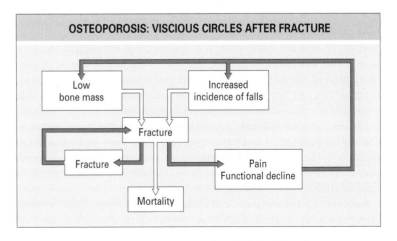

Fig. 197.1 **Clinical features of osteoporosis** include the clinical consequences of fractures (clinical outcome) and the clinical predisposition (clinical risk factors) for osteoporosis and fractures. The clinical consequences of fractures in survivors include physical and functional limitations, reduced quality of life and an increased risk for subsequent fractures, resulting in a vicious circle of new fractures and increasing morbidity[11].

(Chapter 198). In principal, fractures should be easily diagnosed because they usually present as an acute pain episode after trauma, with clinical signs of a fracture. Nevertheless, the clinical picture can be overlooked or hidden, especially in the case of vertebral fractures, which are the most frequent fractures in postmenopausal women[2].

Fractures of long bones commonly result in acute pain with one or more clinical signs of fracture (swelling, hematoma, deformation, local crepitations, localized pain on pressure), and are easily confirmed radiographically. Some fractures, such as stress fractures, are difficult to diagnose, and local clinical signs can be confounded by arthritis or tendinitis[3]. The clinical symptoms of vertebral fractures are variable. Only about one third of all people with radiographic vertebral fractures are diagnosed clinically[2,4]. Although as many as half of people with vertebral fractures seen on radiographs in population surveys do not report having had an episode of acute pain, such fractures are associated with morbidity such as chronic back pain and loss of function[5].

The clinical consequences of fractures are related to the short- and long-term outcomes and differ according to fracture location (Table 197.1) and patient characteristics. Although individual fractures often resolve without severe long-term complications, many studies indicate that, overall, fractures are associated with increased morbidity and mortality. Fractures of the hip and clinical vertebral fractures are associated with increased mortality[6,7]. After a mean time of 7 years, patients with any osteoporosis-related fracture have a doubling of the risk for physical limitations in movement and an even higher risk for functional limitations in daily activities[8]. The clinical consequences of fractures in survivors include physical and functional limitations, reduced quality of life (QoL)[8,9], and an increased risk for subsequent fractures[10], resulting in a vicious cycle of new fractures and increasing morbidity (Fig. 197.1)[11].

Before the first fracture occurs, bone loss is asymptomatic; this fact has led to the description of osteoporosis as a 'silent thief'[12]. This asymptomatic nature of bone loss suggests that osteoporosis cannot be detected clinically before the first fragility fracture occurs, unless bone density is measured. Bone densitometry is considered the gold standard for diagnosis of osteoporosis[1]. The clinical question, then, is how to identify patients at risk for osteoporosis before the first fracture has occurred, in order to select the right patients for bone densitometry and treatment[13,14]. Clinical signs and symptoms, together with anthropometric characteristics of the patient, have limited value for estimating women's actual bone density and need for treatment[13,14]. However, clinical risk factors such as age and weight can be used to help decide which patients are more likely to have osteoporosis, and who should have bone density measurements to confirm the diagnosis or rule-out disease[15,16]. Furthermore, clinical risk factors for fracture can be useful in identifying women at high risk of fracture (case finding)[13,14]. Indeed, osteoporosis is a multifactorial disease that includes several risk factors, such age, sex, and body weight, that can be readily recognized in clinical practice before the first fracture occurs. Therefore, osteoporosis can be rather described as a clinically 'hidden' – but still recognizable – disease before the first fracture occurs.

Patients who have already experienced a fragility fracture have twice the risk of subsequent fractures compared with those without a prior fracture[10]. However, osteoporosis often remains undiagnosed and untreated, even in patients that have sustained a clinical fragility fracture of the vertebrae or hip[17].

Patients can benefit from early diagnosis of osteoporosis, because effective therapies are available for the prevention and treatment of osteoporosis and associated fragility fractures[13,14]. For example, the risk of additional fractures can be reduced in patients with a prevalent vertebral fracture (Chapter 198). In addition, treatment can prevent the occurrence of a first fracture in patients with low bone density (Chapter 198). Furthermore, fracture prevention is associated with preservation of quality of life[18].

CLINICAL FEATURES OF FRACTURES: SHORT- AND LONG-TERM OUTCOMES

Wrist fractures

Wrist fractures occur after a fall. In women, the incidence of wrist fracture increases from approximately 0.1% per year below age 45 to approximately 0.7% per year at ages 65 and older[19]. Functional outcome after fracture has been studied in clinical case studies ranging in duration from weeks up to a decade[20–23]. Persisting hand pain (29–44% of patients), weakness (36–40%), and algodystrophy are the most commonly reported consequences[20–23]. Mortality is not increased after wrist fracture[6].

Impairment of activities of daily living (ADL) is reported in one population-based cohort[8]. Seven years after a wrist fracture, women with fracture were three times more likely than women without fracture to report difficulty in shopping for groceries or clothing[8]. They were nine times more likely to report difficult cooking and 2–3 times more likely to report difficult getting in and out a car or descending stairs than women who had never fractured their wrist[8]. The true frequency of reported algodystrophy is unknown with reports varying from 0.1–47%. This high variability is due to differences in diagnostic criteria, patient selection, and measures[24]. Prospective studies indicate that several symptoms of algodystrophy still persist after 10 years[21,23].

Patients with a wrist fracture have an increased risk of having osteoporosis and approximately twice the risk for sustaining other fractures compared with patients without wrist fractures[10]. However, only a small proportion of women with a wrist fracture currently receive osteoporosis follow-up care or treatment[25].

Hip fractures

Hip fractures are the most serious consequence of osteoporosis in terms of disability, mortality, and use of hospital and institutional care[26]. Hip fractures usually occur after a fall to the side or straight down[27], but only 1% of falls among the elderly result in a hip fracture. The frequency of spontaneous insufficiency hip fractures is low (0.27% in a survey in nursing homes)[28]. Clinical signs of hip fracture include severe, acute functional restriction resulting in immobilization and hospitalization. Typically, the leg is shortened and in exorotation. Almost all hip fractures require urgent surgical intervention for optimal recovery[29].

The immediate clinical consequences of hip fracture can be dramatic. Many patients are unable to move or summon help after falling, and may be hypothermic when found. Hospital complications are common (occurring in more than 30% of patients)[30,31] and are often related to the implants used (dislocation, fixation failure, infection) or to anesthetic stress.

Patients with hip fracture are particularly prone to complications. General complications (cardiovascular, pulmonary and cerebral problems, and infections) and local complications (wound and prosthetic problems) also occur in the post-fracture period. These complications have been reported to affect more than 30% of patients 4 months after hip fracture and more than 10% of patients 1 year after hip fracture[30]. Similard data are available from a 2-year follow-up study[31].

Mortality

In-hospital mortality ranges between 1 and 9%[32,33] but can be as high as 55% in patients with end-stage dementia or pneumonia[34]. Approximately 20–25% of hip fracture patients die within the first year[32] and 19% more hip fracture patients than controls die within 5 years[6]. After adjustment for many other predictors of hip fracture, women with a hip fracture are still 2.4 times more likely to die than women without fracture[6].

Hospitalization and institutionalization

The number of hospital bed days for patients with hip fracture is higher than that for patients with stroke, diabetes, or myocardial infarction in at least one survey[35] (Fig. 197.2). The combined costs of hospitalization and medical care during the 12 months after a hip fracture are approximately three times higher than for patients without hip fractures[36].

The wide variation in practice patterns and availability of services make it difficult to estimate the proportions of patients who are transferred to nursing homes[32]. The duration of stay in nursing homes after hip fracture was 1 month in 24% of patients, 6 months in 10%, and more than 1 year in 34%[37].

Morbidity

Substantial short- and long-term morbidity has been documented in survivors of a hip fracture, both in terms of suffering and cost. Functional competence and physical functioning markedly diminish after hip fracture[30,32,33,38–44]. After 3 months, physical performance had decreased by 51%, vitality by 24% and social function by 26% compared with pre-fracture levels[44]. After 6 months, only 24% of patients had returned to prefracture walking competence, and only 43% had returned to prefracture basic ADL[38]. Little further improvement occurred after 1 year[30,41].

Of the women who could dress independently before fracture, only 60% were able to do so after hip fracture, and only two thirds were able to resume independent transferring (from bed to chair or standing from chair) (Fig. 197.3)[39]. The proportion of women that could walk across a room independently dropped from 75% before the hip fracture to 15% 6 months after the fracture. Similarly, the proportions of women able to walk one half mile dropped from 41% before fracture to 6% 6 months after fracture, while the proportion of women able to climb stairs dropped from 63% to 8%[39]. Only 38% of women reporting independence in several ADL and basic mobility measures (including transfer from bed to chair and toilet, putting on socks and shoes, and indoor walking) recovered independence in all functions after a hip fracture[40]. Further limitations were found in cooking, performance of housework, use of transportation, grocery shopping, carrying bundles, taking medication, visiting friends, managing money, and engaging in community activities[32,41].

Indirect evidence for morbidity comes from a prospective case-controlled study of survivors of hip fracture[36]. The medical and non-medical needs were significantly higher in fracture patients than in age- and sex-matched controls. These needs were reflected in an increased number of physician contacts, increased use of physiotherapy, more days of new hospitalizations and home care, and a longer stay in nursing homes (Fig. 197.4)[36].

Fracture risk

Patients with a hip fracture have approximately twice the risk for further fractures, including a second hip fracture, compared with patients without a fracture[10].

Predictors of mortality and morbidity after hip fracture

Many of the predictors of death and long-term physical disability after hip fracture include clinical features related to the patient's health before the fracture occurs.

The elderly tend to have co-morbid conditions (such as other diseases and functional limitations); thus, hip fracture is not the sole factor leading to mortality and functional decline[32]. Indeed, outcome depends largely on the prior condition of individuals who suffer the fracture. Mortality is higher in patients who are living in an institution[31] than in other patients. Most studies evaluate physical function or mortality separately, but it appears that prefracture level of function may influence both outcomes. In a study adjusting for known risk factors, mortality at 6 months after fracture was significantly associated with pre-fracture locomotion, a score of health evaluation, and the use of paid help at home prior to fracture[33]. Furthermore, mortality and functional recovery differed between hospitals, probably because of differences in the type of care provided to patients[33]. Men have more complications than women, on average[31,32]. Longer hospital stay is associated with older age, male sex,

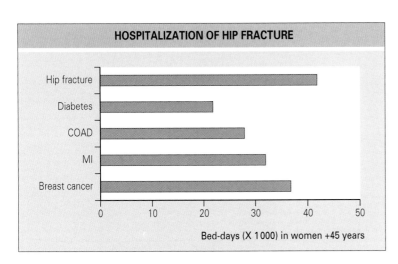

Fig. 197.2 Hospitalization for hip fracture. Number of bed-days for hip fracture or other diseases in women older than 40 years[35].

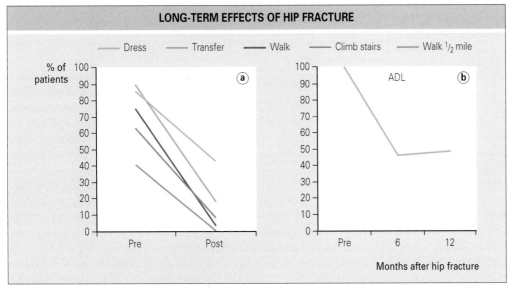

Fig. 197.3 Long-term effects of hip fracture. (a) Proportion of subjects able to perform each activity independently before hip fracture and at 6 months after sustaining a hip fracture[39]. (b) ADL during 1 year[41].

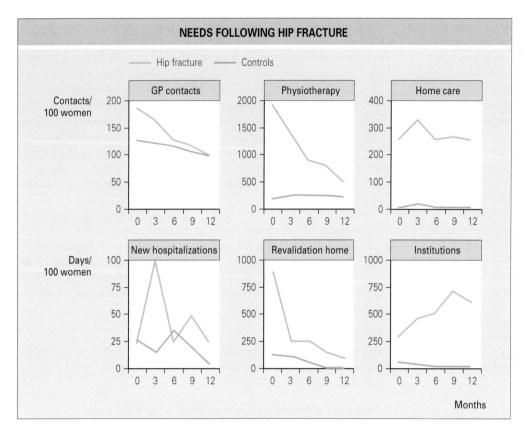

Fig. 197.4 Needs following hip fracture. The medical and non-medical needs during 12 months following a hip fracture in women were significantly higher than in age matched controls. These needs included increased number of physician contacts, increased use of physiotherapy and home care, and more days of new hospitalizations and stay in nursing homes[36].

and poorer general health[32]. Patients living in an institution have a higher risk for pressure sores, surgical complications, and pulmonary and urinary infections than patients living independently before the fracture[31]. Morbidity after hip fracture is higher after an intertrochanteric fracture than after a fracture of the femoral neck but the reason for this is uncertain[32]. Although the level of prefracture condition of the patient is a major determinant for recovery, even patients with good prefracture functioning often recover only partially[39].

Other appendicular fractures

With the exception of fractures in patients with metastatic bone disease, almost all fragility fractures occurring after the age of 40 years are associated with the presence of osteoporosis[4]. Apart from fractures of the vertebrae, wrist, and hip, the most frequent other fractures are those of the ribs, proximal humerus, pelvis, and legs[8]. No data are available concerning the risk of mortality after these fractures. Morbidity, however, can be substantial in the elderly and is associated with complications of the fracture, such as soft tissue lesions and incomplete recovery of adjacent joint function (e.g. in the shoulder after fracture of the proximal humerus)[29].

Furthermore, the risk for new fractures is approximately twice as high in patients with these fractures than in patients without a history of fracture[10].

VERTEBRAL FRACTURES

Hippocrates discussed the diagnosis and treatment of vertebral fractures approximately 2000 years ago, but the fractures he described presumably occurred after severe trauma[45,46]. It was only recently that Albright et al. reported that the majority of vertebral fractures in postmenopausal women are a result of relatively minor trauma[46,47].

The clinical features of osteoporotic vertebral fractures are quite different from other osteoporotic fractures. Only one in three vertebral fractures comes to clinical attention and is diagnosed (Fig. 197.5)[4,46]. The reasons for this low rate of diagnosis are not fully understood, but may be related to the variable degree of preceding trauma[47,48], the variable

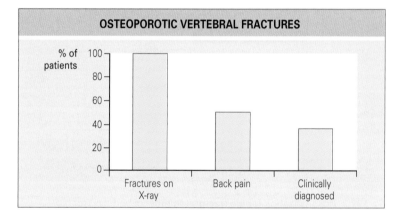

Fig. 197.5 Osteoporotic vertebral fractures. In population-based studies of patients with radiographically identified vertebral fractures, 50% have back pain and only one in three come to clinical attention and diagnosis[2].

degree of pain intensity and duration[49,50], and the frequency of back pain in the population[2].

An evaluation of the clinical outcomes of vertebral fracture is further complicated by differences in the criteria for defining a prevalent or incident vertebral fracture and differences in study populations. Furthermore, 'wedge' vertebral fractures are sometimes difficult to differentiate from wedging associated with other diseases such Scheuermann's disease, remodeling in osteoarthritis[51], and metastatic bone disease[4].

The consequences of vertebral fracture have been extensively reviewed[52–55] and studied from two perspectives: studies in patients with clinical fractures with or without controls (clinical cases)[4,56–64] or surveys of radiographic deformities in which patients with vertebral fractures were compared to those without such fractures[5,18,50,65–72]. A limited number of prospective studies are available using serial spine radiographs[5,18,69,71]. Many studies used a variety of measures that are not specific for evaluation of the outcomes of vertebral fractures. Recently, however, more uniform evaluation of outcomes was introduced with the development of osteoporosis-specific measures of quality of life (QoL; Table 197.2).

Mortality

Mortality is increased after vertebral fractures by 19% compared with the general population[6], and by 23–60% compared with people without vertebral fractures in other studies[7,73–75]. The age-adjusted relative risk for dying after vertebral fracture is as high as 8.6[7]. Increased mortality is observed shortly after the fracture and has been attributed to poor physical condition and acute medical consequences[6,46]. However, an increased risk of death compared with people without vertebral fracture persists for at least 5 years after a vertebral fracture[46]. In one study, the increased risk of death was associated with clinical problems such as pulmonary disease and cancer[73]. The rate of death among vertebral fracture cases is highest in patients with multiple vertebral fractures[73] and in patients who required hospitalization because of vertebral fracture[76].

Fracture risk

Patients with a prevalent (pre-existing) vertebral fracture have approximately 4 times greater risk for new vertebral fracture[77,78], and twice the risk of hip and other non-vertebral fractures as patients without prevalent fracture[10,75,79,80]. This relationship is independent of bone density; patients who have both low bone density and an existing vertebral fracture have a higher risk of subsequent fractures than those with only low bone density or only an existing vertebral fracture, who in turn have a higher risk than those without either low BMD or prevalent vertebral fracture[10,77]. The risk of additional vertebral fracture is extremely high among those patients with multiple past vertebral fractures[18,77]. For example, the risk of an additional vertebral fracture is 12 times higher among those with two or more vertebral fractures at baseline, compared to women without existing vertebral fracture[77]. More than half of women with five or more vertebral fractures at baseline experienced additional fractures within the subsequent 3.8 years of observation[18]. Importantly, after experiencing an initial vertebral fracture, additional vertebral fractures will occur within 1 year in one in five postmenopausal women with osteoporosis (Fig. 197.6)[78]. Osteoporosis is, therefore, a quickly progressive disease in many postmenopausal women. The clinical message is that vertebral fracture should be recognized and treated early in order to prevent future vertebral fractures.

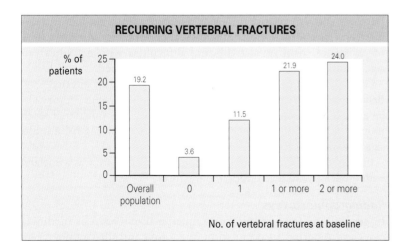

Fig. 197.6 Recurring vertebral frature. Incidence of new vertebral fractures in the year following vertebral fracture. After experiencing an initial vertebral fracture, additional vertebral fractures will occur within one year in one in five postmenopausal women with osteoporosis[78].

Back pain in clinically diagnosed (symptomatic) cases

In patients with severe osteoporosis, vertebral fractures often occur after minimal trauma. In patients with clinically diagnosed vertebral fractures, 14% followed severe trauma, 83% followed moderate or no trauma, and 3% were pathologic[4]. In another study, pain onset was sudden in 73% of women with vertebral fracture, compared with 21% in women with chronic low back pain without fractures[56]. The vertebral fracture occurred after an accident at home (such as a fall or stumble) in 13% of cases, after lifting a heavy load in 24% of cases, and without any evident reason in 44% of cases. A total of 19% of women reported a more gradual beginning of complaints[56]. Severe back pain (71%) and height reduction (10%) were the most common events that triggered further investigation[56]. The mean duration of symptoms before fracture diagnosis was 7 days, but 25% of fractures were diagnosed clinically after more than 1 month[4].

Acute back pain episode

As noted above, not all vertebral fracture patients report having acute pain, and the severity of back pain varies substantially among patients who do experience pain. Symptoms of an acute clinical vertebral fracture include sudden moderate to severe lancing back pain, which worsens on movement and is often relieved by rest[48]. The pain can be sufficiently severe to cause breathlessness, pallor, nausea, and vomiting, and is exacerbated by coughing or sneezing. The pain often radiates laterally following the dermatomal distribution and is often accompanied by spasms of the paraspinal muscles. On clinical examination, tenderness can be elicited over the affected vertebrae and paraspinal muscles and mobility of the spine is restricted and painful. However, pain is sometimes diffuse and not localized to the fractured vertebra. Variable degrees of kyphosis of the thoracic spine can be found in the case of a thoracic vertebral fracture, and flattened (reduced) lumbar lordosis in the case of a lumbar vertebral fracture. This acute, severe pain episode gradually subsides within 2–6 weeks.

Chronic back pain

Restoration of normal spinal anatomy is not possible following vertebral fracture. Therefore, even vertebral fractures without acute symptoms contribute to chronic morbidity[81]. Patients with clinical vertebral fracture are at increased risk for chronic back pain[65]. Pain is most commonly reported as deeply localized and bone- or muscle-related[48]. It is described variously as tearing, burning, piercing, drilling, dull, convulsive, or dragging[48].

The most frequent triggers for pain are sitting, standing, staying in the same position for a long time, bending, walking, and sudden movements[48]. In many patients, pain is relieved by lying, sitting, changing position, application of warmth, gymnastics, drugs, or aversion[48]. Compared with patients with chronic low back pain without fractures, chronic back pain after a vertebral fracture is more effectively relieved by lying down, is more aggravated by doing housework, and is more frequently only present during physical activity[48]. No specific circadian rhythm of pain is found. The frequency of pain is variable (several times per week or per day, permanent, or dependent on physical stress)[48].

Back pain after an acute pain episode can last for many years and decreases over time[48,69]. One study surveyed patients with chronic back pain 4 years after an acute painful fracture; back pain was mild in 27%, moderate in 44% and severe in 29% of these patients[62]. In another study, half of the patients with symptomatic clinically-diagnosed vertebral fracture reported slight to moderate chronic pain after 4 years, the other half reported severe to intolerable pain[48].

In clinical cases, chronic back pain is related to the number and severity of vertebral fractures[48,59,63], but not to small reductions in vertebral height (minor vertebral deformities)[62]. In some studies, pain was related to the degree of kyphosis[59] and height loss[82,83].

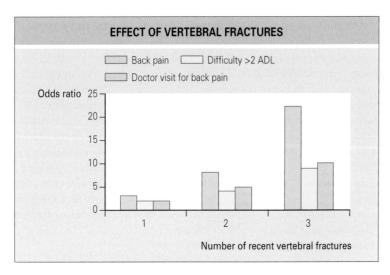

Fig. 197.7 Effect of vertebral fractures. Odds ratio for pain and disability increase by number of recent vertebral fractures[70,71].

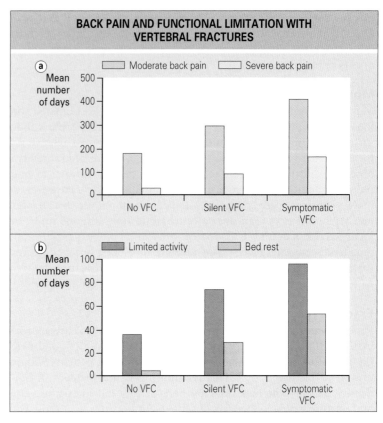

Fig. 197.8 Back pain and functional limitation with vertebral fractures. New vertebral fractures (VFC), even those not recognized clinically, are associated with substantial increases in (a) back pain and (b) functional limitation due to back pain in older women[5].

Back pain in fractures derived from radiographic surveys

In cross-sectional population studies measuring vertebral dimensions on radiographs, chronic back pain was related to the number and severity of vertebral fractures in some studies[50,65,68]. Other studies failed to detect an association, perhaps because of methodologic problems such as less stringent morphometric vertebral fracture criteria[66], or a relatively small number of women with severe deformities[83].

In prospective studies using serial radiographs to detect new vertebral fractures, a single new vertebral fracture increased the odds for back pain (reported at the end of the study, not at the time of the vertebral fracture) threefold, whereas two and three fractures increased the odds of back pain by eight and 22 times, respectively[70,71] (Fig. 197.7). The pain frequency index increased approximately threefold relative to prefracture levels and pain was long lasting (twofold increase of pain frequency index after 3.5 years)[65]. New vertebral fractures, even those not recognized clinically, are associated with substantial increases in back pain in older women (Fig. 197.8)[5].

In contrast to these studies in which radiographic deformities were meticulously documented, radiographic vertebral fractures are often overlooked in daily clinical practice. A survey of 934 hospitalized older women with an available chest radiograph was used to evaluate the frequency with which vertebral fractures were identified and treated by clinicians[84]. Moderate-to-severe vertebral fractures were identified in 132 (14.1%) of the study subjects, but only 1.7% had a discharge diagnosis of vertebral fracture[84]. Of these, 50% were recorded in the radiology reports and only 17% had a fracture noted in the medical record or discharge summary[84].

Physical and functional outcomes of vertebral fractures

Pain, hyperkyphosis, and loss of spinal mobility result in multiple forms of disability[32]. Pain and disabilities cause a spiralling decline in function, mobility, and muscle strength[58,64,85]. This decline in function, in turn, contributes to pain and to an increased risk of falls[86], bone loss[87], fractures[10], and loss of independence[48,56] (Fig. 197.1).

Clinical cases

Vertebral fractures were associated with increased kyphosis in several studies[56,88–90], but not in one study that analyzed only severe vertebral fractures[50]. Hyperkyphosis results in the typical clinical presentation of a 'dowager's hump' (Fig. 197.9).

Vertebral fractures are associated with height loss[54,56]. During a follow-up period of 8 years, standing height decreased by approximately 1cm with each new wedge or crush vertebral fracture, but not with endplate fractures[72]. Significant height loss has also been described in women with

postmenopausal osteoporosis in control groups of clinical trials and was three times greater (4.6mm/year) in women with new vertebral fractures than in women without vertebral fracture (1.8mm/year)[91].

Hyperkyphosis and height loss also reduce the distance between the iliac crest and ribs[48], resulting in problems with digestion and a protruding abdomen that makes fitting clothes difficult and detracts from appearance[54]. Loss of spinal mobility due to vertebral fracture has been associated with difficulty in dressing, fixing hair, standing, laying down, moving in bed, doing housework, walking, climbing stairs, washing, bathing, using the toilet, and getting to the floor[48,54,59]. Lung function progressively decreases with increasing number of vertebral fractures and the degree of kyphosis, perhaps as a result of increased abdominal pressure[92,93].

Functional disability was higher in patients with two or more vertebral fractures and was related to height reduction, kyphosis, and distance between ribs and iliac crest[48]. Functional performance measures (level of assistance, pain on activity and difficulties with activities) are significantly reduced in patients with vertebral fracture[58].

General measures of health and ADL are significantly affected[48,56–58]. Balance capability, an important risk factor for hip fracture[94], may also be affected[54]. Physical performance measures such as functional reach, mobility skills, and 6 minute walk[58] and muscle strength[58] are also significantly decreased.

Increased dependency with need for help in self-care was associated with moderate and severe vertebral fractures[56,57].

Radiographic surveys

In general, the same physical and functional outcomes as in clinical cases are reported in population and case-controlled radiographic surveys[50,54,59,65,95]. In the Study of Osteoporotic Fractures (SOF), the odds of impaired function (difficulty with more than two ADL) was 2.3 times higher among elderly women with a history of clinically diagnosed vertebral fracture[95]. New vertebral fractures, even those not recognized

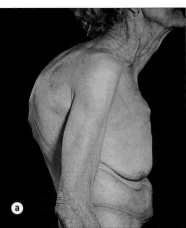

Fig. 197.9 Dowager's hump.
(a) Marked thoracic kyphosis due to multiple osteoporotic fractures in an elderly woman with (b) corresponding radiograph.

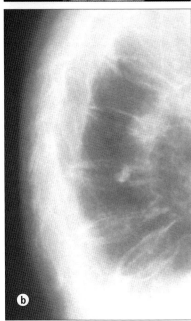

DISCRIMINATORY CAPACITY OF QUALITY OF LIFE QUESTIONAIRES

Fig. 197.10 Discriminatory capacity of quality of life questionnaires (disease targeted QUALEFFO and generic SF-36) in a radiographic survey comparing patients with and without vertebral fracture[96]. *$p < 0.05$ between QUALEFFO and SF-36.

clinically, are associated with substantial increases in functional limitation due to back pain in older women (Fig. 197.8)[5].

A multidimensional and validated osteoporosis-targeted quality of life questionnaire (QUALEFFO) has been used in another population study to assess the impact of vertebral fractures[68]. Patients with vertebral fracture had a higher QUALEFFO score than patients with low BMD without a vertebral fracture indicating more. The total score and its sub-domains (pain, physical function, general health and physical mobility) correlated with the number of vertebral fractures (Fig. 197.10)[68]. Lumbar vertebral fractures led to greater impairment of physical function than thoracic vertebral fractures, and were associated with lower physical function, lower general health, and a lower total QUALEFFO score[68].

Effect of pharmacologic treatment on quality of life (QoL) related to vertebral fracture

One of the earliest clinical observations in the prevention of osteoporosis is a cross-sectional study that found that hormone replacement therapy protected against height loss in postmenopausal women (Chapter 198). More convincing evidence of fracture efficacy comes from several prospective, randomized, placebo-controlled studies using raloxifene or bisphosphonates (Chapter 198).

In a preliminary study with raloxifene, the occurrence of new vertebral fracture was associated with significant deterioration in QUALEFFO score[96].

In patients of the Fracture Intervention Trial, the number of days with limited activity or bed rest rose immediately and sharply after an incident vertebral fracture, most prominently in patients with clinical

vertebral fracture but also in patients with morphometric vertebral fracture without acute pain (Fig. 197.8)[18]. Treatment with alendronate significantly reduced the number of days of bedrest and disability; during 3 years of follow up, there were more than 3000 additional days affected by back pain among the 1005 women randomized to placebo compared with the 1022 women in the alendronate group[18]. These findings indicate that effective fracture prevention using bone-specific treatments helps to prevent reductions in QoL associated with osteoporotic fractures.

Psychosocial outcomes of vertebral fractures

Psychosocial consequences may not be evident clinically or may be excluded from the medical history because patients themselves are reluctant to discuss or complain about them[32]. Psychosocial outcome has been studied using a variety of measures, including individual questions, general measures, or osteoporosis-specific measures of psychosocial status[32]. Unfortunately, many studies did not include a control group.

Psychiatric symptoms were significantly worse after vertebral fracture in one study[58], but no effect of vertebral fracture on social and mental function was found in another study[68]. As is the case for pain symptoms, psychosocial outcomes vary with the time after vertebral fracture. Social extroversion and well-being were significantly decreased during the first 2 years after a new vertebral fracture than later on, in spite of similar spine deformity index and height reduction[64]. Even patients with a diagnosis of osteoporosis before fracture have a higher incidence of fear of falling (38% versus 2% in controls) and a higher proportion of patients said that they limited their activities in an attempt to avoid falling (24% versus 2%) following vertebral fracture[98].

Vertebral fractures are associated with depression[32]. Depression is the most prevalent mental health problem of older adults and can be a major problem in osteoporosis[32,99]. Depression is associated with low bone mass throughout the skeleton[100]. Some patients feel angry or depressed because the physical deformity from hyperkyphosis detracts from their appearance. Women with osteoporosis have a score three

TABLE 197.3 EVALUATION OF QUALITY OF LIFE

Instrument	No. of questions	Time (min)	Reliability to clinical	Longitudinal correlation
OFDQ[63]	56	25	yes	NA
OPAQ[102]	71	30	yes	NA
QUALEFFO[103]	54	20	yes	Yes
OPTOQOL[60,62]	26	NA	yes	NA

NA, Not available.

Disease-targeted questionnaires for clinical evaluation of quality of life in osteoporosis.

times higher and prevalence of depression compared to those without osteoporosis[100]. Depression score is related to the number and severity of vertebral fractures[63], and parameters of mood are related to the severity of vertebral fracture[48]. Loss of self-esteem can occur, presumably as a result of deformity, disability, and pain, but no studies are available on the prevalence and relation of self-esteem to vertebral fracture[99]. Many patients with vertebral fractures reported emotional problems, but no comparison with a control group was reported[57].

EVALUATION OF QUALITY OF LIFE (QoL) IN OSTEOPOROSIS

Emphasis on the number of fractures provides an incomplete accounting of the clinical consequences of osteoporosis, given the many non-skeletal consequences of fracture. As discussed above, common physical and social outcomes, such as loss of height, kyphosis, chronic back pain, digestive problems, decreased mobility, loss of independence and depression lead to a chronic decrease in QoL. QoL measures can therefore be helpful in clinical studies, and are applicable in daily clinical practice[101].

QoL includes the functioning and performance of individuals in their daily lives and their subjective perception of well-being[102]. These aspects can be assessed by performance measures and questionnaires (self-reporting or by interview).

Examples of generic (not disease-targeted) questionnaires used in osteoporosis are the SF-36, the AIMS2, the Nottingham Health Profile (NHP), the Sickness Impact Profile (SIP), and the Health Assessment Questionnaire (HAQ)[102]. Generic measures may, however, be unresponsive to changes in a specific disease.

Several disease-targeted measures of QoL in osteoporosis are available (Table 197.3). These include the Osteoporosis Functional Disability Questionnaire (OFDQ)[63], the QoL Questionnaire for Osteoporosis (OPTOQLQ)[60,62], the Osteoporosis Assessment Questionnaire (OPAQ)[102], and the QoL Questionnaire of the European Foundation for Osteoporosis (QUALEFFO)[103]. The use of QoL measures in osteoporosis was reviewed by a working group of the Outcome Measures in Rheumatology Clinical Trials (OMERACT)[104–106]. Several of these QoL measures have been shown to have discriminant value (Table 197.4). Studies on minimal clinically important differences (MCID) of these measures are in progress[106]. Only limited prospective data are available on validated multidimensional QoL measures in the natural course and during therapy of osteoporosis[102,104–106]. Studies are, at the time being, underway[96,105].

QUALEFFO was shown to be more discriminative than SF-36 for pain and social function, indicating that this questionnaire is useful in osteoporosis patients with vertebral fracture (Fig. 197.10)[103]. Postal administration of the QUALEFFO has been shown to be reliable, and comparable to nurse-supported administration[107].

CLINICAL FEATURES BEFORE THE FIRST FRACTURE: CLINICAL RISK FACTORS

A fracture is the result of an overload of the mechanical competence of the skeleton. The risk for fractures is therefore related to the degree of osteo-

TABLE 197.4 CLINICAL RISK FACTORS INCLUDED IN QUESTIONNAIRES

	SCORE[60]	OST[15]	SOFSURF[111]	ORAI[110]
Age	X	X	X	X
Weight	X	X	X	X
History of fracture	X	–	X	–
Smoking	–	–	–	X
Race	X	–	–	–
Rheumatoid arthritis	X	–	–	–
Estrogen intake	X	–	–	X

X, Evaluated; –, Not evaluated.

These are the risk factors included in various questionnaires for the clinical diagnosis of osteoporosis.

porosis and to the risk of trauma, most commonly a fall. The etiology of osteoporotic fragility fractures is thus multifactorial, including a number of clinical risk factors. This fact is best illustrated in studies of risk factors for hip fracture[94,108,109]. These studies have shown that some risk factors are associated with low bone density, others to trauma, and others to both. Furthermore, it has been demonstrated that the number of clinical risk factors is associated with hip fracture risk, independent of and in addition to bone density (Fig. 197.11)[108]. In clinical studies of the effects of bisphosphonates in glucocorticoid-induced osteoporosis, the incidence of vertebral fractures was substantially higher in elderly postmenopausal women than in premenopausal women (Chapter 198).

Clinical risk factors of osteoporosis (e.g. low body weight, age) can be present long before the first fracture occurs, but some risk factors (e.g. use of high-dose glucocorticoids) have dramatic effects within a short time. Some risk factors have a high prevalence (e.g. hip fracture in the mother) but are associated with moderate fracture risk; others are rather rare (e.g. glucocorticoid use after transplantation) but are associated with a high risk for fractures. Among the most common clinical risk factors are the menopause (type I, postmenopausal osteoporosis), age (type II, senile osteoporosis), and the use of glucocorticoids or other drugs known to be associated with bone loss (type III, secondary osteoporosis). Additional common and strong risk factors are history of previous fracture, low body weight, and family history of fractures. Less common risk factors for osteoporosis are primary hypogonadism, anorexia nervosa, mal-absorption, primary hyperparathyroidism, gastrectomy, Cushing's syndrome, organ transplantation, rheumatoid arthritis, epilepsy, Parkinson's disease, dementia, and previous cardiovascular accident.

Clinical evaluation of risk factors

Bone densitometry is the golden standard for the diagnosis of osteoporosis[1]. However, there is no justification for screening the whole population using densitometry[13,14]. Clinical case finding of patients at risk for osteoporosis is therefore advocated[13,14].

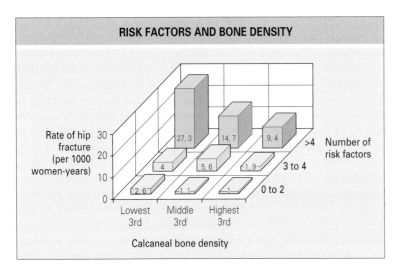

RISK FACTORS AND BONE DENSITY

Rate of hip fracture (per 1000 women-years)

Number of risk factors: >4, 3 to 4, 0 to 2

Calcaneal bone density: Lowest 3rd, Middle 3rd, Highest 3rd

Fig. 197.11 Risk factors and bone density. Annual risk of hip fracture according to the number of risk factors and the age-specific calcaneal bone density. The number of clinical risk factors is associated with hip fracture risk, independent and additive to bone density[108].

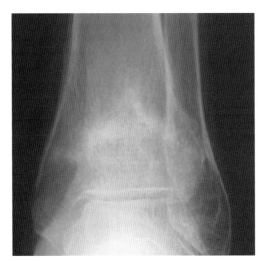

Fig. 197.12 Stress fractures of the distal tibia in a patient with rheumatoid arthritis during methotrexate therapy.

Several questionnaires focusing on the clinical recognition of risk factors for osteoporosis have been studied (Table 197.4). The purpose of these indices is not to diagnose osteoporosis or low BMD, but rather to identify women who are more likely to have low BMD, for the purpose of identifying individuals who could then undergo BMD measurement for a definitive assessment. The simplest questionnaire is the Osteoporosis Self-assessment Tool (OST), which is based on age and weight[15]. Other indices, such as the Simple Calculated Osteoporosis Risk Estimation (SCORE)[60], the Osteoporosis Risk Assessment Index (ORAI)[110], and SOFSURF (derived using data from the Study of Osteoporotic Fractures, SOF)[111], involve 1–4 other risk factors in addition to age and weight. They are based on a combination of risk factors, selected on the basis of the available evidence of their relationhip to osteoporosis and fracture risk.

It is important for the rheumatologist to be aware of the common risk factors and those that may be rare in the general population but more common among patients seen in the rheumatological practice. Indeed, recent data indicate that many patients with metabolic bone disease consult a rheumatologist[112], and that rheumatologists thus are in a favorable position to identify patients with primary and secondary osteoporosis. In a survey of 669 patients with osteoporotic vertebral fractures diagnosed in a rheumatology department over a period of 10 years, one in five women and one in two men had secondary osteoporosis[113]. The conditions most commonly associated with secondary osteoporosis in this setting were glucocorticoid use, chronic obstructive lung disease, and rheumatoid arthritis.

Evaluation of clinical risk factors (with the exception of a history of a fragility fracture) is no substitute for measuring bone density when bone-directed therapy is started. Indeed, in the absence of a prevalent vertebral fracture, a proven low bone density is a prerequisite for patient selection for therapy with bisphosphonates such as alendronate and risedronate (Chapter 198)[114,115]. Risedronate was shown to decrease the risk of hip fracture in elderly postmenopausal women known to have osteoporosis, but no effect could be found in elderly postmenopausal women with mainly fall-related clinical risk factors for hip fracture without proven low bone density in the hip[115].

CLINICAL FEATURES OF OSTEOPOROSIS IN MEN

Osteoporosis is less frequent in men than in women because men develop a higher peak bone mass and lose less bone during later life than women. However, osteoporotic fractures in men are far from uncommon. The clinical features of osteoporosis in men are less well documented than those in women. The available data indicate that osteoporosis in men has some specific features that are different from osteoporosis in women.

Vertebral fractures

The prevalence of vertebral fractures in men is as high as in women at the age of 50 years[116]. In radiographic surveys, however, these radiographic fractures have not been related to back pain[116]. In contrast, in men with clinical vertebral fracture, back pain can last more than 5 years[113] and height loss of more than 2.5cm is common (more than 50%)[117]. Many men with clinical vertebral fracture have decreased QoL, as measured by NHP, a score that assesses energy, pain, emotion, sleep, social function, and mobility[117].

In contrast to women, half of men with clinical vertebral fractures have secondary osteoporosis[113,118]. Men with symptomatic vertebral fracture are usually younger than women[113]. Therefore, causes of secondary osteoporosis should always be evaluated in men with vertebral fracture (Table 197.5).

Hip fractures

As in women, hip fracture risk in men is associated with reduced bone mass and trauma[119]. In a population survey, an increased risk for hip fracture in men was associated with metabolic disease and disorders of movement or balance[120]. The risk for hip fracture was higher in individuals with a history of thyroidectomy, gastric resection, pernicious anemia, chronic bronchitis, or emphysema[120]. Movement and balance disorders associated with an increased risk for hip fracture include neurological disorders (hemiplegia, Parkinsonism, dementia), vertigo, alcoholism, anemia, blindness and use of a cane or walker[120]. The prognosis of men with hip fracture is worse than in women and mortality is higher[31].

STRESS FRACTURES

Stress fractures (also called fatigue fractures) are a particular presentation of fractures related to fatigue damage of bone[3] (Fig. 197.12). Stress fractures have multifactorial causes, including activity level and intensity, bone geometry and bone density. There are two types of stress fracture. *Insufficiency fractures* occur in diseased bone that is involved in routine activity. There are several reports of these fractures in rheumatoid arthritis, some of which are associated with the use of methotrexate[121]. *Fatigue fractures* occur in normal healthy bone repeatedly subjected to high-level stress. Fatigue fractures typically occur after repetitive strain, such as walking, jogging and jumping, especially in young healthy persons involved in new activities, e.g. military recruits[3].

TABLE 197.5 CAUSES OF OSTEOPOROSIS IN MEN

Endocrine diseases	Hypogonadism*
	Cushing's syndrome
	Hyperthyroidism
	Primary hyperparathyroidism
	Hyperprolactinemia
	Idiopathic renal hypercalciuria*
Accompanying osteomalacia	
Neoplastic disease	Multilple myeloma
	Myelo- and lymphoproliferative disease
	Systemic mastocytosis
	Diffuse bony metastases*
	Vertebral metastasis
Drugs/toxins	Glucocorticoids*
	Alcohol abuse*
	Excessive thyroid hormone replacement
	Heparin
	Anticonvulsants*
Genetic collagen disorders	Osteogenesis imperfecta
	Ehlers–Danlos syndrome
	Marfan's syndrome
	Homocystinuria
	Hemochromatosis
Other disorders	Skeletal sarcoidosis
	Gaucher's disease
	Adult hypophosphatasia
	Hemoglobulinopathies
Other factors	Chronic illness (rheumatoid arthritis, liver/renal disease)
	Prolonged immobilization
	Malnutrition (including calcium deficiency and scurvy)
	Gastrectomy*
	Aging*
Idiopathic	Juvenile
	Adult*

* Most frequent causes.

Clinical recognition of stress fractures is often difficult, as they can occur in skeletal sites that are unexpected for classical osteoporosis. They often are difficult to diagnose clinically and not readily recognizable on plain radiographs. Other imaging techniques, such as bone scintigraphy, computer tomography or magnetic resonance imaging, may be needed to identify stress fractures.

DIFFERENTIAL DIAGNOSIS OF VERTEBRAL FRACTURES

Only one in three vertebral fractures comes to clinical attention and diagnosis (Fig. 197.5)[4,46]. Clinical symptoms of vertebral fractures are highly variable. Some vertebral fractures are readily recognizable because of an acute pain episode, with typical irradiating pain and localized pain on pressure. Other patients may have no or mild symptoms and can be overlooked[2]. In contrast to most non-vertebral fractures, many vertebral fractures do not occur as a result of a specific trauma such as a fall, but occurr spontaneously or after trivial activities such as bending or lifting[47,48]. Vertebral fractures are common among elderly women, but are often overlooked – perhaps because patients and physicians may accept symptoms of back pain as a normal phenomenon of age and osteoarthritis[2]. Back pain is common in the population, and symptoms of different back conditions are non-specific, making it difficult to distinguish osteoporotic vertebral fracture from other underlying causes of pain[2]. Moreover, an individual can suffer from more than one type of back problem, either at different times or simultaneously[2]. Some patients with acute back pain can be diagnosed erroneously as having an acute fracture, when in fact the deformity had been present on earlier films. Indeed, the duration of pain is difficult to establish, and additional fractures or a progression of an exisiting vertebral deformity can occur, leading to new episodes of pain[49]. In cross-sectional studies, vertebral deformities probably have developed years before the examination, so that acute back pain and disability could have been missed[50].

Once a vertebral fracture is diagnosed, its cause remains to be determined. Vertebral fractures occurring as a result of osteoporosis should be differentiated from wedging associated with other diseases such Sheurmann's disease, remodeling in osteoarthritis[51], and metastatic bone disease[4].

When a vertebral fracture is caused by osteoporosis, it has to be determined if the fracture is due to primary or secondary osteoporosis. In men in particular, causes of secondary osteoporosis should be carefully assessed, as one in two men with vertebral fracture have secondary osteoporosis (Table 197.5). The incidence of secondary osteoporosis in women in the population has not been established. In women attending an osteoporosis clinic, 11% had a new, unsuspected diagnosis associated with bone loss[121]. The proportion of women with previously undiagnosed conditions may even be higher in osteoporotic women without major risk factors for osteoporosis[81]. In one study, 31% had new diagnoses, such as hypercalciuria, vitamin D deficiency, hyperthyroidism, hyperparathyroidism, gluten-enteropathy, myeloma, Cushing's syndrome and Paget's disease[81]. Thus, a careful history and physical examination are indicated in every patient with osteoporosis. Vigorous pursuit of other diagnoses is appropriate for an osteoporotic woman without major risk factors, with atypical pain or persistence of severe pain for more than 10–12 weeks, or general symptoms (weight loss, diffuse bone pains). In such case, malignant bone diseases, such as osteolytic bone metastases, multiple myeloma and malignant lymphoma of bone, need to be excluded. Further differential diagnoses include osteomalacia, other marrow dysplasias or infiltration, connective tissue diseases, and gastrointestinal and renal disorders. Additional laboratory testing and more sophisticated imaging, such as bone scintigraphy, computer tomography, or magnetic resonance imaging, are then indicated.

REFERENCES

1. World Health Organization. Assessment of fracture risk and its application to screening for postmenopausal osteoporosis. Geneva: World Health Organization Technical Report Series no. 843; 1994.
2. Ross PD. Risk factors for osteoporotic fracture. Endocrinol Metab Clin North Am 1998; 27: 289–301.
3. Parfitt AM. Bone age, mineral density, and fatigue damage. Calcif Tissue Int 1993; 53 (suppl 1): S82–85; discussion S85–86.
4. Cooper C, Atkinson EJ et al. Incidence of clinically diagnosed vertebral fractures: a population-based study in Rochester, Minnesota, 1985–1989. J Bone Miner Res 1992; 7: 221–227.
5. Nevitt MC, Ettinger B et al. The association of radiographically detected vertebral fractures with back pain and function: a prospective study. Ann Intern Med 1998; 128: 793–800.
6. Cooper C, Atkinson EJ et al. Population-based study of survival after osteoporotic fractures. Am J Epidemiol 1993; 137: 1001–1005.
7. Cauley JA, Thompson DE et al. Risk of mortality following clinical fractures. Osteoporos Int 2000; 11: 556–561.
8. Greendale GA, Barrett-Connor E et al. Late physical and functional effects of osteoporotic fracture in women: the Rancho Bernardo Study. J Am Geriatr Soc 1995; 43: 955–961.

9. Greendale GA, DeAmicis TA *et al*. A prospective study of the effect of fracture on measured physical performance: results from the MacArthur Study–MAC. J Am Geriatr Soc 2000; 48: 546–549.

10. Klotzbuecher CM, Ross PD *et al*. Patients with prior fractures have an increased risk of future fractures: a summary of the literature and statistical synthesis. J Bone Miner Res 2000; 15: 721–739.

11. Siris E. Alendronate in the treatment of osteoporosis: a review of the clinical trials. J Womens Health Gend Based Med 2000; 9: 599–606.

12. Dequeker J. Prevention and treatment of osteoporosis. Ned Tijdschr Geneesk 1992; 136: 1188–1192.

13. Osteoporosis: review of the evidence for prevention, diagnosis and treatment and cost-effectiveness analysis. Osteoporosis Int 1998 (suppl 4).

14. Kanis JA, Delmas P *et al*. Guidelines for diagnosis and management of osteoporosis. The European Foundation for Osteoporosis and Bone Disease. Osteoporosis Int 1997; 7: 390–406.

15. Koh LK, Sedrine WB *et al*. Osteoporosis Self-Assessment Tool for Asians (OSTA) Research Group. A simple tool to identify Asian women at increased risk of osteoporosis. Osteoporos Int 2001; 12: 699–705.

16. van der Voort DJ, Dinant GJ *et al*. Construction of an algorithm for quick detection of patients with low bone mineral density and its applicability in daily general practice. J Clin Epidemiol 2000; 53: 1095–1103.

17. Pal B. Questionnaire survey of advice given to patients with fractures. Brit Med J 1999; 318: 500–501.

18. Nevitt MC, Thompson DE *et al*. Effect of alendronate on limited-activity days and bed-disability days caused by back pain in postmenopausal women with existing vertebral fractures. Fracture Intervention Trial Research Group. Arch Intern Med 2000; 160: 77–85.

19. Melton LJ, Cooper C. Magnitude and impact of osteoporosis and fractures. In: Marcus R, Feldman D, Kelsey J, eds. Osteoporosis, 2nd ed. London: Academic Press; 2001.

20. Atkins RM, Duckworth T *et al*. Features of algodystrophy after Colles' fracture. J Bone Joint Surg 1990; 72: 105–110.

21. Field J, Warwick D *et al*. Long-term prognosis of displaced Colles' fracture: a 10-year prospective review. Injury 1992; 23: 529–532.

22. Warwick D, Field J *et al*. Function ten years after Colles' fracture. Clin Orthop 1993; 295: 270–274.

23. Gartland JJ, Werley CW. Evaluation of healed Colles' fractures. J Bone J Surg 1951; 33A: 895–907.

24. Geusens P, Santen M. Algodystrophy. Baillière's Best Pract Res Clin Rheumatol 2000; 14: 499–513.

25. Khan SA, de Geus C *et al*. Osteoporosis follow-up after wrist fractures following minor trauma. Arch Intern Med 2001; 161: 1309–1312.

26. Schurch MA, Rizzoli R *et al*. A prospective study on socioeconomic aspects of fracture of the proximal femur. J Bone Miner Res 1996; 11: 1935–1942.

27. Nevitt MC, Cummings SR. Type of fall and risk of hip and wrist fractures: the study of osteoporotic fractures. The Study of Osteoporotic Fractures Research Group. J Am Geriatr Soc 1993; 41: 1226–1234.

28. Martin-Hunyadi C, Heitz D *et al*. Spontaneous insufficiency fractures of long bones: a prospective epidemiological survey in nursing home subjects. Arch Gerontol Geriatr 2000; 31: 207–214.

29. Obrandt K, ed. Management of fractures in severely osteoporotic bone. Heidelberg: Springer 2000.

30. Koot VC, Peeters PH *et al*. Functional results after treatment of hip fracture: a multicentre, prospective study in 215 patients. Eur J Surg 2000; 166: 480–485.

31. Baudoin C, Fardellone P *et al*. Clinical outcomes and mortality after hip fracture: a 2-year follow-up study. Bone 1996; 18(suppl): 149S–157S.

32. Greendale GA, Barrett-Connor E. Outcomes of osteoporotic fractures. In: Marcus R, Feldman D, Kelsey J, eds. Osteoporosis, 2nd ed. London: Academic Press; 2001.

33. Hannan EL, Magaziner J *et al*. Mortality and locomotion 6 months after hospitalization for hip fracture: risk factors and risk-adjusted hospital outcomes. J Am Med Assoc 2001; 285: 2736–2742.

34. Morrison RS, Siu AL. Survival in end-stage dementia following acute illness. J Am Med Assoc 2000; 284: 47–52.

35. Lippuner K, von Overbeck J *et al*. Incidence and direct medical costs of hospitalizations due to osteoporotic fractures in Switzerland. Osteoporos Int 1997; 7: 414–425.

36. Haentjens P, Autier P *et al*. Belgian Hip Fracture Study Group. The economic cost of hip fractures among elderly women. A one-year, prospective, observational cohort study with matched-pair analysis. J Bone Joint Surg Am 2001; 83-A: 493–500.

37. US congress office.

38. Katz S, Heiple K *et al*. Long-term course of 147 patients with fracture of the hip. Surg Gybecol Obstet 1967; 124: 1219–1230.

39. Marottoli RA, Berkman LF *et al*. Decline in physical function following hip fracture. J Am Geriatr Soc 1992; 40: 861–866.

40. Michel JP, Hoffmeyer P *et al*. Prognosis of functional recovery 1 year after hip fracture: typical patient profiles through cluster analysis. J Gerontol A Biol Sci Med Sci 2000; 55: M508–515.

41. Magaziner J, Simonsick EM *et al*. Predictors of functional recovery one year following hospital discharge for hip fracture: a prospective study. J Gerontol 1990; 45: M101–107.

42. Hall SE, Criddle RA *et al*. A case-control study of quality of life and functional impairment in women with long-standing vertebral osteoporotic fracture. Osteoporos Int 1999; 9: 508–515.

43. Cummings SR, Phillips SL *et al*. Recovery of function after hip fracture. The role of social supports. J Am Geriatr Soc 1988; 36: 801–806.

44. Randell AG, Nguyen TV *et al*. Deterioration in quality of life following hip fracture: a prospective study. Osteoporos Int 2000; 11: 460–466.

45. Adams F. The genuine works of Hippocrates. Baltimore: Williams and Wilkins; 1939: 237–234.

46. Cooper C. Epidemiology of vertebral fractures in Western populations. Spine: State of the Art Reviews 1994; 8: 1–12.

47. Albright F, Smith PH *et al*. Postmenopausal osteoporosis. J Am Med Assoc 1941; 1116: 2465–2474.

48. Leidig G, Minne HW *et al*. A study of complaints and their relation to vertebral destruction in patients with osteoporosis. Bone Miner 1990; 8: 217–229.

49. Lyritis GP, Mayasis B *et al*. The natural history of the osteoporotic vertebral fracture. Clin Rheumatol 1989; 8(Suppl 2): 66–69.

50. Ettinger B, Black DM *et al*. Contribution of vertebral deformities to chronic back pain and disability. The Study of Osteoporotic Fractures Research Group. J Bone Miner Res 1992; 7: 449–456.

51. Abdel-Hamid Osman A, Bassiouni H *et al*. Aging of the thoracic spine: distinction between wedging in osteoarthritis and fracture in osteoporosis – a cross-sectional and longitudinal study. Bone 1994; 15: 437–442.

52. Silverman SL. The clinical consequences of vertebral compression fracture. Bone 1992; 13(suppl 2): S27–31.

53. Kanis JA, McCloskey EV. Epidemiology of vertebral osteoporosis. Bone 1992; 13(suppl 2): S1–10.

54. Gold DT. The clinical impact of vertebral fractures: quality of life in women with osteoporosis. Bone 1996; 18(suppl): 185S–189S.

55. Ross PD. Clinical consequences of vertebral fractures. Am J Med 1997; 103(2A): 30S–42S; discussion 42S–43S.

56. Leidig-Bruckner G, Minne HW *et al*. Clinical grading of spinal osteoporosis: quality of life components and spinal deformity in women with chronic low back pain and women with vertebral osteoporosis. J Bone Miner Res 1997; 12: 663–675.

57. Cook DJ, Guyatt GH *et al*. Quality of life issues in women with vertebral fractures due to osteoporosis. Arthritis Rheum 1993; 36: 750–756.

58. Lyles KW, Gold DT. Association of osteoporotic vertebral compression fractures with impaired functional status. Am J Med 1993; 94: 595–601.

59. Ryan PJ, Blake G *et al*. A clinical profile of back pain and disability in patients with spinal osteoporosis. Bone 1994; 15: 27–30.

60. Lydick E, Zimmerman SI *et al*. Development and validation of a discriminative quality of life questionnaire for osteoporosis (the OPTQoL). J Bone Miner Res 1997; 12: 456–463.

61. Lips P, Cooper C *et al*. Quality of life in patients with vertebral fractures: validation of the Quality of Life Questionnaire of the European Foundation for Osteoporosis (QUALEFFO). Working Party for Quality of Life of the European Foundation for Osteoporosis. Osteoporos Int 1999; 10: 150–160.

62. Cook DJ, Guyatt GH *et al*. Development and validation of the mini-osteoporosis quality of life questionnaire (OQLQ) in osteoporotic women with back pain due to vertebral fractures. Osteoporosis Quality of Life Study Group. Osteoporos Int 1999; 10: 207–213.

63. Helmes E, Hodsman A *et al*. A questionnaire to evaluate disability in osteoporotic patients with vertebral compression fractures. J Gerontol A Biol Sci Med Sci 1995; 50: M91–98.

64. Begerow B, Pfeifer M *et al*. Time since vertebral fracture: an important variable concerning quality of life in patients with postmenopausal osteoporosis. Osteoporos Int 1999; 10: 26–33.

65. Ross PD, Ettinger B *et al*. Evaluation of adverse health outcomes associated with vertebral fractures. Osteoporos Int 1991; 1: 134–140.

66. Nicholson PH, Haddaway MJ *et al*. Vertebral deformity, bone mineral density, back pain and height loss in unscreened women over 50 years. Osteoporos Int 1993; 3: 300–307.

67. Chandler JM, Martin AR *et al*. Reliability of an osteoporosis-targeted quality of life survey instrument for use in the community: OPTQoL. Osteoporos Int 1998; 8: 127–135.

68. Oleksik A, Lips P *et al*. Health-related quality of life in postmenopausal women with low BMD with or without prevalent vertebral fractures. J Bone Miner Res 200l; 15: 1384–1392.

69. Ross PD, Davis JW *et al*. Pain and disability associated with new vertebral fractures and other spinal conditions. J Clin Epidemiol 1994; 47: 231–239.

70. Huang C, Ross PD *et al*. Vertebral fracture and other predictors of physical impairment and health care utilization. Arch Intern Med 1996; 156: 2469–2475.

71. Huang C, Ross PD *et al*. Vertebral fractures and other predictors of back pain among older women. J Bone Miner Res 1996; 11: 1026–1032.

72. Huang C, Ross PD *et al*. Contributions of vertebral fractures to stature loss among elderly Japanese-American women in Hawaii. J Bone Miner Res 1996; 11: 408–411.

73. Kado DM, Browner WS *et al*. Vertebral fractures and mortality in older women: a prospective study. Study of Osteoporotic Fractures Research Group. Arch Intern Med 1999; 159: 1215–1220.

74. Ensrud KE, Thompson DE *et al*. Prevalent vertebral deformities predict mortality and hospitalization in older women with low bone mass. Fracture Intervention Trial Research Group. J Am Geriatr Soc 2000; 48: 241–249.

75. Ismail AA, Cockerill W *et al*. Prevalent vertebral deformity predicts incident hip though not distal forearm fracture: results from the European Prospective Osteoporosis Study. Osteoporos Int 2001; 12: 85–90.

76. Johnell O, Oden A *et al*. Acute and long-term increase in fracture risk after hospitalization for vertebral fracture. Osteoporos Int 2001; 12: 207–214.

77. Ross PD, Davis JW *et al*. Pre-existing fractures and bone mass predict vertebral fracture incidence in women. Ann Intern Med 1991; 114: 919–923.

78. Lindsay R, Silverman SL *et al*. Risk of new vertebral fracture in the year following a fracture. J Am Med Assoc 2001; 285: 320–323.

79. Kotowicz MA, Melton LJ 3rd *et al*. Risk of hip fracture in women with vertebral fracture. J Bone Miner Res 1994; 9: 599–605.

80. Burger H, van Daele PL *et al*. Vertebral deformities as predictors of non-vertebral fractures. Brit Med J 1994; 309: 991–992.

81. Primer on the metabolic bone disorders of mineral metabolism, 4th ed. Baltimore: Lippincott Williams & Wilkins; 1999.

82. Finsen V. Osteoporosis and back pain among the elderly. Acta Med Scand 1988; 223: 443–449.

83. Spector TD, McCloskey EV et al. Prevalence of vertebral fracture in women and the relationship with bone density and symptoms: the Chingford Study. J Bone Miner Res 1993; 8: 817–822.

84. Gehlbach SH, Bigelow C et al. Recognition of vertebral fracture in a clinical setting. Osteoporos Int 2000; 11: 577–582.

85. Sinaki M, Khosla S et al. Muscle strength in osteoporotic versus normal women. Osteoporos Int 1993; 3: 8–12.

86. Nevitt MC, Cummings SR et al. Risk factors for recurrent nonsyncopal falls. A prospective study. J Am Med Assoc 1989; 261: 2663–2668.

87. Ulivieri FM, Bossi E et al. Quantification by dual photonabsorptiometry of local bone loss after fracture. Clin Orthop 1990; 250: 291–296.

88. Cortet B, Houvenagel E et al. Spinal curvatures and quality of life in women with vertebral fractures secondary to osteoporosis. Spine 1999; 24: 1921–1925.

89. Ensrud KE, Black DM et al. Correlates of kyphosis in older women. The Fracture Intervention Trial Research Group. J Am Geriatr Soc 1997; 45: 682–687.

90. Ettinger B, Black DM et al. Kyphosis in older women and its relation to back pain, disability and osteopenia: the study of osteoporotic fractures. Osteoporos Int 1994; 4: 55–60.

91. Kleerekoper M, Nelson DA et al. Outcome variables in osteoporosis trials. Bone 1992; 13(suppl 1): S29–34.

92. Leech JA, Dulberg C et al. Relationship of lung function to severity of osteoporosis. Am Rev Respir Dis 1990; 141: 68–71.

93. Schlaich C, Minne HW et al. Reduced pulmonary function in patients with spinal osteoporotic fractures. Osteoporos Int 1998; 8: 261–267.

94. Lord SR, Sambrook PN et al. Postural stability, falls and fractures in the elderly: results from the Dubbo Osteoporosis Epidemiology Study. Med J Aust 1994; 160: 684–685, 688–691.

95. Ensrud KE, Nevitt MC et al. Correlates of impaired function in older women. J Am Geriatr Soc 1994; 42: 481–489.

96. Oleksik AM, Ewing SK et al. Three years of health related quality of life in postmenopausal women with osteoporosis: impact of incident vertebral fractures, age and severe adverse events. JBMR 2000; 1: S168.

97. Cook DJ, Guyatt GH et al. Development and validation of the mini-osteoporosis quality of life questionnaire (OQLQ) in osteoporotic women with back pain due to vertebral fractures. Osteoporosis Quality of Life Study Group. Osteoporos Int 1999; 10: 207–213.

98. Rubin SM, Cummings SR. Results of bone densitometry affect women's decisions about taking measures to prevent fractures. Ann Intern Med 1992; 116: 990–995.

99. Gold DT, Bales CW et al. Treatment of osteoporosis: the psychological impact of a medical education program in older patients. JAGS 1989; 37: 417–422.

100. Coelho R, Silva C et al. Bone mineral density and depression: a community study in women. J Psychosom Res 1999; 46: 29–35.

101. Michelson D, Stratakis C, Hill L et al. Bone mineral density in women with depression. N Engl J Med 1996; 335: 1176–1181.

102. Silverman SL, Cranney A. Quality of life measurement in osteoporosis. J Rheumatol 1997; 24: 1218–1221.

103. Lips P, Cooper C et al. Quality of life in patients with vertebral fractures: validation of the Quality of Life Questionnaire of the European Foundation for Osteoporosis (QUALEFFO). Working Party for Quality of Life of the European Foundation for Osteoporosis. Osteoporos Int 1999; 10: 150–160.

104. Cranney A, Tugwell P et al. Osteoporosis clinical trials endpoints: candidate variables and clinimetric properties. J Rheumatol 1997; 24: 1222–1229.

105. Cranney A, Welch V et al. Responsiveness of endpoints in osteoporosis clinical trials – an update. J Rheumatol 1999; 26: 222–228.

106. Cranney A, Welch V et al. Discrimination of changes in osteoporosis outcomes. J Rheumatol 2001; 28: 413–421.

107. Murrell P, Todd CJ et al. Postal administration compared with nurse-supported administration of the QUALEFFO-41 in a population sample: comparison of results and assessment of psychometric properties. Osteoporos Int 2001; 12: 672–679.

108. Cummings SR, Nevitt MC et al. Risk factors for hip fracture in white women. Study of Osteoporotic Fractures Research Group. N Engl J Med 1995; 332: 767–773.

109. Dargent-Molina P, Poitiers F et al. EPIDOS Group. In elderly women weight is the best predictor of a very low bone mineral density: evidence from the EPIDOS study. Osteoporos Int 2000; 11: 881–888.

110. Cadarette SM, Jaglal SB et al. Development and validation of the osteoporosis risk assessment instrument to facilitate selection of women for bone densitometry. CMAJ 2000; 162: 1289–1294.

111. Black DM, Palermo L et al. SOFSURF: A simple, usefull risk factor system can identify the large majority of women with osteoporosis. Bone 1998; 23(suppl): S605.

112. Vanhoof J, Declerck K, Geusens P. Prevalence of rheumatic diseases in a rheumatological outpatient practice. Ann Rheum Dis 2002; 61: 453–455.

113. Nolla JM, Gomez-Vaquero C et al. Osteoporotic vertebral fracture in clinical practice. 669 Patients diagnosed over a 10 year period. J Rheumatol 2001; 28: 2289–2293.

114. Cummings SR, Black DM et al. Effect of alendronate on risk of fracture in women with low bone density but without vertebral fractures: results from the Fracture Intervention Trial. J Am Med Assoc 1998; 280: 2077–2082.

115. McClung MR, Geusens P et al. Effect of risedronate on the risk of hip fracture in elderly women. Hip Intervention Program Study Group. N Engl J Med 2001; 344: 333–340.

116. Johnell O, O'Neill T et al. Anthropometric measurements and vertebral deformities. European Vertebral Osteoporosis Study (EVOS) Group. Am J Epidemiol 1997; 146: 287–293.

117. Scane AC, Sutcliffe AM, Francis RM. The sequelae of vertebral crush fractures in men. Osteoporos Int 1994; 4: 89–92.

118. Seeman E. Osteoporosis in men. Osteoporos Int 1999; 9(suppl 2): S97–S110.

119. Riggs BL, Melton LJ 3rd. Involutional osteoporosis. N Engl J Med 1986; 314: 1676–1686.

120. Poor G, Atkinson EJ et al. Predictors of hip fractures in elderly men. J Bone Miner Res 1995; 10: 1900–1907.

121. Alonso-Bartolome P, Martinez-Taboada VM, Blanco R, Rodriguez-Valverde V. Insufficiency fractures of the tibia and fibula. Semin Arthritis Rheum 1999; 28: 413–420.

122. Johnson BE, Lucasey B, Robinson RG, Lukert BP. Contributing diagnoses in osteoporosis. The value of a complete medical evaluation. Arch Intern Med 1989; 149: 1069–1072.

198 Management of osteoporosis

Anthony D Woolf and Kristina Åkesson

- Osteoporosis is the structural failure of the skeleton with increased risk of fracture. There is low bone mass and microarchitectural deterioration of bone tissue leading to increased bone fragility. This manifests itself as fracture following low energy trauma
- Fracture is associated with increased mortality and significant short- and long-term morbidity
- The management of osteoporosis must encompass all these components of the condition. Bone mass should be maximized, fractures should be prevented and those who have already sustained a fracture should be rehabilitated to minimize the associated pain, limitation of activities and restriction of participation

INDIVIDUAL VERSUS POPULATION MANAGEMENT

The management of osteoporosis can either be focused on the individual or be targeted at the population. We need to know what the best strategy is for the individuals in the clinic to avoid an osteoporotic fracture in the future, or what to advise the person who has already sustained a low energy fracture to prevent a further fracture and how to rehabilitate them. However, osteoporosis is also a public health issue because of the high incidence and cost of fractures and strategies are needed to reduce the number of osteoporotic fractures in the population. This can be accomplished by reducing the risk for the population as a whole irrespective of their individual risk (primary prevention), or by targeting those who are known to be at high risk of future fracture and who may already have early features of osteoporosis with a low bone mass and may have sustained a fracture (secondary prevention).

Targeting the population as a whole or those at high risk are not mutually exclusive strategies and both approaches are recommended in parallel–general measures to reduce the population risk in conjunction with specific therapies aimed at those who are at most risk of future fracture. There is a move towards the use of specific therapy at a later stage in those at highest risk. This is for two reasons; firstly, there is better identification of those who will gain most because of their high absolute risk of fracture at the time of the treatment effect, and secondly, treatments have an early onset of benefit, with fracture prevention within a year[1]. There are several evidence-based guidelines for the prevention and treatment of osteoporosis[2–5] but the application of them in routine clinical practice still remains a challenge.

WHO TO TREAT?

The main targets for therapy are individuals at increased risk of fracture, in particular if they are likely to have a poor outcome following a fracture. The difficulty is to identify such individuals.

Who is at high risk of future fracture?

The risk of fracture increases with age and is greater in women than men, and the frail elderly have the worst outcome. In addition, the strongest risk factors for fracture include low bone density and falling. There are data on which risk factors can be used to try and identify those who may have low bone density (Table 198.1) or may fall. These

TABLE 198.1 RISK FACTORS FOR FRACTURE RELATED TO LOSS OF BONE MASS		
High risk (RR ≥2)	**Moderate risk (1 <RR <2)**	**No risk (RR ≤1)**
Aging (>70–80 years)	Gender (female)	Consumption of caffeine
Low body weight	Smoking (active)	Consumption of tea
Weight loss	Low sunlight exposure (low or none)	Menopause
Physical inactivity	Family history of osteoporotic fracture	Nulliparity
Corticosteroids	Surgical menopause	Consumption of fluoridated water
Anticonvulsants	Early menopause (<45 years)	Thiazide diuretics
Primary hyperparathyroidism	Short fertile period (<30 years)	
Diabetes mellitus type I	Late menarche (>15 years)	
Anorexia nervosa	No lactation	
Gastrectomy	Low calcium intake (<500–850mg/day)	
Pernicious anemia	Hyperparathyroidism (N/S)	
Prior osteoporotic fracture	Hyperthyroidism	
	Diabetes mellitus (type II or N/S)	
	Rheumatoid arthritis	
(Adapted from Espallargues et al.[9])		

various risk factors can be used to aid clinical decision-making about whom to treat.

Bone mineral density (BMD) measured by dual energy X-ray absorptiometry (DXA) accounts for 75–90% of the variance of bone strength[6] and for each decrease of one standard deviation in bone density at the proximal femur or lumbar spine there is a two- to three-fold increase in fracture risk[5]. Nomograms are being developed to estimate absolute fracture risk for any given bone density at any given age over a relative time interval. Measurement of BMD at the total hip is regarded as most reliable because of changes in disc spaces and joints of the lumbar spine with advancing age.

Fracture risk can also be assessed by measurements at other skeletal sites using different techniques. Quantitative ultrasound has a demonstrated role in elderly women[7] but is less established in other age groups and there are problems of standardization of machines and sites of assessment. Forearm densitometry is also used to assess risk[8]. Their specificity is less than DXA of the lumbar spine or proximal femur for predicting fractures at these sites.

Previous fracture of the vertebrae, hip, distal radius and other sites over the age of 40 if a clinical manifestation of existing osteoporosis is an important predictor for future fracture[9]. At present osteoporosis is undiagnosed and untreated in many people who have sustained such fractures. Osteoporosis should thus be suspected following a low energy fracture or in someone who has lost height with kyphosis. A coincidental X-ray of the spine may reveal a vertebral deformity or suggest demineralization.

Fracture is not only a result of bone fragility but also is a consequence of an abnormal force, usually due to a fall. Risk factors for falls thus need to be identified. The best predictors of future falls are a fall in the previous year and abnormality in neuromuscular function, measured simplest as inability to rise unaided from a chair without using the arms.

There are other risk factors for fracture, which are principally mediated either through bone density[9] (Table 198.1) and/or falls[10]. Risk factors identified by systematic review that carry a high risk of osteoporosis, in addition to aging and female gender, include previous low energy fracture, glucocorticosteroid therapy, reduced lifetime estrogen exposure, anorexia nervosa, low body mass index, maternal hip fracture, smoking, low levels of physical activity and certain diseases such as rheumatoid arthritis and diabetes mellitus[9]. Although these factors are associated with increased personal risk, they cannot predict who will fracture and are of limited value alone in deciding who will benefit most from an intervention. They can however be used to identify who should be assessed for their future risk of fracture by bone densitometry[5] and this can form part of a high-risk strategy (see Chapter 197).

Bone loss may be predicted by biochemical markers of high bone turnover. They may be independent measures of future fracture risk but their predictive power for the individual is poor. Used in combination with bone density, biochemical bone markers are more predictive of fracture and may strengthen the indication for treatment[11].

Identification of those at highest risk of fracture

The decision to intervene must consider the balance between the benefits, risks and costs of the intervention, and the level of risk for osteoporosis and future fracture. For example, a well tolerated intervention with additional health benefit outside the skeleton needs only a low level of increased risk of osteoporosis and fracture to justify its recommendation, whereas a treatment that only benefits the skeleton needs greater justification for its use. Any decision by the person around this balance of risk and benefit will be influenced by other factors such as the individual's personal experiences and subsequent anxieties about sustaining a fracture or suffering side effects from treatment. It is not possible to predict for the individual whether they will sustain a fracture or benefit from a treatment but we can estimate probabilities by the

application of knowledge of the above risk factors to the individual. Once the level of risk is estimated, it requires careful explanation to have any meaningful value for the patient.

There are different approaches to identifying those at risk of osteoporosis and fracture at different ages. At the younger ages, predictors of low bone density are the major determinants of future fracture. With a person over 70 years, the prevalence of low bone density is greater and other factors, such as falling, are more important in discriminating those at high risk of fracture.

No method of assessing risk of osteoporosis and fracture has both optimal sensitivity and specificity, and there have to be trade offs in any strategy to identify those at risk. Bone density at the site of a potential fracture is the best predictor of fracture at that site and osteoporosis is defined in terms of bone density. It is generally agreed however that population screening for osteoporosis by bone densitometry is not appropriate. This is because it is not cost-effective, there is poor uptake of the measurements, limited specificity for future fracture and low compliance with the therapeutic recommendations[12]. A two stage process is proposed with the use of the strongest clinical indicators for osteoporosis (Table 198.1) as a first stage with bone densitometry restricted to the second stage, as a more cost-effective approach. The indicators proposed vary between guidelines from just being a women over 65 years[4] to having a variety of known risk factors[5]. Simple self-administered questionnaires can be used to help identify those at potential risk for further assessment. There is a move towards assessing an individual's needs at an older age for bone-specific treatments when the absolute risk of fracture is highest. The 5-year risk of fracture in a 50-year-old women is 3.4%, whereas it is 14.5% in a 75-year-old[13]. Thresholds of bone density T-scores have been recommended for treatment[14]. Clinical indicators for osteoporosis could be used alone to target interventions that are well tolerated, inexpensive or have additional benefits outside the skeleton such as lifestyle changes or estrogen replacement therapy. The presence of multiple vertebral deformities is diagnostic of osteoporosis providing other causes are excluded and treatment with a bone specific agent could be considered. However osteoporosis should ideally be confirmed in most cases by bone density using DXA before using a bone specific treatment. Most intervention studies have specifically shown fracture prevention in the context of low bone mass and/or prevalent vertebral fractures.

Once osteoporosis is confirmed, any underlying cause should be looked for but osteoporosis is idiopathic in most cases, although comorbidities that can affect the outcome are common. If a fracture is the presentation, then other causes of fracture must be considered.

INVESTIGATIONS

Osteoporosis should be assessed and managed in the context of the person's general health. All those with osteoporosis, with or without fracture, should have a diagnostic evaluation including a careful history, physical examination and laboratory investigations to exclude conditions that can mimic osteoporosis, to elucidate secondary causes of osteoporosis and contributory factors, and to identify any comorbidities that will influence outcome. This evaluation also includes an estimate of severity and prognosis to enable the development of an appropriate plan of management. Repeat DXA measurement may be needed to monitor treatment. Much can be learnt from a good history and examination in combination with clinical experience and intuition.

Identifying cause of fracture

If the person presents with sudden onset back pain or loss of height with stoop, then X-ray is first needed to confirm the presence of vertebral deformity. If vertebral deformity is confirmed or if the person presents with a low energy fracture of another site, then causes other than osteoporosis should first be excluded (Tables 198.2 & 198.3).

TABLE 198.2 DIFFERENTIAL DIAGNOSIS OF FRACTURE AND VERTEBRAL DEFORMITY

- Osteoporosis
- Primary malignancy including myeloma
- Metastatic malignancy – breast, prostate, lung and renal most common
- Osteomalacia
- Paget's disease
- Osteomyelitis
- Traumatic vertebral fracture earlier in life
- Scheuermann's osteochondritis of the spine

TABLE 198.3 INVESTIGATION OF FRACTURE OR BONE PAIN

Baseline

- Full examination, in particular breasts or prostate
- X-ray of affected site
- Hematology
  - Full blood count
  - Viscosity or ESR
- Biochemistry
  - Serum calcium, phosphate
  - Serum alkaline phosphatase
  - Serum creatinine
  - Serum albumen
  - Testosterone and SHBG in men

Further assessment

- Further imaging
  - Isotope bone scan – if any concern of metastases
  - CT scan or MRI to characterize lesion
- Biochemistry
  - Liver function tests
  - Serum protein electrophoresis
  - Thyroid function tests
  - Urine Bence-Jones protein
  - PSA in men with vertebral fractures

Investigations need to be tailored to the individual depending on site of fracture and whether other findings suggest a pathological cause.

TABLE 198.4 CAUSES OF GENERALIZED OSTEOPOROSIS

Cause	Example
Age	
Endocrine	Primary and secondary hypogonadism including early menopause (<45years) Hyperparathyroidism Hyperthyroidism Cushing's syndrome Hyperprolactinemia
Specific conditions	Anorexia nervosa Over-exercise syndrome Osteomalacia Pregnancy Rheumatoid arthritis Chronic obstructive airways disease Cystic fibrosis Gastrointestinal disease – postgastrectomy, celiac disease, Crohn's disease, ulcerative colitis Chronic liver disease Chronic renal failure Post-transplantation Immobility related to paraplegia, multiple sclerosis, etc.
Malignant disease	Metastatic malignancy Myeloma Leukemia, lymphoma Mastocytosis
Drugs	Glucocorticosteroids Thyroxine in excess Anticonvulsants Heparin
Lifestyle factors	Smoking Alcohol in excess Lack of physical activity
Hereditary connective tissue disorders	Osteogenesis imperfecta Marfan's syndrome Ehlers–Danlos syndrome Homocystinuria

Imaging

Although a plain X-ray cannot be used to diagnose osteoporosis as 30% of bone mass can be lost before it is evident, such imaging should be used to confirm the presence of a vertebral fracture. Vertebrae may show endplate deformities, anterior wedging or crush fractures. The X-ray may reveal bone destruction or lytic lesions and a PA view of the spine may demonstrate pedicles that have been destroyed by metastases. The X-ray of any non-vertebral fracture, including hip fracture, should be carefully viewed for abnormalities to suggest malignancy or osteomalacia. Pathological fractures are however not very likely at some sites such as the distal radius. Stress fractures may not be visible on the plain X-ray and require bone scintigraphy, CT scan, or MRI. Radiographs cannot by themselves tell if the fracture is recent.

Bone density measurement should be considered to confirm underlying osteoporosis. Bone mineral density may be reduced compared to peak bone mass but fractures occur in the presence of bone density within the normal range for their age, particularly in the very old.

Bone scintigraphy will show increased uptake for several weeks after a fracture and can indicate timing of a vertebral fracture but there is rarely reason to obtain such close temporal relationship. Bone scintigraphy,

CT scan or MRI is used when a fracture of non-osteoporotic origin is suspected. Multiple lesions on bone scintigraphy will suggest metastatic disease but it may be normal in myeloma. MRI scan may be necessary to exclude malignancy particularly of the spine, but it is difficult to distinguish myeloma from an osteoporotic vertebral fracture.

Identifying cause of osteoporosis

Osteoporosis is idiopathic in the majority of women but secondary causes are identified in up to 55% of men. The underlying causes of bone loss should be sought (Table 198.4). They often manifest long before presentation with osteoporosis. Comorbidities that affect outcome of osteoporosis and fracture should be identified. These are common in the more elderly and should be treated where present and possible.

Identifying avoidable causes of falls

Fracture usually relates to trauma and causes of that trauma, most often a fall, must also be addressed (Table 198.5). Falls are most effectively prevented by recognizing those most at risk of falling, identifying any intrinsic or extrinsic risk factors and co-ordinating appropriate intervention. Intrinsic risk factors should be sought by a general

TABLE 198.5 CAUSES OF FALLS IN THE ELDERLY

Intrinsic factors

General deterioration associated with aging	Poor postural control
	Defective proprioception
	Reduced walking speed
	Weakness of lower limbs
	Slow reaction time
Balance, gait or mobility problems	Joint disease
	Cerebrovascular disease
	Peripheral neuropathy
	Parkinson's disease
	Alcohol
Multiple drug therapy	Sedatives
	Hypotensive drugs
	Various comorbidities
Visual impairment	Impaired visual acuity
	Cataracts
	Glaucoma
	Retinal degeneration
Impaired cognition or depression	Alzheimer's disease
	Cerebrovascular disease
'Blackouts'	Hypoglycemia
	Postural hypotension
	Cardiac arrhythmia
	TIA, acute onset cerebrovascular attack
	Epilepsy
	Drop attacks ? VBI

Extrinsic factors

Bad lighting
Steep stairs
Slippery floors
Loose rugs
Inappropriate footwear or clothing
Tripping over pets, grandchildren's toys, etc.
Uneven pavements
Bad weather
Lack of safety equipment such as grab rails

examination including checks on pulse, postural blood pressure, vision and neuromuscular function. A careful description of the fall from the patient or an eyewitness is essential. The drug history is important. A formal home assessment for extrinsic risk factors may be necessary, for example by an occupational therapist.

WHAT ARE THE TREATMENT OPTIONS?

Treatments should be evaluated separately for their effect on bone mass and on fracture rate. These effects may be independent for some interventions and the evidence should be considered separately. Primary prevention studies are usually performed in unselected women with normal bone density or in those with osteopenia (bone mineral density T score between −1 and −2.5) and in whom the absolute risk of fracture is low. Subsequently the antifracture efficacy cannot be easily tested, but bone mass is used as an intermediate endpoint. Studies of those at high risk of fracture enable the assessment of anti-fracture efficacy. Such studies are usually of those with osteoporosis (bone mineral density T score below −2.5) with or without a prevalent fracture.

In general pharmacological agents either decrease bone resorption leading to a secondary gain in bone mass or are anabolic with a direct increase of bone mass. Preferably these agents also increase bone strength and quality. Since the turnover of bone is slow, the time from initiating intervention to assessing effect on bone mass or fracture is

extended over years. This has an impact on design of trials – the selection of appropriate subjects (relative risk within duration of study) and duration of study (to ensure intended outcome is measurable within time frame). In addition, few trials assess the duration of effect beyond the treatment period – the offset of effect – which may be either prolonged or be lost soon after termination. This is clearly of clinical importance and influences effectiveness.

Some of these problems are obvious in evaluating intervention studies and hampers their reliability. The reporting of, for example, main outcome as in exact number of fractures or statistical corrections for persons partially completing or non-completers are not always transparent, unfortunately decreasing the quality of a study. A further difficulty is related to the fact that appropriately powered randomized controlled trials have not been made with fracture as end-point for all agents. In the following section the major interventions are briefly described and in some cases the difficulties in interpreting data are pointed out.

PHARMACOLOGICAL INTERVENTIONS

Calcium and vitamin D

Serum calcium levels are tightly regulated as calcium is essential for transmembrane transportation and cell communication for all cell types throughout the body. Bone tissue is the main calcium reservoir, and the bone mineral content is regulated through feedback systems that involve parathyroid hormone (PTH), calcium and vitamin D. PTH initiates bone resorption in response to low serum levels of ionized calcium. Consequently, insufficient calcium intake or absorption may provoke a continuous upregulation of PTH release causing increased bone loss. This low-grade secondary hyperparathyroidism is not uncommon in the elderly. This mechanism provides the rationale for calcium and vitamin D treatment as part of a strategy to prevent bone loss, particularly in the elderly.

Calcium – monotherapy

Calcium is the basic requirement for bone mineralization. The developing skeleton unequivocally needs calcium, while the effectiveness of calcium in the treatment of osteoporosis remains debated, particularly concerning fracture as outcome. Studies using calcium supplement alone as an anti-resorptive agent have shown conflicting results. In a recent Cochrane review[15] that included 15 studies and a total of 1806 women, a small but significant effect on bone density was seen at all measured sites. The anti-fracture effect was estimated at a relative risk of 0.77 (95%CI 0.54–1.09) for vertebral fracture and 0.86 (95%CI 0.43–1.72) for non-vertebral fracture. In an earlier meta-analysis evaluating the association between calcium and hip fracture, the estimates varied between a 3% to 12% fracture risk reduction from an increase in calcium intake of between 300 and 1000mg[16]. Benefits are greatest in those with a low calcium intake[17]. In almost all randomized controlled trials for bone specific anti-resorptive agents, calcium supplementation (400–800mg) is included in the placebo group and typically show a 0.5–2% gain in bone mass at the lumbar spine.

Calcium dietary enrichment or supplementation has also shown beneficial effects on the growing skeleton, with increasing bone density in young girls on additional calcium intake[18].

Vitamin D monotherapy

Vitamin D plays a central role in calcium regulation. It is either provided through food intake or by exposure of the skin to sunlight. Vitamin D, in the ingested form or from dermal conversion of 7-dehydrocholesterol by ultraviolet light, is biologically inactive until metabolized through several stages in the liver and kidneys. Vitamin D insufficiency is common in the elderly, particularly in northern latitude countries with few hours of sunlight.

TABLE 198.6 COMPARING THE FRACTURE EFFECT IN STUDIES OF CALCIUM AND VITAMIN D						
Substance	Indication for treatment	Total no. of patients (incl. placebo)	Mean age	Duration (years)	Type fracture	NNT (95% CI)
Calcium[26]	Osteoporosis + fracture	78	58	4	Fractures, various sites	NS
Vitamin D3[27]	Non-specific inclusion criteria	2578	80	3.5	Hip fracture	NS
					Other fractures	NS
Calcium + vitamin D3[24]	Non-specific inclusion criteria: institutionalized patients	1505	84	1.5	Hip fracture	47 (24–429)
					Fracture ≠ vertebra	24 (14–90)

Vitamin D3 supplement of 10μg/day (400IU/day) alone, with the assumption of adequate dietary calcium intake, has not been shown to reduce the incidence of fractures in studies of elderly men and women living in the community[19] or in nursing homes[20]. A recent Cochrane review[21] concluded that the fracture preventive effect from vitamin D supplementation alone was yet to be proven.

Vitamin D has, nevertheless, been shown to increase femoral neck bone density (0.2–2.6%) and reduce the rate of loss in elderly women after 2 years of treatment, while the effect on other skeletal sites remain similar compared to the placebo groups[22,23]. The dose required to obtain a measurable bone effect over this period was between 10–20μg/day.

Duration of treatment in a clinical setting will greatly exceed that of trials, and a long term additive fracture sparing effect directly related to the vitamin D intake cannot be ruled out, in addition to acting as an enhancer of calcium bioavailability.

Combined calcium and vitamin D

Calcium and vitamin D in combination is an accepted baseline treatment for osteoporosis and also as a preventive measure, in particular in the frail elderly. In a large randomized controlled study of elderly French nursing home patients given calcium (1200mg) and vitamin D (20μg, 800IU) there was significant reduction in new hip 0.70 (95% CI 0.62–0.78) and all non-vertebral fractures 0.70 (95% CI 0.51–0.91) after 3 years treatment, with significant benefit at 18 months[24,25] (Table 198.6). A smaller study of community dwelling men and women above age 65 showed a significant reduction in non-vertebral fractures on 17.5μg vitamin D3 and 500mg calcium[28]. It is also possible to give vitamin D as a yearly injection, an advantageous route of administration in institutionalized settings. In a Finnish study, elderly patients were given a yearly dose of 150 000–200 000IU of vitamin D with a significant reduction in fracture risk[29]. Data pooled from epidemiological studies also suggest a small anti-fracture effect of combination treatment[16,30].

These agents have shown an effect on bone mass both in the femoral neck[28], and in the spine in early postmenopausal women[31]. Furthermore in large randomized controlled trials of other agents, calcium and vitamin D supplementation is commonly used in both the placebo with a typical increase of 1–2% on bone density in comparison to baseline after 3–4 years and with a 10–20% decrease in bone turnover markers apparent after 3–6 months of treatment. In a RCT involving men, no effect was seen on spinal bone density after three years with 25μg vitamin D and 1000mg of calcium, but the subjects had a high baseline calcium intake which may obscure the effect or suggests that above a certain intake no additional advantages are evident.

Recommended supplementation

- Calcium 50–1000mg depending on dietary intake to reach above a total of 1200–1500mg/day
- Vitamin D 10–20μg (400–800IU) daily – the higher dose is indicated for institutionalized persons or those receiving equivalent care or during the winter in northern latitude countries

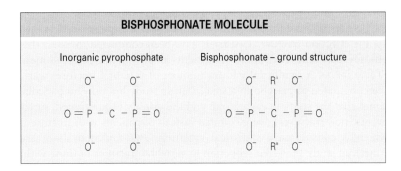

BISPHOSPHONATE MOLECULE

Inorganic pyrophosphate

Bisphosphonate – ground structure

Fig. 198.1 Bisphosphonate molecule.

Calcitriol

The active metabolite calcitriol (1,25 dihydroxyvitamin D) has theoretical therapeutic advantages compared to cholecalciferol, as metabolic activation is surpassed and, for example, an age-dependent decreasing kidney function becomes less important. Side effects include hypercalcemia and nephrolithiasis, which demands close monitoring of serum calcium.

The effectiveness of calcitriol and 1α (OH)-vitamin D is uncertain[4]. The effect on fracture is unclear as only one large one year study, with a much criticized methodology, has been performed[32]. The study was single blinded, included postmenopausal women with one or more vertebral fractures at baseline and it suggested an effect on new vertebral fractures. Other studies have shown inconsistent results, which in part may be related to variable calcium intakes[33,34].

Bisphosphonates

Bisphosphonates are chemically developed from pyrophosphates, compounds that inhibit precipitation of calcium carbonate and have industrial applications. Bisphosphonates are characterized by two C-P bonds (Fig. 198.1). When the bonds are on the same carbon atom as a P-C-P binding structure, it allows for large side chain variation which gives each compound specific physiologic and biochemical properties.

Bisphosphonates have bone anti-resorptive activity with little effect on other organ systems. Bisphosphonates act on bone by binding to the hydroxyapatite and inhibiting osteoclasts. Osteoclast numbers are reduced by inhibition of osteoclast recruitment and increased apoptosis, and osteoclast activity is reduced with decreased ruffled border, alterations of the cytoskeleton, decreased acid production and decreased production of lysosomal enzymes and prostaglandins[35]. Nitrogen-containing bisphosphonates, such as alendronate, risedronate and ibandronate inhibit the mevalonate pathway, while non-nitrogen containing bisphosphonates, such as etidronate, tiludronate or clodronate are metabolized in the cell into cytotoxic ATP analogues.

Bisphosphonates are poorly absorbed from the gastrointestinal tract. Only about 0.5–5% of a given dose is absorbed which is further decreased by food intake (particularly calcium containing foods) or even drinks such as coffee or juice, and is the reason why these drugs must be taken after a food free interval.

The plasma half-life of bisphosphonates is very short and the drug is displaced into bone tissue within 30 min to 2 hours, whereas the half-life of bisphosphonates deposited in bone is probably up to 10 years or more[35].

Side-chain substitution results in different bisphosphonates having up to 1000-fold different potency, which is clinically obviated by giving smaller doses, although variations may also be seen in clinical effects. The following section will therefore describe the main clinical studies related to each compound (see also Hochberg[36]).

Etidronate

Etidronate was the first available bisphosphonate for treatment of osteoporosis. Etidronate is taken cyclically, 400mg for 2 weeks every 3 months, since over dosage may cause mineralization defects.

There are no randomized controlled trials primarily powered to evaluate the effect on fracture. Two trials have been conducted to assess the efficacy of cyclic etidronate treatment in postmenopausal women (Table 198.7). A significantly lower number of vertebral fractures were seen compared to placebo in a small Danish study but only 20 patients completed the study in each group and the validity is questioned, since events (new fractures), were counted instead of patients with fractures, which is considered a statistical violation. *Post-hoc* analysis of an American study showed a reduction in vertebral fractures in those with the most severe osteoporosis[38]. In clinical practice, using prescription data from the British General Practice Research Database, patients on etidronate appear to have fewer non-vertebral fractures compared to patients not treated, however the study also indicates that the treated patients may have a different health situation[39].

Alendronate

Alendronate, a second generation bisphosphonate, was the first bisphosphonate for which a clear anti-fracture effect was seen in large randomized controlled trials. Three major trials have shown a reduction in vertebral deformities of about 50%, and prevention of non-vertebral fractures has been demonstrated.

The first study, which included postmenopausal women with low bone density (T-score ≤ 2.5) with or without prevalent vertebral deformity[40], found the effect was most pronounced in women above age 65 and with at least one vertebral fracture at entry. In the Vertebral Fracture Arm of the Fracture Intervention Trial 1 (FIT 1)[41] 2027 women with at least one prevalent vertebral fracture were included. Alendronate treatment over 3 years gave a highly significant reduction in the number of new radiographic and clinical vertebral fractures ($P = 0.0001$) (Table 198.8) and a significant reduction of hip ($P = 0.0001$) and wrist fractures ($P = 0.0001$), albeit the number of fractures was small. In the Clinical Fracture Arm of FIT (FIT 2) over 4000 women were included on the basis of low BMD (T-score femoral neck < -1.6) in a 4 year trial[42]. The reduction of radiographically verified vertebral deformities was significant, but not for clinically presented vertebral fractures (Table 198.7). In a pre-planned sub-group analysis, all clinical fractures were reduced in women with bone density below the WHO threshold for osteoporosis (T-score of -2.5). In an international multicenter study of alendronate, the number of non-vertebral fractures was reduced in postmenopausal women with a T-score below -2.0[1]. In a randomized placebo controlled study of men with osteoporosis ($n = 241$) treated with alendronate 10mg/day, the incidence of vertebral deformities was lower after two years of treatment (0.8% versus 7.1%, $P = 0.022$)[43] with a corresponding increase in bone mass ($P = 0.001$).

These findings imply that treatment with alendronate is most efficient in reducing fracture in those at highest risk of new fractures by having a prevalent vertebral fractures or bone density confirming osteoporosis (T score of -2.5 or below). Treatment of women at lower risk appears less beneficial with fracture prevention as the end point.

Bone density increases at all sites during alendronate treatment. When comparing with placebo the mean increase over three years is about 6%

in the lumbar spine, 4–4.5% in the femoral neck and 4.5–5.0% in the total hip measure. A significant 50–65% decrease of bone markers, particularly resorption markers such as N-telopeptide (NTx), is evident after 6–8 weeks of therapy[44].

Long-term treatment is often recommended, but data is still sparse concerning the continued anti-fracture effect. However, a sustained increase in BMD has been shown at all skeletal sites with 10mg/day of alendronate over 7 years in 235 postmenopausal women, which may suggest a concomitant anti-fracture effect[45]. The off-set of treatment after termination of alendronate therapy is not rapid as with hormone replacement but delayed over several years[46]. With the long-term deposition of alendronate in the skeleton, re-exposure at a site with new cycles of bone turnover is not excluded.

Treatment with alendronate 10mg/day has in clinical practice been linked to gastrointestinal side effects not identified in the randomized controlled trials of which esophageal erosions is the most serious. Side effects and the strict dosing routines for optimal absorption have lowered compliance.

A 70mg once weekly dosing regimen is now available which has been shown to give a similar increase in bone mass as daily or biweekly dosing in a study of 1258 postmenopausal women with osteoporosis. The fracture effect is assumed to be consistent with the reduction seen in earlier studies[47]. No increase in adverse GI events was experienced despite the higher dose, and there may even be a lower risk of serious GI events.

Estrogen and bisphosphonates act through different mechanisms on bone. A possible approach for those failing to gain enough bone on estrogen treatment alone or in those fracturing despite treatment would be to combine estrogen with a bisphosphonate. Two studies suggest an additive effect on BMD when combining estrogen treatment with alendronate in postmenopausal women over 1 or 2 years[48,49], but were not powered to evaluate the effect on fracture.

Risedronate

Risedronate is a third generation bisphosphonate with a 1000-fold higher potency than etidronate that has also been shown to prevent vertebral and non-vertebral fractures.

The number of radiographically diagnosed vertebral fractures was reduced by 41% and non-vertebral fractures reduced by 39% in a 3 year randomized controlled trial of 2458 postmenopausal women with one or more prevalent radiographic vertebral deformities[50] (Table 198.7). The study completion rate was only 55–60% as the 2.5mg group was discontinued prematurely and a high number of patients did not complete for other reasons. However, in the similar European and Australian arm of the trial which included women with two or more vertebral deformities ($n = 1226$), vertebral fractures were reduced by 49% and non-vertebral fractures by 33%[51].

Recently, results of a study to specifically evaluate the effect on hip fractures has been published[52]. Women aged 70–79 with low bone density ($n = 5445$) or women over 80 years with at least one risk factor for hip fracture ($n = 3886$) were randomized to risedronate or placebo. A 49% reduction in hip fracture was evident only in women with low bone density, while no effect was seen in the group of very elderly women aged 80–89 included on risk factors alone. Again this study points out that low bone density is a major determinant for clinical effect of anti-resorptive agents.

The effect on bone density is similar to that of alendronate producing about 4–6% increase in spinal and femoral bone mass after 3 years of treatment.

Risedronate has also become available in a once-weekly formula containing 35mg of active substance to be taken one day a week and thereby simplifying for the patients and enhance adherence to therapy[53].

Risedronate as other bisphosphonates, must be taken according to instructions. It appears to be well tolerated both in the studies and clinically with no serious side effects reported.

TABLE 198.7 THE EFFECT OF PHARMACOLOGICAL TREATMENT ON FRACTURE

Substance (reference)	Indication for treatment	No. of patients; mean age (range)	Duration (years)	Type of fracture; relative risk (95% CI)	NNT (95% CI)	Comments
Alendronate (FIT 1)[41]	Bone mineral density (−2.1) + vertebral fracture	2027; 71 years (55–81)	3	Vertebral fracture (X-ray) ε1; 0.53 (0.41–0.68)	15 (11–25)	A study of adequate design. In patients with prevalent vertebral fracture incident fractures are reduced. Because of small number of other fractures, only one additional hip fracture might have changed the result
				Vertebral fracture (X-ray) ε2; 0.10 (0.05–0.22)	24 (18–35)	
				Hip fracture; 0.49 (0.23–0.99)	90 (43–8949)	
				Vertebral fracture, symptomatic; 0.72 (0.58–0.90)	37 (23–89)	
Alendronate (FIT 2)[42]	Bone mineral density (−1.6) Subgroup: BMD ≤2.5	4432; 68 years (55–81) 266	4	Clinical fractures (all types); 0.86 (0.73–1.01)	NS	A study of adequate design. In patients without earlier fracture, only effect on radiographic vertebral fractures. Subgroup analysis showed effect also on other clinical fractures in women with BMD < −2.5SD. In women with BMD > −2.5SD no fracture reduction
				Vertebral fractures; 0.64 (0.50–0.82)	15 (10–35)	
Risedronate[50]	Osteoporosis + fracture	2458; 69 years (?–84)	3	Vertebral fractures; 0.59 (0.43–0.82)	20 (12–62)	The study is of adequate design, but suffers from a high discontinuation rate
				Non-vertebral fractures; 0.6 (0.39–0.94)	44 (22–640)	
				Hip fracture	NS	
Risedronate[51]	Osteoporosis + fracture	1226; 71 years (?–85)	3	Vertebral fractures; 0.51 (0.36–0.73)	10 (7–24)	The study is of adequate design, but suffers from a high discontinuation rate
				Non-vertebral; 0.67 (0.44–1.04)		
Risedronate[52]	Osteoporosis + fracture	5445; 71 years (?–85)		Hip fracture; 0.6 (0.4–0.9)	99 (52–421)	A study specifically designed to evaluate the effect on hip fracture. Indicates that risk factors alone are insufficient indicators for treatment
	Osteoporosis + risk factor	3886; 83 years	3	Hip fracture; 0.8 (0.6–1.2)	NS	
Etidronate[37]	Osteoporosis + fracture	66; 69 years	≤3	Vertebral fractures	NS	Not significant reduction when analyzed according to intention to treat
Etidronate[38]	Osteoporosis + fracture	378; 65 years	2	Vertebral fractures	NS	Not significant reduction when analyzed according to intention to treat
Raloxifene 60mg[69]	Osteoporosis	3012	3	Vertebral fractures 0.5 (0.4–0.8)	48 (29–120)	A large and well-done study with effect only on vertebral fractures
	Osteoporosis + fracture	1539		Vertebral fractures 0.7 (0.6–0.9)	16 (10–38)	
	Osteoporosis + fracture	7705 67 years (31–80)		Non-vertebral fractures 0.9 (0.8–1.1)	NS	
Estradiol + medroxy-progesterone[54]	Osteoporosis + fracture	75; 65 years	1 year	Vertebral fractures	NS	Limited from small size and short duration
Estradiol + norethisterone or estradiol alone[55]	Post-menopause	1006; 50 years	5 years	All types of fractures	NS	Reduction in wrist fractures when randomized and open label patients were pooled
Calcitonin[71]	Vertebal fracture	1255 70 yrs	5 yrs	Vertebral fractures 0.67 (0.47–0.97)	13 (7–77)	Only effect in the 200IU dose and not the higher dose. The study suffers from a high discontinuation rate
Parathyroid hormone[76]	Vertebal fracture	1637 70 yrs	21 mo	Vertebral fractures 0.31 (0.22–0.55)	11 (8–18)	Fracture reduction in high risk patients.
				Non-vertebal fractures 0.47 (0.25–0.88)		The study was prematurely ended, planned for 24 mo

Summary of major randomised controlled trials with fracture as primary end-point. The table includes number needed to treat (NNT). The interpretation of NNT must consider the specific conditions of the study and the values are therefore not necessarily directly comparable. From the perspective of evidence-based medicine, NNT is nevertheless the best way to obtain an overall comparison.

Sex hormones

The balance between bone resorption and bone formation in adulthood is, at least in part dependent on intact estrogen levels (see Chapter 192). The rapidly decreasing estrogen levels at menopause may lead to increased activation frequency, that is the number of active resorption sites increase while the capacity to refill the site with new bone diminishes causing bone loss. By substituting for estrogen loss or manipulating the estrogen receptor activity, the rate of bone turnover should remain in balance. This is the rationale for the use of ERT and for the development of new drugs that modify the ER.

TABLE 198.8 OPTIONS FOR PREVENTING OSTEOPOROSIS AND FRACTURE

For the population	Individuals at high risk of fracture
Health education	**Education**
• Raising awareness	Self management
• General health promotion	Exercise
	Physiotherapy
Promote healthy lifestyle	Rehabilitation
• Encourage physical activity	Calcium and vitamin D supplements
• Dietary calcium and vitamin D	Estrogen replacement therapy
• Avoid excess dieting	SERMs
• Avoid smoking	Fluoride
• Avoid excess alcohol	Calcitonin
	Bisphosphonates
Avoid premature estrogen deficiency	PTH
• Raising awareness of risks associated with estrogen deficiency	
	Fall prevention
	Targeted at the individual
Fall prevention	Hip protectors
• Promote physical activity	
• Reduce environmental hazards	

These can be considered for the population or for the individual.

Estrogen replacement

The initial indication for estrogen substitution to alleviate post-menopausal symptoms related to estrogen withdrawal, with the additional effect on bone turnover and bone mass have lead to wide use.

Unfortunately, the effect on fracture by ERT has only been evaluated in two prospective randomized controlled trials[54,55] (Table 198.7) with still inconclusive results and evidence of fracture efficacy relies on epidemiological or case-control studies[30,56–60] in which a 25–50% fracture risk reduction is seen. In the Danish Osteoporosis Prevention study ($n = 2016$) the number of fractures was not significantly reduced in the randomized groups, while pooling with the open label group showed a reduction in wrist fracture. In a meta-analysis identifying 22 studies, data on fractures suggests an overall reduction in non-vertebral fractures, which was more pronounced on women below age 60 (RR 0.67, 95% CI 0.46–0.98) after at least 12 months of HRT[61]. The analysis included both placebo and non-placebo controlled trials, published and unpublished reports and fractures caused by high energy trauma or malignancy, rendering the results less certain but nevertheless indicative.

Numerous studies have indicated the beneficial effect of ERT on bone mass, with an increase of between 2–4% over 3 years in the spine but less in the hip. Even lower doses of estrogen, which may be better tolerated in elderly women, appear to prevent bone loss, particularly in the spine, but there is no fracture data on reduced dosage[62–64].

Estrogen should be given opposed with either cyclic or continuous progestogen to women with intact uterus.

The major concern for most women deciding to start on HRT is regarding the risk of breast cancer. An increase in breast cancer incidence in women taking HRT was seen in a recent large meta-analysis[65]. The relative risk increase was RR 1.023 (95% CI 1.011–1.036) or equal to a 2.3% risk of breast cancer with each year of HRT, but the aggressiveness of identified tumors or mortality was not increased. The findings were recently comfirmed in the large randomized controlled trial as part of the Women's Health Initiative, specifically designed to evaluate the overall health benefits and risks of hormone treatment[66]. This trial included 16 608 postmenopausal women randomized to equine estrogen or placebo. At the 5.2-years safely monitoring, the risk estimates for breast cancer and cardiovascular events were significantly increased. On the other hand the study confirmed a risk reduction for hip fracture

(0.66, CI 0.45–0.98) and fracture in total. Duration of HRT should stay within 5–10 years or the risks may outweigh the benefits.

There is no upper age limit for initiating estrogen treatment, although it is better tolerated in recently postmenopausal women, in the elderly dose adjustments are normally necessary. If started in the early post-menopausal years an effect on vertebral fractures is more likely. The mean age for women with hip fracture is about 80 years of age and beginning HRT at later ages may then also confer protection of non-vertebral fractures, but other agents with proven fracture efficacy may be the treatment of choice in this situation. After discontinuation, the bone density effect of HRT rapidly disappears at a loss rate similar to that of normal menopause. Consequently, long-term effects on fracture cannot be assumed.

Raloxifene

Selective estrogen receptor modulators (SERM) have been developed related to the identification of estrogen receptors. Binding of raloxifene to the ERα blocks the conformational changes of the receptor and by this modulation alters its gene activation and subsequent protein production.

Raloxifene reduces the urinary calcium excretion, conferring a positive calcium balance[67] and decreases bone turnover assessed by bone markers[68].

In the Multiple Outcomes of Raloxifene Effectiveness (MORE) trial that enrolled 7705 osteoporotic women with and without vertebral fractures, there was an overall risk reduction of vertebral fractures (RR 0.70, 95% CI 0.50–0.80) with 60mg/day of raloxifene over 3 years[69] (Table 198.7). No effect was seen on non-vertebral fractures. Bone mass increased with 2.1% in the spine and 2.6% in the femoral neck on 60mg of raloxifene. The side effects were usually mild and mostly short lasting vasomotor symptoms. The more serious side effect was thromboembolic events, both deep vein thrombosis and pulmonary embolism, with a relative risk of 3.1 (95% CI 1.5–6.2) in the MORE trial, which corresponds to the risk with HRT.

New breast cancer cases were lower in the treated groups in the MORE study[70], despite the fact that the study was not powered to study breast cancer and at the 4-year follow up the risk reduction persisted[71]. Among the 5129 women treated with raloxifene 13 new cases were diagnosed, and in the placebo group of 2576 women 27 cases, giving an overall relative risk of 0.24 (95% CI 0.13–0.44). This apparent protective effect on the development of breast cancer is limited to those cancers that are estrogen receptor-positive; no reduction was noted in estrogen receptor-negative tumors.

Tibolone

Tibolone is a synthetic steroid with estrogenic, androgenic and gestagenic properties also exerting its effect by binding to the estrogen receptor. Tibolone relieves climacteric symptoms, without causing menstrual bleeding and with less breast tenderness compared to ERT. Two years of tibolone treatment in early postmenopausal women has shown a bone density response similar to that of ERT, but no data on fracture prevention is available[72,73].

Non-sex hormones

Calcitonin

Calcitonin is a peptide hormone with hypocalcemic and hypophosphatemic properties that acts as a physiologic antagonist to parathyroid hormone. Calcitonin is a 32 amino acid polypeptide synthesized in the parafollicular or C-cells of the thyroid gland, but under little pituitary control. Receptors for calcitonin are primarily present in bone and kidney. Calcitonin reduces bone resorption by acting on osteoclasts, rendering the cells smaller and less mobile, elevated serum calcium levels decrease and the renal excretion of calcium, sodium and phosphate increase. The bone effects have been extensively studied with hopes of obtaining a physiologic anti-resorptive agent. In addition, an analgesic effect from administration has been observed.

Calcitonin is available as subcutaneous or intramuscular injections or as nasal spray, developed from salmon calcitonin. Salmon calcitonin is about 10 times more potent than normally produced human calcitonin with a higher affinity for the receptor. Salmon calcitonin fragments may induce antibody production, a side effect more likely when using the parenteral route of administration. True allergic reactions or resistance are rare, while hot flushes and nausea are common transient side effects.

The potential of preventing vertebral fractures by nasal calcitonin in postmenopausal women is unclear. In a large study ($n = 1255$), postmenopausal women with one or more vertebral deformity were randomized to receive 100IU, 200IU or 400IU of calcitonin for 5 years. Fracture reduction assessed by X-ray was only seen in women treated with 200IU [RR 0.67 (95% CI 0.47–0.97)], while the higher dose 400IU did not significantly affect the fracture rate[74]. Radiographs were available in 88% of the women at one occasion, but only 511 (41%) of the included women completed the 5 year trial. Spinal bone mineral density increased between 1–1.5% from baseline.

In an earlier meta-analysis examining the efficacy of calcitonin in maintaining bone mass, eighteen clinical trials of various length were identified[75]. The mean increase in spinal BMD was 1.97% (CI 1.77–2.17) and in the femoral neck 0.32% (CI 0.27–0.91). The analysis also suggested an effect on vertebral fracture incidence.

In conclusion, present data suggest a relatively smaller effect on bone mineral density from calcitonin treatment compared to other anti-resorptive agents, while a reduction in vertebral fractures may still be induced. It has been speculated that the anti-fracture effect may be related to enhanced bone quality, which is not identified from DEXA measurements.

Parathyroid hormone

The physiological function of parathyroid hormone (PTH) is to maintain extracellular calcium levels. Rapid changes in the plasma calcium levels results from hormonal effects on bone and to a lesser extent on the kidney with change in renal calcium clearance. The effects are either direct on target cells or indirectly mediated through synthesis of 1,25 dihydroxyvitamin D. There is evidence for a dual action on bone and both osteoblasts and osteoclasts are responsive to PTH. Osteoblast differentiation and activity is stimulated as is the recruitment of lining cells and osteoclasts increase in number and activity. The resorptive effect predominates during sustained elevation of PTH, as is also seen in primary or secondary hyperparathyroidism, while an anabolic effect on bone is seen with intermittent dosing.

PTH consists of a single-chain peptide of 84 amino acids. The sequence and structure is well defined and it has been found that the N-terminal 1–34 amino acid residues are essential for the hormonal activity.

Utilizing the anabolic properties of PTH on bone has therefore been an attractive concept in order to obtain larger increases in bone mass than possible with anti-resorptive agents. PTH has been shown to primarily increase the cancellous or trabecular bone, hence the most pronounced effects have been seen in spinal bone density[76]. However, a smaller effect is also seen on the endosteal surface of cortical bone, including increased breaking strength in animal studies[77,78].

Recombinant human PTH (rhPTH) given as subcutaneous injection has been tested in patients with osteoporosis. Postmenopausal women with prevalent vertebral fractures ($n = 1637$) receiving 20 or 40μg of rhPTH 1–34 experienced a 65–69% (95% CI 0.22–0.55 and 0.19–0.50) reduction in new vertebral fractures and 53–54% (95% CI 0.25–0.88 and 0.25–0.86) reduction in non-vertebral fractures over 21 months[79]. There was a dose dependent increase in spinal and femoral neck BMD of 9–13% and 6–9%, respectively. Other studies have shown marked

increases in predominantly spinal BMD and suggested reduction in vertebral fractures, particularly when PTH has been combined with agents reducing bone resorption[80,81].

The availability of PTH, as an anabolic agent, opens up the treatment options for severe cases of osteoporosis, unresponsive to other agents or possibly when side effects prohibits their use. Since PTH needs to be more closely monitored because of risk for hypercalcemia, cyclic combination therapy of PTH with for example a bisphosphonate may be a future alternative for longer term treatment.

Other substances

Fluoride

Fluoride is a potent anabolic agent acting directly on the osteoblast by altering intracellular signal transduction. The effect of fluoride on bone was initially identified as endemic fluorosis in regions of high natural fluoride content in drinking water, causing dental and skeletal deformities and increased bone fragility. Fluoride has been shown to promote incremental increases in bone formation and this anabolic effect can be utilized in the treatment of osteoporosis if the dose is titrated to stay within a therapeutic window. However this is without a demonstrated reduction in fracture rate[82–84]. Further development of fluoride treatment is not anticipated without clear evidence of an anti-fracture effect and the continued suspicion of a detrimental effect on bone quality and bone strength.

Novel therapies

Increasing knowledge of mechanisms regulating bone cell activity provides potential sources for new therapeutic strategies. The unique ability of osteoclasts to dissolve and degrade bone tissue includes production of numerous substances both for mineral dissolution and the enzymatic degradation of matrix. The degradation of matrix is mediated by cathepsin K, an osteoclast protease which appears to specifically act on bone collagen[85]. Animal models confirm the important effect of cathepsin K and deletion of the cathepsin K gene results in an osteopetrotic bone in mice[86]. An inhibitor of cathepsin K may therefore have potential use as an anti-resorptive drug. Recent knowledge on cell differentiation and cell activity shows that cytokines are important regulators on the local level. In addition, molecular biology has provided novel insight about the intracellular signaling and transcellular communication. Most cytokines are implicated as enhancers of osteoclast activity and subsequently bone resorption. Blockage of cytokine activity has already gained success with the anti-TNFα treatment of rheumatoid arthritis (RA), which may have additional effects on bone turnover, since TNFα has been shown to be one of the more important cytokines modifying bone resorption. Bone resorption markers significantly decrease in patients with RA treated with infliximab[87]. This may allow for development of inhibitors to other bone active cytokines, such as IL-1 or IL-6. The relative non-specificity and subsequent effects on other organs may limit the usefulness.

Identification of factors acting on receptors for osteoclast attachment or function, such as the $\alpha_v\beta_3$integrin, RANKL (receptor activator of nuclear factor κB ligand) or the soluble ligand osteoprotegerin may be fertile ground for development of antagonists. Clinical testing of osteoprotegerin indicates a positive effect on bone density in postmenopausal women[88].

NON-PHARMACOLOGICAL INTERVENTION

Physical exercise

Physical activity is of benefit for the well-being and general health of every person. Mechanical loading of the skeleton is one of the mechanisms by which bone remains physiologically intact as it is an important signal for bone remodeling. Bone mass increases in response to increased load. The question is whether the beneficial effect on bone of physical exercise is maintained beyond active training or through periods of inactivity and if a risk reduction of falls and fracture is measurable.

Evaluating current and lifetime effects on exercise retrospectively indicates higher total and hip BMD in persons exercising[89]. Exercise programs appear to increase bone mass by a few percent in the post-menopausal and elderly women[90]. This is consistent with a meta-analysis which separately estimated the effect from impact and non-impact training in randomized controlled trials[91]. Impact exercise conferred a 0.9–1.6% non-significant net gain in spine or femoral neck bone density in pre- and postmenopausal women. The effect from non-impact exercise was 1.0–1.2% in the spine and not calculable in the femoral neck because of too few trials. Evidence suggests a stronger effect of exercise in childhood prior to sexual maturation and achievement of peak bone mass[92].

Longitudinal and cross-sectional studies suggest a protective effect against fracture in women with a higher physical activity level[93–95]. Since physical activity only gives a small percentage increase in bone mass, it is likely that a significant contribution of an anti-fracture effect is related to improvement of balance, co-ordination and muscle strength. These factors may not only reduce the risk of falls by tripping or misplacing steps, but also reduce the impacts by increased ability to protect and counteract a fall.

Prospective studies indicate that it is possible in the elderly to increase muscle strength[96] and to improve balance with a concomitant decrease in the number of falls[97–99] through exercise programs.

In these studies, as in studies evaluating the effect on bone mass, an effect induced by sampling or participation bias cannot be excluded, and it remains a challenge to determine the full effect of physical activity.

Smoking cessation

Numerous epidemiological studies indicate an independent risk increase of osteoporosis from smoking, the relative risk being between 1.2–1.8[100,101]. Smokers often have additional risk factors and comorbidities such as chronic pulmonary obstruction or emphysema.

The adverse effect of smoking is more pronounced in current smokers and dose dependent with a greater impact in men compared to women[102] with an overall bone mass reduction of 0.1 SD, but most pronounced at the hip and with a positive effect on bone mass with cessation. In addition, an increased risk of hip fracture is seen in both sexes (RR 1.36–1.59), with a higher risk in male smokers[103]. After 5 years male ex-smokers had a decreased risk of hip fracture, while no risk reduction was seen in women, suggesting a longer lasting negative effect of smoking in women.

Hip protectors

Hip fracture, the most debilitating fragility fracture, occurs predominantly in the elderly. An estimated 25% of fracture patients are admitted from institutions or various forms of residential care, indicating the frailty and morbidity of these patients. Hip fractures usually result from a sideways fall with maximum impact on the trochanter to which the faller is unable to take any protective measures. Hip fracture patients are often thin with only minimal cushioning from subcutaneous tissue over the hip. External hip protectors have been developed to reduce the impact on the fall and subsequently the incidence of hip fracture.

An external hip protector has a hard external surface with an underlying soft padding close to the body and it is formed to fit over the trochanter. They are either attached to the underwear or by Velcro belts and worn under clothes.

Studies to evaluate the efficacy of external hip protectors have been made on institutionalized patients of high age (mean 80–85 years), acknowledged frequent fallers and at high risk of hip fracture[104–106] and a Cochrane review concludes that hip protectors reduce the risk of hip fracture in selected populations[107]. One problem has been the low acceptance by the users which has been down to 30–40%.

Fall prevention

The vast numbers of non-vertebral fractures are related to falls, and measures to prevent falls and to reduce the impact of a fall are first line interventions to prevent fractures in those at risk. Fall preventive strategies are aimed at external or environmental factors, both in the home and in society, and at internal or patient related factors. Such factors are described in Table 198.5.

Falls become increasingly common with aging. About 30% of individuals over 65 years fall each year, increasing to 50% over 80 years, most common amongst residents of long-term care institutions. Most falls occur indoors where the majority of hip fractures occur. The likelihood of an elderly person falling is increased if he or she has fallen already. Although not all falls result in fracture, many result in impaired health, hospitalization and permanent disability. There will be an identifiable treatable cause of the fall in 10% of cases; an identifiable environmental cause in a further 10% but the cause of most falls is multifactorial and relates to general ill-health – more specifically, to sensory and musculoskeletal decline with lower limb weakness, unsteadiness and loss of protective mechanisms. The inability to rise unaided from a chair without using the arms is an important risk factor of falls and is common in institutionalized people.

The role of exercise in reducing falls has been discussed above. Interventions to reduce the risk of falling at home are aimed at minimizing known hazards related to falls, such as loose carpets, electrical cords, abundance of furniture or insufficient indoor light. Numerous studies have described the hazards and indicate the attributable risks. Prevention programs, both self-assessed through check-lists or carried out by home care providers, have been developed[10]. The long-term efficacy of fall prevention programs is difficult to evaluate and information is lacking with regards to fracture. Available studies suggest that modification of home hazards particularly in the elderly with a history of falling can reduce the risk of additional falls by 30–40%[108,109], while the evidence is not conclusive in unselected populations.

Preventive steps to reduce hazards in other areas of society should also result in a reduced risk of falls and of fracture, but there is little evidence. Elderly persons sustain falls and fracture in traffic areas without being directly related to traffic accidents for example from slippery or uneven side-walks and curbs, buses starting or breaking abruptly or inadequate snow and ice removal[110].

Rehabilitation following osteoporotic fracture

An important part of the management of osteoporosis is the rehabilitation of subjects following a fracture.

Fracture treatment aims to restore anatomical continuity allowing the patient to regain function or minimize the loss of function and to diminish associated pain. With either conservative or operative treatment the rehabilitation period may last up to a year.

For patients returning to their home a multidisciplinary team-approach often gives a superior result[111]. Hip fracture patients should have a complete assessment of their pre-fracture situation with respect to physical functioning, home and social situation. Based on this assessment an individual rehabilitation plan should be developed including a 'best-outcome' estimate. The plan should be developed with the patient so that he or she has an understanding of the goals, in order to make it successful.

Rehabilitation after hip fracture is often undertaken in the home with support from community health professionals. It is imperative that the care givers are educated in and have an understanding of the different aspects involved in the rehabilitation and healing process after fracture. Walk training, use of walking aids and later adapted exercise programs need to be monitored, but most of all, the patient needs to be encouraged.

The severely disabled elderly women who have previously suffered from multiple fractures including vertebral fractures may need rehabilitative efforts. The main goal should be to preserve the remaining physical function to allow as much independence of self-care as possible. The ability to stand with or without support is an important functional divide in the most frail and the main objective of lower limb fracture treatment. Long periods of non-weight bearing are often detrimental to the standing and walking capability in the elderly, therefore it is equally important to achieve stable fracture fixation in the elderly. With upper extremity fracture early motion training leads to better long term function. Even if full range of motion is not regained the functional impairment may not be perceived as detrimental.

Rehabilitation should also include preventive measures against future fracture. Simple training programs of balance, co-ordination and muscle strength can accomplish improvement even in the eldest[112].

MANAGEMENT STRATEGIES

The principles of fracture prevention are to maximize bone strength and to prevent falls at the age when fracture risk is greatest, that is in later life, and prevention must be considered at all stages of life to achieve this. In addition, those who have already sustained a fracture must be appropriately managed to ensure the best possible outcome.

Strategies will be discussed for the population as a whole and for the individual (Fig. 198.2), relating evidence-based interventions with clinical experience.

Fracture prevention at the population level

Fracture prevention requires addressing all factors that can modify fracture risk throughout life (Fig. 198.2). These recommendations must be supported by raising public awareness of osteoporosis and of what factors should raise their concern about personal risk and the potential health gain to be achieved by its prevention.

Peak bone mass is the major determinant of bone mass in later stages of life. A total of 60–80% of peak bone mass is genetically determined, the rest depending on factors such as nutrition, physical activity and adequate sex hormone levels. The skeleton consolidates in young adults and then turnover is in balance to maintain a relatively stable bone mass. Prevention entails establishing and maintaining a lifestyle that ensures maximum bone mass at all times of life. Exercise increases bone density but the effect is dependent on continued loading so that any activity needs to be sustainable throughout life. Calcium intake influences peak bone mass achieved (Table 198.9). Smoking and excess alcohol are associated with low bone density as is over-exercise and over-dieting leading to hypogonadism and amenorrhea. There needs to be greater awareness of the risk of future osteoporosis associated with reduced exposure to female sex hormones, such as with primary hypogonadism or secondary amenorrhea to encourage early recognition and management.

Bone mass starts to decline in the 5th and 6th decades, slowly in men; however, the menopause marks the onset of rapid bone loss in some women. Regular physical activity, exercise and avoidance of smoking and excess alcohol are recommended. The rate of bone loss may be slowed down at any stage by ERT. Its use is a balance between the individual's risk and the potential benefit and risks from ERT and any decision needs to be made at the level of that individual. Health promotion campaigns should make all women aware of these options and of factors that may influence their own risks of future fracture.

Most fractures occur above the age of 65 years. Over this age there is also the clearest separation between the fit and the unfit aging population. Apart from specific conditions, the level of physical activity is one of the best discriminators of this and much effort needs to be put into trying to encourage people to increase their level of physical activity in a way that is sustainable throughout old age. This will have a small effect on bone mass but the benefit of exercise at this age is more directly related to improving muscle strength, lower limb function, co-ordination and balance with a reduction in risk of falls. At this age bone mass is low in an increasing number and the occurrence of falls is an important discriminator of who does and who does not fracture. Awareness must also to be raised of risk factors for falls and environmental causes should be removed. In addition, dietary dairy intake often reduces as age increases and calcium intake must be improved by reversing this trend or by encouraging the use of supplements (Table 198.9). Lack of going outdoors with consequent low sunlight exposure and as well as poor diet can lead to vitamin D insufficiency with secondary hyperparathyroidism, and these trends need reversing.

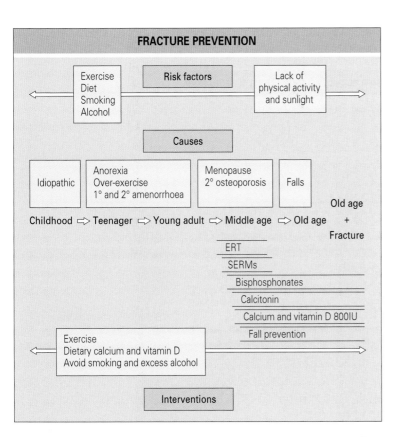

Fig. 198.2 Fracture prevention. Fracture prevention requires addressing all factors that modify fracture risk at all stages of life.

TABLE 198.9 RECOMMENDED DAILY DIETARY ALLOWANCE FOR CALCIUM

Group	Age (years)	Range (mg)
Newborn	0–0.5	400
Children	1–3	400–600
	4–6	450–600
	7–10	550–700
Men	11–24	900–1000
	25–65	700–800
	65–	700–800
Women	11–24	900–1000
	25–50	700–800
	50–65	800
	65–	700–800
Pregnant		700–900
Lactating		1200
(Adapted from European Community Report[3].)		

Fracture prevention in the individual

The prevention of a fracture in an individual requires treating those at highest risk of fracture and addressing all risk factors linked to fracture with low bone mass being one of the most important. It also means preventing fracture in those already with osteoporosis. In addition, any one who has sustained an osteoporotic fracture needs appropriate management to ensure the best outcome.

Who to treat

Those at highest risk of osteoporosis and future fracture need to be recognized at all stages of life.

In childhood and early adulthood the commonest specific cause relates to gonadal hormone deficiency which can affect both sexes. Females with late menarche and secondary amenorrhea need to be identified, the underlying cause found and treated. Anorexia nervosa and over-exercise syndrome are common causes. Infertility is often associated with low estrogen levels that need to be treated beyond the management of infertility. Pregnancy can be rarely associated with osteoporosis with rapid loss of spinal bone mass and fracture. Adequate nutrients during the growth phase are important and lactose intolerance can result in lifelong low calcium intake. Other conditions include celiac disease, causes of prolonged immobility, and steroid treated inflammatory conditions such as juvenile idiopathic arthritis, asthma, inflammatory bowel disease, or rheumatoid arthritis. Cystic fibrosis now has a better prognosis but is often complicated by osteoporosis and may present with fracture. Osteogenesis imperfecta often manifests as childhood fractures. Diagnosis of osteoporosis is difficult by bone density in the growing skeleton as it is dependent on stage of puberty and the relationship of T or Z score with fracture risk is not established at this age.

From mid-life and onwards idiopathic osteoporosis becomes increasingly common. Those who will benefit most from an intervention can be identified by the combination of risk factors (Table 198.1) and bone densitometry. Identification and investigation is only appropriate if the person is prepared to and capable of taking any recommended treatment for long enough to achieve its goal of fracture prevention (Fig. 198.3). Women and men at high risk can either be found by a systematic approach at a midlife health check or opportunistically when being seen for an intercurrent problem. Risk factors may be documented on health records. A low trauma fracture at this age, such as a Colles fracture, is a strong risk factor for future fracture. Many are however not in routine contact with their family physicians and public awareness campaigns are needed to encourage them to inquire about their individual needs for preventive therapy for osteoporosis.

In the more elderly, it is important to target those who are frail and with an adherent risk of falling, as well as those with other risks for fracture. The benefit from any intervention is greater at this age because of the increased incidence of fractures in the later decades of life. The opportunities for case finding are greater at this age as many will be in contact with health professionals for routine procedures such as flu vaccination or as a result of various intercurrent problems. Indeed, an unique opportunity for case finding is the patient who presents with a low trauma fracture.

The person may present with a low energy fracture of the limb bones or pelvis, a sudden onset of back pain or a gradual loss of height and stoop.

The management of osteoporosis once confirmed

When osteoporosis has been diagnosed the appropriate management must be considered.

Education and support

Osteoporosis must be fully explained to the individual so they understand what the risks are and what they can do to reduce them. They may not have sustained a fracture and one must be careful not to give them a 'disease' when it is a risk they have for a possible future fracture. A bone-healthy lifestyle must be encouraged and unnecessary fear avoided.

Maximize bone strength

Bone mass must be maximized to increase strength and reduce risk of fracture.

In the developing skeleton and younger adults, as these situations are all uncommon, there is little evidence as yet for different interventions, and it is unlikely that fracture prevention data will become readily available. The principles are to treat the underlying condition effectively,

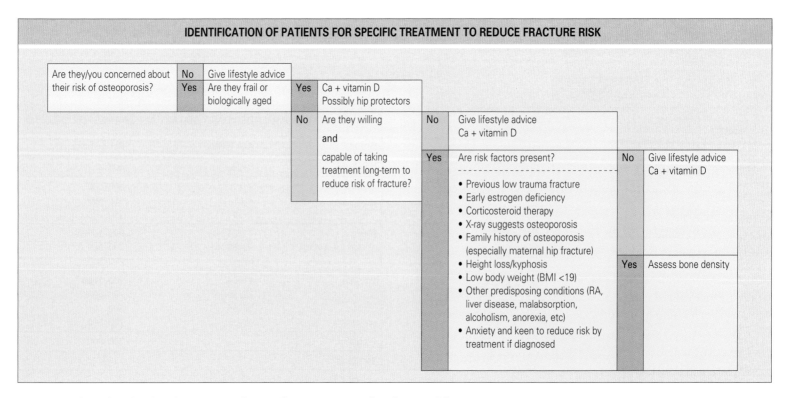

IDENTIFICATION OF PATIENTS FOR SPECIFIC TREATMENT TO REDUCE FRACTURE RISK

Fig. 198.3 A flow chart for identifying patients for specific treatment to reduce fracture risk.

TABLE 198.10 RECOMMENDATIONS FOR MANAGEMENT BASED ON HIP–BONE DENSITY	
T > –1	Lifestyle advice
T –1 to –2.5	Lifestyle advice HRT
T –1 to –2.5 and low-energy fracture	Investigate for causes of fracture Treat • Lifestyle advice *and one of* • Bisphosphonate • SERM • HRT • Intranasal calcitonin
T < –2.5	Investigate for causes of osteoporosis Treat • Lifestyle advice *and one of* • Bisphosphonate • SERM • HRT • Intranasal calcitonin
T < –2.5 and low-energy fracture	Investigate for causes of osteoporosis Investigate for causes of fracture Treat • Lifestyle advice *and one of* • Bisphosphonate • SERM • HRT • Intranasal calcitonin

TABLE 198.11 PRINCIPLES OF FALL PREVENTION

- Identify treatable causes (Table 198.5)
- Maintenance of fitness, balance and alertness
- Maintenance of vision and hearing
- Reduction of environmental hazards
- Reduce impact of falls

TABLE 198.12 PRINCIPLES OF TREATMENT OF ESTABLISHED OSTEOPOROSIS

- Explanation to and education of the patient and partner or care-giver
- Fracture management
- Pain management
- Functional assessment and practical advice
- Physiotherapy advice and exercise regimes
- Prevention of falls and of their impact
- Prevention and attempted reversal of bone loss

ensure adequate estrogen levels and avoid any excessive use of corticosteroids where relevant. Specific treatments have to be considered on the merits of the individual case. There is increasing experience of the effective use of bisphosphonates in children and young adults, mainly in the management of osteogenesis imperfecta[113].

At mid-life, in addition to recommending a bone health promoting lifestyle, bone loss may also be slowed down by ERT, SERM or bisphosphonates. There is little comparative data between the different treatment options. The intervention chosen and duration of treatment may be based on estimated fracture risk from the T-score measured by bone densitometry (Table 198.10). Because of offset of effect, treatment will have to be taken long-term to prevent fracture at the age they are most prevalent, that is over 70 years. The risks and health economics of this approach have to be considered. From an evidence based point of view the anti-fracture effect is significant only in those with osteoporosis or prevalent vertebral fracture. That is why any specific intervention at this age is targeted at those who are at highest risk of future fracture and why interventions that have broader benefits than just on bone mass and fracture risk should be first considered.

Over 65 years a bone healthy promoting lifestyle is recommended as there is most evidence at this age that correcting calcium deficiency and increasing physical activity are effective. Calcium and vitamin D should be the baseline treatment and have been shown to prevent hip fracture in the institutionalized elderly[24,25]. Bisphosphonates, SERM and calcitonin reduce bone loss and can prevent fracture. There is little comparative data between the different treatment options in this situation. Bisphonates are clearly most effective in those with osteoporosis.

Prevent falls and their impact

Falls can be prevented by identifying those most at risk of falling (Table 198.5) and coordinating appropriate preventive action (Table 198.11).

Interventions are most effective that target both the multiple intrinsic risk factors for the individual and environmental hazards[10].

The likelihood of an elderly person falling is increased if he or she has fallen already. It is therefore important to look for the causes of a fall and to try and prevent further falls in future from that or any other correctable cause. Structured home visits can be effective in identifying and modifying both intrinsic and extrinsic causes of the fall. Falls can be reduced by exercise programs that concentrate on improving lower limb strength, co-ordination and balance. Exercises can also improve protective responses.

Hip protectors can prevent fracture of the hip and should be considered in recurrent fallers who have osteoporosis.

The management of established osteoporosis

Once a fracture has occurred in the presence of low bone density, it is called established osteoporosis. Management is directed at the prevention of further fracture and the control of pain and the rehabilitation of the person. Fractures are typically of the distal radius, proximal femur or vertebral bodies, but low bone mineral density is associated with low trauma fractures at all sites except the head.

The aims of treatment are to relieve symptoms, by controlling pain and appropriate fracture treatment, to improve quality of life by tackling functional and practical problems, and to prevent further fractures by prevention of falls and reversal of bone loss (Table 198.12).

Education and support

A patient can cope much better with a chronic painful disabling disease if they have a good understanding of it and know what to expect. Information is available from support organizations and programs that teach self-management but can with advantage be developed locally.

Fracture management

Survival and future independence depends on proper management of the acute fracture. Comorbidity affects outcome and many are frail and confused when they fracture their hip. For the best outcome it is recommended[114] that hip fracture cases should be rapidly transferred to hospital, receive adequate pain relief and pressure area protection, and have surgery if possible within 24 hours. Antibiotic prophylaxis and anticoagulation to prevent thromboembolism are part of routine care. Postoperative pain management, adequate hydration, early mobilization followed by a structured rehabilitation program are important.

Pain management

Pain management is essential for the effective rehabilitation of the person with an acute or previous fracture. Patients tend to avoid analgesics and hence undertreat their pain. Analgesics should be selected according to severity of pain and response to previous treatment.

Acute vertebral fracture may require short-term use of opiate analgesics and bed rest for the first few days to get the pain under control and allow early mobilization. This should be on a background of simple analgesics such as paracetamol, dextropropoxyphene, tramadol or a NSAID. If NSAIDs are used, COX 2 selective inhibitors are recommended in view of age and likely presence of other risk factors for serious upper gastrointestinal complications. It is important to use sufficiently high and regular doses of analgesics to avoid peaks of pain and optimize pain control. If this is inadequate, calcitonin (100IU on alternate days by injection for up to 6 weeks) has some analgesic effects but can be associated with nausea, vomiting, flushing and dizziness. As the pain improves, opiate analgesics should be discontinued. The early introduction of antiresorptive therapy with bisphosphonates will decrease bone fragility and may reduce pain.

Chronic pain may require long-term treatment with analgesics which may need to be used regularly and in combination to gain maximum effect but full pain relief is an optimistic outcome. Tricyclic antidepressants may improve pain control but need to be used with caution to avoid daytime sedation with increased risk of falling. Heat, ultrasound, and massage can help to reduce muscle spasm. Corsets seldom help as they constrict an already compressed abdomen and chest. Surgical vertebroplasty, lifting and augmenting the collapsed vertebra, may be a future possibility to decrease pain.

Functional and practical problems and advice

A multidisciplinary approach is needed to assess and discuss problems of everyday life and provide solutions where possible. Many older people lose independence following a limb fracture. Rehabilitation may need to include everything from simple walking aids to home assessment or advanced home care.

Physiotherapy advice and exercise in osteoporosis

The aim of physiotherapy is to reduce symptoms and disability related to the fracture often worsened by comorbidity. Early mobilization is necessary to avoid pressure sores, constipation, venous thromboembolism, disorientation and dependency. Physiotherapy may be used to increase body awareness, encourage pain avoiding behavior, improve balance and coordination and reduce risk and fear of falls. An individualized exercise program is often needed because of pain and comorbidities. Additional benefits of motivation and social interaction can be gained if the program can be performed in a group setting, which also may improve compliance. Any exercise must not increase the risk of falling. Hydrotherapy is especially suitable if in pain and mobility is restricted.

Specific exercises for vertebral osteoporosis should also be encouraged. These should include relaxation to relieve muscle spasm; breathing exercises; and strengthening of postural (legs, back, and abdominals), pelvic floor, shoulder girdle and neck muscles. The exercises should be tried cautiously at first, preferably under supervision, and then performed regularly if they do not aggravate symptoms and are not too exhausting. Height and posture should be monitored. Manipulation should be avoided.

Prevention of further bone loss and fracture

Osteoporosis should be confirmed by bone densitometry, although multiple vertebral fractures are almost always diagnostic of osteoporosis. Bone loss cannot be fully restored at this stage but further bone loss can be slowed or reversed as recommended above with reduction in risk of further fracture. Falls should be prevented where possible by looking for and modifying causes and risk factors. Consideration should be given to the use of hip protectors.

MONITORING TREATMENT

Bone mineral density

Bone mineral density is a surrogate end-point for fracture, but it is the effect measure that is possible to evaluate in the individual patient. Because of the precision error of available bone densitometers and the low rate of change in bone mass even with pharmacological treatment options, reevaluation of the patients is usually not meaningful in clinical practice until after 2 years of anti-resorptive therapy. At the time of remeasurement of bone mass, a change less than 2% in the individual patient it is most likely not clinically significant. The estimated rate of loss of 0.5–1.0% per year that might have occurred without any intervention may be considered at reevaluation.

Follow-up measurements by DXA of the hip or spine are validated, while treatment response has not been followed long term by ultrasound of the heel.

Bone markers

Bone markers are extensively studied and used as early markers of effect in pharmaceutical trials. Most therapies act by repressing bone resorption, consequently the major effect is seen on bone resorption markers, such as deoxypyridinoline, N- or C-telopeptide (NTx, CTx,). A 40–60% decrease is commonly observed after 6–12 weeks of specific anti-resorptive therapy with bisphosphonates. The problem in using bone markers is related to the analytical and biological variability, particularly the relatively high intra-individual variability. Part of these problems can be reduced by standardized sampling procedures. If used properly, bone markers have potential in monitoring treatment and evidence suggests that markers can predict the BMD response to treatment for 2–3 years[11].

Quality of life

Osteoporosis with either vertebral or non-vertebral fractures influence quality of life and this should be monitored to ensure optimal management. Pain and loss of physical function, especially mobility, are the common problems with limitation of activities and restricted participation along with anxiety about future fracture. A number of validated instruments are available to measure outcome such as the EFFOQOL[115] which includes questions in the domains pain, physical function, social function, general health perception and mental function. Such instruments are however often too complex to use in regular practice. A simple 4-5-questionnaire would be of advantage for the practising physician to provide a simple, rapid and systematic evaluation of the quality of life that could be used on a regular basis in the clinic. This questionnaire should consider pain that affects function; self care such as washing and dressing; independent activities such as going out; and well-being – are you happy. Suggestions for questions are; (1) "Have you experienced pain that limited your daily activities during the past week?"; (2) "Are you able to wash and dress your-self?"; (3) "Have you walked outside for pleasure or shopping during the past 2 weeks?"; and (4) "Are you satisfied with your current living situation?".

CONCLUSION

- Patients with fracture or with background factors associated with high risk of fracture should be assessed for osteoporosis.
- Patients with high risk of fracture should be considered for specific treatment to reduce the risk of fracturing, dietary assessment and supplementation with calcium and vitamin D.
- Non-pharmacological interventions to prevent falls and to improve bone mass should be encouraged throughout life, emphasizing that the effect is sustained only in those currently training.

REFERENCES

1. Pols HA, Felsenberg D, Hanley DA et al. Multinational, placebo-controlled, randomized trial of the effects of alendronate on bone density and fracture risk in postmenopausal women with low bone mass: results of the FOSIT study. Foxamax International Trial Study Group. Osteoporos Int 1999; 9: 461–468.
2. Genant HK, Cooper C, Poor G et al. Interim report and recommendations of the World Health Organization Task Force for Osteoporosis. Osteoporos Int 1999; 10: 259–264.
3. Report on osteoporosis in the European Community: action for prevention. Luxembourg: European Communities Report; 1998.
4. National Osteoporosis Foundation. Osteoporosis: review of the evidence for prevention, diagnosis and cost-effectiveness analysis 11. Osteoporos Int 1998; 8: S1–S88.
5. Osteoporosis: clinical guidelines for prevention and treatment. London: Royal College of Physicians; 1999.
6. Lauritzen JB. Hip fractures: incidence, risk factors, energy absorption, and prevention. Bone 1996; 18(suppl): 65S–75S.
7. Hans D, Dargent-Molina P, Schott AM et al. Ultrasonographic heel measurements to predict hip fracture in elderly women: the EPIDOS prospective study. Lancet 1996; 348: 511–514.
8. Gardsell P, Johnell O, Nilsson BE, Gullberg B. Predicting various fragility fractures in women by forearm bone densitometry: a follow-up study. Calcif Tissue Int 1993; 52: 348–353.
9. Espallargues M, Sampietro-Colom L, Estrada MD et al. Identifying bone-mass-related risk factors for fracture to guide bone densitometry measurements: a systematic review of the literature. Osteoporos Int 2001; 12: 811–822.
10. Department of Health. National service framework for older people. London: DoH; 2001.
11. Ebeling PR, Åkesson K. Role of biochemical markers in the management of osteoporosis. In: Sambrook P, Woolf A, eds. Clinical rheumatology. London: Baillière Tindall, 2001: 385–400.
12. Torgerson DJ, Donaldson C, Reid DM. Bone mineral density measurements: are they worthwhile? J R Soc Med 1996; 89: 457–461.
13. Doherty DA, Sanders KM, Kotowicz MA, Prince RL. Lifetime and five-year age-specific risks of first and subsequent osteoporotic fractures in postmenopausal women. Osteoporos Int 2001; 12(1): 16–23.
14. Osteoporosis: Clinical guidelines for prevention and treatment. Update on pharmacological interventions and an algorithm for management. London: Royal College of Physicians; 2000.
15. Shea B, Rosen CJ, Guyatt GH et al. A meta analysis of calcium supplementation for the prevention of postmenopausal osteoporosis. Osteoporos Int 2000; 11(suppl 2): S114.
16. Cumming RG, Nevitt MC. Calcium for prevention of osteoporotic fractures in postmenopausal women. J Bone Miner Res 1997; 12: 1321–1329.
17. Dawson-Hughes B, Dallal GE, Krall EA et al. A controlled trial of the effect of calcium supplementation on bone density in postmenopausal women. N Engl J Med 1990; 323: 878–883.
18. Bonjour JP, Carrie AL, Ferrari S et al. Calcium-enriched foods and bone mass growth in prepubertal girls: a randomized, double-blind, placebo-controlled trial. J Clin Invest 1997; 99: 1287–1294.
19. Lips P, Graafmans WC, Ooms ME et al. Vitamin D supplementation and fracture incidence in elderly persons. A randomized, placebo-controlled clinical trial. Ann Intern Med 1996; 124: 400–406.
20. Meyer HE, Falch JA, Kaavik E et al. Can vitamin D supplementation reduce the risk of fracture in the elderly? Osteoporos Int 2000; 11(suppl 2): S114–S115.
21. Gillespie WJ, Henry DA, O'Connell DL, Robertson J. Vitamin D and vitamin D analogues for preventing fractures associated with involutional and post-menopausal osteoporosis. Cochrane Database Syst Rev 2000; CD000227.
22. Ooms ME, Roos JC, Bezemer PD et al. Prevention of bone loss by vitamin D supplementation in elderly women: a randomized double-blind trial. J Clin Endocrinol Metab 1995; 80: 1052–1058.
23. Dawson-Hughes B, Harris SS, Krall EA et al. Rates of bone loss in postmenopausal women randomly assigned to one of two dosages of vitamin D. Am J Clin Nutr 1995; 61: 1140–1145.
24. Chapuy MC, Arlot ME, Duboeuf F et al. Vitamin D3 and calcium to prevent hip fractures in elderly women. N Engl J Med 1992; 327: 1637–1642.
25. Chapuy MC, Arlot ME, Delmas PD, Meunier PJ. Effect of calcium and cholecalciferol treatment for three years on hip fractures in elderly women. Brit Med J 1994; 308: 1081–1082.
26. Reid IR, Ames RW, Evans MC et al. Long-term effects of calcium supplementation on bone loss and fractures in postmenopausal women: a randomized controlled trial. Am J Med 1995; 98: 331–335.
27. Lips P. Vitamin D supplementation and fracture incidence in elderly persons. A randomized, placebo-controlled clinical trial. Ann Intern Med 1996; 124: 400–406.
28. Dawson-Hughes B, Harris SS, Krall EA, Dallal GE. Effect of calcium and vitamin D supplementation on bone density in men and women 65 years of age or older. N Engl J Med 1997; 337: 670–676.
29. Heikinheimo RJ, Inkovaara JA, Harju EJ et al. Annual injection of vitamin D and fractures of aged bones. Calcif Tissue Int 1992; 51: 105–110.
30. Kanis JA, Johnell O, Gullberg B et al. Evidence for efficacy of drugs affecting bone metabolism in preventing hip fracture. Brit Med J 1992; 305: 1124–1128.
31. Baeksgaard L, Andersen KP, Hyldstrup L. Calcium and vitamin D supplementation increases spinal BMD in healthy, postmenopausal women. Osteoporos Int 1998; 8: 255–260.
32. Tilyard MW, Spears GF, Thomson J, Dovey S. Treatment of postmenopausal osteoporosis with calcitriol or calcium. N Engl J Med 1992; 326: 357–362.
33. Aloia JF, Vaswani A, Yeh JK et al. Calcitriol in the treatment of postmenopausal osteoporosis. Am J Med 1988; 84: 401–408.
34. Falch JA, Odegaard OR, Finnanger AM, Matheson I. Postmenopausal osteoporosis: no effect of three years treatment with 1,25-dihydroxycholecalciferol. Acta Med Scand 1987; 221: 199–204.
35. Fleisch H. Bisphosphonates in bone disease. From laboratory to man. London: Academic Press; 2000.
36. Hochberg MC. Bisphosphonates. In: Cummings SR, Cosman F, Jamal S, eds. Osteoporosis. Philadelphia: American College of Physicians; 2002, in press.
37. Storm T, Thamsborg G, Steiniche T et al. Effect of intermittent cyclical etidronate therapy on bone mass and fracture rate in women with postmenopausal osteoporosis. N Engl J Med 1990; 322: 1265–1271.
38. Watts NB, Harris ST, Genant HK et al. Intermittent cyclical etidronate treatment of postmenopausal osteoporosis. N Engl J Med 1990; 323: 73–79.
39. van Staa TP, Abenhaim L, Cooper C. Use of cyclical etidronate and prevention of non-vertebral fractures 2. Br J Rheumatol 1998; 37: 87–94.
40. Liberman UA, Weiss SR, Broll J et al. Effect of oral alendronate on bone mineral density and the incidence of fractures in postmenopausal osteoporosis. The Alendronate Phase III Osteoporosis Treatment Study Group. N Engl J Med 1995; 333: 1437–1443.
41. Black DM, Cummings SR, Karpf DB et al. Randomised trial of effect of alendronate on risk of fracture in women with existing vertebral fractures. Fracture Intervention Trial Research Group. Lancet 1996; 348: 1535–1541.
42. Cummings SR, Black DM, Thompson DE et al. Effect of alendronate on risk of fracture in women with low bone density but without vertebral fractures: results from the Fracture Intervention Trial. J Am Med Assoc 1998; 280: 2077–2082.
43. Orwoll E, Ettinger M, Weiss S et al. Alendronate for the treatment of osteoporosis in men. N Engl J Med 2000; 343: 604–610.
44. Greenspan SL, Parker RA, Ferguson L et al. Early changes in biochemical markers of bone turnover predict the long-term response to alendronate therapy in representative elderly women: a randomized clinical trial. J Bone Miner Res 1998; 13: 1431–1438.
45. Tonino RP, Meunier PJ, Emkey R et al. Skeletal benefits of alendronate: 7-year treatment of postmenopausal osteoporotic women. Phase III Osteoporosis Treatment Study Group. J Clin Endocrinol Metab 2000; 85: 3109–3115.
46. Stock JL, Bell NH, Chesnut CH III et al. Increments in bone mineral density of the lumbar spine and hip and suppression of bone turnover are maintained after discontinuation of alendronate in postmenopausal women. Am J Med 1997; 103: 291–297.
47. Schnitzer T, Bone HG, Crepaldi G et al. Therapeutic equivalence of alendronate 70mg once-weekly and alendronate 10 mg daily in the treatment of osteoporosis. Alendronate Once-Weekly Study Group. Aging (Milan) 2000; 12: 1–12.
48. Lindsay R, Cosman F, Lobo RA et al. Addition of alendronate to ongoing hormone replacement therapy in the treatment of osteoporosis: a randomized, controlled clinical trial. J Clin Endocrinol Metab 1999; 84: 3076–3081.
49. Bone HG, Greenspan SL, McKeever C et al. Alendronate and estrogen effects in postmenopausal women with low bone mineral density. Alendronate/Estrogen Study Group. J Clin Endocrinol Metab 2000; 85: 720–726.
50. Harris ST, Watts NB, Genant HK et al. Effects of risedronate treatment on vertebral and nonvertebral fractures in women with postmenopausal osteoporosis: a randomized controlled trial. Vertebral Efficacy With Risedronate Therapy (VERT) Study Group. J Am Med Assoc 1999; 282: 1344–1352.
51. Reginster JY, Minne HW, Sorensen OH et al. Randomised trial of the effects of risedronate on vertical fractures in women with established postmenopausal osteoporosis. Osteoporos Int 2000; 11: 83–91.
52. McClung MR, Geusens P, Miller PD et al. Effect of risedronate on the risk of hip fracture in elderly women. Hip Intervention Program Study Group. N Engl J Med 2001; 344: 333–340.
53. Gordon MS, Gordon MB. Response of bone mineral density to once-weekly administration of risedronate. Endocr Pract 2002 May–Jun; 8(3): 202–207.
54. Lufkin EG, Wahner HW, O'Fallon WM et al. Treatment of postmenopausal osteoporosis with transdermal estrogen. Ann Intern Med 1992; 117: 1–9.
55. Mosekilde L, Beck-Nielsen H, Sorensen OH et al. Hormonal replacement therapy reduces forearm fracture incidence in recent postmenopausal women – results of the Danish Osteoporosis Prevention Study. Maturitas 2000; 36: 181–193.
56. Maxim P, Ettinger B, Spitalny GM. Fracture protection provided by long-term estrogen treatment. Osteoporos Int 1995; 5: 23–29.
57. Cauley JA, Seeley DG, Ensrud K et al. Estrogen replacement therapy and fractures in older women. Study of Osteoporotic Fractures Research Group. Ann Intern Med 1995; 122: 9–16.
58. Kiel DP, Felson DT, Anderson JJ et al. Hip fracture and the use of estrogens in postmenopausal women. The Framingham Study. N Engl J Med 1987; 317: 1169–1174.
59. Grady D, Rubin SM, Petitti DB et al. Hormone therapy to prevent disease and prolong life in postmenopausal women. Ann Intern Med 1992; 117: 1016–1037.
60. Michaelsson K, Baron JA, Farahmand BY et al. Hormone replacement therapy and risk of hip fracture: population based case-control study. The Swedish Hip Fracture Study Group. Brit Med J 1998; 316: 1858–1863.
61. Torgerson DJ, Bell-Syer SE. Hormone replacement therapy and prevention of nonvertebral fractures: a meta-analysis of randomized trials. J Am Med Assoc 2001; 285: 2891–2897.
62. Ettinger B, Genant HK, Cann CE. Postmenopausal bone loss is prevented by treatment with low-dosage estrogen with calcium. Ann Intern Med 1987; 106: 40–45.

63. Genant HK, Lucas J, Weiss S et al. Low-dose esterified estrogen therapy: effects on bone, plasma estradiol concentrations, endometrium, and lipid levels. Estratab/Osteoporosis Study Group. Arch Intern Med 1997; 157: 2609–2615.

64. Recker RR, Davies KM, Dowd RM, Heaney RP. The effect of low-dose continuous estrogen and progesterone therapy with calcium and vitamin D on bone in elderly women. A randomized, controlled trial. Ann Intern Med 1999; 130: 897–904.

65. Beral V, Bull D, Doll R et al. Familial breast cancer: collaborative reanalysis of individual data from 52 epidemiological studies including 58,209 women with breast cancer and 101,986 women without the disease. Lancet 2001; 358: 1389–1399.

66. Rossouw JE, Anderson GL, Prentice RL et al. Writing Group for the Women's Health Initiative Investigators. Risks and benefits of estrogen plus progestin in healthy postmenopausal women: principal results from the Women's Health Initiative randomized controlled trial. JAMA. 2002 Jul 17; 288(3): 321–333.

67. Draper MW, Flowers DE, Huster WJ et al. A controlled trial of raloxifene (LY139481) HCl: impact on bone turnover and serum lipid profile in healthy postmenopausal women. J Bone Miner Res 1996; 11: 835–842.

68. Delmas PD, Bjarnason NH, Mitlak BH et al. Effects of raloxifene on bone mineral density, serum cholesterol concentrations, and uterine endometrium in postmenopausal women. N Engl J Med 1997; 337: 1641–1647.

69. Ettinger B, Black DM, Mitlak BH et al. Reduction of vertebral fracture risk in postmenopausal women with osteoporosis treated with raloxifene: results from a 3-year randomized clinical trial. Multiple Outcomes of Raloxifene Evaluation (MORE) Investigators. J Am Med Assoc 1999; 282: 637–645.

70. Cummings SR, Eckert S, Krueger KA et al. The effect of raloxifene on risk of breast cancer in postmenopausal women: results from the MORE randomized trial. Multiple outcomes of raloxifene evaluation. J Am Med Assoc 1999; 281: 2189–2197.

71. Cauley JA, Norton L, Lippman ME et al. Continued breast cancer risk reduction in postmenopausal women treated with raloxifene: 4-year results from the MORE trial. Multiple outcomes of raloxifene evaluation. Breast Cancer Res Treat 2001; 65: 125–134.

72. Berning B, Kuijk CV, Kuiper JW et al. Effects of two doses of tibolone on trabecular and cortical bone loss in early postmenopausal women: a two-year randomized, placebo-controlled study. Bone 1996; 19: 395–399.

73. Beardsworth SA, Kearney CE, Purdie DW. Prevention of postmenopausal bone loss at lumbar spine and upper femur with tibolone: a two-year randomised controlled trial. Br J Obstet Gynaecol 1999; 106: 678–683.

74. Chesnut CH III, Silverman S, Andriano K et al. A randomized trial of nasal spray salmon calcitonin in postmenopausal women with established osteoporosis: the prevent recurrence of osteoporotic fractures study. PROOF Study Group. Am J Med 2000; 109: 267–276.

75. Cardona JM, Pastor E. Calcitonin versus etidronate for the treatment of postmenopausal osteoporosis: a meta-analysis of published clinical trials. Osteoporos Int 1997; 7: 165–174.

76. Cann CE, Roe EB, Sanchez S et al. PTH effects in the femur: envelope-specific responses by 3DQCT in postmenopausal women. J Bone Miner Res 1999; 14: S137.

77. Mosekilde L, Danielsen CC, Sogaard CH et al. The anabolic effects of parathyroid hormone on cortical bone mass, dimensions and strength-assessed in a sexually mature, ovariectomized rat model. Bone 1995; 16: 223–230.

78. Zanchetta JR, Bogado CE, Ferretti JL et al. Effects of LY333334 recombinant parathyroid hormone (1–34) on cortical bone strength indices as assessed by peripheral quantitative computed tomography. Bone 2001; 28: S86.

79. Neer RM, Arnaud CD, Zanchetta JR et al. Effect of parathyroid hormone (1–34) on fractures and bone mineral density in postmenopausal women with osteoporosis. N Engl J Med 2001; 344: 1434–1441.

80. Lindsay R, Nieves J, Formica C et al. Randomised controlled study of effect of parathyroid hormone on vertebral-bone mass and fracture incidence among postmenopausal women on oestrogen with osteoporosis. Lancet 1997; 350: 550–555.

81. Rittmaster RS, Bolognese M, Ettinger MP et al. Enhancement of bone mass in osteoporotic women with parathyroid hormone followed by alendronate. J Clin Endocrinol Metab 2000; 85: 2129–2134.

82. Riggs BL, Hodgson SF, O'Fallon WM et al. Effect of fluoride treatment on the fracture rate in postmenopausal women with osteoporosis. N Engl J Med 1990; 322: 802–809.

83. Meunier PJ, Sebert JL, Reginster JY et al. Fluoride salts are no better at preventing new vertebral fractures than calcium-vitamin D in postmenopausal osteoporosis: the FAVO Study. Osteoporos Int 1998; 8: 4–12.

84. Pak CY, Sakhaee K, Adams-Huet B et al. Treatment of postmenopausal osteoporosis with slow-release sodium fluoride. Final report of a randomized controlled trial. Ann Intern Med 1995; 123: 401–408.

85. Drake FH, Dodds RA, James IE et al. Cathepsin K, but not cathepsins B, L, or S, is abundantly expressed in human osteoclasts. J Biol Chem 1996; 271: 12511–12516.

86. Gelb BD, Shi GP, Chapman HA, Desnick RJ. Pycnodysostosis, a lysosomal disease caused by cathepsin K deficiency. Science 1996; 273: 1236–1238.

87. Dimai HP, Muller T, Eder S et al. Effects of the TNF-alfa antibody imfliximab on serum markers of bone turnover and mineral metabolism in patients with rheumatoid arthritis. Bone 2001; 28: S179.

88. Bekker PJ, Holloway D, Nakanishi A et al. The effect of a single dose of osteoprotegerin in postmenopausal women. J Bone Miner Res 2001; 16: 348–360.

89. Greendale GA, Barrett-Connor E, Edelstein S et al. Lifetime leisure exercise and osteoporosis. The Rancho Bernardo study. Am J Epidemiol 1995; 141: 951–959.

90. Kelley GA. Aerobic exercise and bone density at the hip in postmenopausal women: a meta-analysis. Prev Med 1998; 27: 798–807.

91. Wallace BA, Cumming RG. Systematic review of randomized trials of the effect of exercise on bone mass in pre- and postmenopausal women. Calcif Tissue Int 2000; 67: 10–18.

92. Karlsson M, Bass S, Seeman E. The evidence that exercise during growth or adulthood reduces the risk of fragility fractures is weak. Baillière's Clin Rheumatol 2001; 15: 429–450.

93. Gregg EW, Cauley JA, Seeley DG et al. Physical activity and osteoporotic fracture risk in older women. Study of Osteoporotic Fractures Research Group. Ann Intern Med 1998; 129: 81–88.

94. Paganini-Hill A, Chao A, Ross RK, Henderson BE. Exercise and other factors in the prevention of hip fracture: the Leisure World study. Epidemiology 1991; 2: 16–25.

95. Johnell O, Gullberg B, Kanis JA et al. Risk factors for hip fracture in European women: the MEDOS Study. Mediterranean Osteoporosis Study. J Bone Miner Res 1995; 10: 1802–1815.

96. Lord SR, Ward JA, Williams P, Strudwick M. The effect of a 12-month exercise trial on balance, strength, and falls in older women: a randomized controlled trial. J Am Geriatr Soc 1995; 43: 1198–1206.

97. Wolf SL, Barnhart HX, Kutner NG et al. Reducing frailty and falls in older persons: an investigation of Tai Chi and computerized balance training. Atlanta FICSIT Group. Frailty and injuries: cooperative studies of intervention techniques. J Am Geriatr Soc 1996; 44: 489–497.

98. Campbell AJ, Robertson MC, Gardner MM et al. Falls prevention over 2 years: a randomized controlled trial in women 80 years and older. Age Ageing 1999; 28: 513–518.

99. Tinetti ME, McAvay G, Claus E. Does multiple risk factor reduction explain the reduction in fall rate in the Yale FICSIT Trial? Frailty and injuries: cooperative studies of intervention techniques. Am J Epidemiol 1996; 144: 389–399.

100. Lunt M, Masaryk P, Scheidt-Nave C et al. The effects of lifestyle, dietary dairy intake and diabetes on bone density and vertebral deformity prevalence: the EVOS study. Osteoporos Int 2001; 12: 688–698.

101. Huopio J, Kroger H, Honkanen R et al. Risk factors for perimenopausal fractures: a prospective study. Osteoporos Int 2000; 11: 219–227.

102. Ward KD, Klesges RC. A meta-analysis of the effects of cigarette smoking on bone mineral density. Calcif Tissue Int 2001; 68: 259–270.

103. Hoidrup S, Prescott E, Sorensen TI et al. Tobacco smoking and risk of hip fracture in men and women. Int J Epidemiol 2000; 29: 253–259.

104. Lauritzen JB, Petersen MM, Lund B. Effect of external hip protectors on hip fractures. Lancet 1993; 341: 11–13.

105. Ekman A, Mallmin H, Michaelsson K, Ljunghall S. External hip protectors to prevent osteoporotic hip fractures. Lancet 1997; 350: 563–564.

106. Kannus P, Parkkari J, Niemi S et al. Prevention of hip fracture in elderly people with use of a hip protector. N Engl J Med 2000; 343: 1506–1513.

107. Parker MJ, Gillespie LD, Gillespie WJ. Hip protectors for preventing hip fractures in the elderly (Cochrane Review). Cochrane Database Syst Rev 2001; 2: CD001255.

108. Cumming RG, Thomas M, Szonyi G et al. Home visits by an occupational therapist for assessment and modification of environmental hazards: a randomized trial of falls prevention. J Am Geriatr Soc 1999; 47: 1397–1402.

109. Gillespie LD, Gillespie WJ, Robertson MC et al. Interventions for preventing falls in elderly people (Cochrane Review). Cochrane Database Syst Rev 2001; 3: CD000340.

110. Ytterstad B. The Harstad injury prevention study: the characteristics and distribution of fractures amongst elders – an eight year study. Int J Circumpolar Health 1999; 58: 84–95.

111. Thorngren KG, Ceder L, Svensson K. Predicting results of rehabilitation after hip fracture. A ten-year follow-up study. Clin Orthop 1993; 287: 76–81.

112. Kronhed AC, Moller M. Effects of physical exercise on bone mass, balance skill and aerobic capacity in women and men with low bone mineral density, after one year of training – a prospective study. Scand J Med Sci Sports 1998; 8: 290–298.

113. Glorieux FH, Bishop NJ, Plotkin H et al. Cyclic administration of pamidronate in children with severe osteogenesis imperfecta. N Engl J Med 1998; 339: 947–952.

114. Prevention and management of hip fracture in older people. A national clinical guideline. Scottish Intercollegiate Guidelines Network 2002.

115. Lips P, Cooper C, Agnusdei D et al. Quality of life in patients with vertebral fractures: validation of the Quality of Life Questionnaire of the European Foundation for Osteoporosis (QUALEFFO). Working Party for Quality of Life of the European Foundation for Osteoporosis. Osteoporos Int 1999; 10(2): 150–160.

199 Glucocorticoid-induced osteoporosis

Philip N Sambrook

- Glucocorticoids are effective agents in many rheumatic diseases but glucocorticoid-induced bone loss is common because of :
  - complex effects of glucocorticoids on gene expression in osteoblasts
  - inhibition by glucocorticoids of bone formation and enhancement of bone resorption
- Glucocorticoids can cause rapid bone loss and increase the risk of fracture throughout the skeleton, but especially in trabecular rich sites such as the spine and ribs
- Glucocorticoid bone loss can be effectively prevented or reversed by therapy with bisphosphonates, PTH and vitamin D metabolites

PATHOPHYSIOLOGY OF GLUCOCORTICOID BONE LOSS

It is currently believed that most of the biological activities of glucocorticoids are mediated via binding to the glucocorticoid receptor (GR). By this classic genomic mechanism, lipophilic glucocorticoid passes across the cell membrane, attaches to the cytosolic GR and after dimerization (Fig. 199.1), the GR binds to conserved sequence motifs (glucocorticoid response elements or GRE) to positively or negatively regulate specific gene transcription[1]. However it is also now recognized certain biological activities of glucocorticoids may be mediated via other transcription factors, such as activated protein (AP)-1 and nuclear factor κB (NFκB), independent of GR binding to DNA but dependent upon interaction with these factors[1].

Glucocorticoids affect bone metabolism through multiple pathways, influencing aspects of both bone formation and bone resorption in the remodeling cycle (Fig. 199.2). However the most important effects of glucocorticoids in relation to bone loss appear to be on bone formation. For the most part, the decreased bone formation is due to direct effects on cells of the osteoblastic lineage although indirect effects related to sex steroid production are also important. Glucocorticoids have complex actions on gene expression in bone cells, dependent on the stage of

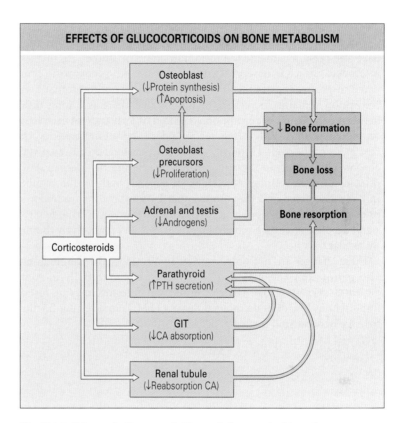

EFFECTS OF GLUCOCORTICOIDS ON BONE METABOLISM

Fig. 199.2 Schematic diagram of effects of glucocorticoids on bone metabolism. The thicker arrows for effects on bone formation indicate this is more important than effects on bone resorption.

osteoblast growth and differentiation[2]. Thus they decrease cell replication and repress type I collagen gene expression by the osteoblast by decreasing the rates of transcription and destabilizing type 1 collagen mRNA. They also have complex and unique effects on collagen degradation and regulate the synthesis of matrix metalloproteinases.

In addition to direct actions on the collagen gene, glucocorticoid effects on skeletal cells may be indirect and involve effects on the synthesis, release, receptor binding or binding proteins of locally produced growth factors. Bone cells synthesize insulin growth factors (IGF) I and II. These molecules are among the most important local regulators of bone cell function because of their abundance and anabolic effects to increase type I collagen synthesis by the osteoblast and bone formation. Glucocorticoids decrease IGF I synthesis in osteoblasts by transcription mechanisms and inhibit IGF II receptor expression in osteoblasts[2]. Glucocorticoids have also been shown to decrease mRNA levels encoding for osteoblast products such as osteocalcin.

Enhanced osteocyte apoptosis has also been implicated as an important mechanism of glucocorticoid osteoporosis[3]. Glucocorticoids have

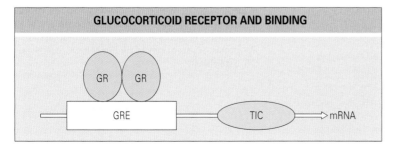

GLUCOCORTICOID RECEPTOR AND BINDING

Fig. 199.1 Schematic diagram of the glucocorticoid receptor and binding. Dimers of GR bind to GRE followed by interaction with the transcriptional initiation complex (TIC) to activate transcription.

been shown to reduce the birth rate of osteoblasts and osteoclasts and cause earlier death of osteoblasts[3]. The effect of glucocorticoids to promote apoptosis in osteocytes as well as in osteoblasts could account for the rapid increase in fracture susceptibility.

Although there have been many reports that bone resorption is increased in glucocorticoid treated patients, this is probably only true during the first 6 or 12 months of therapy. This early, temporary increase in bone resorption is probably due to increased osteoclast production from the effects of glucocorticoids on osteoprotegerin and its ligand[4]. In addition, osteoclast apoptosis may be postponed, contributing to rapid bone loss. It has been hypothesized that in some patients, secondary hyperparathyroidism increases bone turnover and expands the remodeling space, but this does not usually persist. Indeed with longer term glucocorticoid use, bone turnover is reduced.

The direct inhibitory effects of glucocorticoids on bone formation have also been documented in histomorphometric studies. An increase in eroded surface is observed with glucocorticoid osteoporosis compared to postmenopausal osteoporosis[5]. This does not mean that bone resorption remains increased but rather that there is a long delay between completion of resorption and onset of formation in each basic multicellular units (BMU) (Fig. 199.3). Indeed activation frequency, the best index of the overall intensity of bone remodeling, is decreased with chronic glucocorticoid therapy. At any time during the lifespan of an osteoid seam the number of osteoblasts depends both on the number initially assembled and the number that have escaped entrapment as osteocytes or death by apoptosis. Even with fewer cycles of remodeling, a significant loss after each remodeling cycle leads to progressively thinner trabeculae.

These changes are not only associated with trabecular thinning, but also perforation and major loss of trabecular connectivity in some patients[6], suggesting that changes in microarchitecture may be just as important as loss of bone mineral density (BMD) in assessing fracture risk in glucocorticoid treated patients (Fig. 199.4).

An additional effect of glucocorticoids is to decrease intestinal absorption of calcium[7]. Glucocorticoids increase urinary phosphate and calcium loss by direct effects on the kidney[8] which, together with impaired calcium absorption, may lead to secondary hyperparathyroidism[8] and increased bone resorption as an early but temporary phenomenon as noted above (Fig. 199.2).

Epidemiology

Glucocorticoids are effective, widely used, agents in rheumatology practice but glucocorticoid-induced osteoporosis is a common associated problem, first recognized by Cushing[9]. The risk of developing osteoporosis with glucocorticoid therapy remains unclear, but has been reported to occur in up to 50% of persons who require long term therapy. Fractures can occur rapidly with a predilection for sites rich in trabecular bone such as the spine and ribs, however prospective epidemiological fracture data in glucocorticoid bone loss is generally lacking. The largest study is a retrospective cohort study of 244,236 subjects on glucocorticoids identified from a general practice registry in the UK matched with 244 235 control patients[10]. The relative risks during oral glucocorticoid therapy for clinical vertebral fracture was 2.6, for hip fracture was 1.6 and for non-vertebral fracture was 1.3 (Fig. 199.5). Fracture risk increased with increasing daily doses of glucocorticoids[10] and on discontinuation, the fracture risk appeared to return to baseline.

The cumulative prevalence of vertebral fracture with glucocorticoids has been derived from cross-sectional studies and rates as high as 28% have been reported[11,12]. Estimates of vertebral fracture incidence with glucocorticoids, derived from the calcium treated control arms of recent randomized trials[13–16] range from 13–22% in the first year of therapy. The incidence appears to be particularly low in premenopausal women, intermediate in men and consequently highest in postmenopausal women.

Fracture risk with glucocorticoids is determined by several factors[17] (Fig. 199.6) including:

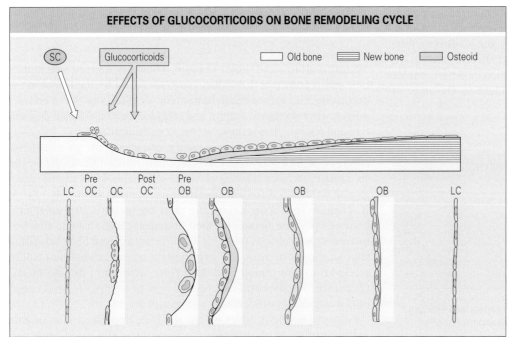

EFFECTS OF GLUCOCORTICOIDS ON BONE REMODELING CYCLE

SC   Glucocorticoids   ☐ Old bone   ▤ New bone   ☐ Osteoid

LC   Pre OC   OC   Post OC   Pre OB   OB   OB   OB   LC

Fig. 199.3 Schematic diagram of the effects of glucocorticoids on bone remodeling cycle. A trabecular BMU is depicted in a longitudinal section (upper panel) and at selected transverse sections (lower panels). Successive stages of quiescence, activation, resorption, formation and quiescence occur. Corticosteroids may enhance activation early, but later delay the interval between completion of resorption and onset of formation. Histomorphometric studies, being cross-sectional in nature, would show an apparent increase in resorptive surfaces, in this situation when resorption is in fact reduced due to decreased recruitment of osteoclast precursors and enhanced osteoblast apoptosis. SC, stem cell; LC, lining cell; OC, osteoclast; OB, osteoblast.

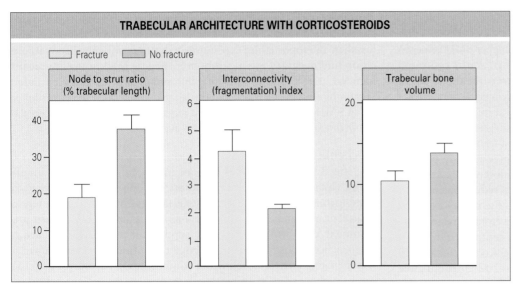

Fig. 199.4 Trabecular architecture with corticosteroids. Histomorphometry of glucocorticoid effects on trabecular connectivity. (Adapted with permission from Chappard *et al.*[6])

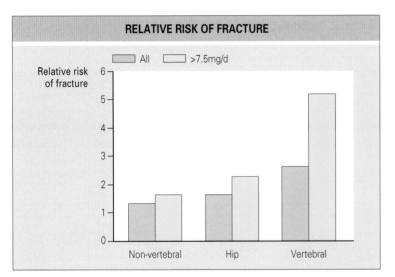

Fig. 199.5 Relative risk of fracture. Relative risk of different types of fracture with glucocorticoids. (Adapted with permission from Van Staa *et al.*[10])

- age: this is a risk factor for vertebral fracture, independent of bone mineral density (BMD)[12]
- BMD: both the initial value before glucocorticoid therapy and the amount of subsequent glucocorticoid-induced loss are important. Thus bone loss of 10% from a baseline T score of zero (as in a pre-menopausal woman) has a weaker influence on fracture risk than a similar bone loss from a baseline T score of −2 (as for example in a postmenopausal woman). Indeed the greatest risk of vertebral fracture is in older postmenopausal women
- glucocorticoid dose: bone loss is dependent both on cumulative and mean daily dosage[10]
- duration of exposure, i.e. a short course of glucocorticoids will cause bone loss that is largely reversible on ceasing glucocorticoids, but long term therapy causes a sustained reduction in BMD due to decreased bone formation increasing the likelihood that a fracture will occur eventually
- the underlying disease for which glucocorticoids are prescribed, which may be independently associated with increased fracture risk[18,19].

Bone density and fracture risk

In postmenopausal women, a decrease of one standard deviation in BMD is associated with an approximate doubling of fracture risk.

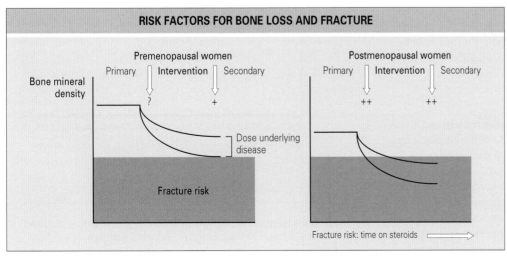

Fig. 199.6 Risk factors for bone loss and fracture. Schematic diagram of how the degree of bone loss and risk of fracture from glucocorticoids varies according to age, dose and underlying disease. The case for early intervention (primary prevention) is strongest in postmenopausal women and older men with low BMD. As fracture risk is a function of time on glucocorticoids, secondary prevention is appropriate to consider in men and pre- and postmenopausal women on long term glucocorticoids with low BMD.

However, this relationship may underestimate fracture risk in patients treated with glucocorticoids. Indeed some studies[11,20] have suggested that vertebral fractures due to glucocorticoids occur at higher BMD values to that observed in other types of osteoporosis. Luengo *et al.*[20] compared fractured thresholds (determined as the 90th percentile of the mean BMD) between 32 asthma patients with steroid related vertebral fractures and 55 postmenopausal patients with vertebral fractures. Fracture thresholds were 1.17 and 0.98 g/cm² respectively, suggesting that glucocorticoid treated patients sustained fractures at significantly higher BMD values. Peel *et al.*[11] examined vertebral deformity prevalence in patients with rheumatoid arthritis (RA) treated with low dose glucocorticoids, compared to age matched controls. There was a reduction in mean BMD of 0.8 SD in the RA patients. Compared to the overall expected doubling in risk of fracture, the authors found a fivefold increase in the prevalence of vertebral fractures (28 versus 6%). In contrast, Selby *et al.*[21] observed no increased risk of vertebral fracture in glucocorticoid treated patients compared to other causes of osteoporosis when cumulative fracture prevalence was compared to BMD.

Dose, duration and formulation of therapy and bone loss

Bone loss with glucocorticoids is most rapid in the first 6 to 12 months after starting therapy, followed by a slower decline in patients on chronic glucocorticoids[13–16]. When high dose glucocorticoids are used, rates of spine bone loss range between 5–10% per annum[22]. A serial histomorphometric study of patients treated with prednisone (10–25mg/day) demonstrated a 27% decrease in iliac crest cancellous bone volume by 6 months, however no further decline was observed at re-biopsy after 19 months[23]. In patients on chronic low dose prednisone therapy, bone loss continues at a much slower rate[16]. The overall reduction in BMD and change in microarchitecture with chronic glucocorticoid therapy still increases the likelihood that a fracture will occur eventually. Glucocorticoid bone loss appears reversible at least in part in young patients and recovery in bone density has been reported, for example, following successful treatment of Cushing's syndrome[24].

Although glucocorticoid osteoporosis is dose dependent[10], 'low dose' glucocorticoid may still cause rapid initial bone loss in some patients. A longitudinal study observed loss averaging 9.5% over 20 weeks from spinal trabecular bone in patients receiving a mean dose of 7.5mg prednisone per day[25].

Inhaled steroids are less likely to have systemic effects than oral glucocorticoids, but in higher doses result in adrenal suppression, growth impairment and reduced bone density. Wong *et al.*[26] reported a large cross-sectional study in patients receiving long term inhaled glucocorticoids for asthma. They found a significant inverse relationship between glucocorticoid dose and duration of glucocorticoid therapy and bone density at the spine and hip. Analysis of 170 818 inhaled glucocorticoid users from the general practice registry in the United Kingdom matched against an equal number of controls observed the relative risk of vertebral, hip and non-vertebral fracture was 1.5, 1.2 and 1.2 respectively but no differences were found between inhaled and bronchodilator groups[27].

Investigations

Bone mineral density

Effects of glucocorticoids on BMD can be measured precisely and accurately using dual energy X-ray absorptiometry (DXA) of the lumbar spine, hip and distal forearm or quantitative computerized tomography (QCT) for the lumbar spine. The earliest changes of glucocorticoid-induced bone loss are seen in the lumbar spine because of its high content of trabecular bone and can be quantitated by QCT or DXA. Since the radiation exposure with QCT is higher than with DXA, it is recommended to obtain a DXA measurement of the lumbar spine (anteroposterior scan) and femoral neck when subjects are initiating glucocorticoid treatment or

soon thereafter. Lateral DXA measurement has also been used to assess glucocorticoid treated patients as it is more sensitive to trabecular bone loss than anteroposterior DXA, however due to positioning issues, its precision and accuracy are much poorer. Repeat DXA scans are recommended at 12 monthly intervals, but should not be repeated before 12 months even in glucocorticoid treated patients because the errors inherent in BMD measurement mean that repeating a scan at a time interval of less than 12 months may not reflect a real change.

Biochemical markers

The effects of glucocorticoids on bone metabolism are reflected in profound changes in biochemical markers of bone turnover. Markers of bone formation such as serum osteocalcin fall within a few hours of treatment with glucocorticoids (Fig. 199.7) to as low as 30% of their pre-treatment level[8] with the degree of suppression significantly related to glucocorticoid dose[28]. Markers of bone resorption have been shown to rise following acute glucocorticoid administration[8]. However the exact role of such markers in diagnosis and management remains unclear.

TREATMENT OF GLUCOCORTICOID OSTEOPOROSIS

The most rapid bone loss occurs in the first 6–12 months in patients commencing high dose glucocorticoids. It is thus important to consider two different strategies:

● primary prevention in patients starting glucocorticoids who have not yet lost bone and

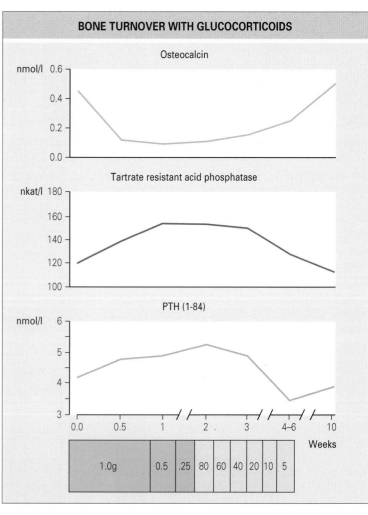

Fig. 199.7 Bone turnover with glucocorticoids. Effects of glucocorticoids on biochemical markers of bone turnover. (Adapted with permission from Cosman *et al.*[8])

- treatment (or secondary prevention) in patients on chronic glucocorticoids who will almost certainly have some significant degree of existing glucocorticoid related bone loss, with or without fractures.

Current therapeutic approaches to preventing glucocorticoid-induced bone loss include:

- use of the lowest glucocorticoid dose possible
- minimize lifestyle risk factors (e.g. smoking, low dietary calcium intake)
- consider individualized exercise programs with the help of a physical therapist to prevent muscle loss and fall.

In addition there are a number of drugs that have been used both to prevent osteoporosis but also to treat those with established bone loss. A number of agents have been investigated for potential benefit, including calcium, vitamin D and its metabolites, calcitonin, hormone replacement therapy, PTH and bisphosphonates. Agents such as the bisphosphonates have shown most consistent efficacy in clinical trials of glucocorticoid osteoporosis, as discussed below. Although by definition, anti-resorptive therapy should only operate within the bone remodeling envelope (which represents only a small proportion of the bone surface at any given time), their efficacy suggests other effects, such as to reduce osteoblast and osteocyte apoptosis are also important.

Hormone replacement therapy

Hormone replacement therapy is frequently recommended for glucocorticoid treated patients but the evidence supporting its use is limited. There has been only one controlled trial in 15 men receiving chronic glucocorticoids for asthma comparing testosterone 250mg/month with calcium 1000mg in a crossover design. After 12 months, testosterone increased lumbar BMD by 5%, which was significant compared to calcium, but the calcium group had no significant loss[29]. For estrogen there has also been one randomized controlled trial of the effect of estrogen on disease activity and BMD in postmenopausal women with RA. In a small subgroup of patients who were receiving chronic low dose glucocorticoids, lumbar BMD increased by 3.8% over 2 years compared to 0.6% loss in the calcium treated control group[30]. No fracture data are available from these studies. No randomized trials have been performed in glucocorticoid treated premenopausal women.

Calcium and vitamin D

Several studies suggest a benefit of calcium supplementation for secondary prevention in patients receiving chronic low dose glucocorticoids. However primary prevention trials in patients starting glucocorticoids, where calcium alone was used in the control arm, have still observed rapid rates of loss[15,31]. Therefore calcium alone is insufficient to prevent rapid bone loss in patients starting high dose glucocorticoids.

The evidence supporting the use of calcium in combination with vitamin D in glucocorticoid osteoporosis is mostly based upon older studies. One study examined treatment with calcium 500 mg/day and vitamin D 50 000 units per week in patients on chronic glucocorticoids[32]. This showed a significant increase in forearm bone density, but the study was not randomized and the patients were on chronic glucocorticoid treatment. Bone density was also only measured in the radius, whereas the greatest and most rapid bone loss occurs from the spine with glucocorticoids, so the clinical significance of these results is unclear. The only primary prevention study of combination calcium and vitamin D examined the use of 1000mg calcium daily plus 50 000 units vitamin D weekly against placebo over 3 years in 62 patients starting glucocorticoids[33]. Bone loss at the lumbar spine was not significantly different between calcium/vitamin D and placebo. Further, the amount of bone loss observed in the first year with the calcium/vitamin D combination

(4.9%) was similar to that seen in the calcium treated control groups in other primary prevention studies[15,31]. In contrast, a secondary prevention study in patients receiving chronic low dose glucocorticoids for RA[34] observed an annual spinal loss of 2.0% in placebo treated patients compared to 0.7% gain in calcium/vitamin D3 treated patients (1000mg + 500 IU/day respectively). As the patients were on chronic low dose glucocorticoid, the BMD rise may have been a 'remodeling transient' and the results are not necessarily applicable to patients commencing high dose glucocorticoids, i.e. primary prevention.

The term vitamin D covers both the calciferols and active metabolites, but these two groups of agents have quite distinct therapeutic effects. The most commonly used active hormonal forms of vitamin D, are calcitriol (1,25 dihydroxy vitamin D) and alfacalcidol (1α hydroxy vitamin D). Two studies have examined their use in primary prevention of glucocorticoid osteoporosis. One study examined the effect of 12 months of calcium, calcitriol or calcitonin in 103 patients starting glucocorticoids[31]. Patients treated with calcium lost bone rapidly at the lumbar spine (−4.3% in the first year) whereas patients treated with either calcitriol or calcitriol plus calcitonin lost at a much reduced rate (−1.3% and −0.2% per year respectively). The loss in both these latter groups was significantly different from the calcium group. Another randomized double blind controlled trial in 145 patients starting glucocorticoids compared alfacalcidol with calcium[35]. After 12 months, the change in spinal BMD with alfacalcidol was +0.4% compared to −5.7% with calcium. Hypercalcemia occurred in only 6.7% of alfacalcidol treated patients[35] compared to 25% with calcitriol[31]. The exact mechanism of this possible benefit of active metabolites compared to simple vitamin D for primary prevention is unclear, but may relate to reversal of the early temporary secondary hyperparathyroidism.

One secondary prevention study has evaluated the efficacy of active vitamin D metabolites compared with simple vitamin D in patients on chronic glucocorticoids[36]. A total of 85 patients on long-term glucocorticoid therapy were randomized to either 1μg alfacalcidol or 1000IU vitamin D3 with both groups also receiving 500mg calcium. Over 3 years, a small but significant increase was seen in lumbar spine BMD in the alfacalcidol group (+2.0%, $P < 0.0001$) with no significant changes at the femoral neck. In the vitamin D3 group, there were no significant changes at either site. By the end of the study, 12 new vertebral fractures had occurred in 10 patients of the alfacalcidol group and 21 in 17 patients of the vitamin D3 group. The alfacalcidol group showed a significant decrease in back pain ($P < 0.0001$) whereas no change was seen in the vitamin D3 group. This study also suggests active vitamin D metabolites are superior to simple vitamin D in the treatment of established glucocorticoid osteoporosis.

Calcitonin

Calcitonin has been studied both in patients starting glucocorticoids and in those receiving chronic glucocorticoids. In two primary prevention studies, there was no statistically significant evidence of additional benefit of adding calcitonin to calcitriol or cholecalciferol[31,37]. In the latter study, incident vertebral fractures occurred in 11% of calcitonin and 14% of calcium/vitamin D treated controls. No significant spinal bone loss was observed in either group suggesting the high vertebral fracture rate observed was more explained by underlying disease and the largely postmenopausal sample studied rather than the glucocorticoid use.

Bisphosphonates

A number of trials have examined the efficacy of bisphosphonates on glucocorticoid-induced bone loss and vertebral fractures. In 141 patients initiating glucocorticoids (i.e. primary prevention) who received prophylaxis with either cyclical etidronate or 500mg of calcium[13], mean lumbar BMD change with etidronate was +0.6% compared to −3.2% in the calcium group at the end of 12 months. For post menopausal women only, there was a significant reduction in the incidence of new vertebral fractures in the patients treated with etidronate (22 versus 3%).

The combined results of two trials in 477 glucocorticoid treated subjects who received prophylaxis with alendronate or placebo plus calcium/vitamin D (800–1000mg daily plus 250–500 IU daily respectively) have also been reported[14]. Patients were stratified according to the duration of their prior glucocorticoid treatment. Over 12 months of follow up, the mean change in lumbar spine BMD in patients in the primary prevention group (i.e. those who received glucocorticoids for < 4 months) was +3.0% for alendronate 10mg/day compared to –1% in the placebo group. In those who had received chronic glucocorticoids for > 12 months, the increase with alendronate was +2.8% but also +0.2% for calcium. These latter data suggest calcium/vitamin D might be able to prevent further bone loss in patients on chronic low dose glucocorticoids (secondary prevention). Interestingly the spinal bone loss was relatively minor (–1%/year) in patients enrolled within 4 months of initiating glucocorticoids and treated with calcium/vitamin D. These results contrast with the only study with a true untreated control group[35], in which cumulative doses of glucocorticoids were higher and spinal bone loss averaged 4.9%/year despite treatment with calcium with vitamin D. A *post-hoc* analysis of incident vertebral fractures favored alendronate in postmenopausal women (13 versus 4.4%). A 12 month extension of this trial in 212 patients to evaluate the effects of alendronate over 2 years in glucocorticoids osteoporosis has been reported[38]. This showed treatment with either 5 or 10mg of alendronate daily preserved bone mass at all sites compared to placebo over 2 years. No new vertebral fractures occurred in any alendronate treated patients in the second year.

The effects of alendronate on bone histomorphometry has been assessed in 88 patients (52 women and 36 men aged 22–75 years) from the above studies[39]. Iliac bone biopsies were obtained after tetracycline double-labeling at the end of the first year of treatment. Alendronate treatment did not influence osteoblastic activity, which is already low in glucocorticoid-induced osteoporosis. Alendronate also did not impair mineralization at any dose as assessed by mineralization rate. Osteoid thickness and volume were significantly lower in alendronate-treated patients, irrespective of the dose; however, mineral apposition rate was not altered. Significant decreases of mineralizing surfaces, activation frequency and bone formation rate were also noted with alendronate treatment.

Bisphosphonates may act to decrease glucocorticoid-induced apoptosis. Studies have shown etidronate, alendronate and pamidronate can prevent glucocorticoid-induced apoptosis of murine osteocytic cells and alendronate abolished the increased prevalence of apoptosis in vertebral cancellous bone osteocytes and osteoblasts that follows prednisolone administration to mice[40].

The results of primary prevention trial in 224 glucocorticoid treated subjects who received prophylaxis with either risedronate or placebo plus calcium 500mg daily have also been reported[15]. Risedronate 5mg per day prevented spinal bone loss (+0.6%) compared to calcium (–2.8%) over 12 months. Incident vertebral fracture rates were 17.3% with calcium and 5.7% for risedronate 5mg ($P = 0.072$). Vertebral fractures were only seen in postmenopausal women and men, not in premenopausal women. The effects of risedronate in 290 patients receiving chronic glucocorticoid treatment (prednisone > 7.5mg/day for > 6 months) have also been reported[16]. Approximately one third of patients had vertebral fractures as baseline. The control group, who were treated with calcium (1000mg) plus vitamin D (400IU) daily, showed a stable BMD over 12 months. However treatment with risedronate 5mg/day significantly increased lumbar spine (+2.9%) and femoral neck (+1.8%) BMD. Although not powered to show fracture efficacy, 15% of patients in the control group versus 5% in the risedronate groups sustained new vertebral fractures suggesting a 70% reduction in fracture

rate. A combined analysis of 518 patients in these two trials showed risedronate 5mg was associated with a 70% reduction in vertebral fracture risk compared to placebo ($P = 0.01$)[41].

Intermittent intravenous pamidronate has also been studied as a primary prevention agent in glucocorticoid treated patients[42]. A regimen involving 90mg for the first infusion, then 30mg every 3 months plus calcium 800mg/day found nearly a 4% increase in lumbar spine bone mass and a 3% increase in femoral neck bone mass over 12 months while the placebo group has a –6% at the lumbar spine and –4.1% at the femoral neck.

Parathyroid hormone

Parathyroid hormone is an important hormone in calcium metabolism. Large randomized placebo controlled clinical trials have demonstrated daily low dose injections of human parathyroid hormone (hPTH)(1–34) for 21 months can increase bone density by 14% at the spine[43]. The mechanism for the anabolic effect is not known, however the PTH receptor is located on the bone marrow stromal, preosteoblast cell. In vitro work has found that PTH may increase the lifespan of osteoblasts and osteocytes. It is thought that PTH has the potential to increase osteoblast numbers by increasing both their replication rate and by decreasing apoptosis.

A randomized controlled trial has been performed in postmenopausal women with glucocorticoid-induced osteoporosis[44] comparing hPTH(1–34) and estrogen with estrogen alone. This found that patients treated with hPTH (1–34) and estrogen had significant increases in bone mass (+35% for lumbar spine QCT, +11% by lumbar spine DXA, 1% hip) after 1 year compared to the minimal changes observed in the estrogen alone group. All study patients were followed for an additional year after the hPTH(1–34) was discontinued and total hip and femoral neck bone mass increased about 5% above baseline levels[45]. Treatment with PTH resulted in a dramatic increase in biochemical markers of bone turnover. Osteocalcin increased more than 150% above baseline levels within one month of starting the therapy and remained elevated for the remainder of the treatment period. Bone resorption increased to the same levels as osteocalcin after 6 months of therapy. The study was not powered to determine if hPTH(1–34) could reduce new vertebral fractures in glucocorticoid treated patients.

Based upon the summary evidence reviewed above, an algorithm for the diagnosis and management of glucocorticoid osteoporosis is shown in Figure 199.8.

SUMMARY

Evidence from randomized controlled trials suggests that postmenopausal women receiving glucocorticoids are at the greatest risk of rapid bone loss and consequent vertebral fracture and should be actively considered for prophylactic measures. In men and premenopausal women receiving glucocorticoids, the decision to use anti-osteoporosis prophylaxis is less straightforward and will depend upon a number of factors including BMD, anticipated dose and duration of glucocorticoids and other risk factors. Guidelines for the management of glucocorticoid osteoporosis are continuing to evolve as new evidence from randomized controlled trials become available[46]. Based upon available evidence the rank order of choice for prophylaxis would be a bisphosphonate followed by a vitamin D metabolite or an estrogen type medication. Calcium alone appears unable to prevent rapid bone loss in patients starting glucocorticoids. If an active vitamin D metabolite is used, calcium supplementation should be avoided unless dietary calcium intake is low. HRT should clearly be considered if hypogonadism is present. In patients receiving chronic low dose glucocorticoids, treatment with calcium and vitamin D may be sufficient to prevent further bone loss. However since fracture risk is a function of

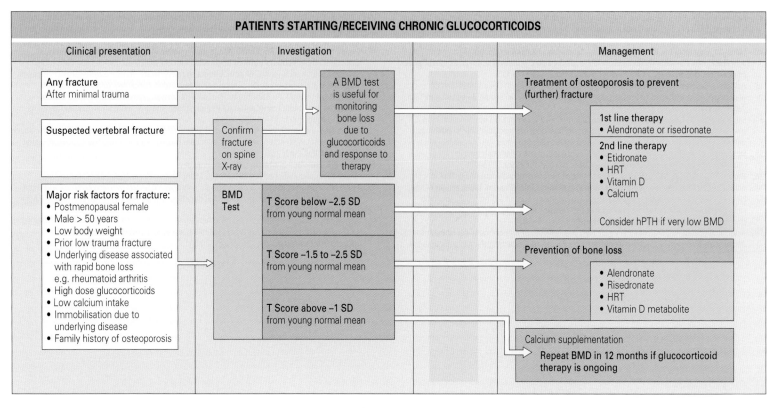

Fig. 199.8 Patients starting/receiving chronic glucocorticoids. Algorithm for the diagnosis and management of glucocorticoid osteoporosis.

multiple factors including the severity of low bone density as well as the duration of exposure, treatment with therapy to increase bone density will further reduce fracture risk in patients receiving chronic low dose glucocorticoids. In patients with severe reductions in bone density, treatment with hPTH (1–34) followed by an anti-resorptive would be appropriate.

REFERENCES

1. Karin M. New twists in gene regulation by glucocorticoid receptor: is DNA binding dispensable? Cell 1998; 93: 487–490.
2. Canalis E. Mechanisms of glucocorticoid action in bone: implications to glucocorticoid induced osteoporosis. J Clin Endocr Metab 1996; 81: 3441–3447.
3. Weinstein RS, Jilka RL, Parfitt AF et al. Inhibition of osteoblastogenesis and promotion of apoptosis of osteoblasts and osteocytes by glucocorticoids. J Clin Invest 1998; 102: 274–282.
4. Hofbauer LC, Gori F, Riggs BL et al. Stimulation of osteoprotegerin ligand and inhibition of osteoprotegerin production by glucocorticoids in human osteoblastic lineage cells: potential paracrine mechanisms of glucocorticoid-induced osteoporosis. Endocrinology 1999; 140: 4382–4389.
5. Carbonare LD, Arlot ME, Chavassieux PM et al. Comparison of trabecular bone microarchitecture and remodeling in glucocorticoid-induced and postmenopausal osteoporosis. J Bone Miner Res 2001; 16: 97–103.
6. Chappard D, Legrand E, Basle MF et al. Altered trabecular architecture induced by glucocorticoids: a bone histomorphometric study. J Bone Miner Res 1996; 11: 676–685.
7. Klein RG, Arnaud SB, Gallagher JC et al. Intestinal calcium absorption in exogenous hypercortisolism. Role of 25-hydroxyvitamin D and glucocorticoid dose. J Clin Invest 1977; 60: 253–259.
8. Cosman F, Nieves J, Herbert J et al. High-dose glucocorticoids in multiple sclerosis patients exert direct effects on the kidney and skeleton. J Bone Miner Res 1994; 9: 1097–1105.
9. Cushing H. The basophil adenomas of the pituitary body and their clinical manifestations. Bull Johns Hopkins Hospital 1932; 50: 137–195.
10. Van Staa TP, Leufkens HGM, Abenhaim L et al. Use of oral glucocorticoids and risk of fractures. J Bone Miner Res 2000; 15: 993–1000.
11. Peel NFA, Moore DJ, Barrington NA et al. Risk of vertebral fracture and relationship to bone mineral density in steroid treated rheumatoid arthritis. Ann Rheum Dis 1995; 54: 801–806.
12. Naganathan V, Jones G, Nash P et al. Vertebral fracture risk with long term glucocorticoids: prevalence, relationship to age, bone density and glucocorticoid use. Arch Int Med 2000; 160: 2917–2922.
13. Adachi JD, Bensen WG, Brown J et al. Intermittent etidronate therapy to prevent glucocorticoid-induced osteoporosis. New Engl J Med 1997; 337: 382–387.
14. Saag K, Emkey R, Schnitzler TJ et al. Alendronate for the prevention and treatment of glucocorticoid induced osteoporosis. New Engl J Med 1998; 339: 292–299.

15. Cohen S, Levy RM, Keller M et al. Residronate therapy prevents glucocorticoid-induced bone loss. Arthritis Rheum 1999; 42: 2309–2318.
16. Reid DM, Hughes RA, Laan RFJM et al. Efficacy and safety of daily risedronate in the treatment of glucocorticoid induced osteoporosis in men and women: a randomised trial. J Bone Miner Res 2000; 15: 1006–1013.
17. Sambrook PN. Glucocorticoid osteoporosis: practical implications of recent trials. J Bone Miner Res 2000; 15: 1645–1649.
18. Gough AK, Lilley J, Eyre S et al. Generalised bone loss in patients with early rheumatoid arthritis. Lancet 1994; 344: 23–27.
19. Pearce G, Ryan PF, Delmas PD et al. The deleterious effects of low-dose corticosteroids on bone density in patients with polymyalgia rheumatica. Brit J Rheumatol 1998; 37: 292–299.
20. Luengo M, Picado C, Del Rio L et al. Vertebral fractures in steroid dependent asthma and involutional osteoporosis: a comparative study. Thorax 1991; 46: 8063–8065.
21. Selby PL, Halsey JP, Adams KRH et al. Glucocorticoids do not alter the threshold for vertebral fractures. J Bone Miner Res 2000; 15: 952–956.
22. Sambrook PN, Kempler S, Birmingham J et al. Glucocorticoid effects on proximal femur bone loss. J Bone Miner Res 1990; 5: 1211–1216.
23. LoCascio V, Bonnucci E, Imbimbo B et al. Bone loss in response to long-term glucocorticoid therapy. Bone Mineral 1992; 8: 39–51.
24. Pocock NA, Eisman JA, Dunstan CR et al. Recovery from steroid-induced osteoporosis. Ann Intern Med 1987; 107: 319–323.
25. Laan RFJM, Van Riel PLCM, Van de Putte LBA et al. Low dose prednisone induces rapid reversible axial bone loss in patients with rheumatoid arthritis. Ann Int Med 1993; 119: 963–968.
26. Wong CA, Walsh LJ, Smith CJP et al. Inhaled glucocorticoid use and bone mineral density in patients with asthma. Lancet 2000; 355: 1399–1403.
27. Van Staa TP, Leufkins HG, Cooper C. Use of inhaled glucocorticoids and risk of fractures. J Bone Miner Res 2001; 16: 581–588.
28. Kotowicz MA, Hall S, Hunder GG et al. Relationship of glucocorticoid dosage to serum bone Gla-protein concentration in patients with rheumatologic disorders. Arthritis Rheum 1990; 33: 1487–1492.
29. Reid IR, Wattie DJ, Evans MC, Stapleton JP. Testosterone therapy in glucocorticoid-treated men. Arch Intern Med 1996; 156: 1173–1177.
30. Hall GM, Daniels M, Doyle DV, Spector TD. The effect of hormone replacement therapy on bone mass in rheumatoid arthritis treated with and without steroids. Arthritis Rheum 1994; 37: 1499–1505.

31. Sambrook PN, Birmingham J, Kelly PJ *et al*. Prevention of glucocorticoid osteoporosis; a comparison of calcium, calcitriol and calcitonin. New Engl J Med 1993; 328: 1747–1752.

32. Hahn TJ, Halstead LR, Bran DT *et al*. Effects of short term glucocorticoid administration on intestinal calcium absorption and circulating vitamin D metabolite concentrations in man. J Clin Endocr Metab 1981; 52: 111–115.

33. Adachi J, Bensen W, Bianchi F *et al*. Vitamin D and calcium in the prevention of glucocorticoid-induced osteoporosis: a three year follow up study. J Rheumatol 1996; 23: 995–1000.

34. Buckley LM, Leib ES, Cartularo KS *et al*. Calcium and vitamin D3 supplementation prevents bone loss in the spine secondary to low dose glucocorticoids in patients with rheumatoid arthritis. Ann Intern Med 1996; 125: 961–968.

35. Reginster JY, Kuntz D, Verdicht W *et al*. Prophylactic use of alfacalcidol in glucocorticoid-induced osteoporosis. Osteoporosis Int 1999; 9: 75–81.

36. Ringe JD, Coster A, Meng T *et al*. Treatment of glucocorticoid-induced osteoporosis with alfacalcidol/calcium versus vitamin D/calcium. Calcif Tiss Int 1999; 65: 337–340.

37. Healey J, Paget S, Williams-Russo P *et al*. Randomised trial of salmon calcitonin to prevent bone loss in glucocorticoid treated temporal arteritis and polymyalgia rheumatica. Calcif Tiss Int 1996; 58: 73–80.

38. Adachi JD, Saag KG, Delmas PD *et al*. Two year effects of alendronate on bone mineral density and vertebral fracture in patients receiving glucocorticoids. Arthritis Rheum 2001; 44: 202–211.

39. Chavassieux PM, Arlot ME, Roux JP *et al*. Effects of alendronate on bone quality and remodeling in glucocorticoid-induced osteoporosis: a histomorphometric analysis of transiliac biopsies. J Bone Miner Res 2000; 15: 754–762.

40. Plotkin LI, Weinstein RS, Parfitt AM *et al*. Prevention of osteocyte and osteoblast apoptosis by bisphosphonates and calcitonin. J Clin Invest 1999; 104: 1363–1367.

41. Wallach S, Cohen S, Reid DM *et al*. Effects of risedronate on bone density and vertebral fracture in patients on corticosteroid therapy. Calcif Tissue Int 2000; 67: 277–285.

42. Neer RM, Arnaud CD, Zanchetta JR *et al*. Effect of parathyroid hormone(1–34) on fractures and bone mineral density in postmenopausal women with osteoporosis. N Engl J Med 2001; 344: 1434–1441.

43. Boutsen Y, Jamart J, Esselinckx W *et al*. Primary prevention of glucocorticoid-induced osteoporosis with intermittent intravenous pamidronate: a randomized trial. Calcif Tissue Int 1997; 61: 266–271.

44. Lane NE, Sanchez S, Modin GW *et al*. Parathyroid hormone treatment can reverse glucocorticoid-induced osteoporosis. J Clin Invest 1998; 102: 1627–1633.

45. Lane NE, Pierini E, Modin G *et al*. Bone mass continues to increase after parathyroid hormone treatment is stopped in glucocorticoid-induced osteoporosis. J Bone Min Res 2000; 15: 944–951.

46. American College of Rheumatology Ad Hoc Committee on Glucocorticoid-Induced Osteoporosis. Recommendations for the prevention and treatment of glucocorticoid-induced osteoporosis: 2001 update. Arthritis Rheum 2001; 44: 1496–1503.

METABOLIC BONE DISEASES

200 Rickets and osteomalacia

Peter Selby

- Rickets is a defect of mineralization affecting the growing skeleton whereas osteomalacia is abnormal mineralization of the mature skeleton

- The commonest cause of both conditions is vitamin D deficiency

- Other causes include hypophosphatemia, either inherited or acquired, renal tubular acidosis and inherited abnormalities of vitamin D metabolism

- The clinical features of rickets include growth failure, skeletal deformity and proximal myopathy. In osteomalacia the main features are bone pain, fracture and muscle weakness

- The radiological appearance of rickets with widening of the epiphyses and loss of distinction of the growth plate is pathognomonic. In osteomalacia diagnosis may require bone biopsy but the characteristic radiological lesion is the Looser's zone

- Treatment of vitamin D deficiency is based on replacement of physiological amounts of native vitamin D. Hypophosphatemia requires the use of phosphate supplements with additional supraphysiological vitamin D supplementation. Osteomalacia due to systemic acidosis may respond to treatment of the underlying metabolic abnormality

INTRODUCTION

Although frequently linked together, it is important to remember that rickets and osteomalacia are separate conditions. The former is a defect of growing (modeling) bone in which there is an abnormality of the growth plate brought about by abnormal mineralization, and the latter can be seen in either growing or mature bone and results from the production of abnormal bone in which there is inadequate mineralization of the matrix. Clinically the conditions have several areas of similarity, including:

- hypotonia, muscle weakness and bowing of long bones.
- bone tenderness and pain
- pelvic deformities and a waddling gait

Children, the elderly, those who are disabled and some ethnic groups, such as south Asian women, who have a reduced exposure to sunlight or reduced intake or absorption of vitamin D are most at risk.

HISTORY

Rickets has been recognized since the Middle Ages and there are probable descriptions from antiquity[1]. It was common in 19th century urban Europe and its prevalence in Vienna after World War I provided the basis for one of the most detailed descriptions of the disease. The histologic appearances of adult osteomalacia were first described in 1885 but clinical appreciation of the disease was slower. A large concentration of adult osteomalacia in China then provided the basis for detailed study in the 1930s, Maxwell estimating that there may have been 100 000 cases at that time[2]. Nevertheless, in 1948 Albright and Reifenstein were 'cognizant of no single case of osteomalacia in the United States due to simple vitamin D lack'[3].

EPIDEMIOLOGY

Rickets and osteomalacia due to vitamin D deficiency have long been endemic in certain regions – northern China, India, North Africa and the Middle East. Industrialization spread the disease in 19th century urban Britain, deprivation made it prevalent in Germany and Austria after World War I, and dietary restrictions introduced it to France and The Netherlands during World War II.

The principal cause of hypovitaminosis D responsible for privational osteomalacia is lack of sunshine exposure. This is a particular problem among women and children whose cultural mores lead to extensive covering with clothes or remaining indoors. In some groups this may be compounded by low vitamin D consumption in the diet, possibly together with phytic acids of cereals that could also reduce calcium absorption.

In modern times osteomalacia is frequently seen in south Asian populations, in particular when they come to live in north-west Europe, where sunshine is less abundant. Although it had been believed that these conditions were declining in a prosperous economic climate, there is evidence that this is not the case, with increasing numbers of children with rickets being reported[4]. Sporadic osteomalacia is mostly due to gastrointestinal diseases with malabsorption of vitamin D. The main cause is celiac disease but it can also be seen in Crohn's disease and following gastric surgery.

Although the vast majority of cases of rickets and osteomalacia are related to vitamin D deficiency there are also several other causes of impairment of mineralization. These are discussed in more detail below and their rarity means that it is difficult to describe their epidemiology other than in terms of simple information regarding prevalence.

VITAMIN D

Given the importance of vitamin D metabolism for normal bone mineralization and the observation that the majority of cases of osteomalacia and rickets are associated with vitamin D deficiency it seems appropriate to consider the endocrinology, biochemistry and metabolism of vitamin D at this stage in order to understand how alterations in this process can impact on the skeleton.

The designation 'vitamin D' is somewhat of a misnomer, implying as it does that this is a compound that is primarily derived from the diet. The situation is more complex than that: only a small proportion of the vitamin D requirements are met from this source and the vast majority are satisfied by endogenous production (Fig. 200.1). Furthermore, vitamin D itself is relatively inactive biologically and must undergo two further biochemical steps for the production of calcitriol (1,25-dihydroxy vitamin D – the active form of vitamin D). Its production is under tight

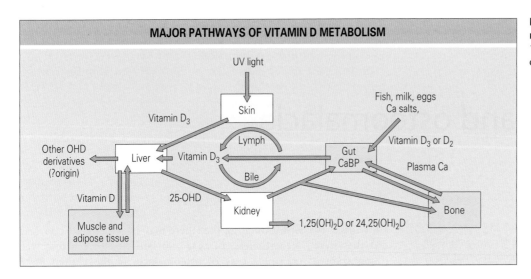

Fig. 200.1 Major pathways of vitamin D metabolism. 25-OHD,25-hydoxyvitamin D; 1,25(OH)$_2$D, 1,25-dihydroxyvitamin D, CaBP, calbindin.

feedback control and this compound is therefore best thought of as a hormone rather than a vitamin[5,6].

The basic precursor for vitamin D synthesis, 7-dehydrocholesterol, is stored in the malpighian layer of the epidermis (Fig. 200.2). Irradiation cleaves the steroid B ring to form previtamin D, which isomerizes under thermal influence to vitamin D$_3$ (cholecalciferol), one of a family of compounds chemically designated, by the broken B ring, as secosteroids. In contrast to cholecalciferol, the true prohormone, previtamin D in skin has low affinity for the circulating vitamin D binding protein. which therefore selectively transports the former either to muscle and adipose tissue for storage or to liver, where it undergoes microsomal 25-hydroxylation to form 25-hydroxycholecalciferol (25-OHD), the chief circulating metabolite under physiologic conditions. Most circulating 25-OHD is bound to a specific globulin.

Dietary vitamin D

The only significant dietary source of vitamin D in a western diet is oily fish. In some countries fortification of food products is used to increase the intake and reduce the risk of vitamin-D-deficient rickets and osteomalacia. For instance, in the USA vitamin D is added to milk. This has its own problems, since excessive vitamin D intake can lead to toxicity and hypercalcemia, which has been reported in America as a result of inadequate quality control of milk supplementation[7].

In the UK the average dietary intake of vitamin D between the ages of 16 and 64 is only 3.4μg per day. This contrasts with the USA recommended dietary intake of 5μg daily up to the age of 50, 10μg daily from 50–70 and 15μg daily over that age. Furthermore, this indicates the importance of sunlight for ensuring vitamin repletion in those countries where there is no dietary supplementation. Indeed, in the UK there is no specific recommended dietary intake as it is acknowledged that most individuals obtain their requirement from sunlight.

Vitamin D measurements

Prior to the development of radioassays for 25-hydroxyvitamin D in 1971[8], all information on vitamin D content was derived solely from tedious bioassays of antirachitic activity in rats, leading to expression of potency in international units (IU) and promulgation of recommended intakes in these terms. One IU is contained in 0.025μg cholecalciferol

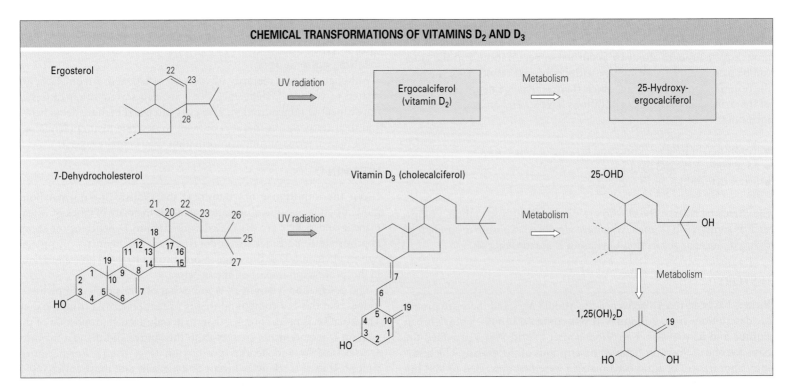

Fig. 200.2 Chemical transformations of vitamins D$_2$ and D$_3$. The only difference between these two forms is in the side chain illustrated here.

(i.e. 1μg vitamin D contains 40IU). In terms of receptor affinity, however, the IU is meaningless: cholecalciferol has virtually no affinity and must be converted to 25-OHD, whose affinity in turn is about two orders of magnitude less than that of calcitriol. The receptor affinity of 25-OHD, however low, nevertheless explains why pharmacologic doses of vitamin D (and 25-OHD) are effective substitutes in the virtual absence of 25-OHD 1α-hydroxylase (e.g. in renal failure, the anephric state, vitamin-D-dependent rickets type I – see below – and hypoparathyroidism).

Since solar irradiation is the major determinant of vitamin D production, recommended daily vitamin D intakes are only valid in the absence of sunlight exposure. Nutrition is best evaluated in individuals by measurement of circulating 25-OHD; under physiologic conditions, the serum concentration of cholecalciferol is negligible. Winter sunshine contains insufficient amounts of ultraviolet light of the appropriate wavelength for vitamin D synthesis in temperate latitudes; plasma levels of 25-OHD therefore show marked seasonal variation[9]. The mean maximum level of approximately 20–25ng/ml is achieved in the UK in September and a mean minimum of about 10ng/ml occurs in March. Levels below 5ng/ml are associated with a high risk of osteomalacia/rickets. However, recent work has suggested that, even at levels higher than this, there is a substantial risk of secondary hyperparathyroidism and associated bone loss leading to osteoporosis and fracture[10,11].

The 25-hydroxylation of cholecalciferol is inhibited by calcitriol, which also hastens the hepatic inactivation of vitamin. Hence evolution seems to have ensured a mechanism for abundant synthesis and storage of vitamin D in summer, followed by slow release and utilization in winter.

Calcitriol

In the kidney, 25-OHD is converted to calcitriol in the proximal renal tubular cell under tight endocrine feedback. The enzyme responsible, 25-OHD 1α-hydroxylase, is a mitochondrial mixed function oxidase of the cytochrome P450 family. It is stimulated chiefly by parathyroid hormone (PTH) and secondarily by low inorganic phosphate levels. Calcitriol also regulates its own synthesis in an uncertain fashion. Other hormones can stimulate calcitriol production. These include growth hormone, prolactin and estrogens; the mechanisms of action and biological significance of these remain unclear.

In the presence of low PTH and high phosphate levels, 25-OHD is converted instead to 24,25-dihydroxyvitamin D, which is probably inactive in humans. Other metabolites of vitamin D include 25,26-dihydroxy vitamin D from liver and 1,24,25-trihydroxy vitamin D; these too are probably of little if any biological importance. Degradative pathways involve both side-chain cleavage to a C-23 calcitroic acid and lactone production. Metabolic inactivation of vitamin D may be enhanced independently by both PTH and calcium deficiency.

Degradation of vitamin D is increased in conditions such as the post-gastrectomy syndrome, where there is failure of calcium absorption with secondary hyperparathyroidism. This probably accounts for the high rate of osteomalacia seen in these patients. A similar process may also explain the osteomalacia seen in patients with celiac disease. A variety of different drugs that interfere with vitamin D metabolism have been described[12]. These include enzyme-inducing agents such as the majority of antiepileptic drugs. These increase the rate of breakdown of vitamin D and add to the likelihood of deficiency in patients whose underlying disease may cause them to have lower exposure to sunlight.

Molecular biology of calcitriol

Receptor proteins for calcitriol are present in cells throughout mammalian systems. They belong to the same superfamily as all steroid hormone receptors. Calcitriol diffuses into the cell, where it combines with the receptor protein, which contains a hormone-binding domain at the carboxy terminus and a DNA-binding domain. Once it has bound calcitriol, the receptor migrates to the nucleus, where it binds specific regions of DNA and regulates gene transcription. One of the most important genomic effects of vitamin D is to promote the synthesis of calcium-binding proteins or calbindins[13].

In the intestine, the main action of calcitriol is to stimulate calcium transport[14]. In the main this is undertaken by the stimulation of calbindin production. Calbindin in intestinal cells serves two functions: in the first place it rapidly complexes calcium entering the cells from the luminal border; this ensures that there is a low intracellular calcium concentration, which in turn facilitates calcium diffusion from within the bowel lumen. The calbindin–calcium complex is then transported to the basolateral aspect of the cell where the calcium is transported into the interstitial fluid. Part of this activity appears too rapid to involve DNA transcription and is probably a direct effect leading to passive diffusion through the tight junctions between cells.

In bone, calcitriol stimulates resorption experimentally, with rapid calcium released *in vitro*, but any net *in vivo* effect is less obvious and difficult to evaluate[14]. Calcitriol stimulates osteoblastic production of specific proteins, it is established as a maturation and/or differentiation factor in a wide variety of normal and malignant cell lines and it regulates the pancreatic insulin response to glucose/arginine. Calcitriol is also produced by placenta and, under certain circumstances, by endothelium and by activated macrophages. Evidence suggests that, in addition to its role as a hormone in the classic sense, calcitriol also acts as an autocrine or paracrine regulator, although understanding of its role outside the intestine remains limited. In humans, the normal range of serum calcitriol is broad, numerous laboratories reporting a lower limit of 15–19pg/ml and an upper limit of 45–58pg/ml. Normal levels are higher among children and adolescents. Persistently low levels are found in some forms of 'vitamin-D-resistant' hypophosphatemic osteomalacia. In privational disease, levels rise so briskly after a small amount of administered vitamin D that they are of no diagnostic significance. In this situation the renal 1α-hydroxylase is so primed by hyperparathyroidism that a small dose of calciferol may produce calcitriol levels more than double those achieved by 1mg calcitriol daily (Fig. 200.3).

OTHER CAUSES OF RICKETS AND OSTEOMALACIA

Although the vast majority of cases of rickets and osteomalacia encountered in clinical practice are the result of vitamin D deficiency, other causes are recognized and need to be considered.

Abnormal vitamin D metabolism

Abnormalities of both of the enzymes involved in the activation of vitamin D have been described. Contrary to expectations, 25-hydroxylase activity is rarely reduced in liver disease. There is sufficient hepatic reserve of this enzyme that 25-hydroxylation of vitamin D is not compromised until the final stages of liver disease. Two cases of apparent deficiency of hepatic 25-hydroxylase causing rickets have been described[16,17] but it has not been described as a cause of osteomalacia presenting in adulthood.

The major cause of loss of activity of the renal 1α-hydroxylase is renal failure. This is an important contributory factor in renal bone disease but is outside the scope of this chapter.

Inherited deficiency of 1α-hydroxylase is known as vitamin-D-dependent rickets type I (VDDR I or pseudovitamin-D-deficiency rickets). This is an autosomal recessive trait that presents with severe rickets early in life with associated myopathy and enamel hypoplasia[18,19]. In the absence of effective treatment the condition is fatal through a combination of rib cage deformity and myopathy leading to respiratory failure.

Abnormal vitamin D action

After the biochemistry of vitamin D had been elucidated it became apparent that there were some patients with severe rickets and osteomalacia in whom there was an elevated level of 1,25-dihydroxyvitamin D.

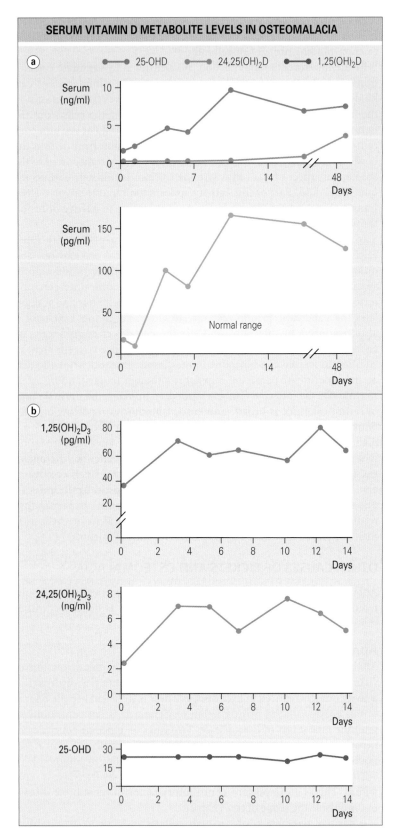

Fig. 200.3 Serum vitamin D metabolite levels in osteomalacia. The response in vitamin D metabolites in (a) an osteomalacic patient treated with 450 units of vitamin D daily and (b) a normal subject given 1μg calcitriol daily. (Adapted with permission from Mawer[15])

This was presumed to be due to defective vitamin D receptors and subsequent genetic analysis has revealed a variety of different mutations that lead to receptor inactivation[20,21]. The condition is known as vitamin-D-dependent rickets type II (VDDR II).

There is considerable heterogeneity in the presentation of this condition. The majority of affected individuals are normal at birth and

develop bone disease early in childhood. However, the first reported case did not present with osteomalacia until the age of 22 and the oldest reported case presented at age 45. About two-thirds of affected individuals have alopecia; this tends to occur with the more severe bone disease. The variety is known as vitamin-D-dependent rickets type IIA while that form of the disease with normal hair growth is termed vitamin-D-dependent rickets type IIB. The condition is inherited in an autosomal recessive manner.

Hypophosphatemia

Phosphate is an important component for skeletal mineralization. It is therefore little surprise to find that conditions leading to phosphate deprivation are associated with osteomalacia and rickets. In contrast to vitamin D deficiency, where low phosphate levels are the result of secondary hyperparathyroidism, these conditions are not associated with parathyroid overactivity until late in the disease process.

Inherited hypophosphatemia

The commonest form of hypophosphatemic rickets is X-linked hypophosphatemia (vitamin-D-resistant rickets; VDRR). This is a syndrome of renal phosphate wasting caused by mutations on the *PHEX* gene on the short arm of the X chromosome[22]. It is transmitted in an X-linked dominant manner. Interestingly, heterozygous females appear to be less severely affected than do hemizygous males (males whose X chromosome carries the mutant allele). The explanation for this observation appears to lie in the random inactivation of one X chromosome in each female cell, leading to half the cells in an affected female having a normal gene.

PHEX is predicted to encode for a metalloproteinase with homology with several well-recognized enzymes. How defects in what was thought to be a degradative enzyme could lead to hypophosphatemia was initially unclear. A clue to the possible mechanism was recently obtained when it was discovered that the similar condition autosomal dominant hypophosphatemic rickets was caused by a mutation in the gene encoding a new fibroblast growth factor (FGF23) on the short arm of chromosome 12[23]. The mutation leads to increased levels of FGF23. A variety of different observations have suggested that FGF23 is capable of stimulating phosphate loss in the kidney. The overarching hypothesis to explain both these conditions is that in X-linked hypophosphatemia the absence of the enzyme needed to cleave FGF23 leads to its increase with associated hypophosphatemia, while in autosomal dominant hypophosphatemic rickets the mutated FGF23 is resistant to degradation and also results in phosphate loss[24].

Children affected with X-linked hypophosphatemia have normal body habitus at birth but develop bowed legs as they start to walk[25]. Unlike privational rickets, X-linked hypophosphatemia does not normally lead to myopathy[26]. Affected individuals are eventually of short stature and as they go through adult life tend to develop new bone formation at a variety of different sites. This occurs particularly at the entheses, where it can lead to disabling restriction of movement[26,27] (Figs 200.4 & 200.5). It can also occur in the ligamentum flavum and the longitudinal ligaments of the spinal canal, where it can lead to spinal cord compression, which may progress to cause neurological deficit[28].

Acquired hypophosphatemia

Phosphate depletion by itself can lead to osteomalacia. This is perhaps best illustrated by the fact that phosphate-binding antacids can lead to osteomalacia if given for long enough. In such cases the hypophosphatemia stimulates renal 1α-hydroxylase, which leads to high levels of calcitriol. This causes increased calcium absorption and a characteristic of such patients is the presence of hypercalciuria[29].

Over the past 40 years there have been several reports of hypophosphatemia being associated with the presence of tumors (oncogenic osteomalacia). Generally, the associated tumors are small, benign,

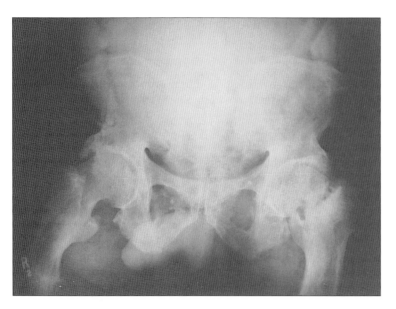

Fig. 200.4 Radiograph of the pelvis in X-linked hypophosphatemia to illustrate periarticular calcification.

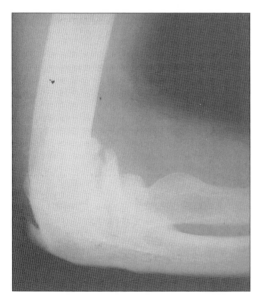

Fig. 200.5 Radiograph of the elbow in X-linked hypophosphatemia to illustrate calcific enthesopathy.

mesenchymal lesions but oncogenic osteomalacia has also been reported with carcinoma of the prostate, breast and lung as well as with hematological malignancy. A similar condition is also seen in some cases of neurofibromatosis and polyostotic fibrous dysplasia[30]. The mechanism by which tumors could cause the metabolic disturbance was unclear until recently. Some tumors associated with oncogenic osteomalacia have now been show to generate high levels of FGF23[31] and it is believed that a similar situation holds as in autosomal dominant hypophosphatemic rickets (see above).

In addition to features of bone disease such as pain and fracture, patients with oncogenic osteomalacia frequently suffer from profound muscle weakness. This appears to be due to marked reduction in the circulating levels of calcitriol despite the presence of normal vitamin D nutrition.

Renal tubular dysfunction
Renal tubular acidosis

It is not clear why systemic acidosis can lead to defective skeletal mineralization but osteomalacia is a well-recognized feature of renal tubular acidosis. It can also occur following ureterocolic anastamosis where there is a systemic acidosis resulting from the colonic reabsorption of chloride from the urine. Several different varieties of abnormality

leading to renal tubular acidosis are recognized. Of these the two most common varieties are type I, in which there is a failure of hydrogen ion secretion in the distal tubule and type II, in which there is excess loss of bicarbonate in the proximal tubule. Type I renal tubular acidosis is infrequently associated with osteomalacia or rickets. Type II renal tubular acidosis, on the other hand, is frequently associated with osteomalacia. This is particularly true if there are other tubular abnormalities coexisting with the bicarbonate wasting (see Fanconi's syndrome, below).

Fanconi's syndrome

This term applies to a constellation of abnormalities affecting renal tubular transport mechanisms. In particular there is excessive loss of phosphate, bicarbonate, glucose and amino acids. In addition to this there may also be reduced activity of 1α-hydroxylase, leading to reduction in calcitriol production. Many of these abnormalities are individually associated with rickets and osteomalacia and so it is not surprising that defective mineralization is common in Fanconi's syndrome.

Toxicity

Certain drugs or poisons inhibit mineralization and, for example, histologic appearances of osteomalacia (excess osteoid and/or defective mineralization fronts) have been reported following chronic fluoride ingestion[32], etidronate overdosage[33], aluminum[34] and gallium toxicity.

CONDITIONS RESEMBLING RICKETS AND OSTEOMALACIA

A few uncommon conditions resemble rickets or osteomalacia on clinical, radiologic or histologic grounds but are not associated with obvious disturbances of the parathyroid and vitamin D endocrine systems.

Hypophosphatasia is a hereditary deficiency of bone alkaline phosphatase that is inherited as either an autosomal recessive or a dominant form. The recessive form presents in infancy with gross rickets, clinically and radiologically, and survival is limited. The dominant form may not present until adult life, usually with pathologic fractures complicated by non-union; chondrocalcinosis and even a syndrome of diffuse hyperostosis resembling Forestier's disease may also occur. Urinary excretion of an unusual metabolite, phosphoethanolamine, is a characteristic feature.

Osteopetrosis (Albers-Schönberg's disease) may show ragged epiphyses in childhood, especially during attempted therapeutic calcium depletion, although overall appearances should not give rise to confusion. **Metaphyseal dysostosis** (or chondrodysplasia), type Schmidt, shows grossly disorganized and rachitic-looking growth plates and children may develop severe bow legs; vitamin D treatment is unavailing but osteotomies heal normally in any case. **Blount's disease** is another cause of pathologic bow legs in children; it is essentially a fracture dislocation of the medial tibial condyles.

In adult life, **stress fractures** may have the appearance of a Looser's zone. Such fractures occurring as a consequence of Paget's disease rarely cause confusion, but sporadic stress fracture might be misdiagnosed. **Osteoid osteoma** may rarely appear in this guise, for example in the femoral neck, and be cured by excision biopsy.

Fibrogenesis imperfecta ossium is a rare acquired disease of middle age onwards characterized by defective bone collagen. Collagen fibrils become attenuated and 'disappear' histologically into an amorphous background. The skeleton is radiologically osteopenic, usually with very coarse trabeculation, pathologic fractures develop and histology superficially suggests gross osteomalacia. However, when viewed under polarized light the collagen is seen to have lost its lamellar birefringence and this appearance is diagnostic[35].

CLINICAL FEATURES

The main clinical features of rickets and osteomalacia are bone pain and tenderness, skeletal deformity and muscle weakness. Occasionally, signs

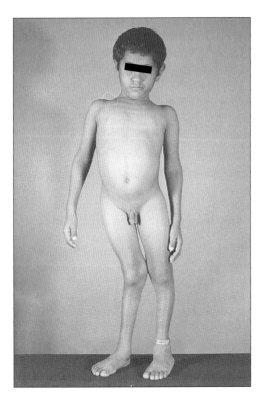

Fig. 200.6 'Windswept' appearance of legs in 8-year-old boy with rickets secondary to Fanconi syndrome.

of tetany from associated hypocalcemia may also be present. These symptoms generally provide no clue as to the cause.

Rickets

Rickets only occurs, by definition, during growth. It is characterized by defective mineralization, most prominent in those areas where bone growth is most rapid; usually in the metaphyseal region of the long bones[21]. Hence many of the physical (and radiologic) signs of rickets are found at these sites. The areas of most rapid bone growth vary with age and the signs of rickets therefore vary similarly. At birth, the skull's growth is most rapid and neonatal rickets may therefore show craniotabes, the cranial vault being softened. In the first year of life rickets becomes manifest in the swollen epiphyses at the wrist and in swelling ('beading') of the costochondral junctions, the so-called 'rickety rosary'. The inward pull of the diaphragm produces a groove in the rib cage, Harrison's sulcus. Rickets in the toddler tends to produce bow-leg deformities while knock-knees are characteristic of rickets in later childhood. Occasionally, both can occur together, producing a 'windswept' appearance of the legs (Fig. 200.6).

Rickety myopathy is part of the differential diagnosis of the 'floppy baby'. If muscle weakness is severe enough to prevent walking, it may limit deformity of the lower limbs. Conversely, one form of childhood rickets that is not associated with myopathy, the X-linked dominant hypophosphatemic syndrome, tends to produce early severe bow legs. A variable degree of dwarfism is another obvious feature of rickets. Pathologic fractures in the shafts of long bones only occur in very severe forms.

MAIN BIOCHEMICAL FEATURES IN RICKETS, OSTEOMALACIA AND RELATED BONE DISEASES

Legend: ↑ High   ↓ Low   □ Normal   ▣(low half shaded) Low normal   ▣(high half shaded) High normal   Occ Occasionally or rarely

Diagnosis	Plasma Ca	Plasma P	Plasma alkaline phosphatase	Plasma TCO₂	Plasma urea, creatinine	Plasma 25–OHD	Plasma 1,25(OH)₂D	Plasma PTH	Urine Ca (24h or Ca/creatinine)
Chondrodystrophies	Normal	Normal	Normal	Normal	Normal	Normal	Normal	Normal	Normal
Osteoporosis or osteogenesis imperfecta	Normal	Normal	Normal	Normal	Normal	Normal	Normal	Normal	Normal
Privational rickets/osteomalacia	↓ or Low normal	↓ or Low normal[a]	↑ occ High normal	↓ or High normal	Normal	↓ or High normal[b]	Low normal or Normal[c]	↑	↓ or High normal
Hypophosphatemic rickets/osteomalacia	Normal occ Low normal	↓	↑ or Normal[d]	Normal	Normal	Normal	High normal or Normal	Normal[e]	Normal
Acidotic forms of rickets/osteomalacia	↓ or Low normal	↓ or Low normal	↑ occ Low normal	↓	High normal or Normal	Normal	Normal[f]	↑ or Normal	↑ or High normal
Renal glomerular osteodystrophy	↓ or Low normal	↑ or High normal	↑	↓	↑	↓ or Normal	↓ or High normal	↑	↓
Primary hyperparathyroidism	↑	↓ or Low normal	↑ or Normal	Normal or High normal	↑ occ Normal	Normal or High normal	Normal	↑	↑ or Normal
Hypophosphatasia	↑ or Normal	Normal	↓	Normal	Normal	Normal	Normal[f]	Normal[f]	↑ or Normal
Hypoparathyroidism	↓	↑ or High normal	Normal	High normal	Normal	Normal	↓ or High normal	↓	↓
Pseudo-hypoparathyroidism	↓	↑ or High normal	↑ or Normal	Normal	Normal	Normal	↓ or High normal	↑	↓

a. Paradoxically ↑ if calcium is very low (in children), and rises rapidly in early healing stage.
b. Depending on seasonal variation.
c. Levels rise too briskly with recent vitamin D intake to provide diagnostic value.
d. Depends on disease activity, i.e. adults usually normal.
e. ↑ with large phosphate supplements, rarely spontaneously.
f. Insufficient data for certainty.

Fig. 200.7 Main biochemical features in rickets, osteomalacia and related bone diseases.

If hypocalcemia is present at the time of development of the permanent teeth, enamel hypoplasia may persist into adulthood.

Osteomalacia

Symptoms of osteomalacia in the adult tend to be more vague. Bone pain usually occurs in the axial skeleton, spine, shoulders, ribs and pelvis. Localized pain, for example in the groin, may be due to fracture or may be associated with an underlying pseudofracture (Looser's zone) on radiography, although the latter may not produce symptoms. Tenderness may be elicited by spinal percussion or by sternal and lateral rib compression; the most painful bones are generally those with the thinnest cortices. When adult osteomalacia occurs as a recrudescence of childhood rickets, stigmata of previous dwarfism, deformity or even scars of long-forgotten osteotomies may be a helpful sign in the differential diagnosis. In severe cases, vertebrae become compressed.

Osteomalacic myopathy has a characteristic proximal distribution, the reason for which is unknown. It may be difficult clinically to ascertain myopathy in the presence of pain, even when it is undoubtedly present. Electromyographic abnormalities are non-specific and may be absent. Associated hypocalcemia may lead to symptoms of latent tetany (Chvostek's and Trousseau's signs). The often vague nature of osteomalacic pain and muscle weakness can easily lead to missed diagnosis.

DIAGNOSIS

Biochemistry

Even in patients with vitamin D deficiency, hypocalcemia is only present in 50% because of secondary hyperparathyroidism, and rarely occurs in the hypophosphatemic syndromes. In vitamin D deficiency serum phosphorus levels are almost always towards or below the lower limit of normal, but may be paradoxically high if hypocalcemia is severe. Serum phosphorus is always abnormally low in hypophosphatemic syndromes. Serum alkaline phosphatase is generally high. It is important to remember that alkaline phosphatase levels in healthy adolescents, at peak height velocity, may reach three times the upper normal adult limit. A small proportion of affected adults may have serum alkaline phosphatase within the normal adult range. Markers of bone resorption such as type 1 collagen cross links in serum or urine and urinary hydroxyproline excretion may be elevated. Raised immunoreactive PTH levels are almost invariable in vitamin D deficiency and may be present in other osteomalacic syndromes. The different causes of osteomalacia are associated with a variety of different biochemical abnormalities that are summarized in Figure 200.7.

Specific investigations are available for some of the rarer forms of osteomalacia. For instance, renal tubular acidosis is diagnosed by the failure of the urine to acidify following an oral load of ammonium chloride. In addition, the presence of glycosuria and aminoaciduria should also be sought in patients with hypophosphatemic osteomalacia to exclude the presence of Fanconi's syndrome.

Radiology

In rickets the growth plate is characteristically widened, splayed and concave, holding the epiphysis in the 'cup': it is also frayed and ragged (Figs 200.8 & 200.9). The metaphysis may be rarefied by resorption due to secondary hyperparathyroidism and such changes also occur in membranous bone when the defect is severe. The severity of rickets in any given bone is directly related to its growth rate. One subtlety, for example, is at the wrist where the ulna is usually more affected than the radius because its growth rate there is almost double that of the radius – the radius grows at both ends while the proximal ulna is incorporated into the elbow joint and does not have an epiphysis in early childhood.

Healing of rickets with vitamin D tends to follow a pattern, with a clean line of ordered calcification forming first at the outer edge of

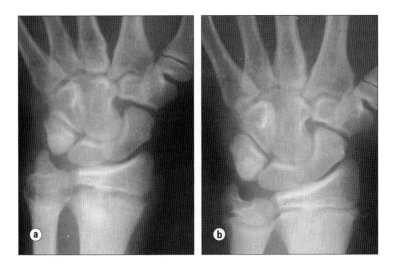

Fig. 200.8 Radiographs of the wrist of a 14-year-old Asian boy. (a) shows the presence of typical changes of rickets. (b) shows healing of these features following a holiday in India but no medication.

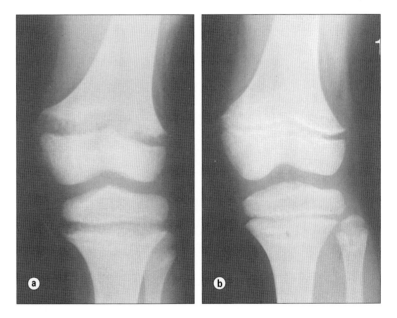

Fig. 200.9 Radiographs of the knee of a 9-year-old girl with X-linked hypophosphatemic rickets. (a) shows the typical appearances of rickets and (b) healing of these appearances following treatment with alfacalcidol and microcrystalline hydroxyapatite.

defective calcification, suggesting that vitamin D is acting 'early' in the zone of provisional calcification (zone of hypertrophy plus zone of maturation). The region may become denser than the subjacent metaphysis until normal growth and remodeling incorporate this region into the healing shaft.

Once the epiphyses have disappeared after fusion, the radiologic signs of vitamin D insufficiency must be sought elsewhere, although persisting 'fuzziness' of unfused ischial and iliac apophyses may be noted after growth has ceased. Bone texture may show no abnormal features. The characteristic abnormality is the 'Looser's zone', or pseudofracture, seen as one or more ribbon-like zones of decalcification that may be noted almost anywhere in the skeleton except in the skull (Figs 200.10 & 200.11). Their significance was obscure until their establishment as a general feature of osteomalacia by Albright and Reifenstein. Looser's zones in chronic forms of osteomalacia may show callus on the surface, which may be partially calcified. The common sites at which Looser's zones are seen include the medial border of the upper femora, pubic and

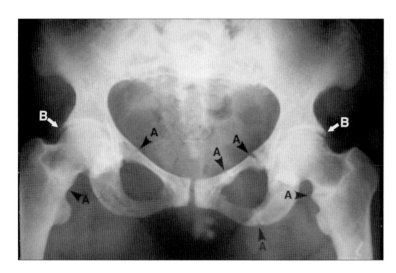

Fig. 200.10 Radiograph of the pelvis showing multiple Looser's zones in an asymptomatic woman with X-linked hypophosphatemia. The Looser's zones are arrowed (A) and arrows (B) point to early heterotopic ossification.

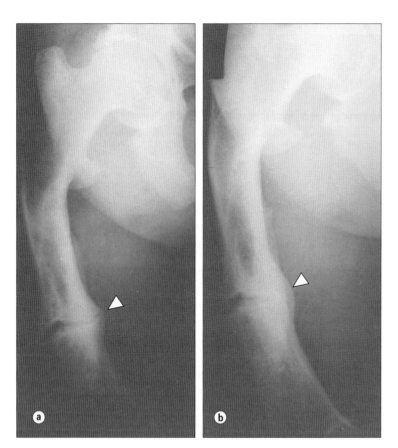

Fig. 200.11 Looser's zones. (a) A Looser's zone in the femur of a man with X-linked osteomalacia. (b) This only incompletely responded to treatment with vitamin D.

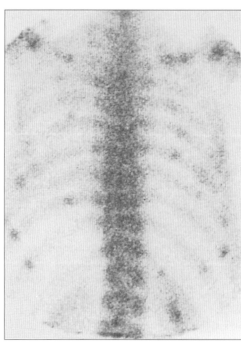

Fig. 200.12 Isotope bone scan in a 37-year-old man with severe osteomalacia associated with intestinal malabsorption. The majority of the 'hot spots' were not evident as Looser's zones radiologically.

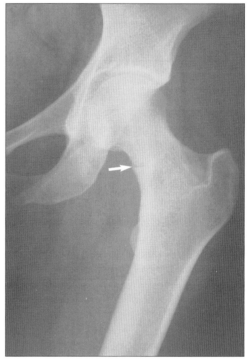

Fig. 200.13 Radiograph showing stress fracture of the femoral neck (arrow), with all the appearances of a Looser's zone, in an otherwise healthy woman of 27 years who presented with pain in the hip.

ischial rami and ribs, with scapulae and other long bones following next in order of frequency. Scintigraphy may be valuable in indicating developing Looser's zones before they are apparent radiologically (Fig. 200.12) and the whole skeleton may have a metabolic 'glow'. In very severe cases, the softened vertebrae develop an evenly biconcave outline from pressure transmitted through the intervertebral discs (called 'codfish' vertebrae, from the anatomic configuration of these teleosts). Occasionally, a stress fracture with all the characteristics of a Looser's zone is unrelated to osteomalacia (Fig. 200.13).

In vitamin D deficiency, but not necessarily in other causes of osteomalacia, secondary hyperparathyroidism is frequently present.

Radiological signs of hyperparathyroidism, including subperiosteal erosions in the phalanges (often best seen along the radial border of the middle phalanx of the index finger) and erosion of the outer ends of the clavicles and of the symphysis pubis, may contribute to the diagnosis of osteomalacia (Fig. 200.14). Areas of increased density, particularly in the vertebral endplates, where the colloquial term 'rugger-jersey spine' has been applied, are often presumed to result from secondary hyperparathyroidism, although the precise cause is unknown.

The causative tumors in oncogenic osteomalacia are frequently small and difficult to identify. Although a variety of different imaging modalities have been advocated these have frequently met with only limited success. The observation that the underlying mesenchymal tumors frequently exhibit somatostatin receptors has led to the use of radiolabeled octreotide as an imaging modality to detect these lesions. Preliminary reports suggest that this may be successful in several instances[36] (Figs 200.15 & 200.16).

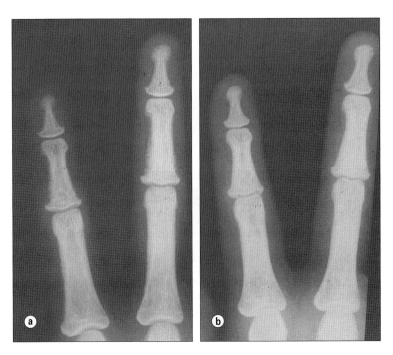

Fig. 200.14 Radiograph showing subperiosteal erosions of hyperparathyroidism (a) before and (b) after healing.

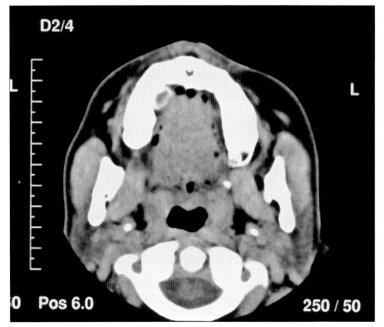

Fig. 200.16 CT scan of jaw in same patient as in Figure 200.15 revealing a tumor of the mandible. Removal of this tumor resulted in resolution of symptoms.

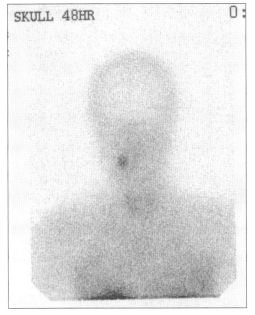

Fig. 200.15 Octreotide scanning. Octreotide scan of patient with oncogenic osteomalacia showing increased uptake in the region of the mandible.

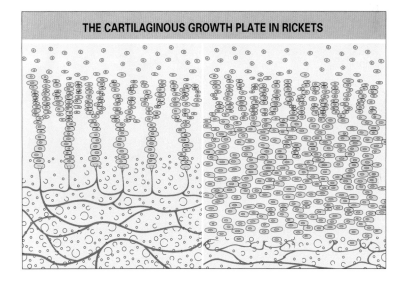

Fig. 200.17 The cartilaginous growth plate in rickets. The diagram illustrates the normal epiphyseal growth plate (left) and that in rickets (right). The top of the diagram faces towards the epiphysis. The elongation and distortion of the normal columnar arrangement of chondrocytes in rickets is readily apparent.

Histopathology

Although the diagnosis of rickets and osteomalacia is frequently made without recourse to bone biopsy, this remains necessary in difficult cases as osteomalacia is essentially a disease of abnormal bone mineralization and the diagnosis may sometimes be impossible to establish without direct measurement of mineralization. In rickets the diagnosis is usually established on the basis of clinical, biochemical and, most importantly, radiological findings.

Histologically, rickets is characterized by elongation and distortion of the normal columnar arrangement of chondrocytes in the zone of hypertrophy of the cartilaginous growth plate. In the underlying zone of maturation, provisional calcification is delayed or absent and vascularization via defective or obliterated channels is impaired and irregular (Fig. 200.17). The primary spongiosa is also abnormal.

The diagnosis of osteomalacia in adults may be confirmed by biopsy through the iliac crest. A standard trephine obtains a transiliac speci-

men, 8mm in diameter, of trabecular bone bounded by cortex at each end. The procedure can be undertaken using local anesthesia with i.v. sedation and usually causes little more than minor discomfort. It is important that specimens are handled correctly to maximize the information from this procedure. In particular, sections should be undecalcified to accurately assess the width and extent of unmineralized collagen (osteoid). Prior administration of fluorochromes, such as tetracycline, is essential to establish defective mineralization. These compounds are bound at sites of active mineralization and produce linear fluorescence under ultraviolet light (Fig. 200.18). This line of fluorescence is termed the calcification front. If two courses of oral tetracycline are given, separated by approximately 10 days, they will show up as two parallel lines; measurement of the mean distance between these lines allows the rate of bone mineralization to be measured. The mineralization rate can be related to the width of prevailing osteoid by dividing

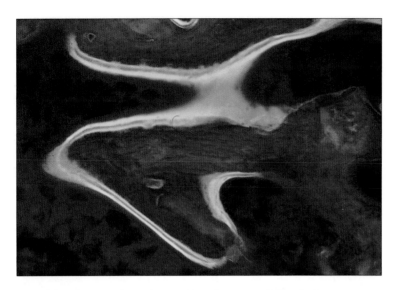

Fig. 200.18 Iliac crest bone biopsy viewed under UV light. The fluorescent bands are made by the presence of previously administered tetracycline, which accumulates in mineralizing osteoid.

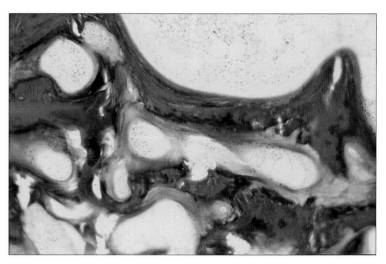

Fig. 200.20 Microscopic appearance of osteomalacia showing abnormally wide osteoid seams covering all the bone surfaces.

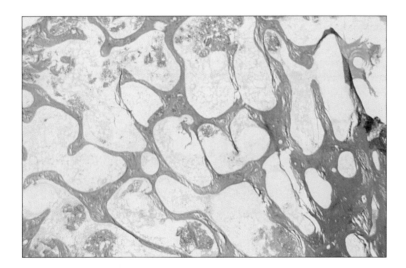

Fig. 200.19 Microscopic appearance of a normal iliac crest bone biopsy.

the latter by the former, to give the 'mineralization lag time'. This is prolonged in osteomalacia and a normal mineralization lag time excludes the diagnosis.

Excessive osteoid is typical of osteomalacia, but 'false-positive' pictures occur wherever collagen synthesis is increased, e.g. in thyrotoxicosis, hyperparathyroidism, Paget's disease and osteosclerotic malignancies. Coverage of trabecular bone surfaces of unmineralized osteoid is normally less than 27% (Fig. 200.19) and can spread to 100% in osteomalacia (Fig. 200.20). In all, 80–90% of normal osteoid shows tetracycline fluorescence. As severity increases, so osteoid thickness, or volume, increases. There is usually evidence of increased resorption due to secondary hyperparathyroidism which also produces peritrabecular fibrosis and increased synthesis of immature 'woven' bone. When marked, these changes are termed osteitis fibrosa.

Even with tetracycline labeling, caution is required. Wide and irregular labels are a feature of some forms of 'vitamin-D-resistant' osteomalacia but also occur when calcification, or turnover, is rapid; however, these situations are not associated with an increase in mineralization lag time. Rapid or normal mineralization is a rule once treatment of vitamin D deficiency is begun – excessive osteoid may be the last feature to disappear with healing.

Specific stains are available to demonstrate the presence of metals such as aluminum within the skeleton. This is useful in the identification of toxic causes of osteomalacia.

TREATMENT

Vitamin D deficiency

Vitamin D deficiency can be treated with vitamin D supplementation or by the administration of ultraviolet radiation to improve endogenous vitamin D production.

Simple vitamin D deficiency is best treated with the native vitamin itself. The more potent hydroxylated metabolites (calcitriol and alfacalcidol) are no more effective and are much more costly. Furthermore, their potency increases the risk of hypercalcemia during treatment. Finally, they do not contribute to repletion of the body's stores of vitamin D and so the deficiency may recur soon after therapy is stopped.

In adults it is usually possible to heal osteomalacia with a dose of 25µg (1000IU) ergocalciferol (vitamin D_2) or cholecalciferol (vitamin D_3) daily. In patients with gastrointestinal disease, higher doses may be necessary to overcome problems with absorption. Under such circumstances it may be necessary to a give a dose of 1.25mg (50 000IU) calciferol daily for 10 days or even a single dose of 7.5mg (300 000IU) calciferol. If possible, it is preferable to give this as an oral dose, which can be given under medical supervision rather than the often suggested intramuscular preparation, which has variable bioavailability[37]. Single doses at these levels are not associated with the development of vitamin D toxicity, which only occurs with prolonged administration of high doses of calciferol (usually in excess of 250µg (10 000IU) daily).

A single dose of 2.5mg of calciferol has been shown to maintain vitamin D stores of elderly infirm patients for about 6 months and so such a dose would need to be given twice a year to ensure that the deficiency does not recur[38]. Generally speaking, it is prudent to ensure that vitamin D deficiency does not recur by giving regular doses of calciferol of 10–20µg (400–800IU) daily. This represents little more than a dietary supplement and does not necessitate monitoring of plasma calcium levels.

In infants with rickets it is usual to employ similar doses of vitamin to those used in treating adults with vitamin D deficiency.

In addition to replacing the low levels of vitamin D it is important to seek out a cause for this deficiency and to remedy that. In particular, celiac disease should be sought in adults presenting with vitamin D deficiency and no obvious underlying cause.

Vitamin D resistance

Failure of hydroxylation of vitamin D responds to treatment with the potent hydroxylated metabolites of vitamin D. Treatment with calcitriol generally requires doses of 0.5–2µg per day. Unlike physiological doses of calciferol, this treatment is accompanied by a risk of hypercalcemia and all patients receiving calcitriol need regular measurement of plasma calcium.

Vitamin-D-dependent rickets type II (i.e. the receptor defect) may respond to very large doses of calcitriol. Patients needing a daily dose of 60µg daily have been reported. In addition it is usually necessary to give large doses of oral calcium (up to 3g daily) and in some cases intravenous calcium infusion is needed.

Hypophosphatemia

Hypophosphatemia as a result of phosphate-binding antacids will respond to withdrawal of that treatment. If the tumor responsible for oncogenic osteomalacia can be identified and removed, the bone lesions will heal. It is possible to use plasma phosphate as a marker for tumor recurrence. In other cases of hypophosphatemia it is usually necessary to give phosphate replacement.

In the case of X-linked hypophosphatemia up to 3g of elemental phosphorus (96mmol phosphate) per day may be needed to restore plasma phosphate levels to normal. This is poorly tolerated and can lead to diarrhea. This amount of phosphate will tend to stimulate parathyroid hormone production, which can lead to the development of osteitis fibrosis cystica. In order to minimize this, it is usual to give large doses of vitamin D or, more usually, supraphysiological, doses of its hydroxylated metabolites (such as calcitriol 2–4µg daily, titrated against calcium and PTH). Unfortunately, this treatment may result in nephrocalcinosis

and it is vital that patients receiving such therapy have regular monitoring of their plasma calcium.

Such treatment can lead to healing of the bone disease and restoration of Looser's zones to normal (Fig. 200.21). However the other benefits of treatment are less clear-cut. There is little evidence that aggressive treatment in childhood leads to improved adult height and in adults treatment of the hypophosphatemia does not diminish the tendency to heterotopic bone formation. In view of this, the poor acceptability of treatment and its associated hazards, it is our practice to reserve treatment in affected adults for those with symptomatic bone disease.

If it is not possible to identify or remove the causative tumor in oncogenic osteomalacia it is generally possible to use a similar regimen of phosphate and calcitriol to heal the bone disease.

Acidosis

Treatment with sodium bicarbonate, which may need to be given in a dose of up to 7.2g daily, will lead to normalization of blood pH and healing of the bone lesions. With such high doses of alkali there is a risk of hypokalemia, which needs to be treated with potassium supplementation. If this is given as potassium citrate or bicarbonate this will tend to increase the degree of alkalinization. In Fanconi's syndrome, potassium replacement is mandatory and supplementation with physiological doses of calcitriol (0.5–2µg daily) may be necessary to heal the skeletal lesions.

Other causes

Toxic causes will usually respond slowly following withdrawal of the toxic agent. In the case of aluminium it is possible to remove this directly by chelation with desferrioxamine. In general, toxic osteomalacia does not respond to vitamin D.

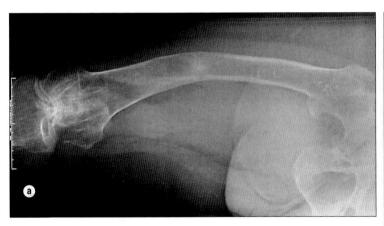
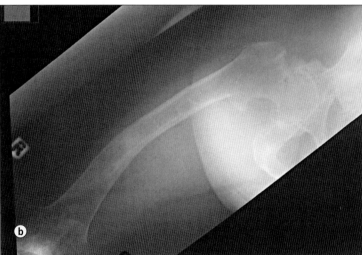

Fig. 200.21 Treatment of hypophosphatemia. (a) Looser's zone in femur of patient with hypophosphatemic osteomalacia. (b) Resolution after 1 year's treatment with phosphate supplements and calcitriol.

REFERENCES

1. Petifor JM, Daniels ED. Vitamin D deficiency and nutritional rickets in children. In: Feldman D, Glorieux FH, Pike JW, eds. Vitamin D. San Diego, CA: Academic Press, 1997: 663–678.
2. Maxwell JP, Pi HT, Liu HAC, Kuo CC. Further studies in adult rickets (osteomalacia) and foetal rickets. Proc Roy Soc Med 1939; 32: 287–297.
3. Albright F, Reifenstein EC. The parathyroid glands and metabolic bone disease: selected studies. Baltimore, MD: Williams & Wilkins; 1948.
4. Mughal MZ, Salama H, Greenaway T et al. Lesson of the week: florid rickets associated with prolonged breast feeding without vitamin D supplementation. Br Med J 1999; 318: 39–40.
5. Horst RL, Reinhardt TA. Vitamin D metabolism. In: Feldman D, Glorieux FH, Pike JW, eds. Vitamin D. San Diego: Academic Press, 1997: 13–31.
6. Holick MF. Photobiology of vitamin D. In: Feldman D, Glorieux FH, Pike JW, eds. Vitamin D. San Diego, CA: Academic Press, 1997: 33–39.
7. Jacobus CH, Holick MF, Shao Q et al. Hypervitaminosis D associated with drinking milk. N Engl J Med 1992; 326: 1173–1177.
8. Haddad JG, Chyu KJ. Competitive protein binding assay for 25-hydroxycholecalciferol. J Clin Endocrinol Metab 1971; 33: 992–995.
9. Stamp TC, Round JM. Seasonal changes in human plasma levels of 25-hydroxyvitamin D. Nature 1974; 247: 563–565.
10. Peacock M, Selby PL, Francis RM et al. Vitamin D deficiency, insufficiency, sufficiency and intoxication. What do they mean? In: Vitamin D. A chemical, biochemical and clinical update. Berlin: Walter de Gruyter; 1985.
11. Chapuy MC, Arlot ME, Duboeuf F et al. Vitamin D₃ and calcium to prevent hip fractures in elderly women. N Engl J Med 1992; 327: 1637–1642.
12. Bowman AR, Epstein S. Drug and hormone effects on vitamin D metabolism. In: Feldman D, Glorieux FH, Pike JW, eds. Vitamin D. San Diego, CA: Academic Press, 1997: 13–31.

13. Pike JW. The vitamin D receptor and its gene. In: Feldman D, Glorieux FH, Pike JW, eds. Vitamin D. San Diego, CA: Academic Press, 1997: 105–125.

14. Selby PL. Normal calcium homeostasis. Clin Rev Bone Mineral Metab 2002; 1.

15. Mawer EB. Clinical implications of measurements of circulating vitamin D metabolites. Clin Endocrinol Metab 1980; 9: 63–79.

16. Zewerkh JE, Glass K, Jowsey J, Pak CYC. An unique form of osteomalacia associated with end organ refractoriness to 1,25-dihydroxyvitamin D and apparent defective synthesis of 25-hydroxyvitamin D. J Clin Endocrinol Metab 1979; 49: 171–175.

17. Casella SJ, Reiner BJ, Chen TC et al. A possible genetic defect in 25-hydroxylation as a cause of rickets. J Pediatr 1994; 124: 929–932.

18. Prader A, Illig R, Heierli E. Eine besondere Form der primaeren Vitamin-D-resistenten Rachitis mit Hypocalcaemie und autosomal-dominantem Erbgang: die hereditaere Pseudo-Mangelrachitis. Helv Paediatr Acta 1961; 16: 452–468.

19. Dent CE, Friedman M, Watson L. Hereditary pseudo-vitamin deficiency rickets ('pseudo-mangelrachitis'). J Bone Joint Surg 1968; 50B: 708–719.

20. Brooks MH, Bell NH, Love L et al. Vitamin-D-dependent rickets type II: resistance of target organs to 1,25 dihydroxyvitamin D. N Engl J Med 1978; 298: 996–999.

21. Liberman UA, Marx SJ. Vitamin D-dependent rickets. In: Favus MJ, ed. Primer on the metabolic bone diseases and disorders of mineral metabolism, 3rd ed. Philadelphia, PA: Lippincott-Raven, 1996: 311–316.

22. HYP Consortium. A gene (HYP) with homologies to endopeptidases is mutated in patients with X-linked hypophosphataemic rickets. Nat Genet 1995; 11: 130–136.

23. White KE, Jonsson KB, Carn G et al. The autosomal dominant hypophosphatemic rickets (ADHR) gene is a secreted polypeptide overexpressed by tumors that cause phosphate wasting. J Clin Endocrinol Metab 2001; 86: 497–500.

24. Strewler GJ. FGF23, hypophosphatemia, and rickets: has phosphatonin been found? (letter; comment). Proc Natl Acad Sci USA 2001; 98: 5945–5946.

25. Winters RW, Graham JB, Williams TF et al. A genetic study of hypophosphatemia and vitamin D-resistant rickets with a review of the literature. Medicine 1958; 37: 97–142.

26. Davies M, Stanbury SW. The rheumatic complications of metabolic bone disease. Clin Rheum Dis 1981; 7: 595–646.

27. Scriver CR, Tenehouse HS, Glorieux FH. X-linked hypophosphatemia: an appreciation of a classic paper and a survey of progress since 1958. Medicine 1991; 70: 218–228.

28. Adams JE, Davies M. Intra-spinal new bone formation and spinal cord compression in familial hypophosphataemic vitamin D resistant osteomalacia. Q J Med 1986; 61: 1117–1129.

29. Carmichael KA, Fallon MD, Dalinka M et al. Osteomalacia and osteitis fibrosa in a man ingesting aluminium hydroxide antacid. Am J Med 1984; 76: 1137–1143.

30. Drezner MK. Tumor-induced rickets and osteomalacia. In: Favus MJ, ed. Primer on the metabolic bone diseases and disorders of mineral metabolism, 3rd ed. Philadelphia, PA: Lippincott-Raven, 1996: 319–325.

31. Shimada T, Mizutani S, Muto T et al. Cloning and characterization of FGF23 as a causative factor of tumor-induced osteomalacia. Proc Natl Acad Sci U S A 2001; 98: 6500–6505.

32. Compston JE, Chadha S, Merrett AL. Osteomalacia developing during treatment of osteoporosis with sodium fluoride and vitamin D. Br Med J 1980; 281: 910–911.

33. Boyce BF, Smith L, Fogelman I et al. Focal osteomalacia due to low-dose diphosphonate therapy in Paget's disease. Lancet 1984; 1: 821–824.

34. Boyce BF, Eldr HY, Fell GS. Localisation of aluminium in osteomalacic bone using X-ray micro analysis. Scot Med J 1981; 26: 282.

35. Swan CHJ, Shah K, Brewer DB, Cooke WT. Fibrogenesis imperfecta ossium. Q J Med 1976; 45: 223–253.

36. De Beur SMJ, Streeten EA, Civelek AC et al. Localisation of mesenchymal tumours by somatostatin receptor imaging. Lancet 2002; 359: 761–763.

37. Whyte MP, Haddad JG Jr, Walters DD, Stamp TC. Vitamin D bioavailability: serum 25-hydroxyvitamin D levels in man after oral, subcutaneous, intramuscular, and intravenous vitamin D administration. J Clin Endocrinol Metab 1979; 48: 906–911.

38. Davies M, Mawer EB, Hann JT et al. Vitamin D prophylaxis in the elderly: a simple effective method suitable for large populations. Age Ageing 1985; 14: 349–354.

201 Hyperparathyroidism

Michael Kleerekoper and Robert Igwe

Definition

- Primary hyperparathyroidism (PHPT) is characterized by hypercalcemia resulting from excess parathyroid hormone secretion by one or more parathyroid glands.

- Secondary hyperparathyroidism results from prolonged stimulation of the parathyroid glands in response to diminished serum calcium. It may be seen in chronic renal failure as a result of diminished production of calcitriol (1, 25-dihydroxyvitamin D), and in malabsorption or malnutrition as a result of diminished calcidiol (25-hydroxyvitamin D) availability.

Clinical features

- Musculoskeletal manifestations include bone pain, pathologic fractures, selective decrease in cortical bone mass, bone cysts and the classic form of advanced bone disease – osteitis fibrosa cystica. Pseudogout has been reported as an infrequent complication.

- Renal manifestations range from colic, nephrolithiasis and nephrocalcinosis to impairment of renal function.

- Nonspecific symptoms include fatigue, emotional lability and neuropsychiatric abnormalities.

HISTORY

The earliest descriptions of patients with primary hyperparathyroidism were based on the severely progressive bone disease, osteitis fibrosa cystica, as reported by Cope[1]; subsequently, patients were observed with recurrent nephrolithiasis with no evidence of bone disease. Serum calcium levels were less elevated in the latter group of patients. Following these observations, Lloyd[2] classified primary hyperparathyroidism into two types: type 1, in which large parathyroid glands were associated with markedly elevated calcium levels and bone disease, and type 2, with small glands, moderate hypercalcemia and renal stone disease. However, the development of automated biochemistry analyses, 20–25 years ago, led to the detection of hypercalcemia and diagnosis of primary hyperparathyroidism prior to the appearance of any clinical symptoms. It is rare, in current clinical practice, to see patients with advanced bone disease as the initial mode of presentation.

EPIDEMIOLOGY AND RISK FACTORS

Primary hyperparathyroidism is a relatively common endocrine disease. The prevalence in the general population is approximately 1 in 1000 persons[3]. It occurs at all ages, but most frequently in the sixth decade of life, with women being affected more than men by a ratio of 3:2[4]. There are no clearly identifiable risk factors for primary hyperparathyroidism; however, a history of external irradiation to the head and neck region many years prior to the disease has been reported in 15–25% of patients[5].

CLINICAL FEATURES

There are no abnormal physical findings that are specifically related to primary hyperparathyroidism. The most common presentation is hypercalcemia, usually with mild elevations within 1mg/dl (0.25mmol/l) above the upper limits of normal and detected on a biochemical profile obtained for other reasons. Increasingly, as serum calcium has become (perhaps unnecessarily) a routine test ordered in patients with low bone mineral density, identification of the latter is increasingly the precipitating event for diagnosis, even though the two phenomena may be unrelated. Symptoms and signs may be related to features of hypercalcemia. Patients with the disease can be divided, somewhat arbitrarily, into three groups with regard to clinical presentation:

- those with a mild form that is asymptomatic and is detected by routine determination of serum calcium;
- those with symptoms running an insidious course over several years with renal colic as the mode of presentation;
- those with more rapid onset of disease, with significant hypercalcemia, bone pain and occasionally pathologic fractures.

Musculoskeletal

The classic form of parathyroid bone disease is called osteitis fibrosa cystica. It is seen in primary and secondary hyperparathyroidism. Manifestations include generalized osteopenia, with bone pain, increased bone resorption (especially in the subperiosteal regions) and formation of bone cysts. Cyst-like areas may be seen with localized swelling of bone (brown tumors) (Fig. 201.1) and epulis (seen in the jaw area). Bones commonly involved on radiologic examination include the distal phalanges, distal clavicle and skull. There is preferential loss of cortical bone with relative sparing of cancellous bone[6]. Other musculoskeletal features of primary hyperparathyroidism include nonspecific arthralgias involving joints of the hands, sometimes centered in the proximal interphalangeal joints. Gout and chondrocalcinosis may be complicating features.

Renal

Nephrolithiasis and renal colic are the most common renal manifestations of primary hyperparathyroidism due to deposition of calcium containing stones in various parts of the urinary tract. Most stones are calcium oxalate; however, calcium phosphate stones do occur. Nephrocalcinosis, which is deposition of calcium phosphate crystals throughout the renal parenchyma, may also occur.

Other

Neurologic manifestations include a slowing in mental function, poor memory and emotional lability. Easy fatigability is a common manifestation. Patients may complain of muscle weakness, which is more pronounced in the proximal group of muscles. Increased frequency of peptic ulcer disease and exacerbation of pancreatitis have also been reported. Clinical features, more nonspecifically related to hypercalcemia, include

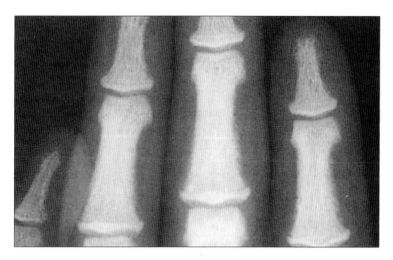

Fig. 201.1 Part of the hand radiograph of a patient with hyperparathyroidism, showing the characteristic subperiosteal resorption of the phalanges and lacelike trabecular pattern. This patient also had lytic lesions ('brown tumors') in the long bones.

polyuria, polydipsia and constipation. Cardiovascular manifestations include shortened Q–T interval and ectopic calcifications of the kidneys and arteries. Hypertension is thought to be associated with hyperparathyroidism and is more evident when the disease is complicated by renal impairment or severe hypercalcemia, or is part of the multiple endocrine neoplasia (MEN) syndrome.

INVESTIGATIONS

Documentation of elevated parathyroid hormone (PTH) levels in the face of hypercalcemia establishes the diagnosis of primary hyperparathyroidism. Clinical features are not very helpful since they are not specific. Serum calcium level is elevated in all cases of primary hyperparathyroidism but may not be elevated on every occasion it is measured. Assay of ionized calcium is preferable to total calcium, especially in those with a borderline elevations. There are, though, many practical problems with precise measurement of ionized calcium; in these patients, serial values of serum calcium yield more useful information than do single measurements. Measurement of PTH levels is essential to help differentiate patients with hyperparathyroidism, where levels are clearly elevated or inappropriately in the high-normal range, from patients with hypercalcemia of malignancy where PTH levels are low or undetectable. Figure 201.2 shows the level of PTH in different disease states, as measured by immunochemiluminometric assay. Different regions of PTH, like the C-terminal and N-terminal portions, have been measured in the past, but the current assay of choice is the intact PTH, and there are few if any clinical indications for measuring any other PTH fragment. With the development of the two-site immunoradiometric assays, yields are highly sensitive and specific.

Other laboratory abnormalities include serum phosphate levels which are usually in the low-normal range, and frankly low in about 25% of patients. Bone mineral density (BMD) has replaced standard skeletal radiography as the 'imaging' modality of choice in patients with primary hyperparathyroidism. In general there is preferential loss of bone from cortical bone sites (e.g. radius mid-shaft) but a significant decrease in

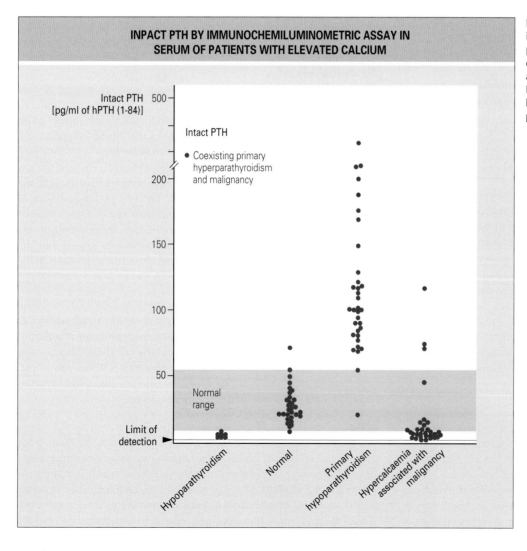

Fig. 201.2 Intact PTH by immunochemiluminometric assay in serum of patients with elevated calcium. There is a clear distinction between primary hyperparathyroidism and hypercalcemia associated with malignancy. Note patients with coexisting primary hyperparathyroidism and malignancy. (With permission from Endres et al.[7])

TABLE 201.1 ETIOLOGIC CAUSES OF HYPERCALCEMIA	
Parathyroid hormone	Primary hyperparathyroidism (adenoma or hyperplasia)
	Parathyroid cancer
	Lithium-induced hypercalcemia
	Thiazide-induced hypercalcemia
PTH-related protein	Solid tissue malignancies (with or without skeletal metastases)
Cytokines	Hematologic malignancies (including myeloma and lymphoma)
	(?) Skeletal metastases
Vitamin D or metabolites	Granulomatous diseases (1,25-dihydroxycholecalciferol D)
	(?) Lymphoma
	Vitamin D intoxication (vitamin D, 25-hydroxycholecalciferol, 1,25-dihydroxycholecalciferol)
(?) Prostaglandin	Renal cell carcinoma
Uncertain (and uncommon)	Hyperthyroidism
	Acute adrenal insufficiency
	Pheochromocytoma
	Immobilization
	Familial (benign) hypocalciuric hypercalcemia

lumbar spine BMD is present in a substantial minority of patients with primary hyperparathyroidism. Standard radiographic investigations have become less helpful in identifying patients with primary hyperparathyroidism. Radiographs of the phalanges may reveal marked periosteal bone erosion in the terminal phalanges. In advanced cases, radiographs will reveal bone cysts, brown tumors and some areas of increased bone density (osteosclerosis). In secondary hyperparathyroidism, interpretation of PTH levels is more complicated as renal failure can cause retention of PTH fragments. Intact PTH is still a sensitive assay and is elevated, but should be correlated with bone histology which usually reveals high bone turnover. These patients typically have elevated serum phosphate levels, 1,25-dihydroxycholecalciferol [1,25(OH)$_2$] D deficiency and hypocalcemia.

DIFFERENTIAL DIAGNOSIS

Hypercalcemia has a wide variety of etiologic factors, as listed in Table 201.1. After primary hyperparathyroidism the most common cause of hypercalcemia is malignancy. This may be the most frequent cause in hospitalized patients. Hypercalcemia of malignancy can easily be excluded by PTH assay which will be low or even undetectable. High or inappropriately elevated PTH levels, in the presence of hypercalcemia, usually establishes a diagnosis of primary hyperparathyroidism. The only other states where PTH levels may be elevated occur with the use of lithium or thiazide diuretics. This can easily be excluded by careful history. In 5–10% of patients with familial hypocalciuric hypercalcemia (FHH), the PTH levels may be modestly elevated. They can be distinguished from primary hyperparathyroidism by obtaining the ratio of calcium clearance to creatinine clearance. The ratio in FHH is one third that in primary hyperparathyroidism and is a more useful index than a 24-h urine collection, since it corrects for variation in glomerular filtration.

ETIOLOGY

Primary hyperparathyroidism results from a single adenoma in 80–90% of cases and hyperplasia of all four glands in most of the remaining cases.

TABLE 201.2 INDICATIONS FOR PARATHYROIDECTOMY IN PRIMARY HYPERPARATHYROIDISM[10]
• Symptoms or signs referable to hypercalcemia
• Active nephrolithiasis
• Fragility fractures
• Serum calcium >12.0mg/dl (3mmol/l)
• Urine calcium >400mg/24h
• Bone mineral density (at any site) >2 SDs below age- and sex-matched reference interval
• Age <50 years

Parathyroid cancer is quite uncommon, accounting for less than 1% of all cases of PTH-mediated hypercalcemia. As the name implies, the precise etiologic diagnosis of primary hyperparathyroidism is uncertain. Recent molecular studies suggest that the majority of adenomas are monoclonal in origin while primary parathyroid hyperplasia has a polyclonal origin[8]. Abnormalities have been observed in the PTH gene, and gene rearrangement between the PTH gene and the PRAD-1 oncogene may play a role in at least a subset of patients with primary hyperparathyroidism[9].

MANAGEMENT

The best available therapy for management of primary hyperparathyroidism is parathyroidectomy. However, there are still conflicting reports as to which patients should be referred for surgery. This dilemma arose because many patients are diagnosed in the asymptomatic stage and, in a proportion of these patients, the risk of development of renal and skeletal complications is unknown. Based on guidelines from the National Institutes of Health Consensus Development Conference (Table 201.2) on the management of asymptomatic primary hyperparathyroidism, the criteria for surgery include:

- serum calcium >12mg/dl (3mmol/l)
- hypercalciuria
- bone mineral density at cortical sites >2 standard deviations below age- and sex-matched controls
- any specific complications (e.g. kidney stones)
- patients younger than 50 years of age[10]

For patients who do not meet any of the above criteria, follow-up is necessary with serum calcium and creatinine determinations every six months, annual 24-h urinary calcium measurements and biannual bone densitometry. Surgical therapy is clearly indicated for patients with symptomatic primary hyperparathyroidism. It is imperative that surgery be performed by a skilled and experienced surgeon because of the potential difficulties in localization of abnormal glands. The glands may be located at ectopic sites such as retro-esophageal, the lateral neck, within the thyroid gland or in the mediastinum. Preoperative localization of the parathyroid glands is not necessary in patients without a history of prior neck surgery but increasing experience with these procedures appears to slightly shorten operative time and hospital length of stay without adding to the cost of care or altering the high success rate of surgery. In patients with a history of previous neck surgery, preoperative imaging studies are almost always performed. Ultrasound, CT scanning, MRI and technetium and/or thallium scintigraphy are various non-invasive imaging modalities utilized alone or as a combination of any two tests. However, most of these procedures have limited sensitivity and specificity, especially in patients with mild disease. More recently improved sensitivity and specificity have been demonstrated with sestamibi scans, and this is improved further when an ultrasound imaging study is also used. Intra-operative use of either ultrasound or sestamibi radio-guided probes are being used more frequently such that a more limited surgical procedure can be performed[11]. Most patients, after successful surgery, will have transient hypocalcemia necessitating postoperative monitoring of serum calcium with replacement warranted if levels fall below 8mg/dl (2mmol/l). In a small group of patients, there may be prolonged periods of hypocalcemia characterized by rapid deposition of calcium and phosphate into bones – hungry bone syndrome – and rarely hypoparathyroidism may complicate parathyroid surgery[12].

REFERENCES

1. Cope O. The study of hyperparathyroidism at the Massachusetts General Hospital. N Engl J Med 1966; 21: 1174–1182.
2. Lloyd HM. Primary hyperparathyroidism: an analysis of the role of the parathyroid tumor. Medicine 1968; 47: 53–71.
3. Palmer M, Akerstrom G, Ljunghall S. Prevalence of hypercalcemia in a health survey: a 14-year follow-up study of serum calcium values. Eur J Clin Invest 1988; 18: 39–46.
4. Fitzpatrick L, Bilezikian JP. Primary hyperparathyroidism. In: Becker KL, ed. Principles and practice of endocrinology and metabolism. Philadelphia: Lippincott; 1990: 430–437.
5. Cohen J, Glerlowski TC, Schneider AB. A prospective study of hyperparathyroidism in individuals exposed to radiation in childhood. J Am Med Assoc 1990; 264: 581–584.
6. Kleerekoper M, Villanueva AR, Parfitt AM et al. PTH mediated bone loss in primary hyperparathyroidism. In: Frame B, Potts J Jr, eds. Clinical disorders of bone and mineral metabolism. Amsterdam: Excerpta Medica; 1983: 200–203.
7. Endres DB, Villanueva R, Sharp CF Jr, Singer FR. Measurement of parathyroid hormone. Endocrinol Metab Clin North Am 1989; 18: 611–629.
8. Backdahl M, Howe JR, Larimore TC et al. The molecular biology of parathyroid disease. World J Surg 1991; 15: 756–762.
9. Arnold A. Molecular basis of primary hyperparathyroidism. In: Bilezikian JP, Marcus R, Levine MA, eds. The parathyroids. New York: Raven Press; 1994: 407–421.
10. Proceedings of the NIH Consensus Development Conference on diagnosis and management of asymptomatic primary hyperparathyroidism: consensus development conference statement. J Bone Miner Res 1991(suppl 2): s9–s166.
11. Lorenz K, Nguyen-Thanh P, Dralle H. Unilateral open and minimally invasive procedures for primary hyperparathyroidism: a review of selective approaches. Langenbecks Arch Surg 2000; 385: 106-117.
12. Aurbach GD, Marx SJ, Spiegel AM. Parathyroid hormone, calcitonin and the calciferols. In: Wilson JD, Foster DW, eds. Williams' textbook of endocrinology. Philadelphia: Saunders; 1992: 1397–1476.

202 Renal bone disease

John B Eastwood and Michaelis Pazianas

Definition

- Osseous abnormalities occurring in patients with chronic renal failure
- The earliest and most classic abnormality is hyperparathyroidism (osteitis fibrosa) and there may be an osteomalacic component which in some patients is due to aluminum toxicity
- Adynamic bone disease has been recognized recently
- In general the bony problems are worst in patients with end-stage renal disease maintained on dialysis
- Bone biopsy is the gold standard when defining the type of bone disease

Clinical features

- Often asymptomatic in adults, except when osteomalacia due to aluminum overload is present
- Children may present with rickets
- Bone pain and loss of height may develop and progress in patients maintained on dialysis
- Soft tissue calcification with itching and conjunctivitis

HISTORY

The term 'renal osteodystrophy' was introduced by Liu and Chu in 1943 to include all the types of bone disease associated with chronic renal failure[1]. It was in reports in the early 1930s that attention was first paid to the frequent occurrence of diffuse parathyroid hyperplasia in renal rickets. Albright et al.[2] pointed out that in adults with nephritis there were sometimes radiologic and histologic features that resembled primary hyperparathyroidism, and they considered the condition to be the 'adult counterpart of so-called renal rickets'.

Later, bone lesions were classified into those that were predominantly due to hyperparathyroidism and those that showed osteomalacia. Currently, renal bone disease includes hyperparathyroidism, osteomalacia, including a special form of resistant osteomalacia caused by aluminum overload, and a newly described form of bone disease, adynamic bone disease. There is also the phenomenon of dialysis arthropathy, caused by deposition of β_2 microglobulin, that occurs particularly in individuals who have been on dialysis for 10 years or longer.

EPIDEMIOLOGY

Hyperparathyroidism

The hyperparathyroidism starts relatively early, when the glomerular filtration rate (GFR) is in the region of 60–90ml/min[3], as shown by increased circulating plasma levels of intact parathyroid hormone (PTH) as well as histological abnormalities in the bone. As uremia progresses abnormalities become more pronounced, so that when the GFR falls to below 10ml/min, and renal replacement therapy is about to be insti-

TABLE 202.1 HYPERPARATHYROIDISM IN END-STAGE RENAL DISEASE

Evidence of hyperparathyroidism	Percentage of patients
Increased circulating PTH	95–100
Hyperparathyroidism on bone histology	85–90
Subperiosteal resorption on radiography of hands	25–30

tuted, most patients have histologic evidence of hyperparathyroidism (Table 202.1). Often the focus for remodeling is in the cortical osteons of long bones, resulting in increased porosity and subperiosteal resorption. In addition, there is uniform enlargement of the parathyroid glands.

Risk factors for the development of radiological subperiosteal resorption in patients with chronic renal failure include duration of renal failure, young age, female gender and certain renal diagnoses, in particular non-glomerular causes of renal failure[4].

Osteomalacia

In a minority of patients with end-stage renal failure, bone histology reveals evidence of a mineralization defect with accumulation of osteoid, i.e. osteomalacia. In the UK, in patients with renal failure who are not yet on dialysis the most likely cause is lack of vitamin D, and such patients usually have low circulating levels of 25-hydroxycholecalciferol (25-OHD)[5]. These data support other European evidence that 25-OHD concentrations are frequently low in chronic renal failure. However, studies in the USA have failed to demonstrate such a relationship, probably because of greater exposure to sunlight and the addition of vitamin D to certain foods.

A number of factors contribute to the vitamin D deficiency. In patients with advanced chronic renal failure dietary restriction may result in inadequate intake, and anorexia is also often a feature. There is also lack of 1,25-dihydroxycholecalciferol [$(1,25(OH)_2D_3)$], the kidney metabolite of vitamin D. Studies of vitamin D administration in patients with the osteomalacia of renal failure have shown no conclusive evidence of any resistance to its action at the bone (i.e. osteoid) level[6]. In other words, the osteomalacia of renal failure, if not associated with aluminum intoxication, is probably not resistant to vitamin D.

Aluminum toxicity

In the early 1970s in Newcastle, England, a particularly disabling form of bone disease was reported among hemodialysis patients. Evidence was produced that a toxin, probably aluminum, was responsible[7]. The osteomalacia was associated with dementia and anemia, and did not respond to vitamin D. The discovery that aluminum in the dialysis fluid was passing across the membrane into the patients' circulation and being deposited in various organs, especially bone and brain, led to stringent measures being adopted in the preparation of water used for dialysis. Dialysis units drawing their water from sources that did not treat water with aluminum sulphate were more fortunate and rarely saw the problem.

For some 25 years it has been realized that aluminum can be absorbed via the gastrointestinal tract in patients with uremia. It is only relatively recently, however, that it has become clear that the aluminum-containing phosphate binders widely used in patients with renal failure also lead to aluminum accumulation in bone and brain. The elimination of aluminum-induced osteomalacia depends upon adequate water purification and upon discontinuing the practice of giving aluminum-containing phosphate binders to patients with chronic renal failure. Currently, around 5% of patients with significantly reduced renal function have stainable bone aluminum. In dialysis patients the proportion can be as high as 50%.

Adynamic bone disease

Some patients with chronic renal failure, especially those undergoing chronic ambulatory peritoneal dialysis (CAPD), exhibit normal amounts of osteoid on bone biopsy, but diminished numbers of osteoblasts and osteoclasts, and low or unmeasurable rates of bone formation. This disorder has been termed 'adynamic' or 'aplastic' bone disease, and aluminum deposition along the trabecular surfaces is not uncommon. It is possible that the condition is a forerunner of overt histologic osteomalacia; bone aluminum concentrations in this group of patients are lower than in patients with the osteomalacia of aluminum toxicity. It is now known that aluminum is not wholly responsible and that other factors may play a part in the genesis of this adynamic form of osteopathy. These factors include overtreatment with calcium and vitamin D of patients with chronic renal failure who have not been dialysed; sustained elevation of serum calcium in patients on CAPD; and factors such as age, diabetes mellitus and hyperphosphatemia. It is claimed in some reports that the condition is particularly common in predialysis patients (prevalence up to 48%)[8] and in CAPD patients (up to 63%)[9].

CLINICAL FEATURES

In patients not on dialysis, symptoms are unusual, although occasionally osteomalacia may present with local pelvic and hip pain and difficulty in walking, and is associated with Looser's zones in the pelvis and femoral necks. It should be stressed that the development of clinical rickets in a child with renal failure usually reflects hyperparathyroidism rather than osteomalacia[10].

In dialysis patients, hyperparathyroidism gives rise to few symptoms, though pruritus and non-specific aches and pains may occur. There may also be loss of height due to compression of the vertebrae. Fractures are unusual. The osteomalacia of vitamin D deficiency is uncommon in dialysis patients as general nutrition improves. Aluminum-induced osteomalacia can be devastating in such patients, however, and if not recognized can lead to the patient being in a wheelchair within 6 months. Knowledge of the association with anemia and dementia is important so that the diagnosis is not overlooked.

In patients whose plasma calcium phosphate product is consistently high, mineral may be deposited in soft tissues. It is most commonly seen radiologically in peripheral arteries, but can give rise to calcified subcutaneous nodules. Such tumoral calcinosis can sometimes be very significant clinically and associated with skin necrosis (calciphylaxis).

Adynamic bone disease can only be diagnosed on bone biopsy as it does not give rise to symptoms. There are now, however, suggestions that there may be a relationship between adynamic bone disease and hip fracture.

INVESTIGATIONS

It is not possible to predict the type or severity of bone disease from plasma levels of calcium and phosphate, and indeed patients with unequivocal bone disease may have normal levels. Typically, however, patients with renal failure have a low plasma calcium and raised plasma phosphate. If the bone disease is severe the plasma alkaline phosphatase may be elevated. Aluminum-induced osteomalacia is usually associated with a normal to high plasma calcium but a low plasma phosphate; the plasma alkaline phosphatase is usually normal or even low.

PTH

Plasma PTH levels are raised in patients with advanced renal failure (unless there is aluminum toxicity), even when there is relatively mild histologic evidence of hyperparathyroidism. In the past, interpretation of the results of different immunoassays has been complicated by the molecular heterogeneity of circulating PTH, i.e. a number of fragments were measured in addition to the whole (1-84) PTH molecule. Assays for intact PTH developed in the late 1980s gave more accurate measurements of active hormone and have been very useful clinically. Recently, it has been realized that these two-site PTH assays cross-react with an inactive fragment (most likely 7-84) which is increased in renal failure[11]. The significance of this finding is that the 7-84 fragment by binding, possibly to a carboxy-terminal PTH receptor, antagonises the effects of PTH and therefore functions as a negative regulator of serum calcium concentration. With the new whole PTH non-cross reactive assays it is likely that we will gain greater understanding of the role of PTH in the investigation and treatment of renal bone disease. Currently, values of PTH significantly ($>4 \times$) above the upper limit of normal are taken to indicate continuing hyperparathyroidism, but values at the lower limit of normal or below normal are indicative of adynamic bone disease. Values in between are more difficult to interpret.

Vitamin D

Levels of 25-OHD are often normal, depending on the state of nutrition and exposure to sunlight, but circulating $1,25(OH)_2D_3$ becomes progressively lower as the GFR falls, so that in dialysis patients it is often undetectable. Therefore, measurements of plasma $1,25(OH)_2D$, if available, are of little discriminatory value in the investigation of the type or severity of bone disease.

Biochemical markers of bone turnover

Plasma total alkaline phosphatase activity is a measurement that is widely available. However, it is composed of both bone and liver elements, and so patients with liver disease may give rise to diagnostic difficulty. The isoenzyme that originates from bone (bone-specific alkaline phosphatase) is produced by osteoblasts and one would expect it to be useful in the separation of the various forms of renal bone disease. Unfortunately, bone alkaline phosphatase can be normal in patients with osteitis fibrosa, and osteomalacia, as well as in low bone turnover states and in those with normal bones. Even a raised concentration of bone alkaline phosphatase is incapable of distinguishing osteitis fibrosa from osteomalacia.

There are now a number of other markers of bone formation – bone γ-carboxylglutamic acid protein (osteocalcin), procollagen type I carboxy-terminal propeptide (PICP) and procollagen type I amino-terminal propeptide (PINP) – that can be measured in blood and/or urine. Similarly, there are potentially useful markers of resorption, such as cross-linked C-telopeptide of type I collagen (ICTP), tartrate-resistant acid phosphatase (TRAP), free and total pyridinoline, free and total deoxypyridinoline, and both the N-and C-telopeptides of collagen cross-links (NTX and CTX). At the moment, however, the place of these markers in the diagnosis and management of patients with renal bone disease is unclear.

Other investigations

Serum aluminum measurements may provide a clue to aluminum overload but give no indication as to severity.

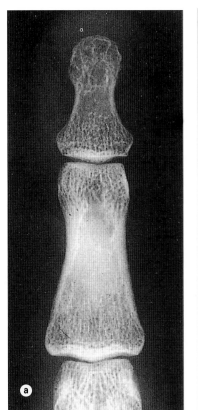
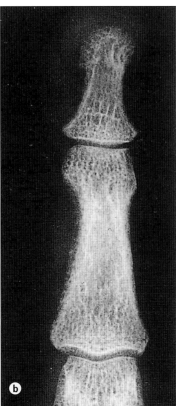

Fig. 202.1 Radiographs of fingers. Comparison of (a) a normal right middle finger with (b) the right middle finger of a patient on maintenance hemodialysis for 6 years. There is marked evidence of subperiosteal resorption of bone, especially on the lateral aspect of the middle phalanx but also involving the terminal phalanx.

The most important investigation in renal bone disease is bone biopsy, for it is only by examining histological sections of bone that the type and severity of bone disease can be ascertained with any certainty.

Radiographs are useful in demonstrating abnormal bone texture and subperiosteal resorption in the fingers, particularly the middle phalanx of the index and middle fingers (Fig. 202.1). It should be remembered, however, that radiologic features appear late, and so individuals with quite marked hyperparathyroidism may have normal radiographs. Patchy osteosclerosis is also common, and this accounts for the classic appearance of 'rugger jersey' spine – (i.e. horizontal bands of alternating intensity – upper vertebral endplate (light), center of vertebra (darker), lower vertebral endplate (light), disc space (dark), upper vertebral endplate (light) etc.) as seen in lateral views, and the 'salt and pepper' appearance of the skull. Cystic lesions may also be a manifestation of hyperparathyroidism ('Brown' tumors), but the presence of cysts in bone should always alert one to the possibility of amyloid deposition.

Isotope bone scanning may be useful if other, particularly focal, osseous diagnoses are being considered, and bone densitometry usually reveals a reduction in the amount of mineral in the skeleton. Imaging, especially ultrasound and thallium–technetium subtraction isotope scans of the parathyroid glands, however, though commonly carried out, does not often produce clinically useful information. However, for individuals with recurrent hyperparathyroidism where a second exploration is being contemplated, the techniques can be most useful. Indeed, this notion is in keeping with the recent recommendations of the group working on calcium metabolism for the European Renal Association[12]. Ectopic glands may be detectable with MRI scanning if isotope techniques are unsuccessful.

DIFFERENTIAL DIAGNOSIS

Hyperparathyroidism and osteomalacia are common accompanying features of renal failure and do not usually produce symptoms. When skeletal symptoms do occur other diagnoses should be sought; in particular, it is important to exclude metastatic disease, myelomatosis and Paget's disease. Another problem for long-term dialysis patients is the occurrence of dialysis amyloid as a result of retention of β_2 microglobulin. In this condition there is both large and small joint arthropathy with erosions and certain associated features, such as carpal tunnel syndrome. The resulting joint symptoms can thus be easily confused with the symptoms of metabolic bone disease. Because the severity of both dialysis-related amyloidosis and hyperparathyroidism increases with time on dialysis, it is important in any patient with arthropathy being considered for parathyroidectomy because of the symptoms, to exclude dialysis-related amyloidosis. Biopsy of periarticular tissues or carpal tunnel is usually diagnostic. Interestingly, a link has recently been established between dialysis-related amyloidosis and renal osteodystrophy, with the finding that β_2 microglobulin may influence the development of renal osteodystrophy by means of a T-cell mediated immune mechanism.

The secondary hyperparathyroidism of chronic renal failure involves all four glands. In the past a distinction has been made between 'four-gland hyperplasia' (which should be suppressible by raising the plasma calcium by giving calcitriol) and 'four-gland hyperplasia with adenomas'. It is this latter group that sometimes does not respond and requires parathyroidectomy. Typically, the glands are unequal in size and there is sometimes hypercalcaemia – so-called 'tertiary' hyperparathyroidism. Recent research suggests that there may be a connection between parathyroid cell clonality and histological findings, i.e. that the cells of diffuse hyperplasia of the parathyroid glands are mostly polyclonal, whereas focal collections of cells (adenomas) are monoclonal. However attractive this suggestion may seem, there is as yet only circumstantial evidence to support it. It is tempting to speculate that monoclonal clusters might arise against a background of polyclonal hyperactivity.

STRUCTURE AND FUNCTION

Disturbances of calcium and phosphate metabolism are central to the development of hyperparathyroidism. It is probable also that lack of $1,25(OH)_2D_3$ is etiologically important. The result of these disturbances is that the parathyroid glands become hyperplastic and may exceed 1 g in weight (normal total parathyroid weight 100–150mg). Whatever the histological type (see above) circulating PTH levels are high, the effect of which is to increase the activity of both osteoblasts and osteoclasts. This hyperactivity leads to an increase in bone turnover. The osteoid formed is primarily of the woven type, and in advanced cases the bone marrow may be more or less completely replaced by fibrous tissue[13]. It is not surprising that in these circumstances an anemia develops that is relatively unresponsive to erythropoietin.

Osteomalacia is essentially a histological diagnosis. There are wide osteoid seams, and dynamic markers (such as demeclocycline) show that osteoid lamellae fail to mineralize appropriately. In the form resulting from vitamin D deficiency there is often parathyroid hyperplasia as well, so the bone may show a mixed picture. In the form associated with aluminum intoxication the histological appearances in the bone are solely those of osteomalacia, and the parathyroids are not overactive. Hence, there is no evidence of increased bone turnover and the plasma alkaline phosphatase is typically normal or low. The lack of osteoclastic resorption is in keeping with the low plasma phosphate.

Like osteomalacia, adynamic bone disease is essentially a histological diagnosis. Typically, bone turnover is low, but the amount of osteoid tissue, though usually low, may be normal. Biochemical bone markers, including $25-(OH)_2D$ and PTH, are unremarkable.

ETIOLOGY AND PATHOGENESIS

Hyperparathyroidism

Phosphate retention has been implicated in the development of hyperparathyroidism in chronic renal failure. Bricker[14], in his widely accepted 'trade-off' hypothesis, suggested that small incremental rises of plasma phosphate occurring in the course of progressive renal insufficiency lead to the formation of $CaHPO_4$ complexes, with a subsequent fall in serum ionized calcium levels and rise in PTH secretion. In early renal failure the PTH-stimulated increase in fractional excretion of phosphate keeps the serum phosphate within the normal range. The plasma calcium also is often normal initially because of increased bone resorption. However, the 'trade-off' hypothesis on its own cannot account for many of the clinical and experimental observations that have been made[15].

Llach[16] has proposed a different explanation for the development of secondary hyperparathyroidism. He suggests that a fall in $1,25(OH)_2D_3$ production (secondary to hyperphosphatemia) leads to impaired intestinal absorption of calcium and increased secretion of PTH. As $1,25(OH)_2D_3$ also interferes with the action of PTH on bone, PTH is relatively less effective at restoring plasma calcium to normal. Therefore, the hypocalcemia remains and there is continued stimulation of the parathyroid glands.

Importantly, $1,25(OH)_2D_3$ has a direct effect on the synthesis of PTH by means of its suppressive effect on the production of PTH mRNA. In patients with chronic renal failure, however, the lack of $1,25(OH)_2D_3$ in combination with the known reduction in the number of $1,25(OH)_2D_3$ receptors in the parathyroid glands leads to a significant reduction in its inhibitory action on the production of PTH. Furthermore, $1,25-(OH)_2D_3$ – normally a potent inhibitor of parathyroid cell hyperplasia – is less effective in this regard because of a reduction in vitamin D receptor expression in individuals with nodular hyperplasia. The lack of $1,25-(OH)_2D$ receptors also explains, at least in part, why administration of $1,25(OH)_2D_3$ itself is often ineffective in the hyperparathyroidism of chronic renal failure.

The suppressive effect of calcium ions at the level of the parathyroid cell, which can sense relatively small changes in Ca^{2+} in the extracellular fluid through the calcium sensing receptor, is also well established[17]. This G-protein coupled cell surface receptor, which is also abundantly expressed in the kidneys, regulates the synthesis of PTH at the post-transcriptional level. It may also be able to reduce parathyroid gland hyperplasia. Interestingly, in chronic renal failure the expression of the calcium-sensing receptor in the parathyroid gland is diminished, as it is also in the kidney. How these changes affect function is not clear.

Interest in the role of phosphate has undergone a recent revival because of new evidence suggesting that phosphate, rather than acting indirectly as suggested originally by Bricker[14], may have a direct effect on the secretion of PTH at the post-transcriptional step. Another possibility is that phosphate may modulate the expression of the calcium-sensing receptor. In addition, a number of cytokines (interleukin 1 (IL-1), IL-6, IL-11) have been implicated in the pathogenesis of hyperparathyroidism in chronic renal failure[18].

Osteomalacia

Osteomalacia in patients with chronic renal failure is of two types. Before dialysis became commonplace, dietary restriction of protein was the mainstay of treatment and it is likely that many patients became nutritionally deficient in vitamin D. In the mid-1970s there were several publications reporting low plasma 25-OHD levels. It was therefore not surprising that these individuals (who were also deficient in calcitriol) developed osteomalacia[5] which was similar in origin to that occurring in other circumstances of vitamin D lack.

Osteomalacia resulting from exposure to aluminum is a direct consequence of the accumulation of aluminum in osteoid lamellae. Such lamellae become mineralized much more slowly than normal and there is a distinct lack of active osteoblasts. Appropriate stains show aluminum both in calcifying and calcified lamellae, but there is no lack of circulating 25-OHD$_3$ and concentrations of $1,25(OH)_2D_3$ are no different from those of other patients with renal failure. PTH levels are not increased and the serum alkaline phosphatase is typically normal or low, in keeping with the lack of active osteoblasts. In the parathyroid cell there is evidence that, at a molecular level, a transferrin receptor is responsible for the uptake of aluminum. The effect is a reduction in the secretion of PTH, but synthesis is unaffected.

Adynamic bone disease

It is perhaps surprising in a population of patients with renal failure (with its high incidence of hyperparathyroidism) that there should be individuals with low bone turnover, and the question arises as to why this should develop. Slatopolsky et al.[11] have found that in patients with chronic renal failure there is a circulating non-1-84 PTH fragment (most probably 7-84 PTH) that accounts for up to 60% of the measured PTH immunoreactivity. Their suggestion is that although this fragment binds to the PTH receptor, it does not activate it. It does, however, prevent the action of PTH at the receptor and effectively reduces the number of available receptors. There is therefore a state of 'PTH resistance' or 'functional uremic hypoparathyroidism'. The clinical importance of this condition is that some individuals with chronic renal failure may need a circulating level of PTH that is higher than the upper limit of normal to preserve adequate bone function.

It has become clear that advances in molecular biology are beginning to enhance our understanding of the pathophysiology of renal osteodystrophy. For example, animal models with gene-targeted deletions, such as the 1α-hydroxylase-deficient mouse produced by Goltzman's[19] group, as well as tissue-specific gene inactivation, should be capable of defining the role of the agents involved and uncovering the sequence of events that lead to the development of this bony complication.

MANAGEMENT

Prevention

It is clear that it is theoretically possible to reduce the incidence and severity of hyperparathyroidism in patients with chronic renal failure. One cannot alter many of the risk factors for individual patients, such as gender, age, renal diagnosis and duration of renal failure, but it should be possible to reduce the plasma phosphate and increase plasma calcium by the measures listed in Table 202.2. It is probable that these measures will increase the plasma bicarbonate, leading to an improvement in the acidosis as well as an increased sensitivity of receptors to vitamin D. These are further reasons why the hyperparathyroidism should improve if managed as summarized in Table 202.2.

In patients on hemodialysis or peritoneal dialysis the above may need some modification, depending on the dialysate calcium and adequacy of dialysis, etc. In general, provided that patients are not hyperphosphatemic, and as the effect on renal function is not of concern, $1,25-(OH)_2D_3$ can be given in appropriate dosage. There is clearly the hazard of hypercalcemia, so until the dose is stable plasma calcium (and phosphate) will need to be measured frequently. The evidence suggests that by judicious use of $1,25-(OH)_2D_3$ the progression of hyperparathyroidism is delayed,

---

TABLE 202.2 PREVENTION OF HYPERPARATHYROIDISM IN CHRONIC RENAL FAILURE

1. Dietary phosphate restriction
2. Administration of calcium salts, e.g. $CaCO_3$
3. Administration of $1,25(OH)_2D_3$ to those most at risk

TABLE 202.3 PREVENTION OF OSTEOMALACIA IN CHRONIC RENAL FAILURE
Patients not on dialysis
1. Avoid all aluminum-containing compounds, i.e. most phosphate-lowering drugs and antacids
2. Ensure adequacy of vitamin D; check plasma 25-OHD and replete with vitamin D₃ as necessary
Patients on dialysis
1. Ensure dialysis fluid aluminum of ,20mg/l
2. Avoid all possible sources of ingested aluminum
3. Measure plasma aluminum levels regularly
4. Confirm sufficiency of vitamin D by measuring 25-OHD levels

if not reversed[20]. The aim is to keep the plasma PTH below four times the upper limit of normal.

A strategy for the prevention of osteomalacia in patients with renal failure is given in Table 202.3.

Treatment

Hyperparathyroidism

In patients not on dialysis it is unusual to need to take steps other than those outlined above. However, occasionally patients show evidence of hyperparathyroidism out of proportion to their degree of renal failure. There may be hypercalcemia, hyperphosphatemia, and progressive bone erosions unresponsive to treatment. Indeed, hypercalcemia is often made worse by giving otherwise appropriate treatment such as $1,25(OH)_2D_3$. In such cases, autonomy of the parathyroid glands is presumed (especially if backed up by radiographic evidence of subperiosteal erosions and raised plasma PTH concentrations) and parathyroidectomy will need to be considered. Clearly, however, it is important to rule out aluminum-related bone disease and other causes of hypercalcemia, as there can be serious implications for the bone if parathyroidectomy is undertaken in a patient who has histologic evidence of aluminum deposition. It is clear that in some individuals the hyperparathyroid state is maintaining bone turnover; removal of the parathyroids can lead to an adynamic bone state. It is important therefore to treat the aluminum intoxication of such individuals before undertaking parathyroidectomy.

In patients dependent on dialysis it is important to keep the serum PTH at an acceptable level. The treatment of choice is one of the active analogs of vitamin D, the most widely used in the USA being $1,25(OH)_2D_3$ (calcitriol). 1α-OHD₃ (alfacalcidol) and the more recently introduced 19-nor-$1\alpha,25(OH)_2D_2$ (doxercalciferol) are also available. Intravenous pulse administration confers no advantage over the oral route, but if compliance is in doubt there could be a role for supervised administration. There is some evidence that those with the highest PTH levels should be given larger doses of $1,25(OH)_2D$ and those with lower levels lower doses. Indeed, as PTH falls with treatment it may be possible to lower the dose of $1,25(OH)_2D_3$. A normal starting dose is 0.25μg/day, and it is unusual to need a maintenance dose of more than 2μg/day; for 1α-OHD₃ the dose is about double that of $1,25(OH)_2D_3$. There is no evidence from published studies that any of the newer metabolites are more effective than $1,25(OH)D_3$ or 1α-OHD₃, and there is no evidence as yet that any of them is any less likely to cause hypercalcemia or hyperphosphatemia.

A major element in the prevention and treatment of the hyperparathyroidism is lowering the plasma phosphate[21]. Dietary restriction is a useful early measure but is not usually effective on its own in dialysis patients. Oral calcium salts (usually carbonate or acetate) will raise the plasma calcium and tend to cause a fall in plasma phosphate but, if ineffective, phosphate binders will usually be necessary. Because of the toxic effect of aluminum on bone, parathyroid and other organs,

aluminum-containing phosphate binders are best avoided completely. In some patients the addition of a magnesium-containing phosphate binder to oral calcium salts may give better control of the plasma phosphate. There is now a phosphate-binding agent free of both aluminum and calcium that has been approved by the US Food and Drug Administration. The drug Sevelamer, an ion-exchange resin, is effective in preventing intestinal phosphate absorption. Because it is not absorbed from the gut it is believed that there will be a low risk of systemic toxicity. An additional benefit is its reported ability to lower cholesterol.

A novel method of treating the parathyroid overactivity in the future may be to use one of the new 'calcimimetic' compounds currently undergoing clinical evaluation[22]. These compounds, which are small phenylalkylamine derivatives, act by making the calcium receptor more sensitive to extracellular calcium. It is likely that, rather than being used on their own, they will find their clinical role as adjuncts and be used alongside drugs such as $1,25(OH)_2D_3$ to enhance their effectiveness.

A comprehensive strategy for the prevention and management of renal osteodystrophy has recently been devised by a Medical Expert Group of the European Renal Association[12].

Parathyroidectomy

For individuals not being considered for a renal transplant it is likely that total parathyroidectomy will give the most benefit, as there will not be the problem of recurrent hyperparathyroidism and the challenging search for a hidden gland. On the other hand, there will be the unknown hazard of being 'aparathyroid', though as yet there is no suggestion that any long-term harm results from chronic hypoparathyroidism. For patients likely to be transplanted, total parathyroidectomy does have the consequence of post-transplant hypocalcemia and the possible need for lifelong vitamin D treatment, and so should be avoided.

Subtotal parathyroidectomy (three and a half glands removed) has been the operation most commonly undertaken for those likely to be transplanted, but although effective in the short term it is often followed by regrowth of the parathyroid remnant.

Total parathyroidectomy involving implantation of parathyroid tissue in the forearm has fallen into disfavor because of reports of invasion by the implanted tissue into the subcutaneous tissues and muscles of the forearm. Likewise, other methods, such as ultrasound-guided alcohol injection into hypertrophic glands, have not entered general clinical practice except in specialized centers. Overall, some 6–10% of dialysis patients will come to parathyroidectomy by the time they have been on dialysis for 10 years[8].

Once patients are transplanted the hyperparathyroidism tends to improve. Nevertheless, bone histology remains abnormal in up to 90% of patients 5 years after transplantation. Whether this is residual bone disease or an effect of the immunosupressant drugs on bone metabolism is not clear, and of course it should be remembered that in some transplant patients renal function will not be normal.

Hypercalcaemia can be quite severe during the first few months after transplantation, and can cause allograft dysfunction. It is unusual, however, for parathyroidectomy to be necessary. After a successful transplant dialysis-related amyloidosis tends to resolve. There is marked improvement in symptoms as well as considerable histologic improvement.

Osteomalacia

In patients not on dialysis, and without evidence of aluminum toxicity, it is important to measure 25-OH vitamin D levels and, if low, to give parent vitamin D (vitamin D₃) to replenish the stores of vitamin D.

Among patients on dialysis, osteomalacia is much more likely to be due to aluminum toxicity. Treatment is with desferrioxamine administered during hemodialysis; it may need to be continued for several months.

Adynamic bone disease

The prevention of adynamic bone disease depends on maintaining bone turnover. This is best achieved by careful monitoring of the plasma PTH to ensure that it is kept no lower than three to four times the upper limit of normal. The plasma phosphate should be kept below 2mmol/l and, in patients on 1,25-$(OH)_2D_3$ particularly, care should be taken to ensure that the plasma calcium does not rise to, and remain, above the upper limit of normal.

REFERENCES

1. Liu SH, Chu HI. Studies of calcium and phosphorus metabolism with special reference to pathogenesis and effects of dihydrotachysterol (AT10) and iron. Medicine (Baltimore) 1943; 22: 103–161.
2. Albright F, Drake TG, Sulkowitch HW. Renal osteitis fibrosa cystica. Report of a case with discussion of metabolic aspects. Bull Johns Hopkins Hosp 1937; 60: 377–399.
3. Reichel H, Deibert B, Schmidt-Gayk H, Ritz E. Calcium metabolism in early chronic renal failure: Implications for the pathogenesis of hyperparathyroidism. Nephrol Dial Transplant 1991; 6: 162–169.
4. Pazianas M, MacRae KD, Phillips ME, Eastwood JB. Identification of risk factors for radiographic hyperparathyroidism in 422 patients with end-stage renal disease. Nephrol Dial Transplant 1992; 11: 1098–1105.
5. Eastwood JB, Harris E, Stamp TCB, de Wardener HE. Vitamin D deficiency in the osteomalacia of chronic renal failure. Lancet 1976; ii: 1209–1211.
6. Memmos DE, Eastwood JB, Harris E, O'Grady A, de Wardener HE. Response of uremic osteoid to vitamin D. Kidney Int 1982; (Suppl 11): S50–54.
7. Ward MK, Feest TG, Ellis HA *et al*. Osteomalacic dialysis osteodystrophy: evidence for a water-borne aetiological agent, probably aluminum. Lancet 1978; i: 841–845.
8. Weinreich T. Prevention of renal osteodystrophy in peritoneal dialysis. Kidney Int 1998; 54: 2226–2233.
9. Sanchez M, Baio A, Selgas R *et al*. Parathormone secretion in peritoneal dialysis patients with adynamic bone disease. Am J Kidney Dis 2000; 36: 953–961.
10. Mehls O. Renal osteodystrophy in children: etiology and clinical aspects In: Fine RN, Gruskin AB, eds. End-stage renal disease in children. Philadelphia: WB Saunders, 1984; 227–250.
11. Brossard J-H, Yamamoto LN, D'amour P. PTH Metabolites in Renal Failure: Bioactivity and Clinical implications. Sem Dialysis 2002; 15: 196–201.
12. Cannata-Andía J, Passlick-Deetjen J, Ritz E (eds) Management of the renal patient: experts' recommendations and clinical algorithms on renal osteodystrophy and cardiovascular risk factors. Nephrol Dial Transplant 2000; 15 (Suppl. 5): 39–57.
13. Hruska KA, Teitelbaum SL. Renal osteodystrophy. N Engl J Med 1995; 333: 166–173.
14. Bricker NS. On the pathogenesis of the uremic state: An exposition of the 'trade off hypothesis'. N Engl J Med. 1972; 286: 1093–1099.
15. Adler JA, Berlyne GM. Phosphate retention and the genesis of secondary hyperparathyroidism. Am J Nephrol 1986; 6: 417–421.
16. Llach F. Secondary hyperparathyroidism in renal failure: the trade-off hypothesis revisited. Am J Kidney Dis 1995; 25: 663–679.
17. Brown EM, McLeod J. Extracellular calcium sensing and extracellular calcium signaling. Physiol Rev 2001; 81: 239–297.
18. González E.A. The role of cytokines in skeletal remodelling: possible consequences for renal osteodystrophy. Nephrol Dial Transplant 2000; 15: 945–950.
19. Panda DK, Miao D, Tremblay ML *et al*. Targeted ablation of the 25-hydroxyvitamin D 1a-hydroxylase enzyme: Evidence for skeletal, reproductive, and immune dysfunction. PNAS 2001; 98: 7498–7503.
20. Schömig M, Ritz E. Management of disturbed calcium metabolism in uraemic patients: 1. Use of vitamin D metabolites. Nephrol Dial Transplant 2000; 15 (Suppl 5): 18–24.
21. Malluche HH, Mawad H. Management of hyperphosphataemia of chronic kidney disease: lessons from the past and future directions. Nephrol Dial Transplant 2002; 17: 1170–1175.
22. Frazã JM, Martins P, Coburn JW. The calcimimetic agents: perspectives for treatment. Kidney Int 2002; 61: 149s–154s.

METABOLIC BONE DISEASES

203 Paget's disease of bone

Jean-Pierre Devogelaer and Charles Nagant de Deuxchaisnes

Definition

- Paget's disease is a localized disorder of bone remodeling. It may be monostotic or pluriostotic
- The process is initiated by dramatic increases in osteoclast-mediated bone resorption with subsequent compensatory increases in new bone formation
- Local bone activity is mediated by large multinucleated osteoclasts and by enlarged blood vessels
- The net result is a disorganized structure of woven and lamellar bone at affected skeletal sites, complicated by bone deformity and an increase in bone fragility
- Paget's disease of bone is sporadic, but a few familial cases have been described

Clinical features

- Paget's disease is predominantly a disease of the elderly
- The main features of Paget's disease are bone pain, brittleness and deformity
- The most frequent localizations, in decreasing frequency of occurrence, are the spine, the pelvis, the lower limbs, the upper extremities and the skull

HISTORY

Sir James Paget is credited with the first description of the disease more than a century ago. He described a chronic inflammation of bone and termed the condition 'osteitis deformans'. There is evidence, though, that the disease has existed since prehistoric times.[1]

EPIDEMIOLOGY

It is difficult to provide a single estimate of the prevalence of Paget's disease because it varies greatly between countries, and even within a country. Moreover, it is a focal disorder, frequently asymptomatic. This simply explains why it is not easy to obtain accurate information concerning its real prevalence. The highest prevalence is probably in the UK, where some 3.6% and 5.4% of the population aged 40 and above and 55 and above, respectively, are affected.[2] In France, the prevalence above the age of 55 is about half of that in the UK, whereas in Ireland, Denmark, West Germany, Spain and Italy, it is about half that in France. It is conspicuously rare in Scandinavia, India, Japan, China, the Arab Middle East and black Africa. In the US, a higher prevalence is seen in the northern part of the country than in the south.[3] In New York, the prevalence is about as high as in the UK. In Australia, the prevalence in British-born immigrants is a little lower than that in the UK (4.0% over the age of 50 years versus 4.5%) but higher than in the natives of Australia (3.2%). Interestingly, the disease is extremely rare in Australian aboriginals. The more recent epidemiological data tend to demonstrate a decline in the prevalence and severity of the condition.[4] This could at least partially be explained by changes in the use of radiographs, the number of plain abdomen films, of intravenous pyelography and barium enemas – the classic source of most epidemiological data in Paget's disease of bone – which have dramatically decreased owing to the shift to other techniques of investigation, such as ultrasonography and endoscopic examinations, devoid of radiological images of the skeleton.

The disease is seldom encountered before the age of 40 years, but its prevalence approximately doubles each decade from the age of 50 onwards,[5] to reach about 10% in the ninth decade. It affects males more than females in a proportion of 3:2. Family clustering has been observed, with parents and siblings of patients with Paget's disease having a 10-fold higher risk than controls. This suggests evidence for a strong genetic contribution.[6]

CLINICAL FEATURES

In most cases Paget's disease is asymptomatic. This does not mean that asymptomatic patients must simply remain ignored and not be treated. Two factors must drive the indication of therapy in asymptomatic cases:

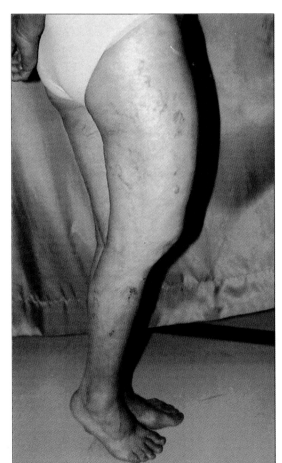

Fig. 203.1 Bowing of the right femur. A forward and lateral deformity provoking excruciating pain, due to varus osteoarthritis of the knee and shortening of the right lower limb.

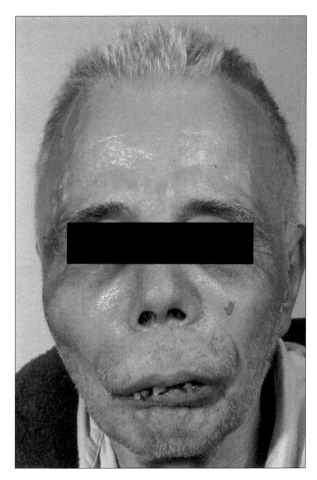

Fig. 203.2 **Paget's disease of the maxilla, provoking the characteristic facial deformity known as leontiasis ossea.** Note also the hypertrophy of the right temporal artery, which can potentially be mistaken for temporal arteritis.

the age of the patient at diagnosis and his or her life expectancy, as well as the localization of the lesion. When symptomatic (about 30% of subjects), pain is the presenting manifestation of Paget's disease. Approximately half complain of joint pain, especially at the knee, hip and spine; in the other half the pain is osseous in origin. This is a classic complication of the condition. Paget's disease may be monostotic (17%), predominantly at the tibia and the iliac bone, or polyostotic, which produces more symptoms than the monostotic form.

Paget's disease can affect every bone in the skeleton. However, the bones mostly implicated are, in descending order of frequency, the

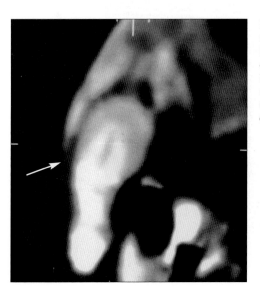

Fig. 203.3 **CT of the maxilla of a patient with leontiasis ossea shows characteristic marked hypercementosis of the root of a tooth (arrow), rendering the tooth extraction difficult.**

pelvis, lumbar spine, femur, thoracic spine, sacrum, skull, tibia and humerus. The resultant deformities may be crippling, particularly in the limbs (Fig. 203.1) and may induce osteoarthritis. The secondary osteoarthritis, of course, will produce pain aggravated by weightbearing, or weight lifting. These deformities may also be unsightly, particularly in the facial bones (leontiasis ossea) (Fig. 203.2) and cause problems for artificial dentures, tooth extraction and prosthetic difficulties (Fig. 203.3). When the skull is involved, it may lead to deafness and cranial nerve involvement, particularly the entrapment of orbital nerves (Fig. 203.4). When the base of the skull is affected there may be platybasia, basilar invagination, basilar impression, hydrocephalus and vertebrobasilar insufficiency. Vertebral involvement may provoke spinal cord lesions, nerve root compressions and cauda equina syndrome. Cord or nerve root symptoms are more frequently encountered when Paget's disease involves the thoracic spine. The explanation could be that the width of the vertebral canal is larger at the cervical level and therefore less prone than at the thoracic level to be significantly deformed by the bony overgrowth. Spinal compression should be suspected when three to five adjacent vertebral bodies are pagetic.[7] The usual complaint consists of a slowly progressive impairment of spinal cord function. The lumbar spine is a more common site for Paget's disease, being affected in up to 50% of patients. In the vast majority of patients the lumbar involvement is asymptomatic. In symptomatic cases the vertebral deformity attributable to the pagetic process (Fig. 203.5) may favor prolapse of the intervertebral disc, eventually leading to entrapment of a nervous root. Alternatively, osteophytosis, favored by disc degeneration, could directly compress nervous tissue, which could also be encroached by a pagetic collapsed vertebra.[8] Fissure fracture (Fig. 203.6), a frequent complication in the convex aspect of long bones, is frequently asymptomatic. When symptomatic, it may represent a harbinger for a complete fracture.

Pagetic bones are brittle and may fracture spontaneously, particularly the femur, the tibia, the humerus and the forearm. Such fractures are typically transverse.

Vascularization

Pagetic bone and the skin overlying the lesion are highly vascularized, which gives rise to local hyperthermia. In the skull, this increased vascularization may divert so much blood from the external carotid artery system that this occurs at the expense of the brain, accounting for hypertrophy and tortuosity of the superficial temporal artery (see Fig. 203.2) which might lead to confusion with temporal arteritis. This

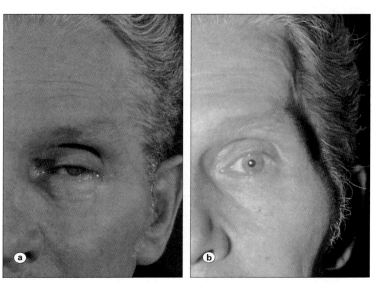

Fig. 203.4 **Entrapment of the left oculomotor nerve in the fissura orbitalis inferior.** This caused ptosis of the eyelid (a); eyelid mobility returned to normal after calcitonin therapy (b).

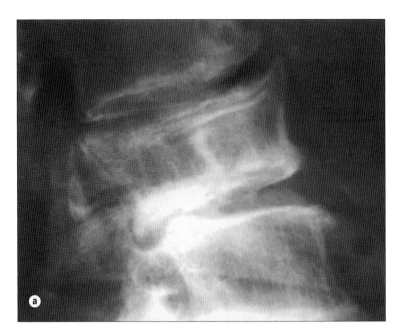

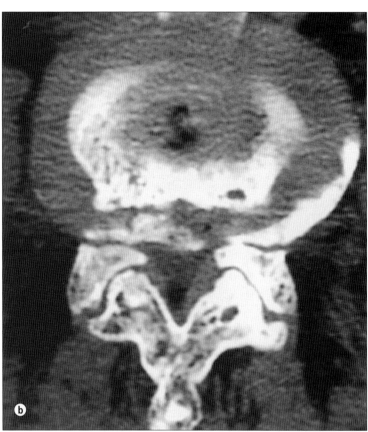

Fig. 203.5 Paget's disease of the spine. (a). Slipped pagetic vertebra narrowing the neuroforamen. (b) Bulging of intervertebral disc leading to spinal stenosis, whereas the stenosis is less severe at the level of the pagetic vertebra. (Courtesy of Professor B. Maldague.)

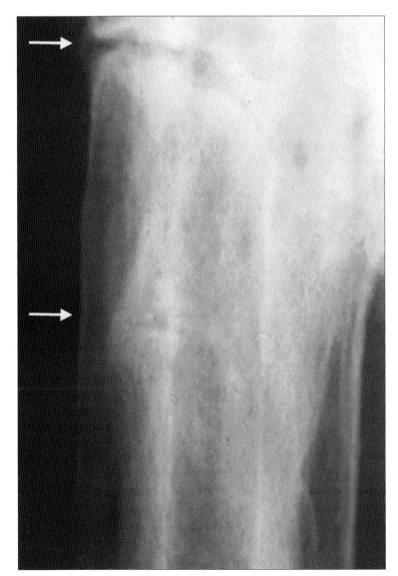

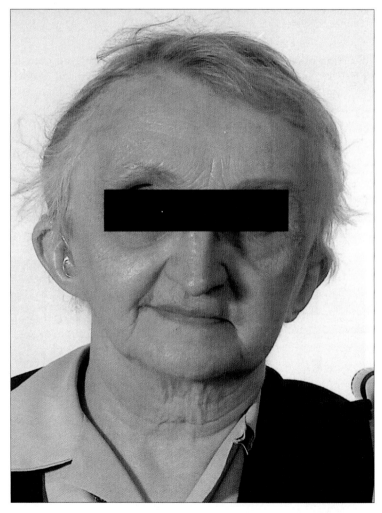

Fig. 203.6 Fissure fractures at the anterior aspect of the tibia. The upper one led eventually to a transverse fracture.

Fig. 203.7 Paget's disease producing a right deformity of the skull, deafness (see hearing amplifier device in the right ear) and apathy due to vascular steal syndrome.

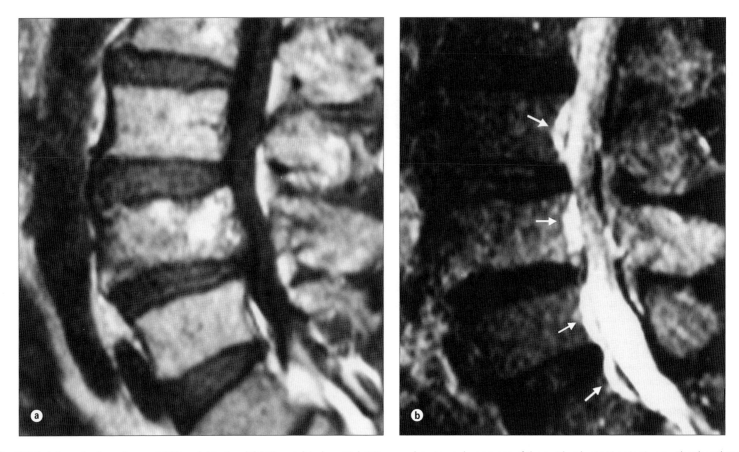

Fig. 203.8 Artery steal syndrome. (a) T1-weighted and (b) T2-weighted sagittal MRI scans showing enlargement of the epidural veins impinging on the thecal sac. (Courtesy of Professor B. Maldague.)

diversion of blood flow may provoke a vascular steal syndrome that affects the brain, rendering patients drowsy, withdrawn and apathetic (Fig. 203.7). Similar problems of artery steal syndrome may also occur at the level of the spinal cord, where diversion of the blood supply may eventually give rise to symptoms of paraparesis or quadriparesis (Fig. 203.8). Furthermore, when Paget's disease affects more than 35% of the skeleton it may cause high cardiac output failure owing to this increased bone blood flow.

Osteosarcomatous degeneration

The most devastating complication of Paget's disease is osteosarcomatous degeneration, which is estimated to occur in 0.2% of cases, although the risk of osteosarcoma is 30 times greater in patients with Paget's disease than in a control population. Usually, the malignancies are osteosarcomas, but fibrosarcomas, chondrosarcomas, reticulosarcomas or other forms of neoplasia may occur (Fig. 203.9). Surprisingly, the location of the sarcoma in Paget's disease does not correspond to the preferential location of the affected bones. For example, the spine is seldom affected, whereas the humerus and the facial bones are affected more frequently than one would expect from the prevalence of Paget's disease in these bones. The prognosis is poor, with most patients dying within 12 months after the diagnosis is established. More aggressive therapy using a combination of radiotherapy, chemotherapy and radical surgical removal might improve prognosis.

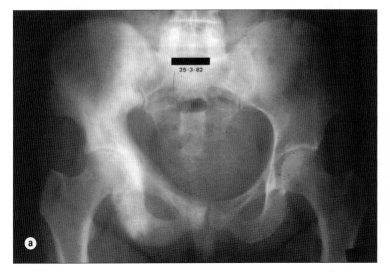

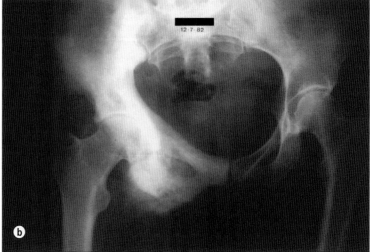

Fig. 203.9 Sarcomatous degeneration. (a) Painful Paget's disease of the right pelvis. (b) Three months later, sarcoma degeneration of the right ischiopubic branch is evident on the plain film.

Miscellaneous

Other associated conditions have been described, and some of them, if not all, probably constitute fortuitous associations, such as calcific periarthritis, gout and cardiovascular complications, hyperparathyroidism, kidney stones and angioid streaks.[9]

INVESTIGATIONS

Biochemistry

Paget's disease is characterized by elevation of the serum alkaline phosphatase (AP). This is the most useful parameter owing to its excellent reproducibility, with, in our experience, a coefficient of variation of $6.5 \pm 1.1\%$ obtained in 22 pagetic patients tested at fortnightly intervals.[10] There is a significant correlation between AP values and the extent of skeletal involvement. However, some bones, notably the skull, are known to give rise to high AP levels. In contrast, some other bones appear to produce proportionally lower levels of AP, notably the pelvis, the sacrum, the lumbar spine and the femoral head. In most clinical circumstances it is not necessary to measure bone-specific isoenzyme in the assessment and follow-up of Paget's disease.

Serum osteocalcin levels are also elevated in Paget's disease, but are a less reliable index of disease activity. During treatment, most notably with bisphosphonates, a rapid fall in the parameters of bone turnover is accompanied by a transient rise in osteocalcin.[11]

More useful indices of bone resorption are the urinary excretion of total hydroxyproline and, more recently, pyridinium cross-links. In contrast to hydroxyproline the latter are not influenced by diet. α and β isomerization of cross-linked C-telopeptides of type I collagen (CTx) could impair the interpretation of the values of this urinary parameter in Paget's disease follow-up, with the elevated ratio α-CTx/β-CTx in the urine of patients with untreated Paget's disease of bone decreasing dramatically after bisphosphonate therapy. Urinary cross-linked N-telopeptides of type I collagen (NTx), as well as serum NTx and CTx, are fortunately devoid of these changes. Assays of these parameters in blood could also be used because they are not dependent on the correction by creatinine urinary excretion. The widespread availability of tests for total AP activity makes it the most widely used test in the clinical assessment and follow-up of Paget's disease of bone. If the patient is immobilized, for example after a fracture, the serum calcium may also be elevated. Otherwise, there is no obvious abnormality in serum calcium in ambulatory patients.

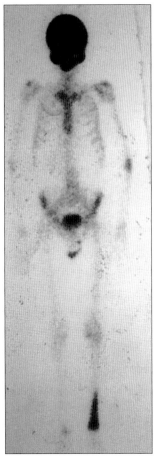

Fig. 203.10 ^{99m}Tc-MDP scan illustrating the utility of scanning the whole skeleton. In this particular case pagetic lesions are confined to the extremities: the skull and the distal tibia.

Imaging

Paget's disease is often detected on routine blood screening because of the elevated serum AP. If this is an isolated finding (no other biological signs of liver disease, for example) and the hydroxyproline or pyridinium cross-links excretion in the urine or serum αCTx or NTx is elevated, the next step is to request a bone scan. Hot spots on the bone scan will show the extent and location of the pagetic lesions (Fig. 203.10), allowing these to be explored further by conventional radiographic techniques and, if necessary, by computerized axial tomography (CT) or magnetic resonance imaging (MRI). However, there is no perfect concordance between the bone scan and the radiographic pictures. About 12% of the

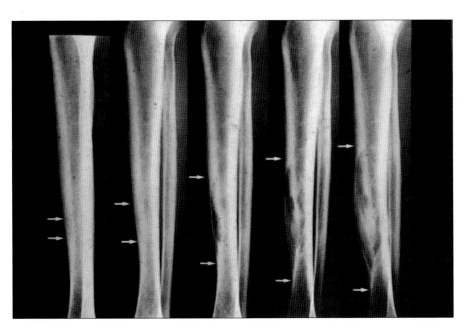

Fig. 203.11 Sequential radiographs of a pagetic tibia demonstrating the natural progression of the advancing osteolytic fronts within the bone.

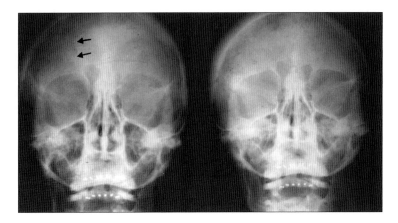

Fig. 203.12 Anteriorposterior radiographs of a pagetic skull. (a) Pagetic osteolytic front (arrows) ('osteoporosis circumscripta'). (b) After 12 months of therapy with oral pamidronate: disappearance of the lytic front.

lesions recorded on bone scans have no radiographic counterpart. Some of the lesions may be in a preradiologic state and appear on radiographs only some years later: a typical example is the skull. However, the reverse is also true, and about 6% of radiographic lesions will not show up on the bone scan. These are typically extinct lesions and histologically paucicellular.

Radiography has the huge advantage over bone scans of showing whether focal bone balance is predominantly osteolytic (which may be important in the choice of therapy, particularly in the lower limbs), predominantly osteoblastic, or mixed. In the long bones, sequential radiographs can document the progression of the advancing osteolytic front within the bone. This progression is usually 8.0 ± 0.5mm/year and is relentless (Fig. 203.11). It is only arrested by the use of second-generation bisphosphonates.[12] Another predominantly osteolytic lesion is the so-called osteoporosis circumscripta in the skull (Fig. 203.12).

Whereas the progression in single bones is relentless, the disease does not spread from one bone to an adjacent one unless there is a bony bridge between the two (e.g. a bridging osteophyte, syndesmophyte or bone graft). The anatomic distribution of the disease remains largely unchanged throughout life.

DIFFERENTIAL DIAGNOSIS

Paget's disease is easily diagnosed on radiography, which reveals enlargement of the affected bone. For example, a pagetic vertebra will be larger and more radiodense than the two adjacent vertebrae, thus distinguishing it from 'ivory vertebrae' of other origins, such as metastases or lymphoma. The same is true of other affected bones. For example, in an affected pelvis there will be significant cortical thickening, one example of which is the so-called 'brim sign'. The cortical thickening is associated with an increased intracortical porosity, whereas the adjacent trabecular bone has thickened trabeculae. This produces the the typical pattern of corticotrabecular dedifferentiation (Fig. 203.13).

The progression of the lesion in Paget's disease is characterized in the first stage predominantly by bone resorption, leading to the so-called lytic, destructive or radiolucent stage. During the second stage, bone resorption is partially compensated by bone formation and the lesion is referred to as mixed. This is followed by a stage where bone construction predominates, resulting in sclerotic lesions. These characteristic changes help in differentiating Paget's disease from other bony osteoblastic metastases, particularly those arising from prostatic carcinoma. More difficult is the situation where metastases disseminate into parts of the skeleton affected by Paget's disease. In these cases, the lytic areas are less well delineated than the lytic area associated with the pagetic process. More troublesome to differentiate is the sarcomatous degeneration of

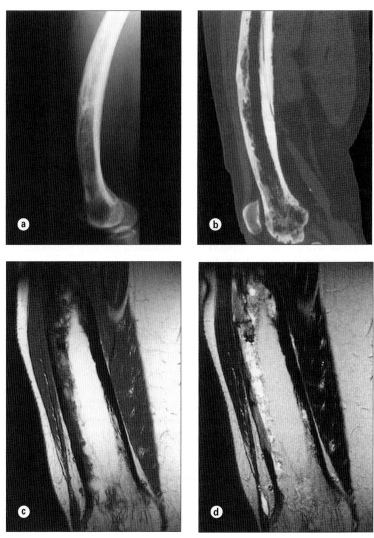

Fig. 203.13 Corticotrabecular dedifferentiation. (a) Plain radiograph of a pagetic right femur. (b) Sagittal reformatted image after spiral CT of the same femur showing irregularities in the cortex. (c) T1-weighted coronal MRI scan of the same femur, showing normal medullary appearance. (d) Corresponding T2-weighted image showing high signal intensity within the cortical bone, suggestive of the presence of fibrovascular tissue. (Courtesy of Professor B Vande Berg.)

the pagetic lesions in its incipient stage, which is accompanied by pain, the appearance of sunray spicules and osteolysis which invades the coarse trabecular pattern typical of uncomplicated Paget's disease. A rapid tumoral extension into the soft tissues is usually observed, and may be associated with a sunburst pattern. On the bone scan there may be an area of decreased uptake.

Another picture that may be misleading is the pseudosarcomatous pattern, sometimes induced by disodium etidronate and which heals typically when calcitonin is administered.[13]

Fissure fractures should not be confused with pseudofractures (Looser's zones). They occur on the convex aspect of the long bones affected by Paget's disease and have dense borders.

STRUCTURE AND FUNCTION

The structure and function of pagetic bone is intimately related to the pagetic process, which evolves in the three phases described on radiography. First, there is invasion of the existing bone by huge multinucleated osteoclasts. Amongst pagetic osteoclasts, 50% have more than seven nuclei and 10% have more than 20. In normal osteoclasts, 50% have more than three nuclei and 10% more than five.[5] This intense bone resorption is accompanied by vascular hypertrophy followed by medullary fibrosis, which is directly related to hyperosteoclastosis. Bone resorption is soon accompanied by the formation of lamellar bone in a disorganized fashion (mixed phase). This is followed, by bone formation without bone resorption, which results in irregular-shaped trabecular bone that characterizes the mosaic pattern of cement lines. In some areas woven bone develops. As a result of this anarchic behavior bone enlargement occurs.

A histomorphometric analysis of pagetic bone reveals the magnitude of the changes taking place in the iliac bone:[14] a twofold increase in trabecular bone volume, a sevenfold increase in the eroded surfaces, a ninefold increase in the number of osteoclasts, a threefold increase in the osteoid volume and a fourfold increase in the osteoid surface. The mineral appositional rate is also increased twofold, but this is a feature that is seen only in woven areas of pagetic bone. In lamellar areas the mineral appositional rate is normal. The histomorphometric analysis is confined to the iliac bone. Elsewhere, the turnover of pagetic bone is more intense. From [47]Ca kinetic analysis it has been calculated that in the areas affected by the pagetic process the turnover of bone may be increased by as much as 46-fold compared to the uninvolved areas of the skeleton.[13]

The very nature of the osteolytic and mixed phases of Paget's disease, as well as the architecture of the so-called sclerotic bone, predisposes pagetic bone to fragility. Indeed, bone fractures do occur and may be the presenting manifestation in some cases.

ETIOLOGY AND PATHOGENESIS

Ever since Rebel *et al.*[15] found, by electron microscopy, intranuclear and intracytoplasmic inclusions resembling nucleocapsids of the paramyxovirus family of RNA viruses in the osteoclasts of pagetic bone, the hypothesis that Paget's disease results from slow virus infection has been prevalent. However, similar structures have also been found in giant cell tumors of bone and in the osteoclasts of some patients with pyknodysostosis and osteopetrosis. The presence of measles virus antigens and/or respiratory syncytial virus antigens has been shown in pagetic osteoclasts. Canine distemper virus antigen has also been detected. However, more recent data have not confirmed the viral hypothesis,[16] and more confirmatory work will be required before it is accepted.

MANAGEMENT

Calcitonin

Salmon and human calcitonin were the first uniformly active therapeutic agents used in the treatment of Paget's disease. Indeed, calcitonin has transformed the life of pagetic patients by alleviating pain, relieving neurologic symptoms resulting from the steal syndrome for a prolonged period, and altering the focal bone balance in a positive way, as seen on radiographs. However, a disadvantage with calcitonin is the plateau phenomenon. For reasons that remain unknown, calcitonin is unable, in most cases, to suppress the turnover to more than 50%. The parenteral mode of administration is associated with unpleasant but harmless side effects. These can be overcome by using a nasal spray or suppositories.[10]

Bisphosphonates

The current mainstay of treatment of Paget's disease is with the second-generation bisphosphonates, which are potent inhibitors of bone resorption. These can be administered orally or parenterally. First-generation bisphosphonate (disodium etidronate) produced mineralization defects at high doses, generalized osteomalacia and, at low doses, focal osteomalacia. Nevertheless, in many countries where second-generation bisphosphonates are not available, disodium etidronate is still widely used. Small doses are recommended (5mg/kg during 6 months), provided no osteolytic lesions are present, especially in the lower limbs.

Second-generation bisphosphonates have greater beneficial effects on the mineralization defect ratio. The best known and oldest in this category are disodium pamidronate and clodronate. Disodium pamidronate[13,17,18] is many times more potent than clodronate. Newer compounds include tiludronate,[19] alendronate,[20] risedronate and dimethyl APD, with, hopefully, more to be developed in the future. In Paget's disease most studies have involved pamidronate, both orally and intravenously, or alendronate or risedronate given orally, with good results.

The greatest advantage of bisphosphonates over calcitonin is the duration of remission, which can last for years, while the resorption front is halted.[12] This new bone is lamellar and replaces woven bone. With bisphosphonates the parameters of bone turnover diminish more strikingly than with calcitonin, although the most severely affected cases may not be normalized. In any event, hydroxyproline decreases in a matter of days, and the AP level in a matter of weeks. One disadvantage of pamidronate, and of the other aminobisphosphonates, chiefly if they are administered intravenously, is the slight rise in body temperature, with flu-like symptoms and a transient leukopenia. On retreatment with aminobisphosphonate, this phenomenon does not in most cases recur. After a long period of weaning from therapy the organism loses this 'memory' and these benign side effects may reappear.

Oral administration can result in esophageal and gastrointestinal irritation,[21] although this phenomenon can be minimized by strongly recommending that the patient drinks a large glass of water with the drug and does not lie down within the next hour. Another drawback is the weak gastrointestinal absorption, which is of the order of 1%. However, with daily doses as large as 600mg of pamidronate, 40mg of alendronate and 30mg of risedronate, this may not matter. These local problems can also be circumvented by administering pamidronate intravenously at 20–120mg/perfusion. With i.v. administration mild thrombophlebitis may occasionally occur.

Following the administration of pamidronate, 600mg/day orally for an average period of 9.5 months, 80% of patients normalized their AP level. Of the 20% who did not, all had a very high initial AP level before treatment started (597 ± 7IU/l; upper limit of normal 60IU/l). Of the 80% with normalized AP levels, 72% remained normalized despite the absence of therapy during a follow-up of 2 years, 16% increased the level towards pretreatment values and 12% increased the level to initial values.[13]

These various treatment modalities have produced a variety of results, including an 82% significant improvement in spontaneous bone pain; a 38% improvement in low back pain; 27% improvement in pain associated with OA of the hip or knee; and a 52% improvement in pain associated with deformity of the femur or the tibia.[18] Good results can also be expected in the steal syndrome. On retreatment, apparent resistance to therapy should be distinguished from a rare but true acquired resistance. Apparent resistance is observed in cases in which the resurgence of alkaline phosphatase activity before retreatment has not been high enough to allow a further full effect of therapy.[22]

In milder cases of Paget's disease single courses of therapy may bring about a prolonged remission for up to 1 year.[23] However, caution should be exercised not to provide excess pamidronate, even if the ratio between therapeutic efficacy and localized inhibition of mineralization is much better than with sodium etidronate. Very high doses of pamidronate can produce focal osteomalacia and endanger the solidity of bone. It has been calculated that 11% of patients with an involved femur sustained a fracture during therapy with etidronate.[13] A number of fractures have been observed with etidronate but none with calcitonin (nor have any been reported in the literature).

On fine radiographic analysis the construction index with calcitonin (ratio of positive to negative radiographic signs) is infinite, i.e. no negative signs were observed. With etidronate it is below 1, as there are more

TABLE 203.1 EFFECT OF THERAPY WITH ETIDRONATE AND TILUDRONATE

Radiological images prior to therapy	After therapy	Etidronate	Tiludronate
Predominantly lytic (n = 3)	Denser		n = 2
	Questionable densification	n = 1	
Mixed lytic + condensing (n = 4)	Questionable densification		n = 1
	Denser		n = 3
Predominantly condensing (n = 9)	Questionable densification	n = 1	n = 2
	Denser		n = 1
	Unchanged	n = 1	
	Questionable increase in resorption	n = 2	
	Clearcut resorption	n = 2	
	Questionable densification	n = 1	
	Unchanged	n = 1	n = 1

Example of a semiquantitative radiological evaluation of pagetic bone lesions during a double-blind study with etidronate or tiludronate. (With permission from Devogelaer et al.[24])

negative signs than positive, and with pamidronate it is 12 (four negative signs were observed versus 48 positive signs).[13] In a double-blind study comparing daily oral tiludronate 400mg with daily oral etidronate 400mg, a significant deterioration of the radiographic aspect was confined to the etidronate group[24] (Table 203.1). Radiographic evaluation is therefore essential, especially when bisphosphonates are studied, because these concentrate in pagetic lesions for a long period of time. The simple evaluation of the biological indices of bone turnover may indeed be misleading, as exemplified with etidronate. The more etidronate that is given, the more the bone turnover is inhibited and bone mineralization

depressed. At 20mg/kg/day, general osteomalacia developed in at least 60% of cases.[25] At 5–8mg/kg/day, focal osteomalacia was seen in 100% of the pagetic lesions rebiopsied after 6 months.[26] This may be corrected by giving subcutaneous salmon calcitonin (50U/day) for 3 months.

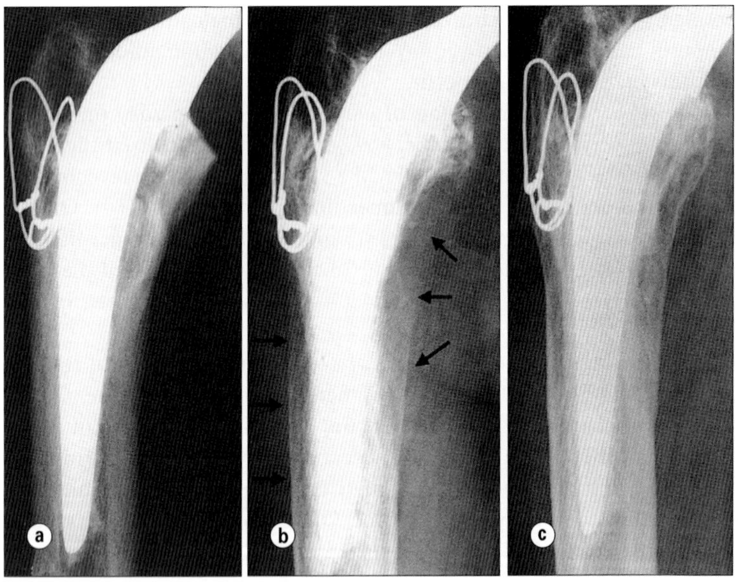

Surgery

Operative procedures are extremely useful, particularly total hip replacement for the relief of pain and for locomotion. However, patients with Paget's disease may present unique intraoperative problems, such as bone deformity (e.g. coxa vara or femoral bowing), acetabular protrusion and bony enlargement, which may cause alterations in the choice of implant or fixation method used.[27] In these cases, surgery must be preceded by antiresorptive therapy to reduce the risk of bleeding and improve bone quality. Further antiresorptive therapy may prove to be necessary in case of bone regional dystrophy after total hip replacement in order to prevent bone fragilization and fracture.[28] This rapid, reactive postoperative osteolysis of pagetic bone should not be mistaken for an infection or a tumor, and reintervention should be avoided (Fig. 203.14). Involvement of the femur or tibia with Paget's disease in secondary knee osteoarthritis may be associated with multiple technical difficulties at operation, and with a final position in suboptimum varus or valgus alignment or suboptimum alignment of the mechanical axis.[29] However, the presence of Paget's disease does not seem to affect the postoperative course nor the rate of loosening of the prostheses.[29]

Fig. 203.14 Total hip prosthesis replacement in a patient suffering from osteoarthritic complication of sclerotic pagetic hip. (a) Immediately after surgical orthopedic operation, dense cortical bone. (b) Dramatic focal osteolysis 4 months after operation, which could be mistaken for prosthesis loosening or periprosthetic infection. (c) Normalization after antiresorptive therapy. (Courtesy of Professor B Maldague.)

SUMMARY

Since the advent of second-generation bisphosphonates, Paget's disease can now be well controlled. More active disease, as witnessed by an elevated AP (up to seven times the upper limit of normal) tends to recur relentlessly, but a second course of therapy remains as effective as the first. All patients in their eighth decade should be treated when symptomatic, and younger patients in their fifth decade should be treated aggressively. What is not clear, however, is whether this therapeutic approach can avoid sarcoma, the most serious complication of Paget's disease.

REFERENCES

1. Nagant de Deuxchaisnes C, Krane SM. Paget's disease of bone. Clinical and metabolic observations. Medicine 1964; 43: 233–266.
2. Detheridge FM, Guyer PB, Barker DJP. European distribution of Paget's disease of bone. Br Med J 1982; 285: 1005–1008.
3. Altman RD, Bloch DA, Hochberg MC, Murphy WA. Prevalence of Paget's disease of bone in the United States. J Bone Miner Res 2000; 15: 461–465.
4. Cundy T, McAnulty K, Wattie D, Gamble G, Rutland M, Ibbertson HK. Evidence for secular changes in Paget's disease. Bone 1997; 20: 69–71.
5. Kanis JA. Pathophysiology and treatment of Paget's disease of bone, 2nd edn. London: Martin Dunitz, 1998.
6. Van Hul W. Paget's disease from a genetic perspective. Bone 1999; 24: 29S–30S.
7. Chen JR, Rhee RSC, Wallach S, Avramides A, Flores A. Neurologic disturbances in Paget disease of bone: response to calcitonin. Neurology 1979; 29: 448–457.
8. Devogelaer JP, Maldague B. Lumbar spinal stenosis in metabolic bone diseases. In : Gunzburg R, Szpalski M, eds. Lumbar spinal stenosis. Philadelphia: Lippincott Williams & Wilkins, 2000; 61–68.

9. Franck WA, Bress NM, Singer FR, Krane SM. Rheumatic manifestations of Paget's disease of bone. Am J Med 1974; 56: 592–603.

10. Nagant de Deuxchaisnes C, Devogelaer JP. Alternative mode of administration of salmon calcitonin in Paget's disease of bone. In: Singer FR, Wallach S, eds. Paget's disease of bone. Clinical assessment, present and future therapy. New York: Elsevier, 1991; 135–165.

11. Papapoulos SE, Frolich M, Mudde AH, Harinck HIJ, Berg HVD, Bijvoet OLM. Serum osteocalcin in Paget's disease of bone: Basal concentrations and response to bisphosphonate treatment. J Clin Endocrinol Metab 1987; 65: 89–94.

12. Maldague B, Malghem J. Dynamic radiologic patterns of Paget's disease of bone. Clin Orthop 1987; 217: 126–151.

13. Nagant de Deuxchaisnes C. Paget's disease of bone. Medical management. In: De Groot LJ, ed. Endocrinology, 2nd edn. Philadelphia: WB Saunders, 1989; 1211–1244.

14. Meunier PJ, Coindre JM, Edouard CM, Arlot ME. Bone histomorphometry in Paget's disease. Arthritis Rheum 1980; 23: 1095–1103.

15. Rebel A, Malkani K, Basle M. Anomalies nucleaires des osteoclastes de la maladie osseuse de Paget. Nouv Presse Med 1974; 3: 1299–1301.

16. Ooi CG, Walsh CA, Gallagher JA, Fraser WD. Absence of measles virus and canine distemper virus transcripts in long-term bone marrow cultures from patients with Paget's disease of bone. Bone 2000; 27: 417–421.

17. Harinck HIJ, Papapoulos SE, Blanksma HJ, Moolenaar AJ, Vermeij P, Bijvoet OLM. Paget's disease of bone: early and late responses to three different modes of treatment with aminohydroxypropylidene bisphosphonate (APD). Br Med J 1987; 295: 1301–1305.

18. Harinck HIJ, Bijvoet OLM, Blanksma HJ, Dahlinghaus-Nienhuys PJ. Efficacious management with aminobisphosphonate (APD) in Paget's disease of bone. Clin Orthop 1987; 217: 79–98.

19. Roux C, Gennari C, Farrerons J et al. Comparative prospective, double-blind, multicenter study of the efficacy of tiludronate and etidronate in the treatment of Paget's disease of bone. Arthritis Rheum 1995; 38: 851–858.

20. O'Doherty DP, McCloskey EV, Vasikaran S, Khan J, Kanis JA. The effects of intravenous alendronate in Paget's disease of bone. J Bone Miner Res 1995; 10: 1094–1100.

21. Lufkin EG, Argueta R, Whitaker MD et al. Pamidronate: an unrecognized problem in gastrointestinal tolerability. Osteoporosis Int 1994; 4: 320–322.

22. Yates AJP, Gray RES, Urwin GH et al. Intravenous clodronate in the treatment and retreatment of Paget's disease of bone. Lancet 1985; i: 1474–1477.

23. Thiebaud D, Jaeger P, Gobelet C, Tacquet AF, Burckhardt P. A single infusion of bisphosphonate AHPrBP (APD) as treatment of Paget's disease of bone. Am J Med 1988; 85: 207–212.

24. Devogelaer JP, Malghem J, Stasse P, Nagant de Deuxchaisnes C. Biological and radiological responses to oral etidronate and tiludronate in Paget's disease of bone. Bone 1997; 20: 259–261.

25. Coindre JM, Edouard CM, Arlot ME, Meunier PJ. Etude histomorphometrique de l'os non pagetique chez le pagetique. Resultats avant et apres diphosphonates. Rev Rhum Mal Osteoartic 1982; 49: 103–109.

26. Boyce BF, Smith L, Fogelman I, Johnston E, Ralston S, Boyle IT. Focal osteomalacia due to low-dose diphosphonate therapy in Paget's disease. Lancet 1984; i: 821–824.

27. Lewallen DG. V. Total hip arthroplasty in special cases. Hip arthroplasty in patients with Paget's disease. Clin Orthop Rel Res 1999; 369: 243–250.

28. Marr DS, Rosenthal DI, Cohen GL, Tomford WW. Rapid postoperative osteolysis in Paget disease. J Bone Joint Surg 1994; 76A: 274–277.

29. Gabel GT, Rand JA, Sim FH. Total knee arthroplasty for ostearthrosis in patients who have Paget disease of bone at the knee. J Bone Joint Surg 1991; 73A: 739–744.

HERITABLE DISEASE AND TUMORS OF BONE AND CONNECTIVE TISSUE

204 Gaucher's disease

Philippe Orcel and Nadia Belmatoug

Definition

- A disease resulting from the accumulation of glucosylceramide in organs and tissues throughout the body in characteristic storage cells, namely 'Gaucher cells'
- The most common inherited glycolipid storage disease
- There are three clinical types:
  - type 1, the adult, non-neuropathic chronic form
  - type 2, the infantile, neuropathic acute form
  - type 3, the juvenile, neuropathic subacute form

Clinical features

- Type 1: organomegaly, hematologic disorders secondary to hypersplenism, bone lesions attributable to the medullary infiltration by Gaucher cells, no involvement of the CNS
- Type 2: early involvement of brain and cranial nerves, fatal by 2 years of age
- Type 3: involvement of visceral organs, bone, and CNS, but neurologic symptoms appear later and are less severe

HISTORY

The disease was first described as 'epithelioma of the spleen' by Philippe Gaucher in 1882, in a patient with massive hepatosplenomegaly and hematologic features suggestive of leukemia[1]. The storage cells were characterized by Marchand in 1907[2]. By 1965, Brady *et al.* had demonstrated that the metabolic defect is a deficiency of the lysosomal enzyme glucocerebrosidase[3], leading to a decreased catabolic pathway of glucosylceramide (Fig. 204.1). Molecular approaches have identified several mutations in the glucocerebrosidase gene[4,5]. The recent use of enzyme replacement therapy has dramatically changed the management and prognosis of the disease[6].

EPIDEMIOLOGY

Type 1 is the most common form of Gaucher's disease (GD) (Table 204.1). It is more frequent in persons of Ashkenazi Jewish heritage, but is pan-ethnic. Types 2 and 3 are rarer and predominantly involve non-Jewish patients. A genetic isolate of type 3 patients has been identified in northern Sweden (Norrbottnian GD, personal communication). No family has been reported with more than one type of the disease, suggesting that the three types of GD are genetically distinct. Each type is inherited as an autosomal recessive trait without sex preponderance. The peak age is variable: any age from birth to elderly for type 1, usually before 6 months of age for type 2, and juvenile (teenage) for type 3[4,7].

CLINICAL FEATURES

This chapter will focus on the clinical manifestations of type 1 GD, the most common form of the disorder. GD is very heterogenous as far as age at presentation and severity of clinical expression are concerned.

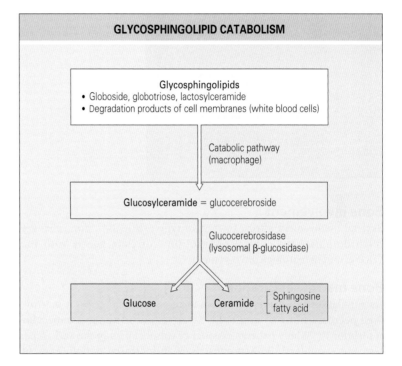

Fig. 204.1 Glycosphingolipid catabolism. The impaired activity of the lysosomal enzyme glucocerebrosidase results in the accumulation into macrophages of glucosylceramide, which is normally catabolized into ceramide and glucose.

Hematologic manifestations

The principal presenting feature is splenomegaly, usually painless. Splenic rupture is rare, but infarction may occur, sometimes as the initial complaint. Primary hypersplenism with thrombocytopenia, anemia and leukopenia is frequent. In most patients these abnormalities are not life-threatening and may go unrecognized for many years. Hepatomegaly is also common but occurs later in the disease course. A moderate increase of cholestatic enzymes is frequent; cytolysis, however, is rare but when present may be associated with the development of an irreversible fibrosis. Liver failure has been reported in a few patients with portal hypertension and extensive fibrosis[8].

TABLE 204.1 EPIDEMIOLOGY OF TYPE 1 GAUCHER'S DISEASE	
Peak age	any age from birth to old age
Sex distribution	1:1
Prevalence rate (/100 000) and geography	15–40 in Ashkenazi Jews; rare (<1) in other populations (panethnic)
Genetic association	?
Transmission	autosomal recessive

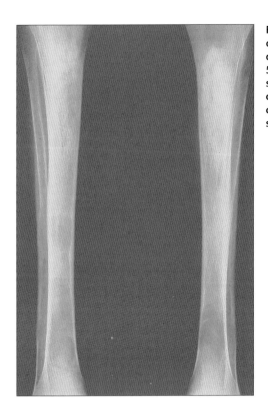

Fig. 204.2 Radiograph of the right tibial diaphysis of a 52-year-old man, showing osteopenia, osteolytic lesions, cortical thinning and scalloping.

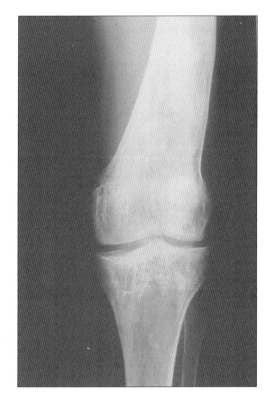

Fig. 204.3 Radiograph of the distal femur and proximal tibia of a 31-year-old man, illustrating the typical Erlenmeyer flask deformity on the distal femur. Note the expansion of the contour of the long tubular bones with convexity of the osseous margins, typical but not pathognomonic of GD.

Bone involvement

Skeletal involvement affects 50–75% of type 1 patients[4,7]. Bone changes often dominate the clinical picture[4] but correlate poorly with the visceral and hematologic involvement[7,9,10].

Bone marrow infiltration

Accumulation of Gaucher cells leads to alterations of both bone marrow (cell necrosis, fibrosis) and bone tissue (endocortical and trabecular resorption)[9,10]. Many patients experience episodic pain in the back, hips, legs and shoulders[8]. Radiographs show an increased radiolucency of bone, and cortical scalloping and thinning[9,10]. These abnormalities predominantly involve the axial skeleton and proximal long bones, where they are often symmetric.[10] They are prominent in the distal portion of the femur and tibia[7] (Fig. 204.2). In some cases they appear as limited massive osteolytic lesions in a metaphysis, resembling a tumor or aneurysmal bone cyst and called 'gaucheroma'.[9]

Fractures

Bone weakening may result in pathologic fractures, most frequently in the vertebral spine, with intraosseous discal displacement, compression fractures or vertebra plana[10]. Fractures of the ribs or long bones are less common. Following fracture, there is prompt callus formation and early osseous union[7].

Failure of modeling

This is the most characteristic and least symptomatic skeletal abnormality[9,10]. It develops progressively throughout the period of rapid skeletal growth, being manifest in about 80% of adults with the disease. Expansion of the contours of long tubular bones results in cortical thinning and loss of the normal concavity of the bony outline, particularly medially (Fig. 204.3). The so-called 'Erlenmeyer flask deformity' is very suggestive of GD, although not pathognomonic (see Differential Diagnosis). Vertebral bodies sometimes show step-like depressions of the superior and inferior margins. This deformity, which has been termed 'H vertebra', is identical to that observed in sickle cell anemia[10].

Osteonecrosis and bony infarctions

These are the most frequent cause of chronic pain and functional limitation. Both are the consequence of sudden ischemia in an infiltrated bone area, resulting in acute-onset episodes (bone crisis). Symptoms include

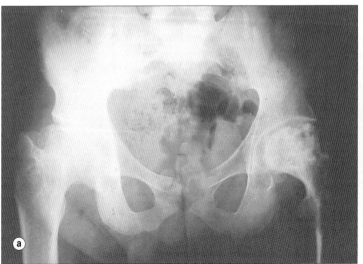

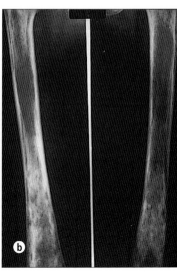

Fig. 204.4 Radiographs of the pelvis (a) and right femoral diaphysis (b) showing the typical aspects of ischemic bone complications in GD. Ischemic osteonecrosis of both femoral heads with collapse of bone and secondary osteoarthrosis, and condensation of pelvic bones with sacroiliac joint involvement simulating sacroiliitis (a). Bony infarction of the femoral diaphyses with a cortical reaction producing a cortical splitting, so-called 'bone-within-bone' appearance (b).

acute pain, tenderness and fever, simulating those of osteomyelitis or septic arthritis[7,9,10]. The typical radiographic appearance of bony infarctions consists of osteosclerotic areas, located nearby or within lytic lesions, and associated with periostitis (Fig. 204.4). In the cortex, an inner layer of new bone formation, which does not merge with the overlying cortical bone, produces a cortical splitting, or 'bone-within-bone' appearance[6]. Epiphyseal osteonecrosis is frequently multiple, affecting femoral heads (Fig. 204.4), humeral heads and, less commonly, femoral condyles and tibial plateaux. Radiographic changes are similar to those seen in other forms of osteonecrosis[10]. Secondary cartilage destruction often appears subsequently, resulting in a disabling arthropathy which may require total arthroplasty.[7]

Osteoarticular infections

Although infectious hazards have been poorly assessed, an increased susceptibility to bone infections has been reported. Septic arthritis is rare, but osteomyelitis occurs in less than 5% of affected patients.[7,9] Clinical features may simulate those of bone crisis. Bacteriologic findings, short-term repeated bone scans, tomodensitometry and magnetic resonance imaging (MRI) facilitate the proper diagnosis.

Miscellaneous osteoarticular manifestations

Sporadic cases of migratory polyarthritis, sacroiliac joint or symphysis pubis involvement, destructive disc alterations, or associations with hypergammaglobulinemia or B-lymphocyte disorders, as well as osteosarcomas, have been reported[9].

INVESTIGATIONS

Biology

The serum levels of several enzymes are elevated in GD: tartrate-resistant acid phosphatase, angiotensin-converting enzyme, lysosomal hydrolases and lysozyme. Partial thromboplastin, prothrombin and bleeding times may be increased because of liver involvement. Plasma glucosylceramide is usually elevated, but is less sensitive than the elevation of the glucocerebrosidase content of leukocytes (obtained from samples of venous blood), cultured fibroblasts or urine[4]. High plasma levels of chitotriosidase and of ferritin seem to be related to abnormal macrophage activation and to reflect the severity of the disease and the efficacy of enzyme replacement therapy[11].

Imaging

Conventional radiographs are usually sufficient to establish the diagnosis[10]. However, the extent and severity of the disease are very variable and poorly evaluated by radiography, computerized tomography (CT) or bone scan. MRI has been shown to be the most sensitive technique for detecting early bone marrow changes and for assessing the extent and severity of marrow involvement[12]. Many sites in the marrow are characterized by a signal of abnormally low intensity, on both T_1 and T_2 sequences (Fig. 204.5). The distribution of the abnormality is heterogeneous: vertebrae are consistently involved, but in the lower extremity the femoral areas are affected more frequently than the tibial sites. The epiphyses are generally spared unless the involvement of bone is extensive. MRI allows early detection of ischemic bone lesions with a high intensity signal on T1 weighted sequences at the time of clinical bone crisis. A decrease in bone mineral density has been reported to correlate with the severity of the skeletal involvement and may be useful to monitor bone changes[13]. Coupling CT and technetium-99m methylene–bisphosphonate bone scan helps in the differential diagnosis between osteonecrosis and osteomyelitis in the clinical setting of sudden bone crisis. The presence of a necrotic soft tissue swelling adjacent to the affected bone is suggestive of an infectious complication. An increased uptake on a bone scan performed a few days after the onset of a bone crisis suggests an acute osteomyelitis, whereas its absence makes an ischemic bone crisis more likely[9].

Histology

Demonstration of Gaucher cells in bone marrow biopsies is key to the diagnosis[4,9]. These large mono- or multinucleated cells have characteristic cytologic features with a typical 'wrinkled tissue paper' appearance of the cytoplasm (Fig. 204.6). Bone tissue alterations are highly variable, but one study suggests that bone turnover might be increased[9].

DIFFERENTIAL DIAGNOSIS

Bone features of GD are not specific and may be observed in other disorders (Table 204.2), particularly the hemoglobinopathies (see Chapter 188)[10]. The diagnosis should be considered in a patient with hepatosplenomegaly who exhibits widespread osteopenia with a coarsened trabecular pattern, focal osteosclerosis, osteonecrosis of the proximal femoral epiphyses and Erlenmeyer flask deformities of the distal portions of the femur.

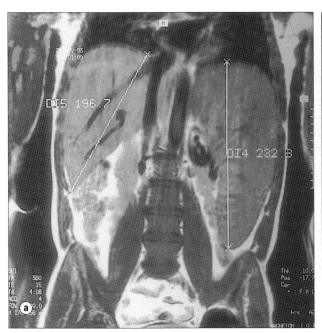

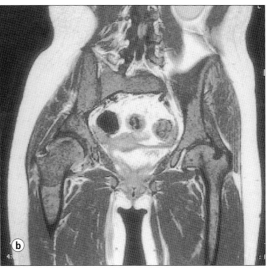

Fig. 204.5 MRI scans of the abdomen and pelvis (a) and of the femoral heads (b) on T1-weighted images obtained from two different patients. Huge hepatomegaly and splenomegaly are clearly observed (a), and could be measured. This index is useful for the follow-up, particularly for the assessment of treatment efficacy. In the same patient the lower lumbar spine vertebral bodies show low intensity signal, characteristic of the bone marrow infiltration by Gaucher cells. The upper femoral extremities of the second patient show a heterogenous signal of low intensity and the irregular shape of both femoral heads, suggestive of osteonecrosis.

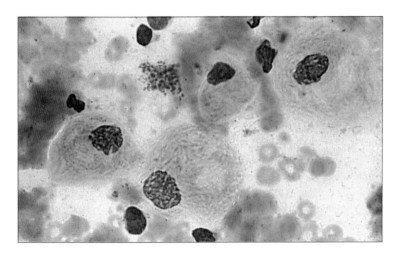

Fig. 204.6 Light microscopy aspect of Gaucher cells in bone marrow. Note the typical 'wrinkled tissue paper' appearance of the cytoplasm. (May–Grünwald–Giemsa, original magnification 1×13 600. Prepared by Dr Mallarmé.)

TABLE 204.2 DIFFERENTIAL DIAGNOSIS OF RADIOLOGIC FEATURES OF TYPE 1 GAUCHER'S DISEASE

Diffuse or localized osteopenia
　Osteoporosis (idiopathic, corticosteroid)
　Hyperparathyroidism
　Hemoglobinopathies
　Neoplastic disorders (multiple myeloma)

Osteosclerosis
　Osteosclerotic skeletal metastasis
　Phakomatosis (tuberous sclerosis)
　Osteopetrosis
　Mastocytosis
　Osteomyelofibrosis
　Hodgkin's disease
　Hemoglobinopathies

Osteonecrosis
　Hemoglobinopathies (sickle cell anemia)
　Hypercorticism
　Caisson disease
　Collagen vascular disorders
　Hyperlipemia
　Pancreatitis

Erlenmeyer flask deformity
　Niemann–Pick disease
　Pyle disease
　Fibrous dysplasia
　Hyperthyroidism
　Hemolytic anemias (thalassemia)
　Leukemia
　Osteopetrosis (Albers-Schönberg disease)
　Heavy metal poisoning
　Rachitism sequellae
　Fracture sequellae

ETIOLOGY

Biochemistry

Gaucher's disease arises from an inherited deficiency of the activity of glucocerebrosidase[4,5], a membrane-associated monomeric glycoprotein with a molecular weight of 65kDa. This enzyme hydrolyses β-glucosidic ester bonds and is specialized for complex lipid substrates[5]. Impairment of its activity results in the accumulation of glucosylceramide, linked by a β-glucosidic bond. Glucosylceramide is at the end of the glycosphin-golipid catabolic pathway and is normally catabolized into ceramide and glucose by glucocerebrosidase[5]. The compounds that contribute to the pool of glucosylceramide are derived from the degradation of membranes, particularly those of white blood cells (see Fig. 204.1).

Molecular biology and genetics

More than 200 genetic mutations have been identified in the β-glucocerebrosidase gene 1q21 that result in the phenotypic expression of GD[5]. There is also a pseudogene that is about 96% homologous with the active gene and which may complicate the pattern of mutations[5]. Mutations include both insertional and point mutations, as well as crossover mutations with the pseudogene. There are four common mutations in 96–98% of the Ashkenazi Jewish population[4,5]: the most common is a A →G point mutation at nucleotide 126, resulting in an asparagines (370) to serine substitution, a decreased catalytic activity of the enzyme, and a mild phenotype. This mutant allele is not observed in patients with neuronopathic type 2 or 3 forms. Other common mutations include: 1) insertion of a guanine at nucleotide 84, inducing a shift in the reading frame with no enzyme production and a severe phenotype; 2) a T→C mutation at nucleotide 1448, producing a leucine (444) to proline substitution, with a severe loss of activity, and a severe phenotype (homozygous patients have a neuronopathic form); and 3) a G →A mutation at nucleotide 1604, resulting in an arginine (496) to histidine substitution, with a very mild phenotype[4].

PATHOGENESIS

Tissue changes are multifocal and located around clusters of storage cells, suggesting that tissue injury results from physical crowding or blood flow impairment[4,9]. The absence of correlation between pathologic or clinical features with the distribution of Gaucher cells, the tissue levels of glucosylceramide or with spleen and liver blood flow rules against this hypothesis, except for the genesis of bone ischemia.

Recently, a 'cellular theory' has emerged[4]: Gaucher cells are considered as 'transformed macrophages', sharing membrane and cytoplasmic markers with macrophages. In vitro, the uptake of glucosylceramide by cultured macrophages causes the release of lysosomal enzymes, interleukins (IL-1 and IL-6) and other macrophage-derived factors, which all could be involved in the pathogenesis of osteolytic bone lesions. Both the alteration of macrophage function and the local release of such agents may have deleterious effects on neighboring cells and tissues, which could take place in any tissue (spleen, liver, bone, central nervous system, CNS), and contribute to the variety of the disease features[4,9].

MANAGEMENT

Enzyme replacement therapy

Macrophage-targeted glucocerebrosidase was first extracted and purified from human placental tissue – 'alglucerase' (Ceredase®) and then produced by recombinant DNA technology (imiglucerase, Cerezyme®, both Genzyme Corporation, Cambridge, MA). Glucocerebrosidase infusions reverse hematologic complications and hepatosplenomegaly within 12–20 weeks[4,16], although bone response requires a longer period. Pain and the frequency of bone crises decrease over 6–9 months, and imaging features improve after 1–2 years[5,9,12,15,16]. Currently recommended therapeutic regimens start with 2-hour intravenous infusions of 60 IU/kg every 2 weeks[4]. Optimal management with enzyme replacement therapy (ERT) in type 1 Gaucher patients is not well defined. Low-dose or intermittent dosing regimens fail to achieve a sustained improvement of bone lesions/symptoms, and treatment for 2–3 years (lifelong in severely affected patients) is currently recommended[5,9].

Splenectomy

Enzyme replacement therapy has considerably limited the indications for splenectomy, as glucocerebrosidase infusions commonly reverse hematologic disorders associated with hypersplenism[2] and because splenectomy has been shown to accelerate the skeletal involvement.

Orthopedic treatments

Relief of bone and joint pain may require strong analgesics. Osteonecrosis or pathologic fractures often require surgery. Improved surgical techniques have increased good results and decreased postoperative complications, which were reported in historical series: bleeding, infection, prosthetic loosening[9]. Infectious complications (e.g. osteomyelitis) require both careful bacteriologic studies, because of the frequency of atypical organisms, and prolonged antibiotic therapy[9].

Experimental therapies

Marrow transplantation has been shown to be curative in some patients, but the risks, which increase with the severity of the disease, do not justify this procedure in patients with relatively mild disease, especially with the development of ERT[5]. An exception may be patients with neuronopathic disease. Somatic cell gene therapy is currently under investigation. Iminosugars such as *N*-butyldeoxynojirimycin are able to decrease substrate synthesis but have limited effects on the symptoms of GD[17].

The treatment and management of GD is a rapidly growing area. It now appears possible to prevent and reverse some of the most devastating and disabling complications of this disease. Prevention and treatment of bone complications will lead to a much higher quality of life for all patients with GD.

REFERENCES

1. Gaucher PCE. De l'epithelioma primitif de la rate, hypertrophie idiopathique de la rate sans leucémie. Thesis, Paris, 1882.
2. Marchand F. Über sogenannte idiopatische Splenomegalie (Typus Gaucher). Münch Med Wochenschr 1907; 54: 1102.
3. Brady RO, Kanfer JN, Shapiro D. Metabolism of glucocerebrosides II. Evidence of an enzymatic deficiency in Gaucher's disease. Biochem Biophys Res Commun 1965; 18: 221–225.
4. Beutler A, Grabowski GA. Gaucher disease. In: Scriver CR, Beaudet AL, Valle D, Sly WS, eds. The metabolic and molecular bases of inherited disease, 8th edn, vol 3. New York: McGraw-Hill; 2001; 3635–3668.
5. Grabowski GA, Horowitz M. Gaucher's disease: molecular, genetic and enzymological aspects. Baillière's Clin Haematol 1997; 10: 635–656.
6. Beutler E. Enzyme replacement therapy for Gaucher's disease. Baillière's Clin Haematol 1997; 10: 751–763.
7. Elstein D, Itzchaki M, Mankin HJ. Skeletal involvement in Gaucher's disease. Baillière's Clin Haematol 1997; 10: 793–816.
8. Lachmann RH, Wight DG, Lomas DJ *et al*. Massive hepatic fibrosis in Gaucher's disease: clinico-pathological and radiological features. Q J Med 2000; 93: 237–244.
9. Mankin HJ, Rosenthal DI, Xavier R. Gaucher disease. New approaches to an ancient disease. J Bone Joint Surg 2001; 83A: 748–762.
10. Resnick D. Lipidoses, histiocytoses and hyperlipoproteinemias. In: Resnick D, ed. Diagnosis of bone and joint disorders, vol 4. Philadelphia, PA: WB Saunders; 1995: 2191–2246.
11. Young E, Chatterton C, Vellodi A, Winchester B. Plasma chitotriosidase activity in Gaucher disease patients who have been treated either by bone marrow transplantation or by enzyme replacement therapy with alglucerase. J Inherit Metab Dis 1997; 20: 595–602.
12. Hermann G, Pastores GM, Abdelwahab IF, Lorberboym AM. Gaucher disease: assessment of skeletal involvement and therapeutic responses to enzyme replacement. Skeletal Radiol 1997; 26: 687–696.
13. Pastores GM, Wallenstein S, Desnick RJ, Luckey MM. Bone density in Type 1 Gaucher disease. J Bone Miner Res 1996; 11: 1801–1807.
14. Pastores GM, Sibille AR, Grabowski GA. Enzyme therapy in Gaucher disease type 1: dosage efficacy and adverse effects in 33 patients treated for 6 to 24 months. Blood 1993; 82: 408–416.
15. Rosenthal DI, Doppelt SH, Mankin HJ *et al*. Enzyme replacement therapy for Gaucher disease: skeletal responses to macrophage-targeted glucocerebrosidase. Pediatrics 1995; 96: 629–637.
16. Terk MR, Dardashti S, Liebman HA. Bone marrow response in treated patients with Gaucher disease: evaluation by T1-weighted magnetic resonance images and correlation with reduction in liver and spleen volume. Skeletal Radiol 2000; 29: 563–571.
17. Cox T, Lachmann R, Hollak C *et al*. Novel oral treatment of Gaucher's disease with *N*-butyldeoxynojirimycin (OGT 918) to decrease substrate biosynthesis. Lancet 2000; 355: 1481–1485.

205 Mucopolysaccharidoses

Pierre Maroteaux

Definition

- Mucopolysaccharidoses are lysosomal storage diseases
- The lysosomal defect is responsible for the deficient degradation of glycosaminoglycans
- These are a complex group of mucopolysaccharidoses with several well-defined types; the most frequent forms are Hurler's disease (type I) and Morquio's disease (type IV)

Clinical features

- The main clinical features of the most common mucopolysaccharidosis (type I) are facial dysmorphism, visceral and corneal storage abnormalities, and skeletal disorders (dysostosis multiplex)
- Neurologic abnormalities are present in several types

HISTORY

In 1917, Hunter reported the cases of two brothers with coarse facies, mental retardation and bone disorders[1]. However, the first detailed description of mucopolysaccharidosis was that of Gertrud Hurler in 1919, inspired by Pfaundler[2]. In 1929, Morquio and Brailsford gave a precise description of type IV mucopolysaccharidosis and in 1963 Sanfilippo defined type III and Maroteaux and Lamy type VI diseases[3–7].

In 1952, Brante reported the identification of the material stored in these patients as mucopolysaccharides[8]. Dorfman and Lorincz documented increased urinary excretion of mucopolysaccharides and Van Hoof and Hers demonstrated that mucopolysaccharides are stored in lysosomes[9,10]. They proposed that a specific lysosomal enzyme deficiency was responsible for the deficient degradation of mucopolysaccharides. Neufeld demonstrated that defective degradation of mucopolysaccharides in cultured fibroblasts is corrected by cocultivation of Hurler's and Hunter's cells[11]. The corrective factors were then purified and their enzyme functions identified (Table 205.1).

CLINICAL FEATURES

Type I

This chapter focuses on the manifestations of Hurler's disease (mucopolysaccharidosis type IH), as this is the most typical of these disorders. The disease usually presents at 2 years of age with facial dysmorphism, dorsal kyphosis or mental retardation. The craniofacial morphology is

	Skeletal dysplasia	Corneal opacities	Mental degradation	Inheritance	Urinary glycosaminoglycans	Enzymatic deficiency	Gene localization
Type IH (Hurler's disease)	+	+	+	Autosomal recessive	Heparan sulfate Dermatan sulfate	I-iduronidase	4p16.3
Type IS (Scheie's disease)	±	+	−	Autosomal recessive	Heparan sulfate Dermatan sulfate	I-iduronidase	4p16.3
Type II (Hunter's disease)	− −	+	±	X-linked recessive	Heparan sulfate Dermatan sulfate	Iduranidate-2-sulfate sulfatase	Xq27.3q28
Type III (Sanfilippo's disease)	±	−	++	Autosomal recessive	Heparan sulfate	(a) Heparan sulfatase	17q25.3
				Autosomal recessive		(b) N-acetyl-D-glucosaminidase	17q21.1
				Autosomal recessive		(c) α-glucosaminide N-acetyl-transferase	14p13
				Autosomal recessive		(d) N-acetyl-glucosamine-6-sulfate-sulfatase	12q14
Type IV (Morquio's disease)	++(a)	+	−	Autosomal recessive	Keratan sulfate	(a) N-acetyl-glucosamine-6-sulfate-sulfatase	16q24.3
	+(b)	+	−	Autosomal recessive		(b) β-galactosidase	3p21p33
Type VI (Maroteaux–Lamy)	+/++	+	−	Autosomal recessive	Dermatan sulfate	Arylsulfatase B	5p11p13
Type VII (Sly)	+	+	+	Autosomal recessive	Chondroitin sulfate	β-glucuronidase	7q11.21q11.22

TABLE 205.1 SUMMARY OF THE MAIN TYPES OF MUCOPOLYSACCHARIDOSIS

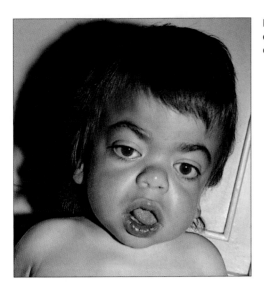

Fig. 205.1 Hurler's disease. Typical facial dysmorphism.

typical, with macrocephaly, broad nasal bridge, full cheeks, thick lips, enlarged tongue, coarse hair and hirsutism (Fig. 205.1). Joint movements are limited, with claw hands (Fig. 205.2). Lumbar kyphosis is frequent. The abdomen is protuberant, with hepatosplenomegaly and hernias. Corneal opacities are visible with slit-lamp examination. Progressive mental and physical deterioration leads to death, often between 10 and 15 years of age.

Scheie's disease (mucopolysaccharidosis type IS) is detected later, usually in childhood, and has a slow evolution[12]. Joint stiffness, claw hand, heart murmur and corneal clouding are the main clinical manifestations of this form. Phenotypes intermediate between those of Hurler's and Scheie's disease are not infrequent[13].

Radiographic features

Radiographs show macrocephaly, sagittal craniosynostosis and an enlarged sella turcica. The ribs are wide, with an 'oar-shaped' deformity. The vertebral bodies are ovoid and hook-like dysplasia is visible at the apex of the gibbus (Fig. 205.3). The midshafts of the long bones are enlarged, with typical tilting of the distal radius and ulna towards each other, together with coxa valga. The epiphyses, carpal and tarsal bones

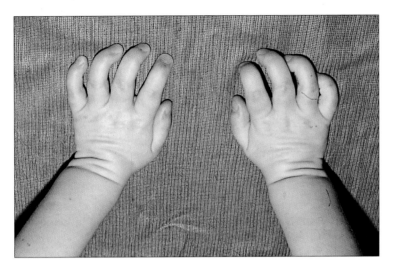

Fig. 205.2 Hurler's disease. Claw hands are a common feature.

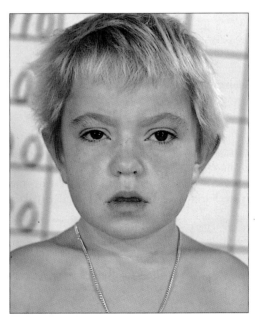

Fig. 205.4 Hunter's disease. Note that the facial dysmorphism is milder than in Hurler's disease.

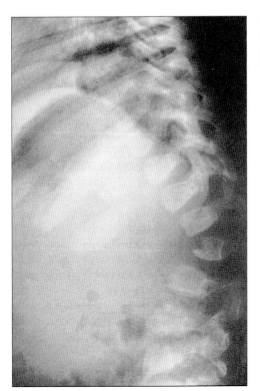

Fig. 205.3 Hurler's disease. Hook-like deformity of the second lumbar vertebral body.

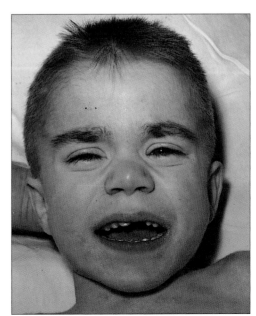

Fig. 205.5 Sanfilippo's disease. Mild coarsening of the facial features.

are small and irregular. The iliac wing is small and subluxation of the femoral head is frequent. The phalanges and metacarpal bones are shortened and enlarged, and the pointed proximal end of the metacarpals gives the characteristic 'sugar loaf' appearance[14–16].

Clinical forms of mucopolysaccharidosis

Type II

Mucopolysaccharidosis type II is an X-linked recessive disorder. Clinical and radiologic manifestations are similar to Hurler's disease but are often more slowly progressive (Fig. 205.4) and the cornea is clear.

Type III

In mucopolysaccharidosis type III (Sanfilippo's disease), the facial features and skeletal deformities are much milder than those in Hurler's syndrome (Fig. 205.5). However, the mental and motor deterioration are precocious and severe.

Type IV

In type IV (Morquio's disease), dwarfism is severe, with short trunk, kyphosis at the thoracolumbar junction, pectus carinatum and knock-knees (Fig. 205.6). Intelligence is normal and no visceral storage is

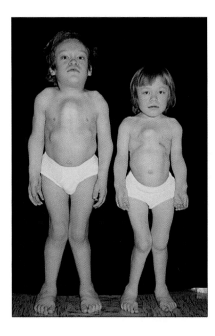

Fig. 205.6 Morquio's disease in a brother and sister. Short trunk with pectus carinatum and knock knees.

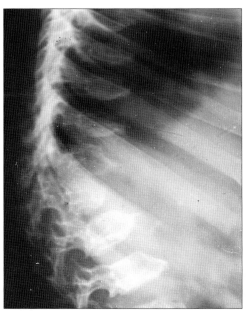

Fig. 205.7 Lateral radiograph of the thoracolumbar spine in a 17-year-old girl with the clinical presentation of Morquio's disease. The vertebral bodies show an anterior breaking which is seen also in association with Hurler's syndrome. Note the associated kyphosis. (With permission from Bullough[17].)

observed (only minimal corneal clouding). Universal platyspondyly (Fig. 205.7) with small odontoid processes, coxa valga, irregularities of the epiphyses and metaphyses, small and irregular carpal bones and pointed proximal ends of the metacarpals are the more typical radiologic manifestations. The spinal cord compression due to atlantoaxial dislocation must be prevented by surgical intervention. The Morquio type B syndrome is similar but with milder deformities.

Type VI

In type VI, the facies is less grotesque than in Hurler's disease. The cornea is cloudy but mental development remains normal. Skeletal changes and dwarfism are variable but often severe.

Type VII

Mucopolysaccharidosis type VII (Sly's disease) is very rare. There are considerable phenotypic and bone deformity variations[18].

HISTOLOGIC MANIFESTATIONS

In type I and type II diseases, vacuolated lymphocytes are found with metachromatic inclusions in the vacuoles (Gasser cells). In addition, reticular cells of the bone marrow contain inclusions that vary from moderately coarse to very thick black–violet (type II Gasser cells)[19]. In type II, lymphocytes have also been described with pink-ringed vacuoles[20]. In mucopolysaccharidosis type III, the Gasser cells are more numerous and plasmocyte cells containing vacuoles with metachromatic inclusions (Buhot cells) are found in the bone marrow. Alder's anomaly is seen in type VI: coarse, dense granules in granulocytes and monocytes and in a large proportion of lymphocytes.

BIOCHEMICAL MANIFESTATIONS

There is increased urinary elimination of dermatan sulfate and heparan sulfate in type I and type II diseases. Heparan sulfate is elevated in type III, keratan sulfate in type IV and dermatan sulfate in type VI. These diseases arise from an inherited deficiency of the activity of lysosomal enzymes. For example, in type I there is an inherited deficiency of α-L-iduronidase (Table 205.1).

PATHOGENESIS

The mucopolysaccharidoses are caused by deficiency of specific lysosomal enzymes that catabolize glycosaminoglycans into shorter subunits for reuse or excretion. The deficiency of these enzymes results in the intracellular accumulation and the increased urinary excretion of the products of incomplete catabolism. As a result, cellular function is altered in the cartilage, connective tissues, heart and central nervous system.

At the present time, the genes of these deficient enzymes have been mapped and cloned (Table 205.1). There are several mutations for each gene. For instance, in mucopolysaccharidosis type IVA, around 40 mutations have been demonstrated to date. The mutation 1113F is common and produces a severe phenotype, whereas the mutation T312S is found in milder patients[21]. However a significant interpopulation variation is observed[22].

MANAGEMENT

The major focus of management of patients with mucopolysaccharidoses is orthopaedic in nature. Procedures include treatment of the lumbar kyphosis by bracing or posterior fusion and decompression of the carpal tunnel syndrome, often reported in types I, II or VI, whereas in type IV correction of genu valgum is required[23,24].

In type IV and in patients with a hypoplastic odontoid process with other types of mucopolysaccharidosis, surgical stabilization of atlantoaxial instability and subluxation is necessary. An assay for correcting the loss of the deficient enzyme in these diseases has been in existence for some years and correction has been demonstrated in tissue culture. Bone marrow transplantation with an identical donor alters the natural evolution, especially in type I: there is regression of hepatomegaly and splenomegaly, improvement of the respiratory and cardiac function and protection of the brain if transplantation is performed early in life. However, the cartilage and bone manifestations are poorly or not prevented or corrected[25]. Bone marrow transplantation is also advisable for type VI (prevention of cardiac and pulmonary complications)[26] but it is not effective in types II, III or type IV.

The correction of human mucopolysaccharidosis type VI and type I fibroblasts or in human bone marrow has been accomplished by retroviral-vector-mediated gene transfer[27–29]. In the future, gene therapy may become a realistic approach to disease management. However, enzyme replacement therapy with recombinant α-L-iduronidase is an other promising possibility[30] but unexpected immunological reactions seem to be frequent. Prenatal diagnosis is also possible through biochemical studies of cultured amniotic cells or analysis of fetal blood.

REFERENCES

1. Hunter C. A rare disease in two brothers. Proc R Soc Med 1917; 10: 104–116.
2. Hurler G. Ueber einen Typ multipler Abartungen, vorwiegend am Skelettsystem. Z Kinderheilk 1919; 24: 220–224.
3. Morquio L. Sur une forme de dystrophie osseuse familiale. Bull Soc Pediatr 1929; 27: 145–152.
4. Brailsford JF. Chondro-osteodystrophy. Am J Surg 1929; 7: 404–410.
5. Sanfilippo SJ, Podosin R, Langer L, Good LA. Mental retardation associated with acid mucopolysacchariduria (heparitin sulfate type). J Pediatr 1963; 63: 837–838.
6. Maroteaux P, Lamy M, Foucher M. La maladie de Morquio. Etude clinique, radiologique et biologique. Presse Med 1963; 71: 2091–2094.
7. Maroteaux P, Leveque B, Marie J et al. Une nouvelle dystostose avec élimination urinaire de chondroitine-sulfate B. Presse Med 1963; 71: 1849–1852.
8. Brante F. Gargoylism: a mucopolysaccharidosis. Scand J Clin Lab Invest 1952; 4: 43–46.
9. Dorfman A, Lorincz AE. Occurrence of urinary acid mucopolysaccharides in the Hurler syndrome. Proc Natl Acad Sci USA 1957; 43: 443–446.
10. Van Hoof F, Hers HG. The abnormalities of lysosomal enzymes in mucopolysaccharidoses. Eur J Biochem 1968; 7A: 34–44.
11. Neufeld EF, Fratantonil JC. Inborn errors of mucopolysaccharide metabolism. Science 1970; 169: 141–146.
12. Scheie HG, Hambrick GW Jr, Barness LA. A newly recognized forme fruste of Hurler's disease (gargoylism). Am J Ophthalmol 1962; 53: 753–769.
13. McKusick VA. Heritable disorders of connective tissue, 15th ed. St Louis, MO: CV Mosby; 1993: 367–499.
14. Eggli KD, Dorst JP. The mucopolysaccharidoses and related conditions. Semin Roentgenol 1986; 21: 275–294.
15. Maroteaux P. Maladies osseuses de l'enfant: autres désordres du métabolisme. Paris: Flammarion Medecine Sciences; 1995: 334–353.
16. Spranger J, Perch HJ, Stoss H. Skelettveranderungen bei angeborenen Stoffwechselstorungen. Monatsschr Kinderheilk 1981; 129: 670–676.
17. Bullough PG. Orthopaedic pathology, 3rd ed. London: Mosby-Wolfe; 1997.
18. Sly WS, Quinton BA, McAlister WH, Rimoin DL. Beta-glucuronidase deficiency: report of clinical, radiologic and biochemical features of a new mucopolysaccharidosis. J Pediatr 1973; 82: 249–257.
19. Hansen HG. Hematologic studies in mucopolysaccharidoses and mucolipidoses. Birth Defects 1972; 8: 115–128.
20. Maier-Redelsperger M, Stern MH, Maroteaux P. Pink rings lymphocytes: a new cytologic abnormality characteristic of mucopolysaccharidosis type II (Hunter disease). Pediatrics 1988; 82: 286–287.
21. Yamada N, Fukuda S, Tomatsu S et al. Molecular heterogeneity in mucopolysaccharidosis IVA in Australia and Northern Ireland: nine novel mutations including T312S, a common allele that confers a mild phenotype. Hum Mutat 1998; 11: 202–208.
22. Rezvi GMM, Tomatsu S, Fukuda S et al. Mucopolysaccharidosis IVA: a comparative study of polymorphic DNA haplotypes in the Caucasian and Japanese populations. J Inher Metab Dis 1996; 19: 301–308.
23. Tandon V, Williamson JB, Cowbie RA, Wraith JE. Spinal problems in mucopolysaccharidosis I (Hurler syndrome). J Bone Joint Surg 1996; 78B: 938–944.
24. Haddad FS, Jones DHA, Vellodi A et al. Carpal tunnel syndrome in the mucopolysaccharidoses and mucolipidoses. J Bone Joint Surg 1997; 79B: 576–582.
25. Field RE, Buchanan JAF, Copplemans MGJ, Aichroth PM. Bone-marrow transplantation in Hurler's syndrome. J Bone Joint Surg 1994; 76B: 975–81.
26. Herskhovitz E, Young E, Rainer J et al. Bone marrow transplantation for Maroteaux–Lamy syndrome (MPS VI): long-term follow-up. J Inher Metab Dis 1999; 22: 50–62.
27. Anson DS, Bielicki J, Hopwood JJ. Correction of mucopolysaccharidosis type I fibroblasts by retroviral-mediated transfer of the human α-L-iduronidase gene. Hum Gene Ther 1992; 3: 371–380.
28. Peters C, Rommerskirch W, Modaressi S, von Figura K. Restoration of arylsulphatase B activity in human mucopolysaccharidosis-type-VI fibroblasts by retroviral-vector-mediated gene transfer. Biochem J 1991; 276: 499–504.
29. Fairbairn LJ, Lashford LS, Spooncer E et al. Long-term in vitro correction of alpha-L-iduronidase deficiency (Hurler syndrome) in human bone marrow. Proc Natl Acad Sci USA 1996; 93: 2025–2030.
30. Kakkis ED, Muenzer J Tiller GE et al. Enzyme-replacement therapy in mucopolysaccharidosis I. N Engl J Med 2001; 344: 182–188.

206 Heritable connective tissue disorders

Joan C Marini

Definition

Osteogenesis imperfecta

- A genetic syndrome of abnormal bone matrix with secondary osteoporosis
- Generalized connective tissue disorder with variable non-osseous features
- Associated with abnormalities of structure or synthesis of type I collagen

Ehlers–Danlos syndrome

- A genetic syndrome affecting primarily joints, skin and blood vessel walls
- Generalized connective tissue disorder
- Heterogeneous group of disorders associated with multiple modes of inheritance and associated with abnormalities of types I, III or V collagen or fibronectin, enzyme deficiencies or abnormalities of copper metabolism

Marfan's syndrome

- A genetic syndrome with abnormalities of the musculoskeletal, cardiovascular and ocular systems
- Generalized connective tissue disorder with variability of clinical expression
- Associated with abnormality of fibrillin, an extracellular matrix protein found in microfibrils

Chondrodystrophies

- A large and strikingly heterogeneous group of heritable skeletal dysplasias with abnormal proportions of limbs, trunk and/or skull, and often with short stature
- Disorders classified according to the Paris nomenclature of 1976
- Some chondrodystrophies are associated with an abnormality of type II collagen. However, in most chondrodystrophies the abnormality of extracellular matrix is unknown

Clinical features

Osteogenesis imperfecta

- 'Brittle bone disease': susceptibility to fractures from mild trauma
- Non-osseous involvement may include abnormal scleral hue, hearing loss, dentinogenesis imperfecta, short stature, macrocephaly, joint laxity and easy bruising
- Forms of osteogenesis imperfecta range from lethal in the perinatal period to barely detectable

Ehlers–Danlos syndrome

- Joint involvement may include hyperextensibility of large or small joints and joint dislocations
- Skin involvement may include soft, velvety texture, hyperextensibility, fragility with stretched or 'cigarette paper' scars
- Vascular and visceral involvement ranges from easy bruising to life-threatening arterial rupture, rupture of the colon or uterus

Marfan's syndrome

- Musculoskeletal involvement may include tall stature, dolichostenomelia (long, thin extremities), arachnodactyly, scoliosis and chest deformities
- Cardiovascular manifestations include aortic root dilatation and mitral valve prolapse
- Ocular manifestations include lens dislocation or subluxation and myopia

Chondrodystrophies

- Skeletal involvement may include short or disproportionate stature, joint and skull abnormalities. Non-skeletal involvement may affect cardiac, ocular or auditory systems
- Achondroplasia, the most common chondrodystrophy, is evident at birth with rhizomelic shortening of limbs, large calvaria with prominent forehead, trident hand and lordosis
- Stickler syndrome presents with ocular, facial and joint involvement

INTRODUCTION

In the past decade, dramatic progress has been made in understanding the molecular genetics of heritable connective tissue disorders. Some types of osteogenesis imperfecta (OI) and Ehlers–Danlos syndrome (EDS) have been shown to be caused by abnormalities of types I, III, or V collagen, some chondrodystrophies have been associated with abnormal type II collagen, and Marfan's syndrome, long classified as a 'collagen disorder', has been associated with abnormality of fibrillin, a component of extracellular matrix.

These discoveries have served to highlight the basic principles that distinguish these disorders. First, they are primary connective tissue disorders, in which there is a heritable defect in a gene coding for a component of matrix. The mutation affects that protein's synthesis, structure or function in the extracellular matrix directly. The 'collagen–vascular' disorders exert their effect on connective tissue indirectly, through autoimmune mechanisms. Second, the pattern of heritability of these disorders is influenced by the multimeric structure of collagen, so that a defect in one allele can inactivate up to 93% of the total product of both alleles. In contrast, enzymatic metabolic disorders are usually symptomatic only when both alleles of a gene are defective. Third, as is true for many genetic disorders, the connective tissue disorders display variability, differences in phenotypic expression among individuals with the same mutation and heterogeneity, different mutations in one gene (or a different gene) causing the same phenotype in different individuals.

OSTEOGENESIS IMPERFECTA

History

The term osteogenesis imperfecta was first used by Vrolik in 1849. The division of OI into 'congenita' and 'tarda' forms by Looser in 1906 has

Type	Genetics	Description
I	Autosomal dominant	Mildest form of OI Mild-to-moderate bone fragility without deformity Associated with blue sclerae, early hearing loss, easy bruising May have mild-to-moderate short stature Type 1A: dentinogenesis imperfecta absent Type 1B: dentinogenesis imperfecta present
II	Autosomal dominant or recessive	Perinatal lethal or recessive Extreme fragility of connective tissue, multiple in utero fractures, usually intrauterine growth retardation Soft, large cranium Micromelia, long bones crumped and bowed, ribs beaded
III	Autosomal dominant or recessive	Progressive deforming phenotype Severe fragility of bones, usually have in utero fractures Severe osteoporosis Relative macrocephaly with triangular facies Fractures heal with deformity and bowing Associated with white sclerae and extreme short stature, scoliosis
IV	Autosomal dominant	Skeletal fragility and osteoporosis more severe than type I Associated with bowing of long bones; light sclerae, ± moderate short stature, ± moderate joint hyperextensibility Type IVA: dentinogenesis imperfecta absent Type IVB: dentinogenesis imperfecta present

TABLE 206.1 SILLENCE CLASSIFICATION OF OSTEOGENESIS IMPERFECTA SYNDROMES[1]

fallen into disuse since the 1979 Sillence genetic classification. In the early 1980s, the Prockop and Byers laboratories demonstrated that OI was caused by abnormalities in type I collagen[2,3].

Epidemiology

The overall frequency for OI identifiable at birth is about 1 per 20 000–30 000, based on birth record surveys in Australia and Scotland[4]. The frequency of mild type I OI has been estimated at 1 in 30 000 in Australia[4]; this is a minimum estimate, since some individuals do not come to medical attention. The prevalence and severity is not influenced by gender, race or ethnic origin.

Clinical features

Sillence classification

The Sillence classification of OI (Table 206.1)[1] is based on genetic, clinical and radiographic data. Type II OI is lethal in the perinatal period. The overwhelming majority of cases are associated with new dominant mutations; most occurrences to clinically normal parents are due to germline mosaicism in one parent. A few exceptional cases appear to be recessive. Type III, the most severe form compatible with long-term survival, has a natural history characterized by extreme short stature, progressive scoliosis and deformity of long bones. Type IV is moderately severe in skeletal features with significant short stature; this form is compatible with assisted ambulation. In some cases of type IV OI, it has not been possible to demonstrate a collagen abnormality. This type is proba-

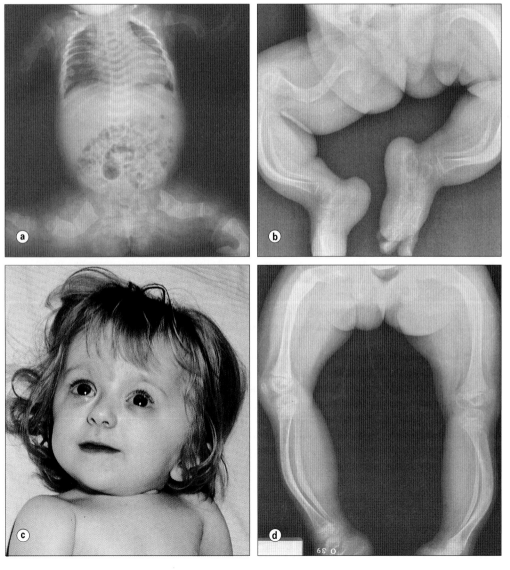

Fig. 206.1 Features of osteogenesis imperfecta. (a) Type II OI has short, crumpled long bones and rib fractures. (b) Type III OI has progressive deformity and osteoporosis of long bones. (c,d) Type IV OI has triangular facies, frontal bossing and shallow orbits and long bones with moderate deformity and osteoporosis.

bly genetically heterogeneous. Individuals with type I OI have mild skeletal disease and often have blue sclerae.

Skeletal dysplasia

Although fracture susceptibility is extremely variable, the skeletal system in OI is characterized by osteoporosis secondary to osseous matrix abnormality, bowing of long bones, compression of vertebral bodies and characteristic triangular facies. Individuals with type II OI (Fig. 206.1a) have prenatal fractures of ribs and long bones, with severe limb shortening and deformity. There is relative macrocephaly, soft membranous skull and wormian bones. Individuals with type III (Fig. 206.1b) experience frequent fractures, progressive scoliosis, long bone deformity and metaphyseal flaring. Type IV (Fig. 206.1d) and type I long bones are generally well modeled although relatively osteoporotic. Fractures usually occur after ambulation, are related to some degree of trauma, heal with minimal deformity, decrease dramatically in number post puberty and recur after menopause[4].

Ocular

Blue scleral hue, caused by decreased scleral thickness, is a common finding in OI and occurs in all types, especially types I and II. Ocular rigidity is lower than normal in OI patients but is unrelated to myopic refractive error.

Dental

Dentinogenesis imperfecta, with grayish opalescent or brown–yellow dentition, may be present. Some dentinogenesis imperfecta leads to easy crumbling and wearing of dentition. Generally, the permanent dentition is less severely affected than the primary dentition[5].

Other systems

Hearing loss is a common feature of OI, occurring in about 50% of patients over their lifetime and being especially prevalent in type I[5]. It generally presents as a conductive or mixed hearing loss in the early adult years. Pulmonary complications may be a significant source of morbidity and mortality. Infants with type II OI generally die of respiratory insufficiency. In types III and IV OI, pectoral deformities, scoliosis and flaring and softness of the rib cage may predispose to frequent pneumonia or eventual cor pulmonale. Mitral valve prolapse may be present, especially in milder, dominant forms of OI. Growth impairment[4] affects virtually 100% of type III patients and 25–50% of types I and IV patients; it is unrelated to fracture frequency or location. Neurologically, types III and IV children often have ventriculomegaly and sulcal prominence, even without macrocephaly[4]. This does not indicate hydrocephalus and is not associated with intellectual impairment.

Investigations

The diagnosis of OI can usually be made clearly on clinical and radiologic bases. The initial radiologic survey should include all long bones, thorax, pelvis and lateral views of skull and vertebral column. For vaginally delivered infants with OI diagnosable at birth, an ultrasound can be useful to rule out intracranial bleeds. A normal serum alkaline phosphatase, calcium and phosphate can rule out metabolic mineralization disorders.

In moderate and severe OI, periodic radiographs of lower long bones and vertebral bodies are useful in adjustment of surgical and orthotic management. Dual X-ray absorptiometry can be used to follow disease progression in both cortical and trabecular bone. Audiologic evaluation and pulmonary functions tests every other year starting in childhood allow anticipatory management. Biochemical analysis of the collagen produced by fibroblasts cultured from a skin biopsy is vital for understanding the genetic inheritance of individual cases, distinguishing different types of OI and providing accurate genetic counseling. A type I collagen abnormality can be demonstrated in about 85% of OI patients. However, data on the osseous consequences of different amino acid

substitutions and locations are insufficient to predict phenotypic outcome.

Prenatal detection of OI by ultrasound is possible in types II and III. Linkage analysis can be applied to the milder dominant forms when there is a family history of OI. Analysis of collagens produced by cultured chorionic villus cells has been accurate in OI types II, III and IV and allows detection by 12–15 weeks gestation[6]. Cultured amniotic fluid cells may yield false-positive diagnoses.

Etiology and pathogenesis

Structure and function

Osteogenesis imperfecta has been associated with defects in the structure or synthesis of type I collagen[2,3] (Fig. 206.2). Type I collagen[2] is the

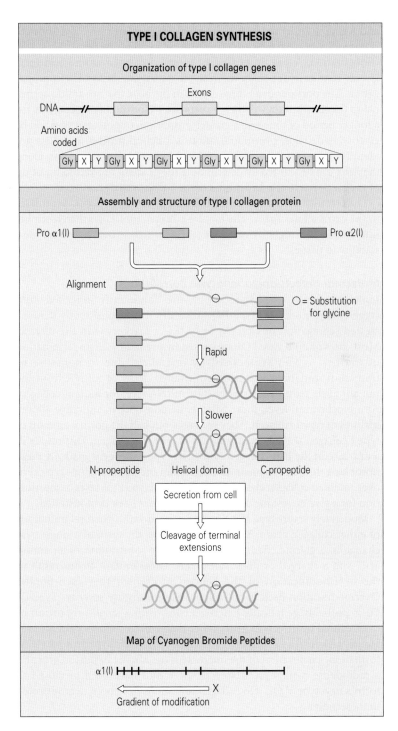

Fig. 206.2 Type I collagen synthesis. Organization of type I collagen genes and protein. Assembly of heterotrimer containing a mutant chain, its effect on glycosylation and cyanogen bromide mapping are shown.

major protein of human extracellular matrix and plays a crucial scaffolding role in bone, skin, ligaments, tendons, sclerae and blood vessel walls. This wide distribution accounts for the generalized nature of OI.

Type I collagen is a heterotrimer, composed of two $\alpha1(I)$ chains and one $\alpha2(I)$ chain twisted around each other in a long, right-handed helix. Each chain is synthesized as a propeptide, with globular extensions at both ends and a central helical domain of 1014 amino acids. The helical domain is composed of repeating triplets of the sequence Gly–X–Y, in which X and Y are often proline and hydroxyproline respectively. The exons of the genes encoding these chains code for an even multiple of triplets; each exon begins with a glycine and ends with a Y codon.

The three chains of the helix initially associate through the globular carboxyl extension. Helix formation then proceeds linearly towards the amino terminus, with glycine residues occupying the core positions inside the helix. Concomitant with synthesis and helix formation, proline and lysine residues along the chain are hydroxylated and glycosylated. The modifying enzymes are not active on residues in the triple helical configuration. A substitution of a charged or a polar amino acid for a glycine residue in one chain will result in a temporal delay of helix propagation. The portions of all three chains in the helix that are amino-terminal to the substitution will then be exposed to the modifying enzymes for a longer period of time and a greater proportion of potential sites will be glycosylated. Thus, overmodification is a helical process and does not identify the mutant chain. The regional location of the mutation along the helix can be learned by determining the gradient of overmodification of the cyanogen bromide peptides of the collagen chains.

The terminal extensions of the helix are cleaved by specific peptidases in the extracellular space. The mature collagen molecules then assemble into fibrils and higher-order structures, which provide strength and stability to tissues.

Molecular defects and phenotypic correlations

Linkage analysis of pedigrees with the dominantly inherited mild (type I) and moderate (type IV) forms of OI has consistently demonstrated segregation of COL1A1 or COL1A2 markers with the disease. Most cases of mild type I OI are caused by premature chain termination of the $\alpha1(I)$ chain synthesized by one allele, due to nonsense or frameshift mutations[7]. Nonsense-mediated decay of mRNA from the mutant allele reduces the steady-state mRNA level for mutant collagen. At a biochemical level, these patients demonstrate quantitative abnormalities of type I collagen. They secrete about half the normal amount of type I collagen and a normal amount of type III collagen. This results in a decrease in the I:III collagen ratio. The type I collagens made by these fibroblasts do not demonstrate electrophoretic abnormalities typical of overmodified collagen chains. In a handful of type I OI cases, a substitution for a glycine residue or a small deletion has been demonstrated.

Moderately severe type IV OI[2,3] is associated with structural mutations of either collagen chain. Most often this takes the form of a single base change in a glycine codon, which causes the substitution of an amino acid with a charged or polar side chain. These mutant chains result in the overmodification of the helices into which they incorporate. Overmodification itself is not responsible for disease severity. Type IV OI is probably genetically heterogeneous, with a small proportion of cases caused by defects in genes other than collagen. Some patients previously classified as Type IV OI and characterized by hypertrophic callus formation, calcification of the interosseus membrane of the forearm and a radiodense metaphyseal band in the radius have been proposed to form a new type V OI[8]. No collagen mutations have been demonstrated in these patients.

Most cases of type III OI are also caused by structural defects of one of the two chains of type I collagen. In one unusual recessive case[3], none of the $\alpha2(I)$ chains of the proband could be incorporated into the triple helix. The proband synthesized only $\alpha1(I)$ homotrimers.

Type II OI, like type IV OI, is associated with structural defects in the chains of type I collagen that result in overmodification of the helices. Most are point mutations causing substitutions for glycine residues, a few are deletions or insertions. On sodium dodecyl sulfate–polyacrylamide gel electrophoresis (SDS-PAGE) collagen analysis, the collagens from patients with types II and IV OI both contain forms with delayed electrophoretic migration and are indistinguishable. The pathophysiologic correlations of the particular substitutions for glycine and their position along the chain are not fully understood. For the $\alpha2(I)$ chain, the outcome of mutations is best explained by a regional model, in which severity is related to the existence of regularly spaced regions along the chain that are crucial for the function of collagen in matrix.

At the molecular level, almost all cases of type II OI have been new dominant mutations in one allele. However, the Sillence classification originally postulated a recessive inheritance based on recurrences to phenotypically normal parents. This apparent discrepancy has been explained by the demonstration in several families of mosaicism for the lethal mutation in the germline of one parent[3]. Parental germline mosaicism may account for 5–7% of type II OI and should be considered in genetic counseling.

Management

Rehabilitation

The goal of physical rehabilitation in OI is to attain age-appropriate physical skills as a child and to retain maximum physical skills in the adult. The specific goals range widely with age and severity, and include independent or assisted ambulation, transfer ability and wheelchair-assisted mobility.

Active physical therapy, with an OI-experienced therapist, should begin in the neonatal period[9]. To prevent deformities and assist respiratory effort, severely affected infants may require a custom-molded seating insert for proper positioning of the head, spine and pelvis. Hydrotherapy[9] should begin in the bath in infancy and continue through life as swimming and water exercises. This improves general conditioning as well as muscular strength for head and trunk control and independent extremity movements.

Children who are not expected to walk should be provided with a powered wheelchair for independent mobility in the preschool years. Children with ambulation potential should receive regular physical therapy to strengthen abdominal, pelvic girdle and lower extremity musculature and to prevent contractures[9]. When they are ready to pull to standing, they are fitted with ultra-lightweight plastic clam-shell braces with a pelvic band and hinged joints[9]. Some children may require surgical correction of lower limb deformities before weight-bearing is attempted. Once in braces, children progress through ambulation aids such as walkers and crutches to independent ambulation. Bracing does not prevent fractures but it may aid in the natural remodeling of tibias.

Women with even mild OI may experience a postmenopausal exacerbation of osteoporosis. Physiologic estrogen provides some protection during the postpubertal years and is a good postmenopausal therapeutic choice in many cases.

Orthopedic management

An orthopedic surgeon experienced with OI is essential to a successful physical outcome. Even in severely affected individuals, fractures should not be allowed to heal without proper alignment and reduction. Fracture healing is generally normal in OI patients; the period of immobilization should be minimized to avoid worsening osteoporosis by disuse.

Intramedullary rod fixation for improving limb appearance is inappropriate. The multiple osteotomy and rod fixation procedure of Sofield and Millar is useful for interrupting rapid refracture sequences and correcting deformity prior to weight-bearing[4]. The extensible Bailey–Dubow rod has been used most often. It has the advantage of extending with bone growth.

Unfortunately, it has the complication of frequent migration into a joint space. Further, because the rod is 30 times stiffer than normal bone, it bears a disproportionate share of the gravity load and causes significant cortical atrophy. To circumvent the problems of rod migration and bone atrophy, a straight Sofield rod or a Rush rod with a crook may be used to stabilize a healing osteotomy in the lower limb. Ideally, these would be removed within a year of placement. The use of plates and screws to stabilize an osteotomy has resulted in increased osteoporosis of bone with poorly healed screw holes and cannot be recommended.

The scoliosis of moderate and severe OI is not responsive to Milwaukee bracing. When scoliosis exceeds 40°, spinal fusion with Harrington instrumentation generally provides good stabilization.

Management of generalized connective tissue symptoms

The bisphosphonate drugs have emerged as a promising treatment for osteogenesis imperfecta[10]. The vertebral bodies appear to have the most positive response, with changes in vertebral height suggesting that bone strength as well as density have been improved. The outcome for long bones is not yet clear. Trials in animal models for OI and controlled trials in children are now under way.

Growth deficiency is one of the most consistent secondary features of OI. In a treatment trial of children with types III and IV OI, half of the children responded to recombinant growth hormone (rGH) with more than a 50% increase in their linear growth rate. The responders had predominantly type IV OI. Responders also experienced increased vertebral bone mineral density as measured by DEXA and positive changes in bone histology. The effect of rGH therapy on final adult stature is unknown, as is the possible synergy between rGH and bisphosphonates.

Mitral valve prolapse is sometimes present in dominant OI and patients should receive prophylactic measures as appropriate. Severely affected infants may have multiple bouts of pneumonia in the first years of life and should be treated promptly with antibiotics. If early signs of desaturation appear, patients should be given oxygen as needed to forestall development of pulmonary hypertension and cor pulmonale.

Some degree of high-frequency hearing loss is characteristic of OI. Functionally significant hearing loss can usually be overcome with amplification. If conductive hearing loss is severe, stapedectomy requires an OI-experienced surgical team to avoid fracturing the stapes or creating a 'floating footplate'.

If dentinogenesis imperfecta is present, dentition may crumble or wear rapidly. Artificial crowns may be necessary to preserve tooth structure and proper occlusion.

EHLERS–DANLOS SYNDROME

History

Ehlers and Danlos each made a contribution to the associations of this syndrome shortly after 1900. Molecular work by Byers, De Paepe, Pope, Steinmann, Ramirez and others has described defects in types I, III and

---

TABLE 206.2 TYPES OF EHLERS–DANLOS SYNDROME

Type	Name	Genetics	Etiology	Clinical
EDS I	Gravis	AD	30% of cases caused by null allele for COL5A1 or COL5A2	Soft skin with scars Hypermobile joints Easy bruising
EDS II	Mitis	AD	30% of cases caused by null allele for COL5A1 or COL5A2	Less severe form of type I EDS
EDS III	Hypermobile	AD	Unknown	Soft skin without scars Marked mobility of large and small joints
EDS IV	Vascular	AD (AR)	Defects of type III collagen	Translucent skin Marked bruising Ruptured arteries, uterus, bowel Normal joint mobility
EDS V	X-linked	XL	Unknown	Similar to EDS II
EDS VI	Ocular-scoliotic VI-A-decreased lysyl hydroxy case type VI-B-decreased lysyl hydroxy case type	AR	Defects in lysyl hydroxylase Unknown	Skin soft and extensible Scoliosis Ocular fragility Hypermobile joints
EDS VII	Arthrochalasis multiplex congenita VIIA-α1 (I) type VIIB-α2 (I) type VIIC-enzyme deficiency	AD AD AR	α1(I) DE6 α2(I) DE6 Deficient procollagen N-proteinase	Congenital hip dislocation Hypermobile joints Skin soft without scars
EDS VIII	Periodontitis type	AD	Unknown	Generalized periodontitis Skin soft and extensible Easy bruising Hypermobile joints
EDS IX	(Vacant)			Soft, lax skin Bladder diverticula and rupture Bony occipital horns
EDS X	Fibronectin	AR	Fibronectin	Mild joint hypermobility Easy bruising Abnormal platelet aggregation

AD, autosomal dominant; AR, autosomal recessive.

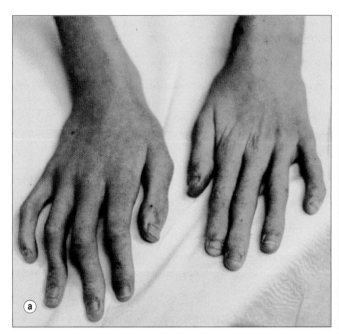
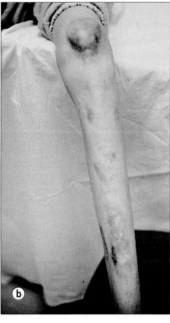

Fig. 206.3 Features of Ehlers–Danlos syndrome.
(a) Hyperextensibility of small joints.
(b) Cigarette-paper scarring. (Courtesy of Dr DK Grange.)

V collagen in EDS patients. The Villefranche nosology updates the recognized genetic heterogeneity of the syndromes[11]. Recently, deletion of tenascin-X has been identified in a patient with EDS findings[12].

Epidemiology

The genetic inheritance and incidence of EDS varies widely with type[11]. Fortunately, severe type IV EDS is rare and occurs in less than 1 in 100 000 births; the diagnosis is often made in childhood. Milder dominant forms of EDS are much more common, with an estimated prevalence of 1 in 20 000 for EDS type I.

Clinical features

The different types of EDS and main clinical features listed in Table 206.2 are based on those of Beighton and Byers[13].

Type I EDS is the gravis form. Patients have velvety and hyperextensible skin, marked joint extensibility, 'cigarette paper' scars and easy bruising (Fig. 206.3). Many are born prematurely or have mitral valve prolapse.

Type II EDS has a less severe presentation of type I clinical associations, except premature degenerative arthritis may develop. In type III EDS, joints dislocate repeatedly and are associated with degenerative joint disease. Scars form normally.

Type IV EDS, the severest form, includes complications that reduce adult life expectancy, such as rupture of arterial walls, colon or pregnant uterus. There is a characteristic facies with large eyes and thin nose and lips. Patients have marked bruisibility, an aged skin appearance on hands and feet, and joint hypermobility limited to the small joints of the hands.

Type VII EDS presents predominantly with joint symptoms, beginning with congenital hip dislocations, usually bilateral, and continuing with striking joint laxity and multiple dislocations. There may be moderate short stature and mild skin bruising and extensibility.

Diagnostic studies

Biochemical studies of types I and III collagen from patient fibroblasts are important to establish the genetics of the EDS and to identify those patients with EDS type IV for anticipatory management. Fibroblast lysyl hydroxylase deficiency can be demonstrated in EDS type VI[14]; low serum copper and ceruloplasmin are present in EDS type IX.

Differential diagnosis

The features of EDS overlap with those of other connective tissue disorders, especially the marfanoid hypermobility syndrome, cutis laxa and mild OI. Neuromuscular disorders and Menkes syndrome are in the differential diagnosis of some childhood EDS.

Etiology and pathogenesis

Type III collagen

Type III collagen is a homotrimer encoded by a gene on chromosome 2q31. The constituent $\alpha 1$(III) chains share with type I collagen their general exon organization and Gly–X–Y repeats. Type III collagen is located in skin, blood vessel walls and pleuroperitoneal lining; bone has a minimal amount of type III collagen.

Molecular defects in types I, III and V collagen in Ehlers–Danlos syndrome

The most consistent molecular correlations in EDS have been of type IV EDS with type III collagen and of type VII EDS with type I collagen defects. Type IV EDS results from defects in the structure or synthesis of type III collagen which dramatically decrease type III collagen secretion. Some defects are similar to those in OI, in which a bulky amino acid replaces a glycine; others have been point mutations causing aberrant splicing of one or more exons. At the molecular level, all cases have been dominant heterozygous lesions, consistent with the fact that a mutation in one allele will result in 93% of homotrimers containing at least one mutant chain.

Type VII EDS involves defects in the processing of the N-terminal peptide of type 1 collagen. Type 1 collagen which retains its N-terminal peptide forms abnormal fibrils. Most cases have been documented to be dominant structural defects in the type I collagen substrate (EDS types VIIA and VIIB). They are due to mutations that cause skipping of exon 6, which contains the N-proteinase cleavage site. More recently, the occurrence of the human equivalent of dermatosparaxis has been documented. In this recessive form of EDS type VII, there is a deficiency of the N-terminal proteinase.

The classical types I and II EDS have been demonstrated to have defects in type V collagen, a quantitatively minor fibrillar collagen of skin. The great majority of these mutations cause haploinsufficiency of the $\alpha 1$(V) chain[15]. However, only 30% of classical EDS is clearly caused by type V defects, so there is most probably genetic heterogeneity of these EDS forms as well.

Management

Joint hypermobility generally decreases with age; sports that hyperextend or otherwise stress joints should be discouraged in childhood. Joint surgery may be performed for pain, instability or poor range of motion. Success in terms of joint stability and pain relief is limited in about half of cases[16]. Joint effusions and hemarthrosis may occur from cumulative minor trauma and require intervention to maintain ambulation.

Skin fragility in EDS necessitates particular attention to closure in even minor surgical procedures. Sutures should be more closely spaced and left in place for a longer period than normal.

Patients with the EDS type IV diagnosis should be taught to communicate all appropriate vascular and visceral symptoms to their physician. The natural history of EDS type IV necessitates prompt evaluation of even vague complaints in pertinent systems, with echocardiography, computed tomography (CT) or laparoscopy as indicated[17]. If pregnancy is attempted in severe EDS, elective cesarean section through the lower uterine segment is essential as it will stress the uterus less than spontaneous vaginal delivery and prevent delivery-related tears.

MARFAN'S SYNDROME

History

This syndrome, first reported by Marfan in 1896, was the first heritable disorder of connective tissue to be described. Its genetic and clinical features were subsequently listed by McKusick and then by Pyeritz[18]. The demonstration that the syndrome was due to molecular defects in fibrillin was made by Byers, De Paepe, Dietz, Godfrey and others and a mouse model was recently generated by Ramirez[18].

Epidemiology

Marfan's syndrome is characterized by autosomal dominant inheritance. Advanced paternal age has been associated with sporadic cases. One of the most common connective tissue disorders, Marfan's syndrome has an approximate prevalence of 1 per 20 000[18]. There is no racial or geographic influence on incidence.

Clinical features

Skeletal

Musculoskeletal features[18], such as stature greater than the 95th percentile and limbs disproportionately long for trunk size (arachnodactyly), may first bring the patient to medical attention. Other skeletal aspects of the Marfan syndrome include scoliosis, pectus excavatum (Fig. 206.4) or carinatum, a high-arched narrow palate and laxity of joints, including flat feet. There may be limited extension of some joints.

Ocular

Non-progressive subluxation of the lens is present in about 60% of cases. It is most commonly bilateral, with the lens displaced upwards. Myopia is frequent and may be severe because of increased axial length of the globe.

Cardiovascular

Mitral valve prolapse and dilatation of the ascending aorta are the most common cardiovascular features. Mitral or aortic regurgitation may develop. Histologically, the aorta demonstrates cystic medial necrosis. Clinically, the progressive dilatation of the aorta is symmetric and begins at the sinus of Valsalva; it predisposes to aortic rupture or dissection.

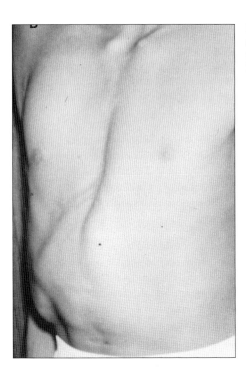

Fig. 206.4 Marfan's syndrome – pectus excavatum. (Courtesy of Dr K Rosenbaum.)

Infantile Marfan's syndrome

There is a severe perinatal subset of Marfan's syndrome patients. Progressive cardiovascular abnormalities and pulmonary disease cause increased morbidity and mortality in the childhood years.

Ghent nosology

The prior diagnostic criteria for Marfan's syndrome were revised to reflect more stringent criteria for diagnosis of Marfan's syndrome in relatives of affected patients and the potential contribution of molecular diagnosis[19]. This Ghent nosology (Table 206.3) uses skeletal features as a major criteria if at least 4 of 8 typical skeletal features are present. A diagnosis of Marfan's syndrome in the index case requires meeting major criteria in at least two organ systems (skeletal, ocular, cardiovascular, skin, family history) and having involvement of a third system. Relatives of an individual with a confirmed case require major criteria in one system and involvement of a second system.

TABLE 206.3 GHENT NOSOLOGY OF MARFAN'S SYNDROME – MAJOR CRITERIA

Skeletal system (four or more of)
- Pectus carinatum
- Pectus excavatum
- Span to height >1.05
- Wrist and thumb signs
- Scoliosis >20°
- Elbow extension <170°
- Pes planus
- Protrusio acetabulae

Dura
- Lumbosacral dural ectasia by CT or MRI

Ocular system
- Ectopia lentis

Cardiovascular
- Dilatation of ascending aorta involving at least sinuses of Valsalva
- Dissection of ascending aorta

Family/genetic history
- First degree relative with Marfan's syndrome
- Presence of FBN-1 mutation

For index case: Diagnosis requires major criteria in at least two different organ systems and involvement of a third organ system
For a relative of an index case: Major criterion in one organ system and involvement of a second organ system

MRI, magnetic resonance imaging.

Prognosis

In the past, cardiovascular complications reduced the mean life span of Marfan patients by 30–40%. Mean life span is now approaching normal, aggressive and anticipatory management of aortic root dilatation helping the majority of patients to have a life span in the 50–70-year range.

Diagnostic studies

Studies essential to establishing the Marfan diagnosis include a slit lamp examination, with fully dilated pupils, and echocardiography focused on mitral valve and aortic root. A radiographic skeletal survey should include limbs, spine, skull and chest. Detection of a fibrillin mutation contributes to the diagnostic criteria but the diagnosis is primarily clinical.

Differential diagnosis

Several other conditions should be considered when making a diagnosis of Marfan's syndrome. Homocystinuria has similar ocular and skeletal manifestations but has a positive urine cyanide–nitroprusside test and downward lens dislocation. Congenital contractural arachnodactyly shares Marfan's skeletal traits but has normal eyes and aorta and congenital contractures that improve with age. In the 'marfanoid' hypermobility syndrome, the lens and aorta are normal and skin and joints are more extensible than in Marfan's syndrome (see Chapter 207). In familial mitral valve prolapse, there is mitral valve prolapse, scoliosis and chest deformity but the eyes and aortic root are normal. In EDS types I, II and III, valvular defects may be present but joint laxity is more severe and skeletal proportions are normal.

Etiology and pathogenesis

Classical Marfan's syndrome is caused by mutations in fibrillin-1, a 350kDa glycoprotein discovered in 1986 and abundant in aortic tunica media, ciliary zonules, periosteum and skin. Decreased microfibrils were demonstrated in Marfan patients, followed by assignment of both fibrillin and the Marfan locus to chromosome 15q15. Mutation screening of all 65 exons of the *FBN-1* gene is available and can detect the majority of mutations[20]. Although several hundred mutations have been delineated, the genotype/phenotype correlations are not straightforward. Mutations causing severe neonatal Marfan's syndrome usually occur in the epidermal growth factor like sequences but there are no apparent mutation clusters causing severe cardiovascular or skeletal manifestations. A second fibrillin gene on chromosome 5 has 80% homology to fibrillin-1 and is linked to cases of congenital contractural arachnodactyly but not to Marfan's syndrome.

Management

Marfan's syndrome patients are best managed at a tertiary center by a multidisciplinary team. Management includes annual ophthalmology and semiannual orthopedic evaluation. Surgical intervention may be needed when scoliosis exceeds 45°. Because deformity may recur, pectus correction is best postponed until growth stops. Cardiovascular care includes annual echocardiography and electrocardiogram until the aortic root exceeds 45mm and more frequently thereafter. Treatment with β-adrenergic blockers may decrease the rate of aortic dilatation. Aortic surgery may be necessary and the outcome of surgical repair can be improved by elective Bentall procedure at about 55mm and by using a composite graft to replace both ascending aorta and aortic valve[21]. In experienced hands, 88% of patients have a greater than 5 year surgical survival. Pregnancy represents a very high risk of a catastrophic cardiovascular event for patients with moderate aortic dilatation.

CHONDRODYSTROPHIES

The chondrodystrophies are classified according to the Paris nomenclature of 1976 using clinical and radiographic criteria, such as different part of long bone involved (epiphyses, metaphyses or diaphyses) and presence of spinal involvement (Table 206.4).[22]

Stickler's syndrome presents with ocular, facial and joint involvement. It is one of the milder phenotypes resulting from mutations in the gene that encodes type II collagen. The mutations in type II collagen that cause Stickler's syndrome result in premature termination codons and presumably in haploinsufficiency. About 25% of Stickler's patients have mutations in the genes encoding type XI collagen. Manifestations of the syndrome include myopia, retinal detachment, midface hypoplasia, midline clefting and hearing loss but their expression is highly variable. Progressive osteoarthritis of large joints may develop in the third or fourth decade.

History

Several studies have revealed the familial nature[23] and more recently the underlying molecular defect in this group of disorders. These advances have led to an attempt to classify the disorders (Table 206.4).

Epidemiology

The most common chondrodystrophy, achondroplasia, occurs in about 1 per 40 000 live births. Some recessive disorders, however, such as McKusick-type metaphyseal dysplasia, are comparatively common among the relatively inbred Old Order Amish in Pennsylvania.

TABLE 206.4 PARIS NOMENCLATURE OF CHONDRODYSTROPHIES

Osteochondrodysplasias

I.	Defects of growth of tubular bones and/or spine
II.	Disorganized development of cartilage
III.	Abnormalities of density of cortical diaphyseal structure and/or metaphyseal modeling

Dysostoses

I.	With cranial and facial involvement
II.	With predominant axial involvement
III.	With predominant involvement of extremities

Idiopathic osteolysis

Primary metabolic abnormalities

I.	Calcium and/or phosphorus
II.	Complex carbohydrates
III.	Lipids
IV.	Nucleic acids
V.	Amino acids
VI.	Metals

(As cited in Rimoin and Lachman[22].)

REFERENCES

1. Sillence DO, Senn A, Danks DM. Genetic heterogeneity in osteogenesis imperfecta. J Med Genet 1979; 16: 101–116.
2. Prockop DJ, Kivirikko KJ. Heritable diseases of collagen. N Engl J Med 1984; 311: 376–386.
3. Byers PH. Brittle bones – fragile molecules: disorders of collagen gene structure and expression. Trends Genet 1990; 6: 293–300.
4. Chernoff E, Marini JC. Osteogenesis imperfecta. In: Allanson J, Cassidy S, eds. Clinical management of common genetic syndromes. New York: John Wiley & Sons; 2001: 281–300.
5. Paterson CR, Monk EA, McAllion SJ. How common is hearing impairment in osteogenesis imperfecta? J Laryngol Otol 2001; 115: 280–282.
6. Pepin M, Atkinson M, Starman BJ, Byers PH. Strategies and outcomes of prenatal diagnosis for osteogenesis imperfecta: a review of biochemical and molecular studies completed in 129 pregnancies. Prenat Diagn 1997; 17: 559–570.
7. Willing MC, Deschenes SP, Slayton RL, Roberts EJ. Premature chain termination is a unifying mechanism for COL1A1 null alleles in osteogenesis imperfecta type I cell strains. Am J Hum Genet 1996; 59: 799–809.
8. Glorieux FH, Rauch F, Plotkin H et al. Type V osteogenesis imperfecta: a new form of brittle bone disease. J Bone Mineral Res 2000; 15: 1650–1658.
9. Gerber LH, Binder H, Weintraub J et al. Rehabilitation of children and infants with osteogenesis imperfecta. Clin Orthop Rel Res 1990; 251: 254–262.
10. Glorieux FH, Bishop NJ, Plotkin H et al. Cyclic administration of pamidronate in children with severe osteogenesis imperfecta. N Engl J Med 1998; 339: 947–952.
11. Beighton P, De Paepe A, Steinmann B et al. Ehlers-Danlos syndromes: revised nosology, Villefranche, 1997. Am J Med Genet 1998; 77: 31–37.
12. Burch GH, Gong Y, Liu W et al. Tenascin-X deficiency is associated with Ehlers–Danlos syndrome. Nat Genet1997; 17: 104–108.
13. Byers PH, Holbrook KA, Barsh GS. Ehlers–Danlos syndrome. In: Emery AE, Rimoin DL, eds. Principles and practice of medical genetics. Edinburgh: Churchill Livingstone; 1983: 836–850.
14. Yeowell HN, Walker LC. Mutations in the lysyl hydroxylase 1 gene that result in enzyme deficiency and the clinical phenotype of Ehlers–Danlos syndrome type VI. Mol Genet Metab 2000; 71: 212–224.
15. Schwarze U, Atkinson M, Hoffman GG et al. Null alleles of the COL5A1 gene of type V collagen are a cause of the classical forms of Ehlers–Danlos syndrome (types I and II. Am J Hum Genet 2000; 66: 1757–1765.
16. Weinberg J, Doering C, McFarland EG. Joint surgery in Ehlers–Danlos patients: results of a survey. Am J Orthop 1999; 406–409.
17. Bergqvist D. Ehlers–Danlos type IV syndrome: a review from a vascular surgical point of view. Eur J Surg 1996; 162: 163–170.
18. Pyeritz RE. The Marfan syndrome. Ann Rev Med 2000; 51: 481–510.
19. De Paepe A, Devereux RB, Dietz HC et al. Revised diagnostic criteria for the Marfan syndrome. Am J Med Genet 1996; 62: 417–426.
20. Hayward C, Porteous ME, Brock DJH. Mutation screening of all 65 exons of the fibrillin-1 gene in 60 patients with Marfan syndrome: report of 12 novel mutations. Hum Mutat 1997; 10: 280–289.
21. Gott VL, Laschinger JC, Cameron DE et al. The Marfan syndrome and the cardiovascular surgeon. Eur J Cardiothorac Surg 1996; 10: 149–158.
22. Rimoin DL, Lachman RS. The chondrodysplasias. In: Emery AE, Rimoin DL, eds. Principles and practice of medical genetics. Edinburgh: Churchill Livingstone; 1983: 703–35.
23. Spranger JW. Pattern recognition in the chondrodystrophies. Prog Clin Biol Res 1985; 200: 315–342.

207 Hypermobility syndrome

Rodney Grahame

Definition

- Occurrence of musculoskeletal symptoms in hypermobile subjects in the absence of demonstrable systemic rheumatologic disease
- The degree of hypermobility relates to the degree of ligamentous laxity
- A profusion and spectrum of common lesions arise, as a result of the hypermobility, over the patient's lifetime. Neurophysiological defects including proprioceptive impairment and autonomic dysfunction occur contributing to the patient's malaise and discomfort

Clinical features

- Range of traumatic and overuse lesions (traction enthesopathy, tenosynovitis, bursitis, rotator cuff lesions, back pain, stress fractures etc.)
- Hyperextensible, thin, soft skin
- Joint instability effects
- Chronic arthritis, either low-grade inflammatory synovitis or osteoarthritis and/or spondylosis
- Secondary chronic pain syndrome, pseudofibromyalgia, chronic fatigue and depression
- Neurophysiological defects involving joint proprioception and autonomic nervous system

DEFINITION

The definition given in the box, 'the occurrence of musculoskeletal symptoms in hypermobile subjects in the absence of demonstrable systemic rheumatologic disease', was suggested by Kirk *et al.*[1] in 1967. Studies over the past 30 years have established that extra-articular manifestations occur, and the syndrome is now considered to be the most common of the heritable disorders of connective tissue and is almost certainly identical with Ehlers–Danlos syndrome – hypermobility type (formerly designated EDS III)[2].

EPIDEMIOLOGY

Generalized ligamentous laxity, the prerequisite of joint hypermobility, is seen in a substantial proportion (perhaps 10%) of healthy individuals (varying according to methodology and to the age, sex and ethnic origin of the population studied), the majority of whom probably suffer few or any ill effects[3].

Hypermobility syndrome, as seen in clinical practice, is a common finding. In one general rheumatology clinic survey 15% of 130 consecutive referrals showed joint hypermobility at three or more sites[4].

Hypermobility diminishes steadily throughout childhood[5] and then more slowly during adult life. Women generally show a greater joint range of motion than men, and Asians a greater range than African blacks, who in turn are more mobile than Caucasians. Surveys among Iraqis, Yoruba Nigerians[6] and Omanis show prevalences of generalized hypermobility of up to 25%. 'Pauciarticular' hypermobility is even more highly prevalent in otherwise healthy subjects than is the generalized variety[7]. Because of their facility to contort their bodies with ease, hypermobile people may gravitate towards such professions as ballet dancers, musicians or circus performers[8,9].

CLINICAL FEATURES

Hypermobility syndrome is a multisystem disorder involving:

- joints and soft tissues, with associated tendency to recurrent sprains, dislocations and eventually, in some cases, secondary osteoarthritis
- skin, with hyperextensible skin, striae atrophicae and paper-thin scars
- skeleton, with features of a marfanoid habitus in approximately one-third of cases
- nervous system, with neurophysiological defects.

Symptoms often commence in childhood and persist and increase in severity throughout adult life[10].

The recognition of joint hypermobility rests on the ability of the person to perform a series of passive joint maneuvers. This is the nine-point scale of Beighton[11] shown in Table 207.1 and Figure 207.1.

Since joint hypermobility is often pauciarticular, the diagnosis is frequently overlooked if reliance is placed on the Beighton scale alone and the clinician fails to observe obvious hypermobility in joints outside the scale. A common source of misunderstanding is the widely held notion that symptoms can only be ascribed to hypermobility when a Beighton score of 4 or more is present. Suggested criteria for the diagnosis of hypermobility syndrome[12] are shown in Table 207.2.

Articular and periarticular features

Patients present with a wide variety of readily identifiable traumatic and overuse lesions, including traction injuries at tendon or ligament insertions, joint, bursa or tendon sheath synovitis, chondromalacia patellae,

---

TABLE 207.1 THE 9-POINT BEIGHTON SCORING SYSTEM FOR JOINT HYPERMOBILITY SCALE

Scoring 1 point on each side
- Passive dorsiflexion of the fifth metacarpophalangeal joint to 90°
- Apposition of the thumb to the flexor aspect of the forearm
- Hyperextension of the elbow beyond 0°
- Hyperextension of the knee beyond 0°

Scoring 1 point
- Forward trunk flexion placing hands flat on floor with knees extended

Maximum score = 9

(Adapted from Beighton *et al.*[11])

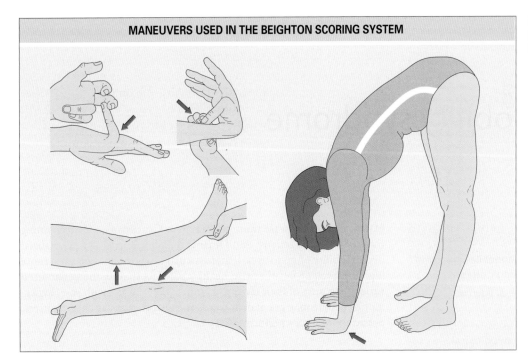

MANEUVERS USED IN THE BEIGHTON SCORING SYSTEM

Fig. 207.1 Maneuvers used in the Beighton scoring system. Relevant scores for joint hypermobility are shown in Table 207.1.

rotator cuff lesions or back pain. Other presentations result from the effects of joint instability, such as flat feet, recurrent dislocation or subluxation – notably of the shoulder, patella, metacarpophalangeal joints or temporomandibular joints. Some patients develop a chronic arthritis – either a low-grade inflammatory synovitis of traumatic origin (misdiagnosed as rheumatoid or juvenile idiopathic arthritis) or osteoarthritis, which is held by many authorities to be a direct complication of hypermobility syndrome[13]. Evidence is emerging of a significant correlation between articular hypermobility and thumb-base OA[14]. Widespread arthralgia or fibromyalgia-like pain in the absence of any demonstrable clinical abnormality (other than hypermobility) is a frequent finding[15]. The recent discovery of impairment of joint proprioception[16], a lack of efficacy of topical anesthetic effects of lidocaine[17] and evidence of dysautonomia[18] add a new neurophysiological dimension and complexity to the syndrome. In one series of hypermobility syndrome patients the marfanoid habitus (as defined as an upper segment:lower segment ratio of less than 0.89) was present in 39% of cases compared with 11.5% of controls ($p < 0.05$)[3].

A recent survey amongst 319 British rheumatologists revealed widely differing perceptions about all aspects of the hypermobility syndrome and its impact[19]. Clinicians unfamiliar with the syndrome were tempted to discount the symptoms or to ascribe them erroneously. The hapless patients, often in chronic pain, are unable to lead a normal life. They feel frustrated by a lack of understanding and help from their doctors, and often are moved to despair[20]. This is an area of neglect in rheumatology and a recently published editorial cautioned fellow pediatric and adult rheumatologists into taking hypermobility syndrome more seriously in both adults and children[10,21].

Extra-articular features

Organs and tissues, which rely on the tensile strength of normal collagen, may also become disordered in hypermobile subjects. The skin may be thin, soft, hyperextensible, brittle and develop striae and papyraceous scars (Figs 207.2–207.4).

TABLE 207.2 1998 BRIGHTON REVISED DIAGNOSTIC CRITERIA FOR THE BENIGN JOINT HYPERMOBILITY SYNDROME

Major criteria

1. A Beighton score of 4/9 or greater (either currently or historically)
2. Arthralgia for longer than 3 months in four or more joints

Minor criteria

1. A Beighton score of 1, 2 or 3/9 (0, 1, 2 or 3 if aged 50+)
2. Arthralgia (>3 months) in one to three joints or back pain (>3 months), spondylosis, spondylolysis/spondylolisthesis
3. Dislocation/subluxation in more than one joint, or in one joint on more than one occasion
4. Soft tissue rheumatism – >3 lesions (e.g. epicondylitis, tenosynovitis, bursitis)
5. Marfanoid habitus: tall, slim, span/height ratio >1.03, upper:lower segment ratio less than 0.89, arachnodactyly (positive Steinberg/wrist signs).
6. Abnormal skin: striae, hyperextensibility, thin skin, papyraceous scarring
7. Eye signs: drooping eyelids or myopia or antimongoloid slant
8. Varicose veins or hernia or uterine/rectal prolapse

The benign joint hypermobility syndrome (BJHS) is diagnosed in the presence of **two** major criteria, or **one** major and **two** minor criteria, or **four** minor criteria. **Two** minor criteria will suffice where there is an unequivocally affected first-degree relative. BJHS is excluded by the presence of Marfan's or Ehlers–Danlos syndrome (EDS) (other than the EDS hypermobility type (formerly EDS III) as defined by the Ghent 1996[25] and the Villefranche 1998[26] criteria respectively. Criteria major 1 and minor 1 are mutually exclusive as are major 2 and minor 2.

(Adapted from Grahame *et al.*[12])

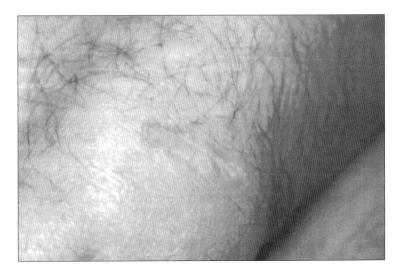

Fig. 207.2 A typical tell-tale papyraceous scar that has resulted from a childhood laceration in a patient with benign joint hypermobility syndrome.

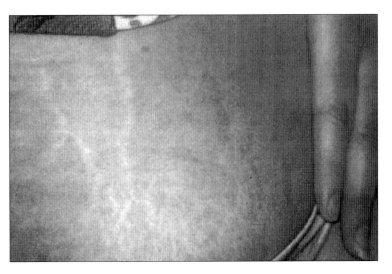

Fig. 207.3 Striae atrophicae on the tight abdomen of a female patient with benign joint hypermobility syndrome. Striae are significant when they are not the result of irreversible skin stretching, as occurs in pregnancy or obesity.

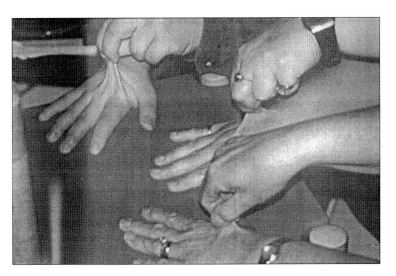

Fig. 207.4 Skin stretch in a three-generation family. Note that the grandmother's skin hyperextensibility (nearest the camera) is markedly reduced compared to that of her granddaughter (furthest from the camera), while the skin of her daughter (middle) is intermediate in degree of stretch.

An association between mitral valve prolapse and the hypermobility syndrome has not been confirmed using the latest echocardiographic technology and diagnostic criteria[22]. Weakness of the musculotendinous supporting structures of the anterior abdominal wall and pelvic floor explains the reported increased findings of abdominal hernia and of both rectal and uterine prolapse, including cystocele and rectocele[23]. Bone mineral density measurements using dual X-ray absorptiometry (DXA) scanning show a tendency towards low bone mineral density with osteopenia rather than osteoporosis[22]. Following vigorous physical activity, however, as occurs in sport and ballet dancing (to which hypermobile subjects are drawn), stress fractures of the metatarsal bones, shins and vertebral bodies and partes interarticulares of the lumbar spine are particularly common. A common contributory factor in females is osteoporosis secondary to exercise- and starvation-induced amenorrhea with hypoestrogenemia[24].

INVESTIGATIONS

Indicators of inflammation or of immunologic reactivity such as a raised erythrocyte sedimentation rate, C-reactive protein, autoantibodies or hypergammaglobulinemia are characteristically absent, except in the presence of coincidental disease.

DIFFERENTIAL DIAGNOSIS

Hypermobility syndrome has to be distinguished from the more severe heritable disorders of connective tissue such as Marfan's syndrome, the vascular form of Ehlers–Danlos syndrome (EDS IV) and osteogenesis imperfecta, with which it shares a number of common features (see Chapter 206). Patients with Marfan's syndrome often have cardiac or ocular features, or a history of a first-degree relative with the classic syndrome. EDS IV has a distinct recognizable phenotype but the classic or rarer subtypes may be more difficult to exclude. Hypermobility syndrome is benign in the sense that life-threatening complications are not a feature[22]. For this reason the term 'benign joint hypermobility syndrome' has largely replaced the earlier 'hypermobility syndrome'.

Since there are currently no readily available laboratory or genetic tests that can reliably distinguish between the different heritable disorders of connective tissue (with the exception of the finding of an absence of collagen 3 in EDS IV), the distinction remains a clinical exercise. Recently refined diagnostic criteria for Marfan's syndrome[25], Ehlers–Danlos syndrome[26] and benign joint hypermobility syndrome are available. The 1998 validated Brighton criteria for the benign joint hypermobility syndrome are shown in Table 207.2[11].

STRUCTURE AND FUNCTION

The multisystem pattern of the clinical features seen in the benign joint hypermobility syndrome points to a widespread disorder of connective tissue. The evidence available points to collagen as being the culprit. Skin biopsies taken from hypermobility syndrome patients and examined by scanning electron microscopy show striking abnormalities in the architecture of the collagen bundles by comparison with controls (Fig. 207.5)[27].

ETIOLOGY

For practical purposes, hypermobility syndrome is a genetically determined heritable disorder of connective tissue. Studies of family

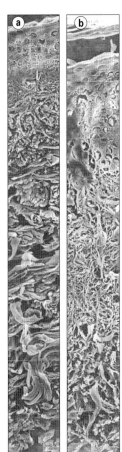

Fig. 207.5 Skin thinning in hypermobility syndrome. (a) Electron micrograph (×1500) of full-thickness flexor forearm skin from a 51-year-old hypermobile female with mitral valve prolapse compared with a normal age- and sex-matched control. The skin is thinner in the hypermobility syndrome patient than in the control. (b) The reticular layer shows a reduction in the thick collagen fibers and an increase in disorganized fine collagen fibers. (With permission from Beighton et al.[3])

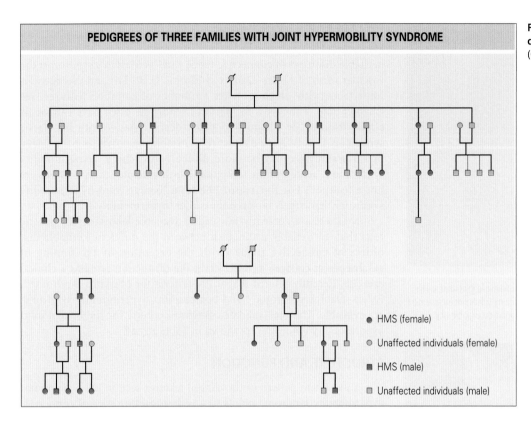

PEDIGREES OF THREE FAMILIES WITH JOINT HYPERMOBILITY SYNDROME

- ● HMS (female)
- ○ Unaffected individuals (female)
- ■ HMS (male)
- □ Unaffected individuals (male)

Fig. 207.6 Pedigrees of three families with dominant benign joint hypermobility syndrome. (Courtesy of Dr A Child.)

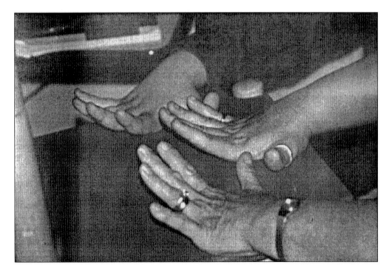

Fig. 207.7 A three-generation family demonstrating finger hyperextensibility (the same as in Fig. 207.4). Note that the grandmother has retained her hypermobility in spite of aging, in comparison with her daughter and granddaughter.

pedigrees have provided evidence for a dominant mode of inheritance, with sex-influenced phenotypic manifestations in most cases of hypermobility syndrome (Fig. 207.6)[3]. Figure 207.7 shows a three-generation family demonstrating their finger joint hyperextensibility.

Acquired polyarticular joint laxity has been reported to occur in a variety of diseased states, including acromegaly, after rheumatic fever (Jaccoud's arthropathy), in hyperparathyroidism and in chronic alcoholism[3].

PATHOGENESIS

Although mutations have been discovered in connection with most families with osteogenesis imperfecta and some with Ehlers–Danlos syndrome, the application of molecular biology techniques to unraveling the mysteries of hypermobility syndromes is still in its infancy and the genetic defect(s) responsible for the benign joint hypermobility syndrome remains to be determined.

MANAGEMENT

A recent evidence-based review of the management of hypermobility syndrome has been published elsewhere[28]. Hypermobility syndrome patients can be helped many ways. Providing a correct diagnosis is a relief to many who fear (or have been told) that they have rheumatoid arthritis, juvenile idiopathic arthritis, Marfan's syndrome or EDS IV, with their less favorable prognoses. They are comforted by knowing that they have a condition that doctors recognize and understand; that their pain and other symptoms are neither imaginary nor neurotic in origin; that these symptoms do not have to be borne without help; and that, although their children may inherit joint hypermobility, this does not necessarily mean that they will inherit the symptoms that constitute the syndrome.

In hypermobility syndrome patients, the tissues, in particular the ligaments, are not only lax but are less robust than in other people, rendering them more vulnerable to the effects of trauma, either in the form of acute injury or chronic 'overuse' injury. Torn or attenuated ligaments lead to joint instability, which in turn may lead over time to osteoarthritis. Where ligament injury occurs, efforts should be directed to promote healing using ultrasonic therapy and other methods, including therapeutic muscle-building exercises (which help to compensate for instability arising from joint laxity). Impaired proprioceptive acuity as referred to above may have therapeutic implications. A randomized clinical trial has shown that proprioceptive enhancement over a 12-week period was significantly more effective than a conventional muscle strengthening programme[29].

Many of the rheumatologic complications listed earlier are easily identified and are treated along conventional lines. More difficult to manage are those pains that are not so easily attributable, such as arthralgia and chronic widespread pain (sometimes attributed to fibromyalgia). Patients should be encouraged to seek out factors in their daily activities that aggravate their symptoms and adjust their lifestyle accordingly. These pains respond poorly to simple analgesics or non-steroidal anti-inflammatory drugs. Conventional physical therapy is also often disappointing, although a program of joint and core stabilizing exercises combined with proprioceptive enhancement techniques are anecdotally effective. Chronic musculoskeletal pain syndrome, when present, is best treated by means of a pain management program, preferably one incorporating cognitive behavioral therapy[30]. Surgical intervention should always be viewed with caution, as sutures may not hold and poor scar tissue formation ensue.

REFERENCES

1. Kirk JH, Ansell B, Bywaters EGL. The hypermobility syndrome. Ann Rheum Dis 1967; 26: 425.
2. Grahame R. Joint hypermobility and genetic collagen disorders: are they related? Arch Dis Child 1999; 80: 188–191.
3. Beighton PH Grahame R, Bird HA. Hypermobility of joints, 3rd ed. London Springer-Verlag; 1999.
4. Bridges AJ, Smith E, Reid J. Joint hypermobility in adults referred to rheumatology clinics. Ann Rheum Dis 1992; 51 : 793–796.
5. Silverman S, Constine L, Harvey W, Grahame R. Survey of joint hypermobility and in vivo skin elasticity in London school children. Ann Rheum Dis 1975; 34: 177–180.
6. Birrell FN, Adebajo AO, Hazleman BL, Silman AJ. High prevalence of joint laxity in West Africans. Br J Rheumatol 1994; 33: 56–59.
7. Larsson LG, Baum J, Mudholkar GS. Hypermobility: features and differential incidence between the sexes. Arthritis Rheum 1987; 30: 1426–1430.
8. Grahame R. Hypermobility – not a circus act. Int J Clin Pract 2000; 54: 314–315.
9. Grahame R. Joint hypermobility and the performing musician. N Engl J Med 1993; 329: 1120–1121.
10. Murray KJ, Woo P. Benign joint hypermobility in childhood. Rheumatology 2001; 40: 489–491.
11. Beighton PH Solomon L, Soskolne C. Articular mobility in an African population. Ann Rheum Dis 1973; 32: 413–417.
12. Grahame R, Bird HA, Child A et al. British Society for Rheumatology Special Interest Group on Heritable Disorders of Connective Tissue. The Revised (Brighton 1998) Criteria for the Diagnosis of the BJHS. J Rheumatol 2000; 27: 1777–1779.
13. Grahame R. How often, when and how does joint hypermobility lead to osteoarthritis? Br J Rheumatol 1989; 28: 320.
14. Jonsson H, Valtysdottir ST, Kjartansson O, Brekkan A. Hypermobility associated with osteoarthritis of the thumb base: a clinical and radiological subset of hand osteoarthritis. Ann Rheum Dis 1996; 55: 540–543.
15. Grahame R. Pain, distress and joint hyperlaxity. Joint Bone Spine 2000; 54: 314–315.
16. Mallik AK, Ferrell WR, McDonald AG, Sturrock RD. Impaired proprioceptive acuity at the proximal interphalangeal joint in patients with the hypermobility syndrome. Br J Rheumatol 1994; 33: 631–637.
17. Arendt-Nielsen L, Kaalund P, Bjerring P, Hogsaa B. Insufficient effect of local analgesics in Ehlers–Danlos type III patients (connective tissue disorder). Acta Anaesthesiol Scand 1990; 34: 358–361.
18. Gazit Y Jacob G. Grahame R, Nahir M. The pathophysiology that underlies autonomic dysfunction in hypermobility syndrome. Arthritis Rheum 2001; 44: S126 (Abstract 444).
19. Grahame R, Bird HA. British consultant rheumatologists' perceptions about the hypermobility syndrome. Rheumatology 2001; 40: 559–562.
20. Gurley-Green S. Living with the hypermobility syndrome. Rheumatology 2001; 40: 487–489.
21. Grahame R. Time to take hypermobility seriously (in adults and children). Rheumatology 2001; 40: 485–487.
22. Mishra MB, Ryan P, Atkinson P et al. Extra-articular features of benign joint hypermobility syndrome. Br J Rheumatol 1996; 135: 861–866.
23. Norton PA, Baker JE, Sharp HC et al. Genitourinary prolapse and joint hypermobility in women. Obstet Gynecol 1995; 85: 225–228.
24. Keay N, Fogelman I, Blake G. Bone mineral density in professional female dancers. Br J Sports Med 1997; 31: 143–147.
25. De Paepe A, Devereux RB, Dietz HC et al. Revised diagnostic criteria for the Marfan syndrome. Am J Med Genet 1996; 62: 417–426.
26. Beighton P, De Paepe A, Steinmann B et al. Ehlers–Danlos syndromes: revised nosology, Villefranche, 1997. Ehlers–Danlos National Foundation (USA) and Ehlers–Danlos Support Group (UK). Am J Med Genet 1998; 77: 31–37.
27. Child A. Joint hypermobility syndrome: inherited disorder of collagen synthesis. J Rheumatol 1986; 13: 239–242.
28. Grahame R. Heritable disorders of connective tissue. In: Balint GP, Bardin T, eds. Baillière's best practice & research in clinical rheumatology. Uncommon non-inflammatory osteoarticular disorders, Vol. 14, No 2. London: Baillière Tindall; 2000: 345–361.
29. Beard DJ, Dodd CA, Trundle HR, Simpson A. Proprioceptive enhancement for anterior cruciate ligament deficiency. A prospective randomised trial of two physiotherapy regimes. J Bone Joint Surg 1994; 76B: 654–659.
30. Williams ACdeC, Nicholas MK, Richardson PH et al. Evaluation of a cognitive behavioural programme for rehabilitating patients with chronic pain. Br J Gen Pract 1993; 43: 513–518.

208 Skeletal dysplasias

Frederic Shapiro

The term 'skeletal dysplasias' refers to a large number of inherited disorders primarily associated with structural abnormalities of the skeletal system. Over 150 developmental disorders of the skeletal system have been described, with most having several variants within each category[1]. If one includes the broader spectrum of developmental disorders in which there are multisystem abnormalities including bone, joint, and limb malformations, then there are as many as 450 different syndromes described[2]. This chapter will provide a brief overview of the skeletal dysplasias encompassing gene and molecular abnormalities, their translation into structural abnormalities of the skeleton, the prominent role of imaging in both defining syndromes and assessing clinically significant deformity, and a discussion of those deformities at specific areas and in specific syndromes that have a disproportionately high incidence of rheumatologic sequelae. A detailed review of the subject has recently been published[3].

The syndromes associated with a high incidence of rheumatologic problems are those characterized by angular deformities of the long bones, joint surface irregularity, joint contractures and joint instability. Some of the skeletal dysplasias are also associated with developmental abnormalities of the axial skeleton ranging from major deforming kyphoscolioses to less apparent cervical vertebral instability or lumbar spinal stenosis.

APPROACHES TO CLASSIFICATION

Skeletal dysplasias have been recognized since antiquity, primarily because many are associated with short stature. Efforts at categorizing them began only about 100 years ago. Classification criteria have been based on clinical, radiographic and molecular approaches. Patient groups were defined clinically based on similar gross appearances, the commonest group being achondroplasia. With the advent of widespread use of radiography to assess skeletal structure during development, many were noted to have not only shortening and deformation of the bones but also abnormalities concentrated in the epiphyseal, metaphyseal or (rarely) diaphyseal regions. Many dysplasias are defined by these localized affected regions such as multiple epiphyseal dysplasia, metaphyseal dysplasia (of Schmid), or diaphyseal dysplasia (of Camurati–Engelmann).

Currently, many dysplasias are increasingly defined by the gene and molecular abnormality affecting connective tissue structure or function. Many spondyloepiphyseal dysplasias (radiographic abnormalities of the spine and epiphyseal regions of long bones) are now known to be due to glycosaminoglycan processing abnormalities and are called mucopolysaccharidoses, while a very large number of skeletal dysplasias are due to underlying collagen abnormalities and are referred to increasingly as collagenopathies.

GENE AND MOLECULAR ASPECTS OF LIMB MORPHOGENESIS

The characteristic histologic appearance of the developing limb from the limb bud stage to skeletal maturation has been known for some time but the increasing knowledge of the timing and position of gene and molecular expression in long bone, epiphyseal, and joint development

---

TABLE 208.1 PARTIAL OUTLINE OF MUTATIONS IN SKELETAL DYSPLASIA SYNDROMES

1. Fibroblast growth factor receptor (FGFR) mutation group
   a) *FGFR3*
      Thanatophoric dysplasia, types I and II
      Achondroplasia
      Hypochondroplasia
   b) *FGFR2*
      Crouzon syndrome
      Apert syndrome
      Jackson-Weiss syndrome
      Pfeiffer syndrome
   c) *FGFR1*
      Pfeiffer syndrome
2. Collagen mutation group
   a) Type I collagen
      COL1A1
      Osteogenesis imperfecta
      COL1A2
      Osteogenesis imperfecta
   b) Type II collagen
      COL2A1
      Achondrogenesis type II
      Hypochondrogenesis
      Spondyloepiphyseal dysplasia congenita (SEDC)
      Kniest dysplasia
      Stickler dysplasia type I
      Spondyloepimetaphyseal dysplasia (SEMD)
      Strudwick dysplasia
   c) Type IX collagen
      COL9A2
      Multiple epiphyseal dysplasia type 2 (EDM2)
      COL9A3
      Multiple epiphyseal dysplasia type 3 (EDM3)
   d) Type X collagen
      COL10A1
      Schmid metaphyseal dysplasia
   e) Type XI collagen
      COL11A1
      Otospondylomegaepiphyseal dysplasia (OSMED) dominant and recessive
      COL11A2
      Stickler syndrome type II
3. Diastrophic dysplasia sulfate transporter mutation group
   DTDST
   Achondrogenesis type 1B
   Atelosteogenesis type 2
   Diastrophic dysplasia
4. Arylsulfatase gene mutation family
   ARSE
   Chondrodysplasia punctata, X-linked recessive
5. Lysosomal enzyme gene mutation family
   Mucopolysaccharidoses (MPS I–VI)
   Mucolipidoses
6. Cartilage oligomeric matrix protein mutation group
   COMP
   Multiple epiphyseal dysplasia type I (EDM 1)
   Pseudoachondroplasia
7. Parathyroid hormone/ parathyroid-hormone-related peptide receptor mutation group
   PTHrPR
   Jansen metaphyseal dysplasia
   Blomstrand lethal chondrodysplasia
8. SOX mutation family
   SOX9
   Campomelic dysplasia
9. Short-stature-homeobox-containing mutation family
   SHOX
   Leri–Weil dyschondrosteosis
   Langer's mesomelic dysplasia
10. Cartilage-derived morphogenic protein mutation family
    CDMP1
    Grebe's dysplasia
    Hunter–Thompson dysplasia
    Brachydactyly type C
11. Cell-surface heparan sulfate proteoglycan mutation group
    EXT1, EXT2
    Hereditary multiple exostoses

---

has led to increased understanding of the interplay between these. We have recently published a histologic study classifying the structural stages of long bone and epiphyseal development into 16 stages[4].

The epiphyseal regions in particular are characterized by a large number of developmental changes occurring both in a relatively small time period and confined to a small space. As a consequence, molecular abnormalities can have major negative effects on the shape of the epiphyses, leading to angular deformity and joint incongruity, and on the structure of the articular cartilage, leading to possible early degeneration. Much of long bone, epiphyseal and joint development can now be correlated with specific genetically determined molecules such as growth factors and structural proteins. Mutations in these genes, moreover, are shown increasingly to underlie specific skeletal dysplasia syndromes. Table 208.1 outlines some of the mutations detected in skeletal dysplasia syndromes. Detailed summary tables have been presented[5,6] and new information is accumulating rapidly.

HISTOPATHOLOGY OF SKELETAL DYSPLASIAS

The role of histopathological analysis has been significantly under-utilized in the skeletal dysplasias. Many studies show, however, that both chondrocyte and matrix abnormalities in epiphyseal and articular cartilage underlie the development of more serious problems. At the ultrastructural level, changes in chondrocyte endoplasmic reticulum include massive dilation with retention of an electron-dense homogeneous material (as in osteogenesis imperfecta and spondyloepiphyseal dysplasia), alternating electron-dense and electron-lucent whorled lamellae (as in pseudoachondroplasia)[7] and alternating electron-dense and electron-lucent parallel lamellae (as in multiple epiphyseal dysplasia, EDM3)[8] (Fig. 208.1). These changes are reflective of abnormal protein processing intracellularly. Matrix studies can show early abnormal aggregation of type II collagen fibrils within the cartilage matrix in diastrophic dysplasia, a precursor finding to cartilage stiffness with diminished physeal growth and premature articular cartilage degeneration[9] (Fig. 208.2). An overview of these features has been presented[10].

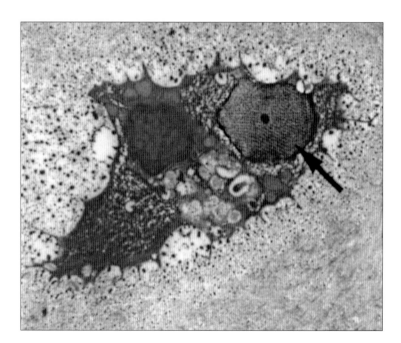

Fig. 208.1 Electron micrograph of iliac crest chondrocyte from biopsy in 10-year-old male with multiple epiphyseal dysplasia. It shows dilated rough endoplasmic reticulum (arrow) containing parallel lamellae of alternating electron-dense and electron-lucent material. There is also pathologic presence of a circular fat inclusion. Studies identified a mutation of the α_3 chain of type IX collagen. The material in the rough endoplasmic reticulum would appear to represent abnormally processed protein.

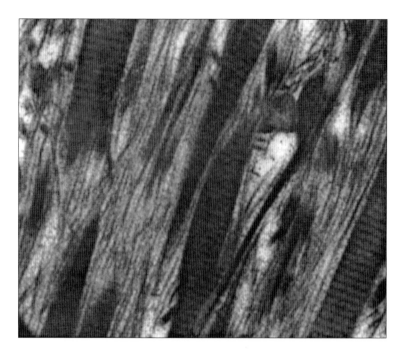

Fig. 208.2 Electron micrograph of iliac crest cartilage from skeletally immature patient with diastrophic dysplasia. Large accumulations of abnormally thickened and aggregated type II collagen can be seen. The crossbanding was due to the thickened type II, since no type I was identified on testing. Type II collagen is normally present in the cartilage matrix as thin, 10–15nm-wide fibrils but the molecular abnormalities in diastrophic dysplasia cartilage allowed fibrils to aggregate.

IMAGING APPROACHES TO ASSESSMENT OF THE SKELETAL DYSPLASIAS

All the most frequently used modalities of imaging currently available play a major role in assessments of patients with a skeletal dysplasia.

Ultrasound

This is particularly valuable for intrauterine assessments in the fetal period. Charts are available from 12 weeks to birth indicating the normal ranges of developing bone lengths for each of humerus, radius, ulna, femur, tibia and fibula[11]. The ultrasound studies document length from one metaphyseal end of the bone to the other. These lengths can serve as an early (16th week on) indicator of a short stature syndrome. The study can also identify major angular deformity, which can lead to diagnosis of some skeletal dysplasias. Ultrasound is particularly valuable in diagnosing lethal perinatal dysplasias in the second trimester owing to the severity of the short stature and long bone abnormalities in this group.

In the postnatal period ultrasound is helpful in assessing the position and shape of the cartilaginous epiphyses prior to the formation of secondary ossification centers.

Plain radiographs

These remain the most frequent and important method for assessing a skeletal dysplasia patient. The skeletal survey defines the type of dysplasia a patient has, based on the characteristic radiographic shapes of the various bones. It also can assess deformity of the spine or appendicular skeleton and indicate the presence of osteoarthritis in specific joints.

Computed tomography

The computed tomography (CT) scan is most valuable in the dysplasias for outlining three-dimensional relationships. These can be significantly altered, for example, in the hip where acetabular dysplasia, subluxation and coxa vara can occur, and in the cervical spine where C1–C2 subluxation is common in some disorders.

Magnetic resonance imaging

Magnetic resonance imaging (MRI) is of extreme importance in assessing patients with skeletal dysplasias owing to its ability to detect and differentiate such soft tissue components as muscle, fibrous connective tissue, cartilage and blood vessels[12,13]. Joint structure, which is often abnormal in the dysplasias, can be assessed in terms of articular cartilage structure, ligamentous continuity, capsular position, meniscal pathology and even the vascularity of the epiphyseal cartilage. Efforts are now under way to assess chondrocyte viability in the epiphyseal cartilage and in the articular cartilage using diffusion-weighted imaging. Gadolinium enhancement is particularly valuable in determining the vascularity of cartilaginous regions.

OCCURRENCE OF ORTHOPEDIC DEFORMITIES

Skeletal dysplasias reach clinical significance in two broad areas – shortness of stature and structural deformity. The latter group can be determined by assessing axial and appendicular regions, since various dysplasias have a characteristic pattern of involvement. There are two general approaches to assess a patient with skeletal dysplasia. One is to determine the specific diagnosis and then look for the known regional abnormalities, the other to assess each region clinically and if necessary by radiographs to define abnormalities of clinical significance and if possible allow for syndromal diagnosis. The latter method is preferable, especially for those who see few patients with these relatively rare disorders, since it is the deformities that have clinical significance rather than the diagnostic categorization. In this section we will outline the deformities that commonly affect the various regions.

Abnormalities of the spine (axial abnormalities)

Cervical spine

The possibility of spinal abnormalities should always be considered in assessing a patient with skeletal dysplasia[3]. Cervical abnormalities can be associated with neurologic compromise. This can be very problematic, if undetected, for induction of general anesthesia owing to the extreme head and neck manipulation often needed for intubation. Abnormalities of the cervical spine occur in approximately 35 of the 150 defined dysplasia syndromes[14]. Symptoms generally develop slowly

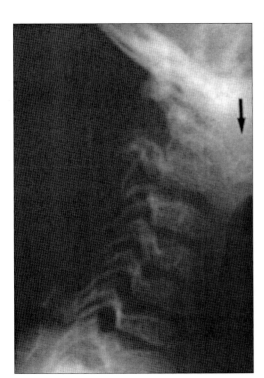

Fig. 208.3 Lateral cervical radiograph from patient with spondyloepiphyseal dysplasia congenita with quadriparesis, showing C1 subluxation anteriorly (arrow) on C2.

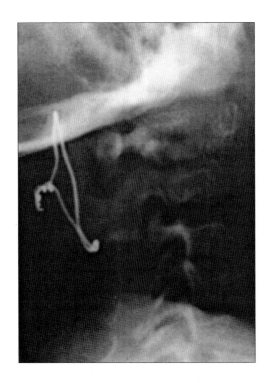

Fig. 208.4 Lateral cervical radiograph following occiput–C2 fusion, showing reduced position of C1 on C2 and posterior bone and wire fusing occiput, C1 and C2. Symptoms resolved almost fully in association with the repair.

and often do not appear until adulthood, even although the deformity has been present since birth. A myelopathy is seen with elements of increased fatigability, motor weakness, sensory diminution and hyper-reflexia.

Maldevelopment of the odontoid process with atlantoaxial instability[15] predisposes to anterior subluxation of the first cervical vertebra on the second (C1–C2 subluxation) with spinal cord pressure (Fig. 208.3). When identified, treatment is generally by C1–C2 posterior fusion or occiput–C2 fusion (Fig. 208.4). This finding is seen almost invariably with Morquio's disease (mucopolysaccharidosis type IV, MPS IV) and is also very common in the type II collagenopathies spondyloepiphyseal dysplasia (SED) congenita, Kniest dysplasia, pseudoachondroplasia, Larsen's syndrome, diastrophic dysplasia and spondylometaphyseal dysplasia.

Midcervical kyphosis is seen commonly with diastrophic dysplasia and occasionally in some of the type II collagenopathies. Some cases resolve with growth in the first few years of life but those that don't can lead to rigid and increasing deformity with cord stretching and compression.

Cervical spina bifida occulta, cervical spinal cord stenosis – usually accompanied by foramen magnum stenosis (achondroplasia) – and spinal cord nerve root compression by exostoses in hereditary multiple exostoses are other disorders seen in the skeletal dysplasias.

Thoracolumbar spine

These regions are affected frequently with deformity, which can be either scoliosis (lateral curvature of the spine), kyphosis (posterior convex angulation of the spine) or a combined kyphoscoliosis. Many of these require spinal fusion in childhood or adolescence but if untreated by surgery they can increase in adulthood, especially with the onset of mid- to late-life osteoporosis.

Lumbar spinal stenosis and lumbar lordosis

Many syndromes are complicated by lumbar spinal stenosis, which can lead to an increased incidence of nerve root compression with intervertebral disc herniation in mid-adult life. These deformities characterize three of the most common skeletal dysplasias: achondroplasia, where they are seen invariably (Fig. 208.5), diastrophic dysplasia and pseudoachondroplasia. They are not problematic alone but their presence predisposes to spinal stenosis, which, in the presence of intervertebral disc herniation, leads to nerve root irritation with pain and paresis.

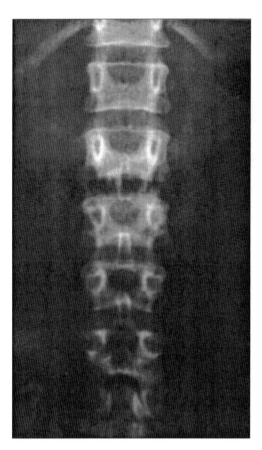

Fig. 208.5 Anteroposterior radiograph of lumbar spine in a patient with achondroplasia, showing progressive narrowing of interpedicular distance from L1 above to S1 below. The distance should normally increase with each descending level.

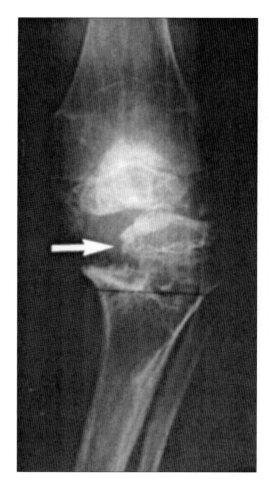

Fig. 208.6 Anteroposterior radiograph of the knee in a patient with pseudoachondroplasia, illustrating the severe structural abnormalities that can occur in some dysplasias. Note the irregular surfaces of distal femur and proximal tibia, varus angulation with lateral subluxation of tibia and fibula, and irregular ossification of medial tibial secondary ossification center and adjacent metaphysis (arrow). The lateral view showed a small, irregularly shaped patella.

Abnormalities of the extremities (appendicular abnormalities)

Abnormalities of the extremities are seen invariably in the skeletal dysplasias[3]. Shortening of the bones is common and most skeletal dysplasias are recognized originally because of short stature. In most dysplasias the shortening is symmetric and one of four patterns generally predominates. Thus the shortening can be:

- micromelic, where all parts of the limb are short
- rhizomelic, where there is proportionally greater proximal shortening (humerus and femur)
- mesomelic, where shortening is concentrated in the midlimb regions (radius, ulna, tibia, fibula)
- acromelic, where the most marked shortening is distally in hands and feet.

Lower extremity length discrepancies with asymmetric right–left shortening occur and are seen most with Ollier's enchondromatosis and hereditary multiple exostoses. Other types of extremity deformity include: angular bone deformity due to growth associated with asymmetric physeal involvement leading to varus, valgus, flexion, extension or rotational malposition; limb deformity due to unequal growth rates of paired long bones in forearm and leg; and joint contractures, instability or articular cartilage/epiphyseal cartilage malformation, all of which can predispose to early osteoarthritis due to abnormal weight bearing.

Abnormalities of the hip

A large number of patients with skeletal dysplasias have hip abnormalities, which predispose to early osteoarthritis, often necessitating total joint arthroplasty in early to mid adult life. There is an increasing tendency in many pediatric orthopedic centers to resort to femoral and acetabular osteotomies during the growing years in an effort to forestall degenerative changes. These often improve the structural relationships of the hip bones and the gait but many of the abnormalities involve either the shape of the femoral head, including the articular surface, and the structure of the cartilage matrix, such that premature osteoarthritis is still destined to occur in many.

One of the most common of the skeletal dysplasias, which is associated with a high number of hip and knee joint arthroplasties in involved families, is multiple epiphyseal dysplasia. Three variants have been defined at a molecular level: EDM 1 is associated with a cartilage matrix oligomeric protein (*COMP*) mutation, EDM 2 with a collagen IX (*COL9A2*) mutation and EDM 3 with a different collagen IX (*COL9A3*) mutation.

There remains a reasonable suspicion that many cases of isolated or idiopathic osteoarthritis will eventually be associated with other, as yet undetected, mutations of genes expressing cartilage matrix proteins.

Structural defects of the hip in skeletal dysplasias with a known predisposition to osteoarthritis include congenital hip dislocation, acetabular dysplasia, coxa vara, hip contractures and primary lack of sphericity of the femoral head.

Abnormalities of the knee

The knee is another joint with a high number of abnormalities in the dysplasias, predisposing to early degenerative change (Fig. 208.6). As in the hip, both structural abnormality leading to abnormal weight-bearing and inherent cartilage abnormality of shape and molecular matrix composition predispose to arthritic change. Genu varum or genu valgum is common in childhood in many syndromes, often with associated rotational and flexion–extension components. These are due to epiphyseal abnormalities of the distal femur or proximal tibia or both including asymmetric growth plate involvement, under- or overdevelopment of condylar cartilage shape, cruciate ligament and meniscal abnormalities and capsular laxity. A tendency to lateral patellar subluxation or full dislocation is common, often with underdevelopment of the lateral femoral condyle.

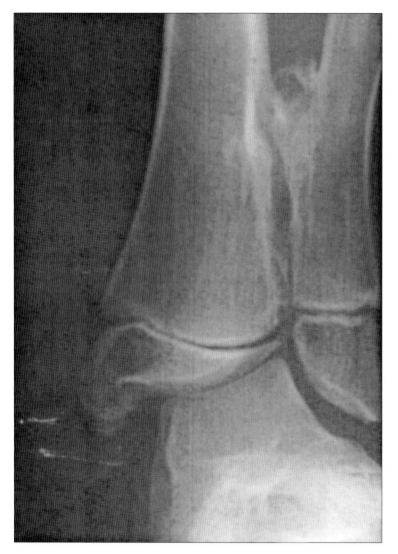

Fig. 208.7 Anteroposterior radiograph of the ankle in a boy with hereditary multiple exostosis. The distal fibula is shorter than the distal tibia, allowing for lateral displacement and lateral tilt of the talus. Osteochondromas of the fibula are present. The pressure of tethering due to abnormal asymmetric growth rates has caused underdevelopment of the secondary ossification center in the epiphysis of the distal lateral tibia.

Ankle and foot abnormalities

Ankle and foot abnormalities are common in some dysplasias but in general are not as problematic as hip or knee involvement. Some disorders, such as hereditary multiple exostosis, have unequal growth of the distal tibia and fibula with the shorter fibula leading to an ankle valgus, which may require surgical correction (Fig. 208.7). The bones of the foot are often misshapen and the foot is shorter and wider than normal, such that shoe fitting can be very difficult.

Upper extremity abnormalities

The upper extremities are also the site of structural defects of bone in many dysplasias but the symptoms are considerably less than in the lower extremities, primarily because of the lack of requirement for weight-bearing. Ostearthritis is relatively infrequent. The most common problems are stiffness of finger joints and problems at elbow and wrist, again due to asymmetric bone segment growth. In hereditary multiple exostosis there can be dislocation of the radial head at the elbow and dorsal prominence and shortening of the distal ulna with ulnar angulation of the hand (Madelung deformity). In distal dysplasias there can be considerable wrist and hand involvement, which generally presents with shortened tips of the fingers, nail dysplasias, and stiffened interphalangeal and metacarpophalangeal joints.

MANAGEMENT APPROACHES IN THE SKELETAL DYSPLASIAS

Medical management

It is ideal to ascertain whether the abnormality affects the articular cartilage surface either directly or indirectly. In many disorders, for example achondroplasia, which is the commonest of the dysplasias, there is rarely any arthritis since the epiphyseal ends of the bone are of a normal or at least mutually congruent shape and the articular cartilage has no molecular matrix abnormalities. In other conditions, such as diastrophic dysplasia, degenerative arthritis is almost invariable in all joints and the combination of epiphyseal malformation, flattening and irregularity of the articular cartilage surface, fibrosis of the cartilage and joint contractures renders many patients either non-ambulatory or ambulatory with extreme difficulty in their late teenage years even with intensive orthopedic management.

Conservative measures are often very helpful for the painful joint or joints in patients with a skeletal dysplasia. Simple measures such as decreased use, rest, crutches, splints and anti-inflammatory medications allow symptoms to diminish.

Surgical treatment

Surgical treatment in the extremities can be of great help even in the growing years before skeletal maturity. These procedures include osteotomies to restore anatomic bone alignment, patellar realignment, and arthroscopy or open arthrotomy to remove degenerative debris from affected joints. On the other hand, it is extremely important not to operate on joints that appear structurally abnormal but are asymptomatic in the hope of preventing or slowing down osteoarthritic changes. Many patients with dysplasia tolerate apparently abnormal structure for decades because the surrounding musculature and soft tissues have developed in that position from the fetal period onwards and are often stressed abnormally by radical surgical repositioning.

Total joint arthroplasty is resorted to with great frequency in these disorders in the adult years. Young and even middle-aged adults present a problem in determining the age at which any prosthetic implant procedure is done, since the need for replacement of a prosthesis is greater the longer it is used. These decisions are based on patient wishes and current practice standards. The initial results are generally favorable because the bone tissue is normal and the patients are healthy. There is increased attention currently, however, in performing osteotomy in the young adult age group if at all possible.

Surgical approaches to spinal problems will not be considered in detail. Those taking care of such patients must be aware when general anesthesia is being given of the high incidence of cervical C1–C2 abnormalities, which are often asymptomatic, even into adulthood[15]. Extreme neck movements in the anesthetized patient may cause neurologic damage. Some centers perform lateral neck radiographs in skeletal dysplasia patients prior to general anesthesia even if no symptoms have been elicited by history.

OVERVIEW OF THE MORE COMMON SKELETAL DYSPLASIAS

Achondroplasia

Achondroplasia is the commonest of the skeletal dysplasias. It is seen in all races. The disorder is due to a mutation in the gene expressing the fibroblast growth factor receptor 3 ($FGFR3$)[5,6]. Disorders in the same mutation group include the lethal thanatophoric skeletal dysplasia and the much milder hypochondroplasia variant.

There is relatively little clinical variability in achondroplasia since the same mutation is present in virtually all patients. The diagnosis is usually made in the first few days of life since the anteroposterior radiograph of the spine and pelvis is characteristic for a progressively narrowed interpedicular distance from L1 to S1 (Fig. 208.5; it should widen with each descending vertebra)[16], a horizontal acetabulum and a small sciatic notch. The childhood appearance is characterized by bow legs and a fixed lumbar lordosis. There is little evidence of osteoarthritis, even in adult life.

Current practice is for some patients to undergo limb lengthening, bilateral femoral and tibial procedures adding several centimeters to their height. Patients with achondroplasia are usually good candidates for the procedure because their joints are normal. Abnormal joints often limit the effectiveness of limb lengthening because of the increased stresses usually placed on the intervening joint cartilage surfaces. The procedures are best done in the second decade. At present, such procedures in the adult have a much higher level of complication, more prolonged healing and less extensive length gained.

Multiple epiphyseal dysplasia

This disorder has many subtypes in the clinical–radiographic classifications and, not surprisingly, different mutation groups are found to underlie it. Although the condition is a true skeletal dysplasia, not all patients are of short stature and many with severe joint involvement are normal to tall in terms of overall height. Those with multiple epiphyseal dysplasia comprise the commonest diagnostic group undergoing total joint arthroplasty. The condition tends to affect certain groups of joints in different families with the differing mutations. Many just have hip involvement and this tends to be bilateral.

The radiographic appearance in those with hip involvement in the first decade resembles the appearance in Legg–Perthes disease. At this time the hips are usually minimally symptomatic or asymptomatic in comparison with Legg–Perthes disease, the range of motion is good, and the bilateral appearance is close to symmetric, whereas in Legg–Perthes disease bilateral involvement occurs in only about 20% with second-side involvement occurring 18–24 months later than the first side. Molecular abnormalities of *COMP* and collagen type IX were referred to above.

Spondyloepiphyseal dysplasia

This common skeletal dysplasia has two clinical variants, a more severe congenita form and a milder tarda form. Both are associated with mutations in type II collagen. The more severe variants have considerable short stature, a high incidence of bilateral coxa vara and a high incidence of C1–C2 subluxation, often with neurogenic deficits (Figs 208.3 & 208.4). In spite of this, most joints within the body are of normal structure.

Kniest dysplasia

This disorder is also associated with mutations in type II collagen but tends to be much more severe than SED congenita or tarda. The abnormalities are evident at birth. There is a high incidence of a depressed nasal bridge and cleft palate. Many develop hearing problems in the second decade and others develop severe eye problems, including myopia, retinal detachment, glaucoma and even eventual blindness. Skeletal deformity is marked and progressive. Moderate to severe kyphoscoliosis is seen. The joints are misshapen and can develop contractures and, by the late second or early third decade, there may be marked clinical and radiographic osteoarthritis. The hips, knees and ankles have considerable involvement. Procedures such as realignment osteotomy, patellar realignment and knee joint debridement have been helpful in allaying symptoms.

Diastrophic dysplasia

This disorder is one of the most deforming of the skeletal dysplasias, with severe short stature worsened by a high incidence of scoliosis and multiple severe fixed joint contractures of hips (flexion), knees (flexion), and feet/ankles (equinus and/or metatarsus adductus). Deformity correction often requires osteotomy but even this can be followed by relent-

less recurrence. The disorder is further worsened by osteoarthritic degeneration of articular cartilage due to misshapen epiphyses and inherent structural abnormality of the cartilage matrix, which is excessively fibrotic, thus limiting normal growth and function of each of physeal, epiphyseal and articular cartilage regions.

The disorder is due to mutation in the gene expressing the diastrophic dysplasia sulfate transporter (*DTDST*) which also is responsible for two lethal dysplasias, atelosteogenesis type 2 and achondrogenesis type 1B. Growth plate cartilage is characterized histologically by increased deposition of fibrous tissue. Electron microscopy shows huge aggregates of crossbanded collagen in the cartilage matrix due to excess aggregation of type II fibrils normally kept apart from one another by surface deposition of normal type IX collagen[9] (Fig. 208.2).

Many patients become partially or totally wheelchair-bound by the end of the second decade. There is also a high incidence of thoracolumbar scoliosis, midcervical kyphosis (some of which resolves with growth, although some cases require posterior fusion), and posterior cervical spina bifida, which is asymptomatic but must be noted if cervical fusion is performed.

Morquio's disease

Morquio's disease – mucopolysaccharidosis (MPS) IV – is the most common MPS syndrome compatible with longevity. The major enzyme deficiency is of galactose-6-sulfatase, leading to imperfect processing of keratan sulfate. The patients are mentally normal and physically healthy but suffer from severe short stature, marked bilateral hip coxa vara/acetabular dysplasia with a waddling gait, genu valgum (knock-knees), a shortened spine with platyspondyly (flattened vertebrae), and an almost invariable incidence of odontoid hypoplasia of C2, leading to C1–C2 instability with myelopathy. Surgical stabilization of the C1–C2 junction is often required[17].

Hereditary multiple exostoses

In this autosomal dominant disorder, multiple exostoses, or osteochondromas, are present at the periphery of the growth plates and metaphyses. They grow from cartilage caps via the endochondral sequence and the bone of the exostosis is continuous with the metaphyseal bone with no cortical bone interposition.

Three genes have been found associated with multiple exostoses, *EXT1*, *EXT2* and *EXT3*. EXT1 and EXT2 are proteins with glycosyltransferase activities needed for the synthesis of heparan sulfate, proteoglycans present both on cell surfaces and in the extracellular matrix. Growth of the exostoses is normally controlled such that it ceases when the adjacent physeal growth stops. Recurrence of growth in adulthood in any of the osteochondromas is a sign of malignant transformation of persisting cartilage, usually to the chondrosarcoma line. The frequency of this has been difficult to determine but is probably in the range of 3–5% of patients[18].

The osteochondromas themselves can cause discomfort, especially at or near skeletal maturation, when involution of the cartilage cap exposes bone tissue to surrounding tendon and surgical excision is often necessary. Asymmetric growth of paired long bones because of the presence of osteochondromas can contribute to angular deformation with the following seen: genu valgum (knee), ankle tilt into valgus (relatively shorter fibula), dislocation of the radial head at the elbow; and wrist deformation with dorsally displaced and shortened ulna (Madelung deformity). Disorders occurring towards the end of growth and early in the adult time period can include pain and swelling behind the knee due to pseudoaneurysm of the popliteal artery caused by a pointed posteromedial exostosis, weakness of the foot/ankle due to stretching of the peroneal nerve with a prominent head of fibula osteochondroma, and radicular nerve symptoms due to an intraspinal osteochondroma growing to press against a nerve root.

SUMMARY

This brief overview of the skeletal dysplasias has highlighted the increasing knowledge gained from gene and molecular findings in the various syndromes. Awareness of clinical problems with these disorders is important, since many impact negatively on the musculoskeletal system and may compromise neurologic function. Osteoarthritis is common in some of the dysplasias. It is often responsive for a considerable time to non-surgical management but many joints in these disorders eventually benefit from arthroplasty. The disorders represent a highly active field of investigation concerning the interplay between molecular abnormality and clinical dysfunction.

REFERENCES

1. International nomenclature and classification of the osteochondrodysplasias. Am J Med Genet 1997; 79: 376–382.
2. Jones KL. Smith's recognizable patterns of human malformation, 5th ed. Philadelphia, PA: WB Saunders; 1997.
3. Shapiro F. Pediatric orthopedic deformities. Basic science, diagnosis and treatment. San Diego, CA: Academic Press; 2001.
4. Rivas R, Shapiro F. Structural stages in the development of the long bones and epiphyses. A study in the New Zealand white rabbit. J Bone Joint Surg 2002; 84A: 85–100.
5. Frezal J, LeMerrer M, Chauvet ML. Osteochondrodysplasia, dysostoses, disorders of calcium metabolism, congenital malformations with skeletal involvement mapped on human chromosomes. Pediatr Radiol 1997; 27: 366–387.
6. Ho NC, Jia L, Driscoll CC et al. A skeletal gene database. J Bone Miner Res 2000; 15: 2095–2122.
7. Cooper RR, Ponseti IV, Maynard JA. Pseudo-achondroplastic dwarfism: a rough-surfaced endoplasmic reticulum storage disorder. J Bone Joint Surg 1973; 55A: 475–484.
8. Bonnemann CG, Cox GF, Shapiro F et al. A mutation in the alpha-3 chain of type IX collagen causes autosomal dominant multiple epiphyseal dysplasia with mild myopathy. Proc Natl Acad Sci USA 2000; 97: 1212–1217.
9. Shapiro F. Light and electron microscopic abnormalities in diastrophic dysplasia growth cartilage. Calcif Tissue Int 1992; 51: 324–331.
10. Shapiro F. Structural abnormalities of the epiphyses in skeletal dysplasias. In: Buckwalter JA, Ehrlich MG, Sandell LJ, Trippel SB, eds. Skeletal growth and development: clinical issues and basic science advances. Rosemont, IL: American Academy of Orthopaedic Surgeons; 1998: 471–490.
11. Hobbins JC, Benacerraf BR. Diagnosis and therapy of fetal anomalies. San Diego, CA: Academic Press; 1989: 174–175.
12. Jaramillo D, Connolly SA, Mulkern RV, Shapiro F. Developing epiphysis: MR imaging characteristics and histologic correlation in the newborn lamb. Radiology 1998; 207: 637–645.
13. Bashir A, Gray ML, Boutin RD et al. Glycosaminoglycan in articular cartilage: in vivo assessment with delayed Gd(DTPA)2-enhanced MR imaging. Radiology 1997; 205: 551–558.
14. Lachman RS. The cervical spine in the skeletal dysplasias and associated disorders. Pediatr Radiol 1997; 27: 402–408.
15. Skeletal Dysplasia Group. Instability of the upper cervical spine. Arch Dis Child 1989; 64: 283–288.
16. Lutter LD, Lonstein JE, Winter RB, Langer LO. Anatomy of the achondroplastic lumbar canal. Clin Orthop Rel Res 1977; 126: 139–142.
17. Lipson SJ. Dysplasia of the odontoid process in Morquio's syndrome causing quadriparesis. J Bone Joint Surg 1977; 59A: 340–344.
18. Black B, Dooley J, Pyper A, Reed M. Multiple hereditary exostoses: an epidemiologic study of an isolated community in Manitoba. Clin Orthop Rel Res 1993; 287: 212–217.

209 Tumors of bone

John Dixon

INTRODUCTION

Rheumatological practice occasionally includes problems of diagnosis and treatment of tumors of the locomotor system. Clinical features common to many rheumatological disorders can also be observed in patients with bone tumors, including joint swelling, tenderness, pain on motion, stiffness and flexion contractures of peripheral joints. In addition, however, there may be muscle atrophy and constitutional symptoms such as fever, loss of weight and anorexia.

The principal aim of this chapter is to raise awareness of these problems to ensure that diagnosis is made early, when effective treatment can be started. These tumors are rare and deceptive in their presentation. Clinical and radiological features are often non-specific, and histological appearances of malignant tumors can easily be confused with benign processes.

It is therefore very important that cases with possible malignancy are referred early to a center familiar with these rare conditions. The center should have specialist surgical, oncological, histopathological and radiological opinions available, as it is only by the interaction of these disciplines that mistakes in diagnosis can be avoided, and optimal treatment begun without delay.[1]

HISTORY

One of the first classifications of bone tumors was by Virchow in 1864–65[2], who divided bone sarcomas into spindle-cell, round-cell and giant-cell types. Since then numerous classifications have been proposed, based on various criteria. The establishment by Codman in 1920[3] of the Bone Sarcoma Registry, under the auspices of the American College of Surgeons, was one of the most important contributions to the advancement of our knowledge and understanding of bone tumors.

In 1930, chondrosarcomas were separated from osteogenic sarcomas; in 1938 the group of giant-cell tumors were divided into benign and malignant forms and in 1939 the reticulum-cell sarcoma of bone was separated from Ewing's sarcoma. The revised classification of 1939 by Ewing has since been modified by others, based on embryogenetic or histogenic concepts. In 1952 Lichtenstein was the first to place Ewing's sarcoma in a separate division on the basis of its derivation from mesenchymal cells. Lichtenstein also created an intermediate group between the benign and malignant tumors. In 1958, HL Jaffe[4] adapted the classification proposed in 1949 by Phemister. Recently, there is evidence that Ewing's sarcoma of bone is a member of the neural tumor family.

In this chapter, the revised World Health Organization (WHO) classification and definitions of bone tumors, as published in 1972 by Schajowicz et al. and revised by Schajowicz in 1994[5], are followed. This classification is based on histologic criteria (Table 209.1).

BENIGN BONE-FORMING TUMORS

Osteoma

World Health Organization definition

An osteoma is a benign lesion consisting of well-differentiated mature bone tissue with a predominantly laminar structure, and showing very slow growth.

Epidemiology

Osteomas are found in all age groups, most frequently between the second and fourth decades. Three different types of osteomas may be distinguished:

- conventional, classic osteomas ('ivory exostosis')
- juxtacortical (parosteal) osteomas
- medullary osteomas (enostosis, bone islands).

TABLE 209.1 REVISED WHO CLASSIFICATION OF BONE TUMORS	
Bone-forming tumors	**Vascular tumors**

Benign
  Osteoma
  Osteoid osteoma and osteoblastoma
	Benign
	  Hemangioma
	  Lymphangioma
	  Glomus tumor (glomangioma)

Intermediate Aggressive (malignant) osteoblastoma	

Malignant
  Osteosarcoma
    Central (medullary)
    Surface (peripheral)
     - Parosteal
     - Periosteal
     - High-grade surface
	Intermediate or indeterminate
	  Hemangioendothelioma
	    (epithelioid–histiocytoid)
	  Hemangiopericytoma

	Malignant
	  Angiosarcoma (malignant
	    hemangioendothelioma)
	  Malignant hemangiopericytoma

Cartilage-forming tumors	**Other connective tissue tumors**

Benign
  Chondroma
    Enchondroma
    Periosteal (juxtacortical)
  Osteochondroma
    Solitary
    Multiple hereditary
  Chondroblastoma (epiphyseal)
  Chondromyxoid fibroma
	Benign
	  Benign fibrous histiocytoma
	  Lipoma

	Intermediate Desmoplastic fibroma

Malignant
  Chondrosarcoma (conventional)
  Dedifferentiated chondrosarcoma
  Juxtacortical (periosteal) chondrosarcoma
  Mesenchymal chondrosarcoma
  Clear-cell chondrosarcoma
  Malignant chondroblastoma
	Malignant
	  Fibrosarcoma
	  Malignant fibrous histiocytoma
	  Liposarcoma
	  Malignant mesenchyma
	  Leiomyosarcoma
	  Undifferentiated sarcoma

Giant-cell tumor (osteoclastoma)	**Other tumors**

Marrow tumors (round cell tumors)	Benign
	  Neurilemoma
	  Neurofibroma

Ewing sarcoma of bone
Neuroectodermal tumor of bone
Malignant lymphoma of bone (primary–secondary)
Myeloma
	Malignant
	  Chordoma
	  Adamantinoma

The conventional classic osteomas involve almost exclusively bones of intramembraneous formation, particularly the external table of the skull and the frontal and ethmoid sinuses. They are found more frequently in women (2:1 ratio). The juxtacortical (parosteal) osteomas are mostly found in long (femur, humerus) or flat bones and more commonly in men. The medullary osteomas (bone islands) are more common in women and are frequently located in the tibia and femur.

Clinical features

Osteomas are often asymptomatic. The appearance of a slowly increasing swelling with a hard consistency is frequently the first complaint. Infrequently this enlargement may lead to obstruction such as of the ostium of a paranasal sinus or proptosis.

Multiple osteomas form part of Gardner's syndrome, a familial autosomal dominant disease consisting of the triad of colonic polyposis, osteomas and soft tissue tumors. The colonic polyposis is premalignant. Bone lesions range from localized, cortical thickening to large osteomas and all parts of the skeleton may be involved. Multiple enostosis is a rare hereditary (autosomal dominant) benign disorder. The disease is also referred to as osteopoikilosis and may be associated with multiple osteochondromatosis and a tendency to keloid formation.

Investigations and differential diagnosis

Radiologically, osteomas are characterized by a dense, radiopaque, structureless, well-defined image, usually less than 3cm in diameter. The borders are often lobular.

On pathologic examination, most osteomas are usually dense compact bone masses adjacent to the underlying cortex, well circumscribed and covered by a thin fibrous membrane. Histologically they consist of thick trabeculae of mature lamellar bone. The absence of cartilaginous tissue on the surface of the lesion, which is found in osteochondromas and in most cases of juxtacortical osteosarcomas, is important. In senescent osteochondromas, the cortex of the lesions flares into the cortex of the bone, a phenomenon not seen in osteomas.

On histologic examination, parosteal osteosarcomas usually show trabeculae of woven bone embedded in a fibroblastic stroma. Periostitis ossificans in its mid-to-late phase can be observed after an injury. Histologically, woven to lamellar bone can be observed.

Management

Treatment is only indicated in patients with clinical symptoms or for aesthetic reasons. Treatment consists of simple excision. Juxtacortical osteomas of long bones should always be excised as it is impossible to exclude juxtacortical osteosarcoma clinically or radiographically.

Osteoid osteoma

World Health Organization definition

Osteoid osteoma is a benign osteoblastic lesion characterized by size (usually less than 1cm), a clearly demarcated outline and the usual presence of a surrounding zone of reactive bone formation. Histologically, it consists of cellular, highly vascularized tissue, made up of immature bone and osteoid tissue[6].

Epidemiology

Osteoid osteomas occur relatively frequently. Among benign tumors of the skeleton only exostosis and histiocytic fibroma are more common. This tumor occurs more frequently in men (2:1) and is typical of late childhood, adolescence and young adult age. It is rarely observed before 5 years of age or after 30.

The most common localizations are in the long bones particularly the femur and tibia. It may occur in the diaphyseal shaft or towards the metaphysis with considerable predilection for the proximal femur (neck and intertrochanteric region). It can also occur in short bones, such as the tarsus, the vertebral column, with a preference for the lumbar region, and the metacarpals and phalanges.

Clinical features

Pain is an almost constant and permanent symptom, not relieved by rest and often more intense at night. Pain is often exacerbated when alcoholic beverages are drunk and is frequently relieved dramatically with aspirin. Pain is not always well localized, which may lead to the attribution of symptoms to the nearby joint or to a radicular irradiation. The pain may be present for several months before radiographic evidence becomes apparent.

Atrophy of muscle, localized swelling and tenderness are frequent findings in superficial lesions. Osteoid osteomas located at a joint may present problems of differential diagnosis with an articular process. Patients may have been treated for arthritis for months before correct diagnosis. Osteoid osteoma of the spine is usually associated with painful scoliosis, with the concavity at the site of the nidus due to paravertebral muscle spasms. Generally, untreated osteoid osteomas increase very little in volume. However, because of the inflammatory reaction around the tumor, deformity of the meta-epiphysis during growth and joint stiffness may be seen.

Investigations and differential diagnosis

Radiologically, three types may be distinguished according to the location of the nidus:

- cortical, the classic type
- medullary or cancellous
- subperiosteal.

The basic element is a small rounded area of osteolysis (nidus), surrounded by a regular halo of hyperostosis (Fig. 209.1). Within the nidus there may be a central and irregular nucleus of bony opacity. This picture may vary considerably, depending on the site and its state of progression.

In the cortical localization there is a fusiform thickening of a single side of the shaft. The osteolytic area of an osteoid osteoma is usually located at the center of the thickening. At times, bony reaction is so pronounced that the small nidus cannot be seen except with a computed tomography (CT) scan or tomographs. In cancellous bone, as in the femoral neck and the vertebrae, the halo of osteosclerosis may be very scarce. A diffuse, intense osteoporosis may be evident. Radiographically, diagnosis may be very difficult. CT and bone scans are very helpful for

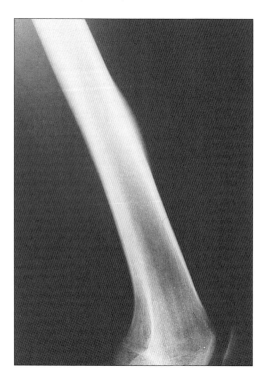

Fig. 209.1 Osteoid osteoma. Lateral radiograph of the shaft of the femur showing reactive bone sclerosis on the outer and inner surface of the anterior femur.

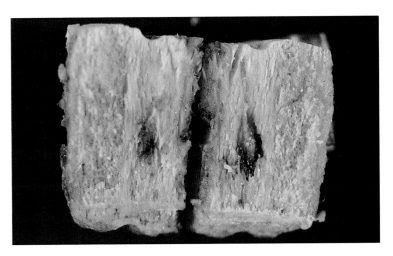

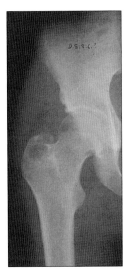
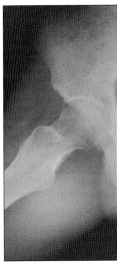

Fig. 209.3 Osteoblastoma. Radiograph of the right proximal femur showing a radiolucent lesion surrounded by reactive bone formation of the greater trochanter.

Fig. 209.2 Osteoid osteoma. Photograph of the resected specimen revealing the hyperemic aspect of the nidus.

diagnosis. Bone scan reveals a surrounding area of increased uptake. A normal bone scan excludes the diagnosis of osteoid osteoma. A CT scan shows the nidus, permitting accurate planning of surgery.

When the tumor is localized in long bones, differential diagnosis includes Brodie's abscess, fatigue fracture and sclerosing osteoperiostitis. Brodie's abscess occurs more often in the metaphyseal region and has a clinical history of intermittent pain. Radiographically it shows a larger, more irregular osteolysis. On surgery, pus is found. In inflammatory osteoperiostitis and in fatigue fracture, there is no nidus.

Management
Treatment consists of complete surgical removal of the nidus (Fig. 209.2) but this treatment can lead to major weakness of the bone and pathological fracture. This is particularly a hazard in the femoral neck and consequently radiologically guided core resection or photocoagulation[7] has become a more popular treatment. Incomplete resection may result in recurrence.

Osteoblastoma (benign)
World Health Organization definition
The basic WHO definition of an osteoblastoma is the same as that of an osteoid osteoma. However, an osteoblastoma is characterized by a nidus greater than 2cm[8].

Epidemiology
Osteoblastomas are less common than osteoid osteomas. Most of the patients are children or young adults. Men are affected more than women (2:1, 3:1). Although encountered in other sites, the tumor most frequently occurs in the vertebral column and the sacrum. In decreasing order, it is distributed in the long bones of the limbs, hands and feet. In long bones, an osteoblastoma is generally observed in the metadiaphysis.

Three types can be distinguished on the basis of their clinical and radiographic characteristics:

- medullary and cortical osteoblastoma
- periosteal osteoblastoma
- multifocal sclerosing osteoblastoma.

Clinical features
Pain is frequently present, sometimes for more than 2 years. Compression of the spinal cord and/or the spinal nerve roots are due to skeletal expansion.

Etiology and pathogenesis
An osteoblastoma is a benign tumor of osteoblasts, similar to osteoid osteomas, osteomas and fibrous dysplasia. Compared to an osteoid osteoma, the osteoblastoma has a high growth potential and provokes less reactive hyperostosis of the host bone.

Investigation and differential diagnosis
The radiographic picture varies, depending on the evolution and maturation of the tumor. The dominant finding is generally a single, roundish area of osteolysis, sometimes marked by moderately reactive osteosclerosis (Fig. 209.3). As well as central and eccentric localizations, the tumor tends to attenuate the cortex and expand the bone, resembling an aneurysmal bone cyst. There is at most only a small amount of periosteal reaction. In some cases, a picture characterized by disseminated or confluent irregular areas of more intense opacity may be seen because of maturation of the neoplastic osteoid. Angiograms show an intense vascularity of the tumor. Bone scans reveal an area of increased uptake, although less intense than in cases of an osteoid osteoma.

There are a few other lesions whose clinical and radiographic appearance may simulate osteoblastomas. These include Brodie's abscess, medullary osteoma and hemangioma. Angiography permits distinction between the former two. Histologic examination easily differentiates a hemangioma from an osteoblastoma. More important is the differential diagnosis from osteosarcomas, giant-cell tumors and aneurysmal bone cysts. An osteoblastoma mistaken for an osteosarcoma results in tragic consequences. To avoid such tragedy a complete clinical, radiographic and extensive microscopic examination of the tumor and the surrounding tissue must be carried out.

Management
Treatment depends on the stage and localization of the tumor. In the vertebral column, near growth plates and near some important joints, curettage should be carried out. In aggressive osteoblastomas marginal or wide excision is indicated, sometimes complemented by radiotherapy.

INTERMEDIATE BONE-FORMING TUMORS

Malignant osteoblastoma
World Health Organization definition
Malignant osteoblastomas differ from benign osteoblastomas by distinct histologic features. In addition to formation of abundant osteoid and immature bone trabeculae, fields with numerous giant cells of the osteoclast type and fields showing formation of bone spicules of irregular shape are found. Also, some nuclear atypism can be found[9].

Epidemiology
This is a rare tumor found in patients aged 6–70 years. The diaphysis or epiphysis of long bones are most frequently affected.

Clinical features

Pain and local swelling are the typical complaints. Osteoblastomas appear only locally aggressive but may recur, especially after incorrect treatment[9].

Investigations and differential diagnosis

Radiologically the appearance can be extremely variable and not diagnostic. The lesions do not have the characteristic appearance of osteosarcomas. Mostly there is a large area of osteolysis with expansion and thinning of the cortex, sometimes showing spotty calcifications[9]. In the more advanced cases, destruction of the cortex and invasion of the surrounding soft tissues can be observed. Histologically, osteoblasts are found more abundantly and are larger in size, often with plump hyperchromatic nuclei, more nuclear atypism and more frequent mitosis than benign osteoblastomas.

Management

Wide excision or block resection is preferred. Amputation is rarely indicated.

MALIGNANT BONE-FORMING TUMORS

Osteosarcoma

World Health Organization definition

An osteosarcoma is a malignant tumor characterized by the direct formation of bone or osteoid tissue by the tumor cells. Different clinicopathologic entities of osteosarcoma with different biologic behavior can be distinguished.

Conventional osteosarcoma

Epidemiology

After myelomas, osteosarcomas are the most frequent primary malignant bone tumor. Nonetheless, osteosarcoma is a relatively uncommon tumor. Its incidence is estimated to be about 2–3 per million. Osteosarcomas occur more often in men (male:female ratio 3:2) and three-fourths of patients are between the ages of 10 and 30 years. Most cases in older patients are secondary to Paget's disease, irradiation, dedifferentiated chondrosarcoma or fibrous dysplasia.

Although any bone may be affected, osteosarcomas are mostly found in long bones, with a predilection for the metaphysis of the lower end of the femur, the upper end of the tibia and the upper end of the humerus.

The upper metaphysis of the femur and the lower metaphysis of the tibia are involved less frequently. Osteosarcomas of the hands or feet and pelvis are rare.

Clinical features

Pain at the tumor site, sometimes radiating to the adjacent joint, is the most common complaint. Usually the pain is mild and intermittent but worsened by activity. Sometimes the pain is attributed to trauma. In the later stages of the disease a palpable mass can be felt (Fig. 209.4). The skin above the tumor tends to be warm, which is due to the intense vascularity of the tumor. Palpation becomes painful. Pathologic fracture is moderately common and is usually found in the more aggressive lesions, making early diagnosis all the more important.

The duration of the symptoms prior to diagnosis varies from a few weeks to not more than a few months. The general condition of the patient is nearly always good at diagnosis. Usually, osteosarcomas have a rapid course, although a slow evolution is rarely seen in osteosarcomas of the sclerosing type. Metastases occur mainly by the hematogenous route, particularly to the lungs. Secondarily, an osteosarcoma may metastasize in the skeleton; rarely, metastases may be seen in internal organs and in the regional lymph nodes.

Investigations and differential diagnosis

Radiographically, the classical osteosarcoma can show different pictures according to the type of tumor-cell differentiation. This can be with predominance of either bone, cartilage or fibroblastic proliferation, associated with more or less reactive bone formation. With bone differentiation, the picture is generally referred to as *sclerotic*. In more cellular or telangiectatic tumors, bone destruction dominates, and a permeative, moth-eaten radiolucent pattern with ill-defined borders is produced (*osteolytic* type).

The most characteristic radiologic features are found after cortical destruction and extension of the tumor into soft tissues. The intraosseous area is always characterized by faded boundaries where the normal trabeculation is replaced by radiolucency or a combination of lucent and radiopaque areas. The periosteum shows reactive bone formation consisting of long, thin, filiform spicules, radiating perpendicularly, giving the typical 'sunburst' pattern (Fig. 209.4c). This picture may also be observed in some benign (hemangioma, meningioma) or other malignant lesions (Ewing's sarcoma). The so-called Codman's triangle is due to reactive bone formation between the elevated periosteum and the

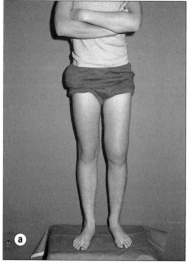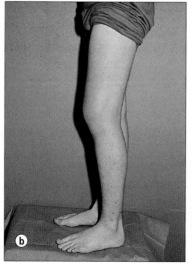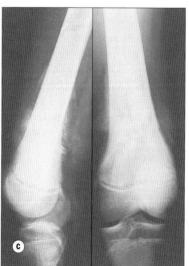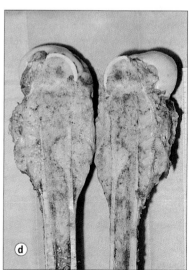

Fig. 209.4 Osteosarcoma. (a,b) A 16-year-old patient complaining of a painful swelling near the left knee joint. (c) Anteroposterior and lateral radiographs of the lower metaphysis of the femur show patchy increased bone density, extension in the soft tissues and typical Codman's triangle. (d) Photograph of the resected specimen, showing the polymorphism of osteosarcoma caused by various stages of differentiation, such as fibroblastic, myxoid, cartilaginous and especially osteoid and reactive processes.

underlying cortex. Codman's triangle may also be seen in osteomyelitis and Ewing's sarcoma.

Computed tomography scans and magnetic resonance imaging (MRI) allow study of the extent of the tumor in the soft tissues, its relationship to the large vessels and nerves, and to the nearby joint and articular structures. MRI is the best method available to evaluate the extent of the tumor in the bone and to detect skip metastasis. Because of the high incidence of pulmonary metastases, radiographs, tomograms and CT scans of the lungs are necessary at the time of diagnosis.

On pathologic examination, osteosarcomas exhibit a wide spectrum of histologic patterns. The production of osteoid or bone by the proliferating tumor cells is essential for diagnosis, depending upon the predominant tissue component. The histochemical demonstration of alkaline phosphatase in tumor cells may help in distinguishing osteoblasts from fibroblasts or chondroblasts.

Radiologically, differential diagnosis with Ewing's sarcoma, lymphoma and sometimes with metastatic disease may be difficult, particularly when the osteosarcoma is located towards the diaphysis or in osteolytic cases. Poorly differentiated osteosarcomas must be differentiated histologically from malignant fibrous histiocytomas or poorly differentiated fibrosarcomas. In osteosarcomas with extensive chondroblastic differentiation, may be difficult to differentiate from high-grade chondrosarcoma.

Management

Treatment consists of pre- and postoperative chemotherapy and surgery. This combination has changed the outcome of this tumor dramatically. Survival after 5 years is now approximately 60–70%. With surgical treatment alone, only 10–20% of patients survived after 5 years. Other forms of adjuvant therapy, such as preoperative irradiation of the tumor, preventive irradiation of the lung fields and immunotherapy, have been abandoned. With preoperative chemotherapy, the percentage of conservative surgery is now approximately 90%, despite most osteosarcomas being extracompartmental (stage IIB according to Enneking[10]).

Juxtacortical parosteal osteosarcoma

World Health Organization definition

A juxtacortical osteosarcoma is a destructive, malignant, bone-forming tumor characterized by an origin on the external surface of a bone and a high degree of structural differentiation. These tumors grow relatively slowly and have a better prognosis than the conventional type of osteosarcoma.

According to this descriptive definition, bone-forming tumors arising on the surface of a bone with a high degree of histologic malignancy are not accepted as juxtacortical osteosarcomas but are rather better classified as a peripheral (conventional) osteosarcoma.

Epidemiology

Juxtacortical osteosarcomas are a relatively rare tumor comprising 2–5% of the primary malignant bone tumors. There appears to be a slight predilection for women. The average age is higher than for typical osteosarcomas, with most patients more than 20 years old. Juxtacortical osteosarcomas are almost exclusively located in long bones, preferentially on the lower end of the femur, especially in the popliteal region. Less frequently the tumor is observed in the upper end of the humerus, the tibia, the fibula and the upper femur[11,12].

Clinical features

The most common clinical symptom is a swelling, sometimes with pain. Symptoms may already exist months or years before diagnosis. Generally, the growth of the tumor is slow. The reported survival rate 5 years after the first treatment is 70–80%[13].

Investigations and differential diagnosis

Radiographically, juxtacortical osteosarcomas have characteristic features, showing a densely ossified mass attached to the underlying cortex, predominantly at the metaphyseal region. The surface is mostly lobulated and less dense than the base of the tumor. A characteristic feature is a linear, translucent zone between the bulk of the tumor and the underlying cortex, except at the site of attachment. Occasionally, cortical thickening under the tumor and a defined surface with spicules on linear extension is observed. A periosteal bone reaction in the form of 'onion peel' or Codman's triangle is not seen.

Pathologically, the tumor is characterized by well-defined lobulated masses varying from a few to more than 20cm. The tumor is hard and primarily osseous. The extensive bone formation has a well-organized trabecular pattern composed of immature bone in different stages of maturation to lamellar bone. The fibrous stroma is composed of numerous spindle cells, forming a moderate amount of collagen fibers.

The differential diagnosis with osteochondromas can be made by studying the cap of the tumor, which never shows the regular continuous cartilaginous cap of osteochondromas.

Management

The treatment of parosteal osteosarcomas consists of segmental block resection and subsequent reconstruction. Local excision is frequently followed by one or more recurrences within 5–10 years.

Periosteal osteosarcoma

Clinically and radiographically, periosteal osteosarcoma and periosteal chondrosarcoma are very similar. Histologically, this tumor is usually predominantly chondroblastic, showing production of fine, lace-like osteoid trabeculae towards the center.

Because of a rather favorable clinical course, wide *en bloc* resection is proposed as therapy.

BENIGN CARTILAGE-FORMING TUMORS

Chondroma
World Health Organization definition

A chondroma is a benign tumor characterized by the formation of mature cartilage but lacking the histologic characteristics of chondrosarcomas.

Epidemiology

Most chondromas are solitary lesions located centrally within the medullary cavity (enchondroma). Rarely, they are found outside the bone in close contact with the underlying cortex, described by Lichtenstein and Hall[14] as 'periosteal chondroma' and by Jaffe as 'juxtacortical chondroma'[15]. Multiple enchondromas (enchondromatosis) affect few or many bones. Cases with predominantly unilateral involvement are termed 'Ollier's disease'. This syndrome associated with soft tissue hemangiomas and pheboliths is termed 'Maffucci's syndrome' (Fig. 209.5).

Chondromas are less common than osteochondromas and nonossifying fibromas. They occur more frequently in older age groups than do osteochondromas, with an obvious predominance after the second decade (80%). There is no gender predilection. The great majority of chondromas are located in the tubular bones of the hands and less frequently the feet. In addition, long bones such as the femur, the humerus, the fibula and the ribs are frequent sites of involvement.

Clinical features

Chondromas often remain asymptomatic. However, if they do cause symptoms it is because they are localized in small and superficial bones. These tumors easily provoke expansion of the bone and produce a visible swelling. Pain is felt in cases with pathologic fracture. In the long bones of the limbs, chondromas are often discovered by chance or for

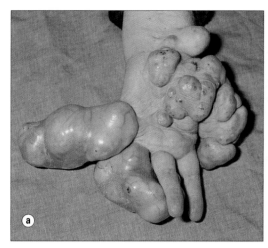
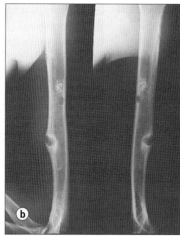
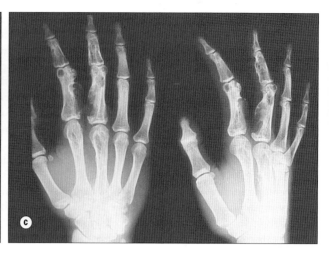

Fig. 209.5 Multiple enchondromatosis. (a) A patient suffering from enchondromatosis with multiple hemangiomas of soft tissue ('Maffucci's syndrome'). Radiographs of (b) the left humerus and (c) the left hand show multiple enchondromas ('Ollier's syndrome').

some other reason, such as a pathologic fracture. If pain occurs without pathologic fracture, malignancy is suspected. In multiple chondromas, the risk of malignant transformation is greater than with any other benign cartilage lesion. A cumulative frequency of 15–30% is reported.

Investigations and differential diagnosis
Radiologically, chondromas appear as small to moderate sized osteolytic round or ovoid areas with well-defined boundaries, expanding and slightly thinning the cortex. The lesion is usually located in the metaphysis and less frequently in the epiphysis. Chondromas in the terminal phalanx often involve the entire extension of the bone and are generally radiologically indistinguishable from the somewhat more frequent epidermal cysts.

Mottled calcifications are characteristic of cartilaginous tumors but may be absent in some cases. Different patterns are described, varying from finely stippled foci to large, coarse conglomerates, the latter mostly occurring in the metaphyseal region of long bones. This pattern has been called 'calcifying and ossifying chondroma'. The most common location is in the upper humerus and distal femoral metaphysis. Radiographically it may be difficult to differentiate these lesions from ischemic bone infarcts, which often exhibit a similar location.

Management
The decision to treat these tumors, which may have been discovered by chance and may not be symptomatic, is difficult.

For most enchondromas of the tubular bones of the hands and feet, curettage, perhaps followed by bone chips, is the treatment of choice. In other bones, block resection or wide excision is indicated. This treatment is also performed in some cases of recurrence after previous curettage.

Osteochondroma
World Health Organization definition
An osteochondroma is a cartilage-capped bony projection on the external surface of a bone.

Epidemiology
Osteochondromas are the most frequently occurring bone tumors (approximately 40% of all benign bone tumors and 20% of all bone tumors). Osteochondromas may be associated with any bone that has been preformed from cartilage. The most commonly involved locations are the long bones in the metaphyseal region of the most active growth plate, i.e. the upper end of the humerus and the tibia and the lower end of the femur. Other bones often involved are the ilium, the scapula, the fibula and the phalanges of hands and feet.

In cases of multiple osteochondromas, growth disturbances such as shortness and deformities of the involved long bones are frequently observed. Most patients are less than 20 years of age at the time of diagnosis. The male:female ratio is about 1.5:1 in most series.

Clinical features
Osteochondromas are frequently discovered on an incidental radiograph or because of a painless bony mass. Sometimes, pain due to pressure on neighboring structures such as bones or neurovascular elements is present. In some cases the development of a painful bursa on the top of the cartilage cap may lead to discovery. Sudden pain can be due to a fracture of the long stalk of a pedunculated osteochondroma. Malignant transformation is rare in solitary osteochondromas, occurring in less than 1% in most series. When this happens, the malignant tumor arising in osteochondromas is generally a chondrosarcoma. Cases of secondary osteosarcoma have also been observed. The risk of sarcomatous transformation is much higher in cases of multiple osteochondromas. The reported percentage varies from 11% to 20% in these tumors and is most common in tumours arising in the axial skeleton.

Investigations and differential diagnosis
Radiologically, osteochondromas may be either *pedunculated* (narrow base) or *sessile* (broad base). The pedunculated type shows a bony projection of different thickness or length, continuous with the cortex and spongiosa around the tumor. The cartilage-capped surface is mostly characterized by irregular calcifications. The diagnosis of a sessile osteochondroma is sometimes difficult and may be misdiagnosed as a parosteal osteoma or hyperostosis. The finding of a superficial layer of irregular calcifications favors the diagnosis of an osteochondroma.

Management
Surgical removal is only indicated in those cases that present with symptoms, especially pain, and in cases where the tumor has increased in size or became painful after the end of the epiphyseal growth period. Recurrence is rare in the pedunculated type, but more frequent in the sessile type because complete removal of the sessile osteochondroma is more difficult. Remnants of the cartilaginous tissue may remain and therefore a wider excision is advised in the sessile type.

Chondroblastoma
A chondroblastoma is a relatively rare benign tumor, characterized by highly cellular and relatively undifferentiated tissue made up of rounded or polygonal chondroblast-like cells with distinct outlines, together with multinucleated giant cells of osteoclast type arranged either singly or in a

group[16–18]. Local pain and tenderness are the most frequent complaints. Later on, local swelling and limitation of movement of the adjacent joint may follow. Sometimes, effusion into the joint caused by destruction of articular cartilage may be observed. With delayed diagnosis, the tumor may grow to an enormous size. Radiographically the most characteristic feature is an oval or rounded, sharply limited area of osteolysis located eccentrically in the epiphysis. Most chondroblastomas are cured with curettage and packing with cancellous bone chips.

Chondromyxoid fibroma

A chondromyxoid fibroma is a rare benign tumor characterized by lobulated areas of spindle-shaped or stellate cells with abundant myxoid or chondroid intercellular material, separated by zones of more cellular tissue rich in spindle-shaped or rounded cells with a varying number of multinucleotic giant cells of different size[19]. Symptoms are not specific and consist of pain, slowly increasing local swelling and sometimes a palpable tumor. Limping may be observed. A pathologic fracture occurs rarely. Radiographically the lesion appears as a transradiant area of variable size. In long bones, the tumor is located eccentrically in the metaphysis, only rarely crossing the epiphyseal line. In small tubular bones, it generally occupies the entire width of the affected bone, producing a fusiform expansion and thinning of both cortices. Differential diagnosis with fibrous dysplasia, chondromas, aneurysmal and simple bone cysts may be radiographically difficult. Block resection or wide excision are the treatment of choice because of the high incidence of recurrences after curettage. Malignant transformation is extremely rare.

MALIGNANT CARTILAGE-FORMING TUMORS

Chondrosarcoma (primary–secondary)
World Health Organization definition
A chondrosarcoma is a malignant tumor characterized by the formation of cartilage, but not bone, by the tumor cells. It is distinguished from a chondroma by the presence of more cellular and pleomorphic tumor tissue, and by appreciable numbers of plump cells with large or double nuclei. Mitotic cells are infrequent.

Epidemiology
Central primary chondrosarcomas comprise 10–13% of malignant bone tumors. In most series men are more affected than women (3:2). Chondrosarcoma is a tumor of adulthood with a peak incidence between 30 and 60 years of age. Secondary chondrosarcomas, as a complication of multiple enchondromatosis, are estimated to occur in 20–50% of cases. The frequency of malignant transformation in a solitary osteochondroma is estimated to be less than 1%, in multiple osteochondromas approximately 10%.

Clinical features
Pain is usually the first symptom of a chondrosarcoma. A firm swelling is noticed in many cases. The duration of complaints may range from a few weeks to years. Occasionally, a pathologic fracture is the first symptom[20,21].

Investigations and differential diagnosis
The radiographic picture of a central chondrosarcoma is of an intraosseous, osteolytic tumor, which often grows slowly. Chondrosarcomas are commonly situated in the metaphysis, often eccentrically. They may extend into the diaphysis along a considerable distance of the medullary cavity, producing a lobular, radiolucent area. They often show thickening and expansion of the cortex. Especially in low-grade chondrosarcomas, stippled or ring-like calcification may appear in the radiolucent areas (Fig. 209.6). Some chondrosarcomas may disrupt the cortex and extend

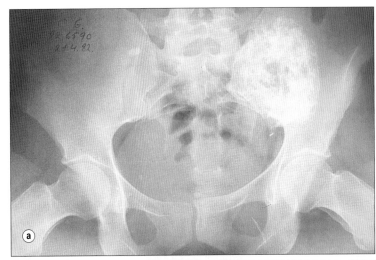

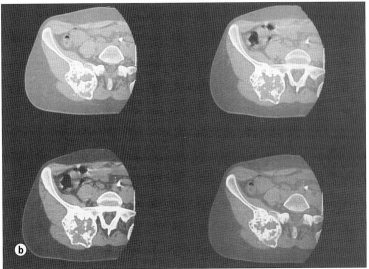

Fig. 209.6 Chondrosarcoma. (a) Radiograph of chondrosarcoma showing an irregular, radiodense area on the left ilium. (b) CT scan demonstrating an intraosseous more calcified tumor and an extraosseous more chondroid mass.

into the extraosseous soft tissues; this indicates a high-grade malignancy. MRI and CT scans are the best method for defining extraosseous involvement, especially in pelvic tumors (Fig. 209.6).

On microscopic examination, chondrosarcomas show a wide range of histologic features. Chondrosarcomas are divided into low-grade, moderate and highly malignant. Low-grade chondrosarcomas comprise approximately 60% of the group[21] and are frequently 'underdiagnosed' by the pathologist.

Management
The preferred primary treatment of chondrosarcomas is surgical and varies, according to grading and local appearance, from local resection with bone graft or prosthesis to amputation. In most series the 5-year survival rate varies from 50% to 60%; the 10-year survival rate is approximately 40%. Chondrosarcomas have a tendency to recur after incomplete excision. The most common site of metastasis is the lung. The results of radiotherapy are disappointing and there is little experience with chemotherapy.

Juxtacortical chondrosarcoma
A juxtacortical chondrosarcoma is a rare malignant cartilage-forming tumor arising from the external surface of a bone, usually characterized by well-differentiated cartilage with extensive areas of enchondral ossification. This tumor must be differentiated from a chondrosarcoma arising in the cartilage, and from an osteochondroma (secondary

chondrosarcoma)[13,22]. Slight pain and a firm swelling are the symptoms encountered. Radiographically, the characteristic appearance is that of a small tumor adjacent to the cortex localized on the metaphysis or towards the end of the diaphysis of a long bone. More often, areas of spotty calcification, sometimes accompanied by radiating bone spicules, and a typical Codman's triangle are observed. The problems in differential diagnosis involve periosteal chondroma, peripheral chondrosarcoma and the so-called periosteal osteosarcoma. In most series, *en bloc* resection of the tumor is the treatment of choice.

Mesenchymal chondrosarcoma

World Health Organization definition

A mesenchymal chondrosarcoma is a malignant tumor characterized by the presence of scattered areas of more or less differentiated cartilage together with highly vascular spindle-celled or round-celled mesenchymal tissue[23].

Epidemiology

Mesenchymal chondrosarcomas are found most commonly in the ribs and jaw but a wide variety of bones can be affected. One-third arise in extraskeletal soft tissue. Less often the long bones are involved. Women seem to be affected more than men. More than half the cases occur in the second and third decades.

Clinical features

Symptoms are not characteristic. Swelling and pain are the main complaints. The duration of symptoms prior to diagnosis varies from a few days to many years.

Investigations and differential diagnosis

Radiographically, mesenchymal chondrosarcoma is an osteolytic tumor with well-defined borders showing irregular calcifications in most cases and sometimes distension or destruction of the cortex. In soft tissues, the tumors are characterized by stippled, relatively heavy calcifications. Pathologically, they generally show areas of frankly cartilaginous aspects, alternating with areas of soft consistency and grayish white or yellowish color. On microscopic examination, three different histologic patterns can be observed: those of conventional chondrosarcomas, a pattern that can cause confusion with Ewing's sarcoma and a characteristic hemangiopericytomatous pattern. This combination of three different histologic patterns induces some to believe that this tumor could be a mixed mesenchymal tumor (mesenchymoma)[23].

Management

Radical surgical treatment appears to give the best results. Metastasis in the lungs may occur after several years.

Clear-cell chondrosarcoma

This is a rare tumor mostly involving the proximal femur or humerus. It is somewhat similar to a chondroblastoma and between grade 1 and grade 2 malignancy of a chondrosarcoma[24]. Radiographically, the tumor resembles an epiphyseal chondroblastoma. It is localized in the epiphysis or apophysis. Histologically, areas similar to those seen in chondroblastoma and prominent aneurysmal bone cyst-like areas are observed but the distinctive findings are the numerous cells with abundant, clear cytoplasm. The treatment of choice is wide excision.

GIANT CELL TUMORS (OSTEOCLASTOMA)

World Health Organization definition

An aggressive tumor characterized by richly vascularized tissue and consisting of rather plump, spindle-shaped or ovoid cells and the presence of many giant cells of the osteoclast type, which are uniformly distributed throughout the tumor tissue[25].

Epidemiology

Giant cell tumors occur relatively frequently, representing 4–5% of all bone tumors. They mainly affect young adults between 20–40 years of age but are also observed in patients aged 15–20 and 40–50. Most series report a slight predilection for women (1.5:1). In 90% of cases the tumors are observed in the long bones. The most frequent locations are the lower end of the femur, the upper end of the tibia, the distal end of the radius and the upper end of the humerus. More than 50% occur about the knee. Rarely, giant cell tumors are encountered in multiple locations. Most of the tumors are located at the epiphyseal end, abutting the articular cartilage and sometimes extending towards the metaphysis.

Clinical features

The most frequent complaint is pain, which increases with time, accompanied by local swelling and tenderness. Limitation of motion of the adjacent joint is present in many cases. Rarely, a pathologic fracture is the first symptom.

Investigations and differential diagnosis

Radiologically, the most common appearance of a giant cell tumor is a radiolucent expanding lesion, located eccentrically in the epiphyseal end of a long bone. The lesion may extend towards the articular cartilage and the metaphyseal region. The cortex is mostly thinned, distended and often partially destroyed. The limits are generally imprecise. Periosteal reaction and a sclerotic bone rim are usually not observed. Sometimes trabeculation is seen, indicating a non-aggressive lesion (Fig. 209.7).

On pathologic examination, the tumor generally shows extensive fleshy areas, alternating in color from gray to a light red or dark hemorrhagic color. Thin septae of connective tissue and small, bright-red or brownish cystic cavities may be observed. A giant cell tumor mostly respects the articular cartilage. Invasion of the joint space is more frequent by way of the synovial and capsular tissues, following destruction of the bone cortex. The margin of the tumor to the cortex consists of a thin bone shell, which is in fact newly displaced cortex caused by the process of constant periosteal bone deposition. The margin of the tumor to the spongiosa is not well defined.

Management

The treatment of choice for giant cell tumors is surgical. For lesions not amenable to surgery, for instance in the spine, the use of irradiation therapy is advocated but there is a high risk of malignant transformation. In most instances complete block resection followed by an autograft, allograft or prosthetic replacement is the preferred procedure. The rate of recurrence after resection is low. An initial treatment of curettage and bone grafting, with or without cauterization of the resulting cavity, has a recurrence rate ranging from 35% to 60%. Amputation is indicated only in advanced lesions with major destruction of bone near a major joint, especially after recurrences or secondary infections.

MARROW TUMORS

Ewing's sarcoma

World Health Organization definition

Ewing's sarcoma is a malignant tumor characterized by tissue with a rather uniform histologic appearance made up of densely packed small cells with round nuclei but without distinct cytoplasmic outlines or prominent nucleoli. The intercellular network of reticulin fibers, which is a feature of reticulosarcoma, is not seen[26].

Epidemiology

Ewing's sarcoma is one of the most frequent malignant bone tumors, accounting for approximately 6–9% of cases. Men are slightly more affected than women (1.5:1) and 90% of the tumors occur before 25 years

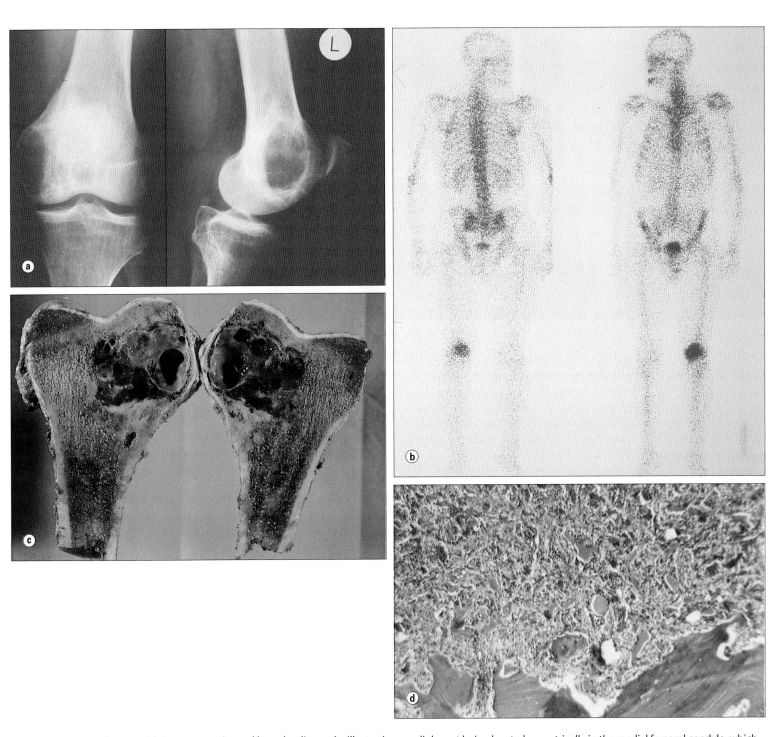

Fig. 209.7 Giant cell tumor. (a) Anteroposterior and lateral radiographs illustrating a radiolucent lesion located eccentrically in the medial femoral condyle, which expands the thinned cortex. Note the ill-defined borders to the medullary cavity. (b) Bone scintigraph revealing increased uptake of the bone-seeking tracer in the tumor. (c) Photograph of the resected tumor, showing that some parts of the tumor are grayish white in color or show fleshy and hemorrhagic areas. (d) Photomicrograph showing the characteristic histologic pattern of giant-cell tumor with numerous multinucleated giant cells, uniformly distributed and separated by mononuclear stromal cells.

of age. The diaphyseal regions of long bones are especially affected. The most common localization in long bones is in the femur, followed by the tibia, humerus, fibula and bones of the forearm. In the skeleton of the trunk, the pelvis is mostly affected, followed by the vertebral column, scapula, ribs and clavicle. No part of the skeleton is immune from Ewing's sarcoma.

Clinical features

Pain, tenderness and later local swelling are the most common complaints. Frequently, the general condition is further impaired by fever,

anemia and leukocytosis. These symptoms may lead to an erroneous clinical diagnosis of osteomyelitis.

Investigations and differential diagnosis

Radiographically the picture varies considerably depending on the age of the patient, the site and degree of expansion of the tumor and the reaction of the endosteum and the periosteum. Generally, the first feature in long bones is an area of bone sclerosis accompanied by irregular central areas of bone destruction and by an enlarged cortex with formation of slightly laminated, periosteal reactive bone or radial spicules. Later, an

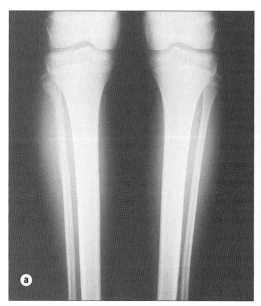
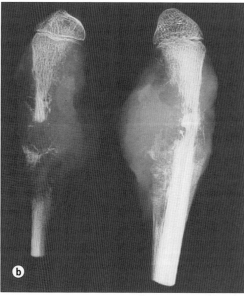

Fig. 209.8 Ewing's sarcoma. (a) Anteroposterior radiograph of the right fibula, showing a mottled area of bone destruction with laminated periosteal reaction ('onion peel') and perpendicular spicules. (b) Radiograph of the resected tumor. Note the large extraosseous tumor mass.

increased central area of osteolysis with ill-defined borders and even partial or complete destruction of the cortex can be observed. At this stage the cortex can be covered by the more evident formation of periosteal lamellated 'onion-peel' reactive bone (Fig. 209.8). In more advanced stages the extraosseous soft tissues may be involved, provoking spicular, perpendicular reactive bone formation of 'sunburst' appearance, as in an osteosarcoma.

Diagnostic problems may be encountered on radiography of some benign lesions such as osteomyelitis or eosinophilic granuloma. The most common diagnostic problem may be presented by osteosarcomas, especially when localized in the diaphysis. On microscopic examination, diagnostic problems may be encountered with metastatic neuroblastomas, which are more common in children under 5 years of age. However, in neuroblastomas, the presence of neurosecretory granules and neurofibrils can be observed under the electron microscope.

Management

Currently, the treatment of choice is intensive preoperative chemotherapy followed by surgery, local radiation and postoperative chemotherapy for 12 months. Surgical treatment involves problems related to the age of the patient. Prosthetic replacement or arthrodesis are less acceptable during childhood. The use of bone grafts is not advised if irradiation must follow surgery. Sometimes, particularly in small children and in sites distal to the knee, the best type of surgery is amputation.

Before chemotherapy was used, the prognosis of Ewing's sarcoma was very poor. The 10-year survival rate was less than 5%. Since the introduction of chemotherapy, the 5-year survival percentage has increased to 50%. However, local recurrence and metastasis may be observed after several years.

PRIMARY NEUROECTODERMAL TUMOR OF BONE

World Health Organization definition

Primary neuroectodermal tumor of bone is a rare and highly malignant tumor that morphologically resembles the peripheral neuroepithelioma of soft tissues.

The clinical, radiologic and histologic features resemble Ewing's sarcoma. The distinction between Ewing's sarcoma, primary neuroectodermal tumor of bone and other small round-cell sarcomas has been based particularly on the results of immunohistochemical staining with neuron-specific enolase (NSE) and other neural markers (HNK-1, HBA-7/1, etc.), although positive staining is also seen in a number of

Ewing's sarcomas. Both tumors share the presence of a reciprocal 11;22 chromosome translocation[27–29].

MALIGNANT LYMPHOMA OF BONE

World Health Organization definition

In malignant lymphoma, the tumor cells are usually round and pleomorphic and may have well-defined cytoplasmic outlines; many of their nuclei are indented or horseshoe-shaped and have prominent nucleoli. In most cases, numerous reticulin fibers are present and are distributed uniformly between the tumor cells[30].

Epidemiology

Primary malignant lymphoma in bone comprises nearly 3% of malignant bone tumors. Men appear to be involved more frequently than women (2–3:1–2). It is a tumor that occurs during adult and advanced age, with most cases observed after age 25–30 years. There is a predilection for the axial skeleton, especially the ilium, vertebrae and scapula, and for long tubular bones, particularly the femur and tibia.

Clinical features

One of the most striking clinical features is the general well-being of the patient, which is very different from the systemic form of lymphoma. The main symptom is pain of variable intensity, generally accompanied by a swelling of the involved bone and local tenderness. The onset is often insidious. Pathologic fracture is frequent in most series. Neurologic symptoms may occur in cases localized in the vertebrae.

The course of the disease is varied and unpredictable. If treated, healing may occur, even in cases with metastases in the regional lymph nodes. In other cases, systemic diffusion follows.

Investigation and differential diagnosis

The radiographic picture resembles that of Ewing's sarcoma. The first changes are usually one or more small areas of bone destruction arising in the metaphysis or diaphysis but rarely in the epiphysis. Later, the radiolucent lesions become confluent; often the bone appears motheaten. Alongside the osteolysis, areas of increased opacity caused by reactive bone formation may be observed. Generally, the cortex is partially or completely destroyed, producing slight periosteal new bone formation. Nevertheless, a typical 'onion-peel' reaction or a 'sunburst' pattern is infrequent. Pathologic fractures occur quite frequently. Destruction of the cortex is invariably accompanied by a soft tissue mass, which can be visualized well by bone scan and MRI.

Lymphography is necessary for study of the regional lymph nodes. Systemic disease can be excluded by total bone scan and by hepatic and splenic isotope scans. On microscopic examination, differential diagnosis with undifferentiated metastatic carcinomas and with poorly differentiated myelomas is sometimes difficult. Biochemical findings may facilitate the diagnosis.

Management

Radiation therapy associated with cyclical and long-lasting combination chemotherapy is the treatment of choice. The 10-year survival rate is 60–80%.

MYELOMA

World Health Organization definition

A myeloma is a malignant tumor, usually showing multiple or diffuse bone involvement, characterized by round cells related to plasma cells but showing varying degrees of immaturity, including atypical forms. The lesions are often associated with the presence of abnormal proteins in the blood and urine, and occasionally with the presence of amyloid or para-amyloid in the tumor tissue or other organs[31].

Epidemiology

Myelomas are the most common primary malignant bone tumors. In most series there is a predilection for men (3:2). They occur mostly in patients after 40–50 years of age and are rarely observed prior to 30 years of age. Myelomas primarily involve the bones that contain red marrow. These are the bones of the trunk, the cranium and the meta-epiphyses, particularly the hip and the shoulder.

Myelomas are primary malignant neoplasms of the bone marrow originating from the B-lymphoid cells. On gross and microscopic appearance they may be classified into several categories: multiple myeloma; disseminated myelomatosis; solitary myeloma; extraskeletal myeloma; and plasma cell leukemia.

Clinical features

The most frequent clinical symptom is bone pain, often remaining vague or not localized and generally referred to the spine. General symptoms such as asthenia, weight loss and moderate anemia are observed. Sudden intense back pain is often a sign of pathologic vertebral fracture and may be accompanied by neurologic symptoms, usually a consequence of nerve root or spinal cord compression. Pathologic fractures of other bones are frequently seen.

In advanced stages of the disease, a swelling of the superficial bones, extraskeletal myelomatous masses, hemorrhagic diathesis and hyperuricemic and hypercalcemic syndromes may be observed. The prognosis of multiple or diffuse myelomatosis is unfavorable. About 50% of patients die within 2 years of diagnosis as a result of infection, anemia, renal insufficiency or amyloidosis. The solitary myelomas have a better prognosis, although dissemination may develop after a long disease-free interval following treatment.

Investigations and differential diagnosis

Laboratory examinations are important for diagnosis of myeloma. Anemia, a high erythrocyte sedimentation rate (ESR), hyperuricemia, azotemia and hypercalcemia are common features. Examination of peripheral blood sometimes reveals a large number of white cells with a high percentage of plasma cells. Common features of plasma cell leukemia are hepatosplenomegaly and an M component in serum protein electrophoresis. Serum and urinary protein electrophoretic patterns show a peak in almost 75% of cases Immunoelectrophoresis shows a monoclonal heavy chain in about 80% and a monoclonal light chain (kappa or lambda) in about 10% of cases. Rarely, 'non-secretory' myelomas are encountered (1–2%). The study of the bone marrow by iliac biopsy is of fundamental diagnostic importance. An increase of only 10% in the number of plasma cells does not permit the diagnosis of myeloma unless several atypical plasma cells are seen, while a 30% increase is diagnostic.

The radiographic appearance of myeloma is variable depending on the clinical type. The most common picture is one of numerous, round or oval osteolytic lesions with a characteristic punched-out aspect (Fig. 209.9). In time, the osteolytic lesions may coalesce and destroy the affected bone and cortex. Sclerosis of the margin of the lesion rarely occurs except following chemo- or radiotherapy. Expansion of the thinned cortex may be seen in long and small bones such as the ribs and

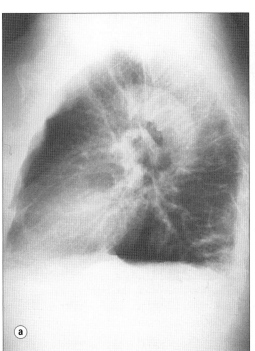
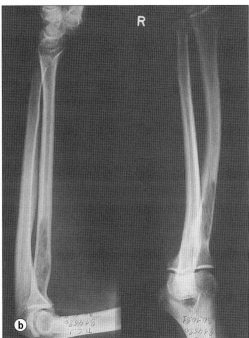
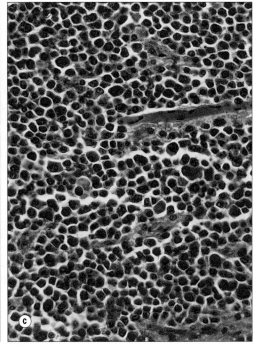

Fig. 209.9 Myeloma. (a) Lateral radiograph of the sternum and vertebrae of a 49-year-old male patient with multiple myeloma, showing destruction of the sternum and 'osteoporosis' of the vertebrae. (b) Radiograph of the right forearm – osteolytic lesions. (c) Photomicrograph of the histologic pattern of myeloma. Some pleomorphism can be seen.

the sternum, and a generalized osteopenia is encountered in cases of diffuse myelomatosis. Pathologic fractures are observed particularly in the vertebrae and the ribs. Sclerosis of the bone lesions, resembling osteoblastic metastatic lesions, is rarely described. Bone scans may be normal, even in areas with massive lesions, because it is a condition of pure osteoclastic bone resorption.

Management

Chemotherapy based on antiblastic drugs (cyclophosphamide, melphalan, vincristine, doxorubicin, etc.) associated with corticosteroids is indicated in disseminated or multiple lesions. In some cases, chemotherapy produces long-term survival. Radiotherapy is often used to relieve pain, to decrease spinal compression or to prevent pathologic fracture. Allogeneic bone marrow transplantation may be used in younger patients.

Surgery is indicated in patients with threatening spinal compression and in treatment of pathologic fractures. In localized lesions, wide excision or block resection with or without previous irradiation may be applied to bones that can be removed without appreciable loss of function.

BENIGN VASCULAR TUMORS

Hemangioma

World Health Organization definition

A hemangioma is a benign lesion consisting of newly formed blood vessels of either a capillary or cavernous type[32].

Epidemiology

Cases with clinical features are rare. Some publications have reported a frequency as high as 60% of all bone tumors. There is no sex predominance in most series and the lesions can be found in all age groups. The most common sites are the spine and the cranium and more rarely in some long or short bones. Sometimes multiple disseminated lesions are found.

Clinical features

Most hemangiomas are asymptomatic. In cranial or long bones, moderate pain or swelling may be noted. In vertebral lesions, neurologic features caused by spinal compression may occasionally occur.

Investigations and differential diagnosis

The radiographic appearance of vertebral lesions is often characteristic, showing rarefaction with prominent vertical striations or a honeycomb appearance. In cranial and long bones the radiographic aspect is uncharacteristic. A radiolucent defect without periosteal reaction, sometimes with a honeycombed area, may be observed. 'Sunburst' or 'sunray' patterns on the skull may be noted. Differential diagnosis with osteosarcoma may be difficult.

Management

Most hemangiomas of the vertebrae are asymptomatic and do not require treatment. Surgery may be necessary in cases with neurologic symptoms or pain. Radiotherapy is sometimes used for relief of pain. Because of diagnostic difficulties hemangiomas of the skull or long bones are best treated by *en bloc* resection.

Lymphangioma

A lymphangioma is a benign lesion consisting of newly formed lymph vessels, usually in the form of dilated cystic spaces. Lymphangiomas of bone are extremely rare and frequently diffuse or multiple. They are probably hamartomas or vascular malformations.

Glomus tumor

A glomus tumor is a benign lesion consisting of rounded uniform cells intimately associated with vascular structures and probably derived from the neuromyoarterial glomus. Glomus tumors of bone are very rare. All are located in a terminal phalanx. They are associated with severe pain. Radiologically they show an osteolytic, well-delineated lesion.

INTERMEDIATE VASCULAR TUMORS

Hemangioendothelioma

An hemangioendothelioma is an aggressive but non-metastasizing tumor characterized by the presence of solid cell cords and vascular endothelial structures. The cells are often prominent and plump but the frankly malignant features of angiosarcoma are lacking[33]. Hemangioendothelioma is a rare tumor, affecting more men than women (3:2). Any age group and any skeletal region may be affected. Most patients complain of pain and/or swelling.

Radiographically, the lesions are osteolytic, sometimes showing permeation with expansion or destruction of the cortex. The evolution of hemangioendotheliomas is unpredictable. They may recur after excision but rarely metastasize. Treatment consists of wide excision or amputation in cases of multiple lesions.

Hemangiopericytoma

This is a low grade malignant tumor characterized by a pattern of vascular spaces lined by a single layer of endothelial cells surrounded by zones of proliferating cells (Fig. 209.10)[34].

It is a rare tumor found in multiple skeletal locations. Hemangiopericytoma structures are observed in several other bone tumors, such as osteosarcomas, fibrosarcomas and in mesenchymal chondrosarcomas. Their behavior is unpredictable and resection is the treatment indicated.

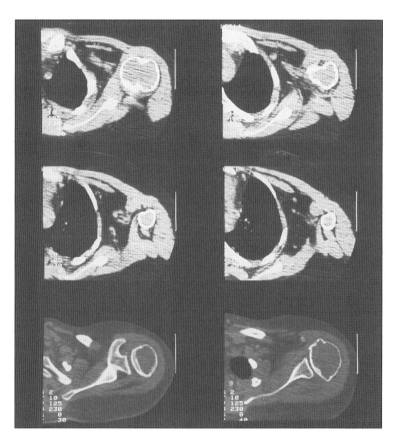

Fig. 209.10 Hemangiopericytoma of bone. CT scan showing an osteolytic lesion, with thinning and destruction of the cortices and some extension into the soft tissues.

MALIGNANT VASCULAR TUMORS

Angiosarcoma

This is a malignant tumor characterized by the formation of irregular vascular channels, lined by one or more layers of atypical endothelial cells, often of immature appearance, and accompanied by solid masses of poorly differentiated or anaplastic tissue.

The clinical, radiographic and pathologic features are similar to those of the other malignant vascular tumors. Angiosarcomas appear to be even rarer than the better differentiated vascular tumors. Multifocal lesions occur in some cases. The prognosis is more ominous. Radical surgery is the treatment of choice. Most patients die less than 2 years after surgery.

BENIGN CONNECTIVE TISSUE TUMORS

Benign fibrous histiocytoma

World Health Organization definition

A benign lesion characterized by the presence of spindle-celled fibrous tissue with a storiform pattern and containing a variable number of multinucleated giant cells, hemosiderin pigment and lipid-bearing histiocytes.

Benign fibrous histiocytoma is a rare lesion, histologically similar to that of non-ossifying fibroma but clinically and radiologically different. Most patients are adults, between 15 and 60 years old. The lesion is generally confined to the diaphysis or epiphysis of long bones.

Clinical features

Pain, without evidence of fracture, is almost always present.

Investigations and differential diagnosis

Radiologically, benign fibrous histiocytoma shows a well-defined radiolucent, sometimes slightly expanding lesion with sclerotic borders. The lesion can be located centrally or eccentrically. If present in the epiphysis, differential diagnosis with a grade 1 giant-cell tumor may be extremely difficult.

Management

En bloc excision is the treatment of choice.

Lipoma

Lipoma is a benign tumor made up exclusively of mature adipose tissue and showing no evidence of cellular atypism.

There are two types of lipoma: parosteal and intraosseous. It is a rare tumor, without predilection for any age group, mostly involving the long bones of the leg. Radiologically, a radiolucent, well-delineated cystic area is mostly observed. Treatment consists of excision of the tumor.

INTERMEDIATE CONNECTIVE TISSUE TUMORS

Desmoplastic fibroma

World Health Organization definition

Desmoplastic fibroma is a benign tumor characterized by the formation of abundant collagen fibers by the tumor cells. The tissue is poorly cellular and nuclei are ovoid or elongated. The cellularity, pleomorphism and mitotic activity noted in fibrosarcomas are lacking.

It is a rare tumor, mostly found in young adults, and frequently localized in long or flat bones. The metaphysis is mostly affected.

Clinical features

Pain or swelling are the most common complaints, sometimes present long before diagnosis. A pathologic fracture may occur.

Investigations and differential diagnosis

Radiographs generally show an extensive radiolucent lesion, often expanding into the thinned cortex. A trabeculated pattern may be observed. Differential diagnosis with osteoblastomas, fibrous dysplasia and well-differentiated fibrosarcomas is sometimes difficult.

Management

The treatment of choice is complete *en bloc* resection, since recurrences after incomplete excision have been reported.

MALIGNANT CONNECTIVE TISSUE TUMORS

Fibrosarcoma

World Health Organization definition

A fibrosarcoma is a malignant tumor characterized by the formation of interlacing bundles of collagen fibers and by the absence of other types of histological differentiation, such as the formation of cartilage or bone.

Epidemiology

Fibrosarcomas are less frequent than osteosarcomas or chondrosarcomas. Both sexes are equally affected in the age range between 20–60 years. The most common locations are in the metaphysis or epiphysis of the femur and tibia (50%). The skull and jaws are also frequently involved.

Clinical features

The most common complaint is pain and swelling. Usually there is a long delay before diagnosis, particularly in slow-growing lesions. Pathologic fracture is a frequent complication.

Investigations and differential diagnosis

Radiologically the tumor is characterized by a radiolucent, often permeative lesion with ill-defined borders, most frequently located in the metaphyseal region with extension into the epiphysis or the diaphysis. Thinning, expansion and disruption of the cortex may be observed according to the rate of growth. In slow-growing lesions, differential diagnosis from a giant cell tumor, chondromyxoid fibroma or dermoplastic fibroma is sometimes difficult. Rapidly growing fibrosarcomas have to be differentiated from osteosarcomas, lymphomas, metastases and myelomas. Arteriography, bone scan, CT and MRI are indicated for evaluation of the extension of the tumor.

Management

According to the histologic grade and the extent of soft tissue invasion, wide resection or radical surgery is indicated. Radiotherapy is indicated only as a palliative measure because fibrosarcomas are resistant. Cyclical and combined chemotherapy using the same protocols as those used for osteosarcomas may be attempted in high-risk cases and in younger patients.

Malignant fibrous histiocytoma

Definition

There is no existing WHO definition of malignant fibrous histiocytoma. However, the same histologic criteria as for the diagnosis of malignant fibrous histiocytoma of the soft tissues are used: bundles of fibers and spindle-shaped, fibroblast-like cells in a uniform pattern; rounded cells with features of histiocytes; and infiltration of inflammatory cells, predominantly lymphocytes[35].

Epidemiology

Malignant fibrous histiocytoma of bone has a predilection for men of adult to advanced age. The long bones such as the femur, the tibia and the humerus are mostly affected, especially in the metaphyseal region.

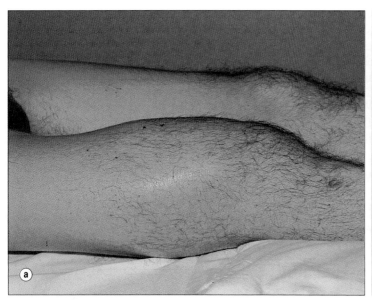

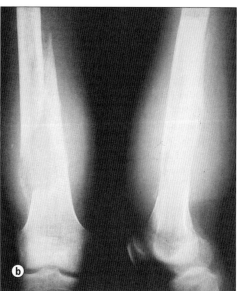

Fig. 209.11 Malignant fibrous histiocytoma. (a) Photograph of the right leg of a 24-year-old male patient admitted because of fracture. (b) Anteroposterior and lateral radiographs of the right femur showing an oblique fracture through an extensive osteolytic lesion.

Clinical features

The most common complaints are pain and swelling, usually of short duration at diagnosis (Fig. 209.11a).

Investigations and differential diagnosis

Radiologically, the lesion is radiolucent with ill-defined borders, mostly localized in the metaphyseal region, usually destroying the cortex and penetrating into the soft tissues. A significant periosteal reaction is usually lacking (Fig. 209.11b). Differential diagnosis with osteosarcoma and fibrosarcoma is frequently difficult. Bone scan (Fig. 209.13), CAT scan and MRI are helpful for evaluation of the intramedullary and extraosseous extension of the tumor.

Management

Pre- and postoperative chemotherapy, as used for osteosarcomas, and wide or radical resection of the tumor is the treatment of choice, which has substantially improved survival. Previously, treatment with curative surgery or irradiation produced only a 2-year survival rate.

OTHER TUMORS

Chordoma

A chordoma is a rare malignant tumor characterized by a lobular arrangement of tissue, which is usually made up of highly vacuolated cells ('physaliphorous cells') and mucoid intercellular material. These tumors are restricted to the axial skeleton[36].

The clinical symptoms vary according to the location (Fig. 209.13). Radiologically, the constant feature of chordoma is a lytic lesion with irregular scalloped margins, associated in 50% of cases with

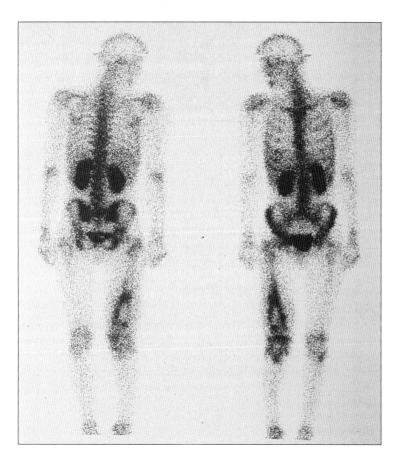

Fig. 209.12 Malignant fibrous histiocytoma. Bone scintigraph demonstrating increased uptake of the tracer around the osteolytic lesion.

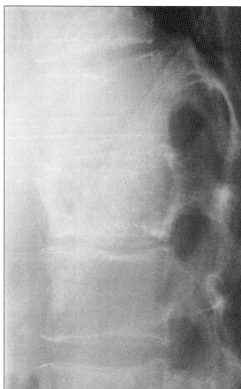

Fig. 209.13 Chordoma. Lateral radiograph of T12, showing an osteolytic lesion with irregular scalloped margins, intratumoral calcifications and extension of the tumor into the spinal space.

intratumoral calcifications. Wide resection is the treatment of choice. In inoperable cases, high-dose radiation may be applied[36].

Adamantinoma

An adamantinoma is a rare malignant, or at least locally malignant, tumor characterized by the presence of circumscribed masses of apparent epithelial cells surrounded by spindle-cell tissue[37,38]. Most cases involve the tibia, although localizations in the fibula, ulna, femur, radius and humerus are observed. The first symptoms are usually complaints of localized swelling or enlargement of the involved bone.

Radiologically, an adamantinoma shows a radiolucent, often well-delineated elongated lesion with osteolytic areas of different sizes, separated by slightly sclerotic bone. The lesion may be located centrally, as is more often the case, moderately expanding the cortex. Wide resection of the tumor and reconstruction by means of auto- or allografts and solid osteosynthesis is the treatment of choice[37,38].

REFERENCES

1. Mankin HJ, Mankin CJ, Simon MA. The hazards of the biopsy, revisited. Members of the Musculoskeletal Tumor Society. J Bone Jt Surg 1996; 78A : 656–663
2. Virchow R. Die krankhaften Geschwulste, vol 2. Berlin: Hirschwald; 1864–65.
3. Codman EA. The registry of cases of bone sarcoma. Surg Gynecol Obstet 1922; 34: 335–343.
4. Jaffe HL. Tumors and tumorous conditions of the bones and joints. Philadelphia, PA: Lea & Febiger; 1958.
5. Schajowicz F. Tumors and tumorlike lesions of bone, 2nd ed. Berlin: Springer-Verlag; 1994.
6. Jaffe HL. 'Osteoid osteoma'. A benign osteoblastic tumor composed of osteoid and atypical bone. Arch Surg 1935; 31: 709–728.
7. Witt JD, Hall-Craggs MA, Ripley P et al. Interstitial photocoagulation for the treatment of osteoid osteoma J Bone Jt Surg 2000; 82B; 1125-1128
8. Jaffe HL. Benign osteoblastoma. Bull Hosp Joint Dis 1956; 17: 141–151.
9. Unni KK, Dahlin DC, Beabout JW, Ivins JC. Parosteal osteogenic sarcoma. Cancer 1976; 37: 2466–2475.
10. Enneking WF, Spanier SS, Goodman MA. Current concepts review: the surgical staging of musculoskeletal sarcoma. J Bone Jt Surg 1980; 62A: 1027–1030.
11. Unni KK, Dahlin DC, Beabout JW. Periosteal osteogenic sarcoma. Cancer 1976; 37: 2476–2485.
12. Farr GH, Huvos AG. Juxtacortical osteogenic sarcoma. An analysis of fourteen cases. J Bone Joint Surg 1972; 54A: 1205–1216.
13. Schajowicz F, Lemos D. Malignant osteoblastoma. J Bone Joint Surg 1976; 58B: 202–211.
14. Lichtenstein L, Hall JF. Periosteal chondroma. A distinctive benign cartilage tumor. J Bone Joint Surg 1952; 34: 691–697.
15. Jaffe HL. Juxtacortical chondroma. Bull Hosp Joint Dis 1956; 17: 20–29.
16. Codman EA. Epiphyseal chondromatous giant-cell tumors of the upper end of the humerus. Surg Gynecol Obstet 1931; 52: 543–548.
17. Jaffe HL, Lichtenstein L. Benign chondroblastoma of bone. A reinterpretation of the so-called calcifying or chondromatous giant cell tumor. Am J Pathol 1942; 18: 969–983.
18. Huvos A, Marcove R, Erlandson R, Mike MD. Chondroblastoma of bone. Cancer 1972; 29: 760–771.
19. Jaffe HL, Lichtenstein L. Chondromyxoid fibroma of bone; a distinctive benign tumor likely to be mistaken especially for chondrosarcoma. Arch Pathol 1948; 45: 541–551.
20. Phemister DV. Chondrosarcoma of bone. Surg Gynecol Obstet 1930; 50: 216–233.
21. Lichtenstein L, Jaffe HL. Chondrosarcoma of bone. Am J Pathol 1943; 19: 553–589.
22. Lichtenstein L. Tumors of periosteal origin. Cancer 1955; 8: 1060–1069.
23. Lichtenstein L, Bernstein D. Unusual benign and malignant chondroid tumors of bone. Cancer 1959; 12: 1142–1157.
24. Unni KK, Dahlin DC, Beabout JW, Sim JH. Chondrosarcoma clear cell variant. A report of sixteen cases. J Bone Joint Surg 1976; 58: 676–683.
25. Bloodgood JC. Benign giant cell tumor of bone. Its diagnosis and conservative treatment. Am J Surg 1923; 7: 105–116.
26. Ewing J. The classification and treatment of bone sarcoma. Cancer. New York: Wood; 1928: 365.
27. Jaffe R, Santamaria M, Yunis EJ et al. The neuroectodermal tumor of bone. Am J Surg Pathol 1984; 8: 885–898.
28. Llombart-Bosch A, Lacombe MJ, Peydro-Olaya A et al. Malignant peripheral neuroectodermal tumors of bone other than Askin's neoplasm: characterization of 14 new cases of immunohistochemistry and electro microscopy. Virchows Arch A 1988; 412: 421.
29. Aurias A, Rimbaut C, Buffe D et al. A. Translocation involving chromosome 22 in Ewing's sarcoma: a cytogenetic study of four fresh tumors. Cancer Genet Cytogenet 1984; 12: 21.
30. Parker F Jr, Jackson H Jr. Primary reticulum cell sarcoma of bone. Surg Gynecol Obstet 1939; 68: 45–53.
31. Kahler O. Zur Symptomatologie des multiplen Myeloms. Wien Med Presse 1889; 30: 209–13; 253–255.
32. Topfer D. Zur Kenntnis der Wirbelangiome. Frankf Z Pathol 1928; 36: 337–345.
33. Hartmann WH, Stewart FW. Hemangioendothelioma of bone. Unusual tumor characterized by indolent course. Cancer 1962; 15: 846–854.
34. Marcial-Rojas RA. Primary hemangiopericytoma of bone. Review of the literature and report of the first case with metastases. Cancer 1960; 13: 308–311.
35. Feldman F, Norman D. Intra- and extra-osseous malignant histiocytoma (malignant fibrous xanthoma). Radiology 1972; 104: 497–508.
36. Stewart MJ, Morin JE. Chordoma: a review with report of a new sacrococcygeal case. J Pathol Bacteriol 1926; 29: 41–60.
37. Fisher B. Uber ein primäres Adamantinom der Tibia. Frankf Z Pathol 1913; 12: 422–441.
38. Maier C. Ein primäres myelogenes Platten-Epithelcarcinoma der Ulna. Bruns Betr Chir 1900; 26: 552–566.

INDEX

Page numbers in **bold** refer to major discussions in the text, and usually include aspects such as epidemiology, clinical features, diagnosis, pathology and treatment.
Page numbers in followed by (i) refer to pages on which tables/figures are to be found.
vs denotes *differential diagnosis, or comparisons*
This index is arranged in *letter-by-letter order*, whereby hyphens and spaces between words are ignored in the alphabetization. Terms in brackets are also ignored from initial alphabetization.
Cross-references in *italics* are either general cross-references (e.g. *see also specific drugs*), or refer to subentries within the same main entry .
Readers are advised that the *categorization* inherent in the contents list is not specifically replicated in the index, owing to space constraints.
Owing to divergent views over *juvenile idiopathic arthritis/juvenile rheumatoid arthritis/juvenile inflammatory arthritis*, entries have mostly been kept to the terminology preferred by individual authors. Readers are advised to refer to all variant arthritis forms beginning *juvenile.*

Abbreviations

ACR - American College of Rheumatology
ANCA - antineutrophil cytoplasmic antibodies
AS - ankylosing spondylitis
ARA - American Rheumatism Association
BCP - basic calcium phosphate

CPPD - calcium pyrophosphate dihydrate
ENT - ear, nose and throat
ESR - erythrocyte sedimentation rate
GFR - glomerular filtration rate
HBV - hepatitis B virus

HCV - hepatitis C virus
OA - osteoarthritis
RA - rheumatoid arthritis
SLE - systemic lupus erythematosus

A

A77 1726, leflunomide metabolite 431, 432(i)
AA amyloidosis *see* amyloidosis, AA
abdominal aneurysm
  low back pain 595
  see also aortic aneurysm
abdominal binder (corset) 523–524
abdominal muscles, role in lumbar spine stability during lifting 563
abdominal pain 325
  adult Still's disease 794–795
  arthritis with 325(i)
  familial Mediterranean fever (FMF) 1719
  Henoch–Schönlein purpura 1676
    management 1679
  hyper-IgD with periodic fever syndrome 1727
  inflammatory bowel disease 326
  rheumatic fever 1137
  TNF-receptor-associated periodic syndrome (TRAPS) 1723
abdominal symptoms 325
  see also gastrointestinal disease/involvement
abductor hallucis muscle, hypertrophy 723
abductor pollicis longus, de Quervain's stenosing tenosynovitis 646, 647
abnormalities, definition 178
abortifacient, methotrexate 425, 502
abortion, spontaneous
  antiphospholipid antibodies and 1450
  antiphospholipid syndrome 1445, 1446, 1449, 1450, 1451
  in SLE pregnancy 1429, 1446
abrasion arthroplasty 249
abrasion chondroplasty 1858
abscess
  Brodie's 1059, 1059(i)
  cold (tuberculous) 1077
  corneal 299, 299(i)
  paraspinal 1078
acanthocytes, in urine 338, 338(i)
acanthosis nigricans, juvenile dermatomyositis and 1020, 1021(i)
accelerations 77, **77**
accessory navicular syndrome 735(i)
ACE inhibitors 151
  hypertension with lupus nephritis 1413
  systemic sclerosis 1460, 1504
    renal disease 1502
acetabular dysplasia, hip osteoarthritis after 1788, 1818
acetabular labrum 651
acetabulum
  anatomy 651, 652(i)
  changes in Legg–Calvé–Perthes disease 988
  development 987
  protrusion *see* protrusio acetabuli deformity
acetaminophen
  community use in rheumatic disease 358, 358(i)
  hepatotoxicity 374
  low back pain management 609
  neck pain treatment 577
  pain management 374
  preoperative pain relief 533
  renal complications 345
  use in osteoarthritis 1856
N-acetyl-β-D-glucosaminidase (NAG)
  excretion, Henoch–Schönlein purpura 1680
  urinary testing 337
acetyl-CoA dehydrogenase deficiency 1568
acetylsalicylic acid (ASA) *see* aspirin
Achilles bursitis **688**, 741, 744
Achilles reflex (ankle jerk), low back pain examination 588
Achilles tendinitis **688**
  children 983
  insertional 688
  nodules in 285
Achilles tendinopathy 740–741
  deep tendinosis 741
  paratendinitis 740
Achilles tendon 682
  calcification 1940, 1941(i)

central necrosis 741(i)
  composition 1185
  deep tendinosis 741
  disorders **688**
  enthesis 1185, 1185(i).
  enthesitis
    ankylosing spondylitis 1163
    psoriatic arthritis 1245(i)
  rupture **688**, 741
    partial 688
    sports injuries 735
  superficial injury (paratendinitis) 740
  xanthomatosis 1988(i)
achondrogenesis 1803
  type 1B 2182
achondroplasia 1819–1820, 2168, **2181–2182**
  cervical spinal cord stenosis 2179
  management 2181
acid-fast bacilli 1044–1045
acid maltase deficiency 1568
  myositis *vs* 1544
acidosis
  management in rickets/osteomalacia 2127
  renal tubular *see* renal tubular acidosis
acid phosphatase 2045
  bone 2045
  tartrate-resistant, plasma levels, bone resorption marker 2045
Acinetobacter 1041
acne conglobata 287
acne fulminans 287
acne rosacea, differential diagnosis 283(i), 284(i)
ACR improvement criteria 896, 897
acroasphyxia *see* Raynaud's phenomenon
acrodermatitis, Lyme disease 1093–1094
acrodermatitis chronica atrophicans 1094
acrolein 440
  hemorrhagic cystitis 443
acromegaly **1967–1972**
  clinical features 1967–1971
    arthropathy 1967, 1969–1971, 1970(i)
    backache 1967
    diabetes development 1967
    myopathy 1967
    neuropathy 1967
    osteoporosis 1968–1969
    skin thickening 1969, 1969(i)
    skull abnormalities 1968, 1968(i)
    vertebral abnormalities 1967, 1968, 1969(i)
  definition 1967
  diagnosis 1967
    hand examination 1970, 1970(i)
  differential diagnosis 1971
    DISH syndrome 1865, 1968, 1971
  DISH-type features 1866
  etiopathogenesis 1971
  facial appearance 1967, 1968(i)
  historical aspects 1967
  management 1971
  radiologic features 1967–1969, 1968(i), 1969(i)
  radiologic–pathologic correlation 1968(i)
acromioclavicular joint
  anatomy 617
  aspiration/injection therapy 240
  dislocation 627
  examination 618
    adduction stress test 619, 619(i)
  osteoarthritis 627–628, 1796
  pain, examination 618
  pain referred to neck 570
  rheumatoid arthritis 773, 803
  strapping and stabilization 627
  trauma 627
acromioclavicular syndromes 627–628
acromion, 'bearded' 1173
acropachy 1763, 1764
  see also hypertrophic osteoarthropathy (HOA)
ACTH 138–139, 138(i)
actinic degeneration, giant cell arteritis association 1623
Actinobacillus 1043–1044
Actinomyces 1042
activated protein C 1598
  activation mechanism 1450, 1450(i)

angiogenesis stimulation 853
activator protein-1 *see* AP-1 proteins
activities of daily living (ADL)
  ankylosing spondylitis, occupational therapy 1213–1214
  compensation for limitations 528(i)
  impairment
    hip fractures in osteoporosis 2083
    history-taking 174
    juvenile idiopathic arthritis 1034, 1034(i)
    wrist fractures in osteoporosis 2082
  rheumatoid arthritis evaluation 766(i), 778(i)
activity, ICF model 517, 517(i)
acupressure 507
  osteoarthritis 1855
acupuncture **506–509**
  analgesia 507, 508
  evidence 507–509
  fibromyalgia 507
  licensing and training (USA) 513(i)
  low back pain 507–508, 610
  meridian theory 507, 508(i)
  osteoarthritis 507, 509, 1855
  philosophy and history 506–507
  randomized controlled trial difficulties 508–509
  rheumatoid arthritis 508
  safety 509
  treatment method 507, 508(i)
acute febrile neutrophilic dermatosis *see* Sweet's syndrome
acute hemorrhagic edema (AHE) of childhood
  clinical features 1691
  Henoch–Schönlein purpura *vs* 1677, 1691
acute lupus pneumonitis, in SLE 322
acute phase proteins **199–201**
  applications 200–201
  clinical relevance 200
  definition 199
  negative reactants 200
  positive reactants 199
  proteins included 199
  rheumatic fever 1137
  undifferentiated spondyloarthropathies 329
  use of multiple tests 200
  see also C-reactive protein (CRP); erythrocyte sedimentation rate (ESR)
acute phase response 199
acylmonoglucuronide 1932
adalimumab 471–472
  Crohn's disease 472
  injection site reactions 472
  monotherapy studies 472
  rheumatoid arthritis 471–472
adamantioma 2199
ADAM proteinases 1806
  cartilage matrix 129
Adams, R., rheumatoid arthritis drawing 753(i)
ADAM-TD4 gene 1806
ADAM-TD5 gene 1806
ADAM-TS 1806
adaptive immunity *see* immune system
addressin, lymphocyte migration 122–123
adducter tendinitis 660
adductor tendon injuries, sports-related 745
ademalysins 487
adenine, structure 1904(i)
adenine phosphoribosyl transferase (APRT) 1906
  deficiency 1907
adenosine, anti-inflammatory effects of methotrexate 418
adenosine A_1 receptor, methotrexate-induced nodulosis 425
adenosine deaminase (ADA) 1906
adenosine triphosphate (ATP), pyrophosphate metabolism and 1944
S-adenosyl-methionine *see* S-adenosyl-methionine (SAM-e)
adenovirus
  gene transfer by 92
    cytokine inhibitors 831
  myositis etiology 1533
adhesion molecules *see* cell adhesion molecules
adhesive capsulitis, shoulder *see* capsulitis (adhesive) of shoulder

adipocytes
  hypertrophy, osteonecrosis pathogenesis 1888
  necrotic 1887(i)
  normal 1887(i)
adipose tissue, inflammation *see* panniculitis
adjuvant-induced arthritis (AIA) 136, 826, **1049**, 2041
  features 1049
  heat shock proteins 1048, 1049
  mechanisms 826(i), 844, 844(i).
  mycobacterial cell wall and 1044, 1049
adolescence
  acute bacterial infections (musculoskeletal) 979
  fibromyalgia 1024
  knee pain 668–670
  menisci (knee) injuries 983
  patellofemoral syndrome 983
  shin splints 983
  tendon injuries 735
α-adrenoceptor, reflex sympathetic dystrophy 729
adrenocorticotropic hormone (ACTH), production/effects in inflammation 138–139, 138(i)
Adson maneuver 714(i)
  in thoracic outlet syndrome 714, 714(i)
adult learning 363
adult-onset Still's disease *see* Still's disease, adult-onset
advanced practice nurse, responsibilities in rheumatic disease care 938(i)
adverse drug reactions (ADR) *see individual drugs/drug groups*
adverse reactions, measurement 26
adynamic bone disease *see* renal bone disease, adynamic
AECA *see* antiendothelial cell antibodies
aerobic exercise *see* exercise, aerobic
affected sibling pairs (ASP) 103, 103(i)
affective disorders
  pain causing 373
  see also depression
'affective spectrum disorders' 707
afferent nerve fibers
  in joint, bone and muscle 370, 371
  mechanically insensitive (MIAs) 370, 371
AG4263 peptide, vaccine 451
agammaglobulinemia, clinical features 1126
age/aging
  bone changes *see* bone, age-related changes
  cartilage changes *see* articular cartilage
  chest expansion changes 1222(i)
  chondrocytes changes 1805
  collagen changes 2034
  CPPD deposition disease 1945
  creatinine clearance 340(i)
  dialysis arthropathy 1986
  disease susceptibility 15–16
  extracellular matrix changes 1803
  fracture incidence 2063, 2064, 2078(i)
  giant cell arteritis etiology and 1630, 1631
  glomerular filtration rate decrease 339
  'gompertization' 2063
  inorganic pyrophosphate formation 1944
  intervertebral disc changes 67
  joint remodelling 1837, 1844
  low back pain 583, 584(i)
  musculoskeletal disorders prevalence 37(i), 39
  musculoskeletal tissue changes 67
  neck pain 567
  nucleus pulposus changes 67, 549
  osteoarthritis incidence 1786(i)
  osteoarthritis *vs* 1805–1806, 1805(i)
  polymyalgia rheumatica etiology 1630
  temporal arteries changes 1629
  TGF-β *vs* osteoarthritis 1805–1806
Agency for Health Care Policy and Research (AHCPR), acute low back pain 590
aggrecan 873, 1803
  ankylosing spondylitis pathogenesis 1185, 1185(i)
  as target antigen (G1 domain) 1185
  autoantibodies, rheumatoid arthritis 835, 844
  cartilage 129, 132(i), 1803
    arthritis model 825–826
  degradation 1806
  depletion 1806
    osteoarthritis 1806
  osteoarthritis pathogenesis 1806, 1812
  structure 1804(i)
  turnover 132(i), 1806

INDEX

angioedema
'allergic,' hereditary angioedema *vs* 211
hereditary 211, 1331–1332
angioendotheliomatosis, CNS vasculitis *vs* 1713
angiogenesis 1594
corneal, assay 1594(i)
definition 851
factors promoting 1594–1595
factors promoting in arthritis 852–853, 852(i)
hypoxia 857
rheumatoid arthritis 857
growth factors 1594
inhibitors *see* anti-angiogenic agents
mechanisms 1594
processes involved 851–852, 852(i)
regulation 1594, 1595
in arthritis 852
rheumatoid arthritis **851–854**
roles in physiology/pathology 851, 851(i)
tumors 851
angiogenic factors 852–853
angiography
benign angiopathy of CNS 1708, 1708(i), 1709
granulomatous angiitis of CNS 1706
hemophilic arthropathy 1992, 1993(i)
polyarteritis nodosa 1614, 1617
reversibility, benign angiopathy of CNS 1712
stroke-like syndromes 1710
superselective, osteonecrosis 1881
vasculitis 1589
angioimmunoblastic lymphadenopathy (AILD) 281, **1753**
angioimmunolymphoproliferative lesions (AIL), CNS vasculitis due to 1713
angiopathy, benign, of CNS *see* benign angiopathy of CNS (BACNS)
angioplasty, percutaneous transluminal, Takayasu's arteritis 1663
angiopoietins 1594
angiosarcoma 2197
angiostatin 1595
antiangiogenic activity 853, 1595
angiotensin-1 converting enzyme (ACE), in sarcoidosis 1737, 1740
angiotensin-converting enzyme (ACE) inhibitors *see* ACE inhibitors
angiotensin II antagonists
Raynaud's phenomenon management 1498(i), 1511
uricosuric effects 1914
animal models
ANCA-associated vasculitis (AAV) 1604–1605
ankylosing spondylitis, target antigens 1185
antiarthritis treatment development 830–831
gene therapy 831
inflammatory cytokine inhibition 830–831
tolerance induction 831
arthritis **1049–1050,** 1049(i)
adjuvant-induced *see* adjuvant-induced arthritis (AIA)
anti-A2/RA33 antibodies 838–839
antigen-induced 826
antigen persistence inducing 827–828
bacterial 1057(i)
bacterial cell wall-induced **1049–1050**
central changes in nociception 372
class II MHC genes and 829
collagen-induced *see* collagen-induced arthritis
gene regulation of specific models 829(i)
glucose-6-phosphate isomerase role 844, 844(i)
hsp60 molecular mimicry 844
IL-1 causing 865
immunoregulation 829–830
leflunomide efficacy 431
lentivirus-induced 827, 827(i)
lipopolysaccharide-induced 1042–1043, 1050
mycoplasmal 827, 1045
non-MHC gene regulation 830
onset and cytokines involved 826
pristane-induced 826(i), 831
proteoglycan-induced 825–826, 825(i)
rheumatoid *see* animal models, rheumatoid arthritis
staphylococcal 826–827, 827(i), 1050
streptococcal cell walls and 827–828
TCR genes and *MIs* regulation 829–830
TNF causing 865
viral 827, 827(i)
Yersinia-associated 1050
arthritis induction mechanisms 825–829
autoimmunity to cartilage 825–826, 825(i)
gene manipulation 828–829
infectious agents 826–828
response to non-specific stimuli 826
transgenic animals 828–829
autoimmune keratitis 1771
Chlamydia trachomatis synovitis 1228
collagen-induced arthritis *see* collagen-induced arthritis
COX-1/COX-2 role in inflammation, evidence 153–154
cutaneous vasculitis 1606
enteropathic arthropathy 1271(i), 1272
genetics, association-based studies 105
giant cell arteritis 1630
gonococcal infections 1074
gout 1914
graft-*vs*-host disease 1351–1352, 1352(i)
IL-1 functions 463
lupus-like diseases 1320–1321
Lyme disease 1092–1093
myositis, central changes in nociception 372
neuropathic arthropathy (Charcot's joints) 1873
nociception 370
ossifying enthesopathy 1185
osteoarthritis *see* osteoarthritis, animal models
rheumatoid arthritis **825–832**
anticomplement therapy 453
non-T-cell depleting anti-CD4 antibodies 450
oral tolerance induction 452
SLE *see* systemic lupus erythematosus (SLE)
systemic sclerosis 1459, 1486
T-cell vaccination 451
transgenic *see* transgenic animals
see also mice; rats
anisotropic behavior, bone 81(i)
anisotropy 2039
Anitschkow cells 1131
ankle **681–692**
anatomy 681–683
bones 681(i)
capsule 681–682
ligaments and tendons 682–683, 682(i)
arthritis, examination 684
arthrodesis 539
arthroplasty 539
articular cartilage
metabolism 1810–1811
thickness 1810
bursae around 683, 683(i)
bursitis 744
corticosteroid injection therapy **242–243,** 243(i)
deformity/abnormalities
hemophilia 1993, 1993(i), 1997
skeletal dysplasia 2181, 2181(i)
disorders 688–691
examination 189(i), 684–687
anterior draw test/sign 687, 687(i)
inspection 684–685
palpation 685–686, 685(i), 686(i)
special maneuvers 686–687
hemorrhagic 'crescent' sign above 775
malalignment, juvenile idiopathic arthritis 1029
movements 189(i), 683
during gait cycle 76(i)
normal range 683, 683(i)
testing 686, 686(i)
neuropathic 1870(i)
night splinting 689
osteoarthritis 1799
pain
children 983
differential diagnosis 687–688, 687(i)
reactive arthritis 1200
referred pain 687(i)
reflex sympathetic dystrophy 728(i)
rheumatoid arthritis *see* rheumatoid arthritis (RA)
sprains 687
surgery 539
synovial hypertrophy, rheumatoid arthritis 805
tenosynovitis 684, 740
valgus 2181
ankle mortise 681
ANK protein 1944, 1944(i), 1957
ankylosing hyperostosis *see* diffuse idiopathic skeletal hyperostosis (DISH)
ankylosing spondylitis (AS) **1153–1159, 1161–1181**
age of onset 1162
in AIDS 1229
amyloidosis in 1210, 2017, 2018(i)
antigens (target)
animal models 1185
human studies 1185–1186
atlantoaxial subluxation 1169, 1169(i), 1219
autoantibodies 1170
candidate target lesion 1184–1185
anatomical predilection 1184–1185
cardiac involvement 309–310, 310(i), 1168
pathology 1209–1210
causes of death 1210
chest involvement 1164
children *see* juvenile ankylosing spondylitis
classification criteria 1150(i), 1151, 1173, 1175(i)
clinical features **1162–1170,** 1162(i)
buttock region pain 1162
cardiac features *see cardiac involvement (above)*
chronic low back pain 1162, 1176
extraskeletal 1167–1170
gastrointestinal 1168
musculoskeletal 1162–1167
neurological 1169
ocular 1167, 1168(i)
pain *see pain (below)*
pattern of joint involvement 179(i)
pulmonary *see below*
renal 1169–1170
sacroiliitis *see* sacroiliitis
skeletal sites 1161(i)
sleep disturbance and fatigue 1162–1163
stiffness 1162
see also specific joints/regions (above/below)
clinical trials
definition of short-term improvement 27–28
measurements 27–28
outcome measures 27(i)
clinical variants 1157, 1157(i)
costotransverse joints 1166
costovertebral joints 1166, 1221–1222, 1221(i), 1222(i)
C-reactive protein 1170
definition 1161
deterioration/improvement determination 1178, 1178(i), 1220–1223
chest expansion monitoring 1166, 1221–1222, 1221(i), 1222(i)
clinical measures 1178, 1221–1222, 1221(i)
enthesitis index 1222
imaging 1222, 1222(i)
patient-centred outcomes 1222–1223
questionnaires and indices 1178, 1222–1223
spinal movement 1167, 1167(i), 1222
diagnosis **1173–1176**
delayed 1173
importance of early diagnosis 1211
post-test (HLA-B27) probability 1175, 1176(i)
probability in terms of features 1175(i)
diagnostic criteria 1150(i), 1151, 1153–1154, 1153(i), 1173
European 1153, 1153(i)
New York 1153(i)
Rome 1153(i)
differential diagnosis 1176–1177
ankylosing hyperostosis 1177, 1177(i)
back pain of other causes 1176
DISH syndrome 1145, 1146, 1865
features comparisons 1174(i)
inflammatory bowel disease 331
ochronotic arthropathy 2013(i)
osteitis condensans ilii 1177
psoriatic arthritis 1250(i)
rheumatoid arthritis 1177
spinal infections 1177
spinal stenosis posture and 1177
disability 1178
diseases associated 1170, 1178, 1219
Sjögren's syndrome 1170
diskitis 1168–1169, 1220(i)
diskovertebral joint imaging 1196–1197, 1197(i)
drug therapy 1214–1217
analgesics 1214
corticosteroids 1216, 1216(i)
cyclophosphamide 1215
disease-modifying 1215–1216
immunosuppressives 1215
indications 1216
methotrexate 421, 1215
NSAID 1212, 1214–1215
NSAID choice 1214–1215
pamidronate 1215
sulfasalazine 1215
sulfasalazine efficacy 410–411, 411(i)
thalidomide 1215
TNF-α blockade 476–477, 1215–1216
employment 1178, 1213–1214
enthesitis 1163
examination 1164–1165
imaging 1172(i)
MRI 1164(i), 1170, 1171(i)
radiotherapy 1216
enthesopathy 1205, 1205(i), 1206(i)
epidemiology **1153–1159**
incidence rate 1157
prevalence *see prevalence (below)*
etiology and pathogenesis **1183–1192**
bacterial role 1190, 1229
cartilage molecule relationships 1185, 1185(i)
environmental influences 1186
future prospects 1191
HLA-B27 and *see HLA-B27 (below)*
immunological effector mechanisms 1190–1191
primary lesion evolution 1183–1184
target antigen 1185–1186
examination, musculoskeletal features 1164–1167
extraskeletal lesions, pathology **1209–1210**
eye disease 1167, 1168(i)
management 1217
familial 1176, 1186
foot 1172(i), 1200
genetics 1176, 1178, 1186, 1188, 1188(i), 1191
genome-wide scan 1228
HLA genes *see HLA associations (below)*
non-HLA-B27 genes 1228
non-HLA genes 1188, 1228
see also HLA-B27 association (below)
glenohumeral joint 1164, 1173
hand 1199
heterogeneity of disease 1178
hip involvement 1163–1164, 1164(i), 1200, 1208(i), 1220
examination 1166, 1166(i)
imaging 1173
prognostic sign 1173
testing 1166(i)
hip replacement 1178, 1220, 1220(i)
histopathology 1183–1184, 1183(i)
historical aspects **1145–1147,** 1145(i), 1146(i), 1161–1162
classification 1146
HLA association 1188(i)
non-HLA-B27 1187–1188
HLA-B27 association 211, 1149, 1154, **1175–1176, 1186–1188,** 1318
as diagnostic aid 1175–1176
discovery 1146–1147
false-positives 1175
frequency 1186, 1226
geographical/ethnic distribution 1186, 1186(i)
HLA-B*2705 1186, 1226
pathophysiological role 1188–1190, 1189(i)
prevalence/frequency 1154, 1154(i), 1175, 1176(i), 1186
racial variations 1175, 1186, 1186(i)
subtypes 1154, 1186–1187, 1225–1226
subtypes and peptide binding capability 1227
transgenic animal models 1189–1190, 1189(i)
see also HLA-B27
HLA-B27-negative 1178
HLA-B39 1228
HLA-B60 1228
imaging 601(i), 1170–1173, 1184, 1193–1194, 1193(i), 1194(i)
MRI 1184, 1184(i)
sacroiliac joint *see sacroiliac joint (below)*
spinal *see spinal involvement (below)*
immunogenetics 1186
inflammatory bowel disease association 1168, 1267, 1268, 1271
investigations **1170–1173**
imaging *see imaging (above)*
laboratory tests 1170
juvenile *see* juvenile ankylosing spondylitis
Klebsiella pneumoniae association 1271
knee 1164
last-joint syndrome 1219, 1219(i), 1220, 1220(i)
life span 1178–1179
malignant disease in 1210
management **1211–1224**
advice and information sources 1211
alternative therapy 1214
breathing exercises 1213, 1217
daily exercise 1213
drug therapy *see drug therapy (above)*
education program 1212–1213
of enthesopathy 1212
hip replacement 1178, 1220, 1220(i)
hydrotherapy 1212
intensive physical therapy 1213
motivation for exercise 1213
multidisciplinary team 521, 1213
objectives 1211
occupational therapy 1213–1214
of osteoporosis 1217
pain relief 1212
patient-run groups 1213
physical therapy 1211–1213, 1212(i), 1214
radiation therapy 1216–1217
regular exercise 1213
surgical *see surgery (below)*
techniques 1211–1213
women 1218–1219, 1218(i)
movement
measurement 1221
spinal, monitoring 1166–1167, 1166(i), 1167(i), 1221, 1222
natural history **1178–1179**
non-locomotor disease 1167–1170, 1217
organisations for 1211
origin of name 1161
osteitis pathophysiology 1186
osteoporosis in 1168, 1216, 1217
pain 1162, 1176
in women 1178, 1218
paleopathology 4, **1145–1147,** 1145(i), 1146(i)
pathology **1205–1210**
cartilaginous joints **1205–1208,** 1206(i), 1207(i), 1208(i)
extraskeletal lesions **1209–1210**
intervertebral discs 1206–1208, 1206(i), 1207(i)
ligamentous attachments **1205,** 1205(i)
manubriosternal joint 1208
symphysis pubis 1208
synovial joints **1208–1209,** 1208(i)
peripheral joints 1164
postpartum 1218
posture 1212(i), 1213
examination 1166, 1166(i)
monitoring 1221, 1221(i)
spinal stenosis posture *vs* 1177
surgery indication 1220
pregnancy 1218
prevalence 1154–1157, 1155(i)
Asian populations 1156(i), 1157
blood donor studies 1155–1156, 1155(i)
European populations 1156–1157, 1156(i)
hospital-based studies 1154–1155, 1155(i)
North American populations 1156, 1156(i)
population surveys 1156–1157, 1156(i)
sex ratios 1155(i), 1156(i)
primary lesion, evolution 1183–1186
prognostic factors 1178, 1216
pubic symphysis 1194, 1194(i)
pulmonary involvement 322, 1168, 1217, 1218(i)
management 1217
pathology 1210
quality of life 1223
recurrence-risk modeling 1186
renal involvement 343(i), 344, 1210
sacroiliac joint 1183(i)
CT and MRI 1170–1171, 1170(i), 1171(i)
examination 1164, 1165, 1165(i)